The Concise Encyclopedia of
FOODS& NUTRITION

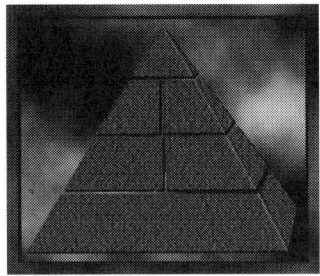

Audrey H. Ensminger
M.E. Ensminger
James E. Konlande
John R.K. Robson

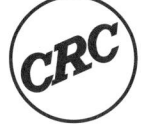

CRC Press
Boca Raton   London   Tokyo

Library of Congress Cataloging-in-Publication Data

The concise encyclopedia of foods and nutrition / Audrey H. Ensminger. . .
   [et al.].
     p.   cm.
   Includes index.
   ISBN 0-8493-4455-7
   1. Nutrition--Encyclopedias.   2. Food--Encyclopedias.
I. Ensminger, Audrey.
TX349.F573 1994
613.2′03--dc20

94-3000
CIP

No claim to original U.S. Government works
International Standard Book Number 0-8493-4455-7
Library of Congress Card Number 94-3000
Printed in the United States of America   1 2 3 4 5 6 7 8 9 0
Printed on acid-free paper

Dedicated to—

the global advancement of food, nutrition, and health

for the benefit of humankind

About the Authors

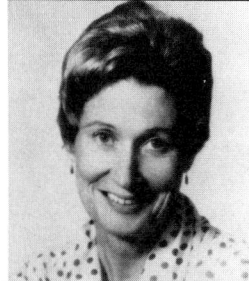

Audrey H. Ensminger, whose expertise is human nutrition, is Adjunct Professor, California State University-Fresno. She (1) completed the B.S. degree in Home Economics, University of Manitoba, Canada, and the M.S. degree in Home Economics, Washington State University; (2) taught at the University of Manitoba, the University of Minnesota, and Washington State University; and (3) served as dietitian for the U.S. Air Force, at Washington State University, during World War II. Audrey Ensminger has lectured throughout the world. She is the senior author of the two widely used human nutrition books, *FOODS & NUTRITION ENCYCLOPEDIA* and *FOOD FOR HEALTH.*

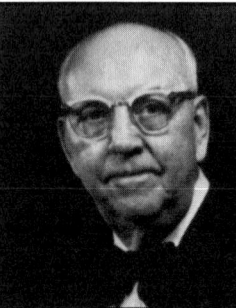

M. E. Ensminger, whose field is nutrition and biochemistry, is President, Agri-services Foundation, a nonprofit foundation serving world agriculture. Dr. Ensminger (1) completed B.S. and M.S. degrees at the University of Missouri, and the Ph.D. at the University of Minnesota; (2) served on the staffs of the University of Massachusetts, the University of Minnesota, and Washington State University; and (3) served as Consultant, General Electric Company, Nucleonics Department (Atomic Energy Commission). Dr. Ensminger is the author or co-author of 21 widely used books that are in several languages and used throughout the world. Dr. Ensminger is Adjunct Professor, California State University-Fresno; Adjunct Professor, the University of Arizona-Tucson; and Distinguished Professor, the University of Wisconsin-River Falls.

James E. Konlande completed the B.A. degree at Brooklyn College, Brooklyn, NY; and the M.S. and Ph.D. degrees at Rutgers University, New Brunswick, NJ, with a major in physiology, biochemistry, and nutrition. Prior to co-authoring *FOODS & NUTRITION ENCYCLOPEDIA,* he served as (1) Assistant Professor, Nutrition, the University of Michigan School of Public Health, Ann Arbor, Michigan; and (2) Head, Foods and Nutrition, Winthrop College (The University of South Carolina), Rock Hill, South Carolina.

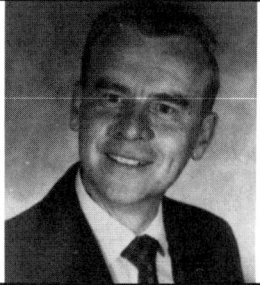

John R. K. Robson, M.D. was educated in England. He completed (1) the Bachelor of Medicine (M.B.) and Bachelor of Surgery (B.S.) degrees at Durham University, Kings College Medical School; (2) the Diploma in Tropical Medicine and Hygiene (D.T.M.&H. Edin.), Edinburgh University Medical School; (3) Diploma in Public Health—Special subject Nutrition (D.P.H. London), London University; and (4) the Doctor of Medicine (M.D.) at the University of Newcastle on Tyne, Medical School, and he is a Certified Specialist in Clinical Nutrition, American Board of Nutrition. Dr. Robson has done human nutrition work throughout the world. Also, he served as Professor of nutrition and Director of Nutrition Program, School of Public Health, University of Michigan; and as Professor of Nutrition and Medicine, Medical University of South Carolina, Charleston; and Executive Editor, *Ecology of Food and Nutrition*—and international journal. He is a Fellow of the Royal Society of Tropical Medicine and Hygiene; and a member of the New York Academy of Sciences, the Nutrition Society of Great Britain, the Scientific Council Population Food Fund, and the American Society of Parenteral and Enteral Nutrition.

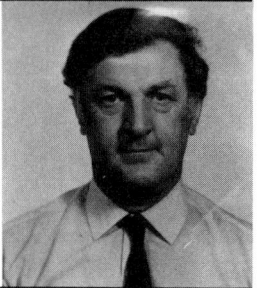

PREFACE

True to its title, *THE CONCISE ENCYCLOPEDIA OF FOODS AND NUTRITION* covers the whole gamut of the three-pronged subject—foods-health-nutrition. A simple definition of each of these terms follows:

> *A food is* any material that is taken or absorbed into the body of an organism for the purpose of satisfying hunger, growth, maintenance, tissue repair, reproduction, work, or pleasure.

> *Health is* the state of complete physical, mental, and social well-being.

> *Nutrition is* the science of food and its nutrients and their relation to health.

IT'S FOR CONSUMERS—ALL

THE CONCISE ENCYCLOPEDIA OF FOODS AND NUTRITION is for all consumers—for everyone who seeks good health, and for those who counsel with them—physicians, dentists, nutritionists, health experts, and others in allied fields. It's for teachers and students. It's for those who produce, process, and market foods. It's for those who wish to know the "why" of foods and nutrition—for those who wish to be educated rather than indoctrinated. It's for those who want the facts—both the pros and cons—on which they may base a judgment. It's for those who wish to know from whence their food comes—from field to table. It's for those who are concerned with getting the most nutrition from their food dollars. It's for those who desire authoritative and pleasurable reading about foods and nutrition, and their relationship to health.

AUTHORITATIVE

The authoritativeness of a work is evidenced by the credentials of those who created it. *THE CONCISE ENCYCLOPEDIA OF FOODS AND NUTRITION* is the team effort of four well-known professionals in the field of foods-health-nutrition.

TOPICS COVERED

The selection of the topics that are covered in *THE CONCISE ENCYCLOPEDIA OF FOODS AND NUTRITION* was based on the authors' professional experiences and perceptions relative to the needs of consumers, with application to many related fields, including medicine, dentistry, nursing, dietetics, teaching, nutritional science, public health, athletics, homemaking, and food production, processing, distribution and marketing. As the authors selected and treated each of the subjects, they were guided by the simple question: "Is it helpful?" If the answer was in the affirmative, they proceeded with the philosophy of "let the chips fall where they may," no matter how complex or how controversial the subject. Also, the authors were ever aware that some contemporary interests are transient; so, they strived to achieve a balance between the timely and the timeless.

COMPREHENSIVENESS

The comprehensiveness of *THE CONCISE ENCYCLOPEDIA OF FOODS AND NUTRITION* is indicated by the following statistics pertaining to it: 1,184 pages; more than 2,700 entries (or topics); more than 1,000 illustrations, of which 96 are in color; more than 200 tables; more than 1,300 food compositions; and a comprehensive index for easy reference.

It covers all aspects of foods-health-nutrition, with adequate historical and interpretive context. Each article includes all relevant aspects of the topic. Also, the entries reflect the whole gamut of foods-health-nutrition. There are precious few items on foods and nutrition not found as a subject entry and/or an index entry in *THE CONCISE ENCYCLOPEDIA OF FOODS AND NUTRITION.*

EASE OF USE

THE CONCISE ENCYCLOPEDIA OF FOODS AND NUTRITION is organized so that the reader may quickly and easily find the desired information. This is achieved through—

1. All topics being arranged alphabetically, using the word-by-word system—the same system that is used in a dictionary or in a library card catalog.

2. Cross referencing to related articles; usually at the end of an article, but within the text of an article when it makes for greater convenience.

3. A comprehensive index, which makes it possible for the reader, easily and quickly, to make a systematic survey of all parts and locations in *THE CONCISE ENCYCLOPEDIA OF FOODS AND NUTRITION* pertaining to a given subject, directly or indirectly. Additionally, where more than one reference page is listed in the index for a particular subject, the main section is listed in bold numbers.

(Continued)

ALTERNATE NAMES

Alternate names are used wherever appropriate, with each name indexed, so that the article can be located under any of the alternate names; for example—

VITAMIN C (ASCORBIC ACID)

FOOTNOTES

Literature pertaining to new and/or controversial material is documented in footnotes wherever possible.

ACKNOWLEDGMENTS

Authoring and publishing a first class book necessitates a first class supporting staff. So, special appreciation is expressed to the following staff members for their commitment to excellence and adhering to a rigid schedule: Joan Wright who deciphered the authors' hieroglyphics and put them through a typewriter; Randall and Susan Rapp, Rapp Typographic Service, who typeset the many changes for the second edition; Margo Williams who prepared the new art that enhances the second edition, and Jean Nelson who proofread the copy. Also, we shall be ever grateful to Robin Spencer Palmisano, who at the time of preparing the first edition was Systems Dietitian, University Hospitals, The Ohio State University, Columbus, Ohio, a very special person and dedicated professional, who contributed so much to Table F-21 Food Compositions. (Presently, Robin Spencer Palmisano is a lawyer and a member of the firm of McGlinchey, Stafford, Cellini & Lang, New Orleans, Louisiana.) Further, we are grateful to Ron Bruce, President, Unisoft Systems Associates, 1340 Dublin Road, Columbus, Ohio, 43215, for permission to continue to use Table F-21 Food Compositions. At appropriate places, due acknowledgment and sincere appreciation is expressed to those who responded so liberally to our call for information and pictures. The unnumbered line drawings in *THE CONCISE ENCYCLOPEDIA OF FOODS AND NUTRITION* were created by Dynamic Graphics, Inc.

If *THE CONCISE ENCYCLOPEDIA OF FOODS AND NUTRITION* ushers a better fed, nourished, and healthier world into the 21st century, the authors will feel amply rewarded.

A. H. Ensminger
M. E. Ensminger
J. E. Konlande
J. R. K. Robson

Clovis, California   (March, 1995)

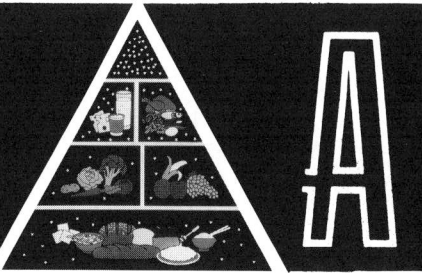

ABERNETHY BISCUIT

A hard biscuit containing caraway seeds, named after an English surgeon who, in the early 1800s, treated maladies with diet.

ABSORPTION

• The transfer of a substance through a membrane or the taking in of nutrients or other substances from an outside source; e.g., the passage of substances into the blood and/or lymph system from the digestive tract, through the skin, or by way of the lungs.

• The uptake of water, fat, or other substances by foods. (Also see DIGESTION AND ABSORPTION.)

ABSORPTION METER

An instrument used to measure the absorption of light, by which a quantitative measure of a colored substance in a solution may be obtained. Many substances, such as minerals, vitamins, and amino acids, will react with a particular reagent to form a colored complex. Since the color developed is proportional to the amount of the substance present, its quantity may be measured by an absorption meter.

ACCLIMATIZE

The process of becoming adjusted to a new environment, especially temperature, altitude, or climate.

ACETATE

A salt of acetic acid. The name also refers to the metabolic product called acetylcoenzyme A.
(Also see METABOLISM.)

ACETIC ACID

An organic acid which is produced by (1) the metabolism of nutrients, and (2) vinegar fermentation. It reacts with alkalis to form acetates.
(Also see VINEGAR.)

ACETOACETIC ACID

This ketone acid is formed when the quantities of fat which are burned for energy greatly exceed the amounts of carbohydrate which undergo metabolism. An excessive accumulation of acetoacetic in the body results in the condition called ketosis.
(Also see ACID-BASE BALANCE.)

ACETOBACTER *Acetobacteriaceae*

A genus of bacteria used aerobically (with air) to convert alcohol to acetic acid. An acetobacter, *Acetobacter pasteurianus*, is used in the making of vinegar.

ACETO-GLYCERIDES (PARTIAL GLYCERIDE ESTERS)

These differ from triglycerides in that either one (or sometimes two) of the long chain fatty acids attached to the glycerol molecule is replaced by acetic acid. They are nongreasy and have lower melting points than the corresponding triglycerides.

Aceto-glycerides are used in shortenings and spreads, as films for coating foods, and as plasticisers for hard fats.

ACETOIN

Acetyl methyl carbinol, $C_4H_8O_2$, precursor of diacetyl, which imparts the flavor to butter. Acetoin is a product of fermentation, produced by bacteria during the ripening of cream for churning and by the action of yeast on diacetyl.

ACETONE

A substance that gives the breath a fruity odor. It may accumulate in the blood, breath, and urine when there is an abnormal metabolism of fats.
(Also see KETONE BODIES.)

ACETONEMIA

A buildup of acetone in the blood. This condition occurs only when there is an impairment in breathing. Under normal circumstances most acetone is removed from the body via the breath.

ACETONURIA

The passing of abnormally large amounts of acetone in the urine. This may be a sign of ketosis, which may be brought on by (1) diets high in fat, and low in carbohydrate; (2) starvation; or (3) diabetes.
(Also see DIABETES MELLITUS; and STARVATION.)

ACETYLCHOLINE

A substance released from the ending of certain nerves which (1) stimulates the digestive functions, and (2) slows the heart rate and lowers the blood pressure. It is noteworthy that digestive disorders characterized by hypersecretion of digestive juices and spasms of the alimentary tract are often treated with medications like atropine and belladonna, which counteract acetylcholine and its effects.
(Also see ATROPINE; BELLADONNA DRUGS; and DIGESTION AND ABSORPTION.)

ACETYLCOENZYME A

A key substance formed during the metabolism of carbohydrates, fats, and proteins. It plays important roles in (1) the production of energy, carbon dioxide, and water from the intermediate products of metabolism; and (2) the synthesis of fatty acids, ketone bodies, acetylcholine, choles-

terol, and related compounds.
(Also see METABOLISM.)

ACHALASIA

A malfunctioning of the muscular coat around the esophagus. There is less than the normal amount of peristalsis and the lower sphincter fails to relax. Hence, solid food tends to remain in the esophagus because it cannot pass into the stomach. The condition may be corrected by surgery, or by stretching the lower sphincter with a dilator.
(Also see DIGESTION AND ABSORPTION.)

ACH INDEX (ARM, CHEST, HIP INDEX)

This refers to the arm girth, chest diameter, and hip width. It is sometimes used as a method of assessing the state of nutrition.

ACHLORHYDRIA

A condition in which there is a lack of hydrochloric acid in the gastric juices.
(Also see AUTOIMMUNITY; DIGESTION AND ABSORPTION; and DISEASES.)

ACHOLIC

An abnormal condition in which there is a deficiency of bile.
(Also see DIGESTION AND ABSORPTION.)

ACHROMOTRICHIA

A lack of pigment or graying of the hair. It occurs in rats as a result of pantothenic acid deficiency. The discovery of this condition led to the designation of pantothenic acid as the antigray hair vitamin. However, there is no evidence that it prevents the graying of hair in people.
(Also see PANTOTHENIC ACID.)

ACID

A substance which has a pH of 6.9 or lower and is capable of turning litmus indicators red. It is responsible for the sour taste of foods such as lemons, pickles, tomatoes, vinegar, etc. Many acids occur naturally in foods, while others are added for flavoring, or to inhibit the growth of certain microorganisms associated with food spoilage. Acids also occur naturally in the body, such as the hydrochloric acid of the stomach.
(Also see ACID-BASE BALANCE; ACID FOODS AND ALKALINE FOODS; ADDITIVES; and PRESERVATIVES.)

ACID-ASH RESIDUE

A mineral residue which is left after (1) the other nutrients in a food have been metabolized or (2) a food has been burned to an ash in a laboratory. Ashes of foods give an acid reaction, when the predominant chemical elements are chlorine, phosphorus or sulfur, because these elements generally form acids. Foods which are most likely to have an acid residue are breads and cereal products, eggs, fish, meats, and poultry. Milk has an alkaline residue.
(Also see ACID FOODS AND ALKALINE FOODS.)

ACID-ASH RESIDUE DIETS

These diets leave an acid residue in the body because they contain foods rich in chlorine, phosphorus and/or sulfur—such as eggs, meat, fish, poultry, bread, and cereal products. They are often prescribed for patients with kidney stones (calculi) that are believed to be formed under alkaline condi-

tions. Sometimes, these stones dissolve in acid. Therefore, acid-ash diets are used to keep the urine acid.
(Also see ACID FOODS AND ALKALINE FOODS; and DISEASES.)

ACID-BASE BALANCE

An acid is a chemical that can release hydrogen ions, whereas a base, or alkali, is a chemical that can accept hydrogen ions. For the pH, or hydrogen ion concentration, of extracellular fluid to remain normal, a balance between acids and bases must be maintained. This equilibrium is known as the acid-base balance; it refers to the hydrogen ion concentration in the body fluids. When the hydrogen ion concentration is high, the fluids are acidic—the condition is acidosis; when the hydrogen ion concentration is low, the fluids are basic—the condition is alkalosis. Since the chemical reactions of the cells depend very greatly on the hydrogen ion concentration, the acid-base balance must be regulated very precisely.

The degree of acidity is expressed in terms of pH. A pH of 7 is the neutral point between an acid and an alkaline (base). Substances with a lower pH than 7 are acid, while substances with a pH above 7 are alkaline. The normal pH of the extracellular fluids of the body is 7.4, with a range of 7.35 to 7.45. Maintenance of the pH within this narrow range is necessary to sustain the life of cells. The extremes between which life is possible are 7.0 to 7.8.

BUFFER. In chemistry, a buffer is a mixture of acidic and alkaline components, which protects a solution against wide variations in the pH, even when strong bases or acids are added to it. A solution containing such a protective mixture is called a buffer solution. A buffer protects the acid-base balance of a solution by rapidly offsetting changes in its ionized hydrogen concentration. It works by protecting against either added acid or base.

ACID-FORMING AND BASE-FORMING FOODS.
The potential acidity or alkalinity of the foods ingested covers a wide range and depends on the minerals present. On combustion, certain foods, such as most vegetables and fruits, leave an ash in which the basic elements (sodium, potassium, calcium, and magnesium) predominate; hence, they are known as base-forming foods. Other foods, such as cereals, meat, and fish, leave an ash in which the acid-forming elements (chlorine, phosphorus, and sulfur) predominate; these are known as acid-forming foods. Although sulfur is present in foods mainly in neutral form in the sulfur-containing amino acids (methionine, cystine, cysteine), it is oxidized in the body to sulfuric acid; hence, it is an acid-forming mineral. Therefore, foods containing a large amount of protein are generally acid-forming. Contrary to popular belief, citrus fruits are not acid-forming. They do contain citric acid and acid potassium citrate, but the citrate radicals are completely metabolized in the body, leaving only potassium. Thus, many acid fruits are really base-forming foods.
(Also see ACID FOODS AND ALKALINE FOODS.)

REGULATION OF ACID-BASE BALANCE. Regulation of the acid-base balance refers to the control of the hydrogen ion concentration in the body fluids. It is very important that the pH of body fluids be maintained within the narrow, slightly alkaline range of 7.35 and 7.45, because variance from this range leads to disruption of normal body processes and activity. The acid-base balance is regulated by chemical buffers, by the lungs (respiratory), and by the kidneys (renal), as follows:

1. **Chemical Buffers.** All of the body fluids contain acid-base buffers. These are chemicals that can combine readily with any acid or base in such a way that they keep the acid or base from changing the pH of the fluids greatly. The three most important chemical buffers are the bicarbonate buffer, phosphate buffers, and protein buffers.

a. **Bicarbonate Buffer.** This buffer, which is present in all body fluids, is a mixture of carbonic acid (H_2CO_3) and bicarbonate ion (HCO_3^-). When a strong acid is added to this mixture, it combines immediately with the bicarbonate ion to form carbonic acid—an extremely weak acid. Thus, this buffer system changes a strong acid to a weak acid and keeps the fluids from becoming strongly acid. However, when a strong base is added to this mixture, the base immediately combines with the carbonic acid to form water and neutral bicarbonate salt.

Loss of the weak acid and the addition of the neutral salt scarcely affect the hydrogen ion concentration in the body fluids. Thus, the carbonic acid-bicarbonate buffer system protects the body fluids from becoming either too acidic or too basic.

b. **Phosphate buffers.** These chemical buffers are especially important for maintaining normal hydrogen ion concentration in the intracellular fluids, because their concentration inside the cells is many times as great as the concentration of the bicarbonate buffer.

c. **Protein buffers.** Like phosphate buffers, protein buffers, including hemoglobin, are especially important within the cells.

In essence, the chemical buffers of the body fluids are the first line of defense against changes in hydrogen ion concentration, for any acid or base added to the fluids immediately reacts with these buffers to prevent marked changes in the acid-base balance.

2. **Lungs (respiratory).** Carbon dioxide combines with water and electrolytes in the extracellular fluid to form carbonic acid in accordance with the following reaction:

$$CO_2 + H_2O \longrightarrow H_2CO_3$$

Ultimately, the lungs control the body's supply of carbonic acid. This is so because, normally, respiration removes carbon dioxide at the same rate that it is formed by all cells of the body as one of the end products of metabolism. However, if respiration decreases below normal, carbon dioxide will not be excreted normally; instead, it will accumulate in the body fluids, causing an increase in the concentration of carbonic acid. As a result, the hydrogen ion concentration rises. On the other hand, if the respiration rate rises above normal, the opposite effect occurs; carbon dioxide is blown off at a more rapid rate than it is formed, thereby decreasing the carbon dioxide and carbonic acid concentrations. It is noteworthy that complete lack of breathing for a minute will reduce the pH of the extracellular fluid from the normal of 7.4 down to about 7.1, while over-breathing can increase it to about 7.7 in a minute. Thus, the acid-base balance of the body can be changed greatly by under- or over-ventilation of the lungs.

In the preceding paragraph, the effect of changing the rate of breathing on the acid-base balance is detailed. In this paragraph, the opposite effect of the acid-base balance on respiration is discussed. A high hydrogen ion concentration stimulates the respiratory center in the medulla of the brain, greatly enhancing the rate of ventilation. Conversely, a low hydrogen ion concentration depresses the rate of ventilation. So, the effect of the hydrogen ion concentration on the activity of the respiratory center affords an automatic mechanism for maintaining a fairly constant pH of the body fluids. That is, an increase in hydrogen ion concentration increases the rate of ventilation, which in turn removes carbonic acid from the fluids. Loss of the carbonic acid decreases the hydrogen ion concentration back toward normal. Conversely, diminished hydrogen ion concentration depresses the ventilation, and the hydrogen ion concentration rises back toward normal. This respiratory mechanism for regulating acid-base balance reacts almost immediately when the extracellular fluids become either too acidic or too basic. Thus, acidosis greatly increases both the depth and rate of respiration, while alkalosis lessens the depth and rate of respiration. This respiratory mechanism is so effective in regulating the acid-base balance that it usually returns the pH of the body fluids to normal within a few minutes after an acid or alkali has been administered.

3. **Kidneys (renal).** In addition to carbonic acid, a number of other acids are continually being formed by the metabolic process of the cells, including phosphoric, sulfuric, uric, and keto acids. On entering the extracellular fluids, all of these can cause acidosis. Normally, the kidneys rid the body of these excess acids as rapidly as they are formed, preventing an excessive build-up of hydrogen ions.

Occasionally, too many basic compounds enter the body fluids, rather than too many acidic compounds. This may occur when basic compounds are injected intravenously or when large quantities of alkaline food or drugs are consumed.

The kidneys regulate acid-base balance by (a) excreting hydrogen ions into the urine when the extracellular fluids are too acidic, and (b) excreting basic substances, particularly sodium bicarbonate, into the urine when the extracellular fluids become too alkaline.

The kidneys also conserve base by eliminating extra hydrogen ions through the production and excretion of ammonia (NH_4):

NH_3 (from deamination + H^+ $\longrightarrow$ NH_4 of amino acids)

If the normal amounts of buffers are present in the blood, and if the lungs and kidneys are normal, one can recover promptly from the effects of severe muscular exercise, intake of acid or base, unbalanced diets (so far as acids and bases are concerned), short periods of starvation, short bouts of vomiting, and other adverse conditions. But there are limits to the adjustments that the body can make; if the capacity is exceeded, the pH changes and the body cells are prevented from performing their functions normally.

ABNORMALITIES OF ACID-BASE BALANCE.
Many disorders of the respiratory system, the kidneys, or the metabolic system for forming acids and bases can cause serious derangement of the acid-base balance. Some of the effects of these conditions, compared with the normal pH of the blood of 7.4, are shown in Fig. A-1; and a brief discussion of each condition follows:

Acidosis generally causes depressed mental activity, and, if unchecked, it may culminate in coma and death. Usually the afflicted person will pass into a coma when the pH of the extracellular fluid falls below 6.9.

Alkalosis causes overexcitability, resulting in excessive initiation of impulses, muscle contraction, and even convulsions.

In acidosis, the ionized hydrogen concentration is above normal. In alkalosis, ionized hydrogen concentration is below normal. Either of these abnormal states initiates compensatory responses of the chemical buffers, lungs, and kidneys, which cause body fluids to accept, to release, or to excrete ionized hydrogen. Increases and decreases in ionized hydrogen concentration are changed so that the pH is not significantly changed from its normal range of 7.35 to 7.45. Failure of either the lungs or the kidneys to carry out this function results in acidosis or alkalosis. If the failure is largely related to the lungs (respiratory), it is called respiratory acidosis or respiratory alkalosis. If the failure is mainly related to the kidneys, it is called metabolic acidosis or metabolic alkalosis.

Examples of diseases that affect the lungs and contribute to the development of respiratory acidosis are: pneumonia, emphysema, asthma, pulmonary edema, barbiturate poisoning, morphine poisoning, and congestive heart failure. Common causes of respiratory alkalosis are: extreme emotion, hysteria, or anxiety (causing hyperventilation); labored breathing in response to hot weather, high altitude, or fever (causing hyperpnea); excessive breathing forced upon a patient by a poorly adjusted mechanical respirator; or overstimulation of the respiratory center in the brain, which may be brought about by aspirin, poisoning, meningitis, or encephalitis.

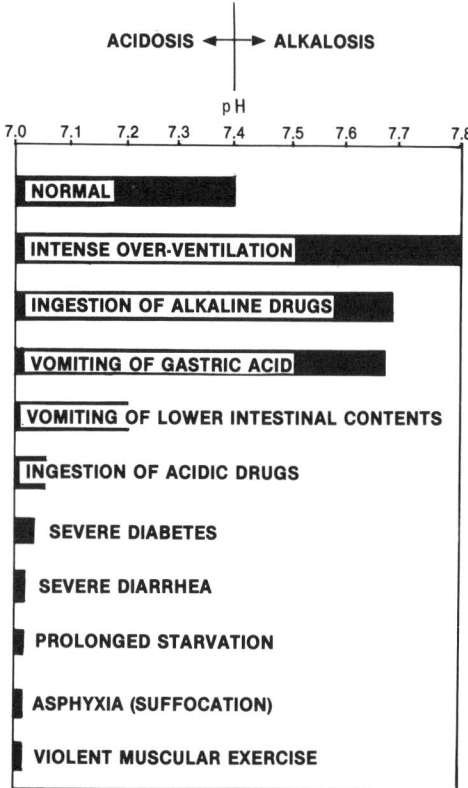

Fig. A-1. pH of the body fluids in various acid-base disorders compared with normal pH.

Examples of metabolic acidosis are: diabetic acidosis, brought about because the body cannot metabolize blood glucose properly and turns for its energy to the catabolism of protein and fat; starvation, when the body turns to its own stores of protein and fat to supply its needs; greatly accelerated metabolism, such as thyrotoxicosis, resulting in the depletion of carbohydrate stores and the burning of protein stores, followed by ketosis; gastrointestinal problems, such as may be caused by prolonged vomiting and the inability to eat, resulting in decreased carbohydrate intake, glycogen

depletion, burning of body protein and fat, and finally ketosis; severe diarrhea, induced because large amounts of bicarbonate (HCO_3) and sodium (Na) are swept away with the intestinal contents; and chronic or acute kidney disease, as the kidneys become unable to cope with excess ionized hydrogen concentrations.

Examples of metabolic alkalosis include: initial vomiting, resulting in loss of ionized hydrogen and chlorine; potassium depletion (caused by insufficient potassium intake, gastrointestinal loss of potassium, or ACTH therapy), inducing alkalosis as ionized hydrogen and sodium move into the cells to replace the lost potassium; and excess intake of alkali powders or sodium bicarbonate, as in long-term ulcer therapy.

In all cases of acid-base imbalance, three basic rules should be followed: (1) rely on a medical doctor for diagnosis and prescribed treatment, (2) treat the primary cause of the acidosis or alkalosis, and (3) make every effort to aid the various compensatory responses of the lungs and kidneys.

ACID-BASE REACTION OF FOODS

This refers to the potential acidity or alkalinity of food, which depends upon the reaction they yield after being broken down (metabolized) in the body, thus releasing their mineral elements. These minerals function in maintaining the acid-base balance in the body. Acid-forming elements are chlorine, phosphorus, and sulfur, while base (alkaline)-forming elements are calcium, sodium, potassium, and magnesium. Foods can be classified as acid foods, alkaline (basic) foods, or neutral foods according to their mineral content.

(Also see ACID-BASE BALANCE; ACID FOODS AND ALKALINE FOODS; and WATER AND ELECTROLYTES, section headed "Acid-Base Balance.")

ACID DETERGENT FIBER (ADF)

The fiber which is extracted from plant foods with acidic detergent, a technique employed to determine indigestible matter. The extract is composed of cellulose and lignin, cell-wall substances which are not digested by man.

(Also see ANALYSIS OF FOODS; CARBOHYDRATES, UNAVAILABLE; and FIBER.)

ACID FOODS AND ALKALINE FOODS

The metabolism of many foods results in a small amount of mineral residue, or ash (so-called because it is similar to the ash remaining after burning material). Only highly refined foods, consisting chiefly of fats, sugars, or starches do not yield an ash. The processing of such foods has resulted in the removal of the mineral elements; the carbon, hydrogen, and oxygen which remain are metabolized to water, carbon dioxide, and energy.

A solution of the mineral residue of a food will, upon testing, give an acid, alkaline (basic), or neutral reaction, depending upon the relative proportions of acid-forming elements (chlorine, phosphorus, and sulfur) and of alkali-forming elements (potassium, sodium, calcium, and magnesium). The type of reaction of the food ash in water is important because it gives an indication of the contribution of the food to the acidity, alkalinity, or neutrality of the body fluids, and, ultimately, to the urine. The kidneys help to maintain the neutrality of the body fluids by excreting the excess acid or alkali in the urine.

FOODS YIELDING AN ACID RESIDUE. The acid-forming elements predominate over the alkali-forming mineral elements in foods containing moderate to large amounts of protein, with the exception of milk and some of the other dairy products which contain sufficient calcium to give an alkaline reaction. Whole grains give an acid reaction disproportionate to their protein content due to the extra phosphorus present in the form of phytates. Although most fruits have an alkaline ash, others like prunes, plums, and cranberries make a net contribution of acid to the body since they contain organic acids that are not metabolized by the body, but which pass unchanged into the urine.

FOODS YIELDING AN ALKALINE RESIDUE. Fruits and vegetables generally contain higher proportions of alkali-forming mineral elements than the acid-forming elements since their protein content is usually low. Corn and lentils, however, are acid forming. Surprising as it may seem, because of their pronounced acid taste, an alkaline residue is formed from tomatoes, citrus fruit, and rhubarb, due to their organic acids (citric, ascorbic, oxalic, and others) being completely metabolized in the body to carbon dioxide, water, and energy. Some nuts (coconuts, almonds, chestnuts) yield an alkaline ash, while others (peanuts, walnuts) yield an acid.

Table A-1 lists foods which yield acid, alkaline, or neutral ashes.

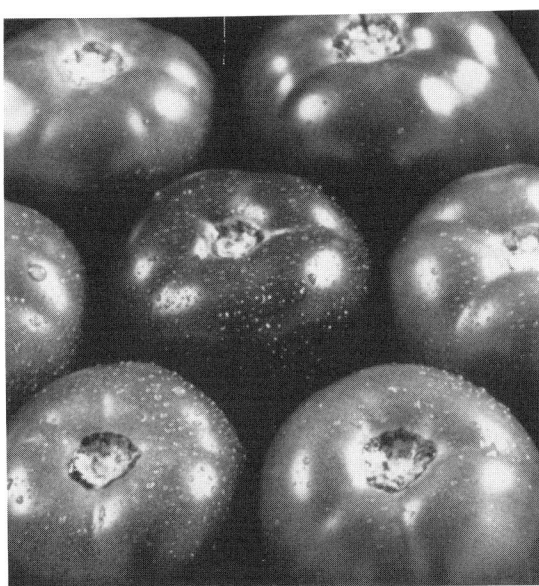

Fig. A-2. Tomatoes produce an alkaline ash in the body. (Courtesy, USDA)

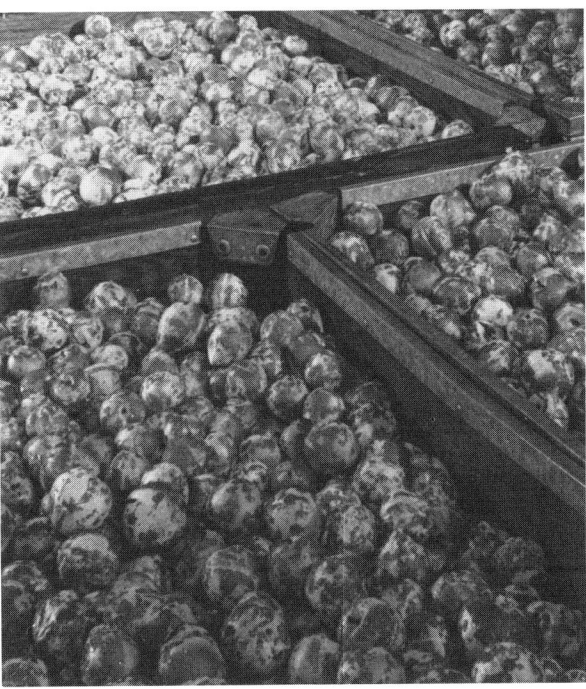

Fig. A-3. Plums, unlike most fruits, produce an acid ash in the body. (Courtesy, California Tree Fruit Agreement, Sacramento)

TABLE A-1
ACID, ALKALINE, OR NEUTRAL FOODS[1]

Acid-Ash Foods	Alkaline (Basic)- Ash Foods		Neutral-Ash Foods
Bread:	**Cheese, American[2]**		**Arrowroot starch**
White	**Cream**		**Butter**
Whole Wheat	**Fruit:**		**Candy, plain**
Rye	Apple	Loganberries	**Coffee**
Cake, plain	Apricots	Mango	**Cornstarch**
Cereal:	Banana	Nectarines	**Lard**
Cornflakes	Blackberries	Olives	**Margarine**
Farina	Blueberries, raw	Orange	**Oil, vegetable**
Macaroni	Cantaloupe	Peach	**Postum**
Oatmeal	Cherries	Pear	**Sugar, white**
Puffed wheat	Currants	Persimmon	**Syrup**
Puffed rice	Dates	Pineapple	**Tapioca**
Rice	Figs	Pineapple juice	**Tea**
Shredded wheat	Gooseberries	Raisins	
Fat, mayonnaise	Grapefruit	Raspberries	
Fruit:	Grapes	Strawberries	
Cranberries	Lemon	Tangerine	
Plums	Lime	Watermelon	
Prunes	**Ice cream**		
Meat:	**Jam**		
Bacon	**Milk**		
Beef	**Nuts:**		
Cheese, cheddar	Almonds		
Cheese, cottage	Chestnuts		
Chicken	Coconut, fresh		
Eggs	**Sweets:**		
Fish	Molasses, medium		
Ham	**Vegetables**		
Lamb	Asparagus	Onions	
Pork	Beans, lima	Parsnips	
Veal	Beans, navy	Peas	
Nuts:	Beans, snap	Peppers	
Brazil nuts	Beets	Potato, white	
Peanut butter	Beet greens	Pumpkin	
Peanuts	Broccoli	Radish	
Walnuts, English	Cabbage	Rutabagas	
Vegetables:	Carrots	Salsify	
Corn	Cauliflower	Sauerkraut	
Lentils, dried	Celery	Squash,	
	Chard, Swiss	summer	
	Cucumber	Squash, winter	
	Dandelion greens	Sweet potato	
	Eggplant	Tomatoes or	
	Endive, curly	juice	
	Kale	Turnip greens	
	Kohlrabi	Turnip	
	Lettuce	Water cress	
	Mushrooms		
	Okra		

[1]Adapted by the authors from data presented in *Mayo Clinic Diet Manual,* 3rd ed., W.B. Saunders Company, Philadelphia, 1961, pp. 182-184.
[2]Ash of this type of processed cheese is alkaline, due to additives such as sodium aluminum phosphate.

GAPS IN INFORMATION CONCERNING ACID FOODS AND ALKALINE FOODS. The classification of a food ash as acid or alkaline has metabolic significance only when there is certainty as to the proportion of the food minerals which are digested and absorbed. This is not the case with dairy products (a variable amount of dietary calcium is excreted in the stool) or with the phosphorus present as phytates in whole grains. Phytates further complicate the picture by binding with alkali-forming minerals and carrying them into the stool. Similar effects might be expected to occur when diets high in fiber are consumed. Certain additives in food mixtures, such as sodium aluminum phosphate used as an emulsifying agent in pasteurized, processed American cheese, may have an unpredictable effect on the food residue, depending upon the net absorption and metabolism of the food and additive combination, which cannot be accurately predicted from a knowledge of the separate components.

Nonetheless, tables of acidic, alkaline, or neutral foods provide, for the dietician, a means of planning menus to accomplish certain metabolic alterations.

DIETARY USES OF ACID FOODS AND ALKALINE FOODS. Under normal circumstances, there is no reason to be concerned about dietary excesses of either acid or alkaline foods, since the neutrality of the blood is maintained by the kidneys, aided somewhat by the lungs. When, however, there are kidney stones or impairment of kidney function, it may be necessary to select foods to obtain an acid, alkaline, or neutral urine.

Kidney stones composed of calcium and magnesium phosphates, carbonates, and oxalates are formed under alkaline conditions; since these salts are insoluble in alkaline solutions. It is, therefore, believed that a diet resulting in an acid urine will help to reduce the formation of such stones. Physicians sometimes recommend that the urine be kept acid by giving the patient cranberry juice (which contains a nonmetabolizable organic acid) several times a day.

Uric acid and cystine stones are formed under acid conditions; hence, a therapeutic diet should, in this case, make the urine alkaline.

Milk is usually allowed in either acid-ash or alkaline-ash diets since much of the calcium is unabsorbed, and it is, therefore, debatable whether this food has an acidic or alkaline reaction.

CAUTION: It is not advisable for people to undertake on their own, without a physician's advice, to change the relative acidity or alkalinity of their body fluids and urine. Overemphasis of certain foods and avoidance of others may result in a deficient or imbalanced diet.
(Also see ACID-BASE BALANCE.)

ACIDOPHILUS MILK

Milk inoculated with *Lactobacillus acidophilus* bacteria for the purpose of establishing this organism in the intestines, where it may have beneficial effects.
(Also see LACTOBACILLUS ACIDOPHILUS; and MILK.)

ACIDOSIS

A disorder characterized by an abnormally high level of acid in the blood, or by a decrease in the blood bicarbonate. The excess acids may consist of ketone bodies, phosphoric acid, sulfuric acid, hydrochloric acid, lactic acid, or carbonic acid.
(Also see ACID-BASE BALANCE.)

ACID TIDE

A short-lived increase in the acidity of the blood and the urine which may occur after eating a protein-rich meal that stimulates a heavy secretion of alkaline juice from the pancreas.
(Also see DIGESTION AND ABSORPTION.)

ACINI

Groups of secretory cells in glands such as the salivary glands, the pancreas, and the liver. *Acini* means shaped like a cluster of grapes, which is indicative of the shape of these organized clusters of cells. Their secretions of enzymes and bile feed into ducts that empty into the digestive tract.

ACNE

An outbreak of pimples or similar eruptions on the face, back, or chest. At one time it was thought that certain foods caused outbreaks of acne, but now this does not seem likely unless the foods cause allergic reactions.
(Also see ALLERGIES; and CHILDHOOD AND ADOLESCENT NUTRITION.)

ACONITASE

This is an enzyme occurring in many animal and plant tissues that accelerates the conversion of citric acids (1) into aconitic acid, and (2) then into isocitric acid.

ACRODYNIA (PINK DISEASE)

A disease, also called pink disease, which occurs in young children, usually between 4 months and 3 years of age. It is characterized by painful red swollen hands and feet, muscular pains that make movement difficult, loss of energy, and general mental and physical sluggishness. Acrodynia may be caused by chronic mercury intoxication. Also, there are other, as yet unknown, causes of the disease. A similar condition occurs in rats on a diet deficient in pyridoxine (vitamin B-6).

ACROLEIN

A bitter substance produced by overheating fats. If consumed in sufficient quantity, it may irritate the stomach and the intestines.

ACROMEGALY

A disorder resulting from the oversecretion of growth hormones by the pituitary after most of the bones have stopped growing. The excess of hormone causes overgrowth of the bones in the face, hands, and feet. It may also lead to a diabetic condition and various other abnormalities.
(Also see ENDOCRINE GLANDS.)

ACTH

An abbreviation for adrenocorticotropic hormone, which is secreted by the pituitary. Under certain stressful conditions, it stimulates (1) the secretion of certain hormones by the adrenal cortex, and (2) a release of free fatty acids from various fatty tissues.
(Also see ENDOCRINE GLANDS.)

ACTIVATE

To convert a substance, such as a provitamin or enzyme, into an active form or different substance.

ACTIVATION OF ENZYMES

In order to function, some enzymes require a metal (such as calcium), or a nonmetal, or both, attached to them, either loosely or tightly; others function independently. For example, calcium activates a number of enzymes including pancreatic lipase, adenosine triphosphatase, and some proteolytic enzymes.

ACTIVATOR

An agent that initiates metabolic activity by another substance. For example, certain trace minerals combine with vitamins to activate some important enzymes. The enzymes may not function unless activated.

(Also see ENZYME; MINERAL[S]; and VITAMIN[S].)

ACTIVE TRANSPORT

The process by which one type of molecule is carried through a membrane by another molecule. Active transport requires energy that is derived from the metabolism of nutrients.

(Also see DIGESTION AND ABSORPTION.)

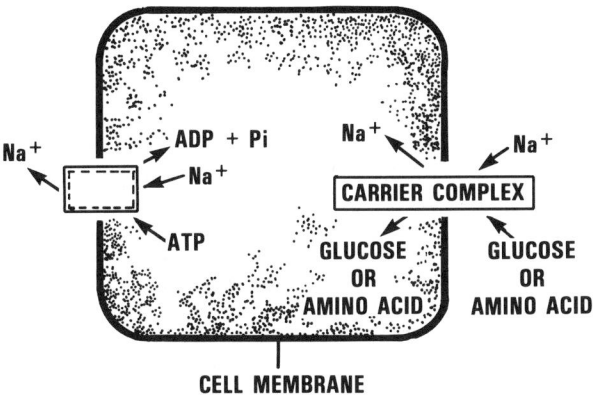

Fig. A-4. Active transport occurs when there is movement against a concentration gradient, thus necessitating the expenditure of energy. A carrier system utilizing Na $^+$ has been implicated in the active transport of glucose and some amino acids.

ACUTE CONDITION

A disease or disorder having a sudden beginning, and lasting a short time. Often, the symptoms are severe.

ADDISON'S DISEASE

A chronic condition resulting from an undersecretion of the adrenal cortical hormones. Usually, there is an inability to adapt to such stresses as low blood sugar (hypoglycemia), infection, dehydration, and chilling.

(Also see ENDOCRINE GLANDS.)

ADDITIVES, FOOD

A food additive is any substance that food manufacturers intentionally add to foods to achieve specific effects during production or processing or to impart or retain desired characteristics. Some additives come from foods. Others are synthesized by scientists in the laboratory.

Some people consider food additives to be dangerous to their health. But processing food without additives would be to go back to the good old days of baking freshness—good today, stale tomorrow—the days when cottage cheese separated, cookies dried up in 2 days, any food with fat or oil in it became rancid, canned vegetables and fruits were soft and mushy, and marshmallows got too hard to toast. Furthermore, quantities available would be less due to spoilage, and convenience foods would be nonexistent

But even in the good old days there were additives! Many additives occur naturally and have been used for centuries. The Egyptians used food coloring made from vegetables; the Romans preserved fruit in honey; Marco Polo searched for food additives—herbs and spices—in his travels; and salting foods was common in the Middle Ages. Also, food additives have long been used in homes; among them, iodine, put in salt to prevent goiter; baking powder, added to dough to make it rise; pectin and sugar added to jams; and vinegar (acetic acid) used in pickling, production of sour milk, salad dressings, and tomato products.

KINDS OF ADDITIVES. Some additives increase the nutritional value of foods. Others keep foods from spoiling. Still others improve the flavor, color, or texture of foods.

There are approximately 3,000 food additives, all of which can be classified into the following six major groups:

1. **Nutritional Supplements.** Many foods are fortified with minerals and vitamins that might otherwise be lacking in the diet or that have been destroyed or lost in processing. Common nutritional additives include iodine in table salt, vitamin D in milk, and vitamin A in margarine. Breads and cereals are enriched with iron and B vitamins, lost or destroyed during the milling and processing of grains. Such fortification has helped eradicate once prevalent deficiency diseases, such as goiter, rickets, beriberi, and pellagra.

(Also see ENRICHMENT.)

2. **Preservatives.** The shelf and refrigerator life of foods has been extended by additives that retard spoilage, preserve natural color and flavor, and keep fats and oils from turning rancid. For example, microbial agents, such as benzoates, propionates, and sorbates are used to retard spoilage by bacteria, yeasts and molds. Nitrates and nitrites protect cured meats, fish, and poultry from contamination by the bacterially produced toxin responsible for botulism, a food poisoning illness. Ascorbic acid (vitamin C) is useful as a means of preventing the discoloration of canned fruits. Antioxidants keep fats and oils from spoiling and prevent discoloration of smoked and canned meats.

Additives save money by preventing spoilage and maintaining freshness. It has been estimated that the removal of additives from bread would cost the consumer $1.1 billion per year; from margarine, $600 million per year; from meats, $600 million per year; and from processed cheese $32 million per year.

3. **Flavoring Agents.** These products, which make up the largest single class of additives, are intended to make foods taste better. This group includes natural and synthetic flavors, spices, essential oils, flavor enhancers such as MSG (monosodium glutamate), and sweeteners. The characteristic flavor of strawberry ice cream may come from real strawberries, or it may come from a chemical flavoring.

4. **Coloring Agents.** These additives are for the purpose of making foods more attractive. Manufacturers add yellow coloring to margarine to make it look like butter; canners add coloring to many canned foods to replace natural colors lost in processing; orange processors add orange color to the skins of oranges to improve the appearance of the fruit; and ice cream manufacturers tint strawberry ice cream pink, because consumers associate strawberries with a reddish color.

5. Emulsifiers, Stabilizers, and Thickeners. A wide variety of products are used to improve texture. For example, lecithin, obtained primarily from soybeans, is used as an emulsifier in dressings and chocolates, to keep ingredients in a processed form from separating. Pectin and gelatin are added to thicken jams and jellies; and gums, dextrins, and starches are used to give more substance to soups and desserts

6. Acids and Alkalis. Additives are used to control the acidity or alkalinity of some foods. For example, when added to fruit juice, citric acid imparts a tart taste; and carbonic acid puts the fizz in soft drinks. Alkalis may be added to neutralize the high acid content of such canned foods as peas and olives.

YEARLY CONSUMPTION. By far, the most consumed additives are sugar, salt, and corn syrup. These three, plus such other substances as citric acid, baking soda, vegetable colors, mustard, and pepper, account for more than 98%, by weight, of all food additives used in this country.

Fig. A-5 shows the yearly per capita consumption of food additives. The majority of additives are consumed at a level of about 1 lb (0.45 kg) per year—0.04 oz (1.12g) per day.

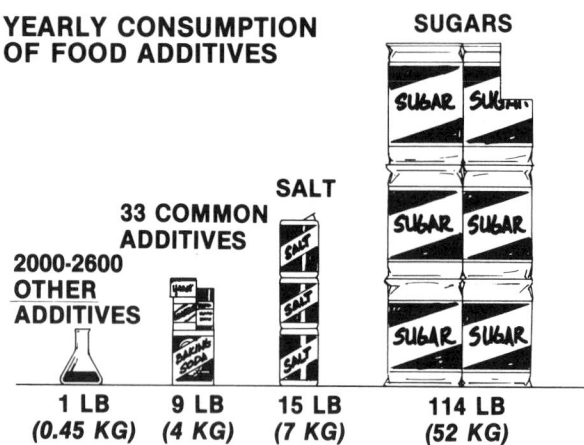

YEARLY CONSUMPTION OF FOOD ADDITIVES

SUGARS

SALT

33 COMMON ADDITIVES

2000-2600 OTHER ADDITIVES

| 1 LB | 9 LB | 15 LB | 114 LB |
| (0.45 KG) | (4 KG) | (7 KG) | (52 KG) |

Fig. A-5. Per capita yearly consumption of food additives.

GOVERNMENT CONTROLS OF ADDITIVES. In the United States, the basic food law is the Federal Food, Drug and Cosmetic Act of 1938. This law sets standards for the food industry and requires truthful labeling. The Food and Drug Administration enforces the act. This act gives the Food and Drug Administration (FDA) primary responsibility for the safety and wholesomeness of our food supply. The three important amendments which follow strengthened the act:

1. **The Miller Pesticide Amendment** of 1954 provides for the establishment of safe tolerances (permissible amounts) for pesticide residues on raw agricultural commodities.

2. **The Food Additives Amendment** of 1958 requires premarketing clearance for substances intended to be added to food and for substances occurring in food during processing, storage, or packaging. This amendment includes the Delaney Clause which states that no chemical can be added to food if, in any amount, it produces cancer when ingested by man or animal.
(Also see DELANEY CLAUSE.)

3. **The Color Additive Amendment** of 1960 regulates the listing and certification of color additives. About 1,700 samples are examined annually by FDA scientists.

Prior to the 1958 Food Additives Amendment, the FDA had to prove that an additive was potentially harmful before it could obtain a court order banning its use. Today, the manufacturer must prove to the FDA that an additive is safe under the conditions of intended use before permission to use it is given. The FDA requires extensive testing on at least two species of laboratory animals but not on humans. The manufacturer must present a petition stating results of studies on organ and tissue function including the liver, brain, kidneys, blood forming organs, excretory and reproductive systems. FDA scientists review the petition. If they judge the proposed additive safe and effective, they issue a regulation permitting its use.

• **Generally Recognized as Safe (GRAS)**—When the Food Additives Amendment of 1958 was adopted, about 200 substances were exempted from the testing requirement because they were judged by experts to be *Generally Recognized as Safe* (GRAS) under conditions of their use in foods at the time. The GRAS list is now much larger. About half of the products are natural flavorings or their derivatives. Vitamins, minerals, and other dietary supplements make up another large group.

In the time since the GRAS list was formulated, better testing methods have been developed. Also, use of some GRAS list items has increased far beyond their use at the time the list was compiled. As a result, several of the items, including cyclamates, were found to be of questionable safety and taken off the market.

(Also see BACTERIA IN FOOD; CARRAGEENAN; COLORING OF FOOD; ENRICHMENT; FLAVORS, SYNTHETIC; GUMS; MEAT, sections headed "Meat Curing," "Sausage Making," and "Meat Preservation"; NITRATES AND NITRITES; ORGANICALLY GROWN FOOD; and POISONS.)

ADENINE AND ADENOSINE

These related substances have metabolic roles as (1) components of chemical messengers that help to regulate metabolic processes, (2) parts of nucleic acids, and (3) components of special compounds that store and release chemical energy.

(Also see ENERGY-UTILIZATION BY THE BODY; METABOLISM; and NUCLEIC ACIDS.)

ADENOHYPHYSIS

The frontal lobe of the pituitary gland. It secretes hormones that stimulate the secretion of the other endocrine glands.

(Also see ENDOCRINE GLANDS.)

ADIPOSE TISSUE

A special connective tissue in which fat is stored for later use to provide energy. It also provides body protection against injury by trauma, insulation against excessive loss of heat from the body, and helps to keep certain organs in place.

(Also see TISSUES OF THE BODY; and FATS AND OTHER LIPIDS.)

ADIPOSITY

Obesity or the excessive accumulation of body fat.
(Also see OBESITY.)

ADIPSIA

A lack of thirst when water is needed by the body.
(Also see APPETITE.)

AD LIBITUM (AD LIB)

This latin term means to take food freely without restriction, in contrast to restrictive feeding where only fixed amounts of food are allowed to be taken.
(Also see APPETITE.)

ADRENAL CORTEX INSUFFICIENCY (ADDISON'S DISEASE)

The cortex or outside of the adrenal gland secretes several hormones which are very important in controlling metabolism. These hormones are broadly called the mineralocorticoids (mineral metabolism) and the glucocorticoids (glucose metabolism). Diseases such as tuberculosis or cancer can cause a destruction of the cortex of the adrenal gland, thereby preventing the proper secretion of its hormones. The resulting condition is characterized by marked pigmentation of the skin, decreased heart size, low blood pressure, and inability to withstand stress.
(Also see ENDOCRINE GLANDS.)

ADRENAL GLAND

One of the endocrine (ductless) glands of the body, located near the kidney, which secretes hormones needed to utilize nutrients.
(Also see ENDOCRINE GLANDS.)

ADRENALIN

A manufacturer's trade name for the hormone adrenaline (epinephrine).
(Also see ADRENALINE; and ENDOCRINE GLANDS.)

ADRENALINE

The common name for the hormone epinephrine, which is secreted by the adrenal glands. Adrenaline stimulates the nervous system and various other tissues—producing effects such as a racing of the heart, elevation of both the blood pressure and blood sugar, and breakdown of the glycogen in muscle to glucose.
(Also see ENDOCRINE GLANDS.)

ADRENERGIC

A drug, nerve transmitter, or similar substance which has the same effects as noradrenaline (norepinephrine).
(Also see ENDOCRINE GLANDS.)

ADRENOCORTICAL HORMONES

The hormones secreted by the adrenal cortex. These hormones help the body to adjust to stresses like low blood sugar, chilling, emotional excitement, and starvation.
(Also see ENDOCRINE GLANDS.)

ADULTERATION

The fraudulent addition of substances to food so as to gain an economic advantage.
(Also see FOOD AND DRUG ADMINISTRATION.)

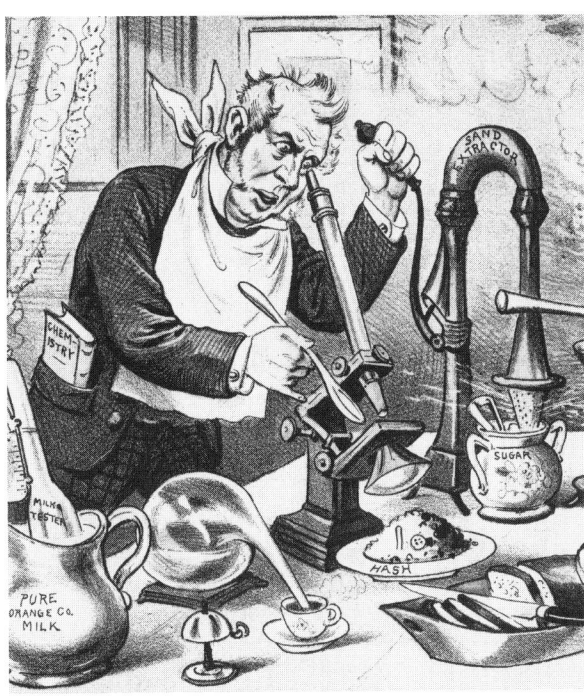

Fig. A-6. Look Before You Eat, and see if you can discover any unadulterated food. (19th century cartoon by Opper. Courtesy, The Bettman Archive, Inc., New York, N.Y.)

ADULT NUTRITION

Many adults are literally *cut down* in the prime of life by one or more degenerative diseases such as atherosclerosis, cancer, coronary heart disease, diabetes, or high blood pressure. Many health professionals and researchers believe that these dreaded conditions result mainly from a combination of hereditary susceptibility and poor health practices such as lack of exercise and unwholesome diets. Others lay some of the blame on the stresses of modern life, since the typical American adult often appears to be caught *in the middle* of the conflicts between the younger and older generations, demands of an employer and his or her family, and putting into practice the principles espoused by leading personalities in health, politics, and religion.

This article details some of the dietary principles that are believed to be helpful in the maintenance of good health during the adult years.
(Also see CANCER; HEART DISEASE; HIGH BLOOD PRESSURE; OBESITY; and STRESS.)

CHANGES IN THE BODY DURING ADULTHOOD.

One of the most notable changes to occur during the adult years is that many people who were fit and trim in their late teens and early twenties become fat and flabby in middle age. One indication of the prevalence and seriousness of this problem is the number of adults who consider themselves to be overweight, as shown in Fig. A-7.

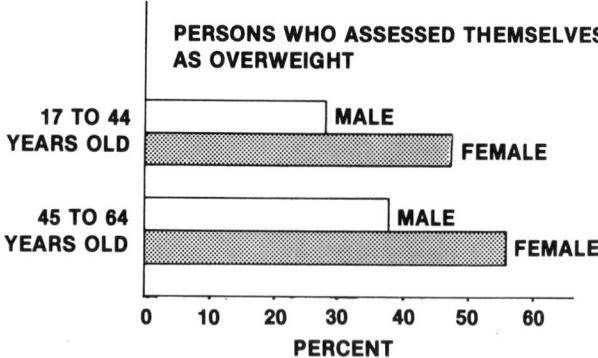

Fig. A-7. Percentages of younger and older adults who consider themselves to be overweight. (Adapted from *Social Indicators III*, U.S. Dept. of Commerce, Chart 2/23)

Fig. A-8 shows that only a few inches of gain around the waist represent quite a few pounds of extra fat.

The onset of these and other important changes generally starts at maturity (following the growth period), then continues ceaselessly until death. But, how fast and how far they develop is determined by a host of factors, including diet, heredity, exercise, stress, etc.

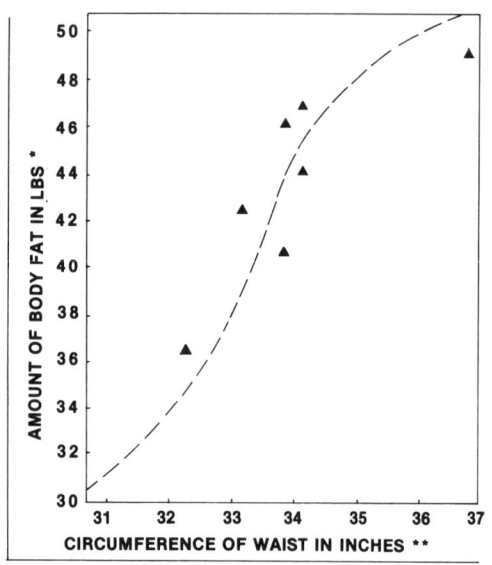

* TO OBTAIN KG, DIVIDE LB BY 2.2

** TO OBTAIN CM, MULTIPLY IN. BY 2.54

Fig. A-8. Correspondence of body fat with waistline measurements in adult males. (The graph was prepared by the authors from data in Krywicki, H. J., et al., "Alterations in Exercise and Body Composition with Age," *Proceedings of the Eighth International Congress on Nutrition*, Excerpta Medica Congress Series No. 213)

Generally speaking, the following body changes and cautions apply more to young adults than to the aged: (1) peak weight is often attained at middle age, after which there may be a gradual decrease in weight; (2) young adults with a family history of cardiovascular disease should be checked regularly for symptoms; (3) if the blood levels of insulin and glucose are not normal after an overnight fast, adult-onset diabetes should be suspected; (4) reduction in the secretion of thyroid hormones usually occurs later in life; and (5) the marked reactions after menopause—accelerated rate of mineral loss from the bones; thinner, less elastic skin; and hot flashes —usually begin in adult women in their 40s.

The changes that begin in the adult body and become evident to various degrees, and which are usually speeded up and accentuated in the aged, do not occur to an equal extent in every older person, since many of the elderly are healthier than some of their juniors.

HEALTH STATUS OF AMERICAN ADULTS.

Surveys have been conducted in which adults in various parts of the United States were asked about their health status. The results of one of these surveys are reported in Fig. A-9, which (1) shows that chronic health-impairing conditions are more prevalent in older adults, and (2) suggests that various tissues deteriorate as adults grow older.

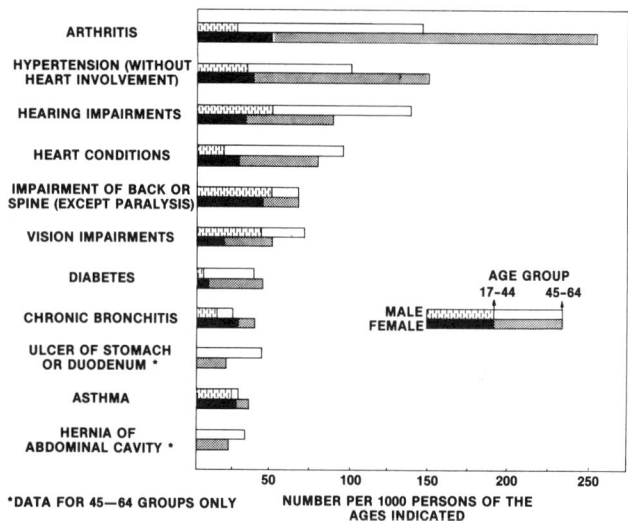

Fig. A-9. Prevalences of selected chronic conditions reported by American adults in health interviews. (Based upon data in *Health, United States*, U.S. Dept. HEW, pp. 481 and 487, Tables CD.III.23 and CD.III.26)

Health workers have attempted to find statistical correlations between degenerative diseases and certain types of dietary patterns. This approach has led to the identification of what are commonly called *risk factors*.

Major Risk Factors for Degenerative Diseases.

The leading killer diseases in the United States are heart diseases, cancer, and strokes, which together account for about two-thirds of all deaths. It is thought that many early deaths from these diseases may be prevented by (1) identifying people who have one or more risk factors, and (2) modifying the risk conditions as much as is feasible under the circumstances. The major risk factors follow.

• **Abnormal electrocardiogram**—This condition is closely associated with the risk of a heart attack because it usually indicates a defective conduction of the heartbeat through the heart muscle. Most of the sudden deaths of middle-aged people from heart attacks are believed to be associated with conductivity defects. Sometimes, the cause of the abnormality may be identified and corrected. For example, deficiencies of magnesium and/or potassium may be responsible for electrolyte imbalances that can be treated by oral or intravenous administration of the appropriate mineral salts.

• **Alcoholism**—Two of the most direct effects of this vice are impairment of the mental processes and damage to the liver.

It is noteworthy (1) that some chronic alcoholics suffer from multiple nutritional deficiencies because of failure to consume adequate diets, and (2) that alcoholism is the number one social problem in the United States.

• **Family history of cancer, diabetes, heart disease, high blood pressure, and/or obesity**—Certain diseases run in families which appear to have hereditary susceptibilities to various metabolic abnormalities. Hence, people whose close relatives have had one or more of these conditions early in life should go to a doctor for regular physical examinations that include the appropriate laboratory tests.

• **High blood cholesterol and lipoproteins**—Total blood cholesterol is an indicator of a heart attack. Even better indicators are the level of the lipoproteins which carry cholesterol in the blood; specifically, high-density lipoproteins (HDL) and low-density lipoproteins (LDL). HDL has a protective role since it transports cholesterol back to the liver, while LDL seems to deposit cholesterol in cells, including blood vessels. Also, evidence indicates that high HDL decreases the risk of heart attack while high LDL increases the risk.

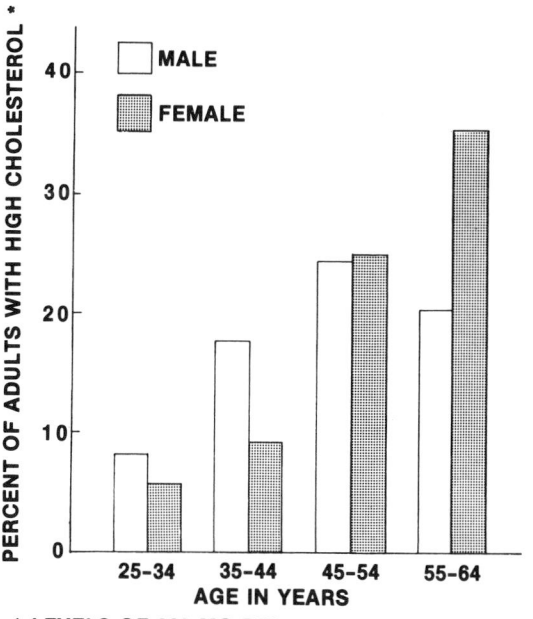

Fig. A-10. Percentages of adults with high blood cholesterol. (Adapted from *Social Indicators III*, U.S. Dept. of Commerce)

• **High blood pressure (hypertension)**—This condition is defined as a systolic pressure of 140 or greater and/or a diastolic pressure of 90 or greater. (See Fig. A-11.)

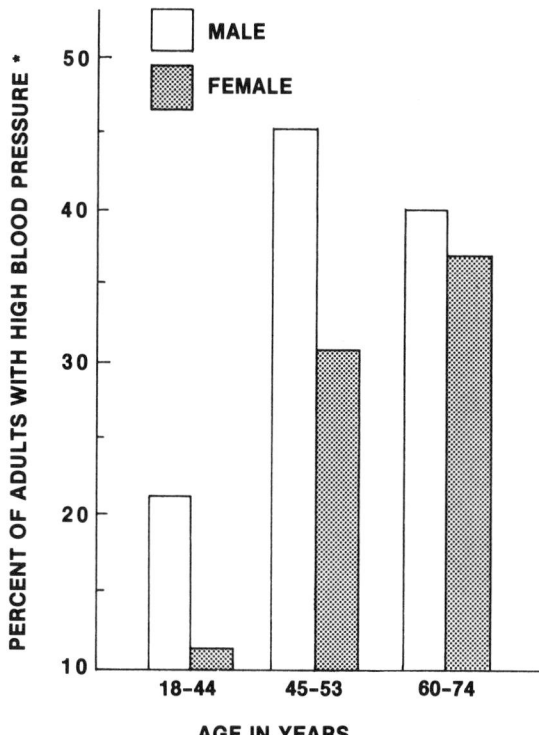

Fig. A-11. Percentages of adults with high blood pressure. (Based upon data from *Health, United States*, U.S. Dept. HEW)

High blood pressure is a dangerous condition because it hastens the development of atherosclerosis and increases the likelihood of an aneurism, heart attack, kidney disease, or stroke. Hence, it has been called the *silent killer*. Prompt treatment by means of dietary salt restriction, drugs, and reduction of overweight will decrease the risks.

• **Impaired glucose tolerance (diabeticlike metabolism of carbohydrates)**—This term designates the failure of the blood sugar level to come down to normal within a specified time after the consumption or injection of a test dose of sugar (glucose). Prolonged elevation of the blood sugar after meals increases the risk of diabetic complications such as arteriosclerosis, atherosclerosis, coronary thrombosis, injuries to the eyes and the kidneys, and stroke. Adults who have no previous history of diabetic symptoms are usually helped considerably by reduction of overweight to normal, since this condition occurs much more frequently in the obese than in people whose weights are normal. It is noteworthy that an impaired glucose tolerance sometimes results from the depletion of the body's supply of the essential mineral chromium. The latter circumstance is confirmed by the improvement of glucose tolerance when either inorganic chromium or the glucose tolerance factor (an organic complex that contains chromium) is administered orally or by injection.

• **Lack of exercise**—About 45% of American adults of age 22 and over fail to engage in physical exercise on a regular basis.[1] Hence, it is not surprising that the rates of various diseases increase steadily with age, since lack of exercise is closely associated with the development of obesity and its dire consequences. Furthermore, regular exercise increases the chances of surviving a heart attack since it enlarges the small blood vessels that may take over some of the task of blood circulation when the major coronary arteries are plugged.

• **Obesity**—Life insurance statisticians have found that notable obesity results in significantly increased risks of coronary heart disease, diabetes, gallbladder disease, high blood pressure, kidney disease, osteoarthritis, and stroke. However, people who are only moderately overweight according to life insurance tables may have little or no increased risk if they are otherwise in good health. Hence, the decision to undertake a stringent program for weight reduction should be made only after consulting a doctor.

• **Poor dietary practices**—Generally, this designation applies to diets that are high in calories from refined carbohydrates, fats, and starches, but low in proteins, minerals, and vitamins. However, even certain reasonably well-balanced diets may be unsuitable for people with greater than normal tendencies to develop such conditions as arteriosclerosis, atherosclerosis, bowel problems, cancer, congestive heart failure, coronary heart disease, diabetes, high blood fats, high blood pressure, kidney disease, or various types of food intolerances. In such cases, normal diets may be potentially harmful—except those specially modified to meet nutritional needs while avoiding factors that may aggravate the degenerative disorder(s). For example, people prone to congestive heart failure, excessive fluid buildup in the tissues, and high blood pressure may have to go to considerable trouble to avoid salt-containing foods that supply too much sodium for such conditions.

• **Rapid and/or irregular heartbeat**—Racing of the heart while at rest may be a sign of one or more disorders such as anemia, congestive heart failure, hyperthyroidism, or an infectious disease. Hence, a doctor should be consulted promptly whenever the pulse remains at 90 beats per minute or greater for prolonged periods of time. Also, an irregular pulse may be a sign of a disorder such as a reaction to a drug or other medication, or a severe deficiency of potassium, magnesium, or thiamin. It is noteworthy that the normal resting pulse rates of trained athletes may be as low as 45 to 60 beats per minute.

• **Smoking**—At least seven potential carcinogens are present in cigarette smoke, but the level of smoking needed to cause lung cancer is uncertain, and may even depend upon the overall resistance to injury of the smoker's lungs. Smoking is also believed to be a major contributor to cardiovascular disease because (1) it reduces the supply of vital oxygen to the tissues, (2) it speeds up the heart rate, and (3) it causes an inflammatory disease of the blood vessels.

• **Stress**—Although brief exposures to certain emotional or physical stresses may be stimulating to the body, prolonged severe stresses may cause irreversible damage to tissues and organs. Therefore, people who find it difficult to cope with day-to-day affairs should seek some help from a competent person such as a clergyman, doctor, friend, or psychologist.

NUTRITIONAL ALLOWANCES OF ADULTS. A complete presentation of nutrient allowances for different age groups, including adults, along with nutrient functions and best food sources of each nutrient, is given in this book in the section on Nutrients: Requirements, Allowances, Functions, Sources, and its accompanying Table N-3; hence, the reader is referred thereto.

DIETARY GUIDELINES. The first dietary guideline is: *Eat enough of proper foods consistently.* To ensure nutritional adequacy, adults (and those responsible for their diets) are admonished to—

1. Read and follow the section on Nutrients: Requirements, Allowances, Functions, Sources, including Table N-3.

2. Eat a daily diet which includes definite amounts of foods from each of the Six Food Groups as detailed in the section on Food Groups.

But, lots of folks don't know what constitutes a good diet; and, worse yet, altogether too many people neglect or ignore the rules even if they know them. In either case, the net result is always the same; we shortchange ourselves on the right amounts of good nutritious foods. As a result, more and more doctors and nutritionists are recommending judicious mineral and vitamin supplementation.

It is noteworthy, too, that those whose diets are restricted for the treatment of certain disorders may need to use supplements as sources of the nutrients that would ordinarily be provided by foods which are not allowed in their diets. For example, people who cannot drink milk or eat cheese may have to take a calcium supplement that provides this mineral.

Planning of Meals. A convenient way of planning meals is to use a food guide that translates the technical language of nutrients into terms of everyday eating. The Six Food Groups does this. It (1) groups foods in categories which reflect their similarities as good sources of specific nutrients, and (2) gives recommended amounts of each.
(Also see FOOD GROUPS.)

Modified Diets and Dietetic Foods. Some people may need to follow diets that restrict certain foods as part of the overall therapy for one or more conditions such as atherosclerosis, cancer, diabetes, gall bladder disease, gout, heart disease, high blood fats, high blood pressure, or obesity. The percentages of adults on the most common types of modified diets are shown in Fig. A-12. However, one should *not* undertake to follow such a diet without the advice of a doctor or a dietitian.

It may be noted from Fig. A-12 that the percentages of people on modified diets are much higher for older adults than for younger adults. The high rates of high blood pressure, high blood cholesterol, and obesity indicate the need for greater use of modified diets by people of all ages.
(Also see MODIFIED DIETS)

---

[1]*Health, United States,* U.S. Dept. HEW, p. 453, Table CD.III.9.

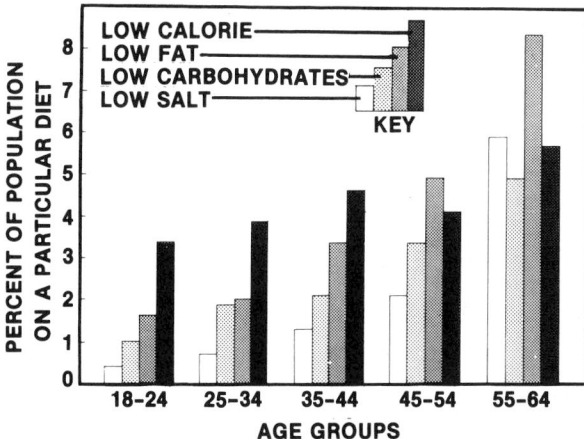

Fig. A-12. Adults of selected age groups who are commonly prescribed modified diets. (Based upon data in *Social Indicators, III*, U.S. Dept. of Commerce, 1980, p. 106, Table 2/24)

SUMMARY. It is generally recognized that there are changes in appearance, mental outlook, and body functions as individuals pass from youth into middle age and then into old age. Behind the outer changes in people as they grow older are changes in the body and its workings. Some of these changes are not due to aging as such, but to impaired nutrition of body cells. So, adult nutrition involves the past, the present, and the future. An adult's nutritional state at any specific age reflects all his/her previous dietary history as well as his/her current food practices. Consequently, a good diet early in life will make for vigorous maturity; and continuance of good adult nutrition will extend the years of usefulness and delay—and, in some instances, even prevent—the appearance of old age. With good nutrition throughout life, it is the privilege of adults to extend their youthful vigor into middle age and beyond and to enjoy buoyant good health.

(Also see NUTRIENTS: REQUIREMENTS, ALLOWANCES, FUNCTIONS, SOURCES.)

ADZUKI BEAN *Phaseolus angularis*

This legume, which ranks next to soybeans in importance among the Chinese and Japanese, recently became known in the United States as a staple food in the Zen Macrobiotic diets.

AEQUUM

This is the food required for body maintenance under usual or specified activity.

AEROBIC

In the presence of air. The term usually applied to microorganisms that require oxygen to live and reproduce.

(Also see METABOLISM.)

AEROPHAGIA

The swallowing of air, a habit commonly found in nervous people.

AESCULIN (Esculin)

This is a glycoside found in chestnuts.

AFLATOXIN

Aflatoxins are the most feared of the mycotoxins—toxin-producing molds. There are four main aflatoxins: B_1, B_2, G_1, and G_2, of which B_1 is the most common and the most toxic. A high incidence of cancer, especially liver cancer, is associated with aflatoxin.

(Also see POISONS, Table P-2 Mycotoxins.)

AGAR-AGAR

This material is extracted from red algae (*Rhodophyceae*) and is known to most people as a medium for growing microorganisms, but it has long been used by Asians for making jellies and other food preparations. Although many people use the term agar-agar, food technologists simply call the substance agar.

Some of the agar-containing seaweed is collected from rocks exposed at low tide along the sea coast of Japan, but the best material is collected under water by specially trained female divers, called *Ama*. Male divers, equipped with diving apparatus, make the collections at depths greater than 60 feet. The algae is sold to commercial processors after it has been dried and partly bleached on the beach.

The seaweed is extracted by boiling in water in open pots or by autoclaving. The extract is then filtered and further bleached, followed by reextracting in order to obtain the maximum yield of agar. After jelling, freezing, and thawing, the gel is dried and pulverized.

USES OF AGAR IN FOODS. Although agar costs more than synthetic and other natural jelling agents, it is usually superior to such products because its gels have greater transparency, strength, stability over a range of acidity and alkalinity, and reversability (gels may be formed and melted without decomposition of the agar). Some of the most common food uses follow.

• **Confections**—Jelly-type candies are still made with agar (it is used at concentrations from 0.3 to 1.8% by weight), although starch and pectin are used whenever a transparency and other characteristics of agar gel are not required.

• **Fish, meat, and poultry products**—Canning of soft animal products, such as various meats, in agar gel prevents them from being broken into pieces during shipment. Other jelling agents are not as satisfactory since they are more likely to melt.

• **Fruit and vegetable gels**—Although other jelling agents have replaced agar in most of these products, it is still used in dietetic and vegetarian preparations (it is noncaloric and may be used in place of gelatin).

USE OF AGAR IN HOME RECIPES. Agar may be used in place of gelatin, but much smaller quantities are needed to produce the same jelling effects.

(Also see ADDITIVES.)

AGEUSIA

The lack of normal tasting ability which may be due to zinc deficiency or other causes.

(Also see TASTE; and ZINC.)

AGING

The process by which certain body functions decline gradually with the passing of time until there may be great impairment(s). The rate of aging depends upon dietary, genetic, and environmental factors.

(Also see GERONTOLOGY AND GERIATRIC NUTRITION; and LONGEVITY.)

AGING MEAT

The process through which meat is made tender and flavor develops. The tenderizing process starts soon after slaughter. Aging is usually accomplished by holding the cuts at a temperature of 38° to 40°F (3° to 4°C) and a relative humidity of 85 to 90%, with a gradual flow of air to provide fresh atmosphere.

ALANINE

One of the nonessential amino acids.
(Also see AMINO ACID[S].)

ALAR (DAMINOZIDE)

Alar is the brand name of the chemical daminozide, and organic acid. It is a growth regulator which enables growers to provide consumers top quality apples that maintain firmness and resist bruising, early decay, and cracking. Alar was formerly applied as a spray on some varieties of apples, including Red Delicious, McIntosh, and Staymen, about 60 days before harvest.

ALBEDO

The white, fibrous material which lies between the segments and the peel of citrus fruits. It constitutes from 20 to 60% of the whole fruit, and is used in the production of pectin. The albedo is rich in fiber and bioflavonoids.

(Also see BIOFLAVONOIDS; CITRUS FRUITS; FIBER; and PECTIN.)

ALBINISM

A lack of pigment in the eyes, hair, and skin due to an inborn error of metabolism. People who have this trait are called albinos. Their hair and skin are white, while the corneas of their eyes are pink.

(Also see INBORN ERRORS OF METABOLISM.)

ALBUMEN

The watery material which comprises the white of eggs and which consists mainly of the protein albumin.
(Also see ALBUMIN.)

ALBUMIN

A type of protein which is easily digested and which contains a good proportion of the essential amino acids. It is present in the tissues and body fluids of animals and man as plasma albumin. It is also in milk, as lactalbumin, and in egg white, as egg albumin. Albumin is soluble in water, and is coagulated and solidified by heat. It is the principal type of protein in the blood, where it plays a major role in regulating the fluid flow between the blood and tissues. However, lactalbumin and egg albumin provoke allergies in some people.

(Also see ALLERGIES; and PROTEIN[S].)

ALBUMIN INDEX

A measure of egg quality and freshness; the ratio of the height of the albumin to the width when an egg is broken onto a flat surface. As the egg deteriorates, the albumin index decreases, i.e., the egg white spreads.

ALBUMINOIDS

Fibrous proteins that have supporting or protective function in the animal, of which there are three types: (1) collagens in the skin, tendons and bones, which are resistant to pepsin and trypsin, and are converted to water-soluble gelatin by boiling with water; (2) elastins in the tendons and arteries, which are not converted to gelatin; and (3) ceratins, which comprise the horns, hoofs, feathers, scales, and nails, and which are insoluble in dilute acids and alkalis and are not attacked by any animal digestive enzymes.

ALBUMINURIA

A condition in which some of the albumin in the blood escapes through the kidney's filtering membrane into the urine. Albuminuria often accompanies kidney diseases.

ALCAPTONURIA (ALKAPTONURIA)

A rare inborn (recessive) abnormality of metabolism in man marked by the inability to complete the degradation of tyrosine and phenylalanine; their metabolism ceases at homogentisic acid, which is excreted in the urine. The homogentisic acid oxidizes to black melanoid pigment; hence, the urine of alcaptonurics slowly turns black. The defect appears to be harmless.

ALCOHOL AND ALCOHOLIC BEVERAGES

Broadly speaking, the term alcohol refers to the hundreds of colorless, volatile, flammable organic compounds formed by the fermentation of starch, sugar, and other carbohydrates. As commonly used, however, the term alcohol refers to one particular member of the alcohol group—it refers to ethyl alcohol, or ethanol, which has the formula C_6H_6O, most of which is used in alcoholic beverages.

HISTORY. Anthropologists believe that alcoholic beverages were produced by almost every prehistoric society that had access to fermentable substances such as fruits or starchy products. (It appears that only the Eskimos lacked the means to produce these drinks.) The processes for making the beverages were easy to discover because (1) fruits and beverages that contained honey fermented spontaneously, (2) some starchy grains (notably barley, rye, and wheat) contained enzymes that converted starch to sugar during the process of sprouting (germination), and (3) human saliva supplied a starch splitting enzyme that was made to work on starchy foods by chewing them briefly prior to fermentation.

The first widespread use of alcohol by people in ancient societies appears to have been for religious ceremonies and social rites of passage such as those marking birth, puberty, marriage, and death. Many of the writings from the ancient civilizations contain admonitions against drunkeness, while tolerating or even encouraging the drinking of alcoholic beverages. For example, orthodox Jews have long used wine as a ceremonial drink, yet the rate of alcoholism for these people is about the lowest for any ethnic or religious group that consumes this type of drink. However, other cultural groups have accepted drinking to intoxication as a normal occurrence on certain occasions, as evidenced by the literature of Greece and Rome, and the observations anthropologists have made of certain Latin American Indian tribes.

ETHYL ALCOHOL (ETHANOL; GRAIN ALCO-HOL). Ethyl alcohol is obtained by fermenting sugar or such starchy products as corn, barley, wheat, rye, rice, and potatoes. Beverage alcohol may also be obtained by distilling fermented mashed fruit or grain.

Most ethyl alcohol is used primarily as beverages. Other uses include denatured alcohol, solvent in laboratories and industries, pharmaceuticals, perfumery, and organic synthesis.

Any beverage that contains ethyl alcohol in intoxicating quantities is classed as an alcoholic drink. People drink alcohol in the following three main kinds of beverages:

1. **Beers**, which are made from grain through brewing and fermentation and contain 2 to 8% alcohol.
(Also see BEERS AND BREWING.)

2. **Distilled beverages** (spirits) such as whiskey, gin, and vodka, which contain an average of 45 to 50% alcohol.
(Also see DISTILLED LIQUORS.)

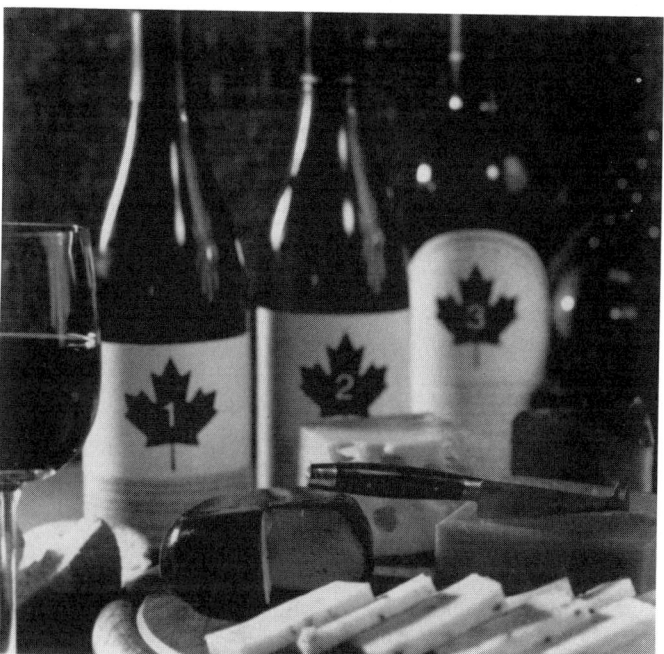

Fig. A-13. Canadian wine and cheese. (Courtesy, Agriculture Canada, Ottawa, Canada)

3. **Wines**, which are fermented from grapes and other fruits and contain 8 to 12% alcohol.
(Also see WINE.)

EFFECTS OF ALCOHOL. When ingested in moderate amounts, alcohol acts on the central nervous system and higher centers of the brain, lowering inhibitions and affecting judgment. Large amounts may produce a loss of muscular control, unconsciousness, and even death. Also, people may become addicted to any alcoholic beverage.

OTHER ALCOHOLS. Other important alcohols, in addition to ethyl alcohol, include methyl alcohol (wood alcohol), butyl alcohol, ethylene alcohol, methol, and

glycerol or glycerin. Most of these alcohols have commercial importance. They are used as solvents and in the preparation of dyes, pharmaceuticals, antifreeze, esters, and other compounds. Some alcohols are very toxic; for example, methyl alcohol (wood alcohol) affects the optic nerve and causes blindness, and as little as 1 oz (*30 ml*) has caused death.
(Also see ALCOHOLISM AND ALCOHOLICS; BEERS AND BREWING; DISTILLED LIQUORS; and WINE.)

ALCOHOL, DENATURED

This refers to ethyl alcohol, which is made *unfit* for drinking, though its usefulness for other purposes is not affected. The following are some of the most commonly used denaturants: methanol, camphor, amyl alcohol, gasoline, isopropanol, terpineol, benzene, castor oil, acetone, nicotine, aniline dyes, ether, pyridine, cadmium iodine, sulfuric acid, kerosene, and diethyl phthalate. These may be used either alone or in combination. One of the prime reasons for denaturing ethyl alcohol is taxation purposes.

ALCOHOLISM AND ALCOHOLICS

Alcoholism is a disease in which the drinking of an alcoholic beverage becomes a compulsion. People who have this urge to drink are called alcoholics. It is noteworthy that 12 to 14% of regular drinkers become problem drinkers and that at least 5% become alcoholics. It is the major form of substance abuse that occurs in the United States and the former U.S.S.R.

HARMFUL EFFECTS OF ALCOHOLISM. Chronic, excessive drinking often has dire consequences that result from the alteration of normal physiological functions by alcohol, and from the disruptrive effects of alcohol behavior on personal functioning and interpersonal relationships. For example, alcoholics have a mortality 2½ times greater than average, a suicide rate 2½ times greater than average, and an accident rate 7 times greater than average. Details relative to the major physiological, emotional, and behavioral disorders associated with chronic alcoholism follow.

• **Cardiovascular problems**—Alcohol affects the cardiovascular system by (1) causing vasodilation of the peripheral vessels, producing flushing, heat loss, and a sense of warmth; and (2) promoting vasoconstriction of the central blood vessels, producing resistance to the flow of blood, and increasing the work load on the heart.

• **Central nervous system disorders**—Long-term excessive use of alcohol can result in premature aging of the brain. Whereas some difficulties with cognitive function clear up after a period of abstinence, residual problems can remain, usually due to a combination of nutritional deficiencies, repeated alcohol-related convulsions, head injuries, and degeneration of nerve and tissue cells.

• **Decreased immunity to infections and impaired healing of injuries**—Alcohol-dependent persons frequently have a lowered resistance to infections of all types because of the depressing effect of alcohol on the immunological system, especially white blood cells. Upper respiratory infections and pneumonia are common. Injuries, including surgical wounds, require longer to heal.

• **Development of an addiction to alcohol**—Consuming large quantities of alcohol over extended periods of time results in a decreased sensitivity of the brain to the effects of the alcohol. As a person continues to drink, an increased intake of alcohol is needed to achieve a desired effect. Many alcohol-dependent people do not seem to be intoxicated after drinking large amounts. Their bodies can tolerate higher continuous blood alcohol concentrations without noticeable signs or symptoms of intoxication. The risk of greatly increased tolerance and development of addiction seems greater in those who consume an average of about six or more drinks per day. The increase in tolerance and the development of addiction are gradual processes that usually progress over a period of many years. However, some individuals may experience these developments over a period of only a few years or months.

• **Emotional disturbances**—Alcohol decreases cognitive functions and allows the emotions to predominate. Anger or rage, sadness, and euphoria are commonly experienced during heavy drinking and often displayed in an exaggerated manner. Hence, the person who drinks may become argumentative, hostile, or intent on fighting; tearful and maudlin; or the *life of the party*. In contrast, some people drink to dull or escape their feelings. Drinking to lessen the pain of guilt, rage, or sorrow usually provides only temporary relief, and when the effects of the alcohol are gone, the painful feelings return, often with increased intensity. In certain situations, with mental judgment diminished by alchohol and normal fears dampened, a person may take unaccustomed risks. Accidents, homicide, and suicide are serious consequences of alcohol's effect on emotions.

• **Fetal addiction and the fetal alcohol syndrome (FAS)**—When the mother is an active alcoholic, her child may be born addicted and experience withdrawal symptoms within the first week of life.

Heavy drinking during pregnancy can also cause the fetal alcohol syndrome. Most common in the FAS are prenatal growth deficiencies, usually more severe with respect to birth length than birth weight, and postnatal growth deficiencies persisting through early childhood. Failure to thrive is reported despite adequate calorie intake and excellent foster care in the first year of life. Often, the infant has an abnormally small head. Mental deficiency or developmental delay are almost always present. Fine motor dysfunction including tremulousness, weak grasp, and poor eye-hand coordination are present in most children with FAS.

Craniofacial malformation are common features of FAS, which impairs the normal development of the skull, jaws, teeth, nose, eyes, and facial skin. Sometimes variable anomalies of limbs and joints are present, including congenital hip dislocations, abnormalities of the toes, and inability to extend completely the elbows or metacarpal phalangeal joints. Cardiac malformations syndrome encompasses an atrial septal defect, a patent ductus arteriosis, and cardiac murmurs representing ventricular septal defects. Anomalies of external genitalia have also been noted.

There are still a number of unanswered questions about fetal alcohol syndrome, such as the risk of moderate drinking, whether the risk to the fetus is greater at particular times during pregnancy, and the influence of other factors such as smoking and nutrition. While research continues on these and other issues, caution is advised. The recommended guideline for alcohol consumption during pregnancy is no more than 1 oz (28 g) of ethanol per day (two drinks).

• **Gastrointestinal disorders**—Alcohol is an irritating chemical and in strong solution can damage the mucosa and result in esophagitis and gastritis. Increased capillary fragility can result in gastric bleeding. Erosion and ulceration of the mucosa can occur, and gastric or duodenal ulcers are a frequent result. The severity of these problems is related to the extent and duration of alcohol misuse.

• **Increased risk of cancer**—An excessive intake of alcohol increases the risk of cancer, particularly of the mouth, pharynx, larynx, and esophagus. In addition, alcoholic patients with cancer show lower survival rates and higher rates of developing another primary tumor when compared to other patients with the same cancer. The highest risk occurs when heavy alcohol intake is combined with heavy smoking, especially for esophageal cancer. One study reported the risk of esophageal cancer as 44 times higher for individuals who took more than six drinks per day and smoked a pack or more of cigarettes per day than for individuals who used little or none of either substance.

• **Liver disease**—Enlargement of the liver occurs with prolonged heavy alcohol use, probably as a result of accumulation of triglycerides in the hepatic cells. This fatty liver condition is usually reversible with abstinence from alcohol and a nutritional diet. Alcohol-induced hepatitis and cirrhosis are more serious disease processes. Each of these ailments is thought by some to be due largely to the direct effects of alcohol on the liver tissue and may occur even in the presence of adequate diet. With cirrhosis, death usually results from hepatic failure, hemorrhage from esophageal varices, portal vein thrombosis, or infection. Approximately 85 to 90% of deaths from cirrhosis are alcohol related.

• **Nutritional deficiencies**—A number of alcohol-related neurological disorders are due to nutritional deficiencies—primarily the B vitamins, including thiamin. These deficiencies result from decreased taste for food, decreased appetite (alcohol is high in calories and suppresses the appetite), and malabsorption of nutrients due to the irritated lining of the stomach and small intestine. A common nutritional deficiency disorder, peripheral polyneuropathy, is characterized by weakness, numbness, partial paralysis of extremities, pain in the legs, and impaired sensory reaction and motor reflexes. This condition is reversible with adequate diet and supplemental thiamin and other B vitamins.

If the polyneuropathy is left untreated, it may progress to Wernicke's encephalopathy. This more serious disorder is also reversible. It is characterized by ophthalmoplegia, nystagmus, ataxia, apathy, drowsiness, confusion, and inability to concentrate. Without treatment, it can be fatal. Another disease, often manifested after improvement from Wernicke's encephalopathy is Korsakoff's psychosis. This condition is characterized by disorientation and memory defect, usually with filling of the gaps with fictitious details, and often polyneuropathy. Many of those who develop this disorder show only limited improvement with treatment and generally require placement in psychiatric institutions or nursing homes. For obvious reasons, these persons require close supervision and assistance with activities of daily living.

• **Pancreatitis**—Acute pancreatitis, which may develop from prolonged alcohol misuse, exhibits symptoms ranging in severity from a gastritislike sensation to severe pain with nausea and vomiting and rigidity of the abdominal musculature. The most serious consequences of this condition include necrosis and hemorrhaging of the organ. Usually all that is required to alleviate the problem is abstinence from alcohol, maintenance of nutrition and fluid balance, and treatment of symptoms.

• **Personality changes**—With long misuse, alcohol alters the personality. The particular changes caused by alcohol misuse are related to the person's basic personality structure and his individual response to the long-term effects of alcohol. For example, a fun-loving, outgoing person who enjoys life and the company of others may, with problem drinking, become irritable, belligerent, defiant, hostile, isolated, rigid, or stubborn. The preteen or teen-ager may misuse alcohol to avoid the painful aspects of adolescence, a critical period of psychosocial growth and development. Bypassing the *growing up* process leaves the person handicapped as an adult. This is one possible explanation for the emotional immaturity and juvenile behavior often seen in the alcohol-dependent adult.

• **Sensory impairments**—For some people, alcoholic beverages, such as wine, may serve to enhance the flavor of some foods. For others, alcohol reduces the sensitivity to taste and odors, making food less appealing. Tactile response is not affected, but sensitivity to pain is decreased. This is one factor in the increased incidence of burns, cuts, scrapes, and bruises among problem drinkers. At high doses, vision is impaired in terms of decreased resistance to glare (i.e., the eyes take longer to readjust after exposure to bright lights), and there is a narrowing of the visual field (tunnel vision). These effects are particularly significant when a person attempts to drive while under the influence of alcohol. Normal function returns when alcohol is no longer present in the body.

• **Sexual difficulties**—It is a popular notion that alcohol acts as a sexual stimulant. While it may assist in overcoming guilt and lack of self-confidence, promote a feeling of sexiness or amorousness, and release inhibitions, actual performance is impaired. Chronic heavy use of alcohol can result in sexual frigidity or impotency. Generally, the disturbance in sexual function disappears with abstinence from alcohol over a period of several months or more.

• **Sleep disturbances**—While low doses of alcohol induce relaxation and sleepiness, large doses produce sleep disturbances.

• **Violent and destructive behavior (pathological alcohol reaction)**—After drinking only a small amount of alcohol, some people lose contact with reality, get out of control, and become violent and physically destructive. Such persons may smash windows, throw things, break furniture, or assault another person. The episode may last several hours. The victim usually collapses in a state of exhaustion and awakens with no memory of what occurred. Pathological alcohol reaction is differentiated from blackout because of the extremely violent behavior which characterizes it. There is no way of predicting who will develop this disorder or when. A person in this state may attempt homicide. The mechanism of pathological alcohol reaction, a rare condition, is unknown.

SIGNS AND SYMPTOMS OF ALCOHOLISM. Early indications that a person is heading down the path towards alcoholism are often overlooked by his or her relatives and friends, which is unfortunate because at least 5% of all drinkers become alcoholics, and it is much easier to treat the disorder in its early stages than after it has become well established. Therefore, some noteworthy signs and symptoms of alcoholism follow:

• **Drinking enough to be moderately high several times a week**—This pattern includes the *martinis for lunch bunch* as well as those who sip continuously at home most afternoons, have extended cocktail hour every night, or settle down for almost daily TV and six-pack sessions.

• **Drinking enough to get really drunk once a week**—The weekend heavy drinkers are in this category: those who think parties are a reason to get drunk and find a party once a week; and workers to whom every Friday means happy hour. The latter are prone to reason: "I can really get drunk tonight because I can sleep late tomorrow."

• **Drinking to oblivion once a month**—Generally referred to as spree drinking, this pattern is often followed by the heavy drinkers who try to cram all the drinks they didn't have on other days into one long drinking session.

• **A tolerance to alcohol is developed**—Greater amounts must be consumed to obtain the desired effects. Often, the increased tolerance to alcohol is accompanied by increased tolerances to drugs such as barbiturates.

• **Occasional periods of temporary amnesia or *blackouts** drinking*—During these periods, the drinker remains conscious but does not remember what happened during the blackout. (Nondrinkers may also have blackouts, but for different reasons such as fatigue, reduced blood flow to the brain, and emotional stress.)

The drinker who regularly drinks to the point of intoxication or sickness has already become an alcoholic, because other people who can control their drinking behavior will usually be able to stop before these undesirable effects occur.

TREATMENT OF ALCOHOLISM. The two major phases of the treatment of alcoholism are (1) correcting the medical, nutritional, and psychological problems brought on by this disorder; and (2) alleviating or curing the dependency on alcohol. These treatments are in many respects interdependent in that total recovery requires that the alcoholic be helped to function as normally as possible. However, they are covered separately in order to simplify the various aspects of the treatment.

Correction of Medical, Nutritional, and Psychological Disorders. Doctors and other health professionals are likely to be called upon to assist alcoholics in various stages of debilitation and/or intoxication. Naturally, the highest priority should be given to the life-threatening aspects of the disorder before attending the less critical problems of the patient. Brief discussions of the most commonly encountered conditions follow:

• **Mild to moderate intoxication**—Although most patients can recover from this condition without outside intervention, prompt treatment ensures that the intoxicated persons will not inflict injuries on themselves or other people. Usually, a cold shower, strong coffee, forced walking, and/or induced vomiting will help to speed the return to full consciousness; although, in some cases a doctor may have to administer a stimulant drug. (None of these measures hasten the oxidation of alcohol by the body. Rather, they act as stimulants to the central nervous system, which has been depressed by alcohol.)

• **Alcoholic stupor**—The need for intervention depends upon whether or not the vital signs (body temperature, heart rate, and rate of breathing) are normal since alcohol may depress the centers of the brain that control these functions. When the vital signs are normal, most people can be allowed to return to normal gradually, although someone should be present to check the vital signs at regular intervals.

• **Violent and aggressive behavior**—This condition is sometimes referred to as *pathological intoxication*. It may be necessary for the doctor to quiet the patient with a sedative such as one of the barbiturates.

• **Coma**—Sometimes, comatose patients may appear to be asleep, but in fact do not respond to external stimuli in normal ways. The treatment depends upon the depth of the coma and the status of the vital functions.

• **Abstinence or withdrawal disorders**—Alcoholics who have interrupted their pattern of drinking may have the *shakes,* hallucinations, convulsive seizures, and/or delirium tremens. Treatment requires medical detoxification and close observation until this critical period has passed. Sometimes, patients may be in shock and require intravenous infusions of saline solutions.

Also, these disorders may be aggravated by severe nutritional deficiencies that damage the nervous system. Hence, some doctors may inject large doses of the B vitamins.

• **Nutritional deficiencies**—Many alcoholics eat poorly and are likely to have multiple nutritional deficiencies. However, the most appropriate nutritional therapy can only be chosen after the patient's medical status has been determined by means of close observations and laboratory tests. For example, an alcoholic fatty liver may be treated with a normal-fat, normal-protein, vitamin-enriched diet, whereas more severe liver disease may require restriction of the protein intake to prevent a coma from being induced. Other medical problems such as salt and water retention in the tissue, kidney failure, central nervous system disorders, anemias, and alcoholic heart disease may also require special medical *and* nutritional therapies.

• **Psychological disturbances**—Depending upon the type of disorder, the patient may require institutionalization or may be treated on an outpatient basis. For example, some alcoholics suffer from paranoia and are potentially dangerous to themselves and others. Nevertheless, great strides have been made in the use of medications to control psychological disorders.

Alleviation or Curing of Dependence on Alcohol.

In the United States, the aim of therapists seeking to treat alcoholics in recent years has been the achievement of complete abstinence. Before the emergence of Alcoholics Anonymous, it was generally conceded that alcoholics could continue to drink, and the alcoholic was therefore usually advised to drink in moderation. This treatment was characteristically unsuccessful. After the A.A. experience, the prevailing contemporary view has generally been that the alcoholic must not only abstain from the use of alcohol but must also alter his self-concept, changing his image from that of a drinker to an abstainer. The demand for complete abstinence which the American culture tends to impose upon the arrested alcoholic shapes the prevailing treatment philosophy and is generally reflected in the orientation of the institutions providing this treatment. (Therapists in certain other countries such as Japan do not attempt to achieve complete abstinence.)

A recently developed alcoholism therapy is known as the *total push*. It subjects the patient to a variety of treatments such as Alcoholics Anonymous meetings, correction of nutritional deficiencies, drug therapy, group sessions, hypnosis, individual psychological and religious counseling, lectures, and physiotherapies in order to identify those which best meet the patient's needs. Then, the patient is encouraged to continue those deemed most suitable on a long-term outpatient basis. However, there is little objective evidence on the effectiveness of the various therapies. Therefore, many of the treatment programs around the country still rely on drug therapy and various types of group sessions.

• **Drug therapy**—Antabuse (trade name for disulfiram) is a drug widely recommended by a number of clinicians. Its effect is to make the patient violently nauseated whenever he drinks alcohol. It has been found that it works much more effectively if patients are asked to give it to themselves. The drug alone is claimed not to be effective, and it is generally recommended that it be combined with psychotherapy. It is also observed that patients who come to psychotherapy in the first place, who stay with it, and are willing to take antabuse, constitute a highly motivated group. Their high level of motivation is viewed as an important factor in treatment success.

• **Group sessions (Alcoholics Anonymous)**—Various programs have been developed in which the psychotherapy is oriented towards (1) the alcoholic and his or her family; or (2) groups of alcoholics who share their trials and tribulations. So far, the most successful programs have been those of Alcoholics Anonymous and the separate organizations that were founded along similar lines.

Alcoholics Anonymous (AA), founded in 1935 in Akron, Ohio, by two desperate alcoholics, a stock broker and a surgeon, now claims 2 million participants in 136 countries. AA is a remarkable fellowship of mutual and spiritual support that has endured in simplicity. It has no dues, no bureaucracy, no minutes; the only requirement for membership is a desire to stop drinking. The cornerstone of the program is *abstinence*.

Two of the organizations that operate on principles similar to those of Alcoholics Anonymous are (1) Al-Anon Family Groups, which are fellowships of wives, husbands, relatives, and friends of problem drinkers; and (2) Alateens, which is strictly for teen-age children of alcoholics.

SUMMARY. Alcoholism, a compulsive addiction to heavy and frequent drinking, is a behavior over which the afflicted individual has little, if any, control. Untreated alcoholism may cause extensive and severe physical and mental damage and may eventually result in psychosis and/or death.

Although various treatment methods have been recommended, and although there has been considerable activity in some states to develop a variety of treatment and training facilities, there is very little adequate research to indicate that any of these various intervention strategies significantly reduce alcoholism in groups of alcoholics, over time periods of a year or more. Individual cases of cures are reported, especially by members of Alcoholics Anonymous. However, scientifically precise studies of the impact of this organization have not been carried out, partly because of the principle of the anonymity of its members.

Therefore, prevention of alcohol misuse before it occurs would seem to be one of the best ways to reduce the incidence of alcoholism in the United States. Some examples of alcoholism prevention programs are education of people in schools, churches, and other community settings; guidelines for responsible advertising of alcoholic beverages; public service messages on alcoholism prevention and treatment in the mass media; and legislation to control the availability of alcoholic beverages.

(Also see ALCOHOL, AND ALCOHOLIC BEVERAGES.)

ALDEHYDE

Any of a large group of organic compounds containing the grouping -CHO and holding an intermediate position between the alcohols and acids; for example, formaldehyde, acetaldehyde, and benzaldehyde.

ALDOHEXOSE

A 6-carbon sugar (such as glucose or mannose) containing a -CHO grouping.

ALEURONE

The protein-rich layer(s) of cells which lie(s) just inside the branny seed coats of cereal grains. These cells contain enzymes that become active when the grains sprout. The activated enzymes digest starch and protein which is stored in the seed so that there is an ample supply of sugars and amino acids for the growth of the embryonic plant. Hence, the enzyme actions in the aleurone layer(s) of sprouted grains are highly useful for the production of alcoholic beverages, because the enzymatically-liberated sugars may be fermented by yeast to produce alcohol.

(Also see BEERS AND BREWING; CEREAL GRAINS; and DISTILLED LIQUORS.)

ALGAE

Algae are primitive plants. They contain chlorophyll and are capable of photosynthesis—converting the sun's energy into food. As part of the food chain, many algae provide food for fish. They vary in size and shape. Some consist of individual microscopic cells while others form flat sheets of narrow filaments or stem-like structures that may be more than 100 ft (30 m) long. Algae are able to live almost anywhere—salt water, fresh water, hot springs, polar snow, soil, trees, and rocks. Probably the best known algae are the seaweeds, specifically kelp. Algae are classified as green, brown, or red.

(Also see ADDITIVES, FOOD; AGAR-AGAR; CARRAGEENAN; SEAWEED; and SINGLE-CELL PROTEIN.)

ALGINATES

Salts of alginic acid, found in many seaweeds (kelp). They hold large amounts of water and are used (1) as thickeners, stabilizers, and emulsifiers in various foods, and (2) to provide bulk and smoothness in ice cream, synthetic cream,

and evaporated milk.

(Also see ADDITIVES.)

ALGINIC ACID

An acid [$(C_6H_8O_6)n$] obtained from seaweeds, used by the food industry as a thickener and emulsifier.

ALIMENTARY TRACT (DIGESTIVE TRACT)

The tubular, and in part sacculated, passage that serves the functions of digestion, absorption of food, and elimination of residual waste products.

(Also see DIGESTION AND ABSORPTION.)

ALKALI

A substance which neutralizes acids. It usually refers to a soluble salt or a mixture of soluble salts present in some of the residues of food which remain after complete burning or metabolism of the organic matter.

(Also see ACID FOODS AND ALKALINE FOODS.)

ALKALINE-ASH RESIDUE

A mineral residue which is left after (1) the other nutrients in a food have been metabolized, or (2) a food has been burned to an ash in a laboratory. Ashes of foods give an alkaline reaction when the predominant chemical elements in the ash are sodium, potassium, calcium, and/or magnesium; because these elements generally form alkali. Milk has an alkaline-ash residue because of its high calcium content. Fruits and vegetables are most likely to have an alkaline-ash residue, whereas breads, cereals, eggs, fish, meats, and poultry are most likely to have an acid-ash residue.

(Also see ACID FOODS AND ALKALINE FOODS.)

ALKALINE TIDE

A temporary increase in the alkalinity of the blood and urine that may occur after the ingestion of a meal which stimulates the secretion of large amounts of hydrochloric acid into the stomach.

(Also see DIGESTION AND ABSORPTION.)

ALKALI RESERVE

This term designates the substances in the blood and body fluid which will neutralize acids. The main alkali in the blood is the bicarbonate ion. The alkali reserve protects the body against the damaging effects of the acids which arise from metabolism. The most significant of these acids are the ketone bodies, phosphoric acid, sulfuric acid, hydrochloric acid, and lactic acid.

(Also see ACID-BASE BALANCE.)

ALKALOIDS

Alkaline, druglike substances found in certain plants. All alkaloids contain nitrogen in a nonprotein form. Some of the important alkaloids used in medicine are atropine, cocaine, morphine, quinine, and strychnine.

(Also see ATROPINE; and BELLADONNA DRUGS.)

ALKALOSIS

A disorder characterized by a rise in the alkaline content of the blood, or a fall in the blood acid. Alkalosis may result from vomiting, overuse of alkalizing preparations such as sodium bicarbonate, or excessively deep breathing.

(Also see ACID-BASE BALANCE.)

ALKANET

A dye extracted from the root of *Alkanona tinctoria*, which grows in Asia, Hungary, Greece, and the Mediterranean region. It is used to color wines, cosmetics, and confectionery. In the United States, alkanet is approved for coloring sausage casings, margarine, shortening, and for marking or branding products.

ALKAPTONURIA

An inherited metabolic disorder in which the urine turns dark upon exposure to air. The abnormality is due to the presence in the urine of abnormally large amounts of homogentisic acid, a compound resulting from the incomplete metabolism of certain amino acids. Usually, the disorder is treated with a low protein diet in order to reduce the amount of homogentisic acid which is formed.

(Also see INBORN ERRORS OF METABOLISM.)

ALLERGEN

Any of a wide variety of substances, or environmental conditions which may provoke an allergic reaction such as asthma, hives, or runny nose, when they come in contact with certain tissues. Some of the most common allergens are beverages, foods, spices, pollen, dust, cosmetics, drugs, vaccines, exposure to cold or heat, sunlight, and various emotional states.

(Also see ALLERGIES.)

ALLERGIES

An allergy may be defined as any unusual or exaggerated response to a particular substance, called an allergen, in a person sensitive to that substance. Formerly, the condition was called hypersensitivity, but allergy is now the preferred term. Allergies are the result of reactions of the body's immunological processes to *foreign* substances (chemical substances in such items as foods, drugs, and insect venom) or to physical conditions.

Every person has some protection from infections and diseases. This is called immunity. The body develops immunity by forming antibodies to overcome viruses, bacteria, or other substances that are not normally found in the tissues. Likewise, most people have little or no trouble

ALLERGIC REACTION

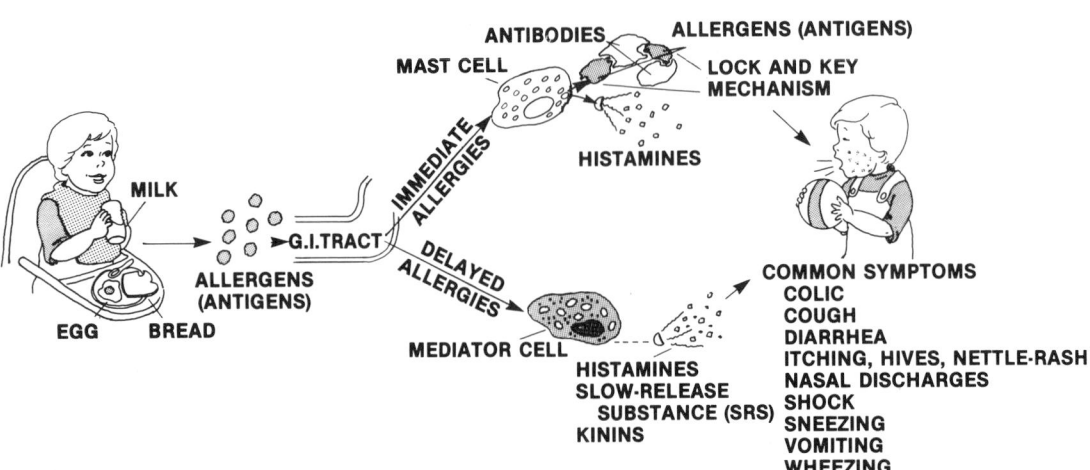

Fig. A-14. The cause and mechanisms of food allergies. Note that different mechanisms are involved in (1) immediate allergies and (2) delayed allergies. In immediate allergies, antibodies *lock* onto an allergen (antigen), effectively immobilizing and neutralizing the allergen, thereby preventing it from damaging body tissues. In delayed allergies, there are no antibodies; instead, allergens are mediated by special cells.

with allergies because antibodies or special mediator cells respond normally to protein-type substances to which they are exposed. However, the allergy-prone person has a protective mechanism which overreacts (it gets out of control) to certain substances; resulting in allergy symptoms.

Allergy specialists classify allergies into two broad categories: (1) immediate, and (2) delayed.

Immediate allergies, as implied by the name, are those that occur almost immediately (within minutes) after a person is exposed to the allergen (the allergy-producing agent). Examples of immediate allergies are: some food allergies, hay fever, bronchial asthma, hives, many drug allergies, and sensitivity to insect venom.

Delayed allergies occur hours (at least 4 hours) or days after exposure to the allergen. Examples of delayed allergies are: some food allergies, poison ivy, cosmetics, metals, soaps, solvents, and rejection of skin grafts and organ transplants.

PREVALENCE AND COST. Allergic diseases are among the most common and most costly health problems, afflicting an estimated 40 million Americans, and making for total annual costs in excess of $1.5 billion.[2] These are prevalence figures of patients actually afflicted at the time; they do not include those who have had the condition and recovered. Another noteworthy statistic is that approximately 9% of all patients seeking medical care at a physician's office do so for one of the allergic diseases.[3]

CAUSES. Allergies can be caused by an innumerable variety of substances, including foods, pollens, dust, molds, animal dander, drugs, cosmetics, toilet articles, dyes, chemicals, fabrics, and poison ivy. Thus, allergies may be caused by substances eaten or drunk (foods), inhaled (dust, pollen, and animal dander), touched (soap, wood, and cosmetics), and injected (insect bites). Sunlight and heat or cold may aggravate allergic response, as may bacteria or parasites in the intestine.

Foods. Foods are frequent causes of allergic reactions. Some are more likely to produce allergic reactions than others, but practically all foods can produce an allergic reaction in some people. The only exceptions to which scientists have yet to find anyone who is allergic are most fats (although not all), refined sugar, and salt. Also, people may be sensitive to single or multiple foods. Protein is especially likely to cause an allergy, and even a minute amount may be enough to cause difficulty. The most common food allergens—that is, the foods which cause allergic reactions most frequently—are milk, eggs, wheat, corn, legumes, nuts, and seafoods. Also, many people are allergic to strawberries, citrus fruits, tomatoes, chocolate, and berries.

Foods are seldom the only factors affecting the allergic patient. Inhalant allergy is almost always present, and contact and drug allergies are likely.

Stress. There is substantial evidence that psychological factors contribute to allergic reactions in hypersensitive individuals, and that both physical and emotional stress increase the sensitivity of a person through allergic attacks. Among the types of emotions that increase the probability of an allergic response are: anger, fear, resentment, worry, and lack of self-confidence.

Heredity. For many years, scientists have recognized that certain allergies tend to be hereditary—that they are handed down from parent to child.

It is suggested that parents with a history of allergies in their families exercise the following precautions to reduce their child's risk, although these recommendations are not based on rock-solid evidence: breast-feed the infant as long as possible; avoid cow's milk and cow's milk products for at least 6 months; delay giving eggs, fish, and citrus juices; don't keep pets; don't have wool fabrics or feathers in the house; minimize dust and mold; and don't smoke. And good luck!

Inhalants (Hay Fever). This refers to allergic symptoms—sneezing, itching, and weeping—caused from substances inhaled through breathing, such as dust, pollen, and animal dander.

Hay fever is caused by the action of histamine that has been released from mast cells. Antihistamines are drugs that prevent the released histamine from causing symptoms. They are the main treatment for hay fever and help more than two-thirds of the people who try them.

Insects. Insect allergy affects four out of every 1,000 Americans. This refers to the allergic reactions suffered by most everyone from the sting of bees, wasps, hornets, yellow jackets, mosquitoes, bedbugs, fire ants, and other insects.

Drugs. It is estimated from 1 to 4% of persons receiving drugs experience an allergic reaction.

Among the many drugs that can produce allergic reactions are sulfa drugs, antibiotics, aspirin, tranquilizers, diuretics, antituberculosis drugs, anticonvulsants, phenobarbital, insulin, and quinine. Also, some people are allergic to the horse serum present in certain antitoxins and other immunity-producing agents.

It is noteworthy that drug allergies greatly resemble food allergies. Note, too, that drug allergies are especially common in patients with multiple food allergies.

Contactants. This refers to materials which can cause allergic skin reactions in persons who come in contact with them by touching or by external physical contact. Among contactant allergens are such everyday substances as cosmetics, perfumes, soaps, shampoos, face lotions, shaving lotions, deodorants, mouthwashes, fabrics (wool and silk, but not cotton and synthetic fibers), and solvents. Also, included in this group are such plants as poison ivy, poison oak, and poison sumac; about 70% of the population develops some sort of skin reaction, such as inflammation and blistering, from contact with the causative agents in these plants.

In a highly sensitive person, contactants can cause inflammation, itching, swelling, and blistering.

Physical Agents. These include heat, cold, and ultraviolet light. In some people, these agents cause a pronounced, localized rash on the exposed area.

Bacteria and Fungi. Bacteria and fungi are known to be sources of allergies in some people.

[2]*Asthma And The Other Allergic Diseases*, NIAID Task Force Report, U.S. Department of Health, Education, and Welfare, Public Health Service, National Institute of Health, NIH Publication No. 79-387.

[3]*Ibid.*

SYMPTOMS. A wide variety of symptoms are caused by allergies; among them, nasal congestion, acne, cough, chest/throat mucus, wheezing, constipation, diarrhea, stomachache, bloating, poor appetite, eczema, hives, headache, tension, fatigue, breath odor, and sweating. Many of these symptoms are also characteristic of other disorders. For these reasons, in treating an allergy, it is first necessary that the diagnosis definitely establish the cause.

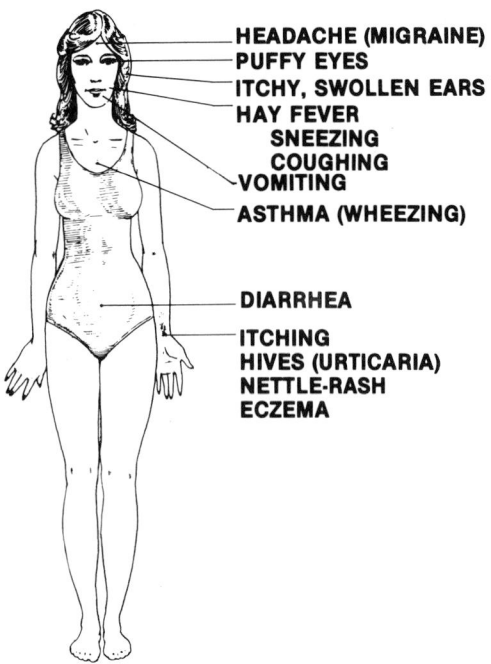

Fig. A-15. Common areas and symptoms of allergic reactions.

Allergic manifestations may occur within a few minutes of the patient coming in contact with the allergen, or they may be delayed for many hours or even for several days. With food allergies, the time lapse between consumption and the appearance of symptoms is determined by the rapidity with which the food is absorbed from the gastrointestinal tract. The quicker the absorption, the more rapidly the symptoms will develop after eating.

Allergic reactions may be trivial and local, e.g., a mild nettle-rash or hives (urticaria), or they may be general and so serious as to result in sudden death. Serious reactions are known as anaphylactic shock. Anaphylaxis can be caused by drugs (penicillin and others), horse serum, insect stings, foods (shellfish, nuts, eggs), pollen extracts, and various other agents.

How Food and Inhalant Allergies Differ. In order to identify and manage food allergies, it is first necessary to recognize the differences between food allergies and inhalant allergies. These differences may be summarized as follows:

1. Food allergies may be present at birth or begin in early childhood, whereas inhalant allergies are unusual under the age of 2 years and rare under the age of 1 year.

2. Reactions to food allergies are usually delayed for several hours and last for several days, whereas reactions to inhalants tend to develop within minutes and to disappear with an hour or so if exposure is not continued.

3. Food allergies tend to cause a wide variety of manifestations, often constituting a systemic disturbance,

whereas inhalant allergies tend to be limited in scope, affecting principally (but not exclusively) the respiratory tract.

4. Food allergies usually cause gastrointestinal disturbances, whereas inhalant allergies seldom do.

5. Except in severe cases (and not always then), food allergies may not be revealed by skin tests or other objective methods, whereas these procedures are usually accurate in inhalant allergies.

6. Desensitization (reduced sensitivity), a common method of treating inhalant allergies, is ineffective in food allergies.

7. Detection of most food allergies depends on clinical methods, chiefly, elimination and challenge, which are not adapted to inhalant allergies.

DIAGNOSIS OF FOOD ALLERGIES. First, the physician determines by the symptoms whether the patient has an allergic disease. If the presence of an allergy is confirmed, he then proceeds to identify the allergen(s) causing the trouble.

Detection of food allergies may involve one or more of the following diagnostic procedures.

Dietary History. The physician will usually take a food history. In case of doubt, the physician will usually give the patient a diary in which to record with great care and detail over a period of many days or even weeks, all the food which he eats and the time of his meals. He should record in the diary any disturbances which he believes may be due to food allergy, noting the nature and intensity of the symptoms and the time of the occurrence. If a study of the diary suggests a relationship between the intake of a certain food and the onset of allergic manifestations, the doctor will usually carry out additional tests.

Skin Test (Patch Test). This test has been used much in the past. A minute quantity of an extract of the suspected food (or other substance) is injected into the skin or rubbed into a scratch. If temporary hivelike wheals of varying sizes appear, it is indicative of sensitivity to the food in question.

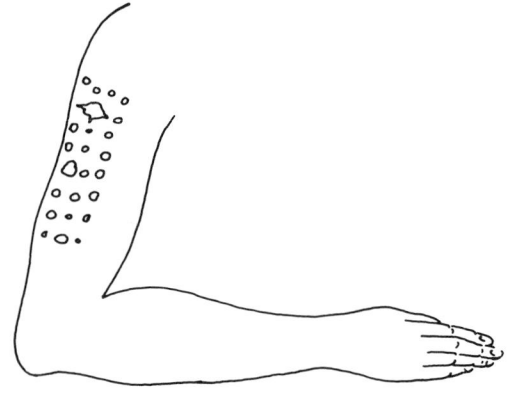

Fig. A-16. The skin test used on a patient to detect the allergic substance and the degree of hypersensitivity. Graded dilutions of the suspected substance are injected into the skin, following which the temporary hivelike wheals of varying sizes appear, indicating an allergy to the substance tested.

Provocative Food Test. This consists in giving the patient a small quantity of the suspected food camouflaged in a dish in such manner that he is unaware that he is eating the food to which he thinks he may be allergic. If, at the appropriate interval after the meal, the patient records in his diary the typical symptoms, this strongly suggests that the food is responsible. Because of the variability of allergic responses, however, the test should be repeated three times before either a positive or negative result is accepted. If a negative result is obtained on three occasions, it can be concluded that the symptoms are not due to the suspected food. On the other hand, if the tests are positive, then appropriate treatment should be undertaken.

Elimination Diets; Rowe Elimination Diets. If the dietary history, skin tests, and provocative food tests fail to detect the causative food, elimination diets may be helpful. With infants and young children, it is easy to administer strict elimination diets. Thus, it is possible to eliminate from a childs' diet separately, and in order, the common causes of children's food allergies: milk, eggs, and wheat. In adults, the procedure is much more difficult because of the number of foods to which sensitivity may develop. Also, patients may have to be fed on such diets for many weeks before the offending article of food is discovered. And, as the diets are complicated, they are normally only suited for the investigation of patients in the hospital with a dietetic department and a physician experienced in the subject of allergies. Because such elimination tests are tedious and time-consuming for both patient and doctor, they should be used as a last resort only when symptoms believed to be due to food sensitivity cannot be detected by other tests and are seriously inconveniencing the patient.

Various types of elimination diets have been devised with the object of discovering the offending article. The most widely used elimination diets are those formulated by Rowe. However, the choice and use of an elimination diet should be left to the physician.

The Pulse Test. Some physicians report that the pulse speeds up following the consumption of foods to which the patient is allergic. The pulse-testing technique is conducted as follows: For one week, the patient should (1) record everything that he eats at every meal; and (2) take his pulse (a) before rising each morning, (b) just before each meal, (c) three times (at 30-minute intervals) after each meal, and (d) just before going to bed. This is a total of 14 pulse counts daily for a week.

If the highest pulse count everyday for a week is not over 84, and if it is the same each day, the person may not be allergic to any food. On any given day, the range from the lowest to the highest count will probably not be more than 16 beats. A count greater than 84, points to a food allergy. Also, if the highest count varies more than two beats from day to day the person may be allergic; for example, if on Monday the count is 72, on Tuesday 78, Wednesday 76, and Thursday 71.

TREATMENT OF FOOD ALLERGIES. Basically, treatment consists of determining the allergen, then avoiding it as much as possible, but, at the same time, following a superior nutritional program.

Elimination of the Causative Food. If the food can be identified and eliminated from the diet, the symptoms will not recur. If the responsible item of food is one which is not consumed regularly (e.g., strawberry, walnut, chocolate, or shrimp), it can easily be avoided. But such avoidance is far more difficult in the case of milk, eggs, and wheat, which are present in so many foods.

Avoidance of offending food may not need to be absolute. Thus, tolerance level is important in the management of food allergy.

Denaturation of the Protein. Sometimes a protein ceases to act as an allergen if it is denatured by heat. Thus, a patient sensitive to raw milk may be able to take with impunity boiled milk and milk in cooked products. Also, a patient sensitive to lightly boiled eggs may be able to take eggs which have been boiled for at least 10 minutes; and patients who are sensitive to eggs may be able to eat the yoke, especially if well cooked, although the whites may continue to cause symptoms.

Drug Treatments. Drug treatments had best be by prescription of a physician. Such drugs as antihistamines, adrenalin, and ephedrine, and some newer drugs, are often effective in relieving allergic symptoms, but they do not cure the condition. In severe cases the hormonal substances ACTH and cortisone may be used, but their adverse effects limit their long-term use, especially in children. Tranquilizers and sedatives are often indicated because of the close connection between emotion and allergy.

Desensitization (Reduced Sensitivity). Many attempts have been made to desensitize patients who suffer from food allergy by repeatedly injecting or giving by mouth increasing quantities of the allergen. Generally speaking, this method is regarded as of little or no value in food allergies.

Keep Healthy. Physicians have long known that good health will lessen allergies. So, persons subject to allergies should eat a superior nutritional diet, practice good hygiene, get enough rest and sleep, and avoid extreme fatigue.

Avoid Stress. Allergies often appear to involve emotional factors, as well as organic factors; and conversely the allergy may induce tensions which did not originally exist. So, the doctor must determine the place of these emotional factors in the patient's condition. Sometimes, all treatments for the condition fail until the psychological problems are determined and alleviated.

Maintain Good Nutrition. Persons suffering from allergies should eat a balanced diet, containing adequate minerals and vitamins, to insure maximum good health. They should consult the family doctor or a nutrition specialist if they feel they are lacking in nutrients.

Unfortunately, many intelligent allergic patients, knowing something of the nature of their disease, go to extremes to avoid any foods that may aggravate it. Some avoid so many kinds of food that they become severely undernourished or malnourished. This is particularly true in the case of growing children. So, it is emphasized that allergic patients should not be subjected to dietary restrictions without good evidence that their symptoms are due to a food allergen.

Eat a variety of foods rather than concentrating on a limited number. Eat a moderate amount and try to avoid food jags. Eat regularly without overeating at a particular meal or time of day.

Know Botanical Families. There is evidence that all foods of the same botanical family are likely to produce allergic reactions; that is, if one member of the family produces such a response, all of them will likely do so. Since many food items not normally associated are members of the same botanical family, such as asparagus and onions, a careful study of the botanical family of an identified allergen is advised.

Read Labels. Labels tell what is in the food package. So, those suffering from allergies should become inveterate label readers. They should read labels continually to make sure that the products which they purchase do not contain ingredients to which they are allergic. However, consideration should be given to the fact that refinement or extensive processing may modify food enough so that it can be tolerated, especially if the allergy is a mild one.

Treatment of Food Allergies in Children. Food allergies in children are of particular concern to parents. If, upon being given a new food, a child responds with wheezing, coughing, running of the nose, colic, vomiting, diarrhea, constipation, or eczema, the new food should be avoided for at least a week or two, then it may be tried again.

Fortunately, children tend to outgrow their sensitivity to food allergens. Foods known to have caused reactions in infancy may be tried months or years later when perhaps they can be taken with impunity.

ALLERGY-PRODUCING FOODS. In this section, we turn to the most important aspect of food allergies—the foods themselves. Because of space limitations, the discussion will be limited to the most common offenders; namely, milk, eggs, wheat, corn, legumes, nuts, and seafoods. It is unfortunate that these foods are allergy-producing because most of them are also essential foods; hence, their avoidance becomes a serious problem in undernourished people and in children or infants.

People may be sensitive to a single food or to multiple foods. When a patient is sensitive to one or two foods only, it is not difficult for him to realize it himself. The difficulty arises, however, when he is allergic to many foods.

Also, allergy to a food may be of various degrees of severity. Symptoms of asthma or hives may not arise if only one food is eaten, provided the sensitivity is mild. However, if a number of such foods are ingested at one time, the symptoms may be pronounced. Another factor which is important in connection with the production of symptoms is the readiness with which a food is absorbed from the gastrointestinal tract. The more quickly the absorption, the more rapid will the symptoms develop after eating.

In addition to the foods themselves, some food additives may cause allergic reactions. An example is tartrazine, an azo dye, which is added to many foods and soft drinks, and which may cause urticaria and asthma. The food preservatives sulphur dioxide and sodium benzoate, present in many orange drinks, have also been responsible for attacks of asthma.

MILK ALLERGY. Although the word *milk* ordinarily means cow's milk, it also applies to milk from any mammal, including human milk and goat's milk. Also, in various parts of the world, milk is obtained from ewes, buffalos, mares, yaks, camels, and reindeers.

Cow's milk is the most common food allergen. Studies show that, among patients known to have food allergies, 65% are allergic to milk. It is not only the most common in all age groups, but it also causes an unusually large variety of symptoms, including nasal stuffiness, hives, eczema, migraine headache, vomiting, diarrhea, or a serious attack of asthma. Also, there are some reports that bed-wetting may be an allergic reaction to milk. Since it ordinarily does not cause severe reactions, at least in patients over 1 year of age, milk allergy is easily overlooked. But the physician or nutritionist who watches constantly for a milk allergy will find that it is amazingly common.

People who must avoid milk do so for different reasons; some have an inherent inability to digest milk properly, known as a lactose intolerance, others have a milk protein allergy. (For information relative to lactose intolerance, see MILK AND MILK PRODUCTS, section headed "Lactose Intolerance.")

• **Protein Allergy**—Milk contains two proteins, casein and lactalbumin, either or both of which can cause an allergic reaction. If a person is allergic only to the casein protein, milk from animals other than cows, such as goats, may sometimes be substituted. Also, heat treatment of cow's milk (as well as dried and evaporated milk preparations) is sometimes helpful in decreasing allergic symptoms, but may not be completely satisfactory because of some cross-reactive milk proteins.

EGG ALLERGY. The hen's egg (and eggs from other birds) is an excellent food; it is nourishing, delicious, and a valuable source of protein, vitamins, and iron. Also, it has many uses in cookery. Unfortunately, however, it is also a common allergen, capable of producing any of the reactions known to be caused by food allergies. Also, it is often said that egg allergy is always severe.

Like milk, egg has several different protein fractions which may induce an allergic reaction. They are vitellin, livetin, ovalbumin and other conjugated proteins. The egg white contains the larger amount of protein and is usually a greater offender than the egg yolk. Since the yolk is rich in iron and fat-soluble vitamins, sometimes it may be fed to infants allergic to whole eggs. Sometimes, heating destroys the allergy causative factor(s) of the egg white by coagulating it, with the result that some people who are allergic to eggs may be able to eat hard-boiled eggs without developing symptoms.

One of the great dangers of egg allergy is that its victims, no matter how slight their degree of sensitivity, tend to have violent reactions to certain vaccines grown on chicken embryos (influenza, spotted fever, yellow fever). Some of these vaccines seem to be entirely free of egg protein contamination, whereas others, notably influenza vaccine, are not to be trusted.

WHEAT ALLERGY. Wheat is not the only cereal grain to produce allergies. But, because it is found in such a large variety of foods, it is the most burdensome to its victims and to those who prepare their meals.

• **Gluten allergy**—The chief causative factor in wheat is gluten protein. Wheat gluten is extremely versatile because it provides the strong foundation for the leavening action of yeast. For this reason, wheat gluten or wheat flour is frequently used in the baked products made from other grains, including soy flour. Anyone having a wheat allergy should be extremely suspicious of a label that includes *other flours,* for they will likely include at least some wheat flour or wheat flour derivatives.

• **Celiac disease** (*Celiac sprue*)—Celiac disease is due to a genetically-inherited intolerance to wheat gluten, a main constituent of wheat flour, which is also present to a small extent in rye, barley, and oats, but not in rice. Such persons develop lesions of the small intestine which lead to diarrhea and malabsorption. It is not known why gluten causes intestinal damage. Symptoms usually arise during the first 3 years of life, but it may affect adults. Patients are relieved if gluten is excluded completely from the diet.

CORN ALLERGY. Corn is another common allergy-inducing food. Since it is extremely versatile, it is found in cereals, oils, sweeteners, and starches. It is also used as a filler, extender, and thickener. For these reasons, some form of corn is found in many foods.

Patients vary as to the type of corn to which they are allergic. Some cannot take it in any form but pure corn sugar (glucose). Others have no trouble with immature corn; that is, corn-on-the-cob or canned (either kernel or cream-style) corn. Some patients can eat popcorn and other whole corn products, but they cannot consume corn syrup. For unknown reasons, corn syrup is the most potent offender; corn oil the least.

LEGUME ALLERGY. Legumes include such foods as peas, beans, and peanuts. A patient with an allergy to legumes, should be extremely careful in selecting food since the legume family includes the following foods:

Acacia
Alfalfa
Arabic
Beans (green, kidney, lima, mung, navy, wax; soybean, including soya flour and oil)
Carob
Cassia
Karaya
Lentils.
Licorice
Locust bean gum
Peas (black-eye, chick, green, split)
Peanuts (includes oil)
Tragacanth

Patients allergic to nuts are often allergic to legumes, also. Yet, some patients tolerate legumes, such as peanuts, despite being allergic to most nuts.

• **Soybean allergy**—An allergy to soybeans is becoming increasingly difficult to live with, since soybeans have become so versatile. They provide oil, flour, and protein. Spun soybean protein concentrate is being used as extenders and replacements for some meats. Soybean products also find extensive use as binders, fillers, and emulsifiers.

NUT ALLERGY. The term *nut* is applied to a variety of seeds, not all of which are true nuts. Those most likely to act as allergens are peanut (actually a legume), walnut, pecan, Brazil nut, hazelnut (filbert), and coconut. Less common offenders are almond, cashew, pistachio, macadamia nut, and pinyon nut.

Patients on a nut-poor diet, should avoid nuts of all types; nut crumbs on cookies, cake icings, and ice cream; candies containing nuts; and oils from nuts used in salad oils, lard substitutes, and margarines. Patients allergic to nuts may be allergic to cottonseed meal and oil, also. (Olive oil is permitted.)

A variety of symptoms may result from the eating of nuts, including asthma, nose allergy, hives, or headaches.

SEAFOOD ALLERGY. Fish is a strong antigen, which usually produces severe symptoms. Some patients develop asthma if they are merely exposed to the odor of fish that is being cooked. Hence, no fish-sensitive patient is unaware of his problem.

Patients on a seafood-free diet should avoid fish and shellfish—fresh, canned, smoked, or pickled; fish liver oils and concentrates in vitamin preparations; fish and shellfish stews, bisques, broths, soups, salads, hors d'oeuvres, and caviar. Also, they should avoid licking labels, which may contain a fish glue adhesive; and they should avoid injections of fish origin in the treatment of varicose veins.

Those allergic to fish may be able to eat oysters, shrimp, and lobster. Also, patients unable to eat one type of fish may be able to eat others.

OTHER ALLERGY-PRODUCING FOODS. Many other foods produce allergies in some people; among them, certain spices—especially mustard and oil of wintergreen; cottonseed; castor bean; strawberries, chocolate, and sulfites.

ALLERGY-FREE PRODUCTS LIST. The following companies will send lists of their products which are free of particular allergy-producing ingredients:

Akins Special Foods, Inc.
P.O. Box 2747
6947 East 13
Tulsa, OK 74119

Chicago Dietetic Supply, Inc.
405 E. Shawmut Avenue
La Grange, IL 60525

Ener-G Foods, Inc.
1526 Utah Avenue South
Seattle, WA 98134

Frito-Lay, Inc.
P.O. Box 660634
Dallas, TX 75266-0634

General Foods Kitchen
250 N. Street
White Plains, NY 10625

General Mills
Nutrition Department
1 General Mills Blvd.
Minneapolis, MN 55426

ALLERGY-FREE RECIPES. Generally, the physician will either provide allergy-free receipes or tell the patient where to obtain them.

(**Note well**: For a more complete discussion of allergies, including elimination diets and foods to avoid, see the two-volume *Foods & Nutrition Encyclopedia,* a work by the same authors as *Food For Health*.)

ALLICIN

An antibacterial substance extracted from garlic, *Allium sativum.*

ALLIGATOR SKIN

A roughening of the skin which may be the result of nutritional deficiencies (particularly the lack of vitamin A), poor liver function, poor hygiene, and/or a hot, dry, environment.

ALLOTRIOPHAGY (PICA)

Depraved, or abnormal, appetite characterized by the desire to eat such substances as dirt, chalk, pencils, etc. This condition is usually caused by nutritional deficiencies.
(Also see GEOPHAGIA.)

ALMONDS *Prunus amygdalus*

The almond is a small deciduous, nut-bearing tree which is closely related to the peach, apricot, and cherry tree—all belong to the genus *Prunus,* and bear stone fruits. Edible almonds are also called sweet almonds because there is a variety which is inedible and called bitter almonds. The fruit of the almond is classified botanically as a drupe, like that of the peach but the outer fleshy layer of the almond is astringent, tough, and becomes dry at maturity. This fleshy layer—the hull—splits and releases the nut.

ORIGIN AND HISTORY.   The almond tree is native to Asia and Africa. Since Biblical times, the sweet almond has been one of the world's most popular nuts. Today, almonds are grown in most temperate regions.

WORLD AND U.S. PRODUCTION.   Almonds are the third leading nut crop in the world. Worldwide, about 1.3 million metric tons are produced annually; and the leading producing countries, by rank, are: United States, Spain, China, Italy, and Iran.[4]

In the United States, almonds are grown on a commercial basis only in California, where about 660 million pounds are produced annually.[5]

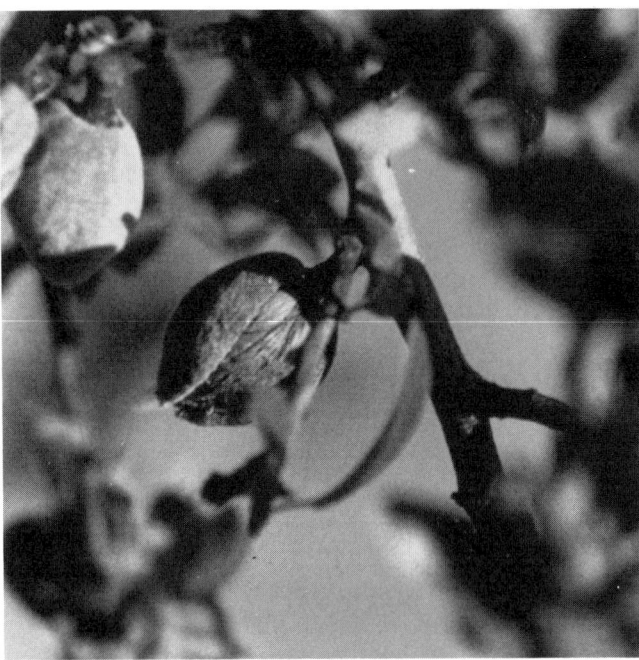

Fig. A-17. Almonds are grown for their fragrant blossoms as well as for their nuts. A leathery hull encases the woody shell of the nut, and splits open when the kernel is ripe. The somewhat flat, oval, brown kernel is one of the most popular nuts. (Courtesy, Anderson/Miller & Hubbard Consumer Services, San Francisco, Calif.)

PROCESSING.   Almonds are sold unshelled or shelled. They are shelled mechanically, and then the kernels are electronically sorted for defects, graded for size, and packaged. Shelled almonds may also be salted and roasted, blanched, ground into a meal or made into a paste.

• **Almond Oil**—Oil of almond is obtained by expression or distillation of the kernels of sweet (edible) or bitter almonds; primarily, bitter almonds are used for this purpose. The prussic acid (hydrocyanic acid) contained in bitter almonds is eliminated during the process. Almond oil is used in flavoring extracts.

---

[4]Based on data from *FAO Production Yearbook 1990*, FAO/UN, Rome, Italy, Vol. 44, p. 172, Table 76. **Note well:** Annual production fluctuates as a result of weather and profitability of the crop.

[5]Based on data from *Agricultural Statistics 1991*, USDA, p. 220, Table 340. **Note well:** Annual production fluctuates as a result of weather and profitability of the crop.

SELECTION, PREPARATION, AND USES.   Almonds in shells should be free from splits, cracks, stains, or holes. Moldy nuts should be discarded. Nutmeats should be plump and fairly uniform in color and size. Limp, rubbery, dark, or shriveled kernels are likely to be stale. If antioxidants are added to delay the onset of rancidity, thus extending the shelf life of packaged nutmeat, they are listed on the package.

Because of their oil content, almonds need protection from air and high temperatures. Whole almonds become rancid less quickly than nut pieces, and unroasted almonds keep better than roasted ones. For prolonged storage, almonds should be kept cool and dry. Shelled almonds will stay fresh for several months stored in tightly closed containers in the refrigerator. For longer storage, almonds can be frozen in tightly closed freezer containers at 0°F *(-18°C)* or lower.

Bitter almonds contain prussic acid and should not be eaten; but sweet almonds are popular eaten alone when dried, or when roasted and salted. Almonds are also used in a variety of products, including candies and rich pastries. Additionally, other imaginative uses for almonds may be found, such as waffles, biscuits, muffins, vegetable salads, topping for baked goods, or as additions to meats, poultry, or seafood salads. Almond oil is used in flavoring extracts.

NUTRITIONAL VALUE.   Almonds are very nutritious. Dried almonds contain only about 5% water and each 100 g (about 3½ oz) are packed with 598 Calories (kcal) of

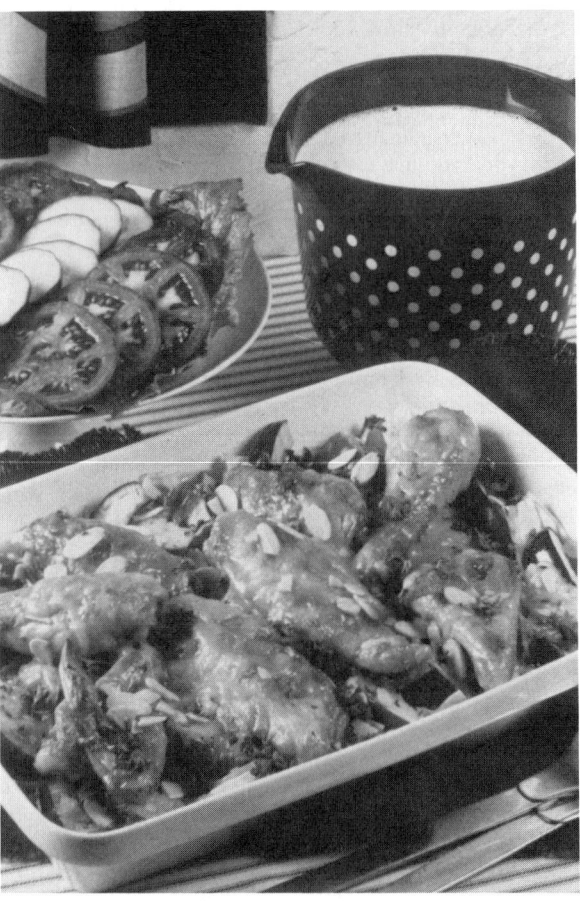

Fig. A-18. Hungarian baked chicken with cabbage and almonds. (Courtesy, United Dairy Assoc., Rosemont, Ill.)

energy. Almonds are high in calories primarily because they are 54% fat (oil) which contains $2\frac{1}{4}$ times more calories per unit of weight than does protein or carbohydrate. Even with the fat content, each 100 g of almonds also contains 19 g of protein, 20 g of carbohydrate, 773 mg of potassium, 5 mg of iron, 3 mg of zinc, and 28 mg of vitamin E. Unsalted almonds have only 3 mg of sodium per 100 g. More complete information regarding the nutritional value of dried or roasted and salted almonds, almond meal, and almond paste is provided in Food Composition Table F-21.

ALOPECIA

Loss of hair. Sometimes, the condition is due to a nutritional deficiency.

Also, there are various other causes of hair loss such as disorders of the scalp, reaction to certain drugs or chemicals, venereal disease, and infection. Loss of hair also occurs in thyroid deficiency (myxedema) and in certain types of pituitary disorders.

(Also see BALDNESS.)

ALPHA-CHOLESTEROL

This term is a layman's designation for blood cholesterol which is carried on alpha-lipoproteins, in contrast to that carried on beta-lipoproteins. However, the cholesterol molecule itself does not vary, only the lipoprotein which carries it in the blood.

(Also see ALPHA-LIPOPROTEINS; BETA-LIPOPROTEINS; CHOLESTEROL; and HEART DISEASE.)

ALPHA-KETOGLUTARIC ACID

One of the intermediary products in the Krebs cycle; also the product of oxidative deamination of glutamic acid.

ALPHA-LIPOPROTEINS

Special fat-carrying proteins which are produced in the liver. Alpha-lipoproteins are also called high density lipoproteins (HDL). Normally, they contain from 5 to 8% triglycerides, 17 to 30% cholesterol, 21 to 29% phospholipid, and 33 to 57% protein. Cholesterol which is carried in the blood by these proteins is much less likely to be deposited in the blood vessels than that borne by the beta-lipoproteins. Hence, it is desirable for one to have a high blood level of alpha-lipoproteins, and a low one of beta-lipoproteins. It appears that the former may be increased, and the latter reduced by (1) loss of excess body weight, (2) strenuous physical exercise, (3) a diet low in animal fats and cholesterol, and (4) drugs such as clofibrate and niacin (the latter vitamin must be administered in large doses in order to achieve the desired effect). **NOTE:** Measures designed to alter the levels of blood fats should be undertaken under the supervision of a physician.

(Also see BETA-LIPOPROTEINS; CHOLESTEROL; and HEART DISEASE.)

ALVEOGRAPH

An instrument used to measure the stretching quality of dough; it indicates the stability, extensibility, and strength of doughs.

ALZHEIMER'S DISEASE Senile Dementia

This affliction was named after Alois Alzheimer, a German physician, who first described the disease in one of his patients in 1906. It is estimated that about 4 million Americans have Alzheimer's disease.

The disease is characterized by a decreased mental acuity. There is increased forgetfulness, failing judgment, a decreased capacity to do simple calculations, and sometimes a disorientation in time and place. The ailment is more prevalent in middle-aged women than in men, but may occur occasionally at an earlier age. In many cases it does not appear until the individual reaches the 70s.

Currently, there is no cure. However, some work has indicated that niacin may be helpful in stimulating blood circulation to the brain. Also, during the last five years, a significant neurochemical abnormality has been found in senile patients. There is a definite deficiency of acetylcholine, which is known to be involved in learning and memory. The precursor of the neurotransmitter, acetylcholine, is choline, one of the vitamin B complex. Some reports have shown that dietary choline may improve learning and behavior.

As in the case of most degenerative diseases, prevention, if at all possible, is better than cure. Thus, a conclusion may be drawn that consumption of choline may be helpful. It is also suggested that adequate trace elements and vitamins may be helpful in the diet throughout life.

Along with a superior diet, it has been found that remaining active and involved, with a positive rather than a negative attitude to life, can be helpful in delaying any onset of senile dementia, whether it develops prematurely or in old age.

AMARANTH Amaranthus

Amaranth, a relative of pigweed, is a tall, bushy plant with broad leaves and a showy flower or seed head. Amaranth is grown for the leaves as a green vegetable and for the seed as a grain. It is a high-protein grain, with 15 to 18% protein which is high in the amino acids lysine and methionine. Amaranth is available in many health food stores.

AMEBIASIS

Infestation with harmful amoebas, particularly *Entamoeba histolytica*. Cysts of the amoeba may be ingested in contaminated food or water. Also, flies and infested animals may carry the organisms to foods.

(Also see DISEASES.)

AMELOBLASTS

Special epithelial cells surrounding tooth buds in gum tissue, which form cup-shaped organs for producing and depositing the enamel on the surfaces of developing teeth. Vitamin A deficiency results in faulty production of ameloblasts and makes for unsound teeth.

AMERICAN DIETETIC ASSOCIATION (ADA)

This is a professional organization of more than 40,000 dietitians. Its goals are: (1) to improve the nutrition of human beings, (2) to advance the science of dietetics and nutrition, and (3) to promote education in these allied areas. The ADA was founded in 1917 during World War I. In 1925, the ADA began publication of the *Journal of the American Dietetic Association*, which it continues today. Furthermore, the ADA publishes other educational material for nurses, doctors, teachers, and other related professionals.

AMERICAN INSTITUTE OF NUTRITION (AIN)

This is a professional society for nutrition scientists, which publishes the *Journal of Nutrition*. The AIN was founded in 1928 to (1) develop and extend nutrition knowledge, and (2) promote personal contact between researchers in nutrition and related fields. Only individuals who have published research and who are engaged in the field of nutrition may be elected to membership.

AMERICAN SOCIETY FOR CLINICAL NUTRITION (ASCN)

This society is a division of the American Institute of Nutrition (AIN), which publishes the *American Journal of Clinical Nutrition*. The aims of the ASCN are (1) to promote education about human nutrition in health and disease, (2) to promote the presentation and discussion of research in human nutrition, and (3) to publish a journal devoted to experimental and clinical nutrition. Members of the American Institute of Nutrition with publications in the field of clinical nutrition may become members of ASCN.

(Also see AMERICAN INSTITUTE OF NUTRITION [AIN].)

AMIDASE

The enzyme which removes amino groups from amino acids and related compounds.

AMINATION

The taking up of an amine group (NH_2) by an amino acid resulting in the amine form of that acid. Amination is one means by which toxic nitrogenous products such as ammonia (NH_3) are removed from the system and made ready for excretion.

AMINE

A substance derived from an amino acid by (1) the action of certain intestinal bacteria, or (2) enzymatic action within the cells of the body.

(Also see AMINO ACID[S].)

AMINO ACID(S)

These are the structural units of protein. The term *amino* indicates the presence of the NH_2 group—a base—while the term *acid* indicates the presence of the COOH groups or carboxyl group—an acid. Since all amino acids possess this unique chemical feature of containing both an acid and a base, they are capable of both acid and base reactions in the body. Thus, they are said to be amphoteric. There are 22 amino acids.

HISTORY. In studies conducted from 1935 to 1955, Dr. W.C. Rose and coworkers at the University of Illinois were the first to determine the essentiality of the amino acids and the minimum requirements of each. Using rats, Rose found that 10 different amino acids must be supplied in adequate amounts in the food to support the normal growth of young rats; and using his graduate students in nitrogen balance studies (nitrogen in the food minus that in the urine and feces), Rose found that only 8 of these amino acids were essential for the maintenance of nitrogen equilibrium in fully grown young men. Subsequently, it was shown that a ninth amino acid (histidine) is essential to human infants and, in longer term studies, to adults as well.

PEPTIDE BONDS. In the formation of protein from amino acids, amino acids are linked to each other by peptide bonds. These peptide bonds are formed by the combination of the HN_2 group of one amino acid, and the COOH groups of another, with the elimination of water. Since all amino acids contain both NH_2 and COOH groups, long chains of amino acids may be formed. These long chains are called peptides or proteins. Therefore, digestion of protein involves breaking protein into individual amino acids by enzymatic hydrolysis of the peptide bonds. Amino acids are then absorbed and distributed by the bloodstream to the cells of the body. On the other hand, protein synthesis involves the systematic linking of individual amino acids to form body proteins. The nature of protein is determined by the types of amino acids in the protein, and also by the order in which they are joined.

ESSENTIAL AND NONESSENTIAL. In order for a protein to be synthesized in the body, all of its constituent amino acids must be available. Some of the amino acids can be synthesized within the body. These are called nonessential or dispensable amino acids. If the body cannot

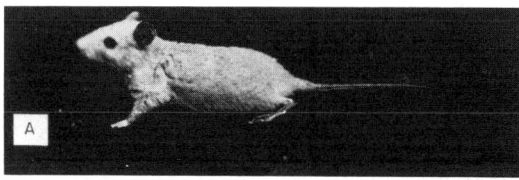
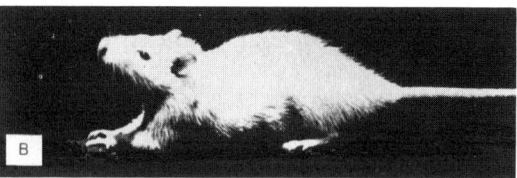

Fig. A-19. Stunting of growth due to feeding and incomplete protein. The two rats were the same age (140 days old) and were fed the same diets except for the protein. Rat A received gliadin from wheat—an incomplete protein, deficient in the amino acid lysine, whereas rat B received casein from milk—a complete protein. (From experiements by Osborne and Mendel. Courtesy, The Connecticut Agricultural Experiment Station, New Haven, Conn.)

synthesize an amino acid from materials normally available, at a speed that will meet the physiological needs of the body for normal growth and development, and it must be supplied in the diet, it is referred to as an essential or indispensable amino acid. The essential and nonessential amino acids are:

Essential (indispensable)	Nonessential (dispensable)
Histidine	Alanine
Isoleucine	Arginine
Leucine	Asparagine
Lysine	Aspartic acid
Methionine (some used for the synthesis of cysteine)	Cysteine
	Cystine
	Glutamic acid
Phenylalanine (some used for the synthesis of tyrosine)	Glutamine
	Glycine
	Hydroxyproline
Threonine	Proline
Tryptophan	Serine
Valine	Tyrosine

NOTE WELL: Arginine is not regarded as essential for humans, whereas it is for animals; in contrast to human infants, most young mammals cannot synthesize it in sufficient amounts to meet their needs for growth.

An amino acid is nonessential (dispensable from the diet) if its carbon skeleton can be formed in the body, and if an amino group can be transferred to it from some donor compound available, a process called transamination.

REQUIREMENTS. Proteins differ in nutritive value mainly due to their amino acid composition. If one essential amino acid is missing from the diet, a certain protein or proteins will not be formed, and an adult will enter a state of negative nitrogen balance while a child or infant will cease to grow. These two facts provide the basis for experimentally determining amino acid requirements. The estimated essential amino acid requirements shown in Table A-2 may serve as a guide for the selection of dietary protein sources.

TABLE A-2
ESTIMATED AMINO ACID REQUIREMENTS[1]

Amino Acid	Requirement, mg/kg Body Weight/Day		
	Infants	Children	Adults
	(3–4 mo)	(–2 yr) (10–12 yr)	
Histidine	28	? ?	8–12
Isoleucine	70	31 28	10
Leucine	161	73 42	14
Lysine	103	64 44	12
Methionine plus cystine	58	27 22	13
Phenylalanine plus tyrosine	125	69 22	14
Threonine	87	37 28	7
Tryptophan	17	12.5 3.3	3.5
Valine	93	38 25	10

[1]*Recommended Dietary Allowances*, 10th ed., 1989, NRC–National Academy of Sciences, p. 57.

These requirements are adequate only (1) if the body cells have the ability to synthesize the necessary carbon skeletons (alpha-keto acids) to which the amino nitrogen can be attached; and (2) if the diet provides enough nitrogen for the synthesis of the nonessential amino acids so that essential amino acids will not be used to supply amino groups for the nonessential amino acids.

Even in infants the essential amino acids make up only about 35% of the total need for protein. In adults, essential amino acids account for less than 20% of the total protein requirement. Most proteins contain plenty of dispensable amino acids; usually, the concern is to meet the essential amino acid needs, particularly of infants and children.

It should be noted from Table A-2 that on a weight basis infants and children require larger amounts of essential amino acids by virtue of their higher rate of protein synthesis. There is no information on amino acid requirements for pregnancy and lactation.

All proteins are not created equal. Plant foods often contain insufficient quantities of lysine, methionine and cystine, tryptophan, and/or threonine. When a protein source is low in some essential amino acid, that amino acid is termed the limiting amino acid. Lysine is the limiting amino acid of many cereals, while methionine is the limiting amino acid of beans

(legumes). In general, the proteins of animal origin—eggs, dairy products, and meats—provide mixtures of amino acids that are well suited for human requirements of maintenance and growth. The egg provides all of the essential amino acids in sufficient quantities and balance to meet the body's requirements without excess. Frequently, the essential amino acid pattern of the egg is used to evaluate the amino acid pattern of other foods by assigning a chemical score or amino acid score. A score of 100 indicates that the food has the same amino acid pattern as eggs, while a score of

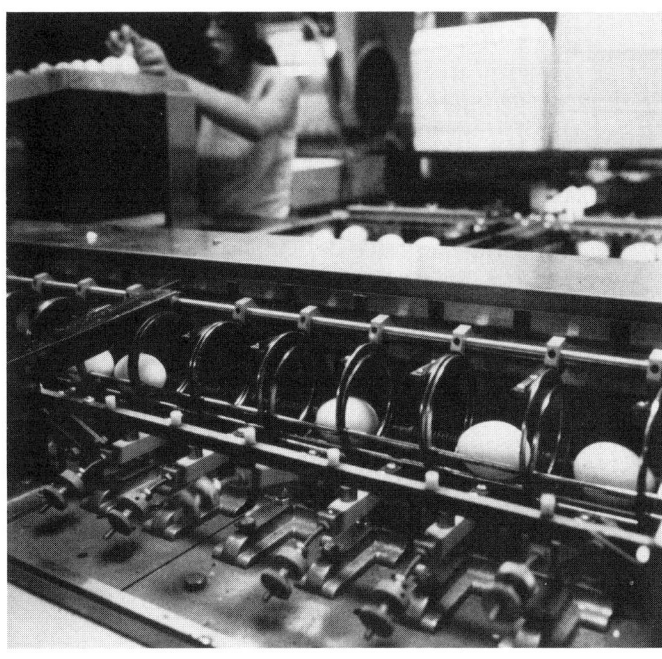

Fig. A-20. Frequently eggs are used to evaluate the amino acid pattern of other foods, with eggs assigned a score of 100. (Courtesy, Univ. of Maryland, College Park, Md.)

60 indicates that the most limiting amino acid is 60% of the amount contained in an egg. Often proteins in the diet which are low in some amino acid can be complemented by the addition of protein from another source. That is, proteins having opposite strengths and weaknesses are mixed. For example, many cereals are low in lysine, but high in methionine and cystine. On the other hand, soybeans, lima beans, and kidney beans are high in lysine but low in methionine and cystine. When eaten together, the deficiencies are corrected. Rather than eating more of a protein low in some amino acid(s) it is much better to supplement with a protein that complements the deficiency. This avoids the possibility of creating an amino acid imbalance which may reduce the utilization of or increase the need for other amino acids. Complementary protein combinations are found in almost all cultures. In the Middle East, bread and cheese are eaten together. Mexicans eat beans and corn, Indians eat wheat and pulses (legumes). Americans eat breakfast cereals with milk. This kind of supplementation works only when the deficient and complementary proteins are ingested together or within a few hours of each other. For those who are interested, the protein and amino acid content for a

variety of foods are given in Proteins and Amino Acids in Selected Foods, Table P-16.

(Also see DIGESTION AND ABSORPTION; INBORN ERRORS OF METABOLISM; METABOLISM; NITROGEN BALANCE; PROTEIN[S]; and REFERENCE PROTEIN.)

AMINO ACID ANTAGONISM

Interference with the utilization of certain amino acids by others which are chemically similar.

AMINO ACID IMBALANCE

A condition in which the dietary supply of amino acids is poorly utilized in meeting the body's requirements. An amino acid imbalance usually occurs when the total protein intake is low, and there are excesses of certain amino acids while others are deficient.

(Also see AMINO ACID[S].)

AMINO ACID REFERENCE PATTERN

The amounts of each of the essential amino acids which in combination are believed to meet the body's protein needs in the most efficient manner. Patterns are usually based upon the minimum requirements for infants and young children; or they may be based upon the proportions in which the amino acids occur in such well utilized foods as eggs and human breast milk.

(Also see AMINO ACID[S].)

AMINOACIDURIA

A condition in which abnormally large amounts of amino acids are excreted in the urine. This disorder is usually due to one or more defects in the processes by which the kidneys prevent such urinary loss.

AMINOPEPTIDASE

An enzyme, produced by the intestinal glands, which digests peptides, especially polypeptides, by splitting off the amino acids containing free amino groups.

(Also see DIGESTION AND ABSORPTION.)

AMINOPTERIN

This is a yellow crystalline compound used clinically as an antagonist to folic acid in the treatment of certain leukemias.

AMINO SUGAR

A sugar which contains an amino group. Amino sugars are important constituents of compounds in connective tissues.

(Also see CARBOHYDRATE[S].)

AMMONIA

A potentially toxic alkaline gas which is formed from amino acids or urea by (1) intestinal bacteria, or (2) metabolic activities of cells. Normally, the accumulation of ammonia in the body is prevented by enzymes which convert the ammonia to safer compounds such as urea or amino acids. However, ammonia intoxication is a common occurrence in certain liver diseases.

(Also see DIGESTION AND ABSORPTION; METABOLISM; and PROTEIN[S].)

AMMONIUM

A singly charged positive ion formed during protein metabolism. Under alkaline conditions, the ammonium ion may be converted to ammonia gas; under acid conditions, it forms salts. Also, the ammonium ion is a nontoxic means by which the kidney excretes excess acid.

(Also see METABOLISM; and PROTEIN[S].)

AMPHETAMINES

Drugs which are used as both stimulants and appetite depressants. They are habit forming and create a false sense of well being, which makes it easy for users to increase the dosage and to become dependent on these substances. Also, people with various ailments may suffer severe side effects which are sometimes fatal. Therefore, amphetamines should be used only under a doctor's close supervision.

(Also see APPETITE; and OBESITY.)

AMPHOTERIC

A compound having properties of both an acid and a base and therefore able to function as either. Amino acids and proteins have this dual chemical nature—they contain both an acid group (carboxyl, COOH) and a basic group (amino, NH_2).

AMYDON

This starch preparation was used for many centuries to thicken liquids. It was made by soaking wheat in water, then sun-drying the liquid, which left the amydon.

AMYLASE

Any one of several enzymes which convert starch to maltose, such as pancreatic amylase (amylopsin) and salivary amylase (ptyalin).

(Also see DIGESTION AND ABSORPTION.)

AMYLODYSPEPSIA

Inability to digest starch.

AMYLOPECTIN

A complex carbohydrate molecule made up of glucose units linked together in a branched chain. Amylopectin is the major component of starches from corn, rice, and barley in which it often comprises the outer layer of the starch granules. These starches make excellent thickeners for cream soups, gravies, puddings, and white sauces.

(Also see STARCH.)

AMYLOPSIN

A digestive enzyme secreted by the pancreas. It helps to break down (digest) starch to the sugar, maltose. Another name for this enzyme is pancreatic amylase.

(Also see DIGESTION AND ABSORPTION.)

AMYLOSE

A complex carbohydrate molecule made up of glucose units linked together in straight chains. It occurs together with amylopectin in many food starches.

(Also see AMYLOPECTIN; CARBOHYDRATE[S]; and STARCH.)

ANABOLISM

A process involving the conversion of simple substances into more complex substances of living cells (constructive metabolism).
(Also see METABOLISM.)

ANACIDITY

A lack of hydrochloric acid in the stomach.
(Also see DIGESTION AND ABSORPTION.)

ANAEROBIC

A type of metabolism which occurs in the absence of oxygen.
(Also see METABOLISM.)

ANALOG

Anything that is analogous or similar to something else. (Also spelled analogue.)

ANALYSIS OF FOODS

Nutritional science owes much of its rapid growth during the 20th century to the continual improvement of biological, chemical, and physical analyses of foods.

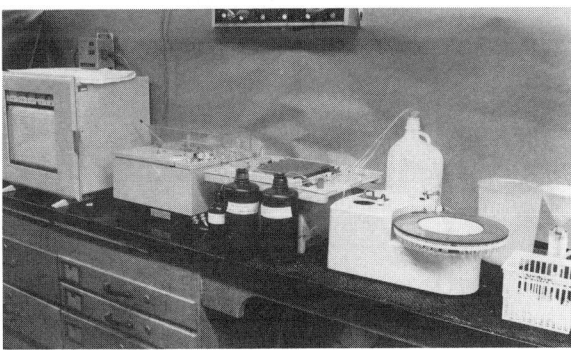

Fig. A-21. An automated analysis of digested samples for percent nitrogen or crude protein. (Courtesy, C.W. Gehrke, University of Missouri)

HISTORY. Today, many good methods of food analysis are available, but the cost of equipment, labor, and supplies limits the use of certain ones to well funded research projects. Hence, the current trend is toward the development of pro-

cedures that may be automated and carried out on many samples at a time. Similarly, bioassays that utilize animals are very expensive and are gradually being replaced by those employing microorganisms whenever it is feasible to do so. Yet, much needs to be done to fill the present gaps in our knowledge regarding the composition of our common foods.

ANALYTICAL PROCEDURES. Foods are analyzed by chemical, biological, microscopic, and/or physical procedures. Each type of procedure has its advantages and disadvantages.

Chemical Analyses. Today, many foods are being analyzed routinely by highly sophisticated chemical procedures. The laboratories in government agencies, universities, and large food manufacturing concerns are often equipped to perform these analyses when needed to determine nutrient compositions in order to (1) enforce or comply with the laws on nutrient labelling; or (2) provide data for nutritional research.

PROXIMATE ANALYSIS. This group of chemical analyses, which has been utilized for over 100 years, still forms the basis for much of our nutrient composition data. A summary of the analytical scheme is given in Table A-3.

TABLE A-3
THE FRACTIONS OF PROXIMATE ANALYSIS

Fraction	Major Components	Procedure[1]
Moisture (dry matter by difference)	Water and any volatile compounds (100% − H_2O = % dry matter)	Heat chopped or pulverized sample to constant weight at a temperature just above boiling point of water. Loss in weight equals water.
Ash (mineral matter)	Mineral elements	Burn at 930° to 1,110°F (*500° to 600°C*) for 2 hr.
Crude protein (protein averages 16% N; hence, N x 6.25 = crude protein)	Proteins, amino acids, nonprotein nitrogen	Determine nitrogen by Kjeldahl sulphuric acid digestion.
Ether extract (fat)	Fats, oils, waxes, fat-soluble vitamins, coloring matter	Extraction with ether
Crude fiber[2]	Cellulose, hemicellulose, lignin	Organic portion[3] of the residue after boiling a dried, defatted sample in weak acid and weak alkali
Available carbohydrate Also known as nitrogen-free extract (NFE).	Starch, sugars, some cellulose, hemicellulose, pectins, and lignin	Remainder; i.e. 100 minus sum of the other fractions

[1]Each procedure is applied to a separate, chopped or pulverized, sample of standard weight of the food to be analyzed.
[2]Total carbohydrate = crude fiber + available carbohydrate (NFE).
[3]Organic portion is measured by the loss in weight of the residue after ashing.

Usefulness of the Proximate Analysis. As with all analytical techniques, there are advantages and disadvantages in the use of the proximate analysis for the evaluation of foods.

The **advantages** of the system should not be minimized. They are:

1. **Most laboratories are equipped to run this type of analysis.** Expensive and sophisticated equipment is not needed.

2. **It provides a good general evaluation of the food.** A food that is high in crude fiber will probably be inferior in nutritional value to one that is very low in crude fiber. Likewise, a food with a high percentage of ether extract is likely to be high in calories.

3. **Much of the data available on food composition is reported in terms of proximate analysis.**

Some of the **disadvantages** of the proximate analysis are:

1. **The system does not define the individual nutrients of the food.** Rather, the fractions represent mixtures of the various nutrients.

2. **It is not accurate.** Crude protein, crude fiber, and available carbohydrates are rough estimates of their respective fractions.

3. **The procedure is time-consuming.** There is little possibility for automation in the proximate analysis. Many of the fractionations involve several weighings of samples and other procedures which must be done by the laboratory technician.

4. **It does not tell how much indigestible material there is in a food.** Unfortunately, the acid-alkali treatment dissolves much of the crude fiber of plant products, making it impossible to predict accurately how much indigestible matter there is in the food. The method overestimates the nutritive value of some foods, underestimates that of others, and fails to indicate how the constituents of the indigestible residue are related to each other or the function(s) some of them perform in digestion.

5. **It does not go far enough.** Proximate analysis does not provide any information relative to palatability, texture, toxicity, digestive disturbances, or nutritional availability. Thus, further steps need to be taken to evaluate a food.

It is likely that the use of proximate analysis will decline in the future as new techniques are utilized, but, for the present, it offers a means of estimating the water, ash, protein, fat, fiber, and carbohydrate contents of food.

VAN SOEST ANALYSIS FOR FIBER. This procedure separates and classifies the digestible and undigestible parts of plant cells.

The food sample is initially boiled in a neutral detergent solution to separate the neutral detergent soluble fraction (cell contents) and the neutral detergent insoluble fraction (cell walls). The cell contents are highly digestible (about 98%) and include various sugars, starches, pectins, proteins, lipids, nitrogenous compounds, soluble carbohydrates, and water-soluble minerals and vitamins. Cell walls can be further fractionated by boiling in an acid detergent solution. Hemicellulose is solubilized during this procedure, while the lignocellulose fraction of the food remains insoluble. Cellulose is then separated from lignin by the addition of sulfuric acid. Only lignin and acid-insoluble ash remain upon the completion of this step. This residue is then ashed, and the difference of the weights before and after ashing yields the amount of lignin present in the sample.

(Also see FIBER, section on ''Analysis of Cell Wall Consitituents''.)

BOMB CALORIMETRY. When compounds are burned completely in the presence of oxygen, the resulting heat is referred to as gross energy or the heat of combustion. The bomb calorimeter is used to determine the gross energy of foods, waste products from the body (for example, feces and urine), and tissues.

The unit of measurement of food energy is the kilogram-calorie (commonly designated as the Calorie or kilocalorie) which is defined *as the amount of heat required to raise the temperature of 2.2 lb (1 kg) of water 1°C (precisely from 14.5° to 15.5°C).* With this fact in mind, we can readily see how the bomb calorimeter works.

Briefly stated, the procedure is as follows: An electric fuse wire is attached to the sample being tested, so that it can be ignited by remote control; 2,000 g of water are poured around the bomb; 25 to 30 atmospheres of oxygen are added to the bomb; the material is ignited; the heat given off from the burned material warms the water; and a thermometer registers the change in temperature of the water.

However, some of the heat liberated from the food is absorbed by the metal parts of the calorimeter and is not available for heating the water. This error is corrected for by burning a sample of a benzoic acid standard which will emit a known amount of heat. Other corrections are made for the burning of the fuse wire and the acids produced during the combustion.

(Also see BOMB CALORIMETER.)

CHROMATOGRAPHY. In 1903, Tswett, a Russian botanist, first described his attempts to separate colored substances; hence, the origin of the term chromatography. Today, many of the compounds that are separated and identified by chromatographic techniques are colorless; but new refinements in these techniques enable the food analyst to measure extremely minute amounts of many compounds.

Chromatography separates compounds through the use of two phases—a stationary or fixed phase and a mobile phase. The differences between the various chromatographic techniques lie in the variation of the materials used in these phases. The stationary phase can be either solid or liquid material, while the mobile phase or *carrier* can be either gas or liquid in nature. The various types of chromatography are listed in Table A-4.

TABLE A-4
TYPES OF CHROMATOGRAPHY

Stationary Phase	Mobile Phase	Chromatographic Procedure
Solid	Liquid	Thin-layer chromatography. Ion exchange chromatography. Gel chromatography. Absorption-column chromatography.
Liquid	Gas	Gas-liquid chromatography. Capillary-column chromatography.
Solid	Gas	Gas-solid chromatography
Liquid	Liquid	Paper chromatography. Partition chromatography. Zone electrophoresis.

Numerous materials from foods, such as proteins, amino acids, sugars, fatty acids, minerals, and many other components, are routinely identified and measured by this type of analytical procedure. In addition to nutrient analysis, chromatography can be adapted to the detection of drug residues, hormones, pesticides, and other food contaminants.

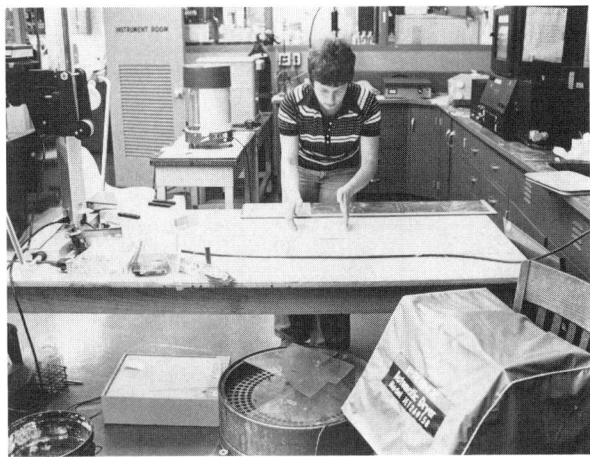

Fig. A-22. Preparation of thin-layer chromatographic plates for food analysis. (Courtesy, University of Illinois at Urbana-Champaign)

The **advantages** of chromatography are numerous; among them, the following:

1. **Extreme sensitivity.** Many compounds can be detected and measured when present in amounts as small as parts per billion (mcg/kg of sample).

2. **Inexpensive.** Many chromatographic techniques can be adapted by almost any laboratory. Relatively little equipment is needed for many chromatographic procedures.

3. **Rapid.** In techniques such as thin-layer chromatography, a large number of samples can be done simultaneously in a relatively short period of time.

4. **Readily adaptable.** Chromatography can be adapted readily to almost any chemical compound.

On the other hand, there are several **disadvantages**, such as:

1. **Complexity of operation.** Many of the newer techniques involve sophisticated equipment which require the operator to be familiar with the theory and the *art* of chromatography.

2. **Sample preparation.** Most samples require some sort of preparation before they can be chromatographed. This may involve such procedures as extraction, hydrolysis, and/or evaporation.

3. **Sample size.** Samples must be small in order to be chromatographed. This means that the sampling procedure must be carefully planned if the results are to be valid.

(Also see CHROMATOGRAPHY.)

COLORIMETRY AND SPECTROPHOTOMETRY. These procedures are chemical analyses in which light is passed through solutions to yield information about the concentration of certain compounds. A particular wavelength of light is passed through the samples, and the amount of light absorbed by the sample gives an indication of the concentration of the compound being tested. Colorimetry differs from spectrophotometry in that colorimetry is useful for measuring wavelengths in the visible region of the light spectrum whereas spectrophotometry utilizes wave lengths in the ultraviolet, visible, and infrared regions of the spectrum.

Many nutrients are analyzed by chemical procedures which involve either colorimetry or spectrophotometry. Vitamin A analysis is a good example of a colorimetric procedure. The standard assay for vitamin A determination involves the treatment of the sample with antimony trichloride. A deep blue-colored solution is produced, the intensity of which is dependent on the amount of vitamin A in the sample. The solution of unknown concentration is measured in the colorimeter and compared to a series of standards of known concentrations. Spectrophotometric assays are essentially the same as colorimetric assays except the researcher has a more versatile machine with which to work.

The atomic absorption spectrophotometer is one of the most widely used instruments for mineral analysis, having the ability to detect many minerals at concentrations less than 1 part per billion (1 mcg/kg of sample). In addition to its high sensitivity, this machine is readily adaptable to automation, thus presenting the chemist with a rapid, accurate method of food analysis. The atomic absorption spectrophotometer works on a slightly different principle than the regular spectrophotometer. The main principle behind this machine is that when certain compounds (for example, minerals) are volatilized, they emit light of a characteristic wavelength. The machine is calibrated to detect this light.

Mass spectrometry is one of the most recently developed procedures for the analysis of foods. Fig. A-23 shows the instruments used in this type of analysis.

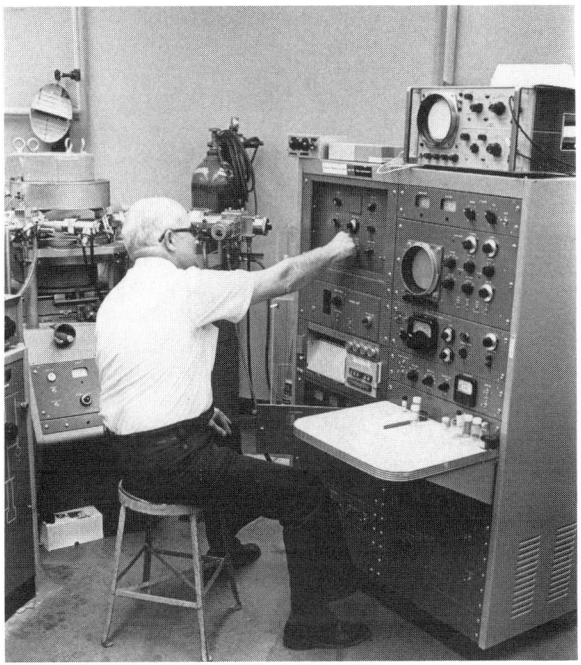

Fig. A-23. A mass spectrometer and its accessories being used to make food analyses. (Courtesy, University of Illinois at Urbana-Champaign)

In this procedure, the substance to be analyzed in the spectrometer is usually subjected to various preliminary treatments such as solvent extraction and gas-liquid chromatography in order to isolate the constituents for identification and measurement. Then, the sample is introduced into the spectrometer, where it is ionized by bombardment with electrons, or by other means such as chemical ionization. The ions are passed through electrical and magnetic fields which separate them into a spectrum of light to heavy masses. Electrical instruments then detect and record the ion masses, which are literally *fingerprints* of the substances analyzed.

Mass spectrometry offers a means of certain identification of substances whose identity might otherwise be uncertain when assayed by other analytical procedures. (Many of the procedures of colorimetry, spectrophotometry, and gas-liquid chromatography identify only general classes of compounds.)

PROTEIN AND AMINO ACID ANALYSES. In the past, the Kjeldahl procedure was considered to be the most efficient way to measure the protein content in food. In recent years, several other means of protein determination have been developed.

When colorimetric techniques for the determination of total protein nitrogen are used, a certain degree of automation can be designed, thereby offering distinct advantages over the Kjeldahl procedure. However, the various procedures which measure the total nitrogen content give only a rough indication of the total protein content because many foods contain nonprotein nitrogen compounds. Therefore, nutritionists and biochemists have developed techniques that yield estimates of the total true protein. A few of these procedures follow:

1. **Biuret assay.** This calorimetric assay compares light absorbence of the unknown protein solution to the absorbences of standard protein concentrations. A biuret reagent is reacted with the protein to produce a colored solution.

2. **Lowry assay.** This colorimetric assay is based on the presence of tyrosine and tryptophan in protein.

3. **Turbidity measurements.** This assay utilizes turbidity measurements after precipitation has been accomplished in a controlled manner.

4. **Peptide bond method.** This spectrophotometric assay is based on the fact that peptide bonds absorb light in the 195 to 225 nanometer region of the spectrum.

5. **Warburg-Christian assay.** This spectrophotometric assay utilizes ultraviolet absorption analysis after all nonprotein material has been removed by fractionation or dialysis.

In planning certain diets, the amino acid composition of the foods must be considered. While most procedures for determining the amino acid patterns of foods are automated to a considerable degree, much time and labor is still involved in sample preparation. For example, the protein within the food must be completely hydrolyzed into its constituent amino acids. In many cases 6N HC1 is used. Unfortunately, this and many other hydrolysis procedures make for the following problems:

1. Some amino acids are destroyed in the process.

2. Some amino acids are chemically altered during hydrolysis.

3. Some of the peptides remain incompletely hydrolyzed, thereby tying up amino acids which should be measured. Following the hydrolysis of the protein, the resulting amino acids are commonly separated by ion-exchange chromatography and subsequently measured by colorimetric techniques or by gas-liquid chromatography.

This procedure may be simplified somewhat if the levels of only the few limiting amino acid(s) in the foods have to be measured. Then, the sample is hydrolyzed and portions of the hydrolyzate are analyzed by procedures that are specific for the amino acids sought. For example, it is most useful to analyze grains for lysine, which is almost always the limiting amino acid in this type of food. Fig. A-24 shows a typical analysis.

Biological Analyses. Chemical analyses do not always provide information about the biological availability of nutrients. For example, the amino acid analysis of hair indicates that it contains sufficient quantities of certain essential amino acids to make it a high-quality protein. Yet, it is not

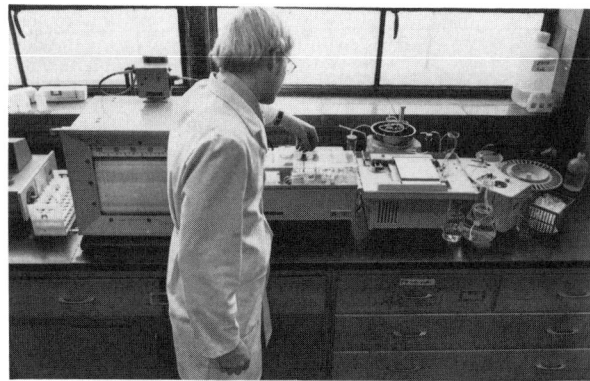

Fig. A-24. Automated analysis of lysine in grain hydrolysates. (Courtesy, C.W. Gehrke, University of Missouri)

digestible by people, pigs, or poultry. Similar circumstances may limit the utilization of other nutrients such as minerals and vitamins, which may be present in poorly utilized forms in certain foods. Therefore, it is sometimes necessary to utilize biological analyses to fill the gaps in the information provided by chemical analyses.

Biological assays tend to be laborious and time-consuming. Large numbers of samples are needed to produce statistically reliable results, and quite often data obtained from these assays is highly variable. For example, some people do not digest cellulose at all, while others apparently harbor microorganisms in their colon which convert some of it into other substances. In the latter cases, only 60 to 80% of an oral dose of cellulose is recovered in the feces. Hence, digestibility data provides only a crude approximation of the percent absorption of certain complex carbohydrates. The assay utilizing nutrient-deficient animals—rats, mice, guinea pigs, pigeons, or chicks—is particularly cumbersome because (1) the animals should be of approximately the same age, sex, and weight, and (2) time is required to induce deficient conditions in these animals.

(Also see VITAMIN[S], section headed "Biological [Animal] Assay.")

DIGESTIBILITY TRIALS. A digestibility trial is made by determining the percentage of each nutrient in the food through chemical analysis; giving the food to human subjects or test animals for a preliminary period, so that all residues of former foods will pass out of the digestive tract; giving weighed amounts of the food during the test periods; collecting, weighing, and analyzing the feces; determining the difference between the amount of the nutrient fed and the amount found in the feces; and computing the percentages of each nutrient digested. The latter figures are known as the *coefficients of digestibility* for those nutrients.

NUTRIENT-DEFICIENT ANIMALS. In this assay, animals, such as the rat or the chick, are fed diets deficient in a specific nutrient. Growth response curves are developed by the feeding of known amounts of the nutrient to some of the deficient animals. Other deficient animals are given the product to be assayed, and their responses are compared to the growth curves. In addition, the evaluator can observe changes in specific tissues as various levels of the specific nutrients are supplied.

(Also see VITAMIN[S], section headed "Biological [Animal] Assay"; VITAMIN D, section headed "Measurement/Assay.")

MICROBIOLOGICAL ASSAYS. In this type of assay, a micoorganism is selected that is known to require the nutrient in question. Therefore, if the nutrient is unavailable, the selected microorganism will not grow. The growth medium is prepared so that it is nutritionally complete except for the nutrient to be tested. Graded levels of the nutrient are then added to the media and a growth response curve is prepared. The sample to be assayed can then be tested and compared to the growth response curve to determine the concentration of the nutrient. Many of the micronutrients, such as the B complex vitamins, are assayed in this manner.

(Also see VITAMIN[S], section headed "Microbiological Assay.")

Microscopic Analyses for Filth and Other Adulterants or Contaminants. *Filth* in foods is considered by the U.S. Food and Drug Administration to consist mainly of insect fragments, and rodent feces and hairs, which are present at higher levels than are consistent with good manufacturing practices. Therefore, special analyses have been developed for the detection of these extraneous materials.

Microscopic analyses are also used to detect adulterants and/or contaminants such as husks, particles of shell, dirt, and sand in dried herbs and spices. Usually, the herbs or spices are ground finely, and placed in a microscope slide with a few drops of water and glycerine. It is usually necessary for the analyst conducting the microscopic examination to refer to authentic samples, photographs, and/or drawings of the herbs or spices and of the most commonly occurring extraneous materials in order to be certain of making correct judgments about the presence or absence of adulteration or contamination. The presence of large amounts of dirt and sand may be confirmed by ashing the sample and examining the ash.

Physical Methods of Analyses. More rapid and less expensive methods of analyses are being sought. Among the more promising procedures are: (1) infrared reflectance spectroscopy for the analysis of nutrients in foods and feeds; and (2) ultrasonics (special sound waves) to measure the thickness of fat in livestock prior to slaughter.

USE OF FOOD COMPOSITION DATA FOR PLANNING MENUS AND DIETS. Most of the procedures used by dietitians and home economists in their planning of meals and modified diets are based, at least in part, on the nutrient data obtained by food analysis. Basic food exchange lists (based upon the values for protein, carbohydrate, fat, and food energy) have been developed by a joint committee of the American Dietetic Association, the American Diabetes Association, and the United States Public Health Service. These lists give portion sizes of foods within each of several categories of foods (milk, vegetables, fruits, bread, cereals, meats, and fats). The portion sizes have been calculated so as to be approximately equal in nutritive value (with respect to the major nutrients, but not in regard to mineral and vitamin contents). For example, one slice (3″ x 2″ x ⅛″) of meat or poultry is approximately equivalent to one all-meat frankfurter (when there are 8 or 9 per pound).

An intelligent lay person, however, may refer directly to a table of food compositions to obtain information for selecting the foods most appropriate for his individual preferences and health needs.

It is noteworthy that the storage of nutrient composition

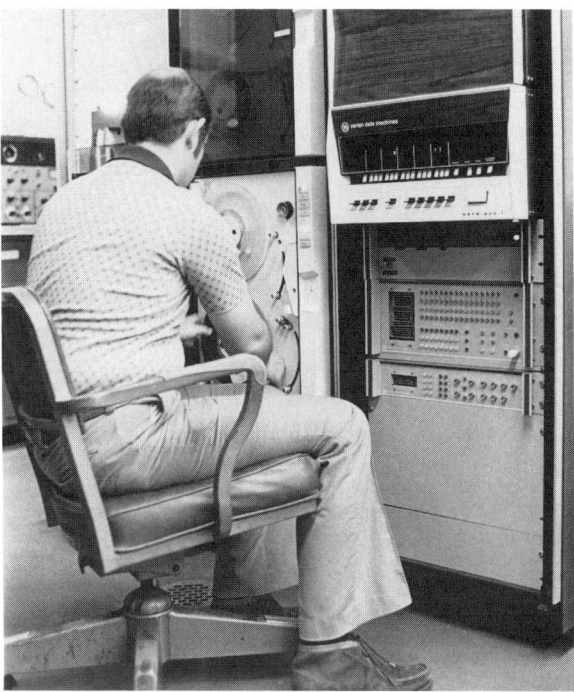

Fig. A-25. Computer analyses of the content of foods. (Courtesy, University of Illinois at Urbana-Champaign)

data on computer tapes has made it possible for more thorough analyses of diets and menus to be made by busy dietitians. Hence, it is hoped that more attention will be paid to the mineral and vitamin contents of hospital menus when computer printouts of nutrient composition are readily available to all dietitians.

ANAPHYLAXIS

A severe allergic reaction which often leads to shock and sometimes to death. The extreme reaction is due to a massive release of histamine which causes the blood vessels to dilate and the blood pressure to fall.

(Also see ALLERGIES.)

ANCHOVY PEAR *Grias cauliflora*

A West Indian tree related to the Brazil nut which bears a fruit resembling the mango. This tree and the fruit are referred to as the anchovy pear. It is an oval fleshy fruit that grows 2 to 3 in. (5 to 8 cm) long with eight grooves on its brown skin. Anchovy pears are usually eaten pickled.

ANDROGENS

Hormones secreted by the testes which promote the development of male sexual characteristics. They also promote the buildup of tissues such as muscle and bone. The secretion of these hormones from the testes is responsible in large part for the larger body mass of males compared to females.

(Also see ENDOCRINE GLANDS.)

ANDROSTERONE

One of the hormones secreted by the testes.
(Also see ENDOCRINE GLANDS.)

ANEMIA

One of the most common disorders which saps the vitality of many persons around the world is a condition where the blood is deficient in either the quantity and/or quality of red cells (erythrocytes). The overall effect of any type of anemia is a reduced supply of oxygen to the tissues of the body. Symptoms and clinical signs of this disorder are paleness of skin and mucous membranes, weakness, frequent tiredness, dizziness, sensitivity to cold, shortness of breath after exercise, loss of appetite, dyspepsia, tingling sensations in the extremities, rapid heartbeat, brittleness and dryness of the nails, soreness and cracks at the corners of the mouth, and atrophy of the tongue papillae, giving it a glossy appearance.

Many studies have shown that the highest prevalence of anemia is in infants and women of reproductive age. A high prevalence is also found in preschool children and adolescents, particularly those from low-income families.

PRODUCTION OF RED BLOOD CELLS (Erythropoiesis). Fig. A-26 outlines the major processes in the life cycle of erythrocytes (red blood cells).

Insufficient oxygen in tissues and blood (hypoxia) is the most important of the various factors which stimulate the production of red cells (other factors are alkalosis which develops at high altitudes, cobalt salts, adrenal cortical and sex hormones, and thyroxine). The process begins with the synthesis and secretion by the liver of a *protein substrate* (PS) in response to a subnormal level of oxygen in the blood circulating in the organ. Similarly, the kidneys produce an enzymelike substance (renal erythropoietic factor or REF) which converts PS to *erythrocyte stimulating factor (ESF)*. Formation of ESF is increased in anemia and after hemorrhage, and decreased when the blood contains a sufficient amount of red cells (regulation of ESF production is altered in disorders such as polycythemia in which there is overproduction of red cells).

Stem cells (embryonic blood cells) in the bone marrow are stimulated by ESF to differentiate into erythrocytes. There are several stages in the transformation of stem cells into red blood cells where nutrient deficiencies may lead to abnormalities in the quality and quantity of mature erythrocytes. Lack of protein, iron, or pyridoxine (vitamin

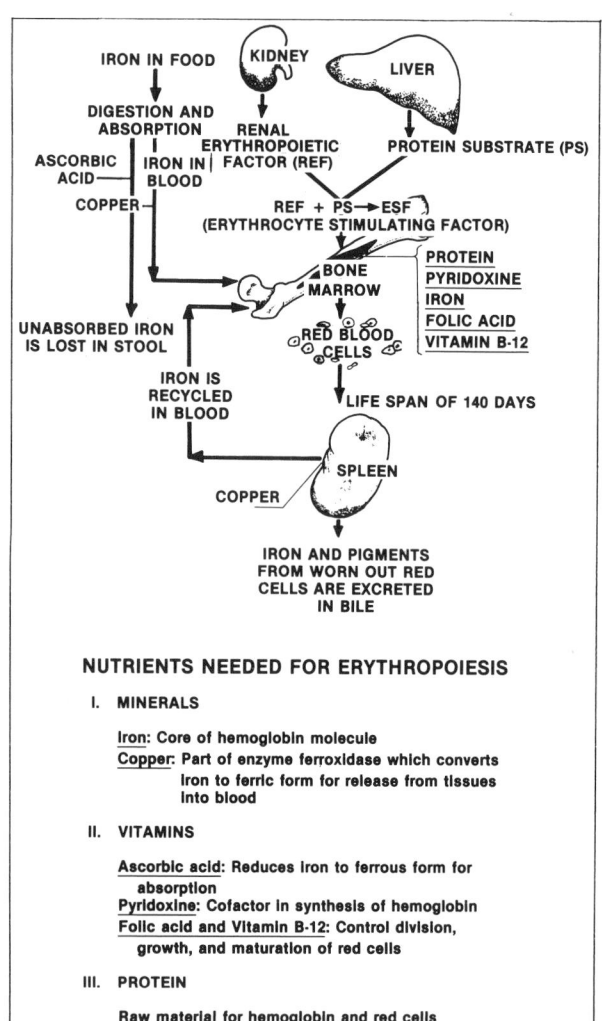

NUTRIENTS NEEDED FOR ERYTHROPOIESIS

I. **MINERALS**

   <u>Iron</u>: Core of hemoglobin molecule
   <u>Copper</u>: Part of enzyme ferroxidase which converts
     iron to ferric form for release from tissues
     into blood

II. **VITAMINS**

   <u>Ascorbic acid</u>: Reduces iron to ferrous form for
     absorption
   <u>Pyridoxine</u>: Cofactor in synthesis of hemoglobin
   <u>Folic acid and Vitamin B-12</u>: Control division,
     growth, and maturation of red cells

III. **PROTEIN**

   <u>Raw material for hemoglobin and red cells</u>

Fig. A-26. Formation of red blood cells (erythropoiesis).

B-6) limits the synthesis of hemoglobin, while copper has an indirect, but similar, effect (as part of an enzyme which converts iron to a form suitable for transport in the blood). Availability of iron for hemoglobin synthesis is also affected by dietary ascorbic acid (vitamin C), which helps to promote the absorption of dietary iron. Limitation of hemoglobin synthesis leads to the formation of abnormally small, or microcytic, cells. Cell division requires folic acid and vitamin B-12. Lack of either nutrient results in increased numbers of *megaloblasts*—immature blood cells enlarged in size and containing segmented nuclei.

Mature red cells lose their nuclei within a day or two of their release into the blood from the bone marrow. The average life span of these cells is about 140 days, but nutrient deficiencies may shorten this period. There is an increased rate of red cell breakdown by hemolysis (liberation of hemoglobin from red blood cells) when there is a deficiency of vitamin E, which protects the cell membrane against substances which cause it to rupture. Similarly, riboflavin (vitamin B-2) deficiency is accompanied by increased hemolysis due to lack of a protective compound generated by an enzyme containing riboflavin.

Iron from the fragments of red cells is stored in the spleen, liver, and bone marrow (reticuloendothelial system). Recycling of this iron requires the action of a copper-containing enzyme.

Maintenance of an adequate supply of erythrocytes, therefore, depends not only on the supply and utilization of iron, but also, to a lesser degree, on ascorbic acid, copper, folic acid, protein, pyridoxine, riboflavin, vitamin B-12, and vitamin E.

FUNCTIONS OF RED BLOOD CELLS.

The toroidal (donutlike) shape of erythrocytes helps to ensure their survival, since their travel through the bloodstream might be compared to the passage of a rubber inner tube through a river full of rapids. This shape also provides a large surface area for picking up and releasing oxygen and carbon dioxide by the hemoglobin present in these cells. Red cells also contribute most of the buffering capacity of the blood. (*Buffering is the process by which a substance, present in a solution, prevents excessive changes in the acidity or alkalinity of the solution.*)

The Role of Iron In Red Blood Cells.

Transport of oxygen by erythrocytes depends upon an atom of iron attached within the core of each molecule of hemoglobin, and the protective shell provided by the protein part of the molecule. Thus, iron in hemoglobin may loosely bind oxygen whereas other forms of iron may bind oxygen so that it cannot be released readily. The presence of iron-containing hemoglobin in the red cells allows the blood to carry approximately 40 times as much oxygen as could be carried solely by a simple solution of iron in the fluid part of the blood. Only 0.5 ml of oxygen can be carried by a simple solution in 100 ml of blood, while approximately 19.5 ml of oxygen can be transported by the red cells which are normally present in the same volume of blood. Likewise, only about 3 ml of carbon dioxide dissolves in 100 ml of blood, but a total of 56 ml of carbon dioxide is actually transported by this volume of blood. Approximately 70% of the carbon dioxide transported in the blood is in the form of bicarbonate ions which are synthesized and broken down within the red cells through the action of an enzyme. About 20% of the carbon dioxide is bound to hemoglobin. The remainder is dissolved in water solution as carbonic acid.

Buffering action is required in the blood because carbon dioxide, formed during energy metabolism in tissues, reacts with water to form carbonic acid. Most of this action is contributed by red cells because oxygenated hemoglobin releases acid in the form of hydrogen ions and deoxygenated hemoglobin picks them up. Thus, the oxygenated hemoglobin furnishes hydrogen ions to compensate for the loss of acid when carbon dioxide is expired from the lungs, while the deoxygenated hemoglobin binds the additional acid formed by metabolism in the tissues. The two-part system of buffering by red blood cells is outlined in the equations which follow:

1. **Buffering in the lungs.**

$$H^+ + (HCO_3)^- \rightarrow H_2CO_3 \rightarrow H_2O + CO_2$$

| Acid (hydrogen ion) is released from oxyhemoglobin. | Bicarbonate ion in the blood is picked up by red cells. | Carbonic acid (breakdown is accelerated by carbonic anhydrase enzyme in red cells) | Water | Carbon dioxide is eliminated in expired air. |

2. **Buffering in other tissues.**

$$CO_2 + H_2O \rightarrow H_2CO_3 \rightarrow H^+ + (HCO_3)^-$$

| Carbon dioxide is generated by metabolism in the tissues. | Water | Carbonic acid (formation is accelerated by carbonic anhydrase enzyme in red cells) | Acid (hydrogen ion) is picked up by deoxygenated hemoglobin. | Bicarbonate ion is released from red cells into blood. |

THE MAJOR CAUSES OF ANEMIA.

Factors which reduce the quality or quantity of hemoglobin are: (1) loss of blood from the body as in menstruation, or within the body as in internal hemorrhages; (2) increased destruction of red blood cells due to genetic defects, deficiencies of protective nutrients, toxic agents, or Hodgkin's disease (cancer of the lymph nodes); (3) reduced production of hemoglobin and/or red cells in disorders affecting iron utilization (deficiency of gastric acid or disease of the bone marrow), or as a result of deficiencies of nutrients which are needed for red blood cell production; and (4) abnormal hemoglobins or red cells (Mediterranean or Cooley's anemia, and sickle cell anemia).

Types of Anemia.

Identification of the correct cause of an anemia is important because indiscriminate use of iron therapy may make some conditions worse (such as hemolytic anemia due to vitamin E deficiency, or anemia due to infectious organisms which thrive on iron). In order to help with such identification, the various types of anemia are described in Table A-5.

GROUPS OF PERSONS SUSCEPTIBLE TO NUTRITIONAL ANEMIAS.

Most of the anemias are likely to be more severe in population groups that have high metabolic requirements, or that are subjected to various stresses. A discussion of these groups follows:

• **Infants**—Both human milk and cow's milk are very poor sources of iron. The full-term newborn infant enters life with a store of iron and red cells which should prevent for several months the development of anemia on a diet containing only milk. However, the premature infant is likely to have a much smaller store of iron, and is much more susceptible to hemolytic anemia. Even healthy infants, however, may be depleted of iron (due to small, daily losses in the stool and urine) after several months on a low-iron diet. Also, pasteurized milk has been found to induce, in some infants and children, a small but regular loss of blood from the gastrointestinal tract; evaporated milk does not seem to have this effect (heating during evaporation alters the protein).

• **Children**—Low income, lack of education, or other problems of parents may result in a poor diet for some growing children. There may also be stress factors, such as infestation with worms, chronic infections, diarrheal disease, or milk-induced loss of blood from the gastrointestinal tract.

• **Adolescents**—Adolescent females are more likely to be deficient in iron than adolescent males. A survey by the U.S. Department of Agriculture showed that, on the average, intakes of iron were low for this group (about 50% of Recommended Dietary Allowance).[6] The reasons for poor diets among this group include erratic eating patterns, skipping meals to lose weight, and low socioeconomic status. Although both male and female adolescents from ages 15 to 18 have the same allowance for iron, the energy allowances are 3,000 Calories (kcal) for males but only 2,200 Calories (kcal) for females; making it more difficult for the latter to obtain sufficient iron without consuming excess calories. Furthermore, menstrual blood losses plus the possibility of early marriage and pregnancy for females make their iron nutrition critical.

---

[6]*Dietary Levels of Households in the United States, Spring, 1965*, USDA Ag. Res. Serv. Bull. No. 62, 1969, p. 17.

TABLE A-5
TYPES OF ANEMIAS

Type	Description	Effects on the Body	Possible cures
A. *Nutritional in origin:* **Hemolytic anemia resulting from vitamin E deficiency**	Red blood cells have an abnormal membrane (results from a deficiency of vitamin E) which makes them extra sensitive to hemolysis. Most often found in premature infants given milk formulas containing polyunsaturated fats without adequate vitamin E. Also found in adults with a deficiency of the vitamin.	An increased rate of destruction of red cells, resulting in anemia. Edema and some of its consequences (swollen legs, noisy breathing, and puffy eyelids). Severe deficiency of vitamin E in infants may also be accompanied by encephalomalacia (softening of the brain).	Administration of 25 IU of vitamin E daily. (Water soluble forms of the vitamin are more effective than fat-soluble forms.) Avoid administration of iron (interferes with the utilization of vitamin E).[1]
Iron-deficiency anemia	The most common form of anemia. Red cells are reduced in size (microcytic) and contain a subnormal amount of hemoglobin (hypochromic). Also, the cell count is subnormal, due to a decreased production of hemoglobin. Most prevalent in infants, children, and pregnant women.	Deficiency of hemoglobin and its consequences (paleness of skin and mucous membranes, fatigue, dizziness, sensitivity to cold, shortness of breath, rapid heartbeat, and tingling in fingers and toes).	Therapeutic oral doses of iron (60–180 mg/day). Injections of iron dextran or similar compounds may be necessary in severe cases. Care should be taken to avoid excessive doses which might result in toxicity (hemochromatosis).
Megaloblastic anemia	Enlarged and immature red cells (megaloblasts) which are irregular in shape and size but contain normal concentration of hemoglobin (normochromic). Subnormal cell count. There are two major types of megaloblastic anemia; one due to a deficiency of folic acid, and the other due to a deficiency of B-12.	Megaloblastic reaction in the bone marrow (abnormalities of red cells, white cells, and platelets). Macrocytic anemia. Folate deficiency is frequently accompanied by diarrhea. Vitamin B-12 deficiency may lead to gastrointestinal and nervous disorders. (Also see effects given below under pernicious anemia.)	First test for the possibility of pernicious anemia. If there is no deficiency of vitamin B-12, then therapeutic oral doses of 0.1–1.0 mg of folic acid per day are usually effective. Daily injections of 0.01 mg of folic acid in cases due to malabsorption. Include good food sources of folic acid in the diet.
Pernicious anemia[2]	Same as above description of megaloblastic anemia. Additionally, there are gastrointestinal disosrders (glossitis, achlorhydria, and lack of intrinsic factor for vitamin B-12 absorption) and neurologic damage (shown by abnormal electroencephalogram).[2] Caused much more frequently by autoimmunity (antibodies to intrinsic factor for vitamin B-12) than by dietary deficiency of the vitamin.	Megaloblastic anemia. Abnormalities of cells lining the gastrointestinal tract. Atrophy of gastric parietal cells and achlorhydria. Synthesis of abnormal fatty acids and their deposition in nerve tissue. Mental dysfunction.	Administration of 100 mcg per day of vitamin B-12 by injection (may be given orally *only* in those cases where absorption is known to be good). Lifelong maintenance injections (100 mcg per month) may be necessary for patients lacking intrinsic factor. *Caution*: Megadoses (1,000 mcg per day) have sometimes resulted in blood clots after the first week of therapy.[3] Include good food sources of vitamin B-12 in the diet.
Pica associated with iron-deficiency anemia	Abnormal craving for nonfood items leads to the eating of clay, dirt, plaster, paint chips, and ice. Iron deficiency is believed to be one cause of this disorder.	Certain nonfood items (some types of clays) interfere with iron absorption and make the condition worse.	Treat iron deficiency (as described above for iron deficiency anemia). The possibility of chronic blood loss should also be investigated.
Pregnancy anemia	The added requirements of a developing fetus produce in most cases an iron-deficiency anemia, although there may also be a folic acid deficiency.	Effects are the same as those of iron deficiency, except that the anemia may develop more rapidly in the pregnant woman, making her very vulnerable to the effect of blood loss during childbirth.	Therapeutic doses of iron, and folic acid if required (the latter should be considered in the case of women who were taking oral contraceptives prior to pregnancy and who may have had folic acid depletion as a result of the drug). (Also see cure given above for iron-deficiency anemia.)
Siderotic anemia due to deficiency of pyridoxine (vitamin B-6)	Microcytic, hypochromic anemia similar to that caused by iron dificiency; except that serum iron is normal or at an elevated level. Vitamin B-6 deficiency impairs synthesis of hemoglobin.	(See effects given above for iron-deficiency anemia.)	Oral doses of 50–200 mg of vitamin B-6 per day. **Note**: The disorder may have nonnutritional causes (factors that interfere with synthesis of hemoglobin).
B. *Nonnutritional in orgin:* **Aplastic anemia**	Cessation of blood cell production in the bone marrow due to toxic agents, reaction to drugs, and unknown causes.	Great decrease in all blood cells produced in the bone marrow (red cells, white cells, and platelets). All the complications of anemia plus hemorrhages (due to lack of platelets needed for clotting).	No cures are available, but there may be gradual recovery if the causative factor is eliminated. Patients may be maintained on blood transfusions. There have been some successful bone marrow transplants from close relatives
Blood loss	Restoration of the full complement of red cells after blood loss is slower than repletion of other constituents of blood.	Effects are the same as those of iron deficiency, but may be more severe, depending upon extent of blood loss.	Same as for iron deficiency, except in severe cases, where transfusion of packed red cells may be necessary.

Footnotes at end of table.

(Continued)

TABLE A-5 *(Continued)*

Type	Description	Effects on the Body	Possible cures
Nonnutritional in origin, *(continued)* **Familial hemolytic jaundice** (spherocytic anemia)	A hereditary disorder in which the red cells are shaped like spheres instead of being of toroidal (donutlike) shape. Jaundice results from excessive destruction of the abnormal cells by the spleen.	Yellowish color of the skin and whites of the eyes (jaundice). Reduction in the number of circulating red cells.	There is no cure for the hereditary disorder, but surgical removal of the spleen is a cure of the effects of jaundice and excessive red cell destruction.
Hemolytic anemia due to deficiency of G6PD enzyme	Increased hemolysis of red cells due to the effects of drugs, toxic agents, and compounds in foods such as fava beans. This disorder is due to an increased susceptibility of red cells in persons who have hereditary deficiencies of Glucose-6-phosphate dehydrogenase (G6PD).	Anemia and jaundice (due to excessive hemolysis). Men are more likely to have the effects since the trait is sex-linked.	Avoidance of the substance(s) which causes hemolysis. Sometimes treatment with hormones such as ACTH and cortisone is helpful. This disease might be confused with spherocytic anemia, which has similar symptoms.
Hemolytic anemia of the newborn due to Rh factor incompatibility	Rh-negative mothers develop antibodies against Rh-positive blood towards the end of pregnancy with an Rh-positive fetus (due to some transfer of blood from the fetus). The first child is not usually affected (unless the mother was previously sensitized by abortion or blood transfusion), but there are likely to be blood problems (caused by the transfer of antibodies from the mother) in the infants from subsequent pregnancies.	Destruction of red cells in the newborn infant. In severe cases, there may be almost complete destruction of the infant's red cells and damage to the brain by the accumulation of bilirubin (pigment resulting from the breakdown of hemoglobin).	A severely affected infant may require a total exchange of blood by transfusion. The antibody production by the mother may be blocked by a substance called RhoGam[TM],[4] which should be administered to Rh-negative women when they first show signs of sensitization (usually after first pregnancies and abortions).
Hookworm or tapeworm infestation	Infestation of the gastrointestinal tract by parasitic worms which feed on blood (hookworm) or nutrients (tapeworm). Anemia may be due to blood loss; deficiencies of folic acid, iron, and/or vitamin B-12.	Anemia, fatigue, irritability, fever, abdominal discomfort, nausea, or vomiting	Treatment with an antiworm drug to eliminate parasite. Nutritional therapy (iron in the case of the hookworm; iron, folic acid, and/or vitamin B-12 in the case of the tapeworm).
Infection	The production of red cells by the marrow is sometimes inhibited by toxins from an infectious agent.	Anemia and weakness.	Elimination of the infection. Not helped by extra folic acid, iron, or vitamin B-12.
Leukemia	A form of cancer in which there is overproduction by the body of white cells. Normal production of other blood cells (red cells, platelets, normal white cells) is prevented by the overgrowth of abnormal leukocytes in the bone marrow and other blood-forming organs (liver, spleen, and lymphatic tissues).	Grayish-white color of blood with a large excess of leukocytes. Death often results from the acute form of the disease and from the chronic form when it is not treated.	Drugs which prevent the growth of the abnormal cells.
Mediterranean anemia (also called thassalemia and Cooley's anemia)	A hereditary disease which is most prevalent in persons whose ancestors came from the Mediterranean basin (Italy, Sicily, Sardinia, Greece, Crete, Cyprus, Syria, or Turkey). Red cells are fragile and contain abnormal hemoglobin.	An increased rate of destruction of red cells. Bone abnormalities, enlargement of the spleen, leg ulcers, and jaundice.	Blood transfusions provide temporary relief, but eventually there is a toxic accumulation of iron (due to increased breakdown of red cells).
Sicle cell anemia	A hereditary disease in which the red cells have a sickle shape due to the presence of abnormal hemoglobin. Sickle cells cannot carry as much oxygen as normal red cells, and they have a shorter than normal lifetime.	Anemia. Pain in the joints and extremities. Limited ability to perform strenuous exercise. Death may occur if sickle cells clump together and clog blood flow in tissues, such as the brain.	There is no known cure for the hereditary disorder. Transfusions and/or iron and folic acid therapy may be helpful in cases of severe anemia. Pregnant women with the disease are at high risk due to blood loss during childbirth.

[1]"Vitamin E Therapy in Premature Babies," *Nutrition Reviews*, Vol. 33, 1975, p.206.
[2]"Pernicious Anemia and Mental Dysfunction," *Nutrition Reviews*, Vol. 34, 1976, p. 264
[3]"A Qualitative Platelet Defect in Severe Vitamin B-12 Deficiency," *Nutrition Reviews*, Vol. 32, 1974, p. 202
[4]RhoGam[TM] is a product recently developed by Ortho Pharmaceutical Corp., Raritan, N.J., which acts by transferring protective antibodies (passive immunity) to the sensitized woman, blocking her production of antibodies against Rh-positive blood.

• **Athletes and others engaged in strenuous activity**—A sedentary person may not experience symptoms of a mild anemia, while a person who attempts hard work or vigorous exercise may feel handicapped by such a condition (due to the increased requirement for oxygen during such activities).

• **Nonpregnant women**—It has been established that there are many healthy, nonanemic, young women who have negligible amounts of iron stores (the liver, bone marrow, and spleen may contain some unused iron which may be drawn upon to meet physiological requirements). These women have no reserves to meet increased needs due to such events as blood loss, pregnancy, and other stresses. Furthermore, some women who use the contraceptive pill may become depleted of folic acid and, therefore, have increased susceptibility to megaloblastic anemia (hormones present in oral contraceptives reduce the utilization of dietary folic acid).

• **Pregnant women**—During the course of pregnancy, there is, on the average, about a 50% expansion of the blood volume compared to that existing prior to the pregnancy. This means that for the average woman who has a blood volume of 9 to 10 pt (about *4 to 5 liters*), the blood volume expands to 13 or 14 pt (about *6 or 7 liters* of blood). The hemoglobin will then be diluted as it becomes distributed in a larger volume of blood. There is, in pregnancy, some increase in synthesis of red blood cells by the body, but the amount of increase in red blood cell production is proportionately less than the expansion of the total blood volume. In almost all pregnant women, the hemoglobin concentration, or amount of hemoglobin found in a given volume of blood, will, therefore, drop below the level found prior to the start of pregnancy. It has been estimated that the total amount of additional iron required in pregnancy is about 540 mg (or about 2 mg of extra iron per day). While this does not seem like a difficult requirement to meet, it must be noted that there might have to be a daily dietary increase of 20 mg or more of iron due to the low efficiency of iron absorption by the body (10% or less of dietary iron may be absorbed, except when there is a severe deficiency and percent absorption is increased). These women also run increased risk of developing megaloblastic anemia due to folic acid deficiency since the growing fetus also needs this vitamin. Those who become pregnant right after stopping longterm use of oral contraceptives may have had a folic acid deficiency from the start of pregnancy. This makes for concern, since some congenital malformations in infants have been traced to deficiencies of folic acid in the mother.

• **Aged persons**—The elderly (age 65 and older) have higher incidences of iron-deficiency anemia and pernicious anemia. First of all, atrophy of gastric secretory cells occurs more frequently, and, as a result, they are more likely to have deficiencies of hydrochloric acid (aids in the absorption of iron) and of intrinsic factor (required for vitamin B-12 absorption). Second, reduced incomes and decreased energy requirements make it more difficult to select an adequate diet. Finally, many elderly persons live alone and are, therefore, not as likely to prepare well-balanced meals.

DIAGNOSIS OF NUTRITIONAL ANEMIAS. Advertisements in the mass media suggest to their audiences that a ''tired, run-down feeling'' is a sign of anemia. Although such a diagnosis may apply to some persons, the symptom of fatigue may have other causes. It is, therefore, necessary to have greater accuracy in the diagnosis of anemia. The

two major diagnostic approaches are observation of signs and symptoms and laboratory tests of the blood.

Signs and Symptoms. Anemic persons often have pale skin and mucous membranes along with feelings of tiredness. There usually is a low tolerance to strenuous exercise, and the anemic person quickly becomes *out-of-breath*. Often the heart works harder to deliver more blood to the tissues (shown by rapid pulse). These characteristics may indicate, however, any one of several different anemias (including some with nonnutritional causes). It is, therefore, often necessary to confirm diagnosis of signs and symptoms with laboratory tests.

Laboratory Tests. Usually, determination of the quantity and quality (size, color, shape) of red blood cells is sufficient to confirm the general diagnosis of anemia and to identify the specific type of anemia. Occasionally, it is necessary to perform tests on other body tissues or fluids, particularly when anemias other than that due to iron deficiency is suspected.

A number of reliable laboratory tests are available from which the physician may select.

Interpretation of Signs, Symptoms, and Laboratory Tests. Most cases of anemia are due to iron deficiency, although there are several other causes for anemia. The other types of anemia constitute only a small minority of cases. Nevertheless, they need to be considered when persons with anemia do not respond to iron therapy, or when the symptoms of their anemia differ from those normally found in iron deficiency. One of the problems in the diagnosis of iron-deficiency anemia is the disagreement among both scientists and health practitioners as to the levels of hemoglobin which indicate the presence of the disorder.

The World Health Organization considers anemia to be present when blood levels of hemoglobin are below the following values (g/100 ml of venous blood): children aged 6 months to 6 years, 11; children aged 6 to 14 years, 12; adult males, 13; adult females, nonpregnant, 12; adult females, pregnant, 11.[7]

Anemia, like other diseases, is accompanied by specific symptoms; yet, a number of investigators have reported that there does not seem to be a direct correlation between these symptoms and marginal blood levels of hemoglobin. It follows that diagnosis is difficult for borderline cases of iron-deficiency anemia, but serious cases are easily detected.

TREATMENT AND PREVENTION OF IRON-DEFICIENCY ANEMIA. Once anemia has been diagnosed, the patient should be given some form of supplemental iron since treatment consisting only of additional dietary iron takes a long time to cure anemia.

Oral Administration of Iron. Iron-containing tablets are a more stable form of ferrous iron than tonics because iron in solution might become oxidized to the ferric form, the absorption of which is very poor.

TABLETS. Ferrous sulfate is the best-utilized form of iron available. Ferrous iron in the form of other salts (fumarate, gluconate, and succinate) is equal in effectiveness to ferrous sulfate, but they are more expensive. There is some evidence

---

[7]*Nutritional Anemia*, WHO: Technical Report Series No. 405, Geneva, 1968.

of an increased effectiveness of so-called *chelated iron* (iron in chemical combination with well-absorbed organic compounds such as amino acids) compared to ferrous sulfate. The usual dose of the latter compound is 200 mg in tablets taken three times a day. Although most forms of oral iron produce at least a mild irritation of the gastrointestinal tract, enteric-coated tablets are not a good solution to the problem since the iron from these tablets is released farther down in the intestine than that from uncoated tablets; consequently, absorption is reduced. Also, tablets may not disintegrate soon enough in the intestines of persons who have diarrhea or abnormally rapid motions of the intestines.

TONICS. These preparations may be preferable to tablets when there are problems concerning the disintegration of the latter. Some of these tonics contain alcohol, but there is disagreement as to its effect on the absorption of iron (some think it produces an improved absorption).

Parenteral Administration of Iron (Injections).
This form of medication is generally used for persons unable to benefit from orally administered iron due to disorders of the digestive tract or an intolerance to oral iron. Occasionally, there are persons who do not have any problems with oral iron, but cannot be relied upon to take their medication regularly. Three commonly used preparations for injection are iron dextran, iron sorbitol, and dextriferron.

Dangers of Therapeutic Administration of Iron.
Accumulation of excess iron in tissues may result from chronic ingestion or injection of therapeutic doses of iron, particularly when there are abnormal conditions of iron absorption and utilization such as the following: (1) an increased rate of destruction of red cells, (2) transfusion of a large amount of blood, and (3) an abnormally high rate of absorption such as occurs in chronic alcoholism and chronic disease of the liver or pancreas. An increase in nontoxic tissue storage of iron is called *hemosiderosis*, while that resulting in tissue damage is called *hemochromatosis*. Tissue damage from excess iron is most frequently found in the liver (produces fibrosis and cirrhosis), pancreas (results in *bronze diabetes*) and the heart muscle.

Some clinicians are concerned over the possibility that routine administration of therapeutic doses of iron to pregnant women might lead to the accumulation of an iron overload in the tissues of the mothers and/or the fetuses. This situation was found to exist in Bantu women who drank large quantities of a beer very rich in iron. Autopsies of Bantu infants showed an excess of iron in their tissues. The infants, however, had died from other causes. Very few studies have been made of the metabolism of therapeutic iron administered during pregnancy.

Good Food Sources of Iron.
The uncertainties associated with the diagnosis and treatment of anemia make it desirable to make special efforts to prevent development of the disorder. There is a wide variety of both plant and animal foods supplying iron in quantities sufficient to prevent anemia. Some of the best food sources of iron are listed in Table A-6.

It should be noted that unrefined foods usually contain more iron than unenriched, highly processed foods. For example, unenriched white flour contains only about ¼ as much iron as whole wheat flour, and unenriched white rice only about ½ as much iron as brown rice (enrichment of the refined grains with iron restores the amount lost in processing). Much has been said about the iron-binding

TABLE A-6
GOOD FOOD SOURCES OF IRON[1]

Source	Iron	Energy
	(mg/100 g)	(kcal/100 g)
Liver, hog, fried in margarine	29.1	241
Wheat-soy blend (WSB)/bulgur flour or straight grade wheat flour	21.0	365
Molasses, cane, blackstrap	16.1	230
Wheat bran, crude commercially milled	14.9	353
Liver, calf, fried	14.2	261
Kidneys, beef braised	13.1	252
Soybean flour, defatted	11.1	326
Liver, chicken broiler/fryer, simmered	8.5	165
Oyster, fried	8.1	239
Eggs, raw yolk, fresh	5.5	369
Apricots, dehydrated, sulfured, uncooked	5.3	332
Sardines, Pacific, canned in brine or mustard, solids/liquid	5.2	186
Prunes, dehydrated, uncooked	4.4	344
Peaches, dried, sulfured, uncooked	3.9	340
Beef, all cuts[2]	3.8	300
Nuts, mixed, dry roasted	3.7	590
Pork, all cuts[2]	3.2	325
Beans, lima, mature, seeds, dry, cooked	3.1	138
Rice, white, enriched, raw	2.9	363
Wheat flour, all-purpose or family, enriched	2.9	365
Raisins, natural, uncooked	2.8	289

[1]These listings are based on the data in Food Composition Table F-21. Some good food sources may have been overlooked since some of the foods in Table F-21 lack values for iron.

Whenever possible, foods are on an "as used" basis, without regard to moisture content; hence, certain high-moisture foods may be disadvantaged when ranked on the basis of iron content per 100 g (approximately 3½ oz) without regard to moisture content.

[2]Values for different cuts range from 3.9 to 2.5 mg/100 g.

effects of phytates in whole grains, but it should be noted that these compounds are broken down by a phytase enzyme in yeast when it is used as a leavening agent in baking. Even the choice of a sweetening agent affects the iron content of the diet. For example, the third extraction (or blackstrap molasses) contains (1) 4 times as much iron as the first extraction (or light molasses), (2) 4½ times as much iron as brown sugar, (3) 12 times as much iron as maple sugar, (4) 32 times as much iron as honey, and (5) 160 times as much iron as white sugar.

Factors Affecting the Utilization of Iron in Foods.
One of the limitations of tables giving iron content of various foods is that there are differences in the percent utilization of the iron present in these foods. Iron present as heme (in blood-containing foods such as liver and muscle meats) is probably the most efficiently used form of iron from foods. In general, iron from plant foods does not seem to be as well utilized as iron from animal foods. Other food ingredients may aid or hinder the absorption of iron, but only a few such effects are well understood.

Substances which promote the absorption of iron are:
(1) vitamin C (helps to keep iron in the ferrous or reduced state); (2) hydrochloric acid from the stomach (neutralizes some of the alkalinity in the small intestine and thereby increases the solubility of iron); (3) lactose or milk sugar (ferments to lactic acid, which acts similarly to gastric acid in the small intestine); (4) iron-containing foods from animal sources (reasons for this effect are not known); and (5) alcohol (a major ingredient in several proprietary remedies for iron-deficiency anemia).

Iron absorption is inhibited by the following: phytates (whole grains, bran), oxalates (spinach and rhubarb), raw soybeans, large excesses of calcium in the diet, protein from egg yolks, and antacids.

The cooking of acid-containing foods in iron pots has been shown to add significant amounts of iron to the food. For example, it was found that spaghetti sauce, cooked for 3 hours in an iron skillet, contained 87.5 mg of iron per 100 g of sauce, compared to 3.0 mg of iron in an equal amount of sauce cooked in a glass dish.[8] In most developed countries, however, pots and pans made of iron have been replaced by those made from aluminum, stainless steel, and other materials.

Enrichment and Fortification of Foods with Iron. From time to time, the Food and Drug Administration (FDA) has been pressured to promulgate new standards for the fortification of grain products and flour with iron. Present practices, however, should be examined before new measures are considered. These follow.

NOTE WELL: Originally, the FDA differentiated between enrichment and fortification, but now the two terms are used interchangeably.

(Also see enrichment standards in the following sections: ENRICHMENT, Table E-11, Enrichment levels of Cereal Products; and WHEAT, section on "Enriched Flour.")

ENRICHMENT. *This term refers to the restoration of some of the nutrients lost during the processing of foods.* At the present time, about ¾ of the states in the United States have laws requiring the enrichment of flour and certain grain products with iron, thiamin, riboflavin, and niacin according to the standards of the FDA (requires that 12 mg of iron be added to each pound of flour). Not all states, however, require that enriched flour be used for the production of all baked goods. Also, some ethnic groups (notably, Afro-Americans from the South) use rice as a staple food (although required by law in but a few states, about ½ of the rice available in retail markets is enriched). It should be noted that the highest incidence of anemia is among Afro-American females (according to the Ten State Nutrition Survey). One of the problems with the enrichment of flour and baked goods is that the form of iron used for this purpose is not well absorbed (iron sodium pyrophosphate is presently being used since other forms discolor white flour products). However, recent research has shown that the bioavailability of certain iron salts can be more than doubled by reducing the particle size of the iron compound to about ¼ of that commonly used.[9]

FORTIFICATION. *This means the addition to food of nutrients in such amounts that their final levels in the food are greater than those that were naturally present.* Some of the common foods which are presently fortified with iron are commercial infant formulas, infant cereals, and breakfast cereals.

In 1971, the FDA proposed that the enrichment standards for flour and grain products be revised so that iron might be added at a level of fortification (40 mg of iron per pound of flour). The proposal met with considerable opposition from some physicians who argued that the level of iron (designed to protect most women against anemia) might have a toxic effect on men (who require *less* iron than women, but eat more food, and therefore, consume *more* iron). Hemochromatosis is found mainly in alcoholic men, but it is not known what might be the effect of longterm ingestion by normal men of increased amounts of iron. Finally, the FDA withdrew the proposal in 1977 because there was lack of evidence that the benefits of the iron fortification would outweigh the risks.

Although there have been suggestions that white sugar be enriched or fortified with iron, it seems to be more appropriate to add iron to flour and grain products for the following reasons: (1) many nutritionists are trying to persuade people to cut down on their intake of sugar; and (2) there is a substantial and predictable consumption of flour and grain products by low-income groups.

There has also been a great amount of discussion relative to providing iron-fortified milk formulas for infants. However, these formulas may be too expensive for low-income families. Also, pediatricians and nutritionists usually advise parents to start feeding meats, cereals, and other iron-containing foods to infants by the time they are 3 months of age (when the iron stores from birth may be depleted). Like the iron used to enrich flour and bread, the iron used to fortify cereals has a low bioavailability. Meats provide the most available form of iron, but their cost sometimes limits their use. Perhaps some of the newly engineered foods, like textured vegetable protein, will provide suitable vehicles for iron fortification.

(Also see IRON.)

ANEMIA, MEGALOBLASTIC

This disorder is characterized by enlarged and immature red cells (megaloblasts) which are irregular in shape and size but contain the normal concentration of hemoglobin. However, the total amount of hemoglobin circulating in the blood is subnormal, since there are fewer red cells. White blood cells and platelets are often abnormal, since there is a general megaloblastosis of all of the blood cells formed in the bone marrow. Although nowhere near as prevalent as anemia due to iron deficiency, the effects of megaloblastic anemia are as debilitating and, until recently, frequently fatal.

There are two major types of nutritonal megaloblastic anemia; one is due to a deficiency of folic acid, and the other is due to a deficiency of vitamin B-12.

(Also see ANEMIA; FOLACIN; and VITAMIN B-12.)

ANEMIA, PERNICIOUS

The characteristics of this disease are as follows: (1) megaloblastic anemia (enlarged and immature red cells, and a reduced number of normal blood cells); (2) disorders of the bone marrow (impaired formation of red cells, platelets, and white cells); (3) prolonged bleeding time (resulting from deficiency and abnormality of platelets); (4) inflammation and atrophy of stomach lining (lack of gastric acid and intrinsic factor may result from destruction of stomach lining cells by antibodies); (5) glossitis (smooth, shiny, and inflamed tongue) and bowel disorders; (6) impairment of fatty acid metabolism (accumulation of abnormal fatty acids in the myelin sheath of nerves, and elevated urinary excretion of propionic and methylmalonic acids); and (7) degeneration of the spinal cord and cerebral damage (indicated by abnormalities in an electroencephalogram). Although the blood disorders in pernicious anemia are very similar to those in megaloblastic anemia due to folic acid deficiency, the abnormalities of the nerves, tongue, and stomach are unique in pernicious anemia.

Most cases of this disease are found in persons over 40 years of age. If not promptly treated, death may result in about 3 years after diagnosis of the disease.

(Also see ANEMIA; and VITAMIN B-12.)

[8]Moore, C. V., "Iron," *Modern Nutrition in Health and Disease,* 5th Ed., Lea and Febiger, 1973, p. 300, Table 6C-2.

[9]"Physical Acceptability and Bioavailability of Iron Fortified Foods," *Nutrition Reviews,* Vol. 34, 1976, p. 298.

ANEURINE

The name given to vitamin B-1 (called thiamin in the U.S.) by the British.
(Also see THIAMIN.)

ANEURYSM

A bulging out of (1) a small segment of an artery such as the aorta or one of the cerebral arteries, or (2) the wall of the heart. Little is known about the cause(s) of aneurysms, but nutritional deficiency is suspicioned. The rupture of an aneurysm often leads to sudden death from a massive hemorrhage. Rupture may be prevented by surgery in which one or more dacron patches are sewn onto the artery or the heart.

ANGINA PECTORIS

A sharp pain felt on the breastbone over the heart which may spread to the left arm and to the fingers. It may occur after strenuous exercise, emotional excitement, or other factors that cause the heart to work harder.
(Also see HEART DISEASE.)

ANGIOGRAM

A means of visualizing certain blood vessels through the injection of a medium which may be seen on x rays.

ANGIOTENSIN

A substance formed in the blood from angiotensinogen, a protein which is synthesized in the liver. Angiotensin constricts blood vessels and raises the blood pressure.

ANGIOTENSINOGEN

A protein that is synthesized by the liver and circulates in the blood. Under certain conditions, it is converted to angiotensin which causes blood vessels to constrict and the blood pressure to rise.

ANGULAR STOMATITIS

An infection of the skin at the angles of the mouth, characterized by the epithelium protruding into ridges, giving the appearance of fissures. This is a symptom of riboflavin deficiency and of other diseases. But it can also be produced by poorly fitting dentures.

ANIMAL FATS

These are the fats that are isolated from animal tissues and animal sources. Primarily, animal fats include lard, tallow, and butter fat. Overall, animal fats are saturated. That is, the carbon atoms of fatty acids joined to the glycerol molecules in their triglycerides contain all possible hydrogen atoms. The iodine value, a measure of the degree of unsaturation, is low (under 80) for animal fats. The most common long-chain saturated fatty acids of animal tissues are palmitic acid and stearic acid. The saturated short-chain fatty acids—butyric, caproic, and caprylic acid—are common to butter fat. Since animal fats are high in saturated fatty acids they are usually solid, and have fairly high melting temperatures. Certain oils from fishes and marine animals remain liquid at low temperatures. Also, like all fats, they contain about two and one-fourth times as much energy as do proteins or carbohydrates. Each 100 g of animal fat contains about 850 to 900 Calories (kcal) of energy. All of the following are considered animal fats and may exist in a separate form: bacon fat, beef tallow, butter fat, chicken fat, duck fat, goose fat, mutton tallow, turkey fat, lard, pork backfat, and suet. Of course, the meat of animals contains fats similar to these extracted fats.
(Also see FATS AND OTHER LIPIDS; LARD; and MEAT[S].)

ANIMAL PRODUCTS

Meat, milk, eggs, and other products derived from animals, including four-footed animals, poultry, and fish.

ANIMAL PROTEIN FACTOR (APF)

The term formerly used to refer to an unidentified growth factor essential for poultry and swine and present in protein feeds of animal origin. It is now known to be the same as vitamin B-12.
(Also see VITAMIN B-12.)

ANIMAL STARCH

This name has been given erroneously to glycogen which is a storage form of carbohydrate found in animal tissues such as liver and muscle. It is not starch, however, since true starch is found only in plant materials.
(Also see CARBOHYDRATE[S]; and STARCH.)

ANION

A negatively charged ion. Examples are: hydroxyl, OH^-; carbonate, CO_3^-; phosphate, PO_4^-.
(Also see WATER AND ELECTROLYTES.)

ANORECTIC (ANOREXIGENIC) DRUGS

Drugs that depress the appetite and are used as an aid in weight reduction. Amphetamine is the most common anorectic drug.
(Also see AMPHETAMINES.)

ANOREXIA

A lack or loss of appetite for food.
(Also see ANOREXIA NERVOSA.)

ANOREXIA NERVOSA

A condition most frequently found in adolescent girls or young adult single women, characterized by pitiful emaciation resulting from self-inflicted voluntary starvation. The term implies that the condition is a neurosis, which is true in the majority of cases. Occasionally, however, it is caused by endocrine imbalances, usually resulting from disorders within the pituitary gland.

In extreme cases, the loss of weight may be so great that death may ensue if the malady is not corrected in time. Both psychological and medical treatment are necessary, accompanied by dietary regulation and diet therapy. Psychotherapy is necessary in order to enable the patient to realize the problem and to recognize the need for food consumption; hence, it should be continued until recovery is complete. Medical treatment may include small doses of insulin before meals to stimulate need and desire for food. Diet therapy may consist of a nurse giving support to the patient by offering intimate personal attention at meals, such as feeding the patient in an unhurried and acceptable manner and gradually encouraging self-feeding. However, some patients will require tube feeding. If tube feeding must be used as a last life-saving resort, the procedure should be done in a therapeutic manner—never in a punitive manner.

ANOREXIGENIC DRUG

A medication which takes away the appetite. Such drugs are useful in programs designed to reduce the body weight. (Also see APPETITE.)

ANOSMIA

This is the loss or impairment of the sense of smell, which may be permanent or temporary, depending on whether or not the olfactory nerves are damaged or destroyed completely beyond hope of healing. Such a condition makes it quite difficult for afflicted persons to derive enjoyment from eating.

ANOXIA

Lack of oxygen, or hypoxia, in the blood or tissues. This condition may result from various types of anemia, reduction in the flow of blood to tissues, or lack of oxygen in the air at high altitudes.
(Also see ANEMIA.)

ANTABUSE

This is a drug used in the treatment of alcoholism, for the purpose of producing a distaste for alcohol. When antabuse is administered to an alcoholic, extreme discomfort, severe nausea, vomiting, and flushing develops, with intolerance to alcohol.

Antabuse should never be given without the full knowledge and consent of the person; and it should never be given to a person who is intoxicated. The drug is best used along with psychotherapy.
(Also see ALCOHOLISM.)

ANTACIDS

These compounds are usually nonabsorbable basic substances or buffers used to treat indigestion and to soothe discomfort associated with this problem. The wide range of disorders referred to under the general term *indigestion* are generally believed by the public to be related, in one way or another, to gastric hyperacidity; hence, there is very wide usage of antacid preparations. Among such disorders are peptic ulcer, gastritis, gastric hyperacidity, heartburn, excessive gas, stomach irritation (from corticosteroid drugs, food intolerance, excessive smoking, or alcoholic stimulation), pylorospasm (spasm of the sphincter between the stomach and the small intestine), nervous dyspepsia, bleeding ulcers, colitis, hiccups, hypermotility (for which an antacid may be used with an antispasmodic drug), diverticulitis, after gallbladder surgery, before Caesarean sections, and anxiety (for which an antacid may be used with a sedative drug). More than likely, anyone watching television for 2 hours or more at a time will see an antacid commercial promising relief from indigestion due to nervous irritation and/or overeating.

CAUTION: Antacids are not to be chewed like candy, even though they are often flavored with sugar and peppermint. Also, there is need for a person suffering from chronic indigestion to obtain a correct diagnosis of his disorder so that there is neither hyperacidity nor hypoacidity, both of which may give rise to similar discomfort. There is also the possibility that a person with chronic distress may be suffering from some such a condition as hiatus hernia.

(Also see HIATUS HERNIA.)

Often, nonantacid demulcent preparations (usually mucilaginous substances such as mucin or psyllium seed gel) might be used in place of part of the dose of antacid since these substances have coating and soothing effects. The role of food proteins as buffers of stomach acid are well known, but these substances also stimulate acid secretion by an unpredictable amount.

Finally, persons who have indigestion due to anxiety and other psychological problems might well seek treatment of these underlying disorders.
(Also see DYSPEPSIA; HEARTBURN; and ULCERS, PEPTIC.)

ANTAGONIST

In nutrition, this term refers to a substance which counteracts the beneficial effects of one or more vital nutrients. For example, the substance avidin from raw egg white binds the vitamin biotin. Sometimes, cooking eliminates or reduces antagonistic effects.

ANTHOCYANINS

These are violet, red, and blue flavonoid pigments contained in many fruits, vegetables, flours, and leaves, such as delphinin, pelargonidin, and cyanidin. They are pH sensitive and water soluble, and they contain glucose and anthocyanidins. They become more violet in alkali mediums and more red in acidic mediums. Due to the fact that they are water soluble, they leak out of cut fruits and vegetables during processing and cooking. Anthocyanins will react with metals and become more blue or violet. Therefore, cans must be lined if the natural color of the canned fruit and vegetable containing anthocyanins is to be maintained. Anthocyanins are found in grapes, berries, cherries, beets, and eggplants.

ANTHROPOMETRIC MEASUREMENTS

Simple measurements of the various parts of the human body. They include weight, height, shoulder width, arm circumference, leg circumference, head circumference, etc. These measurements are useful in assessing nutritonal status and weight condition.
(Also see OBESITY.)

ANTI–

A prefix meaning against or opposing; e.g., antiscorbutic means preventing scurvy.

ANTIBIOTICS

Contents   Page

Antibiotics are chemical substances produced by living organisms which inhibit the growth of or kill other organisms.

As a group, antibiotics exhibit selective antimicrobial activity. Some are active against many gram-positive bacteria, others predominantly against gramnegatives, and a few, the *broad-spectrums,* are inhibitors of members of both groups. Others are antifungal only.

The search for effective and nontoxic antibiotics is unceasing. Since the discovery of penicillin in 1928, thousands of antibiotics have been isolated and studied. But relatively few are in active use. The following are among the better known and more widely used antibiotics: bacitracin, chlortetracycline (Aureomycin), erythromycin, neomycin, nisin, nystatin, oxytetracycline (Terramycin), penicillin, pimaricin, streptomycin, and tylosin.

MODE OF ACTION OF ANTIBIOTICS.

Numerous theories, each with convincing support, have been hypothesized with respect to the mode of action of antibiotics. No one theory has proven to be the total answer. Rather, the true mechanism is most likely the result of the additive effects from the various proposed mechanisms.

One fact is well substantiated. Antibiotics are effective in controlling certain environmental stresses, as evidenced by the fact that animals raised under germ-free conditions exhibit no improved responses to them.

The proven or probable modes of action of antibiotics follow:

1. They may spare certain nutrients. Studies have indicated that antibiotics can replace inadequate intakes of certain vitamins and amino acids.

2. They may selectively inhibit growth of nutrient-destroying organisms while promoting growth of nutrient-producing organisms.

3. They may increase food and/or water intake.

4. They may inhibit growth of organisms which produce toxic waste products or toxins.

5. They may kill or inhibit pathogenic organisms (a) in foods (when used as preservatives), (b) within the gastrointestinal tract, or (c) systemically. Each antibiotic has a distinct mode of disrupting cellular life.

6. They may improve the digestion and subsequent absorption of certain nutrients.

ANTIBIOTICS IN FOODS.

Antibiotics may occur in foods in the following three ways:

1. **Naturally.** Nisin, for example, is a naturally-occurring antibiotic, which is sometimes found in milk. Thus, it is noteworthy that gassy fermentations in raw cheese made with milk containing clostridia are controlled by the use of nisin-producing starter cultures.

2. **Through direct addition.** Antibiotics may occur in foods through direct addition as a food additive to aid in keeping quality of the food. Nisin, for example, is permitted as a direct food additive in many countries.

3. **As an unintentional food additive.** This can result from the carryover of the antibiotic in milk, meat, or eggs as a result of the addition of antibiotics to the feed of animals for growth promotion, or from animal medication for the prevention or treatment of animal diseases. In the case of all antibiotics used in animals, either a zero tolerance or a *negligible residue* in the products has been established. Also, in granting approval for the use of antibiotics in animal feeds and animal medication, the FDA establishes withdrawal periods—the required legal withdrawal period for the antibiotic between the time last received by the animal and the animal's slaughter or product use. Also, where antibiotics are used for intramammary application in mastitis control, the amount of antibiotic that may be used is limited per infusion and the milk must be discarded for a period of 48 to 96 hours following treatment, depending upon the excretion pattern of the antibiotic in the vehicle employed.

The direct addition of antibiotics to foods is not permitted in the United States. In the past, the limited use of tetracyclines (chlortetracyline and oxytetracycline) to extend the shelf life of poultry and fish was permitted. However, questions about development of antibiotic-resistant pathogenic and other microorganims in consumers who were repeatedly exposed to low concentrations of antibiotics led to withdrawal by the U.S. Food and Drug Administration of even this limited usage of these antibiotics as preservatives in poultry and fish.

But many countries favor the use of antibiotics as food preservatives. The FAO/WHO Expert Committee on Food Additives favors the use of nisin as a direct additive to foods.

SOME ANTIBIOTIC CONCERNS.

When properly used, antibiotics enhance human health; when improperly used, they may be a health hazard. Among the concerns are: (1) allergic reactions, (2) indirect additives, (3) vitamin K deficiency, (4) side effects, and (5) resistance to bacteria.

Allergic Reactions. About 10% of the population of the United States is sensitive to various drugs, with antibiotics heading the list. For this reason, the addition of antibiotics to foods must be carefully controlled; and only small amounts of antibiotics may be employed. It is noteworthy, however, that antibiotic residues in foods are destroyed in cooking.

Indirect Additives. Indirect antibiotic additives may be contained in foods derived from animals treated with or fed antibiotics. The use of antibiotics (1) for the prevention or treatment of diseases like mastitis in lactating cows or blackhead and coccidiosis in poultry, and (2) as growth promotants for animals, involves the risk that residues may be transmitted to foods (meat, milk, and eggs) derived from animal sources. For this reason, regulations for the use of drugs take into consideration the safety of residues of the drugs in food for man. Where relevant, withdrawal periods are required on meat animals prior to slaughter and on milk cows and poultry prior to the food use of milk and eggs, respectively.

Vitamin K Deficiency. The prolonged use of antibiotics may adversely affect the normal bacterial flora of the intestine, with the result that vitamin K deficiency occurs.

Side Effects. In some instances, antibiotics have produced such undesirable side effects as diarrhea, nausea, vomiting, abdominal cramps, and damage to the kidneys or other organs.

Resistance to Bacteria. There has been concern lest the indiscriminate use of antibiotics may lead to increased resistance of certain strains of bacteria which could ultimately render antibiotics ineffective for the treatment and control of diseases.

The controversy is centered around the ability of certain bacteria to develop resistance to antibiotics and to spread this resistance to other bacteria, a phenomenon known as *episome*. This well-documented ability involves what are termed resistance factors (RF). *An episome is an independent genetic element occurring in addition to the normal cell genetic makeup, which can be transmitted to other bacteria, and which can replicate either as an incorporated piece of the host's genome (chromosomal material) or as a separate unit within the bacteria.* This means that an episome can be fused with the chromosomal material of the host bacteria or can be a separate piece of genetic material in the cytoplasm.

Plasmids are episomes which never become part of the host chromosome; rather, they become a self-replicating unit. Plasmids are responsible for the synthesis of resistance transfer factors (RTF).

Resistance factors are transferred among bacteria via three mechanisms—transformation, transduction, and conjugation.

• **Transformation**—In transformation, the resistance to antibiotics is transferred and incorporated directly to the genome of the host organism. As shown in Fig. A-27, the re-

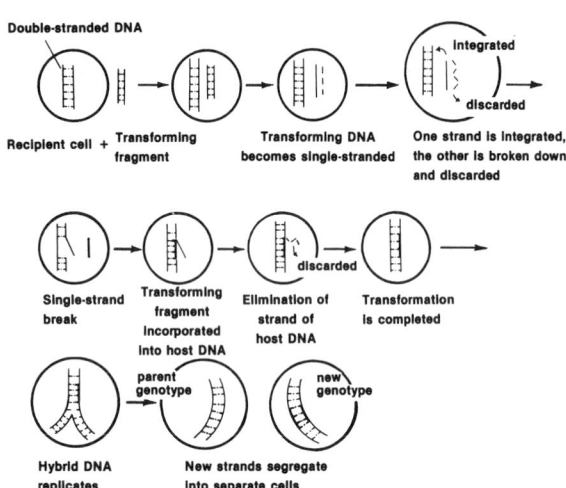

Fig. A-27. Transformation mechanism of genetic recombination.

cipient cell incorporates a piece of double stranded DNA which contains the genetic information resistance. Once inside the cell, the transforming DNA becomes single-stranded with the other strand being broken down and discarded. A break in the host's chromosome then occurs and the transforming fragment then replaces a piece of the host's DNA, thereby producing a hybrid organism. When the cell replicates and divides, one daughter cell has the parent genotype and the other has the newly formed genotype.

• **Transduction**—Transduction, as illustrated in Fig. A-28,

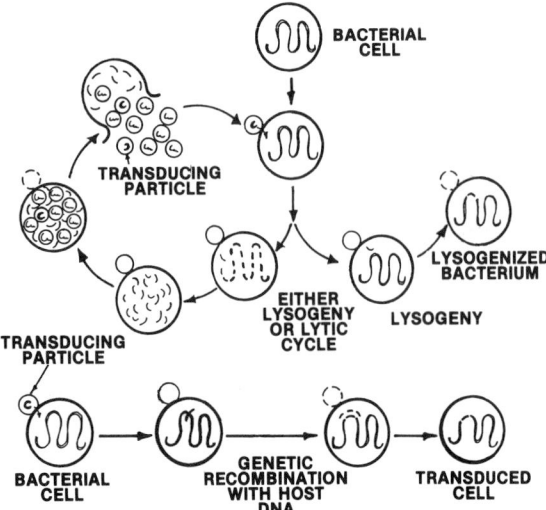

Fig. A-28. Mechanism of transduction.

involves the formation of transducing particles in the donor cell. When the cell lyses (breaks open), these particles are released and eventually come into contact with other bacteria, whereupon the material inside the particle can either be incorporated into the chromosomes of the host bacteria or stimulate lyses of the newly involved cell.

• **Conjugation**—Conjugation (Fig. A-29) can be described as being similar to the act of mating in higher animals. An extension, referred to as a pilus (plural, pili) joins the donor bacteria to the recipient. Genetic material is then passed from the donor to the recipient. Resistance transfer factors are transferred by this mechanism.

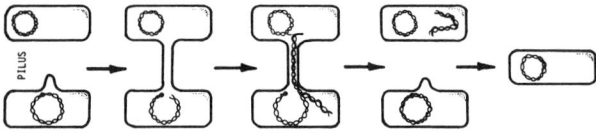

Fig. A-29. Conjugation of bacteria.

FUTURE OF ANTIBIOTICS.   Today, more and more antibiotics are less and less effective in the treatment of infections, due to more resistant bacteria. When first used, penicillin was nearly 100% effective against the most prevalent *Staphylococci aureus* that spread hospital-related infection among patients; presently, the drug is far less effective. Both tetracycline and penicillin, once used to cure gonorrhea, now have a failure rate of more than 20% against certain strains. A growing body of evidence indicates that the overuse of antibiotics is helping to make the miracle drugs less effective in treating infections, and that there may come a time when many infections are resistant to all known antibiotics. Before such a disaster strikes, some groups urge setting international standards for prescription, distribution, and advertising.

Also, pressure from consumer groups and many medical people may result in banning many of the antibiotics that are primarily used for medicinal purposes in humans from the list of approved production promoters for animals. However, in the future, an increasing number of antibiotics will likely be developed specifically for the purpose of improving livestock performance. One example is that of bambermycins. This antibiotic was developed solely for use as a production promoter, serving to increase rate of gain and feed efficiency in chickens and swine; it has no medical application. Bambermycins has no toxic effect; does not result in tissue residue—so, no withdrawal period is required; and has a molecular structure completely different from other antibiotics—hence, no cross-resistance to other antibiotics has been found. Strains of bacteria resistant to bambermycins are susceptible to other antibiotics.

ANTIBODIES

Special proteins produced by the body as a defense against invasion by foreign substances called antigens—which may be (1) components of certain drugs or food; (2) infectious microorganisms or parasites; (3) substances from the environment, such as chemicals, dusts, pollen grains, etc; or (4) tissues of the body itself. Normally, antibodies react with antigens and render them harmless. However, certain antibodies may attack body tissue. This abnormal condition is called autoimmunity. Generally, repeated exposure to a specific type of antigen increases the rate at which antibodies against the substance are produced. Antibody production may be impaired under such conditions as (1) advanced aging; (2) inherited inability to produce certain antibodies; (3) oversecretion of stress hormones; or (4) malnutrition.

(Also see ALLERGEN; ALLERGIES; ANTIGEN; AUTO-IMMUNITY; DISEASES; and MALNUTRITION.)

ANTICOAGULANT

A substance that interferes with one or more of the processes in the blood clotting mechanism. Such agents may be useful in preventing the formation of unwanted clots, and in the breaking up of such clots once they have formed.

(Also see BLOOD; and VITAMIN K.)

ANTIDIURETIC HORMONE (ADH)

A hormone secreted by the pituitary gland. It acts to reduce the excretion of water in the urine so that the supply of body water is conserved.

(Also see ENDOCRINE GLANDS.)

ANTIDOTE

A substance that counteracts another substance which is poisonous. Sometimes the antidote is as toxic as the poison it counteracts, but the two agents may counteract each other. For example, selenium in tuna fish greatly reduces the toxicity of any mercury which may be present in the fish.

ANTIFOAMING AGENTS (DEFOAMING AGENTS)

These substances suppress or inhibit the formation of foam in systems where it may interfere with processing. Foaming occurs due to the presence of proteins, gases, or nitrogenous materials. Examples of antifoaming agents include octanol, sulfonated oils, organic phosphates, or silicone fluids.

ANTIGEN

Any substance capable of stimulating the production of antibodies against itself. The most common antigens are animal danders, chemicals, dusts, foods, microorganisms, and pollens. Tissue or proteins from the body itself, which are normally enclosed within cells or other structures, may become antigens if they escape into the blood as a result of disease or injury.

(Also see ANTIBODIES.)

ANTI-GRAY HAIR VITAMIN

This designation was once given to pantothenic acid, one of the members of the vitamin B complex. In 1940, when pantothenic acid was first synthesized, it received widespread attention as a possible preventive for gray hair, since it had been observed that the black hair of a rat would turn gray when the animal was deprived of the vitamin, but subsequent studies did not reveal any such benefits to accrue to humans.

(Also see PANTOTHENIC ACID.)

ANTIHEMORRHAGIC

Preventing hemorrhage. A term often applied to vitamin K.

(Also see VITAMIN K.)

ANTIHISTAMINES

Any of various compounds used to treat certain allergic reactions in the body.

ANTIKETOGENESIS

The prevention of ketosis by similating the tricarboxylic acid cycle and thereby bringing about oxidation of the ketone bodies. Fatty acids and ketogenic amino acids are precursors of ketone bodies. The antiketogenic factors are precursors of glucose; these include the carbohydrates, glucogenic amino acids, and the glycerol portion of fat.

ANTIMETABOLITE

A substance bearing a close structural resemblance to one required for normal physiological functioning, which exerts its effect by replacing or interfering with the utilization of the essential metabolite.

ANTIMYCOTICS

Substances that are added to foods to inhibit mold growth, such as sodium and calcium propionate, methyl hydroxy-benzoate, quaternary ammonium chloride, sodium benzo-ate, and sorbic acid.

ANTINEURITIC

A substance used for preventing or treating neuritis.

ANTIOXIDANT

A substance which prevents the reaction of various food constituents with oxygen. This protective effect is desirable because many substances become discolored or spoil when oxidation takes place. A wide variety of synthetic antioxidants is now available. Some of the better known natural antioxidants are vitamins C and E, and the bioflavonoids.

ANTISIALAGOGUES

Substances that stop the flow of saliva.

ANTISTALING AGENTS

These agents slow or prevent the loss of softness, flavor, and consistency of baking products.

(Also see STALING.)

ANTITOXIN

A substance produced within the body which has the power to neutralize a toxin. Sometimes antitoxins produced by cattle, horses, or rabbits are injected into man to combat fast-acting, potent toxins.

(Also see DISEASES, section on "Vaccination.")

ANTIVITAMIN

A substance which interferes with the action of a vitamin.

(Also see VITAMIN[S], Section on "Factors Influencing the Utilization of Vitamins.")

ANURIA

Lack of, or defective, excretion of urine.

ANUS

The opening at the posterior end of the digestive tract.

(Also see DIGESTION AND ABSORPTION.)

AORTA

The major blood vessel which carries blood away from the heart and down to the lower parts of the body. There are various branches from the aorta which connect with the arteries that carry blood to the arms and to the head.

APASTIA

Refusal to take food.
(Also see ANOREXIA NERVOSA.)

APATHY

Indifference; lack of interest or concern. A type of behavior sometimes found in a deficiency disease.

APHAGOSIS

The inability to consume food.

APHRODISIACS

Substances or foods used to promote sexual desire. Through the years, the following foods have been consumed for this purpose: anise, artichokes, avocados, beans, caraway seed, carrots, chocolate, clams, cloves, cola drinks, fish, garlic, honey, hot sauces, various mushrooms and cheeses, mutton, nutmeg, olives, oysters, peas, peppermint, pistachio nuts, radishes, saffron, shellfish, thyme, tomatoes, vanilla, along with such exotic items as hyena eyes, eel's eggs, bird's nest soup, shark fin soup, and truffles. However, there is no scientific evidence that any food item possesses such powers.

APOENZYME

The protein part of an enzyme to which the prosthetic group or coenzyme is attached. The coenzyme may be a vitamin.

APOFERRITIN

The protein base in intestinal mucosa cells, which binds with iron (from food) to form ferritin, the storage form of iron.
(Also see IRON, section headed "Absorption, Metabolism, Excretion".)

APOLLINARIS WATER

A highly aerated alkaline water, containing sodium chloride and calcium, sodium, and magnesium carbonates. It is obtained from a spring in the valley of the Ahr (Prussia).

APOPLEXY

Another name for a stroke, which may be either a hemorrhage in the brain (cerebral hemorrhage) or a blockage of the flow of blood to the brain (cerebral infarct). In either case, the effect is that certain vital parts of the brain are deprived of a supply of blood.
(Also see CEREBRAL HEMORRHAGE; CEREBRAL INFARCT; and HIGH BLOOD PRESSURE.)

APOSIA

Absence of the sensation of thirst.

APOSITIA

Lack of desire for food.

APPENDICITIS

An inflammation of the appendix, which is often accompanied by (1) pain in the lower right side of the abdomen, (2) a low fever, (3) an elevated white blood cell count, (4) nausea, and (5) tightening of the muscles of the abdominal wall. Appendicitis almost always requires prompt surgery, because the appendix may rupture and the lining of the abdominal cavity become inflamed, producing the condition called peritonitis. The latter condition is very dangerous because it may result in shock, systemic poisoning, and other complications.

It is risky to administer a laxative or an enema to a person who complains of abdominal pain suggestive of appendicitis because these treatments may cause an inflamed appendix to rupture. However, such pain may also be due to constipation, ileitis or ileocolitis, infection of the kidneys, inflamed pouches on the wall of the colon (the condition called diverticulitis), or certain pelvic disorders in women.

(Also see APPENDIX; COLITIS; DIGESTION AND ABSORPTION; and ILEITIS.)

APPENDIX

A narrow, wormlike tube of tissue, closed at one end, with its open end attached to the cecum. Fig. A-30 shows the location of the appendix.
(Also see APPENDICITIS.)

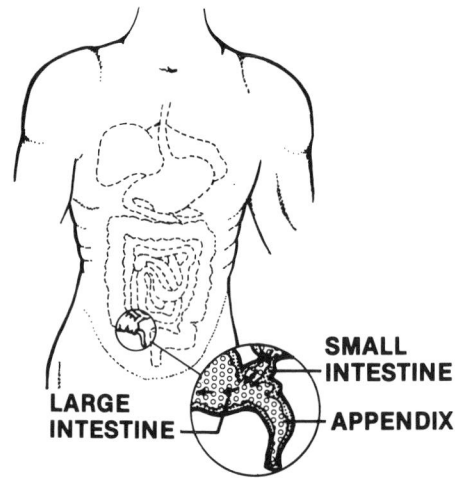

Fig. A-30. The appendix, a nonfunctional tissue which may be very troublesome if it becomes inflamed and appendicitis results.

APPESTAT

A nerve center in the hypothalamus (a small structure at the base of the brain) believed to regulate appetite.
(Also see DIGESTION AND ABSORPTION, section headed "Hunger and Appetite.")

APPETITE

This is the desire for food. A good appetite, which is a sign of good health, is characterized by eating with relish.

A distinction needs to be made between appetite and hunger. Hunger is a physiological desire for food following a period of fasting. Hunger pangs result from contractions of an empty stomach and are rarely felt by anyone who regularly eats adequate amounts of food (especially protein). Appetite, on the other hand, is a learned or habitual response, which arises with the customary intervals of eating and may be influenced by numerous external and internal phenomena. It can become excessive or subject to distorted impulses.

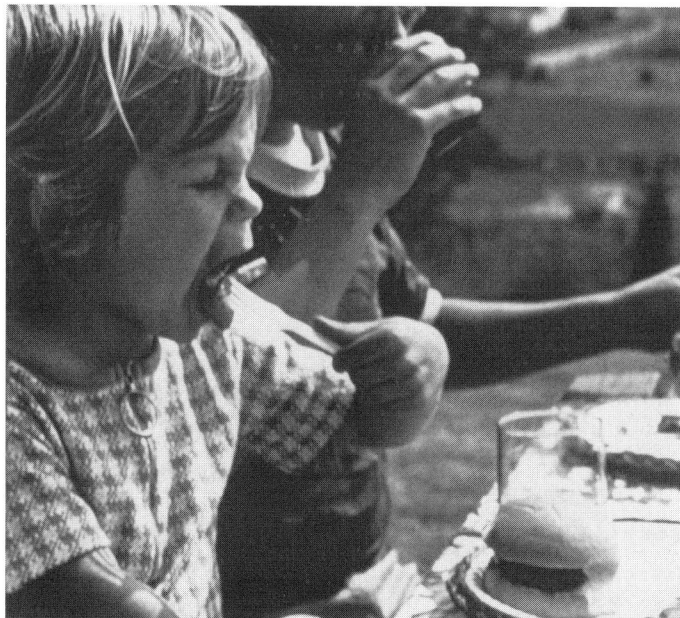

Fig. A-31. Children often eat too much or too little. If the condition persists, parents should consult a doctor. (Courtesy, New Mexico State University, Las Cruces, N.M.)

• **Hypothalamic control of appetite**—The hypothalamus (derived from the terms *hypo* meaning below, and *thalamus*, a region of the brain)—a structure in the ventral region of the diencephalon—has been implicated as one of the major control centers of appetite regulation.

(Also see DIGESTION AND ABSORPTION, section on "Hunger and Appetite.")

• **Gastric influences on appetite regulation**—When the gastrointestinal tract is distended, there is normally a cessation of eating. Thus, the actual physical limit of the digestive system has a direct influence on appetite. If a person eats a bulky salad, he may become satiated, even though it does not fulfill his energy requirements.

• **Sociological and psychological factors affecting appetite**—Appetite is affected by such sociological factors as habits, family customs, education, cultural background, environment, and social customs; and by such psychological factors as emotional need, stress, and anxiety.

It is known that the amount of physical activity indirectly influences the appetite. Likewise, it is believed that idleness and boredom stimulate the appetite and produce snacking as a means of breaking the monotony.

It is believed that psychological attitudes can either promote or suppress appetite. Various associations with past pleasures of food consumption and the desirable appearance, odor, and flavor of foods are known to stimulate the appetite. Children are apt to develop cravings for food without realizing the cause. Eating may be a form of compensation for a major loss or disappointment; or a means of securing attention from adults who otherwise might not notice them.

• **Physiological factors**—Various physiological factors, such as mild thiamin deficiency, illness, and infection have been associated with anorexia, or loss of appetite. Occasionally people suffering from specific disorders, such as diabetes, gastric ulcers, or chronic gastritis, develop an appetite out of proportion to their needs. In pregnancy or hysteria, unusual and specialized cravings may develop for particular kinds of food, or even for injurious substances.

Persons with duodenal ulcer seem to have a special form of appetite. Their pain is apt to rise and fall with the stomach's desire for food and content of hydrochloric acid. In such cases, eating tends to relieve the pain, at least temporarily.

Diminution or loss of appetite accompanies many disordered conditions. It is usually one of the symptoms of tuberculosis and anemia. Also, loss of appetite and refusal to eat anything characterizes *anorexia nervosa*, a disease ordinarily related to some form of emotional instability and observed more frequently in women than in men.

The loss of sensitivity to flavors and odors, which often accompanies aging, appears to be related to a concommitant reduction in appetite.

• **Drugs, alcohol, tobacco, and empty calories**—Appetite can be artificially decreased by taking such drugs as Benzedrine and Dexedrine. These drugs are sometimes prescribed for weight reduction, but they should be taken only on the advice of a doctor.

Small amounts of an alcoholic drink will increase appetite. On the other hand, overconsumption of alcohol usually results in loss of appetite. Excessive use of tobacco appears to reduce the appetite; for this reason, addicted smokers often gain weight when they break the habit.

The consumption of empty calories, such as candy and soft drinks, inhibits the appetite.

APPETIZER

A substance that stimulates the appetite.

APPLE *Malus pumila*

The apple, which belongs to the rose family, *Rosaceae*, is a pome—a fruit consisting of firm, juicy, flesh surrounding a core that contains several seeds. It is a close relative of the pear and the quince. With about 7,500 varieties grown worldwide and 2,500 varieties in the United States, size, sweetness, aroma, and crispness vary greatly from one variety to another, as does the color which ranges from shades of red to yellow or green.

Apple trees grow everywhere except in the very coldest and the very hottest climates of the world. They do not thrive in the tropics because they need a period of cold and dormancy to grow properly. Apple trees are a medium-sized

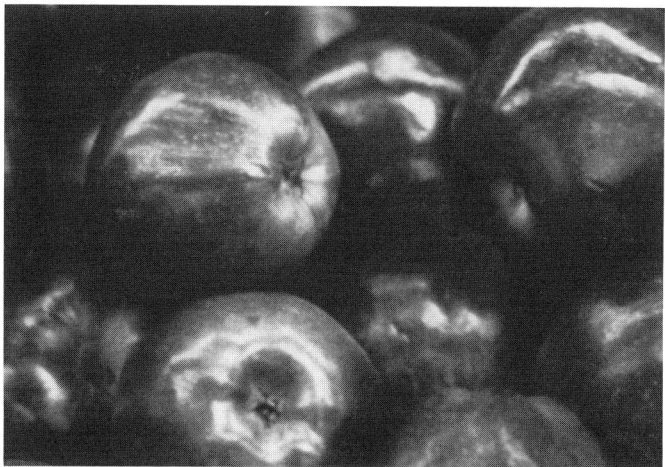

Fig. A-32. Apple—the king of the fruits. (Courtesy, USDA)

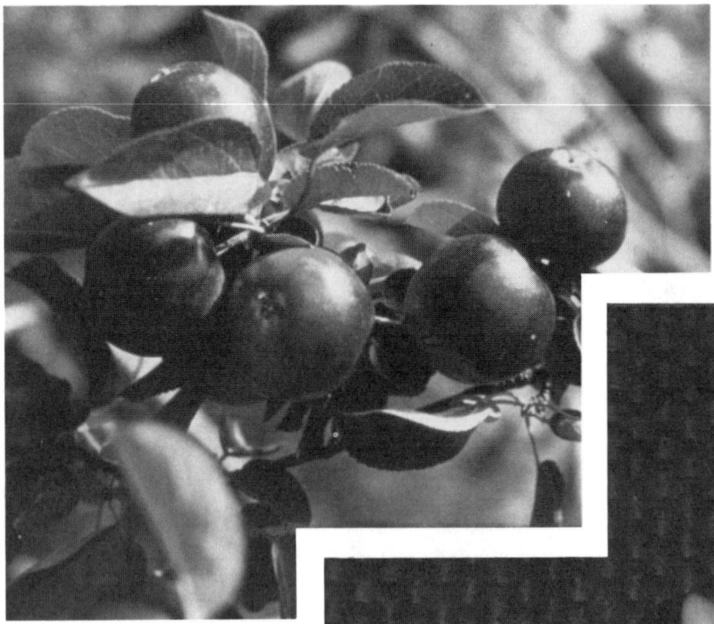

Fig. A-33. McIntosh Apples. (Courtesy, National Film Board of Canada)

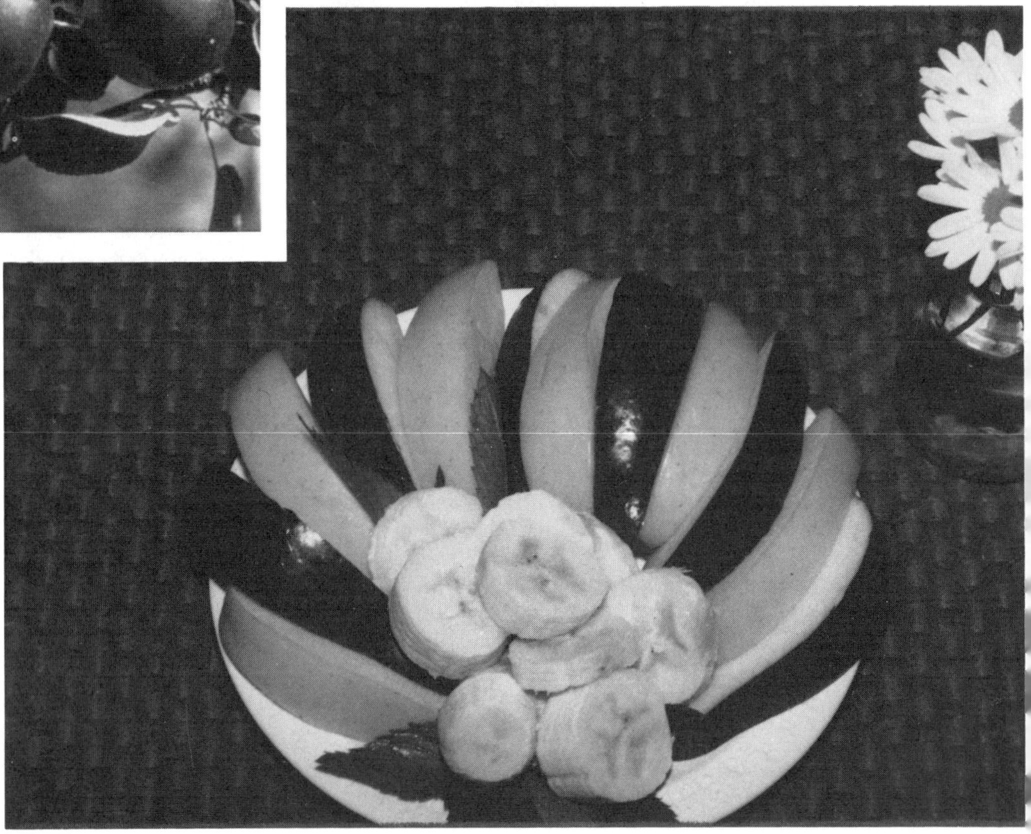

Fig. A-34. Apples are a great snack food. (Courtesy, North Dakota State Cooperative Extension Service)

tree, with unpruned trees on good soil reaching a height of 30 to 40 ft (9.2 to 12.2 m). Their trunks may be 2 ft (0.6 m) or more in diameter. Branches of the apple tree are twisted and spreading, and the tree is about as broad as it is high.

The leading variety of apple in the United States is the Delicious, which originated from a mutation on a farm in Peru, Iowa about 1881.

ORIGIN AND HISTORY. The apple is native to western Asia and/or eastern Europe. Apples were grown by the Greeks as early as the 4th century B.C.

Mention of the apple in mythology suggests man's long relationship with it; in Greek mythology, Hercules traveled to the end of the world to bring back the golden apples of the Hesperides.

Supposedly, the Romans took apples with them when they conquered England, and apple growing became popular in England and other parts of Europe thereafter.

During the 1620s, the colonists introduced the apple to North America.

WORLD AND U.S. PRODUCTION. Apples are the third leading fruit crop of the world, and the third ranking fruit crop of the United States.

Worldwide, about 40 million metric tons of apples are produced annually; and the leading apple-producing countries are: U.S.S.R., China, United States, Germany, France, and Italy.[10]

In the United States, about 4.8 million short tons of apples are produced annually; and the leading states, by rank, are: Washington, New York, California, Michigan, Pennsylvania, North Carolina, and Virginia. Washington alone produces 49.5% of the U.S. apple crop.[11]

PROCESSING. More than half (55%) of the apples in

[10]Based on data from *FAO Production Yearbook 1990*, FAO/UN, Rome, Italy, Vol. 44, pp. 160-161, Table 69. **Note well:** Annual production fluctuates as a result of weather and profitability of the crop.

[11]Based on data from *Agricultural Statistics 1991*, USDA, p. 178, Table 255. **Note well:** Annual production fluctuates as a result of weather and profitability of the crop.

the United States are marketed on a fresh basis. The remaining 45% is processed as canned, dried, or frozen apples, or as vinegar, cider, and juice. Only 16% is canned; 3% is dried; and 2% is frozen. Twenty-three percent is crushed and used to make vinegar, cider, and apple juice.

Apples are canned, sliced or cubed, as pie filling or as applesauce. Slices are usually packed without syrup. However, applesauce is the most important canned apple product.

Dried apples are trimmed, peeled, cored and sliced, and sulfured prior to drying. They are generally cut in rings or quarters, and they are dried to 25 to 33% moisture. Some apples are dehydrated to 2 to 3% moisture.

Frozen apples are sliced and packed with dry sugar or in a sugar syrup. The major problem with frozen apples is the prevention of enzymatic browning during storage and especially after thawing.

• **Apple juice and cider**—These products are gaining in popularity. Apple juice refers to the product preserved by heat (pasteurization) and packed in hermetically sealed containers. Cider is the unfermented fresh juice from apples. Originally fresh cider was sold at roadside markets, but now it can be purchased in supermarkets. Fresh cider rapidly spoils without the addition of some chemical preservative such as potassium sorbate, or exposure to ultraviolet radiation, though refrigeration slows spoilage extending the storage life of fresh cider to 1 or 2 weeks.

Other products from apples include cider vinegar, jelly, and apple butter. In Europe, much of the apple crop pressed for cider is fermented to make brandy or wine.

(Also see PRESERVATION OF FOOD; and VINEGAR.)

SELECTION, PREPARATION, AND USES. The many varieties of apples differ widely in appearance, flesh characteristics, seasonal availability, and suitability for different uses. For good eating as fresh fruit, the commonly available varieties are: Delicious, McIntosh, Stayman, Golden Delicious, Jonathan, and Winesap. Tart or slightly acid varieties such as Gravenstein, Grimes Golden, Jonathan, and Newton make good pies and applesauce. For baking, the firmer-fleshed varieties—Rome Beauty, Northern Spy, Rhode Island Greening, Winesap, and York Imperial—are widely used.

Fresh apples should be firm, crisp, and well-colored. Flavor varies in apples and depends on the stage of maturity at the time the fruit is picked. Apples must be mature when picked to have a good flavor, texture, and storing ability.

Most apples are marketed by grade, and many consumer packages show the variety, the grade, and the size. U.S. grades for apples are U.S. Extra Fancy, U.S. Fancy, U.S. No. 1, and combinations of these grades. U.S. No. 2 is a less desirable grade. Apples from the far western states are usually marketed under state grades which are similar to federal grades. The qualities of color, maturity and lack of defects—appearance in general—determine the grade.

After washing, apples may be served fresh without further preparation; or they may be baked, stewed, dipped in batter and fried (apple fritters).

Apples may be used as fresh fruit dishes, desserts, jams, jellies, juices, pies, salads, or syrups; and in the production of alcoholic beverages and vinegar.

NUTRITIONAL VALUE. Fresh apples contain 85% water. Each 100 g (about 3½ oz) contains about 60 Calories (kcal) of energy. One average apple weighs about 150 g. Calories in the fresh apple are derived from the naturally-

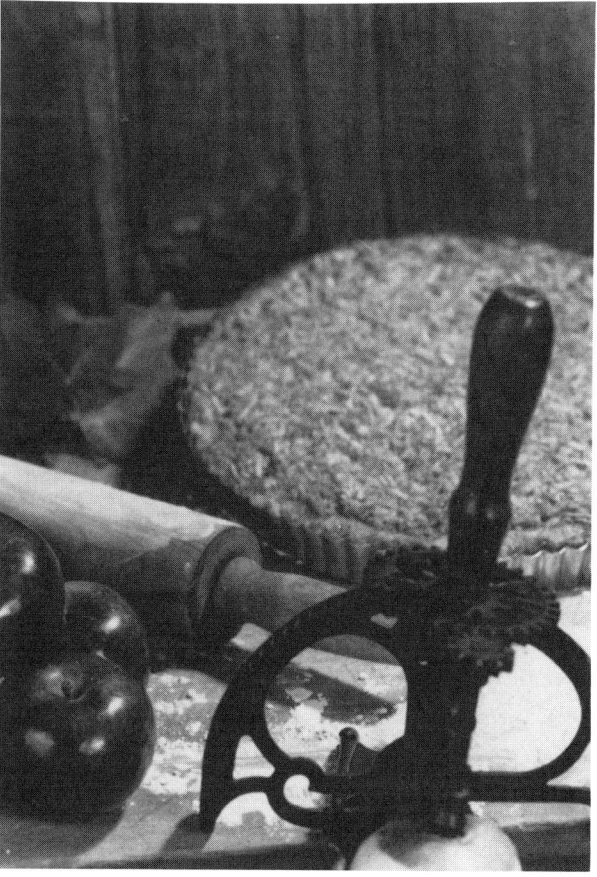

Fig. A-35. An old fashioned apple tart makes good use of the fruits of autumn. (Courtesy, Agriculture Canada, Ottawa, Canada)

occuring sugars (carbohydrate) which give the apple its sweet taste. Their taste is also due to small amounts of organic acids. Overall, apples possess minor amounts of the minerals and vitamins. Dried apples contain only 33% water; hence, concentrating the nutrients, including calories. Each 100 g of dried apples contains 239 Calories (kcal) of energy, 3 g of fiber, 405 mg of potassium, and 1.7 mg of iron. More complete information regarding the nutritional value of fresh, baked, canned, and dried apples, apple juice, cider, and applesauce is presented in Food Composition Table F-21.

APPLE BUTTER

A spread for bread which is made by the prolonged cooking of a mixture of apple pulp and sugar until it turns to a dark brown color and has a caramel flavor. The rural people of Colonial America sometimes added apple cider, orange peels, and quinces to their apple butter. About 2½ lb (*1.1 kg*) of cored, peeled apples (which is equivalent to 3 lb [*1.35 kg*] of fresh apples) are required to make 1 lb (*0.45 kg*) of apple butter.

The nutrient composition of apple butter is given in Food Composition Table F-21.

(Also see APPLE.)

APPLE CIDER

In the United States, this term usually refers to freshly prepared apple juice that is bottled without pasteurization. Products labeled *apple juice* have usually been pasteurized during bottling. Sometimes, pasteurized apple juice is marketed as cider during the fall, when the demand for cider is great. Unpasteurized cider will ferment within a few days unless preservatives such as sodium benzoate or potassium sorbate are added to it. In Europe, cider means fermented apple juice, whereas Americans call fermented cider hard cider.

It is noteworthy that 100 lb (*45 kg*) of apples yield 65 to 70 lb (*31 kg*) of apple cider or apple juice.

The residue of apple pulp which remains after the juice has been extracted is called pomace and is used as (1) a material for the production of pectin, and (2) an animal feed.

Hard cider contains less alcohol (the content ranges from 0.5 to 8.0%) than wine. It may be plain or sparkling (sparkling cider is made by allowing some fermentation to take place after bottling).

The nutrient composition of unfermented apple cider is given in Food Composition Table F-21.

(Also see APPLE.)

APPLE, DRIED

Pieces of apple (usually slices from peeled and cored fruit) which have been dried by artificial means to a moisture content of 24% or less. Discoloration during drying is prevented by treating the pieces with sulfur dioxide. Compared to fresh apples, dried pieces of apple contain about 5 times the level of calories, carbohydrates, and potassium. About 5 lb (*2.3 kg*) of peeled, cored apples (equivalent to between 5½ and 6 lb of fresh apples) are required to make 1 lb (*0.45 kg*) of dried apple pieces. Certain other dried apple products may contain added sugar or syrup.

The nutrient compositions of various forms of dried apples are given in Food Composition Table F-21.

(Also see APPLE.)

APPLE JACK (APPLE BRANDY)

This is the American term for apple brandy. It is called *Calvados* in Europe. This brandy, which contains from 55 to 65% alcohol by volume, is produced by distilling fermented apple cider. Most of the world's supply of apple brandy comes from France, where the annual rate of production is usually several times that of the United States.

(Also see DISTILLED LIQUORS.)

APRICOT *Prunus armeniaca*

The apricot, which belongs to the rose family, *Rosaceae*, is classified as a drupe—a fleshy, one-seeded fruit not splitting open by itself and containing a seed enclosed in a stony endocarp. As the genus name suggests, the apricot is a close relative of the almond, cherry, peach, and plum. Ripe apricots are orange or yellow, round, and about 1¼ to 2 in. (*3 to 5 cm*) in diameter. Their skin is smoother than that of a peach and their edible flesh is sweet, but dry compared to other fruits.

ORIGIN AND HISTORY. The apricot originated in eastern Asia (China). From there, it spread to Europe, thence to North America.

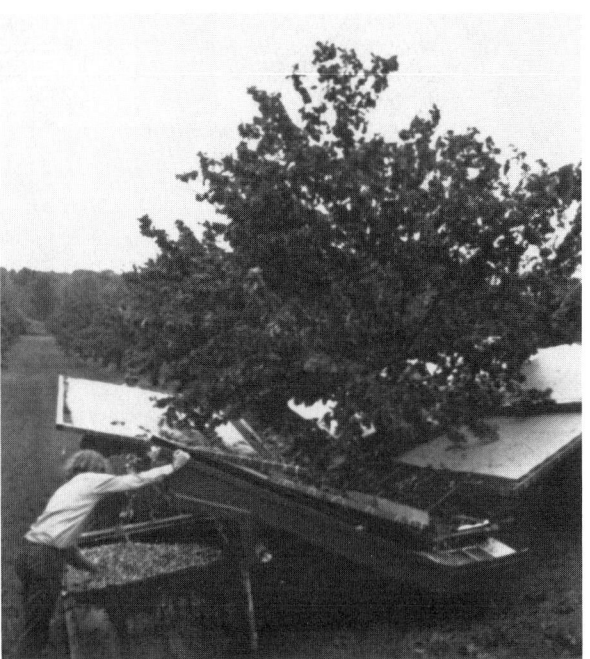

Fig. A-36. Harvesting equipment aids large apricot producers. (Courtesy, USDA)

WORLD AND U.S. PRODUCTION. Worldwide, about 2.1 million metric tons of apricots are produced annually; and the leading apricot-producing countries, by rank, are: Turkey, Italy, U.S.S.R., Spain, and Greece.[12]

The United States produces about 122.5 short tons of apricots annually; and the leading states, by rank, are: California, Utah, and Washington, with California alone accounting for 94% of the crop.[13]

PROCESSING. Apricots are marketed as fresh, canned, dried, or frozen fruit. Utilization of the apricot crop in the United States is as follows: 8% fresh, 58% canned, 26% dried, and 7% frozen.

SELECTION, PREPARATION, AND USES. Apricots should be plump and juicy in appearance, with a uniform, golden-orange color. The fruit develops its flavor and natural sweetness on the tree. It should be mature—but firm—at the time of picking.

Apricots can be eaten fresh out of the hand or prepared in fresh fruit dishes. Canned apricots are eaten as a dessert dish or also used to add a piquant flavor to sauces, salads, or baked goods. Both fresh and dried apricots are cooked to make jam, pies, and puddings. Dried apricots are also a good snack. Frozen apricots are used in confections and baked goods. Also, apricots may be used to produce alchoholic beverages.

---

[12]Based on data from *FAO Production Yearbook 1990*, FAO/UN, Rome, Italy, Vol. 44, pp. 165-166, Table 72. **Note well:** Annual production fluctuates as a result of weather and profitability of the crop.

[13]Based on data from *Agricultural Statistics 1991*, USDA, p. 183, Table 266. **Note well:** Annual production fluctuates as a result of weather and profitability of the crop.

NUTRITIONAL VALUE. Fresh apricots contain 85% water. Additionally, each 100 g (about 3½ oz) provides 51 Calories (kcal) of energy, 319 mg potassium, 2,700 IU of vitamin A, and only 1 mg of sodium. The calories in apricots are derived primarily from sugars (carbohydrate) which give them their sweet taste. When canned in syrup, apricots contain more calories due to the addition of sugar. Dried apricots contain only 32% water; hence, many of the nutrients are more concentrated, including the calories. In dried form, they contain 236 Calories (kcal), 1,422 mg potassium, 4.8 mg of iron, and 7,147 IU of vitamin A in each 100 g. Frozen apricots are similar to fresh, with slightly more calories due to the sugar added before freezing. More complete information regarding the nutritional value of fresh, canned, dried and frozen apricots is presented in Food Composition Table F-21.

APRICOT LEATHER

A chewy sheet of dried apricot pulp that is made by: (1) deskinning and pureeing the fruit, (2) adding a little sweetening and spices, (3) boiling the mixture for about 3 minutes, and (4) drying the puree on a sheet of plastic wrap in a drying tray. The leather makes a nutritious, easily carried, nonperishable snack for between meals, and for camping and hiking trips.
(Also see APRICOT.)

AQUEOUS EMULSION

A stable mixture of two or more immiscible liquids held in suspension by an emulsifier is called an emulsion. An oil and water emulsion is known as an aqueous emulsion, e.g., milk.

ARABINOSE

A five-carbon sugar found mainly in certain root vegetables. It has no known function in man.
(Also see CARBOHYDRATE[S].)

ARACHIDONIC ACID

A 20-carbon unsaturated fatty acid with four double bonds, which occurs in most animal fats and is considered essential in the nutrition of man.
(Also see FATS AND OTHER LIPIDS.)

ARACHIS OIL

Arachis is the genus name for peanut; hence, arachis oil is sometimes used to designate peanut oil.
(Also see PEANUT.)

ARBUTUS BERRY (STRAWBERRY TREE)
Arbutus unedo

The fruit of an ornamental shrub of the family *Ericaceae* which grows in North America, Mexico, Europe, and Africa.
Although the berries are not very palatable when fresh, they may be made into confections, distilled liquors, liqueurs, and wine. The alcoholic beverages are produced in Algeria, France, Italy, and Spain.

ARGINASE

An enzyme present in most animal cells, which splits arginine to urea and ornithine, the last state of urea synthesis from the amino groups of the amino acids. A deficiency of arginase produces elevated arginine levels in the blood and an accumulation of ammonia in the body, which may result in spastic diplegia (Little's disease), epileptic seizures, and severe mental retardation.

ARGININE

An amino acid which participates in the formation of the waste product urea and the muscle constituent creatine. In certain species such as chickens, pigs, and rats, arginine appears to be essential for growth. It is noteworthy that this amino acid is a potent stimulator for the secretion of growth hormones.
(Also see AMINO ACID[S].)

ARIBOFLAVINOSIS

The term given to a set of symptoms produced by a deficiency of riboflavin (vitamin B-2) or by the presence of a factor which interferes with the absorption and utilization of riboflavin over a period of several months. Ariboflavinosis is characterized by swollen, cracked, bright red lips (cheilosis); enlarged, tender, purplish or bright red tongue (glossitis); cracking at the corners of the mouth (angular stomatitis); congestion of the blood vessels of the conjunctiva; flaking and irritation of the skin in the folds around the nose and in the groin area (seborrheic dermatitis); and ocular disorders, such as vascularization of the cornea, irritation and sensitivity of the eyes, inflammation of the eyelids, watering and mattering of the eyes, abnormal pigmentation of the iris and intense photobia. But, since none of these symptoms are unique to ariboflavinosis, diagnosis is quite difficult. In general, however, ariboflavinosis is associated with lower plasma and urinary riboflavin levels. Less than 14 mcg of riboflavin per 100 ml of plasma and/or less than 200 mcg of riboflavin per gram of creatinine in the urine are indicative of a deficiency condition.

Deficiency symptoms often occur during periods of physiological stress, such as pregnancy, lactation, and rapid growth. Also, ariboflavinosis is often associated with such diseases as pellagra, rheumatic fever, tuberculosis, subacute bacterial enteritis, chronic congestive heart failure, hyperthyroidism, malignancy, chronic fever conditions, and cirrhosis of the liver. Abnormalities of riboflavin metabolism result from all types of severe injuries; and degradation of riboflavin coenzymes appear to be related to shock. Surgical removal of sections of the gastrointestinal tract and chronic diarrhea have both produced malabsorption of riboflavin, followed by ariboflavinosis.

Ariboflavinosis is best prevented dietarily by an adequate diet containing riboflavin rich foods, such as milk, liver, meat, eggs, and certain green leafy and yellow vegetables. Milk is the best common source of riboflavin; one quart will more than fulfill the daily riboflavin requirement. Seeds and whole-grain cereals are not good sources of riboflavin, unless they are enriched and fortified. Enrichment of these products has done a great deal in preventing ariboflavinosis in the United States.

Ariboflavinosis is treated with an adequate diet and administration of 5 mg of riboflavin 3 to 4 times daily. The riboflavin supplement is usually administered orally. However, it is sometimes given intramuscularly, particularly when problems of absorption exist.
(Also see RIBOFLAVIN.)

ARRHYTHMIA

A nonrhythmic, irregular beating of the heart which is sometimes an early warning of a heart attack. However, some people have a slightly nonrhythmic heartbeat for most of their lives. When an arrhythmia causes a serious disturbance of the heart rhythm, the heart is generally inefficient in pumping blood.

(Also see HEART DISEASE.)

ARROWROOT

There are two sources of arrowroot:

1. *C. angustifolia* is found in the Himalayan region and has long been used by the natives of India. It has a slight yellow color, but it is a good substitute for the West Indian arrowroot.

2. *Maranta arundinacea* is grown in South America, the West Indies, Mexico and Florida. The American Indians used it to heal wounds made by poisoned arrows, which probably accounts for its name.

The starch made from the root is used in foods prepared for children and invalids. Other similar starches which can be substituted for arrowroot are obtained from several other plants of the same genus, *Maranta*, or other genera such as *Zamia*, *Curcuma*, *Tacca*, *Canna*, and *Musa*.

(Also see FLOURS, Table F-13 Special Flours.)

ARTERIOLE

A blood vessel which delivers blood from an artery to the capillaries. Arterioles are smaller in diameter than the arteries, yet bigger than the capillaries.

ARTERIOSCLEROSIS

A hardening and thickening of the normally elastic walls of arteries so that they no longer respond readily to changes in the blood pressure. Often, there are calcium deposits in the walls of the arteries which make them brittle. Arteriosclerosis is often accompanied by atherosclerosis.

(Also see HEART DISEASE.)

ARTERY

A large blood vessel carrying blood from the heart to various parts of the body.

ARTHRITIS

Arthritis is an inflammation of the joints of the body. The term refers to all the conditions that cause stiffness, swelling, soreness, or pain in the joints.

Arthritis is among the oldest diseases known to affect human beings. Evidence of its occurrence has been found in the mummies and excavations of ancient civilizations. Also, Hippocrates (460-377 B.C.), the Greek physician, called the Father of Medicine, described arthritis graphically.

Arthritis is a dreaded and feared crippling disease. The Arthritis Foundation estimates that more than 13 million Americans are afflicted by some form of this condition, and that a quarter of a million more become victims of this disease every year. The human suffering from arthritis is awesome; and the cost in dollars is almost impossible to comprehend. Figures show that arthritis sufferers lose an estimated 115 million days a year from work, which is equivalent to 470,000 persons on sick leave for an entire year. This is more days lost from work than is caused by any other malady except nervous and mental diseases.

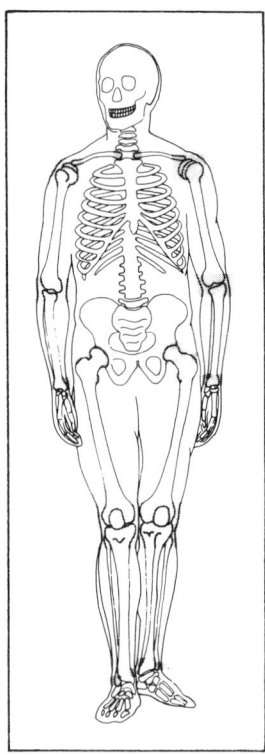

Fig. A-37. Arthritis. The shaded areas show the joints which are most subjected to the wearing away of the linings of the cartilages which reduce friction and serve as *bearings* for the moveable parts of the body.

There are many different types of arthritis. Some are caused by infections, some by injury, some by aging, and still others by entirely unknown causes. Infectious arthritis may follow influenza, typhoid fever, tuberculosis, syphilis, or gonorrhea. Arthritis of unknown cause is common, the worst form of which is rheumatoid arthritis.

There are three main kinds of arthritis: (1) osteoarthritis, (2) rheumatoid arthritis, and (3) gout.

OSTEOARTHRITIS (DEGENERATIVE JOINT DISEASE, OR HYPERTROPHIC ARTHRITIS). Osteoarthritis, which is the most common type of arthritis, results from the wear and tear on the joints. Most persons over 50 years of age have osteoarthritis to some degree; for this reason it is often called *old-age rheumatism*. However, it often follows injuries, infections and/or diseases afflicting the joints, and it can occur in relatively young people.

Causes. Osteoarthritis is usually produced by a constant strain on a joint which produces a wearing away of the articular cartilage within the joint, especially the weight-bearing joints—the knees, hips, ankles, and spine. Overweight and stress can aggravate the disease. (See Fig. A-38.)

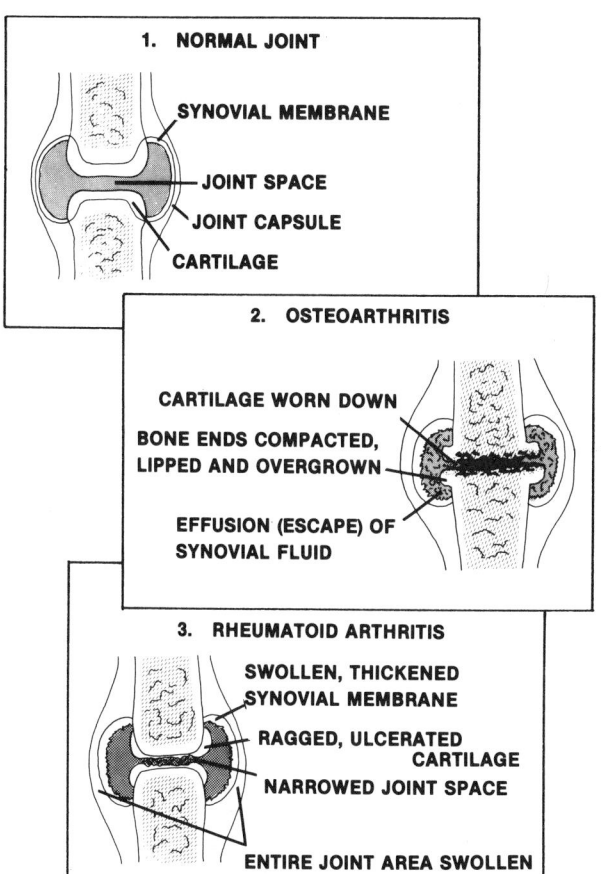

Fig. A-38. Schematic drawings of: (1) A normal joint. (2) Osteoarthritis joint, showing the cartilage worn down; the bone ends compacted, lipped, and overgrown; and effusion (escape) of synovial fluid. (3) Rheumatoid arthritis joint, showing swollen, thickened synovial membrane; ragged, ulcerative cartilage; and narrowed joint space. (See Fig. A-40 for gout.)

Symptoms (diagnosis). Osteoarthritis is the most common cause of painful knees, backs, and fingers. But it seldom causes deformity of the joints or crippling. Affected joints may *creak* and grate on movement. Typically, pain is increased by exercise and relieved by rest. Unlike rheumatoid arthritis, osteoarthritis does not produce any nodes under the skin and is not accompanied by constitutional symptoms such as fever and weight loss.

Treatment. The treatment of osteoarthritis consists of weight reduction if overweight, moderation of activity, use of heat, taking aspirin, and, in severe cases, the physician may resort to the injection of cortisone or ACTH into the painful joints and the use of braces to relieve strain. People with osteoarthritis seem to feel better in warm dry climates, like Arizona, California, and New Mexico; wet or damp environments may aggravate the condition.

Diet may be significant. Osteoarthritis is more common among those who are past middle age—when there is a tendency to put on extra weight, to deposit less calcium in the bones, and sometimes to develop a mild form of anemia. Although these conditions are not caused by the osteoarthritis as such, they can be improved by sound nutrition. So, the doctor will probably advise the person suffering from osteoarthritis to eat more foods rich in calcium, such as milk and milk products, as well as foods containing iron and vitamins; and he will advise the patient to lose weight without deprivation of any of the essential nutrients.

Obesity is to be avoided because extra weight places additional stress on the weight-bearing joints. Patients lose weight more happily on a high-protein, low-carbohydrate, modest-fat, low-caloric diet.

Prevention. An essential element of prevention of osteoarthritis is the avoidance of excessive weight gain, which adds to the wear and tear of weight-bearing joints. Secondary preventive measures are directed at reducing the strain on affected joints by use of a back brace, abdominal support of a sagging abdomen (to take the strain off the back), a neck brace, and adequate rest.

RHEUMATOID ARTHRITIS (ARTHRITIS DEFORMANS, OR ATROPHIC ARTHRITIS). Rheumatoid arthritis, often called the great crippler, is a progressive, debilitating, and chronic disease that manifests itself primarily by joint pain and inflammation, usually leading to deformities. Studies show that about one out of three arthritic patients have this type. Although this form of arthritis can develop in people of any age, including children just a few months old, it most commonly attacks middle-aged persons. Three times as many women as men get rheumatoid arthritis. Patients with rheumatoid arthritis are usually underweight and undernourished. Rheumatoid arthritis is not related to rheumatic fever, with which it may be confused due to the similarity of names.

People afflicted with rheumatoid arthritis normally have negative nitrogen and calcium balances and reduced tolerances to carbohydrates (starches and sugars). Reduced carbohydrate tolerances are believed to result from the chronic inflammatory state, rather than from any defect in carbohydrate metabolism.

Causes. Although medical science is learning more and more about rheumatoid arthritis, no known cause has been identified and documented. Some experts believe that it results from a generalized infection and that pain, swelling and inflammation in the joints is only one of its manifestations. Others believe that an emotional component influences the course of the disorder. Other possible causes that have been suggested include a cold, damp climate; a bacterium or virus; injury, accident, fatigue, strain to a joint (for example, *housemaid's knee*), shock, allergy, heredity, metabolic disorders, and/or metabolic deficiencies.

Symptoms (diagnosis). Rheumatoid arthritis is progressive and involves many joints. The most common symptoms are swelling and pain of the joints of the fingers, wrists, knees, ankles, or toes, alone or in combination, although other joints may be involved. One hallmark of the disease is that usually both sides of the body are affected; both hands or both ankles, for example. Eventually, the joints stiffen in deformed positions, producing crippling. Other common symptoms are: fever, fatigue, stiffness of joints, weakness of muscles, anemia, anorexia (loss of appetite), and loss of

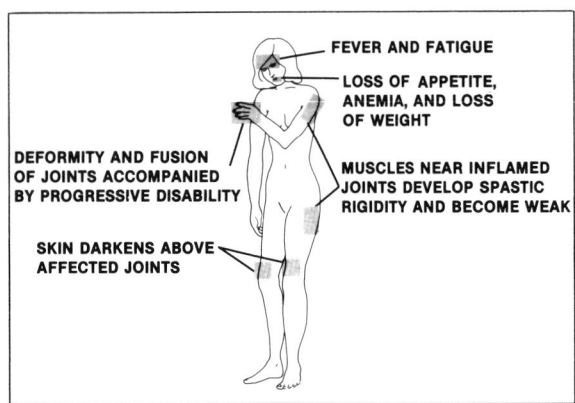

FEVER AND FATIGUE

LOSS OF APPETITE, ANEMIA, AND LOSS OF WEIGHT

DEFORMITY AND FUSION OF JOINTS ACCOMPANIED BY PROGRESSIVE DISABILITY

MUSCLES NEAR INFLAMED JOINTS DEVELOP SPASTIC RIGIDITY AND BECOME WEAK

SKIN DARKENS ABOVE AFFECTED JOINTS

Fig. A-39. Characteristics of rheumatoid arthritis in later stages.

weight. In about 10% of the cases, nodules may appear under the skin, especially around the elbows, wrists, fingers, and occasionally the ankles. Diagnosis in the early stage of the disease may involve x-ray studies; confirmation consists of characteristic changes of bones and joints.

About ¼ of the people who get rheumatoid arthritis recover from the first attack without serious symptoms; ½ suffer only minor discomfort; while the remaining ¼ develop chronic, progressive, disabling arthritis.

Treatment. The treatment of rheumatoid arthritis is difficult and prolonged. But, in most cases, deformity can be prevented. Helpful treatments include a well-balanced diet, adequate rest along with enough physical exercise to prevent stiffening, the application of heat on the joints, maintaining inflamed joints in nondeforming positions (this may require the use of splints and braces), and taking aspirin and other pain-killing drugs as recommended by the physician. Injection of gold salts (gold chloride and gold with sodium thiosulfate) and the use of ACTH or cortisone drugs over long periods of time have helped certain persons through this chronic disease with little or no crippling. Also, intravenous injection of antimalarial drugs is sometimes of benefit in lessening the symptoms in younger persons. In some cases, replacement of patients' joints with plastic or rubber joints enables them to move without pain. There is no cure for rheumatoid arthritis, but more than half of the patients recover eventually.

Due to the chronic disability and severe pain produced by rheumatoid arthritis, afflicted people often fall prey to food faddists and charlatans who offer quick and easy cures. Numerous diets have been devised and promoted as a treatment for rheumatoid and other forms of arthritis; based on low carbohydrate levels, high protein levels, low protein levels, acid-ash, alkaline-ash, low fat levels, high levels of B-complex vitamins, high levels of vitamin C, high levels of sulfur, and/or high levels of vitamin A. Claims are even made that a bowl of cherries will help some gouty patients. In the past, sometimes massive doses of vitamin D were prescribed and used, but this treatment is seldom recommended today, because excess vitamin D has been demonstrated to produce severe, and sometimes even fatal, calcification of the kidneys, through disruption of normal calcium and phosphorus metabolism.

Although food will neither cause nor cure rheumatoid arthritis, good nutrition can affect the way the patient feels, how well he responds to treatment, and how successfully he can resist the ravages of inflammation.

The diet of rheumatoid arthritis patients should be rich in proteins, minerals, and vitamins—all vital to tissue resistance and repair. This calls for plenty of meat, fish, and dairy products, fruits, and vegetables. Liberal amounts of milk and other sources of calcium are recommended. The extra supply of dietary calcium helps avoid the adverse effects of the disease on (1) tissue repair and growth, and (2) bone metabolism; and such a diet helps fortify the body against the general debilitation and possible anemia that may accompany rheumatoid arthritis.

Since rheumatoid arthritis is a chronic, progressive, inflammatory tissue disorder, many patients lose weight and become undernourished. Thus, a high-protein, high-calorie diet, with adequate minerals and vitamins, is recommended until a normal nutritional state is achieved. Also, since anorexia, or loss of appetite, normally accompanies rheumatoid arthritis, it is important that attractive meals be served.

Prevention. There is no known preventive for rheumatoid arthritis. But deformities should be avoided if possible.

GOUT (GOUTY ARTHRITIS). To many people mention of gout conjures up a stereotyped picture of a fat old aristocrat sitting with his flannel-wrapped foot propped up on a stool, crippled because of his chronic indulgence in alcohol and food, particularly beef.

In reality, gout is an inherited disorder of metabolism in which uric acid in excessive amounts appears in blood and tissues and produces a painful swelling of the joints of the hands or feet, especially the big toe.

Causes. Gout is caused by a defect in the body's natural process of breaking down *purines* (nucleoproteins, which are compounds of one or more proteins and nucleic acid). This results in the production of too much uric acid, which accumulates in the blood, where it combines with sodium to produce sodium urate. Crystals of uric acid are deposited in tissues around the joints. These deposits cause sudden attacks of swelling, most commonly in the feet.

It is not known why the excess of uric acid appears in the blood, why the excess is not destroyed, or why urates are deposited in the tissue.

Gout tends to be familial; about 25% of the relatives of patients suffering from gout have the disease. Also, it is noteworthy that there is a high prevalence of gout in certain populations, including the Maoris of the Pacific area, and the Blackfoot and Pima Indians of the United States.

Attacks can be brought on by excesses in eating or drinking, or by certain acute medical or surgical problems.

Symptoms (diagnosis). The major symptoms of gout are those of severe arthritis, a singularly dramatic and painful type of joint inflammation which comes on without warning in acute and recurrent attacks. Ordinarily gout first appears in men in middle or early old age, but it sometimes occurs in young people, also. It affects women infrequently, only about one case in 50. Hippocrates observed the age-sex relationship of gout, and noted that eunuchs were not affected. Typically, an attack of gout begins very suddenly, often at night, with the onset of excruciating pain in a single joint. Most frequently it involves the *bunion joint*—where the big toe joins the foot, but the ankle, the instep, the knee, or virtually any other joint may occasionally be the site of the attack. Usually only one joint or tendon or bursa is affected at a time. If the disease continues uncontrolled, multiple joints may be affected. Bumps (crystalline deposits of urates,

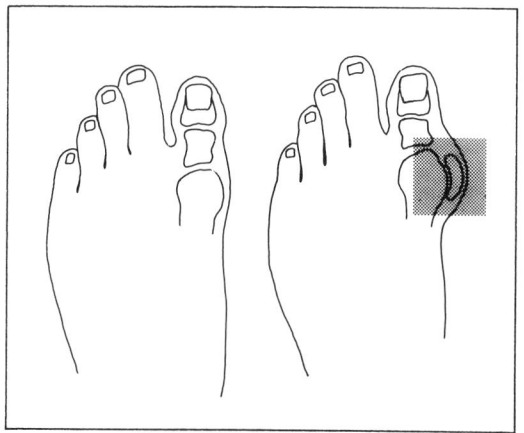

Fig. A-40. Gout, showing (1) normal toe (left) vs (2) swollen big toe (bunion) where the big toe joins the foot.

known as tophi) on the cartilage of the ear appear in about half of all gout victims. Gout may also begin with the sudden appearance of kidney stones.

Unlike the dull deep-seated ache of rheumatoid arthritis or osteoarthritis, the pain of gout tends to be sharp and agonizing, accompanied by sudden swelling of the affected joint and marked redness of the overlying skin. The pain may be so severe that the victim cannot even bear the touch of light bedclothes on the affected area. If untreated, the attack may last for three or more days before it gradually subsides, followed by the skin of the affected joint peeling and a completely symptom-free period. Typically, early in the disease, an attack may occur once every 4 or 5 months or even at longer intervals, usually affecting just one joint. Later, the attacks become more frequent and multiple joints may be involved. Gout finally becomes chronic.

People in sedentary work are more likely to have gout than manual laborers.

Patients with gout often have increased amounts of uric acid (as urates) in their blood, but such increases occur under a number of other circumstances. Thus, a test that shows an elevated concentration of uric acid in the blood does not necessarily indicate the presence of gout.

Treatment. Treatment consists of limiting the amount of purines in the diet, and of taking drugs under the supervision of a physician. Among the drugs used in the treatment of gout are aspirin, salicylic acid, cortisone, ACTH, Butazolidin, Benemid, uricosuric agents, and colchicine (the alkaloid from the autumn crocus, Colchicum atumnale, L, used to treat gout since the 5th century).

It is recognized that dietary measures are effective in reducing the incidence and severity of acute gout attacks. The diet should largely exclude foods that are rich in the white crystalline substances known as purines, which includes liver, sweetbreads, kidneys, brains, and anchovies. Also, alcohol and fats should be avoided. Milk, eggs, cheese, cereals, fruits, green vegetables, cocoa, tea, coffee, sweets, and nuts are relatively low in purines.

Gout is not curable, but it may be controlled by proper treatment.

Prevention. In a family where there is gout, men should routinely be given a blood test for uric acid. A diet may be suggested to delay the onset of gouty symptoms, since there are foods which are thought to predispose the

formation of uric acid. However, it has not been established that this approach is effective.

ADVICE TO ALL ARTHRITICS. Evidence exists that different forms of arthritis may result from overwork, allergy, exposure to extreme cold conditions, accidents, injuries, infections, diseases, malnutrition and/or severe mental stress. However, none of these causes has been fully documented. Therefore, the specific cause of most forms of arthritis is presently unknown. It is also known that administration of calcium, vitamins A, C, D, E, K, and/or the B-complex vitamins does not uniformly alter arthritic symptoms or the course of the disorder.

Contrary to popular belief, there is no such thing as an arthritis diet—a diet that will cure arthritis. However, certain adjustments in the diet of arthritics may be desirable, depending on the kind of arthritis, the treatment and medicines used, and the weight and overall state of health. There is overwhelming evidence that nutritionally balanced meals eaten regularly benefit anyone's overall health, muscle tone, and, in the case of arthritis, build ability to resist the wear and tear of the disease. Although some minor adjustments in specific items may be required, in general the good diet for anyone, whether they have arthritis or not, is based on a selection from six food groups—the bread, cereal, rice, and pasta group; the vegetable group; the fruit group; the meat, poultry, fish, dry beans, eggs, and nuts group; the milk, yogurt, and cheese group; and the fats, oils, and sweets group.

Doctors lament the money that is spent on useless and extravagantly advertised preparations. If some of this money were spent on nutritionally adequate and pleasurable meals, it would help fortify the patient's body and emotions against the pain and crippling of the disease.

The following suggestions provide the soundest advice to arthritics:

1. Consume a nutritious, well-balanced diet.
2. Avoid everyday tensions and get plenty of rest.
3. Maintain proper weight; do not overeat or undereat.
4. Pay no attention to the free advice from well-meaning but unqualified friends, relatives, and self-styled food experts.
5. Do not be taken in by the false claims and fancy cures of food faddists, makers of quack medicines, or unscrupulous drug purveyors; they benefit (profit) only those who produce and market them.
6. Consult the family physician or an established arthritis clinic, and follow the advice obtained.
7. Use corticosteroid therapy and/or other medication only under the direction of a reliable physician.

ARTICHOKE, GLOBE *Compositae*

This vegetable, which is considered to be a delicacy, is a thistlelike plant. The edible flower bud is characterized by green leaflike scales (bracts) that enclose it. Both the bracts and the base of the flower (receptacle), which is called the heart, are eaten. In some places, the tender young leaf stalk may also be consumed. Fig. A-41 depicts a typical globe artichoke.

ORIGIN AND HISTORY. The globe artichoke is native to the Mediterranean region. It was an important crop of ancient Greece and Rome.

WORLD AND U.S. PRODUCTION. World production of artichoke is about 1,353,000 metric tons annually. Most of the world's artichoke crop is produced in the coun-

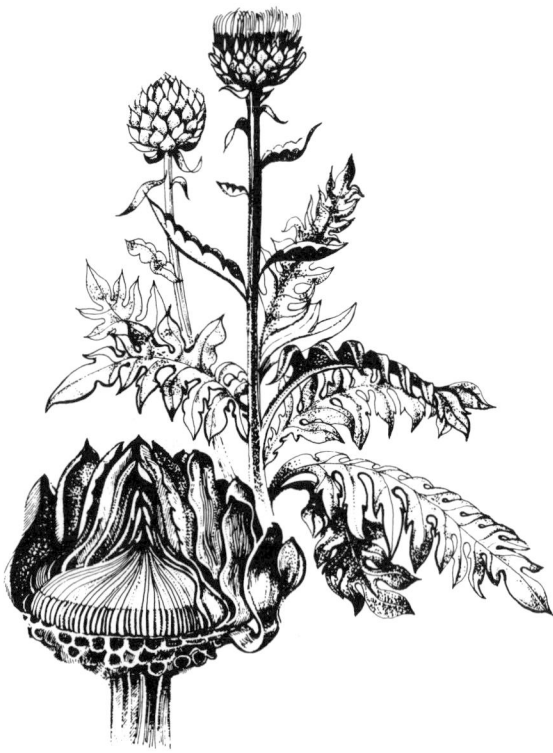

Fig. A-41. Globe artichoke.

tries bordering the Mediterranean Sea. The six leading artichoke producing countries, by rank, are: Italy, Spain, France, Argentina, United States, and Egypt. More than 80% of the world's artichoke crop comes from Italy, Spain, and France.[14]

Artichoke is a minor crop in the United States, only about 58,000 metric tons are produced annually.[15]

PROCESSING. About 60% of the U.S. crop is marketed fresh; the rest is processed.

SELECTION, PREPARATION, AND USES. The most desirable globe artichokes are compact, plump, heavy in relation to size, somewhat globular, and with large, fresh, fleshy, tight-clinging green leaf scales. Freshness is indicated by the green color, which with age or injury become partially brown. Overmature artichokes have hard-tipped leaf scales that are opening or spreading; also, the center formation may be fuzzy and dark pink or purple in color. Leaf scales on such overmature specimens are tough and woody when cooked and may be undesirably strong in flavor.

Some of the most common ways of preparing artichokes are: (1) boiling the whole vegetable; (2) stuffing parboiled artichokes with ground meat, bread crumbs, bacon bits, and/or anchovies, and baking; (3) breading and deep frying the parboiled vegetable; and (4) cooking artichoke hearts together with fish, meat, or poultry in a cream sauce.

The vegetable may be served hot or cold with a well-seasoned sauce. Often, artichoke sections are held by the fingers and dipped into the sauce. The tender inner portion is eaten and the remainder is discarded.

---

[14]Based on data from *FAO Production Yearbook 1990*, FAO/UN, Rome, Italy, Vol. 44, p. 130, Table 51. **Note well:** Annual production fluctuates as a result of weather and profitability of the crop.

[15]*Ibid.*

NUTRITIONAL VALUE. The nutrient composition of the globe artichoke is given in Food Composition Table F-21.

Globe artichokes may contain some nonnutritive substances which exert medicinal effects, because they have been thought useful in (1) stimulating the flow of bile and other digestive juices, (2) promoting the urinary loss of excessive water from the body, and (3) lowering the blood sugar. (**NOTE:** The authors make no claim that any of the beliefs regarding the medicinal effects of globe artichokes are accurate; rather, it is hoped that mentioning these claims will encourage further research relative thereto.)

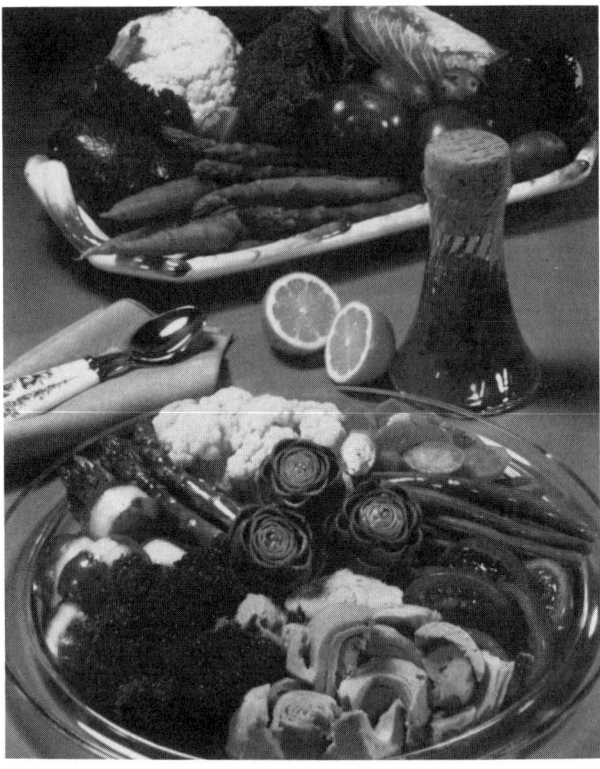

Fig. A-42. Globe artichokes served with a summer salad. (Courtesy, United Fresh Fruit and Vegetable Association)

ARTICHOKE, JERUSALEM

The Jerusalem artichoke, which is native to America, is a close relative of the sunflower. It is cultivated for the edible tubers, which grow underground and look like ginger root or misshapen potatoes. Jerusalem artichoke is often recommended for diabetics, as it has no starch; the carbohydrate of fresh tubers is in the form of inulin rather than sugar. But if they are stored for a long period of time, the inulin converts to sugar.

ARTIFICIALLY DRIED

Dried, or dehydrated, by other than natural means, usually by heat.

(Also see PRESERVATION OF FOOD.)

ARTIFICIAL SWEETENERS

Numerous naturally occurring chemicals have a sweet taste. Man, too, can create chemicals which have a sweet taste. Examples of artificial sweeteners include saccharin and aspartame—products of the laboratory. Generally, artificial sweeteners impart sweetness without adding calories.

(Also see SWEETENING AGENTS.)

ASCARIDS

Roundworms, ranging from 8 to 12 in. (20 to 30 cm), which may infest the human intestine. The infection enters the body through the mouth, by the ingestion of unclean or contaminated fruits or vegetables and impure drinking water containing eggs of the parasite. A female ascarid lays about 200,000 eggs per day, most of which pass into the feces. Ascarid eggs may remain alive for several years on moist earth in a warm climate such as that in the southeastern United States. In the body, sometimes the worms migrate to the gallbladder, throat, lungs, liver, heart or nose.

(Also see DISEASES.)

ASCITES

An accumulation of fluid in the abdomen. This disorder may be due to high blood pressure, sodium retention, heart failure, or a severe protein deficiency.

ASCORBIC ACID (VITAMIN C)

Ascorbic acid is another name for vitamin C, the very important substance, first found in citrus fruits, which prevents scurvy, one of the oldest scourges of mankind.

(Also see VITAMIN C.)

ASCORBIN STEARATE

This is a fat-soluble ester of ascorbic acid (vitamin C) and stearic acid. It is often added to food as an antioxidant at concentrations of about 0.1%.

ASCORBYL PALMITATE ($C_{22}H_{38}O_7$)

A derivative of ascorbic acid (vitamin C) and palmitic acid. It is a white or yellowish white powder with a citruslike odor, which is used as an antioxidant for fats and oils and as a source of vitamin C. In amounts of 0.1 to 0.4% by weight of the flour, it serves as an antistaling agent in bakery products. It will retard staling for 2 to 4 days.

–ASE

A suffix used in naming an enzyme; for example, peptidase.

ASH

The minerals in a food. Also, the residue that remains after complete burning or metabolism of the organic matter.

(Also see ANALYSIS OF FOODS.)

ASPARAGINE

A derivative of aspartic acid, a nonessential amino acid. Asparagine is formed in protein metabolism and is found both in tissues and in the blood.

(Also see AMINO ACID[S].)

ASPARAGUS *Asparagus officinalis*

The spears (young shoots) of asparagus, which is a member of the Lily (*Liliaceae*) family, are a popular vegetable

It is often served with butter or a sauce such as hollandaise. Asparagus tips au gratin with sliced hard-boiled egg on toast is appealing when served as an hor d'oeuvre with an accompanying dip or sauce, or when toasted in a salad with grated cheese, oil, and/or a well seasoned dressing. Fig. A-43 shows a typical asparagus salad.

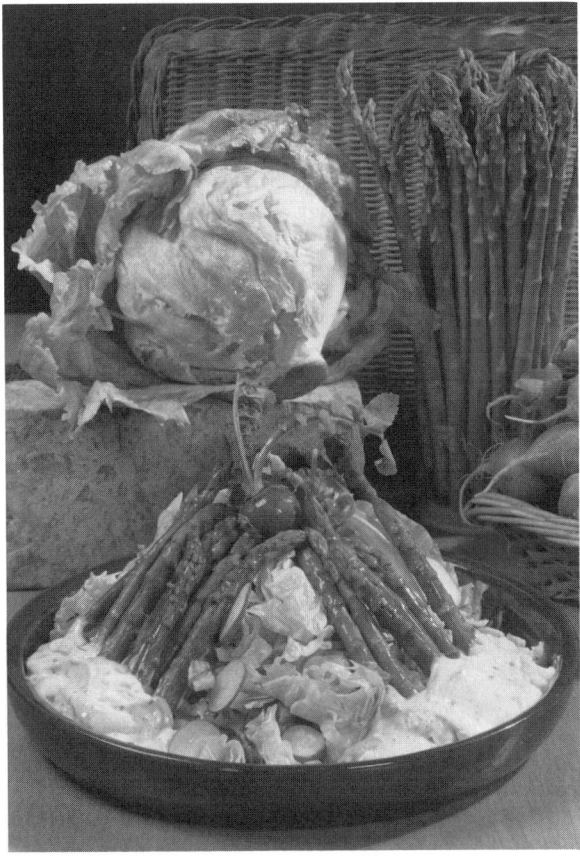

Fig. A-43. Iceberg asparagus salad. An appetizing combination of asparagus, iceberg lettuce, and a dressing which contains mayonaise, tarragon, chervil (dill may be substituted), and a touch of garlic. (Courtesy, California Iceberg Lettuce Commission, San Rafael, Calif.)

NUTRITIONAL VALUE. Asparagus is low in calories and carbohydrates, but 1 cup (240 ml) contains more protein (3 to 6 g) than a cup of cooked cornmeal (2.6 g) or a cup of cooked rice (3 to 5 g). Also, the vegetable is a fair source of the vitamins thiamin, riboflavin, and niacin.

(Also see VEGETABLE[S], Table V-2, Vegetables of the World.)

ASPARTAME

A low calorie artificial sweetener which was approved for human consumption by the Food and Drug Administration (FDA) in mid-August 1981. It is manufactured by G. D. Searle and Company of Skokie, Illinois, and sold under a different brand name. Chemically, aspartame is the combination of the two amino acids, aspartic acid and phenylalanine—a dipeptide. It is about 180 times sweeter than table sugar. Therefore, it provides the same sweetness as sugar with fewer calories. Furthermore, it does not promote tooth decay, nor does it have an after taste.

Aspartame is sold to food processors for use in cold cereals, drink mixes, gelatin, puddings, dairy products, and toppings. Consumers can purchase aspartame in tablets or powder for use on or in their foods. Aspartame loses its sweetness during long periods of storage. Also, aspartame is not suitable for baking, since heat causes the loss of sweetness.

NOTE WELL: Aspartame is safe for diabetics, but the phenylalanine released during its metabolism may affect individuals with phenylketonuria. Foods manufactured with aspartame are required to carry a warning for phenylketonurics.

(Also see SWEETENING AGENTS.)

ASPARTIC ACID

A nonessential amino acid which provides amino groups that help to conserve the body's supply of protein. Also, it is involved in the formation of urea and other compounds in the body.

(Also see AMINO ACID[S].)

ASPERGILLUS

A genus of fungi that are commonly-occurring food spoilage organisms. (The name is derived from *aspergillum*, the device used for sprinkling holy water in Roman Catholic rituals, because the head and stalk of the fungi are shaped like the device.) These fungi grow readily on breads and other grain products, legumes, and meats. Certain species even infest such parts of the body as the feet, lungs, and the external opening of the ear.

However, man has learned to utilize certain species of *Aspergillus* for such beneficial purposes as (1) sources of enzymes which convert starches or proteins to sugars or amino acids, respectively; and (2) production of antibiotics, and of organic acids used as food additives. Conversely, *Aspergillus flavus* produces the deadly aflatoxins, which cause liver cancer and other disorders.

(Also see AFLATOXIN; POISONS, Table P-2, Mycotoxins.)

ASSAY

Determination of (1) the purity or potency of a substance, or (2) the amount of any particular constituent of a mixture.

ASSIMILATION

A physiological term referring to a group of processes by which the nutrients in food are made available to and used by the body; including digestion, absorption, distribution, and metabolism.

(Also see DIGESTION AND ABSORPTION; and METABOLISM.)

ASSOCIATION OF OFFICIAL AGRICULTURAL CHEMISTS (AOAC)

The AOAC is a voluntary organization of chemists that sponsors the development and testing of methods for analyzing nutrients, foods, food and color additives, animal feeds, liquors, beverages, drugs, cosmetics, pesticides, and many other commodities. Periodically, they publish methods which are acceptable for these analyses.

ASTHMA

A condition characterized by difficulty in breathing due to obstruction of the bronchial tubes. Usually, it is due to an allergic reaction.

(Also see ALLERGIES.)

ASYMPTOMATIC

Without symptoms.

ATAXIA

A general term which means a lack of coordination of muscular movement. It may be due to various disorders such as damage to certain parts of the nervous system, nutritional deficiencies, intoxication, or a congential disorder.

ATHEROMA

A deposit of fat on or in the walls of arteries. (Also see HEART DISEASE.)

ATHEROSCLEROSIS

A degenerative disease, characterized by the buildup of abnormal patches (plaques) on the walls of arteries, thought to be the main cause of heart attacks.

(Also see HEART DISEASE, Section headed "Atherosclerosis.")

ATHLETICS AND NUTRITION

Many athletes and their coaches believe that certain foods and diets help to build strength and endurance for superior performances.

HISTORY. Primitive peoples realized that courage and physical fitness were required for success in hunting wild game and fighting neighboring groups that threatened their security. Hence, they sometimes prepared themselves for these occasions by (1) participating in religious ceremonies to win the favors of their tribal gods, (2) eating the hearts and other parts of animals that were thought to impart courage and strength, and (3) performing feats of ability and endurance. It is noteworthy that certain modifications of these practices have been passed down through the ages and are still utilized by some modern athletes. Furthermore, some of the long-standing controversies over the effects of diet on performance, such as the one regarding meat consumption vs vegetarianism, continue to be the subjects of heated debates. However, one should consider the historical circumstances under which the various diets were consumed before jumping to conclusions about the merits and demerits of various foods.

The diets of American Indians who engaged in sporting events usually were based upon the foods that were readily available from their environments. For example, the Iroquois Indians, who played lacrosse, ate a varied diet of wild game, fish, vegetables, nuts, berries, and other wild plants because they lived in the bounteous Eastern Woodlands of North America.

On the other side of the world, sports contests became important events in the ancient civilizations of Greece and Rome. The first renowned Greek athletes who participated in the running competitions of the early Olympic Games (which are believed to date back to the 13th century B.C.) ate mainly fruits, grains, legumes, and vegetables like the rest of the people, because the hilly, rocky soil supported

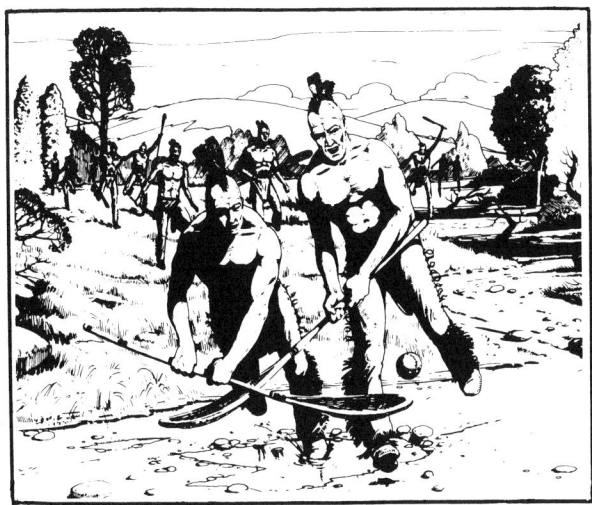

Fig. A-44. Iroquois Indians playing lacrosse.

only limited crops and small numbers of goats and sheep. Only one province in the northern part of the Greek peninsula had land suitable for raising cattle.

Later, the sports-loving Greeks introduced wrestling and boxing, but there were no weight classes. Hence, the heavier athletes had an advantage over the lighter ones. At that time, some of the champions were hefty-built meat eaters who consumed rather large amounts of food. This led to criticism by philosophers who claimed that an athlete was a slave to his jaw and belly. Recent research findings suggest that the consumption of large amounts of meats and other high protein foods enhanced the appetite so that extra food may be eaten.

Unfortunately, many athletes and other lay people are often misled by profit hungry promoters of tonics and other nostrums into believing that certain secret products will improve performance in athletic events. Facts follow.

HEALTH BENEFITS FROM PARTICIPATION IN SPORTS.
It is generally believed that athletes are healthier than nonathletes. This is attributed to the following health benefits from participation in sports:

1. Augmented collateral circulation in the heart muscles.
2. Added output of blood by the heart.
3. Lowered resting heart rate.
4. Reduced diastolic and systolic blood pressure.
5. Increased endurance.
6. Enlarged aerobic capacity.
7. Strengthened muscles.
8. Improved carbohydrate utilization.
9. Accelerated loss of excess body fat.

Details relative to the latter two benefits follow.

• **Normalization of carbohydrate utilization**—Physical exercise increases the rate at which the sugar in the blood is utilized. For example, the blood sugar levels of well-trained males were found to be about one-third lower after an oral dose of glucose than those in untrained males. Hence, athletes may safely consume greater amounts of dietary carbohydrates than nonathletes. Furthermore, diabetic athletes do not usually require as much insulin as sedentary diabetics.

• **Loss of excess body fat**—Strenuous exercise performed

several times a week helps to speed the loss of unwanted body fat, provided that the caloric intake is held constant or moderately reduced. For example, the expenditure of an additional 500 Calories (kcal) per day, 3 times a week in sports such as basketball, handball, jogging, racketball, swimming, or tennis will result in the loss of about 2 lb (0.9 kg) per month. If, in addition to exercising, the dietary caloric intake is cut by 500 Calories (kcal) per day, there will be an additional loss of about 4 lb (1.8 kg) per month. It is noteworthy that athletes sometimes gain weight during training, but this gain is likely to be almost entirely muscle protein and water. Each pound of body protein is associated with approximately 3 lb (1.4 kg) of water.

METABOLISM DURING ATHLETICS.
The utilization of food energy for muscular work involves (1) the production of energy-rich adenosine triphosphate (ATP) from carbohydrates, fats, and proteins by means of a series of tightly linked oxidative (aerobic) processes, and (2) the contraction of the muscle fibers which is induced by ATP. High rates of muscular work which exceed the aerobic capacity, such as those performed in sprinting, may also be sustained in part by nonoxidative (anaerobic) processes that produce ATP and lactic acid. However, the accumulation of lactic acid often results in heavy breathing and fatigue which persists for a while after the work has been completed. This condition is called an *oxygen debt* because the elimination of the lactic acid buildup requires extra oxygen.

It is noteworthy that athletic training speeds up the metabolism of lactic acid and retards the development of fatigue. Furthermore, the feeding of salts of lactic acid (lactates) during training apparently stimulates the processes that reduce the lactate accumulation. Therefore, some trainers have conjectured that it may be helpful for athletes in training to consume liberal amounts of fermented milk products such as buttermilk and yogurt which are rich in lactic acid.

(Also see ENERGY UTILIZATION BY THE BODY; and METABOLISM.)

NUTRIENT REQUIREMENTS OF ATHLETES DURING TRAINING AND COMPETITION.
One of the most convenient means of estimating the nutritional needs of an athlete is to consider the needs to be the sums of basic requirements for nonathletic people of the same age, sex, height, and body build; plus, the extra nutrients needed to cover the cost of the work performed in playing the sport.

The most important nutritive requirements of athletes are (1) the extra calories to cover the energy cost of the physical activity (unless he or she is trying to lose some body fat by means of caloric restriction), and (2) water to replace that which is lost in sweat. Data on the energy expenditure for various sports are given in Table A-7 (next page).

The extra energy that is required for most sports may be provided by one or more nutritious snacks such as those shown in Table A-8 (next page).

It should be noted that the snacks in Table A-8 provide minerals and vitamins in addition to calories. For example, the orange furnishes potassium (a mineral that is very important to the heart muscle and other tissues) and vitamin C (which may improve performance). The other items are good sources of additional minerals and vitamins. Therefore, a variety of nutritious snacks should be consumed, in addition to the well-balanced meals that are desirable for all people. Generally, it is better to obtain nutrients from wholesome foods than to consume *junk foods* that furnish mainly

TABLE A-7
ENERGY EXPENDITURES FOR
SELECTED ATHLETIC ACTIVITIES[1]

Energy Expenditure	Activity[3]
(kcal per hour)[2]	
170 to 240	Bicycling slowly (6 m.p.h.), table tennis, volleyball, walking slowly (2 m.p.h.).
250 to 350	Bowling, golf, swimming slowly (25 yd per minute), tennis doubles, walking moderately fast (3 m.p.h.).
360 to 500	Bicycling moderately fast (12 m.p.h.), dancing, football, handball, hockey, ice skating, roller skating, skiing (downhill), squash, swimming moderately fast (50 yd per minute), tennis singles, and walking fast (4½ m.p.h.).
510 to 750	Cross-country skiing, jogging (5½ m.p.h.), jumping rope, and running in place.
760 to 1,000	Jogging (7 m.p.h.), and running (8 m.p.h.).

[1]Adapted by the authors from *Exercise and Your Heart*, U.S. Dept. of Health and Human Services, 1981, p. 7; and *Food*, Home and Garden Bull. No. 228, USDA, p. 15.

[2]A range of caloric expenditures is given for each level of activity because the values for individual participants vary according to the intensity of play, body build, and skill of playing. The low end of the range is probably a better estimate for small persons and most women, whereas, the upper end of the range is most applicable to large persons and most men.

[3]To convert to metric see WEIGHTS AND MEASURES.

TABLE A-8
CALORIC VALUES OF SELECTED
POPULAR SNACK FOODS[1]

Food	Calories (kcal)
1 small, 2 3/8 in. (5.9 cm), navel orange	45
2 medium graham crackers	55
2 Tbsp (30 ml) fruit-nut snack[2]	70
2 Tbsp (30 ml) peanuts	105
1 cup (240 ml) plain low-fat yogurt	145
1 cup (240 ml) split-pea soup	195
1 cup (240 ml) fruit-flavored yogurt	225
½ cup (120 ml) granola cereal[3]	280
1 hamburger, 3 oz (85 g) patty, on bun	365
12 oz (360 ml) chocolate milkshake	430

[1]Adapted by the authors from *Food*, Home and Garden Bull. No. 228, USDA, p. 14.

[2]A mixture of salted Spanish peanuts, raisins, and chopped dates.

[3]A slow-baked mixture of quick-cooking rolled oats, unsweetened wheat germ, unsweetened shredded coconut, coarsely chopped nuts, raisins, vegetable oil, honey, and almond or vanila flavoring.

empty calories because the former practice minimizes the likelihood that nutritional supplements will be needed.

(Also see NUTRIENTS: REQUIREMENTS, ALLOWANCES, FUNCTIONS, SOURCES; and RECOMMENDED DIETARY ALLOWANCES.)

Water and Salt Requirements. Excessive losses of water (dehydration) and mineral salts (electrolyte depletion) by athletes exercising strenuously in hot environments are believed to be mainly responsible for the heat stroke deaths that occur among high school and college football players. Players who begin practice during the hot, humid *dog days* of August are highly susceptible to dehydration and heat injury because (1) they are often out of condition when they start their training, (2) the protective gear and uniform prevents the escape of heat from the body, and (3) they may fail to consume sufficient water and mineral salts. Runners may also be at risk due to their becoming accustomed to

dehydration during practice sessions and failing to drink enough fluid. Finally, wrestlers may deliberately dehydrate themselves in order to lose sufficient weight to qualify for a lower weight class. Often, there is a period as long as 5 hours between weighing in and the beginning of the match. Hence, the wrestlers expect to rehydrate themselves during that interval.

Therefore, players, coaches, and trainers should be aware that the excessive loss of water from the body may have consequences such as fatigue, fever, heat stroke, impairment of sweating, an increased heart rate, and permanent damage to the physiological mechanisms which regulate the body temperature. These consequences may be prevented by the procedures which follow:

1. Athletes should be encouraged to consume from 8 to 10 8-oz glasses (*1.9 to 2.4 liter*) of fluids per day. This includes milk, soups, stews, etc. The liberal consumption of liquids has been shown to boost athletic performances by conferring benefits such as a lower heart rate, increased sweating, and a lower rectal temperature (a measure of overheating in the body).

2. Water should be available during practice sessions and matches that last for two or more hours and for shorter ones that involve intense activity in a warm environment.

3. Athletes, coaches, and trainers should monitor the loss of body water during exercise by weighing participants before and after practice sessions or matches. Each pound of weight loss is equivalent to 1 pint (*0.47 liter*) of water.

4. Salt tablets may not be needed if athletes salt their food liberally. However, it may be better to use the tablets when needed rather than to salt food heavily since the habitual use of excessive amounts of this seasoning may lead to high blood pressure in certain susceptible people. A good rule of thumb is for athletes to use one 7 grain salt tablet for each pound of weight loss *after* 5 to 6 lb have been lost. Furthermore, each tablet should be taken with at least 1 pint (*0.47 liter*) of water. Taking salt without water aggravates dehydration and may cause nausea.

5. Sport drinks which contain sugar, salt, and other mineral salts (electrolytes) may be suitable for use during practice sessions and contests, provided that overconcentrated products are diluted with water. Coaches should obtain the compositions of these products from the manufacturers or other authoritative sources.

MEALS TAKEN BEFORE AND DURING COMPETITION. Some athletic competitors place great value on pregame meals and on the types of refreshments consumed during competition.

Many athletes are tense prior to the start of competition; hence, they may become nauseous if the wrong types of foods are eaten. Also, the meal should be cleared rapidly from the stomach and be low in undigestible material such as plant fiber. Carbohydrates are the most rapidly utilized and promote the best short-term performances from athletes, whereas fats and proteins require much longer for digestion and are best suited for slower paced events that are conducted over longer periods of time.

A typical pregame meal for an event lasting only an hour or two might consist of cereal, milk, and sugar with toast, butter, and/or jam. Another meal might be an instant breakfast powder mixed with milk. Generally, coaches tell their players to avoid condiments, fatty foods, gravies, and pies.

FOODS AND NUTRIENTS WHICH ARE BELIEVED TO HELP PERFORMANCES. Food fads are prevalent among athletes who are ever in search of an item that will give them an edge in competition. Nevertheless, some foods appear to be better boosters of energy (ergogenic aids) than others. Therefore, details on some of the more popular items follow:

• **Alcoholic beverages**—Beer and champagne have long been consumed by athletes in Europe. In America, the drinking of beer is common after practice sessions and informal competitions. Even the more serious athletes may take beer to relax and sleep well during the night before competition and occasionally on the day of the event to remove inhibitions over extending themselves fully. However, performances that require finely tuned perceptual and motor skills may be impaired by alcohol.

• **Caffeine-containing beverages**—Coffee, tea, and cola beverages are widely consumed by athletes around the world. Nevertheless, it is still uncertain whether these drinks impair or improve athletic performances. Furthermore, caffeine-containing beverages increase the loss of water in urination (caffeine is a diuretic) and may contribute to dehydration if excessive amounts are consumed.

• **Carbohydrate-rich diets**—Recent studies have shown that the consumption of high carbohydrate diets for 3 or 4 days prior to an athletic event improves performances in sports that require considerable aerobic capacity. The effect of this type of diet is greatest when it is preceded by 3 days of strenuous exercise while consuming a high fat, high protein, low carbohydrate diet that empties the muscles of the stored carbohydrate (glycogen). This practice, which is called glycogen loading, may not be advisable for all athletes on all occasions, since some competitors may develop cardiac irregularities while overzealously adhering to such a dietary program.

• **Dextrose (glucose)**—The ingestion of sugar prior to or during contests improves performances provided that it is taken with sufficient water to prevent irritation of the digestive tract.

• **Honey**—This form of sugar does not appear to offer any advantage over other forms.

• **Iron**—Women athletes may need iron supplementation, particularly when they have heavy losses of blood during their menstrual periods.

• **Orange juice**—The Russians claim that the outstanding performances of their athletes in the 1960 Olympics in Rome were due in part to the consumption of liberal amounts of orange juice, which is rich in potassium (an essential electrolyte) and vitamin C. They won more gold medals than any other country. However, it is still uncertain whether orange juice is an ergogenic food.

• **Protein-rich diets**—These diets help to build muscle during training for events such as weight lifting and wrestling that require great strength. However, they do *not* help performances of trained athletes, and may even impair endurance in certain types of sports.

• **Thiamin**—Where a deficiency of thiamin exists, a thiamin supplement may be advisable for athletes who consume highly refined carbohydrates or sugar such as dextrose and honey to obtain extra calories.

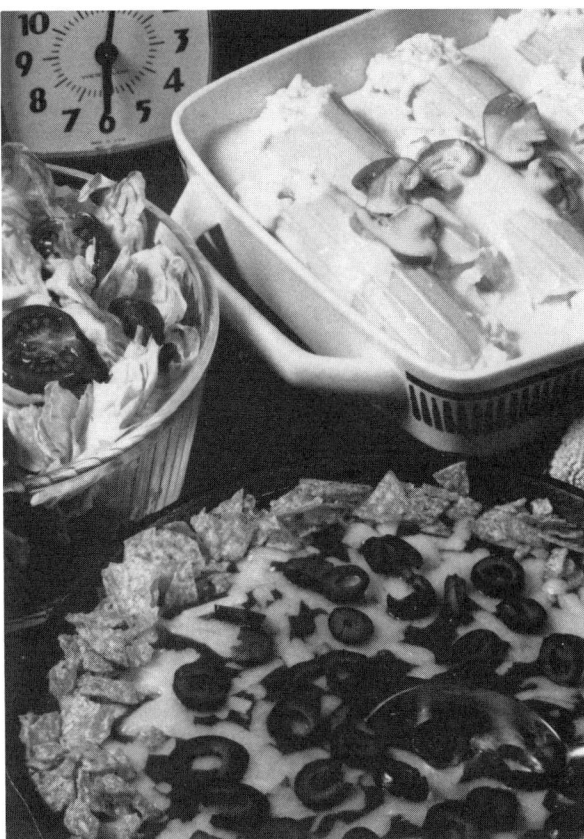

Fig. A-45. Athletes need to eat well to perform well. (Courtesy, Carnation Co., Los Angeles, Calif.)

• **Vitamin C**—Present findings indicate that massive doses of vitamin C are not only ineffective in improving the performance of athletes, but may have a negative effect on athletic performance by disturbing the equilibrium between oxygen transport and oxygen utilization.

• **Vitamin E**—Unfortunately, many of the studies of the use of this vitamin by athletes were poorly controlled. Nevertheless, vitamin E has been helpful in the treatment of some cases of muscle cramping.

• **Wheat germ oil**—This food may have an effect that is unrelated to the vitamin E which it contains, but to date, athletic performance studies involving the use of wheat germ oil have been inconclusive.

STEROID ALTERNATIVES. Steroids, which increase muscle mass, and which have been used in both people and animals, are based on the hormones secreted by the testes, ovaries, and adrenal glands, and are known as *anabolic steroids.*

In human athletic events, the use of anabolic steroids is being curbed by both legislative and educational efforts. but many manufacturers of dietary supplements are now promoting products as substitutes of anabolic steroids, or as *steroid alternatives.*

Before taking dietary supplementation of anabolic alternatives, an athlete should seek the counsel of a health professional—a physician, a physical therapist, or nutritionist—even if they advise against these products until more is known about them.

ATONIC CONSTIPATION

A condition characterized by retention of material in the digestive tract, particularly in the bowel. It is believed to be due to a weakening of the muscular coat surrounding the intestine, which results in a lack of peristaltic waves. It is common in elderly and/or obese people, following surgery, and in conjunction with pregnancy and fevers.

(Also see CONSTIPATION.)

ATONY

Lack of tone or tension. The term is usually applied to muscles which have become flabby and weak.

ATRIA

The upper chambers of the heart which receive blood from the veins and transfer it to the lower chambers (ventricles). Atria are also referred to as auricles.

ATROPHY

Failure of growth, or a wasting of one or more tissues of the body due to such causes as nutritional deficiencies, aging, disease, or injury.

ATROPINE

One of several similar substances, collectively known as the belladonna alkaloids, which are extracted from the deadly nightshade plant (*Atropa belladonna*). Atropine is used mainly to treat disorders of the digestive tract such as excessively rapid movements of the stomach and bowel, overacidity, and ulcers, because it (1) reduces the amounts of digestive secretions, and (2) slows the motions of the digestive organs. Some common side effects are dryness of the mouth and constipation.

(Also see BELLADONNA DRUGS; and DIGESTION AND ABSORPTION.)

ATWATER VALUES (or ATWATER FACTORS)

These are average physiologic fuel values of carbohydrates, proteins, and fats, based on experiments conducted by W. O. Atwater, at Wesleyan University, Middletown, Connecticut. Professor Atwater, who is thought of as the father of American nutrition, published the first extensive table of food values in 1896. Atwater values reflect the number of kilocalories of energy physiologically available from a gram of food. They were derived by Atwater from the heat of combustion and corrected for energy losses from unabsorbed nutrients in the feces and urine. Atwater approximated that on a typical American diet each gram of carbohydrate, fat, and protein will yield 4, 9, and 4 Calories (kcal), respectively. The Atwater values are used extensively in dietary calculations and food analysis.

AURICLES

Another name for the two upper chambers of the heart, called atria.

(Also see ATRIA.)

AUTOIMMUNITY

The presence in the blood of antibodies that attack one or more tissues of the body.

Autoimmune disorders are characterized by the breakdown of various connective tissues (the collagen diseases), such as lupus erythematosus, polyarteritis nodosa, rheumatoid arthritis, and rheumatic fever. Also, it is suspected that autoimmune reactions may be responsible in part for certain abnormalities associated with (1) diabetes, when there has been an unexplainable deterioration of the cells of the pancreas that secrete insulin; (2) insufficient secretion of adrenal cortical hormones (Addison's disease) due to wasting of the glandular tissue; (3) lack of stomach acid (achlorhydria) and/or lack of intrinsic factor resulting in pernicious anemia, because antibodies have attacked the cells of the stomach which secrete the deficient substances; and (4) ulcerative colitis, when the lesions are much more severe than might be expected under the circumstances.

Therapeutic measures for autoimmune disorders include (1) anti-immune drugs like ACTH and cortisone, (2) replacement of hormones and other secretions that are lacking, and (3) optimal nutrition to slow the rate of tissue deterioration.

(Also see ACHLORHYDRIA; ADDISON'S DISEASE; and ANEMIA.)

AVAILABLE NUTRIENT

A nutrient that is available and can be absorbed from the intestine into the blood. Not all nutrients are available or fully available; e.g., when calcium combines with phytic acid to form calcium phytate, the calcium cannot be absorbed.

AVIDIN

A proteinaceous substance in raw egg white which ties up the vitamin biotin so that it is unavailable. Cooking egg white inactivates avidin.

(Also see BIOTIN.)

AVITAMINOSIS

Literally, this means without vitamins. The condition may be due to inadequate intake of vitamins, deficient absorption, increased body requirements, or injection of antivitamins. When referring to a specific vitamin deficiency, avitaminosis is used as a prefix; for example, avitaminosis A.

AVOCADO (ALLIGATOR PEAR) *Persea americana*

The Avocado belongs to the laurel family, *Lauraceae*, which also includes cinnamon, camphor, and sassafras.

The avocado tree is an evergreen, subtropical tree which bears oval or round, green, or black fruits containing a single large seed. The fruit is called an avocado, and it may range in weight from ½ to 3 lb (.2 to 1.4 kg). The edible portion is the yellow-green pulp which is soft like butter and has a rather nutty flavor.

ORIGIN AND HISTORY. Avocados are native to Central America. Today, avocados are grown in most tropical and subtropical countries.

WORLD AND U.S. PRODUCTION. Annually, about 1.5 million metric tons of avocados are produced worldwide; and the leading producing countries, by rank, are: Mexico, United States, Dominican Republic, Brazil, Colombia, and Indonesia.[16]

---

[16]Based on data from *FAO Production Yearbook 1990*, FAO/UN, Rome, Italy, Vol. 44, p. 167, Table 73. **Note well:** Annual production fluctuates as a result of weather and profitability of the crop.

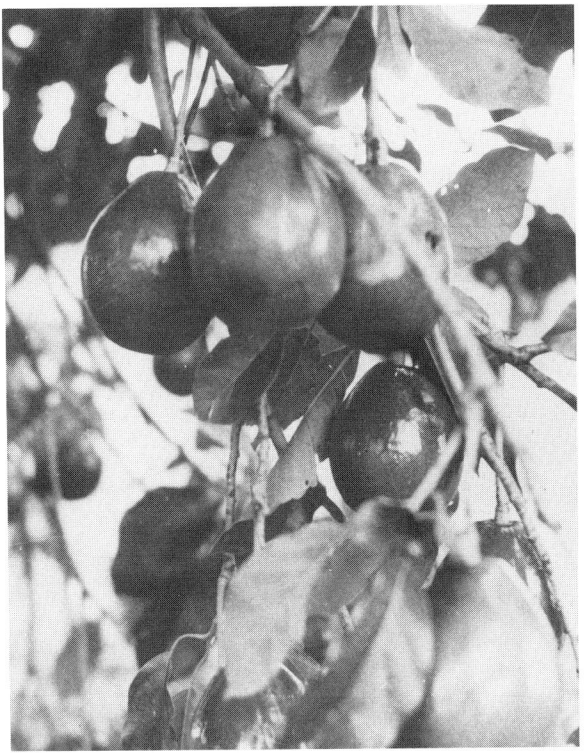

Fig. A-46. Avocados on the tree. Avocados are the *fat fruit*. The buttery flesh contains 16 to 25% fat. (Courtesy, USDA)

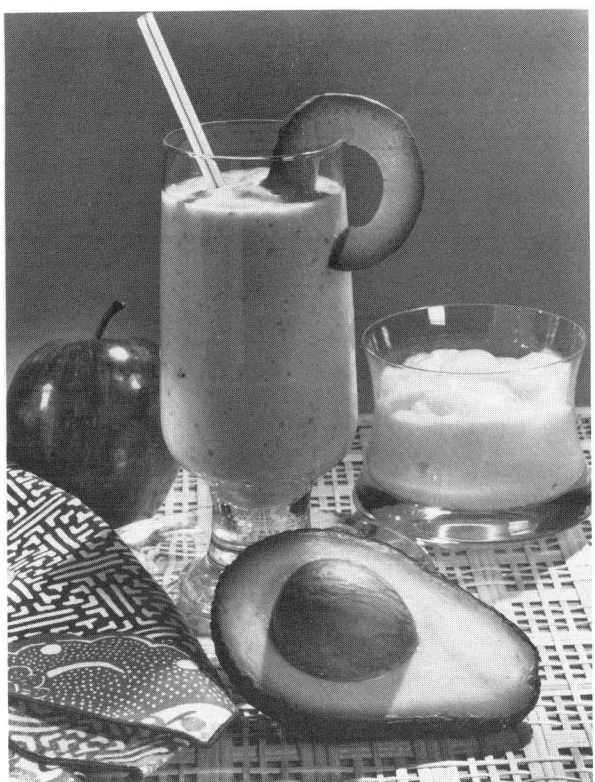

Fig. A-47. Avocados are good with other fruits. The avocado-yogurt *blenderable* breakfast contains lemon-flavored yogurt, avocado, ice, and apple, blended until smooth. (Courtesy, Harshe-Rotman & Druck, Inc., Public Relations, Los Angeles, Calif.)

The U.S. commercial production of avocados totals about 145,000 short tons annually, all of which is in California and Florida, with California alone accounting for 86% of the crop.[17]

SELECTION, PREPARATION, AND USES.
Ripened fruits are slightly soft, yielding to a gentle pressure on the skin. Avocados that do not yield to the squeeze test may be ripened during 3 to 5 days at room temperature.

Avocados are peeled and seeded, and then used in a variety of fruit dishes, cocktails, dips, salads, salad dressings, and sandwiches. Bacon and avocado sandwiches are a favorite. To avoid the brownish color of avocado flesh that develops when exposed to the air, peeled fruit should be placed immediately in lemon juice until used. Avocados may also be eaten alone, served as halves with lemon juice, vinegar, Worchestershire sauce, and salt and pepper.

NUTRITIONAL VALUE.
Nutritional data on several varieties of fresh avocados is given in Food Composition Table F-21.

The fat content of avocados ranges from 11 to 25%. Thus, avocados contain 128 to 233 Calories (kcal) per 100 g (about 3½ oz), depending primarily on their fat content. No other fruit has an energy value as high as avocados. Additionally, each 100 g of avocados provides about 1 to 2 g of protein, 500 to 700 mg of potassium, and 300 to 400 IU of vitamin A.

AVOIRDUPOIS WEIGHTS AND MEASURES

Avoirdupois is a French word, meaning to *weigh*. The old English system of weights and measures is referred to as the Avoirdupois System, or U.S. Customary Weights and Measures, to differentiate it from the Metric System.

(Also see WEIGHTS AND MEASURES.)

AZAROLE (NEOPOLITAN MEDLAR)
Crataegus azarolus

The crab apple like fruit of a tree (of the family *Rosaceae*) that grows in Algeria, Spain, France, and Italy.

Azaroles are usually yellow-orange to red in color and have a red flesh with a sweet, applelike flavor when they're ripe. However, only the fruit grown in the warmer areas of the countries bordering the Mediterranean ripens fully. In other areas, azaroles may reach maturity, but not ripeness. Unripe fruit must undergo a slight deterioration called *bletting* to become palatable. Azaroles are usually made into jam, jelly, a liqueur, or marmalade.

AZOTEMIA

An accumulation in the body of excessive amounts of urea and other nitrogenous wastes due to failure of the kidneys to excrete these products in the urine. The condition is characterized by an abnormally high level of urea in the blood.

(Also see KIDNEYS.)

AZOTOBACTER

A bacterium of the genus *azotobacter*, which is capable of synthesizing protein from atmospheric nitrogen.

---

[17]Based on data from *Agricultural Statistics 1991*, USDA, p. 177, Table 254. **Note well:** Annual production fluctuates as a result of weather and profitability of the crop.

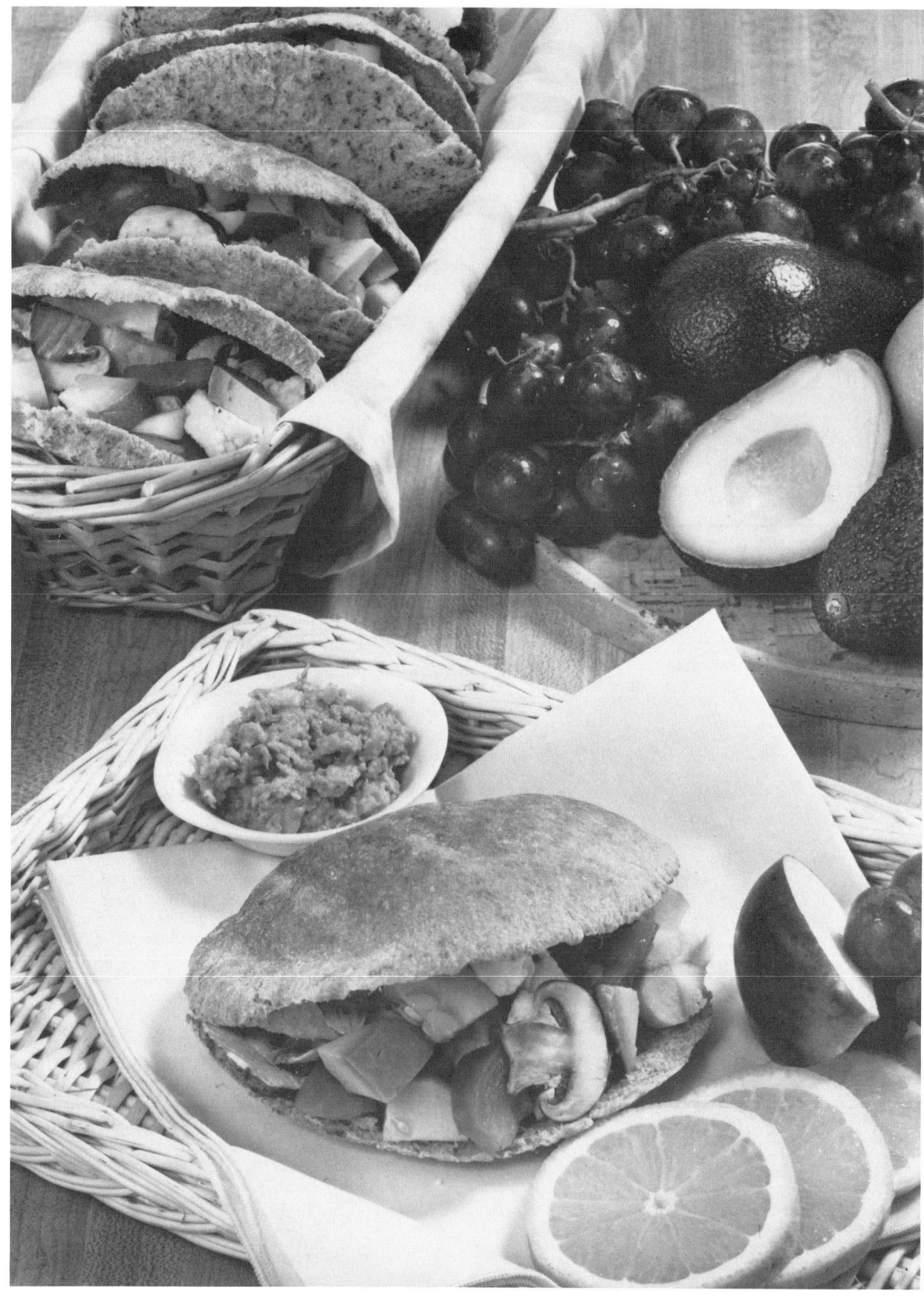

Fig. A-48. To ensure nutritional adequacy, the daily diet should include an item from each of the Food Groups. (Courtesy, The California Avocado Advisory Board, Los Angeles, Calif.)

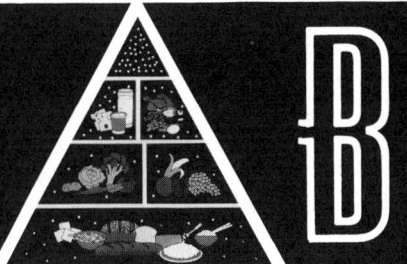

BABASSU OIL

The babassu is a type of palm which grows all over Brazil. A nondrying edible oil similar to coconut oil may be expressed from the kernels. It is usable in foods and soapmaking, but export from Brazil is small and supplies are limited.

BABCOCK TEST

This is a simple, rapid, accurate, and inexpensive test for determining the fat content of milk and cream, developed by Dr. S. M. Babcock of the University of Wisconsin in 1890.

A fat test is needed in order to establish the market value of milk and cream. Also, a fat test is important for numerous other purposes. For example, in Cheddar cheese 50% of the dry matter must be fat; hence, a fat test provides a means of standardizing milk for the production of such cheese. Similarly, fat content must be known for the production of nonfat dry milk from skim milk, butter from cream, ice cream from numerous possible sources of fat, and evaporated milk from milk.

BABY FOODS

Contents	Page

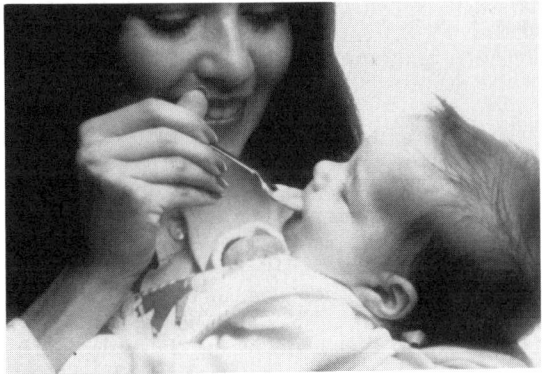

Fig. B-1. Baby foods are a specialty food item today. (Courtesy, Gerber Products Company)

The term *baby foods* usually refers to foods other than milk or formula that are fed to infants during the first year of life. Baby foods are generally used during the period between the time an infant first requires supplementation of milk or formula and the age when he or she is ready to eat the foods served to the rest of the family.

HISTORY. It was long thought that infants in prehistoric societies received only breast milk for the first year or two of life. However, there is now evidence from studies of primitive peoples that supplementation of breast-feeding was often started early in infancy. For example, anthropologists have found (1) that Eskimos traditionally gave their babies bits of raw fish and meat; (2) that Australian aborigines supplemented breast-feeding with honey, turtle eggs, fish, meat, fruits, and vegetables; and (3) that Masai tribes in Africa fed blood drawn from their cattle.

The spread of subsistence agriculture and the decline of nomadic hunting, fishing, gathering, and the herding of livestock eventually led to the weaning of infants on diluted gruels made from grains, starchy roots and tubers, and occasionally, legumes. Diets limited to these plant products have often been responsible for the development of protein-energy malnutrition in children. Hence, the settling of people in farming societies may not have resulted in an impoverishment in the health of children, unless sufficient amounts of animal products were produced. Therefore, it is noteworthy that even in recent times the agriculturists who fed their infants dairy products, eggs, and meat from cattle, goats, pigs, poultry, and sheep had much healthier children than those who utilized mainly cultivated grain and root crops.[1]

The baby food industry was born in 1928 in response to a challenge of Mrs. Dan Gerber to her husband, whose family owned the Fremont Canning Company in Fremont, Michigan. She asked him if strained food for babies could be produced at the cannery so that mothers might be spared the tedious chore of straining foods at home. He investigated the possibility, and soon tins of strained carrots, peas, prunes, spinach, and vegetable soup were being produced and promoted by salesmen who toured the country in Austin automobiles. Other companies soon entered the competition for a share of the growing market, and new products were developed.

IMPORTANCE OF SUPPLEMENTING MILK OR FORMULAS AT AN EARLY AGE. Baby foods, which were once viewed as luxury items, are now seen in a new perspective as a result of the discovery that mothers in primitive societies often fed their babies supplemental foods (some of which were prechewed by the mother) soon after birth.[2] Furthermore, health professionals working with people in the developing countries are now recognizing that there is usually need to supplement mother's milk when the infant reaches 3 months of age. In the United States, many pediatricians recommend that solid foods may be introduced at 4 to 6 months of age, although many mothers do so much earlier. It appears that mothers in Europe start supplementary foods at 6 to 10 weeks of age. Some of the major reasons for supplementing breast milk or evaporated milk prepara-

[1]Price, W. A., *Nutrition and Physical Degeneration*, Paul B. Hoeber, Inc., 1939.
[2]Raphael, D., "Margaret Mead—A Tribute," *The Lactation Review*, 1979, Vol. 4:1, p. 2.

tions may be deduced from comparisons of the nutrient composition data of these items with the Recommended Daily Allowances (RDAs) for infants, which are shown in Fig. B-2.

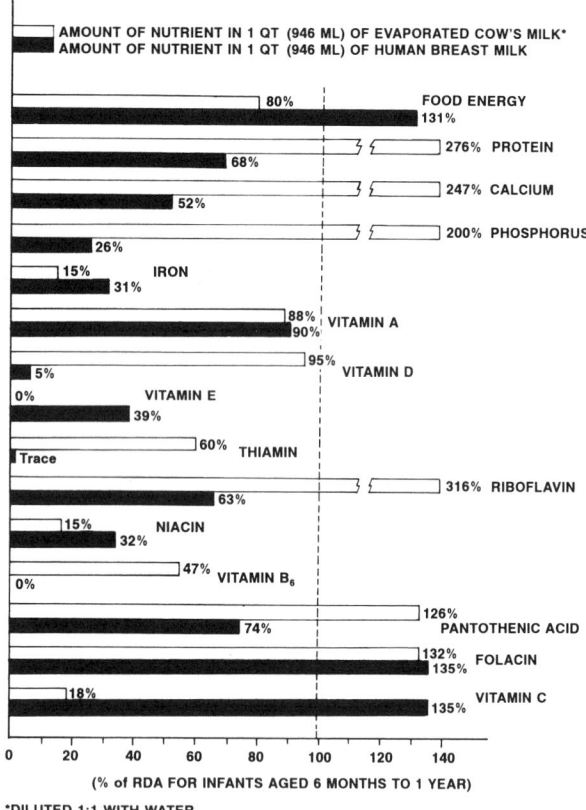

Fig. B-2. Percentages of the RDAs for infants which are supplied by 1 qt (0.95 liter) of either human milk or evaporated milk diluted 1:1 with water. (Based upon data from *Recommended Dietary Allowances*, 10th rev. ed., National Academy of Sciences, 1989, and Table F-21, Food Compositions, p. 450 of this book.)

It may be seen from Fig. B-2 that for infants at age 6 months, a quart (0.95 liter) of diluted evaporated milk provides very high levels of protein, calcium, and phosphorus. Some nutritionists and specialists in infant growth believe that large excesses of these nutrients may be harmful because (1) the infant's kidneys may be taxed in ridding the body of the metabolic waste products, and (2) an excessively rapid and stressful rate of growth may be stimulated since calves that are fed cow's milk double their birth weight in 5 to 10 weeks, whereas infants require about 21 weeks. Furthermore, the evaporated milk falls far short of providing the allowances for iron, vitamin E, and vitamin C; and is moderately low in calories, thiamin (vitamin B-1), and vitamin B-6 (pyridoxine). Therefore, greater dilution of evaporated milk to lower the levels of protein, calcium, and phosphorus would make the deficiencies of the other nutrients even worse.

Human breast milk provides far too little phosphorus, iron, vitamin D, vitamin E, thiamin, and vitamin B-6; and is low in calories, protein, calcium, riboflavin, niacin, and pantothenic acid. Hence, reliance solely on this food for the feeding of infants aged 6 months and older is likely to result

in slower than optimal rates of growth that may be accompanied by various nutritional deficiencies such as anemia.

Although commercially produced infant formulas now provide the proper amounts and proportions of nutrients for infants up to 1 year of age, it is better to introduce solid foods early than to rely solely on the formulas, because some nutritionists, pediatricians, and psychologists fear that failure to give infants solid foods shortly after they have learned to chew may lead to great difficulty in getting them to accept solids later. (Psychologists believe that certain types of learning and behavioral advances are most likely to occur during the periods when the body undergoes the developmental changes that allow the new learning or behavior to be practiced. It is noteworthy that chewing strengthens an infant's throat muscles for the development of speech.) Also, the feeding of sweetened milk or formulas in nursing bottles to infants after some of the teeth have erupted (this stage usually starts at about 6 months of age) may lead to *nursing bottle syndrome,* which is tooth decay initiated by prolonged contact of the sweetened mixture with the teeth. This undesirable condition is most likely to result from habitually giving a bottle to an infant at bedtime when the rate of sucking is very slow and the flow of saliva is minimal.

GUIDELINES FOR INTRODUCING BABY FOODS DURING THE FIRST YEAR.
While still meeting individual needs, the baby's first year should be a gradual transition to the following *broad* pattern—a working toward including in the daily diet suitable portions of foods from *each* of the following groups:

Milk group, including milk products, cheese, and ice cream.

Meat group, including beef, veal, pork, lamb, liver, poultry, fish, eggs (occasionally dry beans, peas and nuts for older children and adults).

Vegetable-fruit group, including a dark-green or deep-yellow vegetable (for vitamin A value) and a citrus fruit or other good vitamin C source, daily.

Bread-cereal group, emphasizing whole grain, fortified or enriched varieties.

Babies grow and develop at different rates. Some babies need more nutrients at an earlier time than breast milk or a formula can provide. The age for introduction will be variable but most doctors choose sometime within the baby's first month to start fruit juice, and by the third or fourth month to start infant cereals and/or strained foods.

It is noteworthy that some pediatricians consider that an infant is ready for semisolid foods when (1) his or her weight is 11 to 13 lb (5 to 6 kg), or double the birth weight; (2) more than a quart of milk or formula is consumed daily; (3) breast feeding fails to meet his or her demands for at least 3 hours after each feeding, and (4) he or she seems to be chronically hungry or dissatisfied. Usually, one or more of these signs are present before there's a possibility of nutritional deficiency. Therefore, parents can offer the first supplementary beverages and foods in a relaxed frame of mind, not worrying whether they're accepted the first day, the first week or even the first month they're offered.

Suggestions for introducing these items are given in Table B-1.

(Also see BREAST FEEDING; and INFANT DIET AND NUTRITION.)

TABLE B-1

SUGGESTIONS FOR INTRODUCING SUPPLEMENTARY BEVERAGES AND FOODS DURING THE FIRST YEAR

Beverage or Food	Stage at Which Supplementary Item is Introduced	Comments
Fruit juices	Fruit juices are usually started *between 2 and 4 weeks of age*. Use juices that are naturally high in vitamin C or those that have vitamin C added. Use fresh, canned, or frozen orange juice or a noncitrus fruit juice fortified with vitamin C. Fresh juice should be strained to remove the pulp.	At first, juices are usually given in small amounts in a nursing bottle. They are prepared by mixing with cool water that was boiled to kill germs. The amount of water may be decreased each day until undiluted juice is fed (usually within a week or so of starting the item). Once weaning has been started, the juices may be given in a cup.
Cereals	Cereals with iron are usually started *between 2½ and 3 months of age*. Iron is needed to prevent iron-deficiency anemia. Read the label. Look for *iron-fortified* cereals. Special baby cereal (in the box) has extra iron added. Quick or instant Cream of Wheat has extra iron added. Grits and cornmeal are not good sources of iron unless enriched with iron. Use an iron-fortified cereal each day. Cereal is usually offered at the morning and evening feeding. Try rice cereal first as there is less chance of the baby having an allergic reaction. Then try oat or barley cereals. Wheat cereals may then be added. Mixed cereals should not be started until all of the single-grain cereals have been accepted by the baby without any allergic reaction.	These items are usually the first solid foods fed to a baby. They should be *fed by spoon rather than putting them into the baby's bottle because the* swallowing of semisolids is an important function to be developed at 2½ to 3 months of age. (At first, it is natural for infants to reject solids by thrusting the tongue out, which is an inborn reflex that protects against choking. However, the tongue thrust reflex disappears as the baby learns to swallow solids.) Swallowing is made easier by holding an infant with its head tipped back slightly and by placing the food near the back of the tongue. The mother should hold the baby in a relaxed manner and refrain from *force feeding* since eating should be a pleasant experience.
Vegetables	Vegetables are usually started *between 3 and 4 months of age*. They provide vitamins and minerals needed for growing. Dark yellow and leafy green vegetables provide vitamin A which helps keep the eyes and skin healthy. Vegetables also add color and new flavors to the baby's meals. Bulk from vegetables helps promote regular bowel movements.	Start with a teaspoon (5 ml) or so of a mild-tasting vegetable such as beets, carrots, green beans, green peas, or squash. Then, increase the amount gradually to about ½ of a small jar daily, but reduce the amount if the baby develops loose stools. It is desirable for infants to receive at least two different vegetables each day. Therefore, vegetables should have priority over fruits when the baby's appetite is small.
Fruits	Fruits are usually started *between 3 and 4 months*. This is a new *sweet taste* for the baby. Fruits supply vitamins and minerals. They also provide bulk to prevent constipation. Include a serving of fruit each day.	Begin with 1 tsp (5 ml) and gradually increase until the baby is getting 2 to 3 Tbsp (30 to 45 ml). Do not use raw fruit except ripe bananas until the baby is older. If the infant's stools become soft and *runny*, stop the fruit for a few days; then add a small amount gradually.
Cottage cheese	Strained cottage cheese and fruit mixtures may be introduced *between 3 and 4 months of age*, provided that the infant has already been fed iron-fortified cereals and other semisolid foods on a regular basis. Ordinary cottage cheese may be fed after the baby has been given junior foods.	The nutritive value of cottage cheese is similar to that of milk or formula. Hence, it should be fed in combination with other types of foods so that an excessive emphasis on dairy products is avoided. Only very fresh cottage cheese should be fed to infants since they are very susceptible to diarrhea caused by spoilage microorganisms.
Yogurt	Yogurt may be introduced *between 3 and 4 months of age*, provided that the infant has already been fed iron-fortified cereals, fruits, and vegetables on a regular basis. Plain yogurt mixed with a little strained fruit or juice is better than the sweetened, flavored varieties.	Yogurt has essentially the same nutritive value as the milk (whole or skim) from which it is made. Hence, the feeding of milk or formula plus yogurt without other foods places too much emphasis on dairy goods. Some doctors have treated infant diarrhea successfully by substituting yogurt for milk or formula.
Meats	Meats are usually started *by 6 months of age*. They supply protein needed to build and repair muscles and other body tissues, and iron that is needed to prevent the baby from getting anemic. Meat also supplies minerals and vitamins needed to keep the body healthy. Begin with 1 tsp (5 ml) of meat gradually increase to 2 or 3 Tbsp (30 to 45 ml) daily. Start with one meat and feed it several days before adding a new flavor. This gives the baby a chance to learn to like the taste. It also gives the mother a chance to see if her baby is allergic to the meat.	Plain meats are best for babies with small appetites because they are more concentrated sources of protein than the meat and vegetable mixtures. However, the latter products may be more suitable for hearty eaters since the feeding of excessive amounts of protein should be avoided. Furthermore, the mixtures teach babies to like blends of flavors that will be encountered later in stews and other mixed dishes.
Egg yolks	Egg yolks are usually started *between 4 and 6 months of age*. Egg yolks (yellows) give an infant iron needed to make red blood. They also give the baby a new taste and texture. Begin with 1 tsp (5 ml) and gradually increase until he or she is getting one yolk each day. If a rash develops, see your doctor before giving egg yolk again.	Egg whites should not be used until recommended by your doctor. They may cause the baby to have an allergic reaction.
Baked goods	Dry toast is a good food to develop chewing at *5 to 7 months of age*. To prepare, cut small strips of bread and put in a low (200 °F or 93°C) oven for 1 hour. Store this hard toast in an airtight container. Commercially made teething biscuits are especially shaped for easy grasping. They are hard-baked for biting and to prevent crumbling. The latter is a safety factor since crumbs can choke a baby. That's why babies shouldn't be allowed to eat breads or other dry foods while lying down or unattended. Animal-shaped cookies are also hard-baked and have a thin glaze fortified with several B vitamins.	These products are best suited for use as snacks or desserts after the major food items have been consumed. Therefore, the amounts fed should be limited in order to prevent spoiling of the baby's appetite for other items. Although the first baked goods given infants are usually made from enriched white flour, items made from whole wheat flour should be introduced by age 1, so that the growing child learns to eat more nutritious products.

BACILLARY DYSENTERY (SHIGELLOSIS)

An acute infection of the bowel with *Shigella bacilli*. It is characterized by fever; abdominal pain; vomiting; and diarrhea which contains fluid and mucus, blood and pus, if the organisms have ulcerated the intestines. Often the victim becomes dehydrated and loses weight. There is a high death rate in infants from bacillary dysentery. Even when treated with antibiotics, the condition may continue for a long time.

Due to the loss of nutrients, mineral salts, and water, it is essential that nutrients and fluids be consumed by the afflicted person. Frequent small meals with an adequate caloric content, but which are high in protein and low in fat and carbohydrate, are usually most successful. It may be necessary to give fluids intravenously to combat the dehydration.

The source of infection is infected human feces, which is a potential source of contamination in food or water. It is noteworthy that flies may carry the organism to areas where foods are prepared.

(Also see BACTERIA IN FOOD; and FOODBORNE DISEASE.)

BACILLUS

A rod-shaped form of bacteria. These organisms are commonly found in soil, milk, and the intestine of man and animals. Most of the bacilli found in the colon are harmless, but a few species such as *Bacillus cereus* and *Shigella* may cause illness.

(Also see BACTERIA IN FOOD; and FOODBORNE DISEASE.)

BACON

Cured and smoked sides of pork carcasses.
(Also see MEAT.)

BACON, FLITCH OF

A side of cured and smoked bacon.

BACTERIA

Microscopic, single-cell plants, found in most environments; some are beneficial, others are capable of causing disease.
(Also see BACTERIA IN FOOD.)

BACTERIA IN FOOD

Bacteria—microscopic, single-celled plants—are very small. Most of them are of the order of one to a few microns in cell length and somewhat smaller than this in diameter. (A micron is 1/25,000 of an inch or 1/1000 of a millimeter.) They can penetrate the smallest opening, many of them can even pass through the pores of an eggshell once the natural bloom of the shell is worn or washed away.

Bacteria may enter food during production, handling, processing, or serving. Since they require nutrients, moisture, and temperatures conducive to their growth, not all bacteria will grow in food; and one species may thrive where another will not. Some bacteria require oxygen from the air—they are known as *aerobic*; others grow in the absence of oxygen—they are *anaerobic*. Some bacteria like temperatures below freezing, others higher temperatures. The minimum temperature for most bacteria is 10°F (-12°C), the maximum 140° to 190°F (60° to 88°C).

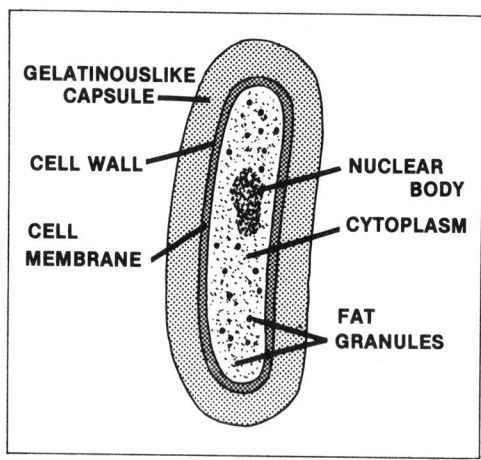

Fig. B-3. Diagram of typical cell structure of bacteria. Although some bacteria have certain special structures, almost all of them have the basic parts shown above.

BACTERIA MAY BE HELPFUL OR HARMFUL. Most bacteria are helpful—they're benefactors of mankind; without them, no life on earth could exist. But some bacteria are harmful—they're agents of disease and death.

Helpful Food Bacteria. Fortunately, many bacteria benefit foods and are widely used in biological oxidation reactions and in fermentation processes. Butter and cheese, for example, depend on bacteria for the development of their characteristic flavors. Bacteria are indispensable for making pickles, sauerkraut, olives, yogurt, buttermilk, beer, and wine. They are also employed in the manufacture of corn beef and rye bread. Bacteria are used to enhance the flavor of coffee, being introduced just prior to the roast. Also, a bacterium of the genus *Acetobacter* is used in making vinegar.

In recent years, bacteria have been employed to produce protein. Grown on petroleum-based raw materials—heavy oils, long chain paraffins, etc.—these bacteria, which contain 45 to 85% protein, may eventually have an important role in food production. Good progress has been made in petroprotein production for animals. Product purity, nutritive quality, and gastrointestinal tolerance stand in the way, at present, of the use of petroprotein as human food.

In addition to their role in foods, other helpful bacteria are found in the gastrointestinal tracts of ruminants (cattle, sheep, etc.) and pseudoruminants (horses, rabbits, etc.) which synthesize most, if not all, of the B vitamins and vitamin K; the nitrogen-fixing bacteria which grow in nodules (small bumps) on the roots of legume plants and convert nitrogen gas in the air into chemical forms that can be used by plants and animals; the bacteria that are used in sewage treatment plants to purify water; and the bacteria that are important in the cycling of chemicals in nature—for example, after a plant or animal dies, bacteria help break down the dead organisms into simple molecules that can be used by living plants and animals.

Harmful Food Bacteria. Many bacteria are harmful—they may cause food spoilage or foodborne diseases.

Bacteria are involved in many, but not all, types of food spoilage. The stale, putrid odor of spoiled meat, the foul odor of spoiled egg, and the sour odor of spoiled milk are examples of bacteria food spoilage. Both fresh and canned foods are subject to food spoilage. Some types of food spoilage are caused by enzymes, and others are caused by chemical reactions—for example, by nonenzymatic browning. The control of bacterial spoilage has received a tremendous amount of research attention since the days of Louis Pasteur, who pioneered in the study of bacteria.

Foodborne diseases are of two types: (1) food infections (bacterial), and (2) food poisonings (bacterial toxins). The most common diseases in each of these categories will be discussed briefly in the sections that follow.

FOOD INFECTIONS (bacterial). Each year, more than 24 million Americans suffer from botulism, salmonellosis, and other foodborne illnesses. When unreported, untreated, and misdiagnosed cases are added, the number may exceed 70 million. Victims often experience little more than an upset stomach, but nearly 9,000 cases prove fatal.

Food infections result from the ingestion of food with large amounts of viable bacteria, which multiply inside the host (man) and cause infectious diseases. Each disease is caused by a specific organism. Because incubation and multiplication of the bacteria take time, symptoms of food infection develop relatively slowly, usually 12 to 24 hours or more after the infected food has been eaten.

Foodborne infections are especially prevalent in poor urban communities with inadequate facilities for storing foods and unsanitary water supplies and lavatories. Under such circumstances, food-related infections are common and contribute to a high sickness and death rate, especially in children.

The usual diet therapy for a bacterial food infection includes: providing small amounts of cracked ice, barley water, and tea until the gastrointestinal disturbance stabilizes. Then, custards, gelatin, eggs, milk, toast, broth and/or cream soups can be given. Solid foods can usually be tolerated on the second or third day and the usual diet can be resumed.

The common bacterial food infections are summarized in Table B-2.

TABLE B-2
FOOD INFECTIONS (BACTERIAL)

Disease	Disease Organism	Signs and Symptoms	How Disease Is Transmitted	Prevention and Treatment	Remarks
Bacillus cereus	*Bacillus cereus*, a saprophytic, (bacteria that obtain food by absorbing dissolved organic material) spore-bearing organism widely found in nature.	Severe vomiting 1 hour after ingestion, or diarrhea later. Recovery is rapid.	Usually, the disease occurs among those who eat in Chinese restaurants. The spore may survive normal cooking and produce vegetative forms during cooling.	Do not allow cooked rice to cool over a long period without refrigerating.	*Bacillus cereus* occurs in many samples of uncooked rice.
Brucellosis (Bang's disease, undulant fever, Malta fever)	*Brucella abortus. Brucella melitensis. Brucella suis.* The genus *Brucella* is named after Sir David Bruce, a British army doctor, who, working in Malta in 1887, first isolated the organism from goats and from soldiers who had been drinking goat's milk.	A recurrent or undulating fever, which may rise to 104° to 105°F (*40° to 41°C*) in the evening, then drop to normal each morning; sweating; fatigue; muscle ache; constipation. If untreated, symptoms may persist for months.	From consuming infected milk or milk products, or from infected animals.	Pasteurizing milk; testing animals and slaughtering reactors. Treatment with sulfonamides or antibiotics and with heat may be helpful.	The disease affects cattle, sheep (rarely), goats, swine, and man.
Cholera	*Vibrio comma*, a comma-shaped bacillus	Fever, severe diarrhea, abdominal cramps, vomiting, intense thirst, followed by collapse. If untreated, a 50% death rate is common. Cholera is one of the most acute and violent infections known to man.	From infected persons and fecal-contaminated food and water	Isolation of cholera patients, destruction by fire of material passed by patient, well cooked food, chlorinated water, and vaccination. Treatment consists in replacing body fluids and electrolytes.	Epidemics of cholera are rather common in India, Pakistan, and Southeast Asia.
Clostridium perfringens food infection	*Clostridium perfringens* (also known as *Clostridium welchii* or the gangrene organism), a spore-forming anaerobe widely distributed in soil, sewage, and unsanitary food processing plants.	Diarrhea, which is often accompanied by abdominal pain; and headache. Vomiting and fever are uncommon The incubation period of the disease is 8 to 24 hours. Most patients recover in 24 hours, or at the most within a few days. Rarely fatal.	Infected foods, especially meats and gravies that have been allowed to cool slowly for several hours after cooking. The spores are resistant to heat and will survive boiling for as long as 5 hours.	Cook meats adequately. Do not allow foods, especially meats and gravies, to cool slowly after cooking—refrigerate them promptly	This is the bacterium that causes gas gangrene when it infects deep wounds.

(Continued)

TABLE B-2
FOOD INFECTIONS (BACTERIAL) *(Continued)*

Disease	Disease Organism	Signs and Symptoms	How Disease Is Transmitted	Prevention and Treatment	Remarks
Escherichia coli (E. coli) food infection	*Escherichia coli.* (*E. coli*) *Escherichia* was named for the German physician, T. Escherichia, who first studied it.	Acute gastroenteritis in infants, and traveler's disease; characterized by severe watery diarrhea. In these instances, the victims may not have built up an immunity to a particular serotype (a group of closely related microorganisms distinguished by possessing a common set of antigens).	*E. coli* are one of the predominate bacterial flora of the gut. They are excreted in human feces (and urine to some extent). Thence infection is spread to foods and food utensils by flies and human hands. Baby formulas prepared under unsanitary conditions are the usual route of infection.	Avoid contaminated food and water. Avoid overindulgence with food and alcohol. Treatment with sulfa drugs and antibiotics supplemented by kaolin or pectin preparations will often afford speedy relief. Lomotil, a synthetic drug.	This disease occurs worldwide. Sometimes it is known as *tourist diarrhea* or *traveler's dysentery.*
Leptospirosis	*Leptospira,* so named because it is the smallest and most delicately formed of the spirochetes (spiral-shaped bacteria).	High fever and intense, hemorrhagic jaundice and hepatitis.	By polluted water—from drinking it or swimming in it, or through cuts or scratches on the skin. From exposure to animals or people with leptospirosis. By consuming food or water that has been polluted, usually by rats.	Prevention consists of avoiding polluted food or water, along with control of rats.	Infected dogs, cattle, horses, swine, rats, and wild animals may pollute water. Leptospirosis is most common among persons who work in foul, watery places such as sewers, rice fields, wartime trenches, and poorly built mines.
Salmonellosis It is named for the American bacteriologist and veterinarian, Daniel E. Salmon, who first isolated the organism in 1885. This is one of the most common foodborne infections in the U.S.; sometimes single outbreaks involve thousands of people.	*Salmonella typhimurium* is the organism most commonly responsible. But there are more than 1,600 types of the genus *Salmonella.*	Diarrhea, abdominal cramps, and vomiting, which usually lasts for 2 to 3 days. The incubation period is 12 to 36 hours. Salmonellosis is rarely fatal except in elderly people and infants.	*Salmonella* bacteria grow rapidly in such cooked foods as meats, eggs, custards, and salads, which have been left unrefrigerated several hours. It may also be transmitted by sewage-polluted water. The organisms may be eliminated 2 to 3 days after the symptoms subside, thereby providing a continuing source of contamination for others.	Refrigerating foods at temperatures below 40°F (4°C); hand washing by food handlers; scrupulous cleaning of food processing equipment; and avoiding use of cracked eggs unless thoroughly cooked. *Salmonella* in food is destroyed by a temperature of 140°F (60°C) for 20 minutes or 149°F (65°C) for 3 minutes. Prevent flies, cockroaches, and rodents from coming into contact with food.	An accurate bacteriological diagnosis of the cause of an outbreak is essential to establish its source.
Shigellosis (bacillary dysentery)	*Shigella* bacteria. The *Shigella* genus is named for the Japanese physician, Kiyoshi Shiga, who was the first to discover a species of the organism during an epidemic in Japan in 1898.	Fever, loss of appetite, vomiting, severe abdominal cramps, and massive diarrhea. Young children and frail adults may become dehydrated; hence, care must be taken to maintain their balance of mineral salts.	Spread by fecal contamination of food, water, clothing, and household objects by infected individuals. House flies are also an active agent in its spread.	Good public sanitation and personal hygiene; control of flies; boiling food and water and pasteurizing milk; washing hands before handling foods or eating; and isolation of patients and carriers, especially if they are handling foods. Sulfa drugs or antibiotics are used in treatment.	Epidemics of the disease most commonly occur where large groups are crowded together without adequate sanitation, such as refugee camps.
Tuberculosis (TB)	*Mycobacterium bovis* (tubercle bacillus). Robert Koch identified the causative organism in 1892.	Chronic coughing, usually fever and night sweats, extreme fatigue, loss of appetite and, eventually, coughing up blood. Enlargement of the cervical and mesenteric lymph nodes.	The bacteria are spread by particles of dust or droplets expelled by a tubercular patient, especially when coughing or sneezing; or introduced into the digestive tract by contaminated foods—such as milk from tuberculin cows or objects placed in the mouth.	Avoid contact with infected people and foods; testing, followed by slaughter of tubercular animals; pasteurization of milk; adequate and nutritious diet, comfortable living quarters; and sufficient daily rest. Successful treatment involves early detection by x-rays or by the tuberculin test—a skin test. Once the diagnosis is established, the physician will likely prescribe an antibiotic. In 1943, Dr. Selman Waksman discovered streptomycin which would kill or slow down the tubercle bacilli, for which discovery he later received the Nobel Prize.	Studies of human mummies have shown that the disease was active in the earliest Egyptian civilizations.
Tularemia (rabbit fever) It was first described in Tulare, California in 1911 (from whence came the name).	*Francisella tularensis*	An ulcerlike sore at the point where the germs enter the skin, followed by headache, aching muscles and joints, weakness, chills, and fever.	About 90% of the reported cases can be traced to handling infected wild rabbits. But the disease has been found in almost every type of small wild animal. Cats and sheep have also been known to be infected.	Prevention consists of wearing protective rubber gloves when handling wild rabbits, and thoroughly cooking meat from wild rabbits. Broad-spectrum antibiotics are effective treatment.	Those who hunt rabbits should remember that a slow-running rabbit is probably a sick rabbit, and had best be ignored.

(Continued)

TABLE B-2 *(Continued)*

Disease	Disease Organism	Signs and Symptoms	How Disease Is Transmitted	Prevention and Treatment	Remarks
Versinia entero-colitica (formerly known as *Pasteurella pseudo-tuberculosis*) food infection		Gastroenteritis	The first human cases reported in 1963 were contracted from infected chinchillas		
Vibrio parahaemo-lyticus food infection	*Vibrio parahaemolyticus*, an organism related to the cholera vibrio which grows in sea water.	Profuse diarrhea and dehydration	Consumption of raw or undercooked sea foods.	Avoid contaminated foods. Cook foods well.	

FOOD POISONINGS (bacterial toxins). Food poisoning is caused by the ingestion of bacterial toxins that have been produced in the food by the growth of specific kinds of bacteria before the food is eaten. The powerful toxins are ingested directly, and symptoms of food poisoning develop rapidly, usually within 1 to 6 hours after the food is eaten.

The common bacterial food poisons are summarized in Table B-3.

TABLE B-3
FOOD POISONINGS (BACTERIAL TOXINS)

Disease	Disease Organism	Signs and Symptoms	How Disease Is Transmitted	Prevention and Treatment	Remarks
Botulism This severe form of food poisoning was first described in Germany, in 1817 as *sausage poisoning* (the Latin word for sausage is *botulus*), the first food in which it was found.	*Clostridium botulinum* A saprophyte (bacteria that obtain food by absorbing dissolved organic material) which is widespread and found in soils, It forms heat-resistant spores. If the latter are not destroyed by heat in cooking, vegetative forms may grow anaerobically and produce one of the most powerful toxins known. According to one authority on poisons, botulism type A—the most lethal—is 10,000 times as deadly as cobra venom and millions of times more potent than strychnine or cyanide.	Weakness of the eye muscles and difficulty in swallowing, followed by paralysis of the muscles of respiration and death. Symptoms usually begin 18 to 36 hours after the food is eaten. Formerly, about 65% of all instances of botulism were fatal. Today, with early diagnosis, improved emergency hospital care, and the advent of antitoxins, the death rate is much lower. In 1988, only 84 cases of botulism were reported in the U.S.A.	Primarily by eating inadequately cooked home-canned meat, and non-acid vegetables (beans, asparagus, corn, and peas).	Adequate cooking. The toxin is inactivated in 10 minutes by heat at 176° F (80°C), but the spore is not destroyed. The food lindustry uses nitrites as a preservative to prevent the anaerobic growth of *C. botulinum*. Do not use food that shows gas production or change in color or consistency. Burn such foods; otherwise, animals may be poisoned by eating them. Discard canned food that shows bulging in one end of the can. The only known treatment is an antitoxin, which must be of the right type.	The toxin blocks transmission of the neuro-muscular junctions. Today, botulism is very rare in the U.S. Botulinus-infected foods do not necessarily taste or smell spoiled.
Staphylococcal food poisoning This is by far the most common form of food poisoning observed in the U.S. It is caused by a toxin formed in the food before ingestion.	*Staphylococcus aureus*, primarily	Vomiting and diarrhea, which may be severe and accompanied by collapse due to dehydration. Ingestion of contaminated food may be followed by symptoms within minutes to 6 hours. Usually, the illness lasts only 1 to 3 days. Mortality is low.	Ingestion of food or water containing the enterotoxin. Many healthy people are carriers of staphylococcal infections, specifically *Staphylococcus aureus*. Foods are readily contaminated by carriers and may, under suitable conditions, provide a good culture medium for growth of the organism. A wide variety of foods have been implicated, but the most common ones are ham, poultry, cream, and custard-filled baked products.	Prevent carriers from contaminating food. Prompt refrigeration of foods at 40°F (4°C) or below. Eliminate flies. *Staphylococcus* can be killed by heating to boiling temperature, but toxins may not be destroyed by boiling.	Some strains of *Staphylococcus* produce a powerful enterotoxin which is resistant to heat.

BACTERIAL CONTROL METHODS. From time immemorial, one of man's major food problems has been that of controlling the bacteria of food. Fortunately, bacteria are extremely sensitive to the conditions under which they live; hence, they are relatively susceptible to complete control. Various methods have been practiced through the ages, the most common of which are: (1) chemicals, (2) antibiotics, (3) phages, and (4) physical methods.

1. **Chemicals.** Chemicals are the chief source of bacterial control agents. The list of such agents begins with salt, its use as a preservative for fish and meat dating far back into antiquity. Sugar in high concentrations inhibits the growth of bacteria (and also yeasts and molds). Sugar in solution apparently dehydrates the bacteria as a result of osmosis. Acetic acid acts as a preservative, although it is seldom used alone as is true of other acids. Benzoates and nitrites have long been used as preservatives; their effect is bacteriostatic.

2. **Antibiotics.** The use of antibiotics in foods, and their application in food technology, has been known and studied for many years. Antibiotics may occur in foods (a) naturally, (b) through direct addition as a food additive to aid in production and keeping quality of the food, or (c) as an unintentional food additive resulting from the carry over of the antibiotic in milk, meat, or eggs, as a result of the addition of antibiotics to the feed of animals for growth promotion or medication in the treatment of diseases.

(Also see ANTIBIOTICS, section headed "Antibiotics in Foods.")

3. **Phages.** This refers to a group of organisms that attack bacteria. They are capable of destroying disease-producing bacteria and living organisms, and they have specific effects on bacteria and food—sometimes good, sometimes bad. Bacteriophages appear to be viruses composed of nucleoproteins, with capacity to multiply. They pass through bacterial filters readily.

(Also see BACTERIOPHAGE.)

4. **Physical methods.** Physical means comprise another category of bacterial control. Heat, of course, is the chief physical control method. Freezing retards proliferation. Also, the preservation of food by radiation has received much study, the goal being to sterilize foods and preserve them indefinitely.

Both high and low temperatures usually inhibit bacterial growth and multiplication. However, some bacteria, referred to as thermophils, grow at relatively high temperatures and produce what is called *flat sour* in canned foods. Other bacteria produce spores, which are quite resistant to heat, as well as other sterilizing agents. Nevertheless, all pathogens may be destroyed by heat; thus, food which has been properly cooked and handled is safe. But, in cooking, the heat may not penetrate the food sufficiently, particularly a large cut of meat (use a meat thermometer to ensure that the desired internal temperature is reached in large cuts of meat); and undercooked foods are dangerous. Furthermore, foods may be contaminated after cooking. Meat, milk, and eggs are excellent growth media for bacteria; hence, foods which have been cooked, improperly stored, then warmed up are especially dangerous. A very important group of bacteria is referred to as psychrophils, which grow and reproduce at the usual refrigeration temperatures. These bacteria are responsible for most of the fresh food spoilage that occurs. Very little bacterial growth occurs in frozen foods, and freezing temperatures bring about a very slow and usually incomplete death to most bacteria. Since the death of bacteria in frozen foods is incomplete, it must be remembered not to allow frozen foods to stand at room temperature after thawing.

Bacteria multiply by cell division at a very rapid rate. Within the temperature range of 50° to 140°F (*10° to 60° C*), the growth rate increases tenfold for each 18°F (*10°C*) increase in temperature, and under favorable conditions bacteria can double their numbers every 30 minutes. Therefore, bacterial numbers can become astronomical in foods left at room temperature for a period of 3 to 4 hours. In fact, it has been estimated that if a single *Escherichia coli* cell were given enough food under optimum conditions it could produce a mass of bacteria larger than the earth in a relatively short period of time. Of course, it would be impossible to supply enough food to keep the bacteria multiplying at the maximum rate.

PREVENTION OF BACTERIAL INFECTION AND FOOD POISONING. Prevention of infections spread by food and the fecal-oral route depends on scrupulous attention to cleanliness along the whole food chain—meat packers, slaughter houses, food manufacturers, retail shops, caterers, restaurants, and kitchens. In all these places care is required to prevent rodents and flies from getting access to food. All food handlers should be scrupulously clean in their personal habits and be provided with clean lavatories and opportunities for washing their hands. Some persons harbor a pathogen and excrete it continuously in their feces and/or urine without having any symptoms of disease. Such carriers are particularly dangerous and have been responsible for many outbreaks of disease. Public health authorities are responsible for inspecting commercial food establishments, and they have the legal right to close any premises that are not up to acceptable standards of hygiene.

A general program for preventing bacterial food infections and food poisonings follows:

1. Keep food handling areas spotlessly clean.

2. Wash hands often with soap and water, especially after using the restroom, dressing a wound, and before handling any food; this will help get rid of transient bacteria which can cause disease.

3. Wash raw fruits and vegetables thoroughly in clean water.

4. Don't handle food with hands that have cuts, bruises, or sores on them, *unless* covered by gloves.

5. Don't sneeze or cough on food or in areas where food is being prepared; wear a mask if a nose, throat, or sinus infection is present.

6. Keep body and clothes clean.

7. Wear a hairnet or a cap when handling food.

8. Keep rats, cockroaches, flies and other insects out of areas where food is processed, stored, prepared, or served.

9. Don't use wooden cutting boards—they can't be cleaned properly.

10. Sanitize cutting tools used on raw food before using them on cooked food.

11. Don't smoke in areas where food is processed, stored, prepared, or served.

12. Cook meats to the following minimum internal temperatures: fresh beef, 140°F (*60°C*); fresh veal, pork, and lamb, 170°F (*77°C*); turkey, 180°F (*82°C*) (Use a meat thermometer when cooking large cuts of meat.)

13. Keep cooking and eating equipment clean.

14. Keep perishable foods in refrigerator when not being prepared, cooked, or consumed.

15. Avoid consumption of contaminated or partially deteriorated foods.

16. Burn completely all canned foods with abnormal color or composition, putrid odor, or in bulged cans.

BACTERIAL COUNT (PLATE COUNT)

Two methods are commonly employed in determining the degree of bacterial contamination of a sample of material: (1) the plate method, and (2) the direct microscopic count.

• **Plate count method**—In the plate method, a diluted sample (such as milk) is poured onto a standard agar (which is obtained from the stems of certain seaweeds) in a Petri dish where each bacterial cell or group of cells multiplies to produce a colony which is visible to the naked eye. A count of the number of colonies gives the number of bacteria in that portion of the sample that was taken. This is the method most frequently used to estimate the bacterial count of milk. The bacterial count plays a major role in the sanitary quality of milk upon which grades are largely based. Grade A raw milk should not exceed 100,000 bacteria per milliliter; and the bacterial count of Grade A pasteurized milk should not exceed 20,000 bacteria per milliliter.

• **Direct microscopic count method**—In the direct microscopic count method for determining milk quality, 0.01 ml of milk is deposited in 1 sq cm of a glass slide, which is then dried and stained. The number of bacteria is determined by using a calibrated microscope. In addition to providing a bacterial count, this method permits recognition of the type of bacteria present and serves as a general guide to the way the milk was handled prior to sampling. Since the leucocytes and other somatic cells present will also be stained, the direct microscopic count also provides information about possible udder troubles among cows in the herd. Because dead bacteria are stained and may be counted in this method, and because in the plate count each colony is counted as if it developed from a single organism (which isn't always true), direct microscopic counts are usually 3 to 4 times greater than the figures obtained by the plate count method.

BACTERIAL ENDOTOXIN (ENDOTOXIN)

Poisonous substance present inside bacteria which separates from the cell upon its disintegration.

BACTERIAL EXOTOXIN (EXOTOXIN)

Poisonous substance that is liberated during the growth of certain bacteria. Botulism is caused by a bacterial exotoxin.

BACTERIAL SPOILAGE OF FOOD

Certain types of bacteria are involved in many, but not all, types of food spoilage. The stale odor of spoiled meat, the foul odor of a spoiled egg, the souring of milk, and the rotting of fruits and vegetables are familiar examples of bacterial spoilage. Also, the spoilage of canned foods is usually traced to bacterial causes.
(Also see BACTERIA IN FOOD.)

BACTERICIDE

A product that destroys bacteria.

BACTERIOPHAGE

The word *bacteriophage* means bacteria-eater. It refers to a substance that makes living bacteria disintegrate or dissolve. Most scientists believe that phages are viruses; but some believe that phages may be self-reproducing proteins, bacterial enzymes, or hereditary factors in bacteria. What-ever they may be, phages dissolve many kinds of bacteria, particularly those in the intestines. Also, it is noteworthy that bacteriophages exhibit a considerable degree of specificity with respect to the kind of bacteria attacked.

Bacteriophages cause considerable trouble in milk starter cultures. (A culture [starter] is a controlled bacterial population that is added to milk or milk products to produce acid and/or flavorful substances which characterize cultured milk products.) For this reason, commercial suppliers of cultures recognize the need for bacteriophage inhibitors in starter media.

(Also see BACTERIA IN FOOD, section headed "Bacterial Control Methods.")

BAKING POWDER AND BAKING SODA

These convenience leavening powders have brought about many advances in the baking industry, because they have made it possible to bake certain doughs right after mixing, instead of having to wait for the action of yeast to take place. Hence, the products made with baking powder, baking soda, or similar leavening agents are commonly called *quick breads*. Also, the use of these powders in baking is referred to as *chemical leavening* in order to distinguish it from the biological leavening obtained with sourdough starters or yeast.

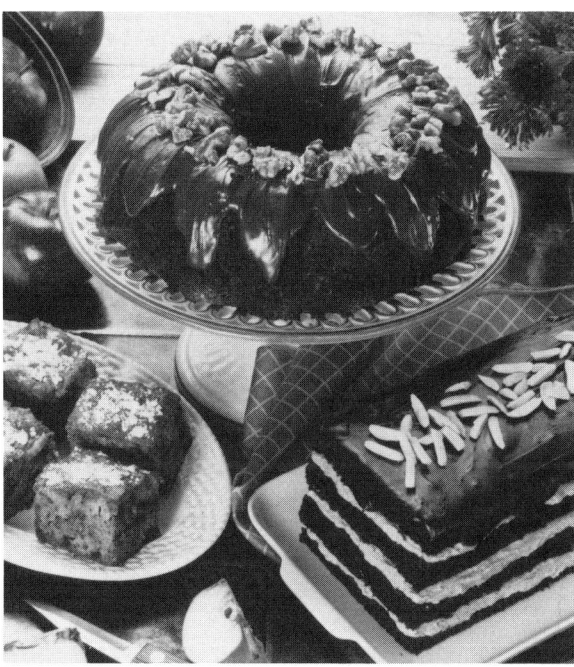

Fig. B-4. Cakes and other quick breads are usually made with baking powder, baking soda, or similar leavening agents. (Courtesy Hershey Foods Corp., Hershey, Pa.)

In addition to saving time, baking powder or baking soda allows for the use of a wide variety of ingredients in baked goods. For example, softer, weaker flours may be used in quick breads; whereas, strong flours are usually required for good yeast breads.

THE BASIC PRINCIPLES OF CHEMICAL LEAVENING.
The actual leavening agent in most baked goods is carbon dioxide gas, whether it be generated from baking powder, sourdough, or yeast. However, chemical leavening agents such as baking powder and baking soda produce carbon dioxide by means of the chemical breakdown of bicarbonate salts rather than by biological means. Some of the basic facts about bicarbonates follow:

1. Baking soda is the common name for sodium bicarbonate, a white powder which yields carbon dioxide when it is (a) dissolved in water and heated, or (b) reacted with an acid. The latter means of leavening is more desirable because reaction with an acid may convert all of the bicarbonate to carbon dioxide and water, whereas heating alone converts most bicarbonates to carbonates, carbon dioxide, and water. Residues of carbonates in baked goods are undesirable because of their bitter and soaplike taste.

2. Household baking powders usually contain a mixture of baking soda and one or more acidic salts, which may be (a) fast-acting, (b) slow-acting, or (c) a combination of (a) and (b). The leavening reaction takes place only when the powders are wetted with water or a liquid containing water.

3. Some recipes call for baking soda plus an acidic soured dairy product, rather than for baking powder.

4. Baking ammonia (ammonium bicarbonate) is sometimes used by commercial bakers in the preparation of cookies or crackers. This salt is totally decomposed into ammonia and carbon dioxide by heating.

NUTRITIONAL VALUES OF CHEMICAL LEAVENING AGENTS.
Although most batters and doughs contain only small amounts of baking powder (from 1 to 2%, on the average), this type of leavening agent contributes significant amounts of calcium, phosphorus, sodium, and/or potassium to baked products. Table B-4 gives the amounts of these minerals which are present in some commonly used baking powders and preleavened mixes.

It may be seen from Table B-4 that many of the products, when used in the amounts indicated, contribute from ¼ to ½ of the Recommended Daily Allowances (RDAs) of calcium and phosphorus (the RDA for adults for each of these minerals is 800 mg). This contribution is very important because many people may drink coffee, tea, beer, or other nondairy beverages at their meals. Hence, quick breads may make up for some of the lack of dietary calcium. Nevertheless, it pays for the consumer to read the labels on these products, because there is a wide variation in their calcium contents. For example, tartrate baking powders contain no calcium.

Some people may have to use a special, low-sodium baking powder because they have been advised to restrict dietary sodium. Fortunately, baking powders are available in which the sodium salts have been replaced by potassium salts that serve similar functions.

Most baking powders contain cornstarch. Thus, if an individual suffers from an allergy to corn, a homemade baking powder can be made by sifting together several times: 9 Tbsp (135 ml) of cream tartar and 4 Tbsp (60 ml) of baking soda.

Other Nutritive Benefits Which May Be Obtained From the Use of Baking Powders.
The fast leavening action of most baking powders eliminates some of the need for a highly elastic dough to trap carbon dioxide, because there is less time for the gas to escape prior to baking, which then stiffens the dough. Therefore, flours used for quick breads may be weaker than those that are required for good yeast breads.

Baking powder breads are often strengthened by the addition of eggs because the protein of the egg white acts as a binder. (Egg protein does not work as well in yeast breads because it loses some of its effect during the long time required for the dough to rise.) Strengthening of quick breads allows greater amounts of highly nutritious ingredients to be used without producing a heavy baked product. For example, the maximum amount of liquid skim milk which

TABLE B-4
MAJOR CONTENT OF SOME COMMON BAKING POWDERS AND PRELEAVENED PRODUCTS[1]

Leavening Agent or Preleavened Product	Quantity		Minerals			
	Measure	Weight	Calcium	Phosphorus	Sodium	Potassium
		(g)	(mg)	(mg)	(mg)	(mg)
Baking powders, classified by ingredients:[2]						
Sodium aluminum sulfate (SAS), and monocalcium phosphate, monohydrate (MCP)	1 tsp (5 ml)	3.0	58	87	329	5
SAS, MCP, and calcium carbonate	1 tsp (5 ml)	3.0	173	44	349	0
SAS, MCP, and calcium sulfate	1 tsp (5 ml)	3.0	190	47	300	0
MCP, anhydrous (coated)[3]	1 tsp (5 ml)	3.0	188	283	246	5
Cream of tartar, and tartaric acid	1 tsp (5 ml)	3.0	0	0	219	114
Low-sodium preparation[4]	1 tsp (5 ml)	3.0	145	219	0	328
Cornmeal, self-rising	1 cup (240 ml)	145.0	1,631	760	2,001	164
Flour, self-rising	1 cup (240 ml)	114.0	302	531	1,230	103

[1]Data from Food Composition Table F-21 of this book.
[2]All of the powders also contain sodium bicarbonate, except for the low-sodium product, which contains potassium bicarbonate.
[3]This product is commonly referred to as *straight phosphate* baking powder.
[4]Sodium-containing salts have been replaced by potassium salts that serve the same functions.

may be used in yeast breads is about ⅓ cup (*80 ml*) per cup of flour, whereas standard recipes for various baking powder (or baking soda) breads call for greater amounts of milk (from ½ cup [*120 ml*] to 1 cup [*240 ml*] per cup of flour). Similarly, greater amounts of such ingredients as bran, cheese, chopped dates, cornmeal, nuts, raisins, rolled oats, shortening, soy flour, and wheat germ may be added to quick breads.

(Also see BREADS AND BAKING, section headed "Quick Breads Made With Baking Powder or Baking Soda.")

BALANCED DIET

One which provides a person with the proper proportions and amounts of all the required nutrients for a period of 24 hours. In practical use, the term *diet* refers to the foods eaten by a person or a group of people without limitation to the time in which they are consumed.

BALANCE STUDY

A determination of the amount of a nutrient retained by the body under specified conditions. Measurements are made of (1) the amount of the nutrient consumed in food, and (2) amounts lost in the feces, urine, and/or sweat. The body is said to be in positive balance with respect to the nutrient when the intake is greater than the sum of the excretion products. It is in negative balance when the excretion products exceed the intake. At equilibrium, nutrient intake equals excretion.

BALDNESS

This condition, which is known in medical circles as alopecia, is a loss of hair on the skull to the extent that formerly hairy areas have become bare.

It is noteworthy that research on various species of hairy animals has established that the nutrients which might be helpful in the prevention of excessive hair loss are: amino acids, particularly those which contain sulfur (cystine and methionine); the essential, polyunsaturated fatty acids; iodine and zinc; many members of the vitamin B complex; and vitamins A, C, and E. The best way to obtain these nutrients is from a wide variety of nutritious foods such as dairy products, eggs, fish and seafood, fruits and vegetables, meats and poultry, vegetable oils, and whole-grain breads and cereal products.

BALSAM APPLE *Momordica balsamina*

The orange-red, egg-shaped fruit of a vine (of the family *Cucurbitaceae*) that originated in Africa or Asia, and was brought to the American tropics in the latter part of the 16th century. It is closely related to the balsam pear (*M. charantia*), which is shaped more like a banana. The unripe fruits are usually preferred to the ripe ones, because they grow more bitter with age. Although the very young fruits are sufficiently palatable to eat raw, balsam apples are usually made into pickles and curries, or used as flavoring for fish and meat dishes.

(Also see BALSAM PEAR.)

BALSAM PEAR (BITTER MELON)
Momordica charantia

The orange-red, furrowed, banana-shaped fruit of a vine (of the family *Cucurbitaceae*) that originated somewhere in Africa or Asia, and was taken to the West Indies and Brazil during the early days of slave trading.

Usually the bitter-flavored unripe fruits, which range from 2 to 10 in. (*5 to 25 cm*) long, are used as a vegetable, or to make curries and pickles. However, the Chinese add the fruit to fish and meat dishes, and the people of India use the seeds of the ripe fruit as a seasoning. The tender shoots and leaves of the plant may also be utilized as vegetables.

(Also see BALSAM APPLE.)

BANANA *Musa paradisiaca*, variety *sapientum*

Bananas belong to the banana family, *Musaceae*, which also includes plantains.

The slightly curved, yellow or red fruit with firm creamy flesh—the banana—is familiar to many people. It represents one of the world's leading fruit crops, and the number one seller in the produce department of American supermarkets. Americans are most familiar with the large yellow, smooth skinned banana known as *Gros Michel* (*Big Mike*) or *Martinique*, and the Cavendish varieties. A smaller red-skinned variety is known as the *Red Jamaica* or *Baracoa* banana. Plantains are also a type of banana which are used more like a vegetable than a fruit.

ORIGIN AND HISTORY. Bananas originated primarily in Malaysia about 4,000 years ago, thence they spread over an area from India to the Philippines and New Guinea. They were taken to Africa by Indonesian migrants.

WORLD AND U.S. PRODUCTION. Bananas are raised in the tropics of both the Eastern and Western Hemispheres. However, Latin America is the most important commercial banana-producing region.

Bananas are the second leading fruit crop of the world. Worldwide, about 45.8 million metric tons of bananas are produced annually; and the leading producing countries by rank, are: India, Brazil, Philippines, Ecuador, Indonesia, China, Burundi, Costa Rica, Tanzania, and Colombia.[3]

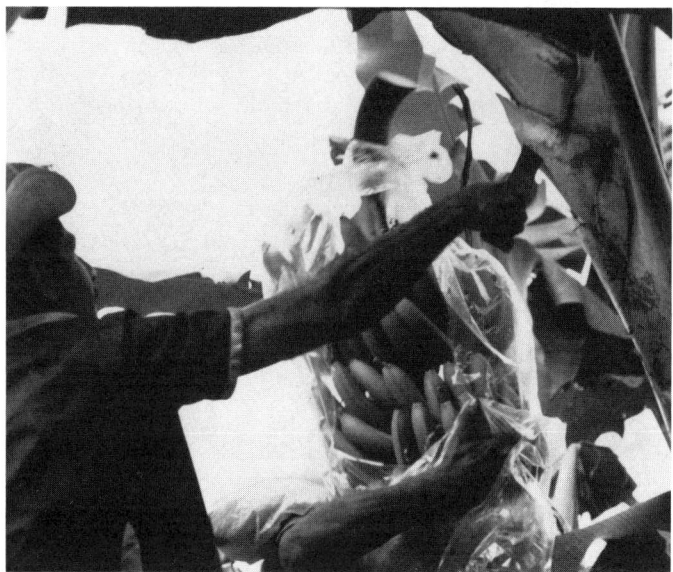

Fig. B-5. Bananas grow in bunches, weighing 60 to 100 lb (*27 to 45 kg*). Each bunch is comprised of 9 to 16 clusters of fruit called *hands*, containing 12 to 20 separate bananas or *fingers*. (Courtesy, Castle and Cooke, Inc.)

[3]Based on data from *FAO Production Yearbook 1990*, FAO/UN, Rome, Italy, Vol. 44, p. 169, Table 74. **Note well:** Annual production fluctuates as a result of weather and profitability of the crop.

Small quantities of bananas are produced in the United States; in Hawaii, and in Florida along the Gulf of Mexico. Hawaii produces about 6,000 short tons of bananas each year.[4]

PROCESSING. Almost all bananas are consumed fresh—after removing the skin—nature's unique packaging. In most areas of the United States, they can be purchased year round. Only a small amount is dried into banana flakes or chips. However, more wide use is being made of banana flour from the dried ground unripened fruit. In the tropics where bananas are grown, some are fermented to make beer.

SELECTION, PREPARATION, AND USES. Fresh bananas are at their best when the peel is solid yellow and speckled with brown and still quite firm. Bananas with green tips, or with practically no yellow color, have not developed their full flavor potential. When purchased, bananas should be firm, bright in appearance, and free from bruises or other injury. They will continue to ripen at room temperature. Bananas may be refrigerated, and they will remain good for 3 to 5 days, though the peel will turn dark.

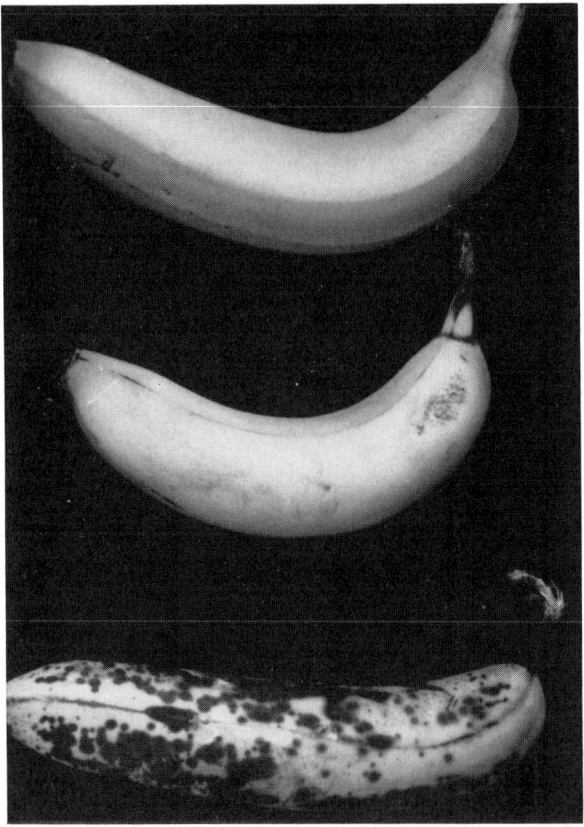

Fig. B-6. Stages of ripeness of bananas, with most ripe at the bottom. (Courtesy, University of Minnesota, St. Paul, Minn.)

Ripe bananas are peeled and then eaten whole, sliced, mashed, baked, or dipped in batter and fried. Starchy green bananas and plantains may be made digestible by cooking—baking, boiling or frying.

---

[4]Based on data from *Agricultural Statistics 1991*, USDA, p. 177, Table 254.
Note well: Annual production fluctuates as a result of weather and profitability of the crop.

Bananas may also be used in combination with other foods in fresh fruit dishes, ice cream, pies, gelatin desserts, salads, cookies and cakes.

NUTRITIONAL VALUE. Fresh bananas contain about 70 g of water, 1 g of protein, and 25 g of carbohydrate per 100 g (3½ oz; about one banana), and contribute about 85 to 100 Calories (kcal) of energy. They are good sources of potassium and vitamin A, and a fair source of vitamin C. Dried banana flakes contain only 3% water; hence, many of the nutrients, including calories, are more concentrated. Each 100 g of banana flakes contains 340 Calories (kcal) of energy, 2.8 mg of iron, and 760 IU of vitamin A. More complete information regarding the nutritional value of several varieties of bananas, banana flakes, banana powder and plantains is presented in Food Composition Table F-21.

(Also see PLANTAIN.)

BANANA FIG

Peeled bananas that have been halved lengthwise and dried without sulfuring. (The latter treatment usually prevents darkening of the fruit.) Hence, the product is darkly colored and sticky like figs.

(Also see BANANA.)

BANNOCKS

These are flat, round cakes of oat, rye or barley meal, baked on a griddle or in the oven.

BAOBAB (MONKEY BREAD) *Andansonia digitata*

Fruit of the largest tree in tropical Africa, which belongs to the family *Bombaceae* and is one of the longest lived trees in the world.

The fruit pulp is made into refreshing drinks and is also used as a condiment. It is high in calories (290 kcal per 100 g) and carbohydrates (77%), and very rich in fiber, iron, and vitamin C. Surprisingly, the fruit pulp contains more calcium (284 mg per 100 g) than milk, and the calcium to phosphorus ratio is 2.4:1.

BARBADOS GOOSEBERRY *Pereskia aculeata*

A very acidic tropical fruit (of the family *Cactaceae*) that is usually cooked and sweetened before it is consumed.

The Barbados gooseberry has a very high water content (97%) and is low in calories (11 kcal per 100 g) and carbohydrates (2%). It is a good source of vitamin A, but a poor source of vitamin C.

BARBECUE

• To roast or broil red meat, poultry, or fish on a rack or revolving spit before, over or under a source of cooking heat, usually basting with a highly seasoned sauce.

• Red meat, poultry, or fish cooked in or served with a barbecue sauce.

BARBECUE, PIT

A pit (trench) in which wood is burned to make a bed of hot coals over which meat is barbecued. Large cuts of meat are wrapped in paper and burlap, dipped in water, placed over a bed of hot coals, covered with damp soil, and cooked for 12 to 24 hours. Actually the meat is steamed.

BARBITURATES

Sedative drugs which are often used as sleeping pills or anesthetics. The chronic use of barbiturates leads to stepping up of the liver's metabolism of drugs, with the result that greater amounts of drugs are needed to produce a given effect. The need to increase the dosage of a regularly used drug is said to constitute a *tolerance* to the drug.

BARDING

The process of tying a thin sheet of bacon over lean meat.

BARFOED'S TEST

A test for all monosaccharides which gives a red precipitate of cuprous oxide when mixed with Barfoed's solution (copper acetate in acetic acid) and heated in a boiling water bath.

BARIUM MEAL

A mixture of buttermilk or malted milk with a small amount of barium sulfate. The fluid is given orally or as an enema after an overnight fast. The parts of the digestive system containing the barium sulfate can then be seen on a fluoroscope.

BARLEY *Hordenum vulgare*

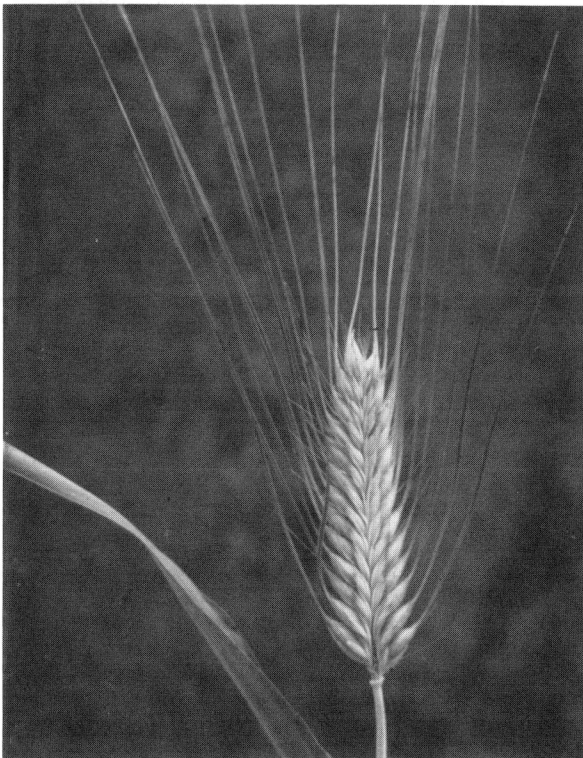

Fig. B-7. A closeup look at a barley head. (Courtesy, USDA)

This important cereal grain belongs to the grass family, *Gramineae*. It is classed as genus *Hordenum*, species *H. vulgare*. The barley plant resembles wheat.

Barley has long been used as a human food and beverage in the Asian countries. It produces the most satisfactory malt of all cereals, and is the basis of the best beers and much whiskey in many countries.

(Also see CEREAL GRAINS.)

ORIGIN AND HISTORY. Barley was formerly believed to have originated as early as 7000 B.C. in the dry lands of southwestern Asia, where wild strains of the grain may still be found. Apparently, the primitive people of this area used barley as food for man and beast, and fermented it to make an alcoholic beverage, as evidenced by the oldest known recipe for barley-wine found engraved on a Babylonian brick dated about 2800 B.C.

More recent research points to two primary centers of origin of barley: (1) the highlands of Ethiopia, and (2) southeastern Asia. In any case, barley is one of the oldest cultivated grains, as old as agriculture itself.

WORLD AND U.S. PRODUCTION. Barley is grown throughout the world. It is the most dependable cereal crop where drought, summer frost, and alkali soils are encountered. Barley is the fourth ranking cereal crop of the world, being exceeded only by wheat, corn, and rice. World production totals 180 million metric tons; and the ten leading barley-producing countries, by rank, are: U.S.S.R., Germany, Canada, France, Spain, United States, United Kingdom, Turkey, Denmark, and Czechoslovakia.[5]

Barley is the fourth leading cereal grain in the United States. The United States produces about 9,047,290 metric tons (*418,856,000 bu*), annually; and the ten leading states, by rank, are: North Dakota, Montana, Idaho, Minnesota, South Dakota, Washington, Colorado, California, Wyoming, and Oregon.[6]

PROCESSING BARLEY. The most important uses of barley are for human food, beverages, and livestock feed. In 1990, 47% of the U.S. barley supply was used for food, alcohol, and seed, and 53% was used for feed.

Barley is processed for human use by milling and malting as follows:

Milling. Like oats and rye, barley grains are covered with hulls or husks, while wheat, rye, and corn have naked seeds. The structure of the dehusked barley grain is similar to that of wheat—both grains have an outer seed coat covering an aleurone layer (the bran layer), a large starchy endosperm, and an oil-containing germ.

Most of the barley used for human food in the United States, and in some other parts of the world, is in the form of whole kernels from which the outer hull or husk and part of the aleurone layer (the bran layer) have been removed. Different types of machines provide scouring or abrasive actions, called pearling, to remove the indigestible hull and all or part of the bran layer. After three successive pearlings,

---

[5]Based on data from *FAO Production Yearbook 1990*, FAO/UN, Rome, Italy, Vol. 44, pp. 77-78, Table 19. **Note well:** Annual production fluctuates as a result of weather and profitability of the crop.

[6]Based on data from *Agricultural Statistics 1991*, USDA, p. 45, Table 58. **Note well:** Annual production fluctuates as a result of weather and profitability of the crop.

all of the hull and most of the bran are removed; the remaining kernel part is known as pot barley. Two or three additional pearlings, followed by sizing with a grading wheel, produce pearl barley—small, round, white grains of uniform size, from which most of the embryo has been removed. From 100 lb (*45 kg*) of barley, about 65 lb (*29 kg*) of pot, or 35 lb (*16 kg*) of pearl, barley are produced. It is estimated that six pearlings remove 74% of the protein, 85% of the fat, 97% of the fiber, and 88% of the mineral of the original barley.

A variety of products is produced by the milling of whole barley grains to different percentages of extraction. These are listed and described in Table B-5.

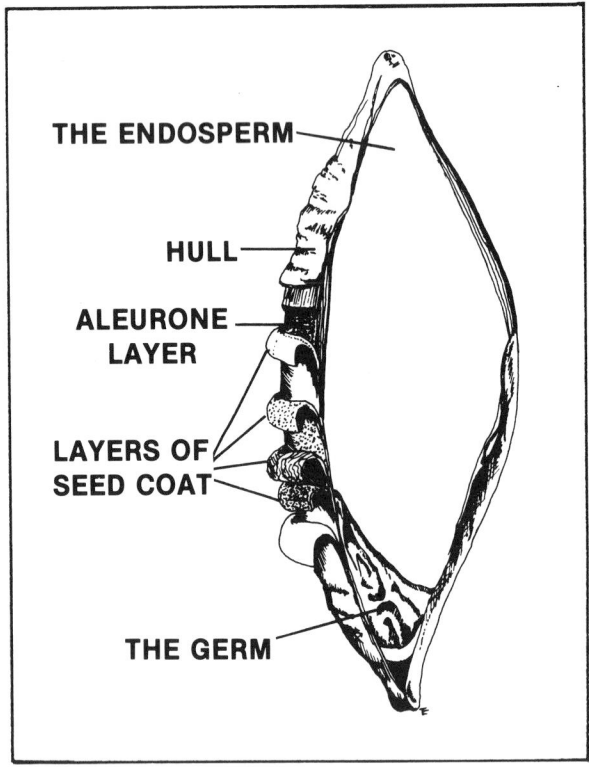

Fig. B-8. Cross section of a barley grain.

Malting (Sprouting).   Barley occupies a unique position in malting and brewing, stemming from the fact that the aleurone layer is 3 to 4 cells thick in barley, while most other cereals have only a single layer of aleurone cells. These cells contain the protein that is converted to enzymes during germination of the grain. It follows that barley is better suited for malting than the other cereal grains.

The malting process involves the germination (sprouting) of barley in a controlled state, followed by drying under conditions that retain enzymatic activity.

Malting depends upon development of various enzymes within the aleurone layer of the intact grain of barley when it is germinated under suitable conditions. Failure of grains to germinate results in loss of profit to the malter, so care is taken to select whole, undamaged grains. Also, freshly harvested barley is usually stored for at least 3 weeks prior to malting because there is more likely to be a high rate of germination of barley which has been stored for a short time.

During malting, enzymatic action converts part of the starch to maltose (a disaccharide sugar like lactose and sucrose) and some of the insoluble proteins to soluble proteins. The germination process is stopped by careful heating and drying of the grain (so as to retain enzyme activity) before an excess amount of sprouting has taken place, following which the sprouts are removed from the malted grain by passing the dried malt through revolving sets of wire screens.

Malted barley is usually subjected to further processing steps which yield the products listed and described in Table B-5.

NUTRITIONAL VALUE.   In comparison with corn, barley contains approximately the same percentage of carbohydrates, about 3% more protein, and slightly less fat. Because of the hull, it contains 5% less digestible material.

Malting and milling of barley yield a variety of products which differ widely in their nutrient compositions. Food Composition Table F-21 gives nutrient data for selected barley products.

Pearling barley is a refining process. It removes protein, fiber, minerals, and vitamins. Thus, the decrease in nutrient content which results from the milling of barley are similar to those resulting from the milling of rice, wheat, corn, and other grains.

During the malting of barley, there is an increase in the levels of the vitamin B complex and a decrease in the starch content. Thus, there are more nutrients per calorie in the malted grain. Also, part of the carbohydrate and protein of the original barley grain is digested by the action of enzymes produced during malting. So, the malted product has both increased digestibility and greater palatability due to the roasted malt flavor.

The production of beer and whiskey from barley malt yields such by-products as brewers' grains, brewers' yeast, distillers' grains, and distillers' solubles, all of which are good sources of the B vitamins and various other nutrients.

(Also see BEERS AND BREWING; CEREAL GRAINS; DISTILLATION; FERMENTATION; MALT; and UNIDENTIFIED FACTORS.)

BARLEY PRODUCTS AND USES.   Broadly speaking, barley is used in two ways: (1) commercially in foods, beverages, and feeds; and (2) in home recipes.

The production of foods and beverages from barley is almost always linked to the production of animal feeds since the foods and beverages consumed by man are usually produced by milling the whole grain to remove the hull, seed coat, aleurone layer, and embryo; or by malting the grain to make beer or whiskey.

Barley finds little use for human food in North America and Europe, but it is widely used for this purpose in Asia. In the developed countries, the predominant use of barley for human food is the production of beer from malted grain. In the developing countries, however, a considerable amount of the grain is used as a cereal and for bread making. It is inevitable that world food shortages and increased population will force the developing nations to divert even greater amounts of barley and other grains to human use, rather than share precious grain with animals.

Table B-5 presents in summary form the story of barley products and uses for human food.

(Also see BREADS AND BAKING; CEREAL GRAINS; and FLOURS, Table F-12 Major Flours.)

TABLE B-5
BARLEY PRODUCTS AND USES FOR HUMAN FOOD

Product	Description	Uses	Comments
Barley 1. Pot barley (Scotch barley)	The remaining kernel following three pearlings, with all of the hull and most of the bran removed.	Commonly used in mushroom and barley soup (a favorite of Jewish and Russian peoples), Scotch broth (a hearty soup), stews, vegetable dishes, and dressings.	*Caution:* It is hazardous to cook barley in a pressure cooker unless a small amount of oil or fat is added to the barley and water mixture prior to cooking. Barley forms a starchy foam which may clog the safety valve of the pressure cooker. This may cause a buildup of pressure until the counter weight is blown from the vent. This hazard may be alleviated by first obtaining drippings of fat from either lamb shanks or short-ribs of beef by browning them in the open pressure cooker, then cooking the ingredients together (the meat is placed on a rack over the mixture of barley, drippings, and water) under pressure for 15 min., after which the heating is stopped and the pressure is allowed to drop by itself until it is safe to open the cooker (about 20 min. after the cessation of heating).
2. Pearl barley	The remaining kernel after 2 to 3 additional pearlings beyond the pot barley stage, followed by sizing—small, round, white grains of uniform size, from which most of the embryo has been removed.	Immigrants to the U.S. from Northern Europe and the Middle East brought with them many recipes for tasty dishes which contained refined barley. Some suggestions for preparing barley dishes follow. Barley, which has a flavor that is stronger than polished rice but not as strong as brown rice, may be substituted for rice in many recipes such as casseroles, porridges, puddings, and soups. Also, when cooked in water (use 4 cups [*960 ml*] of water per cup [*240 ml*] of barley), its cooking time is about the same as that for brown rice—about 45 min. The flavor of barley blends well with the flavors of such legumes as soybeans, split peas, or lentils; and with the flavors of other vegetables such as cabbage, carrots, onions, or mushrooms. A typical mixture might contain 1 cup (*240 ml*) of legumes to 3 cups (*720 ml*) of barley. The starchy cooking water from barley has long been used as a broth in invalid diets, to stop diarrhea, and to relieve indigestion.	
Barley flakes	Barley groats that have been soaked, steamed, and rolled.	Cereal in Europe, but not in the U.S.	
Barley flour (also see MALT FLOUR; WHEAT MALT FLOUR.)	There are two kinds of barley flour: 1. Coarse barley flour milled from barley groats. 2. Patent barley flour, a highly refined flour milled from pearled barley.	Quick-rising doughs (leavened with baking powder) to make biscuits, muffins, and pancakes. Baby foods and food specialties. Small amounts of diastatic malt flours (or the equivalent in malt syrups) may be used by bakers because the enzymes present in these malt products convert the starch of dough to sugars. Patent barley flour is used to make items which are well tolerated by persons with certain digestive disorders.	Doughs made from barley flour lack sufficient elasticity (because of their low gluten content) for making yeast-leavened breads. However, barley flour may be substituted for wheat flour in recipes for muffins, biscuits, and pancakes which are normally leavened with baking powder. Also, the use of eggs in baked products helps to make up for the lack of gluten in barley flour. These products are useful where an allergy to wheat is encountered. (Also see BREADS AND BAKING.)
Barley groats	Kernels from which the outer hulls and seed coats have been removed	Porridges in the developing countries	Usually the kernels are crushed for porridges. (Also see BREAKFAST CEREALS.)
Infant cereals (Also see INFANT DIET AND NUTRITION.)	Usually made from coarse barley flour, produced by milling the de-hulled, whole grain, with added ingredients such as yeast, tricalcium phosphate, salt, iron, niacin, and thiamin.	For human infants	Many of these items are more nutritious than the ready-to-eat breakfast cereals eaten by older children and adults. (Also see BREAKFAST CEREALS.)
Malted barley cereals	Cooked and ready-to-eat cereals which contain malted barley that has been coarsely ground and then toasted to bring out its full flavor.	Breakfast cereals	Malted barley cereal may also be used to make muffins, pancakes, and other quick breads. (Also see BREADS AND BAKING.)

FERMENTATION PRODUCTS
(Also See BEERS AND BREWING; DISTILLED LIQUORS; and FERMENTATION.)

Product	Description	Uses	Comments
Beer	The product resulting from a two-step process— 1. Malting 2. Brewing	Alcoholic beverage	Barley was one of the first foods used for the production of beers and whiskeys, because it was readily available, easily malted, and rapidly fermented. Even today, when other materials have replaced part of the barley in these uses, it still has a major role in the production of malts for brewers and distillers. The manufacture of beer from barley comprises two major processes: 1. Malting, a controlled germination process which produces enzymes that are able to convert cereal starch to fermentable sugars. 2. Brewing, which is the process of converting the starch to an alcoholic solution, first by transforming the starch to sugar, then by fermenting the sugar to alcohol by means of yeast.
Brewers' yeast	The yeast that is produced in the brewing of beer. (One lb [*0.45 kg*] of yeast increases to 4 lb [*1.8 kg*] during fermentation.)	Nutrient supplement which provides proteins, nucleic acids, selenium, and the B complex vitamins (exclusive of vitamin B-12).	Brewers' yeast was once distributed by public health nurses in southeastern U.S. to prevent pellagra. It was also given to malnourished refugees after World War II. Presently, there is considerable interest in the selenium content of brewers' yeast, because it is one of the best food sources of this essential mineral. (Also see BREWERS' YEAST; SELENIUM.)

(Continued)

TABLE B-5 *(Continued)*

Product	Description	Uses	Comments
Gin	Distilled spirit flavored with juniper or some other flavoring.	Dutch gin is made by distilling a mash of which at least ⅓ is barley.	
Malt	The product secured by germinating (sprouting) barley in a controlled state, followed by (1) drying under conditions that retain enzymatic activity, and (2) removing of the sprouts.	Malts for brewers and distillers, special breads, extracts, flours, and malted milk	Starchy materials that are cheaper than malt are sometimes used as brewing *adjuncts* to replace a part of the malt. Among them, unmalted barley flakes, unmalted corn and wheat starches, rice grits, wheat flour, etc. Malt contains various enzymes.
Whiskey	The product resulting from the distillation of fermented mash cereal grain, followed by aging in wooden barrels from 2 to 8 years. Scotch pot-still or malt whiskey is made only from malted barley. Scotch patent-still or grain whiskey is made from barley and other unmalted cereal grains. Irish whiskey is made from malted barley alone or from malted barley with an admixture of unmalted barley, wheat, rye, or oats. Canadian whiskey is produced from barley, corn, wheat, or rye.	Alcoholic beverage	It is noteworthy that an early American nickname for whiskey was *John Barleycorn*. The distinctive smokey flavor of Scotch whiskey is due to the peat used for firing the malt kilns, and to the characteristics of the water used.

BARM

Yeast formed during the fermentation of alcoholic beverages.

BASAL DIET

A diet common to all groups of experimental subjects to which the experimental substance(s) is added. This type of diet is often used in research studies.

BASAL METABOLIC RATE (BMR)

The heat produced by a person during complete rest (but not sleeping) following fasting, when using just enough energy to maintain vital cellular activity, respiration, and circulation, the measured value of which is called the basal metabolic rate (BMR). Basal conditions include thermoneutral environment, resting, postabsorptive state (digestive processes are quiescent), consciousness, quiescence, and sexual repose. It is determined 14 to 18 hours after eating and when at absolute rest. It is measured by means of a calorimeter and is expressed in calories per square meter of body surface.

(Also see CALORIC [ENERGY] EXPENDITURE.)

BASAL METABOLISM

The energy expended by the body when (1) the subject is awake, but there is complete physical and mental rest; and (2) from 14 to 18 hours have elapsed after the last meal. Also, the environmental temperature must be in the comfort zone (usually 70° to 80°F [21° to 27°C]) so that no extra work is being done by the body either to heat or to cool itself. The energy expenditure which is measured under these conditions is taken to represent the minimal energy required to sustain the life of a healthy person. The extra energy expended over and above that used for basal metabolism is called the activity increment.

(Also see CALORIC [ENERGY] EXPENDITURE.)

BASE

Any of a large class of compounds with one or more of the following properties: bitter taste, slippery feeling insolution, ability to turn litmus blue and cause other indicators to take on characteristic colors, ability to react with (neutralize) acids to form salts. Bases include both hydroxides and oxides of metals.

BASE BICARBONATE

In the term *base bicarbonate*, the word *base* refers to any base that might be combined with bicarbonate. In the main buffer system of the human body, this base is sodium bicarbonate ($NaH\,CO_3$).

BASEDOW'S DISEASE

This disorder—which is also called exophthalmic goiter, Graves' disease, hyperthyroidism, or toxic goiter—is characterized by protrusion of the eyeballs (exophthalmos), swelling of the thyroid gland, breathlessness, an abnormally rapid heartrate, loss of weight despite an increased appetite and hearty eating, high blood pressure, an oversensitivity to heat, increased sweating, nervousness, muscle weakness, and fatigue. Basedow's disease results from an overproduction of hormones by the thyroid gland, and is more likely to occur in females than males.

Treatment consists of such measures as (1) surgical removal of part of the thyroid gland; (2) administration of radioactive iodine, which destroys some of the tissue of the gland; and/or (3) drugs which block the production of thyroid hormones.

It is noteworthy that Basedow's disease may be produced by the administration of iodine supplements to people living in iodine-poor areas. This phenomenon is called the Jod-Basedow effect.

(Also see GOITER.)

BASES

Another name for substances known as alkalis. They may be used to neutralize acids. Some common household bases are ammonia, baking soda, and lye.

(Also see ALKALI.)

BATAAN EXPERIMENT

A study conducted in 1947 on the Bataan Peninsula of the Philippines which established that enrichment of rice and the substitution of enriched rice for highly-polished rice effectively prevents beriberi and similar disorders.

(Also see ENRICHMENT, section headed "The Bataan Experiment;" and THIAMIN.)

BDELYGMIA

The severe dislike for food.

BEACH PLUM *Prunus maritima*

A small fruit of a native American bush (of the family *Rosaceae*) that grows wild on the beaches of the Atlantic Coast from New Brunswick to Virginia.

Beach plums are about ½ in. *(1 to 1.5 cm)* in diameter and vary in color from dark red to dull purple when they ripen in the late summer or early fall. The fruit is too sour for eating raw, but it makes good jam and jelly. In most cases the plums may be picked freely by visitors to the beaches, but in the resort areas of Cape Cod, Martha's Vineyard, and Nantucket they are harvested by local residents and sold to the tourists.

BEAN(S)

The name *bean* denotes several related plants of the legume family, *Leguminosae*. Both the edible pods and the seeds of these plants are called beans. They are among the most nourishing vegetables eaten by man. Being legumes, beans also enrich the soil with nitrogen that their bacteria take from the air.

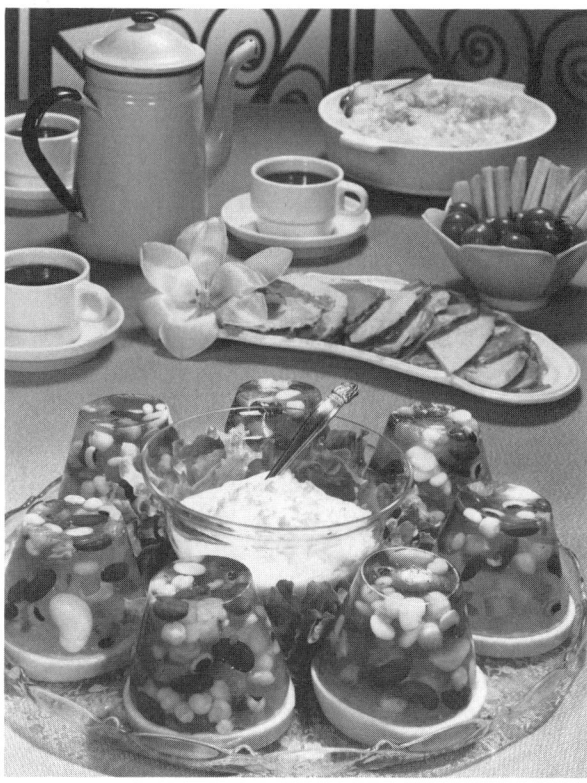

Fig. B-9. Jellied bean salad containing eight varieties of beans: dark red kidney beans, chickpeas, pink beans, light red kidneys, black-eyes, small whites, baby limas. (Courtesy, California Dry Bean Advisory Board, Dinuba, Calif.)

ORIGIN AND HISTORY. Beans are native to Central America, where, even today, cultivated forms and wild forms are found growing together. Archeological evidence indicates that beans were first cultivated 7,000 years ago. From Central America, beans were spread northward and southward by the Indians; and, from the Americas, they were taken to Europe by the Spanish explorers.

WORLD AND U.S. PRODUCTION. Statistically, dry beans and green beans are reported separately, and common beans and lima beans are grouped together.

Dry beans rank third among the legume crops of the world, and green beans rank eighth.

Worldwide, about 16.3 million metric tons of dry beans are produced annually; and the leading countries, by rank, are: India, Brazil, China, United States, and Mexico.[7]

Globally, about 3.1 million metric tons of green beans are produced annually; and the leading producers, by rank, are: China, Turkey, Spain, Italy, and France.[8]

Dry beans rank third among the legume crops of the United States, and green beans rank fourth.

The United States produces about 1.6 million short tons of dry beans annually; and the leading states, by rank, are: Michigan, North Dakota, Nebraska, Colorado, Idaho, and California.[9]

The United States also produces about 795,550 tons of green (snap) beans; and the leading states, by rank, are: Wisconsin, Oregon, Michigan, New York, and Illinois.[10]

KINDS OF BEANS. Some 100 or more species of beans are cultivated throughout the world.

Fig. B-10 shows the leading kinds of dry beans produced in the United States.

TYPES OF DRY BEANS PRODUCED IN USA

	(1,000 METRIC TONS)
PINTO	609
PEA (NAVY)	297
GREAT NORTHERN	127
RED KIDNEY	106
PINK	54
BLACK TURTLE SOUP	49
SMALL RED	29
BABY LIMA	25
LARGE LIMA	21
SMALL WHITE	15
CRANBERRY	14
CALIFORNIA BLACKEYE	4

= 50,000 MT

0 50 100 150 200 250 300 350 400 450
(1,000 METRIC TONS)

Fig. B-10. The leading varieties of dry beans produced in the United States. Based on data from *Agricultural Statistics 1991*, USDA, p. 240, Table 374.

[7]Based on data from *FAO Production Yearbook 1990*, FAO/UN, Rome, Italy, Vol. 44, p. 100, Table 32. **Note well:** Annual production fluctuates as a result of weather and profitability of the crop.

[8]*Ibid*, p. 144, Table 60.

[9]*Agricultural Statistics 1991*, USDA, p. 241, Table 375.

[10]*Ibid*, p. 147, Table 204.

In the United States and Canada, the most important kinds are (1) varieties of the Common Bean, and (2) the Lima Bean. Separate sections are devoted to each of them. (See BEAN, COMMON; and LIMA BEAN.)

UTILIZATION. Beans are consumed as food in several forms. Lima beans and snap beans are used as fresh vegetables, or they may be processed by canning or freezing. Limas are also used as a dry bean. Mung beans are utilized as sprouts.

The use of dry beans for food is dependent upon the seed size, shape, color, and flavor characteristics, and is often associated with particular social or ethnic groups. Popular uses include soups, mixed-bean salads, pork and beans, beans boiled with meat or other vegetables or cereals, baked beans, precooked beans and powder; and, in the Peruvian Andes, parched or roasted beans.

Most dry beans contain from 23 to 25% protein, 61 to 63% carbohydrate, and about 1½% fat. They may be eaten as a substitute for meat. Green shell beans are rich in both proteins and vitamins. Stringless or snap beans are a fair source of energy, but a rich source of vitamins A, B, and C.

Many foods contain components which are harmful at certain stages if they are not processed properly; and uncooked, mature beans are no exception. Fortunately, soaking until the seeds begin to swell, followed by thorough cooking, with water discarded after each step, renders most of these factors harmless. Also, it is known that acid treatment followed by incubation, and various types of fermentation and sprouting alleviate much of the gas problem by breaking down the indigestible carbohydrates. But those who suffer discomfort from excess gas may be well advised to eat only immature (green) beans.

(Also see LEGUMES, Table L-2, Legumes Of The World.)

BEAN, COMMON (FRENCH BEAN; KIDNEY BEAN; NAVY BEAN; PEA BEAN; PINTO BEAN; SNAP BEAN; STRINGLESS BEAN; OR GREEN BEAN)
Phaseolus vulgaris

(NOTE WELL: See BEAN[S] for the "Origin and History" and "World and U.S. Production" of beans.)

The common bean is very versatile; the immature pods and seeds may be picked and used as snap beans (also called string beans or green beans), or they may be left on the plant until fully mature for use as dried beans. In the latter case, the pods become too tough for eating.

PROCESSING. The demand for convenience foods made from dried beans and snap beans has increased steadily while the use of fresh, unprocessed bean products has declined, because many homemakers go to work and have only limited time for the preparation of meals at home.

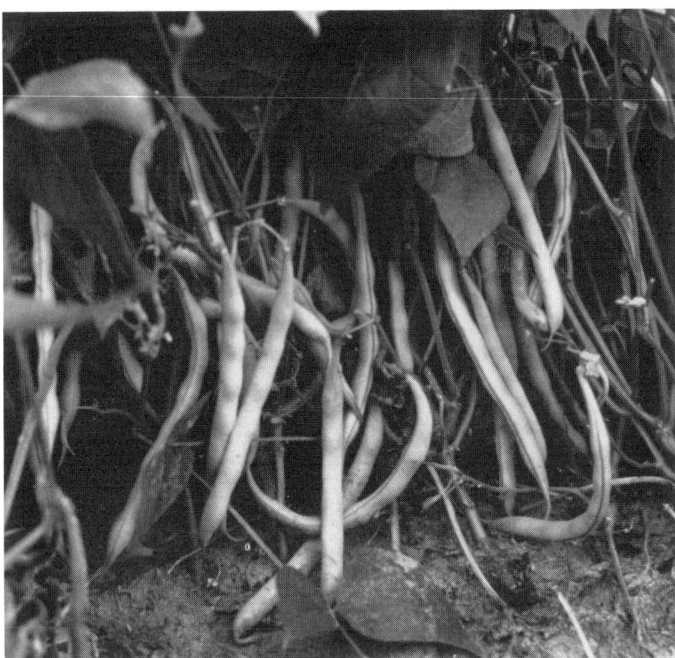

Fig. B-11. A close-up view of green bush bean plants with their seed pods. (Courtesy, USDA)

Dried Beans. Much of this crop is stored and utilized throughout the year for the production of canned items such as beans and pork in tomato sauce, Boston style baked beans, chili con carne and similar products, soups, and dips.

Snap Beans. About 16% of this crop is marketed fresh, 64% is canned, and 20% is frozen.

Commercially canned beans are much safer than those canned at home because (1) this vegetable is susceptible to the growth of *Clostridium botulinum*, a species of bacteria which produces a highly lethal toxin; and (2) commercial canning procedures are more certain to destroy spoilage organisms.

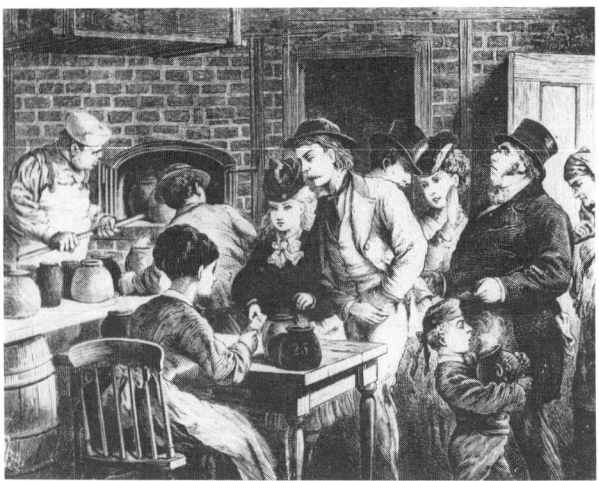

Fig. B-12. Sunday morning in a Boston bakery. Waiting in line for the ever popular baked beans. (Courtesy, The Bettmann Archive, Inc., New York, N.Y.)

SELECTION, PREPARATION, AND USES. Dry beans are often used in a main dish, whereas snap beans are usually served as a vegetable. Hence, the selection and preparation of these items will be treated separately.

Dried Beans. Money may be saved by purchasing dried beans and cooking them, instead of using canned beans, because (1) each cup of dried beans yields about three times as much cooked beans, and (2) the prices per pound of the various types of uncooked dried beans are close to those of the corresponding canned products. Furthermore, cooking beans at home allows the choice of sauces and seasonings, which are very important in enhancing the appeal of bean dishes. Finally, the soaking and cooking times may be shortened considerably by utilizing the procedures that follow:

• **One-hour hot soak**—This method may be substituted for 15 hours of cold soaking. A pound of dry beans is placed in a saucepan with 8 cups (*1.9 liter*) of water, then heated to boiling and boiled for 2 minutes, then allowed to soak in the water for about an hour. The initial boiling softens the skins of the beans so that water penetrates them much more readily than when they are placed in cold water. However, the water should be soft; otherwise, the bean skins may be toughened to the extent that longer soaking is required. If only hard water is available, it must be softened by adding not more than $1/_8$ to ¼ tsp (*0.625 to 1.25 ml*) of baking soda per cup (*240 ml*) of dry beans.

• **Pressure cooking**—Although beans cooked with water in a pressure cooker may produce enough foam to clog the vent, foaming may be reduced to a minimum by the addition of a tablespoon (*15 ml*) of oil or melted fat per cup (*240 ml*) of dried beans. Most beans may be cooked within 30 minutes in a pressure cooker, but it is advisable to consult the directions supplied with the cooker which is used.

The most nutritious dishes are those which are mixtures of beans with cheeses, grains, fish or seafood, meats, poultry, and/or other vegetables. Figs. B-13 and B-14 show some typical items.

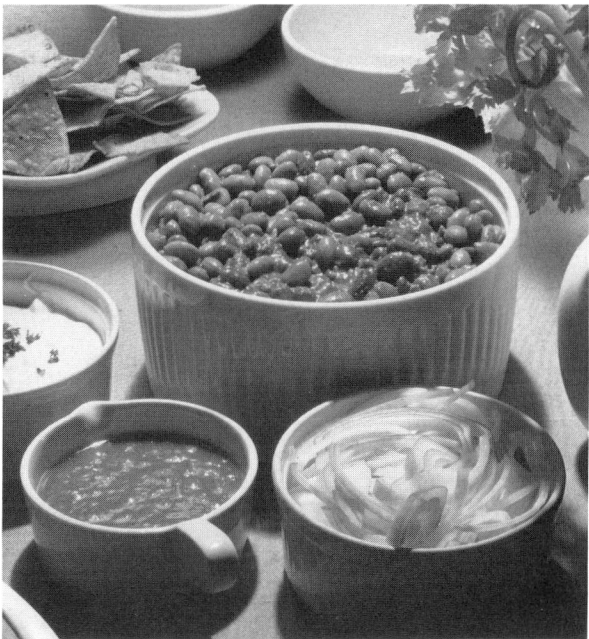

Fig. B-13. Chili beans con carne. This dish, which is popular in the California-Arizona-Mexico border areas, is made from dried pink beans, tomato sauce, onion, melted fat or oil, garlic, salt, chili powder, and cumin seed or powder. (Courtesy, The California Dry Bean Advisory Board, Dinuba, Calif.)

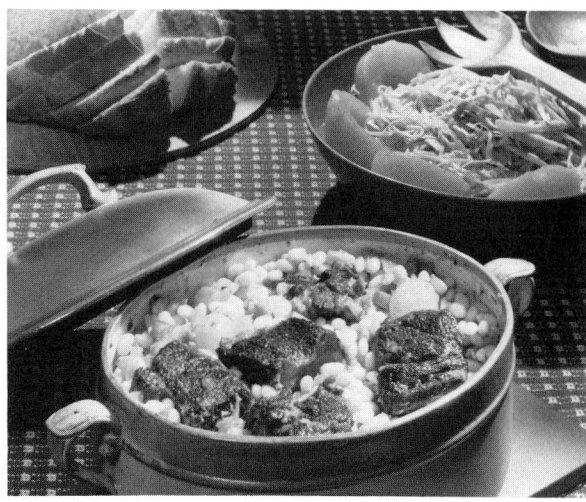

Fig. B-14. Beef-and-bean pot. This hearty main dish, which may be served with a tossed green salad and hard, crusty bread, contains short ribs of beef, small white beans, onions, celery, and garlic. (Courtesy, The California Dry Bean Advisory Board, Dinuba, Calif.)

• **Beans without gas**—Some people avoid eating beans because of the gas that they produce.

The effect of beans on gas (flatus) formation in the GI tract has been confirmed in experiments, with the following results:[11]

1.   Beans are powerful producers of gas in the GI tract.
2.   The CO_2 in the gas is 3 to 6 times higher on bean diets than on a basal diet.
3.   Different kinds of beans differ in their capacity to produce gas.
4.   When an antibacterial preparation is administered to the subjects, gas production is suppressed, thus showing the influence of bacterial action on gas production.
5.   The clostridial group of anaerobes is responsible for flatus formation.
6.   Oligosaccharides (carbohydrates containing from 2 to about 8 simple sugars linked together; beyond eight they are called polysaccharides. Raffinose contains three simple sugars linked together; stachyose contains four) are largely responsible for the flatulent properties of beans. Raffinose is a trisaccharide containing one molecule each of galactose, glucose, and fructose whereas stachyose is a tetrasaccharide containing one molecule of glucose, one molecule of fructose, and two molecules of galactose.

The excess gas (flatulence) following consumption of beans is due to the presence of raffinose and stachyose in beans. The intestinal tract does not produce enzymes capable of splitting these oligosaccharides (raffinose and stachyose), with the result that they pass to the colon where they are fermented by anaerobic microflora and produce gaseous products. This is an unfortunate characteristic of beans, for otherwise, they are one of nature's most perfect foods. They are an excellent low fat source of protein, and they are a good source of important minerals.

The gassiness of beans can be greatly lessened by the following treatments:

[11]Strong, Frank M., Chairman, Subcommittee on Naturally Occurring Toxicants in Foods, *Toxicants Occurring Naturally in Foods*, National Academy of Science, 1973, pp. 487-489. Summary of results adapted by the authors of this book.

1. **Acid treatment, followed by incubation.** When beans (whole, crushed, or ground) are mixed with water, the mixture will have a natural pH of 6.0 to 6.5. To activate the enzymes in the seeds, the pH of the mixture is reduced below 6.0, preferably to a pH of 5.0 to 5.5. The pH adjustment is made by adding appropriate amounts of food-grade hydrochloric, sulfuric, phosphoric, or acetic acid. The acid treatment should be followed by incubation in a warm environment at 113° to 149°F *(45° to 65°C)* for 1 to 2 days.

2. **Eliminating the sugars by soaking–discarding soaking water; cooking–discarding cooking water.** This consists in eliminating most of the tri- and tetra-sugars by (a) soaking the beans at least 3 hours, then discarding the soaking water; (b) covering the beans with boiling water and cooking for 30 minutes, then discarding the water again, followed by rinsing the beans well; and (3) adding fresh water and finishing the cooking process.

3. **Fermentation and sprouting.** Various types of fermentation and sprouting alleviate much of the gas problem by breaking down the indigestible carbohydrates.

People who are greatly bothered with gas should not eat beans unless (1) mature beans have been treated, or (2) they are immature (green).

• **Antinutritional and toxic factors**—Many foods contain components which are harmful at certain stages if they are not processed properly; and beans are no exception. *Uncooked, mature* common beans contain the following antinutritional and toxic factors: antivitamin E, inhibitors of trypsin, and red blood cell clumping agents (hemagglutinins). Soaking until the seeds begin to swell, followed by cooking (steaming, pressure cooking, or extrusion cooking) until the beans are tender, renders these factors harmless. Also, these components in bean flour are inactivated by pressure cooking prior to grinding. It is noteworthy, too, that various types of fermentation and sprouting, which have been utilized by Asian peoples for centuries, are an effective means of detoxifying beans.

Snap Beans. There are many varieties of both green and wax (yellow pod) snap beans. Some are flat, while others are oval or round. Most varieties of snap beans now grown for market are stringless when fully mature, but some develop stringiness as they pass the best stage for harvest. Overmature pods may become fibrous and tough whether stringless or not.

To be of the best quality, snap beans should be fresh in appearance, clean, firm but tender, crisp, free from scars, and reasonably well shaped. All beans in a selected lot should be at approximately the same stage of maturity so that they will cook uniformly. Firm, crisp, tender beans will snap readily when broken. Pods in which the seeds are very immature are the most desirable. Length is generally unimportant if the beans meet the requirements for quality. If seeds are half-grown or larger, pods are likely to be tough or fibrous. Stringiness can be detected by breaking the bean and gently separating the two parts. A dull, lifeless, or wilted appearance indicates that beans have been held too long after picking. Decay appears as a soft, watery, or moldy condition.

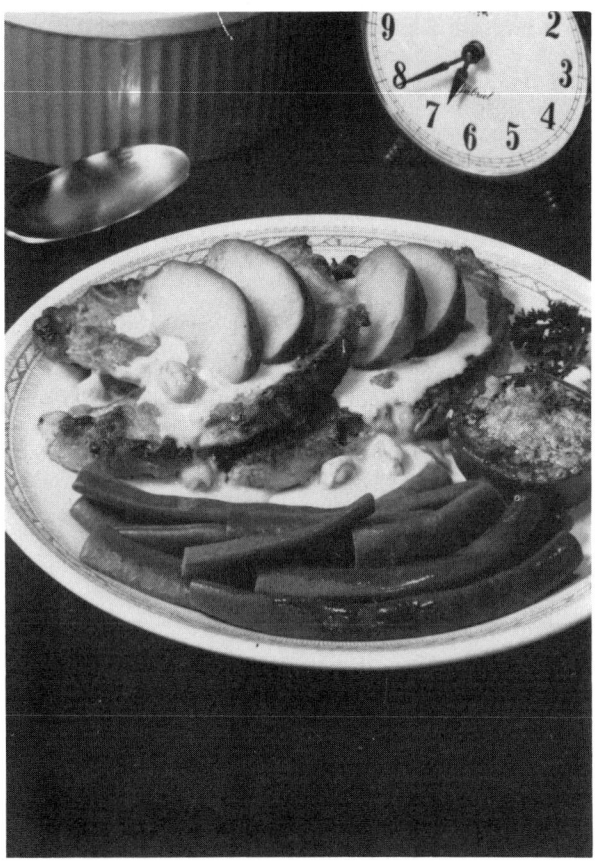

Fig. B-15. Green (snap) beans with apple-raisin pork chop. (Courtesy, Carnation Co. Los Angeles, Calif.)

The older methods of cooking snap beans are no longer applicable because the modern varieties have been selected for tenderness. Hence, a pound of crosscut pieces will be thoroughly cooked after 13 to 15 minutes in boiling water. Some other ways of preparing snap beans are: (1) tossing in hot oil or fat with minced onion or garlic and/or bits of bacon, (2) boiling French style pieces (thin strips prepared by cutting the beans lengthwise or diagonally) for only 7 to 10 minutes, and (3) cooking them in casseroles, soups, and stews. (The beans should be added near the end of the cooking period when incorporated in dishes requiring much longer cooking.)

NUTRITIONAL VALUE. The nutritive composition of common beans is given in Food Composition Table F-21.

Some noteworthy observations regarding the nutritive value of common beans follow:

1. Cooked dried beans contain about three times as many calories and protein per cup *(240 ml)* as cooked snap beans, because the former have three times the solid content of the latter (snap beans contain more than 90% water). Hence, people trying to lose weight should be encouraged to eat plenty of snap beans, which are filling but not fattening.

2. One cup *(240 ml)* of cooked dried beans contains about the same amount of protein (14 g) as 2 oz *(56 g)* of cooked lean meat, but the beans contain from 50 to 100% more calories.

3. Dried beans contain about one-third as much calcium as phosphorus, but snap beans contain more calcium than phosphorus. It is suspected that an excessively

low ratio of dietary calcium to phosphorus might limit the utilization of calcium by the body.

4. Both dried and snap beans provide ample amounts of iron and potassium per calorie.

5. Snap beans are a much better source of vitamins A and C than dried beans.

6. Commercial bean products which contain various meat ingredients are usually much higher in calories, but only slightly higher in protein than similar products without meat. The disproportionate increase in calories is due to the use of high-fat meats.

Protein Quantity and Quality. People are likely to substitute beans for meat in their diets when the latter becomes scarce or expensive. Therefore, certain facts concerning the quantity and quality of the protein in cooked dried beans follow:

1. Cooked beans furnish less protein per gram of food and per calorie than low and medium fat types of cheeses, eggs, fish, meats, milk, and poultry. For example, 3½ oz (*100 g*) of cooked common beans supplying 118 Calories (kcal) are required to provide the same amount of protein (about 7 g) as 1¾ oz (*50 g*) of cottage cheese (53 kcal) or one large egg (82 kcal). Also, the protein quality of the legumes is lower than that of the animal foods.

2. Cooked beans contain from 2 to 4 times the protein of most cooked cereals. For example, a cup of cooked dried beans (*approx. 185 g*) supplies from 14 to 15 g of protein, whereas a cup of cooked rice (*130 g to 205 g*) provides from 3 to 5 g of protein.

3. The protein in beans is moderately low in the sulfur-containing amino acids, methionine and cystine. However, the importance of this deficiency has been exaggerated, because the tests of protein quality have been conducted with rats, which have a higher requirement for these amino acids than people. The feeding of a little extra protein by serving ample portions of beans usually ensures that adequate amounts of the deficient amino acids are provided.

4. Mixtures of beans and cereals have a protein quality which comes close to that of meat, milk, and other animal proteins. The highest protein quality is usually achieved in mixtures comprised of 50% bean protein and 50% cereal protein because the amino acid patterns of the two types of foods complement each other. Some examples of food combinations utilizing this principle are corn tortillas and refried beans, baked beans and brown bread, and rice and beans.

5. Beans may be used to upgrade the protein quantity and quality of diets based mainly on cereals and/or starchy foods such as bananas, cassava, and sweet potatoes. The latter foods are the mainstays of people in the developing countries in the tropics. For example, a protein-enriched flour or meal may contain about ⅓ bean flour or meal, and about ⅔ cereal flour made from corn, rice, or wheat. Highly starchy diets may be upgraded considerably by mixing bean flour with the starchy food. For example, impoverished people in the tropical areas of Latin America might well be encouraged to prepare mixtures of bean flour and bananas.

6. Animal protein foods may be extended by the use of legumes. Some approximate *equations* of protein value follow:

(a) 1 frankfurter + ½ cup (*120 ml*) cooked beans = 2 frankfurters.

(b) 10% bean flour + 5% skim milk powder + 85% cereal flour = 10% skim milk powder + 90% cereal flour.

Both examples show that the requirement for expensive animal protein may be halved by the judicious use of legume products. However, it should be noted that the substitution of legumes for animal foods may raise the caloric value of the diet.

(Also see LEGUMES, Table L-2, Legumes of the World.)

BEAN FLOUR

Lima beans and soybeans are the two most common beans from which flour is made, but flour can be made from any bean.

(Also see FLOURS.)

BEATEN BISCUIT OR SOUTHERN BEATEN BISCUIT

This is an unleavened bread made with flour, shortening, water and milk. The stiff dough is beaten with a rolling pin and folded over many times, then rolled out and cut with a biscuit cutter. When baked, it should be light, even textured, and crack at the edges like crackers.

BEECHWOOD SUGAR (XYLOSE)

Wood sugar is the pentose—five-carbon—sugar which is widely distributed in plant material, especially wood.

(Also see CARBOHYDRATE[S]; and XYLOSE.)

BEEF AND VEAL

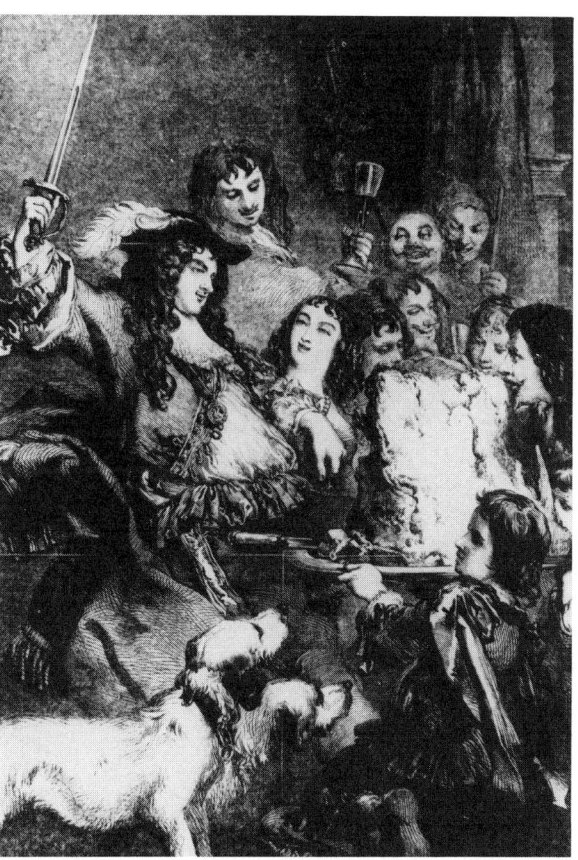

Fig. B-16. King Charles II was so impressed with a platter of beef that was served at one of his feasts, that—according to an old English legend—he ceremoniously arose, touched his sword to the steaming platter and said, "A noble joint it shall have a title. Loin, I dub thee Knight—henceforth thou shall be Sir Loin." (Courtesy, Picture Post Library, London, England)

Beef is the flesh of adult cattle, whereas veal is the flesh of calves.

FEDERAL GRADES OF BEEF AND VEAL.
The quality and yield grades of beef and veal are summarized in Table B-6.

TABLE B-6
FEDERAL QUALITY AND YIELD GRADES
OF BEEF AND VEAL[1]

Beef		Calf and Veal
Quality Grades	Cutability (Yield) Grades	(Quality Grades Only)
1. Prime[2]	1. Yield Grade 1	1. Prime
2. Choice	2. Yield Grade 2	2. Choice
3. Select	3. Yield Grade 3	3. Select
4. Standard	4. Yield Grade 4	4. Standard
5. Commercial	5. Yield Grade 5	5. Utility
6. Utility		
7. Cutter		
8. Canner		

[1]In rolling meat, the letters *USDA* are included in a shield with each Federal Grade name. This is important, as only government-graded meat can be so marked. For convenience, however, the letters *USDA* are not used in this table or in the discussion which follows.

[2]Cow beef is not eligible for the prime grade. The quality grade designations for bullock carcasses are Prime, Choice, Select, Standard, and Utility.

BEEF CUTS AND HOW TO COOK THEM.
In order to buy and/or process beef and veal wisely, and to make the best use of each part of the carcass, the consumer should be familiar with the types of cuts and how each should be processed.

Every grade and cut of meat can be made tender and palatable provided it is cooked by the proper method. Also, it is important that meat be cooked at the proper temperature.

Fig. B-19 shows the retail cuts of beef and gives the recommended method(s) of cooking each.

(Also see MEAT, section headed "Meat Cooking.")

U.S. BEEF PRODUCTION.
The dominant position of beef production in the United States is attested to by the following statistics:

1. It has 4.9% of the world's human population.
2. It has 8.0% of the world's cattle population.
3. It produces 22.2% of the world's beef and veal.
4. It consumes 16.6% of the world's beef and veal.

Thus, 8.0% of the world's cattle population produces 22.2% of the world's beef. This points up the tremendous efficiency of the U.S. cattle industry.

In 1989, 23.4 billion pounds (*10.7 billion kg*) of beef and veal were produced in the United States; and on January 1, 1991, there were 99.4 million cattle and calves in the United States.

PER CAPITA BEEF AND VEAL CONSUMPTION.
In 1990, the U.S. per capita consumption of beef (carcass basis) was 64 lb (*29 kg*), and the per capita consumption of veal was 0.9 lb (*0.4 kg*).

BEEF AS A FOOD.
Beef is a favorite American food; it's good eating, and it's good nutritionally, too.

Beef provides high-quality protein; it contains all the amino acids, and the proportion of the amino acids almost exactly parallels that in human protein. Beef is a good source of several minerals, but it is an especially rich source of iron, phosphorus, copper, and zinc. Beef is also a good source of vitamin A, and of the B vitamins—vitamin B-12, vitamin B-6, biotin, niacin, pantothenic acid, and thiamin. The calories in meat are dependent largely upon the amount of fat it contains.

(Also see MEAT[S].)

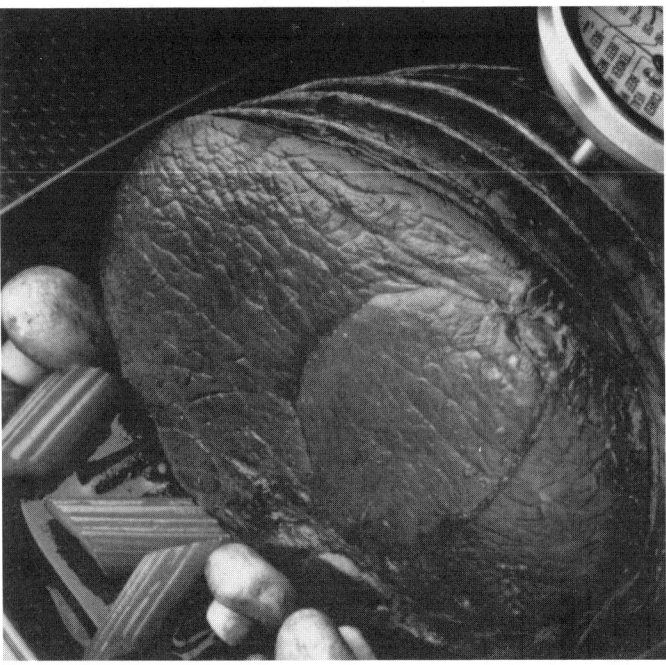

Fig. B-17. Beef round tip roast. (Courtesy, National Live Stock and Meat Board, Chicago, Ill.)

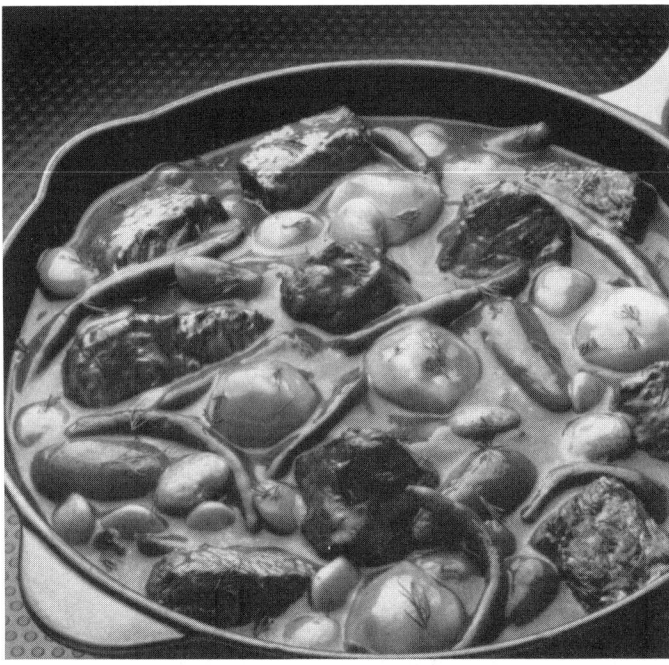

Fig. B-18. Beefstew. (Courtesy, National Live Stock and Meat Board, Chicago, Ill.)

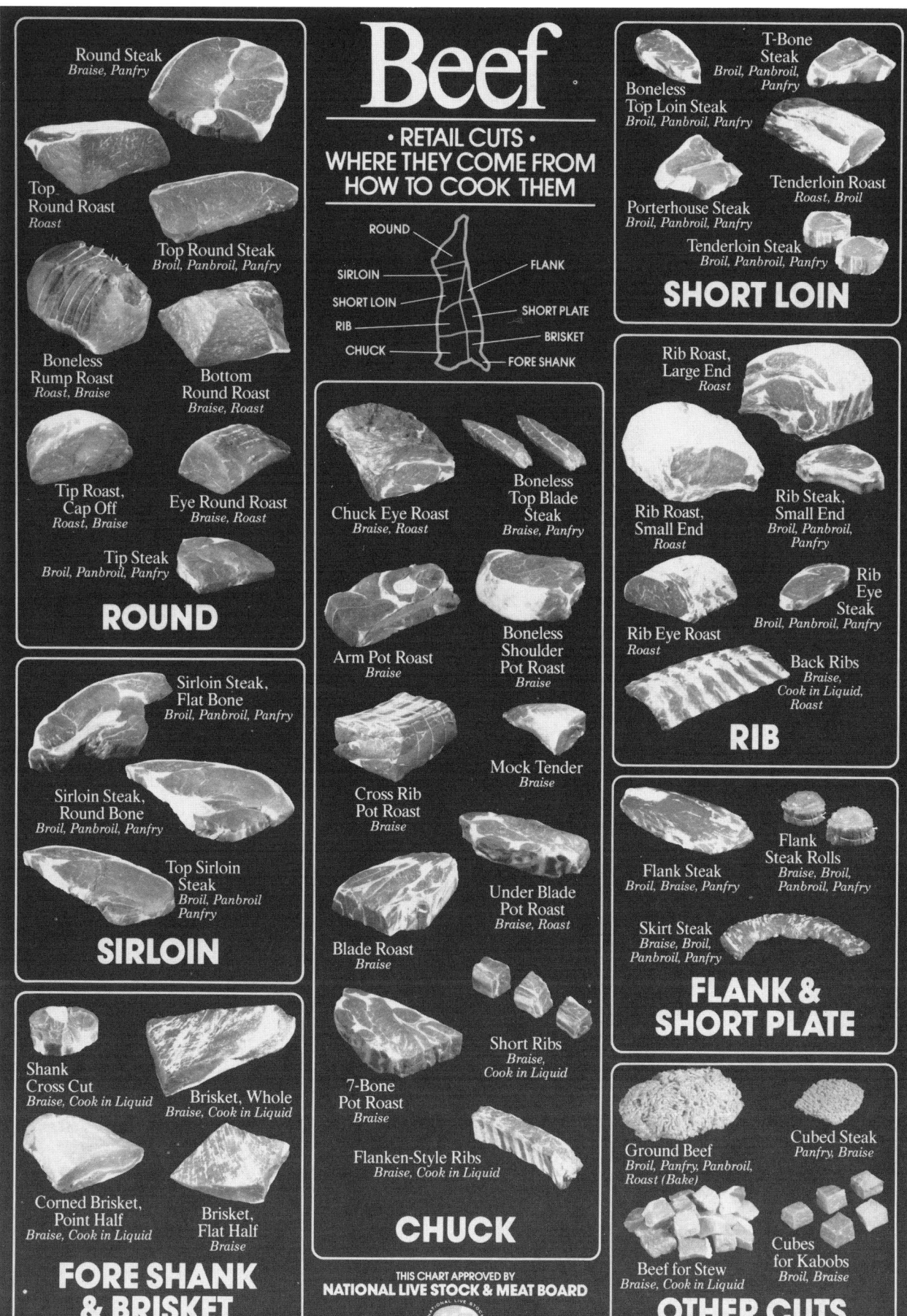

Beef

• RETAIL CUTS •
WHERE THEY COME FROM
HOW TO COOK THEM

ROUND
SIRLOIN
SHORT LOIN
RIB
CHUCK
FLANK
SHORT PLATE
BRISKET
FORE SHANK

ROUND

Round Steak
Braise, Panfry

Top Round Roast
Roast

Top Round Steak
Broil, Panbroil, Panfry

Boneless Rump Roast
Roast, Braise

Bottom Round Roast
Braise, Roast

Tip Roast, Cap Off
Roast, Braise

Eye Round Roast
Braise, Roast

Tip Steak
Broil, Panbroil, Panfry

SIRLOIN

Sirloin Steak, Flat Bone
Broil, Panbroil, Panfry

Sirloin Steak, Round Bone
Broil, Panbroil, Panfry

Top Sirloin Steak
Broil, Panbroil Panfry

FORE SHANK & BRISKET

Shank Cross Cut
Braise, Cook in Liquid

Brisket, Whole
Braise, Cook in Liquid

Corned Brisket, Point Half
Braise, Cook in Liquid

Brisket, Flat Half
Braise

CHUCK

Chuck Eye Roast
Braise, Roast

Boneless Top Blade Steak
Braise, Panfry

Arm Pot Roast
Braise

Boneless Shoulder Pot Roast
Braise

Cross Rib Pot Roast
Braise

Mock Tender
Braise

Under Blade Pot Roast
Braise, Roast

Blade Roast
Braise

Short Ribs
Braise, Cook in Liquid

7-Bone Pot Roast
Braise

Flanken-Style Ribs
Braise, Cook in Liquid

SHORT LOIN

T-Bone Steak
Broil, Panbroil, Panfry

Boneless Top Loin Steak
Broil, Panbroil, Panfry

Porterhouse Steak
Broil, Panbroil, Panfry

Tenderloin Roast
Roast, Broil

Tenderloin Steak
Broil, Panbroil, Panfry

RIB

Rib Roast, Large End
Roast

Rib Roast, Small End
Roast

Rib Steak, Small End
Broil, Panbroil, Panfry

Rib Eye Steak
Broil, Panbroil, Panfry

Rib Eye Roast
Roast

Back Ribs
Braise, Cook in Liquid, Roast

FLANK & SHORT PLATE

Flank Steak
Broil, Braise, Panfry

Flank Steak Rolls
Braise, Broil, Panbroil, Panfry

Skirt Steak
Braise, Broil, Panbroil, Panfry

OTHER CUTS

Ground Beef
Broil, Panfry, Panbroil, Roast (Bake)

Cubed Steak
Panfry, Braise

Beef for Stew
Braise, Cook in Liquid

Cubes for Kabobs
Broil, Braise

THIS CHART APPROVED BY
NATIONAL LIVE STOCK & MEAT BOARD

Fig. B-19. The wholesale and retail cuts of beef, and the recommended methods of cooking. (Courtesy, National Live Stock and Meat Board, Chicago, Ill.)

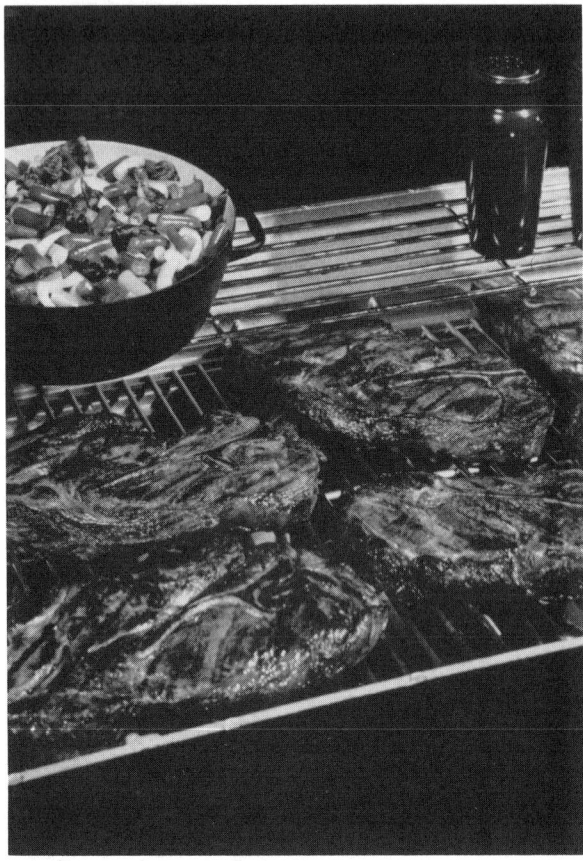

Fig. B-20. Chuck Steak on Grill. (Courtesy, National Live Stock and Meat Board, Chicago, Ill.)

BEEF BREAD

The pancreas of a mature animal used for food.

BEEF EXTRACT (MEAT EXTRACT)

An extract of the soluble constituents of beef, made by cooking beef.

BEEF TEA

A beverage made by extracting finely cut lean beef with hot water. Also, there are commercial beef extracts and cubes that can be used for beef tea. Beef tea, bouillon, and consomme, are different designations for the same beverage.

BEERS AND BREWING

The word *beer* is derived from *baere*, the German word for barley, which is the major grain used in the brewing of beer. Brewers make beers and similar alcoholic beverages by fermenting sugary extracts of cereal grains. Usually, the alcoholic content of these beverages ranges from 2 to 8%. Sometimes, other drinks made from such diverse items as fruits, roots and tubers, and herbs are called beers. However, this article is limited to beers made from grains.

HISTORY OF BREWING. The brewing of cereal beers is probably about as old as grain farming, as evidenced by fermented grains found in clay pots unearthed at the sites of ancient agricultural settlements. Also, it seems likely that various types of brewing were developed independently by native peoples in many places around the world because fermentation may occur wherever there are (1) food-fermenting microorganisms in the air, (2) fermentable foods exposed to the microorganisms, or (3) temperatures warm enough to encourage fermentation. Hence, a wide variety of substances and methods of brewing were used to make primitive beers.

Many historians believe that the first grain beers were brewed before 5000 B.C. by the ancient Chaldeans (the people who settled at the southern ends of the Tigris and Euphrates rivers in what is now Iraq) and the Egyptians. These first beers, made from barley—a grain uniquely suited for brewing, were the forerunners of those now produced in all of the developed countries of the West.

The latest chapter in the story of how brewing has contributed to human welfare began in Germany right after World War II when medical scientists studied the nutritional effects of brewers' yeast. They found that experimental diets based on the European strains of yeast produced liver disorders in laboratory rats. Then, in 1951 the German medical scientist Schwarz came to the United States to work as a visiting scientist at the National Institute of Health, where he and his coworker, Foltz, discovered that the American type of brewers' yeast prevented the liver disorder observed in Germany. This work led to their discovery in 1957 that the American yeast contained a complex compound of the element selenium, which they showed to be an essential nutrient. (Perhaps, the nutritional superiority of the American brewers' yeast is due to the growing of grains used for brewing on soils which have a moderately high selenium content.) Two years later, Schwarz and Mertz (Mertz was a German medical scientist who came to the United States) discovered that chromium was an essential nutrient and that the most biologically active form of this element was the glucose tolerance factor from brewers' yeast.

BASIC BEER BREWING STEPS. The art of brewing has evolved over the centuries into a highly scientific profession, which provides us with a variety of beers and similar products. Brewers also help to put meat, milk, and eggs on the table because the by-products of brewing are fed to livestock. Therefore, the major processes which constitute brewing are noteworthy.

Pertinent steps of the major brewing operations follow.

Malting. Yeast fermentation produces alcohol from sugars, but not from starch. Hence, the most common method of making beer involves the conversion of the starch in cereal grains to sugars by the enzymes produced in the operation called malting.

During malting, whole grain barley, or a similar cereal, is allowed to sprout (germinate) under controlled conditions so that certain enzymes in the grain are activated. The sprouting is stopped at the desired point by careful heating which allows the enzyme activity to be retained. Then, the sprouts are removed from the malted grain by passage through revolving sets of wire screens. Usually, the malt is ground before it is used by brewers.

(Also see MALT.)

Mashing. This process is used to prepare the sugary broth, or wort, which is fermented by yeast. Certain brewers around the world rely solely upon malted barley to yield the sugars in mashing, whereas others use malt plus other unmalted grains called *adjuncts*, which supply starch and cost less than malt.

Mashing begins with the precooking of the malt and adjuncts in separate vessels to form watery porridges. Then, the cooked malt is combined with the cooked adjuncts in a mash tub, where the mixture is heated slowly so that the enzymes in the mash convert almost all of the starch to sugars. The sugary extract which results is called a *wort*. After mashing has been completed, the mixture of spent grains (brewers' grains) and wort is piped to a lauter tub (a large tank with a slotted or perforated false bottom) where the grains settle to the bottom. The hot wort is then filtered through the brewers' grains into the brew kettle. Hot water, used to rinse the grains, is also added to the brew kettle. The rinsed brewers' grains are used as ingredients in livestock feeds.

Hopping. Hops (dried flowers of the hop vine) are added to the wort in the brew kettle to impart to beer its traditional odor and bitter taste. The mixture is then boiled to extract the aromatic components of the hops, and to sterilize and concentrate the wort prior to fermentation. After boiling, the hops are removed by passing the mixture through a strainer. The hopped wort is held in a tank where the excess protein settles out. Tannins from the hops react with the protein so that it comes out of solution. Otherwise, it might cause clouding of the beer. The spent hops are saved for use as a livestock feed ingredient. After the protein has been removed, the wort is piped to a cooler, then to an open fermentation tank.

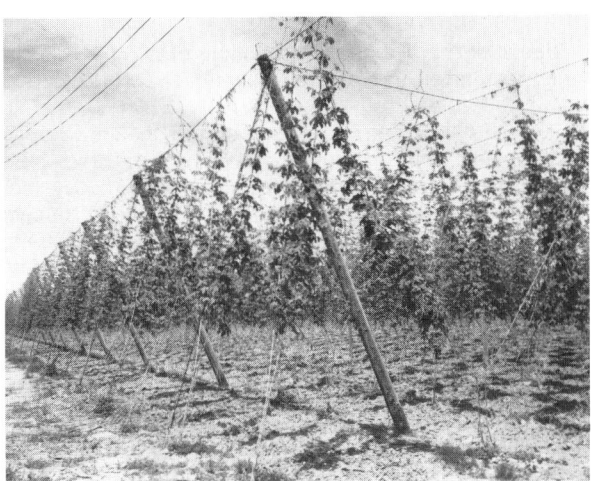

Fig. B-21. Hops are grown for the making of beer. (Courtesy, Union Pacific Railroad Company, Omaha, Neb.)

Fermentation. This process is started by the addition of yeast to the hopped wort in the open fermentation tank.

Once fermentation is underway, the mixture is transferred to a closed fermentation tank, where it is kept for a week or more. The carbon dioxide produced in the fermentation is pumped off and stored in pressurized tanks. Next, the newly formed beer is pumped to a storage tank where it is aged for weeks or months, depending upon the brewery's procedure. The yeast residue, which is known as brewers' yeast, is used as a nutritional supplement for people or as an ingredient of livestock feeds.

Finishing. Some unfermented wort may be added to the beer in storage to produce a mild fermentation which gives the beer a tangy quality. This process is called *krausening*. When the storage period is over, the beer is filtered to remove all residue, and a small amount of carbonation is added.

By-products of Malting and Brewing. Typically, a barrel of beer (31 gal [*117.8 liters*]) which is produced in the United States may be made from the following raw materials: 30 lb (*13.5 kg*) of barley, 10 lb (*4.5 kg*) of corn, 5 lb (*2.25 kg*) of rice, ½ lb (*225 g*) of hops, and ¼ lb (*113 g*) of yeast.[12] However, beer contains from 85 to 90% water, so it may be readily seen that much of the solids in the grains used as raw materials end up in the by-products which remain after the fermentable matter has been extracted.

The main by-products derived from malting and brewing beer are: malt sprouts and hulls, brewers' grains, spent hops, and brewers' yeast. As feed for cattle and sheep, the first three by-products help to lower the cost of producing valuable, high protein animal foods for people. Brewers' yeast is used as a nutritional supplement for both people and animals.

• **Brewers' yeast**—The ¼ lb (*112 g*) of yeast used to brew each barrel of beer grows to 1 lb (*454 g*) during fermentation.[13] Hence, there is a net gain of ¾ lb (*338 g*) of yeast per barrel of beer produced, for a total of 148.5 million pounds (*67.5 million kg*) of yeast gained in the U.S. annual beer production of 198 million barrels. The surplus brewers' yeast, which is high in both protein and the vitamin B complex, is used mainly as a nutritional supplement for both man and animals. Perhaps, this yeast also contains some unidentified, nutritionally beneficial factors. For example, research conducted at Rockefeller University showed that it protected laboratory animals against the carcinogenic effects of butter yellow, a synthetic dye which is no longer allowed in foods.

TYPES OF BEERS AND RELATED DRINKS. The name beer has long been given to a wide variety of undistilled, alcoholic beverages made from fermented extracts of mashed grains. For example, the name itself was derived from the German word for barley, but beers have also been brewed from (1) wheat by the Germans, (2) rice by the Chinese and Japanese, (3) sorghums and millets by the African tribes, (4) rye by the Russians, and (5) corn by the American Indians. Even when beer is made mainly from malted barley plus hops, yeast, and water, the flavor, aroma, and color of the product depend upon other factors such as (1) the type of malt used (various roasting treatments are used after malting to produce the various types); (2) amounts and types of adjuncts, if any; (3) the temperatures and the lengths of time used for mashing, hopping, fermentation,

[12]Couch, J. R., "Review of Nutrition Papers from Brewers Feed Conference," *Feedstuffs*, December 5, 1977, p. 8.
[13]*Ibid.*

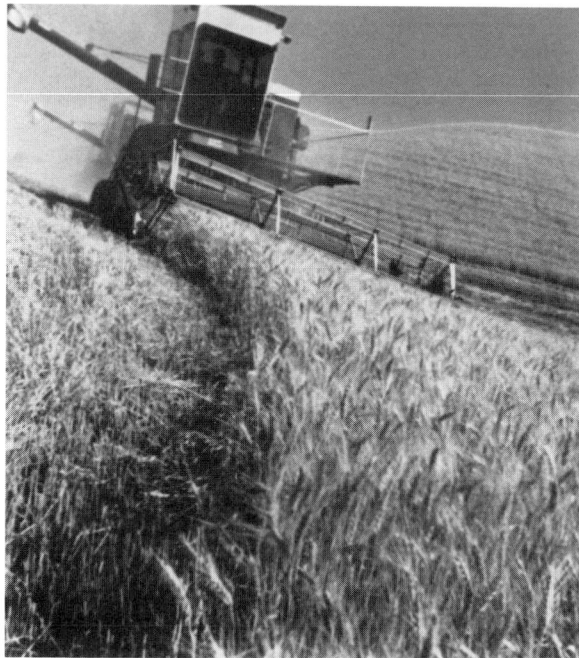

Fig. B-22. Harvesting barley, the major grain used in the brewing of beer. (Courtesy, USDA.)

and storage; and (4) the strains of yeast used for fermentation (the identities of many of these strains are well-kept company secrets). Descriptions of some of the most common types of beers and related beverages follow:

• **Ale**—The pilgrims brought ale, rather than beer, to America. Both beverages are made from malted barley, adjuncts, hops, yeast, and water, but ale is stronger and contains more alcohol than beer. Another difference is that production of ale utilizes strains of yeast which rise to the top of the fermentation tank. Hence, it is said to be a *top-fermented* beverage.

• **Beer**—What is commonly called beer in the United States is known as lager in Europe. The process for brewing lager beers was brought to America by the German immigrants who arrived in the 1840s. These beers are made with yeasts which drop to the bottom of the fermentation tank; so, they are said to be *bottom-fermented*. Lagers are lighter, lower in alcohol, and contain less hop extract than ales.

• **Bitter**—This British draft beer is one of the driest and most heavily hopped. Generally, the British use from 2 to 3 times more hops to brew their beers than the Americans. When bottled, the beverage is called light ale or pale ale.

• **Bock beer**—At one time, this beer was sold in the spring, when, for unknown reasons, it was associated with the symbol of the goat. Darker, heavier, and sweeter than most other beers, it has long been thought to be more nutritious. The dark color comes from the use of a highly toasted, dark malt.

• **Lager**—The name of this type of beer is derived from the German word *lagern*, which means *to store*. It seems that when monks operated many of the breweries in Germany they stored their newly made beer in cool caves during the summer to keep it from spoiling. A lager is a light-colored,

mild-tasting beer which was made so popular by the German immigrant brewers that it now claims most of the market for beer in the United States.

• **Light ale or pale ale**—When made in Great Britain, this product is one of the driest and most heavily hopped. The British give it the name *bitter* when it is dispensed as a draft beer.

• **Malt liquor**—American labeling regulations provide that brewed beverages which contain more than 5% alcohol cannot be called beers, but must be designated as malt liquors, ales, porters, or stouts. Usually, malt liquors are higher alcoholic versions of the lager types of beer.

• **Pilsner**—Once, this name applied only to a highly regarded lager beer from Pilsen, Czechoslovakia. Now, it merely signifies that a certain product may bear a similarity to the premium beer from Pilsen.

• **Porter**—This alelike beverage got its name because it was favored by London market porters. It was designed by an enterprising brewer to embody the desirable qualities of several different brews, because customers often asked bartenders to mix them together in a single glass. The name porterhouse steak was later given to the special cut of beef which was served in establishments which dispensed porter.

• **Shandy**—This British drink is a mixture of beer and ginger beer, or a mixture of beer and lemonade—called lemon shandy.

• **Stout**—Some time ago, a demand arose in Great Britain for an *extrastout* porter. Hence, this very dark and slightly bitter ale came to be brewed from a dark malt. A burnt taste may be evident when the brewer has used carmelized sugar.

• **Weisse**—The Germans make this cloudy beer from wheat, barley malt, hops, yeast, and water. It is fermented in the bottle, which makes the beer cloudy because some of the particles of yeast remain suspended. The presence of yeast in the beer raises its nutritional value above other beers, particularly with respect to the vitamin B complex.

Beers of the World. Descriptions of selected brewing practices and beers in various parts of the world follow:

• **African sprouted grain beers**—Although the brewing procedures used by the various tribal peoples of Africa resemble those used elsewhere to make beer from malted barley, they differ in that much of the conversion of the grain starches to sugars is due to the action of enzymes from wild strains of the fungus *Aspergillus oryzae*, in addition to the conversion which results from sprouting alone. Furthermore, there are many different native beers made by various tribes in Africa. Hence, only a few of the more common brewing practices can be described here.

In the mid-continent regions of Africa, corn, millet, or sorghum are sprouted alone or in a mixture by first soaking in water; then, the grain is covered with leaves or soil for a day or so. The sprouted grain may be (1) dried and ground into a flour, (2) cooked with water to make a gruel, or (3) put directly into a vessel containing water, and fermented. Some tribes mix a portion of sprouted grain flour with water to form a paste. Then, they make a yeasty froth from the paste by exposing it to the wild yeasts that are in the air and/or on the surface of the brewing vessel. Other tribes initiate fermentation by adding a soured sweet potato to a watery gruel made from malted grain. Sometimes, cassava (manioc) paste or crushed sugar cane may be added to the fermentation mixture. Fermentation is usually completed within a few days, after which the beer may be boiled, sieved, or consumed.

• **Sake (Japanese rice beer)**—Many people call sake *rice wine* because it has an alcohol content of 14 to 16%, which is more comparable to wine than most beers. However, it is truly a cereal beer because the starches in the rice must be converted to sugars before fermentation can take place. It is noteworthy that the fungus *Aspergillus oryzae*, which is used by the Japanese to convert rice starch to sugars, is the same species which acts on the sprouted grains used to make African native beers. This is no coincidence, since *Aspergillus* fungi are common spoilage organisms that attack grains and legumes around the world.

Sake differs from most beers in (1) containing from 2 to 3 times as much alcohol, (2) being almost colorless, (3) lacking carbonation, and (4) being more desirable when served warm, whereas other beers are better when served cold.

• **Latin American chewed corn beer (chicha)**—It is not known where the practice of using chewed corn to make beer originated, but it appears to have been spread throughout the Americas by the Indians because Columbus observed it in the Caribbean, and it is still found in the more primitive regions of South America. Certain groups of Indians even have professional chewers who prepare the corn for fermentation into chicha.

• **Russian rye bread beer (kvass or quass)**—This refreshing beverage, which contains not more than 0.7% alcohol, is made by (1) pressure cooking a brown rye bread, (2) treating the cooked bread mash with rye malt, (3) fermenting the malt-treated mash with a combination of yeast and *Bacillus lactis*, and (4) filtering the beer. The drink is usually dispensed cold from special tank trucks which tour the cities during the summer.

NUTRITIVE VALUE OF ORDINARY BEER.

The nutritive composition of beer and ale is given in Food Composition Table F-21. The modern preference for a highly clarified beer which is unclouded by protein hazes or yeast sediment appears to have been responsible for a reduction in the nutritive value of this beverage compared to more primitive types of beer. For example, various studies have shown that the African native beers may make significant nutritive contributions to the diets of tribes who rely mainly upon cereal grains and starchy roots and tubers. However, these beers are subjected to only minimal filtration because they are usually consumed from opaque drinking vessels made from clay.

One of the few unclarified beers produced in the developed countries is the German beverage *weisse*, which ranks about the highest in nutritive value among the commercial beers because it is fermented in the bottle and the yeast is left in the product. However, even the ordinary beers are nutritionally superior to nonalcoholic, carbonated drinks. The extent to which some people regard beer as a source of nutrients is evidenced by the fact that females who normally abstain from alcoholic beverages may consume it after childbirth in the belief that it helps to stimulate the flow of breast milk. Hence, the nutrient composition of beer presented in Table B-7 is noteworthy.

TABLE B-7
NUTRIENT COMPOSITION OF BEER[1]

Nutrient and Unit of Measurement	Amount in 12 oz (360 ml) of Beer	RDA For Adult Male[2]	Percent of RDA Furnished By 12 oz (360 ml) of Beer
Major constituents:			
Food energy, Calories .. (kcal)	151	2,900	5.2
Protein ....g	1.1	63	.02
Fat ....g	0	—[3]	—
Carbohydrates ....g	13.7	—	—
Water ....ml	332	2,900	11.4
Alcohol (4.5% by volume) . ml	16.2	—	—
Minerals:			
Calcium ....mg	18	800	2.2
Phosphorus ....mg	108	800	13.5
Sodium ....mg	25	500	5
Magnesium ....mg	36	350	10.3
Potassium ....mg	90	2,000	0.5
Vitamins:			
Folate (folic acid) ....mcg	21.6	200	10.8
Niacin .... mg NE	2.2	19.0	11.6
Pantothenic acid (B-3) ....mg	0.29	4–7	5.3
Riboflavin (B-2) ....mg	0.11	1.7	6.5
Vitamin B-6 (pyridoxine) ...mg	0.21	2	10.5

[1]Data from Food Composition Table F-36.

[2]The RDAs are from *Recommended Dietary Allowances*, 10th rev. ed. NRC—National Academy of Sciences, 1989.

[3]Blank means that no allowance has been set.

It may be seen from Table B-7 that beer supplies liberal amounts of phosphorus, magnesium, riboflavin, vitamin B-6, and niacin.

Although 12 oz (360 ml) of beer furnishes only about 9% of the estimated allowance for chromium, few foods other than brewers' yeast supply this mineral in such a readily utilized form, since all of the chromium in beer is alcohol extractable. Recent research has shown that the biological activity of chromium is associated with an alcohol soluble factor which appears to promote better utilization of carbohydrates by the body. Hence, certain chromium-deficient people with diabeticlike tendencies might benefit from drinking beer.

(Also see CHROMIUM.)

The thiamin (vitamin B-1) and pantothenic acid content of beer is low in proportion to its caloric content. Hence, deficiencies of these vitamins might be aggravated by heavy beer drinking, unless other foods rich in the vitamin B complex are consumed.

There is only a small amount of sodium in beer. Thus, it does not seem to be responsible for the water logging effect attributed to it. Rather, the excessive water retention which afflicts some heavy beer drinkers might be due to the salty foods often consumed while drinking. Generally, the consumption of alcoholic beverages is likely to cause the loss of water from the body since alcohol promotes copious urination.

Ounce for ounce, beer contains about the same number of calories as the nonalcoholic, sweetened, carbonated beverages. Hence, anyone who consumes large quantities of any of these beverages might expect to gain excess weight since each 8-oz (240 ml) glass supplies about 100 Calories (kcal).

MENTAL AND PHYSICAL EFFECTS OF BEER

DRINKING. It is difficult to ascribe specific effects to the drinking of specified quantities of beer because (1) the alcohol of the common beers and ales varies widely, (2) higher blood levels of alcohol are reached when beer is consumed on an empty stomach than when it is taken with a meal, and (3) habitual heavy drinkers who are otherwise well nourished metabolize alcohol much more rapidly than light-to-moderate drinkers. Nevertheless, it is important to have some guidelines for distinguishing between safe and dangerous amounts of beer consumption.

Beneficial Effects. The consumption of a few glasses of beer may calm jittery people because small amounts of alcohol slow the activity of the areas of the brain which govern the thought processes, while the areas associated with the other functions are unaffected. Therefore, it is noteworthy that overexcitable persons may be able to improve their performance of both mental and physical tasks after having a few beers. Psychologists have found that optimal performance of mental activities depends upon just the right amount of arousal. Both overarousal and underarousal reduce concentration and performance. Hence, the counteraction of overarousal by small amounts of alcohol or other substances may help to promote a more effective utilization of one's mental abilities.

A few beers may also help to promote sociability by calming feelings of apprehension toward others. The business luncheon is a prime example of how food and drink are employed to bring about a spirit of mutual understanding.

Finally, beer and other alcoholic beverages appear to promote health and well being in ways which are not well understood. For example, a study of over 7,000 Japanese men living in Hawaii showed that those who drank one or two alcoholic drinks per day had only one-half the rate of cardiovascular disorders as those who abstained from these beverages.[14] These findings attest to the wisdom of doctors who prescribe a daily drink for patients suffering from clogged blood vessels (atherosclerosis or arteriosclerosis). Apparently, alcohol relaxes the walls of blood vessels so that their openings are enlarged (it is a vasodilator) and the flow of blood is increased.

Harmful Effects. A few people may fly into violent rages after only a few drinks. It is suspected that they may suffer from a combination of a personality disorder and a tendency to develop low blood sugar. Perhaps, some of these people harbor strong antisocial feelings which they have great difficulty in suppressing. Hence, the diminishing of inhibitions by alcohol causes their violent dispositions to emerge under the slightest provocation. Needless to say, those with such antisocial tendencies would be better off abstaining from all alcoholic drinks.

Fortunately, it is much more difficult to drink too much alcohol in the form of beer than by imbibing wine or distilled liquors which contain much more alcohol. For example, four 8-oz (240 ml) glasses of beer provide a quart of fluid, which is about as much as most people may feel comfortable drinking in a short period of time. The alcohol in this quantity of beer will produce only the mildest impairment of mental and physical functions. However, drinking too much beer, or any other beverage for that matter, may interfere with the normal nutritive processes by (1) causing feelings of

fullness before sufficient food is consumed, (2) provoking diarrhea or vomiting, or (3) causing excessive urination which flushes vitamins and minerals out of the body.

Finally, drinking to the point of intoxication is a very dangerous thing because (1) it may become habitual, (2) control of behavior is lost, and (3) the drinker becomes highly prone to accidents.

(Also see ALCOHOL; ALCOHOLIC BEVERAGES; and ALCOHOLISM AND ALCOHOLICS.)

MEALS AND SNACKS TO ACCOMPANY BEER. It

makes good sense to eat food while drinking beer because (1) food reduces the effects of the beer since it slows the rate at which the stomach empties its contents into the small intestine, where most of the alcohol in the beer is absorbed; (2) the tendency to drink too much beer may be curtailed somewhat by slowing the rate at which the stomach empties; and (3) food may provide the protein, minerals, and vitamins lacking in beer so that better nutrition is achieved.

Most beers contain about the same number of calories as the popular brands of sweetened, carbonated soft drinks, although a few special *light* beers may be significantly lower in calories. Hence, the best foods to eat with beer are those rich in protein, minerals, and vitamins, but low in carbohydrates and fats. Also, it is better *not* to eat salty, spicy, or sugary foods with beer because they may provoke excessive thirst and overconsumption of beer. Crafty owners of bars have long supplied such snacks free of charge in order to encourage a greater consumption of their beverages. Some good accompaniments to beer are: (1) cheeses and other dairy products; (2) eggs, fish, meats, poultry, and seafood; (3) fruits, vegetables, and salads; (4) pretzels, whole grain breads, and other baked goods; and (5) beans, peas, nuts, and other seeds.

BEET SUGAR

Table sugar—sucrose—extracted from the sugar beet. (Also see SUGAR, section headed "Sugar Beet.")

BEETURIA

A harmless condition characterized by red pigmented urine which may occur after the consumption of beets.

BEHAVIOR AND DIET

Behavior is the manner in which individuals handle or manage themselves in relation to other individuals and their surroundings; or an individual's response to specific conditions. Normal and abnormal behavior are subjective classifications. What is normal or abnormal may be merely a matter of degree and the manner in which a person's behavior is perceived by family, friends, and professionals. There are, however, some general classifications of abnormal behavior, including disruptive behavior, failure to develop learning skills and motor skills, and behavior which breaks moral and

[14]Yano, K., G. G. Rhoads, and A. Kagan, "Coffee, Alcohol and Risk of Coronary Heart Disease Among Japanese Men Living in Hawaii," *The New England Journal of Medicine*, Vol. 297, 1977, p. 405.

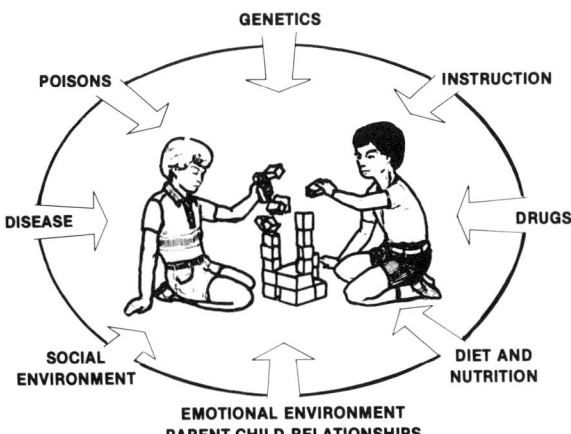

Fig. B-23. Behavior results from a complex interaction of many factors.

social values and laws of the land. Diet—all nutrients entering the body through the mouth, and nutrition—the body processes nutrients undergo after ingestion,have been implicated in forms of abnormal behavior.

BEHAVIORAL PROBLEMS. There are numerous forms of specific behavioral problems, but primarily hyperactivity (hyperkinesis), learning disabilities, and juvenile delinquency and crime have in some way been linked to diet, whether correctly or incorrectly. In some cases, diet is suggested as both the cause and the cure, while in other cases dietary modifications are suggested as cures for abnormal behavior of unknown origin.

• **Hyperactivity**—*Hyperactive,* or in medical terminology *hyperkinetic,* is a label that has been applied to between 5 and 20% of all school-age children in the United States. Unfortunately, hyperactivity is a vague term and some ill-mannered children have been conveniently labeled as hyperactive. Hyperactive children are described as being significantly more restless, easily distracted, inattentive and emotionally labile relative to their peers. Attention is drawn to hyperactive children in situations which require sedentary and attentive behavior; thus, these children usually come under medical and psychological evaluation because of behavioral problems and learning difficulties at school. Furthermore, the hyperactive child may be physically sound but have difficulty with motor skills and coordination.

Many theories on the cause of hyperactivity have been presented, including genetics, brain damage, crowded homes, environmental pollutants, parent-child interactions, fluorescent lights, and diet.

A variety of treatments have been tried with mixed results. These have included stimulants, elimination of fluorescent lighting in the classrooms, determination of allergies, restriction of diet, and, recently, behavioral modification programs. Popular treatments are diet oriented.

• **Learning disabilities**—Life is a learning process involving motor skills, speech, reading, writing, and social skills. The inability to learn may appear at various stages of life, and, due to the many things to be learned, the disabilities are given various labels. Many causes of learning disabilities have genetic roots; others involve social and environmental deprivation, or injury and disease, while still others have

nutritional causes. Regardless of the cause, some dietary treatments have been proposed.

• **Juvenile delinquency and crime**—Recently, there have been attempts to lay a large share of the blame for juvenile delinquency and crime upon poor diet. While diet may have a role in emotional well-being, so do many other factors. Moreover, moral behavior and respect for the law are taught rather than fed.

DIETARY CAUSES AND CURES. Possible causes and cures are almost as numerous as specific behavioral problems. However, some are more important than others due to their popularity or validity. Among the dietary causes and cures of behavior problems being promulgated by different theorists are those which follow.

Feingold or K-P Diet. In 1973, Dr. Ben Feingold, an allergist from the Kaiser-Permanente (K-P) Medical Center in San Francisco, California, introduced his solution to hyperactivity. Dr. Feingold suggested that the elimination of certain chemical compounds in the diet would prevent and treat hyperactivity. Originally, Dr. Feingold believed that salicylates (chemicals related to aspirin), naturally-occurring substances present in many foods—including many fruits, caused hyper-activity. Gradually, Dr. Feingold added (1) artificial food colors and flavors with a chemical structure similar to salicylates, (2) all artificial colors and flavors, and (3) preservatives such as butylated hydroxytoluene (BHT) and butylated hydroxyanisole (BHA). The Feingold or K-P diet is an elimination diet which seeks to remove these chemicals from the diet. Since most all commercially processed and prepared foods contain artificial colors, flavors or preservatives, and since salicylates are present naturally in many fruits and vegetables, it becomes nearly impossible to eliminate them totally from the diet.

Dr. Feingold recommends that many common foods be excluded; among them, all manufactured baked goods, luncheon meats, ice cream, powdered puddings, candies, soft drinks, and punches. Also, teas, coffee, margarine, butter, and many commercially produced condiments are barred. Additionally, many nonfood items such as mouthwash, toothpaste, cough drops, perfume, and some over-the-counter and prescription drugs are taboo. Obviously, eating in restaurants and school cafeterias becomes impossible for a child adhering to the Feingold plan. Foods for the Feingold diet must be prepared from *scratch* in the home. Therefore, Dr. Feingold recommends that the entire family become involved in following the diet plan thereby lessening temptation to stray and preventing the child from feeling different. Following the diet becomes a family affair.

Since its introduction in 1973, numerous professionals have tested, evaluated and/or studied the Feingold or K-P Diet, with the doubters outnumbering the believers. Nevertheless, Dr. Feingold's hypothesis has stimulated awareness and research of the problem.

Sugar Elimination. Sugar, primarily sucrose or table sugar, has been blamed for a variety of ills including behavior problems. Some popular theories suggest that the consumption of refined sugar causes hyperactivity, mental illness, juvenile delinquency, and crime.

Supporters of the *sugar-undesirable behavior theory* explain that consumption of excess sugar leads to the development of reactive or functional hypoglycemia—low blood sugar. Then, undesirable behavior results from the mental changes induced by the low blood sugar, or in the case of hyperactive children, their behavior results from the release of hormones from the adrenal gland which attempt to increase blood sugar.

Although most nutritionists would agree that Americans eat too much sugar, the overall result of such indulgence is that it displaces more nutritious foods from the diet, possibly creating a diet low in other essential nutrients, which could possibly affect the mental attitude. Also, all the sugary between meal snacks play havoc with dental health. But blaming sugar *per se* for behavioral problems is based primarily on anecdotes— not scientific facts.

(Also see HYPOGLYCEMIA; METABOLISM; and SUGAR.)

Food Allergies. A food allergy is an immunologically mediated adverse reaction to food. Some suggestion has been made that a food allergy may be responsible for behavioral disturbances ranging from hyperactivity to a feeling of tiredness to criminal behavior.

Without doubt, many of the symptoms of food allergies may alter the behavior of afflicted persons by making them uncomfortable. But any direct connection between a food allergy and some undesirable behavior remains obscure, and for the time being, hypothetical. Scientists, however, maintain an open mind and continue to conduct well-controlled studies further to elucidate any connection between food allergies and behavior.

(Also see ALLERGIES.)

Megavitamin Therapy. Another popular idea is that massive doses of vitamins may cure hyperactivity and other behavioral abnormalities. Advocates of megavitamin therapy, or orthomolecular psychiatry, propose that optimum molecular concentrations of vitamins are essential for proper mental functioning. No one will argue that dietary deficiencies of such vitamins as thiamin, riboflavin, niacin, pantothenic acid, vitamin B-6 and vitamin B-12 will modify sensory functions (nervous functions), motor ability, and personality. However, most of the reported efficacy of megavitamin therapy results from anecdotal observations. Studies investigating the benefits of megavitamins with proper scientific protocol have failed to demonstrate improved behavior with megavitamins.

Currently, the American Academy of Pediatrics and the American Psychiatric Association feel that megavitamin therapy is unproved in terms of safety and efficacy. Nevertheless, hope should not be abandoned. There are certain genetic disorders for which megavitamin therapy can be justified and future research may find its justification in other disorders. For example, nine studies reported in the world literature show that megadoses of vitamin B-6 are helpful in treating autism, though more experimental work is needed.[15]

(Also see VITAMIN[S].)

Brain Transmitters and Diet. Brain function, hence behavior, relies upon the ability of the cells of the brain to synthesize and release normal amounts of transmitters which control brain function by modifying the conduction and transmission of nervous impulses. An exciting area of new research is that the possibility exists that the availability of certain nutrients in the food can raise or lower the formation of brain transmitters thereby modifying brain function. The transmitters subject to dietary control include: serotonin, norepinephrine, and acetylcholine.

Serotonin is derived from dietary tryptophan, an essential amino acid. A high carbohydrate (simple sugar) diet increases the serotonin level in the brain of rats and humans. However, there is no direct evidence that an increased concentration of serotonin in the brain affects behavior. Neurologists claim that cells in the brain that release serotonin influence sleep. Tryptophan supplements have been used to treat various sleep disorders, and to improve the mood in depressed patients.

Norepinephrine is also derived from an amino acid— tyrosine. The administration of tyrosine to rats with high blood pressure dramatically reduces blood pressure. This effect seems to be caused by the stimulation of norepinephrine synthesis in the brain. Some have conjectured that, in the future, tyrosine may be used in the treatment of behavioral disorders such as depression.

Choline is the dietary precursor of the neurotransmitter *acetylcholine*. Variations in the daily intake of choline also modify the brain levels of choline and acetylcholine. Some preliminary reports have shown that dietary choline may improve learning and behavior. Recently, clinical trials have shown choline to be successful in the treatment of *tardive dyskinesia*, a disorder of the central nervous system.

The story of the effect of diet on brain transmitters is still incomplete, but it is an area of exciting research—where sound scientific protocol has been followed. Important discoveries ahead may help in understanding the relationship between diet, brain chemistry, and behavior.

(Also see AMINO ACID[S]; and CHOLINE.)

Malnutrition. In humans, it is difficult to say whether nutrition *per se* contributes to behavioral abnormalities, since conditions of malnutrition and a deprived social and emotional environment often coexist. Studies have demonstrated the importance of the mother-child relationship to learning and behavior, and malnutrition may adversely affect this interaction. While the effects of malnutrition are uncertain, the following points deserve consideration:

1. The brain and spinal cord grow rapidly during the last of pregnancy, and continue rapid growth during infancy.

2. Malnutrition during the early life of animals and humans alters the number of brain cells, brain cell size and/or other biochemical parameters, depending upon the time of onset and the duration of the malnutrition.

3. Malnourished animals demonstrate impaired learning abilities.

4. Teachers have observed that hungry, undernourished children are apathetic and lethargic.

5. Children suffering from kwashiorkor are apathetic, listless, and withdrawn; and they seldom either (a) resist examination or (b) wander off when left alone.

6. Children who recover from marasmus have a reduced head circumference—brain size—even after 5 years of rehabilitation.

7. Numerous studies suggest that infants subjected to acute malnutrition during the first years of life develop irreversible gaps in mental development, and thus never attain their full genetic potential.

(Also see INFANT DIET AND NUTRITION; MALNUTRITION; and MALNUTRITION, PROTEIN-ENERGY.)

OVERLOOKED FACTORS. A host of factors are involved in determining behavior. Too often popularized theories are the result of *witch hunts*; hence, caution should be exercised when entertaining them. To blame only the

[15]Rimland, Bernard, Ph.D., Letters to the editor, *Science News*, Vol. 119, No. 16, April 18, 1981, p. 243.

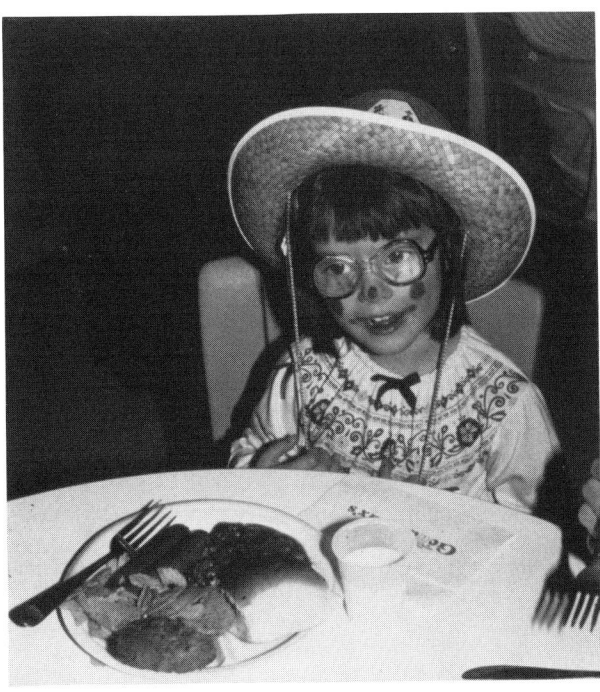

Fig. B-24. In humans, abnormal behavior may be due to heredity and/or environment, including nutrition. (Courtesy, Louisiana Cooperative Extension Service, Louisiana State University, Baton Rouge, La.)

diet and nutrition for undesirable behavior is to take an attitude of *the devil made me do it*. Human behavior is far too complex even to hint that only one condition in the environment determines it. Rather, individuals would be well advised to consider the effects of such things as (1) smoking and alcohol use during pregnancy, (2) drug abuse during pregnancy and lactation, (3) stress and nutrition during pregnancy, (4) genetic background and genetic errors, (5) family interactions, and (6) social environment.

Unfortunately, blaming the diet for behavior is attractive since it is more palatable to believe undesirable behavior results from conditions outside the individual rather than inherent problems, lack of instruction, or social interactions.

(Also see MINERAL[S]; NERVOUS SYSTEM DISORDERS; PREGNANCY AND LACTATION NUTRITION, section headed "Factors That May Warrant Special Counseling of Pregnant Women;" and VITAMIN[S].)

BELCHING

The bringing up of gas from the stomach. Excessive belching may be due to (1) swallowing of large amounts of air as a result of nervousness, (2) the drinking of carbonated beverages, (3) a heavy consumption of caffeine-containing beverages such as coffee and tea, or (4) force of habit. In certain countries, belching after a meal is considered to be a sign to the host that the food was greatly appreciated. However, frequent and uncomfortable belching may mean that a person has a digestive disorder which requires treatment by a doctor.

BELLADONNA DRUGS

This group of drugs, which is extracted from plants of the Nightshade family, is so named because at one time they were used by ladies to dilate the pupils of their eyes, since ladies with large pupils were considered to be more glamorous. (*Bella donna* in Italian means beautiful lady.) These drugs are now used mainly to reduce the amount of gastrointestinal secretions and to calm the digestive tract in the treatment of such conditions as peptic ulcers, spasms of the gallbladder, diarrhea, stomach and bowel irritation, ulcerative colitis, and heartburn. However, people given these drugs may have such side effects as convulsions, drowsiness, dryness of the mouth, constipation, and blurring of the vision. Hence, they should only be used under a doctor's supervision, even though certain preparations which contain these drugs may be obtained without a prescription.

(Also see ATROPINE.)

BENEDICT'S TEST

A chemical test for determining the presence of reducing sugars; for example, glucose and maltose. Heating with Benedict's reagent—copper sulfate, sodium citrate, and sodium carbonate—gives a green, yellow, or orange-red precipitate, depending upon the amount of reducing sugar present. Benedict's test is used to test for the presence of sugar in the urine.

BENGAL QUINCE (BEL FRUIT; GOLDEN APPLE) *Aegle marmelos*

This fruit grows on a thorny tree (of the family *Rutaceae*) that is native to India and is now found throughout Southeast Asia and the East Indies. The yellow fruit ranges from 2 to 7 in. (5 to 17.5 cm) in diameter and has a hard skin and a soft flesh. It is usually eaten fresh, dried, or made into an ice or a sherbet.

Bengal quince is moderately high in calories (133 kcal per 100 g) and carbohydrates (35%). It is a good to excellent source of fiber and potassium, but it is a poor source of vitamin C.

BENIGN DISORDERS

Mild illnesses or other abnormal conditions which do not generally endanger life. Benign is also used to describe a tumorous growth that is not cancerous.

BENZEDRINE

A member of the amphetamine family of drugs used as both a stimulant and an appetite depressant.

(Also see AMPHETAMINES; and APPETITE.)

BERGAMOT ORANGE *Citrus bergamia*

A small citrus fruit (of the family *Rutaceae*) that is believed to have arisen from a natural crossbreeding (hybridization) of the sour orange (*Citrus aurantium*) with another species of citrus fruit.

The flesh of the bergamot is highly acid and of little commercial importance, but the oil from the peel has a distinctive aromatic odor and taste which suits it well for use in candies, medicines, and perfumes. Sometimes, the whole peel is candied. It is also noteworthy that bergamot peel oil is the aromatic base for eau de cologne. Most of the crop is grown in Italy.

(Also see CITRUS FRUITS.)

BERIBERI

This ancient nutritional disease results from a severe deficiency of thiamin (vitamin B-1). It is usually found in areas of the world where diets are high in carbohydrate, but low in thiamin. However, chronic abuse of alcohol may precipitate the disease in persons who might otherwise have access to a balanced diet. A typical victim of beriberi is shown in Fig. B-25.

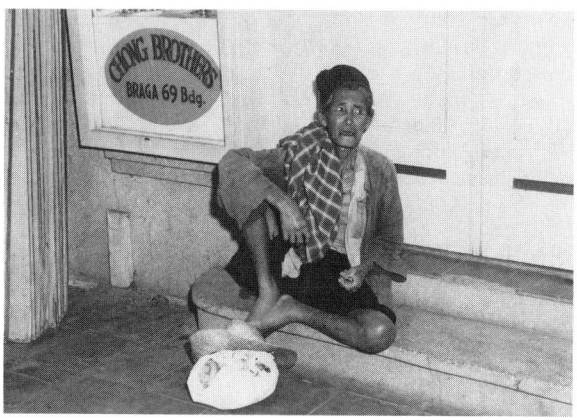

Fig. B-25. Beriberi, a deficiency disease due to a lack of vitamin B-1 (thiamin) in the diet. Note the cracked skin and swollen legs (edema). In the Far East, beriberi is largely due to the almost exclusive use of polished rice. (Courtesy, FAO, Rome, Italy.)

HISTORY OF BERIBERI. A historical record of beriberi, along with a chronolgy of the experimenters and experiments involved in the cause, cure, and prevention of the disease, is presented in the section on thiamin; hence, the reader is referred thereto.

CAUSES OF BERIBERI. The disease is regularly found in populations whose diets contain less than 0.3 mg of thiamin per 1,000 nonfat Calories (kcal). Diets which may cause beriberi are those in which the staple foods are either highly refined, such as white rice, white flour, or degerminated cornmeal, or where there are starchy items like cassava.

Occasionally, beriberi may be precipitated by stress factors such as pregnancy, lactation, strenuous exercise, or by restoration of growth after protein-energy deficiencies. Thus, pregnancy may be debilitating, or even fatal, to a thiamin-deficient woman. Even if the woman herself escapes such morbid consequences, her child may develop beriberi as a result of a low level of thiamin in her milk. Thiamin-deficient men may also be prone to beriberi if they engage in hard labor, since a heightened energy metabolism is likely to hasten the depletion of the body's limited supply of thiamin. (This supply consists of the small amount of thiamin which is present in the body fluids.)

Chronic alcoholism may also precipitate beriberi since alcohol cannot be converted to fat in the body, but must be metabolized by the same thiamin-dependent processes as carbohydrate and protein. Furthermore, alcohol increases urinary excretion of water (diuretic effect) and water-soluble vitamins. A similar, but lesser, effect may result from the heavy consumption of caffeine (in beverages such as coffee, colas, and tea) coupled with a diet chronically high in refined foods which are rich in carbohydrates. (Like alcohol, caffeine is a diuretic. Also, it stimulates the utilization of stored carbohydrate for energy.)

FORMS OF BERIBERI. The disease may appear in any one of several forms which may resemble other diseases. Also, there may be a sudden change from one form to another. Therefore, the features of each form are discussed in the sections which follow.

Dry Beriberi. This form is characterized by signs of multiple nervous disorders such as sensations of pins and needles on the legs, muscle pain, delayed pain response, and foot drop, which may indicate the beginning of a brain disorder known as *Wernicke's encephalopathy* (typical signs are double vision, squint-eyedness, disorientation, delusions, and loss of memory). The psychotic effects of the brain disorder are collectively called *Korsakoff's psychosis*, which is particularly distinguished by confused thinking and the making up of stories to fill in gaps of memory (confabulation). This aspect of the disease may eventually result in a stupefied state. These effects may commonly be found in chronic alcoholics, diabetics whose disease has been out of control, and semistarved persons such as prisoners of war.

Wet Beriberi. The presence of edema distinguishes this form from dry beriberi. Other features are extreme loss of appetite, breathlessness, and disorders of the heart which range from palpitation and rapid heart rate to dilation of the heart muscle (myocardium) and congestive heart failure. When the cardiac disorders are severe, the disease may be called *cardiac beriberi*, or *Shoshin beriberi* (a name used in Asia).

Infantile Beriberi. This form is usually found in infants living in areas of endemic beriberi who have been breast-fed by mothers whose milk is deficient in thiamin. Signs of the disorder are weakness of voice during bawling (complete lack of sound in severe cases), lack of appetite, vomiting, diarrhea, rapid pulse, and cyanosis (in severe cases). The disease results in a high death rate of infants from 2 to 5 months of age. There may be a rapid course of the disease from mild disorders to death.

Juvenile Beriberi. The feeding of extra protein without extra thiamin to protein-deficient children who are stunted in their growth may bring on beriberi because (1) growth resumes and the need for thiamin is increased, and (2) part of the dietary protein may be converted in the body to carbohydrates and/or other substances which require thiamin for their metabolism.

TREATMENT AND PREVENTION OF BERIBERI. Intramuscular injections of from 5 mg to 50 mg of thiamin per day are more effective during the first few days of the therapy for severe beriberi than oral doses of the vitamin since gastrointestinal absorption may be less efficient. Such therapy is usually followed by prompt remission of the cardiac disorders, but the neurological disorders may persist for a while. Oral doses of from 20 mg to 30 mg of thiamin may be given in place of the injections as soon as the patient shows signs of improvement. The last stage of therapy consists of supplying foods or special supplements which are rich in thiamin, such as dried brewers' yeast, dried torula yeast, liver, liver extract, rice polishings, wheat germ, or legumes such as beans and lentils.

The enrichment of white flour with thiamin has been effective in lessening thiamin deficiency in the United States, and elsewhere where practiced. It is more difficult, however, to obtain widespread enrichment of rice which requires impregnation of the individual grains with vitamin mix; the enriched rice takes on the yellow color of riboflavin which is objectionable to some rice eaters.

The age old practice in some rice eating areas, such as certain parts of India, of parboiling rice before milling is at least partly effective in preventing beriberi. Parboiling is now done on a commercial basis by first soaking the unhulled grains of rice in water, then parboiling them until their hulls split open. This process causes such water-soluble vitamins as thiamin to migrate deeper into the grain from the outer layers. Hence, these vitamins are retained within the grain when the outer layers are removed by milling.

(Also see RICE; THIAMIN; WHEAT, section on "Enriched Flour;" and VITAMIN[S], Table V-5, Vitamin Table.)

BERRY

A type of fleshy fruit in which the seeds are enclosed within the pulp. Some of the most common berries are blackberries, blueberries, currants, cranberries, gooseberries, grapes, raspberries, and strawberries. However, the term is often applied to various fruits which are not strictly berries from a botanical point of view.

(Also see FRUIT[S], Table F-23, Fruits of the World.)

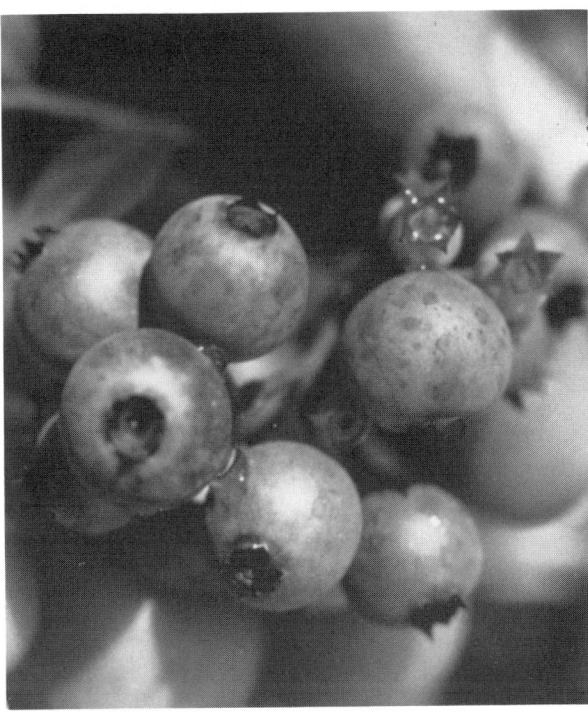

Fig. B-26. Blueberries, a popular berry. (Courtesy, University of Minnesota, St. Paul, Minn.)

BETA

Second letter in the Greek alphabet, corresponding to the letter B in our alphabet. In chemistry and nutrition, the prefix beta is used with a hyphen to indicate the second member of a closely related series of substances.

BETA-CAROTENE

A yellow-orange plant pigment which may be converted in the body to vitamin A. The best food sources of beta-carotene are the yellow, orange, or red fruits and vegetables, or the green leafy vegetables. In the latter, the intense green color of chlorophyll masks the color of the underlying carotene.

(Also see VITAMIN A.)

BETA CELLS OF THE PANCREAS

The cells which synthesize, store, and secrete the hormone insulin.

(Also see ENDOCRINE GLANDS.)

BETA-CHOLESTEROL

This term is a layman's designation for blood cholesterol which is carried on beta-lipoproteins, in contrast to that carried on alpha-lipoproteins. However, the cholesterol molecule itself does not vary, only the lipoprotein which carries it in the blood.

It is important to differentiate between the ways in which cholesterol is conveyed in the blood, because that carried on beta-lipoproteins is much more likely to be deposited in the walls of blood vessels than that borne by alpha-lipoproteins.

(Also see ALPHA-LIPOPROTEINS; BETA-LIPOPROTEINS; CHOLESTEROL; and HEART DISEASE.)

BETA-HYDROXYBUTYRIC ACID

One of the ketone bodies which accumulates in the blood and is passed in the urine when fat is incompletely metabolized.

(Also see ACIDOSIS; and DIABETES MELLITUS.)

BETAINE

A substance closely related to choline. It may serve as a raw material from which the body synthesizes choline. Betaine has been shown in animal experiments to prevent fatty livers when diets high in fat, cholesterol, and/or sugar are consumed. The best sources of betaine are plant foods, particularly beets.

(Also see CHOLINE.)

BETA-LIPOPROTEINS

Special fat-carrying proteins which are produced in the liver. Beta-lipoproteins are also called low density lipoproteins (LDL). Normally, they contain from 10 to 50% triglycerides, 22 to 46% cholesterol, 18 to 22% phospholipid, and 9 to 21% proteins. It is not desirable for one to have a high blood level of beta-lipoproteins because the cholesterol they carry may be deposited in the blood vessels. However, alpha-lipoproteins (HDL) convey cholesterol in a much more stable complex, so that there is little risk of cholesterol deposits when the blood levels of these proteins are elevated. It appears that the levels of beta-lipoproteins may be reduced, and those of alpha-lipoproteins raised by (1) loss of excess body weight, (2) strenuous physical exercise, (3) a diet low in animal fats and cholesterol, (4) drugs such as clofibrate and niacin (this vitamin must be administered in large doses to achieve the desired effects), and (5) moderate amounts of alcohol.

NOTE: Measures designed to alter the levels of blood fats should be undertaken under the supervision of a physician.

(Also see ALPHA-LIPOPROTEINS; CHOLESTEROL; and HEART DISEASE.)

BETA-OXIDATION

A major means by which fatty acids are metabolized in the body.

(Also see FATS AND OTHER LIPIDS; and METABOLISM.)

BETEL LEAVES

Leaves from a creeping plant (*Piper betel*) which are chewed in some parts of the world for a stimulating effect.

(Also see BETEL NUTS.)

BETEL NUTS

The nuts produced by the areta palm (*Areta catethu*), which are chewed in order to obtain stimulating effects.

(Also see BETEL LEAVES.)

BEVERAGES

Any liquid used or prepared for drinking is a beverage. Numerous beverages have been invented, but most of them can be included in one of the following categories.

1. Aromatic and stimulating infusions such as herbal tea, tea, coffee, and roasted grain drinks.

2. Fruit juices, including lemonade and fruit-flavored drinks.

3. Fermented beverages such as beer, wine, and cider.

4. Distilled liquors.

5. Soft drinks or carbonated beverages.

6. Water.

Some noteworthy statistics relative to the consumption of soft drinks in the United States follow:

1. Per capita consumption of soft drinks is estimated at more than 40 gal.

2. Yearly consumption of soft drinks surpasses all other beverages including milk, beer, coffee, or water (22% for water vs 23.8% for soft drinks).

3. Total annual wholesale value of soft drinks is more than $20 billion.

For information about specific beverages, consult the individual articles, and Food Composition Table F-21 of this book.

(Also see ALCOHOLIC BEVERAGES; BEERS AND BREWING; COFFEE; DISTILLED LIQUORS; SOFT DRINKS; WATER; and WINE.)

BEZOAR

A hard, gummy ball which forms in the stomach and which may block the intestines. A bezoar may form when foods rich in gums are swallowed without adequate chewing.

BIBULOUS

Refers to a person who is fond of alcohol beverages.

BICARBONATE

Name used by lay people to designate antacids that contain baking soda or sodium bicarbonate. The chemical definition of bicarbonate is a salt produced by the reaction of carbonic acid with an alkali. Sometimes, the term bicarbonate is used to designate the major alkali present in the blood. However, the correct term for the so-called alkali reserve is bicarbonate ion.

(Also see ACID-BALANCE; ALKALI RESERVE; BAKING POWDER AND BAKING SODA; and BICARBONATE ION.)

BICARBONATE ION

A negatively charged alkali ion derived from bicarbonate salts, or from carbonic acid. It helps to regulate acid-base balance.

(Also see ACID-BASE BALANCE; ALKALI RESERVE; BAKING POWDER AND BAKING SODA; and CARBONIC ACID.)

BICARBONATE OF SODA

Another name for baking soda or sodium bicarbonate.
(Also see BAKING POWDER AND BAKING SODA.)

BICYCLE ERGOMETER

A machine, similar to an ordinary bicycle, but fixed to a stand, which is equipped to measure the work performed during pedaling. It is often used in metabolic studies, and in tests of cardiovascular efficiency.

BIFIDUS FACTOR

A substance found in human breast milk which promotes the growth of *Lactobacillus bifidus* in the intestines of infants. *L. bifidus* protects infants against various types of bacterial infections in the digestive tract.

(Also see INFANT DIET AND NUTRITION; and MILK AND MILK PRODUCTS.)

BILBERRY *Vaccinium myrtillus*

The fruit of a wild shrubby plant (of the family *Ericaceae*) that grows wild in the northern parts of Europe and Asia. This berry is closely related to the North American varieties of blueberries. Furthermore, bilberries are sometimes referred to as blaeberries (in Iceland), huckleberries, whortleberries, or windberries.

The fruit has a tart flavor which is improved by sweetening. Also, it makes good jams and pies.

BILE

A yellowish-green fluid produced by the liver and stored in the gallbladder, which empties through the bile duct into the duodenum of the small intestine, where it participates in the digestion of fats. It is considered to be one of the digestive juices of the intestinal tract.

(Also see DIGESTION AND ABSORPTION; and GALLBLADDER.)

BILE ACIDS

A group of several similar compounds present in bile, a digestive fluid secreted by the liver, and stored in the gallbladder. Bile acids are (1) produced by the breakdown of cholesterol in the liver, and (2) converted into bile salts by the alkaline constituents of the bile.

(Also see BILE; BILE SALTS; DIGESTION AND ABSORPTION; and GALLSTONES.)

BILE DUCTS

This designation includes (1) the hepatic ducts which collect the bile formed in the liver, (2) the common bile duct connecting the hepatic ducts with the small intestine, and (3) the cystic duct which connects the gallbladder and the common bile duct.

(Also see DIGESTION AND ABSORPTION; and GALLSTONES.)

BILE PIGMENTS

Breakdown products of red blood cells, which are excreted in the bile and the feces. Bile pigments may accumulate in the blood when various liver disorders prevent their excretion in the bile. In such cases, the skin may turn yellow, a condition known as jaundice.

(Also see DIGESTION AND ABSORPTION; and GALLSTONES.)

BILE SALTS

These important components of bile are formed by the reactions between the bile acids and the alkaline substances present in the bile. After the various constituents of bile have been mixed and secreted by the liver, the bile is stored in the gallbladder until food is consumed. Then, the passage of food from the stomach into the small intestine triggers the release of bile from the gallbladder into the duodenum. There, the bile salts help to emulsify the fatty materials in the diet so that they may be digested and absorbed.

Almost all of the bile salts are reabsorbed from the intestine and returned to the liver via the blood. However, certain undigestible carbohydrates, collectively called fiber, bind bile salts so that greater amounts are lost in the stool. This effect tends to reduce the body's content of cholesterol because increased amounts of the sterol are converted to bile salts to replace those which are excreted.

(Also see BILE; CHOLESTEROL; DIGESTION AND ABSORPTION; FIBER; and GALLSTONES.)

BILHARZIASIS

This condition, often called *schistomiasis* at the present time, is an infestation of the body with small flat worms (flukes). It is most common in Asia, Africa, and in parts of Europe where sanitation is poor. Usually the larvae of the flukes penetrate the skin when people wade into contaminated water. However, the flukes may also be present in food.

BILIARY

Pertaining to the bile or to the gallbladder.
(Also see BILE; and DIGESTION AND ABSORPTION.)

BILIARY CALCULI

A disorder in which stones are formed in various parts of the biliary system (the liver, bile ducts, gallbladder, and small intestine.) Another name for this condition is gallstones. The condition is usually more common in people who manifest one or more of the four Fs: female, fat, forty, and fair complexion.

(Also see GALLSTONES.)

BILIARY CIRRHOSIS

A disorder of the liver which is due to blockage of the bile duct(s) and accumulation of bile in the liver and the blood. The condition is characterized by fever, abdominal pain, jaundice, gas, nausea, itching, and an elevated count of white cells in the blood. Prompt surgery is needed to correct the condition.

(Also see BILIARY OBSTRUCTION; and GALLSTONES.)

BILIARY COLIC

A spasm of the muscle surrounding the gallbladder due to (1) blockage of a bile duct by a gallstone; or (2) contraction of the gallbladder against a closed sphincter. Biliary colic is usually accompanied by an attack of severe cramping pain which occurs in the right side of the abdomen just below and in front of the ribs. A doctor should be called at once, when this type of pain is present.

(Also see BILIARY DYSKINESIA; and GALLSTONES.)

BILIARY DYSKINESIA

A malfunctioning of the gallbladder in which (1) it contracts but fails to empty properly because the sphincter does not relax and allow the bile to pass; or (2) the muscles around the gallbladder which cause it to contract lack tone and, therefore, fail to do their job.

(Also see BILIARY COLIC; and GALLSTONES.)

BILIARY OBSTRUCTION

A blockage somewhere in the system of bile ducts that (1) prevents bile from passing into the small intestine, and (2) causes it to accumulate in the liver and in the blood.

(Also see BILE DUCTS; and GALLSTONES.)

BILIMBE (CUCUMBER TREE) *Averrhoa bilimbe*

The green, cucumberlike fruit of a tree (of the family *Oxalidaceae*) that is native to Malaysia and now grows in many tropical areas of the world. Bilimbe fruits are usually between 2 and 3 in. (*5 to 7.5 cm*) long and contain a sour, seedy pulp which makes them good for curries, pickles, jams, jellies, and sweetened juices.

The fruit is high in water content (94%) and low in calories (20 kcal per 100 g) and carbohydrates (5%). It is a good source of iron and a fair source of fiber and vitamin C.

BILIOUSNESS

A digestive disorder which is usually attributed to some type of malfunctioning of the liver. It is characterized by headache, nausea and vomiting, constipation, lack of appetite, furred tongue, and occasionally slight jaundice.

(Also see DIGESTION AND ABSORPTION.)

BILIRUBIN

One of the bile pigments which results from the breakdown of hemoglobin. Normally, it is excreted into the intestine with the bile. However, blockage of the biliary tract leads to accumulation of bile in the liver and blood. The buildup of pigment often imparts a yellow color to the skin (a condition called jaundice). Newborn babies are particularly prone to brain damage by elevated blood levels of bilirubin.

(Also see DIGESTION AND ABSORPTION.)

BILIRUBINURIA

The presence of the bile pigment bilirubin in the urine. This pigment colors the urine dark. Bilirubinuria is often accompanied by jaundice.

(Also see BILIRUBIN.)

BILIVERDIN

A green pigment resulting from the breakdown of hemoglobin. The pigment is converted to bilirubin in the liver.

(Also see BILE PIGMENTS; and BILIRUBIN.)

BIO-

A prefix denoting life.

BIOASSAY

Determination of the relative effective strength of a substance (as a vitamin, hormone, or drug) by comparing its effect on a test organism with that of a standard preparation.

BIOCHEMISTRY

The study of chemical processes which take place in living organisms.

BIOFLAVONOIDS (VITAMIN P)

At this time, no evidence exists that bioflavonoids serve any useful role in human nutrition or in the prevention or treatment of disease in humans; hence, this presentation is for two purposes: (1) informational, and (2) stimulation of research.

Bioflavonoids, also known as vitamin P, are a group of natural pigments in vegetables, fruits, flowers, and grains. They appear as companions of natural vitamin C, but they are not present in synthetic vitamin C. Because of the basic yellow color of most of them, they are called flavonoids, after the Latin, *flavus*, for yellow. (Some of these substances are naturally occurring dyes.) To date, about 800 different flavonoids have been identified, of which more than 30 are in the genus *Citrus* alone. Three of the better known bioflavonoids are *hesperidin*, *naringin*, and *rutin*.

Hesperidin is found in the blossom, in the small unripe fruit, and in the peel of the mature sweet orange. Also, it is found in lemons, mandarins, bitter oranges, and citrons. Each mature sweet orange contains almost 1 g of hesperidin-like material of which approximately half can be recovered by commercial procedures. Hesperidin is used extensively as a therapeutic agent in the pharmaceutical industry.

Naringin is the predominant flavonoid in grapefruit. It is distinguished readily from hesperidin by its extreme bitterness, which it sometimes imparts to grapefruit products. Naringin is used in the preparation of beverages and to enhance the piquant flavor of high class confections.

Rutin was first prepared in 1842 by a German pharmacist-chemist, who obtained it from garden rue, *Ruta graveolens*; hence, the name *rutin*. Since then, chemists have found rutin in a number of plants, including tobacco and buckwheat (in the green or dehydrated leaves). Many pharmaceutical laboratories are now marketing dosage forms of rutin, principally in tablets, for the treatment of capillary fragility—a condition in which the smallest blood vessels (1) become abnormally fragile and rupture, so that small hemorrhages occur, or (2) become abnormally permeable, so that they allow substances to pass from the blood into the tissue spaces in larger quantities or of different kinds than normally filter through the capillary walls. Where either of these faults is present, there is increased danger of retinal hemorrhage or apoplexy, particularly in people with high blood pressure.

Claims are made that rutin, taken by mouth, will correct these capillary faults in a large proportion of cases. Diabetics frequently have complications of this sort, with loss of vision and even blindness. Some reports indicate that the use of rutin results in arresting progress in the loss of sight, and sometimes improvement of vision, especially in young patients. Rutin has also been used in treating certain types of glaucoma, in treating injury from x-ray irradiation, in treating cold injury (frostbite), and in lessening the severity of the symptoms in cases of hemophilia—the hereditary disease characterized by failure of the blood to clot normally after injury.

HISTORY. In the mid-1930s, Szent-Gyorgyi, the Hungarian scientist, who subsequently (in 1937) won a Nobel Prize in medicine for his work with vitamin C, isolated a material in citrus rind that he called *citrin*, and which he showed consisted of a mixture of flavonoids. His initial test of the new substance with scorbutic guinea pigs, reported in 1936, seemed to indicate that, in combination with ascorbic acid, it was effective in strengthening the body's smallest blood vessels, the capillaries, and in curing scurvy. From this and subsequent work arose the concept of vitamin P, a substance or a group of substances of a flavonoid nature involved in regulation of permeability and maintenance of capillary integrity.

Soon, the race was on! Research was stimulated; studies involving vitamin C and vitamin P were conducted on both humans and animals all over the world; and journal articles attested to clinical successes. Vitamin P (usually in combination with vitamin C) was rushed in to treat a whole host of disorders believed to be related to faulty capillary function; among them, habitual and threatened abortion, postpartum bleeding, nosebleed, skin disorders, diabetes retinitis, bleeding gums, heavy menstrual bleeding, hemorrhoids, and many others.

But the earlier hopes held for vitamin P did not materialize. In 1938, Szent-Gyorgyi reported that subsequent tests failed to confirm the results of his earlier experiments. Similar work in other laboratories verified his conclusions. Although the observation that flavonoids display a synergistic action towards ascorbic acid was demonstrated, the initial claim that some or all of the flavonoids are indispensable food components equivalent to vitamins was not substantiated. As a result, in 1950 the Joint Committee of Biochemical Nomenclature of the American Society of Biological Chemists and the American Institute of Nutrition recommended that the term *vitamin P* be dropped. Following this, the name *bioflavonoids* came into use except in France and the U.S.S.R., where the term *vitamin P* persisted. Then, in the late 1960s, the U.S. Food and Drug Administration (FDA) concluded that, not only were the bioflavonoids not a vitamin, they were without any nutritional value whatsoever.

In the two decades following Szent-Gyorgyi's original work, numerous researchers studied the effects of the flavonoids on capillary fragility, infections, the common cold, hypertension, and various hemorrhagic disorders. But no therapeutic value was demonstrated. Also, for flavonoids to be classified as vitamins requires proof (1) that they are essential and indispensable food constituents, and (2) that deficiency syndromes are known which can be cured specifically by their administration. But neither of these prerequisites was fulfilled. So, two schools of thought evolved; those who believed, and those who doubted—with few undecided.

There is a logical explanation, according to the believers, why little therapeutic or nutritive value of bioflavonoids has been demonstrated. They point out that most fruits (especially citrus fruits) and vegetables are rich in bioflavonoids, and that almost everyone gets sufficient of these foods to prevent vitamin P deficiency. It is not that vitamin P is not required, they argue; it's already in the diet.

CHEMISTRY, METABOLISM, PROPERTIES.

- **Chemistry**—The chemical structure of two important bioflavonoids is given in Fig. B-27.

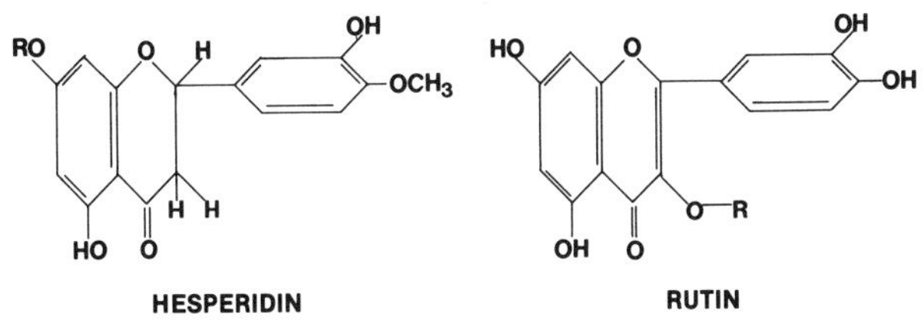

HESPERIDIN   RUTIN

Fig. B-27. Structure of two bioflavonoids. *Hesperidin* is found in citrus fruit; *rutin* is found in buckwheat leaves.

- **Metabolism**—The absorption, storage, and excretion of the bioflavonoids are very similar to vitamin C. They are readily absorbed into the bloodstream from the upper part of the small intestine. Excessive amounts are excreted primarily in the urine.

- **Properties**—Bioflavonoids are brightly colored water-soluble substances. They are relatively stable compounds, resistant to heat, oxygen, dryness, and moderate degrees of acidity, but they are rather quickly destroyed by light.

MEASUREMENT. Dosages of bioflavonoids are given in milligrams (mg).

FUNCTIONS. Bioflavonoids are promoted chiefly because of their function in capillary fragility and permeability. Thus, a knowledge of the physiology of the capillary system is requisite to an understanding of this particular role.

Since all body cells depend on the capillaries to bring them everything they need and to take away wastes, they are important.

The entire cardiovascular system—heart, arteries, and veins—is dependent upon the capillaries. These minute-sized vessels, averaging about 1/2,000 of an inch in diameter, are a part of the microcirculation system—the connecting link between the smallest branches of the arteries and the connecting veins. The segments of this small vessel system in order from the arterial to the venous side are: (1) arteriole, (2) terminal arteriole, (3) metarteriole, (4) capillary, and (5) venule (see Fig. B-28).

The capillaries (1) receive from the bloodstream the oxygen, nutrients, hormones, and antibodies; and (2) take up the wastes. All the rest of the circulatory vessels (the arteries that carry oxygenated blood from the heart to all parts of the body, and the veins that carry the used blood back to the heart for reoxygenation in the lungs) are impermeable. It is only at the capillary level (the network that links the tiniest arteries [arterioles] and the tiniest veins [venules]) that fluid from the bloodstream seeps out of this otherwise closed system and mingles with the fluid that surrounds all the body cells, then seeps back again. For this seepage to take place, the walls of the capillaries must be permeable—but not too permeable. When capillaries are too fragile and break, or

become too permeable, blood passes out into the intercellular fluid.

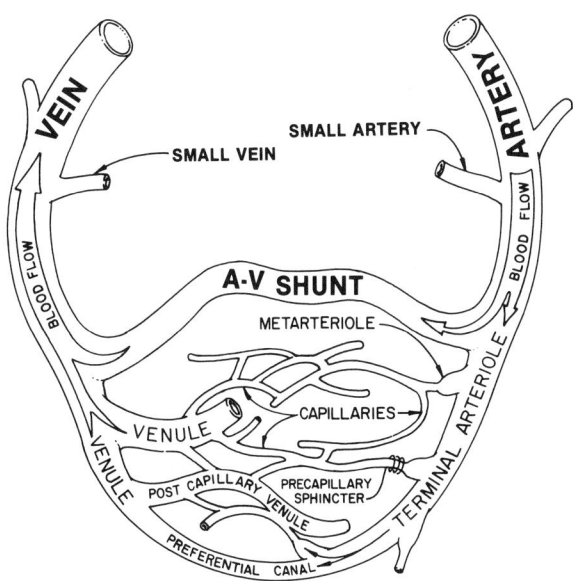

Fig. B-28. Schematic diagram of terminal vascular bed. Arrows indicate direction of flow.

Bleeding into the skin (evidenced by red spots under the skin) and bruises are a sign of capillary breakage and an indication that the capillaries are fragile. Edema (the accumulation of fluid in the tissue) can also result from weak capillaries that are too permeable—capillaries that allow the escape of blood proteins that are needed for retaining the proper osmotic pressure to draw accumulated intercellular fluid back into the bloodstream.

The mechanism by which bioflavonoids exert their claimed influence on capillary fragility and permeability is not fully understood. It is known that capillary breakage is characteristic of the vitamin C deficiency disease, scurvy; and that vitamin C has a vital role in maintaining capillary health. Since bioflavonoids and vitamin C are found together in nature, it is conjectured that they function together in increasing the strength of the capillaries and regulating their permeability. These actions help prevent hemorrhages and ruptures in the capillaries and connective tissues and build a protective barrier against infection.

Although flavonoids are not classified as vitamins for higher animal life because of lack of proof that they are essential food constituents, and that deficiency symptoms can be cured by their administration, there are strong indications that they are essential for lower stages of animal life—butterflies, silkworm larvae, crickets, and some species of beetles. Moreover, there are indications that similar essential effects may exist in higher animals and man, too. For example, rutin has been shown to exert a growth-promoting action on young rats and on bacteria. Some authorities believe that a vitaminlike effect of flavonoids may manifest itself only under stress conditions. Moreover, food flavonoids have been shown to exhibit in mammals a great number of specific effects contributing to buoyant good health. Further research on the essentiability of flavonoids as an essential food factor is needed.

In addition to their reputed effect on capillary fragility and permeability on the health, it is claimed that food flavonoids function as follows:

1. **They are active antioxidant compounds in food**, ranking second only to the fat-soluble tocopherols in this regard. This antioxidant effect protects the flavonoid-containing vegetable and fruit foodstuffs from oxidative deterioration, prolongs their shelf life and keeping quality, and improves taste, acceptability, and wholesomeness of mixed dishes by inhibiting the oxidation of the accompanying animal lipids.

2. **They possess a metal-chelating capacity**; and they affect the activity of enzymes and membranes.

3. **They have a synergistic effect on ascorbic acid**, and they appear to stabilize ascorbic acid in human tissues.

4. **They possess a bacteriostatic and/or antibiotic effect**, which is sufficiently high to account for their measurable anti-infectious properties in normal daily food.

5. **They possess anticarcinogenic activity in two ways**; a cytostatic effect against malignant cells (stopping or inhibiting the growth of cells), and a biochemical protection of the cell from damage by carcinogenic substances.

DISORDERS TREATED WITH BIOFLAVONOIDS.
Despite the controversial status of bioflavonoids and the lack of experimental evidence of their value, they are being used in the prevention and treatment of the following:

1. Capillary fragility and bleeding.
2. Bleeding gums.
3. Bleeding into the retina of the eye.
4. Certain types of glaucoma.
5. Hemorrhage into the brain.
6. Bleeding kidneys.
7. Female problems, including heavy menstrual bleeding.
8. Varicose veins.
9. Hemorrhoids.
10. Ulcers.
11. Habitual and threatened miscarriages.
12. Bruises that occur in contact sports, like football.
13. Injury from x-ray irradiation.
14. Frostbite.
15. Diabetes and diabetic retinopathy.
16. Thrombosis (a blood clot which may form in the veins of the leg, and subsequently block a major blood vessel—and even cause death). It appears that the bioflavonoids are natural and helpful antithrombosic agents.

No claims are made that the bioflavonoids are the total answer in treating the above disorders or that they should replace established treatments. Rather, they are being used as supplemental preventives and treatments where capillary fragility and permeability are involved.

DEFICIENCY SYMPTOMS.
Symptoms of bioflavonoid deficiency are closely related to those of a vitamin C deficiency. The tendency to bleed (hemorrhage) or bruise easily is especially claimed.

RECOMMENDED DAILY ALLOWANCE OF BIO-FLAVONOIDS.
There are no NRC-National Academy of Sciences recommended daily allowances (RDA) of bioflavonoids, similar to vitamin C.

Since synthetic vitamin C does not contain the bioflavonoids, and since bioflavonoids occur with vitamin C in natural food sources, a daily allowance would seem to be indicated. Moreover, most researchers who have worked with the bioflavonoids have found (1) that they are most beneficial when taken with vitamin C; and (2) that in some

cases where vitamin C alone is ineffective, the combination of the two may be helpful. Thus, the label on a rather typical vitamin C-bioflavonoid supplement reads as follows:

Each tablet contains:	
	mg
Rose hips powder	500
Vitamin C (ascorbic acid)	500
Lemon bioflavonoid*	500
Rutin (buckwheat)*	50

*NOTE: Need in human nutrition not established.

• **Bioflavonoid intake in average U.S. diet**—It is noteworthy that the average daily intake of flavonoids in the American diet amounts to about 1 g, of which one-half (0.5 g) is absorbed from the gut.

TOXICITY. Bioflavonoids are nontoxic.

BIOFLAVONOID LOSSES DURING PROCESSING, COOKING, AND STORAGE.
Bioflavonoids are not greatly damaged by food processing or by food preparation in the kitchen unless these are done in strong light. Likewise, losses in storage are minimal, provided they are not exposed to strong light.

SOURCES OF BIOFLAVONOIDS.
Bioflavonoids were first discovered in citrus peel. The white pulp of citrus fruits is also a rich source. Citrus fruits contain the bioflavonoids hesperidin and naringin.

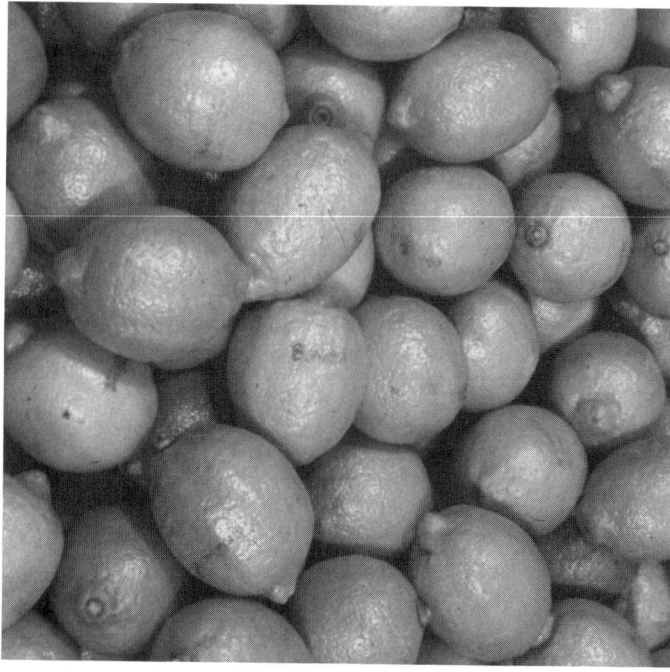

Fig. B-29. Lemons, skins, and pulp, are rich in bioflavonoids (Courtesy, USDA)

Tangerine juice is a very rich source of tangeretin and nobiletin. But frozen orange juice is a poor source of bioflavonoids; the bioflavonoids impart an off-taste to the juice, so squeezing of the pulp is carefully controlled.

Citrus bioflavonoids, made by extracting the pulp which remains after juicing oranges and lemons, are available in concentrated form. Sometimes, rose hips, obtained from roses, and rutin, obtained from buckwheat leaves, are included with the citrus bioflavonoids.

Animals are unable to synthesize flavonoids. Moreover, they are quickly metabolized in the body of higher animals. Hence, vegetables constitute the top food sources of the bioflavonoids given in the boxed list herewith.

It is noteworthy that a great deal of flavonoids enter the human body by means of beverages and drinks. Tea, coffee, cocoa, wine (particularly red wine), beer, and even vinegar are important flavonoid sources, accounting for at least 25 to 30% of the total flavonoid intake.

(Also see VITAMIN[S], Table V-5.)

TOP SOURCES OF BIOFLAVONOIDS

Although no standard food composition tables are available showing the bioflavonoid content of foods, the following foods are generally recognized as the richest sources:

Rose hips	Broccoli
Buckwheat leaves	Cantaloupe
Oranges and	Cherries
lemons (skin and	Grapes
pulp, especially	Green peppers
the little white	Onions with colored
core that runs	skins
down the middle)	Papaya
Tangerine (juice)	Plums
Grapefruit	Tea, coffee, cocoa,
Apricots	red wine
Blackberries	Tomatoes
Black currants	

BIOLOGICAL VALUE (BV) OF PROTEINS

The percentage of the protein of a food or feed mixture which is usable as a protein by a growing child, or an animal. It can be determined by a balance experiment in which a measured intake of nitrogen (N) in food (or feed) is compared to the measured excretion of N in the feces and urine. Then, BV is calculated by the formula which follows:

$$\text{Biological value} = \frac{\text{N intake} - (\text{fecal N} + \text{urinary N})}{\text{N intake} - \text{fecal N}} \times 100$$

The biological value of a protein is a reflection of the kinds and amounts of amino acids available to the animal after digestion. A protein which has a high biological value is said to be of *good quality*.

(Also see PROTEIN[S].)

BIOLOGY

The study of living organisms which includes (1) plants under the branch of botany, and (2) animals under the branch of zoology.

BIOPSY

The removal of a small piece of tissue for purposes of diagnosis.

BIOS

Initially, this was the designation given to a factor which stimulated the growth of yeast. Later, it was shown that the factor consists of two fractions, bios 1 (inositol) and bios 2 (biotin).

(Also see BIOTIN; and INOSITOL.)

BIOTIN

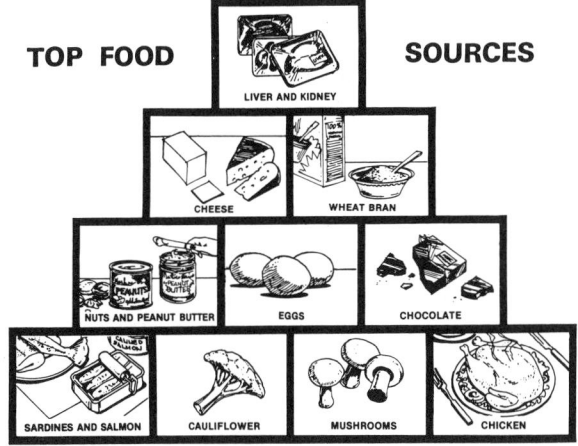

Fig. B-30. Good sources of biotin.

Biotin, a member of the vitamin B complex, is a water-soluble, sulfur-containing vitamin that is widely distributed in nature and essential for the health of many animal species, including man. It plays an important role in the metabolism of carbohydrates, fats, and proteins.

HISTORY. The history of biotin is the history of the merging of investigations, a chronological record of which follows:

In 1901, Wildiers expressed the belief that yeast required for its nutrition an organic substance which he called *bios*.

In 1916, Bateman reported that raw egg white had a detrimental effect on rats, but that the raw egg white was rendered *innocuous* by heat coagulation.

In 1927, Boas in England reported that feeding egg white to rats produced a dermatitis.

In 1933, Allison and co-workers isolated a nitrogen-fixing bacteria in legume nodules, which they named coenzyme R.

In 1936, Kogl and Tonnis of Germany isolated a crystalline substance from boiled yolks of duck eggs, which they called *biotin,* since they believed it to be identical to the *bios* factor needed for yeast growth.

In 1937, Gyorgy, the Hungarian scientist, found that a substance which he named vitamin H, would prevent the pathological condition that resulted from feeding rats and chicks raw egg white.

In 1940, Gyorgy and associates obtained conclusive experimental evidence that coenzyme R, biotin, and vitamin H were the same substance.

In 1942, du Vigneaud and associates, at Cornell, suggested the correct structural formula for biotin based on a study of its degradation products.

In 1943, Harris and his co-workers of Merck and Company synthesized biotin.

Looking back, it is now known that the deficiency (once called egg-white injury) occurs when the biotin in food combines with a factor in the protein of uncooked egg white (called avidin, because of its avidity for biotin); and that when egg white is cooked, avidin is inactivated. This also explains why, in early studies, liver and yeast offered protection against egg-white injury. (Both of them contain sufficiently large amounts of biotin to saturate the avidin completely and leave a surplus of biotin available to meet the needs of experimental animals.)

CHEMISTRY, METABOLISM, PROPERTIES.

• **Chemistry**—Biotin, like thiamin, is a sulfur-containing vitamin. It is a cyclic derivative of urea with an attached thiophene ring. Its structure is given in Fig. B-31.

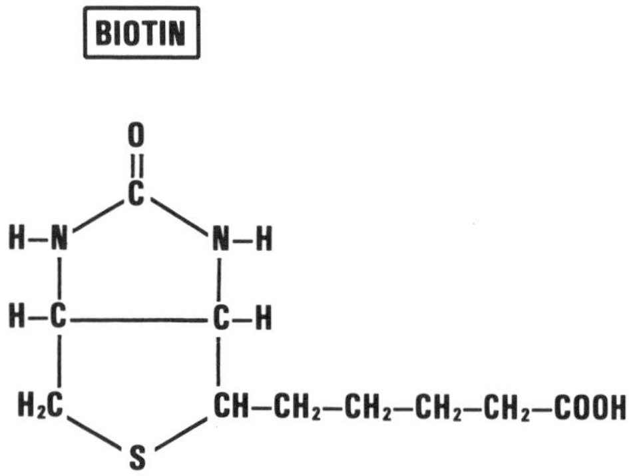

BIOTIN

Fig. B-31. Structure of biotin.

• Metabolism—Biotin is absorbed primarily from the upper part of the small intestine. However, avidin, a protein found in raw egg white, binds biotin and prevents its absorption from the intestinal tract. Fortunately, cooking inactivates avidin so that it no longer has the ability to bind biotin.

A considerable amount of biotin is synthesized by human intestinal bacteria, as evidenced by the fact that 3 to 6 times more biotin is excreted in the urine and feces than is ingested. But synthesis in the gut may occur too late in the intestinal passage to be absorbed well and play much of a direct role as a biotin source. Also, several variables affect the microbial synthesis in the intestines, including the carbohydrate source of the diet (starch, glucose, sucrose, etc.), the presence of other B vitamins, and the presence or absence of antimicrobial drugs and antibiotics.

Following absorption, biotin enters the portal circulation. It is stored primarily in the liver and kidneys, although all cells contain some biotin.

Excretion is mainly in the urine. Only traces of biotin are secreted in milk.

Determination of biotin levels in the blood and urinary excretion levels of biotin both provide evidence of biotin status in human beings.

• **Properties**—Biotin is a colorless, odorless, crystalline substance. It is readily soluble in hot water, but only slightly soluble in cold water; and it is stable to heat. It is destroyed by strong acids and alkalis and by oxidizing agents. Also, it is gradually destroyed by ultraviolet light.

MEASUREMENT/ASSAY. No International Units have been defined for the biological activity of biotin.

Analytical results are generally expressed in terms of weight units of pure d-biotin. Purified, high potency solutions of biotin may be assayed by a photometric method based on splitting of an avidin dye complex by biotin. Also, gas-liquid chromatography is sometimes used. However, the microbiological assay is the method of choice for biotin assay of foods. The biotin content of foods can also be determined by using the rat or the chick. Biological assays with rats or chicks are more reliable than the other methods because of determining availability; for example, it has been shown that the biotin in milo, oats, and wheat is less available to the chick than the biotin in corn.

FUNCTIONS. Biotin is required for many reactions in the metabolism of carbohydrates, fats, and proteins. It functions as a coenzyme mainly in decarboxylation-carboxylation and in deamination.

Biotin serves as a coenzyme for transferring CO_2 from one compound to another (for decarboxylation—the removal of carbon dioxide; and for carboxylation—the addition of carbon dioxide), as shown in Fig. B-32.

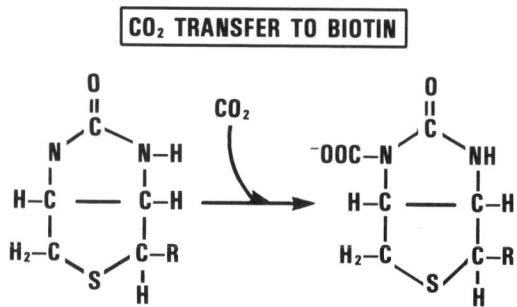

CO_2 TRANSFER TO BIOTIN

Fig. B-32. Transfer of CO_2 by biotin.

Numerous decarboxylation and carboxylation reactions are involved in carbohydrate, fat, and protein metabolism; among them, the following:

1. Interconversion of pyruvate and oxaloacetate. The formation of oxaloacetate is important because it is the starting point of the tricarboxylic acid cycle (TCA), known also as the Krebs cycle, in which the potential energy of nutrients (ATP) is released for use by the body.

2. Interconversion of succinate and propionate.

3. Conversion of malate to pyruvate.

4. Conversion of acetyl CoA to malonyl CoA, the first step in the formation of long chain fatty acids (fat synthesis).

5. Formation of purines, an essential part of DNA and RNA, and for protein synthesis.

6. Conversion of ornithine to citrulline, an important reaction in the formation of urea.

Biotin also serves as a coenzyme for deamination (removal of -NH₂) reactions that are necessary for the production of energy from certain amino acids (at least aspartic acid, serine, and threonine); for amino acids to be used as a source of energy, they must first be deaminated—the amino group must be split off.

Biotin is closely related metabolically to folacin, pantothenic acid, and vitamin B-12.

DEFICIENCY SYMPTOMS. Deficiency symptoms in humans (and in some animals) can be produced (1) by feeding large amounts of raw egg white, containing the biotin-binding glycoprotein known as *avidin;* or (2) by feeding a biotin-free diet in conjunction with a sulfa drug. *Avidin* renders the vitamin nutritionally unavailable, whereas the sulfa drug prevents intestinal synthesis. Deficiency symptoms in man include: a dry scaly dermatitis, loss of appetite, nausea, vomiting, muscle pains, glossitis (inflammation of the tongue), pallor of skin, mental depression, a decrease in hemoglobin and red-blood cell levels, a high cholesterol level, and low excretion of biotin; all of which respond to biotin administration.

There is now substantial evidence that *seborrheic dermatitis* (an abnormally oily skin, which results in chronic scaly inflammation) of infants under 6 months of age is due to nutritional biotin deficiency. In such cases, blood levels and urinary excretion of the vitamin are depressed. Prompt improvement occurs with therapeutic doses of the vitamin, about 5 mg/day, given intravenously or intramuscularly.

Biotin Dependency. A rare inherited disease called *biotin dependency* is known. In people with the disease, the body's use of biotin, the B vitamin necessary for certain metabolic processes, is somehow disrupted. Symptoms include loss of hair, lethargy, coma, and susceptibility to infections. The only treatment is daily doses of biotin. In 1981, medical researchers at the University of California in San Francisco reported successfully (1) diagnosing a biotin deficiency of an unborn baby by examining the amniotic fluid (the fluid was extracted from the womb by a procedure called amniocentesis, then cells from the fluid were grown in various nutrients and compared with normal cells); and (2) giving the mother massive doses of biotin, enough of which passed through the placenta so that the baby was born healthy.

NOTE WELL: Treating an unborn baby via the mother is an important new concept that could be applicable and very beneficial in treating other genetic diseases.

RECOMMENDED DAILY ALLOWANCE OF BIOTIN. It is difficult to obtain a quantitative requirement for biotin, for the reason that intestinal microflora make a significant contribution to the body pool of available biotin; often humans excrete via the feces and urine considerably more biotin than they have ingested. However, the estimated safe and adequate intakes of biotin are given in the section on VITAMIN(S), Table V-5, Vitamin Table.

In general, the combined urinary and fecal excretion of biotin exceeds the dietary intake. It seems likely that the fecal excretion of biotin is an indication of intestinal synthesis, whereas urinary excretion is a reflection of the dietary intake. Published reports of normal values of biotin in blood vary too widely for diagnostic use without carefully controlled observations.

The biotin content of human milk varies widely, but averages about 10 mcg/1,000 kcal. Most formulas provide at least 15 mcg/1,000 kcal, as recommended by the National Research Council (NRC).

An intake of 50 mcg/1,000 kcal should provide adequate biotin intake for infants and older children.

The NRC recommended daily allowance of biotin for adults is 30 to 100 mcg per day.

• **Biotin intake in average U.S. diet**—Mixed American diets are thought to provide a biotin intake of 100 to 300 mcg/day for adults. In western Europe, the dietary intake of biotin has been calculated to be between 50 and 100 mcg/day.

TOXICITY. There are no known toxic effects from biotin.

BIOTIN LOSSES DURING PROCESSING, COOKING, AND STORAGE. Considerable biotin is lost in the milling of cereal grains; hence, whole grains are a good source of the vitamin, whereas refined cereal products are a poor source.

Since biotin is stable to heat, cooking losses are not great.

SOURCES OF BIOTIN. Biotin is widely distributed in foods of both plant and animal origin; and it occurs in both the free state and in a form bound to protein. It occurs in the free state in fruits, vegetables, milk, and rice bran; and

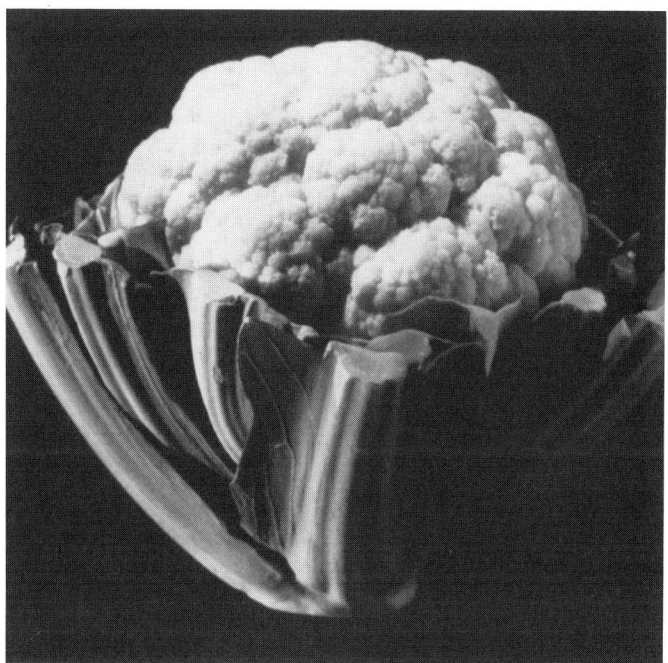

Fig. B-33. Cauliflower is a good source of biotin (Courtesy, Field Museum Of Natural History, Chicago, Ill.)

it occurs partly in a form bound to protein in meats, egg yolk, plant seeds, and yeast. Wide differences exist in the availability of biotin from food sources; for example, the biotin of corn and soybean meals is completely available to test animals, whereas the biotin of wheat is almost completely unavailable. Much needs to be learned about biotin availability. Sources of biotin are given in the section on VITAMIN(S), Table V-5, Vitamin Table.

For additional sources and more precise values of biotin, see Food Composition Table F-21 of this book.

It is noteworthy that the amount of avidin in raw egg white exceeds the amount of biotin in the whole egg. But, since avidin is destroyed by cooking, the usual diet includes little of the biotin-interfering substance.

In addition to food sources, biotin is available in pure synthetic form.

Also, considerable biotin is synthesized by the microorganisms in the intestinal tract, as evidenced by the fact that 3 to 6 times more biotin is excreted in the urine and feces than is ingested.

(Also see VITAMIN[S], Table V-5.)

BIRCH BEER

This is not really a beer, but an old-fashioned soft drink like ginger beer, lemon beer, and root beer. It is flavored with the oil of wintergreen, or oil of sweet birch and oil of sassafras. These old-fashioned soft drinks were fermented briefly with yeast, bottled, and stored. The fermentation served only to provide the carbonation.

BITTERS

• An alcoholic beverage flavored with extracts of bitter substances like quinine.

• A tonic containing bitter matters from such substances as aloes, bitter orange peel, cinchona bark, gentian, or quassia.

BIURET TEST

A chemical test for determining the presence and amount of protein in a solution. The biuret reagent containing copper sulfate is a bright blue. When the biuret reagent is added to a protein in a strong alkali solution, a blue-violet color is formed due to the reaction of the biuret reagent with the peptide bonds. The intensity depends upon the amount of protein.

(Also see PROTEIN[S].)

BLACK BREAD

A dark-colored bread made with rye, which is popular in central and northern Europe.

BLACKSTRAP MOLASSES

In the extraction of sugarcane, blackstrap molasses is the third and final extraction. It has more of the minerals than light or medium molasses. Blackstrap has a strong flavor, so usually only small amounts are eaten. The nutrient composition of blackstrap molasses is given in Food Composition Table F-21.

(Also see SUGAR, section headed "Sugarcane.")

BLACK TONGUE

A nutritional disorder in dogs which is similar to human pellagra, a disease due to a deficiency of the vitamin niacin. Dogs with black tongue were used in the experiments which identified niacin as the cure for this condition.

(Also see NIACIN.)

BLADDER

A hollow saclike organ in which the urine is stored before it is voided. The bladder is surrounded with a muscular coat which contracts when it is stretched. Hence, a full bladder is likely to be emptied by this muscular reflex. However, people can train themselves to delay the emptying of the bladder.

BLAND DIETS

Diets which have long been prescribed for people with disorders such as colitis, hiatus hernia, ileitis, inflammation of the esophagus, and ulcers—illnesses that are commonly characterized by (1) irritation and excessively rapid motions of one or more digestive organs; and (2) oversecretion of digestive juices such as stomach acid and bile. Hence, in an attempt to avoid, or lessen, gas and/or diarrhea, the doctor or dietitian is likely to recommend foods which (1) are soft in consistency and nonirritating, (2) do not overstimulate the flow of gastric acid or other digestive juices, and (3) are relatively low in fermentable carbohydrates and undigestible matter.

Bland diets may be nutritionally deficient and lead to constipation, so their use should be limited to the acute stages of digestive disorders.

(Also see MODIFIED DIETS, Table M-28, Modified Diets.)

BLEEDING TIME

An approximate measure of the blood clotting ability. In this test, either the end of the finger or the earlobe is pricked so that it bleeds, and a piece of filter paper is touched to the wound every 20 seconds. The measure of clotting time is taken to be the length of time after which the filter paper no longer becomes stained with blood. This may be a very rough indicator of nutritional status, and a test for other disorders such as impairment of blood clotting. For example, blood clotting takes an abnormally long time in vitamin K deficiency. However, there are much more sensitive tests of blood clotting time which may be performed when suitable laboratory facilities are available.

(Also see VITAMIN K.)

BLENDED

Combined or mixed so as to render the constituent parts indistinguishable from one another, such as when two or more food ingredients are mixed.

BLETTING

The overripening and softening of certain fruits in storage.

BLIND LOOP SYNDROME

A disorder characterized by (1) distention of a section of the small intestine so that a blind loop is formed; (2) stagnation of the flow of digesta in the loop; and (3) an overgrowth of certain bacteria in the loop. Blind loop syndrome may develop after certain types of intestinal surgery or when there are multiple diverticula (outpouchings of the intestinal wall). The syndrome is characterized by abdominal pain (especially after meals), gas, weight loss, diarrhea, constipation, nausea, vomiting, and malabsorption of vitamin B-12 and other essential nutrients. Usually, surgery is needed to correct the condition.

BLINDNESS DUE TO VITAMIN A DEFICIENCY (XEROPHTHALMIA)

On a worldwide basis, blindness due to vitamin A deficiency is the most prevalent type of blindness. This condition is very common in some parts of the developing countries of Asia, the Middle East, Africa, and Latin America, where diets contain practically no vegetable or animal sources of vitamin A. Fetuses, infants, and preschool children are the most affected due to a high requirement for the vitamin during the development of the tissues of the eye.

(Also see DEFICIENCY DISEASES, Table D-1, Major Dietary Deficiency Diseases; and VITAMIN A.)

BLOATERS

Herrings (fish) that have been salted less and smoked for a shorter period of time than red herring. (The latter are well salted and smoked for about 10 days.)

BLOOD

The fluid that circulates in the vascular system of vertebrate animals, carrying nourishment and oxygen to all parts of the body and taking away waste products for excretion. Blood consists of liquid plasma containing dissolved nutrients, waste products, and other substances and suspended red blood cells, leukocytes, and blood platelets.

BLOOD CELLS

Three classes of blood cells (corpuscles) are recognized—red cells, white cells, and platelets. All these cells are suspended in the fluid called plasma.

BLOOD CHOLESTEROL LEVEL

This measurement is often used for assessing the risk of heart disease. However, it is sometimes misinterpreted because cholesterol does not travel by itself in the blood, but is carried by complex molecules called lipoproteins. For example, beta-lipoproteins, when elevated in the blood, are associated with increased risks of heart disease and stroke; whereas, a high level of alpha-lipoproteins is apparently a good sign. Hence, the measurement of blood cholesterol alone is at best a very crude measurement of the status of cholesterol metabolism in the body.

(Also see ALPHA-LIPOPROTEINS; BETA-LIPOPROTEINS; CHOLESTEROL; and HEART DISEASE.)

BLOOD FATS (LIPIDS)

The type of fatty substances which are most commonly found in the blood are: triglycerides, fatty acids, cholesterol, phospholipids, lipoproteins, and the fat-soluble vitamins A, D, E, and K.

(Also see FATS AND OTHER LIPIDS.)

BLOOD PLATELETS (THROMBOCYTES)

These cells, which are also called thrombocytes, are involved in blood clotting. There may be too few platelets when certain nutritional deficiencies result in anemia. Hence, the blood clotting time may be prolonged in these blood disorders.

BLOOD PRESSURE

The force which the blood exerts against the wall of the blood vessels, due to the pumping action of the heart. When the blood pressure is measured, two readings are generally taken. The higher reading, which is called *systolic blood pressure*, is that which occurs when the heart exerts its maximum force of contraction. The lower reading, which is called the *diastolic blood pressure*, occurs when the heart rests between contractions. Normal blood pressure values center around readings of 120 systolic, and about 80 diastolic. Generally, blood pressure increases a few points with age, but a large increase is indicative of *high blood pressure*, a condition which greatly increases the risk of kidney disease and stroke. High blood pressure probably has multiple causes such as (1) the loss of elasticity in the blood vessel walls, making it necessary for the heart to pump harder to force the blood through these vessels; (2) retention of sodium and water, which increases the blood volume; and (3) clogging of blood vessels so that the openings are smaller. *Low blood pressure may be a sign of heart weakness and it may make the person susceptible to fainting.*

(Also see HIGH BLOOD PRESSURE.)

BLOOD SAUSAGE

A variety of cooked sausage containing a large proportion of blood, usually formulated with pork (skins, cured ham fat, and/or pork snouts and lips) and stuffed in a casing.

BLOOD SUGAR

Although several different sugars circulate in the blood, the main blood sugar is glucose. Hence, the blood sugar level is usually considered to mean the same thing as the blood glucose level. In healthy people, the blood sugar is maintained within a narrow range. In diabetes, the blood sugar may be abnormally high; in the condition called low blood sugar (hypoglycemia), the blood sugar is too low.

(Also see DIABETES MELLITUS; and HYPOGLYCEMIA.)

BLOOD SUGAR TEST

Various tests of the blood sugar may be given in order to diagnose certain metabolic disorders such as diabetes and low blood sugar (hypoglycemia). One of the simplest tests is called a fasting blood sugar which is usually made on a sample of blood taken after an overnight fast. Another commonly used test is the glucose tolerance test in which a fasting blood sugar is measured; then a test dose of glucose is given by mouth or by vein and the blood sugar is measured at regular intervals. Diagnoses are not always based upon blood sugar tests alone because there are many causes of blood sugar abnormalities. Hence, many doctors measure other factors along with the blood sugar, such as the level of insulin in the blood.

(Also see DIABETES MELLITUS; and HYPOGLYCEMIA.)

BLOOD VASCULAR SYSTEM

The vessels that transport blood throughout the body.

BLOOM

A state of beauty, freshness, and vigor.

BLUE CHEESE

A type of cheese characterized by visible blue-green veins of mold throughout the cheese and by a sharp, piquant flavor. In the family of blue-mold cheese, there are varietal names, but the products differ appreciably only where the milk source varies. For example, roquefort is made only in the Roquefort area of France from sheep's milk; its cow's milk counterpart is known as bleucheese in other areas of France, blue in the United States, Stilton in England, and Gorgonzola in Italy.

BLUE VALUE

• When referring to vitamin A, it is a color indicator of the vitamin A; the depth of the transient blue color produced by reaction of the substance with antimony trichloride is proportional to the amount of vitamin A present.

• When referring to starch, it is an index of the free soluble starch present; for example, the amylose present in cornstarch.

BOBOLINK (REEDBIRD; RICEBIRD)
Dolichonyx oryzivorus

A North American songbird related to the blackbird and oriole, named for the sounds of its lovely song—*bob-o-lee, bob-o-link*. The bobolink was formerly regarded as a table delicacy.

BOBWHITE (QUAIL)

This game bird is classified as *Colinus virginianus*, family *Phasianidàe* (which includes pheasants and partridges). The bobwhite gets its name from its whistling call, which sounds like *ah bob White*. It is the only kind of quail native to the area east of the Mississippi River. It usually lives in the region of southern Ontario to the Gulf states.

The bobwhite is called a quail in northern and eastern United States and in Canada; and in the South it is called a partridge.

The flesh of the bobwhite makes for good eating.

BODY BUILD

(See BODY TYPES.)

BODY COMPOSITION

Nutrition encompasses the various chemical and physiological reactions which change food elements into body elements. It follows that knowledge of body composition is useful in understanding the individual's response to nutrition.

Based on studies that have been made, there is a wide range in body composition according to age and nutritional state (degree of fatness). Fig. B-34 shows the changes in body composition from infancy to adulthood.

The following conclusions can be made from these figures:

1. **Water.** On a percentage basis, the water content shows a marked decrease with advancing age and maturity.

2. **Fat.** The percentage of fat normally increases with growth and age. There is considerable difference in the amount of fat in men as compared to women. Men average 12% fat, but women may have as high as 29 to 33% fat.

3. **Fat and water.** As the percentage of fat increases, the percentage of water decreases.

4. **Protein.** The percentage of protein increases slightly during growth, but may decrease if the individual puts on excess weight.

5. **Ash.** The percentage of ash shows a slight increase with age.

There is a very small amount of carbohydrates (mostly glucose and glycogen) present in the body, found principally in the liver, muscles, and blood.

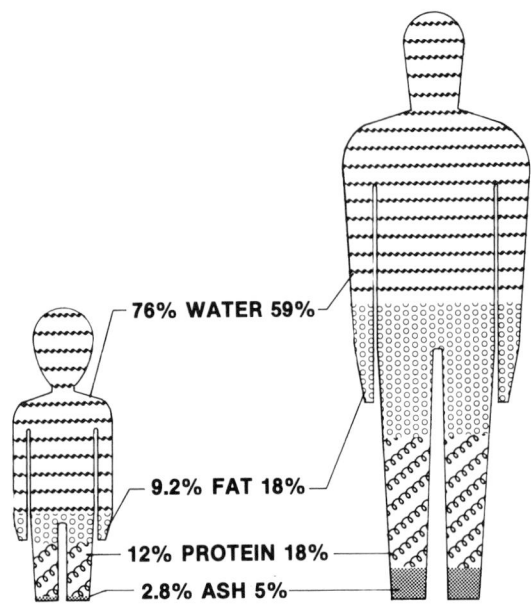

Fig. B-34. This shows the changes in body composition from the infant on the left to the adult on the right.

BODY FLUIDS

These are contained in two major compartments within the body. The extracellular fluid, the *internal sea* that bathes the cells, is comprised of the blood plasma and the *interstitial* (between the cells) *fluid*. A larger part of the body fluid is contained in the second compartment, the *intracellular* (inside the cell) compartment. Fluids in each compartment have a different chemical composition. Lymph, cerebrospinal, pericardial, pleural and peritoneal fluids are specialized interstitial fluids.

(Also see WATER AND ELECTROLYTES.)

BODY SURFACE AREA

The area covered by the exterior of the body, which determines the heat lost from the body, and therefore basal metabolism.

The body surface area is estimated by plotting a person's height and weight on a standard chart developed by DuBois, based on the following formula:

Surface (cm²) = weight (kg) .425 × height (cm) .725 × 71.84

BODY TEMPERATURE

The heat produced by metabolism is usually distributed throughout the body. Hence, a good indication of the body temperature may be secured by taking either the oral or the rectal temperature. Body temperature is normally maintained within a narrow range; hence, the normal temperature is usually within a degree or so of 98.6°F (37°C). An elevated body temperature—more than 2°F (1°C) above normal—suggests that a fever may be present. However, strenuous exercise may raise the body temperature by that amount or more. A subnormal body temperature may mean that there is a circulatory disorder or a metabolic problem such as malnutrition.

BODY TISSUE

An aggregate of cells of a particular kind or kinds together with their intercellular substance that form one of the structural materials out of which the body is built, such as connective tissue, epithelium tissue, muscle tissue, and nerve tissue.

BODY TYPES

This much used system of body typing was devised by Dr. W. H. Sheldon, an American physical anthropologist, in 1940. He recognized three major types of physiques, which he described as follows:

• **Ectomorph**—This type of body is tall and slender, with a delicate bone structure. The trunk is short in proportion to the arms and legs. Furthermore, the fingers, hands, and toes are disproportionately long. Finally, the muscles are wiry, rather than bulky.

Life insurance companies have found that people with this physique live the longest, so their tables of ideal weights for various heights favor ectomorphs over the two other body types (endomorphs and mesomorphs).

• **Endomorph**—People with this body build are often described as chubby or pleasingly plump, because they appear to be round and soft. Also, they usually have large abdomens, long trunks, and short, but heavily fleshed arms and legs. Lastly, their body measurements from front to back are likely to be greater than their dimensions from side to side.

• **Mesomorph**—This so-called *masculine* physique is characterized by (1) bulky muscles; (2) heavy bones with large joints; (3) and a large chest and broad shoulders, which are notably more prominent than the abdomen or hips. Most people consider the proportions between the trunk and the arms and legs to be ideal. It is noteworthy that some women may have this body build, yet be truly feminine in every respect.

(Also see OBESITY.)

BODY WATER

This term generally designates the total water content of the body. However, the distribution of water within the human body is not uniform. It is distributed between two major compartments: extracellular water, which is outside of the cells; and intracellular water, which is inside the cells. The extracellular water is present in the fluid which bathes the cells (interstitial fluid), blood plasma, cerebrospinal fluid, synovial fluid, and lymph. Normally, the water content in the bodies of adults averages about 60% of the body weight. However, human infants may contain up to 77% water right after birth. Also, as the percentage of fat increases, the percentage of water decreases.

(Also see BODY FLUIDS; WATER AND ELECTROLYTES; and WATER BALANCE.)

BOILING POINT

The temperature at which the vapor pressure of a liquid equals the atmospheric pressure.

BOLOGNA

A large moist sausage, usually made of beef, veal, and pork, that is chopped fine, seasoned, enclosed in a casing, boiled and smoked.

BOLTING OF FOOD

People who eat too rapidly or greedily are said to be bolting their food.

BOLUS

The name given to the mass of food that is swallowed after chewing.

(Also see DIGESTION AND ABSORPTION.)

BOMB CALORIMETER

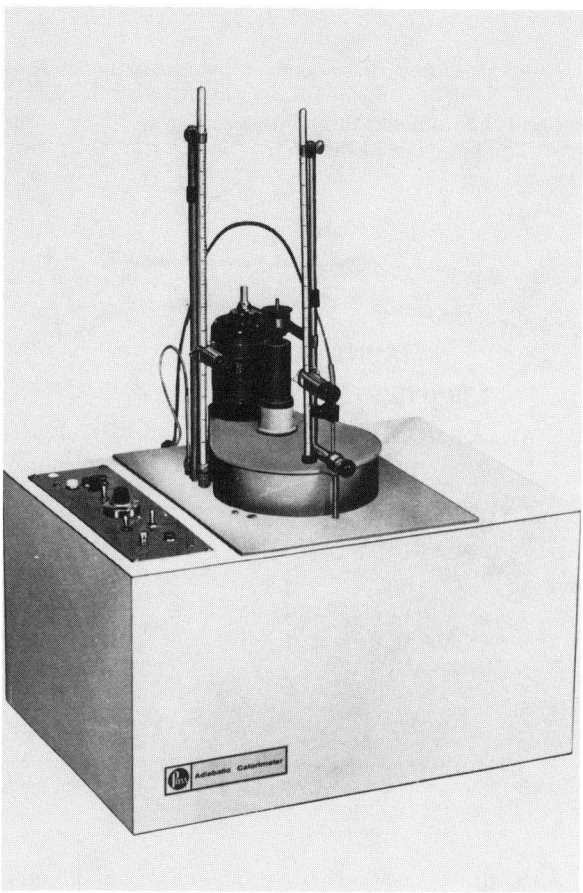

Fig. B-35. Bomb calorimeter for the determination of gross energy. (Courtesy, Parr Instrument Company, Moline, Ill.)

The bomb calorimeter is an instrument for measuring the energy value of food and other materials. It consists of an inner chamber that contains the food sample surrounded by a double-walled insulated jacket that holds water. It works as follows: An electric wire is attached to the material being tested, so that it can be ignited by remote control; 2,000 g of water are poured around the bomb; 25 to 30 atmospheres of oxygen are added to the bomb; the material is ignited; the heat given off from the burned material warms the water; and a thermometer registers the change in temperature of the water.

A *calorie* is the amount of heat required to raise the temperature of 1 g of water 1 °C (precisely from 14.5° to 15.5 °C).

The heat liberated by burning a food in the bomb calorimeter is referred to as the gross energy or heat of combustion. It will coincide with the metabolizable energy in that food only if it can be completely metabolized. For example, proteins liberate 5.65 kcal/g in the bomb calorimeter, but only 4.4 kcal/g in the body where the nitrogen is excreted as urea and uric acid (containing 1.25 kcal/g).

BONE

Contents   *Page*

There are 206 separate bones in the human body. They form the skeleton, the framework of hard structures which supports and protects the soft tissues. Fig. B-36 shows the parts and structure of the bone.

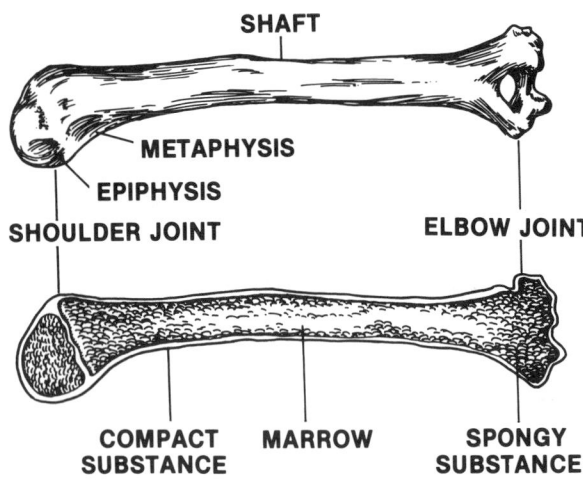

Fig. B-36. The humerus bone—the long bone of the upper arm.
Top: Humerus bone, showing the three parts: (1) the shaft—the long part of the bone; (2) the metaphysis—the end of the shaft, or diaphysis, where it joins the epiphysis, and (3) the epiphysis—the rounded end.
Bottom: The humerus bone split open to show the inside.

CHEMICAL COMPOSITION OF BONE. Chemically, bone consists of organic and inorganic matter in the approximate ratio of 1:2.

The organic matter, which accounts for about one-third of the weight of bone and gives toughness and elasticity, consists largely of collagen in a gel of cementing substance. It may be separated out by immersing a bone for considerable time in dilute mineral acid, following which it comes out exactly the same shape as before, but so flexible that a long bone (one of the ribs, for example) can be easily tied into a knot.

The mineral part, which gives bone its hardness and rigidity, may be obtained by heating bone to a high temperature, completely burning out the organic part and reducing its weight by about one-third. Five-sixths of the mineral part is calcium phosphate, the remainder consists of calcium carbonate, calcium fluoride, calcium chloride, and magnesium phosphate, with small amounts of sodium chloride and sulfate.

BONE GROWTH AND METABOLISM. Growth in length of the long bones normally occurs at the band of epiphyseal cartilage (growth band) lying between the epiphysis and the diaphysis (shaft). The epiphyseal cartilage is a temporary formation which grows by the multiplication of its own cells at the epiphysis end, while at the diaphysis end it degenerates and is replaced by calcified bone. When the epiphyseal cartilage ceases to regenerate and is entirely replaced by bone, the epiphysis unites with the diaphysis and growth ceases. This is referred to as the closing of the epiphysis, or ossification. In the process of ossification, cartilage is replaced by osteoid, which is then calcified (see Fig. B-37).

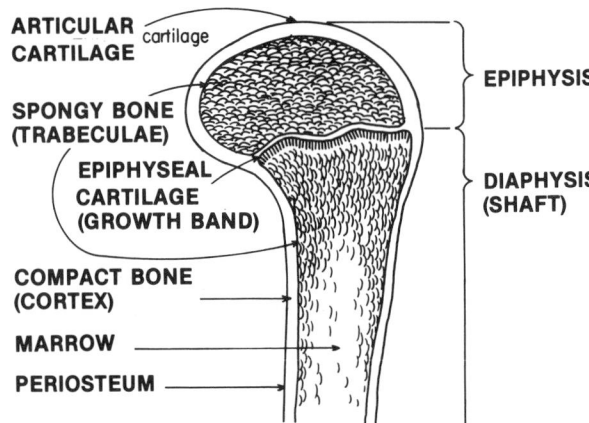

Fig. B-37. Diagram of the longitudinal section of a long growing bone.

In addition to serving as structural material, bones serve as a storehouse for calcium and phosphorus which may be mobilized when the assimilation of these minerals is inadequate to meet body needs. Thus, if the dietary intake of calcium does not meet the requirements, the body can draw upon its bone reserves, which are found in the spongy bone. The exact mechanism involved in the mobilization of bone calcium during periods of stress, i.e., during formation of milk or of fetal bones, is not fully understood. But, it is known that, in some manner, it is under the influence of the parathyroid hormone, and perhaps it is also affected by vitamin D. The phosphorus which is released simultaneously with the calcium does not appear to be used to meet nutritional phosphorus requirements, but is promptly excreted in the urine.

BONE DISORDERS. Bones are subject to numerous disorders, including fractures, congenital defects, infections, tumors, and nutritional diseases. The major bone nutritional diseases are osteomalacia, osteoporosis, and rickets.

(Also see DEFICIENCY DISEASES, Table D-1, Major Dietary Deficiency Diseases; OSTEOMALACIA; OSTEOPOROSIS; and RICKETS.)

BONE CHARCOAL

The residue from charring bones in a closed retort; sometimes referred to as bone black. It has excellent absorbent properties; therefore, it is used to remove impurities from food items such as crude sugar solutions and vodka.

BONE, COMPACT

A dense type of bone, which forms the outer layer of the long bones.

BONE COMPARTMENT

The total sketetal tissue in the body. For example, the bone compartment contains 99% of the body's total metabolic calcium pool.

BONE DENSITY

The mineral compactness of bone, which gives it hardness and rigidity.

BONE MATRIX

The protein *network* (fibers of collagen) of bone in which minerals are deposited.

BONE MEAL

Packinghouse bones are degreased and processed into valuable products.

Bone meal, which is nature's own formulation, is fresh, degreased, ground animal bone. It is used as a mineral supplement for both humans and animals, and as a source of calcium, phosphorus, and needed trace elements. For human use, it is available in both powder and tablet form. It is noteworthy that (1) bone meal never contains toxic levels of the essential trace elements, whereas these are sometimes exceeded in man-made mineral formulations; and (2) bone meal trace elements rate high in biological availability, physical and chemical compatability, and storage life.

(Also see MINERAL[S].)

BONE, SPONGY

A porous type of bone, which forms most short bones and the ends of long bones.

BONITO (THE ATLANTIC BONITO: *Sarda sarda*; THE PACIFIC BONITO: *Sarda chiliensis*)

An open-sea fish closely related to the larger tuna and the smaller mackerel. They are found worldwide in warm and tropical waters, but are more coastal in distribution than the tunas. Bonitos have torpedo-shaped bodies, with narrow dark blue lines running from the head toward the back and a silvery underside. Most bonitos weigh about 6 lb (*2.7 kg*), although some weigh as much as 40 lb (*18 kg*) and are over 3 ft (*91 cm*) long. They travel in large schools.

Bonitos are important game and commercial fish and are considered good eating. They are usually canned.

BOOKS

Books pertaining to foods, nutrition, and health abound! Generally speaking, they can be classified as *recommended* and *not recommended*. Unfortunately, it's not easy to distinguish between the two.

The *not recommended* books are usually well written. But some are sheer nonsense; others are downright hazardous to your health. Many of them promote a product or a program. The authors of most of them are charming—some are even TV personalities.

For authoritative and sound books pertaining to foods, nutrition, and health, the layman should seek the advice of an able and reputable professional nutritionist or rely on the review of a respected scientific journal.

BORAX (SODIUM BORATE, SODIUM TETRABORATE)

This is a colorless crystalline substance (chemical formula: $Na_2B_4O_7 \cdot 10\ H_2O$) found in major quantity in the salt deposits of California, Chile, Tibet, Peru, and Canada. Sodium borate was once extensively used as a chemical food preservative, but in many countries, including the United States, its use for this purpose was discarded when it was shown to be potentially toxic in the amounts used.

BORON

Boron is a biologically dynamic element that affects numerous metabolic processes in higher animals including humans. Further research is needed relative to the nutritional, biochemical, and physiological effects of boron.

BOSTON BROWN BREAD

This is quick bread which was formerly very popular in New England and the standard fare on Saturday evenings, along with baked beans. It is made with whole wheat flour, rye flour, and cornmeal, plus molasses, milk and baking soda, and raisins may be added. Traditionally, it is steamed.

BOUT

A term used to designate an episode of an acute illness.

BOWEL

Another name for the small and large intestines.
(Also see DIGESTION AND ABSORPTION.)

BRADYCARDIA

A slower than normal resting heart rate. Bradycardia may be a sign of physical training, because, following training, the heart is able to deliver more blood with each beat. Hence, it does not have to beat as rapidly as it did before training. However, bradycardia may also be due to a disorder of the heart muscle, or other abnormalities.

BRADYPHAGIA

A term meaning abnormally slow eating.

BRAINS

A very tender and delicately flavored meat by-product. The covering membrane should be removed. Brains may be sauteed, creamed, breaded, or used in salads.

BRAN

The outer coarse coat (pericarp) of grain which is separated in milling. Wheat, oat, rice, and corn bran are most common. Bran contains a large part of the valuable nutrients found in grains. It is the most popular food for the purpose of increasing bulk in the diet. Most nutritionists recommend that healthy adults get 20 to 35 g of fiber per day.

(Also see CEREAL GRAINS; FIBER; and FLOURS.)

BRAWN

A British term for a pork dish made from the chopped, cooked, and molded edible parts of pig's head, feet, legs, and sometimes tongue. Mock brawn differs in that other meat by-products are used.

BRAZILIAN CHERRY (PITANGA; SURINAM CHERRY) *Eugenia uniflora*

A small ribbed fruit of a shrub or a small tree (of the family *Myrtaceae*) that is eaten fresh or made into jams and pies. Brazilian cherries are red to almost black in color and ¾ to 1½ in. (*2 to 4 cm*) in diameter, and contain one or two seeds. They are now grown throughout the tropics and subtropics, including Florida. They may also be grown as hedges.

Some noteworthy observations regarding the nutrient composition of the Brazilian cherry follow:

1. The raw fruit has a low to moderately high content of calories (51 kcal per 100 g) and carbohydrates (12½%).

2. Brazilian cherries are an excellent source of vitamin A and a good source of vitamin C.

BREADNUT

The nut of a tree (*Brosimum alicastrum*) of Jamaica and Mexico that is roasted and ground into a flour from which bread is made.

BREADROOT *Psoralea esculenta*

The root of a densely hairy plant of western United States used for food.

BREADS AND BAKING

To most people, breads are doughs that have been baked in the shape of loaves. However, the term may also refer to any type of baked product, either leavened or unleavened, that is prepared from a flour or a meal mixed with water and other ingredients. Baking means the cooking of a food by dry heat, whether in an oven, or on a flat, heated surface such as a frying pan or a griddle. Occasionally, breads may also be cooked by other processes, such as steaming or frying in deep fat.

Bread is a favorite food all over the world. For taste, texture, and social significance, it is unsurpassed. *Breaking bread together* is a well known figure of speech, indicative of people sharing a meal; and the foundation of the Christian church is the Last Supper, when Christ broke bread with his disciples. Hence, it is of more than passing historical

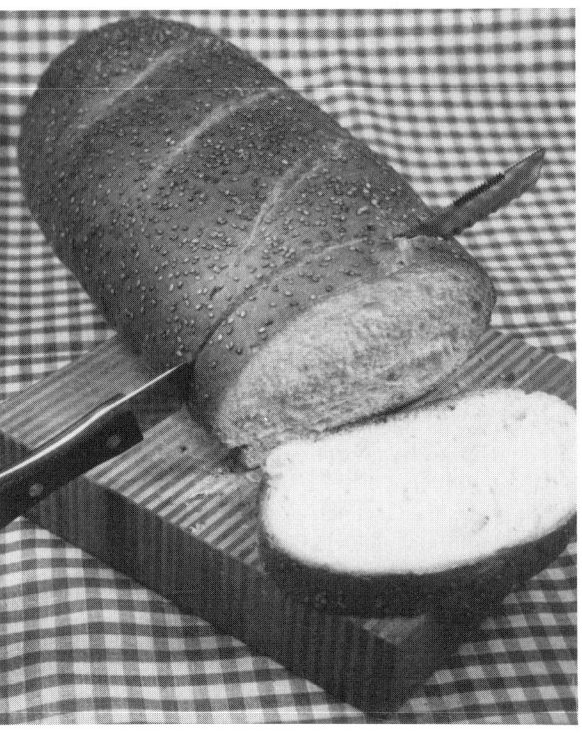

Fig. B-38. Slicing fresh bread. (Courtesy, Univ. of Maryland, College Park, MD.)

interest to determine how ingenious bakers and cooks transformed cereal flours and meals, plus a few other simple ingredients, into tasty products such as bagels, biscuits, breads, cakes, chapaties, cookies, crackers, danish pastry, doughnuts, dumplings, muffins, pancakes, pie pastry, pizza, popovers, puff pastry, rolls, tortillas, turnovers, and waffles.

HISTORY OF BAKING. The Egyptians were the first people to become experts in the leavening of bread. Legend has it that leavening was discovered by an Egyptian baker who set some wheaten dough aside in a warm place. The dough, having been contaminated with wild yeasts and/or bacteria, rose significantly as the microorganism grew and multiplied. No doubt, the person who sampled the accidentally leavened dough after baking was favorably impressed with its light airy texture. Hence, the Egyptians became the first professional bakers. They also invented ovens shaped like beehives, with both a fuel compartment and a compartment for baking.

The type of leavening first used by the bakers of Egypt was a sourdough, made by exposing fresh dough to the wild yeasts and bacteria in the air. Later, they cultivated yeasts in order to obtain greater uniformity in their baked products. It appears that the ancient Hebrews learned to leaven breads from the Egyptians before the 13th century B.C., when they were led out of Egypt by Moses. The flight of the Jews from Egypt is commemorated in the Jewish Passover by the use of an unleavened, crackerlike bread called *matzo*, because there had not been time for the use of leavening during the exodus.

Eventually, the ancient Romans adopted the baking practices of the Egyptians and spread them throughout their empire during the early Christian Era.

The use of a crude type of baking soda had its beginning in the United States in the 1790s, when it was discovered that potassium carbonate prepared from wood ashes gave off carbon dioxide gas when heated. Thus, it became possible to shorten the time required for making breads, because the new powder acted much more rapidly than yeast. Improvements were made in this early type of baking powder, so that, by the 1850s, it was used by bakers around the world.

A steam-driven roller mill for crushing grain was first tested in Switzerland in 1834. But it took almost 50 years for it to be developed for commercial use because the iron rollers wore out too soon. Finally, it was discovered that porcelain rollers did a better job and lasted much longer. As a result of this invention, the baking industry was provided with a large supply of white flour. Roller mills rapidly replaced all other mills because the rollers broke the grain so that the white, starchy part could be separated more easily from the branny seedcoats and the oily germ.

Today, much of the baking industry is mechanized so that only a few people are needed to operate machines that turn out thousands of loaves daily. However, there are still many small bakeries which cater to local needs and turn out special breads that are not produced by the large baking companies. Furthermore, food technologists are ever busy searching for ways to improve breads and to develop new breads for the future.

BASIC PRINCIPLES OF BAKING.

The basic principles and operations of baking consist of the following:

1. Mixing the flour with a liquid, a leavening agent (a substance used to make doughs rise), and other ingredients such as salt, sugar, fat, eggs, raisins, nuts, etc.

2. Allowing the dough to rise if yeast or a sourdough starter has been used as the leavening agent. *Yeast* and other microorganisms leaven bread by fermenting sugars in the dough to carbon dioxide gas and water. Hence, carbon dioxide gas is the actual leavening agent. Breads made with baking powder or baking soda do not usually require any rising time before baking because rapid leavening occurs when the doughs are heated.

3. Baking the dough in a pan placed in an oven. Some doughs may be cooked on hot griddles, fried in hot fat, or steamed. Sometimes the baker opens the oven door and is dismayed to find a product that is notably inferior to what is usually expected. For example, the dough may have started to rise, then collapsed as the leavening gas escaped. Fallen doughs are too heavy and too moist. Therefore, doughs must have sufficient elasticity to expand, and they must be strong enough to prevent the escape of the leavening gases. This means that the flour used in baking should contain enough of the protein *gluten*, which imparts elasticity and strength, or else other measures should be taken to make up for lack of this substance in a flour. Wheat contains the most gluten of all the grains, while rye is a poor second in this respect. All of the other flours are very low in gluten. One of the ways to compensate for the lack of gluten is to add eggs to a dough, because the protein of the egg white acts as a binder. Another way is to use a high baking temperature so that a tough crust is formed rapidly enough to prevent the escape of the leavening gas. Details of the application of these and other principles are given in the section which follows.

TYPES OF BREADS AND BAKED DOUGHS.

Through the centuries, many types of baked products were developed by various peoples who attempted to make the best uses of the cereal grains and the baking equipment available to them. Although many diverse items have been prepared, breads and baked doughs may be classed according to the following types: (1) unleavened breads, (2) breads leavened with yeast and other microorganisms, (3) quick breads made with baking powder and baking soda, or (4) products leavened with air or steam.

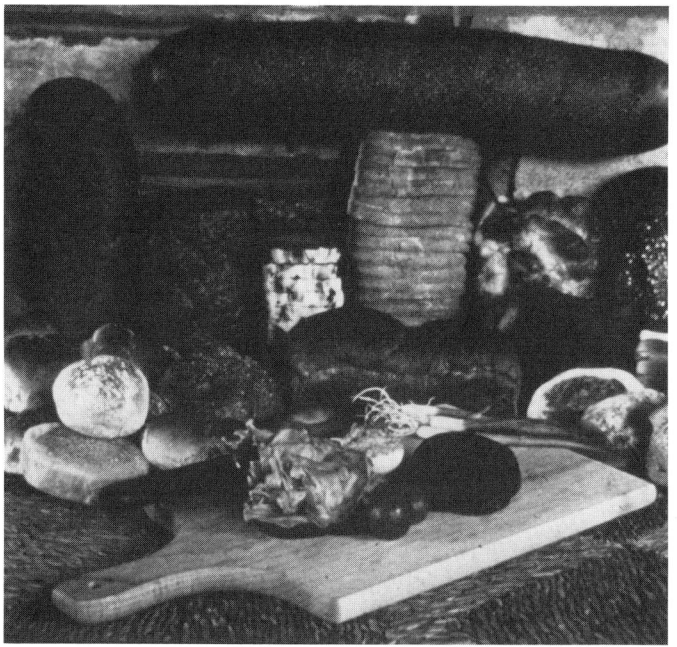

Fig. B-39. A variety of baked products. (Courtesy, USDA)

Unleavened Breads. These items were made about 10,000 years ago by the first grain farmers. Yet, certain similar products are still popular today. Generally, the most favored ones are made from thin layers of unleavened dough. Among the unleavened breads are: (1) chapaties, circles of whole wheat dough which are eaten in India, Pakistan, and Iran; (2) Matzo, the unleavened bread which the Jews eat during passover; (3) pastry, used in pie crusts and pastry shells; and (4) tortillas, the popular Mexican bread, made of corn or wheat flour and baked on a hot griddle.

Breads Leavened with Yeast and other Microorganisms. Among the special nutritional benefits attributed to leavening doughs with yeast are: (1) the bread contains extra vitamins and other nutrients synthesized by the yeast; (2) certain essential minerals, such as chromium, are converted into forms that are well utilized by the body; and (3) phytates (phosphorus compounds found in whole grains and certain legumes, which bind minerals and impede their absorption) are broken down during fermentation.

Among the yeast- and bacteria-leavened products are the following: (1) bagels—doughnut-shaped rolls; (2) Danish pastry; (3) Jewish challah bread; (4) malt breads; (5) pita or *pocket* bread; (6) pizza; (7) raised doughnuts; (8) salt-rising bread; (9) sourdough bread; and (10) whole wheat bread.

Quick Breads made with Baking Powder or Baking Soda. The development of various types of chemical leavening agents, called baking powders, make it possible to prepare breads and other baked items in a much shorter time than is required for yeast-leavened breads. Hence, products leavened with these powders are often called *quick breads* because there is no need for allowing the dough to rise before baking.

The type of leavening agent is only one of the factors responsible for the characteristics of various baked doughs. Additional important factors are the amounts and types of other ingredients such as flour, liquid, fat, eggs, sugar, and salt; and, the time and temperature used in baking.

Some of the common types of quick breads made with baking powder or baking soda are: biscuits, cookies, cornbread, crackers, doughnuts, dumplings, gingerbread, muffins, pancakes, plain cake, soda bread, and waffles.
(Also see BAKING POWDER AND BAKING SODA.)

Products Leavened with Air or Steam. A few baked products are leavened mainly with air or steam, and little, if any, baking powder. The success of such leavening is uncertain unless the batters or doughs are mixed and baked in ways which ensure the retention of the gases. Some long-time favorites of this type are: angel food cake, chiffon cake, cream puffs, popovers, and sponge cake.

Figs. B-40, B-41, and B-42, show that the levels of selected nutrients in various baked products vary considerably.

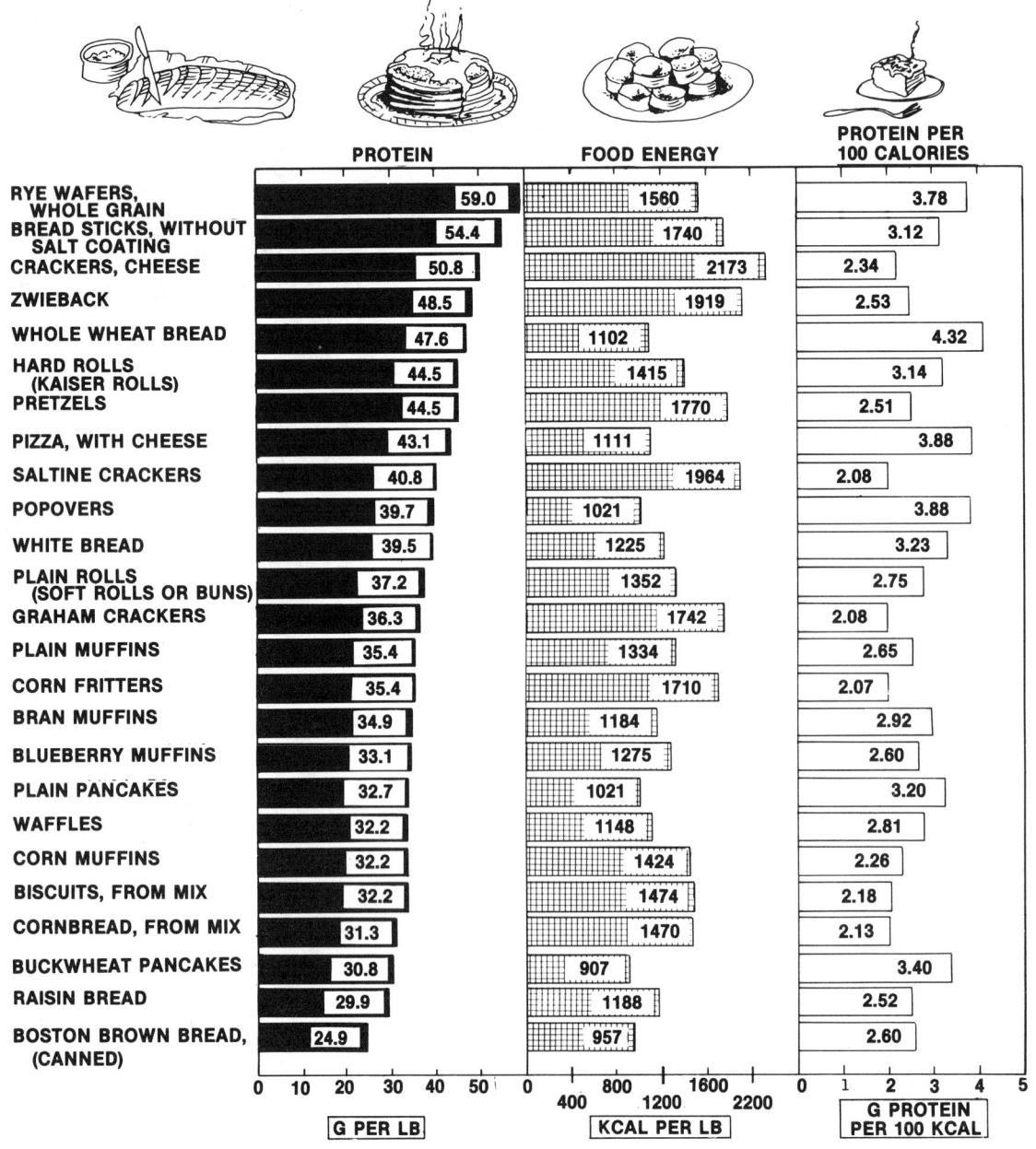

	PROTEIN (G PER LB)	FOOD ENERGY (KCAL PER LB)	PROTEIN PER 100 CALORIES (G PROTEIN PER 100 KCAL)
RYE WAFERS, WHOLE GRAIN	59.0	1560	3.78
BREAD STICKS, WITHOUT SALT COATING	54.4	1740	3.12
CRACKERS, CHEESE	50.8	2173	2.34
ZWIEBACK	48.5	1919	2.53
WHOLE WHEAT BREAD	47.6	1102	4.32
HARD ROLLS (KAISER ROLLS)	44.5	1415	3.14
PRETZELS	44.5	1770	2.51
PIZZA, WITH CHEESE	43.1	1111	3.88
SALTINE CRACKERS	40.8	1964	2.08
POPOVERS	39.7	1021	3.88
WHITE BREAD	39.5	1225	3.23
PLAIN ROLLS (SOFT ROLLS OR BUNS)	37.2	1352	2.75
GRAHAM CRACKERS	36.3	1742	2.08
PLAIN MUFFINS	35.4	1334	2.65
CORN FRITTERS	35.4	1710	2.07
BRAN MUFFINS	34.9	1184	2.92
BLUEBERRY MUFFINS	33.1	1275	2.60
PLAIN PANCAKES	32.7	1021	3.20
WAFFLES	32.2	1148	2.81
CORN MUFFINS	32.2	1424	2.26
BISCUITS, FROM MIX	32.2	1474	2.18
CORNBREAD, FROM MIX	31.3	1470	2.13
BUCKWHEAT PANCAKES	30.8	907	3.40
RAISIN BREAD	29.9	1188	2.52
BOSTON BROWN BREAD, (CANNED)	24.9	957	2.60

Fig. B-40. Protein and caloric contents of selected breads and baked products.

NUTRITIVE VALUES OF BREADS AND RELATED ITEMS.

Bread has often been called the *staff of life*. This implies that it supplies most of the required nutrients. While this characterization might have had some basis when it was applied to the ancient types of coarse, whole grain breads that sometimes contained malted or sprouted grains, it does not seem to be very applicable to the modern types of breads made from highly refined flours.

Comments on Figs. B-40, B-41, and B-42 follow:

1. The items which are highest in protein—both on a per pound basis, and a per calorie basis—are those made from whole grains, such as rye wafers and whole wheat bread. However, products made from highly refined flours may be equally high in protein if they contain milk, eggs, or cheese. For example, Fig. B-40 shows that buckwheat pancakes, popovers, and cheese pizza furnish almost as much protein per calorie as rye wafers.

2. Low moisture items, such as crackers and zwieback (a type of toast), may be good snacks for hikers to carry because they furnish about twice as many calories per pound as a high-moisture item such as Boston brown bread. On the other hand, the latter item may be more filling to people trying to lose weight.

3. Whole grain products generally contain the greatest amounts of minerals and vitamins, although certain items made with white flour plus bran or wheat germ may be close rivals because the latter ingredients are exceptionally rich in these nutrients.

4. The baked products which rank near the bottom of the mineral and vitamin rankings are those made from white flour plus large amounts of fat and sugar. They are rich in calories, but poor in other nutrients. For example, in comparison with whole wheat bread, pound cake contains only ⅓ as much magnesium and ¼ as much vitamin B-6.

There are other pitfalls in relying upon breads to supply much of one's nutritive needs, since even whole grain products may be very deficient in certain minerals and vitamins. Fig. B-43 shows the nutritional merits and demerits of whole wheat bread.

It may be seen from Fig. B-43 that whole wheat bread contains none of the vitamins A, D, C, or B-12. Furthermore, it is a poor source of vitamin E. While a few men might be able to meet their needs for most of the other essential nutrients by eating 2 lb (*0.9 kg*) or more of whole wheat bread per day, most women would gain weight from eating so much bread. This amount of bread would furnish 2,482 Calories (kcal), whereas the energy requirement of most adult females is 2,000 Calories (kcal).

Therefore, it would seem preferable that both men and women (1) limit their consumption of bread and cereals, and (2) obtain a substantial portion of their daily food energy allowance from milk and dairy products, fruits and vegetables, and meats, poultry, fish, eggs, and legumes. In this manner, they would be more likely to meet their needs for the nutrients that are deficient in the breads and cereals.

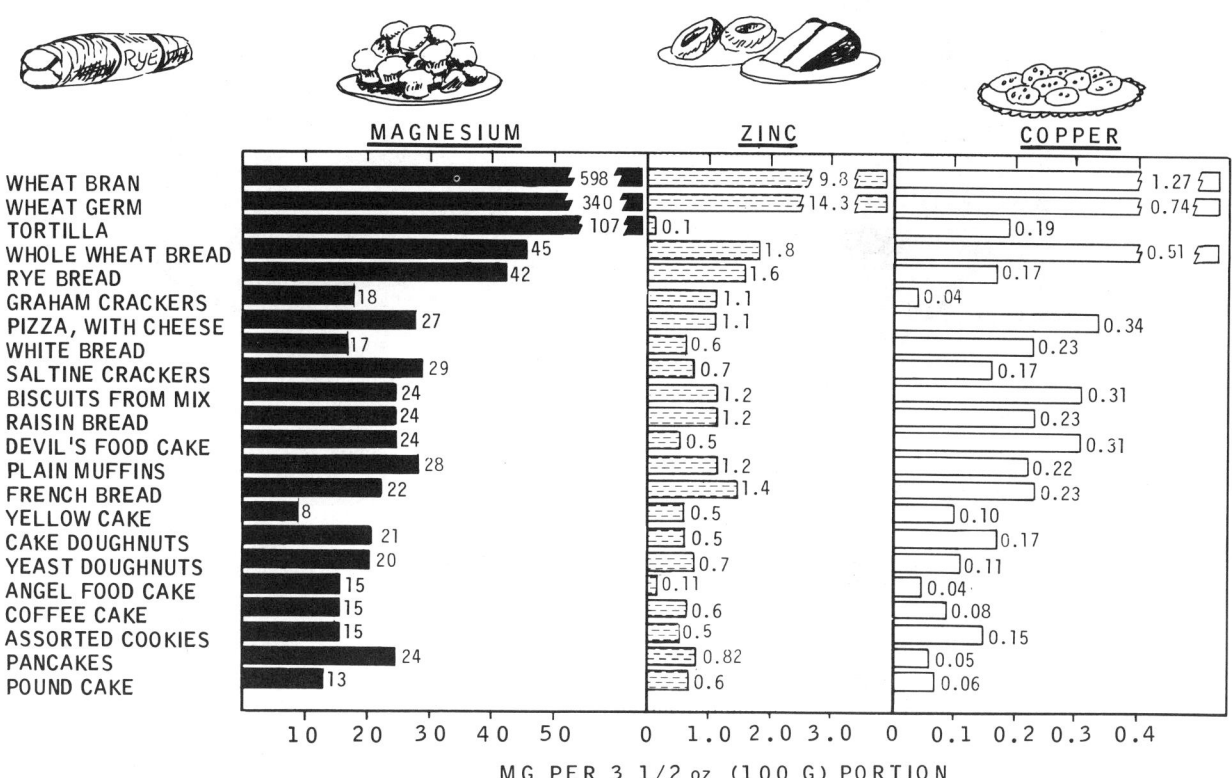

MG PER 3 1/2 oz (100 G) PORTION

Fig. B-41. Magnesium, zinc, and copper contents of selected breads and baked products.

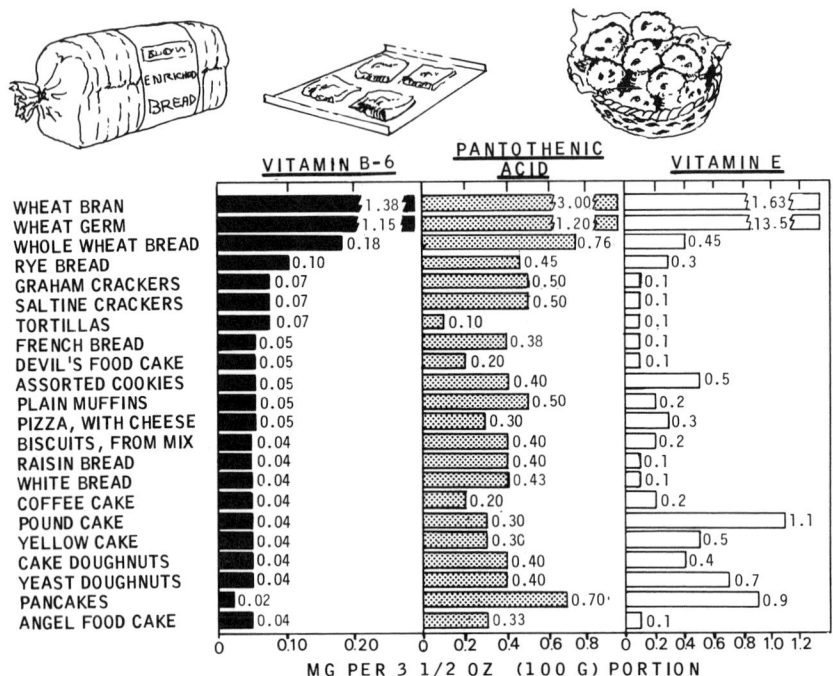

Fig. B-42. Vitamin B-6, pantothenic acid, and vitamin E contents of selected breads and baked products.

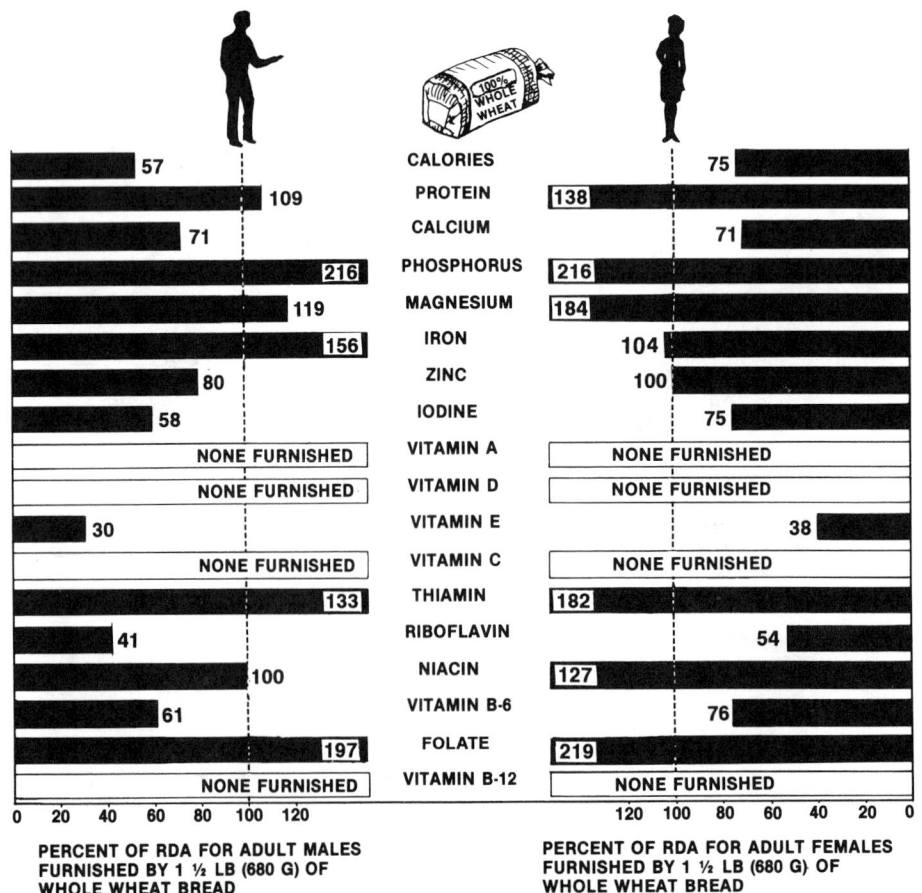

Fig. B-43. The percentages of the Recommended Dietary Allowances (RDAs) for adult (25 to 50 year) males and females furnished by 1½ lb (680 g) of whole wheat bread. (Based upon RDAs given in *Recommended Dietary Allowances*, 10th ed., NRC—National Academy of Sciences, 1989; and upon nutrient data in Food Composition Table F-21 of this book.)

Special Bread Products for Modified Diets. Many people have been advised by their doctors to modify their diets in order to treat or prevent certain diseases. Furthermore, they may be accustomed to eating plenty of bread with their meals. Hence, it may be beneficial for them to eat modified breads and bakery products which have been prepared in accordance with their dietary prescriptions because these items may make it easier for them to avoid other foods that are not allowed in their diets. Table B-8 lists some of the more common dietary modifications, and the special products that are in accordance with them.

NOTE: The data on special dietetic products are not to be considered as recommendations for people with various health problems to use these products for self treatment. It is the responsibility of the patient's doctor or dietitian to decide which foods best fill a dietary prescription. Therefore, the details which follow are given so that the patient might be better informed in discussions with his or her professional health counselor.

(Also see MODIFIED DIETS.)

TABLE B-8
SPECIAL BAKERY PRODUCTS

Dietary Prescription	Reasons for the Dietary Prescription	Ingredients in Special Dietetic Bakery Products	Comments
Carbohydrate restriction	Sometimes, disorders such as diabetes, dumping syndrome, high blood triglycerides, low blood sugar, and obesity are improved if the foods which raise the level of blood sugar are restricted.	The carbohydrate content is reduced by replacing some of the flour with nonstarchy ingredients such as bran, cellulose, Jerusalem artichoke flour, ground seed-coats from edible seeds, and nondigestible vegetable gums.	Often, restriction of dietary sugars alone works as well or better than the restriction of carbohydrates in general.
Cholesterol and saturated fat restriction	People who are extra susceptible to atherosclerosis, coronary heart disease, diabetes, or high blood levels of fats such as cholesterol and triglycerides might benefit from this diet.	Products which would normally contain whole eggs are made with egg white, lecithin, and vegetable gums. Also, solid animal fats are replaced with liquid vegetable oils, but not with coconut oil.	Imitation, yolk-free egg products are now sold in most supermarkets. Liqluid oils might be unsatisfactory for items such as pastries and pie crusts.
Egg free	It is necessary to eliminate all forms of egg from the diets of those who are allergic to this food.	Special *egg replacers*, which are mixtures of various starches, may be used instead of eggs in certain recipes.	Egg replacers are sold by health food stores and dietetic supply companies.
Electrolyte restriction	Patients with high blood levels of certain mineral salts (electrolytes) due to kidney failure require diets low in the salts and low in proein, since some of the products of protein metabolism are electrolytes.	These items are essentially starch cakes made from wheat starch, yeast, mineral-free water, sugar, unsalted margarine with the nonfat solids removed, and a cellulose derivative or a vegetable gum. Sometimes, artificial flavorings and colorings are added.	This type of product provides calories, but no protein, minerals, or vitamins. It is used only during the critical stage of kidney failure.
Energy restriction	Reduction of excess body weight may be aided by the consumption of foods high in bulk and low in calories.	Poorly digested fibrous materials such as bran, cellulose, and seedcoats are added to give bulk and to reduce the caloric content. Vegetable gums, gluten, or gluten flour may be added to strengthen the dough.	The taste and texture of these items may be unappealing when the nondigestible fiber content exceeds 30%. These items may also have a laxative effect.
Fat restriction	A few people lack the means for removal of fats from the blood, so there is a need for a drastic restriction of dietary fat in order to prevent the buildup of dangerously high levels of blood fats.	Most breads and other bakery products may be prepared from modified home recipes which eliminate fats. Commercial mixes for biscuits, muffins, cornbread, rolls, and cakes usually contain too much fat for this diet.	Sometimes, small amounts of special fats called medium-chain triglycerides may be allowed, because they do not accumulate in the blood.
Fiber enrichment	Diets high in fiber might help to prevent constipation, diverticulitis, and other bowel disorders. Sometimes, they may even help to lower elevated blood levels of fats and sugars.	High-fiber items are usually made with whole grain flours plus extra fiber in the form of bran, cellulose, and/or seedcoats. They are also used in carbohydrate restricted diets and in energy restricted diets.	Plenty of water should be taken with high-fiber products in order to prevent the formation of dried, hard masses in the lower bowel.
Fiber restriction	Very bland, low-fiber diets are recommended in order to avoid irritating lesions of the digestive tract such as those which occur in bleeding ulcers, after gastrointestinal surgery, in the acute stages of gastritis or colitis, and when hemorrhoids are either bleeding or severely inflamed.	All baked goods must be made from white flours rather than whole grain flours, and there should be no other fibrous, irritating, or spicy ingredients.	These diets are now used only when critical conditions are present because people with healed lesions appear to tolerate fiber well.
Gluten free	Dietary sources of gluten—a protein abundantly present in wheat, rye, oats, and barley—must be eliminated from the diets of people who cannot tolerate it. This condition sometimes occurs after gastrointestinal surgery, or severe diarrhea.	Only products containing flours made from corn, rice, starchy vegetables like potatoes, or legumes such as soybeans and lima beans may be used. Egg whites and special vegetable gums may be used in place of gluten to strengthen doughs.	People who cannot tolerate gluten must use a minimum gluten diet for the rest of their lives.

(Continued)

TABLE B-8 *(Continued)*

Dietary Prescription	Reasons for the Dietary Prescription	Ingredients in Special Dietetic Bakery Products	Comments
Hypoallergenic	In certain allergic conditions, such as asthma, which may be due to a sensitivity to one or more foods, it is best to eliminate the most common sensitizing foods until the actual offenders are identified.	Hypoallergenic breads are generally made without any cereal flours, milk, eggs, or yeast. Generally, the ingredients of these products consist of bean or potato flour, baking powder, sugar, fat, salt, and water. Even vegetable gums may provoke allergies in some people.	Sometimes, cornmeal, corn flour, cornstarch, potato flour, or rice flour may be used to make hypoallergenic items, because only a few people are allergic to these ingredients.
Iron enrichment	Children and women who have iron-deficiency anemia might be better off eating iron-rich foods than taking iron supplements in pill form because the latter may cause digestive upsets and interfere with dietary vitamin E.	Iron-rich ingredients for baked goods include whole grain flours, enriched white flours, soybean flour, wheat germ, molasses, nuts, raisins, and egg yolks.	Whole grain flours, bran, and soybean flour contain phytates which interfere with iron absorption. Yeast fermentation breaks down some of the phytates in whole grain breads.
Milk free	Milk must be eliminated from the diets of people who have milk allergies.	Many types of baked items may be made from water as well as from milk, but it may be better to use imitation milks made from soybeans because they are rich in protein and and other nutrients.	Nondairy creamers and coffee whiteners sometimes contain protein derived from milk, so they may aggravate allergies.
Phosphorus restriction	Dietary phosphorus must be kept low for people whose blood level of the mineral is too high. Usually, this condition results from the failure of the kidneys to excrete excesses of phosphorus via the urine.	Only refined flours may be used in baking because whole grains and bran are too rich in phosphorus. Yeast or baking soda may be used for leavening, but baking powders which contain phosphate salts may not be used.	The overall diet should provide enough calories, protein, and calcium to prevent soft tissues and bones from breaking down and releasing phosphorus into the blood.
Potassium restriction	There is a danger of the heart stopping if the kidneys fail to excrete excesses of potassium via the urine. Protein and sodium are also restricted in kidney failure.	Breads low in potassium, sodium, and protein are made from wheat starch, yeast, mineral-free water, sugar, unsalted margarine with the nonfat solids removed, and a cellulose derivative or a vegetable gum.	Tissue breakdown releases potassium into the blood, so it should be minimized by providing adequate calories.
Protein enrichment	Extra dietary protein is needed by patients who are recovering from extensive surgery, severe burns, malnutrition, loss of blood, prolonged illnesses and broken bones.	Even whole grain flours contain only moderate amounts of protein, so baked products may be fortified with high-protein ingredients such as soy flour, bean flours, eggs, nonfat dry milk or evaporated milk, and debittered brewers' yeast powder.	Gluten, gluten flour, vegetable gums, or other additives may be used to strengthen the dough so that it rises properly. Gluten-rich products also provide extra protein.
Protein restriction	Even moderate amounts of dietary protein may be toxic when (1) the liver loses its ability to detoxify the ammonia generated in protein metabolism, or (2) the kidneys fail to excrete nitrogenous wastes from protein metabolism.	A low protein, energy-rich bread may be made from wheat starch, yeast, water, sugar, margarine or butter, and a vegetable gum or other type of nonprotein additive to serve as a binder in place of gluten.	The diet is high in calories in order to minimize the breakdown of body protein. Sometimes, eggs are used because their metabolism produces little nitorgenous waste when low protein diets are consumed.
Purine restriction	High blood levels of urates, or even gout, may result from (1) the abnormal metabolism of dietary substances called purines, and (2) diets which produce ketosis.	All of the common ingredients except wheat germ and bean flours may be used in low-purine breads. Excessive growth of yeast in dough (2 or 3 prolonged periods of rising) may raise the purine content, because yeast is rich in these substances.	Diets high in protein and fat, but low in carbohydrates, may cause ketosis and elevation of the blood level of uric acid.
Sodium restriction	People who lack the ability to get rid of excess sodium in the urine may develop disorders such as water retention in their tissues, high blood pressure, and congestive heart failure.	No salt or any other sodium compound should be added to items allowed in low-sodium diets. Therefore, yeast should be used for leavening unless a special sodium-free baking powder is available.	A pharmacist may prepare a sodium-free baking powder from certain potassium salts.
Sugar restriction	The limiting of rapidly utilized dietary sugars such as fructose (fruit sugar), glucose (grape sugar), lactose (milk sugar), maltose, and sucrose (cane or beet sugar) may be of some benefit to people with disorders such as diabetes, dumping syndrome, high blood fats, low blood sugar, and obesity.	Breads should be made without any sugary ingredients such as honey, molasses, sugar, syrups, malt, etc. However, items like angel food cake and certain types of cookies cannot be made without sugars, because the textures of these products depend upon the effects of such ingredients.	Certain artificial sweeteners should be used cautiously as sugar substitutes because (1) they do not have the effects on texture that sugars do, and (2) an undesirable flavor may result if their bitter taste is not masked by flavorings and spices such as lemon, orange, cinnamon, and strongly flavored cocoa or chocolate.
Wheat free	Even small amounts of wheat flour may provoke severe allergic reactions in susceptible people.	Flours from any materials other than wheat may be used in baking.	Bakers sometimes develop allergies to wheat as a result of inhaling flour in the air of their bakeries.

Many of the special dietetic items listed in Table B-8 are intended only for people who are on restricted diets which have been ordered by their doctors. It would not be wise for normal, healthy people to eat them because they might develop nutritional deficiencies unless they take pains to obtain the missing nutrients from other foods. Therefore, some suggestions for preparing more nutritious products are given in the sections which follow.

(Also see MODIFIED DIETS.)

IMPROVING THE NUTRITIVE VALUES OF BREADS AND BAKED GOODS.

Many attempts have been made to produce special fortified breads which may be both acceptable to most consumers and as nutritious as they are practical. Some suggestions are given in the sections that follow.

Cornell Bread. One of the notable achievements in the improvement of white bread was the development of a special bread by the renowned nutritionist, Dr. McCay and his colleagues at Cornell University.

The bread is made by the Cornell Triple Rich Formula—which is so named because it contains soy flour, skim milk powder, and wheat germ. Table B-9 shows how the nutritive values of breads made according to this formula compare with those made from standard recipes.

TABLE B-9
SELECTED NUTRIENTS FURNISHED BY 1-LB LOAVES OF BREADS MADE FROM VARIOUS INGREDIENTS[1]

Nutrient and Unit of Measurement	White Bread		Whole Wheat Bread	
	Standard Recipe[2]	Cornell Bread[3]	Standard Recipe[4]	with Cornell Ingredients[5]
Calories .... (kcal)	1,065	1,050	1,097	1,082
Protein .... (g)	32	42	38	48
Protein per unit of food energy .... (g per 100 kcal)	3.0	4.0	3.5	4.4
Minerals:				
Calcium .... (mg)	60	305	122	367
Magnesium .... (mg)	84	167	300	383
Iron .... (mg)	8.9	9.8	10.5	11.4
Vitamins:				
Vitamin B-6 .... (mg)	.6	.7	2.5	2.6
Pantothenic acid .... (mg)	2.2	2.7	3.7	4.2
Folic acid .... (mg)	.2	.2	.2	.3

[1]The nutrient contents of the baked items were calculated by summing up the contents of the individual ingredients. It was assumed that each of the finished breads contained 35% moisture. Nutrient data for the ingredients were obtained from various USDA sources.
[2]Made from enriched white flour, yeast, sugar, butter, salt, and water.
[3]Same ingredients as Standard Recipe plus soy flour, nonfat dry milk, and wheat germ in the proportions developed by Dr. McCay and his associates at Cornell University.
[4]Made from whole wheat flour, yeast, sugar, butter, salt, and water.
[5]Same ingredients as standard whole wheat bread, plus soy flour, nonfat dry milk, and wheat germ in the same proportions as the ingredients used in the Cornell bread.

It may be seen from Table B-9 that the addition of soy flour, skim milk, and wheat germ to the standard recipe white bread raises the protein, calcium, and magnesium contents by significant amounts. However, the greatest improvement is made by substituting whole wheat flour for the white flour, *and* adding the special ingredients of the Cornell formula. Then, the fortified whole wheat bread produced by this means contains about half again as much protein, over six times the calcium, over 4½ times the magnesium and vitamin B-6, 1⅓ times the iron, and almost double the pantothenic acid and folic acid as the unfortified standard recipe white bread. White bread has been used for comparison in order to dramatize the differences between the popular bread which contains mainly white flour and water, and those made with more nutritious ingredients. Additional details on this subject are given in the section which follows.

Suggestions for Adding Highly Nutritious Ingredients to Baked Goods.

Some suggestions for adding various types of nutritious ingredients to home baked goods are given in the next two sections. (Nutrient composition data for the suggested additives are given in Food Composition Table F-21.)

SPECIAL NUTRITIONAL SUPPLEMENTS ADDED TO BAKED GOODS.

A little of each of these products goes a long way because they are concentrated sources of nutrients. For example, only ½ cup *(120 ml)* of soy flour, ¾ cup of skim milk powder, and 3 tablespoons *(45 ml)* of wheat germ added to 6 cups of white flour make Cornell Bread much more nutritious than ordinary white bread. (See Table B-9 for details.) Suggestions for adding other nutritional supplements follow:

1. From ¼ to ¾ cup each of bland-flavored items such as alfalfa (leaf) powder, bran, rice polishings, and/or dried whey may be used for every 6 cups of flour, provided that the total amount of these ingredients combined is not more than 1 cup. Larger quantities may make the baked product too heavy and too moist.

2. Ingredients such as blackstrap molasses, bone meal, brewers' yeast, carob powder, dolomite, lecithin granules, and liver powder have unusual tastes and textures. Therefore, it is unwise to use more than 1 teaspoon *(5 ml)* of each of them per cup of flour.

3. Some of the special supplements may interfere with the development of gluten strands in yeast-leavened breads; so, it is best to mix them gently into the dough after it has risen at least once and has been kneaded.

4. The supplements may be mixed right in with the other dry ingredients when breads are leavened with baking powder or baking soda.

COMMON FOODS THAT MAY BE ADDED TO BAKED GOODS.

People who eat a lot of bread may appreciate some variety in taste and texture, as well as the nutritional gains which result from fortifying breads with nutritious ingredients. Such variety may be achieved by mixing some of the common foods into bread doughs; among them, the following: (1) adding beverages and other liquids such as beer, fruit juice, and wine instead of milk or water in doughs; (2) adding cereals and grain products (such as infant cereals, instant cooking hot cereals, and ready-to-eat breakfast cereals) directly to the other bread ingredients (noninstant hot cereals should be cooked first)—adding 1 to 2 cups of cereal for each 6 cups of flour; (3) adding any of the cheeses, except those that have been mold-ripened (blue, Camembert, or Roquefort, which are mold-ripened, may contribute moldy flavors)— add 2 cups of grated cheese per 6 cups of flour; (4) adding dairy products, except those high in fat (butter and sweet or sour cream), replacing not more than 1/3 to 1/2 of the required liquid in the recipe— to increase the protein, minerals, and vitamins; (5) adding eggs, egg white, or egg yolks (egg white foams and holds lots of air, and also strengthens weak doughs; egg yolks help to disperse the added fat uniformly throughout the product); (6) adding fruits and fruit products, to increase the minerals and vitamins; (7) adding meats, poultry, and fish to increase the quantity and quality of proteins; (8) adding nuts and seeds to enhance the quality of proteins, and increase the minerals and vitamins; (9) adding sprouted seeds to provide extra fiber and vitamins, along with active enzymes which digest the starch and protein in flours; or (10) adding various vegetables and legumes—securing added vitamins from the vegetables and increased proteins from the legumes.

RECENT DEVELOPMENTS IN BAKING TECHNOLOGY.

Bakers and food technologists have long experimented with new ingredients and procedures in order to produce the high quality baked products expected by consumers. In their quest for quality, they have worked towards objectives such as (1) reduction of staling and spoilage (bread is usually taken out of supermarkets, or sold at reduced prices, if it has not been sold within 2 to 3 days after delivery); (2) modification of recipes so as to improve nutritive values or meet special dietetic requirements; (3) overcoming of the problems inherent in the mass production of standard products from ingredients which may vary in their baking characteristics; and (4) development of convenience items for consumers who wish to do their own baking. Some recent applications of food technology to the baking industry are: (1) air classification of flours into high-protein and low-protein fractions; (2) artificial sweeteners; (3) bulking agents; (4) chemical combinations of fats and sugars; (5) emulsifying agents; (6) enzymes; (7) imitation egg products; (8) Jerusalem artichoke flour; (9) microwave ovens; (10) mixes for quick, yeast-leavened breads; (11) preservatives; (12) seedcoat flours that are rich in fiber; (13) vegetable gums; and (14) xanthan gum.

There seems to be an almost endless variety of baked goods which may be produced by varying the amounts and types of ingredients. Hence, just about everyone should be able to enjoy some of these products, since they may be tailored to fit many types of modified diets. This wide selection of items has been made possible by the persistent efforts of researchers who have sought to improve on what nature has to offer, and who have often succeeded in their quest.

BREAD SPREADS

A slice of fresh whole wheat bread with butter and a sweet spread make a wonderful nutritious addition to any meal, between-meal, or bedtime snack. Down through the ages, breads have been the foundation of most western diets. In ancient days, some of the breads were unleavened; and they still are in some parts of the undeveloped countries. But whether unleavened or leavened, breads may be eaten with a sweet spread made from the fruits available during the summer months; among such spreads are: conserves, fruit butters, lemon butter or lemon curd, jams, jellies, marmalades, and preserves.

BREAKFAST CEREALS

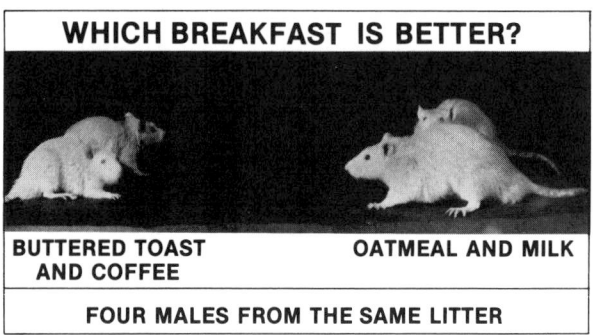

Fig. B-44. Which breakfast is better? Four male rats from the same litter. The two on the left had a breakfast of buttered toast and coffee. The others had oatmeal and milk. This advertisement, which was used in the early 1900s, was based on an experiment conducted by Thomas B. Osborne, of the Connecticut Agricultural Experiment Station, and LaFayette B. Mendel, of Yale University, who, in 1911, formed a brilliant partnership and pioneered in protein, mineral, and vitamin studies. (Courtesy, The Connecticut Agricultural Experiment Station, New Haven)

This term covers a wide variety of grain products that are usually cooked or processed to improve their texture, flavor, and digestibility. Although these products are often made from flours, they differ from breads and other baked goods in that they are not usually leavened; instead, they may be toasted to crispiness like crackers. In the United States and Great Britain, cereals are considered suitable for breakfast primarily, even though certain items like cooked rice may be the basis of every meal in Southeast Asia.

Recently, there has been a lot of controversy in the United States over the nutritional merits and demerits of various breakfast cereals. Therefore, some background information on these products is provided so that consumers might be better informed regarding the types of cereals which are best suited for their particular circumstances.

EFFECTS OF A GOOD BREAKFAST ON MENTAL AND PHYSICAL PERFORMANCE.

Many children and adults go to school or work after having had little or no food for breakfast. Some of these people may take only coffee or tea. However, the well-known research studies conducted at the University of Iowa showed that the eating of at least a light breakfast increased the speed of mental response and improved the perfomance of physical work during the late morning hours.[16] Furthermore, the skipping of breakfast sometimes resulted in adverse reactions such as muscle tremors, fatigue, dizziness, nausea, and vomiting when strenuous physical activity was undertaken in the morning.

Most of the researchers who have studied the effects of eating a good breakfast have suggested that the benefits are due mainly to the protein that is eaten at this meal, because high-protein breakfasts were found to be better than low-protein breakfasts in helping to maintain a normal blood sugar level between midmorning and lunch.[17] It is noteworthy that breakfasts consisting chiefly of vegetable protein foods (breads, cereals, peanut butter, and soybean milk) were found to be as effective as those consisting chiefly of animal protein foods (eggs, meat, and milk) in keeping the blood sugar at normal levels.[18] The level of protein eaten at breakfast may depend partly upon the amount supplied by a cereal, because ready-to-eat breakfast cereals are included in about one-fourth of all the breakfasts eaten by Americans.[19] Hot cereals also may make a contribution, particularly in areas such as the southern United States, where hot grits (cornmeal) are still served at many breakfasts. Unfortunately, the degermed meal used to make grits is nutritionally inferior to the whole grains first used by ancient peoples.

HISTORY OF CEREALS.

The modern types of ready-to-eat breakfast cereals—which are less than 150 years old—owe their development to Seventh-day Adventists, an American religious sect. This religion was officially founded in 1863 by a small group of people which included an Adventist preacher's wife who later came to be known as Mother White. In 1866, this zealous lady established the Western Health Reform Institute (later known as the Battle Creek Sanitarium, or simply the San) at Battle Creek, Michigan. People who came to the sanitarium for a health cure were given austere vegetarian diets based mainly upon minimally refined grain products and fresh fruits and vegetables, because this was in keeping with the dietary principles taught by Mother White. Subsequently, Dr. J. H. Kellogg—who had been hired by Mother White to manage

the San—invented a granolalike, ready-to-eat breakfast cereal for the Adventists who shunned the traditional American breakfast of ham and eggs. Later, Dr. Kellogg and his brother, W. K. Kellogg, founded the cereal company which still bears their name.

Another pioneer of the breakfast cereal industry was C. W. Post, who had been a patient at the Battle Creek Sanitarium. Among his inventions were (1) a cereal-based, caffeine-free beverage called Postum for use by the Adventists, who avoided stimulants such as coffee and tea; and (2) a granular cereal called Grape-Nuts.

By the beginning of World War II, cereal companies had started to enrich their products with thiamin, riboflavin, niacin, and iron. *Enrichment means the restoration of some of the nutrients that are removed during the processing of a food.* Later, in about 1955, fortification of cereals was started. *Fortification means the addition of certain nutrients to foods in order to provide higher levels of such nutrients than are normally present in the natural, unprocessed foods.*

The steady trend towards the fortification of more and more foods with more and more nutrients spurred the U.S. Food and Drug Administration to make several attempts during the 1960s and the early 1970s to regulate the amounts and types of nutrients that were added to foods. At about the same time, the consumer movement got underway, and some of the leading activists began to attack certain cereals which they classified as vitamin- and mineral-fortified confections. One of the reactions to these controversies was the production of so-called *granolas* or *natural cereals* which in many ways were similar to the first product developed by Dr. Kellogg.

There seems to be every indication that there will be a steady increase in the consumption of commercial cereal products around the world as the developing countries attempt to feed their burgeoning populations. It is noteworthy, too, that certain American cereal and milling companies have assisted in the development of marketing of nutritive cereal mixtures for needy peoples.

PRODUCTION OF BREAKFAST CEREALS.

Few people in the world today eat whole, raw grains because (1) they are too chewy; (2) the raw starch which comprises the greater part of the grains is not very tasty; and (3) they are poorly digested. It is noteworthy that the starch which is present in grains and many other plant foods is often in the form of hard granules that are very resistant to the digestive juices. Cooking starchy foods in water causes the granules to swell and form a pasty mass which is more readily digested. Dry heating or roasting, which alters starch granules by breaking them down into dextrins, enhances the taste of the food. Therefore, some type of cooking or processing is needed to give cereal products the characteristics which are most beneficial and desirable to man.

Hot Cereals. In comparison with ready-to-eat cereals, these products are less processed in the factory, but they require more preparation time in the home. The grains or grainlike seeds which have husks (rice, barley, oats, and buckwheat) are dehulled to produce groats. Naked or huskless grains (corn, wheat, and rye) do not require any special processing prior to cooking, although the cooking time is much longer when they are left whole than when they are broken up into smaller particles. However, many of the products currently on the market contain small pieces of grains which have had the branny layers removed. Quick-cooking cereals are made by precooking the grains and/or cutting them into fine pieces or flakes. Flake-type hot cereals

[16]Tuttle, W. W., M. Wilson, and K. Daum, ''Effect of Altered Breakfast Habits on Physiologic Response,'' *Journal of Applied Physiology,* Vol. I, 1949, p. 558.

[17]Coleman, M. C., W. W. Tuttle, and K. Daum, ''Effect of Protein Source on Maintaining Blood Sugar Levels After Breakfast,'' *Journal of the American Dietetic Association,* Vol. 29, 1953, p. 239.

[18]*Ibid.,* p. 243.

[19]Hayden, E. B., ''Breakfast and Today's Lifestyles,'' *The Journal of School Health,* Vol. XLV, 1975, p. 84.

are made by steaming the grain, then passing it between rollers.

Ready-to-Eat Breakfast Cereals. These items are designed to be eaten without cooking; hence, they are cooked at one of the stages in their processing. Usually, grains in the form of a meal or a flour are cooked with added flavorings and other ingredients such as malt, syrups, and heat-stable vitamins and minerals. Then, the cooked cereals are further processed by flaking, puffing, shaping, shredding, sugar-coating, or other operations. Vitamins and other nutrients that may be altered by heating are sprayed on the cereals after the hot processing operations have been completed.

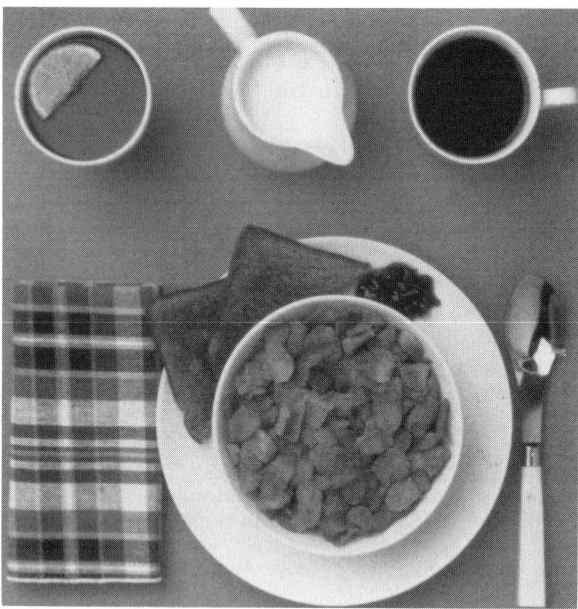

Fig. B-45. A 300 calorie breakfast. (Courtesy, USDA)

Infant Cereals. These items have a bland taste because they are not toasted or flavored like the ready-to-eat breakfast cereals. However, they are easy to prepare by mixing with infant formula or milk and they generally cost less per serving than the other pre-cooked cereals.

Infant cereals are produced by mixing bolted flours (*bolting is the removal of seed coat particles from a flour by passing it through a cloth or a fine sieve*) with water and other heat-stable ingredients to form a paste. The paste is cooked, then spread on a drying drum. Flakelike particles of dried cereal are scraped from the drum as it revolves. Vitamins and other ingredients which might be altered by heating are then added to the dried cereal.

SELECTING THE MOST NUTRITIOUS CEREALS AT THE LOWEST COST. Most of the packaged cereals sold in supermarkets have nutritional labeling, but it may not be easy for the average consumer to evaluate rapidly all of the data on the label while shopping in a crowded store. Table B-10 shows the percentages of the Recommended Dietary Allowances (RDAs) for elementary schoolchildren that are furnished by a bowl of cereal and milk, while Fig. B-46 illustrates the distribution of nutrients contributed by the cereal and the milk.

TABLE B–10
AMOUNTS OF SELECTED NUTRIENTS FURNISHED BY 1 OZ OF A TYPICAL READY-TO-EAT CEREAL PLUS 4 OZ OF MILK

Nutrient	Amount in 1 Oz Cereal plus 4 Oz Milk	Percent of RDA[1] for 7- to 10-Year-Old
Calories	192 kcal	10
Protein	6.2 g	22
Calcium	157.4 mg	20
Phosphorus	167.6 mg	21
Magnesium	38.3 mg	23
Iron	3.3 mg	33
Vitamin A	451 mcg RE	64
Vitamin D	5 mcg	50
Niacin	3.4 mg	26
Riboflavin	0.61 mg	51
Thiamin	0.37 mg	37
Vitamin B-6	0.72 mg	51
Vitamin B-12	2.16 mcg	154
Vitamin C	11 mg	24

[1]From *Recommended Dietary Allowances*, 10th ed., NRC–National Academy of Sciences, 1989, pp. 33, 284.

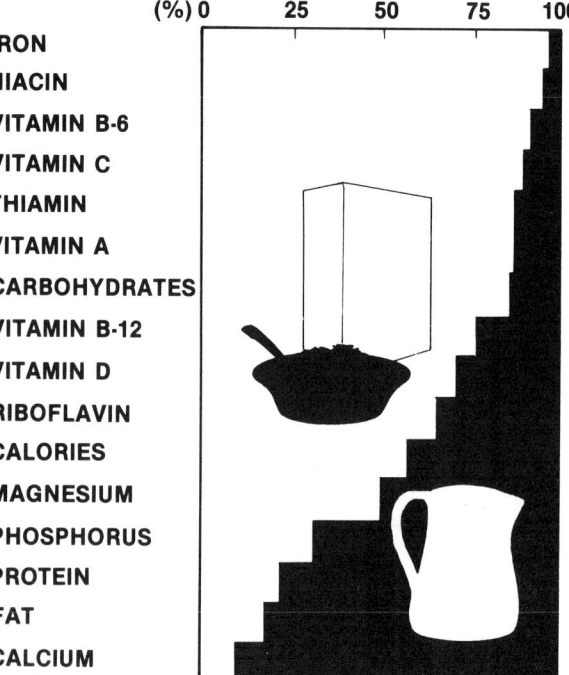

Fig. B-46. The distribution of nutrients contributed by 1 oz of a typical ready-to-eat cereal (shown by white) and 4 oz of milk (shown by black).

As shown in Table B-10, the combination of the typical ready-to-eat cereal and milk supplies ¼ or more of the RDAs for many essential nutrients, but it furnishes only about 30% of the allowance for protein. This means that some additional protein should be provided at breakfast, from foods such as extra cereal and milk, eggs, meat, and/or bread.

Fig. B-47, ranks major types of breakfast cereals by their protein contents, without regard to their vitamin and mineral contents. For additional information regarding the nutritive value of cereals, see Food Composition Table F-21 of this book.

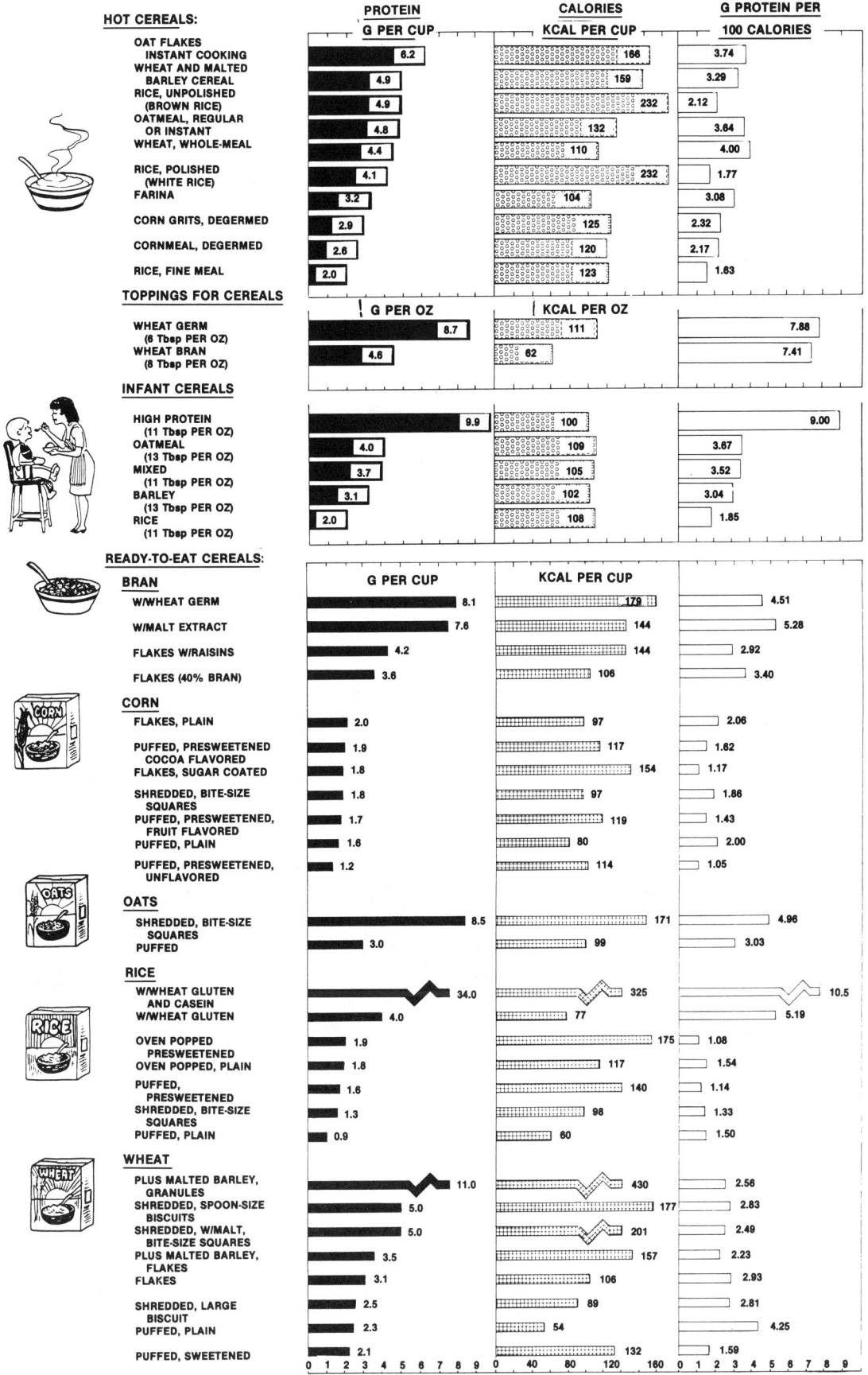

Fig. B-47. Rankings of the major types of breakfast cereals by their protein contents.

Discussions of each of the types of cereal shown in Fig. B-47 follow:

• **Hot cereals**—The oat and wheat cereals supply the most protein per calorie, while the rice and corn cereals supply the least. Cooked grains of rice furnish more calories and protein per cup than the hot corn cereals, because the water content of the cooked rice is less than that of the cooked corn. In general, hot cereals cost less than either ready-to-eat items or infant cereals because they require less commercial processing.

• **Nutritious toppings for cereals**—Bran and wheat germ are natural accompaniments to cereals because they (or the similar parts of other grains) are usually removed during milling. It is noteworthy that these by-products of milling provide more protein per calorie than most of the grain products, which is a boon for people trying to lose weight.

The cereals which are high in bulk, but low in nutrients—such as farina, and the unsugared puffed cereals—might be good items for filling up heavy eaters who need to watch their weight. Also, the dry, ready-to-eat cereals make good snacks which are less fattening than salted nuts or some types of crackers.

• **Infant cereals**—Except for the rice cereal, these products equal or top the hot cereals and the ready-to-eat cereals in protein content. However, babies may not receive very much of these cereals because mothers usually mix from 2 to 6 Tbsp (30 to 90 ml) (equivalent to from 1/6 to 1/2 oz) of cereal with approximately 1 to 3 oz (30 to 90 ml) of formula or milk. Even so, older children and adults may consume larger quantities of these cereals if they do not mind the bland taste.

• **Ready-to-eat cereals**—Certain items in this category are unusually high in protein because they have been fortified with protein-rich ingredients such as wheat gluten, casein (derived from milk), wheat germ, and malt. It is noteworthy that two of these cereals—rice with wheat gluten and casein, and wheat and malted barley granules—are concentrated sources of both protein and energy, so that servings of 1/2 cup (120 ml) or less equal or exceed the protein and caloric values of 1-cup servings of the other cereals.

The best protein sources among the cereals not fortified with this nutrient are the wheat and oat products, since the unfortified rice and corn cereals are low in protein. The presweetened or sugarcoated cereals provide significantly less protein per unit of food energy than their nonpresweetened counterparts. Furthermore, it is much cheaper for people to add their own sugar than it is to pay for it as part of the weight of the cereal, which costs much more per pound than sugar. Finally, the puffed cereals contain only about half as much protein and energy per cup as the nonpuffed products.

THE ROLE OF CEREAL MIXTURES IN THE TREATMENT AND PREVENTION OF MALNUTRITION.
Relief operations in areas of widespread malnutrition often distribute cereals, because these foods are among the most convenient for such operations, and most people will eat them. Sometimes cereals are mixed with other ingredients

that supply the nutrients lacking in the grains. Such relief measures often result in at least a temporary improvement in the nutritional status of the people they serve, which shows that rather simple cereal-based diets may be quite adequate.

The use of cereal mixtures for the improvement of nutritional status was demonstrated in a 24-week feeding trial in Tanzania, in which groups of schoolchildren who normally ate only one meal per day (in the late afternoon) were given various types of midday snacks that contained 25 g of protein.[20] The groups of children who received the special snacks in school had greater gains in height, weight, and hemoglobin than a group which received no snack. Apparently, a mixture of cornmeal and nonfat dry milk was as effective as meat powder in promoting growth, except that the latter stimulated a greater increase in hemoglobin.

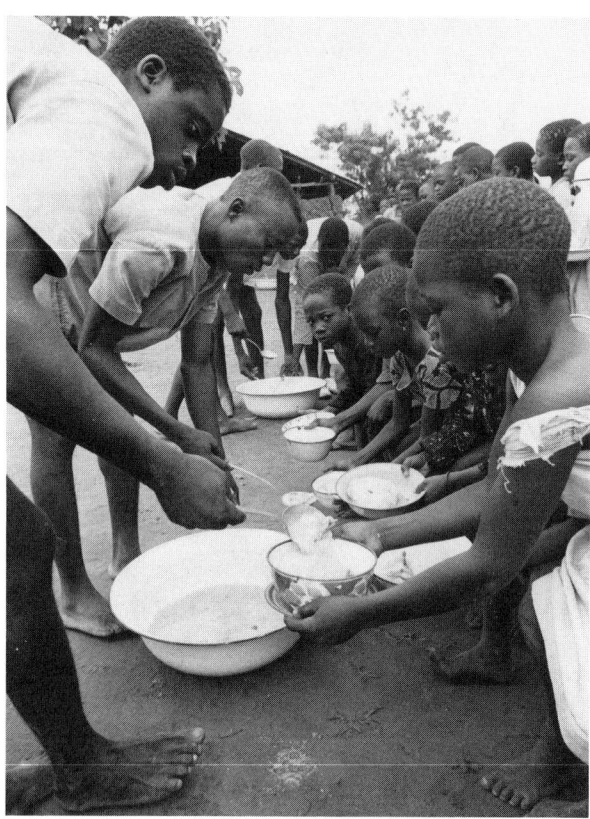

Fig. B-48. Lunchtime for school children in a rural village in the West African nation of Togo. The cereal mixture was provided by a program operated by the government of Togo and the Food and Agriculture Organization of the United Nations. (Courtesy, FAO, Rome, Italy)

At the present time, a variety of cereal-based, high-protein food products is being tested throughout the world to determine whether they might help to prevent malnutrition. The products contain grain derivatives such as wheat flour, corn flour, cornmeal, and rice flour; plus other ingredients

---

[20]Latham, M. C., and J. R. K. Robson, "A Trial to Evaluate the Benefit of Different Protein Rich Foods to African School Children," *Nutritio et Dieta*, Vol. 7, 1965, pp. 28-36.

such as nonfat dry milk, fish protein concentrate, soybean derivatives, lentils, chick-peas, yeast, sugar, starch, minerals, and vitamins. Some of the products were developed with the assistance of American cereal companies. Certainly, cereal grains are one of the least expensive ways of furnishing both protein and calories.

(Also see CEREAL GRAINS.)

THE SUGARED-BREAKFAST-CEREAL BINGE. The ready-to-eat breakfast cereals of the United States were developed by health food advocates of whom it may be said: They meant to do good, and they did well (financially). In the spirit of the founders, enrichment (restoration of nutrients) followed at the time of World War II, and fortification (the addition of certain nutrients) was introduced in about 1955. Soon the race was on! In an attempt to capture more and more of the market, the sugar content of many breakfast cereals went up and up, ushering in breakfast cereals which have been referred to as *empty calories.*

In a study reported in 1979, the U.S. Department of Agriculture revealed that only 3 out of 62 ready-to-eat breakfast cereals contained less than 1% sugar, and that two of the cereals tested contained more than 50% sugar. The USDA analyses, which examined sugars from five different sources, showed that manufacturers used far more table sugar than any other kind.

BREAST FEEDING

Contents   *Page*

There is abundant evidence that nutrition during pregnancy and early infancy is of great importance in the baby's development and later adjustment to the world in which it must live. For example, the entire period of brain growth begins during the third month of pregnancy and ends around the second or third year of life. Protein, folic acid, and iron intake are especially important, as they are crucial to normal brain development. Inadequate supplies of protein or folic acid will result in fewer brain cells and a small brain. Iron deficiency is a prime consideration, too, because children with anemia show learning disabilities and lack of concentration at school. Also, growth during the first year is greater than during any other period—birth weight triples by 1 year of age; hence, nutritive requirements are critical at this time.

Peasant women, like other mammals, lactate easily and naturally. For them it is a normal part of life and a natural experience from which they derive emotional satisfaction. Both urban life and wealth brought distractions, and for many women they made lactation difficult and sometimes distasteful. The decline in breast feeding was marked. In the decade 1960-70, fewer than 15% of infants in the United States and most of Europe, and among the wealthy of Africa and Asia, were breast fed.

Both working away from home and social life are obstacles to lactation. Fashion, advertisements for artificial milks, and greater convenience for staff in obstetrical wards all mitigate

against natural feeding. Among many of the elite there is a taboo against suckling except in strictest privacy. Also, many mothers who start breast feeding switch to bottle feeding because they feel that their baby is not getting sufficient milk. Whatever the reasons for not breast feeding, if it is to be successful, the advantages must be sold to mothers early in pregnancy.

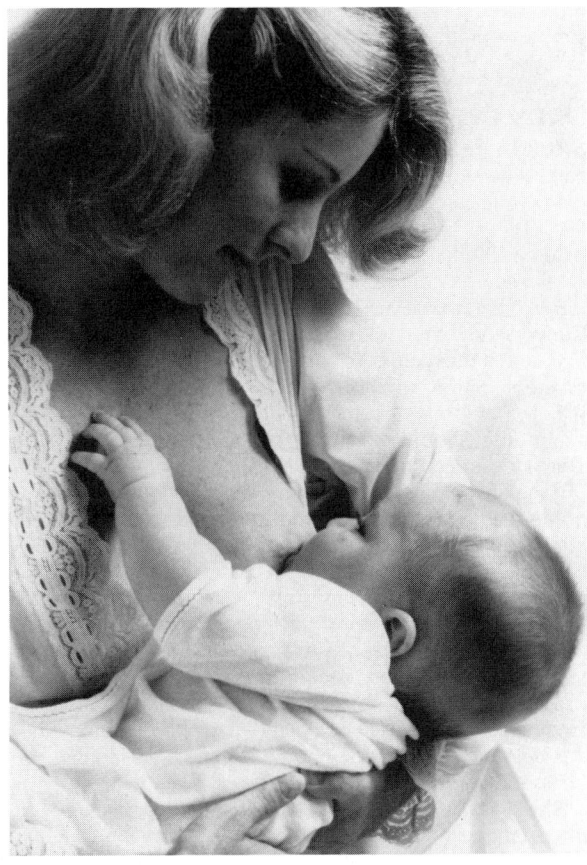

Fig. B-49. Breast feeding (Courtesy, Gerber Products Company)

During the first 6 months of life, human milk with an initial supplement of vitamin K and daily supplements of vitamin D, iron, and fluoride is regarded by the authors of this book as the best source of nourishment for the young infant. Alternatives to breast feeding include milk- or soy-based commercially prepared formulas, evaporated milk formulas, or cow's milk.

There is considerable controversy regarding the necessity of vitamin and mineral supplements for the exclusively breast fed infant. For the newborn, an injection of vitamin K is generally recommended, because the vitamin K content of human milk is low. To avoid a vitamin D deficiency, particularly when exposure to sunlight is limited, supplementation with 400 IU of vitamin D per day is advocated. The question of iron supplementation is debated, but the authors recommend 7 mg of iron daily during the first 6 months. There are also opposing views concerning fluoride supplementation. Because the fluoride content of human milk is low, the authors recommend a supplement of 0.25 mg of fluoride per day, dispensed with a dropper, beginning at 2 weeks of age.

Breast feeding may continue into the second year of life. But after the first 6 months, the energy needs of the infant may exceed those that can be met by breast feeding; so, the addition of solid foods is desirable at this time.

Unfortunately, there are many gaps in our present knowledge regarding infant nutritional needs and the appropriateness of various feeding regimens. As a result, opinions and practices of infant feeding differ. So, in arriving at a choice between dietary regimens—breast feeding versus formula feeding—and in deciding on the mineral and vitamin supplementation, each mother is admonished to seek and follow the counsel of her pediatrician.

ADVANTAGES AND DISADVANTAGES OF BREAST FEEDING.

There is much evidence that the earliest experiences of the newborn baby are of great importance in its later adjustment to the world in which it must live. This is particularly true of feeding, and it applies whether the baby is breast fed or bottle fed. If the mother is relaxed and confident, the baby will respond to her and, through her, to the world about it with trust and confidence. Conversely, if the mother is tense and radiates anxiety and fear, and if the feeding is hurried, the baby becomes aware of the situation; and there may be fretfulness or crying, which may prevent it from taking the food that it needs.

A mother should be encouraged to breast feed her baby. This is best accomplished in early pregnancy by pointing out the advantages and disadvantages of breast feeding vs bottle feeding. Then, if the mother decides to breast feed her infant, instructions for the preparation of her breasts prior to delivery should be given by the doctor or nurse. Likewise, she must be well informed relative to the importance of proper diet and rest during the rigors of lactation.

Despite what has been said, a mother should not be made to feel guilty if there are circumstances, such as mothers not producing sufficient milk or being ill, which favor bottle feeding. If the baby is cuddled and made comfortable when it is being fed, whether by bottle or breast, its feelings will be those of warmth and comfort.

Also, it is noteworthy that breast feeding is of greater importance in the developing countries than in the developed countries with more affluent societies.

Although not all the advantages or disadvantages herein ascribed to breast feeding apply to a particular circumstance, all of them have been pertinent in one case or another; hence, they are important when deciding between breast feeding and bottle feeding.

The **advantages** of breast feeding are:

• **Presence of colostrum**—Although scientists have improved upon nature's product, milk, they have not yet learned how to formulate a synthetic product that will replace colostrum.

• **Most nutritive requirements are met**—The nutritive composition and certain nutritive interactions of human milk are suited to infant needs.

• **Nutrient availability**—Protein and iron are more readily available from human milk than from prepared formulas.

• **Less obesity**—The low calorie content of human milk, along with the lack of maternal concentration of feedings, are important factors in the uncommonness of infantile obesity in breast-fed infants.

• **Lessened risks**—Breast feeding reduces risk of neonatal tetany, hypertonic dehydration, allergy to cow's milk, constipation, and certain other hazards.

• **Immunization**—Through antibodies received in the mother's milk, it imparts immunization to the baby against certain infectious diseases.

• **Fewer diseases and less mortality**—It lessens gastroenteritis and protein-energy malnutrition, which inevitably make for increased infant mortality in the developing countries.

• **Safer**—It is bacteriologically safer than a poor formula unhygienically prepared.

• **Freedom from contamination**—It is free from contamination.

• **Ease of preparation**—It eliminates preparation of the formula with special utensils and sterilized bottles and nipples; and the milk is available at proper temperature and without errors of calculation and formula preparation. (Of course, ready bottled commercial formulas are available today.)

• **Alleviates space and equipment needs**—It does not require space and equipment to prepare each feed in a hygienic manner—an important consideration in developing countries.

• **Economical**—It is more economical; it takes money to buy formula products.

• **Alleviates dependence on availability**—It is not dependent on the availability of high quality formula foods, an important consideration in some of the developing countries.

• **A comforting and satisfying experience**—It provides a natural part of the life cycle for both mother and baby, which may be a comforting and satisfying experience.

• **Psychological effects on the mother**—Many mothers derive satisfaction from knowing that they are the source of their baby's food.

• **Enhances mother-child relationship**—It permits an early mother-child bonding.

• **Birth control**—Continued lactation tends to delay the resumption of ovulation and increase birth spacing, an important consideration in developing countries. It is not, however, a reliable method of contraception.

• **Some speculations**—It has been speculated, without proof, that the use of unnatural foods in the first months of life may sow seeds which appear later as chronic disorders such as allergies, atherosclerosis, hypertension, and diabetes.

The following **disadvantages** have been attributed to breast feeding at one time or another:

• **Milk is not the perfect food**—It is deficient in iron, copper, and vitamin D. In addition to correcting these deficiencies, formulas for bottle feeding may be fortified with other minerals and vitamins.

• **Time out from work for breast feeding**—It necessitates that women who work away from home take time out to breast feed their babies.

• **It curbs social life**—Breast feeding is an obstacle to a full social life.

• **Mother must give adequate milk**—The mother must supply at least half the infant's needs; otherwise, breast feeding isn't practical. It should be added that it is unusual for a healthy woman with no disease of the breast to fail to produce enough food for her baby.

• **Subject to being discontinued**—Breast feeding must be discontinued when any of the following conditions arise:
1. When chronic illnesses—such as heart disease, tuberculosis, severe anemia, nephritis, epilepsy, insanity, or chronic fevers—strike the mother.
2. When another pregnancy ensues.
3. When it is necessary for the mother to return to employment away from home.
4. When the infant is weak and unable to nurse because of cleft palate or harelip.
5. When the mother acquires a long-lasting infection which the infant has not yet had.

COLOSTRUM. During pregnancy, the breast is prepared for lactation. The alveoli enlarge and multiply, and toward the end of the pregnancy period, secrete a thin yellowish fluid called colostrum. After delivery, colostrum is secreted for 2 to 4 days, following which regular milk is produced. Colostrum contains more protein, minerals, and vitamin A than regular milk, but less carbohydrate and fat. In addition, it also contains helpful antibodies which confer to the newborn an immunity to certain infections during the first few months.

FEEDING TECHNIQUE. Breast feeding should be initiated within 24 to 48 hours after birth.

The rooting reflex of the newborn, its oral need for sucking, and its basic hunger drive make breast feeding easy for the healthy relaxed mother whose diet meets lactation requirements. Nevertheless, the suggestions that follow may be helpful:
1. The mother must be comfortable and relaxed; she not only feeds, but she talks and smiles. At first she will probably hold the baby cradled in her arms in a semireclining position against the breast while reclining on and supported by pillows. Later, she should sit in a comfortable chair with armrests—perhaps a rocker; preferably, with a footstool to support her feet.
2. The warm touch of the breast on the baby's cheek will stimulate the natural rooting reaction, causing it to turn its head in the direction of the touch and to begin sucking motions with its mouth. Stroke the cheek nearest the nipple, and the baby will turn toward it. (Never touch the cheek furthest from the nipple, as it will cause the baby to turn its head in that direction—away from the nipple.) If necessary to get the baby started, press a little milk onto its lips. The baby should grasp most of the nipple in its mouth, not merely the outer tip.
3. In the beginning, the baby may get enough food by emptying one breast, but if it is still hungry it should be offered the other breast. After lactation is established, alternate breasts may be used for each feeding.

4. Usually, a hungry baby will get its fill of milk in about 5 minutes of nursing, but some will continue as long as 20 minutes. When the infant has had sufficient milk and is satisfied, it will stop nursing and become disinterested in more feeding.

5. After each feeding (and sometimes during the feeding), the baby should be *burped*, to expel any air that it may have swallowed during nursing. This may be accomplished (a) by holding the baby over the shoulder and patting it on the back, (b) by laying it, stomach down, across the knee, and patting its back.

INTERVALS AND ADEQUACY OF FEEDING. Although there is not full agreement, most authorities subscribe to the following thinking relative to the frequency of feeding and the amount to feed:

1. Feedings may be given according to the hunger needs of the baby, sometimes referred to as *self-demand feeding*. The very young infant may require feeding every 2 to 3 hours, but it soon establishes a rhythm of feeding at 3- to 4-hour intervals. After the second month, the night feeding usually may be discontinued.

2. About 2.5 oz of human milk per pound of body weight results in satisfactory weight gain. The baby is getting enough milk (a) if it is satisfied and falls asleep after feeding; and (b) if it is making satisfactory gains as determined by weighing each week, at the same time and with the same amount of clothing. Also, by weighing the baby before and after feeding, a mother can get a pretty good idea of how much milk it is getting.

Insufficient milk is indicated when the baby is not satisfied at the completion of feeding, or is restless and either fails to fall asleep quickly after nursing or awakens frequently. In such cases, the physician may recommend adding a supplemental food, or replacing one or more of the breast feedings with bottle feeding.

3. After lactation is established, an occasional bottle feeding may replace breast feeding if the mother so desires or has to be away.

MOTHER'S LACTATION DIET. The lactating mother requires more food and more nutritious food than a nonlactating woman, with the amount of such increases dependent upon the quantity of milk secreted. Under normal conditions, a mother produces approximately ⅓ oz (*10 g*) of milk on the 1st day, and 33 oz (*1,000 g*) per day on the 24th week.

Lactating mothers need to increase their daily energy intake by 600 Calories (kcal), and more if they are doing a lot of housework or are employed in a factory. They may also draw upon stores of fat laid down during pregnancy for additional energy. A weekly weighing is the best way to determine if the food intake is sufficient.

The extra protein and calcium for lactation are most conveniently provided by drinking a minimum of 1 pt (*470 ml*) of milk daily.

The mother's diet determines the pattern of fatty acids and the concentration of vitamin A, thiamin, riboflavin, vitamin C, and vitamin B-12.

Coffee, tea, beers, and wines may be taken in moderation and do not alter the quality of the milk. But most drugs are excreted in the milk, although they are usually in such small amounts as to cause no ill-effects to the baby. However, all drugs are potentially harmful if taken in large amounts. Most authorities recommend against the use of the following drugs while breast feeding: anticoagulants, antithyroid drugs, atrophine, diuretics, morphine, oral contraceptives, radioactive preparations, reserpine, and steroids.

Fortunately, women can store up body reserves of certain nutrients before and during the pregnancy period, to be drawn upon following birth. Here is how this phenomenon works: When properly fed before and during pregnancy, certain nutrient deposits are made in the body. Then, during lactation when the demands may be greater than can be obtained from the food, the mother draws from the stored body reserves. Thus, maternal stores of energy in the form of subcutaneous fat are laid down; and both calcium and phosphorus can be stored in the bones, then withdrawn during early lactation when milk production is at its peak. Of course, if there hasn't been proper body storage, something must *give*—and that something will be the mother, for nature ordained that the growth of the fetus, and the lactation that follows, shall take priority over the maternal requirements. Hence, when there is a nutrient deficiency, the mother's body will be deprived, or even stunted if she is young, before the developing fetus or milk production will be materially affected.

Even for a healthy woman on a good diet, providing sufficient milk to meet all the demands of a rapid-growing infant is a physiological strain. So, supplemental feeding, i.e., the substitution of a bottle feed for one or more breast feeds and/or the early introduction of solid foods, may be indicated. Also, it is important that the mother's hemoglobin should be checked during the period between childbirth and the return of the uterus to its normal size. Iron deficiency anemia is rather common at this time, especially if blood loss was excessive at or after delivery.

It is noteworthy, too, that fetal stores of iron and vitamin A are made during pregnancy, provided the mother's nutritional status during pregnancy is adequate.

WEANING THE BABY. Weaning is the process whereby feeding from the breast or bottle is replaced by other foods, usually pasteurized cow's milk and solid foods. Except in an emergency, it should be started during the 5th to 9th month, and it should take place gradually. Weaning is usually accomplished by substituting a cup feeding for the breast or bottle feeding one period daily. When the baby has become accustomed to this—after about 4 to 5 days—the second cup feeding daily may be offered. Subsequent increases of cup feedings should be offered until the baby is entirely weaned. Weaning usually requires a period of 2 to 3 weeks.

(Also see BABY FOODS; INFANT DIET AND NUTRITION; and NUTRIENTS: REQUIREMENTS, ALLOWANCES, FUNCTIONS, SOURCES.)

BREATHING RATE

Normal breathing rates per minute are: men, 18; women, 20; children, 25; and infants, 35. It varies under different conditions of health and disease. Breathing increases on exertion and excitement, and in case of fever, asthma, and heart disease. It slows down during rest and sleep.

BREWERS' YEAST

Brewers' yeast, which is usually dried (the fresh form spoils quickly), is the nonfermentative, nonextracted yeast of the botanical classification, *Saccharomyces*, derived as a by-product from the brewing of beer and ale. It is used primarily as a rich supplemental source of the B vitamins and unidentified factors. It is also an excellent source of protein (it contains a minimum of 35% crude protein) of good quality.

When irradiated with ultraviolet light, it also provides vitamin D.

BREWING

• The process of making malt beverages such as beer and ale.

• A process of preparation, or a concoction, such as teas and herbal teas.
(Also see BEERS AND BREWING.)

BRIGHT'S DISEASE

This term is commonly used to designate kidney disease in general. However, the types of kidney disease vary greatly in terms of their causes and their effects on the rest of the body. Depending upon the disease, there are various therapeutic diets.
(Also see MODIFIED DIETS.)

BRISKET

A cut of meat consisting of the breast.
(Also see BEEF AND VEAL, Fig. B-19.)

BRITISH GUMS

These are formed by modifying starch with high temperatures and possibly a little acid. The glucose molecules forming the starch rearrange under these conditions, and become highly branched molecules. British gums are used as carriers for food flavors.
(Also see STARCH.)

BRITISH THERMAL UNIT (BTU)

The amount of energy required to raise 1 pound of water 1°F; equivalent to 252 calories.

BRIX

A term used to express the sugar (sucrose) content of molasses, and of syrups used in canned fruits.

BROCCOLI *Brassica oleracea*, **variety** *italica*

Broccoli, which is closely related to the cauliflower, is a member of the mustard family, *Cruciferae*.

Because the edible parts of this vegetable (flower heads and stalks) resemble miniature trees, the ancient Romans named it broccoli, from the Latin word *Brachium*, meaning arm or branch. Fig. B-50 shows the edible portion of this vegetable.

ORIGIN AND HISTORY. Broccoli developed from the wild cabbage that was native to coastal Europe, which had spread to the Orient at an early date. The ancient plant resembled modern-day collards in that the leaves did not clump together to form a head.

WORLD AND U.S. PRODUCTION. Broccoli is not an important vegetable worldwide. However, it is important in the United States, where it ranks eleventh among the leading vegetable crops, with about 617,250 short tons produced annually. California produces more than 90% of the U.S. broccoli.[21]

---

[21]Based on data from *Agricultural Statistics 1991*, USDA, p. 148, Table 206.
Note well: Annual production fluctuates as a result of weather and profitability of the crop.

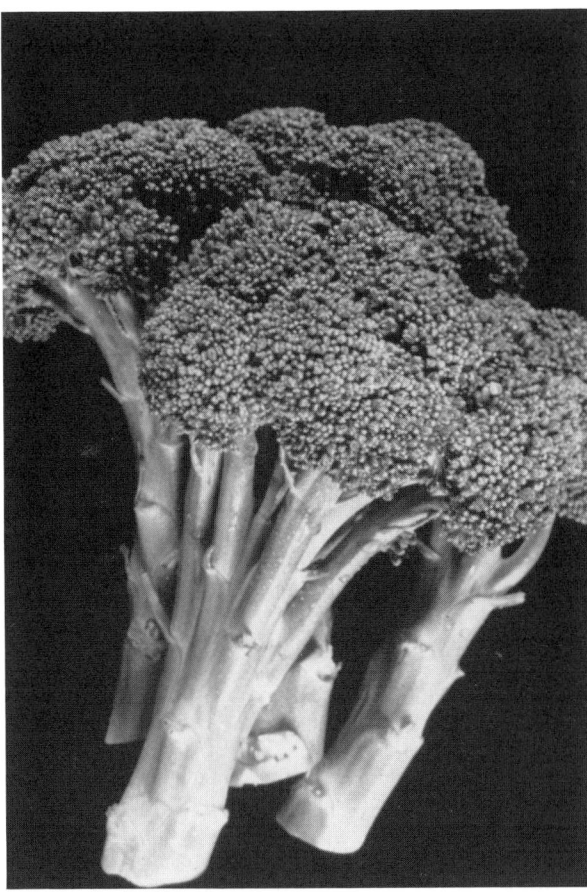

Fig. B-50. Broccoli. (Courtesy, USDA)

PROCESSING. A little over ½ of the U.S. broccoli crop is processed by freezing, and the rest is marketed fresh.

SELECTION, PREPARATION, AND USES. Good quality broccoli is fresh and clean, with compact bud clusters which have not opened to the extent that the flower color is evident. The general color should be dark-green, deep sage-green, or purplish-green, depending on variety. Stalks and stem branches should be tender and firm.

Most recipes for broccoli dishes utilize the cooked vegetable. Fresh broccoli requires from 9 to 12 minutes cooking in boiling water, depending on the size of the pieces, whereas frozen broccoli requires 6 to 8 minutes. Frozen broccoli is cooked partially by blanching prior to freezing.

Once cooked, the vegetable may, or may not, be sauteed briefly in oil or bacon fat, with or without bits of browned garlic, capers, coriander, crisp bacon, curry powder, pepper, and/or pimiento. Broccoli may also be served on toast with a cheese sauce, hollandaise sauce, or a white sauce containing sliced hard-cooked eggs. Finally, pureed broccoli makes an excellent soup.

NUTRITIONAL VALUE. The nutrient composition of broccoli is given in Food Composition Table F-21.

Some noteworthy observations regarding the nutrient composition of broccoli follow:

1. It is high in water content (over 91%), and low in calories. Only about 39 Calories (kcal) are provided by 1 cup (*240 ml*) of the cooked vegetable.

2. A 1-cup serving of cooked broccoli supplies about the same amount of protein (4.7 g) as a cup of cooked corn or rice, but less than one-third as many calories (less than 40 kcal, vs 150 to 200 kcal in the cooked cereals).

3. Approximately equal amounts of calcium and phosphorus are furnished by broccoli, which is an ideal dietary ratio between the two essential minerals. The vegetable is also a fair to good source of iron, and it is an excellent source of potassium.

4. Broccoli is an excellent source of vitamins A and C. A cup of the cooked vegetable supplies as much vitamin C as two oranges.

5. Broccoli is also a good source of bioflavonoids, substances that appear to act along with vitamin C in strengthening the smallest blood vessels (capillaries) against breakage or leakage of fluid into the surrounding tissues.

Broccoli contains small amounts of goitrogens. (See GOITROGENS.)

BROILERS (FRYERS)

Meat-type chickens that are 6 to 8 weeks of age. (Also see POULTRY.)

BROMATOLOGY

The science of foods (from the Greek *broma*—food).

BROMELIN

This is a protein-digesting and milk-clotting enzyme isolated from fresh pineapple juice. Bromelin is used in biochemical research, and for tenderizing meat. Because bromelin will digest gelatin, pineapple cannot be used to make gelatin dishes unless it has been canned or heated.

(Also see MEAT[S], section headed "Meat Tenderizing.")

BROMINATED VEGETABLE OILS

These are made by adding bromine to the unsaturated fatty acid component of the vegetable oil. The major use of brominated vegetable oils is the production of stable flavor emulsions for use in citrus-flavored soft drinks. They are considered a food additive, and the Food and Drug Administration (FDA) allows citrus and other fruit-flavored beverages to contain only 15 parts per million (ppm).

BRONCHIAL ASTHMA

A serious and often chronic condition in which the bronchial tubes which bring air into the lungs become clogged with mucus so that little air may pass through them. Usually, broncial asthma is due to allergic reactions provoked by one or more of a wide variety of different allergens. Some of the most common allergens are house dust, mold, pollens, ordinary foods, various medicines, or even hair or flakes of skin from house pets. Emotional upset, extreme fatigue, changes in temperature or humidity, or moving to a new climate may also bring on or aggravate bronchial asthma. The best preventive measures are identification and avoidance of the allergens responsible for the condition.

(Also see ALLERGIES.)

BRONCHIECTASIS

A condition in which the bronchial tubes and a portion of the lungs are stretched and dilated. Bronchiectasis is characterized by continuous coughing and the bringing up of a puslike secretion. It may be caused by chronic bronchitis, dust, infections, asthma, and/or malnutrition. If the disorder lasts long enough, respiratory acidosis and a coma may develop because the lungs cannot get rid of the excess carbon dioxide produced in metabolism.

(Also see ACID-BASE BALANCE; and BRONCHITIS.)

BRONCHITIS

An inflammation of the mucous lining of the bronchial tubes which bring air into the lungs. Bronchitis is often accompanied by a slight fever and a dry rasping cough. It is usually caused by a bacterial infection and may occur suddenly after chilling, exposure to irritants in the air, or upon the development of a common cold. If the condition is not treated promptly, it may develop into bronchopneumonia. Therefore, acute bronchitis should be treated with (1) bed rest in a warm room with a vaporizer; (2) small but nutritious meals; and (3) plenty of hot liquids. Bronchitis may be aggravated by very dry air, smoking, excessive use of alcohol, a dusty environment, and obesity.

BRONZE DIABETES

A disorder in which (1) the skin has a bronzelike hue, and (2) there is a loss of function of the liver and/or the pancreas. It results from the abnormal accumulation of iron in these tissues due to some unknown disorder of iron metabolism, or to the absorption of a great excess of iron. One of the conditions under which a great excess of iron may be absorbed is the consumption of iron in alcoholic beverages, such as the beer made by the Bantu tribes of Africa. (The Bantu tribes brew their acid beer in iron pots.) Also, iron overload can be caused by high intakes of iron supplements.

(Also see IRON.)

BROWN RICE

Paddy rice from which the husk has been removed.

BROWN SUGAR

Brown sugar, technically known as *soft* sugar, is a mass of fine crystals covered with a film of highly-refined, colored, molasses-flavored syrup. It is valued primarily for flavor and color. Brown sugar does contain several minerals at levels higher than refined sugar. Still, the energy content is similar to refined sugar, 385 kcal/100 g for granulated refined sugar and 373 kcal/100 g for brown sugar. Lighter types are used in baking and making butterscotch, condiments, and glazes for ham. The dark brown sugar, with its rich flavor, is desirable for gingerbread, mince meat, baked beans, plum pudding, and other full-flavored foods.

(Also see SUGAR.)

BRUCELLA

A family of microorganisms which chiefly affect livestock and cause pregnant females to abort their young. Man is also susceptible to the organism, which may be transmitted in defective meat or milk. However, such transmission may be prevented by pasteurizing milk and cooking meat.

(Also see DISEASES, ''Brucellosis.'')

BRUNNER'S GLANDS

Duodenal glands that secrete mucus which protects the mucosa from irritation and erosion by the strongly acid gastric juices entering from the stomach. Emotional stress inhibits mucous secretion, which may lead to an ulcer.

BRUSH BORDER

Microscopic bristlelike projections (microvilli) which line the villi of the small intestine and which function in the absorption of nutrients. These cells are also the sources of certain intestinal enzymes which aid in digestion.

(Also see DIGESTION AND ABSORPTION.)

BUCKWHEAT *Fagopyrum*

There are three species of buckwheat: common buckwheat, *F. esculentum*; Tartary buckwheat, *F. tataricum*; and winged buckwheat, *F. emarginatum*.

ORIGIN AND HISTORY. Buckwheat is a native of Asia. It was cultivated widely in China during the 10th and 13th centuries. From China it was taken to Europe via Turkey and the U.S.S.R. during the 14th and 15th centuries, thence to Great Britain and the United States during the 17th century.

WORLD AND U.S. PRODUCTION. World production of buckwheat is estimated at 3 million tons annually. The U.S.S.R. is the leading producer, followed by Poland. In both countries, buckwheat is a basic food item, consumed mainly as porridge and soup. Currently, U.S. production amounts to less than 30,000 tons annually, most of which is in the North Central and Northeastern states.

MILLING BUCKWHEAT. Buckwheat is milled into flour by a roller milling process, much like wheat flour is produced. The flour yield ranges from 60 to 80%.

To make buckwheat groats, the grain is passed between two mill stones adjusted to crack the hull without grinding the seed.

NUTRITIONAL VALUE. The nutritive composition of buckwheat grain and flour are given in Food Composition Table F-21.

The gluten content of buckwheat is low; the principal protein is globulin. The profile of essential amino acids of buckwheat shows that it is high in lysine and low in methionine; the amino acid pattern of buckwheat complements the major cereal grains. The carbohydrate is mostly starch.

BUCKWHEAT PRODUCTS AND USES. The chief food use of buckwheat in the United States and Canada is griddle cakes made from the flour, often mixed with wheat flour. Buckwheat cakes are brown, palatable, and nutritious. Groats, which are sometimes sold under the name kasha, are used as breakfast food and in soups.

Buckwheat is also an important honey plant. It blossoms profusely over an extended period of a month or more, and the flowers contain a rich store of nectar, which attracts bees. Buckwheat honey has a dark color and a pleasant flavor.

Buckwheat is also used to a limited extent for medicinal purposes. It contains 1 to 6% rutin (formerly called vitamin P) a flavonoid which is used in the treatment of certain kinds of hemorrhage, frostbite, x-ray burns, and exposure to atomic radiation.

(Also see CEREAL GRAINS; and FLOURS, Table F-12 Major Flours.)

BUERGER'S DISEASE

This disorder, which is also known as *thromboangiitis obliterans,* is a blockage of the veins and small arteries in the feet, legs, hands, and arms by blood clots. The characteristic symptoms and signs of Buerger's disease are: (1) pain in the feet and legs which is brought on by walking (doctors call this condition intermitten claudication); (2) blanching of the skin on the limbs when they are elevated, but reddening of the skin when they hang down; (3) coldness, numbness, and tingling in the extremities; and (4) inflammation and swelling of the veins (phlebitis). Sometimes, the affected tissues develop gangrene and require amputation.

Most of the victims of Buerger's disease are men who have been heavy smokers, although a few nonsmokers develop the condition after their legs have been chilled. The disease appears to run in certain families.

Measures which slow the worsening of the condition are: (1) immediate cessation of smoking, (2) avoidance of chilling and injury to the limbs by wearing warm and protective clothing, (3) mild exercises to keep the blood vessels open, and (4) administration of vitamin E under a doctor's supervision, because this measure has relieved the pains brought on by walking.

BUFFALO BERRY *Shepherdia argentea*

The small scarlet berry of the shrub (of the family *Eleagnaceae)* which grows wild in the Great Plains and the western United States.

Sweetening is sometimes needed to offset the sour taste of the fruit. However, the acidity is reduced somewhat after the berries have been exposed to a frost. The Indians used this fruit in mushes and stews, and the early settlers made the berries into jams and jellies.

BUFFALO HUMP

An abnormal, humplike deposit of fat under the skin of the upper back, which is seen in people who have chronic oversecretion of certain adrenal cortical hormones. The medical name for this disorder is *Cushing's Syndrome.*

(Also see CUSHING'S SYNDROME; and ENDOCRINE GLANDS.)

BUFFER

A substance in a solution that makes the degree of acidity (hydrogen-ion concentration) resistant to change when an acid or base is added. Buffers such as bicarbonate ion help to maintain neutrality in body fluids.

(Also see ACID-BASE BALANCE.)

BULIMAREXIA (BULIMIA NERVOSA; GORGE PURGE)

Bulimarexia (from the Greek words for ox and hunger), an eating disorder, is anorexia's opposite. Bulimarexia is characterized by eating binges, whereas anorexia nervosa is distinguished by self-inflicted voluntary starvation.

Some bulimarectics gorge themselves four to five times a week; and they always follow each eating binge by self-induced vomiting or heavy use of laxatives. They have chosen this way to handle stress, just as alcoholics use alcohol.

Treatment, which consists of group therapy, individual psychotherapy, or behavior modification, lessens the frequency of the binges, but, to date, cures are unknown.

It is noteworthy that bulimarectics dislike cooking for friends. The reason: They're afraid that they will eat all the food before the guests arrive.

BULIMIA

This refers to an insatiable appetite.
(Also see APPETITE.)

BULK

The undigestible residue from foods which passes unabsorbed through the intestine and acts as a stimulus for bowel movement. Usually, bulk is provided by fruits, vegetables, and whole grains, but not by dairy products, eggs, fish, meats, or poultry. However, tough connective tissue from meat may also provide bulk.

(Also see FIBER.)

BULKING AGENT

This term generally refers to nonfood materials, such as methylcellulose, which may be added to foods so that the diet contains greater amounts of undigestible matter. The purpose of this addition is to (1) provide a greater feeling of fullness so that less food is eaten; or (2) help control constipation.

(Also see CONSTIPATION; and FIBER.)

BURGOO

In times past, this word was applied to different things. Today, it is not used very extensively, but it can mean any one of the following:

• Oatmeal gruel—a thick porridge which was the mainstay of a ship's mess.

• Hardtack (giant soda crackers) and molasses cooked together, also popular ship's fare.

• A savory, highly seasoned stew or thick soup containing several kinds of meats and vegetables. It became associated with Kentucky, and, because it was easy to prepare, it was served at political rallies, group picnics, and other large gatherings, which were sometimes referred to as *burgoos.*

BURN

An injury to the skin most commonly due to the application of excessive heat. However, similar injuries may also be due to chemicals, friction, electricity, or radiation. In severe burns, the skin may be broken so that fluids escape. In such cases, special treatment is required to replace the fluid and salts which have been lost. Furthermore, prompt healing requires a diet rich in protein, calories, and vitamins.

(Also see DISEASES, section headed "Nutritional Therapies or Adjuncts.")

BURNING FEET SYNDROME

A dietary deficiency disease which is usually due to very poor diets that lack protein and the B-complex vitamins. The disease is characterized by a burning in the feet that becomes worse as the condition progresses.

(Also see DEFICIENCY DISEASES.)

BURP

Another name for a belch.
(Also see BELCHING.)

BUSHEL

A unit of capacity equal to 2,150.42 cubic inches (approximately 1.25 cu ft).
(Also see WEIGHTS AND MEASURES.)

BUTT (SIRLOIN)

• The sirloin portion of a full beef loin that has been separated from the short loin.
(Also see BEEF AND VEAL, Fig. B-19.)

• The upper end of a ham, now more correctly termed the rump portion.
(Also see PORK.)

BUTTER, BLACK

Butter that has been browned by heating, then vinegar, salt, pepper or other seasoning added; used as a sauce.

BUTTERMILK

• The residue from churning cream to make butter.

• A cultured skim milk.
(Also see MILK AND MILK PRODUCTS.)

BUTTER, MOWRAH (VEGETABLE BUTTER)

This includes a number of vegetable butters, such as cocoa butter (made from the cocoa bean), Borneo tallow or green butter (made from Malayan, an East Indian plant), shea butter (made from an African plant), and Mowrah fat or illipe butter (made from an Indian plant and used for soap and candles).

BUTTER STOOLS

Stools with a high fat content. The condition usually occurs in infants and children, and is due to a malabsorption of dietary fats. The underlying cause may be (1) a lack of pancreatic enzymes which digest fat, (2) a sensitivity to dietary gluten, or (3) a disorder of the liver which reduces the flow of bile.
(Also see DIGESTION AND ABSORPTION.)

BUTYLATED HYDROXYANISOLE (BHA)

An antioxidant (see Fig. B-51) that prevents oxidative rancidity of polyunsaturated fats, used to prevent rancidity in foods.
BHA is considered GRAS (Generally Recognized As Safe) by the Food and Drug Administration (FDA) for addition to edible fats and oils and to foods containing them. The FDA limitation on its use is: 0.02% (200 ppm) of fat or oil content, including essential (volatile) oil content, of the food.

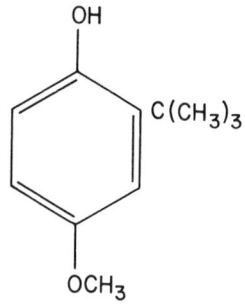

Fig. B-51. Chemical structure of butylated hydroxyanisole.

BUTYLATED HYDROXYTOLUENE (BHT)

Like BHA, BHT is a phenol (see Fig. B-52), is considered GRAS, and is limited in its use to 0.02% (200 ppm) of fat or oil content, including essential (volatile) oil content, of the food.

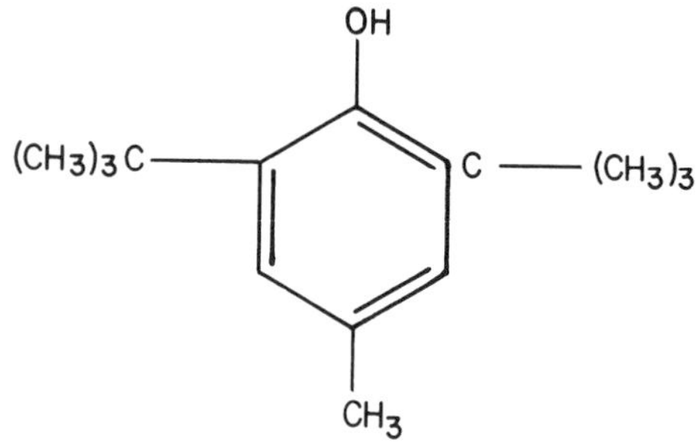

Fig. B-52. Chemical structure of butylated hydroxytoluene.

BUTYRIC ACID

One of the volatile fatty acids with the formula $CH_3CH_2CH_2COOH$, commonly found in butter and certain products of microbial action.
(Also see FATS AND OTHER LIPIDS; and MILK AND MILK PRODUCTS.)

BUTYROMEL

A home remedy consisting of a mixture of butter and honey, which is given to weakened, underweight people to help them gain weight.

BY-PRODUCT

Secondary products produced in addition to the principal product; often refers to wastes which have a productive use.

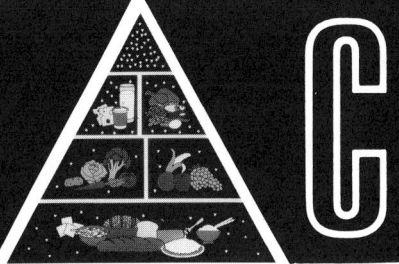

CABBAGE Brassica oleracea, family Cruciferae

This vegetable has been used for many centuries in Europe and Asia, although it originally differed considerably from its present form. It is a member of the mustard family (Cruciferae).

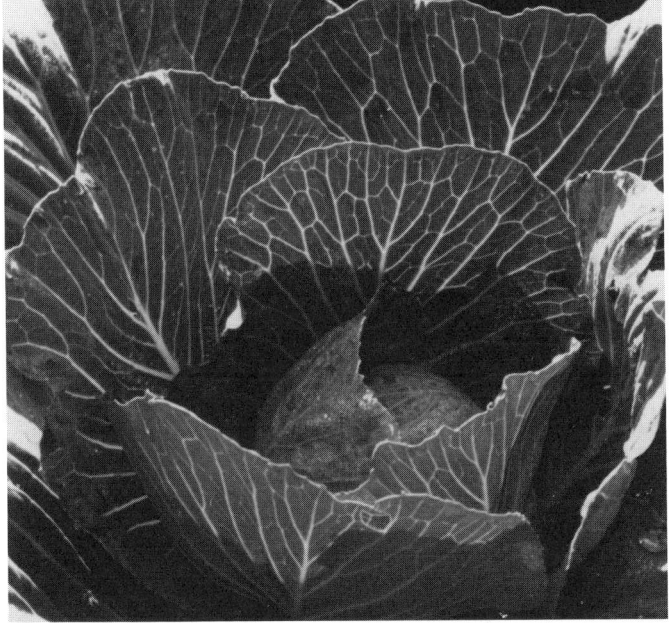

Fig. C-1. Head of a cabbage, one of the world's leading vegetable crops. (Courtesy, University of Minnesota, St. Paul, Minn.)

ORIGIN AND HISTORY. Cabbage developed from wild cabbage that is indigenous to the coastal areas of western Europe and Great Britain. Wild cabbage does not form heads; it more closely resembles collards and kale than domesticated cabbage.

WORLD AND U.S. PRODUCTION. Cabbage ranks fifth among the vegetable crops of the world, with an annual production of about 39 million metric tons; and the leading cabbage-producing countries, by rank, are: U.S.S.R., China, South Korea, Japan, Poland, and U.S.A.[1]

Cabbage ranks sixth among the vegetable crops of the United States, with annual production of about 1.4 million short tons. The leading cabbage markets of the United States, by rank, are: Los Angeles, Chicago, New York, Atlanta, Boston, Baltimore, San Francisco, and Philadelphia.[2]

---

[1]Based on data from *FAO Production Yearbook 1990*, FAO/UN, Rome, Italy, Vol. 44, p. 128, Table 50. **Note well:** Annual production fluctuates as a result of weather and profitability of the crop.

[2]Based on data from *Agricultural Statistics 1991*, USDA, pp. 167-168, Table 242-243.

PROCESSING (Sauerkraut). About 1/6 of the cabbage produced in the United States is made into sauerkraut, while most of the rest is marketed fresh. Sauerkraut is made by mixing shredded cabbage with salt, then allowing lactic acid fermentation to occur. A considerable amount of the sauerkraut now sold in supermarkets is canned, although some is also sold in sealed plastic bags kept under refrigeration. (Also see SAUERKRAUT.)

SELECTION, PREPARATION, AND USES. Prime quality heads of cabbage should be reasonably solid, hard, or firm; heavy or fairly heavy in relation to size, and closely trimmed (stems cut close to the head and only three or four outer or wrapper leaves remaining). Early cabbage need not be as solid or firm as late crop cabbage.

Raw cabbage is often shredded and made into cole slaw, which is a mixture of the vegetable with French dressing, mayonnaise, salad dressing, sour cream, and/or vinegar. Usually, sugar and other seasonings are added to the slaw.

Cooked cabbage goes well with a wide variety of meats, potato dishes, poultry, and other vegetables. The usual ways of cooking cabbage are boiling, frying, sauteeing, and stuffing and baking. However, overcooking drives off the pleasant odorous components and intensifies the unpleasant ones. It also reduces the nutritional value greatly. Hence, cabbage should be added near the end of the cooking period when it is to be part of mixed dishes such as casseroles, soups, and stews. Many of these cabbage dishes were invented by the peoples of Europe.

Sauerkraut has long been served as an accompaniment to meat dishes such as pig knuckles, roasts, and sausages. (Also see SAUERKRAUT.)

NUTRITIONAL VALUE. The nutrient composition of cabbage is given in Food Composition Table F-21.

Some noteworthy observations regarding the nutrient composition of cabbage follow:

1. Cabbage is high in water content (over 90%) and low in calories (29 Calories [kcal] per cup [*240 ml*]) when cooked in a small amount of water. However, most types of cole slaw contain about five times as many calories as cabbage alone because the slaw usually contains a dressing that is rich in fat. Hence, dieters would be wise to make their own cole slaw with a low-calorie dressing.

2. Sauerkraut is about as nutritious as the various forms of unfermented cabbage, except that the former has a high sodium content.

3. All forms of cabbage are good sources of potassium and vitamin C.

Cabbage contains small amounts of goitrogens. (See GOITROGENS.)

• **Antiulcer factors**—Starting in the 1940s and continuing into the 1950s, American medical researchers demonstrated that the juice from raw cabbage speeded up the healing of peptic ulcers. The unidentified therapeutic substance was called *vitamin U*, because of its effect on ulcers. Recently, it was found that vitamin U contains the amino acid methionine, but that methionine alone does not have this effect.

The problem in treating people with cabbage juice is that the antiulcer factor is present in only minute amounts in cabbage, so that it is necessary to drink about 1 qt *(0.95 l)* of fresh cabbage juice (the equivalent of about 3 lb *[1.35 kg]* of raw cabbage) per day in order to obtain a noticeable improvement in healing. Therefore, scientists have developed various nondestructive means of concentrating the juice. (Heat destroys *vitamin U.*)

CACHEXIA

A term which indicates a severe weight loss and wasting of body tissues—a general lack of nutrition. Frequently, cachexia occurs in the course of a chronic disease; for example, in many forms of cancer.

CADMIUM

A widely used industrial metal which may get into air, food and water; and ultimately into the human body where it may have toxic effects. It appears that regions which have high levels of cadmium in the environment are likely to have greater than normal incidences of high blood pressure because cadmium causes damage to the kidneys. Fortunately, certain dietary minerals, such as selenium and zinc, may counteract the effects of cadmium.

(Also see MINERAL[S].)

CAFFEINE $(C_8H_{10}N_4O_2)$

Caffeine is a drug with stimulating effects. It is found in foods, beverages, and medicines, and it occurs naturally in plant products such as coffee, tea, cacao beans, kola nuts, mate drink, and guarana paste. More than 63 species of plants growing in all parts of the world contain caffeine in their leaves, seeds, or fruit. Pure caffeine is obtained (1) as a by-product from the manufacture of decaffeinated coffee, (2) from the extraction of coffee bean and tea leaf waste, and (3) from the methylation of theobromine obtained from cocoa waste. Most Americans consume some caffeine. Recently, there has been considerable concern as to the effect of caffeine on health.

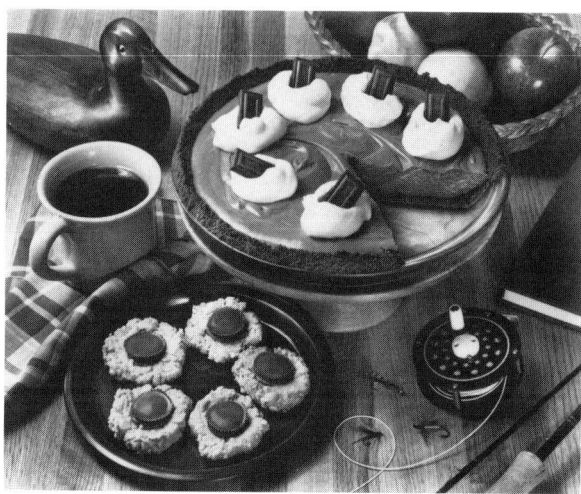

Fig. C-2. Coffee served with chocolate bar pie and peanut butter cup cookies. (Courtesy, Hershey Foods Corporation, Hershey, Pa.)

CHEMISTRY AND METABOLISM. Caffeine is an organic chemical belonging to a class of chemicals called purines—some of which are constitutents of the nucleic acids, RNA and DNA.

Ingested caffeine is rapidly absorbed from the intestine and within a few minutes caffeine enters all organs and tissues. Within one hour after ingestion, it is distributed in the body tissues in proportion to their water content. The metabolic half-life of caffeine is about 3 hours; hence, there is no day-to-day accumulations as it almost completely dissapears from the body overnight. Most of the ingested caffeine is excreted in the urine.

EFFECTS ON THE BODY. A pharmacologically active dose of caffeine is about 200 mg, depending upon the individual. In the body, caffeine demonstrates the following actions:

1. Stimulates the central nervous system (brain) thereby prolonging wakefulness with alert intellectual facilities.
2. Stimulates the heart action.
3. Relaxes smooth muscle—the type of muscle found in the digestive tract and blood vessels.
4. Increases urine flow—a *diuretic.*
5. Stimulates stomach acid secretion.
6. Increases muscle strength and the amount of time a person can perform physically exhausting work.

While the effects of caffeine vary from person to person, a dose of 1,000 mg or more will generally produce adverse effects such as insomnia, restlessness, excitement, trembling, rapid heart beat with extra heart beats, increased breathing, desire to urinate, ringing in the ears, and heartburn. A fatal dose of caffeine appears to be more than 10 g or 170 mg/kg of body weight—about 80 to 100 cups of coffee in one sitting.

SOURCES AND CONSUMPTION. In the United States, about 75% of all the caffeine consumed as food comes from coffee while 15% comes from tea and the remaining 10% comes from soft drinks, cocoa, and chocolate. Additionally, many over-the-counter medications contain caffeine. Table C-1 shows the caffeine content of some sources.

One survey showed the average intake of caffeine from coffee to be about 186 mg or 2 cups *(480 ml)* of coffee, but some individuals within the survey drank as much as 8 cups of coffee or about 676 mg of caffeine. Some individuals may

TABLE C-1
CAFFEINE CONTENT IN FOOD AND DRUGS

Item	Measure[3]	Caffeine
		(mg)
Percolated roasted and ground coffee[1]	cup	76-155
Instant coffee	cup	66
Decaffeinated coffee	cup	2-5
Tea[1]	cup	20-100
Instant tea	cup	24-131
Hot cocoa	cup	5
Soft drinks[2]	12 oz can	26-34
Milk chocolate candy	2 oz	12
Sweet or dark chocolate	2 oz	40
Baking chocolate	2 oz	70
Alertness tablets	tablet	100-200
Pain relievers	tablet	32-65
Cold allergy relief remedies	tablet	15-32

[1]The longer coffee or tea is brewed, the greater its caffeine content.
[2]Primarily cola and pepper drinks, but other flavors of soft drinks may also contain caffeine.
[3]One cup = 240 ml; one oz = 30ml

even consume more. Users of the over-the-counter drugs may receive substantially more than coffee drinkers.

HEALTH CONCERNS. In the amounts normally consumed, caffeine acts as a drug, indeed much of its popularity is owed to its stimulant effect on the central nervous system. Like many drugs, users develop a dependence on caffeine when consumed in amounts equivalent to more than 4 cups of coffee per day. Furthermore, abstinence from caffeine-containing substances for a day or two may cause the development of withdrawal symptoms—headaches, irritability, restlessness, or fatigue. Everyone responds to any drug differently and some individuals using caffeine may experience mood changes, anxiety, depression, and irritability. Large amounts of caffeine may cause heartburn, upset stomach, and irregular heartbeats.

Overall, caffeine, as consumed in foods, beverages, and over-the-counter drugs, does not seem to represent a threat to the health of most Americans. However, some sensitive individuals who consume large amounts may experience insomnia, chronic headaches, rapid heart beat, anxiety, and upset stomach.

(Also see COFFEE; SOFT DRINKS; and TEA.)

CALAMONDIN *Citrus mitis; C. madurensis*

A small citrus fruit (of the family *Rutaceae*) that looks like a miniature orange and is native to China.

CALCEMIA (HYPERCALCEMIA)

An abnormally high level of calcium in the blood. This condition may be dangerous because it can lead to calcium deposits in various soft tissues. The condition is also called hypercalcemia.

CALCIFEROL

Another name for vitamin D_2 or ergocalciferol. Both vitamin D_2 and vitamin D_3 have equal activity for people, but chickens, turkeys, and other birds utilize vitamin D_3 more efficiently than vitamin D_2.

(Also see VITAMIN D.)

CALCIFICATION

The process by which organic tissue becomes hardened by a deposit of calcium salts.

CALCITONIN (OR THYROCALCITONIN)

A hormone secreted by the parafollicular or C cells of the thyroid gland. When the calcium level of the blood rises above normal, calcitonin is secreted, which prohibits further release of calcium from the bones. Thus, the effect of this hormone is opposite to that of the parathyroid hormone which removes calcium from bone. However, it appears that the action of calcitonin occurs mainly during the growing years and that it does not have much effect in adulthood.

(Also see CALCIUM; PHOSPHORUS; and ENDOCRINE GLANDS.)

CALCIUM (CA)

Contents   Page

Everyone needs calcium, which constitutes about 2% of the body. Calcium gives strength and structure to bones and teeth. Additionally, it controls the heartbeat—the heart could not keep up its continuous alternate contraction and relaxation were it not for calcium; it has a role in the transmission of nerve impulses; it is related to muscle contraction—without calcium, muscles lose their ability to contract; it is necessary for blood clotting—calcium prevents fatal bleeding from any break in the wall of a blood vessel; and it activates a number of the enzymes, including lipase—the fat-splitting enzyme.

Ninety-nine percent of the calcium of the body is present in the bones and teeth, where calcium salts (chiefly calcium phosphate) held in a cellular matrix provide the rigid framework of the body. The bones also furnish the reserves of calcium to the circulation so that the concentration in the plasma can be kept constant at all times. It has been estimated that in an adult man about 700 mg of calcium enter and leave the bones each day. Teeth are similar to bone in chemical composition, but, in comparison with bone, enamel is much harder and lower in water content—containing only about 5%. The calcium in teeth, unlike that in bone, cannot be replaced; therefore, teeth cannot repair themselves.

CALCIUM, builds bones, teeth, and is needed by all tissues of the body

Rats from same litter 22 weeks old.

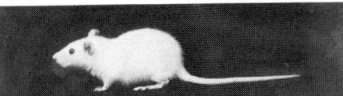

This rat did not have enough calcium. Note the short, stuffy body, due to poorly formed bones. It weighed 91 g.

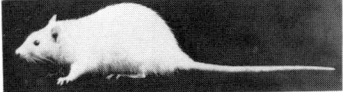

This rat had plenty of calcium. It has reached full size, and its bones are well-formed. It weighed 219 g.

TOP FOOD SOURCES

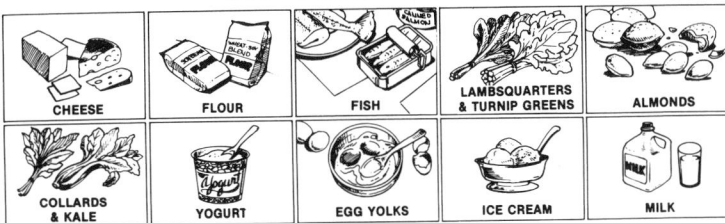

Fig. C-3. Calcium made the difference! *Left:* Rat on calcium-deficient diet. *Right:* Rat that received plenty of calcium. Note, too, top sources of calcium. (Adapted from USDA sources.)

The remaining 1% of the calcium—about 10 g in an adult—is widely distributed in the soft tissues and the extracellular fluids. The vital role of this small amount of calcium is reflected in the precision with which plasma calcium is regulated, a narrow range of 9 to 11 g that is controlled by the parathyroid hormone and calcitonin.

Obviously, all of the calcium in the body comes from food. Because this element is both a body builder and a body regulator, everyone needs dietary calcium.

HISTORY. Calcium was among the first materials known to be essential in the diet. As early as 1842, Chossat, a Frenchman, showed experimentally that pigeons developed poor bone on a diet low in calcium. When fed wheat alone, the birds died after 10 months; and, on autopsy, the bones were found very much depleted. Calcium carbonate prevented the trouble. In later studies, Chossat also used chickens, rabbits, frogs, eels, lizards, and turtles. But well-controlled experiments with man were not made until recent years.

ABSORPTION OF CALCIUM. Calcium salts are more soluble in acid solution; hence, absorption occurs largely in the upper part (proximal part, or the duodenal area) of the small intestine, where the food contents are still somewhat acidic following digestion in the stomach. An increase in the passage of food through the gastrointestinal tract also decreases the percentage of absorption.

Not all the calcium in food becomes available to the body. Normally, depending on the intake, only 20 to 30% of the calcium in the average diet is absorbed from the intestinal tract and taken into the bloodstream. Calcium absorption is dependent upon the calcium needs of the body, the type of food, and the amount of calcium ingested. Growing children and pregnant-lactating women utilize calcium most efficiently—they absorb 40% or more of the calcium in their diets. Also, the body's need is greatest and the absorption of calcium is relatively more efficient following long periods of low calcium intake and body depletion and during healing of bone fractures.

It follows that utilization of calcium is much more efficient in countries where the diet is low in calcium than in the United States where diets are high in calcium.

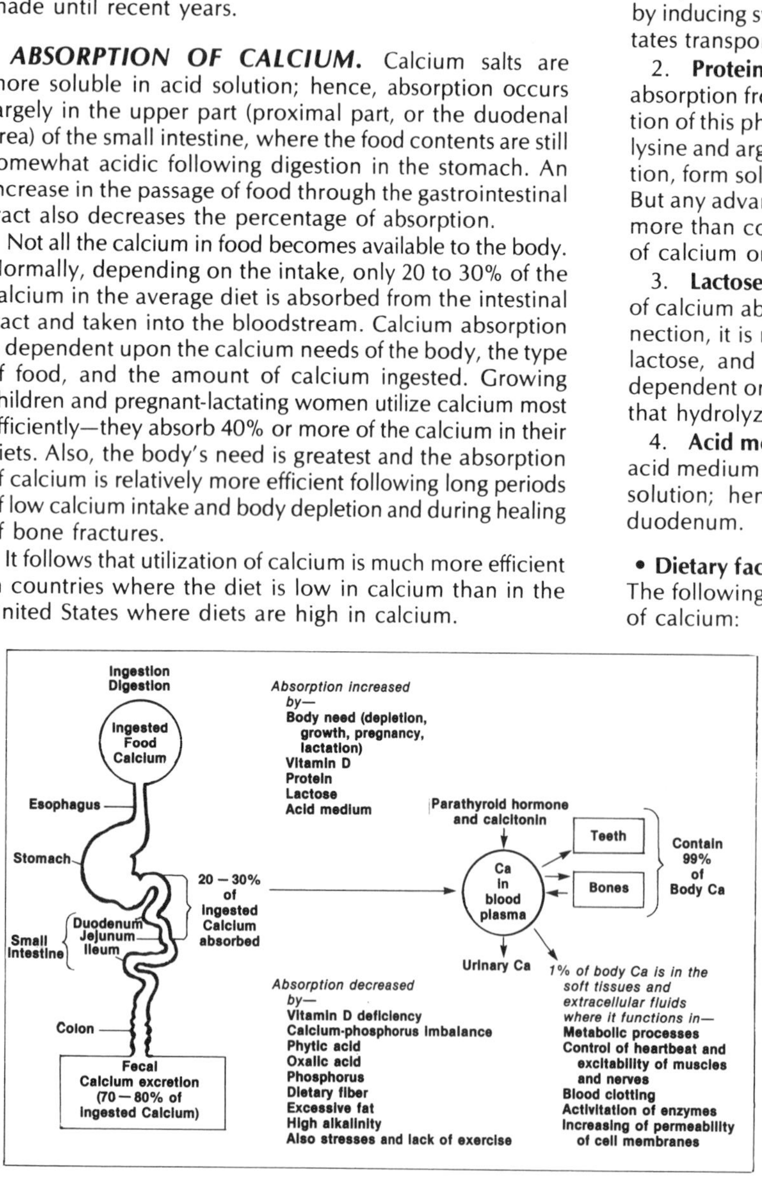

Thus, the relative amounts of calcium retained in the body vary according to (1) the age and the pregnancy-lactation status of the person, (2) the previous dietary habits, and (3) the level of current supply.

By increasing the absorptive capacity of the gut and by regulating the renal (kidney) excretion, the body can either adapt itself to (1) reduced dietary intakes of calcium, or (2) increased requirements for calcium.

A number of dietary factors in addition to need and the amount of calcium ingested influence calcium absorption; some enhancing it, others interfering with it.

• **Dietary factors enhancing absorption of calcium**—The following dietary factors increase the absorption of calcium:

1. **Vitamin D.** One of the most important factors affecting calcium absorption is an adequate supply of vitamin D, whether from the diet or exposure to ultraviolet radiation of the sun. Vitamin D or its derivative (metabolite), 25-hydroxycholecalciferol (25-HCC), increases calcium absorption by inducing synthesis of a calcium-binding protein that facilitates transport of the calcium through the intestinal walls.

2. **Protein.** Dietary protein increases the rate of calcium absorption from the small intestine. The probable explanation of this phenomenon is that the amino acids, especially lysine and arginine, liberated in the course of protein digestion, form soluble calcium salts which are easily absorbed. But any advantage from increased absorption will likely be more than counterbalanced by the increased urinary loss of calcium on high-protein diets.

3. **Lactose.** Dietary lactose (milk sugar) enhances the rate of calcium absorption from the small intestine. In this connection, it is noteworthy that (1) milk is the only source of lactose, and (2) the improved absorption of calcium is dependent on the activity of intestinal lactase, the enzyme that hydrolyzes lactose.

4. **Acid medium.** Absorption of calcium is favored in an acid medium (a lower pH) because it keeps the calcium in solution; hence, most of the absorption occurs in the duodenum.

• **Dietary factors interfering with absorption of calcium**—The following dietary factors interfere with the absorption of calcium:

1. **Vitamin D deficiency.** Insufficient levels of vitamin D depress the amount of the calcium-binding protein that is essential for the absorption of calcium. Thus, in northern latitudes and/or in smoggy cities where ultraviolet radiation is limited or blocked, the dietary source of vitamin D becomes very important.

2. **Calcium-phosphorus imbalance.** A great excess of either calcium or phosphorus interferes with the absorption of both minerals and the increased excretion of the lesser mineral. This is why a certain ratio between them in the diet is desirable. The Ca:P ratio in U.S. diets has been estimated to be 1:1.5 to 1:1.6, while the most desirable ratio is thought to be 1.5:1 in infancy, decreasing to 1:1 at 1 year of age, and remaining at 1:1 throughout the rest of life; although man can tolerate a much wider Ca:P ratio—between 2:1 and 1:2.

Fig. C-4. Calcium utilization. Note that healthy adults absorb only 20 to 30% of the calcium contained in their food, and that 70 to 80% is excreted in the feces. Note, too, the factors that increase and decrease absorption.

3. **Phytic acid**. Phytic acid, found in the outer hulls (bran) of many cereal grains, forms an insoluble salt with calcium—calcium phytate—which prevents the absorption of calcium. But the effect of phytic acid is important only when whole grain cereals comprise a major part of the diet and/or the calcium intake is low.

Phytin can be split by the enzyme phytase, which has been identified in several cereal grains. The presence of this enzyme may explain why calcium is more available in leavened than in unleavened breads.

4. **Oxalic acid**. This compound can inhibit the absorption of calcium because of the formation of calcium oxalate, a relatively insoluble compound. Oxalic acid is high in only a few foods; among them, spinach, beet tops, swiss chard, cocoa, and rhubarb. But the amount of oxalic acid present in typical American diets is not sufficiently great to interfere seriously with the absorption of calcium.

5. **Dietary fiber**. The fiber in plants low in phytate binds calcium in proportion to its uronic acid content. Since uronic acids can be digested by bacteria in the colon, this may be part of the process whereby calcium absorption is increased slowly after a change from a low-fiber to a high-fiber diet.

6. **Excessive fat**. Excessive levels of fat, especially those that are saturated, depress calcium absorption because the fats combine with calcium to form insoluble soaps, a process called *saponification*. These insoluble soaps are excreted in the feces, with consequent loss of the incorporated calcium. (They may also carry with them fat-soluble vitamin D.) This explains why patients with chronic intestinal disorders, such as sprue and celiac disease, leading to increased fat in the feces (steatorrhea) may develop osteomalacia in due time.

7. **High alkalinity**. Calcium is insoluble in an alkaline medium, and is poorly utilized under such conditions.

8. **Other factors**. Stresses and lack of exercise have an important bearing upon the calcium balance; several studies have shown that persons who are under extreme nervous strain or worry or who do not exercise sufficiently have negative calcium balances even when the dietary intake is good. Also, aging appears to decrease the rate of calcium absorption.

METABOLISM OF CALCIUM. Fig. C-5 shows the factors affecting the metabolism of calcium. Normally, the small intestine acts as an effective control and prevents an excess of calcium from being absorbed. Body requirement is the major factor governing the amount of calcium that will be absorbed; growing children and pregnant and lactating women absorb 40% or more of the calcium in their diets.

After absorption through the intestinal wall, most of the calcium is stored in the bones, especially the spongy bones (trabeculae), from which it is withdrawn in time of need. (Also see BONE.)

• **The endocrine glands and hormones**—The calcium concentration in the blood is kept relatively constant primarily by two endocrine glands—the parathyroids which secrete parathyroid hormone, in response to *hypocalcemia* (low blood calcium), and the parafollicular or C cells of the thyroid gland which release calcitonin during *hypercalcemia* (high blood calcium). (The parafollicular or C cells of the mammal are of ultimobranchial origin.) Secretion or release of both hormones (parathyroid hormone and calcitonin) is determined by the level of calcium in the blood. When the calcium level of the blood drops, the parathyroid releases its hormone, which acts in three ways to restore the normal calcium level: (1) it increases calcium absorption from the intestine; (2) it withdraws calcium from the bone; and (3) it causes the kidney to lessen excretion of calcium in the urine. When the calcium level of the blood rises, the secretion of the parathyroid hormone is decreased and calcitonin, which prohibits further release of calcium from the bones, is secreted.

The pituitary growth hormone may influence calcium metabolism indirectly through its action on longitudinal bone growth. The adrenocortical hormones control calcium movements at three sites: (1) at the renal level—calcium excretion is increased; (2) at the gastrointestinal level—calcium absorption may be inhibited; and (3) at the skeletal level—both bone formation and bone resorption are inhibited, with the greater effect on bone formation. The role of the sex hormones in calcium metabolism is less clear, but the major evidence to date suggests that neither androgens nor estrogens have much effect on calcium metabolism.

EXCRETION OF CALCIUM. The quantity of calcium excreted by adults in good nutritional state tends to equal the intestinal absorption. The body disposes of the calcium

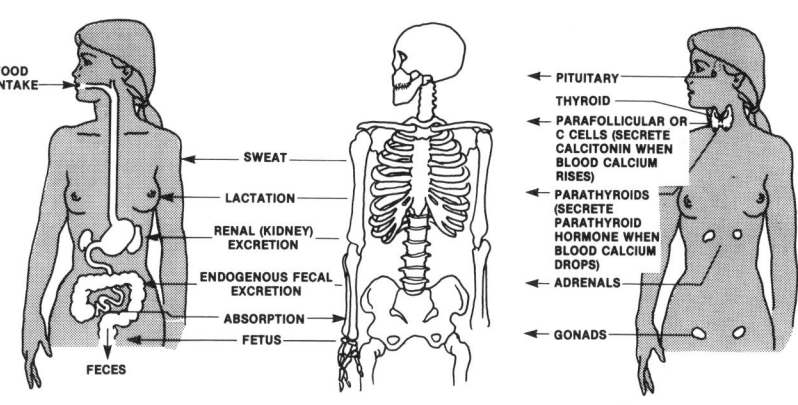

SKELETAL CALCIUM STORES (99%)
EXTRACELLULAR FLUID CALCIUM (1%)

Fig. C-5. Factors involved in calcium metabolism. To maintain a constant extracellular fluid calcium concentration, calcium is excreted through the kidneys and gut when the concentration increases, or is recruited by increased absorption from the gut or resorption from the skeleton when the concentration decreases. These movements of calcium are regulated by the endocrine system. Calcium is also lost through sweating, pregnancy, and lactation.

that it does not need in three ways—in the feces, in the urine, and in the sweat. Also, about 30 g of calcium is passed from the mother to the fetus during gestation; and during lactation the mother excretes as much as 250 mg of calcium daily in her milk.

• **Calcium in the feces**—Calcium is excreted mainly in the feces, most of which is dietary intake that is not absorbed (see Fig. C-4). The remainder, called endogenous fecal calcium (which ranges between 125 and 180 mg per day) comes from shed epithelial cells and the digestive juices (bile and pancreatic juice). As shown in Fig. C-4, approximately 70 to 80% of food calcium is unabsorbed and excreted in the feces.

A recent study suggests that excessive intakes of phosphorus may lead to increased bone resorption and increased calcium loss in the feces.

• **Calcium in the urine**—Urinary calcium excretion varies widely among individuals, ranging anywhere from 100 to 200 mg per day. But, under most conditions, it appears to be relatively constant for any given individual. Major changes in calcium intake produce little change in the quantity of urine calcium, whereas fecal calcium, by contrast, is highly correlated with calcium intake, indicating that the gut exercises considerable control over calcium absorption.

The amount of calcium excreted in the urine is related to skeletal size, the acid-base regulation of the body, and the dietary protein intake. Urinary excretion of calcium rises when dietary protein is increased and falls when dietary protein is decreased. It appears that calcium losses can be substantial when protein intake is high; hence, if this type of diet is continued for a prolonged period, it could result in a considerable loss of body calcium and even osteoporosis. However, studies show that a high protein intake from a high meat diet has little effect on calcium excretion, possibly because of the high phosphate intake with the meat diet. A recent study suggests that increased phosphorus intakes reduce urinary excretion of calcium and lower serum calcium levels.

• **Calcium in the sweat**—Normally, the loss of calcium in perspiration amounts to only 15 mg per day and is insignificant. However, persons working in extreme heat may lose over 100 mg of calcium per hour in the sweat—which may approximate 30% of the total calcium output.

• **Calcium losses in pregnancy and lactation**—In the female, there are two other possible losses of calcium. Approximately 30 g of calcium is deposited in the fetal skeleton, and during lactation, 250 mg of milk calcium per day may be secreted in the milk.

FUNCTIONS OF CALCIUM. The physiologic function of 99% of the calcium in the body is to build the bones and teeth, and to maintain the bones. The remaining 1% of the calcium controls the vital physiologic functions which are summarized in the section on MINERAL(S), Table M-25, Mineral Table.

DEFICIENCY SYMPTOMS. The most dramatic symptoms of calcium deficiency are manifested in the bones and teeth of the young of all species. Such a deficiency during the growth period is evidenced in one or more of the following ways:
1. Stunting of growth.
2. Poor quality bones and teeth.
3. Malformation of bones—rickets.

The clinical manifestations of calcium related diseases are rickets, osteomalacia, osteoporosis, hypercalcemia, tetany, and renal calculi, or kidney stones.

(Also see section on MINERAL[S], Table M-25, Mineral Table.)

INTERRELATIONSHIPS. Calcium is involved in a number of relationships, the most important of which follow:

• **Calcium-phosphorus ratio and vitamin D**—Without doubt, the best known relationship pertaining to minerals is the calcium-phosphorus ratio, along with vitamin D. Generally speaking, nutritionists recommend a calcium-phosphorus ratio of 1.5:1 in infancy, decreasing to 1:1 at 1 year of age, and remaining at 1:1 throughout the rest of life; although they consider ratios between 2:1 and 1:2 as satisfactory. However, the ratio of calcium to phosphorus is less critical when adequate amounts of vitamin D are present.

• **Fats**—An excessive intake of dietary fats or poor absorption of fats results in an excess of free fatty acids which unite with calcium to form insoluble soaps that are excreted in the feces.

• **Protein intake**—Dietary protein increases the rate of calcium absorption from the small intestine, probably because the amino acids, especially lysine and arginine, liberated in the course of protein digestion, form calcium salts which are easily absorbed. But any advantage from increased absorption is likely more than counterbalanced by the increased urinary loss of calcium on high-protein diets.

• **Excess calcium intake**—Excessive calcium intake (intake much higher than body requirements) will combine with phosphorus to form insoluble tricalcium phosphate, and thus interfere with the absorption of phosphorus. Also, excessive calcium intake may reduce the absorption of magnesium, iron, iodine, manganese, zinc, and copper, particularly when the intake of one of these minerals is borderline in terms of need.

• **Other factors enhancing absorption of calcium**—Absorption of calcium is increased by adequate vitamin D, dietary lactose (milk sugar), and an acid medium (a low pH). (See earlier section headed "Absorption of Calcium.")

• **Other factors interfering with absorption of calcium**—Absorption of calcium is decreased by vitamin D deficiency, phytic acid, oxalic acid, fiber, high alkalinity, stress, and lack of exercise. (See earlier section headed "Absorption of Calcium.")

RECOMMENDED DAILY ALLOWANCE OF CALCIUM. The National Research Council recommended daily dietary allowances, with provision for individual variation, of calcium are given in the section on MINERAL(S), Table M-25, Mineral Table.

Note that the recommended daily allowances for calcium range from 400 mg to 1,200 mg. Note, too, that the allowances vary according to age, and that provision is made for added allowances for pregnant and lactating females.

• **Infants and children**—For infants, the calcium intake requirements may well be stated in terms of the amount of milk, since this is the chief source of food. Also, it is noteworthy that the proportion of calcium to phosphorus in milk is about the same as it is in the skeleton.

A breast-fed infant receives about 60 mg of calcium per kilogram of body weight (300 mg/liter of milk) and retains about two-thirds of this. By contrast, an infant fed a standard cow's milk formula containing added carbohydrate (600 to 700 mg of calcium per liter) receives about 170 mg of calcium per kilogram but retains 25 to 30%. Although the breast-fed infant has less calcium available, its calcium needs are fully met. Thus, the NRC recommended allowance for infants to 6 months is set at 400 mg per day.

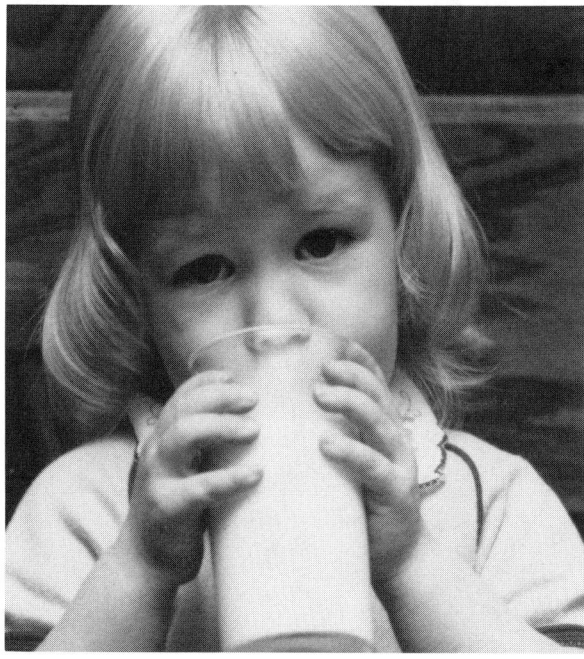

Fig. C-6. The calcium need of children is most easily met by drinking milk. (Courtesy, University of Minnesota, St. Paul, Minn.)

For children 1 to 10 years of age, the recommended NRC calcium allowances are 800 mg/day. Per unit of weight, growing children may need two to four times as much calcium as does an adult.

During the rapid growth that characterizes preadolescence and puberty (10 to 18 years), a higher intake of calcium is recommended, i.e., 1,200 mg/day.

For older children, the requirements are most easily met by including a quart of milk a day or its equivalent in milk products.

During all periods of growth, vitamin D (or sunshine) is essential for the most efficient absorption and utilization of calcium.

• **Recommended calcium level for adults**—In view of the high levels of protein and phosphorus provided by U.S. diets, an allowance of 800 mg of calcium per day is recommended for healthy adults.

• **Recommended calcium intake for the elderly**—Special attention should be given to the calcium intake for the elderly, those at high risk for development of osteoporosis. Because they have a tendency to decrease their intake, and because they absorb calcium less efficiently, some eminent scientists who have done extensive research on the calcium requirements of the aged feel that the Recommended Daily Allowances (RDA) for the elderly made by the National Academy of Sciences are too low. Most of these researchers recommend 1,000 to 1,200 mg of calcium per day as optimum intake for the prevention of osteoporosis.

Even though osteoporosis may not be preventable by increasing calcium intake, there are reports that calcium supplements have induced calcium retention and relieved symptoms. This may reflect the fact that, although the efficiency of absorption decreases with the amount of calcium in the diet, the total amount of calcium actually retained increases.

Collectively, the possible effects of high dietary intakes of protein and phosphate on urinary calcium excretion and enhanced bone resorption, respectively, along with the possibility of reduced calcium absorption with advancing age, argue for recommending an ample intake of calcium.

• **Recommended calcium level during pregnancy and lactation**—Calcium accumulation during pregnancy totals approximately 30 g, nearly all related to calcification of the fetal skeleton in the last third of pregnancy. To meet this need, and to provide for individual variation, an additional allowance of 400 mg of calcium/day (for a total allowance of 1,200 mg/day) is recommended during gestation. An intake of this magnitude is recommended throughout pregnancy, rather than just during the last third of pregnancy when needs are greatest, because of the likelihood that calcium is stored in the skeleton in early gestation. Diets deficient in calcium (as well as in energy and protein) during pregnancy have been associated with decreased bone density in newborn infants.

The calcium content of breast milk averages 300 mg/liter. Assuming a daily production of 850 ml, this makes for a daily yield of approximately 250 mg of milk calcium. To meet this need, a total allowance of 1,200 mg of calcium daily is recommended for the lactating woman. Such an intake should prevent maternal demineralization, which otherwise accompanies lactation. A greater allowance may be necessary for women with a very high production of milk.

Also it is important to remember that, in addition to age and to pregnancy and lactation of women, calcium requirements are affected by the several factors that influence calcium absorption and excretion. Calcium is a good example, therefore, of a nutrient whose requirement cannot be decided on its own; the factors that influence calcium absorption and excretion must also be considered. For this reason, calcium supplementation should be determined by a knowledgeble nutritionist or M.D.

• **Calcium intake in average U.S. diet**—Of the nutrients that must be provided by the food we eat, studies show that calcium is most likely to be lacking.

The calcium available for consumption in foods in the United States amounts to approximately 890 mg per day, 75% of which is from dairy products, excluding butter.

TOXICITY. Normally, the small intestine acts as an effective control and prevents excess calcium from being absorbed. However, a breakdown of this control may raise the level of calcium in the blood and lead to pathological calcification of the kidneys and other internal organs. This may occur in infants who have been fed on artificial foods fortified with excessive amounts of vitamin D and calcium.

Continuous high dietary calcium intake may cause a hypersecretion of calcitonin and bone abnormalities such as *osteopetrosis* (dense bone). High calcium intakes have also been reported to cause the formation of kidney stones.

CALCIUM RELATED DISEASES. Diseases may be caused by (1) inadequate intake of calcium or (2) factors inhibiting its absorption or excretion. The clinical manifestations of calcium related diseases are rickets, osteomalacia, osteoporosis, hypercalcemia, tetany, and renal calculi (kidney stones).

(Also see Table M-25, Mineral Table; BONE, section headed "Bone Disorders;" RICKETS; OSTEOPOROSIS; and KIDNEY STONES.")

CALCIUM-PHOSPHORUS RATIO AND VITAMIN D. When considering the calcium and phosphorus requirements, it is important to realize that the proper utilization of these minerals of the body is dependent upon three factors: (1) an adequate supply of calcium and phosphorus in an available form, (2) a suitable ratio between them, and (3) sufficient vitamin D to make possible the assimilation and utilization of the calcium and phosphorus.

Generally speaking, nutritionists recommend a calcium-phosphorus ratio of 1.5:1 in infancy, decreasing to 1:1 at 1 year of age, and remaining at 1:1 throughout the rest of life; although they consider ratios between 2:1 and 1:2 as satisfactory. However, if plenty of vitamin D is present (provided either in the diet or by sunlight), the ratio of calcium to phosphorus becomes less critical. Likewise, less vitamin D is needed when there is a desirable calcium-phosphorus ratio.

The dietary Ca:P ratio is particularly important during the critical periods of life—for children, and for women during the latter half of pregnancy and during lactation.

The most recent estimates indicate that the Ca:P ratio in the United States diet is approximately 1:1.5 to 1.6.

CALCIUM LOSSES DURING PROCESSING, COOKING, AND STORAGE. Homogenization, pasteurization, heating, drying, or acidifying does not reduce availability of calcium. However, when milk is heated, a precipitate of calcium phosphates usually settles on the bottom of the pan. To reduce the loss of both calcium and phosphorus, the milk should be stirred as it heats to incorporate the calcium salts into the liquid.

Calcium losses in the cooking of vegetables can be minimized by using small amounts of water, by keeping the size of the pieces as large as possible to avoid excessive surface exposure, and by cooking with the skins on when practical, since minerals occur in greatest concentration near the skin. Cooking dried fruits and vegetables in the liquid in which they are soaked decreases calcium loss.

SOURCES OF CALCIUM. Among common foods, the milk and milk products group contains many of the richest sources of calcium. Some leafy green vegetables and some fish are also rich sources of calcium. However, in the United States, more than 70% of the calcium intake is derived from milk and milk products. Other foods contribute smaller amounts.

Furthermore, the total quantity of calcium available for absorption is augmented by the calcium in intestinal secretions.

The calcium-phosphorus ratio is determined by the total intake of each of the minerals. For the most part, this means foods, for few people take calcium and/or phosphorus mineral supplements.

Groupings by rank of common sources of calcium are given in the section on MINERAL(S), Table M-25, Mineral Table.

For additional sources and more precise values of calcium, see Food Composition Table F-21 of this book.

It is difficult to meet the recommended daily allowances for calcium without including milk and/or milk products in the diet. If the average American diet contained no dairy products, one would be hard pressed to obtain more than 300 mg of calcium daily. Two cups (*480 ml*) of milk are sufficient to meet the daily calcium needs of adults. Children need 3 or more cups daily, whereas adolescents need 4 cups or more.

(Also see MINERAL[S], Table M-25; and PHOSPHORUS.)

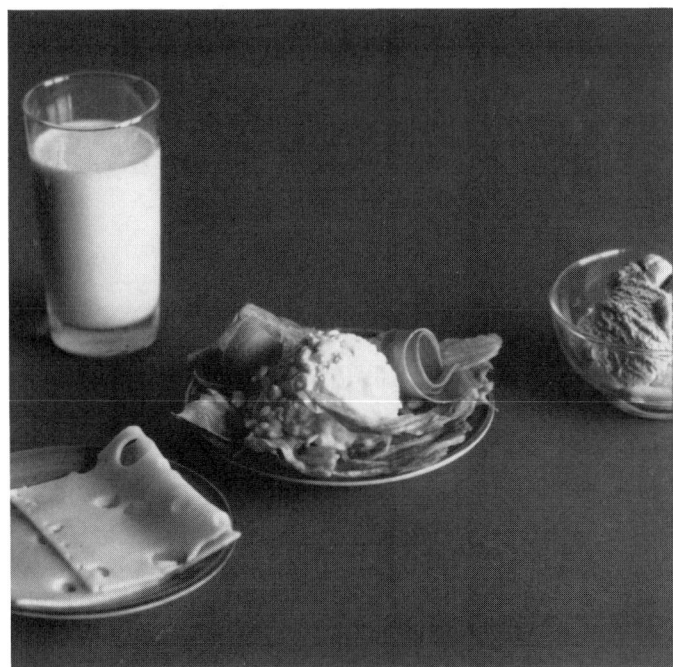

Fig. C-7. Milk and milk products top the list of sources of calcium. (Courtesy, University of Minnesota, St. Paul, Minn.)

CALCIUM ACETATE

An approved food additive sometimes employed as an antimicrobial or sequestering agent. Calcium acetate will prevent the formation of *ropy* bread.

(Also see ROPE.)

CALCIUM ACID PHOSPHATE

An acid-tasting major calcium salt, composed of approximately 16% calcium and 21% phosphorus, which is soluble in the acid environment of the stomach. It is used as the leavening ingredient of baking powder and of self-rising flour as it reacts with bicarbonate of soda to liberate carbon dioxide. Also, it is used in mineral supplements, to control the pH in malt, as a buffer in foods, as a firming agent in foods, and in fertilizers.

CALCIUM GLUCONATE ($Ca[C_6H_{11}O_7]_2 \cdot H_2O$)

A tasteless, odorless, water soluble salt of calcium. It may be administered intravenously for the relief of tetany, caused by an abnormal decrease in blood serum calcium and characterized by cramplike involuntary muscle spasm. Also, calcium gluconate is used as a food additive, buffer, and firming agent, and in some vitamin tablets.

CALCIUM-PHOSPHORUS RATIO

The proportional relation that exists between calcium and phosphorus is known as the calcium-phosphorus ratio. Generally speaking, nutritionists recommend a calcium-phosphorus ratio of 1:1, although they consider ratios between 2:1 and 1:2 as satisfactory. An excess of either can hinder absorption, however, the normal variation encountered in dietary calcium to phosphorus ratios does not significantly affect absorption from the intestine. If plenty of vitamin D is present (provided either by the diet or by sunlight), the ratio of calcium to phosphorus is less critical.

(Also see CALCIUM, section headed "Calcium-Phosphorus Ratio and Vitamin D;" and PHOSPHORUS, section headed "Calcium-Phosphorus Ratio and Vitamin D.")

CALCULUS

Another name for stones formed in one or more passages or organs of the body. It is believed that many types of stones are formed when various substances come out of solution from the body fluids. Hence, some of the therapeutic measures consist of attempts to redissolve the stones.

(Also see KIDNEY STONES.)

CALIPER

An instrument, which usually has movable jaws, that is used to measure the thickness or diameter of various objects. Special types are used by nutritionists for measuring skin-fold thickness, as part of the assessment of nutritional status, and in judging leanness or fatness.

(Also see OBESITY, section headed "Pinch Tests for Hidden Fat.")

CALORIC (Energy) EXPENDITURE

There has been a recent growth of worldwide interest in the application of calorimetry in the fields of human medicine and nutrition, exercise and sports physiology, and space exploration. Furthermore, new technological developments have made it possible to transmit physiological measurements via radio or telephone to distant diagnostic centers. Hence, many investigators around the world are currently engaged in modern versions of the calorimetric studies that were first conducted over 200 years ago. Fig. C-8 shows a typical study in progress.

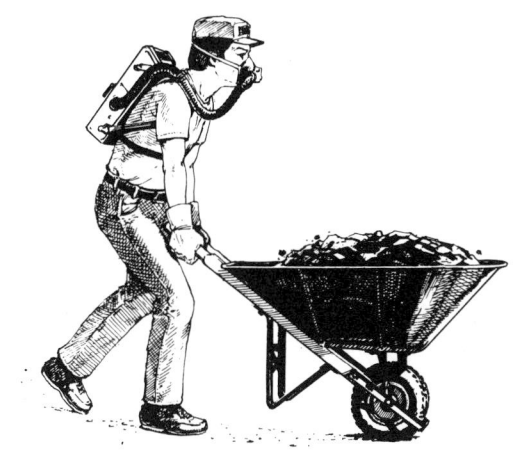

Fig. C-8. Measurement of energy expenditure during physical work. The man pushing the loaded wheelbarrow is exhaling into a Max Planck respirometer which measures and records the volume of air and collects a sample for subsequent analysis of its composition.

HISTORY OF CALORIMETRY. The French chemist Antoine Lavoisier (1743 to 1794) demonstrated in the 1770s that in the processes of combustion and respiration oxygen gas was consumed and carbon dioxide was produced. Other researchers of his era conducted similar experiments, but they made erroneous interpretations—based upon the cumbersome phlogiston theory that Lavoisier discredited by his work. Then, in 1780 Lavoisier and the mathematician La Place measured the oxygen consumption, carbon dioxide production, and heat emitted from guinea pigs. The exchange or respiratory gases was measured in a bell jar, whereas, the emission of heat was measured in an ice calorimeter. Five years later, Lavoisier studied the respiration of his associate Sequin, whose body was enclosed in a specially constructed bag. This experiment showed that the rate of metabolism, which was measured at normal room temperature after an overnight fast, was increased significantly by (1) exposure to cold, (2) consumption of food, and (3) physical work. Unfortunately, Lavoisier, who is credited with having founded the science of nutrition, went to the guillotine at age 50 because he was a tax collector during the French Revolution. (He was accused of having collected taxes on the water content of tobacco.)

In 1862, Liebig's former associates Max von Pettenkofer and Carl von Voit constructed a large roomlike open-circuit calorimeter in which they measured the metabolism of human subjects at rest, while fasting, and during the performance of various types of work.

In 1892, Atwater and the physicist Rosa began construction of a calorimeter at the Connecticut Agricultural Experiment Station in New Haven, and in 1899 published tables of food composition which had been prepared with the aid of data obtained in their calorimeter. Atwater was the first to deduct the energy losses which occurred in both the feces and urine from the gross energy obtained by the combustion of the foods. Francis Benedict, who had worked with Atwater starting in 1896, became the head of the Carnegie Nutrition Laboratory in Boston, where he continued the work started by Atwater. During World War I, Benedict found that fasting male students who had lost 12% of their body weight had a lowering of their basal metabolic rates which averaged about 19%.

A renewed interest in human caloric expenditures developed during World War II when food supplies had to be rationed. Studies conducted in Germany showed that the production of both coal and steel dropped significantly when the caloric intakes of the workers in these industries were restricted. In the United States, Ancel Keys and his co-workers at the University of Minnesota studied the effects of semistarvation on a group of conscientious objectors. After consuming approximately 1,600 Calories (kcal) per day for 22 weeks the subjects resembled prisoners of war and had an average reduction in basal metabolism of about 18%. They also expended subnormal amounts of energy while performing various exercises.

After the war, calorimetric studies were made of various groups suffering from protein-energy malnutrition, and of healthy people engaged in various activities. The use of the basal metabolic rate as a diagnostic measure for thyroid disorders was replaced in many hospitals by more specific tests of thyroid hormonal status. By the 1960s, there was renewed interest in the basal metabolism of normal and obese people, since statistics showed that obesity was sometimes associated with various degenerative and fatal diseases. Subsequently, studies of the specific dynamic action (thermogenesis) due to food consumption have suggested that this effect may play an important role in the regulation of the body weights of some people.

(Also see CALORIC VALUES OF FOODS.)

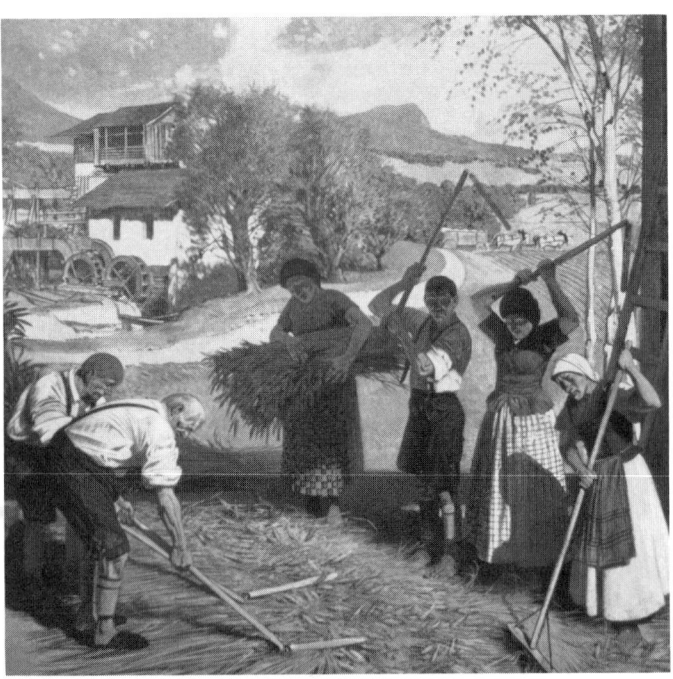

Fig. C-9. Prior to the advent of machines, much energy (calories) was expended in human power, such as threshing with flails. (Courtesy, Field Museum of Natural History, Chicago, Ill.)

UTILIZATION OF DIETARY ENERGY BY THE BODY.
The total heat content of the foods which constitute a diet may be determined by burning representative samples in a bomb calorimeter. However, some of the food energy cannot be utilized by the body because it is present in one or more substances that are not completely digested and absorbed, or if they are absorbed, are not metabolized completely. Unabsorbed materials are excreted in the feces,

whereas those that are absorbed, but not metabolized, are excreted in the urine. The utilizable and nonutilizable forms of dietary energy are illustrated in Fig. C-10.

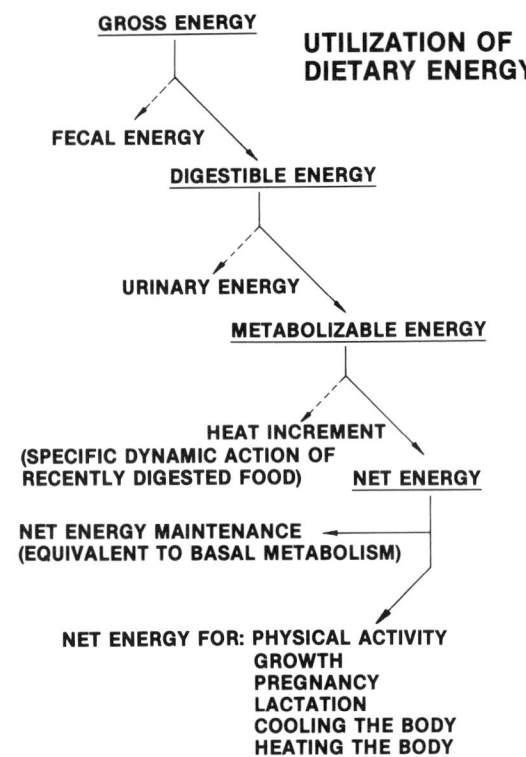

Fig. C-10. Utilization of dietary energy by the body.

Definitions of the parts of the outline shown in Fig. C-10 follow:

- **Gross energy (Heat of combustion)**—This is the total heat released from a food when it is burned in a calorimeter. This value may be considerably larger than the amount of energy that is available for utilization by the body since it does not take into account the unavailable part of the food energy. For example, 1 lb (0.45 kg) of corncobs contains about the same amount of gross energy as 1 lb of corn grain.

- **Fecal energy**—This fraction represents the energy content of the food constituents that are not asorbed in the digestive tract. The most common contributor to fecal energy in the human diet is cellulose and the related carbohydrates that collectively constitute the crude fiber of plant foods. Certain lipids and nitrogenous substances also contribute to the fecal energy.

- **Digestible energy**—This is the energy present in the food constituents that is absorbed by the body. It is determined by subtracting the fecal energy from the gross energy.

- **Urinary energy**—This fraction represents the energy content of the metabolic products that is excreted in the urine. Most of this energy is present in the nitrogenous waste products of metabolism such as urea, uric acid, creatine, and creatinine.

- **Metabolizable energy**—This is the energy that is released from food constituents during metabolism. It is determined by subtracting both the fecal and urinary energy fractions from the gross energy. The Atwater caloric conversion factors of 4, 9, and 4 Calories (kcal) represent the average metabolizable energy content of each gram of the dietary carbohydrate, fat, and protein, respectively.

• **Heat increment**—This fraction corresponds to the heat that is lost from the body after the consumption of a meal. It is generally considered to be wasted, except when it contributes to the maintenance of the body temperature in a cold environment. The heat increment varies in magnitude with the composition of the meal that is consumed, since dietary protein generally yields more waste heat than equicaloric amounts of carbohydrate and fat. However, the heat increment also varies among different people who have consumed the same meal. It is noteworthy that the heat increment of the diet has often been referred to as the *specific dynamic action,* or more recently as the *thermic effect.*

• **Net energy**—This is the energy that is available in a useful form for doing the work of the body. It is determined by subtracting the heat increment (usually assumed to be 10% of the metabolizable energy, since it cannot be measured readily) from the metabolizable energy.

• **Net energy for maintenance**—This fraction of the net energy is that which is required to keep the body in a state of balance; that is, with no net loss or gain of energy in the body tissues. Hence, it corresponds to what is considered to be the basal metabolism in healthy, nonpregnant, nonlactating adults.

• **Net energy for physical activity, growth, pregnancy, lactation, cooling the body, and heating the body**—This is the energy cost of body functions over and above those of maintenance. Values for these incremental energy expenditures range from next to nothing for certain awake, but resting, adults to amounts that greatly exceed the basal metabolism when the various functions other than those of maintenance are operative.

(Also see ENERGY UTILIZATION BY THE BODY.)

CONSEQUENCES OF TOO FEW OR TOO MANY CALORIES.

People may be weakened significantly and made extra vulnerable to disease by either undernourishment or overnourishment. A recent statistical analysis of mortality data from around the world has shown that the minimum mortality occurs in the middle range of body weights and that mortality increases for both lower and higher weights.[3] Discussion of caloric imbalances follow:

Caloric Deficiencies. Many Americans tend to overlook the possible consequences of underweight because they are exposed to a steady stream of propaganda on the virtues of being slim. However, the older generation seemed to know better since they employed many different dietary measures to ensure that the members of their families maintained adequate body weights. Standards for defining underweight vary, but the condition is said to exist when one is more than 10% below the average weight for his or her height, body build, sex, and age. Therefore, it is worth reviewing some of the consequences from the lack of sufficient food energy.

[3]Keys, A., "Overweight, Obesity, Coronary Heart Disease and Mortality," *Nutrition Reviews,* Vol. 38, September, 1980, pp. 297-307.

• **Failure of growth and development in infants, children, and adolescents**—Adequate energy intake is required for efficient utilization of dietary protein, growth, and sexual development during adolescence. Furthermore, even mild energy deficiencies may delay the various stages of growth and sexual development. More severe deficiencies may stunt growth permanently and bring the normal sexual development to a halt. It is well known that stringent dieting by adolescent girls sometimes stops menstruation.

• **Greater susceptibility to chilling and infections**—Heat escapes from the bodies of overly thin people much more rapidly than it does from those who are heavier because layers of fat act as insulation against heat loss. Also, the heat production by the body is diminished in caloric undernutrition. Studies of malnourished children in the developing countries have shown that caloric deficiencies may be accompanied by reduced immunity to infection. Furthermore, the effects of infections are likely to be more severe and longlasting due to the lack of energy reserves for the maintenance of the body tissues.

• **Lack of energy for physical activities**—Many studies have shown that the failure to provide sufficient dietary energy to cover the cost of muscular work usually results in apathy and lack of drive. It is believed that the caloric undernutrition somehow alters the normal patterns of hormonal secretion which promote physical vigor.

(Also see MALNUTRITION; and UNDERWEIGHT.)

Caloric Excesses. It is well known that the chronic consumption of excessive amounts of food energy leads to obesity. Fig. C-11 shows an extraordinary gain in weight which occurred throughout the life of the heaviest medically weighed human.

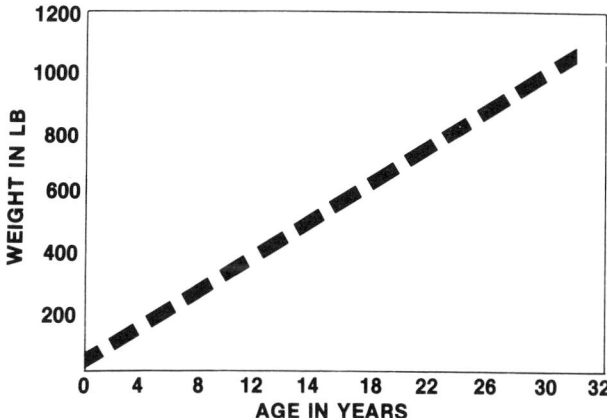

Fig. C-11. The continuous gain in weight of one of the world's heaviest humans. (Plotted from data given in McWhirter, N., *Guinness Book of World Records,* 16th ed., Bantam Books, Inc., New York, N.Y., 1978, pp. 21-22)

The man whose weight record is plotted in Fig. C-11 gained an average of 33.3 lb (*15 kg*) per year over his lifespan of 32 years. This pattern of weight gain can be accomplished by the consumption of as few as 318 excess Calories (kcal) per day since approximately 3,500 Calories (kcal) are equivalent to a pound of body weight. In terms of extra food, this means an extra hamburger, or a piece of cake or pie each day. Fortunately, there are some poorly understood biological mechanisms by which most overeaters are protected from the extreme results shown in Fig. C-11. Nevertheless, the disorders which may be associated with obesity are noteworthy. (Insurance companies consider a person to be obese when his or her weight is more than 20% greater than that deemed to be appropriate for his or her height, body build, and age.)

(Also see OBESITY, section headed "Height-Weight Tables.")

• **Disorders of the heart and circulation**—The relationship between obesity and these disorders is not simple, since susceptibility also depends upon many other factors such as age, body build, climate, heredity, metabolic disorders, physical activity, sex, and smoking. Even so, obesity often aggravates conditions such as angina pectoris (sharp pain in the chest or shoulder which regularly accompanies physical exertion), coronary heart disease, enlargement of the heart, excessive numbers of red cells and abnormal clotting of the blood, high blood pressure, high levels of fats in the blood, stroke, and sudden death resulting from a heart attack.

• **Increased susceptibility to heat exhaustion**—Layers of body fat slow the escape of heat from the body. Experiments have shown that exercising in a hot environment usually results in a greater elevation of body temperature in the obese than in the nonobese.

• **Kidney diseases**—Insurance company statistics show that obese policyholders have about twice the death rate from kidney diseases as the nonobese, but it is not certain whether obesity is a direct cause of the disease, or whether they result from conditions that may be associated with obesity.

• **Metabolic abnormalities**—Patterns of hormonal secretion and metabolism are sometimes altered in obesity and may be responsible in part for the greater susceptibility of some obese people to diabetes, gallstones, gout and/or hyperuricemia (high blood levels of uric acid), hypoglycemia (low blood sugar), and toxemia of pregnancy. However, obesity may not necessarily be the direct cause of the metabolic problems but rather the result of an acquired or an inhibited abnormality that predisposes the people to both the disorder and the obesity.

• **Physical handicaps**—The workload that is imposed upon the body by a great amount of extra weight may increase the likelihood of breathing difficulties, easy fatigability, hernia, osteoarthritis, and sleepiness in spite of what seems to be adequate sleeping time.

(Also see OBESITY.)

MEASUREMENT OF ENERGY EXPENDITURES.
The dangers of underweight and overweight which were discussed in the preceding section show the need for accurate data for estimating caloric requirements of people in various circumstances. These data are obtained by the means which follow:

Direct Calorimetry. In this procedure, the subject is confined to a well-insulated chamber and the heat losses (by radiation, convection, and conduction from the body surface; by evaporation of water from the skin and lungs; and by excretion of urine and feces) are measured either by (1) the increase in temperature of a known volume of water, or (2) electrical current generated as heat passes across thermocouples (gradient layer calorimetry). About ¼ of the heat lost by the body results from moisture vaporization. The remaining ¾ of the body heat is lost by radiation,

conduction, and convection.

Direct calorimetry is the most accurate method of measuring the heat production of people, but it is costly and arduous. The machine itself is very expensive to build and maintain; and considerable labor is involved in running the machine and analyzing the results. For these reasons, indirect calorimetry is usually the method of choice for the measurement of energy expenditures.

Indirect Calorimetry. In this procedure, heat production is calculated from measurement of the respiratory exchange—the O_2 consumption, and usually the CO_2 production—of the subject. This method is based on the fact that O_2 consumption and CO_2 production are closely related to heat production. Measurement of the respiratory exchange of a person may be made with an open circuit mask system or an automated system for metabolic measurements.

• **Open circuit mask system**—The nose is clamped, and the subject is told to exhale through an expiratory tube for a short period so that all of the exhaled air may be collected in a bag or spirometer for analysis.

• **Automated system for metabolic measurements**—This type of system usually includes an infrared CO_2 analyzer, a high-speed O_2 analyzer, electronic temperature and pressure transducers, a turbine volume meter, and an automated system for sample handling, data collection, computation, and printout.

The operation of this type of system is shown in Fig. C-12.

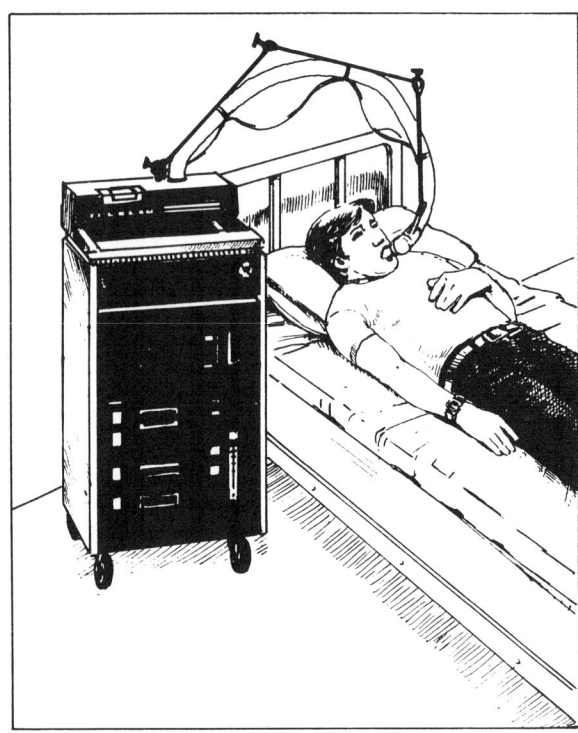

Fig. C-12. An automated system for metabolic measurements. Before the test, the operator enters the program that will control data collection on a magnetic program card which controls the operation of the system.

The most commonly made calorimetric tests are the measurements of the basal metabolic rate and the respiratory quotient. Details follow:

BASAL METABOLIC RATE (BMR).

This test provides a measure of the minimum daily energy expenditure required to maintain the essential functions of the body. Doctors have often ordered BMR tests to determine whether excessive fatness or thinness is due to hypometabolism or hypermetabolism, respectively. The simplest determination consists of measuring the oxygen consumption of the subject for two 6-minute periods, then averaging the results. Sometimes the CO_2 production is also measured. The following conditions are necessary for the accurate measurement of BMR:

1. A minimum fasting period of 12 hours prior to measurement, so as to guarantee the absence of the specific dynamic action which accompanies food consumption. For this reason measurement of the BMR is usually made in the morning before the subject has had breakfast.

2. The subject should be awake and relaxed, but lying down and in a calm state of mind.

3. The temperature of the room should be within the range of 70 to 80°F (*21 to 27°C*) so that no extra work is being done by the body to heat or cool itself.

The result of a BMR determination is usually calculated in terms of Calories (kcal) per square meter of body surface per hour. Body surface values are given in charts and tables as functions of height and weight. Then, the result is compared with standard BMR values for age and sex and expressed as a percentage deviation from the standard value which is appropriate for the subject under consideration. For example, a 47-year-old female who has a basal metabolic rate of 30 Calories (kcal) per square meter per hour would be given a rating of −14. This means that her BMR is 14% below the standard value for her age. The interpretation of the measurement may vary among different physicians, but generally the range from −15 to +15 is considered normal, because it covers about 95% of normal, healthy people.

Among the factors that may lower the BMR are: depression, glandular deficiencies, malnutrition, obesity, or sedative drugs.

Factors that may raise the BMR include: anemia, anxiety, cardiovascular disorders, fever, glandular oversecretions, lactation, lung disorders, Parkinson's disease, pregnancy, stimulant drugs, stress, thinness, or trauma.

RESPIRATORY QUOTIENT (RQ).

This measurement may be made as part of the determination of the basal metabolic rate, or it may be measured separately in order to provide other information, such as the amounts and types of the nutrients which are metabolized under various circumstances. The noted American physiologist Eugene DuBois made many determinations of the RQ for the latter purpose.

The ratio of carbon dioxide produced to oxygen consumed, which is known as the respiratory quotient (RQ), is distinctive for each of the three major types of energy-yielding nutrients; hence, it serves to indicate the type(s) of nutrient being metabolized. Respiratory quotient can be determined through the following equation:

$$RQ = \frac{CO_2 \text{ produced}}{O_2 \text{ consumed}}$$

Therefore, if we utilize the equation for the catabolism of carbohydrates, we can calculate a respiratory quotient:

1. $C_6H_{12}O_6 + 6\ O_2 \rightarrow 6\ CO_2 + 6\ H_2O + \text{heat}$

2. $RQ = \dfrac{6\ CO_2}{6\ O_2} = 1$

The RQ for fat would be less than 1, as seen in the following example:

1. Palmitic acid $(C_{16}H_{32}O_2) + 23\ O_2 \rightarrow 16\ CO_2 + 16\ H_2O + \text{heat}$

2. $RQ = \dfrac{16\ CO_2}{23\ O_2} = .70$

Most mixed fats have RQ values of about .7, while short-chained fatty acids have higher values (about .8). Proteins have values intermediate between carbohydrates and fats—about .81.

It should be noted that in stress conditions, the RQ value can be greater than 1. This can occur when there is hyperventilation where large quantities of carbon dioxide are exhaled while an oxygen debt exists in the body. Metabolic acidosis creates an excess exhalation of carbon dioxide as a compensatory mechanism.

RECOMMENDED CALORIC (Energy) INTAKES.

In lieu of individual calorimetric studies, it is possible to establish daily caloric allowances by utilizing standard data that have been compiled by the leading authorities. A good

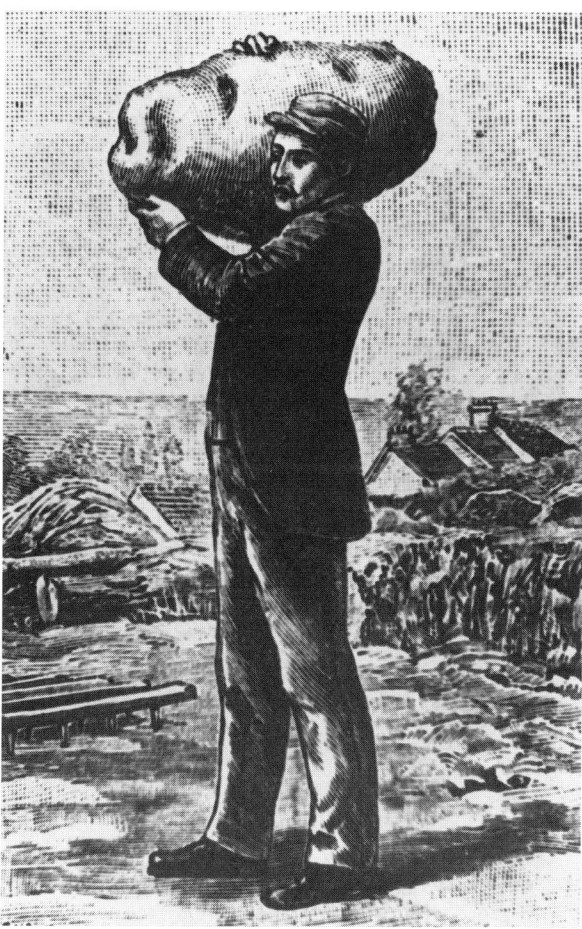

Fig. C-13. One acre of potatoes meets the annual energy requirement of more than 10 people. (Courtesy, The Bettmann Archive, Inc.)

way to begin this procedure is to consider the recommended energy intakes that have been published by the Food and Nutrition Board, which are shown in Table C-2.

These data are only very rough approximations which

may be refined somewhat by a close scrutinizing of the major factors that influence total energy expenditures. Adult needs will be considered first, then those of infants, children, and adolescents, followed by the special circumstances that may also influence the energy expenditures.

TABLE C–2
MEAN HEIGHTS AND WEIGHTS AND RECOMMENDED CALORIC (ENERGY) INTAKES[1,2]

Category	Age	Weight		Height		Energy Needs	
	(years)	(lb)	(kg)	(in.)	(cm)	(kcal/kg)	(per day)
Infants	0.0–0.5	13	6	24	60	108	650
	0.5–1.0	20	9	28	71	98	850
Children	1–3	29	13	35	90	102	1300
	4–6	44	20	44	112	90	1800
	7–10	62	28	52	132	70	2000
Males	11–14	99	45	62	157	55	2500
	15–18	145	66	69	176	45	3000
	19–24	160	72	70	177	40	2900
	25–50	174	79	70	176	37	2900
	51+	170	77	68	173	30	2300
Females	11–14	101	46	62	157	47	2200
	15–18	120	55	64	163	40	2200
	19–24	128	58	65	164	38	2200
	25–50	138	63	64	163	36	2200
	51+	143	65	63	160	30	1900
Pregnancy	2nd & 3rd trimester						+300
Lactation							+500

[1]Adapted by the authors from *Recommended Dietary Allowances*, 10th ed., 1989, NRC–National Academy of Sciences, p. 33, Table 3–5.

[2]The data in this table have been assembled from the observed median heights and weights of children, together with desirable weights for adults based on the mean heights of men (70 in., or *178 cm*) and women (64 in., or *163 cm*) between the ages of 18 and 34 years as surveyed in the U.S. population (HEW/NCHS data).

The energy allowances for the young adults are for men and women doing light work.

Allowances for Adults. In many cases, the energy need of adult males and females are determined mainly by the average daily expenditure of energy in physical activities. Special allowances have to be made for females who are either pregnant or lactating. Table C-3 shows how the average amounts of time spent engaged in various energy-consuming activities may be utilized in the estimation of daily energy needs.

It may be seen from Table C-3 that the estimated daily expenditures of typical American men and women are based entirely on sedentary, light, and moderate levels of activity. However, increases in the energy allowances should be made from persons who are both larger than the reference persons and more active than shown in the example. For example, people who spend significantly more time in activities requiring moderate, vigorous, and/or strenuous energy expenditure may be allowed 300 or more extra Calories (kcal) daily.

Allowances for Infants, Children, and Adolescents.
It is difficult to determine the caloric needs of individuals within these groups because of the great variations in heights, weights, and participation in physical activities. This is particularly true in the case of older adolescents because differences in the rates of growth are accentuated with the passage of time. For example, 18-year-old boys in the 95th

percentile on the growth charts by the National Center for Health Statistics (NCHS) weigh about 210 lb (96 kg), whereas those in the 5th percentile weigh about 119 lb (54 kg). Furthermore, many children are transported to school and have only minimal exercise, where others engage in strenuous activities for an hour or more daily.

One way of coping with the uncertainty of caloric allowances for our youth has been the derivation of formulas such as the one which follows:

Calories/kg = 100 – (3 × age in years).[4]

In terms of pounds, this formula may be expressed as follows:

Calories/lb = 45 – (1.4 × age in years).

The formula is suitable for predicting the allowances of boys up to 14 years of age, and for girls up to 12. After that, other formulas which may be used are as follows:

I. **Boys**—Calories/lb = 19 (Appropriate for boys from ages 15 to 18)

II. **Girls**—Calories/lb = 35 – (1.1 × age in years from 13 to 18)

[4]Wallace, W. M., "Quantitative Requirements of the Infant and Child for Water and Electrolyte Under Varying Conditions," *The American Journal of Clinical Pathology*, Vol. 23.

TABLE C-3
ESTIMATION OF DAILY CALORIC (ENERGY) NEEDS OF ADULTS[1]

Type of Activity[2]	Time	Man, 154 lb (70 kg)		Woman, 123 lb (56 kg)	
		Rate	Total	Rate	Total
	(hr)	(kcal/hr)	(kcal)	(kcal/hr)	(kcal)
Sleeping	8	75	600	60	480
Sedentary .... Reading, writing, watching TV, sewing, typing, or miscellaneous work or games while seated	12	100	1,200	80	960
Light .... Food preparation, dusting, ironing, washing dishes, walking slowly (2½ to 3 mph), or shopping	3	160	480	110	330
Moderate .... Walking at 3½ to 4 mph, making beds, sweeping floors, washing clothes in a machine, or table tennis	1	240	240	170	170
Vigorous .... Gardening, bowling, golfing, scrubbing or waxing floors, or other heavy work	0	350	—	250	—
Strenuous .... Work with pick and shovel, running, dancing, swimming, tennis, skiing, or bicycling (7 mph)	0	350+	—	350+	—
Total	24		2,520		1,940

[1]Based mainly upon data in *Food, Home and Garden Bull.* No. 228, USDA, pp. 14-15.
[2]One mi equals 1.6 km.

The formulas are all based upon the concept of feeding growing youth on the basis of their body weights. Unfortunately, the thin person may receive too little and the obese one too much. Nevertheless, the prevailing belief among nutritionists today is that this approach, while faulty, is not as bad as stuffing thin children with food and starving the obese. Severe nutritional deprivation of obese children while they are growing rapidly may result in a reduction in growth and poor development of essential body functions. Furthermore, children who are obviously at either of these extremes should be examined by a pediatrician to make certain that they are not suffering from any metabolic or other disorders. Those who are moderately overweight according to their age, sex, and body build should be encouraged to engage in more vigorous activities, rather than restrict their diets drastically. It is noteworthy that the caloric allowances for children established by the Food and Agriculture Organization (FAO) of the UN are considerably higher than those of the U.S. Food and Nutrition Board. The main reason for this difference is that children in the developing countries expend much more energy in physical activities than American children.

(Also see CHILDHOOD AND ADULT NUTRITION; and INFANT DIET AND NUTRITION.)

Resting Energy Expenditures (REE). Unless levels of physical activity are very high, resting energy expenditure (REE) is the largest component of total energy expenditure. REE represents the energy expended by a person at rest under conditions of thermal neutrality. Basal metabolic rate (BMR) is more precisely defined as the REE measured soon after awakening in the morning, at least 12 hours after the last meal. REE is not usually measured under basal conditions. REE may include the residual thermic effect of a previous meal and may be lower than BMR during quiet sleep. In practice, BMR and REE differ by less than 10%, and the terms are used interchangeably. The values used in Table C-4 were derived from equations published by WHO (1985). These equations take into account age, sex, and weight, but ignore height.

Special Circumstances that Affect Energy Requirements. The major conditions which require adjustment of energy allowances follow.

PREGNANCY. The National Research Council Committee on Maternal Nutrition recommends that women, who start pregnancy with a normal body weight, eat sufficient calories to bring about a weight gain of about 24 lb (*11 kg*). Teenagers who become pregnant should gain this amount of weight *plus* whatever they would normally gain during this time if they were not pregnant. Women who are underweight when they conceive should also gain more than the recommended 24 lb. However, women who are overweight at the time of conception should *not* attempt to gain less than 24 lb. Physiologists have determined that the daily caloric intake of healthy pregnant women should be at least 16 Calories (kcal) per lb (*36 kcal per kg*) of pregnant body

TABLE C-4
CALCULATING REE (RESTING ENERGY EXPENDITURE) USING BODY WEIGHTS[1]

Males		Females	
Age-years	REE-kcal/day	Age-years	REE-kcal/day
0–3	(60.9 × wt)[2] − 54	0–3	(61.0 × wt) − 51
3–10	(22.7 × wt) + 495	3–10	(22.5 × wt) + 499
10–18	(17.5 × wt) + 651	10–18	(12.2 × wt) + 746
18–30	(15.3 × wt) + 679	18–30	(14.7 × wt) + 496
30–60	(11.6 × wt) + 879	30–60	(8.7 × wt) + 829
60+	(13.5 × wt) + 487	60+	(10.5 × wt) + 596

[1]Adapted from *Recommended Dietary Allowances*, 10th ed., 1989, National Research Council, p. 26, Table 3–1.
[2]Weight of person in kilograms.

weight. Normally, meeting this requirement would require the consumption of 300 *extra* Calories (kcal) per day through pregnancy, or about 150 Calories (kcal) daily during the first trimester and 350 Calories (kcal) daily during the second and third trimesters.

LACTATION. It has been estimated that the production of about 30 oz (*850 to 900 ml*) of breast milk daily expends from 750 to 900 Calories (kcal) per day. However, it is expected that most healthy women who consume adequate food energy during pregnancy will have gained from 4 to 9 lb (*2 to 4 kg*) of extra body fat which will furnish some of the extra calories for lactation. Therefore, the Recommended Dietary Allowances specify that about 500 extra Calories (kcal) should be consumed daily during lactation.

ENVIRONMENTAL STRESSES. Recently, the traditional concepts regarding the need to make special caloric allowances for climate have been revised significantly. The latest thinking in this regard is that working in a cold environment requires only about 2 to 5% increase in the caloric allowance, which is mainly to compensate for the extra work of physical activity while encumbered somewhat by heavy clothing. On the other hand, the energy allowances for people living in warm climates should be about the same as those for the more moderate environments. However, physical work at temperatures over 85°F (*30°C*) requires an extra energy allowance of about 0.5% for each degree centigrade above this temperature because the heart has to work harder to keep the body cool.

DISEASES, INJURIES, AND SURGERY. It is very important to make certain that people in these circumstances receive adequate food energy so that dietary protein is utilized efficiently to promote healing and recovery. Furthermore, the basal metabolic rate may be increased significantly. For example, for each °F of fever, the metabolic rate is increased by about 7%. Multiple fractures may increase the resting energy expenditure from 10 to 30%, and recovery from surgery may involve up to a 10% increase in metabolism.

People who are in any way hobbled by having to use crutches or various prosthetic devices may expend extra energy in normal activities. Victims of cerebral palsy and Parkinson's disease are also likely to require extra food energy when they are ambulatory.

SUMMARY: BALANCING ENERGY INTAKES AND EXPENDITURES. The U.S. Food and Nutrition Board has recommended that, whenever feasible, efforts to reduce excessive body weight should include only a moderate restriction of dietary calories which is accompanied by increased physical activity, because it is difficult to ensure the nutritional adequacy of diets that are too low in energy content (less than 1,800 to 2,000 kcal daily). Therefore, the authors recommend that healthy people step up their activity so that they may continue to eat a well-balanced diet containing a variety of foods. Some guidelines on the exercise equivalents of various foods are given in Fig. C-14. (Also see OBESITY.)

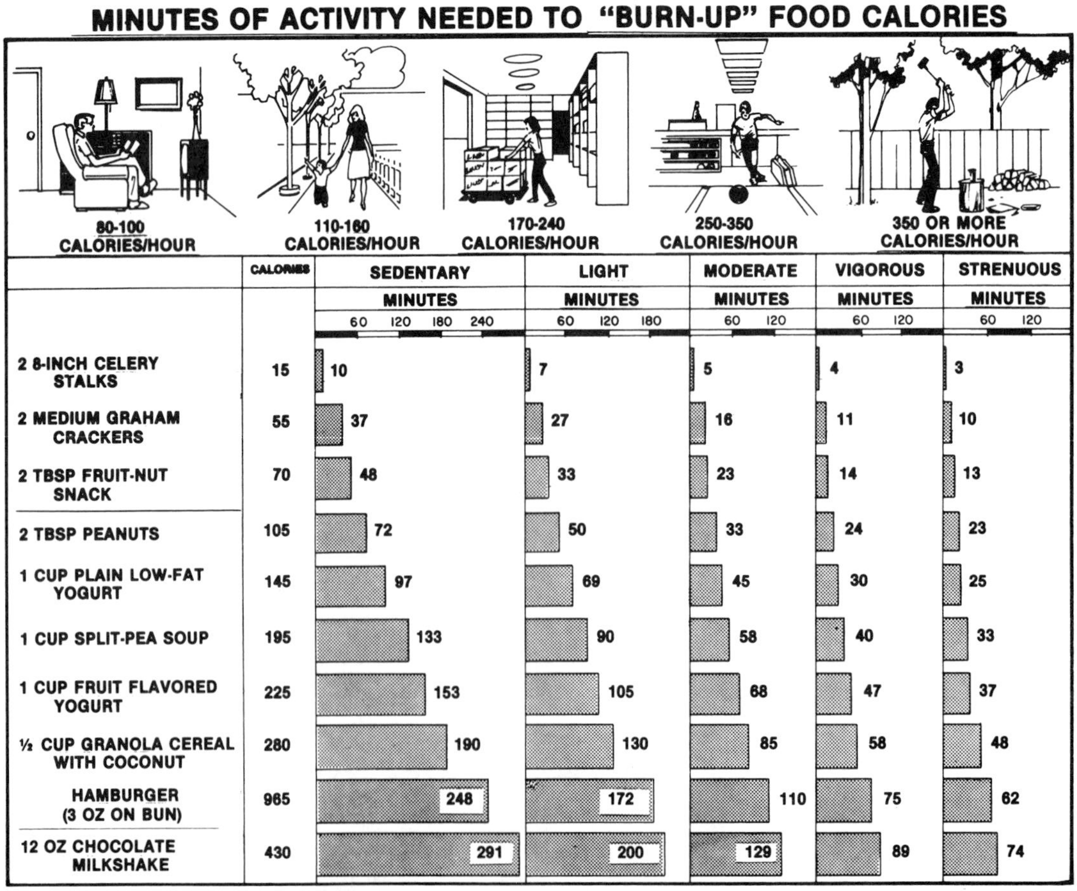

MINUTES OF ACTIVITY NEEDED TO "BURN-UP" FOOD CALORIES

	CALORIES	SEDENTARY 80-100 CALORIES/HOUR MINUTES	LIGHT 110-160 CALORIES/HOUR MINUTES	MODERATE 170-240 CALORIES/HOUR MINUTES	VIGOROUS 250-350 CALORIES/HOUR MINUTES	STRENUOUS 350 OR MORE CALORIES/HOUR MINUTES
2 8-INCH CELERY STALKS	15	10	7	5	4	3
2 MEDIUM GRAHAM CRACKERS	55	37	27	16	11	10
2 TBSP FRUIT-NUT SNACK	70	48	33	23	14	13
2 TBSP PEANUTS	105	72	50	33	24	23
1 CUP PLAIN LOW-FAT YOGURT	145	97	69	45	30	25
1 CUP SPLIT-PEA SOUP	195	133	90	58	40	33
1 CUP FRUIT FLAVORED YOGURT	225	153	105	68	47	37
½ CUP GRANOLA CEREAL WITH COCONUT	280	190	130	85	58	48
HAMBURGER (3 OZ ON BUN)	965	248	172	110	75	62
12 OZ CHOCOLATE MILKSHAKE	430	291	200	129	89	74

Fig. C-14. Exercise equivalents of the Calories provided by some common foods. (Based upon data in *Food*, Home and Garden Bull. No. 228, USDA, pp. 14-15.)

CALORIC VALUES OF FOODS

It is necessary for nutritionists to obtain accurate estimates of the caloric values of various diets in order to help people avoid the consumption of too little or too much food energy. For example, a chronic dietary deficit of calories may result in the wasting of muscles and other body tissues and a temporary or permanent impairment of certain functions. On the other hand, long-term dietary excesses of food energy may lead to obesity which is believed to increase the risk of diabetes, heart disease, and high blood pressure.

The caloric contents of diets are usually calculated by the use of *Atwater caloric conversion factors* which were derived for the mixed diets consumed by Americans around the turn of the century. These factors are based upon the assumptions that each gram of carbohydrate, fat, and protein in the diet will yield 4, 9, and 4 Calories (kcal), respectively. However, the Atwater factors were not intended to be used for single foods or for mixed diets that differed markedly in composition from those for which they were derived. Today, there are a wide variety of diets that have been drastically modified from the average American dietary pattern. Therefore, it is important that dietary planners understand the basic principles of food calorimetry.

The Atwater procedure, in brief, was to adjust the heats of combustion (gross calories) of the fat, protein, and carbohydrate in a food to allow for the losses in digestion and metabolism found for human subjects, and to apply the adjusted caloric factors to the amounts of protein, fat, and carbohydrate in the food. The contents of protein and fat were determined by chemical analysis, and the percentage of carbohydrate was obtained by difference; that is, it was taken as the remainder after the sum of the fat, protein, ash, and moisture had been deducted from 100. This so-called total carbohydrate, therefore, included fiber (an all-inclusive term for carbohydrates that are not digested by people) as well as any noncarbohydrate residue present.

(Also see CALORIC [Energy] EXPENDITURE; and FOOD GROUPS, section on "Calorie Counting.")

CALORIE (cal)

This unit, which is always written with a small c, is the amount of energy heat required to raise the temperature of 1 gram of water 1°C (precisely from 14.5 to 15.5°C). It is equivalent to 4.184 joules. In popular writings, especially those concerned with human caloric requirements, the term *calorie* is frequently used erroneously for the *Kilocalorie* (kcalorie or kcal).

(Also see CALORIMETRY; and KILOCALORIE.)

CALORIES, EMPTY

A term identifying foods that supply energy (calories) only, while other nutrients such as minerals, vitamins and proteins are missing or present in very low levels. For example, table sugar made from sugarcane or sugar beets is almost pure carbohydrate and provides calories only.

(Also see BREAKFAST CEREALS, section headed "The Sugar-Breakfast-Cereal Binge.")

CALORIMETER

In nutrition, this term designates any apparatus used for measuring (1) the heat content of food, or (2) the heat given off by living organisms.

(Also see BOMB CALORIMETER; CALORIE [Energy] EXPENDITURE; and CALORIC VALUES OF FOODS.)

CALORIMETRY

• **Direct calorimetry**—The following two methods of direct calorimetry are employed; the first one for foods, the second one for people:

1. The heat content of foods is determined by burning them in a bomb calorimeter.

2. The heat given off by a person engaged in various activities is determined by placing the subject in an insulated chamber that contains pipes carrying circulating water. The heat given off by the subject is calculated from the rise in temperature of a fixed quantity of water that enters and leaves the chamber. In a more recent type, the *gradient layer calorimeter*, the quantity of heat is measured electrically as it passes through the wall of the chamber.

• **Indirect calorimetry**—In indirect calorimetry, the heat produced in metabolism is calculated by measuring, in a fixed period of time, the respiratory exchange of the person—the oxygen consumed, and usually the CO_2 exhaled.

(Also see BOMB CALORIMETER; CALORIC VALUES OF FOODS; CALORIE [Energy] EXPENDITURE; and METABOLISM.)

CAMOMILE

This is a member of the daisy family. Its flowers have been touted as a minor complaint cure-all for centuries in Europe. It is a popular folk remedy for mild stomach upset, menstrual cramps, throat sprays, inhalants, ointments, creams, and lotions.

CAMU-CAMU *Myrciaria paraensis*

The small grapelike fruit of a bush (of the family *Myrtaceae*) that is native to Peru. Camu-camu berries are red-colored, and about 1 in. (3 cm) in diameter. They may be eaten fresh, or made into jam, jelly, or wine.

CANADIAN BACON

Bacon made from pork loins, which are given a light cure and smoked.

CANCER

Americans have reason to worry about cancer! In 1991, 1,100,000 people in the United States were told that they had a life-threatening malignancy; and that same year 514,000 people died from cancer.

The characteristic of cancer is wild uncontrolled growth of cells which can arise in any organ or tissue of the body. Cancer cells have a rather primitive appearance when compared to normal cells. They are quite irregular in shape and they have large irregular nuclei. Fig. C-15 illustrates the difference between normal cells and cancer cells under the microscope.

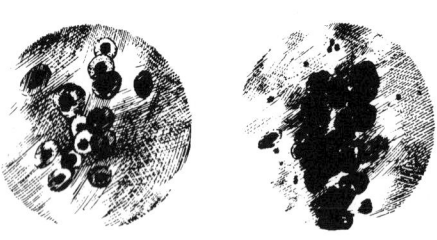

Fig. C-15. Microscopic views of normal cells on the left and cancer cells on the right.

All cells have the capacity to divide. This process is called *mitosis*—one cell becomes two, two cells become four, four cells become eight, and so on. When a cell divides, it goes through a cell cycle and the cell receives some sort of signal that starts and stops this process. Cancer cells divide more often. Out of 100 cancer cells, 10 or 20 of them will continuously be going through division and many cells pile up. The cancer cell, then, has an apparent autonomy due to some abnormality in the chromosomes. It will continue to grow regardless of the size of the mass it creates. As cancers continue to grow, they interfere with body function by crowding normal organs and outstripping the food supply available to the patient, eventually killing the patient.

TYPES OF CANCER. Tumors formed from rapidly dividing cells are of two types: benign and malignant. Benign tumors are those that cannot invade the surrounding tissues and remain as strictly local growths. The more dreaded malignant tumors or cancers are those that spread from their site of origin and, therefore, can reach the bloodstream and lymphatic system. These cancers are divided into three broad groups:

1. **Carcinomas,** which arise in the epithelial tissues—the sheets of cells covering the surface of the body and lining the various glands.

2. **Sarcomas,** which are rather rare, and which arise in supporting structures such as fibrous tissue or connective tissue and blood vessels.

3. **Leukemias** and **lymphomas,** which arise in the blood-forming cells of the bone marrow and lymph nodes.

Cancers are further classified by the organ in which they originate and by the kind of cell involved. Considered this way, there are 100 or more distinct varieties of cancer. Most of these are rare.

COMMONLY AFFLICTED ORGANS AND MORTALITY RATES. Most new cases of cancer and cancer mortality can be accounted for by considering a fairly short list. Twelve leading cancer sites are shown in Fig. C-16.

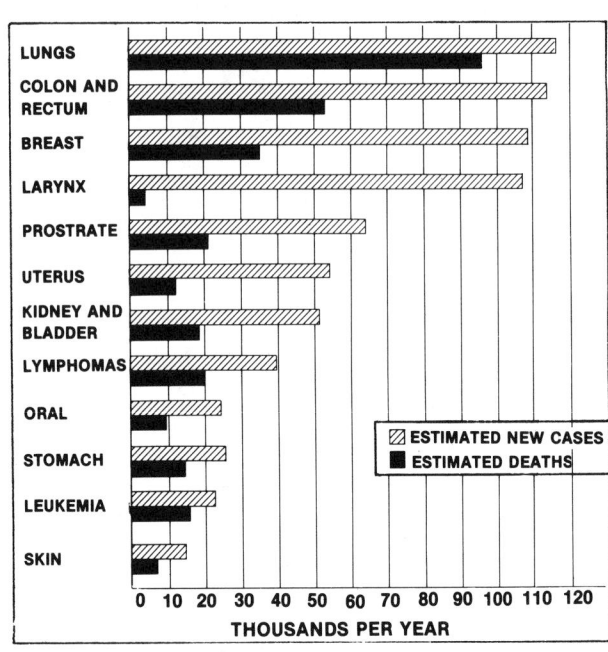

Fig. C-16. Leading cancer sites.

In terms of total deaths, cancers are responsible for about 22% of the deaths in the United States. A majority of the people, 78%, die from some other cause. Of the cancers, roughly half of the deaths are caused by cancer of three organs: the lungs, the colon or rectum, and the breast. Leukemia and lymphomas—cancers of the blood and immune system—are important mainly because they often affect children and young adults. While the estimated new cases is a useful statistic, mortality is the most accessible and reliable indicator of the impact of cancer. Too many variables influence the diagnosis of cancer to make new cases a reliable statistic. Death from cancer is a cold hard fact.

Over the years, several of the cancers have demonstrated mortality rate patterns. Fig. C-17 illustrates some trends.

As shown in Fig. C-17, the most common sites of cancer in men, by rank, are: prostate, lung, and colon, with lung cancer being the leading cause of deaths from cancer.

In women, breast cancer is by far the leading site of cancer, with death from cancer highest from lung cancer, followed in order by breast cancer and colon cancer.

It is noteworthy that lung cancer is the leading cause of deaths from cancer in both men and women.

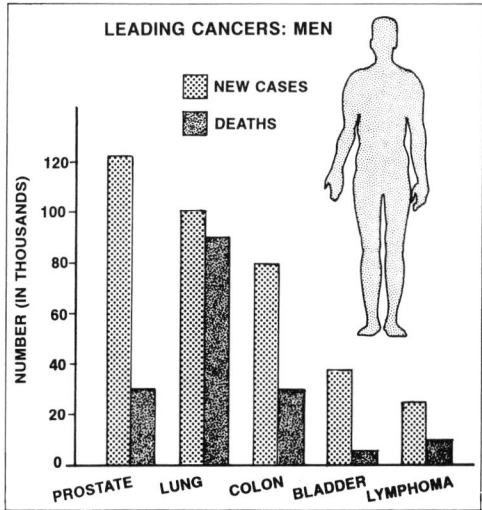

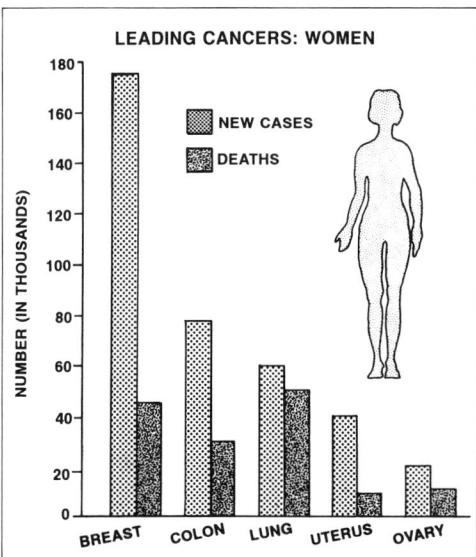

Fig. C-17. Leading cancer sites in (a) men and (b) women, with new cases and deaths of each. (Source: *American Cancer Society Facts and Figures*, 1991)

For unknown reasons, cancer of the pancreas is increasing in incidence. In 1990, an estimated 5% of both males and females in the United States died from cancer of the pancreas.

CAUSES OF CANCER—CARCINOGENS. *Any cancer-producing substance or agent is known as a carcinogen.*

At times we all may feel that everything we enjoy is either illegal, immoral, fattening, or causes cancer. Indeed, the list of suspected carcinogens continues to grow. Still the cause of cancer is more complex than just the exposure to a carcinogen. Many factors must be considered, including chemical agents, physical agents, heredity, viruses, emotions and stress, and diet and nutrition.

Chemical Agents. Chemicals have long been a fact of life; by no means are they a creation of the 20th century.

However, the word *chemical* has been given a negative connotation by some, as if all chemicals or anything containing chemicals causes cancer. Some chemicals do cause cancer, but *not* all chemicals.

Numerous chemicals are scrutinized for carcinogenic activity in an effort to help us make decisions about the chemicals we swallow, inhale, or rub on our skin. To do this, mice, rats, hamsters, or sometimes larger animals, are used by researchers to test for carcinogens. Hence, animals are *stand-ins* for humans.

A brief discussion of some of the more important carcinogens follows.

TOBACCO. At the top of the list of substances that contain carcinogens is tobacco. Chemists have isolated and identified at least a dozen carcinogenic chemicals of the hydrocarbon type in the "tars" from tobacco smoke. There is general agreement—and good evidence—that cigarette smoking contributes to a large proportion of cancer in both men and women—especially lung cancer. Although estimates of the number of lung cancer deaths caused by smoking vary, most experts agree that at least 80% and perhaps 90% of lung cancer deaths are the result of cigarette smoking. But smoking acts to increase cancer risks for body sites in addition to the lungs. Tobacco smokers have greater risks than nonsmokers for cancers of the mouth, throat, bladder, pancreas, and kidney. Scientists have estimated that cigarette smoking and other tobacco use is responsible for about 30% of all cancers, and that cigarette smoking causes one out of every five deaths in the United States. Also, it is noteworthy that secondhand smoke is a health hazard to nonsmokers.

ALCOHOL. It is well established that there is an association between excessive alcohol consumption and cancer of the mouth, throat, and esophagus. Furthermore, persons drinking large quantities of alcohol may develop nutritional deficiencies leaving them more susceptible to the action of tobacco, alcohol, and other possible carcinogens.

NATURALLY OCCURRING CHEMICALS. Cancer-producing chemicals also occur in nature in plants and in molds. Exposure to these naturally occurring carcinogenic chemicals may be largely attributed to geographical location and culture. The nut of the *Cycas circinalis* palm used as food in the Pacific islands contains cycasin, a compound that produces cancer of the kidney and other organs in the rat. Alkaloids of *Senecio jacobaes*, a plant used by the African natives in their diet, and chili peppers, lead to the development of liver cancer in rats. While it is generally not a problem for humans in the United States, a common mold, *Aspergillus flavus*, which grows on wet peanuts, corn and other foods, forms potent liver carcinogens—the aflatoxins. Nitrosamines, another group of potent liver carcinogens, can be found in some plants, and some bacteria cause the formation of nitrosamines in foods. Safrole and related compounds, which are components of essential oils such as sassafras, produce liver cancer in rats. Antithyroid compounds found in plants such as turnips, kale, cabbage, and rapeseed produce thyroid tumors in test animals. The above are some of the more important potential carcinogens that occur in nature. There are more, and the list will undoubtedly grow as more information based on human population studies and animal studies is collected.

FOOD ADDITIVES. Food additives and their potential dangers can best be discussed by dividing food additives into two groups—intentional and incidental. Intentional are, of course, those added during the processing of a food to improve, maintain, or stabilize some characteristic of the food. Incidental additives are environmental chemicals of known origin and anticipated use; for example, pesticides, antibiotics, and growth stimulants. Due to the wording in the Delaney Clause of the Federal Food Drug and Cosmetic Act, the occurrence of additives, whether intentional or incidental, has created a dilemma. On the one hand, we hear that anything shown to cause cancer in man or animal shall not exist in the food supply at any level. On the other hand, we need to consider the risks versus the benefits in light of sound scientific judgment.

(Also see ADDITIVES; DELANEY CLAUSE; and SACCHARIN.)

AIR AND WATER POLLUTION. About 10% of all cases of lung cancer occur in nonsmokers. This may in part be due to air pollution and other environment factors. Densely populated and industrialized areas have higher mortality rates from cancer of the lung and digestive system than rural areas. Numerous factors may account for this, but air and water pollution are suspect. Some of the common indices of air pollution are measures of suspended particulates, sulfates, nitrogen oxides, carbon monoxide, and hydrocarbons. Thus far, all attempts to define and measure the effects of air pollution on the incidence of cancer have not resolved a clear cut association.

From a list of organic compounds found in the drinking water in the United States, about two dozen suspected carcinogens have been identified. One group of organic contaminants, the trihalomethanes, may be related to increases in cancer of the urinary bladder and large intestine. There is no evidence to suggest that drinking fluoridated water, whether natural or artificial, increases the risk of cancer.

Physical Agents. Throughout our life we are exposed to numerous physical agents which may elicit some biochemical change in a cell and eventually lead to the development of cancer.

AGE. Although aging involves biochemical processes, it is observed as a physical occurrence. Aging definitely increases the risk of cancer as Fig. C-18 illustrates.

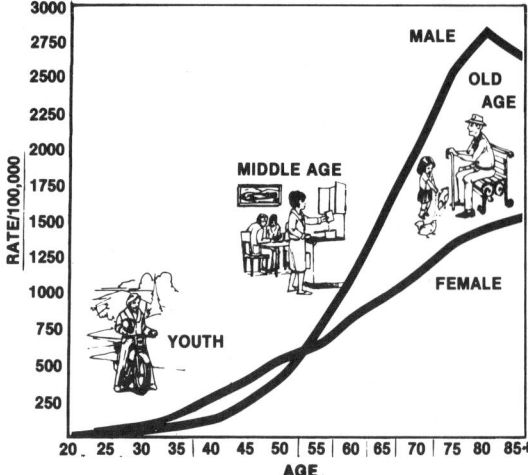

Fig. C-18. Age-specific cancer incidence rates in the United States by sex.

The incidence of almost all forms of cancer increases dramatically with advancing age. With age, cells accumulate damage to their genetic material—the chromosomes. The reason for this accumulated damage seems to be that the repair processes of the cell just slow down. This damage, may eventually lead to the development of cancer. Some other physical agents such as radiation and irritation may contribute to the genetic damage.

RADIATION. There is clear evidence that radiation can cause cancer in humans. Exposure comes from two sources, (1) natural and (2) man-made.

• **Natural**—The sun—the energy source upon which life itself depends—is a cancer-inducing stimuli. The incidence of skin cancer is highest in the white populations of the southern and western part of the United States. Furthermore, skin cancer occurs more frequently among people who work outdoors.

• **Man-made**—Exposures, or at least the chance of exposures, to man-made radiation is a hotly debated issue. It is believed that no level of radiation is entirely without risk; the concern is just how much risk?

Heredity. The role of heredity seems two-fold. Heredity is a predisposing factor in the development of cancer, and there are some cancers which are directly hereditary.

PREDISPOSING FACTORS. Susceptibility to some cancers seems to run in families. However, it is not easy to determine whether or not genetic factors are truly involved since close relatives also are likely to share the same environment. Of the common cancers, the one with the strongest likelihood to run in families is breast cancer, which is found at about twice the normal frequency in close relatives of patients with cancer of the breast. Recent studies have pinpointed some chromosomal changes which appear related to the development of breast cancer. Cancer of the rectum and lung may also aggregate in families. Furthermore, animal studies demonstrate that animals can be selected for their susceptibility to certain cancers.

Some inborn disorders lead to cancer. These include the following: modularity syndromes such as neurofibromatosis and tuberous sclerosis; genetic skin disorders such as albinism; chromosome breakage disorders such as Down's, Bloom's, and Fanconi's syndrome; and immune deficiency syndromes such as agammaglobulinemia.

(Also see INBORN ERRORS OF METABOLISM.)

DIRECTLY HEREDITARY. Some known hereditary cancers of man include: retinoblastoma; multiple polyps of the colon; Gardner's syndrome; chemodectoma; pheochromocytoma; and thyroid cancer. Fortunately, all these are relatively rare and contribute little to the total cancer causes. However, study of these cancers may help determine the actual importance of genetic susceptibility to cancer.

Viruses. Again, from animal studies comes the idea that viruses may be involved in carcinogenesis. Certain leukemia-like diseases of chickens, cats, and inbred strains of mice can be induced in young animals by inoculating them with viruses isolated from leukemic animals. If the same is true for some human cancers, then there is the hope of developing a vaccine to prevent the cancer. Unfortunately, no human cancer, or for that matter animal cancer, has proven that simple. As of yet, there is no hard evidence that any class of human cancers is caused by a virus. Still the search continues, and there is some evidence linking perhaps one of the most common of all the viruses—the Epstein-Barr virus—to two types of cancer, a carcinoma and a lymphoma. The future will tell.

Emotions and Stress. Think happy thoughts and avoid or cure cancer! If it were only that simple. There is one popular theory suggesting that destructive emotions—*stress*, or rather *distress*—can weaken the surveillance mechanism of the body—the immune system—which is constantly destroying abnormal cells that may otherwise cause cancer. Furthermore, there is also increased interest in the possibility that healthy emotions and good thoughts can be directed by a cancer patient to fight the disease. While there is no doubt that a holistic approach and the will to live are strongly tied to overcoming any disease, there is no hard evidence to support this position. On the other hand, our mental state, our response to our environment should not be disregarded. Physiological processes are influenced by sociologic and psychologic factors.

(Also see DISEASES; ENDOCRINE GLANDS; and STRESS.)

Nutrition and Diet. There is substantial scientific evidence that diet may be an important factor in human cancer development. However, the exact roles played by specific aspects or components of the diet are still very uncertain. Also, it is recognized that cancer is *not* caused by any single item, but by an interaction of such things as genetics, lifestyle, cultural patterns, health status, nutrition, and diet. A direct cause-effect relationship between diet and cancer has not been established. The sources of information implicating diet in the formation of cancer include epidemiological surveys, animal experiments, and a few controlled studies in humans. From all of these studies emerge some patterns, which in general seem to be that dietary and nutrient excesses, deficiencies, or imbalances are related to the development of cancers in the stomach, colon, pancreas, liver, and breast. Nutrition and diet appear to modify rather than to initiate the carcinogenic processes. Based on numerous studies there are some hints and guidelines which may be gleaned.

• **Caloric intake**—Many animal studies have shown that caloric restriction generally inhibits cancer formation and increases life expectancy. Conversely, obesity seems to be associated with uterine (endometrial) and kidney cancer in women.

• **Nutrient deficiencies**—Many animal studies have linked nutrient deficiencies, especially of the trace elements, to the development of cancer. Furthermore, deficiencies of vitamins A, C, E, and the B-complex vitamins have been associated with the increased susceptibility of chemically-induced tumors in animals, as have protein, iodine, iron, magnesium, and selenium deficiencies.

• **Foodborne carcinogens**—These have already been mentioned under the section headed "Chemical Agents." Foodborne carcinogens may occur as naturally occurring, intentionally added, or incidentally added chemicals. The known hazards have been eliminated from our foods, while other unknown possible hazards are continually monitored and tested.

• **Dietary fiber**—Lack of fiber in the American diet has been implicated by some as the sole cause of cancer of the colon. Population studies have shown that in countries where dietary fiber intake is high, such as Africa and Finland, the risk of colon cancer is lower than in countries like the United States and Western Europe. The theory: Fiber binds potential carcinogens in the bowel, making them inactive and promoting rapid removal from the large intestine, thus reducing the time carcinogens are in contact with the wall of the colon. In the other direction, studies of both Mormons and non-Mormons in Utah show a lower colon cancer incidence than that of the American population, but little difference in fiber consumption.

(Also see FIBER.)

• **Bile acids**—The diet—in particular fat—may have a role in the development of colon cancer. A current hypothesis is that high dietary fat intake (1) increases bile secretion, and (2) influences the composition and the metabolic activity of the intestinal microfloral so that the anaerobic clostridia increase. These microorganisms—clostridia—are capable of converting, by dehydrogenation, bile acids and neutral sterols (primary bile acids) to carcinogens or cocarcinogens—secondary bile acids. There is substantial evidence in experimental animal studies to implicate dietary fat and secondary bile acids as colon cancer related.

• **Cholesterol**—Studies have indicated that low blood levels of cholesterol appear to *correlate* with a modest increase in cancer risk. So, individuals with levels of blood cholesterol less than 180 mg/100 ml should possibly avoid further reductions until the connection between low cholesterol and cancer is resolved.[5]

• **Hormone production**—Nutritional status, nutrient intake and dietary components play a role in determining an individual's hormone profile. A greater risk of breast cancer has been associated with other conditions which influence endocrine status—increased body height and weight, age of menarche and late menopause. Diet may, in turn, affect these conditions. For example, it is known that over the last 100 years or so the age at menarche of girls in developed countries has declined dramatically; presently, in the United States it is about 11 or 12 years of age. The level of nutrition in developed countries is undoubtedly related to this decline in age at menarche. Breast cancer, a hormone-dependent malignancy of the mammary gland, is the leading cause of cancer mortality in developed countries with the exception of Japan. Furthermore, diet may promote or inhibit breast cancer by modifying the levels or actions of hormones like androgens, prolactin, and estrogens.

After two decades of relative neglect, attention is again being focused upon the role of diet and nutrition in the development of cancer. While there seems to be no doubt that diet can and does influence the development of cancer, diet and nutrition should not be considered the sole causative factors.

DETECTION. The most curable cancers are those that have not progressed to the stage of producing symptoms. Hence, the best detection methods are those that are able to determine cancerous growths in their early stages.

Most cancers are diagnosed because an individual becomes aware of certain symptoms or signs, or because

[5]*The Harvard Medical School Health Letter*, published by the Department of Continuing Education, Harvard Medical School, October, 1981, p. 1.

a physician suspects that certain symptoms or signs exhibited by a patient suggest cancer.

A wide variety of biochemical tests on urine and blood is available for hormones, enzymes and antigens, some of which are used to detect and follow the development of cancer.

An actual biopsy—a small piece of living tissue—of the suspected organ or tissue is necessary for a definite diagnosis of cancer. Biopsies must be taken expertly from the right spot and then examined under a microscope by a pathologist with the experience and judgment necessary for a correct interpretation.

THERAPY—TREATMENT. Successful treatment of cancer is, or course, entire removal from the body. The indicated therapy depends upon (1) the type of cancer, (2) the extent of the cancer, (3) location of the cancer, (4) the age of the patient, and (5) the general health of the patient. Generally three types of therapy are employed in the United States. One type of therapy, or a combination, may be used on a patient. The three methods of treatment that produce the most curative results are surgery, radiation, and chemotherapy. Nutrition plays a role in each of these forms of treatment. Furthermore, there are some suggestions that nutritional therapy can provide some relief from cancer.

Research on treatment of cancer is directed toward developing and evaluating new and improved methods, minimizing toxicity and avoiding the injury of the more radical procedures required to treat advanced stages. Many advances have been made on the traditional three—surgery, radiation, and chemotherapy. In 1991, the National Cancer Institute reported that 51.1% of cancer patients live 5 years or longer.

Surgery. The hope of surgical therapy is the removal of all cancerous tissue. It is the primary form of treatment for cancer of the lung, and most effective for cancer of the colon and rectum. Cancer of the breast is also treated primarily by surgery. Other cancers may also require surgery depending upon their nature.

Some cancer surgeries create the need for specialized nutrition and diet therapy.

Radiation. The principle is to encompass total cancerous tumor with a dose of radiation large enough to destroy cancer cells, but not so large as to seriously damage normal tissue and prevent healing. Various sources of radiation may be used, but the two most familiar sources of radiation are x rays and cobalt-60.

Radiation therapy can create nutritional problems depending upon the general area of the body exposed. These problems and some approaches to these problems are discussed subsequently in the section headed "Nutrition and Diet in Cancer Therapy."

Chemotherapy. Cancer which has spread—metastasized—or cancer of the blood or blood-forming tissues, such as leukemia, are treated with drugs or chemicals. These drugs or chemicals supposedly hunt out and destroy cancer cells. Unfortunately, most chemotherapeutic agents, except the hormones, act to inhibit one or more of the key intermediary metabolism steps in normal as well as cancerous cells. Chemical agents may be classified into three general groups: alkylating agents, metabolic antagonists, and hormones.

Still under criticism and study are such compounds as bioflavonoids, pangamic acid, and Laetrile.

Nutrition And Diet In Cancer Therapy. Nutrition may be considered as an adjunct to the current therapies, or as a therapy. Furthermore, good nutrition of the cancer patient (1) improves sense of well-being, (2) preserves tissue function and repair, (3) improves the immune function, and (4) increases the tolerance to the side effects of chemotherapy, radiation and surgery.

STATUS PRIOR TO AND DURING THERAPY. Many cancers adversely affect the nutritional status of the victim before any treatment has been started. Depending on the type of cancer some of the following may be observed:

1. Malnutrition resulting from anorexia—failure to eat.

2. Malnutrition caused by an obstruction which impairs food intake.

3. Malabsorption associated with (a) a deficiency of pancreatic enzymes or bile, (b) infiltration of the small intestine by the cancer, (c) gastric hypersecretion as in the Zollinger-Ellison syndrome, (d) blind loop syndrome caused by obstruction in upper part of the small intestine, or (e) hypoplasia—regression of the villi of the small intestine.

4. Protein-losing malabsorption associated with stomach cancer or lymphatic obstruction.

5. Disturbances in the electrolyte and fluid balance of the body which are associated with (a) persistent vomiting due to an obstructive growth, (b) vomiting due to pressure from a brain tumor, (c) diarrhea induced by hormone secreting cancers and cancer of the colon, (d) cancers which disrupt the release of antidiuretic hormone from the posterior pituitary, and (e) tumors causing excessive secretion of corticotropin or corticosteroid which results in hyperadrenalism.

For the above reasons, and probably others yet unknown, cancer patients often exhibit cachexia—a general lack of nutrition. Hence, steps should be taken to correct the malnutrition and fluid and electrolyte imbalances in order for other therapeutic measures to proceed—and succeed.

• **Nutritional problems following cancer treatment**—Radiation, surgery, and chemotherapy—predispose the cancer patient to nutritional problems. Obviously, each case is different and the dietary adjustments required differ; hence, the patient should follow the advice of the physician and/or dietician.

(Also see DIGESTION AND ABSORPTION.)

AS A THERAPY. While clinical studies have shown that a nutritionally balanced patient has a much improved chance of undergoing successful treatment and withstanding the rigors of cancer, no conclusive evidence exists to indicate that reduced or excessive amounts of any nutrients have a beneficial role in the treatment of cancer in humans. Still, the role of nutrition as a cancer therapy may be viewed as three-fold depending upon the need of the patient: (1) supportive, (2) adjunctive, and (3) definitive. To this end, some current research is aimed at increasing the appetite and food utilization in cancer patients.

• **Supportive**—Cancer victims who, because of malnutrition caused by cancer, are a poor risk for other forms of therapy; for example, surgery. The risk of this type of cancer patient can be clinically lowered by nutritional means before undertaking other forms of therapy.

• **Adjunctive**—In this case nutrition becomes part of the therapy—a complement. Improved nutrition will (1) improve the immune status, (2) allow better adherence to a proposed antitumor therapeutic program, and (3) induce healing.

• **Definitive**—This type of nutrition therapy occurs when adequate nutrition becomes the means of longer term existence for the cancer patient. Definitive nutrition is the employment of special oral, tube, or intravenous programs which allow the survival of the patient in good condition. Intravenous hyperalimentation has recently received attention as a viable means for supplying the much needed nutrition. Definitive nutrition is required by patients who have had a massive bowel resection and/or extensive radiation treatment of the abdomen.

(Also see INTRAVENOUS [PARENTERAL] NUTRITION, SUPPLEMENTARY.)

PREVENTION. If the factors causing cancer can be identified, then individuals can avoid, eliminate, or counteract their effects. Environmental factors are now generally thought to play a major role in causing cancer. However, the exact nature of environmental factors needs to be considered.

Environment. The statistic that 60 to 90% of all cancer is related to environmental factors is often quoted. People immediately take this figure to mean that cancer is being caused by synthetic chemicals or air pollution. This is not correct. Environment includes smoking, alcohol, diet, sunlight, background radiation, health, hygiene and pollution. On the basis of facts and sound judgment, we must determine our exposure to carcinogenic substances in the environment and take the necessary steps to counteract, avoid, or eliminate. As has been pointed out, levels of exposure and risk following exposure to a carcinogen are difficult to assess. Every individual responds differently to his environment. Factors which should be considered when assessing an individual's exposure to carcinogens are listed in Table C-5.

TABLE C-5
FACTORS WHICH CAUSE CANCER DEATHS

Factor	Percentage of All Cancer Deaths	
	(average)	(range)
Tobacco	30	25 – 40
Diet	35	10 – 70
Infection	10	1 – ?
Reproductive and sexual behavior	7	1 – 13
Occupation	4	2 – 8
Geographical[1]	3	2 – 4
Alcohol	3	2 – 4
Pollution	2	<1 – 5
Medicine and medical procedures	1	.5 – 3
Food additives[2]	<1	–5 – 2
Industrial products	<1	<1 – 2
Unknown	?	?

[1]Actually geographical factors cause more nonfatal cancers due to the importance of ultraviolet light causing the relative nonfatal carcinomas of sunlight exposed skin.

[2]Some food additives may actually exert a protective effect; hence, the range from –5 to 2.

Nutrition And Diet In Cancer Prevention. Many epidemiological studies have been conducted which suggest correlation between certain dietary habits or nutritional imbalances. From these studies some individuals have drawn rather exacting dietary recommendations, failing to recognize that epidemiologic correlations do not establish causation. Furthermore, there is no possible way that epidemiological studies can pinpoint carcinogenic agents. Therefore, when an epidemiological study says meat consumption was correlated with the incidence of cancer of the large intestine, this does not mean that meat causes cancer. The number of dresses a woman owns may also be correlated to the incidence of cancer of the large intestine. *Thus,* epidemiological studies may provide leads, but not definitive scientific evidence.

Based on all current information from epidemiological studies, animal studies, and case studies, foods and nutrients appear to modify rather than initiate the carcinogenic process. There is no proof that a certain diet will cause cancer. Conversely, no diet will prevent cancer. Furthermore, the role that foodborne carcinogens have in causing human cancers remains to be ascertained. Although, no specific diet can be recommended that will prevent cancer, the following salient points deserve mention:

1. Some studies have shown that persons with a higher vitamin A (carotene) intake or blood level are less susceptible to cancer. Nontoxic vitamin A analogs have been successfully used to prevent cancer in animals.

2. Obesity seems to be associated with cancer of the uterus and of the kidneys in women.

3. Various indoles present in vegetables of the *Brassicaceae* family—Brussels sprouts, cabbage and broccoli—induce drug metabolizing enzymes in the lining of the digestive tract which inactivate carcinogens.

4. Long-standing deficiencies of vitamins A, C, and E, as well as of most of the B-complex vitamins, have been shown to increase the susceptibility of animals to chemically induced tumors.

5. Minerals appear to have an optimum range, and an intake above or below this range may increase susceptibility to cancer. For example, high levels of selenium may be carcinogenic, while selenium deficiency has been associated with an increased incidence of cancer.

6. Some new studies suggest that while a low cholesterol diet may protect against heart attacks, it may also increase vulnerability to cancer.

7. Antioxidants, such as vitamin C, have been shown to prevent the formation of nitrosamines. It is noteworthy that some individuals attribute the decline in stomach cancer to the increased availability of vitamin C.

8. Restriction of energy intake or underfeeding decreases the development of transplanted or spontaneous tumors in animals.

9. Dietary fats—saturated and polyunsaturated—have been implicated in colon and breast cancer through population studies; but this has not been confirmed by properly designed and well-controlled experiments.

10. In some areas of the world where foods are likely to be stored under warm damp conditions, there is a high incidence of liver cancer. This may be due to the formation of aflatoxins during storage.

11. Population studies indicate that fiber may lessen cancer of the bowel by increasing the rate of food passage, and by altering the types and amounts of microorganisms. But this theory has not been tested in controlled experiments.

12. It has been suggested that coffee may be contributing to cancer of the pancreas. Although this remains unproved, moderation in the use of coffee is recommended—limiting it to 2 cups a day.

13. Foods which contain bioflavonoids may provide protection against cancer, but this is without proof. Currently, studies are in progress to determine the efficacy of bioflavonoids in this regard.

14. Protease inhibitors, compounds found in foods such as soybeans and lima beans, appear to have antitumor activity. They have been suggested as a possible factor in the lowered incidence of cancers among vegetarians. But further studies are needed.

An "anticancer" diet exists for almost every one of the above points. All of the above points contain an element of truth which can contribute—but cannot stand alone—to our overall understanding of carcinogenesis. As for food or diet which prevents cancer, the best recommendations that can be made are: (1) eat less fat, (2) eat more fiber-containing foods, (3) eat fruit and vegetables every day, (4) eat a well balanced diet and maintain your ideal weight, (5) consume adequate minerals and vitamins, and (6) avoid the known carcinogens, particularly tobacco and excessive alcohol.

THE FUTURE. While a pill or injection that will prevent cancer has not been discovered, more is known and victory is a reasonable expectation. In the battle against cancer, research continues in a number of important directions; among them nutrition and diet.

• **Nutrition and diet**—The use of such nutrients as vitamin A (carotene), folic acid, vitamin C, and other vitamins, along with a general supplemental program of minerals, may be significant for cancer treatment. Perhaps, even more important in the long run is the apparent success of nutrients of many kinds in strengthening the body's immune system—as preventives.

(Also see BIOFLAVONOIDS; DEFICIENCY DISEASES; LAETRILE; NITRATES AND NITRITES; OBESITY; and PANGAMIC ACID.)

CANCRUM ORIS

A decaying of the flesh around the mouth, due to a combination of malnutrition and infection. However, the infectious organism responsible for this condition has not been isolated.

CANDY

The story of candy is the story of sugar. In fact, the word *candy* comes from both an Arabic word *qandi*, meaning *candied*, and the Persian word *qand*, meaning *sugar*. About the middle of the 1400s, a candymaker in Venice learned to refine sugar for making confections. But it wasn't until the cultivation of sugarcane became worldwide that the candy industry developed into one of major significance. Today, the United States is the leading manufacturer of candies (a dubious honor).

The basic candy-making principle is simply the boiling of sugar; and the temperature to which it is cooked determines whether it will be a fondant (236°F [113.3°C]) or a toffee (300°F [148°C]). Today, candy manufacturing plants are equipped with every conceivable machine for each step in the manufacture of over 2,000 different kinds of sweets. There are continuous cookers, cooling tunnels, crystallizers, forming machines, chocolate coaters, and taffy-pulling machines.

The annual candy consumption in the United States is over 17 lb (or almost *8 kg*) per person, which ranks us number 11 in world candy consumption. Switzerland and the United Kingdom share in the top consumption of about 27.5 lb (*12.5 kg*) per person.

The U.S. Food and Drug Law requires that all candy be made with pure ingredients and nonpoisonous flavorings and colorings. In addition to the sugar(s) and syrups, candies may contain eggs, fats, gelatin, gums, lecithin, milk products, cooked starches, and every kind of fruit, nut, or flavoring. Although these are all good, wholesome food ingredients, the high sugar content makes candy less desirable for consumption in large amounts. Candy should be eaten very sparingly and is not recommended as a source of quick energy. A much more desirable food for quick energy is fresh fruit. In addition to the fact that sugar is being increasingly incriminated in the degenerative diseases, there is also the well-documented fact that sugar produces tooth decay. So a *sweet tooth* may eventually mean *no teeth*.

CANE SUGAR

Table sugar—sucrose—recovered from the juice of the sugarcane plant.
(Also see SUGAR, section headed "Sugarcane.")

CANKER

A small ulcer in the mouth around the lips, which may be due to a virus or to digestive disorders.

CANOLA (RAPE)

Canola was created from selected rape by Canadian scientists in the 1970s. In comparison with rape seeds, canola seed is lower in glucosinolates and erucic acid (a long-chain fatty acid).
(Also see RAPE.)

CANTALOUPE (MUSKMELON) *Cucumis melo*

The cantaloupe (muskmelon) belongs to the gourd family, *Cucurbitaceae*.

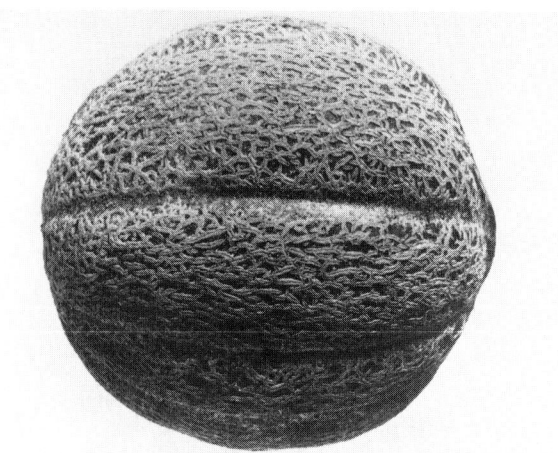

Fig. C-19. A cantaloupe, also called muskmelon. The edible, juicy pulp is 6 to 8% sugar when ripe and is encased in a hard netted rind. Cantaloupe belong to the same family as cucumbers, squash, pumpkins, gourds, and watermelons. (Courtesy, USDA)

True cantaloupes are seldom grown in the United States. Correctly speaking, the term *cantaloupe* should be applied only to a rough, scaly fruit with deep vein tracts, grown in Europe and Asia. These true cantaloupe bear the scientific name of *Cucumis melo*, variety *cantalupensis*. In the United States, the term cantaloupe is applied to melons with the scientific name *Cucumis melo*, variety *reticulatus*, which are more correctly muskmelons. Herein, the term *cantaloupe* is used to refer to the familiar fruit with a yellowish-brown, netted rind and orange pulp, and with seeds attached to a netlike fiber in a central hollow. Ripe cantaloupe have a distinctive sweet flavor and a musky odor. The plant producing cantaloupe is an annual trailing vine with 3 to 5 runners that may reach 10 to 12 ft (*3 to 3.6 m*) in length, with lobed leaves and small yellow flowers.

ORIGIN AND HISTORY. The place of origin of cantaloupe is lost in antiquity. Some experts believe that the cantaloupe was first grown in India. Others feel that it originated in Africa. Wild plants have never been discovered with certainty anywhere.

WORLD AND U.S. PRODUCTION. A world total of about 9.5 million metric tons of cantaloupes is produced annually; and the leading producing countries, by rank, are: China, Spain, United States, Egypt, Iran, Japan, and Mexico.[6]

About 735 thousand metric tons of cantaloupes are produced annually in the United States. Most of the U.S. commercial crop is produced in California, Arizona, and Texas.[7]

PROCESSING. Most cantaloupes are consumed as fresh fruit. The only processed product of any significance is frozen cantaloupe balls. These are processed by (1) washing and sorting, (2) cutting into halves, (3) removing seeds, (4) scooping out round balls, and (5) freezing in a sugar syrup. Melon balls may be frozen as only cantaloupe or as a mixture of cantaloupe, watermelon, or honeydew.

SELECTION, PREPARATION, AND USES. Cantaloupe should be mature and ripe. There are three major signs of full maturity: (1) no stem, with a smooth, symmetrical, shallow basin (*full slip*) at the point of the stem attachment; (2) thick, coarse and corky netting or veining, which stands out in bold relief over some part of the surface; and (3) yellowish-buff, yellowish-gray, or pale yellow skin color (ground color) between the netting.

For fresh consumption, cantaloupes are halved and the seeds are scooped out. They may be served in the rind, or they may be cut into smaller sections and the rind removed before serving.

Cantaloupes are enjoyed alone as a breakfast fruit or a dessert. Also, cantaloupe can be used in a variety of fruit dishes and salads. It is good with a scoop of ice cream, too.

NUTRITIONAL VALUE. The sweetness of cantaloupe is attributed to the 6 to 8% sugar it contains, but the water content is around 90% so each 100 g (about $3\frac{1}{2}$ oz of cantaloupe contains only 30 Calories (kcal). The salmon-colored flesh is an excellent source of vitamin A, containing about 3,400 IU per 100 g, and a good source of potassium, vitamin C, and bioflavonoids. Additional details of the nutritive value of cantaloupe are listed in Food Composition Table F-21.

CAPE GOOSEBERRY *Physalis peruviansa*

Fruit of a perennial shrub (of the family *Solanaceae*) that is native to the American tropics, and is closely related to the ground cherry and the strawberry tomato, and more distantly related to the common tomato (*Lycopersicon esculentum*). It is called the Cape gooseberry because it had become an important fruit on the Cape of Good Hope by the end of the 18th century.

The husk-covered yellow berries, which resemble gooseberries, but are not related to them, are about ½ in. (*1 to 2 cm*) in diameter and have a slightly acid flavor.

The fruits are usually stewed or made into preserves. Raw Cape gooseberries are moderately high in calories (73 kcal per 100 g) and carbohydrates (20%). They are a good source of fiber, iron, vitamin A, and vitamin C.

CAPER *Capparis spinosa* L.

The caper bush is a spiny, straggling, vine-like shrub, up to 3 ft high, with round to ovate, deciduous leaves. The buds are pickled in strong vinegar and used as pickles or in sauce.

CAPILLARIES

The tiny blood vessels which (1) deliver fresh, oxygenated blood from the arteries to the tissues; and (2) carry used, deoxygenated blood from the tissues to the veins.

CAPILLARY EXCHANGE MECHANISM

This is the process that controls the movement of water and small molecules in solution (electrolytes, nutrients) between the capillaries and the surrounding interstitial area.

CAPILLARY RESISTANCE TEST

A test which determines the ability of capillaries to resist breaking down and producing small hemorrhages under the skin. Usually, pressure is applied to the arm and the number of minute blood spots in the skin due to ruptured capillaries are noted. A lowering of capillary resistance is suspected as being due to deficiencies of vitamin C and other nutrients such as the bioflavonoids.

(Also see BIOFLAVONOIDS; and VITAMIN C.)

CAPRIC ACID ($CH_3[CH_2]_8COOH$)

A fatty acid, which is so named because in pure form it has a goatlike smell. (The Latin name for goat is *caper*.) Capric acid is found in coconut oil, cow's milk, and goat's milk. It is a short-chain fatty acid containing only ten carbon atoms, and it is very well absorbed and utilized by the body.

(Also see FATS AND OTHER LIPIDS.)

CAPROIC ACID; HEXANOIC ACID ($CH_3[CH_2]_4COOH$)

A naturally occurring saturated fatty acid normally found as a triglyceride in cow and goat butter, and in coconut and palm oils.

(Also see FATS AND OTHER LIPIDS.)

CAPRYLIC ACID; OCTANOIC ACID ($CH_3[CH_2]_6COOH$)

A naturally occurring rancid-tasting saturated fatty acid found in butter (cow and goat) and coconut oil and used as an intermediary in the manufacture of perfumes and dyes.

(Also see FATS AND OTHER LIPIDS.)

CARAMBOLA *Averrhoa carambola*

The fruit of a tree (of the family *Oxalidaceae*) that grows wild in Indonesia and other tropical areas.

Carambola fruit is yellow when ripe, from 3 to 5 in. (*8*

---

[6]Based on data from *FAO Production Yearbook 1990*, FAO/UN, Rome, Italy, Vol. 44, p. 151, Table 64. **Note well:** Annual production fluctuates as a result of weather and profitability of the crop.

[7]*Ibid.*

to 12 cm) long and from 1 to 3 in. *(3 to 6 cm)* in diameter, with a star-shaped cross section. It may be used fresh, or made into jam, jelly, juice, or tarts.

CARBOHYDRASES

A general name for all of the enzymes which act on complex carbohydrate molecules and break them down into smaller, simple molecules such as dextrins and sugars.

(Also see CARBOHYDRATE[S].)

CARBOHYDRATE(S)

The carbohydrates are organic compounds composed of carbon (C), hydrogen (H), and oxygen (O). They are one of three main classes of foods essential to the body; the others are proteins and fats.

No appreciable amount of carbohydrate is found in the animal body at any one time, the blood supply being held rather constant at about 0.05 to 0.1% for most animals. However, this small quantity of glucose in the blood, which is constantly replenished by changing the glycogen of the liver back to glucose, serves as the chief source of fuel with which to maintain the body temperature and to furnish the energy needed for all body processes. The storage of glycogen (so-called animal starch) in the liver amounts to 3 to 7% of the weight of that organ.

HISTORY. Long before anything was known about the chemical nature or the formation of carbohydrates, primitive people made good use of them. They lived on carbohydrates—they ate what fruits, seeds, and roots they could find. They fueled their fires with them. They fermented them. They fed them to their animals. They built with them. They wrote about them.

Considering all of the uses made of carbohydrates of many kinds, they are truly an important and versatile group of chemicals. Furthermore, they will continue to be important in the future since their formation relies on the ultimate source of all energy—the sun, through the process known as photosynthesis.

(Also see PHOTOSYNTHESIS.)

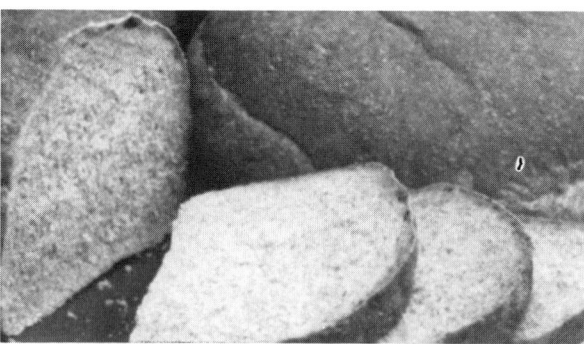

Fig. C-20. Wheat bread. Wheat is the leading source of carbohydrates in the American diet. (Courtesy, National Film Board of Canada)

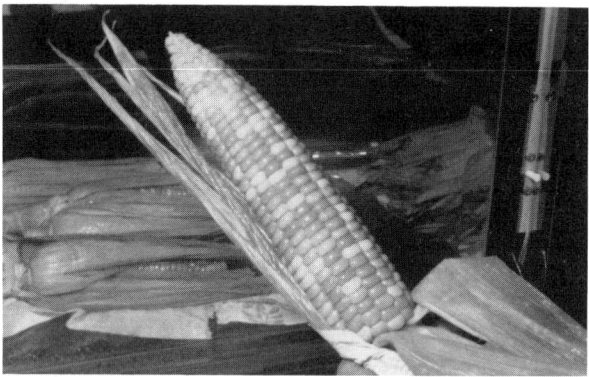

Fig. C-21. Corn ranks second to wheat as the leading source of carbohydrates in the American diet. Shown above: Sweetcorn going into the microwave oven. (Courtesy, University of Minnesota, St. Paul, Minn.)

CLASSIFICATION. Carbohydrates are extremely abundant in plants, occurring in a wide variety of forms. Table C-6 lists the types of carbohydrates that are commonly found in nature.

Monosaccharides. The term *saccharide* is derived from the Latin word *Saccharum,* meaning sugar. Monosaccharides, or single sugars, are seldom found free in nature. Rather, they constitute the building blocks of more complex carbohydrate molecules. Simple sugars are classified as to the number of carbon atoms within the molecule. For example, a triose is a sugar containing 3 carbons, and a tetrose is a 4-carbon molecule. While monosaccharides of various lengths are integral to the metabolism of carbohydrates, the pentoses (5-carbon sugars) and hexoses (6-carbon sugars) are of paramount importance. Furthermore, there are some derivatives of these monosaccharides which are also important—the sugar alcohols, amino sugars, and sugar acids.

PENTOSES (5-Carbon Sugars). Very limited amounts of this type of sugar are found in a free form in plants. All pentoses have the same chemical formula, $C_5H_{10}O_5$, but a slightly different structure.

TABLE C-6
CLASSIFICATION OF CARBOHYDRATES

Monosaccharides		Oligosaccharides[1]			Polysaccharides		
Pentoses $(C_5H_{10}O_5)$	Hexoses $(C_6H_{12}O_6)$	Disaccharides $(C_{12}H_{22}O_{11})$	Trisaccharides $(C_{18}H_{32}O_{16})$	Tetrasaccharides $(C_{24}H_{42}O_{21})$	Pentosans $(C_5H_8O_4)n^2$	Hexosans $(C_6H_{10}O_5)n^2$	Mixed Polysaccharides
Arabinose Ribose Xylose	Fructose Galactose Glucose (Dextrose) Mannose	Lactose Maltose Sucrose Trehalose	Maltotriose Melezitose Raffinose	Stachyose Maltotetrose	Araban Xylan	Cellulose Dextrins Glycogen Inulin Mannan Starch (amylose and amylopectin)	Agar Alginic acid Carrageenan Chitin Hemicelluloses Pectin Vegetable gums
Derivatives of monosaccharides: Sugar alcohols Amino sugars Sugar acids							

[1]Includes compounds that may be 2 to 10 sugar units.

[2]The "n" indicates any number of sugar units greater than 10.

Generally, pentoses are polymerized (combined chemically into very large molecules) to form pentosans. Arabinose is a 5-carbon sugar found in large amounts in gums. When a number of arabinose molecules are linked together, the pentosan, araban, is formed.

Ribose plays a major role in many physiological systems. When it is joined with pyrimidines and purines, nucleosides are formed. When phosphoric acid is esterified with the nucleosides, nucleotides are formed. These compounds are then used in the formation of ribonucleic acid (RNA) and deoxyribonucleic acid (DNA). The nucleotides of adenosine monophosphate (AMP), adenosine disphosphate (ADP), and adenosine triphosphate (ATP) are compounds that are essential to cellular energy metabolism. Ribose is also a constituent of the vitamin riboflavin.

Xylose is a pentose produced upon the hydrolysis—breakdown—a number of roughages and woody material. When polymerized, xylose forms the pentosan xylan.

HEXOSES (6-Carbon Sugars). Four hexoses are found in physiological systems: fructose, galactose, glucose, and mannose. All hexoses have the same chemical formula, $C_6H_{12}O_6$, but a slightly different structure. In nature, only two—fructose and glucose—occur in free form. Galactose, together with glucose, forms the disaccharide, lactose, or milk sugar. Mannose is found in the polysaccharide mannan.

DERIVATIVES OF MONOSACCHARIDES. Some of the monosaccharides possess a slightly altered chemical structure yielding sugar alcohols, amino sugars, and sugar acids. Mannose is not found free in food, but it is a component of some glycoproteins and mucoproteins of the body.

Sugar Alcohols. Monosaccharides reduced by having a hydroxyl group (OH) replace the aldehyde or ketone group (C = O) are known as sugar alcohols. One of these alcohols, glycerol, is important in the metabolic process, while other sugar alcohols such as galactitol, inositol, mannitol, sorbitol, and xylitol, are present in some foods.

Amino Sugars. The amino sugars have an amino (NH_2) group substituted for a hydroxyl (OH) group. More than 60 of these have been identified. Possibly these sugars give antibiotics their activity. Two important representatives are galactosamine and glucosamine.

Sugar Acids. These compounds contain an acid group (COOH) in their chemical structure. Familiar sugar acids are gluconic acid, gluconolactone, glucuronic acid, and ascorbic acid (vitamin C).

Oligosaccharides. The prefix oligo means *few*. Oligosaccharides contain 2 to 10 monosaccharides chemically bonded. Most oligosaccharides result from the partial breakdown of polysaccharides. The three most important oligosaccharides are all disaccharides—lactose, maltose, and sucrose. In 1990, the per capita consumption of sucrose in the United States was 64.2 lb (*29 kg*).

DISACCHARIDES. Disaccharides are compound sugars composed of two monosaccharides (see Table C-6). This group includes the first sugar eaten—lactose, and the sugar eaten to excess—sucrose.

(Also see MILK AND MILK PRODUCTS, Section headed "Carbohydrates in Milk"; and SUGAR.)

TRISACCHARIDES. Trisaccharides, 3-sugar polymers, are not abundant in nature, but two trisaccharides—melezitose and raffinose—are found in limited amounts in certain plants. Melezitose, a component of sap in some coniferous plants, contains 2 molecules of glucose and 1 of fructose. Raffinose, which is found in sugar beets, molasses, beans, and cottonseed meal, consists of glucose, fructose, and galactose. Enzymes of the digestive tract are not capable of splitting melezitose and raffinose into monosaccharides.

Maltotriose is a trisaccharide which is formed during the digestion of starch; it contains 3 glucose molecules which are eventually split and absorbed during the digestive processes.

TETRASACCHARIDES. Stachylose is a tetrasaccharide composed of 2 molecules of galactose, 1 molecule of glucose, and 1 molecule of fructose. Beans produce gas in the digestive tract—flatulence—due to microbial action on stachylose and raffinose which are not split into monosaccharides by enzymes of the digestive tract. Maltotetrose is formed during the digestion or breakdown of starch. It consists of four molecules of glucose, which the digestive enzymes of the body can break.

Polysaccharides. Polysaccharides are large sugar complexes that contain repeating sequences of simple sugars—chains of monosaccharides. In plants and animals they are used either for carbohydrate storage or structural support.

PENTOSANS. These polysaccharides yield pentose sugars upon hydrolysis—breakdown to individual sugars. Some common pentosans include araban, a chain of arabinose molecules; and xylan, a chain of xylose molecules. These pentosans are widely distributed plant polysaccharides.

HEXOSANS. Hexosans are polysaccharide sugars which contain hexoses as their respective repeating units.

Several polymers of glucose are found in plants or animals. The difference among the various compounds results from the linkages between the glucose molecules. The chief polymers—long chains—of glucose are cellulose, dextrins, glycogens, inulin, mannan, and starch.

MIXED POLYSACCHARIDES. A number of complex mixed polysaccharides are found in nature, many of them serving structural or protective functions. These include agar, alginic acid, carrageenan, chitin, hemicelluloses, pectins, and vegetable gums. Man has adapted some of these for use in foods as thickening and stabilizing agents.
(Also see ADDITIVES.)

DIGESTION, ABSORPTION, AND METABOLISM. The digestion of starch begins in the mouth and continues in the small intestine. Eventually, most all available carbohydrates are converted, by enzymes, to the monosaccharides galactose, glucose, and fructose, absorbed into the bloodstream and distributed to the tissues of the body. Metabolism of carbohydrates involves primarily glucose, which can be metabolized directly to yield energy or it can be stored as glycogen in the liver and muscle. Liver glycogen is used constantly to replenish blood glucose as it is depleted between meals. Excess glucose may also be stored as fat.
(Also see DIGESTION AND ABSORPTION; and METABOLISM.)

FUNCTIONS. Although carbohydrates comprise only about 1% of the human body, they now account for about 47% of the caloric intake of Americans.

Carbohydrates in the diet make the important contributions shown in Fig. C-22 and detailed in the sections which follow.

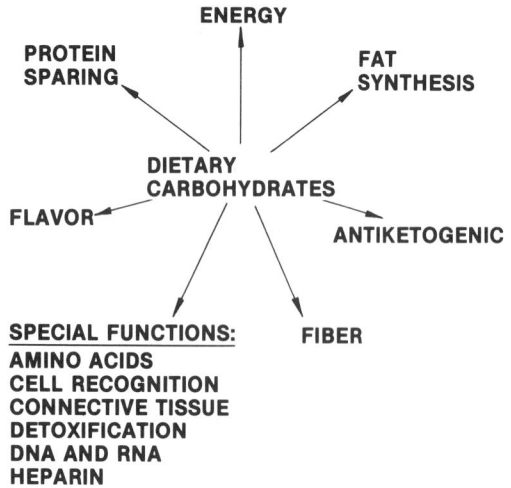

Fig. C-22. Functions of dietary carbohydrates.

Energy. Carbohydrates are the fuel of life. Each gram of carbohydrate provides about 4 Calories (kcal) of energy—the same as protein but less than fat. Following digestion and absorption, available carbohydrates may be (1) used to meet immediate energy needs of tissue cells, (2) converted

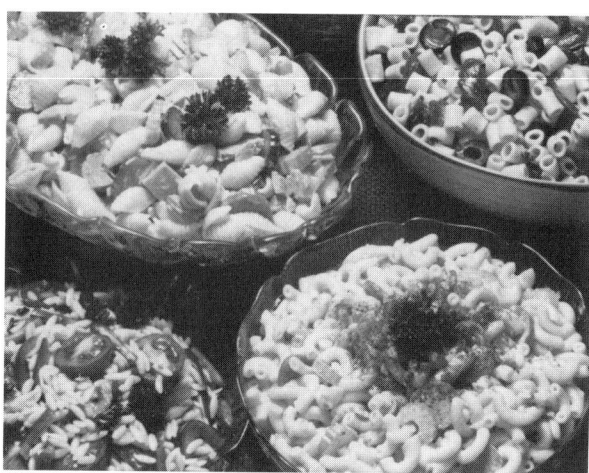

Fig. C-23. Carbohydrates are the fuel (energy) of life. A variety of carbohydrate dishes is shown above. (Courtesy, Hershey Foods Corp., Hershey, Pa.)

to glycogen and stored in the liver and muscle for later energy needs, or (3) converted to fat as a larger reserve for energy.

1. **Immediate energy.** Glucose can be used directly by all tissues of the body. However, about one-fifth of the basal metabolic rate is due to the brain. The major source of energy for the brain appears to be carbohydrate (glucose) since it does not possess any store or reserve of energy.

2. **Glycogen.** Although glycogen is a stored form of glucose, there is only enough glycogen stored in the body to meet about one half of a day's energy requirements. Furthermore, exercise such as a walk for 2 to 3 hours without food depletes the glycogen stores of the body. Glucose is released from liver glycogen when needed to maintain the blood glucose levels, while muscle glycogen is available for the energy needs of the muscle but is not available for the regulation of blood glucose. Glycogen storage and release are controlled by the hormones glucagon, insulin, and epinephrine.

3. **Fat.** Once the energy needs of the body have been fulfilled, excess carbohydrate is converted to fat and stored in adipose tissue. As many people can testify, this type of storage seems to be unlimited.
(Also see ENERGY UTILIZATION BY THE BODY.)

Protein Sparing Action. Meeting the energy needs of the body takes priority over other functions. Thus, any deficiency of energy will be made up by energy yielding reactions involving protein and adipose. When available carbohydrates are supplied in sufficient quantities by the diet, the body uses carbohydrates first as a source of energy. This spares protein for tissue building. Eating 50 to 100 g of digestible carbohydrate daily prevents the excessive breakdown of tissue protein. Most American diets include 200 to 300 g of carbohydrate daily.

Regulation of Fat Metabolism. If carbohydrate intake is very low, fats are not completely utilized. Fat metabolism occurs faster than the body can take care of the intermediate products of fat metabolism—ketones. As ketones accumulate, the individual is said to be in a state of ketosis. If the production of ketones goes unchecked, the serious condition of acidosis occurs. This can be prevented by the ingestion of a minimum of 50 to 100 g of digestible carbohydrate per day. Since the metabolism of adequate amounts of carbohydrate allows the ketone forming substances to be completely metabolized, carbohydrates are said to have an antiketogenic effect.

(Also see METABOLISM.)

Provide Fiber. Not all carbohydrates yield nutrients to the body. Cellulose, gums, hemicelluloses, pectins, and pentosans are such carbohydrates. Collectively, they are referred to as dietary fiber or roughage. These substances absorb water and lend bulk to the intestinal contents, thereby

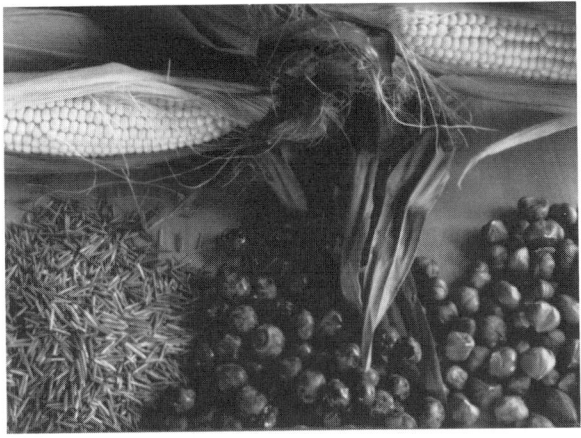

Fig. C-24. The Native Americans (Indians) ate a high-fiber diet, including corn, wild rice, blueberries, and hazel nuts. (Courtesy, University of Minnesota, St. Paul, Minn.)

stimulating the peristaltic movements of the digestive tract and reducing the passage time through the bowel. There is no metabolic requirement for fiber. Recently, much has been attributed to the amount of or lack of fiber in the diet; for example, (1) constipation, (2) diverticular disease, (3) irritable bowel syndrome, (4) bowel cancer, (5) inflammatory bowel disease, (6) atherosclerosis, (7) gallstones, (8) dental caries, (9) hemmorrhoids, and (10) ulcers.

Currently, it is not possible to recommend a specific intake of fiber; more research is needed. However, dramatic increases in dietary fiber should be avoided since the absorption of minerals may be reduced by high dietary fiber intakes. Moderate increases in the consumption of fiber can be easily achieved by increasing the consumption of nuts, vegetables, fruits, and whole grain cereal products. The fiber content of various foods is given in Food Composition Table F-21.

(Also see FIBER.)

Flavor. Foods are often accepted or rejected on the basis of their flavor. Some carbohydrates flavor food. Their flavor is interpreted by our taste buds as sweet, one of the four taste sensations. Sweeteners of any kind, whether nutritive or nonnutritive, are commonly compared to the carbohydrate, sucrose. Table S-18, in the section headed SWEETENING AGENTS, gives a comparison of the sweetness of some sweet-tasting substances to sucrose—table sugar.

(Also see ADDITIVES; SOFT DRINKS; SUGAR; SWEETENING AGENTS; and TASTE.)

Special Functions. Some carbohydrates and carbohydrate derivatives perform special duties in structure and function. These carbohydrates include (1) glucuronic acid which detoxifies chemicals and bacterial by-products, and inactivates hormones in the liver prior to their excretion; (2) hyaluronic acid and chondroitin sulfate which are components of connective tissue; (3) the compounds deoxyribonucleic acid (DNA) and ribonucleic acid (RNA) which possess and transfer genetic information; (4) heparin which prevents clotting of blood; (5) carbon skeletons for certain amino acids; (6) those which associate with lipids in nerve tissues; and (7) those which serve as biological markers and provide information for cell recognition and antigen antibody reactions of the immune system. A familiar example of the last special function is that the difference between blood type A and blood type B lies in a single sugar unit that sticks out from the end of a carbohydrate chain of a glycoprotein or glycolipid on the surface of the red blood cell. This small difference is sometimes a matter of life and death since using the wrong type of blood in a transfusion can have fatal results.

REQUIRED INTAKE. There is no specific dietary requirement for carbohydrate. Nonetheless, it is generally agreed that a reasonable proportion of the caloric intake should be derived from carbohydrates. A diet devoid of carbohydrates is likely to lead to ketosis, excessive breakdown of tissue protein, loss of cations—especially sodium, and involuntary dehydration. These effects, produced by high-fat diets or fasting, can be prevented by the ingestion of 50 to 100 g of digestible carbohydrate per day. However, intakes considerably above this minimal level are desirable. Foods such as fruits, vegetables, and whole-grain cereals provide energy principally from carbohydrates and are generally good sources of other nutrients such as vitamins and minerals.

SOURCES. The carbohydrate content of various foods is given in Food Composition Table F-21. No specific level of carbohydrate intake is most conducive to health. Furthermore, foods vary in their carbohydrate content, and the relative prominence of carbohydrate-rich foods in the diet varies widely in individuals, and in different parts of the world. A diet consisting of chiefly carbohydrate-rich foods need be no health hazard provided those foods are not lacking in proteins, minerals, and vitamins. In most cases, a country's staple food is its primary source of carbohydrate, and it must serve as the principal source of protein in poor countries. Total protein consumption and total calorie intake increase with income.

Plant. Plants provide the major source of carbohydrates. Among the plants, the cereal grains, fruits, nuts, and vegetables are the most important source of available carbohydrates for man. The total carbohydrate content of numerous foods is given in Food Composition Table F-21.

CEREAL GRAINS. Much of the world is dependent upon calories supplied by a single cereal staple which supplies carbohydrate in the form of starch. For example, in Afghanistan and Pakistan the staple is wheat, and in Mexico and Central America it is corn (maize). In China and southeastern Asia, regions of the world with the largest population, the staple is rice. Annually, world production of these three cereals dwarfs the production of all other plant foods. American diets derive carbohydrates from wheat, corn, and rice because they appear in so many forms. Other cereal grains include barley, millet, oats, rye, sorghum, and triticale. The grains and the products made from them have variable water content, with the result that their carbohydrate content ranges from 10 to 85%.

(Also see BARLEY; CEREAL GRAINS; CORN; MILLET; OATS; RICE; RYE; SORGHUM; TRITICALE; and WHEAT.)

FRUITS. Because of their high water content, fruits represent a less concentrated source of carbohydrates than cereals. In fresh fruits, the carbohydrate is mainly in the form of monosaccharides—glucose and fructose—and some disaccharide—sucrose. Canned fruits often contain added sucrose or glucose unless specifically labeled as being canned with no added sugar.

In fresh fruits, the sugar—availabale carbohydrate—content may range from about 6 to 25%. Cantaloupe and watermelon contain 3 to 7% while bananas contain about 20%. The degree of ripeness also influences the sugar content of fruits. Ripe fruits have a higher sugar content. Dried fruits possess a much higher sugar content. Dried dates, figs, raisins, prunes, and apricots may contain 50 to 90% sugar due to their low water content. Thus, the energy value of fruits, whether fresh or canned, is determined largely by their sugar (monosaccharide and disaccharide) content.

(Also see FRUIT[S]; and SUGAR.)

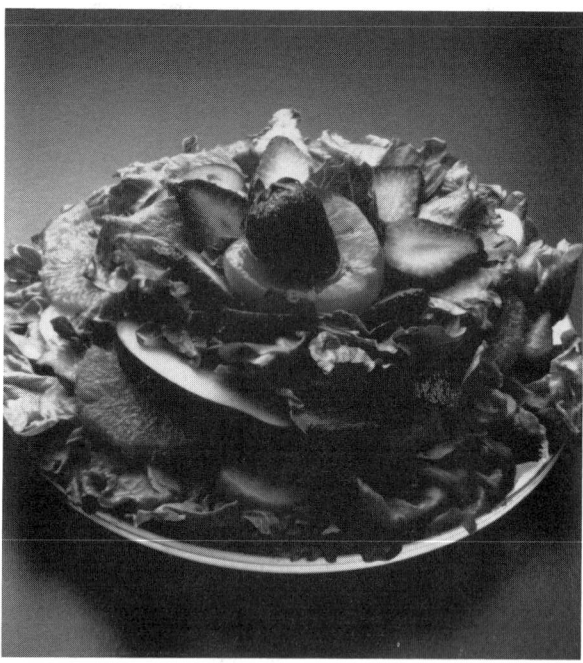

Fig. C-25. Fruit and vegetable salad, high in carbohydrates. (Courtesy, California Iceberg Lettuce Commission, Monterey, Calif.)

NUTS. Due to their low moisture content, nuts contain from 10 to 27% carbohydrate. Furthermore, nuts contain from 1 to 3% fiber. However, because of their high protein and high fat content, nuts are not usually thought of as a carbohydrate source.

(Also see NUT[S].)

VEGETABLES. Almost every part of the plant used for food—leaves, stems, seeds, seed pods, flowers, fruits, roots and tubers—has been grouped under the term vegetable. For this reason, the carbohydrate content of vegetables may range from 3 to 35%, and the carbohydrate may be present as starch, sugar, and fiber. Leaf, flower, and stem vegetables contain high levels of water and cellulose and few calories. The root, tuber, and seed vegetables have a high starch and sugar content and low water content, thus providing more calories per unit of weight. Freshly picked vegetables—sweet corn, young peas, and young carrots—contain more sugar and less starch than mature vegetables—just the opposite of fruits.

(Also see VEGETABLE[S].)

Animal. Most animal foods contain little, if any, carbohydrate. When an animal is slaughtered, the glycogen stored in the liver and muscles is rapidly broken down to lactic acid and pyruvic acid. Oysters and scallops may contain some glycogen but the amount is not significant to the diet. Milk is the only animal food, or at least the only animal-produced food, that is an important carbohydrate source. Milk provides the carbohydrate lactose or milk sugar.

(Also see MEAT[S]; and MILK AND MILK PRODUCTS.)

Other. Actually, the other sources of carbohydrate are plant sources. However, they represent an important, but rather specialized, source of carbohydrate. These consist of common table sugar, molasses, maple syrup and sugar, corn syrup, honey, and sorghum syrup. These sources of carbohydrate are extremely concentrated. They provide mainly calories and little else.

FERMENTATION. Many carbohydrate sources may be fermented; for example fruit juices, palm juice, cactus juice, molasses, sugar, honey, milk, potatoes, or cereal grains. Fermentation is the production of ethanol or ethyl alcohol by the action of yeast on carbohydrate as shown in Fig. C-26.

$$C_6H_{12}O_6 \xrightarrow{\text{YEAST}} 2C_2H_5OH + 2CO_2$$

HEXOSE (SUGAR)   **ETHYL ALCOHOL**   **CARBON DIOXIDE**

Fig. C-26. The action of yeast on sugar to produce ethyl alcohol—the alcohol of beers, distilled liquors and wine.

Throughout history, most cultures have learned to use and control the process of fermentation. Regardless of the carbohydrate source used, the ethanol produced is the same, while the taste may vary with the carbohydrate source. Hard liquors are those produced by distillation which concentrates the ethanol and separates it from the starting material. Beer and wine contain some of the nutrients present in the malted barley or fruit juice.

Alcohol contains calories. It is metabolized at a fixed rate in the liver and yields about 7 Calories (kcal) per gram. Therefore, the intake of alcoholic beverages must be accounted for when counting calories. When alcohol is consumed faster than can be metabolized, then the level of alcohol in the body tissues builds up and intoxication follows. Upon drinking, alcohol is rapidly absorbed from the stomach and the small intestine. It requires no digestion. Excessive drinking of alcoholic beverages creates many problems, one of which is low intake of minerals and vitamins. In many cases the calories of alcoholic drinks are empty calories. Furthermore, the evidence is mounting that any level of intake during pregnancy may be harmful to the developing child.

(Also see ALCOHOL AND ALCOHOLIC BEVERAGES; ALCOHOLISM AND ALCOHOLICS; BEERS AND BREWING; and DISTILLED LIQUORS.)

CARBOHYDRATE INTOLERANCE

A digestive disorder due to (1) the lack of one or more enzymes which digest carbohydrates, or (2) other conditions which prevent the absorption of certain sugars. The unabsorbed sugars provide nutrients for bacterial growth and have a laxative effect which often results in diarrhea.

CARBOHYDRATES, AVAILABLE

These are carbohydrates—products of photosynthesis—which provide nourishment to humans and other monogastric animals. They may be digested and absorbed. Included are the sugars, dextrins, and starches.

(Also see CARBOHYDRATE[S]; and DIGESTION AND ABSORPTION.)

CARBOHYDRATES, UNAVAILABLE

These are carbohydrates which do not provide nourishment to humans. Man and other monogastric animals lack the enzymes necessary to breakdown such carbohydrates as cellulose, hemicellulose, and pectin. Often these carbohydrates are referred to as dietary fiber or roughage. Because of the microbial action in the rumen, ruminant animals—cattle, sheep, and goats—can utilize carbohydrates that are unavailable to man and other monogastrics.

(Also see CARBOHYDRATE[S].)

CARBON DIOXIDE (CO₂)

A gas formed in the cells of the body during the production of energy by the metabolism of nutrients. It is carried in the blood to the lungs, where it is exhaled.

(Also see METABOLISM.)

CARBONIC ACID (H₂CO₃)

A weak acid formed by the reaction of carbon dioxide gas with water. Under certain conditions carbonic acid may release the bicarbonate ion which helps to maintain the neutrality of the blood and body fluids.

(Also see ACID-BASE BALANCE.)

CARBONIC ANHYDRASE

An enzyme which contains an atom of zinc in each molecule. It is present in various tissues, and in red blood cells, where, depending upon the circumstances, it promotes either (1) the formation of carbonic acid from carbon dioxide, or (2) the breakdown of carbonic acid to carbon dioxide and water. These reactions facilitate the picking up of carbon dioxide from the tissues by the red blood cells, and the transfer of carbon dioxide from the red blood cells to the lungs, where it is exhaled.

(Also see ACID-BASE BALANCE.)

CARBOXYLASE

A general term for an enzyme that promotes the breakdown of organic acids, such as amino acids, to carbon dioxide and compounds that contain fewer carbon atoms.

(Also see ENZYMES.)

CARBOXYMETHYL CELLULOSE (CMC) (SODIUM CARBOXYMETHYL CELLULOSE; CM CELLULOSE)

A preparation of cellulose, made from the pure cellulose of cotton or wood, which absorbs up to 50 times its weight of water to form a stable mass. Because of this unique characteristic, it is used as a whipping agent in confectioneries, jellies and ice cream, and as an inert food filler in slimming aids. Ethyl methyl cellulose and hydroxyethyl-cellulose are examples of other cellulose derivatives with similar properties.

CARBOXYPEPTIDASE

A digestive enzyme secreted by the pancreas via the pancreatic juice into the small intestine where it digests protein.

(Also see DIGESTION AND ABSORPTION.)

CARCASS

The body of an animal without the viscera, and usually without the head, skin, and/or lower legs.

CARCINOGEN

Any cancer-producing substance or agent.
(Also see CANCER.)

CARCINOGENIC

Cancer producing.

CARDIA

• The heart.

• The region extending from the lower portion of the esophagus to the upper part of the stomach.

Hence, pains coming from the region under the breastbone may originate from (1) the heart or (2) the digestive tract. Therefore, a heart attack may be mistaken for indigestion, or vice versa.

(Also see DIGESTION AND ABSORPTION; and HEART DISEASE.)

CARDIAC

A term which refers to the heart.

CARDIOSPASM

• A fluctuation in the beating of the heart.

• A spasm occurring anywhere between the lower portion of the esophagus and the upper part of the stomach.

CARDIOVASCULAR

Relating to or involving the heart and blood vessels.
(Also see HEART DISEASE.)

CARDIOVASCULAR DISEASE

A general term which is used to denote a large number of disorders that affect the heart and/or the blood vessels. The disorders which are most common are atherosclerosis, heart disease, high blood pressure, and stroke. Currently, there is a tendency to attribute these disorders to faulty diets. However, nondietary factors may be responsible for many cases of cardiovascular disease.

(Also see HEART DISEASE; and HIGH BLOOD PRESSURE.)

CARDOON (CARDON) *Cynara cardunculus*

A large thistlelike plant related to the artichoke, the blanched leaves and stalks and the thick main roots of which are used as food.

CARIOGENIC AGENT

A food, or a food ingredient, which promotes the formation of dental caries.

(Also see DENTAL HEALTH, NUTRITION, AND DIET.)

CARMINATIVE

A substance that helps in the expulsion of gas from the stomach or intestine, or prevents the formation of gas.

(Also see DIGESTION AND ABSORPTION.)

CARNITINE (VITAMIN B$_T$)

Carnitine, a vital coenzyme in animal tissues and involved in fat metabolism, is a vitaminlike substance that has received much attention recently. It is similar to a vitamin with the exception that under normal conditions higher animals synthesize their total requirement within their bodies; hence, it is unnecessary to supply this substance in food on a daily basis. However, recent studies suggest (1) that synthesis of body carnitine may be inadequate for some individuals, and (2) that a number of diseases alter levels of carnitine in body fluids and tissues. This prompts two questions: (1) Are carnitine needs met adequately by body synthesis to assure buoyant good health; and (2) what role, if any, does carnitine play in certain diseases?

HISTORY. Carnitine was first isolated from meat extract in 1905, but its structure was not established until 1927. Then, another 20 years elapsed before Fraenkel, in 1947, while investigating the role of folic acid in the nutrition of insects, found that the meal worm *(Tenebrio molitor)* required a growth factor present in yeast. Frankel called this factor *Vitamin B$_T$*; vitamin B because of its water-soluble property, and the T standing for *Tenebrio*. Because of not being recognized as a vitamin, the name was subsequently changed to carnitine.

CHEMISTRY, METABOLISM, PROPERTIES.

• **Chemistry**—Carnitine has the following molecular structure:

$$(CH_3)_3 \ N\text{-}CH_2\text{-}CH\text{-}CH_2\text{-}COOH$$
$$\overset{|}{O}H$$

• **Metabolism**—Like the water-soluble vitamins, it is believed that carnitine is easily and rather completely absorbed. However, the form of carnitine (free or esterified) which is absorbed, the exact mechanism of absorption across the mucosa, and the site of the absorption are unknown.

It is not known how carnitine is transported in the blood from the gut to tissues.

In addition to being obtained from food, carnitine is synthesized in the liver.

In the rat, the highest concentrations of carnitine are found in the adrenal gland, followed by the heart, skeletal muscle, adipose tissue, and liver. Smaller concentrations are found in the kidney and brain. In humans, skeletal muscle has about 40 times the concentration of carnitine found in the blood.

Free carnitine is excreted in the urine.

• **Properties**—Carnitine is very hygroscopic (it absorbs water readily), and is easily soluble in water and ethanol.

MEASUREMENT/ASSAY. Several different assay procedures for determining the carnitine content of foods and tissues have been developed, but the two most common methods are: (1) bioassay, based on the growth or survival of meal worm *(Tenebrio molitor)* larvae; and (2) enzymatic techniques. Comparisons of carnitine values between studies are made difficult by lack of uniformity of assay procedures.

FUNCTIONS. Carnitine plays an important role in fat metabolism and energy production in mammals. It functions as follows:

1. **Transport and oxidation of fatty acids.** Carnitine plays an important role in the oxidation of fatty acids by facilitating their transport across the mitochondrial membrane.

Carnitine is part of the shuttle mechanism whereby long-chain fatty acids are made into acyl carnitine derivatives and transported across the mitochondrial membrane, which is impermeable to long-chain fatty acids *per se* and to their coenzyme A esters. Once across the membrane, the acyl carnitines are reconverted to their fatty acid CoA form and undergo beta-oxidation to liberate energy.

2. **Fat synthesis.** Although this role is controversial, carnitine appears to be involved in transporting acetyl groups back to the cytoplasm for fatty acid synthesis.

3. **Ketone body utilization.** Carnitine stimulates acetoacetate oxidation; thus, it may play a role in ketone body utilization.

Currently, the main emphasis of research is on the role of carnitine in fatty acid oxidation. Carnitine metabolism is being studied with increasing frequency (1) where there are changes in fat catabolism with changes in physiological state (fasting, exercise, extensive burns, pregnancy, cold adaptation), or (2) where there is disease (hyperthyroidism or hypothyroidism, diabetes, muscle fat storage disease, atherosclerosis, etc.).

DEFICIENCY SYMPTOMS. If carnitine is to be considered an essential dietary nutrient, it must be possible to show that a lack in the diet results in a reproducible deficiency disease in humans. To date, carnitine has not met this criterion.

RECOMMENDED DAILY ALLOWANCE OF CARNITINE. Under normal conditions, there is no dietary requirement for carnitine. However, where a metabolic abnormality exists which inhibits synthesis, interferes with use, or increases catabolism of carnitine, illness may follow, which is sometimes relieved by dietary supplement.

There is need for further research on the dietary role of carnitine in human health and disease.

CARNITINE LOSSES DURING PROCESSING, COOKING, AND STORAGE.
Since carnitine is water-soluble, cooking procedures using moist-heat methods will likely result in loss of free carnitine.

SOURCES OF CARNITINE.
Generally speaking, carnitine is high in animal foods and low in plant foods. Few foods have been assayed for carnitine, but, based on available data, the sources of carnitine given in the section on VITAMIN(S),Table V-5, Vitamin Table, may be helpful.

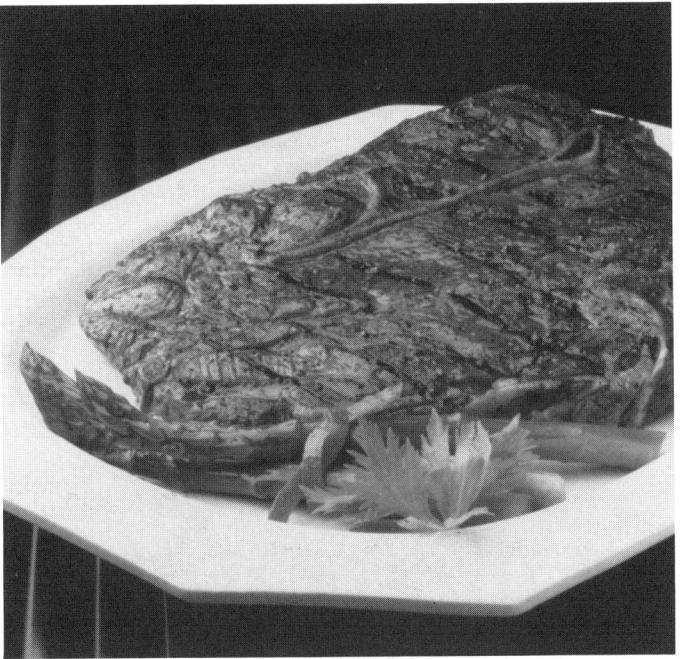

Fig. C-27. Steak, a muscle meat, a source of carnitine. (Courtesy, National Live Stock and Meat Board, Chicago, Ill.)

The lower level of carnitine in plant foods in comparison with animal foods is explainable on the basis that plant materials are most likely deficient in the essential amino acids, lysine and methionine, precursors of carnitine. Thus, a vegetarian diet will likely be low in carnitine, in both preformed carnitine and the amino acid precursors of carnitine.

Man and other higher animals appear to be able to synthesize their total needs within the body. But the mechanism of carnitine synthesis in humans is unknown. Very likely, carnitine is synthesized in humans from lysine and methionine—two essential amino acids which are low in plant foods.

(Also see VITAMIN[S], Table V-5.)

CAROTENE

This is the counterpart of vitamin A, found in fruits and vegetables. Since the animal body transforms carotene into vitamin A, it is often referred to as *provitamin A.*

Carotene derives its name from the carrot, from which it was first isolated 100 years ago. It is the yellow-colored, fat-soluble substance that gives the characteristic color to carrots and butter.

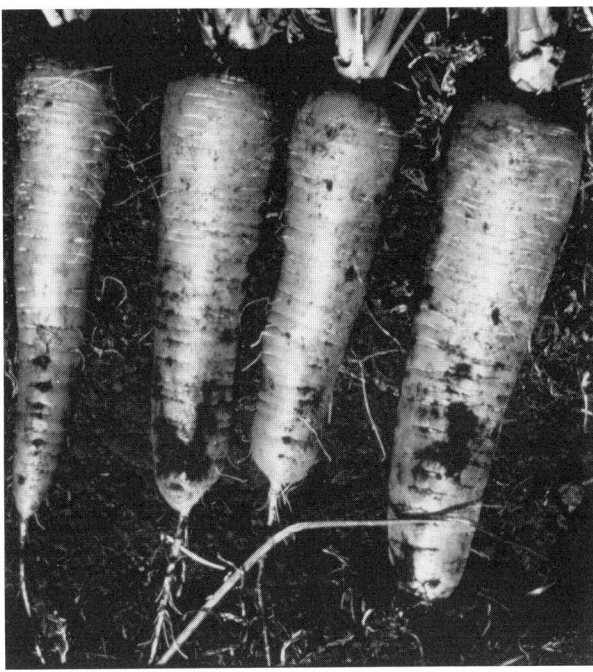

Fig. C-28. Carotene derives its name from carrots from which it was first isolated. (Courtesy, USDA)

Several of the cartenoids found in plants can be converted with varying efficiencies to vitamin A. Of the group, beta-carotene has the highest vitamin A activity.

Different species of animals convert beta-carotene to vitamin A with varying degrees of efficiency. The conversion rate of the rat is used as the standard value, with 1 mg of beta-carotene equal to 1,667 IU of vitamin A. Man is only one-third as efficient as the rat in making the conversion—1 mg of beta-carotene being equal to only 556 IU of vitamin A.

(Also see VITAMIN A.)

CAROTENEMIA

A yellowish discoloration of the skin, which appears first on the palms of the hand and the soles of the feet. It is due to a heavy consumption of food rich in carotene. It may sometimes be mistaken for jaundice. However, carotenemia differs from jaundice in that the whites of the eyes and the urine are not discolored.

CAROTENOID PIGMENTS

A group of substances with yellow, orange, and red colors. Many of the pigments have vitamin A activity. They are present in a wide variety of fruits and vegetables.

(Also see VITAMIN A.)

CARRAGEENAN

This naturally occurring food gum is obtained from several related species of red seaweed (algae), of which the best known is *Chondrus crispus,* or Irish moss. These algae are found along the Atlantic coasts of Europe and North America. The seaweed and its gums were first exploited on a commercial basis by the people who lived in the vicinity of Carragheen, !reland; hence, the names Carrageenan and Irish moss.

Chondrus crispus is mostly reddish-brown, but it also has hues of green, purple, and black. Although a cluster of these plants looks like a bed of moss when viewed from a distance, a closer look reveals a mass of short, flat, branching stems which are attached to underwater rocks.

SPECIAL PROPERTIES OF THE DIFFERENT TYPES OF CARRAGEENAN.

Most commercial carrageenan is derived form the algae species of *Chondrus, Gigartina, Eucheuma, Irideae,* and *Hypnea.* The characteristics of a batch of the commercial gum depend upon the species of seaweed used as a source, because there are three types of naturally occurring carrageenan molecules present in varying proportions in the different algae. These giant molecules have molecular weights ranging fom 100,000 to 500,000, and are polysaccharides made up of chains of galactose (a 6-carbon sugar like glucose) units. Some of the galactose units have attached sulfate groups, while others are unsulfated. The three types of gum molecule are designated as iota, kappa, or lambda carrageenan. They differ by (1) the types of linkages between the galactose units, and (2) the points of attachment of the sulfate groups to the galactose units. These small differences in chemical constitution and structure make major differences in the properties of each type of molecule. Therefore, a food technologist should know the makeup of his batch of carrageenan so that he may obtain the desired properties in his products.

USES OF CARRAGEENAN IN FOODS.

Most of the food applications of carrageenans are concerned with gelling, thickening, and/or prevention of separation (stabilization) of food mixtures. Some of these applications follow:

• **Batters, doughs, and pastas**—Strengthening of proteins in flour by carrageenan results in (1) better batters for coating chicken and fish prior to frying, (2) elimination of shrinkage in breads due to the addition of nonfat dry milk, and (3) greater resistance of spaghetti to breakdown during cooking.

• **Dairy products**—Carrageenan prevents separation of the fat, protein, and water phases during the processing of milk, and imparts smoothness and a sensation of richness to cheeses, ice creams, and eggless (blanc mange) milk puddings. It even gives evaporated skim milk a consistency like that of cream.

• **Fish, meat, and poultry**—These products may be protected from spoilage during shipment by antibiotic ice containing carrageenan as a stabilizer. Also, the canned products may be cushioned against breakage during transit by carrageenan gels which, unlike gelatin, do not melt at room temperature.

• **Fruit products**—The addition of carrageenan to the packing syrup prior to the freezing of fruits results in better quality of the fruits upon thawing. Carrageenan may be substituted for some or all of the pectin in jams and jellies, particularly in the low-caloric types where pectin is not an effective jelling agent because the sugar content is drastically reduced.

• **Gelled desserts**—Mixtures of carrageenan and carob (locust bean) gum may be used for clear fruit gels which do not melt or soften at room temperature. Also, the viscous solutions of the gums keep fruit ingredients suspended until gelling has occurred.

• **Relishes, salad dressings, and sauces**—Relishes retain water better when carrageenan is used in the recipe. Also, salad dressings and sauces may be stabilized by carrageenan. However, care must be taken to prevent degradation of carrageenan during the processing of acidic sauces. Whenever possible, acidic ingredients should be added after heating.

• **Special dietary products**—Carrageenan is nonnutritive, so it may be used in low-caloric recipes in place of emulsifiers, thickeners, and stabilizers, such as egg, flour, and lecithin.

(Also see ADDITIVES, FOOD; and SEAWEED [KELP].)

CARRIER

• A substance that carries one or more nutrients, such as the carrying of fat-soluble vitamins by fat.

• A filler material which is mixed with some of the minerals and/or vitamins required in a diet. The mix, which is sometimes called a premix, makes it easier to measure the correct amounts of the trace nutrients providing that they are homogenously distributed in the carrier material.

• An animal, or a person that carries and transmits disease-germs, but does not show any signs of a disease.

CARROT *Dacus carota*

The edible roots of this plant are one of the world's leading vegetable crops. They are also the richest source of vitamin A among the commonly-used vegetables. Carrots are a member of the parsley family (*Umbelliferae*) of plants. Other well-known members of this family are caraway, celery, dill, fennel, parsley, and parsnips.

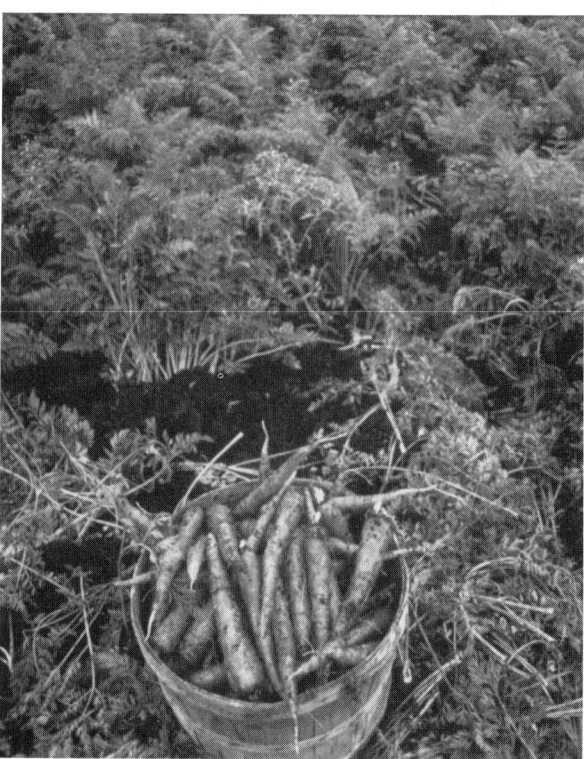

Fig. C-29. A field of carrots at harvest time. (Courtesy, National Film Board of Canada)

ORIGIN AND HISTORY. Carrots are believed to have originated in the Near East and central Asia, where they were cultivated for thousands of years. However, the ancient ancestors of this vegetable were not yellow-orange—they were purplish, ranging from lavender to almost black. Apparently, the yellow roots arose from a mutant variety which lacked the purple pigment.

WORLD AND U.S. PRODUCTION. Carrots rank eighth among the vegetable crops of the world, and seventh among the vegetable crops of the United States.

Worldwide, about 13.4 million metric tons are produced annually; and the leading carrot-producing countries, by rank, are: China, United States, Poland, Japan, France, United Kingdom, and Germany.[8]

About 1.5 million short tons of carrots are produced annually in the United States, of which California alone produces 869,550 short tons, which is about 59% of the U.S. crop.[9]

PROCESSING. A little less than half of the U.S. carrot crop is processed. The leading type of processing is freezing (over 148,000 metric tons annually), followed by canning. However, there is a steadily growing utilization of dehydration and juice production.

SELECTION, PREPARATION, AND USES. Carrots of good quality are firm, fresh, smooth, well-shaped, and generally well-colored.

The mild, sweet flavor of carrots blends well with those of many other foods. Hence, this vegetable enhances a wide variety of mixed dishes.

Grated raw carrots may be (1) added to salads made predominantly from fruits such as chopped apples, pineapple slices and raisins; (2) used in vegetable salads along with raw cabbage, chopped celery, hard-boiled eggs, sliced onions, and chopped green peppers; (3) mixed with peanut butter to make a filling for sandwiches; (4) baked in a carrot cake; or (5) combined with eggs, bread crumbs or flour, milk or water, and grated onions, then formed into patties and fried.

Cooked carrots are often used in casseroles, soups, and stews. However, they are also good when boiled and served with butter, margarine, or a special sauce.

Pureed cooked carrots may be used in cookies, puddings, and souffles. (Baby food purees may be convenient to use when only small amounts of carrot puree are needed.)

Candied or glazed carrots are prepared by steaming whole carrots briefly, cooling, scrubbing off the skin with a stiff brush, and simmering the scrubbed roots in a mixture of melted butter or margarine, brown sugar or orange marmalade, salt, and pepper.

Carrot pickles are prepared by soaking the briefly steamed and deskinned vegetables in a mixture of vinegar, water, sugar, and seasonings.

NUTRITIONAL VALUE. The nutrient compositions of various forms of carrots are given in Food Composition Table F-21.

---

[8]Based on data from *FAO Production Yearbook 1990*, FAO/UN, Rome, Italy, Vol. 44, p. 147, Table 62. **Note well:** Annual production fluctuates as a result of weather and profitability of the crop.

[9]Based on data from *Agricultural Statistics 1991*, USDA, p. 149, Table 207. **Note well:** Annual production fluctuates as a result of weather and profitability of the crop.

Some noteworthy observations regarding the nutrient composition of carrots follow:

1. Most forms of carrots are high in water content (88 to 92%) and low in calories (29 to 42 kcal per 100 g). However, they are excellent sources of vitamin A, since a 3½ oz *(100 g)* serving provides more than double the Recommended Dietary Allowance (RDA) for adults.

2. Baby food purees and cooked carrots furnish only ⅔ of the calories supplied by raw carrots and carrot juice. The former items have a higher water content than the latter ones.

3. Dehydrated carrots furnish almost as many calories and about ¾ of the protein supplied by dried forms of corn and rice. It is noteworthy that each ounce *(28 g)* of this product also provides about ¼ of the calcium and phosphorus content of a cup *(240 ml)* of milk and almost 6 times the RDA for vitamin A. Hence, dehydrated carrots may be added to various dishes to increase their nutritional values.

CARTILAGE

The gristle or connective tissue attached to the ends of bones.

CASAL'S NECKLACE

A sunburnlike rash seen around the collar where the neck is exposed to the sun. These lesions are characteristic of severe niacin deficiency or pellagra. Apparently this deficiency makes the skin extra sensitive to the sun.

(Also see NIACIN; and PELLAGRA.)

CASSAVA (TAPIOCA; MANIOC; YUCCA)
Manihot esculenta

This is a small tropical shrub, the roots of which are eaten or used to make tapioca. Cassava belongs to the same family (*Euphorbiaceae*) as the tung tree (noted for its oil-bearing nuts), rubber tree, and castor bean. There are two main kinds of cassava—bitter cassava (*Manihot esculenta*) which is used to make tapioca, and sweet cassava (*M. dulcis; M. aipi;* or *M. utilissima*) which is eaten like potatoes. Fig. C-30 shows a typical cassava plant.

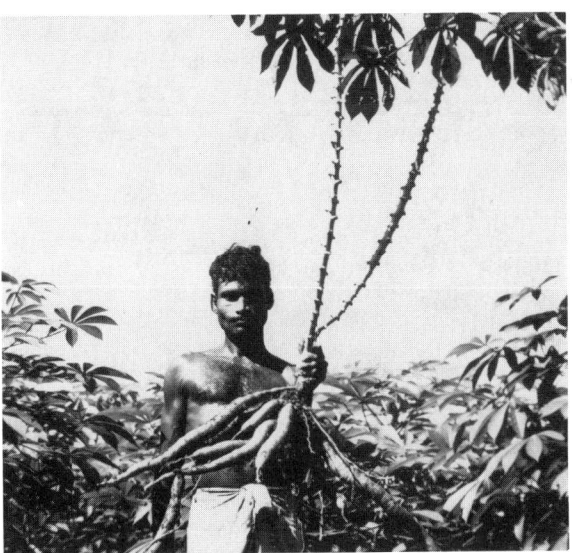

Fig. C-30. The cassava, a valuable food plant of the tropics. (Courtesy, International Development Research Centre, Ottawa, Canada)

ORIGIN AND HISTORY. Cassava is native to the humid tropics of northeastern Brazil and the low-lying western and southern sections of Mexico. It was taken to Africa in the 16th century, by the Portuguese.

WORLD AND U.S. PRODUCTION. Cassava ranks third among the vegetable crops of the world. Worldwide, about 157 million metric tons of cassava are produced annually; and the leading cassava-producing countries are: Nigeria, Brazil, Thailand, Zaire, and Indonesia.[10] A small amount of cassava is produced in the southern part of the United States.

PROCESSING. The moist tubers keep for only a few days following digging; hence, processing should not be delayed.

The different varieties contain variable amounts of linamarin, a substance that may be converted into toxic prussic (hydrocyanic) acid by an enzyme present in the plant tissues. The tubers which contain moderate to large amounts of linamarin usually have a bitter taste, whereas those that are low in the toxicant are likely to be slightly sweet. Also, the outer layer (rind) of a tuber of the bitter variety has a notably higher level of linamarin than the inner layers. Nevertheless, all varieties of cassava should be processed to minimize the likelihood of toxicity, which varies according to the local soil and climatic conditions.

Among the most common ways of processing cassava tubers are: soaking the peeled or unpeeled roots in water; boiling or roasting whole or cut tubers; drying whole, cut up, or grated cassava; expressing the juice from cassava; or fermenting cassava into a beer.

SELECTION, PREPARATION, AND USES. Fresh unbruised cassava tubers of a sweet variety should be selected. The most common processing consists in peeling the tubers; washing the peeled tubers under running water; cooking the vegetable in fresh water in an open pot; and discarding the water.

Tapioca may be made by gentle heating of the cassava starch to cause clumping. Flour or meal may be made by grinding the dried roots.

Cassava may be used as a starchy vegetable in much the same way as Irish potatoes. As a flour, it may be used as a thickener for gravies, soups, and stews. Also, it may be used in tapioca puddings and fruit pies.

NUTRITIONAL VALUE. The nutrient composition of various cassava products is given in Food Composition Table F-21.

Some noteworthy observations regarding the nutrient composition of cassava follow:

1. Cassava tubers are rich in carbohydrates (mostly starch), but low in proteins and most other nutrients. The raw roots are lower in water content and higher in calories than the other leading roots and tubers. Also, the various dried forms of cassava tubers are about as rich in food energy as the common cereal flours. Nutritional deficiencies may result if cassava is the predominant food in the diet unless the missing nutrients are obtained by consuming adequate amounts of certain other foods. For example, the Brazilians, who can afford to do so, mix cassava flour with meats and vegetables.

2. The leaves of the cassava plant are nutritionally superior to the tubers with respect to protein, calcium, phosphorus, iron, vitamin A, the vitamin B complex, and vitamin C. However, the leaves often contain sufficient amounts of cyanide compounds to warrant special processing to make them safe.

3. Growth studies using laboratory animals show that breads made from cassava starch and peanut flour, and from cassava starch and soy flour, contain higher quality protein than a standard bread made from wheat flour alone. An acceptable bread may be made from 70% wheat flour and 30% cassava flour.

4. Common cassava meals consisting of porridgelike mixtures of cereal grains, legumes, and other ingredients may be improved nutritionally by fortification with soy flour, skim milk powder, sugar, minerals, and vitamins.

CAUTION: Cassava must be washed thoroughly (or boiled, dried, expressed, or fermented) to remove the prussic (hydrocyanic) acid. Because of this acid, the bitter cassava root cannot be eaten raw. Also, a cassava-rich diet should be supplemented with animal protein foods (rich in vitamin B-12) to assure that any residual traces of prussic acid are handled safely by the body.

CASTOR OIL

A very strong laxative (also called a cathartic or a purgative) obtained from castor beans (*Ricinus communis*). It is one of the oldest household remedies for constipation.

CATABOLISM

The oxidation of nutrients, liberating energy (exergonic reaction) which is used to fulfill the body's immediate demands. Catabolism is the reverse of anabolism.

(Also see METABOLISM.)

CATALASE

An enzyme which splits hydrogen peroxide into water and oxygen. This reaction prevents a buildup of the dangerous peroxide which may harm sensitive cell membranes.

CATALYST

Any substance which speeds up the rate of a chemical reaction without being destroyed or inactivated in the process. Enzymes are catalysts.

(Also see ENZYME.)

CATALYZE

To speed up the rate of a chemical reaction through the action of a catalyst.

CATARACT

Cataract is a clouding over of the lens of the eye due to the formation of certain types of crystals and deposits. When the lens becomes completely opaque, no longer allowing light to pass through to the retina, sight is lost. The disease may start in one eye, but eventually both eyes are affected.

This clouding of the lens is seen most frequently after middle age. But some people are born with cataracts. Various causes have been implicated. Some people appear to inherit the disease or a tendency toward it. Cataracts may also be caused by nutritional deficiencies, diabetes, certain drugs, or radiation.

---

[10]Based on data from *FAO Production Yearbook 1990*, FAO/UN, Rome, Italy, Vol. 44, pp. 94–95, Table 28. **Note well:** Annual production fluctuates as a result of weather and profitability of the crop.

Once cataracts have developed, treatment consists of surgically (1) removing the clouded lens, followed by wearing special glasses or contact lenses, or (2) replacing the clouded lens with a lens made of plastic.

CATECHOLAMINES

These compounds, which are also called biogenic amines, are transmitters of impulses in the nervous system and in the brain. The three principal catecholamines found in the body are dopamine, norepinephrine (also called noradrenaline), and epinephrine (adrenaline). They have strong effects on body movement and balance, the emotional state, heart rate, and blood pressure.

CATHARTIC

A strong laxative.

CAULIFLOWER *Brassica oleracea*, VARIETY *botrytis*

This vegetable, which is grown for its whitened flower head, is practically a gourmet item, because it sells for several times the price of cabbage. Cauliflower was derived from the wild cabbage, *B. oleracea.* Fig. C-31 shows a cauliflower with a large edible flower head (commonly called a curd).

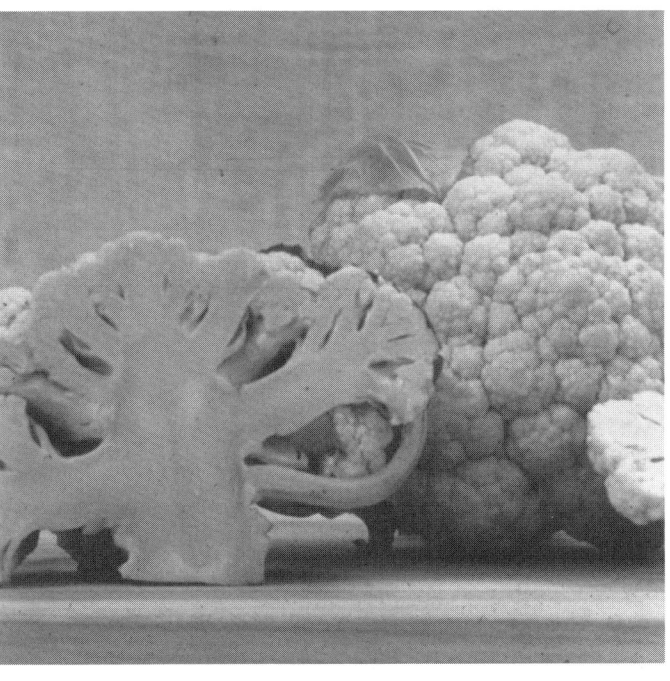

Fig. C-31. Cauliflower, a high-class relative of the common cabbage. (Courtesy, USDA)

ORIGIN AND HISTORY. Primitive forms of cauliflower were in cultivation in the Near East in pre-Christian times. From these ancient plants, selections adapted to the cooler climates of northern Europe were developed.

WORLD AND U.S. PRODUCTION. Cauliflower ranks thirteenth among the vegetables of the world. World production of cauliflowers totals about 5,356,000 metric tons annually; and the leading countries, by rank, are: China, India, France, Italy, United States, and United Kingdom.[11]

Cauliflower ranks twelfth as a U.S. vegetable crop. About 392,750 short tons of cauliflower are produced annually in the United States with 78% of the production in California.[12]

PROCESSING. About half of the cauliflower grown in the United States is processed. The leading form of processing is freezing, but pickling is also a major means of preservation.

SELECTION, PREPARATION, AND USES. Good quality in cauliflower is indicated by white or creamy-white, clean, firm, compact curd, with the *jacket leaves* (outer leaf portions remaining) fresh, turgid, and green. Small leaves extending through the curd do not affect edible quality. Large or small heads, equally mature, are equally desirable. A slightly *ricy* or granular appearance is not objectionable unless the flower clusters are spreading.

Raw cauliflower may be served in a relish tray or a salad, or it may be dipped into well-seasoned sauces before eating.

Cooked cauliflower goes well with a wide variety of cheese or cream sauces, egg dishes, meats, poultry, and other vegetable. Also, pieces of the cooked vegetable may be dipped into an egg batter, then fried in deep fat.

Cauliflower pickles are very good appetizers or accompaniments to cold meat sandwiches.

NUTRITIONAL VALUE. The nutrient composition of cauliflower is given in Food Composition Table F-21.

Some noteworthy observations regarding the nutrient composition of cauliflower follow:

1. Boiled cauliflower is low in calories (23 to 32 kcal per cup) because it contains over 90% water. Hence, it is filling, but not fattening for people trying to lose weight.

2. The blanching (whitening) of cauliflower makes it low in vitamin A, compared to most of the other cabbage vegetables. However, the purple-headed varieties which turn green when cooked contain much more of the vitamin.

3. A 1-cup (240 ml) serving of cooked cauliflower provides about the same amount of vitamin C as a medium size orange. Raw cauliflower provides at least 20% more vitamin C than the cooked vegetable.

Cauliflowers contain small amounts of goitrogens. (See GOITROGENS.)

CAVY (GUINEA PIGS)

South American rodents constituting the family *Cavidae*, the best known of which are guinea pigs. Cavy flesh is edible.

CECUM (CAECUM)

A blind sac or pouch located at the junction of the small and large intestines, often considered to be part of the large intestine. A valve at the ileocecal junction allows the products of digestion to flow from the ileum to the cecum, but

---

[11]Based on data from *FAO Production Yearbook 1990*, FAO/UN, Rome, Italy, Vol. 44, p. 133, Table 53. **Note well:** Annual production fluctuates as a result of weather and profitability of the crop.

[12]Based on data from *Agricultural Statistics 1991*, USDA, p. 151, Table 210. **Note well:** Annual production fluctuates as a result of weather and profitability of the crop.

not in the opposite direction. The nonfunctional appendix is attached to the cecum.

CELERY Apium graveolens, VARIETY dulce

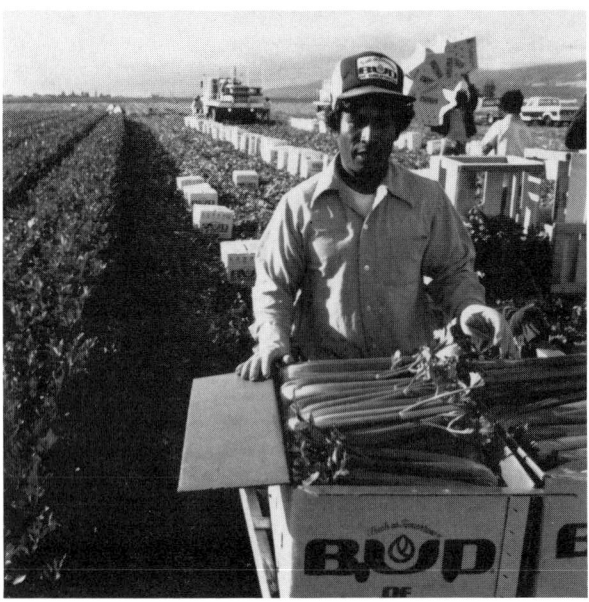

Fig. C-32. Celery being packed in the field immediately following harvest. (Courtesy, Castle and Cooke, Inc.)

This vegetable, which has edible leafstalks, leaves, and seeds, is a leading salad crop of the United States. Celery is a member of the Parsley family (Umbelliferae), which also includes caraway, carrots, celeriac, dill, fennel, parsley, parsnips and certain lesser known vegetables.

ORIGIN AND HISTORY. Celery was developed from wild celery, which was native to the marshy areas of the Mediterranean region. It is thought to have been domesticated in either France or Italy.

WORLD AND U.S. PRODUCTION. On a worldwide basis, celery is of minor importance. In the United States, celery ranks eighth among the vegetable crops, with about 989,750 short tons produced annually, 75% of which is produced in California.[13]

PROCESSING. Most of the celery crop is marketed fresh. However, small but steadily increasing amounts of this vegetable are processed into forms such as (1) canned celery hearts, (2) other canned items that contain celery, and (3) dried celery, which can be rehydrated to 16 times its dried weight.

Celery seed is dried and sold in whole or ground form as a seasoning agent, or the ground seed may be mixed with (1) table salt to make celery salt, a product that may not legally contain more than 75% salt, (2) ground black pepper to make celery pepper, which may not contain more than 70% pepper, or (3) various other products such as bouillon preparations, salad dressings, and vegetable juices.

---

[13]Based on data from *Agricultural Statistics 1991*, USDA, p. 151, Table 211. **Note well:** Annual production fluctuates as a result of weather and profitability of the crop.

SELECTION, PREPARATION, AND USES. Best quality celery is fresh, crisp, and clean, of medium length, thickness, and density, with good heart formation, and branches that are brittle enough to snap easily.

Raw celery should be washed well to remove any sand or soil. Then, the leaves should be removed for immediate use. The stalks may be stored for 1 to 2 weeks in a refrigerator.

• **Celery leaves**—Although this part of the plant is often discarded, it is very nutritious and useful for flavoring or garnishing various dishes.

• **Celery seeds**—This item is quite expensive. Hence, it is used sparingly in (1) dishes such as casseroles, chicken loaf, sauces, soups, and stews; and (2) mixtures with other seasoning agents such as pepper and salt.

• **Celery stalks**—Raw celery can be used for (1) dunking in cold or hot dips; (2) relish trays or salads; (3) hors d'oeuvres in which the stalks are stuffed with fillings such as cheese spreads, chopped or pureed cooked beans, eggs, fish, meats, poultry, or seafood, fruit butters or purees, mashed banana, or peanut butter; or (4) making celery juice or a mixture of vegetable juices.

Celery stalks are also good when cooked in soups or stews, with stewed tomatoes, stir-fried in Chinese dishes, or as an individual vegetable dish served with butter or margarine and various seasonings, or with a special sauce.

NUTRITIONAL VALUE. The nutrient compositions of various forms of celery are given in Food Composition Table F-21.

Some noteworthy observations regarding the nutrient composition of celery follow:

1. Celery stalks have a high water content (94%) and a low caloric content (17 kcal per 100 g). They are an excellent source of potassium, but only a fair source of vitamins A and C. It is noteworthy that the white varieties of the vegetable and the green ones which have been blanched have a much lower vitamin A content than the unblanched green varieties. Whenever possible, celery stalks should be eaten with the leaves on because the leaves are much richer than the stalks in calcium, iron, potassium, vitamin A, and vitamin C.

2. Celery seeds are among the tiniest vegetable seeds; 72,000 seeds weigh only 1 oz (28 g). Nevertheless, they are very rich in calories (392 kcal per 100 g), protein, fat, fiber, calcium, phosphorus, magnesium, potassium, iron, and zinc.

3. Herbalists have long used celery to treat a wide variety of ailments, of which the most common is dropsy (an accumulation of excess water in the tissues) because consumption of the stalks or roots is thought to increase urination. (The authors are not aware of any research confirming or contradicting this belief. Hence, it is presented for purposes of (1) information, and (2) in order to stimulate research on the subject.)

CELIAC DISEASE

A rare metabolic disorder of children, sometimes called *Malabsorption Syndrome*, which appears to run in families and, therefore, may be due to a genetic defect. The disease results from a sensitivity to gluten, a protein found in wheat, rye, and several other—but not all—grains. Affected children are unable to absorb fats, certain starches, and some sugars.

Symptoms include recurrent diarrhea, severe cramps, a pale, foul-smelling stool containing large amounts of fat, distended abdomen, stunted growth, anemia, irritability and susceptibility to infection. Therapy evolved during World War II when a Dutch scientist observed improvement in affected children when bread was unavailable. Treatment is now based on a diet low in high gluten foods, but high in protein. Buckwheat, rice, corn, and soybean flours are substituted for wheat, rye, barley, and oat flours, and fruit sugars are used to replace milk sugars. Once the symptoms disappear, a fuller diet is achieved by adding one food at a time to the diet and then monitoring its effects. Celiac disease is similar to an adult disease called sprue.

(Also see ALLERGIES, section headed "Wheat Allergy"; and SPRUE.)

CELL MEMBRANE

The thin layer of tissue that encloses the cell and restricts the entry and exit of various substances.

CELLOBIOSE

A sugar formed by the partial breakdown of cellulose.

CELLULASE

The general name given to an enzyme which breaks down cellulose. Cellulases are present in certain intestinal bacteria and in various other microorganisms such as those which inhabit the digestive tract of grazing animals (cattle, goats, and sheep).

CELL WALL

The outer layer of plant and animal cells. Plant cell walls are made up mainly of cellulose plus other complex carbohydrates; hence, they are poorly digested by man.
(Also see FIBER.)

CEMENTUM

The calcified portion covering the root of the tooth.

CENTIGRADE (CELSIUS)

A thermometer scale on which the interval between the two standard points, the freezing point and the boiling point of water, is divided into 100°, with 0° representing the freezing point and 100° the boiling point. To convert Centigrade to Fahrenheit multiply by 9/5 and add 32.
(Also see WEIGHTS AND MEASURES.)

CENTRAL NERVOUS SYSTEM

The brain and spinal cord in vertebrates. It is that part of the nervous system to which sensory impulses are transmitted and from which motor impulses pass out; it supervises and coordinates the activity of the entire nervous system.

CENTRIFUGE

A machine for whirling fluids rapidly, which exerts a pull many times stronger than gravity. It is used to separate two liquids of different densities; e.g., cream from milk—the Babcock Test. Also, specimens of blood, urine, and other substances are centrifuged to separate the sediment or solid constituents from the liquid.
(Also see BABCOCK TEST.)

CEPHALIN

A group of phospholipids; associated with lecithins found in brain tissue, nerve tissue, and egg yolk.

CEREAL GRAINS

Contents   *Page*

Cereal grains denote the seeds or fruits from cereal plants—members of the grass family *Gramineae*—which are used as food for man and animals. The word cereal is derived from Ceres, the Roman goddess of agriculture.

Grains, and the products made from them, are the *staff of life* for many peoples around the world. Fig. C-33 shows that a large part of the world's food crop production— 40% of it—is represented by cereal grains.

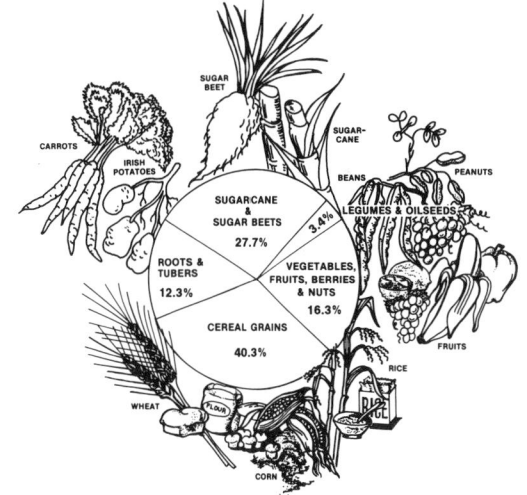

WORLD PRODUCTION OF FOOD PLANTS

Fig. C-33. Major food crops of the world. (Data from *FAO Production Yearbook 1990*, FAO/UN, Rome, Italy, Vol. 44)

The principal cereal grain crops of the world, in descending order of production, are wheat, corn, rice, barley, sorghum, oats, rye, and millet. The cereals supply most of the carbohydrates in human diets throughout the world; and the proteins, oils, minerals, and vitamins contained in cereals are also of considerable nutritional importance.

HISTORY. The development of the ancient civilizations was spurred by man's cultivation of grains, which made it possible for many more people to be fed from the food produced on a given amount of land.

Archeological evidence indicates that wild varieties of barley and wheat were used as food as early as 10,000 B.C. by the peoples living in the *Levant*—the eastern coastal region of the Mediterranean which extends from Greece to Egypt. However, the first cultivation of these crops by man appears to have occurred in an area east of the Levant (the countries of the eastern Mediterranean) called *The Fertile Crescent*, a broad, crescent-shaped area that curved northward and eastward from what is now the eastern border of Egypt, to the Taurus Mountains of southern Turkey, across to the Zagros Mountains of western Iran, and down to the Persian Gulf. (See section on WHEAT, "Origin and History.")

One of the earliest agricultural villages excavated in this region was Jarmo, a small settlement about 150 miles (*240 km*) north of Baghdad, Iraq. It appears that by around 7000 B.C. the people of Jarmo had domesticated several types of wild barley and wheat. Crops were first irrigated in this area around 5000 B.C.

WORLD AND U.S. PRODUCTION OF CEREAL GRAINS. The world production of cereal grain averages about 1,955 million metric tons, of which the United States accounted for 312,708,000, or 16%.[14] Fig. C-34 shows the leading cereals grains of the world, and the annual production of each. Fig. C-35 shows the leading cereal grains of the United States, and the production of each.

---

[14]*FAO Production Yearbook 1990*, FAO/UN, Rome, Italy, Vol. 44, p. 67.

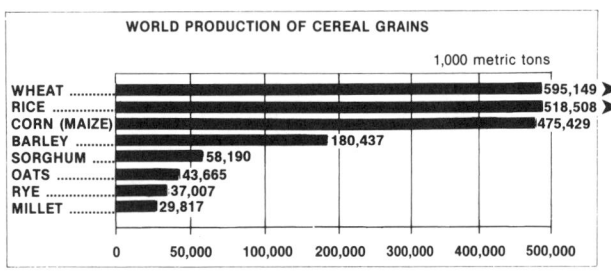

Fig. C-34. Leading cereal grains of the world. (Data from *FAO Production Yearbook 1990*, FAO/UN, Rome, Italy, Vol. 44)

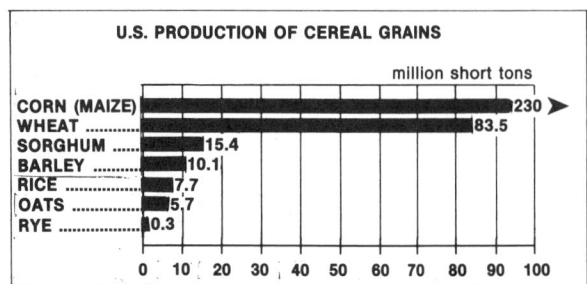

Fig. C-35. Leading cereal grains of the U.S. (Data from *Agricultural Statistics 1991*)

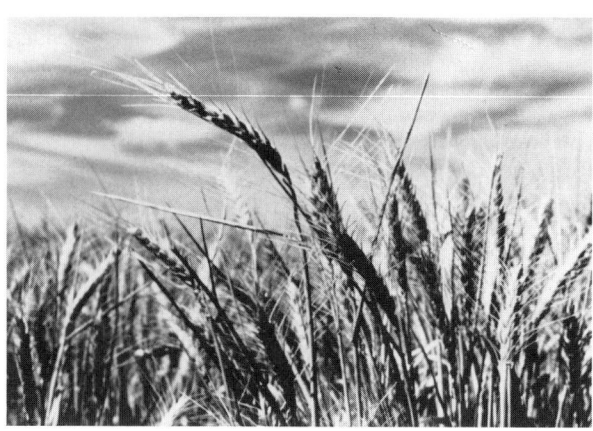

Fig. C-36. Wheat, leading cereal grain of the world. (Courtesy, USDA)

PRODUCTION OF BEVERAGES, FOODS, AND FEEDS FROM GRAINS. Cereal technology around the world is directed mainly towards the processing of wheat, corn, rice, and barley, because these four grains account for over 90% of the world's grain production. However, products are also made from sorghum, oats, rye, and millet, particularly in those countries where these crops are of greater than average importance. Fig. C-37 shows the proportion of the world grain production contributed by each of the major cereal crops.

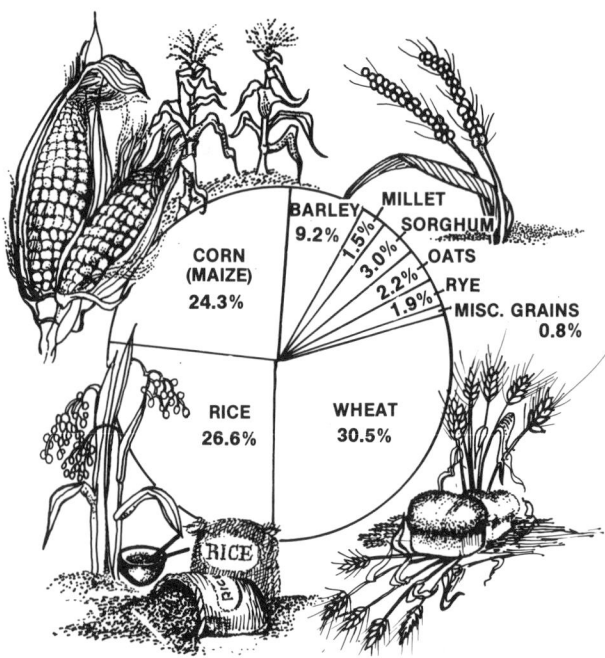

Fig. C-37. Contributions of the major cereal crops to world grain production. (Data from *FAO Production Yearbook 1990*, FAO/UN, Rome, Italy, Vol. 44)

Details of the major types of cereal technology follow.

Malting (Sprouting). In this process the germination of grains is started by soaking them in water—for the purpose of activating certain enzymes that are useful in baking, brewing, and the production of distilled alcoholic beverages. The enzymes activated during sprouting digest the stored carbohydrates and proteins in the grains to sugars and amino acids which support the growth of the embryonic plant. Usually the malt producer stops the germination right after the emergence of sprouts by careful heating and drying so as to retain the desired enzyme activity. Then, the sprouts are removed from the malted grain by passing them through revolving sets of wire screens. The term malt may be applied to any grain which has been so treated. However, it is generally understood that when the term malt is used alone (without indicating the grain source) it refers to malt from barley.

(Also see BARLEY; and MALT.)

Brewing. This process consists of a series of operations in which (1) starchy gruels are prepared by cooking crushed grains; (2) the gruels are digested or *mashed* with malted grains or other sources of enzymes in order to produce sugary solutions; and (3) the sugary solutions are filtered, flavored with hops or other substances, and fermented with yeast to yield a beverage which contains about 4% alcohol (ale, beer, lager, porter, stout, etc.). Most commercial brewers now use malted barley as the source of the starch-digesting enzymes, and other grains or *adjuncts* such as corn, rice, sorghum, and wheat to prepare the starchy gruels. Nevertheless, it is noteworthy that beers have been brewed from (1) wheat by the Germans, (2) rice by the Chinese and the Japanese, (3) sorghums and millets by African tribes, (4) rye by the Russians, and (5) corn by the American Indians.

(Also see BEERS AND BREWING.)

Distilling. Distilled alcoholic beverages are produced by distilling fermented mashes which are prepared like those used for making beer. Most of these beverages are produced from corn, rye, and malted barley.

(Also see DISTILLATION; DISTILLED LIQUORS; and FERMENTATION.)

Milling. The term milling refers to various processes of grinding and/or rolling which are applied to grains for the purposes of (1) removing fibrous hulls, branny seed coats, and oily embryos (germs); (2) altering their sizes and shapes, as in the pearling of barley; and (3) reducing the size of grain

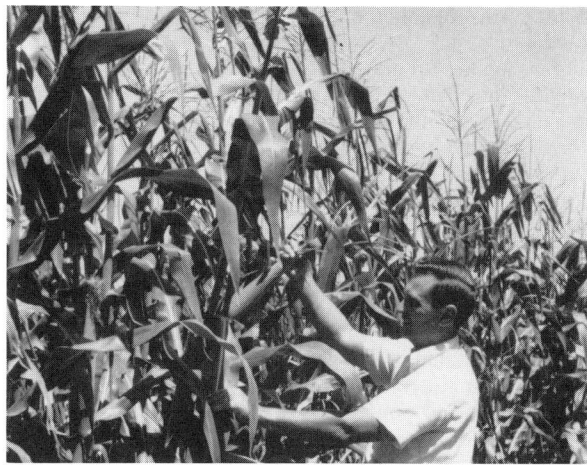

Fig. C-38. Corn, leading cereal grain of the U.S. (Courtesy, New Jersey Department of Agriculture)

particles to meal or flour. *Meal* denotes particles like grains of sand, whereas *flour* denotes a fine powder. Table C-7 provides a guide to the main products of milling which may be used as foods.

(Also see BARLEY; CORN; MILLETS; OATS; RICE; SORGHUM; TRITICALE; WHEAT; and WILD RICE.)

Baking. The first breads were made by mixing grain meals with water and baking the resulting dough over hot coals. They were flat, heavy, and unleavened until the ancient Egyptians and the Hebrews learned how to use sourdough cultures for leavening. The Egyptians soon went a step further and cultivated yeast, which they sometimes dried for later use. However, it was not until the end of the 18th century that a crude baking powder made from wood ashes was developed in the United States. Now, breads leavened with baking powder are called *quick breads* because this type of leavening takes place much more rapidly than the production of gas by yeast fermentation. Brief descriptions of the major types of bread leavening follow:

TABLE C-7
CEREAL BY-PRODUCTS

Cereal Product	Description	Grain(s)	Comments
Bran	The coarse outer covering of the grain kernel in the form of tiny flakes.	Corn, oats, rice, wheat.	High in water-absorbing fiber which has a laxative action.
Flour	Soft, powdery product derived mainly from the inner portion of the grain kernel.	Barley, corn, oats, rice, rye, wheat.	Consists mostly of starch and protein. Low in fiber. Used to make bread.
Germ	Embryo of the seed.	Corn, rice, wheat.	Rich in fat and protein.
Gluten	Tough, elastic protein which remains when flour is washed to remove the starch.	Wheat	Imparts elasticity to doughs, thereby enabling them to be leavened with yeast.
Grits (hominy)	Coarsely ground deskinned grain from which the bran and germ have been removed.	Corn	Usually cooked in water and used as a cereal or a side dish.
Groats	Grain from which the hulls have been removed.	Barley, oats.	Usually cooked in water and used as a cereal or in soups.
Meal	Particles of ground grain that are larger than those in flour.	Corn, oats, rice, wheat.	Usually cooked in water and used as a breakfast cereal.
Polishings	Soft, fine residue obtained by polishing brown rice to make white rice.	Rice	Added to infant cereals to increase the content of minerals and vitamins.

• **Unleavened breads**—These items, which in their simplest forms consist of baked doughs made from flour and water, are the most palatable when they are thin and crackerlike, such as the Jewish matzo, made from wheat flour, and the Mexican tortilla. There is usually a slight leavening of the so-called unleavened breads when some of the water in the dough is converted to steam and trapped within the bread during baking. This effect is most likely to occur when the dough is placed in a very hot oven so that there is a rapid formation of a crust which prevents the steam from escaping.

• **Sourdough breads**—Generally, the leavening agent for these products is a species of bacteria such as *Lactobacilli* that produces (1) carbon dioxide which leavens the bread, and (2) lactic acid which gives it a sour taste. The bacteria is provided in the form of either a dried, pure culture of the organism; or as a component of a *starter*, which is usually a portion taken from a batch of previously fermented dough. Sometimes, both bacteria and yeast are present in the starter so that two types of fermentation occur, such as in the production of San Francisco sourdough breads. Rye breads are often leavened with sourdough cultures; typical ingredients of these breads are sourdough, rye flour, white flour, yeast, sugar, shortening, and flavorings.

• **Yeast-leavened breads**—Wheat flours rich in gluten are required for these breads. Because the yeast fermentation is slow and a strong, elastic dough is needed to trap the bubbles of carbon dioxide. However, the leavening process may be speeded up by (1) adding sugar to hasten the growth of the yeast, and (2) using double or triple the amount of yeast. Too much yeast produces a sticky, stringy texture in the bread. Excess sugar slows the growth of yeast. Usually, these breads contain flour, water, yeast, salt, sugar, and a small amount of shortening.

• **Quick breads**—Flours made from any of the grains may be used in these breads when eggs are added to the dough, because the inelasticity due to lack of gluten is compensated for by the protein in egg white. The leavening action results from one or more chemical reactions between the baking powder and the water in the dough. Sometimes, a combination of an acidic food, such as a soured dairy product and baking soda, is used for leavening. These breads usually contain variable amounts of flour, water or milk, egg, sugar, and shortening.

(Also see BREADS AND BAKING; and FLOUR.)

Miscellaneous Grain Processes. Many of these processes are used in the production of breakfast cereals and snack foods. Hence, the basic principles underlying these processes are noteworthy. Details follow.

(Also see BREAKFAST CEREALS; and SNACK FOODS.)

• **Canning**—Cooked sweet corn is the only commonly used canned grain in the United States. However, cooked rice and bulgur wheat are also available in cans.

• **Cracking**—Breakfast cereals which require cooking often contain cracked grains, which cook faster than whole grains. Also, limited amounts of cracked grains are added to certain breads to give them a nutty flavor and texture.

• **Extruding**—In cereal technology this term denotes the process of forcing doughs through a die to form pellets, ribbons, rods, tubing, etc. After extrusion, the shaped dough is cut to an appropriate length and either dried or cooked, so that (1) a strengthened product is formed which does not readily break upon handling, and (2) the moisture content is reduced to the point where the product keeps well when stored for prolonged periods at room temperature. The various forms of pasta (macaroni, noodles, shells, etc.) are the best-known products of this type of processing.

• **Flaking**—The flake types of ready-to-eat breakfast cereals are usually prepared by (1) cooking whole grains or partially milled pieces of grain in water with added flavorings such as sugar, salt, and malt; (2) drying the cooked grains to the desired moisture content; (3) forming flakes by passing the grains between rollers; and (4) drying or toasting the flakes. Sometimes, flakes are rolled from pellets of cooked doughs prepared from various flour mixtures.

• **Oil extraction**—The oils which are present in the various grains may be extracted in connection with the milling operations. Corn oil is by far the leading grain oil produced in the United States; the amounts of oil extracted from wheat and rice are small by comparison. The oil of corn is extracted by a combination of heating, pressing, and solvent extraction —after the separation of the germ in either the dry milling or wet milling process.

• **Parboiling**—Both rice and wheat grains may be cooked in water prior to milling. Parboiled rice requires longer cooking than ordinary white rice because parboiling followed by drying makes the grain harder. However, the parboiled rice is higher in vitamins than unenriched white rice and it is less likely to stick when cooked. Most parboiled wheat is used to produce bulgur wheat, a product which is cracked into small pieces after parboiling and light milling. Bulgur wheat, unlike parboiled rice, requires considerably less cooking than whole grains of untreated wheat.

• **Pearling**—This process is applied mainly to barley grains after the hulls have been removed. The dehulled kernels or *groats* are polished into rounded shapes by an abrasive action.

• **Popping**—Although most people are familiar with the application of this process to popcorn (a special variety of corn), few realize that it is also applied to rice, sorghum, and wheat. The success of this procedure requires that grains of appropriate moisture content be heated rapidly so that the moisture changes to steam, which literally causes the starchy, inner portion of the grains to explode.

• **Puffing**—Special puffing guns—consisting of heated, rotating cylinders that shoot out puffed grains—have long been used by the makers of breakfast cereals. A newer development is the puffing of dough mixtures rather than whole grains or pieces. In the latter process, the doughs are expanded by forcing them through dies. Sometimes, grains are cooked in water with sugar, salt, and flavorings; then, they are puffed by tumbling in a hot oven.

• **Rolling**—Rolled oats are the best-known example of grains which have been compressed into flat pieces (flakes) by passing through rollers. The oats are prepared for rolling by (1) removal of their hulls; and (2) steaming to destroy enzymes which might cause deterioration, and to condition them for rolling. Other grains are also rolled into flakes, but they are usually subjected to more preliminary processing than oats.

• **Shredding**—This process dates back to the end of the 19th century, when it was first patented. Whole grain wheat is converted into shredded wheat biscuits by (1) cooking and drying to the desired moisture content; (2) squeezing into long, slender strands by passage through very closely spaced, grooved rolls; and (3) forming the strands into biscuits and baking them in an oven. Similar types of biscuits may also be made from corn, oats, and rice.

• **Sprouting**—Sometimes, grains may be sprouted for use as a vegetable, rather than for the production of malt. Hence, it is noteworthy that special equipment is now available for sprouting grains by hydroponics—a process in which the grain is sprouted by immersion in a water solution of essential nutrients.

• **Starch extraction**—Corn is the leading grain used as a source of starch in the United States, followed by sorghum, wheat, and rice. Starch is extracted by (1) soaking the grains in water containing small amounts of sulfur dioxide or sodium hydroxide; (2) grinding of the soaked kernels to free the germs and the fibrous components; and (3) flotating and centrifuging to separate the other components from the starch. A newer process for obtaining wheat starch involves the milling of wheat into flour, followed by the washing of the starch from the dough prepared by mixing the flour with water.

NUTRITIVE VALUES. Many people tend to regard cereal products solely as starchy foods that are rich in calories, yet these items may provide substantial amounts of protein, minerals, and vitamins—depending upon such factors as the type of grain and the degree of refining. Food Composition Table F-21 of this book gives the nutrient composition for the commonly used grain products.

Based on the data presented in the Food Composition Table F-21 and other sources in this book, the following conclusions may be drawn:

1. The cereal grains are rich in carbohydrates, which makes them good sources of calories. For example, 1 lb (*0.45 kg*) of raw, dried grain supplies from 1,550 to 1,750 Calories (kcal). Cooked cereals supply much fewer calories because of their higher water content.

2. Although grains may serve as the main source of dietary protein for adults, young growing children also need protein from other sources, because most grains are low in the amino acid lysine.

3. Most grain products are low in fat, except for rice polish and wheat germ, which are good sources of polyunsaturated fats.

4. Milling lowers the fiber content of grains, making them more digestible but less filling.

5. Grains contain only small amounts of calcium compared to much greater quantities of phosphorus, but much of the latter element may be in the form of unavailable phytates—which bind with minerals such as calcium, iron, and zinc so as to hinder their absorption. It is noteworthy that the yeast leavening of breads breaks down some of the phytates. (Whole grains contain more phytates than milled grains.)

6. Most cereals are very poor sources of vitamins A and C, unless they have been sprouted. However, yellow corn contains about 490 IU of vitamin A per l00 g.

7. Removal of the outer layer of grain by milling reduces the levels of essential minerals and vitamins because the inner, starchy portion of the kernel contains less of the nutrients than the outer layers. Hence, by-products of milling such as rice polish, wheat bran, and wheat germ are good sources of the minerals and vitamins lost in milling.

(Also see BREADS AND BAKING; BREAKFAST CEREALS; FLOUR; and MACARONI AND NOODLE PRODUCTS.)

Protein Quality of Grains. The people of southeastern Asia whose diets consist mainly of rice are usually short of stature, but the children of those who immigrated to the United States are often taller than their parents. It appears that the higher quantity and quality of protein in the American diet is largely responsible for the taller children, because cereal grains alone do not provide sufficient amounts of lysine and other amino acids needed for optimal growth. Fig. C-39 shows the lysine and protein content of the major grains in comparison with cow's milk.

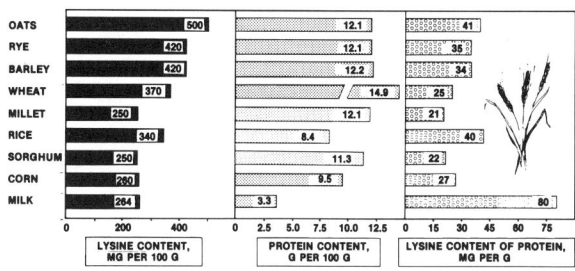

Fig. C-39. The amounts of lysine and protein in some of the major grains in comparison with cow's milk.

It may be seen from Fig. C-39 that the proportion of lysine to protein in the cereal grains is only about half that of cow's milk, which is almost an ideal source of protein for growing children. The amino acid lysine is much more essential for growing children than it is for adults, because it is required for the growth of the tissues such as bone, cartilage, and muscle. For this reason, the protein in most cereal grains is poorly utilized by infants and children.

The nutritional quality of diets based on cereals may be improved by adding higher quality protein in the form of (1) animal products or (2) legumes, both of which contain proportionately more lysine than grains. Other means of overcoming the problems of protein quality in cereal products are described in the sections that follow.

(Also see INFANT DIETS AND NUTRITION; LYSINE; and PROTEIN[S].)

Enriched or Fortified Cereals. Cereal products are often the mainstay of emergency feeding programs designed to serve large numbers of people, because they are less expensive than many of the other foods which provide calories and protein. However, it is well known that the prolonged consumption of a diet consisting mainly of grains may lead to multiple nutritional deficiencies, because cereals fail to supply sufficient amounts of certain other essential nutrients. Nevertheless, it may cost less to enrich or fortify simple mixtures of grains, legumes, and a few other ingredients—with amino acids, minerals, and vitamins—than it would to provide these nutrients from a wide variety of foods. Details of some typical measures follow:

• **Amino acids**—These nutrients—which are provided in the form of pure, white powders—are usually added to flours or meals prior to their incorporation into various products. In certain cases, increased amounts should be added because heat processing by baking and/or toasting renders some of the lysine and other amino acids unavailable.

• **Minerals**—Iron has frequently been added to grain products, particularly those that have been highly milled. However, the milling of grains into refined flours removes large percentages of many of the other essential minerals, but they are rarely replaced by enrichment. Calcium is deficient in grains, but it is seldom added to cereal products because of certain technical difficulties; although calcium salts are added to flour in Great Britain, Denmark, and Israel, and to certain breakfast cereals in the United States.

• **Vitamins**—Thiamin, riboflavin, and niacin are often added to white flour and breakfast cereals, and sometimes to white rice. Milling also removes much of the other B-complex vitamins present in whole grains. Vitamins A, C, and D are not always added to cereal products; so, other sources of the vitamins should be consumed along with the cereal products.

New and Improved Varieties of Grains. Some of the limitations in the protein quality of the most important cereal grains have been overcome by cross-breeding them with mutant varieties so as to obtain new hybrids which have higher contents of both lysine and protein. Fig. C-40 shows how the new high-lysine and high-protein varieties compare with some of the older, more common varieties of the major grains.

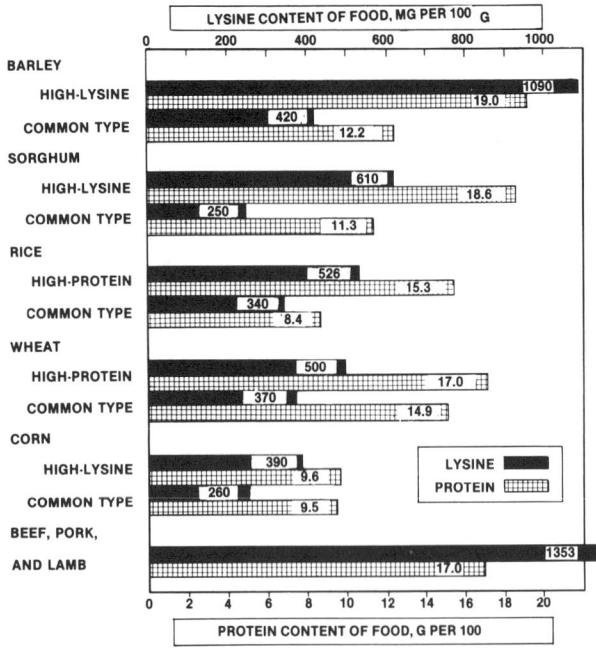

Fig. C-40. The amounts of lysine and protein supplied by hybrid and common types of the major grains in comparison with red meats—beef, pork, and lamb.

It may be seen from Fig. C-40 that the new, improved hybrids are notably higher in lysine and/or protein than the more common types of cereals which are presently grown around the world. For example high-lysine barley contains 81% as much lysine as the red meats (beef, pork, and lamb), and has a slightly higher protein content. However, farmers are reluctant to grow the hybrid varieties because they yield from 10 to 15% less grain per acre than the more common varieties. Hence, their margin of profit would shrink drastically if both types of grains were bought at the same

price. Certain agricultural economists and nutritionists believe that higher prices for the high-protein, hybrid cereals are justified because (1) they may be used to feed people who have high protein requirements—such as infants, children, and pregnant and lactating women—without much need for additional protein from eggs, legumes, fish, meats, milk, nuts, or poultry; and (2) providing the other protein foods is much more expensive in terms of energy, land, and money than paying a higher price for the hybrids in order to give farmers an incentive to grow them.

Sprouted Grains. During World War II, people were advised to use sprouted seeds as sources of vitamin C in the event that the supplies of fresh produce became limited. Nevertheless, few people are aware of the other improvements in nutritive value which result from the sprouting of the cereal grains. Table C-8 shows how the sprouting of oats in a special nutrient solution (the process known as hydroponic sprouting) affects the level of nutrients.

TABLE C-8
NUTRIENT COMPOSITION OF OAT GRAIN VS SPROUTED OATS

Nutrient or Other Constituent	Oat Grain	Sprouted Oats
		(2 oz dry = 1 lb sprouted)[1]
Water ....(g)	7	404
Dry Matter ....(g)	50	50
Protein ....(g)	7.5	10.5
Fat ....(g)	2.1	2.6
Carbohydrate, available ....(g)	32.9	21.4
Energy[2] ....(kcal)	181	151
Fiber ....(g)	5.9	13.1
Ash ....(g)	1.6	2.0
Calcium ....(mg)	32	119
Phosphorus ....(mg)	180	254
Vitamin A[3] ....(IU)	0	3,039
Vitamin E ....(mg)	0.9	2.4
Niacin ....(mg)	0.9	5.2
Riboflavin ....(mg)	0.1	1.1
Thiamin ....(mg)	0.2	0.6
Vitamin C ....(mg)	0	10.9

[1]Approximately 1 lb (*0.45 kg*) of fresh sprouts may be obtained from 2 oz (*56 g*) of grain.

[2]Calculated by allowing 4 Calories (kcal) per gram of protein, 9 Calories (kcal) per gram of fat, and 4 Calories (kcal) per gram of carbohydrate.

[3]The vitamin A equivalent of the carotene content, considering 1 mg of carotene to be equivalent to 1,667 IU of Vitamin A.

It may be seen from Table C-8 that the hydroponic sprouting of oats results in (1) great increases in fiber, water, vitamin A, and bulk (1 lb [*0.45 kg*] of sprouts is obtained from 2 oz [*56 g*] of grain); (2) moderate increases in protein, fat, total minerals (ash), calcium, phosphorus, vitamin E, vitamin C, and the vitamin B complex; and (3) decreases in carbohydrate and calories. Therefore, sprouted grains make a satisfactory vegetable supplement to diets when fresh fruits and vegetables may not be available. Unfortunately, the large amounts of water and fiber that they contain make them very filling, so consumption is limited.

USES OF GRAINS AND CEREAL PRODUCTS.
The cereal products that people eat are derived from only a small portion of the grain plants. Likewise, hardly any of the by-products from the brewing and distilling industries are consumed by people. Therefore, the greater part of the

vegetable matter from these crops may go to waste unless arrangements are made to feed the surplus materials to livestock. The efficient utilization of grain by-products for the feeding of farm animals has helped to keep the prices of meats, poultry, and dairy products within the reach of most American families. Uses of some of the major cereal products follow. Additional details regarding the products made from each of the major grains are given in the separate articles covering each of these items.

(Also see BARLEY; CORN; MILLET; OATS; RICE; RYE; SORGHUM; TRITICALE; WHEAT; and WILD RICE.)

Beverages and Foods. Most of the people who eat minimally processed grains do so because of either sheer necessity or long-standing custom. Even the most primitive cultures devised ways of converting the rather bland and chewy raw grains into more appealing beverages and foods.

• **Alcoholic beverages**—These drinks are the basis of popular social institutions such as the *pub* (short for public house) in Great Britain and the *bar* in the United States. Beer and grain whiskeys are the leading beverages served in these establishments. Home consumption of beer and liquor also account for much of the usage of these grain-based beverages, which may be produced from a wide variety of different cereals.

(Also see BEERS AND BREWING; and DISTILLED LIQUORS.)

• **Alimentary pastes (pasta)**—Macaroni, noodles, and spaghetti—which probably originated in China, but came to the United States by way of Europe—are often used as the main course of low cost dinners. Most of these products are made from durum wheat, which imparts to the pasta a great resistance to disintegration in boiling water. However, a few American food companies have developed special macaronis that are made from various combinations of corn, soy, and wheat flours. These products have higher protein quality than those made from wheat flour alone.

(Also see MACARONI AND NOODLE PRODUCTS.)

• **Breads**—Although the total consumption of all types of breads in the United States has declined steadily since the beginning of the 20th century, the use of specialty bread products such as hero or submarine sandwiches, hamburgers, and pizza has increased. There are now fast food restaurants which serve a variety of these products. Also, sandwiches of all types appear to be among the most popular lunch items for Americans, whether they carry a *bag lunch* from home or eat out. Furthermore, a wide variety of breads and related products are now available in frozen forms which require only baking.

The predominant grain used for breads in the United States is wheat, but recent innovations in baking technology have made it possible to use almost any type of flour to produce appealing products.

(Also see BREADS AND BAKING; and GLUTEN.)

• **Breakfast cereals**—Most of the impetus for the development of ready-to-eat breakfast cereal came from certain members of the Seventh-Day Adventist Church who founded the Western Health Reform Institute at Battle Creek, Michigan in 1866. They sought a meatless substitute for the traditional American breakfast of meat (usually bacon or ham) and eggs. It is noteworthy that the Kellogg brothers, who later founded the cereal company that bears their name, invented a granola-type of ready-to-eat breakfast while they were on the staff of the Battle Creek Sanitarium in Michigan. Mr. Post, who was one of their patients, also developed a cereal and founded another company in Battle Creek. Lately, there has been rising interest in so-called *natural cereals* which bear a close resemblance to their early forerunners.

(Also see BREAKFAST CEREALS.)

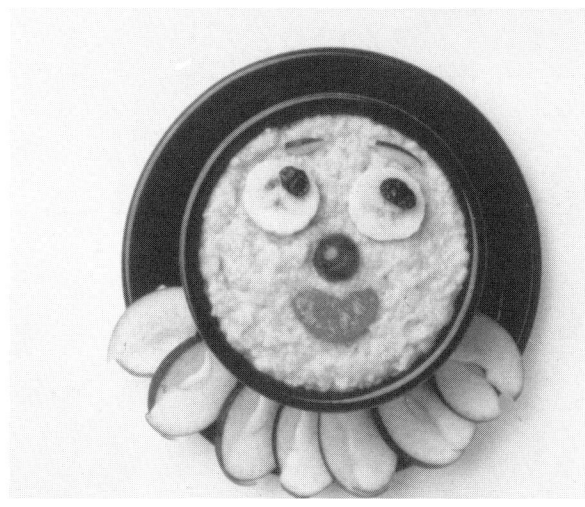

Fig. C-41. Cereal for breakfast can be made interesting for everyone. (Courtesy, USDA)

• **Flours**—Any of the major grains may be milled into flour, but people still prefer baked goods made from the traditional type of white flour that is derived from wheat. Nevertheless, food technologists have recently developed some new additives which impart good leavening characteristics to a wide variety of flours.

(Also see FLOURS.)

• **Infant cereals**—These items account for only a small fraction of the total consumption of grain products in the United States, yet they represent a nutritious group of fortified cereal products that might be used profitably by people of all ages. However, some mothers may feed their babies excessive amounts of cereals, milk, and other foods in the belief that if a little is good, more is better. Overfed infants may become afflicted with lifelong obesity.

(Also see INFANT DIETS AND NUTRITION.)

• **Snacks**—Many processes have been invented for turning grains into such tempting snacks as biscuits, cakes, cookies, corn chips, crackers, popcorn, pretzels, and similar items. These tidbits usually supply some of the daily nutrient requirements, except that they are often overloaded with fat, salt, and/or sugar. Therefore, some of the unsugared, ready-to-eat breakfast cereals might make more nutritious snacks, particularly when they are taken with milk.

(Also see SNACK FOODS.)

• **Vegetable dishes**—Many peoples around the world prepare cooked grains as vegetable side dishes, or in mixed dishes like stews and casseroles. For example, cooked corn grits are a regular accompaniment to meals in the southeastern United States, whereas cooked fresh sweet corn often serves a similar function in the Midwest. Likewise, most southeastern Asians have cooked rice with their meals.

(Also see BARLEY; CORN; MILLET; OATS; RICE; SORGHUM; TRITICALE; WHEAT; and WORLD FOOD.)

ECONOMICAL AND NUTRITIOUS MEALS BASED UPON COOKED CEREALS.

Economical and nutritious meals, which are not fattening despite their starchiness, may be based upon cooked cereals. This is evidenced in Table C-9. The nutritive values of the products not covered in Table C-9 are given in other articles and/or in Table F-21 Food Compositions.

Table C-9 shows that the cooking of cereals in water results

TABLE C-9
NUTRITIVE VALUES OF COOKED CEREAL PRODUCTS[1]

Product	Amount of Uncooked Cereal Which Yields 1 Cup of Cooked Cereal[2] (oz)	(g)	Yield of Cooked Cereal from 1 Lb of Uncooked Cereal (cups)	Weight of 1 Cup of Cooked Cereal[3] (oz)	(g)	Composition of 1 Cup of Cooked Cereal Product				Carbohydrate		Minerals			Vitamins		
						Water (g)	Cal- ories (kcal)	Pro- tein (g)	Fat (g)	Total (g)	Fiber (g)	Cal- cium (mg)	Phos- phorus (mg)	Iron (mg)	Thia- min (mg)	Ribo- flavin (mg)	Niacin (mg)
Corn, sweet, on-the-cob[4] ...	10.6	300	1.5	5.8	165	125	137	5.3	1.7	31.0	1.2	5	147	1.0	0.2	0.2	2.1
Cornmeal, degermed, enriched	1.2	34	13.5	8.4	240	211	120	2.6	0.5	25.7	0.2	2	34	1.0	0.1	0.1	1.2
Macaroni, elbow, enriched[5] .	1.5	42	10.8	4.9	140	102	155	4.8	0.6	32.2	0.1	11	70	1.3	0.2	0.1	1.5
Noodles, egg, enriched	1.8	52	8.8	5.6	160	113	200	6.6	2.4	37.3	0.5	16	94	1.4	0.2	0.1	1.9
Oats, rolled[6]	1.2	35	12.8	8.4	240	208	132	4.8	2.4	23.3	0.5	22	137	1.4	0.2	0.1	0.2
Popcorn, large kernel, without oil[7]	0.2	6.4	70.6	0.2	6	—	23	0.8	0.3	4.6	0.1	1	17	0.2	Trace	Trace	0.1
Rice, brown[8]	2.3	66	6.9	6.9	195	137	232	4.9	1.2	49.7	0.6	23	142	1.0	0.2	Trace	2.7
Rice, white, enriched[8]	2.2	64	7.1	7.2	205	149	223	4.1	0.2	49.6	0.2	21	57	1.8	0.2	Trace	2.1
Spaghetti, enriched[5]	1.5	42	10.8	4.9	140	102	155	4.8	0.6	32.2	0.1	11	70	1.3	0.2	0.1	1.5
Wheat, farina, quick cooking enriched	1.1	30	15.1	8.6	245	218	105	3.2	0.2	21.8	Trace	147	162	12.3	0.1	0.1	1.0
Wheat, rolled	1.9	54	8.4	8.4	240	192	180	5.3	1.0	40.6	1.2	19	182	1.7	0.2	0.1	2.2
Wheat, whole grain	1.2	34	13.5	8.6	245	215	110	4.4	0.7	23.0	0.7	17	127	1.2	0.2	0.1	1.5

[1]From Food Composition Table F-21, which also contains further composition data on these cereal products. One cup equals 240 ml and 1 lb equals 454 g.

[2]The amount of uncooked cereal is calculated from the weight (wt) and dry matter content (dm) of 1 cup of the cooked cereal, by the following formula:

$$\text{Wt uncooked cereal (g)} = \frac{\text{wt cooked cereal (g)} \times \text{dm of cooked cereal (\%)}}{\text{dm of uncooked cereal (\%)}}$$

[3]Weight is that of the freshly cooked, hot cereal.

[4]The weight of the kernels cut from the cob represents 55% of the weight of the uncut cob.

[5]Cooked to the tender stage.

[6]Data apply to either the regular or the instant-cooking product.

[7]Small, popped kernels pack together more closely. Hence, a cup of the small variety may weigh up to twice as much as one of the large variety, and the nutrients will be increased proportionately.

[8]Long grain variety.

in great increases in their water content and bulk. For example, 1 lb (0.45 kg) of uncooked wheat farina yields 15.1 cups (3.6 liter) of cooked cereal which weigh 8.6 oz (241 g) each, for a total yield of 8.1 lb (4 kg). Similarly, 1 lb of dry cornmeal cooks up to 7.1 lb. Fortunately, few people rely on either cooked wheat or cornmeal alone for their dietary energy, because it would be difficult for most people to eat enough of these items to meet their needs. On the other hand, large numbers of low income people around the world rely heavily on rice and various types of pasta, which cook up to only about three times their original bulk. Therefore, it is noteworthy that cooked cereals alone are not fattening—since it takes from 7 to 15 cups (1.7 to 3.6 liter) of the various items to meet the minimum caloric needs of most adults. (Most sedentary adults require between 1,600 and 2,800 Calories [kcal] per day.) Usually, obesity in cereal eaters is due to the fatty and sugary foods consumed along with the grain products.

Another important consideration in deciding which cereals are the best buys is the amounts of protein supplied by these items. The most nutritious products are those which supply the maximum protein per pound and per calorie. Fig. C-42 gives these data for some of the most commonly used cereal items on an as-purchased basis.

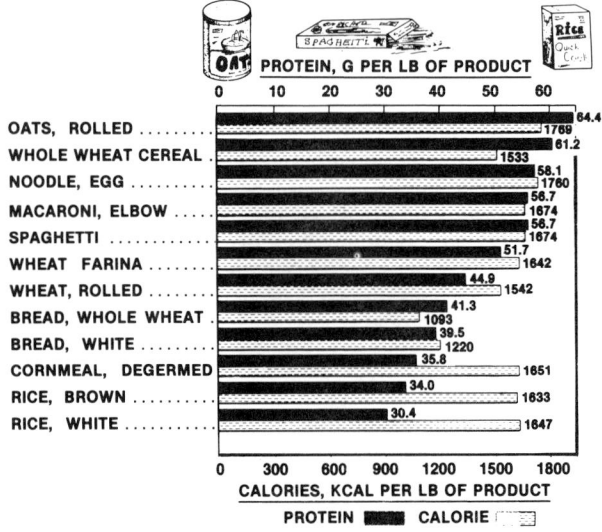

Fig. C-42. Protein and caloric contents of 1-lb (0.45 kg) packages of selected cereal products. (Values are from Food Composition Table F-21 of this book)

It may be seen from Fig. C-42 that rolled oats and whole wheat cereal provide the most protein per pound; whereas brown and white rice provide the least. Also, the oat and wheat products provide about twice as much protein per calorie as the rice products.

Finally, it is not desirable for people to attempt to eat the quantities of cereals which might completely meet their protein needs, because they would have little appetite left for the foods that supply the other essential nutrients. Hence, it is necessary to plan for the use of other protein-containing foods. Methods of accomplishing this are detailed in this book in the section devoted to Food Groups.

(Also see BREADS AND BAKING; BREAKFAST CEREALS; FLOUR; and MACARONI AND NOODLE PRODUCTS.)

FUTURE OF CEREAL GRAINS. It seems likely that the worldwide demand for cereal grains will continue to rise along with the steady growth in population. However, not much land is left for expansion of the acreage which is presently allotted to grain crops. Therefore, certain other measures have been either instituted, or are under consideration, so that additional supplies of grain may be made available to prevent malnutrition and starvation from occurring on a massive scale.

• **Grain reserves**—There is a great need to establish reserve supplies of grains which may be used when adverse conditions in some countries reduce crop production below the levels needed to feed people adequately. The details of such a program still need to be worked out, especially who will pay for it and where it will be stored.

• **The Green Revolution**—This term refers to the development and utilization of special, high-yielding varieties of rice and wheat. The effect of this breakthrough has been the doubling and tripling of the yields of these popular grains so that more people might be fed by the crops grown on fixed acreages.

(Also see GREEN REVOLUTION.)

• **High-lysine and high-protein varieties of grain**—Special, new hybrid varieties of grains have been developed which have markedly higher protein quality and quantity than the older, more common types. These new varieties meet the amino acid and protein requirements of growing children and pregnant mothers better, so that there is less need to supplement their diets with other protein-containing foods. Much more land is required to produce high-quality animal protein foods such as eggs, legumes, meats, milk, and poultry than is required to produce cereal protein.

• **Less grain for livestock and more for people**—Mounting demands for grains are likely to make it increasingly expensive to feed these crops to livestock. Fortunately, grazing animals—cattle, goats, and sheep—can be fed rations based mainly on forage crops and various by-products, whereas pigs and poultry require more readily digestible feeds such as grains and certain by-products from food processing. Therefore, the diversion of corn and other feed grains from animals to people may not cause any reduction in the supplies of beef, lamb, and milk, but it may lessen pork, chicken, turkey, and eggs.

• **Increased utilization of crops which provide the nutrients that are lacking in grains**—Attempts to cope with world food shortages by utilization of the high-yielding varieties of grains should allow for measures that provide the nutrients lacking in grains. For example, legumes and oilseeds are often used to supplement the protein of cereals. Therefore, the production of the required amounts of grains on fewer acres of land might make it possible to shift some of the acreage now devoted to corn, rice, and wheat to other crops such as peanuts, soybeans, and green leafy vegetables.

Another approach would be to promote the cultivation of lesser known species such as *Amaranth* and *Chenopodium*. The grainlike seeds of these plants have long been used as food by the native peoples of Latin America. It is noteworthy that the amino acid patterns of these seeds, which contain about 13% protein, resemble those of the legumes and oilseeds, and that they complement those of the major cereals. Furthermore, the leaves of *Amaranth* and *Chenopodium* are rich in vitamin A, a nutrient that is lacking in the grains. Finally, it has been reported that cultivated stands of *Amaranth* have yielded more seeds per acre than corn.

(Also see WORLD FOOD.)

CEREAL GRAINS OF THE WORLD. Four cereal grains—wheat, corn, rice, and barley—account for over 89% of the world's grain production. However, sorghum, oats, rye, and millet are important in countries where they are better adapted than the major cereal grains.

The better known cereal grains of the world are listed in Table C-10, Cereal Grains of the World. Additionally, the most important cereal grains (those produced in greatest quantity), worldwide and/or in the United States are accorded detailed narrative coverage, alphabetically, whereas cereal grains of lesser importance are presented in summary form only in Table C-10, Cereal Grains of the World.

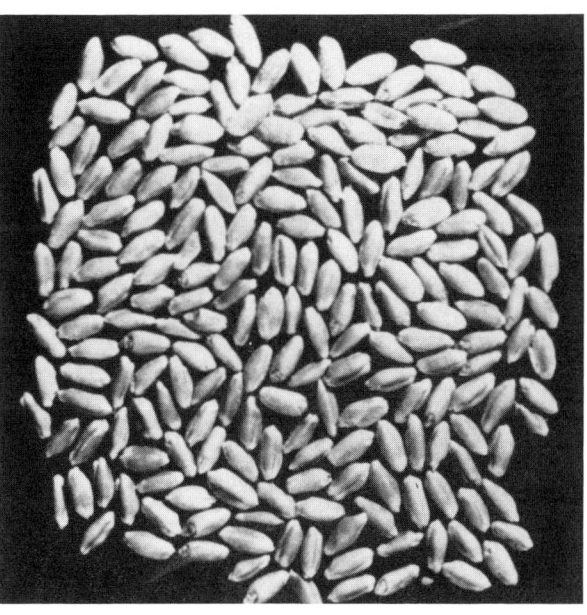

Fig. C-43. Wheat, leading cereal grain of the world. (Courtesy, J. I. Case Company, Racine, Wisc.)

TABLE C-10
CEREAL GRAINS OF THE WORLD

Popular Name(s); Scientific Name Origin and History	Importance Principal Areas Growing Conditions	Processing Products and Uses	Nutritional Value Comments
Adlay (Job's Tears) *Coix lachrma-jobi* Shaped like a large drop of fluid; hence, the form has suggested the name, Job's Tears. **Origin and History:** Native to India.	**Importance:** As a food crop for the poorer people in eastern Asia and in the Philippines. **Principal Areas:** Throughout the tropical world. **Growing Conditions:** Marshy areas; tropical rain forests.	**Processing:** The grain may be parched, boiled whole, or milled into flour. **Products and Uses:** As a cereal food in parts of eastern Asia and in the Philippines. The seeds are also used as beads and for rosaries.	**Nutritional Value:** The grain has a higher protein-to-carbohydrate ratio than most cereals. **Comments:** It is claimed that Adlay seed has anti-asthma and diuretic properties.
Barley (See BARLEY.)			
Buckwheat (See BUCKWHEAT.)			
Corn (See CORN.)			
Emmer *Triticum dicoccum* **Origin and History:** Cultivated by ancient Mediterranean people; and identified in ancient archeological diggings.	**Importance:** Minor. **Principal Areas:** Cultivated in some of the mountainous areas of Europe. Formerly grown in the Dakotas of the U.S. **Growing Conditions:** Dry soils of mountainous regions.	**Processing:** The Indians often ground it into bread flour. **Products and Uses:** Baking breads, and as a livestock feed.	**Nutritional Value:** Similar to barley and oats; 12–13% protein on a dry basis. **Comments:** Presently, emmer is primarily of historic interest.
Indian Ricegrass *Oryzopsis hymenoides* **Origin and History:** Native to western U.S.	**Importance:** Minor importance for human food. **Principal Areas:** From the Dakotas south to Texas, and west to the Pacific Ocean. **Growing Conditions:** Dry, sandy soils but it also tolerates alkali soils and drought.	**Processing:** The American Indians ground the grain into flour. **Products and Uses:** The Indians baked it into bread.	**Nutritional Value:** Similar to the other cereal grains. **Comments:** Used primarily as a livestock forage.
Millet (See MILLET.)			
Oats (See OATS.)			
Rice (See RICE.)			
Rye (See RYE.)			
Sorghum (See SORGHUM.)			
Spelt *Triticum spelta* **Origin and History:** Probably originated in the Mediterranean area.	**Importance:** Minor. **Principal Areas:** Northern Spain. Formerly grown in the Dakotas of the U.S. **Growing Conditions:** Cold areas and dry soils.	**Processing:** Threshed for feed grain. Hulls not removed in threshing. **Products and Uses:** Primarily as a livestock feed and forage.	**Nutritional Value:** Similar to barley and oats; 12–13% protein on a dry basis. **Comments:** Presently, spelt is of historic interest.
Teff (See TEFF.)			
Teosinte *Euchlaena mexicana* **Origin and History:** A wild cereal of Mexico. It is suspected that it crossed on primitive corn (maize) about 1500 B.C.	**Importance:** Minor. **Principal Areas:** In Mexico, and sparingly in southern U.S. **Growing Conditions:** Tropical, with long days; and a rich, moist soil.	**Processing:** Similar to corn. **Products and Uses:** Similar to corn.	**Nutritional Value:** Similar to corn. **Comments:** In Mexico, hybrids of teosinte and maize are found, giving rise to the view that the two plants developed from a common ancestor.
Triticale (See TRITICALE.)			
Wheat (See WHEAT.)			
Wild Rice (See WILD RICE.)			

CEREBRAL

Pertaining to the cerebrum, the largest part of the human brain.

(Also see TISSUES OF THE BODY.)

CEREBRAL HEMORRHAGE

This condition, which is commonly called stroke or apoplexy, results from a breaking of a blood vessel in the brain. A hemorrhage is more likely to occur when the blood pressure is elevated, than when it is normal. A stroke is often followed by a loss of consciousness and/or partial paralysis. The diagnosis of a cerebral hemorrhage may be confirmed by finding of blood in the cerebrospinal fluid, which bathes both the brain and the spinal cord. If blood is absent from the cerebrospinal fluid, the stroke was most likely due to the blockage of blood flow to the brain (cerebral infarct).

(Also see CEREBRAL INFARCT; CEREBROSPINAL FLUID; and HIGH BLOOD PRESSURE.)

CEREBRAL INFARCT

A blockage of the blood flow to the brain, which is usually due to a clot lodged within an artery serving the brain. The consequences of this mishap are essentially the same as those of a cerebral hemorrhage (loss of consciousness and partial paralysis.) Hence, both conditions are commonly referred to as *strokes*. An infarct is most likely to occur in people afflicted with atherosclerosis and/or congestive heart failure. Also, it may take place when the blood pressure is normal or subnormal. This condition is distinguished from a cerebral hemorrhage by the absence of blood in the cerebrospinal fluid.

(Also see CEREBRAL HEMORRHAGE; CEREBROSPINAL FLUID; and HEART DISEASE.)

CEREBROSPINAL FLUID

A clear fluid secreted by the ventricles of the brain, which bathes both the brain and the spinal cord. It serves to (1) act as a medium for the exchange of nutrients and metabolic products with the nerve cells; (2) regulate the fluid content and pressure within the brain and spinal cord; and (3) protect the tissues of the brain against injury. Doctors may withdraw some of the cerebrospinal fluid from the spine (spinal tap) in order to diagnose certain diseases.

CERIMAN *Monstera deliciosa*

The conelike fruit of a vine (of the family *Araceae*) that is native to Mexico.

Cerimans are usually about 8 in. (*20 cm*) long and are suitable for eating only if they are fully ripe, when the flavor is like that of a mixture of bananas and pineapple. The unripe fruit contains acid crystals that burn the mouth.

CEROID

A type of brownish pigment found in clogged arteries (such as in atherosclerosis), the intestinal lining, and in various types of disorders where polyunsaturated fats are abnormally oxidized. The accumulation of ceroid pigment appears to be associated with deficiencies of selenium and vitamin E.

CERULOPLASMIN

A protein which transports copper in the blood. When there is a deficiency of ceruloplasmin, copper is not efficiently utilized. Hence, there may be certain types of anemia, or deposits of copper in various tissues.

CERVELAT (CERVELET; CHERVELAS)

Sausage of several regional kinds made of varying proportions of pork and beef with added fat and spices, stuffed into casings, and smoked.

CHAFF

Glumes, husks, or other seed coverings, together with other plant parts, separated from seed in threshing or processing.

CHARCOAL, ACTIVATED

This is an antidote for many types of poisons. Poison centers commonly use activated charcoal as a follow-up measure after doctors induce vomiting with syrup of ipecac or pump the patient's stomach.

CHARQUI (CHARQUE)

Dried meat; jerked meat.

CHEDDARING

After whey is drained and curds have knit together suf-ficiently, slabs are cut from the curd. These are turned and piled, then repiled, to induce matting of the curd and expel most of the whey. This turning and stacking technique, known as *cheddaring*, helps give the cheese its characteristic body.

CHEILITIS

A soreness of the lip, that is sometimes due to a riboflavin deficiency.

(Also see CHEILOSIS.)

CHEILOSIS

Cracks at the corners of the mouth that often signify a riboflavin deficiency. However, this disorder may also be due to badly chapped lips, particularly when the victim has been exposed to a cold or windy environment.

(Also see RIBOFLAVIN.)

CHELATE

The word *chelate* is derived from the Greek word meaning *claw*. It refers to a cyclic compound which is formed between an organic molecule and a metallic ion, the latter being held within the organic molecule as if by a claw. Examples of naturally occurring chelates are the chlorophylls, cytochromes (respiratory enzymes), hemoglobin, and vitamin B-12. The addition to foods and mineral supplements of a chelating agent, such as ethylenediaminetetraacetic acid (EDTA), may in some cases improve the availability of the mineral elements.

(Also see MINERAL[S], section on "Food Additives.")

CHELATION

The processing chelating—the formation of a bond between an organic molecule and a metallic ion.

CHEMICAL BONDING

The attachment of various chemical elements to form chemical compounds. The chemical bonds that hold the elements of a compound together consist of stored potential energy, which is released to do body work when the compound is broken into parts.

CHEMICAL REACTION

A chemical reaction that may occur by (1) combination, (2) replacement, (3) decomposition, or (4) some modification of the first three, the process may either require energy or yield it.

CHERRY *Prunus* spp

Cherries, which belong to the rose family, are a small round fruit of certain species of trees belonging to the genus *Prunus*—a group which also includes the plum, peach, nectarine, apricot, and almond.

The three basic kinds of cultivated cherry trees are (1) sweet cherry, (2) sour cherry, and (3) the Duke. However, the sweet cherry and sour cherry are of prime importance in the United States. The Duke is a hybrid resulting from a cross between the sour and the sweet cherry.

ORIGIN AND HISTORY. Some kinds of cherry trees are native to America. Others came from Europe and the Middle East. The cherry was one of the first fruits to be brought to the new world by the colonists.

WORLD AND U.S. PRODUCTION. Approximately

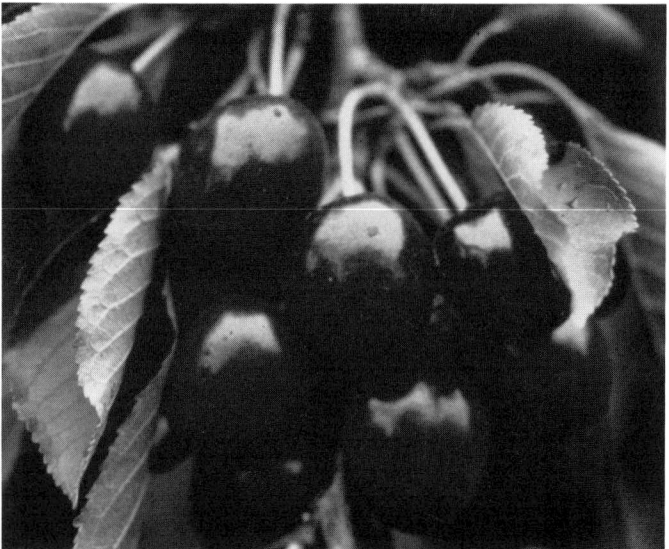

Fig. C-44. Cherries, a cherished summer fruit. (Courtesy, USDA)

850,000 metric tons of cherries are produced annually in the 11 leading cherry-producing countries of the world; and the leading countries, by rank, are: United States, Germany, Italy, France, Spain, and Greece.[15]

The United States produces about 236,000 short tons of all varieties of cherries (sweet and tart combined) annually; and the leading states, by rank, are: Michigan, Washington, Oregon, and California. Michigan produces 77% of the nation's sour cherries.[16]

PROCESSING. In the United States, 54% of the sweet cherries are sold fresh, 10% frozen, 7% canned, and 30% brined (maraschino or confectionery use). Of the sour cherries, 3% are sold fresh, 35% are canned, 59% are frozen, and 3% are brined. Cherries sold fresh include cherries sold for home use.

At processing plants, cherries are graded, sorted, and pitted before being canned, frozen, juiced, or brined. Some sour cherries are water-packed; others are canned as ready-to-use pie filling; still others are canned as cherry sauce and jellied cherry sauce containing spices. Sweet cherries are canned in syrup, with or without pits. The pitted sour cherry is one of the most satisfactory fruits for freezing, with or without sugar. A few sour cherries are pressed fresh or frozen for juice extraction. Brined cherries are used for the production of maraschino cherries, and for candied and glaceed cherries. Brine contains sulfur dioxide to bleach cherries to a uniform white or yellowish-white, and lime or calcium salt to firm or toughen the fruit.

• **Maraschino**—Maraschino cherries are sweetened, dyed, given maraschino flavoring, packed and canned in syrup. The original maraschino flavoring was obtained from the fruits and leaves of Marasca cherry trees grown in Yugoslavia. However, today, most maraschino flavoring is made from bitter almond oil, neroli oil, and vanilla extract.

• **Candied and glaceed cherries**—The candying process consists essentially of slowly impregnating the fruit with syrup until the sugar concentration in the fruit is high enough to prevent growth of microorganisms. Following impregnation, the fruit is washed and dried and sold as candied fruit. For glaceed fruit, the washed and dried candied fruit is coated with a thin transparent layer of heavy syrup that dries to a more or less firm texture.

SELECTION, PREPARATION, AND USES. Bing, Black Tartarian, Schmidt, Chapman, and Republican varieties should range from deep maroon or mahogany red to black, for richest flavor. Lambert cherries should be dark red. Good cherries have bright, glossy, plump-looking surfaces and fresh-looking stems.

Cherries may be washed and served raw, or they may be cooked and used as a topping for various dishes. Served alone, sweet cherries, fresh or canned, are an excellent dessert fruit, or they may be used in sauces, fresh fruit dishes, gelatin desserts, and ice cream. Sour cherries are used primarily in cooked desserts. Cherry pie is an all-time favorite, but there are other baked goods requiring sour cherries. Maraschino cherries are used as an accent on other desserts or toppings and in cocktails. They are available with or without stems. Candied cherries are used in baked goods.

NUTRITIONAL VALUE. Fresh cherries are 80 to 84% water. Fresh sweet cherries contain 70 Calories (kcal) per 100 g (about 3 ½ oz), while fresh sour cherries contain 58 Calories (kcal) per 100 g. When either type is canned in water they contain fewer calories than the fresh cherries. When cherries are canned in a syrup, the calories per serving increase. Calories in the fresh cherries are derived primarily from the natural sugars (carbohydrate). Cherries contain small amounts of minerals and vitamins. Per 100 g, sour cherries contain 1,000 IU of vitamin A while sweet cherries contain only 110 IU of this vitamin. Candied cherries contain only 12% water but they are packed with 339 Calories (kcal) per 100 g and little else. They are higher in calories due to the added sugar. More detailed information regarding the nutritional value of fresh or canned sour and sweet cherries, frozen sour cherries, candied cherries and maraschino cherries is provided in Food Composition Table F-21.

CHIEF CELLS

Cells in the stomach lining which secrete (1) pepsinogen, an enzyme that begins the digestion of protein; and (2) lipase, an enzyme that splits fatty acids from fat. These enzymes only start the digestive process which is finished by the pancreatic enzymes secreted into the small intestine. However, the partially digested products from the stomach trigger the release of hormones from the small intestine, which (1) stimulate the pancreas to secrete digestive juices, (2) slow the rate at which the stomach empties its contents into the intestines, and (3) cause the gallbladder to expel its bile.

(Also see DIGESTION AND ABSORPTION; and ENZYME.)

CHILDHOOD AND ADOLESCENT NUTRITION

---

[15]Based on data from *Agricultural Statistics 1991*, USDA, p. 186, Table 273. **Note well:** Annual production fluctuates as a result of weather and profitability of the crop.

[16]*Ibid.,* Table 274.

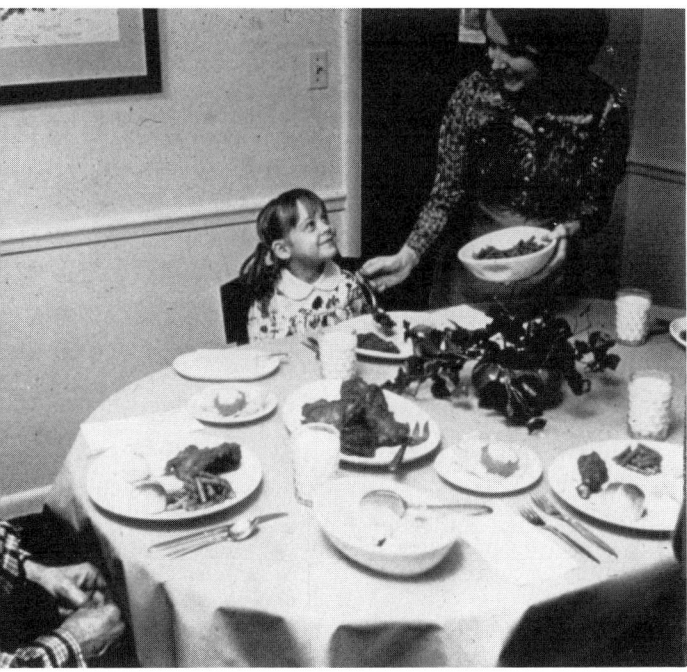

Fig. C-45. Mealtime should be a happy time for children. (Courtesy, Louisiana State Cooperative Service)

The early nutrition of children has major effects on the physical and mental well-being in later years. Furthermore, each young person develops important habits of food selection and consumption as he or she progresses from infancy to adolescence and adulthood. Therefore, nutrition during both childhood and adolescence is covered in this article since these stages of physical, mental, and emotional growth usually occur within the same family setting.

HISTORY. Even today children in some parts of the world live precarious existences because their nutritional needs are high in relation to their size, yet they often receive only a meager share of the available food. In many societies, the male heads of families receive the largest shares. This situation has existed for countless centuries, as evidenced by the disproportionate number of skeletons of children aged 14 years and younger which have been found at various archeological sites that were occupied by prehistoric peoples. However, not all primitive societies fared so poorly with their children since there is much evidence that well fed, healthy young people have had the innate biological capacities to adapt to a wide range of environments, ranging from the frigid arctic region to the hot, humid tropics or the dusty, dry deserts.

CHILDHOOD GROWTH AND ITS MEASUREMENT.
Some parents may be dismayed when the appetite of their toddler declines considerably from what it was during infancy. However, it is noteworthy that the average rates of growth for children during their second and third years are only about one-third of the rate for the first year of life, when the birth weight is tripled. For example, the average gain in weight from birth to age 1 is between 14 and 15 lb (*6.5 to 7.0 kg*), whereas only 10 lb (*4.5 kg*) are gained between ages 1 and 3.

Standard growth curves for girls and boys aged 2 to 18 years are presented in Figs. C-46 through C-51.

(Also see INFANT DIET AND NUTRITION.)

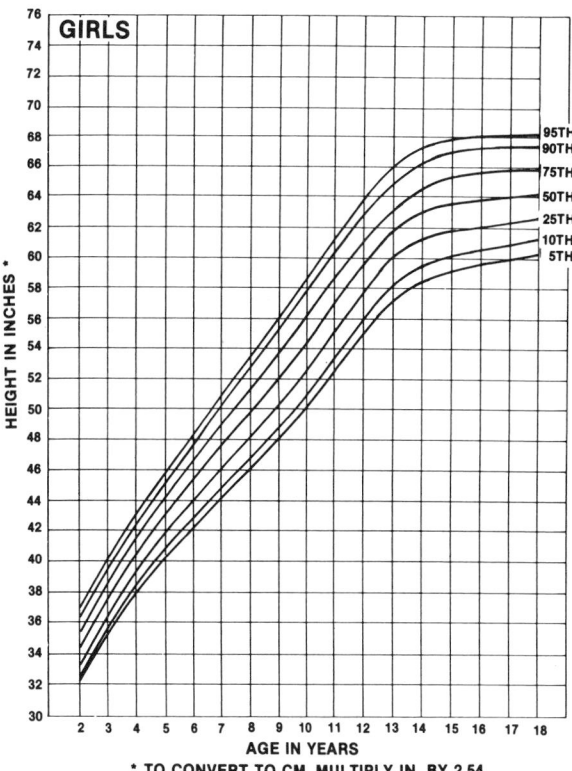

Fig. C-46. Heights of girls by age percentiles from 2 to 18 years. (Source: *NCHS Growth Curves for Children, Birth–18 Years, United States,* U.S. Dept. HEW)

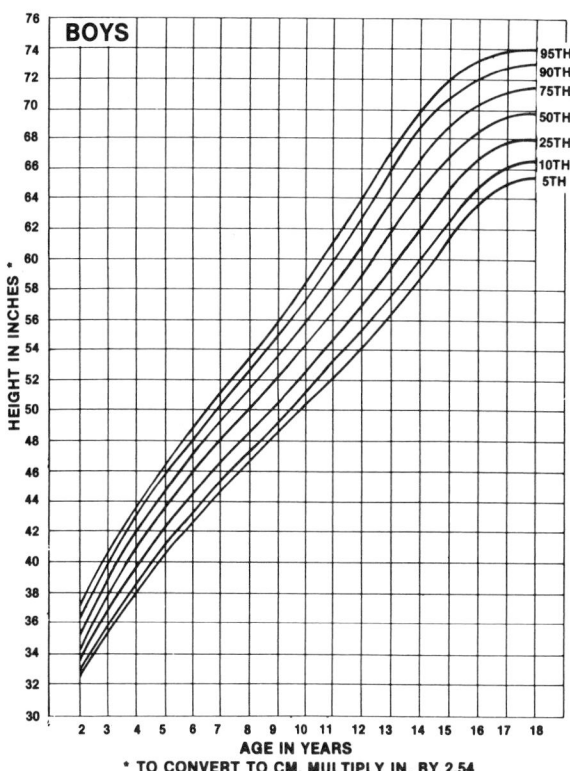

Fig. C-47. Heights of boys by age percentiles from 2 to 18 years. (Source: *NCHS Growth Curves for Children, Birth–18 Years, United States,* U.S. Dept. HEW)

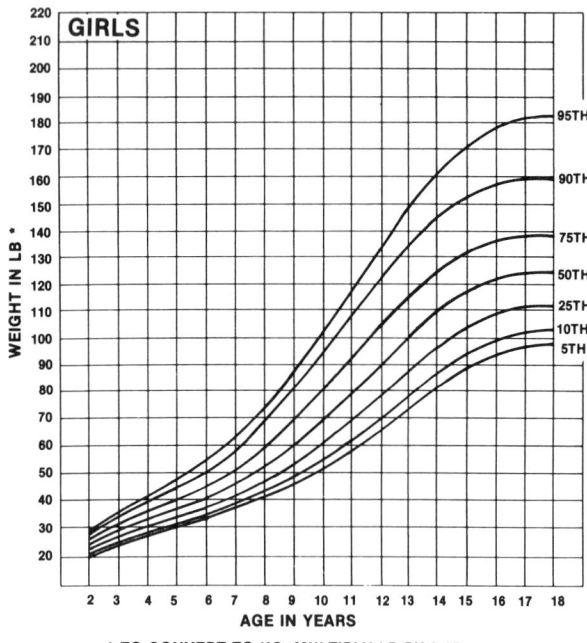

Fig. C-48. Weights of girls by age percentiles from 2 to 18 years. (Source: *NCHS Growth Curves for Children, Birth–18 Years, United States,* U.S. Dept. HEW)

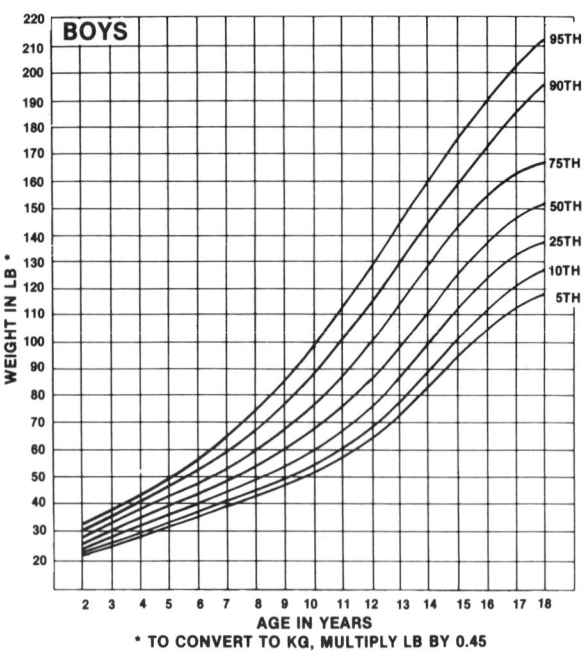

Fig. C-49. Weights of boys by age percentiles from 2 to 18 years. (Source: *NCHS Growth Curves for Children, Birth–18 Years, United States,* U.S. Dept. HEW)

To use the growth curves shown in Figs. C-46 through C-51, it is necessary to determine the percentiles which correspond most closely to the data from the girl or boy that was measured. A simple procedure follows:

1. Locate and mark the height or weight of the child on the vertical scale in the left margin of the appropriate chart. If the value of the measurement falls between the values marked on the scale, its placement should be estimated as accurately as possible.

2. With the aid of a ruler draw a light, horizontal line across the chart, starting from the marked value for height or weight.

3. Using a procedure similar to that in Step 1, locate and mark the age of the child on the horizontal scale at the bottom of the chart.

4. Draw a vertical line on the chart, starting from the marked value for age.

5. Circle the point at which the horizontal and vertical lines intersect on the chart and note the percentile curve which is closest to the intersection.

Values which fall between the 5th and 95th percentiles are considered to be within the normal range. However, there should not be a wide discrepancy between the percentiles for height and weight. Sometimes, a pediatrician will not diagnose and treat an otherwise healthy girl or boy until a clear-cut trend of growth abnormality is indicated by measurements taken at two or more consecutive monthly or bimonthly visits.

GROWTH AND DEVELOPMENT IN PUBESCENCE AND ADOLESCENCE. The period of growth and development between childhood and adulthood is commonly called adolescence, although it is more accurate to divide this interval into two phases that are referred to as pubescence and adolescence.

Pubescence, which occurs first and usually lasts for 2 to 3 years, begins with the initial appearance of secondary sex characteristics such as pubic hair and ends with the attainment of reproductive capability. This phase begins around 10 to 11 years of age in girls, and at about 12 to 13 years of age in boys, although it may occur one or more years earlier or later in early-maturing or late-maturing children. It is noteworthy that the maximum rate of growth of pubescent girls is about 3 in. (*8 cm*) in a single year, whereas boys may grow as much as 4 in. (*10 cm*) during the growth spurt.

Adolescence extends from the end of pubescence to the completion of physical growth. Growth in height is usually completed between 16 and 18 years of age in girls, and around 18 to 21 in boys, although some people continue to grow in height up to age 30. During adolescence, females gain a considerable amount of body fat, whereas males gain less fat, but more muscle. Accumulation of fat in adolescent females serves the purpose of supplying extra calories to meet the high demands of pregnancy and lactation. Hence, many adolescent girls may begin to consider themselves too fat, and attempt to lose weight by going on stringent diets. On the other hand, adolescent boys often consider themselves too slender, and may gorge themselves with food to become heavier.

The growth curves shown in Figs. C-46 through C-51 provide some general guidelines for evaluating the progress of girls and boys during pubescence and adolescence. However, the ranges of normal values for height and weight grow wider with age, with the result that it becomes increasingly difficult to detect deviations from normal. Sometimes, doctors or other health professionals will assess excessive fatness or slenderness by skinfold measurements, since

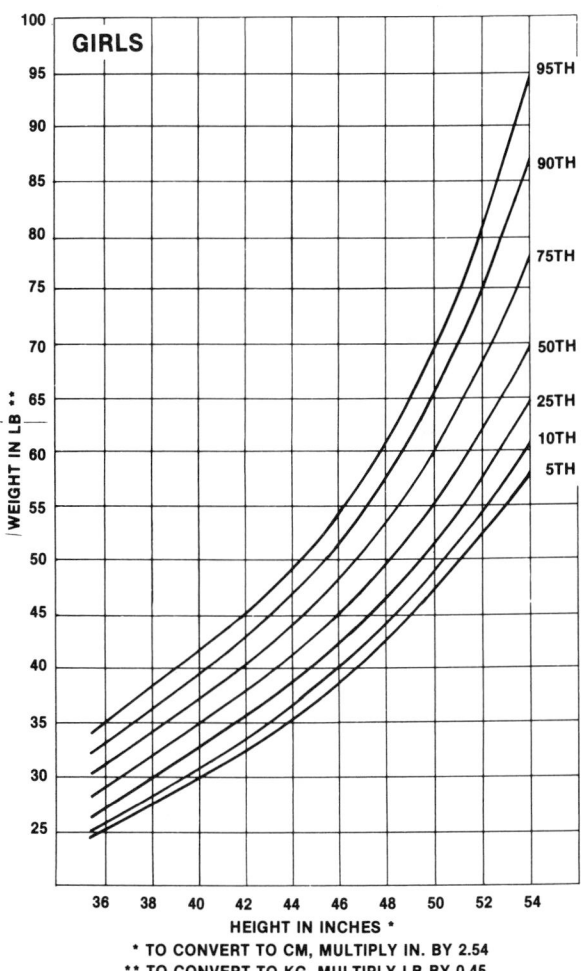

Fig. C-50. Weight by height percentiles for prepubescent girls. (Source: *NCHS Growth Curves for Children, Birth–18 Years, United States,* U.S. Dept. HEW)

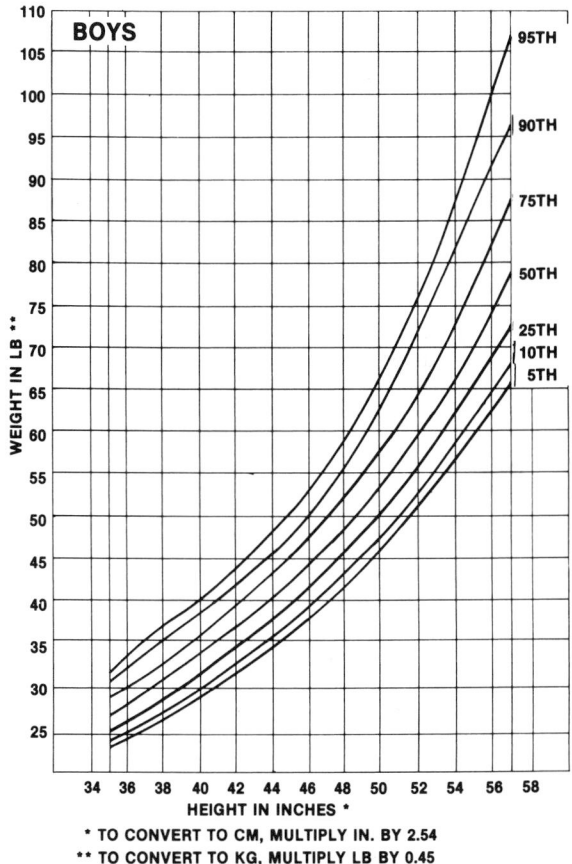

Fig. C-51. Weight by height percentiles for prepubescent boys. (Source: *NCHS Growth Curves for Children, Birth–18 Years, United States,* U.S. Dept. HEW)

weight gain alone gives little indication of the gain in fat, bone, and muscle. Furthermore, pediatricians can usually judge the growth and development status of adolescents better than most other people because they are experienced in observing the sequence of physical changes during pubescence and adolescence. The growth spurts which are accompanied by significant gains in weight often occur in conjunction with certain stages of sexual development.

NUTRIENT ALLOWANCES. Growing children and adolescents need a highly nutritious diet to meet the requirements for the growth and development of their body tissues. For example, dietary protein should supply from 8 to 10% of the calories, depending upon the rate of growth. Poor diets during these stages of life may have consequences that cannot be overcome later. Thus, a poorly nourished female during childhood and adolescence may bear weakened babies and have a gradual deterioration in health during childbearing. A male may be so physically and/or mentally handicapped from a poor diet in childhood and adolescence that he makes a poor breadwinner, husband, and father.

Meeting the allowances of growing children and adolescents requires the consumption of foods that are rich in protein, minerals, and vitamins in proportion to the calories

that are provided. However, it is not expected that many parents will attempt to check the composition of their children's diets in detail; rather, they will teach and guide them to make intelligent food choices.

The nutrient allowances by age groups, including children and adolescents, along with nutrient functions and best food sources of each nutrient, are fully covered in this book in the section on NUTRIENTS: REQUIREMENTS, ALLOWANCES, FUNCTIONS, SOURCES, and in its accompanying Table N-3; hence, the reader is referred thereto.

DIETARY GUIDELINES. Parents should help their children to make wise food choices as soon as possible, because there are many influences that encourage bad eating habits. Furthermore, most children, adolescents, and adults can spare little room in their diets for *empty calories* without risking the development of obesity. (The term *empty calories* refers to the food energy that is obtained from highly refined foods that are rich in carbohydrates and fats and furnish little else in the way of nutrients; for example, sugar.) Table C-11 gives some guidelines for daily food patterns.

(Also see FOOD GROUPS.)

TABLE C-11
DAILY FOOD GUIDE FOR CHILDREN AND ADOLESCENTS[1]

Type of Food	Each Day
Meat and Meat Substitutes	2 or more servings
Include—	
Meat, poultry, fish, shellfish, or eggs	
Dried beans or peas, peanut butter, or nuts can be used as meat substitutes.	
Milk Group	
Milk (fluid whole), evaporated (diluted 50:50 with water), skim, buttermilk, nonfat dry milk	
Children under 9	2 to 3 cups[2]
Children 10 to 12	3 or more cups[2]
Teenagers	4 or more cups[2]
Dairy products such as:	
Cheddar cheese, cottage cheese, ice cream, or yogurt	May sometimes be used in place of milk
Vegetable-Fruit Group	5 or more servings
Include—	
A fruit or vegetable that contains a high amount of vitamin C: grapefruit, oranges, cantaloupe, tomatoes (whole or in juice), raw cabbage, green or sweet red pepper, broccoli, or fresh strawberries.	
A dark green or deep yellow vegetable or a yellow fruit for vitamin A: broccoli, spinach, greens, cantaloupe, apricots, carrots, pumpkin, sweet potatoes, or winter squash.	
Other vegetables and fruits, including potatoes.	
Breads and Cereals	6 or more servings
Whole grain, enriched, or restored bread and cereals or other grain products such as cornmeal, grits, macaroni, noodles, spaghetti, or rice.	
Plus Other Foods	
To round out meals and to satisfy the appetite, many children will eat more of these foods, and other foods not specified will be used, such as butter, margarine, other fats, oils, sugars, or unenriched refined grain products. These *other* foods are frequently combined with the suggested foods in mixed dishes, baked goods, desserts, or other recipe dishes. They are a part of daily meals, even though they are not stressed in the food plan.	

[1]Adapted by the authors from *Your Child from 6 to 12*, Children's Bureau, U.S. Dept. HEW, Pub. No. 324.

[2]Or equivalent in nonfat dry milk (usually, about 1/4 cup of dry milk powder is equivalent to a cup of fluid milk). One cup equals 240 ml.

SCHOOL LUNCH AND BREAKFAST PROGRAMS.

This refers to the noon and morning meals served to children in schools.

The School Lunch Program was initiated in the 1930s, followed by the addition of the School Breakfast Program in 1966. The program expanded rapidly in response to (1) more children being transported to schools greater distances from their homes, (2) more mothers working away from home, (3) the desire of people and government to provide improved nutrition to the children of the poor, and (4) low-cost, subsidized meals.

A good understanding of the School Lunch Program is important to parents and teachers who influence the child's eating habits.

(Also see GOVERNMENT FOOD PROGRAMS; and SCHOOL LUNCH PROGRAM.)

COMMON NUTRITION-RELATED PROBLEMS.

Most of these problems may be dealt with successfully if the appropriate dietary measures are used without undue delay. If this is done, then only minor changes need be made in the diet of the child or adolescent. It is often wise to play down minor health problems in order to avoid creating excessive concern, or perhaps even hypochondria. Nevertheless, a doctor should be consulted whenever an abnormal condition persists for more than a few days. Therefore, the information which follows is presented mainly to foster better communication between parents, patients, and doctors; rather than to encourage an excessive reliance on home remedies.

Among the childhood and adolescent nutrition-related problems are the following: (**NOTE WELL:** those that are preceded by an asterisk are covered under similar headings elsewhere in this book [see Index]; the others are detailed in the sections which follow.)

*ADOLESCENT PREGNANCY
*ANEMIA
*ANOREXIA NERVOSA
*COLITIS
*CONSTIPATION
*DENTAL CARIES (CARIES; TOOTH DECAY)
*DIARRHEA
 Food Preferences and Aversions
 Overweight and/or Obesity
 Skin Blemishes
*ULCERS, PEPTIC
 Underweight

Food Preferences and Aversions. The food likes and dislikes that are developed in childhood may have far-reaching effects on one's health throughout life. For example, preferences for refined, sweet, or fatty foods combined with aversions to fresh fruits and vegetables may lead to the chronic consumption of a diet excessively high in calories, but low in the other essential nutrients. This problem is not new to our times, since many ancient cultures had deeply ingrained prejudices regarding the foods deemed suitable and unsuitable. Even when a wide variety of foods is available at reasonable cost, many people adhere to nutritionally imbalanced diets based upon their early eating experiences. It seems that everytime the cooks in the schools prepare broccoli for lunch, most of the vegetable ends up in the garbage pails, yet the serving of hamburger, hot dogs, and pizza is greeted enthusiastically. The latter foods are good sources of calories, protein, and some other nutrients, but they alone do not constitute a nutritionally balanced diet.

One of the solutions to this problem appears to be the introduction of a variety of foods to youngsters as soon as they are able to eat them. Sometimes, the parents of a child are the source of the poor eating habits that are acquired at an early age since children are very observant of parental reactions to foods. Recently, there have been many attempts by educators to make youngsters in day care centers and elementary schools more nutrition conscious. However, parental cooperation is needed to ensure that students receive a variety of nutritious, tasty foods at home.

Overweight and/or Obesity. Because excessive gain in weight represents an imbalance between food energy intake and energy needs, prevention of obesity cannot be concerned only with energy intake. Energy needs are determined by the basal metabolic rate and by energy requirements for activity and growth. After infancy, energy requirements for growth represent a small percentage of the total energy requirements. Basal metabolic rates vary from child to child but are more or less fixed in a particular child. The balance therefore depends primarily on the relation between energy intake and expenditures of energy in activity.

Imbalance between energy intake and expenditure leading to excessive gain in weight may result from abnormally high intake, unusually low expenditure, or from a combination of the two. Relatively small excesses of energy, accumulating day after day, year after year, are the common factor leading to obesity. A common pattern for children is an excess gain of about 4 to 5 lb (2 kg) in a year, representing an excess of from 35 to 50 Calories (kcal) per day.

Consumption of an amount of food that is barely adequate for one child may represent overeating for another. Not only do energy expenditures at rest vary from individual to individual but activity patterns are also widely different. There is reason to believe that highly active children may be at relatively low risk of developing obesity. In a society in which food is readily available, nearly all children are likely to eat at times for reasons other than satisfying energy requirements—because of social pressures, or merely because irresistibly attractive food is at hand. Under these circumstances, the child with high activity and consequent large energy expenditures seems likely to be at less risk from overeating than the inactive child whose energy needs are readily met.

A number of measures may be suggested for prevention of obesity:

1. Parents should be educated about the dangers of overfeeding during infancy and early childhood because of the possibility that habits of overeating may be established and persist into childhood and adult life.

2. Breast feeding should be encouraged and the introduction of supplementary foods should be delayed at least until 3 months of age.

3. Vigorous physical activity should be encouraged on a regular basis.

4. Efforts to develop appropriate community facilities for year-round physical activity of children (and adults) are important.

5. Several smaller meals are more effective in preventing obesity than 1 or 2 large meals providing the same energy intake.

6. When one or both parents are obese, the child is at greater risk of obesity than are most other children. Therefore, children from families with an obese parent should be identified and given particular guidance with respect to avoidance of excess weight gain.

(Also see OBESITY.)

Skin Blemishes (Acne). Although various types of skin blemishes may be signs of nutritional deficiencies, the most common skin imperfection found in American children and adolescents is acne, which occurs on the face, chest, and back. It is believed to result mainly from an inflammation of the sebaceous glands of the skin due to (1) external irritation from dirt, cosmetics, soap, or other agents; (2) changes in hormonal secretion that occur during pubescence; and/or (3) intolerances to foods such as chocolate, fats, iodized salt, peanut butter, soft drinks, or sugars. However, restriction of the latter foods does not always result in improvement.

Prevention or treatment of acne should involve skin care, good nutritional habits, and the use of topical preparations for the inflammation. There is little evidence that large doses of vitamin A are beneficial to those who already receive sufficient amounts of the vitamin in their diets. Furthermore, excesses of vitamin A are accumulated in the body and can cause toxic effects such as increased intracranial pressure which has symptoms like those of a brain tumor.

(Also see ALLERGIES.)

Underweight. The current concerns about obesity have led some people to pay insufficient attention to children and adolescents who may be underweight. Therefore, it is noteworthy that the very thin child is likely to be chilled easily, have a lowered resistance to infection, and a tendency to tire easily from physical activity. Excessive slenderness in adolescent females should keep teachers and parents on the watch for anorexia nervosa, because the female sex hormones which are secreted during this period normally promote the deposition of fat when the diet is adequate. Fortunately, most boys wish to avoid excessive slenderness, and are likely to seek means of gaining weight.

Underweight is best treated with a diet that contains abundant amounts of calories, protein, minerals, and vitamins. The diet should provide from 500 to 1,000 Calories (kcal) more than is needed for the maintenance of body weight. It may be a problem for the thin person to eat sufficient food, unless it is apportioned among frequent small meals. Finally, mild outdoor exercise may enhance the appetite, providing that it is done more than ½ hour before meals. Also, strenuous activity should be avoided for at least an hour after a meal because the increased flow of blood to the skeletal muscles during exercise decreases the circulation to the digestive organs.

MODIFICATION OF CHILDREN'S AND ADOLESCENT'S DIETS. It is generally recognized (1) that the early nutrition of children and adolescents has major effects on their physical and mental well-being later in life, and (2) that habits of food selection and consumption firmly established at a young age are likely to remain throughout a lifetime. Thus, the meals of children and adolescents, both at home and at school, should be closely linked to an educational program for better health. This should include a balanced diet, along with reduced sugar and salt and increased whole grains and raw fruits and vegetables.

(Also see NUTRIENTS: REQUIREMENTS, ALLOWANCES, FUNCTIONS, SOURCES.)

CHINESE RESTAURANT SYNDROME

The name given to a set of transient symptoms noted after dining on Chinese food or other highly flavored foods. The symptoms include headache, neck and chest pain, palpitations, and numbness. Monosodium glutamate (MSG), a food additive in high favor in most such restaurants, is the cause. An estimated 30% of consumers are affected. Sufferers soon learn to avoid excess consumption of highly flavored Chinese foods (especially the soup course).

CHIPOLATA

A small spicy sausage which is used as a garnish or as an hors d'oeuvre. Sometimes the name is used for a dish that contains such sausages.

CHIPPED BEEF

Thinly sliced dried beef.

CHITIN

A complex nitrogen-containing carbohydrate which is a major component of the cuticles or shells of insects, lobsters, shrimp, crayfish, and similar animals. It is not digestible in the human digestive tract. Therefore, it provides mainly bulk to those who eat the chitinous membranes.

CHITTERLING

The term chitterling applies only to the large intestine of swine. If the large intestine of young bovine is used, it must be identified as *veal chitterling* or *calf chitterling*.

CHLORIDE SHIFT (HAMBERGER SHIFT)

The exchange process of bicarbonate and chloride between plasma and red blood cells is referred to as the chloride shift, or Hamberger shift, after the Dutch physiologist.

CHLORINE DIOXIDE (ClO_2)

A chemical used to age or bleach flour, to impart to it the desirable characteristics of flour stored for weeks. Also chlorine dioxide is used to bleach organic materials such as cellulose, flour, fats and oils, and to act as a bacteriocide and antiseptic in water purification.

(Also see ADDITIVES.)

CHLORINE OR CHLORIDE (Cl)[17]

Chlorine, which is a strong-smelling, greenish-yellow gas, is never found in nature as an individual element. But its compounds, such as sodium chloride (common salt), are widespread.

Chlorine is an essential mineral, with the special function of forming the hydrochloric acid (HCl) present in gastric juice. The body contains approximately 100 g of chlorine, which represents about 0.15% of the weight of an average person, most of which is combined with sodium or potassium. It is found mainly in the extracellular fluids of the body, but it is present to some extent in red blood cells and to a lesser extent in the cells of other tissues. The blood contains 0.25% chlorine, 0.22% sodium, and 0.02% to 0.22% potassium; thus, the chlorine content of the blood is higher than that of any other mineral.

HISTORY. Carl Wilhelm Scheele, a Swedish chemist, discovered chlorine in 1774 by treating hydrochloric acid with manganese dioxide. A few years later Antoine Lavoisier, a French chemist, concluded that all acids contained oxygen. It followed that chlorine was called oxymuriatic acid gas because chemists believed that it also contained oxygen. In 1810, Sir Humphrey David, the English chemist, determined that chlorine was an element (further, he showed that muriatic acid itself contains only hydrogen and the new element, chlorine), which he named *chloros*, a Greek word meaning greenish-yellow.

ABSORPTION, METABOLISM, EXCRETION. Chloride from foods and from gastric juice is absorbed chiefly from the small intestine.

During digestion some of the chloride of the blood is used for the formation of hydrochloric acid in the gastric glands and is secreted into the stomach where it functions temporarily with the gastric enzymes and is then reabsorbed into the bloodstream with other nutrients.

The highest concentrations of body chlorine are found in the gastric juice and in the cerebrospinal fluid.

Excessive chlorine in the diet is excreted via the urine. Additional losses occur in sweating, vomiting, and diarrhea. Excreted chlorine is usually accompanied by excess sodium or potassium, unless the body has need to conserve base; in the latter case, the ammonium ion accompanies the chloride ion.

FUNCTIONS OF CHLORINE. Chlorine, in the form of the chloride ion which is negatively charged, plays a major role in the regulation of osmotic pressure, water balance, and acid-base balance. The chloride ion is also required for the production of hydrochloric acid by the stomach. This acid is necessary for proper absorption of vitamin B-12 and iron, for the activation of the enzyme that breaks down starch, and for suppressing the growth of microorganisms that enter the stomach with food and drink.

Chloride is a normal constituent of extracellular (between cells) rather than intracellular (within cells) fluid. However, in erythrocytes (red blood cells), chloride crosses the cell membrane rapidly to establish an equilibrium between cell contents and the extracellular fluids to aid in minimizing fluid shifts. The ability of the chloride to pass readily from the erythrocytes into the blood plasma (known as the chloride shift) enhances the ability of the blood to carry large amounts of carbon dioxide to the lungs.

Some cities add chlorine to drinking water to kill harmful bacteria. Opponents of chlorinated drinking water argue (1) that chlorine is a highly reactive chemical and may join with inorganic minerals and other chemicals to form substances that may be harmful, (2) that chlorine in drinking water destroys vitamin E, and (3) that chlorine destroys many of the intestinal flora that help in the digestion of food.

DEFICIENCY SYMPTOMS. Deficiencies of chloride may develop from prolonged or severe vomiting, diarrhea, pumping the stomach, injudicious use of diuretic drugs, or strict vegetarian diets used without salt. Severe deficiencies may result in alkalosis (an excess of alkali in the blood), characterized by slow and shallow breathing, listlessness, muscle cramps, lack of appetite, and occasionally, by convulsions.

INTERRELATIONSHIPS. Loss of chloride, generally parallels that of sodium. When sodium chloride intake is restricted, the chlorine level in the urine falls, followed by a drop in tissue chloride levels. Increased losses of sodium that occur with sweating or diarrhea result in concurrent losses of chloride.

---

[17]Chlorine exists in the body almost entirely as the chloride ion. The two terms—chlorine and chloride—are used interchangeably.

RECOMMENDED DAILY ALLOWANCE OF CHLORINE.
The are no recommended dietary allowances for chlorine because the average person's intake of 3 to 9 g daily from foods and added table salt easily meets the requirements. Also, diets that provide sufficient sodium and potassium provide adequate chlorine.

The body's requirement for chlorine is approximately half that of sodium.

Estimated safe and adequate intakes of chloride are given in the section on MINERAL(S), Table M-25, Mineral Table.

TOXICITY. An excess of chlorine ions is unlikely when the kidneys are functioning properly.

SOURCES OF CHLORINE. Chlorine is provided by table salt (sodium chloride) and foods that contain salt. Also, a number of chloride-containing salt substitutes are available.

(Also see MINERAL[S], Table M-25.)

CHLOROPHYLL

The green pigment of plants which permits them to manufacture foodstuffs from simple salts and carbon dioxide with energy derived from sunlight; i.e., photosynthesis.

(Also see PHOTOSYNTHESIS.)

CHLOROPHYLLASE

An enzyme present in all green plants which removes a chemical group from the chlorophyll molecule, producing a chlorophyllide and phytol.

(Also see PHOTOSYNTHESIS.)

CHLOROPHYLLIDE

A water soluble, green colored substance resulting from the chemical or enzymatic removal of a portion of the chlorophyll molecule. It is responsible for the green color of water after cooking certain vegetables.

(Also see CHLOROPHYLLASE; and PHOTOSYNTHESIS.)

CHLOROPHYLLIN COPPER

This is a synthetic version of chlorophyll, the substance that makes plants green. It is most commonly used for its deodorant qualities. Chlorophyllin copper tablets are sometimes given to incontinent patients in nursing homes to help neutralize odors. Sometimes, they are used for the same purpose by people who have had a colostomy or ileostomy. Chlorophyllin copper tablets are available without prescription.

CHLOROPHYLLINS

These are chemically prepared salts of chlorophyll used commercially in food coloring, dyes, breath and body deodorants, and medicine.

CHLOROSIS ("GREEN SICKNESS")

A type of anemia, formerly found in young women, characterized by a large reduction of hemoglobin in the blood, but only a slight diminution of the number of red blood cells. The symptoms are a greenish color to the skin, due to iron deficiency. Today, chlorosis has almost completely disappeared because of increased knowledge of the role of iron in the diet.

CHLORTETRACYCLINE (AUREOMYCIN)

An antibiotic.
(Also see ANTIBIOTICS.)

CHOKING

When food or some other object becomes lodged in the throat or larynx, resulting in blocking the air passage, the condition is known as choking. When the air passage is blocked, the person turns bluish-gray, and unconsciousness and death can result within 4 to 6 minutes.

The hallmarks of choking are excitement and attempted speech, but the inability to speak. Often the victim will point to his mouth or his throat. In contrast, a person may be excited, but he is usually able to speak.

When total blockage of the airflow occurs, immediate action is necessary. While emergency medical help is on the way, first aid may include any or all of the following:

1. The Heimlich Maneuver, named for Dr. Henry J. Heimlich of Cincinnati, is a first aid technique for choking victims. It is performed by (a) grabbing the victim from behind with both arms, (b) making a fist with one hand, (c) placing the fist near the navel but just below the rib cage, and (d) using the other hand to pull the fist quickly upward toward the victim's diaphragm. The maneuver may be repeated several times, and it can be applied with the victim sitting in a chair or lying down. The Heimlich maneuver rushes air out of the lungs with a sudden burst of pressure, thereby popping the obstruction out of the airway.

2. With the victim upside down or with his head lowered, a pound on the back *may* dislodge the object. However, this should never be done with the victim in the upright position, as the obstruction may fall further down the trachea.

3. There are devices for removing material from the back of the throat, which many restaurants have available. These are effective in trained hands. Furthermore, a finger may be used to dislodge the object. However, blind and frantic attempts to reach into the back of the throat should be avoided, as this may only serve to push the blockage further down the air passage.

CHOLAGOGUE

A food, nutrient, or similar substance that brings about expulsion of bile from the gallbladder. Most cholagogues act by stimulating the lining of the duodenum to release the hormone cholecystokinin-pancreozymin which travels via the blood to the gallbladder and triggers its contraction. Egg yolk and fats are considered to be the most potent cholagogues, although it seems likely that dairy products, fish, meat, and poultry have similar effects.

(Also see DIGESTION AND ABSORPTION; and GALLSTONES.)

CHOLANGITIS

An inflammation of the bile ducts.
(Also see GALLBLADDER.)

CHOLECALCIFEROL (VITAMIN D)

Another name for vitamin D_3. Both vitamin D_2 and vitamin

D_3 have equal activity for people, but chickens, turkeys, and other birds utilize vitamin D_3 more efficiently than vitamin D_2.

(Also see VITAMIN D.)

CHOLECYSTITIS

An inflammation of the gallbladder due to such causes as (1) infection, (2) trapped bile which cannot be secreted due to some type of blockage in the bile duct, (3) a tumor, or (4) adhesions of the walls of the gallbladder. It is characterized by a sharp pain under the breastbone which may travel to the shoulder and/or the lower abdomen. It may also be accompanied by vomiting, chills and fever, and jaundice.

(Also see GALLSTONES.)

CHOLERTIC AGENT

A substance that stimulates the liver to produce and secrete bile. The most potent cholertic agents appear to be protein, corn oil, and olive oil. Also, the entry of partially digested food and stomach acid into the duodenum has a cholertic effect.

(Also see DIGESTION AND ABSORPTION.)

CHOLESTEROL ($C_{27}H_{46}O$)

Cholesterol is found in all body tissues, especially the brain and spinal cord. Also, it is present in many animal food products—egg, meat, dairy products, poultry, fish, lard, and other fats. Further, cholesterol is an essential ingredient for certain biochemical processes, including the production of sex hormones in humans.

CHEMISTRY. Chemically, cholesterol is a fatlike compound—actually an alcohol—which in its pure form appears as pearly flakes. It is composed of 27 carbon atoms which form 3 fused cyclohexane (6-carbon) rings, a cyclopentane (5-carbon) ring and a side chain of 8 carbon atoms.

HISTORY. The cholesterol-heart disease debate was officially opened when, in 1953, Dr. Ancel Keys at the University of Minnesota reported a positive correlation between the consumption of animal fat and the occurrence of atherosclerosis in humans. Subsequently, other studies correlated high blood levels of cholesterol with increased incidence of atherosclerosis in humans. In 1964, the American Heart Association recommended that the general public reduce cholesterol intake to 300 mg/day. Subsequently, various government and health agencies around the world have followed suit. Thus, attention was, and still is, centered on cholesterol.

BLOOD LEVELS. Cholesterol is present in both free and esterified forms in the blood. From birth, blood cholesterol increases throughout life as shown in Table C-12. The

moderate risk category in Table C-12 includes large numbers of people with elevated blood cholesterol due, in part, to their diet. The high risk category in Table C-12 includes individuals with hereditary forms of high blood cholesterol which require the most aggressive treatment.

TABLE C-12
AGE AND CHOLESTEROL CONCENTRATION OF MEN AND WOMEN AT MODERATE AND HIGH RISK[1]

Age	Moderate Risk	High Risk
(years)	(mg/dl)	(mg/dl)
2 to 19	Greater than 170	Greater than 185
20 to 29	Greater than 200	Greater than 220
30 to 39	Greater than 220	Greater than 240
40 and over	Greater than 240	Greater

[1]National Insitute of Health guidelines of moderate and high risk levels of blood cholesterol as measured in milligrams per deciliter (mg/dl).

Since cholesterol is insoluble in a water-based medium such as blood, it is transported in blood as a lipoprotein. Primarily, two types of lipoproteins are involved in cholesterol transport. Low-density lipoproteins—LDL—transport cholesterol from the liver to the cells, while high-density lipoproteins—HDL—transport cholesterol from the tissue cells to the liver. Current research suggests that measuring HDL and LDL may be the most accurate means of assessing one's blood cholesterol level. Regardless of whether total cholesterol, the HDL, and/or LDL are measured in the blood of an individual, one should be aware that just a single determination on a blood sample is far from adequate for evaluating the cholesterol status. Factors such as (1) age, (2) time of day, (3) physical condition, (4) stress, (5) genetic background, (6) laboratory expertise may all affect the determination.

METABOLISM. Cholesterol in the body arises from two sources: (1) that from the diet—exogenous cholesterol; and (2) that manufactured in the body—endogenous cholesterol. Cholesterol in the blood reflects the overall cholesterol metabolism—that derived from both sources.

Digestion and Absorption. The average individual ingests between 500 and 800 mg of cholesterol each day. Dietary fat aids the absorption of cholesterol. Moreover, absorption is dependent upon the availability of bile acids from the liver, and pancreatic cholesterol esterase. Also, the absorption of cholesterol depends upon the amount eaten. Increasing intake decreases the percentage absorbed. At high levels, man absorbs less than 10%, and the remainder leaves the body via the feces. Initially, dietary cholesterol enters the blood as chylomicrons which are eventually converted to the cholesterol-containing lipoproteins—LDL and HDL. About 2 to 4 hours after eating, the cholesterol in the blood which came from the food is indistinguishable from that synthesized in the body.

Synthesis. Most all tissues, except possibly the brain, are capable of manufacturing—synthesizing—cholesterol. However, the liver is the major site of synthesis. The entire cholesterol molecule can be synthesized from 2-carbon units called acetate. In the whole metabolic scheme, acetate can be derived from the breakdown of carbohydrates, proteins (amino acids), and of course, fats. Each day the body manufactures 1,000 to 2,000 mg of cholesterol. However, on a day-to-day basis the synthesis and metabolism of cholesterol is controlled by such factors as (1) fasting, (2) caloric intake, (3) cholesterol intake, (4) bile acids, (5) hormones, primarily the thyroid hormones and estrogen, and (6) disorders such as diabetes, gallstones and hereditary high blood cholesterol—hypercholesterolemia. Control of cholesterol synthesis by cholesterol intake is important, since this means that when intake is high then synthesis is low and vice versa.

Functions. Cholesterol is vital to the body. Its primary importance concerns tissues, bile acids, and hormones.

Excretion. Removal from the body occurs primarily via the conversion of cholesterol to bile acids. About 0.8 g of cholesterol is degraded daily by this method. Also, a minor amount is converted to the above mentioned hormones. Additionally, some cholesterol is never digested, and hence, excreted via the feces, particularly when the intake is high.

THE RISK—HEART DISEASE.[18] High blood cholesterol is one of the three major modifiable risk factors for coronary heart disease (CHD); the other two are high blood pressure and cigarette smoking. Approximately 25% of the adult population 20 years of age and older has high blood cholesterol levels—levels that are high enough to need intensive medical attention. More than half of all adult Americans have a blood cholesterol level that is higher than desirable.

The following seven changes should be made in the diet of persons having high blood cholesterol:

1. **Eat less high-fat food.** The intake of total fat should constitute less than 30% of the calories.

Note: Eating less total fat is an effective way to eat less saturated fat and fewer calories.

2. **Eat less saturated fat.** The intake of saturated fat should constitute less than 10% of the calories.

Note: Saturated fats are found primarily in animal products. But a few vegetable fats and many commercially processed foods also contain saturated fat. Read labels carefully. Choose foods wisely.

3. **Substitute unsaturated fat for saturated fat.** Unsaturated fats (polyunsaturated and monounsaturated fats) should be substituted for saturated fat to the extent practical.

Note: Unsaturated fats lower blood cholesterol levels when substituted for saturated fats.

4. **Eat less high-cholesterol food.** The intake of cholesterol should be less than 300 mg/day. Dietary cholesterol can raise the blood cholesterol level. Therefore, it is important to eat less food that is high in cholesterol. (See Table C-14, Cholesterol Content of Some Common Foods.)

Note: There is very little cholesterol in low-fat dairy foods like skim milk and no cholesterol in food from plants, like fruits, vegetables, vegetable oils, grains, cereals, nuts, and seeds.

5. **Substitute complex carbohydrates for saturated fats.** Breads, pasta, rice, cereals, dried peas and beans, fruits, and vegetables are good sources of complex carbohydrates (starch and fiber). They are excellent substitutes for foods that are high in saturated fat and cholesterol.

Note: Foods that are high in complex carbohydrates, if eaten plain, are low in saturated fat and cholesterol as well as being good sources of minerals, vitamins, and fiber.

6. **Maintain a desirable weight.** People who are overweight frequently have higher blood cholesterol levels than people of desirable weight.

Note: To achieve or maintain a desirable weight, caloric intake must not exceed the number of calories the body burns.

7. **Eat foods that are high in soluble fiber.** Among such foods is oat bran.

Note: Basically, there are two types of fibers: water soluble fiber (like oat bran) and non-soluble fiber (like wheat bran). Only soluble fiber is effective in lowering cholesterol. Soluble fiber dissolves in water.

All of the above indicate that the development of atherosclerosis is not just a simple matter of eating too much cholesterol. Moreover, these recommendations encompass accepted measures of good health—cessation of smoking, normal blood pressure, ideal weight, exercise, control of stress, and awareness of family history. Each of the recommendations complement the others and contribute to decreasing the risks of atherosclerosis and heart disease.

(Also see HEART DISEASE; and HYPERLIPOPROTEINEMIAS.)

SOURCES. The following information is presented for those individuals who wish to reduce their cholesterol intake for personal reasons or who require cholesterol restriction as part of a control measure in cases of hyperlipoproteinemias.

Table C-13 indicates the foods in the American diet which supply cholesterol and their relative contribution to the total cholesterol available.

TABLE C-13
AMOUNT OF CHOLESTEROL AVAILABLE
PER PERSON PER DAY IN THE UNITED STATES[1]

Food Source	Year	
	1967–1969	1988
	(mg)	(mg)
Meat, poultry, fish	183.3	207.2
Eggs	239.6	144.0
Dairy products	73.9	67.0
Fats and oils	28.8	21.0
Animal sources	525.6	440.0
Vegetable sources	0	0

[1]*Agricultural Statistics 1991*, USDA, p. 478.

Table C-14 which follows provides a ranking of the cholesterol levels of some common foods. This is provided for informational purposes only—not to encourage or discourage consumption of certain foods by the general public. Rather, each individual should consider his or her own case.

Information on the cholesterol levels of more foods is given in Fats and Fatty Acids in Selected Foods, Table F-4 in the article entitled FATS AND OTHER LIPIDS.

(Also see EGGS; and HEART DISEASE.)

---

[18]In this section, the authors drew heavily from the following authoritative publication: *The Surgeon General's Report on Nutrition and Health*, U.S. Department of Health and Human Services, Public Health Service, DHHS (PHS) Publication No. 88-50211, 1988.

TABLE C-14
CHOLESTEROL CONTENT OF SOME
COMMON FOODS[1]

Food	Cholesterol
	(mg/100 g)
Egg yolks, chicken	1602
Kidneys, beef, braised	804
Liver, chicken or turkey, simmered	615
Eggs, fried, poached or hard cooked	540
Sweetbread (thymus), braised	466
Liver, beef, calf, or pork, fried	438
Kidneys, calf, lamb, or pork, raw	375
Roe, salmon, sturgeon, or turbot, raw	360
Heart, beef, braised	274
Butter	219
Shrimp, canned	150
Sardines, canned	140
Whipping cream, 37.6% fat	133
Cream cheese	111
Beef tallow	109
Cheddar cheese	106
Turkey, roasted	105
Veal	101
Beef and lamb, variety of cuts	95
Swiss cheese	92
Chicken, roasted	90
Pork, variety of cuts	89
Frankfurter	62
Ice cream, 12% fat	60
Tuna, canned	55
Milk, evaporated	31
Milk, whole	14
Milk, 2% fat	8
Yogurt	6
Cottage cheese	4
Milk, 1% fat	4

[1]Values are approximate and they are for foods in Food Composition Table F-21.

CHOLESTYRAMINE

A drug which binds bile salts and causes them to be excreted in the stool. By this effect, it tends to reduce blood cholesterol because a more rapid breakdown of cholesterol is needed to produce bile acids that are lost in the stool. Under certain conditions cholestyramine may also help to dissolve gallstones.

(Also see CHOLESTEROL; and GALLSTONES.)

CHOLIC ACID ($C_{24}H_{40}O_5$)

The most abundant bile acid, which is synthesized from cholesterol in the liver, and is then combined chemically with the amino acids glycine and taurine.

(Also see DIGESTION AND ABSORPTION.)

CHOLINE

Contents   Page

Choline, which is a key part of the constituent of lecithin, is vital for the prevention of fatty livers, the transmitting of nerve impulses, and the metabolism of fat. The classification of choline as a vitamin is debated, however, because it does not meet all the criteria for vitamins, especially those of the B vitamins.

The following facts favor classifying choline as an essential nutritional factor with vitaminlike activity, and *not* a vitamin:

1. Specific deficiency symptoms have not been observed in man.

2. The body can synthesize considerable choline, thereby reducing the need for dietary supplementation.

3. Choline is used in much larger quantities than any of the known vitamins.

4. Choline serves as a structural component of fat and nerve tissue, rather than a catalytic role characteristic of the vitamins.

5. It does not share the common ability of B vitamins to support the growth of microorganisms; only a very few require it.

On the other hand, the following biological roles favor classifying choline as a vitamin:

1. Although the need by man has not been established, choline is required for the growth of the young of many animal species; and deficiencies, evidenced primarily by liver and kidney damage, have been produced in rats, mice, dogs, chicken, pigs, hamsters, guinea pigs, rabbits, calves, ducklings, and monkeys.

2. Although choline can be synthesized in the body from serine and methionine with the aid of vitamin B-12 and folacin as coenzyme factors, it is not made fast enough and in sufficient quantity for many animal species—especially the young; besides, adequate building materials—serine, methionine, vitamin B-12, and folacin—must be present.

3. Choline is a key component of the phospholipid lecithin and is present in sphingomyelins, the principal bound forms of choline, which together make up 70 to 80% of the phospholipids in the body. Lecithin is important in the metabolism of fat by the liver, whereas sphingomyelin is involved in brain and nerve tissue. Choline also serves as a precursor of acetylcholine, which is physiologically important in the transmission of nerve impulses.

HISTORY. In 1844 and 1846, N. T. Gobley isolated a substance from egg yolk, which he called lecithin (from the Greek, *lekithos*, egg yolk. Choline is a basic constituent of lecithin).

In 1940, Sure, and Gyorgy-Goldblatt, working independently, reported that choline is essential for growth of rats, thereby indicating its vitamin nature.

By 1942, the vitamin nature of choline was fully confirmed by many other workers, who used the rat, chicken and turkey as experimental animals.

CHEMISTRY, METABOLISM, PROPERTIES.

• **Chemistry**—Structurally, choline ($C_5H_{15}NO_2$) is a relatively simple molecule, containing three methyl groups (CH_3-) (see Fig. C-52).

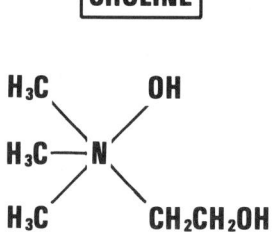

Fig. C-52. Structure of choline.

• **Metabolism**—Choline is absorbed in the small intestine.

• **Properties**—It is a colorless, bitter-tasting, water-soluble white syrup that takes up water rapidly on exposure to air (hygroscopic) and readily forms more stable crystalline salts with acids such as choline chloride or choline bitartrate. It is fairly stable to heat and storage, but unstable to strong alkali. It exists in all foods in which phospholipids occur liberally.

MEASUREMENT/ASSAY.

The activity of choline and choline chloride is expressed in grams and milligrams of the chemically pure substances.

Choline content of foods is usually determined by a colorimetric method or by microbiological assay. Recent assay techniques include: fluorometric enzyme assay, enzymatic radioisotopic assay, and gas chromatography.

FUNCTIONS.

Choline has several important functions in the body. As a constituent of several phospholipids (primarily lecithin), it prevents fatty livers through the transport and metabolism of fats; as a constituent of acetylcholine, it has a role in nerve transmission; and by a phenomenon known as *transmethylation*, it serves as a source of labile methyl groups, which facilitate metabolism.

1. **Prevention of fatty livers.** Choline is a *lipotropic agent*; lipotropic means *having an affinity for fat*. In this role, choline prevents the abnormal accumulation of fat in liver (fatty liver) by promoting its transport as lecithin or by increasing the utilization of fatty acids in the liver itself. Without choline, fatty deposits build up inside the liver, blocking its hundreds of functions and throwing the whole body into a state of ill health.

2. **Nerve transmission.** Choline combines with acetate to form acetylcholine, a substance which is needed to jump the gap between nerve cells so that impulses can be transmitted.

3. **Facilitation of metabolism.** When the methyl group (CH_3-) is present in such form that it can be transferred within the body from one compound to another, it is called a labile methyl group and the process is called transmethylation. The body has a pool of labile methyl groups, which it uses for such purposes as (a) the formation of creatine (important in muscle metabolism), (b) methylating certain substances for excretion in the urine, and (c) the synthesis of several hormones, such as epinephrine. Among the dietary sources of labile methyl are choline (and related substances), the amino acid methionine, and the vitamins folacin and vitamin B-12. Of the related substances that can replace choline, the primary one is betaine (which derives its name from the Latin word *beta*—the beet family, which is a rich source). Each of these sources of a labile methyl group serves to *spare* (or partially make up for the shortage of) one of the others. Thus, choline can be fully replaced by betaine in preventing fatty liver in some species; in other species, betaine can only supplement choline. To some extent, methionine and vitamin B-12 can also spare choline in certain animal species.

Thus, the metabolic needs for choline can be supplied in either of two ways: by dietary choline as such, or by choline synthesis in the body which makes use of labile methyl groups. But the synthesis in the body cannot take place fast enough to meet the choline needs for rapid growth; hence, the symptoms of deficiency may result.

DEFICIENCY SYMPTOMS.

Poor growth, fatty livers, and hemorrhagic kidney damage are the common deficiency symptoms in mammals. Chickens and turkeys develop slipped tendons (perosis). In young rats, choline deficiency produces hemorrhagic lesions in the kidneys and other organs.

RECOMMENDED DAILY ALLOWANCE OF CHOLINE.

Experimental deficiency of choline in humans has not been produced. Of course, methionine can completely eliminate the mammalian requirements for choline, but not those for young birds.

Fatty infiltration of the liver is common in chronic alcoholics and in persons on very low protein diets (e.g., in children with kwashiorkor). But treatments of these disorders with choline have been inconsistent and disappointing.

The requirement for choline is influenced by the amounts of methionine, folacin, and vitamin B-12 in the diet, plus the growth rate of the individual, the energy intake and expenditure, the amount and type of dietary fat, the type of carbohydrate eaten, the total amount of protein in the diet, and possibly the amount of dietary cholesterol. As a result, the exact human requirement has not been established.

It is noteworthy, however, that a Committee of the American Academy of Pediatrics recommends that choline be added to infant formulas in amounts equivalent to breast milk. Human milk contains about 145 mg of choline per liter, nearly 0.1% of total solids.

• **Choline intake in average U.S. diet**—It is estimated that an average mixed diet for adults in the United States contains 400 to 900 mg of choline per day.

TOXICITY.

No toxic effects have been observed. However, oral pharmacologic doses of up to 20 g per day of choline chloride used for periods of several weeks in the treatment of fatty liver, alcoholism, and kwashiorkor have caused some patients to experience dizziness, nausea, and diarrhea.

CHOLINE LOSSES DURING PROCESSING, COOKING, AND STORAGE.

Choline is heat-stable; hence, little of it is lost in processing and cooking.

Choline remains at nearly a constant level in dried foods when stored over long periods.

SOURCES OF CHOLINE.

Choline is widely distributed in foods. Sources are given in the section on VITAMIN(S), Table V-5.

Lecithin, of which choline is a basic constituent, is a rich source of choline. Soybean lecithin and egg yolk lecithin have been used as natural concentrates of choline for dietary supplementation.

Also, the body manufactures choline from methionine, with the aid of folacin and vitamin B-12 as coenzymes. So, the needs for choline can be supplied in two ways: (1) by dietary choline, and/or (2) by body synthesis through transmethylation.

Choline values are not given in Food Composition Table F-21 of this book, simply because few such values are available. So, the top food sources are given in Table C-15.

(Also see VITAMIN[S], Table V-5.)

TABLE C-15
TOP FOOD SOURCES OF CHOLINE ALONG WITH ENERGY VALUES

Food	Choline	Energy
	(mg/100 g)	(kcal/100 g)
Eggs	527	157
Brewers' yeast	408	283
Liver (beef, pork, lamb)	356	136
Wheat germ	306	391
Soybean seeds	290	405
Torula yeast	289	277
Potatoes, dehydrated	262	334
Cabbage, raw	254	24
Soybean flour	225	386
Wheat bran	188	353
Navy beans, dried	168	340
Buttermilk, dehydrated	167	387
Alfalfa leaf meal, dehydrated	150	215
Milk, skim, dehydrated	139	360
Rice polish	122	265
Rice bran	122	276
Oats, whole grain	101	283
Wheat, whole grain	101	360
Hominy	99	358
Rice, whole grain	93	363
Turnip greens	91	30
Barley, whole grain	90	305
Wheat flour	80	361
Blackstrap molasses	74	230
Sorghum, whole grain	63	339
Corn, whole grain	54	348

CHOLINERGIC

A type of nerve fiber which utilizes acetylcholine as a transmitter. Some of these nerves stimulate the secretion of digestive juices and the movement of the digestive tract. Also, they slow the heart.

(Also see DIGESTION AND ABSORPTION.)

CHOLINESTERASE

An enzyme which breaks down the nerve transmitter acetylcholine at the nerve junction. The breakdown of the transmitter is necessary to restore the nerve to its resting state so that it is made ready to transmit another impulse. Certain foods contain cholinesterase inhibitors, which may produce toxic effects when eaten by man or animals.

CHONDROITIN SULFATE

A mucopolysaccharide which is an important component of cartilage.

CHOP SUEY

This is a favorite Chinese dish containing chicken, bean sprouts, onion, bamboo shoots, and mushrooms; cooked and served with a Chinese gravy.

CHOWCHOW

• Consisting of several kinds mingled together: hodgepodge, assorted, or mixed.

• A Chinese preserve or confection of ginger, fruits, and peels in heavy syrup.

• A spicy relish of chopped mixed pickles in mustard sauce.

CHOWDER

Chowder is a word of French origin, derived from the French word *chaudiere,* the vessel in which the French of the coastal regions cooked fish soups and stews.

Chowder is a thick soup or stew of seafood (like clams or white-fleshed sea fishes), usually made with milk and containing salt pork or bacon, onions, potatoes, and sometimes other vegetables.

CHROMATIN

The part of the cell nucleus that stains most intensely; it contains the chromosomes.

CHROMATOGRAPHY

A method used in analytical chemistry first employed by a Russian botanist in 1903. Initially, the technique was used to separate colored substances; hence, the name chromatography, from the Greek meaning *color writing.* Today, many of the compounds separated by chromatography are colorless, so the name no longer relates to the underlying principles.

There are a number of variations of the general chromatographic technique. Partition chromatography was introduced in 1941, paper chromatography in 1944, gas chromatography in 1952, and thin-layer chromatography in 1958.

Numerous materials from foods, such as proteins, amino acids, sugars, fatty acids, minerals, coffee aroma, and many other components, are routinely identified and quantitated through this analytical technique. In addition to nutrient analysis, chromatography can be adapted to the detection of drug residues, hormones, pesticides and other food contaminants, smog, and cigarette smoke.

CHROMIUM (Cr)

The mention of this chemical element makes most people think of the *chrome* plating on the bumpers and body trim of their automobiles. However, it was recently discovered that the shiny metal may also exist in forms which function as (1) an essential element, (2) a hormone, (3) a vitamin, and (4) a poison.

HISTORY. Chromium was discovered by the French chemist Vauquel in 1797, while he was studying the properties of crocoite, an ore which is rich in lead chromate. Its common name of chrome was derived from the Greek word *chroma,* which means color, because the element is present in many different colored compounds. These compounds have long been used as pigments in dyeing, and in the tanning of leather. In the early 1900s, chromium became an important ingredient of corrosion-resistant metals—a use which has increased to the present. Because of this use, people living in or near industrialized areas are likely to be exposed to air, food, and water contaminated by traces of chromium compounds. Unfortunately, much of the inorganic chromium in the environment is harmful rather than helpful to the body, because certain compounds of the element injure body tissues.

It was not until 1959 that the medical scientists W. Mertz and K. Schwarz—who came to the United States from Germany—discovered that the feeding of chromium salts corrected the abnormal metabolism of sugar in rats which resulted from the feeding of diets based upon torula yeast. Later work by these researchers, and by H. Schroeder of the Dartmouth Medical School, established chromium as a cofactor with insulin, necessary for normal glucose utilization and for growth and longevity in rats and mice. (Dr. Schwarz had long studied the nutritional effects of various types of yeasts; in 1957, he had discovered that selenium was present as a vital factor in the American type of brewers' yeast.) Shortly thereafter, it was found that the inorganic salts of chromium were utilized poorly, compared to an organically bound form of chromium present in brewers' yeast which was utilized well by both animal and man. The chromium-containing substance from yeast was named the *glucose tolerance factor* (GTF), because it sometimes restored the metabolism of sugars to normal when diabeticlike tendencies were present. (The term *glucose tolerance* denotes the ability of the body tissues to take the sugar glucose from the blood. Hence, it is measured by the rate at which the blood sugar drops back to normal after a test dose of the sugar has been administered to the patient. The blood sugar of diabetics remains abnormally high during the test of glucose tolerance.) Diabetic animals and people were *not* always helped by either inorganic chromium or the glucose tolerance factor because their disease may have been caused by factors other than a deficiency of chromium.

Recently, evidence was found which suggested that other disorders such as atherosclerosis, cataracts, and high blood fats might be the results of prolonged deficiencies of chromium. Details of these discoveries are given in the sections which follow.

ABSORPTION, METABOLISM, EXCRETION. Further studies are needed to determine chromium's role in metabolism and its nutritional significance. Nevertheless, current thinking is reflected in the sections that follow.

• **Absorption**—Studies have shown that only about 1%, or less, of the dietary intake of inorganic chromium is absorbed, whereas as much as 10 to 25% of the GTF-chromium may be absorbed. Chromic oxide, an inorganic form of the mineral, is so insoluble that it has found wide application as a *marker* for determining the digestibility of components of the diet and of feed intakes by grazing livestock. (All of the marker which is put into the feed appears in the feces—it is not absorbable or degradable. Hence, when used as an indicator, chromic oxide provides a quick, indirect way of determining the digestibility of feed.)

(Also see DIGESTIBILITY.)

• **Age**—It appears that the ability of the body to utilize inorganic salts of chromium decreases with aging. The problem appears to be related to the metabolism of chromium in the tissues as well as with its absorption because tissue levels in older experimental animals have been found to be half those of younger ones, after both groups have been injected

with chromium. (The injections bypassed the absorptive processes.)

• **Alkalinity of the intestinal contents and the blood**—One of the reasons for the poor absorption and utilization of the common inorganic forms of chromium is that they are converted in the intestine and elsewhere in the body to triply charged chromium ions, which react with alkali ions to form insoluble masses that are biologically inactive. Furthermore, both the intestinal contents and the blood are mildly alkaline. Hence, it is noteworthy that the binding of inorganic chromium by substances such as (1) oxalates (present in rhubarb and spinach), (2) phosphates (occur naturally or are present as additives in many foods), or (3) tartrates (in grapes and other fruits, baking powders, and wines) prevents the formation of the insoluble masses and helps to keep chromium in solution so that it might be more readily absorbed and transported in the blood under alkaline conditions.

Chromium which is found in certain organic molecules, such as the glucose tolerance factor, appears to be much better absorbed and utilized by the body because it is protected against adverse chemical reactions which affect inorganic chromium.

• **Anemia**—Anemic people, or those who consume diets low in iron, may have better utilization of inorganic chromium because both elements are carried in the blood by the same protein, transferrin. These people have less than normal amounts of iron bound to their transferrin, so the protein has a greater capacity for carrying chromium.

Inorganic chromium is also carried in the blood by the protein albumin, whereas organically-bound chromium is carried in the blood as a component of the glucose tolerance factor. These forms of chromium do not appear to be affected by the iron nutritional status.

• **Chelating agents**—Other molecules that bind (chelate) mineral elements may alter the amounts of chromium which are absorbed and retained within the body. For example, oxalate (occurs in spinach and rhubarb) increases, while phytate (present in whole grains and legumes) decreases the absorption of chromium salts. However, the feeding of oxalate also causes a great increase of chromium in the urine.

• **Diabetes**—When other conditions are similar, diabetics absorb a greater percentage of inorganic chromium than normal people, but they also excrete much more of the element in their urine.

• **Dietary carbohydrate**—It is suspected that overconsumption of low-chromium, high-carbohydrate foods such as white flour and white sugar may rapidly deplete the body's stores of chromium by overstimulating both the release of the mineral from the tissues and its subsequent loss in the urine.

• **Fats**—One way in which dietary fat may reduce the absorption of chromium is by stimulating the flow of bile, which is an alkaline secretion. Alkaline substances tie up inorganic chromium in soluble masses that cannot be absorbed.

• **Infant malnutrition**—A diabeticlike disorder of metabolism is often found in malnourished infants and children around the world. Therefore, it is noteworthy that this disorder was promptly corrected by the administration of chromium salts to young victims of malnutrition in Jordan, Nigeria, and Turkey. However, malnourished Egyptian children apparently did not benefit from chromium supplements, because they had already received adequate amounts of the mineral in their diets.

• **Intestinal microorganisms**—It has been suggested that the unusually good utilization of inorganic chromium by malnourished infants may be due to its conversion to the glucose tolerance factor by microorganisms present in their intestines. This idea is supported by the finding that chromium stimulates the growth of *Aerobacter aerogenes*—a bacteria found in foods such as cereals, soured dairy products, and vegetables; and present in the human intestine. Perhaps, people eat the foods which contain this bacteria and it gets into the intestine where it converts inorganic chromium to a more biologically active form (like the way in which brewers' yeast synthesizes the glucose tolerance factor from chromium).

• **Other dietary minerals**—Zinc-deficient animals absorb five times as much inorganic chromium as those given zinc supplements. Other minerals that appear to interfere with the absorption and/or the utilization of chromium are calcium, iron, and manganese. Thus, the taking of supplements which contain large doses of these minerals may contribute to the development of a chromium deficiency.

• **Pregnancy**—The unborn child draws chromium from its mother, as evidenced by the fact that the hair of newborn infants contains about 2½ times the level of chromium as the hair of their mothers. There is evidence that chromium content of hair may be a good indicator of the chromium present in other tissues such as the liver. Furthermore, the levels of chromium in the hair of women who had borne children were found to be much lower than those in women who were childless. Hence, it appears that pregnant women may not consume enough readily available chromium to meet both their own needs and those of their unborn children. Perhaps, chromium deficiency is responsible for some of the cases of diabetes in women which appear to have been brought on by pregnancy.

Other studies have produced evidence that most of the chromium loss from the mother is likely to occur during the first pregnancy, since the chromium content of the mother's hair does not appear to decrease further during subsequent pregnancies. If such is the case, then it leads one to speculate whether children other than the firstborn begin life with an adequate supply of chromium in their bodies.

• **Storage of chromium in the body**—The storage of chromium by the body may provide insurance against the development of diabeticlike disorders at times when the requirements for the glucose tolerance factor (GTF) exceed the amounts which (1) are supplied preformed in the diet, or (2) are synthesized from dietary inorganic chromium. However, animal studies have shown that a greater proportion of a given dose of chromium is stored in the liver when it is supplied as GTF, than when it is supplied as an inorganic salt. Furthermore, chromium in the liver has been shown to have GTF activity. Next to the liver, the kidneys appear to be one of the best sources of GTF-chromium. Finally, it is noteworthy that diabetics were found to have had only about two-thirds as much chromium in their hair and their liver as normal, healthy people.

• **Stresses**—Various stressful conditions, such as malnutrition and loss of blood, have long been known to impair the body's utilization of sugars, or even to bring on diabetes. Likewise, it seems that the chromium needs of the body become more critical under such conditions. For example, studies on animals have shown that the effects of (1) low-protein diets accompanied by controlled exercise, and (2) the withdrawal of measured amounts of blood were more severe in the chromium-deficient groups than in those given supplements containing the mineral.

• **Excretion of chromium**—The predominant route of excretion of endogenous chromium is the urine. The average daily loss is about 7 to 10 mcg.

FUNCTIONS OF CHROMIUM. Identifying functions is difficult because this essential element does not do its work by itself; rather, it appears to act cooperatively with other substances that control metabolism, such as (1) a hormone—insulin, (2) various enzymes, and (3) the genetic material of the cell—DNA and RNA. Chromium has a variety of functions, including (1) component of the glucose tolerance factor (GTF), (2) activator of certain enzymes, (3) stabilizer of nucleic acids (DNA and RNA), and (4) formation of fatty acids and cholesterol. Details follow.

• **Component of the glucose tolerance factor (GTF)**—The complete identity of this hormonelike agent is not yet known, although it is certain that it contains chromium and the vitamin niacin, and perhaps amino acids such as glycine, glutamic acid, and cysteine.

Chromium in the form of the GTF is released into the blood—from perhaps the liver, kidneys, or other tissues which store chromium—whenever there is a marked increase in the blood levels of sugar (glucose) and/or of insulin. *Hence, the GTF might be considered to behave like a hormone.* It, along with insulin, acts in making it easier for amino acids, fatty acids, and sugars to pass from the blood into the cells of various tissues. It also promotes the metabolism of the nutrients within the cells. Much more insulin is required to accomplish these tasks when GTF is lacking; but GTF does not have any effect when insulin is absent. (Some types of diabetes are caused by lack of insulin.) Other noteworthy actions which are jointly promoted by GTF and insulin are (1) utilization of amino acids for the synthesis of proteins, (2) improvement in the ability of germ eating (Phagocytic) white blood cells to search out noxious bacteria (this function of the cells is impaired in diabetics), and (3) utilization of glucose by the lens of the eye.

Each time that the GTF is called upon to do its work, there is a corresponding rise in the amount of chromium excreted in the urine. Apparently, the GTF is utilized less efficiently by diabetics who need injections of insulin than it is by normal, healthy people. Hence, diabetics might have above average needs for this factor.

Various experimental studies have produced evidence that the bodies of many people are able to convert inorganic chromium into the GTF, but that the speed of this conversion slows with aging. For example, the impaired sugar metabolism in a group of malnourished Jordanian infants was corrected overnight by a chromium supplement, whereas from 1 to 3 months were required for noticeable improvement in sugar metabolism to be achieved in elderly people.

Pregnant women and diabetics, who appear to have above average requirements for the GTF, may not be able to synthesize adequate amounts of this factor from the inorganic chromium that is supplied in their diets. Hence, they may need dietary sources of preformed GTF in order to avoid the depletion of the limited supplies of this factor in their bodies. Furthermore, the results of studies in animals suggest that GTF, but *not* inorganic chromium, passes through the placenta from the mother to her unborn child.

• **Activator of certain enzymes**—Chromium is the spark plug which *fires up* certain enzymes into vigorous metabolic activity. Most of these enzymes are involved in the production of energy from carbohydrates, fats, and proteins. However, some of these enzymes may also be activated by other metal elements such as aluminum, iron, manganese, and tin. Similarly, chromium activates the digestive enzyme trypsin; although here, too, other metals may act as substitutes. Hence, the activities of these enzymes may not be noticeably depressed when there is a chromium deficiency.

• **Stabilizer of nucleic acids (DNA and RNA)**—Chromium and certain other essential elements appear to stabilize nucleic acids (mainly RNA) against distortions of their structures. Hence, it is tempting to speculate that these elements may help to prevent mutations of the genetic material within cells, and thereby prevent the development of cancer and similar diseases. However, there is little evidence either to support or refute this speculation.

• **Formation of fatty acids and cholesterol**—Chromium is a stimulator of synthesis of fatty acids and cholesterol in the liver.

DEFICIENCY SYMPTOMS. Chromium deficiency, which is believed to be relatively common in the United States, is manifested by impaired glucose tolerance, which may be accompanied by high blood sugar and the spilling of sugar into the urine. It is seen especially in older persons, in maturity-onset diabetes, and in infants with protein-calorie malnutrition.

There are *no* clear-cut signs or symptoms of the early stages of chromium deficiency because it appears that tissue stores are drawn upon to meet the needs of the body. Even after the body's reserves have been exhausted, it may take time before any signs or symptoms of a deficiency appear, because enough extra insulin may be secreted to compensate for the reduced effectiveness of the hormone which occurs in chromium deficiency. However, an excessive secretion of insulin is thought to be undesirable, because it may lead to low blood sugar, unhealthy fattening, atherosclerosis, or even exhaustion and damaging of the insulin-secreting cells of the pancreas. Thus, diabetes—accompanied by the usual signs or symptoms of impaired growth in children, sugar in the urine, frequent and excessive urination, abnormal thirst, increased hunger, loss of weight, nausea, and tiredness—may develop if the pancreas is overstressed by chromium deficiency and/or other conditions. Chromium deficiency is also characterized by disturbances in lipid and protein metabolism.

Diagnosis of Chromium Deficiency. The morbid consequences of chromium deficiencies make it desirable to detect them before there is irreparable damage to body tissues. However, the laboratory tests which provide the most information regarding chromium nutritional status are expensive and inconvenient for the patient. The screening of patients according to their recent dietary histories is of little value because (1) there is a lack of information regarding the chromium content of the various foods eaten by people in the United States; (2) such information tells little about the body stores of chromium, even if the recent chromium intakes could be determined; and (3) other conditions such as intestinal microorganisms and stresses may have altered the utilization of dietary chromium.

Several laboratory tests may be used to diagnose chromium deficiency. Most likely, a combination of two or more tests will be needed.

• **Analysis of hair samples**—It is hoped that this test may serve at least as a screening method to identify people whose body stores of chromium are low because (1) the levels of the mineral in hair appear to parallel, roughly, the levels in other body tissues, and (2) extracts of hair have been found to act like the glucose tolerance factor (GTF). People whose hair levels of chromium are found to be low might then be given sugar and chromium metabolism tests.

• **Blood sugar test (glucose tolerance test)**—The term *glucose tolerance* refers to the speed at which an elevated level of blood sugar—produced by feeding or injecting glucose—drops back to normal as the cells of the body remove the sugar from the blood. Both insulin and chromium are needed to facilitate the passage of sugar and other nutrients from the blood into the cells, so an abnormally slow return of an elevated blood sugar level to normal may be indicative of a deficiency of insulin and/or of chromium. Hence, blood levels of insulin may also have to be determined if the glucose tolerance test is to be used to diagnose chromium deficiency; unless the glucose tolerance test is given on two separate occasions, both before and after the administration of chromium. An improvement in glucose tolerance after one or more doses of chromium may mean that the patient has a deficiency of the mineral.

(Also see HYPOGLYCEMIA, section headed "Glucose Tolerance Test.")

• **Chromium in the urine**—Normally, only small amounts of chromium are excreted in the urine. However, the administration of a test dose of glucose usually causes a marked increase in the amount of the mineral in the urine, unless the patient happens to be chromium deficient. Hence, the use of this test requires that the urine be collected and analyzed for chromium content both before and after the administration of the sugar. The test is not valid for diabetics who require injections of insulin, because they usually excrete abnormally high amounts of chromium in the urine.

Evidence of Chromium Deficiencies. Evidence suggesting that many Americans might have various degrees of chromium deficiency began to accumulate in the 1960s when it was found that some people who showed diabetic tendencies benefited from chromium supplementation. It was concluded that the people who showed improvement after receiving chromium had suffered from a deficiency which aggravated the disease.

Further evidence of chromium deficiencies in the United States is provided by the low chromium levels found in the tissues obtained from deceased persons of various ages and nationalities, and of both sexes. Also, it was found that people from Europe, Africa, and Asia had, on the average, several times as much chromium in their aortas, hearts, kidneys, livers, and spleens as the average American.

Disorders Which May Result from a Chromium Deficiency. Much of the evidence of the role of chromium deficiency in the disorders that follow is circumstantial. Nevertheless, some current concerns are presented, in order that readers may (1) be alerted to the dangers of low chromium diets, and (2) make special efforts to plan their diets so as to obtain sufficient chromium.

• **Adult-onset diabetes**—People who have this disease—which occurs mainly in obese people, and is characterized by an abnormal metabolism of sugar in spite of an apparently adequate secretion of insulin—may sometimes be helped by supplemental chromium in the form of either inorganic salts or the glucose tolerance factor (usually provided as brewers' yeast, or as a special extract of this substance). Perhaps, some of the people who developed this disease after having had an apparently healthy childhood underwent a gradual depletion of their body stores of chromium, which brought on the abnormal condition.

• **Atherosclerosis**—This disorder—which is the buildup of abnormal patches or *plaques* on the walls of arteries—has been produced by making animals chromium deficient, and it has been prevented by chromium supplementation. Researchers have also found that chromium cannot be detected in the aortas of people who die from atherosclerosis, whereas it is almost always present in the aortas of people who die accidently.

• **Cloudy spots on the lens of the eye (cataracts)**—Diabetics have an above-average likelihood of developing cataracts because their abnormally slow utilization of carbohydrates allows unmetabolized sugars to accumulate in the lens of the eye. Studies of the lenses removed from the eyes of rats showed that, although insulin causes a slight speedup of sugar metabolism in these tissues, a much greater effect was obtained by the administration of chromium along with insulin.

• **Growth retardation in children**—It has long been known that diabetic children may be stunted in growth due to lack of insulin, one of the hormones which promotes the synthesis of protein for the building up of body tissues. However, even children with metabolic abnormalities that are milder than diabetes may also suffer from growth retardation. Therefore, it is noteworthy that chromium supplementation of diets promotes better growth, both in rats fed low-protein diets and in children suffering from protein-energy malnutrition.

• **Heart Disease**—The Framingham study of the risk factors associated with heart disease—which was conducted from 1949 to 1969 on over 5,000 men and women, aged 30 to 62, in Framingham, Massachusetts—showed that people

with diabetic tendencies had a much higher risk of heart disease than those without such tendencies. Hence, it appears that chromium might be linked in various ways to heart disease, because (1) lack of this mineral results in an abnormal metabolism of sugars, like that which occurs in diabetes; and (2) hearts obtained from deceased people in countries with low rates of heart disease contained several times as much chromium as the hearts of deceased Americans.

(Also see HEART DISEASE, section headed, "The Framingham Study of Risk Factors.")

• **High blood fats (cholesterol and triglycerides)**—Diabetes and other disorders of sugar metabolism are often accompanied by high blood levels of fatty substances such as cholesterol and triglycerides. Researchers report that a group of people with these conditions had lower levels of blood fats after their diets were supplemented with either inorganic chromium, or with brewers' yeast containing the glucose tolerance factor. However, the declines in the blood fats due to chromium therapy averaged only about 14%.

• **Impotence and frigidity**—These problems might be the first signs of unsuspected diabetes because they are sometimes due to impairment of the nerves which usually accompany this disease. Occasionally, chromium deficiency may contribute to the development of diabetes.

• **Low resistance to infections**—People who have diabetes may be overly susceptible to infections because their germ-eating white blood cells may have lost some of their power to locate and engulf infectious microorganisms. However, the addition of small amounts of inorganic chromium to samples of these weakened cells in test tubes has been shown to restore their vitality for fighting infections.

• **Neurological disorders**—Although it is common knowledge that disorders of the nerves often develop in diabetics, recently doctors learned that chromium deficiency alone may sometimes be the cause of this problem, judging from the case of a 38-year-old female whose sole source of nourishment for more than 3 years was intravenous feedings.[19] The feedings had supposedly furnished all of her nutrient requirements, but she lost weight and developed various other signs of diabetes, such as abnormal sugar metabolism and disorders of the nervous system. The addition of insulin to her intravenous formula was ineffective. Analysis of her blood and hair for chromium revealed severely deficient levels. Thereupon, an inorganic chromium salt was added to her intravenous feedings, and the insulin was withdrawn. The diabetic condition was corrected within 2 weeks, but it took about 5 months for the normal functioning of her nervous system to be restored.

• **Unexpected loss of weight**—The inability to maintain body weight when sufficient dietary energy is consumed may be a sign of uncontrolled diabetes, or, in some cases, of an unsuspected deficiency of chromium. Furthermore,

[19]Jeejeebhoy, K. N., *et al.*, "Chromium Deficiency, Glucose Intolerance, and Neuropathy Reversed by Chromium Supplementation, in a Patient Receiving Long-term Total Parenteral Nutrition," *The American Journal of Clinical Nutrition*, Vol. 30, 1977, p. 531.

chromium supplements have been found to increase the weight gain of infants undergoing treatment for protein-energy malnutrition.

TREATMENT AND PREVENTION OF CHROMIUM DEFICIENCY.
The treatment of chromium deficiency is strictly a job for the physician because he/she will have to decide on the form of chromium which is most suitable for the patient. Very ill people may even require injections of the mineral.

The prevention of chromium deficiency requires the application of such information as (1) the daily needs of various types of people, (2) food sources of well-utilized forms of the mineral, and (3) the maximum amounts of chromium which may be taken without toxic effects. Unfortunately, there is a paucity of information on this subject.

INTERRELATIONSHIPS.
The following interrelationships are pertinent:

1. Chromium functions best in the body when it is in the form of the GTF.

2. Diets rich in carbohydrates may cause the supply of GTF-chromium to be depleted.

3. Inorganic chromium is utilized by many people, but less efficiently than that in GTF.

4. The absorption of chromium is impeded by oxalates (in rhubarb and spinach), and phytates (present in whole grains).

5. Zinc and vanadium antagonize the effects of chromium.

RECOMMENDED DAILY ALLOWANCE OF CHROMIUM.
A normal healthy adult loses about 1 mcg (microgram) of chromium daily in his/her urine. The dietary intake of chromium needed to replace this loss ranges from 4 mcg of GTF-chromium in brewers' yeast (as much as 25% of this form may be absorbed) to 200 mcg of chromium from an inorganic salt (as little as 0.5% of this form may be absorbed).

It is difficult to establish an allowance for this mineral, because of the limited amount of data regarding its availability from various food sources. Therefore, some intakes that have been estimated to be suitable by the National Academy of Sciences are presented in the section on MINERAL(S), Table M-25, Mineral Table.

• **Chromium intake in average U.S. diet**—Chromium intake from typical Western diets varies between 25 to 200 mcg per day, but in the most recent international studies, intakes below 100 mcg per day were reported.[20]

CONSERVING THE BODY'S SUPPLY OF CHROMIUM.
Although the present evidence is mainly circumstantial, some researchers suspect that cardiovascular diseases and diabetes may be more severe in people who have very low body stores of chromium. Therefore it is important to prevent excessive urinary excretion of this essential element, while also making every effort to obtain adequate amounts of dietary chromium to replace the daily losses. Some dietary measures which may help to reduce the urinary losses of chromium follow.

NOTE: It is not known for certain whether these measures are effective in cutting down the loss of chromium in the urine, since very little research has been performed on this subject. Nevertheless, all of the recommendations represent good nutritional practices, so their application may bring other benefits.

• **Avoidance of excessive amounts of highly refined sugars**—The object of this practice is to avoid the sudden burdening of the body with large loads of readily available sugars which may overstimulate the secretion of both insulin and glucose tolerance factors (GTF), since these conditions tend to increase the amount of chromium lost in the urine. This means that it is better to take dietary carbohydrate in the form of starches combined with fiber, such as occurs in legumes and whole grain products, than it is to rely largely on foods rich in simple sugars.

• **Maintenance of an appropriate body weight**—People who are markedly underweight or overweight may be troubled with an abnormal carbohydrate metabolism, so efforts should be made—with the help of a doctor and/or a dietitian when necessary—to attain the weight which is normal for one's age, sex, height, and body build. *Crash* or semistarvation diets are not recommended, because they may promote the tearing down of vital protein tissues in the body (such as the heart, kidneys, muscles, and liver), which are believed to store much of the body's supply of chromium. The sudden release of large amounts of chromium into the blood is likely to result in the copious loss of this element in the urine.

TOXICITY.
It is unlikely that people will get too much chromium in their diets because (1) only minute amounts of the element are present in most foods, (2) the body utilizes it poorly, and (3) there is a wide range of safety between the helpful and the harmful doses of chromium (the toxic dose is about 10,000 times the lowest effective medicinal dose). However, the taking of chromium in the form of inorganic salts may cause a reduction in the absorption of other trace elements, as evidenced by the fact that doses of inorganic chromium reduce the absorption of zinc in experimental animals. **NOTE WELL:** Under no conditions should a lay person take an inorganic chromium salt without the prior advice of a doctor, because certain types of these compounds—which are readily available for nonmedicinal uses—may be deadly poisons. Finally, the administration of chromium in the form of the glucose tolerance factor (GTF) to diabetics who require injections of insulin may cause their blood sugar levels to drop to dangerously low levels because the GTF enhances the effects of insulin. Certain researchers have even speculated that perhaps some of the diabetics who find it difficult to manage their disease might have a highly variable dietary intake of both chromium and glucose tolerance factor. Thus, the effects of a regular dose of insulin may vary from day to day.

(Also see DIABETES; MINERAL[S]; and POISONS.)

SOURCES OF CHROMIUM.
Groupings by rank of some common food sources of chromium are given in the section on MINERAL(S), Table M-25, Mineral Table.

For additional sources and more precise values of chromium, see Table C-16, The Chromium Content of Some Foods, which follows.

---

[20]*Recommended Dietary Allowances,* 10th ed., NRC-National Academy of Sciences, 1989, p. 241.

TABLE C-16
THE CHROMIUM CONTENT OF SOME FOODS[1]

Food	Chromium
	(mcg/100 g)
Dried liver	170
Brewers' yeast	118
Blackstrap molasses	115
Eggs	52
Cheese	51
Liver	50
Wheat bran	40
Beef	32
Wheat, whole grain	29
Apple peel	25
Wheat germ	25
Potatoes	24
White flour	23
White bread	20
Oysters	20
Brown sugar	18
Butter or margarine	15
Chicken	14
Cornflakes	14
Vegetable oils	13
Cornmeal	11
Banana	11
Spinach	9
Carrots	8
Orange	5
Green beans	4
Strawberries	3
Mushrooms	3
White sugar	2
Milk	1

[1]These values represent the total amount of chromium present in a food, and not the amount available to the body.

NOTE WELL: The content and/or availability of chromium in foods may be affected by the following:

1. **The chromium content of the soil.** Soil content of chromium affects the chromium content of plants grown therein.

2. **The processing of grains.** As with other essential minerals, there is much more chromium in the outer layers of grains—the branny layers which are usually removed—than there is in the inner layers.

3. **The refining of molasses.** Generally, the darker the color (and the less the refinement), the richer the chromium content of molasses.

4. **The type of cooking utensil.** The heating of acid foods—such as tomato sauce—in stainless steel equipment may result in some of the chromium content of the stainless steel being leached out into the food.

5. **Fermentation.** Brewers' yeast converts inorganic chromium into a highly active organic substance—the glucose tolerance factor. Thus, beer, which is produced through the action of brewers' yeast, may have (a) much of its chromium in the form of the glucose tolerance factor, and (b) all of its chromium content in an alcohol-extractable form, which has a high level of biological activity.

Other fermented foods which also may be good sources of glucose tolerance factor are: wine, apple cider, cider vinegar, wine vinegar, root beers, yeast-leavened whole grain breads, pickles, summer sausages, cheeses and their derivatives, and sauerkraut.

6. **The alcohol-extractable fraction.** A close correlation appears to exist between the amount of chromium in the alcohol-extractable fraction and the level of GTF activity. Therefore, it is tempting to speculate that the alcohol-extractable fraction is an organically bound form that might be more readily absorbed and utilized than the chromium which cannot be so extracted. This might mean that the chromium in such alcoholic beverages as beer and wine is highly available to the body. Of course, Table C-16, The Chromium Content of Some Foods, like most food composition tables, gives only the total chromium content of foods. At this time, the relationship between total chromium, alcohol-extractable chromium, and the human dietary requirement is uncertain; hence, further research in this area is needed.

(Also see MINERAL[S], Table M-25; and POISONS, Table P-2. Some Potentially Poisonous [Toxic] Substances.)

CHRONIC DISORDER

A long-lasting disorder, in contrast to one that is acute.

CHUTNEY

The word *chutney* is derived from an East Indian word meaning to taste or lick. Chutneys are either like a sweet pickle or a condiment—with the consistency of jam. They are highly seasoned and contain a variety of chopped fruits and vegetables. Chutneys are served with cold meats, sausages, or stews.

CHYLE

The globules of emulsified fat which are formed in the small intestines as a result of digestion, and which are transported as chylomicrons via the lymphatics.

CHYLOMICRON

Complex molecules of protein and fats which are (1) synthesized in the intestinal mucosa, (2) carried by the lymphatics to the blood, and (3) circulated in the blood until metabolized by the liver or other tissues. After a meal high in fat, the blood plasma has a milky appearance due to the large number of circulating chylomicrons. However, after an overnight fast, very few of the chylomicrons should be present and the plasma should be clear, unless there is a disorder of fat metabolism called hyperchylomicronemia (also called Type I-Hyperlipoproteinemia), in which clearing is impaired due to the lack of substance called *clearing factor.*

(Also see CLEARING FACTOR; FATS AND OTHER LIPIDS; and HYPERLIPOPROTEINEMIAS.)

CHYME

The mixture of partially digested food and gastric juice which passes from the stomach into the small intestine.
(Also see DIGESTION AND ABSORPTION.)

CHYMOTRYPSIN

A digestive enzyme secreted by the pancreas, which acts on proteins.
(Also see DIGESTION AND ABSORPTION.)

CIBOPHOBIA

Another name for sitophobia, an abnormal fear of eating. Cibophobia differs from anorexia since appetite may persist but the person fears eating because of some associated or subsequent discomfort.

CIDER

In the United States this term usually refers to unfermented, unpasteurized, fresh apple juice; whereas, in Europe it means apple juice that has been fermented. Americans call fermented cider *hard cider*. Unpasteurized cider will begin to ferment in a few days unless it is kept from doing so by the addition of a preservative such as sodium benzoate or potassium sorbate.

Europeans also make a fermented cider from pears, which is called *perry*.

(Also see APPLE; and PEAR.)

CIEDDU (FERMENTED MILK)

A type of fermented milk in Italy.

CIRCULATORY SYSTEM

The system of blood, blood vessels, lymphatics, and heart concerned with the circulation of the blood and lymph.

CIRRHOSIS

A disorder in which functioning liver tissue is replaced by a type of scar tissue. Cirrhosis may be due to (1) alcoholism, (2) infections, (3) disorders of the biliary tract, or (4) nutritional deficiencies. People may recover from mild cases of cirrhosis with only a small loss of liver function. However, advanced cases usually result in liver failure and death.

CISSA

A craving for and eating of unnatural substances (such as chalk, hair, dirt, or sand) that sometimes occurs in nutritional deficiencies during pregnancy, or in children (in which it is a recurrence of the natural tendency to put everything in the mouth).

(Also see ALLOPRIOPHAGY; and PICA.)

CITRAL

A constituent of orange peel that is suspected of causing damage to blood vessels when large amounts are consumed. Orange peel is present in such food products as marmalade, fruit juices, and fruit drinks. However, it is not known whether many people are affected by the small amount of citral that is usually consumed.

CITRIC ACID

An acid that is (1) present in citrus fruits, and (2) formed during metabolism in the body. Citric acid is used as a flavoring agent in foods, carbonated beverages, and pharmaceuticals.

(Also see METABOLISM.)

CITRIC ACID CYCLE (KREBS CYCLE)

This oxygen-requiring (aerobic) metabolic process, which is also known as the Krebs cycle, is the means by which metabolic products of fats, carbohydrates, and protein are converted to water and carbon dioxide, plus energy. The citric acid cycle operates in the mitochondria of cells, where the appropriate enzymes are located.

(Also see METABOLISM.)

CITRIN

A substance from citrus fruits which has a vitaminlike activity. It was originally designated as vitamin T. Now, it is classified among substances called bioflavonoids.

(Also see BIOFLAVONOIDS.)

CITRON MELON (STOCKMELON)
Citrullus vulgaris

This is a variety (*Citroides*) of watermelon that is not as palatable as the commonly used varieties of the fruit because it has a hard white flesh. However, the rind may be candied or pickled. It is noteworthy that the candied *citron* sold in many American stores is often made from the citron melon rather than from the peel of the citrus fruit citron, which is much more expensive and has a more distinctive flavor.

(Also see WATERMELON.)

CITROVORUM FACTOR (FOLINIC ACID)

A form of the vitamin folic acid.
(Also see FOLIC ACID.)

CITRULLINE

A nonessential amino acid formed in the urea cycle. It was first isolated from the juice of watermelon.

(Also see METABOLISM; and UREA CYCLE.)

CITRUS FRUITS *Citrus spp*

These subtropical fruits, which together constitute a major part of U.S. fruit production, are members of the rue family (*Rutaceae*).

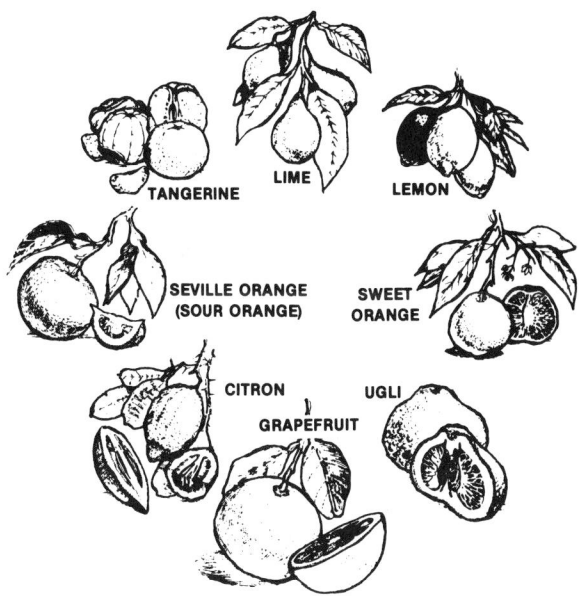

Fig. C-53. The major types of commercially grown citrus fruits.

The processing, selection, preparation, and nutritional value of each specie of citrus fruits is detailed in separate articles pertaining to each of them. However, nutritional aspects of citrus fruits as a whole follow.

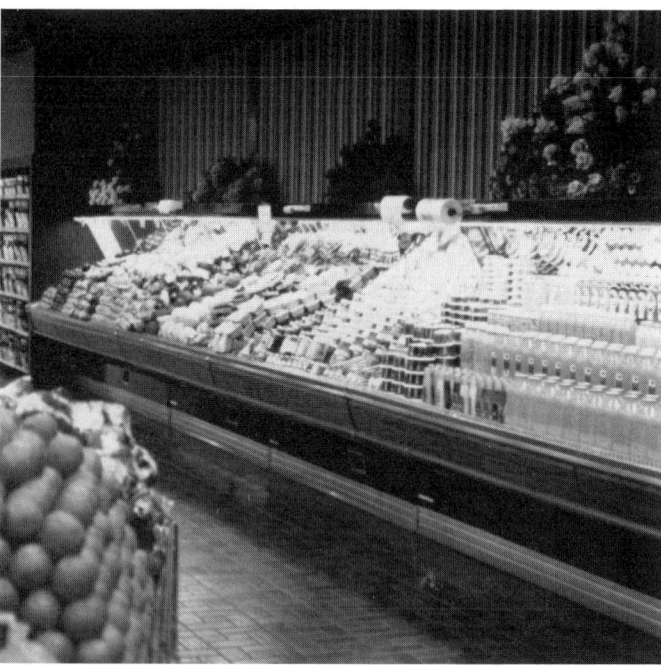

Fig. C-54. Oranges and orange juice in a supermarket. (Courtesy, Univ. of Minnesota, St. Paul, Minn.

NUTRITIONAL VALUE. The nutrient compositions of various citrus fruits and citrus products are given in Food Composition Table F-21.

Some general facts relative to the overall nutritional merits of citrus fruits and related products follow:

1. Fresh citrus fruits are low in calories and sugars, but they are good to excellent sources of fiber, pectin, potassium, vitamin C, inositol, and bioflavonoids (vitaminlike substances). They are also fair sources of folic acid.

2. Citrus juices are not as nutritious as the whole edible portion of the fruits including all but the seeds and the peel, because substances such as fiber, pectin, and bioflavonoids are present mainly in the peel and the membranes which surround the segments of fruit.

3. More of the vitamin C is likely to be retained in juices packed in bottles or cartons, or in those prepared from concentrates, than in canned juices which are heated strongly during canning, then stored at room temperature for extended periods of time.

4. Citrus peel contains citral, an aldehyde that antagonizes the actions of vitamin A. Hence, people should make certain that their dietary supply of the vitamin is adequate before consuming large amounts of the peel from citrus fruits.

CAUTION: Some people are allergic to one or more constituents of citrus peel. When such allergies are suspected, neither the peel nor products containing it should be consumed, and juice from citrus fruits should be extracted gently to avoid squeezing the oil and other substances from the peel into the juice. It is noteworthy that some of the commercially prepared citrus juices and citrus drinks may contain peel and/or the substances extracted from it, but that prepared citrus juice products for infants contain little or none of the peel constituents.

(Also see FRUIT[S], Table F-23; Fruits of the World; PECTIN; and the separate articles devoted to each of the following citrus fruits: GRAPEFRUIT; LEMON; LIME; ORANGE, SWEET; SEVILLE ORANGE; and TANGERINE.)

CLARIFICATION

Means of making a cloudy liquid clear by such processes as filtration, centrifugation, or allowing the particles which cause cloudiness to settle out upon standing.

CLARIFIXATION

A method of homogenizing milk. First the cream is separated and homogenized, then it is remixed with the milk in a clarifixator.

(Also see HOMOGENIZATION.)

CLAUDICATION

Weakness and pain in the leg which cause limping and difficulty in walking.

CLAUDICATION, INTERMITTENT

Soreness of the calf muscles in the leg due to lack of blood resulting from blockage or constriction of the blood vessels. This condition has been helped by the administration of therapeutic amounts of vitamin E.

(Also see HEART DISEASE, section headed "Easily Recognizable Abnormalities"; BUERGER'S DISEASE; and VITAMIN E.)

CLEARING FACTOR

An enzyme which helps to clear the fat from the blood after a meal. This is demonstrated by the disappearance of the milky color of blood several hours after eating. Clearing factor appears to act together with a complex carbohydrate called heparin, but it also requires calcium and magnesium as activators.

CLIMACTERIUM (CLIMACTERIC)

The combined phenomena accompanying cessation of the reproductive function in the female—the menopause; and the corresponding phenomena of reduced sexual activity and potency in the male.

CLOD

This is an English term for the cuts of beef made from what is known as the chuck in the United States; it's the shoulder of beef, or of the neck near the shoulder. This is a cheaper and less tender cut, usually used in roasts or stews.

CLOFIBRATE

A drug used to lower the blood levels of both cholesterol and triglycerides.

CLOUDBERRY *Rubus chamaemorus*

A species of raspberry (a fruit of the family *Rosaceae*) that grows in the swampy areas of Alaska, northern Canada, northern Europe, Asia, and as far north as the Arctic Circle.

(Also see FRUIT[S], Table F-23 Fruits of the World—"Raspberry".)

COAGULATED

Curdled, clotted, or congealed, usually brought about by the action of a coagulant.

COARSE-BOLTED

Separated from its parent material by means of a coarsely woven bolting cloth.

COARSE-SIFTED

Passed through coarsely woven wire sieves for the separation of particles of different sizes.

COB

The fibrous inner portion of an ear of corn (maize) from which the kernels have been removed.

COBALT (CO)

This element is an essential constituent of vitamin B-12 and must be ingested in the form of the vitamin molecule inasmuch as humans synthesize little of the vitamin. No other function of cobalt has been established.

The body of an average adult human contains about 1.1 mg of cobalt.

HISTORY. The word cobalt is derived from the German word *kobold*, meaning goblin or mischievous spirit. The term originated in the 16th century, when arsenic-containing cobalt ores were dug up in the silver mines of the Harz Mountains. Believing that the ores contained copper, miners heated them and were injured by the toxic arsenic trioxide vapors that were released. These evils were attributed to the goblin or kobold. George Brandt, the Swedish chemist, first isolated the element in 1742, although cobalt had been used for centuries for the blue color in decorative glass and pottery.

The discovery, in 1948, that vitamin B-12 (cyanocobalamin) contains 4% cobalt (Co) proved this element to be an essential nutrient for man. It is noteworthy that cobalt's essential role in ruminant animal nutrition was known much earlier. In 1935, Australian scientists discovered that lack of cobalt, resulting from its deficiency in the soil and thus in the herbage grazed, produced a wasting disease. Much earlier, and long before the cause was known, stockmen in different areas of the world learned that this peculiar malady could be prevented and/or cured by transferring animals from *sick* to *healthy* areas.

ABSORPTION, METABOLISM, EXCRETION. Cobalt is readily absorbed in the small intestine. But the retained cobalt serves no physiological function since human tissues cannot synthesize vitamin B-12.

Most of the absorbed cobalt is excreted in the urine; very little of the element is retained—only small amounts are concentrated in the liver and kidneys.

Vitamin B-12, of which cobalt is a component, is synthesized by *E. coli*, a species of bacteria commonly found in the human colon. But the microorganisms of the colon do not make sufficient B-12 to meet human requirements; besides, very little of the vitamin can be absorbed past the small intestine.

FUNCTIONS OF COBALT. The only known function of cobalt is that of an integral part of vitamin B-12, an essential factor in the formation of red blood cells.

DEFICIENCY SYMPTOMS. A cobalt deficiency as such has never been produced in humans. The signs and symptoms that are sometimes attributed to cobalt deficiency are actually due to lack of vitamin B-12, characterized by pernicious anemia, poor growth, and occasionally neurological disorders.

A cobalt deficiency in soils has been reported in Australia, western Canada, and in many of the eastern and midwestern states of the United States.

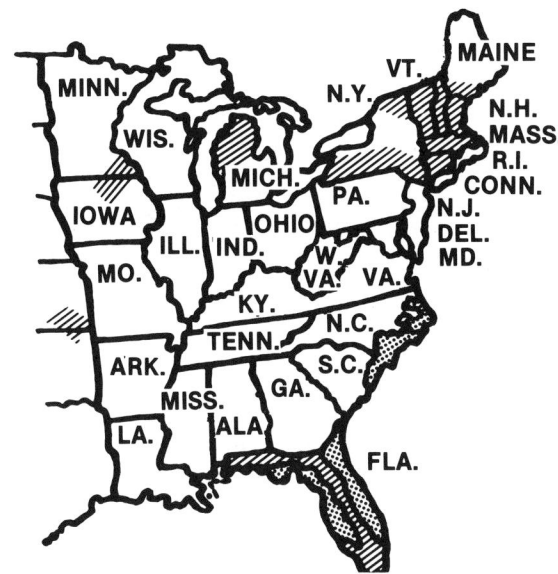

Critical cobalt-deficient areas, where soils and crops are very low in cobalt.

Marginal cobalt areas, where soils and crops are often low in cobalt.

Fig. C-55. Cobalt-deficient areas in eastern United States, resulting from its deficiency in the soil and thus in the herbage produced thereon.

INTERRELATIONSHIPS. Cobalt is a component of vitamin B-12.

RECOMMENDED DAILY ALLOWANCE OF COBALT. There is no known human requirement for cobalt, except for that contained in vitamin B-12.

• **Cobalt intake in average U.S. diet**—Estimates of the average cobalt intake of adults in the United States range from 0.14 to 0.58 mg per day.

TOXICITY. Cobalt toxicity is not likely to result from the consumption of normal foods and beverages, because there is a very wide margin between essential and harmful levels. Excess cobalt intake in man results in an increase in the number of red blood cells, a disorder known as polycythemia.

SOURCES OF COBALT. Cobalt is present in many foods. However, the element must be ingested in the form of vitamin B-12 in order to be of value to man; hence, a table showing the cobalt content of human foods serves no useful purpose. Instead, some rich sources of vitamin B-12 are shown in Table C-17.

(Also see MINERAL[S], Table M-25; and VITAMIN B-12.)

TABLE C-17
SOME RICH SOURCES OF VITAMIN B-12
(COBALAMINS)[1]

Food	Vitamin B-12 (Cobalamins)
	(mcg/100 g)
Beef liver	111
Clams	98
Lamb kidneys	63
Turkey liver	48
Calf kidneys	25
Chicken liver	19
Beef pancreas	16
Roe	15
Oysters	15
Crab	10
Sardines	10
Pork kidneys	10
Mozzarella cheese	8
Herring	8
Salmon	7

[1]Data from Food Composition Table F-21.

COCARBOXYLASE

A thiamin-containing enzyme; it is the key substance in decarboxylation (removal of the carboxyl group [COOH]), an energy-producing reaction in the body.

COCCI

A spherical type of bacteria. Various species of cocci are responsible for human illnesses such as strep throat (streptococci), boils and similar infections (staphylococci), gonorrhea (gonococci), and meningitis (meningococci). Unsanitary practices of food handlers may result in the contamination of beverages and foods by these microorganisms.

COCKLE

A common edible European bivalve mollusk of the family *Cardiidae* that has a shell with radial ribs. It is boiled and eaten with a variety of condiments.

COCOA AND CHOCOLATE

Through different processing, cocoa and chocolate are derived from the seeds of the cacao tree or *Theobroma cacao*—its scientific name. The Swedish botanist, Carolus Linnaeus, must have been familiar with the pleasant flavor of cocoa or chocolate when he classified it in the 1700s, since the Latin term *theobroma* means *food of the gods*. This pleasant chocolate flavor develops during processing.

Chocolate liquor, formed by grinding the roasted, cracked cacao bean, is the base for cocoa and chocolate products. To make cocoa, the chocolate liquor is put under pressure and most of the cocoa butter (fat) is squeezed out leaving a cake that is pulverized and sifted into a powder. Alkalizing cocoa produces Dutch cocoa. While cocoa butter is removed in the making of cocoa, it is added in the making of chocolate. Chocolate is a combination of chocolate liquor, sugar, cocoa butter, and vanilla or some other added flavor. Chocolate may be light, dark, sweet, semisweet, or milk chocolate.

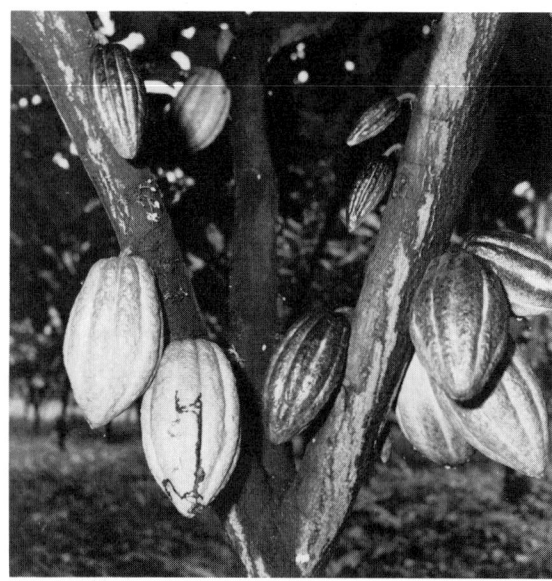

Fig. C-56. Fruiting cacao tree. The cacao tree is unique in that the flowers and the pods (fruit) grow on both the trunk and older branches. (Courtesy, Chocolate Manufacturers Association of the United States of America, McLean, Va.)

ORIGIN AND HISTORY. Milton Snavely Hershey, who opened a factory in Lancaster, Pennsylvania in 1888, was largely responsible for the peak development of cocoa and chocolate in the United States. In fact, a Hershey bar is synonymous to a chocolate bar. Americans now rank tenth among the world's chocolate eaters. The Swiss hold first place.

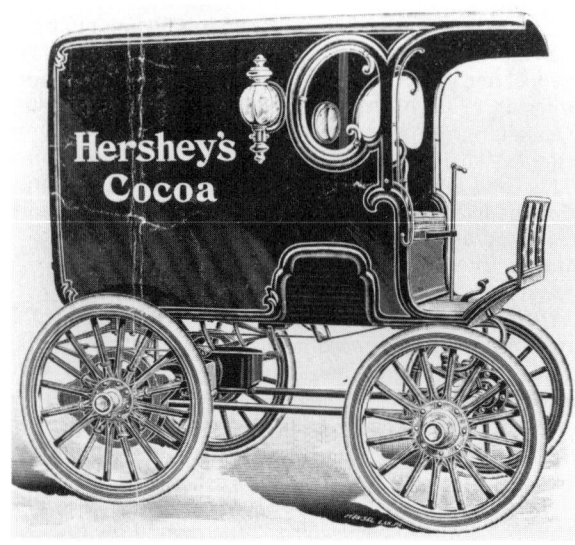

Fig. C-57. The first automobile seen in Lancaster, Pennsylvania—a Riker Electric. The vehicle was purchased in 1900 to attract attention and "make people think the chocolate company was modern and up-to-date." After the people in Lancaster became accustomed to its presence, the automobile was sent to other Pennsylvania cities manned by salesmen with orderbooks in hand. (Courtesy, Hershey Food Corporation, Hershey, Pa.)

PRODUCTION. Cacao trees grow best in a warm, moist climate. Therefore, most cacao trees are grown within an area 20° latitude north and south of the equator. Most cacao beans come from small farms in West Africa and Brazil.

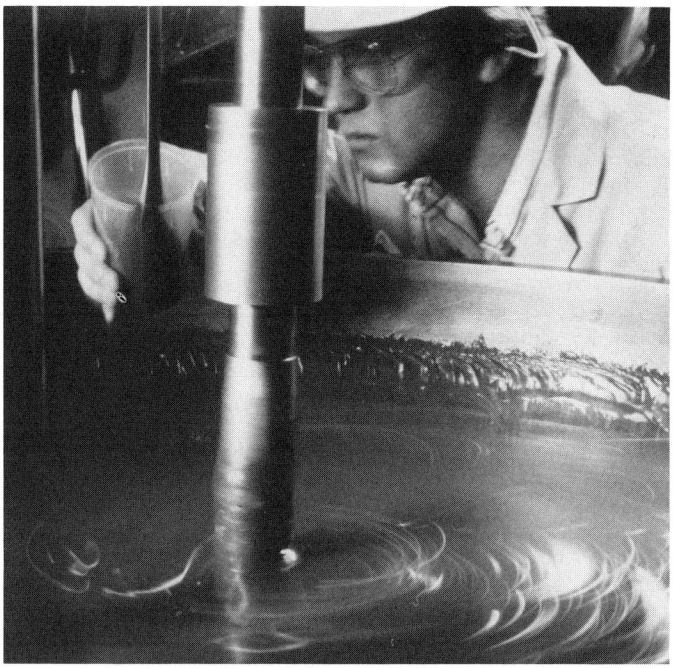

Fig. C-58. Chocolate being processed and sampled. (Courtesy, Hershey Foods Corporation, Hershey, Pa.)

NUTRITIONAL VALUE. Because of their fat content, cocoa and chocolate are high in calories. One hundred grams, or about 3 ½ oz, of chocolate (sweet or semisweet) provides about 470 to 528 Calories (kcal) of energy, since it contains 40 to 53% fat. Cocoa powders contain about 215 to 300 Calories (kcal) per 100 g (3½ oz), depending upon their fat content. Cocoa and chocolate also supply some carbohydrate and protein as well as significant amounts of some minerals such as chromium, iron, magnesium, phosphorus, and potassium. More complete information on the composition of cocoa powder (high, medium, and low fat) and chocolate (bitter, candy, and semisweet) may be obtained in Food Composition Table F-21 of this book.

The theobromine and caffeine content of cocoa and chocolate produce a mild stimulating effect.

USES. The major products manufactured from the chocolate liquor include cocoa, baking chocolate, milk chocolate, and sweet and semisweet chocolate. Each product has some specific uses.

• **Cocoa**—Whether regular or Dutch, and whether high, medium, or low fat, cocoa powder is used to flavor milk drinks, candy, baked goods, ice cream, syrups, and pharmaceuticals.

• **Baking chocolate**—This is the commercial form of the chocolate liquor. It is cooled and formed into cakes. Home use of baking chocolate, which is bitter and unsweetened, includes many baked products.

• **Milk chocolate**—Milk chocolate is probably the most popular of the chocolate products. It is sold directly to the consumer in a variety of solid bars or chocolate coated candy bars or other coated candies.

• **Sweet and semisweet chocolate**—Sweet chocolate is usually dark colored and contains sugar, added cocoa butter, and flavorings. Semisweet contains less sugar. Confectioners use the sweet and semisweet chocolate for making chocolate covered candies. Home use includes cookies, candy, cakes, and a variety of other items.

Recently, carob powder, a product obtained from the bean of a leguminous evergreen tree, *Ceratonia siliqua*, has gained attention as a possible substitute for cocoa. Carob is grown in the United States, contains no stimulants, and may be used without additional sweetening.

(Also see CAROB in Table L-2, Legumes of the World.)

COCOA BUTTER

Fat pressed from the roasted cacao bean (cocoa bean) is known as cocoa butter. It is yellow and possesses a slight chocolate flavor. It consists primarily of triglycerides (three fatty acids bonded to glycerol) of the fatty acids palmitic, stearic, and oleic acids. This fatty acid composition causes cocoa butter to be solid at room temperature but to melt at near body temperature. Most of the cocoa butter is used in the manufacture of chocolate.

(Also see COCOA AND CHOCOLATE.)

COCONUT (COCONUT PALM) *Cocos nucifera*

ORIGIN AND HISTORY. The coconut palm probably originated in the New Guinea-Fiji area. Through the centuries, however, coconuts were distributed by water (coconut fruits float readily) and man from continent to continent and island to island to all the tropical and subtropical parts of the world, where they became the *staff of life* of the natives.

WORLD AND U.S. PRODUCTION. The world production of coconuts averages 42.1 million metric tons annually; and the leading producing countries, by rank, are: Indonesia, Philippines, India, Sri Lanka, Thailand, and Mexico.[21]

Coconut trees thrive best in tropical areas near the coast.

The United States does not produce coconuts commercially.

---

[21]Based on 1990 data from *FAO Production Yearbook 1990*, FAO/UN, Rome, Italy, Vol. 44, p. 122, Table 47. **Note well:** Annual production fluctuates as a result of weather and profitability of the crop.

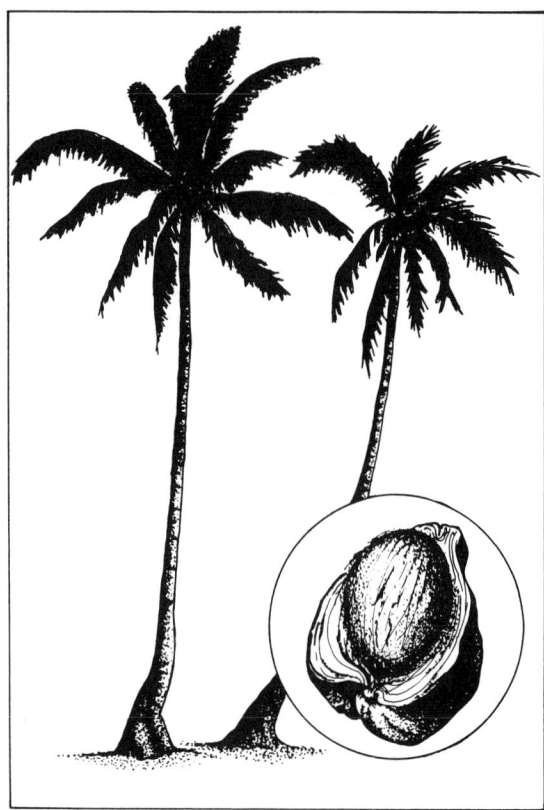

Fig. C-59. Coconut palm tree. A tall (up to 100 ft [30 m] high), graceful tree that produces fruits called coconuts. The fruits yield (1) a refreshing sugary liquid called coconut milk and (2) a sweet tasting meat, which yields coconut oil and is eaten raw or dried for baking or garnishing.

PROCESSING COCONUTS. The first step in processing is to reduce whole coconut to copra, the dried meat of the coconut from which coconut oil, the most important commercial product of the coconut palm, is obtained. In the production of copra, the nuts are husked, opened, and dried, to separate the oil-bearing meat from the shell and to prevent spoilage. The primitive, and still-used, system of drying consists of splitting the nuts open and drying the meat either in the sun or in a kiln heated by burning coconut shells. Copra of better and more uniform quality is produced by hot air drying, in which the copra is conveyed slowly through a heated tunnel or oven.

In general, 1,000 coconuts will yield about 500 lb (225 kg) of copra and 25 gal (95 liter) of oil.

Most of the world production of coconut oil is obtained from copra by the use of the continuous mechanical screw presses. Sometimes solvent extraction is employed following the preliminary compressing in screw presses. In some areas, hydraulic cage and hot presses are still used.

SELECTION, PREPARATION, AND USES. Coconut fruits should be selected that measure 8 to 12 in. (20 to 30 cm) long and from 6 to 10 in. (15 to 25 cm) across. The shell should be hard and strong and covered with a fibrous husk.

Except for local use by the natives, the preparation of coconut products is done commercially. It varies according to (1) the part of the nut, and (2) the desired end product. For these reasons, preparation is presented along with the uses which follow.

About 200 different food uses have been made of coco-

nuts for centuries; among them, the following:

1. **Whole Coconuts.** These may be either green or mature.

Green coconuts are harvested when the meat is soft and rubbery. At this stage, the husk and shell can be cut with a heavy knife or saw, and the meat can be easily scooped out of the shell with a spoon. It is eaten unseasoned, sometimes with a scoop of ice cream added. Also, the meat of green coconuts may be removed and chipped, then used in ice cream, pies, cakes, or cookies, to which it imparts excellent flavor and texture.

Mature coconuts are harvested after the shell is hard and the meat is firm. The *eyes* are punched out and the sugary liquid (called coconut milk) is drained off for subsequent adding to the ground product; the shell is broken by striking; the meat is removed, hand peeled, and ground in a food chopper; then the liquid that was drained off is added to the ground meat. This product is used in salads, desserts, puddings, candies, toppings, cakes, pies, ices, and ice cream.

2. **Copra.** This is the dried meat of the coconut from which the oil is to be extracted, yielding coconut oil and coconut meal or copra meal. The oil is generally extracted by either (a) continuous mechanical screw presses, or (b) hydraulic presses.

3. **Coconut oil.** Because of the high degree of saturation and long stability of coconut oil, it is one of the most desirable oils for confections, bakery goods, deep fat frying, and candies. It is also used in shortening, oleomargarines, soaps, shampoos, and detergents. Minor uses of coconut oil include filled milk, imitation milk, lotions, rubbing creams, prepared flours and cake mixes, and pressurized toppings.

(See OILS, VEGETABLE, Table O-5, Vegetable Oils.)

4. **Desiccated or shredded coconut.** About 70% of the desiccated or shredded coconut is sold directly to bakery and confectionary manufacturers without further processing. The other 30% is further processed to produce (1) white sweetened coconut, by adding powdered sugar, propylene glycol, salt, and moisture; (2) toasted coconut, by adding powdered sugar, dextrose, and salt, then belt-conveying through toasting ovens; or (3) creamed coconut, by grinding, aerating, chilling, and whipping desiccated coconut to a smooth consistency. Desiccated coconut is used primarily for the following purposes: topping agent, bulking agent, nutmeat, or flavoring.

Additional uses of coconuts include: a refreshing and palatable drink obtained from green coconuts; in the treatment of diarrhea, to replace body fluid and provide some electrolytes; toddy, a beverage which is consumed either fresh or fermented as an intoxicating palm wine, obtained from the unopened flower stalks; and palm cabbage, a salad made from the delicate young buds cut from the top of the tree.

NUTRITIONAL VALUE OF COCONUTS. The nutritional value varies according to the coconut product. The nutritive composition of some coconut products is given in Food Composition Table F-21.

The fresh nut contains about 50% water and 30 to 40% oil. Coconut oil has the highest percentage of saturated fatty acids of all common food oils. The chief fatty acids of coconut oil are: lauric (45%), myristic (18%), palmitic (9.5%), oleic (8.2%), caprylic (7.8%), capric (7.6%), and stearic (5%).

The high content of lauric, caprylic, and capric acids is a nutritional asset because these medium and short chain fatty acids are very useful in the dietary treatment of certain digestive disorders. However, the high degree of saturation of coconut oil may raise the blood cholesterol in some people, even though the oil itself contains no cholesterol.

The high degree of saturation imparts long stability to coconut oil.

(Also see FATS AND OTHER LIPIDS; and OILS, VEGETABLE Table O-5.)

COCONUT MILK

This is the clear or whitish, sugar fluid contained inside of coconuts. It is good to drink, and has some nutritional value. Each cup of coconut milk contains about 57 Calories (kcal) of energy, 0.7 g of protein, 0.5 g of fat, and 12 g of carbohydrate, as well as some minerals and vitamins. However, the coconut milk listed in Food Composition Table F-21 of this book is actually liquid squeezed from a mixture of grated coconut meat and water. Therefore, it has a different composition, primarily higher fat and protein content. This type of coconut milk contains about 615 Calories (kcal) of energy, 8 g of protein, 61 g of fat, and 13 g of carbohydrate per cup. The natural sugary fluid contained inside of coconuts is referred to as coconut water in Food Composition Table F-21 of this book.

(Also see COCONUT.)

CODDLE

• To cook very gently, just below boiling point, such as coddled eggs (also referred to as the 3-minute egg).

• To pamper or to treat with excessive care.

COD-LIVER OIL

The oil obtained from the liver of the cod and related fishes, used for its medicinal properties long before vitamins were discovered. Cod-liver oil is an important supplemental source of vitamins A and D. Also, it is a fair source of vitamin E. Each 100 g provides approximately 85,000 IU of vitamin A, 8,500 IU of vitamin D, and 20 mg of vitamin E. (See Food Composition Table F-21, "Food Supplements section.")

Cod-liver oil, along with the vitamins therein, is easily oxidized and destroyed; hence, it should be protected from strong light and stored air-tight.

(Also see FATS AND OTHER LIPIDS.)

COEFFICIENT OF DIGESTIBILITY

The percentage value of a food nutrient that is absorbed. For example, if a food contains 10 g of nitrogen and it is found that 9.5 g are absorbed, the digestibility is 95%.

COENZYME

A substance whose presence is required for the activity of an enzyme. Coenzymes usually contain vitamins as part of their structure, and they may contain a mineral element (metal ions) as the activator. Coenzymes resist breakdown by heat. (They're heat-stable.) It is noteworthy that the same coenzyme may be used in different enzyme systems; it is the protein molecule that gives an enzyme its particular specificity.

COENZYME I (Co I)

An old name for a coenzyme employed as an electron transporter in biological oxidations. Following the recommendation of the International Commission on Nomenclature, it is more frequently called nicotinamide adenine dinucleotide or NAD.

(Also see NICOTINAMIDE ADENINE DINUCLEOTIDE.)

COENZYME II (Co II)

An old name for a coenzyme employed as an electron transporter in biological oxidations. Following the recommendation of the International Commission on Nomenclature, it is more frequently called nicotinamide adenine dinucleotide phosphate or NADP.

(Also see NICOTINAMIDE ADENINE DINUCLEOTIDE PHOSPHATE.)

COENZYME A (CoA)

A key coenzyme which contains the vitamin pantothenic acid. Its combining with two-carbon fragments from fats, carbohydrates, and certain amino acids to form acetyl coenzyme A is an essential step in their complete metabolism, because the coenzyme enables these fragments to enter the citric acid cycle. The combination of acetyl group and coenzyme A is commonly referred to as acetyl CoA.

(Also see KREBS CYCLE.)

COENZYME Q (UBIQUINONE)

Coenzyme Q, or ubiquinone, is a collective name for a number of ubiquinones—lipidlike compounds that are chemically somewhat similar to vitamin E.

Coenzyme Q is found in most living cells where it seems to be concentrated in the mitochondria. Because it is synthesized in the cells, it cannot be considered a true vitamin.

HISTORY. In 1957-58, coenzyme Q (ubiquinone) was discovered independently at Liverpool (England) and Madison (Wisconsin) via two different routes; in the one case via the study of the fat-soluble vitamins, and in the other via enzymatic processes in mitochondria.

In 1958-59, the structures of the ubiquinones were proved jointly by the Liverpool and Madison groups.

CHEMISTRY, METABOLISM, PROPERTIES. The ubiquinones consist of a basic quinone ring structure to which between 30 and 50 carbon atoms are attached in a side chain. Differences in properties are due to the difference in length of the side chain. The 50-carbon side chain occurs exclusively in mammalian tissues (see Fig. C-60).

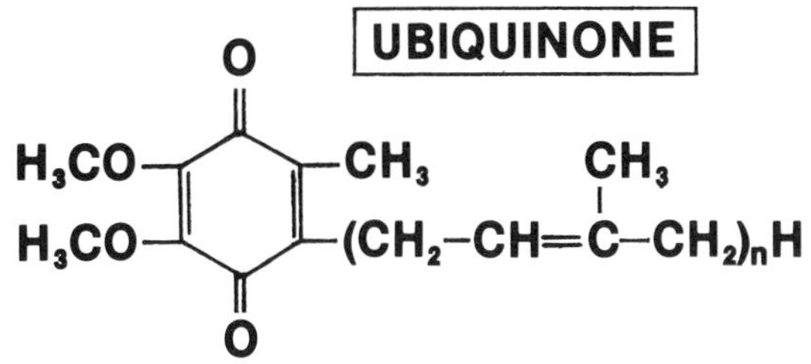

Fig. C-60. Structure of ubiquinones (coenzymes Q). The "n" in the formula varies according to the source—it varies from 6 in some yeasts to 10 in mammalian liver.

Coenzyme Q is present in all cell nuclei and microsomes. It is concentrated in the mitochondria.

FUNCTIONS. Coenzyme Q functions in the respiratory chain in which energy is released from the energy-yielding nutrients as ATP.

There is evidence that specific ubiquinones function in

the remission (prevention) of some of the symptoms of vitamin E deficiency.

SOURCES OF COENZYME Q. Quinones occur widely in aerobic organisms, from bacteria to high plants and animals. Because they are synthesized in the body, they cannot be considered a true vitamin.

The entire series of ubiquinones has been prepared synthetically.

CONCLUSION. The importance of coenzyme Q as a catalyst for respiration imparts status as an essential metabolite. It may have other significant roles. For man and other higher animals a simple precursor substance with an aromatic ring may have vitaminlike status, but dietary ubiquinone seems, on the whole, to be unimportant unless it provides the aromatic nucleus for endogenous (body) synthesis.
(Also see VITAMIN[S], Table V-5.)

COENZYME R

An out-of-date name for the vitamin biotin.
(Also see BIOTIN.)

COFACTOR

A nonprotein substance which is a part of an enzyme and is needed for the full functioning of the enzyme. A cofactor may consist of an organic compound, e.g., a vitamin derivative; or a metallic ion, e.g., potassium, manganese, magnesium, calcium, or zinc. In the latter case, the metals are usually activators of the enzymes to which they become attached.

COFFEE *Coffea arabica*

Coffee is the beverage made from the roasted and ground beans of the coffee tree. It is the favorite drink in almost every country in temperate or cold climates. It is noteworthy, too, that the coffee break has become an integral part of the business world.

The coffee bean is the world's most valuable agricultural commodity. Among natural commodities in international trade, coffee usually ranks second only to petroleum in dollar value.

ORIGIN AND HISTORY. According to legend, coffee was discovered in Ethiopia when Kaldi, an Arabian goatherder, who lived in that part of Africa now known as Ethiopia in about the 3rd century A.D., noticed his goats prancing and cavorting on their hind legs after eating coffee berries. Being an adventuresome sort and needing a lift, he decided to try the fruit himself. Soon thereafter, the abbot

of a nearby monastery passed that way and was astonished to see the herder and his goats merrily dancing together in a meadow. The whimsical story goes on to say that the abbot decided to test the power of the berries on himself. So, he poured boiling water on them to make a brew. When he drank it, he found that he could stay awake for hours on end. From that time forward, he and the monks drank the berry liquid so that they could stay awake during the long hours of evening prayers.

Coffee was first used as a food, rather than as a beverage. African tribes crushed ripe cherries from wild coffee trees with stone mortars, added animal fat, mixed this exotic blend and fashioned it into round balls, which they ate at their war parties. The food filled two needs: (1) the animal fat and the protein of raw coffee beans (the protein is lost when coffee is prepared as a beverage) provided concentrated nourishment; and (2) the caffeine of the coffee served as a stimulant to spur the warriors to greater heights of savagery.

Later, African tribes made wine from coffee, by fermenting the ripe berries and adding water to the juice.

Coffee reached Yemen about 1000 A.D., where the ingenious Arabs stirred up the first *bean broth* from the cherry's agreeable seed. Soon, its popularity perked across all Arabia. For teetotal Muslims, it became an integral part of religious and secular life. Coffee moved from Arabia to Turkey during the 1500s, where it quickly acquired such importance that Turkish law permitted a wife to divorce her husband for failing to keep the family *ibrik* (pot) filled. Merchants of Venice carried their first cargo of coffee from Constantinople to Italy in 1615. Coffeehouses, where people met for serious discussions, sprang up all over Europe in the 1600s. But, some devout Catholics denounced it as the drink of infidels, and therefore sinful. Before committing himself, Pope Clement— so it's said—tried a cup of coffee and became an instant convert. He settled the matter by baptizing the brew in order to give it Christian status. Coffee probably came to America in the 1660s. Coffee-growing was introduced into Brazil in the 1700s.

THE COFFEE PLANT.

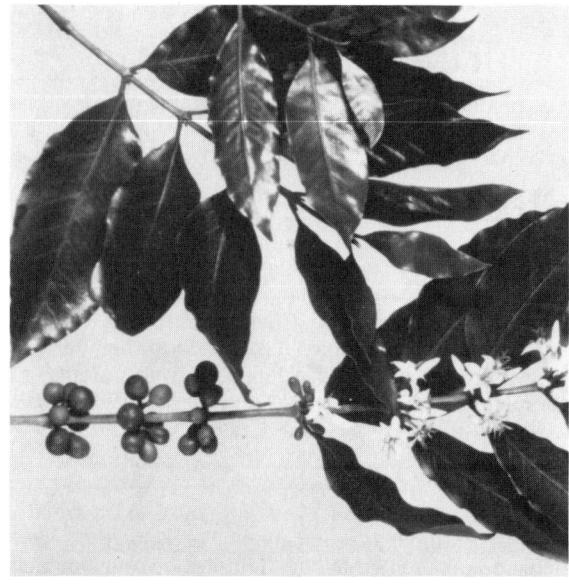

Fig. C-61. Coffee *(coffea arabica)*, indigenous to Ethiopia. (Courtesy, Field Museum of Natural History, Chicago, Ill.)

The coffee plant belongs to the genus *Coffea,* species *C. arabica,* evergreen shrub or small tree, which is propagated from seed.

The desirable flavor in coffee seems to result more from the location in which the coffee is grown than from the kind and amount of care. Colombian, Blue Mountain Jamaican, and highland Central American coffees are usually considered superior to African coffees.

The vast majority of cherries are harvested by hand. If the dry method of processing is to be used, all the cherries are stripped from the branches at once—green, partially ripe, ripe, and overripe. If the wet method is to be used, only ripe cherries are picked.

WORLD AND U.S. PRODUCTION.

The world production of coffee totals about 5.5 million metric tons annually, of which nearly one-third is grown in Brazil.

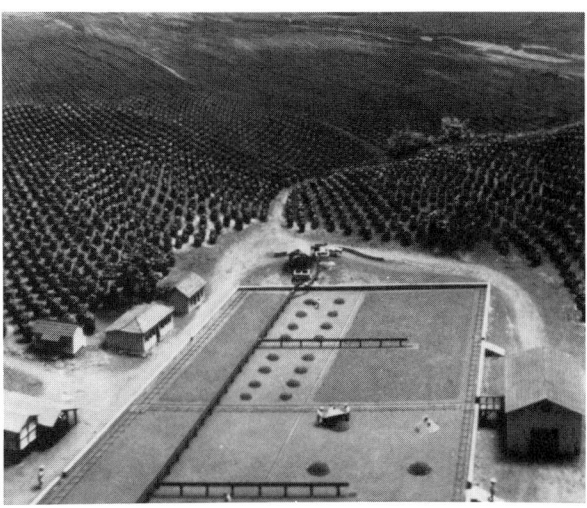

Fig. C-62. Coffee plantation in Brazil. (Courtesy, Field Museum of Natural History, Chicago, Ill.)

Brazil and Colombia dominate the world's coffee production, which they have done for many years. But some of the old coffee-producing countries are again active, and new countries are making inroads on the supremacy of Brazil and Colombia. The ten leading coffee-producing countries of the world, by rank, are shown in Fig. C-63.

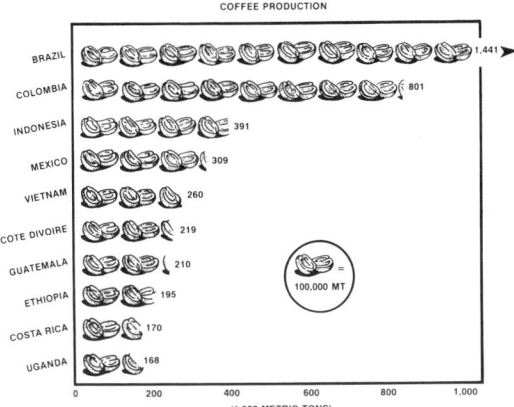

COFFEE PRODUCTION

BRAZIL 1,441
COLOMBIA 801
INDONESIA 391
MEXICO 309
VIETNAM 260
COTE DIVOIRE 219
GUATEMALA 210
ETHIOPIA 195
COSTA RICA 170
UGANDA 168

= 100,000 MT

0   200   400   600   800   1,000
(1,000 METRIC TONS)

Fig. C-63. Leading coffee-producing countries of the world in 1990. (Source: *FAO Production Yearbook 1990,* FAO/UN, Rome, Italy, Vol. 44, pp. 174-175, Table 78)

Hawaii grows the only U.S. coffee. This premium bean, started from imported Brazilian trees in 1825, is produced in small quantities. Complex production methods are required due to the hard volcanic soil of the island. Its flavor is excellent and it commands high prices wherever coffee is sold. In 1990/91, Hawaii produced 2,700,000 lb (*1,225,800 kg*) of coffee, which sold at $2.60 per pound and had a total value of $7,020,000.

PROCESSING COFFEE.

The flavor of the coffee is determined by the variety, by where and how the coffee was grown, by the method of preparation for market and by the roasting.

At the roasting plant, the beans are emptied into chutes leading from the upper to the lower floor. An air-suction device removes dust and other materials. The coffee may then go to the blending machine, a cylinder that mixes different types of coffee. From the blender, the beans flow by gravity to storage bins, then to roaster ovens.

Roasting.

Roasting brings about both physical and chemical changes in coffee beans. When coffee is roasted, it shrinks about 16% in weight (up to 20% for the darkest Italian roast), doubles in volume, turns from pale green to a rich brown in color, and develops characteristic coffee taste and aroma. The resulting chemical composition differs radically from that of the green beans.

In continuous roasting, hot air (400° to 500°F [*200° to 260°C*]) is forced through small quantities of beans for a 5-minute period. In batch mixing, much larger quantities of beans are roasted for a longer time.

The longer coffee is roasted, the darker it gets. From light to dark are a variety of roasts all tasting like coffee, each appealing to a particular taste.

Unblended Coffee.

Two species provide most of the world's commercial coffee; namely, *Coffea arabica* and *Coffea robusta.* A third species, *Coffea liberica,* provides about 5% of American coffee. As a rule, only *arabica* coffee, which possesses finer aroma, flavor, and body than *robusta,* is offered unblended. *Robusta* coffee, which is neutral in the cup, is widely used in commercial blends.

The growing demand for unblended coffees is indicative of the desire of people to experience the distinctive qualities of some of the world's great varieties and types of coffee, along with their disenchantment of *nothing much* blends. There's magic in such names as Kona, Jamaican, Mocha, and Java.

Blended Coffee.

Almost all of the coffee brought into, and marketed in, the United States is blended by the major packers. Although the proportion of unblended coffee is less in other countries than in the United States, blended coffee predominates throughout the world.

Today, brand name coffees are promoted in the United States, with little or no attempt made to identify the species or place where grown. Coffee brands are extolled on the basis of being richer, coffee-er, good to the last drop, mountain grown, tree-ripened, or hand-picked.

The art of blending coffees was born because coffee men found that, by blending various coffees, they could create a single coffee with an aggregate of delightful traits. Nature provides beans possessing taste, aroma, and body in varying degrees, but unblended coffees rarely possess these qualities in the most desirable proportions. So, the job of the blender is to combine these qualities in a balanced coffee. Not only that, the blender of commercial coffee must, from month to month, be able to find suitable replacements for coffees that cease to satisfy the requirements of his blend.

Chicory.
Sometimes, chicory, which is also known as French endive or witloof, is added to coffee to reduce the cost. In New Orleans, where the Creole influence is strong, chicory blended coffee is widely used. Also, to economize, many European immigrants learned to use chicory in the old country; some never switched to pure coffee because they came to prefer the flavor of the chicory additive.

Chicory is the perennial turnip-shaped vegetable the tops of which are commonly used as a salad green and the young roots of which may be boiled and eaten like carrots. The roots are also kiln dried, then roasted and ground; it then looks like ground coffee. Coffee with chicory additive is more bitter, heavier, and darker than pure coffee.

The United States imports chicory from Central Europe. Some is also grown in Michigan.

Instant Coffee.
Instant coffee entails the extraction of ground coffee with warm water to form a concentrated liquid brew, followed by removal of the water from the brew by some method of dehydration. The residue which is left is instant coffee.

Instant coffee, which constitutes about one-fifth of all coffee sold, is prepared in either of the following ways:

1. By forcing an atomized spray of very strong coffee extract through a jet of hot air. This evaporates the water in the extract and leaves dried coffee particles, which are packaged as instant, or soluble, coffee.

2. By freeze-drying, which results in a product that looks somewhat like ground roasted coffee and retains some of coffee's aroma.

Decaffeinated Coffee.
Decaffeinated coffee is made by removing the caffeine from the green beans as follows: The green, unroasted beans are softened by steam and water; flushed with a solvent, usually containing chlorine, which soaks through all parts of the beans; agitated in the solvent to cause the caffeine from the beans to be drawn in combination with the chlorine; drained of the solvent, then heated and blown with steam to evaporate all traces of solvent. To obtain a product that is 97% caffeine-free, this process must be repeated up to 24 times. In addition to removing caffeine, the process removes some of the coffee's oils and waxes.

During the decade of the 70s, the consumption of decaffeinated coffee more than doubled.

WORLD AND U.S. CONSUMPTION.
Reports on per capita coffee consumption for any given year are estimates, based on annual imports of green beans, without consideration of changes in inventory levels at the beginning and the end of the year, and on population figures, which for some of the coffee-consuming areas are uncertain. However, estimates of daily per capita coffee consumption are given in Fig. C-64.

Note that Finland, top per capita coffee consumer, downs 5.3 cups (1.3 liter) a day for every man, woman, and child. By contrast, the United States averages less than half that much per person.

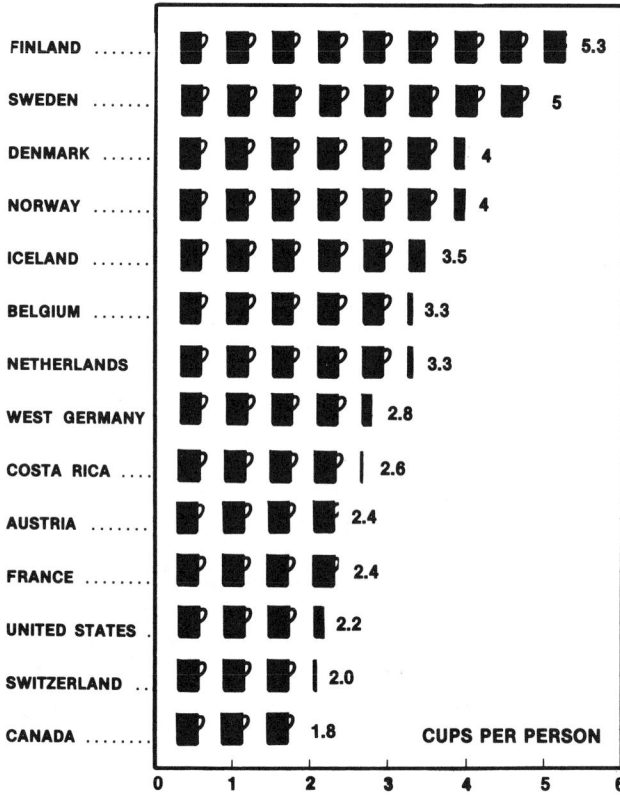

COFFEE CONSUMPTION

	CUPS PER PERSON
FINLAND	5.3
SWEDEN	5
DENMARK	4
NORWAY	4
ICELAND	3.5
BELGIUM	3.3
NETHERLANDS	3.3
WEST GERMANY	2.8
COSTA RICA	2.6
AUSTRIA	2.4
FRANCE	2.4
UNITED STATES	2.2
SWITZERLAND	2.0
CANADA	1.8

Fig. C-64. World's coffee drinkers. (One cup = 240 ml)

COFFEE, CAFFEINE, AND HEALTH.
Various accusations have been leveled at coffee, including that it causes heart attacks, high blood pressure, pancreatic cancer, peptic ulcers, hypoglycemia, fetal malformations, cystic breast disease, and nervousness; and that it shortens life.

Increasingly, the debate has focused on caffeine, most of which comes from coffee, although headache and cold remedies also contain caffeine. The two major varieties of coffee beans, arabica and robusta, contain 1 and 2% caffeine, respectively. Brewed coffee contains 80 to 120 mg of caffeine per cup (240 ml), usually about 85 mg; tea contains about one-half this amount per cup, and cola beverages about 30 mg per cup. Instant coffee has about 65 to 75 mg of caffeine per cup and decaffeinated coffee about 1 to 6 mg per cup. Caffeine is absorbed readily and reaches peak levels in the body about 1 hour after ingestion.

The question is whether caffeine does any real harm. The accusation and fact of each case against coffee follow:

• **Coffee causes heart attacks?**—In the early 1970s, heavy coffee drinkers were shaken by certain research reports linking coffee with heart attacks.

Fact. Later, it was found that the studies indicating that heavy coffee drinking was a causative factor in heart disease did not take into account the fact that heavy coffee drinkers were often heavy smokers.[22]

---

[22]Kannel, W. B., "Coffee, Cocktails and Coronary Candidates," *The New England Journal of Medicine,* Vol. 297, 1977, p. 443.

The famed Framingham study, conducted in Framingham, Massachusetts, from 1949 to 1969, on 5,209 males and females, ages 30 to 62 showed that when cigarette smoking was held constant, the association of coffee consumption with coronary heart disease ceased to exist.

Since 1968, the IBM Corporation has conducted a voluntary health testing, or screening, study of its employees above 35 years of age. At the time of the reported results which follow, 92,000 initial and 48,000 follow-up examinations had been done, for a total of 140,000. One of the questions in the questionnaire concerns coffee, and the question is divided as follows: Do you regularly take 0 cups per day, 1 to 3 cups (*240 to 720 ml*), 4 to 8 cups, or 9 or more cups per day? Using the abnormal electrocardiogram as an index of heart disease, IBM also did a univariate analysis of coffee vs the abnormal electrocardiogram. They reported that *there was no relationship whatsoever between coffee consumption and the electrocardiogram.*

In summary, there is no convincing evidence that coffee causes heart attacks. However, protracted abuse of coffee drinking appears responsible for arrhythmia (an alteration in the rhythm of the heartbeat either in time or force) in a small percent of the population.

• **Coffee causes high blood pressure?**—In the January 26, 1978 issue of *The New England Journal of Medicine*, Robertson *et al.* reported that, after 250 mg of caffeine (roughly the amount of caffeine in 3 cups of coffee) was given, there was a modest rise, of rather short duration, in blood pressure of 14/10. Then the article concluded with this statement: "Further investigation into the effects of chronic caffeine use and caffeine use in hypertensive subjects is needed."

Fact. The short-duration rise in blood pressure of a mean figure 14/10, as reported above, is not significant. Almost any individual may, for example, experience a rise in blood pressure of from 30 to 60 mm of mercury when he becomes nervous and excited such as (1) when watching a sports event, or (2) when having an argument with his wife.

In the IBM study described under "Coffee causes heart attacks?," the blood pressure was also taken on all participants. The IBM researchers concluded that, "it is clear that there was no specific relationship between daily coffee consumption and blood pressure in those studied." It is noteworthy, too, that the IBM study included 72,100 chronic coffee drinkers.

It may be concluded, therefore, that man apparently adapts well to coffee, even in fairly large amounts, and chronic coffee use is not a cause of high blood pressure.

• **Coffee causes pancreatic cancer?**—It has been suggested that coffee may be contributing to cancer of the pancreas. This disease has been increasing in frequency for about 50 years. In 1990, an estimated 5% of both males and females in the United States died from cancer of the pancreas.

Fact. U.S. coffee consumption has been decreasing since 1946. Besides, the case remains unproved.

Of two recent studies, one implicated *decaffeinated* coffee and the other made no distinction; neither study was regarded as conclusive. Meanwhile, moderation in the use of coffee is suggested—limiting to 2 cups (*480 ml*) a day in any form. An estimated 5 million Americans take upward of 10 cups a day. But drinkers of coffee (with caffeine) may find that they have trouble cutting back because they have become dependent on the caffeine and suffer from headache, muscle tension, sleepiness, and other symptoms when they experience withdrawal. These individuals should try

to taper off on coffee and perhaps switch to tea (1 cup of tea supplies about a third of the caffeine of a cup of coffee). Further studies are indicated.

• **Coffee causes peptic ulcers?**—The possible relationship between caffeine and peptic ulcers has long been debated. Stimulation of gastric secretion by caffeine has been shown in several experimental animals and with human subjects in single dose experiments.

Fact. A variety of studies have failed to establish a clear-cut cause and effect relationship between caffeine ingestion and peptic ulcer. Nevertheless, coffee is known to cause acidosis (sourness) of the stomach. So, when a patient has an ulcer, most internists recommend that coffee be eliminated.

• **Coffee causes hypoglycemia (low blood sugar)?**—This condition, characterized by an abnormally low concentration of sugar in the blood, may be associated with excess coffee.

Fact. Low blood sugar may be associated with a number of disorders; among them, alcoholism, allergies, behavior problems, brain damage in infants, depression, diabetes, drug addiction, fatigue, high blood pressure, impotency, obesity, ulcers, underachievement, and coffee.

Coffee gives a temporary lift in energy and sharpens mental acuity, but some individuals experience a let down feeling later. The reason for the lift is that caffeine stimulates the central nervous system and promotes the breakdown of glycogen to glucose in the liver, which raises the blood sugar level. However, the elevation of blood glucose may be short lived in some people, because their pancreas reacts by secreting insulin. Hence, they may feel let down due to a drop in their blood sugar.

If excess coffee (caffeine) is the cause of hypoglycemia, recommended treatment is to lessen or eliminate the coffee.

• **Coffee causes fetal malformations?**—There have been reports that pregnant women who drink caffeine-containing substances may be increasing the risk of birth defects. Also, it is known that transfer of caffeine across the placental barrier occurs readily.

Fact. After evaluating thousands of studies, the American Council on Science and Health (ACSH) concluded: "There is no evidence from human studies to support the belief that the use of coffee or cola is harmful to the fetus." Dr. Elizabeth Whelan of the ACSH continued: "Use some common sense. People who drink 10 cups of coffee a day should realize that they are over-doing it. In the case of pregnant women, it's been found that they don't metabolize caffeine as well as those who are not pregnant. Another reason why pregnant women shouldn't drink too much coffee, or other caffeine-containing drinks, is that it may keep them awake during a time when they need their rest."[23]

Although more evidence is needed, there does appear to be sufficient reason to caution pregnant women, or soon to be pregnant women, about their coffee consumption.

• **Coffee causes cystic breast disease?**—Cystic breast disease—a noncancerous condition—affects about 50% of American women, most of them under age 45. One study, involving about 50 women, indicated that caffeine consumption may increase the incidence of cystic breast disease.

---

[23]*American Council on Science and Health*, Update, Fall 1981, p. 16.

Fact. There is no conclusive evidence to link cystic breast disease to caffeine consumption. More research is needed.

• **Coffee causes nervousness, tremors, insomnia, and gastric symptoms; withdrawal symptoms?**—With excessive coffee intake, some individuals develop untoward nervous system effects from caffeine, such as nervousness, tremors, and insomnia. In rare cases, there may be gastric symptoms such as heartburn, abdominal discomfort, or diarrhea; but generally such gastrointestinal effects occur with excessive coffee consumption. Also, some experience headaches with the withdrawal of caffeine, beginning about 12 to 16 hours after the last dose of caffeine.

Fact. Such adverse effects as the above are rare with moderate intakes of coffee. Rather, the nervous system is stimulated agreeably—there is enhanced alertness and wakefulness, increased energy, and elevated mood. Of course, those who experience gastric distress from minimal amounts of coffee should abstain from it. Two remedies for caffeine withdrawal headaches are suggested: (1) a gradual decrease in coffee consumption—a weaning period of about a week; and (2) the use of a suppository containing 150 mgm of caffeine.

• **Coffee drinking shortens life?**—Creative people have long sworn by, and occasionally at, the heavenly brew. Typical are the experiences of three Frenchmen-of-letters.

Balzac, one of the most important novelists of the 1800s, gave this description of what coffee did for him: "Everything becomes agitated; ideas are set in motion like army battalions on the battlefields, and then the battle begins. Memories charge forward, banners flying; the light cavalry of comparisons progresses at a magnificent gallop; the artillery of logic hastens into the fray with its cannons and cartridges...." Balzac often wrote more than 16 hours a day, keeping himself awake with countless cups of black coffee, kept hot over the flame of a spirit lamp in his studio. But he died in 1850 at age 51. His death was immediately attributed to the gradual accumulation of coffee poisons in his system.

Fact. Caffeine doesn't accumulate in the human body; it's metabolized at the rate of 15% an hour and rapidly excreted. Moreover, in addition to writing and drinking black coffee, Balzac filled his life with wild money-making schemes and affairs with women. So, there could have been other reasons than coffee for his relatively early demise. Besides, what of Voltaire, French author and philosopher, who a century earlier drank 50 cups (*12 liter*) a day and lasted, still vigorous, into his middle eighties? Even more arresting is the case of a third French writer, Bernard de Fontenelle, who on his hundredth year (in 1757) attributed his long life to coffee.

Whatever explanations for their longevity centenarians make, it's unlikely that coffee drinking prolongs life. But not many think it shortens life, either.

SUMMARY. While individual tolerances vary, up to 200 or 300 mg of caffeine, which is equivalent to 3 to 4 cups of coffee per day, seems to be a mild stimulant helpful in relieving minor fatigue and boredom, with little risk of any harmful effects. This was substantiated in a nationwide survey, conducted by the U.S. Department of Health and Human Services, from which it was concluded that: "There is no evidence that heavy coffee drinking—5 or more cups (*1.2 liter*) per day—is related to poor health."

• **The confession of a coauthor**—I have a confession. I am addicted to coffee. Some people say that I drink too much of the stuff. Maybe I do. But if I didn't drink coffee, I would write less. Besides, I wonder how I would feel were I to drink 20 cups of either orange juice or milk daily! So, at my age, I side with Voltaire, who reportedly drank 50 cups of coffee a day and said of the brew: "It is a poison, certainly—but a slow poison, for I have been drinking it these eighty-four years." Pass me a cup of that poison-laden coffee. M.E.E.

(Also see CAFFEINE.)

COFFEE ESSENCE

Concentrated extract of coffee. Not less than 4 lb of coffee must be used to prepare 1 gal (*3.8 liter*).

COGNAC

A brandy produced in southern France from special varieties of grapes.

COHUNE NUT

This is the nut from a Central American palm. The shells of the nut are made into ornaments, and the meat yields an oil resembling coconut oil.

COLD STERILIZATION

Large doses of radiation are capable of destroying the bacteria in food. However, doses sufficient to destroy bacteria only slightly elevate the temperature of the food, hence, the term cold sterilization.

(Also see RADIATION PRESERVATION OF FOOD.)

"COLD STORE" BACTERIA

Microorganisms that survive and may even thrive at the usual refrigeration temperatures (40°F [3 to 4°C]).

(Also see BACTERIA IN FOOD, section headed "Bacterial Control Methods," point No. 4; and PSYCHROPHILIC BACTERIA.)

COLIC

A severe indigestion, which causes abdominal discomfort.
(Also see INFANT DIET AND NUTRITION.)

COLIFORM BACTERIA

A term which refers to a group of intestinal tract bacteria which can survive with or without air. *Escherichia coli* is the most important member of the group. Most coliform bacteria are disease-causing only under special circumstances, but their presence in food, and particularly in water, suggests fecal contamination.

(Also see BACTERIA IN FOOD, Table B-5 Food Infections [Bacterial]—"*Escherichia coli*.")

COLITIS

This is an inflammation of the large intestine (colon) which may be accompanied by abdominal pain, constipation or diarrhea, passage of bloody stools, weakness, and/or weight loss. Although it may seem that most of those afflicted with colitis are either middle-aged or elderly, the various types of the disorder afflict people at all ages. Hemorrhages, malnutrition, and other consequences sometimes result if treatment is delayed too long. Also, the chances of developing cancer of the colon increase greatly with the duration of ulcerative colitis, so prompt treatment is a good preventative measure. For these reasons, the characteristics of the different forms of colitis are noteworthy. Fig. C-65 shows the parts of the digestive tract where colitis is likely to occur.

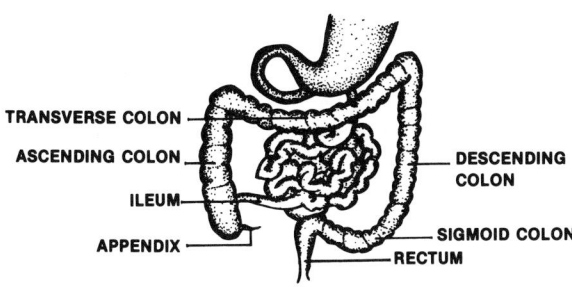

Fig. C-65. Colitis may strike anywhere between the ileum and the rectum.

• **Ileocolitis**—This condition affects the lower part of the small intestine (ileum) and the adjoining part of the colon. It occurs commonly in children, adolescents, and young adults. They may have pain or tenderness on the lower right side of the abdomen which is similar to that of appendicitis. Other characteristics of ileocolitis are (1) partial obstruction of the intestine by scar tissue; (2) anemia, fatty stools, lack of appetite, and weight loss due to malabsorption; and (3) inflammation and fever.

• **Mucous colitis**—Abdominal cramps, along with the passage of large amounts of mucus with dry, hard stools characterize this disorder, which is thought to result from (1) food intolerances or other allergic conditions; and/or (2) emotional disturbances.

• **Spastic colitis**—The main sign of this condition, which is also called irritable colon, is irregular, abnormally rapid movements of the bowels. The most common symptoms are (1) various types of abdominal pain, ranging from a dull ache to cramps; (2) lack of appetite, nausea, and vomiting; and (3) heartburn. Often, mucous colitis and spastic colitis are considered to be essentially the same disorder because their characteristics are similar. Together, they constitute the most prevalent digestive disturbances.

• **Ulcerative colitis**—Young adults who strive hard to conform to others' expectations may be afflicted with this disorder, which is indicated by (1) ulcers of the colon that bleed from time to time, (2) a recurring, crampy diarrhea, (3) abdominal pains of variable severity and duration, (4) formation of scar tissue which sometimes blocks the intestine, (5) lack of appetite and vomiting, and (6) fever. The condition is somewhat unpredictable, in that the acute attacks may occur at irregular intervals over periods of 20 years or more. Often, the attacks coincide with emotional distress.

Various studies have shown that as many as two-thirds of the patients who have had chronic ulcerative colitis for many years die from either its direct effects or its complications. Nevertheless, total recovery without recurrence of the condition is possible, thanks to recent advances in dietary therapy, anti-inflammatory drugs, and certain surgical procedures.

CAUSES OF COLITIS. Any discussion of the causes of colitis is bound to be controversial because of great variations in susceptibility among people who appear to be exposed to the same environmental factors. It might be that some people have an inherited tendency to develop one or more of the forms of colitis when certain provocative conditions are present. Some of the factors which are generally thought to be responsible for attacks of colitis are:
1. Allergic conditions
2. Cold or hot environments
3. Constipation
4. Diarrhea
5. Drugs
6. Emotional upsets
7. Immune reactions against one's own body tissues (autoimmunity)
8. Infectious microorganisms
9. Irritating drinks, foods, and spices
10. Lack of rest
11. Laxatives and enemas
12. Nutritional deficiencies
13. Parasitic infections
14. Smoking
15. Strenuous exercise right after eating
16. Surgery

DIAGNOSTIC, PREVENTATIVE, AND THERAPEUTIC MEASURES. Many people have long been afflicted with mild forms of mucous or spastic colitis without ever developing either ileocolitis or ulcerative colitis. Nevertheless, it is wiser to take certain preventive measures at the first sign of bowel trouble, than to suffer needless anxiety and pain at a later time. Hence, some common diagnostic, preventive and therapeutic measures follow.

G.I. Series (Fluoroscopic Examination Of The Digestive Tract). This diagnostic procedure is used to detect various abnormalities of the gastrointestinal tract by means of fluoroscopy, which consists of the placing of the patient between a source of x rays and a fluorescent screen that displays a picture of the organs outlined by the x rays. Usually, a series of photographs are taken of various parts of the digestive tract. There are two types of G.I. series.

• **Upper G.I. series**—In this series, the patient swallows a chalky suspension of barium sulfate (sometimes called a barium meal) which fills the esophagus, stomach, and small intestine so that they may be seen in x-ray photographs.

• **Lower G.I. series**—This series requires that the patient be given a barium-containing enema to outline his or her colon. X-ray photographs are then taken before and after the enema is expelled.

The diagnosis of colitis may require both upper and lower G.I. series, because ileocolitis often affects both the small intestine and the colon.

Modified Diets. The dietary measures used to relieve the symptoms and signs of colitis should be selected carefully, because the characteristics of the disorder vary widely from patient to patient. Furthermore, there is uncertainty regarding the diets which may prevent even the mildest forms of colitis, because some people can eat highly irritating foods from infancy to old age without developing the disorder, whereas others are afflicted after only the briefest exposures to an irritant or a stress factor. Therefore, modified diets for the most critical cases are presented first, following which dietary guidelines are given for the milder forms of colitis.

CAUTION: The dietary information which follows is given only for the purpose of illustrating certain dietary principles, because the selection of a patient's diet is strictly the responsibility of his or her attending physician and of the consulting dietitian.

ACUTE STAGES OF ILEOCOLITIS OR ULCERATIVE COLITIS.
Patients who are critically ill with these disorders may be badly malnourished because (1) they reduced their food consumption drastically in order to avoid aggravating their condition; or (2) chronic diarrhea prevented absorption of nutrients, while also causing the loss of the gastrointestinal secretions that are rich in protein and mineral salts. Therefore, it is sometimes necessary to resort to special medical measures such as hyperalimentation (feeding a liquid formula rich in nutrients through a vein at the base of the neck) or nasogastric tube feeding (a tube is passed up through the nose and down through the throat and the esophagus to the stomach) until the patient is well enough to take food by mouth.

It may be necessary to eliminate the carbohydrate in the diets of patients on oral feedings until diarrhea has been brought under control.[24] In these cases, the minimum requirement for sugar (glucose) may be met by intravenously administered solutions of dextrose. Usually, the ability of the patient to tolerate carbohydrates improves as malnutrition is corrected and the damaged intestinal lining is healed. Sometimes, wheat protein (gluten) is tolerated poorly and has to be eliminated from the diet.

Hence, therapeutic diets should be designed so that they are (1) very well digested and absorbed, and contain only minimal amounts of undigestible residue; (2) rich in calories and protein; (3) free from foods which commonly cause allergic or other digestive disturbances; and (4) soft in texture and bland. These criteria are best met by elemental diets, followed by diets containing low-residue foods.

• **Elemental diets**—These liquids and powders (intended for mixing with water), which have recently been marketed by certain pharmaceutical companies, usually contain (1) predigested protein, or a mixture of individual amino acids; (2) sugar, and/or partially digested starch; (3) small amounts of special fats (medium-chain triglycerides); and (4) supplemental minerals, vitamins, and flavoring. The undigestible residue content of elemental diets is so low that the bowel movements of patients are smaller than normal and occur only about once every 5 days. The results obtained with these products have generally been favorable, since prompt healing and gains in weight have often occurred. Unfortunately, elemental diets may become monotonous to patients as they begin to feel better, because (1) the products come in only a few flavors, and (2) drinking liquids is not as enjoy-

able as eating solid foods. However, the manufacturers of the dietary preparations now provide recipes for varying the ways in which their products are served.

(Also see LIQUID DIETS.)

• **Diets containing selected, low-residue foods**—The doctor may recommend that the first foods to be given be limited to those low in residue, such as clear broth, weak tea, toasted white bread, small amounts of butter (which should be immediately discontinued if fatty, frothy stools are produced), soft cooked eggs, custards, gelatin desserts, and bland cooked cereals like cream of rice and cream of wheat. Milk and items made from it are often barred from these diets because there is a high incidence of milk intolerance in patients with ulcerative colitis. The digestive problems which follow the consumption of milk or milk-containing foods may be due to (1) an intolerance to milk sugar, which may disappear after the intestine has healed, and/or (2) a sensitivity to milk protein that makes it necessary to eliminate these foods from the patient's diet. If milk is not allowed, calcium supplements should be taken to prevent weakening of the bones. Extra calories may be obtained from moderate amounts of sugar, hard candies, honey, and syrups, as long as there is no laxative effect from these items.

If improvement continues, the next step is to add (1) tender cooked fish, meats, and poultry (providing that the fat content is low); and (2) baked or boiled white potatoes without skins. After that, canned fruits and cooked vegetables may be added, a little at a time; but they should be discontinued immediately if watery stools are passed. It is noteworthy that many people who have recovered from acute attacks of ulcerative colitis may have relapses if they attempt to eat raw fruits and vegetables. Hence, these items may have to be restricted permanently.

CAUTION: The elimination of certain foods, such as raw fruits and vegetables, from low residue diets makes it advisable for people following these recommendations to take mineral and vitamin supplements. Most doctors and dietitians will advise their patients regarding the products best suited to their needs.

MILD AND CHRONIC FORMS OF COLITIS.
People who are prone to develop various forms of colitis may have to avoid irritating foods for the rest of their lives, particularly at times when they are likely to have emotional stress. However, they must also avoid dietary extremes which may lead to constipation, diarrhea, or nutritional deficiencies because these conditions make colitis worse. Therefore, it is necessary to eat a wide variety of nutritious, nonirritating foods.

CAUTION: The information which follows is for illustrative purposes only, because individual diets to control colitis must be designed to meet the specific needs of the patient. For example, a mildly alcoholic drink such as a small glass of table wine diluted 50/50 with water may help tense people to relax. However, no forms of alcoholic beverages are allowed when certain medicines are taken. Table C-18 gives some general guidelines for the selection of nonirritating foods.

SPECIAL DIETARY PRODUCTS.
The dietary recommendations in Table C-18 list a few special products which may be substituted for the ordinary foods that may aggravate colitis. Brief descriptions of these items follow.

[24]Coale, M.S., and J. R. K. Robson, "Dietary Management of Intractable Diarrhea in Malnourished Patients," *Journal of the American Dietetic Association*, Vol. 76, May 1980, pp. 444-450.

TABLE C-18
DIETARY GUIDELINES FOR PEOPLE WHO ARE LIKELY TO DEVELOP COLITIS

Foods That Are Allowed	Foods That Are Not Allowed
Beverages (other than fruit juices or milk)	
Caffeine-free coffee substitutes; carob drinks; decaffeinated coffee; herb teas; mildly carbonated soft drinks (carbonation may be weakened by allowing to stand in a warm place after opening); weak coffee and tea; and table wine diluted to half strength with water.	Beer; boiling hot or ice-cold drinks; cocoa; distilled liquors; highly carbonated soft drinks; and strong coffee. All alcoholic beverages (including wine) when certain medications are taken.
Breads and cereal products	
Breads and cereal products made from refined flours, without added fibrous substances. Yeast-raised doughnuts baked in an oven.	Items made from bran, candied fruits, coconut, nuts, pie crust, raisins, seeds, wheat germ and whole grain flour; doughnuts fried in fat.
Cheeses	
American cheese, cottage cheese, cream cheese; and other mild flavored items; providing that milk products are well tolerated.	Strongly flavored cheeses, such as those aged for long periods, and those ripened with molds.
Desserts	
Bread pudding, cakes, and cookies (of low to moderate fat content), cornstarch puddings, custards, gelatin desserts, junket puddings (if milk is well tolerated), rice pudding without raisins, and sherbets (must be eaten slowly).	Desserts containing candied or dried fruits, coconut, nuts, peel, pie crust, seeds, whole grain products, and large amounts of fats or oils. Sugary items when diarrhea occurs.
Eggs	
Boiled or poached (medium to hard cooked); soft scrambled in a double boiler with a minimum of fat.	Fried, hard scrambled, or raw eggs.
Fats	
Butter, lard, margarine, vegetable oils, and mild flavored mayonnaise. (In the event of diarrhea these items should be eliminated temporarily.) It is noteworthy that medium-chain triglycerides (MCT, a special dietetic fat derived from coconut oil) does not aggravate diarrhea as ordinary dietary fats do.	Spicy mayonnaise, salad dressings, and sandwich spreads—particularly those similar to relishes and tartar sauce.
Fish, meats, poultry, and seafood	
Baked or broiled with visible fat removed. Canned fish or seafood without bones or skin.	Cured, fatty, fried, pickled, or smoked items; luncheon meats; sausages; skins from meats, poultry, and seafood. Certain canned meat products such as hash may contain sufficient fat to cause diarrhea.
Fruits and fruit juices	
Baby food purees; canned or cooked items without seeds or skin; all juices (it might be wise to dilute citrus products and similar acid juices to half strength with water). Citrus fruits should be eaten at the end of a meal (one such item per day is sufficient).	Berries; candied fruit or peel; canned or cooked fruits with seeds or skin; canned grapefruit, orange, or pineapple; dried fruits, unless pureed; and fresh or frozen raw fruits other than avocado or ripe banana.
Herbs, seasonings, and spices	
Cinnamon, lemon, salt, and vanilla. Other items as recommended by the doctor or dietitian.	Coarsely textured or pungent products such as chili, garlic, green and red peppers, horseradish, mustard, pepper, vinegar, and Worchestershire sauce.
Milk	
Small amounts of various products should be tried to see if they are tolerated. Some patients may have to use nondairy substitutes.	In the event that a milk intolerance is diagnosed, all forms of this food may have to be eliminated from the diet.
Nuts, nut products, and seeds	
Smooth style nut butters (amounts should be limited because of the high fat content).	Chunk style nut butters; nuts and seeds.
Potatoes	
Baked or boiled sweet or white (Irish) potatoes without skins.	Any form of fried potatoes; potato chips; and skins of potatoes.
Sugar and other sweeteners	
Honey, molasses, sugar, and syrups; confections such as gumdrops, hard candies, and marshmallows; and strained cranberry sauce. Products which contain milk sugar (lactose) should be used cautiously.	Jams and preserves; sauce containing whole cranberries. All sugars may have to be restricted greatly if diarrhea occurs (particularly, molasses).
Vegetables	
Baby food purees; canned or soft cooked items without seeds or skins; and juices without seasonings other than salt. Whole cooked beans, kernels of corn, lentils, and peas may have to be mashed and strained in order to be tolerated by some extra sensitive people.	Any forms of broccoli, Brussels sprouts, cabbage, cauliflower, kale, and turnips; beans, if they produce excessive gas; fried onions; pickles; raw vegetables other than finely shredded lettuce.

• **Nondairy substitutes for milk**—Soybean derivatives are commonly used in formulas for infants who have an intolerance to cow's milk. The infants who cannot tolerate soybean protein may be given a formula based upon pureed beef heart. Therefore, it might be useful for some colitis patients to try one or more of these milk substitutes.

• **Medium-chain triglycerides (MCT)**—This item, which is an ingredient of certain commercial dietary formulations, is made from coconut oil by a special process. MCT is useful in the treatment of various disorders of fat absorption because under such conditions it is much more readily digested, absorbed, and utilized than ordinary dietary fats.

• **Baby food purees**—Many of these products are useful for people who are recovering from bowel problems because (1) they are designed for infants, who have sensitive intestines; (2) their contents of fat, fiber, and irritating seasonings are low; and (3) little or no preparation is required.

• **Water-soluble derivatives of vitamins A, D, E, and K**—The fat-soluble vitamins may not be well absorbed when ileocolitis or ulcerative colitis is accompanied by disorders of fat absorption. Therefore, it may be necessary for the patient to take water-soluble derivatives of these vitamins.

Drugs And Other Therapeutic Agents. Each of the medications commonly used in treating colitis has some undesirable effects, so it is essential that they be used only under a doctor's supervision. Hence, the information which follows is presented so that patients may recognize the need for careful selection of medications.

• **Antidiarrheal agents**—One of the long used remedies is a mixture of finely powdered clay (kaolin) and pectin, a gummy substance extracted from apple skins and the white membranes of oranges. However, its effectiveness in stopping infectious diarrhea is uncertain, unless an antibiotic is added to the mixture.

Another old remedy is paregoric (camphorated tincture of opium), which drastically slows the motion of the intestine.

Finally, one of the newer preparations which many people take with them on trips out of the country is a mixture of (1) a neuromuscular blocking agent (diphenoxylate hydrochloride); and (2) atropine, an antispasmodic drug.

The antidiarrheal agents should be used cautiously, because they may have such unwanted side effects as abdominal discomfort and nausea. Occasionally, intestinal obstruction occurs when intestinal movements are slowed excessively.

(Also see ATROPINE; and DIARRHEA.)

• **Bulking agents for constipation**—The low-residue diets which are often used in the treatment of colitis may not provide sufficient bulk to stimulate normal bowel movements. Therefore, the doctor or dietitian may recommend that the patient take certain nonirritating, bulking agents. These undigestible substances increase the bulk of the intestinal contents by binding large amounts of water. Some typical preparations are (1) agar-agar, a seaweed derivative; and (2) refined, psyllium seed powder. It is noteworthy that plenty of water should be taken with these substances because there have been cases in which certain bulking agents formed hard, dry masses in the colon, and did more harm than good.

(Also see CONSTIPATION; and FIBER.)

• **Medicated enemas and suppositories**—Rectal administration of medication is not new, since herbal enemas have long been used as *natural cures* for various ailments. These measures treat the bowel directly, and avoid any interference with the normal functioning of the rest of the body. (Medications given by mouth are likely to be absorbed and carried in the blood to all of the body tissues.) A medicated enema or suppository may contain (1) belladonna drugs which reduce the secretions and slow the movements of the intestine, or (2) hydrocortisone, an anti-inflammatory steroid drug. Unfortunately, the long-term use of anti-inflammatory steroids may render the small and large intestines extra susceptible to ulcers, hemorrhages, and perforation.

• **Orally-administered, anti-inflammatory steroids**—These substances are usually identical, or at least similar, to the adrenal cortical hormones secreted by the body in stressful situations. They may be administered orally in the treatment of colitis—even though their absorption exposes the whole body to their effects—because (1) they counteract inflammation elsewhere in the body, which may indirectly cause agitation of the bowels via the nerves; and (2) their protein-degrading actions throughout the body raise the blood level of amino acids so that these nutrients become more available for the healing of the intestines. However, the long-term administration of these steroids is risky because of such side effects as (1) weakening of the bones and muscles, and (2) thinning of the digestive tract so that it becomes extra susceptible to ulceration and/or rupture.

• **Sedatives and tranquilizers**—These drugs are sometimes useful in treating people whose bowels are continually agitated as a result of their chronic anxiety and nervous tension. Nevertheless, they are only stopgap measures in critical situations, since they do not remove the underlying cause(s) of the emotional distress. Furthermore, some patients may become so dependent upon the drugs that they cannot function normally without them.

Surgery. Surgical removal of highly inflamed portions of the intestines may be necessary in certain cases of ileocolitis or ulcerative colitis when there is a deterioration due to (1) obstruction of the intestinal opening, (2) bleeding or diarrhea which is difficult to stop, (3) continuous pain, or (4) tumors which may become cancerous. Fortunately, recent advances in surgical techniques and supportive measures have reduced the risks of such operations.

A typical surgical procedure (a colectomy) may involve (1) removal of the lower portion of the colon and attachment of the upper portion to an artificial opening (stoma) on the abdomen (this operation is called a colostomy); or (2) removal of the upper portion of the colon and/or the lower ileum so that the remaining end of the ileum is connected to a stoma (an ileostomy). Sometimes, the upper end of the remaining colon or ileum is connected to the rectum, so that a stoma is unnecessary.

Many people have had these operations and are able to live normal lives. Furthermore, moral support is provided by members of local chapters of the United Ostomy Association to those who have undergone this type of surgery.

Psychological Measures. Attacks of colitis sometimes follow events which produce anger, anxiety, fear, or resentment. Therefore, certain patients may benefit from being taught how to modify their behavior and control their emotions. Such instruction requires an understanding of the underlying causes of unhealthy reactions to ordinary circumstances like delays in traffic and disagreements with other people. Few amateurs are able to provide much help with such matters, so it would seem best for easily aggravated, colitis-prone people to obtain either professional counseling or to participate in group therapy which is conducted by a well-trained leader.

(Also see ELEMENTAL DIETS; LIQUID DIETS; and MODIFIED DIETS.)

COLLAGEN

A protein which forms the major part of the connective tissue. It forms gelatin when heated with water.

(Also see BODY TISSUE.)

COLLOID

A substance (as gelatin, albumin, or starch) dispersed through another medium. Colloids are larger than crystalline molecules, but not large enough to settle out; and they are incapable of passing through an animal membrane.

COLLOIDAL

Having the properties of a colloid.

COLLOIDAL OSMOTIC PRESSURE

The pressure exerted by the protein molecules in the plasma and in the cell. Because proteins are large molecules, they do not pass through the separating membranes of the capillary cell walls; hence, they remain in their respective compartments, producing a constant osmotic pull that protects vital plasma and cell fluid volumes in these compartments.

COLLOP

• A small slice of meat made tender by beating

• A rasher of bacon

• A fold of fat flesh

• An Irish measure of land based on the grazing requirements for one year, of a beef animal, a horse, or the equivalent in sheep.

COLON

A term used to designate a portion or all of the large intestine.

(Also see DIGESTION AND ABSORPTION.)

COLORING OF FOOD

The eyes are involved in eating, since the appearance is the first judgment passed on a food. Except under dire circumstances, foods which are unappealing to the eye will often be rejected. It's the color of a food that's eye catching first, then association with flavor, texture, nutritive value, and wholesomeness follow. For example, individuals are taught color associations: dark green vegetables, yellow vegetables, white potatoes, yellow egg yolks, and yellow butter and margarine. These associations and many others are then related to the quality of a food. Furthermore, color contributes to the attractiveness of food, which, in turn, adds to its enjoyment.

Of all the food additives, perhaps the addition of colors is the hardest to justify. Many people feel that foods have a natural color, so why tamper with it. Indeed, color additives have met strong opposition; and regulations have been passed banning some and restricting the use of others. Most of the opposition and regulation involves the synthetic colors, while the natural colors receive less attention. However, 90% of the colors used in food come from a small group of synthetic colors, while the diverse group of natural color sources is used in about 10% of foods only.

REGULATION OF FOOD COLORS. The Food and Drug Act of 1906 listed seven dyes which could be used in food. Subsequently, eight more colors were tested and approved. Therefore, at the time of the passage of the Food, Drug, and Cosmetic Act of 1938, 15 synthetic dyes were approved for use in foods. Also, under the new Act the common names of the dyes were no longer employed, but the color prefix FD&C, plus a number were used to designate the dyes. For example, orange 1 became FD&C orange No. 1, erythrosine became FD&C red No. 3; fast green became FD&C green No. 3; and so on. In 1950, an unfortunate incident occurred which cast a shadow on use of dyes in food. The overuse of color in candy and on popcorn resulted in a number of cases of diarrhea in children. This incident, along with some additional toxicity tests in animals, led to the delisting of three synthetic dyes, and to additional legislation. In 1960, the Color Additives Amendment became law. This gave the FDA the authority to impose limits on the amounts of color used in foods, drugs, and cosmetics. Furthermore, the new Amendment placed the onus of establishing safety of food dyes upon industry. Undoubtedly, some manufacturers will shift to the less functional and more expensive natural food colorings which have not been scrutinized as rigorously.

SYNTHETIC FOOD COLORS. In the past, the synthetic dyes were commonly referred to as coal tar dyes of which there are about 700. Because of the effectiveness of the synthetic dyes, only exceedingly small amounts—parts per million—are required to color foods. Also, the synthetic dyes are generally much more stable than natural food colorings, resisting breakdown in air, light, or heat, or by interacting with the other food components. Table C-19 lists the synthetic dyes and the guidelines for their use.

TABLE C-19
SYNTHETIC COLOR ADDITIVES
APPROVED FOR FOOD USE

Coloring Compound		Restriction in Use[1]
Color Prefix and Number	Common Name	
Citrus Red No. 2		Skins of oranges at 2 ppm.
FD&C Blue No. 1	Brilliant blue FCF	No specific limitations or restrictions on use.
FD&C Blue No. 2	Indigo carmine	No specific limitations or restrictions on use.
FD&C Green No. 3	Fast green FCF	No specific limitations or restrictions on use.
FD&C Red No. 4	Ponceau	Maraschino cherries at levels not exceeding 150 ppm.
FD&C Red No. 40	Allura Red AC	No specific limitations or restrictions on use.
FD&C Yellow No. 5	Tartrazine	No specific limitations or restrictions on use.
FD&C Yellow No. 6	Sunset yellow FCF	No specific limitations or restrictions on use.
Orange B		Sausage casings at 150 ppm.

[1]*Code of Federal Regulations*, 1975, Title 21, Parts 1-9.

NATURAL FOOD COLORS. Colors abound in the plant and animal kingdom which can be used for coloring foods. None of these require batch certification. Some are nutrients in their own right, others are spices, and still others fall under the general classification of carotenoids—a product of which nature makes about 400 million lb (*180 million kg*) annually. Table C-20 lists most of the more common approved naturally-occurring color compounds, and indicates their source and use.

USES OF FOOD COLORS. Not all foods contain added coloring agents. Major staple foods like bread, meat, potatoes, vegetables, and fruits are not colored. Moreover, all color additives, synthetic or natural (uncertified), are designated on the label as artificial color. The general classes of food making the greatest use of food colors follow:

• **Beverages**—One of the largest users of the certified colors (FD&C) is the beverage industry. Most of the fruit-type beverages contain single or combinations of certified color additives while colas and root beers are colored with caramel.

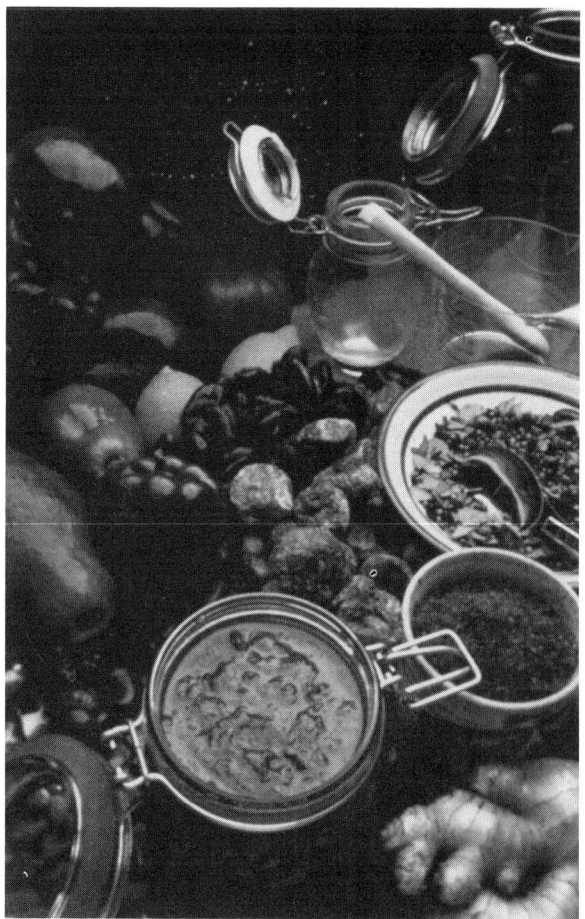

Fig. C-66. Some foods and ingredients are used because they add color, as well as flavor. (Courtesy, National Film Board of Canada)

TABLE C-20
COMMON NATURALLY-OCCURRING COLOR ADDITIVES APPROVED FOR FOOD USE[1]

Substance	Source	Restriction on Use
Algae meal, dried	Algae	Chicken feed to promote yellow skin and egg color
Alkanet	Roots of *Alkanna tinctoria*	Sausage casings, oleomargarines, and shortenings
Annatto	Seed pods of *Bixa orellana*	No limitations or restrictions on use
Aztec marigold (Tagetes meal)	Flower petals of Aztec marigold	Chicken feed to promote yellow skin and and egg color
Beets, dry powder	Beets	No limitations or restrictions on use
Beta-apo-8'-cartenal	Fruits, vegetables	Not to exceed 15 mg per lb (*0.45 kg*) or pt (*0.47 liter*) of food
Beta-carotene	Fruits, vegetables	No limitations or restrictions on use
Canthaxanthin	Fruits, vegetables	Not to exceed 30 mg per lb (*0.45 kg*) or pt (*0.47 liter*) of food
Caramel	Heated sugars	No limitations or restrictions on use
Carmine (cochineal)	Female insects, *Coccus cacti*	No limitations or restrictions on use
Carrot oil	Carrots	No limitations or restrictions on use
Chlorophyll	Green leaves	Sausage casings, margarine, and shortening
Corn endosperm oil	Corn	Chicken feed to promote yellow skin and egg color
Cottonseed flour partially defatted, cooked, toasted	Cottonseed	No limitations or restrictions on use
Ferrous gluconate	Iron salt of gluconic acid	Ripe olives
Fruit juice	Fruit	No limitations or restrictions on use
Grape skin extract	Grapes	No limitations or restrictions on use
Iron oxide (ferric oxide)	Hematite	Dog and cat foods not to exceed 0.25% by weight of finished product
Paprika	Plant *Capsicum annum*	No limitations or restrictions on use
Paprika oleoresin	Plant *Capsicum annum*	Not for use on fresh meat or ground fresh meat products except chorizo sausage and Italian brand sausage and other meats as specified by USDA
Riboflavin (vitamin B-12)	Plant and animal sources	No limitations or restrictions on use
Saffron	Stigmas of *Crocus sativus*	No limitations or restrictions on use
Titanium dioxide	Found in the minerals —rutile, titanite anatase, brookite, almenite	Not to exceed 1.0% by weight of food
Tumeric and oleresin	Rhizome of *Curcuma longa*	No limitations or restrictions on use
Ultramarine blue	Mineral, lapis lazuli	Animal feed, not to exceed 0.5% by weight of salt
Vegetable juice	Vegetables	No limitations or restrictions on use

[1]*Code of Federal Regulations*, 1974, Title 21, Parts 1–9.

• **Bakery products**—Bakery items which employ color additives include dough products, cookies, sandwich fillings, icings, coatings, and ice cream cones.

- **Candy**—With the wide variety of candies available, the use of color additives is extremely important to their desired appearance.

- **Dairy products**—Most all ice creams and sherbets contain artificial color. Chocolate ice cream may be the exception. Annatto and beta-carotene are used in cheese, since the certified colors are not sufficiently stable. Margarine and butter are also colored with annatto and beta-carotene.

- **Dry mix products**—Products such as gelatin desserts, puddings, cake mixes, doughnut mixes, and pancake mixes depend on proper color blends for their desired appearance.

- **Pet foods**—Although not for human consumption, pet food coloring is under the jurisdiction of the Food, Drug, and Cosmetic Act. Traditionally, iron oxide has been used to color pet foods because of its stability during the retorting operation. However, the certified colors are used extensively in dry extruded pet foods.
(Also see ADDITIVES; and BEHAVIOR AND DIET.)

COLOSTOMY

An operation in which an artificial opening (a stoma) from the colon to the outside of the body is placed on the abdomen. This type of surgery is performed when the lower part of the intestines must be removed or closed off because of a disease.
(Also see DIGESTION AND ABSORPTION.)

COLOSTRUM

The first secretion of a mammal (human or animal) after childbirth. Colostrum is valuable to the newborn because it is high in protein and it contains antibodies which transfer some of the immunity of the mother to the newborn.
(Also see BREAST FEEDING, section headed "Colostrum.")

COMA

A prolonged state of unconsciousness. The two most common types of nutritionally related comas follow:

- **Diabetic coma**—This condition is usually brought on by the combination of acidosis and ketosis which occurs when diabetes is (1) out of control; or (2) aggravated by failure to eat, the stress of infection, or the failure to take insulin when it is needed.

- **Hepatic coma**—In this condition the brain is intoxicated by an excess of ammonia which accumulates in the blood during liver failure. Normally, the liver converts the ammonia formed in protein metabolism to urea which may be excreted safely in the urine.

COMFIT

A confection consisting of a solid center, such as a piece of fruit or a nut, which is preserved by covering with layers of sugar.

COMPETITIVE INHIBITION

This refers to the inhibition of enzyme action, which causes the rate of enzyme-catalyzed reactions to decrease. Competitive inhibition occurs when a foreign molecule becomes tightly bound to the active site of an enzyme,

preventing the binding of the normal substrate (the substance acted on by the enzyme). Many of the *nerve gases* manufactured as chemical warfare agents act by inhibiting enzymes of the body in this manner.

COMPOTE

A dish of fresh, canned, or stewed fruit served in a syrupy liquid that may be flavored with grated peel, a liqueur, and/or various spices. The caloric content of compotes varies considerably since the liquid medium may be solely the liquid in which dried fruit has been stewed, or, at the other extreme, it may contain a heavy syrup or jelly. Fruit compotes are best when made from a mixture of mildly and strongly flavored fresh fruits such as sliced bananas and citrus fruits.

COMPOUND

- In chemistry, a substance formed by the intimate chemical union of two or more elements.

- In pharmacy, a preparation containing several ingredients as distinguished from one of the same name containing one or a few.

CONALBUMIN

A protein of the white of an egg which may combine with iron salts to form a red iron-protein complex. This accounts for the pinkish color resulting when eggs are stored in rusty containers.

CONGENITAL

Malformation existing at birth; acquired during development in the uterus and not through heredity. Sometimes, congenital defects in newborns are the result of (1) the administration of drugs during pregnancy, or (2) maternal deficiencies of nutrients such as folic acid.

CONJUNCTIVA

The membrane which lines the eyeball and the eyelid. Certain nutritional deficiencies cause conspicuous abnormalities of the conjunctiva.
(Also see DISEASES; and DEFICIENCY DISEASES.)

CONJUNCTIVAL HEMORRHAGES

Hemorrhages in the membranes that line the eyelids and cover the eyeball.

CONNECTIVE TISSUE

The name given to the types of tissues which hold the body together or give it structural support. Bones, muscles, tendons, ligaments, adipose tissue, and teeth are typical connective tissues.

CONSTIPATION

An excessively long retention of the stool within the lower bowel. Also, difficulty may be encountered in moving the bowel. Two major types of constipation follow:

- Atonic constipation is due to the lack of tone in the muscle around the lower bowel. This condition may occur because there is insufficient bulk or fluid in the diet. It also may be due to lack of sufficient exercise or activity.

• Spastic constipation is characterized by irregular movements (spasms) of the bowel which may be painful. It may be due to various nervous disorders, irritating foods, excessive smoking, and/or obstruction in the bowel itself. The stools are small, and very slender.

Only the doctor can safely outline the measures to be followed to rectify constipation. In the absence of any illness that might be causative, most cases of constipation can be alleviated by embarking upon a program of good eating habits combined with proper exercise and regular time for elimination. Common treatments include:

1. Exercise.
2. Foods.
3. Water.
4. Vitamins.
5. Drugs.

Constipation in infancy is not infrequent, especially in formula-fed babies. Usually, the condition may be corrected by changing the type of sugar used in the formula, or by giving prune juice or strained prunes once or twice daily.

CONSUMER ADVOCATES

This refers to those who take it upon themselves to plead the causes of consumers; presumably, they protect consumers, usually by protesting.

Today, consumer-protection laws exist at the local, state, and federal levels. Chief among the federal agencies that act to protect and serve the consumer are the Food and Drug Administration, the Federal Trade Commission, The U.S. Public Health Service, and the Consumer and Marketing Service of the U.S. Department of Agriculture.

CONVENIENCE AND FAST FOODS

These two types of products, convenience foods and fast foods, are closely related, because both were developed to save considerable time in food preparation. However, they may also differ in certain aspects. Hence, some commonly accepted definitions follow.

• **Convenience foods**—These are partially or fully prepared items that have been combined, processed, and/or cooked by the manufacturer and/or the distributor so that only minimal amounts of preparation time are required in the home. Some of the old standbys in this category are baby foods in jars, baking mixes, canned fruits and vegetables, and ready-to-eat breakfast cereals.

• **Fast foods**—This term refers to ready-to-eat items that are dispensed by commercial establishments which may or may not have accommodations for eating on the premises. The hallmark of these operations is that there is little or no waiting time between the time the food is ordered and when it is served. This speedy handling of orders may be the result of (1) using commercial types of convenience foods, and/or (2) cooking the unprocessed food item well in advance and keeping it warm (or cold, if necessary to prevent spoilage) until it is purchased.

CONVENIENCE FOODS. Among the major types of convenience foods that are replacing their homemade counterparts are the following:

1. Baby foods.
2. Bakery products (breads, cakes, cookies, and pies).
3. Beverages.
4. Cheese products.
5. Egg substitutes.
6. Entrees (canned and frozen main dishes).
7. Fish and seafood.
8. Fruits.
9. Juices.
10. Legumes.
11. Meats.
12. Milk (dried and evaporated).
13. Pizza.
14. Poultry.
15. Puddings.
16. Salads.
17. Soups.
18. Vegetables.

The modern age of food production and food processing dawned in the 18th century as a result of such developments as (1) the establishment of guilds of bakers and cooks by the king of France for the purpose of providing high quality cooked meals to those who could afford them, (2) the opening of the first "restaurant" in Paris, which was actually a small soup shop operated for the common people by a man named Boulanger, and (3) the development of a safe canning process by the French confectioner Nicholas Appert. Nevertheless, canning was not utilized widely until the latter part of the 19th century, when the explanation of food spoilage was given by the French microbiologist Louis Pasteur. The Civil War in America provided the major impetus for the utilization of canning in the United States, whereas the Franco-Prussian War did the same for France.

During the 20th century, the migration of people from the country to the cities continued at a rapid pace and created a growing need for foods in the urban areas. At first, horse-drawn trucks conveyed all foods, ice, and other commodities, but within a few years motorized vehicles appeared. The first ones were limited in size by their small engines and served mainly as transportation for street vendors and deliverymen.

A great demand was created for canned foods by World War I, which broke out shortly after the modern type of "sanitary" can had been developed. Similarly, World War II spurred the growth of the fledgling frozen foods industry which was started by the experiments of Clarence Birdseye in the 1920s. The war also fostered the use of convenience foods at home and eating out in restaurants as large numbers of homemakers went out to work in factories to help the war efforts.

The life-style of the American consumer in the 1990s is moving steadily towards the expenditure of more time at work and play, and less at home. Despite inflation, more income is being spent on leisure activities. The daily three-meal schedule has changed because population mobility has increased, eating patterns have become more individualistic, and more time is used in traveling to work and to recreation areas. Because people are eating away from home more often, the traditional family gathering at the dinner table has become less frequent. Social mobility has given rise to hamburger and fried chicken chains, the steak and seafood restaurant, and other fast-food chains.

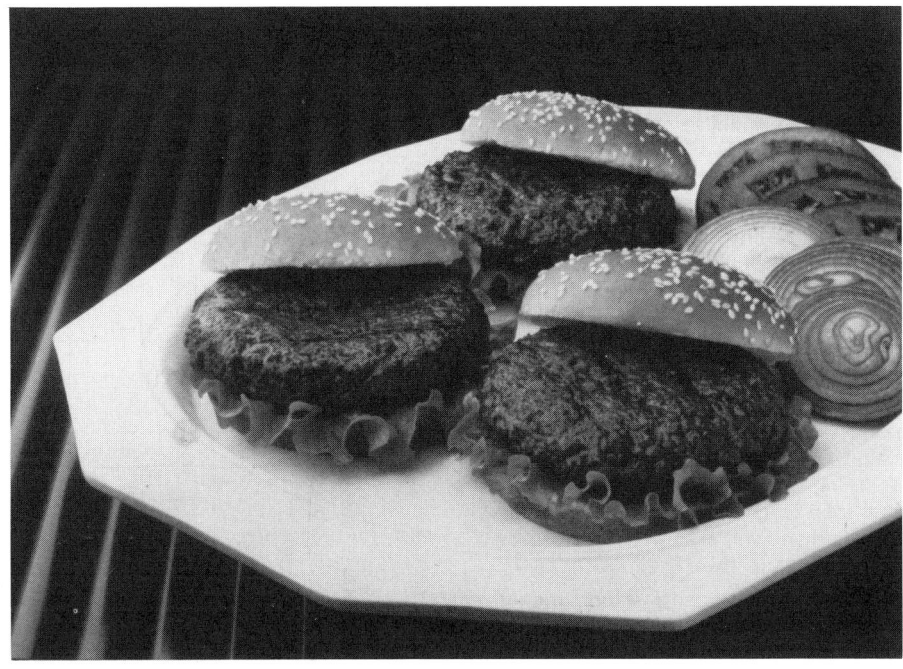

Fig. C-67. Hamburgers, the leading fast food of America. (Courtesy, National Live Stock and Meat Board, Chicago, Ill.)

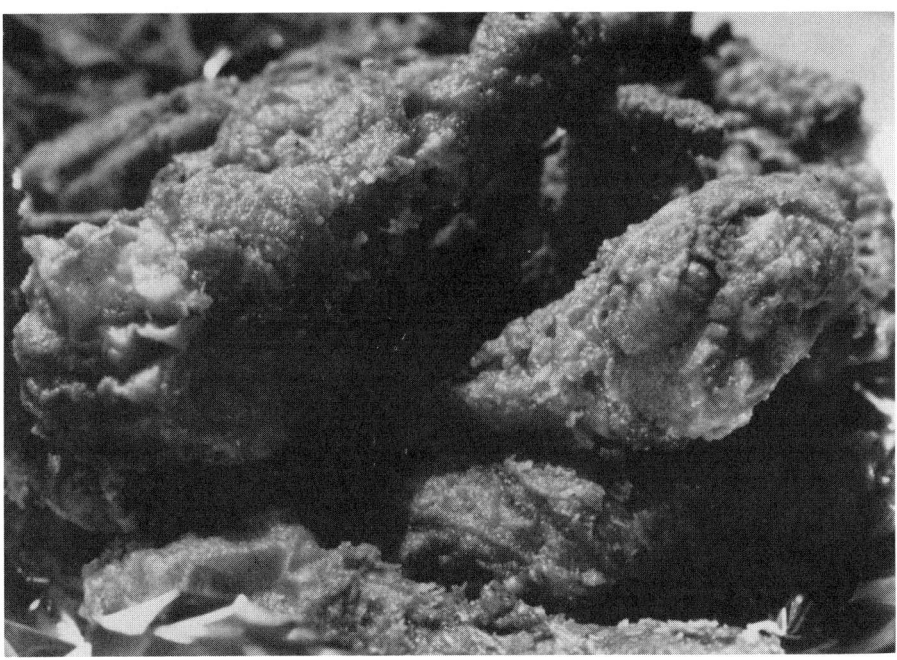

Fig. C-68. Fried chicken, the second most popular food in America. (Courtesy, USDA)

FAST FOODS. Fast-food establishments date back to 1905, when the Sears and Roebuck mail-order firm in Chicago opened a restaurant for their employees which could feed 8,400 people in 1 hour and 20 minutes. An automatic machine washed the dishes and an artificial ice maker provided 1 ton of ice per day. Franchising (the selling of individual food service units by a food service chain to investors who own and operate their units under the name of the chain) originated with the A & W Corporation which started a small root beer stand in 1919.

The fast food industry has enjoyed a phenomenal growth. In 1955, McDonald's one and only fast-food restaurant was located in Des Plaines, Illinois. In 1992, McDonald's had over 12,000 restaurants, in more than 59 countries, worldwide. The U.S. National Restaurant Association estimates that 45.8 million people eat at fast-food restaurants each day; and that the typical American eats 1 out of 12 meals at a fast-food restaurant.

As time becomes increasingly valuable, more and more Americans will rely on fast foods. So, it is important that nutrient compositions be available to enable people to make more healthful food choices. To the latter end, the nutritional analyses of items served at some of the leading fast-food chains are presented in Table C-21.

Through the years, convenience and fast-food menus have reflected current health concerns as they worked to meet the demand of consumers and public interest groups. In the 1960s, Americans were urged to eat less sugar. Sugar substitutes were soon produced and made available in the food industry. Nearly all restaurants now offer diet beverages and sugar substitutes. In the 1970s, Americans were advised to increase the amount of fiber in their diets to reduce the risk of developing certain types of cancer. Salad bars and take-out salads quickly appeared on the menus.

Today, the dietary "culprit" is fat. An estimated 35 million Americans are considered to be obese. Obesity is connected with a higher incidence of diabetes, hypertension, osteoarthritis, gallbladder disease, and some types of cancer. Additionally, high blood lipid levels are a major risk factor for heart disease. So, convenience and fast-food menus currently reflect consumer concern about the amount and type of dietary fat they are eating. For example, McDonald's "McLean Deluxe" is a low-fat ground beef patty that is 91% fat free, and contains only 310 calories and 10 grams of fat.

SUMMARY. Convenience and fast foods are now used by a substantial number of Americans. These items may make significant nutritional contributions to the diet when the purchaser knows enough about their nutrient composition to make wise selections. Furthermore, many products are economical in terms of their overall cost, which includes the purchase price, and the costs of fuel for heating (or electricity for cold storage) and labor for preparing.

Today, some convenience and fast-food chains publish pamphlets listing the nutrient content of their menu items. In the future, more and more of them will include values for saturated fat, cholesterol, and fiber.

(Also see FAST FOODS.)

TABLE C-21. NUTRITIONAL ANALYSIS OF FAST FOODS[1]

NUTRIENTS PER SERVING

ITEM	SERVING SIZE (oz)	SERVING SIZE (g)	Calories	Protein (g)	Carbohydrate (g)	Dietary Fiber (g)	Total Fat (g)	Unsaturated Fatty Acids Poly (g)	Unsaturated Fatty Acids Mono (g)	Saturated Fatty Acids (g)	Cholesterol (mg)	Sodium (mg)	Potassium (mg)	Vitamin A (IU)	Vitamin A (% US RDA)	Vitamin C (mg)	Vitamin C (% US RDA)	Iron (mg)	Iron (% US RDA)	Calcium (mg)	Calcium (% US RDA)
Restaurant: Arby's®																					
Regular Roast Beef	5	147	353	22.2	31.6	1	14.8	2.4	5.1	7.3	39	588	368	0	0	1.2	2	3.6	20	80	8
Beef 'N Cheddar	7	197	455	25.7	27.7	1	26.8	7.1	12.1	7.6	63	955	335	400	8	0.0	0	3.6	20	60	6
Chicken Breast Sandwich	7	184	493	23.0	47.9	1	25.0	10.3	9.6	5.1	91	1019	330	0	0	4.8	8	3.6	20	80	8
Roast Chicken Club	8	234	610	31.0	40.0	1	33.0	14.0	11.0	8.0	80	1500	430	0	0	0.0	0	3.6	20	150	15
Turkey Deluxe	7	197	375	23.8	32.5	2	16.6	7.8	4.7	4.1	39	1047	346	300	6	4.8	0	2.7	15	80	8
Ham 'N Cheese	6	156	292	22.9	19.2	1	13.7	2.7	6.3	4.7	45	1350	312	250	5	0.0	0	2.7	15	200	20
Super Roast Beef	8	234	501	25.1	50.4	1	22.1	5.4	8.2	8.5	40	798	503	750	15	36.0	60	4.5	25	100	10
French Fries	3	71	246	2.1	29.8	2	13.2	4.7	5.5	3.0	0	114	240	0	0	0.0	0	1.1	6	0	0
Potato Cakes	3	85	204	1.8	19.8	1	12.0	4.3	5.5	2.2	0	397	289	0	0	21.0	35	1.4	8	0	0
Jamocha Shake	12	326	368	9.3	59.1	2	10.5	1.6	6.4	2.5	35	262	525	300	6	2.4	4	2.7	15	250	25
Restaurant: Arthur Treacher's Fish & Chips'																					
Chicken Sandwich	6	156	413	16.2	44.0	1	19.2	6.7	7.7	2.8	32	708	173	117	2	19.0	32	1.7	9	59	6
Fish Sandwich	6	170	440	16.4	39.4	1	24.0	6.9	8.1	4.2	42	836	223	117	0	2.0	3	1.5	8	89	8
Chicken	5	147	369	27.1	16.5	1	21.6	5.6	9.1	3.5	65	495	221	102	2	2.0	3	0.8	4	11	0
Coleslaw	4	107	123	1.0	11.1	3	8.2	4.4	1.9	1.1	7	266	346	170	5	59.0	99	0.2	0	24	2
Lemon Luvs™	3	83	276	2.6	35.1	2	13.9	1.9	5.9	2.2	0	314	68	64	0	0.9	0	0.9	5	10	0
Krunch Pups™	3	74	203	5.4	12.0	1	14.8	2.2	6.2	3.7	25	446	101	43	0	4.0	6	0.6	3	8	0
Chips	4	113	276	4.0	34.9	3	13.2	2.7	5.9	2.3	1	39	597	85	0	6.0	10	0.5	3	12	0
Shrimp	4	106	381	13.1	27.2	1	24.4	6.2	11.0	3.3	93	538	128	86	0	1.0	2	0.6	4	57	6
Fish	5	153	355	19.2	25.4	1	20.1	5.6	9.0	2.8	56	450	255	111	0	2.0	3	0.6	4	15	0

Restaurant: Burger King*

Item																					
Whopper®/Everything	10	270	628	27.0	46.0	2	36.0	13.0	11.0	12.0	90	545	880	678	14	12.0	19	5.0	28	84	8
Whopper/Cheese	10	294	706	32.0	47.0	2	43.0	13.0	15.0	17.0	113	568	1164	1061	21	12.0	19	5.0	28	215	21
Hamburger	4	108	272	15.0	29.0	1	12.0	5.0	5.0	4.0	37	235	509	150	3	3.0	5	3.0	16	37	4
Cheeseburger	4	121	318	17.0	30.0	1	15.0	1.0	6.0	7.0	48	247	651	341	7	3.0	5	3.0	16	102	10
Bacon Double Cheeseburger	6	160	515	33.0	27.0	1	31.0	2.0	.13.0	15.0	104	363	728	384	8	0.0	0	4.0	21	168	17
Hamburger Deluxe	5	138	344	15.0	30.0	1	17.0	7.0	6.0	6.0	41	275	486	296	6	6.0	10	3.0	16	40	4
Cheeseburger Deluxe	5	151	390	17.0	31.0	2	20.0	7.0	7.0	8.0	52	287	628	488	10	6.0	10	3.0	16	105	11
Ocean Catch Filet	7	194	488	19.0	45.0	2	25.0	13.0	6.0	4.0	77	369	592	36	1	0.0	0	2.0	9	46	5
Chicken Specialty Sandwich	8	229	685	26.0	56.0	2	40.0	20.0	11.0	8.0	82	685	1423	126	3	0.0	0	3.0	16	79	8
Chicken Tenders™	3	90	236	20.0	10.0	1	10.0	3.0	5.0	2.0	47	200	636	375	2	0.0	0	1.0	7	18	2
French Fries	4	111	341	3.0	24.0	3	13.0	0.0	9.0	7.0	14	360	160	95	0	0.0	0	1.0	7	0	0
Onion Rings	3	86	302	4.0	28.0	2	16.0	4.0	8.0	3.0	0	173	665	0	0	0.0	0	1.0	7	124	12
Breakfast Croissan'wich™/Bacon	4	118	355	14.0	20.0	1	24.0		8.0	8.0	249	182	762	426	9	0.0	0	2.0	9	136	14
Breakfast Croissan'wich/Sausage	6	159	538	20.0	20.0	1	40.0	5.0	20.0	13.0	293	285	1042	426	9	0.0	0	3.0	16	145	15
Breakfast Croissan'wich/Ham/Egg/Cheese	5	144	346	19.0	19.0	1	21.0	2.0	11.0	7.0	241	256	962	426	10	0.0	0	2.0	11	136	15
Breakfast Bagel Sandwich/Bacon	6	169	438	20.0	46.0	2	20.0	4.0	7.0	7.0	274	202	905	426	9	0.0	0	3.0	16	124	12
Breakfast Bagel Sandwich/Sausage/Egg/Cheese	7	210	626	27.0	49.0	2	36.0	6.0	15.0	12.0	318	305	1137	426	10	0.0	0	4.0	21	135	14
Breakfast Bagel Sandwich/Ham/Egg/Cheese	7	196	418	23.0	46.0	2	15.0	4.0	6.0	6.0	287	276	1130	426	9	3.0	5	3.0	16	125	12
Scrambled Egg Platter	7	211	549	17.0	44.0	3	30.0	6.0	18.0	9.0	370	487	808	375	7	3.0	5	3.0	16	101	12
Scrambled Egg Platter/Sausage	9	260	768	26.0	47.0	3	53.0	8.0	30.0	15.0	412	623	1271	375	7	5.0	9	4.0	21	120	12
Scrambled Egg Platter/Bacon	8	221	610	21.0	44.0	3	39.0	7.0	20.0	11.0	373	532	1043	375	22	5.0	9	3.0	16	110	11
French Toast Sticks	5	141	538	10.0	53.0	2	32.0	11.0	15.0	5.0	80	126	537	0	0	0.0	0	3.0	16	77	8
Great Danish	3	71	500	5.0	40.0	3	36.0	11.0	15.0	23.0	6	116	288	94	2	2.0	0	2.0	9	91	9
Vanilla Shake	10	284	334	9.0	51.0	0	10.0	0.0	3.0	6.0	39	505	205	157	64	0.0	0	0.0	9	295	29
Chocolate Shake	10	284	326	9.0	49.0	1	10.0	0.0	4.0	6.0	33	567	202	108	2	2.0	0	2.0	9	262	26
Apple Pie	4	125	311	3.0	44.0	2	14.0	1.0	8.0	4.0	4	122	412	0	0	5.0	8	1.0	7	0	0
Chicken Salad	9	258	142	20.0	8.0	2	4.0	1.0	1.0	1.0	50	630	440	4742	90	20.0	35	1.0	7	44	4
Chef Salad	10	273	178	17.0	7.0	2	9.0	3.0	3.0	4.0	120	550	570	4889	100	14.0	23	2.0	9	158	16
Garden Salad	8	223	95	6.0	8.0	2	5.0	1.0	1.0	3.0	15	440	125	5143	100	34.0	60	1.0	7	147	15
Side Salad	5	135	25	1.0	5.0	0	0.0	0.0	0.0	0.0	0	230	20	2495	50	11.0	17	1.0	7	21	2
Thousand Island Dressing	2	63	290	5.0	15.0	3	26.0	14.0	5.0	23.0	36	470	600	157	64	2.0	17	1.0	7	11	0
Bleu Cheese Dressing	2	59	300	3.0	2.0	0	32.0	16.0	10.0	6.0	40	600	108	23	2	0.0	0	0.0	0	58	6
Reduced Calorie Italian	2	59	170	0.0	3.0	0	18.0	10.0	5.0	3.0	3	762	6	0	0	0.0	0	0.0	0	0	0
French Dressing	2	64	290	0.0	23.0	1	22.0	8.0	10.0	3.0	2	400	70	237	31	0.0	0	0.0	0	0	0
Bacon Bits	0.1	3	16	1.0	0.0	0	1.0	0.0	0.0	0.0	5	1	30	0	0	0.0	0	0.0	0	0	0
Croutons	0.3	7	31	1.0	5.0	0	1.0	0.0	0.0	0.0	0	90	10	0	1	1.0	0	0.0	0	0	0

Restaurant: Dairy Queen*

Item																					
Cone, Small	3	85	140	3.0	22.0	0	4.0	0.1	0.9	1.7	10	146	45	100	2	0.0	0	0.4	2	100	10
Cone, Regular	5	142	240	6.0	38.0	0	7.0	0.2	1.5	3.1	15	252	80	200	4	0.0	0	0.7	4	150	15
Cone, Large	8	213	340	9.0	57.0	0	10.0	0.3	2.6	5.2	25	417	115	400	8	0.0	0	1.4	8	250	25
Cone, Small, Chocolate-Dipped	3	92	190	3.0	25.0	2	9.0	0.3	2.3	4.2	10	179	55	100	2	0.0	0	0.4	2	100	10
Cone, Regular, Chocolate-Dipped	6	156	340	6.0	42.0	3	16.0	0.5	4.1	7.8	20	312	100	200	4	0.0	0	0.7	4	150	15
Cone, Large, Chocolate-Dipped	8	234	510	9.0	64.0	4	24.0	0.7	6.2	11.8	30	473	145	400	8	0.0	0	1.4	8	250	25
Chocolate Sundae, Small	4	106	190	3.0	33.0	1	4.0	0.1	1.0	2.2	10	215	75	100	2	0.0	0	0.4	2	100	10
Chocolate Sundae, Regular	6	177	310	5.0	56.0	1	8.0	0.2	1.8	3.8	20	370	120	200	4	0.0	0	0.7	6	200	20
Chocolate Sundae, Large	9	248	440	8.0	78.0	2	10.0	0.3	2.6	5.6	30	530	165	400	8	0.0	0	1.4	8	250	25
Chocolate Shake, Small	9	241	409	8.0	69.0	1	11.0	0.5	3.8	7.8	30	530	150	500	10	0.0	0	1.8	10	300	30
Chocolate Shake, Regular	15	418	710	14.0	120.0	2	19.0	0.7	6.0	12.4	50	708	260	750	15	0.0	0	2.7	15	450	45
Chocolate Shake, Large	17	489	831	16.0	140.0	2	22.0	0.8	6.9	14.2	60	809	304	1000	20	0.0	0	3.6	20	550	55
Chocolate Malt, Small	9	241	438	9.0	77.0	2	10.0	0.5	3.1	6.5	30	416	150	500	10	0.0	0	2.7	15	300	30
Chocolate Malt, Regular	15	418	760	14.0	134.0	3	18.0	0.8	5.4	11.2	50	711	260	750	15	0.0	0	4.5	25	450	45
Chocolate Malt, Large	17	489	889	16.0	157.0	3	21.0	0.9	6.4	13.1	60	828	304	1000	20	0.0	0	5.4	30	550	55
Float	14	397	410	5.0	82.0	0	7.0	0.2	1.6	3.5	20	270	85	200	4	0.0	0	1.1	6	200	20
Peanut Buster Parfait*	11	305	740	16.0	94.0	6	34.0	4.0	11.6	14.1	30	759	250	300	6	0.0	0	1.8	10	250	25
Parfait	10	283	430	8.0	76.0	1	8.0	0.3	2.2	5.8	30	379	140	400	8	0.0	0	1.4	8	250	25
Freeze	14	397	500	9.0	89.0	2	12.0	0.4	3.3	7.0	30	532	180	400	8	0.0	0	1.8	10	300	30
Mr Misty*, Small	9	248	190	0.0	48.0	0	0.0	0.0	0.0	0.0	0	4	10	0	0	0.0	0	0.0	0	0	0
Mr Misty, Regular	12	330	250	0.0	63.0	0	0.0	0.0	0.0	0.0	0	6	10	0	0	0.0	0	0.0	0	0	0
Mr Misty, Large	16	439	340	0.0	84.0	0	0.0	0.0	0.0	0.0	0	8	10	0	0	0.0	0	0.0	0	0	0
Mr Misty Kiss	3	89	70	0.0	17.0	0	0.0	0.0	0.0	0.0	0	2	10	0	0	0.0	0	0.0	0	60	6
Mr Misty Freeze	15	411	500	9.0	91.0	2	12.0	0.4	3.3	7.0	30	532	140	400	8	0.0	0	1.4	8	300	30
Mr Misty Float	15	411	390	5.0	74.0	0	7.0	0.2	1.6	3.5	20	269	95	200	4	0.0	0	0.7	4	200	20
Buster Bar	5	149	448	10.0	41.0	6	29.0	5.9	12.0	8.9	10	485	175	300	6	0.0	0	1.8	10	100	10
Fudge Nut Bar	5	142	406	8.0	40.0	2	25.0	3.2	6.3	11.3	10	226	167	100	2	0.0	0	1.1	6	100	10
Dilly Bar	3	85	210	3.0	21.0	0	13.0	0.3	1.1	11.1	10	179	50	100	2	0.0	0	0.4	2	100	10
DQ Sandwich	2	60	140	3.0	24.0	0	4.0	0.3	1.5	2.0	5	105	40	0	0	0.0	0	0.0	0	60	6
Chipper Sandwich	4	113	318	5.0	56.0	0	7.0	0.5	3.0	5.7	13	368	170	100	2	1.0	2	2.7	15	100	10
Heath* Blizzard, Regular	14	404	800	15.0	125.0	3	24.0	0.8	6.8	13.8	65	1009	325	300	6	5.0	8	2.7	15	500	50

(Continued)

TABLE C-21 (Continued)

NUTRIENTS PER SERVING

ITEM	Serving Size (oz)	(g)	Calories	Protein (g)	Carbohydrate (g)	Dietary Fiber (g)	Total Fat (g)	Unsaturated Fatty Acids — Poly (g)	Mono (g)	Saturated Fatty Acids (g)	Cholesterol (mg)	Sodium (mg)	Potassium (mg)	Vitamin A (IU)	Vitamin A (% US RDA)	Vitamin C (mg)	Vitamin C (% US RDA)	Iron (mg)	Iron (% US RDA)	Calcium (mg)	Calcium (% US RDA)
Dairy Queen (cont'd)																					
Single Hamburger	5	148	360	21.0	33.0	1	16.0	1.4	6.2	5.7	45	630	328	100	2	0.0	0	3.6	20	100	10
Double Hamburger	7	210	530	36.0	33.0	1	28.0	1.9	11.4	10.6	85	660	546	100	2	0.0	0	6.3	35	100	10
Triple Hamburger	10	272	710	51.0	33.0	1	45.0	2.3	16.5	15.4	135	690	763	200	4	0.0	0	9.0	50	100	10
Single Hamburger/Cheese	6	162	410	24.0	33.0	1	20.0	1.6	7.5	8.5	50	790	351	200	4	0.0	0	3.6	20	200	20
Double Hamburger/Cheese	8	239	650	43.0	34.0	1	37.0	2.2	14.0	16.1	95	980	592	400	8	0.0	0	6.3	35	350	35
Triple Hamburger/Cheese	11	301	820	58.0	34.0	1	50.0	2.6	19.1	21.0	145	1010	809	400	8	0.0	0	9.0	50	350	35
Hot Dog	4	100	280	11.0	21.0	1	16.0	2.2	8.5	6.7	45	830	133	0	0	0.0	0	1.4	8	80	8
Hot Dog/Chili	5	128	320	13.0	23.0	1	20.0	2.2	9.2	7.4	55	985	215	0	0	0.0	0	1.4	8	80	8
Hot Dog/Cheese	5	114	330	15.0	21.0	1	21.0	2.3	9.7	9.4	55	990	156	100	2	0.0	0	1.4	8	150	15
DQ Hounder	5	151	480	16.0	21.0	1	36.0	3.7	16.2	12.8	80	1800	227	0	0	0.0	0	4.5	25	150	15
DQ Hounder/Chili	7	208	575	22.0	25.0	1	41.0	4.0	18.6	14.9	89	1900	489	0	0	0.0	0	4.5	25	200	20
DQ Hounder/Cheese	6	165	533	19.0	22.0	1	40.0	3.8	17.4	15.5	89	1995	250	0	0	0.0	0	4.5	25	250	25
Super Hot Dog	6	175	520	17.0	44.0	1	27.0	3.5	13.0	10.2	80	1365	218	0	0	0.0	0	2.7	15	150	15
Super Hot Dog/Chili	8	218	570	21.0	47.0	2	32.0	3.7	14.7	11.8	100	1595	405	100	2	0.0	0	2.7	15	150	15
Super Hot Dog/Cheese	7	196	580	22.0	45.0	1	34.0	3.7	14.9	14.4	100	1605	253	100	2	0.0	0	1.4	8	250	25
Fish Filet	6	177	430	20.0	45.0	1	18.0	4.9	6.4	5.4	40	674	259	0	0	0.0	0	3.6	20	150	15
Fish Filet/Cheese	7	191	483	23.0	46.0	1	22.0	4.4	7.9	9.4	49	870	291	500	10	0.0	0	3.6	20	250	25
Chicken Breast Filet	7	202	608	27.0	46.0	2	34.0	12.6	9.7	8.4	78	725	284	100	2	2.4	4	5.4	30	150	15
Chicken Breast Filet/Cheese	8	216	661	30.0	47.0	2	38.0	11.6	11.2	12.2	87	921	318	750	15	2.4	4	5.4	30	250	25
All White Chicken Nuggets	4	99	276	16.0	13.0	1	18.0	2.4	6.6	6.1	39	505	166	750	15	0.0	0	1.1	6	0	0
BBQ Nugget Sauce	1	28	41	0.0	9.0	0	0.7	0.1	0.3	0.3	0	130	72	750	15	9.0	15	0.4	2	20	2
French Fries, Small	3	71	200	2.0	25.0	2	10.0	0.2	4.4	4.4	10	115	416	0	0	9.0	15	0.4	2	0	0
French Fries, Large	4	113	320	3.0	40.0	3	16.0	1.3	7.0	7.1	15	185	675	0	0	15.0	25	1.1	6	0	0
Onion Rings	3	85	280	4.0	31.0	3	16.0	1.3	6.7	6.7	15	140	336	0	0	2.4	4	0.7	4	0	0
Restaurant: Domino's Pizza® (2 slices of each pizza)																					
Cheese Pizza	6	168	376	21.6	56.3	6	10.0	1.2	3.3	5.5	19	483	364	374	7	0.5	0	2.8	13	221	17
Pepperoni Pizza	7	187	460	24.1	55.6	5	17.5	1.9	7.3	8.4	28	825	423	482	7	0.6	0	3.1	17	239	19
Sausage/Mushroom Pizza	7	200	430	24.2	55.3	8	15.8	1.8	6.3	7.7	28	552	418	488	8	0.5	0	3.0	17	227	20
Veggie Pizza	9	261	498	31.0	60.0	8	18.5	1.7	6.6	10.2	36	1035	537	529	10	0.3	0	4.7	26	435	39
Deluxe Pizza	8	234	498	26.7	59.2	7	20.4	2.2	8.9	9.3	40	954	616	468	9	0.8	0	4.7	26	233	23
Double Cheese/Pepperoni Pizza	8	227	545	32.1	55.2	8	25.3	2.2	9.9	13.3	48	1042	529	472	9	1.0	2	4.0	22	459	45
Ham Pizza	7	186	417	23.2	58.0	2	11.0	1.3	3.8	5.9	26	805	485	242	0	0.6	2	4.6	19	226	19
Restaurant: Kentucky Fried Chicken®																					
Nuggets	1	16	46	2.8	2.2	0	2.9	0.3	1.3	0.7	12	140	23	100	2	1.0	0	0.1	0	2	0
Barbeque Sauce	1	28	35	0.3	7.1	0	0.6	0.3	0.4	0.1	0	450	98	370	7	0.0	0	0.2	0	6	0
Sweet & Sour Sauce	1	28	58	0.1	13.0	0	0.6	0.3	0.0	0.1	0	148	12	100	2	0.0	0	0.2	0	5	0
Honey	1	14	49	0.0	12.1	0	0.0	0.0	0.0	0.0	0	15	9	0	0	0.0	0	0.1	0	1	0
Mustard	1	28	36	0.9	6.0	0	0.9	1.1	0.2	0.1	0	346	37	100	0	0.0	0	0.3	0	10	0
Chicken Littles™ Sandwich	2	47	169	5.7	13.8	0	10.1	3.4	3.2	2.0	18	331	61	100	0	0.0	0	1.7	9	23	2
Buttermilk Biscuit	2	65	235	4.5	28.0	1	11.9	2.2	6.0	3.2	1	655	78	100	0	0.0	0	1.6	9	95	10
Mashed Potatoes/Gravy	4	98	71	2.4	11.9	1	1.6	0.2	0.5	1.6	0	339	217	100	2	0.0	0	0.4	2	22	2
French Fries, Regular	3	77	244	3.2	31.1	2	11.9	0.7	6.1	2.6	2	139	519	100	0	16.0	26	0.6	3	13	0
Corn-on-the-cob	5	143	176	5.1	31.9	7	3.1	1.5	1.3	0.5	0	21	307	272	5	2.0	3	0.8	4	7	0
Coleslaw	3	91	119	1.5	13.3	1	6.6	3.4	1.5	1.0	5	197	161	310	6	22.0	36	0.2	0	33	3
Original Recipe Chicken																					
Wing	2	55	178	12.2	6.0	0	11.7	1.8	4.5	3.0	64	372	9	100	0	1.0	0	1.2	6	48	4
Breast	4	115	283	27.5	8.8	0	15.3	2.0	6.8	3.8	93	672	242	100	0	1.0	0	1.0	5	36	3
Drumstick	2	57	146	13.1	4.2	0	8.5	1.3	3.4	2.2	67	275	122	100	0	1.0	0	1.1	5	21	2
Thigh	4	104	294	17.9	11.1	1	19.7	3.1	9.3	5.3	123	619	164	104	2	1.0	0	1.3	7	65	6
Extra Crispy Chicken																					
Wing	2	65	254	12.4	9.3	0	18.6	2.5	9.8	4.0	67	422	116	100	2	0.0	0	0.5	2	21	2
Breast	5	135	342	33.0	11.7	1	19.7	2.0	8.9	4.8	114	790	298	100	0	0.0	0	0.8	4	33	3
Drumstick	2	69	204	13.6	6.1	0	13.9	1.7	6.3	3.4	71	324	127	100	0	0.0	0	0.6	4	13	1
Thigh	4	119	406	20.0	14.4	1	29.8	4.2	14.6	7.7	129	688	193	100	3	0.0	0	1.2	6	46	4

Restaurant: Long John Silver's® Seafood Shoppe

Food																				
Three-piece Fish Light/Paprika (Baked)	5	134	120	28.0	1.0	0	1.0	0.4	0.4	110	120	395	44	43	0.0	0	0.4	2	21	2
Three-piece Fish Light/Lemon Crumb (Baked)	5	141	150	29.0	4.0	0	1.0	0.7	0.4	110	370	409	45	44	0.0	0	0.6	3	24	2
Three-piece Fish/Lemon Crumb (Baked)	5	148	170	28.0	2.0	0	5.0	0.9	2.9	110	270	396	195	19	0.0	0	0.4	2	22	2
Three-piece Fish/Scampi Sauce (Baked)	5	148	120	15.0	2.0	0	5.0	0.5	2.9	110	610	143	351	35	1.7	3	2.4	13	32	3
Shrimp/Scampi Sauce (Baked)	4	117	140	25.0	1.0	0	4.0	1.2	3.2	205	670	234	12	5	0.0	1	1.0	5	15	1
Chicken Light/Herbs (Baked)	5	142	210	5.0	43.0	1	2.0	0.6	0.3	70	570	113	5	0	0.5	1	1.9	10	33	3
Rice Pilaf	4	113	30	1.0	6.0	3	6.0	0.1	1.2	5	30	534	6148	53	8.3	14	0.8	4	46	4
Green Beans	4	113	120	4.0	16.0	5	6.0	2.0	1.2	5	95	233	91	100	4.4	7	1.1	6	36	3
Garden Vegetables	3	98	140	1.0	20.0	1	6.0	3.8	1.0	15	260	152	155	9	28.2	47	0.4	2	7	1
Coleslaw	1	34	110	3.0	18.0	1	3.0	1.0	0.6	0	120	27	1056	15	5.3	9	0.2	1	7	0
Breadstick	2	54	8	1.0	2.0	1	0.0	0.1	0.0	0	0	109	100	0	0.0	9	0.3	1	8	0

Restaurant: McDonald's®

Food																				
Egg McMuffin®	5	138	290	18.2	28.1	1	11.2	1.3	3.8	226	740	469	499	10	0.0	0	2.8	15	256	25
Hotcakes/Butter/Syrup	6	176	410	8.2	74.4	2	9.2	2.5	3.7	21	640	168	173	4	0.0	0	2.1	10	114	10
Scrambled Eggs	4	100	140	12.4	1.2	0	9.8	1.4	3.3	399	290	121	518	10	0.0	0	2.1	10	57	6
Pork Sausage	2	48	180	8.4	0.0	0	16.3	1.9	5.9	48	350	175	0	0	0.0	0	0.7	4	8	0
English Muffin/Butter	2	59	170	5.4	26.7	1	4.6	0.5	2.4	9	270	319	122	2	1.6	2	1.1	8	151	15
Hashbrown Potatoes	2	53	130	1.4	14.9	2	7.3	0.4	3.2	9	330	328	0	0	0.0	0	0.3	8	6	0
Biscuit/Biscuit Spread	3	75	260	4.6	31.9	1	12.7	0.6	3.4	1	730	82	0	0	0.0	0	1.3	8	75	8
Biscuit/Sausage	4	123	440	13.0	31.9	1	29.0	2.5	9.3	49	1080	323	0	0	0.0	0	2.0	10	83	8
Biscuit/Sausage/Egg	6	180	520	19.9	32.6	1	34.5	3.4	11.2	275	1250	293	294	6	0.0	0	3.2	20	116	10
Biscuit/Bacon/Egg/Cheese	6	156	440	17.5	33.3	1	26.4	2.0	8.2	253	1230	215	534	10	0.0	0	2.6	15	185	20
Sausage McMuffin®	4	117	370	16.5	27.3	1	21.9	2.4	7.8	64	830	487	240	4	0.0	0	2.3	15	235	25
Sausage McMuffin/Cheese	6	167	440	22.6	27.9	1	26.8	3.2	9.5	263	980	548	499	10	0.0	0	3.3	20	263	25
Apple Danish	4	115	390	5.8	51.2	2	17.9	2.0	3.5	25	370	76	115	0	16.1	25	1.4	8	14	0
Iced Cheese Danish	4	110	390	7.4	42.3	1	21.8	1.8	6.0	47	420	83	188	4	1.1	2	1.4	8	33	4
Cinnamon Raisin Danish	4	110	440	6.4	57.5	1	21.0	1.6	4.2	34	430	130	110	0	3.2	6	1.8	10	35	4
Raspberry Danish	4	117	410	6.1	61.5	1	15.9	1.1	3.1	26	310	84	117	0	3.2	6	1.5	8	14	0
Apple Bran Muffin	3	85	190	5.0	46.0	1	0.0	0.0	0.0	0	230	251	7	0	0.7	2	0.6	3	31	3
Blueberry Muffin	3	85	170	3.0	40.0	1	0.0	0.0	0.0	65	220	180	136	15	1.2	2	1.0	6	13	0
Chicken McNuggets®	4	113	290	19.0	16.5	1	16.3	1.8	4.1	65	520	136	157	15	1.2	2	0.6	3	81	8
Hot Mustard Sauce	1	30	70	0.5	8.2	0	3.6	1.9	0.5	5	250	7	16	0	0.5	4	0.2	2	15	2
Barbeque Sauce	1	32	50	0.3	12.1	0	0.5	0.2	0.1	0	340	126	153	4	2.3	4	0.3	0	13	0
Sweet & Sour Sauce	1	32	60	0.2	13.8	0	0.2	0.1	0.0	0	190	13	324	6	0.6	0	0.2	0	11	0
Honey	1	14	45	0.0	11.5	0	0.0	0.0	0.0	0	0	7	0	0	0.1	0	0.1	0	1	0
Hamburger	4	102	260	12.3	30.6	1	9.5	0.8	3.6	37	500	221	152	4	2.2	4	2.3	15	122	10
Cheeseburger	4	116	310	15.0	31.2	1	13.8	0.9	5.2	53	750	244	392	8	2.2	4	2.3	15	199	20
McLean Deluxe™	7	203	310	20.0	34.0	2	10.0	1.2	4.6	49	650	404	493	49	7.2	12	3.8	21	145	14
Quarter Pounder®	6	166	410	23.1	34.0	1	20.7	1.2	8.1	86	660	392	223	4	3.2	4	3.7	20	142	15
Quarter Pounder®/Cheese	7	194	520	28.5	35.1	1	29.2	1.5	16.5	118	1150	438	703	15	3.2	6	4.0	20	296	30
Big Mac®	8	215	560	25.2	42.5	2	32.4	1.8	20.9	103	950	361	352	8	1.7	2	4.0	25	256	25
Filet-O-Fish®	5	142	440	13.8	37.9	1	26.1	10.8	5.2	50	1030	217	146	2	0.1	0	1.8	10	165	15
McD.L.T.®	8	234	580	26.3	36.0	1	36.8	8.5	11.5	109	990	480	754	15	7.4	10	3.9	20	225	25
McChicken®	7	190	490	19.2	39.8	1	28.6	11.6	5.4	43	780	245	104	2	2.4	4	2.6	15	143	15
Chef Salad	10	283	230	20.5	7.5	2	13.3	0.9	5.9	128	490	572	4114	80	13.6	20	2.6	8	256	25
Chicken Salad Oriental	9	244	140	23.1	5.0	2	3.4	0.5	0.9	78	230	492	3625	70	11.0	20	1.3	6	149	15
Side Salad	4	115	60	3.7	3.3	1	3.3	0.3	1.5	41	85	194	2173	45	7.4	10	0.7	4	76	8
Bleu Cheese Dressing	1	14	70	0.5	1.2	0	6.9	3.8	1.3	6	150	6	18	0	0.0	0	0.0	0	15	0
French Dressing	1	14	58	0.1	2.7	0	5.2	3.1	0.8	0	180	12	15	0	0.0	0	0.0	0	2	0
Ranch Dressing	1	14	83	0.2	1.3	0	8.6	5.1	1.4	5	130	35	11	0	0.5	0	0.0	0	7	0
1000 Island Dressing	1	14	78	0.2	2.4	0	7.5	4.4	1.2	8	100	22	49	0	0.4	0	0.1	0	3	0
Lite Vinaigrette Dressing	1	14	15	0.2	2.0	0	0.5	0.3	0.1	0	75	2	92	2	0.4	0	0.2	0	3	0
Oriental Dressing	1	14	24	0.2	5.8	0	0.1	0.0	0.0	0	180	10	28	0	0.6	0	0.2	0	6	0
Red French Reduced Calorie Dressing	1	14	40	0.1	5.2	0	1.9	1.1	0.3	0	110	74	13	10	0.6	0	0.2	0	3	0
Caesar Dressing	1	14	60	0.4	0.6	0	6.1	3.5	1.1	7	170	5	9	0	2.4	4	0.6	0	13	0
Peppercorn Dressing	1	14	80	0.2	0.5	0	8.7	5.2	1.4	7	85	5	0	0	7.4	10	0.7	4	3	0
French Fries, Small	2	68	220	3.1	25.6	2	12.0	0.5	6.5	9	110	390	306	6	8.2	15	0.5	2	10	2
French Fries, Medium	3	97	320	4.4	36.3	3	17.1	0.7	9.2	12	150	571	306	6	11.6	20	0.7	4	14	4
French Fries, Large	4	122	400	5.6	45.9	3	21.6	0.9	11.6	16	200	701	306	6	14.6	25	0.9	6	18	4
Apple Pie	3	83	260	2.2	30.0	2	14.8	0.9	4.8	6	240	72	0	0	11.4	20	0.7	4	110	4
Vanilla Lowfat Milk Shake	11	293	290	10.8	60.0	0	1.3	0.1	0.6	10	170	510	306	6	0.0	0	0.1	0	327	35
Chocolate Lowfat Milk Shake	11	293	320	11.0	66.0	1	1.7	0.1	0.9	10	240	552	306	6	0.0	0	0.9	0	332	35
Strawberry Lowfat Milk Shake	11	293	320	10.7	67.0	0	1.3	0.1	0.6	10	170	635	306	25	0.0	0	0.1	0	327	35
Soft Serve Cone	3	86	140	3.9	21.9	0	4.5	0.2	2.1	16	70	152	128	2	1.3	2	0.2	0	11	10
Strawberry Sundae	6	171	210	5.7	49.2	1	1.1	0.0	0.6	5	95	298	214	4	1.3	2	0.2	0	191	20

(Continued)

TABLE C-21 (Continued)

NUTRIENTS PER SERVING

ITEM	Serving Size (oz)	Serving Size (g)	Calories	Protein (g)	Carbohydrate (g)	Dietary Fiber (g)	Total Fat (g)	Unsat. Poly (g)	Unsat. Mono (g)	Saturated Fatty Acids (g)	Cholesterol (mg)	Sodium (mg)	Potassium (mg)	Vitamin A (IU)	Vitamin A (% US RDA)	Vitamin C (mg)	Vitamin C (% US RDA)	Iron (mg)	Iron (% US RDA)	Calcium (mg)	Calcium (% US RDA)
McDonald's (cont'd)																					
Hot Fudge Sundae	6	169	240	7.3	50.5	1	3.2	0.1	0.8	2.4	6	170	323	214	4	0.0	0	0.5	2	235	25
Hot Caramel Sundae	6	174	270	6.6	59.3	0	2.8	0.1	1.2	1.5	13	180	297	291	6	0.0	0	0.1	0	222	20
McDonaldland Cookies	2	56	290	4.2	47.1	1	9.2	0.5	6.8	1.8	0	300	181	0	0	0.0	0	2.1	10	9	0
Chocolaty Chip Cookies	2	56	330	4.2	41.9	0	15.6	0.4	10.2	5.0	4	280	43	0	0	0.0	0	2.2	10	24	2
Restaurant: Pizza Hut																					
Pan Pizza, 2 slices																					
Cheese	7	205	492	30.0	57.0	5	18.0	0.7	4.2	9.3	34	940	320	450	9	7.2	12	5.4	30	630	63
Pepperoni	8	211	540	29.0	62.0	5	22.0	1.5	6.8	10.9	42	1127	405	500	10	8.4	14	6.3	35	520	52
Supreme	9	255	589	32.0	53.0	7	30.0	1.6	7.3	11.6	48	1363	580	600	12	9.6	16	5.0	28	500	50
Super Supreme	9	257	563	33.0	53.0	6	26.0	1.5	7.0	11.1	55	1447	532	600	12	10.8	18	6.7	37	540	54
Thin 'n Crispy Pizza, 2 slices																					
Cheese	5	148	398	28.0	37.0	4	17.0	0.7	4.6	10.2	33	867	261	350	7	4.8	8	3.2	18	660	66
Pepperoni	5	146	413	26.0	20.0	4	20.0	1.5	7.3	8.9	46	986	287	350	7	6.0	10	3.2	18	450	45
Supreme	7	200	459	28.0	41.0	5	22.0	1.2	5.7	9.0	42	1328	544	500	10	9.6	16	5.9	33	430	43
Super Supreme	7	203	463	29.0	44.0	5	21.0	1.2	5.8	9.3	56	1336	463	500	10	8.4	14	4.9	27	460	46
Hand-Tossed Pizza, 2 slices																					
Cheese	8	220	518	34.0	55.0	7	20.0	0.8	4.5	9.9	55	1276	396	500	10	9.6	16	5.4	30	750	75
Pepperoni	7	197	500	28.0	50.0	6	23.0	1.4	6.4	10.2	50	1267	415	500	10	7.2	12	5.0	28	440	44
Supreme	8	239	540	32.0	50.0	7	26.0	1.5	7.0	11.1	55	1470	578	550	11	12.0	20	8.0	45	480	48
Super Supreme	9	243	556	33.0	54.0	7	25.0	1.5	7.1	11.4	54	1648	516	550	11	12.0	20	6.8	38	440	44
Personal Pan Pizza, 1 pizza																					
Pepperoni	9	256	675	37.0	76.0	8	29.0	1.8	8.6	13.7	53	1335	408	600	12	10.2	17	5.8	32	730	73
Supreme	9	264	647	33.0	76.0	9	28.0	1.8	8.3	13.2	49	1313	487	600	12	10.8	18	6.7	37	520	52
Restaurant: Taco Bell																					
Bean Burrito/Red Sauce	7	191	356	13.1	54.4	5	10.2	2.0	4.0	2.9	9	888	428	353	7	53.0	87	3.5	19	147	14
Beef Burrito/Red Sauce	7	191	403	22.5	39.1	3	17.3	2.0	8.6	7.4	57	1051	313	504	10	2.0	2	3.7	20	114	11
Burrito Supreme/Red Sauce	9	241	413	18.0	46.6	4	17.6	2.0	7.2	7.7	33	921	434	876	17	26.0	42	3.6	19	153	15
Double Beef Burrito Supreme/Red Sauce	9	255	457	23.7	41.7	4	21.8	2.1		10.1	57	1053	431	952	19	9.0	14	4.0	21	145	14
Tostada/Red Sauce	6	156	243	9.5	26.6	6	11.1	0.8	4.4	4.1	16	596	401	668	13	45.0	75	1.5	8	179	17
Enchirito/Red Sauce	8	213	382	19.8	30.9	4	19.7	1.5	6.9	9.3	54	1243	423	965	19	28.0	46	2.8	15	269	26
Cinnamon Crispas	2	47	259	2.7	27.5	2	15.3	1.2	7.4	3.7	1	127	36	3	0	0.0	0	1.3	6	37	3
Pintos & Cheese/Red Sauce	5	128	191	9.0	19.0	4	8.7	0.8	3.8	3.6	16	642	384	441	8	52.0	86	1.4	7	156	15
Nachos	4	106	346	7.5	37.5	4	18.5	1.5	8.1	5.7	9	399	159	564	11	2.0	3	0.9	5	191	19
Nachos Bellgrande	10	287	649	21.6	60.6	7	35.3	2.6	14.3	12.3	36	997	674	1137	22	58.0	96	3.5	19	297	29
Taco	28	778	183	10.3	11.0	1	10.8	0.8	4.0	4.6	32	276	159	327	6	1.0	0	1.1	5	84	8
Taco Bellgrande	6	163	355	18.3	17.7	2	23.1	1.3	8.2	11.0	56	472	334	845	16	5.0	9	1.9	10	182	18
Taco Light	6	170	410	19.0	18.1	2	28.8	5.4	11.2	11.6	56	594	316	662	13	5.0	7	2.4	12	155	15
Soft Taco	3	92	228	11.8	17.9	1	11.9	5.4	4.6	5.4	32	516	178	213	4	1.0	2	2.3	12	116	11
Soft Taco Supreme	4	124	275	12.6	19.1	1	16.3	1.2	7.1	8.1	32	516	225	440	8	3.0	4	2.3	12	142	14
Taco Salad/Salsa	21	595	941	36.0	63.1	10	61.3	12.1	26.6	18.7	80	1662	1212	2958	59	77.0	128	7.1	39	398	39
Taco Salad/Salsa Without Shell	19	530	520	30.6	30.0	6	31.4	1.7	9.8	14.4	80	1431	1151	3024	60	76.0	126	5.1	28	367	36
Taco Salad Without Shell	19	530	520	29.5	26.3	6	31.3	1.7	9.8	14.4	80	1056	988	1906	38	74.0	123	4.5	25	331	32
Mexican Pizza	8	223	575	21.3	39.7	6	36.8	9.7	16.7	11.4	52	1031	408	984	19	31.0	51	3.7	20	257	25
Taco Sauce	<1	<1	2	0.1	0.4	0	0.1	0.0	0.0	0.0	0	126	13	185	3	0.0	0	0.0	0	2	0
Hot Taco Sauce	<1	<1	3	0.1	0.3	0	0.1	0.0	0.0	0.0	0	82	14	147	2	1.0	2	0.1	0	2	0
Salsa	3	10	18	1.1	3.6	1	0.1	0.0	0.0	0.0	0	376	376	1120	22	2.0	3	0.6	3	36	3
Ranch Dressing	4	74	236	1.7	1.5	0	24.9	13.8	6.6	4.6	36	571	44	240	4	0.0	0	0.5	2	29	2
Jalapeno Peppers	5	100	20	1.0	4.0	1	0.2	0.0	0.0	0.1	0	1370	110	250	5	2.0	3	0.3	0	40	4
Steak Fajita	5	135	234	14.6	19.5	1	10.9	1.1	5.1	4.8	14	485	207	560	11	3.0	4	3.0	16	118	11
Chicken Fajita	1	135	226	13.6	19.8	1	10.2	2.1	5.2	3.7	44	619	201	721	14	4.0	6	2.1	11	123	12
Sour Cream	1	21	46	0.6	0.9	0	4.4	0.2	1.3	2.7	16	10	31	168	3	0.0	0	0.0	0	6	2
Pico De Gallo	1	28	8	0.3	1.1	0	0.2	0.1	0.0	0.0	1	88	0	546	10	2.0	2	0.2	0	0	0
Guacamole	4	21	34	0.4	3.0	1	2.3	0.4	1.6	0.4	0	113	110	116	2	3.0	5	0.2	0	10	0
Meximelt	4	106	266	12.9	18.7	1	15.4	1.5	5.6	7.9	38	689	114	811	16	2.0	2	2.0	10	247	24

Restaurant: Wendy's Old Fashioned Hamburgers

Item																					
Junior Hamburger	3	104	260	15.0	32.0	1	9.0	1.1	3.7	3.3	35	570	205	100	2	1.2	2	2.7	20	100	10
Junior Cheeseburger	3	116	300	18.0	33.0	1	13.0	1.3	5.1	6.4	35	770	205	100	2	1.2	2	2.7	20	100	10
Small Hamburger	4	111	260	15.0	33.0	1	9.0	1.2	3.7	3.4	34	570	215	100	2	2.4	4	2.7	20	100	10
Small Cheeseburger	4	125	310	18.0	33.0	1	13.0	1.4	5.3	7.2	34	770	215	100	2	2.4	4	2.7	20	100	10
Chicken Sandwich	8	219	430	26.0	41.0	2	19.0	7.2	7.3	4.6	60	725	390	500	2	500.0	8	14.4	80	100	10
Big Classic/Cheese	10	295	640	30.0	46.0	4	38.0	7.0	12.6	12.5	100	1370	590	1000	20	15.0	25	5.4	30	150	15
Plain Single	4	126	340	24.0	30.0	1	15.0	1.5	7.0	6.4	65	500	275	0	0			4.5	25	100	10
Single/Everything	8	210	420	25.0	35.0	1	21.0	4.3	7.3	6.4	70	890	430	750	15	15.0	25	4.5	30	100	10
Plain Single/Cheese	5	137	410	25.0	29.0	1	22.0	1.7	8.9	10.6	80	710	265	0	0			4.5	25	100	10
Garden Salad (Take-Out)	10	227	102	7.0	9.0	4	5.0	0.4	1.1	5.2	0	110	560	5500	110	66.0	110	1.8	10	200	20
Chef Salad (Take-Out)	12	331	180	15.0	10.0	4	7.0	0.6	3.1	2.9	120	140	590	5500	110	66.0	110	2.7	15	250	25
New Chili	9	256	220	21.0	23.0	7	7.0	2.4	3.2	15.9	45	750	495	1000	15	9.0	15	4.5	35	60	8
Taco Salad	28	791	660	40.0	46.0	9	37.0	2.4	13.9	4.6	35	1110	1330	4000	80	48.0	80	6.3	35	800	80
French Fries, Small	3	97	240	3.0	33.0	2	12.0	0.8	8.0	4.6	15	145	510	0	0	0.0	10	0.7	4	0	0
Salad Bar Items																					
Creamy Peppercorn Dressing	1	15	80	0.0	0.0	0	8.0	4.3	1.9	1.5	100	135	5	1250	25	1.2	2	0.0	0	100	10
Hidden Valley Ranch Dressing	1	15	50	0.0	0.0	0	6.0	2.9	1.6	1.0	5	115	15	0	0	0.0	0	0.0	0	0	0
Thousand Island Dressing	1	15	70	0.0	2.0	0	7.0	3.1	1.3	0.9	5	105	15	0	0	0.0	0	0.0	0	0	0
French Dressing	1	15	60	0.0	4.0	0	6.0	3.4	1.3	1.5	0	190	25	100	2	0.0	0	0.0	0	0	0
Sweet Red French Dressing	1	15	70	0.0	5.0	0	6.0	2.7	1.0	1.2	0	130	20	0	0	0.0	0	0.0	0	0	0
Italian Caesar Dressing	1	15	80	0.0	0.0	0	8.0	4.1	1.7	1.0	0	125	5	0	0	0.0	0	0.0	0	0	0
Blue Cheese Dressing	1	15	80	0.0	0.0	0	9.0	4.3	1.9	1.5	10	90	5	0	0	0.0	0	0.0	0	0	0
Celery Seed Dressing	1	15	70	0.0	3.0	0	6.0	3.1	1.3	0.9	5	65	10	0	0	0.0	0	0.0	0	0	0
Golden Italian Dressing	1	15	45	0.0	3.0	0	4.0	3.4	1.3	1.5	0	260	10	0	0	0.0	0	0.0	0	0	0
Reduced Calorie Italian Dressing	1	15	25	0.0	2.0	0	2.0	0.6	0.2	0.1	0	180	10	0	0	0.0	0	0.0	0	0	0
Reduced Calorie Bacon & Tomato Dressing	1	15	45	0.0	3.0	0	4.0	0.9	1.1	0.4	0	190	15	0	0	0.0	0	0.0	0	0	0
Alfredo Sauce	2	56	50	2.0	7.0	0	2.0	0.1	0.6	1.3	0	300	80	0	0	0.0	0	0.0	0	60	6
Cheese Sauce	2	56	50	1.0	8.0	0	2.0	0.1	0.7	1.4	0	420	260	0	0	0.0	0	0.4	0	60	6
Spaghetti Sauce	2	56	30	1.0	7.0	1	0.1	0.1	0.0	0.0	0	345	95	200	4	0.0	0	0.4	2	0	0
Deluxe Three Bean Salad	2	57	60	1.0	13.0	2	0.1	0.1	0.0	0.0	10	15	55	750	15	15.0	25	0.0	0	20	2
California Coleslaw	2	57	60	0.0	9.0	1	6.0	1.5	1.7	0.6	10	140	95	150	10	6.0	10	0.4	2	0	0
Red Bliss Potato Salad	2	57	110	0.0	6.0	0	9.0	4.8	2.3	1.3	10	265	150	200	4	0.0	0	0.4	2	0	0
Old Fashioned Corn Relish	2	57	35	2.0	9.0	1	0.0	0.1	0.0	0.1	0	205	30	0	0	18.0	30	0.4	2	0	0
Pasta Deli Salad	2	57	35	2.0	6.0	0	0.0	0.9	0.5	0.3	0	120	88	0	0	0.0	0	0.4	2	0	0
Sliced Pepperoni	1	28	140	5.0	2.0	0	12.0	1.2	6.0	4.6	30	450	95	0	0	0.0	0	0.4	2	60	6
Cheddar Chips	1	28	160	3.0	12.0	0	11.0	2.7	4.0	3.3	11	445	34	0	0	9.0	15	2.7	15	20	2
Crushed Red Peppers	1	28	120	5.0	15.0	7	4.0	2.4	0.8	1.0	0	5	571	10,000	200	0.0	0	0.0	0	500	50
Imitation Parmesan Cheese	1	28	80	9.0	4.0	0	3.0	0.1	1.9	4.1	trace	410	95	1000	20	0.0	0	0.0	0	200	20
Shredded Imitation Cheese (Salad Bar)	1	28	90	6.0	4.0	0	6.0	2.3	2.7	1.0	2	120	135	300	6	0.0	0	0.0	0	200	20
Potato Chili Cheese	1	28	100	6.0	6.0	0	8.0	0.3	2.5	5.6	27	130	50	500	10	18.0	30	0.4	2	0	0
Picante Sauce	2	56	18	<1.0	4.0	0	<1.0	0.0	0.2	5.0	0	5	40	0	0	0.0	0	0.0	0	20	2
Imitation Sour Topping	1	28	45	<1.0	2.0	0	5.0	3.0	3.0	1.3	0	30	trace	0	0	0.0	0	0.0	0	1	0
Country Crock* Spread	1	14	70	0.0	0.0	3	7.0	3.8	4.1	1.5	38	100	79	200	4	0.0	0	0.7	4	80	8
Taco Chips	1	40	260	4.0	40.0	1	10.0	0.6	0.5	1.0	0	20	28	0	0	0.0	0	0.0	0	20	2
Taco Shells	<1	11	45	<1.0	8.0	1	2.0	0.3	1.3	1.1	3	trace	37	0	0	0.0	0	0.4	2	80	8
Flour Tortilla	1	37	110	3.0	19.0	1	3.0	0.3	1.3	0.5	trace	220	99	0	0	9.0	0	0.4	2	150	15
Chocolate Pudding	2	57	90	0.0	12.0	1	4.0	1.1	1.3	0.5	trace	70	54	0	0	2.6	0	0.4	2	60	6
Butterscotch Pudding	2	57	90	1.0	11.0	0	4.0	1.1	1.3	0.5	trace	85	54	0	0	13.5	0	0.4	2	60	6

Restaurant: White Castle

Item																			
Hamburger	2	58	161	5.9	15.4	2	7.9	0.7	3.0	2.8	18	266	86	0	0.0	0	1.1	44
Cheeseburger	2	65	200	7.8	15.5	3	11.2	0.8	4.0	4.9	28	361	103	130	0.0	0	1.1	98
Fish Sandwich Without Tartar Sauce	2	59	155	5.8	20.9	1	5.0	1.2	2.2	1.2	8	201	111	9	0.2	0	1.0	49
Sausage/Egg Sandwich	3	96	322	12.6	16.1	3	22.0	4.3	9.4	6.4	151	698	193	543	0.7	0	1.5	69
Sausage Sandwich	2	49	196	6.7	13.3	2	12.3	2.2	5.2	3.7	22	488	117	155	0.5	0	0.8	44
Chicken Sandwich	2	64	186	8.0	20.5	2	7.5	2.1	2.9	1.6	19	497	87	17	0.0	0	1.2	47
French Fries	3	97	301	2.5	37.7	5	14.7	5.6	6.3	2.3	0	193	597	0	13.5	4	0.6	15
Onion Rings	2	63	246	2.9	26.6	3	13.4	5.3	5.9	2.1	0	566	112	0	2.6	2	1.4	80
Onion Chips	3	93	329	3.7	38.8	4	16.6	5.6	6.3	2.3	0	823	597	0	13.5	2	0.6	15

Dietetic Currents, Vol. 18, No. 4, 1991, Ross Laboratories, Columbus, Ohio 43216, Division of Abbott Laboratories, USA, with the permission of Ross Laboratories.

CONVULSION

A violent involuntary contraction or series of contractions of the voluntary muscles.

COPPER (Cu)

Contents   Page

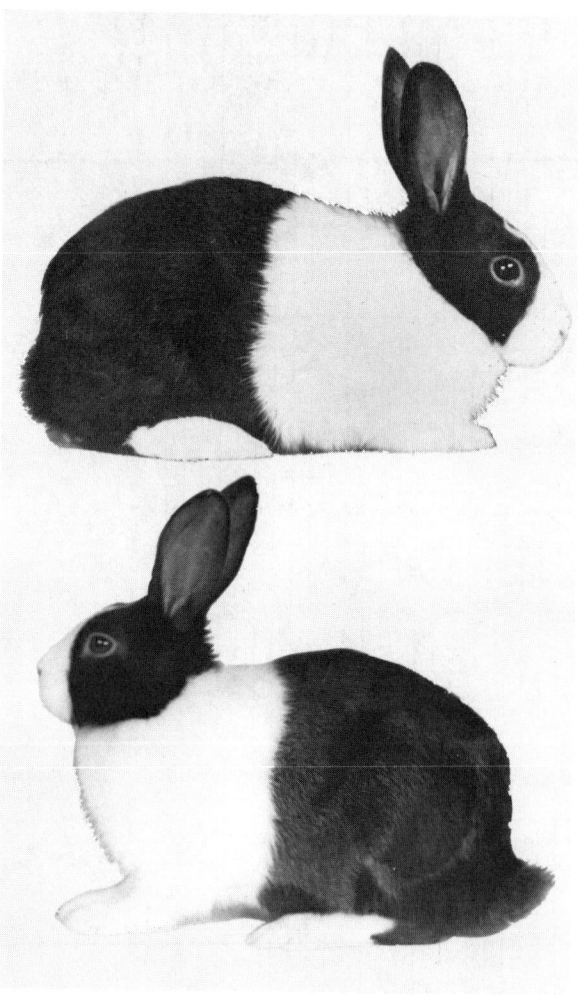

Fig. C-69. Copper is required for normal pigmentation of hair. Top: Rabbit reared on a diet adequate in copper. Bottom: Rabbit reared on a copper-deficient diet, showing graying of hair. (Courtesy, Sedgwick E. Smith, Cornell, University)

HISTORY. Copper was discovered and first used by neolithic man during the late Stone Age. The exact date of this discovery will probably never be known, but it is believed to have been about 8000 B.C. The late Bronze Age (3000 to 1000 B.C.) takes its name from the use during this period of bronze, an alloy of copper and tin.

In ancient times, the chief source of copper for the people near the Mediterranean Sea was the island of Cyprus. As a result, the metal became known as *Cyprian metal.* Both the word copper and the chemical symbol for the element, *Cu,* come from *cuprum,* the Roman name for Cyprian metal.

As a result of a series of studies beginning in 1925 (and reported in 1928), Hart and associates at the University of Wisconsin discovered that a small amount of copper is necessary, along with iron, for hemoglobin formation.[25] Then, in 1931, Josephs found that copper was more effective than iron alone in overcoming the anemia of milk-fed infants. Today, copper is considered as an essential nutrient for all vertebrates and some lower animal species.

ABSORPTION, METABOLISM, EXCRETION. The site of copper absorption depends on the specie of animal; it's primarily in the stomach and the upper part of the small intestine in man. Of the intake, about 30% is absorbed.

After absorption in the intestine, copper reaches the bloodstream where most of it (80% or more) becomes bound to ceruloplasmin, a protein (globulin-copper) complex. The rest is loosely bound to albumen and transported to various tissues.

FUNCTIONS OF COPPER. The role of copper in hemoglobin formation is generally recognized as that of facilitating the absorption of iron from the intestinal tract and releasing it from storage in the liver and the reticuloendothelial system. Although it is not a part of the hemoglobin as such, copper is essential for the formation of hemoglobin. Also, copper is a constituent of several enzyme systems required for normal energy metabolism and its many ramifications; is essential for the development and maintenance of skeletal structures (bones, tendons, and connective tissue); is necessary for the development of the aorta and vascular system; and is required for the formation and functioning of the brain cells and the spinal cord. Additionally, copper is required for normal pigmentation of the hair. Also, a number of important copper-containing proteins and enzymes have been identified; some of which are essential for the proper utilization of iron.

DEFICIENCY SYMPTOMS. Dietary copper deficiency is not known to occur in adults under normal circumstances, but it has been diagnosed in Peru in malnourished children; and in the United States in premature infants fed exclusively on modified cow's milk and in infants breast fed for an extended period of time. Fortunately, the liver of newborn babies contains 5 to 10 times as much copper as the liver of adults—a reserve which is drawn upon during the first year of life.

Copper deficiency leads to a variety of abnormalities, including anemia, skeletal defects, demyelination and degeneration of the nervous system, defects in the pigmentation and structure of hair, reproductive failure, and pronounced cardiovascular lesions.

Recent animal experiments have shown that a mild copper deficiency can result in elevated serum cholesterol levels, particularly in the presence of high zinc intakes, and

[25]Hart, E. B., *et al.,* Iron in Nutrition, VII, Copper as a supplement to iron for hemoglobin building in the rat, *Journal of Biological Chemistry,* Vol. 77, 1928, p. 792.

epidemiological studies have postulated a positive correlation between the zinc-to-copper ratio in the diet and the incidence of cardiovascular disease.[26,27]

INTERRELATIONSHIPS. Copper, along with certain vitamins, is involved in iron metabolism.

Dietary excesses of cadmium, calcium, iron, lead, molybdenum plus sulfur, silver, and zinc reduce the utilization of copper.

RECOMMENDED DAILY ALLOWANCE OF COP-PER. The estimated copper requirement of man is based on balance studies. On the basis of such studies, and in order to allow for a margin of safety, the National Academy of Sciences–National Research Council, recommends a daily copper intake of 1.5 to 3 mg for adults. The requirement for infants and children has been estimated at between 0.4 and 2.0 mg per day. It is emphasized, however, that intake of copper at this level may be too low for the premature infant, who is always born with low copper reserves. It is suggested that infant bottle formulas contain sufficient copper to furnish 100 micrograms/kg of body weight per day.

Estimated safe and adequate intakes of copper are given in the section on MINERAL(S), Table M-25, Mineral Table.

• **Copper intake in average U.S. diet**—Ordinary varied U.S. diets supply from 2.5 to 5 mg per day.

TOXICITY. Copper is relatively nontoxic to monogastric species, including man. A FAO/WHO Expert Committee has stated that no deleterious effects in man may be expected from a copper intake of 0.5 mg/kg of body weight per day. Usual diets in the United States rarely supply more than 5 mg/day. In order to provide for a margin of safety, the National Academy of Sciences–National Research Council recommended copper intake for adults is in the range of 1.5 to 3 mg/day. Daily intakes of more than 20 to 30 mg/day over extended periods would be expected to be unsafe.

Most cases of copper poisoning, which are rare, result from drinking water or beverages that have been stored in copper tanks and/or that pass through copper pipes.

Wilson's disease, a genetically determined inborn error of metabolism, is characterized by a marked reduction in blood ceruloplasmin and greatly increased deposits of copper in the liver, brain, and other organs. The excess copper leads to hepatitis, renal malfunction, and neurologic disorders. The condition can be reversed by controlling dietary copper intake and by administering chelating agents to bind the free copper and excrete it in the urine.

(Also see POISONS, Table P-2, Some Potentially Poisonous [Toxic] Substances.)

SOURCES OF COPPER. Copper is widely distributed in foods. The contribution of drinking water to copper intake varies with the type of piping and the hardness of water. Milk is a poor source of copper. Cow's milk ranges from 0.015 to 0.18 mg/liter; and human milk ranges from 1.05

mg/liter at the beginning of lactation to 0.15 mg/liter at the end.

Groupings by rank of common food sources of copper are given in the section on MINERAL(S), Table M-25, Mineral Table.

For additional sources and more precise values of copper, see Food Composition Table F-21.

(Also see MINERAL[S], Table M-25; and POISONS, Table P-2, Some Potentially Poisonous [Toxic] Substances.)

COPPER (Cu) TOXICITY

Although the incidence of copper toxicity is rare, it may occur in diets rich in the mineral, but low in other minerals which counteract its effects.

(Also see MINERAL[S]; COPPER; and POISONS.)

COPROPHAGY

The ingestion of fecal material. This constitutes normal behavior among many insects, birds and other animals. But in man it is indicative of some form of behavioral disorder.

(Also see PICA.)

CORI CYCLE

The series of reactions which (1) break down muscle glycogen to blood glucose, or (2) convert blood glucose to muscle glycogen.

(Also see CARBOHYDRATE[S]; and GLYCOGEN.)

CORN (MAIZE) *Zea mays*

Contents | Page

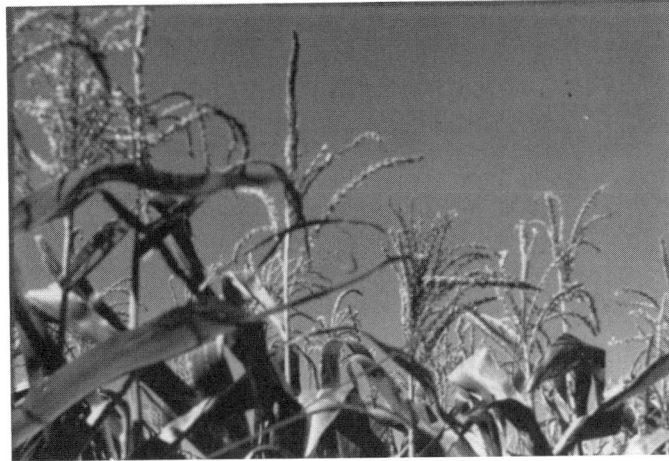

Fig. C-70. Corn as high as an elephant's eye and climbing clear up to the sky—has long been the most important U.S. cereal grain. (Courtesy, USDA)

[26]Murphy, L., E. O'Flaherty, and H. G. Petering, Effect of Low Levels of Copper and Zinc on Lipid Metabolism, *Report on Center of Environmental Health*, University of Cincinnati, Cincinnati, Ohio, 1973, p. 35.

[27]Klevay, L. M., Hypercholesterolemia in Rats Produced by an Increase of the Ratio of Zinc to Copper Ingested, *American Journal of Clinical Nutrition*, 1973, Vol. 26, pp. 1060–1068.

Corn or maize (Indian corn, *Zea mays*) is a plant of the tribe Maydea of the grass family (*Gramineae*).

The word *maize* is preferred in international usage because in many countries the term *corn,* the name by which the plant is known in the United States, is synonymous with the leading cereal grain; thus, in England *corn* refers to wheat, and in Scotland and Ireland it refers to oats.

(Also see CEREAL GRAINS.)

ORIGIN AND HISTORY.

Corn is indigenous to America. Fossilized pollens, estimated to be 80,000 years old, have been found in soil profiles near Mexico City; and ears of corn about the size of strawberries, estimated to be 3,000 years old, have been discovered in Mexico. Archeological discoveries almost as ancient as those in Mexico have been found in South America, causing postulation of another locus of domestication.

The Indians, from Canada to Chile, grew all the main types of corn that are raised today. They prized corn with colorful kernels—red, blue, pink, and black, or with bands, spots, or stripes. They often used fish as a fertilizer; various rituals

WORLD AND U.S. PRODUCTION.

Corn (maize) ranks second only to wheat among the leading cereal grains of the world, and it ranks first by a wide margin as the leading U.S. cereal grain.

North America has always been the center of corn production. In 1990, it accounted for 48% of the total world production of 475,429,000 metric tons annually; the United States alone produces 42% of the world total.[28]

The leading corn-growing countries of the world, in descending order, are: United States, China, Brazil, Romania, France, South Africa, Mexico, and Yugoslavia.[29]

Although corn is grown throughout the United States, the greatest production is in an area of the Midwest called the Corn Belt, consisting of the seven states of Illinois, Indiana, Iowa, Kansas, Missouri, Nebraska, and Ohio. About two-thirds of the corn grown for grain is produced in Illinois and Iowa. The United States produces about 8 billion bushels of corn annually; and the ten leading corn-growing states of the nation, in descending order, are: Iowa, Illinois, Nebraska, Minnesota, Indiana, Ohio, Wisconsin, Michigan, South Dakota, and Missouri.[30]

[28]Based on data from *FAO Production Yearbook 1990*, FAO/UN, Rome, Italy, Vol. 44, p. 79, Table 20. **Note well:** Annual production fluctuates as a result of weather and profitability of the crop.

[29]*Ibid.*

[30]Based on data from *Agricultural Statistics 1991*, USDA, p. 33, Table 41. **Note well:** Annual production fluctuates as a result of weather and profitability of the crop.

KINDS OF CORN.

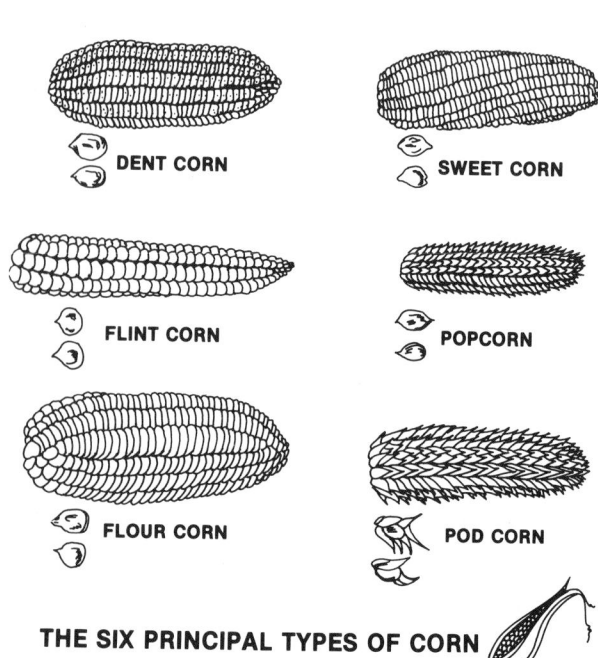

DENT CORN

SWEET CORN

FLINT CORN

POPCORN

FLOUR CORN

POD CORN

THE SIX PRINCIPAL TYPES OF CORN

Fig. C-72. The six principal types (races) of corn.

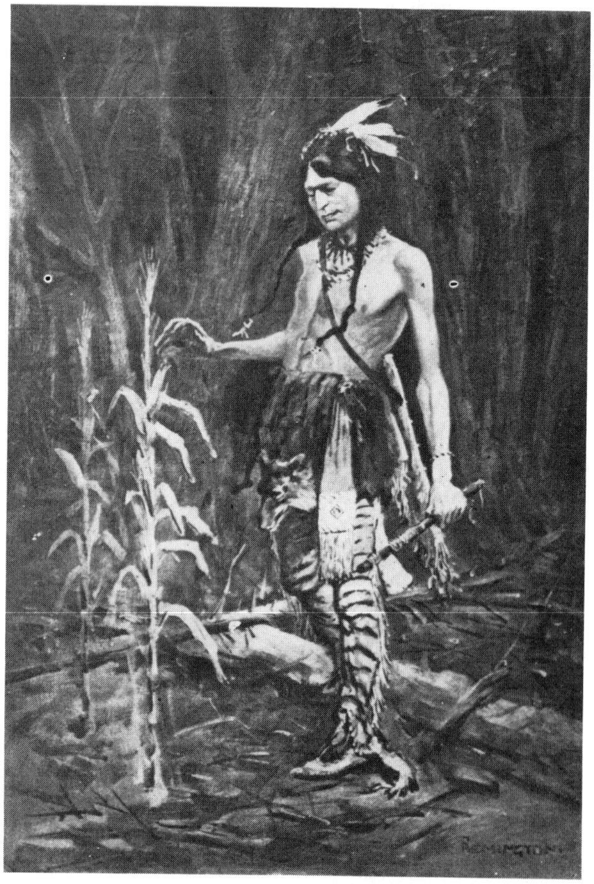

Fig. C-71. Indian observing the growth of corn (maize). After a painting by Frederick Remington. (Courtesy, The Bettmann Archive, Inc., New York, N.Y.)

were carried out to ward off evil spirits; and human sentries were stationed to discourage pilfering by birds and animals. Also, they used corn patterns to decorate pottery, sculpture, and other works of art.

The many kinds or varieties of corn can be grouped into six different categories based on types of kernels: (1) dent corn, (2) sweet corn, (3) flint corn, (4) popcorn, (5) flour corn, and (6) pod corn.

• **Dent corn**—This is the most common variety. It accounts for about 95% of all the corn grown in the United States. Each kernel of dent corn has a small dent on top, caused by the hard and soft starch in the kernel shrinking unequally in drying. Dent corn may be yellow, white, or red. Most of the corn grown commercially is yellow, although white corn is preferred for the manufacture of cereals. Most of the dent corn is fed to livestock, although some of it is sold to manufacturers who make many food and industrial products from it.

• **Sweet corn**—Sweet corn is grown chiefly for human food and is harvested at an immature stage. The kernels are relatively high in sugar at the time they are canned, frozen, or eaten as corn on the cob. Most of the sweet corn is grown for the canning industry, but some is grown by truck gardeners and almost all home gardeners. Practically all varieties of sweet corn are white or yellow. Upon maturity, the kernels are characterized by their wrinkled, caramelized appearance.

Unless it is kept refrigerated after harvesting, sweet corn quickly loses its flavor. This happens because heat turns the sugar in the kernels to starch. Refrigerated trucks make it possible to carry fresh sweet corn far from the places where it is grown. Canned and quick-frozen sweet corn lasts indefinitely and can be shipped throughout the world. The leading states in producing sweet corn for processing are Wisconsin, Minnesota, Washington, Oregon, Illinois, Idaho, and New York. Florida supplies most of the fresh sweet corn for the winter, spring, and fall markets. Several states produce a substantial amount of fresh sweet corn for the summer markets, with New York and California leading.

Sweet corn is a good source of energy. It contains twice as much sugar as dent corn. Also, it is a good source of vitamins A (if yellow) and C.

• **Flint corn**—The corn that the Indians taught the early settlers to grow was flint corn. The kernels of flint corn are comprised of small amounts of soft starch completely surrounded by a large quantity of hard starch. Flint corn makes a good quality corn meal. There is less spoilage than with dent corn when flint corn is shipped overseas, because the hard seed absorbs less moisture. Also, it is more resistant to corn weevil damage. Argentina, which exports a large proportion of its corn crop, produces mostly flint corn.

Compared to dent corn, most flint corn varieties mature earlier, and their seeds germinate better in cold, wet soil in the spring. For the latter reason, they are grown farther north than the dent types. Flint corn comes in many colors—white, yellow, red, blue, and variable.

• **Popcorn**—This is a favorite *fun food* of Americans. It is eaten plain with salt and butter, or covered with caramel or white sugar syrup.

The kernels of popcorn are smaller than flint corn. When heated rapidly, the moisture inside the kernels turns to steam and builds up a great pressure. This pressure bursts the outer shell, and the entire inside of the kernel puffs out into a mass of flaky starch. Upon popping, the volume is 25 to 30 times greater than the original kernel.

• **Flour corn**—Flour corn, or soft corn as it is sometimes called, has soft, starchy kernels. Because the kernels can be easily ground into flour by hand, flour corn is popular with the Indians of the southwestern United States. Also, it is grown in the warm areas of South America. White and blue are the most common colors, although numerous other colors are found. Flour corn ripens late in the season.

• **Pod corn**—Each kernel of pod corn is enclosed within a separate pod or husk; and the entire ear is surrounded by a large husk similar to that found on other types of corn. Some scientists believe that pod corn may be the ancestor of all other types of corn. Pod corn is of no commercial importance in the United States; it is grown only as a curiosity and for use in breeding and related studies.

PROCESSING OF CORN. Most of the corn crop goes directly into animal feed uses, much of it right on the farm where it is grown. But each day of the year corn refiners process over a million bushels of corn, producing ingredients vital to innumerable food and industrial products. Of the 94 supermarket items that go into most grocery carts, over a quarter contain one or more ingredients from the corn refining industry.

Corn Milling.

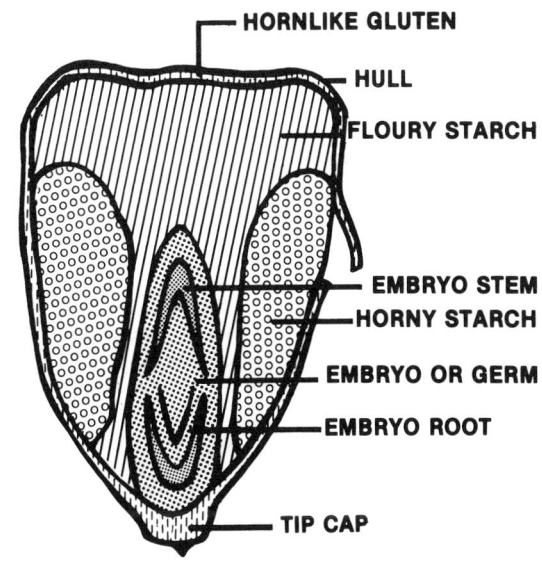

Fig. C-73. Part of a kernel of dent corn.

In order to understand corn milling and corn by-products, it is first necessary to know the composition of the different parts of the corn kernel. Each year, about 6% of the U.S. corn crop is milled. Corn is wet milled for the production of starch, sweeteners, and oil; or is dry milled for the production of grits, flakes, meal, oil, and feeds.

WET MILLING. Before storage, shelled corn (mostly yellow dent) intended for wet milling is cleaned to remove all foreign matter, such as insects, rocks, and trash. When it is taken from storage, it is cleaned again, then soaked in water—swelling the kernels. In the soaking (or steeping) process, nutrients are absorbed by the water (steepwater). When the steeping is complete, this water is drawn off and concentrated.

During the subsequent milling process, the corn germ is separated from the kernel. The germ is further processed to remove oil, and the remaining germ meal is isolated for later use.

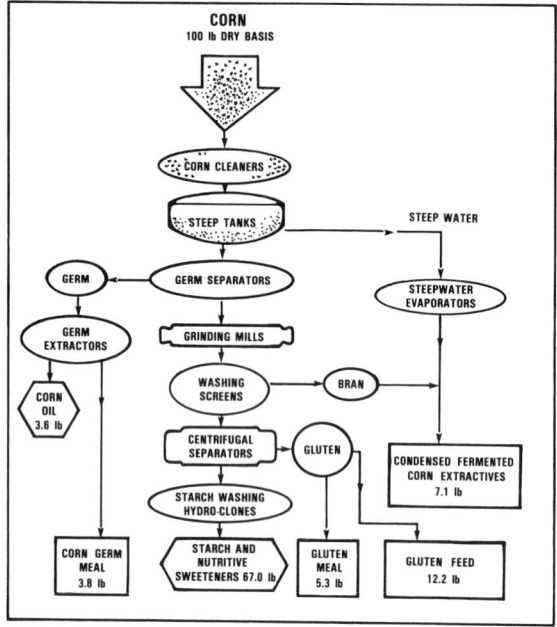

Fig. C-74. Schematic outline of the corn wet milling process.

After the germ has been removed, the rest of the corn kernel, containing starch, gluten, and bran (the outer hull of the kernel) is screened, and the bran is removed. The remaining mixture of starch and gluten is separated by centrifugal action. The starch portion is either dried, or modified and dried, and sold to the food, paper, and textile industries, or is further converted into various sweeteners.

Thus, the following four major ingredients are isolated during the production of starch, sweeteners, and oil: steepwater, germ, bran, and gluten. From these substances come the refining industry's four major feed ingredients: corn gluten meal, corn gluten feed, corn germ meal, and condensed fermented corn extractives—commonly known as corn steepwater. Thus, while the corn refiners primarily produce corn starch, corn sweeteners (sugar and syrup), and corn oil, 25 to 30% of their output is livestock feed ingredients.

DRY MILLING. The dry milling of corn is generally less involved than wet milling. Two basic processes—degerming and nondegerming—are used extensively.

In the degerming process, the hull, germ, and endosperm are separated before milling. This process is used for the production of grits, flakes, meal, flour, oil, and feeds.

The entire kernel is ground intact in the nondegerming process of dry milling. The resulting product is an oily flour which is subsequently used in baked products. Although some hulls and germs sift out in this process, the quantity of by-products is too insignificant to be considered as a reliable source of animal feed.

Dry millers produce cornmeal by either of two methods; the *old process*, or the *new process*. In the old process, the germ is left in the meal. This improves the flavor and nutritional value, but it limits the time that the meal stays fresh. Most commercial cornmeal is made by the new process, from hulled corn kernels with the germ removed.

Distilling And Fermentation. The corn distilling and fermentation industries include manufacturers of ethyl and butyl alcohols, acetone, and whiskey.

• **Alcohol**—Malt converts corn starch to sugar, which is fermented by yeast to ethyl alcohol and carbon dioxide. The grain that remains is used as livestock feed.

The current fuel shortage has sparked much interest in *gasohol,* a mixture of 10% anhydrous ethyl alcohol and 90% gasoline; with the ethyl alcohol manufactured from corn, wheat, sorghum, and other agricultural products).

(Also see BEERS AND BREWING; and DISTILLED LIQUORS.)

• **Industrial products**—Manufacturers allow bacteria to ferment cornmeal to produce acetone and butyl alcohol, which are used in manufacturing rayon, plastics, and other products.

The by-products of distilling and fermentation of corn include carbon dioxide, corn oil, vitamin and protein concentrates, and grain germ mixtures.

NUTRITIONAL VALUE. Corn is palatable, nutritious, and rich in the energy-producing carbohydrates (starch) and fats. It is higher in fat than rice or wheat (4% vs 2%). The caloric values of these 3 cereal grains are: cornmeal, whole-ground, 1,610 Calories (kcal) per pound (0.45 kg); rice, brown, 1,633 Calories (kcal) per pound (0.45 kg); and wheat grain, 1,497 Calories (kcal) per pound (0.45 kg). But corn has certain limitations! It lacks quantity of protein (8 to 11%) and quality of protein (being especially low in the amino acids, lysine and tryptophan), and it is deficient in minerals, particularly calcium, and in the vitamin niacin. White corn is also low in carotene (the precursor of vitamin A). However, when vitamin A is added, white corn and yellow corn are equal in nutritive value. It is noteworthy that the carotene content of yellow corn decreases with storage; about 25% of its original vitamin A value may be lost after 1 year of storage, and 50% after 2 years.

The nutritive value of different forms of corn and corn products is given in Food Composition Table F-21.

The amino acid composition of corn warrants careful consideration (see Table C-22). In countries where high corn diets prevail, the amino acid profile can be used as a basis to determine what protein supplement to add.

TABLE C-22
PROFILE OF ESSENTIAL AMINO ACIDS IN CORN COMPARED TO MILK—A HIGH-QUALITY PROTEIN[1]

Amino Acid	Whole Corn	Cow's Milk
	(mg/g protein)	
Histidine	27	27
Isoleucine	38	47
Leucine	133	95
Lysine	27	78
Methionine plus cystine	41	33
Phenylalanine plus tyrosine	92	102
Threonine	37	44
Tryptophan	9	14
Valine	46	64

[1]*Recommended Dietary Allowances*, 10th ed. 1989, NRC–National Academy of Sciences, p. 67, Table 6-5.

Although corn contains about 10% protein, half of the protein consists of zein, which is especially poor in lysine and tryptophan, essential amino acids which people must get from food (see Table C-22).

In 1944, researchers at the Connecticut Agricultural Experiment Station induced starvation in laboratory rats by feeding them generous helpings of corn. Further, it was found that rats could be restored to health by supplementing the high-corn diet with two protein fractions—the amino acids lysine and tryptophan.

Children Cannot Live By Corn Alone.

Corn alone will not keep weaning infants alive. They will develop the disease kwashiorkor, primarily due to protein deficiency; and they may develop pellagra, due to a deficiency of the vitamin niacin.

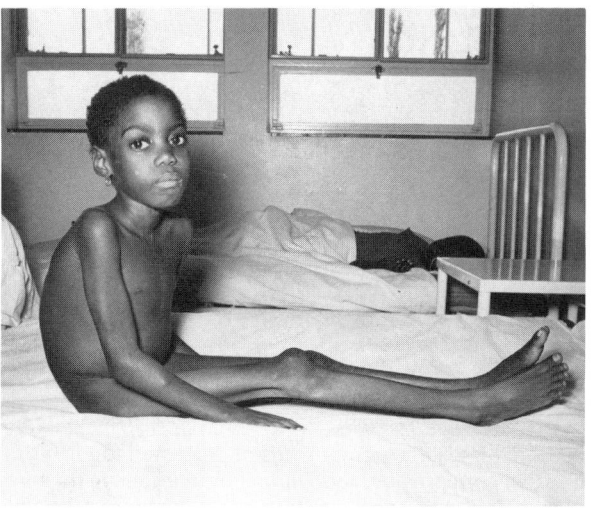

Fig. C-75. Kwashiorkor, due to a protein deficiency. Note enlarged stomach and knees of this 9-year-old girl. (Courtesy, FAO and United Nations Children's Fund)

The disease *pellagra*, caused by a deficiency of niacin, is prevalent among peoples who rely on corn for a large proportion of their daily food. Although corn contains niacin, 50 to 80% of it occurs in a bound form as niacytin, which is biologically unavailable. It is noteworthy that pellagra is not suffered by Mexicans who consume cornmeal in the form of tortillas. The explanation: tortillas are made by mixing cornmeal with lime water, creating an alkaline condition which releases the bound niacin and makes it available.

In Colombia, corn grain is pounded with potash and a little water is added, in the preparation of cornmeal. Although the primary purpose of the potash is to loosen the bran, the alkaline reaction is effective in unbinding the bound niacin.

The quantity of protein provided by the diet depends both on the amount of food consumed and on the concentration of protein in the food. Foods with low concentrations of protein, such as corn, may provide useful amounts of protein provided enough of them are eaten. There is, however, a limit to consumption, since the amount of food eaten is determined largely by the requirement for calories, rather

than the requirement for protein. Also, the stomach can hold just so much. For example, to meet the energy requirements (1,200 kcal/day) of a 2-year old, 30 lb (13.6 kg) child from cornmeal would necessitate the consumption of about 3 ½ lb (1.6 kg) per day of a gruel or dough—a physical impossibility. Even if this large amount of corn cereal could be consumed, it would still fall short of meeting the child's protein requirements by about 18%.

Also, corn lacks quality of protein. It is deficient in lysine and tryptophan, amino acids that are essential for all single-stomached creatures, such as humans and pigs.

High-Lysine Corn (Opaque-2, or O₂).

It has been known for many years that corn, the world's third most important human food after rice and wheat, is nutritionally inadequate.

Although normal corn contains about 10% protein, half of it is locked up in the fraction zein, which is poorly utilized by man. Moreover, normal corn is especially poor in lysine and tryptophan, essential amino acids that the human body cannot manufacture and must get from food.

This deficiency of corn shows up in people wherever corn is a major source—if not the only source—of protein in the diet. Known by the name kwashiorkor, this nutritional deficiency disease is the leading cause of mortality among infants and children in many parts of the world.

For years, plant scientists assayed the world's corn varieties one by one, looking for a strain with more nutritionally balanced protein. Finally, in 1963, a Purdue University team headed by biochemist Edwin T. Mertz analyzed an odd group of corns characterized by soft, floury endosperm inside an opaque, chalk-white kernel. The Purdue scientists found that the opaque characteristic of corn, which had been noted for years without exciting much scientific interest, is associated with a recessive gene that replaces some of the kernel's amino acid deficient zein with other protein higher in the needed lysine and tryptophan. The mutant—routinely labeled opaque-2, or O₂ for short—had a lysine

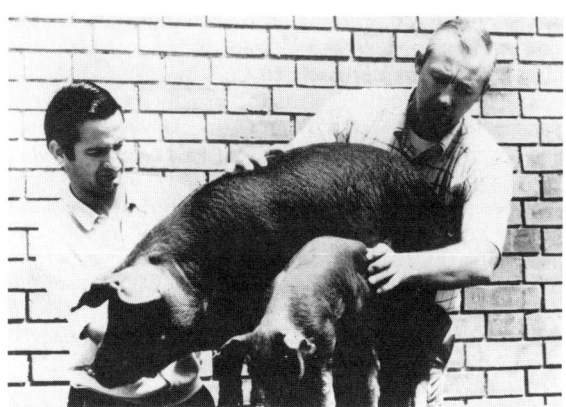

Fig. C-76. Lysine made the difference! These littermate pigs were started on test at weaning, at a weight of 20 lb (9 kg). The only difference in their ration was the kind of corn. The pig (left) received high-lysine corn; the little pig (right) got regular corn. During the 130-day trial, the pig fed opaque-2 gained a respectable 73.2 lb (33 kg), whereas the pig eating ordinary corn gained only 6.6 lb (3 kg). Lysine is essential for growing children as it is for growing pigs. (Courtesy, The Rockefeller Foundation, New York, N.Y.)

content of 3.4%, compared to 2.0% for normal corn. Additionally, opaque-2 showed higher levels of tryptophan and other amino acids.

But the millenium that seemed so near with the discovery of opaque-2'corn has remained frustratingly out of reach. Although the nutritional value of the high-lysine corn is recognized, two major hurdles between discovery and application must yet be overcome: (1) The mutant gene is linked to opaque-2's soft, floury kernel, which is both light in weight and vulnerable to pest attacks, producing lower yields for farmers; and (2) opaque-2 has not been accepted by the majority of consumers, who are accustomed to the harder *flint* or *dent* kernels with a deeper, translucent color. But the need is great—human lives are at stake. So, plant breeders have set about crossing the opaque-2 gene on corn varieties that better meet the demands of farmers and consumers.

Supplementing Corn.

Corn, which is the basic human food in many parts of the Americas, is an excellent energy food when properly supplemented. Zein, the principal protein in corn, which forms about half of the total protein in the whole grain, is an imperfect protein; its biological value is about 60 (vs biological values of 94 and 85 for whole eggs and milk, respectively), it is almost devoid of lysine, and it contains very little tryptophan. As a result, kwashiorkor is altogether too common among children subsisting on high corn diets. Also, most of the niacin (nicotinic acid) in corn is in bound form and unavailable; for this and other reasons, pellagra is associated with high corn diets.

In the new mutant corn, opaque-2, the ratio between the protein fractions is changed, with the zein content lowered from about 50% to less than 30% of the protein. The net result of this changed ratio is that opaque-2 has a higher content of lysine and tryptophan than regular corn. For this reason, corn of this type can supply a larger part of the protein requirement in the diets of people than ordinary corn.

Fortunately, man does not normally derive protein from a single source; rather, he gets protein from a variety of sources. Moreover, it is well recognized that proteins of different sources mutually supplement each other; hence, blends of two or more protein sources usually possess a higher nutritive value than a single source protein. In most parts of the world, corn-based diets traditionally include small amounts of pulses—the seeds of leguminous plants. Pulses contain more protein than corn (beans, 20-28%; soybeans, 39-45%; corn, 8-11%), and usually they supply the amino acids not provided by corn, especially lysine. Hence, diets based on corn and a pulse possess a nutritive value that is significantly higher than those based on corn alone.

Also, as people prosper, their diet becomes more varied and the consumption of part of the corn is replaced by animal protein foods—meat, fish, milk, and eggs. Animal proteins have a significant supplemental value in relation to corn; they provide added protein, along with increased lysine, tryptophan, and niacin. Thus, animal protein can be used to supplement corn-based diets effectively.

CORN PRODUCTS AND USES.

Corn is used as food for man, for fermentation, for feed for livestock, and for industrial purposes. The U.S. annual supply of corn is used about as follows: livestock feed, 87%; human food, 11%; alcohol, 1.5%; and seed, 0.5%.

In one form or another, corn makes up more of our diet than any other farm crop. Corn-derived products are used

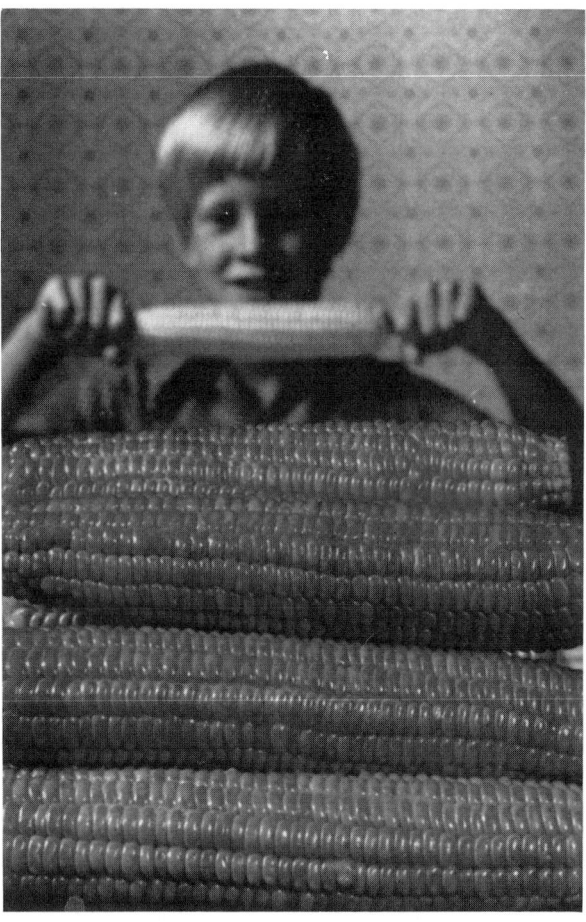

Fig. C-77. Sweet corn, grown chiefly for human food. (Courtesy, USDA)

in more than 800 different kinds of processed foods. Additionally, corn provides food indirectly; we eat it in the form of meat, milk, and eggs—products that come from animals raised on corn.

At the present time, few of the developing countries outside Latin America or Africa produce or utilize much corn as human food. However, these circumstances could change dramatically in the future, as the demand for cereals in the densely populated emerging nations continues to spiral and the great potential of corn becomes more fully appreciated. For example, the average corn yield in the United States is 2.5 tons per acre, compared to 0.9 tons per acre for wheat and 2.2 tons per acre for rice. Therefore, some special fortified foods, based on corn products, for use as low cost staple foods in developing countries are noteworthy (see Table C-23, section headed "Fortified Foods, Based on Corn Products, For Developing Countries."

Corn grain is fed to all classes of animals. It accounts for about 12% of all U.S. livestock feeds. Additionally, about 116 million tons of corn silage and enormous quantities of corn by-products are fed to animals each year.

The corn distilling and fermentation industries manufacture ethyl and butyl alcohols, acetone, and whiskey; and factories manufacture hundreds of nonedible corn products.

Table C-23 presents, in summary form, the story of corn products and uses for human food.

(Also see CEREAL GRAINS; FLOURS, Table F-12, Major Flours; OILS, VEGETABLE, Table O-5; and VEGETABLE[S], Table V-2, Vegetables of the World.)

TABLE C-23
CORN PRODUCTS AND USES FOR HUMAN FOOD

Product	Description	Uses	Comments
Corn grain, whole Corn on the cob	This is the whole grain, on or removed from the cob.	Roasted or boiled, freshly picked corn on the cob. Whole grain removed from the cob is consumed as succotash, chowder, pudding, popcorn, fritters, and parched corn.	Americans eat about 50 lb (22.7 kg) of corn per person per year. Corn kernels are a rich source of carbohydrates and fats. One lb or 0.5 kg (about 3 ears) of sweet corn on the cob contains about 240 Calories (kcal). Also, the kernels on four 5 in. (12.5 cm) ears of corn are about equal to the contents of one 12-oz (360-ml) can of vacuum packed corn.
Corn flakes	Manufactured from hominy by flavoring, rolling, and toasting.	Ready-to-eat breakfast cereal.	
Corn flour	The smallest particles of ground corn.	Pancake mixes, as a filler in various meat products, and as a substitute for wheat flour in baking.	Doughs made from corn flour lack sufficient elasticity (because of their low-gluten content) for making yeast-leavened breads.
Corn grits	Hominy ground into large particles.	Cooked cereal or starchy vegetable.	Grits were long served in one or more forms with almost every meal in southeastern United States. They are still served at many breakfasts, with a pat of butter and a dab of jam or jelly.
Corn, hominy	Deskinned, degerminated kernels of soaked dried corn. Hominy may be left whole and canned or frozen. Usually, it is ground into large particles (grits).	Starchy vegetable or cooked cereal.	Hominy is prepared from a hard type of corn (Dent or Flint) that is (1) dried on the cob; (2) shelled; (3) soaked in a solution of baking soda, lime, lye, or wood ashes (each of which is an alkali that can burn the skin); and (4) deskinned and degermed by rubbing. Whole hominy requires long soaking and cooking. Generally, it is served with butter.
Cornmeal	Whole or degerminated corn grain coarsely ground.	Corn bread, cooked cereal, cookies, tamales, tortillas, griddlecakes, and waffles.	Whole grain cornmeal spoils readily because of the high oil content of the germ. Hence, it should be kept in a freezer or refrigerator. Degerminated cornmeal serves well in most recipes. One pound (0.45 kg) of uncooked cornmeal yields about 13½ cups (3 l) of cooked cereal.
Cornmeal, enriched	Degerminated cornmeal with added thiamin, riboflavin, niacin, and iron.	Corn bread, cooked cereal, cookies, tamales, tortillas, griddlecakes, and waffles.	The federal standards for enriched cornmeals and enriched corn grits are: Ingredient — Required lb/(0.45 kg) of Cornmeal or Grits Thiamin . . . 2.0– 3.0 mg Riboflavin . . . 1.2– 1.8 mg Niacin . . . 16.0– 24.0 mg Iron . . . 13.0– 26.0 mg Calcium . . . 500.0–750.0 mg* *(optional)
Cornmeal, self-rising	Whole or degerminated cornmeal with added baking soda, salt, and one or more acidic salts such as monocalcium phosphate.	Corn bread, cookies, griddlecakes, and waffles.	Self-rising cornmeal contains its own leavening. Hence, no baking powder is required. One cup (0.24 l) of this product may contain up to 412 mg of calcium and 859 mg of phosphorus, depending upon the types and amounts of acidic salts that are added. The federal standards for enriched self-rising cornmeal are: Ingredient — Required lb/(0.45 kg) of Self-rising Cornmeal Thiamin . . . 2.0– 3.0 mg Riboflavin . . . 1.2– 1.8 mg Niacin . . . 16.0– 24.0 mg Iron . . . 13.0– 26.0 mg Calcium . . . 500.0–1750.0 mg* *(optional)
Corn oil (Also see OILS, VEGETABLE; and FATS AND OTHER LIPIDS.)	Corn oil is extracted from the germ of the kernel.	Salad dressings and cooking oil; and in such products as margarine and shortenings.	The oil is rich in essential fatty acids and contains moderate amounts of vitamin E.
Cornstarch	A white, odorless, tasteless, granular or powdery material.	Thicken puddings, gravies, and sauces; and in such products as candy, chewing gum, and baked goods.	The first step in the production of cornstarch involves the soaking of the corn in water and sulfur dioxide for 24 hours. This liquor is called corn steep liquor.
Corn sugar (dextrose) (Also see SUGAR.)	Converted from cornstarch.	Used in ice cream, frozen fruits, jams and jellies, bakery products, candy, carbonated beverages, many canned foods, and some meat products.	Dextrose (glucose) is the sugar present in the human bloodstream. Corn sugar is not as sweet as either honey or table sugar, because the latter items also contain fructose—one of the sweetest of the common sugars.
Corn syrup (Also see SYRUPS.)	Made by heating cornstarch with acid in closed tanks.	To sweeten many foods, and as a spread for bread, pancakes, and waffles.	Recently, a process was developed for converting some of the dextrose in corn syrup into fructose, thereby resulting in a sweeter syrup.

(Continued)

TABLE C-23 *(Continued)*

Product	Description	Uses	Comments
FORTIFIED FOODS, BASED ON CORN PRODUCTS, FOR DEVELOPING COUNTRIES			
CSM (corn-soy-milk)	A finely ground mixture of corn, soybean flour, skim milk powder, soybean oil, minerals, and vitamins. Contains 22% protein.	Substitute for milk.	Developed by the American Corn Millers' Federation in cooperation with the U.S. Department of Agriculture for use in the U.S. Food for Peace Program. On a par with the best of the cereal-based products for feeding young children. It may be supplemented with extra calories in the form(s) of sugar and/or peanut oil.
Golden elbow macaroni	Macaroni made with corn flour, soy flour, wheat flour, minerals, and vitamins. It contains about 20% protein.	Replacement for conventional macaroni products used as staple foods.	Developed by General Foods and test marketed in Brazil, where it was well accepted. Protein quality equals that of milk protein (casein).
Incaparina	Mixture of corn flour, cottonseed flour, torula yeast, minerals, and vitamins. It has a protein content of about 25%.	Cereal for weaning infants and young children.	Developed by the Institute of Nutrition of Central America and Panama (INCAP) with the aid of funds from Central American governments, Kellogg Foundation, Rockefeller Foundation, and several other foundations. Test marketed in Nicaragua, El Salvador, Guatemala, and Colombia.
Pronutro	A finely ground mixture of corn, skim milk powder, peanuts, soybeans, wheat germ, sugar, salt, minerals, vitamins, and flavoring(s). It has a protein content of about 22%.	Cereals, soups, gravies, beverages, and chocolate bars.	Developed without any governmental or international assistance by Hind Brothers, a private food firm in Natal, South Africa. Effective as skim milk powder in the rehabilitation of infants suffering from severe protein-energy malnutrition (kwashiorkor).
FERMENTED PRODUCTS **(Also see BEERS AND BREWING; DISTILLED LIQUORS)**			
Corn grain, whole	Cleaned, whole corn.	Bourbon whiskey.	Each year, about 1.5% of the U.S. corn crop is used by the fermentation processors. Whiskey is obtained from the distillation of fermented mash of cereal grain, and is aged in wooden barrels 2 to 8 years before sale. Bourbon whiskey is made from at least 51% corn. The rise of the whiskey industry in Kentucky dates to a time when it was easier and more profitable for a farmer to ship his corn east over the mountains in the form of whiskey rather than in sacks of grain.
Corn and other cereal grains	Cleaned, whole corn, wheat, rye, or barley.	Canadian whiskey.	
Cornstarch	Malt converts cornstarch to sugar, which is fermented by yeast to ethyl alcohol and carbon dioxide.	1. Ethyl alcohol, used largely for beverages. 2. Denatured alcohol for industrial purposes. (This is ethyl alcohol which has been rendered unfit for human consumption as a beverage by the addition of a denaturant.) 3. Gasohol (10% anhydrous ethanol/90% gasoline) a motor fuel.	
	Cornstarch, mostly in the form of grits, is used as a brewing adjunct, providing up to 40% of the mash.	Beer.	The Indians brewed beer from corn before Columbus discovered America. Certain African tribes consume about 40% of their corn supply in the form of beer, thereby receiving substantially greater amounts of the B vitamins than they would receive by consuming their corn in unfermented form.

CORNEA

The transparent circular membrane which covers the front of the eyeball. Good nutrition is important for corneal function. Hence, nutritional deficiencies may be indicated by abnormalities such as the appearance of tiny blood vessels at the edge of the cornea (corneal vascularization).

(Also see DEFICIENCY DISEASES.)

CORNED BEEF

Beef that has been cured in brine. Boneless cuts of brisket, plate, chuck, and round usually are used in making corned beef.

CORN STEEPWATER (CORN STEEPLIQUOR)

When corn is wet milled to make starch, sweeteners, and

oil, the first step is to soften or condition the kernel for grinding. This is accomplished by soaking the grain in a sulfurous acid steep for 28 to 48 hours. This liquor is called corn steepwater or corn steepliquor. When concentrated, steepwater is excellent for growing the mold that produces penicillin, because it contains a biochemical precursor of penicillin. It is also used in animal feeds.

(Also see CORN, section headed "Wet Milling," Fig. C-74 Schematic outline of the corn wet milling process.)

CORN, WAXY (MAIZE, WAXY)

Corn high in amylopectin, a starch which is used in the paper industry and as a coating or sizing in the fabrication of woven fiber glass.

CORONARY

A term referring to the heart and certain blood vessels that serve it.

CORONARY HEART DISEASE

A type of heart disease resulting from an obstruction in a coronary artery that reduces the flow of blood to the heart muscles. However, other types of disorders may be diagnosed as coronary heart disease. For example, the failure of diseased heart muscles to pump sufficient blood may result in a stagnation of blood flow, the formation of a clot, and a blockage of the coronary artery. In the latter case, the heart muscle weakness leads to the problem in the coronary artery rather than vice versa.

(Also see HEART DISEASE.)

CORTEX

The outside layer(s) of a gland or a special tissue, in contrast to the inner layers or medulla. For example, the adrenal cortex secretes steroid hormones; whereas, the adrenal medulla secretes catecholamine hormones (adrenaline and noradrenaline). However, the most important cortex is the cerebral cortex, which is the outer layer or thinking part of the human brain.

CORTICOSTEROIDS

A group of organic compounds secreted by the outside layer (cortex) of the adrenal gland in response to starvation and other stresses.

(Also see ENDOCRINE GLANDS.)

CORTICOSTERONE

A steroid hormone secreted by the adrenal cortex. Corticosterone promotes the formation of carbohydrate from protein and the breakdown of glycogen to glucose.

(Also see ENDOCRINE GLANDS.)

CORTICOTROPIN

Another name for ACTH, a hormone secreted by the pituitary gland.

(Also see ENDOCRINE GLANDS.)

CORTISOL

The major hormone from the adrenal cortex which raises the blood sugar through the conversion of glycogen and protein to glucose. Cortisol also counteracts the effect of insulin

so that there is a reduction in the rate at which glucose in the blood is picked up by the muscles and the fatty tissues of the body. However, it does not seem to slow the rate at which glucose is used by the brain. Hence, the net effect of the hormone is to ensure that there is a continuous supply of blood sugar for the brain.

(Also see ENDOCRINE GLANDS.)

CORYZA

An inflammation of the membranes in the nose that is often accompanied by a watery secretion. This disorder may be due to an allergy, an infection, or hay fever.

(Also see ALLERGY.)

COSTIVENESS

A type of constipation due to lack of sufficient water in the bowels. It is usually due to insufficient water-binding bulk in the diet. Hence, it may often be corrected by increasing the fiber content of the diet and drinking plenty of water.

(Also see CONSTIPATION.)

COTTONSEED *Gossypieum*

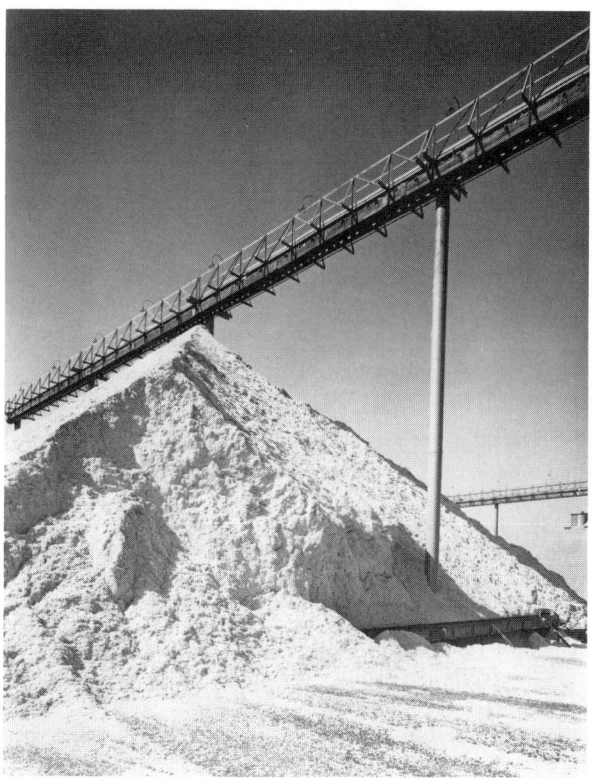

Fig. C-78. Cottonseed stored at mill, showing screw conveyer (above) which distributes the seed. (Courtesy, Rancher's Cotton Oil, Fresno, Calif.)

Cotton belongs to the genus *Gossypieum,* of which there are about 20 species, only four of which are cultivated. The four cultivatrd species are: *G. hirsutum,* American upland cotton; *G. barbadense,* Egyptian and Sea Island cottons; *G. herbaceum* and *G. arboreum,* the Asiatic cottons. Each of the four species embraces several varieties.

Cottonseed is the seed of the cotton plant, and cotton is the white fluff that grows attached to the seed. Cotton is grown primarily for its fiber (lint), which is used in making textiles, while the seed is used in making food for man and feed for livestock. Because this book pertains to food, the rest of this article will be devoted primarily to a discussion of cottonseed.

Cottonseed is a by-product of fiber production. With each 100 lb (*45 kg*) of fiber, the cotton plant yields approximately 170 lb (*77 kg*) of cottonseed.

The cottonseed, once largely wasted, is now converted into food, feed, and many other useful products. Oil is the most important product made from cottonseed; meal ranks second in importance.

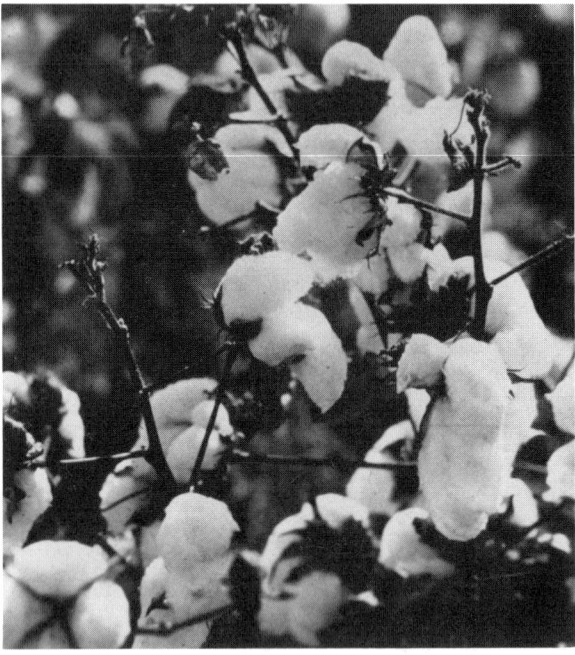

Fig. C-79. Cotton bolls: fully opened, mature cotton—one of the most beautiful and useful gifts of nature to man. (Courtesy, USDA)

ORIGIN AND HISTORY. Cotton has been grown for fiber for centuries. The Aztec Indians of Mexico grew cotton for textile purposes nearly 8,000 years ago. Record of cotton textiles, dating back about 5,000 years, was found in the Indus River Valley in what is now Pakistan. Excavations in Peru have uncovered cotton cloth identified as 4,500 years old. Cotton fabrics have also been found in the pueblo ruins in Arizona and in the ruins of some of the early civilizations of Egypt. The ancient peoples used cotton for clothing, and for many other necessities—ranging from bindings for sandals to elephant harnesses.

Although cotton was grown for its fiber for centuries, extensive use of the seed is of relatively recent origin. The ancient Hindus and Chinese developed crude methods for obtaining oil from cottonseed, using the principal of the mortar and the pestle. They used the oil for their lamps and fed the remainder of the processed seed to their cattle.

During the first part of the 19th century, mills in Europe began to crush Egyptian cottonseed on a limited scale. However, it remained for American machinists and chemists to transform cottonseed into useful products. For the most part, the oil came to be used for human food, and the meal and hulls were fed to cattle and sheep.

WORLD AND U.S. PRODUCTION. Worldwide, the production of cottonseed, from which cotton oil may be extracted, totals about 33,824,000 metric tons; and the ten leading cottonseed-producing countries, by rank, are: China, United States, U.S.S.R., India, Pakistan, Brazil, Turkey, Egypt, Australia, and Greece.[31]

U.S. production of cottonseed, from which oil may be extracted, totals about 5,966,500 short tons; and the ten leading U.S. cottonseed-producing states, by rank, are: Texas, California, Mississippi, Louisiana, Arkansas, Arizona, Tennessee, Oklahoma, Georgia, and Alabama.[32]

PROCESSING COTTONSEED. The usual steps in processing are:

1. **Cleaning.** Seeds are cleaned to remove any leaves, twigs, bolls, or dirt.

2. **Delinting.** The cleaned seeds are conveyed to the lint room where the short fibers, known as linters, are removed. The delinting machines use a series of circular saws designed to cut the short fibers. The linters are then collected and pressed into bales. Most mills run the seed through the delinting machine twice.

3. **Hulling.** Hulling is accomplished by a machine that employs a series of knives which cut the leathery hull and loosen it from the meat, following which the seeds are passed through a series of beaters, shakers, and separators which separate the loosened hulls from the meats.

4. **Removing oil.** The oil is removed by either of three methods. The methods, along with the proportion of the U.S. cottonseed production processed by each, are: screw processing, 40%; prepress solvent extraction, 28%; and direct solvent extraction, 32%.

NUTRITIONAL VALUE OF COTTONSEED. Typically, cottonseed is comprised of about 10% linters, 35% hull, and 55% kernels (meats). The kernels, from which food and feed are obtained, contain about 7% moisture, 30% oil, 30% crude protein, 24% nitrogen-free extract, 4.8% crude fiber, and 4.4% ash.

Cottonseed oil is classified as a polyunsaturated vegetable oil. Linoleic acid, its principal fatty acid, comprises about 47 to 50% of the total fatty acids. Its unique crystalline properties result from the presence of about 26% palmitic acid. Its good flavor is generally attributed to the absence of linoleic acid.

Table C-24 shows the composition of two defatted cottonseed flours that are suitable for human consumption—glandless (direct solvent) and glanded (liquid cyclone). Presently, neither product is available commercially on a large scale; nevertheless, they are feasible, and it is expected that supplies will increase with demand and price.

---

[31]Based on data from *FAO Production Yearbook 1990,* FAO/UN, Rome, Italy, Vol. 44, p. 120-121, Table 46. **Note well:** Annual production fluctuates as a result of weather and profitability of the crop.

[32]Based on data from *Agricultural Statistics 1991,* USDA, p. 106, Table 140. **Note well:** Annual production fluctuates as a result of weather and profitability of the crop.

TABLE C-24
COMPOSITION OF GLANDLESS AND GLANDED
COTTONSEED FLOURS[1]

	Glandless Direct Solvent	Glanded Liquid Cyclone
	(%)[2]	(%)[2]
Moisture	9.5	3.8
Crude fat	2.4	1.2
Crude fiber	3.3	2.3
Total gossypol	.06	.06
Free gossypol	.04	.02
Protein (N × 6.25)	54.7	66.2
Available lysine (g/16gN)	3.9	4.0
Nitrogen solubility	95.7	99.6

[1]Martinez, W. H., L. C. Berardi, and L. A. Goldblatt, Southern Regional Research Laboratory, New Orleans, La. "The Potential of Cottonseed: Products, Composition, and Use," paper presented at the Third International Congress of Food Science and Technology, Washington, D.C., August 9–14, 1970.

[2]All values in percent except lysine. The latter is in grams/16 grams of nitrogen.

Cottonseed flour, protein concentrates, and protein isolates are also obtained from the processing of cottonseed. The quality of the flour, therefore, is important not only from the standpoint of its edible use, but also as the raw material for the production of cottonseed concentrates and isolates.

The protein quality of cottonseed is inherently high. However, the effects of protein fractionation and processing techniques on amino acid availability must be recognized and balanced in the final food product. Lysine will probably be the major deficiency; and the limiting amino acid in cottonseed-cereal mixtures used for human food in some of the developing countries. Preservation of the existing lysine content by careful processing becomes one of the means of improving the nutritive potential of cottonseed protein.

As is true in any food formulation, the manufacturer will utilize the protein product which provides the most advantageous compromise between end-use functional requirements and cost; and each country must decide which use of its oilseed resources provides the most advantageous route toward an adequate supply of protein for its people. In some instances, the best route may be to use the oilseed proteins as feed for animals; in others the best use will be as food for man. If the need for protein becomes critical, food not feed should be the dominant course; and the potential of cottonseed is available to fulfill this need.

COTTONSEED PRODUCTS AND USES FOR HUMAN FOOD.
Of the four primary products of cottonseed—oil, cake or meal, hulls, and linters—oil is the most valuable. On the average, it accounts for slightly more than half of the total value of the four products. Cottonseed meal, the second most valuable product of cottonseed, accounts for 30 to 35% of the total product value.

In recent years, industry-wide yields of products per ton of seed have averaged 336 lb (151 kg) of oil, 936 lb (421 kg) of meal, 460 lb (207 kg) of hulls, and 168 lb (76 kg) of linters, with manufacturing loss of 100 lb (45 kg) per ton. These figures vary from area to area and from mill to mill, depending on the character of the seed, the type of process used, and the marketing practices.

Scientists and technologists are convinced that, because of its unique properties, the prospective new markets for cottonseed are food-oriented. Without doubt, this time will be hastened by the perfection and wide production of glandless cottonseed.

Table C-25 presents in summary form the story of cottonseed products and uses for human food.

(Also see OILS, VEGETABLE, Table O-5.)

Fig. C-80 shows cottonseed food uses.

TABLE C-25
COTTONSEED PRODUCTS AND USES FOR HUMAN FOOD

Product	Description	Uses	Comments
Cottonseed flour (Also see FLOURS, Table F-13, Special Flours.)	Finely ground cottonseed meal, containing 48 to 60% protein. Concentration to 70% protein can be achieved by extraction or particle classification.	In the bakery trade; to increase shelf life (because of its capacity to bind water), reduce fat absorption (especially in doughnuts), improve mixing and machining properties of the dough, and, in some cases, to impart a rich golden color to the bakery product. In meat products, such as hot dogs, luncheon meats, hamburger, sausage, and meat loaf; to retain fat and natural juices in the product, bind and hold the ground meat products together, and minimize shrinkage during cooking. In improving the diets of undernourished populations in the developing countries.	When the hulls are completely removed in the dehulling operation, cottonseed flour will contain substantially in excess of 50% protein. The presence of gossypol has been a major deterrent in the direct food utilization of cottonseed flour. Nevertheless, a food grade cottonseed flour, specially processed to minimize the toxicological properties of the gossypol, has been marketed for many years. In the future, meat analogs may be created from the protein of cottonseed flour.
Cottonseed oil	A high quality vegetable oil, processed from cottonseed and used primarily for human food, preferred because of its flavor stability. The crude oil extracted from the seed is usually subjected to the following processes: (1) refined, resulting in a clear yellow oil; (2) bleached to remove the color pigments, resulting in a clear white oil, preferred especially for shortening and margarine; (3) deodorized by exposing to steam under partial vacuum; and (4) winterized by reducing the temperature to 38° to 40°F (3° to 4°C), then removing the portion of the stearine that crystallizes or solidifies.	Salad oil, shortening, margarine, and mellorine. The principal use of cottonseed oil in the U.S. is in salad and cooking oils.	Cottonseed oil is one of the most important food oils, both in the U.S. and elsewhere. It is the third most widely consumed vegetable oil in the U.S., being exceeded only by soybean oil and palm oil. Mellorine is a frozen dessert that is comparable to ice cream in appearance and nutritive value. The fat content of this product is provided by vegetable oil. In the production of margarine, oil is hydrogenated.
Cottonseed linters	The short fibers removed from the seed after ginning.	Sausage casings	

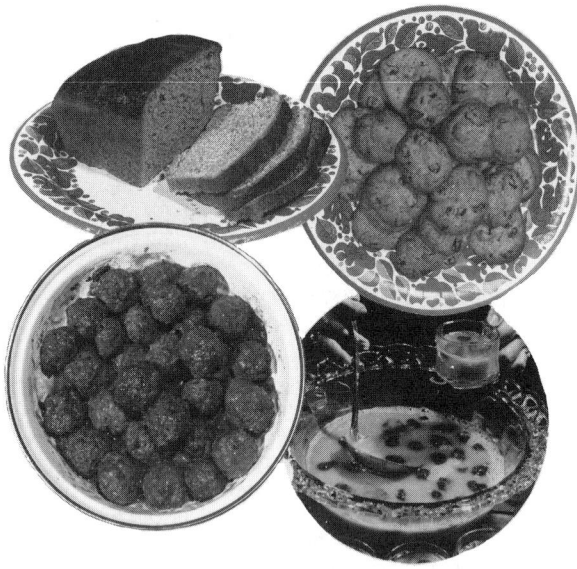

Fig. C-80. Foods fortified with cottonseed protein: top left, bread; top right, cookies; bottom left, meatballs; bottom right, Rio punch with strawberries. (Courtesy, USDA)

COUMARIN

Coumarin is found in certain plants, including sweet clover. During the process of spoiling, the natural coumarin in sweet clover is converted to dicoumarol (bishydroxycoumarin). Coumarin was formerly used in the synthesis of dicoumarol, but most dicoumarol is made synthetically today.

Coumarin was previously used as an anticlotting agent and as a flavor for tobacco, butter, and medicines. Today, it is used as a deodorizing and odor-enhancing agent, in perfumery and soap. Presently, the use of coumarin in food and feed products is prohibited by the Food and Drug Administration.

The properties and uses of coumarin and dicoumarol are very dissimilar. Today, coumarin is not used as an anticlotting agent, whereas the primary use of dicoumarol is for this purpose.

CRACKLINGS

The term applied to pressed, rendered pork fat remaining after the lard has been extracted.

CRANBERRY Vaccinium spp

This berry type of fruit grows on viny plants that belong to the heath family *Ericaceae,* which also includes bilberries, blueberries, huckleberries, and certain nonedible plants such as azaleas, heathers, mountain laurel, and rhododendrons.

Most Americans associate cranberries with the celebration of Thanksgiving and Christmas, although many people now consume them in one form or another throughout the year.

ORIGIN AND HISTORY. Cranberries are native to the bogs and marshes of the northern United States. They were first cultivated in Massachusetts.

WORLD AND U.S. PRODUCTION. The cranberry is almost exclusively an American product, little known to the rest of the world. Approximately 170 short tons of cranber-

ries are produced annually in the United States; and the leading cranberry-producing states, by rank, are: Wisconsin, Massachusetts, New Jersey, Oregon, and Washington.[33]

PROCESSING. About 80% of the cranberry crop is processed. Some of the processed berries are made directly into cranberry juice drinks and the traditional types of cranberry sauces (mainly those made from either pureed or whole berries). The rest of the processed berries are frozen in bulk for later production of these items.

SELECTION, PREPARATION, AND USES. Good quality in cranberries is indicated by a fresh, plump appearance, combined with high luster and firmness.

Fresh cranberries can be stored in a refrigerator for several months, or they may be kept in deep-freeze storage for several years with only minimal loss of moisture. However, the frozen berries become very soft upon thawing and should be utilized immediately in order to avoid spoilage.

The various cranberry products may be utilized in ways such as those which follow:

1. Fresh cranberries may be made into an uncooked relish by chopping them in a food grinder with quartered oranges (after removal of any seeds), apples, and/or other raw fruit. The chopped fruit mixture should be sweetened with honey or sugar and stored in a refrigerator until it is used.

2. The fruit is good when cooked and sweetened in preparations such as gelatin desserts, jam, jelly, pies (cranberries alone or in combination with apples, mincemeat, or peaches), and sauces.

3. Canned cranberry sauce (pureed or whole berry) is not only good with meats or poultry, but also when substituted for the fillings, spreads, and toppings commonly added to baked products, ice cream, puddings, and other desserts.

4. Cranberry juice cocktails may be used alone or when mixed with unflavored soda water or gingerale.

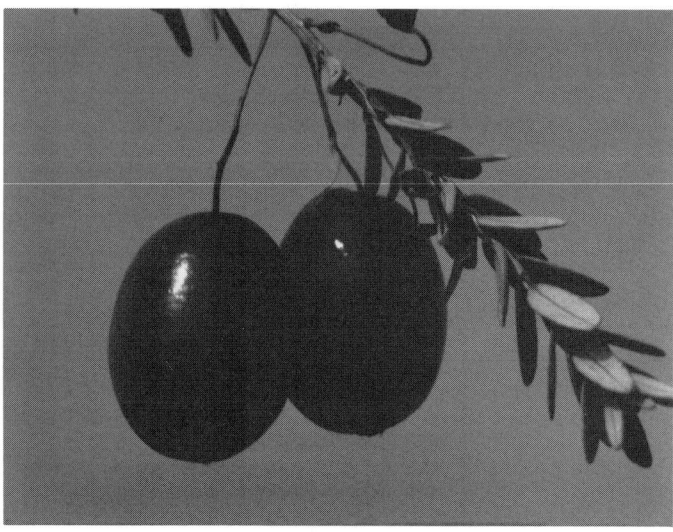

Fig. C-81. Cranberries. (Courtesy, Rutgers, The State University of New Jersey, New Brunswick, N.J.)

[33]Based on data from *Agricultural Statistics 1991,* USDA, p. 195, Table 289. **Note well:** Annual production fluctuates as a result of weather and profitability of the crop.

NUTRITIONAL VALUE. The nutrient compositions of various cranberry products are given in Food Composition Table F-21.

Some noteworthy observations regarding the nutrient composition of some of the more common cranberry products follow:

1. Raw cranberries are fairly low in calories (46 kcal per 100 g) and carbohydrates (11%). They are a good source of fiber and bioflavonoids, and a fair source of potassium and vitamin C. Hence, they may be sweetened with an artificial sweetener and used in various low calorie dishes.

2. Cranberry-orange relish that has been sweetened with a caloric sweetener (corn syrup, honey, sugar, etc.) usually contains about four times the calories and carbohydrates that are present in raw cranberries, but the levels of the other nutrients are approximately the same in the relish and the raw fruit.

3. Canned cranberry sauce is high in calories (145 kcal per 100 g) and carbohydrates (38%), and is low in most other nutrients.

4. Most types of cranberry juice drinks are sweetened with caloric sweeteners and fortified with added vitamin C. Hence, they are likely to contain moderate amounts of calories (about 60 kcal per 3½ oz [100 g]) and carbohydrates (about 15%), and to be good sources of vitamin C. It is noteworthy that artificially sweetened cranberry drinks and unsweetened juices are available which contain only about ¼ of the calories and carbohydrates of the beverages that contain added caloric sweetener(s).

5. Cranberry juice has long been prescribed by some doctors to reduce the likelihood that calcium phosphate stones will form in the urinary tract. (Cranberries contain quinic acid which is not broken down in the body but is excreted unchanged in the urine. Hence, it serves to make the urine mildly acidic, a condition that keeps calcium and phosphate ions from forming insoluble stones. Some doctors also believe that in certain cases stones already formed may be dissolved.)

6. New England folk medicine has it that a mixture of boiled cranberries and seal oil will reduce the severity of a gallbladder attack. The truth of this belief has not been confirmed by medical science, but it is noteworthy that acid (amply present in cranberries) and fat (seal oil) stimulate the release of bile from the gallbladder, thereby preventing the stagnation of bile that sometimes leads to the formation of gallstones.

7. The color of ripe cranberries is due mainly to anthocyanin pigment(s) (anthocyanins are a type of bioflavonoid) that certain European researchers have found to (a) accelerate the regeneration of visual purple (the pigment in the eyes that is involved in vision), (b) aid in the adaptation of the eyes to the dark, and (c) inhibit the formation of tumors. **NOTE:** These findings have not been confirmed by researchers in the United States. Hence, the authors make no claims regarding the benefits of consuming foods that contain anthocyanins; rather, the findings are reported (1) for informational purposes, and (2) in order to stimulate interest in additional research.

(Also see BIOFLAVONOIDS; and FRUIT[S].)

CREAM, CLOTTED (DEVONSHIRE CREAM)

This is a high fat content cream, prepared by allowing cream to rise on milk, setting it by heating and cooling then skimming it from the underlying skim milk.

CREAM, CORNISH

This is a high fat content cream, similar to clotted cream or Devonshire cream. But it is prepared by scalding the cream alone, not floated on a layer of milk.

CREAM LINE

The place where the risen cream meets the milk.

CREAM LINE INDEX

This is the ratio of the percentage cream layer to the percentage of fat in the milk. It is used as a test of the milk. In ordinary bulk milk it is about 1:7.

CREAM OF TARTAR (POTASSIUM BITARTRATE, ACID TARTRATE, ACID TARTRATE OF POTASH [$KHC_4H_4O_6$])

Take your choice of name, but whatever you call it, this acid is a white odorless powder with an acid taste. Besides its use in leavenings, it can be used as a diuretic and to neutralize alkaline urine.

(Also see BAKING POWDER AND BAKING SODA.)

CREAM, PLASTIC

Cream that has been centrifuged at high speed causing it to form an oil-in-water emulsion; used for preparation of cream cheese and whipped cream.

CREATINE

A nitrogenous compound formed in the liver, which is converted to phosphocreatine in muscle, where it serves as a source of high energy phosphate for muscle contraction. Greater than normal amounts of creatine are excreted in the urine when muscle disorders and other abnormal conditions are present. In muscular dystrophy, the muscle is unable to accept creatine, and it is excreted in the urine.

The anhydride of creatine is creatinine, in which form it is found in urine. Changes in the excretory function of the kidneys are reflected in plasma urea and creatinine concentrations. Glomerular filtration rate (GFR) and overall kidney function is conveniently estimated by measuring creatinine clearance in the volume of urine excreted in 1 minute. Its value is about 125 ml/minute in healthy young men. It is usually a little less in young women; and at 70 years of age it is about 75% of the value in youth. Kidney failure rarely produces symptoms until the GFR falls below 30 ml/minute.

CREATININE

A nitrogenous compound arising from protein metabolism and excreted in the urine.

(Also see PROTEINS.)

CREATININE COEFFICIENT

The amount of urinary creatinine excreted in 24 hours divided by the body weight in kilograms. Creatinine is formed from phosphocreatine in muscle and is excreted in fairly constant amounts each day. Hence, the amount of urinary creatinine which is excreted under uniform conditions may be taken as an indication of the total muscle mass.

CREME

Cream or cream sauce as used in cookery.

CROHN'S DISEASE (REGIONAL ENTERITIS)

This mysterious and frustrating intestinal disorder goes by a variety of names, including Crohn's Disease (after the New York physician who first described it), regional enteritis, ileitis, and granulomatous colitis, depending on which part of the intestinal tract is affected. It is an intermittent and chronic inflammation of the small and large intestines, in which hardening, thickening, and eventual ulceration of parts of the bowel lining occur.

The cause is unknown, although researchers suspect that a virus or a flaw in the body's immune system may be involved.

CROQUETTES

Croquettes can be made from chopped beef, chicken, crab, egg, fish, ham, lobster, oyster, salmon, sweetbreads, or veal. The chopped, cooked meat is mixed with seasonings and flour, egg, etc. This mixture is formed into the traditional croquette shape, which is like a small cone. They are rolled in crumbs, dipped in beaten egg, rolled in crumbs again, and fried in deep fat. They are served with or without a sauce, depending on the recipe of choice.

CROUTONS

Dried cubes of bread, seasoned or unseasoned, homemade or commercially manufactured, which are added to soups and salads.

CROWDIES

A type of fermented milk in Scotland.

CRUCIFEROUS VEGETABLES

Vegetables belonging to or having the characteristics of the mustards or related plants, including broccoli, Brussels sprouts, cabbage, cauliflower, mustard, rutabagas, and turnips.

CRYPTOXANTHIN

A yellow pigment which may be converted to vitamin A in the body. It is found mainly in such foods as corn, oranges, and paprika.
(Also see VITAMIN A.)

CUCUMBER AND GHERKIN Cucumis spp

These crops together rank among the top nine vegetable crops of the world, although in the developed countries they are used more as condiments than as vegetables. The cucumber (C. sativus) is long and cylindrical, whereas the closely-related gherkin (C. anguria) is much smaller and is shaped more like a miniature football. Gherkins are thought to be a mutant of the African wild species, C. longipes. Sometimes, small cucumbers are erroneously called gherkins. However, the growing, processing, preparation, and nutritional values of the two vegetables are sufficiently similar to warrant their joint coverage here. Both species belong to the gourd or melon family (Cucurbitaceae), which also includes pumpkins and squashes. Only the immature fruits of these plants are commonly consumed, but some peoples in Southeast Asia also eat the young leaves and the seeds of the mature fruit.

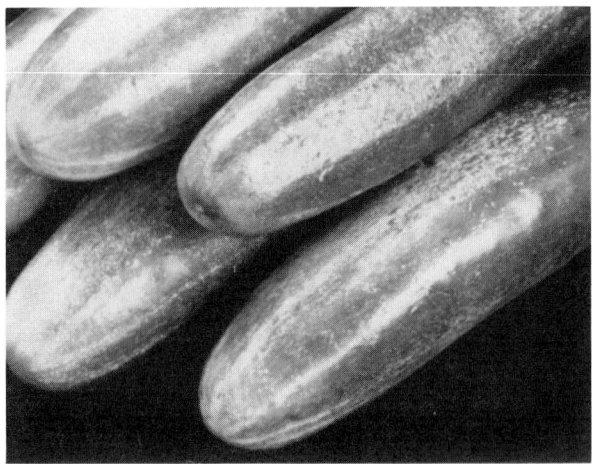

Fig. C-82. Cucumbers. (Courtesy, USDA)

ORIGIN AND HISTORY. Both the cucumber and the gherkin are tropical plants. However, the modern form of the cucumber is not found growing wild. Hence, it must have been developed from a wild ancestor. Present thinking is that the cucumber did not originate in India or Africa as was first thought, but that it originated in Southeast Asia where seeds judged to be about 12,000 years old have been found. Perhaps the cucumber was brought from the Far East to Central Asia and India by ancient land travelers, or by the seafaring peoples who migrated as far as Madagascar. However, the gherkin appears to have been developed from a wild plant that is native to Africa.

The ancient Egyptians ate cucumbers and/or gherkins, for it is recorded that the Hebrews longed for them while being led out of Egypt by Moses. Cucumbers were also highly esteemed by the ancient Greeks and Romans, as evidenced in their writings. It is not certain when the fruit was first pickled, but it is noteworthy that Roman emperors had pickles imported from Spain. Gherkins were brought to the New World during the early days of African slave trading and became an important crop in the West Indies.

In recent times, the English have developed seedless varieties of cucumbers that set fruit without pollination and are grown exclusively in greenhouses from which bees are excluded. Pollination of these varieties results in seedy, bitter fruit that is unsuitable for marketing.

WORLD AND U.S. PRODUCTION. Cucumbers and gherkins rank ninth among the leading vegetable crops of the world. About 13.3 million metric tons of cucumbers and gherkins are produced worldwide, annually. The leading cucumber and gherkin-producing countries, by rank, are: China, Japan, Turkey, United States, Romania, Netherlands, Iraq, Poland, Egypt, and Spain.[34]

Cucumbers rank ninth among the vegetable crops of the United States, with a production of about 656,570 short tons annually.[35]

---

[34] Based on data from *FAO Production Yearbook 1990*, FAO/UN, Rome, Italy, Vol. 44, p. 136, Table 55. **Note well:** Annual production fluctuates as a result of weather and profitability of the crop.

[35] Based on data from *Agricultural Statistics 1991*, USDA, p. 154, Table 216. **Note well:** Annual production fluctuates as a result of weather and profitability of the crop.

Cucumber seeds are planted in the field when there is no longer any danger of frost and the temperature ranges from 60° to 75°F (16° to 24°C). Furthermore, the plants grow best when the daytime temperature is around 85°F (30°C) and the night temperature ranges from 65° to 70°F (19° to 22°C). Hence, production of this crop during the winter is limited to the warmest areas of the southern states. In the northern states, the seeds may be planted early in the spring in greenhouses or hotbeds, then the seedlings may be transplanted in the field when the weather warms up. Elsewhere, cucumbers are grown in the field from spring to fall.

The soil should be deeply cultivated, well drained, neutral to mildly alkaline, and rich in both inorganic and organic nutrients. Therefore, many growers may find it necessary to add lime, nitrogen, phosphorus, potassium, and compost or manure. However, compost should not be made from the residues of plants belonging to the gourd or melon family, because diseases may be spread among the different species of this family.

Irrigation is often needed when the crop is grown commercially. Furrow irrigation is the best way to water the plants because sprinklers wet the leaves and increase the likelihood of disease.

Many home gardeners and greenhouse producers of cucumbers (in Great Britain, the entire crop is grown in greenhouses) train the vines to climb trellises or special wire frameworks so that the maximum production of fruit per unit of land may be obtained. One vine may yield 100 cucumbers.

The fruit is ready for picking in about 2 months after planting. Removal of the cucumbers allows the vines to set more fruit, whereas the vines stop fruiting if the fruit is not picked. Cucumbers are rarely allowed to reach maturity because the development of mature seeds requires large amounts of nutrients and stresses the vines excessively. The worldwide average yield of cucumbers is 12,856 lb per acre (14,413 kg/ha) but yields as high as 265,000 lb per acre (296,800 kg/ha) are obtained in British greenhouses. In comparison, the U.S. average yield per acre is 11,319 lb (12,689 kg/ha), but yields as high as 31,600 lb (35,392 kg/ha) are obtained in California fields.

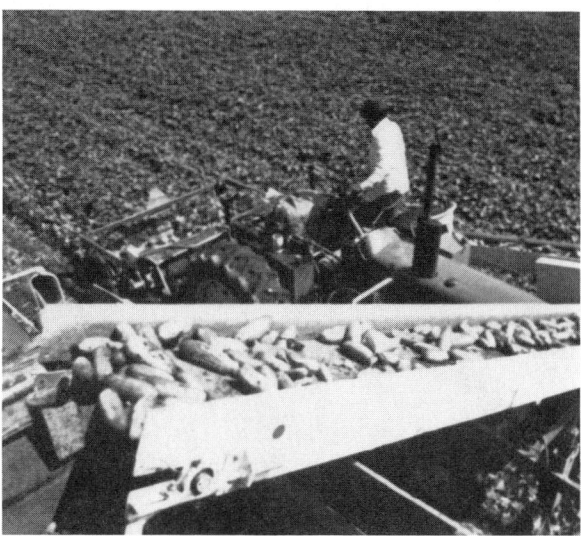

Fig. C-83. Harvesting cucumbers. (Courtesy, USDA)

PROCESSING. Over 70% of the U.S. cucumber and gherkin crop is made into pickles. The major operations utilized in the production of cucumber pickles are (1) fermentation of whole or sliced cucumbers in a concentrated salt solution called a brine; (2) soaking of the pickles in hot water to remove some of the salt; and (3) canning the pickles in a mixture of vinegar and various seasonings.

SELECTION, PREPARATION, AND USES. Cucumbers should be firm, fresh, bright, well-shaped, and medium to dark green in color. A small amount of whitish green color at the tip and on the ridged seams is not objectionable in certain varieties. The flesh should be firm and the seeds immature.

Raw cucumbers or pickles may be diced or sliced and added to relish trays, salads, and sandwiches. It is noteworthy that the slightly bitter flavor of the raw vegetable is improved by dressing with acid-flavored items such as lemon juice, mayonnaise, sour cream, vinegar, and yogurt; whereas pickles are acid-flavored to begin with, and have no need for such dressing.

Although cucumbers are rarely cooked, they are an adventure in good eating when (1) boiled and served with a special sauce; (2) grated and added to a soup; (3) stewed or roasted with meat; (4) sliced, dipped in egg batter or flour, and fried; (5) stewed with tomatoes; and (6) hollowed out by removal of the seeds, stuffed with bread crumbs, cheese, chopped eggs, meat, nuts, or poultry, and baked.

NUTRITIONAL VALUE. The nutrient compositions of various forms of cucumbers are given in Food Composition Table F-21.

Some noteworthy observations regarding the nutrient composition of cucumbers follow:

1. Fresh cucumbers have a very high water content (95%), and they are low in calories (15 kcal per 100 g) and most other nutrients. However, they are a fair source of iron, potassium, vitamin A, and vitamin C. Most of the vitamin A is in the rind. Hence, peeled cucumbers contain only traces of this vitamin.

2. The different types of cucumber pickles and relishes vary widely in their compositions, which depend mainly upon the ingredients and procedures used in processing. For example, dill pickles, sour pickles and sour relishes contain from 93 to 95% water and only 10 to 19 Calories (kcal) per 3½ oz (100 g) serving, whereas the sweet pickles and relishes contain on the average only 62% water and a whopping 142 Calories (kcal) per 100 g. The much higher caloric contents of the sweet items are due mainly to the sugar and/or other sweeteners that are used in their production.

It is noteworthy that the nutrient compositions of pickles differ from that of fresh cucumbers in that the former generally have a high sodium content and are poor sources of vitamins A and C. Sour pickles contain much more sodium and iron than sweet pickles. Some types of dietetic pickles are very low in sodium.

3. Practitioners of herbal medicine have long held that the consumption of cucumbers induces copious urination, which may be helpful in ridding the body of excessive water and purging the blood of potentially harmful substances such as uric acid. However, pickles would be more likely to induce retention of water in the body by virtue of their high sodium content. **NOTE:** The authors make no claim regarding the veracity of these beliefs. Rather, they are presented here to stimulate further research on the subject.

CURD

The coagulated or thickened part of milk. Curd from whole milk consists of casein, fat, and whey, whereas curd from skim milk contains casein and whey, but only traces of fat.

(Also see MILK PRODUCTS.)

CURD TENSION

A measure of toughness of the curd formed from milk by the digestive enzymes and used as an index of the digestibility of the milk.

CUSHING'S SYNDROME

A group of symptoms associated with Cushing's disease, first described in 1932 by Dr. Harvey Williams Cushing, famous American brain surgeon. The disease, which seems to affect women primarily, is due to the oversecretion of adrenocortical hormone. Excesses of these hormones promote obesity of the trunk, face, and buttocks. It also produces a weakening of the muscles, because the protein in muscle is broken down and converted to sugar in the blood. Hence, there may also be a diabetic condition. Older people who have had this condition for a long time tend to develop a hump on their back (buffalo hump) which results from an abnormal deposit of fat, and they also develop a rounded face (moon face). Women with Cushing's disease develop excessive hair growth, such as mustaches and beards.

If the diagnosis is made relatively early, before the onset of heart and kidney involvement, a patient can be helped. When the adrenal gland becomes enlarged, a cure may be effected by surgery. In a third to a half of the cases where the pituitary gland is involved, x-ray therapy may halt or slow the progress of the disease.

(Also see ENDOCRINE GLANDS.)

CYCLAMATES

Compounds which were formerly used as artificial sweeteners. Their use for this purpose was banned by the FDA because it was found that toxic metabolites were sometimes formed. However, cyclamates were reclassified as drugs so that they might be used under medical supervision.

CYSTEINE

A nonessential, sulfur-containing amino acid. However, it may to a limited degree spare the essential amino acid methionine. Furthermore, it is converted in the body to the amino acid cystine, an important constituent of hair.

(Also see AMINO ACID[S].)

CYSTIC DUCT

The tube between the gallbladder and the common bile duct, through which the gallbladder discharges its bile to the small intestine. Occasionally, gallstones may lodge in the cystic duct and block the flow of bile from the gallbladder.

(Also see GALLSTONES.)

CYSTIC FIBROSIS

A disease characterized by general malfunctioning of various secretory glands in the body. It usually results in death unless a combined therapy is undertaken immediately. The therapy involves (1) a special diet which provides missing enzymes in purified form, (2) treatment of digestive disorders, and (3) careful control of respiratory infections.

(Also see DISEASES.)

CYSTINE

One of the nonessential amino acids. It is sulfur-containing and may be used in part to meet the need for methionine.

(Also see AMINO ACID[S].)

CYSTOLITHIASIS

The presence of stones in the urinary bladder. The condition is usually treated with a special diet, and medication to dissolve the stones.

(Also see KIDNEY STONES.)

-CYTE

Suffix meaning cell.

CYTOCHROME

A class of iron-porphyrin proteins of great importance in cell metabolism.

CYTOLOGY

The anatomy, chemistry, pathology, and physiology of the cell.

CYTOPLASM

Substance within the cell exclusive of the nucleus.

CYTOSINE

One of the nitrogenous bases in nucleic acid.
(Also see NUCLEIC ACIDS.)

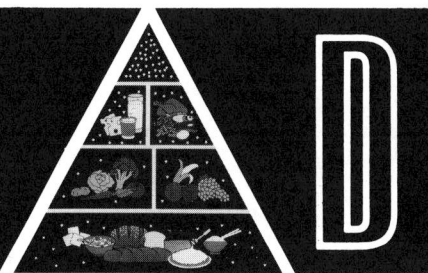

DADHI

A type of fermented milk in India.

DAIRY PRODUCTS

This generally refers to all products made from milk.

DARK ADAPTATION

The rate at which a person's eyes adapt to a change from bright light to darkness. A slower than normal rate may indicate a vitamin A deficiency.

(Also see VITAMIN A.)

DATE *Phoenix dactylifera*

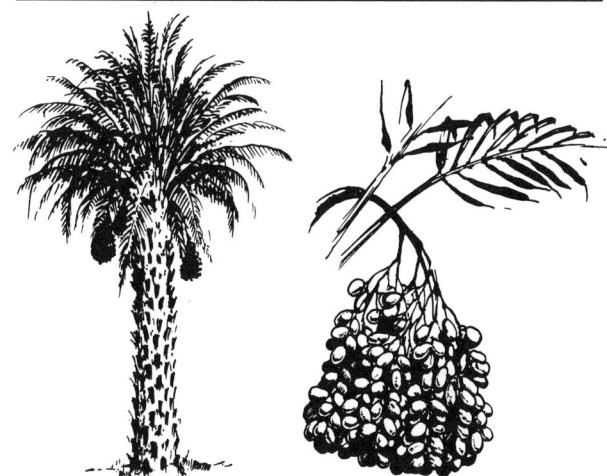

Fig. D-1. Clusters of dates that may have up to 200 dates each hanging from a palm tree.

The date palm belongs to the palm family, *Palmae.*

Next to the coconut palm, the date palm is the most useful tree in the palm family. It produces the fruit that provides one of the chief articles of food in North Africa and the Middle East.

Fruits of the date palm, *Phoenix dactylifera,* are over 1 in (2.5 cm) long, sweet, fleshy, oblong, and contain a single seed. They grow in clusters that contain up to 200 dates and weigh up to 25 lb (11 kg). While hanging on the tree, dates are a rich red to golden brown.

ORIGIN AND HISTORY. The date palm is native to the dry areas of southwestern Asia. It was likely the first cultivated tree in history; it has been under cultivation in the Holy Land for at least 8,000 years. About 1,700 years ago, it was introduced into China from Iran. Then, in the 17th century, the Spanish took it to California.

WORLD AND U.S. PRODUCTION. Worldwide, about 3.4 million metric tons of dates are produced annu-

ally; and the leading producing countries, by rank, are: Egypt, Iran, Saudi Arabia, Iraq, Pakistan, and Algeria.[1]

Dates are a minor fruit in the United States. California, which accounts for most of the commercial crop, produces about 24,000 short tons each year.[2]

SELECTION, PREPARATION, AND USES. The fruit should be fleshy and rich in color.

Dates are served alone, fresh or dried, or used in various dishes such as fruit dishes, baked goods, candies, ice cream, salads and syrups.

In the Arab world, dates are commonly consumed with milk products which bolster the protein content.

A fermented maceration of dates yields an alcoholic beverage called *arrak,* which Pedro Texeira, a 16th century traveler, described as, "the strongest and most dreadful drink ever invented." The date pits are roasted, ground and used as a coffee substitute in some countries. Additionally, like many other palms, date palms provide a food supply from the sugary sap which can be obtained by tapping the crown of the plant. This can be boiled down to provide sugar, or it can be fermented to make palm wine or toddy. When the tree is cut down, the tender terminal bud is eaten as a vegetable or salad.

NUTRITIONAL VALUE. The chief nutritional value of dates is their high sugar content, which varies from about 60% in soft dates to as much as 70% in some dry types. Most varieties contain glucose or fructose sugar, but one variety, Deglet Noor, grown primarily in California, contains only sucrose sugar. The dried fruit contains about 271 kcal per 100 g, 2.3% fiber, 1.0 mg iron per 100 g, 666 mg potassium per 100 g, and 2.2 mg niacin per 100 g. But dates contain little or no vitamin C. Complete nutritional information on dates may be found in Food Composition Table F-21.

DEAERATION

Removal of air, without removing moisture. In the processing of milk, it refers to vacuumization for removal of undesirable volatile substances that impart odors.

DEAMINATION

A process in protein metabolism whereby an amino group is removed from an amino acid through the action of an enzyme called deaminase. This reaction occurs in the liver and in the kidneys.

(Also see METABOLISM, Section on Protein "Catabolism".)

---

[1]Based on data from *FAO Production Yearbook 1990,* FAO/UN, Rome, Italy, Vol. 44, p. 155, Table 66. **Note well:** Annual production fluctuates as a result of weather and profitability of the crop.

[2]Based on data from *Agricultural Statistics 1991,* USDA, p. 177, Table 254. **Note well:** Annual production fluctuates as a result of weather and profitability of the crop.

DEBILITY

Weakness.

DECALCIFICATION

A loss of calcium from the bones and teeth which may occur when (1) the diet contains too little calcium to replace the daily losses of the mineral in the urine and the stool, or (2) overactivity of the parathyroid glands causes demineralization.

(Also see CALCIUM; and OSTEOPOROSIS.)

DECARBOXYLATION

A metabolic reaction in which a decarboxylase enzyme brings about the removal of carbon and oxygen from a molecule.

(Also see METABOLISM.)

DECIDUOUS TEETH

Another name for the baby teeth which are lost in the early years of life and replaced by the permanent teeth.

(Also see DENTAL HEALTH, NUTRITION, AND DIET.)

DECORTICATION

• Removal of the bark, hull, husk, or shell from a plant, seed, or root.

• Removal of portions of the cortical substance of a structure or organ, as in the brain, kidney, and lung.

DEFIBRILLATION

Any means by which an irregular beating of the heart muscle fibers is brought back to normal.

(Also see HEART DISEASE.)

DEFIBRILLATOR

An electrical device which converts an irregular beating of the heart muscle fibers to a normal rhythmic pattern.

(Also see HEART DISEASE.)

DEFICIENCY DISEASES

Contents   Page

These diseases result from dietary shortages of one or more essential nutrients. They may be prevented or cured by the administration of the missing nutrient(s), except when there is irreparable damage to vital tissues of the body.

EATING PATTERNS WHICH LEAD TO DIETARY DEFICIENCIES. Although hunger due to a lack of a sufficient quantity of food often causes a deficiency disease(s), the factors which lead to this problem are discussed elsewhere. (See HUNGER, WORLD; MALNUTRITION, PROTEIN-ENERGY; POPULATION, WORLD; and WORLD FOOD.) Herein, the dietary patterns which may cause deficiency diseases even though sufficient quantity of food is available are identified as follows:

1. Lack of sufficient variety of foods.
2. Use of highly refined foods.
3. Dependence on starchy fruits and vegetables.
4. Foods containing substances which interfere with nutrient utilization.
5. Destruction or loss of nutrients during cooking.
6. Foods grown in mineral-deficient soils.
7. Protein-deficient diets.

TYPES OF DIETARY DEFICIENCY DISEASES. It is common practice to classify deficiency diseases according to the ways in which they are produced. Thus, diseases directly due to deficient levels of dietary nutrients are said to be *primary deficiencies,* while those due to substances which interfere with utilization of marginal to adequate levels of nutrients are called *secondary deficiencies.*

Primary deficiencies are often divided into two groups: The *major deficiency diseases* where there are severe impairments of vital functions such as heart action, vision, energy metabolism, or tissue growth; and the *minor deficiency disorders* which are characterized by irritating and/or unsightly conditions such as skin lesions, loss of ankle and knee reflexes, or mottled teeth. The features of each group of deficiencies are outlined in Tables D-1 and D-2.

Secondary deficiencies result from some type of interference with what otherwise might be adequate intakes of nutrients. The end results of such interferences are essentially the same as those outlined under primary deficiencies.

PREVENTION AND TREATMENT OF DIETARY DEFICIENCIES. There are several basic approaches to preventing and treating dietary deficiency diseases. These follow.

• **Adhering to dietary patterns based upon food groups—** The aim of this approach is to encourage people to select a variety of foods from among such designated food groups as bread, cereal, rice, and pasta; vegetables; fruit; meat, poultry, fish, dry beans, eggs, and nuts; milk, yogurt, and cheese; and fats, oils, and sweets.

• **Enriching and fortifying preferred foods**—The aim here is either to restore some of the nutrients removed during processing (this action is called *enrichment*), or to add nutrients in amounts which were not present in the foods in the first place (the process of *fortification*).

(Also see ENRICHMENT; and FORTIFICATION.)

• **Increasing the use of special food products which are high in nutrients**—Livestock are fed the *lion's share* of the highly nutritious by-products of food processing like brewers' yeast, distillers' grains, wheat germ, bran, whey, and blackstrap molasses. While it would be wrong to overemphasize these items (dietary excesses of any concentrated source of nutrients may lead to nutritional problems), perhaps there should be more effort to promote their incorporation into such food items as breads, buns, cakes, drinks, and ice cream.

• **Producing new, fabricated foods**—Food technologists have recently begun to use the term *nutrification* to denote the addition of nutrients to fabricated foods. What is often overlooked in this approach is the possibility that processing alters, destroys, or removes nutrients or other beneficial substances which are not replaced by enrichment or fortification. For example, some of the totally synthetic orange drink powders contain such ingredients as sugar, citric acid, ascorbic acid (vitamin C), artificial flavoring, and artificial coloring. These items may replace orange juice which contains such additional constituents as potassium and the bioflavonoids.

• **Increasing mineral and vitamin supplements**—This might be the least expensive way to cover nutrient deficiencies in ordinary diets. However, nutritionists are concerned that the promotion of nutrient supplements in the forms of pills or tonics might lead the public away from selecting foods which are good sources of the essential nutrients.

(Also see MINERALS; and VITAMINS.)

• **Using megadoses of certain nutrients periodically**—Some of the outlying areas of Africa, Asia, and Latin America are inhabited by people suffering from deficiency diseases; yet public health personnel can pay only infrequent visits to those areas. These conditions have led to the development of types of nutritional therapy which have long-term effects and which need only periodic administration. For example, goiter may be prevented in regions where there are scarcities of iodine-containing foods by the periodic injection (as infrequently as once every 4 years) of iodized oil.[3] Likewise, injections of megadoses of vitamin A (200,000

IU every 6 months) have been used in India, Asia, and Latin America.[4]

Finally, monthly injections of vitamin B-12 are the only practical means of treating people who lack the intrinsic factor which is required for the intestinal absorption of this vitamin.

Treatment of severe deficiencies may require therapeutic amounts of nutrients which are many times the normal physiological requirements. It is best to use purified forms of nutrients so that the dosage is accurately known. When absorption is poor, the nutrients should be injected rather than given orally. See Tables D-1 and D-2 for the treatments used for various deficiency diseases.

(Also see MALNUTRITION, PROTEIN-ENERGY.)

DEFICIENCY DISEASES OF THE WORLD. Dietary deficiency diseases provide a dramatic and vivid way in which to relate the story of undernutrition and malnutrition. Tables D-1 and D-2 list most of the nutritional diseases and ailments of people. Pertinent information relative to the less common and/or less well known deficiency diseases, worldwide and/or in the United States, is summarized in D-2. The most common and/or better known diseases are merely listed in Table D-1; then, in addition, they are accorded detailed narrative coverage, alphabetically, in this book.

---

[3]Kevany, J., and J.G. Chopra, "The Use of Iodized Oil in Goiter Prevention," *American Journal of Public Health*, Vol. 60, 1970, p. 919.

[4]Reddy, V., "Vitamin A Deficiency in Children," *Indian Journal of Medical Research*, Vol. 54, 1969, p. 54.

TABLE D-1
MAJOR DIETARY DEFICIENCY DISEASES

Disease	Cause	Signs & Symptoms	Distribution[1]	Treatment	Prevention	Remarks
Anemia, nutritional (See ANEMIA.)						
Beriberi (See BERIBERI.)						
Blindness due to vitamin A deficiency (See VITAMIN A.)						
Cretinism (Also see GOITER; and IODINE.)	Failure of the fetal thyroid to develop fully. It may be due to a maternal deficiency of thyroid hormones, or perhaps an inherited lack of a thyroid protein factor.	Congenital retardation of thyroid development, stunted growth, mental retardation, deaf-mutism, flat nose, thick lips, enlarged tongue, underdeveloped gonads, obesity, and dry skin.	Worldwide, particularly in mountainous regions and areas subjected to the action of glaciers. In some areas, it may affect 4% of the population.	Daily administration of thyroid extract (120 mg) or 0.2 mg of thyroxine. Treatment should be initiated at the first sign of the disorder, and continued for the lifetime of the patient. Some or all of the developmental defects may be incurable, particularly when there is a delay in diagnosis and treatment.	Special efforts should be made to detect thyroid deficiencies in females during their reproductive years. Newborn children should be carefully scrutinized for signs of cretinism, since early treatment may prevent some of the development defects, such as mental retardation.	There seems to be a higher incidence of cretinism in areas of endemic goiter, and where there are close kinship marriages.
Goiter (See GOITER; and IODINE.)						
Hemolytic anemia of the newborn (Also see ANEMIA; and VITAMIN E.)	Vitamin E deficiency which may be aggravated by milk formulas which contain vegetable oils.	Increased susceptibility of red blood cells to hemolysis.	Found mainly in premature infants who were fed formulas containing vegetable oils (sources of polyunsaturated fats).	Oral administration of 25 IU water-soluble vitamin E per day (use of the water-soluble form avoids problems due to disorders of fat absorption).	Supplementation of all infant formulas with 8–12 IU vitamin E per qt (0.95 liter), particularly those which contain polyunsaturated fats.	Avoid unnecessary iron supplementation (iron interferes with the utilization of vitamin E).

Footnote at end of table

(Continued)

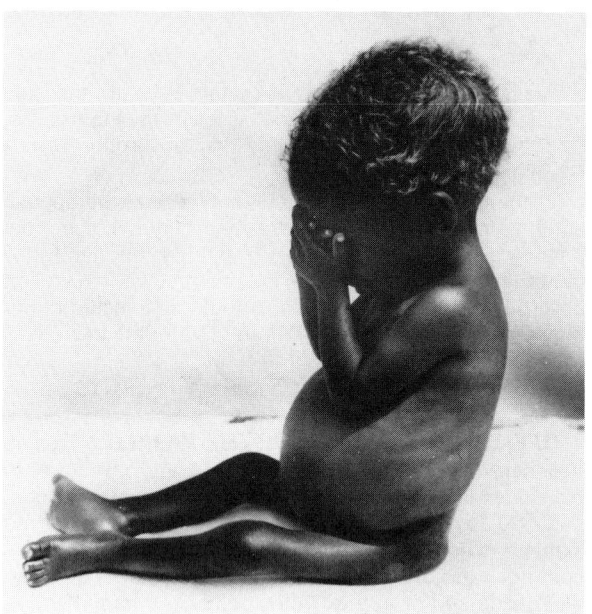

Fig. D-2. A little African boy suffering from "hidden hunger"—a lack of protein in this case, the African name for which is Kwashiorkor. (Courtesy, FAO, Rome, Italy)

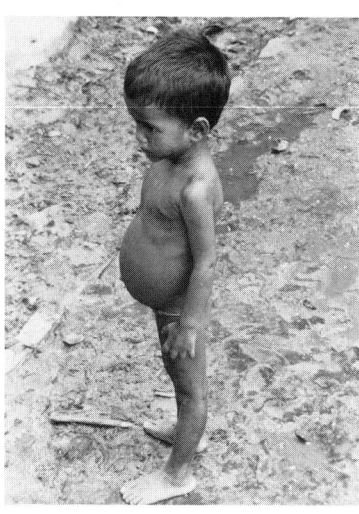

Fig. D-3. The swollen stomach of this youngster is a symptom of serious malnutrition. For millions of children throughout the world, food is needed to save them from permanent mental and physical damage that can be caused by lack of essential nutrients in their early years. (Courtesy, CARE, 660 First Avenue, New York, NY)

TABLE D-1 *(Continued)*

Disease	Cause	Signs & Symptoms	Distribution[1]	Treatment	Prevention	Remarks
Hemorrhagic disease of the newborn (Also see VITAMIN K.)	Impairment of blood clotting due to a deficiency of vitamin K, which is needed by the baby for synthesis of clotting factors.	Bleeding of infant in various tissues such as the brain, skin, nervous system, peritoneal cavity, gastrointestinal tract; or excessive bleeding by boys upon circumcision.	Occurs mainly in newborn infants during the first week of life.	Intramuscular injection of 1 mg of vitamin K.	Administration of 5 mg per day vitamin K to pregnant women just prior to childbirth.	Synthetic water-soluble analogs of vitamin K should *not* be given to premature newborns because of their susceptibility to hemolytic anemia, jaundice, and brain damage.
Iron-deficiency anemia (Also see ANEMIA; and IODINE.)	Dietary deficiency of iron, and/or factors which interfere with its absorption or utilization.	Paleness of the gums and mucous membranes, easy tiring, shortness of breath, light headedness, rapid heartbeat, and red blood cells which are subnormal in color, size, and numbers.	Millions of persons worldwide. The highest incidences are in infants, children, women in their reproductive years, and elderly persons.	Administration of therapeutic doses of iron (orally or by injection). Severe cases may require 60-180 mg of iron per day.	Provide foods rich in iron and the other nutrients needed for the production of red blood cells (meats, fish, legumes, nuts, fresh fruits and vegetables, and whole grains).	Care should be exercised in the administration of therapeutic doses of iron since excessive iron intake can lead to the deposition of iron in tissues.
Keratomalacia (Also see VITAMIN A.)	Vitamin A deficiency.	Softening and perforation of the cornea leading to loss of lens, infection and scarring of the eye, and blindness.	Occurs in most developing countries, but there are higher incidences in South Asia and East Asia.	Immediate administration of 100,000 IU of vitamin A per day. Injection of a water-soluble form is the most effective therapy when there is severe malnutrition.	Foods which contain good sources of vitamin A or carotene (animal livers, fish-liver oil, green and yellow vegetables, butter, or fortified margarine).	Victims of protein-energy malnutrition may develop the disease during their rehabilitation, particularly when they are given nonfat dry milk.
Kwashiorkor (See KWASHIORKOR.)						
Marasmus (See MARASMUS.)						
Osteomalacia (See OSTEOMALACIA.)						
Osteoporosis (See OSTEOPOROSIS.)						
Pellagra (See PELLAGRA.)						

Footnote at end of table

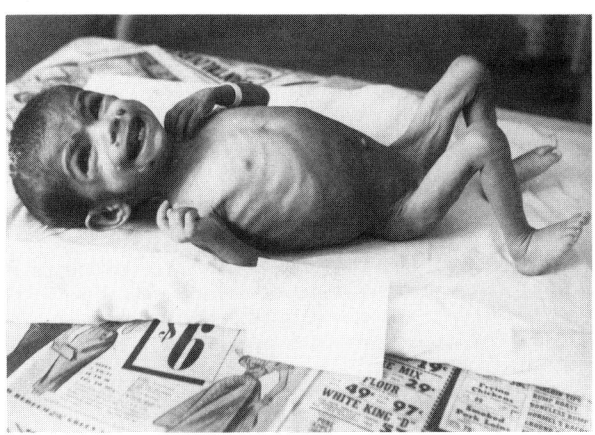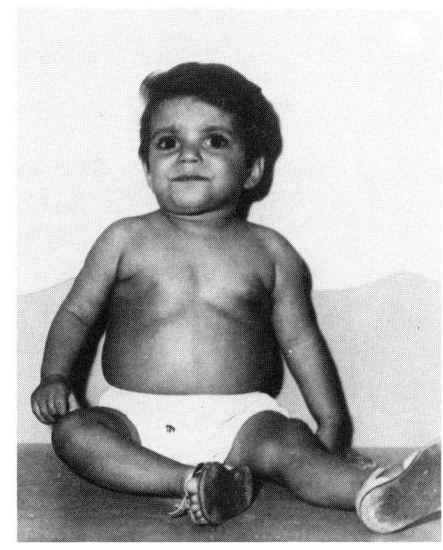

Fig. D-4. Hunger and malnutrition claim increasing numbers.
Left: Sheila at 20 months of age and weighing 10.8 lb.
Right: Same little girl after 10 months' treatment, weighing 22.7 lb.
(Courtesy, Public Health Dept., Iran; Issued by FAO)

TABLE D-1 *(Continued)*

Disease	Cause	Signs & Symptoms	Distribution[1]	Treatment	Prevention	Remarks
Pernicious anemia (See ANEMIA, PERNICIOUS.)						
Protein-energy malnutrition (Also see KWASHIORKOR; MALNUTRITION, PROTEIN-ENERGY; MARASMUS; and STARVATION.)	Deficiency of energy and/or protein due to intake of low-quality protein or insufficient amounts of food.	Growth failure (less than expected height for age, and subnormal weight for height and age), anemia, weakness, apathy, gastrointestinal disturbances, and increased susceptibility to infectious disease.	Occurs mainly in children under 5 years of age.	Provide 50 kcal energy and 1 g protein per pound *(0.45 kg)* of body weight. Vitamin and/or mineral supplementation may also be required.	Promotion of breast feeding. Food supplementation for vulnerable groups of pregnant women, infants, and children.	The various types of protein-energy malnutrition may require different therapies.
Rickets (See RICKETS.)						
Scurvy (See SCURVY; and VITAMIN C.)						
Starvation (See STARVATION.)						
Wernicke's disease	Thiamin deficiency, and, in some cases, deficiencies of other B-complex vitamins.	Lack of appetite, nausea, vomiting, failing vision, poor balance in walking, and wrist drop, apathy, confusion, and delusions.	Prevalent among prisoners of war and others living on a very poor diet and among chronic alcoholics.	Intramuscular injection of 25 mg doses of thiamin twice a day followed by supplements rich in the vitamin B complex (such as yeast) during convalescence.	Nutritional surveillance of persons subject to thiamin deficiency (alcoholics; diabetics; toxemic, pregnant women; patients with chronic gastrointestinal disease).	The severe psychiatric disorders which accompany this disease constitute *Korsakoff's psychosis.*
Xerophthalmia (See VITAMIN A.)	Vitamin A deficiency.	Drying and pigmentation of the conjunctival membranes of the eyes; opacity of the cornea.	Occurs in areas where the diet is lacking in whole milk, butter, green or yellow vegetables.	Administer 100,000 IU doses of vitamin A. If there are disorders of fat absorption, then intramuscular injections of water-soluble form of vitamin A should be used.	Supply dietary sources of vitamin and/or carotene (see BLINDNESS). Fortify margarine with vitamin A.	The signs of dryness and pigmentation of the conjunctival membranes may sometimes be due to irritants such as dust and glare.

[1]The estimated incidence of disease figures given under the column headed "Distribution" are from Aykroyd, W. R., *Conquest of Deficiency Diseases*, WHO, Geneva, Switzerland.

TABLE D-2
MINOR DIETARY DEFICIENCY DISORDERS

Disorders	Cause	Signs & Symptoms	Treatment	Prevention	Remarks
Eyes					
Angular blepharocon- junctivitis	A combination of pyridoxine (vitamin B-6) deficiency and a bacterial infection (*Hemophilus duplex*).	Inflammation of the lining of the eyelid.	Administration of 10 mg of vita- min B-6 per day.	Provision of food sources of vitamin B-6 (eggs, fish, leg- umes, meats, milk, nuts, and whole grains).	Although the inflamation is caused by the bacterial infec- tion, it is much more likely to occur when there is a vitamin B-6 deficiency.
Bitot's spots (Also see VITAMIN A.)	Deficiency of vitamin A. How- ever, Bitot's spots have been observed when there is ade- quate vitamin A, indicating that other nutritional deficien- cies may be responsible for this condition.	Foamy patches on the white portion of the eyes.	Immediate administration of from 25,000–100,000 IU of vitamin A per day until condi- tion improves (injection of water-soluble forms should be used to treat patients suffering from any type of malabsorp- tion).	Diets containing carotene (pro- vitamin A found in deep-green and dark-yellow fruits and vegetables) or vitamin A (but- ter, fortified margarine, or fish- liver oils).	Neglect of this early sign of vita- min A deficiency could lead to xerophthalmia and possible blind- ness.
Corneal vascularization	Riboflavin (vitamin B-2) defi- ciency.	Invasion of cornea by capillaries (Usually seen only under mag- nification). However, dilated blood vessels may often be readily seen in the neighboring conjunctiva (mucous membrane covering the eyeball).	Administration of 5 mg of ribo- flavin per day until condition improves.	Provision of food sources of riboflavin (cereal products from whole or enriched grains, fish, meats, and milk).	Patients may also have photo- phobia (aversion to light), mak- ing examination difficult.
Night blindness (Also see BLINDNESS due to vitamin A defi- ciency; and VITAMIN A.)	Deficiency of vitamin A.	An abnormally long time is re- quired for adaptation from vision in strong light to vision in dim light or darkness.	Administration of from 25,000– 100,000 IU vitamin A per day until condition improves.	Diets containing food sources of vitamin A. (Also see BITOT'S SPOTS.)	This disorder may also result from emotional disturbances and tired- ness.
Pigmentation of the conjunctiva	May sometimes be due to vita- min A deficiency.	Abnormal pigmentation (coloring in the whites of the eyes or in the lower eyelid).	Administration of from 25,000– 100,000 IU vitamin A per day until condition improves.	Plant and/or animal foods contain- ing vitamin A. (Also see BITOT'S SPOTS.)	
Xerosis of the conjunctiva (Also see VITAMIN A.)	Vitamin A deficiency.	Dryness and thickening of the conjunctiva.	Immediate administration of 100,000 IU of vitamin A orally (or by injection in cases of malabsorption) for 3 days, then 30,000 IU per day until condi- tion improves.	Diets containing food sources of vitamin A. (Also see BITOT'S SPOTS.)	This condition may also be caused by environmental irritants such as dust and bright light, or by infections. (Also see BITOT'S SPOTS.)
Glands					
Parotid enlargement	Deficiency of protein and/or the B-complex vitamins.	Swelling of the parotid gland.	Provide sources of high-quality protein and B-complex vitamins (eggs, fish, legumes, meats, milk, and nuts).	Same as Treatment.	There may be temporary parotid enlargement during the rehabili- tation of victims of malnutrition This condition should be distin- guished from mumps.
Gums					
Bleeding gums	Vitamin C deficiency.	Gums may be bleeding and swollen.	Administer 4 daily doses of 250 mg of ascorbic acid (vitamin C) per day for a week.	Diets containing fresh fruits and vegetables.	May also be caused by lack of dental hygiene or certain drugs.
Periodontal disease	In some cases, deficiency of cal- cium.	Teeth fall out of gums, which may be inflamed. In calcium deficiency there may be loss of the underlying (alveolar) bone in the jaw.	Administer daily doses of calcium (1,000 mg) and vitamin D (1,000 IU).	Calcium-containing foods, such as dairy products and green, leafy vegetables.	May also be caused by bacterial infections (*Pyorrhea alveolaris*).
Hair					
Discoloration and early pluckability (Also see HAIR ANAL- YSIS.)	Protein and/or energy deficiency.	Light-colored hair turns dirty- brown, dark hair becomes lighter in color (reddish brown to white or grey). Hair may be plucked without pain.	Provide adequate dietary protein (eggs, fish, legumes, meats, milk, and nuts).	Same as Treatment.	May also be due to deficiency of thyroid hormones such as in cre- tinism and myxedema.
Loss of hair in patches (Also see ALOPECIA.)	Uncertain in man. Lack of ribo- flavin or inositol in various animal species.	Hair falls out in patches from various parts of the body (dif- ferent from male pattern bald- ness).	Uncertain in man. Some have been helped by various mineral and vitamin supplements.	Provide food sources of essential fatty acids, minerals, protein, and vitamins.	This condition may also be due to hormone deficiencies or the side effects of certain drugs.
Internal Organs					
Liver enlargement (hepa- tomegaly)	Deficiencies of protein, methionine, and/or choline.	An enlarged liver which may be felt by touching the abdomen.	Provide adequate dietary protein (eggs, fish, meats, and milk).	Same as Treatment.	May also be due to chronic alco- holism and the toxic effects of chemicals and drugs.

(Continued)

TABLE D-2 *(Continued)*

Disorders	Cause	Signs & Symptoms	Treatment	Prevention	Remarks
		Internal Organs *(Continued)*			
Racing heartbeat (tachycardia)	Anemia (lack of iron) or thiamin deficiency. This disorder may also be due to emotional stress or excessive secretion of thyroid hormones.	Heart rate is over 100 beats per minute.	First, confirm the nature of the deficiency; then administer iron or thiamin.	Foods containing iron and thiamin (eggs, fish, legumes, liver, muscle meats, nuts, and whole grains).	Nutritional tachycardia should be distinguished from that due to other causes (anxiety, heart disease, drug effects, etc.).
		Lips			
Angular fissures (stomatitis)	Often due to riboflavin deficiency, but may also be due to lack of iron, niacin, or pyridoxine (vitamin B-6).	Skin is broken at the corners of the mouth (the condition often occurs along with cheilosis).	Provide a multivitamin and mineral supplement which contains riboflavin, niacin, pyridoxine, and iron.	Foods rich in the B-complex vitamins and minerals, such as eggs, fish, legumes, meats, nuts, green vegetables, and whole grains.	This condition may also be caused by herpes infection, various irritants, chapping, or hot and dry environments.
Cheilosis	Often due to deficiency of riboflavin or niacin.	Lips are swollen and puffed out. In some cases, the lining of the inside of the mouth may be exposed (eversion of buccal membrane).	Provide vitamin supplement containing niacin and riboflavin.	Same as for Angular fissures.	Same as for Angular fissures.
		Mouth and Tongue			
Dry mouth (xerostoma)	Prolonged deficiency of vitamin A.	Lack of saliva which may be accompanied by dried patches on the mucous membranes. Often accompanied by signs of vitamin A deficiency in the eyes.	Administration of 7,500 IU vitamin A per day, until condition improves.	Dietary sources of carotene (provitamin A present in dark-green and deep-yellow fruits and vegetables) or vitamin A (butter, fortified margarine, and fish-liver oils).	Any form of vitamin A deficiency should be treated immediately so as to avoid permanent damage to the eyes. However, dry mouth may also be caused by emotional distress, various medical treatments, or disorders of the salivary glands.
Glossitis	Deficiencies of folic acid, iron, niacin, pyridoxine (vitamin B-6), riboflavin, tryptophan, and/or vitamin B-12.	Tongue is inflamed and shiny, with atrophy of the nipplelike projections (papillae). Fissures may also be present. Often accompanies anemia.	Provide a supplement containing vitamin B-complex and iron, together with high-quality protein.	Foods rich in iron, protein, and the vitamin B-complex (eggs, fish, legumes, meats, nuts, green vegetables, and whole grains).	May also be present in nonnutritional anemias, uremia, and infections.
		Muscles			
Wasting and flabbiness	Deficiency of protein and/or calories.	Muscles are subnormal in size (as determined by measurements) and lack firmness when flexed.	Provide sufficient protein and calories.	Same as Treatment.	Other wasting diseases (like cancer) may produce similar effects.
		Nails			
Spoon nails (koilonychia) (Also see NAILS.)	Iron deficiency.	Nails are spoonlike (concave).	Administration of iron.	Foods rich in iron (eggs, fish, legumes, meats, nuts, vegetables).	May also be a sign of a cardiac defect.
		Nervous System			
Peripheral neuropathies	Deficiencies of the vitamin B-complex, particularly thiamin and vitamin B-12.	Absence of vibratory sense in the feet, aching, burning, or throbbing in the feet, lack of ankle and tendon reflexes, and tender calf muscles.	Provide a supplement containing the vitamin B-complex.	Foods containing the B-complex vitamins (eggs, fish, legumes, meats, milk, nuts, and whole grains).	These conditions may also result from toxic substances in foods, or from nonnutritional causes.
		Skeleton			
Misshapened bones	Deficiencies of calcium and/or vitamin D, or interference with their utilization.	Bossing (a rounded swelling) of the skull, bowing of the legs, enlarged wrists, and beaded ribs.	Provide a daily supplement containing 1,000 mg calcium and 1,000 IU vitamin D.	Adequate dietary calcium (milk products and deep-green vegetables) plus vitamin D (dietary and/or by exposure of skin to sunlight).	These conditions may also be produced by low blood levels of phosphate (a rare disorder characterized by excessive excretion of the mineral).
		Skin			
Atrophy of the skin	Starvation	Skin is drawn taut over the bones.	Provide sufficient quantity and quality of food.	Same as Treatment.	Care should be taken to avoid injury to atrophied skin, since healing of lesions may be greatly impaired.
Discoloration	Various nutritional deficiencies.	Skin may have darkened areas (as in pellagra), lightened patches (protein-energy malnutrition), or it may be pale (as in anemia).	First establish diagnosis of specific deficiencies; then provide missing nutrients.	Diets containing adequate amounts of all essential nutrients.	Color changes are most likely to be detected on the parts of the body normally exposed to sunlight.

(Continued)

TABLE D-2 (Continued)

Disorders	Cause	Signs & Symptoms	Treatment	Prevention	Remarks
		Skin (Continued)			
Dryness of the skin (xeroderma)	Lack of essential fatty acids and/or vitamin A.	Dry skin which is lined and flaky.	Administer vitamins A and E and vegetable oils. Although vegetable oils contain vitamin E, the losses in processing are uncertain.	Foods containing vitamin A, such as dark-green and deep-yellow fruits and vegetables, butter, fish-liver oils, and fortified margarine (the latter usually contains the essential fatty acids which should also be provided).	The condition may also be caused by poor hygiene, excessive washing of the skin with soap, hypothyroidism, uremia, and poor circulation.
Easy bruising (ecchymosis)	Deficiency of vitamin C or vitamin K.	Bruises occur where there is only slight pressure or trauma.	After suitable diagnostic tests, give either vitamin C or vitamin K.	Diets containing fresh fruits and vegetables (sources of vitamins C and K).	Other causes are nonnutritional blood disorders and trauma.
Eczema	Sometimes caused by lack of essential fatty acids and/or pyridoxine (vitamin B-6).	Skin eruptions which may be dry or moist, and may be accompanied by burning or itching.	Administer vegetable oils with pyridoxine (large doses of the vitamin [10 mg or more per day] have sometimes been used in such therapy).	At least 1 tsp of vegetable oil per day plus foods containing pyridoxine (eggs, fish, legumes, meats, milk, nuts, and whole grains).	It is generally believed that the majority of cases of this condition are caused by sensitivities to foods and other substances rather than by dietary deficiencies.
Elephant skin (pachyderma)	It is believed to be due to a vitamin A deficiency.	Skin like that of an elephant in such areas as the elbow, knee, and instep.	Administration of 7,500 IU of vitamin A per day.	Foods containing vitamin A. (Also see Dryness of the skin.)	The condition may be aggravated by diet and other irritating factors.
Flaky paint dermatosis	Protein-energy malnutrition.	Darkening and flaking of the skin.	Diets containing high-quality protein (eggs, fish, legumes, meats, milk, nuts) and sufficient energy.	Same as Treatment.	Amino acid supplementation may be required for people whose major sources of protein are cereal grains.
Follicular hyperkeratosis (toad-skin or phrynoderma)	May be due to deficiencies of vitamin A, essential fatty acids, and/or pyridoxine (vitamin B-6).	The hair follicles are plugged with a hardened material (keratin) which may project from the skin and gives it a bumpy appearance like the skin of a toad.	Provide vitamin A, essential fatty acids, and pyridoxine.	Diets containing vitamin A (also see Dryness of the skin), essential fatty acids (vegetable oils) and pyridoxine (also see Eczema).	A similar condition occurs in secondary syphilis.
Naso-labial seborrhea	Deficiencies of niacin, pyridoxine, and/or riboflavin.	Plugging of the follicles around the nose with a yellow, fatty material.	Provide a supplement containing the vitamin B-complex.	Diets containing sources of the B-complex vitamins (eggs, fish, legumes, meats, milk, nuts, and whole grains).	Dried brewers' yeast or non-fat dry milk may be useful in areas where food sources of the vitamin B-complex are scarce.
Orogenital syndrome	Deficiencies of the B-complex vitamins.	Angular fissures of the lips plus inflammation of the lining inside the mouth. There may also be dermatitis around the eyes, ears, and genital areas.	Provide a supplement containing the vitamin B-complex.	Diets containing vitamin B-complex. (Also see Naso-labial seborrhea.)	May often occur along with corneal vascularization and naso-labial seborrhea.
Tropical ulcer (jungle rot)	Believed to be caused by a poor diet plus environmental conditions in hot, humid areas.	Ulcers of the skin on the legs. These lesions may be infected with such organisims as *Treponema vincenti*, staphylococci, and streptococci.	Provide an adequate diet and proper hygiene (prompt disinfection and treatment of skin lesions).	Same as Treatment.	The condition may be precipitated by debilitating diseases like dysentery and malaria.

DEGENERATION

• Deterioration—a sinking from a higher to a lower level or type.

• A worsening of physical or mental qualities.

• A retrogressive pathological change in cells or tissues as a result of which the functioning power is lost.

DEHYDRATE

To remove most or all moisture from a substance for the purpose of preservation, primarily through artificial drying.

DEHYDRATION

The removal of water from a material. In nutrition, dehydration generally means one or both of the following:

• Drying of a beverage, food, or tissue of the body.

• A state in which the body lacks sufficient fluids to carry out its normal function. If it is not corrected this condition may result in death.

(Also see WATER AND ELECTROLYTES.)

DEHYDROASCORBIC ACID (C₆H₆O₆)

The oxidized (hydrogen removed) form of ascorbic acid (vitamin C). In the body, it readily reverts to ascorbic acid; thus, it is utilized as such.
(Also see VITAMIN C.)

DEHYDROCHOLESTEROL

A substance produced by the body, and found in or on the skin. It is converted to vitamin D by ultraviolet radiation from the sun or from another source, such as a sun lamp.
(Also see VITAMIN D.)

DEHYDROGENASES

Enzymes that accelerate oxidation by transferring hydrogen to a hydrogen acceptor and thus play an important role in biological oxidation-reduction processes.

DEHYDRORETINOL

One of the forms of vitamin A.
(Also see VITAMIN A.)

DELANEY CLAUSE

In 1958, the food additives amendment, better known for its Delaney Clause (named after the congressman who sponsored it), was passed. This bill has proven to be one of the most controversial pieces of legislation ever to affect American producers and consumers. The Delaney Clause states:

"Provided, That no additive shall be deemed safe if it is found to induce cancer when ingested by man or animal, or if it is found, after tests which are appropriate for the evaluation of the safety of food additives, to induce cancer in man or animals . . ."

This clause gave rise to the policy of *zero tolerance*—that is, no substance can be used as a food additive, even in miniscule amounts, if it has been, in any way, implicated as an inducer of cancer in either man or beast. What, at the time, appeared to be a well-intentioned law aimed at protecting the consumer from potential health hazards proved to be a nightmare for the drug industry and livestock producers. The manufacturers must now prove a negative hypothesis which many feel is impossible. That is, a new drug must be demonstrated to be 100% noncarcinogenic. Unfortunately, the lawmakers are in a tenuous position because, to repeal the Delaney Clause, they run the risk of being accused of supporting the addition of cancer-causing drugs to our food supply.

The Delaney Clause will, in all likelihood, be modified, but the debate of how safe is *safe* will probably continue without end.
(Also see FEDERAL FOOD, DRUG, AND COSMETIC ACT; and FOOD AND DRUG ADMINISTRATION.)

DELIRIUM TREMENS

A condition which occurs in alcoholics. It is characterized by mental confusion, trembling, loss of appetite, and nausea.
(Also see ALCOHOLISM AND ALCOHOLICS.)

DEMENTIA

A mental disorder characterized by serious mental impairment and deterioration.

DEMINERALIZATION

The loss of calcium and phosphorus from the bones.
(Also see OSTEOPOROSIS.)

DEMOGRAPHY

The study of the statistical characteristics of human population. Such statistics may be useful in determining the need for certain types of health services.

DEMULCENT

A material which soothes mucous membranes. Certain mucilaginous gums such as psyllium and tragacanth have long been used as herbal remedies to soothe the digestive tract. Some of these gums also have a laxative effect because they absorb water.

DEMYELINATION

A process by which the protective sheath around nerve endings breaks down.

DENATURATION

A chemical (acid, base, detergent, organic solvent, salt, urea) or physical (heating, shaking, whipping) process which alters the nature of a substance. In biology the substance is often protein. Two examples of denaturation are: (1) the coagulation of egg white (albumen) by heating, and (2) the formation of meringue by beating egg white.

DENDRITIC SALT

A structurally different form of ordinary table salt (sodium chloride; NaCl). Normally table salt crystals are cubes. Dendritic crystals are branched or star-like, hence the term dendritic. The following advantages are listed for dendritic salt: lower bulk density, rapid solution, and an unusual capacity for absorbing moisture before becoming wet.

DENSITY

The weight of a given volume of a substance. For example, the weight of 1 ml of water at 39°F (4°C) is 1 g. Hence, the density of water at that temperature is 1 g per milliliter. Objects that are less dense than water (such as the human body) will float in water, whereas those that are more dense will sink in water.

DENTAL CARIES

The conventional name for tooth decay or *cavities,* caused by the bacterial breakdown of sugars to lactic acid, which occur mainly at contact points between teeth, at the gum margins, or in pits and fissures of posterior teeth. Eventually the lactic acid erodes the tooth enamel, which cannot regenerate, and a *cavity* is formed. Up to this point the whole process is usually quite painless and may continue to be so until the decay process passes through the dentin and approaches the tender pulp. Several factors determine the amount of dental caries a person will experience: (1) the bacterial flora of the mouth; (2) the level of sugar (carbohydrate) in the diet, or the eating habits; (3) oral hygiene, including brushing, flossing, and dental checkups; (4) resistance of the teeth due to genetic influences and adequate dietary amounts of protein, calcium, phosphorus, and vitamins A, C, and D; and (5) fluoride in the drinking water. Fig. D-5 illustrates the structure of teeth and the stages of tooth decay.

(Also see DENTAL HEALTH, NUTRITION, AND DIET.)

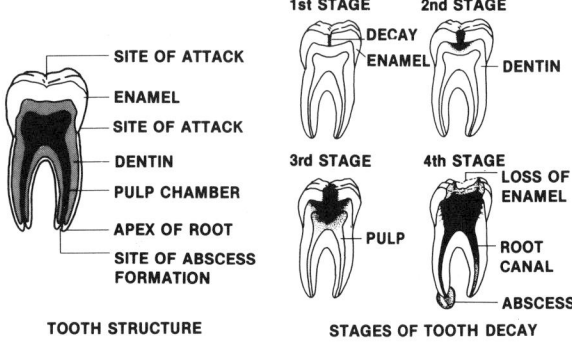

Fig. D-5. Tooth structure and dental caries.

DENTAL FLUOROSIS

Although very low levels (1 ppm) of fluoride in the drinking water help prevent dental caries (tooth decay), higher levels (3 to 5 ppm) can cause mottling or dental fluorosis of the permanent teeth during their formation. This mottling is characterized by rough enamel without luster and brown pigmentation separated by chalk white patches. In areas where it is known that the fluoride content of the water is naturally high, dental fluorosis can be prevented by treating the water supply with phosphate.

(Also see FLUORINE.)

DENTAL HEALTH, NUTRITION, AND DIET

A complementary relationship exists between nutrition and dental health. Good nutrition is necessary for the development of sound healthy teeth and gum structures, while healthy teeth and gum structures are needed so that a nutritious diet may be eaten.

Except for the common cold, tooth decay is the most prevalent disease in the United States. More than 95% of all Americans have decayed teeth by the time they become adults. In 1989, the annual bill for dental care totaled $31.4 billion. But more than money is involved! Tooth decay results in lost time, pain, and if it leads to loss of teeth, there is impaired chewing, speech, appearance, and general well-being. However, since no one dies of tooth decay, people generally do not get overly excited about it, as they do heart disease or cancer. Overall, dental health is viewed indifferently by the general public.

Good dental health depends upon (1) nutrition and diet, (2) care of the teeth, and (3) fluoride.

DEVELOPMENT AND ANATOMY OF TEETH.

Humans grow two sets of teeth. The first set—the one formed in the womb—is called the primary teeth. These are also known as the baby teeth, deciduous teeth, or milk teeth. Primary teeth appear—erupt—in the mouth when a baby is from 6 to 30 months old. Twenty teeth—ten uppers and ten lowers—make a complete set of primary teeth. Next, the permanent teeth begin appearing in the mouth at about 6 years of age and continue to appear until about 21, though calcification begins in the jaw near the time of birth. There are 28 to 32 permanent teeth, depending upon whether or not the four wisdom teeth appear. Table D-3 lists the primary and permanent teeth and the approximate ages at which they appear or erupt in the mouth.

TABLE D-3
APPROXIMATE AGE AT THE TIME OF ERUPTION OF PRIMARY TEETH AND PERMANENT TEETH

Primary Teeth (Baby Teeth)	Approximate Eruption Age	Permanent Teeth	Approximate Eruption Age
	(months)		(years)
Upper Teeth		**Upper Teeth**	
Central incisor	7.5	Central incisor	7– 8
Lateral incisor	9	Lateral incisor	8– 9
Cuspid (canine or		Cuspid (canine or	
eyetooth)	18	eyetooth)	11–12
First molar	14	First bicuspid	
Second molar	24	(premolar)	10–11
		Second bicuspid	
Lower Teeth		(premolar)	10–12
Central incisor	6	First molar	6– 7
Lateral incisor	7	Second molar	12–13
Cuspid (canine or		Third molar (wisdom	
eyetooth)	16	tooth)	17–21
First molar	12		
Second molar	20	**Lower Teeth**	
		Central incisor	6– 7
		Lateral incisor	7– 8
		Cuspid (canine or	
		eyetooth)	9–10
		First bicuspid	
		(premolar)	10–12
		Second bicuspid	
		(premolar)	11–12
		First molar	6– 7
		Second molar	11–13
		Third molar (wisdom	
		tooth)	17–21

The anatomy of a tooth and the supporting tissues is shown in Fig. D-6. A tooth is composed of four separate tissues:

1. Enamel.
2. Dentin.
3. Pulp.
4. Cementum.

Other tissues called the periodontal tissues make up the gums and tissue which hold the tooth in place. Fig. D-6 shows the structure of a tooth and gum (gingiva) area.

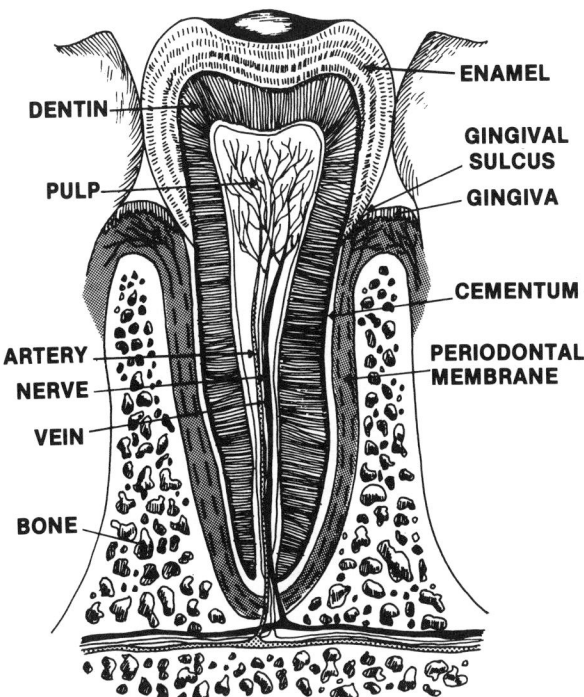

Fig. D-6. The structure of a tooth and adjacent gum (gingiva) area, and the cementum, periodontal membrane, and bone which hold the tooth in place.

ENAMEL

GINGIVAL SULCUS

GINGIVA

CEMENTUM

PERIODONTAL MEMBRANE

DENTIN

PULP

ARTERY

NERVE

VEIN

BONE

ROLE OF NUTRITION AND DIET. Nutrition and diet have a role in dental health throughout life—starting in the womb during embryonic and fetal life. Although dental caries (tooth decay) and periodontal disorders are influenced by the interaction of (1) tooth resistance or supporting structures, (2) bacteria in contact with the oral tissues, and (3) the oral environment, the quality, quantity, physical consistency of foods, and the frequency of food intake further interact with these three items.

Development. Since teeth are largely formed during pregnancy and childhood, deficiencies of calcium, phosphate, vitamins A, D, or C, proteins, calories, or fluoride may enhance the susceptibility of teeth to decay-promoting factors. A well-planned diet, providing good nutrition, is necessary for optimal tooth development—chemical composition, size, shape, and possibly time of eruption. While the relationship of the nutritional status of the pregnant or lactating woman to the subsequent dental health of her child is not well understood, the following points indicate the importance of nutrition to dental health during pregnancy and childhood:

1. Any deficiency of calcium during the formation of the teeth and jaws is likely to cause malformed teeth, teeth crowded too closely together in a narrow jaw, and/or poor quality teeth.

2. Calcium for the formation of teeth (and bones) during pregnancy is derived from the mother's diet, not her teeth. The *loss of a tooth for every child* is a popular notion, but false.

3. The calcium-phosphorus ratio is important to the proper utilization of these minerals, as is adequate vitamin D.

4. The growth and proper mineralization of teeth requires vitamin D. Teeth of vitamin D-deficient children have thin, poorly calcified enamel, with pits and fissures, and are especially prone to decay.

5. Excessive vitamin D causes misshapen jaws in the offspring.

6. Vitamin A is essential for optimal development of the enamel. Vitamin A-deficiency results in enamel with fissures and pits, and poorly formed dentin.

7. Prolonged periods of subclinical vitamin A-deficiency may cause inadequate bone growth patterns resulting in misalignment of teeth which further increases the susceptibility of teeth to attack by bacteria.

8. Normal formation of the dentin requires vitamin C.

9. In rats, low protein and high carbohydrate diets have been shown to be associated with reduction in the size of molars, delay in eruption and increased susceptibility to caries.

10. The prevalence of protein-calorie malnutrition in less affluent societies suggests an explanation for the relatively high incidence of dental caries found in the primary teeth of children.

11. Fluoride strengthens the enamel during its formation.

During pregnancy and lactation, extra energy, protein, calcium, phosphorus, and vitamins A, D, and C in the diet are recommended.

(Also see NUTRIENTS: REQUIREMENTS, ALLOWANCES, FUNCTIONS, SOURCES.)

Dental Caries (Tooth Decay). Before the age of 35, the primary reason for loss of a tooth is dental caries. Moreover, it is estimated that 96% of all high school students—those at the halfway mark between birth and age 35—have tooth decay. Dental caries is the conventional name for tooth decay or cavities, caused by the bacterial breakdown of sugars to an acid, which occur mainly at contact points between teeth, at the gum margins, or in pits and fissures of posterior teeth. Eventually, the acid erodes the tooth enamel, which cannot regenerate, and a cavity is formed. Up to this point, the whole process is usually quite painless, and it may continue to be so until the decay process passes through the dentin and approaches the tender pulp where the nerves are located.

CAUSATIVE FACTORS. No single factor is involved in causing tooth decay. Rather, tooth decay requires the interaction of (1) susceptible teeth, (2) microbiology of the mouth (bacteria), (3) nutrition and diet, and (4) passage of time.

Susceptible Teeth. A small portion, probably less than 2%, of the American people appear immune to caries. As already pointed out, general nutrition knowledge, animal studies, and some population studies of protein-calorie malnutrition suggest that the availability of nutrients such as protein, energy, vitamins A and D, calcium, phosphorus and fluoride influence the mineralization and formation of teeth; hence, the susceptibility of teeth. The vulnerability of teeth also depends on their spacing and shape, which can encourage food particles to collect between or on them. Furthermore, although not directly related to the teeth, the salivary glands influence the susceptibility of teeth to tooth decay. Anytime the salivary glands quit functioning or markedly reduce their function—the formation of saliva, rampant tooth decay usually develops. This is evidenced when salivary glands are removed from rats or when salivary gland function is markedly reduced in individuals receiving radiation treatment for head or neck cancer. Normally, saliva washes away food particles, bacteria and acids, and neutralizes acids.

Microbiology of the Mouth.   Tooth decay does not develop in germ-free animals, but unfortunately this is an unrealistic situation for humans. Decay-promoting bacteria live in the mouth and adhere to the tooth surfaces forming sticky colorless masses called dental plaque.

Overall, it is the ability of bacteria in the mouth to produce organic acids, primarily lactic acid, which contributes to the formation of dental caries in susceptible teeth, given the right diet and length of time. The acids produced decompose the hydroxyapatite in the enamel by removing calcium and phosphate, allowing bacteria entry inside the tooth—and a cavity is born.

Diet and Nutrition.   Diet is highly influential in caries development. Certain diets enhance the activity of cariogenic bacteria, and the formation of plaques.

• **Plaques**—Plaques vary in thickness, and are composed of about 70% bacteria, with the remaining 30% being polysaccharides, enzymes, and acids. Unless a tooth has been thoroughly cleaned, the bacteria colonies in plaques continue to grow, particularly near the gum line (gingival sulcus). A thin organic layer, the pellicle, between the tooth enamel and the plaque is formed when proteins in the saliva are adsorbed on the enamel. It seems that the pellicle promotes the attachment of bacteria to the teeth and influences the transport of acids into the enamel and diffusion of calcium and phosphate out of the enamel. Accumulations of plaques are implicated in caries and periodontal disease.

• **Sugar and carbohydrates**—Dietary carbohydrates, in particular sugar (sucrose), are prime contributors to the bacterial colonization of the teeth and the production and support of tooth decay. Bacteria in the plaque act on sucrose to produce lactic acid.

The following points demonstrate the role of sucrose in the development of dental caries:

1.   Dental caries dropped significantly 2 years after sugar consumption was severely restricted in Europe during World War II. The incidence of caries returned to the prewar levels when sugar intake increased.

2.   Nursing caries are observed in infants and young children who are allowed to fall asleep suckling on a bottle of fruit juice or milk with sugar. This continuously bathes the upper front teeth—the four incisors—with sugar. Eventually rampant caries destroy these four teeth.

3.   In the classical Vipeholm, Sweden study, various diets were examined for their ability to produce caries. Over a 5-year period, those individuals who ate sticky toffee several times a day demonstrated 12 times more caries than those individuals who were not exposed frequently to sugar.

4.   In rats, it has been shown that fructose, glucose, lactose, and maltose are less cariogenic (caries-causing) than sucrose (sugar).

5.   In countries where sugar intake is low, such as China and Ethiopia, the incidence of caries is low, while in areas where the intake of sugar is high, such as Australia, Hawaii, and French Polynesia, there is a very high incidence of tooth decay.

6.   Studies, which have subsituted nonfermentable sugar alcohols or polyols such as sorbitol or xylitol for some or all of the sweeteners (sugar) used in the diet, have shown a reduction in caries.

7.   People with the genetic defect called fructose intolerance, avoid all sucrose-containing foods since sucrose (sugar) is comprised of a molecule of glucose and a molecule of fructose. These people display excellent dental health.

8.   Sugar consumption in England has increased from 20 lb (*9 kg*) per person to over 110 lb (*149.5 kg*) per person in the last 100 years. There has been a nearly parallel rise in the incidence of dental caries.

9.   Sucrose (sugar) is used in the formation of the extracellular polysaccharides or glucans which contribute to plaque formation. Maltose, lactose, fructose, and glucose cannot be used for this purpose.

Sucrose is not the only culprit carbohydrate. The other sugars—glucose, fructose, lactose, and maltose—and even starch, contribute to acid formation, though starchy foods seem the least offensive.

• **Physical properties of foods**—Foods that stick to tooth surfaces and that are slowly soluble promote caries. Liquid foods, in comparison to sticky or retentive foods, tend to have lower cariogenicity. Therefore, honey and the sugars of dried fruits can contribute to dental caries as well as refined sugar and the products made from it. Sometimes, raw fibrous foods are recommended for between meal snacks. These foods generally require more chewing and stimulate saliva flow, but they do not clean the teeth. Increased saliva flow is beneficial. Also, fats, which produce a protective oily film on the surface of the teeth serve as a barrier of acid penetration to the enamel.

• **Nutritional factors**—Adequate, balanced nutrition is essential for all tissues to grow, develop, and remain healthy. Nutrition is an ally to good oral health which depends upon the health of the salivary glands, the bones of the face, periodontal tissues, and the immune system. Moreover, nutrients in the food contribute to the environment in the mouth by stimulating or inhibiting caries-producing bacteria in the dental plaque. Some trace minerals, other than fluorine, may increase the resistance of the enamel or change the properties of the saliva or plaque, while other minerals may promote caries. Dietary phosphates seem to prevent caries, but copper and lead may be cariogenic. More research is needed to determine the effects of specific nutrients on the growth, development, and maintenance of the teeth and supporting structures.

Passage of Time.   One to two years are necessary for a small area of decalcified enamel to progress to clinical caries. But if preventative dietary and oral hygiene measures are taken, the development of the decay may be stopped, though the decalcified area will never return to normal.

New teeth are more susceptible to decay than older teeth, since 2 to 4 years after eruption the enamel is in the final stages of maturation. Therefore, individuals with new primary or permanent teeth are more susceptible; hence, young children and teen-agers have a higher incidence of caries.

The more frequent the exposure to sugar, the longer the acid levels are elevated in the mouth, thus increasing the incidence of caries. This also relates to sticky foods which stay in contact with the teeth for long periods and are not washed away by the saliva. Therefore, snacking on sugary foods is not good, but snacking on sticky sugary foods is worse.

Periodontal Disease.   An inflammatory disease of the gums and of the bones that support the teeth is called periodontal disease, because it involves structures surrounding the teeth. Periodontal disease is the major cause of tooth loss in adults. The exact cause of periodontal disease is unknown, but several local factors may be involved in its initiation. The primary factor is poor oral hygiene, since bacterial plaques near the gum line (gingival sulcus) (see Fig. D-6) are a prime initiating factor. Rates of periodontal disease are the highest in populations where oral hygiene is the poorest. Plaques cause the inflammation of the gingiva (gingivitis) resulting in red swollen gums (gingiva). As the bacteria continue to invade the sulcus, they secrete toxins that cause pockets of pus to form. Eventually, the disease reaches the bone and results in demineralization. Reabsorption or loss of the bone supporting the teeth results in loose teeth which eventually fall out.

Nutrition and diet have been widely studied as possible causative factors in periodontal disease, but there does not seem to be a direct relationship. Nutritional deficiencies do not initiate periodontal disease. The diet is, however, the source of all nutrients necessary for the health of the periodontal tissues that are resistant to disease. Dietary restriction of sugars, especially those in sticky foods, is important, due to the role of sugar in the formation of dental plaques.

GOOD DENTAL HEALTH. Disregarding some genetic defect, most tooth decay and periodontal disease is preventable through sound nutrition and diet, proper care of the teeth, and fluoride treatment.

Nutrition And Diet. Teeth form during a prolonged period, beginning 7 months before birth, continuing through childhood and adolescent years, and not ending until the formation of the wisdom teeth is complete. Like any other developing structure, the teeth require that all nutrients be supplied in adequate amounts. Of prime importance are energy (calories), protein, calcium, magnesium, phosphate, fluoride, and vitamins A, C, and D, which ensure the development of teeth with a rigid structure and increased resistance to decay. Therefore, proper nutrition during pregnancy, lactation, infancy, childhood, and adolescence contributes to good dental health.

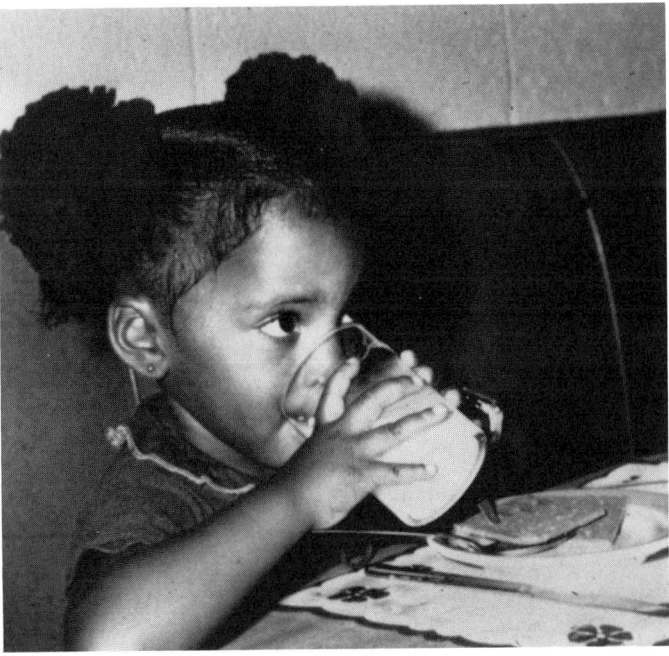

Fig. D-7. Proper nutrition during childhood contributes to good dental health. (Courtesy, Louisiana State University, Baton Rouge, La.)

High incidence of dental caries is associated with dietary carbohydrates, primarily the monosaccharides (glucose and fructose) and the disaccharides (sucrose and lactose). But more important than their intake is the frequency and their form; therefore, for good dental health the following should be practiced:

1. Sticky sugary snack foods should be avoided; for example, caramel, dried fruits, bread and butter with honey, honey, cookies, chewing gum, jams and jellies, and syrups.

2. Snacking should be confined to foods such as nuts, popcorn, raw fruit and vegetables, and cheeses.

3. Sweets and carbohydrates should be consumed in conjunction with meals. Even starch, if allowed to remain on the teeth long enough, will release glucose molecules which bacteria will convert to acid.

The use of foods containing artificial sweetening agents such as saccharin and aspartame, and the use of polyols like mannitol, sorbitol, and xylitol, may decrease the incidence of caries, since bacteria of the mouth cannot ferment these sweeteners to acids.

(Also see CHILDHOOD AND ADOLESCENT NUTRITION; INFANT DIET AND NUTRITION; PREGNANCY AND LACTATION NUTRITION; and SWEETENING AGENTS.)

Care Of The Teeth. Good dental hygiene is important. Proper tooth brushing along with flossing breaks up the plaque before the underlying enamel begins to decalcify. A daily routine is necessary. It is especially important to brush before going to sleep since less saliva is secreted and, therefore, bacterial acids are less diluted. Brushing following a meal is not always feasible, but a thorough rinsing of the mouth with just plain water is helpful.

Visits to the dentist help maintain good oral health. Dentists may remove plaque from teeth, or fill cavities to prevent further decay. Also, a dentist may apply a plastic sealant to the chewing surfaces of decay-free teeth as a preventative measure.

Fluoride. Fluoride is the most effective agent available for strengthening tooth resistance to acid demineralization. The mechanism by which fluorine increases caries resistance of the teeth is not fully understood. However, it appears that crystals of fluoroapatite can replace some of the calcium phosphate crystals of hydroxyapatite that are normally deposited during tooth formation, and that it may also replace some of the carbonate normally found in the tooth. Apparently these fluoride substances are more resistant to mouth acids. Fluorine may also inactivate oral bacterial enzymes which create acids from carbohydrates.

The fluoride ion, at proper levels of intake, assists in the prevention of dental caries. When children under 9 years of age consume drinking water containing 1 part per million of fluorine, the teeth have fewer dental caries in childhood, adolescence, and throughout life. This has led to the fluoridation of water supplies in many countries. Fluoridation of water supplies to bring the concentration of fluoride to 1 ppm (one part of fluorine to a million parts of water) has proved to be safe, economical, and an efficient way to reduce tooth decay—a highly important public health measure in areas where natural water supplies do not contain this amount. Extensive medical and public health studies have clearly demonstrated the safety and nutritional advantages that result from fluoridation of water supplies. In communities in which fluoridation has been introduced, the incidence of tooth decay in children has been decreased by 50% or more.

The concentration of fluoride in public water supplies should be adjusted slightly to allow for differences in water consumption with seasonal temperature changes.

In areas where water supplies are not fluoridated, fluoride supplements are available as drops, tablets, and mouth rinses. A physician or dentist can prescribe a supplement appropriate for each individual and provide instructions for its use. Generally, drops are prescribed for infants until they are old enough to use the tablets. Older children and teen-agers use tablets or mouth rinses, or both. Dentists sometimes recommend a fluoride mouth rinse for adults with tooth decay problems. Also, about 80% of all toothpaste sold in the United States contains fluoride.

Because fluoride is so effective against tooth decay, many states have established school fluoridation programs in which schools with independent water supplies fluoridate their water through the use of special equipment. In addition, schools in some areas of the country have adopted programs that provide fluoride tablets or a mouth rinse to children in the schools. The procedure takes only a few minutes each day and is supervised by someone trained to administer the supplement, usually the teacher.

(Also see FLUORIDATION; FLUORINE; and MINERALS, Table M-25.)

Although the future may hold a vaccine which will prevent dental caries, dental health, including dental caries prevention, requires lifelong dedication of an individual who understands and incorporates into daily habits the benefits to be derived from the combined effects of nutrition and diet, oral hygiene (care of the teeth and supporting structures), and fluoride.

(Also see CALCIUM; PHOSPHORUS; VITAMIN A; VITAMIN C; and VITAMIN D.)

DEOXYPYRIDOXINE

A compound with similar structure to pyridoxine but which is antagonistic (opposes or neutralizes) to the action of pyridoxine.

DEOXYRIBONUCLEIC ACID (DNA)

The main chemical substance of the genes (chromosomes), which are located in the nucleus of cells. Hence, DNA and similar substances such as RNA are called nucleic acids. It is a complex molecule which varies in composition from species to species. The individual constituents of DNA determine the characteristics which are passed down from generation to generation of living organisms. DNA also governs the metabolic processes which take place during the life of an organism.

(Also see NUCLEIC ACIDS.)

DEPOT FAT

The body fat which is stored in the adipose tissues.

DERMATITIS

An inflammation or irritation of the skin which may be accompanied by flaking, itching, redness, or swelling. Dermatitis may result from contact with irritants, from drugs or foods which have been ingested, or from various types of nutritional deficiencies.

DERMATOLOGY

The medical specialty which is concerned with the diseases of the skin.

DERMIS

The inner layer of skin which is just inside the outer layer or epidermis. It is much more sensitive than the epidermis, so a wound in the skin which exposes the dermis may be quite painful.

DESICCATE

To dry.

DESSERTS

Such adages as *sweets for the sweet* and *sugar and spice and everything nice* indicate that many· people look on desserts as a delightful and romantic conclusion to each meal. Special occasion meals would not be considered proper unless the traditional desserts were served; for example, pumpkin pie for Thanksgiving, and mincemeat pie or plum pudding for Christmas. And what would a birthday party be without a birthday cake?

Although, as children, all of us were persuaded to eat our vegetables so that we could have some dessert, our love for desserts should be curbed, because we now know that too much sugar can be counterproductive to continued buoyant good health. However, it is not recommended that 100% of the sugar or sweetening be eliminated from the diet. Even when on a reducing diet, it is recommended that some dessert be eaten, but it should be a considerably reduced portion—like ½ or ⅓ of the average serving.

A small amount of sweet food may help digest a meal. Many of our grandmothers used warm sweetened water to ease the infant's colic. In addition, desserts containing milk, eggs, fruit, whole wheat flour and honey or molasses do contribute important nutrients to the diet.

For the composition of the various desserts see Table F-21, Food Composition Table, the sections on Bakery Products, Desserts & Sweets, and Milk and Products.

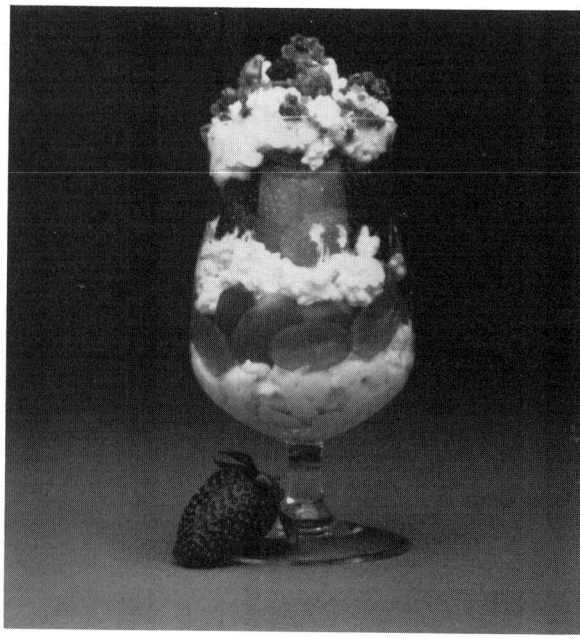

Fig. D-8. Parfait featuring fruits. (Courtesy, USDA)

The basic types of desserts are:

1.	Cakes	13.	Meringues
2.	Candies	14.	Milk
3.	Charlottes	15.	Mousses
4.	Cheesecakes	16.	Parfaits
5.	Cobblers	17.	Pastries
6.	Cookies	18.	Puddings
7.	Crepes or pancakes	19.	Sherbets
8.	Custards	20.	Shortcakes
9.	Eclairs and cream puffs	21.	Souffles
10.	Frozen desserts	22.	Tortes
11.	Fruits	23.	Trifles
12.	Ice cream		

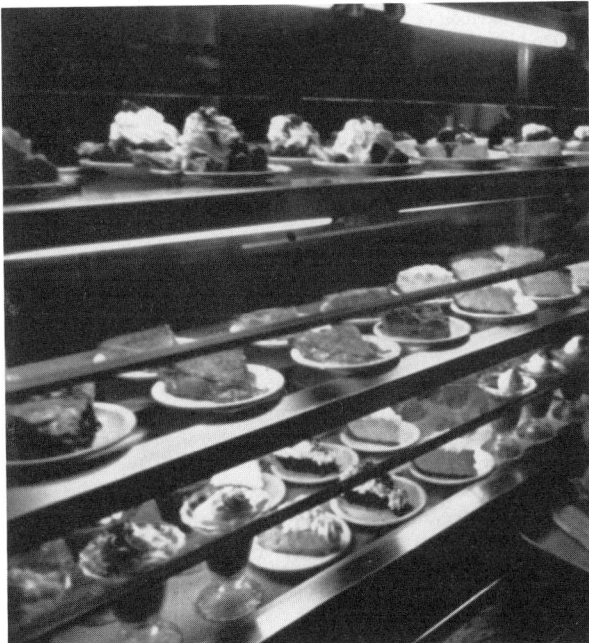

Fig. D-9. Assorted pies. (Courtesy, USDA)

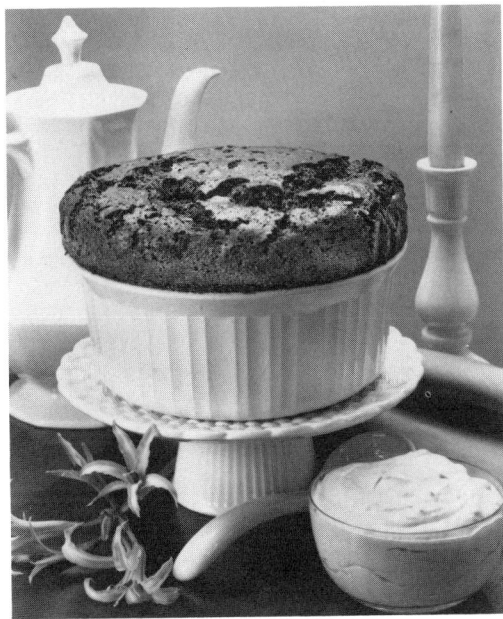

Fig. D-10. Baked chocolate souffle with raspberry cream. (Courtesy, Hershey Food Corporation, Hershey, Pa.)

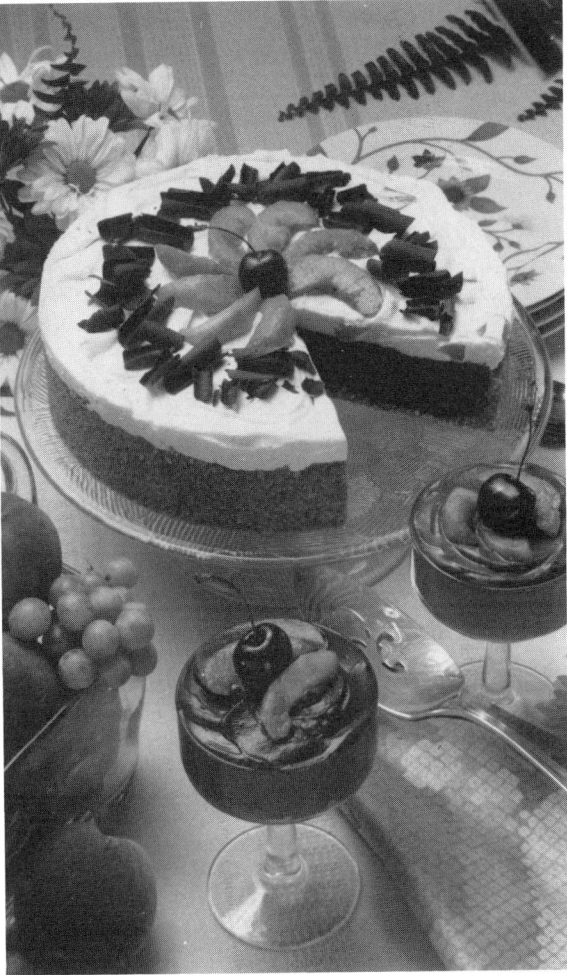

Fig. D-11. No-Bake Chocolate Cheesecake (top), Chilled or Frozen Chocolate Mousse (bottom). (Courtesy, Hershey Foods Corporation, Hershey, Pa.)

DETOXICATION

A process by which poisonous substances are rendered less harmful. Most of the detoxication reactions in the body take place in the liver.

DEVELOPMENT

As applied to humans, it generally denotes the series of changes by which the embryo becomes a mature organism; for example, the replacement of skeletal cartilage by calcified bone in the growing child.

DEWBERRY *Rubus baileyanus*

A trailing type of blackberry (a fruit of the family *Rosaceae*) that is grown in the eastern United States. The drupes of the berries are soft and less closely joined together than those of the other blackberries.

Dewberries are good fresh (especially when sweetened a little) and in jams, jellies, pies, and sauces.

DEXTRAN

A gummy substance which is produced by the action of certain microorganisms on sugar (sucrose). It may be dissolved in water to make an intravenous solution which is used for the treatment of hemorrhage or severe burns when blood plasma is unavailable.

DEXTRIMALTOSE

A mixture of dextrins and maltose prepared from cornstarch by acid treatment or by digestion with enzymes. It is used mainly in milk formulas for infants.

DEXTRIN

An intermediate polysaccharide, formed during the partial breakdown of starch.

(Also see CARBOHYDRATE[S].)

DEXTROSE (GLUCOSE; $C_6H_{12}O_6$)

Dextrose is the commercial name for glucose.

Since it rotates polarized light to the right (dextrorotatory), the industrial name for the simple sugar, glucose, is dextrose or corn sugar. It is made commercially from starch by the action of heat and acids, or enzymes. Two types of refined dextrose are available commercially: (1) dextrose hydrate, containing 9% by weight of water of crystallization and 426 kcal/100 g; and (2) anhydrous dextrose, containing 366 kcal/100 g and less than 0.5% water. Both are very soluble in water, but only 74% as sweet as sugar. However, dextrose acts synergistically with other sweeteners. Due to the following properties, dextrose is used in many food products: browning, fermentability, flavor enhancement, osmotic pressure, sweetness, humectancy (prevention of drying), hygroscopicity (moisture absorption), viscosity, and reactivity. The major users of dextrose are the confection, wine, and canning industries. In medicine, various concentrations of glucose (dextrose) are utilized for intravenous administration. *Example:* A 5% sterile dextrose solution or "D5W."

(Also see CARBOHYDRATE[S]; GLUCOSE; and SUGAR.)

DEXTROSE EQUIVALENT VALUE

During the conversion of corn starch to corn syrup, dextrins, maltotetrose, maltotriose, maltose, and dextrose are formed. As the process continues, more and more dextrose is formed. If the process is stopped at any given point a corn syrup of certain dextrose equivalent (DE) is produced. The longer the conversion process, the higher the DE and the sweeter the syrup. Pure dextrose has a DE of 100.

DIABETES, ALLOXAN

Diabetes experimentally induced in animals by the administration of the chemical alloxan, which preferentially damages the insulin-producing cells of the pancreas. Alloxan diabetes provides a useful animal model for the study of diabetes mellitus.

(Also see DIABETES MELLITUS.)

DIABETES INSIPIDUS

An unusual form of diabetes (the term means the passage of an excessive amount of urine) in which large quantities of water are lost in the urine. This disorder leads to dehydration and excessive thirst. Diabetes insipidus differs from ordinary diabetes in that it has no connection with the blood sugar, but is due to an abnormality of the pituitary gland.

(Also see ENDOCRINE GLANDS.)

DIABETES MELLITUS

Contents

This disease is a collection of disorders which result from either lack of insulin (a hormone secreted by the pancreas) or factors which interfere with the actions of this hormone. Most of the tissues in the body depend upon insulin for the promotion of the flow of sugars, fats, and amino acids into cells. The untreated diabetic literally starves to death in the midst of abundance since his or her blood may be loaded with nutrients which cannot get into the cells where they are needed. Diabetes is now the fifth leading cause of death by disease in the United States. There are two major forms in which the disease usually appears: adult-onset diabetes, and juvenile diabetes. Brief descriptions follow.

• **Adult-onset diabetes**—This form, which is by far the most common, may also be called *obesity diabetes* because it is found mainly in obese adults, and often it may be treated successfully by the reduction of body weight. There may be many adults who are free from symptoms, yet who have an early stage of this disease since the complications may develop very slowly. Sometimes, the pathological changes develop over several decades of life. Other characteristics of this form of diabetes are (1) victims are resistant to the development of ketoacidosis, except under conditions of stress; (2) persons over 40 years are the most likely to have the disease, although it sometimes occurs in children; (3) the various disorders develop slowly; (4) injections of insulin may *not* be needed when the early stages are successfully controlled by diet and/or oral drugs; and (5) most deaths from the disease are now due to degenerative disorders of the blood vessels, brain, kidneys, and heart, rather than to diabetic coma.

• **Juvenile diabetes**—In contrast to the adult-onset form, this type accounts for only about 10% of all cases of diabetes, yet it is much harder to control, and severe ketoacidosis is common. Other characteristics of this form are (1) oral drugs are not suitable, so injections of insulin are required; (2) its victims are often underweight rather than obese; (3) progress of the disease may be very rapid; (4) symptoms of excessive urination, unusual thirst, and overeating are common features; and (5) it usually strikes young people (under 25 years). This form is believed to originate from a genetic defect in the pancreas. The tendency to develop diabetes is passed along as a recessive trait, but it appears that as many as 20% of the world's people may carry the gene.

HISTORY OF DIABETES.
This disease has apparently plagued man for a very long time, since the writings from the earliest civilizations (Asia Minor, China, Egypt, and India) refer to boils and infections, excessive thirst, loss of weight, and the passing of large quantities of a honeysweet urine which often drew ants and flies. (The term *diabetes* is derived from the Greek word meaning *siphon*, or *the passing through of water*; while *mellitus* is Latin for *honeysweet*.) For example, the *Papyrus Ebers*, an Egyptian document dated about 1550 B.C., recommended that those afflicted with the malady go on a diet of beer, fruits, grains, and honey, which was reputed to stifle the excessive urination. Indian writings from the same era attributed the disease to overindulgence in food and drink.

In 1921, Banting and Best, physiologists who were working at the University of Toronto, discovered that they could obtain biologically active insulin from the pancreases of dogs provided (1) they first tied off the pancreatic duct so as to cause degeneration of the cells that secreted digestive juices, or (2) they used embryonic pancreases from fetal pups, since the insulin-secreting cells develop before the digestive cells. The insulin they obtained cured the diabetes of depancreatized dogs. Following many other tests on dogs, the hormone was administered to a male diabetic human, who experienced a remarkable recovery. Banting was awarded the Nobel Prize for the discovery, but Best was not even considered for the award because he held only an undergraduate degree at the time. However, Banting shared the money with him.

About the same time as the initiation of the use of oral drugs, medical researchers discovered that adult-onset diabetics secreted approximately normal amounts of insulin, but that the action of the hormone was somehow impaired. It was then discovered that obesity is a major contributing factor to this type of diabetes, and that a great improvement in the utilization of glucose often follows a reduction in body weight. It seems that the distended fat-containing cells found in obese people are resistant to the effects of insulin. Other researchers have recently suggested that it is wise to have strict dietary control in diabetes so as to minimize the need for extra insulin. Excessive insulin may accelerate the development of cardiovascular lesions. Hence, it appears that some of the strict dietary measures which were used in the preinsulin days are still useful for the treatment of adult-onset diabetes.

METABOLIC ABNORMALITIES IN DIABETES.
Many of the deadly complications of uncontrolled diabetes can be traced to the metabolic disorders which accompany advanced stages of the disease. Many of these disorders may be absent in mild cases of adult-onset diabetes. Nevertheless, it is important for all diabetics to recognize the consequences of poor control of their disease. These disorders follow:

1. **Abnormal appetite.** Diabetics usually have an excessive appetite and overeat.

2. **Excessive hormones in the small intestine.** There may be excess secretion of hormones by the small intestine.

3. **Abnormal secretion of insulin by the pancreas.** The secretion of insulin may be deficient (juvenile diabetes); or the secretion of insulin may be delayed or required in greater amounts due to *insulin resistance* (adult diabetes).

4. **Disorders of metabolism in the liver.** The liver may contribute to elevated levels of ketones, cholesterol, glycoproteins, glucose, and fat; and there may be reductions in the synthesis of carbohydrate reserves (glycogen) and in the utilization of carbohydrate for energy.

5. **Abnormal blood chemistry.** There may be elevated levels of cholesterol and other fatty materials.

6. **Impaired brain.** Abnormal carbohydrate metabolism may affect the structure and function of the brain.

7. **Altered metabolism in the muscles.** Lack of insulin results in reduced muscle cell uptake of amino acids, fatty acids, and glucose, followed by deterioration of muscles.

8. **Altered metabolism in adipose (fatty) tissues.** Without insulin, adipose tissues can not take up the nutrients that they need with the result that these fatty tissues break down and release fatty acids and glycerol in the blood.

9. **Disorders involving the kidneys.** Severe diabetes provokes the kidneys to convert amino acids to ammonia and glucose, which are released to the blood. Also, the diabetic excretes a large volume of urine containing glucose, ketone bodies, and mineral salts.

10. **Damaged eyes.** Elevated blood levels of fats and glucose may result in damage to the retina and cause cataracts.

11. **Damaged nerves.** High levels of fats and glucose may damage the nerves, and result in loss of their functions.

12. **Damaged blood vessels.** Excessive bloodborne fats and glucose result in thickening of the lining and the formation of plaques in blood vessels.

FACTORS WHICH MAY PRECIPITATE OR AGGRAVATE DIABETES.
Many doctors have observed that diabetes seems to be more prevalent in certain families than others, so they have concluded that the tendency to develop the disease is an inherited trait. Support for this theory is found in studies of twins who originate from a single, fertilized egg cell (identical or monozygotic twins). Identical twins have identical genes, so they should also have the same susceptibility to hereditary diseases; whereas fraternal twins (which originate from two separate, fertilized eggs) have no greater similarity in their heredity than brothers or sisters born at different times. A study revealed that 70% of the identical twins of known diabetics had the disease, while only 10% of the fraternal twins of known diabetics were diabetic.[5] The fact that fewer than 100% of the identical twins of diabetics had the disease showed that environmental factors also played a role in its development.

Another study showed that about 25% of the nontwin brothers and sisters of diabetics might be expected to develop either the insulin-requiring form, or the milder adult-onset form sometime in their lifetime.[6]

The strong evidence for hereditary susceptibility to diabetes leads many health professionals to believe that for diabetes-prone families, the potential to become diabetic is present in all members at the time of their birth. Whether or not they develop clinical signs of the disease depends upon their exposure to factors which may precipitate or aggravate the disease. If this concept is correct, then heredity is the single *cause* of diabetes. Therefore, it is important to

[5]Gottlieb, M. S., and H. F. Root, "Diabetes Mellitus in Twins," *Diabetes*, Vol. 17, 1968, p. 693.

[6]Kobberling, J., "Studies on the Genetic Heterogeneity of Diabetic Mellitus," *Diabetologia*, Vol. 7, 1971, p. 46.

be aware of the more common factors which may trigger the clinical features of diabetes. These follow.

1. Autoantibodies in the blood causing the insulin to be ineffective—a phenomenon called autoimmunity.
2. Chronic hypoglycemia (low blood sugar).
3. Damage to the pancreas by an iron overload (hemochromatosis).
4. Deficiencies of essential minerals, especially calcium, chromium, magnesium, manganese, potassium, and zinc.
5. Excessive secretion of diabetogenic hormones (hormones that maintain or raise blood sugar), including adrenocorticotropic hormone (ACTH) and a growth hormone from the pituitary; adrenalin, noradrenalin, and adrenal cortical hormones (mainly cortisol) from the adrenals; glucagon from the pancreas; and thyroid hormone from the thyroid.
6. Fasting or starvation.
7. Fever.
8. High-fat diets.
9. High-protein diets.
10. High-sugar diets.
11. Infections.
12. Irregular patterns of eating, exercising, and sleeping.
13. Ketosis.
14. Lack of exercise.
15. Lack of fiber.
16. Larges meals.
17. Obesity.
18. Oral contraceptives (birth control pills).
19. Pancreatitis.
20. Pregnancy.
21. Pregnancy diabetes due to a deficiency of pyridoxine (vitamin B-6).
22. Protein-energy malnutrition.
23. Stress diabetes.
24. Thiazide diuretics (water pills).

COMPLICATIONS OF DIABETES.

Good diabetic control requires much more than the prevention of the spilling of sugar into the urine. The other factors which need to be controlled are the blood levels of cholesterol, free fatty acids (these come from the body's fat stores), glucose, insulin, ketones, and triglycerides (this is the main form of fat carried by lipoproteins in the blood). Failure to control these factors may result in some of the following complications:

1. Alcoholic diabetics may react to insulin treatment similar to an overdose of insulin.
2. Atherosclerosis.
3. Birth defects in children of diabetic mothers.
4. Blindness.
5. Blood clots.
6. Bone disorders.
7. Brain damage.
8. Cloudy spots on the lens of the eyes (cataracts).
9. Death of tissue (gangrene).
10. Dehydration (excessive loss of body water).
11. Diabetic coma.
12. Digestive disorders.
13. Dizziness when standing up (postural hypotension).
14. Excessive loss of essential minerals in the urine.
15. Fatty liver.
16. Heart failure due to ventricular fibrillation.
17. Heavy babies.
18. High blood fats.
19. High blood pressure (hypertension).
20. Impotence and other sexual problems.
21. Infections.

22. Ketoacidosis.
23. Ketosis.
24. Kidney disease.
25. Lacticacidosis.
26. Loss of sensation in the feet.
27. Loss of weight.
28. Muscle wasting.
29. Nerve disorders.
30. Pains in the chest and shoulder (angina pectoris).
31. Pancreatic deterioration and the worsening of diabetes.
32. Skin disorders.
33. Spontaneous abortion.
34. Stroke.

DIAGNOSIS OF DIABETES.

The ways in which diabetes is diagnosed have changed in recent years, from those with a major emphasis on examination for overt signs of the disease to those used to detect the early stages which are present prior to the appearance of clinical signs. Therefore, it is of interest to note the stages of development of the disease, since the earlier the disease is found, the better the prognosis.[7]

1. **Prediabetes.** The widespread belief that there is a hereditary basis for diabetes leads to the classification of close kin of diabetics (usually the nondiabetic identical twins of diabetics and the children of two diabetic parents) as prediabetics, even though these people may show no signs of the disease. Although it is not inevitable that those so classified will eventually develop the disease, there is a high probability that this may be the case. Hence, these people should be watched for the early signs of the disease.

2. **Subclinical or *stress* diabetes.** This stage, where clinical signs are absent, is characterized by a diabeticlike utilization of carbohydrate under stress, but a normal utilization when the stress is removed. The utilization of carbohydrate is assessed by measuring the fasting blood sugar, or by giving a glucose tolerance test. Typical stresses which provoke abnormal carbohydrate metabolism are emotional disturbances, fever, infections, and pregnancy. The diagnosis of subclinical diabetes is based upon giving the patient a dose of a stress hormone, such as cortisone, prior to the glucose tolerance test. This test determines whether the pancreas has sufficient reserve capacity to meet the challenge imposed by stress situations where there may be greater than normal secretion of diabetogenic hormones.

3. **Chemical or latent diabetes.** Unlike the preceding stages, the utilization of carbohydrate in this stage is clearly abnormal, even when no stress factors are present. However, clinical signs, such as sugar in the urine, are not usually present unless there is some type of stress. Nevertheless, the abnormal glucose tolerance is a sign that there will most likely be a further development of the disease if treatment is not started promptly.

4. **Clinical, or overt, diabetes.** In this stage, there are both chemical and clinical signs of diabetes such as excessive urination, sugar in the urine, and occasional bouts of ketosis or ketoacidosis.

The progression of diabetes to the overt stage may be rapid, particularly in the cases of juvenile diabetics. Regression of diabetes to a less severe stage also occurs in significant numbers of people, so there is almost always hope for victims of this disease.

[7]Goodkin, G., "How Long Can a Diabetic Expect to Live?" *Nutrition Today*, Vol. 6, May/June 1971, p. 21.

Signs and Symptoms of Diabetes. These signs are usually present only in the overt diabetic, but they may sometimes be seen in latent diabetics. Hence, their absence does *not* eliminate the possibility of diabetes. The signs are sugar in the urine, frequent and excessive urination, abnormal thirst, increased hunger, loss of weight, nausea, and tiredness. People who repeatedly have these signs should go to a doctor. Symptoms of hypoglycemia may also be early signs of diabetes.

(Also see HYPOGLYCEMIA.)

Tests of Blood and Urine. A markedly elevated fasting blood sugar in the absence of unusual stress is a strong indicator of diabetes. (Usually, this test is conducted on a sample of blood drawn after an overnight fast.) However, the glucose tolerance test provides more specific information as to the severity of the disease.

The repeated spilling of sugar into the urine is another strong indicator of diabetes. Often young people spill sugar without being diabetic. On the other hand, older diabetics with high blood sugar levels may fail to spill sugar in their urine, particularly if their kidney function is partially impaired. Therefore, the test for sugar in the urine has its limitations for the detection of diabetes, but it may be useful to diabetics as a rough indicator of the control of their disease.

Glucose Tolerance Test (GTT). This test is considered to be the most reliable of those available for the evaluation of carbohydrate utilization by the body. The term *glucose tolerance* literally means the rate at which the cells of the body take up glucose from the blood. An abnormal and/or prolonged rise in the blood sugar after a test dose of glucose is interpreted as a sign that the utilization of carbohydrate by the cells is somehow impaired. Diabetes is the most likely cause of this abnormality because insulin is required for the passage of glucose and other nutrients from the blood into the cells.

(Also see HYPOGLYCEMIA, section headed "Glucose Tolerance Test.")

Detection of Diabetes in Children. The development of diabetes in children may be very rapid; so, the earlier that it is detected, the better the outcome. Sometimes, children in certain families develop the juvenile form of the disease well in advance of the time that the disease is detected in its adult-onset form in older relatives such as grandparents. At present, no one knows why juvenile diabetes may suddenly appear in a family with no apparent history of the disease.

The most common signs of juvenile diabetes are excessive urination (it may be almost impossible to stop some children from wetting their beds), unusual thirst, unexplainable weight loss, tiredness, and increased appetite. A negative test for sugar in the urine does not rule out the disease, nor does a positive test confirm it. Blood tests (fasting blood sugar and/or glucose tolerance) are the only certain means of diagnosis. However, it might be wise to apply the tests for sugar and ketones to the urine of a child with a fever, particularly if his or her breath smells like acetone (a rotten, fruity odor, like that noticed after the drinking of alcoholic beverages). The fever may be a sufficient stress to bring out a hidden diabetic tendency. (Specially treated paper strips and tablets for testing urine are sold in most drug stores.)

TREATMENT AND PREVENTION OF DIABETES.

One of the great medical achievements of our time is the successful treatment of diabetics so as to give those so afflicted many trouble-free years of life, an almost impossible task prior to the discovery of insulin. Many highly successful people, and even some celebrities, have been lifelong diabetics, yet they have not let the disease prevent them from enjoying life. An entire book has been written on this subject.[8] However, what is unique in diabetes, compared to most other diseases, is that the diabetic is literally his or her own doctor, since most of the therapeutic measures have to be self-administered on a day-to-day basis. Therefore, careful attention should be paid to the treatments which follow.

Emergency Treatments. There are two life-threatening crises which may occur in diabetes: diabetic coma, and hypoglycemia. The measures to be taken depend upon the correct identification of the critical condition, since the wrong treatment may do more harm than good. The characteristics of each condition are presented in Table D-4.

TABLE D-4
DIAGNOSTIC FEATURES OF DIABETIC COMA AND HYPOGLYCEMIA

Feature[1]	Diabetic Coma	Hypoglycemia
Signs and symptoms:		
Abdomen	Pain is often present.	Pain is **not** usually present.
Blood chemistry ..	Acidosis (bicarbonate is low) sugar is elevated.	Normal bicarbonate, low sugar level.
Blood pressure ...	Low.	Normal to high.
Breathing	Deep and labored.	Normal or shallow.
Digestive system ..	Vomiting often occurs.	Occasional vomiting.
Emotional status ..	Apathetic.	Anxious and irritable.
Mouth	Dry.	Moist.
Odor of breath ...	Fruity (acetone).	Normal.
Pulse	Slow and weak.	Rapid.
Reflexes	Slow.	Normal.
Skin	Dry, warm.	Moist, cool.
Urine, characteristics[2]	Contains ketones and sugar; volume may be greater than normal.	Normal composition and volume.
History of the patient:		
Control of the disease	Usually not very good.	May be either good or poor.
Insulin status	Too little (dose may have been skipped).	Too much.
Previous infection .	Often brings on condition.	Not usually present.
Skipping of meals .	Sometimes.	Often brings on condition.
Strenuous exercise	Not usually.	Often brings on condition.
Time required for development of condition	There may be a gradual deterioration over several days.	Onset is usually rapid, and often occurs between meals.

[1]It is not always easy to distinguish between diabetic coma and hypoglycemia because (a) vigorous treatment of the coma may lead to hypoglycemia, (b) prolonged hypoglycemia causes brain abnormalities which have many features like those of diabetic coma, and (c) the metabolic reaction to hypoglycemia (increased secretion of diabetogenic hormones) in severe diabetes may lead to diabetic coma.

[2]Has diagnostic value only when it represents metabolism over the past few hours. Sometimes, urine has been retained in the bladder so long that it represents an earlier metabolic state.

Treatments for diabetic coma and hypoglycemia follow.

[8]Biermann, J., and B. Toohey, *The Diabetic's Sports and Exercise Book*, J. B. Lippincott Co., Philadelphia, Pa., 1977.

DIABETIC COMA. The acetone breath which accompanies this condition has often led to the mistaken identification of a comatose diabetic as a drunk. Subsequent confinement in a prison has sometimes resulted in severe complications, and in a few cases, death. Therefore, a diabetic should always *wear* an identification tag. (Purses or wallets are often lost or stolen during emergency situations.) A doctor should be immediately summoned, since attempts at first aid by lay persons may be ineffective, or even dangerous. The family of a diabetic should *not* attempt to administer insulin unless the doctor so advises, since the injection of insulin may be fatal to a person suffering from hypoglycemia.

HYPOGLYCEMIA (Insulin Shock). All diabetics should have available at all times a source of readily available sugar for use in case of hypoglycemia (low blood sugar). Convenient sources of sugar are items such as soft candy (hard candy may dissolve too slowly), cubes or paper packets of table sugar, dextrose tablets (a form of pure glucose which is sold in certain health foods stores and pharmacies), and malted milk tablets. If a diabetic is at home, he or she may drink a glass of fruit juice. However, nothing should be placed in the mouth of an unconscious person. In the latter case, a doctor should be called immediately.

Some doctors recommend that diabetics keep home supplies for the injection of glucagon, and that family members be instructed in its administration in the event that emergency care is not available. Each of these emergency measures should be used with great discretion, for the rapid raising of the blood sugar may worsen diabetes. Hence, each diabetic should be very familiar with the specific symptoms of hypoglycemia, and should refrain from using these measures for getting a lift from feelings of depression or tiredness.

(Also see HYPOGLYCEMIA, section headed "Signs and Symptoms.")

Dietary Measures. In 1986, the American Diabetes Association (ADA) revised its dietary guidelines for only the second time in more than 25 years. It is noteworthy that these guidelines are similar to those of the American Heart Association and the National Cancer Institute. The revised ADA nutritional recommendations follow:[9]

1. **Calories.** Calories should be prescribed according to energy needs and to achieve and maintain a desirable body weight.

2. **Carbohydrates.** The amount of carbohydrate intake should be liberalized to 55–60% of daily total calories. Whenever possible, substitute unrefined carbohydrates high in fiber (such as whole grain bread and cereal) for highly refined foods.

3. **Fat.** Lower the fat intake to 30% or less of the total daily calories; and limit saturated fat to 10% of the total calories.

4. **Cholesterol.** Limit cholesterol in the diet to 300 mg/day or less.

5. **Sweeteners.** The use of nutritive and nonnutritive sweeteners is not encouraged, but is acceptable in diabetes management.

6. **Salt.** The limitation of salt intake is highly recommended in most circumstances.

7. **Protein intake.** The recommended daily allowance

for adults is 0.8 g/kg body weight.

8. **Alcohol.** Preferably, drinking of alcohol should be avoided; otherwise, drink in moderation.

The control of blood sugar also involves the maintenance of the body weight which is appropriate for age, body build, height, and sex. This means that obese diabetics should make every effort to lose weight in a medically approved manner, but not by crash diets which may aggravate their disease.

Finally, the diet should help to prevent rather than promote atherosclerosis. (There is growing concern that the traditional practice of replacement of dietary carbohydrate with fat in diets has been at least partly responsible for the high rate of cardiovascular disease.)

TYPES OF DIETS. The three basic types of diets which are currently being prescribed for diabetics are (1) a moderately low-carbohydrate diet which restricts mainly simple sugars and alcohol, for those who have high blood levels of triglycerides (Type IV Hyperlipoproteinemia), (2) the most commonly used diabetic diet which has from 45 to 55% of its calories supplied by carbohydrate, and (3) a recently tested high-carbohydrate, low-fat diet for people who have high blood levels of cholesterol and/or other fats (Type II and other types of hyperlipoproteinemias). However, the selection of diets to combat the various types of hyperlipoproteinemia is still somewhat controversial, so doctors tend to rely on special laboratory tests for guidance in selecting a diet. Some typical diets and their compositions are given in Table D-5.

(Also see HYPERLIPOPROTEINEMIAS.)

SPECIAL FOODS WHICH ARE LOW IN ENERGY (kilocalories). One of the major problems of obese diabetics is that of sticking to a diet low in calories. Whether they are taking insulin or not, they must lose weight because neither their own nor the various insulins which may be injected have maximum effectiveness in obesity. Thus, they are faced with the problem of selecting foods that are not only low in energy, but also palatable and satisfying. There are several ways to accomplish these objectives. Suggestions follow.

The most common foods which are filling but not fattening are high-fiber, low-energy fruits and vegetables such as blackberries, bean sprouts, cabbage, greens, and string beans.

(Also see FIBER.)

Less common, but also useful, are special low-energy foods like Jerusalem artichoke tubers which contain inulin, a starchlike carbohydrate which cannot be utilized by man. The floury material obtained by drying and pulverizing these tubers is used to replace all or part of the wheat flour in dietetic noodles and spaghetti. Although these products are sold in many health food stores, they are seldom labeled as to their content of available carbohydrate or energy.

Some other special food items are agar-agar (a nonnutritive gelling agent), fruits canned in water instead of sugar syrup, gluten flour (low in starch, high in protein), and low-fat salad dressings. While these items were once available only in health food stores or pharmacies, they are now sold in many supermarkets. Also, materials like agar-agar may be purchased for incorporation in recipes prepared at home. Greater detail as to the use of these and other similar products is presented elsewhere in the book.

---

[9]These recommendations were developed by a task force of the American Diabetes Association, chaired by Aaron I. Vinik, M.D.; published in *Nutrition Today*, January/February, 1987, pp. 29–30.

TABLE D-5
TYPICAL MENUS FOR VARIOUS TYPES OF DIETS

Types of Food Exchanges (used for each meal or snack)[1]	Number of Exchanges per Meal (based upon daily energy requirements)					
	Moderately Low-Carbohydrate, High-Protein Diet		Standard Diet (50% carbohydrate)		High Carbohydrate, Low-Fat Diet	
	1,800 kcal/day	2,400 kcal/day	1,800 kcal/day	2,400 kcal/day	1,800 kcal/day	2,400 kcal/day
Breakfast:						
Bread (or biscuits, cereals, crackers, muffins, pancakes, waffles, etc.)	1	2	2	2	2	3
Fat (bacon, butter, coffee whitener, margarine, mayonnaise, etc.)[2]	1	3	2	2	1	2
Fruit (or its equivalent in juice)	1	1	1	2	1	1
Lean meat (or low-fat cheese, fish, fowl, etc.)	2	2	1	1	1	1
Milk, nonfat (if whole milk products are used, deduct 2 servings of fat from the day's allowance)	0	0	0	0	1	1
Optional beverage: bouillon (fat free), clear broth, club soda, coffee, herb tea, tea, water	Any amount, but limit sweetener.					
Mid-morning snack:						
Bread	1	1	1	1	2	2
Fat	2	2	0	2	0	1
Fruit (or juice)	0	0	0	0	0	0
Meat	0	1	0	0	0	0
Milk or yogurt, plain, nonfat	1	1	1	1	0	0
Optional beverage (see Breakfast)	Any amount, but limit sweetener.					
Lunch:						
Bread	1	2	2	3	3	3
Fat	1	3	2	3	1	2
Fruit	0	0	1	1	1	1
Meat, lean (see Breakfast)	3	4	3	3	2	3
Optional beverage (see Breakfast)	Any amount, but limit sweetener.					
Raw vegetable, or salad w/o dressing	1	1	1	1	1	1
Mid-afternoon snack:						
Bread	1	1	1	1	2	2
Fat	2	2	0	2	0	1
Fruit (or juice)	0	0	0	0	0	0
Meat	0	1	0	0	0	0
Milk, nonfat	1	1	1	1	1	1
Optional beverage (see Breakfast)	Any amount, but limit sweetener.					
Supper:						
Bread	1	1	2	4	2	4
Fat	2	4	3	3	2	2
Fruit	1	1	1	2	1	2
Meat, lean (see Breakfast)	4	4	3	3	3	3
Optional beverage	Any amount, but limit sweetener.					
Raw vegetable, or salad w/o dressing	1	1	1	1	1	1
Nonstarchy vegetable, cooked	1	1	1	1	1	1
Late evening snack:						
Bread	1	1	1	2	1	2
Fat	2	2	1	1	0	0
Fruit	0	1	1	1	1	2
Meat	1	1	0	0	0	0
Milk, nonfat	1	1	1	1	1	1
Optional beverage	Any amount, but limit sweetener.					

[1]Exchanges are groups of foods which may be substituted for each other because they contain similar proportions of carbohydrate, fat, protein, and calories.

[2]The total day's allowance for fat plus the distributing of fat at meals and snacks may have to be adjusted so as to compensate for foods which contain considerably less or more fat than the amounts which are typical for their exchange groups. Also, doctors generally recommend that as many as possible of the fat exchanges be chosen from polyunsaturated fats (salad oils and soft margarines) because ample amounts of saturated fats are provided by the meat exchanges.

PREVENTION OF NUTRITIONAL DEFICIENCIES IN DIABETICS. It was mentioned earlier that diabetes may be brought on and/or aggravated by deficiencies of the essential nutrients chromium, manganese, potassium, pyridoxine (vitamin B-6), or zinc. This is *not* to say that the basic nutrient requirements of diabetics are significantly different from nondiabetics; it is only to note that (1) a few people may show diabetic tendencies due to deficiencies of various nutrients, (2) diabetes may impair the utilization and/or increase the urinary excretion of certain nutrients and so create a need for higher dietary levels of such substances, and (3) diets made up mainly of highly refined foods may be lacking in nutrients.

However, information as to the incidence of nutritional deficiencies is lacking, since the appropriate diagnostic tests are rarely performed, except in a few research studies.

Although the widespread use of such tests might be objected to on the grounds of increased costs of health care, the ultimate cost of disabilities due to severe deficiencies might be much greater.

A good start towards the prevention of the various deficiencies might be made if doctors would take more dietary histories from their patients, since many medical centers now have computers programmed to translate food patterns into the nutrients which are consumed. Once patients on deficient diets have been identified, the next step is to use such tests as those for pyridoxine (vitamin B-6) deficiency, and/or the analysis of hair for such trace minerals as chromium, manganese, and zinc.

While mineral and vitamin pills may be purchased without a prescription, it would be better for most people to obtain all of the nutrients they need from minimally processed foods such as dairy products, fish, fresh or frozen vegetables, legumes (beans and peas), meats, and whole grain products. Each of the plant foods is also a good source of fiber, which helps to control overeating by providing a feeling of fullness.

(Also see FIBER; MINERALS; and VITAMINS.)

Insulin.   This hormone has proved to be a lifesaver for many diabetics. The current thinking is that injections of insulin may not be necessary for some adults with mild diabetes, but that this therapy is almost always necessary for juvenile diabetics and adult diabetics whose insulin secretion is inadequate. Sometimes, insulin-dependent diabetics may appear to have a remission of their disease so that it may seem that injections of the hormone are no longer necessary. It is believed that injections of insulin reduce the stress on the few insulin-secreting cells which remain functional. Thus, the *rested* pancreatic cells may be able to cope for a while on their own. However, many doctors believe it is wise to continue the administration of insulin throughout temporary periods of remission so as to keep the insulin-dependent diabetic in a consistent pattern of regulation.

Like many other therapies, injections of insulin have their drawbacks. First of all, it is not always easy for the doctor to determine the dose that is needed. Too little gives poor control, which is still better than no control, while too much may produce hypoglycemia (low blood sugar). Second, it was mentioned earlier that some doctors suspect that excessive insulin might accelerate the buildup of fatty materials in atherosclerotic plaques, since insulin promotes the uptake of fat by cells and the synthesis of storage fat. Finally, some diabetics develop various types of physiological blocks against the actions of the hormone. It is now suspected that occurrence of these problems might be greatly curtailed if the requirements for insulin were to be lowered in many diabetics by strict dietary control and regular programs of moderate to vigorous physical activity.

Determination of the amounts and types of insulin to be administered is the responsibility of the attending physician. Likewise, the choice of a diet to be used by an insulin-dependent diabetic must also be determined by the doctor who usually asks a dietitian to work out the details. Although this situation differs from that of the mild diabetic treated by diet alone (where the dietary prescription may merely be to consume less energy so as to lose weight), extra precautions are necessary in order to coordinate the effects of both diet and insulin injections (and, in some cases, the added effects of strenuous exercise). It is with this in mind that Fig. D-12, types of insulin and their characteristics, is presented.

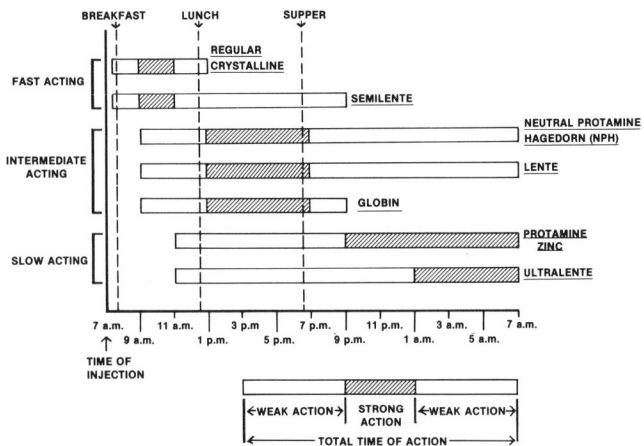

Fig. D-12. Types of insulin and their characteristics.

MEAL PATTERNS FOR DIFFERENT TYPES OF INSULIN.
Fig. D-12 shows that each type of insulin has specific characteristics relating to its speed and duration of action. Hence, meal patterns must be coordinated so that carbohydrate feedings throughout the day correspond with the times of maximum action of the injected insulin(s). Typical patterns follow.

• **Mixtures of regular and slow-acting insulins**—The injection is usually given before breakfast, so about 2/5 of the day's allowance of carbohydrate is assigned to that meal because of the early effect of regular insulin; only 1/5 is assigned to lunch when there is a lull in insulin activity, and the remaining 2/5 is assigned to dinner when the slow-acting insulin begins to take effect.

• **Slow-acting insulins**—In this case there is little insulin action in the morning, so only 1/6 of the carbohydrate is allotted to breakfast, 2/6 to lunch, 2/6 to dinner, and 1/6 to a late evening snack. This pattern has most of the carbohydrate assigned to the afternoon and evening because most of the insulin action occurs late in the day.

• **Intermediate-acting insulins**—The effects of these insulins peak in the afternoon; hence, only 1/6 of the carbohydrate allowance for the day is given at breakfast, 2/6 at lunch, 1/6 at a mid-afternoon snack to counteract a tendency for low blood sugar to develop at that time, and 2/6 at dinner.

Oral Drugs.   These drugs are effective in lowering the blood sugar *only* when the diabetic is able to secrete sufficient insulin. They are *not* usually effective for either juvenile or adult-onset diabetics who are dependent upon injections of insulin, nor do they help much where there has been a history of ketosis or acidosis. Hence, they are mainly used to treat adult-onset diabetics who are unable to control their disease by diet alone, but who may be able to use these drugs in lieu of injections of insulin. Some doctors believe that when patients secrete adequate insulin it is best to avoid giving injections of extra insulin provided oral drugs reduce the high blood sugar levels and stop the spilling of sugar in the urine.[10] The reason for avoiding extra insulin is that

---

[10]Fineberg, S. K., "Obesity-Diabetes," *Nutrition Today*, Vol. 1, September 1966, p. 16.

this hormone stimulates the production of fat from carbohydrate, and most adult-onset diabetics already have too much body fat. There are two main types of oral antidiabetic drugs, descriptions of which follow.

SULFA-TYPE DRUGS (SULFONYLUREAS). The main action of these compounds is stimulation of the pancreatic cells to release insulin. Some, like tolbutamide are short acting (6 to 12 hours), while others like acetohexamide and tolazamide are intermediate acting (12 to 24 hours), and chlorpropamide is long acting (24 to 72 hours). These drugs sometimes cause hypoglycemia, which may be prolonged in the case of chlorpropamide, particularly when given to elderly people who eat poorly or who have kidney disorders. In the latter case, the drug may not be excreted from the body, so the patient may require dialysis in order to correct the low blood sugar.

NOTE: People who are receiving tolbutamide should avoid alcoholic beverages because the drug may interfere with alcohol metabolism to the extent that they become nauseous and feel poorly.

PHENFORMIN. This drug slows the rate of glucose absorption from the intestine (which results in a slowing in the rise of blood sugar after meals) and increases the utilization of carbohydrate. Its disadvantages are that its effects are short lived (4 to 6 hours), it may irritate the gastrointestinal tract, and occasionally it may be the cause of lacticacidosis. Hence, the dosage level of this drug has to be limited. However, it works well in combination with the sulfa-type drugs, since the antidiabetic effects of the two agents are additive.

Foot Care. Too many diabetics have sustained permanent, but often preventable, damage to their feet and legs from what may have started out as such minor problems as cuts and infections. The reasons why the lower limbs of diabetics are so vulnerable is that (1) nerve disorders result in the dulling of the sense of pain; (2) the reduction in the circulation through the small blood vessels is greatest in the feet because the force of gravity on the circulating blood produces the greatest pressure there and, hence, the greatest

thickening of capillary membranes; (3) the feet and legs bear the weight of the rest of the body, which in most adult diabetics is greater than normal; and (4) infections spread more rapidly in diabetics.

Exercise. Physical activity may be a form of therapy for the diabetic (since it may make it easier to lose weight, and it may also lower the blood levels of both fats and glucose), or it may cause such problems as low blood sugar. Therefore, it is worthwhile for diabetics to try and anticipate in advance any change in their customary level of activity. Although it is well known that increases in energy expenditures by diabetics usually lower their requirements for insulin, most doctors prefer that patients who are dependent upon such injections adjust their food intake to correspond with changes in activity, rather than change their doses of insulin. If such increased energy expenditure becomes a regular part of a diabetic's life, then the doctor will explain how to change the dose of insulin.

NOTE: Any diabetic who is thinking of trying to increase greatly his or her level of physical activity should first have a thorough examination by a doctor since hidden cardiovascular weaknesses may be present. However, many diabetics benefit from well-planned exercise programs.

It is simple enough to add food to the diet so as to replace the extra energy expended in additional physical activity. The best foods for this purpose are those high in carbohydrate—like bread, fruits, and vegetables. People who are trying to lose weight may not wish to replace all of the energy spent in extra exercise, but it might be wise for them to eat at least a little more food (about half of the equivalent of exercise) so that they do not develop low blood sugar. The extra food should be taken between meals, and prior to the activity. The food equivalents of various types of exercise are given in Table D-6.

(Also see ATHLETICS AND NUTRITION, Table A-7, Energy Expenditures For Selected Athletic Activities.)

(For a more complete discussion of DIABETES MELLITUS, the reader is referred to *Foods & Nutrition Encyclopedia,* a two-volume work by the same authors.

TABLE D-6
FOOD EQUIVALENTS OF VARIOUS ACTIVITIES

Description of Activity	Time Spent in Activity	Total Energy Expenditure[1]	Bread Exchanges	Food Equivalents[2]		
				Fruit Exchanges	Vegetables, B Group	
	(minutes)	(kcal)	(70 kcal)	(40 kcal)	(35 kcal)	
Dishwashing	30	30	½	1	1	
Jogging (running alternated with walking)	10	100	1½	2½	3	
Riding a bicycle (7 miles [*11.2 km*] per hour)	20	130	2	3	4	
Sweeping floors	60	110	1½	3	3	
Swimming (30 yards [*21 m*] per minute)	20	170	2½	4	5	
Walking (3½ to 4 miles [*5.6 to 6.4 km*] per hour)	30	156	2	4	4	

[1]Based upon the performance of the activity by a 154-lb (*69.3-kg*) man.

[2]Approximate amount of each food = total energy expenditure ÷ energy per exchange.

DIABETES, RENAL

An older term for renal glucosuria.

(Also see RENAL GLUCOSURIA.)

DIABINASE

A brand name for a form of sulfonylurea called chlorpropamide, a long-acting oral drug used to stimulate the pancreatic cells of a diabetic to release insulin. The drug is only effective when the diabetic has some insulin secreting ability remaining in the pancreas. Other brand names include Adiaben, Asucrol, Catanil, Chloronase, Diabechlor, Diabenal, Diabetoral, Melitase, Millinese, Oradian, and Stabinol.

(Also see DIABETES MELLITUS.)

DIACETYL

A substance produced by the action of micro-organisms on butter fat. It is responsible for the distinct taste of butter which has been ripened. However, it may be produced artificially and used as an additive to margarine.

DIALYSIS

A process in which certain substances in a solution are removed by the passage of the solution through a membrane. Dialysis is used to purify the blood of patients who suffer from kidney disease, when the kidneys are unable to perform this function.

DIAPHYSIS

A shaft of a long bone, such as is found in the arms and legs. During the growth of the long bones the diaphyses are separated from the ends of the bones (epiphyses) by a plate of cartilage. When growth ceases during maturity, the diaphyses fuse with the epiphyses.

(Also see BONE.)

DIARRHEA

Rapid movement of the fecal matter through the digestive system producing frequent, watery stools. It may be caused by a wide variety of disorders, including bacterial contamination of food, virus infection, allergy, nervous reaction, as well as various serious and chronic ailments.

The discomfort of mild cases of diarrhea can be eased by various home remedies. Stomach cramps may be relieved by the application of heat. Dehydration can be prevented by consuming fluids such as tea, soup, and ginger ale. Bland and nourishing solid foods, such as boiled or poached eggs, rice pudding, cottage cheese, and/or toast, should be eaten as soon as possible.

Prompt medical attention is advised (1) when a diabetic has diarrhea, or (2) when diarrhea is chronic.

DIASTASE

The general name given to any of the enzymes which digest starch to smaller molecules of carbohydrate.

DIASTOLE

A period in which the heart fills up with blood. During this time it is in a relaxed state so that the blood pressure is at its lowest point.

(Also see BLOOD PRESSURE.)

DICOUMAROL

A chemical compound found in spoiled sweet clover hay or made synthetically. It is an antagonist of vitamin K and thus an anticoagulant of blood. Medically it is used to prevent blood clots. Other names include Dicoumarin, Dicumol, Dufalone, and Melitoxin.

(Also see VITAMIN[S], section headed, "Vitamin K"; and VITAMIN K.)

DIET

The beverages and foods normally consumed by a person. However, most people take the term diet to mean specially designated foods and beverages to be taken in measured amounts, while other items are restricted.

(Also see MODIFIED DIETS.)

DIETARY GUIDELINES FOR AMERICANS

Americans need to make changes in their eating habits. Dietary guidelines follow:

1. Reduce total fat consumption to 30% or less of total daily calorie intake.
2. Reduce cholesterol intake to less than 300 mg a day.
3. Increase the amount of starches and other complex carbohydrates in the daily diet.
4. Increase the amount of fiber in the diet.
5. Increase the amount of fruits and vegetables eaten daily.
6. Avoid drinking alcohol, especially during pregnancy. If abstaining is impossible, drink in moderation.
7. Reduce the daily intake of sodium to 6 g or less.
8. Maintain desirable body weight through prudent diet and regular exercise.

DIETETIC FOODS

Foods which have been produced so that they conform to the requirements of certain modified diets. For example, canned fruits may be made with little or no sugar, or with artificial sweeteners. In many cases dietetic foods are lower in fat and sugar than the food they are designed to replace.

DIETITIAN; DIETETICS

A dietitian is a person trained in nutrition and dietetics (the science that deals with the relationship of food to health) who plans menus and supervises the preparation of food. Dietitians work in hospitals, industrial food services, restaurants, schools, universities, and in many other areas.

Over half the professionally trained dietitians work in hospitals, where they plan diets and supervise the preparation of food, and help patients plan and understand the diets prescribed for them. Others work in educational and research programs.

To become a dietitian, a student must complete a prescribed course of study leading to a bachelor's, or higher, degree, followed by serving an internship in dietetics work.

(Also see AMERICAN DIETETIC ASSOCIATION [ADA]; and NUTRITIONIST.)

DIETS OF THE WORLD

Worldwide, the diet (the food and drink) of people are similar in one respect—everyone eats foods from plants and/or animals. Until very recently in the history of mankind, the type and amount of plant food and animal food available for eating depended upon the area. For early man, this meant reliance on wild plants and game. Later, man learned to garden, farm, and domesticate animals. Still, the diet of man depended upon the kinds of crops that the climate, geography and soil allowed, and upon the species of animals available for domestication. This, in part, created the difference in the diets of people. Then, based on the foods available, customs, economics, social patterns and religious beliefs, the diet of a country or area developed. As time passed, the diet changed as foods from other countries or areas were introduced. Despite outside influence, however, many diets have remained traditional over the years, particularly in Europe and Asia where there are still well-defined nationalities, or where the food supply is largely controlled by that produced within the country. Countries like the United States and Canada have been influenced by the diets of people from many nations. Moreover, these countries have a plentiful and varied food supply.

Overall, the diet of an individual depends upon where he or she lives; and even when the foods available are similar, they are often prepared differently. The following are some examples of worldwide diets from the food groups:

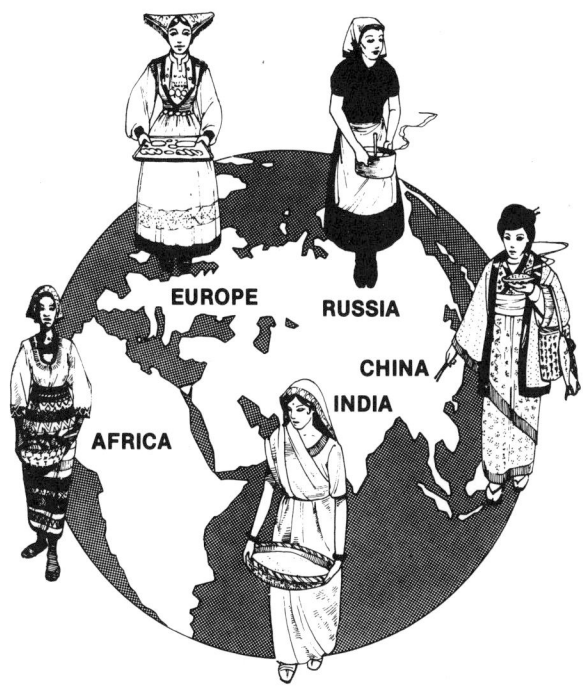

Fig. D-13. Diets vary according to where an individual lives. Many diets of the Old World have influenced those of the New World.

1. **Meat, poultry, fish, dry beans, eggs, and nuts.** Most people in the United States would include in this group beef, lamb, pork, chicken, turkey, goose, and duck, along with some common seafoods like fish, clams, lobsters, oysters, and shrimp. In some countries, people may eat meat from other domestic animals. For example, some Belgian and French people eat horsemeat, and some Greeks and Japanese enjoy goat meat. Hunters in almost all countries seek wild animals for food, as well as for sport. Favorite game meats in the United States include deer, opossum, rabbit, raccoon, squirrel, bear, and such wild fowl as duck, grouse, partridge, pheasant, and quail. In other countries, people may hunt baboons, caribou, elk, elephants, gazelles, monkeys, and snakes for meat. They may also eat ants, grasshoppers, locusts, and other insects.

Eggs from chickens and ducks are an important food almost everywhere. Some people eat the eggs of such birds as emus, gulls, ostriches, plovers, and penguins. In many countries, people enjoy the eggs of alligators, crocodiles, iguanas, turtles, and other reptiles.

In Mexico, beans are a popular food; in China, wide use is made of soybeans.

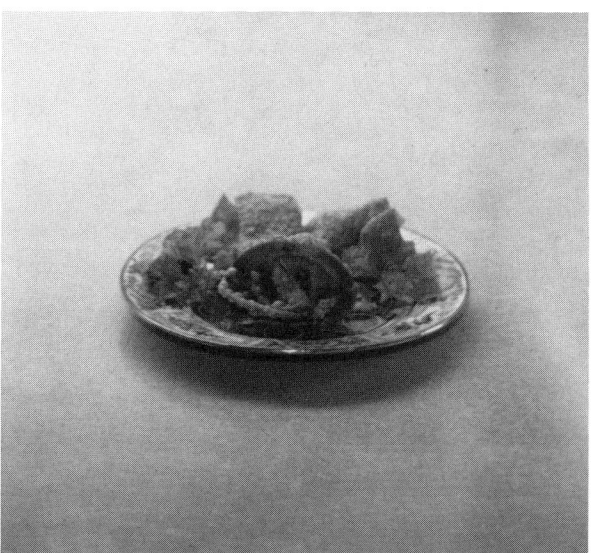

Fig. D-14. Won Ton, an Oriental dish (deep fried thin flour wrapper with seasoned ground pork filling). (Courtesy, Department of Food Science and Human Nutrition, University of Hawaii)

2. **Milk and milk products.** In the United States, Canada, and some other countries, cows provide most of the milk. But in southern Europe and the Middle East, the goat furnishes much milk. In Asia, sheep are often milked. People in India drink buffalo milk, and Laplanders enjoy reindeer milk. The yak furnishes milk in Tibet, the Arab herdsmen milk camels, and mares are milked for human food in different parts of the world. From milk, countless forms of cheese have been developed in many countries.

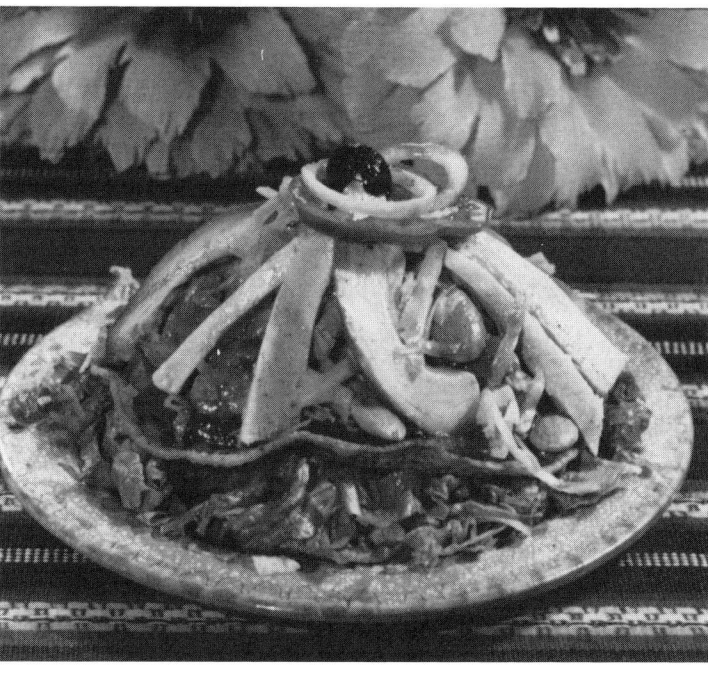

Fig. D-15. Tostada salad, a Mexican favorite. (Courtesy, Anderson/Miller and Hubbard Consumer Services, San Francisco, Calif.)

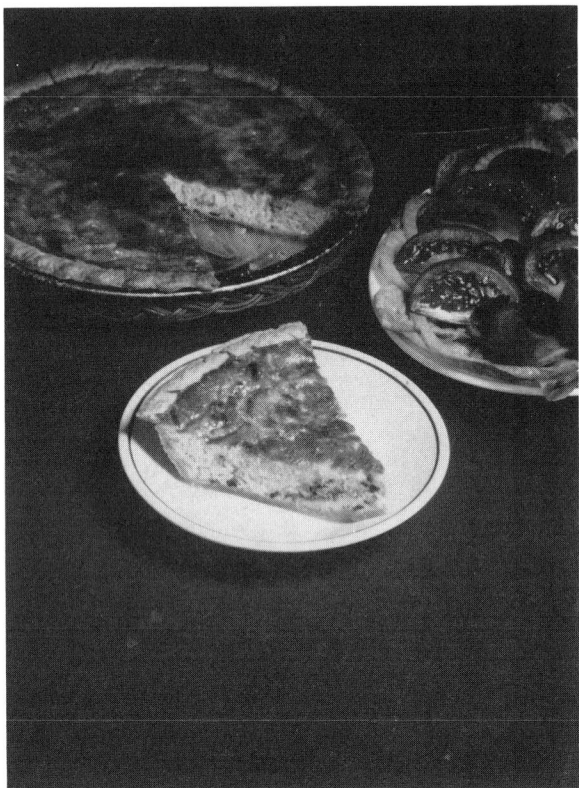

Fig. D-16. Quiche, ethnic food from Europe. (Courtesy, Carnation, Los Angeles, Calif.)

3. **Vegetables and fruits.** Many of the vegetables and fruits eaten today had their origin in specific areas or countries where they became an important component of the diet. Chinese cabbage, eggplant, rhubarb, soybean, and water chestnut came from China. The cowpea, okra and yam came from Africa, while the beet, carrot, lentil, onion, and turnip came from Asia. Corn, beans, potatoes and tomatoes are New World vegetable crops.

Numerous fruits, including the apricot, orange, peach, persimmon, plum, and tangerine, originated in China. The akee, cantaloupe, tamarind, and watermelon originated in Africa. Berries were common fruits of Europe and North America. Acerola, avocados, and papaya come from Central America, while cherimoya, custard apples, guava, and pineapple are native to South America. Today, many regions still grow vegetables and fruits which are unique to them.

4. **Breads and cereals.** Grains—wheat, rice, barley, rye and oats—are the largest single food item used throughout the world. The methods of preparing the grains for consumption vary widely, but almost everyone in the world eats some kind of bread, either English *graham bread*, Scottish *bannocks*, Finnish *tunnbrod*, German *pumpernickel*, Latin-American *arepas*, or Swedish *hardtack*. Worldwide, breads may be sweet or sour, brown or white, heavy or light, and raised or flat. In addition, grains are cooked in a variety of dishes or processed to make such products as macaroni, spaghetti, or breakfast cereals.

Condiments also vary from country to country—olives from Greece, malt vinegar from England, spices from the Far East, and maple sugar and syrup from North America. Every country has its favorite flavorings and seasonings.

EATING HABITS AND PATTERNS. Eating habits and patterns vary between countries or regions. Many factors, such as economics, religion, customs, and fads, influence eating habits and patterns, as well as individual preferences.

Economics inside a country, and those directly relating to an individual, determine the types of foods available. In general, the poorer nations and individuals buy less food and less variety, which limits their diet. People in highly developed industrial nations generally have the most varied diets, because they have money to buy different kinds of food. Also, they eat the greatest amount of animal foods, which are the most costly to produce and the most expensive to buy.

(Also see INCOME, PROPORTION SPENT FOR FOOD; and WORLD FOOD.)

Religions and diets have been closely connected for a long time. The ancient Greeks and Romans worshiped gods and goddesses who ruled over agriculture and hunting. The word *cereal* comes from *Ceres*, the Roman goddess of fruits and grains. The Bible tells of the early use of food as religious offerings.

Many religions do not permit their followers to eat certain foods. Buddhists are not allowed to eat any meat. Moslems can eat no pork. Hindus consider the cow sacred, and eat no beef. Some Hindus consume no animal foods except milk and dairy products, because their belief forbids them to kill animals. Orthodox Jews avoid certain kinds of foods, including pork, nonkosher meats, and shellfish, such as shrimp and lobsters. The Seventh-Day Adventists promote ovolacto-vegetarianism.

(Also see RELIGIONS AND DIETS.)

Customs influence the way people eat, and to some extent what they eat. Most Americans and Europeans eat from individual plates, using knives, forks, and spoons. Arabs use only their right hands to spoon foods from a central bowl. Chinese and Japanese use chopsticks to pick up food from a small bowl held close to the mouth. Many Orientals sit on the floor and eat from low tables.

Most persons eat at least three meals a day—breakfast, lunch, and dinner. The English and some other Europeans eat a fourth meal, supper, late at night. Meals vary in different countries. For example, breakfast in the United States, may include fruit or fruit juice, coffee, toast, and a choice of cereal or bacon and eggs. Some people like pancakes or meat and potatoes for breakfast. In rural areas, families usually have their big meal at noon and a lighter meal in the evening. In many areas, families and groups enjoy outdoor meals, such as picnics, corn roasts, clambakes, and backyard barbecues.

Continental Europeans sometimes have an early breakfast of sweet rolls and coffee or hot chocolate, and eat a second breakfast later in the morning. English breakfasts often include *kippers* (salted, smoked herring), or such meat as kidneys or sausage; cooked porridge; toast and marmalade; fresh or stewed fruit; and tea. Another English tradition, tea or *tiffin*, provides an extra meal served in the late afternoon. Its simplest menu usually includes tea and special tea cakes such as crumpets and scones, or biscuits with jam.

Some people choose their diet on the basis of fads and myths. Eating habits have long been partly controlled by beliefs about what is fit to eat. For example, some people once thought that tomatoes were poisonous, and refused to eat them. Today, some persons avoid white bread or processed foods, because they fear that substances added during flour milling or processing make these foods impure. Others, eat *natural* or organically grown food to ensure a healthy diet. Still others think that certain foods should not be eaten together, such as orange juice and milk, or starches and proteins. Some fad groups have encouraged strict vegetarianism for the purpose of achieving a certain *spiritual* level. Many of these faddish diets are based on misinformation—they are reminiscent of some ancient food practices such as eating a bull's tail for bravery, or eating brains for wisdom.

In areas where a wide variety of foods are abundantly available, people may not eat certain foods simply because they do not like them. Many areas of the world, however, cannot afford this luxury.

(Also see FOOD MYTHS AND MISINFORMATION.)

MEALTIME IN THE UNITED STATES. The diets of the United States have grown out of the customs of many peoples from many different lands, since people immigrating to America brought their diets with them. Moreover, the climatic and geographical conditions of the United States are so varied that almost every food known to man can be produced within its borders. With modern technology, the produce of one section of the country can be enjoyed in any other. But there are still special dishes that certain localities claim as their own. To mention a few: baked beans and brown bread belong to Boston; lobster stew to Maine; fried chicken, hominy grits, and pecan pie are at home south of the Mason-Dixon line; roast pork tastes best in Iowa; and New Orleans is where one finds the best Creole cooking. Furthermore, in most large cities in the United States one can find restaurants representing almost every country in the world. In New York City of Los Angeles, for example, one can order a dinner in any language—Rumanian mushk steak, Japanese sukiyaki, Italian antipasto, French hors d'oeuvres, or Swedish smorgasbord. The menus in the restaurants that serve foreign foods can be the magic carpet that whisks one to faraway places.

The life-style of the American consumer beginning in the 1960s, with more time at work and play and less time at home, gave rise to a fast-food industry peculiar to America, dedicated to eating as quickly as possible for as little money as possible. The most common fast-foods: hamburgers, french fries, and shakes; pizza and cola; fried chicken and slaw; fish and chips; roast beef sandwiches; tacos; and hot dogs—all very American.

DIFFUSE

Not localized.

DIFFUSION

The process by which particles (as molecules and ions) in solution spread throughout the solution and across separating membranes from the places of highest concentration to lowest concentration.

DIGESTIBLE NUTRIENT

The part of each food nutrient that is digested or absorbed by man.

Digestible nutrients are computed by multiplying the percentage of each nutrient in the food (protein, fiber, nitrogen-free extract, and fat) by its digestion coefficient. The result is expressed as digestible protein, digestible fiber, digestible NFE, and digestible fat. For example, if corn contains 8.9 percent protein of which 77 percent is digestible, the percent of digestible protein is 6.9.

DIGESTIBILITY

The proportion of a nutrient absorbed from the digestive tract into the bloodstream. It is determined by the difference between the nutrients consumed and the nutrients excreted, expressed as a percentage of the nutrients consumed. The digestibility for most foods is 90-95%.

(Also see DIGESTION AND ABSORPTION.)

DIGESTIBILITY, APPARENT

An approximate measure of digestibility, determined by the difference between intake and fecal output without considering the part of the feces not derived from undigested food. For example, the feces also contains shed lining cells of the digestive tract, bacteria, and digestive juice residues. These items are considered when the true digestibility is determined.

(Also see DIGESTION AND ABSORPTION.)

DIGESTION AND ABSORPTION

Digestion is the process by which food is broken down into smaller particles, or molecules, for use in the human body.

Absorption is the process of moving the nutrients from the digestive system into the circulation where they can be distributed to the cells of the body.

Humans eat because of the sensation of hunger, and they eat certain foods, partially due to learned responses and partially due to the anatomy and physiology of their digestive system. Moreover, the digestive tract has certain controls which affect digestion and absorption. Also, some foods influence digestion and absorption. Like any system, however, there are functional problems which can occur.

HUNGER AND APPETITE. Hunger is the physiological desire for food following a period of fasting. Appetite, on the other hand, is a learned or habitual response to the presence of food. An individual that is extremely hungry may not have an appetite for a type of food that it deems undesirable. Conversely, if the food is of a desirable nature, an individual may have an appetite for it in spite of the fact that he is not hungry. If a food is extremely high in nutrients but is refused by an individual because he does not have an appetite, its value is nil. On the other hand, many individuals eat only the foods they like. This may lead to a poor selection of foods, particularly in children.

(Also see HUNGER; and APPETITE.)

ANATOMY OF THE DIGESTIVE SYSTEM.

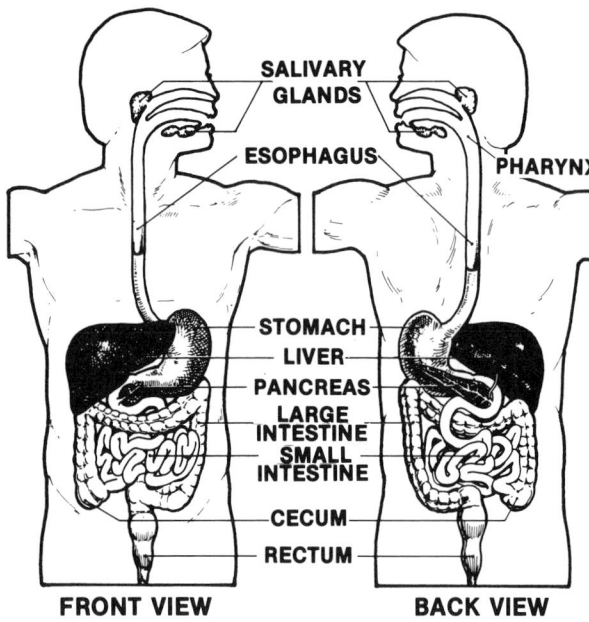

Fig. D-17. Anatomy of the human digestive tract.

Basically, the digestive system consists of a tube which courses internally from the lips to the anus. In the adult human, it is a 25 to 30 ft (7.5 to 9 m) long tube, through which food passes following consumption. At prescribed intervals, it becomes specialized in regions called the mouth, esophagus, stomach, small intestine, large intestine, rectum, and anus. Protruding along the way are the salivary glands, gallbladder, liver, and the pancreas, which provide essential secretory products for digestion. Based on the anatomy of the digestive system, man belongs to the group of animals called nonruminants. Furthermore, man's digestive system does not possess a functional cecum; hence, he has a limited capacity and limited microbial action and fiber digestion.

PHYSIOLOGY OF DIGESTION. In discussing the digestive process in the sections that follow, events ocurring in the various structures are considered in the order that food passes through them—mouth, esophagus, stomach, small intestine, and large intestine.

Mouth. Three physical processes occur in the mouth region: (1) prehension, (2) mastication, and (3) the initiation of deglutition.

Prehension can be defined as the act of bringing food into the mouth.

Mastication is the act of chewing food.

Deglutition is the act of swallowing.

In the mouth, the teeth, tongue, and salivary glands aid these physical processes.

• **Teeth**—The teeth serve primarily as a mechanical aid for mastication. By tearing and grinding the food, they provide a means whereby a large surface area is created which can be exposed effectively to the digestive fluids of the tract.

• **Tongue**—Throughout the process of mastication, the tongue serves a threefold purpose. First, movement of the tongue transports the food to the various areas of the mouth to be torn and ground. While doing this, the tongue is also mixing the food with the various secretions of the mouth, ultimately forming a bolus. Secondly, the presence of taste buds on the tongue provides a neurological control for food selection and intake. If the food is bitter or unpalatable, as determined by the taste buds, the food may be rejected. Finally, the tongue initiates the process of deglutition. When the bolus has been adequately prepared, the tongue moves it to the back of the mouth where nerves are stimulated, and swallowing commences.

• **Salivary glands**—The salivary glands represent a network of accessory structures which are essential to digestion. Three pairs of salivary glands are of primary importance—parotid, submaxillary, and sublingual. Fig. D-18 illustrates the location of these glands.

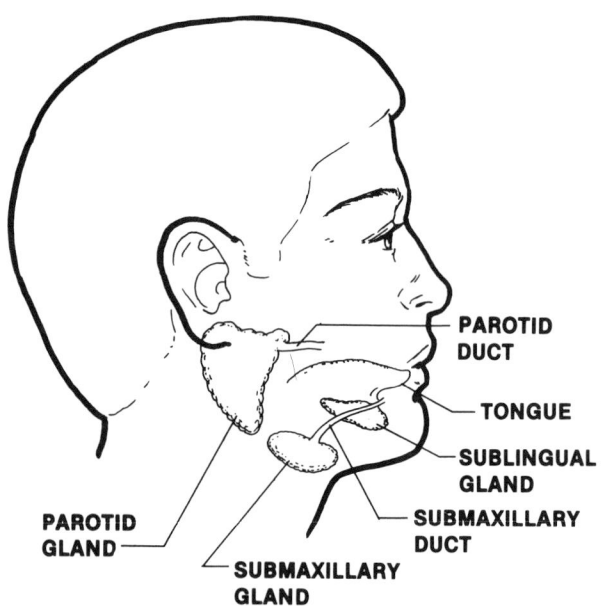

Fig. D-18. Location of the salivary glands.

The uses of saliva in digestion are manyfold. Saliva acts as a lubricant and aids in mastication, the formation of the bolus, and swallowing. Without this moisture, swallowing would be extremely difficult. The enzyme amylase, or ptyalin, in the saliva begins the digestion of starch. A large quantity of bicarbonate in the saliva serves as a buffer. The saliva solubilizes the chemicals in food so that bitter, sweet, sour, and salt taste can be detected by the taste buds on the tongue. Finally, the saliva keeps the membranes within the mouth moist, thus keeping them viable.

Esophagus. Upon swallowing, gravity and unidirectional peristaltic waves move the bolus through the esophagus and down to the stomach. Travel time is about 7 seconds.

Stomach. Secretions of the stomach amount to about 2 liters each day. Two specialized types of cells in the stomach provide the gastric secretions needed for the initial stages of digestion. The parietal cells, located in the fundic region, secrete hydrochloric acid. Hydrochloric acid hydrolyzes a limited amount of protein, but its main function is to establish an acid environment conducive to the activity of certain hormones and enzymes. The second cell type is called the chief cell or peptic cell. These cells secrete the enzyme pepsinogen. When pepsinogen is secreted in an acid environment (pH of 1.6 to 3.2), the proenzyme is activated forming pepsin—an enzyme that hydrolyzes certain peptide bonds. In addition, rennin is secreted by the stomach of young mammals, including babies; it coagulates milk and is important to their nutrition. Apparently, rennin is absent from the gastric secretions of adults.

Mucus is secreted by cells in the stomach lining. This secretion provides protection for the lining of the stomach. If there is a malfunction in the secretion of mucus, the stomach can digest itself—resulting in an ulcer.

Two types of motility have been observed in the stomach. The first type is that of peristalsis whereby food is moved toward the duodenum of the small intestine. Tonic contractions, the second type of motility, churn and knead the ingesta to ensure thorough mixing, but do not propel the food from one end of the stomach to the other.

The rate of passage of food depends largely on the nutrient composition of the diet. Carbohydrates pass through the stomach faster than either proteins or fats, with proteins being intermediate in rate of passage. Water can pass directly through to the small intestine, spending very little time in the stomach.

Intrinsic factor, a protein necessary for proper absorption of vitamin B-12, is produced in the parietal cells of the stomach. If there is a malfunction in the production of this protein, a condition called pernicious anemia results. Quite often, people suffering from this condition eat amounts of dietary vitamin B-12 that are normally considered adequate, but the vitamin has no means of being absorbed—thus, pernicious anemia develops.

Small Intestine. The small intestine is the primary site of both digestion and absorption. In normal individuals, 90 to 95% of all absorption occurs in the first half of the small intestine. The structure, both visible and microscopic, contributes to the absorptive capacity of the small intestine, and to the mechanical processes of digestive physiology.

• **Mechanical digestion**—Throughout the luminal surface—the inside surface of the small intestine—lies an extensive network of fingerlike projections called villi. Moreover, the surface is thrown into folds called mucosal folds. In the human, there are about 20 to 40 of these projections per square millimeter of intestine, each one being from 0.5 to 1.0 mm long. Each villus contains a lymph vessel called a lacteal and a series of capillary vessels. On the surface of the villi are cells which possess a great number of microvilli and provide further surface area for absorption. These microvilli form the brush border, which contains high concentrations of digestive enzymes.

Constant motion of the small intestine (1) mixes food with secretions, (2) exposes new villi surfaces for absorption, and (3) moves the chime (intestinal contents) down the tract.

PANCREAS. The pancreas secretes a digestive fluid directly into the small intestine via the pancreatic duct. This digestive fluid produced by the pancreas is clear and alkaline and consists of two phases—an aqueous phase and an organic phase. Being rich in bicarbonate, the aqueous phase serves primarily to neutralize the highly acid chyme produced in the stomach and passed on to the small intestine. In the organic phase, enzymes produced in the acinar cells of the pancreas are transported to the duodenum. These enzymes are stored as granules in the pancreas and are secreted from the cells through the process of emeiocytosis (cell vomiting). This process is sometimes called reverse pinocytosis because the granule fuses with the cell membrane, followed by a breakdown of the membrane and the evacuation of the granule. A listing of the composition and function of pancreatic fluids is given in Table D-7.

TABLE D-7
COMPOSITION AND FUNCTION OF PANCREATIC SECRETIONS

Composition	Function
Proteolytic enzymes: Trypsin Chymotrypsin A Chymotrypsin B Carboxypeptidase A Carboxypeptidase B	Splits proteins into peptides and amino acids
Lipolytic enzymes: Phosphorolipase A Pancreatic lipase Cholesterol esterase	Breakdown of lipids. Esterification of cholesterol to fatty acids.
Nucleolytic enzymes: Ribonuclease Deoxyribonuclease	Breakdown of nucleic acids
Amylolytic enzymes: Pancreatic amylase	Breakdown of starch
Cations: Sodium (Na^+) Potassium (K^+) Calcium (Ca^{++}) Magnesium (Mg^{++})	Buffers; cofactors; osmotic regulators
Anions: Bicarbonate (HCO_3^-) Chloride (Cl^-) Sulfate ($SO_4^=$) Phosphate ($HPO_4^=$)	Buffers; osmotic regulators
Proteins: Albumin Globulin	Buffers

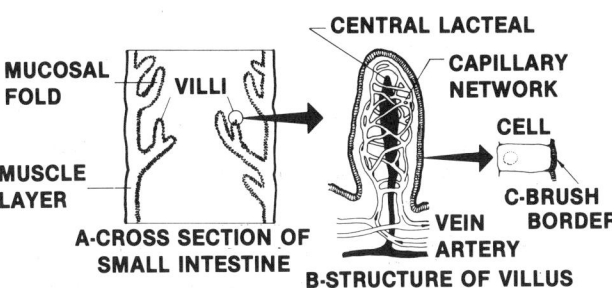

Fig. D-19. Three views of the small intestine structure. (A) Mucosal folds studded with numerous villi. (B) A villus containing capillaries and a central lacteal which transport absorbed nutrients. (C) The brush border on a cell like those covering each villus.

LIVER. The hepatic region includes the liver, gallbladder, and bile duct.

In addition to the salivary glands and pancreas, the liver is an indispensable accessory organ of the gastrointestinal tract. From the stomach and small intestine, most of the absorbed nutrients travel through the portal vein to the liver—the largest gland in the body. The liver not only plays an important part in nutrient metabolism and storage, but also forms bile, a fluid essential for lipid absorption in the small intestine. The numerous physiological functions of the liver follow:

1. Secretion of bile.
2. Detoxification of harmful compounds.
3. Metabolism of proteins, carbohydrates, and lipids.
4. Storage of vitamins.
5. Storage of carbohydrates.
6. Destruction of red blood cells.
7. Formation of plasma proteins.
8. Inactivation of polypeptide hormones.
9. Urea formation.

The primary role of the liver in digestion and absorption is the production of bile. Bile facilitates the solubilization and absorption of dietary fats and also aids in the excretion of certain waste products such as cholesterol and by-products of hemoglobin degradation. The greenish color of bile is due to the end products of red blood cell destruction—biliverdin and bilirubin. Bile contains a number of salts resulting from the combination of sodium and potassium with bile acids. There are four types of bile acids: cholic acid, deoxycholic acid, chenodeoxycholic acid, and lithocholic acid. These salts combine with lipids in the small intestine to form micelles. *Micelles are colloidal complexes of monoglycerides and insoluble fatty acids that have been emulsified and solubilized for absorption.* When the micelle has been formed, the lipid can be digested and the resulting products (fatty acids and glycerol) can cross the mucosal barrier of the small intestine and enter the lymphatic system. Bile salts, however, do not travel with the lipid; rather, they are reabsorbed in the intestine and then excreted again by the liver. This recycling process is termed enterohepatic circulation.

Large Intestine. The large intestine is composed of several layers of muscle. There is a circular layer of muscle that forms the basic tube of the colon and facilitates movement. In addition to this layer of muscle, there are three strips of longitudinal muscle which form the taenia coli. These strips form a series of pouches or sacculations throughout the colon which are called haustrae. Ingesta are held in these saclike structures to facilitate the removal of water. Subsequently, the feces generally take on the shape of the haustrae. Numerous mucous-secreting goblet cells can be found in the colon, but villi, such as the type that are found in the small intestine, are absent. The large intestine performs no digestive functions. Movement through the large intestine is much slower than in all other parts of the digestive system. Movement from the stomach to the end of the small intestine may require 30 to 90 minutes while passage through the large intestine may require 1 to 7 days. Three types of motility can be observed in the colon: (1) haustral contractions, (2) massive peristalsis, and (3) defecation.

The large intestine contains a dense population of bacteria of predominantly *Escherichia coli*. These bacteria affect the color and odor of the stool. Those food components not acted upon by digestive processes may be altered or digested by the bacteria. Thus, some complex polysaccharides or a few simple carbohydrates such as stachyose (four sugar) or raffinose (three sugar) will be converted to hydrogen, carbon dioxide and short-chain fatty acids. Nondigestible protein residues are converted to odorous compounds by the bacteria. Additionally, the bacteria synthesize vitamin K, biotin, and folacin, though it is not known for sure how much or how important these vitamin sources are to the individual.

PROCESS OF ABSORPTION. Once the various nutrients have been adequately digested, several modes of absorption can occur. These modes are dependent on the chemical nature of the nutrient and the site of absorption. Virtually no absorption takes place before the food enters the stomach; and very little absorption occurs in the stomach. The primary site for the absorption of most nutrients is in the small intestine. For the most part, absorption in the large intestine is restricted to water and electrolytes.

Mechanisms of Absorption. The four basic mechanisms of absorption are: (1) diffusion, (2) osmosis, (3) active transport, and (4) pinocytosis.

(Also see DIFFUSION; OSMOSIS; ACTIVE TRANSPORT; and PINOCYTOSIS.)

Nutrient Carriers. When the nutrients have been digested and absorbed, they must be transported to tissues that either have an immediate demand for them or can store them for later use. Lymph and blood are the primary transport media for the nutrients which have been absorbed.

LYMPH. Within the membranes of the intestinal tract there is a capillary network of lymph vessels. Cholesterol, water, long-chain fatty acids, and some proteins are picked up by this system and transported through a series of larger vessels which ultimately empty into the venous system just before the heart.

Since the immune system of the newborn baby is not well developed, it is essential that it receive colostrum from its mother as soon as possible. Through this intake of colostrum, antibodies are passed from the mother to the newborn, imparting a certain degree of immunity to stress and disease which will last for the first critical days of the life of the young. Many of these antibodies are absorbed intact in the newborn and transported via the lymphatic system.

BLOOD. Most of the low molecular weight (small) products of digestion are absorbed and transported by the blood. These nutrients include water, salts, glycerol, amino acids, short-chain fatty acids, monosaccharides, and certain vitamins. These materials are absorbed into the capillary system of the intestine. The capillary network drains into the venous system, eventually entering the portal vein of the liver. From the liver, the nutrients then travel through the hepatic veins which, in turn, enter the main systemic vein—the vena cava.

CHEMICAL DIGESTION AND ABSORPTION OF NUTRIENTS. *Chemical digestion is the process whereby proteins, fats, and complex carbohydrates are broken down into units that are of small enough size to be absorbed from the digestive tract into the circulation and distributed to the cells of the body.*

The process of digestion is accomplished primarily through the action of digestive enzymes, though mechanical events such as chewing and mixing are also important. Enzymes are organic catalysts produced by certain cells within the body. They speed biochemical reactions at ordinary body temperatures without being used up in the process. Enzymatic activity is responsible for most of the chemical changes occurring in foods as they move through the digestive tract. Many of the digestive enzymes are stored in an inactive form. In this state, they are called zymogens or proenzymes. Once secreted into a favorable environment for digestion, generally governed by activators such as pH or other enzymes, these inactive enzymes *turn on* and perform their specific digestive function. A summary of the enzymatic digestion of carbohydrates, fats, and proteins is presented in Table D-8.

From this point, the final digestion and absorption events are best discussed as they relate to the general classes of nutrients—carbohydrates, proteins, lipids (fats), and minerals and vitamins.

Carbohydrates. The digestion and absorption of most carbohydrates occurs in the small intestine, though it starts in the mouth. Such intestinal enzymes as sucrase, maltase, and lactase split carbohydrates—maltose, sucrose, lactose—into monosaccharides, whereupon absorption takes place. These enzymes are located on the surface of the cells lining the villi in the brush border. Of course, sugars ingested as monosaccharides, primarily glucose and fructose, do not require digestion. Sugar absorption takes place in the duodenum and jejunum of the small intestine. Glucose and galactose are absorbed through an active transport mechanism somehow tied to the active transport of sodium. Sodium ion concentration within the intestinal contents has been shown to be critical in this mechanism. A high sodium ion (Na^+) concentration will facilitate rapid absorption of these sugars while a low Na^+ concentration will reduce the rate of absorption. Some pentoses (5-carbon sugars) and other hexoses are absorbed through diffusion—a process considerably slower than that of active transport.

TABLE D-8
ENZYMATIC DIGESTION OF CARBOHYDRATES, FATS, AND PROTEINS

Source (secretion)	Enzyme	Activator	Substrate (substance acted upon)	Catalytic Function or Products
Salivary glands (saliva)	Salivary amylase (ptyalin)	—	Starch	Produces dextrins, maltotriose, and maltose.
Stomach (gastric juice)	Pepsins (pepsinogens)[1] Rennin[2]	HCl (hydrochloric acid) —	Proteins and polypeptides Casein	Cleave peptide bonds adjacent to aromatic amino acids. Clots the milk protein casein.
Pancreas (pancreatic juice)	Trypsin (trypsinogen)[1]	Enterokinase	Proteins and polypeptides	Cleaves peptide bonds adjacent to the amino acids arginine or lysine.
	Chymotrypsins (chymo-trypsinogens)[1]	Trypsin	Proteins and polypeptides	Cleave peptide bonds adjacent to aromatic, large, hydrophobic amino acids.
	Elastase (proelastase)[1]	Trypsin	Elastin, some other proteins	Cleave peptide bonds adjacent to the amino acids alanine, glycine, or serine.
	Carboxypeptidases (pro-carboxypeptidase)[1]	Trypsin	Proteins and polypeptides	Cleaves terminal amino acids.
	Pancreatic lipase Cholesterol esterase	Emulsifying agents (bile) —	Triglycerides Cholesterol and fatty acids	Di- and monoglycerides and fatty acids. Joins cholesterol and fatty acids before absorption.
	Pancreatic anylase	Cl⁻ (chloride ion)	Starch	Same as salivary amylase.
	Ribonuclease	—	RNA	Nucleotides
	Deoxyribonuclease	—	DNA	Nucleotides
	Phospholipase A (pro-phospholipase A)[1]	Trypsin	Lecithin	Lysolecithin (one fatty acid removed).
Small intestine (intestinal juice)	Enterokinase	—	Trypsinogen	Trypsin
	Aminopeptidases	—	Polypeptides	Cleave terminal amino acid from peptide.
	Dipeptidases	—	Dipeptides	Two amino acids.
	Maltase	—	Maltose, maltotriose	Glucose
	Lactase	—	Lactose	Galactose and glucose.
	Sucrase	—	Sucrose	Fructose and glucose.
	Isomaltase	—	Limit dextrins	Glucose
	Nucleases and related enzymes.	—	Nucleic acids	Pentoses and purine and pyrimidine bases.
	Intestinal lipase	—	Monoglycerides	Glycerol, fatty acids.

[1] The corresponding proenzyme.

[2] Present in infants and other young mammals.

Carbohydrates are 98% digested. However, this figure refers only to the digestion of starch, sucrose, and lactose, and not to those carbohydrate components of the diet called fiber. While fiber includes a number of polysaccharides, cellulose, the most abundant carbohydrate in nature, is a component of the diet. It is composed of glucose molecules, but man lacks the enzymes necessary to break cellulose down into glucose. Cellulose and other nondigestible polysaccharides contribute bulk to the diet and intestinal contents. Collectively these carbohydrates are termed unavailable carbohydrates, while those carbohydrates which are digested and absorbed are termed available carbohydrates.

The whole process of digestion is dependent upon enzymes which are specific for the reaction they catalyze. Interestingly, many individuals lack the enzyme lactase which is necessary for the conversion of lactose—milk sugar—to glucose and galactose. Hence, lactose is not digested or absorbed. This leads to diarrhea, bloating, and flatulence (gas) after ingesting lactose (milk). In most mammals and many races of humans, intestinal lactase is high at birth and declines to low levels during childhood, remaining low in adulthood. Lactose intolerance is uncommon among individuals with a European background. However, it occurs among 72 to 77% of the blacks in North America.

(Also see CARBOHYDRATE[S]; and FIBER.)

Lipids. Lipids (fats) are digested and absorbed primarily in the upper part of the small intestine, but considerable absorption can take place as far down as the ileum. Fats are not water soluble. Since enzymatic reactions of the body occur in water-base solution, fats must be emulsified for digestion to occur. Bile salts from the gallbladder play two roles in fat digestion: (1) they act as a detergent decreasing the surface tension, and (2) they transport the end-products of digestion away from fat globules in water soluble micelles which are absorbed. It is the detergent action which allows the mixing movements of the intestines to break the fat globules into very finely emulsified (water/oil mixture) particles with a greatly increased surface area on which the water soluble enzymes—lipases— can act. When lipids, emulsified by bile salts, come into contact with the various lipases that are found in the duodenum, they are broken down into diglycerides, monoglycerides, fatty acids, and glycerol. Short-chain fatty acids, less than 10 to 12 carbon atoms, are absorbed directly into the mucosa—lining—of the small intestine and are transported to the portal circulation of the liver. Monoglycerides and insoluble fatty acids are emulsified by bile salts, forming micelles. By attaching to the surface of the epithelial cells, the micelles enable these components to be absorbed into the intestinal cells. Once inside these cells, the long-chain fatty acids are reesterified (joined to the alcohol, glycerol) to form triglycerides. Triglycerides then combine with cholesterol, lipoproteins, and phospholipids to form chylomicrons—minute fat droplets. The chylomicrons are then passed into the lymphatic circulatory system via the central lacteal of the villi. Eventually these chylomicrons dump into the blood. After a fatty meal, the level of chylomicrons circulating in the blood reaches a maximum about 2 to 4 hours after a meal and may give blood a cloudy appearance. Within 2 to 3 hours, they disappear—having been deposited in the fat tissue or liver.

Fats are about 95% digestible. When fats are not digested due to lack of lipase or bile, absorption does not take place and a fatty stool, or steatorrhea, results.

(Also see CHOLESTEROL; FATS AND OTHER LIPIDS; and MALABSORPTION SYNDROME.)

Proteins. While protein digestion is initiated in the stomach, most digestion and absorption occurs in the small intestine. Numerous pancreatic and intestinal enzymes split proteins into proteoses, peptones, polypeptides, and finally their constituent amino acids, which are subsequently absorbed. In humans, it has been estimated that 50% of the digested protein comes from the diet, 25% from the proteins in the digestive fluids, and the remaining 25% from sloughed cells of the gastrointestinal tract. The rate of turnover of mucosal intestinal cells is extremely rapid—1 to 3 days—thereby giving an excellent source of recyclable protein. Overall, about 92% of the dietary protein is digested. The digestibility of vegetable protein is 80 to 85% while that of animal protein is about 97%.

Amino acid absorption is not clearly understood; but an active transport mechanism involving sodium ions ($Na+$), similar to that of glucose absorption, has been implicated. Amino acids are rapidly absorbed in the duodenal and jejunal segments, but are poorly absorbed in the ileum.

A limited amount of absorption of protein can occur, especially in the newborn. This mechanism of absorption, pinocytotic in nature, facilitates the passage of antibodies from the colostrum of the mother to her young. Additionally, this may contribute to allergic reactions which infants, and some adults, develop after eating certain food. Presumably, these individuals are capable of absorbing whole proteins, which then provoke an antigen-antibody reaction—an allergic reaction.

(Also see PROTEIN[S].)

The intestine also contains enzymes capable of digesting the nucleic acids—ribonucleic acid (RNA) and deoxyribonucleic acid (DNA). Pancreatic nucleases split nucleic acids into nucleotides (purine or pyrimidine base, sugar, and phosphoric acid), and the nucleotides are split into nucleosides (purine or pyrimidine base and a sugar), and phosphoric acid. These nucleosides are then split into their constituent sugar (pentoses), purine (adenine or guanine) and pyrimidine (cytosine, uracil, or thymine) bases. These bases are then absorbed by active transport.

Minerals and Vitamins. Mineral absorption occurs throughout the small and large intestines, with the rate of absorption depending on a number of factors—pH, carriers, diet composition, etc. Numerous mechanisms of mineral absorption have been elucidated. Many minerals, for example, iron and sodium, require active transport systems. Others, such as calcium, utilize both carrier proteins and diffusion mechanisms. Moreover, vitamin D is required for calcium absorption, and vitamins C and E favor the absorption of iron.

Most of the vitamins are absorbed in the upper portion of the intestine; vitamin B-12, which is an exception, is absorbed in the ileum. Water-soluble vitamins are rapidly absorbed, but the absorption of fat-soluble vitamins relies heavily on the fat absorption mechanisms which are generally slow.

(Also see MINERAL[S]; and VITAMIN[S].)

Water. Water moves freely across the membranes of the digestive tract—from inside the digestive tract to inside the cells lining the digestive tract. It's movement is via diffusion and osmosis. As the products of digestion—sugars, amino acids, and minerals—are actively transported out of the intestine, they create an osmotic gradient, also causing water to move out of the intestine and into the cells. In the large intestine sodium ions ($Na+$) are actively pumped out of the large intestine and again water moves out following the concentration gradient. The amount of water moved is considerable when one considers that the water in foods and in the digestive secretions entering the digestive tract amount to about 10,000 to 12,000 ml per day, and that the water lost in the feces only amounts to 150 to 200 ml per day.

(Also see WATER; and WATER AND ELECTROLYTES.)

CONTROL OF THE DIGESTIVE TRACT.

Like any system in the body, control is exerted over the functioning of the digestive tract in an effort to maintain the status quo of the body. The digestive tract is under neurological and hormonal control.

Neurological Control. The nervous system can be divided into two anatomical systems—the somatic nervous system, and the autonomic nervous system. The somatic nervous system enables the body to adapt to stimuli from the external environment. Various stimuli, such as touch, are perceived by specialized receptors within this system, and the body responds accordingly. The autonomic system involves the maintenance of homeostasis—the internal environment of the body. This is the system that controls the gastrointestinal tract.

The autonomic system can be further divided into (1) the sympathetic nervous system, and (2) the parasympathetic nervous system. The sympathetic system is generally associated with the traditional *fight or flight* response, and the parasympathetic system is usually associated with routine integration of normal activity.

When the sympathetic system is stimulated, there is a need for large amounts of blood in peripheral tissues, such as skeletal muscle. In order to accommodate this need, blood is shunted from the gastrointestinal tract, resulting in reduced digestive activity. For the most part, salivation ceases, and the mouth becomes dry. Secretions from the digestive glands are inhibited as well as peristalsis throughout the tract. The various sphincters of the gastrointestinal tract contract in response to sympathetic stimulation.

Stimulation of the parasympathetic system induces increased gastrointestinal activity. Generally, the parasympathetic system is stimulatory to the gastrointestinal system during rest and normal activity.

With the knowledge of the action of the sympathetic and parasympathetic autonomic systems, one can understand the action of certain drugs. When acute diarrhea is encountered, sympathetic-type drugs or parasympathetic depressant drugs are often used. Drugs that act as parasympathetic stimulators are frequently used as laxatives.

Hormonal Control. Chemical substances, known as hormones, are secreted by a number of ductless—endocrine—glands throughout the body. Hormones control a variety of body functions. Several areas of the digestive tract secrete hormones which act as chemical messengers on other areas of the digestive tract to control the process of digestion. Their secretion is a well-planned concert directed by the passage of foods through the gastrointestinal tract. A number of hormones have been isolated and characterized from the gastrointestinal tract. Gastrointestinal endocrinology is a very recent area of study; and new hormones are being found and chemically identified. Table D-9 lists the gastrointestinal hormones, and gives their site of origin, signal for release, and action.

Some other hormones, not of gastrointestinal origin, also influence digestion. Glucocorticoids from the cortex of the adrenal gland may increase stomach secretions, while epinephrine from the medulla of the adrenal gland inhibits stomach secretions. Thyroid hormones stimulate the motility of the intestines.

(Also see ENDOCRINE GLANDS.)

FOOD FACTORS AFFECTING DIGESTION AND ABSORPTION.

Most people believe that some foods are hard to digest, that others are easy to digest, or that still others are irritating. In many cases the foods cannot be blamed, but the functions of the digestive tract can be blamed. However, there are some food factors which are known to alter digestion and absorption; among them, the following:

• **Alcohol and caffeine**—Both alcohol and caffeine act directly on the lining of the stomach and stimulate gastric secretion. The use of alcohol for this purpose has been known since ancient times.

TABLE D-9
GASTROINTESTINAL HORMONES[1]

Hormone	Origin	Mechanism of Release	Physiological Function
Gastrin	Antral portion of gastric mucosa; pancreatic islets.	Distension of stomach; presence of proteins and polypeptides; alcohol; caffeine; stimulation of vagus nerve.	Stimulates gastric acid (HCl) and pepsin secretion; stimulates gastric motility.
Enterogastrone	Duodenum	Presence of fats.	Inhibits gastric acid (HCl) secretion and motility.
Cholecystokinin-Pancreozymin (cholecystokinin)	Duodenum	Presence of fats and products of protein digestion.	Contraction of gallbladder and secretion of pancreatic enzymes.
Secretin	Duodenum	Presence of acid and protein.	Stimulates secretion of aqueous pancreatic fluid (high in bicarbonate).
Enterocrinin	Duodenum	Presence of chyme.	Increases secretion of enzyme containing intestinal fluids.
Villikinin	Duodenum	Presence of chyme.	Increases contractions of villi.
Glucagonlike immunoreactive factor (GLI)	Wall of small intestine	—	Stimulates insulin secretion.

[1]Other gastrointestinal hormones have been proposed to exist, but their existence has not yet been proven.

• **Fiber**—Diets consisting of unrefined cereals and containing large amounts of fiber decrease the digestibility of proteins and increase the loss of protein in the feces.

• **Liquids and fine foods**—Since chewing increases the surface area for enzyme action and is necessary for the digestive processes to proceed, it stands to reason that finely divided foods would be easily digested. Some food processing can divide foods into much finer particles than chewing; for example, a puree. Liquids are also rapidly handled by the digestive tract. Fat foods, especially fats mixed with protein and introduced into the digestive tract in large chunks, are hard to digest and require time.

• **Chelates**—Chelates are formed when certain organic molecules combine with metallic ions to form cyclic compounds. These chelated complexes possess different solubility characteristics than unbound metallic ions. By this binding, certain minerals may be more readily or less readily absorbed in the gastrointestinal tract. Several naturally-occurring chelating agents are: chlorophylls, cytochromes, hemoglobin, ascorbic acid, vitamin B-12, and some amino acids. The most commonly used synthetic chelating agent is EDTA (ethylenediamine tetraacetic acid).

• **Phytic acid**—Phytic acid is a hexaphosphoric acid ester of inositol. When the acid form is combined with a cation (a positively charged ion) to form a salt, the compound is referred to as phytin. More than 50% of the phosphorus in mature seeds is in the form of phytin. In man, phytic acid may combine with calcium, thus making the calcium less available for absorption.

• **Oxalic acid**—Oxalic acid, a compound present in certain leafy plants, may interfere with calcium absorption. The acid precipitates calcium and renders it less available for absorption. Spinach has a high oxalic acid content, which may subsequently tie up substantial portions of its calcium.

(Also see MINERAL[S].)

DYSFUNCTIONS OF THE DIGESTIVE TRACT.

Some rather common and general disorders include diarrhea, gastritis, malabsorption, ulcers, and vomiting.

(Also see DIARRHEA; GASTRITIS; MALABSORPTION; ULCERS; and VOMITING.)

DIGESTION COEFFICIENT (COEFFICIENT OF DIGESTIBILITY)

The difference between the nutrients consumed and the nutrients excreted expressed as a percentage.

DIGESTIVE JUICES

A broad term which includes the secretions of the salivary glands, the stomach, the intestine, the pancreas, and the gallbladder, all of which aid the process of digestion.

(Also see DIGESTION AND ABSORPTION.)

DIGESTIVE SYSTEM (ALIMENTARY CANAL)

Consists of a tube which courses internally from the lips to the anus. In the adult, it's a 25 to 30 ft (7.5 to 9 m) long tube, through which food passes following consumption.

(Also see DIGESTION AND ABSORPTION.)

DIGLYCERIDE

A fat containing two fatty acid molecules.

DIPEPTIDE

The name given to two amino acids chemically linked together. It is a final stage in the digestion and absorption of proteins or an initial step in protein synthesis.

(Also see DIGESTION AND ABSORPTION; and PROTEIN[S].)

DIPSOGEN

An agent which causes the sensation of thirst.
(Also see THIRST.)

DIPSOMANIA

An uncontrollable urge to overindulge in alcoholic drinks.
(Also see ALCOHOLISM AND ALCOHOLICS.)

DIPSOSIS

Excessive thirst, or a longing for certain unusual forms of drink.

DISACCHARIDASE

An enzyme which splits double sugars (disaccharides) such as lactose, maltose, and sucrose into single sugar units (monosaccharides) such as fructose, galactose, and glucose.

(Also see CARBOHYDRATE[S].)

DISEASES

This term denotes harmful disorders in the normal structures and functions of one or more parts of the body. The consequences of disease depend upon (1) the parts of the body which are affected; (2) the amount of impairment of normal functions; and (3) the characteristics of the diseased person, such as previous state of health, age, sex, and temperament. For example, small, benign tumors of the skin may have no more than a cosmetic effect. Conversely, a heart attack may cause rapid deterioration and death in an overweight, quick-tempered, elderly person.

The purpose of this article is to put foods and nutrition in their proper perspectives with regard to the various types of diseases. Keeping healthy requires an understanding of the relationship between diets and nutrition-related disorders. Resistance to disease, and the ability to make a fast recovery from a disease or an injury, depend to a large extent upon one's nutritional status. Hence, each of the major causes of disease will be briefly discussed, along with what is known concerning the influence of food and nutrition thereon. The common diet-related diseases will be covered in greater detail in the articles noted in the cross references.

Data compiled by the U.S. government and published in the Surgeon General's report on *Nutrition and Health* in 1988 warned the nation that many of its top causes of death and chronic diseases—including heart disease, cancer, stroke, diabetes, intestinal disease, and osteoporosis—are linked to diet. The National Academy of Sciences echoed this warning and admonished Americans to make changes in their eating habits. (See section on "Dietary Guidelines for Americans" for the recommended dietary guidelines.)

CAUSES OF DISEASES.

Any agent which adversely alters the harmonious balance between the body's processes may be the cause of disease. This is not to say that any exposure to a harmful agent will inevitably result in disease. Whether or not disease develops depends upon (1) the potency or severity of the injurious agent, and (2) the ability of the body's defenses to counter the effects of the injurious agent.

It is important to be aware of each of the basic factors which may cause disease, along with the preventative measures. These follow.

Abnormal Growths.

Various cells within the body may start to grow abnormally and spread throughout the body, because they have escaped the controls which regulate their growth. When such abnormal growth (neoplasia) occurs, disease may result from pressure on neighboring tissues, competition for vital nutrients by cancer cells, and other pathological effects. Tissues in aging persons appear to be more susceptible to tumorous growths than those in growing children, although certain types of cancer are leading causes of death in teenagers.

Medical scientists have long known that trace contaminants such as asbestos, coal tar, dyes, and hydrocarbons in air, food, and water may cause cancer in man.

(Also see CANCER.)

Aging and Degeneration of Tissues.

For reasons not well understood, many of the tissues of the body undergo degenerative changes with aging. Thus, certain disorders, such as arthritis, bowel lesions, bone loss (osteoporosis), cancer, diabetes, hardening of the arteries (arteriosclerosis), and high blood pressure (hypertension), are found more frequently in persons over 50 years of age than in younger persons.

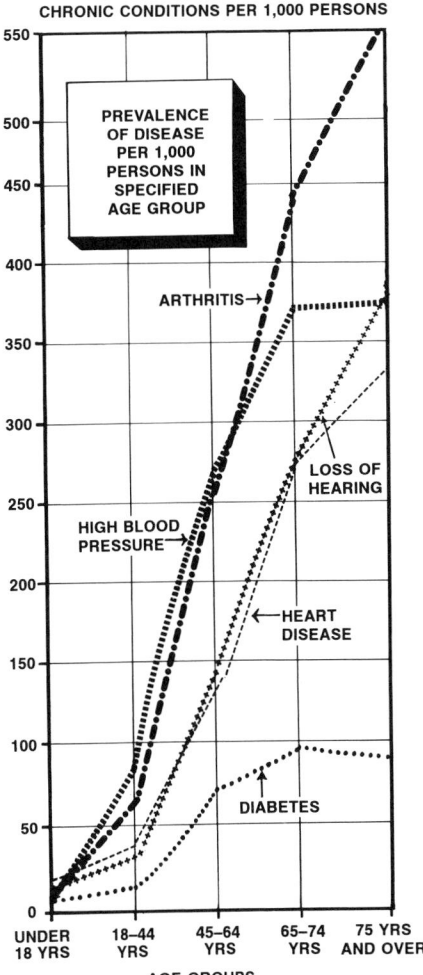

CHRONIC CONDITIONS PER 1,000 PERSONS

Fig. D-20. The prevalence of selected chronic disorders in people of various ages in the U.S. for each of the diseases or conditions. (*Statistical Abstract of the United States, 1991*, U.S. Dept. of Commerce, p. 120, Table 195)

Fig. D-20 shows how the prevalence of various chronic diseases and conditions increases with aging.
(Also see GERONTOLOGY AND GERIATRIC NUTRITION.)

Allergies and Other Disorders of Immunity.

An allergy is considered to be a disorder of the process(es) by which immunity is produced in that it is an overreaction (hypersensitivity) to one or more mildly irritating substances which may occur in the air, on one's clothing, or in certain foods. Some people have such a hypersensitivity to certain antigens or other irritants that they may develop hives, asthma, dermatitis, diarrhea, or even severe shock which sometimes leads to death. Occasionally, these disorders may also be provoked by chilling of the body, or by various emotional stresses. Many of the unpleasant signs of hypersensitivity result from the body's overproduction of histamine, a substance which is synthesized from the amino acid histidine.

(Also see ALLERGIES.)

Congenital and Genetic Disorders.

Abnormalities which are present at birth are said to be congenital. They may result from inherited (genetic) traits, or they may have been induced by environmental factors during either fetal development or the birth process itself.

Inborn errors of metabolism are inherited physiological defects which interfere with the normal utilization of nutrients by the body. For example, phenylketonuria (PKU) may cause mental retardation due to the accumulation of phenylpyruvic acid, which is derived from the incomplete metabolism of the amino acid phenylalanine. Sometimes, permanent damage from these disorders may be prevented by restricting the dietary content of the nutrients which give rise to the harmful products of metabolism. In other cases, it may be necessary to provide extra amounts of certain nutrients to people who have a genetic defect which leads to poor utilization of these nutrients.

(Also see GENETIC DISEASES; and INBORN ERRORS OF METABOLISM.)

Endocrine and Metabolic Disorders. The secretions of the endocrine glands (hormones) are in many ways the switches that turn metabolic processes on or off. Therefore, disorders involving one or more of these glands are likely to produce corresponding abnormalities of metabolism. Conversely, impairment of almost any aspect of metabolism usually triggers some type of endocrine response.

For example, excessive secretion of hormones by the thyroid gland may overstimulate energy metabolism and other functions to the extent that there is loss of weight, a rapid heartbeat, and extreme nervousness. On the other hand, victims of protein-energy malnutriton may have markedly subnormal thyroid functions, so that they always feel cold, even in the tropics.

In other situations, stress factors such as emotional disturbances, fasting, starvation, or diabetes, are signals to the pituitary gland to release adrenocorticotropic hormone (ACTH), which acts both alone on tissues and stimulates secretion of other stress hormones by the adrenal glands. The net effects of these stress-responsive hormones are the tearing down (catabolism) of fat, muscle, and/or bone tissues, so as to provide essential nutrients for metabolism.

Finally, malnutrition, or even the administration of sex hormones, may inhibit the stimulation of the sex glands by the pituitary, so that there is a weakening of these glands. For example, atrophy of the testes has occurred in men who have been severely deprived of food, or who have regularly taken testosterone for the purpose of accelerating the development of their muscles.

(Also see ENDOCRINE GLANDS.)

Injuries from Physical Agents. Both acute and chronic injuries may result from cold, electric shock, heat, mechanical forces, radiation, or sunlight. Such injuries to cells and tissues may be difficult to heal or may lead to other problems such as infections. Sometimes, these injuries cause disfiguration or deformity.

The human body has a limited ability to resist injury from physical agents, by virtue of the innate strength of such tissues as skin, muscle, and bone. However, people whose tissues have been previously weakened by poor nutrition may be badly hurt by even the mildest of injurious agents. For example, older people may have bones which are easily broken, due to long subsistence on a diet low in calcium, vitamin D, and/or protein. Some of the other ways in which nutritional factors affect susceptibility to injury follow.

• **Heat exhaustion**—This disorder results from the over-taxing of the body's mechanisms for keeping cool, and for maintaining the balance between body water and various mineral salts. It has been found that lack of sufficient potassium in the body renders it more susceptible to heat

exhaustion and heat stroke. Of course, it is well known that lack of sufficient salt is also a major contributor to heat exhaustion, as evidenced by the practice of giving extra salt to people working in hot environments.

(Also see HEAT EXHAUSTION.)

• **Radiation injury**—People who are deficient in iodine are more susceptible to damage to their thyroid glands by radioactive iodine (I-131), an atmospheric contaminant which results from the testing of nuclear weapons. The reason for the increased susceptibility is that iodine deficiency causes the thyroid gland to increase the rate of its uptake of both normal and radioactive iodine.

Radiation may also cause cellular damage by triggering the body to produce free radicals—highly reactive chemical fragments which may deform the membranes and nuclei of cells. Injury to tissues by free radicals is enhanced by deficiencies of selenium and vitamin E.

Diet may also play a role in the susceptibility of the digestive tract to radiation injury. Animal studies have shown that a given dose of radiation in the form of x rays is more likely to be fatal if there is a large population of coliform bacteria in the intestine.[11] The growth and multiplication of *E. coli* appears to be encouraged by diets rich in protein. On the other hand, animals fed laboratory chow—which is made up mainly of unrefined cereal grains—have much fewer coliform bacteria in their intestines and are more likely to survive radiation. Many other studies have shown that milk sugar (lactose) promotes the growth of lactobacilli that make the intestinal contents acid so that the growth of *E. coli* is inhibited.

Stresses. Chilling, overheating, exhaustion, starvation, dehydration, emotional stress, or even overeating, may trigger the oversecretion of the endocrine glands, particularly the adrenals, thyroid, pancreas, and pituitary, as the body attempts to counter the threats to its harmonious function. Stresses which are mild and short lasting can be beneficial when they tone up the body and its functions, but prolonged stress may lead to upsetting of the balance between the processes of the body.

Some health scientists believe that hardening of the arteries and high blood pressure are the end result of long-term exposure to various stress factors. However, it seems that the stresses have different effects on different people since some people experience many hardships over a lifetime, yet live to ripe old ages, while others succumb to disease by middle age.

(Also see STRESS.)

Toxic Substances. This designation applies to a large number of substances, including some of the otherwise beneficial nutrients, such as several of the trace minerals and vitamins A and D, which are potentially harmful or poisonous at high levels. Thus, toxicity is relative rather than absolute, since the harmful level of a poisonous substance depends upon a person's size, weight, genetic traits, metabolic activity, and overall health status.

Toxic substances may be inhaled while breathing, ingested with food or drink, taken as medications, absorbed through the skin or mucous membranes, or produced in the body as products of the normal metabolic processes. These substances produce their effects by attacking tissues and

---

[11]Klainer, A. S., S. Gorback, and L. Weinstein, "Studies of Intestinal Microflora VII. Effect of Diet and Fecal Microflora on Survival of Animals Exposed to X Irradiation," *Journal of Bacteriology*, Vol. 94, 1967, p. 383.

cells, by disrupting physiological processes, or by interfering with the utilization of vital nutrients. A discussion of several different toxicants follows.

(Also see POISONS.)

Chemicals and Drugs. The chemical industry has developed many products which contribute to both our exceptionally high rate of agricultural productivity and the attractiveness of our homes, meals, and personal appearances. Hand in hand with this development, there has been increased public concern over the use of these products, for fear of human poisoning.

For example, farmers may use insecticides, rodent killers, weed killers, fertilizers, disinfectants, solvents, and petroleum products, some of which may be toxic under certain circumstances. When properly used, agricultural chemicals are an important adjunct to providing food for people and feed for animals. However, improper use may result in the chemical contamination of food plants, eggs, meats, and dairy products.

The hazards associated with the commonly used chemicals and drugs underscore the need for the accurate labeling and use of these products.

(Also see POISONS.)

Constituents of Foods. There have been many scare stories concerning the potentially toxic effects of a wide variety of food constituents which have been administered to experimental animals in grossly abnormal ways. For example, even a naturally occurring substance such as cholesterol may cause tumors when it is *injected* under the skin. However, findings which demonstrate potential toxicity are most likely to be relevant when the test substance has been *fed* in quantities which might be consumed under normal circumstances. Foodborne toxicants may fall into one or more of the categories which follow.

• **Naturally occurring toxicants**—Through trial and error, man has usually learned of the animals and plants which are either acutely poisonous or are safe to eat. However, mildly toxic effects are more difficult to detect. For example, such vegetables of the *Brassicae* (cabbage family) as rutabaga, turnip, cabbage, and kale contain substances (goitrogens) which interfere with the utilization of iodine by the thyroid gland. Hence, eating large amounts of these items may cause goiter when the dietary level of iodine is low.

(Also see GOITER.)

• **Products of deterioration or of spoilage**—Foods which go bad may often be identified by discoloration, disagreeable odors, and peculiar tastes, unless such characteristics are masked by added colorings or flavorings. However, certain food-contaminating organisms produce deadly toxins which may cause such diseases as aflatoxin poisoning, botulism, or staphyllococcal food poisoning, even though the contaminated foods appear to be normal in all respects. It is noteworthy that the botulism toxin, produced by the bacteria *Clostridium botulinum,* is one of the most potent poisons known to man. Outbreaks of this type of food poisoning usually result from foods that have been improperly canned.

Even readily recognizable types of contamination, such as ergotism on grains of rye, may be concealed when the contaminated grain is ground into flour and baked into bread.

(Also see BACTERIA IN FOOD, Table B-2, Food Infections (Bacterial); POISONS, Table P-2, Mycotoxins; and PRESERVATION OF FOOD.)

• **Toxicants which result from the cooking or processing of foods**—Recently, it has been found that certain members of a group of compounds called *nitrosamines* are carcinogens. These substances may be formed in the chemical reactions between the amines (breakdown products of amino acids and proteins), which occur naturally in foods, and the nitrites that are added to certain meats to prevent discoloration and botulism. The foods most likely to contain such carcinogens are various types of smoked fish (which are believed to be responsible for the high rates of stomach cancer in Iceland and Japan), sausages, and bacon (the high cooking temperature of bacon may be a factor in the formation of nitrosamines).

(Also see NITRATES AND NITRITES; and NITROSAMINES.)

• **Substances added to improve the characteristics of foods**—Foods may often have slight deviations from optimal color, odor, and taste which render them less desirable to consumers, even though they are safe and wholesome. The wholesale rejection of these items by shoppers could result in considerable financial losses by farmers, processors, shippers, and merchants. Therefore, it has become common practice to add a wide variety of substances to foods for the purpose of enhancing their appeal to consumers; among them, preservatives, spices and other flavorings, artificial and natural coloring agents, sweeteners, emulsifying agents to prevent separation of various components, nutritional supplements, air, and water.

The United States and the other developed countries have strict governmental regulation of *intentional food additives* so that cases of acute poisoning from these substances are rare, if not nonexistent. Nevertheless, a few additives are suspected of having subtle toxic effects over long periods of use. Then, too, small bakeries, restaurants, and other establishments, which mainly serve local clientele, occasionally deviate from acceptable practices of food preparation, with the result that there may be sporadic outbreaks of poisonings.

(Also see ADDITIVES.)

• **Trace contaminants of food**—Toxic or otherwise undesirable materials may get into foods when contaminants such as lead, cadmium, and mercury are present in the environment, equipment, or containers with which the foods come in contact during their production, processing, packaging, or shipping. Likewise, minute traces of pesticides are occasionally found in various farm commodities. Occasionally, traces of plastics and antioxidants used to treat packaging materials seep into food products that are stored for long periods. But, like the use of the intentional additives, there are also strict governmental regulations concerning substances which may get into foods accidentally.

(Also see POISONS; and POISONS, CHEMICAL.)

Environmental Pollutants. For centuries, most of man's activities were conducted on such a small scale that their impact on local environments was limited. However, the Industrial Revolution, which began in the late 18th century, led to steady increases in the populations of cities, and in the discharge of waste products into the environment. At first, these products were promptly dissipated by the natural processes of rain, winds, and percolation through the soil. Now, it seems that in certain heavily industrialized areas there are likely to be persistent accumulations of toxicants in the air, water, and some types of foods. Hence, it is believed that the higher incidence of such diseases as cancer, lung disorders, and kidney disease found in urban areas than in rural areas may be partly due to various pollutants.

(Also see POISONS; and POISONS, CHEMICAL.)

Essential Nutrient Excesses. Most well-informed people know that eating too much carbohydrates and/or fat may bring on obesity, and perhaps a host of other ills. However, many of those who take various types of nutritional supplements might be surprised to learn that even excesses of proteins, minerals, and vitamins may be the cause of disorders such as those which follow.

• **Protein overload effect(s)**—This term designates the combination of (1) excessive urinary loss of water, and (2) accumulation of the products of protein metabolism in the blood which may result from diets overly rich in protein. These diets might be hazardous for such vulnerable groups as infants, people with liver or kidney disorders, and those prone to dehydration and gouty arthritis (where there is a buildup of uric acid in the blood).

(Also see PROTEIN.)

• **Mineral imbalances and toxicities**—There is still considerable controversy regarding the optimal amounts of various essential mineral elements because dietary excesses of certain elements may interfere with the utilization of others. Furthermore, almost every one of the nutritionally essential minerals has potential toxicity at high levels. However, these toxicities are not as likely to result from eating unfortified foods, as they are from special circumstances such as (1) the taking of mineral supplements; (2) contamination of food and water by environmental factors such as containers, piping, and airborne dusts; and/or (3) fortification of foods with minerals.

It is noteworthy that there are only small margins of safety between beneficial and hazardous doses for (1) fluoride, which may cause severe defects of teeth and bones; and (2) selenium, which is suspected of being a cause of liver damage and tooth decay.

(Also see MINERAL[S].)

• **Vitamin overdoses (hypervitaminoses)**—The best known vitamin toxicities are those which result from vitamin A and vitamin D, because (1) these vitamins are fat soluble, (2) small amounts of them have strong effects, and (3) they tend to accumulate in the liver. Toxic effects do not occur so readily with vitamins E and K, which are also fat-soluble, unless high potency supplements are taken.

Excesses of water-soluble vitamins (vitamin C and the vitamin B complex) are not stored in the body to any great extent, so toxicities from food sources of these nutrients are rare. However, people who take very large doses (megadoses) in the form of supplements run the risk of dangerous, druglike effects.

Additional information on vitamin toxicities is provided in the general article on vitamins and in the separate articles dealing with the individual vitamins.

(Also see VITAMIN[S].)

Poisonous Animals and Plants. Many people around the world know that certain animals and plants may cause severe poisoning, yet they often take their chances on eating these items if they know of someone else who has escaped drastic consequences. Therefore, it is noteworthy that, although certain animals and plants are poisonous under all circumstances, others are variable in their toxicities because (1) the animal or plant is poisonous only when it acquires the toxic principle from its food or its environment; (2) certain types of processing either develop or eliminate the toxicity in the food; (3) the development of poisoning in man depends upon the actions of microorganisms, special enzymes, or other processes which occur in the food or in the human body; or (4) only certain stages of maturity in the animal or plant are toxic. Some examples of such variable toxicities follow.

• **Poisonous quail**—Throughout history there have been sporadic outbreaks of poisoning when people have eaten quail that have consumed the seeds of poison hemlock. Normally, quail eat these seeds only when other more favored foods are not available.

• **Seleniferous wheat**—Wheat may contain dangerous levels of selenium when it has been grown in high-selenium soils, such as those in the Great Plains of the United States, where *selenium converter plants* such as *Astragalus racemosus* have grown, died, and decayed for several years. Utilization of selenium from the soil by the converter plants, followed by the return of this mineral to the soil when the plants decay, results in its conversion from a form not readily picked up by wheat to one that is much more absorbable. Hence, high selenium soils alone will *not* yield wheat containing toxic levels of selenium, unless the mineral is in a form which is available to the growing wheat.

(Also see SELENIUM.)

• **Raw fish toxicity**—Various species of freshwater fish (such as carp) and crustaceans contain an enzyme (thiaminase) which destroys thiamin (vitamin B-1). Hence, persons eating these items raw may develop thiamin deficiencies, particularly if the rest of their diets are rich in carbohydrates and/or alcohol which raise the requirement for thiamin. However, thorough cooking destroys the enzyme, but leaves the thiamin intact.

(Also see THIAMIN.)

• **Cassava poisoning**—Cassava (*Manihot utilissima*) is a staple food for many people who live in the hot, humid areas of Africa, Asia, and Latin America. However, some varieties of this tuberous plant contain a toxic principle which is greatly reduced by proper processing—soaking, boiling, drying, expression, or fermentation.

(Also see CASSAVA.)

• **Cyanide-containing lima beans**—Some varieties of lima beans, such as those that are native to the Caribbean, and which are usually colored, contain harmful levels of cyanide-releasing glucosides. Fortunately, soaking and cooking the beans releases much of the toxic principle. Anyhow, the varieties grown in the United States contain only negligible amounts of cyanide. Besides, U.S. law prohibits the marketing of lima beans that contain harmful amounts of this toxic factor.

(Also see LIMA BEANS.)

• **Irish potato poison**—Green (unripened) or sprouted potatoes may contain toxic levels of solanine, an alkaloidal substance which may bring on headache, vomiting, abdominal pain, diarrhea, slowing of the heart and breathing, and occasionally, death.

(Also see POTATO.)

Toxicants from Metabolism. The human body, like a factory, requires a suitable means of getting rid of the waste products which are produced during its operations. Even excess sugar in the blood, which often occurs in diabetes, has harmful effects, particularly when this condition is prolonged or chronic in nature. The failure of the kidneys to excrete urea and uric acid may also result in illness due to the accumulation of these toxins in the blood and tissues. Furthermore, the presence of excessive amounts of fat in the blood (hyperlipoproteinemia) has come to be regarded as dangerous to health. Perhaps there are other little known ways in which the body may poison itself.

Malnutrition. In the discussion that follows, malnutrition is typed as subclinical, dietary deficiency, or dietary excess.

Subclinical malnutrition is the stage of malnutrition which precedes the appearance of specific signs of disease. However, there may be subnormal levels of minerals or vitamins in the blood or urine. Other indicators of such malnutrition might be elevations in blood levels of such substances as cholesterol, triglycerides, glucose, uric acid, urea, or bilirubin.

(Also see MALNUTRITION.)

Dietary deficiency diseases are those whose major features are due to the lack of one or more nutrients. They are often characterized by specific signs of abnormalities, such as discoloration of the hair or skin, bleeding gums, swollen glands, etc. One of the major causes of such diseases is the consumption of a diet which does not contain sufficient amounts and varieties of foods. For example, young children fed mainly cereals in the form of watery gruels may develop either protein-energy malnutrition, and/or blindness, due to vitamin A deficiency.

(Also see DEFICIENCY DISEASES.)

Dietary excess of certain nutrients may also cause disease when (1) such excesses are toxic, or (2) they create imbalances.

Vitamin D poisoning, for example, results from excessive dietary intake and/or production in the body of excessive amounts of this nutrient. The latter situation may be caused by overexposure of the skin to light from the sun or a sunlamp.

(Also see VITAMIN D.)

Another example of dietary excess is the storage of surplus dietary energy as fat when there is chronic overeating. Normally, fattening is a natural activity of the body. However, if the deposition of fat results in marked obesity, there may be some pathological deviations from normal metabolism. For example, some obese persons have a diabeticlike underutilization of carbohydrates, fats, and proteins. They seem to secrete normal amounts of insulin, but the effects of the hormone appear to be hampered. Eventually, the pathology of diabetes may develop.

(Also see OBESITY.)

Three of the leading causes of death in the United States—heart disease, cancer, and diabetes—are believed to be at least partly associated with obesity and related dietary factors. However, it also seems that there are other factors—such as stress, heredity, smoking, and environmental pollu-

tants—which may affect one's susceptibility to these diseases. Therefore, poor nutrition may be only one of the multiple factors which cause certain diseases.

What constitutes good nutrition under one set of circumstances may mean malnutrition in others since nutrient needs may vary according to age, sex, environmental conditions, amount of physical activity, and inherited traits which influence the metabolism of nutrients. Furthermore, it may be difficult to detect some types of malnutrition since their features may not be evident until there has been noticeable damage to the body.

Food Related Infectious and Parasitic Diseases. The invasion of the body by bacteria, protozoa, or viruses, or by larger organisms such as worms, can lead to disease when the invading species secretes toxins, carries other disease organisms, feeds on body tissues, or competes with its host for essential nutrients. The severity of the disease depends upon the type and the numbers of the infectious or parasitic organisms which are present in the host.

Pertinent information relative to various types of infectious and parasitic dieases which may be food related follow:

1. **Infectious types of organisms.** The principal types of infectious organisms that may cause disease are: bacteria, molds (fungi), mycoplasmas (PPLO), rickettsiae, and viruses. The defenses of the human body vary. They may be weak or entirely lacking, especially under conditions of malnutrition or poor hygienic practices.

(Also see BACTERIA; and DEFICIENCY DISEASES.)

2. **Parasites.** *Broadly speaking, parasites are organisms living in, on, or at the expense of another living organism.*

People may harbor a wide variety of internal and external parasites. They include fungi, protozoa (unicellular animals), arthropods (insects, lice, ticks, and related forms), and helminths (worms).

Some people tolerate parasites better than others. Also, the better the nutrition the greater the resistance to parasitism.

Table D-10 lists and summarizes the most common food related and parasitic diseases.

SIGNS AND SYMPTOMS OF DISEASES. Often, the first signs of disease are abnormalities like fever, rashes, swelling, pallor, diarrhea, vomiting, or discoloration of parts of the body such as the hair, face, eyes, nose, lips, tongue, teeth, gums, throat, glands, skin, or nails. The patient may also have lack of appetite, dizziness, fatigue, headache, pains in muscles or joints, or tingling in the hands and feet. However, these signs and symptoms may sometimes be present when there is no disease. Hence, the doctor or nurse will most likely check some of the vital functions. Details follow.

(Also see HEALTH, sections headed "Signs of Ill Health" and "Signs of Good Health.")

WAYS IN WHICH DISEASES AND PARASITES ARE SPREAD. Infectious and parasitic diseases may be spread in a variety of ways; among them, the following:

1. **Direct contact** with diseased animals or people in which the infected host actually touches the susceptible person and transmits the disease.

2. **Indirect contact,** such as (a) by susceptible people touching infected animal's or people's excretions or secretions, like feces, urine, blood, pus, or saliva; or (b) by susceptible people breathing airborne infected droplets exhaled from the nose and mouth of infected people.

TABLE D-10
FOOD RELATED INFECTIOUS AND PARASITIC DISEASES[1]

Disease	Disease Organism	Signs & Symptoms	How Disease is Transmitted	Preventative Measures	Remarks
Infectious diseases: Amoebic dysentery	*Entamoeba histolytica* (An amoeba is a microscopic one-celled animal organism.)	Diarrhea may occur anytime from several days to 4 weeks after consuming contaminated food or water. Symptoms are: unexplained fatigue, low grade fever, and recurrent diarrhea.	Cysts of the amoeba are ingested in contaminated food or water, particularly those which are uncooked when eaten. Flies may carry the organism to foods.	Prevention of sewage contamination of water supply. Avoidance of drinking cold water, use of ice, or eating cold foods in places with poor sanitation.	Infection is most likely to occur in warm climates. An infected person with no apparent signs of the disease may spread the organism to other people.
Brucellosis (See Table B-2, Food Infections [Bacterial].)					
Cholera (See Table B-2, Food Infections [Bacterial].)					
Diphtheria	*Corynebacterium diphtheriae*	Fever accompanied by running nose and sore throat which occur from 1–6 days after exposure. Death by suffocation has resulted from a membrane which sometimes forms in the throat.	Usually by contact with nose or throat discharges from an infected person. Epidemics have been spread through the use of raw milk.	Immunization of all young children, plus booster shots when necessary. Disinfection of all articles which were in contact with infected persons.	The disease organisms produce a toxin which may travel through the body and cause damage to the heart, nerves, and kidneys.
Epidemic diarrhea of the newborn	Unknown virus	A marked change in the infant's stool pattern towards more frequent, watery, and unformed stools.	It is not certain whether the infant picks up the virus from its food or from direct contact with others. However, people handling the infant may infect the food of others.	Scrupulous sanitation in the preparation of milk formulas for bottle-fed babies. Hand washing by people in contact with the infant. Disinfection of infant's clothing and bedding.	Many infants around the world—including a few in the U.S.—die from the dehydration which may result from severe diarrhea.
Epidemic gastroenteritis (intestinal flu) (Also see GAS-TROENTERITIS.)	Unidentified virus.	Diarrhea, nausea, and vomiting which last for a few hours.	Possibly in food handled by infected persons. More likely by personal contact, contaminated water, or discharge from the nose and throat of the infected persons.	Persons with this disease should *not* handle food until all signs have disappeared. Protection of food against airborne droplets by *sneeze shields* at serving counters. Protection and disinfection of water supply.	Measures should be taken to stop diarrhea and/or vomiting which last for more than a few hours so that severe dehydration may be prevented.
Hepatitis, infectious	Type-A hepatitis virus	Yellowing of the skin and whites of the eyes (jaundice), nausea, lack of appetite, and weakness. Signs may not appear until more than a month after infection.	The virus is carried in secretions and excretions from the digestive tract. Hence, it may be spread by personal contact, sewage-contaminated water or shellfish, or poorly handled food.	Hand washing by food handlers. Protection and/or disinfection of the drinking water supply, and avoidance of shellfish (mainly clams and oysters taken from polluted waters).	The recovery period may be as long as several months, so prolonged use of sanitary precautions may be needed for those in contact with the patient.
Poliomyelitis (infantile paralysis)	Polio viruses—types I, II, and III.	Sore throat and/or diarrhea, fever, nausea, and vomiting.	Mainly by personal contact, contaminated water, or secretions and excretions from the digestive and respiratory tracts. It is suspected that the viruses may be borne in foods.	Immunization of all young children and food handlers. Protection of foods and drinking water against contamination.	Most infected persons do *not* become paralyzed. However, such persons, with barely noticeable symptoms, may be carriers of the disease.
Salmonellosis (See Table B-2, Food Infections [Bacterial].)					
Scarlet fever	*Streptococcal* bacteria	Fever, vomiting, sore throat, and characteristic rash (which appears only in certain susceptible people). Occurs mainly in children.	Usually by direct contact or airborne droplets from infected people. However, food may occasionally be contaminated by infected people.	Disinfection of personal articles from infected people. Use of the Dick test to confirm disease, since it may be necessary to treat the patient so as to prevent the spread of the disease.	Scarlet fever is now uncommon in the U.S. Treatment with various antibiotics eliminates the ability of the patient to transmit the disease.
Shingellosis (bacillary dysentery) (See Table B-2, Food Infections [Bacterial].)					
Strep throat	*Streptococcus pyogenes*	Fever, vomiting, and sore throat. Sometimes, related bacteria are the cause of communicable skin infections.	Organisms may get into foods from infected handlers since they are carried on airborne droplets from the respiratory tract of infected people who may sneeze or cough on food. Likewise, the causative organism may be spread directly from person to person through the air.	Protection of foods against coughs and sneezes, and against contamination by handlers with skin infections.	Occasionally, there may be such complications as rheumatic fever, or infections of the bones and the kidneys. Penicillin and other antibiotics are effective against this disease.

Footnote at end of table

(Continued)

TABLE D-10 *(Continued)*

Disease	Disease Organism	Signs & Symptoms	How Disease is Transmitted	Preventative Measures	Remarks
Tuberculosis (TB) (See Table B-2, Food Infections [Bacterial].)					
Tularemia (See Table B-2, Food Infections [Bacterial].)					
Typhoid fever	*Salmonella typhi,* or *Salmonella paratyphi.*	Fever, nausea, headache, and loss of appetite.	Contamination of food or water by sewage, flies, or infected persons. Direct contact with patients or symptomless carriers of the disease. Shellfish (mainly oysters and clams) from polluted waters may carry the disease.	Protection and disinfection (chlorination) of drinking water. Finding and curing carriers of the disease. Sanitary food handling practices.	The bacteria which cause the disease may live in the gallbladder for long periods of time and be gradually shed in the feces. Antibiotics have greatly reduced the number of deaths from this disease.
Parasitic diseases: Beef tapeworm (beef measles)	*Taenia saginata*	Often, the infested person is free of symptoms. Occasionally there may be anemia, nausea, vomiting, or diarrhea, alternating with constipation. There may be some discomfort when the worm segments are passed in the stool.	Deposition of feces from infested humans in water, feeds, or pastures causes infestation of cattle with eggs. The eggs hatch in cattle and the larvae invade tissues used for meat. Man picks up live larvae from undercooked beef.	Cooking of beef until well done. Enforcement of the use of proper sanitary facilities by help on cattle farms. Protection of pastures, feeds, and cattle from contamination by human feces or sewage. Where possible, protection of feedlots against flooding. Barring of hobos and hunters from farms and feedlots.	This problem is confined largely to the four states which border Mexico—Texas, New Mexico, Arizona, and California. However, it may be spread to other states by animals, feeds, meats, and people that are infested with the parasite.
Dwarf tapeworm	*Hymenolepis nana*	Usually there are no symptoms unless the infestation is massive. Then, there may be abdominal pains, nausea, or vomiting.	Contamination of foods with feces from infested mice, rats, and people—all of whom may harbor the parasite for its entire life cycle. Sometimes, people pick up the worm eggs from foodborne insects such as grain beetles.	Control of rats, mice, and insects, and protection of foods from their contamination.	Infestation is very common in areas of the world which abound with rats. However, few cases appear in the U.S.
Fish tapeworm	*Diphyllobothrium latum*	Often, an infested person has no symptoms; but there may eventually be pernicious anemia due to the worm(s) consuming most of the host's dietary vitamin B-12.	Newly hatched tapeworm larvae are first eaten by waterfleas, which are then ingested by freshwater fish. Man becomes infested by eating the living worm in raw fish. The tapeworm also infests dogs, cats, polar bears, and sea lions.	Cooking of all fresh-water fish. Freezing of fish for several days at 0°F (−17.8°C) will also kill the parasite.	Many of the fresh-water fish in northern European lakes and in the U.S. Great Lakes contain fish tapeworms. However, regular microscopic examination of these fish is not feasible.
Liver flukes	*Clonorchiasis*	Digestive disturbances and eventually liver damage.	Eggs of flukes from infested people are shed via feces into fresh water where they are ingested by snails. Fish become infested by eating the snails, while man picks up living parasites from undercooked fish.	Thorough cooking of all fish, whether fresh, dried, salted, or pickled. Prevention of contamination of lakes and ponds by human feces.	Infestations with liver flukes affect many people in the crowded areas of eastern Asia. However, there are few deaths, and some people carry flukes for more than 20 years.
Pinworms (seat worms, thread worms)	*Enterobius vermicularis*	Itching of the anal region. Sometimes there is also lack of appetite, irritability, and loss of weight.	Usually the eggs are spread from the human anal region to other people through the air, on clothing, or on furniture. However, food is sometimes contaminated by fecal material, or by unhygienic food handlers.	Sanitary disposal of human wastes. Daily bathing by infested people. Elimination of worms from the patient(s) by medical means. Hand washing by food handlers.	This is the most common parasite found in U.S. children. White people appear to be more susceptible than other races.
Pork tapeworm	*Taenia solium*	Symptoms may range from mild digestive disturbances to serious disorders when larvae invade the heart, brain, eyes, or nerves.	Swine pick up worm eggs from eating matter contaminated with human feces. The larvae from the hatched eggs invade the muscles. Man becomes infested by (1) eating the eggs on raw vegetables grown in soils fertilized with human feces, and (2) undercooked pork which contains the larvae.	Avoidance of the use of untreated human wastes as fertilizer for vegetables eaten raw. Thorough cooking of all forms of pork (fresh pork, hams, sausages, luncheon meats, frankfurters, etc.). Cooking of all vegetables grown in soils fertilized by human wastes.	Many deaths are caused by this parasite in countries where there is poor sanitation.
Round worms	*Ascaris lumbricoides*	Often, there are no symptoms of this infestation. Occasionally, there is nausea, fever, loss of weight, and allergiclike irritation of the nose and throat due to the presence of the worms in these places.	The eggs are spread by unhygienic practices of food handlers, use of human wastes to fertilize vegetables which are eaten raw, or when there is cesspool or sewage contamination of drinking water.	Sanitary disposal of human wastes. Careful washing of vegetables to be eaten raw, although in areas where infestation is common, it might be best to cook all foods thoroughly and to boil drinking water.	It is believed that as many as ⅔ of the world's people may be infested with these worms. The worms may migrate to the liver, heart, lungs, nose, and Eustacian tubes (which connect the throat and the ears).

Footnote at end of table

(Continued)

TABLE D-10 *(Continued)*

Disease	Disease Organism	Signs & Symptoms	How Disease is Transmitted	Preventative Measures	Remarks
Trichinosis	*Trichinella spiralis*	The first symptoms of intestinal infestation may appear as early as a day after eating parasitized meat. They are: abdominal pain, diarrhea, nausea, and vomiting. About a week later, when the larvae have migrated to various tissues, there may be severe muscle pain, difficulty in breathing, swollen eyelids, and sometimes death (when the heart muscle is infected).	Swine become infested by eating contaminated garbage or infested rats. (Other meat-eating animals, such as bears, may become infested by similar means.) The larvae of the worms migrate from the pig's intestine to its muscles where they form cysts. Man may become infected by eating raw or undercooked pork (or bear meat) which contains trichina larvae.	Thorough cooking of pork (until the last trace of pink in the meat disappears), or freezing the meat continuously for not less than 20 days at a temperature not higher than 5°F (−15°C). (The meat of wild carnivores, such as bears, should be similarly treated.) Destruction of all rats on the farm. Cooking of all garbage and slaughterhouse by-products fed to swine.	This disease is not often found in the U.S. or in the developed countries of Europe, where the laws governing the sanitary feeding and handling of swine are strictly enforced. However, the disease is common in the developing countries where pork is eaten.

¹Also see BACTERIA IN FOOD; FOODBORNE DISEASE; FOOD POISONING; PRESERVATION OF FOOD; and SPOILAGE OF FOOD.

3. Contaminated items, including beverages, foods, water, kitchen utensils, dishes, silverware, counters and sinks, dish cloths and towels, bedding, clothing, etc. Gastrointestinal diseases, such as parasitic worms and salmonellosis (a bacterial infection which causes intestinal inflammation) are often transmitted in contaminated foods. Table D-10 summarizes various ways in which certain common diseases and parasites are spread by means of contaminated foods and water.

4. Carriers (also called disease vectors) which include insects, mites, ticks, and snails. In some cases, transmission of the agent by carrier is purely mechanical; for example, a biting fly serves as a "flying needle." In other cases, a stage of development, or part of the life cycle, of the infectious agent in the carrier is actually necessary before it may be passed on to the new host.

The term *carrier* may also be applied to a person who is infected with a disease organism, but who shows no signs of the disease. *Typhoid Mary* was a cook in New York City who appeared to be healthy although she carried the typhoid bacillus. An investigation showed that she transmitted typhoid fever to at least 100 other people before it was discovered that she was a carrier.

5. Carrion feeders (flesh eaters, such as rats, cats, dogs, foxes, or birds) may serve as reservoirs of infectious organisms or of parasites such as trichina, which they may spread to people by means of direct contact or by infecting pork.

PREVENTION OF DISEASES. The prevention of disease not only involves the minimization of exposure to injurious agents, but also the building up of maximum resistance by suitable health practices. It is next to impossible to avoid all of the disease-causing factors. One should keep medical records of close relatives, since susceptibility or resistance to certain diseases may be inherited. Often, preventive measures may be instituted early if a disease is suspected; for example, if there is a family tendency to diabetes. However, each type of preventive action should be designed so as to be in harmony with the body's natural defenses.

Immunization Against Infectious Diseases. While it is not within the scope of this book to cover immunization procedures fully, a brief presentation is made so that the reader may be informed about some of the nondietary protective measures against infectious diseases.

The artificial or natural process by which a person acquires sufficient antibodies to be immune to one or more diseases is called immunization. For example, an unborn child receives antibodies from its mother through the placenta. Additionally, antibodies may be received if the child is fed colostrum and/or breast milk. In these cases, the infant is said to have *passive immunity* since the antibodies were preformed outside of the infant's body. This type of immunity lasts for only a short time. Longer lasting *active immunity* is that type which results from antibodies being produced within the body in response to the introduction of a weakened or dead disease organism.

Brief descriptions of some common types of artificial immunizations follow.

VACCINATION. This procedure may be defined as the injection or oral administration of some agent (such as a serum or vaccine) for the purpose of preventing disease.

In regions where a disease, such as measles, appears season after season, it is advised that healthy susceptible people be vaccinated before they are exposed, and before there is a disease outbreak, because (1) it takes time to produce an active immunity, and (2) some people may be about to be infected with the disease. Descriptions of the most common types of vaccinations or *shots* follow.

• **Serums**—These agents, which are obtained from the blood of animals (often horses), are used for the protective nature of the antibodies that they contain, which stop the action of an infectious agent or neutralize a product of that agent. They give an immediate, but passive, immunity. Among the serums that have proved successful are those for Rocky Mountain spotted fever, tetanus, and typhus.

• **Toxoids (or antitoxins)**—A toxoid is a *tamed* toxin which is treated chemically so that it loses the poisonous or toxic properties but still retains the power to stimulate the body cells to form the appropriate antibody. Typical toxoids are diphtheria toxoid and tetanus toxoid.

• **Vaccines**—Usually these agents consist of suspensions of live microorganisms (bacteria or viruses) or microorganisms that have had their disease-causing properties removed but their antibody-stimulating properties retained. Examples are smallpox vaccine, Salk (injected) and Sabin (oral) types of polio vaccines, and measles vaccine.

It is noteworthy that the ability of the body to form antibodies against disease appears to be related to nutritional status since it has been shown that various forms of malnutrition, particularly protein deficiency, are accompanied by both subnormal levels of antibodies and increased susceptibility to infection.

Hence, various types of immunizations may not be fully effective when they are given to malnourished people.

Sanitary Measures. Disease epidemics are most likely to occur in densely populated areas, particularly when certain sanitary measures fall short of what is needed. Hence, the sanitation measures which follow are pertinent.

FOOD SANITATION. Opportunities for the contamination of foods are present at the various points between their production on farms or factories, and the serving of them at meals. Hence, the following sanitary measures should be observed:

1. Raw fruits and vegetables should be washed before using.

2. All meats should be thoroughly cooked, particularly hamburger and pork, which are the most susceptible to contamination.

3. Dairy products should be made from pasteurized milk unless the dairy has been certified to produce raw milk.

4. Food handlers should be free of contagious disease; and they should be required to conform to recommended food sanitation practices.

5. Perishable foods should not be kept at room temperatures between 40° and 140°F (*4.4° and 60°C*) (the range where most microorganisms thrive) for more than a few hours.

6. Frozen foods which have been allowed to thaw completely so that they no longer contain ice crystals should not be refrozen for continued storage.

7. Cracked or broken eggs should *not* be used for the dishes which require short cooking times at low temperatures because they may contain Salmonella organisms. These eggs are safe only when they have been heated to at least 160°F (*71.1°C*) for 20 minutes or longer.

(Also see BACTERIA IN FOOD; FOODBORNE DISEASE; FOOD POISONING; POISONS; and PRESERVATION OF FOOD.)

OTHER SANITARY MEASURES. In addition to the sanitary handling of food, other measures are necessary to prevent the spread of communicable diseases. Hence, the practices which follow are noteworthy.

• **Waste Disposal**—In the distant past, when people lived in small and widely scattered villages, there was little spread of disease. Today, much of the world's population is crowded into areas where accumulations of garbage, sewage, and other wastes provide fertile breeding grounds for disease. Hence, in these places there may be a need for more efficient sewage treatment, better waste disposal, control of pests, and perhaps tougher laws to prevent air, land, and water pollution.

• **Disinfection**—Dishes and eating utensils which have been in contact with diseased persons, or which may have somehow been contaminated with germs or parasites, should either be disposed of or disinfected. Unfortunately, there is no one best germ killer, nor is there anything like a general disinfectant that is effective against all types of microorganisms and parasites under all conditions. However, the application of heat by steam, by hot water or by boiling is an effective method of disinfection.

• **Quarantine**—This term refers to the regulation of movement of people, food, animals, or plants by either agricultural or health authorities so as to prevent the spread of infectious diseases, parasites, insects, and other disease agents.

Today, strict quarantines are rarely applied to people in their homes, except in the cases of a few diseases like diphtheria. It is more common for school authorities to bar children who may lack evidence of having had certain immunizations.

• **Ventilation**—This term refers to the circulation of air through buildings with the objective of supplanting foul air with fresh air containing needed oxygen. Generally, moist air is a more favorable medium for the existence of microorganisms than dry air, thus lending itself well to the transmission of contagious diseases. However, excessively dry air, which is present in certain heated buildings during the winter months, may irritate the nose, throat, and lungs and increase susceptibility to respiratory infections. This problem might be overcome by introducing small amounts of moisture into the air with humidifiers.

Healing Of Injuries From Physical Agents. It is well known that some people heal more rapidly than others, which suggests that good nutrition plus other health-promoting factors—like fresh air, sunshine, and adequate rest—may be responsible. Additional vitamin A, vitamin C, protein, and energy may be required for the formation of new connective tissue. Also, the building up and maintenance of abundant muscle through diet and exercise is important. The protein in muscle is often an emergency source of amino acids needed for the synthesis of protein during healing. Most injuries from physical agents involve a stress response where there is an elevated secretion of adrenal cortical hormones. These stress hormones promote the breakdown of muscle protein and the release of amino acids into the blood where they are available for the repair of tissue. However, unnecessary stresses should be avoided, as they may retard healing.

Recently, the mineral element zinc has been shown to promote healing. Also, it has been claimed that vitamin E has similar effects.

It is noteworthy that diabetics heal poorly, so it is important to be ever watchful for signs of this disease.

Prevention of Malnutrition. Reaching this goal requires more than the consumption of sufficient food from each of the food groups. It also requires a recognition of individual needs which may vary according to heredity and the special circumstances of individual life-styles. When sufficient food and the incentive to eat are present, there must be considerable self-discipline to avoid overeating of the high-energy foods. People who have great appetites should eat foods which fill, but do not fatten, such as low-calorie fruits and vegetables which contain liberal amounts of fiber.

Some scientists suggest that there may be widespread subclinical malnutrition due to deficiencies of the trace elements, like chromium and selenium, which are removed during the refining of grains and other foods. When the refined foods comprise much of the diet, it may be necessary either to enrich them with the missing elements or to provide some type of mineral supplement.

(Also see MALNUTRITION.)

Reduction Of Stress. Some stress is inevitable, and may even be beneficial. However, situations which provoke the secretion of stress hormones also cause marked reduction in the vitamin C content of the adrenals. Therefore, it has been suggested that supplemental ascorbic acid might be helpful in meeting the demands of stress. Also, multiple mineral and vitamin capsules which are supposedly beneficial in counteracting stresses are available, but their effectiveness is uncertain.

The best policy seems to be to avoid, or to minimize, stresses whenever they may be anticipated. For example, much of the stress from cold weather may be reduced by wearing protective clothing. Emotional stresses may often be alleviated when one develops a new set of responses to problem situations. Although the evidence is vague, it has been assumed that regular exercise helps hard-pressed executives to overcome their emotional stresses.

Finally, a simple, but helpful principle is to try, whenever possible, to help the body to cope with unavoidable stresses. This means that the treatment of a taxing, infectious disease should include good nutrition and rest.

Detoxification Of Poisonous Substances. A healthy liver has at its disposal many chemical reactions for the detoxification of poisonous substances. These reactions rely on the presence of enzymes whose activity depends in part on the level of dietary protein, and in part on the need to detoxify substances such as alcohol and various drugs. Therefore, protein-deficient persons may have heightened susceptibility to the undesirable side effects of certain medications. Chronic abuse of alcohol may also impair liver function since it may promote fatty degeneration. In addition to protein, other nutrients which promote liver function are the B-complex vitamins, methionine, choline, and lecithin.

HEALTH AND NUTRITION FUNCTIONS OF GOVERNMENT.

The welfare of a nation is dependent upon the health of its citizens. Hence, it is often necessary that the various levels of government within a country provide both assistance and regulation in health- and nutrition-related areas such as (1) the prevention and treatment of disease, (2) the production and distribution of foods and drinking water, and (3) other activities and conditions which may affect the health of the people. Some noteworthy functions of government agencies in disease prevention and nutrition follow.

U.S. Department Of Health And Human Services.

This department is made up of agencies that have responsibility for public health, education, and economic security. The health agencies come under the jurisdiction of the U.S. Public Health Service (USPHS). Brief descriptions of these agencies follow.

• **Alcohol, Drug Abuse, and Mental Health Administration** —Programs concerned with the prevention and treatment of alcoholism, drug addiction, and mental illness are conducted by this agency.

• **Center for Disease Control (CDC)**—This agency, whose initials originally stood for *Communicable Disease Center* was established to conduct programs dealing with the causes and the control of contagious disease. Its name was changed to the present one when its mission was expanded to include noninfectious diseases resulting from environmental, nutritional, and occupational factors.

• **Food and Drug Administration (FDA)**—The FDA is charged with the responsibility of safeguarding American consumers against injury, unsanitary food, and fraud. It also protects industry against unscrupulous competition. It

inspects and analyzes samples and conducts independent research in fields such as contamination of food by insects, microorganisms, and other unsanitary items; toxicity (using laboratory animals); disappearance curves for pesticides; and long-range effects of drugs.

• **Health Resources Administration**—The programs conducted by this agency are concerned with (1) the training of health professionals, (2) collection of data on health problems in the United States, and (3) research designed to evaluate and improve health services.

• **Health Services Administration**—This agency either provides or oversees (1) health care for American Indians and merchant seamen, (2) family planning, (3) improvement of maternal and child health, and (4) community health programs.

• **National Institutes of Health (NIH)**—The NIH is composed of the following nine sister institutes: the National Cancer Institute, the National Heart Institute, the National Institute of Allergy and Infectious Diseases, the National Institute of Arthritis and Metabolic Diseases, the National Institute of Dental Research, the National Institute of Mental Health, the National Institute of Neurological Diseases and Blindness (including multiple sclerosis, epilepsy, cerebral palsy, and blindness), the National Institute of Child Health and Human Development, and the National Institute of General Medical Science. In addition to its own research program, the NIH provides grants for health-related research at many universities and research institutes in the United States.

(Also see U.S. DEPARTMENT OF HEALTH AND HUMAN SERVICES.)

U.S. Department of Agriculture (USDA).

The following eight divisions of this department have primary responsibility in the areas of human health and nutrition.

• **The Agricultural Research Service**—This agency is the main research division of the USDA. A considerable amount of its resources and staff are committed to the development of new food products, human nutrition, the nutrient composition of foods, and protection of foods against spoilage.

• **The Animal and Plant Health Inspection Service**—This division is charged with maintaining the wholesomeness and safety of meats processed in packing plants that ship meat and meat products, including poultry and poultry products, interstate.

• **The Consumer and Marketing Service**—The major responsibility for the federal grading of foods is assigned by law to this division. Butter, cheese, eggs, fresh produce, processed fruits and vegetables, grains, legumes, meats, nonfat dry milk, and poultry are inspected and graded according to their desirability for consumers. Also, the safety of certain items is checked by means of bacterial and mold counts, and chemical analyses.

This agency has established standards of identity for meat and poultry products such as breaded items, frankfurters, hash, pot pies, and soups. The standards specify (1) the minimum amounts of meat and poultry which must be present; and (2) the maximum allowable amounts of breading, fat, fillers, sweeteners, and water.

- **The Cooperative State Research Service**—This agency is charged with administering the funds for the research projects which are conducted by the state agricultural experiment stations. Periodically, staff from the experiment stations in various parts of the United States work together in regional projects which study the status of health and nutrition of selected groups within their respective states.

- **The Federal Extension Service**—The function of this division is to teach people how to make better use of agricultural and community resources. Much of their current educational work involves the promotion of better dietary practices. Also, some of the staff are professional dietitians who advise people on the dietary modifications which are necessary in the treatment and prevention of various diseases. The federal extension workers participate in cooperative programs with their counterparts in state and local extension services.

- **The Food and Nutrition Service**—This division provides the means for better nutrition through programs such as (1) distribution of surplus agricultural commodities, (2) food stamps, and (3) reimbursement to schools for the operation of breakfast and lunch programs.

- **The Labeling and Registration Section**—This section has responsibility for the proper labeling and safe use of pesticides. Manufacturers of pesticides must present new products with their proposed labels for approval before they are authorized to sell them.

  It is the responsibility of the FDA, however, to set legal tolerances for pesticides on or in raw agricultural products. Also, it sets the *safe* interval between last application of the insecticide and the time of harvest of the crop or the slaughter of the animal.

  Thus, through the cooperative supervision of the USDA and the FDA, both the pesticide user and the consumer of the product are safeguarded.

- **The Veterinary Services Division (VSD)**—This division is responsible for programs to control and eradicate (if possible) certain diseases of livestock; e.g., brucellosis, tuberculosis, scabies, and hog cholera.

  (Also see U.S. DEPARTMENT OF AGRICULTURE [USDA].)

State And Local Government Agencies. State departments of health and agriculture often perform functions similar to the federal counterparts of these agencies. Some overlapping of activities is unavoidable because the federal government does not have the authority to intervene in matters within the jurisdictions of individual states. However, it is often necessary to delegate further authority to county units such as extension offices and boards of health. Most local units maintain good relations with the state and federal authorities in the event that it might be necessary to call on them for assistance with such problems as epidemics of communicable diseases, and the occurrence of harmful substances in foods or drinking water.

INTERNATIONAL ORGANIZATIONS IN HEALTH AND NUTRITION.

The governments of many of the developing countries lack the resources needed to cope with their widespread health and nutritional problems. Hence, it may often be necessary for them to seek help from the World Health Organization (WHO) and the Food and Agriculture Organization (FAO). Also, sometimes assistance may be obtained from voluntary relief organizations like CARE, or from private nonprofit foundations such as the Ford Foundation and the Rockefeller Foundation.

Even the developed countries—whose peoples and governments contribute generously to the support of the United Nations and other international agencies—may benefit from the activities of these organizations. Typically, the various types of nongovernmental programs serve to (1) call attention to the urgency and scope of worldwide health problems; (2) demonstrate that there may be simpler and less expensive ways of meeting basic health and nutritional needs; (3) provide help with problems that are not adequately met by the activities of the governmental agencies; and (4) mobilize people and resources at the grass-roots level.

The many types of voluntary organizatons engaged in health and nutrition activities are too numerous for inclusion in this article; thus, only a few well-known and noteworthy examples follow.

- **Groups sponsored by private industry**—The best-known organizations in this category are the National Dairy Council and the National Live Stock and Meat Board. Generally, these groups engage in educational and public relations activities, which are intended for a wide audience, ranging from lay persons to highly educated professionals.

- **Professional organizations**—Usually, dentists, dietitians, doctors, health educators, nurses, and public health workers belong to professional groups which (1) may help to set and maintain the standards of practice, (2) hold yearly national meetings to discuss current issues, (3) publish scholarly journals, and (4) otherwise promote the interests of the profession. These activities all help to improve the level of health care received by the patient.

- **Private social or charitable agencies and church-sponsored groups**—These organizations often obtain their operating funds from private contributions and/or endowments. They may engage in activities such as health education, providing food to the needy, operating lunch programs for senior citizens, sending out visiting nurses and/or homemakers to the homebound, and referring their clients to other private and public services. Some typical organizations are the Red Cross, March of Dimes, Salvation Army, visiting nurse associations, settlement houses, and the agencies operated by the major religious denominations. It is noteworthy that the establishment of hospices for the sick poor was one of the major missions of the Franciscan Order which was established by Francis of Assisi around the end of the 12th century.

- **Civic and fraternal organizations**—Long before the governments of nations got into the business of looking after the welfare of their citizens, people from local communities joined together to promote their interests. For example, the forerunners of our present-day chambers of commerce were groups of businessmen in the days of the Roman Empire. Today, civic clubs work with fraternal and charitable organizations such as Elks, Lions, Rotarians, and Shriners to raise funds to provide hospitals, care for the blind, homes for the aged, and other services for the needy. These groups provide settings within which physicians, business people, and others from various walks of life may pool their talents for the improvement of the health and welfare of their community.

  (Also see NUTRITION EDUCATION.)

DISINFECTION

The process of destroying harmful microorganisms in or on items which come in contact with foods by means of (1) exposure to sunlight or other ultraviolet radiation, (2) treatment with chemicals, or, (3) application of dry or moist heat.

(Also see DISEASES.)

DISORDER

A derangement of function; an abnormal physical or mental condition; sickness, ailment, malady.

DISTAL

That part of a structure farthest from the point of attachment.

DISTILLATION

A procedure in which desired substances such as alcohol or water are separated from undesired materials by boiling, followed by condensation and collection of the vaporized liquid in a separate vessel.

(Also see DISTILLED LIQUORS.)

DISTILLED LIQUORS

These alcoholic beverages are made by some of the same processes used to make beers and wines, except that liquors contain more alcohol because they have been distilled. Alcoholic distillation is a process in which (1) a dilute solution of alcohol in a boiler (still) is heated to a temperature above the boiling point of alcohol, but below the boiling point of water, (2) the alcohol vapor produced in the still is led through a condenser where it is converted back into a liquid, and (3) the liquid alcohol (distillate) is caught in a receiving vessel.

Distilled liquors are called *spirits* because, poetically speaking, they represent the spirit or soul of the fermentation mixture. The different types of spirits vary considerably in their characteristics because, in addition to alcohol and water, they contain the volatile substances called congeners, which contribute aroma, color, and taste. The professional distiller is an artist of sorts, who controls the process conditions in order to obtain the desired characteristics in the final product.

• **Proof**—The numerical value of this term is twice the percent alcohol (by volume) in the liquor. For example, 80 proof means that the product contains 40 percent alcohol. Both the government tax and the selling price are pegged to the alcoholic content of the product. Hence, the lower proof variety of a given brand costs less than one with a higher proof.

RAW MATERIALS AND TYPES OF LIQUORS. Alcohol is usually produced by the yeast fermentation of sugars. Hence, the major raw materials may be (1) sugary items such as fruit juices or fruit by-products, honey, sugar or molasses, or the sap from certain trees; or (2) starchy foods such as grains, roots, and tubers. However, starches require conversion to sugar by the enzymes from germinated grains (malts), or from the appropriate microorganisms.

The major types of distilled liquors, along with the source(s) of sugar for fermentation of each type, follow:

• **Brandy**—Made from fruits: apples, apricots, blackberries, cherries, elderberries, grapes, pears, pineapples, plums, raspberries, or strawberries.

• **Gin**—Made from mixtures of grain and malt similar to those used in making beers and whiskies.

• **Liqueur or Cordial**—Made from mixtures of grains, malt, and/or sugar.

• **Rum**—Made from sugarcane; primarily molasses, but juice or syrup may be used.

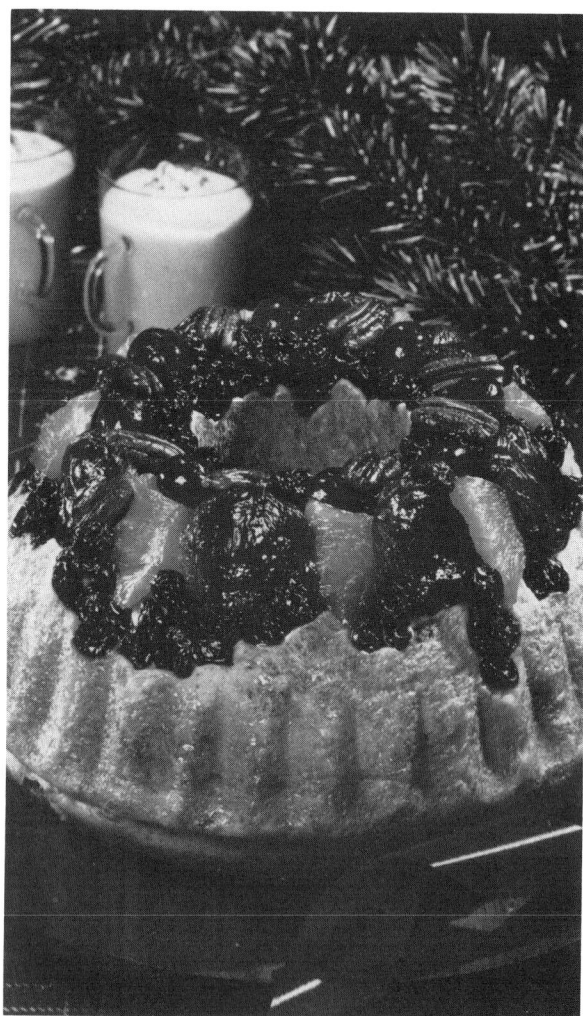

Fig. D-21. Rum-soaked raisin coffee cake. (Courtesy, Siegel/Ketchum, San Francisco, Calif.)

• **Vodka**—Made from starchy materials such as potatoes and/or grain.

• **Whiskey**—Made from malted and unmalted grains, of which the main types are: Bourbon, from corn; Canadian, from barley, corn, rye, and wheat; Irish, from barley, corn, oats, rye, and wheat; Rye, from rye; and Scotch, from barley.

Some less common, but highly regarded liquors, along with their sources are:

• **Aquavit (Akavit)**—Made from barley and potatoes.

• **Bitters**—Made from refined alcohol flavored with aromatic and bitter plant materials.

• **Okolehao**—Made from roots of the sacred ti plant (*Cordyline australis*) of Hawaii.

• **Tequila**—Made from the mezcal plant (a species of *agave*) native to Mexico.

NUTRITIONAL AND MEDICINAL EFFECTS OF SPIRITS.

Food Composition Table F-21 lists a variety of alcoholic beverages—beers, wines, and liquors. In contrast to beers and wines, which contain certain minerals and vitamins, distilled liquors are so highly refined that they supply mainly *empty calories*. For example, the caloric content of 1 oz (*29.6 ml*) of gin, rum, vodka, or whiskey ranges from 65 Calories (kcal) for 80-proof spirits to 83 Calories (kcal) for 100-proof spirits. Furthermore, other beverage spirits such as brandies, cordials, liqueurs, and mixed drinks may contain sufficient added sugar to make their caloric values much higher than the unsweetened spirits. (Most of the liqueurs sold in the United States contain from 100 to 120 Calories [kcal] per ounce.) Hence, heavy drinkers may obtain too much of their caloric requirement from liquor, and too little from the foods which furnish essential nutrients. It is well documented that chronic alcoholics often suffer from various types of malnutrition.[12]

On the other hand, the light to moderate use of spirits may indirectly confer nutritional benefits. A drink of liquor taken before a meal may help to insure that optimal amounts of foods are consumed because its calming effect relaxes those who (1) cannot eat enough because of jitters, or (2) are nervous, compulsive eaters. Also, small amounts of brandies, cordials, or liqueurs are thought to aid digestion.

Some of the other medicinal benefits of alcohol are: alleviation of minor aches and pains, inducement of sleep, dilation of blood vessels so that more blood reaches the tissues, warming of the skin, and relaxation of sexual and social inhibitions. However, there is always the danger that one may become dependent on these effects, and that excessive drinking may result.

(Also see ALCOHOL AND ALCOHOLIC BEVERAGES; and ALCOHOLISM AND ALCOHOLICS.)

MISCELLANEOUS USES OF DISTILLED LIQUORS AND THEIR BY-PRODUCTS.

Many people are unaware of the other uses of the products of alcoholic distillation. These uses (1) help to lower the cost of spirits, since they promote the most efficient use of the raw materials, and (2) provide a boost to the production of nutritious animal foods such as dairy products, eggs, meats, and poultry. A summary of some of the most important of these uses follows:

• **Human foods**—Neutral spirits, used as solvents for dissolving extracts of flavoring agents; distillers' protein concentrate (DPC), used in snack foods and as a meat extender; and neutral spirits, used as a base in certain medications and tonics.

• **Animal feeds**—Distillers grains, used as an energy and protein feed; Distillers' solubles, used as an energy, protein, and vitamin supplement; and Grain distillers dried yeast, used as a protein and vitamin supplement.

[12]Stone, O. J., "Alcoholic Malnutrition and Skin Infections," *Nutrition Today*, Vol. 13, November/December 1978, pp. 6-10, 27-30.

DIURESIS

The passage of more than the normal amount of urine. It may be caused by drinking large quantities of water, coffee, or alcoholic beverages, or by nervous tension.
(Also see WATER BALANCE.)

DIURETIC

An agent that increases the flow of urine.

DIVERTICULA

Small pouches which are formed in the wall of the large intestine because of abnormally high pressures that develop during the passage of the intestinal contents. It is suspected that diverticulitis may result from diets low in fiber.
(Also see DIVERTICULITIS; and FIBER.)

DIVERTICULITIS

Inflammation of the diverticular sacs (outpouchings) often occurring in the colon of middle-aged or elderly persons. Its cause is the mechanical failure of these outpouchings to empty undigested food and bacteria. Attacks of diverticulitis have symptoms similar to acute appendicitis—generalized abdominal pain, nausea, sometimes vomiting, fever, and elevation of the white cell count. Most cases respond to bed rest, liquid diet, and a broad spectrum antibiotic. Occasionally, diverticulitis progresses to the point of perforation of the colon wall or hemorrhage, and surgery may be required.

DNA

The abbreviation for deoxyribonucleic acid, a constituent of the nuclear material of cells.
(Also see NUCLEIC ACIDS.)

DOCK (SORREL; SOUR GRASSES) *Rumex*, spp

This is the name given to several plants of the genus *Rumex* of the buckwheat family, *Polygonaceae*. All of them have juicy leaves and stems that contain oxalic acid. This gives them a sour taste.

In the Northern Hemisphere, most docks are common weeds that thrive in acid soils; hence, their presence in a meadow indicates that the land needs lime. The leaves of curly docks (*R. crispus*) are used in soups and salads, like spinach.

DOLOMITE

This mineral, which is also known as dolomitic limestone, is a major ingredient in several antacids, and food supplements. It is a mixture of approximately equal parts of calcium carbonate and magnesium carbonate. Dolomitic limestone contains about 5 times as much magnesium, and about ⅝ as much calcium as ordinary limestone. A typical analysis of dolomite follows: calcium, 22.30%; chlorine, 0.12%; iron, 0.08%; magnesium, 9.99%; phosphorus, 0.04%; and potassium, 0.36%. Dolomite is sometimes used as a calcium supplement for humans; however, it should be tested and found free of lead and other impurities.

Even though dietary supplementation with dolomite may be indicated, no one should take therapeutic doses of dolomite without first consulting a physician. A therapeutic dose is one which supplies more than 1,500 mg of calcium per day, or the upper limit of the U.S. RDA for this mineral for adults other than pregnant or lactating women.

(Also see ANTACIDS; CALCIUM; and MAGNESIUM.)

DOPAMINE

A nerve transmitter in the brain, the lack of which is believed to be responsible for the symptoms of Parkinson's Disease. It is produced from the amino acid tyrosine, and it, in turn, is converted in the brain to noradrenaline (norepinephrine) and adrenaline (epinephrine).

DOUGLAS BAG

A rubber bag used to collect exhaled air in metabolism studies. It is light enough to be strapped onto a person and permits freedom of movement. After the study is completed the carbon dioxide content of the bag is analyzed, because this measurement may be used to calculate the metabolic rate.

(Also see CALORIE [ENERGY] EXPENDITURE.)

DOVE

This is the common name for various species of birds in the family *Columbidae*—the family that also includes pigeons. Generally, the term dove refers to the smaller members of the family, and pigeon to the larger ones. Doves live throughout the world. In most countries, they are considered a game bird and are hunted.

Doves are drawn (eviscerated), prepared for cooking, and cooked like pigeons of similar ages. The flesh is much esteemed by gastronomes.

DPN

The abbreviation for diphosphopyridine nucleotide, an out-of-date name for nicotinamide adenine dinucleotide (NAD).

DRESSING

Dressing of animals, poultry, game, and fish is a *disassembly* operation—usually on-the-rail, whereas automobile manufacturing is an assembly line procedure. Dressing refers to the skinning of animals and the plucking (removing of the feathers) of birds, along with removing parts other than the carcass—the viscera, feet, head, etc.

DRIED MILK

See MILK.

DRIPPINGS

Juices and melted fat that remain in the pan after meat has been cooked by dry heat.

DROOLING

The dribbling of saliva from the mouth. It is common in most babies and also occurs in some older people.

DROPSY

An abnormal accumulation of fluid in one or more parts of the body.

(Also see WATER AND ELECTROLYTES.)

DRUPES

Fruits which have a single seed that is enclosed in a stony shell, which, in turn, is surrounded by the flesh and skin of the fruits. Almonds, apricots, cherries, peaches, and plums are the best known drupes. These fruits are sometimes referred to as *stone fruits*. It is noteworthy that blackberries and raspberries are aggregate fruits made up of many tiny drupes or drupelets.

(Also see FRUIT[S], Table F-23, Fruits of the World.)

DRY FRYING

The frying of foods without the use of fat, either in a nonstick pan or by using an antisticking agent.

DRY ICE

A solid carbon dioxide (CO_2) used as a refrigerant. The name comes from the fact that solid carbon dioxide does not return to liquid form when it melts; it changes directly into a gas. Dry ice is much colder than ordinary ice; it sometimes reaches a temperature as low as -112°F (*-80°C*). Dry ice can be used to ship perishable foods by parcel post, because it cannot melt.

Dry ice is made by compressing carbon-dioxide gas to a liquid, then cooling. Some of the cold liquid is evaporated to make carbon-dioxide snow, then machines compress the snow into blocks of solid dry ice.

DRY MATTER

That part of a food which is not water. Dry matter is found by determining the percentage of water and subtracting the water content from 100%.

(Also see ANALYSIS OF FOODS.)

DUCT

A tube which carries glandular secretions away from the gland to another part of the body. For example, the bile duct carries bile from the liver and gallbladder to the small intestine.

(Also see DIGESTION AND ABSORPTION.)

DUCTLESS GLAND

A gland which secretes directly into the blood stream. Hence, all parts of the body may be affected by the secreted substances.

(Also see ENDOCRINE GLAND.)

DUMPING SYNDROME

This disorder is a physiological response occurring 10 to 15 minutes after ingestion of a meal by a person who has a gastrectomy (partial or complete surgical removal of the stomach). The symptoms are rapid pulse, rapid breathing, weakness, trembling, pallor, cold sweating, and abdominal fullness and distention. In some cases, there may also be nausea, vomiting, and fainting. Another set of reactions may occur about 2 hours later, due to the onset of hypoglycemia (low blood sugar accompanied by mental confusion, double vision, weakness, hunger, faintness, dizziness, headache, sweating, sleepiness, trembling, and rapid pulse). Another name for this disorder is *jejunal hyperosmolic syndrome*.

CAUSES OF DUMPING SYNDROME. The term *dumping* refers to the rapid deposition of food into the small intestine, which usually occurs in persons part or all of whose stomachs are missing. By contrast, a normal, intact stomach usually releases food, diluted by gastric juice, rather slowly into the intestine. One cause of the symptom is a high concentration in the jejunum of soluble materials in proportion to the amount of water (also known as *hypersomolality*). This condition results in a flow of water into the intestine from the plasma and extracellular fluid (contributed by the intestinal tissue and blood flowing through it). Loss of water from the circulatory system results in decreases in blood volume and blood pressure leading to the symptoms associated with *cardiac insufficiency* (the heart is an inefficient pump when a reduction in the blood volume prevents its filling to capacity). The circulatory changes lead to a response by the sympathetic nervous system (resulting in rapid heart rate, sweating, and weakness). *Distention of the jejunum* (by the volume of food, by fluids taken with the meal, and/or by the fluid originating from the blood and tissues) probably helps to stimulate the set of troublesome physiological responses.

Hypoglycemia is more likely to occur when the meal contains a moderate to large proportion of easily digested carbohydrate. Rapid absorption of sugars, the digestion products of carbohydrate, results in an elevation of the blood sugar level, which in turn stimulates the pancreatic release of a large amount of insulin (temporary *hyperinsulinism*). The net effect is a rapid drop in the blood sugar level due to the action of insulin (which enhances the rate of sugar passage from the blood into cells).

Persons with normal stomachs may also experience symptoms similar to dumping syndrome when they have rapid emptying of gastric contents into the small intestine, such as may occur with (1) a large amount of food and fluid that is rich in carbohydrates, or (2) hyperactivity of the stomach due to other factors such as nervousness.

PREVENTION OF DUMPING SYNDROME. The best approach is to minimize the factors responsible for the conditions. This means that meals should be planned according to the rules which follow:

1. Select meals containing moderate to liberal amounts of protein and fat, and use only small portions of foods high in carbohydrate.
2. Avoid foods high in sugars such as soft drinks, candy, cake, cookies, syrups, honey, and molasses.
3. Take frequent small meals or snacks (5 to 6 per day) instead of eating 2 or 3 large meals.
4. Do not take beverages with meals, but have them about an hour before or after meals.
5. Allow foods that are boiling hot or ice cold to approach room temperature before eating.
6. Avoid emotionally exciting situations at mealtimes.
7. Restrict salt and such seasonings as soy sauce and monosodium glutamate.

(Also see HYPOGLYCEMIA; and ULCERS, PEPTIC.)

DUODENUM

The upper portion of the small intestine which extends from the stomach to the jejunum.
(Also see DIGESTION AND ABSORPTION.)

DUTCH COCOA

The addition of an alkali (the carbonates or hydroxides of sodium, potassium, ammonium, or magnesium) during the processing of cocoa from the cacao bean causes the cocoa flavor to become milder and the color darker, yielding a product called Dutch cocoa. Dutching of cocoa originated in Holland; hence, the name.
(Also see COCOA AND CHOCOLATE.)

DUTCH OVEN

• A metal utensil with shelves and one open side which can be placed close to the fire.

• A cast iron pot with three legs and a lid on which coals can be placed. It is used for baking in an open fire.

• A heavy pot with a tight, domed cover which is used for braising, steaming, or baking, either in the oven or on top of the stove.

DWARFISM

An abnormal condition in which the affected person is much shorter in height than other individuals of the same age, sex and ethnic group. In most cases dwarfism is due to an undersecretion of growth hormone(s) by the pituitary gland, although other metabolic disorders may also be responsible.
(Also see ENDOCRINE GLANDS.)

DYMELOR

A brand name for a form of sulfonylurea called *acetohexamide*, an intermediate-acting oral drug used to stimulate the pancreatic cells to release insulin. The drug is only effective for the treatment of diabetes when some insulin secreting ability remains in the pancreas. Other brand names are Dimelor, Dimelin, and Ordimel.
(Also see DIABETES, section headed "Sulfa-type Drugs [Sulfonylureas]".)

DYS–

A prefix conveying the idea of bad or difficult.

DYSENTERY

An inflammation of the mucous membrane of the large intestine resulting from infection of bacteria, protozoa, or virus, and characterized by the appearance of blood and mucus in the stools, severe diarrhea, cramps, and fever.

DYSENTERY, AMOEBIC

(See DISEASES.)

DYSGEUSIA

Perverted sense of taste; a *bad* taste.

DYSINSULINISM

An abnormality in which the blood sugar after a meal or after a test dose of sugar stays abnormally high for an hour or two, then drops to an abnormally low level. Hence, the blood sugar pattern appears to be a combination of those which are found in both diabetes (the high blood sugar level) and hypoglycemia (the low blood sugar level). It is thought to be due to an abnormally slow release of insulin by the pancreas in response to an elevated blood sugar.
(Also see DIABETES; and HYPOGLYCEMIA.)

DYSOSMIA

Impaired sense of smell; an obnoxious odor.

DYSPEPSIA

The general term used to describe any of a variety of

disorders which occur in the upper part of the digestive tract after food has been taken. Dyspepsia is sometimes referred to as indigestion, which is a rather vague term for these complaints. For example, some typical symptoms of dyspepsia are abdominal pain, chest pain, belching, excessive gas, heartburn, nausea, and an uncomfortable feeling of fullness.

(Also see DIGESTION AND ABSORPTION.)

DYSPHAGIA

A disorder of the esophagus which makes it difficult to swallow.

DYSPNEA

Abnormal breathing characterized by shortness of breath, difficulty in breathing, or an undue awareness of the act of breathing.

DYSSEBACIA

An oily flaking of the skin which may often be due to a lack of riboflavin or other essential nutrients.
(Also see RIBOFLAVIN.)

DYSTROPHY

One or more defects in body tissues due to such causes as poor nutrition, heredity, or a degenerative disease.

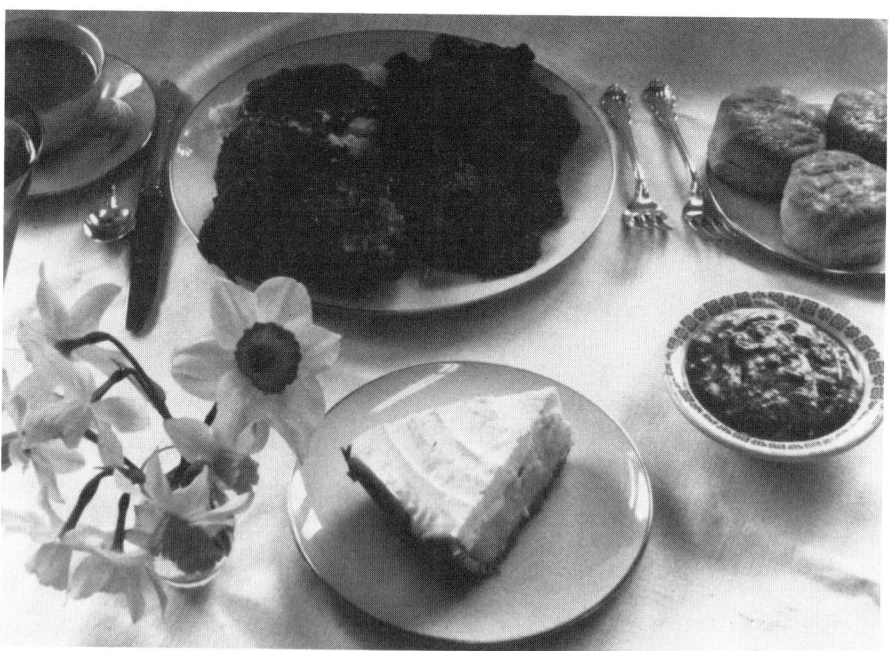

Fig. D-22. A Company meal. (Courtesy, University of Tennessee, Knoxville, Tenn.)

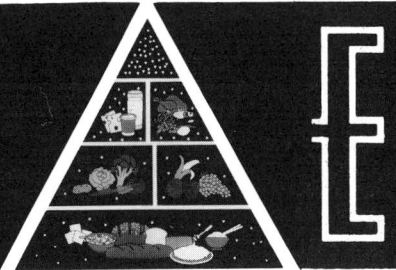

EARTH-EATING

The abnormal practice of eating dirt and/or clay, which is also called *geophagia*. It is suspected that the reasons for this bizarre practice are: (1) a need for a nutrient which is lacking in the diet, and (2) an irritation of the digestive tract which is soothed by the earth which is ingested.

(Also see PICA.)

EBERS' PAPYRUS

An ancient Egyptian medical paper, dated about 1500 B.C., which was found by the German Egyptologist George Ebers in 1872. Ebers' Papyrus is of great interest to those studying the history of dietetics and medicine because it describes the ancient treatment of such diseases as (1) diabetes, for which a diet of beer, fruits, grains, and honey was recommended; and (2) goiter, in which the thyroid gland was removed surgically.

ECLAMPSIA

A toxemia of late pregnancy characterized by excessive retention of water, high blood pressure, passage of protein in the urine, convulsions, and coma. Fortunately, the incidence of this disorder has declined greatly in recent years. A milder toxemia without the convulsions and coma is called preeclampsia. The causes of eclampsia and preeclampsia are uncertain although it is suspected that nutrition and/or the amount of weight gain in pregnancy might be important factors.

EDEMA

Swelling of a part or all of the body due to the accumulation of excess water.

EDIBLE PORTION

The part of an animal or plant food which is commonly eaten, in contrast to refuse portions such as bones, gristle, peels, and seeds which are normally discarded.

EDTA

A chelating agent that is added to certain foods to bind with trace minerals which are responsible for the development of off colors and flavors in the food. It may also be given orally or by injection to tie up excesses of certain trace minerals and draw them out of the body via the urine and/or the stool.

EFFERVESCENT

A term used to describe a liquid that is bubbling because it is giving off bubbles of gas. A common effervescent liquid is a solution of baking soda, which releases carbon dioxide. (The latter solution is used mainly as an antacid or a leavening agent in baking.)

EGG(S)

Contents

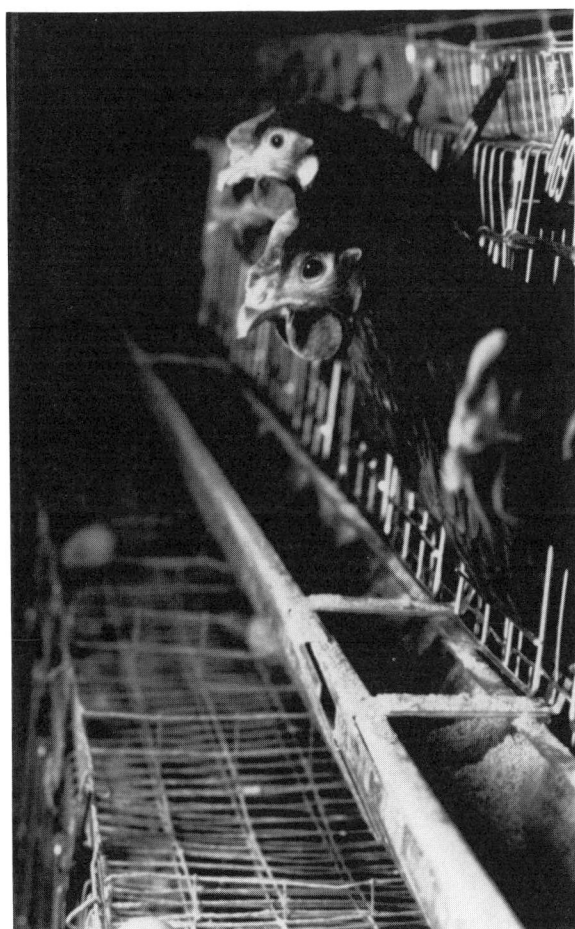

Fig. E-1. Pampered layers producing eggs. (Courtesy, Univeristy of Minnesota, St. Paul, Minn.)

The bird egg is a marvel of nature. It's one of the most complete foods known to man, as evidenced by the excellent balance of proteins, fats, carbohydrates, minerals, and vitamins which it provides during the 20-day in-the-shell period when it serves as the developing chick's only source of food. Also, the egg is one of the few foods that is produced in prepackaged form. Not only that, it is the reproductive cell (ovum) of the hen. Upon fertilization by the male's reproductive cell (sperm), the egg will develop into a chick when incubated properly.

HISTORY. Ancient man persuaded chickens to live and produce near his abode. It is not known exactly when this happened, but it's obvious that chickens were domesticated at a remote period. The keeping of poultry was probably contemporary with the keeping of sheep by Abel and the tilling of the soil by Cain. Chickens were known in ancient Egypt, and they had already achieved considerable status at the time of the Pharaohs, because artificial incubation was then practiced in crude ovens resembling some that are still in use in that country.

The American poultry industry had its humble beginning when chickens were first brought to this continent by the early settlers. Small home flocks were started at the time of the establishment of the first permanent homes at Jamestown in 1607. For many years thereafter, chickens were tenderly cared for by the farmer's wife, who fed them on table scraps and the unaccounted-for grain from the crib.

Since World War II, changes in poultry and egg production and processing have paced the whole field of agriculture. Practices in all phases of poultry production—breeding, feeding, management, housing, marketing and processing—have become very highly specialized. The net result is that more products have been made available to consumers at favorable prices, comparatively speaking.

WORLD AND U.S. PRODUCTION. Worldwide, eggs are an important food. Table E-1 shows the leading egg-producing countries for which reliable data exist.

TABLE E-1
AVERAGE YEARLY EGG PRODUCTION IN SPECIFIED COUNTRIES[1]

Country	Eggs
	(millions)
China	158,920
U.S.S.R.	82,000
United States	67,919
Japan	39,850
Mexico	18,040
Germany	16,800
France	14,629
Brazil	13,454
United Kingdom	12,352
Italy	11,454

[1]*Agricultural Statistics*, 1991, p. 350, Table 521.

In the United States, since 1940 the number of eggs per chicken per year has increased from 134 to 252 as shown in Table E-2. Furthermore, commercial egg production is accomplished on a large scale. Some production units—flocks of layers—consist of 1 million or more chickens. The

overall result of scientific egg production is reflected by the 67.8 billion eggs produced in the United States in 1990.

TABLE E-2
EGG PRODUCTION HISTORY IN THE UNITED STATES[1]

Year	Layers Producing	Eggs per Layer	Eggs Produced
	(thousands)		(millions)
1940	296,595	134	39,695
1945	369,356	151	55,858
1950	339,540	174	58,954
1955	309,297	192	59,526
1960	294,662	209	61,491
1965	301,058	218	66,560
1970	312,759	218	68,212
1975	278,101	232	64,626
1980	287,705	242	69,686
1985	277,592	247	68,645
1990	271,631	252	67,832

[1]*Agricultural Statistics*, USDA, 1949, p. 473, Table 590; 1965, p. 426, Table 619; 1980, p. 412, Table 592; and 1991, p. 351, Table 523.

In the United States, all 50 states report some egg production, but the ten leading states indicated in Table E-3 are responsible for 61% of the eggs produced. California is the leading egg-producing state by a considerable margin. However, the heaviest concentration of layers is in the southeastern United States.

TABLE E-3
TEN LEADING EGG-PRODUCING STATES, 1990[1]

States	Eggs Produced
	(millions)
California	7,472
Indiana	5,445
Pennsylvania	4,976
Ohio	4,667
Georgia	4,302
Arkansas	3,620
Texas	3,317
North Carolina	2,986
Florida	2,586
Alabama	2,206

[1]*Agricultural Statistics*, 1991, USDA, p. 351, Table 524.

PHYSICAL CHARACTERISTICS OF THE EGG AND GRADING. Consumers demand a superior product even from *Mother Nature*; hence, eggs are graded.

The grading of eggs involves their sorting according to quality, size, weight, and other factors that determine their relative value. U.S. standards for quality of individual shell eggs have been developed on the basis of such interior quality factors as condition of the white and yolk, the size of the air cell, and the exterior quality factors of cleanliness and soundness of the shell. These standards cover the entire range of edible eggs.

Eggs are also classified according to weight (or size), expressed in ounces per dozen.

Egg grading, then, is the grouping of eggs into lots according to similar characteristics as to quality and weight. Although color is not a factor in the standards of grades, eggs are usually sorted for color and sold as either *whites* or *browns*.

Four sets of grades, based on the quality standards for individual shell eggs, are used in this country: (1) consumer grades—used in the sale of eggs to individual consumers; (2) wholesale grades—used in the wholesale channels of trade; (3) U.S. Procurement Grades—used for institutional buying and Armed Forces purchases; and (4) U.S. Nest Run Grade—which is also used in wholesale channels of trade.

Structure. A schematic side view of an egg is shown in Fig. E-2 with the various parts labeled in their normal position.

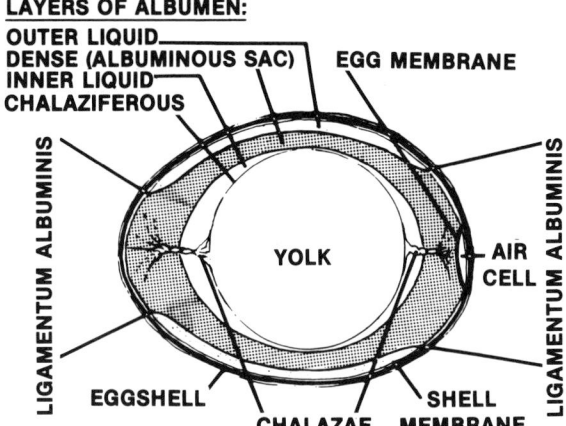

LAYERS OF ALBUMEN:
OUTER LIQUID
DENSE (ALBUMINOUS SAC)
INNER LIQUID
CHALAZIFEROUS
EGG MEMBRANE
LIGAMENTUM ALBUMINIS
YOLK
AIR CELL
LIGAMENTUM ALBUMINIS
EGGSHELL
CHALAZAE
SHELL MEMBRANE

Fig. E-2. Structure of the egg.

The protective covering, known as the shell, is composed primarily of calcium carbonate, with 6,000 to 8,000 microscopic pores permitting transfer of volatile components. The air cell, located in the large end of the egg, is formed when the cooling egg contracts and pulls the inner and outer shell membranes apart. The cordlike chalazae holds the yolk in position in the center of the egg. As shown, the egg is surrounded by a membrane, known as the vitelline membrane. The germinal disc, a normal part of every egg, is located on the surface of the yolk. Embryo formation begins here only in fertilized eggs. For most individuals the two most familiar parts of the egg are (1) the white, and (2) the yolk.

Size. Laying chickens produce eggs of varying sizes, and commercially produced eggs are classified by size according to their weight per dozen, following the guidelines of Table E-4. It is not unusual for the price of medium size eggs to be 5 to 10¢ lower per dozen than the price of large eggs. Egg size (weight) is separate and distinct from egg quality.

Shape. Eggs differ considerably in shape. Although many are truly ovate, some are nearly spherical, whereas others are elongated. Some eggs are almost equally pointed or rounded at both ends; others taper sharply from the large end to the small end. The eggs laid by birds of the same species resemble each other in shape, but they are not identical; nor are all eggs of a particular bird alike.

Color. The shell color of eggs of the domestic hen may be white, many shades of brown, or yellow. One breed lays blue green eggs. Sometimes very small, dark flecks are present on the shell, especially if it is brown.

TABLE E-4
U.S. WEIGHT CLASSES FOR CONSUMER GRADES FOR SHELL EGGS[1]

Size or Weight Class	Minimum Net Weight per Dozen	Minimum Net Weight per 30 Dozen	Minimum Weight for Individual Eggs at Rate per Dozen
	(oz)[2]	(lb)[3]	(oz)
Jumbo	30	56	29
Extra large	27	50½	26
Large	24	45	23
Medium	21	39½	20
Small	18	34	17
Peewee	15	28	—

[1]*United States Standards, Grades, and Weight Classes for Shell Eggs,* Agricultural Marketing Service, Poultry Division, USDA.

[2]One oz = 28.35 g.

[3]One lb = 0.45 kg.

Among domestic fowl, the color of the egg is peculiar to the breed, though tinted eggs occasionally appear in breeds that ordinarily lay white eggs.

Egg color often assumes economic importance, as there are numerous local prejudices in favor of certain shell tints. However, shell color does not alter the nutritional value of the egg.

Abnormalities. Periodically, a deviation in the mechanics of egg laying will create abnormal eggs, including double-yoked eggs, blood spots, meat spots, yokeless eggs, dented eggshells, and soft-shelled eggs.

From the above discussion it is evident that numerous factors are involved in the production of top quality eggs for the consumer. Many of these factors are judged in order to separate those eggs which can be marketed. Eggs are judged for quality through three sets of criteria; (1) external appearance, (2) candling, and (3) samples of eggs broken out to judge internal characteristics.

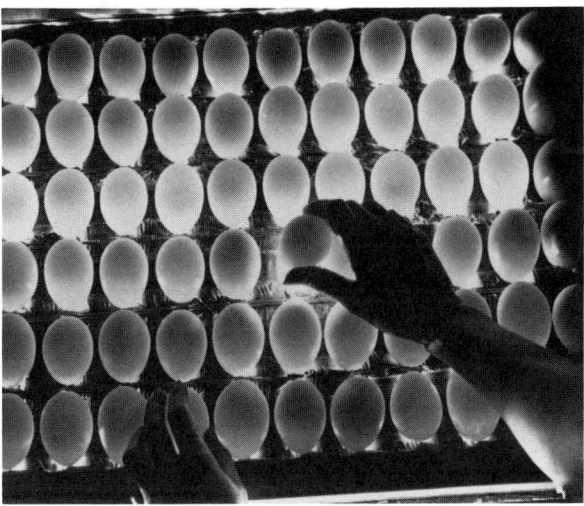

Fig. E-3. Candling. Eggs with defective shells, blood spots, or meat spots are removed in this egg-candling darkened curtain booth as eggs move from the washer to the grading and sizing machine. The eggs are rotated over a bank of high-wattage lights making any defect in them more easily seen by the person doing the candling work. (Courtesy, DEKALB AgResearch, Inc., DeKalb, Ill.)

EGG USES. Eggs serve as the basis for an extraordinarily wide range of uses—a fact emphasized by the large number of food products that contain eggs. Eggs can be eaten scrambled, fried, poached, shirred, baked, soft-boiled, hard-boiled, or coddled as a food. Furthermore, they can be curried, deviled, whipped and variously molded. Eggs are necessary for a good dough—whether for bread, pasta, pie crust, cakes, pancakes, crepes or waffles. Mayonnaise, hollandaise and bernaise sauces depend on the egg. Cosmopolitan dishes such as Frittata, Scotch Woodcock, Egg Foo Young, and Broccoli Timbale all feature the egg—a truly versatile product of nature.

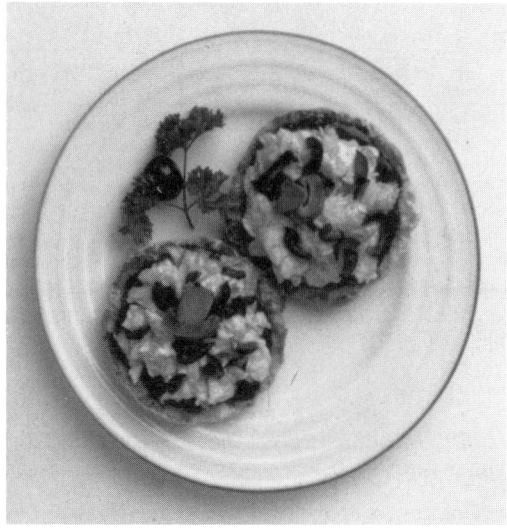

Fig. E-4. Pizza eggs. (Courtesy, USDA)

The popularity of the egg is due to several unique features—functional properties.

• **Coagulation**—Coagulation is a change in the structure of egg protein that results in the loss of solubility and thickening, or in other words, a change from fluid to a solid or semisolid. It may be brought about by heat, mechanical means, salts, acids or alkalis. The success of many cooked foods is dependent upon the coagulation of egg protein. Both the egg white and the yolk are utilized because of their ability to bind foods together. The ability to coagulate on heating is used in custards and pie fillings.

• **Foaming**—When egg white is beaten, air bubbles are trapped in the albumen and a foam is formed—a gas phase dispersed in a liquid phase. This foaming power of the egg white—albumen—makes it useful as a carrier of air for leavening; hence, it contributes to the lightness of certain foods. For example, meringues, angel cakes, souffles, omelets, some candies, and sponge cakes all depend upon eggs for their lightness.

• **Emulsification**—The egg yolk is a dispersion of oil droplets in water—an emulsion. Hence, the yolk is an efficient emulsifying agent. The emulsifying components of egg yolks are lecithin, cholesterol, lipoproteins and proteins. As an emulsifier, egg yolk or whole egg is an essential ingredient in mayonnaise (65-75% oil) and important in foods such as cake batter containing shortening, cream puffs, and hollandaise sauce, or wherever eggs are used with fats and oils.

• **Control of crystallization**—In candies, egg white controls the growth of sugar crystals, thus serving as a *sugar doctor*.

• **Color**—The naturally occurring pigment of egg yolk—xanthophylls, lutein, and zeaxanthin—contribute color to foods. In some foods, their acceptance is determined by the visual impression of egg yolk. For example, egg yolk pigments contribute a pleasing yellow color to baked products, noodles, ice cream, custard sauces, and omelets. In eggs alone, preference has been shown for gold or lemon-colored yolks. It is, however, rare for eggs to be used as an ingredient in food products for only their color contribution.

• **Flavor**—No one component of eggs can be determined as responsible for the characteristic flavor of eggs. The flavor of eggs has been described as fresh, mild, sweet, earthy, and musty. Some of the flavor is imparted to baked goods, and eggs are enjoyed by themselves for their distinct flavor.

• **Nutrition**—Last but not least, eggs contain many nutrients and their addition to any food contributes to the quality of that food. A complete discussion of the nutritional value of eggs is presented elsewhere in this article.

Eggs usually perform more than one function in a food. Table E-5 presents a summary of the functions eggs serve in foods.

TABLE E-5
SUMMARY OF THE USE AND FUNCTION OF EGGS IN FOOD

Food Item	Coagulation	Foaming	Emulsification	Control of Crystallization	Color	Flavor
Angel cake	•	•				
Custards	•				•	•
Divinity		•		•		
Eggs[1]	•				•	•
Fondant				•		
Mayonnaise			•			
Meringues	•	•				
Salad dressing			•			
Sponge cake	•	•			•	

[1]Cooked in shell, fried, scrambled or poached.

Due to the wide variety of uses and the high demand by food institutions and food industry, a large number of the eggs produced become processed eggs—frozen, liquid, or dried eggs. This segment of the egg industry was originally developed as an outlet for soiled, cracked, and abnormal

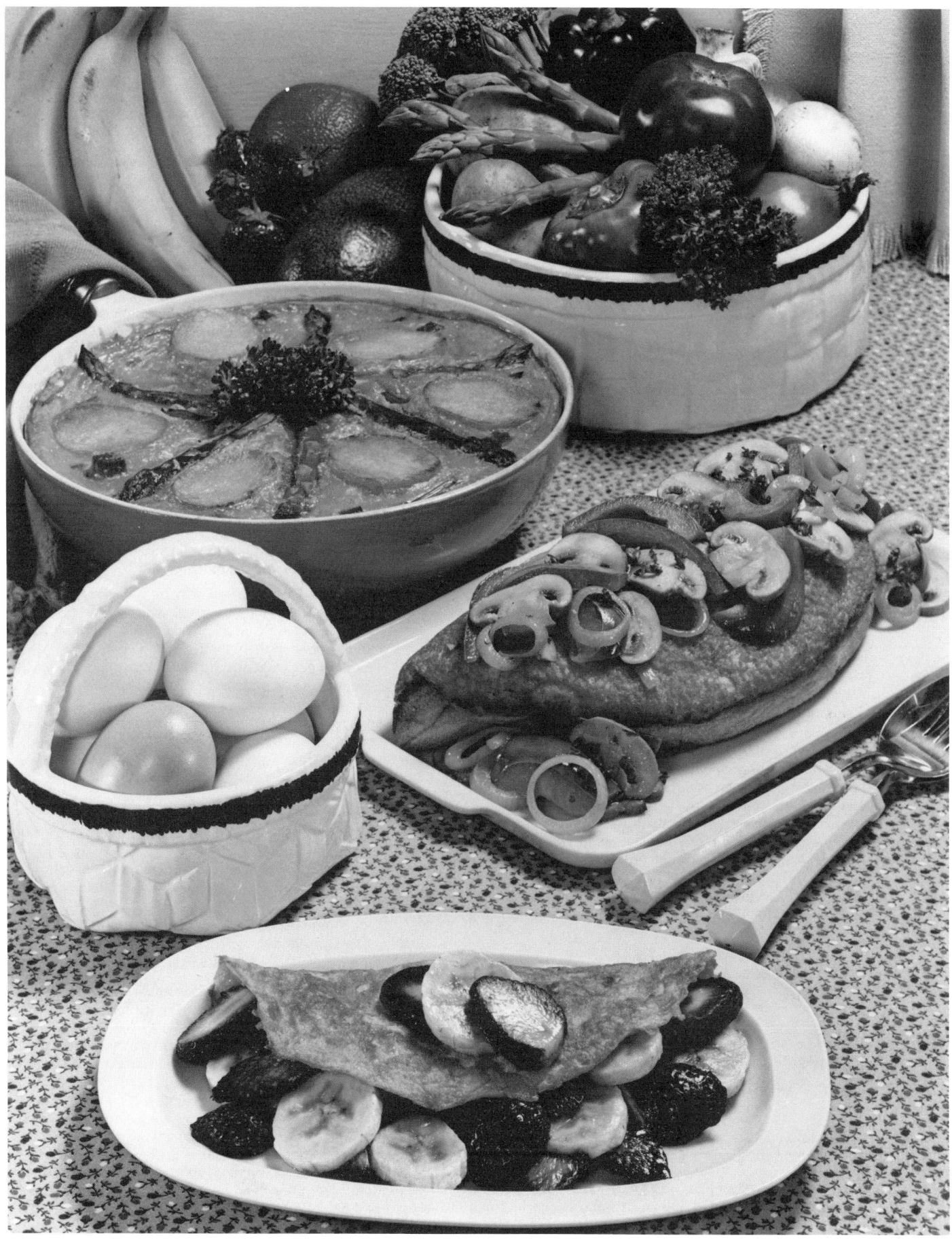

Fig. E-5. Eggs are used in a variety of dishes. (Courtesy, United Fresh Fruit & Vegetable Assoc.)

eggs unsuitable for marketing as shell eggs. Today, many quality eggs are being broken for processed eggs—about 13%.

The advantages of processed eggs are numerous when compared to shell eggs and include the following:

1. Less storage space is involved.
2. Quality of frozen and dried eggs is preserved longer.
3. Packaging is facilitated.
4. Processed eggs are cheaper than shell eggs.
5. Less labor is involved in the egg-breaking industry.
6. One can choose specific parts of the egg for a particular need.

Almost all egg-breaking operations are automated. After the eggs are mechanically broken, they are checked for abnormalities and odor. The broken eggs can then be processed whole or separated into yolks and whites. Whole eggs are mixed and strained before packaging. Yolks are also mixed and strained. Additionally, in frozen yolks, salt or sugar is often added to improve the rubbery consistency of the yolk after freezing and defrosting. Glycerin, molasses, or honey may also be used. Whites are strained to remove the chalazae, meat spots, blood spots, and broken shells, and may be passed through a chopper to homogenize the product. Of the three processed forms—frozen, liquid, and dried eggs—dried eggs have the longest shelf life and require the lowest expense for storage, since refrigeration is not needed. However, the vacuum spray processing of drying incurs additional costs.

Bakeries use about 50% of the processed eggs; food manufacturers about 40% and institutions about 10%.

Nutritional information for many of the various processed egg products is listed in Food Composition Table F-21.

(Also see EGG, DEHYDRATED [Dried].)

CONSUMPTION OF EGGS.

Eggs are used chiefly for human food. In 1990, the U.S. per capita consumption of eggs was 234. Table E-6 illustrates the downward trend of per capita consumption of eggs since 1960. This is an alarming trend for the poultry producer. It can be largely attributed to the cholesterol controversy and the development of egg substitutes that are low in fat and have no cholesterol. From Table E-6 one could make a reliable guess as to the year the cholesterol controversy started. In 1964 the American Heart Association recommended that the general public reduce cholesterol intake to 300 mg/day. One egg contains about 213 mg of cholesterol. Thus, the elimination of eggs from the diet was singled out as a means of reducing cholesterol intake.

TABLE E-6
PER CAPITA CONSUMPTION OF EGGS[1]

Year	Per Capita Number of Eggs Consumed
1960	335
1965	314
1970	311
1975	277
1980	272
1985	256
1990	234

[1]Source: USDA.

HEALTH PROBLEMS ATTRIBUTED TO EGGS.

Americans are becoming more and more health and diet conscious. Unfortunately, much of the nutritional information that they receive is not authoritative, and the facts are not presented objectively. Worse yet, passions and prejudices sometimes trigger such charges as "poultry products cause allergies, heart disease, and salmonellosis." Such accusations must be answered by more than simple denial. To this end, sections on "Allergies," "Cholesterol," and "Salmonellosis" follow.

Allergies. Occasionally, a child exhibits an allergic sensitivity to eggs. In most cases, the white of the egg is the portion that creates the reaction, and the yolk is generally readily tolerated. In highly sensitive individuals, the diet must be totally devoid of eggs. However, these cases are rare, and most infants and children allergic to eggs can follow a diet that provides for some heat-treated or cooked eggs.

(Also see ALLERGIES.)

Cholesterol. In recent years, the attention of the American public has been focused on heart disease—the leading killer in the United States.

That cholesterol is implicated in atherosclerosis is well documented by unbiased, controlled experiments; but research indicates that it is not the sole cause. Rather, a number of factors enters into the cause of heart disease; among them, stress, heredity, hypertension, diabetes mellitus, smoking, lack of exercise, and obesity.

It is noteworthy that eggs contain 22% less cholesterol than previously believed—213 mg instead of 274 mg per large egg. Also, they are low in saturated fat—only 1.5 g per large egg.

(Also see CHOLESTEROL; HEART DISEASE; and HYPER-LIPOPROTEINEMIAS [Hyperlipidemias].)

Salmonellosis. Salmonellosis may be a concern in eggs and egg products unless they are handled properly, as follows:

1. Store eggs at 45°F (7.2°C), or lower, until they are used; and do not keep them longer than 3 to 4 weeks.
2. Never use eggs that are cracked, contain blood spots, or have pinpoint holes in them.
3. Use pasteurized eggs, rather than raw eggs, as ingredients of uncooked, ready-to-eat menu items such as Caesar salad, eggnog, ice cream, milk shakes and other egg-fortified beverages, and freshly prepared mayonnaise, hollandaise, and bearnaise.
4. Do not pool or comingle eggs that are out of their shells unless they are cooked immediately.
5. Cook individual eggs so that all parts reach temperatures of at least 140°F (60°C).
6. Maintain cooked eggs requiring holding (such as those in breakfast buffets) at an internal temperature of at least 140°F (60°C).
7. Cook home-prepared eggs until the white is thoroughly coagulated and the yolk starts to thicken.

(Also see SALMONELLA; and SALMONELLOSIS.)

NUTRITIONAL VALUE.

Eggs contain an abundance of proteins, vitamins, and minerals. The protein fraction of eggs is highly digestible and of high quality, having a biological value of 94 on a scale of 100, the highest rating of any food. The reason for this high quality of protein is that egg proteins are complete proteins; that is, they contain all the essential amino acids required to maintain life and promote growth and health. Additionally, eggs are a good source of iron; phosphorus; trace minerals; vitamins A and E, and most of the B vitamins, including vitamin B-12. Eggs are second only to fish-liver oils as a natural source of vitamin D. Eggs are moderate from the standpoint of calorie content, a medium-size egg containing about 75 Calories (kcal).

Overall, eggs provide a well-balanced source of nutrients for persons of all ages. During the rapid growth of infants, children, and teenagers, eggs can contribute significantly to the body's nutrient needs. They make good therapeutic diets. Eggs are acceptable and valuable for older people whose caloric needs are lower and who sometimes have problems chewing certain foods. Table E-7 shows the nutritive value of eggs.

TABLE E-7
NUTRIENT VALUE OF TWO MEDIUM SIZED EGGS

Nutrient	Amount per Egg[1]	Daily Dietary Recommendations[2]
		(%)
Calories	75.4 kcal	4.2
Protein	6.1 g	9.7
Amino Acids[3]		
Isoleucine	364.0 mg	46.1
Leucine	512.0 mg	46.3
Lysine	394.0 mg	41.6
Methionine and cystine	327.0 mg	31.8
Phenylalanine and tyrosine .	572.0 mg	51.7
Threonine	286.0 mg	51.7
Tryptophan	93.0 mg	33.6
Valine	420.0 mg	53.2
Vitamin A	75 mcg RE	7.5
Vitamin D	0.6 mcg	8.0
Thiamin	0.42 mg	28.0
Riboflavin	0.144 mg	8.5
Niacin	0.030 mg	1.6
Vitamin B-6	0.058 mg	2.9
Folate	31.2 mcg	15.6
Vitamin B-12	0.743 mcg	37.2
Calcium	25.4 mg	3.2
Phosphorus	86.4 mg	10.8
Magnesium	5.8 mg	1.7
Iron	1.104 mg	11.0
Zinc	0.69 mg	4.6

[1]Values obtained from the Proteins and Amino Acids in Selected Foods, Table P-16 and the Food Composition Table F-21.
[2]Daily dietary recommendations for a male age 25 to 50, weighing 174 lb (*79 kg*), and 70 in. (*178 cm*) tall, based on the *Recommended Dietary Allowances*, 10th ed., NRC–National Academy of Sciences, 1989.
[3]The essential amino acids for an adult based on the *Recommended Dietary Allowances*, 10th ed., NRC–National Academy of Sciences, 1989, p. 57, Table 6-1.

Most nutrition programs can be improved by the inclusion of eggs. Eggs are of the highest nutritional quality and are marketed at prices that even the poor can afford.

Notwithstanding the high nutritive value of eggs, millions of Americans routinely eat eggs for breakfast each morning simply because they like them.

NUTRITIONAL MISCONCEPTIONS. Rumors still persist concerning the factors affecting the nutritional value of eggs.

• **Shell color**—Some individuals are willing to pay more for eggs of a certain shell color believing it to be an indication of quality or nutritive value. As pointed out, the color of the shell—whether brown, white, or blue—is directly related to the breed or strain of chicken; and it has no effect on the nutrient composition of the eggs.

• **Yolk color**—Xanthophyll is the major substance causing yolks to have a deeper yellow color. It has no nutritive value. Years ago when chickens ran freely on the farm they ate grass which contains xanthophyll. Modern production units put enough xanthophyll in the ration of chickens to produce a medium-yellow yolk.

• **Fertile eggs**—Some people feel that fertile eggs—eggs from hens mated to roosters—are more nutritious than nonfertile eggs. There is no scientific proof of this fact. Furthermore, infertile eggs are of more economic value, since there is no danger of loss through development of the embryo.

• ***Organic*** **eggs**—Organic eggs are of no higher nutritional value than commercial eggs. In fact, if the diet of an *organic* hen is not well-balanced the nutritive value of her eggs tends to be lower then that of the commercial laying hen fed a balanced diet. Moreover, fewer *organic* eggs are produced; hence, they are more expensive than commercially produced eggs.

• **Digestibility**—Some individuals consider raw eggs more digestible. Cooked eggs are more readily digested, but both are very completely digested and absorbed.

NOTE WELL: Raw egg white contains an antivitamin, a protein called avidin, which binds to biotin and renders it unavailable. However, avidin is denatured when eggs are cooked, thus making biotin available.

(Also see AMINO ACID[S]; DIGESTION AND ABSORPTION; METABOLISM; POULTRY; PROTEIN[S]; and REFERENCE PROTEIN.)

EGG, DEHYDRATED (Dried)

Dehydration—removing the water from foods to a level low enough to slow chemical reactions and stop the growth of microorganisms—is a successful way of preserving eggs. Dried or dehydrated eggs offer the following advantages:

1. Less storage space is involved, and storage space is less expensive.

2. Transportation cost is less.

3. Dried eggs have a long shelf life.

4. One can choose specific parts of the egg for a particular need.

Eggs can be divided into three categories on the basis of the drying methods employed: (1) egg whites, (2) egg yolks, and (3) whole eggs.

1. **Egg whites.** Before drying, egg whites are pasteurized, and a small amount of free glucose must be removed by enzymatic action (glucose oxidase) to prevent the Maillard reaction—a chemical reaction responsible for brown color and off-odors. Often a whipping aid such as sodium lauryl sulfate is added to help whites retain their high whipping ability following drying. Then, after the adjustment of the pH the whites are spray-dried and packaged in 150, 50, or 25 lb (*68, 23, or 11 kg*) containers. Some egg whites are air-dried where the whites are poured in thin layers on trays. This produces flakes of albumen.

2. **Egg yolks.** Egg yolks are pasteurized and then spray-dried, or stabilized by removing the free glucose with the enzyme glucose oxidase and then spray-dried. Often dried egg yolk is converted to a free-flowing powder by the addition of anticaking agents such as silicon dioxide or sodium silicoaluminate.

3. **Whole egg.** Whole eggs are handled in a manner similar to yolks and whites. However, carbohydrates such as sucrose or corn-syrup solids are added before drying to improve or maintain some of the functional qualities like flavor, foaming and emulsifying. Dried whole eggs may also be converted into a free-flowing product by adding anticaking agents.

Overall, the important functional properties of eggs—whipping, emulsifying, coagulation, flavor, and color—are maintained, or in some cases improved, through drying, providing there has been proper processing and storage. Moreover, the nutritional value of dehydrated eggs has been found to be essentially the same as fresh eggs.

Dehydrated egg products are employed in cake mixes, mayonnaise, salad dressings, noodles, candies and all types of baking products.

(Also see EGG[S].)

EGG FRUIT (CANISTEL) *Lucuma bifera; L. mervosa*

The yellow egg-shaped fruit of an evergreen tree (of the family *Sapotaceae*) that is native to northern South America. It is 2 to 4 in. *(5 to 10 cm)* long and has a yellow, mealy flesh. Egg fruit appears to have been a staple food of the ancient Peruvians since it has often been found at archaeological sites.

The fruit is moderately high in calories (140 kcal per 100 g) and carbohydrates (36%). It is a good source of iron and vitamin C.

EGGPLANT (AUBERGINE) *Solanum melongena*

This vegetable is known as eggplant because the fruit of many varieties resemble a large egg.

The eggplant, like chili peppers, the Irish potato, sweet peppers and the tomato, is a member of the nightshade family (*Solanaceae*).

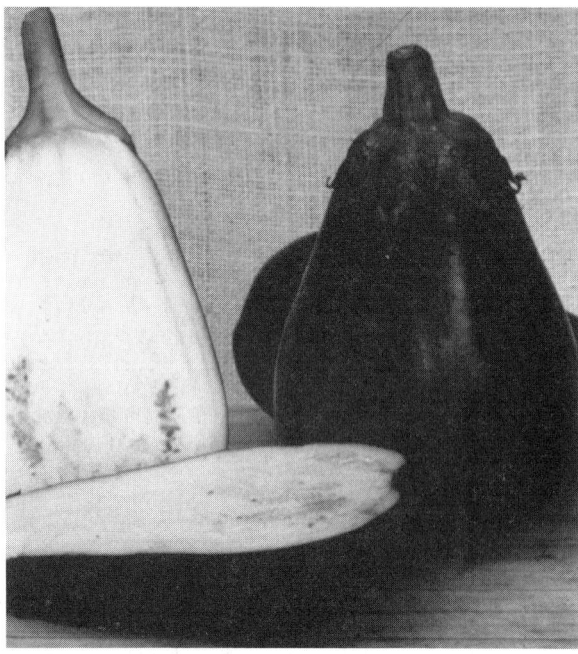

Fig. E-6. Eggplant. (Courtesy, USDA)

ORIGIN AND HISTORY. The eggplant is native to India and China. It was introduced to Europe by the Arabic traders.

WORLD AND U.S. PRODUCTION. The eggplant ranks twelfth among the leading vegetable crops of the world, with a worldwide production of about 5,761,000 metric tons annually. The leading eggplant-producing countries of the world, by rank, are: China, Turkey, Japan, Egypt, and Italy.[1]

The eggplant is not a major vegetable crop in the United States; only 25,695 metric tons were shipped by rail, truck, and air in 1990.[2]

PROCESSING. Most of the eggplant crop is sold on the fresh market. However, a small portion of the production is made into such items as canned eggplant cubes stewed into a tomato sauce, eggplant appetizer (cooked pieces of eggplant mixed with onions and other vegetables) which is sold in small glass jars, frozen eggplant parmigiana, and frozen fried eggplant slices.

SELECTION, PREPARATION, AND USES. A good quality eggplant is firm, heavy in relation to size, with a uniform dark rich purple color, and free from scars or cuts.

The greatest variety of eggplant dishes were developed in the countries of the Mediterranean region and western Asia where the climatic conditions favor the production of this vegetable.

In the United States, eggplant is commonly baked or fried (after dipping in batter). The vegetable may also be stuffed with various combinations of bread crumbs, ground meat, cheese, and/or vegetables before being baked. It is commonly used as a vegetable dish, entree, or ingredient of various mixed dishes.

NUTRITIONAL VALUE. The nutrient composition of cooked eggplant is given in Food Composition Table F-21.

Some noteworthy observations regarding the nutrient composition of eggplant follow:

1. Cooked eggplant is high in water content (94%), and low in calories (only 19 kcal per 100 g). However, it is a fair to good source of iron and potassium.

2. Eggplant has been used as a medicinal plant since ancient times because of the belief that it is effective in (a) stimulating the flow of bile, and (b) increasing urination to rid the body of excess water. (**NOTE:** This report is presented for two purposes: [1] informational, [2] stimulation of research.)

Eggplant contains small amounts of solanine. (See SOLANINE.)

EGG PROTEINS

Proteins comprise 11.8% of the chemical composition of eggs. This protein fraction of eggs is highly digestible and of high quality, having a biological value of 94 on a scale of 100, the highest rating of any food. The reason for this high quality of protein is that egg proteins are complete proteins. They contain all the essential amino acids required to maintain life and promote growth and health. In fact, the amino acid content of eggs is employed as a reference for evaluating the completeness of other proteins. Proteins of the egg white include ovalbumin, conalbumin, ovomucoid, globulins, ovomucin, flavoprotein, ovoglycoprotein, and avidin. The yolk contains the proteins phosvitin, a nonlipid phosphoprotein, and lipovitellins and low-density lipoproteins (LDL)—both lipid-protein complexes.

(Also see EGG[S]; PROTEIN[S]; and REFERENCE PROTEIN.)

---

[1]Based on data from *FAO Production Yearbook 1990*, FAO/UN, Rome, Italy, Vol. 44, p. 138, Table 56. **Note well:** Annual production fluctuates as a result of weather and profitability of the crop.

[2]Data from *Agricultural Statistics 1991*, USDA, p. 169, Table 244.

EGG WHITE

In the shell, the egg white or albumen surrounds the yellow yolk. It is comprised of four layers: (1) the outer thin or liquid white; (2) the dense or thick white; (3) the inner thin or liquid white; and (4) the inner thick white or chalaziferous layer. Water is the major constituent of egg white, amounting to about 88%. The proteins of egg white account for about 11% of the composition.

The unique foaming property of egg white is due to its proteins. When egg white is beaten, air bubbles are trapped in the albumen and a foam is formed—a gas phase dispersed in a liquid phase. This foaming power of the egg white—albumen—makes it useful as a carrier of air for leavening; hence, it contributes to the lightness of certain foods. For example, meringues, angel cakes, souffles, omelets, some candies, and sponge cakes all depend upon eggs for their lightness. Furthermore, these proteins of the white contribute to binding and thickening properties of eggs employed in a number of foods. As foods containing eggs cook, these proteins coagulate—a change in the stucture of egg protein that results in the loss of solubility and increased thickening. The coagulating property of eggs is important to custards and pie fillings.

Last but not least, the proteins of egg white contribute to the nutritional value of eggs.

Egg white is often used as an indicator of egg quality. It must be firm with a rather clear demarcation between the thin and thick albumen. Egg albumen quality is routinely measured in Haugh units—units determined by a micrometer that measures albumen height. This height is then compared to a chart listing the weights of eggs and Haugh units can then be derived. As eggs age, the firmness of the white decreases, and when broken, the contents spread and flatten. Also, the process of candling eggs determines the firmness of egg white—hence the quality of the egg. The pH (hydrogen concentration) of the egg white is another means whereby egg quality is determined. The pH of a freshly layed egg is about 7.62 to 8.2. As the egg ages, carbon dioxide is lost, and the pH increases to as high as 9.5.

(Also see EGG[S]; and EGG PROTEINS.)

EGG WHITE INJURY

A disorder which results from the binding of the vitamin biotin by a substance called avidin which is present in raw egg white. Egg white injury is characterized by shedding of flakes of skin, lack of appetite, loss of weight, and pains in the muscles. However, this disorder is rare in humans because (1) they do not normally eat sufficient amounts of raw egg white to bring about this condition; and (2) most people cook eggs before eating them.

(Also see BIOTIN.)

EKG

Abbreviation for electrocardiogram, because in German, cardiogram is spelled with a K.

(Also see ELECTROCARDIOGRAM.)

ELASTASE

An enzyme which digests the connective tissue protein-elastin.

(Also see ELASTIN.)

ELASTIN

A connective tissue protein which is present in ligaments,

lung tissue, and the walls of blood vessels. This protein is synthesized mainly during the years of rapid growth. It is rich in lysine, so the lysine needs of growing children are high compared to those of adults.

(Also see PROTEIN[S].)

ELECTROCARDIOGRAM

The tracing made by the heartbeat on an electrocardiograph used to determine abnormality in the heart muscle.

(Also see HEART DISEASE, section headed "Special Diagnostic Procedures For Cardiovascular Problems.")

ELECTROENCEPHALOGRAM

This printed record, which is sometimes called a brain wave pattern, shows the fluctuations of electrical charges in the brain. It is commonly used in the diagnosis of such disorders as brain tumors and epilepsy.

ELECTROLYTE

The name given to a substance which when dissolved in water enables the resulting solution to conduct an electric current. The most common electrolytes in the human body are salts of such minerals as sodium, potassium, magnesium, calcium, phosphate, sulfate, and chloride.

(Also see ACID-BASE BALANCE.)

ELECTRON

A negatively charged particle, which is responsible for the various chemical reactions that occur in matter.

ELECTRON MICROSCOPE

A powerful microscope which magnifies the object from 150,000 to 300,000 times, thereby permitting visualization of cellular structure.

ELECTRON TRANSPORT CHAIN

A connected series of chemical reactions which occur within the energy generating part (mitochondria) of cells. The electron transport chain provides the means by which the intermediate products of carbohydrate, fat, and protein metabolism are converted to carbon dioxide, water, and energy.

(Also see METABOLISM.)

ELECTROPURE PROCESS

A technique of pasteurizing milk utilizing a low frequency alternating current.

ELEMENTAL DIETS (SEMISYNTHETIC FIBER-FREE LIQUID DIETS)

These dietary preparations are free of fiber and other undigestible substances, but contain most of the essential nutrients in forms that require little or no digestion and which may be absorbed completely. Hence, little or no residue from the diet reaches the large intestine. The term *elemental* means that the nutrients are present in their most *elemental* or simple chemical forms, although the diets sometimes contain complex forms of certain nutrients. Similarly, the term *semisynthetic* means that the products contain mainly pure chemical compounds rather than the more complex natural food materials. It is noteworthy that the recent development of elemental diets has made it possible to provide much more nutritious diets for people who cannot tolerate normal diets, but can utilize these preparations.

INDICATIONS FOR THE USE OF ELEMENTAL DIETS.

These products are therapeutic preparations which are employed for the treatment of patients with conditions that make feeding with ordinary types of foods unadvisable. Furthermore, they are much more expensive than other dietary formulas. Hence, the decision to give a patient an elemental diet should be made only by a doctor, although an experienced dietitian can usually provide considerable guidance in the selection of the appropriate product.

Generally, elemental diets are indicated when oral feeding is permitted, but it is necessary to have maximal ease of digestion and absorption and only minimal passage of undigestible matter into the large intestine. These requirements are most commonly associated with the following circumstances:

1. Preparation of the bowel for surgery or a barium enema.

2. After surgery on the digestive tract, as an adjunct to or substitute for, intravenous feedings until normal foods or formulas can be consumed.

3. Rehabilitation of severely malnourished patients who cannot tolerate a normal diet.

4. Treatment of certain types of diarrheal diseases. (A product with a low osmolality would be most suitable for these cases.)

5. Nourishment of burn victims who have high metabolic needs. (In these cases, high-nitrogen [or high protein] products should be used.)

6. Tube feedings. It is noteworthy that elemental dietary preparations are less viscous and require smaller bore tubing than ordinary tube feeding preparations because the danger of clogging the tubing is reduced greatly by the low viscosity and the absence of substances that may come out of solution.

7. Inflammation and/or bacterial infection of the bowel resulting from chemotherapy, radiation treatments, or other factors.

8. Fistulae of the digestive tract, which heal more rapidly when the dietary bulk and stimulation of peristalsis are minimal.

9. Pancreatitis, because pancreatic secretions are reduced greatly on these diets.

However, the consumption of an elemental diet may result in certain noteworthy changes in normal physiological functions.

CONTRAINDICATIONS.

Elemental diets should *not* be given to infants under 3 months of age, and older infants should be given *only* diluted diets. The diets are unsuitable also when patients have diseases of the kidneys and the liver in which the metabolism and excretion of nutrients is impaired. Furthermore, they should not be given to people with intestinal stasis of various types, and they should be used with great caution in cases of insulin-dependent diabetes. Finally, it may be preferable to use intravenous hyperalimentation when a jejunal fistula is present.

(Also see HYPERALIMENTATION, INTRAVENOUS.)

PREPARATION AND ADMINISTRATION.

A key to successful use of elemental diets is their gradual introduction to permit patients to become accustomed to their flavors and any feelings of fullness or discomfort that may occur. It is noteworthy that elemental diets may be fed via the normal oral route or through a tube introduced into the digestive tract. (**NOTE:** Elemental diets are *never* used for intravenous feedings.)

Normal Feeding.

Most manufacturers recommend that their formulas be fed only at one-half strength the first day and that the full day's allotment not be fed until several days have passed. Also, many preparations are more palatable if they are served chilled. (Pure amino acids have peculiar and somewhat nauseating tastes that are accentuated in warm solutions.) Usually, individual feedings are packaged in separate packets that contain from 2 to 3 oz (56 to 85 g) of powder to be mixed with 8 to 10 fluid ounces (240 to 300 ml) of water. However, an entire day's supply may be mixed at one time and kept refrigerated until used. These nutrient solutions are ideal culture mediums for microorganisms. Hence, the prepared diets should not be kept at room temperature or stored in a refrigerator for longer than a day. For variety, the diets may be served as broths, frozen slushes, or puddings. Each manufacturer provides instructions for using his particular products.

Tube Feeding.

Although problems of palatability are overcome by tube feeding, the effects of the high solute concentration (hyperosmolality) will be similar to those encountered in normal oral feeding. Hence, the solution should be only one-half strength when fed initially, and the rate of feeding by gravity drip or pumping should be limited to 1 to 2 oz (40 to 60 ml) per hour. Furthermore, not more than 1 to 2 pt (500 to 1,000 ml) should be kept in the reservoir at one time and the solution should be kept chilled. Finally, the external tubing and fluid reservoir should be changed daily to prevent microbial contamination.

(Also see LIQUID DIETS.)

SUMMARY.

Elemental diets are a recent development in dietetics and medicine that can be lifesaving when used properly. As in the case of other therapies which may alter the normal physiology of the body, patients given these diets should be monitored carefully for signs and symptoms of abnormalities. It is noteworthy that patients have done well when given elemental diets as the sole source of nutrients for as long as 1 year.

(Also see MODIFIED DIETS; and LIQUID DIETS.)

EMACIATED

An excessively thin condition of the body.

(Also see MARASMUS; STARVATION; and UNDERWEIGHT.)

EMBDEN-MEYERHOF PATHWAY

The initial stage of metabolism by which carbohydrates are partially converted into energy by living cells. The Embden-Meyerhof Pathway is the part of energy metabolism which takes place without the presence of oxygen. However, only a limited amount of energy may be produced in this pathway. Therefore, it is necessary for the products of this pathway to enter into oxygen-requiring metabolism (respiration) which takes place in the electron transport chain.

(Also see METABOLISM.)

EMBLIC (INDIAN GOOSEBERRY; MALACCA TREE) *Emblica officinalis*

The fruit of a large tree (of the family *Euphorbiaceae*) that is native to southeastern Asia. Its yellowish fruits are 1 to

2 in. (2.5 to 5 cm) in diameter and are very sour. They are consumed raw or preserved, and are sometimes used in baked goods. The emblic tree was recently introduced into Florida as a potential source of tannin.

Emblic fruit is moderately high in calories (81 kcal per 100 g) and carbohydrates (22%). It is very rich in vitamin C and is a good source of fiber.

EMBOLISM

A clogging of a blood vessel by materials such as air, blood clots, cellular debris, fat, or microorganisms.

EMBRYO

The earliest stage of development in which a newly formed animal or plant is recognizable. The term embryo usually designates an organism which arises from sexual reproduction.

EMETIC

Any substance which is given by mouth to induce vomiting.

–EMIA

Suffix that denotes a condition of the blood; for example, leukemia.

EMPHYSEMA

A lung disease which is characterized by a stretching and/or rupture of some of the air cells (alveoli) of the lungs. Emphysema greatly limits the amount of exercise the afflicted person may take without having difficulty in breathing. Also severe, chronic emphysema can lead to heart failure because of the extra work required to pump blood through diseased lungs. Some of the factors which may bring on or aggravate emphysema are (1) air pollution, (2) allergies such as hay fever, (3) cigarette smoking, and (4) infectious respiratory diseases. It is not certain regarding the role that nutrition might play in the prevention of emphysema, although recent research has shown that vitamins A and E apparently protect lung tissue against damage from airborne pollutants.

EMPTY CALORIES

The designation given to foods which supply mainly calories. These foods are usually rich in carbohydrates and/or fats, but contain low levels of proteins, minerals, and vitamins. Some examples of such foods are the various candies and carbonated beverages.

(Also see BREAKFAST CEREALS, section headed "The Sugar-Breakfast-Cereal Binge.")

EMULSIFY

To disperse small drops of one liquid into another liquid, e.g., mayonnaise and hollandaise sauce.

(Also see EMULSIFYING AGENTS.)

EMULSIFYING AGENTS

Food additives, some natural and some synthetic, used in a wide variety of food products to create emulsions. Glycerol monostearate, mono- and diglycerides, gums, egg yolk, albumen, alginate, lecithin, and carrageenan (Irish moss) are all examples of common emulsifying agents. Advantages of these agents are: (1) maintenance of homo-geneity; (2) more economical use of fats; (3) improved volume uniformity; (4) improved whipping properties; and (5) improved keeping qualities. Emulsifiers are used in such foods as baked goods, cake mixes, confectionery products, frozen desserts, ice cream, margarine, salad dressings, etc. In many foods the emulsifier and the stabilizer are inseparable. By law, these agents must be listed on the package or label.

(Also see CARRAGEENAN; EMULSION; ADDITIVES; and STABILIZER.)

EMULSIFYING SALTS

Food additives, commonly the sodium salts of citrate, phosphate, and tartrate, used as emulsifiers in the manufacture of cheese and evaporated and powdered milk. These salts may also serve as sequestering agents (substances that combine with a metal ion or acid radicle and render it inactive) in some foods.

(Also see EMULSION; ETHYLENEDIAMINE TETRA-ACETIC ACID; and ADDITIVES.)

EMULSION

An intimate mixture of two liquids; for example, oil and water, which do not normally stay mixed unless constantly stirred. With the addition of an emulsifying agent, one liquid becomes suspended in the other as fine droplets. Foods such as shortenings, margarines and mayonnaise are emulsions.

(Also see EMULSIFYING AGENTS; EMULSIFYING SALTS; and STABILIZER.)

ENAMEL

The hard, mineralized material that covers the tooth.
(Also see DENTAL HEALTH, NUTRITION AND DIET.)

ENCEPHALOMALACIA

A term which means softening of the brain. Generally, this condition is seen more in livestock than in man. However, there have been a few reports of encephalomalacia in infants fed vitamin E-deficient diets and large quantities of vegetable oils.

(Also see VITAMIN E.)

ENCEPHALOPATHY

Any degenerative disease of the brain.

ENDEMIC

A term referring to a disease that is continually present in a given population. It is in contrast to the word epidemic which refers to the type of disease that suddenly appears in a given area. Certain types of nutritional deficiencies, such as goiter, are endemic in the regions which lack particular nutrients in the soil or water.

ENDERGONIC

Chemical reactions occurring in living cells that require an input of energy; for example, the synthesis of protein.
(Also see EXERGONIC; and METABOLISM.)

ENDO–

Prefix meaning inner or within.

ENDOCRINE

Pertaining to glands that produce secretions that pass

directly into the blood or lymph instead of into a duct (secreting internally). Hormones are secreted by endocrine glands.

(Also see ENDOCRINE GLANDS.)

ENDOCRINE GLANDS

Ductless glands that secrete hormones (chemical messengers) directly into the bloodstream. These hormones then travel via the blood to various organs and tissues where they exert necessary, and sometimes profound, control over such bodily functions as skeletal and sexual development, growth, metabolism, mineral and water balance, and reproduction. Fig. E-7 indicates the location and names of the major endocrine glands, and Table E-8 outlines the origin, names, actions, and associated diseases of the various major hormones.

Secretion of the hormones should never be viewed as a single event, but as a concert. As one hormone comes into play, another may fade out; or one hormone may cause the secretion of another, or the action of one may complement the action of another. Furthermore, the brain or nervous system in many cases acts as the conductor by signaling the proper time for increased or decreased secretion of a hormone.

NOTE WELL: Hormone therapy for whatever reason, and whether oral or by injection, should always be under the direction of a physician.

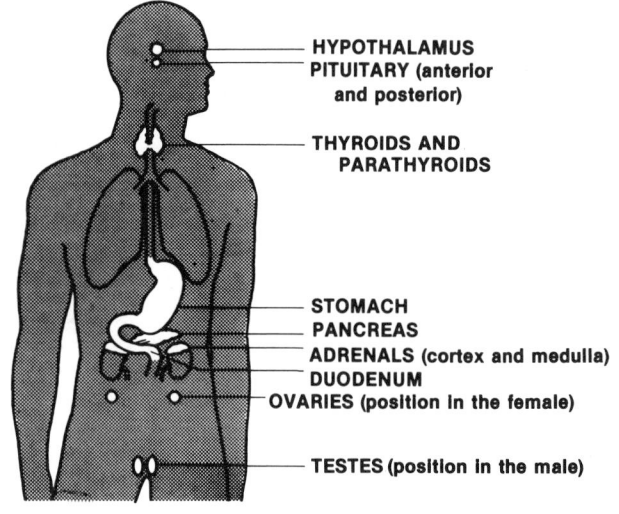

Fig. E-7. The approximate location of the major endocrine glands.

TABLE E-8
HORMONES OF THE ENDOCRINE GLANDS[1]

Hormone	Origin	Mechanism of Release	Physiological Functions	Associated Diseases	Comments
Corticotropin releasing hormone (CRH)	Hypothalamus	The hypothalamic hormones, sometimes called the neurohormones, provide the link between the nervous system and the endocrine system. Thus, such things as stress, nutritional status, emotions, nursing, time of day, season of the year, etc. may manifest themselves as disruptions in bodily function. The hypothalamus acts like a *switchboard* by *plugging in* the proper neurohormone in response to a variety of nervous stimuli received by the brain. Also, other hormones act on the hypothalamus to alter the release of the neurohormone—feedback control.	Releases adrenocorticotropin (ACTH) from the pituitary.	Tumors in the hypothalamus may alter the secretion of any or all of the hypothalamic hormones, then ultimately affect the pituitary, thyroid, adrenals, ovaries, and testes.	So far only GHRIH, TRH, and LRH have been isolated and their chemical nature determined. The presence of other hypothalamic hormones is only suggested by experimental evidence. Much research remains to be done on the hormones of the hypothalamus. Sometimes FRH and LRH are considered one releasing hormone called gonadotropin releasing hormone (GnRH) which controls both LH and FSH. Presently, LRH (GnRH), TRH, and GHRIH are commercially available. LRH (GnRH) offers new hope as a means of fertility control in humans.
Follicle stimulating hormone, releasing hormone (FSHRH or FRH)	Hypothalamus		Releases follicle stimulating hormone from the anterior pituitary.		
Growth hormone, releasing hormone (GHRH; somatotropin releasing hormone, SRH)	Hypothalamus		Releases growth hormone (GH) from the anterior pituitary.		
Growth hormone, release-inhibiting hormone (GHRIH; somatosstatin; somatotrophic release-inhibiting hormone, SRIH)	Hypothalamus		Prevents the release of growth hormone (GH) from the anterior pituitary.		
Luteinizing hormone, releasing hormone (LRH)	Hypothalamus		Releases luteinizing hormone (LH) from the anterior pituitary.		
Prolactin releasing hormone (PRH)	Hypothalamus		Releases prolactin from the anterior pituitary.		
Prolactin release-inhibiting hormone (PRIH or PIH)	Hypothalamus		Prevents prolactin release from the anterior pituitary.		
Thyrotropin releasing hormone (TRH)	Hypothalamus		Releases thyroid stimulating hormone (TSH) from the anterior pituitary.		
Adrenocorticotropic hormone (ACTH)	Anterior pituitary[2]	Corticotropin releasing hormone from the hypothalamus.	Synthesis and release of hormones from the adrenal cortex, mainly the glucocorticoids. ACTH acts directly on fat tissue to liberate free fatty acids into the blood.	Cushing's syndrome; Addison's disease.	ACTH exercises little, if any, control over aldosterone secretion. The effects of stress mediated through the hypothalamus cause increased release. (Also see STRESS.)
Follicle stimulating hormone (FSH)	Anterior pituitary	Follicle stimulating releasing hormone from the hypothalamus.	Stimulation of follicle growth and estrogen secretion in the female; sperm production in the male.	Impaired sexual development or function.	In the female, levels of FSH in the blood rise and fall with each menstrual cycle.

Footnotes at end of table

(Continued)

TABLE E-8 *(Continued)*

Hormone	Origin	Mechanism of Release	Physiological Functions	Associated Diseases	Comments
Growth hormone (GH; somatotropin, STH)	Anterior pituitary	Growth hormone releasing hormone and inhibition of growth hormone release-inhibiting hormone from the hypothalamus.	Growth of all tissues; protein synthesis; mobilization of fats for energy while conserving glucose.	Dwarfism; gigantism; acromegaly.	Over secretion of GH in an adult causes acromegaly—excessive growth of the lower jaw, feet, and hands.
Luteinizing hormone (LH)	Anterior pituitary	Luteinizing hormone releasing hormone from the hypothalamus.	Ovarian follicle rupture and egg release, and progesterone secretion in the female; testosterone secretion and sperm production in the male.	Impaired sexual development or function.	In the male this hormone is called interstitial cell stimulating hormone (ICSH). Together with FSH in the female it acts to control events of the menstrual cycle.
Oxytocin	Posterior pituitary[2]	Stimulation of the breasts, genitals, and uterus.	Milk *let down*, uterine contractions aiding birth process and possibly sperm transport at the time of mating.		There are no known functions in the male. See comment for vasopressin. (Also see BREAST FEEDING.)
Prolactin	Anterior pituitary	Prolactin releasing hormone and inhibition of prolactin release-inhibiting hormone from the hypothalamus.	Formation of milk by the mammary glands by stimulating breast growth and secretory activity.		A variety of nervous stimuli can cause the release of prolactin, but the reason for this is not clear. (Also see BREAST FEEDING.)
Thyroid stimulating hormone (TSH; thyrotropin)	Anterior pituitary	Thyrotropin releasing hormone from the hypothalamus.	Manufacture and release of thyroxin and triiodothyronine from the thyroid gland.	Myxedema; hypothyroidism; goiter.	When the pituitary fails to secrete TSH, the thyroid gland becomes completely nonfunctional.
Vasopressin (antidiuretic hormone; ADH)	Posterior pituitary	Stimulation of special nerves in the hypothalamus which detect the concentration of the body fluids.	Acts on the kidneys to reduce urine volume and conserve body water thus preventing body fluids from becoming too concentrated.	Diabetes insipidus.	Actually, oxytocin and vasopressin originate in the hypothalamus, then they are stored in the posterior pituitary. (Also see WATER BALANCE.)
Calcitonin (thyrocalcitonin)	Thyroid	High calcium level in the blood.	Decreases the level of calcium in the blood by reducing release of calcium from the bones; increases the excretion of calcium in the urine and deposition of calcium in the bones.	Hypocalcemia (low blood calcium).	Some calcitonin may come from the thymus gland. In the thyroid it actually comes from the C-cells. (Also see CALCIUM.)
Parathyroid hormone (PTH; parathormone)	Parathyroid glands	Low calcium level in the blood.	Elevates blood calcium by increasing the rate of calcium absorption from the kidney and intestine and activating vitamin D; stimulating calcium release from the bones.	Parathyroid tetany (hypoparathyroidism); hyperparathyroidism (osteitis fibrosa cystica).	Hyperfunction of the parathyroid glands results in brittle bones. (Also see CALCIUM.)
Triiodothyronine (T_3)	Thyroid	Release of thyroid stimulating hormone (thyrotropin) from the anterior pituitary.	Both hormones have similar actions, however, triiodothyronine is more potent, and its actions are noted faster. Steps up metabolic rate; increases heart performance; increases nervous system activity; stimulates protein synthesis; increases motility and secretion of gastrointestinal tract.	Hypothyroidism (Myxedema or cretinism). Hyperthyroidism (exophthalmos or Graves' disease); goiter.	Thyroxin has 1 more iodine atom than triiodothyronine, otherwise they are the same. Many tissues possess an enzyme capable of removing an iodine from thyroxin thus providing a source of T_3 other than the thyroid. Increased blood levels during cold-adaptation. Decreased blood levels during starvation. (Also see METABOLISM.)
Thyroxin (T_4)	Thyroid				
Gastrin	Antral portion of gastric mucosa; pancreatic islets.	Distension of stomach; presence of proteins and polypeptides; alcohol; stimulation of vegas nerve.	Stimulates gastric acid (HCl) and pepsin secretion; stimulates gastric motility.	The Zollinger-Ellison syndrome is caused by a gastrin secreting tumor. However, for the most part it is not known what role the hormones of the digestion system play in digestive diseases.	The isolation and chemical nature of enterocrinin, glucagonlike immunoreactive factor and villikinin have not been determined. Cholecystokinin-pancreozymin is sometimes referred to as just cholicystokinin or pancreozymin. Injections of cholecystokinin may provide a means of treating obesity. (Also see DIGESTION AND ABSORPTION; and ZOLLINGER-ELLISON SYNDROME.)
Cholecystokinin-pancreozymin	Duodenum	Presence of fats and products of protein digestion.	Contraction of gallbladder and secretion of pancreatic enzymes.		
Enterocrinin	Duodenum	Presence of chyme.	Increases secretion of intestinal fluids.		
Enterogastrone	Duodenum	Presence of fats.	Inhibits gastric acid secretion and motility.		
Glucagonlike immunoreactive factor (GLI)	Wall of small intestine.		Stimulates insulin secretion.		

Footnotes at end of table

(Continued)

TABLE E-8 *(Continued)*

Hormone	Origin	Mechanism of Release	Physiological Functions	Associated Diseases	Comments
Secretin	Duodenum	Presence of acid and protein.	Stimulates secretion of aqueous pancreatic fluid (high in bicarbonate).		
Villikinin	Duodenum	Presence of chyme.	Stimulates alternating contractions and extensions of the villi, which stirs and mixes the chyme and exposes additional material for absorption.		
Glucagon	Pancreas (alpha cells of islets of Langerhans)	Low blood glucose (sugar) level.	Mobilizes glucose from liver glycogen; increases the formation of glucose from proteins—gluconeogenesis.		The important role of glucagon is to keep glucose high enough to prevent hypoglycemic convulsions or coma. (Also see DIABETES MELLITUS; and HYPOGLYCEMIA.)
Insulin	Pancreas (beta cells of islets of Langerhans)	High blood glucose (sugar) level.	Causes transport of glucose from the blood into the cells, and increases protein synthesis in cells.	Diabetes mellitus; hypoglycemia.	In the absence of insulin, blood glucose reaches dangerously high levels. (Also see DIABETES MELLITUS; and HYPOGLYCEMIA.)
Aldosterone (mineralocorticoid)	Adrenal gland (cortex)	Increased potassium concentration in the blood and blood flow through the kidneys; decreased sodium intake; decreased extracellular fluid volume.	Stimulates kidneys to excrete potassium into the urine, and to conserve sodium.	Conn's syndrome, or primary aldosteronism.	Aldosterone accounts for 95% of the mineralocorticoid activity. Renin release from the kidney controls its secretion. (Also see WATER AND ELECTROLYTES.)
Cortisone, corticosterone, and cortisol (glucocorticoids)	Adrenal gland (cortex)	Adrenocorticotropic hormone (ACTH) from the anterior pituitary.	Causes glucose production from protein and fats; makes amino acids available for use wherever needed; stimulates protein synthesis in the liver; mobilizes fats for energy; prevents self-destruction of cells.	Androgenital syndrome; Cushing's syndrome; Addison's Disease.	Necessary for individuals to combat stress; exposure to stress results in increased release of ACTH from the pituitary. The effects of stress are mediated through the hypothalamus. (Also see INBORN ERRORS OF METABOLISM; and STRESS.)
Epinephrine (adrenaline), Norepinephrine (noradrenaline), or Catecholamines	Adrenal gland (medulla)	A variety of nervous stimuli such as surprise, fright, shock, etc.	Both hormones alter heart output, dilate or constrict blood vessels, elevate blood pressure, release free fatty acids into the blood, stimulate the brain, increase heat production, and release glucose from the liver.	Hypertension (high blood pressure).	Epinephrine prevents the action of oxytocin. In the human, 80% of the secretion from the adrenal medulla is epinephrine. Thyroid hormones are required for action of catecholamines. (Also see HIGH BLOOD PRESSURE.)
Estrogens	Ovary	Follicle stimulating hormone from the anterior pituitary.	Deposition of protein and fat for the development and maintenance of feminine charateristics and sex organs; involved in monthly uterine changes.	Female hypogonadism; menopause.	There are actually 3 estrogens: estradiol, estriol, and estrone, and levels rise and fall with each menstrual cycle.
Progesterone	Ovary (corpus luteum)	Luteinizing hormone from the anterior pituitary.	Increases secretory activity in the glands of the breasts and uterus; maintains pregnancy by preventing the uterus from contracting.		During pregnancy, progesterone also comes from the placenta. Progesterone levels also reach high and low levels during the menstrual cycle.
Relaxin	Ovary (corpus luteum)	Associated with the advanced stages of pregnancy.	Believed to be involved in softening of the cervix and relaxation of the pubic ligament.		Sometimes found in the placenta, but its exact role is still quite unclear.
Testosterone (androgen)	Testes (interstitial cells)	Luteinizing hormone from the anterior pituitary, but called interstitial cell stimulating hormone (ICSH) in the male.	Necessary for sperm production; develops and maintains the male sex organs and masculine characteristics; increases the deposition of protein in the muscles.	Male hypogonadism.	Cholesterol is the chemical ancestor of testosterone, progesterone, and estrogens. Removal of the testes, castration, results in an individual with rather feminine appearance. For centuries, adolescent boys were castrated to work in harems, and choir boys were castrated to preserve their soprano voices. Anabolic steroids used by athletes are derivatives of testosterone.

[1]Kidneys, pineal gland, and thymus may also be considered by some as endocrine glands, and during pregnancy, the placenta has some endocrine functions.

[2]The anterior pituitary is also called the adenohypophysis, while the posterior pituitary may be called the neurohypophysis.

ENDOCRINOLOGY

The study of the ductless glands and the effects of their secretion on the various tissues of the body.
(Also see ENDOCRINE GLANDS.)

ENDOGENOUS

Originating within the body, e.g., hormones and enzymes.

ENDOPEPTIDASE

An enzyme which splits the central portions of protein molecules.

ENDOPLASMIC RETICULUM

The more or less continuous network of small channels present in the cytoplasm of nearly all cells which transport nutrients and their breakdown products (metabolites) throughout the cytoplasm.

ENDOSPERM

The starchy part of the seed which surrounds the embryo or germ. When a seed sprouts, enzymes that develop in the seed break the starch down to sugar which may be used by the embryonic plant. It is noteworthy that man has domesticated plants with seeds that have large, starchy endosperms.

ENDOSPERM OIL

Oil obtained from the endosperm of the seed.

ENDOTOXIN

A poison (toxin) that remains inside the microorganism which produced it. The toxicity is noted only when the bacterial cells are ruptured by mechanical or chemical means. *Escherichia coli, Salmonella typhi* and *Shigella dysenteriae* bacteria are known to form endotoxins.
(Also see BACTERIA IN FOOD; and DISEASES.)

ENEMA

The injection of a liquid into the intestines by way of the anus.

ENERGY BALANCE (EB)

Energy balance is the difference between the gross energy intake and the energy output. Fattening results when the intake exceeds the output, while a loss of body fat, and usually a loss of body weight, follows a dietary deficit of energy.
(Also see CALORIC EXPENDITURE.)

ENERGY REQUIRED FOR FOOD PRODUCTION

When considering the energy required to produce food products, it is insufficient to focus entirely on energy use on the farm.

There are two other important steps in the food line as it moves from the producer to the consumer; namely, processing and marketing, both of which require higher energy inputs than to produce the food on the farm (see Table E-9.)

TABLE E-9
MODERN FOOD PRODUCTION
IS INEFFICIENT IN ENERGY UTILIZATION—
THE STORY FROM PRODUCER TO CONSUMER[1]

Year	On the Farm	Food Processing	Marketing and Home Cooking	Total/ Person/ Year
1940[2]				
Million kcal	0.9	2.2	2.1	5.2
Percent	18.0	42.0	40.0	100.0
1990[3]				
Million kcal	2.8	5.7	4.6	13.1[4]
Percent	21.4	43.5	35.1	100.0
Increase, times, 1940–1990	3.1	2.6	2.2	2.5

[1]Energy in million kcal used per capita to produce one million kcal of food in the United States.
[2]Values from Borgstrom, G., "The Price of a Tractor," Ceres, FAO of the U.N., Rome, Italy, Nov.-Dec., 1974, p. 18, Table 3.
[3]Authors' estimate based on several reports detailing trends in energy usage.
[4]This means that in 1990, it required 13.1 million kcal to produce 1 million kcal of food for each person, a daily consumption of 2,740 kcal (1,000,000 ÷ 365 = 2,740).

Table E-9 points up the increasing drain that modern food production is putting on the energy supply. In 1990, U.S. farms put in 2.8 calories of fuel per calorie of food grown, 3.1 times more than the on-farm energy input in 1940.

Table E-9 also shows that, in the United States in 1990, a total of 13.1 calories were used in the production, food processing, and marketing-cooking for every calorie of food consumed, with a percentage distribution of the total cost of energy at each step from producer to consumer as follows: on the farm, 21.4%; food processing, 43.5%; and marketing and home cooking, 35.1%. In 1940, it took only 5.2 calories—about 40% of the 1990 figure—to get 1 calorie of food on the table. It is noteworthy, too, that more energy is required for food processing and marketing-home cooking than for growing the product; and that, from 1940 to 1990, the on-the-farm energy requirement increased by 3.1 times, in comparison with an increase of 2.6 and 2.2 times for each of the other steps—processing and marketing-home cooking.

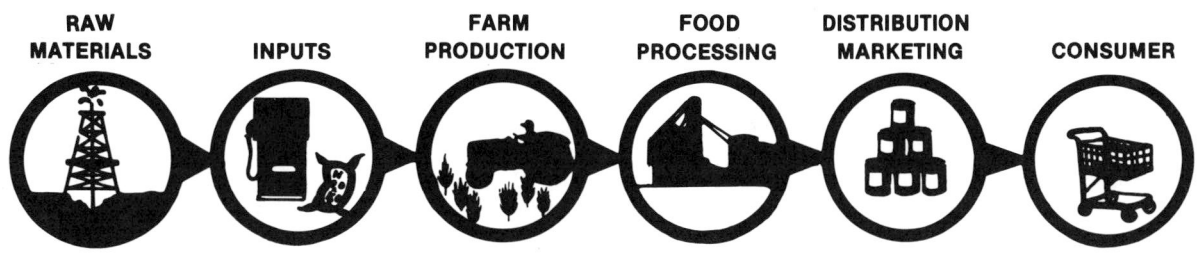

Fig. E-8. Energy use in the food system.

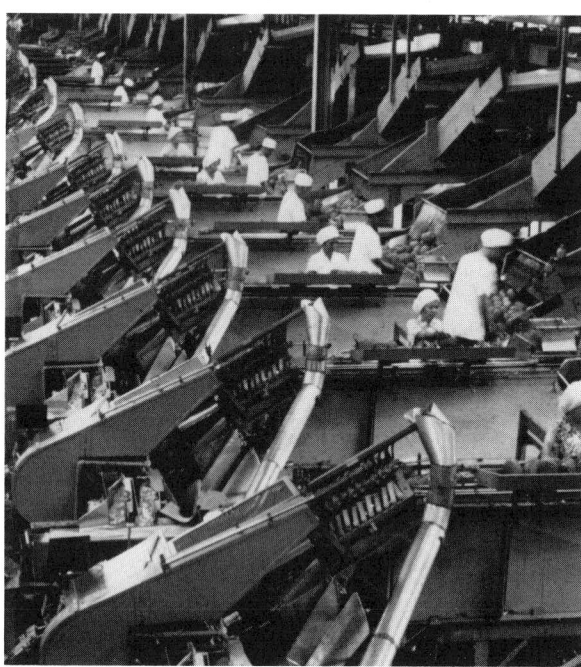

Fig. E-9. Processing foods requires much energy. This shows a battery of machines processing pineapples. The machines cut away the outer shell, remove the fibrous inner core, and produce a perfect hollowed cylinder of fruit. (Courtesy, Castle and Cooke, Inc.)

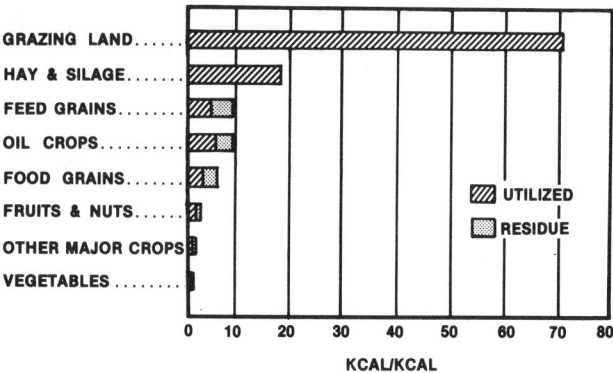

Fig. E-10. Energy output per unit of cultural energy input (kcal/kcal) for production of food, feed, and fiber crops. (Adapted by the authors from *American Society of Agricultural Engineers*, St. Joseph, Mich., paper No. 75-7505, p. 10, Fig. t, prepared by Nelson, L. F., W. C. Burrows, and F. C. Stickler, Deere & Company, Moline, Ill.)

Prior to the advent of machines and fuel in crop production, 1 calorie of energy input on the farm produced about 16 calories of food energy. Today, on the average, U.S. farms put in about 2.8 calories of fuel per calorie of food grown; hence, to produce a daily intake of 3,000 calories of edible food from cultivated crops may require 8,400 calories of energy from fossil fuels—an exhaustible source. It is more surprising yet—and thought-provoking—to know that, even today in the poorer or developing countries, it takes only 1 calorie to produce each 10 calories of food consumed. The Oriental wet rice peasant uses only 1 unit of energy to produce 50 units of food energy. This gives the Orientals a favorable position among the major powers as the energy crisis worsens.

The following additional points are pertinent to the future of the energy required for food production.

1. **Photosynthesis fixes energy.** Photosynthesis is by far the most important energy-producing process. But currently only about 1% of the solar energy falling on an area is fixed by photosynthesis; and only 5% of this captured energy is fixed in a form suitable as food for man. Thus, (a) man's manipulation of plants for increased efficiency of solar energy conversion, and (b) converting a greater percentage of total energy fixed as chemical energy in plants (the other 95%) into a form available to man would appear to hold great promise in solving the future food problems of the world.

Crops vary in their return of captured solar energy per unit of cultural energy input. Fig. E-10 shows that grazing land is highly efficient in the capture of solar energy—requiring little input of energy for a high return. Hay and silage rank second in energy return, followed by feed grains and oil crops. For the most part, these efficient capturers of solar energy are not captured in a form available to man.

2. **Animals step up energy.** Grazing land and hay-silage far outrank the other crops in efficiency of capturing solar energy (see Fig. E-10). It follows that ruminants—cattle, sheep, and goats—which utilize grazing land, hay, and silage (feeds not suitable for human consumption), offer the best means of stepping up and storing energy for man. Petroleum is not required to produce beef, mutton, and wool. Also, dairy cattle are extremely efficient converters of energy to food (milk). Thus, ruminants represent a renewable resource, whereas it takes thousands of years to create coal, oil, and natural gas—longer than any of us can wait. Also, animals perpetuate themselves through their offspring. The 887 million acres (*359 million ha*) of pasture and grazing land of continental United States, as well as the vast acreages of grass and browse throughout the world, are converters of solar energy par excellence. Despite energy shortages, there will always be grazing land and ruminants.

3. **Crop residues contain energy.** Crop residues left in the field, above or below the ground surface, may well constitute four to five times more energy than is harvested. Increasingly, this potential source of added feed and organic fertilizer will be utilized in the future.

4. **Other factors.** Other factors that should be considered to meet the future energy needs are the conservation of energy, elimination of food waste, and the development of other energy sources.

Increasing consideration will be given to the conservation of our fossil energy bank account. Farmers will conserve energy by using minimum tillage techniques, and by switching to fuel-conserving diesel tractors which use approximately 73% as much fuel as gasoline tractors in performing the same work. Also, up to a point, big farms utilize energy more efficiently than little farms. Hence, energy shortages favor the trend to bigness.

Food waste caused by a variety of pests such as plant disease, insects, weeds, rats, and birds represent an estimated 30% annual loss in worldwide food production. By eliminating these wastes, the world food supply can be increased by nearly one-third.

Among the energy sources which could be developed, the most abundant and basic source is the sun. Photosynthesis is by far the *most* important energy-producing process, yet only a small fraction of solar energy is fixed in a form available to man. It should, therefore, be possible to increase the effectiveness of this process. To do this, three approaches are suggested: (a) increasing the amount of photosynthesis on earth, (b) manipulating plants for increased efficiency of solar energy conversion, and (c) converting a greater percentage of the total energy fixed as chemical energy in plants to a form available to man. As already indicated, ruminants provide a solution to the latter approach. In addition to the above, the oceans, which cover more than two-thirds of the earth's surface, receive a proportionate amount of all the solar energy, and their potential to provide food could be dramatically increased by learning to farm them. Also, the wind is being harnessed to supply electricity.

(Also see ENERGY UTILIZATION BY THE BODY; PHOTOSYNTHESIS; and WORLD FOOD.)

ENERGY UTILIZATION BY THE BODY

Contents | Page

One of the major reasons why people around the world strive to obtain food, clothing, shelter, and fuel is that each of these items plays an important role in the body's utilization of energy, which sustains life and human activities.

Energy is defined as the ability to do work. Work is generally thought of as the application of a force in order to produce the motion of one or more masses or energy waves against an opposing force or a natural tendency. For example, the throwing of a ball into the air requires work to overcome the effect of gravity. The maintenance of a body at a temperature higher than that of its surroundings also requires work (an input of heat energy) to replace the heat that flows out of the object into the surroundings.

MAJOR FORMS OF ENERGY.
The various forms of energy are interconvertible. Therefore, it is noteworthy that the Law of Conservation of Energy is that energy can neither be created nor destroyed. This statement must be modified to include "energy and its equivalent in matter," since nuclear reactions involve the interconversion of energy and matter. Furthermore, heat energy can never be totally converted into other forms of energy, but the other forms are totally convertible into heat. The reason for this limitation is that every type of work that is done is accompanied by the release of some heat.

Food energy, which is the chemical energy present in nutrients, is by far the major source of the energy that is utilized by the human body. Nevertheless, few people base their lives on this form of energy alone. Furthermore, the utilization of other forms of energy—chemicals, electrical, heat, light, mechanical, nuclear, and solar—reduces the need for food energy, which is fortunate because there are certain circumstances that would otherwise require the consumption of enormous amounts of food.

THE BIOLOGICAL ENERGY CHAIN.
The rapid rise in energy costs which occurred in the 1970s and early 1980s led to studies of the energy used for food production. Some analysts of this situation have made oversimplified generalizations regarding the overall merits of plants vs animals as foods, without sufficient consideration of (1) the types of foods which best meet the energy needs of people

at various stages of life and in a variety of circumstances, and (2) some of the potentially useful products and by-products of food production. Hence, an overview of biological energy utilization is presented in Fig. E-11.

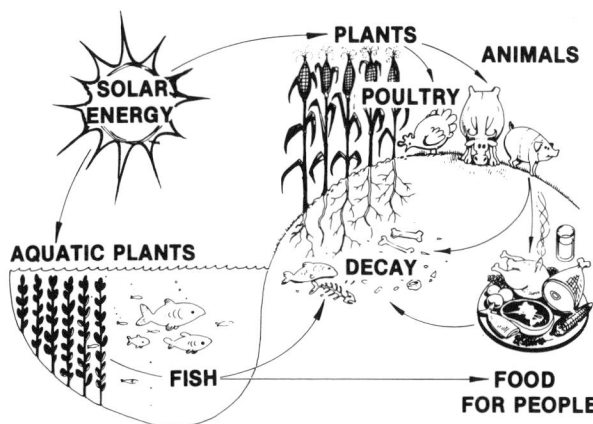

Fig. E-11. The biological energy chain by which energy from the sun is converted into food energy for people.

Details of the various links in the biological energy chain follow:

• **Solar energy**—Although less than 1% of the sun's energy which reaches the earth is converted to chemical energy by photosynthesis in plants, a much larger amount of this energy heats up the atmosphere so that plants, animals, and people can live on this planet. For example, people who live near the equator where the sun's rays are the strongest need little in the way of clothes or shelter to slow the loss of heat from their bodies. As a result, their basal metabolic rates are about 10% lower than those of people living in the North or South Temperate Zones.

• **Photosynthesis by plants**—The chemical energy that is produced in photosynthesis is equivalent to the caloric needs of about 1.2 trillion people, which is almost 280 times the present population of the world. However, the percentages of *plant energy* which are utilizable by the human body as food energy vary considerably for the various types of plant tissue. For example, many types of grasses are high in undigestible fiber that is very poorly utilized by people, but is better utilized by grazing animals such as buffaloes, cattle, goats, and sheep. It is noteworthy that the grazing crops yield an average of 70 Calories (kcal) of total plant energy for each kcal invested by man in their production, whereas the major food crops yield from 1 to 10 Calories (kcal) for each kcal of cultural energy input. Furthermore, even the cereal grains that are favored by man contain large amounts of roots, stems, and leaves that are unsuitable for human food. Hence, there is a need to convert the energy that is present in nonedible plants and plant residues into forms that people can utilize more readily.

(Also see PHOTOSYNTHESIS.)

• **Conversion of plant products into animal products**—Man has long depended upon various members of the animal kingdom to convert plants into more appetizing types of food. Dairy cows, which are at present the most efficient means of converting forages to food, convert about one-sixth of the energy of grasses into the energy of milk. According to most archaeological evidence, primitive peoples consumed many types of animals, birds, fishes, insects, and reptiles when these foods could be obtained readily. These items were supplemented by the edible parts of wild plants.[3] It might have been the pursuit of wild game which led Asian hunters of the Stone Age to cross what was then a land bridge (now, the Bering Strait) between the Asian and American continents. Therefore, it is noteworthy that the prodigious labors of the primitive peoples of the northern lands were fueled mainly by the energy from fishes and meats which contained ample amounts of fats. Even today, most investigations show that diets rich in animal products may lead to the storage of more food energy in the form of body fat than predominantly vegetarian diets because, on the average, animal products are higher in calories than most vegetables. Unfortunately, the stored energy which once was almost always a great asset is now often a liability because most people lead sedentary lives. Nevertheless, the conversion of vegetable foods into animal foods continues to be essential to man, whether it takes place in the lactating mother or in livestock and poultry. The problem is to select the means of conversion that result in the most efficient uses of energy inputs, agricultural land, and critical raw materials.

• **A diet containing both plant and animal foods ensures the best nutrition for people**—The caloric needs of most people can be met by diets consisting mainly of grains and/or legumes. However, those consuming these diets may develop various disorders due to deficiencies of amino acids, minerals, and vitamins because a wide variety of plant foods must be consumed to ensure that vegetarian diets are nutritionally adequate. The nutrient compositions of most plants differ from the nutrients that are required by the human body. Also, less variety is required when ample amounts of dairy products, eggs, fish, meats (both muscles and organs), and poultry are consumed. The animal foods are generally good sources of the nutrients required by people. However, only the milk and bones of animals contain sufficient calcium to meet human needs.

• **Plant and animal wastes yield energy**—The energy that is present in inedible plant and animal wastes need not be wasted, since some of these materials release combustible gases and heat when they undergo fermentation, or are burned. Only limited use was made of these materials until the recent energy crisis made it profitable to do so. Now, there are a growing number of locations at which plant and/or animal materials are fermented in closed chambers so that the gases produced may be collected. After fermentation, the residues may be dried and used as feeds or fertilizers. Another development in this field is the production of hot water, steam, and/or electricity by burning agricultural wastes and municipal garbage.

UTILIZATION OF FOOD ENERGY FOR THE WORK OF THE BODY.

Although the end products and the amounts of energy released are the same, the oxygen-consuming metabolism of carbohydrates, fats, and proteins in the body, which occurs in the process called respiration, differs from the combustion of these substances in a calorimeter in that the energy is released under much more strictly controlled conditions in respiration. The utilization of food energy in the body involves a chain of closely linked

chemical reactions in which the energy of the nutrients is passed from one substance to the next with small leakages of heat occurring at various points in the chain. Consequently, the major end products of energy metabolism are carbon dioxide, water, chemical energy in the form of certain organic phosphates, and heat. Some urea is also formed from the metabolism of protein.

Over one-half of the energy produced in nutrient metabolism is the heat which helps to maintain the body temperature, and most of the rest is contained in the organic phosphates, the most important of which is adenosine triphosphate (ATP). Hence, respiration in the mitochondria of cells throughout the body provides much of the energy to operate the work of the body.

Details of the major energy utilizing processes follow.

Maintenance Of Body Temperature. In the absence of chilling, the heat that is released during the normal functioning of the body is sufficient to maintain the body temperature. Heat is produced whenever chemical, mechanical, or electrical energy is utilized because the processes of the body operate against various types of opposing forces, which, like friction, cause some of the useful energy to be converted into heat. Also, heat escapes from various linkages in the metabolic chain which produces ATP. When chilling does occur, the body temperature is maintained by (1) shivering (involuntary contractions of the skeletal muscles that bring about the conversion of ATP into mechanical energy and heat), and (2) increased rates of secretion of thyroid hormones, epinephrine (adrenalin) and nor-epinephrine (nor-adrenaline), which bring about the production of a greater proportion of heat energy and a lesser proportion of ATP energy for each unit of food energy that is metabolized.

Certain conditions may overwhelm the processes that help to maintain the body temperature so that dangerously low or high internal temperatures result. For example, an unclothed body in a cold windy environment is likely to lose heat more rapidly than it can be generated by metabolism. Hence, people living in such environments need protective clothing, shelter, and fuel to keep warm. On the other hand, the dissipation of body heat can occur only to a limited extent in hot humid environments. Therefore, these circumstances limit the amount of physical work which can be done in the tropics because increased muscle activity results in increased heat production.

Synthesis Of Essential Substances. The maintenance, repair, and growth of body tissues require energy to synthesize large molecules and related structures. For example, the synthesis of a molecule of glycogen (the storage form of carbohydrate), which contains about 10,000 units of glucose, requires the energy that is derived from 20,000 molecules of ATP. This energy is later released when glycogen breaks down to meet the body's need for sugar. Similarly, an average protein molecule requires about 1,500 molecules of ATP energy for its synthesis. When the food energy intake of the diet yields more energy than is needed to fuel the body's essential functions, the surplus ATP energy is utilized to synthesize fats (lipids). The synthesis of each molecule of a typical phospholipid such as lecithin requires the energy from 8 molecules of ATP.

Active Transport Of Substances Across Cell Membranes. The use of metabolic energy to move substances across membranes against concentration gradients is called active transport. Normally, the substances which can pass

---

[3]Robson, J. R. K., "Foods from the Past—Lessons for the Future," *The Professional Nutritionist,* Spring, 1976, pp. 13-15.

through the various membranes in the body can be expected to flow in the directions that will equalize their concentrations on both sides of the membranes. However, the essential functions of the body often require that gradients in the concentrations of many substances be maintained within and without cells. For example, the concentration of potassium ions must be kept higher within cells than in the surrounding medium, whereas the concentration of sodium ions must be kept higher outside of cells. Therefore, it is necessary for energy to be used to pump out the sodium ions which leak into cells, and to pump back in the potassium ions which leak out.

It is noteworthy that the active transport of sodium and potassium across the membranes of nerve cells establishes the conditions required for generating the electric potential that conducts the nerve impulses. After the nerves have *fired* their impulses, the electric potential must be regenerated with the aid of additional active transport.

Some of the other functions which utilize active transport are (1) the secretion of saliva, gastric juice, and pancreatic juice during digestion; (2) absorption of glucose and amino acids from the intestine; (3) accumulation of calcium, manganese, magnesium, and phosphate ions within the mitochondria of cells; and (4) reabsorption of glucose and amino acids from the kidney tubules.

(Also see ACTIVE TRANSPORT.)

Muscle Contraction. The utilization of metabolic energy in muscle differs from that in other cells and tissues in that some of the ATP energy is used to synthesize phosphocreatine, which is a reserve source of the energy used in muscle contraction. Then, when the supply of ATP runs out, it may be replenished rapidly from the phosphocreatine. Respiration is normally required to generate ATP, but the phosphocreatine provides a means of generating it rapidly without respiration. The ATP brings about muscular movement by causing the thick and thin filaments of the muscle fibers to slide past each other so that shortening of the fibers occurs.

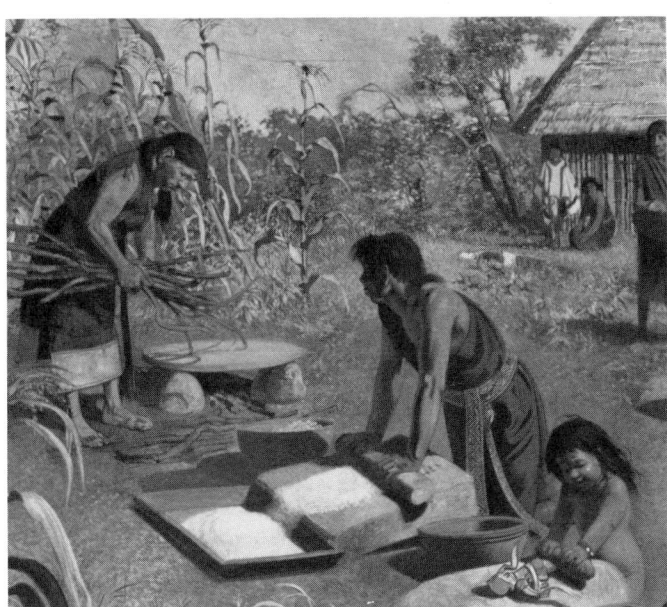

Fig. E-12. Heavy work requires large amounts of energy for muscle contraction. The above picture shows Indians hand grinding corn in ancient Mexico. (Courtesy, Field Museum of Natural History, Chicago, Ill.)

Heavy work may require the consumption of large amounts of food to provide sufficient energy for muscle contraction. The lumberjacks who worked in Wisconsin and Minnesota in the 1920s consumed about 9,000 Calories (kcal) per day.[4] Much of this food energy was provided by large servings of bacon, butter, cheese, cream, eggs, fish, meat, and milk. However, it now may be more practical to utilize machine-powered tools than to rely upon the consumption of large quantities of moderately expensive foods to provide energy for muscular work that is done with only hand-powered tools.

SUMMARY. The human body performs its vital functions with the help of energy that originates in the nuclear reactions in the sun, and is trapped within the chemical substances synthesized by plants during photosynthesis. Animals, which eat the plants, convert the vegetable constituents into animal foods that are often more useful and more palatable sources of food energy for people. Although the energy costs of producing animal foods are sometimes higher than those for vegetable foods, the utilization of both plant and animal wastes as sources of energy helps to keep energy wastage to a minimum. Finally, the utilization of other forms of energy by man for heating, transportation, and the performance of work spares the body from having to use very large quantities of food energy.

(Also see CALORIC [ENERGY] EXPENDITURE; CALORIC VALUES OF FOODS; ENERGY REQUIRED FOR FOOD PRODUCTION; and METABOLISM.)

ENRICHMENT (FORTIFICATION, NUTRIFICATION, RESTORATION)

In foods, enrichment and fortification refer to the addition of vitamins, minerals, and/or protein to raise the nutritive value.

NOTE WELL: Originally, the FDA differentiated between enrichment and fortification, but now the two terms are used interchangeably. Nevertheless, the following differentiations between the terms persist:

• **Enriched**—This refers to the addition of specific nutrients to a food *as established in a federal standard of identity and quality.* The amounts added generally are moderate and include those commonly present at even lower levels.

• **Fortified**—This refers to the addition to foods of specific nutrients. The amounts added are usually in excess of those normally found in the food because of the importance of providing additional amounts of the nutrients to the diet. Some foods are selected for fortification because they are an appropriate carrier for the nutrient.

However, most dictionaries are not able to draw a distinction between enriched and fortified. In fact, according to

[4]Cooley, A. C. J., "Paul Bunyan's Cook," *Nutrition Today*, Vol. 5, Spring 1970, pp. 24-25.

dictionary definitions, to fortify is to enrich with vitamins and minerals. In January 1980, the U.S. Government also decided to delete separate definitions for enrichment and fortification and use the words interchangeably unless another regulation specified which term to use. In the following discussion enrichment and fortification will be used interchangeably unless noted otherwise. Two more terms may be employed as synonyms to enrichment or fortification:

• **Restoration**—This is the replacement of nutrients lost in processing foods.

• **Nutrification**—This is the practice of adding a proportion of vitamins and minerals (1) to a formulated or fabricated food; or (2) to a grouping of foods marketed as a meal or meal replacer—for example, infant formulas and instant breakfast foods.

HISTORY. In the United States, the bread-and-flour-enrichment program has been a controversial one. Some have maintained that the public should be educated to the use of natural foods that would supply all nutrients, but experience of centuries has shown that people are reluctant to change their food habits and that education regarding food choices is a slow process. A classical, pioneering rice enrichment experiment in the Philippines demonstrated how an action program can combat a widespread deficiency disease.

Beriberi In The Philippines. The experimental program of rice enrichment in the Philippines was singularly appropriate for the reason that it was in the Philippines, in 1910, that Dr. Robert R. Williams' attention was first focused on the beriberi problem, and it was there that he found the clue which started him on the 26-year search that culminated in the first successful synthesis of thiamin (vitamin B-1) in 1936. This paved the way for its commercial manufacture on a scale that would within a few years lower the price to the point where enrichment of cereal grains would be economically feasible. By 1946, when peace had come and the Philippine experiment could be considered,

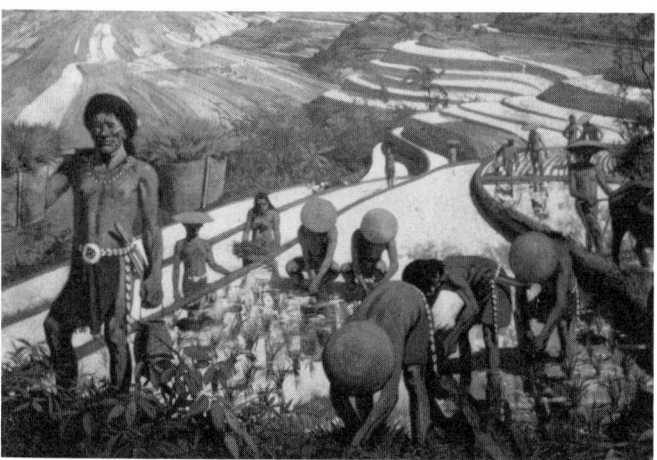

Fig. E-13. Rice growing in the Philippines, where Dr. Robert R. Williams, who was the first to synthesize thiamin (vitamin B-1), conducted the classical, pioneering rice enrichment experiment to combat the deficiency disease, beriberi. (Courtesy, Field Museum of Natural History, Chicago, Ill.)

a process had been developed by the pharmaceutical house of Hoffmann-La Roche, Inc., for adding thiamin, niacin, and iron to rice. By this time, the effectiveness of the technique of premix fortification had also been established.

The Bataan Experiment. The scene of the experiment was to be an area better known to the world for a different reason—the Bataan Peninsula, where early in 1942 the joint Filipino-American forces made their gallant stand.

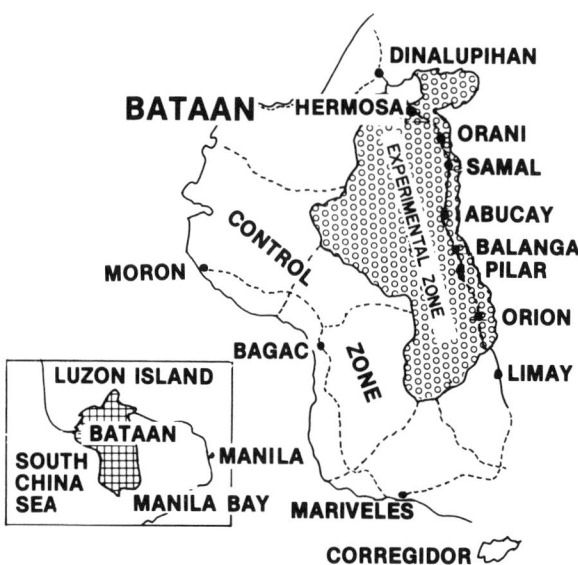

Fig. E-14. Rice enrichment and control areas. All Bataan was divided into two areas for the enrichment project: the experimental zone of smaller but more populous municipalities on the Manila Bayside, which received the enriched rice; and the control zone of the remaining municipalities, which continued to receive ordinary white rice.

It was the combination of the factors of isolation, uniformity of conditions, and rice self-sufficiency, in addition, of course, to the considerable beriberi death rates, that led to the selection of Bataan as the site of the field trials in which, for the first time, a whole population's entire rice supply would be enriched.

In the summer of 1946, Dr. Williams went to the Philippines with a plan for the combat of beriberi. The specific objectives of the mass nutritional feeding experiment were fourfold: (1) to determine to what extent beriberi in the Philippines could be alleviated by substitution of fortified rice for ordinary white rice; (2) to test the feasibility of the practice in the channels of the rice trade; (3) to inaugurate and test practical inspection systems to insure that only fortified rice is sold; (4) to popularize enriched rice with the people and to provide a basis for consideration of the use of fortification throughout the Philippine Islands under adequate government controls.

For purposes of accurately measuring the effects of rice enrichment, the Province of Bataan was divided into two areas, an experimental zone and a control zone. The seven more populous municipalities on the east coast were in the experimental zone, and the remainder of the province served as a control area. Enriched rice would be made available only to the 63,000 people in the experimental zone; the other 29,000 in the control zone would continue to get their customary supply of rice.

• **Thiamin requirements met by enrichment**—It seemed reasonable to fortify the enriched rice with enough thiamin to bring the average daily intake of the vitamin to nearly 2 mg from the rice alone, based on an estimated daily adult consumption of 400 g of rice, and allowing for losses of thiamin in washing and cooking. Other foods were expected to contribute another 0.45 mg of thiamin daily, bringing the total for the experimental zone well above the minimum levels recommended.

For this purpose, rice fortified to the same levels as enriched white wheat flour in the United States seemed appropriate. As distributed, each pound of the product contained 2 mg of thiamin, 16 mg of niacin, and 13 mg of iron.

• **Beriberi deaths decrease**—The mortality figures soon began to show the influence of the enrichment program.

The figures for the first full year of enrichment were startling (see Table E-10). There was a decline of 67.3% in beriberi deaths in the experimental zone, and an increase of 2.4% in the control area, as compared to the year immediately prior to enrichment. In the experimental area, enriched rice had apparently saved the lives of 111 people in 1 year.

TABLE E-10
EFFECT OF RICE ENRICHMENT ON BATAAN MORTALITY RATE

Municipality	Oct. 1, 1947 to Sept. 30, 1948[1]	Oct. 1, 1948 to Sept. 30, 1949[2]	Decrease or Increase (+)
	(per 100,000)	(per 100,000)	(%)
Experimental zone			
Abucay	289.7	23.7	91.9
Balanga	325.0	137.3	57.7
Hermosa	314.2	47.4	84.9
Orani	233.6	55.0	76.4
Orion	234.9	114.7	51.2
Pilar	69.5	0.0	100.0
Samal	156.3	157.3	+ .6
Entire experimental zone	246.2	80.4	67.3
Control zone			
Bagac	180.8	182.1	+ .7
Dinalupihan	166.8	118.5	28.9
Limay	112.3	199.6	+ 77.9
Mariveles	.0	44.8	+ —
Moron	330.1	389.7	+ 18.0
Entire control zone	152.7	156.5	+ 2.4

[1]Ordinary white rice consumed by all people in both experimental and control zones.

[2]Enriched rice consumed by people in experimental zone; ordinary rice by people in control zone.

The results that were shown as the enrichment project went into its second year were even more impressive. In the experimental zone, beriberi deaths decreased again in the fifth and sixth quarters; in the seventh quarter they reached zero. For the 3 months from April 1 to June 30, 1950, not 1 death from beriberi was recorded in any of the 7 municipalities. It appeared that enrichment saved the lives of some 220 people, mostly babies, in Bataan.

Other Enrichment Programs. Enrichment of salt with iodine in 1924 was the first essential nutrient to be added to a consumer product. This enrichment program successfully decreased the incidence of simple goiter in the United States. For example, a survey of the school children in four

Michigan counties indicated that the incidence of goiter dropped from 38.6% in 1924 to 1.4% in 1951.

The discovery of vitamin D as the antirachitic vitamin and the recognition of fish-liver oils as a potent source led to the advice that babies should receive cod-liver oil or some concentrate of vitamin D. Prevention of rickets and development of strong bones in young children depend on an adequate intake of calcium and phosphorus, as well as vitamin D, and therefore fortification of milk with vitamin D was begun in the early 1930s. The Council on Foods and Nutrition of the American Medical Association approved the fortification of milk.

(Also see VITAMIN[S].)

The Danes first realized the need for adding vitamin A to a food. During World War I, practically all the butter of Denmark was exported. Subsequently, an eye ailment was observed in young children and was recognized as a vitamin A deficiency. As a preventive measure, vitamin A concentrates were added to margarine. Other countries adopted the practice. The Council on Foods and Nutrition of the American Medical Association approved it in 1939, and it has since been advocated by the Food and Nutrition Board.

In 1940, the National Academy of Sciences-National Research Council appointed a Committee on Food and Nutrition (later called the Food and Nutrition Board) to develop a table of *Recommended Daily Allowances for Specific Nutrients*. This committee proposed the use of the term *enriched* and set up minimum and maximum limits for the enrichment of bread and flour with thiamin, riboflavin, niacin, and iron. With the support of the millers, enriched flour became available to the public and was used by the Army and Navy.

The enrichment of salt with iodine, the fortification of milk with vitamin D, and the start of the thiamin, riboflavin, niacin, and iron, grain enrichment program in 1941, have played a significant role in the practical elimination of the following deficiency diseases: simple goiter, rickets, beriberi, ariboflavinosis, pellagra and simple iron-deficiency anemia. The average American receives approximately 40% of his thiamin, 25% of his iron, 20% of his niacin, and 15% of his riboflavin from enriched foods.

ENRICHED FOODS. Consumers will find a variety of enriched foods, and at times it is difficult to differentiate between the use of a nutrient for enrichment or as an additive. Indeed, nutrients—minerals, vitamins, and amino acids—are a class of food additives. The commonly enriched foods are: salt, milk, margarine, cereals, and cereal products. Additionally, a variety of other foods may be enriched or fortified with vitamins and minerals to maintain or improve the nutritional value. There are reasons for enriching foods, and principles of enrichment to follow when considering the value of enrichment. Moreover, once it has been determined to enrich food, there are guidelines, standards, and labeling practices to follow for enrichment practices.

Reasons For Enrichment. The prime reason for enrichment is public health so that diets can be nutritionally improved without trying to change food habits. People are usually adverse to changing food habits, and in some populations, the foods creating the nutritional deficiency may be the only foods available. Other reasons for the ingestion of an inadequate diet, thus necessitating enrichment, include (1) lack of interest in nutrition, (2) meals eaten away from home, (3) snacking, (4) poverty, (5) reduced energy expenditure, hence, reduced caloric requirements, (6) lack of knowledge concerning nutrients present in foods, (7) weight control and fad diets, and (8) selection of foods with diminished nutrient content as compared to the raw product.

The function of fresh fruits, vegetables, fresh meat, poultry, and fish in a balanced diet is well established and understood by the public. There is no reason to add nutrients to these foods. Also, it is inappropriate to fortify snack foods such as candies and carbonated beverages.

Guidelines For Enrichment. In January 1980, the Food and Drug Administration (FDA), set forth guidelines to follow when nutrients are added to foods. The new guidelines were designed to provide a sensible set of principles for adding minerals, vitamins, and protein to foods in order to achieve a balance of nutrients—not to encourage widespread enrichment. Enrichment is permissible under the following conditions:

1. To overcome a nutritional deficiency in a particular population group, such as the addition of iodine to salt to prevent goiter and vitamin D to milk to prevent rickets in children.

2. To restore nutrients which have been lost in the storage, handling, and processing of foods. All nutrients in all amounts lost, including protein must be considered.

3. To fabricated foods, in proportion to the total calories.

4. To foods that substitute for and resemble traditional foods so that they will not be nutritionally inferior.

5. To meet nutritional standards which are required or permitted by existing FDA regulations—the standards of enrichment.

• **Standards of enrichment**—While enrichment is not required by law, certain enriched foods must meet established standards. The Food and Drug Administration (FDA) standards for enrichment include iodine, vitamin D, vitamin A, thiamin, riboflavin, niacin, iron, and calcium in some foods.

• **Foods**—Currently, the FDA has standards for the enrichment of the following:

1. Iodine is added to salt at the level of 0.5 to 1 part in 10,000 or 7.6 mg/100 g.

2. Vitamin D is added to milk at the level of 400 IU per qt (*0.95 liter*) of fluid milk or large can of evaporated milk (1⅔ cups or *400 ml*).

3. Vitamin A is added to margarine at the level of 15,000 IU per pound (*0.45 kg*). This is the year-round average for the vitamin A content of butter.

4. Enrichment levels prescribed by federal standards of identity for flour and other cereal products are listed in Table E-11.

TABLE E-11
ENRICHMENT LEVELS OF CEREAL PRODUCTS

Product	Thiamin		Riboflavin		Niacin		Iron		Calcium[1]	
	(mg/lb)	(*mg/100 g*)	(mg/lb)	(*mg/100 g*)	(mg/lb)	(*mg/100 g*)	(mg/lb)	(*mg/100 g*)	(mg/lb)	(*mg/100 g*)
Flour	2.9	*.64*	1.8	*.40*	24	*5.3*	13–16.5	*2.87–3.64*	960	*212*
Flour, self-rising	2.9	*.64*	1.8	*.40*	24	*5.3*	13–16.5	*2.87–3.64*	960	*212*
Bread, rolls, and buns	1.8	*.40*	1.1	*.24*	15	*3.3*	8–12.5	*1.76–2.76*	600	*136*
Cornmeal, corn grits	2.0–3.0	*.44–.66*	1.2–1.8	*.26–.40*	16–24	*3.53–5.29*	13–26.0	*2.87–5.73*	500– 750	*100–165*
Cornmeal, self-rising	2.0–3.0	*.44–.66*	1.2–1.8	*.26–.40*	16–24	*3.53–5.29*	13–26.0	*2.87–5.73*	500–1,750	*110–385*
Macaroni and noodles	4.0–5.0	*.88–1.10*	1.7–2.2	*.37–.48*	27–34	*5.95–7.50*	13–16.5	*2.87–3.64*	500– 625	*110–138*
Farina	2.0–2.5	*.44–.55*	1.2–1.5	*.26–.33*	16–20	*3.53–4.41*	13[2]	*2.87*	500[2]	*110*
Rice, milled	2.0–4.0	*.44–.88*	1.2–2.4[3]	*.26–.53*	16–32	*3.53–7.05*	13–26.0	*2.87–5.73*	500–1,000	*110–220*

[1]The addition of calcium is optional.

[2]No maximum level established.

[3]The addition of riboflavin is feasible but the requirement was stayed many years ago since its addition colors the rice yellow; hence, rice may or may not be enriched.

Today, enrichment is required in about two-thirds of the states and Puerto Rico. In practice, however, all family flour is enriched, and about 90% of all commercially baked standard white bread is enriched.

It is noteworthy that England, Canada, and a few other countries have enrichment programs somewhat similar to the United States, but that France forbids enrichment.

Labels And U.S. RDA. Whenever products are labeled *enriched,* or a food product has added nutrients, or a nutritional claim is made for a product, the FDA requires that the nutritional content be listed on the label. In addition, many manufacturers put nutrition information on products when not required to do so in order to make their product competitive.

Nutrition labels list how many calories and how much protein, carbohydrate, and fat are in a serving of the product. They also list the percentage of the U.S. Recommended Daily Allowances (U.S. RDAs) of protein and seven important minerals and vitamins that each serving of the product contains.

• **Nutrition labels**—At the top, the nutrition labeling panel is identified as *Nutrition Information.*

Nutrition information is given on a per serving basis. The label tells of a serving; for example, 1 cup (*0.45 kg*), 2 oz (*60 ml*), 1 Tbsp (*15 ml*); the number of servings in the container, the number of calories per serving, and the amounts in grams of protein, carbohydrate, and fat per serving.

The lower part of the nutrition label must give the percentages of the U.S. Recommended Daily Allowances (U.S. RDA) of protein and seven vitamins and minerals in a serving of the product, in the following order: protein, vitamin A, vitamin C, thiamin, riboflavin, niacin, calcium, and iron. The listing of 12 other vitamins and minerals, and of cholesterol, fatty acid, and sodium content is optional—for now. Nutrients present at levels less than 2% of the U.S. RDA may be indicated by a zero or an asterisk which refers to the statement, "contains less than 2% of the U.S. RDA of these nutrients."

• **U.S. RDAs**—These allowances are guides to the amounts of vitamins and minerals an individual needs each day to stay healthy. They were set by the FDA as nutritional standards for labeling purposes. The U.S. RDAs are *based* on the Recommended Dietary Allowances established by the Food and Nutrition Board of the National Academy of Sciences-National Research Council. For practical purposes, the many categories of dietary allowances for males and females of different ages were condensed to as few as nutritionally possible for labeling. Generally, the highest values for the ages combined in a U.S. RDA were used. For example, the U.S. RDAs for adults and children over 4 years are representative, generally, of the dietary allowances recommended for a teen-age boy.

There are four groupings of the U.S. RDAs. (See NUTRIENTS: REQUIREMENTS, ALLOWANCES, FUNCTIONS, SOURCES.) The best known, and the one that will be used on most nutrition information panels and most mineral and vitamin supplements, is for adults and children over 4 years of age, shown in Table E-12. The second is for infants up to 1 year, and the third is for children under 4 years. These two will be used on infant formulas, baby foods, and other foods appropriate for these ages as well as vitamin-mineral supplements intended for their use. The fourth is for pregnant women or women who are nursing their babies.

TABLE E-12
UNITED STATES RECOMMENDED
DAILY ALLOWANCES (U.S. RDA),
THE MOST COMMONLY USED GROUPING

Nutrient	Adults and Children 4 Years or Older[1]
Required on labels:	
Protein .... g	59
Vitamin A .... mcg RE	1000
Vitamin C .... mg	60
Thiamin .... mg	1.5
Riboflavin .... mg	1.8
Niacin .... mg	20
Calcium .... mg	1200
Iron .... mg	12
Optional on labels:	
Vitamin D .... IU	400
Vitamin E .... IU	10
Vitamin B-6 .... mg	2
Folate .... mcg	200
Vitamin B-12 .... mcg	2
Phosphorus .... mg	1200
Iodine .... mcg	150
Magnesium .... mg	400
Zinc .... mg	15
Copper .... mg	2
Biotin .... mcg	60
Pantothenic acid .... mg	6

[1]U.S. RDA taken from *Recommended Dietary Allowances*, 10th ed., 1989, National Research Council.

Many foods today are manufactured into products that are different from traditional foods. Some classes of these foods include frozen dinners; breakfast cereals; meat replacements; noncarbonated breakfast beverages; and main dishes such as macaroni and cheese, pizzas, stews, and casseroles. Nutrients may be added to these foods.

Nutritional labeling allows consumers to select foods that are a particularly good source of a specific nutrient, and to determine whether newly introduced products are as nutritious as their familiar counterparts.

NUTRITION INFORMATION
SERVING SIZE: 1 OZ. (28.4 g, ABOUT ⅔ CUP) CEREAL ALONE OR WITH ½ CUP VITAMIN D FORTIFIED WHOLE MILK.
SERVINGS PER PACKAGE: 13

	CEREAL	WITH MILK
CALORIES	110	190
PROTEIN	2 g	6 g
CARBOHYDRATE	24 g	30 g
FAT	1 g	5 g
SODIUM	185 mg (660 mg per 100 g)	245 mg (165 mg per 100 g)

PERCENTAGE OF U.S. RECOMMENDED DAILY ALLOWANCES (U.S. RDA)

	CEREAL	WITH MILK
PROTEIN	4	10
VITAMIN A	25	30
VITAMIN C	25	25
THIAMIN	25	30
RIBOLAVIN	25	35
NIACIN	25	25
CALCIUM	*	15
IRON	4	4
VITAMIN D	10	25
VITAMIN E	25	25
VITAMIN B₆	25	30
FOLIC ACID	25	25
VITAMIN B₁₂	25	30
PHOSPHORUS	8	20
MAGNESIUM	4	8
ZINC	25	30
COPPER	4	4

*CONTAINS LESS THAN 2% OF THE U.S. RDA OF THIS NUTRIENT.

Fig. E-15. An example of a nutritional label from an enriched ready-to-eat breakfast cereal.

On the basis of the nutritional label and the U.S. RDA in Fig. E-15, one serving of the cereal contains 2 g of protein, 1,250 IU of vitamin A, 15 mg of vitamin C, 0.38 mg of thiamin, 0.43 mg of riboflavin, 5 mg of niacin, less than 20 mg of calcium, 0.72 g of iron, 40 IU of vitamin D, 0.5 mg of vitamin B-6, 0.1 mg of folic acid, 1.5 mcg of vitamin B-12, 80 mg of phosphorus, 16 mg of magnesium, 3.8 mg of zinc, and 0.08 mg of copper.

Aside from the labels of many products which are purchased, nutritional information in Food Composition Table F-21 identifies the enriched products. Furthermore, it should be realized that the nutritional information on any fabricated food represents enrichment, since these foods are literally pieced together; for example, breakfast bars and powders, and meat analogs.

SUMMARY. Enrichment is not a panacea—only a tool. All nutrient requirements cannot be ensured with any enrichment program. Rather, to be sure people receive adequate amounts of the 45 to 50 nutrients required for good nutrition, the best advice is sound nutrition education so individuals will choose from a variety of nutritious foods. Moreover, people's eating habits change as do their nutrient intakes; hence, relying on enrichment to cope with malnutrition would require constant re-evaluation of enrichment levels. Another problem with enrichment is manipulation for economic benefit. Unscrupulous manufacturers may boast of a product with a much higher content of some nutrient due to enrichment, or may boast of the *perfect* food and charge consumers a disproportionate price. Currently, some ready-to-eat breakfast cereals are enriched to 100% of U.S. RDAs for many of the vitamins and minerals. Consumption of a fortified food will not ensure a complete or nutritionally sound diet.

Many people are poorly nourished because of (1) lack of interest in nutrition, (2) inadequate information about the role of foods, and (3) economic deprivation. In cultures where dietary patterns are simple and based on a limited number of commodities, one is able to identify which food could be a carrier for an enrichment program. Traditionally, staples such as wheat, rice, and corn have served as vehicles for niacin, riboflavin, thiamin, iron, and calcium. Milk has been as reliable a carrier of vitamin D, as table salt has been a carrier of iodine. Also, water is employed as a carrier for fluorine.

(Also see ADDITIVES; CEREAL GRAINS, section headed "Enriched or Fortified Cereals"; CORN, Table C-23 Corn Products and Uses for Human Food; FLOURS, section headed "Enrichment and Fortification of Flours"; IRON, section headed "Sources of Iron"; NIACIN, section headed "Sources of Niacin"; NUTRIENTS: REQUIREMENTS, ALLOWANCES, FUNCTIONS, SOURCES; RIBOFLAVIN, section headed "Sources of Riboflavin"; RICE, section headed "Nutritional Value"; THIAMIN, section headed "Sources of Thiamin"; and WHEAT, section headed "Enriched Flour.")

ENTERIC

Relating to the small intestine.

ENTERITIS

Inflammation of the intestines.

ENTERO–

A prefix denoting intestinal.

ENTEROHEPATIC CIRCULATION

This refers to the continuous circulation of the bile from the liver to the gallbladder, then into the intestine, from which it is absorbed and carried by the blood back to the liver to be returned to the circulation. This recycling conserves the bile; of the 20 to 30 g of bile used daily, only about 0.8 g is actually eliminated in the feces and must be replenished by the liver.

ENTEROKINASE

An enzyme which converts the inactive form of the enzyme trypsin to the active form.
(Also see DIGESTION AND ABSORPTION.)

ENTEROSTOMY

The general name given to an operation which connects a piece of the intestine to an artificial outlet on the abdominal wall called a stoma.

ENVIRONMENT

The forces and conditions, both physical and biological, that (1) surround an individual and (2) interact with heredity to determine behavior, growth, and development. Air qual-ity, food supply, lighting, noise, other people, and weather are some of the many factors that make up an individual's environment. Extremes or alterations in the environment may subject an individual to stress.
(Also see STRESS.)

ENZYMATIC

Related to an enzyme.

ENZYME

Complex protein compounds produced in living cells which speed biochemical reactions without being used up in the process. They are organic catalysts.
(Also see DIGESTION AND ABSORPTION.)

EPIDEMIC

An outbreak of a disease in an area where it does not normally occur, in contrast to the term endemic which refers to a disease regularly occurring in a certain locality.
(Also see ENDEMIC.)

EPIDEMIOLOGY

The study of the various factors responsible for the presence or absence of diseases in populations.

EPIDERMIS

The outer horny layer of skin which serves as a protection for the underlying layer called the dermis.

EPIGASTRIC

The upper central region of the stomach.

EPIGLOTTIS

A flap of tissue which covers the windpipe and prevents food from getting into the bronchial tubes.

EPILEPSY

A disorder of the nervous system characterized by convulsions and/or loss of consciousness. Special ketogenic diets are sometimes used in the treatment of epilepsy.
(Also see MODIFIED DIETS, Table M-28, Modified Diets—Ketogenic diet.)

EPINEPHRINE

The hormone commonly called *adrenalin*, which is secreted by the adrenal medulla. The hormone epinephrine is secreted in larger than normal amounts when certain emotional states such as anger, fear, and pain cause emotional upsets.
(Also see ENDOCRINE GLANDS.)

EPIPHYSIS

The end of a long bone which during the growing years is separated from the shaft of the bone by a plate of cartilage. When the growth of the long bone stops, the epiphyses are fused to the shafts of the bone (diaphyses).
(Also see BONE.)

EPITHELIAL

Refers to those cells that form the outer layer of the skin and other membranes.

EPSOM SALT

The common name for magnesium sulfate, a mineral salt which is used as a strong laxative. It is also injected into pregnant women to prevent toxemia of pregnancy. However, care must be used in this use of the salt because an excessive amount may cause sedation in the unborn child.

ERGOCALCIFEROL

A substance which is formed from ergosterol, a plant substance that is converted into vitamin D by the action of sunlight or other forms of ultraviolet radiation.
(Also see VITAMIN D.)

ERGOMETER

An instrument used to measure the amount of work done under controlled conditions of time, rate, and resistance.

ERGOSTEROL

A plant sterol which, when activated by ultraviolet rays, becomes vitamin D_2. It is also called provitamin D_2 and ergosterin.
(Also see VITAMIN D.)

ERUCIC ACID

A very long chain fatty acid with one double bond, found in rapeseed oil and mustardseed oil. It has been found that when large amounts of rapeseed oil (50% of the total energy) are fed to experimental animals, fatty changes occur in heart muscle. This is because erucic acid enters the myocardial cells, but is oxidized more slowly than other fatty acids; so, it accumulates intracellularly in triglycerides. Geneticists have now produced strains of rape that produce seed oil with less than 1% erucic acid.
(Also see RAPESEED.)

ERYTHORBIC ACID

A derivative of vitamin C, which is used as an antioxidant in food products to prevent rancidity, to prohibit browning of fruit, and to preserve the red color of meats. It is poorly absorbed and has little antiscorbutic activity.

ERYTHROCYTES

The red blood cells, which carry oxygen to the tissues.
(Also see ANEMIA.)

ERYTHROPOIETIN

The hormone which stimulates the formation of red blood cells.
(Also see ANEMIA.)

ESOPHAGITIS

An inflamation of the esophagus, the tube that leads from the mouth to the stomach. Esophagitis may be a dangerous condition if it is caused by the reflux of acid from the stomach because the esophagus is not very well protected against irritating substances.
(Also see DIGESTION AND ABSORPTION.)

ESSENTIAL FATTY ACID

A fatty acid that cannot be synthesized in the body or that cannot be made in sufficient quantities for the body's needs.
(Also see FATS AND OTHER LIPIDS.)

ESSENTIAL OILS

A large class of volatile, odoriferous oils secured from various parts of certain plants, such as the flowers, the seeds, the leaves, the bark, or the roots. These oils are usually obtained either by (1) steam distillation, (2) expression, or (3) extraction (using a solution that will dissolve out the oil). Essential oils are used in flavoring materials, perfumes, and pharmaceutical preparations. They are called *essential oils* to distinguish them from *fatty oils*.

ESTER

The chemical term applied to any combination of an organic acid and an alcohol. An ester holds the position in organic chemistry that a salt holds in inorganic chemistry. *Example*: ethyl alcohol and acetic acid yield ethyl acetate—an ester.

ETHANOL

The type of alcohol which is present in alcoholic drinks. It is also called ethyl alcohol.
(Also see ALCOHOL AND ALCOHOLIC BEVERAGES.)

ETHER EXTRACT (EE)

Fatty substances of foods that are soluble in ether.
(Also see FATS AND OTHER LIPIDS.)

ETHNIC

This term refers to the characteristics which distinguish certain national and racial groups of people from others. Hence, ethnic characteristics may include social customs, food patterns, character and physical traits of the various peoples.

ETHYLENE

A sweet-smelling gas found in ripening fruit and used commercially to accelerate the ripening of fruit. Green lemons stored where the concentration of ethylene is 0.05% will become yellow in one week.

ETHYLENEDIAMINE TETRA-ACETIC ACID (EDTA; VERSENE)

An organic chemical capable of *tying up* metallic ions such as calcium, copper, iron, and zinc, and thus preventing them from reacting with other compounds. Chemicals that possess this property are called chelating or sequestering agents. A variety of EDTA salts exist; and all are sequestering agents, many of which are used as food additives. EDTA and its salts stabilize and maintain the color, freshness, and flavor of oils, fats, fruits, vegetables, fish, shell fish, dairy, and meat products, and vitamin preparations. In pharmacy and medicine, EDTA is used in the treatment of lead poisoning.
(Also see CHELATE.)

ETHYL FORMATE

An ester with a pleasant odor, made from the chemical combination of ethyl alcohol and formic acid. In the food industry, it is valuable as (1) a fungicide and larvicide for cereals and dried fruits; (2) an ingredient of synthetic flavors such as lemon and strawberry; and (3) a chemical intermediate in the synthesis of thiamin (vitamin B-1).

ETIOLOGY

The causes of disease or disorder.

EVAPORATION, FLASH

A rapid application of superheated steam which quickly distills off a small volume, 1% of the liquid being condensed. This flash distillate carries the volatile flavor constituents. Later, these flavors are added back to the concentrate. This process is employed in the production of concentrated fruit juices.

EXACERBATION

The intensification or aggravation of a disease or painful condition, usually because of something other than the original cause; for example, peptic ulcer is exacerbated by alcoholic beverages.

EXCHANGE LIST (FOOD EXCHANGES)

A grouping of similar foods by serving sizes which provide essentially equivalent nutritive value in terms of calories, carbohydrates, fats, and proteins. This type of system is designed so that people on modified diets might select foods which fit their dietary prescriptions. The most commonly used exchange lists are those for diabetics, because they are also useful for weight control.
(Also see MODIFIED DIETS.)

EXCIPIENT

An inert ingredient added to a medication for the purpose of making the dosage form more convenient to take. For example, excipients such as calcium carbonate are added to tablets to give them bulk.

EXCRETION

The process of eliminating the waste products of metabolism from the body, chiefly in the urine and sweat.

EXERGONIC

Chemical reactions occurring in living cells that produce energy; for example, the breakdown of carbohydrates or fats.
(Also see ENDERGONIC; and METABOLISM.)

EXOGENOUS

Originating or produced from the outside.

EXOPEPTIDASE

An enzyme which digests protein.

EXPERIMENT

The word experiment is derived from the Latin experimentum, meaning proof of experience. It is a procedure used to discover or to demonstrate a fact or general truth.

EXTENSOMETER

In general, extensometers are instruments used for measuring the degree of expansion, contraction, or deformation produced in a substance under an applied stress. An extensometer can be designed to measure the stretching strength of dough, an index of baking quality.

EXTRACELLULAR FLUID

The fluid outside the cells; it comprises about one-third of the total body fluid, and includes tissue fluid, blood plasma, cerebrospinal fluid, fluid in the eye, and the fluid of the gastrointestinal tract.
(Also see BODY FLUIDS.)

EXTRACT

In nutrition, this term generally has one of the meanings which follow:

• A component which has been removed from a mixture by means of treating the mixture with a solvent in which the component is soluble. For example, tea beverage is a water extract of tea leaves. Alcohol, oil, and water are the solvents most commonly used to prepare edible extracts.

• The process by which an extract is made.

EXTRACTION RATIO (EXTRACTION)

The percentage of a grain that is converted to flour. For wheat, high extraction (95 to 100%) flours such as whole wheat contain more bran and germ than low extraction (80% or less) or white flours.
(Also see FLOURS; and WHEAT.)

EXTREMITIES

The medical name given to the limbs. The upper extremities are the hand, arm and shoulder. The lower extremities are the foot, leg, thigh and hip. This term is used mainly to designate blood flow because in chilling there is often less blood flow to the extremities than there is in the central portion of the body.

EXTRINSIC FACTOR

A dietary substance, now known to be vitamin B-12, which was formerly thought to interact with the intrinsic factor of the gastric secretion to produce the antianemic factor.
(Also see INTRINSIC FACTOR; and VITAMIN B-12.)

EXUDATE

A fluid discharge into the tissues or any cavity.

EXUDATIVE DIATHESIS

The accumulation of fluid in subcutaneous tissues, muscles, or connective tissues, caused by the escape of plasma from the capillaries.

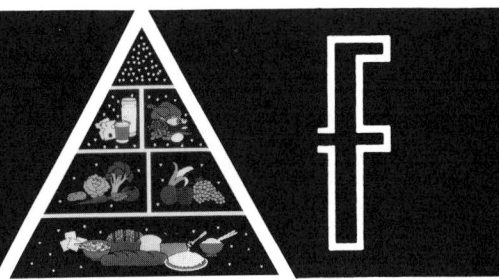

FAGOT (FAGGOT)

Besides meaning a bundle of sticks or pieces of wrought iron, this word is used in two different culinary ways as follows:

• Another term for *Bouquet Garni*—a herbal mixture added to foods during the cooking process.

• A pork product composed of hog livers, hearts, fresh pork, onions, salt, pepper, sweet marjoram, and hog caul fat (fat surrounding the stomach and intestines). The meat is thoroughly ground up, seasoned, then molded in 6-oz (*170 g*) balls. The caul fat is cut into approximately 7-in. squares (*45 cm²*) into which the meat balls are placed and encased, then baked in an oven for 45 minutes.

FAHRENHEIT

A thermometer scale on which the interval between the two standard points, the freezing point and the boiling point of water, is divided into 180°, with 32° representing the freezing point and 212° the boiling point. To convert Fahrenheit to Centigrade subtract 32 and multiply by 5/9.
(Also see WEIGHTS AND MEASURES.)

FAMILIAL

Common to a family.

FARINA

• A general term for starch.

• In the United States, it refers to a breakfast cereal, popularly known as *Cream of Wheat,* which consists of the granulated endosperm of wheat other than Durham wheat. (A similar product produced from Durham wheat is called semolina.) The term may also be applied to any flour made from cereal grains, nuts, or sea moss.

• In Italy, a flour made from dried chestnuts is called *farina dolce.*

FAST FOODS

This refers to eating establishments that serve ready-to-eat foods, with little or no waiting time from ordering to serving. This speedy handling of orders is accomplished by (1) using commercial types of convenience foods, and/or (2) by cooking the foods well in advance and keeping them warm (or cold, if necessary to prevent spoilage) until they are sold. Fast food places may or may not have accommodations for eating on the premises.

The most common fast foods are: hamburgers, french fries, and shakes; pizza and cola; fried chicken and slaw; fish and chips; roast beef sandwiches; tacos; hot dogs; and other mass-produced and mass-served quickie meals.

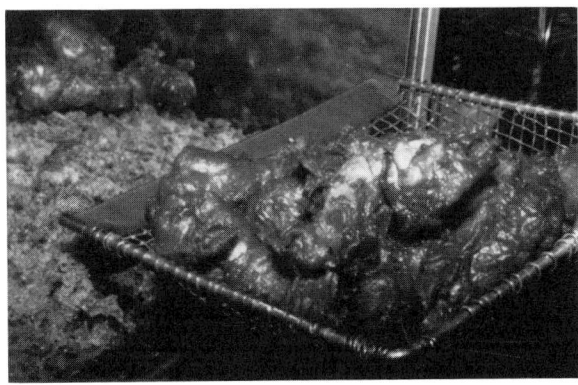

Fig. F-1. Frying chicken in deep fat for the fast food industry. (Courtesy, American Soybean Assoc., St. Louis, Mo.)

Fast foods appeal to the younger set because (1) they are an important feature of their life-style, and (2) they fit their limited spending money. In 1989, Americans spent 43% of their food dollar on meals away from home, which cost a total of $156.4 billion. That same year, the typical American ate 1 out of every 12 meals at a fast-food restaurant.

The American Council of Science and Health (ACSH), a non-profit, independent educational association of scientists, made a study of fast foods and the American diet (*ACSH Media Update,* Spring 1982). *Note well:* Since that time, in response to consumers searching for fitness and long life, most fast-food restaurants have made their menus more healthful, as is detailed in this book in the section on "Convenience and Fast Foods." But, in 1982, The ACSH reported as follows about fast foods:

• **Fast foods contribute to good nutrition**—Fast food meals can make a significant contribution to good nutrition if they are properly incorporated into a varied diet.

• **Known nutritional shortcomings of fast foods and how to compensate**—By knowing the nutritional shortcomings of fast food menus and how to compensate for them, you can eat at a fast food establishment several times a week without compromising your nutritional well being.

• **High in calories and fat**—For the amount of nutrients provided, fast food meals are usually too high in calories and saturated fat. A simple fast food meal may total more than half your daily calories. For example, the calories in a fast food meal may add up as follows: two pieces of Kentucky Fried Extra Crisply Chicken, 765 Calories (kcal); a Burger King Whopper, 630 Calories (kcal); and a McDonald's chocolate shake, 383 Calories (kcal).

• **High protein of good quality**—Fast food establishments get high marks for protein. Such animal products as beef, fish, chicken, pork, cheese, and milk are excellent protein sources. Even a small hamburger supplies 25% of the Recommended Daily Allowance (RDA) of protein for an adult man and 33% of a woman's or child's protein; while a large hamburger topped with cheese, or a shake, will fulfill 60 to 100% of the protein RDA.

• **Mixed marks on vitamins**—Most fast food meals are notoriously low in vitamin A, the best sources of which are dark green, leafy vegetables, yellow or orange vegetables and fruits, whole milk, fortified nonfat dairy products and liver. To assure an adequate amount of vitamin A in your diet on the days you eat fast food, you should balance eating at home with fruit, salad, enriched grains, or milk.

The B-complex vitamins are found in most fast foods in varying amounts. Most fast food meals provide adequate amounts of thiamin (B-1), riboflavin (B-2), niacin, vitamin B-6, and vitamin B-12.

Vitamin C can be gotten from orange juice, sold at some fast food places for breakfast, and, in limited amounts, from cole slaw and french fries.

The addition of salads to some fast food menus has increased the available source of vitamins A and C.

• **High salt**—Fast food is high in sodium. An average fast food meal may contain three-fourths of your recommended daily salt intake. People on a salt-restricted diet will have a problem at a fast food establishment.

• **Low fiber**—Fast food menu items are generally low in fiber, needed in most diets to aid digestion. Fiber is found primarily in fresh fruits and vegetables and in whole grain breads and cereals, most of which are not included on fast food menus.

Some fast food establishments have added salad and cole slaw to their menus, which should provide a source of fiber.

• **Limited selection of items**—A nutritional drawback of fast foods, particularly for frequent consumers, is the limited number of items on many fast food establishment menus, because variety is important for good nutrition. For this reason, meals eaten at fast-service restaurants should be incorporated into a varied diet that includes many other food choices.

From the above, it may be concluded that the good news about fast foods is that it's not all bad news.

(Also see CONVENIENCE AND FAST FOODS.)

FASTING

This is the act of abstaining from food, or of limiting food intake, often by choice. Starvation is to perish from the absence or restriction of food intake, but not always by choice. People who fast do so for a variety of reasons, but whatever the reason, fasting elicits certain metabolic changes, most of which are controlled by hormones.

Actually, everyone fasts day-to-day between meals. Other reasons for fasting include weight loss, religious, medical, and protest.

As always, the prime purpose of the metabolic machinery of the body is to maintain an adequate energy supply to carry on life processes. The major energy source for cells of the body is the carbohydrate, glucose. Without a dietary

source of carbohydrate, the liver reserves of glycogen are adequate for maintaining blood glucose levels for only a few hours. The brain and contracting skeletal muscle require a continuous supply of glucose from the blood, which is normally maintained within very narrow limits—even during fasting. Hence, the body does two primary things during fasting: (1) changes energy sources, and (2) reduces energy expenditures.

(Also see ENDOCRINE GLANDS; HYPOGLYCEMIA; METABOLISM; and STARVATION.)

FAT

The term fat is frequently used in a general sense to include both fats and oils, or a mixture of the two. Both fats and oils have the same general structure and chemical properties, but they have different physical characteristics. The melting points of most fats are such that they are solid at ordinary room temperatures, while oils have lower melting points and are liquids at these temperatures.

(Also see FATS AND OTHER LIPIDS.)

FAT BACK

Solid, relatively uniformly shaped, rectangular fat slabs removed from the surface of the pork loin.

(See PORK.)

FAT, BLOOD

Refers to the total lipid (fat) content of the blood plasma or serum, which is usually 500 to 600 mg/ml.

(Also see BLOOD FATS; and FATS AND OTHER LIPIDS.)

FATS AND OTHER LIPIDS

Fat is easily recognized when it accumulates on the body, but the chemical or technical definitions of fats and lipids are more difficult. Not all lipids are fats but, all fats are lipids, so the two words are often used interchangeably. Like carbohydrates, lipids—fats and fatlike substances, contain the three elements—carbon, hydrogen, and oxygen, but in different proportions—a larger proportion of carbon and hydrogen. As a food, fats function much like carbohydrates in that they serve as a source of heat and energy and contribute to the formation of body fat. Because of the larger pro-

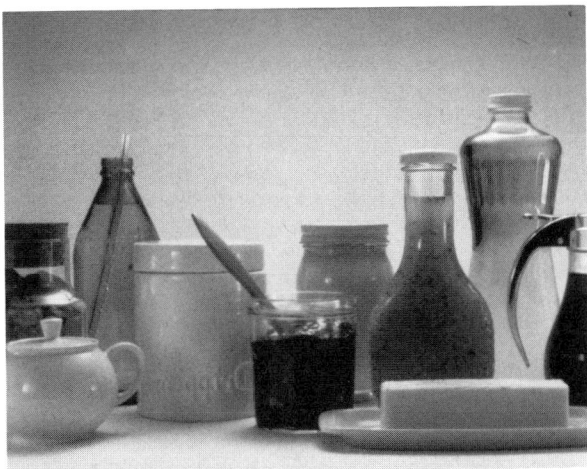

Fig. F-2. Fats and other lipids. (Courtesy, USDA)

portion of carbon and hydrogen, fats liberate more heat—or energy—than carbohydrates or proteins. Upon oxidation, fats liberate approximately 2.25 times as much heat or energy per pound as do carbohydrates or proteins. Hence, they are concentrated energy sources—high in calories, about 900 kcal/100 g.

The general term lipid includes fats, oils, and waxes. Fats are esters (alcohol and acid combinations) of glycerol and fatty acids that are solid at room temperature, while oils are glycerol esters that are liquid at room temperature. However, the term *fats* is often employed for both, to avoid confusion with essential oils and petroleum oils. Waxes are esters of fatty acids with alcohols other than glycerol.

HISTORY. Fats and oils were recognized and used by mankind even before recorded history. Man used fats and oils for food, for soapmaking, for lubrication, for fuel (light and heat), and for cosmetics and medicines. Numerous Biblical passages refer to fats and oils. Indeed, the use of animal fat and oils in cooking was common in Old Testament times (Leviticus 1:8-12 and 2:4-7). Also, the records of the early Egyptians attest to the use of fats and oils. Egyptians used oil preparations from almonds, castor, lettuce seed, linseed, olive, radish seed, safflower seed, and sesame.

SYNTHESIS. Basically, fat synthesis is a process of combining 2-carbon units called *acetyl CoA* into long chains and then adding hydrogen. Acetyl CoA is a step in carbohydrate, protein, and fat metabolism. While a limited amount of fat synthesis occurs in the mitochondria of the cell, most synthesis takes place in the microsomes of adipose (fat) tissue, liver, and many other tissues. Following synthesis, fats may combine with other compounds such as alcohols, proteins, carbohydrates, or phosphorus.

(Also see METABOLISM.)

CLASSIFICATION. Lipids are often classified into three major groups: (1) simple lipids; (2) compound lipids; and (3) derived lipids. When fatty acids are esterified with alcohols, simple lipids result. If compounds such as choline or serine are esterified to alcohols in addition to fatty acids, compound lipids result. The third type of lipid, derived lipids, results from the hydrolysis or enzymatic breakdown of simple and compound lipids.

CHARACTERISTICS OF FATS. Triglycerides—the combination of three fatty acid molecules and a glycerol molecule—account for about 98% of the fats in our foods and over 90% of the fat in the body. The remainder of the diet and body fats is comprised primarily of phospholipids and cholesterol. Since triglycerides and their component fatty acids are so abundant in the diet and body, the discussion which follows centers around fatty acids and triglycerides.

Fatty Acids. Fatty acids are key components of lipids. They are called acids because of the organic acid group (COOH) which they contain. Their degree of saturation and the length of their carbon chain determine many of the physical characteristics of lipids. Numerous triglycerides exist due to the variety of fatty acids which may bind with glycerol.

• **Saturation**—This refers to the ratio of hydrogen atoms to carbon atoms. The backbone of the fatty acid consists of a chain of carbon atoms joined by chemical bonds. When a single bond joins each carbon atom, carbon atoms within the chain have two hydrogen atoms joined to them and carbons at the end of the chain have three hydrogens. When carbon atoms are joined by double bonds, these carbon atoms within the chain are only able to have one hydrogen bound to them. Therefore, saturated fatty acids contain all possible hydrogen and no double bond between carbon atoms. Unsaturated fatty acids contain at least one double bond within the carbon chain (monounsaturated) or two or more double bonds within the carbon chain (polyunsaturated). Therefore, unsaturated fatty acids contain the same number of carbon atoms, but fewer hydrogen atoms than their saturated counterparts. Fig. F-3 illustrates the concept of saturated and unsaturated.

SATURATED

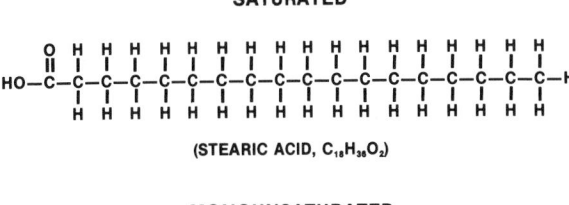

(STEARIC ACID, $C_{18}H_{36}O_2$)

MONOUNSATURATED

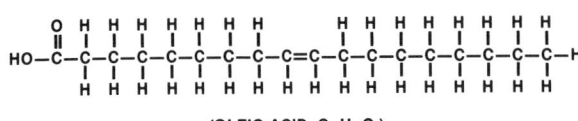

(OLEIC ACID, $C_{18}H_{34}O_2$)

POLYUNSATURATED

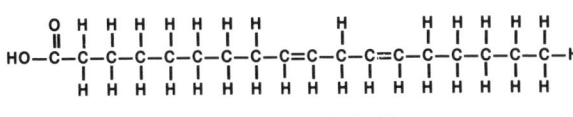

(LINOLEIC ACID, $C_{18}H_{32}O_2$)

Fig. F-3. Three fatty acids all composed of 18 carbons but different degrees of saturation or unsaturation. The = indicates a double bond and C stands for carbon, H for hydrogen, and O for oxygen.

• **Iodine number**—Unsaturated fat readily unites with iodine; two atoms of this element are added to each double bond. Thus, in experimental work, the number of grams of iodine absorbed by a hundred grams of fat—the iodine number—is an excellent criterion of the degree of unsaturation. In the past, the iodine test was commonly used when studying the soft pork problem—a problem caused when pigs are fattened on feeds rich in unsaturated fats, such as peanuts or soybeans. At the present time, the chief measure used in such determinations is the refractive index, as determined by a refractometer.

Fatty acids that are unsaturated have the ability to take up oxygen or certain other chemicals. This presents both advantages and disadvantages. The value of linseed oil and varnish is due to their high content of unsaturated fatty acids, by virtue of which oxygen is absorbed when they are exposed to air, resulting in a tough, resistant coating. On the other hand, because of their unsaturation fats often become rancid through oxidation, resulting in disagreeable flavors and odors which lessen their desirability as foods.

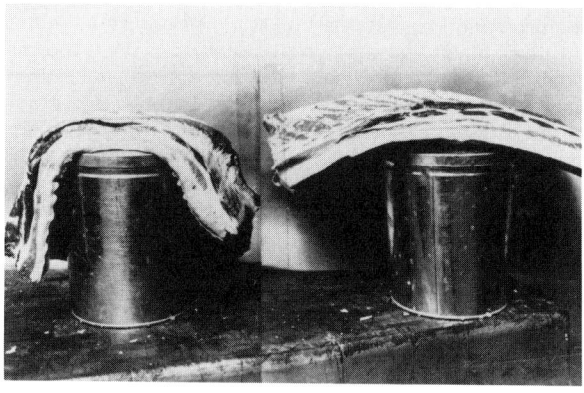

Fig. F-4. Soft pork. The bacon belly on the left came from a hog liberally fed on soybeans. Feed fats affect body fats. (Courtesy, University of Illinois)

• **Rancidity**—This is the oxidation (decomposition) primarily of unsaturated fatty acids resulting in disagreeable flavors and odors in fats and oils. This process occurs slowly and spontaneously, and it is accelerated by light, heat, and certain minerals. Rancidity may be prevented through proper storage and/or the addition of antioxidants such as sodium benzoate. Some fats are naturally protected from oxidation due to the presence of vitamin E. Hydrogenation of fats (adding hydrogen to unsaturated fatty acids) also lessens the threat of rancidity. This process has been used to improve the keeping qualities of vegetable shortenings and lard.
(Also see ADDITIVES.)

• **Effects of heat**—*Acrolein* is a pungent compound produced from glycerol. It is especially irritating to the lining of the gastrointestinal tract and it may be produced by excessive heating of fats. However, normal home or commercial frying usually does not represent a hazard.

• **Hydrogenation**—This process adds hydrogen to the double bonds of unsaturated fatty acids. It is accomplished with hydrogen gas in the presence of a nickel catalyst. The result of hydrogenation is a harder fat since adding hydrogen increases the melting temperature. It may be used on animal or vegetable fats to produce fats with a desired hardness. Many vegetable oils are converted into a solid or semisolid form for use in shortenings and margarines. Not surprisingly, hydrogenation is also known as hardening.

Hydrogenation may have one drawback. It converts the naturally-occurring *cis* fatty acids to *trans* fatty acids. The prefixes *cis* and *trans* refer to the orientation of the atoms around the double bond. The *trans* form of essential fatty acids does *not* function as an essential fatty acid in the body. Also, some researchers have found that (1) *trans* fatty acids are not as effective as their *cis* analogs in lowering blood cholesterol, and (2) fats rich in *trans* fatty acids appear to promote atherosclerosis.[1]

The content of *trans* fatty acids generally increases with the extent to which a vegetable oil has been hydrogenated. For example, hard sticks of vegetable oil margarines may contain from 25 to 35% of *trans* fats, whereas lightly hydrogenated liquid oils usually contain 5% or less of these fats.
(Also see TRANS FATTY ACIDS.)

• **Carbon chain length**—Another variable factor in the makeup of fatty acid molecules is the number of carbon atoms. Fatty acids are designated as having (1) short chains when the number of carbon atoms is 6 or less, (2) medium chains when there are 8 or 10 carbon atoms, and (3) long chains when there are 12 or more carbon atoms. In most cases, naturally-occurring fatty acids contain an even number of carbon atoms.

Together, the degree of saturation and the length of the carbon chain, influence the melting point of fats. The melting points of fats are very important in nutrition, since fats that remain solid in the digestive tract are poorly utilized. Furthermore, the melting points are important to food processors because (1) consumers expect certain items to be solid at ordinary room temperatures, and others to be liquid; and (2) most shortenings should be at least semisolid at room temperature because flakiness of pastry depends upon the production of layers of solid fat.

The melting points of fatty acids are highly dependent on the length of the carbon chain and the degree of unsaturation of the molecule. Short fatty acids tend to be more volatile. In fact, acetic, propionic, and butyric acid are collectively called volatile fatty acids (VFA). There is a steady rise in melting point as the chain lengths increase. However, as the number of double bonds increases, the melting point decreases.

• **Saponification**—The combination of a fatty acid with a cation such as potassium or sodium forms soap. This reaction is called *saponification*. Besides forming soap, it is a method of evaluating the average length of carbon chain in the fatty acids which constitute a fat. The test is performed by reacting fats with potassium hydroxide (an alkali). The saponification number, or value, is the number of milligrams of potassium hydroxide required for the complete saponification of 1 g of the fat. A high saponification value signifies a short chain length and vice versa.

Saponification may also occur in the alkaline medium of the intestine. For example, calcium may combine with free fatty acids.

• **Emulsification**—Fats (oils) and water do not stay mixed, but often it is desirable for them to do so. Therefore, fats are often emulsified. Minute droplets of fats or oils are evenly distributed throughout a water-based solution. Emul-

---

[1]"Newer Concepts of Coronary Heart Disease," *Dairy Council Digest*, Vol. 45, 1974, p. 33.

sions are essential for the digestion, absorption, and transport of fats in the body. Furthermore, emulsification is employed in homogenized milk and other products containing fats or oils such as mayonnaise. Emulsifying agents used to create emulsions include some fatlike and fat-derived substances such as monoglycerides (glycerol with one fatty acid), diglycerides (glycerol with two fatty acids), lecithin and the bile salts.

Other Lipids. Other important lipids include primarily the phospholipids, lipoproteins, and cholesterol. All cells contain phospholipids. They are structural compounds found in cell membranes and in the blood. The brain, nerves, and liver contain particularly high levels. Lecithin is one of the most abundant phospholipids in the diet and the body. Phospholipids are powerful emulsifying agents. Lipoproteins are the primary vehicle for lipid transport in the blood. There are four main types: chylomicrons; very low density lipoproteins (VLDL); low density lipoproteins (LDL); and high density lipoproteins (HDL). Cholesterol is derived from the diet or synthesized in the body. It is necessary for the formation of hormones and bile salts. These will all be discussed in sections which follow.

(Also see CHOLESTEROL.)

DIGESTION, ABSORPTION, AND METABOLISM.
Compared to the digestion of carbohydrates and proteins, the digestion of fats is unique. Before the enzymes of the pancreas and intestine can act on the fats, they are mixed with bile. Fats are not water-soluble. Since enzymatic reactions of the body occur in water-based solution, fats must be emulsified for digestion to occur. Bile salts from the gallbladder play two roles in fat digestion: (1) they act as a detergent decreasing the surface tension, and (2) they form micelles which are colloidal complexes of monoglycerides and insoluble fatty acids that have been emulsified and solubilized for absorption. It is the detergent action of bile which allows the mixing movements of the intestines to break the fat globules into very finely emulsified (water-oil mixture) particles with a greatly increased surface area on which the water-soluble enzymes—lipases—can act. When lipids, emulsified by bile salts, come into contact with the various lipases that are found in the small intestine, they are broken down into diglycerides, monoglycerides, fatty acids, and glycerol. Short-chain fatty acids, less than 10 to 12 carbon atoms, are absorbed directly into the mucosa—lining—of the small intestine and are transported to the portal circulation of the liver. Monoglycerides and insoluble fatty acids are emulsified by bile salts, forming micelles. By attaching to the surface of epithelial cells, the micelles enable these components to be absorbed into the intestinal cells. Once inside these cells, the long-chain fatty acids are reesterified (joined to the alcohol, glycerol) to form triglycerides. Triglycerides then combine with cholesterol, lipoproteins, and phospholipids to form chylomicrons—minute fat droplets. The chylomicrons are then passed into the lymphatic system. Eventually these chylomicrons enter the blood where they are transported to the tissues of the body. Adipose tissue (fat) is the major site for the removal of chylomicron triglycerides. Here the fatty acids are cleaved by the enzyme lipoprotein lipase and taken into the cells. Also, chylomicrons, phospholipids, free fatty acids, cholesterol, and proteins are transported to the liver and formed into other lipoproteins, which provide the major vehicle for the transport of fat in the blood. These lipoproteins include the following: (1) prebeta lipoproteins or very low-density lipoproteins (VLDL); (2) beta lipoproteins or low-density lipoproteins (LDL); and (3) alpha lipoproteins or high-density lipoproteins (HDL).

Fat provides energy to the body. The free fatty acids (FFA) transported in the blood can be oxidized by most cells to release energy. The final products of oxidation are water and carbon dioxide. Dietary fats, carbohydrates, and protein may all contribute to the synthesis of fats within the body.

(Also see CHOLESTEROL; DIGESTION AND ABSORPTION; and METABOLISM.)

FUNCTIONS. In general, fat performs four functions in the body. It provides (1) energy, (2) essential fatty acids, (3) structural components, and (4) regulatory functions.

1. **Energy.** The cells of the body, except for red blood cells and those of the central nervous system, can utilize fatty acids directly as a source of energy. Although carbohydrate (glucose) is the energy source normally used by the nervous system, the brain can utilize ketone bodies that are formed from fatty acids during a period of fasting.

Most food fats are triglycerides, but some also contain phospholipids and cholesterol. Regardless of the fat type, fats are readily digested by healthy individuals. Any excess of energy, whether derived from dietary carbohydrate, protein, or fat, is stored as triglycerides within the adipose cells of the body. Adipose cells are found beneath the skin, between muscle fibers, around abdominal organs and their supporting structures called mesenteries, and around joints. As an energy storage form, it stores in the same weight 2.25 times as much energy as protein or carbohydrate. Fat or adipose is in a continuous turnover state—a dynamic state—which is controlled by the hormones: insulin, growth hormone, epinephrine, adrenocorticotropic hormone (ACTH), and glucagon.

The immediate sources of energy for the body are the free fatty acids in the circulation liberated from adipose triglycerides by the enzyme lipase. These free fatty acids are oxidized or burned by a systematic process called beta-oxidation, whereby 2-carbon fragments are successively cleaved from the fatty acid molecule to form acetyl CoA which releases energy upon completing the Krebs cycle (TCA cycle).

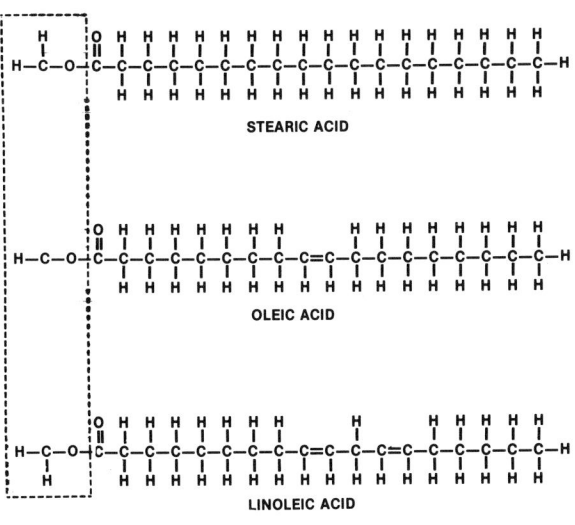

Fig. F-5. A triglyceride containing a saturated, a monosaturated, and a polyunsaturated fatty acid.

2. **Essential fatty acid.** The body has a remarkable ability to synthesize many compounds, and, as has already been pointed out, excess protein and carbohydrates can be converted to fat. However, in 1929, G. M. Burr and M. M. Burr at the University of Minnesota, reported that rats fed a fat-free diet (the diet was adequate in all other nutrients) failed to grow, lost weight, developed scaly skin and kidney damage, and eventually died. These conditions could be prevented or reversed if linoleic acid was added to their diet. Similarly, Hansen found that the inclusion of essential fatty acids in the diet of infants who had eczema led to improvement in the skin and to greater gains in weight (see Fig. F-6). Thus, the concept of essential—not synthesized by the body—fatty acids was introduced.

For many years, three polyunsaturated fatty acids—linoleic acid, linolenic acid, and arachidonic acid—were considered essential fatty acids because they are essential for certain body functioning, and because it seemed that the body could not synthesize them. However, recent research has shown (1) that linolenic acid has relatively little effect in relieving the skin lesions originally associated with a deficiency of essential acids, and (2) that arachidonic acid can be synthesized by the body from linoleic acid and, therefore, does not have to be supplied as such in the diet. (It is noteworthy, however, that recent work indicates that members of the cat family may require arachidonic acid.) So, presently, linoleic acid, the 18-carbon polyunsaturated acid with two double bonds, found widely in foods of both plant and animal origin, may be considered as the only essential fatty acid; it cannot be synthesized in the body and must be present in the diet. Nevertheless, the three fatty acids—linoleic, linolenic, and arachidonic—serve important functions in the body. Deficiency symptoms of these fatty acids have been observed in human infants, and in dogs, guinea pigs, mice, poultry, and swine. Depending on the type of animal, numerous manifestations of these deficiencies are seen; among them, dermatitis, reduced growth, increased water consumption and retention, impaired reproduction and increased metabolic rate.

In the body, linoleic acid is converted to longer-chain fatty acids with three, four, and five double bonds, which are essential components of membranes. In infants fed formulas, the primary symptom noted in essential fatty acid deficiency is drying and flaking of the skin. A fatty acid deficiency in adult humans was unknown until recently. In the past several years, there have been numerous reports of such deficiency being produced inadvertently in hospitalized patients, both infants and adults, fed exclusively by intravenous fluids not containing fat.

Fatty acids in phospholipids are important for maintaining the function and integrity of cellular and subcellular membranes. These acids also play a role in the regulation of cholesterol metabolism—especially its transport, breakdown, and ultimate excretion. In addition, fatty acids have been shown to be the precursors for a group of hormonelike compounds called prostaglandins, which are important in the regulation of widely diverse physiological processes.

(Also see the subsequent section headed, "Essential Fatty Acids.")

3. **Structural components.** Although excessive storage of fat becomes unsightly and burdensome, some body fat is necessary. Indeed, the feminine features owe much to the proper amounts and locations of fat deposits. Body fat (1) holds organs in place, (2) absorbs shock, and (3) insulates the body against rapid temperature changes or excessive heat loss. Furthermore, lipids, in particular phospholipids, have an important role in the structural integrity of the cell membrane. Phospholipids are water soluble and may aid in the transport of other fats in and out of cells.

4. **Regulatory functions.** Often the acceptance of food and its palatability depends upon flavor and aroma. Although triglycerides in the pure state are relatively tasteless, they absorb and retain flavors of foods. Furthermore, in combination with other nutrients, fats provide a texture that enhances palatability, and they delay emptying of the stomach and contribute to a feeling of satiety. Cholesterol is a fatlike compound with a rather sordid history, but it is the chemical ancestor of the hormones of the adrenal glands, ovaries and testes—the steroid hormones—and the bile salts. The prostaglandins are fatlike, hormonelike substances derived from the essential fatty acids and involved in the control of reproduction and circulation. Finally, dietary fat serves as a carrier for the fat-soluble vitamins A, D, E, and K, and as an aid to their absorption in the intestine.

(Also see CHOLESTEROL; DIGESTION AND ABSORPTION; ENDOCRINE GLANDS; METABOLISM; and VITAMIN[S].)

REQUIRED INTAKE. There is no required intake of fats and other lipids, and it seems that the body is capable of adapting to a wide range of intakes. During World War II, the fat intake of Japanese soldiers amounted to only 3% of their total energy intake. Worldwide, fat intake varies dramatically. In many developing countries fat intake is, and has been for many generations, 10 to 20% of the energy intake, while in developed countries dietary fat intake ranges from 35 to 45% of the total energy intake. In general, the consumption of fat increases with increasing per capita income. This observation probably contributed to such expressions as "living off the fat of the land," "fat cat," and

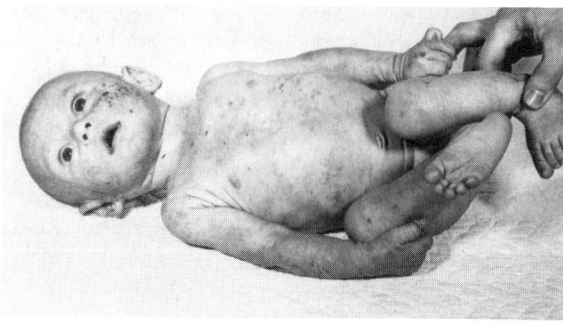

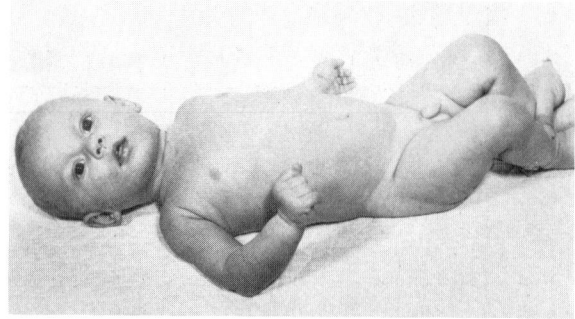

Fig. F-6. Fatty acid made the difference! Above, infant with very resistant eczema (eruption of the skin) since 2½ months of age. Below, the same child 1 month later, after adding linoleic acid (fresh lard) to the diet. (Courtesy, Dr. A. E. Hansen, University of Texas, Medical Branch, Galveston, Tex.)

"fat city." In the United States, fat consumption has increased since the turn of the century, and now amounts to about 42% of the total calories.

Dietary fats are mainly triglycerides composed of fatty acids of varying chain length and degree of saturation or unsaturation. The proportion of saturated fat and unsaturated fat in the diet has shifted. Vegetable fats are a major source of the increase in unsaturated fatty acids.

Recommended Fat Intakes. Many nutritionists and physicians believe that the health of a significant proportion of the United States population could be improved by changes in life style, including dietary modifications. Although some of the proposed changes in diet are currently controversial, there is sufficient evidence to support some recommendations for dietary changes that would be consonant with better health. It should be emphasized that most chronic or degenerative diseases have a number of contributing factors, only one of which may be diet. Changes in diet only, without consideration of measures to alter other risk factors—heredity, smoking, stress, high blood pressure and obesity—will probably have minimal desirable effects.

Associated with diet and nutritional practices is the problem of obesity and general overweight. In the Ten State Nutrition Survey conducted by the U.S. Department of Health, Education, and Welfare, it was found that up to 25% of adult males and 42% of females are classified as obese. Reduction in body weight to the desirable level is considered to be one of the most beneficial measures related to diets that the U.S. population could implement. For much of the U.S. population, maintenance of desirable body weight could be achieved most readily by controlling caloric intake and increasing physical activity. Since fat has the highest caloric density (kcal/g) of the nutrients, a decrease in fat consumption can produce the greatest change in dietary energy.

The Food and Nutrition Board's Committee on Diet and Health recommends that the fat content of the U.S. diet not exceed 30% of caloric intake, that less than 10% of the calories should be provided from saturated fatty acids, and that dietary cholesterol should be less than 300 mg/day.

• **Ketogenic diets**—At times an increased fat intake is recommended. Diets high in fat and low in carbohydrate are termed ketogenic since they cause the accumulation of ketone bodies—acetoacetic acid, beta hydroxybutyric acid and acetone—in the tissues. These diets eliminate carbohydrate sources such as breads, cereals, fruits, desserts, sweets, and sugar-containing beverages, while foods high in fat such as butter, cream, bacon, mayonnaise, and salad dressing are eaten in generous amounts. Ketones are produced from the breakdown (oxidation) of fats. When the ratio of fatty acids to available glucose in the diet exceeds 2:1, ketosis occurs. It is the metabolism of glucose that normally allows fatty acids to be completely oxidized to water and carbon dioxide rather than to ketone bodies. A ketogenic diet is considered monotonous, unpalatable, and most times undesirable. However, a ketogenic diet may be prescribed to control epilepsy, if drugs prove ineffective. Recently, medium chain triglycerides (MCT) have been shown to induce ketosis more readily than regular fats.

(Also see MODIFIED DIETS, Table M-28, Modified Diets—Ketogenic diet.)

Essential Fatty Acids. Past editions of the *Recommended Dietary Allowances* by the Food and Nutrition Board of the NRC have not proposed a recommended intake of essential fatty acid other than that needed to meet the requirement of 1 to 2% of calories. However, the American Academy of Pediatrics has recommended that infant formulas provide at least 2.7% of energy as linoleic acid.[2] For the average adult, a minimally adequate intake of linoleic acid is 3 to 6 g/day. This level is more than met by diets in the United States, since most vegetable oils are particularly rich sources of linoleic acid. In several studies, linoleic acid has been found to range from 5 to 10% of calories in diets providing 25 to 50% of energy as fat. For those consuming diets high in fat, there is evidence that a higher intake of linoleic acid may have beneficial health effects for a significant fraction of the population. These health effects relate to the possible prevention of atherosclerosis, coronary heart disease, and elevated blood lipids. Some rich sources of linoleic acid are listed in Table F-1.

TABLE F-1
RICH SOURCES OF THE ESSENTIAL FATTY ACID LINOLEIC ACID

Source	Linoleic Acid
	(g/100 g)
Safflower oil	73
Corn oil	57
Cottonseed oil	50
Soybean oil	50
Sesame oil	40
Black walnuts	37
English walnuts	35
Sunflower seeds	30
Brazil nuts	25
Margarine[1]	22
Pumpkin and squash seeds	20
Spanish peanuts	16
Peanut butter	15
Almonds	10

[1]May vary depending upon the source of oil used.

Until recently, linoleic acid, an N-6 fatty acid, commonly found in vegetable oils and many other foods, was deemed to be the primary essential fatty acid, together with its derivative N-6 fatty acids, of which arachidonic acid was the most important. However, recent studies indicate that two classes of fatty acids are essential for health; that, in addition to the N-6 fatty acids, the highly polyunsaturated N-3 fatty acids are needed, including alpha linolenic acid and its longer-chained, more polyunsaturated derivative, docosahexaenoic acid. The N-3 fatty acids are also contained in a wide variety of natural foodstuffs, including soybean oil and rapeseed (canola) oil, and in green leafy vegetables. The higher derivative, docosahexaenoic acid, is found in shellfish and fish. Docosahexaenoic acid is abundant in the brain, retina, and spermatozoa.

(Also see FISH AND SEAFOOD[S] section on "Nutritive Qualities of Fish and Seafood.")

[2]*Recommended Dietary Allowances*, National Research Council, 10th ed., National Academy Press, 1989, p. 48.

Polyunsaturated vs Saturated. Some studies have shown that increasing the amount of polyunsaturated (PUFA) fat—linoleic acid, linolenic acid, and arachidonic acid—in the diet while reducing the saturated fat sometimes promotes a modest drop in blood cholesterol and a reduction in the tendency of blood to clot. Of greater importance than increased PUFA intake, however, is the ratio of polyun-

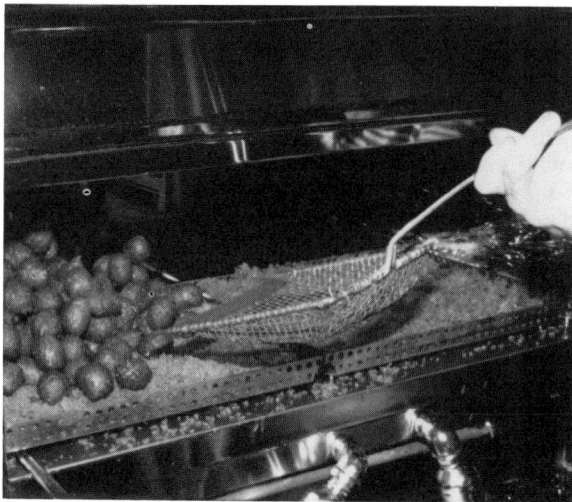

Fig. F-7. Donut holes being fried in soybean oil, a polyunsaturated fat. (Courtesy, American Soybean Assn., St. Louis, Mo.)

saturated fats to saturated fatty acids—the P/S ratio. Currently, the recommendation is for a P/S ratio ranging from 1:1 to 2:1. The basis for this recommendation is that some studies demonstrate increased blood cholesterol levels when the intake of saturated fatty acids is high, and that increasing the linoleic acid counteracts this effect. In all types of hyperlipoproteinemias—conditions of elevated blood lipids—an increase in PUFA is recommended. However, increasing the PUFA in the diet is not without possible problems; among them, the following should be considered:

1. Arachidonic acid, a polyunsaturated fatty acid, found mainly in peanut oil, promotes clotting.

2. The effects of polyunsaturated fatty acids on the heart muscle are uncertain, since it has been found that the lifetime feeding of corn, cottonseed, or soybean oils produced more heart lesions in rats than beef fat, butter, chicken fat, or lard.

3. The drop in blood cholesterol may be due mainly to a shifting of the cholesterol from the blood to the tissues.

4. Polyunsaturated fats cause an increase in the amount of cholesterol secreted in the bile, a condition that sometimes leads to the formation of cholesterol gallstones.

5. Extra vitamin E is required to prevent the formation of toxic peroxides in the body when the dietary level of polyunsaturated fats is raised. However, diets containing ample amounts of the essential trace mineral selenium, which is a part of the enzyme that breaks down the peroxides, may also help to offset this danger. The formation of peroxides may contribute to the cocarcinogenic activity observed in some animal studies.

To date, the National Research Council has not established Recommended Daily Allowances for PUFA. However, an upper limit of 10% of the dietary energy as PUFA is considered safe. For a man consuming 2,700 Calories (kcal) or a woman consuming 2,000 Calories (kcal), this translates to 30 g and 22 g per day, respectively.

For individuals interested in determining or altering their saturated and polyunsaturated intake, Table F-4, Fats & Fatty Acids in Selected Foods, at the end of this article gives values for a variety of common foods. Table F-2 lists common food sources for saturated and polyunsaturated fats.

NOTE WELL: As a rule of thumb, animal fats are traditionally considered as containing high levels of saturated fat. However, Table F-2 shows some exceptions. Palm oil and coconut oil—both vegetable fats—contain high levels of saturated fats while cod liver oil, an animal fat, contains a high level of polyunsaturated fat.

(Also see HYPERLIPOPROTEINEMIAS.)

SOURCES. Worldwide, soybean oil is the world's largest volume oil product, palm oil is the second largest, and rapeseed (canola) oil ranks third.

In 1990, the average U.S. per capita consumption of fats from all sources—visible sources—was about 63 lb *(29 kg)*, or in terms of energy about 261,000 Calories (kcal). This figure includes butter, margarine, lard, shortening, and salad and cooking oils.

Visible and Invisible. Visible fats are those which have been separated from their source and can be readily identified and measured; for example, lard, butter, margarine, shortening, and salad and cooking oils. Invisible fats are those which are not separated from their source. Sometimes these are called hidden fats. Invisible fats includes the fats of meats, eggs, cheese, milk, nuts, and cereals. Thus, the total fat consumed by an individual is at best a good estimate. The fat content of those foods with invisible fat is given in Food Composition Table F-21 for numerous foods.

TABLE F-2
SOME COMMON FOOD SOURCES OF SATURATED AND POLYUNSATURATED FATS[1]

Food Source	Saturated Fats	Food Source	Poly-unsaturated Fats
	(g/100 g)		(g/100 g)
Coconut oil	87	Safflower oil	75
Butter	51	Sunflowerseed oil	66
Palm oil	49	Wheat germ oil	62
Beef tallow	48	Corn oil	59
Mutton tallow	47	Soybean oil	58
Lard	39	Cottonseed oil	52
Baking chocolate	30	Cod liver oil[2]	50
Chicken fat	30	Walnuts	42
Shortening[1]	25	Peanut oil	32
Cream cheese	22	Shortening[1]	26
Cheddar cheese	21	Brazil nuts	25
Pasteurized process cheese	20	Chicken fat	20
Beef, rib cuts	19	Margarine	18
Margarine	19	Peanuts	14
Brazil nuts	17	Peanut butter	12
Peanut oil	17	Lard	11
Lamb chops	16	Almonds	10
Soybean oil	14	Palm oil	9
Olive oil	14	Olive oil	8
Sour cream	13	Mutton tallow	8
Pork sausage	12	Wheat germ	7
Pork chops	11	Beef tallow	4
Hamburger	10	Pork chops	4

[1]Household shortening made from hydrogenated soybean and cottonseed oil.

[2]Primarily contains polyunsaturated fats with carbon chain lengths of 20 and 22 carbons.

Table F-4, Fats & Fatty Acids In Selected Foods, at the end of this article, also lists a variety of foods and gives their saturated, polyunsaturated, oleic, linoleic, and cholesterol content. Table F-3 provides examples of the hidden fat in some foods.

TABLE F-3
HIDDEN FAT OF SOME FOODS

Food	Fat	Food	Fat
	(%)		(%)
Brazil nuts	67	Lamb roast	19
Walnuts	61	Avocado	16
Almonds	54	Ice cream	13
Peanuts	50	Herring	12
Sunflower seeds	47	Poached eggs	11
Pork sausage	44	Tuna, canned	8
Pork roast	30	Poultry, dark meat	7
Cheese	30	Oatmeal, dry	7
Bologna	28	Salmon	6
Beef roast	25	Whole milk	4
Ham, cured	22	Poultry, light meat	4
Hamburger	20	Shredded wheat cereal	2

Animal and Vegetable. Fats in the diet are derived from either animal sources or plant—vegetable—sources. Both are comprised mainly of mixtures of triglycerides.

The comparative food value of animal fats and vegetable oils has long been a stormy issue, particularly in regard to the relative merits of butter vs oleomargarine and of lard vs vegetable shortenings. In general, except for the vitamins that they carry, there is no experimental work to indicate that, as a source of fatty acids, animal fats are superior to vegetable oils. There is reason to believe that margarine, when fortified with vitamins A and D, is— from the nutritional standpoint—just as effective as butter in promoting growth, good health, reproduction, and lactation.

Fats or oils, regardless of their origin from animals or vegetables, furnish about 9 Calories (kcal) per gram. They are all concentrated energy sources containing 2.25 times more energy than carbohydrates or protein. The major differences between plant and animal fats are: (1) plant fats or vegetable oils are higher in polyunsaturated fatty acids, and (2) plant fats do not contain cholesterol. However, there are several exceptions. Cocoa butter, coconut oil, and the palm oils, contain high levels of saturated fats. Marine animals and fish may be rich in unsaturated fats.

Over the years, consumption patterns for vegetable and animal fats have shifted as illustrated in Fig. F-10. While total fat consumption has risen a little, there has been a marked drop in the consumption of animal fat with a corresponding rise in vegetable oil consumption. These shifts may, in part, be explained by (1) educational and media programs encouraging consumers to cut back on saturated fats and cholesterol, (2) changing tastes, and (3) increased availability of vegetable oils such as corn, soybean, peanut, safflower, sunflower, and coconut. Additionally, vegetable oils are the best food source of the natural antioxidant, vitamin E. For example, the amount of vitamin E, in mg per 100 g of oil, supplied by some typical oils are as follows: wheat germ, 150; safflower, 34; cottonseed, 35; peanut, 12; corn, 14; and soybean, 11.

(Also see MEAT[S]; OILS, VEGETABLE; and VITAMIN E.)

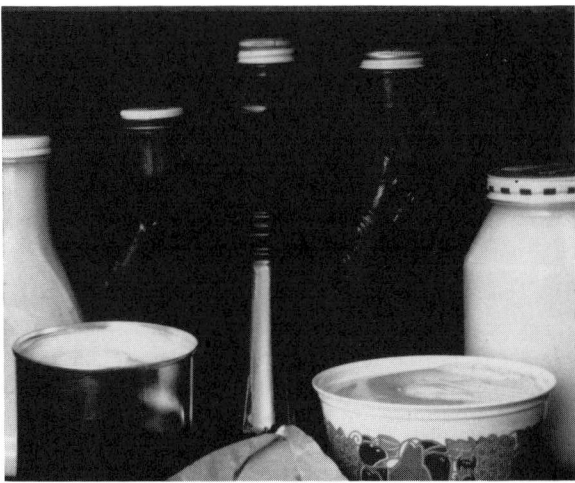

Fig. F-8. Some vegetable fats. (Courtesy, American Soybean Assn., St. Louis, Mo.)

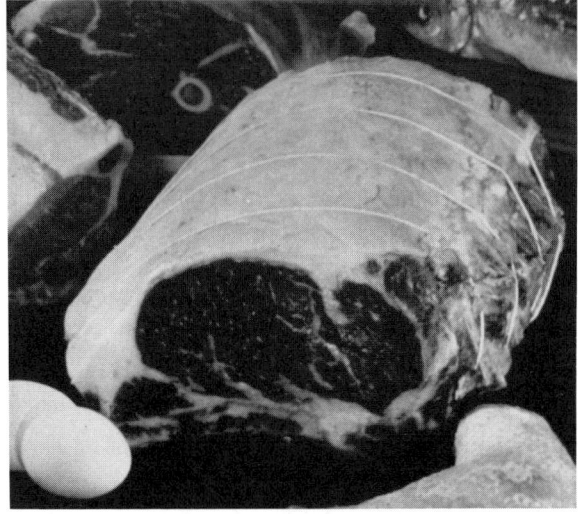

Fig. F-9. Some animal fats. (Courtesy, National Live Stock and Meat Board)

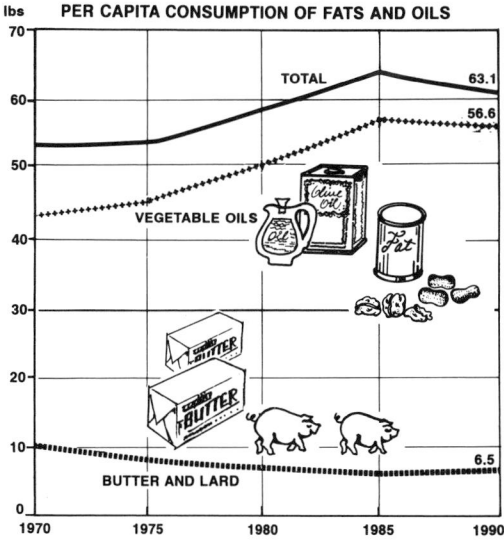

Fig. F-10. Per capita consumption of fats and oils. Animal fats include butter and lard. (Courtesy, USDA)

Medium-Chain Triglycerides (MCT). This is a special dietary product. It is made from coconut oil by (1) steam and pressure hydrolysis of the oil into free fatty acids and glycerol, (2) fractionation of the resulting hydrolysate into medium-chain and long-chain fatty acids, and (3) recombination of the medium-chain fatty acids with glycerol to form MCT oil, which is made up of about ¾ caprylic acid (a saturated fatty acid containing 8 carbon atoms) and about ¼ capric acid (a saturated fatty acid containing 10 carbon atoms). The special nutritive values of this product are as follows:

1. It is much more readily digested, absorbed, and metabolized than either animal fats or vegetable oils which contain mainly long-chain triglycerides. Hence, MCT oil is valuable in the dietary treatment of fatty diarrhea and other digestive disorders in which the absorption of fat is impaired—malabsorption syndrome.

2. Medium-chain triglycerides, unlike other saturated fats, do *not* contribute to a rise in blood cholesterol. Hence, they are used in the treatment of some hyperlipoprotein-emias.

At the present time, MCT oil is used almost exclusively for special dietary formulations in the United States, but it is also available in various nonmedical consumer products in Europe.

Nonnutritive Oils. Mineral oils are lubricating oils derived from petroleum and hydrocarbons—hydrogen and carbon-containing—but completely indigestible. In the past, mineral oil has been used to replace other digestible fats in low-calorie diets, and as a laxative. Its use is discouraged because it interferes with the absorption of the fat-soluble vitamins from the intestine.

FAT AND HEALTH PROBLEMS. Fats either cause heart disease or cancer—or so it seems.[3] As for coronary heart disease, the blame on fats arises primarily from two factors: (1) atherosclerotic deposits in blood vessels are composed of cholesterol and other fatty substances; and (2) increases in certain fat components of the blood contribute to atherosclerosis. Fats are transported in the blood in the form of lipid-protein complexes—lipoproteins. It is the blood levels of cholesterol, triglycerides, and certain lipoproteins which are considered risk factors in the development of heart disease.

Fats in the Blood. Fats are not very soluble in the blood. Therefore, they are transported in the blood as water soluble lipoproteins, all of which contain phospholipids, triglycerides, and cholesterol.

Levels of lipoproteins in the blood are controlled by (1) diet, (2) a number of hormones, (3) age, (4) weight change, (5) emotions and stress, (6) exercise, (7) drugs, (8) illness, and (9) heredity. Excessive concentration of one or more of the lipoproteins is termed hyperlipoproteinemia. There are six of these: (1) hyperchylomicronemia; (2) hyperbeta-lipoproteinemia or hypercholesterolemia; (3) hyperlipidemia or hypercholesterolemia with hyperglyceridemia; (4) broad beta; (5) hyperbetaliproteinemia; and (6) mixed hyperlipidemia. These hyperlipoproteinemias cause numerous health problems; among them, heart disease and accelerated atherosclerosis.

(Also see HYPERLIPOPROTEINEMIAS.)

The Lipid Hypothesis. The lipid hypothesis is based on the following observations:

1. Plaques are rich in cholesterol.

2. Populations with a high average serum cholesterol level tend to have a higher rate of coronary heart disease (CHD).

3. When fed a high cholesterol diet, some laboratory animals develop a type of arterial disease.

The basic assumption underlying this hypothesis is that high serum cholesterol levels cause infiltration of cholesterol into the inner lining of the artery (*intima*) where it causes plaque development. The cholesterol is thought to initiate migration of smooth muscle cells and accumulation of other substances, such as lipids and calcium, which eventually lead to protrusion of a plaque into the artery.

In 1980, Dr. Keys suggested that, depending on the cholesterol levels in the blood, we may have the choice of two fates: (1) high cholesterol and die from a heart attack; or (2) low cholesterol and die from cancer—the second leading cause of death.[4]

Fat and Health Summary. That the form of dietary fat is implicated in atherosclerosis is well documented by unbiased, controlled experiments stemming from the research initiated by Dr. Ancel Keys.

In summary, the following dietary fats are health related:

Cholesterol: A sterol found in animal tissue, synthesized in the body, and consumed in the diet. High cholesterol increases coronary heart disease (CHD) risk.

Saturated fat: Fatty acids with no double bonds, such as stearic and palmitic acids, which increase serum cholesterol along with increased CHD risk.

Monounsaturated fat: Fatty acids with one double bond, such as oleic acid, which has a favorable effect on CHD risk, because they lower the harmful low density lipoproteins (LDL) without affecting the protective high density lipoproteins (HDL).

Polyunsaturated fat: Fatty acids with two or more double bonds, such as the essential fatty acids linoleic and alpha-linolenic acids, which should be consumed in moderation, because they lower both the harmful LDL and the beneficial HDL cholesterol.

Other fats: This includes the saturated and polyunsaturated fatty acids that are outside the above definitions.

(Also see CANCER; CHOLESTEROL; and HEART DISEASE.)

FATS AND FATTY ACIDS IN SELECTED FOODS. Table F-4, Fats & Fatty Acids in Selected Foods, provides information on the total fat, animal fat, plant fat, saturated fat, polyunsaturated fat, oleic acid, linolenic acid, and cholesterol content of a variety of foods. As with any food composition data, the values contained in this table are not absolutes, but guidelines. They are meant to aid individuals who must or wish to alter or control their dietary fat intake.

[3]Kolata, G. B., "Data Sought on Low Cholesterol and Cancer," *Science,* Vol. 211, 1981, pp. 1410-1411.

[4]"HDL's: Possible Role In Cancer," *Science News,* Vol. 118, 1980, p. 246.

TABLE F-4
FATS & FATTY ACIDS IN SELECTED FOODS[1]

Food Name—100 Gram (3.5 oz) Portion	Water	Food Energy Calories	Total Fat	Animal Fat	Plant Fat	Saturated Fat	Polyunsaturated Fat	Fatty Acids Oleic Acid	Linoleic Acid	Cholesterol	Choline
	(g)	(kcal)	(g)	(g)	(g)	(g)	(g)	(g)	(g)	(mg)	(mg)
EGGS & SUBSTITUTES											
EGG, WHOLE, fresh & frozen, raw	74.6	158	11.1	11.1	0	3.4	1.5	4.1	1.2	548	—
WHITE, fresh & frozen, raw	88.1	49	Trace	Trace	0	0	0	0	0	0	—
YOLK, fresh, raw	48.8	369	32.9	32.9	0	9.9	4.3	12.1	3.7	1602	—
WHOLE, FRIED, in butter	71.9	180	13.9	13.9	0	5.2	1.5	4.7	1.3	534	—
WHOLE, HARD-COOKED	74.6	158	11.1	11.1	0	3.4	1.5	4.1	1.2	548	—
OMELET, made w/one large egg, butter & milk	76.3	148	11.1	11.1	0	4.4	1.1	3.7	0.9	388	—
WHOLE, POACHED	74.3	157	11.1	11.1	0	3.3	1.4	4.1	1.2	545	—
WHOLE, SCRAMBLED, w/butter & milk	76.3	148	11.1	11.1	0	4.4	1.1	3.7	0.9	388	—
WHOLE, DRIED	4.1	594	41.8	41.8	0	12.6	5.4	15.3	4.6	1918	—
WHOLE, DRIED, stabilized	1.9	615	44.0	44.0	0	13.2	5.7	16.1	4.9	2017	—
EGGNOG	74.4	135	7.5	7.5	0	4.4	0.3	2.0	0.2	59	—
DUCK EGG, whole, fresh, raw	70.8	185	13.8	13.8	0	3.7	1.2	6.1	0.6	884	—
GOOSE EGG, whole, fresh, raw	70.4	185	13.3	13.3	0	3.6	1.7	5.4	0.7	—	—
QUAIL EGG, whole, fresh, raw	74.3	158	11.1	11.1	0	3.6	1.3	3.9	0.9	844	—
TURKEY EGG, whole, fresh, raw	72.5	171	11.9	11.9	0	3.6	1.7	3.9	1.2	933	—
EGG SUBSTITUTE, frozen, made w/ egg white, corn oil, nonfat dried milk	73.1	160	11.1	0	11.1	1.9	6.2	2.4	6.2	2	—
liquid, made w/egg, white, soy oil, protein	82.8	84	3.3	0	3.3	0.7	1.6	0.9	1.4	1	—
powder	3.9	444	13.0	—	—	3.8	1.7	4.8	1.4	572	—
ENTREES											
BEEF											
CHILI CON CARNE W/BEANS, canned	72.4	133	6.1	2.5	3.6	3.0	—	3.0	Trace	—	—
CHOP SUEY W/MEAT, home recipe	75.4	120	6.8	—	—	3.0	—	2.0	Trace	—	—
CHOP SUEY, canned	85.5	62	3.2	—	—	1.0	—	1.0	Trace	—	—
DRIED, CHIPPED, creamed	72.0	154	10.3	9.1	1.2	6.0	—	3.0	Trace	27	—
GREEN PEPPER STUFFED W/BEEF & crumbs	63.1	170	5.5	—	—	—	—	—	—	—	—
MEAT LOAF, cooked	64.1	200	13.2	12.8	0.4	—	—	—	—	—	—
POT PIE, home prepared, baked	55.1	246	14.5	3.2	11.3	4.0	—	9.0	1.0	21	—
STEW W/VEGETABLES, home recipe, w/o salt	82.4	89	4.3	2.4	1.9	2.0	—	2.0	0.1	26	—
STEW W/VEGETABLES canned	82.5	79	3.1	—	—	—	—	—	—	14	—
CHICKEN											
A LA KING, creamed	68.2	191	14.0	4.9	9.1	5.0	—	7.0	1.0	76	—
CHOW MEIN, w/o noodles, home recipe	78.0	102	4.0	3.0	1.0	1.0	—	1.0	1.0	31	—
CHOW MEIN, w/o noodle, canned	88.8	38	0.1	0.1	0	—	—	—	—	3	—
FRICASSEE	71.3	161	9.3	6.5	2.8	3.0	—	4.0	2.0	40	—
POT PIE, home recipe, baked	56.6	235	13.5	4.5	9.0	5.0	—	7.0	1.0	31	—
HAM CROQUETTE, pan fried	54.0	251	15.1	—	—	6.0	—	7.0	1.0	—	—
LOBSTER NEWBURG	64.0	194	10.6	5.3	5.3	—	—	—	—	182	—
PIZZA W/CHEESE & SAUSAGE, home recipe w/enriched flour	43.0	282	13.3	—	—	3.4	—	4.7	1.2	—	—
PIZZA W/CHEESE, frozen-type, baked, made w/enriched flour	45.3	245	7.1	—	—	2.0	—	3.0	Trace	—	—
TURKEY POT PIE, cooked	56.2	237	13.5	4.5	9.0	4.0	—	7.0	1.0	31	—
FATS & OILS											
LARD	0	902	100.0	100.0	0	39.6	15.2	40.9	10.0	95	5.0
MARGARINE, regular, soft, whipped, or unsalted	15.5	720	81.0	0	81.0	14.8	—	41.4	22.2	0	5.0
OIL											
CORN	0	884	100.0	0	100.0	12.7	58.4	24.6	57.4	0	5.0
COTTONSEED	0	884	100.0	0	100.0	26.1	51.5	18.1	50.3	0	5.0
OLIVE	0	884	100.0	0	100.0	14.2	9.9	71.5	8.2	0	5.0
PEANUT	0	884	100.0	0	100.0	17.4	31.0	45.6	31.0	0	5.0

Footnote at end of table

(Continued)

TABLE F-4 *(Continued)*

Food Name—100 Gram (3.5 oz) Portion	Water	Food Energy Calories	Total Fat	Animal Fat	Plant Fat	Saturated Fat	Polyunsaturated Fat	Fatty Acids Oleic Acid	Linoleic Acid	Cholesterol	Choline
	(g)	(kcal)	(g)	(g)	(g)	(g)	(g)	(g)	(g)	(mg)	(mg)
OIL *(Continued)*											
SAFFLOWER	0	884	100.0	0	100.0	9.4	74.3	11.9	73.3	0	5.0
SESAME	0	884	100.0	0	100.0	15.2	41.3	39.1	40.0	0	5.0
SOYBEAN	0.0	884	100.0	0	100.0	14.3	50.3	23.5	50.3	0	5.0
SHORTENING, vegetable, hydrogenated	0.0	884	100.0	0	100.0	23.0	—	65.0	7.0	0	—
FISH & SEAFOODS											
COD, cooked	64.6	129	0.7	0.7	0	0.1	0.3	0.1	—	50	—
CRAB, all varieties, steamed whole	78.5	93	1.9	1.9	0	0.3	0.6	0.2	Trace	100	—
CRABMEAT, canned	77.2	101	2.5	2.5	0	—	—	—	—	101	—
CRAB LEG, steamed in shell	78.5	93	1.9	1.9	0	0.3	0.6	0.2	Trace	100	—
CRAB IMPERIAL	71.9	147	7.6	—	—	—	—	—	—	140	—
FLOUNDER, baked	58.1	140	1.3	1.3	0	0.3	0.6	0.1	Trace	50	—
HADDOCK, cooked	66.3	90	0.7	0.7	0	0.1	0.2	0.1	Trace	60	—
HALIBUT, cooked	66.6	130	2.4	2.4	0	0.3	0.6	0.2	Trace	50	—
HERRING											
plain, canned	62.9	208	13.6	13.6	0	2.6	—	—	2.6	97	—
pickled	59.4	223	15.1	15.1	0	2.9	—	—	2.9	85	—
smoked, kippered, canned	61.0	211	12.9	12.9	0	2.4	—	—	2.4	85	—
canned w/tomato sauce	66.7	176	10.5	9.5	1.0	2.0	—	—	2.0	97	—
LOBSTER, meat, cooked	76.8	95	1.5	1.5	0	—	—	—	—	85	—
OCEAN PERCH, Atlantic, cooked, piece	59.0	92	1.3	1.3	0	0.4	0.9	0.4	Trace	—	—
OYSTER, eastern, raw	84.6	66	1.8	1.8	0	0.5	0.7	0.1	Trace	50	—
OYSTER, canned	82.2	76	2.2	2.2	0	—	—	—	—	45	—
SALMON											
broiled or baked w/butter or margarine	63.4	182	7.4	7.4	0	1.3	2.9	1.3	0.1	47	—
COHO, SILVER, canned	69.3	153	7.1	7.1	0	2.2	2.8	2.3	0.1	—	—
HUMPBACK, PINK, canned	70.8	141	5.9	5.9	0	1.5	—	1.4	0.1	—	—
SOCKEYE, RED, canned	67.2	171	9.3	9.3	0	0.8	4.3	0.8	0.2	35	—
CHUM, canned, low sodium	70.8	139	5.2	5.2	0	—	—	—	—	35	—
SARDINE											
ATLANTIC, canned, w/oil	61.8	203	11.1	—	—	—	—	—	—	140	—
PACIFIC, canned, w/mustard sauce	64.1	196	12.0	—	—	—	—	—	—	120	—
PACIFIC, canned, w/tomato sauce	64.3	197	12.2	—	—	—	—	—	—	120	—
SCALLOP, bay & sea, steamed	73.1	112	1.4	1.4	0	—	—	—	—	53	—
SHRIMP, canned	70.4	116	1.1	1.1	0	—	—	—	—	150	—
TUNA, canned, w/oil	60.6	197	8.2	8.2	0	3.0	2.0	2.0	2.0	65	—
WHITEFISH, lake, cooked	63.2	125	7.3	7.3	0	0.9	2.0	1.3	0.3	—	—
MEATS											
BEEF											
BRISKET, cooked	36.0	474	42.8	42.8	0	14.6	4.2	14.1	0.8	94	—
CHUCK BLADE STEAK, braised	40.3	427	36.7	36.7	0	15.3	4.5	14.8	0.9	—	—
GROUND, cooked	49.4	327	23.9	23.9	0	8.0	2.4	7.7	0.5	94	—
POT ROAST, braised	53.0	289	19.2	19.2	0	8.0	2.4	7.7	0.5	94	—
STEW MEAT, braised	49.4	327	23.9	23.9	0	8.0	2.4	7.7	0.5	94	—
CUBED STEAK, cooked	54.7	261	15.4	15.4	0	6.3	1.8	5.9	0.4	94	—
DRIED, CHIPPED, uncooked	47.7	203	6.3	6.3	0	3.0	—	3.0	Trace	—	—
FLANK STEAK, braised	61.4	196	7.3	7.3	0	3.1	0.9	2.7	0.3	91	—
HAMBURGER, (GROUND BEEF), cooked	54.2	286	20.3	20.3	0	9.5	2.8	9.1	0.6	94	—
HEART, cooked	61.3	188	5.7	5.7	0	1.8	1.3	1.3	0.7	274	—
KIDNEY, braised	53.0	252	12.0	12.0	0	—	—	—	—	804	—
LIVER, fried in margarine	—	229	10.6	4.8	5.8	2.9	2.0	4.1	1.1	438	—
MINUTE STEAK, cooked	54.7	261	15.4	15.4	0	6.3	1.8	5.9	0.4	94	—
PLATE SHORT RIBS, cooked	36.0	474	42.8	42.8	0	17.8	5.3	17.5	0.9	94	—
PORTERHOUSE STEAK, broiled	37.2	465	42.2	42.2	0	17.6	5.1	17.3	0.9	94	—
RIB ROAST, roasted	40.0	440	39.4	39.4	0	16.5	4.7	16.0	0.9	94	—
RIB STEAK, broiled	40.0	440	39.4	39.4	0	16.5	4.7	16.0	0.9	94	—
ROAST BEEF, canned	60.0	224	13.0	13.0	0	6.3	1.8	5.9	0.4	91	—

Footnote at end of table

(Continued)

TABLE F-4 *(Continued)*

Food Name—100 Gram (3.5 oz) Portion	Water	Food Energy Calories	Total Fat	Animal Fat	Plant Fat	Saturated Fat	Polyunsaturated Fat	Oleic Acid	Linoleic Acid	Cholesterol	Choline
	(g)	(kcal)	(g)	(g)	(g)	(g)	(g)	(g)	(g)	(mg)	(mg)
Beef *(Continued)*											
ROUND, GROUND, cooked	54.7	261	15.4	15.4	0	6.3	1.8	5.9	0.4	94	—
RUMP ROAST, roasted	48.1	347	27.3	27.3	0	11.4	3.4	11.0	0.7	94	—
STEAK, boneless, cooked	54.7	261	15.4	15.4	0	6.3	1.8	5.9	0.4	94	—
TIP, ROAST (SIRLOIN), roasted	35.1	487	44.9	44.9	0	13.3	3.9	13.1	0.7	94	—
SIRLOIN, GROUND, cooked	43.9	387	32.0	32.0	0	13.3	3.9	13.1	0.7	94	—
STEAK, broiled	43.9	387	32.0	32.0	0	13.3	3.9	13.1	0.7	94	—
SWEETBREADS, braised	49.6	320	23.2	23.2	0	—	—	—	—	466	—
T-BONE STEAK, broiled	36.4	473	43.2	43.2	0	18.0	5.3	17.7	0.9	94	—
TENDERLOIN STEAK, broiled	57.9	223	10.3	10.3	0	4.4	1.2	3.8	0.4	91	—
TOP LOIN STEAK (CLUB), broiled	37.9	454	40.6	40.6	0	17.6	5.1	17.3	0.9	94	—
TOP LOIN (STRIP) STEAK, broiled	36.4	473	43.2	43.2	0	18.0	5.3	17.7	0.9	94	—
CHICKEN											
ONE-HALF WHOLE, w/skin, roasted	57.0	248	14.7	14.7	0	4.2	4.5	4.3	3.1	87	—
DARK MEAT, w/o skin, roasted	64.4	176	6.3	6.3	0	2.7	2.9	2.7	1.9	91	—
LIGHT MEAT, w/o skin, roasted	63.8	166	3.4	3.4	0	1.0	1.0	0.8	0.6	79	—
FRYER, BACK, fried in vegetable fat	40.5	347	21.2	13.9	7.3	6.5	—	8.8	4.5	91	—
BREAST, half, fried in vegetable fat	58.4	203	6.4	3.8	2.6	1.9	—	2.8	1.3	80	—
DRUMSTICK, fried in vegetable fat	55.0	235	10.2	5.7	4.5	3.0	—	4.4	2.1	91	—
SKIN, fried in vegetable fat	32.5	419	28.9	—	—	9.0	—	12.0	5.0	—	—
THIGH, fried in vegetable fat	55.8	237	11.4	8.6	2.8	4.0	—	4.0	2.0	91	—
WING, fried in vegetable fat	52.6	268	14.8	5.4	9.4	4.6	—	6.2	3.0	91	—
GIZZARD, simmered	68.0	148	3.3	3.3	0	—	—	—	—	195	—
HEART, cooked	66.7	173	7.2	7.2	0	—	—	—	—	231	—
LIVER, simmered	65.0	165	4.4	4.4	0	—	—	—	—	746	—
CANNED	65.2	198	11.7	11.7	0	4.0	—	4.0	2.0	85	—
CORNISH HEN, roasted, whole	71.0	136	3.8	3.8	0	1.0	1.0	0.8	0.6	—	—
LAMB											
GROUND, cooked	54.0	279	18.9	18.9	0	9.5	1.4	7.9	0.8	98	—
LEG ROAST, roasted	62.2	186	7.0	7.0	0	4.0	0.7	3.4	0.4	100	—
LOIN CHOP, broiled	47.0	359	29.4	29.4	0	15.1	2.3	12.4	1.2	98	—
RIB CHOP, broiled	42.9	407	35.6	35.6	0	16.8	2.5	13.8	1.4	98	—
SHOULDER CHOP OR ROAST, broiled	49.6	338	27.2	27.2	0	12.6	1.9	10.3	1.0	98	—
LUNCHEON MEATS											
BOLOGNA	56.2	304	27.5	27.5	0	11.9	15.3	12.4	0.7	62	60.0
BRAUNSCHWEIGER (smoked liver sausage)	52.6	319	27.4	27.4	0	10.0	—	12.0	2.0	62	—
CORNED BEEF, cooked	43.9	372	30.4	30.4	0	15.0	—	13.0	1.0	94	—
canned	59.3	216	12.0	12.0	0	6.0	—	5.0	Trace	94	—
hash w/potato, canned	67.4	181	11.3	4.0	7.3	5.0	—	5.0	Trace	—	—
HAM, boiled	59.1	234	17.0	17.0	0	5.9	2.6	7.3	1.6	89	—
deviled, canned	50.5	351	32.3	32.3	0	12.0	—	14.0	3.0	—	—
minced	61.7	228	16.9	16.9	0	6.0	—	7.0	2.0	89	—
HEAD CHEESE	58.8	268	22.0	22.0	0	4.5	2.4	6.7	1.4	—	—
LIVERWURST	53.9	307	25.6	25.6	0	—	—	—	—	105	—
PATE DE FOIS GRAS, canned	37.0	462	43.8	43.8	0	—	—	—	—	—	—
PORK/HAM LOAF TYPE LUNCHEON MEAT	54.9	294	24.9	24.9	0	10.7	4.7	13.2	3.1	89	—
SALAMI, BEEF, cooked	51.0	311	25.6	25.6	0	8.7	10.6	8.4	0.6	62	—
SALAMI, BEEF, hard	29.8	450	38.1	38.1	0	—	—	—	—	62	—
SPICED LUNCHEON MEATS, pork/ham type	54.9	294	24.9	24.9	0	10.7	4.7	13.2	3.1	89	—
VIENNA SAUSAGE	63.0	240	19.8	19.8	0	9.4	3.3	11.1	1.6	—	—
PORK											
BACON, cooked	8.1	611	52.0	52.0	0	17.0	—	25.0	5.0	—	—
CANADIAN BACON, broiled or fried, drained	49.9	277	17.5	17.5	0	5.9	2.7	7.3	1.4	88	—
CURED HAM, roasted	53.6	289	22.1	22.1	0	7.8	3.4	9.6	2.1	89	—
CURED PORK SHOULDER (PICNIC), roasted	48.8	323	25.2	25.2	0	8.8	3.9	10.9	2.4	89	—

Footnote at end of table

(Continued)

TABLE F-4 *(Continued)*

Food Name—100 Gram (3.5 oz) Portion	Water	Food Energy Calories	Total Fat	Animal Fat	Plant Fat	Saturated Fat	Polyunsat- urated Fat	Fatty Acids Oleic Acid	Linoleic Acid	Cholesterol	Choline
	(g)	(kcal)	(g)	(g)	(g)	(g)	(g)	(g)	(g)	(mg)	(mg)
PORK *(Continued)*											
GROUND PORK, cooked	45.2	373	30.6	30.6	0	10.8	—	13.2	2.4	89	—
LEG (FRESH HAM) ROAST, roasted	45.5	374	30.6	30.6	0	10.8	—	12.0	2.4	89	—
LOIN CHOP, broiled	42.3	391	31.7	31.7	0	11.4	4.9	13.3	2.8	89	—
LOIN ROAST, roasted	45.8	362	28.5	28.5	0	9.8	4.4	12.1	2.6	89	—
LOIN TENDERLOIN, cooked	55.0	254	14.2	14.2	0	4.7	2.2	5.8	1.2	88	—
PICKLED PIGS FEET	66.9	199	14.8	14.8	0	5.0	—	6.0	1.0	—	—
RIB CHOP, broiled	42.3	391	31.7	31.7	0	11.4	4.9	13.3	2.8	89	—
SHOULDER, simmered	60.3	212	9.8	9.8	0	3.2	—	4.8	1.6	88	—
SHOULDER, BOSTON BUTT ROAST, cooked	48.1	353	28.5	28.5	0	11.7	5.1	14.0	3.0	89	—
SHOULDER, PICNIC ROAST, cooked	45.7	374	30.5	30.5	0	8.7	3.9	10.7	2.3	89	—
SPARE RIB, braised	39.7	440	38.9	38.9	0	13.5	6.0	16.6	3.5	89	—
SAUSAGES											
COUNTRY-STYLE SAUSAGE, link	49.9	345	31.1	31.1	0	11.0	—	13.0	3.0	89	—
FRANKFURTER OR WIENER, cooked	57.3	304	27.2	27.2	0	11.2	15.8	12.3	0.9	62	—
ITALIAN SAUSAGE, cooked	49.9	345	31.1	31.1	0	11.0	—	13.0	3.0	89	—
KNOCKWURST, pork	57.6	278	23.2	23.2	0	—	—	—	—	62	—
POLISH SAUSAGE/KOLBASSI, cooked	53.7	304	25.8	25.8	0	—	—	—	—	89	—
PORK SAUSAGE, cooked	34.8	476	44.2	44.2	0	11.7	5.0	14.1	3.4	89	—
SUMMER SAUSAGE/THURINGER/ CERVELAT, beef	48.5	307	24.5	24.5	0	11.0	14.4	11.2	0.8	62	—
TURKEY											
DARK MEAT, w/o skin, roasted	60.5	203	8.3	8.3	0	1.6	1.8	1.1	1.1	101	—
LIGHT MEAT, w/o skin, roasted	62.1	176	3.9	3.9	0	0.7	0.8	0.5	0.5	77	—
DRUMSTICK, w/o skin, roasted	60.5	203	8.3	8.3	0	1.6	1.8	1.1	1.1	101	—
THIGH, w/o skin, roasted	60.5	203	8.3	8.3	0	1.6	1.8	1.1	1.1	101	—
WING, w/o skin, roasted	60.5	203	8.3	8.3	0	—	—	—	—	101	—
CANNED	64.9	202	12.5	12.5	0	4.0	—	5.0	3.0	89	—
VEAL											
CUTLET, braised or broiled	60.4	216	11.1	11.1	0	4.7	1.1	4.0	0.5	101	—
LOIN, CHOP OR ROAST, cooked	58.9	234	13.4	13.4	0	5.7	1.3	4.9	0.6	101	—
RIB CHOP, cooked	54.6	269	16.9	16.9	0	7.1	1.1	4.0	0.5	101	—
ROUND, GROUND, cooked	60.4	216	11.1	11.1	0	4.7	1.2	4.6	0.5	101	—
SHOULDER ARM ROAST, cooked	58.5	235	12.8	12.8	0	5.4	1.6	6.0	0.7	99	—
MILK & PRODUCTS											
BUTTER, salted or unsalted	15.9	717	81.1	81.1	0	50.5	3.0	20.4	1.8	219	—
BUTTERMILK, cultured	90.1	40	0.9	0.9	0	0.6	Trace	0.2	Trace	4	—
CHEESE											
AMERICAN, pasteurized process	39.2	375	31.3	31.3	0	19.7	1.0	7.5	0.6	94	—
AMERICAN CHEESE FOOD, cold pack	43.1	331	24.5	24.5	0	15.4	0.7	6.0	0.5	64	—
pasteurized process	43.2	328	24.6	24.6	0	15.4	0.7	6.1	0.5	64	—
AMERICAN CHEESE SPREAD, pasteurized process	47.7	290	21.2	21.2	0	13.3	0.6	5.2	0.4	55	—
BLUE	42.4	353	28.7	28.7	0	18.7	0.8	6.6	0.5	75	—
BRICK	41.1	371	29.7	29.7	0	18.8	0.8	7.4	0.5	94	—
BRIE	48.4	334	27.7	27.7	0	—	—	—	—	100	—
CAMEMBERT	51.8	300	24.3	24.3	0	15.3	0.7	5.8	0.5	72	—
CHEDDAR	36.8	403	33.1	33.1	0	21.1	0.9	7.9	0.6	105	—
CHESHIRE	37.7	387	30.6	30.6	0	—	—	—	—	103	—
COLBY	38.2	394	32.1	32.1	0	20.2	1.0	7.8	0.7	95	—
COTTAGE CHEESE, creamed, small or large curd	79.0	103	4.5	4.5	0	2.9	0.1	1.1	0.1	15	—
creamed, w/fruit added	72.1	124	3.4	3.4	0	2.2	0.1	0.8	0.1	11	—
dry curd	79.8	85	0.4	0.4	0	0.3	Trace	0.1	Trace	7	—
lowfat, 2% fat	79.3	90	1.9	1.9	0	1.2	0.1	0.5	Trace	8	—
lowfat, 1% fat	82.5	72	1.0	1.0	0	0.6	Trace	0.2	Trace	4	—
CREAM	53.8	349	34.9	34.9	0	22.0	1.3	8.4	0.8	110	—

Footnote at end of table

(Continued)

TABLE F-4 *(Continued)*

Food Name—100 Gram (3.5 oz) Portion	Water	Food Energy Calories	Total Fat	Animal Fat	Plant Fat	Saturated Fat	Polyunsaturated Fat	Fatty Acids		Cholesterol	Choline
								Oleic Acid	Linoleic Acid		
	(g)	(kcal)	(g)	(g)	(g)	(g)	(g)	(g)	(g)	(mg)	(mg)
CHEESE *(Continued)*											
EDAM	41.6	357	27.8	27.8	0	17.6	0.7	6.9	0.4	89	—
FETA, made from sheep's milk	55.2	264	21.3	21.3	0	15.0	0.6	4.0	0.3	89	—
FONTINA	37.9	389	31.1	31.1	0	19.2	1.7	7.1	0.9	116	—
GJETOST, made from goat's & cow's milk	13.4	466	29.5	29.5	0	19.2	0.9	7.0	0.5	—	—
GOUDA	41.5	356	27.4	27.4	0	17.6	0.7	6.4	0.3	114	—
GRUYERE	33.2	413	32.3	32.3	0	18.9	1.7	8.6	1.3	110	—
LIMBURGER	48.4	327	27.3	27.3	0	16.8	0.5	7.2	0.3	90	—
MOZZARELLA	54.1	281	21.6	21.6	0	13.2	0.8	5.7	0.4	78	—
low moisture	48.4	318	24.6	24.6	0	15.6	0.8	5.9	0.6	89	—
part skim	53.8	254	15.9	15.9	0	10.1	0.5	3.9	0.3	58	—
low moisture, part skim	48.6	280	17.1	17.1	0	10.9	0.5	4.2	0.4	54	—
MUENSTER	41.8	368	30.0	30.0	0	19.1	0.7	7.3	0.4	96	—
NEUFCHATEL	62.2	260	23.4	23.4	0	14.8	0.7	5.7	0.5	76	—
PARMESAN, grated	17.7	456	30.0	30.0	0	19.1	0.7	7.7	0.3	79	—
hard	29.2	392	25.8	25.8	0	16.4	0.6	6.7	0.3	68	—
PIMIENTO, pasteurized process	39.1	375	31.2	—	—	19.7	1.0	7.5	0.6	94	—
PORT DU SALUT	45.5	352	28.2	28.2	0	16.7	0.7	8.1	0.4	123	—
PROVOLONE	41.0	351	26.6	26.6	0	17.1	0.8	6.2	0.5	69	—
RICOTTA, made w/whole milk	71.7	174	13.0	13.0	0	8.3	0.4	2.9	0.3	51	—
made w/part skim milk	74.4	138	7.9	7.9	0	4.9	0.3	1.9	0.2	31	—
ROMANO	30.9	387	26.9	26.9	0	—	—	—	—	104	—
ROQUEFORT, made from sheep's milk	39.4	369	30.6	30.6	0	19.3	1.3	7.5	0.6	90	—
SWISS	37.2	376	27.5	27.5	0	17.8	1.0	6.0	0.6	92	—
pasteurized process	42.3	334	25.0	25.0	0	16.0	0.6	5.9	0.3	85	—
SWISS CHEESE FOOD, pasteurized process	43.7	323	24.1	24.1	0	—	—	—	—	82	—
TILSIT, made w/whole milk	42.9	340	26.0	26.0	0	16.8	0.7	6.1	0.4	102	—
CREAM											
heavy whipping	57.7	345	37.0	37.0	0	23.0	1.4	9.3	0.8	137	—
light whipping	63.5	292	30.9	30.9	0	19.3	0.9	7.7	0.6	111	—
medium, 25% fat	68.5	244	25.0	25.0	0	15.6	0.9	6.3	0.6	88	—
light, coffee or table	73.8	195	19.3	19.3	0	12.0	0.7	4.9	0.4	66	—
half & half, milk & cream	80.6	130	11.5	11.5	0	7.2	0.4	2.9	0.3	37	—
imitation sour cream, non-dairy	71.2	208	19.5	0	19.5	17.8	0.1	0.6	0.1	0	—
sour cream, cultured	70.9	214	21.0	21.0	0	13.1	0.8	5.3	0.5	44	—
sour half & half, cultured	80.1	135	12.0	12.0	0	7.5	0.5	3.0	0.3	38	—
whipped cream topping, pressurized	61.3	257	22.2	22.2	0	13.8	0.8	5.6	0.5	76	—
CREAM SUBSTITUTES											
COFFEE WHITENER, non-dairy liquid w/hydrogenated vegetable oil & soy protein	77.3	136	10.0	0	10.0	1.9	Trace	7.6	Trace	0	—
non-dairy liquid w/lauric acid oil & casein	77.3	136	10.0	0	10.0	9.3	Trace	—	Trace	0	—
non-dairy, powdered	2.2	546	35.5	0	35.5	32.5	Trace	1.0	Trace	0	—
ICE CREAM											
FRENCH VANILLA, ice cream, soft serve	59.8	218	13.0	—	—	7.8	0.6	3.4	0.4	89	—
VANILLA, ice cream, rich, 16% fat, hardened	58.9	236	16.0	16.0	0	10.0	0.6	4.0	0.4	59	—
regular, 10% fat, hardened	60.8	202	10.8	10.8	0	6.7	0.4	2.7	0.2	45	—
VANILLA ICE MILK, hardened	68.6	140	4.3	4.3	0	2.7	0.2	1.1	0.1	14	—
soft serve	69.6	128	2.6	—	—	1.6	0.1	0.7	0.1	8	—
ORANGE SHERBET	66.1	140	2.0	2.0	0	1.2	0.1	0.5	Trace	7	—
MILK											
WHOLE MILK, 3.7% fat	87.7	64	3.7	3.7	0	2.3	0.1	0.9	0.1	14	—
3.3% fat	88.0	61	3.3	3.3	0	2.1	0.1	0.8	0.1	14	—
evaporated, canned	74.0	134	7.6	7.6	0	4.6	0.2	2.1	0.2	29	—
low sodium	88.2	61	3.5	3.5	0	2.2	0.1	0.9	0.1	14	—
dry	2.5	496	26.7	26.7	0	16.7	0.7	6.2	0.5	97	—

Footnote at end of table

(Continued)

TABLE F-4 *(Continued)*

Food Name—100 Gram (3.5 oz) Portion	Water	Food Energy Calories	Total Fat	Animal Fat	Plant Fat	Saturated Fat	Polyunsat- urated Fat	Fatty Acids Oleic Acid	Linoleic Acid	Cholesterol	Choline
	(g)	(kcal)	(g)	(g)	(g)	(g)	(g)	(g)	(g)	(mg)	(mg)
MILK *(Continued)*											
LOWFAT MILK, 2% fat	89.2	50	1.9	1.9	0	1.2	0.1	0.5	Trace	8	—
2% fat w/nonfat milk solids added	88.9	51	1.9	1.9	0	1.2	0.1	0.5	Trace	8	—
2% fat, protein fortified	87.7	56	2.0	2.0	0	1.2	0.1	0.5	Trace	8	—
1% fat	90.1	42	1.1	1.1	0	0.7	Trace	0.3	Trace	4	—
1% fat w/nonfat milk solids added	89.8	43	1.0	1.0	0	0.6	Trace	0.2	Trace	4	—
1% fat, protein fortified	88.7	48	1.2	1.2	0	0.7	Trace	0.3	Trace	4	—
SKIM MILK	90.8	35	0.2	0.2	0	0.1	Trace	Trace	Trace	2	—
evaporated, canned	79.4	78	0.2	0.2	0	0.1	Trace	0.1	Trace	4	—
protein fortified	89.4	41	0.3	0.3	0	0.2	Trace	0.1	Trace	2	—
w/nonfat milk solids added	90.4	37	0.3	0.3	0	0.2	Trace	0.1	Trace	2	—
NONFAT DRY MILK POWDER, non-instantized	3.2	362	0.8	0.8	0	0.5	Trace	0.2	Trace	20	—
instantized	4.0	358	0.7	0.7	0	0.5	Trace	0.2	Trace	18	—
SWEETENED CONDENSED MILK, canned	27.2	321	8.7	8.7	0	5.5	0.3	2.2	0.2	34	—
CHOCOLATE MILK, whole, 3.3% fat	82.3	83	3.4	3.4	0	2.1	0.1	0.9	0.1	12	—
2% fat	83.6	72	2.0	2.0	0	1.2	0.1	0.5	0.1	7	—
1% fat	84.5	63	1.0	1.0	0	0.6	Trace	0.3	Trace	3	—
HOT CHOCOLATE SWEETENED MIX, (powdered)	3.1	392	10.6	0	10.6	6.0	—	4.0	Trace	0	—
COCOA POWDER, high fat/breakfast, plain	3.0	299	23.7	0	23.7	13.0	—	9.0	Trace	0	—
HOT COCOA, homemade w/whole milk	81.6	87	3.6	—	—	2.2	0.1	0.9	0.1	13	—
MALTED MILK powder, natural flavor	2.6	411	8.5	—	—	4.2	1.2	—	—	20	—
beverage, natural flavor	81.2	89	3.8	—	—	2.3	0.2	—	—	14	—
powder, chocolate flavor	2.0	396	4.5	—	—	2.2	0.6	—	—	5	—
beverage, chocolate flavor	81.2	88	3.4	—	—	2.1	0.2	—	—	13	—
MILKSHAKE, vanilla flavor, thick type	74.4	112	3.0	—	—	1.9	0.1	0.8	0.1	12	—
chocolate flavor, thick type	72.2	119	2.7	—	—	1.7	0.1	0.7	0.1	10	—
GOAT MILK, whole	87.0	69	4.1	4.1	0	2.7	0.2	1.0	0.1	11	—
HUMAN MILK, whole	87.5	70	4.4	4.4	0	2.0	0.5	1.5	0.4	14	—
YOGURT											
plain	87.9	61	3.3	3.3	0	2.1	0.1	0.7	0.1	13	—
plain, lowfat	85.1	63	1.5	1.5	0	1.0	Trace	0.4	Trace	6	—
plain, skim milk	85.2	56	0.2	0.2	0	0.1	Trace	Trace	Trace	2	—
coffee & vanilla varieties, lowfat	79.0	85	1.3	1.3	0	0.8	Trace	0.3	Trace	5	—
fruit varieties, lowfat (9g protein/8oz)	75.3	99	1.1	1.1	0	0.7	Trace	0.3	Trace	4	—
fruit varieties, lowfat (10g protein/8oz)	74.5	102	1.1	1.1	0	0.7	Trace	0.3	Trace	4	—
fruit varieties, lowfat (11g protein/8oz)	74.1	105	1.4	1.4	0	0.9	Trace	0.3	Trace	6	—
NUTS & SEEDS											
ALMONDS	4.7	598	54.2	0	54.2	4.3	10.5	36.5	9.9	0	—
BRAZIL NUTS	4.6	654	66.9	0	66.9	17.4	25.7	22.2	25.4	0	—
CASHEW NUTS	5.2	561	45.7	0	45.7	9.2	7.7	26.2	7.3	0	—
CHESTNUTS	52.5	194	1.5	0	1.5	0.4	1.1	1.0	0.9	0	—
COCONUT, dried, shredded, sweetened	3.3	548	39.1	0	39.1	34.0	0.3	3.0	Trace	0	—
COCONUT, fresh	50.9	346	35.3	0	35.3	31.2	0.8	2.0	0.7	0	—
FILBERTS (HAZELNUTS)	5.8	634	62.4	0	62.4	4.6	6.9	49.8	6.6	0	—
HICKORY NUTS	3.3	673	68.7	0	68.7	6.0	12.7	47.0	12.0	0	—
MACADAMIA NUTS	3.0	691	71.6	0	71.6	11.0	16.3	43.2	1.2	0	—
PEANUTS, roasted & salted Spanish	1.6	585	49.8	0	49.8	9.6	16.1	20.5	16.1	0	162.0
roasted & salted, Virginia	1.6	585	49.8	0	49.8	8.3	12.2	24.1	12.2	0	162.0
roasted in shell, w/skins	1.8	582	48.7	0	48.7	8.6	13.3	23.5	13.3	0	162.0
PEANUT BUTTER	1.8	581	49.4	0	49.4	10.5	15.1	23.1	15.1	0	145.0
PECANS	3.4	687	71.2	0	71.2	6.1	18.3	42.9	17.0	0	50.0
PINENUTS (PIGNOLIAS)	5.6	552	47.4	0	47.4	6.2	22.8	19.0	22.2	0	—
PISTACHIO NUTS	5.3	594	53.7	0	53.7	7.4	7.3	36.0	6.8	0	—
PUMPKIN OR SQUASH SEEDS	4.4	553	46.7	0	46.7	8.0	—	17.0	20.0	0	—
SUNFLOWER SEEDS, hulled	4.8	560	47.3	0	47.3	6.0	—	9.0	30.0	0	—

Footnote at end of table

(Continued)

TABLE F-4 *(Continued)*

Food Name—100 Gram (3.5 oz) Portion	Water	Food Energy Calories	Total Fat	Animal Fat	Plant Fat	Saturated Fat	Polyunsaturated Fat	Fatty Acids Oleic Acid	Fatty Acids Linoleic Acid	Cholesterol	Choline
	(g)	(kcal)	(g)	(g)	(g)	(g)	(g)	(g)	(g)	(mg)	(mg)
NUTS (Continued)											
WALNUTS, BLACK	3.1	628	59.3	0	59.3	5.1	40.9	10.7	36.6	0	–
ENGLISH	3.5	651	64.0	0	64.0	6.9	42.0	9.7	34.9	0	–
SNACK FOODS											
PEANUT BUTTER & CHEESE CRACKER SANDWICH	2.4	491	23.9	–	–	6.3	–	11.0	5.6	–	–
POPCORN, plain	4.0	386	5.0	0	5.0	1.0	–	1.0	3.0	0	–
POPCORN, popped in coconut oil, w/salt	3.1	456	21.8	0	21.8	15.0	–	2.0	2.0	0	–
POTATO CHIPS	1.8	568	39.8	0	39.8	9.9	–	8.3	19.9	–	–
POTATO CHIPS, salt free	1.8	568	39.8	0	39.8	9.9	–	8.3	19.9	–	–
POTATO STICKS	1.5	544	36.4	0	36.4	9.0	–	8.0	18.0	–	–
PRETZELS	4.5	390	4.5	0	4.5	1.0	–	–	–	–	–

¹The authors gratefully acknowledge that these food compositions were obtained from the HVH-CWRI Nutrient Data Base developed by the Division of Nutrition, Highland View Hospital, and the Departments of Biometry and Nutrition, School of Medicine, Case Western Reserve University, Cleveland, Ohio.

FATS, HYDROGENATED (HYDROGENATED OILS)

Fats and oils containing polyunsaturated fatty acids can be hardened and turned into solid fats by the addition of hydrogen in the presence of a catalyst, which is usually nickel. The process is called hydrogenation since it adds hydrogen to the double bond linkages of unsaturated fatty acids and converts them to saturated fatty acids. Hydrogenated fats are of commercial importance, since vegetable oils can be converted into a solid form and used as shortenings and margarine.

(Also see FATS AND OTHER LIPIDS.)

FAT-SOLUBLE VITAMINS

These vitamins are stored in appreciable quantities in the body, whereas the water-soluble vitamins are not. Thus, vitamin A and/or carotene may be stored by a person in his (her) liver and fatty tissue in sufficient quantities to meet the body requirements for a period of 6 months or longer. The fat-soluble vitamins are: A (carotene), D, E, and K.

(Also see VITAMIN[S]; VITAMIN A; VITAMIN D; VITAMIN E; and VITAMIN K.)

FATTENING

The deposition of unused energy in the form of fat within the body tissues.

FDA

Food and Drug Administration, a Federal regulatory agency.

(Also see FOOD AND DRUG ADMINISTRATION.)

FEBRILE

Feverish.

FEDERAL FOOD, DRUG AND COSMETIC ACT

On the same day that the Meat Inspection Act was passed, the Food and Drug Act of 1906 was signed. This act was designed to prevent the use of poisonous preservatives and dyes in foods, and to regulate the sales of patent medicines.

In 1927, the Food, Drug, and Insecticide Administration, later to be named the Food and Drug Administration (FDA), was created. In 1938, the Federal Food, Drug, and Cosmetic Act of 1938 was signed, broadening the scope of the Food and Drug Act of 1906 to include (1) coverage of cosmetics and devices; (2) requirements for predistribution clearance for the safety of new drugs; (3) provisions for tolerances for unavoidable poisonous substances; (4) standards of identity, quality, and fill of food containers; (5) authorization for factory inspections; and (6) provision for court injunctions in matters of seizures and possession. With its numerous amendments, the Federal Food, Drug and Cosmetic Act is probably the most extensive law of its kind in the world.

(Also see FOOD AND DRUG ADMINISTRATION.)

FEED ADJUVANTS

An adjuvant is a substance which facilitates or enhances the effectiveness of any process. Feed adjuvants such as antibiotics, hormones, and hormonelike substances alter digestion, absorption, or metabolism of meat producing animals, thus increasing feed efficiency and stimulating growth. Usually these substances are called feed additives, implants, or growth stimulators in the livestock industry.

FEEDBACK MECHANISM

The mechanism that regulates the production and secretion by an endocrine gland of its hormone, which, in turn, stimulates another endocrine gland to produce its hormone. Example: The anterior pituitary secretes thyroid-stimulating hormone (TSH), which, in turn, stimulates the thyroid to secrete thyroxin. When the blood level of thyroxin reaches optimum, the anterior pituitary ceases to secrete TSH; and, thereupon, the thyroid stops secreting thyroxin, and the blood level of thyroxin falls.

FENNEL *Foeniculum vulgare*, **var.** *dulce*

(See VEGETABLE[S], Table V-2, Vegetables of the World.)

FERMENTATION

A gradual chemical change brought about by the enzymes of some bacteria, molds, and yeasts. These chemical changes are usually the acidulation of milk, the decomposition of starches and sugars to alcohol and carbon dioxide, or the oxidation of nitrogenous organic compounds. The three main types of industrial fermentation are (1) bacterial fermentation of carbohydrates, (2) bacterial fermentation of alcohol to acetic acid, and (3) yeast fermentation. In general, the requirements of greatest importance for fermentation are the media, temperature, salt, acidity, the culture container for fermentation, and the time involved. Production of breads, beers, wines, cheeses, yogurts, and antibiotics, to name a few, depends upon the process of fermentation.

(Also see BEERS AND BREWING; BREADS AND BAKING; DISTILLED LIQUORS; MILK AND MILK PRODUCTS; and VINEGAR.)

FERMENTATION PRODUCT

Product formed as a result of an enzymatic transformation of organic substrates.

(Also see FERMENTATION.)

FERMENTED

Acted upon by yeasts, molds, or bacteria in a controlled aerobic or anaerobic process in the manufacture of such products as alcohols, acids, vitamins of the B-complex group, or antibiotics.

(Also see FERMENTATION.)

FERRITIN

The iron-protein complex in which iron is stored, particularly in the cells of the liver, spleen, and bone marrow.

(Also see IRON.)

FIBER

This term designates the complex of carbohydrates and other substances that are present mainly in the cell walls of the plants used as foods. Fiber includes cellulose, hemicelluloses, gums, mucilages, pectic substances, and lignin. These substances are poorly digested by humans and have little nutritional value. However, they appear to have important physiological effects in the digestive tract; hence, the term *nonnutritive fiber.* Other terms used to designate fiber are *crude fiber, unavailable carbohydrates* (although lignin is not a carbohydrate), *bulk, roughage,* and *undigestible residue.* Almost all of the undigestible matter in the human diet now comes from plant foods.

The food industry now uses many types of natural, semi-synthetic (natural materials altered by man), and totally synthetic carbohydrates having effects similar to naturally occurring nonnutritive components of food. These materials are used (1) as dispersing agents—to keep dissimilar food ingredients well mixed; (2) as thickening agents—to increase viscosity or stiffness of mixtures; and (3) as gelling agents. Furthermore, some of these substances are now added to foods solely to increase the fiber content. It is noteworthy

that food technologists have also developed processing techniques for removal of the fiber present in certain foods so that they may be more suitable for people who cannot tolerate much of this substance. Infants and young growing children require highly digestible sources of nutrients. Likewise, people who have impaired digestion and/or absorption should be given diets that are low in fiber. Therefore, many people may benefit from more knowledge of this subject.

HISTORY. Although it was long believed that prehistoric peoples ate mainly animal foods that they obtained by hunting and scavenging, recent archaeological studies have shown that the human diet also contained large amounts of high fiber plant foods. For example, the diets of the Indians who lived in the Great Basin area of the American West contained about 25% fiber.

It is noteworthy that throughout the early 1800s health and religious concerns fired up certain advocates of diets based mainly on whole grains, vegetables, and fruits. These concerns were motivated in part by the high consumption of alcoholic beverages during the 1820s and 1830s. Sailors and laborers often received part of their wages in the form of liquor, and children were encouraged to drink hard cider, which was safer than the drinking water. One of the earliest and most notable of the health reformers was a former Presbyterian minister named Sylvester Graham (1794-1851), after whom graham flour and graham crackers are named, who promoted vegetarianism, abstinence from alcoholic beverages, and the use of coarse, unbolted flour for the making of bread with a high-fiber content. Mother Ellen Harmon White, who was a leader of the Adventists, was influenced considerably by the dietary ideas of Reverend Graham. Hence, whole grains were important items in the diets of the patients at the famous Battle Creek Sanitarium, which was established by Mrs. White and managed by Dr. John Harvey Kellogg, who, with his brother, Will, developed the first ready-to-eat breakfast cereals. However, the work of the 19th century health reformers was offset by the development of large scale roller milling of wheat in the 1870s. This was the first time in history that large supplies of white flour were made available at prices that even the poor could afford.

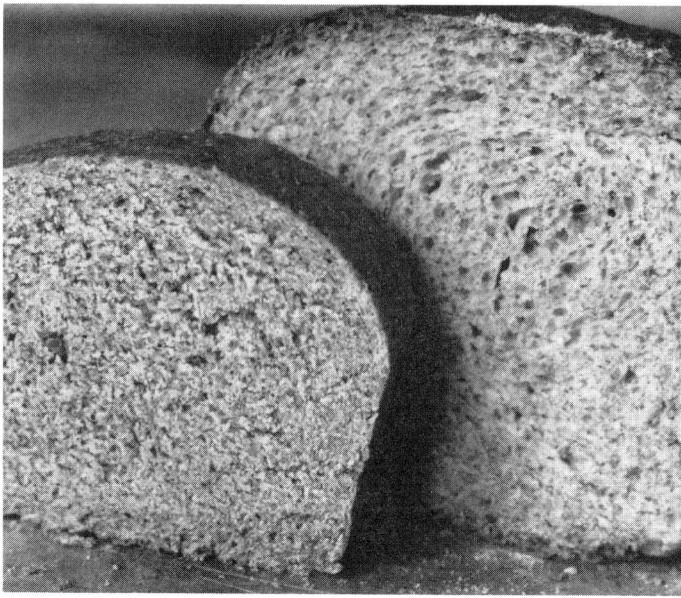

Fig. F-11. Homemade whole wheat breads are a good source of fiber. (Courtesy, University of Minnesota, St. Paul, Minn.)

Interest in whole grain breads and vegetarianism declined steadily in 20th-century America until World War I. The governments of Great Britain and Denmark made the use of high extraction wheat flours mandatory during the war in order to make the fullest possible use of the limited supplies of grain. However, the use of highly refined flours resumed in these countries after the war. Similarly, increased use was made of whole grain flours during World War II, but this salutory practice went out of style in the postwar period.

It was not until the 1960s that the current interest in dietary fiber was stimulated by the reports of several British physicians (mainly Drs. Denis Burkitt, Peter Cleave, Neil Painter, and Hugh Trowell) who noted that certain African peoples who consumed high fiber diets had much lower rates of certain diseases than the people of Great Britain and the United States. The average daily intake of crude fiber in developed nations has been estimated to be about 4 grams, compared with as much as 30 grams in some developing countries. Many other investigations and reports followed, with the result that some new high fiber products appeared in supermarkets.

KINDS OF FIBER. Fiber may be obtained from diverse sources, such as grains, vegetables, fruits, nuts, seaweed, gum trees, and the laboratory of the organic chemist. Therefore, it is worthwhile to consider the plant constituents that comprise most of the fiber in the human diet.

Fibrous Substances in Common Foods. Most unrefined vegetable foods contain variable amounts of the materials which follow:

- **Cellulose**—This compound is the most abundant polysaccharide found in the cell walls of plants. Its molecule is made up of glucose units joined together in a chainlike structure. Cellulose differs from starch (also a polysaccharide consisting of glucose units) in that it is not digested by the enzymes secreted by the human digestive system. Ruminants (such as cattle, sheep, and goats) digest cellulose fairly effectively, but it is poorly digested by humans, pigs, and chickens. However, the three latter species may harbor intestinal microorganisms that digest small amounts of the dietary cellulose.

- **Hemicelluloses**—These polysaccharides, which are closely associated with cellulose in cell walls, are composed mainly of sugar units containing 5- or 6-carbon atoms (pentoses or hexoses). They are insoluble in water, but soluble in alkali. Thus, the cooking of vegetables in water containing baking soda (an alkali) may result in a mushy texture because the alkaline solution extracts the hemicelluloses from the cell walls, resulting in a loss of rigidity.

- **Gums**—Originally, the term *gum* designated the highly viscous and sticky substances that were exuded by various types of plants. Now, gums are considered to be a large class of substances that may be dissolved or dispersed in water to give a gelling or a thickening effect. However, plants having a high content of gummy material are not often used as food sources; rather, they're used as sources of gums for food additives. Some of the most common natural sources of gums are (1) plant exudates (which yield gum arabic, gum karaya, and gum tragacanth); (2) seeds (the sources of locust bean gum and guar gum); (3) seaweeds (such as those which furnish agar, algin derivatives, and carrageenan); and (4) various other plant extracts such as larch gum.

- **Mucilages**—Presently, these substances are usually classified under gums, since they have many of the same properties. Formerly, mucilages were considered to be the plant polysaccharides which readily formed sticky, slimy (mucilagenous) solutions in water. Two of the most familiar examples of these substances are those that may be extracted from flax seeds and psyllium seeds. Various products made from these seeds have long been used as laxatives. It is noteworthy that ladies used to set their hair in curls or waves with a solution obtained by steeping flax seeds in hot water.

- **Pectic substances**—These polysaccharides are made up mainly of chains of galacturonic acid (a derivative of galactose) units. The individual units may be modified by attachments of methyl and other chemical groups. Some of these compounds are water-soluble. Pectins, which are the best known of these materials, form gels with sugar and acid. The pectin present in apples is partly responsible for the crispy texture (a decrease in pectin content after picking results in mealiness). The leading commercial sources of pectin are citrus peel and apple pomace (the residue that remains after juice extraction).

- **Lignin**—Although included under the categories of crude fiber and unavailable carbohydrate, lignin is not a true carbohydrate. Like carbohydrates, however, it contains carbon, hydrogen, and oxygen; but the proportion of carbon is much higher than in carbohydrates, and nitrogen may also be present. Lignin is found in plant cell walls in intimate association with cellulose, to which it imparts rigidity. It increases in amounts with plant maturity; hence, vegetables, such as cabbage and peas, that are eaten before maturity are low in lignin content.

- **Miscellaneous polysaccharides**—This includes compounds that are undigestible, but which are not likely to be detected by the procedures usually employed in the analyses of foods for fiber content. Examples of such compounds are *inulin,* a water-soluble polysaccharide made up of fructose units and found in various roots and tubers such as the Jerusalem artichoke, and *galactan*, a galactose polysaccharide found in agar, a material obtained from seaweed.

Food Additives. The use of various types of nonnutritive carbohydrates in foods is increasing as food manufacturers find new ways to produce the characteristics sought by the consumer. Thanks to these materials, mixtures can be kept from separating, thickening can be achieved without increasing the energy content of foods, and jams gel easily. Some examples follow:

- **Natural materials**—These are generally the gums and pectic substances that are derived from various types of land and sea plants. However, cellulose produced from wood chips is sometimes used to increase the fiber content of foods.

- **Semisynthetic materials**—This includes modified celluloses (microcrystalline, carboxymethyl, and methyl), modified gums (derivatives of pectin, alginates, locust bean gum, and guar gum), and microbial fermentation gums (dextran and xanthan).

- **Synthetic materials**—The principle members of this class are polymers of polyvinylpyrrolidone (PVP), ethylene oxide, carboxyvinyl, and methyl vinylether maleic acid.

DETERMINATION OF THE FIBER CONTENT OF FOODS.

Nutritionists have long been interested in fiber mainly from a negative point of view; that is, it has been necessary to know to what extent the carbohydrate fractions of foods or feeds are unavailable for energy production in the body (burning these materials in a calorimeter gives only the total energy content, rather than that available for metabolism). Also, food inspectors have long used fiber as a measure of adulterants and contaminants, such as husks and shells in ground spices and cocoa.

Much of the current interest in the fiber content of foods stems from reports of its beneficial effects. With this, has come renewed interest in fiber analysis. The most widely used procedures for determining the fiber contents of foods follow.

Proximate Analysis.

This term is used to designate a series of chemical analyses which yield an estimate of food or feed values in terms of water, ash, crude protein, crude fat, available carbohydrate, and crude fiber.

The residue of crude fiber contains much of the cellulose and lignin, but little of the hemicelluloses, gums, mucilages, and pectic substances present in the original sample of food. The latter components are extracted by cooking in acid solution. Thus, the values obtained in this determination represent only part of the total fiber content and should be used mainly for making comparisons between foods that have similar chemical compositions. For example, the types of nuts with the highest contents of crude fiber are likely the richest in total fiber content, also. However, crude fiber values for nuts are not strictly comparable to crude fiber values for green leafy vegetables because the chemical compositions of the two types of foods are quite different.

(Also see ANALYSIS OF FOODS, section headed "Proximate Analysis.")

Digestibility Studies.

Another basis for apportioning the total carbohydrate content of a food into digestible and undigestible fractions is the percent digestibility of the carbohydrate. (100 − % digestibility of carbohydrates = % of total carbohydrates which are undigestible.) The percent digestibility of the carbohydrates in a food may be determined by feeding weighed amounts of the material to be tested. During the test period the feces are collected, weighed, and dried. Percent digestibility is the percent disappearance of carbohydrates (on a moisture-free basis) in the digestive tract (food carbohydrates − fecal carbohydrates = disappearance of carbohydrates). Plant foods usually contain at least small amounts of indigestible crude fat and crude protein, so most studies include proximate analyses of both the food and the feces in order to partition the digestible and undigestible components among the major nutrients (carbohydrates, fats, and proteins).

(Also see ANALYSIS OF FOODS, section headed "Digestibility Trials.")

Van Soest Analysis For Fiber.

Another approach to the problem of measuring indigestible components of plant materials is the determination of percent cell wall in the dried food.[5]

---

[5]Van Soest, P. J., "Development of a Comprehensive System of Feed Analysis and Its Application to Forages," *Journal of Animal Science*, Vol. 26, 1967, p. 119.

The procedure involves the digestion of a dried, pulverized sample in a buffered solution of a neutral detergent such as sodium laurel sulfate. Then, the digest is filtered and the dried residue is taken to represent most of the cell wall material (small amounts of pectic substances are extracted during the digestion), or *neutral detergent fiber* (NDF). Although this analysis might be carried further by the fractionation of NDF into hemicelluloses, cellulose, and lignin, such an extensive analysis of foods for fiber would not always be necessary, since neutral detergent fiber is by itself a better measure of total undigestible carbohydrate for man than is crude fiber.

(Also see ANALYSIS OF FOODS, section headed "Van Soest Analysis For Fiber.")

PHYSIOLOGICAL ACTIONS OF DIETARY FIBER.

Although man has long known about some of the beneficial and harmful effects of roughage in the digestive tract, evidence which suggests that there may be other important physiological actions of cell wall constituents has been found recently. It has even been suggested that fiber may soon be classified as an essential nutrient. Discussions of some of these effects follow.

Beneficial Effects.

There is still considerable uncertainty regarding certain potentially beneficial effects of dietary fiber. The most controversial and hypothetical of the benefits are followed by a question mark to indicate that hard evidence is lacking.

• **Antidiarrheal actions**—The gums, which are generally soothing to the digestive tract, may act against diarrhea by (1) coating inflamed surfaces, and (2) undergoing microbial fermentation to organic acids which inhibit the growth of pathogenic microorganisms. One of the popular remedies for diarrhea is a mixture of pectin and finely powdered clay (kaolin) in a water suspension.

• **Cancer prevention?**—Population studies in Africa and Finland indicate that fiber may help to prevent cancer of the bowel by increasing the rate of food passage (allowing less time for contact of carcinogens with the tissue in the bowel), and by altering the types and amounts of microorganisms (some of which may degrade bile salts to potential carcinogens). This theory, however, has not yet been tested in controlled experiments with humans or animals.

(Also see CANCER, section on "Nutrition and Diet.")

• **Constipation remedy**—The best known effect of fiber in food is the prevention, or correction, of constipation by the stimulating effect of bulk (undigested material) on the colon. Many of the carbohydrates classified under *fiber* absorb and hold water in the bowel, thereby adding to the volume of the stool and helping to prevent the contraction of the bowel in small segments. The latter function is important because it is believed that such contraction leads to the development of diverticuli, or small pouches, in the wall of the large intestine.

Another means by which fiber may help to correct constipation is by undergoing microbial fermentation to organic acids which stimulate the peristaltic movements of the colon.

NOTE WELL: It is very important to consume plenty of fluids with the water-absorbing bulking agents so that soft,

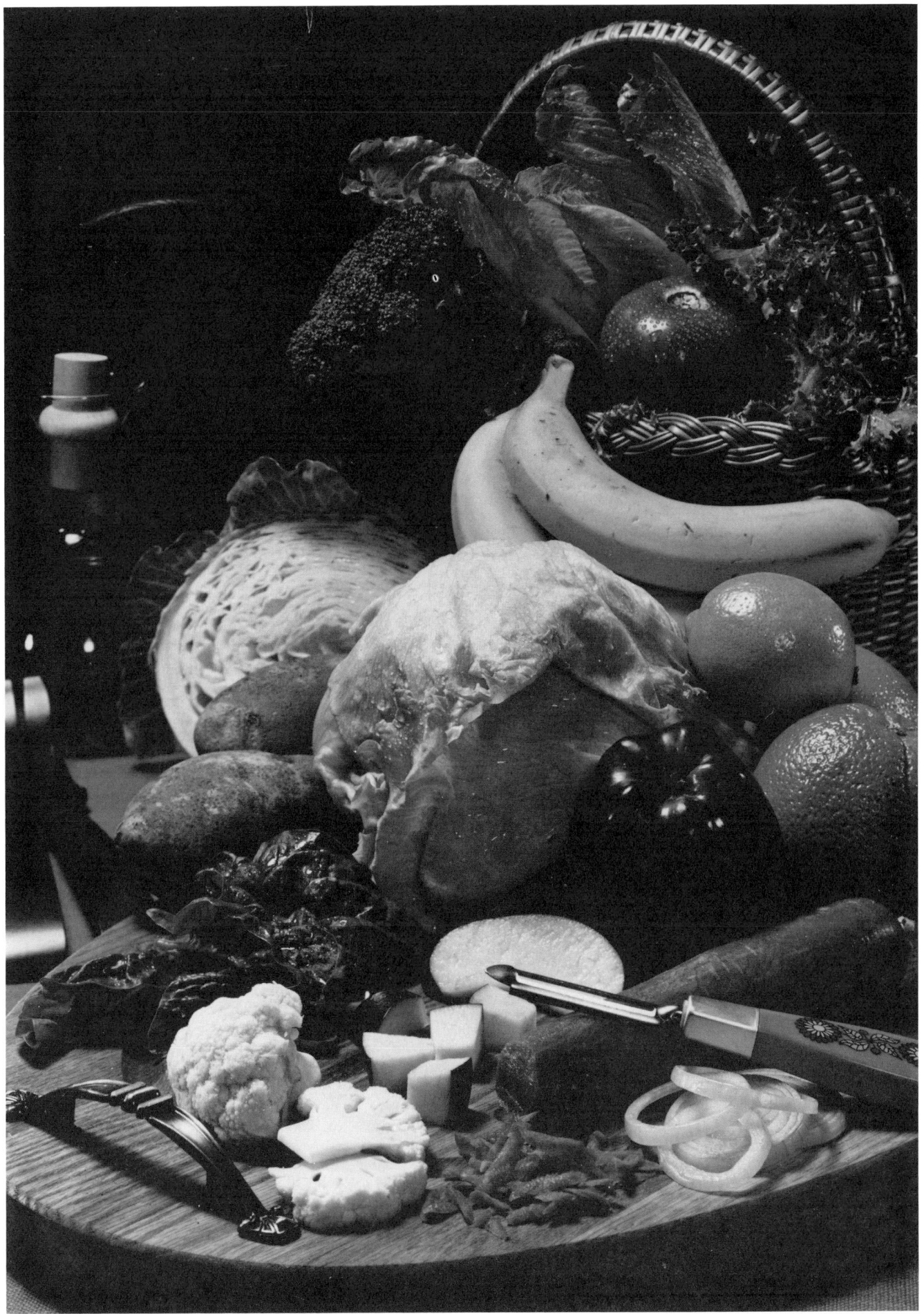

Fig. F-12. A variety of whole fruits and vegetables rich in fiber. (Courtesy, United Fresh Fruit and Vegetable Association, Alexandria, Va.)

smooth masses of fecal material pass through the colon. Otherwise, hard dry masses which can damage the intestinal tissue may be formed.

• **Detoxifying actions?**—It is suspected that various types of dietary fiber may bind potentially harmful substances that originate (1) in foods, or (2) from the action of intestinal microorganisms on the constituents of foods. Hence, a high-fiber intake may help to prevent toxicants from being absorbed, or from acting upon the tissues of the digestive tract.

• **Diabetes therapy?**—A high carbohydrate diet that is rich in fiber and other complex carbohydrates lowers the fasting blood sugar levels of adult male diabetics to significantly lower values.[6] Also, such a diet lowers the blood cholesterol and triglycerides, and reduces the requirements for oral diabetic drugs and insulin.

• **Diverticular disease prevention and therapy**—Diverticula are small pouches that form in the wall of the colon as a result of overly forceful peristaltic contractions in small segments.

It is believed that chronic constipation is a major cause of this disorder, which may become very painful if the pouches become inflamed. The inflammation is called diverticulitis. Although it was once thought that a low-fiber diet was an appropriate treatment, it has recently been found that a high-fiber diet is the best means of both prevention and treatment.

(Also see VEGETARIAN DIETS, section headed " • Diverticular disease.")

• **Gallstone therapy?**—Certain types of dietary fiber alter the composition of the bile by binding one or more of the bile salts that would otherwise be absorbed and recirculated. The altered bile is a better solvent for cholesterol (a major constituent of gallstones) than the unaltered bile. However, further tests of this dietary therapy are needed to confirm that it is both effective and safe.

• **Lipid-lowering agents?**—Recently, it was discovered that some types of dietary fiber lower the blood levels of cholesterol and triglycerides. This effect is believed to take place by the binding of bile salts and dietary lipids (mainly cholesterol and triglycerides) to the fiber. Normally, from 95 to 99% of these compounds are absorbed and transported to the liver. When, however, the absorption of bile salts and lipids is reduced by their binding to fiber and their losses in the stool, the turnover of those substances in the body is accelerated to compensate for the losses. Thus, the overall effect of fiber is to reduce the blood levels of cholesterol and triglycerides. However, food sources of fiber are not as effective in treating elevated levels of blood lipids as some of the drugs designed for this purpose.

(Also see Gallstones, section headed " • Fiber.")

• **Soothing of gastrointestinal irritation**—Mucilagenous types of fiber, such as the water-dispersible gums present in psyllium seed, okra, carob, and quince seed, coat and soothe irritated areas, particularly mucous surfaces.

• **Weight control adjunct**—Eating a diet high in fiber is likely to result in the consumption of less food energy because the digestive tract becomes full sooner. Normally, appetite is diminished by the distention of the gastrointestinal tract. Food plants consumed by prehistoric Indians in Mexico have been found to have been very high in fiber (as determined by analysis of present day plants which matched the dried specimens found in the caves inhabited by the Indians). Anthropologists believe that the prehistoric Mexicans may have had enlarged digestive tracts as a result of regular consumption of such fibrous food plants.

(Also see OBESITY, section headed " • Fiber" and "Water; substances that fill, but do not fatten.")

Potentially Harmful Effects. High-fiber diets which contain seed coats (rich in phytates) and other undigestible substances, may interfere with the absorption of minerals and other nutrients since the fibrous materials accelerate the flow of food through the digestive tract and bind certain nutrients and carry them into the stool. For example, digestibility studies have shown that high levels of dietary fiber reduce the digestibility of fat and protein. Also, people with severe inflammation of the lower bowel, and those recovering from gastrointestinal surgery, often need to eat low-fiber diets until they have sufficient healing. Finally, the consumption of excessive amounts of fiber may lead to enlargement and twisting of the sigmoid colon (the condition called volvulus).

DIETARY FIBER RECOMMENDATIONS. People who are unaccustomed to high-fiber diets should eat just enough fiber to ensure the regularity of bowel movements. Studies with human subjects have shown that there is a relationship between the degree of laxative effect and the proportion of dietary fiber per unit of body weight.[7] It was found that the passage of 1 stool per day may be ensured for most persons by the consumption of 0.02 to 0.03 g of crude fiber per pound of body weight. Persons with a tendency towards constipation may require 0.04 to 0.05 g of fiber per pound (*0.45 kg*) of body weight. Thus, a 160-lb (*72-kg*) man, who has a tendency to be constipated, may require as much as 8.0 g of crude fiber per day to ensure his regularity. It is not unusual for populations consuming mainly plant foods to eat as much as 25 g of fiber per day.

SELECTION AND PREPARATION OF FOODS HIGH IN FIBER. Although there has been selective cultivation by man of plant varieties low in fiber (more succulent and tender), there is still available a wide range of foods with moderate to high fiber content. The crude fiber contents of a large number of foods are given in Food Composition Table F-21. In order to help the reader identify the leading fiber-rich foods, the crude fiber and energy contents of selected items are presented in Table F-5.

To use the data on fiber content, select the basic types of foods desired for a meal or a diet (breakfast cereal, fruit, bread, etc.). Then identify the items with the desired fiber contents, note the amounts provided by 100 g (about 3 ½ oz) of the foods and calculate the fiber supplied by the

[6]Kiehm, T. G., et al., "Beneficial Effects of a High Carbohydrate, High Fiber Diet on Hyperglycemic Diabetic Men," *The American Journal of Clinical Nutrition*, Vol. 29, August 1976, pp. 895-899.

[7]Cowgill, G. R., and W. E. Anderson, "Laxative Effects of Wheat Bran and 'Washed Bran' in Healthy Men. A Comparative Study," *Journal of the American Medical Association*, Vol. 98, 1932, p. 1866.

TABLE F-5
TOP SOURCES OF CRUDE FIBER AND THEIR CALORIC CONTENT[1]

Top Sources[2]	Crude Fiber	Energy
	(mg/100 g)	(kcal/100 g)
Coriander seed	29.1	298
Bay leaves	26.3	313
Pepper, red	24.9	318
Cinnamon	24.4	261
Chili powder	22.2	314
Allspice	21.6	263
Dill Seed	21.1	253
Paprika, domestic	20.9	289
Rosemary leaves	19.0	331
Thyme	18.6	276
Marjoram, dried	18.1	271
Sage	18.1	315
Basil	17.8	251
Rosemary, ground	17.7	331
Curry powder	16.3	325
Fennel seed	15.7	345
Savory	15.3	272
Oregano	15.0	306
Pumpkin pie spice	14.9	342
Anise seed	14.6	337
Pepper, black, ground	13.1	255
Caraway seeds	12.7	333
Parsley, dried	10.3	276
Wheat bran	9.1	350
Pepper, hot chili, mature, red, raw, pods and seeds	9.0	93
Carob flour	7.7	180
Bran breakfast cereals, average of several types	7.6	239
Pears, dried, uncooked	6.3	268
Peppers, hot chili, mature, red, dried pods	6.2	321
Cocoa powder, low fat	5.8	187
Raspberries, black, raw	5.1	73
Figs, dried, uncooked	4.7	274
Onions, mature, dehydrated flakes	4.4	350
Cocoa powder, high and medium fat	4.3	280
Blackberries, raw	4.1	58
Coconut meat, average of several products	4.0	519
Apples, dehydrated, uncooked	3.8	353
Olives, ripe, cured, Greek style	3.0	338
Bran flakes with raisins	3.0	287
Raspberries, red, raw	3.0	57
Almonds, unsalted	3.0	598
Apricots, dried, uncooked	3.0	260

[1]These listings are based on the data in Food Composition Table F-21. Some top or rich sources may have been overlooked since some of the foods in Table F-21 lack values for crude fiber.

Whenever possible, foods are on an *as used* basis, without regard to moisture content; hence, the fiber content of certain high-moisture foods may be misleading when ranked on the basis of crude fiber content per 100 g (about 3½ oz) without regard to moisture content.

[2]Listed without regard to the amount normally eaten.

a product by drying, or adds less digestible materials, such as the addition of bran to breads or cereals. For example, on an equal weight basis (pound for pound), dried fruits contain from 3 to 7 times the calories, fiber, and other nutrients of fresh fruits.

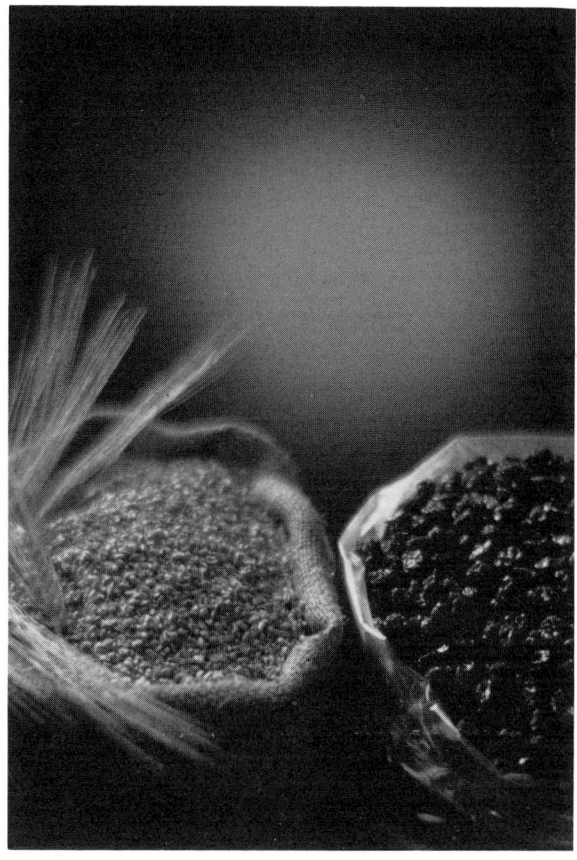

Fig. F-13. Whole cereal grain and whole fruit, two high-fiber foods. (Courtesy, Siegel/Ketchum, San Francisco, Calif.)

amounts of foods to be consumed. For example, a 1 oz (28 g) serving of a bran breakfast cereal furnishes about 2.2 g of fiber (7.6 g per 3½ oz ÷ 3½ = 2.2 g per oz). (The food energy values may be used similarly to make choices between the various items within each of the basic food groups.)

For those who do not wish to bother with calculations of fiber and energy contents, some suggestions for the selection and preparation of foods high in fiber follow:

1. All plant foods are likely to contain at least small amounts of fiber, while animal foods (meat, eggs, fish, dairy products) are almost totally digestible (unless they have been made less digestible by improper cooking).

2. Fresh, unrefined food usually contains more fiber than processed food, except when the processor concentrates

3. Green leafy vegetables and stems of plants are higher in fiber than starchy roots and tubers. An exception to this rule is the inulin-containing roots and tubers, such as those of dandelions, chicory, globe artichokes, Jerusalem artichokes, and salsify. Although inulin is not classified as crude fiber, it is undigestible. However, long storage of inulin-containing roots and tubers may result in conversion, by enzymes in the plant, of inulin to fructose, which is completely utilized by man.

4. Seed coats of grains and legumes are high in fiber, as are the skins and peels of fruits and vegetables.

5. The sprouting of seeds results in more fiber and less food energy.

6. Whole fruits and vegetables usually contain more nonnutritive carbohydrate than the juices extracted from them, since juice extraction generally involves removal of the fiber by straining or other means.

7. The pulpy residue from the juicing of oranges and other fruits may be added to dishes such as biscuits, muffins, puddings, and sauces.

8. Pureed cooked vegetables such as beans, beets, carrots, peas, spinach, squash, sweet potatoes, and turnips may be used to thicken sauces and soups.

CAUTION: Although it is possible to select a diet low in calories and very high in fiber, a sudden change from a low-fiber diet to a high-fiber diet may result in digestive problems such as bowel pains, excessive gas (flatulence), and diarrhea. Also, liberal amounts of water should be ingested, particularly when dried, fibrous foods (bran, dried fruits, dehydrated vegetables) are eaten. There have been reports of distention and pain of the esophagus, and blockage, irritation, and perforation of the colon and rectum resulting from the consumption of dried cellulosic materials without sufficient fluid.

It is also noteworthy that, throughout their lives, many people consume diets which are low in fiber, yet they appear to be healthy and live to ripe old ages. There is a possibility that some of these people have considerable amounts of friendly bacteria in their bowels. Bacterial cell walls are high in fiber and thereby contribute to the bulk of the stool. Diets high in milk and dairy products, for example, may encourage an intestinal growth of lactic acid producing bacteria which apparently stimulate peristalsis by various means. There are also people who cannot tolerate high-fiber diets because of diarrhea or various bowel troubles.

SPECIAL PRODUCTS FOR DIETETIC AND THERAPEUTIC USES.

Although a diet high in fiber may be readily achieved by people who shop in supermarkets and prepare most of their meals at home, it is more difficult for those who eat much of their food in restaurants to consume such a diet regularly. Furthermore, some people do not care to eat the natural foods which are high in fiber. Finally, dietitians and physicians may wish to recommend diets of known fiber content or special low-energy recipes. Therefore, it is desirable in many of these cases to be able to prepare meals where forms of semipurified fiber could be added in known amounts of refined foods. Examples of some special high-fiber products follow:

• **Agar (agar-agar)**—This nonnutritive seaweed gum, called *kanten* by the Japanese, is used to prepare low-calorie recipes, such as jellies, candies, and gelled salads (agar is used by strict vegetarians in place of gelatin). Although the purified flakes are costly (a dollar or so per ounce, or *28 g*), a little goes a long way (1 tsp or 5 g may be used with a pint or 500 ml of hot water).

• **Alfalfa flour**—This is a highly nutritious item (it is rich in protein, fiber, minerals, and vitamins). Usually, alfalfa flour is added in small amounts to (1) the batters or doughs used to prepare various types of baked goods, and (2) sauces or soups.

• **Bran**—This product is well known for its laxative effect and is one of the cheapest sources of food fiber since it is a by-product (seed coat) of the milling of wheat and other cereals. Although not very appetizing by itself, it mixes well in cereals and baked goods. However, it is noteworthy that bran has caused gastrointestinal irritation in some people.

• **Dehydrated onion flakes**—A little of this product goes a long way in that small amounts exert a moderately strong laxative action. On a dry weight basis, onions produce from 2 to 3 times as much intestinal gas as beans.

• **Flax seed**—These nutlike seeds are tasty additions to grain products. Like bran, flax seed is an effective laxative. In addition to being available as seeds, flax seeds are an ingredient of certain ready-to-eat breakfast cereals.

• **Pectin**—This material is extracted from citrus peel and apple pomace (the residue after extraction of juice). It is available in pure form, or in mixtures that contain added sugar and acid and are used to prepare jams and jellies. Although pure citrus pectin has been given orally in the powdered form (1 or 2 tsp [*5 or 10 ml*] per day) to counteract the effects of dietary cholesterol, a more desirable use for it is in low-calorie recipes such as imitation or eggless mayonnaise, tomato aspic, fruit desserts, and pie filling. It is also used in antidiarrheal preparations.

• **Psyllium seed**—Although there are several important varieties of psyllium, the blond variety from India (*Plantago ovata*) is used the most because of its high content of colorless gum. The powdered form (pulverized material from the seeds) swells in water and yields a mucilaginous mixture which is useful as a demulcent (an agent that soothes and protects the lining of the digestive system), a stopping-up agent against diarrhea (the powder is taken with only a small amount of fluid so that a gummy substance is formed in the intestine), or a laxative (the powder is taken with a large amount of water to produce a soft bulk which also lubricates the bowel). A gel is formed when a 1% solution (a teaspoon of psyllium in a pint of water) is heated to 195°F (90°C) and allowed to cool. Like agar and pectin, there are potential uses for psyllium in various recipes. This material also helps to counteract the effects of dietary cholesterol.

Although the nutrition counselor should be aware of the possible role of fiber in the maintenance of buoyant good health, the importance of fiber in the human diet will finally be determined by additional clinical and experimental observations.

(Also see CARBOHYDRATE[S], section headed "Provide Fiber.")

FIBRIN

The insoluble fibrous strands of protein essential to the clotting of blood, derived from fibrinogen by the action of the enzyme thrombin.

FIBRINOGEN

A protein in blood, which, through the action of enzyme thrombin, is converted to fibrin.

FIBROUS

High in cellulose and/or lignin content.
(Also see CARBOHYDRATES, UNAVAILABLE; and FIBER.)

FIBROUS PROTEINS (ALBUMINOIDS, SCLERO-PROTEINS)

Those proteins which form long chains bound together in a parallel fashion are called fibrous proteins. They are the proteins of connective tissue, elastic tissue, and hair, or specifically collagen, elastin, and keratin. Fibrous proteins are not very digestible.
(Also see PROTEIN, section headed "Classification.")

FIG *Ficus carica*

Fig trees belong to the mulberry family, *Moraceae.*

The fig tree is a deciduous bush or tree which grows in the subtropical regions of Asia, Africa, Europe, and the United States.

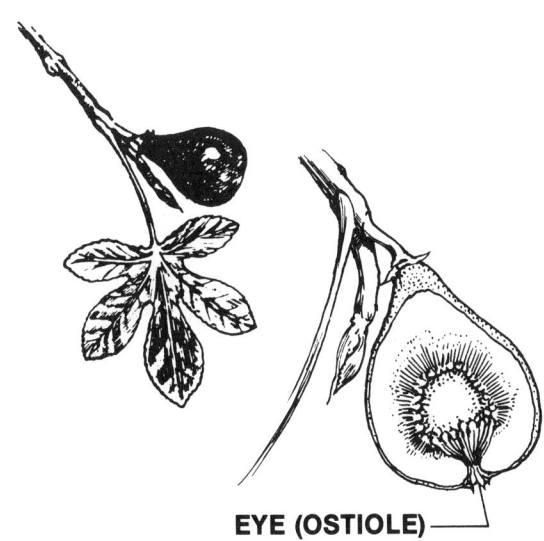

EYE (OSTIOLE)

Fig. F-14. The common orchard fig showing the deeply lobed leaves, and the fleshy fruit with its seedy interior.

ORIGIN AND HISTORY. The Fig is native to the eastern Mediterranean and southwestern Asian regions where its cultivation began. From here, it spread to warm, semiarid areas throughout the world.

WORLD AND U.S. PRODUCTION. Most of world fig production is in Turkey, Greece, United States, Portugal, and Spain.

The United States produces about 46,000 short tons of figs, annually. California produces 99% of the U.S. commercial fig crop.[8]

PROCESSING. About 90% of the fig crop is utilized as dried figs, while the rest is sold fresh or canned.

Upon receipt of fruit, processors hold it under fumigation until processing. Varieties tending to darken, such as Calimyrna and Adriatic, are held in cold storage if facilities are available. Highest quality figs are used whole as *package stock*, while other figs are sliced and ground into *fig paste* and a limited quantity is used for fig juice or *concentrate*. Processing begins by sizing the fruit, passing the figs through a mechanical washer, and then through a retort filled with hot water and steam. This cleans the fruit and increases the moisture content. In the preparation of paste the figs are sliced and then refrigerated to prevent darkening and spoilage. They are maintained under refrigeration until ground into paste.

SELECTION, PREPARATION, AND USES. Figs should be plump, well colored, free from damage, and clean.

Most figs are eaten dried but they may also be eaten fresh, canned, preserved, or pickled. Figs are eaten alone or in fruit dishes, baked goods, jams, relishes, or salads. Bakers use the fig paste in fig bars, fig filled cookies, and other bakers products.

[8]Based on data from *Agricultural Statistics 1991*, USDA, p. 195, Table 290. **Note well:** Annual production fluctuates as a result of weather and profitability of the crop.

NUTRITIONAL VALUE. Raw and canned figs contain 65 to 80 Calories (kcal) of energy per 100 g (about 3½ oz), while dried figs contain 266 Calories (kcal) per 100 g. Dried figs are about 60% sugar—glucose, fructose, and sucrose. Furthermore, dried figs are a good source of calcium, potassium, and iron, containing 152 mg, 773 mg and 2.1 mg/100 g, respectively. More complete nutritional data regarding raw, canned, or dried figs and fig cookies is presented in Food Composition Table F-21.

FIGS, DRIED

The major types of dried figs available in the United States are: (1) light tan Adriatic or Greek string; (2) black Mission; and (3) golden brown Turkish Smyrna and Calimyrna (a California variety developed from the Smyrna fig). Usually, a Smyrna type sells for a much higher price than either the Greek or Mission types because it has a distinctive honey flavor and requires a special type of pollination in its production. Recently, there has been a trend away from the production of the dry, tough figs of the past to moister, more tender products that are protected from spoilage by treatment with potassium sorbate.

Dried figs are high in calories, sugar, fiber, and potassium. They are also good sources of calcium and iron. Many people find that the liberal consumption of dried or stewed figs helps to promote regularity of bowel movements.

(Also see FIG.)

FINELY GROUND

Reduced to very small particle size by impact, shearing, or attrition.

FINES

Any material which will pass through a screen whose openings are immediately smaller than the specified minimum size.

FINISH

To fatten a slaughter animal. Also, the degree of fatness of such an animal.

(Also see MEAT.)

FIRELESS COOKER OR HAYBOX

A tight box packed with hay as insulation, in which food that has been cooked for a short time is placed, and where it continues to remain hot for several hours.

FISH AND SEAFOOD(S)

Fish are vertebrate animals which live exclusively in water, breathe through gills, and have limbs which take the form of fins. Fish make up more than half of all known species of vertebrates. Scientists have named and described more than 20,000 kinds of fish.

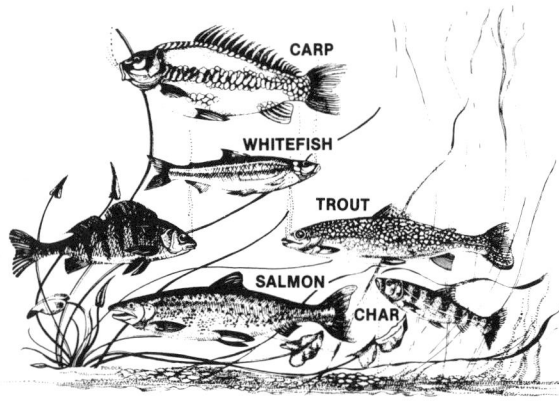

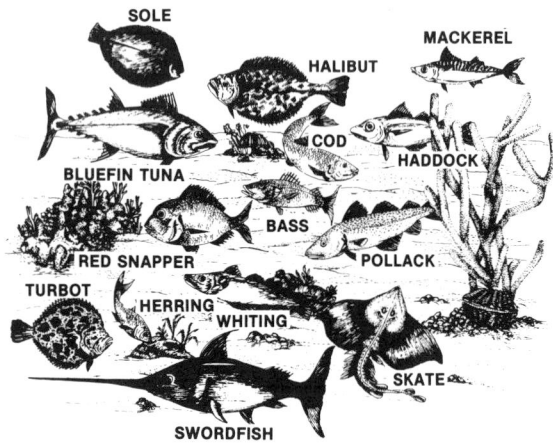

Fig. F-15. Fishes of the world. The upper sketches show freshwater fish, whereas the lower sketches show saltwater fish.

Millions of tons of fish and seafood are taken from the seas, rivers, lakes, and ponds every year. Fish and seafood serve as food and they are also used in manufacturing numerous industrial products.

Fish are classified as freshwater or saltwater fish. Freshwater fish live in the lakes, streams and ponds on land, while the saltwater fish live in the oceans which cover more than 70% of the earth's surface.

Catfish, carp, pike and pickerel, sturgeon, and white fish are popular freshwater fish.

Saltwater fish are often classified in the fishing industry as anadromous, groundfish, or pelagic fish.

• **Anadromous fish**—These fish are born in fresh water, swim to the ocean as adults, and return to their birthplace to spawn. The alewife, American shad, and salmon are examples of anadromous fish.

• **Groundfish or demersal fish**—These fish live near the bottom of the ocean. Fish of the cod family, flatfish family, the mullet, the pompano, the porgy, the red snapper, and sea bass are groundfish.

• **Pelagic fish**—These fish stay in the upper layers of the ocean. Fish of the herring family and the mackerel family are classified as pelagic fish.

Seafood also includes shellfish—which is a commercial, rather than a scientific classification. Shellfish refers to hard-covered, edible, mostly marine animals from two different groups: the mollusks (oysters, clams, mussels) and the crustaceans (crabs, lobsters, and sometimes shrimp). Among the important mollusk species, harvested from both wild and cultivated stocks, are oysters, hard clams, surf clams, quahogs, soft-shell clams, razor clams, and horse clams.

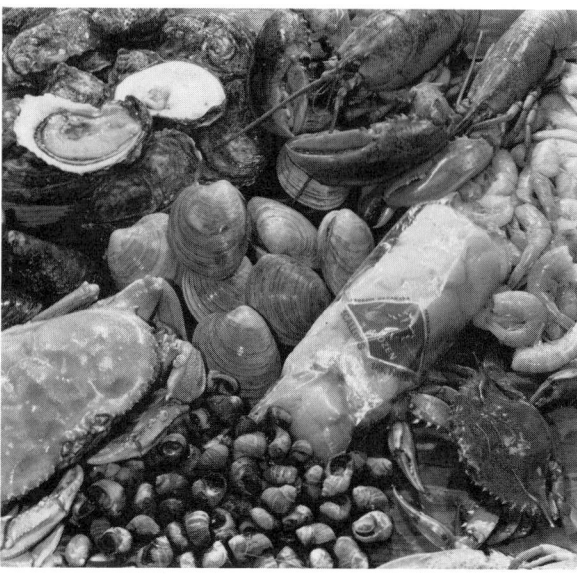

Fig. F-16. Some examples of shellfish harvested by fishermen. (Courtesy, Department of Fisheries and Oceans, Canada)

In addition, octopus, squid, sea turtles, and possibly other foods are taken from the seas, depending upon the area and culture.

HISTORY OF FISHING. Fishing is one of the oldest and most important activities of man. Ancient remains of spears, hooks, and fishnets have been found in ruins of the Stone Age. The people of early civilizations drew pictures of nets and fishermen lines in their art. Through the ages, men wrote about fishing, used fish in exchange for services, and even learned to fish farm.

Commercial fishing on the North American continent started over 300 years ago—with the first colonists. So many fish were close to shore that the colonists did not have to build large sailing vessels as the Europeans did. Instead, the colonists followed the Indians' example and fished from small boats. Some fish were caught in traps and weirs (brush fences) set in the mouths of rivers and harbors. Shore fishermen used nets or, when the tide had gone out, searched the rocks and sand for shellfish.

As colonization progressed, fishermen began sailing farther out to sea to find enough fish for a good catch. They sailed for months as they worked the fishing banks off Canada, and northeastern United States. Many of the early houses along the coast in colonial America had a walk around the roof so that the family could watch for returning ships. Many ships did not return, and this walk became known as the widow's walk.

As ships grew larger and fishing methods were developed and refined, the success of fishing voyages and the types of fish and seafood increased. Like other commercial opera-

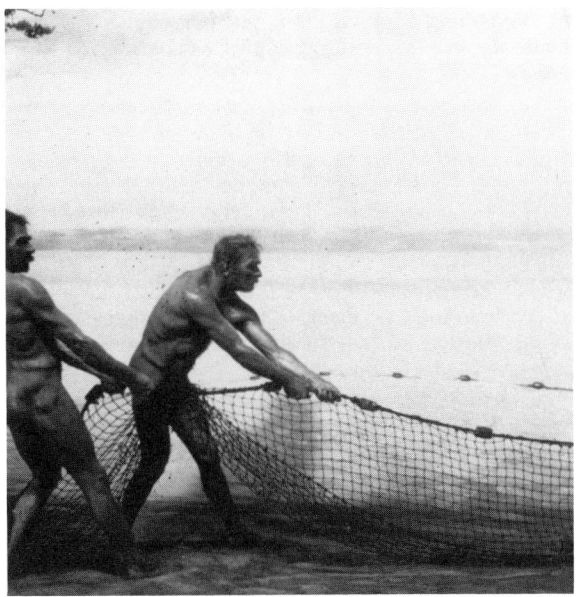

Fig. F-17. Swiss lake dwellers seining, 2800 B.C. (Courtesy, Field Museum of Natural History, Chicago, Ill.)

tions, the fishing industry became mechanized. Today, such technologies as airplane spotters, radar, radio-telephones, sonar, and long-range radio navigation (LORAN), are employed in the fishing industry. Some fishing fleets have a factory ship with equipment on board for fileting and freezing or canning. With all of these new developments, ships were able to find new fishing grounds by sailing farther from port and returning safely—loaded with fish. During the 60 years or so between 1900 and the late 1960s, the world fish catch increased by 27 times.

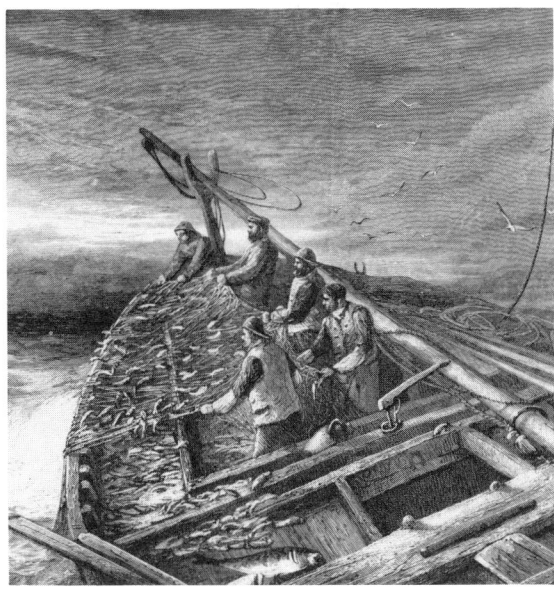

Fig. F-18. Commercial fishing in the early 1800s was hard work—fighting rough seas and handling large catches. (Courtesy, The Bettmann Archive, Inc., New York, N.Y., from an 1875 engraving.)

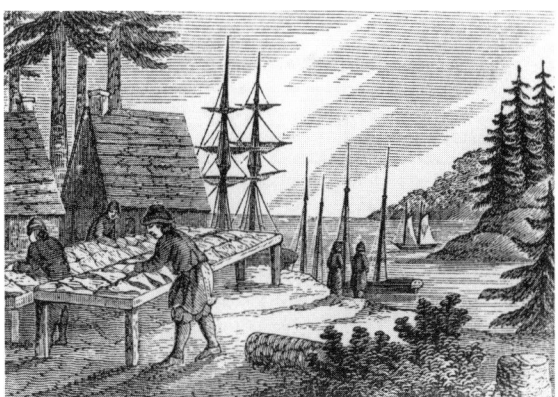

Fig. F-19. To the first colonists of Maine, fishing was the most common occupation since it was easy and profitable. The products of fishing could be bartered for food from other colonies or from England. (Courtesy, The Bettmann Archive, Inc., New York, N.Y.)

FISHING INDUSTRY. As a fishing nation, the United States has declined. As shown in Table F-6, the United States ranked fourth in fish catch in 1984, with Japan and the U.S.S.R. far in the lead, followed by China. In 1988, the United States ranked fifth.

TABLE F-6
CATCH OF FISH
OF FIVE MAJOR FISHING COUNTRIES[1]

Country	Year 1984	Year 1988	Percent of 1988 World Catch
	(billion lb)		(%)
Japan	26.5	26.2	12.1
U.S.S.R.	23.4	25.0	11.5
China	13.1	22.8	10.5
Peru	7.4	14.6	6.7
U.S.A.	10.6	13.3	6.1
Total World Catch	183.2	216.9	

[1]Based on data from *Statistical Abstract of the United States*, 1991, U.S. Department of Commerce, p. 857, Table 1478.

Distant fishing ranks as one of the most energy-consuming methods of producing food. Each calorie of food energy gained by distant fishing requires an input of about 11 Calories (kcal) of energy.

U.S. Species Fish Catch. A relatively few species of fish and shellfish comprise the majority of the catch in the United States. These species and their catch in selected years since 1970 are shown in Table F-7.

With the exception of tuna, and a few lobsters and shrimp, the fish and shellfish listed in Table F-7 are caught within 200 miles (*320 km*) of the U.S. shores. Most tuna, 94%, are caught at distances over 200 miles (*320 km*) from U.S. shores.

In terms of dollars, the U.S. fishing industry's catch is worth more than $3.2 billion. The average price per pound (*0.45 kg*) for the overall catch increased from 2.4¢/lb in 1940 to 38.3¢/lb in 1989. Pacific Salmon is the most valuable catch, worth $591 million, and shrimp is next, being worth $468 million. The crab catch is valued at about $414 million, and tuna at about $104 million. Alaska pollock has become a valuable catch, worth $187 million.

TABLE F-7
CATCH OF PRINCIPAL SPECIES FROM U.S. FISHERIES BY SELECTED YEARS[1]

Species	Yearly Catch		
	1970	1980	1989
	◄──── (million pounds) ────►		
Fish:			
Cod, Atlantic	53	118	78
Flounder	169	217	203
Haddock	27	55	4
Halibut	35	19	75
Herring, sea	79	291	200
Jack mackerel	47	44	28
Menhaden	1,837	2,497	1,989
Ocean perch, Atlantic	55	24	2
Pollock, Atlantic	9	43	23
Salmon, Pacific	410	614	786
Tuna	393	399	89
Whiting	45	36	39
Shellfish:			
Clams	99	95	138
Crabs	277	523	458
Lobsters, American	34	37	53
Oysters	54	49	32
Scallops	11	30	42
Shrimp	367	340	331

[1]Data from *Statistical Abstract of the United States*, 1980, U.S. Department of Commerce, p. 744, Table 1315; 1984, p. 704, Table 1252; and 1991, p. 686, Table 1202. To convert to kg divide by 2.2.

Table F-8 indicates the values of the principal species from U.S. fisheries for 1989.

TABLE F-8
VALUE OF PRINCIPAL SPECIES FROM U.S. FISHERIES ON A LIVEWEIGHT BASIS EXCEPT WHERE INDICATED[1]

Species	Catch	Value	Price per Pound[3]
	(million lb)[2]	($ million)	($)
Fish:			
Cod, Atlantic	78	48	.61
Flounder	202	120	.59
Haddock	4	5	1.19
Halibut	75	85	1.13
Herring, sea	209	29	.14
Jack mackerel	28	1	.07
Menhaden	1,989	84	.04
Ocean perch, Atlantic ..	1	.9	.66
Pollock	23	10	.43
Salmon, Pacific	786	591	.75
Tuna	89	104	1.16
Whiting	39	9	.24
Shellfish:			
Clams	138	135	.98
Crabs	458	414	.90
Lobsters, American	53	149	2.82
Oysters	30	84	2.79
Scallops	40	138	3.43
Shrimp	352	468	1.33

[1]Based on data from *Statistical Abstract of the United States*, 1991, U.S. Department of Commerce, p. 686, Table 1202.

[2]To convert to kg divide by 2.2.

[3]Average price paid to the fisherman.

Fish Farming. This is the raising of food fish and other aquatic life in protected enclosures or controlled natural environments.

Although recent research has shown the advantages of fish farming as an alternative type of livestock production, aquaculture—the science of fish farming—is by no means a newly discovered science. Evidence of fish farming dates back 4,000 years to China, Japan, and Egypt. The practice of fish culture can be found in the societies of India and Java 3,000 years ago, and of Europe 2,500 years ago. Through the years, most of the progress in fish farming has evolved from trial and error. In the United States, it is still a small industry, but new methods and technologies will likely spur its development.

Aquaculture can be divided into two types of production—freshwater and marine water.

PROCESSING FISH AND SEAFOOD. Once caught, the fish must be processed for preservation and for consumer consumption. This includes fish packaged fresh and frozen, canned, or cured (salted, smoked, or dried). In addition to the edible products for humans, some fish are caught solely for industrial purposes. Also, there are a number of by-products from the edible fish industry.

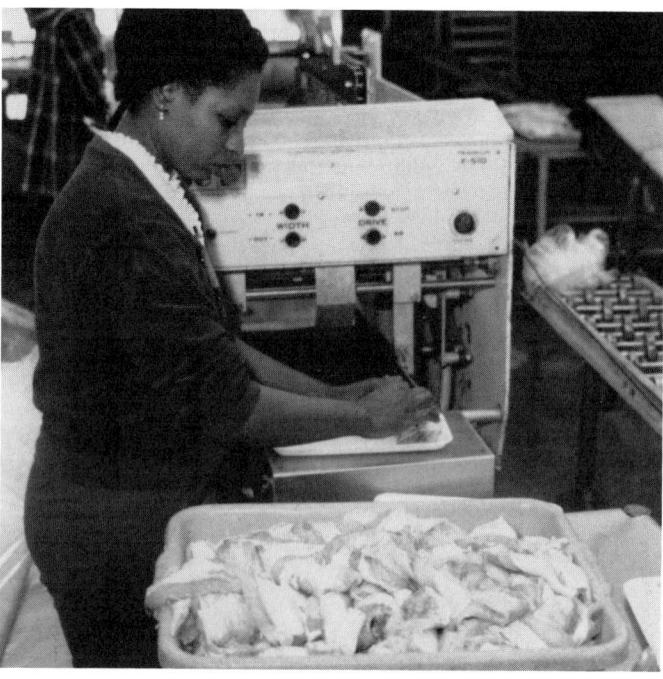

Fig. F-20. Packaging fresh farm-raised catfish fillets. (Courtesy, Mississippi Cooperative Extension Service, MSU, USDA)

Products and Preservation. Of the U.S. catch, 26% is marketed fresh and frozen; 43% is canned; and the remaining 31% becomes by-products and bait. A fully equipped factory ship will have machinery on board for fish filleting and freezing or canning. Fish fillets are often frozen at sea into large blocks weighing up to 100 lb (*45 kg*), which are later reprocessed on shore into individual portions. Some ships may also have facilities for drying and grinding fish into fish meal. The U.S.S.R. pioneered in the development of factory ships, which are often huge vessels operated by crews of 500 to 650, and accompanied by their own fleets of smaller ships called catcher boats.

Some of the details of canning vary for the different species of fish but the fundamental process is the same. Fish are prepared by grading, cleaning, and cutting for the filling machines or for hand packing. After the fish are packed and seasoned, the air is exhausted from the cans, which are then sealed and cooked. Some oily fish, such as sardines and tuna, are precooked before packing. Specialty products, such as fish soups, require more preparation.

Curing fish includes drying, smoking, salting, and pickling. Methods of drying fish by blowing warm, dry air on them have replaced sun-drying in some areas. Herring, salmon, smelt, and mackerel are commonly smoked. The cleaned fish is salted, washed, and drained in preparation for smoking. It is then partially dried and hung in the smokehouse for curing. Producers of salted or pickled fish develop their own characteristic flavor. The process consists of salting, draining, and drying.

Besides being sold whole for fileted, fresh, or frozen, many processors also make breaded fish sticks and meal-sized portions of breaded fish that are sold frozen cooked or ready to cook.

(Also see PRESERVATION OF FOOD.)

• **Shellfish**—Seafood items falling in this category are handled somewhat differently than fin fish. Because of great susceptibility to spoilage, such species are often kept alive during a part of their commercial handling. Oysters and clams should be alive until shucked and crab and lobster until cooked. A considerable portion of the U.S. shrimp is beheaded (usually at sea), washed and graded ashore, and packaged and frozen in the shell usually in institution-sized packages. For the ultimate consumer's use, shrimp is peeled and deveined, often by machine, and then packaged and frozen. A considerable portion is breaded after peeling and then packaged and frozen. Crab are cooked in the shell and the meat picked by hand. Sometimes, especially in the Chesapeake Bay area, the picked meat is pasteurized by raising the temperature of the meat to 170°F (77°C) for 1 minute, thereby greatly extending the storage life of the refrigerated product. Much of the East Coast blue crab and the Pacific Coast dungeness crab is marketed unfrozen, but a considerable portion of the more recently developed Alaskan king crab is sold as a frozen product. The crab is cooked in the shell and the meat removed from the shell by passing through rubber rollers. The meat is then usually frozen in large blocks which are ice glazed and later sawed into consumer sized units. Some king crab is cut in sections and frozen in the shell.

Industrial Products. The commercial value of fish is not limited to its use as food. Various industrial products contain fish parts or fish by-products. For example, manufacturers make shoes from the skins of sharks. Abalone shells are made into buttons. Other manufacturers use by-products to make glue. A kind of gelatin called *isinglass* is made from the air bladders of certain fish. Menhaden, sardines, herrings, and sharks produce valuable oils. These oils are used in making paints and varnishes, in tanning leather, and in the manufacture of linoleum and synthetic materials.

• **Fish flour or fish protein concentrate**—Scraps and waste from fish contain much protein. Much of this waste is processed into dried meal and concentrates that are used for animal feeds. During the early 1970s, many nations sought ways to convert fish waste into food for human beings. They worked to develop an odorless, tasteless fish flour or fish protein concentrate that could be added to foods in parts of the world where people lack sufficient protein in their diets. Fish protein concentrate is prepared through the solvent extraction processing of clean, undecomposed whole fish or fish cuttings.

(Also see FLOURS, Table F-13 Special Flours.)

BUYING FISH AND SEAFOOD. Fish and seafood are marketed in several forms, and buyers should be aware of these forms. Fresh and frozen fish are marketed in various forms or cuts. The following are the best known market forms:

• **Whole**—This is fish as they come from the water. Before cooking, the fish must be scaled and eviscerated—usually the head, tail, and fins are removed. The fish may then be cooked, fileted, or cut into steaks or chunks.

• **Dressed**—These are fish with scales and entrails removed, and usually the head, tail, and fins are removed. The fish may then be cooked, fileted, or cut into steaks or chunks. The smaller size fish are called pan dressed and are ready to cook as purchased.

• **Filets**—Filets are the sides of the fish cut lengthwise away from the backbone. They are ready to cook as purchased. A filet cut from one side of a fish is called a single filet. This is the type most generally available on the market. The filets may or may not be skinless.

The two sides of the fish cut lengthwise away from the backbone and held together by the uncut flesh and skin of the belly are referred to as butterfly filets.

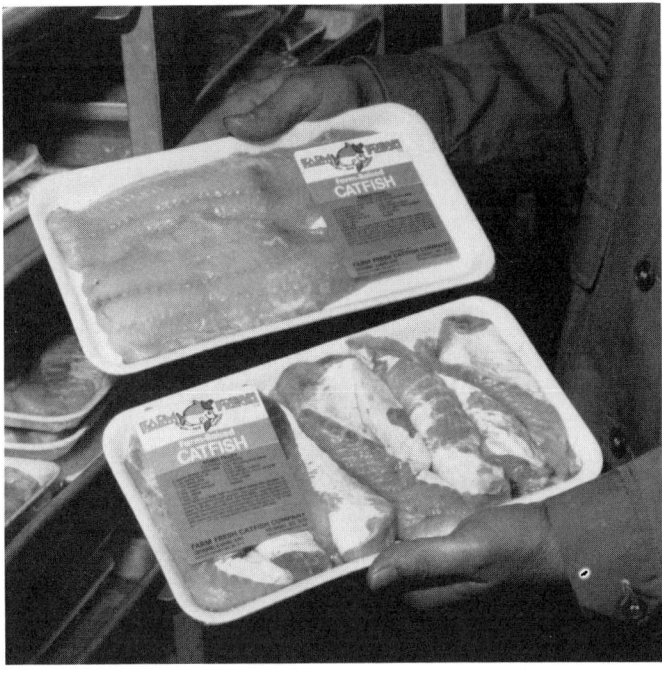

Fig. F-21. Tray-packed catfish filets ready for market. (Courtesy, Mississippi Cooperative Extension Service, MSU, USDA)

• **Steaks**—Steaks are cross section slices from large dressed fish cut 5/8 to 1 in. *(1.6 to 2.5 cm)* thick. A cross section of the backbone is the only bone in a steak. They are ready to cook as purchased.

• **Chunks**—Chunks are cross sections of large dressed fish. A cross section of the backbone is the only bone in a chunk. They are ready to cook as purchased.

• **Raw breaded fish portions**—Portions are cut from frozen fish blocks, coated with a batter, breaded, packaged, and frozen. Raw breaded fish portions weigh more than 1½ oz *(42 g)*, are at least ³/₈ in. *(0.9 cm)* thick, and must contain not less than 75% fish. They are ready to cook as purchased.

• **Fried fish portions**—Portions are cut from frozen fish blocks, coated with a batter, breaded, partially cooked, packaged, and frozen. Fried fish portions weigh more than 1½ oz *(42 g)*, are at least ³/₈ in. *(0.9 cm)* thick, and must contain not less than 65% fish. They are ready to heat and serve as purchased.

• **Fish sticks**—Sticks are cut from frozen fish blocks, coated with a batter, breaded, partially cooked, packaged, and frozen. Fried fish sticks weigh up to 1½ oz *(42 g)*, are at least ³/₈ in. *(0.9 cm)* thick, and must contain not less than 60% fish. They are ready to heat and serve as purchased.

Some shellfish are marketed alive. Other market forms, depending on the variety, include cooked whole in the shell, headless, shucked or fresh meat, cooked meat, breaded, and canned. The following descriptions apply to shellfish:

• **Live in the shell**—Crabs, lobsters, clams, and oysters are available live in their shells. Shellfish purchased live in the shell must be kept alive until it is served or cooked.

• **Cooked in the shell**—Crabs and lobsters are available cooked in the shell either chilled or frozen.

• **Headless**—The shrimp tail is the only part that is sold. Spiny lobster tails are also a common market form. These are ready to cook.

• **Shucked or fresh meat**—Clam, oyster, and scallop meats are available without the shells, either fresh or frozen.

• **Cooked meat**—The cooked meat is picked from the shell of cooked crab, lobster, and shrimp and is available either fresh, frozen, or canned.

• **Breaded**—Frozen raw, breaded or frozen fried clams, oysters, scallops, and shrimp are available. These shellfish are ready to cook or heat as purchased.

• **Canned**—Clams, crabs, lobsters, and shrimp are available canned. They are ready to serve or use as purchased.

Once a person is familiar with the various forms in which fish and seafood can be purchased, there are a few guidelines to follow when buying fresh fish, frozen fish, and shellfish:

• **Fresh fish**—The flesh is firm and elastic and not separating from the bones. In buying filets and steaks, look for a fresh-cut appearance and color that resembles freshly dressed fish.

Odor is fresh and mild. A fish just taken from the water has practically no *fish* odor. Eyes are bright, clear, transparent, full, and often protruding. Gills are red in color and free from slime. Skin is shiny and with color that has not faded.

• **Frozen fish**—The flesh is solidly frozen. The flesh should have no discoloration, brownish tinge, or white cottony appearance. Odor is not evident or is slight. Wrapping in which the fish is packaged is moisture-vapor-proof; there is little or no air space between the fish and the wrapping and there has been no damage to the package. Glazing of ice (used to protect shrimp, salmon, and halibut steaks or whole fish frozen in the round or dressed form against drying out) is present on these forms of frozen fish.

• **Shellfish**—The clams and oysters in the shell are alive and the shells close tightly when tapped. Gaping shells indicate that the clam or oyster is dead and not edible. Shucked oysters are plump and have a mild odor with usually a creamy color and a clear liquor or nectar. Cooked crabs and lobsters are bright red with no disagreeable odor. Fresh shrimp have a mild odor and their meat is firm. Cooked shrimp have red in their shells and their meat has a reddish tint. Scallops have a sweetish odor and they are free of excess liquid when purchased in packages.

Fishery products are voluntarily inspected. By contrast, beef and poultry, as well as many other perishable food items, are federally inspected and graded at various stages of processing to ensure buyers of a safe, wholesome, acceptable quality product. There is no similar mandatory federal inspection program for fishery products. The U.S. Department of Commerce (USDC) provides a voluntary inspection program for fishery products. The program is voluntarily subscribed to by processors, packers, brokers, and seafood users interested in having USDC inspect their products. Inspection service users pay fees for USDC inspectors to evaluate their raw materials, to ensure the hygienic preparation of products—and to certify final product quality and condition. The USDC inspector functions as an objective observer in evaluating processing techniques and product quality and condition. Products packed in plants under USDC inspection can carry marks for easy consumer identification. When displayed on product labels, these marks signify that federal inspectors of the Department of Commerce inspected, graded, and certified the products as having met all the requirements of the inspection regulations, and have been produced in accordance with official U.S. grade standards or approved specifications.

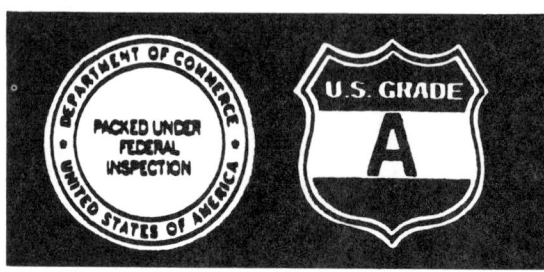

Fig. F-22. The United States Department of Commerce (USDC) makes available a voluntary inspection service which permits processors of inspected seafoods to display official USDC grade or inspection shields on their labels. Only those firms that process fishery products under federal inspection are permitted to use these emblems.

HANDLING AND COOKING FISH AND SEA-
FOOD. Because seafood, like many other food products
will spoil easily if not handled with care, certain procedures
must be followed:

• **Fresh fish and shellfish**—Fresh fish should be placed in
the refrigerator in their original leakproof wrapper immediately after they are received, and stored at 35° to 40°F (1.7°
to 4.4°C) for no longer than a day or two before cooking.
Shellfish should be stored at approximately 32°F (0°C), but
it is a good practice to eat fresh shellfish the day they are
purchased.

• **Frozen fish and shellfish**—To maintain quality, commercially packaged-frozen fishery products should be placed
in the freezer, in their original moisture-vapor-proof wrapper, immediately after purchase. Store in the freezer to 0°F
(-18°C), or lower. At a temperature above 0°F (-18°C),
chemical changes cause the fish to lose color, flavor, texture,
and nutritive value.

When fish is to be frozen, it should be wrapped and sealed
in moisture-vapor-proof materials. Do not freeze fish which
has been wrapped only in wax paper, parchment paper,
or polyethylene materials which are not moisture-vapor-
proof.

Storage time should be limited in order to enjoy the optimum flavor of the frozen fish (see Table F-9). It is a good
practice to date the packages as they are put in the freezer.

When fish thaws, it should be cooked immediately. Any
premature thawing lowers quality because it reduces the
natural moisture and flavor. Never refreeze fish.

TABLE F-9
APPROXIMATE STORAGE LIFE OF FROZEN FISH
AND SHELLFISH HELD AT 0°F (−18°C)

Type	Species	Months
Fat fish	Mackerel, salmon, tuna, etc.	3
Lean fish	Haddock, cod, swordfish, etc.	6
Shellfish	Lobsters and crabs (meat)	2
	Shrimp	6
	Oysters, scallops, clams (shucked)	3 to 4

• **Cooked seafood**—This can be stored in the refrigerator
or freezer. When stored in the refrigerator, seafood should
be placed in covered containers and not held longer than
2 or 3 days. When stored in the freezer, seafood should be
packaged in a moisture-vapor-proof material, and not held
longer than 3 months.

• **Canned fishery products**—Canned products should be
stored in a cool dry place for not longer than a year.

There are endless recipes and preparation techniques for
fish and seafoods. However, they are cooked by using the
basic cookery techniques—baking, pan frying, deep-fat frying, steaming, broiling, oven frying, poaching, or planking.
Fish are cooked when the flesh loses its translucent appearance and becomes opaque. The flesh flakes easily when
pierced with a fork. Cooking fish at too high a temperature
or for too long a time toughens, dries, and destroys the
flavor. There is just one basic rule of seafood cookery to
remember: *Don't overcook!*

(Also see FOOD-BUYING, PREPARING, COOKING, AND
SERVING; and MEAT[S].)

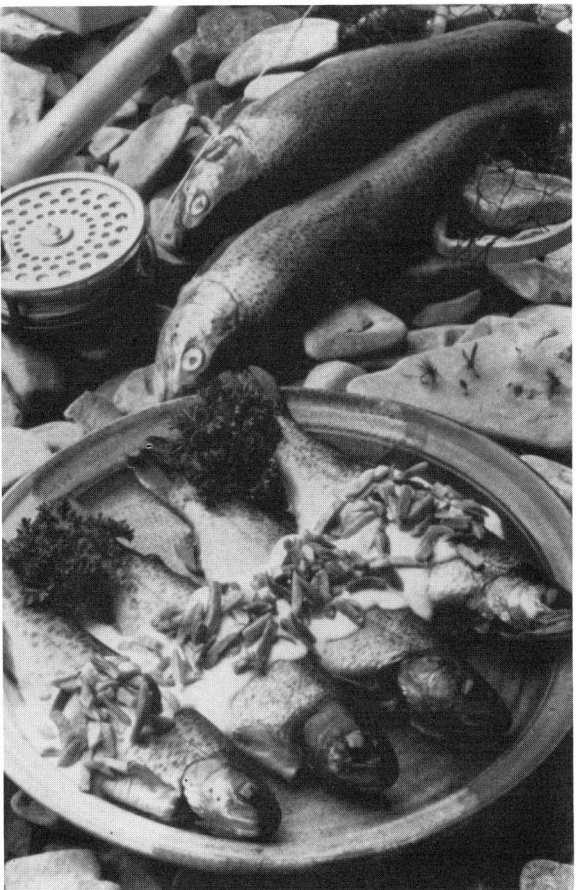

Fig. F-23. Fish attractively prepared. (Courtesy, National Film Board of
Canada)

NUTRITIVE QUALITIES OF FISH AND SEAFOOD.
A prime source of protein, fish and fishery products are
among the most nutritious foods available to the consumer.
Among those foods that provide the best in nutrition, fish
and seafood are at the top right along with meat, milk, and
eggs. Seafoods contain *complete protein.* This means the
protein in seafood supplies the essential amino acids, those
the body cannot manufacture and must get from the foods.
Most fish contain 18 to 20% protein, which is 85 to 95%
digestible.

Fish oil has been shown to slow the formation of arterial
deposits which cause heart attacks and strokes. Most fish
are low in total fat, low in saturated fat, and low in cholesterol. Fish oils, which are rich in unsaturated fats called
omega-3 fatty acids, change the chemistry of the blood; they
increase the high density lipoproteins (HDL) and decrease
the low density lipoproteins (LDL), they lower the level of
triglycerides, they make platelets (the cells involved in clotting) less sticky, and they make the red blood cells less rigid.

Fish and shellfish are rich in vitamins. Varieties of *fat* fish
are rich in vitamins A, D, and K. An average serving of these
fish gives 10% of the daily adult vitamin A requirement and
50% of the vitamin D requirement. The important B complex vitamins are present in seafoods, too. A serving of lean
or fat fish or shellfish, yields about 10% of the thiamin, 15%
of the riboflavin, and 50% of the niacin required each day.

The most common minerals found in fish are iodine, magnesium, calcium, phosphorus, iron, potassium, copper, and

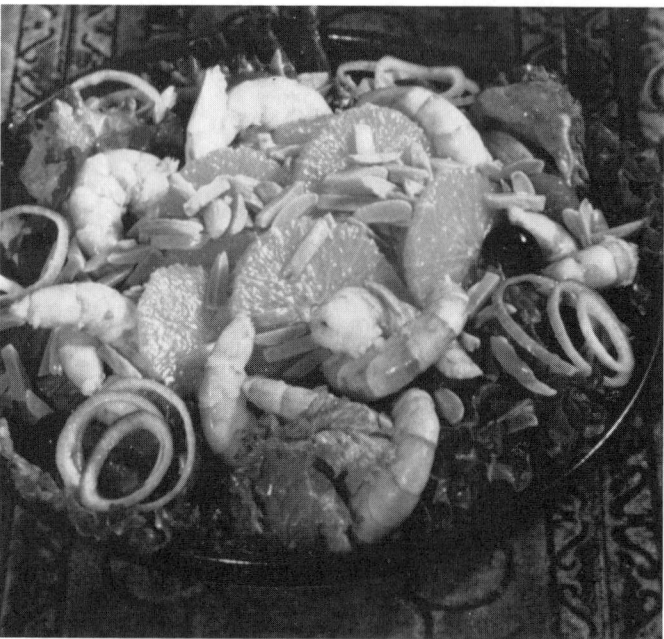

Fig. F-24. A shrimp salad. (Courtesy, Anderson/Miller & Hubbard Consumer Services, San Francisco, Calif.)

fluoride. Shellfish are particularly rich in minerals.

Fish can play a major role in the low-cholesterol diet because the fatty acids present are polyunsaturated. Also, fish can be safely used in the low-sodium diet, unless salt has been added during preparation.

Specific details regarding the nutritional value for a wide variety of fish and seafood may be obtained from Food Composition Table F-21.

Despite all of the good nutrition packed in seafood, the major concern is that most people do not eat enough to contribute significantly to their diet. Table F-10 presents a historical account of the per capita consumption of the fishery products. Total consumption has increased since 1950, and it now stands at about 15.7 lb (7.1 kg). The consumption of meats, and poultry is considerably greater.

TABLE F–10
THE PER CAPITA CONSUMPTION OF FISHERY PRODUCTS
FOR SELECTED YEARS, SINCE 1950[1]

Product	Year		
	1950	1970	1989
	(lb)		
Fresh and frozen	6.3	6.9	10.4
Fish[2]	4.7	4.5	N/A
Shellfish	1.6	2.4	N/A
Canned	4.9	4.5	5.0
Tuna	1.1	2.5	3.9
Salmon	1.4	0.7	N/A
Shellfish	0.4	0.5	N/A
Sardines	1.4	0.4	N/A
Other	0.6	0.4	N/A
Cured	0.6	0.4	0.3
Total	11.8	11.8	15.7

[1]Data from *Statistical Abstract of the United States*, 1980, U.S. Department of Commerce, p. 744, Table 1317; 1988, p. 114, Table 184; and 1991, p. 126, Table 207. To convert to kg divide by 2.2.

[2]Beginning 1973, includes catfish from fish farming.

Table F-11 shows the contribution of meat, poultry, and fish, combined, to the Recommended Dietary Allowances based on the per capita consumption per day. This table points up the small contribution made by fish due to its low level of consumption.

(Also see NUTRIENTS: REQUIREMENTS, ALLOWANCES, FUNCTIONS, SOURCES.)

TABLE F–11
CONTRIBUTIONS OF MEAT, POULTRY, AND FISH TO THE
RECOMMENDED NUTRIENT ALLOWANCES IN THE UNITED STATES[1]

Nutrient	United States Recommended Daily Allowance (RDA)[2]	Contribution from Meat-Poultry-Fish, Combined	
		Total Amt/Day[3]	RDA[4]
			(%)
Energy	2,300–3,100 (2,700) kcal	677 kcal	25.1
Carbohydrate	Not established	0.4 g	—
Fat	Not established	53.3 g	—
Protein	63 g	45.5 g	72
Calcium	800 mg	35 mg	4.4
Phosphorus	800 mg	450 mg	56
Magnesium	350 mg	51 mg	14.6
Copper	2–3 mg	0.3 mg	15
Iron[5]	10 mg	3.8 mg	38
Zinc	15 mg	6.0 mg	40
Vitamin A (R.E.)[6]	1,000 mcg	336 mcg	34
Folate	200 mcg	28 mcg	14
Niacin	19 mg	12 mg	63
Riboflavin	1.7 mg	0.6 mg	35
Thiamin	1.5 mg	0.6 mg	40
Vitamin B-6	2.0 mg	0.9 mcg	45
Vitamin B-12	2.0 mcg	7.0 mcg	35
Vitamin C	60 mg	3.0 mg	5

[1]Data from *Agricultural Statistics 1991*, USDA, pp. 474–478.
[2]National Research Council (1989).
[3]USDA.
[4]Calculated as follows: % RDA = $\dfrac{\text{Av. daily per capita intake}}{\text{Minimum RDA}}$

[5] RDA value used for iron based on adult male, whereas, adult premenopausal female has an RDA of 15 mg/day.

[6]Vitamin A is given in terms of retinol equivalents (R.E.), one R.E. = 3.3 IU of vitamin activity, which was assumed to be the predominant form in meat, poultry, and fish.

FISH PROTEIN CONCENTRATE (FPC)

This term refers to fish protein processed for human consumption. It is produced from types of fish that are not popular in the usual channels of fresh fish trade, such as Menhaden. The fish are extracted to remove oil, dried, and ground to make a bland meal containing about 80% protein, 0.2% fat, and 13% mineral.

(Also see FISH AND SEAFOOD[S], section headed "Industrial Products.")

FISTULA

A tubelike passage from some part of the body to another part or to the exterior—sometimes surgically made.

FLASH-PASTEURIZATION (HIGH TEMPERATURE-SHORT TIME METHOD; HTST)

In flash-pasteurization, the material to be pasteurized is held briefly at a temperature well above that normally required for batch (vat) pasteurization. For milk, the flash process at 161°F (71.7°C) requires at least 15 seconds of holding at this temperature for pasteurization. Conventional batch (vat) pasteurization of milk needs 145°F (63°C) for 30 minutes. Flash-pasteurization is widely used in the food industry. However, time and temperature employed vary according to the needs of the different foods.

(Also see MILK AND MILK PRODUCTS, Section headed ''Processing Milk''; PASTEURIZATION; and ULTRAHIGH TEMPERATURE STERILIZATION.)

FLAT SOURS

A type of canned food spoilage characterized by the production of acid without gas formation. The food becomes sour but the ends of the can remain flat since no gas is formed. Low-acid foods such as peas, corn, beans, and greens are more likely to have flat sour spoilage than other vegetables. Thermophilic bacteria are responsible for flat sours. Hence, this type of spoilage occurs when foods are not cooled quickly after canning, or are held at too high storage temperatures.

(Also see THERMOPHILES.)

FLATULENCE

Excessive gases in the stomach and intestines causing discomfort, bloating, rumblings, and gas removal via the mouth (belching) or anus (passing wind). Foods such as apples, beans, cabbage, turnips and carbonated drinks may produce flatulence. The habit of swallowing air during eating is also a common cause. Sensible eating habits and closing the mouth while chewing provide the best preventative measures, unless it is caused by some diseased condition.

FLAVEDO

The colored, oily outer layer of the peel of citrus fruits, which is also called the *zest*.

There is now a process for recovery of the colored pigment from citrus peel after the juice has been extracted from the fruit. The extracted pigment may be added to pale-colored juices to make them more attractive to consumers.

The oil which is present in the oil glands of the flavedo may be extracted by pressing the peel. It is used for imparting a strong flavor to diluted and sweetened citrus drinks. However, the oil may be oxidized readily and become bitter flavored. Hence, it is not usually added to products that are heated during processing.

FLAVIN ADENINE DINUCLEOTIDE (FAD)

A highly active coenzyme consisting of riboflavin and adenosine diphosphate required in many reactions that affect amino acids, glucose, and fatty acids.

FLAVIN MONONUCLEOTIDE (FMN)

A riboflavin-containing coenzyme involved in the deamination of certain amino acids.

FLAVOPROTEIN

A conjugated protein that contains riboflavin and is involved in tissue respiration.

FLAVOR POTENTIATOR

A substance which enhances the flavor of a food without contributing a flavor of its own. Monosodium glutamate (MSG) is a familiar example.

(Also see ADDITIVES.)

FLAVORINGS AND SEASONINGS

Although the distinctions are not always clear-cut, the following terms and definitions are pertinent to an understanding of flavorings, seasonings, condiments, herbs, and spices.

• **Flavorings**—*These are the substances that stimulate the senses of taste and/or smell.* With the exception of the four primary sensations—sweet, bitter, salty, and sour—flavor characteristics are the result of our perception of odor; the difference between flavor and fragrance is in large part only a semantic distinction. Thus, a substance that provides an odor in perfumes may also be used to add flavoring to a food.

Most natural flavorings, with the exception of common salt, are derived from plant substances—either from the aromatic, volatile vegetable oils known as essential oils, or from the nonvolatile plant oils called resins. But some are derived from synthetics which resemble the natural products.

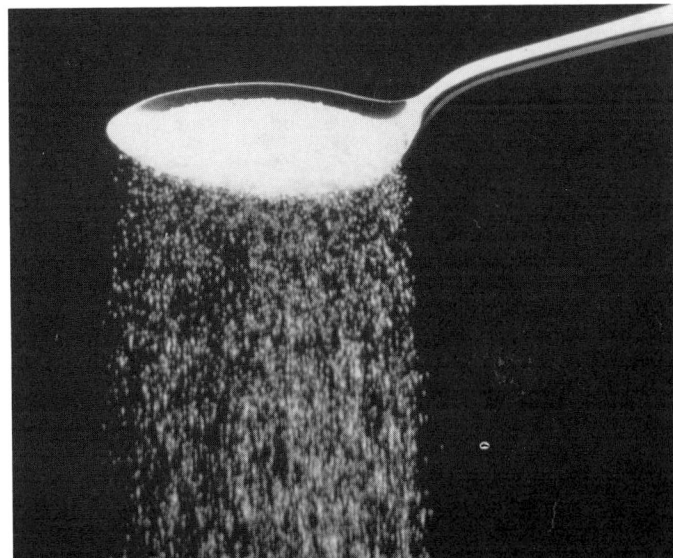

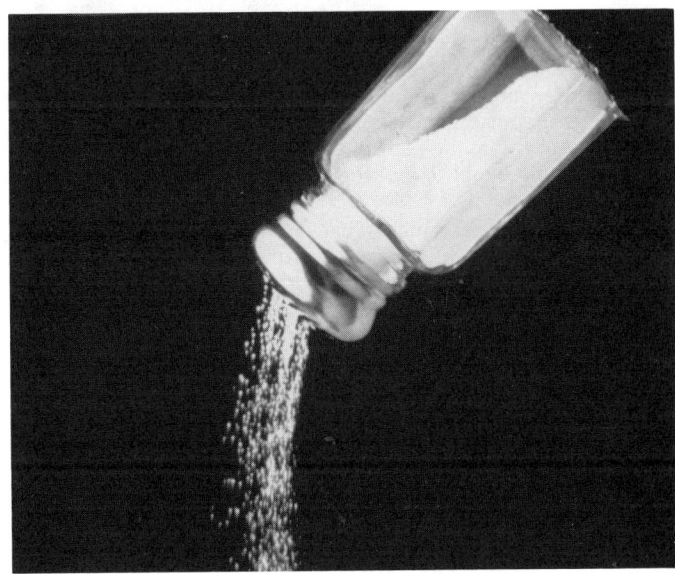

Fig. F-25. Sugar (top) and Salt (bottom) are popular flavorings. (Courtesy, USDA)

• **Seasonings**—*These are ingredients, such as flavorings, condiments, herbs, spices, or extracts, that are added to foods primarily for the savor that they impart.* The imaginative use of these ingredients can lead to highly palatable and interesting flavors.

Salt, or sodium chloride, is the most commonly used seasoning, as well as an essential body mineral. Pepper ranks next to salt as a common seasoning. Herbs, spices, and extracts (including vanilla, almond, and fruit extracts—such as lemon and orange) are also used as seasonings.

• **Condiments**—*This refers to something pungent, acid, salty, or spicy added to or served with food to enhance its flavor or to give added flavor.* They are useful in helping to make certain foods palatable and easier to digest. All condiments should be used sparingly and in such proportions that they do not spoil the natural flavors of other ingredients.

• **Herbs**—*This refers to the fragrant leaves and flowers of certain plants grown in temperate climates.*
(Also see HERB.)

• **Spices**—*Generally, these are products of tropical and subtropical trees, shrubs, or vines and are characterized by highly pungent odors or flavors.*
(Also see SPICES.)

So, take your choice: flavorings, seasonings, condiments, herbs, or spices. The presence of one or more of them makes the difference between the enjoyment of eating and the necessity of eating.
(Also see PALATABILITY.)

HISTORY OF FLAVORINGS AND SEASONINGS.
The quest in far off lands for new and different flavorings and seasonings is ages old. Explorations, wars, and conquests were a part of their history.

Herbs and spices were valued for flavoring and seasoning foods and drinks, for medicinals, and for making cosmetic oils and perfumes. Many romantic legends, beliefs, and superstitions revolved around spices and herbs. Many were reputed to have magical powers: thyme was considered to be a source of courage, and tansy and sesame were associated with immortality.

As early as 3500 B.C., the Egyptian queen, Hatshepsut, used cinnamon as an aromatic. And in 3000 B.C., history records that the gods of the Mesopotamian peoples drank sesame wine, one of the products for which this popular seed was used.

The Bible also makes many references to spices beginning with the Book of Genesis, Chapter 37. Some of the spices mentioned throughout the good book are not familiar today, but many are still used. In the Revelation of St. John the Divine, Chapter 18, we see how distressed the merchants of the world became at the loss of the rich spice market when Babylon fell.

Both the Bible and historical records reveal that spices and aromatics were held in high esteem, and a gift of spices was greatly prized.

In days of yore, many of the noble, as well as the not so noble, had their own herb garden, sometimes formal and sometimes informal. Many were works of art. But whether the cook had a few pots of herbs on the kitchen windowsill, or a formal classic 16th century herbal knot garden, fresh herbs were considered far superior to dried.

POPULAR FLAVORINGS AND SEASONINGS.
An alphabetical listing of flavorings and seasonings follows:

Ajowan *(Carum ajowan)*
Allspice *(Pimenta officinalis)*
Almond, bitter *(Prunus amygdalus amara)*
Almond, sweet *(Prunus amygdalus dulcis)*
Aloe vera *(Aloe barbadensis)*
Anchovy
Angelica *(Angelica archangelica)*
Angostura bitters
Aniseseed *(Pimpinella anisum)*
Anise-pepper *(Xanthoxylum pipesitum)*
Asafoetida *(Ferula asafoetida)*
Balm
Basil, sweet (See Sweet Basil)
Bay leaves *(Laurus nobilis)*
Beer
Bouquet garni
Caper *(Caparris rupestris)*
Caraway *(Carum carvi)*
Cardamom seed *(Elettaria cardamomum)*
Cassia *(Cinnamomum Cassia)*
Cayenne pepper *(Capsicum frutescens)*
Celery salt
Celery seed *(Apium graveolens)*
Chervil garden *(Anthriscus cerefolium)*
Chinese Five Spices

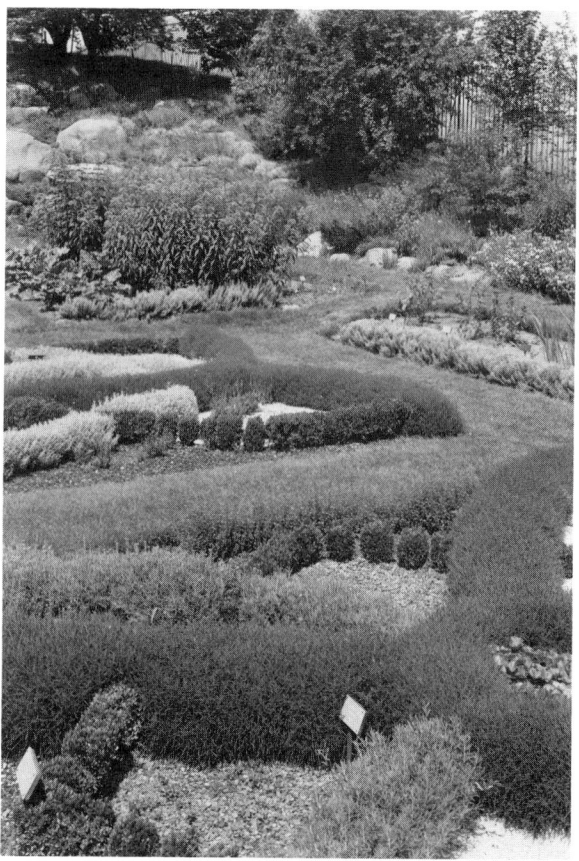

Fig. F-26. An interesting garden of herbs. (Courtesy, Brooklyn Botanic Garden, Brooklyn, N.Y.)

Chives *(Allium schoenoprasum)*
Chocolate *(Theobroma cacao)*
Cinnamon *(Cinnamomum zeylanicum)*
Citron *(Citrus medica)*
Cloves *(Syzygium aromaticum)*
Cola *(Cola acuminata)*
Coriander *(Coriandrum sativum)*
Cress
Cumin *(Cuminum cyminum)*
Curry (powder or sauce)
Dill *(Anethum graveolens)*
Fennel *(Foeniculum vulgare)*
Fenugreek seed *(Trigonella foenumgraceum)*
Fines herbes
Garlic *(Allium sativum)*
Ginger *(Zingiber officinale)*
Horseradish *(Armoracia rusticana)*
Leek *(Allium porrum)*
Lemon *(Citrus limon)*
Licorice *(Glycyrrhiza glabra)*
Lime *(Citrus aurantifolia)*
Lovage *(Levisticum officinale)*
Mace *(Myristica fragrans)*
Marjoram
Mint
Monosodium glutamate (MSG)
Mixed whole spice
Mustard
Noyeau
Nutmeg *(Myristica fragrans)*
Onion *(Allium cepa)*
Oregano *(Origanum vulgare)*
Paprika *(Capsicum tetragonum)*
Parsley *(Petroselinum crispum)*
Pepper *(Piper nigrum)*
Poppy seed *(Papaver somniferum)*
Poultry seasonings
Rosemary *(Rosmarinus officinalis)*
Saffron *(Crocus sativus)*
Sage *(Salvia officinalis)*
Savory
Sesame seed *(Sesamum indicum)*
Shallot *(Allium ascalonicum)*
Soy sauce *(Glycine max)*
Star anise *(Illicium verum)*
Sweet basil *(Ocimum basilicum)*
Sweet cicely *(Myrrhis odorata)*
Tabasco sauce
Tarragon *(Artemesia dracunculus)*
Thyme *(Thymus vulgaris)*
Turmeric *(Curcuma longa)*
Vanilla *(Vanilla planifolia)*
Verbena *(Verbena hybrida)*
Wine
Wintergreen *(Gaultheria procumbens)*
Worcestershire sauce

Where available, the nutrient content of flavorings and seasonings is given in Food Composition Table F-21, under the section, Flavorings and Seasonings. In general, herbs and spices are high in fiber and minerals, but, because of the minute quantities consumed, they do not make any significant contribution to the daily requirement.

WHY, WHEN, AND HOW MUCH FLAVORING TO USE. "Variety is the spice of life," as the old saying

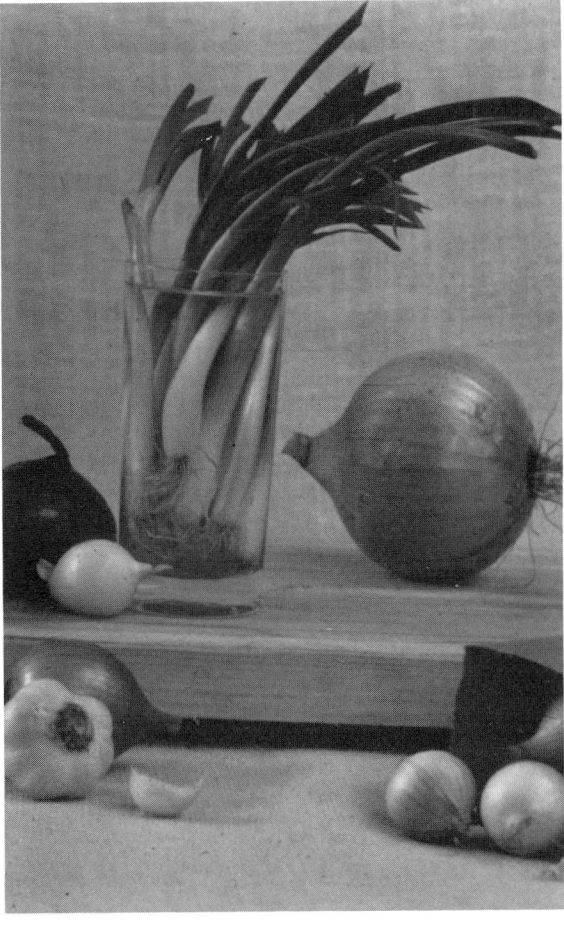

Fig. F-27. Garlic and onions, two popular flavorings and seasonings. (Courtesy, USDA)

goes. This is certainly true in the diet. Not only is life more interesting when meals are varied with different foods, delicately flavored with herbs or spices, but there is an added bonus to your health for it carries out the *Golden Rule of Eating,* which is: "the greater the variety of foods you eat, the greater your chances of getting everything you need."

It is important to keep spices and herbs relatively fresh. If spices have been used only a few times each year, chances are they have become stale. Some of the spices deteriorate with age, with heat, and with exposure to the air. So get rid of the old and stock up on the new. The results of your culinary prowess will be more dramatic with fresh spices.

Any flavoring can be used singly, or two or more may be combined. This is where the cook's daring experimentation can produce just the right effect, and result in delicious food. Sometimes the taste buds have to be educated to new flavorings. The package label usually recommends and suggests how much and when to use. The flavorings and seasonings should always enhance the flavor of the main ingredient, rather than completely mask it. But tastes differ, so, in the final analysis, it is up to the cook to decide.

Flavorings are usually better added the last hour of cooking. But, as the delicate perfume of marjoram or the *pep* of pepper are easily lost in cooking, add them very shortly before serving.

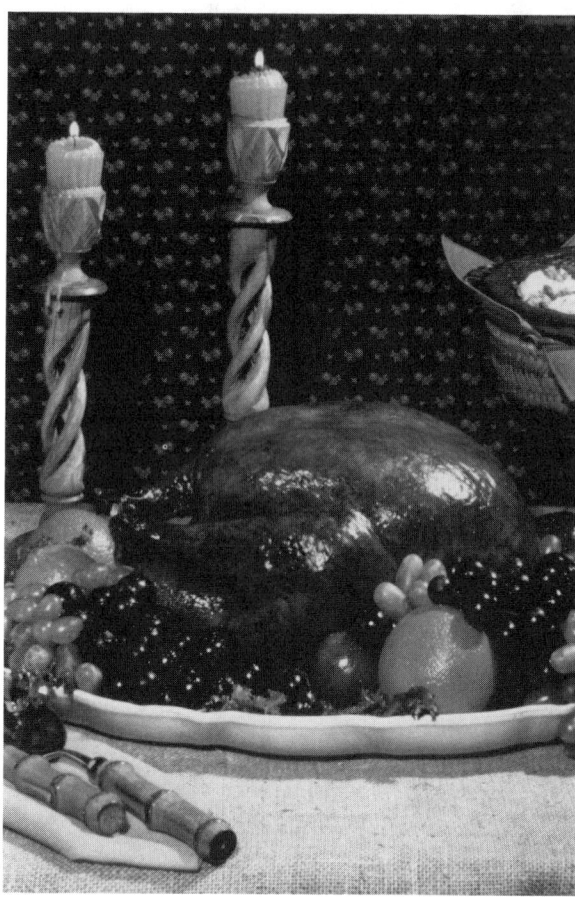

Fig. F-28. Seasonings are a matter of personal choice, but don't forget that a little seasoning goes a long way. (Courtesy, National Turkey Federation, Reston, Va.)

WINES AND LIQUEURS. Wines, sauterne, vermouth, and sherry, etc., all give a distinctive flavor to foods. When added during cooking, they lose their alcoholic content, but still impart an interesting flavor. They can be added to cream soups, and to almost any meat dish, casserole, stew, etc.

Fish is especially good when cooked in a white wine sauce with butter and almonds. Sole is excellent when cooked in vermouth.

Red wines are the best for marinades, and for cooking the red meats. A very good marinade consists of red wine, garlic salt, and rosemary or a herb mix of thyme, oregano, sage, rosemary, marjoram and basil.

Liqueurs add zest to many desserts; for example, ice cream, with a tablespoon of a liqueur, along with nuts, macaroons, grated chocolate, or other topping, makes a simple, but elegant, party dessert. Cointreau can be used with almost all fruit desserts, including fresh fruits.

This is not the end, but just the beginning, of the fun you will have creating new and interesting foods for yourself and your family. Any therapeutic value that these condiments may have will be an added dividend.

NOTE WELL: (For more complete discussion of Flavor-ings and Seasonings, including (1) an extensive table listing and summarizing flavorings and seasonings, and (2) a table giving different food and flavoring combinations, see the two-volume *Foods & Nutrition Encyclopedia,* a work by the same authors as *Food For Health.)*

FLAVORS, SYNTHETIC

With the exception of the four primary taste sensations—sweet, bitter, salty, and sour—food flavors are the result of our sense of smell. Today, chemists can make chemicals in the laboratory which alone or in various combinations can imitate many of the natural food flavors. These are synthetic flavors. In many cases the synthetic flavors are superior to natural flavors in terms of (1) withstanding processing, (2) cost, (3) availability, and (4) consistent quality. Synthetic flavors may be substances that are prepared in the laboratory but chemically identical to those found in nature, or substances prepared in the laboratory which as yet have not been found to occur in nature but which produce familiar aromas.

Flavor, regardless of whether it is naturally occurring or created from synthetic chemicals, often results from a complex mixture of chemicals in the proper proportion. Hence, the vast number of synthetic compounds can be employed to create endless flavor formulations. Creating flavors is a science.

Since there are hundreds of synthetic flavor compounds, a listing is not within the scope of this book.

In the labeling of food products, the term *artificial flavor* is a requirement for all food products to which flavor has been added regardless of its origin.

(Also see FLAVORINGS AND SEASONINGS.)

FLAX (LINSEED) *Linum usitatissimum*

This is a herbaceous annual which originated in the Mediterranean region in prehistoric times. The Abyssinians first used flax for food—they roasted and ate the oval, shiny seeds. Although the seed contains a toxic glucoside, it is detoxicated by heating.

Flax is grown primarily (1) for its fibers, which lie inside the bark of the plant next to the woody core and which are processed and spun into linen cloth; and (2) for its seed, which is processed for oil and meal. The oil is used in the manufacture of varnishes, linoleum, oilcloth, soap, and leather; and the meal is used as livestock feed.

Today, whole flax seed is sold in many health food stores; and certain high-fiber, ready-to-eat breakfast cereals contain whole flax seed. The whole seed contains 24% crude protein, 38% oil, and 6% fiber. The availability of carbohydrates and/or energy is uncertain, as no studies have been made on this subject. More nutritional information is given in Food Composition Table F-21.

An excellent tea, said to be effective in the treatment of colds, may be made with 8 oz (224 g) each of seed and rock candy; 3 lemons paired and sliced; added to 2 qt (1.9 liter) of boiling water; then strained after cooling. The usual infusion is made with 1 tsp (5 ml) of seed steeped in 1 cup (240 ml) of boiling water. Also, the mucilage obtained by infusing the whole seed in boiling water, in the proportion of ½ oz (14 g) to 1 pt (480 ml), is said to be helpful in alleviating constipation, dysentery, catarrh, and other inflammatory affections of the respiratory tract, intestines, and urinary passages. Where any of these problems are serious or persistent, those so afflicted are admonished to see a medical doctor.

FLORIDIAN STARCH

A granular carbohydrate obtained from red algae (*Florideae*), which in several respects resembles glycogen rather than starch.

FLOURS

Contents | Page

Generally, *a flour is considered to be a dry powder produced by the grinding of one or more cereal grains.* A more coarsely ground product is called a *meal.* However, the term may also be applied to similar powders obtained by the grinding of other types of seeds, such as legumes and nuts, or even the dried roots, tubers, or leaves of food plants. Although flours were first used by some of the most primitive peoples, food technologists are ever busy developing new ways of altering the characteristics of the various flours, so that the items made from them may be more appealing and nutritious. Fig. F-29 shows some of the many foods from which flours are made.

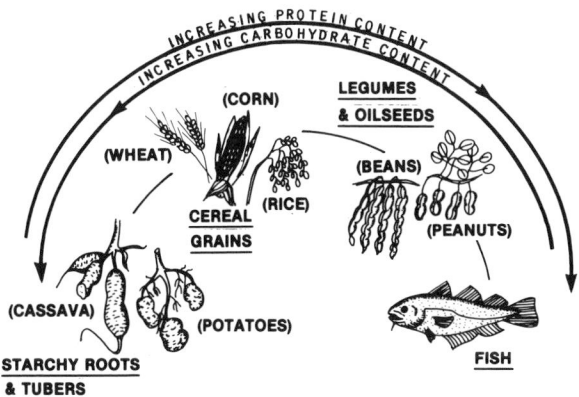

Fig. F-29. Fish, legumes, grains, tubers, and other natural foods comprise the raw materials for man's many flours.

THE HISTORY OF FLOURS. It appears that crude flours and meals were prepared as early as 75,000 years ago, when people obtained their foods solely by fishing, hunting wild game, and gathering wild plants. At that time, edible seeds were roasted, then crushed between two rocks. Sometime between then and the beginnings of agriculture 10,000 years ago, man first made a paste from a grain flour and cooked it on a heated rock to make a crude bread. Although only a few of the North American Indian tribes were agriculturalists, almost all of them prepared flours from various seeds and dried roots and tubers. However, the major grain of the Americas was corn (maize), which produced quite a heavy bread. The development of lighter breads occurred elsewhere in the world, where other grains were available.

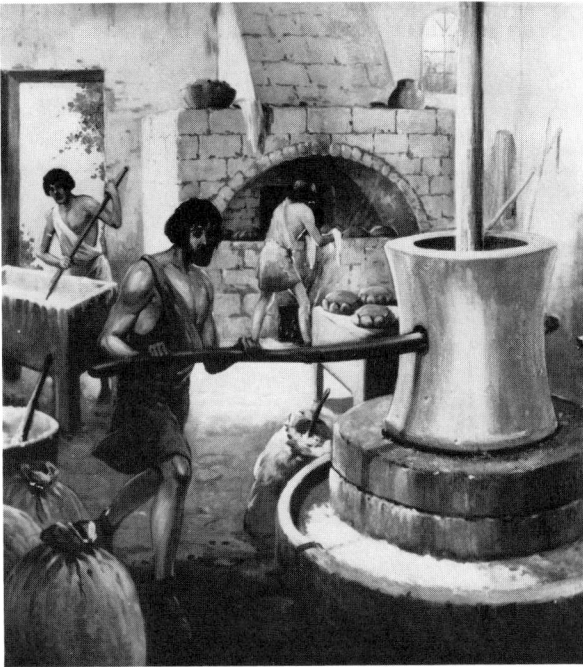

Fig. F-30. Grinding grain and making bread in Pompeii, an ancient city in southern Italy. Note the hand-powered lever and the hopper of the top stone. (Courtesy, The Bettmann Archive, Inc., New York, N.Y.)

In 1929, the per capita consumption of wheat flour was 171 lb. By 1970, with a greater variety of foods on the grocery shelf, the per capita consumption of wheat flour had dropped to a low of 110 lb. But food technologists developed a variety of new products and all baked goods became increasingly popular, so by 1990 the per capita consumption had risen to 137.8 lb.

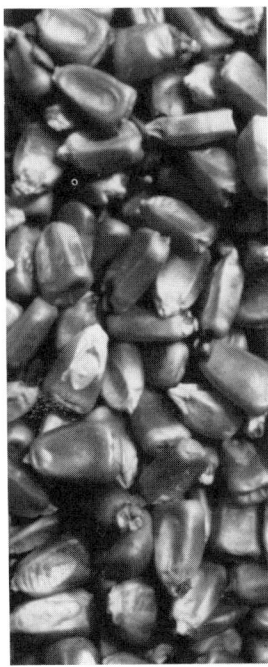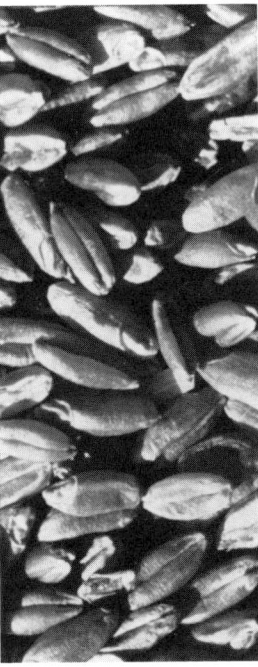

Fig. F-31. Corn (left) and wheat (right) two common sources of cereal flours. (Courtesy, USDA)

PRODUCTION AND PROCESSING. Basically, flour production is the grinding of a dried food material, but the details of processing vary somewhat for each of the different flours. Fig. F-32 shows the modern equipment used in the milling of flour.

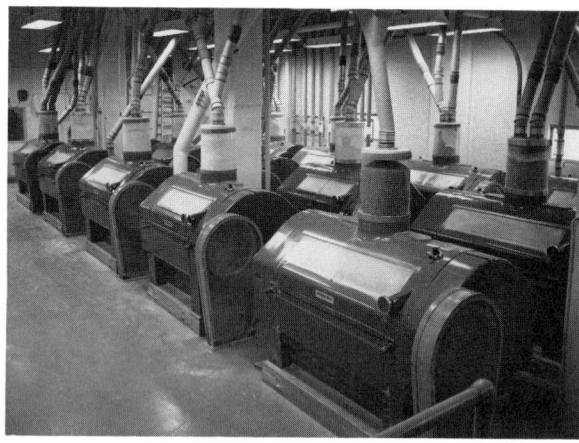

Fig. F-32. Flour milling machines. The whole grain enters the tops of the machines through the cylindrical glass hobbers. (Courtesy, Union Pacific Railroad Company, Omaha, Nebr.)

Major Flours. The American homemaker is most familiar with the flours made from wheat. But there are other important flours.

Pertinent information relative to the major flours is summarized in Table F-12. (Additional details on flour sources are given in the articles dealing with the individual grains. For example, major treatment on the production of wheat flours is given under WHEAT.)

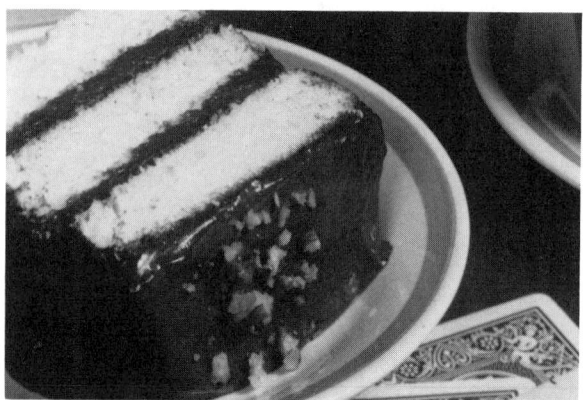

Fig. F-33. Chocolate angel torte made from wheat flour. (Courtesy, Carnation, Los Angeles, Calif.)

TABLE F-12
MAJOR FLOURS

Type of Flour	Production	Characteristics
Barley (Also see BARLEY.)	Dehulled grain (groats) may be (1) milled directly into a course flour, or (2) pearled, then milled into a fine flour.	Bland flavored, white colored. Produces tender baked goods. Not strong enough for yeast leavening.
Buckwheat (Also see BUCKWHEAT.)	Groats may be milled into a high extraction[1] (dark colored) flour, or a low extraction (light colored) flour.	Strongly flavored, with a trace of bitterness; light to dark brown in color. Not suitable for yeast-leavened doughs.
Corn (Also see CORN.)	Most flour is made from degerminated white or yellow dent corn.	Mild, sweet flavor, white or yellow colored. May be gritty if not ground finely. Produces tender baked goods that readily dry out and become crumbly. Flour is too weak for making yeast-leavened products.
Rice (Also see RICE.)	Flour is made from broken pieces of polished, dehulled grain.	Bland flavored, white colored. May be gritty if not ground finely. Baked goods may dry out and crumble. Too weak for yeast leavening.
Rye (Also see RYE.)	Milling is similar to that for wheat. Flour may be of high extraction (dark colored), medium extraction (medium colored), or low extraction (light colored).	Distinctive flavor; color varies. May be used with yeast leavening, but dough is denser and moister than that made from wheat flour.
Wheat (Also see WHEAT.) Cake	Low extraction flour, sometimes bleached, milled from soft wheat.	Bland, white, and soft in texture. Not suitable for yeast leavening.
Gluten	A mixture of 45% gluten (produced by washing the starch from white flour), and 55% white flour.	Bland, white, and high in protein. A very strong, high-protein flour which may be mixed with weak flours to impart sufficient strength for yeast leavening.
High ratio flour	Flour of very fine and uniform particle size, treated with chlorine to reduce the gluten strength.	It is possible to add up to 140 parts of sugar to 100 parts of this flour. High ratio flour makes excellent cakes.
Self-rising	White flour to which a dry leavening acid and baking soda have been added.	Needs no additional leavening. Products may have a slightly bitter taste.
White	A flour of about 80% extraction, which may be milled from soft, medium, or hard wheats.	Most white flours, with the exception of cake flour, may be leavened with yeast.
Whole wheat	A flour of from 95 to 100% extraction, which contains all or most of the bran and germ from the original grain.	Light brown color, may be speckled with bits of bran and germ. May be used for yeast-leavened doughs, but baked products may be heavier and moister than those made from white flours.

[1]Extraction refers to the precentage of the grain that is converted to a flour. High extraction flours contain more bran and germ than low extraction flours.

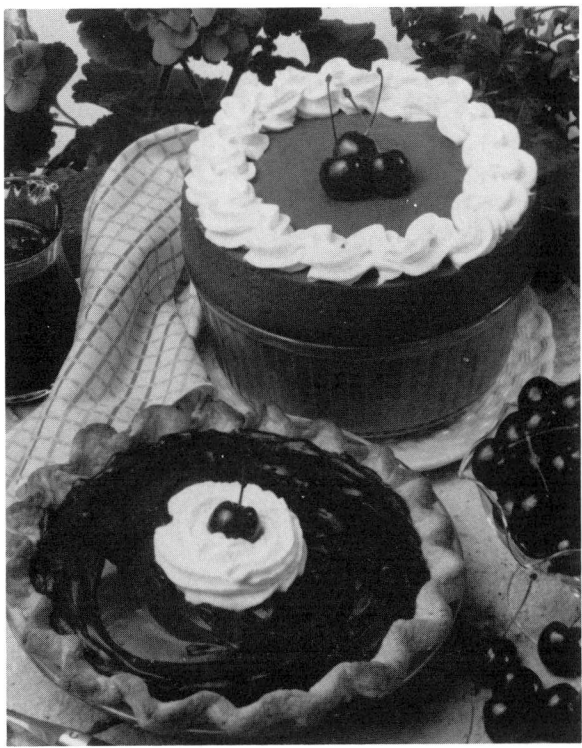

Fig. F-34. Chocolate souffle (upper), and chocolate cream pie (lower) both contain wheat flour. (Courtesy, Hershey Foods Corp., Hershey, Penn.)

Special Flours. Many of the plant materials that ancient peoples used to make flour and meals are once again serving this purpose as food technologists seek new ways to feed exploding populations. Also, these special flours may be used in dietetic foods. It is noteworthy that each of the special flours lacks gluten, the protein in wheat flours which imparts elasticity to doughs and enables them to be leavened with yeast. Therefore, these nonwheat flours are best suited for making baked goods leavened with baking powder or baking soda, the details of which are given in the articles— BAKING POWDER AND BAKING SODA; and QUICK BREADS. The more common special flours are described briefly in Table F-13. (Additional details on flour sources are given in the articles dealing with the individual food materials.)

NUTRITIVE VALUE OF FLOURS. In general, flours are more concentrated sources of nutrients than the plants (or animals, in the case of fish flour) from which they have been made because much water has been removed. Sometimes, large amounts of fat have also been removed. Hence, most flours keep well without refrigeration. Food Composition Table F-21 gives the nutrient composition of the major cereal flours, and of special flours.

TABLE F-13
SPECIAL FLOURS

Type of Flour	Production	Characteristics
Arrowroot (Also see ARROWROOT.)	Ground tubers are mixed with water, then screened to remove fibrous matter. The starchy particles are then allowed to settle out, so they may be removed and dried.	Tasteless white powder that is almost all starch. When heated with water, forms a clear, thick paste which gels upon cooling.
Carob (Also see CAROB.)	After removal of the seeds, the pods are finely ground and sieved.	Chocolate colored powder with a mildly sweet taste. Blends well with various cereal flours.
Cottonseed (Also see COTTONSEED.)	The seeds are dehulled and the oil is extracted. Then, the meal is ground into a flour. Cottonseed which contains gossypol requires a special treatment.	Color varies from very light cream color to dark brown (when degossypolized). Toasted cottonseed has a pleasant flavor. The flour may contain 50% or more protein.
Fish	Whole fish are dried and extracted with a solvent to remove the oil. The meal is then ground.	Tasteless, odorless, tan colored powder. Fish flour may contain about 75% protein.
Lima bean (Also see LIMA BEAN.)	Dried, mature lima beans are ground into a flour.	Bland, white colored powder.
Malt (Also see MALT.)	Malted barley or wheat is dehulled, dried, and ground into flour.	Light to dark colored powder. Contains starch-digesting enzymes.
Millet (Also see MILLET.)	Usually, the flour is made from whole grains of millet. Sometimes, the grain is debranned before milling.	Light yellow powder with a bland taste.
Oat (Also see OATS.)	Cleaned oats are dried, dehulled, cut into granules, steamed, and rolled into flakes. Then, the flakes are ground into flour.	A white powder with a bland taste.
Pea (Also see PEAS, GARDEN.)	The flour may be made from either cooked or uncooked dried peas.	Yellow or green powder which has a bland, pleasant taste. The color of green pea flour usually bleaches out during baking.
Peanut (Also see PEANUTS.)	Defatted peanut meal is ground into a flour.	Pleasant tasting, light cream colored powder.
Potato (Also see POTATOES.)	Pieces of raw or cooked skinned potato tubers are pulverized to a pulpy mass, dried and ground into flour.	A white powder with a bland taste. Forms thick pastes when heated with water. Flour blends well with other flours.
Soybean (Also see SOYBEANS.)	Heat treated, dehulled soybeans are usually defatted to varying degrees before grinding to a flour.	Light tan powder with a beany flavor. The flour may contain up to 50% protein.
Sunflower seed (Also see SUNFLOWERS.)	Dehulled seed is ground, and some or all of the fat extracted. The remaining pulp is ground into a flour.	Grey-brown powder with slightly bitter taste.
Tapioca (Also see CASSAVA.)	Cassava roots are washed, peeled, and ground. The pulp is mixed with water, passed through a screen and the starch allowed to settle out. The starch is then dried.	Tasteless white powder that is almost all starch. Forms thick gels when cooked with water.

Some noteworthy facts relative to the nutritive value of flours follow:

1. The darker colored flours are richer in essential nutrients than the lighter colored ones, as exemplified by the different flours made from buckwheat, rye, and wheat.

2. The reduction in the water content of a food during the production of a flour may make it more nearly possible to use the food as a major dietary source of calories and protein. For example, it would take almost 7 lb (3.14 kg) of boiled potatoes to furnish the recommended daily per capita allowance of 2,385 Calories (kcal) established by WHO and FAO of the UN, whereas only 1½ lb (0.68 kg) of potato flour would be required. Hence, there is much current interest in the utilization of various vegetable flours for feeding people in the developing countries.

3. Flours made from defatted products are rich in nutrients and comparatively low in calories. For example, defatted soybean flour contains ¼ more protein and ⅓ more calcium, but only ¾ as many calories as undefatted soybean flour.

4. One cup (125 g) of self-rising white wheat flour, which contains monocalcium phosphate as a leavening acid, supplies more than ⅓ of the Recommended Daily Allowances (RDA) for calcium, and more than ½ of that for phosphorus. Hence, items baked with this flour may be an important source of these minerals for people who fail to eat sufficient amounts of dairy products.

5. A mere 0.6 oz (17.3 g) of fish flour provides the entire RDA for calcium (800 mg). The same amount of this flour provides more than half of the daily iron allowance for an adult male.

6. The flours highest in protein are those made from defatted fish and from the defatted oilseed meals (cottonseed, peanut, soybean, and sunflower). It is noteworthy that these flours are currently being used around the world as protein supplements.

7. Two other important observations regarding flours, which are not apparent from Food Composition Table F-21, are that (a) the cereal flours are deficient in the amino acid lysine, which is supplied abundantly by the noncereal flours (with the exceptions of arrowroot and tapioca flours, which are almost all starch); and (b) many of the noncereal flours are deficient in the sulfur-containing amino acids (cysteine, cystine, and methionine), which are supplied in greater proportions by the cereal flours. Therefore, it makes good sense to use combinations of cereal and noncereal flours, so that there might be optimal utilization of the proteins in these foods.

Enrichment and Fortification of Flours. People around the world have strived for thousands of years to produce white, soft flours. Hence, the present dominance of flour production by white flours is not the outcome of a recent *conspiracy* by the flour industry; rather, it is the response to an age old public demand. Nevertheless, it is important that appropriate measures be taken to offset the nutritional shortcomings of highly refined flours, particularly in circumstances where these items are relied upon to furnish much of the caloric and protein requirements. The most widely employed measures have been enrichment and fortification.

NOTE WELL: Originally, the FDA differentiated between enrichment and fortification, but now the two terms are used interchangeably. Nevertheless, the following differentiations between the terms persist:

"Enrichment is a term which refers to the addition of specific nutrients to a food *as established in a federal standard*

of identity and quality (for example: enriched bread). The amounts added generally are moderate and include those commonly present at even lower levels."[9]

"Fortified is a term which refers to the addition to foods of specific nutrients. The amounts added are usually in excess of those normally found in the food because of the importance of providing additional amounts of the nutrients to the diet. Some foods are selected for fortification because they are appropriate carriers for the nutrient. Example: Milk is frequently fortified with vitamin D."[10]

It is noteworthy that the FDA regulations for the enrichment and fortification of flours[11] apply to products with labeling that utilizes these terms. Examples of how enrichment and fortification affect the nutrient composition of some typical wheat flours are given in Table F-14. (For additional details, see WHEAT.)

TABLE F-14
MINERAL AND VITAMIN CONTENTS OF
SELECTED FLOURS[1]

Type of Flour	Calcium	Iron	Thiamin	Riboflavin	Niacin
(1 lb, or *0.45 kg*)	(mg)	(mg)	(mg)	(mg)	(mg)
Whole wheat	186	15.0	2.49	.54	19.7
White, 80% extraction, unenriched	109	5.9	1.16	.33	9.3
White, enriched[2]	109	13.0–16.5	2.90	1.80	24.0
White, self-rising, enriched[3]	960[4]	13.0–16.5	2.90	1.80	24.0

[1]Values are from Food Composition Table F-21 of this book.
[2]Enriched according to *Code of Federal Regulations*, Title 21, Revised 4/1/78, Section 137.165.
[3]According to *Code of Federal Regulations*, Title 21, Revised 4/1/78, Section 137.185.
[4]This level of calcium is usually equaled or exceeded when calcium monophosphate is used as the leavening acid.

It may be seen from Table F-14 that the milling procedures used to make white flour result in a product containing much less calcium, iron, thiamin, riboflavin, and niacin than whole wheat flour. However, enrichment of white flour restores the iron, thiamin, riboflavin, and niacin to levels equaling or slightly exceeding those in whole wheat flour. The use of calcium monophosphate in self-rising flour constitutes calcium fortification because it raises the level of this mineral so that it greatly exceeds the calcium content of whole wheat flour.

The calcium content of breads made from whole grain flours may not always be well utilized because the whole grains contain phosphorus compounds called phytates, which interfere with the absorption of calcium and other essential minerals such as iron and zinc. Therefore, it is noteworthy that British nutritionists learned about this effect in the early 1940s and that they also found that removal of phytates restored the availability of calcium in whole grain breads.

More recent research has shown that much of the phytates present in whole grain flours may be destroyed if there is

[9]"Nutrition Labeling—Terms you Should Know," *FDA Consumer Memo,* DHEW Publication No. 74-2010, 1974, p. 2.

[10]*Ibid.,* p. 3.

[11]*Code of Federal Regulations,* Title 21, Revised 4/1/78, Sections 137.160, 137.165, and 137.185.

a considerable amount of yeast fermentation during the leavening of bread doughs.[12]

There are no FDA standards of identity for the enrichment or fortification of nonwheat flours. Instead, there are some standards for macaroni and noodle products made mainly from wheat flour, but nutritionally enhanced by the addition of nonwheat flours such as those derived from other grains or from oilseeds (usually cottonseeds, peanuts, soybeans, or sunflowers).

(Also see ENRICHMENT.)

USES OF FLOURS AND THE BY-PRODUCTS OF MILLING.
Modern technology has made it possible to produce a wide variety of flours with great efficiency

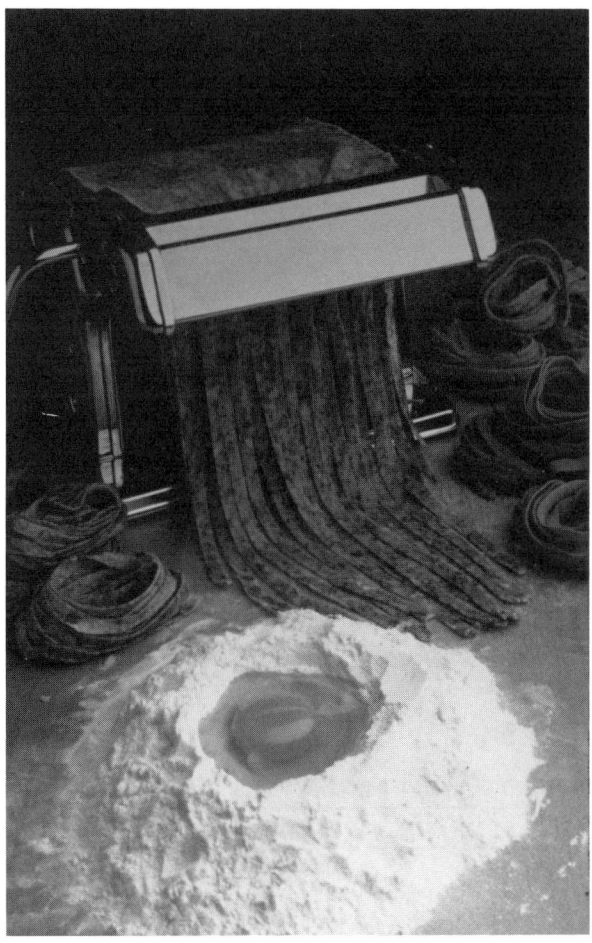

Fig. F-35. Wheat flour being processed into noodles. (Courtesy, National Film Board of Canada)

because only negligible amounts of the original raw materials are wasted. The soft, inner tissues of seeds, roots, and tubers yield the flours used in human foods, whereas the highly fibrous outer tissues are fed to animals. By-products intermediate in fiber are utilized in both human foods and animal feeds. Therefore, the uses of various products are briefed in the sections which follow. (Baking procedures are described in the article BREADS AND BAKING.)

---

[12]"Zinc Availability in Leavened and Unleavened Bread," *Nutrition Reviews*, Vol. 33, January 1975, p. 18.

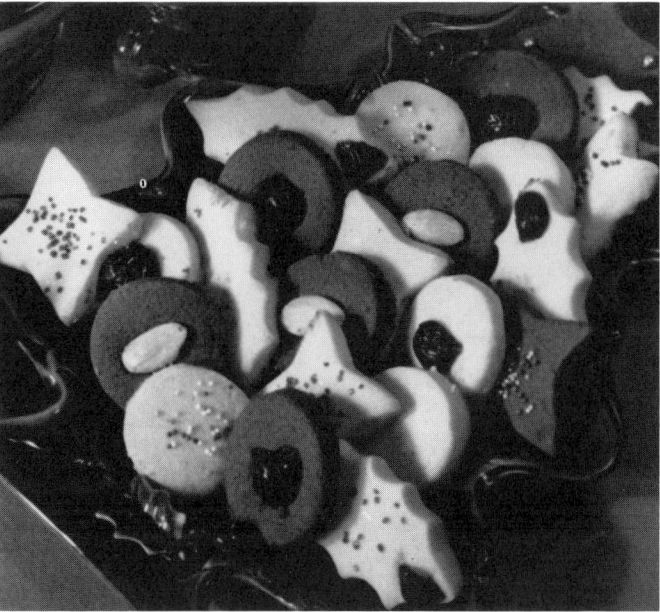

Fig. F-36. Scottish shortbread cookies are traditional Christmas treats. (Courtesy, Agriculture Canada, Ottawa, Ontario, Canada)

Major Cereal Flours. Some of the more important uses of these items are given in Table F-15.

TABLE F-15
USES OF MAJOR CEREAL FLOURS

Flour	Uses
Barley	Infant cereals; substitute for wheat flour when there is an allergy to wheat; biscuits, muffins, and pancakes; and for making a starchy broth that is well tolerated by people who have digestive disturbances.
Buckwheat[1]	In the U.S., most buckwheat flour is used in pancake mixes. In Japan, it is mixed with wheat flour and made into noodles (Soba).
Corn	Ingredient of ready-to-eat breakfast cereals, snack foods, baking mixes (biscuits, muffins, and pancakes); and a meat extender. Replacement for wheat flour in hypoallergenic and low-gluten products.
Rice	Thickening agent in gravies and sauces; and for imparting crispness and tenderness to biscuits, cookies, and crackers. Replacement for wheat flour in hypoallergenic and low-gluten products.
Rye[2]	Alone or mixed with wheat flour in breads, biscuits, crackers, and pancakes. (Commercial baked goods made with rye flour keep fresh longer than those made with wheat flour.) Thickener for sauces, soups, and custard powders.
Wheat: Cake	Soft-textured and tender baked goods leavened with baking powders.
Gluten	High-protein and other types of yeast-leavened breads, macaroni and noodle products, and strengthening agent for mixing with weaker flours.
Self-rising	Mainly for biscuits, cookies, muffins, pancakes, and waffles. Greatest use is in the southeastern U.S. Elsewhere, this product has been replaced by special mixes.
White, 80% extraction	Most baked goods. Well suited for either baking powder or yeast leavening. Thickener for gravies, puddings, and sauces.
Whole wheat	Well suited for making all types of baked goods (products tend to be heavier and moister than those made with white flour) and cereal products.

[1]Dark and light flours are available. The former contains more nutrients per calorie.

[2]Dark, medium, and light flours are available. The darkest contains the most nutrients per calorie.

Special Flours. Major uses of these products are given in Table F-16.

TABLE F-16
USES OF SELECTED SPECIAL FLOURS

Flour	Uses
Arrowroot	Special low-protein baked goods and other items for people with failure of the liver and/or the kidneys or with certain allergies. An ingredient of biscuits that is easily digested by infants and invalids.
Carob	Substitute for chocolate or cocoa in baked goods, confections, drinks, frozen desserts, and puddings.
Cottonseed	Source of complementary protein for mixtures containing cereal flours.
Fish	A high-protein ingredient (also known as fish protein concentrate or FPC) for raising the nutritive values of baked goods, cereals, flour, and macaroni and noodle products.
Lima bean	Dry soup mixes; and an ingredient in products made from cereal flours, where it raises the quantity and quality of protein.
Malt	Production of malted milk powder; and in baked goods (the enzymes present in malt flours convert the starch of the dough into sugars), breakfast cereals, coffee substitutes, confections, and infant foods.
Millet	Brewing of beers (mainly in Africa); and an ingredient of breads, porridges, and soups.
Oat	Ingredient of ready-to-eat breakfast cereals and infant cereals. Popular in Scotland for making oatmeal scones.
Pea	Dry soup mixes; and an ingredient in products made from cereal flours, where it raises the quantity and quality of protein.
Peanut	Production of peanut milk, peanut cheese, and peanut protein concentrate.
Potato	Ingredient of baked goods, snacks and soups. Thickening agent. (Potato starch thickens better than any of the other common food starches. Hence, only small amonts are required.)
Soybean	Added to baked goods, breakfast cereals, confections, dietetic foods, infant foods, macaroni and noodles, and meat products (as an extender and moisturizer).
Sunflower	Source of complementary protein for mixtures containing cereal flours. As such, it is presently being tested for use in baked goods, cereals, desserts, imitation milks, and macaroni and noodle products.
Tapioca	Thickening agent for fruit pies, puddings, and soups.

By-Products. These items are usually rich in fiber, minerals, and vitamins. Their major human food uses are given in Table F-17.

RECENT DEVELOPMENTS IN FLOUR TECHNOLOGY.
The high rates of grain and legume production in the United States have spurred food technologists to develop new ways of utilizing these foods in processed forms such as flours because then the financial return is much greater than that obtained from selling the unprocessed items. Also, wastage due to pests and spoilage is reduced by conversion of the foods into flours. Hence, the American consumer reaps the benefits of (1) lower costs due to more efficient utilization of foods, and (2) a saving of food preparation time because modern flour products are designed for maximum convenience. Most of the developments which follow are still undergoing testing. Nevertheless, they are noteworthy as indicators of the recent trends in flour technology.

• **Air classification of flour fractions**—This process uses swirling streams of air to separate very finely ground flour into fractions which are (1) high in carbohydrate and low in protein, and (2) low in carbohydrate and high in protein. The high-carbohydrate flour is suitable for cakes, cookies, and pastries, whereas the high-protein flour may be used alone or to fortify low-protein flours made from soft wheats. Blending permits a miller to tailor a flour of exact protein value to a buyer's specifications.

• **Corn germ**—Until recently, almost all of this product was utilized in livestock feeds, because its high oil content rendered it susceptible to the development of rancidity while standing on supermarket shelves. Now, this problem has been eliminated by a special process that includes toasting as a final step.

• **Dustless (agglomerated) flour**—The older types of flour were very dry and dusty, and tended to ball up in large masses when mixed with liquids. Furthermore, it is believed that many professional bakers developed allergies to wheat as a result of the chronic inhalation of airborne flour dust.

TABLE F-17
BY-PRODUCTS OF FLOUR PRODUCTION USED IN HUMAN FOODS

Product	Description	Uses	Comments
Bran (corn, rice, wheat)	Outer coarse coat of grain (beneath the hull) removed during milling into flour.	High-fiber ingredient of baked goods and breakfast cereals.	Good source of protein (9 to 18%), fiber (10 to 14%), minerals, and vitamins. Contains phytates which interfere with mineral absorption. Products containing large amounts of bran may have a laxative effect.
Germ (corn, rice, wheat)	Embryo or sprouting part of the seed.	Enrichment or fortification of baked goods and breakfast cereals.	Excellent source of protein (20 to 27%), essential fatty acids, fiber (3 to 12%), minerals, and vitamins. May turn rancid unless kept refrigerated.
Germ oil (corn, rice, wheat)	Oil extracted from germ.	Nutritional supplement.	Rich in essential fatty acids and vitamin E. Maximum nutritional value is obtained when kept refrigerated and used cold (heating destroys vitamin E).
Middlings (rye, wheat)	A mixture of bran, germ, and adhering particles of endosperm.	High-fiber ingredient of *natural* breakfast cereals.	Good source of protein (18 to 20%) and fiber (4 to 8.5%). Rye middlings and wheat middlings cannot contain more than 8.5% crude fiber and 7% crude fiber, respectively.
Polishings (rice)	Finely powdered material removed in the conversion of brown rice into white rice (prior to the milling of the latter into flour).	In many baby foods. To prevent and cure beriberi. In certain baked goods and breakfast cereals.	Contains 10 to 15% protein and 3 to 4% fiber. Rich in essential fatty acids, minerals, and the vitamin B complex (should be stored in a refrigerator to prevent rancidity). Gives baked goods a soft texture and makes them more moist (too much may produce heavy, soggy items).

The newer, dustless, easier-to-mix flours are made by a process which involves (1) wetting the flour to make the individual particles stick together (the process of agglomeration), and (2) drying the agglomerated particles to the desired moisture content. Agglomerated flours are free-flowing and may be mixed into batters or doughs without prior sifting.

• **Gluten-free, low-calorie flour**—Gluten-free baked goods are usually made from corn, rice, or soybean flours. The corn and rice product tend to dry out and become crumbly upon standing, whereas the soybean items are heavy, moist, and have an objectionable beany flavor. These problems have not been encountered in a new type of gluten-free baked product made from a low-calorie flour (about half as high in calories as wheat flour) containing starch, cellulose, and small amounts of special gums derived from cellulose. The very low protein content of the special flour also permits its use in protein restricted diets, such as those employed in the treatment of liver failure or kidney failure.

• **Imitation cheeses made from flour**—Flours (wheat, malted barley, and soy) are the major ingredients of a line of newly developed, dried, imitation cheese products designed for institutional food service. The products contain from 15 to 19% of high quality protein because the flour proteins are complemented by those in the dried buttermilk, dried cheese, and dried whey ingredients. They may be stored at room temperature for up to a year without losing their quality.

• **Pea flour**—Legume flours contain from 2 to 4 times as much protein as the common grain flours. Hence, the addition of legume flours to grain flours raises both the quantity and quality of protein. (The amino acid patterns of legumes are complementary to those of grains. Hence, mixtures have a higher protein quality than either type of flour alone.) However, many legumes impart undesirable characteristics, such as a beany flavor. Therefore, it is noteworthy that USDA scientists have recently found that flours made from green or yellow peas may replace up to 15% of the wheat flour in a loaf of bread without reducing its acceptability. Furthermore, the color of green pea flour is apparently bleached out during baking.

• **Replacement of enzymes lacking in certain flours**—Flours normally contain enzymes which digest starch. These enzyme actions provide sugar for the growth of yeast. When certain flours lack the enzymes, they must be supplied by other ingredients or added in purified form. European bakers have long depended upon malts made from germinated barley or wheat to supply them, but American bakers are now beginning to use pure enzyme preparations derived from various microorganisms.

• **Rice bran derivative**—Protex (trademark of Food Engineering International, Inc.) is a specially processed defatted mixture of rice bran, rice germ, and rice polishings which may be used in baked goods, breakfast cereals, macaroni and noodle products, and milklike beverages. It contains between 17 and 21% protein, plus minerals and vitamins present in the outer layers of the rice grain.

• **Seed coat flours**—The seed coats of grains and legumes are high in fiber and low in calories, so there have been attempts to replace part of the cereal flours used in baking with various seed coat flours. However, yeast-leavened breads made with large amounts of these materials are too heavy and have poor flavors, odors, and textures. Researchers have recently discovered that the seed coat flours may be improved by treating the seed coats with an acid before grinding them into flour.

SUMMARY. Flours have served man for many millennia. Although the major flours now used in the developed countries are made from cereal grains, attempts to improve the nutrition of peoples in these countries have resulted in the utilization of legume flours. It seems likely that in the future a greater variety of flours will be utilized in attempts to feed the burgeoning world population.

FLUID BALANCE

In the body, it is a closely regulated equilibrium between water intake and water output.
(Also see WATER BALANCE.)

FLUID, BODY

This refers to the water and associated dissolved substances within the body. Well known body fluids are: digestive juices, blood, lymph, urine, and perspiration.
(Also see BODY FLUIDS; BODY WATER; and WATER BALANCE.)

FLUMMERY

• A dessert made with stewed fruit, toasted bread, and honey—baked in the oven.

• A soft jelly or porridge made with flour or meal.

FLUORIDATION

This refers to the addition of trace amounts (0.5 to 1.0 parts per million) of fluoride, usually as the sodium salt, to drinking water, for the purpose of providing protection against dental caries. This has proved to be a safe, economical, and efficient way in which to reduce tooth decay—a highly important public health measure in areas where natural water supplies do not contain sufficient fluoride. Extensive medical and public health studies have clearly demonstrated the safety and nutritional advantages that result from fluoridation of water supplies. In communities in which fluoridation has been introduced, the incidence of tooth decay in children has been decreased by 50% or more.
(Also see DENTAL CARIES; FLUORINE OR FLUORIDE; and MINERAL[S].)

FLUORINE OR FLUORIDE[13] (F)

Fluorine is present in small but widely varying concentrations in practically all soils, water supplies, plants, and animals. It is therefore a constituent of all normal diets. Also,

---

[13]Fluoride is the term for the ionized form of the element fluorine, as it occurs in drinking water. The two terms—fluorine or fluoride—are used interchangeably.

fluorine is one of the atmospheric contaminants of industries which use coal, ore, or earthy phosphates.

The adult human contains less than 1.4 mg of fluorine, most of which is in the bones and teeth. In small amounts, fluorides help develop strong bones and teeth, but in excessive amounts bones become porous and soft and teeth become mottled and easily worn down.

A proper intake of fluorine is essential for maximum resistance to dental caries (tooth decay), a beneficial effect that is particularly evident during infancy and early childhood, and which persists through adult life.

HISTORY.
Fluorine was first isolated in 1886 by Henri Moissan, a Frenchman, who obtained it by the electrolysis of anhydrous hydrogen fluoride containing dissolved potassium fluoride. The name fluorine is derived from the Latin *fluo,* meaning to flow, because until 1500 A.D. it was used as a flux in metallurgy.

ABSORPTION, METABOLISM, EXCRETION.
A large proportion (about 90%) of ingested fluorine is normally absorbed, primarily from the small intestine.

That portion of absorbed fluorine which is not taken up by the bones and teeth (50% or more of the fluorine absorbed) is excreted mainly in the urine (although small amounts are excreted in the sweat and the feces), with the result that the level of fluoride in the blood plasma is quite constant.

FUNCTIONS OF FLUORINE.
Although fluorine is found in various parts of the body, it is particularly abundant in bones and teeth; it normally constitutes 0.02 to 0.05% of these tissues. Fluorine is necessary for sound bones and teeth.

The fluoride ion, at proper levels of intake, assists in the prevention of dental caries. When children under 9 years of age consume drinking water containing 1 part per million of fluorine, the teeth have fewer dental caries in childhood, adolescence, and throughout life. This has led to the fluoridation of water supplies in many countries.

The mechanism by which fluorine increases caries resistance of the teeth is not fully understood. However, it appears that crystals of fluoroapatite can replace some of the calcium phosphate crystals of hydroxyapatite that are normally deposited during tooth formation, and that it may also replace some of the carbonate normally found in the tooth. Apparently these fluoride substances are more resistant to mouth acids. Fluorine may also inactivate oral bacterial enzymes which create acids from carbohydrates.

Early attempts to demonstrate that fluorine is essential for growth were unsuccessful, but recent studies with rats raised in isolation units and fed diets containing less than 0.04 ppm fluorine responded with improved growth when fluorine was added to the diet.[14] Mice fed diets containing low levels of fluorine developed anemia and suffered impaired reproduction.[15]

Increased retention of calcium accompanied by a reduction in bone demineralization has been observed in patients receiving fluoride salts. This indicates the possibility that dietary fluorine is essential for optimal bone structure and prevention of osteoporosis in man. This has prompted some medical doctors to use fluorine therapeutically in the treatment of osteoporosis in the aged.

DEFICIENCY SYMPTOMS.
A deficiency of fluorine results in excess dental caries. Also, there is indication that a deficiency of fluorine results in more osteoporosis in the aged. However, excesses of fluorine are of more concern than deficiencies.

INTERRELATIONSHIPS.
Large amounts of dietary calcium, aluminum, or fat will lower the absorption of fluorine.

Fluorine is a cumulative poison; hence, chronic fluoride toxicity, known as fluorosis, may not be noticed for sometime. The enamel of the teeth will likely lose luster and become chalky and mottled when one of the following conditions prevails: (1) when the fluoride content of the drinking water exceeds 2.5 ppm; (2) when the amount of fluorine ingested exceeds 30 to 40 ppm of the dry matter of the diet; or (3) when a person consumes (in food and water) fluorine in excess of 20 mg/day over an extended period of time. The degree of mottling depends upon the level of fluorine intake and individual susceptibility. Mottling of teeth in children has been observed at fluoride concentrations in the diet and drinking water of 2 to 8 ppm.

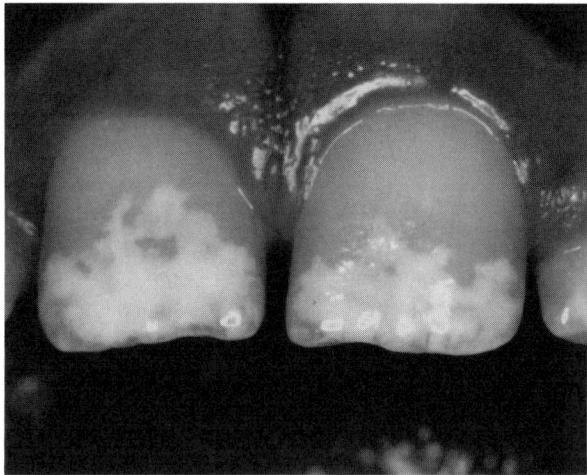

Fig. F-37. Fluorosis of human teeth, showing characteristic change in the enamel—loss of luster, and a chalky mottled appearance. This occurred in a lifetime resident of a community in which the drinking water naturally contained fluoride at concentrations 2 to 3 times greater than the level considered optimal. (Courtesy, Department of Health and Human Services, Public Health Service, National Institute of Health, Bethesda, Md.)

Fluorosis also affects the bones; they lose their normal color and luster, become thickened and softened, and break more easily.

There is no scientific evidence that fluoridation of water has been harmful to anybody at any age, but the effects of fluoride intakes from several sources may be cause for concern. The largest high fluorine area in the United States is the West Texas Panhandle. Also, the soils in some volcanic areas of the world contain large amounts of fluoride, with the result that foods grown in such areas may contain 2 to 3 times more fluoride than foods grown elsewhere.

(Also see POISONS, Table P-2, Some Potentially Poisonous [Toxic] Substances—"Fluorine [F].")

[14]Schwarz, K., and D. B. Milne, "Fluorine Requirement for Growth in the Rat," *Bioinorganic Chemistry,* Vol. 1, 1972, pp. 355-362.

[15]Messer, H. H., W. D. Armstrong, and L. Singer, "Influence of Fluoride Intake on Reproduction in Mice," *Journal of Nutrition,* Vol. 103, 1973, pp. 1319-1326.

RECOMMENDED DAILY ALLOWANCES OF FLU-ORINE. Estimated safe and adequate intakes of fluoride are given in the section on MINERAL(S), Table M-25, Mineral Table.

The ranges suggested in Table M-25 are obtained without difficulty in areas with a water supply containing at least 1 mg/liter of fluoride, either naturally or through fluoridation.

The daily fluoride intake in many areas of the United States is not sufficient to afford optimal protection against dental caries. Fluoridation of water supplies is the simplest and most effective method of providing such added protection, although it is possible to add fluorine to milk, cereals, and salt, or to take it in tablet form as sodium fluoride.

TOXICITY. Fluorine has a small safety range. Yet, the range is wide enough so that the normal fluctuations in the fluoride content of foods poses no risk of excessive intake.

When people or animals consume fluoride concentrations in the diet and drinking water of 2 to 8 ppm (or more) over long periods of time, or when there is environmental contamination, it can result in toxicity (fluorosis), manifested by deformed teeth and bones, and softening, mottling, and irregular wear of the teeth.

SOURCES OF FLUORINE. Fluorine is widely, but unevenly, distributed in nature. It is found in many foods, but seafoods and tea are the richest dietary sources. Table F-18 shows the fluorine content in ppm of some common fluorine sources. (To convert ppm to mcg/g multiply by 1.)

TABLE F-18
SOME FLUORINE SOURCES

Source	Fluorine (ppm)	Source	Fluorine (ppm)
Dried seaweed	326.0	Chicken	1.5
Tea	32.0	Butter	1.5
Mackerel	19.0	Soybeans	1.4
Sardines	11.0	Eggs	1.3
Salmon	6.0	Beef	1.2
Shrimp	4.5	Lamb	1.2
Smoked herring	3.8	Spinach	1.0
Wheat germ	2.4	Parsley	.9
Crab	2.2	Whole wheat	.8
Cheese	1.7	Pork	.7

NOTE WELL: The fluorine content of foods varies widely and is affected by the fluorine content of the environment (the air, soil and/or water) in the areas in which they were produced. Nevertheless, some foods do cumulate and contain more fluorine than others. Remember that it's the total fluorine ingested over an extended period of time that's important. There is hazard of fluorisis (evidenced by mottling of the teeth) (1) when the fluorine content of drinking water exceeds 2.5 ppm; (2) when the amount of fluorine ingested exceeds 30 to 40 ppm of dry matter of the diet; or (3) when a person consumes (in food and water) fluorine in excess of 20 mg/day over an extended period of time.

An average daily diet provides 0.25 to 0.35 mg of fluorine. In addition, the average adult may ingest 1.0 to 1.5 mg daily from drinking and cooking water that contains 1 ppm of fluorine. For children 1 to 12 years old, water may contribute anywhere from 0.4 to 1.1 mg of fluorine per day.

Fluorine tablets and fluorine toothpastes can serve as reliable, though expensive, sources of this element.

• **Fluoridation of water supplies**—Fluoridation of water supplies to bring the concentration of fluoride to 1 ppm (1 part of fluorine to a million parts of water) has proved to be a safe, economical, and efficient way to reduce tooth decay—a highly important public health measure in areas where natural water supplies do not contain this amount. Extensive medical and public health studies have clearly demonstrated the safety and nutritional advantages that result from fluoridation of water supplies. In communities in which fluoridation has been introduced, the incidence of tooth decay in children has been decreased by 50% or more.

The concentration of fluoride in public water supplies should be adjusted slightly to allow for differences in water consumption with seasonal temperature changes.
(Also see MINERAL[S], Table M-25.)

FLUOROSIS

A chronic disease resulting from the accumulation of toxic levels of the mineral fluorine in the teeth and bones. It is a crippling disease characterized by bone overgrowth, brittle bones, stiff joints, weakness, weight loss, and anemia. Mottling of the teeth may occur if exposure occurred during the formation of enamel. Contaminated water and food are the principal sources of excessive fluoride.

(Also see DENTAL FLUOROSIS; FLUORINE OR FLUORIDE; and MINERAL[S].)

FOIE GRAS

Livers of fattened geese and ducks. In cookery, the name *foie gras* is applied only to goose or duck liver from birds fattened by force feeding. The livers of Toulouse and Strasbourg geese sometimes weigh 4.4 lb *(2 kg)*. The finest foie gras comes from geese raised in Alsace and in southwestern France. Duck foie gras is also very delicate, but it has a tendency to disintegrate in cooking.

Foie gras is regarded as one of the greatest delicacies available. The quality of foie gras can be judged primarily by its color and texture; it should be creamy white, tinged with pink, and very firm.

FOLACIN (FOLATE/FOLIC ACID)[16]

There is no single compound vitamin with the name *folacin;* rather, the term *folacin* is used to designate folic acid (pteroylmonoglutamic acid, or PGA) and a group of closely

[16]Although the word *folate* is used in biochemical literature for salts or folic acid, it lacks specificity.

related substances which are essential for all vertebrates, including man, for normal growth and reproduction, for the prevention of blood disorders, for important biochemical mechanisms within each cell, and for the prevention of a variety of deficiency symptoms in different species.

The research work related to folacin is considered to be the most complicated chapter in the story of the B-complex vitamins.

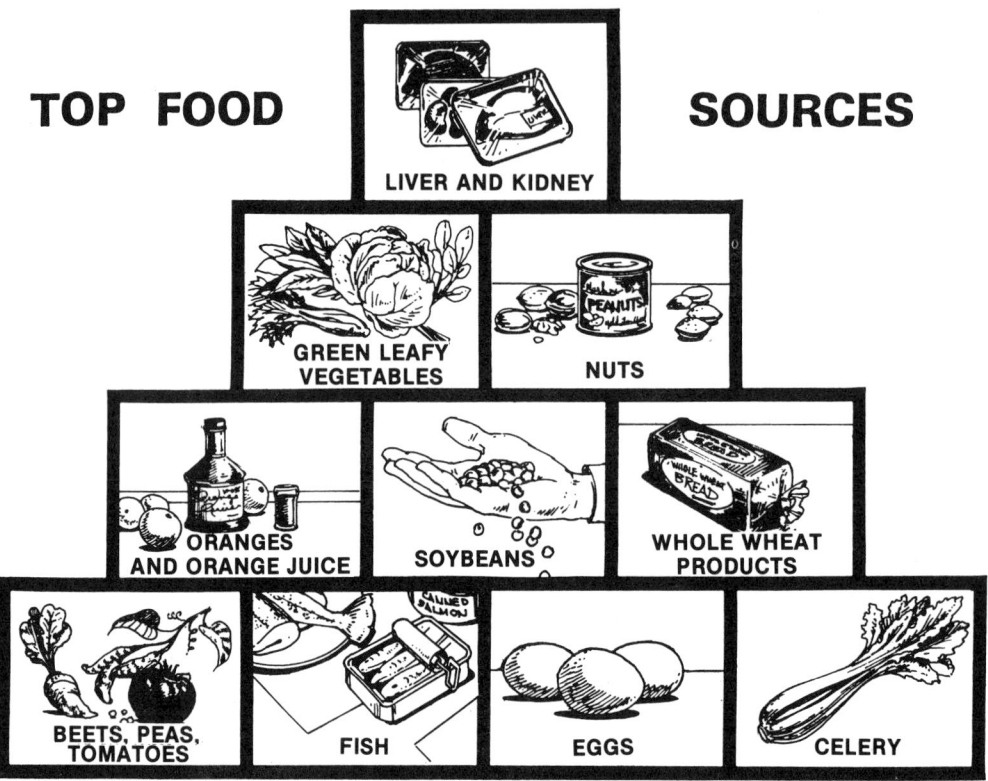

TOP FOOD SOURCES

Fig. F-38. Top food sources of folacin.

HISTORY.   Long before folacin was isolated or synthesized, its deficiency symptoms had been described in humans, animals, and microorganisms. In 1931, while working in a maternity hospital in Bombay, India, Dr. Lucy Wills described a macrocytic anemia in pregnant women which improved when they were given extracts of yeast. Subsequent work showed that the factor in yeast that was effective in curing Dr. Wills' patients was a group of chemically related vitamins with folic acid activity, given the generic name *folacin.*

In 1941, the name *folic acid,* the forerunner of the term *folacin,* was suggested by Mitchell, Snell, and Williams, of Texas, for the growth factor for bacteria that was found in spinach and known to be widely distributed in green leafy plants. The word *folic* is derived from the Latin word *folium,* meaning foliage or leaf.

In 1945, Angier and co-workers isolated and synthesized folic acid. That same year, Dr. Tom Spies showed that folic acid was effective in the treatment of megaloblastic anemia of pregnancy and of tropical sprue.

Through the years, several names other than folacin and folic acid have been given to this vitamin, including: Wills' factor, pteroylmonoglutamic acid, antianemia factor PGA, vitamin M, vitamin Bc, SLR factor, factor R, factor U, vitamin U, *Lactobacillus casei* factor; citrovoram factor (CF); yeast Norit eluate factor, vitamin B-9, vitamin B-10, and vitamin B-11.

CHEMISTRY, METABOLISM, PROPERTIES.

• **Chemistry**—This vitamin exists in several different forms in nature, making up the folacin group of compounds. All forms have similar activity when fed to man and other higher animals, but they have widely different activities as growth factors for microorganisms. The parent compound, folic acid (known chemically as pteroylglutamic acid [PGA]), which probably does not exist free in nature, consists of three linked components: *pteridine* (a yellow phosphorescent pigment related to the yellow pigment in butterfly wings [the Greek word for wing is *pteron*]); *para-aminobenzoic acid* (a growth factor for bacteria)[17]; and *glutamic acid* (an amino acid commonly found in proteins of foods and body tissues). Folic acid may consist of one, three, or seven glutamate groupings; designated as mono-, tri-, or hepta-pteroylglutamate. These conjugated forms serve as the major precursors of the vitamin in the diet. The coenzyme form, tetrahydrofolic acid, the most common form in the body, is also widely distributed in foods. The structural formula of pure folic acid (pteroylmonoglutamic acid) is given in Fig. F-39. If the parent molecule (consisting of pteridine, para-aminobenzoic acid, and glutamic acid) is broken, nutritional activity is lost. The biologically active form of folacin is a reduction product called tetrahydrofolic acid.

---

[17]In addition to having activity as a growth factor for bacteria, para-aminobenzoic acid has considerable folacin activity when fed to deficient animals in which intestinal synthesis of folacin takes place. For example, for rats and mice, para-aminobenzoic acid can completely replace the need for a dietary source of folacin. This explains why para-aminobenzoic acid was once considered to be a vitamin in its own right.

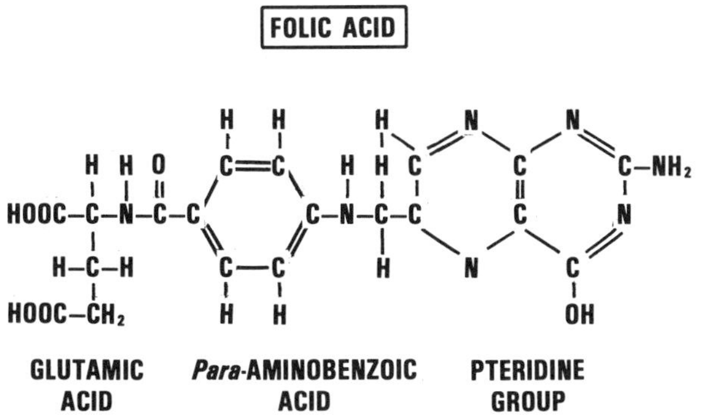

FOLIC ACID

GLUTAMIC ACID — *Para*-AMINOBENZOIC ACID — PTERIDINE GROUP

Fig. F-39. Structure of folic acid (pteroylmonoglutamic acid).

• **Metabolism**—Wide variation exists in the absorption of folates from different foods, with a low of about 10% for yeast to a high of about 80% for eggs and liver. One study showed that only 31% of the folate in orange juice was absorbed, whereas 82% of the folate in bananas was absorbed. It is thought that the number of glutamic acid molecules in the folates affect the rate of absorption.

Folate is absorbed by active transport and by diffusion, mainly in the upper part of the small intestine, although some is absorbed along the entire length of the small intestine; glucose, ascorbic acid, and some antibiotics facilitate its absorption.

Folacin occurs in food in two forms—free folates and bound folates (polyglutamates). The free folates (which account for about 25% of the food intake) are readily absorbed in the intestinal tract. Before polyglutamates can be absorbed, excess glutamates (all but one) must be removed from the side chain of the molecule by conjugase, an enzyme. It is not known whether the conjugase acts in the lumen of the small intestine or in the intestinal wall. The absorption of folic acid is thus controlled by the deconjugating mechanism which, in turn, may be affected by conjugase inhibitors in the food; i.e., yeast. The rate of absorption of conjugated folates appears to be related to chain length.

Folate, bound to protein, is transported in the blood to the liver. There it is methylated and carried to the bone marrow cells, the maturing red blood cells, and perhaps to other cells. Methyl-folate seems to be the chief form of the vitamin in body tissues. Serum levels of folacin range from 7 to 16 nanograms per milliliter of serum. The total body stores of folate normally range between 5 and 12 mg, about half of which is in the liver. The measurement of folacin levels in both blood serum and red blood cells is the procedure used to evaluate folacin nutriture in human beings.

Some folate is excreted in the bile as well as the urine.

• **Properties**—Folic acid is a bright yellow crystaline powder, slightly soluble in water, unstable in acid solution, relatively unstable to heat, and rather easily destroyed upon exposure to light.

MEASUREMENT/ASSAY. Folic acid is measured in micrograms or nanograms (ng, millimicrograms).

Folic acid in food is usually assayed either biologically by chick or rat growth tests, or microbiologically with *L. casei* or another suitable microorganism. Larger quantities of folacin activity may be measured chemically, fluorometrically, or by paper and thin-layer chromatography.

FUNCTIONS. Following absorption, folic acid is changed, by a number of reduction reactions that require niacin, to at least five active coenzyme forms, the parent form being tetrahydrofolic acid. The principal function of these coenzymes is the transfer of single carbon units from one compound to another; the one carbon unit can be formyl, forminino, methylene, or methyl groups.

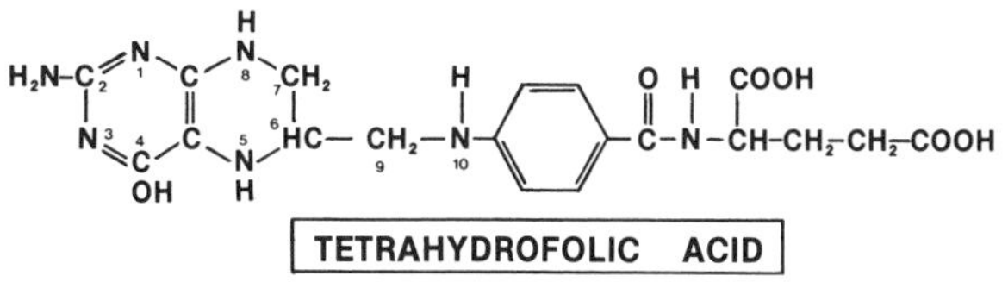

TETRAHYDROFOLIC ACID

Fig. F-40. Structures of tetrahydrofolic acid. The N-5 and N-10 nitrogen atoms participate in the transfer of one-carbon groups.

Folacin coenzymes are responsible for the following important functions:

1. The formation of purines and pyrimidines which, in turn, are needed for the synthesis of the nucleic acids DNA (deoxyribonucleic acid), and RNA (ribonucleic acid), vital to all cell nuclei. This explains the important role of folacin in cell division and reproduction.

2. The formation of heme, the iron-containing protein in hemoglobin.

3. The interconversion of the three-carbon amino acid serine from the two-carbon amino acid glycine.

4. The formation of the amino acids tyrosine from phenylalanine and glutamic acid from histidine.

5. The formation of the amino acid methionine from homocysteine.

6. The synthesis of choline from ethanolamine.

7. The conversion of nicotinamide to N^1-methylnicotinamide, one of the metabolites of niacin that is excreted in the urine.

Ascorbic acid, vitamin B-12, and vitamin B-6 are essential for the activity of the folacin coenzymes in many of these metabolic processes; again and again pointing up the interdependence of various vitamins.

• **Clinical application of folic acid**—The following clinical applications of folic acid are noteworthy:

1. **Nutritional megaloblastic and macrocytic anemias.** These types of anemias, which occur in infancy (megaloblastic anemia) and pregnancy (macrocytic anemia) and are usually due to simple folic acid deficiency, respond rapidly to treatment with folic acid, without vitamin B-12. It is possible that in some cases these anemias are due to an unknown metabolic defect in the production of the folacin enzymes.

2. **Leukemia.** *Aminopterin*, a folic acid antagonist or antivitamin, has been used in the treatment of leukemia.

Folic acid is involved in the normal synthesis of nucleic acid within the cell nucleus, which is responsible for cell growth. As an antagonist, aminopterin can fill in for folic acid, without activity. As a result, it is able to block the rapid production of leucocytes (white blood cells) characteristic of leukemia. Unfortunately, with continued use, the leukemic cells seem to develop a resistance to the antagonist and its effectiveness is lost.

3. **Cancer.** Methotrexate (amethopterin), a drug closely related to aminopterin, is currently being used in cancer chemotherapy. Its action is to bind the enzyme dihydrofolate

reductase and thus inhibit the C_1 fixing function of folic acid, thereby preventing synthesis of DNA and purine in the cell.

4. **Sprue.** Folic acid is effective in the treatment of sprue, a gastrointestinal disease characterized by intestinal lesions, malabsorption of food, diarrhea, stools containing large amounts of fat, macrocytic anemia, and general malnutrition.

DEFICIENCY SYMPTOMS. Folacin deficiency in man may result in megaloblastic anemia (of infancy), also called macrocytic anemia (of pregnancy), in which the red blood cells are larger and fewer than normal, and also immature. The anemia is due to inadequate formation of nucleoproteins, causing failure of the megaloblast (young red blood cells) in the bone marrow to mature. The hemoglobin level is low because of the reduced number of red blood cells. Also, the white blood cell, blood platelet, and serum folate levels are low.

Other symptoms include a sore, red, smooth tongue (glossitis), disturbances of the intestinal tract (diarrhea), and poor growth. Also, recent observations suggest that there may be mental deterioration.

A deficiency of folacin may be caused by inadequate dietary intake, impaired absorption or utilization, or an unusual need (caused by increased losses or requirements) by the body's tissues.

The administration of folic acid to patients with megaloblastic anemia brings about dramatic recovery. But folacin is not a substitue for vitamin B-12 in the treatment of pernicious anemia; although it will alleviate the anemia, only vitamin B-12 will cure the neurologic symptoms.

Man, monkeys, chicks, turkeys, fox, and mink must have folacin supplied in the food in order to avoid deficiency symptoms. Rats, dogs, rabbits, and pigs can meet their need for this vitamin through bacterial synthesis in the intestine.

RECOMMENDED DAILY ALLOWANCE. The Food and Nutrition Board (FNB) of the National Research Council (NRC) recommended daily allowances of folacin (folate) are given in Table F-18a. It should be noted, however, that stress, such as disease, increases the requirement.

● **Infants and children**—The daily folacin requirements for (1) infants and (2) children have been estimated at 25 to 35 mcg and 50 to 100 mcg, respectively (see Table F-18a). Since human and cow's milk contain approximately 2 to 3 mcg/100 ml and most of the folic acid is in an absorbable form, these needs can be met by a milk diet.

CAUTIONS: (1) Boiling destroys folacin in cow's milk, so infants receiving boiled formulas prepared from pasteurized, sterilized, or powdered cow's milk should receive additional folacin to assure an adequate intake; and (2) if the diet consists of goat's milk, folic acid supplementation should be given because of the low content and poor availability of folacin in goat's milk.

● **Adults**—The bulk of the evidence suggests that 25 to 50% of dietary folacin is nutritionally available. Thus, the RDA for adult males is set at 150 to 200 mcg, and for adult females it is 150 to 180 mcg (see Table F-18a).

● **Pregnancy and lactation**—The added burden of pregnancy is known to increase the risk and incidence of folacin deficiency among populations with low or marginal intakes of the vitamin. The RDA for folacin is set at 400 mcg/day during pregnancy (see Table F-18a).

The RDA allowance of folate during lactation is 280 mcg/day during the first 6 months, and 260 mcg/day during the second 6 months (see Table F-18a).

● **Oral contraceptives**—Low tissue folate levels and macrocytic anemia have been found in women taking oral contraceptives. So, higher levels of folacin may be indicated under such circumstances.

● **Folacin intake in average U.S./Canadian diet**—The total folacin of mixed diets varies over a rather wide range. The average folate intake of both U.S. and Canadian populations is about 3 mcg/kg body weight.[18]

Average American intakes of folacin are well over the recommended daily allowances, although low intakes or low tissue levels are often seen in sprue, in infants of low birth weight, in infants on unsupplemented milk diets, in various disease states, in longtime hospitalized patients, in alcoholism, and in pregnancy. Also, it must be remembered that there are large losses of folacin from storage and cooking. So, deficiency of folacin is being found with increasing frequency.

TOXICITY. Normally, folic acid has no adverse effects. However, when it is used to treat megaloblastic anemia secondary to the use of antiepileptic drugs, the epilepsy may be aggravated.

FOLACIN LOSSES DURING PROCESSING, COOKING, AND STORAGE. Although folic acid is present in most common foods, it is subject to storage and cooking losses.

Raw vegetables stored at room temperature for 2 to 3 days lose as much as 50 to 70% of their folate content. But storage in a refrigerator for as long as 2 weeks results in little or no loss of folacin.

TABLE F-18A
RECOMMENDED DAILY FOLACIN (FOLATE) ALLOWANCES[1]

Group	Age	Weight		Height		Folate
	(yr)	(lb)	(kg)	(in.)	(cm)	(mcg)[2]
Infants	0.0–0.5	13	6	24	60	25
	0.5–1.0	20	9	28	71	35
Children	1–3	29	13	35	90	50
	4–6	44	20	44	112	75
	7–10	62	28	52	132	100
Males	11–14	99	45	62	157	150
	15–18	145	66	69	176	200
	19–24	160	72	70	177	200
	25–50	174	79	70	176	200
	51+	170	77	68	173	200
Females	11–14	101	46	62	157	150
	15–18	120	55	64	163	180
	19–24	128	58	65	164	180
	25–50	138	63	64	163	180
	51+	143	65	63	160	180
Pregnant						400
Lactating						280–260

[1]Recommended Dietary Allowances, 10th ed., 1989, NRC-National Academy of Sciences, p. 285.
[2]The RDA are expressed in terms of "total" folacin; that is, the amount of folic acid activity available from all food folates.

[18]Recommended Dietary Allowances, 10th ed., 1989, NRC-National Academy of Sciences, p. 153.

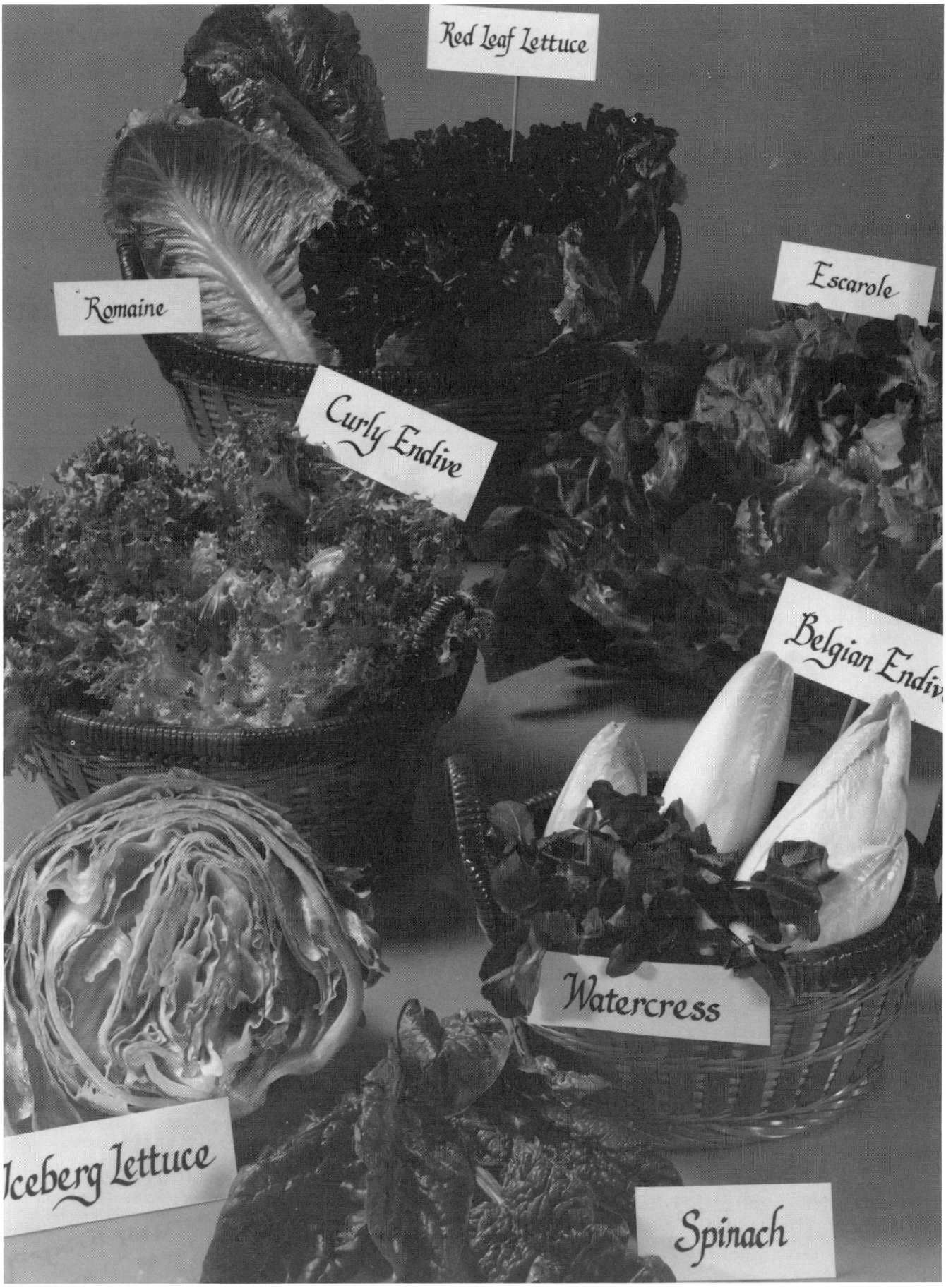

Fig. F-41. Green leafy vegetables, a rich source of folacin, and other essential nutrients. (Courtesy, United Fresh Fruit & Vegetable Assoc., Alexandria, Va.)

Between 50 and 95% of food folate is destroyed by cooking or canning. The losses are greatest when high temperatures, long cooking periods, and large volumes of water are used. Most of the folic acid activity of milk is destroyed in processing dried milk.

Exposure to light also reduces the amount of folacin available in foods.

Foods high in vitamin C tend to lose less folacin than those low in vitamin C; vitamin C protects folates from oxidative destruction.

SOURCES OF FOLACIN. Information relative to the folacin activity of foods for humans is incomplete because of the difficulty of assaying the many different forms of folacin in terms of activity. Nevertheless, the general guides given in the section on VITAMIN(S), Table V-5, Vitamin Table, will help ensure ample folacin in the daily diet.

Intestinal bacteria synthesize folacin. Although this source may be important in man, the amount of folacin produced and absorbed has not been determined.

For additional sources and more precise values of folacin (folic acid), see Food Composition Table F-21 of this book.

NOTE WELL: Tables of folacin composition in foods, especially in the raw state, should be used with discretion because folacin compounds differ in their ability to be absorbed in the intestine depending on (1) the number of glutamic acid molecules in the folates, and (2) the nature of other types of binding—generally with protein.

Folacin deficiency may result from: (1) a shortage of the folacin itself; (2) very considerable storage, processing, and cooking losses; (3) the folacin not being absorbed in the intestine; and/or (4) substances that interfere with the normal function of the folacin enzymes. As a result, folacin deficiencies are thought to be a health problem in this country and throughout the world. Infants (especially those born prematurely, of low birth weight, or on unsupplemented milk diets), adolescents, and pregnant women seem particularly vulnerable. Tropical sprue, certain genetic disturbances, cancer, and parasitic infection increase the folate requirement. Chronic alcoholism is an important cause of folate deficiency; alcohol interferes with folate absorption and transportation from storage sites in the body. Oral contraceptives may also interfere with folate absorption.

It is noteworthy, too, that folacin fortification of corn, rice, and bread among population groups in South Africa has been shown to be an effective measure to prevent the development of macrocytic anemia in pregnancy.

So, dietary supplementation with folacin may be indicated more generally than has been thought necessary in the past.

CAUTION: Vitamin preparations without prescription containing more than 0.1 mg of folacin in a daily dose are prohibited by law. Excessive folacin can mask certain symptoms of pernicious anemia.

(Also see VITAMIN[S], Table V-5.)

FOLINIC ACID $(C_{20}H_{23}N_7O_7)$

Folinic acid is an important metabolite of folic acid and may be the active form in cellular metabolism. Vitamin C and vitamin B-12 are essential for the conversion of folic acid to folinic acid.

FOOD AND AGRICULTURE ORGANIZATION OF THE UNITED NATIONS (FAO)

This is a specialized agency of the United Nations established by 44 countries in 1945 in Quebec, Canada, partially in response to the awareness of world nutrition created

by the War. It now has more than 120 member countries. Headquarters are in Rome, Italy, with a North American office in Washington, D.C. Major objectives of the FAO are (1) elimination of hunger, and (2) betterment of nutrition by improving the production, distribution, and use of food and other products of farms, forest, and fisheries throughout the world. Activities of the FAO include conducting research, providing technical assistance, conducting educational programs, maintaining statistics on world food, publishing reports, and working closely with the World Health Organization (WHO) all over the world. The FAO/WHO Expert Committee on nutrition has produced reports which recommend and encourage work on the assessment of nutritional status, standards of requirement for nutrients, protein-energy malnutrition, nutritional anemia, endemic goiter, xerophthalmia, food technology, and toxicology.

(Also see DISEASES, section headed "International and Voluntary Organizations Engaged in Health and/or Nutrition Activities"; and NUTRITION EDUCATION, section headed "Nutrition Education Sources.")

FOOD AND DRUG ADMINISTRATION (FDA)

This is the federal agency in the Department of Health and Human Services that is charged with the responsibility of safeguarding American consumers against injury, unsanitary food, and fraud. Specifically, the FDA enforces (1) the Federal Food, Drug, and Cosmetic Act with its numerous amendments, (2) the Fair Packaging and Labeling Act, (3) those sections of the Public Health Service Act relating to biological products, and (4) the Radiation Control for Health and Safety Act. Also, the FDA protects industry against unscrupulous competition; and it inspects and analyzes samples, and conducts independent research on such things as toxicity (using laboratory animals), disappearance curves for pesticides, and the long-range effects of drugs.

The FDA began in 1927 as the Food, Drug, and Insecticide Administration. Through the years, it has established rigorous testing policies requiring proof relative to product safety and efficacy. The requirements for new product approval by the FDA have become more rigid, and enforcement has become more unrelenting. In 1962, a new drug could be developed, tested, and approved for a cost of about $1 million—all in a period of 1 to 2 years. In 1990, development to approval of a new drug took 5 to 6 years and cost $10 to $12 million. It is understandable, therefore, why manufacturers resist the threat of a ban on a product in which they have invested.

(Also see DELANEY CLAUSE; DISEASES, section headed "U.S. Department of Health and Human Services"; and FEDERAL FOOD, DRUG, AND COSMETIC ACT.)

FOODBORNE DISEASE

Stated simply, any disease that is transmitted through food is known as a foodborne disease. Because eating is an activity in which all people engage, the risk of obtaining a disease-causing agent from contaminated food is extremely high. Applying a rather broad definition to disease, a foodborne disease may be caused by (1) contamination of food by bacteria, parasites, viruses, fungi and molds, (2) some naturally occurring toxicant, (3) contamination of food by toxic industrial chemicals or radioactive waste, or (4) food allergies. More specifically, foodborne diseases include the familiar examples of typhoid, tapeworm, botulism, brucellosis, tuberculosis, salmonella, hepatitis, and *tourist diarrhea*

—bacterial, parasitic and viral infections—to name only a few. The greatest deterrent to foodborne diseases is scrupulous attention to cleanliness from the production to the consumption of food, since foodborne diseases usually enter the food chain via (1) infected animals or plants, (2) organisms transmitted by flies, roaches or rodents, (3) contact with sewage-polluted water, or (4) food handlers who lack good personal hygiene and/or fail to follow acceptable food handling practices.

(Also see ALLERGIES; BACTERIA IN FOOD; DISEASES, section headed "Food-Related Infectious and Parasitic Diseases;" POISONS; POISONOUS PLANTS; and RADIOACTIVE FALLOUT.)

FOOD—BUYING, PREPARING, COOKING, AND SERVING

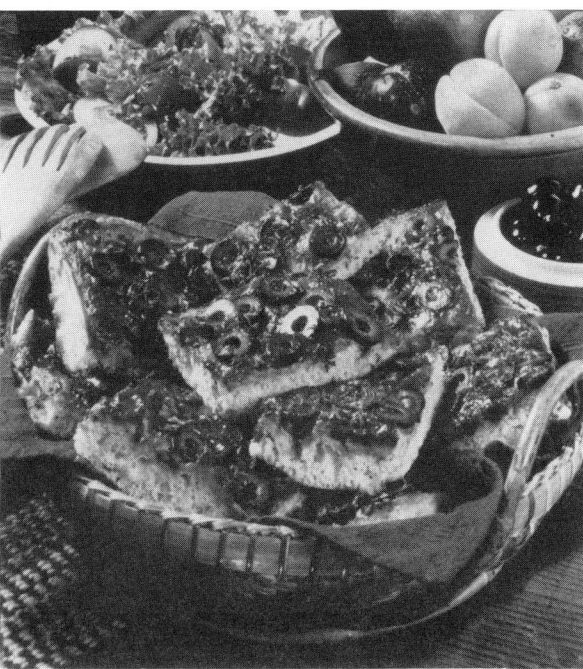

Fig. F-42. Food on the table. Menu planning comes first, followed by buying, preparing, cooking, and serving. (Courtesy, Olive Administrative Committee, Fresno, Calif.)

Legally (according to the Federal Food, Drug, and Cosmetic Act, as Amended, Sec. 201 [f]), *the term food means (1) articles used for food or drink for man or other animals, (2) chewing gum, and (3) articles used for components by any such article.*

Because each step in food preparation is important to the nutritive value of the finished product, consideration should be given to what happens to foods from the time the consumer purchases them in the marketplace to the time they reach the dinner table.

The discussion in this section will deal primarily with the retention of nutrients as they go from raw products to finished in the average home kitchen. In most instances, the correct preparation and cooking not only produces a better product nutritionally, but the psychological advantages to a nicely prepared meal are immeasureable.

(Also see ADDITIVES.)

MEAL PLANNING. Planning the menu is perhaps the most important step in putting food on the table. Once the meal is planned, the purchasing, storing, and preparing of food follow in a more or less automatic sequence. Unfortunately, many shoppers go to the grocery store without a *blueprint* and end up purchasing either more than they need, or not the right things. A menu does not have to be rigid, but it can be used as a guide.

If the marketing is done daily, meals can be planned 1 day at a time. But, if the marketing is done on a weekly basis, about 5 days' meals should be planned, allowing a little leeway for meals eaten outside the home and for leftovers.

The following goals should be considered in meal planning:

1. Balancing the meal nutritionally for all age groups by using the Six Food Groups.
(Also see FOOD GROUPS.)

2. Keeping within the budget.

3. Balancing the flavors, colors, and textures.

4. Managing the available materials, time, and energy efficiently.

5. Considering the family preferences.

THE KITCHEN AND EQUIPMENT. Before the food is purchased at the market, the kitchen and equipment should be considered. It is not necessary to have fancy equipment, but the following items are rather basic: stove, refrigerator, sink, mixing bowls and spoons, measuring cups and spoons, pans, and baking dishes.

No matter how much or how little equipment, it should be conveniently arranged in the kitchen, for ease of preparation. If possible, the work centers should follow a logical sequence from bringing the groceries into the kitchen, to storing in refrigerator or pantry; to sink and preparation center; to stove and/or oven; to serving onto the plates; to dinner table; and, finally, from clearing the table back to the sink, thence to the storage cupboard. These activities should follow in sequence around the room and not be crisscrossing the room.

FOOD BUYING. Food markets have come a long way since the advent of railways, motor freight, and air freight. Years ago, most of the food available was produced locally. The farmers brought their produce to town by horse and wagon, and the customers collected at the wagons to purchase their daily food. These were the first peddlers. Village fairs and town markets evolved when several peddlers banded together for the convenience of the buyer. In those days, there was no refrigeration, so shopping for food was a daily process for the city dweller, as it still is in many parts of the world.

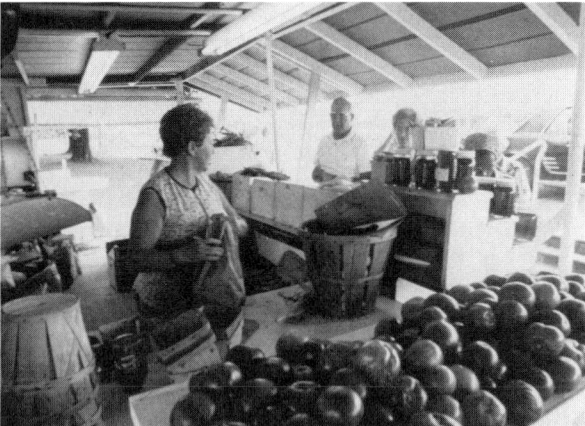

Fig. F-43. Roadside market. (Courtesy, USDA)

By the beginning of the 20th century, the local grocery store was displaying items from many parts of the country. The proprietor was a well-known figure in the community, and a personal friend to all of his customers. However, as cities grew in size, it became increasingly difficult to service all of the grocery store customers with such personalized service. A new concept in marketing came about with the first Alpha Beta store which opened in southern California in 1915. The foods were arranged in alphabetical order (hence its name), so that the customers could find each item easily; and, by the customer serving herself, the proprietor could sell to many more customers at one time.

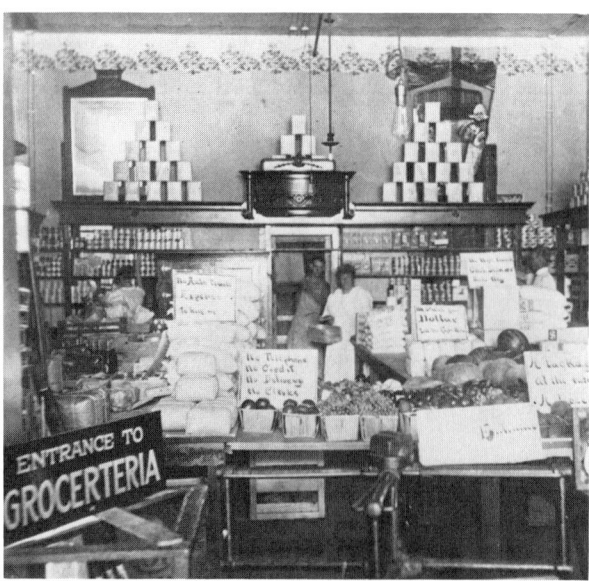

Fig. F-44. Alpha Beta's first self-service *Grocerteria,* in 1915. (Courtesy, Alpha Beta Company, La Habra, Calif.)

Today, the food customer has a wide selection, almost year round. In order to secure maximum nutritive qualities, it is important that perishable foods be as fresh as possible. The produce manager can usually tell from whence most of his fresh foods come; and from this, he can judge how much time has elapsed between picking and marketing.

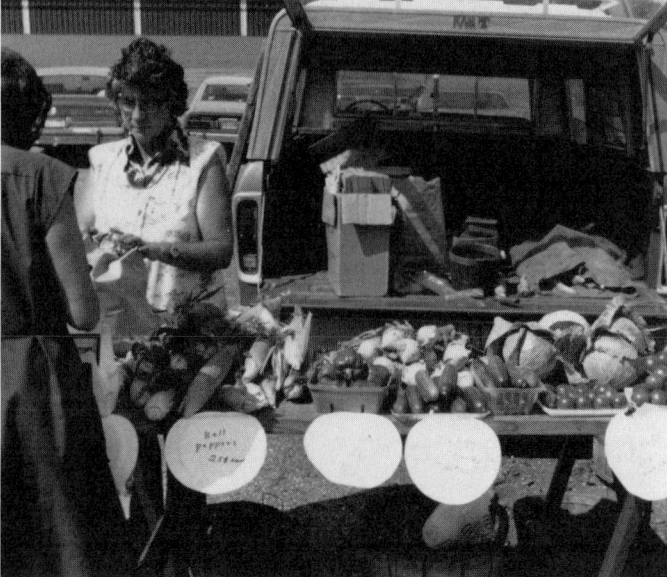

Fig. F-45. Farmers' market. (Courtesy, University of Minnesota, St. Paul, Minn.)

FOOD STORING. The goal in food storage is to prevent food spoilage from microbial decompositions, enzymatic or nonenzymatic chemical changes, or other losses such as may be caused by insects and/or rodents.

Because most spoilage occurs in the presence of moisture and at temperatures between 68° to 131°F (*20° to 55°C*), foods are preserved, both commercially and in the kitchen, by alleviating these conditions. The most popular methods of preservation are canning, freezing, freeze drying, drying, or pickling.

After purchasing the freshest foods available, it is important to get them into refrigeration as soon as possible. As a general rule of thumb, fresh vegetables and fruits can be stored under refrigeration for 1 week. Before storing, to wash or not to wash fruits and vegetables is the question? Possibly the best rule of thumb is to wash those fruits and vegetables that are to be used in salads. Until they are to be used, it is not necessary to wash those fruits and vegetables that eventually will be peeled or prepared in some other way for cooking.

Fresh meats can be stored for only 4 days on the average. If a freezer is not available to freeze part of the week's supply, canned products, dehydrated meats, eggs, cheese, beans, or nuts, can be used for the last meals of the week before the weekly shopping trip for groceries. For those who can get to the grocery store easily, this presents no problem. But for those who live some distance from the store, it requires some planned strategy when a freezer is not available.

Eggs and milk can be kept under refrigeration for about 10 days, without any undue spoilage. The spoilage time depends a great deal on the condition of the item when the consumer purchases it.

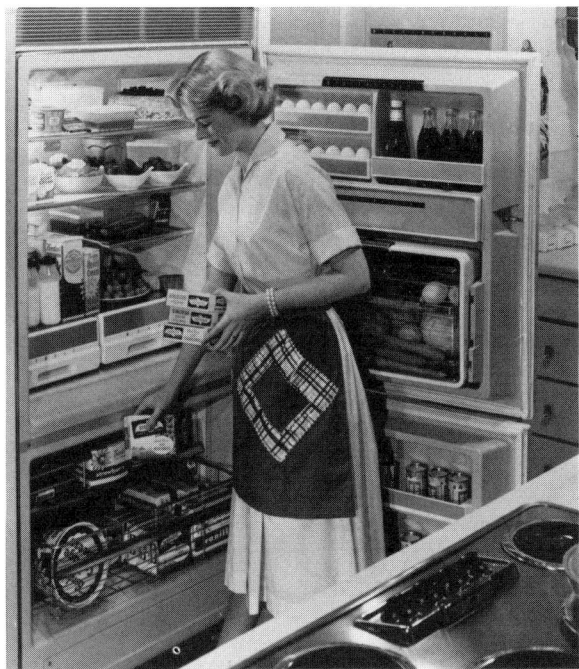

Fig. F-46. Refrigeration revolutionized the marketing of foods and the consumer's purchasing pattern. No longer was it necessary that food be supplied to the grocer, sold to the consumer, and eaten by the family—all in 1 day. The shelf life of perishable foods was extended dramatically. (Courtesy, The Bettmann Archive, Inc., New York, N.Y.)

Frozen foods that are allowed to thaw and then are refrozen usually lose considerable in quality, and possibly some in nutritive value. In addition, it means that the food cannot be held as long in the freezer. When freezing fresh, unfrozen foods, divide into portions that will be needed, so that it is not necessary to thaw the whole piece in order to use a portion of it. The common rule of thumb is to freeze foods only twice. This means that the food can be thawed, prepared and refrozen until it is needed. Or it can be thawed, prepared and served, and any large amount left over can be refrozen to be used at a later date. Foods cannot be held as long if frozen twice as they can if frozen only once.

Cereals and baked goods should be stored in airtight containers. If they contain whole grains or wheat germ, they should be refrigerated or frozen to prevent deterioration and rancidity.

When keeping leftovers in the refrigerator, there are two very important points to remember:

1. Refrigerate the leftover as quickly as possible. Do not let it cool to room temperature first.

2. Store it in an airtight container so that it does not dry out.

(Also see MEAT[S], section headed "Meat Preservation," Table M-11, Storage Time for Refrigerated and Frozen Meats; and MILK AND MILK PRODUCTS, section headed "Care of Milk in the Home," Table M-23, Approximate Storage Life of Milk Products at Specific Temperatures.)

FOOD PROPERTIES. Before plunging into the mixing bowl, some of the basic properties of foods and their ingredients should be understood.

Water And Solutions. There is no substitute for water. It is as indispensable to cooking foods as a match is to

lighting a fire. Water fills a multifaceted role. Here are some of its properties and uses:

1. **Water as a method of cooking.** Water is used for simmering foods such as soup bones, less tender cuts of meats, dried and fresh fruits and vegetables, starches and cereals. However, the more water and the greater the cooking time, the more nutritive value that is lost. This fact makes it important to utilize the liquid left from this method of cookery, with the exception of cured meats. Fortunately, cured meats will lose some of their high salt content through this method of cooking, which is a definite advantage.

2. **Water as an absorbable agent.** Foods that have been dried, such as beans, peas, lentils, fruits, soups, yeast, etc. can be restored to their original condition by soaking and/or cooking in water. Even stale dried bread or rolls can be revived by the addition of water (which they have lost by dehydration), followed by heating. Broadly speaking, these foods are *hydrates* (they take up water) and this process is called *hydration*.

Starches also have the ability, when mixed with water and cooked, to swell and thicken a liquid—gravies, sauces, and soups.

3. **Water as a part of certain chemical changes.** When water is added to dry baking powder, carbon dioxide—the gas that leavens quick breads—is released. The change is accelerated when heat is applied.

4. **Water in foods may cause food spoilage.** Foods containing water will develop molds and other bacterial growths if held at temperatures which favor such growths. That is why, in the prevention of food spoilage, either the moisture should be removed or the food should be stored at a temperature which discourages the growth of molds and bacteria.

5. **Water as a solvent.** Water dissolves flavorings, sugar, and salt. This occurs when making teas, coffee, and sugar drinks. Salt is also dissolved in water to produce a brine, which is used to preserve meats and vegetables. Unfortunately, water also dissolves some minerals and vitamins, either when food is soaked in water or during cooking. This means that fresh vegetables should not be soaked in water for any great length of time. Carrots, celery, and radishes are sometimes soaked in water in order to produce fancy curls, sticks, and fan shapes for relish dishes, but this procedure is not recommended.

Carbohydrates. Plants are composed of 60 to 90% carbohydrates. For the detailed classification and nutritional aspects of these organic foodstuffs, the reader is referred to the section on CARBOHYDRATES.

Monosaccharides (glucose, fructose, galactose) and disaccharides (sucrose, lactose, and maltose) are crystalline, water-soluble, sweet compounds, which are used for sweetening foods. They are found in fruits, honey, milk, maple syrup, sugarcane, and sugar beets, and are digestible without cooking.

The polysaccharides (starches, dextrins, and cellulose) are noncrystalline, and have little taste. The polysaccharide, starch, is used extensively as a thickening agent. Cereal grains are composed mainly of starch, but unlike the sugars, starch is more digestible when cooked. During the cooking process, the starch granules swell and become a soft paste. This is called gelatinization. A starch mixture starts to thicken at 165° to 190°F (73.9° to 87.8°C), but complete gelatinization does not occur until the temperature approaches the boiling point. When using starch for thickening, it is important to remember a few basic rules. Starch added to a hot liquid will form lumps, which can be removed by putting through a sieve or by whirling in the blender. It is better, however, to mix the starch with a cold liquid or fat before adding to the hot liquid. Also, it is important that there be sufficient liquid and heat to obtain the maximum thickening from the starch, otherwise only partial gelatinization occurs.

Starches also change when exposed to dry heat. This process is known as dextrinization. When these dextrins are dissolved in water they have a sweet taste. Slow toasting of cereals will change a portion of the starch to dextrin, and when vegetables are browned slightly they will have the same distinctive flavor. This effect can also be observed in the crusts of baked goods, or when flour is browned when making gravy.

The most important carbohydrates found in the diet are, of course, the cereal grains. Vegetables contain starch, but the vast majority of them are not considered as primary carbohydrate sources. (Also see BREADS AND BAKING; and CEREAL GRAINS.)

Fats And Emulsions. A fat consists of one molecule of glycerol and three molecules of fatty acids. Technically, they can be called *triglycerides*. Fats and oils are the same substance, but a fat is solid at room temperature whereas an oil is a liquid.

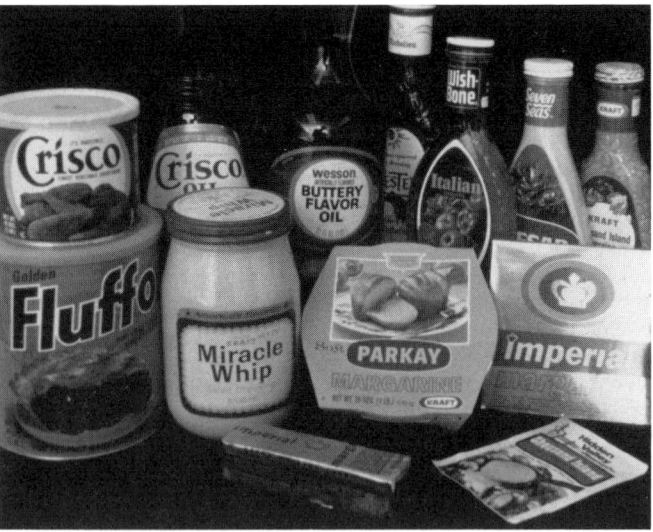

Fig. F-47. There is a wide variety of fats and emulsions on the market. (Courtesy, American Soybean Assoc., St. Louis, Mo.)

Fats and oils have many uses in food preparation. They add flavor and nutritive value to the foods; they prevent foods from sticking to pans; they tenderize batters and doughs; they hold in air which is incorporated when beating a mixture; and they form emulsions in such foods as mayonnaise and Hollandaise sauce.

The choice of fats and/or oils is a personal one, for each cook and each family has its favorites. Whatever fats are used, care should be taken to keep them fresh and to prevent rancidity. The best method is to keep them cold, and exclude light and air. For the same reason, foods that have a high fat content should also be refrigerated; this includes whole cereal products, nuts, fat-rich biscuits and crackers.

There are two methods of frying foods in fat. One is by using a shallow pan with a small amount of fat; the other is by using a large kettle filled with the heated fat, into which the food to be cooked is dropped. It is easy to control the temperature in the deep pan by using a thermometer, but the shallow pan must be temperature controlled to prevent

smoking of the fat. Allowing the fat or oil to smoke will cause deterioration of the oil.

If the fat is not allowed to overheat, it can be used successfully several times. When cooking in deep fat, the temperature of the fat is important. At too low a temperature, the food will absorb too much fat; at too high a temperature, not only will the oil smoke, but the food will be browned on the outside before the inside has had a chance to cook. Thus, it is very important to follow the recommended temperature when frying foods.

An emulsion can be defined as a liquid dispersed in another liquid, without either liquid being dissolved in the other. Most emulsions contain an oil and a liquid, such as water or vinegar. Some emulsions are more permanent than others. For instance, a French dressing is a mixture of oil and vinegar, plus seasonings. When shaken together, an emulsion is formed, but on standing the oil particles reunite; thus, this is a temporary emulsion. Mayonnaise, on the other hand, is also a mixture of oil and vinegar, but it contains egg, which is an emulsifying agent. An emulsifying agent prevents the oil from reuniting. Other common emulsifying agents are: casein, gelatin, mustard, paprika, pectin, and starch.

The most important single factor in producing a stable permanent emulsion is to mix the ingredients together very slowly.

Emulsions can be broken by freezing, by storing at too high temperatures, by agitation, or by storing in an open container.

(Also see FATS AND OTHER LIPIDS.)

Proteins. Protein, *per se*, is covered under the section entitled PROTEIN; hence, the reader is referred thereto for information on proteins other than cooking. In this section, the basic rules for cooking protein foods—meat, fish, poultry, eggs, milk, and cheese—will be covered.

• **Preparing and cooking meat**—The lean part of meat consists of bundles of muscle fibers held together with connective tissue. When the fibers and the bundles are small with minimum connective tissue, the meat is tender. This is usually found in the muscles that are not used to any extent by the animal, which also explains why younger animals produce more tender meat than older animals.

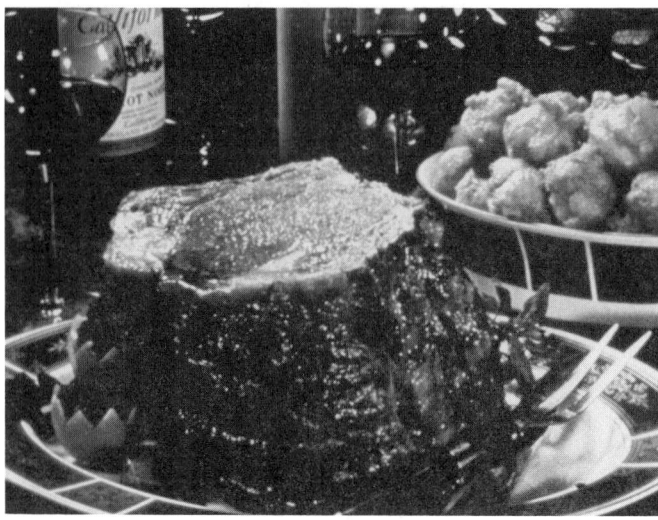

Fig. F-48. Standing rib roast. (Courtesy, USDA)

Tender cuts can be broiled, but the less tender cuts must be stewed or braised. Regardless of the method of cookery, it is a well-known fact that either cooking at too high temperature or overcooking will make the meat tougher, even the more tender cuts.

(Also see MEAT[S], section headed "Meat Cooking.")

• **Preparing and cooking fish (finfish or shellfish)**—Fish is a highly perishable and very delicate product. It cannot be stored long; thus, the fresher the better. It is best when caught and cooked the same day, which illustrates the urgent need to cook it as soon as possible (within 2 days). If it is necessary to hold fish, it should be frozen or canned.

Fish is a tender product which can be cooked by either dry or moist heat methods. Because fish is bland in flavor, the dry-heat method is preferred as it tends to concentrate the flavor. Large fish are baked whole, but filets and steaks can be breaded and either fried or baked. Fish cooked by moist heat is usually served with a sauce to give it added flavor.

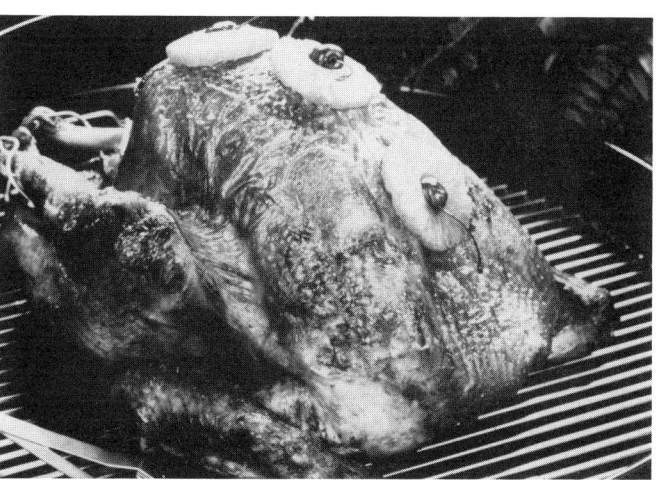

Fig. F-50. Stuffed barbecued turkey. (Courtesy, Cryovac Division, W. R. Grace & Co.)

The same rules that applied to meat cookery, apply also to poultry. These are:

1. Intense heat will toughen the protein and cause considerable shrinkage and loss of juice.

2. The more tender, younger birds can be cooked by dry heat methods.

3. The less tender birds should be cooked by moist heat.

4. When poultry is to be creamed, used in soups, or used in casseroles, there is no advantage to roasting the bird over moist-heat cooking—a point which casserole lovers should keep in mind. In fact, stewed older chickens are superior in flavor to younger birds.

(Also see POULTRY.)

• **Preparing and cooking eggs**—Eggs are the most versatile protein product in the diet, and certainly the cheapest source of high-quality protein. Not only are eggs cooked and eaten as eggs, but they adapt to a multitude of other uses in various dishes; among them, the following:

1. As an emulsifying agent in mayonnaise and ice cream.

2. As a thickening agent in custard sauces.

3. As a gel in baked custards.

4. As a coating agent for fish, pork and veal chops, vegetables, and croquettes, etc.

5. As a leavening in many baked products such as pancakes, muffins, cakes (especially sponge and angel food cakes), cream puffs, and popovers.

6. As a binding agent in meat loaves and croquettes.

7. As a foam for omelets, souffles, meringues, beaten cake frostings, marshmallows, divinity and nougat candy.

8. As a clarifying agent in broths or coffee.

9. As a decorative agent—hard-boiled eggs are used to decorate many buffet dishes, either as slices, or as deviled eggs.

When cooking eggs, the same basic principle for all protein dishes applies. They should be cooked at low to medium temperatures; high temperatures produce a hard, leathery product. The whites coagulate at a lower temperature than the yolks—a point to remember when making custard sauces.

Egg white cookery requires a little skill; hence, it is important to know some of the reasons behind the production of perfect, and other than perfect, results. Meringues can *weep*; souffles will flop; popovers won't pop; and cream puffs won't puff unless certain basic rules are followed.

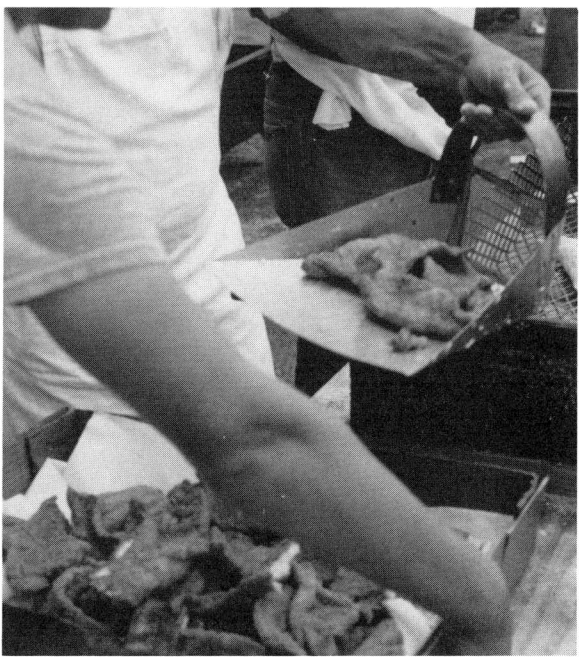

Fig. F-49. Catfish deep-fat fried to a golden brown. (Courtesy, Mississippi Cooperative Extension Service, MSU, USDA)

It is important to cook fish completely, which means it should flake with a fork. Raw fish is not only unpalatable, but it may be unsafe (fish from some localities may be a source of tapeworm). Also, it is important (1) not to cook it at too high a temperature, (2) not to overcook it, and (3) to handle it gently in order to retain its form.

(Also see FISH AND SEAFOOD[S].)

• **Preparing and cooking poultry**—Poultry is probably the most widely used protein food in the world, with few, if any, social or religious restrictions attached to it.

Hard boiled eggs are perhaps one of the most difficult procedures that a novice cook has to learn in order to avoid *green* eggs. A layer of green around the yolk is the result of the hydrogen sulfide in the white combining with the iron in the yolk. What should you do? Should you use cold or hot water; put the pan lid on or take it off; leave the pan on the element or take it off? Whichever method is used, the single most important factor is not to overcook or overheat the eggs. They can be put in either cold or hot water. They can be put on a high heat or a medium heat, as long as they are cooked at a temperature just below the boiling point. The lid can be on or off. If the pan is left on the hot element, it is best not to put the lid on. If the pan is removed from the element, the lid should be put on. The eggs should not stand in the hot water longer than 15 minutes, then they should be chilled under running cold water. The temperature and size of the eggs are both involved, but with a little experimentation, beautiful hard boiled eggs can be produced.

Fried eggs should be fried at a low temperature so that they will not become tough and overly greasy. Here again, a little experience is all that is needed.

Foamy omelets are trickier to produce than souffles. The whites and yolks are beaten separately. The liquid and other ingredients are added to the yolk. Then the yolk mixture is gently folded into the whites. This is poured into a greased pan, which should be hot enough to start coagulation of the egg, but not hot enough to make them tough or to brown them. The top of the omelet can be cooked by one of several methods:

1. Cover the pan, but do not let the top of the omelet touch the lid.

2. When the bottom is partially cooked, the pan can be popped into a 325°F (*180°C*) oven.

3. When the bottom is partially cooked, the pan can be put under the broiler, but with extreme caution, as it is easy to make the top tough, and the whole product collapse.

4. The foamy omelet can be cooked completely in a 325°F (*180°C*) oven for the whole time.

Souffles are easier to produce than foamy omelets, because of the base of white sauce. They are baked for the entire time in the oven, and, like baked custards, the baking dish should be set in a pan of hot water to prevent overheating and a poor product.

Custards consist only of eggs, milk, sugar and flavoring. There is no starch. A baked custard should be firm enough to stand if it is unmolded. When baking custard, it is important to put the custard cups into a pan and add water to prevent overcooking. Too hot an oven produces bubbles of air and an undesirable texture.

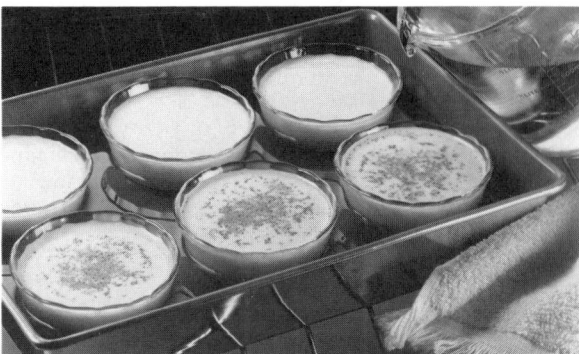

Fig. F-51. Baked custard—a dessert for all ages. (Courtesy, American Egg Board, Park Ridge, Ill.)

Custard sauce should be of the consistency of thick cream, and should be cooked in a double boiler to prevent overcooking and scorching on the bottom of the pan.

Meringues are impressive and look difficult, but they only require some basic knowledge and a little experimentation. Here are some cogent facts:

1. Thin egg whites (usually from older eggs) produce more volume, but the meringue is less stable.

2. Egg whites at room temperature produce more volume, but here again the meringue is less stable.

3. Bowls with small rounded bottoms and straight sides give better meringues when using an electric mixer, because the beater can pick up more of the mass, but bowls with sloping sides are better when using a wire egg beater.

4. Underbeating and overbeating both produce meringues that will break down and *weep*. Meringues should be beaten until just the tips of the peaks fall over and the top shines like satin.

5. Adding any oil (egg yolk, milk, oil, cream, etc.) will prevent the formation of a perfect meringue.

6. Adding salt will inhibit a good meringue.

7. Adding ¼ tsp (*1.25 ml*) cream of tarter aids in the stability of the meringue.

8. Adding sugar to egg whites prolongs the time it requires to whip up a good meringue, but once the sugar is added, it is almost impossible to overbeat it.

Soft meringues for pie toppings require three things to avoid either a tough meringue, or one that *weeps* (little beads of moisture on top).

1. The meringue should be properly beaten.

2. The meringue must be placed on a *hot* pie and spread to the edges.

3. The meringue requires the correct baking temperature—a hot oven of 400°F (*222°C*) requires only 4 to 5 minutes; a slower oven of 375°F (*209°C*) requires 10 minutes, and an oven of 350°F (*195°C*) requires 15 minutes. Above all, the meringue should not be overcooked because it will result in a tough meringue, and it will *weep*.

Hard meringues which are used for desserts, along with fruits, ice cream, sauces, etc., are a different story. This type of meringue is baked in a very slow oven at about 250°F (*139°C*); and, after the heat is turned off, it is left in the oven to dry until it is cool. If this type of meringue is gummy, it is the result of one or more of the following: too much sugar, underbaking, too rapid baking, or baking too long.

(Also see EGG[S].)

• **Using milk in cookery**—Milk, like water, has no adequate substitute. In some cases, the two can be used interchangeably in a recipe. Nutritionally, milk can substitute for water, but water could never substitute for milk. Most milk is consumed in the fluid state, but it adapts to a myriad of uses in food preparation. Because of its excellent nutritive value, it should be included in the diet in some form. Many adults drift away from their childhood habit of drinking a glass of milk with each meal, but, fortunately, milk can be added to many dishes and can substitute for water in some recipes. Here are a few of the many uses of milk and milk products (e.g., canned evaporated and condensed milk, and dry milk solids)—

1. **For beverages.** Milk may be used in malted milk shakes, eggnogs, and hot or cold drinks.

2. **For sauces.** Milk may be included in soups, gravies, white sauce, cream sauces, or dessert sauces.

3. **For entrees.** Milk can be added to meat loaf, casseroles, croquettes, pasta dishes, curry dishes, etc.

4. **For many bakery products.** Milk may be used as a

moistening agent instead of water in many bakery products.

5. **For desserts.** Milk may be used in making many desserts, such as custard, junket, bread pudding, rice pudding, parfaits, cornstarch puddings, and ice creams.

Because milk is a high-protein food, the same principles apply when cooking with milk as with other high-protein foods. Both flavor and texture are adversely affected by too high or too prolonged cooking temperatures.

Milk tends to form a coating on the bottom of the pan and scorches easily, so it is best to heat it either in a double boiler or over a very low heat while stirring constantly. Scalding milk produces a scum, which is a combination of coagulated albumin, some salts, and fat globules. The scum can be prevented by keeping a lid on, or by stirring rapidly.

Curdling is the result of the formation of casein salts (such as casein chloride and casein lactate). Some milk and egg mixtures will curdle if cooked too long. To regain a smooth consistency, cool the mixture and beat or whirl in the blender. When an acid is added to milk, it must be done slowly, so as not to cause curdling. In addition, thickening the mixture helps to prevent curdling.

The following products can be whipped and used for toppings on desserts: thick cream with a minimum of 30% fat, chilled canned evaporated milk, and chilled nonfat dry milk powder. In whipping any of these, the first requisites are a chilled bowl and whipper and icy cold whipping cream or milk. It is important not to overwhip cream as this is the first step in producing butter. Adding sugar before whipping the cream decreases the volume and stiffness and increases the time required to whip it. Add the sugar after the cream is whipped. Whipped cream will be most stable if (1) the cream is whipped as stiff as possible without forming butter, (2) the cream is of optimum (36%) fat, and (3) the cream is held at a cold temperature.

Chilled evaporated milk can be whipped for a topping, but it is not very stable. Stability can be increased by adding a small amount (1 Tbsp/cup of milk) of lemon juice. If the topping is not completely used and it breaks down before the next serving, it can be rewhipped. Nonfat dry milk can also be whipped, but here again it is quite unstable. The stability can be increased by adding a little lemon juice. The evaporated- and dry milk-whipped toppings are best if used immediately.

(Also see MILK AND MILK PRODUCTS.)

• **Using cheese in cookery**—Cheese and nuts are the only two foods that can be found in every course of the meal. The popularity of cheese has been growing in the United States as indicated by the consumption figures.

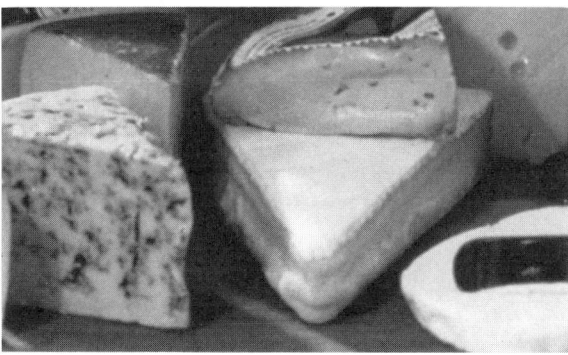

Fig. F-52. Cheese, one of the most versatile foods in the world. (Courtesy, National Film Board of Canada)

Cheese is a concentrated, high fat, high protein food and, therefore, should be cooked at a lower temperature. A high temperature will make the cheese tough and rubbery. When it is necessary to melt cheese, grating will reduce the time required to melt it and, consequently, will reduce the likelihood of overcooking it. Because cheese is so concentrated, it is best when mixed into other foods; indeed, many dishes are improved with a little added cheese.

(Also see MILK AND MILK PRODUCTS, section headed "Cheese.")

Minerals. Some food processing results in loss of minerals. But mineral losses in the kitchen occur mostly by allowing foods to soak in water and then discarding the water. Otherwise, minerals are not lost to any appreciable extent during ordinary cooking methods.

(Also see MINERAL[S].)

Vitamins. The loss of vitamins in food preparation is of prime concern to the nutritionist. If the vitamins present in the raw food are lost during preparation and cooking, it makes it that much more difficult to secure the daily recommended vitamins and minerals.

The fat-soluble vitamins, A, D, E, and K, are not easily lost by ordinary cooking methods. On the other hand, the water-soluble vitamins (B complex and C) are dissolved easily in cooking water, and a portion may be destroyed by heating—thus cooking in as little water as possible, and cooking as short a time as possible is, in general, the best procedure.

(Also see VITAMIN[S], section headed "Vitamin Content of Foods.")

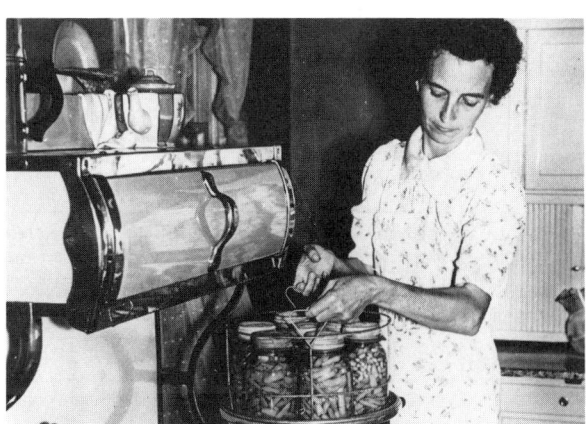

Fig. F-53. Vitamin B-complex and vitamin C losses in processing may be minimized by cooking with as little water as possible and cooking as short a time as possible. (Courtesy, The Bettmann Archive, Inc., New York, N.Y.)

Enzymes. *An enzyme may be defined as a complex protein, produced by living cells, which acts as an organic catalyst to accelerate the rate of a chemical reaction in a wide range of processes, without being used in the action.*

Enzymes are present in all living plant and animal material. They are usually classified into two major categories: (1) those which have a basic reaction which involves the addition of water and the breakdown of larger compounds to smaller, called hydrolytic enzymes; and (2) those which cause a breakdown of a molecule without the addition of water or oxygen. Enzymes are activated by normal physiological processes, such as the destruction of the cell by such processes as grinding or crushing. Enzymes can be inactivated by heat.

Table F-19 lists some of the enzymes pertinent to foods and their preparation, and summarizes their action.

TABLE F-19
ENZYMES PERTINENT TO FOODS AND THEIR PREPARATION

Enzyme	Action
Amylase or diastase	A starch splitting enzyme which is present in flour.
Bromelin	A proteolytic enzyme found in fresh pineapple. Because it will split the protein, gelatin, it prevents the formation of a gel. Pineapple must be cooked or canned for it to be used in gelatin recipes. Bromelin will dissolve or degrade collagen and elastin, action which occurs in tenderizing meat.
Ficin	Obtained from figs. This enzyme is a proteolytic one which is used for tenderizing meat.
Fish enzymes	These enzymes cause rapid spoilage of fish, unless fish are kept icy cold. Fish should not be held longer than 2 days.
Fruit enzymes	Certain fruits turn brown when peeled and cut, and thus exposed to the air. This reaction is halted when the fruit is heated or when acid is present to inactivate the enzyme.
Invertase	This enzyme is used in the production of creamy fondants, or the soft centers in chocolates. It is added to the fondant when it is melted for encasing in a chocolate coating. During storage as some of the sucrose is changed to a liquid, this liquid will dissolve more sucrose and thus produce a soft center. The pH, cooking time, sugar, syrup, water content, and casting temperature all have to be carefully controlled.
Lipase	An enzyme found in fats and oils which can break a fat down into free fatty acids and glycerol. Also, lipases are found in the fat of meat, fish, eggs, milk, and cereals.
Meat enzymes	Meat contains over 50 different enzymes. This is to be expected because of its complex structure and activity.
Milk enzymes	Milk contains a number of enzymes including lipases, phosphatases, xanthine oxidase, amylase, and protease. The enzymes are killed during the pasteurization process.
Papain	A proteolytic enzyme found in the papaya leaf, that is used for meat tenderizing.
Pectinesterase	This enzyme is widely distributed in plant tissue. Many studies have been done without any solution to the question of why or how fruit changes in texture as it ripens.
Phosphatase	Phosphatase, one of the enzymes found in milk, is destroyed by pasteurization; hence, a test for this enzyme has been common practice for 30 years as a means of quality control.
Rennin	Used to coagulate the casein of milk in the production of rennet desserts and cheeses.
Vegetable enzymes	Vegetables contain enzymes which will bring about undesirable chemical changes in canned or frozen products, unless destroyed by heat. Also, some vegetables, such as eggplant, will turn brown when cut and exposed to the air—the same reaction as in fruits.
Wheat enzymes	The enzymes present in wheat (amylases, lipases, oxidases, proteinases) are only a small portion of the total flour protein, but they may influence flour properties. For instance, the lipase present accounts for the rancidity of whole grain flours, and the reason that these flours should be refrigerated.
Yeast enzymes	The production of carbon dioxide in yeast breads is catalyzed by many different enzymes found in the yeast.

Color. Food color means to a cook what paint means to an artist. Without the bright colors of vegetables and fruits, our meals would be a series of brown and white pictures. Synthetic colors are covered in the section on "Coloring of Food"; this section pertains to natural colors.

Sometimes the natural colors of foods are modified with vegetable coloring materials which are obtained from tree bark, fruits, leaves, blossoms, roots, and mosses. Beets contain betanin, a food coloring which is used to intensify the color of tomato soup and tomato sauce. A red food color is also used to intensify the dark brown of chocolate products. Some of the other coloring materials that are used include: alkanet, annatto, caramel, carotene, chlorophyll, saffron, and turmeric. Saffron is popular for coloring bakery products and commercially prepared poultry pies. It imparts a good rich pale yellow color, which looks as though the product contains eggs and butter. Caramel is used to give a richer color to meat gravies, cola, and root beer drinks. The added colors are listed on the container, along with the other ingredients.

Some of the common food colors and the changes that may occur during storage, preparation, and cooking are given in Table F-20.

(Also see COLORING OF FOOD.)

Flavor. If the flavor is not desirable, the food will be left on the platter; and, no matter how important nutritionally, it cannot contribute to the diet unless consumed.

It is noteworthy that it took 40 scientists working since 1920 to segregate out the 80 chemical components of apple flavor. Cocoa has been found to have over 125 basic chemical elements, and coffee has nearly 200.

The food tastes experienced by the eating of foods, is a complex combination of taste, smell, texture, and temperature. Basically, there are just four taste sensations: sweet, salt, sour, and bitter.

Flavor research technology has been rapidly changing with the development of very sensitive instruments capable of identifying ingredients, found in very small amounts, in very complex mixtures. Some of these instruments include: gas-liquid chromatography, infrared spectroscopy, mass spectrometry, and nuclear magnetic resonance.

Texture. Texture is not much easier to evaluate than flavor. Although everyone has a preconceived idea, from past experience, just what the texture of each food should be, it is hard to say just how much deviation from this will be acceptable.

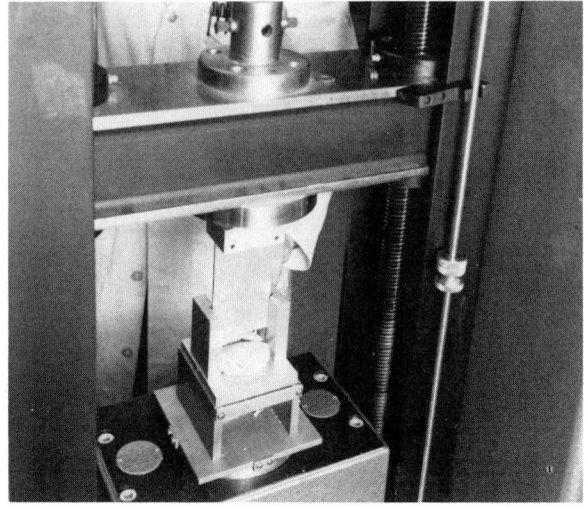

Fig. F-54. This machine simulates teeth biting a bread sample, and thus measures the tenderness of the sample. (Courtesy, Michigan State University)

TABLE F-20
NATURAL COLORS IN FOODS

Food	Color Problems and Pointers
Chocolate	The gloss on chocolate is rapidly lost and changed to a dull, mottled gray called *bloom,* by heat and moisture. This bloom is likely caused by the melting of some of the chocolate and recrystallization on the surface. Although the proper temperature and timing, and the use of stabilizers during production will help retard this development, chocolates are best when stored at a temperature between 60°–70°F (*16°–21°C*) and a relative humidity between 50-65%.
Eggs	The vitamin A content of yolks cannot be predicted by the color of the yolk. Deep-colored yolks are high in vitamin A, however, if the chicken is given a vitamin A supplement because it does not have access to green or yellow feeds, the yolk may be pale in color, yet be high in vitamin A. The predominant yellow pigment in the yolk is xanthophyll, which is not converted to vitamin A in the body.
Fruit	Fruits and vegetables contain the same color pigments. The common ones found in fruits are listed as follows:

Color(s)	Pigment(s)	Solubility	Acid, Alkaline, or Other Reactions
Yellow and orange	*Carotenoid*	Insoluble	Not affected by acid or alkali.
Red, or purple, or blue	*Flavonoids:* Anthocyanins	Very soluble	Acid intensifies the colors. They turn blue or purple in alkaline solutions.
Light or colorless	Flavonols		

Not all colors play the rules of the game. Pineapple juice changes red or purple fruit to blue regardless of acidity. Orange juice is best omitted with red or blue fruits, as it often changes them to brown.

Food	Color Problems and Pointers
Meat	When first cut, meat appears purplish red due to the reduced form of myoglobin. As it combines with oxygen the myoglobin becomes oxymyoglobin, a bright red color. But on further standing, it oxidizes to metomyoglobin, a brownish color. When cooking, the color of the interior of meat changes from bright red, or pink to grayish pink, and finally to grayish brown. During curing, the nitrite reacts with the myoglobin, the red pigment of meat, and the pigment changes to the characteristic pink color of cured meats.
Milk	The white color of milk is the result of the reflection of light by the colloid casein and calcium phosphate dispersed throughout. Also, the two yellow pigments, carotene and riboflavin, impart the creamy color to milk. The carotene is fat soluble and is found in cream and butter. Riboflavin is a greenish-yellow fluorescent color quite easily detected in the whey of milk.
Vegetables	The bright colors of vegetables are a great asset when planning a meal. Without them it would be difficult to make attractive dishes. The vegetable pigments are given in the following summary:

Color(s)	Pigment(s)	Solubility	Acid, Alkaline or Other Reactions
Green	*Chlorophyll*	Most insoluble	During cooking, acid changes chlorophyll to pheophytin, which is a dull olive-green color. If baking soda is added to make it alkaline, the chlorophyll changes to chlorophyllin which is bright green in color.
Yellow and orange	*Carotenoids:* Carotene Xanthophyll	Insoluble	Acid, alkali, and heat have little effect on the carotenoids.
Red	Lycopene		Red of tomato.
Red, or purple, or blue	*Flavonoids:* Anthocyanins	Water soluble	Flavonoids are red in acid and change to purple, then to blue, as the acid changes to alkaline.
White	Flavonols		

There are some mechanical devices for measuring volume, crumb firmness, tenderness of meat, and viscosity of syrups and sauces, but usually, when and if necessary, textures are judged by a panel of experts.

Bacteria. In addition to the many chemical and physical aspects of foods that have been covered in this section, there are the bacteriological reactions. Some are desirable, such as the action of yeast in leavening, and in beers and wines; mold in making cheese; acetic acid bacteria in vinegar; and *acidophilus* in yogurt. But others are undesirable and can cause great discomfort and even death; included in the latter group are *Staphylococcus, Streptococcus, Salmonella,* and the dreaded, *Clostridium botulinum.* Undesirable bacteria can be controlled by—

1. Sanitary food handling.

2. Holding food at refrigerator temperatures until ready to cook.

3. Cooking thoroughly to the center of the product.

4. Refrigerating immediately after the meal is finished.

5. Canning meats and vegetables under pressure, and cooking for 20 minutes any home-canned foods where the method of canning is unknown.

(Also see BACTERIA IN FOOD.)

COOKING. The history of cooking, as it evolved through the ages, like many other things, is not well documented. Archeological finds indicate that food was likely first cooked by hanging it over the open fire; later, food was cooked by rolling it in wet leaves and steaming, or by using hot rocks, or shells. No doubt, the introduction of pottery in the Neolithic Period revolutionized cooking techniques. During this period, the nomads began to settle in little communities, domesticate livestock, and farm the land—civilization was settling down.

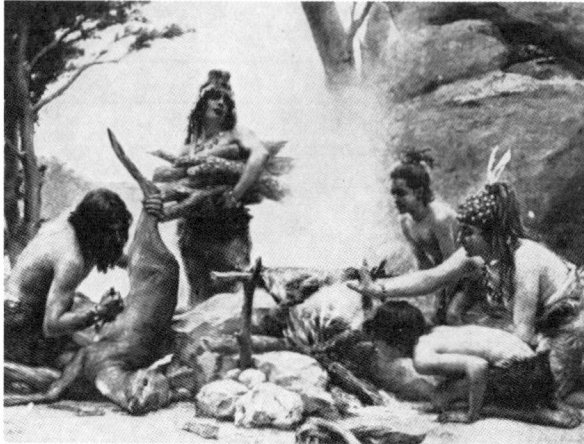

Fig. F-55. A prehistoric family preparing a meal on the caveman's outdoor grill. (Painting by Paul Jamin. Courtesy, The Bettmann Archive, Inc., New York, N.Y.)

Reasons for Cooking. Cooking is the art and the science of applying heat or microwaves to food in order to make it more nutritious, palatable, and flavorful. Today, some people recommend that all foods be consumed raw. Although most raw foods are not harmful, there are several reasons to cook them. There is no question that raw fruits and vegetables are good—and good for you, but some of them are easier to eat and more digestible when cooked. Therefore, foods are cooked for the following reasons:

1. To make available the maximum nutritive value.
2. To improve the digestibility.
3. To increase the palatability or eating quality.
4. To develop the flavor, or to add to the flavor.
5. To destroy any harmful ingredients.

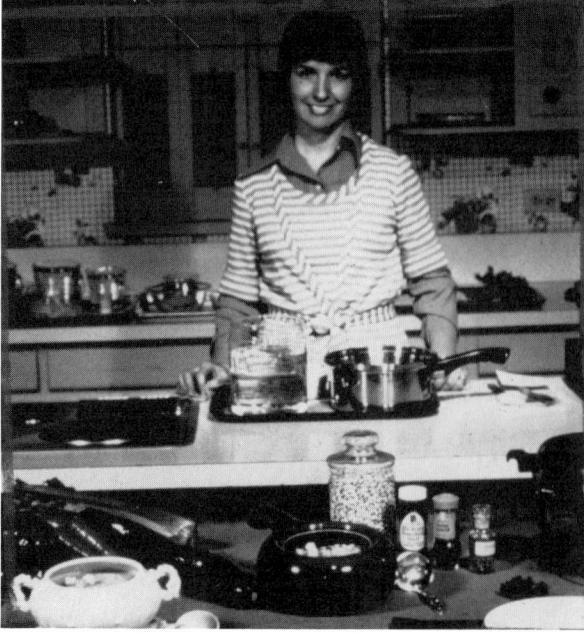

Fig. F-56. Cooking the modern way. (Courtesy, Louisiana Cooperative Extension Service, Louisiana State University, Baton Rouge)

Methods and Media of Cooking. *Cooking may be defined as the application of a force (heat or microwaves) to a substance which results in a higher atomic and molecular activity.* Thus, the temperature of a substance is parallel to the agitation and motility of its atoms and molecules. The higher the temperature, the faster the atoms and molecules bombard each other. It follows that the freezing and boiling points of a substance are related to its molecular structure.

Freezing, melting, evaporation, and condensation are physical changes rather than temperature changes, even though heat brings about the change. For instance, the temperature of melting ice and the water it forms are both 32°F (0°C).

Until the advent of the magnetron tube, which changes electricity into microwaves, the only method of cooking was heat; and, until about 100 years ago, when electricity was developed, this meant by a fire.

Heat is transmitted by means of conduction, convection and radiation. Most cooking methods are a combination of these methods. Heat always travels from the hotter substance to the cooler substance.

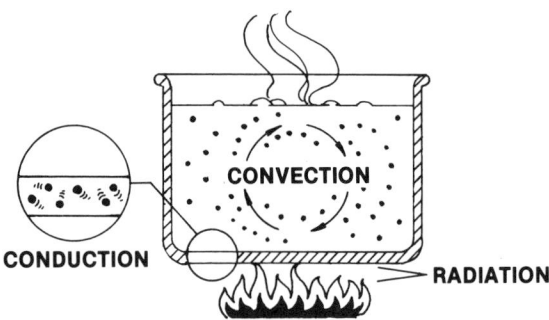

Fig. F-57. A schematic drawing of the three methods of cooking—conduction, convection, and radiation.

Conduction involves the heating of a body (the pan) by the transfer of heat from the element to the bottom of the pan, and within the pan from molecule to molecule.

Convection occurs only in such materials as gases and liquids, where the molecules can move freely from one area to another. The material closest to the heat will warm first, and become less dense.

Radiation involves waves of energy that travel rapidly through space, and heat the surface they strike; they do not penetrate the substance. The rest of the inside of the object is heated by conduction.

Microwave cooking has been available since the 1950s, but, like the electric typewriter, the microwave oven took 20 years to become a common item on the market.

The magnetron tube is a vacuum tube which can convert electricity into electromagnetic energy radiation. The microwaves travel in straight lines.

The media and the various cooking methods are listed below:

Medium	Methods of Cooking
Air	Baking, broiling, roasting.
Water	Boiling, simmering, stewing.
Steam	Steamer, pressure cooker, wrapping in foil.
Fat	Sauteeing, pan and deep-fat frying
Combinations	Braising, fricasseeing, pot roasting

MEALTIME. At least one meal of the day should be a time when all members of the family can gather together around the dinner table and have a good visit.

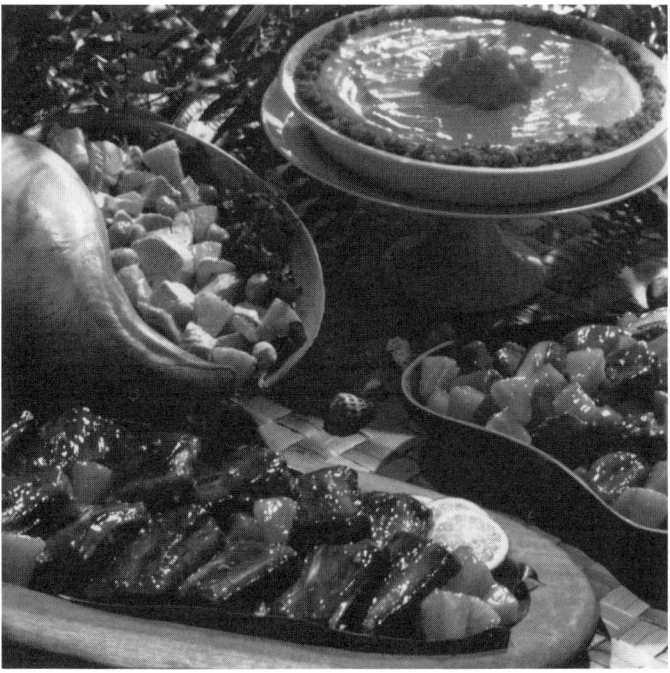

Fig. F-58. Make attractive table settings an every meal occurence. (Courtesy, Castle & Cooke, Inc., San Francisco, Calif.)

FOOD COMPOSITIONS

Food analyses, such as those shown in Table F-21 Food Compositions, have long provided the bases used by human nutritionists and food processors in the evaluation of foods. Additionally, most of the procedures used by dietitians and home economists in planning meals and modified diets are based on food compositions. Also, and most importantly, consumers may refer directly to Table F-21 Food Compositions to obtain information for selecting foods most suitable for their preferences and health needs.

The authors wish to express their gratitude to all those who provided data for Table F-21 Food Compositions, especially Robin Spencer Palmisano, who at the time was Systems Dietitian, University Hospitals, Ohio State University Hospital Nutrient Data Base Catalogue, The Ohio State University, Columbus, Ohio (presently a lawyer and a member of the firm of McGlinchey, Stafford, Cellini & Lang, New Orleans, Louisiana); and Dr. Harold B. Houser, M.D. and Ms. Grace J. Petot, Division of Nutrition, Highland View Hospital, and the Department of Biometry and Nutrition, School of Medicine, Case Western Reserve University, Cleveland, Ohio. We are especially indebted to Robin Spencer Palmisano for her untiring and dedicated effort in the preparation of this table; no one could have done more.

To facilitate quick and easy use, Table F-21 Food Compositions is divided into the following categories:

Baby Foods
Bakery Products
Beverages
Cereals & Flours
Desserts & Sweets
Eggs & Substitutes
Entrees
Fats & Oils
Fish & Seafoods
Flavorings & Seasonings
Food Supplements
Fruits
Gravies & Sauces
Juices
Legumes & Products
Meats
Milk & Products
Nuts & Seeds
Pickles and Relishes
Salads
Salad Dressings
Snack Foods
Soups & Chowders
Vegetables

Where foods fit into more than one category, they are either cross-referenced or listed in more than one category.

Values for each food are given for both (1) approximate serving size, and (2) 100 grams.

With the exception of the footnoted values, the data in this table were supplied by the Ohio State University Hospital Nutrient Data Base Catalogue, Columbus, Ohio. The source of each of the footnoted foods is indicated by the appropriate prefix number from among the following:

[1]Data from the HVH-CWRU Nutrient Data Base developed by the Division of Nutrition, Highland View Hospital, and the Department of Biometry and Nutrition, School of Medicine, Case Western Reserve University, Cleveland, Ohio.

[2]Data from *Composition of Foods*, Ag. Hdbk No. 8–5, USDA.

[3]Data from *Food Composition Table For Use In Africa*, FAO, United Nations, 1968.

[4]Data from *Food Composition Table For Use In East Asia*, FAO, United Nations, 1972.

[5]Data from *Food Composition Table For Use In Latin America*, Institute of Nutrition of Central America & Panama, and National Institutes of Health, USA, 1961.

[6]Footnote 6 and added values in parentheses are from reliable literature sources.

NOTE WELL:

1. The Food Data Bank from which Ohio State University initially provided most of the Table F-21 Food Compositions in this book is now the property of Unisoft Systems Associates, Ron Bruce, President, 1340 Dublin Road, Columbus, Ohio 43215; hence, Table F-21 Food Compositions cannot be reproduced without the permission of Unisoft Systems Associates.

2. Trade and brand names are used for information and identification purposes only.

TABLE F-21 FOOD COMPOSITIONS*

Item No.	Food Item Name	Approximate Measure	Weight (g)	Moisture (%)	Food Energy Calories (kcal)	Protein (g)	Fats (g)	Carbohydrates (g)	Fiber (g)	Minerals (Macro) Calcium (mg)	Phosphorus (mg)	Sodium (mg)	Magnesium (mg)	Potassium (mg)
	BAKED PRODUCTS													
1	ARROWROOT COOKIES, w/enriched flour	1 AVG	6	5.6	26.5	.5	.9	4.3	–	1.9	8.0	20.7	1.3	9.4
			100	5.6	442.0	7.6	14.3	71.2	–	32.0	133.0	345.0	22.0	156.0
2	COOKIES, w/enriched flour, w/nutrients	1 AVG	7	5.9	30.3	.8	.9	4.7	.1	7.1	12.5	13.4	3.4	35.1
			100	5.9	433.0	11.8	13.2	67.1	.4	101.0	179.0	192.0	49.0	501.0
3	PRETZELS, w/enriched flour	1 AVG	6	4.0	23.8	.6	.1	4.9	Trace	1.5	6.6	16.1	1.7	8.2
			100	4.0	397.0	10.8	2.0	82.2	.4	25.0	110.0	269.0	28.0	137.0
4	TEETHING BISCUIT, w/enriched flour	1 AVG	11	6.4	43.1	1.2	.5	8.4	.1	28.9	18.0	39.8	3.9	35.5
			100	6.4	392.0	10.7	4.2	76.4	.5	263.0	164.0	362.0	35.0	323.0
5	ZWIEBACK	1 PIECE	7	4.5	29.8	.7	.7	5.2	Trace	1.4	3.9	16.2	1.0	21.4
			100	4.5	426.0	10.1	9.7	74.2	.2	20.0	55.0	232.0	14.0	305.0
	CEREALS													
6	BARLEY, prepared w/whole milk	1 TBLS	14	74.7	15.5	.6	.5	2.3	Trace	32.2	21.0	6.9	4.2	26.9
			100	74.7	111.0	4.6	3.3	16.3	.2	230.0	150.0	49.0	30.0	192.0
7	CEREAL & EGG YOLKS	1 TBLS	14	88.7	7.3	.3	.3	1.0	Trace	3.4	5.6	4.6	.4	4.9
			100	88.7	52.0	1.9	1.8	7.1	.1	24.0	40.0	33.0	3.0	35.0
8	CEREAL, EGG YOLKS, & BACON	1 TBLS	14	85.9	11.1	.4	.7	.9	Trace	3.9	8.4	6.7	.7	4.9
			100	85.9	79.0	2.5	5.0	6.2	.1	28.0	60.0	48.0	5.0	35.0
9	MIXED CEREAL, prepared w/whole milk	1 TBLS	14	74.6	15.8	.7	.5	2.2	Trace	30.8	19.9	6.6	3.8	27.9
			100	74.6	113.0	4.8	3.5	15.9	.2	220.0	142.0	47.0	27.0	199.0
10	OATMEAL, prepared w/whole milk	1 TBLS	14	74.5	16.2	.7	.6	2.1	Trace	30.8	22.4	6.4	4.9	28.6
			100	74.5	116.0	5.0	4.1	15.3	.2	220.0	160.0	46.0	35.0	204.0
11	RICE, prepared w/whole milk	1 TBLS	14	74.6	16.1	.5	.5	2.3	Trace	33.5	24.5	6.4	6.3	26.6
			100	74.6	115.0	3.9	3.6	16.7	.1	239.0	175.0	46.0	45.0	190.0
	DESSERTS													
12	APPLE BETTY, w/vitamin C	1 TBLS	14	80.5	9.8	.1	0	2.7	–	2.2	–	1.3	–	7.4
			100	80.5	70.0	.4	0	19.0	–	16.0	–	9.0	–	53.0
13	CARAMEL PUDDING	1 TBLS	14	80.4	11.1	1.0	.1	2.4	–	7.7	–	3.9	–	8.1
			100	80.4	79.0	1.4	.9	17.0	–	55.0	–	28.0	–	58.0
14	CHOCOLATE CUSTARD PUDDING	1 TBLS	14	79.9	11.8	.3	.2	2.3	Trace	8.5	6.9	3.2	1.4	12.0
			100	79.9	84.0	1.9	1.7	16.1	.2	61.0	49.0	23.0	10.0	86.0
15	COTTAGE CHEESE & PINEAPPLE, w/vitamin C	1 TBLS	14	80.2	10.9	.4	.1	2.2	.1	4.3	5.5	7.1	.6	5.9
			100	80.2	78.0	3.0	.7	15.9	1.0	31.0	39.0	51.0	4.0	42.0
16	FRUIT DESSERT, w/o vitamin C	1 TBLS	14	82.2	8.8	0	0	2.4	0	1.3	1.1	1.8	.7	13.3
			100	82.2	63.0	.3	0	17.2	.3	9.0	8.0	13.0	5.0	95.0
17	PEACH COBBLER, w/vitamin C	1 TBLS	14	81.2	9.4	0	0	2.6	–	.6	.8	1.3	–	7.8
			100	81.2	67.0	.3	0	18.3	–	4.0	6.0	9.0	–	56.0
18	PINEAPPLE PUDDING, w/vitamin C	1 TBLS	14	76.1	12.2	1.0	.1	3.0	.1	4.8	4.2	3.1	1.3	12.6
			100	76.1	87.0	1.4	.4	21.6	.8	34.0	30.0	22.0	9.0	90.0
19	VANILLA CUSTARD PUDDING	1 TBLS	14	79.4	12.5	.2	.3	2.3	–	7.8	6.3	4.1	.7	8.7
			100	79.4	89.0	1.6	2.3	16.2	–	56.0	45.0	29.0	5.0	62.0
	DINNERS													
20	BEEF & EGG NOODLES	1 TBLS	14	88.6	7.4	.3	.2	1.0	Trace	1.3	4.1	4.1	1.0	6.6
			100	88.6	53.0	2.3	1.7	7.0	.3	9.0	29.0	29.0	7.0	47.0
21	BEEF & RICE	1 TBLS	14	81.9	11.5	.7	.4	1.2	Trace	1.5	4.9	50.0	11.2	16.8
			100	81.9	82.0	5.0	2.9	8.8	.3	11.0	35.0	357.0	80.0	120.0
22	BEEF LASAGNA	1 TBLS	14	82.3	10.8	.6	.3	1.4	Trace	2.5	5.6	63.6	1.5	17.1
			100	82.3	77.0	4.2	2.1	10.0	.2	18.0	40.0	454.0	11.0	122.0
23	BEEF STEW	1 TBLS	14	86.9	7.1	.7	.2	.8	Trace	1.3	6.2	48.3	1.5	19.9
			100	86.9	51.0	5.1	1.2	5.5	.3	9.0	44.0	345.0	11.0	142.0
24	CHICKEN & NOODLES	1 TBLS	14	88.7	7.1	.3	.2	1.1	.1	2.4	3.4	2.4	1.3	4.9
			100	88.7	51.0	1.9	1.4	7.5	.6	17.0	24.0	17.0	9.0	35.0
25	CHICKEN CREAM SOUP	1 TBLS	14	87.1	8.1	.4	.2	1.2	Trace	4.9	4.1	2.7	.8	10.9
			100	87.1	58.0	2.5	1.6	8.4	.3	35.0	29.0	19.0	6.0	78.0
26	COTTAGE CHEESE, w/pineapple	1 TBLS	14	72.0	16.2	.9	.3	2.6	.1	9.1	10.2	20.9	1.0	13.3
			100	72.0	116.0	6.3	2.2	18.9	.9	65.0	73.0	149.0	7.0	95.0
27	HAM, w/vegetables	1 TBLS	14	83.6	10.8	.9	.5	.9	Trace	1.4	7.8	3.1	1.3	22.7
			100	83.6	77.0	6.4	3.3	6.1	.2	10.0	56.0	22.0	9.0	162.0
28	LAMB & NOODLES	1 TBLS	14	86.5	9.1	.3	.3	1.2	–	2.5	–	2.5	–	10.8
			100	86.5	65.0	2.3	2.2	8.7	–	18.0	–	18.0	–	77.0
29	MACARONI & CHEESE	1 TBLS	14	86.5	8.5	.4	.3	1.1	Trace	7.1	8.3	10.6	1.0	6.2
			100	86.5	61.0	2.6	2.0	8.2	.1	51.0	59.0	76.0	7.0	44.0
30	MIXED VEGETABLES	1 TBLS	14	90.6	4.6	.1	0	1.1	–	2.4	–	1.3	–	15.7
			100	90.6	33.0	1.0	0	7.9	–	17.0	–	9.0	–	112.0

*(See notes at end of table)

Item No.	Minerals (Micro)			Fat-Soluble Vitamins			Water-Soluble Vitamins								
	Iron	Zinc	Copper	Vitamin A	Vitamin D	Vitamin E (Alpha Tocopherol)	Vitamin C	Thiamin	Riboflavin	Niacin	Pantothenic Acid	Vit. B-6 (Pyridoxine)	Folacin (Folic Acid)	Biotin	Vitamin B-12
	(mg)	(mg)	(mg)	(IU)	(IU)	(mg)	(mg)	(mg)	(mg)	(mg)	(mg)	(mg)	(mcg)	(mcg)	(mcg)
1	.18	.03	–	–	–	–	.33	.03	.03	.34	–	Trace	–	–	Trace
	3.00	.53	–	–	–	–	5.50	.50	.43	5.74	–	.04	–	–	.07
2	.29	.08	–	1.6	–	–	.49	.10	.23	1.12	–	.41	–	–	.32
	4.18	1.10	–	23.0	–	–	7.00	1.46	3.23	15.97	–	.90	–	–	4.59
3	.23	.05	–	.5	–	–	.22	.03	.02	.21	–	.01	–	–	–
	3.77	.78	–	8.0	–	–	3.80	.46	.36	3.56	–	.08	–	–	–
4	.39	.10	–	12.8	–	–	1.00	.03	.06	.48	–	.01	–	–	.01
	3.55	.93	–	116.0	–	–	9.10	.23	.54	4.33	–	.11	–	–	0.7
5	.04	.04	–	4.1	–	–	.37	.02	.02	.09	–	.01	–	–	–
	.60	.54	–	58.0	–	–	5.30	.21	.24	1.32	–	.08	–	–	–
6	1.73	.12	–	14.7	–	–	.15	.07	.08	.84	–	–	1.25	–	13.44
	12.34	.83	–	105.0	–	–	1.10	.48	.58	5.98	–	–	8.90	–	96.00
7	.07	.04	Trace	20.2	–	–	.10	Trace	.01	.01	–	Trace	.46	–	–
	.51	.29	.02	144.0	–	–	.70	.01	.05	.05	–	.02	3.30	–	–
8	.07	.04	Trace	13.2	–	–	.13	Trace	.01	.04	–	.02	.57	–	Trace
	.47	.27	.02	94.0	–	–	.90	.05	.08	.27	–	.11	4.10	–	.01
9	.46	.10	–	14.7	–	–	.17	.06	.08	.81	–	.01	1.57	–	–
	10.43	.71	–	105.0	–	–	1.20	.43	.58	5.78	–	.07	11.20	–	–
10	1.70	.13	–	14.7	–	–	.18	.07	.08	.84	–	.01	1.40	–	–
	12.14	.92	–	105.0	–	–	1.30	.51	.56	5.93	–	.06	10.00	–	–
11	1.71	.09	–	14.7	–	–	.17	.07	.07	.73	–	.02	1.15	–	–
	12.19	.64	–	105.0	–	–	1.20	.47	.50	5.21	–	.11	8.20	–	–
12	.03	–	–	2.2	–	–	3.79	Trace	.01	.01	–	–	.06	–	–
	.20	–	–	16.0	–	–	27.10	.01	.05	.05	–	–	.40	–	–
13	.02	–	–	4.6	–	–	.31	Trace	.01	.01	–	–	.13	–	–
	.16	–	–	33.0	–	–	2.20	.01	.07	.04	–	–	.90	–	–
14	.05	.06	–	6.4	–	–	.21	Trace	.02	.01	–	Trace	.63	–	Trace
	.38	.32	–	46.0	–	–	1.50	.01	.10	.10	–	.01	4.50	–	.01
15	.02	.03	–	2.2	–	–	3.33	Trace	.01	.01	–	Trace	.71	–	.01
	.13	.16	–	16.0	–	–	23.80	.02	.05	.05	–	.01	5.10	–	.07
16	.03	.01	Trace	33.5	–	–	.42	Trace	Trace	.02	–	.01	.49	–	–
	.21	.05	.03	239.0	–	–	3.00	.02	.01	.14	–	.03	3.50	–	–
17	.01	Trace	–	19.9	–	–	2.87	Trace	Trace	.04	–	Trace	.15	–	–
	.10	.03	–	142.0	–	–	20.50	.01	.02	.26	–	.01	1.10	–	–
18	.03	.03	–	5.2	–	–	3.74	.01	.01	.02	–	Trace	.78	–	.01
	.19	.19	–	37.0	–	–	26.70	.04	.05	.12	–	.04	5.60	–	.06
19	.04	.04	.01	5.0	–	–	.11	Trace	.01	.01	.04	Trace	.87	–	–
	.26	.28	.05	36.0	–	–	.60	.01	.08	.04	.26	.02	6.20	–	–
20	.06	.05	Trace	115.2	–	–	.17	.01	.01	.10	.03	.01	.71	–	.01
	.41	.38	.03	823.0	–	–	1.20	.04	.04	.72	.21	.06	5.10	–	.09
21	.10	.13	.01	70.3	–	–	.55	Trace	.01	.19	–	.03	–	–	–
	.69	.92	.05	502.0	–	–	3.90	.02	.07	1.34	–	.14	–	–	–
22	.12	–	–	162.8	–	–	.27	.01	.13	.19	–	.01	–	–	–
	.87	–	–	1163.0	–	–	1.90	.07	.89	1.35	–	.07	–	–	–
23	.10	.12	–	230.9	–	–	.42	Trace	.01	.18	–	.01	–	–	–
	.72	.87	–	1649.0	–	–	3.00	.01	.07	1.31	–	.07	–	–	–
24	.06	.04	.01	125.3	–	–	.17	Trace	Trace	.07	–	Trace	.74	–	–
	.39	.29	.04	895.0	–	–	1.20	.03	.03	.52	–	.03	5.30	–	–
25	.04	.04	–	101.6	–	–	.18	Trace	.01	.05	–	.01	–	–	.01
	.30	.26	–	726.0	–	–	1.30	.01	.04	.38	–	.04	–	–	.06
26	.01	.04	–	10.8	–	–	.20	.01	.02	.02	–	.01	–	–	.03
	.10	.29	–	77.0	–	–	1.40	.04	.14	.11	–	.05	–	–	.23
27	.08	.15	–	36.4	–	–	.27	.02	.01	.16	.06	.01	.91	–	.04
	.59	1.08	–	260.0	–	–	1.90	.11	.09	.16	.40	.10	6.50	–	.28
28	.05	–	–	109.6	–	–	.27	.01	.01	.09	–	–	–	–	–
	.36	–	–	783.0	–	–	1.90	.04	.07	.67	–	–	–	–	–
29	.04	.05	Trace	1.8	–	–	.18	.01	.01	.08	–	Trace	.21	–	Trace
	.30	.32	.02	13.0	–	–	1.30	.06	.06	.55	–	.02	1.50	–	.03
30	.04	–	–	342.2	–	–	.46	Trace	Trace	.06	–	–	.94	–	–
	.31	–	–	2444.0	–	–	3.30	.01	.02	.41	–	–	6.70	–	–

(Continued)

TABLE F-21 *(Continued)*

Item No.	Food Item Name	Approximate Measure	Weight (g)	Moisture (%)	Food Energy Calories (kcal)	Protein (g)	Fats (g)	Carbo-hydrates (g)	Fiber (g)	Calcium (mg)	Phos-phorus (mg)	Sodium (mg)	Mag-nesium (mg)	Potas-sium (mg)
31	SPAGHETTI, TOMATO & MEAT	1 TBLS	14	85.5	8.8	.4	.2	1.4	.1	2.5	5.2	2.8	–	15.1
			100	85.5	63.0	2.5	1.3	10.1	.4	18.0	37.0	20.0	–	108.0
32	TOMATO SOUP	1 TBLS	14	83.4	7.6	.3	0	1.9	Trace	3.4	7.3	41.2	–	42.0
			100	83.4	54.0	1.9	.1	13.5	.2	24.0	52.0	294.0	–	300.0
33	TURKEY & RICE	1 TBLS	14	89.3	6.9	.3	.2	1.0	Trace	3.2	2.4	2.1	–	4.8
			100	89.3	49.0	1.8	1.4	7.2	.2	23.0	17.0	15.0	–	34.0
34	TURKEY, w/vegetables	1 TBLS	14	82.5	12.6	.8	.7	.8	Trace	9.9	8.8	6.0	1.1	15.0
			100	82.5	90.0	5.9	5.0	5.9	.2	71.0	63.0	43.0	8.0	107.0
35	VEAL, w/vegetables	1 TBLS	14	84.3	10.2	.9	.4	.8	Trace	1.5	7.6	3.5	1.3	22.0
			100	84.3	73.0	6.1	3.1	5.8	.2	11.0	54.0	25.0	9.0	157.0
36	VEGETABLES & BEEF	1 TBLS	14	87.9	7.4	.3	.2	1.0	Trace	1.4	6.0	3.4	.8	14.7
			100	87.9	53.0	2.4	1.7	7.4	.2	10.0	43.0	24.0	6.0	105.0
37	VEGETABLES & CHICKEN	1 TBLS	14	88.2	7.0	.3	.2	1.2	Trace	2.0	3.6	1.3	–	3.6
			100	88.2	50.0	1.9	1.1	8.5	.2	14.0	26.0	9.0	–	26.0
38	VEGETABLES & HAM	1 TBLS	14	88.4	7.3	.3	.2	1.0	Trace	1.1	3.6	2.5	1.0	12.9
			100	88.4	52.0	2.4	1.7	7.0	.2	8.0	26.0	18.0	7.0	92.0
39	VEGETABLES & LAMB	1 TBLS	14	88.6	7.1	.3	.2	1.0	Trace	1.8	6.9	1.8	1.0	13.3
			100	88.6	51.0	2.1	1.7	7.1	.2	13.0	49.0	13.0	7.0	95.0
40	VEGETABLES & LIVER	1 TBLS	14	88.9	6.2	.3	.1	1.1	Trace	1.4	5.3	1.8	–	12.5
			100	88.9	44.0	1.8	.6	8.2	.3	10.0	38.0	13.0	–	89.0
41	VEGETABLES & TURKEY	1 TBLS	14	89.0	6.6	.2	.2	1.1	Trace	1.8	2.7	2.4	–	3.5
			100	89.0	47.0	1.7	1.2	7.7	.2	13.0	19.0	17.0	–	25.0
	FRUITS													
42	APPLESAUCE, w/vitamin C	1 TBLS	14	89.5	5.2	0	0	1.4	.1	.7	.8	.3	.4	10.8
			100	89.5	37.0	0	0	10.3	.6	5.0	6.0	2.0	3.0	77.0
43	APRICOTS, w/tapioca & vitamin C	1 TBLS	14	82.1	8.8	0	0	2.4	.1	1.1	1.4	.8	.6	17.5
			100	82.1	63.0	.3	0	17.3	.5	8.0	10.0	6.0	4.0	125.0
44	BANANAS, w/tapioca & vitamin C	1 TBLS	14	81.5	9.4	.1	0	2.5	Trace	1.1	1.3	1.3	1.7	15.1
			100	81.5	67.0	.4	.2	17.8	.2	8.0	9.0	9.0	12.0	108.0
45	GUAVA, w/tapioca & vitamin C	1 TBLS	14	81.2	9.4	0	0	2.6	.1	1.0	.7	.7	.3	10.2
			100	81.2	67.0	.3	0	18.3	1.0	7.0	5.0	2.0	2.0	73.0
46	MANGO, w/tapioca & vitamin C	1 TBLS	14	77.7	11.2	0	0	3.0	Trace	.6	.8	.6	.6	8.3
			100	77.7	80.0	.3	.2	21.6	.2	4.0	6.0	4.0	4.0	59.0
47	PEACHES, w/vitamin C & sugar	1 TBLS	14	80.1	9.9	.1	0	2.6	.1	.7	1.5	.7	.7	21.7
			100	80.1	71.0	.5	.2	18.9	.7	5.0	11.0	5.0	5.0	155.0
48	PEARS, w/vitamin C	1 TBLS	14	87.8	6.0	0	0	1.6	–	1.1	1.7	.3	1.3	16.1
			100	87.8	43.0	.3	.1	11.6	–	8.0	12.0	2.0	9.0	115.0
49	PLUMS, w/tapioca, w/o vitamin C	1 TBLS	14	79.2	10.4	0	0	2.9	–	.8	.8	1.1	.6	11.6
			100	79.2	74.0	.1	0	20.4	–	6.0	6.0	8.0	4.0	83.0
50	PRUNES, w/tapioca, w/o vitamin C	1 TBLS	14	80.1	9.8	.1	0	2.6	Trace	2.1	2.1	.3	1.4	22.7
			100	80.1	70.0	.6	.1	18.7	.3	15.0	15.0	2.0	10.0	162.0
	FRUIT JUICES													
51	APPLE, w/vitamin C	1 OZ	30	88.0	14.1	0	0	3.5	–	1.2	1.5	.9	.9	27.3
			100	88.0	47.0	0	.1	11.7	–	4.0	5.0	3.0	3.0	91.0
52	MIXED FRUIT, w/vitamin C	1 OZ	30	87.9	14.1	0	0	3.5	–	2.4	1.5	1.2	1.5	30.3
			100	87.9	47.0	.1	.1	11.6	–	8.0	5.0	4.0	5.0	101.0
53	ORANGE, w/vitamin C	1 OZ	30	88.5	13.2	.2	.1	3.1	–	3.6	3.3	.3	2.7	55.2
			100	88.5	44.0	.6	.3	10.2	–	12.0	11.0	1.0	9.0	184.0
	MEATS & EGGS													
54	BEEF	1 TBLS	14	79.9	14.8	2.0	.7	0	0	1.1	10.1	9.2	1.3	26.6
			100	79.9	106.8	14.5	4.9	0	0	8.0	72.0	66.0	9.0	190.0
55	CHICKEN	1 TBLS	14	76.0	20.9	2.1	1.3	0	–	7.7	12.6	7.1	1.5	17.1
			100	76.0	149.0	14.7	9.6	0	–	55.0	90.0	51.0	11.0	122.0
56	EGG YOLKS	1 TBLS	14	70.6	28.4	1.4	2.4	.1	0	10.6	40.2	5.5	1.0	10.8
			100	70.6	203.0	10.0	17.3	1.0	0	76.0	287.0	39.0	7.0	77.0
57	HAM	1 TBLS	14	78.5	17.5	2.1	.9	0	–	.7	12.5	9.4	1.5	29.4
			100	78.5	125.0	15.1	6.7	0	–	5.0	89.0	67.0	11.0	210.0
58	LAMB	1 TBLS	14	79.6	15.7	2.1	.7	0	0	1.0	12.7	10.2	1.4	29.5
			100	79.6	112.0	15.2	5.2	0	0	7.0	91.0	73.0	10.0	211.0
59	LIVER	1 TBLS	14	79.3	14.1	2.0	.5	.2	0	.6	28.4	10.4	1.8	31.8
			100	79.3	101.0	14.3	3.8	1.4	0	4.0	203.0	74.0	13.0	227.0
60	LIVER & BACON	1 TBLS	14	77.0	17.2	1.9	.9	.2	0	.8	22.0	42.3	–	26.9
			100	77.0	123.0	13.7	6.6	1.3	0	6.0	157.0	302.0	–	192.0
61	PORK	1 TBLS	14	74.3	18.8	2.6	.8	0	0	1.1	20.2	33.2	–	29.4
			100	74.3	134.0	18.6	6.0	0	0	8.0	144.0	237.0	–	210.0

Item No.	Minerals (Micro)			Fat-Soluble Vitamins			Water-Soluble Vitamins								
	Iron	Zinc	Copper	Vitamin A	Vitamin D	Vitamin E (Alpha Tocopherol)	Vitamin C	Thiamin	Ribo-flavin	Niacin	Panto-thenic Acid	Vit. B-6 (Pyri-doxine)	Folacin (Folic Acid)	Biotin	Vitamin B-12
	(mg)	(mg)	(mg)	(IU)	(IU)	(mg)	(mg)	(mg)	(mg)	(mg)	(mg)	(mg)	(mcg)	(mcg)	(mcg)
31	.08	.06	–	97.0	–	–	.31	.01	.01	.15	.03	.01	–	–	–
	.55	.42	–	693.0	–	–	2.20	.07	.07	1.10	.18	.06	–	–	–
32	.06	–	–	140.0	–	–	.42	.01	.02	.10	–	–	–	–	–
	.40	–	–	1000.0	–	–	3.00	.05	.12	.70	–	–	–	–	–
33	.04	–	–	148.3	–	–	.17	Trace	Trace	.04	–	Trace	.43	–	–
	.29	–	–	1059.0	–	–	1.20	.01	.03	.28	–	.03	3.10	–	–
34	.11	.13	.01	88.6	–	–	.18	Trace	.01	.11	–	.01	1.39	–	.06
	.78	.91	.04	633.0	–	–	1.30	.01	.07	.81	–	.04	9.90	–	.45
35	.13	.15	.01	59.5	–	–	.24	Trace	.01	.22	.04	.01	–	–	.06
	.89	1.10	.10	425.0	–	–	1.70	.02	.08	1.54	.25	.07	–	–	.46
36	.07	.06	.01	198.0	–	–	.21	Trace	Trace	.09	.02	.01	.69	–	.04
	.47	.41	.04	1414.0	–	–	1.50	.03	.03	.66	.13	.06	4.90	–	.26
37	.04	–	–	167.3	–	–	.20	Trace	Trace	.05	.03	.01	.53	–	–
	.30	–	–	1195.0	–	–	1.40	.01	.02	.33	.24	.04	3.80	–	–
38	.03	.03	0	86.1	–	–	.18	.01	Trace	.05	–	Trace	.74	–	–
	.22	.22	.03	615.0	–	–	1.30	.04	.02	.35	–	.03	5.30	–	–
39	.05	.03	Trace	207.6	–	–	.24	Trace	Trace	.08	.02	.01	.50	–	.02
	.34	.22	.03	1483.0	–	–	1.70	.02	.03	.55	.16	.04	3.60	–	.16
40	.25	–	–	550.1	–	–	.25	Trace	.03	.16	–	.01	4.48	–	–
	1.81	–	–	3929.0	–	–	1.80	.02	.23	1.16	–	.10	32.00	–	–
41	.05	.04	Trace	125.4	–	–	.15	–	–	–	.03	Trace	.41	–	–
	.32	.25	.03	896.0	–	–	1.10	–	–	–	.21	.03	2.90	–	–
42	.03	.01	.01	1.3	–	–	5.29	Trace	Trace	.01	.01	Trace	.24	–	–
	.22	.04	.04	9.0	–	–	37.80	.01	.03	.06	.10	.03	1.70	–	–
43	.04	.01	–	101.2	–	–	2.51	Trace	Trace	.03	.02	Trace	.22	–	–
	.27	.04	–	723.0	–	–	17.90	.01	.01	.28	.14	.03	1.60	–	–
44	.04	.01	.01	6.2	–	–	3.60	Trace	Trace	.03	.02	.02	.90	–	–
	.30	.07	.05	44.0	–	–	25.70	.02	.02	.22	.17	.14	6.40	–	–
45	.03	.01	–	41.9	–	–	10.56	Trace	.01	.05	–	.01	–	–	–
	.20	.08	–	299.0	–	–	75.40	.01	.07	.39	–	.04	–	–	–
46	.01	.01	–	93.1	–	–	17.42	Trace	Trace	.04	–	.02	–	–	–
	.10	.06	–	665.0	–	–	124.40	.02	.03	.25	–	.12	–	–	–
47	.04	.01	.01	24.9	–	–	2.65	Trace	Trace	.09	.02	Trace	.55	–	–
	.27	.06	.05	178.0	–	–	18.90	.01	.03	.65	.13	.02	3.90	–	–
48	.04	.01	.01	4.8	–	–	3.08	Trace	Trace	.03	.01	Trace	.53	–	–
	.25	.08	.08	34.0	–	–	22.00	.01	.03	.19	.10	.01	3.80	–	–
49	.03	.01	.01	13.2	–	–	.11	Trace	Trace	.03	.02	Trace	.13	–	–
	.22	.08	.04	94.0	–	–	.80	.01	.03	.21	.11	.03	.90	–	–
50	.05	.01	–	57.0	–	–	.11	Trace	.01	.07	.02	.01	.03	–	–
	.33	.10	–	407.0	–	–	.80	.02	.08	.53	.14	.09	.20	–	–
51	.17	.01	–	5.4	–	–	17.37	Trace	.01	.03	–	.01	.03	–	–
	.57	.03	–	18.0	–	–	57.90	.01	.02	.08	–	.03	.10	–	–
52	.10	.01	–	12.6	–	–	19.08	.01	Trace	.04	–	.01	2.01	–	–
	.34	.03	–	42.0	–	–	63.60	.02	.01	.12	–	.04	6.70	–	–
53	.05	.02	–	16.5	–	–	18.75	.01	.01	.07	–	.02	7.92	–	–
	.17	.06	–	55.0	–	–	62.50	.05	.03	.24	–	.05	26.40	–	–
54	.23	.28	.01	14.4	–	–	.27	Trace	.02	.46	.05	.02	.80	–	.21
	1.65	2.00	.09	103.0	–	–	1.90	.01	.16	3.28	.35	.12	5.70	–	1.47
55	.14	.14	.01	26.0	–	–	.21	Trace	.02	.48	.10	.03	1.55	–	–
	.99	1.01	.05	186.0	–	–	1.50	.01	.16	3.42	.73	.19	11.10	–	–
56	.39	.27	.01	175.1	–	–	.20	.01	.04	Trace	.30	.02	12.89	–	.22
	2.76	1.92	.07	1251.0	–	–	1.40	.07	.27	.03	2.14	.16	92.10	–	1.54
57	.14	.24	–	4.5	–	–	.29	.02	.03	.40	.07	.03	.29	–	–
	1.01	1.70	–	32.0	–	–	2.10	.14	.19	2.84	.53	.20	2.10	–	–
58	.23	.36	.01	3.8	–	–	.24	Trace	.03	.45	.06	.03	.28	–	.32
	1.66	2.60	.06	27.0	–	–	1.70	.02	.19	3.19	.42	.18	2.00	–	2.27
59	.74	.42	.28	5338.9	–	–	2.70	.01	.25	1.17	–	.05	47.24	–	.30
	5.29	2.98	1.99	38135.0	–	–	19.30	.05	1.81	8.33	–	.34	337.40	–	2.16
60	.59	–	–	3080.0	–	–	.98	.01	.28	1.09	–	–	–	–	–
	4.20	–	–	22000.0	–	–	7.00	.05	1.99	7.80	–	–	–	–	–
61	.17	–	–	–	–	–	.22	.03	.03	.39	–	.07	–	–	.15
	1.20	–	–	–	–	–	1.60	.23	.23	2.80	–	.49	–	–	1.06

(Continued)

TABLE F-21 *(Continued)*

Item No.	Food Item Name	Approximate Measure	Weight	Moisture	Food Energy Calories	Protein	Fats	Carbo-hydrates	Fiber	Calcium	Phos-phorus	Sodium	Mag-nesium	Potas-sium
			(g)	(%)	(kcal)	(g)	(g)	(g)	(g)	(mg)	(mg)	(mg)	(mg)	(mg)
62	TURKEY	1 TBLS	14	77.5	18.1	2.2	1.0	0	0	3.9	13.3	10.1	1.7	25.2
			100	77.5	129.0	15.4	7.1	0	0	28.0	95.0	72.0	12.0	180.0
63	VEAL	1 TBLS	14	79.8	15.4	2.1	.7	0	Trace	.8	13.7	9.7	1.5	33.0
			100	79.8	110.0	15.3	5.0	0	.2	6.0	98.0	69.0	11.0	236.0
	VEGETABLES													
64	BEANS, GREEN	1 TBLS	14	92.5	3.5	.2	0	.8	.1	9.1	2.7	.3	3.1	17.9
			100	92.5	25.0	1.2	0	5.7	.9	65.0	19.0	2.0	22.0	128.0
65	BEETS	1 TBLS	14	90.1	4.8	.2	0	1.1	.1	2.0	2.0	11.6	2.0	25.5
			100	90.1	34.0	1.3	.1	7.7	.8	14.0	14.0	83.0	14.0	182.0
66	CARROTS	1 TBLS	14	91.0	4.5	.1	0	1.0	.1	3.2	2.8	6.9	1.5	28.3
			100	91.0	32.0	.8	.2	7.2	.8	23.0	20.0	49.0	11.0	202.0
67	CORN, creamed	1 TBLS	14	81.4	9.1	.2	.1	2.3	Trace	2.5	4.6	7.3	1.1	11.3
			100	81.4	65.0	1.4	.4	16.3	.1	18.0	33.0	52.0	8.0	81.0
68	MIXED VEGETABLES	1 TBLS	14	89.4	5.7	.2	.1	1.1	.1	1.5	3.5	5.0	–	23.8
			100	89.4	41.0	1.4	.4	8.2	.5	11.0	25.0	36.0	–	170.0
69	PEAS	1 TBLS	14	87.5	5.6	.5	0	1.1	.2	2.8	6.0	.6	2.1	15.7
			100	87.5	40.0	3.5	.3	8.1	1.2	20.0	43.0	4.0	15.0	112.0
70	SPINACH, creamed	1 TBLS	14	88.2	5.9	.4	.2	.9	.1	15.8	6.9	7.7	8.8	30.9
			100	88.2	42.0	3.0	1.4	6.4	.5	113.0	49.0	55.0	63.0	221.0
71	SQUASH	1 TBLS	14	92.8	3.4	.1	0	.8	.1	3.4	2.2	.1	1.7	25.9
			100	92.8	24.0	.8	.2	5.6	.7	24.0	16.0	1.0	12.0	185.0
72	SWEET POTATOES	1 TBLS	14	84.1	8.4	.2	0	1.9	.1	2.2	3.4	3.1	1.7	34.0
			100	84.1	60.0	1.1	.1	13.9	.6	16.0	24.0	22.0	12.0	243.0
	BREADS													
73	BOSTON BROWN	1 SLICE	35	45.0	73.9	1.9	.5	16.0	.3	31.5	56.0	87.9	–	102.2
			100	45.0	211.0	5.5	1.3	45.6	.7	90.0	160.0	251.0	–	292.0
74	CRACKED WHEAT	1 SLICE	25	34.9	65.8	2.2	.6	13.0	.1	22.0	32.0	132.3	8.8	33.5
			100	34.9	263.0	8.7	2.2	52.1	.5	88.0	128.0	529.0	35.0	134.0
75	FRENCH OR VIENNA, enriched	1 SLICE	20	30.6	58.0	1.8	.6	11.1	Trace	8.6	17.0	116.0	4.4	18.0
			100	30.6	290.0	9.1	3.0	55.4	.2	43.0	85.0	580.0	22.0	90.0
76	FRENCH TOAST	1 OZ	28	41.1	51.3	2.3	1.4	7.1	.1	16.6	29.3	32.2	4.5	26.1
			100	41.1	183.3	8.3	5.1	25.5	.1	59.2	104.7	115.1	16.2	93.1
77	HAMBURGER OR WIENER BUN, enriched	1 WHOLE	48	31.0	144.0	3.6	2.4	25.2	–	36.0	–	–	11.0	–
			100	31.0	300.0	7.5	5.0	52.5	–	75.0	–	–	23.0	–
78	RAISIN	1 SLICE	25	35.3	65.5	1.7	.7	13.4	.2	17.8	21.8	91.3	6.0	58.3
			100	35.3	262.0	6.6	2.8	53.6	.9	71.0	87.0	365.0	24.0	233.0
79	ROMAN MEAL	1 SLICE	57	38.0	139.7	6.3	2.3	27.4	.7	60.4	–	342.0	–	–
			100	38.0	245.0	11.0	4.0	48.0	1.3	106.0	–	600.0	–	–
80	RYE, AMERICAN	1 SLICE	23	35.5	55.9	2.1	.3	12.0	.1	17.3	33.8	128.1	9.7	33.4
			100	35.5	243.0	9.1	1.1	52.1	.4	75.0	147.0	557.0	42.0	145.0
81	RYE, PUMPERNICKEL	1 SLICE	32	34.0	78.7	2.9	.4	17.0	.4	26.9	73.3	182.1	22.7	145.3
			100	34.0	246.0	9.1	1.2	53.1	1.1	84.0	229.0	569.0	71.0	454.0
82	STUFFING MIX, stove top, rice	1 OZ	28	6.7	106.1	3.1	1.0	20.9	.2	27.2	28.3	491.1	–	40.9
			100	6.7	379.0	11.0	3.4	74.8	.3	97.0	101.0	1754.0	–	146.0
83	WIENER BUN	1 WHOLE	36	–	108.0	2.7	1.8	18.9	–	27.0	–	–	–	–
			100	–	300.0	7.5	5.0	52.5	–	75.0	–	–	–	–
84	WHITE, enriched, w/1-2% nonfat dried milk	1 SLICE	23	35.8	61.9	2.0	.7	11.6	Trace	16.1	20.0	116.6	3.9	19.6
			100	35.8	269.0	8.7	3.2	50.4	.2	70.0	87.0	507.0	17.0	85.0
85	WHITE, enriched, w/3-4% nonfat dried milk	1 SLICE	23	35.6	62.1	2.0	.7	11.6	Trace	19.3	22.3	116.6	5.8	24.2
			100	35.6	270.0	8.7	3.2	50.5	.2	84.0	97.0	507.0	25.0	105.0
86	WHITE, enriched, w/5-6% nonfat dried milk	1 SLICE	23	35.0	63.3	2.1	.9	11.5	Trace	22.1	23.5	113.9	6.0	27.8
			100	35.0	275.0	9.0	3.8	50.2	.2	96.0	102.0	495.0	26.0	121.0
87	WHOLE WHEAT, made w/water	1 SLICE	23	36.4	55.4	2.1	.6	11.3	.3	19.3	58.4	121.9	13.6	58.9
			100	36.4	241.0	9.1	2.6	49.3	1.5	84.0	254.0	530.0	59.0	256.0
88	WHOLE WHEAT, made w/2% nonfat dried milk	1 SLICE	23	36.4	55.9	2.4	.7	11.0	.2	22.8	52.4	121.2	44.9	62.8
			100	36.4	243.0	10.5	3.0	47.7	1.6	99.0	228.0	527.0	195.0	273.0
89	ZWIEBACK	1 PIECE	7	5.0	29.6	.7	.6	5.2	Trace	.9	4.8	17.5	–	10.5
			100	5.0	423.0	10.7	8.8	74.3	.3	13.0	69.0	250.0	–	150.0
	CAKES													
90	ANGELFOOD	1 PIECE	45	31.5	121.1	3.2	.1	27.1	0	4.1	9.9	127.4	(6.8)	39.6
			100	31.5	269.0	7.1	.2	60.2	0	9.0	22.0	283.0	(15.0)	88.0
91	BANANA OR APPLESAUCE, w/o icing	1 OZ	28	–	98.0	.8	3.7	16.2	–	6.7	12.6	–	3.9	–
			100	–	350.0	2.8	13.1	57.9	–	24.0	45.0	–	14.0	–
92	CARROT	1 OZ	28	–	100.0	1.1	5.3	12.6	.1	10.1	28.0	121.2	–	35.3
			100	–	357.0	4.1	18.8	45.1	.5	36.0	100.0	433.0	–	126.0

Item No.	Minerals (Micro)			Fat-Soluble Vitamins			Water-Soluble Vitamins								
	Iron	Zinc	Copper	Vitamin A	Vitamin D	Vitamin E (Alpha Tocopherol)	Vitamin C	Thiamin	Riboflavin	Niacin	Pantothenic Acid	Vit. B-6 (Pyridoxine)	Folacin (Folic Acid)	Biotin	Vitamin B-12
	(mg)	(mg)	(mg)	(IU)	(IU)	(mg)	(mg)	(mg)	(mg)	(mg)	(mg)	(mg)	(mcg)	(mcg)	(mcg)
62	.19	.25	—	79.5	—	—	.34	Trace	.04	.49	.09	.02	1.69	—	.15
	1.35	1.80	—	568.0	—	—	2.40	.02	.25	3.48	.61	.17	12.10	—	1.07
63	.16	.35	.01	7.0	—	—	.29	Trace	.03	.53	.06	.02	.94	—	.18
	1.25	2.52	.08	50.0	—	—	2.10	.02	.18	3.81	.45	.12	6.70	—	1.30
64	.15	.03	.01	60.6	—	—	1.18	Trace	.01	.05	.02	.01	4.58	—	—
	1.08	.19	.05	433.0	—	—	8.40	.02	.10	.32	.15	.04	32.70	—	—
65	.05	.02	.01	4.6	—	—	.34	Trace	.01	.02	—	Trace	4.31	—	0
	.32	.12	.07	33.0	—	—	2.40	.01	.04	.13	—	.02	30.80	—	0
66	.06	.03	.01	1653.4	—	—	.77	Trace	.01	.07	.04	.01	2.42	—	—
	.39	.18	.05	11810.0	—	—	5.50	.02	.04	.50	.28	.08	17.30	—	—
67	.04	.03	.01	10.8	—	—	.31	Trace	.01	.07	.05	.01	1.78	—	Trace
	.27	.23	.04	77.0	—	—	2.20	.01	.05	.50	.33	.04	12.70	—	.02
68	.06	—	—	587.3	—	—	.35	Trace	Trace	.09	.04	.01	.57	—	—
	.41	—	—	4195.0	—	—	2.50	.03	.03	.67	.26	.08	4.10	—	—
69	.13	.05	.01	79.1	—	—	.97	.01	.01	.14	.04	.01	3.63	—	0
	.96	.35	.06	565.0	—	—	6.90	.08	.06	1.02	.28	.07	25.90	—	0
70	.20	.05	.01	514.6	—	—	.50	Trace	.01	.04	—	.01	9.63	—	—
	1.40	.35	.07	3676.0	—	—	3.60	.02	.09	.26	—	.06	68.80	—	—
71	.05	.01	.01	282.0	—	—	1.09	Trace	.01	.05	.03	.01	2.16	—	—
	.35	.08	.05	2014.0	—	—	7.80	.01	.07	.38	.22	.07	15.40	—	—
72	.06	.02	.01	929.0	—	—	1.34	Trace	.01	.05	.06	.02	1.44	—	—
	.39	.11	.10	6636.0	—	—	9.60	.03	.03	.38	.41	.11	10.30	—	—
73	.67	—	—	0	—	—	0	.04	.02	.42	—	—	—	—	—
	1.90	—	—	0	—	—	0	.11	.06	1.20	—	—	—	—	—
74	.28	—	—	—	—	—	—	.03	.02	.33	.15	.02	—	—	0
	11.0	—	—	—	—	—	—	.12	.09	1.30	.61	.09	—	—	0
75	.44	(.28)	(.05)	—	—	(.02)	—	.06	.04	.50	.08	.01	—	—	0
	2.20	(1.40)	(.23)	—	—	(.10)	—	.28	.22	2.50	.38	.05	—	—	0
76	.55	.21	—	4.6	4.42	—	Trace	.10	.13	.34	.20	.01	10.54	—	.14
	1.96	.73	—	16.4	15.77	—	.01	.34	.45	1.21	.71	.04	37.63	—	.48
77	.96	.29	.12	—	—	—	—	.13	.08	1.08	—	—	—	—	—
	2.00	.60	.25	—	—	—	—	.27	.17	2.25	—	—	—	—	—
78	.33	(.30)	(.05)	—	—	—	—	.01	.02	.18	—	—	—	—	—
	1.30	(1.20)	(.23)	—	—	—	—	.05	.09	.70	—	—	—	—	—
79	1.82	—	—	0	—	—	0	.23	.17	2.00	—	—	—	—	—
	3.20	—	—	0	—	—	0	.40	.30	3.50	—	—	—	—	—
80	.37	.37	.04	0	—	(.07)	0	.04	.02	.32	.10	.02	5.29	—	0
	1.60	1.60	.17	0	—	(.30)	0	.18	.07	1.40	.45	.10	23.00	—	0
81	.77	.38	.05	0	—	—	0	.07	.05	.38	.16	.05	7.36	—	0
	2.40	1.20	.17	0	—	—	0	.23	.14	1.20	.50	.16	23.00	—	0
82	1.18	—	—	0	—	—	—	.16	.06	1.32	—	—	—	—	—
	4.20	—	—	0	—	—	—	.56	.22	4.70	—	—	—	—	—
83	.72	.22	—	—	—	—	—	.10	Trace	.81	—	—	—	—	—
	2.00	.60	—	—	—	—	—	.20	.17	2.25	—	—	—	—	—
84	.55	.14	.05	—	—	.02	—	.20	.13	.53	.10	.01	8.05	.25	—
	2.40	.60	.23	—	—	.10	—	.88	.58	2.30	.43	.04	35.00	1.10	—
85	.58	.14	.03	—	—	.02	—	.20	.13	.55	.10	.01	8.05	.25	—
	2.50	.60	.11	—	—	.10	—	.88	.58	2.40	.43	.04	35.00	1.10	—
86	.58	.14	Trace	—	—	.02	—	.20	.13	.55	.10	.01	8.05	.25	—
	2.50	.60	.02	—	—	.10	—	.88	.58	2.40	.43	.04	35.00	1.10	—
87	.53	.41	.04	—	—	.10	0	.07	.02	.64	.18	.04	13.34	.44	0
	2.30	1.80	.17	—	—	.45	0	.30	.10	2.80	.76	.18	58.00	1.90	0
88	.53	.41	.12	—	—	.10	—	.06	.03	.64	.18	.04	14.26	.25	0
	2.30	1.80	.51	—	—	.45	—	.26	.12	2.80	.76	.18	62.00	1.10	0
89	.04	—	—	2.8	—	—	0	Trace	.01	.06	—	—	—	—	—
	.60	—	—	40.0	—	—	0	.05	.07	.90	—	—	—	—	—
90	.09	.05	(.02)	0	—	(.05)	0	.01	.06	.09	—	—	—	—	—
	.20	.11	(.04)	0	—	(.10)	0	.01	.14	.20	—	—	—	—	—
91	.62	—	—	14.0	—	—	0	.04	.03	.31	—	.02	—	—	.02
	2.20	—	—	50.0	—	—	0	.13	.11	1.10	—	.06	—	—	.07
92	.28	.13	.05	779.5	—	—	.56	.03	.03	.17	—	—	—	—	—
	1.00	.46	.17	2784.0	—	—	2.00	.11	.09	.60	—	—	—	—	—

(Continued)

TABLE F-21 *(Continued)*

Item No.	Food Item Name	Approximate Measure	Weight (g)	Moisture (%)	Food Energy Calories (kcal)	Protein (g)	Fats (g)	Carbo-hydrates (g)	Fiber (g)	Calcium (mg)	Phos-phorus (mg)	Sodium (mg)	Mag-nesium (mg)	Potas-sium (mg)
93	CHOCOLATE CUPCAKE, w/icing	1 AVG	36	22.2	128.9	1.6	4.5	21.3	.1	46.8	70.9	120.6	–	42.1
			100	22.2	358.0	4.5	12.6	59.2	.3	130.0	197.0	355.0	–	117.0
94	CHOCOLATE (DEVIL'S FOOD), w/uncooked icing	1 PIECE	74	21.3	273.1	2.8	10.8	43.8	.1	43.7	78.4	173.2	17.8	81.4
			100	21.3	369.0	3.8	14.6	59.2	.2	59.0	106.0	234.0	24.0	110.0
95	CHOCOLATE (DEVIL'S FOOD), no icing	1 PIECE	40	24.6	146.4	1.9	6.9	20.8	.1	29.6	54.8	117.6	9.6	56.0
			100	24.6	366.0	4.8	17.2	52.0	.3	74.0	137.0	294.0	24.0	140.0
96	CINNAMON COFFEE CAKE	1 PIECE	28	–	105.0	1.5	4.0	15.5	–	–	–	230.0	(4.2)	–
			100	–	375.0	5.4	14.3	55.4	–	–	–	821.4	(15.0)	–
97	COCONUT	1 PIECE	87	–	324.5	2.8	15.2	46.3	.1	25.2	92.2	253.2	8.7	57.4
			100	–	373.0	3.2	17.5	53.2	.2	29.0	106.0	291.0	10.0	66.0
98	FRUITCAKE, dark	1 SLICE	15	18.1	56.9	.7	2.3	9.0	.1	10.8	17.0	23.7	2.4	74.4
			100	18.1	379.0	4.8	15.3	59.7	.6	72.0	113.0	158.0	16.0	496.0
99	FRUITCAKE, light	1 SLICE	15	18.7	58.4	.9	2.5	8.6	.1	10.2	17.3	29.0	2.4	35.0
			100	18.7	389.0	6.0	16.5	57.4	.7	68.0	115.0	193.0	16.0	233.0
100	GERMAN CHOCOLATE	1 PIECE	49	25.1	191.1	2.6	10.0	23.0	.2	28.4	67.1	179.3	7.4	70.1
			100	25.1	390.0	5.4	20.5	47.0	.4	58.0	137.0	366.0	15.0	143.0
101	PINEAPPLE UPSIDE DOWN CAKE	1 SERV	100	41.5	300.0	3.0	13.0	42.0	.2	31.0	67.0	170.0	–	101.0
			100	41.5	300.0	3.0	13.0	42.0	.2	31.0	67.0	170.0	–	101.0
102	PLAIN OR CUPCAKE, w/o icing	1 PIECE	86	24.5	313.0	3.9	12.0	48.1	.1	55.0	87.7	258.0	–	67.9
			100	24.5	364.0	4.5	13.9	55.9	.1	64.0	102.0	300.0	–	79.0
103	PLAIN OR CUPCAKE, w/boiled white icing	1 PIECE	114	22.9	401.3	4.3	12.0	70.5	–	55.9	87.8	298.7	–	73.0
			100	22.9	352.0	3.8	10.5	61.8	–	49.0	77.0	262.0	–	64.0
104	COTTAGE PUDDING, w/strawberry sauce	1 PIECE	70	36.6	204.4	3.6	6.2	33.9	.2	51.1	65.1	163.1	–	65.1
			100	36.6	292.0	5.1	8.8	48.4	.3	73.0	93.0	233.0	–	93.0
105	POUND CAKE, (old fashioned), w/butter & eggs	1 PIECE	30	17.2	141.9	1.7	8.9	14.1	Trace	6.3	23.7	33.0	(3.9)	18.0
			100	17.2	473.0	5.7	29.5	47.0	.1	21.0	79.0	110.0	(13.0)	60.0
106	SHORTCAKE	1 PIECE	25	–	85.8	1.0	2.0	12.2	–	10.3	13.0	–	–	–
			100	–	343.0	3.8	8.1	48.6	–	41.0	52.0	–	–	–
107	SPICE, w/icing	1 OZ	28	–	98.6	1.1	3.0	17.1	–	19.9	54.0	–	5.0	–
			100	–	352.0	4.1	10.8	60.9	–	71.0	193.0	–	18.0	–
108	SPONGE	1 PIECE	33	31.8	98.0	2.5	1.9	17.9	0	9.9	37.0	55.1	4.3	28.7
			100	31.8	297.0	7.6	5.7	54.1	0	30.0	112.0	167.0	13.0	87.0
109	WHITE, w/o icing	1 PIECE	50	24.2	187.5	2.3	8.0	27.0	.1	31.5	45.5	161.5	4.0	38.0
			100	24.2	375.0	4.6	16.0	54.0	.1	63.0	91.0	323.0	8.0	76.0
110	WHITE, w/chocolate icing	1 PIECE	71	21.1	249.2	2.8	7.6	44.6	.1	70.3	127.1	161.2	–	82.4
			100	21.1	351.0	3.9	10.7	62.8	.2	99.0	179.0	227.0	–	116.0
111	YELLOW, w/o icing	1 PIECE	50	23.5	181.5	2.3	6.4	29.1	.1	35.5	56.0	129.0	4.0	39.0
			100	23.5	363.0	4.5	12.7	58.2	.1	71.0	112.0	258.0	8.0	78.0
112	YELLOW, w/chocolate icing	1 PIECE	69	25.6	232.5	2.8	7.8	39.7	.1	62.8	125.6	156.6	–	75.2
			100	25.6	337.0	4.1	11.3	57.6	.2	91.0	182.0	227.0	–	109.0
	COOKIES													
113	ARROWROOT	INDV	4	–	17.3	.2	.4	3.2	–	1.5	4.0	12.0	–	–
			100	–	432.4	5.9	9.9	80.4	–	37.8	100.0	300.0	–	–
114	ASSORTED, commercially packaged	1 AVG	20	2.6	96.0	1.0	4.0	14.2	Trace	7.4	32.6	73.0	–	13.4
			100	2.6	480.0	5.1	20.2	71.0	.1	37.0	163.0	365.0	–	67.0
115	BROWNIE, w/chocolate & nuts, frozen	1 SERV	100	12.0	510.0	6.0	33.0	48.0	.5	30.0	142.0	145.0	–	162.0
			100	12.0	510.0	6.0	33.0	48.0	.5	30.0	142.0	145.0	–	162.0
116	CHOCOLATE CHIP, home recipe	1 AVG	11	3.0	56.8	.6	3.3	6.6	Trace	3.7	10.9	38.3	1.7	12.9
			100	3.0	516.0	5.4	30.1	60.1	.4	34.0	99.0	348.0	15.0	117.0
117	FIG BARS	1 AVG	14	13.6	50.1	.5	.8	10.6	.2	10.9	8.4	35.3	2.1	27.7
			100	13.6	358.0	3.9	5.6	75.4	1.7	78.0	60.0	252.0	15.0	198.0
118	GINGERSNAPS	1 SM	4	3.1	16.8	.2	.4	3.2	Trace	2.9	1.9	22.8	.6	18.5
			100	3.1	420.0	5.5	8.9	79.8	.1	73.0	47.0	571.0	15.0	462.0
119	GRANOLA BAR, honey'n oats	1 BAR	24	–	111.7	2.0	4.1	16.2	–	–	–	–	–	–
			100	–	465.3	8.5	16.9	67.7	–	–	–	–	–	–
120	LADYFINGERS	1 LG	14	19.2	50.4	1.1	1.1	9.0	Trace	5.7	23.0	9.9	2.1	9.9
			100	19.2	360.0	7.8	7.8	64.5	.1	41.0	164.0	71.0	15.0	71.0
121	MACAROONS	1 AVG	14	4.4	66.5	.7	3.2	9.3	.3	3.8	11.6	4.8	–	64.8
			100	4.4	475.0	5.3	23.2	66.1	2.1	27.0	83.0	34.0	–	463.0
122	MOLASSES	1 AVG	33	4.0	139.3	2.1	3.5	25.1	Trace	16.8	27.4	127.4	–	45.5
			100	4.0	422.0	6.4	10.6	76.0	.1	51.0	83.0	386.0	–	138.0
123	OATMEAL	INDV	13	–	59.8	.7	2.3	9.2	–	2.9	16.1	–	–	–
			100	–	460.3	5.7	17.9	70.7	–	22.2	123.8	–	–	–
124	PEANUT BUTTER, prepared	INDV	12	–	54.9	.7	3.1	6.5	–	–	–	75.4	–	–
			100	–	457.1	5.7	25.7	54.3	–	–	–	628.6	–	–
125	RAISIN	1 AVG	15	8.2	56.9	.7	.8	12.1	.1	10.7	23.6	7.8	2.3	40.8
			100	8.2	379.0	4.4	5.3	80.8	.9	71.0	157.0	52.0	15.0	272.0

Item No.	Minerals (Micro)			Fat-Soluble Vitamins			Water-Soluble Vitamins								
	Iron	Zinc	Copper	Vitamin A	Vitamin D	Vitamin E (Alpha Tocopherol)	Vitamin C	Thiamin	Ribo-flavin	Niacin	Panto-thenic Acid	Vit. B-6 (Pyri-doxine)	Folacin (Folic Acid)	Biotin	Vitamin B-12
	(mg)	(mg)	(mg)	(IU)	(IU)	(mg)	(mg)	(mg)	(mg)	(mg)	(mg)	(mg)	(mcg)	(mcg)	(mcg)
93	.29	–	–	61.2	–	.05	–	.01	.04	.07	–	–	–	–	–
	.80	–	–	170.0	–	.14	–	.04	.11	.20	–	–	–	–	–
94	.52	–	–	133.2	–	–	–	.02	.06	.15	.15	–	4.44	–	–
	.70	–	–	180.0	–	–	–	.02	.08	.20	.20	–	6.00	–	–
95	.36	.26	.16	60.0	–	–	–	.01	.04	.08	.08	–	–	–	–
	.90	.65	.41	150.0	–	–	–	.02	.10	.20	.20	–	–	–	–
96	–	(.17)	(.02)	–	–	(.06)	–	–	–	–	(.06)	(.01)	–	–	–
	–	(.60)	(.08)	–	–	(.20)	–	–	–	–	(.20)	(.04)	–	–	–
97	1.22	–	–	87.0	–	–	–	.11	.07	1.13	–	–	–	–	–
	1.40	–	–	100.0	–	–	–	.13	.08	1.30	–	–	–	–	–
98	.39	[6].08	–	18.0	–	–	–	.02	.02	.12	–	–	–	–	–
	2.60	.50	–	120.0	–	–	–	.13	.14	.80	–	–	–	–	–
99	.24	[6].08	–	10.5	–	–	–	.02	.02	.11	–	–	–	–	–
	1.60	.50	–	70.0	–	–	–	.10	.11	.70	–	–	–	–	–
100	.69	–	–	75.5	–	–	.10	.04	.06	.34	–	–	2.94	–	–
	1.40	–	–	154.0	–	–	.20	.09	.12	.70	–	–	6.00	–	–
101	1.50	.20	.12	245.0	–	–	2.00	.07	.06	1.30	–	–	–	–	–
	1.50	.20	.12	245.0	–	–	2.00	.07	.06	1.30	–	–	–	–	–
102	.34	–	–	146.2	–	–	–	.02	.08	.17	–	.03	–	–	–
	.40	–	–	170.0	–	–	–	.02	.09	.20	–	.04	–	–	–
103	.34	–	–	146.2	–	–	–	.02	.08	.23	–	.05	–	–	–
	.30	–	–	130.0	–	–	–	.02	.07	.20	–	.04	–	–	–
104	.84	–	–	84.0	–	–	8.40	.08	.11	.77	–	–	–	–	–
	1.20	–	–	120.0	–	–	12.00	.12	.15	1.10	–	–	–	–	–
105	.24	(.18)	(.02)	84.0	–	.33	0	.01	.03	.06	(.09)	(.01)	–	–	–
	.80	(.60)	(.06)	280.0	–	1.10	0	.03	.09	.20	(.30)	(.04)	–	–	–
106	.13	–	–	84.8	–	–	.25	.03	.03	.10	–	–	–	–	–
	.50	–	–	339.0	–	–	1.00	.13	.11	.40	–	–	–	–	–
107	.36	–	–	44.8	–	–	0	.03	.05	.28	–	.01	–	–	.01
	1.30	–	–	160.0	–	–	0	.12	.16	1.00	–	.04	–	–	.02
108	.40	–	–	148.5	–	–	–	.02	.05	.07	–	–	2.31	–	–
	1.20	–	–	450.0	–	–	–	.05	.14	.20	–	–	7.00	–	–
109	.10	.10	–	15.0	–	–	–	.01	.04	.10	.15	–	–	–	–
	.20	.20	–	30.0	–	–	–	.01	.08	.20	.30	–	–	–	–
110	.36	–	–	42.6	–	–	–	.01	.06	.14	–	–	–	–	–
	.50	–	–	60.0	–	–	–	.02	.08	.20	–	–	–	–	–
111	.20	(.25)	(.05)	75.0	–	(.25)	–	.01	.04	.10	(.15)	(.02)	–	–	–
	.40	(.50)	(.10)	150.0	–	(.50)	–	.02	.08	.20	(.30)	(.04)	–	–	–
112	.41	–	–	96.6	–	–	–	.01	.06	.14	–	–	–	–	–
	.60	–	–	140.0	–	–	–	.02	.08	.20	–	–	–	–	–
113	.10	–	–	–	–	–	–	–	–	–				–	–
	2.43	–	–	–	–	–	–	–	–	–				–	–
114	.14	–	–	16.0	–	(.10)	–	.01	.01	.08	(.08)	(.01)	–	–	–
	.70	–	–	80.0	–	(.50)	–	.03	.05	.40	(.40)	(.05)	–	–	–
115	2.20	–	–	10.0	–	–	2.00	.12	.10	.50	–	–	–	–	–
	2.20	–	–	10.0	–	–	2.00	.12	.10	.50	–	–	–	–	–
116	.23	.11	–	12.1	–	–	–	.01	.01	.10	–	–	.99	–	–
	2.10	.96	–	110.0	–	–	–	.11	.11	.90	–	–	9.00	–	–
117	.14	.09	.04	15.4	–	–	–	.01	.01	.04	–	–	–	–	–
	1.00	.64	.29	110.0	–	–	–	.04	.07	.30	–	–	–	–	–
118	.09	–	–	2.8	–	–	–	Trace	Trace	.02	–	–	–	–	–
	2.30	–	–	70.0	–	–	–	.04	.06	.40	–	–	–	–	–
119	–	–	–	–	–	–	–	–	–	–				–	–
	–	–	–	–	–	–	–	–	–	–				–	–
120	.21	–	–	91.0	–	–	0	.01	.02	.03	–	–	–	–	–
	1.50	–	–	650.0	–	–	0	.06	.14	.20	–	–	–	–	–
121	.13	–	–	0	–	–	0	.01	.02	.08	–	–	–	–	–
	.90	–	–	0	–	–	0	.04	.15	.60	–	–	–	–	–
122	.69	–	–	26.4	–	–	0	.01	.02	.23	–	–	–	–	–
	2.10	–	–	80.0	–	–	0	.04	.06	.70	–	–	–	–	–
123	.30	–	–	–	–	–	–	–	–	–	–	–	–	–	–
	2.30	–	–	–	–	–	–	–	–	–	–	–	–	–	–
124	–	–	–	–	–	–	–	–	–	–				–	–
	–	–	–	–	–	–	–	–	–	–				–	–
125	.32	–	–	31.5	–	–	–	.01	.01	.09	–	–	–	–	–
	2.10	–	–	210.0	–	–	–	.04	.08	.60	–	–	–	–	–

(Continued)

TABLE F-21 *(Continued)*

Item No.	Food Item Name	Approximate Measure	Weight (g)	Moisture (%)	Food Energy Calories (kcal)	Protein (g)	Fats (g)	Carbo-hydrates (g)	Fiber (g)	Minerals (Macro) Calcium (mg)	Phos-phorus (mg)	Sodium (mg)	Mag-nesium (mg)	Potas-sium (mg)
126	**SANDWICH TYPE**	1 AVG	14	2.2	69.3	.7	3.2	9.7	Trace	3.6	33.7	67.6	2.1	5.3
			100	2.2	495.0	4.8	22.5	69.3	.1	26.0	241.0	483.0	15.0	38.0
127	**SHORTBREAD**	1 AVG	7	3.0	34.9	.5	1.6	4.6	Trace	4.9	10.9	4.2	1.1	4.6
			100	3.0	498.0	7.2	23.1	65.1	.2	70.0	156.0	60.0	15.0	66.0
128	**SUGAR,** soft, thick, home, recipe, w/enriched flour	1 AVG	8	7.9	35.5	.5	1.3	5.4	Trace	6.2	8.2	25.4	–	6.1
			100	7.9	444.0	6.0	16.8	68.0	.1	78.0	103.0	318.0	–	76.0
129	**VANILLA WAFERS**	1 SM	4	2.8	18.5	.2	.6	3.0	Trace	1.6	2.5	10.1	.6	2.9
			100	2.8	462.0	5.4	16.1	74.4	.1	41.0	63.0	252.0	15.0	72.0
	CRACKERS													
130	**ANIMAL**	1 AVG	2	3.0	8.6	.1	.2	1.6	Trace	1.0	2.3	6.1	–	1.9
			100	3.0	429.0	6.6	9.4	79.9	.1	52.0	114.0	303.0	–	95.0
131	**CHEESE**	1 AVG	1	3.9	4.8	.1	.2	.6	Trace	3.4	3.1	10.4	.3	1.1
			100	3.9	479.0	11.2	21.3	60.4	.2	336.0	309.0	1039.0	29.0	109.0
132	**GRAHAM,** plain	1 AVG	7	6.4	26.9	.6	.7	5.1	.1	2.8	10.4	46.9	1.3	26.9
			100	6.4	384.0	8.0	9.4	73.3	1.1	40.0	149.0	670.0	18.0	384.0
133	**GRAHAM,** chocolate coated	1 AVG	13	1.9	61.8	.7	3.1	8.8	.1	14.7	26.5	52.9	–	41.6
			100	1.9	475.0	5.1	23.5	67.9	.8	113.0	204.0	407.0	–	320.0
134	**MATZO**	1 PIECE	20	–	78.0	2.1	.2	17.3	–	–	–	–	–	–
			100	–	390.0	10.5	1.0	86.5	–	–	–	–	–	–
135	**MEAL**	1 CUP	128	–	537.6	12.3	12.3	93.1	–	25.6	122.9	–	–	–
			100	–	420.0	9.6	9.6	72.7	–	20.0	96.0	–	–	–
136	**RITZ**	1 AVG	3	2.1	16.1	.2	.9	1.9	–	4.4	7.1	29.1	–	2.3
			100	2.1	535.7	7.1	28.6	64.3	–	147.0	236.0	970.0	–	75.0
137	²**RUSK OR RUSKETT**	1 OZ	28	4.8	117.3	3.9	2.4	19.9	.1	5.6	33.3	68.9	–	45.1
			100	4.8	419.0	13.8	8.7	71.0	.2	20.0	119.0	246.0	–	161.0
138	**RYE WAFERS,** whole grain	1 AVG	7	6.0	24.1	.9	.1	5.3	.2	3.7	27.2	61.7	–	42.0
			100	6.0	344.0	13.0	1.2	76.3	2.2	53.0	388.0	832.0	–	600.0
139	**SODA**	1 AVG	7	4.0	30.7	.6	.9	4.9	Trace	1.5	6.2	77.0	2.0	8.4
			100	4.0	439.0	9.2	13.1	70.6	.2	22.0	89.0	1100.0	29.0	120.0
140	**WHEAT & RYE THINS**	1 AVG	2	–	9.5	.2	.4	1.3	–	.8	3.1	–	.2	–
			100	–	476.0	7.7	20.1	66.1	–	40.0	157.0	–	12.0	–
141	**WHOLE WHEAT**	1 AVG	4	6.9	16.1	.3	.6	2.7	.1	.9	7.6	21.9	–	–
			100	6.9	403.0	8.4	13.8	68.2	2.4	23.0	190.0	547.0	–	–
	DOUGHNUTS													
142	**CAKE-TYPE,** enriched	1 AVG	32	23.7	125.1	1.5	6.0	16.4	Trace	12.8	60.8	160.3	6.7	28.8
			100	23.7	391.0	4.6	18.6	51.4	.1	40.0	190.0	501.0	21.0	90.0
143	**YEAST-LEAVENED,** enriched	1 AVG	30	28.3	124.2	1.9	8.0	11.3	.1	11.4	22.8	70.2	6.0	24.0
			100	28.3	414.0	6.3	26.7	37.7	.2	38.0	76.0	234.0	20.0	80.0
	LEAVENINGS													
	BAKING POWDER													
144	home use, calcium carbonate	1 TSP	3	1.0	2.3	.0	Trace	.6	–	173.3	43.6	348.5	(.3)	(1.5)
			100	1.0	78.0	.1	.2	18.9	–	5778.0	1452.0	11618.0	(9.0)	(49.0)
145	home use, calcium sulfate	1 TSP	3	1.3	3.1	.0	–	.8	–	189.6	46.8	300.0	–	–
			100	1.3	40.0	.1	–	25.1	–	6320.0	1560.0	10000.0	–	–
146	home use, sodium aluminum sulfate	1 TSP	3	1.6	3.9	.0	–	.9	–	58.0	87.1	328.6	–	4.5
			100	1.6	29.0	.1	–	31.2	–	1932.0	2904.0	10953.0	–	150.0
147	home use, tartrate	1 TSP	3	1.0	2.3	.0	–	.6	–	0	0	219.0	–	114.0
			100	1.0	78.0	.1	–	18.9	–	0	0	7300.0	–	3800.0
148	commercial, low sodium	1 TSP	3	2.2	5.2	.0	Trace	1.2	–	144.5	219.2	.2	–	328.4
			100	2.2	72.0	.1	.6	41.6	–	4816.0	7308.0	6.0	–	10948.0
149	**BAKING SODA**	1 TSP	3	–	0	0	0	0	–	–	–	821.4	–	–
			100	–	0	0	0	0	–	–	–	27380.0	–	–
150	**YEAST, BAKER'S,** compressed, unfortified	1 CAKE	12	71.0	10.3	1.5	Trace	1.3	–	1.6	47.3	1.9	7.1	73.2
			100	71.0	86.0	12.1	.4	11.0	–	13.0	394.0	16.0	59.0	610.0
	MUFFINS													
151	**BLUEBERRY,** made w/enriched flour	1 AVG	40	39.0	112.4	2.9	3.7	16.8	.1	33.6	52.8	252.8	10.0	46.0
			100	39.0	281.0	7.3	9.3	41.9	.3	84.0	132.0	632.0	25.0	115.0
152	**BRAN,** made w/enriched flour	1 AVG	40	35.1	104.4	3.1	3.9	17.2	.7	56.8	162.0	179.2	–	172.4
			100	35.1	261.0	7.7	9.8	43.1	1.8	142.0	405.0	448.0	–	431.0
153	**CORN**	1 OZ	28	43.8	77.4	1.7	3.2	10.7	.1	15.0	24.1	59.8	4.9	36.3
			100	43.8	276.3	6.0	11.3	38.1	.2	53.5	85.9	213.7	17.6	129.5
154	**ENGLISH**	1 WHOLE	56	–	137.8	5.3	1.4	28.3	–	–	–	203.3	–	–
			100	–	246.0	9.5	2.5	50.6	–	–	–	363.0	–	–
155	**PLAIN,** made w/enriched flour	1 AVG	40	38.0	117.6	3.1	4.0	16.9	Trace	41.6	60.4	176.4	11.0	50.0
			100	38.0	294.0	7.8	10.1	42.3	.1	104.0	151.0	441.0	27.5	125.0

Item No.	Minerals (Micro)			Fat-Soluble Vitamins			Water-Soluble Vitamins								
	Iron	Zinc	Copper	Vitamin A	Vitamin D	Vitamin E (Alpha Tocopherol)	Vitamin C	Thiamin	Riboflavin	Niacin	Pantothenic Acid	Vit. B-6 (Pyridoxine)	Folacin (Folic Acid)	Biotin	Vitamin B-12
	(mg)	(mg)	(mg)	(IU)	(IU)	(mg)	(mg)	(mg)	(mg)	(mg)	(mg)	(mg)	(mcg)	(mcg)	(mcg)
126	.10	–	–	0	–	–	0	.01	.01	.07	–	–	–	–	–
	.70	–	–	0	–	–	0	.04	.04	.50	–	–	–	–	–
127	.04	.03	–	5.6	–	.03	0	Trace	Trace	.04	–	–	.63	–	–
	.50	.42	–	80.0	–	.46	0	.04	.05	.50	–	–	9.00	–	–
128	.11	.05	.01	8.8	–	–	–	.01	.01	.10	–	–	–	–	–
	1.40	.57	.17	110.0	–	–	–	.16	.16	1.30	–	–	–	–	–
129	.02	.01	–	5.2	–	–	0	Trace	Trace	.01	–	–	–	–	–
	.40	.30	–	130.0	–	–	0	.02	.07	.30	–	–	–	–	–
130	.01	–	–	2.6	–	–	–	Trace	Trace	.01	–	–	–	–	–
	.50	–	–	130.0	–	–	–	.04	.10	.30	–	–	–	–	–
131	.01	–	–	3.6	–	–	0	0	Trace	.01	–	–	–	–	–
	.90	–	–	360.0	–	–	0	.01	.10	.80	–	–	–	–	–
132	.11	.08	Trace	0	–	(.01)	0	Trace	.02	.11	(.04)	(.01)	–	–	–
	1.50	1.10	.04	0	–	(.10)	0	.04	.21	1.50	(.50)	(.07)	–	–	–
133	.34	–	–	7.8	–	–	0	.01	.04	.16	–	–	–	–	–
	2.60	–	–	60.0	–	–	0	.07	.28	1.20	–	–	–	–	–
134	–	–	–	–	–	–	–	–	–	–	–	–	–	–	–
	–	–	–	–	–	–	–	–	–	–	–	–	–	–	–
135	1.41	–	–	0	0	–	0	.08	.06	1.40	–	–	–	–	–
	1.10	–	–	0	0	–	0	.06	.05	1.09	–	–	–	–	–
136	.08	.02	.01	–	–	–	–	.01	.01	.09	–	–	–	–	–
	2.75	.51	.18	–	–	–	–	.39	.35	2.90	–	–	–	–	–
137	.36	–	–	64.4	–	–	Trace	.02	.06	.31	–	.03	–	–	–
	1.30	–	–	230.0	–	–	Trace	.08	.22	1.10	–	.09	–	–	–
138	.27	–	–	0	–	–	0	.02	.02	.08	–	–	–	–	–
	3.90	–	–	0	–	–	0	.32	.25	1.20	–	–	–	–	–
139	.11	–	–	0	–	–	0	Trace	Trace	.07	–	–	–	–	–
	1.50	(.70)	(.17)	0	–	–	0	.01	.05	1.00	–	–	–	–	–
140	.08	–	–	.2	–	–	0	.01	.01	.07	–	Trace	–	–	0
	3.90	–	–	10.0	–	–	0	.58	.37	3.60	–	.08	–	–	0
141	.01	.12	.04	0	–	–	0	Trace	Trace	.04	–	–	–	–	–
	.30	3.04	.87	0	–	–	0	.06	.04	.90	–	–	–	–	–
142	.45	.16	.05	25.6	–	(.12)	–	.05	.05	.38	.12	(.01)	2.56	–	–
	1.40	.50	.17	80.0	–	(.40)	–	.16	.16	1.20	.39	(.04)	8.00	–	–
143	.45	(.21)	(.03)	18.0	–	(.21)	0	.05	.05	.39	.12	–	6.60	–	–
	1.50	(.70)	(.11)	60.0	–	(.70)	0	.16	.17	1.30	.39	–	22.00	–	–
144	Trace	–	Trace	0	0	Trace	0	0	0	0	Trace	Trace	Trace	Trace	0
	Trace	–	Trace	0	0	Tarce	0	0	0	0	Trace	Trace	Trace	Trace	0
145	–	–	–	0	–	–	0	0	0	0	–	–	–	–	–
	–	–	–	0	–	–	0	0	0	0	–	–	–	–	–
146	–	–	–	0	–	–	0	0	0	0	–	–	–	–	–
	–	–	–	0	–	–	0	0	0	0	–	–	–	–	–
147	0	–	–	0	–	–	0	0	0	0	–	–	–	–	–
	0	–	–	0	–	–	0	0	0	0	–	–	–	–	–
148	–	–	–	0	–	–	0	0	0	0	–	–	–	–	–
	–	–	–	0	–	–	0	0	0	0	–	–	–	–	–
149	–	–	–	–	–	–	–	–	–	–	–	–	–	–	–
	–	–	–	–	–	–	–	–	–	–	–	–	–	–	–
150	.59	–	–	–	–	–	–	.09	.20	1.34	.42	.07	–	–	0
	4.90	–	–	–	–	–	–	.71	1.65	11.20	3.50	.60	–	–	0
151	.64	–	–	88.0	–	–	.40	.06	.08	.48	–	–	–	–	–
	1.60	–	–	220.0	–	–	1.00	.16	.20	1.20	–	–	–	–	–
152	1.48	–	–	92.0	.	–	–	.06	.10	1.60	–	–	–	–	–
	3.70	–	–	230.0	–	–	–	.14	.24	4.00	–	–	–	–	–
153	.39	.17	–	51.3	5.34	–	.10	.06	.06	.42	.13	.03	3.81	–	.07
	1.41	.62	–	183.2	19.08	–	.35	.20	.20	1.50	.46	.09	13.59	–	.26
154	–	–	–	–	–	–	–	–	–	–	–	–	–	–	–
	–	–	–	–	–	–	–	–	–	–	–	–	–	–	–
155	.64	(.48)	(.09)	40.0	–	(.08)	–	.07	.09	.56	(.20)	(.02)	–	–	–
	1.60	(1.20)	(.22)	100.0	–	(.20)	–	.17	.23	1.40	(.50)	(.05)	–	–	–

(Continued)

TABLE F-21 *(Continued)*

Item No.	Food Item Name	Approximate Measure	Weight	Moisture	Food Energy Calories	Protein	Fats	Carbo-hydrates	Fiber	Minerals (Macro)				
										Calcium	Phosphorus	Sodium	Magnesium	Potassium
			(g)	(%)	(kcal)	(g)	(g)	(g)	(g)	(mg)	(mg)	(mg)	(mg)	(mg)
	PANCAKES & WAFFLES													
156	PANCAKES, home recipe, enriched	1 AVG	45	50.1	104.0	3.2	3.2	15.3	Trace	45.5	62.6	191.3	11.0	55.4
			100	50.1	231.0	7.1	7.0	34.1	.1	101.0	139.0	425.0	24.4	123.0
157	PANCAKE & WAFFLE MIX, BUCKWHEAT, prepared w/egg & milk	1 AVG	45	57.9	90.0	3.1	4.1	10.7	.2	99.0	151.7	208.8	–	110.3
			100	57.9	200.0	6.8	9.1	23.8	.4	220.0	337.0	464.0	–	245.0
158	WAFFLES, home recipe, enriched	1 MED	75	41.4	209.3	7.0	7.4	28.1	.1	84.8	129.8	356.3	–	108.8
			100	41.4	279.0	9.3	9.8	37.5	.1	113.0	173.0	475.0	–	145.0
	PIES (MADE W/VEGETABLE SHORTENING)													
159	APPLE	1 PIECE	118	47.6	302.1	2.6	13.1	45.0	.5	9.4	26.0	355.2	7.1	94.4
			100	47.6	256.0	2.2	11.1	38.1	.4	8.0	22.0	301.0	6.0	80.0
160	APPLE, DUTCH	1 SERV	200	–	519.5	2.6	21.0	82.0	.6	37.1	31.1	153.1	–	176.4
			100	–	259.7	1.3	10.4	41.0	.3	18.6	15.6	76.6	–	88.2
161	BANANA CUSTARD	1 PIECE	114	54.4	251.9	5.1	10.6	35.0	.2	75.2	93.5	221.2	14.8	231.4
			100	54.4	221.0	4.5	9.3	30.7	.2	66.0	82.0	194.0	13.0	203.0
162	BLACKBERRY	1 PIECE	118	51.0	286.7	3.1	13.0	40.6	2.2	22.4	30.7	316.2	7.1	118.0
			100	51.0	243.0	2.6	11.0	34.4	1.9	19.0	26.0	268.0	6.0	100.0
163	'BLUEBERRY	1 PIECE	114	51.0	275.9	2.7	12.3	39.8	.8	12.5	26.2	305.5	6.8	74.1
			100	51.0	242.0	2.4	10.8	34.9	.7	11.0	23.0	268.0	6.0	65.0
164	BOSTON CREAM, w/powdered sugar topping	1 PIECE	69	34.5	208.4	3.5	6.5	34.4	0	46.2	69.7	128.3	–	61.4
			100	34.5	302.0	5.0	9.4	49.9	0	67.0	101.0	186.0	–	89.0
165	BUTTERSCOTCH	1 PIECE	114	45.1	304.4	5.0	12.5	43.7	–	85.5	92.3	244.0	14.8	108.3
			100	45.1	267.0	4.4	11.0	38.3	–	75.0	81.0	214.0	13.0	95.0
166	CHERRY	1 PIECE	118	46.6	308.0	3.1	13.3	45.3	.1	16.5	29.5	358.7	7.1	123.9
			100	46.6	261.0	2.6	11.3	38.4	.1	14.0	25.0	304.0	6.0	105.0
167	CHOCOLATE CREAM	1 SERV	160	–	362.2	5.6	19.7	43.0	.3	96.6	119.2	169.0	–	192.7
			100	–	226.4	3.5	12.3	26.9	.2	60.4	74.5	105.6	–	120.4
168	COCONUT CUSTARD	1 PIECE	114	55.4	267.9	6.8	14.3	28.4	.2	107.2	132.2	281.6	14.8	185.8
			100	55.4	235.0	6.0	12.5	24.9	.2	94.0	116.0	247.0	13.0	163.0
169	CUSTARD	1 PIECE	114	58.1	248.5	7.0	12.7	26.7	–	109.4	128.8	327.2	–	156.2
			100	58.1	218.0	6.1	11.1	23.4	–	96.0	113.0	287.0	–	137.0
170	LEMON MERINGUE, homemade filling	1 PIECE	105	50.9	251.0	2.8	10.7	37.2	–	14.7	51.5	296.1	–	52.5
			100	50.9	239.0	2.7	10.2	35.4	–	14.0	49.0	282.0	–	50.0
171	MINCE	1 PIECE	118	43.0	319.8	3.0	13.6	48.6	.5	33.0	44.8	528.6	21.2	210.0
			100	43.0	271.0	2.5	11.5	41.2	.4	28.0	38.0	448.0	18.0	178.0
172	PEACH	1 PIECE	118	47.5	305.6	3.0	12.6	45.1	.5	11.8	34.2	316.2	7.1	175.8
			100	47.5	259.0	2.5	10.7	38.2	.4	10.0	29.0	268.0	6.0	149.0
173	PECAN	1 PIECE	103	19.5	430.5	5.3	23.6	52.8	.5	48.4	106.1	227.6	–	126.7
			100	19.5	418.0	5.1	22.9	51.3	.5	47.0	103.0	221.0	–	123.0
174	PINEAPPLE	1 PIECE	118	48.0	298.5	2.6	12.6	45.0	.2	15.3	24.8	319.8	–	85.0
			100	48.0	253.0	2.2	10.7	38.1	.2	13.0	21.0	271.0	–	72.0
175	PUMPKIN	1 PIECE	114	59.2	245.1	4.6	12.8	27.9	.6	58.1	78.7	244.0	14.8	182.4
			100	59.2	215.0	4.0	11.2	24.5	.5	51.0	69.0	214.0	13.0	160.0
176	RAISIN	1 PIECE	118	42.5	318.6	3.1	12.6	50.7	.4	21.2	47.2	336.3	–	226.6
			100	42.5	270.0	2.6	10.7	43.0	.3	18.0	40.0	285.0	–	192.0
177	RHUBARB	1 PIECE	118	47.4	298.5	3.0	12.6	45.1	.7	75.5	30.7	318.6	–	187.6
			100	47.4	253.0	2.5	10.7	38.2	.6	64.0	26.0	270.0	–	159.0
178	STRAWBERRY	1 PIECE	93	58.4	184.1	1.8	7.3	28.7	.7	14.9	23.3	180.4	–	111.6
			100	58.4	198.0	1.9	7.9	30.9	.8	16.0	25.0	194.0	–	120.0
179	PIECRUST, enriched, baked	1 AVG	180	14.9	900.0	11.0	60.1	78.8	.4	25.2	90.0	1099.8	25.2	90.0
			100	14.9	500.0	6.1	33.4	43.8	.2	14.0	50.0	611.0	14.0	50.0
180	PIECRUST, graham cracker, homemade	1 SERV	32	8.2	158.6	1.2	10.0	17.5	.2	8.3	23.7	183.6	2.8	57.3
			100	8.2	495.5	3.8	31.2	54.7	.5	25.8	73.9	573.7	8.6	179.1
	QUICK BREADS (MISCELLANEOUS)													
181	BISCUIT MIX, w/enriched flour & milk	1 AVG	28	28.5	91.0	2.0	2.6	14.6	.1	19.0	65.0	272.4	(6.7)	32.5
			100	28.5	325.0	7.1	9.3	52.3	.2	68.0	232.0	973.0	(24.0)	116.0
182	BISCUITS, BAKING POWDER, w/enriched flour	1 AVG	28	27.4	103.3	2.1	4.8	12.8	.2	33.9	49.0	175.3	6.2	32.8
			100	27.4	369.0	7.4	17.0	45.8	.2	121.0	175.0	626.0	22.0	117.0
183	CORN FRITTERS	1 MED	35	29.1	132.0	2.7	7.5	13.9	.2	22.4	54.3	167.0	–	46.6
			100	29.1	377.0	7.8	21.5	39.7	.5	64.0	155.0	477.0	–	133.0
184	CORNBREAD	1 OZ	28	43.8	77.4	1.7	3.2	10.7	–	15.0	24.1	59.8	4.9	36.3
			100	43.8	276.3	6.0	11.3	38.1	.2	53.5	85.9	213.7	17.6	129.5
185	DUMPLINGS	1 OZ	28	–	37.8	1.0	1.0	6.2	–	29.1	17.4	–	2.8	–
			100	–	135.0	3.6	3.4	22.2	–	104.0	62.0	–	10.0	–
186	EGGROLL	1 AVG	20	–	58.8	–	4.7	–	–	–	–	–	–	–
			100	–	294.0	–	23.6	–	–	–	–	–	–	–
187	GINGERBREAD, homemade	1 PIECE	117	30.8	370.9	4.4	12.5	60.8	.1	79.6	76.1	277.3	–	531.2
			100	30.8	317.0	3.8	10.7	52.0	.1	68.0	65.0	237.0	–	454.0

Item No.	Minerals (Micro)			Fat-Soluble Vitamins			Water-Soluble Vitamins								
	Iron	Zinc	Copper	Vitamin A	Vitamin D	Vitamin E (Alpha Tocopherol)	Vitamin C	Thiamin	Ribo-flavin	Niacin	Panto-thenic Acid	Vit. B-6 (Pyri-doxine)	Folacin (Folic Acid)	Biotin	Vitamin B-12
	(mg)	(mg)	(mg)	(IU)	(IU)	(mg)	(mg)	(mg)	(mg)	(mg)	(mg)	(mg)	(mcg)	(mcg)	(mcg)
156	.59	.37	(.02)	54.0	–	–	–	.15	.10	.59	–	.01	–	–	–
	1.30	.82	(.05)	120.0	–	–	–	.32	.22	1.30	–	.02	–	–	–
157	.59	–	–	103.5	–	–	–	.05	.07	.32	–	–	–	–	–
	1.30	–	–	230.0	–	–	–	.12	.16	.70	–	–	–	–	–
158	1.28	–	–	247.5	–	–	–	.36	.50	.98	–	.03	–	–	–
	1.70	–	–	330.0	–	–	–	.48	.66	1.30	–	.04	–	–	–
159	.35	.11	–	35.4	–	2.95	1.18	.02	.02	.47	.13	–	4.72	–	0
	.30	.09	–	30.0	–	2.50	1.00	.02	.02	.40	.11	–	4.00	–	0
160	2.04	–	–	118.2	–	–	2.40	.13	.08	1.38	–	–	–	–	–
	1.02	–	–	59.1	–	–	1.20	.07	.04	.69	–	–	–	–	–
161	.57	–	–	285.0	–	–	1.14	.05	.15	.34	–	–	–	–	–
	.50	–	–	250.0	–	–	1.00	.04	.13	.30	–	–	–	–	–
162	.59	–	–	106.2	–	–	4.72	.02	.02	.35	.22	–	–	–	0
	.50	–	–	90.0	–	–	4.00	.02	.02	.30	.18	–	–	–	0
163	.14	.01	–	34.2	–	20.18	3.42	.09	.07	.91	.21	–	–	–	–
	1.00	.01	–	30.0	–	17.70	3.00	.08	.06	.80	.18	–	–	–	–
164	.35	–	–	144.9	–	–	–	.02	.08	.14	–	–	–	–	–
	.50	–	–	210.0	–	–	–	.03	.11	.20	–	–	–	–	–
165	.03	–	–	296.4	–	–	–	.03	.11	.23	–	–	–	–	–
	.90	–	–	260.0	–	–	–	.03	.10	.20	–	–	–	–	–
166	.35	.05	–	519.2	–	–	–	.02	.02	.59	–	–	–	–	–
	.30	.04	–	440.0	–	–	–	.02	.02		–	–	–	–	–
167	1.02	–	–	179.2	–	–	.70	.09	.18	1.56	–	–	–	–	–
	.64	–	–	112.0	–	–	.44	.06	.11	.98	–	–	–	–	–
168	.80	–	–	262.2	–	–	0	.07	.22	.34	–	–	–	–	–
	.70	–	–	230.0	–	–	0	.06	.19	.30	–	–	–	–	–
169	.68	–	–	262.2	–	–	0	.06	.18	.34	1.08	–	–	–	0
	.60	–	–	230.0	–	–	0	.05	.16	.30	.95	–	–	–	0
170	.53	–	–	178.5	–	–	3.15	.03	.08	.21	–	–	–	–	–
	.50	–	–	170.0	–	–	3.00	.03	.08	.20	–	–	–	–	–
171	1.18	–	–	–	(.94)	(.94)	1.18	.08	.05	.47	(.12)	(.09)	(5.90)	(1.18)	0
	1.00	–	–	–	(.80)	(.80)	1.00	.07	.04	.40	(.10)	(.08)	(5.00)	(1.00)	0
172	.59	.11	–	861.4	–	–	3.54	.02	.05	.83	.14	–	–	–	0
	.50	.09	–	730.0	–	–	3.00	.02	.04	.70	.12	–	–	–	0
173	2.88	–	–	164.8	–	–	–	.17	.07	.31	–	–	–	–	–
	2.80	–	–	160.0	–	–	–	.16	.07	.30	–	–	–	–	–
174	.59	–	–	23.6	–	–	1.18	.05	.02	.47	–	–	–	–	–
	.50	–	–	20.0	–	–	1.00	.04	.02	.40	–	–	–	–	–
175	.57	–	–	2815.8	–	–	–	.03	.11	.57	.59	–	–	–	0
	.50	–	–	2470.0	–	–	–	.03	.10	.50	.52	–	–	–	0
176	1.06	–	–	–	–	–	1.18	.04	.04	.35	–	–	–	–	–
	.90	–	–	–	–	–	1.00	.03	.03	.30	–	–	–	–	–
177	.83	–	–	59.0	–	–	3.54	.02	.05	.35	.15	–	–	–	0
	.70	–	–	50.0	–	–	3.00	.02	.04	.30	.13	–	–	–	0
178	.65	–	–	37.2	–	–	23.25	.02	.04	.37	–	–	–	–	–
	.70	–	–	40.0	–	–	25.00	.02	.04	.40	–	–	–	–	–
179	3.06	–	–	0	–	.88	0	.36	.25	3.24	–	–	–	–	–
	1.70	–	–	0	–	.49	0	.20	.14	1.80	–	–	–	–	–
180	.24	.12	.05	326.4	0	.19	0	.01	.03	.22	0	0	.32	–	.02
	.76	.36	.15	1019.0	0	.60	0	.02	.10	.68	0	Trace	1.00	–	.05
181	.64	(.34)	(.09)	–	–	(.06)	–	.08	.07	.56	(.11)	(.01)	–	–	–
	2.30	(1.20)	(.31)	–	–	(.20)	–	.27	.25	2.00	(.40)	(.04)	–	–	–
182	.45	–	–	–	–	–	–	.06	.06	.50	–	–	–	–	–
	1.60	–	–	–	–	–	–	.21	.21	1.80	–	–	–	–	–
183	.60	–	–	140.0	–	–	.70	.06	.07	.56	–	–	–	–	–
	1.70	–	–	400.0	–	–	2.00	.16	.20	1.60	–	–	–	–	–
184	.39	.17	–	51.3	5.34	–	.10	.06	.06	.42	.13	.03	3.81	–	.07
	1.41	.62	–	183.2	19.08	–	.35	.20	.20	1.50	.46	.09	13.59	–	.26
185	.22	–	–	8.4	–	–	0	.04	.04	.36	–	.01	–	–	.02
	.80	–	–	30.0	–	–	0	.14	.14	1.30	–	.02	–	–	.07
186	–	–	–	–	–	–	–	–	–	–	–	–	–	–	–
	–	–	–	–	–	–	–	–	–	–	–	–	–	–	–
187	2.69	–	–	105.3	–	–	0	.14	.13	1.05	–	–	–	–	–
	2.30	–	–	90.0	–	–	0	.12	.11	.90	–	–	–	–	–

(Continued)

TABLE F-21 *(Continued)*

Item No.	Food Item Name	Approximate Measure	Weight (g)	Moisture (%)	Food Energy Calories (kcal)	Protein (g)	Fats (g)	Carbohydrates (g)	Fiber (g)	Minerals (Macro) Calcium (mg)	Phosphorus (mg)	Sodium (mg)	Magnesium (mg)	Potassium (mg)
188	POPOVERS, home recipe, enriched, baked	1 AVG	40	54.9	89.6	3.5	3.7	10.3	Trace	38.4	56.0	88.0	–	60.0
			100	54.9	224.0	8.8	9.2	25.8	.1	96.0	140.0	220.0	–	150.0
189	SPOONBREAD, w/white, whole-ground cornmeal	1 AVG	96	–	187.2	6.4	10.9	16.2	.3	92.2	157.4	462.7	–	126.7
			100	–	195.0	6.7	11.4	16.9	.3	96.0	164.0	482.0	–	132.0
190	TACO SHELL	1 AVG	11	–	48.0	.9	2.2	7.6	–	38.2	–	–	–	–
			100	–	436.0	8.3	20.3	68.8	–	347.0	–	–	–	–
191	TORTILLA, lime-treated, yellow corn, 6" in diameter	1 AVG	30	47.5	63.0	1.4	.5	13.6	.2	58.8	41.4	–	(32.1)	–
			100	47.5	210.0	4.6	1.8	45.3	.8	196.0	138.0	–	(107.0)	–
	ROLLS													
192	BAGEL, made w/egg	1 AVG	55	32.0	165.0	6.0	2.0	28.0	–	8.8	–	–	–	–
			100	32.0	300.0	10.9	3.6	50.9	–	16.0	–	–	–	–
193	BROWN & SERVE, enriched, unbrowned	1 AVG	28	33.0	83.7	2.2	1.9	14.2	.1	13.2	23.0	143.6	–	25.5
			100	33.0	299.0	7.9	6.8	50.6	.2	47.0	82.0	513.0	–	91.0
194	CINNAMON	1 AVG	55	31.5	173.8	4.7	5.0	27.1	.1	46.8	58.9	214.0	18.0	68.2
			100	31.5	316.0	8.5	9.1	49.3	.2	85.0	107.0	389.0	32.7	124.0
195	DANISH PASTRY, ready to serve	1 SM	35	22.0	147.7	2.6	8.2	16.0	Trace	17.5	38.2	128.1	8.0	39.2
			100	22.0	422.0	7.4	23.5	45.6	.1	50.0	109.0	366.0	22.9	112.0
196	HARD, enriched, ready to serve	1 AVG	25	25.4	78.0	2.5	.8	14.9	.1	11.8	23.0	156.3	5.7	24.3
			100	25.4	312.0	9.8	3.2	59.5	.2	47.0	92.0	625.0	22.9	97.0
197	SWEET, ready to serve	1 AVG	55	31.5	173.8	4.7	5.0	27.1	.1	46.8	58.9	214.0	18.0	68.2
			100	31.5	316.0	8.5	9.1	49.3	.2	85.0	107.0	389.0	32.7	124.0
198	WHOLE WHEAT, ready to serve	1 AVG	35	32.0	90.0	3.5	1.0	18.3	.6	37.1	98.4	197.4	40.0	102.2
			100	32.0	257.0	10.0	2.8	52.3	1.6	106.0	281.0	564.0	114.3	292.0
199	RUSK OR RUSKETT	1 PIECE	9	4.8	37.7	1.2	.8	6.4	Trace	1.8	10.7	22.1	–	14.5
			100	4.8	419.0	13.8	8.7	71.0	.2	20.0	119.0	246.0	–	161.0
	ALCOHOLIC													
200	ALE, mild	1 CUP	230	–	98.9	1.1	–	8.0	–	29.9	41.4	–	–	–
			100	–	43.0	.5	–	3.5	–	13.0	18.0	–	–	–
201	BEER, natural light	1 CUP	240	–	66.7	.2	0	4.0	–	–	–	–	–	–
			100	–	27.8	.1	0	1.7	–	–	–	–	–	–
202	BEER, 4.5% alcohol by volume	1 CUP	240	92.1	100.8	.7	0	9.1	0	12.0	72.0	16.8	24.0	60.0
			100	92.1	42.0	.3	0	3.8	0	5.0	30.0	7.0	10.0	25.0
203	BRANDY	1 OZ	30	–	72.9	–	–	–	–	–	–	–	–	–
			100	–	243.0	–	–	–	–	–	–	–	–	–
	CORDIAL													
204	ANISETTE	1 CORDIAL	20	–	74.0	–	–	7.0	–	–	–	–	–	–
			100	–	370.0	–	–	35.0	–	–	–	–	–	–
205	APRICOT BRANDY	1 CORDIAL	20	–	64.0	–	–	6.0	–	–	–	–	–	–
			100	–	320.0	–	–	30.0	–	–	–	–	–	–
206	CREME DE MENTHE	1 CORDIAL	20	–	67.0	–	–	6.0	–	–	–	–	–	–
			100	–	335.0	–	–	30.0	–	–	–	–	–	–
207	DAIQUIRI	1 CUP	240	–	292.8	.2	26.9	12.5	–	9.6	7.2	–	–	–
			100	–	122.0	.1	11.2	5.2	–	4.0	3.0	–	–	–
208	GIN/RUM/VODKA/WHISKEY, 80-proof	1 OZ	30	66.6	69.3	0	–	–	0	–	–	.3	0	.6
			100	66.6	231.0	0	–	–	0	–	–	1.0	0	2.0
209	HIGHBALL	1 CUP	240	–	165.6	–	–	–	0	–	–	–	–	–
			100	–	69.0	–	–	–	0	–	–	–	–	–
210	MANHATTAN	1 COCKTAIL	100	–	164.0	–	–	7.9	0	1.0	1.0	–	–	–
			100	–	164.0	–	–	7.9	0	1.0	1.0	–	–	–
211	MARTINI	1 COCKTAIL	100	–	140.0	.1	15.4	.3	0	5.0	1.0	–	–	–
			100	–	140.0	.1	15.4	.3	0	5.0	1.0	–	–	–
212	MINT JULEP	1 OZ	30	–	21.0	–	–	.3	0	–	–	–	–	–
			100	–	70.0	–	–	.9	0	–	–	–	–	–
213	OLD FASHIONED	1 OZ	30	–	53.7	–	–	1.1	0	–	–	–	–	–
			100	–	179.0	–	–	3.5	0	–	–	–	–	–
214	SCOTCH	1 OZ	30	–	67.8	–	–	–	0	–	–	–	–	–
			100	–	226.0	–	–	–	0	–	–	–	–	–
215	TOM COLLINS	1 OZ	30	–	18.0	Trace	1.6	.9	0	.6	.6	–	–	–
			100	–	60.0	.1	5.3	3.0	0	2.0	2.0	–	–	–
216	WHISKEY SOUR	1 COCKTAIL	75	65.3	138.0	.2	0	7.7	0	1.5	3.0	.8	–	93.8
			100	65.3	184.0	.2	0	10.3	0	2.0	4.0	1.0	–	125.0
	WINES													
217	CHAMPAGNE, domestic	WINE GLASS	120	–	84.0	.2	7.9	3.0	0	–	–	–	–	–
			100	–	70.0	.2	6.6	2.5	0	–	–	–	–	–
218	DESSERT, 18.8% alcohol by volume	1 CUP	240	76.7	328.8	.2	0	18.5	0	19.2	–	9.6	21.6	180.0
			100	76.7	137.0	.1	0	7.7	0	8.0	–	4.0	9.0	75.0
219	MUSCATELLE OR PORT	WINE GLASS	100	–	158.0	.2	11.2	14.0	0	8.0	–	4.0	–	75.0
			100	–	158.0	.2	11.2	14.0	0	8.0	–	4.0	–	75.0

Item No.	Minerals (Micro)			Fat-Soluble Vitamins			Water-Soluble Vitamins								
	Iron	Zinc	Copper	Vitamin A	Vitamin D	Vitamin E (Alpha Tocopherol)	Vitamin C	Thiamin	Ribo-flavin	Niacin	Panto-thenic Acid	Vit. B-6 (Pyri-doxine)	Folacin (Folic Acid)	Biotin	Vitamin B-12
	(mg)	(mg)	(mg)	(IU)	(IU)	(mg)	(mg)	(mg)	(mg)	(mg)	(mg)	(mg)	(mcg)	(mcg)	(mcg)
188	.60	–	–	132.0	–	–	–	.06	.10	.40	–	–	–	–	–
	1.50	–	–	330.0	–	–	–	.14	.25	1.00	–	–	–	–	–
189	.96	–	–	278.4	–	–	–	.09	.17	.38	–	–	–	–	–
	1.00	–	–	290.0	–	–	–	.09	.18	.40	–	–	–	–	–
190	.34	.14	.04	5.0	–	–	.01	Trace	.01	.21	–	–	–	–	–
	3.06	1.29	.32	45.0	–	–	.10	.01	.06	1.86	–	–	–	–	–
191	.78	(.03)	(.06)	6.0	–	(.03)	0	.05	.02	.30	(.03)	(.02)	–	–	–
	2.60	(.10)	(.19)	20.0	–	(.10)	0	.15	.05	1.00	(.10)	(.07)	–	–	–
192	1.21	.53	–	30.3	–	–	0	.14	.10	1.20	–	–	–	–	–
	2.20	.96	–	55.0	–	–	0	.25	.18	2.18	–	–	–	–	–
193	.50	–	–	–	–	–	–	.07	.06	.59	.09	.01	–	–	–
	1.80	–	–	–	–	–	–	.24	.20	2.10	.31	.04	–	–	–
194	.44	–	–	38.5	–	–	–	.04	.08	.44	.17	.02	–	–	–
	.80	–	–	70.0	–	–	–	.07	.15	.80	.31	.04	–	–	–
195	.32	–	–	108.5	–	–	–	.03	.05	.23	.11	.01	–	–	–
	.90	–	–	310.0	–	–	–	.07	.15	.80	.31	.04	–	–	–
196	.58	.28	–	–	–	–	–	.07	.06	.68	.08	.01	–	–	–
	2.30	1.13	–	–	–	–	–	.26	.23	2.70	.31	.04	–	–	–
197	.44	–	–	38.5	–	–	–	.04	.08	.44	.17	.02	–	–	–
	.80	–	–	70.0	–	–	–	.07	.15	.80	.31	.04	–	–	–
198	.84	–	–	–	–	–	–	.12	.05	1.05	–	–	–	–	–
	2.40	–	–	–	–	–	–	.34	.13	3.00	–	–	–	–	–
199	.12	–	–	20.7	–	–	–	.01	.02	.10	–	.01	–	–	–
	1.30	–	–	230.0	–	–	–	.08	.22	1.10	–	.09	–	–	–
200	.23	–	–	0	0	–	0	–	.07	.48	–	–	–	–	–
	.10	–	–	0	0	–	0	–	.03	.21	–	–	–	–	–
201	–	–	–	–	–	–	–	–	–	–	–	–	14.40	–	–
	–	–	–	–	–	–	–	–	–	–	–	–	6.00	–	–
202	–	.07	.09	0	–	–	0	–	.07	1.44	.19	.14	14.40	–	0
	–	.03	.04	0	–	–	0	–	.03	.60	.08	.06	6.00	–	0
203	–	.02	.01	–	–	–	–	–	–	–	–	–	–	–	–
	–	.07	.05	–	–	–	–	–	–	–	–	–	–	–	–
204	–	–	–	–	–	–	–	–	–	–	–	–	–	–	–
	–	–	–	–	–	–	–	–	–	–	–	–	–	–	–
205	–	–	–	–	–	–	–	–	–	–	–	–	–	–	–
	–	–	–	–	–	–	–	–	–	–	–	–	–	–	–
206	–	–	–	–	–	–	–	–	–	–	–	–	–	–	–
	–	–	–	–	–	–	–	–	–	–	–	–	–	–	–
207	.24	–	–	0	0	–	19.20	0	0	–	–	–	–	–	–
	.10	–	–	0	0	–	8.00	0	0	–	–	–	–	–	–
208	–	.01	.01	0	–	–	0	0	0	0	–	–	–	–	–
	–	.03	.02	0	–	–	0	0	0	0	–	–	–	–	–
209	–	–	–	–	–	–	–	–	–	–	–	–	–	–	–
	–	–	–	–	–	–	–	–	–	–	–	–	–	–	–
210	–	–	–	35.0	–	–	0	0	0	0	–	–	–	–	–
	–	–	–	35.0	–	–	0	0	0	0	–	–	–	–	–
211	.10	–	–	4.0	–	–	0	0	0	0	–	–	–	–	–
	.10	–	–	4.0	–	–	0	0	0	0	–	–	–	–	–
212	–	–	–	–	–	–	–	–	–	–	–	–	–	–	–
	–	–	–	–	–	–	–	–	–	–	–	–	–	–	–
213	–	–	–	–	–	–	–	–	–	–	–	–	–	–	–
	–	–	–	–	–	–	–	–	–	–	–	–	–	–	–
214	–	.01	–	–	–	–	–	–	–	–	–	–	–	–	–
	–	.02	–	–	–	–	–	–	–	–	–	–	–	–	–
215	0	–	–	0	0	–	2.10	0	0	0	–	–	–	–	–
	0	–	–	0	0	–	7.00	0	0	0	–	–	–	–	–
216	–	–	–	3.8	0	–	7.50	.02	0	–	–	–	–	–	–
	–	–	–	5.0	0	–	10.00	.02	0	–	–	–	–	–	–
217	–	–	–	–	–	–	–	–	–	–	–	–	.60	–	–
	–	–	–	–	–	–	–	–	–	–	–	–	.50	–	–
218	–	–	–	–	–	–	–	.02	.05	.48	.07	.10	.72	–	0
	–	–	–	–	–	–	–	.01	.02	.20	.03	.04	.30	–	0
219	–	–	–	–	–	–	–	.01	.01	.17	–	–	2.00	–	–
	–	–	–	–	–	–	–	.01	.01	.17	–	–	2.00	–	–

(Continued)

TABLE F-21 *(Continued)*

Item No.	Food Item Name	Approximate Measure	Weight (g)	Moisture (%)	Food Energy Calories (kcal)	Protein (g)	Fats (g)	Carbo-hydrates (g)	Fiber (g)	Minerals (Macro) Calcium (mg)	Phos-phorus (mg)	Sodium (mg)	Mag-nesium (mg)	Potas-sium (mg)
	WINES (Continued)													
220	*ROSE	WINE GLASS	100	—	71.5	.1	0	2.8	0	12.3	6.2	4.0	7.3	75.0
			100	—	71.5	.1	0	2.8	0	12.3	6.2	4.0	7.3	75.0
221	SAUTERNE, California	WINE GLASS	100	—	84.0	.2	—	4.0	0	—	—	—	—	—
			100	—	84.0	.2	—	4.0	0	—	—	—	—	—
222	SHERRY, domestic	1 OZ	30	—	42.0	.1	3.6	2.4	0	2.4	(3.0)	1.2	(3.3)	22.5
			100	—	140.0	.3	11.9	8.0	0	8.0	(10.0)	4.0	(10.9)	75.0
223	TABLE, 12.2% alcohol by volume	1 CUP	240	85.6	204.0	.2	0	10.1	0	21.6	24.0	12.0	21.6	220.8
			100	85.6	85.0	.1	0	4.2	0	9.0	10.0	5.0	9.0	92.0
224	VERMOUTH, French	WINE GLASS	100	—	105.0	.1	0	1.0	0	8.0	(7.6)	4.0	(5.8)	75.0
			100	—	105.0	.1	0	1.0	0	8.0	(7.6)	4.0	(5.8)	75.0
	NONALCOHOLIC													
225	CLUB SODA, carbonated, unsweetened	1 CUP	240	100.0	0	0	0	0	0	7.2	—	—	—	—
			100	100.0	0	0	0	0	0	3.0	—	—	—	—
	COFFEE													
226	GROUND, prepared	1 CUP	240	—	7.2	.4	.2	1.1	0	7.2	7.2	Trace	(15.1)	159.1
			100	—	3.0	.2	.1	.4	0	3.0	3.0	Trace	(6.3)	66.3
227	INSTANT, prepared	1 CUP	240	98.1	2.4	—	—	—	—	4.8	9.6	2.4	16.1	86.4
			100	98.1	1.0	—	—	—	—	2.0	4.0	1.0	6.7	36.0
228	DECAFFEINATED, instant, prepared	1 CUP	240	98.1	2.4	Trace	Trace	Trace	Trace	4.8	9.6	2.4	—	86.4
			100	98.1	1.0	Trace	Trace	Trace	Trace	2.0	4.0	1.0	—	36.0
229	COLA	1 CUP	240	90.0	85.7	0	0	24.0	0	7.2	(36.7)	(19.7)	(2.9)	(2.6)
			100	90.0	35.7	0	0	10.0	0	3.0	(15.3)	(8.2)	(1.2)	(1.1)
230	COLA, diet	1 SERV	360	99.6	0	0	0	0	—	35.0	—	50.4	4.0	4.0
			100	99.6	0	0	0	0	—	9.7	—	14.0	1.1	1.1
231	CREAM SODA	1 CUP	240	89.0	103.2	0	0	26.4	0	7.2	—	—	—	—
			100	89.0	43.0	0	0	11.0	0	3.0	—	—	—	—
232	DIET DRINKS, w/artificial sweetener, 1 cal/oz	1 CUP	240	100.0	—	0	0	—	0	24.0	—	—	—	—
			100	100.0	—	0	0	—	0	10.0	—	—	—	—
233	GINGER ALE	1 CUP	240	92.0	74.4	0	0	19.2	0	7.2	—	16.8	—	—
			100	92.0	31.0	0	0	8.0	0	3.0	—	7.0	—	—
234	ICE CREAM SODA	1 CUP	345	—	262.2	2.3	7.2	48.7	—	69.0	55.2	—	—	—
			100	—	76.0	.7	2.1	14.1	—	20.0	16.0	—	—	—
235	QUININE SODA, carbonated, sweetened	1 CUP	240	92.0	74.4	0	0	19.2	0	24.0	—	—	—	—
			100	92.0	31.0	0	0	8.0	0	10.0	—	—	—	—
236	ROOT BEER	1 CUP	240	89.5	98.4	0	0	25.2	0	7.2	—	—	—	—
			100	89.5	41.0	0	0	10.5	0	3.0	—	—	—	—
237	SEVEN-UP	1 CUP	230	—	92.0	0	0	23.0	0	0	0	2.3	—	0
			100	—	40.0	0	0	10.0	0	0	0	1.0	—	0
238	TEA, instant, water-soluble solids	1 CUP	240	99.4	4.8	—	—	1.0	—	16.8	0	2.4	10.1	60.0
			100	99.4	2.0	—	—	.4	—	7.0	0	1.0	4.2	25.0
239	TONIC WATER	1 CUP	240	—	88.0	0	0	22.0	—	—	—	0	—	—
			100	—	36.7	0	0	9.2	—	—	—	0	—	—
	CEREALS													
	ACHITA, AMARANTH													
240	WHOLE GRAIN	1 OZ	28	12.3	100.2	3.6	2.0	18.2	1.9	69.2	140.0	—	—	—
			100	12.3	358.0	12.9	7.2	65.1	6.7	247.0	500.0	—	—	—
241	TOASTED	1 OZ	28	4.3	108.1	3.8	2.3	19.9	2.8	81.8	144.8	—	—	—
			100	4.3	386.0	13.5	8.2	71.1	10.0	292.0	517.0	—	—	—
242	ARROWROOT	1 TBLS	8	—	29.0	0	0	7.0	0	0	0	4.0	—	1.4
			100	—	362.0	0	0	87.5	0	0	0	50.0	—	18.0
243	BARLEY, PEARLED, *light, boiled	1 OZ	28	—	33.6	.8	.2	7.7	Trace	.9	19.0	.3	2.0	1.2
			100	—	120.0	2.8	.6	27.5	.2	3.2	71.0	1.0	7.3	40.0
244	BUCKWHEAT, WHOLE GRAIN	1 CUP	100	11.0	360.0	11.7	2.4	72.9	9.9	114.0	282.0	—	252.6	448.0
			100	11.0	360.0	11.7	2.4	72.9	9.9	114.0	282.0	—	252.6	448.0
245	BULGUR, DRY (from Hard Red Winter Wheat)	1 TBLS	14	10.0	50.5	1.6	.2	10.6	.2	4.1	47.3	.6	22.4	32.1
			100	10.0	361.0	11.2	1.5	75.7	1.7	29.0	338.0	4.0	160.0	229.0
246	CANIHUA (CHENOPODIUM), *WHOLE GRAIN, flakes	1 OZ	28	8.1	102.5	4.9	2.3	17.3	3.1	47.9	138.9	—	—	—
			100	8.1	366.0	17.6	8.3	61.7	11.0	171.0	496.0	—	—	—
247	CORNMEAL, degermed, enriched, cooked	1 CUP	238	87.7	119.0	2.6	.5	25.5	.2	2.4	33.3	—	16.7	38.1
			100	87.7	50.0	1.1	.2	10.7	.1	1.0	14.0	—	7.0	16.0
	GRITS													
248	CORN, degermed, enriched, cooked	1 CUP	242	87.1	121.0	2.9	.2	26.6	.2	2.4	24.2	—	7.3	26.6
			100	87.1	50.0	1.2	.1	11.0	.1	1.0	10.0	—	3.0	11.0
249	HOMINY, enriched, dry	1 CUP	156	10.7	558.5	13.3	1.4	123.4	.8	3.1	121.7	1.6	31.2	166.9
			100	10.7	358.0	8.5	.9	79.1	.5	2.0	78.0	1.0	20.0	107.0
250	*JOB'S TEARS, whole seed, hulled	1 OZ	28	15.0	85.7	3.4	1.9	18.2	.2	12.9	41.4	—	—	61.0
			100	15.0	306.0	12.0	6.7	64.9	.8	46.0	148.0	—	—	218.0
251	MALT EXTRACT, dried	1 TBLS	8	3.2	29.4	.5	—	7.1	—	3.8	23.5	6.4	11.2	18.4
			100	3.2	367.0	6.0	—	89.2	—	48.0	294.0	80.0	140.0	230.0

Item No.	Iron (mg)	Zinc (mg)	Copper (mg)	Vitamin A (IU)	Vitamin D (IU)	Vitamin E (Alpha Tocopherol) (mg)	Vitamin C (mg)	Thiamin (mg)	Riboflavin (mg)	Niacin (mg)	Pantothenic Acid (mg)	Vit. B-6 (Pyridoxine) (mg)	Folacin (Folic Acid) (mcg)	Biotin (mcg)	Vitamin B-12 (mcg)
220	.96	.05	.02	Trace	0	–	0	Trace	.01	.08	.03	.02	.21	0	Trace
	.96	.05	.02	Trace	0	–	0	Trace	.01	.08	.03	.02	.21	0	Trace
221	–	–	–	–	–	–	–	–	–	–	–	–	.50	–	–
	–	–	–	–	–	–	–	–	–	–	–	–	.50	–	–
222	(.12)	–	(.04)	Trace	0	0	0	Trace	Trace	.05	–	Trace	.60	–	Trace
	(.38)	–	(.12)	Trace	0	0	0	.01	.01	.17	–	.01	2.00	–	Trace
223	.96	.24	–	–	–	–	–	–	.02	.24	.07	.10	4.80	–	0
	.40	.10	–	–	–	–	–	–	.01	.10	.03	.04	2.00	–	0
224	(.35)	(.05)	(.06)	0	0	0	0	.01	.01	.17	–	Trace	.50	–	Trace
	(.35)	(.05)	(.06)	0	0	0	0	.01	.01	.17	–	Trace	.50	–	Trace
225	–	–	–	0	–	–	0	0	0	.00	–	–	–	–	–
	--	–	–	0	–	–	0	0	0	.00	–	–	–	–	–
226	.24	.07	Trace	0	0	–	0	0	0	1.20	–	–	–	–	–
	.10	.03	Trace	0	0	–	0	0	0	.50	–	–	–	–	–
227	.24	.07	.01	0	–	0	0	0	–	.72	.01	–	–	–	0
	.10	.03	Trace	0	–	0	0	0	–	.30	Trace	–	–	–	0
228	.24	.02	–	0	–	–	0	0	Trace	.72	–	–	–	–	–
	.10	.01	–	0	–	–	0	0	Trace	.30	–	–	–	–	–
229	Trace	Trace	(.07)	0	0	0	0	0	0	0	0	0	0	0	0
	Trace	Trace	(.03)	0	0	0	0	0	0	0	0	0	0	0	0
230	.20	–	–	0	–	–	75.00	0	0	0	–	–	–	–	–
	.06	–	–	0	–	–	20.83	0	0	0	–	–	–	–	–
231	–	–	–	0	–	–	0	0	0	0	–	–	–	–	–
	–	–	–	0	–	–	0	0	0	0	–	–	–	–	–
232	–	–	–	0	–	–	0	0	0	0	–	–	–	–	–
	–	–	–	0	–	–	0	0	0	0	–	–	–	–	–
233	–	–	–	0	–	–	0	0	0	0	–	–	–	–	–
	–	–	–	0	–	–	0	0	0	0	–	–	–	–	–
234	0	–	–	296.7	0	–	1.04	.04	.10	.07	–	–	–	–	–
	0	–	–	86.0	0	–	.30	.01	.03	.02	–	–	–	–	–
235	–	–	–	0	–	–	0	0	0	0	–	–	–	–	–
	–	–	–	0	–	–	0	0	0	0	–	–	–	–	–
236	–	.02	–	0	–	–	0	0	0	0	–	–	–	–	–
	–	.01	–	0	–	–	0	0	0	0	–	–	–	–	–
237	0	–	–	0	0	0	0	0	0	0	0	0	0	0	0
	0	–	–	0	0	0	0	0	0	0	0	0	0	0	0
238	0	.10	.02	–	–	–	–	–	.02	–	–	–	–	–	–
	0	.04	.01	–	–	–	–	–	.01	–	–	–	–	–	–
239	–	–	–	–	–	–	–	–	–	–	–	–	–	–	–
	–	–	–	–	–	–	–	–	–	–	–	–	–	–	–
240	.95	–	–	0	–	–	.84	.04	.09	.28	–	–	–	–	–
	3.40	–	–	0	–	–	3.00	.14	.32	1.00	–	–	–	–	–
241	.45	–	–	–	–	–	–	0	.09	.31	–	–	–	–	–
	1.60	–	–	–	–	–	–	0	.32	1.10	–	–	–	–	–
242	0	.01	Trace	0	0	Trace	0	0	0	0	–	Trace	Trace	Trace	0
	0	.07	.01	0	0	Trace	0	0	0	0	–	Trace	Trace	Trace	0
243	.08	.02	.01	0	0	Trace	–	–	–	–	–	–	–	–	–
	.30	.07	.05	0	0	Trace	–	–	–	–	–	–	–	–	–
244	3.10	–	.82	0	–	–	0	.60	–	4.40	–	–	–	–	–
	3.10	–	.82	0	–	–	0	.60	–	4.40	–	–	–	–	–
245	.52	–	–	0	–	–	0	.04	.02	.63	–	.03	5.74	–	0
	3.70	–	–	0	–	–	0	.28	.14	4.50	–	.23	41.00	–	0
246	4.20	–	–	–	–	–	.28	.16	.27	.45	–	–	–	–	–
	15.00	–	–	–	–	–	1.00	.57	.95	1.60	–	–	–	–	–
247	.95	.24	–	142.8	–	1.52	0	.14	.10	1.19	1.64	–	21.42	–	–
	.40	.10	–	60.0	–	.64	0	.06	.04	.50	.69	–	9.00	–	–
248	.73	–	–	145.2	–	.75	0	.04	.03	.40	–	–	–	–	–
	.30	–	–	60.0	–	.31	0	.02	.02	.20	–	–	–	–	–
249	4.46	0	.06	0	0	–	0	.69	.41	5.49	0	.19	18.72	6.24	0
	2.86	0	.04	0	0	–	0	.44	.26	3.52	0	.12	12.00	4.00	0
250	.20	–	–	–	–	–	0	.12	.03	.64	–	–	–	–	–
	.70	–	–	–	–	–	0	.41	.10	2.30	–	–	–	–	–
251	.70	–	–	–	–	–	–	.03	.04	.78	–	–	–	–	–
	8.70	–	–	–	–	–	–	.36	.45	9.80	–	–	–	–	–

(Continued)

TABLE F-21 (Continued)

Item No.	Food Item Name	Approximate Measure	Weight (g)	Moisture (%)	Food Energy Calories (kcal)	Protein (g)	Fats (g)	Carbohydrates (g)	Fiber (g)	Calcium (mg)	Phosphorus (mg)	Sodium (mg)	Magnesium (mg)	Potassium (mg)
	MILLET													
252	³BULRUSH, WHOLE GRAIN, dried	1 OZ	28	12.0	95.5	2.9	1.1	20.0	.5	6.2	80.1	–	–	–
			100	12.0	341.0	.4	4.0	71.6	1.9	22.0	286.0	–	–	–
253	PROSO (BROOMCORN, HOG MILLET), WHOLE GRAIN	1 CUP	230	11.8	846.4	22.8	9.4	167.7	7.4	46.0	715.3	–	384.1	989.0
			100	11.8	368.0	9.9	4.1	72.9	3.2	20.0	311.0	–	167.0	430.0
254	OATS, WHOLE GRAIN	1 CUP	80	–	–	–	–	–	–	–	–	–	135.2	–
			100	–	–	–	–	–	–	–	–	–	169.0	–
255	QUINOA (CHENOPODIUM), ⁵WHOLE GRAIN	1 OZ	28	11.0	98.3	3.4	1.7	19.0	1.3	31.4	80.1	–	–	–
			100	11.0	351.0	12.3	6.1	67.7	4.6	112.0	286.0	–	–	–
	RICE													
256	BRAN	1 OZ	28	9.7	77.3	3.7	4.4	14.2	.4	21.3	388.1	–	–	418.6
			100	9.7	276.0	13.3	15.8	50.8	1.5	76.0	1386.0	–	–	1495.0
257	BROWN, cooked	1 CUP	150	70.3	178.5	3.8	1.2	38.3	.5	18.0	109.5	423.0	43.5	105.0
			100	70.3	119.0	2.5	.8	25.5	.3	12.0	73.0	282.0	29.0	70.0
258	WHITE, enriched (all varieties), cooked	1 CUP	150	72.6	160.5	3.0	.3	36.3	.2	15.0	42.0	561.0	12.0	42.0
			100	72.6	107.0	2.0	.2	24.2	.1	10.0	28.0	374.0	8.0	28.0
259	RYE, WHOLE GRAIN	1 CUP	185	12.1	669.7	22.4	4.1	135.8	3.7	70.3	695.6	1.9	246.6	864.0
			100	12.1	362.0	12.1	2.2	73.4	2.0	38.0	376.0	1.0	133.3	467.0
260	SAFFLOWER SEED, KERNELS, dry	1 OZ	28	5.0	172.2	5.3	16.7	3.5	–	–	–	–	–	–
			100	5.0	615.0	19.1	59.5	12.4	–	–	–	–	–	–
261	SEMOLINA, low protein, cooked	1 OZ	28	10.0	95.2	.1	0	23.9	1.1	–	–	2.2	–	.6
			100	10.0	340.0	.5	.1	85.3	4.0	–	–	8.0	–	2.0
262	SORGHUM GRAIN, all types	1 OZ	28	11.0	102.5	3.1	.9	20.4	.5	7.8	80.4	–	–	98.0
			100	11.0	366.0	11.0	3.3	73.0	1.7	28.0	287.0	–	–	350.0
	TEFF													
263	³WHOLE GRAIN, red	1 OZ	28	12.5	91.8	2.7	.7	20.2	.8	48.2	87.6	–	–	–
			100	12.5	328.0	9.6	2.6	72.0	2.7	172.0	313.0	–	–	–
264	³WHOLE GRAIN, white	1 OZ	28	11.3	93.0	2.4	.5	21.1	.6	40.9	106.4	–	–	–
			100	11.3	332.0	8.7	1.9	75.5	2.3	146.0	380.0	–	–	–
265	⁵TEOSINTE, milled	1 OZ	28	12.0	93.5	6.0	.7	17.7	.1	2.5	54.3	–	–	–
			100	12.0	334.0	21.6	2.5	63.1	.4	9.0	194.0	–	–	–
	WHEAT													
266	WHOLE GRAIN, white	1 CUP	198	14.0	706.9	18.6	4.0	149.3	3.8	71.3	780.1	5.9	316.8	772.2
			100	14.0	357.0	9.4	2.0	75.4	1.9	36.0	394.0	3.0	160.0	390.0
267	BRAN, unprocessed	1 TBLS	9	14.0	31.8	1.4	.4	5.6	.8	10.7	114.8	.8	53.8	100.9
			100	14.0	353.0	16.0	4.6	61.9	9.1	119.0	1276.0	9.0	597.9	1121.0
268	GERM, unprocessed	1 TBLS	9	14.0	35.2	2.4	1.0	4.2	.2	6.5	100.6	.3	30.6	74.4
			100	14.0	391.0	26.6	10.9	46.7	2.5	72.0	1118.0	3.0	340.0	827.0
269	GERM, toasted	1 TBLS	6	4.2	23.5	1.5	.7	3.0	.1	2.8	65.0	.1	21.9	56.8
			100	4.2	391.0	25.2	11.5	49.5	1.7	47.0	1084.0	2.0	364.9	947.0
270	WILD RICE, raw	1 CUP	112	8.5	395.4	15.8	.8	84.3	1.1	21.3	379.7	7.8	144.5	246.4
			100	8.5	353.0	14.1	.7	75.3	1.0	19.0	339.0	7.0	129.0	220.0
271	WILD-WHITE RICE MIX	1 CUP	112	4.2	228.5	6.6	1.1	47.3	–	–	–	–	–	–
			100	4.2	204.0	5.9	1.0	42.3	–	–	–	–	–	–
	BREAKFAST CEREALS													
272	BRAN, ALL-BRAN, Kellogg's	1 CUP	56	.03	128.8	6.2	1.1	39.8	4.2	39.2	493.9	566.7	89.6	517.4
			100	.03	230.0	11.0	2.0	71.0	7.5	70.0	882.0	1012.0	160.0	924.0
	CORN													
273	FLAKES, w/added nutrients	1 CUP	25	3.8	96.5	2.0	.1	21.3	.2	4.3	11.3	251.3	2.2	30.0
			100	3.8	386.0	7.9	.4	85.3	.7	17.0	45.0	1005.0	8.7	120.0
274	FLAKES, sugar-covered, w/added nutrients	1 CUP	25	2.2	96.5	1.1	.1	22.8	.1	3.0	6.0	193.8	4.0	–
			100	2.2	386.0	4.4	.2	91.3	.4	12.0	24.0	775.0	16.0	–
275	FARINA, enriched, instant, cooked, w/salt added	1 CUP	245	85.9	134.8	4.2	.2	27.9	.2	188.7	147.0	460.6	9.8	31.9
			100	85.9	55.0	1.7	.1	11.4	.1	77.0	60.0	188.0	4.0	13.0
276	GRANOLA	1 CUP	112	–	480.0	12.0	16.0	76.0	–	–	–	160.0	–	–
			100	–	428.6	10.7	14.3	67.8	–	–	–	142.9	–	–
277	⁵GRAPENUTS	1 SERV	25	–	68.3	3.8	1.4	10.8	–	18.5	60.0	417.5	92.5	267.5
			100	–	273.0	15.1	5.7	43.0	–	74.0	240.0	1670.0	370.0	1070.0
	OATS													
278	GRANULES, maple flavored, quick, cooked	1 CUP	245	85.2	147.0	5.6	1.5	27.9	.5	24.5	154.4	176.4	–	–
			100	85.2	60.0	2.3	.6	11.4	.2	10.0	63.0	72.0	–	–
279	ROLLED (oatmeal), cooked	1 CUP	236	86.5	112.7	4.7	2.4	22.9	.5	21.2	134.5	514.5	49.6	144.0
			100	86.5	52.0	2.0	1.0	9.7	.2	9.0	57.0	218.0	21.0	61.0
	RICE													
280	⁵CREAM OF, cooked	1 OZ	28	87.5	14.0	.2	Trace	3.1	Trace	.6	3.6	49.3	2.2	Trace
			100	87.5	50.0	.8	Trace	11.2	Trace	2.0	13.0	176.0	8.0	Trace

	Minerals (Micro)			Fat-Soluble Vitamins			Water-Soluble Vitamins								
Item No.	Iron	Zinc	Copper	Vitamin A	Vitamin D	Vitamin E (Alpha Tocopherol)	Vitamin C	Thiamin	Riboflavin	Niacin	Pantothenic Acid	Vit. B-6 (Pyridoxine)	Folacin (Folic Acid)	Biotin	Vitamin B-12
	(mg)	(mg)	(mg)	(IU)	(IU)	(mg)	(mg)	(mg)	(mg)	(mg)	(mg)	(mg)	(mcg)	(mcg)	(mcg)
252	5.80	–	–	0	–	–	.84	.08	.06	.48	–	–	–	–	–
	20.70	–	–	0	–	–	3.00	.30	.22	1.70	–	–	–	–	–
253	15.64	–	.54	0	–	.12	0	1.68	.87	5.29	–	–	–	–	–
	6.80	–	.23	0	–	.05	0	.73	.38	2.30	–	–	–	–	–
254	–	–	.03	–	–	1.12	–	–	–	–	–	–	–	–	–
	–	–	.04	–	–	1.40	–	–	–	–	–	–	–	–	–
255	2.10	–	–	0	–	–	.84	.10	.12	.39	–	–	–	–	–
	7.50	–	–	0	–	–	3.00	.36	.42	1.40	–	–	–	–	–
256	5.43	–	–	0	–	–	0	.63	.07	8.34	.78	.70	10.92	16.80	–
	19.40	–	–	0	–	–	0	2.26	.25	29.80	2.77	2.50	39.00	60.00	–
257	.75	.90	–	0	–	.23	0	.14	.03	2.10	2.28	.93	–	–	–
	.50	.60	–-	0	–	.15	0	.09	.02	1.40	1.52	.62	–	–	–
258	1.35	.60	–	0	–	.27	0	.17	.11	1.50	1.13	.06	24.00	7.50	–
	.90	.40	–	0	–	.18	0	.11	.07	1.00	.75	.04	16.00	5.00	–
259	6.85	6.01	.47	0	0	3.05	0	.80	.41	2.96	–	–	–	–	–
	3.70	3.25	.25	0	0	1.65	0	.43	.22	1.60	–	–	–	–	–
260	–	–	–	–	–	–	–	–	–	–	–	–	–	–	–
	–	–	–	–	–	–	–	–	–	–	–	–	–	–	–
261	–	–	–	–	–	–	–	–	–	–	–	–	–	–	–
	–	–	–	–	–	–	–	–	–	–	–	–	–	–	–
262	1.23	–	–	0	–	–	0	.11	.04	1.09	–	–	7.56	–	–
	4.40	–	–	0	–	–	0	.38	.15	3.90	–	–	27.00	–	–
263	21.14	–	–	2.3	–	–	–	.04	.03	.39	–	–	–	–	–
	75.50	–	–	8.3	–	–	–	.13	.12	1.40	–	–	–	–	–
264	5.85	–	–	0	–	–	–	.11	.04	.53	–	–	–	–	–
	20.90	–	–	0	–	–	–	.38	.14	1.90	–	–	–	–	–
265	.92	–	–	0	–	–	0	.04	.02	.20	–	–	–	–	–
	3.30	–	–	0	–	–	0	.14	.07	.70	–	–	–	–	–
266	5.94	4.36	1.05	0	–	2.77	0	1.05	.24	10.49	–	–	102.96	21.78	–
	3.00	2.20	.53	0	–	1.40	0	.53	.12	5.30	–	–	52.00	11.00	–
267	1.34	.88	(.11)	0	–	.15	0	.07	.03	1.89	.27	.12	23.22	5.13	–
	14.90	9.80	(1.27)	0	–	1.63	0	.72	.35	21.00	3.00	1.38	258.00	57.00	–
268	.85	1.29	.07	0	–	(1.22)	0	.18	.06	.38	.11	–	29.52	2.08	–
	9.40	14.30	.74	0	–	(13.50)	0	2.01	.68	4.20	1.20	–	328.00	22.00	–
269	.53	.92	.08	6.6	–	–	.60	.10	.06	.32	.07	.07	25.20	–	0
	8.90	15.40	1.30	110.0	–	–	10.00	1.65	.98	5.30	1.20	1.15	420.00	–	0
270	4.70	–	–	0	–	–	0	.50	.71	6.94	1.14	–	–	–	0
	4.20	–	–	0	–	–	0	.45	.63	6.20	1.02	–	–	–	0
271	–	–	–	–	–	–	–	–	–	–	–	–	–	–	–
	–	–	–	–	–	–	–	–	–	–	–	–	–	–	–
272	8.85	7.39	.51	2469.0	78.96	–	29.68	.74	.84	9.86	–	.99	196.00	–	–
	15.80	13.20	.91	4409.0	141.00	–	53.00	1.32	1.50	17.60	–	1.76	350.00	–	–
273	.35	.08	.01	0	0	.02	0	.11	.02	.53	.05	.02	1.38	–	0
	1.40	.30	.02	0	0	.09	0	.43	.08	2.10	.19	.07	5.50	–	0
274	.25	–	–	0	–	.02	0	.10	.01	.48	.05	.02	–	–	0
	1.00	–	–	0	–	.09	0	.41	.04	1.90	.18	.07	–	–	0
275	15.68	–	–	0	–	–	0	.17	.10	1.23	–	–	–	–	–
	6.40	–	–	0	–	–	0	.07	.04	.50	–	–	–	–	–
276	–	2.35	.95	–	–	–	–	–	–	–	–	–	51.52	–	–
	–	2.10	.85	–	–	–	–	–	–	–	–	–	46.00	–	–
277	1.30	.53	–	–	.88	.40	0	.30	.40	4.25	–	.70	10.25	–	1.25
	5.20	2.10	–	–	3.50	1.60	0	1.20	1.60	17.00	–	2.81	41.00	–	5.00
278	1.47	–	–	0	–	–	0	.15	–	–	–	–	–	–	–
	.60	–	–	0	–	–	0	.06	–	–	–	–	–	–	–
279	1.42	1.18	–	0	0	5.36	0	.20	.05	.24	–	–	–	–	–
	.60	50	–	0	0	2.27	0	.08	.02	.10	–	–	–	–	–
280	.20	–	–	0	–	–	0	.02	Trace	.22	–	–	–	–	–
	.70	–	–	0	–	–	0	.06	.01	.80	–	–	–	–	–

(Continued)

TABLE F-21 *(Continued)*

Item No.	Food Item Name	Approximate Measure	Weight (g)	Moisture (%)	Food Energy Calories (kcal)	Protein (g)	Fats (g)	Carbo-hydrates (g)	Fiber (g)	Minerals (Macro)				
										Calcium (mg)	Phos-phorus (mg)	Sodium (mg)	Mag-nesium (mg)	Potas-sium (mg)
	RICE *(Continued)*													
281	**FLAKES,** w/added nutrients	1 CUP	32	3.2	124.8	1.9	.1	28.1	.2	9.3	42.2	315.8	–	57.6
			100	3.2	390.0	5.9	.3	87.7	.6	29.0	132.0	987.0	–	180.0
282	**PUFFED,** w/added nutrients, no salt	1 CUP	13	3.7	51.9	.8	.1	11.6	.1	2.6	12.0	.3	5.2	13.0
			100	3.7	399.0	6.0	.4	89.5	.6	20.0	92.0	2.0	40.0	100.0
	WHEAT													
283	**CREAM OF,** cooked	1 CUP	245	89.5	102.9	3.2	.2	21.3	–	9.8	29.4	352.8	7.4	22.1
			100	89.5	42.0	1.3	.1	8.7	–	4.0	12.0	144.0	3.0	9.0
284	**PUFFED,** no added salt, w/added nutrients	1 CUP	12	3.4	43.6	1.8	.2	9.4	.2	3.4	38.6	.5	15.5	40.8
			100	3.4	363.0	15.0	1.5	78.5	2.0	28.0	322.0	4.0	129.0	340.0
285	**ROLLED,** cooked	1 CUP	245	79.7	183.8	5.4	1.0	41.4	1.2	19.6	186.2	–	–	205.8
			100	79.7	75.0	2.2	.4	16.9	.5	8.0	76.0	–	–	84.0
286	**SHREDDED,** no salt or other added nutrients	1 MED	22	6.6	83.2	2.2	.4	17.6	.5	9.5	85.4	.7	24.0	76.6
			100	6.6	378.0	10.1	2.0	79.9	2.3	43.0	388.0	3.0	109.0	348.0
	FLOURS													
287	**BUCKWHEAT FLOUR,** dark	1 CUP	100	12.0	357.0	11.7	2.5	72.0	1.6	33.0	347.0	–	–	–
			100	12.0	357.0	11.7	2.5	72.0	1.6	33.0	347.0	–	–	–
288	**CORN, FLOUR**	1 CUP	110	12.0	398.2	8.6	2.9	84.5	.8	6.6	180.4	1.1	–	–
			100	12.0	362.0	7.8	2.6	76.8	.7	6.0	164.0	1.0	–	–
289	**CORNSTARCH**	1 TBLS	8	12.0	28.6	0	0	7.0	Trace	0	0	.3	.2	.3
			100	12.0	357.0	.3	.6	87.6	.1	0	0	4.0	2.2	4.0
290	**COTTONSEED FLOUR**	1 CUP	140	6.1	498.4	67.3	9.2	46.2	2.8	396.2	1556.8	–	910.0	–
			100	6.1	356.0	48.1	6.6	33.0	2.0	283.0	1112.0	–	650.0	–
291	**OAT FLOUR**	1 CUP	133	–	–	–	–	–	–	–	–	–	146.3	–
			100	–	–	–	–	–	–	–	–	–	110.0	–
292	**PEANUT FLOUR,** defatted	1 CUP	60	7.3	222.6	28.7	5.5	18.9	1.6	62.4	432.0	5.4	216.0	711.6
			100	7.3	371.0	47.9	9.2	31.5	2.7	104.0	720.0	9.0	360.0	1186.0
293	**POTATO FLOUR**	1 OZ	28	7.6	98.3	2.2	.2	22.4	.4	9.2	49.8	9.5	–	444.6
			100	7.6	351.0	8.0	.8	79.9	1.6	33.0	178.0	34.0	–	1588.0
294	**RYE FLOUR,** medium	1 OZ	28	11.0	100.0	3.2	.4	20.9	.3	7.6	73.4	.3	20.4	56.8
			100	11.0	357.0	11.4	1.4	74.8	1.0	27.0	262.0	1.0	73.0	203.0
	SOYBEAN													
295	**FLOUR,** full fat	1 CUP	72	8.0	303.1	25.8	14.6	21.9	1.7	143.3	401.8	.7	177.8	1195.2
			100	8.0	421.0	35.9	20.3	30.4	2.4	199.0	558.0	1.0	247.0	1660.0
296	**FLOUR,** defatted	1 CUP	138	8.0	449.9	64.9	1.2	52.6	3.2	365.7	903.9	1.4	427.8	2511.6
			100	8.0	326.0	47.0	.9	38.1	2.3	265.0	655.0	1.0	310.0	1820.0
297	**TORTILLA FLOUR,** white corn, lime treated	1 OZ	28	10.3	103.3	2.3	1.6	20.7	.9	24.9	107.0	–	–	–
			100	10.3	369.0	8.2	5.8	73.9	3.2	89.0	382.0	–	–	–
298	**TRITICALE FLOUR**	1 CUP	130	12.5	426.4	17.2	2.0	92.3	3.3	57.2	900.9	13.0	–	562.9
			100	12.5	328.0	13.2	1.5	71.0	2.5	44.0	693.0	10.0	–	433.0
299	**WHEAT FLOUR,** all purpose, enriched	1 CUP	110	12.0	400.4	11.6	1.1	83.7	.3	17.6	95.7	2.2	–	104.5
			100	12.0	364.0	10.5	1.0	76.1	.3	16.0	87.0	2.0	–	95.0
	PASTAS													
300	**MACARONI,** enriched, cooked firm (8-10 minutes)	1 CUP	140	63.6	207.2	7.0	.7	42.1	.1	15.4	91.0	1.4	28.0	110.6
			100	63.6	148.0	5.0	.5	30.1	.1	11.0	65.0	1.0	20.0	79.0
301	**NOODLES,** cooked	1 OZ	28	3.0	35.0	1.1	.6	6.2	Trace	4.8	15.9	24.2	5.1	11.7
			100	3.0	124.9	3.9	2.0	22.1	.1	17.3	56.7	86.3	18.4	41.8
302	**PASTINAS,** enriched, dry, egg	1 CUP	170	10.4	651.1	21.9	7.0	122.1	.5	59.5	329.8	8.5	–	–
			100	10.4	383.0	12.9	4.1	71.8	.3	35.0	194.0	5.0	–	–
303	**SPAGHETTI,** enriched, cooked firm (8-10 minutes)	1 CUP	146	63.6	216.1	7.3	.7	43.9	.1	16.1	94.9	1.5	29.0	115.3
			100	63.6	148.0	5.0	.5	30.1	.1	11.0	65.0	1.0	19.9	79.0
	DESSERTS AND SWEETS													
304	**APPLE BROWN BETTY**	1 CUP	215	64.5	324.7	3.4	7.5	63.9	1.1	38.7	47.3	329.0	10.8	215.0
			100	64.5	151.0	1.6	3.5	29.7	.5	18.0	22.0	153.0	5.0	100.0
305	**APPLE STRUDEL**	1 SERV	100	43.8	290.0	4.0	14.3	39.0	.4	3.0	19.0	130.0	10.0	74.0
			100	43.8	290.0	4.0	14.3	39.0	.4	3.0	19.0	130.0	10.0	74.0
306	**BANANA SPLIT**	INDV	411	–	580.0	11.0	16.0	97.0	–	–	–	–	–	–
			100	–	141.1	2.6	3.9	23.6	–	–	–	–	–	–
307	**BLINTZES,** cheese	1 SERV	28	–	54.9	–	3.9	–	–	–	–	–	–	–
			100	–	196.0	–	14.1	–	–	–	–	–	–	–
308	**BREAD PUDDING,** w/raisins	1 CUP	220	58.6	411.4	12.3	13.4	62.5	.2	239.8	250.8	442.2	–	473.0
			100	58.6	187.0	5.6	6.1	28.4	.1	109.0	114.0	201.0	–	215.0

Item No.	Minerals (Micro)			Fat-Soluble Vitamins			Water-Soluble Vitamins								
	Iron	Zinc	Copper	Vitamin A	Vitamin D	Vitamin E (Alpha Tocopherol)	Vitamin C	Thiamin	Ribo-flavin	Niacin	Panto-thenic Acid	Vit. B-6 (Pyri-doxine)	Folacin (Folic Acid)	Biotin	Vitamin B-12
	(mg)	(mg)	(mg)	(IU)	(IU)	(mg)	(mg)	(mg)	(mg)	(mg)	(mg)	(mg)	(mcg)	(mcg)	(mcg)
281	.51	.45	–	0	–	.01	0	.11	.02	1.73	.11	.04	2.43	.42	0
	1.60	1.40	–	0	–	.04	0	.35	.05	5.40	.34	.13	7.60	1.30	0
282	.23	.18	.02	0	0	.01	0	.06	.01	.57	.05	.01	.99	.17	0
	1.80	1.40	.17	0	0	.04	0	.44	.04	4.40	.38	.07	7.60	1.30	0
283	.74	–	–	0	0	–	0	.10	.07	.98	–	–	–	–	–
	.30	–	–	0	0	–	0	.04	.03	.40	–	–	–	–	–
284	.50	.31	–	0	0	.07	0	.07	.03	.94	–	.02	–	–	0
	4.20	2.60	–	0	0	.58	0	.55	.23	7.80	–	.17	–	–	0
285	1.72	–	–	0	–	–	0	.17	.07	2.21	–	–	–	–	–
	.70	–	–	0	–	–	0	.07	.03	.90	–	–	–	–	–
286	.77	.62	.13	0	0	.04	0	.05	.02	.97	.16	.05	11.00	–	0
	3.50	2.80	.61	0	0	.19	0	.22	.11	4.40	.71	.24	50.00	–	0
287	2.80	–	–	0	–	–	0	.58	.15	2.90	1.45	.58	44.00	–	0
	2.80	–	–	0	–	–	0	.58	.15	2.90	1.45	.58	44.00	–	0
288	1.98	–	–	374.0	–	–	0	.22	.07	1.54	–	–	–	–	–
	1.80	–	–	340.0	–	–	0	.20	.06	1.40	–	–	–	–	–
289	0	Trace	.01	0	0	–	0	Trace	0	0	–	–	–	–	–
	0	.03	.13	0	0	–	0	Trace	0	0	–	–	–	–	–
290	17.64	–	–	84.0	–	–	–	1.69	1.18	9.10	6.05	1.37	–	–	0
	12.60	–	–	60.0	–	–	–	1.21	.84	6.50	4.32	.98	–	–	0
291	–	–	–	–	–	–	–	–	–	–	–	–	–	–	–
	–	–	–	–	–	–	–	–	–	–	–	–	–	–	–
292	2.10	–	–	–	–	–	0	.45	.13	16.68	–	–	–	–	–
	3.50	–	–	–	–	–	0	.75	.22	27.80	–	–	–	–	–
293	4.82	–	–	–	–	–	5.32	.12	.04	.95	–	Trace	–	–	0
	7.20	–	–	–	–	–	19.00	.42	.14	3.40	–	.01	–	–	0
294	.73	–	.12	0	(1.48)	–	0	.08	.03	.70	(1.85)	(.65)	21.84	(11.10)	0
	2.60	–	.42	0	(1.80)	–	0	.30	.12	2.50	(1.00)	(1.35)	78.00	(6.00)	0
295	6.05	–	–	79.2	0	–	0	.61	.22	1.51	1.26	.41	228.96	50.40	0
	8.40	–	–	110.0	0	–	0	.85	.31	2.10	1.75	.57	318.00	70.00	0
296	15.32	6.72	2.39	55.2	–	–	0	1.50	.47	3.59	3.06	1.00	438.84	96.60	0
	11.10	4.87	1.73	40.0	–	–	0	1.09	.34	2.60	2.22	.72	318.00	70.00	0
297	.73	–	–	1.4	–	–	.28	.10	.03	.53	–	–	–	–	–
	2.60	–	–	5.0	–	–	1.00	.37	.10	1.90	–	–	–	–	–
298	7.02	4.29	–	0	–	–	0	1.05	.35	1.82	–	–	68.90	–	–
	5.40	3.30	–	0	–	–	0	.81	.27	1.40	–	–	53.00	–	–
299	3.19	.77	–	0	–	–	0	.48	.29	3.85	–	–	23.10	–	–
	2.90	.70	–	0	–	–	0	.44	.26	3.50	–	–	21.00	–	–
300	1.54	–	–	0	–	–	0	.25	.14	1.96	–	–	–	–	–
	1.10	–	–	0	–	–	0	.18	.10	1.40	–	–	–	–	–
301	.25	.18	–	18.9	0	–	0	.08	.03	.52	0	.07	0	–	0
	.89	.63	–	67.6	0	–	0	.27	.12	1.84	0	.23	0	–	0
302	4.93	–	–	374.0	–	–	0	1.50	.65	10.20	–	–	–	–	–
	2.90	–	–	220.0	–	–	0	.88	.38	6.00	–	–	–	–	–
303	1.61	–	–	0	–	–	0	.26	.15	2.04	–	–	–	–	–
	1.10	–	–	0	–	–	0	.18	.10	1.40	–	–	–	–	–
304	1.29	–	–	215.0	–	–	2.15	.13	.09	.86	–	–	–	–	–
	.60	–	–	100.0	–	–	1.00	.06	.04	.40	–	–	–	–	–
305	1.20	–	–	10.0	–	–	3.00	.15	.09	.60	–	–	–	–	–
	1.20	–	–	10.0	–	–	3.00	.15	.09	.60	–	–	–	–	–
306	–	–	–	–	–	–	–	–	–	–	–	–	–	–	–
	–	–	–	–	–	–	–	–	–	–	–	–	–	–	–
307	–	–	–	–	–	–	–	–	–	–	–	–	–	–	–
	–	–	–	–	–	–	–	–	–	–	–	–	–	–	–
308	2.42	–	–	660.0	–	–	2.20	.13	.42	.22	–	–	–	–	–
	1.10	–	–	300.0	–	–	1.00	.06	.19	.10	–	–	–	–	–

(Continued)

TABLE F-21 *(Continued)*

Item No.	Food Item Name	Approximate Measure	Weight (g)	Moisture (%)	Food Energy Calories (kcal)	Protein (g)	Fats (g)	Carbo-hydrates (g)	Fiber (g)	Calcium (mg)	Phos-phorus (mg)	Sodium (mg)	Mag-nesium (mg)	Potas-sium (mg)
	CANDY													
309	butterscotch	1 PIECE	5	1.5	19.9	–	.2	4.7	0	.9	.3	3.3	–	.1
			100	1.5	397.0	–	3.4	94.8	0	17.0	6.0	66.0	–	2.0
310	caramels, plain or chocolate	1 MED	10	7.6	39.9	.4	1.0	7.7	Trace	14.8	12.2	22.6	.2	19.2
			100	7.6	399.0	4.0	10.2	76.6	.2	148.0	122.0	226.0	2.0	192.0
311	chocolate coated almonds	1 OZ	28	2.0	159.3	3.4	12.2	11.1	.4	56.8	96.0	16.5	11.2	152.9
			100	2.0	569.0	12.3	43.7	39.6	1.5	203.0	343.0	59.0	40.0	546.0
312	chocolate coated fondant	1 OZ	28	5.8	114.8	.5	2.9	22.7	Trace	16.0	15.1	51.8	–	25.5
			100	5.8	410.0	1.7	10.5	81.0	.1	57.0	54.0	185.0	–	91.0
313	chocolate coated fudge, w/peanuts & caramel	1 OZ	28	7.0	128.5	2.6	6.5	16.4	.2	35.6	53.8	35.8	–	62.2
			100	7.0	459.0	9.4	23.1	58.7	.7	127.0	192.0	128.0	–	222.0
314	chocolate coated nougat & caramel	1 OZ	28	7.7	116.5	1.1	3.9	20.4	.1	35.6	34.4	48.4	–	59.1
			100	7.7	416.0	4.0	13.9	72.8	.2	127.0	123.0	173.0	–	211.0
315	chocolate coated peanuts	1 PIECE	2	1.0	11.2	.3	.8	.8	Trace	2.3	6.0	1.2	–	10.1
			100	1.0	561.0	16.4	41.3	39.1	1.2	116.0	298.0	60.0	–	504.0
316	chocolate coated raisins	1 SM	1	4.8	4.3	.1	.2	.7	Trace	1.5	1.7	.6	–	6.0
			100	4.8	425.0	5.4	17.1	70.5	.6	152.0	174.0	64.0	–	603.0
317	chocolate fudge	1 PIECE	25	8.2	100.0	.7	3.1	18.8	.1	19.3	21.0	47.5	12.5	36.8
			100	8.2	400.0	2.7	12.2	75.0	.2	77.0	84.0	190.0	50.0	147.0
318	chocolate kiss	1 OZ	28	.9	145.6	2.2	9.0	15.9	.1	63.8	64.7	26.3	16.2	107.5
			100	.9	520.0	7.7	32.3	56.9	.4	228.0	231.0	94.0	58.0	384.0
319	chocolate, semi-sweet	1 OZ	28	1.1	142.0	1.2	10.0	16.0	.3	8.4	42.0	.6	27.2	91.0
			100	1.1	507.0	4.2	35.7	57.0	1.0	30.0	150.0	2.0	97.0	325.0
320	chocolate, sweet	1 OZ	28	.9	147.8	1.2	9.8	16.2	.1	26.3	39.8	9.2	30.0	75.3
			100	.9	528.0	4.4	35.1	57.9	.5	94.0	142.0	33.0	107.0	269.0
321	fondant	1 AVG	11	7.6	40.0	0	.2	9.9	–	1.5	.7	23.3	–	.6
			100	7.6	364.0	.1	2.0	89.6	–	14.0	6.0	212.0	–	5.0
322	gum drops, starch jelly pieces	1 SM	1	11.7	3.5	0	.0	.9	0	.1	–	.4	–	.1
			100	11.7	347.0	.1	.7	87.4	0	6.0	–	35.0	–	5.0
323	hard	1 PIECE	5	1.4	19.3	0	.1	4.9	0	1.1	.4	1.6	–	.2
			100	1.4	356.0	0	1.1	97.2	0	21.0	7.0	32.0	–	4.0
324	jelly beans	1 PIECE	3	6.3	11.0	–	.0	2.8	–	.4	.1	.4	–	0
			100	6.3	367.0	0	.5	93.1	–	12.0	4.0	12.0	–	1.0
325	licorice	1 OZ	28	11.7	97.2	0	.2	24.5	0	1.7	Trace	9.1	–	1.4
			100	11.7	347.0	.1	.7	87.4	0	6.0	Trace	35.0	–	5.0
326	Life Savers	1 PIECE	2	1.4	7.7	0	Trace	1.9	0	.4	.1	.6	–	.1
			100	1.4	386.0	0	1.1	97.2	0	21.0	7.0	32.0	–	4.0
327	lollypops	1 MED	28	–	108.1	0	0	28.0	0	0	0	–	–	–
			100	–	386.0	0	0	100.0	0	0	0	–	–	–
328	marshmallows	1 AVG	8	17.3	25.5	.2	–	6.4	0	1.4	.5	3.1	–	.5
			100	17.3	319.0	2.0	–	80.4	0	18.0	6.0	39.0	–	6.0
329	milk chocolate, plain	1 BAR	57	.9	296.4	4.4	18.4	32.4	.2	130.0	131.7	53.6	33.1	218.9
			100	.9	520.0	7.7	32.3	56.9	.4	228.0	231.0	94.0	58.0	384.0
330	milk chocolate, w/almonds	1 BAR	56	1.5	297.9	5.2	19.9	28.7	.4	128.2	152.3	44.8	46.5	247.5
			100	1.5	532.0	9.3	35.6	51.3	.7	229.0	272.0	80.0	83.0	442.0
331	peanut brittle, no added salt or soda	1 PIECE	25	2.0	105.3	1.4	2.6	20.3	.1	8.8	23.8	7.8	–	37.8
			100	2.0	421.0	5.7	10.4	81.0	.5	35.0	95.0	31.0	–	151.0
332	peppermint pattie, chocolate-covered	1 OZ	28	5.8	114.8	.5	2.9	22.7	Trace	16.0	15.1	51.8	–	25.5
			100	5.8	410.0	1.7	10.5	81.0	.1	57.0	54.0	185.0	–	91.0
333	sugar-coated almonds	1 AVG	4	2.3	18.2	.3	.7	2.8	Trace	4.0	6.6	.8	–	10.2
			100	2.3	456.0	7.8	18.6	70.2	.9	100.0	166.0	20.0	–	255.0
334	**CHEWING GUM**	1 PIECE	3	3.5	9.5	–	–	2.9	–	–	–	–	–	0
			100	3.5	317.0	–	–	95.2	–	–	–	–	–	–
335	**CITRON**, candied	1 OZ	28	18.0	87.9	.1	.1	22.5	.4	23.2	6.7	81.2	–	33.6
			100	18.0	314.0	.2	.3	80.2	1.4	83.0	24.0	290.0	–	120.0
336	**COBBLER**, apple cake	1 SERV	100	56.0	195.0	2.0	5.0	37.0	.3	12.0	85.0	135.0	–	50.0
			100	56.0	195.0	2.0	5.0	37.0	.3	12.0	85.0	135.0	–	50.0
337	**CUSTARD**, baked	1 CUP	265	77.2	294.2	14.3	13.3	29.4	0	296.8	310.1	209.4	–	386.9
			100	77.2	111.0	5.4	5.0	11.1	0	112.0	117.0	79.0	–	146.0
338	**ECLAIRS**, w/custard filling & chocolate icing	1 AVG	110	56.2	262.9	6.8	15.0	25.5	0	88.0	123.2	90.2	(17.6)	134.2
			100	56.2	239.0	6.2	13.6	23.2	0	80.0	112.0	82.0	(16.0)	122.0
	GELATIN													
339	dessert, prepared	1 CUP	240	–	146.9	2.8	0	34.0	0	0	0	97.2	–	1.1
			100	–	61.2	1.2	0	14.2	0	0	0	40.5	–	.5
340	all flavors, dietetic	1 SERV	120	–	10.0	2.0	0	0	–	–	–	5.0	–	–
			100	–	8.3	1.7	0	0	–	–	–	4.2	–	–

Item No.	Minerals (Micro)			Fat-Soluble Vitamins			Water-Soluble Vitamins								
	Iron	Zinc	Copper	Vitamin A	Vitamin D	Vitamin E (Alpha Tocopherol)	Vitamin C	Thiamin	Riboflavin	Niacin	Pantothenic Acid	Vit. B-6 (Pyridoxine)	Folacin (Folic Acid)	Biotin	Vitamin B-12
	(mg)	(mg)	(mg)	(IU)	(IU)	(mg)	(mg)	(mg)	(mg)	(mg)	(mg)	(mg)	(mcg)	(mcg)	(mcg)
309	.07	–	–	7.0	0	–	0	0	–	–	–	–	–	–	–
	1.40	–	–	140.0	0	–	0	0	–	–	–	–	–	–	–
310	.14	–	–	1.0	–	–	–	Trace	.02	.02	–	–	–	–	–
	1.40	–	–	10.0	–	–	–	.03	.17	.20	–	–	–	–	–
311	.78	–	–	14.8	9.80	–	.20	.03	.15	.48	–	–	–	–	–
	2.80	–	–	53.0	35.00	–	.70	.12	.53	1.70	–	–	–	–	–
312	.31	–	–	–	–	–	–	.01	.02	.03	–	–	–	–	–
	1.10	–	–	–	–	–	–	.03	.06	.10	–	–	–	–	–
313	.31	–	–	–	–	–	–	.07	.04	1.04	–	–	–	–	–
	1.10	–	–	–	–	–	–	.26	.15	3.70	–	–	–	–	–
314	.45	–	–	11.2	–	–	–	.02	.05	.06	–	–	–	–	–
	1.60	–	–	40.0	–	–	–	.06	.17	.20	–	–	–	–	–
315	.03	–	–	–	–	–	–	.01	Trace	.15	–	–	–	–	–
	1.50	–	–	–	–	–	–	.37	.18	7.40	–	–	–	–	–
316	.03	–	–	1.5	–	–	–	Trace	Trace	Trace	–	–	–	–	–
	2.50	–	–	150.0	–	–	–	.08	.21	.40	–	–	–	–	–
317	.25	–	–	–	–	–	–	.01	.02	.05	–	–	–	–	–
	1.00	–	–	–	–	–	–	.02	.09	.20	–	–	–	–	–
318	.31	.13	.02	75.6	46.76	1.80	.39	.02	.10	.08	–	–	–	17.10	–
	1.10	.46	.07	270.0	167.00	4.20	1.40	.06	.34	.30	–	–	–	30.00	–
319	.73	–	–	5.6	–	–	0	Trace	.02	.14	–	–	–	–	–
	2.60	–	–	20.0	–	–	0	.01	.08	.50	–	–	–	–	–
320	.39	–	–	2.8	–	–	–	.01	.04	.08	–	–	–	–	–
	1.40	–	–	10.0	–	–	–	.02	.14	.30	–	–	–	–	–
321	.12	–	–	0	–	–	0	–	–	–	–	–	–	–	–
	1.10	–	–	0	–	–	0	–	–	–	–	–	–	–	–
322	.01	–	–	0	–	–	0	0	–	–	–	–	–	–	–
	.50	–	–	0	–	–	0	0	–	–	–	–	–	–	–
323	.10	–	–	0	0	–	0	0	0	0	–	–	–	–	–
	1.90	–	–	0	0	–	0	0	0	0	–	–	–	–	–
324	.03	–	–	0	–	–	0	0	–	–	–	–	–	–	–
	1.10	–	–	0	–	–	0	0	–	–	–	–	–	–	–
325	.14	–	–	0	–	–	0	0	Trace	Trace	–	–	–	–	–
	.50	–	–	0	–	–	0	0	Trace	Trace	–	–	–	–	–
326	.04	–	–	0	0	–	0	0	0	0	–	–	–	–	–
	1.90	–	–	0	0	–	0	0	0	0	–	–	–	–	–
327	0	–	–	0	0	–	0	0	0	0	–	–	–	–	–
	0	–	–	0	0	–	0	0	0	0	–	–	–	–	–
328	.13	–	–	0	–	–	0	0	–	–	–	–	–	–	–
	1.60	–	–	0	–	–	0	0	–	–	–	–	–	–	–
329	.63	.06	.04	153.9	95.19	.63	.80	.03	.19	.17	–	–	3.99	17.10	–
	1.10	.11	.07	270.0	167.00	1.10	1.40	.06	.34	.30	–	–	7.00	30.00	–
330	.90	–	–	128.8	39.76	–	.67	.05	.23	.45	–	–	–	–	–
	1.60	–	–	230.0	71.00	–	1.20	.08	.41	.80	–	–	–	–	–
331	.58	–	–	0	–	–	0	.04	.01	.85	–	–	–	–	–
	2.30	–	–	0	–	–	0	.16	.03	3.40	–	–	–	–	–
332	.31	.11	–	Trace	–	–	Trace	.01	.02	.03	–	–	–	–	–
	1.10	.38	–	Trace	–	–	Trace	.03	.06	.10	–	–	–	–	–
333	.08	–	–	0	–	–	0	Trace	.01	.04	–	–	–	–	–
	1.90	–	–	0	–	–	0	.05	.27	1.00	–	–	–	–	–
334	–	–	–	0	–	–	0	0	0	0	–	–	–	–	–
	–	–	–	0	–	–	0	0	0	0	–	–	–	–	–
335	.22	–	–	–	–	–	–	–	–	–	–	–	–	–	–
	.80	–	–	–	–	–	–	–	–	–	–	–	–	–	–
336	.70	–	–	10.0	–	–	0	.10	.04	.60	–	–	–	–	–
	.70	–	–	10.0	–	–	0	.10	.04	.60	–	–	–	–	–
337	.06	–	–	927.5	–	–	1.06	.11	.50	.27	–	–	–	–	–
	.04	–	–	350.0	–	–	.40	.04	.19	.10	–	–	–	–	–
338	.77	(.40)	(.17)	374.0	(1.00)	(1.30)	0	.04	.18	.11	(.33)	(.04)	(4.40)	(1.10)	Trace
	.70	(.40)	(.15)	340.0	(.91)	(1.20)	0	.04	.16	.10	(.30)	(.04)	(4.00)	(1.00)	Trace
339	3.50	.05	–	209.7	–	–	34.23	0	.37	4.32	–	–	–	–	–
	1.46	.02	–	87.4	–	–	14.26	0	.15	1.80	–	–	–	–	–
340	–	–	–	–	–	–	–	–	–	–	–	–	–	–	–
	–	–	–	–	–	–	–	–	–	–	–	–	–	–	–

(Continued)

TABLE F-21 *(Continued)*

Item No.	Food Item Name	Approximate Measure	Weight (g)	Moisture (%)	Food Energy Calories (kcal)	Protein (g)	Fats (g)	Carbo-hydrates (g)	Fiber (g)	Minerals (Macro)				
										Calcium (mg)	Phos-phorus (mg)	Sodium (mg)	Mag-nesium (mg)	Potas-sium (mg)
341	GRAPEFRUIT PEEL, candied	1 OZ	28	17.4	88.5	.1	.1	22.6	.6	–	–	–	–	–
			100	17.4	316.0	.4	.3	80.6	2.3	–	–	–	–	–
	HONEY													
342	ᵇcomb	1 OZ	28	–	78.4	.1	1.2	20.8	–	2.2	8.9	2.0	.6	9.7
			100	–	280.0	.5	4.3	74.3	–	7.9	31.6	7.3	2.2	34.8
343	strained or extracted	1 TBLS	20	17.2	60.8	.1	0	16.5	Trace	1.0	1.2	1.0	.6	10.2
			100	17.2	304.0	.3	0	82.3	.1	5.0	6.0	5.0	3.0	51.0
344	ICES, water, lime	1 CUP	185	66.9	144.3	.7	0	60.3	–	–	–	–	–	5.6
			100	66.9	78.0	.4	0	32.6	–	–	–	–	–	3.0
	ICINGS													
345	caramel	1 SERV	10	14.1	36.0	.1	.7	7.7	0	10.2	6.3	8.3	–	5.2
			100	14.1	360.0	1.3	6.7	76.5	0	102.0	63.0	83.0	–	52.0
346	chocolate	1 SERV	10	14.3	37.6	.3	1.4	6.7	Trace	6.0	11.1	6.1	–	19.5
			100	14.3	376.0	3.2	13.9	67.4	.4	60.0	111.0	61.0	–	195.0
347	coconut	1 SERV	10	15.0	36.4	.2	.8	7.5	.1	.6	3.0	11.8	–	16.7
			100	15.0	364.0	1.9	7.7	74.9	.8	6.0	30.0	118.0	–	167.0
348	white, boiled	1 SERV	10	17.9	31.6	.1	0	8.0	0	.2	.2	14.3	–	1.8
			100	17.9	316.0	1.4	0	80.3	0	2.0	2.0	143.0	–	18.0
349	white, uncooked	1 SERV	10	11.1	37.6	.1	.7	8.2	0	1.5	1.2	4.9	–	1.8
			100	11.1	376.0	.5	6.6	81.6	0	15.0	12.0	49.0	–	18.0
350	JAMS & PRESERVES, red cherry or strawberry	1 TBLS	20	29.0	54.4	Trace	Trace	14.0	.2	4.0	1.8	2.4	–	17.6
			100	29.0	272.0	.6	.1	70.0	1.0	20.0	9.0	12.0	–	88.0
351	JELLY	1 TBLS	20	29.0	54.6	Trace	Trace	14.1	0	4.2	1.4	3.4	–	15.0
			100	29.0	273.0	.1	.1	70.6	0	21.0	7.0	17.0	–	75.0
352	MARMALADE, CITRUS	1 TBLS	20	29.0	51.4	.1	Trace	14.0	0	7.0	1.8	2.8	.8	6.6
			100	29.0	257.0	.5	.1	70.1	.4	35.0	9.0	14.0	4.0	33.0
353	ᵃMINCEMEAT	1 OZ	28	–	66.1	.2	1.2	17.4	1.0	8.5	4.8	39.2	2.9	53.2
			100	–	236.0	.6	4.3	62.0	3.4	30.2	17.3	139.8	10.2	189.8
354	MOLASSES, cane, blackstrap	1 TBLS	20	24.0	46.0	.5	0	11.0	0	136.8	16.8	19.2	41.9	585.4
			100	24.0	230.0	2.4	0	55.0	0	684.0	84.0	96.0	209.3	2927.0
355	POPSICLE	1 AVG	88	80.0	65.1	0	0	16.7	–	0	–	–	–	–
			100	80.0	74.0	0	0	18.9	–	0	–	–	–	–
	PUDDINGS													
356	BUTTERSCOTCH, canned	1 CUP	260	70.5	322.4	6.5	9.4	59.8	0	231.4	176.8	444.6	23.4	306.8
			100	70.5	124.0	2.5	3.6	23.0	0	89.0	68.0	171.0	9.0	118.0
357	CHOCOLATE, canned	1 CUP	227	68.5	297.4	6.8	9.1	52.9	0	215.7	168.0	363.2	52.2	295.1
			100	68.5	131.0	3.0	4.0	23.3	0	95.0	74.0	160.0	23.0	130.0
358	CHOCOLATE, diet	1 OZ	28	89.2	10.7	.9	.1	1.6	0	33.4	27.7	17.6	3.0	45.2
			100	89.2	38.3	3.2	.2	5.6	0	119.3	98.9	63.0	10.7	161.3
359	CUSTARD, instant, prepared w/milk	1 CUP	260	70.0	340.6	8.1	9.1	58.8	–	275.6	213.2	257.4	36.4	335.4
			100	70.0	131.0	3.1	3.5	22.6	–	106.0	82.0	99.0	14.0	129.0
360	LEMON, canned	1 CUP	226	–	305.1	0	5.9	63.3	0	13.6	42.9	282.5	–	20.3
			100	–	135.0	0	2.6	28.0	0	6.0	19.0	125.0	–	9.0
361	RICE, w/raisins	1 CUP	265	65.8	386.9	9.5	8.2	70.8	.3	259.7	249.1	188.2	–	469.1
			100	65.8	146.0	3.6	3.1	26.7	.1	98.0	94.0	71.0	–	177.0
362	TAPIOCA CREAM	1 OZ	28	71.8	37.5	1.4	1.4	4.8	0	29.4	30.5	42.7	–	37.8
			100	71.8	134.0	5.0	5.1	17.1	0	105.0	109.0	156.0	–	135.0
363	VANILLA, made w/whole milk	1 CUP	297	–	351.3	8.2	8.4	61.1	0	298.9	217.2	504.1	0	372.5
			100	–	118.3	2.8	2.8	20.6	0	100.6	73.1	169.7	0	125.4
	SAUCES													
364	CUSTARD	1 TBLS	18	–	21.2	.9	1.0	2.3	–	19.4	20.5	–	–	–
			100	–	118.0	5.1	5.3	12.9	–	108.0	114.0	–	–	–
365	LEMON	1 TBLS	14	–	34.4	0	.7	7.2	–	.7	.6	–	–	–
			100	–	246.0	.2	5.2	51.5	–	5.0	4.0	–	–	–
366	RAISIN	1 TBLS	12	–	31.6	.2	.8	6.5	–	3.7	5.9	–	–	–
			100	–	263.0	1.3	6.3	54.0	–	31.0	49.0	–	–	–
367	SHERBET, orange	1 CUP	193	67.0	258.6	1.7	3.8	59.4	0	104.2	73.3	88.8	12.9	198.8
			100	67.0	134.0	.9	2.0	30.8	0	54.0	38.0	46.0	6.7	103.0
	SUGAR													
368	BEET OR CANE, brown	1 TBLS	14	2.1	52.2	0	0	13.5	0	11.9	2.7	4.2	8.7	48.2
			100	2.1	373.0	0	0	96.4	0	85.0	19.0	30.0	62.0	344.0
369	BEET OR CANE, granulated	1 TSP	8	0.5	30.8	0	0	8.0	0	0	0	.1	Trace	.2
			100	0.5	385.0	0	0	99.5	0	0	0	1.0	.2	3.0
370	BEET OR CANE, powdered	1 TBLS	11	0.5	42.4	0	0	10.9	0	0	0	.1	0	.3
			100	0.5	385.0	0	0	99.5	0	0	0	1.0	0	3.0
371	MAPLE	1 PIECE	15	8.0	52.2	–	–	13.5	–	21.5	1.7	2.1	–	36.3
			100	8.0	348.0	–	–	90.0	–	143.0	11.0	14.0	–	242.0

Item No.	Minerals (Micro)			Fat-Soluble Vitamins			Water-Soluble Vitamins								
	Iron	Zinc	Copper	Vitamin A	Vitamin D	Vitamin E (Alpha Tocopherol)	Vitamin C	Thiamin	Riboflavin	Niacin	Pantothenic Acid	Vit. B-6 (Pyridoxine)	Folacin (Folic Acid)	Biotin	Vitamin B-12
	(mg)	(mg)	(mg)	(IU)	(IU)	(mg)	(mg)	(mg)	(mg)	(mg)	(mg)	(mg)	(mcg)	(mcg)	(mcg)
341	–	–	–	–	–	–	–	–	–	–	–	–	–	–	–
	–	–	–	–	–	–	–	–	–	–	–	–	–	–	–
342	.06	–	.01	0	0	–	Trace	Trace	.01	.07	–	–	–	–	0
	.22	–	.05	0	0	–	Trace	Trace	.04	.26	–	–	–	–	0
343	.10	.02	.04	0	0	–	.20	–	.01	.06	.04	Trace	.60	–	0
	.50	.10	.20	0	0	–	1.00	–	.04	.30	.20	.02	3.00	–	0
344	–	–	–	0	0	–	1.85	–	–	–	–	–	–	–	–
	–	–	–	0	–	–	1.00	–	–	–	–	–	–	–	–
345	.20	–	–	28.0	–	–	–	Trace	.01	–	–	–	–	–	–
	2.00	–	–	280.0	–	–	–	.01	.06	–	–	–	–	–	–
346	.12	–	–	21.0	–	–	–	Trace	.01	.02	–	–	–	–	–
	1.20	–	–	210.0	–	–	–	.02	.10	.20	–	–	–	–	–
347	.05	–	–	0	–	–	0	Trace	Trace	.02	–	–	–	–	–
	.50	–	–	0	–	–	0	.01	.04	.20	–	–	–	–	–
348	–	–	–	0	–	–	0	–	Trace	–	–	–	–	–	–
	–	–	–	0	–	–	0	–	.03	–	–	–	–	–	–
349	–	–	–	27.0	–	–	–	–	Trace	–	–	–	–	–	–
	–	–	–	270.0	–	–	–	–	.02	–	–	–	–	–	–
350	.20	–	–	2.0	0	–	3.00	Trace	.01	.04	–	–	1.60	–	–
	1.00	–	–	10.0	0	–	15.00	.01	.03	.20	–	–	8.00	–	–
351	.30	–	–	2.0	0	–	.80	Trace	.01	.04	–	–	–	–	–
	1.50	–	–	10.0	0	–	4.00	.01	.03	.20	–	–	–	–	–
352	.12	–	(.03)	0	0	Trace	1.20	Trace	Trace	.02	Trace	0	(1.08)	Trace	0
	.60	–	(.13)	0	0	Trace	6.00	.02	.02	.10	Trace	.02	(5.40)	Trace	0
353	.43	.06	.06	.5	0	–	Trace	Trace	.01	.06	Trace	.03	Trace	Trace	0
	1.53	.22	.21	1.7	0	–	Trace	.02	.03	.21	.02	.09	Trace	Trace	0
354	3.22	.44	1.20	0	0	–	0	.02	.04	.40	.07	.04	1.90	1.80	0
	16.10	2.20	6.00	0	0	–	0	.11	.19	2.00	.35	.20	9.50	9.00	0
355	–	–	–	0	–	–	0	0	0	0	–	–	–	–	–
	–	–	–	0	–	–	0	0	0	0	–	–	–	–	–
356	.26	.73	.08	5.2	–	–	2.60	.05	.31	.26	–	–	–	–	–
	.10	.28	.03	2.0	–	–	1.00	.02	.12	.10	–	–	–	–	–
357	.23	1.18	.27	4.5	–	–	2.27	.05	.30	.23	–	–	–	–	–
	.10	.52	.12	2.0	–	–	1.00	.02	.13	.10	–	–	–	–	–
358	.01	.11	8.42	55.4	11.08	–	.27	.01	.04	.02	.09	.01	1.36	–	.11
	.04	.39	30.07	197.9	39.59	–	.97	.04	.14	.09	.32	.04	4.85	–	.38
359	–	–	–	364.0	–	–	–	.05	.36	.26	–	–	–	–	–
	–	–	–	140.0	–	–	–	.02	.14	.10	–	–	–	–	–
360	1.13	–	–	40.7	–	–	2.26	.05	.14	.23	–	–	–	–	–
	.50	–	–	18.0	–	–	1.00	.02	.06	.10	–	–	–	–	–
361	1.06	–	–	291.5	–	–	–	.08	.37	.53	–	–	–	–	–
	.40	–	–	110.0	–	–	–	.03	.14	.20	–	–	–	–	–
362	.11	–	–	81.2	–	–	.28	.01	.05	.03	–	–	–	–	–
	.40	–	–	290.0	–	–	1.00	.04	.18	.10	–	–	–	–	–
363	.34	.83	.08	307.4	100.40	.15	3.36	.10	.44	1.16	.77	.10	12.24	7.57	.89
	.11	.27	.03	103.5	33.80	.05	1.13	.03	.15	.39	.26	.03	4.12	2.55	.30
364	.09	–	–	58.7	–	–	–	.01	.06	.02	–	–	–	–	–
	.50	–	–	326.0	–	–	–	.05	.33	.13	–	–	–	–	–
365	–	–	–	32.2	–	–	.77	0	–	–	–	–	–	–	–
	–	–	–	230.0	–	–	5.50	0	–	–	–	–	–	–	–
366	–	–	–	40.2	–	–	1.25	.01	.01	.15	–	–	–	–	–
	–	–	–	335.0	–	–	10.40	.06	.04	1.25	–	–	–	–	–
367	.19	1.33	.04	185.3	–	–	3.86	.02	.09	.13	.06	.03	13.51	–	.16
	.10	.69	.02	96.0	–	–	2.00	.01	.05	.07	.03	.01	7.00	–	.08
368	.48	Trace	Trace	0	0	–	0	Trace	Trace	.03	–	–	–	–	–
	3.40	.03	.02	0	0	–	0	.01	.03	.20	–	–	–	–	–
369	.01	.01	Trace	0	0	–	0	0	0	0	–	–	–	–	.02
	.10	.05	.02	0	0	–	0	0	0	0	–	–	–	–	.23
370	.01	Trace	Trace	0	0	–	0	0	0	0	–	–	–	–	.03
	.10	.02	.02	0	0	–	0	0	0	0	–	–	–	–	.23
371	.21	–	–	–	0	–	0	–	–	–	–	–	–	–	–
	1.40	–	–	–	0	–	0	–	–	–	–	–	–	–	–

(Continued)

TABLE F-21 *(Continued)*

Item No.	Food Item Name	Approximate Measure	Weight (g)	Moisture (%)	Food Energy Calories (kcal)	Protein (g)	Fats (g)	Carbo- hydrates (g)	Fiber (g)	Calcium (mg)	Phos- phorus (mg)	Sodium (mg)	Mag- nesium (mg)	Potas- sium (mg)
	SYRUPS													
372	CHOCOLATE, thin-type	1 TBLS	20	31.6	49.0	.5	.4	12.5	.1	3.4	18.4	10.4	12.6	56.4
			100	31.6	245.0	2.3	2.0	62.7	.6	17.0	92.0	52.0	63.0	282.0
373	MAPLE	1 TBLS	20	33.0	50.4	0	0	13.0	0	20.8	1.6	2.0	2.0	35.2
			100	33.0	252.0	0	0	65.0	0	104.0	8.0	10.0	10.0	176.0
374	SORGHUM	1 TBLS	20	23.0	51.4	–	–	13.6	0	34.4	5.0	4.0	–	120.0
			100	23.0	257.0	–	–	68.0	0	172.0	25.0	20.0	–	600.0
375	TABLE BLEND OF CANE & MAPLE	1 TBLS	20	33.0	50.4	0	0	13.0	0	3.2	.2	.4	–	5.2
			100	33.0	252.0	0	0	65.0	0	16.0	1.0	2.0	–	26.0
	TOPPINGS													
376	marshallow	1 TBLS	8	17.6	25.3	.1	0	6.4	0	2.6	1.0	4.7	–	2.6
			100	17.6	316.0	1.0	0	80.6	0	32.0	12.0	59.0	–	32.0
377	whipped, non-dairy, Cool Whip	1 TBLS	5	47.3	14.0	0	1.0	1.0	–	0	0	1.0	.1	1.0
			100	47.3	280.0	0	20.0	20.0	–	0	0	20.0	1.0	20.0
378	*TRIFLE	1 SERV (4 OZ)	112	64.5	179.2	3.9	6.8	27.2	0	91.8	97.4	56.0	15.7	91.8
			100	64.5	160.0	3.5	6.1	24.3	0	82.0	87.0	50.0	14.0	82.0
	EGGS AND SUBSTITUTES													
	CHICKEN EGGS													
379	raw, whole, fresh	1 MED	48	73.7	75.4	6.1	5.4	.6	0	25.9	86.4	66.2	5.8	61.9
			100	73.7	157.0	12.8	11.3	1.2	0	54.0	180.0	138.0	12.0	129.0
380	raw whites, fresh & frozen	1 MED	31	87.6	15.8	3.3	0	.4	0	3.4	3.4	45.3	3.1	43.1
			100	87.6	51.0	10.8	0	1.2	0	11.0	11.0	146.0	9.9	139.0
381	raw yokes, fresh	1 MED	17	48.8	62.7	2.8	5.6	0	0	25.8	86.4	8.8	2.6	15.3
			100	48.8	369.0	16.3	32.9	.2	0	152.0	508.0	52.0	15.0	90.0
382	fried	1 MED	48	68.4	100.9	5.6	8.6	.5	0	24.6	79.4	97.6	5.3	57.2
			100	68.4	210.2	11.7	17.9	1.1	0	51.3	165.5	203.3	11.1	119.2
383	hard-cooked	1 MED	48	73.7	75.4	6.1	5.4	.6	0	25.9	86.4	58.6	5.8	61.9
			100	73.7	157.0	12.8	11.3	1.2	0	54.0	180.0	122.0	12.0	129.0
384	poached	1 MED	48	73.3	74.4	6.1	5.4	.6	0	26.4	85.9	140.6	5.8	61.4
			100	73.3	155.0	12.8	11.2	1.2	0	55.0	179.0	293.0	12.0	128.0
385	scrambled	1 MED	65	76.3	96.2	6.1	7.2	1.6	0	52.0	98.2	167.1	7.8	86.5
			100	76.3	148.0	9.3	11.1	2.4	0	80.0	151.0	257.0	12.0	133.0
386	DUCK EGGS, raw, whole, fresh	1 MED	74	70.4	138.4	9.8	10.2	1.1	0	47.4	162.8	90.3	11.8	164.3
			100	70.4	187.0	13.3	13.8	1.5	0	64.0	220.0	122.0	16.0	222.0
387	GOOSE EGGS, raw, whole, fresh	1 MED	144	70.4	260.6	20.0	19.2	1.9	0	–	–	–	–	–
			100	70.4	181.0	13.9	13.3	1.3	0	–	–	–	–	–
388	QUAIL EGGS, raw, whole, fresh	1 MED	9	74.4	14.2	1.2	1.0	0	0	5.8	20.3	–	–	–
			100	74.4	158.0	13.1	11.0	.4	0	64.0	226.0	–	–	–
389	TURKEY EGGS, raw, whole, fresh	1 MED	72	72.6	118.8	9.4	8.5	.8	0	71.3	122.4	–	–	–
			100	72.6	165.0	13.1	11.8	1.2	0	99.0	170.0	–	–	–
390	EGG SUBSTITUTES, egg beaters, Fleischmanns	1 CUP	240	73.0	400.8	26.4	30.0	7.2	–	192.0	168.0	432.0	–	511.2
			100	73.0	167.0	11.0	12.5	3.0	–	80.0	70.0	180.0	–	213.0
	ENTREES													
391	BEANS & FRANKFURTERS, canned	1 CUP	255	70.7	367.2	19.4	18.1	32.1	2.6	94.4	303.5	1374.5	–	668.1
			100	70.7	144.0	7.1	7.1	12.6	1.0	37.0	119.0	539.0	–	262.0
392	BEEF, DRIED, CHIPPED, creamed	1 CUP	240	72.0	369.6	19.7	24.7	17.0	–	252.0	336.0	1718.4	–	367.2
			100	72.0	154.0	8.2	10.3	7.1	–	105.0	140.0	716.0	–	153.0
393	BEEF STEW	1 OZ	28	–	26.7	3.3	.7	1.5	.1	4.1	20.1	58.8	3.1	63.5
			100	–	95.4	11.8	2.6	5.5	.3	14.6	71.7	210.1	11.2	226.8
394	CHEESEBURGER, w/bun	INDIV	105	48.6	258.5	15.5	10.7	25.0	.2	115.5	221.6	664.7	19.7	244.7
			100	48.6	246.2	14.8	10.2	23.8	.2	110.0	211.0	633.0	18.8	233.0
395	CHEESE FONDUE, homemade	1 TBLS	16	54.2	42.4	2.4	2.9	1.6	–	50.7	47.0	86.7	–	26.4
			100	54.2	265.0	14.8	18.3	10.0	–	317.0	294.0	542.0	–	165.0
396	CHEESE SOUFFLE, homemade	1 CUP	150	65.0	327.0	14.9	25.7	9.3	–	301.5	292.5	546.0	–	181.5
			100	65.0	218.0	9.9	17.1	6.2	–	201.0	195.0	364.0	–	121.0
397	CHICKEN A LA KING, homemade, cooked	1 CUP	245	68.2	468.0	27.4	34.3	12.3	–	127.4	357.7	759.5	–	404.3
			100	68.2	191.0	11.2	14.0	5.0	–	52.0	146.0	310.0	–	165.0
398	CHILI CON CARNE, w/beans, canned	1 CUP	230	72.4	305.9	17.3	14.0	28.1	1.4	73.6	289.8	1221.3	–	535.9
			100	72.4	133.0	7.5	6.1	12.2	.6	32.0	126.0	531.0	–	233.0
399	CHITTERLINGS	1 SERV	100	–	335.0	8.6	25.7	–	–	–	–	–	–	–
			100	–	335.0	8.6	25.7	–	–	–	–	–	–	–
400	CHOP SUEY, w/meat, homemade, cooked	1 CUP	250	75.4	300.0	26.0	17.0	12.8	1.3	60.0	247.5	1052.5	–	425.0
			100	75.4	120.0	10.4	6.8	5.1	.5	24.0	99.0	421.0	–	170.0
401	CHOW MEIN, CHICKEN, w/o noodles, homemade, cooked	1 CUP	250	78.0	255.0	31.0	10.0	10.0	.8	57.5	292.5	717.5	–	472.5
			100	78.0	102.0	12.4	4.0	4.0	.3	23.0	117.0	287.0	–	189.0

Item No.	Minerals (Micro)			Fat-Soluble Vitamins			Water-Soluble Vitamins								
	Iron	Zinc	Copper	Vitamin A	Vitamin D	Vitamin E (Alpha Tocopherol)	Vitamin C	Thiamin	Riboflavin	Niacin	Pantothenic Acid	Vit. B-6 (Pyridoxine)	Folacin (Folic Acid)	Biotin	Vitamin B-12
	(mg)	(mg)	(mg)	(IU)	(IU)	(mg)	(mg)	(mg)	(mg)	(mg)	(mg)	(mg)	(mcg)	(mcg)	(mcg)
372	.32	.18	.09	–	0	–	0	Trace	.01	.08	–	–	–	–	–
	1.60	.90	.43	–	0	–	0	.02	.07	.40	–	–	–	–	–
373	.24	–	–	0	0	–	0	–	–	–	–	–	–	–	–
	1.20	–	–	0	0	–	0	–	–	–	–	–	–	–	–
374	2.50	–	–	–	0	–	–	–	.02	.02	–	–	–	–	–
	12.50	–	–	–	0	–	–	–	.10	.10	–	–	–	–	–
375	–	–	–	0	–	–	0	0	0	0	–	–	–	–	–
	–	–	–	0	–	–	0	0	0	0	–	–	–	–	–
376	–	–	–	–	–	–	.80	–	–	–	–	–	–	–	–
	–	–	–	–	–	–	10.00	–	–	–	–	–	–	–	–
377	0	Trace	Trace	0	–	–	–	–	–	–	–	–	–	–	–
	0	.05	.06	0	–	–	–	–	–	–	–	–	–	–	–
378	.78	.45	.10	28.0	.19	.34	1.12	.06	.16	.22	.45	.07	6.72	3.36	Trace
	.70	.40	.09	25.0	.17	.30	1.00	.05	.14	.20	.40	.06	6.00	3.00	Trace
379	1.10	.69	.03	249.6	24.00	(.80)	0	.04	.14	.03	.77	.06	31.20	10.80	.74
	2.30	1.44	.05	520.0	50.00	(1.60)	0	.09	.30	.06	1.60	.12	65.00	22.50	1.55
380	.01	.01	Trace	0	0	0	0	Trace	.08	.03	.06	0	4.96	2.17	.02
	.03	.02	.01	0	0	0	0	.01	.27	.09	.20	0	16.00	7.00	.07
381	.94	.58	0	312.6	26.86	(.78)	0	.04	.08	.01	.75	.05	25.84	8.84	.64
	5.50	3.38	.01	1839.0	158.00	(4.60)	0	.22	.44	.07	4.40	.30	152.00	52.00	3.80
382	1.01	.63	.04	365.1	21.77	.08	0	.05	.26	.03	.70	.04	28.44	9.80	.67
	2.11	1.31	.08	760.7	45.36	.17	0	.10	.54	.06	1.45	.08	59.25	20.41	1.40
383	1.10	.69	–	249.6	22.08	–	0	.04	.13	.03	.83	.06	23.52	–	.63
	2.30	1.44	–	520.0	46.00	–	0	.09	.28	.06	1.73	.11	49.00	–	1.32
384	1.06	.69	–	248.6	25.92	(.80)	0	.04	.12	.03	.83	.05	23.52	(12.02)	.59
	2.20	1.43	–	518.0	54.00	(1.60)	0	.08	.25	.05	1.72	.10	49.00	(25.00)	1.23
385	.95	.72	–	315.9	–	.30	.13	.05	.18	.04	.83	.06	22.75	–	.65
	.46	1.10	–	486.0	–	.46	.20	.08	.28	.07	1.28	.09	35.00	–	1.00
386	2.85	1.04	–	982.7	–	–	0	.13	.22	.07	–	.19	59.20	–	3.99
	3.85	1.41	–	1328.0	–	–	0	.18	.30	.10	–	.25	80.00	–	5.40
387	–	–	–	–	–	–	0	–	–	–	–	–	–	–	–
	–	–	–	–	–	–	0	–	–	–	–	–	–	–	–
388	.33	–	–	27.0	–	–	0	.01	.07	.01	–	.00	–	–	–
	3.65	–	–	300.0	–	–	0	.13	.79	.15	–	.02	–	–	–
389	2.95	–	–	–	–	–	0	.08	.34	.02	–	–	–	–	–
	4.10	–	–	–	–	–	0	.11	.47	.02	–	–	–	–	–
390	4.32	.77	.46	3240.0	103.20	–	–	.31	1.03	–	–	–	–	–	–
	1.80	.32	.19	1350.0	43.00	–	–	.13	.43	–	–	–	–	–	–
391	4.86	–	–	331.5	–	–	–	.18	.15	3.32	–	–	–	–	–
	1.90	–	–	130.0	–	–	–	.07	.06	1.30	–	–	–	–	–
392	1.92	–	–	864.0	4.80	–	–	.14	.46	1.44	–	–	–	–	–
	.80	–	–	360.0	2.00	–	–	.06	.19	.60	–	–	–	–	–
393	.47	.04	–	393.8	0	–	1.20	.02	.03	1.34	.01	Trace	.23	–	0
	1.67	.13	–	1406.6	0	–	4.29	.07	.10	4.79	.04	.01	.81	–	0
394	1.79	2.42	.26	–	–	–	–	–	–	–	–	–	–	–	–
	1.70	2.30	.25	–	–	–	–	–	–	–	–	–	–	–	–
395	.19	–	–	140.8	–	–	–	.01	.05	.03	–	–	–	–	–
	1.20	–	–	880.0	–	–	–	.06	.34	.20	–	–	–	–	–
396	1.50	–	–	1200.0	–	–	–	.08	.36	.30	–	–	–	–	–
	1.00	–	–	800.0	–	–	–	.05	.24	.20	–	–	–	–	–
397	2.45	–	–	1127.0	–	–	12.25	.10	.42	5.39	–	–	–	–	–
	1.00	–	–	460.0	–	–	5.00	.04	.17	2.20	–	–	–	–	–
398	3.91	3.75	–	138.0	–	–	–	.07	.16	2.99	.32	.24	–	–	–
	1.70	1.63	–	60.0	–	–	–	.03	.07	1.30	.14	.10	–	–	–
399	–	–	–	–	–	–	–	–	–	–	–	–	–	–	–
	–	–	–	–	–	–	–	–	–	–	–	–	–	–	–
400	4.75	–	–	600.0	–	–	32.50	.28	.38	5.00	–	–	–	–	–
	1.90	–	–	240.0	–	–	13.00	.11	.15	2.00	–	–	–	–	–
401	2.50	–	–	275.0	–	–	10.00	.08	.23	4.25	–	–	–	–	–
	1.00	–	–	110.0	–	–	4.00	.03	.09	1.70	–	–	–	–	–

(Continued)

TABLE F-21 (Continued)

Item No.	Food Item Name	Approximate Measure	Weight (g)	Moisture (%)	Food Energy Calories (kcal)	Protein (g)	Fats (g)	Carbohydrates (g)	Fiber (g)	Calcium (mg)	Phosphorus (mg)	Sodium (mg)	Magnesium (mg)	Potassium (mg)
402	CORNED BEEF HASH, canned	1 CUP	230	—	457.7	20.4	33.6	18.6	—	59.8	158.7	1994.1	—	—
			100	—	199.0	8.9	14.6	8.1	—	26.0	69.0	867.0	—	—
	FROZEN DINNERS													
403	BEEF POT ROAST, w/whole potato, peas & corn, unheated	1 WHOLE	205	76.3	217.3	26.9	6.6	12.5	.6	20.5	155.8	531.0	—	500.2
			100	76.3	106.0	13.1	3.2	6.1	.3	10.0	76.0	259.0	—	244.0
404	FRIED CHICKEN, w/mashed potato & mixed vegetable, unheated	1 WHOLE	312	66.1	539.8	39.9	26.5	35.3	1.2	127.9	452.4	1073.3	—	349.4
			100	66.1	173.0	12.8	8.5	11.3	.4	41.0	145.0	344.0	—	112.0
405	MEAT LOAF, w/tomato sauce, mashed potato & peas, unheated	1 WHOLE	312	73.7	408.7	25.0	20.9	30.6	.9	59.3	365.0	1226.2	—	358.8
			100	73.7	131.0	8.0	6.7	9.8	.3	19.0	117.0	393.0	—	115.0
406	TURKEY, w/mashed potato & peas, unheated	1 WHOLE	312	74.7	349.4	26.2	9.4	39.6	.9	81.1	271.4	1248.0	—	549.1
			100	74.7	112.0	8.4	3.0	12.7	.3	26.0	87.0	400.0	—	176.0
407	MACARONI & CHEESE, w/margarine, enriched, baked	1 CUP	200	58.2	430.0	16.8	22.2	40.2	.2	362.0	322.0	1086.0	—	240.0
			100	58.2	215.0	8.4	11.1	10.1	.1	181.0	161.0	543.0	—	120.0
408	MEATBALLS, cooked	1 OZ	28	—	78.4	5.0	5.5	1.9	—	11.5	42.0	—	5.6	—
			100	—	280.0	17.9	19.5	6.9	—	41.0	150.0	—	20.0	—
409	MEATLOAF, cooked	1 OZ	28	—	78.4	5.0	5.5	1.9	—	11.5	42.0	—	5.6	—
			100	—	280.0	17.9	19.5	6.9	—	41.0	150.0	—	20.0	—
410	*MOUSSAKA	4 OZ	112	—	218.5	10.4	15.0	11.0	—	99.5	147.1	359.5	23.9	398.0
			100	—	195.1	9.3	13.4	9.8	—	88.8	131.3	321.0	21.3	355.4
	PIZZA													
411	BEEF, ground, frozen, baked	1 PIECE	100	47.0	248.0	6.8	6.4	41.0	—	—	—	—	—	—
			100	47.0	248.0	6.8	6.4	41.0	—	—	—	—	—	—
412	CHEESE, homemade, w/sausage, enriched, baked	1 PIECE	67	50.6	156.8	5.2	6.2	19.8	.2	11.4	61.6	488.4	—	112.6
			100	50.6	234.0	7.8	9.3	29.6	.3	17.0	92.0	729.0	—	168.0
413	PEPPERONI, frozen, baked	1 PIECE	100	44.0	278.0	6.2	10.0	40.7	—	—	—	—	—	—
			100	44.0	278.0	6.2	10.0	40.7	—	—	—	—	—	—
	POTPIES													
414	BEEF, homemade, baked	1 INDV	227	55.1	558.4	22.9	32.9	42.7	.9	31.8	161.2	644.7	—	360.9
			100	55.1	246.0	10.1	14.5	18.8	.4	14.0	71.0	284.0	—	159.0
415	CHICKEN, homemade, baked	1 HALF	116	56.6	272.6	11.7	15.7	21.2	.5	34.8	116.0	297.0	—	171.7
			100	56.6	235.0	10.1	13.5	18.3	.4	30.0	100.0	256.0	—	148.0
416	TURKEY, homemade, baked	1 INDV	227	56.2	538.0	23.6	30.6	42.0	.9	61.3	229.3	619.7	—	449.5
			100	56.2	237.0	10.4	13.5	18.5	.4	27.0	101.0	273.0	—	198.0
417	QUICHE LORRAINE	1 SERV	162	—	494.7	14.6	40.5	18.0	—	256.0	309.4	—	14.6	—
			100	—	305.4	9.0	25.0	11.1	—	158.0	191.0	—	9.0	—
	SANDWICHES													
418	PEANUT BUTTER & JELLY	1 INDV	75	28.0	280.6	9.2	11.3	37.2	.6	54.3	126.8	356.3	46.0	193.1
			100	28.0	374.2	12.3	15.1	49.6	.6	72.3	169.0	475.0	61.3	257.4
419	TUNA, grilled	1 OZ	28	—	77.5	7.0	8.5	10.6	.1	25.2	71.5	239.9	11.0	59.8
			100	—	276.6	25.1	30.5	38.0	.4	89.9	255.3	856.8	39.2	213.4
	SPAGHETTI													
420	w/meatballs in tomato sauce	1 CUP	250	78.1	275.0	10.0	12.5	27.5	.5	47.5	140.0	1150.0	—	440.0
			100	78.1	110.0	4.0	5.0	11.0	.2	19.0	56.0	460.0	—	176.0
421	homemade, cooked	1 CUP	150	78.5	130.5	2.7	2.6	24.9	.8	21.0	59.5	474.0	—	346.5
			100	78.5	87.0	1.8	1.7	16.6	.5	14.0	39.0	316.0	—	231.0
422	SWEDISH MEAT BALLS, frozen	1 PIECE	28	—	58.0	2.5	4.5	1.8	—	20.1	35.0	235.0	—	3.0
			100	—	207.1	9.0	16.0	6.5	—	71.8	125.0	839.3	—	10.7
	VEGETARIAN MAIN DISHES													
423	w/peanuts & soybean, canned	1 OZ	28	55.3	66.4	3.3	4.7	3.8	.3	—	—	—	—	—
			100	55.3	237.0	11.7	16.9	13.4	.9	—	—	—	—	—
424	w/wheat & soy protein, canned	1 OZ	28	73.4	29.1	4.5	.3	2.1	.1	—	—	—	—	—
			100	73.4	104.0	16.1	1.2	7.6	.3	—	—	—	—	—
	FATS AND OILS													
425	BACON	1 TBLS	14	—	126.0	0	14.0	—	—	—	—	—	—	—
			100	—	900.0	0	100.0	—	—	—	—	—	—	—
426	CHICKEN	1 TBLS	14	.2	126.0	0	14.0	0	—	—	—	—	—	—
			100	.2	900.0	0	100.0	0	—	—	—	—	—	—
427	DUCK	1 TBLS	13	.2	117.1	0	13.0	0	0	—	—	—	—	—
			100	.2	900.4	0	99.8	0	0	—	—	—	—	—
428	GOOSE	1 TBLS	13	.2	117.1	0	13.0	0	0	—	—	—	—	—
			100	.2	900.4	0	99.8	0	0	—	—	—	—	—
429	TURKEY	1 TBLS	13	.2	117.1	0	13.0	0	0	—	—	—	—	—
			100	.2	900.4	0	99.8	0	0	—	—	—	—	—
430	LARD, PORK	1 TBLS	13	.0	117.3	0	13.0	0	0	0	0	0	0	0
			100	.0	902.0	0	100.0	0	0	.1	0	0	0	0
	MARGARINES													
431	HARD, salted, hydrogenated vegetable oils	1 TSP	5	15.7	35.9	0	4.0	0	0	1.5	1.1	47.2	.1	2.1
			100	15.7	718.7	.9	80.5	.9	0	29.9	22.9	943.4	2.6	42.4

Item No.	Minerals (Micro)			Fat-Soluble Vitamins			Water-Soluble Vitamins								
	Iron	Zinc	Copper	Vitamin A	Vitamin D	Vitamin E (Alpha Tocopherol)	Vitamin C	Thiamin	Ribo-flavin	Niacin	Panto-thenic Acid	Vit. B-6 (Pyri-doxine)	Folacin (Folic Acid)	Biotin	Vitamin B-12
	(mg)	(mg)	(mg)	(IU)	(IU)	(mg)	(mg)	(mg)	(mg)	(mg)	(mg)	(mg)	(mcg)	(mcg)	(mcg)
402	2.76	–	–	0.0	0	–	0	.07	.32	6.58	–	–	–	–	–
	1.20	–	–	0.0	0	–	0	.03	.14	2.86	–	–	–	–	–
403	3.28	–	–	225.5	–	–	10.25	.12	.21	4.31	–	–	49.20	–	–
	1.60	–	–	110.0	–	–	5.00	.06	.10	2.10	–	–	24.00	–	–
404	3.74	–	–	1840.8	–	–	12.48	.22	.56	16.22	–	–	–	–	–
	1.20	–	–	590.0	–	–	4.00	.07	.18	5.20	–	–	–	–	–
405	4.06	–	–	1341.6	–	–	12.48	.31	.44	5.30	–	–	–	–	–
	1.30	–	–	430.0	–	–	4.00	.10	.14	1.70	–	–	–	–	–
406	3.43	–	–	405.6	–	–	12.48	.22	.28	7.18	–	–	–	–	–
	1.10	–	–	130.0	–	–	4.00	.07	.09	2.30	–	–	–	–	–
407	1.80	–	–	860.0	–	–	–	.20	.40	1.80	–	–	–	–	–
	.90	–	–	430.0	–	–	–	.10	.20	.90	–	–	–	–	–
408	.62	–	–	14.0	–	–	0	.02	.04	.76	–	.12	–	–	.39
	2.20	–	–	50.0	–	–	0	.06	.15	2.70	–	.41	–	–	1.38
409	.62	(.80)	–	14.0	–	–	.28	.02	.04	.76	–	.12	–	–	.39
	2.20	(2.86)	–	50.0	–	–	1.00	.06	.15	2.70	–	.41	–	–	1.38
410	1.52	2.07	.16	40.3	.07	.37	4.60	.07	.17	1.68	.60	.20	9.02	2.39	1.46
	1.36	1.85	.14	36.0	.06	.33	4.11	.06	.15	1.50	.54	.18	8.05	2.13	1.30
411	–	–	–	–	–	–	–	–	–	–	–	–	–	–	–
	–	–	–	–	–	–	–	–	–	–	–	–	–	–	–
412	.54	–	–	375.2	–	–	6.03	.08	.05	.60	–	–	–	–	–
	.80	–	–	560.0	–	–	9.00	.12	.08	.90	–	–	–	–	–
413	–	–	–	–	–	–	–	–	–	–	–	–	–	–	–
	–	–	–	–	–	–	–	–	–	–	–	–	–	–	–
414	4.09	–	–	1861.4	–	–	6.81	.25	.27	4.54	–	–	–	–	–
	1.80	–	–	820.0	–	–	3.00	.11	.12	2.00	–	–	–	–	–
415	1.51	–	–	1542.8	–	–	2.32	.13	.13	2.09	–	–	–	–	–
	1.30	–	–	1330.0	–	–	2.00	.11	.11	1.80	–	–	–	–	–
416	3.18	–	–	3019.1	–	–	4.54	.25	.30	5.68	–	–	–	–	–
	1.40	–	–	1330.0	–	–	2.00	.11	.13	2.50	–	–	–	–	–
417	1.78	–	–	1365.7	–	–	0	.13	.34	.81	–	.28	–	–	1.33
	1.10	–	–	843.0	–	–	0	.08	.21	.50	–	.17	–	–	.82
418	1.77	.84	–	1.5	0	–	.60	.14	.13	4.26	.69	.08	26.66	–	0
	2.36	1.12	–	2.0	0	–	.80	.19	.17	5.68	.93	.11	35.54	–	0
419	.95	.23	–	65.6	3.74	–	.88	.06	.08	2.23	.30	.02	10.65	–	.44
	3.38	.81	–	234.1	13.35	–	3.16	.21	.29	7.96	1.06	.06	38.04	–	1.57
420	3.50	–	–	655.0	–	–	2.75	.23	.20	4.50	–	–	–	–	–
	1.40	–	–	262.0	–	–	1.10	.09	.08	1.80	–	–	–	–	–
421	.90	–	–	990.0	–	–	22.50	.06	.05	1.05	–	–	–	–	–
	.60	–	–	660.0	–	–	15.00	.04	.03	.70	–	–	–	–	–
422	.24	–	–	80.0	–	–	0	.02	.05	.33	–	–	–	–	–
	.86	–	–	285.7	–	–	0	.07	.18	1.18	–	–	–	–	–
423	–	–	–	–	–	–	–	–	–	–	.05	.01	–	–	0
	–	–	–	–	–	–	–	–	–	–	.19	.04	–	–	0
424	–	–	–	–	–	–	–	–	–	–	.02	.02	–	–	0
	–	–	–	–	–	–	–	–	–	–	.06	.07	–	–	0
425	–	–	–	–	–	–	–	–	–	–	–	–	–	–	–
	–	–	–	–	–	–	–	–	–	–	–	–	–	–	–
426	–	–	–	0	–	–	–	–	–	–	–	–	–	–	–
	–	–	–	0	–	–	–	–	–	–	–	–	–	–	–
427	–	–	–	–	–	–	–	–	–	–	–	–	–	–	–
	–	–	–	–	–	–	–	–	–	–	–	–	–	–	–
428	–	–	–	–	–	–	–	–	–	–	–	–	–	–	–
	–	–	–	–	–	–	–	–	–	–	–	–	–	–	–
429	–	–	–	–	–	–	–	–	–	–	–	–	–	–	–
	–	–	–	–	–	–	–	–	–	–	–	–	–	–	–
430	0	.01	.03	0	364.00	.16	0	0	0	0	–	Trace	0	–	0
	0	.11	.26	0	2800.00	1.20	0	0	0	0	–	.02	0	–	0
431	Trace	–	–	165.4	–	–	.01	Trace	Trace	Trace	Trace	0	.06	–	.01
	(.30)	–	–	3307.0	–	–	.16	.01	.04	.02	.08	.01	1.18	–	.10

(Continued)

TABLE F-21 (Continued)

Item No.	Food Item Name	Approximate Measure	Weight	Moisture	Food Energy Calories	Protein	Fats	Carbo-hydrates	Fiber	Minerals (Macro)				
										Calcium	Phos-phorus	Sodium	Mag-nesium	Potas-sium
			(g)	(%)	(kcal)	(g)	(g)	(g)	(g)	(mg)	(mg)	(mg)	(mg)	(mg)
432	SOFT, tub, salted, unspecified oils	1 TBLS	14	16.2	100.3	.1	11.3	.1	–	3.7	2.8	151.0	.3	5.3
			100	16.2	716.4	.8	80.4	.5	–	26.5	20.3	1078.7	2.3	37.7
433	WHIPPED	1 TSP	4	16.0	28.7	.1	3.2	0	–	.8	–	–	–	–
			100	16.0	717.0	1.3	80.3	0	–	20.0	–	–	–	–
434	IMITATION, salted, 40% fat, hydrogenated corn	1 TSP	5	58.1	17.3	0	1.9	0	0	.9	.7	48.0	.1	1.3
			100	58.1	345.2	.5	38.8	.4	0	17.8	13.7	959.6	1.6	25.3
	OILS													
435	ALMOND	1 TBLS	14	.0	123.8	0	14.0	0	0	–	–	–	–	–
			100	.0	884.0	0	100.0	0	0	–	–	–	–	–
436	COCOA (CACAO) BUTTER	1 TBLS	14	.0	123.8	0	14.0	0	0	–	–	–	–	–
			100	.0	884.0	0	100.0	0	0	–	–	–	–	–
437	COCONUT	1 TBLS	14	.0	123.8	0	14.0	0	0	–	–	–	–	–
			100	.0	884.0	0	100.0	0	0	–	.1	–	–	–
438	CORN	1 TBLS	14	.0	123.8	0	14.0	0	0	0	0	0	.1	0
			100	.0	884.0	0	100.0	0	0	0	0	0	.5	0
439	COTTONSEED	1 TBLS	14	.0	123.8	0	14.0	0	0	0	0	0	0	0
			100	.0	884.0	0	100.0	0	0	0	0	0	.1	0
440	LINSEED	1 TBLS	14	.0	123.8	0	14.0	0	0	0	0	–	0	–
			100	.0	884.0	0	100.0	0	0	.1	.2	–	0	–
441	OLIVE	1 TBLS	14	.0	123.8	0	14.0	0	0	0	.2	0	0	0
			100	.0	884.0	0	100.0	0	0	.2	1.2	0	0	0
442	PALM	1 TBLS	14	.0	123.8	0	14.0	0	0	–	0	–	–	–
			100	.0	884.0	0	100.0	0	0	–	.2	–	–	–
443	PALM KERNEL	1 TBLS	14	.0	123.8	0	14.0	0	0	–	–	–	–	–
			100	.0	884.0	0	100.0	0	0	–	–	–	–	–
444	PEANUT	1 TBLS	14	.0	123.8	0	14.0	0	0	0	0	0	0	0
			100	.0	884.0	0	100.0	0	0	.1	0	.1	0	0
445	RAPESEED, low to 30% erucic acid content	1 TBLS	14	.0	123.8	0	14.0	0	0	–	–	–	–	–
			100	.0	884.0	0	100.0	0	0	–	–	–	–	–
446	RAPESEED, 0% erucic acid content	1 TBLS	14	.0	123.8	0	14.0	0	0	–	–	–	–	–
			100	.0	884.0	0	100.0	0	0	–	–	–	–	–
447	SAFFLOWER, over 70% linoleic acid	1 TBLS	14	.0	123.8	0	14.0	0	0	0	0	0	–	0
			100	.0	884.0	0	100.0	0	0	0	0	0	–	0
448	SESAME	1 TBLS	14	.0	123.8	0	14.0	0	0	0	0	0	–	0
			100	.0	884.0	0	100.0	0	0	0	0	0	–	0
449	SOYBEAN	1 TBLS	14	.0	123.8	0	14.0	0	0	0	0	0	0	0
			100	.0	884.0	0	100.0	0	0	0	.3	0	0	0
450	SUNFLOWER, less than 60% linoleic acid	1 TBLS	14	.0	123.8	0	14.0	0	0	0	–	0	0	–
			100	.0	884.0	0	100.0	0	0	.2	–	.1	.2	–
451	WALNUT	1 TBLS	14	.0	123.8	0	14.0	0	0	–	–	–	–	–
			100	.0	884.0	0	100.0	0	0	–	–	–	–	–
452	WHEAT GERM	1 TBLS	14	.0	123.8	0	14.0	0	0	–	–	–	–	–
			100	.0	884.0	0	100.0	0	0	–	–	–	–	–
	SHORTENINGS													
453	SHORTENING, vegetable	1 TBLS	14	.0	123.8	0	14.0	0	0	0	0	0	0	0
			100	.0	884.0	0	100.0	0	0	0	0	0	0	0
	FISH AND SEAFOODS													
454	ABALONE, canned	1 CUP	160	80.2	128.0	25.6	.5	3.7	0	22.4	204.8	–	–	–
			100	80.2	80.0	16.0	.3	2.3	0	14.0	128.0	–	–	–
	ANCHOVY													
455	canned	INDV	4	–	7.0	.8	.4	–	0	6.6	8.3	–	–	–
			100	–	175.0	19.0	10.0	–	0	166.0	208.0	–	–	–
456	paste	1 TSP	7	–	9.0	1.4	.3	.3	0	1.0	15.0	770.0	–	14.0
			100	–	128.0	20.0	3.6	4.0	0	14.0	214.0	11000.0	–	200.0
	BASS													
457	BLACK SEA, stuffed, baked	1 OZ	28	52.9	72.5	4.5	4.4	3.2	0	–	–	–	–	–
			100	52.9	259.0	16.2	15.8	11.4	0	–	–	–	–	–
458	SMALLMOUTH & LARGEMOUTH, raw	1 OZ	28	77.3	29.1	5.3	.7	0	0	13.2	53.8	–	7.6	–
			100	77.3	104.0	18.9	2.6	0	0	47.0	192.0	–	27.0	–
459	STRIPED, broiled	1 OZ	28	67.6	63.8	5.7	3.6	2.2	0	13.2	64.4	–	12.0	–
			100	67.6	228.0	20.2	12.8	7.9	0	47.0	230.0	–	43.0	–
460	BLUEFISH, baked or broiled	1 OZ	28	–	51.0	6.6	2.7	.1	–	7.8	78.1	–	8.1	–
			100	–	182.0	23.5	9.6	.3	–	28.0	279.0	–	29.0	–
461	BUTTERFISH, raw, from northern waters	1 OZ	28	71.4	47.3	5.1	2.9	0	0	–	–	–	–	–
			100	71.4	169.0	18.1	10.2	0	0	–	–	–	–	–

Item No.	Minerals (Micro)			Fat-Soluble Vitamins			Water-Soluble Vitamins								
	Iron	Zinc	Copper	Vitamin A	Vitamin D	Vitamin E (Alpha Tocopherol)	Vitamin C	Thiamin	Ribo-flavin	Niacin	Panto-thenic Acid	Vit. B-6 (Pyri-doxine)	Folacin (Folic Acid)	Biotin	Vitamin B-12
	(mg)	(mg)	(mg)	(IU)	(IU)	(mg)	(mg)	(mg)	(mg)	(mg)	(mg)	(mg)	(mcg)	(mcg)	(mcg)
432	0	–	–	463.0	–	–	.02	Trace	Trace	Trace	.01	Trace	.15	–	.01
	0	–	–	3307.0	–	–	.14	.01	.03	.02	.08	.01	1.05	–	.08
433	0	–	–	131.6	–	–	0	–	–	–	–	–	.08	–	–
	0	–	–	3289.0	–	–	0	–	–	–	–	–	2.00	–	–
434	Trace	Trace	Trace	165.4	(.40)	(.20)	.01	0	Trace	Trace	Trace	0	.04	Trace	Trace
	Trace	Trace	Trace	3307.0	(7.94)	(4.00)	.09	.01	.02	.01	.05	.01	.71	Trace	.06
435	–	–	–	–	–	5.49	–	–	–	–	–	–	–	–	–
	–	–	–	–	–	39.20	–	–	–	–	–	–	–	–	–
436	–	–	–	–	–	.25	–	–	–	–	–	–	–	–	–
	–	–	–	–	–	1.80	–	–	–	–	–	–	–	–	–
437	.01	–	–	–	–	.06	–	–	–	–	–	–	–	–	–
	.04	–	–	–	–	.40	–	–	–	–	–	–	–	–	–
438	0	.02	.03	–	–	2.00	0	0	0	0	–	–	–	–	–
	0	.16	.22	–	–	14.30	0	0	0	0	–	–	–	–	–
439	0	–	.02	0	–	4.94	0	0	0	0	–	–	–	–	–
	0	–	.13	0	–	35.30	0	0	0	0	–	–	–	–	–
440	–	–	–	–	–	–	–	–	–	–	–	–	–	–	–
	–	–	–	–	–	–	–	–	–	–	–	–	–	–	–
441	.05	.01	.05	0	–	1.67	0	0	0	0	–	–	–	–	–
	.38	.06	.32	0	–	11.90	0	0	0	0	–	–	–	–	–
442	Trace	–	–	–	–	2.67	–	–	–	–	–	–	–	–	–
	.01	–	–	–	–	19.10	–	–	–	–	–	–	–	–	–
443	–	–	–	–	–	–	–	–	–	–	–	–	–	–	–
	–	–	–	–	–	–	–	–	–	–	–	–	–	–	–
444	Trace	Trace	.01	0	–	1.62	0	0	0	0	–	–	–	–	–
	.03	.01	.08	0	–	11.60	0	0	0	0	–	–	–	–	–
445	–	–	–	–	–	–	–	–	–	–	–	–	3.99	–	–
	–	–	–	–	–	–	–	–	–	–	–	–	28.50	–	–
446	–	–	–	–	–	–	–	–	–	–	–	–	–	–	–
	–	–	–	–	–	–	–	–	–	–	–	–	–	–	–
447	0	.03	.02	0	–	4.77	0	0	0	0	–	–	–	–	–
	0	.19	.13	0	–	34.10	0	0	0	0	–	–	–	–	–
448	0	–	–	–	–	.20	0	0	0	0	–	–	–	–	–
	0	–	–	–	–	1.40	0	0	0	0	–	–	–	–	–
449	Trace	0	–	0	–	1.54	0	0	0	0	–	–	–	–	–
	.02	0	–	0	–	11.00	0	0	0	0	–	–	–	–	–
450	Trace	–	–	–	–	–	–	–	–	–	–	–	–	–	–
	.03	–	–	–	–	–	–	–	–	–	–	–	–	–	–
451	–	–	–	–	–	.01	–	–	–	–	–	–	–	–	–
	–	–	–	–	–	.04	–	–	–	–	–	–	–	–	–
452	–	.53	.08	–	–	20.92	–	–	–	–	–	–	–	–	–
	–	3.80	.60	–	–	149.40	–	–	–	–	–	–	–	–	–
453	0	–	–	0	–	1.39	0	0	0	0	–	0	0	–	0
	0	–	–	0	–	9.93	0	0	0	0	–	0	0	–	0
454	–	–	–	–	–	–	–	.19	–	–	–	–	–	–	–
	–	–	–	–	–	–	–	.12	–	–	–	–	–	–	–
455	–	6 .13	–	–	–	–	–	–	–	–	–	–	–	–	–
	–	3.20	–	–	–	–	–	–	–	–	–	–	–	–	–
456	–	–	–	–	–	–	–	–	–	–	–	–	–	–	–
	–	–	–	–	–	–	–	–	–	–	–	–	–	–	–
457	–	–	–	–	–	–	–	–	–	–	–	–	–	–	–
	–	–	–	–	–	–	–	–	–	–	–	–	–	–	–
458	–	–	–	–	–	–	–	.03	.01	.59	.14	–	–	–	–
	–	–	–	–	–	–	–	.10	.03	2.10	.51	–	–	–	–
459	.53	–	–	32.5	–	–	0	.04	.04	.81	–	.07	–	–	.42
	1.90	–	–	116.0	–	–	0	.15	.14	2.90	–	.26	–	–	1.50
460	.20	–	–	98.2	–	–	.28	.03	.03	.50	–	.08	–	–	.48
	.70	–	–	322.0	–	–	1.00	.10	.10	1.80	–	.29	–	–	1.71
461	–	–	–	–	–	–	–	–	–	–	–	–	–	–	–
	–	–	–	–	–	–	–	–	–	–	–	–	–	–	–

(Continued)

TABLE F-21 *(Continued)*

Item No.	Food Item Name	Approximate Measure	Weight (g)	Moisture (%)	Food Energy Calories (kcal)	Protein (g)	Fats (g)	Carbo-hydrates (g)	Fiber (g)	Calcium (mg)	Phos-phorus (mg)	Sodium (mg)	Mag-nesium (mg)	Potas-sium (mg)
462	CARP, raw	1 OZ	28	77.8	32.2	5.0	1.2	0	0	14.0	70.8	14.0	–	80.1
			100	77.8	115.0	18.0	4.2	0	0	50.0	253.0	50.0	–	286.0
463	CATFISH, freshwater, raw	1 OZ	28	78.0	28.8	4.9	.9	0	0	3.9	–	16.8	7.6	92.4
			100	78.0	103.0	17.6	3.1	0	0	14.0	–	60.0	27.0	330.0
464	CAVIAR, sturgeon, granular	1 TSP	10	46.0	26.2	2.7	1.5	.3	–	27.6	35.5	220.0	30.0	18.0
			100	46.0	262.0	26.9	15.0	3.3	–	276.0	355.0	2200.0	300.0	180.0
	CLAM(S)													
465	raw, hard & soft, meat only	1 CUP	200	81.7	152.0	25.2	3.2	4.0	–	138.0	324.0	240.0	–	362.0
			100	81.7	76.0	12.6	1.6	2.0	–	69.0	162.0	120.0	–	181.0
466	raw, hard or round, meat only	1 LG	20	79.8	16.0	2.2	.4	1.2	–	13.8	30.2	41.0	17.8	62.2
			100	79.8	80.0	11.1	2.0	5.9	–	69.0	151.0	205.0	89.0	311.0
467	canned, drained solids	1 LG	20	77.0	19.6	3.2	.5	.4	–	–	–	–	–	–
			100	77.0	98.0	15.8	2.5	1.9	–	–	–	–	–	–
468	*COCKLES, sand, raw	1 OZ	28	79.2	22.7	4.7	.3	0	0	60.8	21.8	–	–	–
			100	79.2	81.0	16.8	1.0	0	0	217.0	78.0	–	–	–
	COD													
469	broiled	1 OZ	30	64.6	51.0	8.6	1.6	0	0	9.3	82.2	33.0	–	122.1
			100	64.6	170.0	28.5	5.3	0	0	31.0	274.0	110.0	–	407.0
470	canned	1 OZ	28	78.6	23.8	5.4	.1	0	0	–	–	–	–	–
			100	78.6	85.0	19.2	.3	0	0	–	–	–	–	–
	CRAB													
471	(BLUE, DUNGENESS, ROCK, KING), steamed	1 OZ	28	78.5	26.0	4.8	.5	.1	0	12.0	49.0	65.8	9.5	85.4
			100	78.5	93.0	17.3	1.9	.5	0	43.0	175.0	235.0	34.0	305.0
472	soft shell, fried	1 AVG	107	–	348.8	19.4	21.6	19.2	–	67.4	203.3	–	38.5	–
			100	–	326.0	18.1	20.2	17.9	–	63.0	190.0	–	36.0	–
473	canned	1 OZ	28	77.2	28.3	4.9	.7	.3	0	12.6	51.0	251.4	11.2	54.9
			100	77.2	101.0	17.4	2.5	1.1	0	45.0	182.0	898.0	40.0	196.0
474	CRAYFISH, freshwater & spiny lobster, raw	1 OZ	28	82.5	20.2	4.1	.1	.3	–	21.6	56.3	–	–	–
			100	82.5	72.0	14.6	.5	1.2	–	77.0	201.0	–	–	–
	CROAKER													
475	ATLANTIC, baked	1 OZ	28	71.3	37.2	6.8	.9	0	0	–	–	33.6	–	90.4
			100	71.3	133.0	24.3	3.2	0	0	–	–	120.0	–	323.0
476	WHITE, raw	1 OZ	28	79.7	23.5	5.0	.2	0	0	–	–	–	–	–
			100	79.7	84.0	18.0	.8	0	0	–	–	–	–	–
477	YELLOWFIN, raw	1 OZ	28	79.0	24.9	5.4	.2	0	0	–	–	–	–	–
			100	79.0	89.0	19.2	.8	0	0	–	–	–	–	–
478	DOLLY VARDEN, raw	1 OZ	28	73.1	40.3	5.6	1.8	0	0	–	–	–	–	–
			100	73.1	144.0	19.9	6.5	0	0	–	–	–	–	–
479	EEL, smoked	1 SERV	100	50.2	330.0	18.6	27.8	0	0	–	210.0	–	–	–
			100	50.2	330.0	18.6	27.8	0	0	–	210.0	–	–	–
480	EULACHON (SMELT), raw	1 OZ	28	79.6	33.0	4.1	1.7	0	0	–	–	–	–	–
			100	79.6	118.0	14.6	6.2	0	0	–	–	–	–	–
481	FINNAN HADDIE (SMOKED HADDOCK)	1 OZ	28	72.6	28.8	6.5	.1	0	0	–	–	–	–	–
			100	72.6	103.0	23.2	.4	0	0	–	–	–	–	–
482	FISH, sticks, frozen, cooked	1 PIECE	23	65.8	40.5	3.8	2.0	1.5	–	2.5	38.4	–	–	–
			100	65.8	176.0	16.6	8.9	6.5	–	11.0	167.0	–	–	–
483	FLATFISHES (FLOUNDER/SOLE/SAND DAB), broiled	1 OZ	28	70.7	37.8	5.7	1.9	.1	0	4.1	63.9	26.6	10.2	112.0
			100	70.7	135.1	20.4	6.7	.3	0	14.6	228.2	95.2	36.6	400.1
484	FLOUNDER, w/salt, baked	1 OZ	28	58.1	56.6	8.4	2.3	0	0	6.4	96.3	66.4	8.4	164.4
			100	58.1	202.0	30.0	8.2	0	0	23.0	344.0	237.0	30.0	587.0
485	HADDOCK, broiled	1 OZ	28	70.0	39.5	5.6	1.8	.1	0	3.6	64.5	20.0	9.0	99.6
			100	70.0	141.0	20.1	6.6	.3	0	13.0	230.5	71.4	32.0	355.7
486	HAKE, broiled	1 OZ	28	71.2	39.5	5.6	1.8	.1	0	3.6	62.4	25.3	9.0	118.9
			100	71.2	141.0	20.1	6.6	.3	0	13.0	223.0	90.3	32.0	424.7
	HALIBUT													
487	CALIFORNIA, raw	1 OZ	28	77.8	27.2	5.5	.3	0	0	3.6	(53.5)	23.7	6.4	(74.6)
			100	77.8	97.0	19.8	1.2	0	0	13.0	(191.1)	84.6	23.0	(266.3)
488	GREENLAND, raw	1 OZ	28	74.5	48.7	4.6	3.4	0	0	3.6	58.8	–	6.4	–
			100	74.5	174.0	16.4	12.0	0	0	13.0	210.0	–	23.0	–
489	ATLANTIC & PACIFIC, broiled	1 OZ	28	66.6	45.6	7.1	2.0	0	0	4.5	69.4	37.5	–	147.0
			100	66.6	163.0	25.2	7.0	0	0	16.0	248.0	134.0	–	525.0
	HERRING													
490	PACIFIC, raw	1 OZ	28	79.4	27.4	4.9	.7	0	0	12.0	63.0	20.7	8.7	117.6
			100	79.4	98.0	17.5	2.6	0	0	43.0	225.0	74.0	31.0	420.0
491	ATLANTIC, cooked	1 AVG	85	–	216.8	20.8	14.2	0	0	–	289.9	–	–	–
			100	–	255.0	24.5	16.7	0	0	–	341.0	–	–	–
492	canned, plain, solids & liquid	1 OZ	28	62.9	56.6	5.6	3.8	0	0	41.2	83.2	–	–	–
			100	62.9	202.0	19.9	13.6	0	0	147.0	297.0	–	–	–

Item No.	Minerals (Micro)			Fat-Soluble Vitamins			Water-Soluble Vitamins								
	Iron	Zinc	Copper	Vitamin A	Vitamin D	Vitamin E (Alpha Tocopherol)	Vitamin C	Thiamin	Ribo-flavin	Niacin	Panto-thenic Acid	Vit. B-6 (Pyri-doxine)	Folacin (Folic Acid)	Biotin	Vitamin B-12
	(mg)	(mg)	(mg)	(IU)	(IU)	(mg)	(mg)	(mg)	(mg)	(mg)	(mg)	(mg)	(mcg)	(mcg)	(mcg)
462	.25	–	–	47.6	–	–	.28	Trace	.01	.42	.04	–	–	–	.06
	.90	–	–	170.0	–	–	1.00	.01	.04	1.50	.15	–	–	–	.20
463	.11	–	–	–	–	–	–	.01	.01	.48	.13	–	–	–	.67
	.40	–	–	–	–	–	–	.04	.03	1.70	.47	–	–	–	2.20
464	1.18	–	–	–	–	–	–	–	–	–	–	–	–	–	–
	11.80	–	–	–	–	–	–	–	–	–	–	–	–	–	–
465	12.20	3.00	–	200.0	–	–	20.00	.20	.36	2.60	1.16	–	–	–	38.20
	6.10	1.50	–	100.0	–	–	10.00	.10	.18	1.30	.58	–	–	–	19.10
466	1.50	–	–	22.0	–	–	–	.02	–	.32	.12	–	–	–	–
	7.50	–	–	110.0	–	–	–	.10	–	1.60	.60	–	–	–	–
467	–	–	–	–	–	–	–	–	–	–	–	–	.02	–	–
	–	–	–	–	–	–	–	–	–	–	–	–	.08	–	–
468	.78	–	–	–	–	–	–	–	.04	1.74	–	–	–	–	–
	2.80	–	–	–	–	–	–	–	.15	6.20	–	–	–	–	–
469	.30	–	–	54.0	–	–	–	.02	.03	.90	–	–	–	–	–
	1.00	–	–	180.0	–	–	–	.08	.11	3.00	–	–	–	–	–
470	–	–	–	–	–	–	–	.02	.02	–	–	–	–	–	–
	–	–	–	–	–	–	–	.08	.08	–	–	–	–	–	–
471	.22	1.20	–	607.6	–	–	.56	.05	.02	.78	.17	.08	–	–	2.80
	.80	4.30	–	2170.0	–	–	2.00	.16	.08	2.80	.60	.30	–	–	10.00
472	1.71	–	–	92.0	–	–	2.14	.25	.18	3.42	–	.30	–	–	8.89
	1.60	–	–	86.0	–	–	2.00	.23	.17	3.20	–	.28	–	–	8.31
473	.22	1.01	.08	Trace	Trace	–	Trace	.02	.02	.53	.17	.08	.25	Trace	2.80
	.80	3.60	.27	Trace	Trace	–	Trace	.08	.08	1.90	.60	.30	.90	Trace	10.00
474	.42	–	–	–	–	–	–	Trace	.01	.53	.12	.06	–	–	.76
	1.50	–	–	–	–	–	–	.01	.04	1.90	.41	.21	–	–	2.70
475	–	–	–	19.6	–	–	–	.04	.03	1.82	–	–	–	–	–
	–	–	–	70.0	–	–	–	.13	.10	6.50	–	–	–	–	–
476	–	–	–	–	–	–	–	–	–	–	–	–	–	–	–
	–	–	–	–	–	–	–	–	–	–	–	–	–	–	–
477	–	–	–	–	–	–	–	–	–	–	–	–	–	–	–
	–	–	–	–	–	–	–	–	–	–	–	–	–	–	–
478	–	–	–	–	–	–	–	.02	.02	–	–	–	–	–	–
	–	–	–	–	–	–	–	.06	.06	–	–	–	–	–	–
479	1.00	–	–	2500.0	–	–	–	.14	.07	–	–	.12	–	–	5.60
	1.00	–	–	2500.0	–	–	–	.14	.07	–	–	.12	–	–	5.60
480	–	–	–	–	–	–	–	.01	.01	–	–	–	–	–	–
	–	–	–	–	–	–	–	.04	.04	–	–	–	–	–	–
481	–	–	–	–	–	–	–	.02	.01	.59	–	–	–	–	–
	–	–	–	–	–	–	–	.06	.05	2.10	–	–	–	–	–
482	.09	–	–	0	–	–	–	.01	.02	.37	–	–	–	–	–
	.40	–	–	0	–	–	–	.04	.07	1.60	–	–	–	–	–
483	.26	–	.05	77.3	–	–	.28	.01	.01	.48	.29	.05	–	–	.40
	.91	–	.18	276.0	–	–	1.00	.04	.05	1.70	1.04	.17	–	–	1.44
484	.39	–	–	–	–	–	.50	.02	.02	.70	–	–	–	–	–
	1.40	–	–	–	–	–	2.00	.07	.08	2.50	–	–	–	–	–
485	.14	–	–	77.3	–	–	.84	.01	.02	.59	.05	.06	–	–	.22
	.50	–	–	276.0	–	–	3.00	.03	.07	2.10	.16	.22	–	–	.78
486	.14	–	–	77.3	–	–	.84	.02	.02	.59	–	.06	–	–	.22
	.50	–	–	276.0	–	–	3.00	.09	.07	2.10	–	.22	–	–	.78
487	(.15)	–	(.02)	Trace	Trace	(.26)	Trace	(.02)	(.03)	(1.40)	(.10)	(.06)	(3.36)	(2.00)	(.31)
	(.52)	–	(.06)	Trace	Trace	(.93)	Trace	(.08)	(.10)	(5.00)	(.35)	(.22)	(12.00)	(5.05)	(1.11)
488	–	–	–	–	–	–	–	Trace	–	–	.07	–	–	–	.42
	–	–	–	–	–	–	–	.01	–	–	.25	–	–	–	1.50
489	.22	–	–	190.4	–	–	–	.01	.02	2.32	–	–	–	–	–
	.80	–	–	680.0	–	–	–	.05	.07	8.30	–	–	–	–	–
490	.36	–	–	28.0	–	–	.84	.01	.05	.98	–	–	–	–	.56
	1.30	–	–	100.0	–	–	3.00	.02	.16	3.50	–	–	–	–	2.00
491	1.19	–	–	130.1	–	–	0	.02	.15	3.30	–	–	–	–	–
	1.40	–	–	153.0	–	–	0	.02	.18	3.88	–	–	–	–	–
492	.50	–	–	–	–	–	–	–	.05	–	.20	.05	1.43	–	2.24
	1.80	–	–	–	–	–	–	–	.18	–	.70	.16	5.10	–	8.00

(Continued)

TABLE F-21 *(Continued)*

Item No.	Food Item Name	Approximate Measure	Weight (g)	Moisture (%)	Food Energy Calories (kcal)	Protein (g)	Fats (g)	Carbohydrates (g)	Fiber (g)	Calcium (mg)	Phosphorus (mg)	Sodium (mg)	Magnesium (mg)	Potassium (mg)
	HERRING(Continued)													
493	smoked kippered	1 OZ	28	61.0	59.1	6.2	3.6	0	0	18.5	71.1	—	—	—
			100	61.0	211.0	22.2	12.9	0	0	66.0	254.0	—	—	—
494	**HORSE MACKEREL,** ³raw	1 OZ	28	66.8	40.0	7.0	1.1	0	0	—	—	—	—	—
			100	66.8	143.0	25.0	4.0	0	0	—	—	—	—	—
495	**INCONNU (SHEEPFISH),** raw	1 OZ	28	72.0	40.9	5.6	1.9	0	0	—	—	—	—	—
			100	72.0	146.0	19.9	6.8	0	0	—	—	—	—	—
496	**JACK MACKEREL,** raw	1 OZ	28	71.4	40.0	6.0	1.6	0	0	—	—	—	—	—
			100	71.4	143.0	21.6	5.6	0	0	—	—	—	—	—
497	**JELLY FISH,** ⁴Medusa, raw	1 OZ	28	85.2	8.4	1.1	0	.8	0	7.3	7.6	—	—	23.8
			100	85.2	30.0	4.0	.2	2.9	0	26.0	27.0	—	—	85.0
498	**KINGFISH (SOUTHERN, GULF, NORTHERN WHITING),** cooked	1 OZ	28	67.3	71.4	6.3	3.8	3.3	0	22.4	80.4	28.4	15.7	81.9
			100	67.3	255.0	22.3	13.4	11.7	0	80.0	287.0	101.3	56.0	292.5
499	**LAKE HERRING,** (cisco), raw	1 OZ	28	79.7	26.9	5.0	.6	0	0	3.4	57.7	13.2	4.8	89.3
			100	79.7	96.0	17.7	2.3	0	0	12.0	206.0	47.0	17.0	319.0
	LAKE TROUT													
500	raw	1 OZ	28	70.6	47.0	5.1	2.8	0	0	5.6	66.6	22.4	7.3	93.5
			100	70.6	168.0	18.3	10.0	0	0	20.0	238.0	80.0	26.0	334.0
501	**SISCOWET,** raw, less than 6.5 lb	1 OZ	28	64.9	67.5	4.0	5.6	0	0	—	—	—	—	—
			100	64.9	241.0	14.3	19.9	0	0	—	—	—	—	—
502	**LINGCOD,** raw	1 OZ	28	80.0	23.5	5.0	.2	0	0	—	—	16.5	—	121.2
			100	80.0	84.0	17.9	.8	0	0	—	—	59.0	—	433.0
	LOBSTER													
503	¹tail, cooked	1 OZ	28	76.8	26.6	5.2	.4	.1	0	18.2	53.8	58.8	—	50.4
			100	76.8	95.0	18.7	1.5	.3	0	65.0	192.0	210.0	—	180.0
504	**NORTHERN,** canned or cooked	1 OZ	28	76.8	26.6	5.2	.4	.1	0	18.2	53.8	58.8	(9.8)	50.4
			100	76.8	95.0	18.7	1.5	.3	0	65.0	192.0	210.0	(34.9)	180.0
505	newburg	1 OZ	28	64.0	54.3	5.2	3.0	1.4	—	24.4	53.8	64.1	—	47.9
			100	64.0	194.0	18.5	10.6	5.1	—	87.0	192.0	229.0	—	171.0
	MACKEREL													
506	cooked	1 OZ	28	—	64.4	6.4	4.3	.1	—	1.7	80.6	—	9.5	—
			100	—	230.0	22.9	15.2	.3	—	6.0	288.0	—	34.0	—
507	**ATLANTIC,** canned, solids & liquid, vitamins based on dried solids	1 CUP	210	66.0	384.3	40.5	23.3	0	0	388.5	575.4	—	—	—
			100	66.0	183.0	19.3	11.1	0	0	185.0	274.0	—	—	—
508	**PACIFIC,** canned, solids & liquid, vitamins based on dried solids	1 CUP	210	66.4	378.0	44.3	21.0	0	0	546.0	604.8	—	—	—
			100	66.4	180.0	21.1	10.0	0	0	260.0	288.0	—	—	—
509	**MAHIMAHI,** plain, broiled	1 SERV	100	—	—	—	—	—	—	—	—	120.0	—	267.0
			100	—	—	—	—	—	—	—	—	120.0	—	267.0
510	**MENHADEN, ATLANTIC,** canned, solids & liquid	1 OZ	28	67.9	48.2	5.2	2.9	0	0	—	—	—	—	—
			100	67.9	172.0	18.7	10.2	0	0	—	—	—	—	—
511	**MULLET, STRIPED,** breaded, fried	1 OZ	28	53.7	82.9	6.3	4.9	3.4	—	14.8	72.2	27.7	10.6	95.7
			100	53.7	296.0	22.6	17.4	12.2	—	53.0	258.0	98.8	38.0	341.6
512	**MUSSELS, PACIFIC,** canned, drained solids	1 OZ	28	74.6	31.9	5.1	.9	.4	—	—	—	—	7.0	—
			100	74.6	114.0	18.2	3.3	1.5	—	—	—	—	25.0	—
513	**OCTOPUS,** raw	1 OZ	28	82.2	20.4	4.3	.2	0	0	8.1	48.4	(142.8)	(11.9)	(73.1)
			100	82.2	73.0	15.3	.8	0	0	29.0	173.0	(509.8)	(42.6)	(261.0)
	OYSTER													
514	raw meat only, Pacific and Eastern (Olympia)	1 MED	35	79.1	30.1	3.7	.7	2.2	—	29.8	53.6	—	8.4	—
			100	79.1	86.0	10.6	2.0	6.4	—	85.0	153.0	—	24.0	—
515	fried	1 MED	15	54.7	35.9	1.3	2.1	2.8	—	22.8	36.2	30.9	—	30.5
			100	54.7	239.0	8.6	13.9	18.6	—	152.0	241.0	206.0	—	203.0
	PERCH													
516	**WHITE,** raw	1 MED	100	75.7	118.0	19.3	4.0	0	0	—	192.0	79.0	—	—
			100	75.7	118.0	19.3	4.0	0	0	—	192.0	79.0	—	—
517	**YELLOW,** raw	1 MED	100	79.2	91.0	19.5	.9	0	0	—	180.0	68.0	—	230.0
			100	79.2	91.0	19.5	.9	0	0	—	180.0	68.0	—	230.0
518	filet, fried	1 OZ	28	—	46.5	5.4	2.3	0	0	3.9	48.7	—	—	—
			100	—	166.0	19.2	8.2	0	0	14.0	174.0	—	—	—
519	**ATLANTIC (REDFISH),** fried	1 OZ	28	59.0	63.6	5.3	3.7	1.9	0	9.2	63.3	42.8	—	79.5
			100	59.0	227.0	19.0	13.3	6.8	0	33.0	226.0	153.0	—	284.0
520	**PICKEREL,** chain, raw	1 OZ	28	79.7	23.5	5.2	.1	0	0	—	—	—	—	—
			100	79.7	84.0	18.7	.5	0	0	—	—	—	—	—
	PIKE													
521	**WALLEYE,** raw	1 OZ	30	78.3	27.9	5.8	.4	0	0	—	64.2	15.3	9.3	95.7
			100	78.3	93.0	19.3	1.2	0	0	—	214.0	51.0	31.0	319.0
522	**NORTHERN,** breaded, fried	1 OZ	28	59.2	59.4	5.4	3.3	2.2	—	9.2	65.0	25.6	6.2	114.7
			100	59.2	212.0	19.1	11.8	7.9	—	33.0	232.0	91.5	22.0	409.5

Item No.	Minerals (Micro)			Fat-Soluble Vitamins			Water-Soluble Vitamins								
	Iron	Zinc	Copper	Vitamin A	Vitamin D	Vitamin E (Alpha Tocopherol)	Vitamin C	Thiamin	Ribo-flavin	Niacin	Panto-thenic Acid	Vit. B-6 (Pyri-doxine)	Folacin (Folic Acid)	Biotin	Vitamin B-12
	(mg)	(mg)	(mg)	(IU)	(IU)	(mg)	(mg)	(mg)	(mg)	(mg)	(mg)	(mg)	(mcg)	(mcg)	(mcg)
493	.39	–	–	8.4	–	–	–	–	.08	.92	.29	.07	–	–	.42
	1.40	–	–	30.0	–	–	–	–	.28	3.30	1.04	.25	–	–	1.50
494	–	–	–	–	–	–	–	–	–	–	–	–	–	–	–
	–	–	–	–	–	–	–	–	–	–	–	–	–	–	–
495	–	–	–	–	–	–	–	–	–	–	–	–	–	–	–
	–	–	–	–	–	–	–	–	–	–	–	–	–	–	–
496	–	–	–	–	–	–	–	–	–	–	–	–	–	–	–
	–	–	–	–	–	–	–	–	–	–	–	–	–	–	–
497	.22	–	–	0	–	–	0	.02	Trace	–	–	–	–	–	–
	.80	–	–	0	–	–	0	.06	.01	–	–	–	–	–	–
498	.53	–	–	26.0	–	–	0	.03	.04	.81	–	.08	–	–	.45
	1.90	–	–	93.0	–	–	0	.11	.13	2.90	–	.27	–	–	1.59
499	.14	1.06	–	–	–	–	–	.03	.03	.92	–	–	–	–	–
	.50	3.80	–	–	–	–	–	.09	.10	3.30	–	–	–	–	–
500	.22	1.71	–	3.4	–	–	–	.03	.03	.76	–	–	–	–	–
	.80	6.10	–	12.0	–	–	–	.09	.12	2.70	–	–	–	–	–
501	–	–	–	–	–	–	–	–	–	–	–	–	–	–	–
	–	–	–	–	–	–	–	–	–	–	–	–	–	–	–
502	–	–	–	0	–	–	–	.01	.01	–	–	–	–	–	1.01
	–	–	–	0	–	–	–	.05	.04	–	–	–	–	–	3.60
503	.22	.62	–	–	–	–	0	.03	.02	.62	–	–	–	–	–
	.80	2.20	–	–	–	–	0	.10	.07	2.23	–	–	–	–	–
504	.22	.62	(.49)	77.0	Trace	(.42)	0	.03	.02	.62	(.46)	–	4.76	(1.42)	(.30)
	.80	2.20	(1.76)	275.0	Trace	(1.50)	0	.10	.07	2.23	(1.65)	–	17.00	(5.06)	(1.08)
505	.25	–	–	–	–	–	–	.02	.03	–	–	–	–	–	–
	.90	–	–	–	–	–	–	.07	.11	–	–	–	–	–	–
506	.34	–	–	157.4	–	–	.28	.04	.10	2.35	–	.19	–	–	2.27
	1.20	–	–	562.0	–	–	1.00	.14	.36	8.40	–	.68	–	–	8.12
507	4.41	–	–	903.0	–	–	–	.13	.44	12.18	1.05	.59	–	–	16.17
	2.10	–	–	430.0	–	–	–	.06	.21	5.80	.50	.28	–	–	7.70
508	4.62	–	–	63.0	–	–	–	.06	.69	18.48	.99	.57	1.26	37.80	–
	2.20	–	–	30.0	–	–	–	.03	.33	8.80	.47	.27	.60	18.00	–
509	–	–	–	–	–	–	–	–	–	–	–	–	–	–	–
	–	–	–	–	–	–	–	–	–	–	–	–	–	–	–
510	.36	–	–	–	–	–	–	–	–	–	–	–	–	–	–
	1.30	–	–	–	–	–	–	–	–	–	–	–	–	–	–
511	.66	–	–	26.6	–	–	0	.03	.03	1.43	–	.10	–	–	.06
	2.34	–	–	95.0	–	–	0	.10	.10	5.10	–	.37	–	–	.21
512	–	–	–	–	–	–	–	–	.04	–	–	–	–	–	–
	–	–	–	–	–	–	–	–	.13	–	–	–	–	–	–
513	(1.74)	(12.44)	(2.10)	(2.1)	Trace	(.24)	Trace	.01	.02	.50	(.15)	.10	–	(2.83)	(4.23)
	(6.20)	(44.40)	(7.50)	(7.5)	Trace	(1.86)	Trace	.02	.06	1.80	(.54)	.36	–	(10.10)	(15.11)
514	2.52	52.05	4.80	–	–	–	10.50	.04	–	.46	.09	.02	3.50	–	–
	7.20	148.70	13.71	–	–	–	30.00	.12	–	1.30	.25	.05	10.00	–	–
515	1.22	–	–	66.0	–	–	–	.03	.04	.48	–	–	–	–	–
	8.10	–	–	440.0	–	–	–	.17	.29	3.20	–	–	–	–	–
516	–	–	–	–	–	–	–	–	–	–	–	–	–	–	–
	–	–	–	–	–	–	–	–	–	–	–	–	–	–	–
517	.60	–	–	–	–	–	–	.06	.17	1.70	–	–	–	–	–
	.60	–	–	–	–	–	–	.06	.17	1.70	–	–	–	–	–
518	.31	.70	–	0	–	–	0	.02	.02	1.16	–	–	–	–	–
	1.10	2.50	–	0	–	–	0	.06	.07	4.15	–	–	–	–	–
519	.10	–	–	–	–	–	–	.03	.03	.50	–	–	–	–	–
	.30	–	–	–	–	–	–	.10	.11	1.80	–	–	–	–	–
520	.20	–	–	–	–	–	–	–	–	–	–	–	–	–	–
	.70	–	–	–	–	–	–	–	–	–	–	–	–	–	–
521	.12	–	–	–	–	–	–	.08	.05	.69	–	–	–	–	–
	.40	–	–	–	–	–	–	.25	.16	2.30	–	–	–	–	–
522	.25	–	–	13.7	–	–	0	.06	.05	.64	–	.03	–	–	.42
	.90	–	–	49.0	–	–	0	.21	.19	2.30	–	.11	–	–	1.51

(Continued)

TABLE F-21 *(Continued)*

Item No.	Food Item Name	Approximate Measure	Weight	Moisture	Food Energy Calories	Protein	Fats	Carbo-hydrates	Fiber	Minerals (Macro) Calcium	Phos-phorus	Sodium	Mag-nesium	Potas-sium
			(g)	(%)	(kcal)	(g)	(g)	(g)	(g)	(mg)	(mg)	(mg)	(mg)	(mg)
523	POLLOCK, creamed, cooked	1 SERV	100	74.7	128.0	13.9	5.9	4.0	0	—	—	111.0	—	238.0
			100	74.7	128.0	13.9	5.9	4.0	0	—	—	111.0	—	238.0
524	POMPANO, broiled	1 OZ	28	61.7	79.5	6.4	15.5	0	0	—	—	16.1	—	62.5
			100	61.7	283.9	22.9	55.4	0	0	—	—	57.3	—	223.4
525	PORGY & SCUP, raw	1 OZ	28	76.2	31.4	5.3	1.0	0	0	15.1	70.0	17.6	—	80.4
			100	76.2	112.0	19.0	3.4	0	0	54.0	250.0	63.0	—	287.0
526	*PRAWNS, boiled	1 OZ	28	—	30.0	6.3	.5	0	0	43.5	96.2	442.7	12.1	72.4
			100	—	107.0	22.5	1.9	0	0	155.2	343.3	1580.4	43.3	258.5
	ROE													
527	(SALMON, STURGEON, TURBOT), raw	1 OZ	28	61.3	58.0	7.1	2.9	.4	—	—	—	—	—	—
			100	61.3	207.0	25.2	10.4	1.4	—	—	—	—	—	—
528	(COD, SHAD), baked or broiled	1 OZ	28	71.3	35.3	6.2	.8	.5	0	3.6	112.6	20.4	(3.0)	37.0
			100	71.3	126.0	22.0	2.8	1.9	0	13.0	402.0	73.0	(10.8)	132.0
529	SABLEFISH, raw	1 OZ	28	71.6	53.2	3.6	4.2	0	0	—	—	15.7	—	100.2
			100	71.6	190.0	13.0	14.9	0	0	—	—	56.0	—	358.0
	SALMON													
530	broiled or baked	1 SMALL	100	63.4	182.0	27.0	6.5	0	0	—	414.0	116.0	—	443.0
			100	63.4	182.0	27.0	6.5	0	0	—	414.0	116.0	—	443.0
531	CHUM, canned w/o salt, solids, liquid, & bones	1 OZ	28	70.8	34.7	6.0	1.2	0	0	55.4	59.9	14.8	8.4	94.1
			100	70.8	124.0	21.5	4.2	0	0	198.0	214.0	53.0	30.0	336.0
532	PINK (HUMPBACK), canned, solids, liquid, & bones	1 CUP	250	70.8	352.5	47.0	14.8	0	0	445.0	612.5	967.5	75.0	902.5
			100	70.8	141.0	18.8	5.9	0	0	178.0	245.0	387.0	30.0	361.0
533	SOCKEYE (RED), canned, solids, liquid, & bones	1 OZ	28	67.2	46.8	5.72	2.4	0	0	49.8	60.5	146.2	8.1	96.3
			100	67.2	167.0	20.2	8.4	0	0	178.0	216.0	522.0	29.0	344.0
534	smoked	1 OZ	28	58.9	49.3	6.0	2.6	0	0	3.9	68.6	(560.1)	(8.8)	(118.2)
			100	58.9	176.0	21.6	9.3	0	0	14.0	245.0	(1880.2)	(31.5)	(422.0)
	SARDINES													
535	ATLANTIC, canned in oil, solids & liquid	1 MED	12	50.6	29.5	2.5	2.9	.1	0	42.5	52.1	61.2	—	67.2
			100	50.6	246.0	21.1	24.4	.6	0	354.0	434.0	510.0	—	560.0
536	PACIFIC, canned in tomato sauce, solids & liquid	1 LG	66	64.3	123.4	11.7	8.1	1.1	0	296.3	315.5	264.0	(14.3)	211.2
			100	64.3	187.0	17.7	12.2	1.7	0	449.0	478.0	400.0	(51.2)	320.0
537	SCAD, *raw	1 OZ	28	80.6	21.3	4.9	0	0	0	14.0	32.2	17.1	—	171.9
			100	80.6	76.0	17.5	.1	0	0	50.0	115.0	61.0	—	614.0
538	SCALLOPS, bay & sea, steamed	1 OZ	28	73.1	29.4	6.5	.4	Trace	0	32.2	94.6	74.2	(10.9)	133.3
			100	73.1	105.0	23.2	1.4	Trace	0	115.0	338.0	265.0	(38.8)	476.0
539	SCAMPI, fried	1 OZ	28	—	88.7	3.5	4.7	7.8	0	28.0	88.2	106.4	8.8	109.9
			100	—	316.6	12.5	16.9	27.9	0	99.8	315.0	379.9	31.3	392.2
540	SEABASS, white, raw	1 OZ	28	76.3	26.9	6.0	.1	0	0	—	—	—	—	—
			100	76.3	96.0	21.4	.5	0	0	—	—	—	—	—
541	SHAD, baked, w/butter or margarine & bacon slices	1 OZ	25	64.0	50.3	5.8	2.8	0	0	6.0	78.3	19.8	—	94.3
			100	64.0	201.0	23.2	11.3	0	0	24.0	313.0	79.0	—	377.0
542	SHARK, *raw	1 OZ	28	77.0	28.0	5.8	.4	0	0	9.0	53.8	22.1	—	153.7
			100	77.0	100.0	20.6	1.3	0	0	32.0	192.0	79.0	—	549.0
	SHRIMP													
543	boiled	1 MED	11	—	—	—	—	—	—	—	—	—	5.6	—
			100	—	—	—	—	—	—	—	—	—	51.0	—
544	canned, dry pack or drained solids of wet pack	1 MED	11	70.4	12.8	2.7	.1	.1	0	12.7	28.9	15.4	8.1	13.4
			100	70.4	116.0	24.2	1.1	.7	.2	115.0	263.0	140.0	74.0	122.0
545	SMELT, ATLANTIC, JACK & BAY, canned, solids & liquid	1 MED	23	62.7	46.0	4.2	3.1	0	—	82.3	85.1	—	—	—
			100	62.7	200.0	18.4	13.5	0	—	358.0	370.0	—	—	—
546	SNAPPER, red & grey, raw	1 OZ	28	78.5	26.0	5.5	.3	0	0	4.5	59.9	18.8	7.8	90.4
			100	78.5	93.0	19.8	.9	0	0	16.0	214.0	67.0	28.0	323.0
547	SOLE, *fried	1 OZ	28	—	60.5	4.5	3.9	2.5	0	26.8	67.3	39.3	6.2	70.6
			100	—	216.0	16.0	13.8	9.0	0	95.5	240.2	140.2	22.2	252.0
548	SQUID, raw	1 OZ	28	80.2	23.5	4.6	.3	.4	—	3.4	33.3	—	—	—
			100	80.2	84.0	16.4	.9	1.5	—	12.0	119.0	—	—	—
549	STURGEON, steamed	1 OZ	28	67.5	44.8	7.1	1.6	0	0	11.2	73.6	30.2	—	65.8
			100	67.5	160.0	25.4	5.7	0	0	40.0	263.0	108.0	—	235.0
550	SWORDFISH, broiled, w/butter or margarine	1 OZ	28	64.6	48.7	7.8	1.7	0	0	7.6	77.0	—	—	—
			100	64.6	174.0	28.0	6.0	0	0	27.0	275.0	—	—	—
551	TERRAPIN (DIAMOND BACK), raw	1 OZ	28	77.0	31.1	5.2	1.0	0	0	—	—	—	—	—
			100	77.0	111.0	18.6	3.5	0	0	—	—	—	—	—
552	TILEFISH, baked	1 OZ	28	71.6	38.6	6.9	1.0	0	0	—	—	—	—	—
			100	71.6	138.0	24.5	3.7	0	0	—	—	—	—	—
553	TOMCOD, ATLANTIC, raw	1 OZ	28	81.5	21.6	4.8	.1	0	0	—	—	—	—	—
			100	81.5	77.0	17.2	.4	0	0	—	—	—	—	—
554	TROUT, cooked	1 OZ	28	—	54.9	6.6	3.1	.1	0	61.0	76.2	—	9.8	—
			100	—	196.0	23.5	11.2	.4	0	218.0	272.0	—	35.0	—

Item No.	Minerals (Micro)			Fat-Soluble Vitamins			Water-Soluble Vitamins								
	Iron	Zinc	Copper	Vitamin A	Vitamin D	Vitamin E (Alpha Tocopherol)	Vitamin C	Thiamin	Riboflavin	Niacin	Pantothenic Acid	Vit. B-6 (Pyridoxine)	Folacin (Folic Acid)	Biotin	Vitamin B-12
	(mg)	(mg)	(mg)	(IU)	(IU)	(mg)	(mg)	(mg)	(mg)	(mg)	(mg)	(mg)	(mcg)	(mcg)	(mcg)
523	–	–	–	–	–	–	–	.03	.13	.70	–	–	–	–	–
	–	–	–	–	–	–	–	.03	.13	.70	–	–	–	–	–
524	–	–	–	–	–	–	–	.14	.08	–	–	–	–	–	–
	–	–	–	–	–	–	–	.50	.27	–	–	–	–	–	–
525	–	–	–	–	–	–	–	–	–	–	–	–	–	–	–
	–	–	–	–	–	–	–	–	–	–	–	–	–	–	–
526	.31	.40	.20	Trace	Trace	–	Trace	–	–	–	–	–	–	–	–
	1.10	1.60	.70	Trace	Trace	–	Trace	–	–	–	–	–	–	–	–
527	–	–	–	–	–	–	5.04	.11	.20	.64	–	–	–	–	–
	–	–	–	–	–	–	18.00	.38	.72	2.30	–	–	–	–	–
528	.64	–	–	Trace	.64	(1.90)	7.00	(.36)	(.25)	(.36)	(.73)	(.08)	–	(4.23)	(3.08)
	2.30	–	–	Trace	2.30	(6.80)	25.00	(1.30)	(.89)	(1.29)	(2.61)	(.27)	–	(15.10)	(10.98)
529	–	–	–	–	–	–	–	.03	.03	–	–	–	–	–	–
	–	–	–	–	–	–	–	.11	.09	–	–	–	–	–	–
530	1.20	–	.20	160.0	–	1.35	–	.16	.06	9.80	–	–	–	–	–
	1.20	–	.20	160.0	–	1.35	–	.16	.06	9.80	–	–	–	–	–
531	.20	.16	–	16.8	–	–	0	.03	.01	1.99	.15	.08	5.60	4.20	1.93
	.70	.58	–	60.0	–	–	0	.12	.04	7.10	.55	.30	20.00	15.00	6.89
532	2.00	1.90	–	175.0	–	–	0	.23	.10	15.85	1.38	.75	50.00	37.50	17.23
	.80	.76	–	70.0	–	–	0	.09	.04	6.34	.55	.30	20.00	15.00	6.89
533	.17	.19	.02	46.2	–	–	0	.03	.01	2.04	.15	.08	5.60	4.20	1.93
	.60	.66	.08	165.0	–	–	0	.09	.05	7.30	.55	.30	20.00	15.00	6.89
534	(.17)	(.12)	(.02)	Trace	Trace	–	Trace	(.04)	(.05)	(2.47)	.20	.20	–	–	1.96
	(.60)	(.43)	(.08)	Trace	Trace	–	Trace	(.15)	(.18)	(8.82)	.71	.70	–	–	7.00
535	.42	–	.01	21.6	–	–	0	Trace	.02	.53	.10	.02	1.92	–	1.20
	3.50	–	.11	180.0	–	–	0	.02	.16	4.40	.85	.18	16.00	–	10.00
536	2.71	–	–	19.8	(2.10)	(.15)	Trace	.01	.18	3.50	.26	.15	(3.65)	(1.40)	(3.94)
	4.10	–	–	30.0	(7.52)	(.52)	Trace	.01	.27	5.30	.40	.22	(13.04)	(5.00)	(14.06)
537	.11	–	–	–	–	–	–	.01	.02	.89	–	–	–	–	–
	.40	–	–	–	–	–	–	.03	.08	3.20	–	–	–	–	–
538	.84	–	–	–	Trace	–	Trace	–	–	–	.04	–	4.90	Trace	–
	3.00	–	–	–	Trace	–	Trace	–	–	–	.15	–	17.50	Trace	–
539	.31	.18	.06	Trace	Trace	–	Trace	.03	.02	.37	–	–	–	–	–
	1.11	.63	.23	Trace	Trace	–	Trace	.09	.06	1.32	–	–	–	–	–
540	–	–	–	–	–	–	–	–	–	–	–	–	–	–	–
	–	–	–	–	–	–	–	–	–	–	–	–	–	–	–
541	.15	–	–	7.5	–	–	–	.03	.07	2.16	–	–	–	–	–
	.60	–	–	30.0	–	–	–	.13	.26	8.60	–	–	–	–	–
542	.39	–	–	0	–	–	–	.01	.01	1.23	–	–	–	–	–
	1.40	–	–	0	–	–	–	.02	.03	4.40	–	–	–	–	–
543	–	.23	–	–	–	–	–	–	–	–	–	–	–	–	–
	–	2.10	–	–	–	–	–	–	–	–	–	–	–	–	–
544	.34	.23	.04	6.6	–	–	0	Trace	Trace	.20	.02	.01	1.76	–	–
	3.10	2.10	.40	60.0	–	–	0	.01	.03	1.80	.21	.06	16.00	–	–
545	.39	–	–	–	–	–	–	–	–	–	–	–	–	–	–
	1.70	–	–	–	–	–	–	–	–	–	–	–	–	–	–
546	.22	–	–	–	–	–	–	.05	.01	–	–	–	–	–	–
	.80	–	–	–	–	–	–	.17	.02	–	–	–	–	–	–
547	.34	–	.04	Trace	Trace	–	Trace	–	–	–	–	–	–	–	–
	.20	–	.16	Trace	Trace	–	Trace	–	–	–	–	–	–	–	–
548	.14	–	–	–	–	–	–	.01	.03	–	–	–	–	–	–
	.50	–	–	–	–	–	–	.02	.12	–	–	–	–	–	–
549	.56	–	–	–	–	–	–	–	–	–	–	–	–	–	–
	0	–	–	–	–	–	–	–	–	–	–	–	–	–	–
550	.36	–	–	574.0	–	–	–	.01	.01	3.05	–	–	–	–	–
	1.30	–	–	2050.0	–	–	–	.04	.05	10.90	–	–	–	–	–
551	.90	–	–	–	–	–	–	–	–	–	–	–	–	–	–
	3.20	–	–	–	–	–	–	–	–	–	–	–	–	–	–
552	–	–	–	–	–	–	–	–	–	–	–	–	–	–	–
	–	–	–	–	–	–	–	–	–	–	–	–	–	–	–
553	–	–	–	–	–	–	–	–	.05	–	–	–	–	–	–
	–	–	–	–	–	–	–	–	.17	–	–	–	–	–	–
554	.31	[6].14	–	89.3	–	–	.28	.03	.02	.70	–	.06	–	–	.74
	.10	.50	–	319.0	–	–	1.00	.12	.06	2.50	–	.20	–	–	2.63

(Continued)

TABLE F-21 *(Continued)*

Item No.	Food Item Name	Approximate Measure	Weight	Moisture	Food Energy Calories	Protein	Fats	Carbo-hydrates	Fiber	Minerals (Macro) Calcium	Phos-phorus	Sodium	Mag-nesium	Potas-sium
			(g)	(%)	(kcal)	(g)	(g)	(g)	(g)	(mg)	(mg)	(mg)	(mg)	(mg)
	TUNA													
555	canned in water, solids & liquid, w/salt	1 CUP	200	70.0	238.0	56.0	1.6	0	0	32.0	380.0	1750.0	—	550.0
			100	70.0	119.0	28.0	.8	0	0	16.0	190.0	875.0	—	275.0
556	canned in oil, drained, solids	1 OZ	28	60.6	55.2	8.1	2.3	0	0	2.2	65.5	—	9.4	—
			100	60.6	197.0	28.8	8.2	0	0	8.0	234.0	—	33.4	—
557	**TURTLE**, green, canned	1 OZ	28	75.0	29.7	6.6	.2	0	0	—	—	—	—	—
			100	75.0	106.0	23.4	.7	0	0	—	—	—	—	—
558	**WEAKFISH**, w/salt, broiled	1 OZ	28	61.4	58.2	6.9	3.2	0	0	—	—	156.8	—	130.2
			100	61.4	208.0	24.6	11.4	0	0	—	—	560.0	—	465.0
	FLAVORINGS AND SEASONINGS													
559	**ALLSPICE**	1 TSP	2	8.5	5.3	.1	.2	1.4	.4	13.2	2.3	1.6	2.7	20.9
			100	8.5	263.0	6.1	8.7	72.1	21.6	661.0	113.0	80.0	135.0	1044.0
560	**AMARANTH**, raw	1 OZ	28	86.9	10.1	1.0	.1	1.8	.4	74.8	18.8	—	—	115.1
			100	86.9	36.0	3.5	.5	6.5	1.3	267.0	67.0	—	—	411.0
561	**ANISE SEED**	1 TSP	2	9.5	6.7	.4	.3	1.0	.3	12.9	8.8	.3	—	28.8
			100	9.5	337.0	17.6	15.9	50.0	14.6	646.0	440.0	16.0	—	1441.0
562	**BASIL**	1 TSP	1	6.4	2.5	.1	0	.6	.2	21.1	4.9	.3	4.2	34.3
			100	6.4	251.0	14.4	4.0	61.0	17.8	2113.0	490.0	34.0	422.0	3433.0
563	**BAY LEAVES**	1 TSP	1	5.4	3.1	.1	.1	.7	.3	8.3	1.1	.2	1.2	5.3
			100	5.4	313.0	7.6	8.4	74.7	26.3	834.0	113.0	23.0	120.0	529.0
564	**BRANDY FLAVORING**	1 TSP	5	—	0	—	—	—	—	—	—	—	—	—
			100	—	0	—	—	—	—	—	—	—	—	—
565	**CARAWAY SEEDS**	1 TSP	2	9.9	6.7	.4	.3	1.0	.3	13.8	11.4	.3	5.2	27.0
			100	9.9	333.0	19.8	14.6	49.9	12.7	689.0	568.0	17.0	258.0	1351.0
566	**CARDAMON SEED**	1 TSP	2	8.4	6.2	.2	.1	1.4	.2	7.7	3.6	.4	4.6	22.4
			100	8.4	311.0	10.7	6.7	68.5	11.3	383.0	178.0	18.0	229.0	1119.0
567	°**CAROB POWDER**	2 TBLS	14	—	54.3	.5	Trace	12.9	.8	41.4	—	1.4	—	114.3
			100	—	380.0	3.8	.2	90.6	5.4	290.0	—	10.0	—	800.0
568	**CATSUP**, bottled	1 TBLS	15	68.6	15.9	.3	.1	3.8	.1	3.3	7.5	156.3	3.2	54.5
			100	68.6	106.0	2.0	.4	25.4	.5	22.0	50.0	1042.0	21.0	363.0
569	**CATSUP, LOW SODIUM**	1 TBLS	17	68.7	18.0	.3	.1	4.3	.1	3.7	8.5	3.4	—	61.7
			100	68.6	106.0	2.0	.4	25.4	.5	22.0	50.0	20.0	—	363.0
570	**CELERY SEED**	1 TSP	2	6.0	7.8	.4	.5	.8	.2	35.3	11.0	3.2	8.8	28.0
			100	6.0	392.0	18.1	25.3	41.4	11.9	1767.0	550.0	160.0	440.0	1400.0
571	'**CHERVIL**, dried	1 OZ	28	7.2	66.4	6.5	1.1	13.7	3.2	376.9	126.0	23.2	36.4	1327.2
			100	7.2	237.0	23.2	3.9	49.1	11.3	1346.0	450.0	83.0	130.0	4740.0
572	**CHILI POWDER**	1 TBLS	15	7.8	47.1	1.8	2.5	8.2	3.3	41.7	45.5	151.5	25.5	287.4
			100	7.8	314.0	12.3	16.8	54.7	22.2	278.0	303.0	1010.0	170.0	1916.0
573	**CHILI SAUCE**, regular	1 TBLS	17	68.0	17.7	.4	.1	4.2	.1	3.4	8.8	227.5	—	62.9
			100	68.0	104.0	2.5	.3	24.8	.7	20.0	52.0	1338.0	—	370.0
574	**CHOCOLATE**, bitter or baking	1 OZ	28	2.3	141.4	3.0	14.8	8.1	.7	21.8	107.5	1.1	81.8	232.4
			100	2.3	505.0	10.7	53.0	28.9	2.5	78.0	384.0	4.0	292.0	830.0
575	**CINNAMON**	1 TSP	2	9.5	5.2	.1	.1	1.6	.5	24.6	1.2	.5	1.1	10.0
			100	9.5	261.0	3.9	3.2	79.8	24.4	1228.0	61.0	26.0	56.0	500.0
576	**CLOVES**, ground	1 TSP	2	6.9	6.5	.1	.4	1.2	.2	.1	2.1	5.0	5.3	22.0
			100	6.9	323.0	6.0	20.7	61.2	9.6	6.5	105.0	250.0	264.0	1102.0
	COCOA													
577	powder, w/o milk	1 TBLS	7	1.3	24.3	.3	.1	6.3	.1	2.1	12.0	18.8	29.4	35.0
			100	1.3	347.0	4.0	2.0	89.4	1.0	30.0	171.0	268.0	420.0	500.0
578	mix for hot chocolate	1 TBLS	7	3.1	27.4	.7	.7	5.2	.1	19.3	20.3	26.7	7.7	42.4
			100	3.1	392.0	9.4	10.6	73.9	.8	275.0	290.0	382.0	110.0	605.0
579	**CORIANDER LEAF**, dried	1 TSP	1	7.3	2.8	.2	0	.5	.1	12.5	4.8	2.1	6.9	44.7
			100	7.3	279.0	21.8	4.7	52.1	10.4	1246.0	481.0	211.0	694.0	4466.0
580	**CORIANDER SEED**	1 TSP	3	8.9	8.9	.4	.5	1.7	.9	21.3	12.3	1.1	9.0	38.0
			100	8.9	298.0	12.3	17.7	55.0	29.1	709.0	409.0	35.0	300.0	1267.0
581	**CUMIN SEED**	1 TSP	2	8.1	7.5	.4	.4	.9	.2	18.6	10.0	3.4	7.3	35.8
			100	8.1	375.0	17.7	22.3	44.6	10.5	931.0	499.0	168.0	366.0	1788.0
582	**CURRY POWDER**	1 TSP	2	9.5	6.5	.3	.3	1.2	.3	9.6	7.0	1.0	5.1	30.9
			100	9.5	325.0	12.7	13.8	58.2	16.3	478.0	349.0	52.0	254.0	1543.0
583	**DILL SEED**	1 TSP	2	7.7	6.1	.3	.3	1.1	.4	30.3	5.5	.4	5.1	23.7
			100	7.7	305.0	16.0	14.5	55.2	21.1	1516.0	277.0	20.0	256.0	1186.0
584	**DILL WEED**, dried	1 TSP	1	7.3	2.5	.2	0	.6	.1	17.8	5.4	2.1	4.5	33.1
			100	7.3	253.0	20.0	4.4	55.8	11.9	1784.0	543.0	208.0	451.0	3308.0
585	**FENNEL SEED**	1 TSP	2	8.8	6.9	.3	.3	1.0	.3	23.9	9.6	1.8	7.7	34.0
			100	8.8	345.0	15.8	14.9	52.3	15.7	1196.0	480.0	90.0	385.0	1700.0
586	**FENUGREEK SEED**	1 TSP	4	8.8	12.9	.9	.3	2.3	.4	7.0	11.8	2.7	7.6	30.8
			100	8.8	323.0	23.0	6.4	58.4	10.1	176.0	296.0	67.0	191.0	770.0
587	**GARLIC POWDER**	1 TSP	3	6.5	10.0	.5	0	2.2	.1	2.4	12.6	.8	1.7	33.0
			100	6.5	332.0	16.8	.8	72.7	1.9	80.0	420.0	26.0	58.0	1100.0

Item No.	Minerals (Micro)			Fat-Soluble Vitamins			Water-Soluble Vitamins								
	Iron	Zinc	Copper	Vitamin A	Vitamin D	Vitamin E (Alpha Tocopherol)	Vitamin C	Thiamin	Riboflavin	Niacin	Pantothenic Acid	Vit. B-6 (Pyridoxine)	Folacin (Folic Acid)	Biotin	Vitamin B-12
	(mg)	(mg)	(mg)	(IU)	(IU)	(mg)	(mg)	(mg)	(mg)	(mg)	(mg)	(mg)	(mcg)	(mcg)	(mcg)
555	3.20	[6]1.40	–	–	–	–	–	–	.20	26.60	.64	.85	30.00	6.00	4.40
	1.60	.70	–	–	–	–	–	–	.10	13.30	.32	.43	15.00	3.00	2.20
556	.53	.31	–	22.4	65.00	(1.76)	Trace	.01	.03	3.33	.09	.12	4.20	.84	.62
	1.90	1.10	–	80.0	232.00	(6.30)	Trace	.05	.12	11.90	.32	.43	15.00	3.00	2.20
557	–	–	–	–	–	–	–	–	–	–	–	–	–	–	–
	–	–	–	–	–	–	–	–	–	–	–	–	–	–	–
558	–	–	–	–	–	–	–	.03	.02	.98	–	–	–	–	–
	–	–	–	–	–	–	–	.10	.08	3.50	–	–	–	–	–
559	.14	.02	.01	10.8	–	–	.78	0	0	.06	–	–	–	–	0
	7.06	1.03	.45	540.0	–	–	39.20	.10	.06	2.90	–	–	–	–	0
560	1.09	–	–	1708.0	–	–	22.40	.02	.05	.39	–	–	–	–	0
	3.90	–	–	6100.0	–	–	80.00	.08	.16	1.40	–	–	–	–	–
561	.74	.11	–	–	–	–	–	–	–	–	–	–	–	–	0
	36.96	5.30	–	–	–	–	–	–	–	–	–	–	–	–	0
562	.43	.06	.01	93.8	–	–	.61	.00	Trace	.07	–	–	–	–	0
	42.80	5.83	1.30	9375.0	–	–	61.30	.15	.32	6.90	–	–	–	–	0
563	.43	.04	0	61.9	–	–	.47	.00	.00	.02	–	–	–	–	0
	43.00	3.70	.42	6185.0	–	–	46.60	.10	.42	2.00	–	–	–	–	0
564	–	–	–	–	–	–	–	–	–	–	–	–	–	–	–
	–	–	–	–	–	–	–	–	–	–	–	–	–	–	–
565	.31	.11	.01	7.3	–	–	.24	.01	.01	.07	–	–	–	–	–
	16.23	5.50	.43	363.0	–	–	12.00	.38	.38	3.61	–	–	–	–	–
566	.28	.15	–	0	–	–	.24	.00	Trace	.02	–	–	–	–	0
	13.97	7.47	–	0	–	–	12.00	.18	.18	1.10	–	–	–	–	0
567	.30	–	–	–	–	–	–	–	–	–	–	–	–	–	–
	2.00	–	–	–	–	–	–	–	–	–	–	–	–	–	–
568	.12	.04	–	210.0	–	–	2.25	.01	.01	.24	–	.02	.75	–	0
	.80	.26	–	1400.0	–	–	15.00	.09	.07	1.60	–	.11	5.00	–	0
569	.14	–	–	238.0	–	–	2.55	.02	.01	.27	–	.02	.85	–	0
	.80	–	–	1400.0	–	–	15.00	.09	.07	1.60	–	.11	5.00	–	0
570	.90	.14	–	1.0	–	–	.34	.01	.01	–	–	–	–	–	0
	44.90	6.93	–	52.0	–	–	17.20	.41	.49	–	–	–	–	–	0
571	8.95	2.48	–	–	–	–	–	–	–	–	–	.34	–	–	0
	31.95	8.80	–	–	–	–	–	–	–	–	–	1.23	–	–	0
572	2.14	.41	.19	5239.1	–	–	9.62	.05	.11	1.18	–	–	–	–	0
	14.25	2.70	.60	34927.0	–	–	64.14	.35	.75	7.89	–	–	–	–	0
573	.14	–	–	238.0	–	–	2.72	.02	.01	.27	–	–	–	–	–
	.80	–	–	1400.0	–	–	16.00	.09	.07	1.60	–	–	–	–	–
574	1.88	–	–	16.8	0	–	0	.01	.07	.42	.05	.01	2.52	8.96	0
	6.70	–	–	60.0	0	–	0	.05	.24	1.50	.19	.04	9.00	32.00	0
575	.76	.04	.01	5.2	–	–	.57	Trace	Trace	.03	–	–	–	–	0
	38.07	1.97	.23	260.0	–	–	28.46	.07	.14	1.30	–	–	–	–	0
576	.17	.09	.01	10.6	–	–	1.62	Trace	Trace	.03	–	–	–	–	0
	8.68	4.72	.35	530.0	–	–	80.90	.11	.27	1.46	–	–	–	–	0
577	.15	.39	–	–	–	–	0	Trace	Trace	.04	–	–	–	–	–
	2.10	5.60	–	–	–	–	0	.02	.09	.50	–	–	–	–	–
578	.10	–	–	.7	–	–	.07	.01	.03	.04	–	–	–	–	0
	1.40	–	–	10.0	–	–	1.00	.08	.41	.50	–	–	–	–	0
579	.43	–	–	–	–	–	5.67	.01	.01	.11	–	–	–	–	0
	42.46	–	–	–	–	–	566.71	1.25	1.50	10.71	–	–	–	–	0
580	.49	.14	–	0	–	–	.36	.01	.01	.07	–	–	–	–	0
	16.32	4.70	–	0	–	–	12.00	.24	.29	2.13	–	–	–	–	0
581	1.33	.10	–	25.4	–	–	.15	.01	.01	.09	–	–	–	–	0
	66.35	4.80	–	1270.0	–	–	7.71	.63	.33	4.58	–	–	–	–	0
582	.59	.08	(.21)	19.7	0	–	.23	.01	.01	.07	–	–	–	–	0
	29.59	4.05	(1.03)	986.0	0	–	11.41	.25	.28	3.47	–	–	–	–	0
583	.33	.10	–	1.1	–	–	.24	.01	.01	.06	–	–	–	–	0
	16.32	5.20	–	53.0	–	–	12.00	.42	.28	2.80	–	–	–	–	0
584	.45	.03	.03	–	–	–	–	Trace	Trace	.03	–	0	–	–	0
	44.77	3.30	3.42	–	–	–	–	.41	.28	2.81	–	Trace	–	–	0
585	.37	.07	–	2.7	–	–	.24	.01	.01	.12	–	–	–	–	0
	18.54	3.70	–	135.0	–	–	12.00	.41	.36	6.00	–	–	–	–	0
586	1.34	.10	–	–	–	–	.12	.01	.02	.07	–	–	2.28	–	0
	33.53	2.50	–	–	–	–	3.00	.32	.36	1.64	–	–	57.00	–	0
587	.08	.08	–	0	–	–	.36	,01	.01	.02	–	–	–	–	0
	2.75	2.63	–	0	–	–	12.00	.47	.15	.70	–	–	–	–	0

(Continued)

TABLE F-21 *(Continued)*

Item No.	Food Item Name	Approximate Measure	Weight (g)	Moisture (%)	Food Energy Calories (kcal)	Protein (g)	Fats (g)	Carbohydrates (g)	Fiber (g)	Minerals (Macro) Calcium (mg)	Phosphorus (mg)	Sodium (mg)	Magnesium (mg)	Potassium (mg)
588	GARLIC SALT	1 TSP	5	–	–	–	–	–	–	–	–	–	1.0	–
			100	–	–	–	–	–	–	–	–	–	20.0	–
	GINGER													
589	ROOT, fresh	1 OZ	28	87.0	13.7	.4	.3	2.7	.3	6.4	10.1	1.7	–	73.9
			100	87.0	49.0	1.4	1.0	9.5	1.1	23.0	36.0	6.0	–	264.0
590	ROOT, crystallized (candied)	1 OZ	28	12.0	95.2	.1	.1	24.4	.2	–	–	–	–	–
			100	12.0	340.0	.3	.2	87.1	.7	–	–	–	–	–
591	ROOT, dried, ground	1 TSP	2	9.4	6.9	.2	.1	1.4	.1	2.3	3.0	.6	3.3	26.8
			100	9.4	347.0	9.1	6.0	70.8	5.9	116.0	150.0	30.0	164.0	1342.0
592	HORSERADISH, prepared	1 TSP	6	87.1	2.3	.1	0	.6	.1	3.7	1.9	5.8	–	17.4
			100	87.1	38.0	1.3	.2	9.6	.9	61.0	32.0	96.0	–	290.0
593	KETCHUP—See CATSUP													
594	MACE, ground	1 TSP	2	8.2	9.5	.1	.6	1.0	.1	5.0	2.2	1.6	3.2	9.3
			100	8.2	475.0	6.7	32.4	50.5	4.8	252.0	110.0	80.0	160.0	463.0
595	MARJORAM, dried	1 TSP	1	7.6	2.7	.1	.1	.6	.2	19.9	3.1	.8	3.5	15.2
			100	7.6	271.0	12.7	7.0	60.6	18.1	1990.0	306.0	77.0	346.0	1522.0
596	MONOSODIUM GLUTAMATE, Accent	1 TSP	5	.1	14.4	2.3	0	0	–	–	–	645.0	–	–
			100	.1	288.0	46.8	0	0	–	–	–	12900.0	–	–
	MUSTARD													
597	prepared, brown	1 TSP	5	78.1	4.6	.3	.3	.3	.1	6.2	6.7	65.4	2.4	6.5
			100	78.1	91.0	5.9	6.3	5.3	1.3	124.0	134.0	1307.0	48.0	130.0
598	prepared, yellow	1 TSP	5	80.2	3.8	.2	.2	.3	.1	4.2	3.7	62.6	2.4	6.5
			100	80.2	75.0	4.7	4.4	6.4	1.0	84.0	73.0	1252.0	48.0	130.0
599	NUTMEG	1 TSP	2	6.2	10.5	.1	.7	1.0	.1	3.7	4.3	.3	3.6	7.0
			100	6.2	525.0	5.8	36.3	49.3	4.0	184.0	213.0	16.0	180.0	350.0
600	ONION POWDER	1 TSP	2	5.0	6.9	.2	0	1.6	.1	7.3	6.8	1.1	2.4	18.9
			100	5.0	347.0	10.1	1.1	80.5	5.7	363.0	340.0	54.0	122.0	943.0
601	OREGANO	1 TSP	2	7.2	6.1	.2	.2	1.3	.3	31.5	4.0	.3	5.4	33.4
			100	7.2	306.0	11.0	10.3	64.9	15.0	1576.0	200.0	15.0	270.0	1669.0
602	PAPRIKA, domestic	1 TSP	2	9.5	5.8	.3	.3	1.1	.4	3.5	6.9	.7	3.7	46.9
			100	9.5	289.0	14.8	13.0	55.7	20.9	177.0	345.0	34.0	185.0	2344.0
	PEPPER													
603	BLACK, ground	1 TSP	2	10.5	5.1	.2	.1	1.3	.3	8.0	3.5	.9	3.9	25.2
			100	10.5	255.0	10.4	3.3	66.5	13.1	400.0	173.0	44.0	194.0	1259.0
604	RED	1 TSP	2	8.1	6.4	.2	.3	1.1	.6	3.0	5.9	.6	3.0	40.3
			100	8.1	318.0	12.0	17.3	56.6	24.9	148.0	293.0	30.0	152.0	2014.0
605	WHITE	1 TSP	2	11.4	5.9	.2	0	1.4	.1	5.3	3.5	.1	1.8	1.5
			100	11.4	296.0	10.4	2.1	68.6	4.3	265.0	176.0	5.0	90.0	73.0
606	POPPY SEED	1 TSP	3	6.8	15.9	.5	1.3	.7	.2	43.4	25.4	.6	9.6	21.0
			100	6.8	530.0	18.0	44.7	23.7	6.3	1448.0	848.0	21.0	320.0	700.0
607	POULTRY SEASONING	1 TSP	2	9.3	6.1	.2	.2	1.3	.2	19.9	3.4	.5	4.5	13.7
			100	9.3	307.0	9.6	7.5	65.6	11.3	996.0	171.0	27.0	224.0	684.0
608	PUMPKIN PIE SPICE	1 TSP	2	8.5	6.8	.1	.3	1.4	.3	13.6	2.4	1.0	2.7	13.3
			100	8.5	342.0	5.8	12.6	69.3	14.8	682.0	118.0	52.0	136.0	663.0
609	PURSLANE, leaves & stems, raw	1 CUP	60	92.5	12.6	1.0	.2	2.3	.5	61.8	23.4	–	–	–
			100	92.5	21.0	1.7	.4	3.8	.9	103.0	39.0	–	–	–
610	ROSEMARY, leaves	1 TSP	1	5.7	4.4	0	.2	.7	.2	15.0	.7	.4	–	10.0
			100	5.7	440.0	4.5	17.4	66.4	19.0	1500.0	70.0	40.0	–	1000.0
611	SAFFRON	1 TSP	1	11.9	3.1	.1	.1	.7	Trace	1.1	2.5	1.5	–	17.2
			100	11.9	310.0	11.4	5.9	65.4	3.9	111.0	252.0	148.0	–	1724.0
612	SAGE	1 TSP	1	8.0	3.2	.1	.1	.6	.2	16.5	.9	.1	4.3	10.7
			100	8.0	315.0	10.6	12.7	60.7	18.1	1652.0	90.0	10.0	428.0	1070.0
	SALT													
613	table	1 TSP	5	–	0	0	0	0	–	12.7	–	1940.5	–	.2
			100	–	0	0	0	0	–	253.0	–	38809.0	–	4.0
614	table, iodized	1 PKG	1	.05	0	0	0	0	–	1.0	.4	390.9	0	0
			100	.05	.2	0	0	0	–	100.0	40.0	39090.0	1.4	2.4
615	SAVORY	1 TSP	1	9.0	2.7	.1	.1	.7	.2	21.3	1.4	.2	3.8	10.5
			100	9.0	272.0	6.7	5.9	69.9	15.3	2132.0	140.0	20.0	377.0	1051.0
616	SESAME SEEDS, dry, decorticated	1 OZ	28	4.8	163.0	7.4	15.3	2.6	.8	36.7	217.3	11.2	97.2	114.0
			100	4.8	582.0	26.4	54.8	9.4	3.0	131.0	776.0	40.0	347.0	407.0
617	SOY SAUCE	1 TBLS	15	62.8	10.2	.8	.2	1.4	0	12.3	15.6	1098.8	–	54.9
			100	62.8	68.0	5.6	1.3	9.5	0	82.0	104.0	7325.0	–	366.0
618	TARRAGON	1 TSP	1	7.7	3.0	.2	.1	.5	.1	11.4	3.1	.6	3.5	30.2
			100	7.7	295.0	22.8	7.3	50.2	7.4	1139.0	310.0	62.0	347.0	3020.0
619	THYME	1 TSP	1	7.8	2.8	.1	.1	.6	.2	18.9	2.0	.6	2.2	8.1
			100	7.8	276.0	9.1	7.4	63.9	18.6	1890.0	200.0	55.0	220.0	814.0
620	TABASCO SAUCE	1 TSP	5	87.0	.4	0	0	.1	0	–	–	22.3	–	3.2
			100	87.0	8.1	.9	0	1.1	0	–	–	445.5	–	63.0
621	TOMATO CATSUP OR KETCHUP—See CATSUP													

Item No.	Minerals (Micro) Iron	Zinc	Copper	Fat-Soluble Vitamins Vitamin A	Vitamin D	Vitamin E (Alpha Tocopherol)	Water-Soluble Vitamins Vitamin C	Thiamin	Riboflavin	Niacin	Pantothenic Acid	Vit. B-6 (Pyridoxine)	Folacin (Folic Acid)	Biotin	Vitamin B-12
	(mg)	(mg)	(mg)	(IU)	(IU)	(mg)	(mg)	(mg)	(mg)	(mg)	(mg)	(mg)	(mcg)	(mcg)	(mcg)
588	—	—	—	—	—	—	—	—	—	—	—	—	—	—	—
	—	—	—	—	—	—	—	—	—	—	—	—	—	—	—
589	.59	—	—	2.8	—	—	1.12	.01	.01	.20	.06	—	—	—	0
	2.10	—	—	10.0	—	—	4.00	.02	.04	.70	.20	—	—	—	0
590	—	—	—	—	—	—	—	—	—	—	—	—	—	—	—
	—	—	—	—	—	—	—	—	—	—	—	—	—	—	—
591	.23	.09	.01	2.9	0	—	.24	Trace	Trace	.10	—	—	—	—	0
	11.30	4.72	.32	147.0	0	—	12.00	.05	.19	5.16	—	—	—	—	0
592	.05	.06	—	—	—	—	—	—	—	—	—	—	—	—	—
	.90	1.07	—	—	—	—	—	—	—	—	—	—	—	—	—
593															
594	.28	.05	.05	16.0	—	—	—	.01	.01	.03	—	—	—	—	0
	13.90	2.30	2.47	800.0	—	—	—	.31	.44	1.35	—	—	—	—	0
595	.83	.04	.01	80.7	—	—	.51	.00	Trace	.04	—	—	—	—	0
	82.71	3.60	1.10	8068.0	—	—	51.43	.29	.32	4.12	—	—	—	—	0
596	—	—	—	—	—	—	—	—	—	—	—	—	—	—	—
	—	—	—	—	—	—	—	—	—	—	—	—	—	—	—
597	.09	.01	—	—	—	.09	—	—	—	—	—	—	—	—	—
	1.80	.21	—	—	—	1.75	—	—	—	—	—	—	—	—	—
598	.10	.03	—	—	—	.09	—	—	—	—	—	—	.20	—	—
	2.00	.63	—	—	—	1.75	—	—	—	—	—	—	3.90	—	—
599	.06	.04	.02	2.0	—	—	.24	.01	Trace	.03	—	—	—	—	0
	3.04	2.15	1.03	102.0	—	—	12.00	.36	.06	1.30	—	—	—	—	0
600	.05	.05	—	0	—	—	.29	.01	Trace	.01	—	—	—	—	0
	2.56	2.32	—	0	—	—	14.70	.42	.06	.65	—	—	—	—	0
601	.88	.09	—	138.1	—	—	.24	.01	Trace	.12	—	—	—	—	0
	44.00	4.43	—	6903.0	—	—	12.00	.34	.04	6.20	—	—	—	—	0
602	.46	.08	.01	1212.1	—	—	1.42	.01	.04	.31	—	—	—	—	0
	23.10	4.06	.61	60604.0	—	—	71.12	.65	.74	15.30	—	—	—	—	0
603	.58	.03	.09	3.8	0	—	.24	Trace	Trace	.02	—	—	—	—	0
	28.86	1.42	4.30	190.0	0	—	12.00	.11	.21	1.14	—	—	—	—	0
604	.14	.05	—	832.2	—	—	1.53	.01	.02	.17	—	—	—	—	0
	7.08	2.48	—	41610.0	—	—	76.44	.33	.92	8.70	—	—	—	—	0
605	.29	.02	.02	0	—	—	—	0	Trace	Trace	—	—	—	—	0
	14.31	1.13	.80	0	—	—	—	.02	.13	.21	—	—	—	—	0
606	.28	.31	.05	0	—	.05	.36	.03	.01	.03	—	.01	—	—	0
	9.40	10.23	1.63	0	—	1.80	12.00	.85	.18	.98	—	.45	—	—	0
607	.71	.06	—	52.6	—	—	.24	.01	Trace	.06	—	—	—	—	0
	35.30	3.14	—	2632.0	—	—	11.96	.26	.19	2.97	—	—	—	—	0
608	.39	.05	—	5.2	—	—	.47	Trace	Trace	.05	—	—	—	—	0
	19.71	2.37	—	261.0	—	—	23.38	.13	.14	2.24	—	—	—	—	0
609	2.10	—	—	1500.0	—	—	15.00	.02	.06	.30	—	—	—	—	—
	3.50	—	—	2500.0	—	—	25.00	.03	.10	.50	—	—	—	—	—
610	Trace	—	—	1.8	—	—	.61	.01	0	.01	—	—	—	—	—
	.33	—	—	175.0	—	—	61.30	.51	.04	1.00	—	—	—	—	—
611	.11	—	—	—	—	—	—	—	—	—	—	—	—	—	0
	11.10	—	—	—	—	—	—	—	—	—	—	—	—	—	0
612	.28	.05	—	59.0	—	—	.32	.01	Trace	.06	—	—	—	—	0
	28.12	4.70	—	5900.0	—	—	32.38	.75	.34	4.70	—	—	—	—	0
613	.01	—	—	0	—	—	0	0	0	0	—	—	—	—	—
	.10	—	—	0	—	—	0	0	0	0	—	—	—	—	—
614	Trace	0	Trace	0	0	—	0	0	0	0	0	0	0	0	0
	.10	0	.10	0	0	—	0	0	0	0	0	0	0	0	0
615	.38	.04	—	51.3	—	—	.12	Trace	0	.04	—	—	—	—	0
	37.80	4.30	—	5130.0	—	—	12.00	.37	.04	4.10	—	—	—	—	0
616	2.18	2.87	—	18.5	—	—	0	.20	.02	1.31	.19	.04	—	—	0
	7.80	10.25	—	66.0	—	—	0	.72	.09	4.68	.68	.15	—	—	0
617	.72	.08	.02	0	—	—	0	Trace	.04	.06	—	—	4.20	—	—
	4.80	.53	.13	0	—	—	0	.02	.25	.40	—	—	28.00	—	—
618	.32	.04	—	42.0	—	—	.12	.01	.09		—	—	—	—	0
	32.30	3.90	—	4200.0	—	—	12.00	.25	.34	8.90	—	—	—	—	0
619	1.24	.06	.01	38.0	—	—	.12	.01	Trace	.05	—	—	—	—	0
	123.60	6.40	.86	3800.0	—	—	12.00	.51	.40	4.90	—	—	—	—	0
620	—	—	—	—	—	—	—	Trace	.01	.02	—	—	—	—	—
	—	—	—	—	—	—	—	.03	.10	.32	—	—	—	—	—
621															

(Continued)

TABLE F-21 *(Continued)*

Item No.	Food Item Name	Approximate Measure	Weight (g)	Moisture (%)	Food Energy Calories (kcal)	Protein (g)	Fats (g)	Carbo- hydrates (g)	Fiber (g)	Minerals (Macro) Calcium (mg)	Phos- phorus (mg)	Sodium (mg)	Mag- nesium (mg)	Potas- sium (mg)
622	**TUMERIC**	1 TSP	2	11.4	7.1	.2	.2	1.3	Trace	3.6	5.2	.8	3.9	50.0
			100	11.4	354.0	7.8	9.9	64.9	6.9	182.0	260.0	38.0	193.0	2500.0
	VINEGAR													
623	cider	1 TBLS	15	93.8	2.1	0	0	.9	0	.9	1.4	.2	–	15.0
			100	93.8	14.0	0	0	5.9	0	6.0	9.0	1.0	–	100.0
624	distilled	1 TBLS	15	95.0	1.8	–	–	.8	–	–	–	.2	.2	2.3
			100	95.0	12.0	–	–	5.0	–	–	–	1.0	1.0	15.0
625	**WATER CHESTNUTS,** Chinese, raw	1 PIECE	6	78.3	4.7	.1	0	1.1	Trace	.2	3.9	1.2	.7	30.0
			100	78.3	79.0	1.4	.2	19.0	.8	4.0	65.0	20.0	12.0	500.0
626	**WORCESTERSHIRE SAUCE**	1 TSP	5	70.0	5.9	0	0	.8	Trace	5.3	2.9	48.9	–	40.1
			100	70.0	117.3	.1	.2	16.6	.3	106.0	57.0	977.0	–	802.0
	FOOD SUPPLEMENTS													
627	**ALFALFA LEAF MEAL,** (powder), dehydrated		–	–	–	–	–	–	–	–	–	–	–	–
			100	–	215.0	20.0	3.1	57.8	18.1	1640.0	230.0	60.0	350.0	2070.0
628	**COD LIVER OIL**		–	–	–	–	–	–	–	–	–	–	–	–
			100	–	899.0	0	99.9	0	0	Trace	Trace	Trace	Trace	Trace
	SEAWEED													
629	Irish Moss, (carrageenan),raw	1 OZ	28	19.2	–	–	.5	–	.6	247.8	44.0	809.8	–	796.3
			100	19.2	–	–	1.8	–	2.1	885.0	157.0	2892.0	–	2844.0
630	kelp, raw	1 OZ	28	21.7	–	–	.3	–	1.9	306.0	67.2	842.0	–	1476.4
			100	21.7	–	–	1.1	–	6.8	1093.0	240.0	3007.0	–	5273.0
	YEAST													
631	brewers', tablet form	6 TABLETS	5	–	–	4.0	–	–	–	–	–	–	–	–
			100	–	–	80.0	–	–	–	–	–	–	–	–
632	torula	1 TBLS	10	6.0	27.7	3.9	.1	3.7	.3	42.4	171.3	1.5	16.5	204.6
			100	6.0	277.0	38.6	1.0	37.0	3.3	424.0	1713.0	15.0	165.0	2046.0
	FRUITS													
633	**ACEROLA,** raw, pulp & skin	1 AVG	8	92.3	2.2	0	0	.5	Trace	1.0	.9	.6	–	6.6
			100	92.3	28.0	.4	.3	6.8	.4	12.0	11.0	8.0	–	83.0
	APPLES													
634	raw, fresh, unpared	1 MED	150	84.8	84.0	.3	.9	21.2	1.5	4.5	9.0	1.5	7.2	208.5
			100	84.8	56.0	.2	.6	14.1	1.0	3.0	6.0	1.0	4.8	139.0
635	raw, fresh, pared	1 MED	145	85.3	76.9	.3	.4	20.2	.9	2.9	8.7	1.5	4.6	176.9
			100	85.3	53.0	.2	.3	13.9	.6	2.0	6.0	1.0	3.2	122.0
636	baked, unpared	1 MED	150	–	187.5	.3	.9	–	–	9.0	15.0	1.5	–	165.0
			100	–	125.0	.2	.6	–	–	6.0	10.0	1.0	–	110.0
637	dried, sulfured, uncooked	1 OZ	28	32.9	66.9	.3	.1	18.1	.8	4.2	11.5	25.8	4.5	113.4
			100	32.9	239.0	.9	.3	64.8	2.8	15.0	41.0	92.0	16.0	405.0
	APPLESAUCE													
638	canned, unsweetened or artificial sweetener	1 CUP	244	88.3	102.5	.4	.1	27.6	1.3	9.8	24.4	4.9	7.3	190.3
			100	88.3	42.0	.2	.1	11.3	.5	4.0	10.0	2.0	3.0	78.0
639	canned, sweetened	1 CUP	255	80.0	191.3	.5	.4	49.9	1.1	7.7	17.9	7.7	7.7	153.0
			100	80.0	75.0	.2	.2	19.6	.5	3.0	7.0	3.0	3.0	60.0
	APRICOTS													
640	raw	1 MED	38	85.3	19.4	.4	.1	4.9	.2	3.0	5.7	.4	3.5	121.2
			100	85.3	51.0	1.0	.2	12.8	.6	8.0	15.0	1.0	9.3	319.0
641	canned, water pack, w/o artificial sweetener	1 HALF	33	92.5	8.6	.2	0	2.1	.1	2.6	4.3	1.0	2.3	62.4
			100	92.5	26.0	.7	.1	6.3	.4	8.0	13.0	3.0	7.0	189.0
642	canned, artificial sweetener	1 MED	28	92.5	7.3	.2	0	1.8	.1	2.2	3.6	.8	2.0	52.9
			100	92.5	26.0	.7	.1	6.3	.4	8.0	13.0	3.0	7.0	189.0
643	canned, extra heavy syrup	1 SERV	120	72.9	121.2	.7	.1	31.2	.5	13.2	18.0	1.2	8.4	276.0
			100	72.9	101.0	.6	.1	26.0	.4	11.0	15.0	1.0	7.0	230.0
644	dried, sulfured, uncooked	1 HALF	4	31.5	9.4	.2	0	2.4	.1	2.0	4.8	.4	2.0	56.9
			100	31.5	236.0	3.9	.5	60.8	2.9	51.0	119.0	9.0	50.0	1422.0
645	**AVOCADOS,** all varieties, raw, halved, fruit served w/skin	1 AVG	250	74.0	417.5	5.3	41.0	15.8	4.0	25.0	105.0	10.0	112.5	1510.0
			100	74.0	167.0	2.1	16.4	6.3	1.6	10.0	42.0	4.0	45.0	604.0
	BANANAS													
646	common, yellow, short & thick	1 AVG	100	68.8	110.0	1.2	.2	29.0	.4	7.0	28.0	–	–	–
			100	68.8	110.0	1.2	.2	29.0	.4	7.0	28.0	–	–	–
647	flakes	1 CUP	100	3.0	340.0	4.0	1.0	89.0	–	32.0	–	–	–	–
			100	3.0	340.0	4.0	1.0	89.0	–	32.0	–	–	–	–
648	**ᵃBARBADOS CHERRY,** (acerola) ripe	1 OZ	28	90.3	10.1	.1	.1	2.4	.1	3.4	3.1	–	–	–
			100	90.3	36.0	.4	.4	8.7	.4	12.0	11.0	–	–	–

Item No.	Minerals (Micro)			Fat-Soluble Vitamins			Water-Soluble Vitamins								
	Iron	Zinc	Copper	Vitamin A	Vitamin D	Vitamin E (Alpha Tocopherol)	Vitamin C	Thiamin	Ribo-flavin	Niacin	Panto-thenic Acid	Vit. B-6 (Pyri-doxine)	Folacin (Folic Acid)	Biotin	Vitamin B-12
	(mg)	(mg)	(mg)	(IU)	(IU)	(mg)	(mg)	(mg)	(mg)	(mg)	(mg)	(mg)	(mcg)	(mcg)	(mcg)
622	.83	.09	–	0	–	–	.52	Trace	.01	.10	–	–	–	–	0
	41.42	4.35	–	0	–	–	25.85	.15	.23	5.14	–	–	–	–	0
623	.09	.02	.01	–	0	–	–	–	–	–	–	0	–	–	0
	.60	.10	.08	–	0	–	–	–	–	–	–	Trace	–	–	0
624	–	.02	–	–	–	–	–	–	–	–	–	0	.02	–	0
	–	.10	–	–	–	–	–	–	–	–	–	–	.10	–	0
625	.04	–	–	0	–	–	.24	.01	.01	.06	–	–	–	–	–
	.60	–	–	0	–	–	4.00	.14	.20	1.00	–	–	–	–	–
626	.28	–	–	5.5	–	–	9.15	Trace	.01	.02	–	–	–	–	–
	5.60	–	–	110.0	–	–	183.00	.06	.16	.44	–	–	–	–	–
627	–	–	–	–	–	–	–	–	–	–	–	–	–	–	–
	36.0	1.58	1.0	22940.0	35.6	–	–	.55	1.51	3.90	3.35	–	–	33.00	–
628	–	–	–	–	–	–	–	–	–	–	–	–	–	–	–
	Trace	Trace	Trace	85000.0	8500.0	20.0	0	0	0	0	0	0	0	0	0
629	2.49	–	–	–	–	–	–	–	–	–	–	–	–	–	–
	8.90	–	–	–	–	–	–	–	–	–	–	–	–	–	–
630	–	–	–	–	–	–	–	–	–	–	–	–	–	–	–
	–	–	–	–	–	–	–	–	–	–	–	–	–	–	–
631	0	–	–	–	–	–	–	.48	.16	1.60	.20	.16	13.00	4.00	–
	12.00	–	–	–	–	–	–	9.60	3.20	32.00	4.00	3.20	260.00	80.00	–
632	1.93	.19	–	–	–	–	–	1.40	.51	4.44	1.10	.30	300.00	10.00	0
	19.30	1.85	–	–	–	–	–	14.01	5.06	44.40	11.00	3.00	3000.00	100.00	0
633	.02	–	–	2.6	–	–	104.00	Trace	.01	.03	–	Trace	–	–	0
	.20	–	–	33.0	–	–	1300.00	.02	.06	.40	–	.01	–	–	0
634	.15	.08	.06	135.0	–	.47	10.50	.05	.03	.15	.16	.05	12.00	1.35	0
	.10	.05	.04	90.0	–	.31	7.00	.03	.02	.10	.11	.03	8.00	.90	0
635	.15	.07	.05	58.0	–	–	5.80	.04	.03	.15	.15	.04	11.60	–	0
	.10	.05	.03	40.0	–	–	4.00	.03	.02	.10	.10	.03	8.00	–	0
636	.45	–	–	139.5	–	–	4.50	.05	.03	.20	–	–	–	–	–
	.30	–	–	93.0	–	–	3.00	.03	.02	.13	–	–	–	–	–
637	.48	.05	.05	0	–	–	1.06	0	.05	.26	–	.04	–	–	0
	1.72	.19	.17	0	–	–	3.80	0	.16	.91	–	.14	–	–	0
638	.32	.06	.06	70.8	–	–	40.99	.02	.05	.10	–	–	–	–	–
	.13	.03	.03	29.0	–	–	16.80	.01	.02	.04	–	–	–	–	–
639	.87	.09	.11	28.1	–	–	4.08	.03	.08	.10	.12	.07	2.55	–	0
	.34	.04	.04	11.0	–	–	1.60	.01	.03	.04	.05	.03	1.00	–	0
640	.19	.05	.03	1026.0	0	–	3.80	.01	.01	.23	.09	.03	1.25	–	0
	.50	.12	.08	2700.0	0	–	10.00	.03	.04	.60	.24	.07	3.30	–	0
641	.18	.03	.01	597.3	–	–	1.06	.01	.01	.13	.03	.02	.66	–	–
	.54	.10	.04	1810.0	–	–	3.20	.02	.02	.40	.10	.05	2.00	–	–
642	.15	.03	.01	506.8	–	–	.90	.01	.01	.11	.03	.02	.56	–	–
	.54	.10	.04	1810.0	–	–	3.20	.02	.02	.40	.10	.05	2.00	–	–
643	.36	.14	.05	2064.0	–	–	4.80	.02	.02	.36	.11	.07	2.40	–	0
	.30	.12	.04	1720.0	–	–	4.00	.02	.02	.30	.09	.05	2.00	–	0
644	.19	.03	.02	285.9	0	–	.12	0	.01	.12	.03	.01	.56	–	0
	4.82	.79	.49	7147.0	0	–	3.00	.01	.15	2.99	.75	.17	14.00	–	0
645	1.50	0	1.00	725.0	–	–	35.00	.28	.50	4.00	2.68	1.05	127.50	13.75	0
	.60	0	.40	290.0	–	–	14.00	.11	.20	1.60	1.07	.42	51.00	5.50	0
646	.50	–	–	65.0	–	–	15.00	.04	.04	.70	–	–	–	–	–
	.50	–	–	65.0	–	–	15.00	.04	.04	.70	–	–	–	–	–
647	2.80	–	–	760.0	0	–	7.00	.18	.24	2.80	–	–	–	–	–
	2.80	–	–	760.0	0	–	7.00	.18	.24	2.80	–	–	–	–	–
648	.06	–	–	–	–	–	501.20	.01	.01	.17	–	–	–	–	–
	.20	–	–	–	–	–	1790.00	.03	.05	.60	–	–	–	–	–

(Continued)

TABLE F-21 *(Continued)*

Item No.	Food Item Name	Approximate Measure	Weight (g)	Moisture (%)	Food Energy Calories (kcal)	Protein (g)	Fats (g)	Carbohydrates (g)	Fiber (g)	Calcium (mg)	Phosphorus (mg)	Sodium (mg)	Magnesium (mg)	Potassium (mg)
	BLACKBERRIES													
649	raw	1 CUP	144	84.5	83.5	1.7	1.3	18.6	5.9	20.2	27.4	1.4	28.5	305.3
			100	84.5	58.0	1.2	.9	12.9	4.1	14.0	19.0	1.0	19.8	212.0
650	canned, juice pack, solids & liquid	1 CUP	260	85.8	140.4	2.1	2.1	31.5	7.0	65.0	44.2	2.6	—	442.0
			100	85.8	54.0	.8	.8	12.1	2.7	25.0	17.0	1.0	—	170.0
651	canned, heavy syrup, solids & liquid	1 CUP	250	76.1	227.5	2.0	1.5	55.5	6.5	52.5	30.0	2.5	—	272.5
			100	76.1	91.0	.8	.6	22.2	2.6	21.0	12.0	1.0	—	109.0
	BLUEBERRIES													
652	raw	1 CUP	140	83.2	86.8	1.0	.7	21.4	2.1	21.0	18.2	1.4	8.4	113.4
			100	83.2	62.0	.7	.5	15.3	1.5	15.0	13.0	1.0	6.0	81.0
653	pie filling, canned	1 OZ	28	68.9	35.0	.1	—	8.5	—	1.7	—	—	—	—
			100	68.9	125.0	.2	—	30.4	—	6.0	—	—	—	—
654	**BOYSENBERRIES,** canned, water pack, solids & liquid	1 CUP	140	89.8	50.4	1.0	.1	12.7	2.7	26.6	26.6	1.4	—	119.0
			100	89.8	36.0	.7	.1	9.1	1.9	19.0	19.0	1.0	—	85.0
655	**BREADFRUIT,** raw	1 MED	350	70.8	360.5	6.0	1.1	91.7	4.2	115.5	112.0	52.5	—	1536.5
			100	70.8	103.0	1.7	.3	26.2	1.2	33.0	32.0	15.0	—	439.0
656	**CANTALOUPE,** raw	1 WHOLE	770	91.2	231.0	4.6	.8	57.8	2.3	107.8	123.2	92.4	64.7	1932.7
			100	91.2	30.0	.6	.1	7.5	.3	14.0	16.0	12.0	8.4	251.0
657	**CARAMBOLA,** raw	1 AVG	57	90.4	20.0	.4	.3	4.6	.5	2.3	9.7	1.1	—	109.4
			100	90.4	35.0	.7	.5	8.0	.9	4.0	17.0	2.0	—	192.0
658	**CASABA,** (Golden Beauty), vine ripened	1 WHOLE	850	91.5	272.0	10.2	.9	55.3	4.3	119.0	136.0	102.0	68.0	2133.5
			100	91.5	32.0	1.2	.1	6.5	.5	14.0	16.0	12.0	8.0	251.0
659	**CHERIMOYA,** raw	1 AVG	488	73.5	458.7	6.3	2.0	117.1	10.7	112.2	195.2	—	—	—
			100	73.5	94.0	1.3	.4	24.0	2.2	23.0	40.0	—	—	—
	CHERRIES													
660	sweet, raw	1 CUP	200	80.4	140.0	2.6	.6	34.8	.8	20.0	26.0	4.0	32.4	500.0
			100	80.4	70.0	1.3	.3	17.4	.4	10.0	13.0	2.0	16.2	250.0
661	sweet, canned, light syrup	1 CUP	200	82.0	130.0	1.8	.4	33.0	.6	30.0	26.0	2.0	18.0	256.0
			100	82.0	65.0	.9	.2	16.5	.3	15.0	13.0	1.0	9.0	128.0
662	sweet, canned, heavy syrup	1 CUP	200	77.5	166.0	1.2	.3	42.7	.6	18.0	36.0	6.0	18.0	290.0
			100	77.5	83.0	.6	.2	21.3	.3	9.0	18.0	3.0	9.0	145.0
663	Royal Anne, canned, water pack or artificial sweetener	1 CUP	200	87.1	92.0	1.6	.3	23.5	.4	22.0	30.0	2.0	18.0	262.0
			100	87.1	46.0	.8	.1	11.8	.2	11.0	15.0	1.0	9.0	131.0
664	sour, canned, light syrup	1 CUP	200	80.0	148.0	1.6	.4	37.4	.2	28.0	26.0	2.0	—	252.0
			100	80.2	74.0	.8	.2	18.7	.1	14.0	13.0	1.0	—	126.0
665	sour, canned, heavy syrup	1 CUP	200	76.0	178.0	1.6	.4	45.4	.2	28.0	24.0	2.0	—	248.0
			100	76.0	89.0	.8	.2	22.7	.1	14.0	12.0	1.0	—	124.0
666	candied	1 AVG	4	12.0	13.6	0	0	3.5	Trace	—	—	—	—	—
			100	12.0	339.0	.5	.2	86.7	.5	—	—	—	—	—
667	maraschino, solids & liquid	1 PIECE	8	70.0	9.3	0	0	2.4	Trace	—	—	—	—	—
			100	70.0	116.0	.2	.2	29.4	.3	—	—	—	—	—
668	pie filling, canned	1 OZ	28	71.8	31.4	0	—	7.7	—	2.5	—	—	—	—
			100	71.8	112.0	.1	—	27.4	—	9.0	—	—	—	—
669	**COCONUT**—See Nuts & Seeds													
670	**CRABAPPLES,** raw 1½″ diameter	1 AVG	60	81.1	40.8	.2	.2	10.7	.4	3.6	7.8	.6	—	66.0
			100	81.1	68.0	.4	.3	17.8	.6	6.0	13.0	1.0	—	110.0
	CRANBERRIES													
671	raw	1 CUP	100	87.9	46.0	.4	.7	10.8	1.4	7.0	6.0	2.0	4.5	67.0
			100	87.9	46.0	.4	.7	10.8	1.4	7.0	6.0	2.0	4.5	67.0
672	sauce, homemade, sweetened, whole, unstrained	1 CUP	200	53.9	356.0	.4	.6	91.0	1.4	14.0	10.0	2.0	—	76.0
			100	53.9	178.0	.2	.3	45.5	.7	7.0	5.0	1.0	—	38.0
673	sauce, canned, sweetened, whole	1 CUP	280	61.6	439.6	.6	3.4	101.6	.3	40.0	26.6	79.0	12.6	53.8
			100	61.6	157.0	.2	1.2	36.3	.1	14.3	9.5	28.2	4.5	19.2
	CURRANTS													
674	Black European, raw	1 CUP	132	84.2	71.3	2.2	.1	17.3	3.2	79.2	52.8	4.0	22.6	491.0
			100	84.2	54.0	1.7	.1	13.1	2.4	60.0	40.0	3.0	17.1	372.0
675	red & white, raw	1 CUP	133	85.7	66.5	1.9	.3	16.1	4.5	42.6	30.6	2.7	20.0	341.8
			100	85.7	50.0	1.4	.2	12.1	3.4	32.0	23.0	2.0	15.0	257.0
676	⁶seedless, dried	1 CUP	140	—	394.0	5.8	.4	103.9	2.2	24.4	176.0	9.8	47.6	1262.0
			100	—	283.0	4.1	.3	74.1	1.6	89.0	126.0	7.0	34.0	902.0
677	**CUSTARDAPPLE,** bullocksheart, raw, 3″ diameter	1 AVG	180	71.5	181.8	3.1	1.1	45.4	6.1	48.6	36.0	—	—	—
			100	71.5	101.0	1.7	.6	25.2	3.4	27.0	20.0	—	—	—
678	**DATES,** domestic, natural, dry	1 CUP	178	23.8	482.4	3.5	.9	128.5	4.1	58.7	64.1	1.8	60.5	1185.5
			100	23.8	271.0	1.9	.5	72.2	2.3	33.0	36.0	1.0	34.0	666.0
679	⁵**DURIAN,** civet	1 OZ	28	81.1	18.8	.6	.2	4.1	.4	2.2	10.6	—	—	—
			100	81.1	67.0	2.2	.8	14.8	1.4	8.0	38.0	—	—	—
680	**ELDERBERRIES,** raw	1 CUP	458	79.8	329.8	11.9	2.3	75.1	32.1	174.0	128.2	—	—	1374.0
			100	79.8	72.0	2.6	.5	16.4	7.0	38.0	28.0	—	—	300.0

Item No.	Minerals (Micro)			Fat-Soluble Vitamins			Water-Soluble Vitamins								
	Iron	Zinc	Copper	Vitamin A	Vitamin D	Vitamin E (Alpha Tocopherol)	Vitamin C	Thiamin	Ribo-flavin	Niacin	Panto-thenic Acid	Vit. B-6 (Pyri-doxine)	Folacin (Folic Acid)	Biotin	Vitamin B-12
	(mg)	(mg)	(mg)	(IU)	(IU)	(mg)	(mg)	(mg)	(mg)	(mg)	(mg)	(mg)	(mcg)	(mcg)	(mcg)
649	.58	0	.16	288.0	0	5.00	30.24	.04	.06	.58	.35	.07	19.73	.59	0
	.40	0	.11	200.0	0	3.50	21.00	.03	.04	.40	.24	.05	13.70	.41	0
650	2.34	–	–	390.0	–	–	26.00	.05	.08	.78	.21	.06	36.40	–	–
	.90	–	–	150.0	–	–	10.00	.02	.03	.30	.08	.02	14.00	–	–
651	1.50	–	–	325.0	–	–	17.50	.03	.05	.50	.20	.06	35.00	–	0
	.60	–	–	130.0	–	–	7.00	.01	.02	.20	.08	.02	14.00	–	0
652	1.40	–	.15	140.0	–	–	19.60	.04	.08	.70	.22	.09	8.40	–	0
	1.00	–	.11	100.0	–	–	14.00	.03	.06	.50	.16	.07	6.00	–	0
653	.11	–	–	0	–	–	1.12	Trace	.01	.03	–	–	–	–	–
	.40	–	–	0	–	–	4.00	.01	.03	.10	–	–	–	–	–
654	1.68	–	–	182.0	–	–	9.80	.01	.14	.98	–	–	–	–	–
	1.20	–	–	130.0	–	–	7.00	.01	.10	.70	–	–	–	–	–
655	4.20	–	–	140.0	–	–	101.50	.39	.11	3.15	1.60	–	–	–	0
	1.20	–	–	40.0	–	–	29.00	.11	.03	.90	.46	–	–	–	0
656	3.08	1.08	.11	26180.0	0	1.08	254.10	.40	.26	4.62	1.93	.42	231.00	23.87	0
	.40	.14	.01	3400.0	0	.14	33.00	.05	.03	.60	.25	.06	30.00	3.10	0
657	.86	–	–	684.0	–	–	19.95	.02	.01	.17	–	–	–	–	–
	1.50	–	–	1200.0	–	–	35.00	.04	.02	.30	–	–	–	–	–
658	3.40	–	–	255.0	–	–	110.50	.34	.26	5.10	–	–	–	–	–
	.40	–	–	30.0	–	–	13.00	.04	.03	.60	–	–	–	–	–
659	2.44	–	–	48.8	–	–	43.92	.48	.54	6.34	–	–	–	–	–
	.50	–	–	10.0	–	–	9.00	.10	.11	1.30	–	–	–	–	–
660	.40	0	.27	220.0	–	–	20.00	.10	.12	.80	.52	.06	16.00	–	0
	.20	0	.13	110.0	–	–	10.00	.05	.06	.40	.26	.03	8.00	–	0
661	.60	.22	.12	120.0	–	–	6.00	.04	.04	.40	–	.06	–	–	0
	.30	.11	.06	60.0	–	–	3.00	.02	.02	.20	–	.03	–	–	0
662	.70	.20	.27	304.0	–	–	6.80	.04	.08	.80	–	.06	–	–	0
	.35	.10	.14	152.0	–	–	3.40	.02	.04	.40	–	.03	–	–	0
663	.72	.15	.15	250.0	–	–	4.40	.04	.04	.40	–	–	–	–	–
	.36	.08	.08	125.0	–	–	2.20	.02	.02	.20	–	–	–	–	–
664	.60	–	.10	1320.0	–	–	10.00	.06	.04	.40	.21	.09	16.00	–	0
	.30	–	.05	660.0	–	–	5.00	.03	.02	.20	.11	.04	8.00	–	0
665	.60	–	.10	1300.0	–	–	10.00	.06	.04	.40	.21	.09	16.00	–	0
	.30	–	.05	650.0	–	–	5.00	.03	.02	.20	.11	.04	8.00	–	0
666	–	–	–	8.0	–	–	0	–	–	–	–	–	–	–	–
	–	–	–	200.0	–	–	0	–	–	–	–	–	–	–	–
667	–	–	–	–	–	–	–	–	–	–	–	–	–	–	–
	–	–	–	–	–	–	–	–	–	–	–	–	–	–	–
668	.17	–	–	0	–	–	0	Trace	.01	.03	–	–	–	–	–
	.60	–	–	0	–	–	0	.01	.02	.10	–	–	–	–	–
669															
670	.13	–	–	24.0	–	–	4.80	.02	.01	.06	–	–	–	–	–
	.30	–	–	40.0	–	–	8.00	.03	.02	.10	–	–	–	–	–
671	.20	0	.06	40.0	0	–	11.00	.03	.02	.10	.22	.04	2.00	–	0
	.20	0	.06	40.0	0	–	11.00	.03	.02	.10	.22	.04	2.00	–	0
672	.40	–	–	40.0	–	–	4.00	.03	.04	.20	–	.03	–	–	–
	.20	–	–	20.0	–	–	2.00	.02	.02	.10	–	.01	–	–	–
673	–	–	–	–	–	–	–	–	–	–	–	–	–	–	–
	–	–	–	–	–	–	–	–	–	–	–	–	–	–	–
674	1.45	6.40	(.17)	303.6	0	1.32	264.00	.07	.07	.40	.53	.09	–	(3.00)	0
	1.10	.30	(.13)	230.0	0	1.00	200.00	.05	.05	.30	.40	.07	–	(2.30)	0
675	1.33	–	.15	159.6	0	(.17)	54.53	.05	.07	.13	.09	.05	–	(3.42)	0
	1.00	–	.11	120.0	0	(.13)	41.00	.04	.05	.10	.06	.04	–	(2.57)	0
676	4.54	.93	.66	102.1	–	–	6.44	.22	.20	2.24	–	–	15.40	–	–
	3.24	.66	.47	73.0	–	–	4.60	.16	.14	1.60	–	–	11.00	–	–
677	1.44	.09	–	–	–	–	39.60	.14	.18	.90	.24	–	–	–	0
	.80	.05	–	–	–	–	22.00	.08	.10	.50	.14	–	–	–	0
678	1.85	.52	.50	89.0	0	–	0	.16	.18	3.92	1.39	.35	25.45	–	0
	1.04	.29	.28	50.0	0	–	0	.09	.10	2.20	.78	.20	14.30	–	0
679	.20	–	–	–	–	–	6.72	.10	.06	.20	–	–	–	–	–
	.70	–	–	–	–	–	24.00	.35	.20	.70	–	–	–	–	–
680	7.33	–	–	2748.0	–	–	164.88	.32	.28	.29	.64	1.05	–	–	0
	1.60	–	–	600.0	–	–	36.00	.07	.06	.50	.14	.23	–	–	0

(Continued)

TABLE F-21 *(Continued)*

Item No.	Food Item Name	Approximate Measure	Weight (g)	Moisture (%)	Food Energy Calories (kcal)	Protein (g)	Fats (g)	Carbo-hydrates (g)	Fiber (g)	Minerals (Macro) Calcium (mg)	Phos-phorus (mg)	Sodium (mg)	Mag-nesium (mg)	Potas-sium (mg)
	FIGS													
681	raw	1 MED	41	77.5	32.8	.5	.1	8.3	.5	14.4	5.7	.4	8.2	95.1
			100	77.5	80.0	1.2	.3	20.3	1.2	35.0	14.0	1.0	20.0	232.0
682	canned, light syrup	1 MED	33	82.2	21.5	.2	.1	5.5	.2	4.3	4.3	.7	–	50.2
			100	82.2	65.0	.5	.2	16.8	.7	13.0	13.0	2.0	–	152.0
683	dried, uncooked	1 MED	20	25.8	53.2	.6	.3	13.5	.9	30.4	14.2	2.0	12.2	154.6
			100	25.8	266.0	3.1	1.5	67.5	4.7	152.0	71.0	10.0	61.0	773.0
	FRUIT													
684	cocktail, canned, water pack or artificial sweetener, solids & liquid	1 CUP	256	90.8	81.9	1.1	.1	21.8	1.0	12.8	28.2	10.2	17.9	240.6
			100	90.8	32.0	.4	.1	8.5	.4	5.0	11.0	4.0	7.0	94.0
685	cocktail, canned, light syrup, solids & liquid	1 CUP	256	83.6	153.6	1.0	.3	40.2	1.0	23.0	30.7	12.8	17.9	419.8
			100	83.6	60.0	.4	.1	15.7	.4	9.0	12.0	5.0	7.0	164.0
686	salad, canned, light syrup, solids & liquid	1 CUP	256	83.9	151.0	.8	.3	39.7	1.0	20.5	28.2	2.6	–	348.2
			100	83.9	59.0	.3	.1	15.5	.4	8.0	11.0	1.0	–	136.0
	GOOSEBERRIES													
687	raw	1 CUP	150	88.9	58.5	1.2	.3	14.6	2.8	27.0	22.5	1.5	13.5	232.5
			100	88.9	39.0	.8	.2	9.7	1.9	18.0	15.0	1.0	9.0	155.0
688	canned, heavy syrup	1 CUP	200	76.1	180.0	1.0	.2	46.0	2.4	22.0	18.0	2.0	–	196.0
			100	76.1	90.0	.5	.1	23.0	1.2	11.0	9.0	1.0	–	98.0
689	**GRANADILLA, PURPLE (PASSIONFRUIT)**, pulp & seeds, raw	1 AVG	18	75.1	16.2	.4	.1	3.8	–	2.3	11.5	5.0	5.2	62.6
			100	75.1	90.0	2.2	.7	21.2	–	13.0	64.0	28.0	29.0	348.0
	GRAPEFRUIT													
690	pink-red-white, all varieties	1 WHOLE	482	88.4	197.6	2.4	.5	51.1	1.0	77.1	77.1	4.8	57.8	650.7
			100	88.4	41.0	.5	.1	10.6	.2	16.0	16.0	1.0	12.0	135.0
691	segments, canned, syrup	1 CUP	254	81.1	177.8	1.5	.3	45.2	.5	33.0	35.6	2.5	27.9	342.9
			100	81.1	70.0	.6	.1	17.8	.2	13.0	14.0	1.0	11.0	135.0
	GRAPES													
692	American type, slip skin, raw	1 CUP	153	81.6	105.6	2.0	1.5	24.0	.9	24.5	18.4	4.6	19.9	241.7
			100	81.6	69.0	1.3	1.0	15.7	.6	16.0	12.0	3.0	13.0	158.0
693	European type, adherent skin, raw	1 CUP	153	81.4	102.5	.9	.5	26.5	.8	18.4	30.6	4.6	9.2	264.7
			100	81.4	67.0	.6	.3	17.3	.5	12.0	20.0	3.0	6.0	173.0
694	**'GREENSAPOTE**	1 OZ	28	68.4	30.8	.4	.1	8.0	.5	6.4	7.8	–	–	–
			100	68.4	110.0	1.6	.2	28.6	1.8	23.0	28.0	–	–	–
695	**GROUNDCHERRIES (POHA OR CAPE GOOSE-BERRIES)**, raw	1 CUP	150	85.4	79.5	2.9	1.1	16.8	4.2	13.5	60.0	–	–	–
			100	85.4	53.0	1.9	.7	11.2	2.8	9.0	40.0	–	–	–
	GUAVAS													
696	common, whole, raw	1 MED	100	83.0	62.0	.8	.6	15.0	5.6	23.0	42.0	4.0	13.0	289.0
			100	83.0	62.0	.8	.6	15.0	5.6	23.0	42.0	4.0	13.0	289.0
697	strawberry, whole, raw	1 MED	100	81.8	65.0	1.0	.6	15.8	6.4	23.0	42.0	4.0	–	289.0
			100	81.8	65.0	1.0	.6	15.8	6.4	23.0	42.0	4.0	–	289.0
698	**'HACKBERRY, SPINY**	1 OZ	28	79.5	20.2	.3	.1	5.1	.3	17.6	6.2	–	–	–
			100	79.5	72.0	1.0	.3	18.3	.9	63.0	22.0	–	–	–
699	**HAWS,** scarlet, flesh & skins, raw 1" diameter	1 AVG	35	75.8	30.5	.7	.2	7.3	.7	–	–	–	–	–
			100	75.8	87.0	2.0	.7	20.8	2.1	–	–	–	–	–
700	**HONEYDEW MELON,** vine ripened	1 WHOLE	900	90.6	297.0	7.2	2.7	69.3	5.4	27.0	90.0	108.0	60.3	2259.0
			100	90.6	33.0	.8	.3	7.7	.6	3.0	10.0	12.0	6.7	251.0
701	**INDIANFIG,** 1½″ diameter, 2½″ long	1 AVG	65	81.4	43.6	.7	.3	10.8	.7	37.1	20.8	–	–	–
			100	81.4	67.0	1.1	.4	16.6	1.1	57.0	32.0	–	–	–
702	**JACKFRUIT,** raw, cubed	1 CUP	85	72.0	83.3	1.1	.3	21.6	.9	18.7	32.3	1.7	–	346.0
			100	72.0	98.0	1.3	.3	25.4	1.0	22.0	38.0	2.0	–	407.0
	JUJUBE													
703	**COMMON (CHINESE DATE),** raw	1 MED	20	70.2	21.0	.2	Trace	5.5	.3	5.8	7.4	.6	–	53.8
			100	70.2	105.0	1.2	.2	27.6	1.4	29.0	37.0	3.0	–	269.0
704	**COMMON (CHINESE DATE),** dried	1 AVG	8	19.7	23.0	.3	.1	5.9	.2	6.3	8.0	.2	–	42.5
			100	19.7	287.0	3.7	1.1	73.6	3.0	79.0	100.0	3.0	–	531.0
705	**KUMQUATS,** raw	1 MED	20	81.3	13.0	.2	Trace	3.4	.7	12.6	4.6	1.4	–	47.2
			100	81.3	65.0	.9	.1	17.1	3.7	63.0	23.0	7.0	–	236.0
	LEMONS													
706	pulp w/o peel, raw	1 MED	100	90.1	27.0	1.1	.3	8.2	.4	26.0	16.0	2.0	9.0	138.0
			100	90.1	27.0	1.1	.3	8.2	.4	26.0	16.0	2.0	9.0	138.0
707	peel, candied	1 OZ	28	17.4	88.5	.1	.1	22.6	.6	–	–	–	–	–
			100	17.4	316.0	.4	.3	80.6	2.3	–	–	–	–	–
708	**LIMES,** acid type, raw	1 MED	100	89.3	28.0	.8	.2	9.5	.5	33.0	18.0	2.0	–	102.0
			100	89.3	28.0	.8	.2	9.5	.5	33.0	18.0	2.0	–	102.0
	LOGANBERRIES													
709	raw	1 CUP	150	83.0	93.0	1.5	.9	22.4	4.5	52.5	25.5	1.5	37.5	255.0
			100	83.0	62.0	1.0	.6	14.9	3.0	35.0	17.0	1.0	25.0	170.0
710	canned, light syrup	1 CUP	200	81.4	140.0	1.4	.8	34.4	4.0	46.0	22.0	2.0	22.0	222.0
			100	81.4	70.0	.7	.4	17.2	2.0	23.0	11.0	1.0	11.0	111.0

Item No.	Minerals (Micro)			Fat-Soluble Vitamins			Water-Soluble Vitamins								
	Iron	Zinc	Copper	Vitamin A	Vitamin D	Vitamin E (Alpha Tocopherol)	Vitamin C	Thiamin	Ribo-flavin	Niacin	Panto-thenic Acid	Vit. B-6 (Pyri-doxine)	Folacin (Folic Acid)	Biotin	Vitamin B-12
	(mg)	(mg)	(mg)	(IU)	(IU)	(mg)	(mg)	(mg)	(mg)	(mg)	(mg)	(mg)	(mcg)	(mcg)	(mcg)
681	.16	0	.03	32.8	–	–	.82	.03	.02	.16	.12	.05	5.74	–	0
	.40	0	.07	80.0	–	–	2.00	.06	.05	.40	.30	.11	14.00	–	0
682	.13	–	–	9.9	–	–	.33	.01	.01	.07	.02	–	–	–	0
	.40	–	–	30.0	–	–	1.00	.03	.03	.20	.07	–	–	–	0
683	.41	.10	.06	26.6	0	–	.16	.01	.02	.14	.09	.05	1.80	–	0
	2.06	.50	.28	133.0	0	–	.80	.07	.09	.70	.44	.24	9.00	–	0
684	.64	.22	.16	640.0	–	–	5.38	.05	.03	.92	–	.08	–	–	0
	.25	.09	.06	250.0	–	–	2.10	.02	.01	.36	–	.03	–	–	0
685	1.02	.38	.13	358.4	–	–	5.12	.05	.03	1.28	–	.08	–	–	0
	.40	.15	.05	140.0	–	–	2.00	.02	.01	.50	–	.03	–	–	0
686	.77	–	–	1177.6	–	–	5.12	.03	.08	1.54	–	.08	–	–	0
	.30	–	–	460.0	–	–	2.00	.01	.03	.60	–	.03	–	–	0
687	.75	(.17)	.12	435.0	0	(.59)	49.50	(.06)	(.05)	(.44)	.43	.02	–	(.72)	0
	.50	(.11)	.08	290.0	0	(.39)	33.00	(.04)	(.03)	(.29)	.29	.01	–	(.48)	0
688	.60	[6].20	–	380.0	–	–	20.00	–	–	–	–	–	–	–	–
	.30	.10	–	190.0	–	–	10.00	–	–	–	–	–	–	–	–
689	.29	–	–	126.0	–	–	5.40	–	.02	.27	–	–	–	–	–
	1.60	–	–	700.0	–	–	30.00	–	.13	1.50	–	–	–	–	–
690	1.93	.48	.20	385.6	0	1.21	183.16	.19	.10	.96	1.36	.16	53.02	14.46	0
	.40	.10	.04	80.0	0	.25	38.00	.04	.02	.20	.28	.03	11.00	3.00	0
691	.76	.10	.04	25.4	–	–	76.20	.08	.05	.51	.31	.05	22.86	–	0
	.30	.04	.01	10.0	–	–	30.00	.03	.02	.20	.12	.02	9.00	–	0
692	.61	.06	.05	153.0	–	–	6.12	.14	.09	.46	.12	.19	10.71	2.45	0
	.40	.04	.03	100.0	–	–	4.00	.09	.06	.30	.08	.13	7.00	1.60	0
693	.61	.06	1.45	153.0	–	1.07	6.12	.14	.09	.46	.12	.19	10.71	2.45	0
	.40	.04	.95	100.0	–	.70	4.00	.09	.06	.30	.08	.13	7.00	1.60	0
694	.20	–	–	7.0	–	–	12.04	Trace	.01	.53	–	–	–	–	–
	.70	–	–	25.0	–	–	43.00	.01	.03	1.90	–	–	–	–	–
695	1.50	–	–	1080.0	–	–	16.50	.17	.06	4.20	–	–	–	–	–
	1.00	–	–	720.0	–	–	11.00	.11	.04	2.80	–	–	–	–	–
696	.90	–	–	280.0	–	–	242.00	.05	.05	1.20	.15	–	–	–	0
	.90	–	–	280.0	–	–	242.00	.05	.05	1.20	.15	–	–	–	0
697	.90	–	–	90.0	–	–	37.00	.03	.03	.60	–	–	–	–	–
	.90	–	–	90.0	–	–	37.00	.03	.03	.60	–	–	–	–	–
698	.78	–	–	4.2	–	–	14.28	0	0	.08	–	–	–	–	–
	2.80	–	–	15.0	–	–	51.00	0	0	.30	–	–	–	–	–
699	–	–	–	–	–	–	–	–	–	–	–	–	–	–	–
700	.90	0	.36	360.0	–	–	207.00	.36	.27	5.40	1.86	.50	–	–	0
	.10	0	.04	40.0	–	–	23.00	.04	.03	.60	.21	.06	–	–	0
701	.78	–	–	–	–	–	11.70	.01	.01	.20	–	–	–	–	–
	1.20	–	–	–	–	–	18.00	.01	.02	.30	–	–	–	–	–
702	–	–	–	–	–	–	6.80	.03	–	.34	–	–	–	–	–
	–	–	–	–	–	–	8.00	.03	–	.40	–	–	–	–	–
703	.14	–	–	8.0	–	–	13.80	.00	.01	.18	–	–	–	–	–
	.70	–	–	40.0	–	–	69.00	.02	.04	.90	–	–	–	–	–
704	.14	–	–	3.2	–	–	1.04	.02	.03	.07	–	–	–	–	–
	1.80	–	–	40.0	–	–	13.00	.23	.38	.87	–	–	–	–	–
705	.08	–	–	120.0	–	–	7.20	.02	.02	–	–	–	–	–	–
	.40	–	–	600.0	–	–	36.00	.08	.10	–	–	–	–	–	–
706	.60	–	.26	20.0	–	–	53.00	.04	.02	.10	.19	.08	–	–	0
	.60	–	.26	20.0	–	–	53.00	.04	.02	.10	.19	.08	–	–	0
707	–	–	–	–	–	–	–	–	–	–	–	–	–	–	–
708	.60	–	–	10.0	–	–	37.00	.03	.02	.20	.22	–	4.00	–	0
	.60	–	–	10.0	–	–	37.00	.03	.02	.20	.22	–	4.00	–	0
709	1.80	–	(.21)	300.0	0	(.44)	36.00	.04	.05	.60	(.35)	(.09)	–	–	0
	1.20	–	(.14)	200.0	0	(.29)	24.00	.03	.04	.40	(.23)	(.06)	–	–	0
710	1.60	–	–	260.0	–	–	16.00	.02	.04	.40	–	–	–	–	–
	.80	–	–	130.0	–	–	8.00	.01	.02	.20	–	–	–	–	–

(Continued)

TABLE F-21 *(Continued)*

Item No.	Food Item Name	Approximate Measure	Weight (g)	Moisture (%)	Food Energy Calories (kcal)	Protein (g)	Fats (g)	Carbo-hydrates (g)	Fiber (g)	Minerals (Macro) Calcium (mg)	Phosphorus (mg)	Sodium (mg)	Magnesium (mg)	Potassium (mg)
711	**LONGANS**, raw 1″ diameter	1 AVG	15	82.4	9.2	.2	0	2.4	.1	1.5	6.3	–	–	–
			100	82.4	61.0	1.0	.1	15.8	.4	10.0	42.0	–	–	–
	LOQUATS													
712	raw	1 AVG	12	86.5	5.8	0	0	1.5	.1	2.4	4.3	–	–	41.8
			100	86.5	48.0	.4	.2	12.4	.5	20.0	30.0	–	–	348.0
713	⁴canned, syrup pack	1 OZ	28	76.7	23.5	.1	0	6.4	.1	6.2	.8	–	–	–
			100	76.7	84.0	.3	.1	22.7	.5	22.0	3.0	–	–	–
	LYCHEES													
714	raw	1 AVG	9	81.9	5.8	.1	0	1.5	Trace	.7	3.8	.3	(1.0)	15.3
			100	81.9	64.0	.9	.3	16.4	.3	8.0	42.0	3.0	(9.9)	170.0
715	⁴canned, drained, solids	1 OZ	28	79.7	20.7	.1	.1	5.4	.1	.8	2.8	9.8	–	19.0
			100	79.7	74.0	.3	.4	19.4	.2	3.0	10.0	35.0	–	68.0
716	**MANGOS**, raw	1 WHOLE	200	81.7	132.0	1.4	.8	33.6	1.8	20.0	26.0	14.0	17.6	378.0
			100	81.7	66.0	.7	.4	16.8	.9	10.0	13.0	7.0	8.8	189.0
717	⁴**MANGOSTEEN**, raw	1 OZ	28	84.3	16.0	.1	.1	4.1	1.4	2.8	2.8	.3	–	37.8
			100	84.3	57.0	.5	.3	14.7	5.0	10.0	10.0	1.0	–	135.0
	MELON													
718	CASSABA	1 AVG	874	86.2	445.7	4.4	4.4	109.3	8.7	96.1	96.1	131.1	–	410.8
			100	86.2	51.0	.5	.5	12.5	1.0	11.0	11.0	15.0	–	47.0
719	BALL (CANTALOUPE, HONEYDEW), frozen in syrup	1 CUP	175	83.2	108.5	1.1	.2	27.5	.5	17.5	21.0	15.8	(22.9)	329.0
			100	83.2	62.0	.6	.1	15.7	.3	10.0	12.0	9.0	(13.1)	188.0
720	**MULBERRIES**, ⁴black, raw, pulp and seeds	1 OZ	28	87.9	11.8	.4	.1	2.7	.2	6.7	7.3	8.4	(4.2)	34.4
			100	87.9	42.0	1.4	.3	9.8	.7	24.0	26.0	30.0	(14.9)	123.0
721	**NECTAR, GUAVA**	1 CUP	243	–	–	–	–	–	–	–	–	4.9	–	9.7
			100	–	–	–	–	–	–	–	–	2.0	–	4.0
722	**NECTARINE**, raw	1 MED	50	81.8	32.0	.3	0	8.6	.2	2.0	12.0	3.0	3.1	147.0
			100	81.8	64.0	.6	0	17.1	.4	4.0	24.0	6.0	6.3	294.0
	ORANGES													
723	ALL VARIETIES, w/o peel, raw	1 SM	100	86.0	49.0	.9	.2	12.2	.5	41.0	20.0	1.0	6.7	200.0
			100	86.0	49.0	.9	.2	12.2	.5	41.0	20.0	1.0	6.7	200.0
724	MANDARIN, canned	1 CUP	100	87.0	46.0	.8	.2	11.6	.5	8.0	18.0	2.0	7.0	126.0
			100	87.0	46.0	.8	.2	11.6	.5	8.0	18.0	2.0	7.0	126.0
725	peel, candied	1 OZ	28	17.4	88.5	.1	.1	22.6	–	–	–	–	–	–
			100	17.4	316.0	.4	.3	80.6	–	–	–	–	–	–
726	**PAPAWS**, common North American, raw	1 AVG	98	76.6	83.3	5.1	.9	16.5	–	–	–	–	–	–
			100	76.6	85.0	5.2	.9	16.8	–	–	–	–	–	–
727	**PAPAYAS**, raw	1 MED	300	88.7	117.0	1.8	.3	30.0	2.7	60.0	48.0	9.0	22.8	702.0
			100	88.7	39.0	.6	.1	10.0	.9	20.0	16.0	3.0	7.6	234.0
728	⁴**PASSION FRUIT**, raw	1 OZ	28	–	9.5	.8	Trace	1.7	4.4	4.5	15.1	7.8	10.0	98.3
			100	–	34.0	2.7	Trace	6.1	15.8	16.2	53.8	27.8	38.8	351.1
	PEACHES													
729	raw	1 MED	100	89.1	38.0	.6	.1	9.7	.6	9.0	19.0	1.0	6.6	202.0
			100	89.1	38.0	.6	.1	9.7	.6	9.0	19.0	1.0	6.6	202.0
730	canned, light syrup	1 HALF	50	84.7	28.0	.2	0	7.3	.2	1.5	5.5	2.5	2.5	48.5
			100	84.7	56.0	.5	0	14.5	.3	3.0	11.0	5.0	5.0	97.0
731	dried, sulfured, uncooked	1 CUP	160	32.5	379.2	5.9	1.2	96.8	4.8	44.8	187.2	9.6	68.8	1572.8
			100	32.5	237.0	3.7	.8	60.5	3.0	28.0	117.0	6.0	43.0	983.0
732	frozen, sliced, sweetened	1 CUP	250	74.7	235.0	1.6	.3	60.0	.8	5.0	27.5	15.0	12.5	325.0
			100	74.7	94.0	.6	.1	24.0	.3	2.0	11.0	6.0	5.0	130.0
	PEARS													
733	raw, w/skin	1 AVG	200	83.2	122.0	1.4	.8	30.6	2.8	16.0	22.0	4.0	14.0	260.0
			100	83.2	61.0	.7	.4	15.3	1.4	8.0	11.0	2.0	7.0	130.0
734	⁶raw, peeled	1 MED	182	–	66.4	.5	Trace	17.1	5.1	13.1	27.1	5.3	8.7	184.5
			100	–	36.5	.3	Trace	9.4	2.8	7.2	14.9	2.9	4.8	101.4
735	canned, juice pack	1 HALF	50	86.5	25.0	.2	0	6.5	.2	4.5	6.0	2.0	3.5	48.0
			100	86.5	50.0	.3	.1	12.9	.5	9.0	12.0	4.0	7.0	96.0
736	canned, light syrup	1 HALF	50	84.5	28.5	.1	0	7.6	.3	2.5	3.5	2.5	2.0	32.5
			100	84.5	57.0	.2	0	15.2	.5	5.0	7.0	5.0	4.0	65.0
737	candied	1 OZ	28	21.0	84.8	.4	.2	21.3	–	–	–	–	–	–
			100	21.0	303.0	1.3	.6	75.9	–	–	–	–	–	–
738	dried, sulfured, uncooked	1 CUP	160	26.3	422.4	2.9	1.0	112.4	10.2	51.2	91.2	9.6	52.8	852.8
			100	26.3	264.0	1.8	.6	70.2	6.4	32.0	57.0	6.0	33.0	533.0
739	**PERSIMMONS**, native, raw	1 MED	100	64.4	127.0	.8	.4	33.5	1.5	27.0	26.0	1.0	–	310.0
			100	64.4	127.0	.8	.4	33.5	1.5	27.0	26.0	1.0	–	310.0
	PINEAPPLE													
740	raw	1 CUP	132	85.3	76.6	.4	.3	18.1	.5	22.4	10.6	1.3	17.2	192.7
			100	85.3	58.0	.3	.2	13.7	.4	17.0	8.0	1.0	13.0	146.0
741	canned, water pack	1 SLICE	100	89.1	39.0	.3	.1	10.2	.3	12.0	5.0	1.0	8.0	99.0
			100	89.1	39.0	.3	.1	10.2	.3	12.0	5.0	1.0	8.0	99.0

Item No.	Minerals (Micro)			Fat-Soluble Vitamins			Water-Soluble Vitamins								
	Iron	Zinc	Copper	Vitamin A	Vitamin D	Vitamin E (Alpha Tocopherol)	Vitamin C	Thiamin	Ribo-flavin	Niacin	Panto-thenic Acid	Vit. B-6 (Pyri-doxine)	Folacin (Folic Acid)	Biotin	Vitamin B-12
	(mg)	(mg)	(mg)	(IU)	(IU)	(mg)	(mg)	(mg)	(mg)	(mg)	(mg)	(mg)	(mcg)	(mcg)	(mcg)
711	.18	–	–	–	–	–	.90	–	–	–	–	–	–	–	–
	1.20	–	–	–	–	–	6.00	–	–	–	–	–	–	–	–
712	.05	–	–	80.4	–	–	.12	–	–	–	–	–	–	–	–
	.40	–	–	670.0	–	–	1.00	–	–	–	–	–	–	–	–
713	.01	–	–	56.0	–	–	0	Trace	0	.11	–	–	–	–	–
	.10	–	–	200.0	–	–	0	.01	0	.40	–	–	–	–	–
714	.04	⁶.03	–	–	0	–	3.78	–	.01	–	–	–	–	–	0
	.40	.30	–	–	0	–	42.00	–	.05	–	–	–	–	–	0
715	.22	⁶.06	–	0	–	–	17.36	0	.01	.03	–	–	–	–	–
	.80	.20	–	0	–	–	62.00	0	.05	.10	–	–	–	–	–
716	.80	0	.23	9600.0	0	–	70.00	.10	.10	2.20	.32	–	–	–	0
	.40	0	.12	4800.0	0	–	35.00	.05	.05	1.10	.16	–	–	–	0
717	.14	–	–	0	–	–	1.12	.01	.01	.17	–	–	–	–	–
	.50	–	–	0	–	–	4.00	.03	.02	.60	–	–	–	–	–
718	6.12	–	–	2010.2	–	–	122.36	.18	.35	3.50	.90	–	–	–	0
	.70	–	–	230.0	–	–	14.00	.02	.04	.40	.10	–	–	–	0
719	.53	(.23)	(.05)	2695.0	0	(.23)	28.00	.05	.04	.88	(.39)	(.09)	(51.80)	–	0
	.30	(.13)	(.03)	1540.0	0	(.13)	16.00	.03	.02	.50	(.22)	(.05)	(29.60)	–	0
720	.84	–	(.01)	7.0	0	–	10.92	.01	.02	.20	(.07)	(.02)	–	(.11)	0
	3.00	–	(.05)	25.0	0	–	39.00	.04	.08	.70	(.24)	(.06)	–	(.39)	0
721	–	–	–	–	–	–	–	–	–	–	–	–	–	–	–
	–	–	–	–	–	–	–	–	–	–	–	–	–	–	–
722	.25	.04	.03	825.0	0	–	6.50	(.01)	(.03)	(.55)	(.08)	.01	2.50	–	0
	.50	.08	.06	1650.0	0	–	13.00	(.02)	(.06)	(1.10)	(.16)	.01	5.00	–	0
723	.40	.20	Trace	200.0	0	.23	50.00	.10	.04	.40	.25	.06	46.00	1.90	0
	.40	.20	Trace	200.0	0	.23	50.00	.10	.04	.40	.25	.06	46.00	1.90	0
724	.40	(.24)	.04	420.0	0	Trace	31.00	.06	.02	.10	(.14)	(.03)	(8.03)	(.79)	0
	.40	(.24)	.04	420.0	0	Trace	31.00	.06	.02	.10	(.14)	(.03)	(8.03)	(.79)	0
725	–	–	–	–	–	–	–	–	–	–	–	–	–	–	–
	–	–	–	–	–	–	–	–	–	–	–	–	–	–	–
726	–	–	–	–	–	–	–	–	–	–	–	–	–	–	–
	–	–	–	–	–	–	–	–	–	–	–	–	–	–	–
727	.90	.06	.04	5250.0	–	–	168.00	.12	.12	.90	.65	–	–	–	0
	.30	.02	.01	1750.0	–	–	56.00	.04	.04	.30	.22	–	–	–	0
728	.31	–	.04	4.7	0	–	5.60	Trace	.03	.41	–	–	–	–	0
	1.09	–	.13	16.9	0	–	20.00	Trace	.11	1.48	–	–	–	–	0
729	.50	.20	.07	1330.0	–	–	7.00	.02	.05	1.00	.17	.02	8.00	1.70	0
	.50	.20	.07	1330.0	–	–	7.00	.02	.05	1.00	.17	.02	8.00	1.70	0
730	.18	.04	.03	177.0	–	–	1.20	.01	.01	.30	.03	.01	1.50	.10	0
	.36	.09	.05	354.0	–	–	2.40	.01	.02	.59	.05	.02	3.00	.20	0
731	6.30	.93	.59	3427.2	0	–	8.32	0	.34	6.93	(.05)	.12	(22.37)	–	0
	3.94	.58	.37	2142.0	0	–	5.20	0	.21	4.33	(.03)	.08	(13.98)	–	0
732	.93	.13	.06	710.0	–	–	235.50	.03	.10	1.63	.33	.05	–	–	0
	.37	.05	.02	284.0	–	–	94.20	.01	.04	.65	.13	.02	–	–	0
733	.60	.16	.23	40.0	–	–	8.00	.04	.08	.20	.14	.03	28.00	–	0
	.30	.08	.12	20.0	–	–	4.00	.02	.04	.10	.07	.02	14.00	–	0
734	.40	.15	.18	30.8	0	Trace	5.86	.05	.05	.35	.13	.04	25.48	.20	0
	.22	.08	.10	16.9	0	Trace	3.22	.03	.03	.19	.07	.02	14.00	.11	0
735	.12	.04	.03	0	–	–	.80	.01	.01	.05	.01	.01	–	–	0
	.24	.09	.05	0	–	–	1.60	.01	.01	.10	.02	.01	–	–	0
736	.14	.04	.03	0	–	–	.35	.01	.01	.08	.01	.01	.50	–	0
	.28	.08	.05	0	–	–	.70	.01	.02	.15	.02	.01	1.00	–	0
737	–	–	–	–	–	–	–	–	–	–	–	–	–	–	–
738	3.23	.62	.61	4.8	–	–	11.20	.02	.24	2.21	–	–	–	–	–
	2.02	.39	.38	3.0	–	–	7.00	.01	.15	1.38	–	–	–	–	–
739	2.50	–	–	–	–	–	66.00	–	–	–	–	–	–	–	–
	2.50	–	–	–	–	–	66.00	–	–	–	–	–	–	–	–
740	.66	.28	.19	92.4	0	–	22.44	.12	.04	.26	.21	.12	14.52	Trace	0
	.50	.21	.14	70.0	0	–	17.00	.09	.03	.20	.16	.09	11.00	Trace	0
741	.30	.08	.15	50.0	–	–	7.00	.08	.02	.20	.10	.07	5.00	–	0
	.30	.08	.15	50.0	–	–	7.00	.08	.02	.20	.10	.07	5.00	–	0

(Continued)

TABLE F-21 *(Continued)*

Item No.	Food Item Name	Approximate Measure	Weight (g)	Moisture (%)	Food Energy Calories (kcal)	Protein (g)	Fats (g)	Carbo-hydrates (g)	Fiber (g)	Calcium (mg)	Phos-phorus (mg)	Sodium (mg)	Mag-nesium (mg)	Potas-sium (mg)
	PINEAPPLE (Continued)													
742	canned, juice pack	1 LG	100	83.4	61.0	.4	.1	15.8	.4	20.0	6.0	1.0	14.0	113.0
			100	83.4	61.0	.4	.1	15.8	.4	20.0	6.0	1.0	14.0	113.0
743	canned, light syrup	1 LG	100	83.9	59.0	.3	.1	15.4	.3	11.0	5.0	1.0	8.0	97.0
			100	83.9	59.0	.3	.1	15.4	.3	11.0	5.0	1.0	8.0	97.0
744	candied	1 SLICE	38	18.0	120.1	.3	.2	30.4	.3	–	–	–	–	–
			100	18.0	316.0	.8	.4	80.0	.8	–	–	–	–	–
745	frozen, chunks, sweetened	1 CUP	264	77.1	224.4	1.1	.3	58.6	.8	23.8	10.6	5.3	26.4	264.0
			100	77.1	85.0	.4	.1	22.2	.3	9.0	4.0	2.0	10.0	100.0
746	**PITANGA (SURINAM-CHERRY)**, raw	1 OZ	28	85.8	14.3	.2	.1	3.5	.2	2.5	3.1	–	–	–
			100	85.8	51.0	.8	.4	12.5	.6	9.0	11.0	–	–	–
747	**PLANTAIN (BAKING BANANA)**, green, raw	1 SM	100	66.4	119.0	1.1	.4	31.2	.4	7.0	30.0	5.0	–	385.0
			100	66.4	119.0	1.1	.4	31.2	.4	7.0	30.0	5.0	–	385.0
748	**PLANTAIN**, Maiamaoli, peeled	1 MED	236	67.2	271.4	2.2	.1	72.9	.7	8.7	62.1	–	–	–
			100	67.2	115.0	.9	0	30.9	.3	3.7	26.3	–	–	–
	PLUMS													
749	prune type, raw	1 MED	50	78.7	37.5	.4	.1	9.9	.2	6.0	9.0	.5	4.5	85.0
			100	78.7	75.0	.8	.2	19.7	.4	12.0	18.0	1.0	9.0	170.0
750	Greengage, canned, water pack	1 OZ	28	90.6	9.2	.1	0	2.4	.1	2.5	3.6	.3	–	23.0
			100	90.6	33.0	.4	.1	8.6	.2	9.0	13.0	1.0	–	82.0
751	purple, canned, light syrup	1 MED	50	82.4	31.5	.2	.1	8.3	.2	4.5	5.0	.5	2.5	72.5
			100	82.4	63.0	.4	.1	16.6	.3	9.0	10.0	1.0	5.0	145.0
752	**POMEGRANATE**, pulp, raw	1 MED	100	82.3	63.0	.5	.3	16.4	.2	3.0	8.0	3.0	–	259.0
			100	82.3	63.0	.5	.3	16.4	.2	3.0	8.0	3.0	–	259.0
753	**PRUNES**, dried, softenized, uncooked	1 LG	10	32.4	23.9	.3	.1	6.3	.2	5.1	7.9	.4	4.5	75.4
			100	32.4	239.0	2.6	.5	62.7	2.1	51.0	79.0	4.0	45.0	754.0
754	**PUMPKIN**, canned	1 CUP	250	90.2	82.5	2.5	.8	19.8	3.3	62.5	65.0	5.0	45.0	600.0
			100	90.2	33.0	1.0	.3	7.9	1.3	25.0	26.0	2.0	18.0	240.0
755	**QUINCES**, raw, 2½″ diameter, 3½″ long	1 AVG	155	83.8	88.4	.6	.2	23.7	2.6	17.1	26.4	6.2	(9.8)	305.4
			100	83.8	57.0	.4	.1	15.3	1.7	11.0	17.0	4.0	(6.3)	197.0
756	**RAISINS**, California, Thompson seedless	1 TBLS	10	17.0	28.9	.3	0	7.7	.1	8.6	10.2	1.7	3.5	67.8
			100	17.0	289.0	3.0	.2	77.2	.8	86.0	102.0	17.0	35.0	678.0
757	*RAMBUTAN*, raw	1 OZ	28	82.0	17.9	.3	0	4.6	.3	5.6	4.2	.3	–	17.9
			100	82.0	64.0	1.0	.1	16.5	1.1	20.0	15.0	1.0	–	64.0
	RASPBERRIES													
758	black, raw	1 CUP	123	80.8	89.8	1.8	1.7	19.3	6.3	36.9	27.1	1.2	36.9	244.8
			100	80.8	73.0	1.5	1.4	15.7	5.1	30.0	22.0	1.0	30.0	199.0
759	red, raw	1 CUP	132	84.2	75.2	1.6	.7	18.0	4.0	29.0	29.0	1.3	26.4	221.8
			100	84.2	57.0	1.2	.5	13.6	3.0	22.0	22.0	1.0	20.0	168.0
760	red, frozen, sweetened, not thawed	1 CUP	246	72.6	250.9	1.8	.4	64.3	5.4	39.4	41.8	2.5	32.0	280.4
			100	72.6	102.0	.7	.2	26.1	2.2	16.0	17.0	1.0	13.0	114.0
	RHUBARB													
761	raw	1 CUP	117	94.8	18.7	.7	.1	4.3	.8	112.3	21.1	2.3	13.6	293.7
			100	94.8	16.0	.6	.1	3.7	.7	96.0	18.0	2.0	11.6	251.0
762	cooked w/sugar	1 CUP	266	62.8	375.1	1.3	.3	95.8	1.6	207.5	39.9	5.3	34.6	540.0
			100	62.8	141.0	.5	.1	36.0	.6	78.0	15.0	2.0	13.0	203.0
763	**ROSEAPPLES**, raw, ¾″ diameter	1 AVG	20	84.5	11.2	.1	.1	2.8	.2	5.8	3.2	–	–	–
			100	84.5	56.0	.6	.3	14.2	1.1	29.0	16.0	–	–	–
764	**SAPODILLA**, raw	1 CUP	200	76.1	178.0	1.0	2.2	43.6	2.8	42.0	24.0	24.0	–	386.0
			100	76.1	89.0	.5	1.1	21.8	1.4	21.0	12.0	12.0	–	193.0
765	**SAPOTES (MARMALADE PLUMS)**, raw	1 CUP	200	64.9	250.0	3.6	1.2	63.2	3.8	78.0	56.0	–	–	–
			100	64.9	125.0	1.8	.6	31.6	1.9	39.0	28.0	–	–	–
766	**SOURSOP**, raw, pureed	1 CUP	225	81.7	146.3	2.3	.7	36.7	2.5	31.5	60.8	31.5	–	596.3
			100	81.7	65.0	1.0	.3	16.3	1.1	14.0	27.0	14.0	–	265.0
	STRAWBERRIES													
767	raw	1 CUP	150	89.9	55.5	1.1	.8	12.6	2.0	31.5	31.5	1.5	18.0	246.0
			100	89.9	37.0	.7	.5	8.4	1.3	21.0	21.0	1.0	12.0	164.0
768	frozen, unsweetened	INDV	10	90.0	3.5	0	0	.9	.1	1.6	1.3	.2	1.1	14.8
			100	90.0	35.0	.4	.1	9.1	.8	16.0	13.0	2.0	11.0	148.0
769	frozen, sweetened, sliced	1 CUP	256	74.6	243.2	1.4	.3	62.8	1.6	28.2	30.7	5.1	17.9	250.9
			100	74.6	95.0	.5	.1	24.5	.6	11.0	12.0	2.0	7.0	98.0
770	**SUGARAPPLES (SWEETSOP)**, raw	1 CUP	250	73.3	235.0	4.5	.8	59.3	4.3	55.0	102.5	27.5	–	687.5
			100	73.3	94.0	1.8	.3	23.7	1.7	22.0	41.0	11.0	–	275.0
771	**TAMARINDS**, raw	1 OZ	28	31.4	92.7	5.3	.2	17.5	1.4	20.7	31.6	14.3	–	218.7
			100	31.4	331.0	18.8	.6	62.5	5.1	74.0	113.0	51.0	–	781.0
772	**TANGELOS**, raw	1 MED	170	89.4	39.0	.5	.1	9.2	–	27.2	20.4	1.7	19.0	295.8
			100	89.4	22.9	.3	.1	5.4	–	16.0	12.0	1.0	11.2	174.0

Item No.	Minerals (Micro)			Fat-Soluble Vitamins			Water-Soluble Vitamins								
	Iron	Zinc	Copper	Vitamin A	Vitamin D	Vitamin E (Alpha Tocopherol)	Vitamin C	Thiamin	Riboflavin	Niacin	Pantothenic Acid	Vit. B-6 (Pyridoxine)	Folacin (Folic Acid)	Biotin	Vitamin B-12
	(mg)	(mg)	(mg)	(IU)	(IU)	(mg)	(mg)	(mg)	(mg)	(mg)	(mg)	(mg)	(mcg)	(mcg)	(mcg)
742	.30	.11	.11	27.0	–	–	8.80	.10	.02	.34	.10	.07	.80	–	0
	.30	.11	.11	27.0	–	–	8.80	.10	.02	.34	.10	.07	.80	–	0
743	.30	.08	.15	50.0	–	–	7.00	.08	.02	.20	.10	.07	5.00	–	0
	.30	.08	.15	50.0	–	–	7.00	.08	.02	.20	.10	.07	5.00	–	0
744	–	–	–	–	–	–	–	–	–	–	–	–	–	–	–
	–	–	–	–	–	–	–	–	–	–	–	–	–	–	–
745	1.06	–	–	79.2	–	–	21.12	.26	.08	.79	.28	.20	15.84	–	0
	.40	–	–	30.0	–	–	8.00	.10	.03	.30	.11	.08	6.00	–	0
746	.06	–	–	420.0	–	–	8.40	.01	.01	.08	–	–	–	–	–
	.20	–	–	1500.0	–	–	30.00	.03	.04	.30	–	–	–	–	–
747	.70	–	–	605.0	–	–	14.00	.06	.04	.60	.37	–	16.00	–	0
	.70	–	–	605.0	–	–	14.00	.06	.04	.60	.37	–	16.00	–	0
748	1.06	–	–	915.7	–	–	35.87	.13	.28	1.53	–	–	–	–	–
	.45	–	–	388.0	–	–	15.20	.05	.12	.65	–	–	–	–	–
749	.25	–	–	150.0	–	–	2.00	.02	.02	.25	.09	.04	3.00	–	0
	.50	–	–	300.0	–	–	4.00	.03	.03	.50	.19	.05	6.00	–	0
750	.06	–	–	44.8	–	–	.56	Trace	.01	.08	.02	.01	–	–	0
	.20	–	–	160.0	–	–	2.00	.01	.02	.30	.07	.03	–	–	0
751	.45	–	–	615.0	–	–	1.00	.01	.01	.20	.04	.01	1.50	–	0
	.90	–	–	1230.0	–	–	2.00	.02	.02	.40	.07	.02	3.00	–	0
752	.30	–	–	–	–	–	4.00	.03	.03	.30	.60	–	–	–	0
	.30	–	–	–	–	–	4.00	.03	.03	.30	.60	–	–	–	0
753	.25	.05	.04	199.4	0	–	.33	.01	.02	.19	.05	.03	.40	Trace	0
	2.47	.53	.44	1994.0	0	–	3.30	.08	.22	1.94	.46	.29	4.00	Trace	0
754	1.00	.48	.14	16000.0	–	–	12.50	.08	.13	1.50	1.00	.14	37.50	–	0
	.40	.19	.05	6400.0	–	–	5.00	.03	.05	.60	.40	.06	15.00	–	0
755	1.09	–	(.20)	62.0	0	–	23.25	.03	.05	.31	–	–	–	–	0
	.70	–	(.13)	40.0	0	–	15.00	.02	.03	.20	–	–	–	–	0
756	.21	.02	.04	2.0	0	–	.09	.01	Trace	.06	.01	.02	.40	.45	0
	2.10	.22	.38	20.0	0	–	.88	.10	.03	.60	.06	.23	4.00	4.50	0
757	.53	–	–	0	–	–	14.84	Trace	.02	.11	–	–	–	–	–
	1.90	–	–	0	–	–	53.00	.01	.06	.40	–	–	–	–	–
758	1.11	–	.16	–	–	–	22.14	.04	.11	1.11	.30	.07	6.15	–	0
	.90	–	.13	–	–	–	18.00	.03	.09	.90	.24	.06	5.00	–	0
759	1.19	0	.08	171.6	0	(.41)	33.00	.04	.12	1.19	.32	.08	6.60	(2.52)	0
	.90	0	.06	130.0	0	(.31)	25.00	.03	.09	.90	.24	.06	5.00	(1.91)	0
760	1.72	.44	.26	130.4	–	–	37.15	.05	.10	.54	.37	.08	63.96	–	0
	.70	.18	.11	53.0	–	–	15.10	.02	.04	.22	.15	.03	26.00	–	0
761	.94	0	.01	117.0	0	(.27)	10.53	.04	.08	.35	.10	.04	8.19	–	0
	.80	0	.01	100.0	0	(.23)	9.00	.03	.07	.30	.09	.03	7.00	–	0
762	1.60	.29	–	212.8	–	–	–	–	–	–	–	–	–	–	–
	.60	.11	–	80.0	–	–	–	–	–	–	–	–	–	–	–
763	.24	–	–	26.0	–	–	4.40	Trace	.01	.16	–	–	–	–	–
	1.20	–	–	130.0	–	–	22.00	.02	.03	.80	–	–	–	–	–
764	1.60	–	–	120.0	–	–	28.00	–	.04	.40	.50	–	–	–	0
	.80	–	–	60.0	–	–	14.00	–	.02	.20	.25	–	–	–	0
765	2.00	–	–	820.0	–	–	–	–	–	–	–	–	–	–	–
	1.00	–	–	410.0	–	–	–	–	–	–	–	–	–	–	–
766	1.35	–	–	22.5	–	–	45.00	.16	.11	2.03	.57	–	–	–	0
	.60	–	–	10.0	–	–	20.00	.07	.05	.90	.25	–	–	–	0
767	1.50	0	.04	90.0	0	.20	88.50	.05	.11	.90	.51	.08	24.00	6.00	0
	1.00	0	.02	60.0	0	.13	59.00	.03	.07	.60	.34	.06	16.00	4.00	0
768	.08	–	–	4.5	–	–	4.12	.00	Trace	.05	–	–	1.70	–	–
	.75	–	–	45.0	–	–	41.20	.02	.04	.46	–	–	17.00	–	–
769	1.41	.14	.05	66.6	–	.54	98.30	.05	.15	.97	.28	.07	43.52	10.24	0
	.55	.06	.02	26.0	–	.21	38.40	.02	.06	.38	.11	.03	17.00	4.00	0
770	1.50	–	–	25.0	–	–	85.00	.25	.35	2.50	.57	–	–	–	0
	.60	–	–	10.0	–	–	34.00	.10	.14	1.00	.23	–	–	–	0
771	.78	–	–	8.4	–	–	.56	.10	.04	.34	.04	–	–	–	0
	2.80	–	–	30.0	–	–	2.00	.34	.14	1.20	.14	–	–	–	0
772	.17	0	.06	–	–	–	26.00	–	–	–	–	.09	23.80	–	0
	.10	0	.03	–	–	–	15.29	–	–	–	–	.05	14.00	–	0

(Continued)

TABLE F-21 (Continued)

Item No.	Food Item Name	Approximate Measure	Weight (g)	Moisture (%)	Food Energy Calories (kcal)	Protein (g)	Fats (g)	Carbo-hydrates (g)	Fiber (g)	Calcium (mg)	Phos-phorus (mg)	Sodium (mg)	Mag-nesium (mg)	Potas-sium (mg)
773	TANGERINES, Dancy, raw	1 MED	116	87.0	53.4	.9	.2	13.5	.6	19.7	11.6	2.3	14.3	187.9
			100	87.0	46.0	.8	.2	11.6	.5	17.0	10.0	2.0	12.3	162.0
774	TOMATO—See **VEGETABLES**													
775	TOWELGOURD, raw, cubed	1 CUP	130	94.5	23.4	1.0	.3	5.3	.7	24.7	42.9	–	–	–
			100	94.5	18.0	.8	.2	4.1	.5	19.0	33.0	–	–	–
776	WATERMELON, raw	1 CUP	200	92.6	52.0	1.0	.4	12.8	.6	14.0	20.0	2.0	20.4	200.0
			100	92.6	26.0	.5	.2	6.4	.3	7.0	10.0	1.0	10.2	100.0
777	WAXGOURD (CHINESE PRESERVING MELON), raw, cubed	1 CUP	160	96.1	20.8	.6	.3	4.8	.8	30.4	30.4	9.6	–	177.6
			100	96.1	13.0	.4	.2	3.0	.5	19.0	19.0	6.0	–	111.0
778	⁴WAXGOURD, sugared	1 OZ	28	20.1	79.8	.1	.1	22.2	.1	26.0	4.8	–	–	–
			100	20.1	285.0	.2	.2	79.2	.2	93.0	17.0	–	–	–
	GRAVIES AND SAUCES													
779	GRAVY, BEEF	1 TBLS	18	–	41.0	.3	3.5	2.0	0	0	2.0	–	–	–
			100	–	228.0	1.7	19.4	11.1	0	0	11.0	–	–	–
780	GRAVY, CHICKEN	1 OZ	28	–	63.8	.5	5.4	3.1	0	0	3.1	55.5	.6	2.0
			100	–	228.0	1.7	19.4	11.1	0	0	11.0	198.3	2.1	7.1
	SAUCE													
781	BARBECUE	1 TBLS	16	80.9	14.6	.2	1.1	1.3	.1	3.4	3.2	130.4	–	27.8
			100	80.9	91.0	1.5	6.9	8.0	.6	21.0	20.0	815.0	–	174.0
782	CHEESE	1 TBLS	19	–	34.0	1.5	2.6	1.2	–	44.1	32.5	–	–	–
			100	–	179.0	7.9	13.6	6.3	–	232.0	171.0	–	–	–
783	HARD, medium	1 TBLS	10	–	46.2	0	2.7	5.7	–	.9	.5	–	–	–
			100	–	462.0	.5	27.1	57.1	–	9.0	5.0	–	–	–
784	HOLLANDAISE, true	1 TBLS	13	–	46.8	.6	4.8	.1	–	6.0	20.3	–	–	–
			100	–	360.0	4.4	37.0	.8	–	46.0	156.0	–	–	–
785	WHITE, medium, made w/butter	1 TBLS	15	73.3	24.3	.6	1.9	1.3	–	17.3	14.0	56.9	–	20.9
			100	73.3	162.0	3.9	12.5	8.8	–	115.0	93.0	379.0	–	139.0
786	TARTAR	1 TBLS	20	34.4	106.2	.3	11.6	.8	.1	3.6	6.4	141.4	–	15.6
			100	34.4	531.0	1.4	57.8	4.2	.3	18.0	32.0	707.0	–	78.0
	JUICES													
787	ACEROLA JUICE, raw	100 CC	100	94.3	23.0	.4	.3	4.8	.3	10.0	9.0	3.0	–	–
			100	94.3	23.0	.4	.3	4.8	.3	10.0	9.0	3.0	–	–
788	APPLE, cider	1 CUP	249	–	124.5	.2	0	34.3	0	14.9	27.4	10.0	–	249.0
			100	–	50.0	.1	0	13.8	0	6.0	11.0	4.0	–	100.0
789	APRICOT JUICE, unsweetened	1 CUP	250	–	122.5	1.0	.3	29.3	–	–	–	7.5	–	–
			100	–	49.0	.4	.1	11.7	–	–	–	3.0	–	–
790	APRICOT NECTAR, w/vitamin C added	1 CUP	247	84.6	140.8	.7	.2	36.1	.5	22.2	29.6	–	12.4	373.0
			100	84.6	57.0	.3	.1	14.6	.2	9.0	12.0	–	5.0	151.0
791	BLACKBERRY JUICE, canned, unsweetened	1 CUP	250	90.9	92.5	.8	1.5	19.5	–	30.0	30.0	2.5	52.5	.425.0
			100	90.9	37.0	.3	.6	7.8	–	12.0	12.0	1.0	21.0	170.0
792	CRANBERRY JUICE COCKTAIL, (33% cranberry juice)	1 CUP	250	83.2	162.5	.3	.3	41.3	–	12.5	7.5	2.5	–	25.0
			100	83.2	65.0	.1	.1	16.5	–	5.0	3.0	1.0	–	10.0
	GRAPE JUICE													
793	canned, or bottled	1 CUP	250	82.9	165.0	.5	0	41.5	–	27.5	30.0	5.0	30.0	290.0
			100	82.9	66.0	.2	0	16.6	–	11.0	12.0	2.0	12.0	116.0
794	frozen concentrate, sweetened, diluted	1 CUP	250	86.4	132.5	.5	0	33.3	–	7.5	10.0	2.5	10.0	85.0
			100	86.4	53.0	.2	0	13.3	–	3.0	4.0	1.0	4.0	34.0
	GRAPEFRUIT JUICE													
795	fresh, pink-red-white, all varieties	1 CUP	250	90.0	97.5	1.3	.3	23.0	–	22.5	37.5	2.5	30.0	405.0
			100	90.0	39.0	.5	.1	9.2	–	9.0	15.0	1.0	12.0	162.0
796	canned, unsweetened	1 CUP	247	89.2	101.3	1.2	.2	24.2	–	19.8	34.6	2.5	29.6	400.1
			100	89.2	41.0	.5	.1	9.8	–	8.0	14.0	1.0	12.0	162.0
797	frozen, unsweetened, diluted w/3 parts water	1 CUP	250	89.3	102.5	1.3	.3	24.5	–	25.0	42.5	2.5	22.5	425.0
			100	89.3	41.0	.5	.1	9.8	–	10.0	17.0	1.0	9.0	170.0
798	LEMON JUICE, raw	1 TBLS	15	91.0	3.8	.1	0	1.2	–	1.1	1.5	.2	1.2	21.2
			100	91.0	25.0	.5	.2	8.0	–	7.0	10.0	1.0	8.0	141.0
799	LEMONADE, concentrate, frozen, diluted w/4⅓ parts water	1 CUP	250	88.5	110.0	.3	0	28.5	0	2.5	2.5	–	2.5	40.0
			100	88.5	44.0	.1	0	11.4	0	1.0	1.0	–	1.0	16.0
	LIME JUICE													
800	fresh	1 TBLS	15	90.3	3.9	0	0	1.4	–	1.4	1.7	.2	.8	15.6
			100	90.3	26.0	.3	.1	9.0	–	9.0	11.0	1.0	5.4	104.0
801	canned or bottled, unsweetened	1 TBLS	15	90.3	3.9	0	0	1.4	–	1.4	1.7	.2	–	15.6
			100	90.3	26.0	.3	.1	9.0	–	9.0	11.0	1.0	–	104.0
802	LIMEADE, concentrate, frozen, diluted w/4⅓ parts water	1 CUP	250	88.9	102.5	0	0	27.5	–	2.5	2.5	–	–	32.5
			100	88.9	41.0	0	0	11.0	–	1.0	1.0	–	–	13.0

Item No.	Minerals (Micro)			Fat-Soluble Vitamins			Water-Soluble Vitamins								
	Iron	Zinc	Copper	Vitamin A	Vitamin D	Vitamin E (Alpha Tocopherol)	Vitamin C	Thiamin	Ribo-flavin	Niacin	Panto-thenic Acid	Vit. B-6 (Pyri-doxine)	Folacin (Folic Acid)	Biotin	Vitamin B-12
	(mg)	(mg)	(mg)	(IU)	(IU)	(mg)	(mg)	(mg)	(mg)	(mg)	(mg)	(mg)	(mcg)	(mcg)	(mcg)
773	.46	.17	.03	487.2	0	–	35.96	.07	.02	.12	.23	.08	24.36	–	0
	.40	.15	.03	420.0	0	–	31.00	.06	.02	.10	.20	.07	21.00	–	0
774															
775	1.17	–	–	494.0	–	–	10.40	.04	.05	.52	–	–	–	–	–
	.90	–	–	380.0	–	–	8.00	.03	.04	.40	–	–	–	–	–
776	1.00	.18	.03	1180.0	–	–	14.00	.06	.06	.40	.60	.14	16.00	7.20	0
	.50	.09	.02	590.0	–	–	7.00	.03	.03	.20	.30	.07	8.00	3.60	0
777	.64	–	–	0	–	–	20.80	.06	.18	.64	–	–	–	–	–
	.40	–	–	0	–	–	13.00	.04	.11	.40	–	–	–	–	–
778	.95	–	–	0	–	–	0	0	0	0	–	–	–	–	–
	3.40	–	–	0	–	–	0	0	0	0	–	–	–	–	–
779	.09	–	–	0	0	–	–	.01	.01	0	–	–	–	–	–
	.50	–	–	0	0	–	–	.05	.04	0	–	–	–	–	–
780	.14	.02	1.50	43.0	0	–	.01	.01	.18	.05	.01	Trace	.35	–	0
	.50	.06	5.36	153.7	0	–	.02	.02	.64	.18	.02	Trace	1.23	–	0
781	.13	.02	–	57.6	–	–	.80	Trace	Trace	.05	–	–	.64	–	–
	.80	.13	–	360.0	–	–	5.00	.01	.01	.30	–	–	4.00	–	–
782	.06	–	–	103.0	–	–	–	.01	.04	.05	–	–	–	–	–
	.30	–	–	542.0	–	–	–	.03	.21	.26	–	–	–	–	–
783	0	–	–	110.0	–	–	0	0	0	0	–	–	–	–	–
	0	–	–	1100.0	–	–	0	0	0	0	–	–	–	–	–
784	.23	–	–	267.0	–	–	–	.01	.01	–	–	–	–	–	–
	1.80	–	–	2054.0	–	–	–	.05	.08	–	–	–	–	–	–
785	.03	–	–	69.0	–	–	.06	.01	.03	.03	–	–	–	–	–
	.20	–	–	460.0	–	–	.40	.04	.17	.20	–	–	–	–	–
786	.18	.20	.02	44.0	–	–	.20	Trace	.01	–	–	–	–	–	–
	.90	.98	.12	220.0	–	–	1.00	.01	.03	–	–	–	–	–	–
787	.50	–	–	–	–	–	1600.00	.02	.06	.40	.21	.01	–	–	0
	.50	–	–	–	–	–	1600.00	.02	.06	.40	.21	.01	–	–	0
788	1.25	.08	–	99.6	0	–	2.74	.05	.08	0	–	–	–	–	–
	.50	.03	–	40.0	0	–	1.10	.02	.03	0	–	–	–	–	–
789	–	–	–	–	–	–	–	–	–	–	–	–	5.00	–	–
	–	–	–	–	–	–	–	–	–	–	–	–	2.00	–	–
790	.50	.20	.37	2364.5	–	–	103.74	.03	.03	.50	–	.07	4.94	–	0
	.20	.08	.15	950.0	–	–	42.00	.01	.01	.20	–	.03	2.00	–	0
791	2.25	–	–	–	–	–	25.00	.05	.08	.75	.20	–	–	–	0
	.90	–	–	–	–	–	10.00	.02	.03	.30	.08	–	–	–	0
792	.75	–	–	–	–	–	–	.03	.03	–	–	–	–	–	–
	.30	–	–	–	–	–	–	.01	.01	–	–	–	–	–	–
793	.75	.28	.43	0	–	–	0	.10	.05	.50	.20	.20	5.00	–	0
	.30	.11	.17	0	–	–	0	.04	.02	.20	.08	.08	2.00	–	0
794	.25	.28	.43	–	–	–	10.00	.05	.08	.50	.10	.05	5.00	.75	0
	.10	.11	.17	–	–	–	4.00	.02	.03	.20	.04	.02	2.00	.30	0
795	.50	.25	–	200.0	–	–	95.00	.10	.05	.50	.71	.09	52.50	1.75	0
	.20	.10	–	80.0	–	–	38.00	.04	.02	.20	.28	.04	21.00	.70	0
796	.99	.25	.02	24.7	–	.10	83.98	.07	.04	.50	.32	.03	2.97	1.98	0
	.40	.10	.01	10.0	–	.04	34.00	.03	.02	.20	.13	.01	1.20	.80	0
797	.25	.25	–	25.0	–	–	97.50	.10	.05	.50	.41	.04	52.50	1.75	0
	.10	.10	–	10.0	–	–	39.00	.04	.02	.20	.16	.02	21.00	.70	0
798	.03	0	.01	3.0	–	–	6.90	.01	Trace	.02	.02	.01	.15	–	0
	.20	0	.03	20.0	–	–	46.00	.03	.01	.10	.10	.05	1.00	–	0
799	–	–	–	0	0	–	17.50	.03	.03	.25	.03	.01	12.50	–	0
	–	–	–	0	0	–	7.00	.01	.01	.10	.01	.01	5.00	–	0
800	.03	0	.01	1.5	–	–	4.80	Trace	Trace	.02	.02	.01	–	–	0
	.20	0	.03	10.0	–	–	32.00	.02	.01	.10	.14	.04	–	–	0
801	.03	–	–	1.5	–	–	3.15	Trace	Trace	.02	–	–	1.95	–	–
	.20	–	–	10.0	–	–	21.00	.02	.01	.10	–	–	13.00	–	–
802	–	–	–	–	–	–	5.00	–	–	–	–	–	–	–	–
	–	–	–	–	–	–	2.00	–	–	–	–	–	–	–	–

(Continued)

TABLE F-21 *(Continued)*

Item No.	Food Item Name	Approximate Measure	Weight (g)	Moisture (%)	Food Energy Calories (kcal)	Protein (g)	Fats (g)	Carbo-hydrates (g)	Fiber (g)	Minerals (Macro) Calcium (mg)	Phos-phorus (mg)	Sodium (mg)	Mag-nesium (mg)	Potas-sium (mg)
	ORANGE JUICE													
803	fresh, all varieties	1 CUP	250	88.3	112.5	1.8	.5	26.0	.3	27.5	42.5	2.5	27.0	500.0
			100	88.3	45.0	.7	.2	10.4	.1	11.0	17.0	1.0	10.8	200.0
804	canned concentrate, unsweetened, diluted w/5 parts water	1 CUP	250	88.2	115.0	2.0	.8	25.8	.3	25.0	45.0	2.5	30.0	480.0
			100	88.2	46.0	.8	.3	10.3	.1	10.0	18.0	1.0	12.0	192.0
805	frozen concentrate, unsweetened, diluted w/3 parts water	1 CUP	250	88.1	112.5	1.8	.3	26.8	—	22.5	40.0	2.5	20.5	465.0
			100	88.1	45.0	.7	.1	10.7	—	9.0	16.0	1.0	8.2	186.0
806	**PAPAYA JUICE,** canned	1 CUP	250	—	120.0	1.0	0	30.2	—	45.0	25.0	—	—	—
			100	—	48.0	.4	0	12.1	—	18.0	10.0	—	—	—
807	**PEACH NECTAR,** canned, 40% fruit	1 CUP	250	87.2	120.0	.5	0	31.0	.3	10.0	27.5	2.5	—	195.0
			100	87.2	48.0	.2	0	12.4	.1	4.0	11.0	1.0	—	78.0
808	**PEAR NECTAR,** canned, 40% fruit	1 CUP	250	86.2	130.0	.8	.5	33.0	.8	7.5	12.5	2.5	—	97.5
			100	86.2	52.0	.3	.2	13.2	.3	3.0	5.0	1.0	—	39.0
809	**PINEAPPLE JUICE,** canned, unsweetened	1 CUP	250	85.6	137.5	1.0	.3	33.8	.3	37.5	22.5	2.5	30.0	372.5
			100	85.6	55.0	.4	.1	13.5	.1	15.0	9.0	1.0	12.0	149.0
810	**PRUNE JUICE,** canned or bottled	1 CUP	250	80.0	192.5	1.0	.3	47.5	—	35.0	50.0	5.0	14.5	587.5
			100	80.0	77.0	.4	.1	19.0	—	14.0	20.0	2.0	5.8	235.0
811	**SAUERKRAUT JUICE,** canned	1 CUP	240	94.6	24.0	1.7	—	5.5	—	88.8	33.6	1888.8	—	—
			100	94.6	10.0	.7	—	2.3	—	37.0	14.0	787.0	—	—
812	**TANGELO JUICE,** raw	1 CUP	250	89.4	102.5	1.3	.3	24.3	—	—	—	—	—	—
			100	89.4	41.0	.5	.1	9.7	—	—	—	—	—	—
	TANGERINE JUICE													
813	raw	1 CUP	250	88.9	107.5	1.3	.5	25.3	.3	45.0	35.0	2.5	—	445.0
			100	88.9	43.0	.5	.2	10.1	.1	18.0	14.0	1.0	—	178.0
814	frozen concentrate, unsweetened, diluted w/3 parts water	1 CUP	250	88.1	115.0	1.3	.5	27.0	.3	45.0	35.0	2.5	—	435.0
			100	88.1	46.0	.5	.2	10.8	.1	18.0	14.0	1.0	—	174.0
	TOMATO JUICE													
815	canned or bottled	1 CUP	200	93.5	38.0	1.5	.1	8.7	.4	18.4	34.6	400.0	20.2	454.0
			100	93.5	19.0	.8	.1	4.4	.2	9.2	17.3	200.0	10.1	227.0
816	canned concentrate, diluted w/3 parts	1 CUP	200	93.4	40.0	1.8	.2	9.0	.4	14.0	38.0	418.0	20.0	470.0
			100	93.4	20.0	.9	.1	4.5	.2	7.0	19.0	209.0	10.0	235.0
817	**VEGETABLE JUICE COCKTAIL,** canned	1 CUP	200	94.1	34.0	1.8	.2	7.2	.6	24.0	44.0	400.0	—	442.0
			100	94.1	17.0	.9	.1	3.6	.3	12.0	22.0	200.0	—	221.0
	LEGUMES AND PRODUCTS													
818	**ADZUKI BEAN,** ᵇboiled, sweetened	1 OZ	28	45.3	61.0	.8	0	14.2	.2	7.3	18.5	—	—	—
			100	45.3	218.0	3.0	.1	50.7	.6	26.0	66.0	—	—	—
	BEANS, COMMON, DRY													
819	baked, w/o pork	1 CUP	300	68.5	360.0	18.9	1.5	69.0	4.2	204.0	363.0	1014.0	111.0	804.0
			100	68.5	120.0	6.3	.5	23.0	1.4	68.0	121.0	338.0	37.0	268.0
820	w/tomato sauce, canned	1 CUP	250	68.5	300.0	15.8	1.3	57.5	3.5	170.0	302.5	845.0	182.5	670.0
			100	68.5	120.0	6.3	.5	23.0	1.4	68.0	121.0	338.0	73.0	268.0
821	**BEANS, LIMA,** mature seeds, dry, cooked	1 CUP	169	64.1	233.2	13.9	1.0	43.3	2.9	49.0	260.3	3.4	—	1034.3
			100	64.1	133.0	8.2	.6	25.6	1.7	29.0	154.0	2.0	—	612.0
822	**BROAD BEAN,** ᵇwhole seeds, dried	1 OZ	28	13.8	91.8	7.0	.3	15.9	1.4	29.1	111.2	2.2	—	314.4
			100	13.8	328.0	25.0	1.2	56.9	5.1	104.0	397.0	8.0	—	1123.0
823	**GARBANZOS or CHICK PEAS,** dry, cooked or canned	1 CUP	140	—	250.6	14.3	3.4	42.4	—	105.0	231.0	—	75.6	—
			100	—	179.0	10.2	2.4	30.3	—	75.0	165.0	—	54.0	—
824	**COWPEAS,** mature seeds, dry, cooked, unsalted	1 CUP	250	80.0	190.0	12.8	.8	34.5	2.5	42.5	237.5	20.0	—	572.5
			100	80.0	76.0	5.1	.3	13.8	1.0	17.0	95.0	8.0	—	229.0
825	**HYACINTH BEANS,** raw, mature seeds, dry	1 CUP	184	11.8	621.9	40.8	2.8	112.2	12.7	134.3	769.1	—	—	—
			100	11.8	338.0	22.2	1.5	61.0	6.9	73.0	418.0	—	—	—
826	ᵇ**JACKBEAN,** whole seed, dried	1 OZ	28	11.2	97.4	5.9	.9	17.1	2.1	37.5	84.0	9.8	—	210.0
			100	11.2	348.0	21.0	3.2	61.0	7.6	134.0	300.0	35.0	—	750.0
827	**LENTILS,** dry, whole, cooked	1 CUP	150	72.0	159.0	11.7	(.6)	29.0	1.8	37.5	178.5	(18.9)	(38.1)	373.5
			100	72.0	106.0	7.8	(.4)	19.3	1.2	25.0	119.0	(12.6)	(25.4)	249.0
828	**PEAS,** mature seeds, dry, split, w/o seed coat, cooked	1 CUP	200	70.0	230.0	16.0	.6	41.6	.8	22.0	178.0	26.0	—	592.0
			100	70.0	115.0	8.0	.3	20.8	.4	11.0	89.0	13.0	—	296.0
829	**PIGEON PEAS,** mature seeds, dry, raw	1 OZ	28	10.8	95.8	5.7	.4	17.8	2.0	30.0	88.5	7.3	33.9	274.7
			100	10.8	342.0	20.4	1.4	63.7	7.0	107.0	316.0	26.0	121.0	981.0
	SOYBEANS													
830	**MILK—**see MILK & PRODUCTS													
831	mature seeds, dry, cooked	1 CUP	180	71.0	234.0	19.8	10.3	19.4	2.9	131.4	322.2	3.6	—	972.0
			100	71.0	130.0	11.0	5.7	10.8	1.6	73.0	179.0	2.0	—	540.0
832	**MISO, FERMENTED,** cereal & soybeans	1 OZ	28	53.0	47.9	2.9	1.3	6.6	.6	19.0	86.5	826.0	—	93.5
			100	53.0	171.0	10.5	4.6	23.5	2.3	68.0	309.0	2950.0	—	334.0
833	**NATTO, FERMENTED,** soybeans	1 OZ	28	62.7	46.8	4.7	2.1	3.2	.9	28.8	51.0	—	—	69.7
			100	62.7	167.0	16.9	7.4	11.5	3.2	103.0	182.0	—	—	249.0
834	**PROTEIN**	1 OZ	28	8.2	90.2	21.0	Trace	4.2	.1	33.6	188.7	58.8	—	50.4
			100	8.2	322.0	74.9	.1	15.1	.4	120.0	674.0	210.0	—	180.0

Item No.	Iron (mg)	Zinc (mg)	Copper (mg)	Vitamin A (IU)	Vitamin D (IU)	Vitamin E (Alpha Tocopherol) (mg)	Vitamin C (mg)	Thiamin (mg)	Riboflavin (mg)	Niacin (mg)	Pantothenic Acid (mg)	Vit. B-6 (Pyridoxine) (mg)	Folacin (Folic Acid) (mcg)	Biotin (mcg)	Vitamin B-12 (mcg)
803	.50	.05	.20	500.0	–	.10	125.00	.23	.08	1.00	.48	.10	137.50	.75	0
	.20	.02	.08	200.0	–	.04	50.00	.09	.03	.40	.19	.04	55.00	.30	0
804	.75	.28	–	500.0	–	–	117.50	.20	.05	.75	.33	.06	87.50	2.00	–
	.30	.11	–	200.0	–	–	47.00	.08	.02	.30	.13	.03	35.00	.80	–
805	.25	.28	.02	500.0	–	–	112.50	.23	.03	.75	.41	.07	137.50	.75	0
	.10	.11	.01	200.0	–	–	45.00	.09	.01	.30	.17	.03	55.00	.30	0
806	.75	.13	.20	5000.0	–	–	102.00	.05	.03	.20	–	–	–	–	–
	.30	.05	.08	2000.0	–	–	40.80	.02	.01	.08	–	–	–	–	–
807	.50	–	–	1075.0	–	–	–	.03	.05	1.00	–	–	–	–	–
	.20	–	–	430.0	–	–	–	.01	.02	.40	–	–	–	–	–
808	.25	–	–	–	–	–	–	–	.05	–	–	–	–	–	–
	.10	–	–	–	–	–	–	–	.02	–	–	–	–	–	–
809	.75	.18	.01	125.0	–	–	22.50	.13	.05	.50	.25	.24	57.50	–	0
	.30	.07	.01	50.0	–	–	9.00	.05	.02	.20	.10	.10	23.00	–	0
810	10.25	.30	.05	275.0	–	–	5.00	.03	.03	1.00	–	.17	1.25	–	0
	4.10	.12	.02	110.0	–	–	2.00	.01	.01	.40	–	.06	.50	–	0
811	2.64	–	–	–	–	–	43.20	.07	.10	.48	.29	.60	7.20	–	0
	1.10	–	–	–	–	–	18.00	.03	.04	.20	.12	.25	3.00	–	0
812	–	–	–	–	–	–	67.50	–	–	–	–	–	–	–	–
	–	–	–	–	–	–	27.00	–	–	–	–	–	–	–	–
813	.50	–	–	1050.0	–	–	77.50	.15	.05	.25	–	–	–	–	–
	.20	–	–	420.0	–	–	31.00	.06	.02	.10	–	–	–	–	–
814	.50	–	–	1025.0	–	–	67.50	.15	.05	.25	–	–	–	–	–
	.20	–	–	410.0	–	–	27.00	.06	.02	.10	–	–	–	–	–
815	1.10	.13	.21	1380.0	–	.44	26.80	.14	.07	1.60	.50	.27	52.00	–	0
	.55	.07	.11	690.0	–	.22	13.40	.07	.04	.80	.25	.13	26.00	–	0
816	1.80	–	–	1800.0	–	–	26.00	.10	.06	1.60	.50	.39	19.80	–	0
	.90	–	–	900.0	–	–	13.00	.05	.03	.80	.25	.19	9.90	–	0
817	1.00	–	–	1400.0	–	–	18.00	.10	.06	1.60	–	–	32.00	–	–
	.50	–	–	700.0	–	–	9.00	.05	.03	.80	–	–	16.00	–	–
818	1.09	–	–	–	–	–	0	.01	.00	.02	–	–	–	–	–
	3.90	–	–	–	–	–	0	.05	.01	.10	–	–	–	–	–
819	6.00	–	–	180.0	–	–	6.00	.21	.12	1.80	–	–	–	–	–
	2.00	–	–	60.0	–	–	2.00	.07	.04	.60	–	–	–	–	–
820	5.00	(.22)	(.07)	150.0	0	(.18)	5.00	.18	.10	1.50	–	(.04)	60.00	–	0
	2.00	(.78)	(.24)	60.0	0	(.66)	2.00	.07	.04	.60	–	(.13)	24.00	–	0
821	5.24	1.52	–	–	–	–	–	.22	.10	1.18	–	–	72.67	–	–
	3.10	.90	–	–	–	–	–	.13	.06	.70	–	–	43.00	–	–
822	1.18	–	–	60.7	–	–	0	.13	.05	.67	–	–	–	–	–
	4.20	–	–	216.7	–	–	0	.45	.19	2.40	–	–	–	–	–
823	4.76	[6].39	–	35.0	–	–	0	.21	.10	1.40	–	.38	142.80	–	0
	3.40	.28	–	25.0	–	–	0	.15	.07	1.00	–	.27	102.00	–	0
824	3.25	3.00	–	25.0	–	–	–	.40	.10	1.00	–	–	200.00	–	0
	1.30	1.20	–	10.0	–	–	–	.16	.04	.40	–	–	80.00	–	0
825	9.38	–	–	–	–	–	–	1.14	.33	3.86	2.27	–	–	–	0
	5.10	–	–	–	–	–	–	.62	.18	2.10	1.23	–	–	–	0
826	2.41	–	–	–	–	–	.56	.18	.04	.87	–	–	–	–	–
	8.60	–	–	–	–	–	2.00	.65	.13	31.00	–	–	–	–	–
827	3.15	1.50	(.27)	30.0	0	–	0	.11	.09	.90	(.50)	(.24)	–	–	0
	2.10	1.00	(.18)	20.0	0	–	0	.07	.06	.60	(.33)	(.16)	–	–	0
828	3.40	–	–	80.0	–	–	–	.30	.18	1.80	–	–	14.00	–	–
	1.70	–	–	40.0	–	–	–	.15	.09	.90	–	–	7.00	–	–
829	2.24	–	(.35)	22.4	0	–	Trace	.09	.05	.84	.42	.08	30.80	–	0
	8.00	–	(1.25)	80.0	0	–	Trace	.32	.16	3.00	1.50	.30	110.00	–	0
830															
831	4.86	–	–	54.0	–	–	0	.38	.16	1.08	–	–	–	–	–
	2.70	–	–	30.0	–	–	0	.21	.09	.60	–	–	–	–	–
832	.48	–	–	11.2	–	–	0	.02	.03	.08	–	–	–	–	–
	1.70	–	–	40.0	–	–	0	.06	.10	.30	–	–	–	–	–
833	1.04	–	–	0	–	–	0	.02	.14	.31	–	–	35.28	–	–
	3.70	–	–	0	–	–	0	.07	50	1.10	–	–	126.00	–	–
834	–	–	–	–	–	–	0	–	–	–	–	–	–	–	–
	–	–	–	–	–	–	0	–	–	–	–	–	–	–	–

(Continued)

TABLE F-21 *(Continued)*

Item No.	Food Item Name	Approximate Measure	Weight	Moisture	Food Energy Calories	Protein	Fats	Carbo-hydrates	Fiber	Minerals (Macro)				
										Calcium	Phos-phorus	Sodium	Mag-nesium	Potas-sium
			(g)	(%)	(kcal)	(g)	(g)	(g)	(g)	(mg)	(mg)	(mg)	(mg)	(mg)
	SOYBEANS (Continued)													
835	TOFU, (bean curd)	1 OZ	28	84.8	20.2	2.0	1.2	.7	Trace	35.8	35.3	2.0	31.1	11.8
			100	84.8	72.0	7.0	4.2	2.4	.1	128.0	126.0	7.0	111.0	42.0
	MEATS													
836	[3]ANTELOPE, salted	1 OZ	28	60.2	42.0	8.5	.6	—	—	18.2	84.6	—	—	—
			100	60.2	150.0	30.4	2.2	—	—	65.0	302.0	—	—	—
	BACON													
837	Canadian, broiled or fried, drained	1 SLICE	21	49.9	58.2	5.8	3.7	.1	0	4.0	45.8	536.6	5.0	90.7
			100	49.9	277.0	27.6	17.5	.3	0	19.0	218.0	2555.0	24.0	432.0
838	cured, fried, drained, sliced medium	1 SLICE	7	8.1	40.3	2.1	3.4	.2	0	1.0	15.7	71.5	1.8	16.5
			100	8.1	575.0	30.4	49.0	3.2	0	14.0	224.0	1021.0	25.0	236.0
	BEEF													
839	ARM, Choice, separable lean, cooked w/o bone	1 OZ	28	61.7	54.0	8.5	2.0	0	0	3.9	42.0	16.8	5.0	103.6
			100	61.7	193.0	30.5	7.0	0	0	14.0	150.0	60.0	18.0	370.0
840	BOTTOM SIRLOIN BUTT, Choice, boneless, trimmed, cooked	1 OZ	28	42.1	114.2	6.2	9.7	0	0	2.8	52.1	16.8	5.9	103.6
			100	42.1	408.0	22.2	34.7	0	0	10.0	186.0	60.0	21.0	370.0
841	[1]BRISKET, boneless, lean meat, cooked	1 OZ	28	59.1	62.2	8.3	2.9	0	0	3.6	40.9	16.8	5.0	103.6
			100	59.1	222.0	29.7	10.5	0	0	13.0	146.0	60.0	18.0	370.0
842	CHUCK, entire Choice, total edible, braised, 81% lean, 19% fat	1 OZ	28	49.4	91.6	7.3	6.7	0	0	3.1	39.2	16.8	4.2	102.6
			100	49.4	327.0	26.0	23.9	0	0	11.0	140.0	60.0	15.0	370.0
843	CLUB STEAK, Choice, total edible, boiled, 58% lean, 42% fat	1 OZ	28	37.9	127.1	5.8	11.4	0	0	2.5	49.0	16.8	5.9	103.6
			100	37.9	454.0	20.6	40.6	0	0	9.0	175.0	60.0	21.0	370.0
844	CORNED, boneless, medium fat, cooked	1 OZ	28	43.9	104.2	6.4	8.5	0	0	2.5	26.0	487.2	8.1	42.0
			100	43.9	372.0	22.9	30.4	0	0	9.0	93.0	1740.0	29.0	150.0
845	CORNED, boneless, medium fat, canned	1 OZ	28	59.3	60.5	7.1	3.4	0	0	5.6	29.7	268.0	(4.2)	16.8
			100	59.3	216.0	25.3	12.0	0	0	20.0	106.0	957.0	(15.0)	60.0
846	CUBED STEAK, Choice, cooked	1 OZ	28	54.7	73.1	8.0	4.3	0	0	3.4	70.0	16.8	5.9	103.6
			100	54.7	261.0	28.6	15.4	0	0	12.0	250.0	60.0	21.0	370.0
847	DOUBLE-BONE SIRLOIN STEAK, Choice, total edible, broiled, 66% lean, 34% fat, w/o bone	1 OZ	28	42.1	114.2	6.2	9.7	0	0	2.8	52.1	16.8	5.9	103.6
			100	42.1	408.0	22.2	34.7	0	0	10.0	186.0	60.0	21.0	370.0
848	FLANK STEAK, Choice, cooked, 100% lean	1 OZ	28	61.4	52.6	8.5	2.0	0	0	3.9	42.0	16.8	5.0	103.6
			100	61.4	188.0	30.5	7.3	0	0	14.0	150.0	60.0	18.0	370.0
849	HAMBURGER (GROUND BEEF), cooked, w/21% fat	1 OZ	28	54.2	84.3	6.8	6.4	0	0	3.1	54.3	13.2	5.9	126.0
			100	54.2	301.0	24.2	22.7	0	0	11.0	194.0	47.0	21.0	450.0
850	HAMBURGER (GROUND BEEF), cooked, w/10% fat	1 OZ	28	60.0	61.3	7.7	3.2	0	0	3.4	64.4	13.4	7.0	156.2
			100	60.0	219.0	27.4	11.3	0	0	12.0	230.0	48.0	25.0	558.0
851	HINDSHANK, Choice, total edible, cooked, 66% lean, 34% fat	1 OZ	28	46.1	101.1	7.0	7.9	0	0	3.1	35.0	16.8	4.2	103.6
			100	46.1	361.0	25.1	28.1	0	0	11.0	125.0	60.0	15.0	370.0
852	KNUCKLE, boneless, Choice, cooked	1 OZ	28	46.1	101.1	7.0	7.9	0	0	3.1	35.0	16.8	4.2	103.6
			100	46.1	361.0	25.1	28.1	0	0	11.0	125.0	60.0	15.0	370.0
853	[1]MINUTE STEAK, lean meat & fat, cooked	1 OZ	28	54.7	73.1	8.0	4.3	0	0	3.4	70.0	16.8	7.8	103.6
			100	54.7	261.0	28.6	15.4	0	0	12.0	250.0	60.0	28.0	370.0
854	PORTERHOUSE STEAK, Choice, total edible, broiled, 57% lean, 43% fat, w/bone	1 OZ	28	37.2	128.5	5.5	11.8	0	0	2.5	47.0	16.8	5.9	103.6
			100	37.2	459.0	19.7	42.2	0	0	9.0	168.0	60.0	21.0	370.0
855	RIB, entire, Choice, total edible, roasted, 64% lean, 36% fat, w/o bone	1 OZ	28	40.0	121.5	5.6	11.0	0	0	2.5	52.1	16.8	5.6	103.6
			100	40.0	434.0	19.9	39.4	0	0	9.0	186.0	60.0	20.0	370.0
856	RIBEYE, steak	1 OZ	30	40.0	132.0	6.0	11.8	0	0	2.7	55.8	18.0	6.0	111.0
			100	40.0	440.0	19.9	39.4	0	0	9.0	186.0	60.0	20.0	370.0
857	ROUND, Choice, total edible, cooked, 81% lean, 19% fat, w/o bone	1 OZ	28	54.7	73.1	8.0	4.3	0	0	3.4	70.0	16.8	7.8	103.6
			100	54.7	261.0	28.6	15.4	0	0	12.0	250.0	60.0	28.0	370.0
858	RUMP, Choice, total edible, roasted, 75% lean, 25% fat, w/o bone	1 OZ	28	48.1	95.2	6.6	7.6	0	0	2.8	55.2	16.8	7.8	103.6
			100	48.1	340.0	23.6	27.3	0	0	10.0	197.0	60.0	28.0	370.0
859	SHORT PLATE, Choice, total edible, cooked, 58% lean, 42% fat	1 OZ	28	36.0	131.0	5.8	12.0	0	0	2.5	28.3	16.8	4.2	103.6
			100	36.0	468.0	20.6	42.8	0	0	9.0	101.0	60.0	15.0	370.0
860	SHORT RIBS, Good, cooked	1 OZ	28	39.9	121.0	6.2	10.4	0	0	2.5	30.8	16.8	4.2	103.6
			100	39.9	432.0	22.3	37.3	0	0	9.0	110.0	60.0	15.0	370.0
861	SIRLOIN, GROUND, Choice, 10% fat, cooked	1 OZ	28	42.1	114.2	6.2	9.7	0	0	2.8	52.1	16.8	5.9	103.6
			100	42.1	408.0	22.2	34.7	0	0	10.0	186.0	60.0	21.0	370.0
862	SIRLOIN STEAK, Choice, total edible, cooked, 66% lean, 34% fat, w/o bone	1 OZ	28	43.9	106.4	6.4	9.0	0	0	2.8	53.5	16.8	5.9	103.6
			100	43.9	380.0	23.0	32.0	0	0	10.0	191.0	60.0	21.0	370.0
863	STEW MEAT, Choice, 90% lean, 10% fat, cooked	1 OZ	28	54.7	73.1	8.0	4.3	0	0	3.4	70.0	16.8	5.9	103.6
			100	54.7	261.0	28.6	15.4	0	0	12.0	250.0	60.0	21.0	370.0
864	T-BONE STEAK, Choice, total edible, broiled, 56% lean, 44% fat, w/bone	1 OZ	28	36.4	130.8	5.5	12.1	0	0	2.2	46.5	16.8	5.9	103.6
			100	36.4	467.0	19.5	43.2	0	0	8.0	166.0	60.0	21.0	370.0
865	TENDERLOIN STEAK, broiled	1 OZ	28	—	62.7	7.2	3.5	0	0	4.2	58.0	12.6	6.4	122.1
			100	—	224.0	26.1	12.6	0	0	15.0	207.0	45.0	22.7	436.0
866	TOP SIRLOIN BUTT, Choice, boneless, trimmed, cooked	1 OZ	28	42.1	114.2	6.2	9.7	0	0	2.8	52.1	16.8	5.9	103.6
			100	42.1	408.0	22.2	34.7	0	0	10.0	186.0	60.0	21.0	370.0

Item No.	Minerals (Micro)			Fat-Soluble Vitamins			Water-Soluble Vitamins								
	Iron	Zinc	Copper	Vitamin A	Vitamin D	Vitamin E (Alpha Tocopherol)	Vitamin C	Thiamin	Riboflavin	Niacin	Pantothenic Acid	Vit. B-6 (Pyridoxine)	Folacin (Folic Acid)	Biotin	Vitamin B-12
	(mg)	(mg)	(mg)	(IU)	(IU)	(mg)	(mg)	(mg)	(mg)	(mg)	(mg)	(mg)	(mcg)	(mcg)	(mcg)
835	.53	[6].20	–	0	–	–	0	.02	.01	.03	–	–	–	–	–
	1.90	.70	–	0	–	–	0	.06	.03	.10	–	–	–	–	–
836	.58	–	–	0	–	–	0	.02	.08	2.18	–	–	–	–	–
	2.10	–	–	0	–	–	0	.07	.28	7.80	–	–	–	–	–
837	.86	–	–	0	0	–	0	.19	.04	1.05	–	–	–	–	–
	4.10	–	–	0	0	–	0	.92	.17	5.00	–	–	–	–	–
838	.23	–	–	0	–	.04	0	.04	.02	.36	–	–	.14	–	–
	3.30	–	–	0	–	.53	0	.51	.34	5.20	–	–	2.00	–	–
839	1.06	–	–	2.8	–	.26	–	.02	.06	1.29	–	–	1.12	–	–
	3.80	–	–	10.0	–	.94	–	.06	.23	4.60	–	–	4.00	–	–
840	.61	–	.05	16.8	–	–	0	.02	.05	1.29	–	–	–	–	–
	2.90	–	.18	60.0	–	–	0	.06	.18	4.60	–	–	–	–	–
841	1.06	1.74	–	5.6	–	–	–	.01	.06	1.26	–	–	1.12	–	–
	3.80	6.20	–	20.0	–	–	–	.05	.22	4.50	–	–	4.00	–	–
842	.92	–	–	11.2	–	–	–	.01	.06	1.12	–	–	–	–	–
	3.30	–	–	40.0	–	–	–	.05	.20	4.00	–	–	–	–	–
843	.76	–	.05	19.6	–	–	–	.02	.05	1.20	–	–	–	–	–
	2.70	–	.18	70.0	–	–	–	.06	.17	4.30	–	–	–	–	–
844	.81	–	–	–	–	–	0	.01	.04	.42	–	.04	–	–	–
	2.90	–	–	–	–	–	0	.04	.14	1.50	–	.15	–	–	–
845	1.20	(1.57)	(.07)	0	Trace	(.22)	0	.01	.07	.95	(.12)	(.02)	(.59)	(.58)	.52
	4.30	(5.62)	(.24)	0	Trace	(.77)	0	.02	.24	3.40	(.42)	(.07)	(2.11)	(2.08)	1.84
846	.98	–	.05	8.4	–	–	0	.02	.06	1.57	.15	.14	–	–	–
	3.50	–	.19	30.0	–	–	0	.08	.22	5.60	.52	.50	–	–	–
847	.81	–	.05	16.8	–	–	0	.02	.05	1.29	–	–	–	–	–
	2.90	–	.19	60.0	–	–	0	.06	.18	4.60	–	–	–	–	–
848	1.06	–	–	2.8	–	.26	–	.02	.06	1.29	–	–	–	–	–
	3.80	–	–	10.0	–	.94	–	.06	.23	4.60	–	–	–	–	–
849	.90	–	–	11.2	–	.10	0	.03	.06	1.51	.12	.13	1.12	–	(.50)
	3.20	–	–	40.0	–	.37	0	.09	.21	5.40	.44	.46	4.00	–	(1.80)
850	.98	1.23	–	5.6	–	–	0	.03	.06	1.68	–	–	1.12	–	(.50)
	3.50	4.40	–	20.0	–	–	0	.09	.23	6.00	–	–	4.00	–	(1.80)
851	.92	–	–	14.0	–	–	–	.01	.05	1.09	–	–	–	–	–
	3.30	–	–	50.0	–	–	–	.05	.19	3.90	–	–	–	–	–
852	.92	–	–	14.0	–	–	–	.01	.05	1.09	–	–	–	–	–
	3.30	–	–	50.0	–	–	–	.05	.19	3.90	–	–	–	–	–
853	.98	1.34	–	8.4	–	–	0	.02	.06	1.57	.16	.14	1.12	–	–
	3.50	4.79	–	30.0	–	–	0	.08	.22	5.60	.52	.50	4.00	–	–
854	.73	–	–	19.6	–	–	–	.02	.05	1.18	–	–	–	–	–
	2.60	–	–	70.0	–	–	–	.06	.16	4.20	–	–	–	–	–
855	.73	–	–	22.4	–	–	0	.01	.04	1.01	–	–	–	–	.01
	2.60	–	–	80.0	–	–	0	.05	.15	3.60	–	–	–	–	.03
856	.78	–	–	24.0	–	–	0	.02	.05	1.08	–	–	–	–	–
	2.60	–	–	80.0	–	–	0	.05	.15	3.60	–	–	–	–	–
857	.98	–	–	8.4	–	–	0	.02	.06	1.57	.15	.14	–	–	(.73)
	3.50	–	–	30.0	–	–	0	.08	.22	5.60	.52	.49	–	–	(2.60)
858	.87	–	–	14.0	–	–	0	.02	.05	1.20	–	–	–	–	–
	3.10	–	–	50.0	–	–	0	.06	.18	4.30	–	–	–	–	–
859	.76	–	–	22.4	–	–	–	.01	.05	.90	–	–	–	–	.01
	2.70	–	–	80.0	–	–	–	.04	.16	3.20	–	–	–	–	.02
860	.81	–	–	19.6	–	–	–	.01	.05	.95	–	–	–	–	–
	2.90	–	–	70.0	–	–	–	.04	.17	3.40	–	–	–	–	–
861	.81	1.23	–	16.8	–	–	0	.02	.05	1.29	–	–	–	–	–
	2.90	4.40	–	60.0	–	–	0	.06	.18	4.60	–	–	–	–	–
862	.81	–	.05	14.0	–	–	0	.02	.05	1.32	–	–	–	–	(.50)
	2.90	–	.18	50.0	–	–	0	.06	.18	4.70	–	–	–	–	(1.80)
863	.98	(2.43)	(.07)	8.4	Trace	(.09)	0	.02	.06	1.57	.15	.14	(4.58)	Trace	(.56)
	3.50	(8.70)	(.25)	30.0	Trace	(.31)	0	.08	.22	5.60	.52	.50	(16.00)	Trace	(2.00)
864	.73	–	–	22.4	–	.04	–	.02	.05	1.15	–	–	–	–	–
	2.60	–	–	80.0	–	.13	–	.06	.16	4.10	–	–	–	–	–
865	–	–	–	0	0	–	0	.03	.13	.93	–	–	–	–	–
	–	–	–	0	0	–	0	.10	.46	3.33	–	–	–	–	–
866	.01	–	.05	16.8	–	–	0	.02	.05	1.29	–	–	–	–	–
	2.90	–	.18	60.0	–	–	0	.06	.18	4.60	–	–	–	–	–

(Continued)

TABLE F-21 *(Continued)*

Item No.	Food Item Name	Approximate Measure	Weight	Moisture	Food Energy Calories	Protein	Fats	Carbo-hydrates	Fiber	Minerals (Macro)				
										Calcium	Phos-phorus	Sodium	Mag-nesium	Potas-sium
			(g)	(%)	(kcal)	(g)	(g)	(g)	(g)	(mg)	(mg)	(mg)	(mg)	(mg)
	BEEF (Continued)													
867	**6TH RIB,** Choice, total edible, cooked, 70% lean, 30% fat	1 OZ	28	39.3	122.4	6.2	10.6	0	0	2.8	30.5	16.8	5.6	103.0
			100	39.3	437.0	22.1	38.0	0	0	10.0	109.0	60.0	20.0	370.0
868	**11TH-12TH RIB,** Choice, total edible, cooked, 55% lean, 45% fat	1 OZ	28	36.3	133.3	5.1	12.5	0	0	2.2	42.8	16.8	5.6	103.6
			100	36.3	476.0	18.3	44.7	0	0	8.0	153.0	60.0	20.0	370.0
869	**ROAST BEEF,** canned	1 OZ	28	60.0	62.7	7.0	3.6	0	0	4.5	32.5	—	—	72.5
			100	60.0	224.0	25.0	13.0	0	0	16.0	116.0	—	—	259.0
870	**BRAINS, BEEF,** cooked	1 CUP	140	—	483.7	34.3	38.5	0	0	15.4	254.8	294.0	14.0	266.0
			100	—	345.5	24.5	27.5	0	0	11.0	182.0	210.0	10.0	190.0
871	**⁴BUFFALO, WATER (CARABAO),** meat, raw	1 OZ	28	76.5	33.6	5.0	1.4	0	Trace	3.9	61.9	25.5	—	76.4
			100	76.5	120.0	17.7	4.9	0	Trace	14.0	221.0	91.0	—	273.0
872	**CHEVON**—See **GOAT MEAT**													
	CHICKEN													
	BROILERS—FRYERS													
873	flesh, w/skin, fried, flour coated	1 OZ	28	52.4	75.3	8.0	4.2	.9	Trace	4.8	53.5	23.5	7.0	65.5
			100	52.4	269.0	28.6	14.9	3.2	.01	17.0	191.0	84.0	25.0	234.0
874	dark meat, w/o skin, fried	1 OZ	28	55.7	66.9	8.1	3.2	.7	Trace	5.0	52.4	27.2	7.0	70.8
			100	55.7	239.0	29.0	11.6	2.6	.01	18.0	187.0	97.0	25.0	253.0
875	light meat, w/o skin, fried	1 OZ	28	60.1	53.4	9.2	1.5	.1	0	4.5	64.7	23.7	8.1	73.6
			100	60.1	192.0	32.8	5.5	.4	0	16.0	231.0	81.0	29.0	263.0
876	**CANNED,** meat only w/o bone	1 OZ	28	52.6	55.4	6.1	3.3	0	0	5.9	69.2	152.0	5.3	38.6
			100	52.6	198.0	21.7	11.7	0	0	21.0	247.0	543.0	19.0	138.0
877	**⁴CANNED,** chicken liver pate	1 OZ	28	—	72.0	3.6	5.5	1.9	—	26.6	—	383.6	—	—
			100	—	257.0	12.9	19.5	6.8	—	95.0	—	1370.0	—	—
878	**²FRANKFURTER**	1 OZ	28	—	56.3	3.8	3.7	1.8	—	2.8	—	—	—	—
			100	—	201.0	13.5	13.1	6.6	—	10.0	—	—	—	—
879	**ROASTER,** flesh & skin, roasted	1 OZ	28	62.1	62.4	6.7	3.8	0	0	3.4	50.1	20.4	5.6	59.1
			100	62.1	223.0	24.0	13.4	0	0	12.0	179.0	73.0	20.0	211.0
880	**STEWING,** flesh & skin, stewed	1 OZ	28	53.1	79.8	7.5	5.3	0	0	3.6	50.4	20.4	5.6	51.0
			100	53.1	285.0	26.9	18.9	0	0	13.0	180.0	73.0	20.0	182.0
881	¹**CORNISH HEN,** roasted, whole	1 OZ	28	71.0	38.1	6.7	1.1	0	0	2.5	56.3	18.5	—	76.7
			100	71.0	136.0	23.8	3.8	0	0	9.0	201.0	66.0	—	274.0
	DUCK													
882	²**DOMESTIC,** flesh only, roasted	1 OZ	28	64.2	56.3	6.6	3.1	0	0	3.4	56.8	18.2	5.6	70.6
			100	64.2	201.0	23.5	11.2	0	0	12.0	203.0	65.0	20.0	252.0
883	**WILD,** total edible, raw	1 OZ	28	61.1	65.2	5.9	4.4	0	0	3.4	56.0	—	—	—
			100	61.1	233.0	21.1	15.8	0	0	12.0	200.0	—	—	—
	FRANKFURTERS (Wieners)													
884	all meat, cooked	1 AVG	50	—	124.0	7.0	10.0	1.0	—	3.0	25.0	542.0	—	108.0
			100	—	248.0	14.0	20.0	2.0	—	6.0	50.0	1084.0	—	216.0
885	w/cereal, raw	1 AVG	50	61.7	124.0	7.2	10.3	.1	—	4.0	—	—	8.0	—
			100	61.7	248.0	14.4	20.6	.2	—	8.0	—	—	16.0	—
886	**FROG LEGS,** fried	1 LG	24	—	69.6	4.3	4.8	2.0	0	4.6	38.4	—	—	—
			100	—	290.0	17.9	19.8	8.5	0	19.0	160.0	—	—	—
	GIZZARD													
887	**CHICKEN,** simmered	1 OZ	28	68.0	41.4	7.6	.9	.2	0	2.5	19.9	16.0	—	59.1
			100	68.0	148.0	27.0	3.3	.7	0	9.0	71.0	57.0	—	211.0
888	**GOOSE,** raw	1 OZ	28	73.0	38.9	6.0	1.5	0	0	—	—	—	—	—
			100	73.0	139.0	21.4	5.3	0	0	—	—	—	—	—
889	**TURKEY,** simmered	1 OZ	28	62.7	54.9	7.5	2.4	.3	0	—	—	14.3	—	41.7
			100	62.7	196.0	26.8	8.6	1.1	0	—	—	51.0	—	149.0
890	⁵**GOAT MEAT (CHEVON),** carcass	1 OZ	28	71.0	46.2	5.2	2.6	0	—	3.1	—	—	—	—
			100	71.0	165.0	18.7	9.4	0	—	11.0	—	—	—	—
891	**GOOSE,** total edible, roasted	1 OZ	28	39.1	119.3	6.6	10.1	0	0	3.1	67.2	—	—	—
			100	39.1	426.0	23.7	36.0	0	0	11.0	240.0	—	—	—
892	**GUINEA HEN,** total edible, raw	1 OZ	28	69.0	43.7	6.5	1.8	0	0	—	—	—	—	—
			100	69.0	156.0	23.1	6.4	0	0	—	—	—	—	—
893	⁵**GUINEA PIG,** meat	1 OZ	28	78.2	26.9	5.3	.4	(0)	—	8.1	70.8	—	—	—
			100	78.2	96.0	19.0	1.6	(0)	—	29.0	253.0	—	—	—
	HEART													
894	**BEEF,** lean, w/fat, braised	1 OZ	28	44.4	104.2	7.2	8.1	0	0	—	47.3	—	—	—
			100	44.4	372.0	25.8	29.0	.1	0	—	169.0	—	—	—
895	**CALF,** braised	1 OZ	28	60.3	58.2	7.8	2.5	.5	0	1.1	41.4	31.6	—	70.0
			100	60.3	208.0	27.8	9.1	1.8	0	4.0	148.0	113.0	—	250.0
896	**CHICKEN,** simmered	1 OZ	28	64.9	46.5	7.1	2.0	0	0	1.1	30.0	19.3	—	39.2
			100	64.9	165.0	25.3	7.2	.1	0	4.0	107.0	69.0	—	140.0
897	**TURKEY,** simmered	1 OZ	28	64.2	58.8	6.3	3.7	.1	0	—.	—	17.1	—	59.1
			100	64.2	210.0	22.6	13.2	.2	0	—	—	61.0	—	211.0
898	⁵**HORSE MEAT,** carcass	1 OZ	28	76.0	33.0	5.1	1.1	.3	0	2.8	42.0	—	—	—
			100	76.0	118.0	18.1	4.1	.9	0	10.8	150.0	—	—	—

Item No.	Minerals (Micro)			Fat-Soluble Vitamins			Water-Soluble Vitamins								
	Iron	Zinc	Copper	Vitamin A	Vitamin D	Vitamin E (Alpha Tocopherol)	Vitamin C	Thiamin	Ribo-flavin	Niacin	Panto-thenic Acid	Vit. B-6 (Pyri-doxine)	Folacin (Folic Acid)	Biotin	Vitamin B-12
	(mg)	(mg)	(mg)	(IU)	(IU)	(mg)	(mg)	(mg)	(mg)	(mg)	(mg)	(mg)	(mcg)	(mcg)	(mcg)
867	.81	–	–	19.6	–	–	0	.01	.05	.95	–	–	–	–	–
	2.90	–	–	70.0	–	–	0	.04	.17	3.40	–	–	–	–	–
868	.67	–	–	25.2	–	–	0	.01	.04	.95	–	–	–	–	–
	2.40	–	–	90.0	–	–	0	.05	.14	3.40	–	–	–	–	–
869	.67	–	–	–	–	–	0	.01	.06	1.18	–	–	–	–	–
	2.40	–	–	–	–	–	0	.02	.23	4.20	–	–	–	–	–
870	4.34	2.10	.59	70.0	Trace	3.22	0	.10	.27	7.00	1.96	.14	4.20	4.20	2.52
	3.10	1.50	.42	50.0	Trace	2.30	0	.07	.19	5.00	1.40	.10	3.00	3.00	1.80
871	.92	–	–	5.1	–	–	0	.02	43.40	.98	–	–	–	–	–
	3.30	–	–	18.3	–	–	0	.06	155.00	3.50	–	–	–	–	–
872															
873	.39	.57	.02	24.9	–	–	0	.03	.05	2.52	.30	.11	1.68	–	.09
	1.38	2.04	.08	89.0	–	–	0	.09	.19	8.99	1.08	.41	6.00	–	.31
874	.42	.81	.03	22.1	–	–	0	.03	.07	1.98	.35	.10	2.52	–	.09
	1.49	2.91	.09	79.0	–	–	0	.09	.25	7.07	1.26	.37	9.00	–	.33
875	.32	.36	.01	8.4	–	–	0	.02	.04	3.74	.29	.18	1.12	–	.10
	1.14	1.27	.05	30.0	–	–	0	.07	.13	13.37	1.03	.63	4.00	–	.36
876	.42	–	–	64.4	–	–	1.12	.01	.03	1.23	.24	.08	1.18	–	.22
	1.50	–	–	230.0	–	–	4.00	.04	.12	4.40	.85	.30	4.20	–	.79
877	.56	–	–	–	–	–	–	.02	.03	.87	–	–	–	–	–
	2.00	–	–	–	–	–	–	.07	.12	3.09	–	–	–	–	–
878	2.57	–	–	202.7	–	–	2.72	.02	.39	2.10	–	–	–	–	–
	9.19	–	–	724.0	–	–	9.70	.05	1.40	7.52	–	–	–	–	–
879	.35	.41	.02	23.2	–	–	0	.02	.04	2.08	.26	.10	1.40	–	.08
	1.26	1.45	.06	83.0	–	–	0	.06	.14	7.42	.92	.35	5.00	–	.27
880	.38	.50	.03	36.7	–	–	0	.03	.07	1.62	.21	.07	1.40	–	.06
	1.37	1.77	.10	131.0	–	–	0	.09	.24	5.80	.75	.25	5.00	–	.23
881	.48	–	–	25.2	–	–	–	.01	.05	2.46	–	–	–	–	–
	1.70	–	–	90.0	–	–	–	.05	.19	8.80	–	–	–	–	–
882	.76	.73	.07	21.6	–	–	0	.07	.13	1.43	.42	.07	2.80	–	.11
	2.70	2.60	.23	77.0	–	–	0	.26	.47	5.10	1.50	.25	10.00	–	.40
883	.84	–	–	0	–	–	–	–	–	–	–	–	–	–	–
	3.00	–	–	0	–	–	–	–	–	–	–	–	–	–	–
884	.60	.80	–	0	0	–	0	.08	.09	.60	–	–	–	–	–
	1.20	1.60	–	0	0	–	0	.16	.18	1.20	–	–	–	–	–
885	–	–	–	–	–	–	0	–	–	–	.21	.07	–	–	–
	–	–	–	–	–	–	0	–	–	–	.43	.13	–	–	–
886	.34	–	–	0	0	–	–	.03	.06	.30	–	–	–	–	–
	1.40	–	–	0	0	–	–	.12	.24	1.25	–	–	–	–	–
887	.87	1.20	–	–	–	–	–	.01	.06	1.43	–	–	–	–	–
	3.10	4.30	–	–	–	–	–	.02	.21	5.10	–	–	–	–	–
888	–	–	–	–	–	–	–	–	–	–	–	–	–	–	–
	–	–	–	–	–	–	–	–	–	–	–	–	–	–	–
889	–	1.15	–	–	–	–	–	.01	.04	1.62	–	–	–	–	–
	–	4.10	–	–	–	–	–	.03	.14	5.80	–	–	–	–	–
890	.62	–	–	0	–	–	0	(.05)	.09	(1.57)	–	–	–	–	–
	2.20	–	–	0	–	–	0	(.17)	.32	(5.60)	–	–	–	–	–
891	.59	–	–	0	–	–	–	.02	.07	2.27	–	–	–	–	–
	2.10	–	–	0	–	–	–	.08	.24	8.10	–	–	–	–	–
892	–	–	–	–	–	–	–	–	–	–	–	–	–	–	–
	–	–	–	–	–	–	–	–	–	–	–	–	–	–	–
893	.53	–	–	–	–	–	–	.02	.04	1.82	–	–	–	–	–
	1.90	–	–	–	–	–	–	.06	.14	6.50	–	–	–	–	–
894	–	–	–	–	–	–	–	–	–	–	–	–	–	–	–
	–	–	–	–	–	–	–	–	–	–	–	–	–	–	–
895	1.23	–	–	11.2	–	–	–	.08	.40	2.27	–	–	–	–	–
	4.40	–	–	40.0	–	–	–	.29	1.44	8.10	–	–	–	–	–
896	1.01	1.34	–	8.4	–	–	1.12	.02	.26	1.48	–	–	–	–	–
	3.60	4.80	–	30.0	–	–	4.00	.06	.92	5.30	–	–	–	–	–
897	–	1.34	–	8.4	–	–	1.12	.07	.27	1.60	–	–	–	–	–
	–	4.80	–	30.0	–	–	4.00	.25	.98	5.70	–	–	–	–	–
898	(.76)	–	–	–	–	–	–	.02	.03	(1.20)	–	–	–	–	–
	(2.70)	–	–	–	–	–	–	.07	.12	(4.30)	–	–	–	–	–

(Continued)

TABLE F-21 *(Continued)*

Item No.	Food Item Name	Approximate Measure	Weight (g)	Moisture (%)	Food Energy Calories (kcal)	Protein (g)	Fats (g)	Carbo-hydrates (g)	Fiber (g)	Calcium (mg)	Phos-phorus (mg)	Sodium (mg)	Mag-nesium (mg)	Potas-sium (mg)
	KIDNEYS													
899	**BEEF,** braised	1 OZ	28	53.0	70.6	9.2	3.4	.2	0	5.0	68.3	70.8	(5.3)	90.7
			100	53.0	252.0	33.0	12.0	.8	0	18.0	244.0	253.0	(19.0)	324.0
900	**CALF,** raw	1 OZ	28	77.4	31.6	4.6	1.3	0	0	2.5	47.9	66.6	2.8	67.2
			100	77.4	113.0	16.6	4.6	.1	0	9.0	171.0	238.0	10.0	240.0
	LAMB													
901	**COMPOSITE OF CUTS,** trimmed, Choice, 77% lean, 23% fat	1 OZ	28	61.0	73.6	4.6	6.0	0	0	2.8	41.2	21.0	4.2	82.6
			100	61.0	263.0	16.5	21.3	0	0	10.0	147.0	75.0	15.0	295.0
902	**LEG,** Choice, total edible, roasted, 83% lean, 17% fat, w/o bone	1 OZ	28	54.0	78.1	7.1	5.3	0	0	3.1	58.2	19.6	5.9	81.2
			100	54.0	279.0	25.3	18.9	0	0	11.0	208.0	70.0	21.0	290.0
903	**LOIN,** Choice, chops, total edible, broiled, 66% lean, 34% fat, w/bone	1 MED	46	47.0	165.1	10.1	13.5	0	0	4.1	79.1	32.2	7.8	133.4
			100	47.0	359.0	22.0	29.4	0	0	9.0	172.0	70.0	17.0	290.0
904	**RIB,** Choice, chops, total edible, broiled, 62% lean, 38% fat, w/bone	1 MED	41	42.9	166.9	8.2	14.6	0	0	3.7	64.0	28.7	7.0	118.9
			100	42.9	407.0	20.1	35.6	0	0	9.0	156.0	70.0	17.0	290.0
905	**SHOULDER,** Choice, total edible, roasted, 74% lean, 26% fat, w/o bone	1 OZ	28	49.6	94.6	6.1	7.7	0	0	2.8	48.2	19.6	4.8	81.2
			100	49.6	338.0	21.7	27.2	0	0	10.0	172.0	70.0	17.0	290.0
	LIVER													
906	**BEEF,** fried	1 OZ	28	56.0	62.2	7.4	3.0	1.5	0	3.1	133.3	51.5	5.0	106.4
			100	56.0	222.0	26.4	10.6	5.3	0	11.0	476.0	184.0	18.0	380.0
907	**CALF,** fried	1 OZ	28	51.4	73.1	8.3	3.7	1.1	0	3.6	150.4	33.0	7.3	126.8
			100	51.4	261.0	29.5	13.2	4.0	0	13.0	537.0	118.0	26.0	453.0
908	**CHICKEN,** simmered	1 OZ	28	65.0	46.2	7.4	1.2	.9	0	3.1	44.5	17.1	(6.2)	42.3
			100	65.0	165.0	26.5	4.4	3.1	0	11.0	159.0	61.0	(22.0)	151.0
909	**GOOSE,** raw	1 OZ	28	66.9	51.0	4.6	2.8	1.5	0	–	–	39.2	5.9	64.4
			100	66.9	182.0	16.5	10.0	5.4	0	–	–	140.0	21.0	230.0
910	**HOG,** fried in margarine	1 OZ	28	54.0	68.5	8.4	3.2	.7	0	4.2	150.9	31.1	6.7	110.6
			100	54.0	241.0	29.9	11.5	2.5	0	15.0	539.0	111.0	24.0	395.0
	LUNCHEON MEATS													
911	**BOILED HAM**	1 OZ	28	59.1	65.5	5.3	4.8	0	0	3.1	46.5	–	2.5	–
			100	59.1	234.0	19.0	17.0	0	0	11.0	166.0	–	9.0	–
912	**BOLOGNA,** all samples	1 SLICE	28	56.2	88.5	3.4	8.2	.3	0	2.0	35.8	364.0	4.5	64.4
			100	56.2	316.0	12.1	29.2	1.1	0	7.0	128.0	1300.0	16.0	230.0
913	**BRAUNSCHWEIGER**	1 OZ	28	52.6	101.6	4.3	9.1	.6	0	2.8	68.6	–	4.5	–
			100	52.6	363.0	15.4	32.5	2.3	0	10.0	245.0	–	16.0	–
914	**CAPICCOLA OR CAPACOLA**	1 SLICE	28	26.2	139.7	5.7	12.8	0	0	–	–	–	–	–
			100	26.2	499.0	20.2	45.8	0	0	–	–	–	–	–
915	**DEVILED HAM,** canned	1 TBLS	13	50.5	45.6	1.8	4.2	0	0	1.0	12.0	–	–	–
			100	50.5	351.0	13.9	32.3	0	0	8.0	92.0	–	–	–
916	**HEADCHEESE**	1 SLICE	28	58.8	54.6	4.2	4.1	.3	0	2.5	48.4	–	–	–
			100	58.8	195.0	15.0	14.6	1.0	0	9.0	173.0	–	–	–
917	**LIVERWURST,** fresh	1 OZ	28	53.9	138.9	4.7	9.1	.5	0	2.5	66.6	–	–	–
			100	53.9	496.0	16.7	32.5	1.8	0	9.0	238.0	–	–	–
918	**LIVERWURST,** smoked	1 OZ	28	52.6	89.3	4.1	7.7	.6	0	2.8	68.6	–	–	–
			100	52.6	319.0	14.8	27.4	2.3	0	10.0	245.0	–	–	–
919	**MEAT LOAF**	1 SLICE	70	64.1	140.0	11.1	9.2	2.3	0	6.3	124.6	–	–	–
			100	64.1	200.0	15.9	13.2	3.3	0	9.0	178.0	–	–	–
920	**MINCED HAM**	1 OZ	28	61.7	63.8	3.8	4.7	1.2	0	2.2	24.9	–	–	–
			100	61.7	228.0	13.7	16.9	4.4	0	8.0	89.0	–	–	–
921	**PORK,** cured ham or shoulder, chopped, canned	1 SLICE	28	54.9	94.1	4.2	8.4	.4	0	2.5	30.2	345.5	–	62.2
			100	54.9	336.0	15.0	30.1	1.3	0	9.0	108.0	1234.0	–	222.0
922	**POTTED MEAT,** (beef, chicken, turkey)	1 OZ	28	60.7	78.4	4.5	5.4	0	0	–	–	–	–	–
			100	60.7	280.0	16.1	19.2	0	0	–	–	–	–	–
923	**SALAMI,** cooked	1 OZ	28	51.0	73.1	4.9	5.8	.4	0	2.8	56.0	–	4.5	–
			100	51.0	261.0	17.5	20.6	1.4	0	10.0	200.0	–	16.0	–
924	**SALAMI,** dry	1 SLICE	28	29.8	126.0	6.7	10.7	.3	0	3.9	79.2	(518.3)	4.5	(45.0)
			100	29.8	450.0	23.9	38.1	1.2	0	14.0	283.0	(1850.3)	16.0	(160.8)
925	**SPAM,** Hormel	1 OZ	28	52.6	86.8	3.9	7.4	1.1	.1	3.1	35.3	336.0	–	58.5
			100	52.6	310.0	14.0	26.5	3.8	.2	11.0	126.0	1200.0	–	209.0
926	**°OXTAIL,** stewed	4 OZ	112	–	273.4	34.2	15.1	0	0	15.7	156.8	213.7	20.2	191.4
			100	–	244.1	30.5	13.5	0	0	14.0	140.0	190.8	18.0	170.9
927	**°PARTRIDGE,** roasted	1 OZ	28	54.5	59.4	10.3	2.0	0	0	12.9	86.8	28.0	10.1	114.8
			100	54.5	212.0	36.7	7.2	0	0	46.0	310.0	100.0	36.0	410.0
928	**PATE de FOIS GRAS,** canned	1 TBLS	15	37.0	69.3	1.7	6.6	.7	0	–	–	–	–	–
			100	37.0	462.0	11.4	43.8	4.8	0	–	–	–	–	–
929	**PHEASANT,** total edible, raw	1 OZ	28	69.2	42.3	6.8	1.5	0	0	3.9	73.4	–	–	–
			100	69.2	151.0	24.3	5.2	0	0	14.0	262.0	–	–	–
930	**PIGS FEET,** pickled	1 OZ	28	66.9	55.7	4.7	4.1	0	0	–	–	–	–	–
			100	66.9	199.0	16.7	14.8	0	0	–	–	–	–	–
	PORK, FRESH													
931	**ALL CUTS,** medium fat, total edible, cooked, 77% lean, 23% fat	1 OZ	28	45.2	104.4	6.3	8.6	0	0	2.8	65.0	18.2	6.4	109.2
			100	45.2	373.0	22.6	30.6	0	0	10.0	232.0	65.0	23.0	390.0

Item No.	Minerals (Micro)			Fat-Soluble Vitamins			Water-Soluble Vitamins								
	Iron	Zinc	Copper	Vitamin A	Vitamin D	Vitamin E (Alpha Tocopherol)	Vitamin C	Thiamin	Ribo-flavin	Niacin	Panto-thenic Acid	Vit. B-6 (Pyri-doxine)	Folacin (Folic Acid)	Biotin	Vitamin B-12
	(mg)	(mg)	(mg)	(IU)	(IU)	(mg)	(mg)	(mg)	(mg)	(mg)	(mg)	(mg)	(mcg)	(mcg)	(mcg)
899	3.67	(.84)	(.18)	322.0	—	(.12)	0	.19	1.28	3.00	(.84)	(.08)	(21.01)	(6.72)	(8.68)
	13.10	(3.00)	(.66)	1150.0	—	(.42)	0	.67	4.58	10.70	(3.00)	(.30)	(75.00)	(24.00)	(31.00)
900	1.12	—	—	336.0	—	—	1.66	.07	.67	2.07	1.12	.12	22.40	—	7.00
	4.00	—	—	1200.0	—	—	6.00	.26	2.40	7.40	4.00	.41	80.00	—	25.00
901	.34	—	—	0	0	—	0	.04	.06	1.34	.15	.08	1.12	—	.60
	1.20	—	—	0	0	—	0	.15	.20	4.80	.55	.28	4.00	—	2.15
902	.48	—	—	0	0	—	0	.04	.08	1.54	—	—	.84	—	—
	1.70	—	—	0	0	—	0	.15	.27	5.50	—	—	3.00	—	—
903	.60	[6]1.56	.33	0	0	.07	0	.06	.11	2.30	.27	.15	1.38	—	—
	1.30	3.40	.71	0	0	.16	0	.12	.23	5.00	.59	.33	3.00	—	—
904	.45	—	.29	0	0	.07	0	.05	.09	1.89	—	—	1.23	—	—
	1.10	—	.71	0	0	.16	0	.12	.21	4.60	—	—	3.00	—	—
905	.34	(1.20)	(.04)	0	0	(.03)	0	.04	.06	1.32	(.14)	(.04)	.84	(.28)	(.56)
	1.20	(4.30)	(.15)	0	0	(.12)	0	.13	.23	4.70	(.50)	(.16)	3.00	(1.00)	(2.00)
906	2.46	1.12	(3.36)	14952.0	5.32	.18	7.56	.07	1.17	4.62	—	—	40.60	(26.70)	31.18
	8.80	4.00	(12.00)	53400.0	19.00	.63	27.00	.26	4.19	16.50	—	—	145.00	(96.00)	111.34
907	3.98	1.71	(3.36)	9156.0	3.92	(.14)	10.36	.07	1.17	4.62	(2.47)	(.20)	40.60	(14.85)	(24.37)
	14.20	6.10	(12.00)	32700.0	14.00	(.50)	37.00	.24	4.17	16.50	(8.80)	(.73)	145.00	(53.00)	(87.00)
908	2.38	.95	(.15)	3444.0	18.76	(.09)	4.48	.05	.75	3.28	(1.54)	(.12)	67.20	(47.62)	(13.73)
	8.50	3.40	(.54)	12300.0	67.00	(.33)	16.00	.17	· 2.69	11.70	(5.50)	(.44)	240.00	(170.00)	(49.00)
909	—	—	1.36	—	—	—	—	—	—	—	—	—	—	—	—
	—	—	4.87	—	—	—	—	—	—	—	—	—	—	—	—
910	8.15	(2.32)	(.70)	4172.0	14.28	(.04)	6.16	.10	1.22	6.24	(1.30)	(.18)	40.60	(7.59)	(7.28)
	29.10	(8.29)	(2.50)	14900.0	51.00	(.16)	22.00	.34	4.36	22.30	(4.60)	(.64)	145.00	(27.08)	(26.00)
911	.78	—	—	0	—	—	—	.12	.04	.73	—	—	1.12	—	—
	2.80	—	—	0	—	—	—	.44	.15	2.60	—	—	4.00	—	—
912	.50	.42	.01	Trace	0	.02	0	.05	.06	.73	(.14)	.03	1.40	Trace	(.29)
	1.80	1.50	.02	Trace	0	.06	0	.16	.22	2.60	(.51)	.10	5.00	Trace	(1.03)
913	1.65	.78	—	1828.4	4.20	—	0	.05	.40	2.30	—	—	—	—	—
	5.90	2.80	—	6530.0	15.00	—	0	.17	1.44	8.20	—	—	—	—	—
914	—	—	—	—	—	—	—	—	—	—	—	—	—	—	—
	—	—	—	—	—	—	—	—	—	—	—	—	—	—	—
915	.27	—	—	0	—	—	—	.02	.01	.21	—	—	—	—	—
	2.10	—	—	0	—	—	—	.14	.10	1.60	—	—	—	—	—
916	.64	—	—	0	0	—	0	.01	.03	.25	—	—	.56	—	—
	2.30	—	—	0	0	—	0	.04	.10	.90	—	—	2.00	—	—
917	1.51	—	—	1778.0	4.20	.10	0	.06	.36	1.60	.78	.05	8.40	—	3.89
	5.40	—	—	6350.0	15.00	.35	0	.20	1.30	5.70	2.78	.19	30.00	—	13.90
918	1.65	—	—	1828.4	—	—	—	.05	.40	2.30	—	—	8.40	—	—
	5.90	—	—	6350.0	—	—	—	.17	1.44	8.20	—	—	30.00	—	—
919	1.26	—	—	—	—	—	—	.09	.15	1.75	—	—	—	—	—
	1.80	—	—	—	—	—	—	.13	.22	2.50	—	—	—	—	—
920	.59	—	—	0	—	—	—	.10	.06	.95	—	—	—	—	—
	2.10	—	—	0	—	—	—	.37	.22	3.40	—	—	—	—	—
921	.62	—	—	0	—	—	—	.09	.06	.84	.15	—	—	—	—
	2.20	—	—	0	—	—	—	.31	.21	3.00	.55	—	—	—	—
922	—	—	—	—	—	—	—	.01	.06	.34	—	—	—	—	—
	—	—	—	—	—	—	—	.03	.22	1.20	—	—	—	—	—
923	.73	—	—	—	—	.03	—	.07	.07	1.15	—	—	.56	—	—
	2.60	—	—	—	—	.11	—	.25	.24	4.10	—	—	2.00	—	—
924	1.01	(.50)	(.07)	0	0	(.08)	0	.10	.07	1.48	(.22)	.03	.56	(.87)	.39
	3.60	(1.79)	(.25)	0	0	(.27)	0	.37	.25	5.30	(.80)	.12	2.00	(3.09)	1.40
925	.48	.52	.02	—	—	—	—	.11	.04	.59	—	.06	.90	—	.21
	1.70	1.86	.06	—	—	—	—	.38	.13	2.09	—	.23	3.20	—	.74
926	4.26	9.86	.32	Trace	Trace	.50	0	.02	.31	3.70	1.03	.16	10.14	2.26	2.24
	3.80	8.80	.29	Trace	Trace	.45	0	.02	.28	3.30	.92	.14	9.05	2.02	2.00
927	2.16	—	—	—	—	—	—	—	—	—	—	—	—	—	—
	7.70	—	—	—	—	—	—	—	—	—	—	—	—	—	—
928	—	—	—	—	—	—	0	.01	.05	.38	—	—	—	—	—
	—	—	—	—	—	—	0	.09	.30	2.50	—	—	—	—	—
929	1.04	—	—	—	—	—	—	—	—	—	—	—	—	—	—
	3.70	—	—	—	—	—	—	—	—	—	—	—	—	—	—
930	—	—	—	—	—	—	—	—	—	—	—	—	—	—	—
	—	—	—	—	—	—	—	—	—	—	—	—	—	—	—
931	.81	—	—	0	0	—	0	.14	.06	1.37	—	—	—	—	—
	2.90	—	—	0	0	—	0	.50	.23	4.90	—	—	—	—	—

(Continued)

TABLE F-21 *(Continued)*

Item No.	Food Item Name	Approximate Measure	Weight (g)	Moisture (%)	Food Energy Calories (kcal)	Protein (g)	Fats (g)	Carbo-hydrates (g)	Fiber (g)	Minerals (Macro) Calcium (mg)	Phos-phorus (mg)	Sodium (mg)	Mag-nesium (mg)	Potas-sium (mg)
	PORK, FRESH (Continued)													
932	**BOSTON BUTT,** medium fat, total edible, roasted, 79% lean, 21% fat	1 OZ	28	48.1	98.8	6.3	8.0	0	0	2.8	64.1	10.4	5.9	72.8
			100	48.1	353.0	22.5	28.5	0	0	10.0	229.0	37.0	21.0	260.0
933	**'GROUND,** lean meat & fat, cooked	1 OZ	28	45.2	104.4	6.3	8.6	0	0	2.8	65.0	18.2	6.4	109.2
			100	45.2	373.0	22.6	30.6	0	0	10.0	232.0	65.0	23.0	390.0
934	**HAM,** medium fat, total edible, roasted, 82% lean, 18% fat	1 OZ	28	45.5	76.7	6.4	5.7	0	0	2.8	66.1	18.2	—	109.2
			100	45.5	274.0	23.0	20.2	0	0	10.0	236.0	65.0	—	390.0
935	**HAM,** medium fat, separable lean, roasted	1 OZ	28	58.9	56.0	8.3	2.5	0	0	3.6	86.2	18.2	—	109.2
			100	58.9	200.0	29.7	9.0	0	0	13.0	308.0	65.0	—	390.0
936	**HAM,** thin class, total edible, roasted, 77% lean, 23% fat	1 OZ	28	47.8	96.9	6.8	7.5	0	0	3.1	70.6	18.2	—	109.2
			100	47.8	346.0	24.2	26.9	0	0	11.0	252.0	65.0	—	390.0
937	**LOIN,** fat class, total edible, roasted, 79% lean, 21% fat	1 OZ	28	43.7	108.4	6.6	7.9	0	0	2.8	68.6	18.2	5.6	109.2
			100	43.7	387.0	23.5	28.1	0	0	10.0	245.0	65.0	20.0	390.0
938	**LOIN,** medium fat, total edible, roasted, 80% lean, 20% fat	1 OZ	28	45.8	101.4	6.9	8.0	0	0	3.1	71.7	14.0	5.6	98.6
			100	45.8	362.0	24.5	28.5	0	0	11.0	256.0	50.0	20.0	352.0
939	**'LOIN TENDERLOIN,** lean meat, cooked	1 OZ	28	55.0	71.1	8.2	4.0	0	0	3.6	86.8	18.2	5.6	109.2
			100	55.0	254.0	29.4	14.2	0	0	13.0	310.0	65.0	20.0	390.0
940	**PICNIC,** medium fat, total edible, simmered, 74% lean, 26% fat	1 OZ	28	45.7	104.7	6.5	8.5	0	0	2.8	38.9	—	3.9	—
			100	45.7	374.0	23.2	30.5	0	0	10.0	139.0	—	14.0	—
941	**'SHOULDER BLADE STEAK,** bone-in, lean meat, cooked	1 OZ	28	57.5	68.3	7.6	4.0	0	0	3.4	77.6	18.2	—	109.2
			100	57.5	244.0	27.0	14.3	0	0	12.0	277.0	65.0	—	390.0
942	**'SHOULDER,** boneless, lean meat, cooked	1 OZ	28	60.3	59.4	8.1	2.7	0	0	3.4	49.3	18.2	5.0	109.2
			100	60.3	212.0	29.0	9.8	0	0	12.0	176.0	65.0	18.0	390.0
943	**SPARERIBS,** medium fat, total edible, braised	1 MED	15	39.7	66.0	3.1	5.8	0	0	1.4	18.2	9.8	3.8	58.5
			100	39.7	440.0	20.8	38.9	0	0	9.0	121.0	65.0	25.0	390.0
944	**PORK, CANNED,** w/gravy, 90% gravy, canned	1 OZ	28	56.9	71.7	4.6	5.0	1.8	0	3.6	51.2	—	—	—
			100	56.9	256.0	16.4	17.8	6.3	0	13.0	183.0	—	—	—
	PORK, CURED													
945	**BOSTON BUTT,** medium fat, separable lean, cooked	1 OZ	28	53.9	68.0	7.8	3.9	0	0	3.4	61.0	260.4	—	91.3
			100	53.9	243.0	27.8	13.8	0	0	12.0	218.0	930.0	—	326.0
946	**HAM,** canned	1 OZ	28	65.0	54.0	5.1	3.2	.3	0	3.1	43.7	308.0	—	95.2
			100	65.0	193.0	18.3	11.3	.9	0	11.0	156.0	1100.0	—	340.0
947	**HAM,** dry, long-cure, country-style, medium fat	1 OZ	28	42.0	108.9	4.7	9.8	.1	0	—	—	—	—	—
			100	42.0	389.0	16.9	35.0	.3	0	—	—	—	—	—
948	**HAM,** light-cure, medium fat, separable lean, roasted	1 OZ	28	61.9	52.4	7.1	2.5	0	0	3.1	56.0	260.4	5.6	91.3
			100	61.9	187.0	25.3	8.8	0	0	11.0	200.0	930.0	20.0	326.0
949	**HAM, PICNIC,** medium fat, total edible, roasted, 82% lean, 18% fat	1 OZ	28	48.8	88.5	6.3	7.1	0	0	2.8	51.0	—	—	—
			100	48.8	316.0	22.4	25.2	0	0	10.0	182.0	—	—	—
950	**SALT PORK,** fried	1 SLICE	25	—	170.5	3.0	17.5	0	0	2.0	30.0	—	—	—
			100	—	682.0	12.0	70.0	0	0	8.0	120.0	—	—	—
951	**QUAIL,** total edible, raw	1 OZ	28	65.9	47.0	7.0	1.9	0	0	4.2	75.6	11.2	—	49.0
			100	65.9	168.0	25.0	6.8	0	0	15.0	270.0	40.0	—	175.0
952	**RABBIT DOMESTICATED,** flesh only, stewed	1 OZ	28	59.8	60.5	8.2	2.8	0	0	5.9	72.5	11.5	—	103.0
			100	59.8	216.0	29.3	10.1	0	0	21.0	259.0	41.0	—	368.0
953	**RABBIT, WILD,** flesh only, raw	1 OZ	28	73.0	37.8	5.9	1.4	0	0	—	—	13.2	8.1	116.2
			100	73.0	135.0	21.0	5.0	0	0	—	—	47.0	29.0	415.0
954	**REINDEER,** total edible, 84% lean, 16% fat, raw	1 OZ	28	63.3	60.8	5.7	4.0	0	0	—	—	—	—	—
			100	63.3	217.0	20.5	14.4	0	0	—	—	—	—	—
	SAUSAGES													
955	**BLOOD SAUSAGE,** or blood pudding	1 SLICE	60	46.4	236.4	8.5	22.1	.2	0	4.8	96.0	—	—	—
			100	46.4	394.0	14.1	36.9	.3	0	8.0	160.0	—	—	—
956	**BOCKWURST**	1 OZ	28	61.9	73.9	3.2	6.6	.2	0	—	—	—	—	—
			100	61.9	264.0	11.3	23.7	.6	0	—	—	—	—	—
957	**BROWN & SERVE,** browned	1 OZ	28	39.9	118.2	4.6	10.6	.8	0	—	—	—	—	—
			100	39.9	422.0	16.5	37.8	2.8	0	—	—	—	—	—
958	**COUNTRY STYLE**	1 OZ	28	49.9	96.6	4.2	8.7	0	0	2.5	47.0	—	4.5	—
			100	49.9	345.0	15.1	31.1	0	0	9.0	168.0	—	16.0	—
959	**LINKS OR BULK,** cooked	1 OZ	28	44.6	103.3	5.1	9.1	0	0	2.0	45.4	268.2	4.5	75.3
			100	44.6	369.0	18.1	32.5	0	0	7.0	162.0	958.0	16.0	269.0
960	**POLISH STYLE**	1 OZ	28	53.7	85.1	4.4	7.2	.3	0	2.5	49.3	—	—	—
			100	53.7	304.0	15.7	25.8	1.2	0	9.0	176.0	—	—	—
961	**SCRAPPLE**	1 SLICE	57	61.3	122.6	5.0	7.8	8.3	.1	2.9	36.5	—	—	—
			100	61.3	215.0	8.8	13.6	14.6	.1	5.0	64.0	—	—	—
962	**SOUSE**	1 SLICE	60	70.3	108.6	7.8	8.0	.7	0	4.2	85.2	—	—	—
			100	70.3	181.0	13.0	13.4	1.2	0	7.0	142.0	—	—	—
963	**THURINGER**	1 OZ	28	48.5	86.0	5.2	6.9	.4	0	3.1	59.9	—	—	—
			100	48.5	307.0	18.6	24.5	1.6	0	11.0	214.0	—	—	—

Item No.	Minerals (Micro)			Fat-Soluble Vitamins			Water-Soluble Vitamins								
	Iron	Zinc	Copper	Vitamin A	Vitamin D	Vitamin E (Alpha Tocopherol)	Vitamin C	Thiamin	Riboflavin	Niacin	Pantothenic Acid	Vit. B-6 (Pyridoxine)	Folacin (Folic Acid)	Biotin	Vitamin B-12
	(mg)	(mg)	(mg)	(IU)	(IU)	(mg)	(mg)	(mg)	(mg)	(mg)	(mg)	(mg)	(mcg)	(mcg)	(mcg)
932	.81	–	–	0	0	–	0	.14	.06	1.23	–	–	–	–	–
	2.90	–	–	0	0	–	0	.50	.23	4.40	–	–	–	–	–
933	.81	.85	–	0	–	–	0	.14	.06	1.37	–	–	1.40	–	–
	2.90	3.04	–	0	–	–	0	.50	.23	4.90	–	–	5.00	–	–
934	.84	–	–	0	0	–	0	.14	.06	1.29	.18	.12	–		–
	3.00	–	–	0	0	–	0	.51	.23	4.60	.64	.44	–	–	–
935	1.06	1.12	–	0	0	–	0	.18	.08	1.60	–	–	1.40	–	–
	3.80	4.00	–	0	0	–	0	.64	.29	5.70	–	–	5.00	–	–
936	.90	–	–	0	0	–	0	.15	.07	1.34	.18	.12	–	–	–
	3.20	–	–	0	0	–	0	.54	.25	4.80	.64	.44	–	–	–
937	.87	–	.08	0	0	–	0	.25	.07	1.48	.11	.13	22.40	–	.84
	3.10	–	.30	0	0	–	0	.88	.25	5.30	.40	.48	80.00	–	3.00
938	.90	–	.08	0	0	–	0	.26	.07	1.57	.11	.13	–	–	.84
	3.20	–	.30	0	0	–	0	.92	.26	5.60	.40	.48	–	–	3.00
939	1.06	1.12	.08	0	–	–	0	.30	.09	1.82	.13	.03	1.40	1.40	.84
	3.80	4.00	.30	0	–	–	0	1.08	.31	6.50	.47	.10	5.00	5.00	3.00
940	.84	–	–	0	0	–	0	.15	.07	1.34	–	–	–	–	–
	3.00	–	–	0	0	–	0	.54	.25	4.80	–	–	–	–	–
941	.95	1.26	–	0	0	–	0	.17	.08	1.46	–	–	1.40	–	–
	3.40	4.50	–	0	0	–	0	.59	.27	5.20	–	–	5.00	–	–
942	1.01	1.12	–	0	0	–	0	.19	.08	1.65	–	–	1.40	–	–
	3.60	4.00	–	0	0	–	0	.66	.30	5.90	–	–	5.00	–	–
943	.39	–	–	0	–	–	0	.07	.03	.51	–	–	–	–	–
	2.60	–	–	0	–	–	0	.43	.21	3.40	–	–	–	–	–
944	.67	–	–	0	–	–	–	.14	.05	.98	–	–	–	–	–
	2.40	–	–	0	–	–	–	.49	.17	3.50	–	–	–	–	–
945	1.01	–	–	0	–	–	–	.18	.07	1.40	–	–	–	–	–
	3.60	–	–	0	–	–	–	.64	.25	5.00	–	–	–	–	–
946	.76	6 .64	–	0	–	–	–	.15	.05	1.06	–	.10	–	–	–
	2.70	2.30	–	0	–	–	–	.53	.19	3.80	–	.36	–	–	–
947	–	–	–	0	–	–	0	–	–	–	–	–	–	–	–
	–	–	–	0	–	–	0	–	–	–	–	–	–	–	–
948	.90	–	–	0	–	–	–	.16	.06	1.26	–	–	–	–	–
	3.20	–	–	0	–	–	–	.58	.23	4.50	–	–	–	–	–
949	.81	–	–	0	–	–	–	.15	.06	1.12	–	–	–	–	–
	2.90	–	–	0	–	–	–	.52	.20	4.00	–	–	–	–	–
950	.40	–	–	0	0	–	0	.07	.03	.50	–	–	–	–	–
	1.60	–	–	0	0	–	0	.28	.10	2.00	–	–	–	–	–
951	1.06	–	–	–	–	–	–	–	–	–	–	–	–	–	–
	3.80	–	–	–	–	–	–	–	–	–	–	–	–	–	–
952	.42	–	–	–	–	–	0	.01	.02	3.16	(.22)	(.14)	(1.12)	(.28)	(3.36)
	1.50	–	–	–	–	–	0	.05	.07	11.30	(.80)	(.50)	(4.00)	(1.00)	(12.00)
953	–	–	–	–	–	–	0	–	–	–	.22	.12	–	–	–
	–	–	–	–	–	–	0	–	–	–	.78	.44	–	–	–
954	–	–	–	–	–	–	–	–	–	–	–	–	–	–	–
	–	–	–	–	–	–	–	–	–	–	–	–	–	–	–
955	1.32	–	–	–	0	–	0	–	–	–	–	.02	–	–	–
	2.20	–	–	–	0	–	0	–	–	–	–	.04	–	–	–
956	–	–	–	–	–	–	–	–	–	–	–	–	–	–	–
	–	–	–	–	–	–	–	–	–	–	–	–	–	–	–
957	–	–	–	–	–	–	–	–	–	–	–	–	–	–	–
	–	–	–	–	–	–	–	–	–	–	–	–	–	–	–
958	.64	–	–	–	–	–	–	.06	.05	.87	–	–	3.92	–	–
	2.30	–	–	–	–	–	–	.22	.19	3.10	–	–	14.00	–	–
959	.67	–	–	0	0	.05	0	.22	.10	1.04	–	–	–	–	–
	2.40	–	–	0	0	.16	0	.79	.34	3.70	–	–	–	–	–
960	.67	–	–	0	0	–	0	.10	.05	.87	–	–	–	–	–
	2.40	–	–	0	0	–	0	.34	.19	3.10	–	–	–	–	–
961	.68	–	–	–	0	–	0	.11	.05	1.03	–	–	–	–	–
	1.20	–	–	–	0	–	0	.19	.09	1.80	–	–	–	–	–
962	1.20	–	–	0	0	–	0	–	–	–	–	–	–	–	–
	2.00	–	–	0	0	–	0	–	–	–	–	–	–	–	–
963	.78	–	–	–	–	–	–	.03	.07	1.18	–	–	–	–	–
	2.80	–	–	–	–	–	–	.11	.26	4.20	–	–	–	–	–

(Continued)

TABLE F-21 *(Continued)*

Item No.	Food Item Name	Approximate Measure	Weight (g)	Moisture (%)	Food Energy Calories (kcal)	Protein (g)	Fats (g)	Carbo-hydrates (g)	Fiber (g)	Minerals (Macro)				
										Calcium (mg)	Phos-phorus (mg)	Sodium (mg)	Mag-nesium (mg)	Potas-sium (mg)
	SAUSAGES (Continued)													
964	**VIENNA,** canned	1 OZ	28	63.0	67.2	4.4	5.5	.1	0	2.2	42.8	—	—	—
			100	63.0	240.0	15.8	19.8	.3	0	8.0	153.0	—	—	—
965	**SQUAB (PIGEON),** total edible, raw	1 OZ	28	58.0	78.1	5.2	6.2	0	0	4.8	115.1	—	—	—
			100	58.0	279.0	18.6	22.1	0	0	17.0	411.0	—	—	—
966	**SQUIRREL,** cooked	1 OZ	28	—	60.5	8.2	2.8	0	—	5.9	72.5	—	6.4	—
			100	—	216.0	29.3	10.1	0	—	21.0	259.0	—	23.0	—
	SWEETBREAD (THYMUS)													
967	**BEEF,** yearling, braised	1 OZ	28	49.6	89.6	7.3	6.5	0	0	—	101.9	32.5	—	121.2
			100	49.6	320.0	25.9	23.2	0	0	—	364.0	116.0	—	433.0
968	**CALF,** braised	1 OZ	28	62.7	47.0	9.1	.9	0	0	—	—	—	—	—
			100	62.7	168.0	32.6	3.2	0	0	—	—	—	—	—
969	**¹SWIFTLET NEST,** (used in bird's nest soup), dried	1 OZ	28	12.6	96.6	15.0	.1	8.2	—	131.6	5.0	58.8	—	15.4
			100	12.6	345.0	53.4	.4	29.3	—	470.0	18.0	210.0	—	55.0
	TONGUE													
970	**BEEF,** medium fat, braised	1 OZ	28	60.8	68.3	6.0	4.7	.1	0	2.0	32.8	17.1	4.5	45.9
			100	60.8	244.0	21.5	16.7	.4	0	7.0	117.0	61.0	16.0	164.0
971	**BEEF,** smoked	1 SLICE	20	48.9	—	3.4	5.8	—	0	—	—	—	—	—
			100	48.9	—	17.2	28.8	—	0	—	—	—	—	—
	TRIPE, BEEF													
972	commercial	1 OZ	28	79.1	28.0	5.3	.6	0	0	35.6	24.1	20.2	(4.3)	2.5
			100	79.1	100.0	19.1	2.0	0	0	127.0	86.0	72.0	(15.4)	9.0
973	pickled	1 OZ	28	86.5	17.4	3.3	.4	0	0	—	—	12.9	—	5.3
			100	86.5	62.0	11.8	1.3	0	0	—	—	46.0	—	19.0
	TURKEY													
974	total edible, roasted	1 SLICE	40	55.4	105.2	10.8	6.6	0	0	—	—	—	11.2	—
			100	55.4	263.0	27.0	16.4	0	0	—	—	—	28.0	—
975	²bologna	1 OZ	28	65.1	55.7	3.8	4.3	.3	—	23.5	36.7	245.8	3.9	55.7
			100	65.1	199.0	13.7	15.2	1.0	—	84.0	131.0	878.0	14.0	199.0
976	²frankfurter	1 OZ	28	63.0	63.3	4.0	5.0	.4	—	29.7	37.5	399.3	—	50.1
			100	63.0	226.0	14.3	17.7	1.5	—	106.0	134.0	1426.0	—	179.0
977	**TURTLE,** green, raw	1 OZ	28	78.5	24.9	5.5	.1	0	0	—	—	—	—	—
			100	78.5	89.0	19.8	.5	0	0	—	—	—	—	—
	VEAL													
978	chop	1 OZ	28	54.6	75.3	7.6	4.7	0	0	3.4	69.4	22.4	5.6	140.0
			100	54.6	269.0	27.2	16.9	0	0	12.0	248.0	80.0	20.0	500.0
979	chuck, medium fat, total edible, braised, 85% lean, 15% fat	1 OZ	28	58.5	65.8	7.8	3.6	0	0	3.4	42.3	22.4	—	140.0
			100	58.5	235.0	27.9	12.8	0	0	12.0	151.0	80.0	—	500.0
980	cutlet, total edible, cooked	1 OZ	28	—	77.6	9.3	4.2	0	0	2.8	80.6	15.1	6.4	147.6
			100	—	277.0	33.2	15.0	0	0	10.0	288.0	54.0	23.0	527.0
981	loin, medium fat, total edible, broiled, 77% lean, 23% fat	1 OZ	28	58.9	65.5	7.4	3.8	0	0	3.1	63.0	22.4	—	140.0
			100	58.9	234.0	26.4	13.4	0	0	11.0	225.0	80.0	—	500.0
982	rib, medium fat, roasted, 82% lean, 18% fat	1 OZ	28	54.6	75.3	7.6	4.7	0	0	3.4	69.4	22.4	5.6	140.0
			100	54.6	269.0	27.2	16.9	0	0	12.0	248.0	80.0	20.0	500.0
983	round, w/rump, medium fat, total edible, broiled, 79% lean, 21% fat	1 OZ	28	60.4	64.8	8.1	3.3	0	0	3.3	69.3	24.0	—	150.0
			100	60.4	216.0	27.1	11.1	0	0	11.0	231.0	80.0	—	500.0
984	¹shoulder arm roast, slice, boneless, lean & fat, cooked	1 OZ	28	58.5	65.8	7.8	3.6	0	0	3.4	42.3	22.4	—	140.0
			100	58.5	235.0	27.9	12.8	0	0	12.0	151.0	80.0	—	500.0
985	**VENISON,** lean only, cooked	1 OZ	28	—	48.7	8.4	1.7	0	—	2.5	95.5	—	9.2	—
			100	—	174.0	30.0	6.0	0	—	9.0	341.0	—	33.0	—
	MILK AND PRODUCTS													
	BUTTER													
986	regular, salted	1 TSP	5	15.9	35.9	0	4.1	0	0	1.2	1.2	41.3	.1	1.3
			100	15.9	717.0	.9	81.1	.1	0	24.0	23.0	826.0	2.0	26.0
987	salt free	1 TSP	5	—	35.8	0	4.1	0	0	1.0	.8	.4	.1	1.2
			100	—	716.0	.6	81.0	.4	0	20.0	16.0	8.0	2.0	23.0
988	whipped	1 TBLS	9	16.0	64.0	.1	7.3	0	0	2.2	2.1	74.3	.2	2.3
			100	16.0	711.0	.9	81.0	.1	0	24.0	23.0	826.0	2.0	26.0
989	**BUTTERMILK,** fluid, made from skim milk	1 CUP	244	90.5	87.8	8.4	2.1	11.7	0	295.2	217.2	256.2	26.8	368.4
			100	90.5	36.0	3.4	.9	4.8	0	121.0	89.0	105.0	11.0	151.0
	CARNATION INSTANT BREAKFAST MIX													
990	chocolate	1 PKG	36	—	130.0	7.0	1.0	23.0	—	100.0	150.0	110.0	80.0	380.0
			100	—	361.1	19.4	2.8	63.9	—	277.8	416.7	305.6	222.2	1055.6
991	vanilla	1 PKG	35	—	130.0	7.0	0	24.0	—	100.0	150.0	120.0	80.0	360.0
			100	—	371.4	20.0	0	68.6	—	285.7	428.6	342.9	228.6	1028.6
992	vanilla, in whole milk	1 CUP	276	—	280.0	15.0	8.0	35.0	—	407.0	386.0	242.0	114.4	711.0
			100	—	101.4	5.4	2.9	12.7	—	147.5	139.9	87.7	41.4	257.6

Item No.	Minerals (Micro)			Fat-Soluble Vitamins			Water-Soluble Vitamins								
	Iron	Zinc	Copper	Vitamin A	Vitamin D	Vitamin E (Alpha Tocopherol)	Vitamin C	Thiamin	Ribo-flavin	Niacin	Panto-thenic Acid	Vit. B-6 (Pyri-doxine)	Folacin (Folic Acid)	Biotin	Vitamin B-12
	(mg)	(mg)	(mg)	(IU)	(IU)	(mg)	(mg)	(mg)	(mg)	(mg)	(mg)	(mg)	(mcg)	(mcg)	(mcg)
964	.59	–	–	–	0	–	0	.02	.04	.73	–	.02	–	–	–
	2.10	–	–	–	0	–	0	.08	.13	2.60	–	.08	–	–	–
965	–	–	–	–	–	–	0	.03	.07	1.57	–	–	–	–	–
	–	–	–	–	–	–	0	.10	.24	5.60	–	–	–	–	–
966	.42	–	–	0	–	–	0	.01	.02	3.16	–	.07	–	–	.20
	1.50	–	–	0	–	–	0	.05	.07	11.30	–	.26	–	–	.72
967	–	–	–	–	–	–	–	–	–	–	–	–	–	–	–
	–	–	–	–	–	–	–	–	–	–	–	–	–	–	–
968	–	–	–	–	–	–	–	.03	.08	.81	–	–	–	–	–
	–	–	–	–	–	–	–	.09	.27	2.90	–	–	–	–	–
969	1.20	–	–	0	–	–	0	.014	–	–	–	–	–	–	–
	4.30	–	–	0	–	–	0	.05	–	–	–	–	–	–	–
970	.62	–	–	0	0	.10	0	.01	.08	.98	(.15)	(.03)	(1.41)	(.86)	(1.12)
	2.20	–	–	0	0	.35	0	.05	.29	3.50	(.52)	(.09)	(5.05)	(3.06)	(4.00)
971	–	–	–	–	–	–	–	.01	.04	.60	.12	–	–	–	–
	–	–	–	–	–	–	–	.04	.21	3.00	.60	–	–	–	–
972	.45	(.65)	(.04)	0	0	(.03)	0	Trace	.04	.45	(.07)	Trace	(.28)	(.57)	Trace
	1.60	(2.31)	(.16)	0	0	(.09)	0	Trace	.15	1.60	(.24)	(.02)	(1.00)	(2.02)	Trace
973	–	–	–	–	–	–	–	–	–	–	–	–	–	–	–
	–	–	–	–	–	–	–	–	–	–	–	–	–	–	–
974	–	–	–	–	–	–	–	–	–	–	–	–	–	–	–
	–	–	–	–	–	–	–	–	–	–	–	–	–	–	–
975	.43	.49	.01	–	–	–	–	.02	.05	.99	–	–	–	–	–
	1.53	1.74	.03	–	–	–	–	.06	.17	3.53	–	–	–	–	–
976	.52	–	–	–	–	–	–	.01	.05	1.16	–	–	–	–	–
	1.84	–	–	–	–	–	–	.04	.18	4.13	–	–	–	–	–
977	–	–	–	–	–	–	–	–	–	–	–	–	–	–	–
	–	–	–	–	–	–	–	–	–	–	–	–	–	–	–
978	.95	–	–	0	0	–	0	.04	.09	2.18	–	–	1.40	–	–
	3.40	–	–	0	0	–	0	.13	.31	7.80	–	–	5.00	–	–
979	.98	–	–	0	0	–	0	.03	.08	1.79	–	–	.84	–	–
	3.50	(4.10)	–	0	0	–	0	.09	.29	6.40	–	–	3.00	–	–
980	1.18	–	–	0	0	–	0	.03	.09	1.79	–	–	.84	Trace	(.28)
	4.20	–	–	0	0	–	0	.12	.32	6.40	–	–	3.00	Trace	(1.00)
981	.90	–	–	0	0	–	0	.02	.07	1.51	–	–	.84	–	–
	3.20	–	–	0	0	–	0	.07	.25	5.40	–	–	3.00	–	–
982	.95	–	–	0	0	–	0	.04	.09	2.18	–	–	.84	–	–
	3.40	–	–	0	0	–	0	.13	.31	7.80	–	–	3.00	–	–
983	.96	–	–	0	0	–	0	.02	.08	1.62	–	–	.90	–	–
	3.20	(4.10)	–	0	0	–	0	.07	.25	5.40	–	–	3.00	–	–
984	.98	1.00	–	–	–	–	–	.03	.08	1.79	–	–	.84	–	–
	3.50	3.56	–	–	–	–	–	.09	.29	6.40	–	–	3.00	–	–
985	.62	–	–	0	–	–	0	.01	.07	1.26	–	.11	–	–	.40
	2.20	–	–	0	–	–	0	.02	.24	4.50	–	.38	–	–	1.44
986	.01	0	.02	152.9	(.04)	.08	0	0	0	0	Trace	0	.15	Trace	Trace
	.16	.05	.39	3058.0	(.76)	1.58	0	.01	.03	.04	Trace	0	3.00	Trace	Trace
987	0	–	–	165.0	–	–	0	–	–	–	–	–	.15	–	–
	0	–	–	3300.0	–	–	0	–	–	–	–	–	3.00	–	–
988	.01	.01	–	275.2	–	–	0	0	0	0	–	0	.27	–	–
	.16	.05	–	3058.0	–	–	0	.01	.03	.04	–	.03	3.00	–	–
989	.12	.90	.01	80.5	–	–	2.44	.10	.44	.14	.75	.09	0	0	.54
	.05	.37	0	33.0	–	–	1.00	.04	.18	.06	.31	.04	0	0	.22
990	4.50	3.00	.50	1000.0	0	5.03	24.00	.30	.07	5.00	2.00	.40	100.00	–	600.00
	12.50	8.33	1.39	2777.8	0	13.98	66.67	.83	.19	13.89	5.56	1.11	277.78	–	1666.67
991	4.50	5.00	.50	1000.0	0	5.03	24.00	.30	.07	5.00	2.00	.40	100.00	–	.60
	12.86	14.29	1.43	2857.1	0	14.38	68.57	.86	.20	14.29	5.71	1.14	285.71	–	1.71
992	4.62	3.66	.52	1250.0	100.00	5.19	26.40	.40	.56	5.23	2.66	.51	100.00	–	1530.00
	1.67	1.33	.19	452.9	36.23	1.88	9.57	.15	.20	1.90	.96	.19	36.23	–	554.35

(Continued)

TABLE F-21 (Continued)

Item No.	Food Item Name	Approximate Measure	Weight	Moisture	Food Energy Calories	Protein	Fats	Carbo-hydrates	Fiber	Minerals (Macro) Calcium	Phos-phorus	Sodium	Mag-nesium	Potas-sium
			(g)	(%)	(kcal)	(g)	(g)	(g)	(g)	(mg)	(mg)	(mg)	(mg)	(mg)
	CHEESE FOOD													
993	**AMERICAN**, pasteurized process	1 OZ	28	43.2	91.4	5.5	6.7	2.0	0	159.6	128.5	332.9	8.7	78.1
			100	43.2	326.4	19.6	24.0	7.1	0	570.0	459.0	1189.0	31.0	279.0
994	**SWISS**, pasteurized process	1 OZ	28	43.7	90.4	6.1	6.8	1.3	0	202.4	147.3	434.6	7.8	79.5
			100	43.7	323.0	21.9	24.1	4.5	0	723.0	526.0	1552.0	28.0	284.0
	CHEESE, NATURAL													
995	**BLUE**	1 OZ	28	42.4	100.5	6.0	8.0	.7	0	147.6	109.5	390.3	6.4	71.7
			100	42.4	359.0	21.4	28.7	2.3	0	527.0	391.0	1393.9	22.7	256.0
996	**BRICK**	1 OZ	28	41.0	103.9	6.5	8.2	.8	0	188.7	127.4	156.7	6.7	37.5
			100	41.0	371.0	23.2	29.4	2.8	0	674.0	455.0	559.7	24.0	133.8
997	**BRIE**	1 OZ	28	48.4	93.5	5.8	7.8	.1	0	51.5	52.6	176.1	—	42.6
			100	48.4	334.0	20.8	27.7	.5	0	184.0	188.0	629.0	—	152.0
998	**CAMEMBERT**	1 OZ	28	51.5	83.8	5.5	6.8	.1	0	108.4	97.2	235.8	5.9	52.2
			100	51.5	299.2	19.7	24.2	.5	0	387.2	347.0	842.0	21.1	186.5
999	**CARAWAY**	1 OZ	28	39.3	105.5	7.0	8.2	.9	0	188.3	137.0	193.2	5.9	—
			100	39.3	376.6	25.1	29.1	3.1	0	672.3	489.3	689.9	21.1	—
1000	**CHEDDAR**	1 OZ	28	38.5	112.7	7.0	9.3	.4	0	201.1	142.9	173.5	7.9	27.6
			100	38.5	402.4	24.9	33.1	1.3	0	718.1	510.4	619.5	28.2	98.6
1001	**CHESHIRE**	1 OZ	28	37.7	108.4	6.5	8.6	1.3	0	180.0	129.9	196.0	5.9	26.6
			100	37.7	387.0	23.4	30.6	4.8	0	643.0	464.0	700.0	21.0	95.0
1002	**COLBY**	1 OZ	28	38.2	110.3	6.7	9.0	.7	0	191.8	127.7	169.1	7.5	35.3
			100	38.2	394.0	23.8	32.1	2.6	0	685.0	456.0	604.0	26.8	126.0
1003	**COTTAGE**, large or small curd, uncreamed, 2% fat	1 CUP	226	79.3	203.4	31.1	4.4	8.2	0	153.7	339.0	917.6	13.6	217.0
			100	79.3	90.0	13.7	1.9	3.6	0	68.0	150.0	406.0	6.0	96.0
1004	**COTTAGE**, large or small curd, creamed	1 CUP	225	79.0	232.5	28.1	10.1	6.0	0	135.0	296.8	911.3	11.3	189.6
			100	79.0	103.3	12.5	4.5	2.7	0	60.0	131.9	405.0	5.0	84.3
1005	**CREAM**	1 TBLS	15	54.2	52.4	1.1	5.1	.4	0	12.2	16.2	44.4	.9	18.5
			100	54.2	349.0	7.5	33.8	2.6	0	81.1	108.0	296.3	6.0	123.4
1006	**EDAM**	1 OZ	28	41.6	100.0	6.8	7.8	.4	0	204.7	150.1	270.2	8.4	52.6
			100	41.6	357.0	24.4	27.9	1.4	0	731.0	536.0	965.0	30.0	188.0
1007	**FETA**	1 OZ	28	55.2	73.9	4.0	6.0	1.1	0	137.8	94.4	312.5	5.3	17.4
			100	55.2	264.0	14.2	21.3	4.1	0	492.0	337.0	1116.0	19.0	62.0
1008	**FONTINA**	1 BAR	28	37.9	108.9	7.2	8.7	.4	0	154.0	—	—	3.9	—
			100	37.9	389.0	25.6	31.1	1.6	0	550.0	—	—	14.0	—
1009	**'GOAT'S MILK**	1 OZ	28	65.1	48.4	4.5	2.9	1.0	—	86.8	40.9	—	—	—
			100	65.1	173.0	16.0	10.3	3.7	—	310.0	146.0	—	—	—
1010	**GOUDA**	1 OZ	28	41.5	99.7	7.0	7.7	.6	0	196.0	152.9	299.3	8.1	33.6
			100	41.5	356.0	24.9	27.4	2.2	0	700.0	546.0	819.0	29.0	120.0
1011	**GRUYERE**	1 OZ	28	33.2	115.6	8.3	9.0	.1	0	283.1	169.4	94.1	—	22.7
			100	33.2	413.0	29.8	32.0	.3	0	1011.0	605.0	336.0	—	81.0
1012	**LIMBURGER**	1 OZ	28	48.4	91.8	5.9	7.6	.1	0	139.2	110.0	224.0	5.9	35.8
			100	48.4	328.0	21.2	27.2	.5	0	497.0	393.0	800.0	21.0	128.0
1013	**MONTEREY**	1 OZ	28	—	104.7	6.9	8.5	.2	0	209.4	124.4	150.1	7.9	22.7
			100	—	373.8	24.5	30.3	.7	0	747.7	444.4	536.1	28.2	81.1
1014	**MOZZARELLA**	1 OZ	28	54.1	78.7	5.4	6.0	.6	0	144.8	103.9	104.4	5.3	18.8
			100	54.1	281.0	19.4	21.6	2.2	0	517.0	371.0	373.0	19.0	67.0
1015	**MUENSTER**	1 OZ	28	42.5	103.0	6.5	8.4	.3	0	200.5	131.0	175.8	7.3	37.5
			100	42.5	368.0	23.1	30.0	1.1	0	716.0	468.0	628.0	26.0	134.0
1016	**NEUFCHATEL**	1 OZ	28	62.2	72.8	2.8	6.6	.8	0	21.0	38.1	111.7	2.1	31.9
			100	62.2	260.0	10.0	23.4	2.9	0	75.0	136.0	399.0	7.6	114.0
1017	**PARMESAN**, grated	1 TBLS	5	17.7	22.8	2.1	1.5	.2	0	68.8	40.4	93.1	2.6	5.4
			100	17.7	456.0	41.6	30.0	3.7	0	1376.0	807.0	1862.0	51.0	107.0
1018	**PORT DU SALUT**	1 OZ	28	45.5	98.6	6.7	7.9	.2	0	182.0	100.8	149.5	—	—
			100	45.5	352.0	23.8	28.2	.6	0	650.0	360.0	534.0	—	—
1019	**PROVOLONE**	1 OZ	28	41.3	98.3	7.4	7.3	.6	0	211.7	138.9	245.3	7.6	38.6
			100	41.3	351.0	26.3	26.0	2.1	0	756.0	496.0	876.0	27.3	138.0
1020	**RICOTTA**, part skim	1 OZ	28	75.4	38.6	3.1	2.2	1.4	0	76.2	51.2	35.0	4.2	35.0
			100	75.4	138.0	11.1	7.9	5.1	0	272.0	183.0	125.0	15.0	125.0
1021	**ROMANO**	1 OZ	28	30.9	110.0	9.0	7.6	1.0	0	301.9	214.9	339.9	—	—
			100	30.9	392.7	32.2	27.3	3.7	0	1078.1	767.6	1213.8	—	—
1022	**ROQUEFORT**	1 OZ	28	40.0	103.3	6.0	8.6	.6	0	185.4	109.8	506.5	8.4	25.5
			100	40.0	369.0	21.5	30.6	2.0	0	662.0	392.0	1809.0	30.0	91.0
1023	**SWISS**, domestic	1 OZ	28	38.0	104.2	8.2	7.7	.9	0	269.1	169.4	72.8	10.1	31.1
			100	38.0	372.0	29.2	27.6	3.4	0	961.0	605.0	260.0	35.9	111.0
1024	**TILSIT**, made w/whole milk	1 OZ	28	42.9	95.2	6.8	7.3	.5	0	196.0	140.0	210.8	3.6	17.9
			100	42.9	340.0	24.4	26.0	1.9	0	700.0	500.0	753.0	13.0	64.0
1025	**CHEESE, PASTEURIZED PROCESS**, American	1 OZ	28	39.8	105.0	6.3	8.8	.4	0	172.5	208.6	400.4	6.2	45.4
			100	39.8	375.0	22.5	31.3	1.6	0	616.0	745.0	1430.0	22.0	162.0
1026	**CHEESE SPREAD**, American pasteurized process	1 OZ	28	48.6	80.6	4.5	5.9	2.4	0	158.2	199.4	376.6	8.1	67.2
			100	48.6	288.0	16.0	21.2	8.7	0	565.0	712.0	1345.0	29.0	240.0

Item No.	Minerals (Micro) Iron (mg)	Zinc (mg)	Copper (mg)	Fat-Soluble Vitamins Vitamin A (IU)	Vitamin D (IU)	Vitamin E (Alpha Tocopherol) (mg)	Water-Soluble Vitamins Vitamin C (mg)	Thiamin (mg)	Riboflavin (mg)	Niacin (mg)	Pantothenic Acid (mg)	Vit. B-6 (Pyridoxine) (mg)	Folacin (Folic Acid) (mcg)	Biotin (mcg)	Vitamin B-12 (mcg)
993	.22	.84	—	255.6	—	—	0	.01	.12	.04	.16	—	—	—	.33
	.80	2.99	—	913.0	—	—	0	.02	.44	.14	.56	—	—	—	1.18
994	.17	.99	—	239.7	—	—	0	.0	.11	.03	.14	—	—	—	.64
	.60	3.55	—	856.0	—	—	0	.01	.40	.10	.50	—	.64	—	2.30
995	.09	.74	(.03)	201.9	(.06)	(.20)	0	.01	.11	.28	.50	.05	10.19	.46	.34
	.31	2.64	(.09)	721.0	(.23)	(.70)	0	.03	.38	.02	1.80	.17	36.40	1.64	1.22
996	.12	.73	—	303.2	—	—	0	.0	.10	.03	.08	.02	5.69	.45	.35
	.43	2.61	—	1083.0	—	—	0	.01	.35	.12	.29	.07	20.33	1.59	1.26
997	.14	[6] .62	—	186.8	—	—	—	.02	.15	.11	.19	.07	18.20	—	.46
	.50	2.20	—	667.0	—	—	—	.07	.52	.38	.69	.24	65.00	—	1.65
998	.09	.67	(.02)	258.4	(.05)	(.17)	0	.01	.14	.18	.35	.06	17.42	1.60	.36
	.33	2.39	(.08)	923.0	(.18)	(.60)	0	.03	.49	.63	1.25	.22	62.20	5.70	1.30
999	—	.88	.05	294.7	—	—	0	.01	.13	.05	.05	—	.08	—	.08
	—	23.15	.17	1052.5	—	—	0	.03	.45	.18	.19	—	.27	—	.27
1000	.19	1.12	.06	295.9	(.07)	(.22)	0	.01	.11	.0	.12	.02	5.04	.48	.23
	.67	4.00	.22	1056.7	(.26)	(.80)	0	.03	.38	.01	.41	.07	18.00	1.73	.83
1001	.06	—	—	275.8	—	—	0	.01	.08	—	—	—	—	—	—
	.21	—	—	985.0	—	—	0	.05	.29	—	—	—	—	—	—
1002	.21	.86	.07	289.5	—	—	0	.0	.11	.03	.06	.02	—	—	.23
	.76	3.07	.24	1034.0	—	—	0	.02	.38	.09	.21	.08	—	—	.83
1003	.36	.95	—	158.2	—	—	0	.05	.42	.33	.55	.17	29.38	—	1.61
	.16	.42	—	70.0	—	—	0	.02	.19	.14	.24	.08	13.00	—	.71
1004	.32	.81	.05	366.4	—	—	0	.07	.37	.27	.50	.15	27.86	4.41	1.40
	.14	.36	.02	162.9	—	—	0	.03	.16	.12	.22	.07	12.38	1.96	.62
1005	.18	.08	Trace	214.3	(.04)	(.15)	0	0	.03	.02	.04	.01	1.95	.25	.06
	1.20	.53	(.04)	1428.4	(.28)	(1.00)	0	.02	.20	.10	.27	.05	13.00	1.64	.42
1006	.12	1.05	(.01)	256.5	(.05)	(.22)	0	.01	.11	.02	.08	.02	4.48	.43	.43
	.44	3.75	(.03)	916.0	(.18)	(.80)	0	.04	.39	.08	.28	.08	16.00	1.52	1.54
1007	.18	.81	.04	—	—	—	0	—	—	—	—	—	—	—	—
	.65	2.88	.13	—	—	—	0	—	—	—	—	—	—	—	—
1008	.06	.98	—	328.7	—	—	0	.01	.06	.04	—	—	—	—	—
	.23	3.50	—	1174.0	—	—	0	.02	.20	.15	—	—	—	—	—
1009	.22	—	—	37.3	—	—	0	0	.18	.06	—	—	—	—	—
	.80	—	—	133.3	—	—	0	.01	.63	.20	—	—	—	—	—
1010	.07	1.09	—	180.3	—	—	0	.01	.09	.02	.10	.02	5.88	—	—
	.24	3.90	—	644.0	—	—	0	.03	.33	.06	.34	.08	21.00	—	—
1011	—	—	—	341.3	—	—	0	.02	.08	—	.16	.02	2.80	—	.45
	—	—	—	1219.0	—	—	0	.06	.28	—	.56	.08	10.00	—	1.60
1012	.04	.59	—	358.7	—	—	0	.02	.14	.04	.33	.02	16.10	.63	.29
	.13	2.12	—	1281.0	—	—	0	.08	.50	.16	1.18	.09	57.50	2.26	1.04
1013	.20	.84	—	265.7	—	—	0	—	.11	—	—	—	—	—	—
	.71	3.00	—	948.8	—	—	0	—	.39	—	—	—	—	—	—
1014	.05	.62	.06	221.8	—	—	0	0	.07	.02	.02	.01	1.96	.45	.18
	.18	2.21	.23	792.0	—	—	0	.02	.24	.08	.06	.06	7.00	1.62	.65
1015	.12	.79	—	313.6	—	—	0	0	.09	.03	.05	.02	3.39	.39	.41
	.41	2.81	—	1120.0	—	—	0	.01	.32	.10	.19	.06	12.10	1.39	1.47
1016	.08	.15	.04	317.5	—	—	0	0	.06	.04	.16	.01	3.16	.54	.07
	.26	.52	.15	1134.0	—	—	0	.02	.20	.13	.57	.04	11.30	1.93	.26
1017	.05	.16	—	35.1	(.01)	(.50)	0	0	.02	.02	.07	.01	.40	.10	(.42)
	.95	3.19	—	701.0	(.27)	(.90)	0	.05	.39	.32	.53	.11	8.00	1.70	(1.50)
1018	—	—	—	373.2	—	—	0	—	.07	.02	.06	.02	5.04	—	.42
	—	—	—	1333.0	—	—	0	—	.24	.06	.21	.05	18.00	—	1.50
1019	.15	.90	—	228.2	—	—	0	.01	.09	.04	.13	.02	2.91	.50	.41
	.52	3.23	—	815.0	—	—	0	.02	.32	.16	.48	.07	10.40	1.79	1.46
1020	.12	.38	—	121.0	—	—	0	.01	.05	.02	—	.01	—	—	.08
	.44	1.34	—	432.0	—	—	0	.02	.19	.08	—	.02	—	—	.29
1021	—	—	—	161.9	—	—	0	—	.11	.02	—	—	2.00	—	—
	—	—	—	578.3	—	—	0	—	.38	.08	—	—	7.14	—	—
1022	.14	.58	—	293.2	—	—	0	.01	.16	.21	.48	.03	13.72	—	.17
	.50	2.08	—	1047.0	—	—	0	.04	.59	.73	1.73	.12	49.00	—	.62
1023	.05	1.09	.03	236.6	—	—	0	.01	.11	.03	.12	.02	1.68	.26	.47
	.17	3.90	.11	845.0	—	—	0	.02	.40	.09	.43	.08	6.00	.94	1.68
1024	.06	.98	—	292.6	—	—	0	.02	.10	.06	.10	—	—	—	.59
	.23	3.50	—	1045.0	—	—	0	.06	.36	.21	.35	—	—	—	2.10
1025	.11	.84	(.14)	341.6	(.04)	.19	0	.01	.99	.02	.14	.02	2.18	23.07	.20
	.39	2.99	(.50)	1220.0	(.15)	.67	0	.02	.53	.07	.48	.07	7.80	82.40	.70
1026	.09	.73	(.03)	220.6	Trace	—	0	.01	.12	.04	.19	.03	1.96	23.07	.11
	.33	2.59	(.09)	788.0	(.02)	—	0	.05	.43	.13	.69	.12	7.00	82.40	.40

(Continued)

TABLE F-21 *(Continued)*

Item No.	Food Item Name	Approximate Measure	Weight (g)	Moisture (%)	Food Energy Calories (kcal)	Protein (g)	Fats (g)	Carbo-hydrates (g)	Fiber (g)	Calcium (mg)	Phos-phorus (mg)	Sodium (mg)	Mag-nesium (mg)	Potas-sium (mg)
	CREAM													
1027	whipping, 31.3% fat	1 CUP	240	73.8	468.0	5.2	46.3	7.1	0	165.6	160.8	86.4	16.8	244.8
			100	73.8	195.0	2.2	19.3	3.0	0	69.0	67.0	36.0	7.0	102.0
1028	coffee or table, light, 20.6% fat	1 CUP	240	77.9	511.2	6.4	49.4	8.8	0	228.0	199.2	103.2	21.6	283.2
			100	77.9	213.0	2.6	20.6	3.7	0	95.0	83.0	43.0	9.0	118.0
1029	half-and-half	1 CUP	240	79.7	312.0	7.1	28.1	10.3	0	259.2	228.0	110.4	21.6	309.6
			100	79.7	130.0	3.0	11.7	4.3	0	108.0	95.0	46.0	9.0	129.0
1030	substitute, coffee, rich, liquid	1 TBLS	14	72.8	21.6	0	1.3	1.8	0	.3	5.3	5.6	.1	5.8
			100	72.8	154.0	.3	9.4	12.8	0	2.0	38.0	40.0	1.0	40.0
1031	substitute, dried, w/cream, skim milk, lactose, & sodium hexametaphosphate	1 TSP	3	.9	15.3	.4	.8	1.6	0	14.9	—	17.3	—	—
			100	.9	508.0	8.5	26.7	61.3	0	82.0	—	—	—	—
1032	¹whipped cream topping, pressurized	1 OZ	28	61.3	72.0	.9	6.2	3.5	0	28.3	24.9	36.4	3.1	41.2
			100	61.3	257.0	3.2	22.2	12.5	0	101.0	89.0	130.0	11.0	47.0
1033	**EGGNOG**	1 CUP	254	74.4	342.9	9.7	19.0	3.4	0	330.2	281.9	132.1	45.7	419.1
			100	74.4	135.0	3.8	7.5	1.4	0	130.0	111.0	52.0	18.0	165.0
	ICE CREAM													
1034	regular, 12% fat	1 CUP	135	62.1	282.2	5.4	16.6	27.8	0	166.1	133.7	54.0	18.9	151.2
			100	62.1	209.0	4.0	12.3	20.6	0	123.0	99.0	40.0	14.0	112.0
1035	cone, dipped in chocolate, small	INDIV	85	—	160.0	4.0	7.0	20.0	—	—	—	—	—	—
			100	—	188.2	4.7	8.2	23.5	—	—	—	—	—	—
1036	bar, chocolate coated	1 AVG	47	47.0	149.0	1.6	10.5	12.1	—	55.0	41.8	24.0	6.0	84.1
			100	47.0	317.0	3.4	22.3	25.7	—	117.0	89.0	51.0	12.8	179.0
1037	chocolate	1 CUP	133	—	295.3	5.0	16.0	32.8	—	186.2	167.6	74.5	17.7	—
			100	—	222.0	3.8	12.0	24.7	—	140.0	126.0	56.0	13.3	—
1038	French custard, frozen	1 CUP	133	63.2	256.7	6.0	14.4	27.7	0	194.2	153.0	83.8	10.3	240.7
			100	63.2	193.0	4.5	10.8	20.8	0	146.0	115.0	63.0	7.8	181.0
1039	French vanilla, soft serve	1 CUP	173	59.8	377.1	7.0	22.5	38.3	0	235.3	199.0	154.0	24.2	337.4
			100	59.8	218.0	4.1	13.0	22.1	0	136.0	115.0	89.0	14.0	195.0
1040	strawberry	1 CUP	133	—	250.0	4.3	12.0	31.3	—	146.3	123.7	58.5	19.2	—
			100	—	188.0	3.2	9.0	23.6	—	110.0	93.0	44.0	14.4	—
1041	vanilla	1 CUP	133	61.5	253.5	3.9	13.2	31.3	0	159.6	129.0	81.1	19.2	—
			100	61.5	190.6	2.9	9.9	23.5	0	120.0	97.0	61.0	14.4	—
1042	**ICE MILK,** soft serve	1 CUP	175	67.0	224.0	8.0	4.6	39.0	0	273.0	201.3	162.8	29.8	413.0
			100	67.0	128.0	4.6	2.6	22.3	0	156.0	115.0	93.0	17.0	236.0
1043	**JUNKET,** fruit & vanilla flavors, made w/whole milk	1 CUP	270	—	280.8	11.1	8.9	38.9	.3	321.3	237.6	129.6	38.0	364.5
			100	—	104.0	4.1	3.3	14.4	.1	119.0	88.0	48.0	14.1	135.0
1044	**MILK, BUFFALO OR CARABAO**	1 CUP	245	81.0	281.8	12.7	21.3	10.5	0	514.5	247.5	—	—	—
			100	81.0	115.0	5.2	8.7	4.3	0	210.0	101.0	—	—	—
	MILK, COW'S													
1045	whole, 3.7% fat	1 CUP	244	87.2	161.0	8.0	9.0	11.3	0	285.5	368.4	122.0	31.7	341.6
			100	87.2	66.0	3.3	3.7	4.7	0	117.0	151.0	50.0	13.0	140.0
1046	2% fat	1 CUP	244	89.2	122.0	8.1	4.7	11.7	0	297.7	231.8	122.0	34.2	375.8
			100	89.2	50.0	3.3	1.9	4.8	0	122.0	95.0	50.0	14.0	154.0
1047	partially skimmed, w/2% nonfat milk solids added	1 CUP	245	87.0	125.0	8.5	4.9	12.2	0	313.6	245.0	127.4	34.3	396.9
			100	87.0	51.0	3.5	2.0	5.0	0	128.0	100.0	52.0	14.0	162.0
1048	skim	1 CUP	246	92.0	83.8	8.0	.4	11.9	0	302.6	250.9	127.9	27.1	408.4
			100	92.0	34.1	3.3	.2	4.9	0	123.0	102.0	52.0	11.0	166.0
1049	canned, condensed, sweetened	1 CUP	306	27.1	1003.7	24.8	26.6	166.2	0	868.0	790.5	396.8	76.5	1158.7
			100	27.1	328.0	8.1	8.7	54.3	0	283.7	258.3	129.7	25.0	378.7
1050	canned, evaporated, unsweetened	1 CUP	256	74.0	343.0	17.4	19.4	25.7	0	668.2	517.1	271.4	61.4	775.7
			100	74.0	134.0	6.8	7.6	10.0	0	261.0	202.0	106.0	24.0	303.0
1051	dry, skim solids, instant	1 TBLS	4	4.0	14.1	1.4	0	2.1	0	49.2	39.4	22.0	4.7	68.2
			100	4.0	353.0	34.9	.8	51.6	0	1231.0	985.0	549.0	117.0	1705.0
1052	evaporated	1 CUP	256	73.8	350.7	17.9	20.2	24.8	0	645.1	524.8	302.1	64.0	775.7
			100	73.8	137.0	7.0	7.9	9.7	0	252.0	205.0	180.0	25.0	303.0
1053	¹chocolate, whole	1 CUP	250	82.3	207.5	8.0	8.5	25.8	.2	280.0	250.0	150.0	32.5	417.5
			100	82.3	83.0	3.2	3.4	10.3	.1	112.0	100.0	60.0	13.0	167.0
1054	chocolate, hot, w/cocoa, homemade	1 CUP	250	79.0	217.5	9.5	9.1	25.8	.3	295.0	282.5	127.5	55.0	480.0
			100	79.0	87.0	3.8	3.6	10.3	.1	118.0	113.0	51.0	22.0	192.0
1055	malted beverage	1 CUP	235	81.2	209.2	9.6	8.8	23.6	.1	317.3	286.7	190.4	47.0	470.0
			100	81.2	89.0	4.0	3.8	10.0	.1	135.0	122.0	81.0	20.0	200.0
1056	malted chocolate-flavor beverage	1 CUP	265	81.2	233.2	9.4	9.1	29.2	.1	304.8	265.0	169.6	47.7	498.2
			100	81.2	88.0	3.5	3.4	11.0	0	115.0	100.0	64.0	18.0	188.0
1057	**MILK, GOAT**	1 CUP	244	87.5	163.5	8.1	9.8	11.2	0	314.8	258.6	122.0	34.2	497.8
			100	87.5	67.0	3.3	4.0	4.6	0	129.0	106.0	50.0	14.0	204.0
1058	**MILK, HUMAN,** U.S.A. samples	1 OZ	28	88.3	20.8	.3	1.3	2.1	0	9.9	4.2	4.8	.9	15.3
			100	88.3	69.1	1.0	4.4	6.9	0	33.0	14.0	16.0	2.9	51.0
1059	**MILK, INDIAN BUFFALO,** whole, fluid	1 CUP	244	83.4	236.7	9.2	16.8	12.6	0	412.4	285.5	126.9	75.6	434.3
			100	83.4	97.0	3.8	6.9	5.2	0	169.0	117.0	52.0	31.0	178.0

Item No.	Minerals (Micro)			Fat-Soluble Vitamins			Water-Soluble Vitamins								
	Iron	Zinc	Copper	Vitamin A	Vitamin D	Vitamin E (Alpha Tocopherol)	Vitamin C	Thiamin	Ribo-flavin	Niacin	Panto-thenic Acid	Vit. B-6 (Pyri-doxine)	Folacin (Folic Acid)	Biotin	Vitamin B-12
	(mg)	(mg)	(mg)	(IU)	(IU)	(mg)	(mg)	(mg)	(mg)	(mg)	(mg)	(mg)	(mcg)	(mcg)	(mcg)
1027	.07 / .03	.60 / .25	– / –	2704.8 / 1127.0	120.00 / 50.00	– / –	1.46 / .61	.05 / .02	.29 / .12	.10 / .04	.62 / .26	.07 / .03	9.60 / 4.00	– / –	.48 / .20
1028	.10 / .04	.65 / .27	– / –	1728.0 / 720.0	– / –	– / –	1.82 / .76	.07 / .03	.36 / .15	.14 / .06	.66 / .28	.08 / .03	4.80 / 2.00	– / –	– / –
1029	.17 / .07	1.22 / .51	– / –	1041.6 / 434.0	– / –	– / –	2.06 / .86	.07 / .03	.36 / .15	.19 / .08	.69 / .29	.09 / .04	4.80 / 2.00	– / –	.79 / .33
1030	.02 / .15	0 / .02	0 / .02	22.8 / 163.0	– / –	– / –	0 / 0	0 / 0	0 / 0	0 / 0	0 / 0	– / –	– / –	– / –	– / –
1031	.01 / .30	.02 / .51	– / –	15.6 / 520.0	– / –	– / –	– / –	0 / .14	.02 / .71	.01 / .30	– / –	– / –	– / –	– / –	– / –
1032	.01 / .05	.10 / .37	– / –	255.6 / 913.0	– / –	– / –	0 / 0	.01 / .04	.02 / .07	.02 / .07	.09 / .30	.01 / .04	– / –	– / –	.08 / .29
1033	.51 / .20	1.17 / .46	– / –	873.8 / 344.0	30.48 / 12.00	– / –	3.81 / 1.50	.13 / .05	.46 / .18	.27 / .11	1.06 / .42	.13 / .05	2.54 / 1.00	– / –	1.14 / .45
1034	.14 / .10	.68 / .50	– / –	702.0 / 520.0	– / –	.49 / .36	1.35 / 1.00	.05 / .04	.26 / .19	.14 / .10	– / –	– / –	2.70 / 2.00	– / –	– / –
1035	– / –	– / –	– / –	– / –	– / –	– / –	– / –	– / –	– / –	– / –	– / –	– / –	– / –	– / –	– / –
1036	– / –	– / –	– / –	145.2 / 309.0	1.88 / 4.00	.03 / .07	– / –	.01 / .02	.07 / .14	.38 / .80	– / –	.02 / .04	– / –	– / –	.26 / .55
1037	– / –	– / –	– / –	569.2 / 428.0	– / –	– / –	– / –	.06 / .05	.27 / .20	.15 / .11	– / –	– / –	– / –	– / –	– / –
1038	.13 / .10	– / –	.01 / .01	585.2 / 440.0	– / –	.49 / .37	1.33 / 1.00	.05 / .04	.28 / .21	.13 / .10	– / –	– / –	6.12 / 4.60	– / –	– / –
1039	.43 / .25	1.99 / 1.15	– / –	794.1 / 459.0	– / –	– / –	.92 / .53	.08 / .05	.45 / .26	.18 / .10	1.07 / .62	.10 / .06	8.65 / 5.00	– / –	1.00 / .58
1040	– / –	– / –	– / –	502.7 / 378.0	– / –	– / –	– / –	.05 / .04	.20 / .15	.15 / .11	– / –	– / –	– / –	– / –	– / –
1041	0 / 0	.67 / .50	.04 / .03	631.8 / 475.0	– / –	– / –	1.33 / 1.00	.05 / .04	.27 / .20	.13 / .10	– / –	– / –	2.66 / 2.00	– / –	– / –
1042	.18 / .10	.86 / .49	– / –	175.0 / 100.0	– / –	– / –	1.17 / .67	.09 / .05	.54 / .31	.19 / .11	1.03 / .59	.13 / .08	5.25 / 3.00	– / –	1.37 / .78
1043	.54 / .20	– / –	– / –	337.5 / 125.0	2.70 / 1.00	– / –	– / –	.08 / .03	.43 / .16	.68 / .25	– / –	.08 / .03	– / –	– / –	.54 / .20
1044	.25 / .10	– / –	– / –	408.3 / 166.7	– / –	– / –	2.45 / 1.00	.10 / .04	.39 / .16	.25 / .10	– / –	– / –	– / –	– / –	– / –
1045	.12 / .05	.98 / .40	.08 / .03	336.7 / 138.0	100.04 / 41.00	.15 / .06	3.59 / 1.47	.07 / .03	.42 / .17	.21 / .08	.76 / .31	.10 / .04	12.20 / 5.00	7.56 / 3.10	.87 / .36
1046	.12 / .05	.95 / .39	– / –	500.2 / 205.0	100.00 / 40.98	– / –	2.32 / .95	.10 / .04	.40 / .17	.21 / .09	.78 / .32	.11 / .04	12.20 / 5.00	– / –	.89 / .36
1047	.12 / .05	.98 / .40	– / –	499.8 / 204.0	100.00 / 40.82	– / –	2.45 / 1.00	.10 / .04	.42 / .17	.25 / .10	.82 / .34	.11 / .05	12.25 / 5.00	– / –	.94 / .38
1048	.10 / .04	.98 / .40	.07 / .03	501.8 / 204.0	100.41 / 40.82	Trace / Trace	2.46 / 1.00	.10 / .04	.34 / .14	.22 / .09	.81 / .33	.10 / .04	12.30 / 5.00	– / –	.98 / .40
1049	.58 / .19	2.94 / .96	(.12) / (.04)	1024.1 / 334.7	(.27) / (.09)	.83 / .27	8.12 / 2.65	.25 / .08	1.30 / .42	.61 / .20	2.34 / .77	.16 / .05	34.68 / 11.33	(9.18) / (3.00)	1.36 / .44
1050	.49 / .19	1.97 / .77	.01 / 0	622.1 / 243.0	225.73 / 88.18	.33 / .13	4.81 / 1.88	.13 / .05	.82 / .32	.49 / .19	1.64 / .64	.13 / .05	20.48 / 8.00	11.52 / 4.50	.41 / .16
1051	.01 / .31	.18 / 4.41	0 / .05	94.8 / 2370.0	– / –	.0 / .02	.22 / 5.58	.02 / .41	.07 / 1.78	.04 / .90	.14 / 3.60	.01 / .35	2.00 / 50.00	– / –	.16 / 3.99
1052	.26 / .10	(2.82) / (1.10)	(.10) / (.04)	819.2 / 320.0	(.23) / (.09)	.23 / .09	2.56 / 1.00	.10 / .04	.87 / .34	.51 / .20	1.64 / .64	.13 / .05	20.48 / 8.00	11.52 / 4.50	.41 / .16
1053	.60 / .24	1.03 / .41	– / –	302.5 / 121.0	– / –	– / –	2.28 / .91	.75 / .03	.40 / .16	.33 / .13	.75 / .30	.10 / .04	12.50 / 5.00	– / –	8.3 / .33
1054	1.00 / .40	1.23 / .49	– / –	317.5 / 127.0	– / –	– / –	2.50 / 1.00	.10 / .04	.45 / .18	.36 / .15	.81 / .32	.11 / .04	12.50 / 5.00	– / –	.87 / .35
1055	.26 / .11	1.01 / .43	– / –	333.7 / 142.0	– / –	– / –	2.05 / .87	.14 / .06	.49 / .21	1.13 / .48	.68 / .29	.16 / .07	18.80 / 8.00	– / –	.92 / .39
1056	.50 / .19	1.11 / .42	– / –	326.0 / 123.0	– / –	– / –	2.31 / .87	.14 / .05	.43 / .16	.69 / .26	.77 / .29	.13 / .05	15.90 / 6.00	– / –	.92 / .35
1057	.12 / .05	.73 / .30	.17 / .07	451.4 / 185.0	4.88 / 2.00	– / –	3.15 / 1.29	.10 / .04	.34 / .14	.73 / .30	.78 / .32	.11 / .05	2.44 / 1.00	– / –	.16 / .07
1058	.01 / .02	.05 / .16	.02 / .05	72.0 / 240.0	(.07) / (.03)	.05 / .15	1.50 / 5.00	0 / .01	.01 / .04	.06 / .20	.07 / .22	.00 / .01	1.50 / 1.50	.24 / .80	.01 / .04
1059	.29 / .12	.54 / .22	– / –	434.3 / 178.0	– / –	– / –	5.49 / 2.25	.13 / .05	.33 / .14	.22 / .09	.47 / .19	.06 / .02	14.64 / 6.00	– / –	.89 / .36

(Continued)

TABLE F-21 *(Continued)*

Item No.	Food Item Name	Approximate Measure	Weight	Moisture	Food Energy Calories	Protein	Fats	Carbo-hydrates	Fiber	Calcium	Phos-phorus	Sodium	Mag-nesium	Potas-sium
			(g)	(%)	(kcal)	(g)	(g)	(g)	(g)	(mg)	(mg)	(mg)	(mg)	(mg)
1060	MILK, REINDEER	1 CUP	244	64.1	571.0	26.4	47.8	10.0	0	619.8	483.1	383.1	–	388.0
			100	64.1	234.0	10.8	19.6	4.1	0	254.0	198.0	157.0	–	159.0
1061	MILKSHAKE	1 CUP	345	–	420.9	11.2	17.9	58.0	.3	362.3	320.9	–	–	–
			100	–	122.0	3.2	5.2	16.8	.1	105.0	93.0	–	–	–
1062	chocolate, thick	1 CUP	345	72.2	413.3	11.2	9.3	72.9	.9	455.4	434.7	383.0	55.2	772.8
			100	72.2	119.8	3.2	2.7	21.1	.2	132.0	126.0	111.0	16.0	224.0
1063	vanilla, thick	1 CUP	345	74.5	386.4	13.3	10.5	61.2	.2	503.7	396.8	327.8	41.4	631.4
			100	74.5	112.0	3.9	3.0	17.8	.1	146.0	115.0	95.0	12.0	183.0
1064	MILK, SHEEP, whole, fluid	1 CUP	245	80.7	264.6	14.7	17.2	13.1	0	472.9	387.1	107.8	44.1	333.2
			100	80.7	108.0	6.0	7.0	5.4	0	193.0	158.0	44.0	18.0	136.0
1065	RENNIN DESSERT, chocolate, made from mix, w/milk	1 CUP	255	77.9	260.1	8.7	9.7	36.0	.2	311.1	244.8	132.6	–	318.8
			100	77.9	102.0	3.4	3.8	14.1	.1	122.0	96.0	52.0	–	125.0
1066	SOUR CREAM	1 TBLS	12	71.0	25.7	.4	2.5	.5	0	14.0	10.2	6.4	1.2	17.3
			100	71.0	214.0	3.1	21.0	4.3	0	116.0	85.0	53.0	10.0	144.0
1067	half & half, cultured	1 TBLS	15	80.1	20.3	.4	1.8	.6	0	15.6	14.3	6.0	1.5	19.4
			100	80.1	135.0	2.9	12.0	4.3	0	104.0	95.0	40.0	10.0	129.0
1068	SOYBEAN MILK, fluid	1 CUP	263	92.4	86.8	8.9	3.9	5.8	0	55.2	126.2	–	–	–
			100	92.4	33.0	3.4	1.5	2.2	0	21.0	48.0	–	–	–
	WHEY													
1069	sweet, dry	1 TBLS	8	3.2	28.3	1.0	.1	5.9	0	63.7	74.6	86.3	14.1	166.4
			100	3.2	354.0	12.7	1.0	73.5	0	796.0	932.0	1079.0	176.0	2080.0
1070	acid, dry	1 CUP	57	3.5	193.2	6.7	.3	41.9	0	1170.8	768.4	551.8	113.4	1304.2
			100	3.5	339.0	11.7	.5	73.5	0	2054.0	1348.0	968.0	199.0	2288.0
	YOGURT													
1071	plain, made w/whole milk	1 CUP	227	88.0	138.5	8.0	7.5	10.7	0	274.7	215.7	104.4	27.2	351.9
			100	88.0	61.0	3.5	3.3	4.7	0	121.0	95.0	46.0	12.0	155.0
1072	plain, lowfat, made w/lowfat milk & nonfat milk solids	1 CUP	227	85.1	143.0	12.0	3.6	15.9	0	415.4	326.9	158.9	38.6	531.2
			100	85.1	63.0	5.3	1.6	7.0	0	183.0	144.0	70.0	17.0	234.0
1073	fruit varieties, lowfat, w/nonfat milk solids	1 CUP	227	74.5	231.5	10.0	2.3	43.4	0	345.0	270.1	131.7	34.1	440.4
			100	74.5	102.0	4.4	1.1	19.1	0	152.0	119.0	58.0	15.0	194.0
	NUTS AND SEEDS													
1074	ALFALFA SEEDS	1 OZ	28	7.4	108.9	9.8	3.5	–	2.2	38.1	–	–	–	–
			100	7.4	389.0	35.1	12.6	–	7.9	136.0	–	–	–	–
1075	ALMONDS, shelled	1 CUP	142	–	906.0	26.4	76.5	27.7	20.3	332.3	715.7	4.3	(369.2)	1097.7
			100	–	638.0	18.6	53.9	19.5	14.3	234.0	504.0	3.0	(260.0)	773.0
1076	BEECHNUTS, shelled	1 TBLS	8	6.6	49.0	1.6	4.0	1.6	.3	–	–	–	–	–
			100	6.6	612.0	19.4	50.3	20.3	3.7	–	–	–	–	–
1077	BRAZIL NUTS, shelled	1 CUP	140	4.6	1001.0	20.0	95.5	15.3	4.3	260.4	970.2	1.4	444.5	1001.0
			100	4.6	715.0	14.3	68.2	10.9	3.1	186.0	693.0	1.0	317.5	715.0
1078	BUTTERNUT	1 AVG	3	3.8	18.9	.7	1.8	.3	–	–	–	–	–	–
			100	3.8	629.0	23.7	61.2	8.4	–	–	–	–	–	–
1079	CASHEW NUTS, salted	1 CUP	140	5.2	834.4	24.1	63.8	41.0	2.0	53.2	522.2	280.0	373.8	649.6
			100	5.2	596.0	17.2	45.6	29.3	1.4	38.0	373.0	200.0	267.0	464.0
1080	CHESTNUTS, fresh	1 CUP	200	52.5	408.0	5.8	5.4	84.2	2.2	54.0	176.0	12.0	84.0	908.0
			100	52.5	204.0	2.9	2.7	42.1	1.1	27.0	88.0	6.0	42.0	454.0
	COCONUTS													
1081	meat, fresh, grated	1 CUP	130	50.9	481.9	4.4	46.2	12.2	5.2	16.9	123.5	29.9	59.8	332.8
			100	50.9	370.7	3.4	35.5	9.4	4.0	13.0	95.0	23.0	46.0	256.0
1082	meat, dried, sweetened, shredded	1 CUP	130	3.3	712.4	4.7	50.8	69.2	5.3	20.8	145.6	23.4	100.1	458.9
			100	3.3	548.0	3.6	39.1	53.2	4.1	16.0	112.0	18.0	77.0	353.0
1083	milk	1 CUP	244	65.7	614.9	7.8	60.8	12.7	–	39.0	244.0	129.3	–	463.6
			100	65.7	252.0	3.2	24.9	5.2	–	16.0	100.0	53.0	–	190.0
1084	FILBERTS (HAZELNUTS), whole, shelled	1 CUP	135	5.8	945.0	17.1	87.3	22.5	4.1	282.2	455.0	2.7	234.8	950.4
			100	5.8	700.0	12.7	64.7	16.7	3.0	209.0	337.0	2.0	173.9	704.0
1085	³FLAXSEED, dried	1 OZ	28	6.3	139.4	5.0	9.4	10.4	2.5	75.9	129.4	–	–	–
			100	6.3	498.0	18.0	34.0	37.2	8.8	271.0	462.0	–	–	–
1086	⁴HAZELNUTS	1 OZ	28	–	106.5	2.1	10.1	1.9	1.1	1.23	65.0	.4	15.8	98.1
			100	–	380.2	7.5	35.9	6.9	6.1	43.8	232.1	1.4	56.5	350.3
1087	HICKORY NUTS	1 SM	1	3.3	6.7	.1	.7	.1	0	–	3.6	–	1.6	–
			100	3.3	673.0	13.2	68.7	12.8	1.9	–	360.0	–	160.0	–
1088	MACADAMIA NUTS, shelled	1 CUP	140	3.0	1086.4	10.9	106.0	22.3	3.5	67.2	225.4	–	–	369.6
			100	3.0	776.0	7.8	75.7	15.9	2.5	48.0	161.0	–	–	264.0
1089	MIXED NUTS, shelled	1 AVG	2	–	12.5	.3	1.2	.4	–	1.9	8.9	.3	–	11.2
			100	–	626.0	16.6	59.2	18.0	–	94.0	446.0	14.0	–	560.0
	PEANUTS													
1090	raw, w/skins	1 CUP	150	5.6	846.0	39.0	71.3	27.9	3.6	103.5	601.5	7.5	237.5	1011.0
			100	5.6	564.0	26.0	47.5	18.6	2.4	69.0	401.0	5.0	158.3	674.0

Item No.	Minerals (Micro)			Fat-Soluble Vitamins			Water-Soluble Vitamins								
	Iron	Zinc	Copper	Vitamin A	Vitamin D	Vitamin E (Alpha Tocopherol)	Vitamin C	Thiamin	Ribo-flavin	Niacin	Panto-thenic Acid	Vit. B-6 (Pyri-doxine)	Folacin (Folic Acid)	Biotin	Vitamin B-12
	(mg)	(mg)	(mg)	(IU)	(IU)	(mg)	(mg)	(mg)	(mg)	(mg)	(mg)	(mg)	(mcg)	(mcg)	(mcg)
1060	.24	–	–	–	–	–	–	–	–	–	–	–	–	–	–
	.10	–	–	–	–	–	–	–	–	–	–	–	–	–	–
1061	1.04	–	–	686.6	3.45	–	4.14	.10	.55	.48	–	–	–	–	–
	.30	–	–	199.0	1.00	–	1.20	.03	.16	.14	–	–	–	–	–
1062	1.04	1.66	–	296.7	3.45	–	0	.10	.77	.48	1.25	.09	17.25	–	1.09
	.30	.48	–	86.0	1.00	–	0	.03	.22	.14	.36	.03	5.00	–	.32
1063	.35	–	–	393.3	–	–	–	.10	.67	.50	–	.15	24.15	–	1.79
	.10	–	–	114.0	–	–	–	.03	.20	.15	–	.04	7.00	–	.52
1064	.25	–	–	360.2	–	–	10.19	.16	.87	1.02	1.00	–	–	–	1.74
	.10	–	–	147.0	–	–	4.16	.07	.36	.42	.41	–	–	–	.71
1065	–	–	–	357.0	–	–	2.55	.08	.38	.26	–	–	–	–	–
	–	–	–	140.0	–	–	1.00	.03	.15	.10	–	–	–	–	–
1066	.01	.03	–	94.8	.84	–	.10	0	.02	.01	.04	0	1.32	–	.04
	.06	.27	–	790.0	7.00	–	.86	.03	.13	.07	.36	.02	11.00	–	.30
1067	.01	.08	–	67.8	–	–	.13	.01	.02	.01	.05	0	1.65	–	.05
	.07	.50	–	452.0	–	–	.86	.04	.15	.07	.36	.02	11.00	–	.30
1068	2.10	[6].53	–	105.2	–	–	0	.21	.08	.53	–	–	–	–	–
	.80	.20	–	40.0	–	–	0	.08	.03	.20	–	–	–	–	–
1069	.07	.16	–	4.0	–	0	.12	.04	.18	.10	.45	.04	.96	–	.16
	.88	1.97	–	50.0	–	.03	1.49	.50	2.21	1.26	5.62	.58	12.00	–	2.00
1070	.71	3.60	–	33.1	–	–	–	.36	1.17	.66	3.21	.35	18.81	–	1.43
	1.24	6.31	–	58.0	–	–	–	.62	2.06	1.16	5.63	.62	33.00	–	2.50
1071	.11	1.34	(.09)	279.2	Trace	(.07)	1.20	.07	.32	.17	.88	.07	15.89	–	.84
	.05	.59	(.04)	123.0	Trace	(.03)	.53	.03	.14	.08	.39	.03	7.00	–	.37
1072	.18	2.02	–	149.8	–	–	1.82	.10	.49	.26	1.34	.11	22.70	–	1.28
	.08	.89	–	66.0	–	–	.80	.04	.21	.11	.59	.05	11.00	–	.56
1073	.16	1.68	–	104.4	–	–	1.50	.08	.40	.22	1.11	.09	20.40	–	1.06
	.07	.74	–	46.0	–	–	.66	.04	.18	.10	49	.04	9.00	–	47
1074	3.61	1.93	–	–	–	9.24	7.26	.30	.10	.50	–	–	–	–	–
	12.90	6.90	–	–	–	33.00	26.00	1.08	.58	1.80	–	–	–	–	–
1075	6.67	(4.42)	(.21)	0	0	21.30	–	.34	1.32	4.97	.82	.14	136.32	25.56	0
	4.70	(3.11)	(.15)	0	0	15.00	–	.24	.93	3.50	.58	.10	96.00	18.00	0
1076	–	–	–	–	–	–	–	–	–	–	–	–	–	–	–
	–	–	–	–	–	–	–	–	–	–	–	–	–	–	–
1077	4.76	5.92	3.34	0	0	9.10	14.00	1.34	.17	2.24	.32	.24	5.60	–	0
	3.40	4.23	2.38	0	0	6.50	10.00	.96	.12	1.60	.23	.17	4.00	–	0
1078	.20	–	–	–	–	–	–	–	–	–	–	–	–	–	–
	6.80	–	–	–	–	–	–	–	–	–	–	–	–	–	–
1079	5.32	6.13	–	140.0	–	–	–	.60	.35	2.52	1.82	–	–	–	0
	3.80	4.38	–	100.0	–	–	–	.43	.25	1.80	1.30	–	–	–	0
1080	3.40	[6]1.00	.12	160.0	0	1.00	12.00	.44	.44	1.20	.95	.66	–	(2.62)	0
	1.70	.50	.06	80.0	0	.50	6.00	.22	.22	.60	.47	.33	–	(1.31)	0
1081	2.21	.07	.03	0	0	.91	3.90	.07	.03	.65	.26	.06	31.20	–	0
	1.70	.05	.02	0	0	.70	3.00	.05	.02	.50	.20	.04	24.00	–	0
1082	2.60	–	–	0	0	–	0	.05	.04	.52	.26	–	–	–	–
	2.00	–	–	0	0	–	0	.04	.03	.40	.20	–	–	–	–
1083	3.90	–	–	0	0	–	4.88	.07	–	1.95	–	–	–	–	–
	1.60	–	–	0	0	–	3.00	.03	–	.80	–	–	–	–	–
1084	4.59	3.29	1.73	144.5	0	28.35	4.05	.62	.73	1.21	1.55	.74	97.20	–	0
	3.40	2.44	1.28	107.0	0	21.00	3.00	.46	.54	.90	1.15	.55	72.00	–	0
1085	12.26	–	–	0	–	–	–	.05	.05	.39	–	–	–	–	–
	43.80	–	–	0	–	–	–	.17	.16	1.40	–	–	–	–	–
1086	.31	.67	.62	0	0	5.90	Trace	.12	–	.26	.32	.15	20.18	–	0
	1.11	2.38	.22	0	0	21.10	Trace	.42	–	.92	1.16	.55	72.03	–	0
1087	.02	–	–	–	0	–	0	.01	–	–	–	–	–	–	–
	2.40	–	–	–	0	–	0	.53	–	–	–	–	–	–	–
1088	2.80	2.39	–	0	0	–	0	.48	.15	1.82	–	–	–	–	–
	2.00	1.71	–	0	0	–	0	.34	.11	1.30	–	–	–	–	–
1089	.07	[6].06	–	.4	0	–	–	.01	0	.08	–	–	–	–	–
	3.40	3.10	–	20.0	0	–	–	.59	.13	4.00	–	–	–	–	–
1090	3.15	4.86	1.18	24.0	0	14.55	0	1.71	.20	25.80	4.20	–	–	–	0
	2.10	3.24	.78	16.0	0	9.70	0	1.14	.13	17.20	2.80	–	–	–	0

(Continued)

TABLE F-21 *(Continued)*

Item No.	Food Item Name	Approximate Measure	Weight (g)	Moisture (%)	Food Energy Calories (kcal)	Protein (g)	Fats (g)	Carbo-hydrates (g)	Fiber (g)	Minerals (Macro) Calcium (mg)	Phos-phorus (mg)	Sodium (mg)	Mag-nesium (mg)	Potas-sium (mg)
	PEANUTS (Continued)													
1091	roasted, w/skins, whole	1 AVG	3	1.8	17.5	.8	1.5	.6	.1	2.2	12.2	.2	5.3	21.0
			100	1.8	582.0	26.2	48.7	20.6	2.7	72.0	407.0	5.0	175.0	701.0
1092	roasted, salted	1 CUP	144	1.6	842.4	37.4	71.7	27.1	3.4	106.6	577.4	601.9	252.0	970.6
			100	1.6	585.0	26.0	49.8	18.8	2.4	74.0	401.0	418.0	175.0	674.0
1093	blanched, salted	1 PKG	32	1.4	192.3	8.8	14.6	6.5	–	–	–	–	–	–
			100	1.4	601.0	27.5	45.5	20.2	–	–	–	–	–	–
1094	butter, creamy	1 TBLS	32	–	190.0	8.1	16.2	5.4	(5.9)	(11.8)	105.7	190.0	(57.6)	200.0
			100	–	593.8	25.3	50.6	16.9	(7.6)	(36.8)	330.9	593.8	(180.3)	625.0
1095	**PECANS,** unsalted	1 CUP	108	3.4	797.7	10.2	77.1	15.8	2.5	78.8	312.1	11.9	118.8	651.2
			100	3.4	738.6	9.4	71.4	14.6	2.3	73.0	289.0	11.0	110.0	603.0
1096	**PINE NUTS,** pinon	1 TBLS	7	3.1	41.5	.9	3.6	1.4	.1	.8	42.3	–	–	–
			100	3.1	593.0	13.0	51.0	20.5	1.1	12.0	604.0	–	–	–
1097	**PISTACHIO NUTS,** shelled	1 CUP	125	5.3	793.8	23.6	67.0	23.8	2.4	163.8	625.0	–	197.5	1215.0
			100	5.3	635.0	18.9	53.6	19.0	1.9	131.0	500.0	–	158.0	972.0
1098	²**POPPY SEEDS**	1 TSP	3	6.8	15.9	.5	1.3	.7	.2	43.4	25.4	.6	9.6	21.0
			100	6.8	533.0	18.0	44.7	23.7	6.2	1448.0	848.0	21.0	320.0	700.0
1099	⁹**PUMPKIN & SQUASH SEED KERNELS,** dry	1 CUP	140	–	774.2	40.6	65.4	21.0	2.7	71.4	1601.6	–	–	–
			100	–	553.0	29.0	46.7	15.0	1.9	51.0	1144.0	–	–	–
1100	**SESAME SEEDS,** dry, whole	1 OZ	28	5.4	157.6	5.2	13.7	6.0	1.8	324.8	172.5	16.8	50.7	203.0
			100	5.4	563.0	18.6	49.1	21.6	6.3	1160.0	616.0	60.0	181.0	725.0
1101	**SUNFLOWER SEED KERNELS,** dry, hulled	1 CUP	145	4.8	812.0	33.4	68.6	28.9	5.5	174.0	1213.7	43.5	55.1	1334.0
			100	4.8	560.0	23.0	47.3	19.9	3.8	120.0	837.0	30.0	38.0	920.0
	WALNUTS													
1102	black, shelled, chopped	1 CUP	125	3.1	847.5	25.6	74.5	18.5	2.1	–	712.5	3.8	237.5	575.0
			100	3.1	678.0	20.5	59.6	14.8	1.7	–	570.0	3.0	190.0	460.0
1103	Persian or English, shelled, chopped	1 CUP	120	3.5	832.8	18.0	76.1	19.0	2.5	118.8	456.0	2.4	172.8	540.0
			100	3.5	694.0	15.0	63.4	15.8	2.1	99.0	380.0	2.0	144.0	450.0
1104	**WATERMELON SEEDS,** whole, dried	1 OZ	28	4.6	150.1	6.4	11.5	7.7	.7	23.0	135.2	–	–	169.7
			100	4.6	536.0	22.7	41.2	27.5	2.5	82.0	483.0	–	–	606.0
	PICKLES AND RELISHES													
1105	**CRANBERRY-ORANGE RELISH,** uncooked	1 TBLS	15	53.6	26.7	.1	.1	6.8	–	2.9	1.2	.2	–	10.8
			100	53.6	178.0	.4	.4	45.4	–	19.0	8.0	1.0	–	72.0
1106	**KIM CHEE,** (Vegetable pickle w/garlic, red pepper, & ginger)	1 CUP	133	–	–	–	–	–	–	–	–	904.4	–	203.5
			100	–	–	–	–	–	–	–	–	680.0	–	153.0
	OLIVES													
1107	green	1 MED	5	78.2	5.8	.1	.6	.1	.1	3.1	.9	120.0	1.1	2.8
			100	78.2	116.0	1.4	12.7	1.3	1.3	61.0	17.0	2400.0	22.0	55.0
1108	ripe, Mission	1 LG	5	73.0	9.2	.1	1.0	.2	.1	5.3	.9	37.5	–	1.4
			100	73.0	184.0	1.2	20.1	3.2	1.5	106.0	17.0	750.0	–	27.0
	PICKLES													
1109	relish, sour	1 TBLS	15	93.0	2.9	.1	.1	.4	.2	4.4	3.0	–	–	–
			100	93.0	19.0	.7	.9	2.7	1.1	29.0	20.0	–	–	–
1110	relish, sweet	1 TBLS	15	63.0	20.7	.1	.1	5.1	.1	3.0	2.1	106.8	–	–
			100	63.0	138.0	.5	.6	34.0	.8	20.0	14.0	712.0	–	–
1111	cucumber, dill	1 LG	135	93.3	14.9	.9	.3	3.0	.7	35.1	28.4	1927.8	16.2	270.0
			100	93.3	11.0	.7	.2	2.2	.5	26.0	21.0	1428.0	12.0	200.0
1112	cucumber, fresh, bread & butter	1 SLICE	8	78.7	5.8	.1	0	1.4	0	2.6	2.2	53.8	–	–
			100	78.7	73.0	.9	.2	17.9	.5	32.0	27.0	673.0	–	–
1113	cucumber, sour	1 LG	135	94.8	13.5	.7	.3	2.7	.7	23.0	20.3	1826.6	–	–
			100	94.8	10.0	.5	.2	2.0	.5	17.0	15.0	1353.0	–	–
1114	cucumber, sweet	1 LG	100	60.7	146.0	.7	.4	36.5	.5	12.0	16.0	–	1.0	–
			100	60.7	146.0	.7	.4	36.5	.5	12.0	16.0	–	1.0	–
1115	**SANDWICH SPREAD,** w/chopped pickle, regular	1 TBLS	20	45.4	75.8	.1	7.2	3.2	.1	3.0	4.0	125.2	–	18.4
			100	45.4	379.0	.7	36.2	15.9	.4	15.0	20.0	626.0	–	92.0
	SALADS													
1116	**CARROT & RAISIN SALAD**	1 OZ	28	59.9	22.1	.4	.5	4.5	.2	9.2	10.8	43.2	5.0	29.8
			100	59.9	78.9	1.4	1.7	16.2	.7	32.8	38.5	154.2	17.9	106.3
1117	**CHICKEN SALAD**	1 CUP	200	–	254.0	22.0	15.0	7.8	.6	44.0	136.0	–	–	–
			100	–	127.0	11.0	7.5	3.9	.3	22.0	68.0	–	–	–
1118	**COLESLAW**	1 OZ	28	89.8	7.7	.4	.1	1.6	.2	13.2	8.3	9.9	3.7	65.2
			100	89.8	27.6	1.3	.5	5.7	.8	47.1	29.7	35.3	13.1	232.8
1119	w/salad dressing	1 CUP	120	82.9	118.8	1.4	9.5	8.5	.8	51.6	33.6	148.8	14.4	230.4
			100	82.9	99.0	1.2	7.9	7.1	.7	43.0	28.0	124.0	12.0	192.0
1120	**CRAB SALAD**	1 OZ	28	–	40.6	3.3	2.4	1.4	–	10.6	36.1	–	7.3	–
			100	–	145.0	11.8	8.5	4.9	–	38.0	129.0	–	26.0	–

Item No.	Minerals (Micro)			Fat-Soluble Vitamins			Water-Soluble Vitamins								
	Iron	Zinc	Copper	Vitamin A	Vitamin D	Vitamin E (Alpha Tocopherol)	Vitamin C	Thiamin	Ribo-flavin	Niacin	Panto-thenic Acid	Vit. B-6 (Pyri-doxine)	Folacin (Folic Acid)	Biotin	Vitamin B-12
	(mg)	(mg)	(mg)	(IU)	(IU)	(mg)	(mg)	(mg)	(mg)	(mg)	(mg)	(mg)	(mcg)	(mcg)	(mcg)
1091	.07	−	.01	10.8	0	.29	0	.01	0	.51	.06	.01	3.18	1.02	0
	2.20	−	.27	360.0	0	9.70	0	.32	.13	17.10	2.10	.40	106.00	34.00	0
1092	3.02	(4.26)	(.39)	0	0	13.97	0	.46	.19	24.77	3.02	.58	152.64	48.96	0
	2.10	(2.96)	(.27)	0	0	9.70	0	.32	.13	17.20	2.10	.40	106.00	34.00	0
1093	.63	−	−	−	−	−	−	.02	.05	1.11	−	−	−	−	−
	1.98	−	−	−	−	−	−	.05	.15	3.46	−	−	−	−	−
1094	(.67)	.93	(.22)	0	0	(1.49)	Trace	(.05)	(.04)	(4.89)	(.74)	(.16)	(16.90)	−	0
	(2.09)	2.90	(.69)	0	0	(4.66)	Trace	(.16)	(.11)	(15.30)	(2.32)	(.51)	(52.90)	−	0
1095	2.59	4.43	1.19	140.4	0	1.30	2.16	.93	.14	.97	1.84	.20	25.92	29.16	0
	2.40	4.10	1.10	130.0	0	1.20	2.00	.86	.13	.90	1.71	.18	24.00	27.00	0
1096	.36	6 .46	−	2.1	−	−	−	.09	.02	.32	−	−	−	−	−
	5.20	6.50	−	30.0	−	−	−	1.28	.23	4.50	−	−	−	−	−
1097	9.13	−	−	287.5	−	−	0	.84	−	1.75	−	−	72.50	−	−
	7.30	−	−	230.0	−	−	0	.67	−	1.40	−	−	58.00	−	−
1098	.28	.31	.05	0	−	.05	.36	.03	.01	.03	−	.01	−	−	0
	9.40	10.23	1.63	0	−	1.80	12.00	.95	.18	1.00	−	.45	−	−	0
1099	15.68	−	−	98.0	−	−	−	.34	.27	3.36	−	.13	−	−	0
	11.20	−	−	70.0	−	−	−	.24	.19	2.40	−	.09	−	−	0
1100	2.94	6 1.48	−	8.4	−	−	0	.27	.07	1.51	−	−	−	−	0
	10.50	5.30	−	30.0	−	−	0	.98	.24	5.40	−	−	−	−	0
1101	10.30	6.64	2.57	72.5	−	18.85	−	2.84	.33	7.83	2.03	1.81	−	−	0
	7.10	4.58	1.77	50.0	−	13.00	−	1.96	.23	5.40	1.40	1.25	−	−	0
1102	7.50	−	−	375.0	−	−	−	.28	.14	.88	−	−	−	−	−
	6.00	−	−	300.0	−	−	−	.22	.11	.70	−	−	−	−	−
1103	3.72	3.84	1.68	36.0	−	.48	2.40	.40	.16	1.08	1.08	.88	79.20	44.40	0
	3.10	3.20	1.40	30.0	−	.40	2.00	.33	.13	.90	.90	.73	66.00	37.00	0
1104	2.16	−	−	4.7	−	−	−	.06	.03	.73	−	−	−	−	−
	7.70	−	−	16.7	−	−	−	.22	.10	2.60	−	−	−	−	−
1105	.06	−	−	10.5	−	−	2.70	.01	0	.02	−	−	−	−	−
	.40	−	−	70.0	−	−	18.00	.03	.02	.10	−	−	−	−	−
1106	−	−	−	−	−	−	−	−	−	−	−	−	−	−	−
	−	−	−	−	−	−	−	−	−	−	−	−	−	−	−
1107	.08	0	.08	15.0	0	−	−	−	−	−	0	−	.05	−	0
	1.60	.07	1.60	300.0	0	−	−	−	−	−	.02	−	1.00	−	0
1108	.09	−	−	3.5	0	−	−	−	−	−	0	0	.05	−	0
	1.70	−	−	70.0	0	−	−	−	−	−	.02	.01	1.00	−	0
1109	.17	−	−	−	−	−	−	−	−	−	−	−	−	−	−
	1.10	−	−	−	−	−	−	−	−	−	−	−	−	−	−
1110	.12	−	−	−	−	−	−	−	−	−	−	−	−	−	−
	.80	−	−	−	−	−	−	−	−	−	−	−	−	−	−
1111	1.35	.37	−	135.0	0	−	8.10	−	.03	.10	−	.01	1.35	−	0
	1.00	.27	−	100.0	0	−	6.00	−	.02	.07	−	.01	1.00	−	0
1112	.14	−	−	11.2	−	−	0.72	−	0	−	−	0	−	−	0
	1.80	−	−	140.0	−	−	9.00	−	.03	−	−	.01	−	−	0
1113	4.32	−	−	135.0	−	−	9.45	−	03	−	−	.01	−	−	0
	3.20	−	−	100.0	−	−	7.00	−	.02	−	−	.01	−	−	0
1114	1.20	.14	−	90.0	0	−	6.00	0	.02	−	−	.01	−	−	0
	1.20	.14	−	90.0	0	−	6.00	0	.02	−	−	.01	−	−	0
1115	.14	−	−	56.0	−	−	1.20	0	.01	−	−	−	−	−	−
	.70	−	−	280.0	−	−	6.00	.01	.03	−	−	−	−	−	−
1116	.24	.04	−	2068.8	.34	−	1.54	.02	.02	.14	.06	.03	1.51	−	0
	.85	.16	−	7388.5	1.23	−	5.48	.06	.06	.51	.21	.10	5.40	−	.01
1117	1.80	−	−	398.0	−	−	6.80	.06	.18	4.64	−	−	−	−	−
	.90	−	−	199.0	−	−	3.40	.03	.09	2.32	−	−	−	−	−
1118	.12	.04	−	318.9	0	−	10.98	.01	.01	.09	.07	.04	22.22	−	0
	.42	.14	−	1139.0	0	−	39.20	.05	.05	.33	.23	.15	79.34	−	0
1119	.48	.29	−	180.0	−	−	34.80	.06	.06	.36	−	−	−	−	−
	.40	.24	−	150.0	−	−	29.00	.05	.05	.30	−	−	−	−	−
1120	.17	−	−	27.2	−	−	.56	.02	.02	.36	−	.06	−	−	1.86
	.60	−	−	97.0	−	−	2.00	.06	.06	1.30	−	.21	−	−	6.64

(Continued)

TABLE F-21 *(Continued)*

Item No.	Food Item Name	Approximate Measure	Weight (g)	Moisture (%)	Food Energy Calories (kcal)	Protein (g)	Fats (g)	Carbohydrates (g)	Fiber (g)	Calcium (mg)	Phosphorus (mg)	Sodium (mg)	Magnesium (mg)	Potassium (mg)
	GELATIN SALAD													
1121	w/chopped vegetables	1 SERV	164	—	114.8	2.2	5.7	15.1	.7	24.6	27.9	—	—	—
			100	—	70.0	1.3	3.5	9.2	.4	15.0	17.0	—	—	—
1122	w/fruit cocktail	1 OZ	28	81.6	15.9	2.1	.7	2.1	0	1.3	1.3	11.4	.9	17.2
			100	81.6	56.9	7.3	2.5	7.4	.1	4.8	4.5	40.6	3.1	61.5
1123	**LETTUCE & TOMATO SALAD**	1 SERV	100	—	19.0	1.4	0	4.5	.7	18.0	32.0	—	—	—
			100	—	19.0	1.4	0	4.5	.7	18.0	32.0	—	—	—
1124	**LOBSTER SALAD**	1 SERV	260	80.3	286.0	26.3	16.6	5.0	—	93.6	247.0	322.4	—	686.4
			100	80.3	110.0	10.1	6.4	2.3	—	36.0	95.0	124.0	—	264.0
1125	**MACARONI SALAD,** w/onion & mayonnaise	1 CUP	190	—	334.4	7.7	11.8	48.5	0	20.9	102.6	—	—	—
			100	—	176.0	4.1	6.2	25.5	0	11.0	54.0	—	—	—
1126	**POTATO SALAD**	1 OZ	28	—	42.3	.9	2.3	4.6	1.5	5.2	18.1	50.0	.9	37.3
			100	—	150.9	3.3	8.4	16.4	5.4	18.7	64.7	178.7	3.2	133.2
1127	w/mayonnaise, French dressing, hard cooked egg, & seasoning	1 CUP	250	72.4	362.5	7.5	23.0	33.5	1.0	47.5	157.5	1200.0	—	740.0
			100	72.4	145.0	3.0	9.2	13.4	.4	19.0	63.0	480.0	—	296.0
1128	**TUNA SALAD,** w/celery, mayonnaise, pickle, onion, & egg	1 CUP	200	69.8	340.0	29.2	21.0	7.0	—	40.0	284.0	—	—	—
			100	69.8	170.0	14.6	10.5	3.5	—	20.0	142.0	—	—	—
1129	**TOSSED SALAD**	1 OZ	28	85.2	3.9	.2	.3	.9	.1	5.7	6.0	4.9	2.9	50.5
			100	85.2	13.9	.8	1.0	3.1	.5	20.5	21.4	17.6	10.4	180.4
1130	**WALDORF SALAD**	1 SERV	108	—	137.3	.9	7.5	18.7	.9	18.8	32.7	77.5	—	200.2
			100	—	127.1	.9	7.0	17.3	.8	17.4	30.3	71.8	—	185.3
	SALAD DRESSINGS													
1131	**BLUE & ROQUEFORT,** regular, w/salt	1 TBLS	14	32.3	70.6	.7	7.3	1.0	0	11.3	10.4	153.2	—	5.2
			100	32.3	504.0	4.8	52.3	7.4	.1	81.0	74.0	1094.0	—	37.0
1132	**COOKED,** homemade, w/margarine	1 TBLS	14	69.2	21.8	.6	1.3	2.1	0	11.8	12.2	102.8	—	16.9
			100	69.2	156.0	4.2	9.5	14.9	0	84.0	87.0	734.0	—	121.0
1133	**FRENCH,** regular	1 TBLS	14	38.1	60.2	.1	5.7	2.5	.1	1.5	2.0	191.8	1.4	11.1
			100	38.1	429.7	.6	41.0	17.5	.8	11.0	14.0	1370.0	10.0	79.0
1134	**ITALIAN,** regular	1 TBLS	14	38.4	65.4	.1	6.8	1.4	0	1.4	.7	110.2	—	2.1
			100	38.4	467.3	.7	48.3	10.2	.2	10.0	5.0	787.0	—	15.0
1135	**MAYONNAISE,** regular	1 TBLS	14	39.9	54.6	.1	4.7	3.3	0	2.0	3.6	99.5	.3	1.3
			100	39.9	389.7	.9	33.4	23.9	0	14.0	26.0	710.8	2.0	9.0
1136	**RUSSIAN,** regular	1 TBLS	14	34.5	69.2	.2	7.1	1.5	0	2.7	5.2	121.5	—	22.0
			100	34.5	494.0	1.6	50.8	10.4	.3	19.0	37.0	868.0	—	157.0
1137	**SESAME SEED**	1 TBLS	15	39.2	66.5	.5	6.8	1.3	.1	—	—	150.0	—	—
			100	39.2	443.1	3.1	45.2	8.6	.4	—	—	1000.0	—	—
1138	**THOUSAND ISLAND,** regular	1 TBLS	14	46.1	52.8	.1	5.0	2.1	.3	1.5	2.4	98.0	—	15.8
			100	46.1	377.3	.9	35.7	15.2	2.0	11.0	17.0	700.0	—	113.0
1139	**VINEGAR & OIL,** homemade	1 TBLS	16	47.4	71.8	0	8.0	.4	—	—	—	.1	—	1.2
			100	47.4	448.8	0	50.1	2.5	—	—	—	.5	—	7.5
	SNACK FOODS													
1140	**BACON RINDS**	1 SERV	28	—	144.5	19.2	7.7	.0	—	1.4	.0	217.4	—	—
			100	—	516.2	68.5	27.6	.0	—	5.1	.0	776.5	—	—
1141	**CHEESE PUFFS**	1 CUP	28	—	154.6	2.2	9.7	15.2	.1	15.7	19.9	170.0	3.9	64.1
			100	—	552.0	7.7	34.5	54.3	.5	56.0	71.0	607.0	14.0	229.0
1142	**CORN CHIPS**	1 CUP	40	—	220.4	2.7	14.8	20.9	.4	49.6	73.6	288.0	24.0	32.4
			100	—	551.0	6.8	37.0	52.3	1.0	124.0	184.0	720.0	60.0	81.0
	DIPS													
1143	ENCHILADA	1 OZ	28	—	36.7	1.9	1.5	3.8	.2	17.1	2.5	95.2	15.1	100.0
			100	—	131.0	6.9	5.4	13.6	.8	61.0	9.0	340.0	54.0	357.0
1144	FRENCH ONION	1 TBLS	15	—	24.2	.5	2.0	1.1	—	17.6	13.7	84.2	1.8	26.3
			100	—	161.0	3.3	13.0	7.6	—	117.0	91.0	561.0	12.0	175.0
1145	SOUR CREAM	1 TBLS	15	—	28.1	.4	2.7	1.1	—	21.3	18.1	—	—	—
			100	—	187.5	2.5	17.9	7.5	—	141.7	120.8	—	—	—
1146	**ONION RINGS**	1 SERV	28	—	131.8	.1	5.9	19.3	—	2.8	0	434.9	—	—
			100	—	470.8	.2	21.0	69.0	—	10.1	0	1553.1	—	—
1147	**POPCORN,** popped, w/oil & salt	1 CUP	9	5.6	41.0	.9	2.0	5.3	.2	.7	19.4	174.6	—	—
			100	5.6	456.0	9.8	21.8	59.1	1.7	8.0	216.0	1940.0	—	—
1148	**POTATO CHIPS**	1 CUP	20	1.8	113.6	1.1	8.0	10.0	.3	8.0	27.8	200.0	9.6	226.0
			100	1.8	568.0	5.3	39.8	50.0	1.6	40.0	139.0	1000.0	48.0	1130.0
1149	**PUMPKIN & SQUASH SEED KERNELS,** dry	1 CUP	140	4.4	774.2	40.6	65.4	21.0	2.7	71.4	1601.6	—	—	—
			100	4.4	553.0	29.0	46.7	15.0	1.9	51.0	1144.0	—	—	—
1150	**SUNFLOWER SEED KERNELS,** dry, hulled	1 CUP	145	4.8	812.0	33.4	68.6	28.9	5.5	174.0	1213.7	43.5	55.1	1334.0
			100	4.8	560.0	23.0	47.3	19.9	3.8	120.0	837.0	30.0	38.0	920.0

Item No.	Minerals (Micro)			Fat-Soluble Vitamins			Water-Soluble Vitamins								
	Iron	Zinc	Copper	Vitamin A	Vitamin D	Vitamin E (Alpha Tocopherol)	Vitamin C	Thiamin	Riboflavin	Niacin	Pantothenic Acid	Vit. B-6 (Pyridoxine)	Folacin (Folic Acid)	Biotin	Vitamin B-12
	(mg)	(mg)	(mg)	(IU)	(IU)	(mg)	(mg)	(mg)	(mg)	(mg)	(mg)	(mg)	(mcg)	(mcg)	(mcg)
1121	.49	–	–	1976.2	–	–	7.87	.03	.07	.30	–	–	–	–	–
	.30	–	–	1205.0	–	–	4.80	.02	.04	.18	–	–	–	–	–
1122	.17	0	–	23.5	0	–	1.67	0	0	.04	0	0	0	–	0
	.61	0	–	83.8	0	–	5.97	0	0	.15	0	.01	0	–	0
1123	.70	–	–	1084.0	–	–	19.00	.06	.07	.50	–	–	–	–	–
	.70	–	–	1084.0	–	–	19.00	.06	.07	.50	–	–	–	–	–
1124	2.34	–	–	–	–	–	46.80	.23	.21	–	–	–	–	–	–
	.90	–	–	–	–	–	18.00	.09	.08	–	–	–	–	–	–
1125	.95	–	–	39.9	–	–	2.09	.04	.02	.68	–	–	–	–	–
	.50	–	–	21.0	–	–	1.10	.02	.01	.36	–	–	–	–	–
1126	.23	.05	–	37.2	1.24	–	4.67	.03	.02	.32	.06	.01	1.54	–	.04
	.81	.17	–	132.8	4.41	–	16.68	.10	.06	1.12	.20	.01	5.49	–	.13
1127	2.00	–	–	450.0	–	–	27.50	.18	.15	2.25	–	–	–	–	–
	.80	–	–	180.0	–	–	11.00	.07	.06	.90	–	–	–	–	–
1128	2.60	–	–	580.0	–	–	2.00	.08	.22	10.00	–	–	–	–	–
	1.30	–	–	290.0	–	–	1.00	.04	.11	5.00	–	–	–	–	–
1129	.13	.06	–	52.9	0	–	1.49	.15	.02	.08	.06	.02	4.93	–	0
	.46	.21	–	188.8	0	–	5.31	.53	.05	.29	.20	.06	17.60	–	0
1130	.64	–	–	133.9	–	–	3.34	.07	.04	.23	–	–	–	–	–
	.59	–	–	124.0	–	–	3.09	.06	.04	.21	–	–	–	–	–
1131	.03	–	–	29.4	–	–	.28	0	.01	.01	–	–	–	–	–
	.20	–	–	210.0	–	–	2.00	.01	.10	.10	–	–	–	–	–
1132	.07	.01	–	57.5	–	–	.08	0	.02	.04	–	–	–	–	–
	.50	.11	–	411.0	–	–	.60	.06	.15	.25	–	–	–	–	–
1133	.06	.01	–	–	–	–	–	–	–	–	–	–	–	–	–
	.40	.08	–	–	–	–	–	–	–	–	–	–	–	–	–
1134	.03	.02	–	–	–	–	–	–	–	–	–	–	–	–	–
	.20	.11	–	–	–	–	–	–	–	–	–	–	–	–	–
1135	.03	–	–	30.8	–	–	–	0	0	–	–	–	.42	–	–
	.20	–	–	220.0	–	–	–	.01	.03	–	–	–	3.00	–	–
1136	.08	.06	–	96.6	–	–	.84	0	0	.08	–	–	–	–	–
	.60	.43	–	690.0	–	–	6.00	.05	.05	.60	–	–	–	–	–
1137	–	–	–	–	–	–	–	–	–	–	–	–	–	–	–
	–	–	–	–	–	–	–	–	–	–	–	–	–	–	–
1138	.08	.02	–	44.8	–	–	.42	0	0	.03	–	–	–	–	–
	.60	.14	–	320.0	–	–	3.00	.02	.03	.20	–	–	–	–	–
1139	–	–	–	–	–	–	–	–	–	–	–	–	–	–	–
	–	–	–	–	–	–	–	–	–	–	–	–	–	–	–
1140	.00	–	–	0	–	–	0	.00	0	0	0	0	–	–	0
	.00	–	–	0	–	–	0	.00	0	0	0	0	–	–	0
1141	.10	.00	.04	71.1	–	3.86	0	.01	.03	.20	–	–	–	–	–
	.36	.00	.13	254.0	–	13.80	0	.04	.11	.71	–	–	–	–	–
1142	.44	.11	.18	141.2	–	2.41	0	.01	.03	.42	–	.08	–	–	–
	1.10	.28	.46	353.0	–	6.02	0	.03	.07	1.06	–	.20	–	–	–
1143	.95	.01	.06	112.5	–	–	0	.01	.04	.28	–	–	–	–	–
	3.40	.04	.21	402.0	–	–	0	.03	.15	1.00	–	–	–	–	–
1144	.02	–	–	78.3	.90	.03	0	.01	.02	.13	–	.02	–	–	.08
	.10	–	–	522.0	6.00	.20	0	.03	.16	.83	–	.10	–	–	.54
1145	–	–	–	–	–	–	–	.03	–	–	–	–	–	–	–
	–	–	–	–	–	–	–	.21	–	–	–	–	–	–	–
1146	0	–	–	0	–	–	0	0	0	0	0	0	–	–	0
	0	–	–	0	–	–	0	0	0	0	0	0	–	–	0
1147	.19	.27	–	–	–	–	0	.0	.01	.15	–	–	–	–	–
	2.10	3.00	–	–	–	–	0	.03	.09	1.70	–	–	–	–	–
1148	.36	.16	–	0	–	1.28	3.20	.04	.01	.96	–	.04	–	–	0
	1.80	.81	–	0	–	6.40	16.00	.21	.07	4.80	–	.18	–	–	0
1149	15.68	–	–	98.0	–	–	–	.34	.27	3.36	–	.13	–	–	0
	11.20	–	–	70.0	–	–	–	.24	.19	2.40	–	.09	–	–	0
1150	10.30	6.64	2.57	72.5	–	18.85	–	2.84	.33	7.83	2.03	1.81	–	–	0
	7.10	4.58	1.77	50.0	–	13.00	–	1.96	.23	5.40	1.40	1.25	–	–	0

(Continued)

TABLE F-21 *(Continued)*

Item No.	Food Item Name	Approximate Measure	Weight (g)	Moisture (%)	Food Energy Calories (kcal)	Protein (g)	Fats (g)	Carbo-hydrates (g)	Fiber (g)	Minerals (Macro) Calcium (mg)	Phos-phorus (mg)	Sodium (mg)	Mag-nesium (mg)	Potas-sium (mg)
	SOUPS AND CHOWDERS													
1151	ASPARAGUS SOUP, cream of, made w/= volume milk	1 CUP	240	85.2	165.6	6.5	8.2	17.2	.1	170.4	148.8	1056.0	—	225.6
			100	85.2	69.0	2.7	3.4	7.2	.1	71.0	62.0	440.0	—	94.0
1152	BEAN SOUP, w/ham	1 OZ	28	67.8	36.5	2.4	.8	5.1	.3	11.9	41.3	32.0	1.2	82.4
			100	67.8	130.3	8.7	2.8	18.3	1.2	42.6	147.4	114.4	4.2	294.4
	BEEF SOUP													
1153	broth, bouillon or consomme, canned, made w/= volume water	1 CUP	240	95.8	31.2	5.0	0	2.6	—	—	31.2	782.4	—	129.6
			100	95.8	13.0	2.1	0	1.1	—	—	13.0	326.0	—	54.0
1154	w/vegetable, diluted w/water	1 CUP	244	—	—	2.0	—	—	—	—	—	—	—	—
			100	—	—	.8	—	—	—	—	—	—	—	—
1155	BORSCHT	1 AVG	250	—	80.0	.6	0	19.3	—	—	—	—	—	—
			100	—	32.0	.2	—	7.7	—	—	—	—	—	—
1156	BOUILLON CUBES OR POWDER	1 CUBE	4	4.0	(6.0)	(.6)	(.1)	(.6)	—	—	(8.0)	960.0	(2.0)	(15.0)
			100	4.0	(170.0)	(17.3)	(4.0)	(16.1)	—	—	(225.0)	24000.0	(50.0)	(403.0)
1157	CELERY SOUP, CREAM OF, diluted w/milk	1 CUP	245	85.8	169.0	6.4	9.8	15.5	—	202.1	157.2	1060.6	—	295.0
			100	85.8	69.0	2.6	4.0	6.3	—	82.5	64.2	432.9	—	120.4
	CHICKEN SOUP													
1158	consomme, made w/= volume water	1 CUP	240	96.8	21.6	3.4	.5	1.9	—	12.0	72.0	722.4	—	—
			100	96.8	9.0	1.4	.2	.8	—	5.0	30.0	301.0	—	—
1159	cream of, diluted w/milk	1 CUP	245	85.4	182.7	7.4	11.5	14.5	—	175.6	155.2	1054.0	—	260.0
			100	85.4	74.6	3.0	4.7	5.9	—	71.7	63.3	430.2	—	106.1
1160	gumbo, diluted w/water	1 CUP	241	93.8	55.2	3.1	1.4	7.4	—	190.8	24.1	954.0	—	108.5
			100	93.8	22.9	1.3	.6	3.1	—	79.2	10.0	395.8	—	45.0
1161	noodle, diluted w/water	1 CUP	241	86.6	127.9	3.4	2.4	7.9	—	10.0	36.2	983.1	—	55.2
			100	86.6	53.1	1.4	1.0	3.3	—	4.2	15.0	407.9	—	22.9
1162	w/rice, diluted w/water	1 CUP	241	94.8	48.2	3.1	1.9	5.8	—	7.0	24.1	920.8	—	98.4
			100	94.8	20.0	1.3	.8	2.4	—	2.9	10.0	382.1	—	40.8
1163	CLAM CHOWDER, New England style, condensed & frozen, made w/= volume milk	1 CUP	245	82.8	215.6	8.8	12.6	16.9	.2	235.2	198.5	1127.0	—	411.6
			100	82.8	88.0	3.6	5.2	6.9	.1	96.0	81.0	460.0	—	168.0
1164	⁵LENTIL	1 CUP	250	—	247.8	11.3	9.5	29.5	5.5	100.5	146.5	475.8	40.3	402.5
			100	—	99.1	4.5	3.8	11.8	2.2	40.2	58.6	190.3	16.1	161.0
1165	MINNESTRONE, diluted w/water	1 CUP	244	89.5	104.6	4.9	2.7	14.1	—	36.8	58.8	990.9	—	312.7
			100	89.5	42.9	2.0	1.1	5.8	—	15.1	24.1	406.1	—	128.2
1166	MUSHROOM SOUP, CREAM OF, condensed, diluted w/milk	1 CUP	245	83.2	216.0	6.9	13.7	16.2	—	191.0	169.0	1039.0	—	279.0
			100	83.2	88.2	2.8	5.6	6.6	—	78.0	69.0	424.1	—	113.9
1167	ONION SOUP, ¹canned, made w/= volume water	1 CUP	240	94.5	57.6	3.6	3.4	3.4	.2	9.6	38.4	1108.8	—	115.2
			100	94.5	24.0	1.5	1.4	1.4	.1	4.0	16.0	462.0	—	48.0
1168	OYSTER STEW, homemade, 1 part oysters to 2 parts milk	1 CUP	240	82.0	232.8	12.5	15.4	10.8	—	273.6	266.4	813.6	—	319.2
			100	82.0	97.0	5.2	6.4	4.5	—	114.0	111.0	339.0	—	133.0
1169	PEA, GREEN, SOUP, condensed, made w/= volume milk	1 CUP	200	79.9	170.0	8.4	5.2	23.4	.8	158.0	188.0	786.0	—	306.0
			100	79.9	85.0	4.2	2.6	11.7	.4	79.0	94.0	393.0	—	153.0
1170	PEA, SPLIT, SOUP, homemade	1 OZ	28	63.8	23.2	1.3	.5	3.0	.1	13.9	21.8	111.6	1.3	32.4
			100	63.8	82.9	4.5	1.9	10.8	.3	49.6	77.7	398.5	4.5	115.7
1171	POTATO SOUP, CREAM OF, condensed, diluted w/milk	1 CUP	245	—	—	6.6	—	—	—	—	—	—	—	—
			100	—	—	2.7	—	—	—	—	—	—	—	—
1172	SCOTCH BROTH, condensed, diluted w/water	1 CUP	244	—	—	2.7	—	—	—	—	—	—	—	—
			100	—	—	1.1	—	—	—	—	—	—	—	—
1173	SHRIMP SOUP, CREAM OF, ¹frozen, condensed, made w/= volume milk	1 CUP	250	81.8	250.0	9.5	17.3	14.8	.5	187.5	167.5	1137.5	—	247.5
			100	81.8	100.0	3.8	6.9	5.9	.2	75.0	67.0	455.0	—	99.0
1174	TOMATO SOUP, diluted w/milk	1 CUP	248	84.0	171.6	6.4	6.2	22.3	—	166.7	153.8	1046.6	—	414.7
			100	84.0	69.2	2.6	2.5	9.0	—	67.2	62.0	422.0	—	167.2
1175	TURKEY & NOODLE SOUP, condensed, diluted w/water	1 CUP	241	—	92.7	4.3	2.7	8.4	—	14.1	43.2	1002.2	—	77.3
			100	—	38.5	1.8	1.1	3.5	—	5.8	17.9	415.8	—	32.1
	VEGETABLE SOUP													
1176	condensed, diluted w/water	1 CUP	244	91.7	77.7	2.7	2.2	13.4	—	19.9	38.8	841.6	—	239.0
			100	91.7	31.8	1.1	.9	5.5	—	8.1	15.9	344.9	—	98.0
1177	w/beef broth, condensed, made w/= volume water	1 CUP	245	91.7	78.4	2.7	1.7	13.5	.7	19.6	39.2	845.3	24.5	240.1
			100	91.7	32.0	1.1	.7	5.5	.3	8.0	16.0	345.0	10.0	98.0
	VEGETABLES													
1178	ALFALFA SPROUTS, raw	1 CUP	38	88.3	15.6	1.9	.2	—	.6	10.6	—	—	—	—
			100	88.3	41.0	5.1	.6	—	1.7	28.0	—	—	—	—
1179	⁵AMARANTH LEAVES	1 OZ	28	86.0	11.8	1.0	.2	2.1	.4	87.6	20.7	—	—	—
			100	86.0	42.0	3.7	.8	7.4	1.5	313.0	74.0	—	—	—
1180	⁵ARROWROOT, BERMUDA	1 OZ	28	57.2	44.0	.7	0	10.9	.5	5.6	6.7	—	—	—
			100	57.2	157.0	2.4	—	39.0	1.9	20.0	24.0	—	—	—
1181	ARTICHOKES, Globe or French, boiled, drained	1 LG	100	90.2	38.0	3.4	.1	5.8	1.9	67.0	67.0	30.0	(27.2)	301.0
			100	90.2	38.0	3.4	.1	5.8	1.9	67.0	67.0	30.0	(27.2)	301.0

Item No.	Minerals (Micro)			Fat-Soluble Vitamins			Water-Soluble Vitamins								
	Iron	Zinc	Copper	Vitamin A	Vitamin D	Vitamin E (Alpha Tocopherol)	Vitamin C	Thiamin	Ribo-flavin	Niacin	Panto-thenic Acid	Vit. B-6 (Pyri-doxine)	Folacin (Folic Acid)	Biotin	Vitamin B-12
	(mg)	(mg)	(mg)	(IU)	(IU)	(mg)	(mg)	(mg)	(mg)	(mg)	(mg)	(mg)	(mcg)	(mcg)	(mcg)
1151	1.08	–	–	578.4	–	–	–	.17	.31	1.20	–	–	–	–	–
	.45	–	–	241.0	–	–	–	.07	.13	.50	–	–	–	–	–
1152	.61	.08	–	11.7	.66	–	1.23	.06	.03	.37	.04	0	–	–	.17
	2.18	.29	–	41.9	2.35	–	4.40	.22	.09	1.33	.14	0	–	–	.69
1153	.48	–	–	–	–	–	–	–	.02	1.20	–	–	9.60	–	–
	.20	–	–	–	–	–	–	–	.01	.50	–	–	4.00	–	–
1154	–	–	–	–	–	–	–	–	–	–	–	–	–	–	–
	–	–	–	–	–	–	–	–	–	–	–	–	–	–	–
1155	–	–	–	–	–	–	–	–	–	–	–	–	–	–	–
	–	–	–	–	–	–	–	–	–	–	–	–	–	–	–
1156	(.08)	(.01)	–	–	0	–	0	(.01)	(.01)	(.12)	–	–	–	–	–
	(2.23)	(.21)	–	–	0	–	0	(.20)	(.24)	(3.30)	–	–	–	–	–
1157	.72	–	–	398.1	–	–	2.00	.05	.27	.70	–	–	–	–	–
	.29	–	–	162.5	–	–	.82	.02	.11	.29	–	–	–	–	–
1158	1.20	–	–	–	–	–	–	–	–	–	–	–	–	–	–
	.50	–	–	–	–	–	–	–	–	–	–	–	–	–	–
1159	.51	–	–	610.0	–	–	2.00	.05	.27	.70	–	–	–	–	–
	.21	–	–	249.0	–	–	.82	.02	.11	.29	–	–	–	–	–
1160	.50	–	–	220.9	–	–	5.02	.02	.05	1.21	–	–	–	–	–
	.21	–	–	91.7	–	–	2.08	.01	.02	.50	–	–	–	–	–
1161	.50	–	–	50.2	–	–	0	.02	.02	.70	–	–	–	–	–
	.21	–	–	20.8	–	–	0	.01	.01	.29	–	–	–	–	–
1162	.20	–	–	140.6	–	–	–	0	.02	.70	–	–	–	–	–
	.08	–	–	58.3	–	–	–	0	.01	.29	–	–	–	–	–
1163	1.10	–	–	257.3	–	–	–	.09	.29	.61	–	–	–	–	–
	.45	–	–	105.0	–	–	–	.04	.12	.25	–	–	–	–	–
1164	3.03	1.30	.30	1824.3	.68	–	Trace	.20	.10	.73	–	.15	–	–	0
	1.21	.52	.12	729.7	.27	–	Trace	.08	.04	.29	–	06	–	–	0
1165	1.00	–	–	2340.4	–	–	–	.07	.05	1.00	–	–	–	–	–
	.41	–	–	959.2	–	–	–	.03	.02	.41	–	–	–	–	–
1166	.50	–	–	250.0	–	–	1.00	.05	.34	.70	–	–	–	–	–
	.20	–	–	102.0	–	–	.41	.02	.14	.29	–	–	–	–	–
1167	.63	–	.12	–	–	–	–	.01	.02	.80	–	–	–	–	–
	.25	–	.05	–	–	–	–	.01	.01	.35	–	–	–	–	–
1168	4.56	–	–	816.0	–	–	–	.14	.43	2.16	–	–	–	–	–
	1.90	–	–	340.0	–	–	–	.06	.18	.90	–	–	–	–	–
1169	.80	–	–	420.0	–	–	8.00	.08	.22	1.00	–	–	–	–	–
	.40	–	–	210.0	–	–	4.00	.04	.11	.50	–	–	–	–	–
1170	.19	.03	–	40.6	3.83	–	.27	.01	.02	.15	.03	0	.47	–	.03
	.67	.11	–	145.1	13.67	–	.96	.05	.08	.53	.11	.013	1.67	–	.12
1171	–	–	–	–	–	–	–	–	–	–	–	–	–	–	–
	–	–	–	–	–	–	–	–	–	–	–	–	–	–	–
1172	–	–	–	–	–	–	–	–	–	–	–	–	–	–	–
	–	–	–	–	–	–	–	–	–	–	–	–	–	–	–
1173	.63	–	–	317.5	–	–	–	.09	.28	.50	–	–	–	–	–
	.25	–	–	127.0	–	–	–	.04	.11	.20	–	–	–	–	–
1174	.79	1.07	–	1190.4	–	–	14.88	.10	.25	1.29	–	–	–	–	–
	.32	.43	–	480.0	–	–	6.00	.04	.10	.52	–	–	–	–	–
1175	.70	–	–	190.8	–	–	–	–	–	–	–	–	–	–	–
	.29	–	–	79.2	–	–	–	–	–	–	–	–	–	–	–
1176	.70	1.81	–	3177.0	–	–	–	–	–	–	–	–	–	–	–
	.29	.74	–	1302.0	–	–	–	–	–	–	–	–	–	–	–
1177	.74	–	–	3185.0	–	–	–	.05	.03	1.23	–	–	–	–	–
	.30	–	–	1300.0	–	–	–	.02	.01	.50	–	–	–	–	–
1178	.53	.38	–	–	–	–	6.08	.05	.08	.61	–	–	–	–	–
	1.40	1.00	–	–	–	–	16.00	.14	.21	1.60	–	–	–	–	–
1179	1.56	–	–	448.0	–	–	18.20	.01	.07	.34	–	–	–	–	–
	5.60	–	–	1600.0	–	–	65.00	.05	.24	1.20	–	–	–	–	–
1180	.90	–	–	0	–	–	2.52	.02	.01	.20	–	–	–	–	–
	3.20	–	–	0	–	–	9.00	.08	.03	.70	–	–	–	–	–
1181	.90	.35	(.03)	90.0	0	–	8.40	.07	.03	.93	.21	.07	32.00	4.10	0
	.90	.35	(.03)	90.0	0	–	8.40	.07	.03	.93	.21	.07	32.00	4.10	0

(Continued)

TABLE F-21 *(Continued)*

Item No.	Food Item Name	Approximate Measure	Weight	Moisture	Food Energy Calories	Protein	Fats	Carbo-hydrates	Fiber	Minerals (Macro)				
										Calcium	Phosphorus	Sodium	Magnesium	Potassium
			(g)	(%)	(kcal)	(g)	(g)	(g)	(g)	(mg)	(mg)	(mg)	(mg)	(mg)
1182	ARTICHOKES, Jerusalem, raw	1 SM	25	79.8	10.3	.6	0	4.2	.2	3.5	19.5	–	2.8	–
			100	79.8	41.0	2.3	.1	16.7	.8	14.0	78.0	–	11.0	–
	ASPARAGUS													
1183	fresh, cooked, drained	1 SPEAR	20	93.6	4.0	.4	0	.7	.1	4.2	10.0	.2	(2.9)	36.6
			100	93.6	20.0	2.2	.2	3.6	.7	21.0	50.0	1.0	(10.3)	183.0
1184	green, canned, drained solids	1 CUP	150	92.5	31.5	3.6	.6	5.1	1.2	28.5	79.5	354.0	–	249.0
			100	92.5	21.0	2.4	.4	3.4	.8	19.0	53.0	236.0	–	166.0
1185	frozen spears, boiled, drained	1 SPEAR	22	92.2	5.1	.7	0	.8	.2	4.8	14.7	.2	3.1	52.4
			100	92.2	23.0	3.2	.2	3.8	.8	22.0	67.0	1.0	14.0	238.0
1186	white, canned, drained solids	1 CUP	150	92.3	33.0	3.2	.8	5.4	1.2	24.0	61.5	354.0	–	210.0
			100	92.3	22.0	2.1	.5	3.6	.8	16.0	41.0	236.0	–	140.0
1187	³BAMBARRA-GROUNDNUT, whole seeds, dried	1 OZ	28	10.3	102.8	5.3	1.7	17.2	1.3	17.4	77.3	–	–	–
			100	10.3	367.0	18.8	6.2	61.3	4.8	62.0	276.0	–	–	–
1188	BAMBOO SHOOTS, canned	1 CUP	133	95.0	21.3	1.9	.1	3.5	.9	13.7	20.1	5.1	6.0	128.1
			100	95.0	16.0	1.4	.1	2.6	.7	10.3	15.1	3.8	4.5	96.3
	BEANS, GREEN													
1189	fresh, boiled in small amount of water, drained	1 CUP	125	92.4	31.3	2.0	.2	6.8	1.3	62.5	46.3	5.0	–	188.8
			100	92.4	25.0	1.6	.2	5.4	1.0	50.0	37.0	4.0	–	151.0
1190	frozen, cut, boiled, drained	1 CUP	161	92.1	40.3	2.6	.2	9.2	1.6	64.4	51.5	1.6	32.2	244.7
			100	92.1	25.0	1.6	.1	5.7	1.0	40.0	32.0	1.0	20.0	152.0
	BEANS, LIMA													
1191	immature seeds, boiled, drained	1 CUP	184	71.1	204.2	14.0	.9	36.4	3.3	86.5	222.6	1.8	–	776.5
			100	71.1	111.0	7.6	.5	19.8	1.8	47.0	121.0	1.0	–	422.0
1192	baby, frozen, boiled, drained	1 CUP	173	68.8	204.1	12.8	.3	38.6	3.3	60.6	218.0	223.2	83.0	681.6
			100	68.8	118.0	7.4	.2	22.3	1.9	35.0	126.0	129.0	48.0	394.0
1193	frozen, boiled, drained	1 CUP	160	73.5	158.4	9.6	.2	30.6	2.6	32.0	144.0	161.6	76.8	681.6
			100	73.5	99.0	6.0	.1	19.1	1.6	20.0	90.0	101.0	48.0	426.0
1194	BEANS, MUNG, sprouted seeds, uncooked	1 CUP	210	85.9	111.3	9.0	.4	13.9	1.3	27.3	134.4	10.5	33.6	468.3
			100	85.9	53.0	4.3	.2	6.6	.6	13.0	64.0	5.0	16.0	223.0
1195	BEANS, refried, cooked in iron skillet	1 CUP	210	–	–	–	–	–	–	–	–	–	–	–
			100	–	–	–	–	–	–	–	–	–	–	–
1196	BEAN SPROUTS—See BEANS, MUNG, LENTIL & SOYBEAN SPROUTS													
	BEANS, WAX													
1197	boiled, drained	1 CUP	164	93.4	36.1	2.3	.3	7.5	1.6	82.0	60.7	4.9	–	247.6
			100	93.4	22.0	1.4	.2	4.6	1.0	50.0	37.0	3.0	–	151.0
1198	canned, drained solids	1 CUP	200	92.2	48.0	2.8	.6	10.4	1.8	90.0	50.0	472.0	–	190.0
			100	92.2	24.0	1.4	.3	5.2	.9	45.0	25.0	236.0	–	95.0
1199	frozen, cut, boiled, drained	1 CUP	161	91.5	43.5	2.7	.2	10.0	1.8	56.4	49.9	1.6	33.8	264.0
			100	91.5	27.0	1.7	.1	6.2	1.1	35.0	31.0	1.0	21.0	164.0
1200	BEET GREENS, boiled, drained	1 CUP	200	93.6	36.0	3.4	.4	6.6	2.2	198.0	50.0	152.0	–	664.0
			100	93.6	18.0	1.7	.2	3.3	1.1	99.0	25.0	76.0	–	332.0
	BEETS													
1201	fresh, boiled, drained	1 CUP	200	90.9	64.0	2.2	.2	14.4	1.6	28.0	46.0	86.0	–	416.0
			100	90.9	32.0	1.1	.1	7.2	.8	14.0	23.0	43.0	–	208.0
1202	canned, drained solids	1 CUP	166	89.3	61.4	1.7	.2	14.6	1.3	31.5	29.9	391.8	24.9	277.2
			100	89.3	37.0	1.0	.1	8.8	.8	19.0	18.0	236.0	15.0	167.0
1203	BROADBEAN, ⁴fried & salted	1 OZ	28	7.6	112.6	7.4	4.1	13.3	1.1	20.4	92.7	–	–	278.3
			100	7.6	402.0	26.4	14.8	47.4	3.8	73.0	331.0	–	–	994.0
	BROCCOLI													
1204	spears, cooked	1 CUP	150	91.3	39.0	4.7	.5	6.8	2.4	132.0	93.0	15.0	–	400.5
			100	91.3	26.0	3.1	.3	4.5	1.5	88.0	62.0	10.0	–	267.0
1205	spears, frozen, cooked	1 CUP	188	91.4	48.9	5.8	.4	8.8	2.2	77.1	109.0	22.6	39.5	413.6
			100	91.4	26.0	3.1	.2	4.7	1.1	41.0	58.0	12.0	21.0	220.0
	BRUSSELS SPROUTS													
1206	cooked	1 CUP	150	88.2	54.0	6.3	.6	9.6	2.4	48.0	108.0	15.0	–	409.5
			100	88.2	36.0	4.2	.4	6.4	1.6	32.0	72.0	10.0	–	273.0
1207	frozen, cooked	1 CUP	150	89.3	49.5	4.8	.3	9.8	1.8	31.5	91.5	21.0	31.5	442.5
			100	89.3	33.0	3.2	.2	6.5	1.2	21.0	61.0	14.0	21.0	295.0
1208	CABBAGE, common, shredded, cooked in small amount of water	1 CUP	145	93.9	29.0	1.6	.3	6.2	1.2	63.8	29.0	20.3	–	236.4
			100	93.9	20.0	1.1	.2	4.3	.8	44.0	20.0	14.0	–	163.0
1209	CABBAGE, CHINESE, ⁴salted	1 PKG	183	86.8	71.4	2.0	.5	17.2	3.1	237.9	96.9	1647.0	–	344.0
			100	86.8	39.0	1.1	.3	9.4	1.7	130.0	53.0	900.0	–	188.0
1210	⁵CALABASH GOURD	1 OZ	28	92.2	7.3	.2	.1	1.8	.4	5.0	5.9	–	–	–
			100	92.2	26.0	.7	.2	6.3	1.5	18.0	21.0	–	–	–
	CARROTS													
1211	raw	1 LG	100	59.0	42.0	1.2	.2	9.7	1.0	37.0	36.0	47.0	18.5	341.0
			100	59.0	42.0	1.2	.2	9.7	1.0	37.0	36.0	47.0	18.5	341.0

Item No.	Minerals (Micro)			Fat-Soluble Vitamins			Water-Soluble Vitamins								
	Iron	Zinc	Copper	Vitamin A	Vitamin D	Vitamin E (Alpha Tocopherol)	Vitamin C	Thiamin	Ribo-flavin	Niacin	Panto-thenic Acid	Vit. B-6 (Pyri-doxine)	Folacin (Folic Acid)	Biotin	Vitamin B-12
	(mg)	(mg)	(mg)	(IU)	(IU)	(mg)	(mg)	(mg)	(mg)	(mg)	(mg)	(mg)	(mcg)	(mcg)	(mcg)
1182	.85	.02	—	5.0	—	—	1.00	.05	.02	.33	.02	0	—	—	—
	3.40	.06	—	20.0	—	—	4.00	.20	.06	1.30	.07	0	—	—	—
1183	.12	(.09)	(.06)	180.0	—	(.70)	5.20	.03	.04	.28	(.04)	(.01)	(8.42)	(.13)	0
	.60	(.31)	(.22)	900.0	—	(2.50)	26.00	.16	.18	1.40	(.14)	(.04)	(30.06)	(.46)	0
1184	2.85	—	—	1200.0	—	—	22.50	.09	.15	1.20	—	—	115.00	—	—
	1.90	—	—	800.0	—	—	15.00	.06	.10	.80	—	—	76.00	—	—
1185	.24	—	—	171.6	—	—	5.72	.01	.02	.24	.07	0	17.38	—	—
	1.10	—	—	780.0	—	—	26.00	.07	.10	1.10	.32	.02	79.00	—	—
1186	1.50	—	—	120.0	—	—	22.50	.08	.09	1.05	—	—	—	—	—
	1.00	—	—	80.0	—	—	15.00	.05	.06	.70	—	—	—	—	—
1187	3.42	—	—	9.3	—	—	0	.13	.04	.50	—	—	—	—	—
	12.20	—	—	33.3	—	—	0	.47	.14	1.80	—	—	—	—	—
1188	.36	.65	.01	—	—	—	1.33	.01	.03	.20	—	—	—	—	—
	.27	.49	.01	—	—	—	1.00	.01	.02	.15	—	—	—	—	—
1189	.75	.38	—	675.0	—	—	15.00	.09	.11	.63	—	—	50.00	—	—
	.60	.30	—	540.0	—	—	12.00	.07	.09	.50	—	—	40.00	—	—
1190	1.13	.34	(.10)	933.8	—	.18	8.05	.11	.15	.64	.21	.10	—	—	—
	.70	.21	(.05)	580.0	—	.11	5.00	.07	.09	40	.13	.06	—	—	—
1191	4.60	—	—	515.2	—	—	31.28	.33	.18	2.39	—	—	—	—	—
	2.50	—	—	280.0	—	—	17.00	.18	.10	1.30	—	—	—	—	—
1192	4.50	—	—	380.6	—	—	20.76	.16	.09	2.08	.31	.15	112.45	—	—
	2.60	—	—	220.0	—	—	12.00	.09	.05	1.20	.18	.09	65.00	—	—
1193	2.72	.77	.10	368.0	—	—	27.20	.11	.08	1.60	.29	.16	104.00	—	—
	1.70	.48	.06	230.0	—	—	17.00	.07	.05	1.00	.18	.10	65.00	—	—
1194	4.00	1.89	—	42.0	—	—	42.00	.29	.38	2.31	—	—	—	—	—
	1.90	.90	—	20.0	—	—	20.00	.14	.18	1.10	—	—	—	—	—
1195	3.84	—	—	—	—	—	—	—	—	—	—	—	—	—	—
	1.83	—	—	—	—	—	—	—	—	—	—	—	—	—	—
1196															
1197	.98	—	—	377.2	—	—	21.32	.12	.15	.82	—	—	—	—	—
	.60	—	—	230.0	—	—	13.00	.07	.09	.50	—	—	—	—	—
1198	3.00	.46	—	200.0	—	—	10.00	.06	.10	.60	—	—	—	—	—
	1.50	.23	—	100.0	—	—	5.00	.03	.05	.30	—	—	—	—	—
1199	1.13	—	—	161.0	—	—	9.66	.11	.13	.64	—	—	—	—	—
	.70	.24	.06	100.0	—	—	6.00	.07	.08	40	—	—	—	—	—
1200	3.80	—	—	10200.0	—	—	30.00	.14	.30	.60	—	—	—	—	—
	1.90	—	—	5100.0	—	—	15.00	.07	.15	.30	—	—	—	—	—
1201	1.00	—	—	40.0	—	—	12.00	.06	.08	.60	—	—	156.00	—	.17
	.50	—	—	20.0	—	—	6.00	.03	.04	.30	—	—	78.00	—	.09
1202	1.16	—	—	33.2	—	—	4.98	.02	.05	.17	—	—	39.84	—	—
	.70	—	—	20.0	—	—	3.00	.01	.03	.10	—	—	24.00	—	—
1203	1.98	—	—	4.7	—	—	0	.03	.01	.76	—	—	—	—	—
	7.10	—	—	16.7	—	—	0	.10	.05	1.00	—	—	—	—	—
1204	1.20	.23	—	3750.0	—	—	135.00	.14	.30	1.20	—	—	84.00	1.80	—
	.80	.15	—	2500.0	—	—	90.00	.09	.20	.80	—	—	56.00	1.20	—
1205	1.32	.28	—	3572.0	—	—	137.24	.11	.21	.94	.98	.20	112.80	—	—
	.70	.15	—	1900.0	—	—	73.00	.06	.11	.50	.52	.10	60.00	—	—
1206	1.65	.54	—	780.0	—	—	130.50	.12	.21	1.20	—	—	54.00	—	—
	1.10	.36	—	520.0	—	—	87.00	.08	.14	.80	—	—	36.00	—	—
1207	1.20	.54	(.05)	855.0	—	—	121.50	.12	.15	.90	—	—	132.00	—	—
	.80	.36	(.03)	570.0	—	—	81.00	.08	.10	.60	—	—	88.00	—	—
1208	.44	.58	—	188.5	—	—	47.85	.06	.06	.44	—	—	26.10	—	—
	.30	.40	—	130.0	—	—	33.00	.04	.04	.30	—	—	18.00	—	—
1209	2.0	—	—	—	—	—	9.15	.15	.37	2.40	—	—	—	—	—
	1.1	—	—	—	—	—	5.00	.08	.20	1.30	—	—	—	—	—
1210	.14	—	—	0	—	—	5.32	.01	.00	.17	—	—	—	—	—
	.50	—	—	0	—	—	19.00	.04	.03	.60	—	—	—	—	—
1211	.70	.40	.01	11000.0	—	.45	0	.06	.05	.60	.28	.15	32.00	2.50	0
	.70	.40	.01	11000.0	—	.45	0	.06	.05	.60	.28	.15	32.00	2.50	0

(Continued)

TABLE F-21 *(Continued)*

Item No.	Food Item Name	Approximate Measure	Weight	Moisture	Food Energy Calories	Protein	Fats	Carbohydrates	Fiber	Minerals (Macro)				
										Calcium	Phosphorus	Sodium	Magnesium	Potassium
			(g)	(%)	(kcal)	(g)	(g)	(g)	(g)	(mg)	(mg)	(mg)	(mg)	(mg)
	CARROTS (Continued)													
1212	raw, boiled, drained	1 CUP	150	91.2	46.5	1.4	.3	10.7	1.5	49.5	46.5	49.5	9.3	333.0
			100	91.2	31.0	.9	.2	7.1	1.0	33.0	31.0	33.0	6.2	222.0
1213	CASSAVA, ⁵sweet, root, raw	1 OZ	28	65.2	37.0	.3	.1	9.2	.3	11.2	9.5	–	–	–
			100	65.2	132.0	1.0	.4	32.8	1.0	40.0	34.0	–	–	–
	CAULIFLOWER													
1214	raw	1 CUP	100	91.0	27.0	2.7	.2	5.2	1.0	25.0	56.0	13.0	24.0	295.0
			100	91.0	27.0	2.7	.2	5.2	1.0	25.0	56.0	13.0	24.0	295.0
1215	boiled, drained	1 CUP	120	92.8	26.4	2.8	.2	4.9	1.2	25.2	50.4	10.8	(10.7)	247.2
			100	92.8	22.0	2.3	.2	4.1	1.0	21.0	42.0	9.0	(8.9)	206.0
1216	CELERIAC ROOT, ⁵boiled	1 OZ	28	–	4.0	.4	Trace	.6	.6	13.2	19.7	7.9	3.3	112.0
			100	–	14.1	1.5	Trace	2.3	2.2	47.3	70.5	28.2	11.8	399.8
1217	CELERY, raw	1 SM	20	94.1	3.4	.2	0	.8	.1	7.8	5.6	25.2	1.7	68.2
			100	94.1	17.0	.9	.1	3.9	.6	39.0	28.0	126.0	8.7	341.0
1218	⁵CHAYOTE	1 OZ	28	90.8	8.7	.3	.1	2.2	.2	3.4	8.4	–	–	–
			100	90.8	31.0	.9	.2	7.7	.6	12.0	30.0	–	–	–
1219	fruit, raw	1 HALF	100	91.8	28.0	.6	.1	7.1	.7	13.0	26.0	5.0	14.0	102.0
			100	91.8	28.0	.6	.1	7.1	.7	13.0	26.0	5.0	14.0	102.0
1220	⁵root	1 OZ	28	79.0	22.1	.6	.1	4.5	.1	1.2	9.5	–	–	–
			100	79.0	79.0	2.0	.2	17.8	.4	7.0	34.0	–	–	–
1221	CHERVIL, raw	1 CUP	200	80.7	114.0	6.8	1.8	23.0	–	–	–	–	–	–
			100	80.7	57.0	3.4	.9	11.5	–	–	–	–	–	–
1222	CHICORY GREENS, raw	1 CUP	53	92.8	10.6	.8	.2	2.0	.4	45.6	21.2	9.5	6.9	222.6
			100	92.8	20.0	1.6	.3	3.8	.8	86.0	40.0	18.0	13.0	420.0
1223	CHICORY, Witloof, bleached head, raw	1 CUP	53	95.1	8.0	.5	.1	1.7	–	9.5	11.1	3.7	5.0	96.5
			100	95.1	15.0	1.0	.1	3.2	–	18.0	21.0	7.0	9.4	182.0
1224	CHIVES, raw	1 TBLS	10	91.3	2.8	.2	Trace	.6	.1	6.9	4.4	–	2.4	25.0
			100	91.3	28.0	1.8	.3	5.8	1.1	69.0	44.0	–	24.1	250.0
1225	CHUFA, ⁵flatsedge, tuber, raw	1 OZ	28	32.6	87.1	1.2	4.8	12.3	2.0	16.5	43.4	–	–	–
			100	32.6	311.0	4.4	17.2	43.9	7.1	59.0	155.0	–	–	–
1226	COLLARDS, leaves w/stems, cooked in small amount of water	1 CUP	200	90.8	58.0	5.4	1.2	9.8	1.6	304.0	78.0	50.0	–	468.0
			100	90.8	29.0	2.7	.6	4.9	.8	152.0	39.0	25.0	–	234.0
	CORN, SWEET													
1227	fresh, white & yellow, cooked on cob	1 MED	140	74.1	127.4	4.6	1.4	29.4	1.0	4.2	124.6	(2.5)	(63.3)	274.4
			100	74.1	91.0	3.3	1.0	21.0	.7	3.0	89.0	(1.1)	(45.2)	196.0
1228	canned, creamed, white & yellow, solids & liquid	1 CUP	166	76.3	136.1	3.5	1.0	33.2	.8	5.0	93.0	391.8	31.5	161.0
			100	76.3	82.0	2.1	.6	20.0	.5	3.0	56.0	236.0	19.0	97.0
1229	canned, whole kernel, wet pack, white & yellow, drained solids	1 CUP	166	81.7	102.9	3.2	.9	24.7	1.3	5.8	68.1	350.1	21.2	195.5
			100	81.7	62.0	1.9	.5	14.9	.8	3.5	41.0	210.9	12.8	117.8
1230	canned, whole kernel, vacuum pack, drained solids	1 CUP	166	76.4	134.5	0	1.2	31.9	–	8.0	90.5	439.1	32.0	260.8
			100	76.4	81.0	0	.7	19.2	–	4.8	54.5	264.5	19.3	157.1
1231	frozen, cooked on cob	1 MED	114	73.2	107.2	4.0	1.1	24.6	.8	3.4	109.4	1.1	38.8	263.3
			100	73.2	94.0	3.5	1.0	21.6	.7	3.0	96.0	1.0	34.0	231.0
1232	frozen, cut off cob before cooking	1 CUP	166	77.2	131.1	5.0	.8	31.2	.8	5.0	121.2	1.7	(29.9)	305.4
			100	77.2	79.0	3.0	.5	18.8	.5	3.0	73.0	1.0	(18.0)	184.0
1233	COW PEAS, young pods & seeds, cooked	1 CUP	160	89.5	54.4	4.2	.5	11.2	2.7	88.0	78.4	4.8	–	313.6
			100	89.5	34.0	2.6	.3	7.0	1.7	55.0	49.0	3.0	–	196.0
1234	CRESS, GARDEN, raw	1 AVG	2	89.4	.6	.1	0	.1	0	1.6	1.5	.3	–	12.1
			100	89.4	32.0	2.6	.7	5.5	1.1	81.0	76.0	14.0	–	606.0
1235	CUCUMBERS, raw, pared	1 MED	100	95.7	14.0	.6	.1	3.2	.3	17.0	18.0	6.0	10.0	160.0
			100	95.7	14.0	.6	.1	3.2	.3	17.0	18.0	6.0	10.0	160.0
1236	DANDELIONS, boiled, drained	1 CUP	200	89.8	66.0	4.0	1.2	12.8	2.6	280.0	84.0	88.0	–	464.0
			100	89.8	33.0	2.0	.6	6.4	1.3	140.0	42.0	44.0	–	232.0
1237	DOCK, boiled, drained	1 CUP	200	93.6	38.0	3.2	.4	7.8	1.4	110.0	52.0	6.0	–	396.0
			100	93.6	19.0	1.6	.2	3.9	.7	55.0	26.0	3.0	–	198.0
1238	EGGPLANT, boiled, drained	1 CUP	200	94.3	38.0	2.2	.4	8.2	1.8	22.0	42.0	2.0	–	300.0
			100	94.3	19.0	1.1	.2	4.1	.9	11.0	21.0	1.0	–	150.0
1239	ENDIVE (CURLY & ESCAROLE), raw	1 MED	7	93.1	1.4	.1	0	.3	.1	5.7	3.8	1.0	.7	20.6
			100	93.1	20.0	1.7	.1	4.1	.9	81.0	54.0	14.0	10.0	294.0
1240	FENNEL, common, leaves, raw	1 CUP	60	90.0	16.8	1.7	.2	3.1	.3	60.0	30.6	–	–	238.2
			100	90.0	28.0	2.8	.4	5.1	.5	100.0	51.0	–	–	397.0
1241	GARLIC, clove, raw	1 AVG	3	61.3	4.1	.2	0	.9	0	.9	6.1	.6	.7	15.9
			100	61.3	137.0	6.2	.2	30.8	1.5	29.0	202.0	19.0	23.0	529.0
1242	GRITS, hominy, cooked	1 CUP	242	87.1	123.4	2.9	.2	26.6	.2	2.4	24.2	–	7.3	26.6
			100	87.1	51.0	1.2	.1	11.0	.1	1.0	10.0	–	3.0	11.0
1243	⁵GROUNDCHERRY TOMATO	1 OZ	28	88.3	11.2	.4	.1	–	.5	2.8	9.5	–	–	–
			100	88.3	40.0	1.6	.5	–	1.7	10.0	34.0	–	–	–
1244	HORSERADISH, prepared	1 TBLS	15	87.1	6.0	.2	Trace	1.4	Trace	9.0	5.0	14.0	–	44.0
			100	87.1	38.0	1.3	.2	9.6	2.0	61.0	32.0	96.0	–	290.0
1245	HYACINTH BEANS, raw, young pods	1 CUP	90	88.8	31.5	2.5	.3	6.6	1.6	51.3	47.7	1.8	–	256.5
			100	88.8	35.0	2.8	.3	7.3	1.8	57.0	53.0	2.0	–	285.0

Item No.	Minerals (Micro)			Fat-Soluble Vitamins			Water-Soluble Vitamins								
	Iron	Zinc	Copper	Vitamin A	Vitamin D	Vitamin E (Alpha Tocopherol)	Vitamin C	Thiamin	Ribo-flavin	Niacin	Panto-thenic Acid	Vit. B-6 (Pyri-doxine)	Folacin (Folic Acid)	Biotin	Vitamin B-12
	(mg)	(mg)	(mg)	(IU)	(IU)	(mg)	(mg)	(mg)	(mg)	(mg)	(mg)	(mg)	(mcg)	(mcg)	(mcg)
1212	.90	.45	(.12)	15750.0	0	.17	9.00	.08	.08	.75	(.29)	(.15)	36.00	(.63)	0
	.60	.30	(.08)	10500.0	0	.11	6.00	.05	.05	.50	(.19)	(.10)	24.00	(.42)	0
1213	.39	–	–	0	–	–	2.80	.01	.01	.17	–	–	–	–	–
	1.40	–	–	0	–	–	10.00	.05	.04	.60	–	–	–	–	–
1214	1.10	.34	.14	60.0	0	(.22)	78.00	.11	.10	.70	1.00	.21	55.00	17.00	0
	1.10	.34	.14	60.0	0	(.22)	78.00	.11	.10	.70	1.00	.21	55.00	17.00	0
1215	.84	(.40)	(.04)	72.0	0	(.14)	66.00	.11	.10	.72	(.52)	(.16)	40.80	(1.26)	0
	.70	(.33)	(.03)	60.0	0	(.12)	55.00	.09	.08	.60	(.43)	(.13)	34.00	(1.05)	0
1216	.23	–	.03	0	0	–	1.20	–	.01	.14	–	.03	–	–	–
	.81	–	.12	0	0	–	4.30	.04	.04	.51	–	.11	–	–	–
1217	.06	.01	Trace	48.0	0	.09	1.80	Trace	.01	.06	.09	.01	2.40	(.02)	0
	.30	.07	.01	240.0	0	.46	9.00	.03	.03	.30	.43	.06	12.00	(.10)	0
1218	.16	–	–	1.4	–	–	5.60	Trace	.01	.11	–	–	–	–	–
	.60	–	–	5.0	–	–	20.00	.03	.04	.40	–	–	–	–	–
1219	.50	–	–	20.0	–	–	19.00	.03	.03	.40	.48	–	–	–	0
	.50	–	–	20.0	–	–	19.00	.03	.03	.40	.48	–	–	–	0
1220	.22	–	–	0	–	–	5.32	.01	.01	.25	–	–	–	–	–
	.80	–	–	0	–	–	19.00	.05	.03	.90	–	–	–	–	–
1221	–	–	–	–	–	–	18.00	–	–	–	–	.05	–	–	0
	–	–	–	–	–	–	9.00	–	–	–	–	.03	–	–	0
1222	.48	(.11)	(.07)	2120.0	0	–	11.66	.03	.05	.27	–	.02	27.56	–	0
	.90	(.22)	(.14)	4000.0	0	–	22.00	.06	.10	.50	–	.05	52.00	–	0
1223	.27	–	–	–	–	–	–	–	–	–	–	.02	–	–	0
	.50	–	–	–	–	–	–	–	–	–	–	.05	–	–	0
1224	.17	–	–	580.0	–	–	5.60	.01	.01	.05	–	.02	–	–	0
	1.70	–	–	5800.0	–	–	56.00	.08	.13	.50	–	.18	–	–	0
1225	.67	–	–	–	–	–	–	.03	–	–	–	–	–	–	0
	2.40	–	–	–	–	–	–	.09	–	–	–	–	–	–	0
1226	1.20	–	(.08)	10800.0	–	–	92.00	.28	.40	2.40	–	–	–	–	0
	.60	–	(.29)	5400.0	–	–	46.00	.14	.20	1.20	–	–	–	–	0
1227	.84	.56	(.20)	560.0	0	(.73)	12.60	.17	.14	1.96	(.55)	(.24)	(46.35)	–	0
	.60	.40	(.14)	400.0	0	(.52)	9.00	.12	.10	1.40	(.39)	(.17)	(33.11)	–	0
1228	1.00	.71	.12	547.8	–	–	8.30	.05	.08	1.66	–	.33	13.78	–	0
	.60	.43	.07	330.0	–	–	5.00	.03	.05	1.00	–	.20	8.30	–	0
1229	.37	.66	.04	325.4	0	(.85)	8.30	.046	.10	1.71	.37	.06	59.76	–	0
	.22	.40	.02	196.0	0	(.51)	5.00	.028	.06	1.03	.22	.04	36.00	–	0
1230	.50	.61	.05	343.6	–	–	–	.08	.13	2.13	–	.09	59.76	–	0
	.30	.37	.03	207.0	–	–	–	.05	.08	1.28	–	.06	36.00	–	0
1231	.91	–	–	399.0	–	.22	7.98	.16	.09	1.94	–	–	41.04	–	0
	.80	–	–	350.0	–	.19	7.00	.14	.08	1.70	–	–	36.00	–	0
1232	1.33	(.06)	(.06)	581.0	–	.32	8.30	.15	.10	2.49	–	–	59.76	–	0
	.80	(.04)	(.04)	350.0	–	.19	5.00	.09	.06	1.50	–	–	36.00	–	0
1233	1.12	–	–	2240.0	–	–	27.20	.14	.14	1.28	–	–	–	–	0
	.70	–	–	1400.0	–	–	17.00	.09	.09	.80	–	–	–	–	0
1234	.03	–	–	186.0	–	–	1.48	Trace	.01	.02	–	.01	–	–	0
	1.30	–	–	9300.0	–	–	69.00	.08	.26	1.00	–	.25	–	–	0
1235	.30	[6].10	–	–	–	–	11.00	.03	.04	.20	–	.05	15.00	–	–
	.30	.10	–	–	–	–	11.00	.03	.04	.20	–	.05	15.00	–	–
1236	3.60	–	–	23400.0	–	–	36.00	.26	.32	–	–	–	–	–	–
	1.80	–	–	11700.0	–	–	18.00	.13	.16	–	–	–	–	–	–
1237	1.80	–	–	21600.0	–	–	108.00	.12	.26	.80	–	–	–	–	–
	.90	–	–	10800.0	–	–	54.00	.06	.13	.40	–	–	–	–	–
1238	1.20	–	–	20.0	–	–	6.00	.10	.08	1.00	–	–	32.00	–	–
	.60	–	–	10.0	–	–	3.00	.05	.04	.50	–	–	16.00	–	–
1239	.12	–	–	231.0	–	–	.70	.01	.01	.04	–	–	9.94	–	0
	1.70	–	–	3300.0	–	–	10.00	.07	.14	.50	–	–	142.00	–	0
1240	1.62	[6].30	–	2100.0	–	–	18.60	–	–	–	.15	.06	–	–	0
	2.70	.50	–	3500.0	–	–	31.00	–	–	–	.25	.10	–	–	0
1241	.05	.02	.01	–	–	–	.45	.01	Trace	.02	–	–	–	–	–
	1.50	.59	.32	–	–	–	15.00	.25	.08	.50	–	–	–	–	–
1242	.73	–	–	145.2	–	.75	0	.10	.07	.97	–	–	–	–	–
	.30	–	–	60.0	–	.31	0	.04	.03	.40	–	–	–	–	–
1243	.25	–	–	7.0	–	–	1.68	.03	.01	.67	–	–	–	–	–
	.90	–	–	25.0	–	–	6.00	.09	.04	2.40	–	–	–	–	–
1244	.10	–	–	–	–	–	–	–	–	–	–	–	–	–	–
	.90	–	–	–	–	–	–	–	–	–	–	–	–	–	–
1245	.90	–	–	522.0	–	–	18.00	.08	.10	.81	–	–	–	–	–
	1.00	–	–	580.0	–	–	20.00	.09	.11	.90	–	–	–	–	–

(Continued)

TABLE F-21 *(Continued)*

Item No.	Food Item Name	Approximate Measure	Weight (g)	Moisture (%)	Food Energy Calories (kcal)	Protein (g)	Fats (g)	Carbo-hydrates (g)	Fiber (g)	Minerals (Macro) Calcium (mg)	Phos-phorus (mg)	Sodium (mg)	Mag-nesium (mg)	Potas-sium (mg)
1246	**KALE,** boiled, drained, leaves w/stems	1 CUP	110	91.2	30.8	3.5	.8	4.4	1.2	147.4	50.6	47.3	—	243.1
			100	91.2	28.0	3.2	.7	4.0	1.1	134.0	46.0	43.0	—	221.0
1247	**KOHLRABI,** boiled, drained	1 CUP	149	92.2	35.8	2.5	.1	7.9	1.5	49.2	61.1	8.9	—	387.4
			100	92.2	24.0	1.7	.1	5.3	1.0	33.0	41.0	6.0	—	260.0
1248	**LAMB'S-QUARTER,** boiled, drained	1 CUP	200	88.9	64.0	6.4	1.4	10.0	3.6	516.0	90.0	—	—	—
			100	88.9	32.0	3.2	.7	5.0	1.8	258.0	45.0	—	—	—
1249	**LEEKS,** raw	1 AVG	25	85.4	13.0	.6	.1	2.8	.3	13.0	12.5	1.3	5.8	86.8
			100	85.4	52.0	2.2	.3	11.2	1.3	52.0	50.0	5.0	23.0	347.0
1250	**LENTIL SPROUTS,** raw	1 CUP	130	72.7	135.2	10.9	.4	—	1.4	15.6	—	—	—	—
			100	72.7	104.0	8.4	.3	—	1.1	12.0	—	—	—	—
	LETTUCE													
1251	raw, Butterhead (Boston or Bibb)	1 CUP	66	95.1	9.2	.8	.1	1.7	.3	23.1	17.2	5.9	10.6	174.2
			100	95.1	14.0	1.2	.2	2.5	.5	35.0	26.0	9.0	16.0	264.0
1252	raw, Cos or Romaine, (dark green & white Paris)	1 CUP	66	94.0	11.9	.9	.2	2.3	.5	44.9	16.5	5.9	4.0	174.2
			100	94.0	18.0	1.3	.3	3.5	.7	68.0	25.0	9.0	6.0	264.0
1253	raw, crisphead (iceberg, New York, Great Lakes)	1 CUP	60	95.5	7.8	.5	.1	1.7	.3	12.0	13.2	5.4	6.6	105.0
			100	95.5	13.0	.9	.1	2.9	.5	20.0	22.0	9.0	11.0	175.0
1254	**MIXED VEGETABLES,** frozen, boiled, drained	1 CUP	200	82.6	128.0	6.4	.6	26.8	2.4	50.0	126.0	106.0	48.0	382.0
			100	82.6	64.0	3.2	.3	13.4	1.2	25.0	63.0	53.0	24.0	191.0
	MUSHROOMS													
1255	*Agaricus campestris,* raw	1 SM	10	90.4	2.8	.2	0	.4	.1	.6	11.6	1.5	1.3	41.4
			100	90.4	28.0	2.4	.3	4.4	.8	6.0	116.0	15.0	13.0	414.0
1256	*Agaricus campestris,* sauteed	1 CUP	270	—	299.7	6.5	28.6	10.8	2.7	29.7	313.2	—	—	—
			100	—	111.0	2.4	10.6	4.0	1.0	11.0	116.0	—	—	—
1257	*Agaricus campestris,* canned, drained	1 CUP	270	—	51.3	3.3	.5	6.9	—	21.6	243.0	—	21.0	—
			100	—	19.0	1.2	.2	2.6	—	8.0	90.0	—	7.8	—
1258	**MUSTARD GREENS,** boiled, drained	1 CUP	200	92.6	46.0	4.4	.8	8.0	1.8	276.0	64.0	36.0	—	440.0
			100	92.6	23.0	2.2	.4	4.0	.9	138.0	32.0	18.0	—	220.0
1259	**OKRA,** boiled, drained	1 POD	12	91.1	3.5	.2	0	.7	.1	11.0	4.9	.2	—	20.9
			100	91.1	29.0	2.0	.3	6.0	1.0	92.0	41.0	2.0	—	174.0
	ONIONS													
1260	young green, raw, bulb & entire top	1 MED	20	89.4	7.2	.3	0	1.6	.2	10.2	7.8	1.0	(2.2)	46.2
			100	89.4	36.0	1.5	.2	8.2	1.2	51.0	39.0	5.0	(11.1)	231.0
1261	young green, raw, bulb & white portion of top	1 AVG	8	87.6	3.6	.1	0	.8	.1	3.2	3.1	.4	2.0	18.5
			100	87.6	45.0	1.1	.2	10.5	1.0	40.0	39.0	5.0	25.0	231.0
1262	mature (dry), white, boiled, drained	1 CUP	200	91.8	58.0	2.4	.2	13.0	1.2	48.0	58.0	14.0	(10.4)	220.0
			100	91.8	29.0	1.2	.1	6.5	.6	24.0	29.0	7.0	(5.2)	110.0
1263	mature (dry), yellow, boiled, drained	1 CUP	210	91.8	60.9	2.5	.2	13.7	1.2	50.4	60.9	14.7	—	231.0
			100	91.8	29.0	1.2	.1	6.5	.6	24.0	29.0	7.0	—	110.0
1264	**PARSLEY,** raw	1 TBLS	4	85.1	1.8	.1	0	.3	.1	8.1	2.5	1.8	1.6	29.1
			100	85.1	44.0	3.6	.6	8.5	1.5	203.0	63.0	45.0	41.0	727.0
1265	**PARSNIPS,** boiled, drained	1 CUP	200	82.2	132.0	3.0	1.0	29.8	4.0	90.0	124.0	16.0	25.2	758.0
			100	82.2	66.0	1.5	.5	14.9	2.0	45.0	62.0	8.0	12.6	379.0
	PEAS													
1266	edible, podded, boiled, drained	1 CUP	150	86.6	64.5	4.4	.3	14.3	1.8	84.0	114.0	—	—	178.5
			100	86.6	43.0	2.9	.2	9.5	1.2	56.0	76.0	—	—	119.0
1267	green, immature, sweet, boiled, drained	1 CUP	150	81.5	106.5	8.1	.6	18.2	3.0	34.5	148.5	1.5	(31.8)	294.0
			100	81.5	71.0	5.4	.4	12.1	2.0	23.0	99.0	1.0	(21.2)	196.0
1268	green, immature, frozen, boiled, drained	1 CUP	160	82.1	108.8	8.2	.5	18.9	3.0	30.4	137.6	184.0	38.4	216.0
			100	82.1	68.0	5.1	.3	11.8	1.9	19.0	86.0	115.0	24.0	135.0
	PEPPERS, GREEN													
1269	immature, green, raw	1 MED	40	93.4	8.8	.5	.1	1.9	.6	3.6	8.8	5.2	7.2	85.2
			100	93.4	22.0	1.2	.2	4.8	1.4	9.0	22.0	13.0	18.0	213.0
1270	immature, green, boiled, drained	1 OZ	28	94.7	5.0	.3	.1	1.1	.4	2.5	4.5	2.5	(2.8)	41.7
			100	94.7	18.0	1.0	.2	3.8	1.4	9.0	16.0	9.0	(10.1)	149.0
	PEPPERS, HOT													
1271	chili, immature green pods, no seeds, raw	1 AVG	74	88.8	27.4	1.0	.1	6.7	1.3	7.4	18.5	3.7	17.0	192.4
			100	88.8	37.0	1.3	.2	9.1	1.8	10.0	25.0	5.0	23.0	260.0
1272	chili, mature, red, raw pods, no seeds	1 OZ	28	80.3	18.2	.6	.1	4.4	.6	4.5	13.7	7.0	—	157.9
			100	80.3	65.0	2.3	.4	15.8	2.3	16.0	49.0	25.0	—	564.0
1273	**PIMIENTOS,** canned, solids & liquid	1 MED	40	92.4	10.8	.4	.2	2.3	.2	2.8	6.8	—	—	—
			100	92.4	27.0	.9	.5	5.8	.6	7.0	17.0	—	—	—
1274	***PLANTAIN (COOKING BANANA),** boiled	1 OZ	28	69.1	31.1	.2	.1	8.2	(1.8)	2.5	9.0	(1.2)	(9.6)	(92.6)
			100	69.1	111.0	.8	.3	29.4	(6.5)	9.0	32.0	(4.2)	(34.3)	(330.6)
1275	**POKEWEED (POKEBERRY, POKE),** shoots, boiled, drained	1 OZ	28	92.9	5.6	.6	.1	.9	—	14.8	9.2	—	—	—
			100	92.9	20.0	2.3	.4	3.1	—	53.0	33.0	—	—	—
	POTATOES													
1276	baked in skin	1 MED	100	75.1	93.0	2.6	.1	21.1	.6	9.0	65.0	4.0	(28.8)	503.0
			100	75.1	93.0	2.6	.1	21.1	.6	9.0	65.0	4.0	(28.8)	503.0

Item No.	Minerals (Micro)			Fat-Soluble Vitamins			Water-Soluble Vitamins								
	Iron	Zinc	Copper	Vitamin A	Vitamin D	Vitamin E (Alpha Tocopherol)	Vitamin C	Thiamin	Riboflavin	Niacin	Pantothenic Acid	Vit. B-6 (Pyridoxine)	Folacin (Folic Acid)	Biotin	Vitamin B-12
	(mg)	(mg)	(mg)	(IU)	(IU)	(mg)	(mg)	(mg)	(mg)	(mg)	(mg)	(mg)	(mcg)	(mcg)	(mcg)
1246	1.32	[6].22	–	8140.0	–	–	68.20	–	–	–	–	–	–	–	–
	1.20	.20	–	7400.0	–	–	62.00	–	–	–	–	–	–	–	–
1247	.45	–	–	29.8	–	–	64.07	.09	.05	.30	–	–	–	–	–
	.30	–	–	20.0	–	–	43.00	.06	.03	.20	–	–	–	–	–
1248	1.40	–	–	19400.0	–	–	74.00	.20	.52	1.80	–	–	6.00	–	–
	.70	–	–	9700.0	–	–	37.00	.10	.26	.90	–	–	3.00	–	–
1249	.28	(.03)	(.03)	10.0	0	(.21)	4.25	.03	.02	.13	.03	.05	–	(.40)	0
	1.10	(.12)	(.12)	40.0	0	(.84)	17.00	.11	.06	.50	.12	.20	–	(1.60)	0
1250	3.90	1.95	–	–	–	–	31.20	.27	.12	1.43	–	–	–	–	–
	3.00	1.50	–	–	–	–	24.00	.21	.09	1.10	–	–	–	–	–
1251	1.32	.26	.02	640.2	–	.04	5.28	.04	.04	.20	.13	.04	13.86	2.05	0
	2.00	.40	.04	970.0	–	.06	8.00	.06	.06	.30	.20	.06	21.00	3.10	0
1252	.92	.26	.02	1254.0	–	.04	11.88	.03	.05	.26	.13	.04	118.14	2.05	0
	1.40	.40	.04	1900.0	–	.06	18.00	.05	.08	.40	.20	.06	179.00	3.10	0
1253	.30	.24	.02	198.0	–	.04	3.60	.04	.04	.18	.12	.03	22.20	1.86	0
	.50	.40	.04	330.0	–	.06	6.00	.06	.06	.30	.20	.06	37.00	3.10	0
1254	2.60	–	–	9900.0	–	–	16.00	.24	.14	2.20	.52	.20	–	–	–
	1.30	–	–	4950.0	–	–	8.00	.12	.07	1.10	.26	.10	–	–	–
1255	.08	.01	.01	0	0	Trace	.30	.01	.06	.42	.22	.01	2.30	1.60	0
	.80	.09	.07	0	0	Trace	3.00	.10	.46	4.20	2.20	.13	23.00	16.00	0
1256	2.70	–	–	653.4	–	–	–	.22	1.05	–	–	–	–	–	–
	1.00	–	–	242.0	–	–	–	.08	.39	–	–	–	–	–	–
1257	2.16	2.97	–	0	–	–	–	.05	.65	5.40	–	–	8.10	–	–
	.80	1.10	–	0	–	–	–	.02	.24	2.00	–	–	3.00	–	–
1258	3.60	–	–	11600.0	–	–	96.00	.16	.28	1.20	–	–	–	–	–
	1.80	–	–	5800.0	–	–	48.00	.08	.14	.60	–	–	–	–	–
1259	.06	[6].12	–	58.8	–	–	2.40	.02	.02	.11	–	–	4.56	–	–
	.50	1.00	–	490.0	–	–	20.00	.13	.18	.90	–	–	38.00	–	–
1260	.20	.06	.01	400.0	–	Trace	6.40	.01	.01	.08	.03	(.02)	(8.04)	(.17)	0
	1.00	.30	.06	2000.0	–	Trace	32.00	.05	.05	.40	.14	(.11)	(40.22)	(.93)	0
1261	.05	–	–	26.4	–	–	2.00	.00	Trace	.03	.01	–	2.88	–	0
	.60	–	–	330.0	–	–	25.00	.05	.04	.40	.14	–	36.00	–	0
1262	.80	(.30)	(.16)	0	0	Trace	14.00	.06	.06	.40	(.22)	(.14)	26.00	(1.32)	0
	.40	(.15)	(.08)	0	0	Trace	7.00	.03	.03	.20	(.11)	(.07)	13.00	(.66)	0
1263	.84	–	–	84.0	–	–	14.70	.06	.06	.42	–	–	27.30	–	–
	.40	–	–	40.0	–	–	7.00	.03	.03	.20	–	–	13.00	–	–
1264	.25	.04	0	340.0	0	(.07)	6.88	Trace	.01	.05	.01	.01	4.64	.02	0
	6.20	.92	.02	8500.0	0	(1.84)	172.00	.12	.26	1.20	.30	.16	116.00	.42	0
1265	1.20	(.22)	(.26)	60.0	–	–	20.00	.14	.16	.20	–	–	–	–	–
	.60	(.11)	(.13)	30.0	–	–	10.00	.07	.08	.10	–	–	–	–	–
1266	.75	–	–	915.0	0	–	21.00	.33	.17	–	–	–	–	–	–
	.50	–	–	610.0	0	–	14.00	.22	.11	–	–	–	–	–	–
1267	2.70	1.05	(.24)	810.0	0	.83	30.00	.42	.17	3.45	(.50)	(.17)	–	(.65)	0
	1.80	.70	(.16)	540.0	0	.55	20.00	.28	.11	2.30	(.33)	(.11)	–	(.43)	0
1268	3.04	1.10	(.18)	960.0	0	.40	20.80	.43	.14	2.72	.45	.14	134.40	(.69)	0
	1.90	.69	(.11)	600.0	0	.25	13.00	.27	.09	1.70	.28	.09	84.00	(.43)	0
1269	.28	.01	.02	168.0	0	(.32)	51.20	.032	.03	.20	.09	.10	7.60	–	0
	.70	.03	.04	420.0	0	(.81)	128.00	.080	.08	.50	.23	.26	19.00	–	0
1270	.14	(.06)	(.02)	117.6	0	(.23)	26.88	.017	.02	.14	(.05)	(.04)	(3.11)	–	0
	.50	(.22)	(.06)	420.0	0	(.81)	96.00	.060	.07	.50	(.17)	(.15)	(11.11)	–	0
1271	.52	.02	–	569.8	–	–	173.90	.07	.04	1.26	.51	–	–	–	0
	.70	.02	–	770.0	–	–	235.00	.09	.06	1.70	.69	–	–	–	0
1272	.39	–	–	6048.0	–	–	103.32	.028	.06	.81	.30	–	14.56	–	0
	1.40	–	–	21600.0	–	–	369.00	.100	.20	2.90	1.08	–	52.00	–	0
1273	.60	–	–	920.0	–	–	38.00	.008	.02	.16	.07	–	2.40	–	0
	1.50	–	–	2300.0	–	–	95.00	.020	.06	.40	.17	–	6.00	–	0
1274	.34	(.06)	(.03)	161.0	0	–	3.36	.011	.02	.17	(.08)	(.09)	(5.11)	–	0
	1.20	(.23)	(.12)	575.0	0	–	12.00	.040	.06	.60	(.27)	(.32)	(18.23)	–	0
1275	.34	–	–	2436.0	–	–	22.96	.02	.07	.31	–	–	–	–	–
	1.20	–	–	8700.0	–	–	82.00	.07	.25	1.10	–	–	–	–	–
1276	.70	(.31)	(.18)	Trace	0	.03	20.00	.100	.04	1.70	(.22)	(.17)	(10.11)	Trace	0
	.70	(.31)	(.18)	Trace	0	.03	20.00	.100	.04	1.70	(.22)	(.17)	(10.11)	Trace	0

(Continued)

TABLE F-21 *(Continued)*

Item No.	Food Item Name	Approximate Measure	Weight (g)	Moisture (%)	Food Energy Calories (kcal)	Protein (g)	Fats (g)	Carbohydrates (g)	Fiber (g)	Minerals (Macro) Calcium (mg)	Phosphorus (mg)	Sodium (mg)	Magnesium (mg)	Potassium (mg)
	POTATOES (Continued)													
1277	boiled, pared before cooking	1 MED	100	82.8	65.0	1.9	.1	14.5	.5	6.0	42.0	2.0	(15.3)	285.0
			100	82.8	65.0	1.9	.1	14.5	.5	6.0	42.0	2.0	(15.3)	285.0
1278	mashed, milk added	1 CUP	200	82.8	130.0	4.2	1.4	26.0	.8	48.0	98.0	602.0	—	522.0
			100	82.8	65.0	2.1	.7	13.0	.4	24.0	49.0	301.0	—	261.0
1279	scalloped & au gratin, w/cheese, margarine	1 CUP	245	71.1	355.3	13.0	19.4	33.3	.7	311.2	298.9	1095.2	—	749.7
			100	71.1	145.0	5.3	7.9	13.6	.3	127.0	122.0	447.0	—	306.0
1280	french fried in cottonseed oil	1 PIECE	5	44.7	13.7	.2	.7	1.8	.1	.8	5.6	.3	—	42.7
			100	44.7	274.0	4.3	13.2	36.0	1.0	15.0	111.0	6.0	—	853.0
1281	**PRICKLY PEAR,** raw, 1-½" diameter, 2-½" long	1 AVG	65	88.0	27.3	.3	.1	7.1	1.0	13.0	18.2	1.3	—	107.9
			100	88.0	42.0	.5	.1	10.9	1.6	20.0	28.0	2.0	—	166.0
1282	**PUMPKIN,** canned	1 CUP	243	90.2	80.2	2.4	.7	19.2	3.2	60.8	89.9	12.2	63.2	537.0
			100	90.2	33.0	1.0	.3	7.9	1.3	25.0	37.0	5.0	26.0	221.0
1283	**RADISHES,** raw, common	1 SM	10	94.5	1.7	.1	0	.4	.1	3.0	3.1	1.8	1.5	32.2
			100	94.5	17.0	1.2	.1	3.6	.7	30.0	31.0	18.0	15.0	322.0
1284	**RUTABAGAS,** boiled, drained	1 CUP	200	90.2	70.0	1.8	.2	16.4	2.2	118.0	62.0	8.0	—	334.0
			100	90.2	35.0	.9	.1	8.2	1.1	59.0	31.0	4.0	—	167.0
1285	**SALSIFY,** boiled, drained	1 CUP	150	81.0	61.5	3.9	.9	22.7	2.7	63.0	79.5	(13.2)	(21.5)	399.0
			100	81.0	41.0	2.6	.6	15.1	1.8	42.0	53.0	(8.8)	(14.3)	266.0
1286	**SAUERKRAUT,** canned, solids & liquid	1 CUP	150	92.8	27.0	1.5	.3	6.0	1.1	54.0	27.0	1120.5	(25.5)	210.0
			100	92.8	18.0	1.0	.2	4.0	.7	36.0	18.0	747.0	(17.0)	140.0
1287	**SHALLOT BULBS,** raw	1 OZ	28	79.8	20.2	.7	0	4.7	.2	10.4	16.8	3.4	—	93.5
			100	79.8	72.0	2.5	.1	16.8	.7	37.0	60.0	12.0	—	334.0
1288	**SOYBEAN SPROUTS,** raw	1 CUP	105	86.3	48.3	6.5	1.5	5.6	.8	50.4	70.4	—	—	—
			100	86.3	46.0	6.2	1.4	5.3	.8	48.0	67.0	—	—	—
	SPINACH													
1289	raw	1 CUP	100	90.7	26.0	3.2	.3	4.3	.6	93.0	51.0	71.0	88.0	470.0
			100	90.7	26.0	3.2	.3	4.3	.6	93.0	51.0	71.0	88.0	470.0
1290	boiled, drained	1 CUP	180	92.0	41.4	5.4	.5	6.5	1.1	167.4	68.4	90.0	(106.2)	583.2
			100	92.0	23.0	3.0	.3	3.6	.6	93.0	38.0	50.0	(59.1)	324.0
1291	frozen, chopped, boiled, drained	1 CUP	180	91.9	41.4	5.4	.5	6.7	1.4	203.4	79.2	93.6	117.0	599.4
			100	91.9	23.0	3.0	.3	3.7	.8	113.0	44.0	52.0	65.0	333.0
1292	New Zealand, raw	1 CUP	33	92.6	6.3	.7	.1	1.0	.2	19.1	15.2	52.5	13.2	262.4
			100	92.6	19.0	2.2	.3	.31	.7	58.0	46.0	159.0	40.0	795.0
1293	**SPROUTS**—See **ALFALFA SPROUTS; BEANS, MUNG, SPROUTS; LENTIL SPROUTS**													
1294	**SQUASH, SUMMER,** all varieties, boiled, drained	1 CUP	210	95.5	29.4	1.9	.2	6.5	1.3	52.5	52.5	2.1	(25.2)	296.1
			100	95.5	14.0	.9	.1	3.1	.6	25.0	25.0	1.0	(12.0)	141.0
1295	**SQUASH, WINTER,** all varieties, baked	1 CUP	205	81.4	129.2	3.7	.8	31.6	3.7	57.4	98.4	2.1	—	945.1
			100	81.4	63.0	1.8	.4	15.4	1.8	28.0	48.0	1.0	—	461.0
1296	**SUCCOTASH,** (corn & lima beans)	1 CUP	155	73.0	150.4	6.7	.6	33.3	1.4	21.7	138.0	69.8	54.3	423.2
			100	73.0	97.0	4.3	.4	21.5	.9	14.0	89.0	45.0	35.0	273.0
1297	**SWEET POTATO,** baked in skin	1 SM	100	63.7	141.0	2.1	.5	32.5	.9	40.0	58.0	12.0	—	300.0
			100	63.7	141.0	2.1	.5	32.5	.9	40.0	58.0	12.0	—	300.0
1298	**SWISS CHARD,** boiled, drained	1 CUP	166	93.7	29.9	3.0	.3	5.5	1.2	121.2	39.8	142.8	—	532.9
			100	93.7	18.0	1.8	.2	3.3	.7	73.0	24.0	86.0	—	321.0
1299	**TAPIOCA,** minute	1 TBLS	10	—	36.0	0	0	8.9	Trace	3.5	5.0	.8	—	1.8
			100	—	360.0	.2	.1	89.1	.1	35.0	50.0	8.0	—	18.0
	TARO													
1300	corm, baked	1 CUP	132	—	—	—	—	—	—	—	—	62.0	—	1360.9
			100	—	—	—	—	—	—	—	—	47.0	—	1031.0
1301	⁴leaves, cooked	1 OZ	28	85.7	13.4	.9	.2	2.8	.3	30.8	18.8	—	—	—
			100	85.7	48.0	3.3	.6	9.9	.9	110.0	67.0	—	—	—
1302	⁴tubers, boiled	1 OZ	28	67.3	34.7	.5	.1	7.8	—	13.4	13.4	3.1	—	139.0
			100	67.3	124.0	1.9	.3	28.8	—	48.0	48.0	11.0	—	498.0
1303	³**TEPARY BEAN,** seeds, dried	1 OZ	28	8.6	98.8	5.4	.3	19.0	1.3	31.4	86.8	—	—	—
			100	8.6	353.0	19.3	1.2	67.8	4.8	112.0	310.0	—	—	—
1304	**TOMATO,** paste, canned	1 CUP	249	75.0	204.2	8.5	1.0	46.3	2.2	67.2	174.3	1967.1	49.8	2211.1
			100	75.0	82.0	3.4	.4	18.6	.9	27.0	70.0	790.0	20.0	888.0
	TOMATOES													
1305	ripe, raw	1 SM	100	93.5	22.0	1.0	.2	4.7	.5	13.0	27.0	3.0	17.7	244.0
			100	93.5	22.0	1.0	.2	4.7	.5	13.0	27.0	3.0	17.7	244.0
1306	ripe, boiled	1 CUP	240	92.4	62.4	2.4	.5	13.2	1.4	36.0	76.8	9.6	—	688.8
			100	92.4	26.0	1.0	.2	5.5	.6	15.0	32.0	4.0	—	287.0
1307	**TURNIP GREENS,** boiled, in small amount of water, drained	1 CUP	150	93.2	30.0	3.3	.3	5.4	1.1	276.0	55.5	(11.0)	(15.3)	(116.9)
			100	93.2	20.0	2.2	.2	3.6	.7	184.0	37.0	(7.3)	(10.2)	(77.9)

Item No.	Minerals (Micro)			Fat-Soluble Vitamins			Water-Soluble Vitamins								
	Iron	Zinc	Copper	Vitamin A	Vitamin D	Vitamin E (Alpha Tocopherol)	Vitamin C	Thiamin	Ribo-flavin	Niacin	Panto-thenic Acid	Vit. B-6 (Pyri-doxine)	Folacin (Folic Acid)	Biotin	Vitamin B-12
	(mg)	(mg)	(mg)	(IU)	(IU)	(mg)	(mg)	(mg)	(mg)	(mg)	(mg)	(mg)	(mcg)	(mcg)	(mcg)
1277	.50	.30	(.12)	Trace	0	.04	16.00	.090	.03	1.20	(.21)	(.19)	(10.09)	Trace	0
	.50	.30	(.12)	Trace	0	.04	16.00	.090	.03	1.20	(.21)	(.19)	(10.09)	Trace	0
1278	.80	–	–	40.0	–	–	20.00	.160	.10	2.00	–	–	20.00	–	–
	.40	–	–	20.0	–	–	10.00	.080	.05	1.00	–	–	10.00	–	–
1279	1.23	–	–	784.0	–	–	24.50	.147	.29	2.21	–	–	–	–	–
	.50	–	–	320.0	–	–	10.00	.060	.12	.90	–	–	–	–	–
1280	.07	–	–	–	–	–	1.05	.01	Trace	.16	–	–	1.10	–	–
	1.30	–	–	–	–	–	21.00	.13	.08	3.10	–	–	22.00	–	–
1281	.20	–	–	39.0	–	–	14.30	.01	.02	.26	–	–	–	–	–
	.30	–	–	60.0	–	–	22.00	.01	.03	.40	–	–	–	–	–
1282	.97	.37	.27	66540.7	–	–	12.15	.07	.12	.97	(.97)	(.10)	36.45	–	–
	.40	.15	.11	27383.0	–	–	5.00	.03	.05	.40	(.40)	(.04)	15.00	–	–
1283	.10	0	.01	1.0	0	0	2.60	Trace	Trace	.03	.02	.01	2.40	–	0
	1.00	.02	.13	10.0	0	0	26.00	.03	.03	.30	.18	.08	24.00	–	0
1284	.60	–	–	1100.0	–	–	52.00	.12	.12	1.60	–	–	42.00	–	–
	.30	–	–	550.0	–	–	26.00	.06	.06	.80	–	–	21.00	–	–
1285	1.95	–	(.20)	15.0	0	–	10.50	.05	.06	.30	–	–	–	–	0
	1.30	–	(.13)	10.0	0	–	7.00	.03	.04	.20	–	–	–	–	0
1286	.75	1.22	(.14)	75.0	–	–	21.00	.05	.06	.30	.14	.20	15.00	–	0
	.50	.81	(.10)	50.0	–	–	14.00	.03	.04	.20	.09	.13	10.00	–	0
1287	.34	–	–	–	–	–	2.24	.02	.01	.06	–	–	–	–	–
	1.20	–	–	–	–	–	8.00	.06	.02	.20	–	–	–	–	–
1288	1.05	–	–	84.0	–	–	13.65	.24	.21	.84	–	–	–	–	–
	1.00	–	–	80.0	–	–	13.00	.23	.20	.80	–	–	–	–	–
1289	3.10	.80	.20	8100.0	–	–	51.00	.10	.20	.60	.30	.28	193.00	6.90	0
	3.10	.80	.20	8100.0	–	–	51.00	.10	.20	.60	.30	.28	193.00	6.90	0
1290	3.96	1.26	(.45)	14580.0	0	(3.62)	50.40	.13	.25	.90	(.40)	(.32)	163.80	(.20)	0
	2.20	.70	(.25)	8100.0	0	(2.01)	28.00	.07	.14	.50	(.22)	(.18)	91.00	(.11)	0
1291	3.78	–	–	14220.0	–	–	34.20	.13	.27	.72	.20	.36	194.40	–	–
	2.10	–	–	7900.0	–	–	19.00	.07	.15	.40	.11	.20	108.00	–	–
1292	.86	.26	–	1419.0	–	–	9.90	.01	.06	.20	.10	–	–	–	0
	2.60	.80	–	4300.0	–	–	30.00	.04	.17	.60	.31	–	–	–	0
1293															
1294	.84	(.34)	(.11)	819.0	–	–	21.00	.11	.17	1.68	(.23)	(.12)	35.70	–	–
	.40	(.16)	(.05)	390.0	–	–	10.00	.05	.08	.80	(.11)	(.06)	17.00	–	–
1295	1.64	–	–	8405.0	–	–	26.65	.10	.26	1.44	–	–	–	–	–
	.80	–	–	4100.0	–	–	13.00	.05	.13	.70	–	–	–	–	–
1296	1.71	(.73)	(.10)	465.0	–	–	13.95	.17	.09	2.33	.69	.28	–	–	0
	1.10	(.47)	.06	300.0	–	–	9.00	.11	.06	1.50	.44	.18	–	–	0
1297	.90	–	–	8100.0	–	–	22.00	.09	.07	.70	–	–	18.00	–	0
	.90	–	–	8100.0	–	–	22.00	.09	.07	.70	–	–	18.00	–	0
1298	2.99	–	–	8964.0	–	–	26.56	.076	.18	.66	–	–	–	–	–
	1.80	–	–	5400.0	–	–	16.00	.040	.11	.40	–	–	–	–	–
1299	.10	–	–	0	–	–	–	0	0	0	–	–	–	–	–
	1.00	–	–	0	–	–	–	0	0	0	–	–	–	–	–
1300	–	–	–	–	–	–	–	–	–	–	–	–	–	–	–
	–	–	–	–	–	–	–	–	–	–	–	–	–	–	–
1301	.22	–	–	2191.0	–	–	7.56	.03	.09	.28	–	–	–	–	–
	.80	–	–	7825.0	–	–	27.00	.11	.32	1.00	–	–	–	–	–
1302	.25	–	–	0	–	–	1.12	.02	.01	.17	–	–	–	–	–
	.90	–	–	0	–	–	4.00	.08	.05	.60	–	–	–	–	–
1303	–	–	–	–	–	–	0	.09	.03	.78	–	–	–	–	–
	–	–	–	–	–	–	0	.33	.12	2.80	–	–	–	–	–
1304	8.72	(1.99)	(1.47)	8217.0	–	–	122.01	.50	.30	7.72	1.10	.95	–	–	0
	3.50	(.80)	(.59)	3300.0	–	–	49.00	.20	.12	3.10	.44	.38	–	–	0
1305	.50	.20	.01	900.0	0	.40	23.00	.06	.04	.70	.33	.10	39.00	4.00	0
	.50	.20	.01	900.0	0	.40	23.00	.06	.04	.70	.33	.10	39.00	4.00	0
1306	1.44	.48	–	2400.0	0	–	57.60	.17	.12	1.92	–	–	–	–	0
	.60	.20	–	1000.0	0	–	24.00	.07	.05	.80	–	–	–	–	0
1307	1.65	.62	.23	9450.0	0	(1.50)	103.50	.23	.36	.90	(.47)	(.23)	(165.32)	(.63)	0
	1.10	.41	.15	6300.0	0	(1.00)	69.00	.15	.24	.60	(.31)	(.15)	(110.21)	(.42)	0

(Continued)

TABLE F-21 *(Continued)*

Item No.	Food Item Name	Approximate Measure	Weight (g)	Moisture (%)	Food Energy Calories (kcal)	Protein (g)	Fats (g)	Carbo-hydrates (g)	Fiber (g)	Minerals (Macro) Calcium (mg)	Phos-phorus (mg)	Sodium (mg)	Mag-nesium (mg)	Potas-sium (mg)
	TURNIPS													
1308	raw	1 CUP	132	91.5	39.6	1.5	.3	8.7	1.2	51.5	39.6	64.7	12.5	353.8
			100	91.5	30.0	1.1	.2	6.6	.9	39.0	30.0	49.0	9.5	268.0
1309	boiled, drained	1 CUP	150	93.6	34.5	1.2	.3	7.4	1.4	52.5	36.0	51.0	–	282.0
			100	93.6	23.0	.8	.2	4.9	.9	35.0	24.0	34.0	–	188.0
1310	**VINESPINACH (BASELLA),** raw	1 CUP	52	93.1	9.9	.9	.2	1.8	.4	56.7	27.0	–	–	–
			100	93.1	19.0	1.8	.3	3.4	.7	109.0	52.0	–	–	–
1311	**WATER CHESTNUTS,** sliced, canned	1 PIECE	6	87.8	2.7	.1	0	.6	Trace	.3	1.0	.3	.2	4.2
			100	87.8	45.6	1.1	.1	10.3	.6	5.0	17.1	4.9	3.0	70.4
1312	**WATERCRESS,** leaves & stems, raw	1 PIECE	1	93.3	.2	0	0	0	Trace	1.5	.5	.5	.2	2.8
			100	93.3	19.0	2.2	.3	3.0	.7	151.0	54.0	52.0	20.0	282.0
1313	**YAM,** cooked in skin	1 CUP	200	–	210.0	4.8	.4	48.2	1.8	8.0	100.0	–	–	–
			100	–	105.0	2.4	.2	24.1	.9	4.0	50.0	–	–	–
1314	**YAMBEAN,** tuber, [4]cooked	1 OZ	28	88.6	11.5	.2	0	2.9	.3	2.2	5.0	–	–	–
			100	88.6	41.0	.8	0	10.2	1.2	8.0	18.0	–	–	–

*With the exception of the footnoted values, the data in this table were supplied by the Ohio State University Hospial Nutrient Data Base Catalogue, Columbus, Ohio. These values cannot be reproduced without their permission. Trade and brand names are used only for information. The authors do not guarantee nor warrant the standard of any product mentioned; neither do they imply approval of any product to the exclusion of others which may also be similar.

[1]Data from the HVH-CWRU Nutrient Data Base developed by the Division of Nutrition, Highland View Hospital, and the Departments of Biometry and Nutrition, School of Medicine, Case Western Reserve University, Cleveland, Ohio.

[2]Data from *Composition of Foods*, Agriculture Handbook No. 8-5, USDA, 1979.

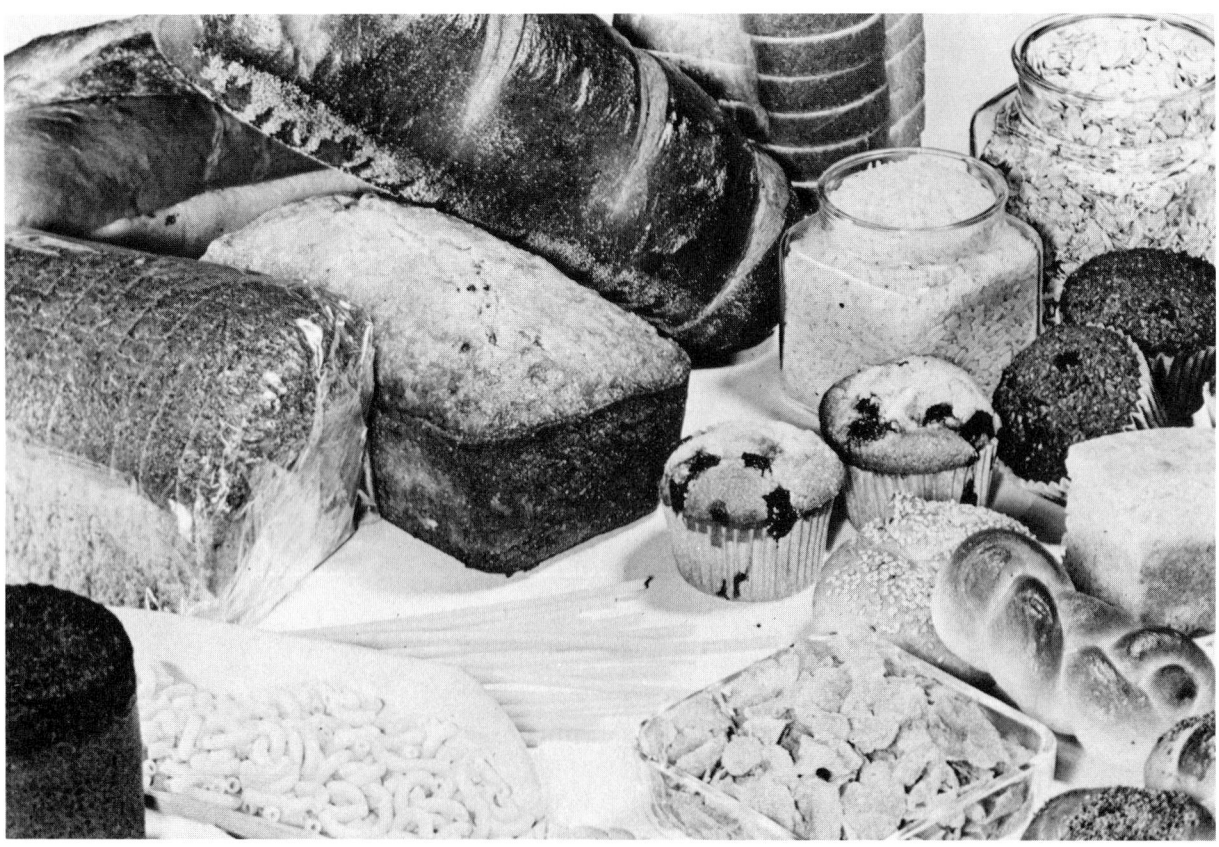

Breads and cereals. (Courtesy, USDA)

Item No.	Minerals (Micro)			Fat-Soluble Vitamins			Water-Soluble Vitamins								
	Iron	Zinc	Copper	Vitamin A	Vitamin D	Vitamin E (Alpha Tocopherol)	Vitamin C	Thiamin	Ribo-flavin	Niacin	Panto-thenic Acid	Vit. B-6 (Pyri-doxine)	Folacin (Folic Acid)	Biotin	Vitamin B-12
	(mg)	(mg)	(mg)	(IU)	(IU)	(mg)	(mg)	(mg)	(mg)	(mg)	(mg)	(mg)	(mcg)	(mcg)	(mcg)
1308	.66	.49	.21	0	0	0	47.52	.05	.09	.79	.26	.12	26.40	(.16)	0
	.50	.37	.16	0	0	0	36.00	.04	.07	.60	.20	.09	20.00	(.12)	0
1309	.60	.42	.12	0	0	0	33.00	.06	.08	.45	(.23)	(.10)	19.50	Trace	0
	.40	.28	.08	0	0	0	22.00	.04	.05	.30	(.15)	(.06)	13.00	Trace	0
1310	.62	–	–	4160.0	–	–	53.04	.03	–	.26	–	–	–	–	0
	1.20	–	–	8000.0	–	–	102.00	.05	–	.50	–	–	–	–	0
1311	.03	.01	.0	–	–	–	–	.00	Trace	.01	–	–	–	–	0
	.46	.17	.03	–	–	–	–	.01	.02	.14	–	–	–	–	0
1312	.02	Trace	0	49.0	0	(.01)	.79	0	.00	.01	Trace	Trace	–	Trace	0
	1.70	(.21)	.04	4900.0	0	(1.00)	79.00	.08	.16	.90	.31	.13	–	(.40)	0
1313	1.20	.62	.44	–	–	–	18.00	.18	.08	1.20	–	–	–	–	–
	.60	.31	.22	–	–	–	9.00	.09	.04	.60	–	–	–	–	–
1314	.11	–	–	0	–	–	2.52	.02	.02	.06	–	–	–	–	–
	.40	–	–	0	–	–	9.00	.08	.06	.20	–	–	–	–	–

[3]Data from *Food Composition Table For Use In Africa*, FAO, United Nations, 1968.
[4]Data from *Food Composition Table For Use In East Asia*, FAO, United Nations, 1972.
[5]Data from *Food Composition Table For Use In Latin America*, Institute of Nutrition of Central America & Panama, and National Institutes of Health, USA, 1961.
[6]Footnote 6 and added values in parentheses are from reliable literature sources.

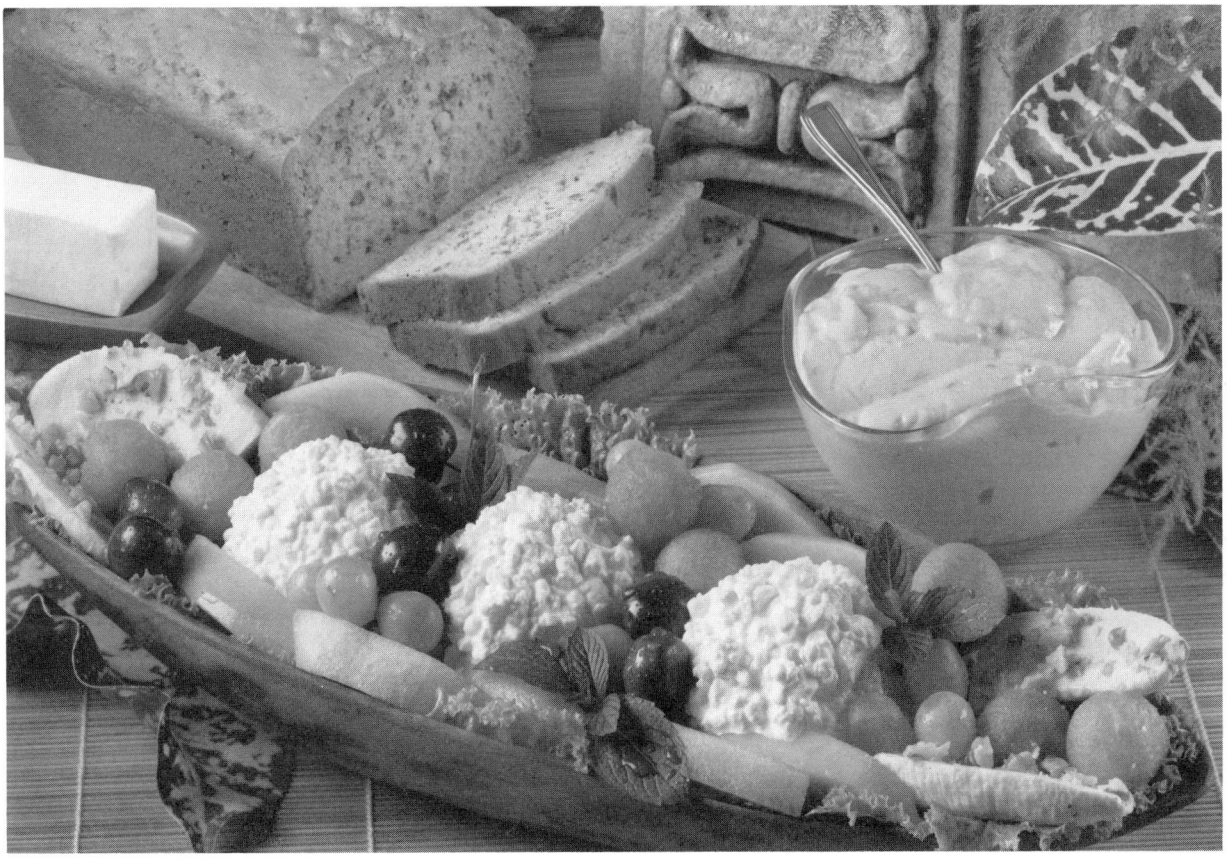

Party food at any time lifts the spirits and adds to the enjoyment of life. (Courtesy, United Dairy Industry Assn., Rosemont, Ill.)

FOOD GROUPS

The Food Groups represent an attempt to list foods together under headings which reflect their similarities as good sources of specific nutrients. Thus, the Food Groups are employed for planning and evaluating diets for nutritional adequacy.

Following World War II, the system of Seven Food Groups was used by most people in public health and nutrition in the United States. Gradually, the Seven Food Groups gave way to the Four Food Groups, to which a fifth group was added. With the introduction of the "Food Guide Pyramid" in 1992, six food groups are now preferred.

FOUR FOOD GROUPS—THE BASIC FOUR. This is the name applied to the daily food guide developed by Harvard's Department of Nutrition (presented at the 38th Annual Meeting of the American Dietetic Association in St. Louis, October 19, 1955, and published in the *Journal of the American Dietetic Association,* November 1955 [31:1103–1107, 1955]).

To ensure nutritional adequacy, use of the Four Food Groups calls for the daily diet to include definite amounts of foods from each of the Four Food Groups: (1) meats, poultry, fish and beans; (2) milk and cheeses; (3) vegetables and fruits; and (4) breads and cereals.

FIVE FOOD GROUPS. The Five Food Groups include the basic four groups plus a fifth group consisting of fats, sweets, and alcohols. Included in the fifth group are such foods as butter, margarine, mayonnaise, salad dressings, and other fats and oils, candy, sugar, jam, jellies, syrups, sweet toppings and other sweets, soft drinks and other highly sugared beverages, and alcoholic beverages. Also included are refined but unenriched breads, pastries, and flour products.

SIX FOOD GROUPS (FOOD GUIDE PYRAMID). For almost 50 years, the Four Food Groups were arranged on a wheel, which was hung in classrooms. In 1992, the U.S. Department of Agriculture released the *Food Guide Pyramid,* featuring Six Food Groups, designed to reflect the changing eating habits of consumers and to give the department's official recommendations of what is good for you. From a broad base, the design narrows progressively toward the top. In the pyramid, the hierarchy and daily servings of the six food groups are as follows: (1) 6 to 11 servings of bread, cereals, and pasta; (2) 3 to 5 servings of vegetables; (3) 2 to 4 servings of fruit; (4) 2 to 3 servings

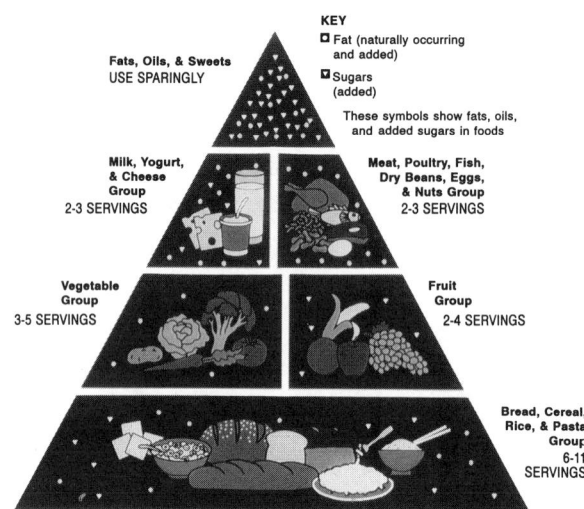

Food Guide Pyramid
A Guide to Daily Food Choices

of milk, yogurt, and cheese; (5) 2 to 3 servings of meat, poultry, fish, dry beans, eggs, and nuts; and (6) at the apex of the pyramid and occupying the smallest space, the fats, oils, and sweets, along with the admonition to use sparingly. (See the Food Guide Pyramid.) Table F-22 is a summary of the Six Food Groups—The Food Guide Pyramid, listing the foods included, the amounts recommended, and the contribution to the diet.

SEVEN FOOD GROUPS. Under the older Seven-Food-Groups' System, the following food groups were recognized: (1) meats, eggs, dried peas and beans; (2) milk, cheese, and ice cream; (3) potatoes, other vegetables, and other fruits; (4) green leafy and yellow vegetables; (5) citrus fruits, tomatoes, and raw cabbage; (6) breads, flour and cereals; and (7) butter and fortified margarine. From these seven groups the number of daily servings of each group were specified to provide a nutritionally adequate diet.

OTHER FOOD GROUPS. The number of food groups—four, five, six, or seven—is not sacred. Also, the groupings may vary in different countries depending upon food habits, economics, and dietary needs. Among the different countries, food grouping systems range from three groups to twelve groups.

The reasons behind the development of these food groups are: (1) the average adult may not use good judgment when it comes to choosing a well-balanced diet; (2) it would be an almost impossible task to calculate and balance a diet with respect to all nutrients involved, flavor, cost, and availability; and (3) the need for a simple but usable guideline for the daily diet.

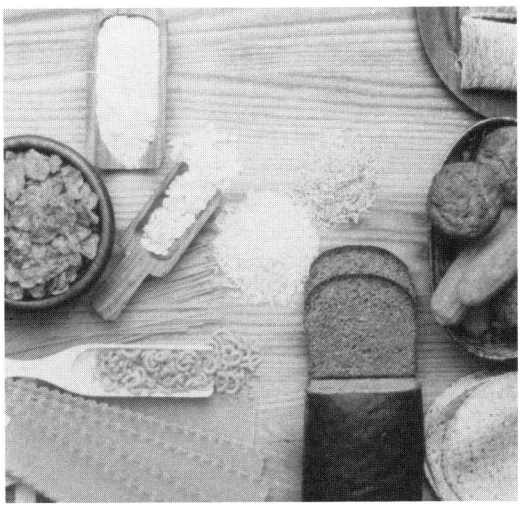

Fig. F-59. Bread, cereal, rice, and pasta group.

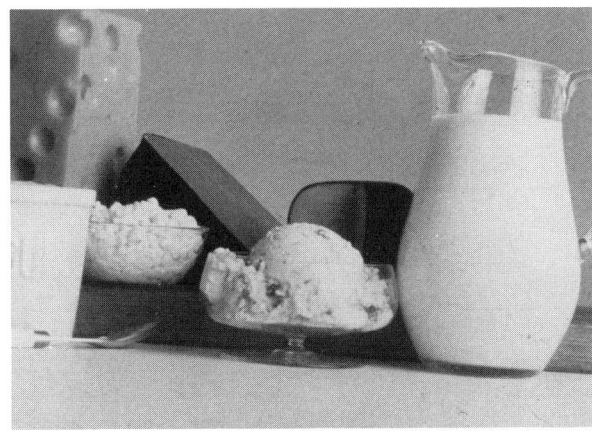

Fig. F-62. Milk, yogurt, and cheese group.

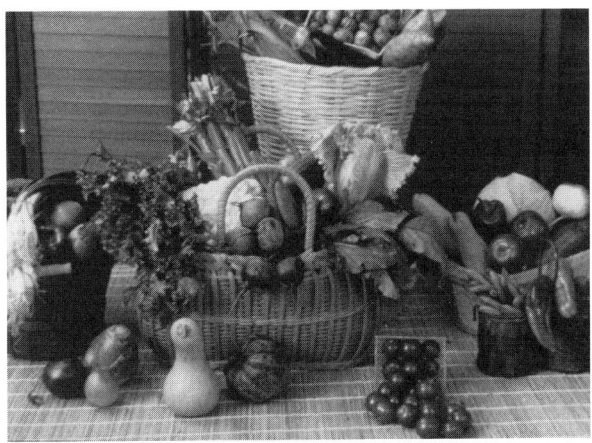

Fig. F-60. Vegetable group.

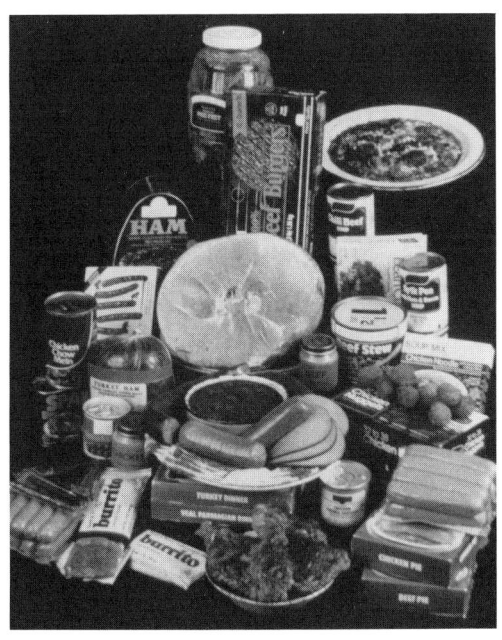

Fig. F-63. Meat, poultry, fish, eggs, dry beans, and nuts group.

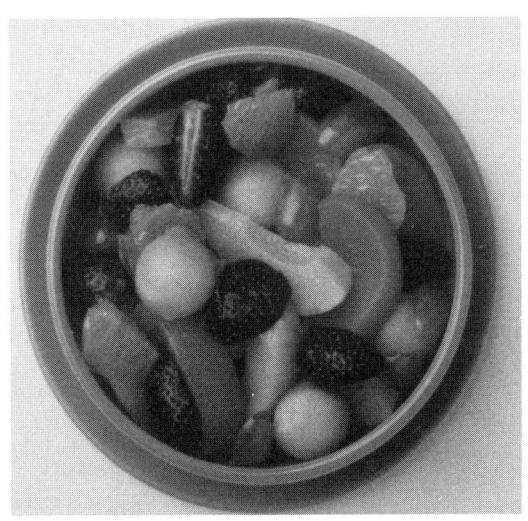

Fig. F-61. Fruit group.

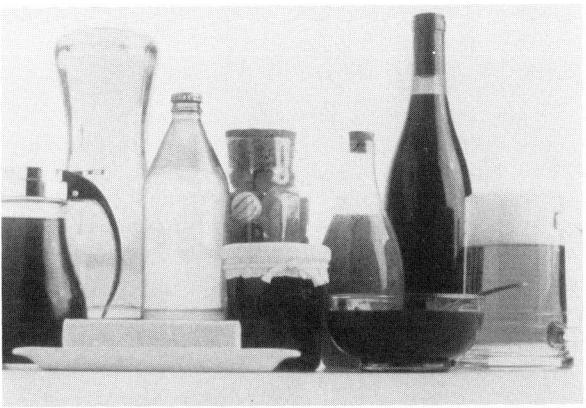

Fig. F-63a. Fats, oils, and sweets group.

TABLE F-22
THE SIX FOOD GROUPS/THE FOOD GUIDE PYRAMID

Group	Foods Included	Amount Recommended[1]	Contribution to the Diet	Comments
Bread, cereal, rice and pasta	All breads and cereals should be whole-grain or enriched products.	6-11 servings daily. 1 serving = 1 slice of bread 1 oz ready-to-eat cereal 1 small muffin 1 small piece of cake	Foods in this group furnish worthwhile amounts of protein, iron, several of the B vitamins, and food energy. Whole-grain products also contribute magnesium, folacin, and fiber.	Includes all products made with whole-grains or enriched flour, or meal. Example: bread, biscuits, muffins, waffles, pancakes, cooked or ready-to-eat cereals, cornmeal, and pastas.
Vegetable	All vegetables, with emphasis on those that are valuable sources of vitamins A and C. (See Table V-1, p. 1034)	3-5 servings daily. 1 serving = 1 c leafy greens ½ c any other vegetable	Vegetables are valuable because of their minerals and vitamins. In addition, they contain fiber.	Should include one or two cruciferous vegetables (broccoli, collards, kale, mustard greens, parsley, and spinach).
Fruit	All fruits. One citrus fruit each day.	2-4 servings daily. 1 serving = 1 medium apple, banana, or orange ½ c other fruits 6 oz fruit juice	Fruits provide fiber, minerals, and vitamins.	All citrus fruits are high in vitamin C. Cantaloupe is high in vitamin A.
Milk, yogurt, cheese	All dairy products: milks, cheeses, ice creams, yogurts.	2-3 servings daily. 1 serving = 1 c milk 8 oz yogurt 1½ oz cheese	Milk and most milk products are our leading source of calcium. They also provide high-quality protein, riboflavin, vitamins A, B-6, and B-12, and vitamin D when fortified with this vitamin.	Milk used in cooked foods—creamed sauces, soups, puddings—can count towards quota for this group.
Meat, poultry, fish, dry beans, eggs, and nuts	Beef, veal, lamb, pork, liver, heart, kidney. Poultry. Fish and shellfish. Dry beans, peas, or lentils. Eggs. Nuts and nut butters.	2-3 servings daily. 1 serving = 2 oz cooked lean meat, poultry, or fish 1 c cooked beans 2 eggs 4 T peanut butter	Foods in this group are valued for their protein. They also provide iron, thiamin, riboflavin, niacin, and phosphorus.	Protein is necessary for growth and repair of body tissues—muscles, organs, blood, skin, and hair. Those of animal origin also supply vitamin B-12.
Fats, oils, and sweets	Butter, margarine, mayonnaise, salad dressing, jams, jellies, syrups, sweetened juices, and alcoholic beverages.	Use sparingly. Less than 30% of calories from fat.	The oils contribute the essential fatty acids, but otherwise, they contribute very little to the diet.	

[1]To convert to metric, see WEIGHTS AND MEASURES

MEAL PLANNING. The Food Groups provide a simple guide for planning the foundation for a day's meals. Choose at least the minimum number of servings from each food group, and select a variety of foods.

CALORIE COUNTING. Calorie counting is almost a national pastime for Americans. The energy (kcal), protein, mineral, and vitamin content of a large number of foods is given in Food Composition Table F-21, which can provide assistance when selecting food. Furthermore, to help count calories, foods and servings of the Food Groups can be classed as low, medium, and high calories.

FOOD INDUSTRY

Today, the U.S. food industry is the largest and most important in the world. It comprises all business operations that are involved in producing raw food material, in processing it, and in distributing it through sales outlets. The entire complex of the industry includes farms, ranches, and feedlots; producers of raw materials, such as fertilizers, for agricultural use; water-supply systems; food-processing plants; manufacturers of packaging materials and food processing and transportation equipment; transportation systems; retail stores; and food-service operations such as restaurants, institutional feeding, and vending machine services.

FOOD MYTHS AND MISINFORMATION

Contents

Without food, medicine as we know it today might never have been born, for until early in the 18th century health treatments were largely based on myths.

The *Papyrus Ebers,* written about 1550 B.C., on paper which the Egyptians made from the papyrus plant, describes scurvy and diabetes and gives a remarkable description of the practice of medicine in Egypt. Foods played many important roles at the time—as medicines, as beauty aids, and as remedies for household problems. Among the recommendations was one for making hair grow, by applying to the bald area either a mixture of honey, palm oil, and fruit juice, or the fat of several wild animals.

A thousand years later, Hippocrates (460 to 377 B.C.), the father of medicine and a contemporary of Socrates, made many wise observations about food and the science of nutrition; among them: Children produce more heat and need more food than adults; persons who are naturally very fat are apt to die earlier than those who are slender; people should exercise; and liver will cure night blindness. But the prescientific era of nutrition was also characterized by a fascinating maze of myths, fallacies, fads, philosophies, taboos, bizarre superstitions, food cults, and religious precepts.

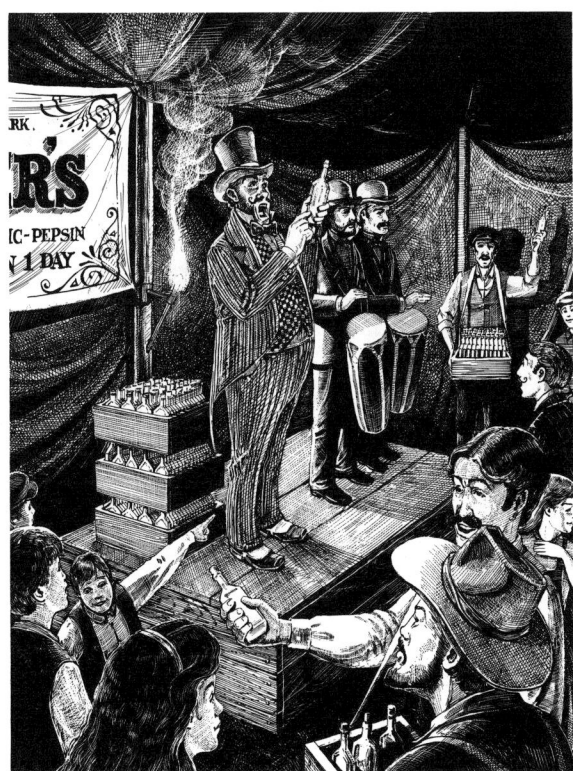

Fig. F-64. The medicine man of old, who, amid tom-toms and torchlights, plied his trade.

THE MEDICINE MAN OF OLD. In frontier America, the medicine man—the doc—plied his trade in a tent, as his show on the road moved from village to village. His potent snake oil and tiger's milk cure-all were always "smuggled out of the sacred tombs of ancient Egypt." Silk-hatted and suave, between band numbers, doc made his pitch:

> "Ladies and gentlemen! Boils and bunions, fevers and fits, gout and gas—these have plagued mankind since life began. But no more! No more for those of you, who for a mere pittance, avail yourselves of this marvelous cure—the guarded secret of health and long life."

Then the band played on while the ushers fanned down the aisles selling their treasures. Their shouts of "all sold out, doc" signaled product number two. Next, the doc gave his soap spiel—a product that would restore glow and youth to dry, harsh skin. Medicine number three was a linament, guaranteed to give relief from all aches and pains. It was a good show, and most of the products were quite harmless.

THE MERCHANT OF MENACE. The top hat and torchlights are gone, but the medicine man is still with us. Today, he's the self-styled scientist or health and nutrition expert, beating the drums for his potions and remedies at your doorstep, on lecture platforms, through the mail, in books, and on the radio and TV. He's the sophisticated salesman who bleats warnings against "that tired feeling"; "subclinical deficiencies"; "devitalized food," "hidden illness," and "aging before your time." Beware of this man! He may be a merchant of menace to you and your health. He has a product—usually an exotic pill, capsule, powder, tonic, special food, or food supplement—which will fortify your diet, increase appetite, build you up, cause you to lose weight, steady your nerves, strengthen your bones, enliven your blood, empty your bladder, roll back the stones from your dying kidneys, and regulate your bowels. Besides, he operates all over the world, from the witch doctors of darkest Africa to plush suites on Park Avenue.

DEFINITIONS. To understand the terms used in this section, several definitions follow:

• **Food myth**—The word *myth* comes from the Greek word *mythos,* meaning *story* or *fable. A food myth is a traditional food story, belief, fable or legend, without proof or determinable basis of fact, which is accepted or used to justify one's own desires, interests, or practices.* To a large extent, food myths represent a reactionary response to advances in scientific agriculture and food technology.

• **Food misinformation**—To misinform is to give incorrect, untrue, or misleading information. *Food misinformation refers to a statement about food that is not in accord with the scientific facts.* Such false information may have arisen out of traditional fallacy, or it may represent belief in magic or folklore, or it may have been fabricated for sales purposes, or it may stem from ignorance.

• **Food fads**—*A food fad is a popular food pursuit or craze, without substantial basis, that is followed with zeal.* Most food fads are short-lived, but a few persist. Some are quite harmless, whereas others may adversely affect the health and welfare of their followers. Two examples of food fads follow:

1. In the early 1600s, coffee drinking became a fad when the brew was first introduced into Europe, and people met at coffeehouses for serious discussions. But the fad passed. Today, coffee drinking is no longer a fad, but a practice widely enjoyed.

2. In the early 1930s, one fad diet, known as the *Hay Diet*, after its promoter Dr. William Howard Hay, stressed the incompatibility of proteins and carbohydrates, and that foods rich in each should be eaten in separate meals.

• **Food faddists**—*A food faddist is a person who takes up a food fad and follows it, usually ardently.* With missionary zeal, most food faddists try to convince others to eat the ingredients to which they attribute their vitality, which may include such things as molasses, wheat germ, yogurt, a *natural vitamin,* soybean oil, etc. Generally speaking, food faddists focus on foods *per se,* not on the chemical agents in them—the nutrients—which are the actual physiologic agents of life and health.

• **Food quack (food charlatan)**—*A food quack is a pretender who claims to have skill, knowledge, and qualifications in foods, nutrition, and/or medicine, which he does not possess.* The quack is the modern counterpart of the medicine man of old. His motive is usually money.

• **Food fallacy**—This refers to a false or mistaken idea or opinion with respect to food and nutrition. A fallacy generally arises through ignorance or through faulty interpretation of the science of food and nutrition as it is applied to the daily diet. For example, an erroneous claim is sometimes made that grapefruit possesses special enzymatic properties that enable it to break down excess fat. This claim may encourage obese persons to eat substantial quantities of grapefruit to the exclusion of other foods.

• **Food folklore (old wives' tales)**—*Folklore refers to the traditional food beliefs and customs held by a people and handed down from generation to generation—the old wives' tales.* For example, the belief that a pregnant woman's appetite for such things as pickles and clay indicate the body's need, and, therefore should be satisfied; or the influence that foods are believed to have on behavior, such as the bravery and courage instilled by eating flesh foods.

• **Folk medicine**—*Folk medicine is the medicine prescribed by nonprofessional people isolated from modern medical services.*

FOOD MYTH AND MISINFORMATION DANGERS.
Food myths and misinformation abound! Most of them are charming, some are sheer nonsense, but others are hazardous. Some myths combine all three; for example, the claim that honey and vinegar will cure an amazing array of ills, ranging from arthritis to the common cold to digestive problems. It has been said that a couple of teaspoons (*10 ml*) of cider vinegar in a glass of water, taken at each meal, will cause the body to burn rather than store body fat. Thus, in easy steps, such pronouncements turn folk medicine into a hazardous practice.

Basically, food fads involve the following hazards, which concern all members of the nutrition and health professions:

1. **They may be a hazard to health.** In some cases, food faddism fosters malnutrition and other health problems. More importantly, self-diagnosis and self-treatment can be dangerous. By following such a course, a person with a serious illness may fail to secure proper medical care; falsely believing that the miraculous properties of this diet will cure their ailment. Many anxious patients with cancer, diabetes, or arthritis have been misled by quacks who fraudulently claimed to have a cure for these diseases, with the result that they postponed effective therapy until it was too late.

2. **They are usually costly.** Most foods and supplements used by faddists are expensive. Each year, Americans spend an estimated $2 billion on special foods, food supplements, and health lectures and literature. Today, conditions are ripe for *fast operators* to make a *quick buck.* Many people have become health conscious. The elderly, the adolescent, the obese, the people whose living depends on their physical appearance, and the sickly are looking for a quick fix; and the charlatans happily accommodate them as they outsell reliable sources of nutrition information. As a result, many quacks, whose products and sales pitches are reminiscent of the medicine men of old, have developed a thriving business, pawning off a myriad of potions, cure-alls, and tonics.

3. **They stymie scientific progress.** The misinformation spread by charlatans hinders scientific progress. Besides, the superstitions that they perpetuate counteract sound nutrition and health teachings.

4. **They create distrust of the food team—the producer, the processor, and the marketer.** A positive program of education in the schools and among the adult population is needed to present the truth about foods and nutrition and to counter the distrust of the food team created by charlatans and faddists.

WHY ARE PEOPLE SO GULLIBLE?
In human folly, facts have never stood in the way of myths and misinformation. Additional reasons for people being so gullible in foods and nutrition follow:

1. **Food is basic, and people's emotions become involved.** Aside from satisfying hunger, food means many things to many people—security, a soothing balm, a means of avoiding idleness, a symbol of success, a sensual appeal. Also, everyone has psychological reactions toward particular foods, determining likes and dislikes. Food quackery plays on these attitudes, plus the powerful incentives of human nature—the desire for health, and the fear of pain, disease, and death. *It is easier to believe a bizarre claim that reassures than a more scientific statement that offers little hope.*

2. **People are sadly uneducated about nutrition and diet.** Because food faddists and quacks talk a good line—they are messiahs and evangelists—it is often difficult for people to recognize what is myth and misinformation and what is fact. *With an informed public, the potential danger of anecdotal information replacing scientific findings can be lessened.*

Thus, there is need for more enlightened information, based on sound research. Additionally, there is need for continued vigilance by the government agencies entrusted to protect the public, especially the Food and Drug Administration, the Federal Trade Commission, and the U.S. Department of Agriculture. Also, several foundations, professional organizations, and trade associations are making monumental contributions through research and education. On a worldwide basis, the following divisions and agencies of the United Nations are engaged in food and nutrition work: Food and Agriculture Organization, World Health Organization, and UNESCO.

(Also see NUTRITION EDUCATION.)

3. **People long for the *good old days.*** The phonies play upon the mistaken notion that our forefathers enjoyed an

ideal food supply and good health. But, the truth is that in the *good old days* things weren't all that good; sickness, crippling diseases, and death rates were higher, and the lifespan was shorter. Just before World War II, for example, rickets, beriberi, pellagra, and goiter—all extremely serious nutrition-deficiency diseases—were, according to the American Medical Association, "common diseases in the United States." Today, these maladies are no longer tabulated as causes of death in this country. Since World War II, more reliable information has been discovered about food production, food composition, and the functions of foods in conserving health than had been established in all previous history. Thus, instead of looking backward, people need to be informed and to look forward in the area of food and nutrition.

FOOD POISONING

Food poisoning is a term which describes a group of illnesses caused by different agents: bacteria, poisonous chemicals, and foods which are intrinsically poisonous, such as certain poisonous plants, certain varieties of mushrooms, rhubarb leaves, the green part of sprouting potatoes, certain clams and mussels, and the puffer fish from which the gland containing neurotoxin tetraodontoxin has not been removed.

America's food supply is the safest in the world. Nevertheless, cases of food poisoning continue to occur.

Prompt and up-to-date information on treatment of poison cases can be obtained by calling the Poison Control Center of the area. When the phone number is not known, (1) ask the operator for the Poison Control Center, or (2) call the U.S. Public Health Service at either Atlanta, Georgia, or Wenatchee, Washington.

In this book, food poisoning is categorized and discussed primarily under the following three sections, to which the reader is referred: BACTERIA IN FOOD; POISONOUS PLANTS; and POISONS.

FOODS, LOW ENERGY

These foods are generally filling, but not fattening. Thus, they contain small amounts of carbohydrates and fats, and great amounts of water and fiber. Many of the fresh fruits and vegetables fall into this category and are used in diets for weight reduction.

(Also see MODIFIED DIETS; and OBESITY, section headed "Selecting Low-Energy Foods.")

FOOD SCIENCE

The study of the physical and chemical characteristics of food is known as food science. Food scientists investigate the chemical, physical, and biological nature of food and apply the knowledge to processing, preserving, packaging, distributing, and storing an adequate, nutritious, wholesome, and economical food supply. About three-fifths of all scientists in food processing are engaged in research and development. Others work in quality control laboratories or in production or processing areas of food plants. Still others teach or do research in colleges and universities.

Food science is taught in more than 60 universities in the United States. Most of the colleges and universities that provide undergraduate food science programs also offer advanced degrees.

The professional organization for food scientists is the Institute of Food Technology.

(Also see INSTITUTE OF FOOD TECHNOLOGY.)

FOOD STAMP PROGRAM

Contents   Page

There are a number of major federal food assistance programs; among them, the Food Stamp Program, the School Lunch Program, the School Breakfast Program, the Milk Program, the Women, Infants, and Children Program, etc. The history, benefits, problems, and costs of all of these programs are given under Government Food Programs; hence, the reader is referred thereto.

Additional and specific information relative to the Food Stamp Program follows:

The Food Stamp Program, which is administered by the U.S. Department of Agriculture, is the nation's primary means for providing food assistance to low-income Americans who meet certain eligibility requirements. Food stamps have been credited with helping to reduce infant deaths and malnutrition in areas of dire poverty. Additionally, food stamps have lessened the surplus food problem. However, the cost and participation in the program have given cause for concerns.

CONCERNS. Two of the major concerns relative to the Food Stamp Program follow:

1. **The increased cost.** Fig. F-65 shows the mounting cost of the program, which in 1989 cost $11.7 billion.

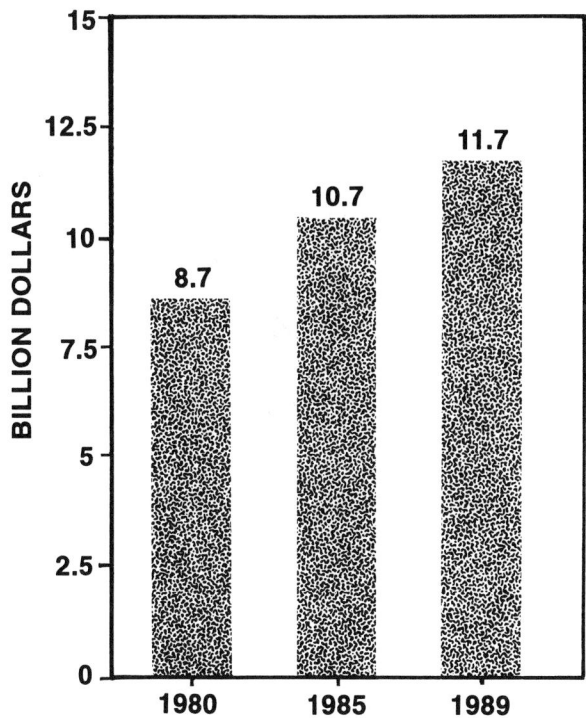

USDA FUNDING FOR FOOD STAMPS

Fig. F-65. The mounting costs of the Food Stamp Program during the 1980s. (Based on data from *Statistical Abstract of the United States 1991*, p. 371, Table 611)

2. **The increased participation.** Fig. F-66 shows that participation in the Food Stamp Program peaked at 21.1 million in 1980, followed by a modest decline.

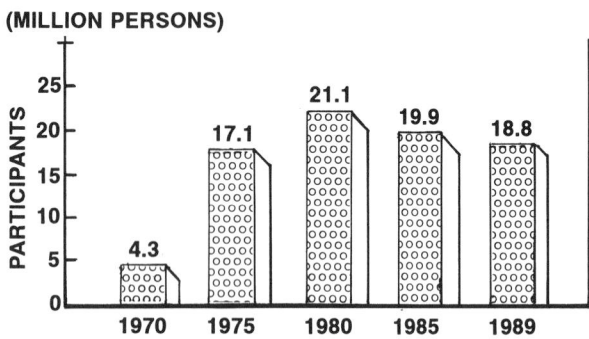

Fig. F-66. Participants in the Food Stamp Program from 1970 to 1989. (Based on data from *Statistical Abstract of the United States 1988*, p. 355, Table 591; *1991*, p. 370, Table 610)

BENEFITS. The value of the food stamps has nearly tripled since 1975, as is shown in Fig. F-67. This increase in food assistance by the government has prompted many people to ask whether there have been any significant benefits from this program. Although there is little hard data on precise cost-to-benefit ratios, some of the more pertinent recent observations follow:

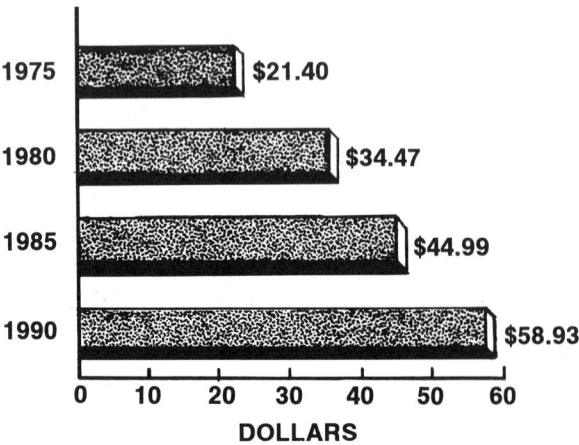

Fig. F-67. Average benefit per person has increased more rapidly than inflation. (*Agricultural Statistics 1991*, USDA, p. 480)

• **Reduction in malnutrition**—In 1979, doctors who had conducted a Field Foundation survey of the urban and rural poor observed that although life in poverty was about as dismal as ever, there were far fewer grossly malnourished people than there were in 1969, thanks to the Food Stamp Program and other federal food assistance programs.[19]

• **Participants consume more animal products and vegetables**—Generally, the proportions of food stamp households with diets that meet the Recommended Dietary Allowances are the same or greater than proportions of households eligible for but not receiving food stamps. It appears that the recipients of food stamps used them to purchase greater quantities of meat, fish, poultry, fruits, and vegetables than people of similar economic status who do not receive the stamps.

• **Lifting people out of poverty**—The extra spending power represented by food stamps raises the incomes of about 30% of the participants who are below the "poverty line" to values which are above this level.[20]

• **Benefits to the overall economy**—A study concluded that the food manufacturing sector business receipts were higher by $589 million in 1972 and by $809 million in 1974 under the Food Stamp Program than they would have been without the program. The study also estimated that between 56,000 and 77,000 new jobs were generated as a result of stimulation of the economy by the Food Stamp Program.

PROBLEMS. Some of the major longstanding problems of the Food Stamp Program follow:

• **Discouragement of needy applicants by bureaucratic procedures**—Some of the most needy people are poorly educated and find it very difficult to comprehend the procedures that are required for certification of eligibility for the program.

• **Loss of dignity of elderly participants**—Many of the elderly just cannot bring themselves to present the coupons in a local store where they may encounter the scorn of their neighbors. Therefore, they go without needed food even though their plight is little due to lack of prudence on their part, but rather to the erosion of the value of their social security and savings that has resulted from the long-term inflationary trend.

• **High costs of administering the program**—The procedures for establishing the eligibility of the applicants are complicated and time-consuming. Hence, they are expensive to execute. Furthermore, some of the regulations cause havoc at local levels, where the circumstances may be quite different from those envisioned by the writers of the regulations.

• **Theft and fraudulent uses of food stamps**—News stories and documentary programs have reported that there is considerable theft and fraudulent use of food stamps.

Sometimes, food stamps have been accepted by unscrupulous merchants from customers offering them as

[19]Vaden, A. G., "Child Nutrition Programs: Past, Present, Future," *The Professional Nutritionist*, Winter 1981, p. 10.

[20]*The Food Stamp Program: Income or Food Supplementation*, Congressional Budget Office, 1977, p. 31.

payment for unauthorized items such as alcoholic beverages and tobacco. There also appears to be criminal networks in some cities which specialize in the circulation of food stamps from liquor stores and other illegal traders in the coupons.

FUTURE PROSPECTS. It seems likely that any new legislation extending the Food Stamp Program will be required to trim the program costs, along with reducing the complexity and vulnerability to abuses.

(Also see GOVERNMENT FOOD PROGRAMS.)

FOOD TECHNOLOGY

Technology, in whatever field, is the application of science and the result of scientific research to the solution of practical problems. *Food technology is the application of science and engineering to the production, processing, packaging, distribution, preparation, and utilization of foods.* As defined by the Institute of Food Technologists, food technology is primarily based on the fundamentals of chemistry, physics, biology, and microbiology.

FOOL

A mashed fruit and cream with or without custard.

FORBIDDEN FRUIT

• The name given to the grapefruit (*Citrus paradisi*) when it was discovered growing on Barbados in 1750. It is believed that the grapefruit arose as either a mutation or a hybrid of the pummelo (*C. grandis*), which had been brought to Barbados in the previous century.

• The fruit of the Ceylonese tree (*Tabernaemontana dichotoma*) that has powerful narcotic seeds.

• An American liqueur of orange color made by grape brandy flavored with shaddock (a variety of citrus fruit).

• The fruit from the Tree of Knowledge in the Garden of Eden which Eve persuaded Adam to eat about 6,000 years ago.

FORMIMINOGLUTAMIC ACID (FIGLU)

An intermediary product of histidine metabolism. Since folic acid is necessary for its breakdown, the measurement of the urinary excretion of FIGLU may be used to determine folic acid status.

FORMULA

• Often a premixed powder or solution for feeding infants, or in some cases special diets for adults, is called a formula.

• A recipe or a prescription may be referred to as a formula.

• In chemical terms, a formula denotes the composition of a compound with symbols and numbers. The formula for table salt is NaCl—one sodium and one chloride atom—while water is H_2O—two hydrogen atoms and one oxygen atom.

• There are formulas which are mathematical expressions used to estimate some characteristic; for example, a formula for body surface area or a formula for a ponderal index, an index of slenderness.

FORTIFICATION

In the food industry, it is the addition of one or more nutrients—vitamins, minerals, amino acids, and/or protein concentrates—to a food thus raising its nutritive value. Enriched bread, and milk fortified with vitamin D, are probably the best well-known examples. Originally, the FDA differentiated between enrichment and fortification, but now the two terms are used interchangeably.

(Also see ENRICHMENT; FLOURS; RICE; and WHEAT.)

FRANGIPANE

• A dessert of almond cream flavored with frangipani (a perfume named after a French nobleman, which is derived from, or imitates, red jasmine flowers).

• A custard cream flavored with almonds and used as a tart filling.

FRANKFURTER (FRANK; WIENER; HOT DOG)

A sausage (made of beef, or of beef and pork, or of a mixture of meats and poultry) that is stuffed in casings or skinless, cured, and cooked. Although frankfurters (franks) and wieners (hot dogs) have merged their identity, it is noteworthy that, originally, wieners were a combination of veal and pork. Today, frankfurters are made of many kinds of meats and seasonings.

FRAPPE

• An iced and flavored semiliquid mixture served in glass.

• An afterdinner drink of liqueur served in a cocktail glass over shaved ice.

• A thick milk shake.

FREE FATTY ACIDS (FFA; UNESTERIFIED FATTY ACIDS, UFA; NONESTERIFIED FATTY ACIDS, NEFA)

A readily available energy source circulating in the blood, and resulting from the enzymatic liberation of fatty acids from triglycerides. Free fatty acids are transported loosely bound to the blood protein, albumin, in a concentration of about 10 mg/100 ml. However, fourfold increases are not uncommon. Liberation of free fatty acids is stimulated by the hormones epinephrine, glucagon, growth hormone, norepinephrine, and glucocorticoids. Insulin inhibits the release of free fatty acids.

(Also see FATS AND OTHER LIPIDS; FATTY ACIDS; ENDOCRINE GLANDS; METABOLISM; and TRIGLYCERIDES.)

FRENCH TOAST

A popular breakfast or supper dish made by dipping bread into beaten eggs and sauteing in a little hot fat. Any kind of bread can be used. French toast can be served with powdered sugar or a syrup, and bacon or sausage.

FROGS' LEGS

Frogs are a web-footed amphibian of which there are about 20 species. In the United States, there is a very large species called the *bull frog*. Only the legs are eaten.

FRUCTOSE

A hexose monosaccharide found abundantly in ripe fruits and honey. It is obtained, along with glucose, from sucrose hydrolysis, and is commonly known as fruit sugar.

(Also see CARBOHYDRATE[S]; and SUGAR.)

FRUIT(S)

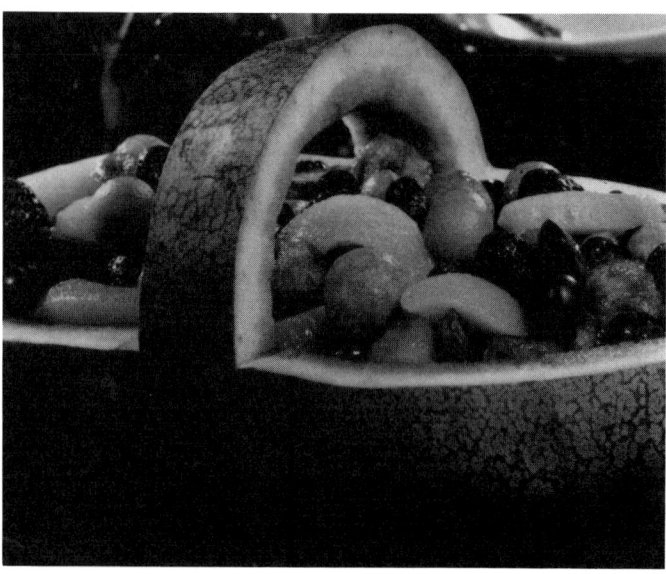

Fig. F-68. Fresh Fruits, (Courtesy, Agriculture Canada, Ottawa, Ontario, Canada)

Botanically, a fruit is a ripened ovary of a female flower. This scientific definition covers both the succulent, fleshy items that lay persons regard as fruits, and the nuts, which are usually encased in hard shells. However, this article deals only with the soft, juicy types of fruits which most people serve raw at (1) breakfast, as accompaniments to the energy and protein foods, and (2) other meals, as appetizers and/or as dessert items. (Vegetables, in contrast to fruits, are usually cooked, and served with the main courses of the major meals other than breakfast. Hence, most people utilize squashes and tomatoes as vegetables rather than as fruits.)

There are various types of fruits, because the ovaries and seeds of the different flowers develop in different ways. Fig. F-69 shows the main types of fruits.

All fruits shown in Fig. F-69 develop from single or multiple ovaries, which are the bulbous bases of the female parts (pistils) of flowers. Sometimes the base of the whole flower (receptacle) also becomes a major part of the fruit.

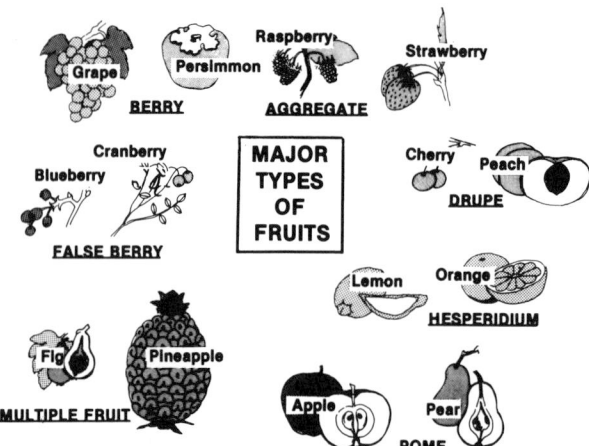

Fig. F-69. Major types of fruits.

Descriptions of each type of fruit follow:

• **Aggregate fruit**—This type consists of many tiny seed-bearing fruits combined in a single mass, which develops from many ovaries of a single flower. In the case of the strawberry, the tiny fruits are embedded on an enlarged, fleshy receptacle.

• **Berry**—These fruits are each derived from a single ovary. They may contain one or more seeds. The banana is a berry which has lost its ability to develop seeds because growers have long propagated it vegetatively with the aim of getting rid of the seeds.

• **Drupe**—In this case the single-seeded stone fruit develops entirely from a single ovary.

• **False berry**—These many-seeded fruits result from the fusion of an ovary and a receptacle.

• **Hesperidium**—The citrus fruits are the most common examples of this type of fruit, which develops from a compound ovary into a many-seeded, multisectioned fruit enclosed in a tough, oily skin.

• **Multiple fruit**—The ovaries and receptacles from multiple flowers on a common base develop into these fruits.

HISTORY. The use of fruits as food dates to the beginning of human existence. According to the Bible, Adam yielded to temptation in the Garden of Eden and was persuaded by Eve to eat of the forbidden fruit from the Tree of Knowledge about 6,000 years ago. From that date forward, the first couple and all their descendants knew but one creed: "In the sweat of thy brow shalt thou eat bread,..."[21]

Early people kept domesticated animals and grew grains, legumes, and/or starchy roots and tubers. In the beginning of this mode of existence, they continued to gather wild fruits, but soon they learned how to propagate their favorite items where they would be close at hand. Dates, figs, and grapes were cultivated and made into wines by about 4000 B.C. in the Near East. However, some of each crop was dried and kept for later use. Fig. F-70 shows where many of the important fruits originated and/or were domesticated.

[21]Genesis 3:19.

FROM WHENCE OUR FRUITS CAME

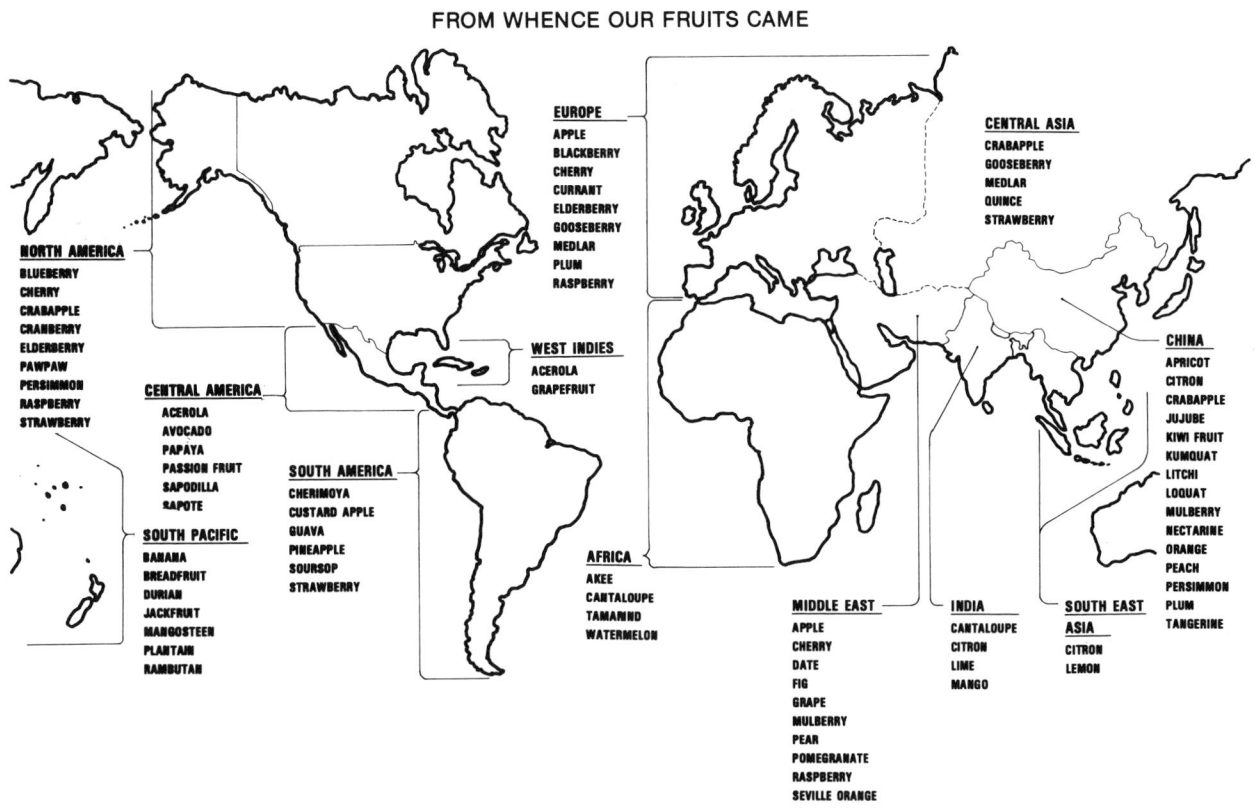

Fig. F-70. Places of origin and/or domestication of fruits.

WORLD AND U.S. PRODUCTION. Data for fruit production in the world and in the United States are shown in Fig. F-71 and F-72.

Fig. F-71 shows that grapes, oranges, bananas, apples, watermelons, and plantains are by far the leading fruit crops of the world. It is noteworthy that most of these crops are produced in subtropical and tropical areas.

Fig. F-72 shows that oranges, grapes, apples, and grapefruits are the leading fruit crops in the United States. The citrus fruits require a subtropical climate. Hence, their production is limited mainly to California, Texas, and Florida. The great growth of the citrus industry after World War II was due in large part to advances in the technology for producing frozen juices from these fruits.

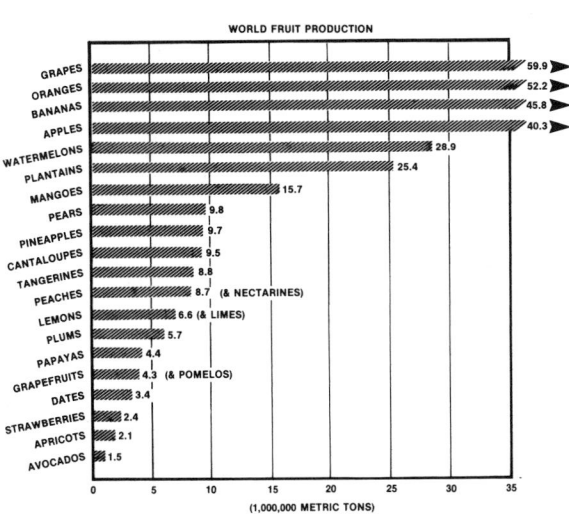

Fig. F-71. World production of the leading fruit crops. (Based on data from the *FAO Production Yearbook 1990*, FAO/UN, Rome, Italy, Vol. 44)

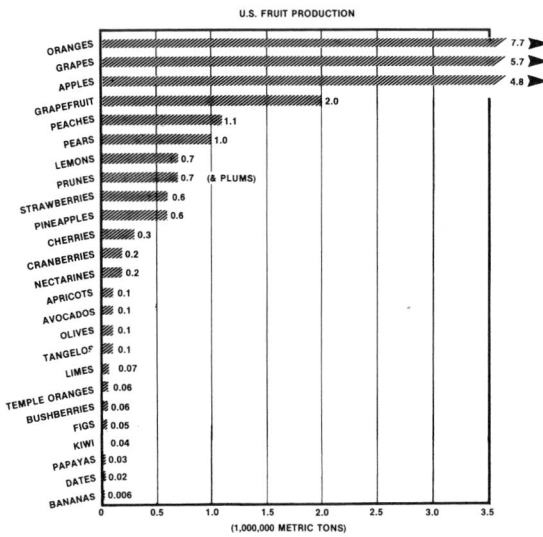

Fig. F-72. U.S. production of the leading fruit crops. (Based on data from *Agricultural Statistics 1991*, USDA, p. 177, Table 254)

PROCESSING. Until recent times, the most common methods of processing fruits were (1) using them to make wines, and (2) drying them in the sun. Now, various other procedures are used to extend the availability of fruits and fruit products over the entire year. Details of the major processes follow.

Canning. In this process, fruits in metal or glass containers are heated to kill the microorganisms that cause spoilage. The more acid the products, the easier any spoilage organisms are destroyed by heat. Fortunately, most fruits are sufficiently acid to be processed safely at the temperature of boiling water in a boiling-water-bath canner. However, the proper procedures must be followed, for if spoilage organisms are not killed by adequate processing, they will continue to grow and reduce the acid content of the canned fruit, thus encouraging the growth of more dangerous organisms, such as *Clostridium botulinum*.

Drying. The drying of freshly harvested fruits in the sun was used as a means of preservation as long as 5,000 years ago by the peoples of the Middle East. Then, the most common items to be dried were apricots, dates, figs, and grapes. Today, fruit drying is a major form of processing in California, which is the leading state for fruit production.

Dried fruits do not spoil readily because they do not contain sufficient water to support the growth of spoilage organisms. Drying requires a means of heating to evaporate the water present in the fruit, and some means of removing the water vapor. The simplest way to accomplish these objectives is to place the fruit in the sun. However, birds, insects, and other pests may eat or contaminate the fruit while drying is underway. Therefore, various types of drying equipment have been developed to insure protection against pests and various contaminants.

Freezing. The U.S. Department of Agriculture first conducted research on the freezing of fruits in 1904, although frozen strawberries were already being used in the production of ice cream. Within a few years, many commercial bakers began to use frozen berries and other fruits for making pies. The early frozen fruit packers learned by trial and error how to avoid deterioration of their product by careful preparation of the fruit before freezing.

Jams And Jellies. It appears that fruits preserved with sugar were used in Roman times, although the original reason for adding the sugar was probably for its sweetening effect. The high sugar content and acidity of fruit preserves prevent the growth of microorganisms. Eventually, cooks developed a variety of heavily sugared products that are similar in their semisolid consistency, but differ with respect to (1) the form(s) of fruit, (2) amounts of sugar and water, and (3) methods of preparation.

The gelling of the various products is due mainly to the substance pectin, which is present in varying amounts in most fruits. Acid is also needed to bring about gelling. If pectin is lacking, a commercial form of it may be added. Extra acid may be added in the form of citric acid or lemon juice. Most items are cooked to bring about the destruction of spoilage organisms. However, strong heating destroys considerable amounts of vitamins.

Juices. There has been a great increase in the production of fruit juices since the end of World War II. The large volumes of these products have tended to keep prices down, so that they have increased much less than the prices for fresh fruits. As a result, shoppers have increased their purchases of juices, while decreasing their consumption of whole fruit.

The production of fruit juices involves (1) extraction of the juice by various types of crushing or squeezing processes, (2) removal of undesired fruit parts (pulp, rind, seeds, etc.) from the juice by passage through screens and/or other equipment, and (3) treatment of the refined juice by filtration, heat, or other means to prevent clouding, fermentation, and other types of deterioration during storage.

FEDERAL STANDARDS FOR PROCESSED FRUIT PRODUCTS. All over the United States, fruit products such as apple butter and frozen cherry pie are essentially uniform with respect to ingredients and quality because food standards, established by the Federal Government set requirements which these products must meet if they move in interstate commerce. There are four major sets of standards which apply to various processed fruit products. These follow:

• **U.S. Department of Agriculture Grade Standards—** These standards, like those for fresh produce, are voluntary. They cover canned, frozen, and dried fruits; and related products such as preserves.

USDA provides official grading services, often in cooperation with State departments of agriculture, for a fee, to packers, processors, distributors, or others who wish official certification of the grade of a product. Also, the grade standards are often used by packers and processors as guidelines for their quality control.

• **Food and Drug Administration Standards of Identity—** These mandatory standards establish what a given food product *is*—for example, what a food must be to be labeled *catsup*. They also provide for the use of optional ingredients, in addition to the mandatory ingredients, that may constitute the product.

Fruit products for which standards of identity have been formulated are canned fruits, canned fruit juices, fruit butters, jellies, preserves, and related products; and frozen cherry pie.

• **Food and Drug Administration Minimum Standards of Quality—**FDA standards of quality are mandatory, as opposed to USDA grade standards of quality, which are voluntary. They have been set for a number of canned fruits to supplement standards of identity, by specifying the minimum acceptable characteristics for such factors as tenderness, color, and freedom from defects.

• **Food and Drug Administration Standards of Fill of Container—**These mandatory standards tell the packer how full a container must be to avoid deception. They prevent the selling of air or water in place of food. For example, the amounts of headspace in cans and jars of fruit products are limited to those consistent with good manufacturing practices.

EFFECTS OF PROCESSING AND PREPARATION. The maximum amounts of essential nutrients are supplied by raw, fresh fruits that have been harvested at just the right stages of maturity. However, it may not be advisable to use only fresh fruits, which are available only at certain times of the year. Therefore, the effects of the various processing and preparation procedures should be taken into account when planning menus that are to be nutritionally adequate.

NOTE: Some of the information which follows is based on relatively few studies and may not be valid in all cases because (1) different fruits are affected in different ways; (2) the effects depend partly upon the condition of the fruits—whether underripe or fully ripe, fresh or taken from long storage, whole or in pieces, and untreated or treated; and (3) information is lacking on some of the effects of commonly used procedures.

• **Artificial ripening**—Most commercially grown apples, apricots, avocados, bananas, and pears are picked before full ripening in order to avoid excessive softness and over-susceptibility to damage and spoilage. (Ripening may be induced artificially just before marketing.) These fruits may have vitamin A and vitamin C contents equal to, or greater than those of tree-ripened fruits, providing that they have been handled properly after picking.

• **Canning**—The vitamin contents of eight commonly canned fruit products (apples, apricots, blueberries, cherries, orange juice concentrate, peaches, raspberries, and strawberries) were found to be considerably lower than those of their fresh counterparts.[22] This study showed that the average vitamin losses were as follows: vitamin A, 39%; vitamin B-1 (thiamin), 47%; vitamin B-2 (riboflavin), 57%; niacin, 42%; and vitamin C, 56%.

• **Chopping, dicing, grating, mashing, mincing, or slicing**—Any process which breaks many cells within fruits is likely to be responsible for significant losses of certain vitamins. The longer the broken pieces of fruit are held, the greater the losses. Therefore, vitamins may be conserved by (1) cutting up fruits just prior to serving, and (2) using a plastic knife for cutting, because metals speed up the destruction of vitamin C.

• **Drying**—Moderate amounts of carotene (provitamin A) and vitamin C may be destroyed in this process, unless the fruits are sulfured before drying. However, sulfuring destroys most of the thiamin content. Vitamin losses are greater during slow processes such as sun drying, than they are for more rapid processes like freeze drying.

• **Fermentation**—The production of wines from grapes and other fruits appears to render minerals like iron more available for absorption. Alcoholic iron tonics have long been used to treat anemia. Also, alcoholic fermentation by yeast may convert the inorganic chromium which is present in various fermentable materials to the glucose tolerance factor (GTF)—an organic form of chromium that acts with insulin to lower the blood sugar.

• **Freezing**—The vitamin contents of eight common frozen fruit products (apples, apricots, blueberries, cherries, orange juice concentrate, peaches, raspberries, and strawberries) were found to be lower than those of their fresh counterparts, but higher than those of canned fruit products.[23] This study showed that the average vitamin losses were as follows: vitamin A, 37%; vitamin B-1 (thiamin), 29%; vitamin B-2 (riboflavin), 17%; niacin, 16%; and vitamin C, 18%.

---

[22]Fennema, O., "Effects of Freeze-Preservation on Nutrients," *Nutritional Evaluation of Food Processing*, 2nd ed., edited by R. S. Harris and E. Karmas, The Avi Publishing Company, Inc., Westport, Conn., 1975, pp. 268-269, Table 10.15.

[23]*Ibid.*

• **Paring**—Removal of the peels or skins of certain fruits may result in disproportionately high losses of nutrients because the outer layers are often richer in minerals and vitamins than the inner layers. Therefore, these measures, which are often performed mainly for cosmetic reasons, should be used only to the extent that is absolutely necessary.

• **Pureeing**—The preparation of purees by homogenizing fruits in water makes the iron in these items more available, because it breaks down the fibrous cell walls which enclose the nutrients. However, the amount of homogenization should be kept to a minimum in order to avoid destruction of vitamins A and C, which occurs upon exposure of the fruit pulp to air.

• **Sulfuring**—This process, which consists of either exposing fruit to fumes from burning sulfur, or dipping them in a sulfate solution, is used to prevent discoloration and spoilage. It is generally utilized before fruit is to be dried. Sulfuring helps to prevent the losses of both carotene (provitamin A) and vitamin C, but it destroys thiamin. Fortunately, fruits are utilized more as sources of the first two vitamins, than as sources of the last one.

• **Thawing**—The thawing of frozen fruits usually results in losses of nutrients in the juices. Freezing foods ruptures cell walls so that the cell contents escape readily during thawing. Although the thawed juices may be used, it may be dangerous to do so if there has been considerable time for the growth of microorganisms during thawing. Hence, it may be desirable to heat frozen fruit carefully, to speed up thawing so that the juices which escape may be used safely. This danger is minimal for fruits packed in sugar or syrup.

Microwave heating may be preferable to other ways of thawing frozen fruits because microwaves penetrate the interior of the product and bring about a rapid and uniform thawing, whereas other means of heating tend to cook the outer layers of the fruit, while the interior remains frozen.

NUTRITIVE VALUES. Fruits are high in water content. However, most fruits are fair to excellent sources of calories (due to their sugars), fiber (poorly digested carbohydrate which stimulates movements of the digestive tract), various essential macrominerals and microminerals, vitamins, and vitaminlike factors. The nutrient composition of common fruits is given in Food Composition Table F-21.

Food Composition Table F-21 does not show the bioflavonoid content of the fruit items because this information is not readily available. Besides, at this time no conclusive evidence exists that bioflavonoids serve any useful role in human nutrition or in the prevention or treatment of disease in humans. However, apricots, cantaloupes, cherries, citrus fruits, grapes, and papayas are believed to be among the richest sources of bioflavonoids.

(Also see BIOFLAVONOIDS.)

FRUITS OF THE WORLD. About 70 or so species of fruit plants account for most of the world's fruit production. Noteworthy information on fruits is presented in Table F-23, Fruits of the World. Additionally, the *most* important and/or better known fruits, worldwide and/or in the United States, are accorded detailed narrative coverage, alphabetically.

NOTE WELL: Where production figures are given in Table F-23, column 2 under "Importance," unless otherwise stated, they are based on 1990 data. Most world figures are from *FAO Production Yearbook 1990*, FAO/UN, Rome, Italy, Vol. 44. Most U.S. figures are from *Agricultural Statistics 1991*. Annual production fluctuates as a result of weather and profitability of the crops.

(Also see WILD EDIBLE PLANTS.)

TABLE F-23
FRUITS OF THE WORLD

Popular and Scientific Name(s); Origin and History	Importance; Principal Areas; Growing Conditions	Processing; Preparation; Uses	Calories; Nutritive Value[1]
Acerola (Barbados Cherry) *Malphigia glabra* **Origin and History:** Native to the West Indies, Mexico, and Central America.	**Importance:** The richest natural source of vitamin C. **Principal Areas:** Puerto Rico and other islands in the Caribbean. **Growing Conditions:** Subtropical or tropical climate.	**Processing:** Most of the crop is processed into fruit products and nutritional supplements (mainly sources of vitamin C). **Preparation:** The fresh fruit, juice, and pulp are prepared as sources of vitamin C. **Uses:** Ingredient of jams, jellies, juices, and vitamin C supplements.	**Calories:** 28 kcal/100 g. **Nutritive Value:** One of the richest known sources of vitamin C (1,000 to 4,000 mg ascorbic acid/100 g); reputed to be excellent source of bioflavonoids.
Akee *Blighia sapida* **Origin and History:** Native to West Africa. Brought to West Indies in the 18th century. The Latin name of the fruit is after Captain Bligh of H.M.S. Bounty.	**Importance:** A popular fruit in Jamaica, W.I. **Principal Areas:** West Africa and West Indies. **Growing Conditions:** Tropical climate.	**Processing:** Only the fresh ripe fruit is eaten. **Preparation:** Serve raw or cooked. **Uses:** Fruit or vegetable dish.	**Calories:** 196 kcal/100 g because of high fat content. **Nutritive Value:** Moderately high in crude fiber (1.6%) and vitamin C (26 mg/100 g); a good source of vitamin A (925 IU/100 g). *Caution:* The unripe fruit is poisonous and should not be eaten. It contains hypoglycin A which lowers the blood sugar and induces vomiting.
Apple *Malus pumila* (See APPLE.)			
Apricot *Prunus armeniaca* (See APRICOT.)			
Avocado (Alligator Pear) *Persea americana* (See AVOCADO.)			
Banana *Musa paradisiaca* (See BANANA.)			
Blackberry (Brambles) *Rubus fructicosus* A plant of the rose family, *Rosaceae*, which has small black fruits called *blackberries*. **Origin and History:** Long gathered from wild plants that were probably native to Europe. Not domesticated until the Middle Ages.	**Importance:** Although they are a minor crop, blackberries grow throughout the world, with the exception of dry desert regions. **Principal Areas:** The largest production is in the Northern Hemisphere. Commercial production in the U.S. is largely limited to Oregon, Texas, Oklahoma, and Arkansas. **Growing Conditions:** Cool, temperate climate.	**Processing:** A small amount of the blackberry crop is consumed fresh, but more than 90% is processed; it's canned, frozen, or used to make other products. **Preparation:** Wash and stem, then serve fresh (alone or with cream), or make into various mixed dishes. **Uses:** Fresh fruit dishes, cakes, gelatin desserts, ice cream, jams, jellies, juices, pies, salads, sherbets, and syrups; and in the production of alcoholic beverages.	**Calories:** 58 kcal/100 g **Nutritive Value:** A good source of fiber (4.1%); a fair source of potassium; a fair to good source of vitamin A, vitamin C, and folic acid; and a rich source of bioflavonoids.
Blueberry *Vaccinium myrtilloides* The blueberry is a member of the family, *Ericaceae*, which also includes bilberries, cranberries, and huckleberries. **Origin and History:** Native to North America, where they have been cultivated since the early 19th century.	**Importance:** Blueberries are a relatively minor crop, worldwide and in the U.S. **Principal Areas:** U.S.A. and Canada. **Growing Conditions:** Cool, moist, temperate climate.	**Processing:** More than ⅔ of the U.S. blueberry crop is processed. More than ½ of the processed blueberries are frozen and the rest are canned. **Preparation:** Wash, then serve raw (alone or with cream), baked in cakes and pies, or prepared in various other dishes. **Uses:** Fresh fruit dishes, baked products, gelatin desserts, ice cream, jams, jellies, pies, and syrups.	**Calories:** 62 kcal/100 g. **Nutritive Value:** A good source of iron (1.0 mg/100g), and bioflavonoids; and a fair source of potassium and vitamin C.
Breadfruit *Artocarpus altillis* The breadfruit belongs to the mulberry family, *Moraceae*. **Origin and History:** Native to Malaysia. In 1787, it was taken from Tahiti to the West Indies by Captain Bligh on his ship the Bounty, on which the well-known mutiny occurred.	**Importance:** A staple food on certain islands in the Pacific and in the Caribbean. **Principal Areas:** South Pacific islands and West Indies. **Growing Conditions:** Tropical climate. Does best when rainfall is abundant.	**Processing:** The fresh fruit is usually cooked and eaten right after harvesting, without processing. **Preparation:** Baked, boiled, or fried. Also, biscuits may be made from the fruit. **Uses:** Fruit or vegetable dish; ingredient of baked products and other mixed dishes.	**Calories:** 103 kcal/100 g. **Nutritive Value:** Good source of crude fiber (1.2%), iron (1.2 mg/100 g), and vitamin C (29 mg/100 g).

Footnote at end of table

(Continued)

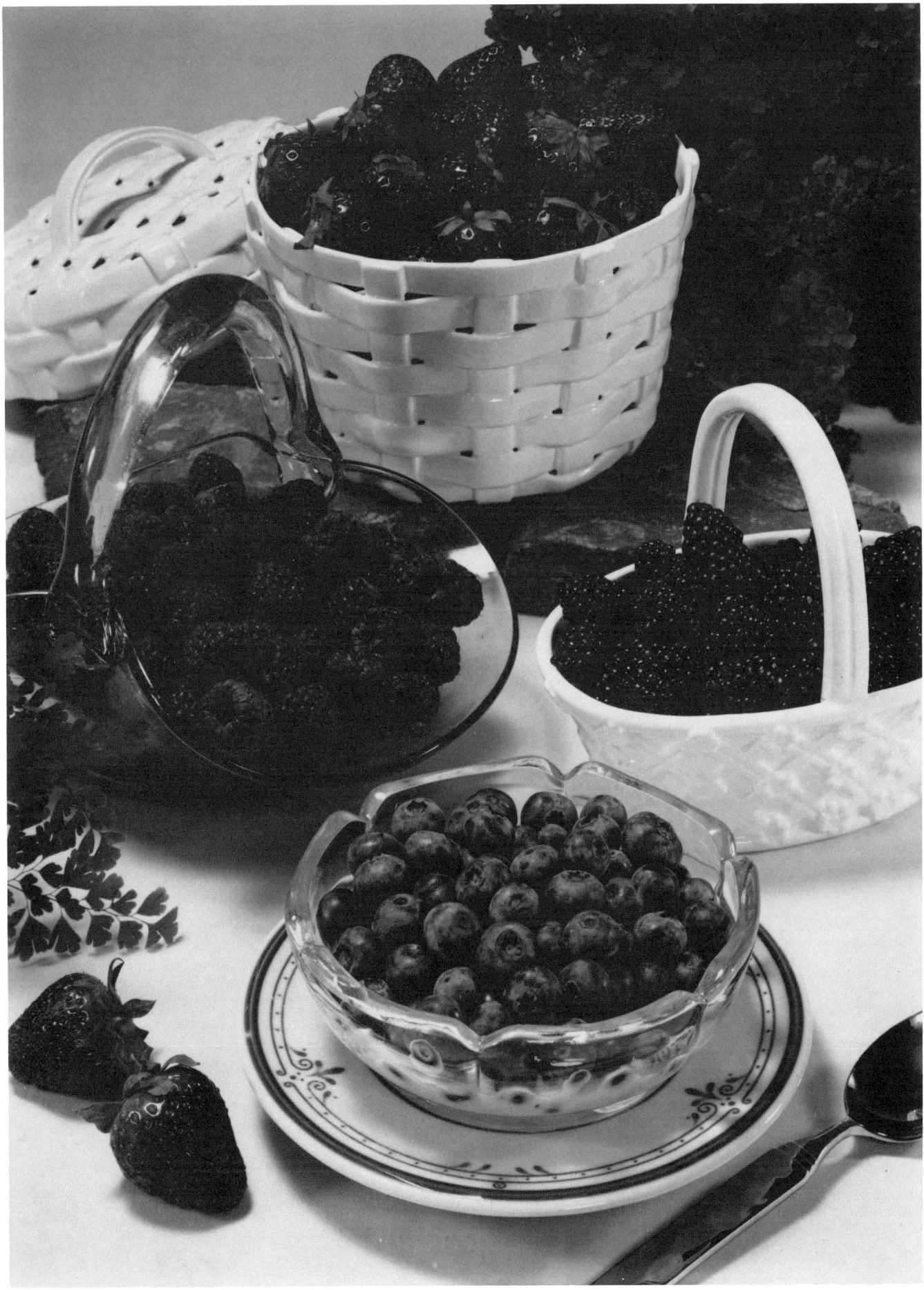

Fig. F-73. Berries (Courtesy, United Fresh Fruit and Vegetable Assn., Alexandria, Va.)

TABLE F-23 *(Continued)*

Popular and Scientific Name(s); Origin and History	Importance; Principal Areas; Growing Conditions	Processing; Preparation; Uses	Calories; Nutritive Value[1]
Cantaloupe (Muskmelon) *Cucumis melo* (See CANTALOUPE.)			
Cherimoya *Annona cherimolia* **Origin and History:** Native to the high valleys in the Andes Mountains of Ecuador and Peru.	**Importance:** Little known outside of native habitat because it does not keep well in shipping. **Principal Areas:** Tropical areas of Central and South America. A small amount is grown in Florida and California. **Growing Conditions:** Higher elevations in the tropics.	**Processing:** Most of the crop is consumed fresh, but some is made into processed fruit products. **Preparation:** The fresh fruit is usually served raw (chilled or unchilled). **Uses:** Desserts, fruit dishes, ice cream, fruit juices, and sherbets.	**Calories:** 94 kcal/100 g. **Nutritive Value:** Moderately high in fiber (2.2%); a poor source of vitamin C.
Cherry *Prunus avium* (sweet cherry) *Prunus cerasus* (sour cherry) (See CHERRY.)			
Citron *Citrus medica* Citron belongs to the rue family, *Rutaceae.* **Origin and History:** Originated in southeast Asia. Domesticated independently in both China and India. Brought to Near East and Mediterranean in ancient times.	**Importance:** Has limited commercial significance. **Principal Areas:** Mediterranean area, West Indies, California, and Florida. **Growing Conditions:** Subtropical or tropical climate. Requires a well-drained soil. May be killed by freezing temperatures.	**Processing:** Grown mostly for the rind, which is sliced and fermented in brine. Then, the rind is desalted and candied. **Preparation:** Candied citron does not require further preparation. **Uses:** Ingredient of cakes, puddings, and candies.	**Calories:** 314 kcal/100 g for candied citron. **Nutritive Value:** Moderately high in fiber (1.4%) and potassium.
Crabapple *Malus ioensis* and *M. floribunda* Crabapple belongs to the rose family, *Rosaceae.* **Origin and History:** Crabapple trees grow wild from Siberia (U.S.S.R.) to northern China, and in North America. Most wild apples are crabapples. The ancestor of many cultivated varieties is the common wild apple of Europe and western Asia.	**Importance:** Not very important commercially. Certain wild species are valuable sources of genetic material which may be bred into commercial varieties of apples. **Principal Areas:** N. America, Europe, and Asia. **Growing Conditions:** Cool, temperate climate.	**Processing:** Most of the limited production is made into jams, jellies, and pickles. **Preparation:** Serve the processed fruit with other items. **Uses:** Appetizers, jams, jellies, pickles, relishes, and spiced fruit mixtures.	**Calories:** 68 kcal/100 g. **Nutritive Value:** A fair source of potassium and a poor source of vitamin C.
Cranberry *Vaccinium macrocarpon* (See CRANBERRY.)			
Currant *Ribes nigrum* (black currants) *Ribes rubrum* (red currants) Currants belong to the saxifrage family, *saxifrageaceae.* **Origin and History:** Currants are native to Europe.	**Importance:** Annual world production of about 500,000 metric tons. **Principal Areas:** West Germany, Poland, U.S.S.R. **Growing Conditions:** Cool, temperate climate.	**Processing:** Marketed fresh or made into various products. **Preparation:** Wash, stem, and serve raw (alone or with other fruits, cream, and/or ice cream). Baked in buns and cake. **Uses:** Baked goods, jams, jellies, juices, and syrups; and in the production of alcoholic beverages.	**Calories:** 54 kcal/100 g for black European currants. **Nutritive Value:** An excellent source of potassium (372 mg/100 g), vitamin C (200 mg/100 g), and bioflavonoids; moderately high in crude fiber (2.4%); and a fair source of calcium, phosphorus, iron, and vitamin A.
Custard Apple (Sweetsop) *Annona squamosa* **Origin and History:** Native to tropical America.	**Importance:** Popularity is limited to the local area of production (too soft for shipping). **Principal Areas:** West Indies and South America. **Growing Conditions:** Higher elevations in the tropics.	**Processing:** Most of this crop is consumed fresh, but some is made into processed fruit products. **Preparation:** Serve the fresh fruit raw (chilled or unchilled). **Uses:** Dessert or fruit dish; an ingredient of ice creams, fruit juices, and sherbets.	**Calories:** 101 kcal/100g. **Nutritive Value:** A fair share of vitamin C.
Date *Phoenix dactylifera* (See DATE.)			

Footnote at end of table

TABLE F-23 *(Continued)*

Popular and Scientific Name(s); Origin and History	Importance; Principal Areas; Growing Conditions	Processing; Preparation; Uses	Calories; Nutritive Value[1]
Durian *Durio zibethinus* Durian is a member of the family *Bombacaceae*. **Origin and History:** Native to the Malay peninsula and nearby areas.	**Importance:** Only the Malays and other southeastern Asians seem to appreciate the peculiar taste and odor of this fruit. **Principal Areas:** Malaysia and other adjoining areas of southeast Asia.	**Processing:** All of the fruit is consumed fresh near where it is grown. **Preparation:** Serve the fresh fruit raw. **Uses:** Dessert or fruit dish.	**Calories:** 81 kcal/100 g **Nutritive Value:** Moderately high in fiber (1.6%); and a good source of vitamin C (24 mg/100 g).
Elderberry *Sambucus canadensis* Elderberries belong to the honeysuckle family, *Caprifoliaceae*. **Origin and History:** Various species are native to North America and Europe.	**Importance:** Not very important commercially. **Principal Areas:** North America, Europe, and Asia. **Growing Conditions:** Cool, temperate climate.	**Processing:** Much of the berries gathered from this wild shrub are used to make wine. **Preparation:** Serve the fresh fruit raw (alone or with cream). **Uses:** Dessert or fruit dish, making jellies, and in the production of brandies and wines.	**Calories:** 72 kcal/100g. **Nutritive Value:** An excellent source of potassium (300 mg/100 g), and fiber (7.0%); a good source of vitamin C (36 mg/100 g), and a fair source of vitamin A.
Fig *Ficus carica* (See FIG.)			
Gooseberry *Ribes grossularia* Gooseberries belong to the saxifrage family, *Saxifragaceae*. **Origin and History:** Native to Europe and western Asia.	**Importance:** More popular in England than elsewhere. **Principal Areas:** England and other European countries; and North America. **Growing Conditions:** Cool, temperate climate.	**Processing:** Much of the crop is canned or frozen, and some is marketed fresh. **Preparation:** Served as fresh fruit or canned in a sugar syrup. **Uses:** Desserts, fruit dishes, jams, jellies, juices, and pies; and in the production of wines.	**Calories:** 39 kcal/100 g. **Nutritive Value:** A good source of fiber (1.9%); potassium (155 mg/100 g), and bioflavonoids; and a fair source of vitamin A.
Grape (Raisin) *Vitus vinifera* (See GRAPES.)			
Grapefruit *Citrus paradisi* (See GRAPEFRUIT.)			
Guava *Psidium guajava* Guava belong to the myrtle family, *Myrtaceae*. **Origin and History:** Native to South America. First cultivated by Inca Indians.	**Importance:** Interest in this crop is increasing steadily around the world. **Principal Areas:** Tropical areas of the Americas and Asia. **Growing Conditions:** Subtropical or tropical climate.	**Processing:** The fruit may be marketed fresh, canned, frozen, or preserved in other ways. **Preparation:** Serve the fresh fruit raw with a little sugar, bake in pies or tarts, or stew. **Uses:** Desserts, fruit dishes, *guava cheese* (a fruit pasta), jams, jellies, juices, *leather* (dried fruit puree), pies and tarts.	**Calories:** 62 kcal/100 g. **Nutritive Value:** High in fiber (5.6%); a good source of potassium (289mg/100 g), and an excellent source of vitamin C (242mg/100 g).
Jackfruit *Artocarpus heterophyllus* **Origin and History:** Believed to have originated in Malaysia.	**Importance:** Used mainly in areas of production. Most popular in Sri Lanka and India. **Principal Areas:** Tropics of Asia and the Americas. **Growing Conditions:** Tropical climate. Does best on well-drained, deep soils.	**Processing:** Little is processed, because most of the fresh fruits are either eaten raw or cooked in the areas where they are grown. **Preparation:** Serve the fresh fruit raw, or cook it briefly. **Uses:** Dessert or fruit dish; ingredient of fruit salads and pickles.	**Calories:** 98 kcal/100 g. **Nutritive Value:** High in potassium (407mg/100g); a poor source of vitamin C.
Jujube (Chinese date) *Zizyphus jujuba* It belongs to the family *Rhamnaceae*. **Origin and History:** Native to China, where it has been cultivated for about 4,000 years.	**Importance:** Minor fruit crop. **Principal Areas:** China, the Mediterranean area, and southwestern United States. **Growing Conditions:** Dry, tropical climate.	**Processing:** The fruits are sold fresh, candied, dried, or made into a juice. **Preparation:** Eaten fresh, dried, or candied. **Uses:** Desserts, fresh fruits, beverages, cakes, and candies.	**Calories:** 105 kcal/100 g. **Nutritive Value:** A good source of potassium (269 mg/100 g); and vitamin C (69 mg/100 g). Dried jujubes contain about 2½ times the solids and calories of the fresh fruit.
Kiwi Fruit (Chinese Gooseberry) *Actinidia chinenesis* **Origin and History:** originated in China.	**Importance:** The present limited cultivation of this crop appears to be increasing steadily. **Principal Areas:** New Zealand and U.S. **Growing Conditions:** Warm, temperate climate or subtropical climate.	**Processing:** All the crop is utilized as fresh fruit **Preparation:** Eaten fresh or cooked. **Uses:** Desserts, fruit dish, jam, jelly, and pies. Like the papaya, kiwi juice may be used as a meat tenderizer.	Nutritional data is not readily available. Like the papaya, kiwi juice may be used as a meat tenderizer.

Footnote at end of table

(Continued)

TABLE F-23 *(Continued)*

Popular and Scientific Name(s); Origin and History	Importance; Principal Areas; Growing Conditions	Processing; Preparation; Uses	Calories; Nutritive Value[1]
Kumquat *Fortunella japonica* and others. Kumquat is a member of the rue family, *Rutaceae*. **Origin and History:** Originated in China. Cultivated in China, Japan, Indochina, and Java for many centuries. Recently introduced into Australia, Europe, and the Americas.	**Importance:** Of much lesser importance than the citrus fruits, to which it is closely related. **Principal Areas:** New Zealand, China, Japan, and Indochina. **Growing Conditions:** Mild, temperate climate. (More cold resistant than any of the other citrus fruits.)	**Processing:** This fruit may be utilized fresh, or it may be preserved by candying, pickling, and other means. **Preparation:** Serve the whole, unpeeled fruit raw, or use the preserved fruit in various dishes. **Uses:** Desserts, fruit dishes, or garnish for roast duck; in candies, pickles, and sauces.	**Calories:** 65 kcal/100 g. **Nutritive Value:** High in fiber (3.7%); a good source of potassium (236 mg/100 g) and vitamin C; and a fair source of calcium and vitamin A.
Lemon *Citrus limon* (See LEMON.)			
Lime *Citrus aurantifolia* (See LIME.)			
Litchi (Lichi nut) *Litchi chinensis* Litchis are members of the soapberry family, *Sapindaceae*. **Origin and History:** Native to southern China. Introduced into tropical areas around the world.	**Importance:** Of minor importance in the U.S. Some plantings were made in Florida in the early 1940s. **Principal Areas:** China, India, Africa, and Florida. **Growing Conditions:** Cool, dry, subtropical climate.	**Processing:** The fleshy part of this fruit is used fresh, canned in syrup, or dried (so that it resembles a large raisin). **Preparation:** Serve the fresh fruit raw. **Uses:** Desserts or fruit dishes. (This fruit is highly esteemed by Chinese people living abroad.)	**Calories:** 64 kcal/100 g. **Nutritive Value:** A good source of potassium (170 mg/100 g) and vitamin C (50 mg/100g). The dried fruit has about 3½ times the solids and calories of the fresh fruit.
Loquat (Japanese Medlar) *Eriobotrya japonica* Loquat belongs to the rose family, *Rosaceae*. **Origin and History:** Native to China and Japan.	**Importance:** Minor, but popular because it bears fruits very early in the year. **Principal Areas:** Japan, China, India, and Mediterranean countries. Also, it is grown commercially in California. **Growing Conditions:** Temperate climate; grows at higher elevations in the tropics.	**Processing:** Usually this fruit is eaten fresh, but it may also be candied, canned, or preserved in other ways. **Preparation:** Serve the fresh fruit raw or stewed, or add the preserved fruit to relishes or salads. **Uses:** Desserts, fruit dishes, candies, jams, jellies, relishes, and salads; and in the production of liqueurs.	**Calories:** 48 kcal/100 g. **Nutritive Value:** An excellent source of potassium (348 mg/100 g) and a good source of vitamin A (670 IU/100 g).
Mango *Mangifera indica* (See MANGO.)			
Mangosteen *Garcinia mangostana* Mangosteens belong to the garcina family, *Guttiferae*." **Origin and History:** Native to Malaysia.	**Importance:** Little known outside native habitat. **Principal Areas:** Malaysia. **Growing Conditions:** Humid tropical climate. (Does not grow well outside of Malaysia).	**Processing:** All of this crop is used fresh in the vicinity of its production. Hence, none is processed. **Preparation:** Serve the fresh fruit raw. **Uses:** Desserts or fruit dishes.	**Calories:** 57 kcal/100 g. **Nutritive Value:** High in crude fiber (5.0%); a fair source of potassium (135 mg/100 g); and a poor source of vitamin C.
Medlar *Mespilus germanica* Medlars are a member of the rose family, *Rosaceae* **Origin and History:** Native to Europe and central Asia. Grown in Europe in Roman times, when it was more popular than it is today.	**Importance:** Grown in some parts of Europe for its acid-flavored, brown-colored, apple-like fruit. **Principal Areas:** European countries. **Growing Conditions:** Temperate climate.	**Processing:** Only the fruit grown in the warmer countries (such as Italy) ripens fully on the trees. Elsewhere, the fruit must be aged in a cool, dry room to become palatable. Some of the crop is also preserved in various ways. **Preparation:** Only properly ripened or aged fruit should be served raw. **Uses:** Desserts, fruit dishes, jams, and jellies.	Nutritional data is not available.
Mulberry, Black *Morus nigra* Mulberries belong to the mulberry family, *Moraceae*. **Origin and History:** Native to the temperate regions of the Northern Hemisphere, and to China and the Middle East.	**Importance:** Has limited commercial importance. **Principal Areas:** China, Iraq, southern U.S.S.R., and various European countries. **Growing Conditions:** Temperate climate.	**Processing:** Most of this fruit is eaten fresh, but a small amount is processed to make preserves, jams, jellies, and wines. **Preparation:** Served as fresh fruit raw (alone or with cream). **Uses:** Desserts, fruit dishes, jams, preserves, and jellies; and in the production of wines (used mainly for its color).	**Calories:** 42 kcal/100 g. **Nutritive Value:** An excellent source of iron (3.0 mg/100 g), a fair source of potassium (123 mg/100 g), and a good source of vitamin C (39 mg/100 g).
Orange (Sweet orange) *Citrus sinensis* (See SWEET ORANGE.)			
Papaw *Asimina triloba* The American papaw belongs to the custard family, *Annonaceae*. **Origin and History:** Native to the woodlands of southeastern U.S.A.	**Importance:** There is only a small scale commercial production in the eastern U.S. **Principal Areas:** Woodlands of eastern U.S. **Growing Conditions:** Temperate climate.	**Processing:** Most of the fruit is eaten in the areas where it is produced, but some is converted to juice. **Preparation:** Serve fresh fruit raw. **Uses:** Desserts, fruit dishes, and in the production of juice.	**Calories:** 85 kcal/100 g. **Nutritive Value:** Over 5.0% protein.

Footnote at end of table

TABLE F-23 *(Continued)*

Popular and Scientific Name(s); Origin and History	Importance; Principal Areas; Growing Conditions	Processing; Preparation; Uses	Calories; Nutritive Value[1]
Papaya *Carica papaya* (See PAPAYA.)			
Passion Fruit (Granadilla) *Passiflora edulis* **Origin and History:** Native to Latin America. Spread throughout tropical areas of the world.	**Importance:** The present limited commercial production of this fruit appears to be increasing steadily around the world. **Principal Areas:** The warmer regions of North and South America; and in Australia, Hawaii, and South Africa. **Growing Conditions:** Tropical highlands with moderate rainfall.	**Processing:** Much of this crop is made into juice, candied fruit, and other products. **Preparation:** People attempting to eat the fresh fruit will find that the seeds cannot be separated, and must be eaten with the fruit. **Uses:** Desserts, fruit dishes, fruit punch, candied fruit, jams, jellies, and juices.	**Calories:** 34 kcal/100 g. **Nutritive Value:** An excellent source of potassium, and a good source of iron (1.09 mg/100 g).
Peach and Nectarine *Prunus persica* (See PEACH and NECTARINE.)			
Pear *Pyrus communis* (See PEAR.)			
Persimmon American Persimmon *Diospyros virginiana* Japanese Persimmon (kaki) *Diospyros kaki* Persimmons belong to the ebony family, *Ebenaceae*. **Origin and History:** The American persimmon is native to southeastern U.S. The Japanese persimmon is native to central and northern China.	**Importance:** A minor crop in the U.S. Only the Japanese persimmon is grown commercially. **Principal Areas:** Subtropical regions of Asia, Europe, and U.S. The Japanese persimmon is the third most important fruit of Japan. **Growing Conditions:** Warm temperate to subtropical climate.	**Processing:** The fruits are very stringent (puckery) unless they are fully ripened. Some persimmons are (1) dried and eaten like candy, or (2) frozen and eaten like popsicles. **Preparation:** Wash, remove skin layer, serve raw, cooked, or candied. **Uses:** Desserts, fruit dishes, jams, jellies, juices, and pies.	**Calories:** Japanese persimmon, 77 kcal/100 g. **Nutritive Value:** Both American and Japanese persimmons are good sources of potassium and vitamin A. The American persimmon is an excellent source of vitamin C, whereas the Japanese persimmon is a poor source of vitamin C.
Pineapple *Ananas comosus* (See PINEAPPLE.)			
Plantain *Musa paradisiaca* (See PLANTAIN.)			
Plum and Prune *Prunus domestica* and others (See PLUM and PRUNE.)			
Pomegranate *Punica granatum* Pomegranates make up the pomegranate family, *Punicaceae*. **Origin and History:** Originated in the Middle East. Long cultivated throughout the Mediterranean world.	**Importance:** A minor fruit crop in the U.S.A., with an annual production of about 16,250 short tons. **Principal Areas:** Subtropical parts of North America but more popular in the Old World than anywhere else. **Growing Conditions:** Subtropical or tropical climate. Does best in areas with cool winters and hot, dry summers.	**Processing:** Marketed fresh or processed. **Preparation:** Cut open and remove the red sac-covered seeds. (The seeds and the white pulp are not eaten.) Serve as raw, fresh fruit. **Uses:** Desserts or fruit dishes; ingredient of alcoholic drinks (used in the form of grenadine syrup or as the fruit juice); jams, jellies, and syrups.	**Calories:** 63 kcal/100 g. **Nutritive Value:** A good source of potassium (259 mg/100 g), but a poor source of vitamin C.
Quince, Pineapple *Cydonia oblonga* Quince belongs to the rose family, *Rosaceae*. **Origin and History:** Believed to have originated in central Asia.	**Importance:** A minor fruit crop. **Principal Areas:** The temperate zones of Europe and Argentina. **Growing Conditions:** Mild, temperate climate.	**Processing:** The fresh fruit is quite acid and not very palatable. Hence, it is usually cooked or processed. **Preparation:** Stewed and sweetened. **Uses:** Desserts, fruit dishes, candies, jams, jellies, juices, and marmalades.	**Calories:** 57 kcal/100 g. **Nutritive Value:** A good source of fiber (1.7%) and vitamin C.
Rambutan *Nephelium lappaceum* **Origin and History:** Native to Malaysia. Seldom grown elsewhere.	**Importance:** Use is limited to native habitat and surrounding areas. **Principal Areas:** Malaysia. **Growing Conditions:** Humid, tropical climate.	**Processing:** There is little or no processing because the fruit is consumed fresh in the areas near where it is grown. **Preparation:** Serve the fresh fruit raw or cooked. **Uses:** Desserts or fruit dishes.	**Calories:** 64 kcal/100 g. **Nutritive Value:** Moderately high in crude fiber (1.1%); a good source of iron (1.9 mg/100 g) and vitamin C (53 mg/100 g).
Raspberry *Rubus idaeus* and others Raspberries belong to the rose family, *Rosaceae*. **Origin and History:** Various species of raspberry are native to eastern Asia, Europe, and North America.	**Importance:** World production of 250 metric tons, annually. **Principal Areas:** U.S.S.R., Yugoslavia, Germany, Poland, U.S.A., and Hungary. **Growing Conditions:** Cool, temperate climate. Does best on light, neutral soils.	**Processing:** The crop is marketed as fresh fruit, canned, frozen, and processed in other ways. **Preparation:** Serve fresh fruit raw (alone or with cream), or in mixed dishes (such as short cakes). **Uses:** Desserts, fruit dishes, baked goods, gelatin desserts, ice cream, ices, jams, jellies, pies, sherbets, soft drinks, and syrups; and in the production of liqueurs and wines.	**Calories:** Red raspberry, 57 kcal/100 g. **Nutritive Value:** Red raspberries, which are the major type grown in the U.S., contain 3.0% fiber, 168 mg potassium/100 g, and are a good source of iron, vitamin C (25 mg/100 g), and bioflavonoids.

Footnote at end of table

(Continued)

TABLE F-23 *(Continued)*

Popular and Scientific Name(s); Origin and History	Importance; Principal Areas; Growing Conditions	Processing; Preparation; Uses	Calories; Nutritive Value[1]
Sapodilla *Manilkara zopota* The sapodilla belongs to the sapodilla family, *Sapotaceae*. **Origin and History:** Originated in Central America and Mexico.	**Importance:** Commercial cultivation throughout the tropics is increasing steadily. **Principal Areas:** Throughout the tropical world. **Growing Conditions:** Tropical climate.	**Processing:** None, because the fresh fruit is consumed in areas near to where it produced. **Preparation:** Serve the fresh fruit raw. **Uses:** Desserts or fruit dishes.	**Calories:** 89 kcal/100 g. **Nutritive Value:** A good source of fiber (1.4%) and potassium (193 mg/100 g); a fair source of vitamin C.
Sapote White Sapote—*Calocarpum sapota* Green Sapote—*Calocarpum viride* The fruits of white and green sapotes are similar. **Origin and History:** Native to Central America and Mexico.	**Importance:** Limited but increasing cultivation. **Principal Areas:** Central America, Mexico, and Caribbean Islands. **Growing Conditions:** Tropical climate.	**Processing:** Some of the crop is marketed fresh, while the rest is made into preserves. **Preparation:** Usually eaten fresh. **Uses:** Desserts, fruit dishes, jams, and jellies.	**Calories:** 125 kcal/100 g. **Nutritive Value:** A good source of fiber (1.9%), iron (1.0 mg/100 g), and vitamins A and C.
Seville Orange (Sour Orange) *Citrus aurantiam* (See SEVILLE ORANGE.)			
Soursop (Guanabana) *Annona muricata* **Origin and History:** Native to the American tropics.	**Importance:** Has a limited commercial production. **Principal Areas:** Puerto Rico and other American areas. **Growing Conditions:** Tropical climate. Very sensitive to cold weather.	**Processing:** Much of the crop is used to make fruit drinks and ice cream, while the rest is marketed fresh. **Preparation:** Serve the fresh fruit raw with a little sugar. **Uses:** Desserts, fruit dishes, fruit drinks, and ice cream.	**Calories:** 65 kcal/100 g. **Nutritive Value:** A good source of fiber (1.1%), and potassium (265 mg/100 g); a fair source of vitamin C.
Strawberry *Fragaria viginiana* and *Fragaria chiloensis* (See STRAWBERRY.)			
Tamarind *Tamarindus indica* The tamarind belongs to the pea family, *Leguminosae*. **Origin and History:** Originated in the savanna zone of tropical Africa. Brought to India in ancient times.	**Importance:** Of minor importance in the U.S. **Principal Areas:** India and other tropical areas throughout the world. **Growing Conditions:** Thrives in moderately dry tropical climates, but tolerates monsoon conditions if the soil is well drained.	**Processing:** This fruit is eaten fresh and made into various products. **Preparation:** Serve the fresh fruit raw (alone or with a little sugar). **Uses:** Desserts, fruit dishes, candied fruit, chutneys, curries, fruit drinks, sauces, and sherbets.	**Calories:** 331 kcal/100 g. **Nutritive Value:** Rich in fiber (5.1%), and potassium (781 mg/100 g); a poor source of vitamin C.
Tangerine (Mandarin Orange) *Citrus reticulata* (See TANGERINE.)			
Watermelon *Citrullus vulgaris* (See WATERMELON.)			

[1]Calories and nutritive values are for fresh, raw fruit, unless stated otherwise. Canned, cooked, or dried fruits usually contain much less vitamin C than the fresh, raw fruits. For more information regarding the nutritive values of fruits the reader is referred to Food Composition Table F-21.

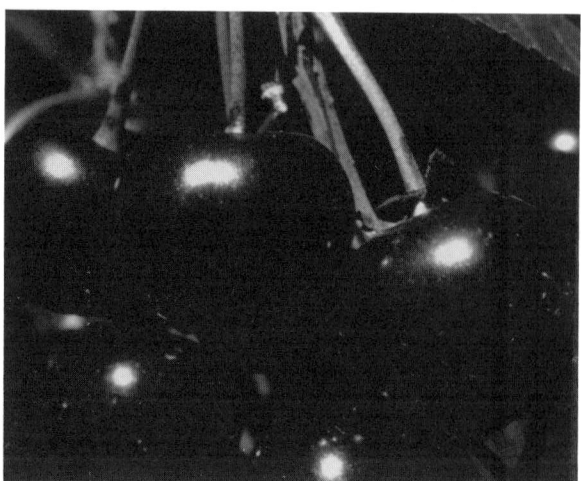

Fig. F-74. A favorite for pie—cherries. (Courtesy, National Film Board of Canada)

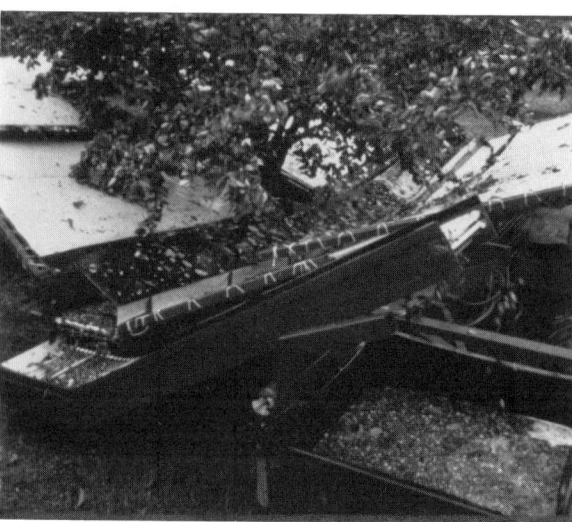

Fig. F-75. Picking pie cherries. (Courtesy, USDA)

FRUIT BEVERAGES

These products range from pure fruit juices to highly diluted, artificially colored and flavored drinks that contain little or no fruit ingredient. Hence, the FDA has issued standards of identity for many types of fruit beverages so that consumers may be assured that certain types of products will contain specified levels of fruit ingredients; for example, *cranberry juice cocktail* must contain at least 25% cranberry juice.

(Also see the articles on the individual fruits for details regarding the various fruit beverages.)

FRUIT, CANNED

Many of the fruits that are grown in the United States are processed by canning, which ensures a supply of the item when fresh fruit is not readily available. Also, canning makes it possible to utilize bumper crops more efficiently since there is a limit to the demand for fresh fruit at harvest time.

Canned fruit is packed in a medium that may vary from plain water or fruit juice to syrups that range in density from "extra light" to "extra heavy." The denser the syrup, the higher its sugar content. Furthermore, the weight of solid fruit in the can or jar (which is called the *drained weight*) may be as low as 50% of the net weight in the cases of grapefruit and whole plums to as high as 78% in the case of "solid pack" crushed pineapple. The FDA standards of identity for canned fruits specify minimum drained weights for certain products.

Canning may reduce the vitamin levels to about one-half of those in fresh fruits, but these fruits are still good sources of some of the vitamins. Minerals remain intact during processing, but some of these nutrients are likely to migrate from the fruit to the packing fluid. Canned fruits may be better tolerated by people with digestive disturbances because some of the fiber is broken down during canning.

(Also see FRUIT[S], section headed "Canning," and the articles on the individual fruits.)

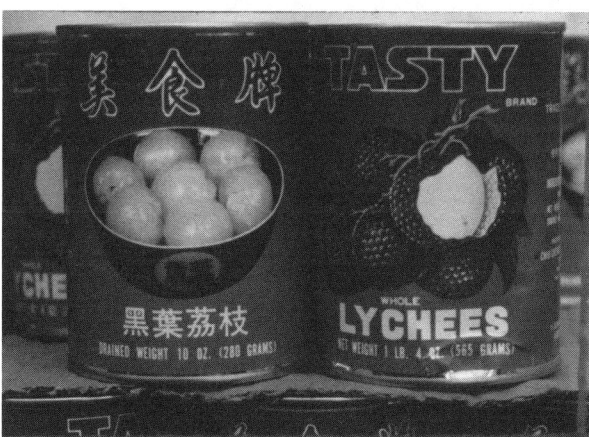

Fig. F-76. Canned lychee (litchi, lichi). Courtesy, Department of Food Science and Human Nutrition, University of Hawaii)

FRUIT, DRIED

The fruits which are most commonly dried in the United States are apples, apricots, dates, figs, nectarines, peaches, plums, prunes, and seedless grapes. Drying reduces the water content of the fruit to about 24%, which is usually low enough to prevent spoilage. Slow drying of fruits in the sun may result in the destruction of much of the vitamin

A and vitamin C contents, unless the fruits are sulfured before drying. However, sulfuring destroys thiamin.

Dried fruits are rich in calories, sugars, fiber, iron, potassium, and various other nutrients because the solids content is about five times that of the fresh fruits. Hence, dried fruit is generally a good buy when it does not cost more than five times the price per pound of the fresh fruit, since the former has no waste in the form of peel and seeds. Furthermore, the consumption of ample amounts of raw or stewed dried fruits may help to promote the regularity of bowel movements.

(Also see the nutrient compositions of fresh and dried fruits which are given in Food Composition Table F-21; and FRUIT[S], sections headed "Drying" and "Effects of Processing and Preparation.")

FRUIT SUGAR

Fructose is found in a free form in some fruits; hence, the name fruit sugar.

(Also see CARBOHYDRATE[S].)

FRUIT SYRUPS

Most of these products are fruit-flavored sugar syrups. For example, apple syrup is made by concentrating apple juice (by boiling or vacuum evaporation), then adding sugar until a syrup of the desired thickness (viscosity) is obtained. Syrups that have citrus fruit flavors may be made in much the same way, except that they may also contain citrus peel and/or essential oil extracted from the peel.

In California, fruit syrups are made from dried figs and dried raisins without added sugar by extracting the chopped fruit with boiling water, then concentrating the resulting juice. However, the fig syrup is rather expensive and is presently sold only in certain health food stores, whereas the raisin syrup is sold only to large food concerns.

Homemakers who would like to utilize other types of syruplike products that are made only from fruits might try thawed, unsweetened frozen fruit juice concentrates such as those made from apple, orange, and pineapple juices.

Also see SYRUPS; and the articles dealing with the individual fruits.)

FRUMENTY

• A dessert made by boiling wheat in milk, flavored with sugar, spice, and raisins.

• A molded cereal dessert.

FUEL FACTOR

The average caloric value of each of three major nutrients is known as its *fuel factor*. One gram of carbohydrate yields 4 calories, 1 g of fat yields 9 calories, and 1 g of protein yields 4 calories.

FUNGI

Plants that contain no chlorophyll, flowers, or leaves, such as molds, mushrooms, toadstools, and yeasts. They may get their nourishment from either living or dead organic matter.

(Also see AFLATOXINS; BACTERIA IN FOOD; MOLDS; MUSHROOMS; and YEAST.)

FUNGICIDE

An agent that destroys fungi.

FUSTIC

A yellow dye derived from the wood of a tropical American tree.

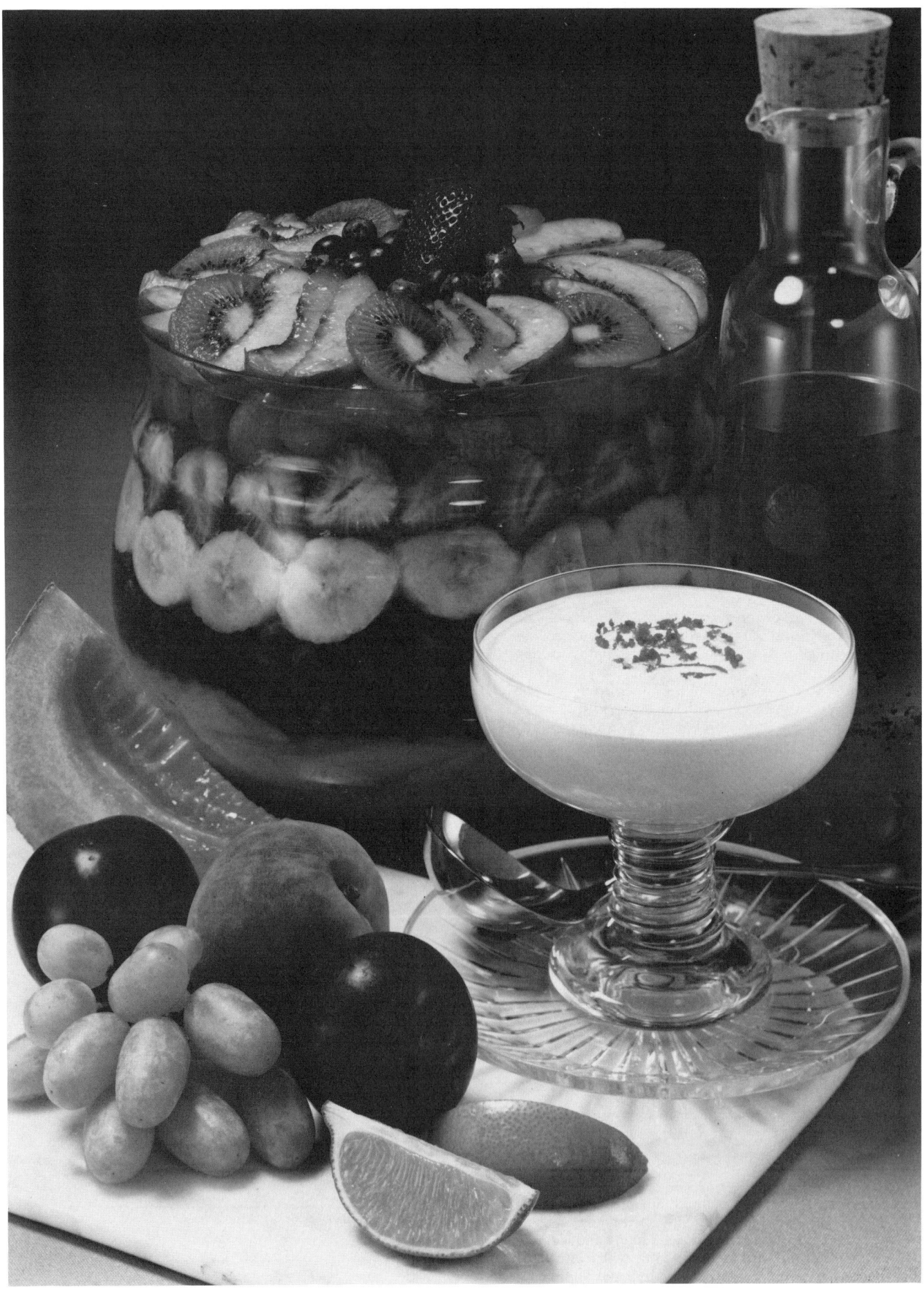

Fig. F-77. Fruits are good for all seasons. (Courtesy, United Fresh Fruit & Vegetable Assn., Alexandria, Va.)

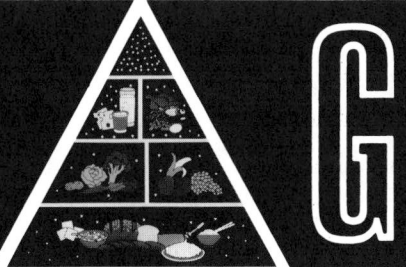

GALACTOSE

A hexose sugar (monosaccharide) obtained along with glucose from lactose hydrolysis.

(Also see CARBOHYDRATE[S].)

GALACTOSEMIA

Literally means a galactose condition of the blood. Galactose builds up in the blood as a consequence of a genetic disorder in metabolism. The enzyme, galactose-1-phosphate uridyl transferase, necessary to change galactose to glucose, is missing; thus, galactose is not metabolized. In the infant, the source of galactose is lactose in the milk.

(Also see INBORN ERRORS OF METABOLISM.)

GALLATES

A class of organic compounds derived from gallic acid and used in the manufacture of writing ink, paper and dyes. In the food industry, propyl, octyl and dodecyl gallates are used as antioxidants, of which propyl gallate is the antioxidant of choice in the United States.

(Also see ADDITIVES; and PROPYL GALLATE.)

GALLBLADDER

The pear-shaped bag located under the right lobe of the liver. Its functions are the storage, concentration, and release of bile, a natural emulsifying agent. The presence of fats and other foods in the digestive tract stimulates the release of the hormone cholecystokinin-pancreozymin which in turn causes the contraction of the gallbladder, releasing bile into the duodenum of the small intestine. Bile is essential for the complete digestion of fats.

(Also see DIGESTION AND ABSORPTION; and GALL-STONES.)

GALLBLADDER DISEASE

In general, it is a disorder in the normal structure and function of the gallbladder and bile ducts. Three types of gallbladder disorders exist: (1) cholecysititis or inflammation (infection) of the gallbladder; (2) cholelithiasis or the formation of gallstones; and (3) although uncommon, tumors or cancer.

Diet is extremely important to persons suffering from a gallbladder disease. The principal aim is to provide a fat-restricted diet, and to reduce the consumption of other foods such as onions, sauerkraut, and alcoholic beverages that may induce the recurrence of the symptoms—mild to severe pain, abdominal distention, nausea, and vomiting. Often persons suffering from gallbladder disorders are obese, and a reduction in total calories to achieve a weight loss is also necessary.

(Also see CHOLECYSITITIS; GALLSTONES; and MODI-FIED DIETS.)

GALLON

A unit of liquid measure in the U.S. Customary System equivalent to 4 quarts or 3.79 liters. The Imperial or British gallon equals 4.55 liters or 1.2 U.S. gallons.

GALLSTONES (CHOLELITHIASIS)

Gallstones—gravellike deposits—are formed when certain substances, which are normally dissolved in the bile, come out of solution as flakelike particles and clump together around a core which may be either tiny bits of sloughed-off lining tissue from the gallbladder, bile salts, calcium carbonate, bile pigments (bilirubin), bacteria, or, in rare cases, such parasites as roundworms (ascarids). Gallstones may vary in their composition from almost pure cholesterol to almost pure compounds of calcium and bile pigments. However, only a few stones may cause problems because most of them are small enough to be easily carried through the bile ducts, and often stones remain in the gallbladder as silent stones. Trouble arises when the stones are too large to pass through the various biliary ducts. Large stones become wedged in the cystic duct, or in the common bile duct—choledocholithiasis—inducing a painful gallbladder attack.

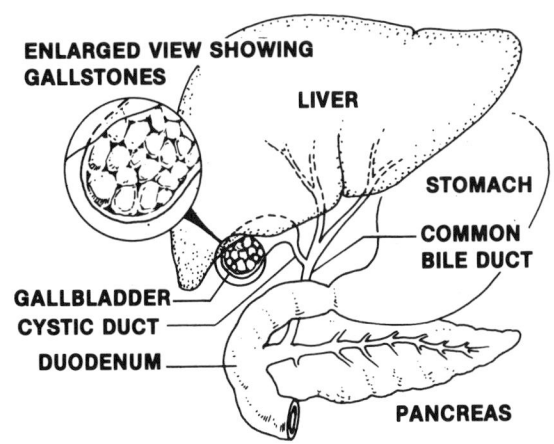

Fig. G-1. The location of the gallbladder with gallstones, the cystic duct and the common bile duct in relation to the liver, intestine, and pancreas.

• **Cholesterol gallstones**—This type of stone is by far the most common—about 85% of the cases in the United States. Cholesterol is a whitish, waxy, fatlike material (lipid) which is almost insoluble in most body fluids unless it is held in solution—emulsified—by means of special complexes. In bile, cholesterol is emulsified and solubilized by a combination of bile salts and lecithin (phosphatidyl-choline). Hence, cholesterol may drop out of the bile when there is a shortage of either of the two types of emulsifying agents.

• **Calcium-containing gallstones**—Normally, both the bile pigments and calcium stay in solution in the bile because (1) the liver usually combines the bile pigments with carbohydrate so as to form soluble, complex molecules, and (2) calcium is present in the bile as a soluble, charged particle or ion. However, certain bacteria, such as E. coli, are sometimes present in the gallbladder. Such bacteria may contain an enzyme which separates the carbohydrate from the bile pigments. Then, the pigments may react with calcium to form the insoluble substances that are found in gallstones.

SYMPTOMS. Generally, stones are undetected—they're silent—until they move and lodge in the bile duct. The hallmark of an acute gallbladder attack is a sharp pain which is felt on the right side of the body just under the rib cage, and sometimes traveling through to the back under the right shoulder blade. Frequently, the pain develops following a meal, when the gallbladder contracts and dumps its stored bile into the duodenum to promote fat digestion. (Pain caused by ulcer is relieved by eating.) Depending upon the location of the stones, jaundice, fever, chills and vomiting may also be symptoms.

(Also see DIGESTION AND ABSORPTION.)

POSSIBLE CAUSES. The exact causes of gallstones are not known. Many people believe that gallstones result from eating lots of fat and/or being fat. Also, there is an old saying that the people who are most likely to have gallstones are characterized by the "4 Fs"—fair, fat, female, and forty. Furthermore, a greater than average susceptibility to gallstones is noted in Jewish people, Pima Indians, and in people with such diseases as cirrhosis of the liver and diabetes. As with many disorders, there are no simple explanations. Various dietary and physiological factors seem to be contributory to stone-forming conditions.

The following discussion deals primarily with cholesterol-containing gallstones, since they are the most common.

Dietary. Deficiencies or excesses of some nutrients may be involved in gallstone formation; among the nutrients implicated are the following:

• **Cholesterol**—This substance is the major constituent of gallstones, so it would seem that eating too much of it may be one of the causes of the stones.

• **Fat**—Excessive consumption of fat over a period of years may lead to the formation of gallstones by stimulating the liver to synthesize greater-than-normal amounts of cholesterol.

• **Fiber**—Gallstones are rare in areas where considerable dietary fiber is eaten—rural Africa, but they are common where diets are low in fiber—the western world.

(Also see FIBER.)

• **Lecithin**—This is an important constituent of bile which helps to keep cholesterol in solution. It is not generally considered to be an essential nutrient because it is thought that the body is able to synthesize the amounts it needs. However, some patients afflicted with gallstones have low levels of lecithin in their bile. Insufficient biliary lecithin may be due to dietary deficiencies of protein, vitamins, choline, and other nutrients which are involved in the synthesis of lecithin by the body.

(Also see CHOLINE; FATS AND OTHER LIPIDS; and LECITHIN.)

• **Protein**—The digestion products of protein may protect against gallstone formation in the following ways:

1. The passage of partially digested proteins from the stomach to the small intestine helps to trigger the mechanism for the emptying of bile from the gallbladder. A static bile favors stone formation.

2. Certain amino acids—serine and methionine—from protein are the raw materials used by the body to make lecithin, which helps to prevent gallstones.

• **Vitamins**—Indirectly, a low intake of some vitamins may contribute to the formation of gallstones. This is demonstrated by the following salient points:

1. Laboratory animals that are deficient in vitamin A develop gallstones due to excessive shedding of the lining cells of the gallbladder, which act as nuclei for the formation of stones.

2. Various B vitamins, such as folacin, vitamin B-6, and vitamin B-12, are required for the production of lecithin by the body.

3. Animal studies suggest vitamin C is required for the conversion of cholesterol in the bile salts, which help to solubilize cholesterol.

4. Vitamin E protects red blood cells against a premature breakdown (hemolysis). Hence, it prevents the production of excessive amounts of bile pigments, which are products of red cell hemolysis. (One type of stone is composed of calcium and bile pigments.) The synthesis of lecithin requires polyunsaturated fatty acids (PUFA). Vitamin E protects these substances against peroxidation. It may also act along with vitamin A in protecting the gallbladder against excessive shedding of its lining cells.

Physiological. Some physiological factors also appear to predispose an individual to gallstone formation; among them, the following have been implicated:

• **Bacteria and inflammation**—Under certain conditions, the small intestine may contain bacteria which convert the primary bile salts which are less effective emulsifying agents. Also, inflammation of the inside lining of the gallbladder resulting from a chronic low grade infection may change the absorptive characteristics of the gallbladder lining, possibly allowing excessive absorption of water, bile salts, or lecithin—the substances necessary to keep cholesterol in solution. As a result, cholesterol begins to precipitate and the small crystals promote the formation of larger and larger crystals.

• **Diabetes**—It is well known that diabetics are more likely to be troubled with gallstones than are nondiabetics. The reasons for this unfortunate situation are that diabetes may often be accompanied by (1) accumulation of cholesterol and fat in the liver, and (2) the growth of intestinal bacteria which degrade bile salts. Furthermore, the administration of insulin increases the cholesterol saturation of bile—a condition which favors stone formation.

• **Disorders of the ileal region of the small intestine**—Gallstones may result from any disorder of the ileum in which the reabsorption of bile salts is drastically reduced so the liver cannot maintain the supply of these salts at the normal level.

(Also see MALABSORPTION SYNDROME.)

• **Hemolysis of red blood cells**—Excessive amounts of bile pigments—bilirubin—may accumulate in the liver and the bile when the rate of breakdown of red blood cells (hemolysis) is considerably more rapid than normal.

• **Hypercholesterolemia**—Hereditary hypercholesterolemia—high blood cholesterol levels—appears to be related to the development of gallstones.

• **Liver disorders**—A logical place to look for abnormalities which may lead to gallstones is the liver—the organ where bile and its components are processed for secretion via the biliary tract. Gallstones occur about 2½ times more often in patients with cirrhosis of the liver—a degenerative disease in which functioning liver tissue is replaced by nonfunctioning fibrous tissue—than in noncirrhotic patients.

Another liver disorder which may be responsible for gallstones is the excessive accumulation of fat in the liver, a condition which is also known as *fatty liver*.

• **Sex and hormones**—Women of child-bearing age are much more likely than men to develop gallstones.

DIAGNOSIS. Proper diagnosis of gallstones is essential so that (1) a potentially hazardous condition is corrected promptly, and (2) unnecessary surgery is avoided if the suspicion of gallstones proves to be unfounded.

The symptomatic pain suggests gallstones. However, these pains may be due to spasms or inflammation of the gallbladder with or without the occurrence of stones. In cases where diagnosis is uncertain, further diagnostic measures such as x rays or ultrasound are employed.

TREATMENT. There is a very strong case for dissolving the stones, or for surgical removal of the gallbladder—cholecystectomy—when (1) large stones are detected by x rays, or other means, (2) gallbladder pain is unremitting, and (3) repeated gallbladder attacks occur.

In 1989, Mayo Clinic researchers reported on a solvent (methyl tert-butyl ether) treatment for gallstones that may eliminate the need for surgery in many cases.

DIET THERAPY. Currently, no sure dietary method exists for preventing or treating gallstones. Possibly, a pill containing chenodeoxycholic acid—a bile acid—may be employed to dissolve small cholesterol gallstones. However, this requires ½ to 2½ years.

Prior to surgery, the diet is restricted in fat to reduce contractions of the gallbladder occurring via the action of the hormone cholecystokinin. Also, fat is often excluded from the diet during acute attacks thereby easing the pain. Following gallbladder removal, a fat-restricted diet may be eaten for several months for wound healing and comfort, but after this time most individuals can eat regular diets. Bile passes directly from the liver to the intestine during the digestive processes in individuals who have no gallbladder.

(Also see FATS AND OTHER LIPIDS; DIGESTION AND ABSORPTION; MODIFIED DIETS; MALABSORPTION SYNDROME; METABOLISM; and OBESITY.)

GAME MEAT

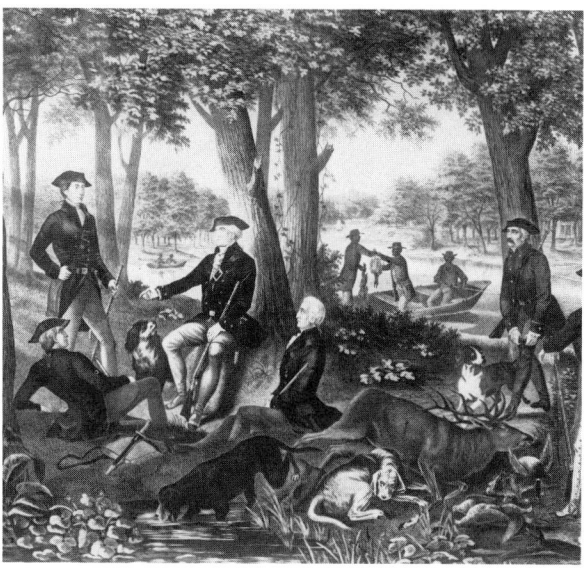

Fig. G-2. Washington (third from left) relaxing with fellow hunters, following the kill of a deer. (Courtesy, General Services Administration, National Archives and Records Service, Washington, D.C.)

Game meat refers to the flesh of wild animals or birds used for food.

Among the wild animals hunted for food are: bear, buffalo, deer, elk, hare, rabbit, roebuck, squirrel, and wild boar.

Among the wild birds hunted for food are: doves, ducks, geese, grouse, partridges, peacocks, pheasants, quails, turkeys, and woodcocks.

GAME FOR GOURMETS. Game meats create romance for good eating. But, contrary to the legendary yarns, there are neither as many secrets relative to game preparation nor as many differences between preparing wild game and domestic animals and birds as most old-time hunters and guides would have us believe. Indeed, neither hunters nor cooks need be terrified about preparing wild game for the table.

The main difference between wild game and domestic animals and birds is that the wild ones are leaner and stronger flavored than a stall-fed ox or a caged bird—they have developed strong muscles from exercising. For this reason, the meat needs a blanket of fat before it is cooked— lard, fat bacon, or salt pork; and it may require tenderizing.

GAMMON

• A ham or a side of cured pork.

• The lower portion of a side of bacon.

GARLIC *Allium sativum*

Garlic, like the other onion vegetables (*Allium genus*), has long been assigned to the lily family (*Liliaceae*), although some botanists now place garlic and its close relatives in the *Alliaceae*. Fig. G-3 shows a typical garlic plant.

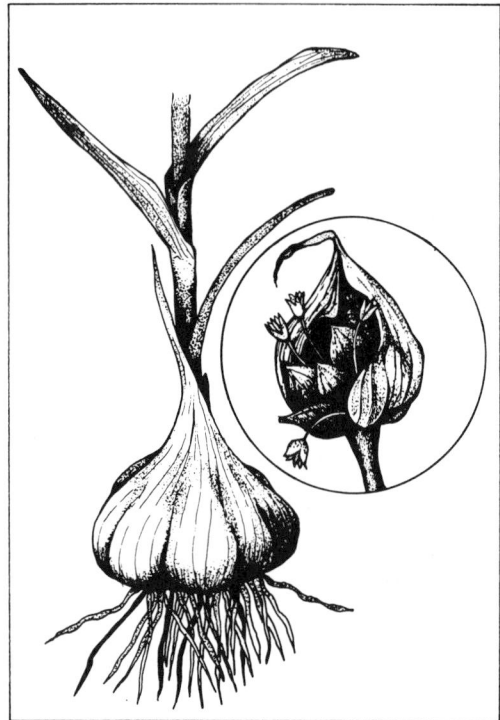

Fig. G-3. Garlic, a herb that has been used as a medicinal agent and a seasoning for many centuries. The flowers (shown in the circle) are often mixed with bulbils (tiny bulbs).

ORIGIN AND HISTORY. Wild varieties of garlic are not found anywhere. The garlic plant originally grew in middle Asia, where it has been cultivated for at least 5,000 years. Egyptian writings attest to its importance as a crop as early as 3200 B.C.; and the Greek historian Herodotus wrote that the laborers who built the Cheops pyramid around 2900 B.C. lived chiefly on onions and garlic.

WORLD AND U.S. PRODUCTION. Garlic ranks fourteenth among the leading vegetable crops of the world, and fifteenth among the vegetable crops of the United States.

About 2.3 million metric tons of garlic are produced worldwide, annually. The leading garlic-producing countries, by rank, are: China, South Korea, India, Spain, U.S.A., Thailand, Egypt, Turkey, and Brazil.[1]

The United States produces 165,000 short tons of garlic annually, most of which is grown in California.[2]

PROCESSING. Much of the U.S. crop is made into dehydrated garlic powder and garlic salt because these forms are more convenient for the food industry than raw garlic bulbs, which are susceptible to spoilage. Somewhat smaller amounts of garlic juice and garlic oil are also produced in the United States.

---

[1]Data from *FAO Production Yearbook 1990*, FAO/UN, Rome, Italy, Vol. 44, p. 143, Table 59. **Note well:** Annual production fluctuates as a result of weather and profitability of the crop.

[2]*Ibid.*

SELECTION, PREPARATION, AND USES. Young, plump cloves of garlic with the outer skin or sheath unbroken are the most desirable.

Raw garlic which is chopped finely or crushed in a garlic press may be mixed with melted butter or margarine for spreading on toasted bread or rolls, or it may be added to relishes, salads, and salad dressing. Cooked garlic loses some of its pungency, yet it still imparts its characteristic taste to casseroles, meats, sauces, soups, and stews.

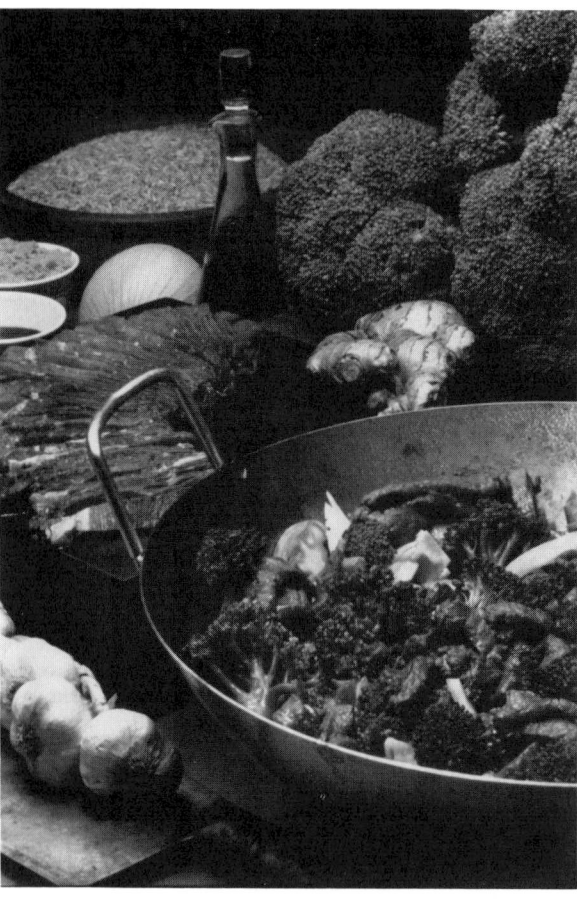

Fig. G-4. Garlic (lower left) imparts its characteristic flavor to many dishes, including meat dishes like the above. (Courtesy, National Film Board of Canada).

NUTRITIONAL VALUE. The nutrient composition of garlic is given in Food Composition Table F-21.

Some noteworthy observations regarding the nutrient composition of garlic follow:

1. It does not usually contribute significant amounts of essential nutrients to human diets because only small amounts are consumed. However, the cooking of garlic in dishes such as casseroles, sauces, soups, and stews eliminates much of its pungency and allows much greater amounts to be consumed. If garlic were to be eaten as an ordinary vegetable, like stewed onions, it would be an excellent source of the essential mineral selenium (it is one of the richest vegetable sources of this nutrient); a good source of calories, protein, phosphorus, iron, and potassium; and a fair source of vitamin C.

2. The therapeutic uses of garlic are as old or older than the use of the vegetable for food. Across the ancient world from Rome to China, the bulbs were considered to be useful in treating deafness, dropsy, intestinal parasites, lack of appetite, leprosy, and respiratory disorders. Although the actual effectiveness of garlic falls short of these expectations, apparently it does possess diuretic and vasodilator properties. These effects alone merit further research into its usefulness in treating certain types of congestive heart failure, excessive fluid retention in the tissues, and high blood pressure.

3. Medical researchers working independently in Great Britain, India, and the United States have recently found that garlic oil contains a substance (*adenosine*) which breaks down the blood-clot-promoting protein called fibrin. This effect suggests that garlic may be helpful in preventing the thrombotic types of heart disease and stroke. Furthermore, the blood cholesterol levels were lowered in volunteers who consumed about 2 oz (56 g) of garlic daily. The latter effect was obtained from cooked garlic as well as raw garlic.

(Also see CHOLESTEROL.)

4. Recently, the age old belief that garlic has germicidal properties has received support by the finding that the allicin it contains retards the growth of certain bacteria.

GAS STORAGE

Primarily a method of storing fresh apples and pears in a controlled atmosphere where the normal 21% oxygen and 0.04% carbon dioxide content of the air is altered. These alterations double the storage life of the fruit. Conditions of storage vary for the different varieties. In general, the objective is to decrease the temperature and oxygen level and increase the carbon dioxide level. McIntosh apples store best at 37°F (3°C), 3% oxygen, 3% carbon dioxide (increased to 5% after one month), and 90% relative humidity. Apples will retain quality for more than 6 months. A high (60%) carbon dioxide concentration is also beneficial for storing eggs for long periods.

Due to the expense and difficulties involved in maintaining apples and pears in a controlled atmosphere, storage in heavy gauge polyethylene liners has proved to be a successful means of increasing the carbon dioxide to oxygen ratio, thereby extending the storage life by reducing the respiration rate similar to gas storage.

(Also see PRESERVATION OF FOOD.)

GASTRECTOMY

The surgical removal of part or all of the stomach.

GASTRIC

Pertaining to the stomach.

GASTRIC JUICE

A clear liquid secreted by the wall of the stomach. It contains hydrochloric acid and the enzymes rennin, pepsin, and gastric lipase.

(Also see DIGESTION AND ABSORPTION.)

GASTRIC MUCOSA

The membrane lining the stomach.

GASTRITIS

This refers to an inflammation of the stomach lining, a condition which most people have experienced, or will experience, during a lifetime. When it involves the intestines, it is called gastroenteritis. Gastritis has a variety of causes some of which are nonspecific. It occurs in three forms: acute, chronic, and toxic or corrosive.

ACUTE GASTRITIS. This type of gastritis, which is experienced by most people, is probably the most common stomach ailment. It arises from a variety of causes, many of which can be summarized in one word—overindulgence.

• **Treatment**—Vomiting and/or diarrhea removes the irritant and often corrects acute gastritis. Other measures may be purely supportive. Small doses of a nonconstipating antacid, coating the stomach with half-and-half milk, and bed rest are recommended. In addition, a liquid of semisolid bland diet consisting of such items as unseasoned eggs, milk, clear soup, and light buttered toast should be eaten for 1 to 2 days following disappearance of the symptoms. Obviously, if the irritant which caused the attack can be identified it should be avoided, at least in excess.

CHRONIC GASTRITIS. This is a mild gastritis which recurs over weeks or months. It is difficult to diagnose, but chronic gastritis is more serious than acute gastritis, as it can signal other more pressing disorders.

Chronic gastritis may be due to repeated exposure to an irritant, as described for acute gastritis, or due to emotional stress, or due to some unknown factors. Although the causes are difficult to sort out, it is often observed in cases of stomach cancer, pernicious anemia, gastric ulcer, gastric polyps, diabetes mellitus, adrenal or pituitary insufficiency, x-ray or surgical treatment of the stomach, and one unavoidable condition—normal aging.

• **Treatment**—Attempts should be made to eliminate the causative factors. However, until this is done the following recommendations are made: (1) avoid alcohol, caffeine, and smoking; (2) eat a bland diet; (3) eat small, but frequent, meals; (4) use a mild antacid or coating agent such as bismuth subnitrate or aluminum hydroxide gel. If symptoms persist, consult a physician.

TOXIC OR CORROSIVE GASTRITIS. This is probably the least common gastritis, but certainly the most dangerous. It often involves children.

The victim, usually by accident, ingests a strong acid, caustic alkali, iodine, or solvent. In the average American home, these chemicals include the powerful cleaning detergents, drain openers, automatic dishwasher compounds, ammonia, paint thinner, turpentine, kerosine, and gasoline.

• **Treatment**—Toxic gastritis is an emergency that demands swift, calm action in order to minimize damage to the victim's esophagus and stomach, and quite possibly prevent death. Immediately give one or two glasses of milk or water to dilute the poison in the stomach. (In 1813, the French chemist Claude Bertrand reported that activated charcoal will absorb poisons like a sponge and prevent them from entering the bloodstream. Similar claims have persisted ever since, but experimental proof is lacking. So, the authors present this report without recommendation, with the hope that it will stimulate research work.) Do not induce vomiting. Vomiting causes further damage. A doctor, the Poison Control Center (ask the operator for the Poison Control Center, or call the U.S. Public Health Service at either Atlanta, Georgia or Wenatchee, Washington), and/or an ambulance should be contacted immediately. When the victim is transported to a doctor or hospital emergency room, the container which held the poison should also be taken.

Prevention is better than treatment. Keep household chemicals inaccessible to small children with big curiosities.

(Also see ANTACIDS; BACTERIA IN FOOD, Table B-2, Food Infections [Bacterial]; INDIGESTION; and POISONS.)

GASTROENTERITIS

Generally, a brief self-limiting inflammation of the stomach and intestines, which is very often caused by a foodborne bacterial infection, bacterial toxin, or viral influenza. However, some of the same agents causing gastritis may also cause gastroenteritis; for example, alcohol overindulgence, and drugs. Common symptoms are nausea, vomiting, cramps, and diarrhea. Treatment depends upon the causative factor, but a bland or liquid diet is recommended until symptoms pass. Some *over-the-counter* preparations may provide symptomatic relief. Bacterial infections may require an antibiotic prescribed by a doctor. Persistent, excessive vomiting and diarrhea are especially dangerous in infants and old people as dehydration can result.

(Also see BACTERIA IN FOODS, Table B-2, Food Infections [Bacterial],—*Escherichia coli*; MODIFIED DIETS; DISEASES, Table D-10, Food Related Infectious and Parasitic Diseases; and GASTRITIS.)

GASTROINTESTINAL

Pertaining to the stomach and intestines.

GASTROINTESTINAL DISEASE

A very broad term suggesting any disorder in the structure or function of the digestive system. Often diets are modified for gastrointestinal tract disorders such as cholecystitis, cirrhosis of the liver, constipation, diarrhea, gastric carcinoma, gastritis, hiatal hernia, ileitis, malabsorption, and peptic ulcers, among others. On the other hand, some diets may be blamed for a specific gastrointestinal disorder, though the cause-and-effect nature of the diet in some cases is only suggestive and not demonstratable.

(Also see BACTERIA IN FOODS; DISEASES; INBORN ERRORS OF METABOLISM; MALABSORPTION SYNDROME; and MODIFIED DIETS.)

GASTROINTESTINAL TRACT

Often this is interchanged with the following terms: digestive tract, digestive system, and alimentary canal, but actually it refers to the stomach and intestines.

(Also see DIGESTIVE SYSTEM.)

GASTROSCOPY

A nonsurgical, diagnostic technique used to view the stomach lining. The instrument used is called a gastroscope, a telescopic system with a light source. The gastroscope is passed down the esophagus to the stomach. No anesthetic is required, but it does cause temporary discomfort.

GAVAGE

Introduction of material (as nutrients) into the stomach by means of a stomach tube.

(Also see TUBE FEEDING.)

GEL

A colloidal suspension which has solidified. It is the abbreviation for gelatinous.

GELATIN

A mixture of proteins not found in nature but derived from connective tissue (collagen) by hydrolytic action—boiling skin, tendons, ligaments and bones. Gelatin is digestible, but it is an incomplete protein. It lacks the essential amino acid tryptophan, and contains only small amounts of other essential amino acids. In its dry form, gelatin is colorless or slightly yellow, transparent, brittle, practically odorless, and tasteless. It is capable of swelling up and absorbing 5 to 10 times its weight of water to form a gel in solutions below 95° to 104°F (35° to 40°C). Gelatin has numerous food and nonfood uses. In foods, gelatin is used as a stabilizer, thickener and texturizer in such foods as confectionery, jellies, and ice cream. The FDA classifies gelatin as a GRAS (generally recognized as safe) additive. Nonfood uses consist of adhesives, capsules for medicinals, inks, plastic compounds, artificial silk, photographic plates and films, sizing of paper and textiles, plasma expander, and hemostasis.

GELOMETER

An instrument used to measure jelly strength.

GENE

A unit of heredity arranged in a definite fashion on a chromosome.

GENETIC DISEASES

Harmful disorders in the normal structure and function of the body caused by an error in the genetic code. The disease is present at birth, though not always evident. It may manifest itself later in life due to some interaction with the environment. Genetic diseases occur (1) as a rare gene mutation; (2) as conditions that *run in the family* or hereditary disorders (dominant and recessive); or (3) as an accidental change in chromosome numbers (Down's Syndrome) or structure. A number of metabolic disorders have genetic origins, and once recognized can be treated by dietary alterations, for example, galactosemia and phenylketonuria (PKU).

Amniocentesis, obtaining fetal cells for genetic analysis, offers some hope for early detection of genetic diseases. However, only when we master genetic engineering will we be able to prevent genetic disorders. For now, the best treatment is early detection.

(Also see INBORN ERRORS OF METABOLISM.)

–GENIC

Suffix, meaning to produce or give rise to; e.g., ketogenic.

GENIPAPO *Genipa americana*

The fruit of a large tree (of the family *Rubiaceae*) that is native to eastern South America and the West Indies. Genipapo trees bear pear-shaped fruits that are about 3 in. (7.5 cm) in diameter and about 4 in. (10 cm) long. The granular pulp of the fruit contains many small seeds. The fruit is used mainly to make fruit drinks, marmalade, or wine.

GEOPHAGIA

The eating of earth, a practice which prevails among some of the population of Africa. *Edible earth*, usually obtained from a particular spot, is commonly mixed with a bean or a green relish and consumed by the whole family. The cause

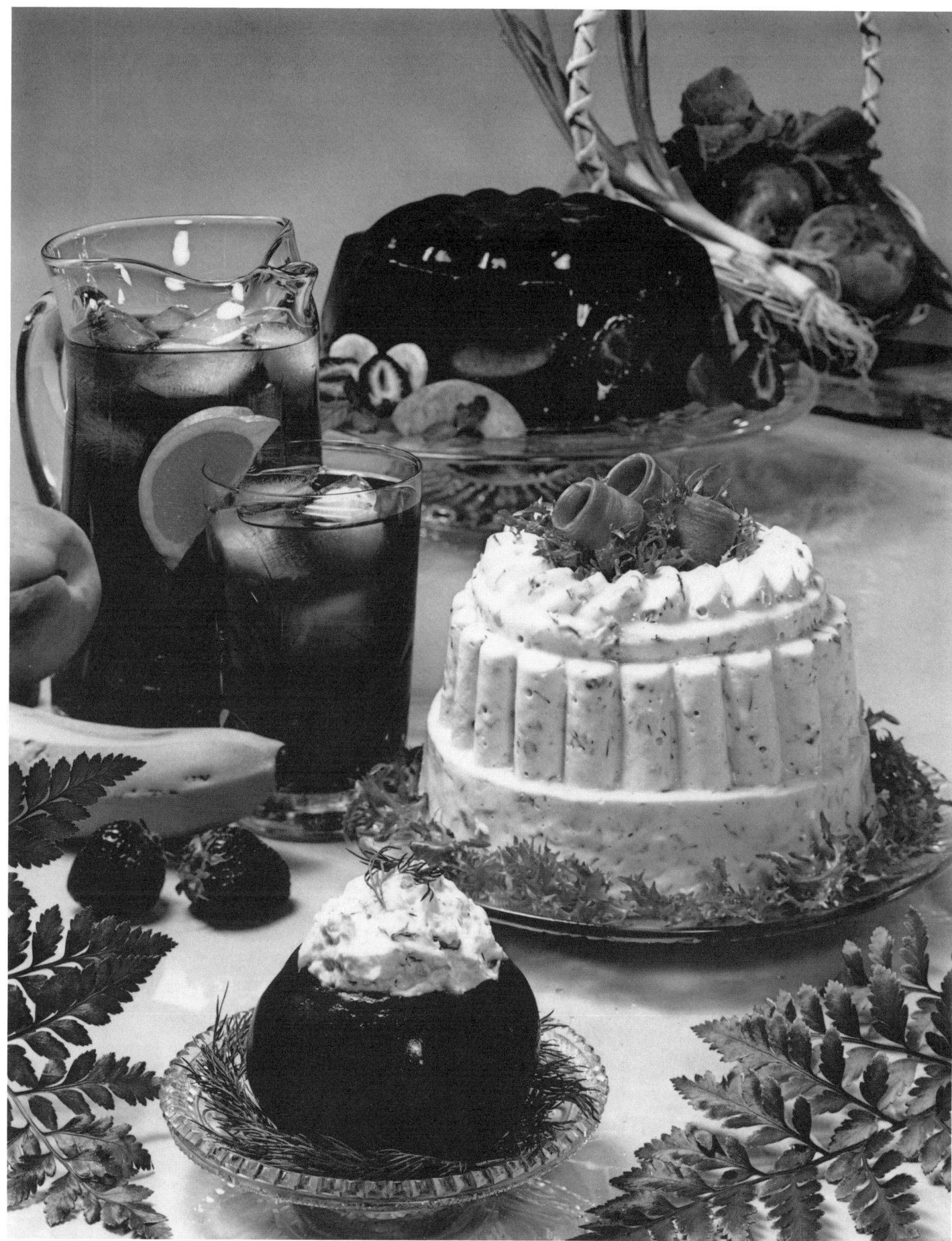

Fig. G-5. Gelatin salads for summer—a cool cook's dream. (Courtesy, United Fresh Fruit and Vegetable Assoc., Alexandria, Va.)

is unclear. It may be a carry-over of a habit acquired in childhood, from the exploratory putting of earth from the hut floor into the mouth; or it may be a means of satisfying hunger and malnutrition.

(Also see ALLOPRIOPHAGY; and PICA.)

GERBER TEST

This is a test for determining the fat content of milk. In principle, it is very similar to the commonly used Babcock test. Sulfuric acid is mixed with milk, releasing the fat and leaving it free to rise. The Gerber bottle, in which this test is performed, has a thin graduated neck. Fat collects in the neck, where it is measured.

(Also see BABCOCK TEST.)

GERM

Embryo of a seed.
(Also see CEREAL GRAINS.)

GERONTOLOGY AND GERIATRIC NUTRITION (SENIOR CITIZENS AGE 65 AND OVER)

People are living longer. But they may not be staying younger. This article is concerned with the latter.

Many people are not as well informed about aging as they might be, considering that both the number and percentage of people 65 years of age or older are increasing steadily, as is shown in Fig. G-6.

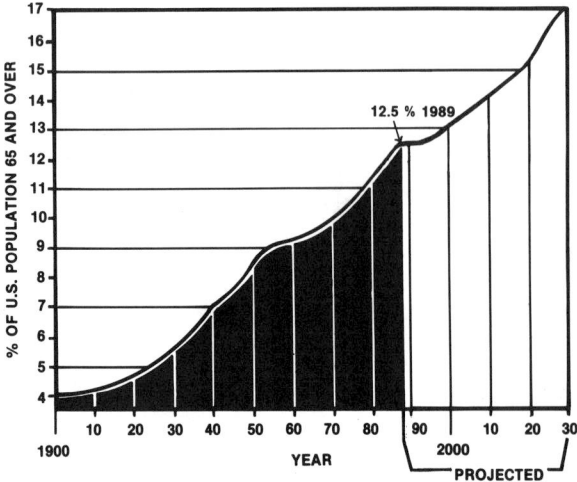

Fig. G-6. The increasing percentage of people aged 65 and over in the United States from 1900 to 1989, with projections for the period 1989 to 2030. (Source: *The Graying of Nations: Implications,* Hearing before the Special Committee on Aging of the U.S. Senate, First Session of the 95th Congress, November 10, 1977, U.S. Government Printing Office, 1978, p. 6, and *Statistical Abstract of the United States 1991,* p. 23)

It may be seen from Fig. G-6 that the percentage of senior citizens is expected to quadruple in the period which began in 1900 and will end in 2030, so that at the latter date this group of people will represent about one-sixth of all Americans.

Better to understand the nutritional needs and other characteristics of our older generation, it is first necessary to clarify some of the terms that are commonly applied to the group.

• **Aging**—Although this term is often applied to people of middle age (40 to 65 years old) and older, in the fullest biological sense it designates the sequences of mental and physical changes that begin at conception and end at death.

• **Elderly**—In common usage, this designation applies to people aged 65 and older.

• **Geriatrics**—This term refers to the medical specialty which deals with the prevention and treatment of the diseases of aging. As such it is one of the areas of concentration within the much broader field of gerontology. Sometimes, the elderly are designated as *the geriatric set.*

• **Gerontology**—This field of study covers many aspects of aging. Hence, it utilizes the methods of such disciplines as anthropology, biochemistry, biology, economics, history, medicine, physiology, psychology, and sociology. However, it should not be confused with geriatrics, which is limited to the medical aspects of aging.

• **Life expectancy**—Many people use this term incorrectly, in that they assume it to have a fixed value throughout a person's life. However, it refers to the number of years that a person may expect to live after having reached a certain age. (Life expectancy data are derived from the vital statistics that have been obtained from various groups of people and national populations.) It is noteworthy that the life expectancy at birth is usually less than that at age 65, because a newborn infant has yet to be exposed to the infectious diseases that threaten life, whereas the 65 year old has already survived many of these hazards.

• **Life-span**—This term usually designates the maximum or optimal amount of time that a person might live, provided that his or her health and life circumstances are quite favorable.

• **Longevity**—Depending upon the context in which it is used, this term means (1) a long life, or (2) the length of life.

• **Retirement age**—Retirement at age 65 is believed to have been first used by Chancellor Otto von Bismarck of Germany in 1889, when he set up the first nationwide old age pension plan. Since then, other nations and certain employers have established retirement ages which vary according to the work performed. For example, people who perform hard, laborious tasks may be allowed to retire as early as age 55, whereas the usual retirement age for Roman Catholic clergy is 75.

• **Senility**—This condition, which is characterized by a marked loss of memory and mental deterioration, is *not* always irreversible as was once thought. Sometimes, the signs of senility are brought on by nutritional deficiencies and/or other correctable conditions such as dehydration, and a reduced flow of blood to the brain.

• **Senior citizens**—It is not known when this term was first applied to the elderly in America, but it appears to have been coined to give greater dignity to older, retired people.

This article is concerned mainly with the conservation of the health, mental acuity, and physical capabilities of older people, rather than the extension of the life-span. The effects of nutrition on longevity are covered elsewhere in this book.

(Also see LIFE EXPECTANCY AND NUTRITION.)

HISTORY. Many ancient writings document man's longstanding search for ways to extend youthful health and vigor into old age. Both the Old and the New Testaments of the Bible tell of miraculous rejuvenations of women who conceived children long after their menses had ceased. Such was the case of Abraham's wife, Sarah (*Genesis* 18:10-14), and of John the Baptist's mother, Elizabeth (*Luke* 1:7-25). Furthermore, the ancient cultures of China, India, and Greece had their legends of the Fountain of Youth that was thought to be located somewhere along the course of a major river. Perhaps, this association was made because the rivers were responsible for bringing new life to the soils they watered.

In the early 1500s, the Spanish explorer Ponce de Leon came to the Americas to search for the Fountain of Youth that was believed to be present on an island in the Caribbean. He never found it, but in the course of his search he explored Puerto Rico and discovered Florida, where many older people now go to escape the ravages of winter and expose themselves to the healing power of the sun.

Interest in diet as a means of maintaining vigor into old age arose at the beginning of the 20th century, when the Russian scientist Metchnikoff advocated the consumption of liberal amounts of yogurt because he believed that this food was responsible for the unusual health and vigor of elderly Bulgarian peasants. The effects attributed to yogurt were believed to result from its content of *Lactobacillus bulgaricus* bacteria which supposedly prevented the formation of certain toxins in the intestine.

Shortly after the early interest in yogurt waned, the era of vitamins began. The dramatic responses that often followed the giving of minute amounts of these nutrients to deficient people led many people to believe that vitamins were potent metabolic stimulators. During and after World War II, military medical personnel administered injections of the vitamin B complex to their fellow servicemen who lined up at the dispensaries on the mornings after nighttime drinking bouts. However, it was ultimately shown by nutritional researchers that excesses of most vitamins have little beneficial effect once nutrient needs have been met.

Recently, a more holistic approach to the retardation of the degenerative changes during aging has emerged, as anthropologists and other social scientists have joined dentists, doctors, and nutritionists in studying various cultural groups in America and abroad to determine why some people age more slowly than others. These studies have focused upon such diverse groups as Mormons, Seventh-day Adventists, and Trappist Monks, and on the apparently long-lived and vigorous inhabitants of isolated mountainous areas such as (1) the valley of the Hunzas in northeast Pakistan, (2) Vilcabamba in the Andes of southern Ecuador, and (3) the Georgian region of the Soviet Union. In almost every case, the most healthy and long-lived people engaged in strenuous work throughout their lives and ate sparingly of reasonably good unrefined diets. However, there are still many unanswered questions regarding the precise physiological means by which above average good health in the elderly is

achieved by diet and exercise. Hence, it is necessary to consider some of the known and postulated factors that may accelerate the aging of cells and tissues.

FACTORS THAT MAY ACCELERATE AGING. The ever-growing percentage of elderly people in the United States and other developed countries has prompted concern over the ability of families, private groups, and governmental agencies to assist the needy seniors. Obviously, slowing of the crippling mental and physical deterioration that occurs in some, but not all, of the aged would help to increase the numbers of these people who could be assets rather than liabilities to society. However, it appears that a number of different factors contribute to the aging of the body tissues. Unfortunately, the physiological processes associated with the aging factors are not understood fully. Some of what is known, along with the relationship of diet and/or hygiene, is presented in Table G-1.

CHANGES THAT MAY OCCUR IN THE BODY DURING AGING. Apparently, Americans are doing some of the things that counter the agents of deterioration discussed in the preceding section, since the death rate for older people from all causes has dropped sharply.

Nevertheless, older people are troubled with various chronic conditions such as those for which data is presented in Fig. G-7.

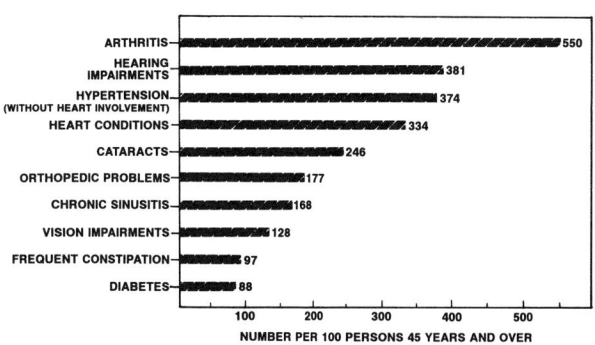

Fig. G-7. The top ten chronic conditions reported in health interviews by persons age 75 and older in 1988. (Based on data from *Statistical Abstract of the United States 1991*, p. 120, Table 195)

Many of the handicapping conditions shown in Fig. G-7 may be the result of one or more of the physiological changes which occur during aging. That is not to say that each type of degeneration occurs to an equal extent in every older person, since many of the elderly are healthier than some of their juniors. Rather, it should be understood that deterioration of body parts occurs at different rates in different people, depending upon their heredity, past medical history, diet, and type of hygiene practiced throughout life.

NUTRITIONAL ALLOWANCES. A complete presentation of nutrient allowances for different age groups, including senior citizens, along with nutrient functions and best food sources of each nutrient, is given in this book in the section on Nutrients: Requirements, Allowances, Functions, Sources, and its accompanying Table N-3; hence, the reader is referred thereto.

TABLE G-1
AGENTS AND PROCESSES THAT MAY CAUSE AGING

Factor	Means By Which Aging is Accelerated	Relationship(s) to Diet and/or Hygiene
Accumulation of residues in cells and tissues	Substances such as amyloid,[1] asbestos, cholesterol, dust, fibrous matter, lipofuschin granules,[2] silica, trace metals, and uric acid may accumulate to the extent that the functioning of cells and tissues is impaired. Sometimes, the tissues are inflamed or irritated and fibrous matter or scar tissue is formed. Also, cancers may start at the sites of certain types of irritating deposits.	Nutritionally imbalanced diets may result in defects of metabolism that produce accumulation of certain residues. Inhalation of particle-laden air may result in deposits of the contaminants in the lung tissues. This may be prevented by the wearing of a respiratory mask.
Autoimmunity	The body develops antibodies that attack its own tissues. It is believed that autoimmune reactions may be responsible for some cases of Addison's disease,[3] arthritis, diabetes, kidney disease, lupus, myocarditis, opthalmia (damage to the eye), and thyroiditis. Sometimes, antibodies against tissues may be the result of mutations of the chromosomes in the antibody-producing cells.	Means for preventing autoimmunity by diet are uncertain. However, experimental animals fed high-protein diets are more prone to autoimmune disorders than those given low to moderate levels of dietary protein. Also, adequate nutrition may help to prevent the breakdown of tissues and the release of fragments into the blood, where autoimmune reactions may occur.
Cell loss from vital tissues	Certain types of cells may be lost more rapidly than they are replaced. Eventually, the tissues are left with too few functioning cells.	Good nutrition may minimize cell loss and maximize cell replacement in some, but not all, tissues.
Chromosome breakage	Radiation and some types of toxic agents cause damage to the chromosomes so that the genetic control of metabolism is altered. Fortunately, human chromosomes can be repaired.	Diets containing nucleic acids (DNA and RNA) or the nucleotide bases such as adenine (abundant in yeast) may help to speed up the repairing of chromosomes.
Collagen stiffening	The protein collagen, which is a major constituent of the blood vessel walls, bones, cartilages, skin, and tendons, gradually loses its elasticity and shrinks in size so that it interferes with the metabolism of cells. Also, collagen is often deposited in the form of fibrous tissue at the sites of inflammation and injury.	Experimental animals that were kept on low-calorie diets for long periods of time after weaning had a much slower rate of collagen stiffening than those given more calorie-rich diets. However, the calorie-deprived animals had retarded growth and development.
Cross-linking of macromolecules	Large molecules such as nucleic acids and proteins may acquire cross-linkages that reduce functioning because of the increased rigidity which results. (DNA and collagen are highly susceptible to cross-linkage.)	It is believed that a heavy consumption of carbohydrates, fats, and/or proteins results in an increased production of aldehydes that form cross-linkages within macromolecules.
Free-radical damage	Polyunsaturated fatty acids that are present in the diet and in the cells are oxidized readily to highly-reactive free radicals that damage the inner and outer membranes of cells and disrupt cellular functions. Free-radical damage is similar to that caused by exposure to radiation.	The formation of free radicals is retarded by liberal amounts of dietary sulfur-containing amino acids, selenium, and vitamin E; and by avoiding an excessive consumption of polyunsaturated fatty acids.
Inborn programming of aging	The cells of the human body have limited life-spans. Hence, tissues age and die when the rates of cell death exceed the rates of replacement. Also, certain cells are not replaced after maturity.	Good nutrition and optimal hygienic practices may prevent the premature deterioration and death of the irreplaceable cells.
Loss of irreplaceable substances	Certain vital substances are produced only during the early stages of growth and development. However, there is a slow but continuous loss of these compounds during the normal functioning of the body throughout life. Rapid aging occurs when the cumulative losses reach critical levels.	Slowing the rates of growth and development of experimental animals by stringent dietary restriction has apparently slowed the metabolism and consequently the rate of loss of irreplaceable substances and aging. It is not certain whether similar results can be obtained in humans.
Mutations	Changes in the genetic material (chromosomes) of cells occur spontaneously and as a result of exposure to radiation and other agents. These changes often produce abnormalities of cell functions. Generally, the rate of mutation increases with age.	The rate of mutations may be slowed somewhat by minimizing exposure to known mutagenic factors such as free radicals and radiation; and by consuming diets containing nucleic acids and other nutrients needed for the maintenance of healthy cells.
Nerve deterioration	The deterioration of nerve cells and/or of the various processes associated with nerve function results in the loss of control of vital functions. Disorders such as diabetes, multiple sclerosis, and certain nutritional deficiencies accelerate the rate of deterioration.	Nerves begin to develop before birth and require adequate nutrition throughout life. Furthermore, conditions in other tissues may ultimately be reflected in the nerves. Hence, a good diet plus the practice of sensible hygiene may prevent the premature deterioration of the nerves.
Radiation	Various types of radiation (neutrons, ultraviolet rays, x rays, etc.) cause damage to the chromosomes in cells that may result in abnormalities in cell function, and in some cases, cancer.	The effects of radiation have been counteracted in experimental animals by low-fat cereal diets that encourage the growth of lactobacilli in the intestine.
Reduced sensitivity of cells and tissues to hormomes	The sensitivity of various tissues to hormones decreases as a result of (1) a reduction in the number of hormone-sensitive areas (receptor sites), and (2) an increase in the processes that counteract the hormonal effects. Hence, the body responds more slowly to stresses such as chilling, fasting, and the need for increased pumping of blood by the heart. The reduced responsiveness makes the body more vulnerable to various types of injury.	Injury to the body may be minimized by (1) eating a nutritionally balanced diet at regularly scheduled meals; (2) avoiding sudden changes in the rate of physical activity; and (3) taking care not to become chilled or overheated. However, moderate mental and physical challenges help to stimulate the functioning of the heart and the other vital organs.
Stress	Stresses that are sufficiently severe and/or prolonged to overtax the body's defense mechanisms may literally exhaust such glands as the adrenals and the pancreas; and/or they may cause the breakdown of tissues such as the stomach lining and the vertebrae.	Some of the destructive effects of stress may be counteracted by (1) a balanced diet that contains moderate amounts of calories, protein, minerals, and vitamins; and (2) sticking to a regular and sensible schedule of exercise and other activities.
Wear and tear on the tissues	Tissues that are subjected to chronic strains of various types may sustain injuries that are not repairable by the natural restorative processes. For example, many older people who have long been obese have a wearing down of their knee joints (osteoarthritis).	The *wearing out* of body tissues may be reduced by avoiding severe or prolonged overloads that may cause injury. Also, obese people should reduce their weight gradually to a more normal, healthy level.

[1]Amyloid deposits are carbohydrate-protein complexes occurring mainly in the tissues of the adrenal glands, digestive tract, kidneys, liver, lungs, muscles, skin, and spleen. They are believed to result from autoimmune reactions in which the tissues are attacked by antibodies. The amount of amyloid usually increases with age.

[2]Lipofuschin granules are yellow pigments (also callded *age pigments*) that accumulate mainly in the heart muscle and the brain. The pigments are the products of the destructive reactions between free radicals and various membranes within cells. These reactions may be minimized by adequate dietary amounts of protective nutrients such as the sulfur-containing amino acids, selenium, and vitamin E. However, diets rich in polyunsaturates promote the reactions.

[3]Addison's disease is an insufficiency of adrenal cortical secretion that may result from (a) diseases such as tuberculosis, (b) an autoimmune disorder, or (c) other causes.

DIETARY GUIDELINES. The first dietary guideline is: *Eat enough of the proper foods consistently.* To ensure nutritional adequacy, the elderly (and those responsible for their diets) are admonished to—

1. Read and follow the section on Nutrients: Requirements, Allowances, Functions, Sources, including Table N-3.

2. Eat a daily diet which includes definite amounts of foods from each of the Six Food Groups as detailed in the section on Food Groups, Table F-22.

But, lots of folks don't know what constitutes a good diet; and, worse yet, altogether too many people neglect or ignore the rules even if they know them. In either case, the net result is always the same; they shortchange themselves on the right amounts of good nutritious foods. As a result, more and more doctors and nutritionists are recommending judicious mineral and vitamin supplementation.

It is noteworthy, too, that those whose diets are restricted for the treatment of certain disorders may need to use supplements as sources of the nutrients that would ordinarily be provided by foods which are not allowed in their diets. For example, people who cannot drink milk or eat cheese may have to take a calcium supplement that provides this mineral.

Menu planning. Nutritionists have found that it is easy to plan menus if the desired foods are put into the Six Food Groups that are easily identified. It is noteworthy, however, that this procedure results in the best nutrition when a wide variety of foods are included in each group. A typical grouping of foods is given in Table G-2.

(Also see FOOD GROUPS, Table F-22, The Six Food Groups/The Food Guide Pyramid.)

A typical menu plan that utilizes the recommended servings of each of the major food groups is given in Table G-3.

Dietary Modifications For Some Common Health Problems. Some of the health problems that affect senior citizens may be remedied by medical treatments prescribed by physicians, assisted by certain types of dietary modifications. However, people should *not* undertake to modify their diets without first consulting a doctor, since conditions other than the most evident problem(s) may require diagnosis and treatment before a dietary change is made. Therefore, the information given in Table G-4 is for the purpose of promoting a better understanding of some common dietary prescriptions.

(Also see MODIFIED DIETS; and NUTRIENTS: REQUIREMENTS, ALLOWANCES, FUNCTIONS, SOURCES.)

TABLE G-2
MAJOR FOOD GROUPS FOR SENIOR CITIZENS

Food Group	Amounts Recommended[1]	Typical Items
Meats, poultry, fish, dry beans, eggs, and nuts	Choose 2-3 servings every day. Count as a serving: 2 to 3 oz (without bone) of lean cooked meat, poultry, or fish. Equivalent in protein to 2 oz meat are 2 eggs; 1 cup cooked beans, dry peas, or lentils; 4 Tbsp peanut butter	Beef, veal, lamb, pork, organ meats such as liver, heart, or kidney; poultry and eggs; fish and shellfish; meat alternates—dry beans, dry peas, lentils, and peanut butter.
Milk, yogurt, and cheese	Use 2-3 cups of milk or the equivalent in a milk alternate, every day. **Note:** Calcium supplements in pill form are *not* the nutritional equivalents of milk and cheese because pills do not supply calories, protein, and the essential nutrients provided by the dairy foods.	Milk: fluid whole, skim, lowfat, evaporated, dry, or buttermilk. Milk alternates on the basis of calcium content are: Cheddar-type cheese, 1-in. cube = ½ cup milk Cream cheese, 2 Tbsp = 1 Tbsp milk Cottage cheese, ½ cup = ⅓ cup milk Ice cream, ½ cup = ⅓ cup milk Ice milk, ½ cup = ⅓ cup milk
Vegetables	Choose 3-5 servings daily including: one vegetable high in vitamin A, and one high in vitamin C. One serving equals: 1 cup of leafy greens, or ½ cup any other vegetable.	Broccoli, carrots, chard, collards, cress, kale, pumpkin, spinach, sweet potato, turnip greens, winter squash, or other dark green leaves are high in vitamin A. Asparagus, broccoli, Brussels sprouts, cabbage, cauliflower, collards, garden cress, green pepper, kale, kohlrabi, mustard greens, potato and sweet potato cooked in the jacket, rutabagas, spinach, sweet red pepper, tomato or tomato juice, and turnip greens are good sources of vitamin C.
Fruits	Two to four servings of any fruit, including those that are valuable for vitamin C and vitamin A. Count as a serving: ½ cup *(120 ml)* of fruit; or a portion as ordinarily served, such as 1 medium apple, banana, or orange, half a medium grapefruit or cantaloupe, or the juice of 1 lemon.	Apples, apricots, berries, cantaloupe, cherries, dates, figs, grapes, grapefruit, guava, lemon, mango, melons, orange, papaya, pear, persimmons, pineapple, plums, prunes, raisins, strawberries, watermelon.
Breads and cereals	Choose 6-11 servings daily. Count as a serving: 1 slice of bread; 1 oz ready-to-eat cereal; ½ to ¾ cup cooked cereal, cornmeal, grits, macaroni, noodles, rice, or spaghetti.	Breads, cooked cereals, ready-to-eat cereals, cornmeal, crackers, flour, grits, macaroni, spaghetti, noodles, rice, rolled oats, parboiled rice and wheat, quick breads, and other baked goods. (The most nutritious products are made from whole grain, or white flour that has been enriched or fortified.)

[1]One cup equals *240 ml*, 1 oz equals *28 g*, and 1 Tbsp equals *15 ml*.

TABLE G-3
A TYPICAL WEEKLY MENU PLAN FOR SENIOR CITIZENS[1]

Sunday	Monday	Tuesday	Wednesday	Thursday	Friday	Saturday
Breakfast						
Grapefruit sections. High-protein pancakes (part whole wheat). Honey or maple syrup.	Cooked prunes. Chicken livers. Whole wheat English muffins.	Tangerine. Scrambled eggs. Bran muffins.	Mixed fruits. French toast with maple syrup.	Applesauce. Cheese omelet. Cornbread.	Canned or stewed figs. Poached egg. Mincemeat coffee cake (part whole wheat).	Orange slices. Whole grain cereal w/milk. Cinnamon rolls (part whole wheat).
Lunch						
Barbecued pork chop. Baked Potato. Spinach. Ice cream—favorite flavor.	Chicken a la king on part whole wheat baking powder biscuit. Asparagus. Homemade chocolate pudding.	Glazed ham logs. Scalloped potatoes. Mixed vegetables. Coconut cream pie.	Meat loaf. Au gratin potatoes. Broccoli. Homemade butterscotch pudding with whipped cream or whipped evaporated milk.	Casserole of broccoli, ham, cream of chicken soup. Cinnamon roll. Pumpkin pie.	Macaroni and cheese. Brussels sprouts. Orange-grapefruit salad. Peanut butter cookies.	Lamb stew. Rice pilaf (brown rice). Cole slaw. Brownie pudding.
Supper						
Creamed dried beef on whole wheat toast. Waldorf salad. Chocolate chip cookies.	Cream of pea soup. Tuna sandwich (part or whole wheat bread). Relish plate. Crushed pineapple or mixed fruit.	Hard-cooked eggs, peas, and white sauce. Celery and peanut sliced salad. Gingerbread.	Salmon, tomato, green onion salad. Whole wheat roll. Baked custard.	Spinach salad w/hard-cooked eggs, bacon, croutons. Cheesecake.	Fish chowder. Carrot and raisin salad. Herb bread. Peach cobbler.	Meat loaf. Baked beans. Steamed brown bread. Apricots with custard sauce.
Evening Snack						
Cheese and whole grain crackers.	Oatmeal-raisin cookies. Milk or buttermilk.	Graham cracker. Milk or buttermilk.	Granola w/milk.	Cinnamon toast. Milk.	Yogurt w/fruit.	Hot chocolate or carob.

[1]Beverages are not included except in the evening snack, because of personal preferences. There are a wide variety of herbal teas, as well as the traditional tea and coffee from which to choose.

TABLE G-4
MODIFIED DIETS FOR SOME COMMON HEALTH PROBLEMS THAT AFFECT SENIOR CITIZENS[1]

Name and Purpose(s) of Diet	Indications for Use	Foods to Use	Foods to Avoid	Comments
Bland (to avoid irritation of inflamed or irritated tissues in the digestive tract by certain types of foods)	Colitis, diverticulitis, duodenal or gastric ulcer, esophagitis, gastritis, heart burn, and hiatus hernia.	Broiled meats, poultry, and fish; boiled eggs; milk drinks and mild cheeses; canned or cooked fruits and vegetables; breads and cereals made from refined flour or grains without hulls or seed-coats; butter, margarine, and mildly flavored mayonnaise and salad dressings; salt, and milk flavoring, herbs, and spices; weakly brewed coffee and tea, and herb tea.	Fried foods; highly seasoned items; aged or ripened cheeses; nuts; raw vegetables and fruits (except ripe bananas), and those with hulls, seeds, and skins; whole grain breads and cereals; and pungent spices.	A mineral and vitamin supplement may be needed if the diet is low in meats, poultry, fish, vegetables and fruits; and rich in refined breads and grains. Some types of soft drinks may be irritating. Some specialists are now recommending high-fiber diets for diverticulitis, with good results.
High calorie (to promote a gain in weight and an efficient utilization of dietary protein for the healing of tissues)	Underweight, malabsorptive disorders, and convalescence after injury, starvation, surgery, and the treatment of cancer.	Meats, poultry, and fish broiled in a little butter, margarine, or salad dressing; eggs in creamy sauces; nuts as snacks; rich milk drinks such as malted milk; cooked vegetables with sauces; stewed dried fruits with honey; breads and cereals with butter, creamy milk products, honey, jam, margarine, and peanut butter; and liberal amounts of ice cream and other wholesome desserts (after other foods have been eaten).	Items that are low in calories and high in bulk such as lean meats, low fat milks and cheeses, raw vegetables and fruits, and whole grain cereal.	It may be easier for some people to eat this diet if it is taken in three small meals plus 2 to 3 daily snacks. Too much fat may be counterproductive in that it may spoil the appetite, interfere with digestion, and be harmful to health.
High fiber (to stimulate more regular bowel movements and/or slow or reduce the absorption of dietary cholesterol, fats, and sugars)	Chronic constipation, gallstones, and high blood levels of cholesterol, triglycerides, and/or sugar (glucose).	Substitute beans and other legumes for some of the meats, poultry, fish, and eggs normally eaten; low-fat milk products and cheeses; raw vegetables and fruits; stewed dried fruits; and whole grain breads and cereal products.	High-fat meats, poultry, fish, egg, nut, and milk products; canned or overcooked vegetables and fruits; and breads or cereal products made from highly refined flours and/or grains.	The fiber content of the diet should be increased gradually to avoid causing diarrhea and irritation of the digestive tract. Fatty foods tend to slow the movements of the digestive tract.

Footnote at end of table

(Continued)

TABLE G-4 *(Continued)*

Name and Purpose(s) of Diet	Indications for Use	Foods to Use	Foods to Avoid	Comments
High protein (to increase the protein content of tissues that are subnormal in this respect)	Convalescence from injury, starvation, surgery, treatment of cancer, or other conditions that result in the wasting of lean body tissue.	Meats, poultry, fish, eggs, nuts, and legumes; milk products and cheeses; canned or cooked fruits and vegetables; and breads and cereal products fortified with eggs, milk, soy flour, and/or wheat germ.	Highly filling, low-protein foods such as fibrous and starchy vegetables, fruits that have a high water content, and bran cereals.	An adequate amount of calories must be consumed to ensure optimal utilization of dietary protein (carbohydrates are more effective than fats).
Lactose restricted (to minimize the amount of milk sugar [lactose] that is consumed)	Lactose intolerance, due to the malabsorption of the milk sugar lactose, caused by a decrease in, or absence of, the enzyme lactase.	Meats, poultry, fish, and egg products that contain *no* milk or cheese; vegetarian analogs of milk and cheese products; vegetables and fruits; and breads, cereals, desserts, and soups without milk.	Processed meats, poultry, and fish that contain milk products; except those that have been fermented; vegetables and fruits in cheese or cream sauces; breads and cereals with added milk; and snacks and desserts made with milk.	Small amounts of lactose taken with other foods may be tolerated by some people who cannot digest this sugar.
Low calorie (to reduce the dietary calories in order to bring about loss of body fat)	Adult-onset diabetes, high blood levels of cholesterol and/or triglycerides, high blood pressure, and obesity (excessive body fat content, *not* merely overweight).	Low-fat meat, poultry, fish, and egg products; milk, and cheese products made from skim milk; vegetables and fruits without high-calorie sauces and syrups; whole grain breads and cereal products containing only minimal amounts of fats and sugars.	Meat, poultry, fish, and egg products that are high in fat; full-fat milk and cheese products; vegetables and fruits with added fat-rich and/or sugar-rich sauces or syrups; breads and cereal products containing more than minimal amounts of fats and sugars; butter, margarine, oils, and other high-calorie dressings, sauces, and spreads; and desserts.	Bulky foods with high contents of water and fiber (legumes, vegetables, fruits, and cooked whole grains) may help to satisfy the appetite.
Low cholesterol and/or saturated fat (to reduce the accumulation of cholesterol and fat in the blood and in certain tissues)	Adult-onset diabetes, arteriosclerosis, atherosclerosis, high blood levels of cholesterol.	Low-fat meat, poultry, and fish products; egg whites; legumes; nuts; milk and cheese products made from skim milk; vegetables and fruits *without* cheese or cream sauces; whole grain breads and cereal products; margarine, mayonnaise, and salad dressings made with vegetable oils, but without egg yolks and animal fats.	High-fat meat, poultry, and fish products; egg yolks; legume dishes with meat fat; full-fat milks and cheeses; vegetables and fruits with cheese or cream sauces; breads and cereals with butter, high-fat milk products; or mayonnaise made with egg yolks; cakes and other desserts made from animal fats.	The benefits of these restrictions to older people are uncertain. However, some evidence suggests that the tendency to have strokes may be reduced somewhat. It may *not* be advisable to substitute polyunsaturated fats for saturated fats.
Low residue (to avoid a laxative effect and distention or irritation of the digestive tract)	Colitis, distention of the digestive tract (indicated by feelings of excessive fullness or by protrusion of the abdomen), acute stage of duodenal or gastric ulcer, lack of appetite, and after surgery of the digestive tract or treatment of cancer by drugs and/or radiation.	Broiled meats, poultry, and fish; boiled eggs; 2 cups (*240 ml*) or the equivalent of milk and mild flavored cheese products; canned or cooked vegetables and fruits without hulls, seeds, or skins; breads and cereal products made from refined flour and/or grains; and ground or very finely chopped herbs and spices.	Fried meats, poultry, fish, and eggs; all beans, legumes, peas, and nuts; milk and cheese products that contain vegetables or fruits; all raw vegetables and fruits except those with minimal fiber content; and breads and cereal products made from whole grains.	Small, frequent meals are tolerated much better than a few large meals.
Low sodium (to restrict the dietary sodium)	Accumulation of excessive fluid in the tissues (edema), congestive heart failure, high blood pressure, and certain kidney disorders.	Meats, poultry, fish, eggs, legumes, nuts, vegetables, fruits, and cereals prepared without salt; milk products; breads and other baked goods leavened with yeast; and seasonings that do not contain salt.	Salted meats, poultry, fish, eggs, legumes, nuts, cheeses; canned vegetables and fruits that contain added salt; baked goods made with baking powder; sauces and soups containing salt or monosodium glutamate (MSG); and desserts, dressings, seasonings, and snack foods that contain salt or MSG.	Various salt substitutes are available. However, a doctor should be consulted before any of them are used. Small amounts of salt in yeast breads and similar products may be acceptable in some cases.
Soft (to provide a diet that is easy to chew and swallow when these functions are weakened or diminished)	Convalescence after a severe illness, stroke, surgery, or treatment of cancer; and the patient finds it difficult to chew and swallow foods.	Tender meats, poultry, and fish that are baked, broiled, creamed, roasted, or stewed; all milk products and cheeses (except those with strong flavors, whole seeds, spices); canned or cooked vegetables and fruits without hulls, membranes, seeds, or skins; breads and baked goods made from refined flour, but without fruits, nuts or seeds; refined cereal products; condiments and seasonings containing finely ground ingredients; and desserts such as custards, dessert gels, and ice creams which do *not* contain coarse fruits or nuts.	Meats, poultry, and fish that are (1) fried, (2) rich in bones or other hard-to-digest connective tissue, and (3) salted or smoked; all legumes, nuts, and seeds other than creamy peanut butter or highly refined soy products; all raw vegetables and fruits except avocados, bananas, and lettuce; fried potatoes; bread stuffing, fried doughs, chow mein needles, wild rice, barley, and whole grain or bran cereals; and candied fruits, nut brittle; popcorn, relishes, and condiments that contain hulls, seeds, and skins.	Sometimes, soft diets are blenderized to make them easier to swallow; or, they may be made sufficiently liquid for tube feeding. Patients who require soft diets often lack sufficient digestive secretions to dilute the food that is consumed. Hence, ample fluids should be provided and excessive amounts of salts and sugars should be avoided because they may cause dehydration, diarrhea, nausea, and/or vomiting.

[1]Also see ELEMENTAL DIETS; HYPERALIMENTATION; LIQUID DIETS; TUBE FEEDING; and MODIFIED DIETS.

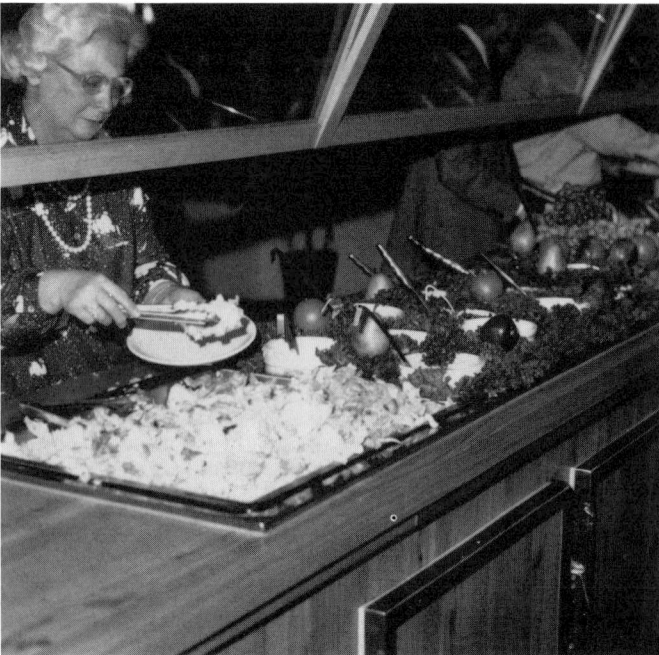

Fig. G-8. Well balanced meals, with something from each of the Six Food Groups, is just as important at age 70 as at age 7. (Courtesy of American Soybean Association, St. Louis, Mo.)

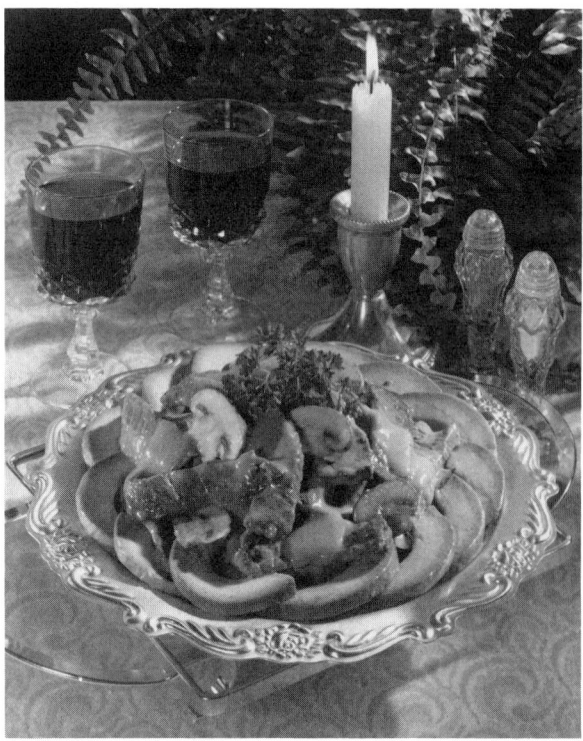

Fig. G-9. Simple but elegant meals can be accomplished easily during the senior citizen years when there is more time to prepare them and more time to savor them. (Courtesy, California Beef Council, Burlingame, Calif.)

GESTATION

The condition of carrying an unborn fetus. Pregnancy.

GHEE

A semifluid butter preparation from the milk of a buffalo, cow, sheep, or goat. It is nearly 100% milk fat and is used mostly in Asia and Africa.
(Also see MILK AND MILK PRODUCTS.)

GIGOT

This is a French word for leg of lamb. The term was also applied to the leg-of-mutton sleeves that were popular in the days of Queen Elizabeth I of England.

GINGER BEER

This is not really a beer but an old time soft drink like root beer. Various recipes exist for making ginger beer, but in general it is made with water, dried gingerroot, sugar, lemon juice, and active yeast. Brief fermentation by the yeast serves to carbonate the drink—to make it fizzy.

GINGIVITIS

Inflammation of the gums.

GINKGO (MAIDENHAIR TREE) *Ginkgo biloba*

Often this tree is described as a *living fossil*, because it so closely resembles its fossilized relatives. It was discovered in northern China, and it has now been transported to many areas of the world where it serves primarily as an ornamental. Ginkgoes are medium sized, deciduous trees growing up to 120 ft (36 m) high, shaped somewhat like a pine tree.

Ginkgo nuts or seeds are good to eat, tasting like mild Swiss cheese. They may be purchased canned in water or they may be gathered in the autumn from the trees; however, it requires special preparation to remove the offensive, fleshy layer. After boiling and removing the shells, ginkgo seeds can be added to a variety of dishes such as duck or chicken. In oriental cooking, ginkgo seeds and chestnuts are often used together. Ginkgo seeds may also be roasted like any other nut or seed.

Ginkgo seeds are listed in Food Composition Table F-21. Overall, they are lower in protein and have fewer calories than most nuts, but they do contain significant amounts of many minerals and vitamins.

GLAND

An organ that produces and secretes a chemical substance in the body.
(Also see DIGESTION AND ABSORPTION; and ENDO-CRINE GLANDS.)

GLIADIN

A protein classified as a prolamine, derived from the gluten of wheat, rye, and other grains. Gliadin and glutenin plus a liquid form the unique protein gluten.
(Also see GLUTEN; and PROTEIN[S].)

GLOBULINS

A type of protein which is abundant in nature. These proteins are slightly soluble in water, but solubility increases with the addition of salts. Globulins are rounded molecules; hence, their name reflects their structure. Upon heating, globulins coagulate. Familiar examples include serum globulins (gamma globulin), muscle globulins, and numerous plant globulins.
(Also see PROTEIN[S].)

GLOMERULONEPHRITIS (NEPHRITIS)

In the kidney the functional unit is called a nephron—a system of tubules and a filter or glomerulus. Each kidney contains about one million of these nephrons. Thus, glomerulonephritis is a diseased condition, an inflammation, of the glomeruli of these functional units. The disease is serious. Glomerulonephritis can be either acute or chronic. It affects mainly children and adolescents, and it often follows a streptococcal infection. Since the disease disrupts the glomeruli—the points where filtration of the blood occurs—signs include albumin (protein) and blood in the urine, edema (water in the tissues), high blood pressure, and sodium retention. When edema, high blood pressure, and reduced urine excretion are noted, the primary dietary adjustments indicated are restriction of water and sodium intake. Sufficient calories in the form of carbohydrates and fat should be supplied in order to prevent the breakdown of the body's own proteins for energy. Protein sources should be rich in essential amino acids—meat, eggs, and milk.

(Also see KIDNEY DISEASES.)

GLOSSITIS

An inflammation of the tongue.

GLUCOASCORBIC ACID ($C_7H_{10}O_7$)

A form of ascorbic acid (vitamin C; $C_7H_{10}O_7$) which has one minor chemical modification. It does not act like vitamin C. Rather, it is an antagonist to the vitamin and can be used experimentally to produce scurvy in animals.

(Also see VITAMIN C.)

GLUCOSE (DEXTROSE; GRAPE SUGAR; $C_6H_{12}O_6$)

Glucose is a monosaccharide—a carbohydrate—which serves as a chief source of fuel for the metabolic fire of life.

Every tissue in the body is capable of removing glucose from the blood and utilizing it for the production of energy needed for body processes. Some tissues rely on the action of insulin for removal of glucose from the blood, while the brain, a large consumer of glucose, does not. All other digestible carbohydrates are eventually converted to glucose for transport in the blood and for utilization by the cells of the body. In the blood, the normal glucose—blood sugar—level ranges between 60 and 100 mg/100 ml, while excess glucose is stored as glycogen in muscles and the liver.

Plants manufacture glucose from carbon dioxide (CO_2) and water (H_2O) by the process of photosynthesis. Some glucose is found free in sweet fruits such as grapes, berries, and oranges, and in some vegetables such as corn and carrots. However, much of the glucose manufactured by plants is converted to other carbohydrate forms. Cellulose and starch are long chains of glucose formed by plants. The disaccharides, sucrose and maltose, and even the nonplant disaccharide lactose, all contain glucose.

Commercially, glucose is employed in the manufacture of confections, in the wine industry, and in the canning industry. Since solutions of glucose rotate polarized light to the right, glucose is often called dextrose, especially in industry.

(Also see CARBOHYDRATE[S]; DEXTROSE; METABOLISM; and PHOTOSYNTHESIS.)

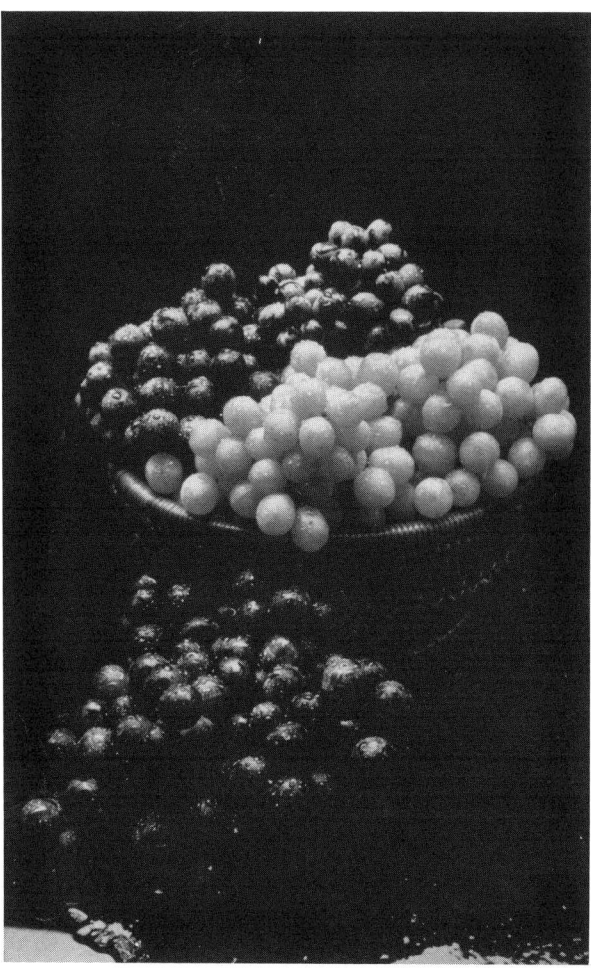

Fig. G-10. Some glucose is found free in sweet fruits such as grapes. (Courtesy, California Table Grape Commission, Fresno, Calif.)

GLUCOSE METABOLISM

Body processes, hence life itself, depends upon a constant supply of energy. Much of this needed energy is derived from the catabolism—controlled combustion—of the sugar, glucose. In the cells of the body, this occurs via a series of enzymatic reactions which permit the orderly transfer of energy from glucose ($C_6H_{12}O_6$) to energy rich compounds, primarily adenosine triphosphate (ATP) as glucose is burned to carbon dioxide (CO_2) and water (H_2O). Then ATP becomes the driving force for those body processes requiring energy. Glucose is transported to the cells by the blood. The source of glucose in the blood is ultimately the diet. All digestible carbohydrate is eventually converted to glucose. However, since (1) eating is an intermittent process, (2) not all glucose is immediately converted to energy, and (3) blood glucose can be rapidly depleted, mechanisms exist for maintaining the level of blood glucose within the narrow limits of about 80 to 100 mg/100 ml. This ensures a constant supply of glucose (energy) to the cells of the body.

Glucose may be converted to two storage forms of energy: (1) muscle and liver glycogen, and (2) fats. Also, the metabolism of glucose cannot be separated from the metabolism of fats and protein. Fats (glycerol) and protein (some amino acids) are potential sources of glucose, and glucose can be converted to glycerol, fatty acids, and certain amino acids. The liver plays a central role in maintaining blood glucose levels by converting (1) glycogen to glucose, (2) some amino acids to glucose, (3) glycerol from fat to glucose, and (4) lactic acid from the muscles to glucose. The brain, muscles, and other tissues consume glucose for the production of energy. Although the brain does not store energy, glucose is its major energy source. The overall direction that glucose metabolism takes depends on the needs of the body. Energy—maintaining the level of glucose in the blood—is a priority need.

Glucose metabolism is primarily directed by the hormones insulin, glucagon, epinephrine, and glucocorticoids. Entry of glucose into most of the cells requires the action of insulin. Glucagon and epinephrine mobilize glucose from liver glycogen. Glucocorticoids and glucagon promote the formation of glucose from protein and fats—gluconeogenesis.

Furthermore, adequate minerals and vitamins must be available for the proper metabolism of glucose. Minerals are cofactors with many of the enzymes involved, and with the B complex vitamins—thiamin, niacin, riboflavin, pantothenic acid, vitamin B-6, biotin, and folacin.

A well-known disorder of glucose metabolism—diabetes mellitus—is the fifth leading cause of death in the United States.

(Also see DIABETES MELLITUS; DIGESTION AND ABSORPTION; ENDOCRINE GLANDS; HYPOGLYCEMIA; METABOLISM, section headed "Carbohydrates"; MINERAL[S]; and VITAMIN[S].)

GLUCOSE OXIDASE

An enzyme produced by a number of fungi. It catalyzes the conversion of glucose plus oxygen to gluconic acid. The important feature of glucose oxidase is that it reacts with only glucose and no other hexoses—sugars. Glucose oxidase is commercially available; it is usually derived from *Aspergillus niger*. In the food industry, the most important application of glucose oxidase is for the removal of glucose from eggs before drying. This prevents the nonenzymatic browning reaction between glucose and proteins during storage, thereby stabilizing dried egg products. Glucose oxidase is also employed to remove oxygen from beverages, canned food products, dried or dehydrated foods, and mayonnaise. This minimizes flavor and color changes during storage.

GLUCOSE TM (GLUCOSE TRANSPORT MAXIMUM)

Glucose is an important substance which the body cannot afford to lose in the urine. Glucose TM is a measure of the ability of the kidneys to *salvage* glucose during the formation of urine. The letters *TM* stand for transport maximum. It is the maximum rate at which glucose can be transported from the filtrate formed in the kidney back into the blood. Healthy human kidneys can transport 320 mg of glucose per min. back into the blood. When this rate is exceeded, glucose *spills over* into the urine (glucosuria). In individuals suffering from diabetes mellitus, blood glucose levels may reach 300 mg/100 ml, thus exceeding the transport maximum, and resulting in glucosuria. Healthy individuals excrete little, if any, glucose in the urine.

(Also see DIABETES MELLITUS; and RENAL GLUCOSURIA.)

GLUCOSE TOLERANCE FACTOR (GTF)

The complete identity of this hormonelike agent is not yet known, although it is certain that it contains the element chromium and the vitamin niacin, and perhaps amino acids such as glycine, glutamic acid, and cysteine. Glucose tolerance factor is released into the blood—from perhaps the liver, kidneys or other tissues which store chromium—whenever there is a marked increase in the blood levels of sugar (glucose) and/or insulin. It, along with insulin, acts in making it easier for amino acids, fatty acids, and sugars to pass from the blood into the cells of the various tissues. It also promotes the metabolism of the nutrients within the cells. Much more insulin is required to accomplish these tasks when GTF is lacking; but GTF does not have any effect when insulin is absent.

(Also see CHROMIUM, section headed "•Component of the Glucose Tolerance Factor.")

GLUCOSURIA (or GLYCOSURIA)

The appearance of glucose (sugar) in the urine. Normally little if any glucose is present in the urine of healthy individuals. However, glucosuria may occur due to (1) a kidney defect; (2) a drug such as phlorhizin; (3) ingestion of a high-carbohydrate meal; (4) excessive stress; or (5) an infection. By far the most common cause of glucosuria is diabetes mellitus.

(Also see DIABETES MELLITUS; and RENAL GLUCOSURIA.)

GLUCURONIC ACID ($C_6H_{10}O_7$)

An acid derived from glucose. It occurs naturally in combination with a variety of chemicals in the urine. It is the body's way of detoxifying many substances, including (1) those normally found in the body, such as hormones, and (2) those introduced into the body, such as drugs and poisons. By combining these substances and glucuronic acid in the liver, they become water soluble and can be eliminated in the urine.

(Also see DISEASES, section headed "Detoxification of Poisonous Substances.")

GLUTAMATE, SODIUM (MONOSODIUM GLUTAMATE; MSG)

This chemical is better known as MSG or monosodium glutamate, the sodium salt of the amino acid glutamic acid (COOH [CH_2]$_2$CH[NH_2]COON$_2$). It is a widely used flavor enhancer, although it does not add any flavor of its own.

For centuries, Japanese cooks used a certain dried seaweed to flavor their soups and other foods. But it was not until the early part of the 20th century that they discovered that this seaweed contained MSG. In 1963, the FDA approved the use of MSG in foods. It is commercially produced (1) from the waste liquor of beet sugar refining, (2) from the hydrolysis of wheat or corn gluten, or (3) by organic synthesis. The worldwide consumption rate of MSG is now more than 150 million pounds (67.5 *million kg*) per year. It has, however, been associated with one minor disease—the Chinese Restaurant Syndrome.

(Also see ADDITIVES; and CHINESE RESTAURANT SYNDROME.)

GLUTAMIC ACID

One of the nonessential amino acids.
(Also see AMINO ACID[S].)

GLUTATHIONE

A tripeptide of cysteine, glutamic acid, and glycine, which can act as a hydrogen acceptor and hydrogen donor.

GLUTEN

A plant protein found mainly in wheat. Rye ranks as a poor second, followed by oats and barley. Corn and rice are low in gluten.

Gluten imparts the properties of elasticity and strength to flours. Actually, two proteins, gliadin and glutenin, form gluten when mixed with liquid. The elastic gluten, developed by kneading the dough, entraps the carbon dioxide, (1) formed during the fermentation of sugars and starches by yeast, (2) released by chemical leavening, or (3) beaten into the mixture. The result is the unique *rising* or expansion characteristics of wheat flour doughs.

Individuals suffering from celiac disease, sprue, or gluten allergy must avoid the numerous foods containing gluten, since it is often used as a food additive.

(Also see ALLERGIES, section headed "Wheat Allergy"; BREADS AND BAKING; CELIAC DISEASE; SPRUE; and WHEAT, section headed "Flour.")

GLUTEN-FREE DIET

Dietary sources of gluten—a protein abundantly present in wheat, rye, oats, and barley—must be eliminated from the diets of people who cannot tolerate it. This condition is characteristic of individuals suffering from celiac disease or sprue, and the condition which sometimes occurs after gastrointestinal surgery or severe diarrhea. Only products containing flours made from corn, rice, starchy vegetables like potatoes, or legumes such as soybeans and lima beans may be used. People who cannot tolerate gluten must use a minimum gluten diet for the rest of their lives.

(Also see ALLERGIES, section headed "Wheat Allergy"; CELIAC DISEASE; MODIFIED DIETS; and SPRUE.)

GLUTEN-FREE FOODS

Those foods manufactured without flour from wheat, rye, barley, or oats, as these flours contain the protein gluten. Due to the versatility of wheat flour and the protein gluten, they are found in a large number of food products. Therefore, a person selecting gluten-free foods should exercise care, read the label, and become familiar with the types of foods likely to contain wheat or gluten.

(Also see ALLERGIES, section headed "Wheat Allergy.")

GLYCERIDES

An ester of glycerol and fatty acids in which one or more of the hydroxyl groups of the glycerol have been replaced by acid radicals. Glycerides may contain one fatty acid (mono-), two fatty acids (di-), or three fatty acids (tri-).

(Also see FATS AND OTHER LIPIDS; and TRIGLYCERIDES.)

GLYCERIN (GLYCERINE)

The popular name for glycerol, an important biochemical and a common food additive.

(Also see GLYCEROL.)

GLYCEROL ($C_3H_5[OH]_3$)

An alcohol containing 3 carbons and 3 hydroxy (OH) groups. It is a colorless, odorless, syrupy, sweet liquid.

Glycerol is most commonly found in chemical combination with fats in compounds called triglycerides. Also, glycerol is a GRAS (generally recognized as safe) food additive employed to prevent drying, a humectant, as well as FDA approved for numerous other uses. Its popular name is glycerine.

(Also see FATS AND OTHER LIPIDS; and TRIGLYCERIDES.)

GLYCEROL-LACTO STEARATE (OLEATE OR PALMITATE)

A USDA approved food additive that is used as an agent to emulsify animal and vegetable fat.

(Also see EMULSIFYING AGENTS.)

GLYCINE

One of the nonessential amino acids.

(Also see AMINO ACID[S].)

GLYCOCHOLIC ACID ($C_{26}H_{43}NO_6$)

The sodium salt of this acid is a normal constituent of bile. Thus, it is a natural emulsifying agent aiding in the digestion of fats. It is a GRAS (generally recognized as safe) food additive employed as an emulsifier.

(Also see DIGESTION AND ABSORPTION; and FATS AND OTHER LIPIDS.)

GLYCOGEN

The storage form of glucose within the liver and muscle cells. It is sometimes referred to as *animal starch* since it is similar to starch—both are composed of numerous glucose units. In a normal adult, there are about 108 g of glycogen in the liver and 245 g of glycogen in all the muscles combined. The storage of glucose as glycogen and the release of glucose from glycogen are hormonally controlled.

Generally, there are no dietary sources of glycogen since it is rapidly converted to pyruvic and lactic acid in the meat and liver of slaughtered animals. Only some seafoods—oysters, mussels, scallops, and clams—which are eaten virtually alive, contain small amounts of glycogen.

(Also see CARBOHYDRATE[S]; and METABOLISM.)

GLYCOGENESIS

Conversion of glucose to glycogen.

(Also see CARBOHYDRATE[S]; and METABOLISM.)

GLYCOGENIC

Of or pertaining to the formation of glycogen, the storage form of carbohydrate in humans and animals.

GLYCOGENOLYSIS

Conversion of glycogen to glucose.

(Also see CARBOHYDRATE[S]; and METABOLISM.)

GLYCOLYSIS

Conversion of carbohydrate to lactate or pyruvate by a series of enzymatic reactions.

(Also see CARBOHYDRATE[S]; and METABOLISM.)

GLYCOPROTEIN

Proteins containing less than 4% carbohydrate. This classification includes such proteins as egg albumin, serum albumins, and certain serum globulins.

(Also see PROTEIN[S].)

GLYCOSIDES

A group of naturally occurring plant toxicants, or poisons. (Not all glycosides are toxic; e.g., several of the common nonphotosynthetic plant pigments.) Specifically, they are various sugars attached to another chemical compound and are designated as glucoside (glucose), mannoside (mannose), galactoside (galactose), etc. Toxic glycosides include cyanogenetic glycosides that yield hydrocyanic (prussic) acid upon hydrolysis, goitrogenic substances that cause acute goiter, irritant oils such as mustard oil, coumarin glycosides, and steroid (cardiac and saponic) glycosides. Symptoms produced by these toxicants range from stomach irritation to cancer, to death. Some common sources of glycosides are choke cherry, peach and apricot pits, and wild black cherries. Two glycosides are familiar to most people: digitalis (digoxin), the heart stimulant; and Laetrile (a brand name), the questionable cancer cure.

(Also see POISONOUS PLANTS.)

GLYCYRRHIZA (LICORICE)

A natural flavoring agent extracted from dried roots of *Glycyrrhiza glabra*. It is a GRAS (generally recognized as safe) food additive.

GOBLET CELLS

Secretory cells on the mucosal surface that produce mucus.

GOITER

Contents   Page

Enlargement of the thyroid gland (which is located in front of the larynx at the base of the neck), known as goiter, is usually the result of dietary deficiencies of iodine. In some cases, however, it may be caused by such things as goitrogenic agents, inflammatory disorders, or tumors. Another type of goiter, called exophthalmic goiter (Graves' disease), is due to overactivity of the thyroid gland, which is usually—but not always—enlarged.

HISTORY OF GOITER. An early Chinese document dated about 3000 B.C. described the symptoms of goiter and blamed the disorder on the poor quality of drinking water, mountainous terrain, or emotional disturbances. The recommended cure consisted of the ingestion of seaweed and burnt sponge, which contained large amounts of iodine. It is known that the Chinese even administered dried thyroid glands of deer as a treatment for goiter. Today, physicians use similar dried glandular extracts from cattle, sheep, or swine.

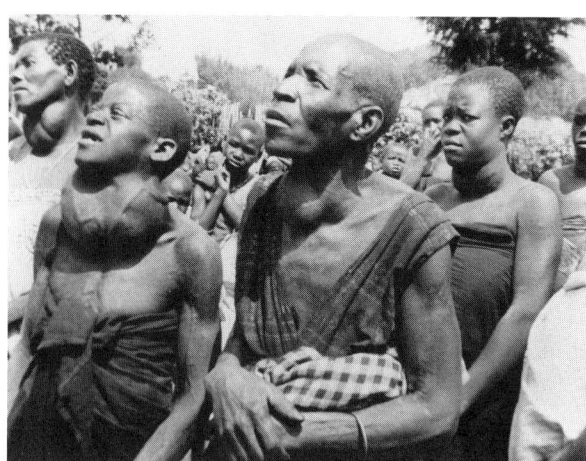

Fig. G-11. Goiter in East Africans. (Courtesy, FAO/UN, Rome, Italy)

The name thyroid (after the Greek word for shield, *thyreos*) was given in a description of the gland by the English physician Wharton in 1656, who determined its location, size, and weight. Although there was much discussion at the time concerning the possible function of the gland, such an understanding required knowledge of the role of the mineral element iodine.

In 1907, Marine, an American medical scientist, studied thyroid disease and iodine deficiency in farm animals and fish. Then, in 1916, he began to apply his findings to the prevention of goiter in humans. His administration of sodium iodide to school girls in the fifth to twelfth grades in Ohio demonstrated that such treatment effectively prevented goiter.

In 1914, Kendall, a scientist at the Mayo Clinic in Minnesota, crystallized thyroxin, one of the thyroid hormones. The chemical structure of thyroxin was described in 1927 by Harrington and Barger, British university scientists. Harrington synthesized thyroxin, thereby paving the way for a more effective therapeutic agent than thyroid extracts which were variable in biological potency.

Chesney and his coworkers at Johns Hopkins Hospital demonstrated, in 1928, that goiter could be produced in rabbits by the feeding of cabbage, which was later found to contain goitrogenic agents. It was also found that the metabolic rate of the animals was lowered. The disorder was corrected by feeding Lugol's solution of iodine, but many animals developed hyperthyroidism and died, a demonstration of the effects of overzealous therapy.

CAUSES OF GOITER AND RELATED DISORDERS. Although simple iodine deficiency goiter is the most common disorder of the thyroid gland, other factors may be responsible for abnormalities of this gland. Therefore, goiter and a group of related disorders are discussed in the sections that follow.

Simple Iodine Deficiency Goiter. The enlargement of the thyroid gland is usually the result of an attempt by the body to adjust to a deficient level of iodine in the diet. An iodine shortage slows the production of thyroid hormones since these hormones contain iodine. Reduced blood levels of thyroid hormones lead to increased secretion by the pituitary of a thyroid-stimulating hormone (TSH) which causes growth and metabolic activity in thyroid tissue. Secretion of TSH by the pituitary is believed to be under constant stimulation by the thyrotropin-releasing hormone (TRH) which flows directly to the pituitary from the hypothalamus. The flow of TRH is shut off when levels of thyroid hormones are adequate, but is operative when additional amounts of thyroid hormones are required, as in cold environments. Stimulation and enlargement of the thyroid results in a more efficient use of the limited supply of iodine for the synthesis of thyroid hormones.

Goiter is more likely to develop during puberty and pregnancy, when there are greater than normal needs for the thyroid hormones. Also, it is more common in females than in males.

It has also been shown in animal studies that joint deficiencies of iodine and vitamin A result in a significant enlargement of the thyroid which ultimately leads to disordered functions of the gland since vitamin A is required for the normal growth and metabolism of the columnar epithelial cells of the thyroid.

AREAS OF ENDEMIC GOITER. There are regions where many persons have goiter (the disorder is said to be endemic when over 20% of adolescent females in an area are affected), due to iodine deficiency in foods produced in the area, or as a result of the ingestion of foods and water which contain goitrogenic agents. Examples of such regions are the western mountains and the Great Lakes and Pacific Northwest regions of the United States; the Andes Mountains of South America; the Alpine areas of Europe; the Himalayas of Asia; and the plains areas in Africa, Asia, and South America.

(Also see IODINE.)

GOITROGENIC AGENTS. A variety of substances produce goiter when they are ingested in food or water. Some sources of these agents are: (1) members of the cabbage family—such as cabbage, turnip, rutabaga, and kale (cooking may inactivate the goitrogenic factor); (2) milk from cows that have eaten plants containing goitrogens; (3) dietary excess of calcium or fluorine (the effect is enhanced by joint excesses of these minerals); (4) raw soybeans; (5) thiocyanate-containing drugs used to treat high blood pressure; (6) arsenic (arsenical ores are used in Alpine regions as a seasoning instead of onions and garlic); and (7) increased levels of indigestible residue (crude fiber) in the diet (unabsorbable fiber may bind the thyroxin secreted in the bile and prevent its reabsorption in the intestine).

Iodine itself may be a goitrogen when it is ingested in large amounts. Excesses of iodine interfere with the synthesis of hormones by the thyroid and have been used clinically in the treatment of hyperthyroidism. Goiters are produced when iodine interference with thyroid function reduces hormone output to subnormal levels.

Toxic Goiter. Hyperthyroidism (excessive secretion of thyroid hormones) is characterized by a goiter which is similar in appearance to a nontoxic goiter, except that there are other accompanying features which help examiners to distinguish between the two conditions. Thyroid enlargement and hypersecretion of hormones, in thyrotoxicosis, is usually accompanied by rapid heartbeat, nervousness, weight loss, fatigue, increased sweating, and sensitivity to heat. The two major types of toxic goiter are (1) diffuse and (2) nodular; both disorders are more common in females than in males.

TOXIC DIFFUSE GOITER (EXOPHTHALMIC GOITER; GRAVES' DISEASE). Most victims of this disorder have protruding eyeballs (exophthalmos). Graves' disease is believed to be caused by a long-acting thyroid stimulator (LATS) produced by lymphocytes (white blood cells which carry antibodies against tissues).

TOXIC NODULAR GOITER. Growth of thyroid nodules sometimes occurs without TSH simulation. In some cases, there may be escape of thyroid hormone production from the control of the pituitary; then, the uncontrolled nodules are described as having become autonomous. This condition is more likely to be found in older persons who may have cardiovascular disorders as a consequence, but have none of the other characteristics of hyperthyroidism.

Cretinism. Congenital deficiency of thyroid function, or cretinism, is characterized by dwarfism, mental retardation, deaf-mutism, and occasionally goiter, which is not present if the defect results in a complete absence of the gland. This condition is found to be more prevalent in areas of endemic goiter and is believed to result from iodine and thyroid hormone deficiencies in the pregnant mother because the developing fetus is dependent during the first 3 months of embryonic life on the maternal supply of thyroid hormones. Cretinism is more common among populations where there are many close kinship marriages. (See Fig. G-12.)

Myxedema. Hypothyroidism (subnormal secretion of thyroid hormones), which is acquired anytime after birth, can develop into the severe clinical disorder of myxedema (named after the fluid accumulation apearing in the face and other areas of the body). Most cases of this disorder are found in females between ages 40 and 60. However, occasionly it is found in young children. Although there seems

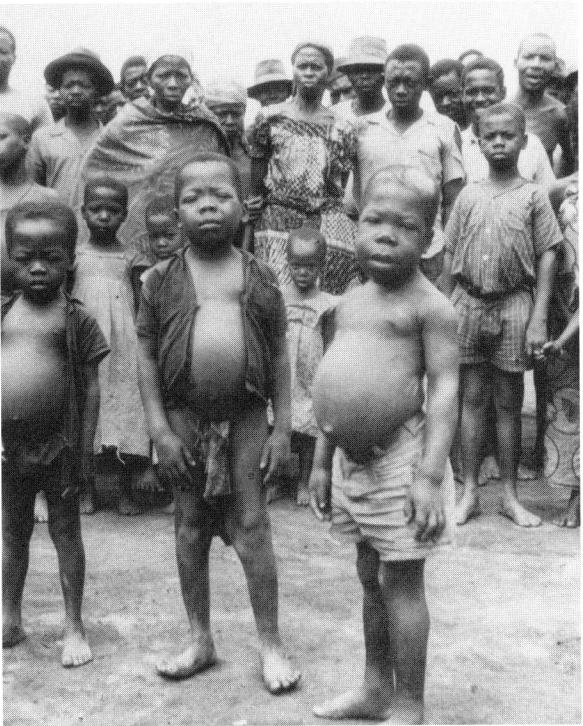

Fig. G-12. Cretins in central Africa. The three children in the foreground show the characteristic signs of lethargy, swollen cheeks (edema), and distended abdomens. (Courtesy, FAO, Rome, Italy.)

to be some evidence that myxedema might be the end result of chronic lymphocytic thyroiditis (Hashimoto's disease), the cause of the chronic condition is not known for certain. It may begin with a slight enlargement of the thyroid. Signs of myxedema are nonpitting edema, impaired mental function (not as severe as in cretinism), increased susceptibility to chills due to a reduction in the basal metabolic rate, overweight, elevated blood cholesterol, constipation, poor circulation of the blood, coarsening of the skin and hair, loss of hair, hoarseness of voice, lack of muscle tone, partial deafness, and enlargement of the heart in severe cases.

TREATMENT AND PREVENTION OF GOITER AND RELATED DISORDERS.
The longterm consequences of most of the chronic disorders of the thyroid gland may be disability or even death. Therefore, any sign of such a disorder should be investigated promptly, and treatment started as soon as the diagnosis is certain. Treatments for these disorders follow.

• **Simple iodine deficiency goiter**—This condition is first treated by the administration of thyroid hormone in doses large enough (0.1 to 0.3 mg of thyroxine per day) to block the secretion of thyroid-stimulating hormone. There may not be regression of the goiter if nodules have developed. After several weeks, the physician may conduct tests of thyroid function to make certain that the goiter does not contain autonomous nodules which could lead to hyperthyroidism. While therapeutic doses of potassium iodine (60 mg per day) may prevent further growth of a simple goiter, this agent is not as effective as thyroxine in obtaining regression of a thyroidal enlargement.

Prevention of goiter may sometimes be achieved in endemic areas of developing countries by the intramuscular injections of iodized oil once every 2 to 3 years. However, prevention of goiter is usually achieved in the developed countries by the use of iodized salt (3 g of which furnishes 228 mcg [micrograms] of iodine or slightly more than the *Recommended Dietary Allowance* [RDA] of 200 mcg per day for lactating women).[3] Most people use more than 3 g of salt per day.

Other dietary sources of iodine are seafoods, food products from animal sources (since all livestock receive iodine in their rations), fruits and vegetables grown on iodine-rich soils, and breads made from iodine-containing flours and/or iodates, which may be used as dough conditioners. However, extra iodine should be given with caution to persons living in iodine-poor environments since it has been frequently observed that persons in areas of endemic goiter are hypersusceptible to iodine and may even develop hyperthyroidism. This phenomenon is called the Jod-Basedow effect, after the man who first described the clinical signs of hyperthyroidism. Such an effect was recently observed in Tasmania where bread was fortified with 2 ppm of potassium iodate.[4] Iodate has been used as a dough conditioner in the commercial production of bread in the United States at levels as high as 12 ppm, resulting in 225 mcg of iodine per ounce of bread.[5] Some large commercial bakers, however, have discontinued the use of this additive.

• **Toxic goiter**—The most commonly used treatments for hyperthyroidism are antithyroid drugs which block the synthesis of thyroid hormones, surgical removal of part of the thyroid gland, and therapy with radioiodine which destroys the cells of the thyroid. It is sometimes necessary to balance these treatments with oral doses of thyroid hormones in order to prevent the effects of hypothyroidism. Administration of large excesses of iodine for the purpose of hormone synthesis is no longer used since the effect is only temporary.

• **Cretinism**—This condition requires lifelong provision of thyroid hormones, in the form of either the pure hormones or of extracts from the thyroid glands of animals such as cattle and sheep. Administration of iodine does not help since there is a lack of functioning tissue in the thyroid gland.

Early diagnosis and treatment of cretinism is important in order to minimize the amount of permanent disability and mental retardation. Some of the signs of the condition in newborn infants are: jaundice, feeding difficulties, respiratory problems, abdominal distention, edema, subnormal body temperature, delay in passing a stool (more than 20 hours after birth), lack of activity, birth weight over 9 lb (*4 kg*), and birth after more than 42 weeks of pregnancy.

• **Myxedema**—This condition, like cretinism, requires lifelong provision of the thyroid hormones which cannot be made in the body. However, the prognosis for the disorder is usually better than that for cretinism, since it occurs at a later age when there has already been some normal growth and development.

(Also see IODINE.)

GOITROGENS

Substances that tend to produce goiter are called goitrogens.

Members of the mustard family *Cruciferae*—including cabbage, turnips, rutabagas, and kale, which are wholesome and nutritious—contain small amounts of substances called goitrogens, which, when consumed in excessive amounts over long periods of time, may interfere with the utilization of iodine by the thyroid gland. As a result, people who eat very large amounts of these vegetables, while on an iodine-deficient diet, may develop an enlargement of the thyroid gland, called a goiter. However, normal consumption of members of the mustard family is in no way harmful. Nevertheless, added protection against this potentially harmful effect may be achieved by the consumption of ample amounts of iodine, which is abundantly present in iodized salt, ocean fish, seafoods, and edible seaweeds such as kelp.

(Also see GOITER.)

GOSSYPOL

The toxic yellow pigment contained in the glands of cottonseeds. Although there are no known cases of gossypol poisoning in humans, it is regarded as a potential toxicant based on animal experimentation. Also, it may cause discoloration of egg yolks during cold storage. Methods have been devised to extract the gossypol from cottonseeds. In the past, extraction was made at the expense of the amino acid content. However, new extraction techniques do not significantly lower the amino acid availability or the yield and quality of the oil. Also, glandless cottonseed, free of gossypol, is now available. As an inexpensive source of protein for humans, the future of cottonseed is bright.

(Also see COTTONSEED.)

[3]*Recommended Dietary Allowances,* 10th rev. ed., Food and Nutrition Board, NRC-National Academy of Science, 1989.

[4]Clements, F. W., et al., "Goiter Prophylaxis by Addition of Potassium Iodate to Bread. Experience in Tasmania," *Lancet,* Vol. 1, p. 489.

[5]Pintauro, N. D., *Food Additives to Extend Shelf Life,* Noyes Data Corporations, Park Ridge, N.J., 1974, p. 174.

GOURDS

• Sometimes the term *gourd* is used to refer to the entire gourd family. The gourd family or cucurbits (*Cucurbitaceae*) includes cucumbers, melons, squash, and pumpkins. Their fruits are usually large, fleshy, and have a thick rind. The plants are vines with broad leaves and trumpet shaped flowers.

• Gourds are also a large and varied group of plants with trailing or climbing vines producing primarily an ornamental fruit, though a few are edible. They are similar to pumpkins and squash. Gourds occur in a variety of odd shapes, sizes and colors. Besides being used for decoration, the hard shells (rinds) are used for making cups, bowls, dippers, and cooking containers. The interior of the dishrag gourd may actually be used as a dishcloth or bath sponge. In India, the bottle gourds are used as sounding boxes for some musical instruments. For decorative purposes, gourds harvested when mature, and then varnished, keep for long periods.

(Also see MELON[S]; PUMPKINS; SQUASHES; and VEGE-TABLE[S].)

GOVERNMENT FOOD PROGRAMS

The major government food programs are those operated by the U.S. Department of Agriculture (USDA) for the purposes of (1) improving the nutritional status of infants, children, and low-income families; and (2) helping to support the income of farmers by providing mechanisms for utilizing surplus foods. The number of participants and the costs of most of the programs have grown rapidly. Recently, many of our elected officials and taxpayers have raised questions as to whether the benefits received have merited the great expenditures. Therefore, the aspects of major programs are noteworthy.

HISTORY. During the early 1930s, the depression led to widespread unemployment and great reduction in the food purchasing power of people in American cities. These unfortunate conditions led to surpluses of food and sharp drops in the incomes of farmers. The paradox of hungry people living in a country which had plenty of food fostered the idea of having the government purchase the surplus food from the farmers and distribute it to the poor. Hence, in 1933 the USDA and the Federal Emergency Relief Administration began the distribution of surplus pork, dairy products, and wheat to needy families.

The early efforts to dispose of farm surpluses led to establishment of the commodity distribution, school lunch, school milk, low-cost milk, and food stamp programs of the 1930s. People employed by the Works Progress Administration (WPA) provided much of the labor for operation of the programs. Some of the programs were discontinued in 1943 because World War II eliminated most of the unemployment together with the surplus since both people and food were needed to sustain the war effort. Thereupon, the USDA started a cash reimbursement to pay schools for food that was purchased locally for the school lunch program. Shortly thereafter, the National School Lunch Act of 1946 was enacted to establish the program on a permanent basis.

After World War II, there was a period of economic expansion that was accompanied by a high birthrate and general prosperity. Nevertheless, there were moderate recessions in the 1950s and farm surpluses reached new highs. So, the USDA reinstated its commodity distribution programs along the lines of those operated just before the outbreak of the war. However, it became evident during the early 1960s that groups of people living in certain areas, such as those in the Appalachian Mountains and Indians on reservations, were receiving poor diets because they depended entirely on the commodities. Shortly thereafter, public interest in families living in *pockets of poverty* became widespread, and new programs were instituted. For example, pilot food stamp programs were started in selected areas in 1961 and the Food Stamp Act was passed in 1964. A little later, the Child Nutrition Act of 1966 established the school breakfast program and added new features to the school lunch program.

The new programs of the 1960s apparently fell short of their goals since the Citizens Board of Inquiry into Hunger and Malnutrition in the United States reported in its 1968 study, *Hunger U.S.A.*, that (1) one-fifth of U.S. households had *poor* diets according to the nationwide survey conducted by the USDA in 1965, (2) 36% of low-income households subsisted on *poor* diets, and (3) people in 266 U.S. counties were living in such distressed conditions that a Presidential declaration called the counties "hunger areas." This report was publicized on a nationwide CBS television program on hunger in America. The national concern which was aroused led to expansion of the food assistance programs during the 1970s. Also, the Special Supplemental Food Program for Women, Infants, and Children, which is commonly known as the WIC program, was started on a pilot basis in 1972 and was expanded in the years that followed.

By the late 1970s, there were widespread concerns that (1) the costs of the food assistance programs would become unmanageable, (2) persons who were not needy were allowed to receive benefits, and (3) a permanent and growing class of dependent people was being fostered. Some of these concerns were addressed in the Food and Agriculture Act of 1977, which contained provisions designed to correct abuses of the food stamp program. Changes in other programs were achieved mainly by the issuance of new regulations.

DETAILS OF THE MAJOR PROGRAMS. Pertinent details of the major federal food assistance programs follow:

• **Food Stamp Program (FSP)**—Stamps that may be used to purchase foods are issued without charge to participants who meet certain criteria of eligibility. The criteria are based upon the net income left after certain costs for shelter, child care, and maintaining or seeking employment are deducted from countable contributions to income. Also, the value of the stamps issued is based upon the amount by which the current cost of the USDA Thrifty Food Plan exceeds 30% of the net income. Physically and mentally fit applicants between the ages of 18 and 60 years must also meet the work registration requirements in order to receive the stamps. In 1990, the Food Stamp Program cost $14.1 billion.

(Also see FOOD STAMP PROGRAM.)

• **School Lunch Program, National (NSLP)**—The USDA assists elementary and secondary schools in providing nutritious lunches through grants-in-aid, donated commodities, nonfood assistance, and technical guidance. Depending upon family income, pupils are served full-price, reduced-price, or free lunches. Each lunch must contain (1) a serving of cooked lean meat, poultry, fish, or a suitable meat alternate; (2) two or more servings of vegetables and/or fruits, one of which may be a fruit or vegetable juice; (3) one or more servings of bread and/or bread alternates such as cereals or pasta products; and (4) a serving of milk (preference is to be given to the serving of unflavored nonfat milk, skim milk, or cultured buttermilk). In 1990, 24,589,000 persons participated in the National School Lunch Program, which cost $3.2 billion.

(Also see CHILDHOOD AND ADOLESCENT NUTRITION, section headed "School Lunch and Breakfast Programs"; and SCHOOL LUNCH PROGRAM.)

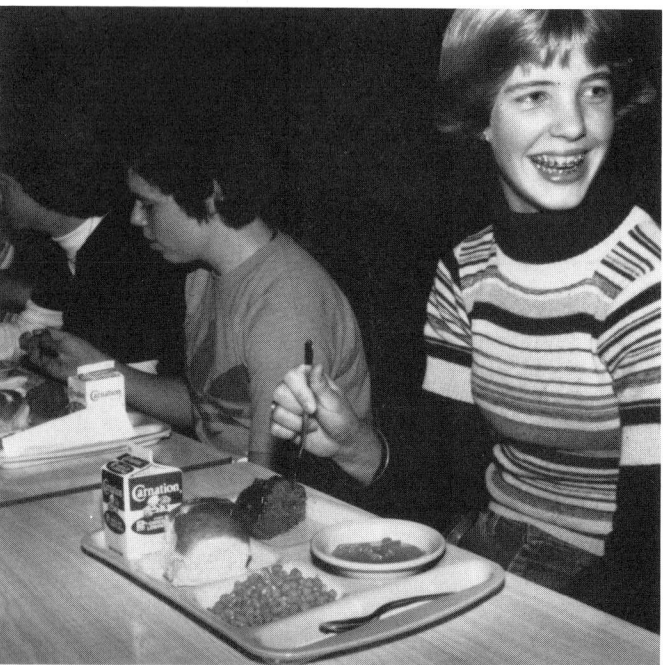

Fig. G-13. The School Lunch is one of the important government food programs. (Courtesy, American Soybean Association, St. Louis, Mo.)

• **School Breakfast Program (SBP)**—Schools that serve breakfasts which meet USDA guidelines may be reimbursed at fixed rates for each full-price, reduced-price, and free breakfast that is served. The criteria of pupil eligibility for the reduced-price or free breakfasts are the same as those for the corresponding types of school lunches. The guidelines require that each breakfast contain as a minimum the following food components in the amounts indicated: (1) ½ pint *(240 ml)* of fluid milk served as a beverage, on cereal, or used in part for each purpose; (2) ½ *(120 ml)* serving of fruit or vegetable or both, or full-strength fruit or vegetable juice; and (3) one slice of whole-grain or enriched bread, or an equivalent serving of cornbread, biscuits, rolls, muffins, etc., made of whole-grain or enriched meal or flour, or ¾ cup *(180 ml)* or 1 oz *(28 g)* (whichever is less) of whole-grain cereal or enriched or fortified cereal, or an equivalent quantity of any combination of these foods. It is further suggested that breakfasts served to children older than 1 year include as often as practicable meat or meat alternates such as a 1 oz serving of meat, poultry, or fish; or 1 oz of cheese; or 1 egg; or an equivalent quantity of any combination of any of these foods. In 1990, 4,235,000 persons participated in the School Breakfast Program, which cost

$596 million.

(Also see CHILDHOOD AND ADOLESCENT NUTRITION, section headed "School Lunch and Breakfast Programs.")

• **Milk Program, Special (SMP)**—This program was established to provide partial reimbursement for milk served at low cost to children in schools where no facilities for serving regular school lunches existed. At the present time, it also promotes the serving of milk in addition to that included in school breakfasts and lunches by providing full or partial reimbursement for the cost of the extra milk. Full reimbursement is given to schools and nonprofit child care institutions for free milk that is supplied to needy children. The type of milk served may be unflavored or flavored whole milk, lowfat milk, skim milk, or cultured buttermilk. In 1990, the Special Milk Program cost $19 million.

• **Special Supplemental Food Program for Women, Infants, and Children (WIC) Program**—Funds are provided to state health departments or comparable agencies for the purpose of supplying supplemental nutritious foods to low-income women, infants, and children who have been judged by health professionals to have special nutritional needs. Hence, the eligibility requirements were established by each of the states rather than by federal authority. Eligible participants receive supplemental food packages via (1) retail purchase with food vouchers, (2) home delivery, or (3) distribution by WIC clinics. In 1990, the WIC Program cost $2.1 billion.

• **Child Care Food Program (CCFP)**—Cash and commodity assistance is provided for meal service for needy and non-needy children in nonprofit day-care centers, as well as in family and group day-care centers. Meals may be provided to participating children free, at a reduced price, or at full price. The assistance covers one or more of the following types of meals: breakfast, lunch, supper, and supplemental food served between meals. However, the center shall not be reimbursed for supplemental food if it also participates in the special milk program. Supper components are the same as those for lunch. Supplemental food must include (1) a serving of fluid milk, full-strength fruit or vegetable juice, a fruit or vegetable, or any combination of these foods; and (2) a serving of whole-grain or enriched breads, cornbread, biscuits, rolls, muffins, etc., or an equivalent quantity of any combination of these foods. In 1990, the Child Care Food Program cost $788 million.

• **Summer Food Service Program for Children (SFSPC)**—All meals served to children by local sponsors of this program are free. Participation is limited to sponsors in areas where at least one-third of the children would qualify for free or reduced-price meals under the National School Lunch and School Breakfast Programs or to institutions providing meals as part of an organized program for children enrolled in camps. Most of the meals are served during the summer months, although some are also served during other approved times. In 1990, the Food Service Program for Children cost $162 million.

• **Commodity Supplemental Food Program (CSFP)**—This program provides surplus agricultural commodities to nutritionally vulnerable groups of needy people such as women, infants, children, and American Indians. However, the number of participants has dropped sharply in recent years as a result of (1) reduced availability of commodities, and (2) serving of the needy people by other federal food assistance programs such as the Food Stamp and WIC Programs.

• **Donation of Foods (commodities) to feeding programs**—This part of the commodity distribution program provides surplus agricultural commodities to schools which participate in the National School Lunch and School Breakfast Programs, child care institutions, nonprofit summer camps, eligible charitable institutions, state correctional institutions for minors, and nutrition programs for the elderly. The last item refers to projects conducted under Title VII

of The Older Americans Act to assist in meeting the nutritional and social needs of persons aged sixty or older.

COSTS. The numbers of participants and the costs for the USDA food assistance programs rose steadily from 1960 to 1989, as is shown in Table G-5.

It is noteworthy that the total cost of the USDA food assistance programs was over $21.7 billion in 1990, with the Food Stamp and National School Lunch Programs accounting for 65% and 15%, respectively, of the total expenditures.

TABLE G–5
NUMBERS OF PARTICIPANTS AND COSTS OF FEDERAL FOOD PROGRAMS[1]

Program	1960	1970	1980	1989
Food Stamp:				
Participants ...... (millons)	—	4.3	21.1	18.8
Federal cost ...... (millions of dollars)	—	550	8,721	11,682
National School Lunch:				
Children participating ...... (millions)	13.8	22.5	26.6	24.2
Federal cost[2] ...... (millions of dollars)	94	300	2,279	3,006
School Breakfast:				
Children participating ...... (millions)	—	0.5	3.6	3.8
Federal cost[2] ...... (millions of dollars)	—	11	288	512
Special Milk:				
Quantity reimbursed ...... (millions of ½ pt)	2,385	2,902	1,796	190
Federal cost ...... (millions of dollars)	81	101	145	19
Women-Infant-Children:[3]				
Participants ...... (millions)	—	0.1	2.0	4.4
Federal cost ...... (millions of dollars)	—	8	603	1,553
Child Care Food:				
Children participating ...... (millions)	—	0.1	0.7	1.4
Federal cost ...... (millions of dollars)	—	6	210	612
Summer Food Service for Children:				
Children participating ...... (millions)	—	0.2	1.9	1.7
Federal cost ...... (millions of dollars)	—	2	106	132
Needy Family Commodity:				
Participants ...... (millions)	3.9	3.8	0.1	0.1
Federal cost ...... (millions of dollars)	59	282	24	52
Donation of Foods:				
Child nutrition ...... (millions of dollars)	132	265	930	795
Charitable institutions ...... (millions of dollars)	16	23	71	136
Emergency feeding ...... (millions of dollars)	—	—	—	265

[1]Adapted by the authors from *Statistical Abstract of the United States 1980*, U.S. Dept. of Commerce, p. 133, Table 214; and *1991*, p. 370, Table 610.

[2]Excludes the cost of commodities donated to the schools, and State contributions to cost of meals.

[3]Covers only special supplemental food program and commodity supplemental food program.

GOVERNOR'S PLUM (RAMONTCHI)
Flacourtia indica

The fruit of a shrub (of the family *Flacourtiaceae*) that is native to the tropics of southern Asia. Governor's plums are purplish red or blackish berries that are about 1 in. (*2 to 3 cm*) in diameter. These fruits contain a red, juicy, seedy pulp that may be eaten fresh or made into jam or jelly. Governor's plums are moderately high in calories (94 kcal per 100 g) and carbohydrates (24%). They are a good source of fiber and potassium, and a poor source of vitamin C.

GRAHAM FLOUR

A whole wheat flour mix, named after Sylvester Graham, an advocate of dietary reform.
(Also see HEALTH FOODS.)

GRAINS

Seeds from cereal plants—members of the grass family, *Gramineae*.
(Also see CEREAL GRAINS.)

GRAM

• A metric unit of weight which equals 1000th of a kilogram or 0.035 oz. Four hundred fifty four grams equal 1 lb, and 1 oz equals about 28 g.

• The name used in the East Indies for any one of several leguminous plants, such as the chickpea and certain beans.

GRANADILLA, GIANT *Passiflora quadrangularis*

This species has the largest fruit of the more commonly known types of passion fruit (family *Passifloraceae*). They usually are from 8 to 12 in. (*20 to 30 cm*) long, and from 4 to 6 in. (*10 to 14 cm*) in diameter.

(Also see FRUIT[S], Table F-23, Fruits of the World—"Passion Fruit.")

GRAPE (RAISINS) *Vitis vinifera*

Grapes belong to the vine family, *Vitaceae*. They are the fruit of the woody vines of the genus *Vitis*. They are classified as berries and they grow in clusters of as few as 6 to as many as 300 berries. The color of grapes can be black, blue, golden, green, purple, red, or white, while the flavors range from fruity to spicy to muscat, depending upon the variety.

Grape vines climb by means of cylindrical-tapering tendrils and bear greenish flowers. Some plants bear perfect flowers, others bear only staminate flowers with rudimentary pistils.

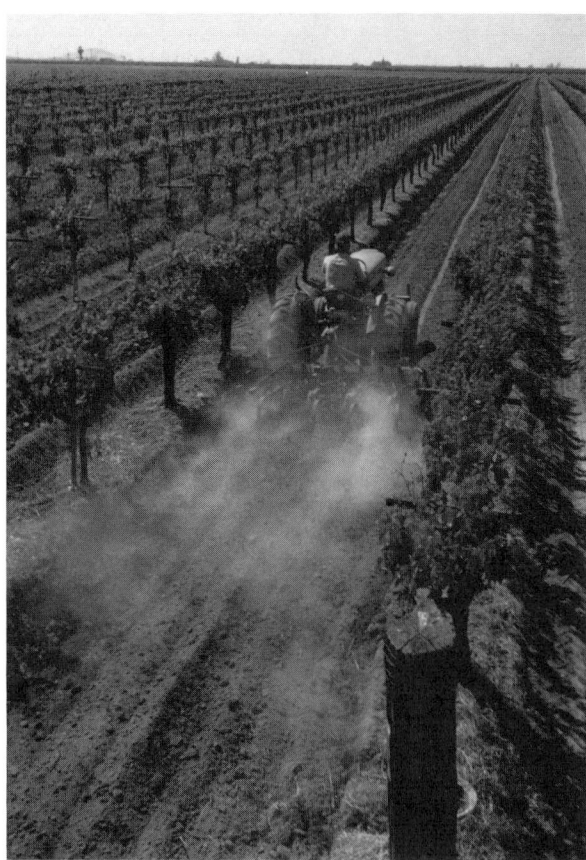

Fig. G-14. Grapes are the fruit of woody vines which are generally supported on trellises. (Courtesy, Table Grape Commission, Fresno, Calif.)

ORIGIN AND HISTORY. Grapes were domesticated in southwestern Asia well before 5,000 B.C. Grape culture then spread to other parts of Asia, thence to Greece and Sicily. Old World grapes were introduced into the New World soon after its discovery.

WORLD AND U.S. PRODUCTION. Grapes are the leading fruit crop of the world. Worldwide, about 60 million metric tons are produced annually; and the leading grape-producing countries are: Italy, France, Spain, United States, Turkey, and Argentina.[6]

In the United States, grapes are the number two crop, outranked only by oranges. About 5.7 million short tons of grapes are produced annually in the United States; and the leading states, by rank, are: California, Washington, New York, Pennsylvania, and Michigan. California produces over 91% of the nation's grapes.[7]

PROCESSING. Harvested grapes reach consumers through several routes: table grapes, canned grapes, juice, jam, jelly, raisins, and wines. In recent years, the U.S. crop has been processed as follows: wines, 48%; raisins, 31%; table grapes, 15%; juice, jam, and jelly, 5.7%; and canned, 0.7%.

• **Wines**—Varieties of the European grape are ideal for alcoholic fermentation. They contain 18 to 24% sugar with only 0.5 to 1.5% acidity. Worldwide, more than 85% of the grape crop is used for wine production.

(Also see WINE.)

• **Raisins**—Raisins are the sun-dried fruit of several varieties of grapes.

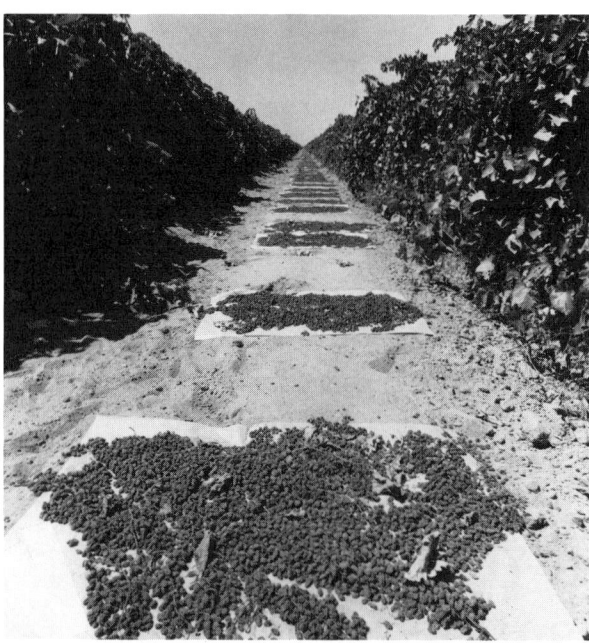

Fig. G-15. Drying grapes in the California sun. Clusters of Thompson Seedless grapes are spread on paper trays laid down between the rows of vines. Two to three weeks of drying reduces about 4½ lb (*2 kg*) of grapes to 1 lb (*0.45 kg*) of raisins. (Courtesy, California Raisin Advisory Board, Fresno, Calif.)

[6]Data from *FAO Production Yearbook 1990*, FAO/UN, Rome, Italy, Vol. 44, p. 153, Table 65. **Note well:** Annual production fluctuates as a result of weather and profitability of the crop.

[7]Data from *Agricultural Statistics 1991*, USDA, p. 197, Table 295. **Note well:** Annual production fluctuates as a result of weather and profitability of the crop.

Sundrying of grapes to produce raisins takes place in the vineyard between the rows of grapevines. Ripe clusters of grapes are picked by hand and placed on the ground on paper trays. Then, depending upon the weather, 2 to 4 weeks are required to dry the grapes to raisins. When the fruit is dry the paper trays are folded to form a package or *roll*. The rolls are collected and transported to a collection site and then further processed.

At the processing plant, the raisins are cleaned, sorted, and fumigated. After washing and inspection, raisins are packaged and shipped.

Most raisins are sun-dried, but golden seedless raisins are fresh Thompson seedless grapes which are picked, washed and then placed on trays and exposed to the fumes of burning sulfur in a closed chamber. Following this treatment, the grapes are dehydrated in forced draft heating chambers. Their finished color is green to golden yellow to amber, since the sulfur dioxide treatment prevents the oxidative darkening that occurs with the sundrying of fruit.

All U.S. raisins are produced in California, and the United States ranks as a leading producer of raisins, along with Turkey and Greece.

• **Table grapes**—Workers cut each cluster, and remove damaged berries. Then, the grapes are carefully packed in the fields, quickly cooled to 40°F *(4°C)*, and treated with sulfur dioxide gas to slow decay. These packed, cooled grapes are shipped via refrigerated railroad cars or trucks to markets. *Caution:* The sulfur dioxide residue on table grapes must be kept below 10 ppm.

• **Juice, jam, and jelly**—The Concord grape is a popular variety for these uses. Juice may be single strength cans, cartons, or bottles of grape juice or drink, or juice may be concentrated and sold as a frozen concentrate.

• **Canned grapes**—Almost all canned grapes are the Thompson Seedless or other seedless varieties. These grapes are mixed with peaches, pears, and pineapple as fruit cocktail or fruit salad.

SELECTION, PREPARATION, AND USES. Table grapes are ripe when shipped to market; grapes do not ripen after harvesting. When purchased, grapes should be well-colored, firmly attached to green, pliable stems, firm and wrinkle-free. Green grapes are sweetest and best flavored when they are yellow-green; red varieties when all the berries are predominantly red; and blue-black varieties when grapes have a full, rich color.

After purchase, fresh grapes should be stored in the refrigerator where they will stay fresh for several days. Just before serving, the clusters are washed under a gentle spray of water and then drained or patted dry. Table grapes are best served slightly chilled to enhance their crisp texture and refreshing flavor.

Since grapes are consumed in a number of forms, there are endless ways to prepare them. A few general suggestions relative to preparation and uses follow:

• **Raisins**—Raisins are excellent as a snack when eaten alone or they may be used in puddings, cakes, candies, cookies, and bread. Chocolate covered raisins are sold as candy. The sultana raisins are used primarily in bakeries. Corinthian raisins are employed mainly to flavor bakery goods.

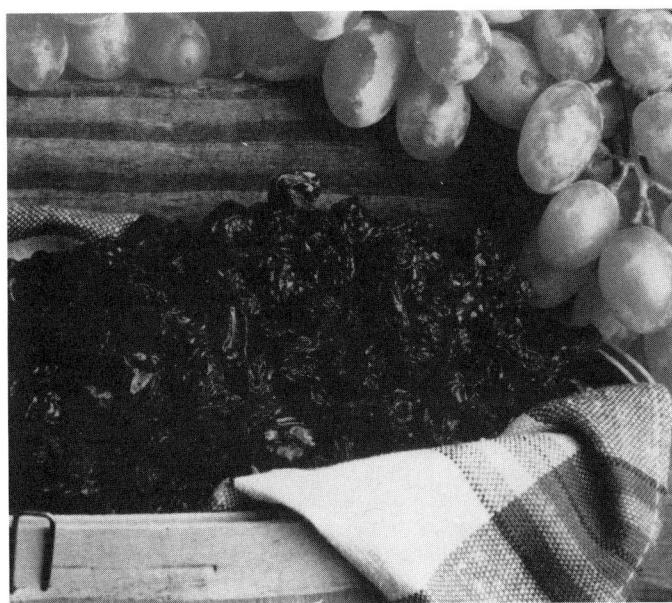

Fig. G-16. Raisins. (Courtesy, Ketchum Public Relations, San Francisco, Calif.)

• **Table grapes**—Aside from being a handy snack, table grapes also offer tantalizing color, flavor, and texture contrasts to all types of recipes. They can be enjoyed in a myriad of ways—in salads, pudding, pies, cakes, tarts, fruit cups, as meat accompaniments, condiments, and relishes, or just as is.

• **Canned grapes**—These are used chilled and directly from the can or they may be incorporated into fruit dishes, gelatin desserts, or baked goods.

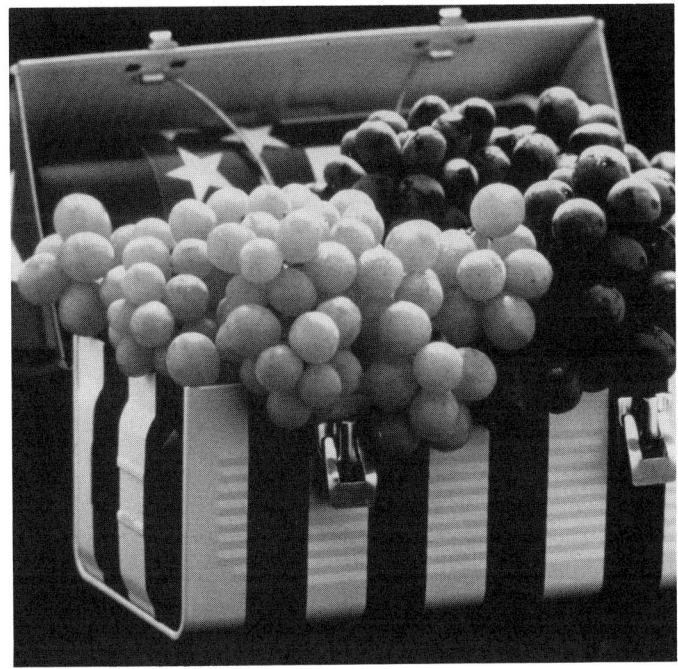

Fig. G-17. Fresh Table Grapes. (Courtesy, California Table Grape Commission, Fresno, Calif.)

NUTRITIONAL VALUE. Grapes are about 80% water, and they contain only about 70 Calories (kcal) per 100 g (about 3½ oz). The calories are derived primarily from the sugars which make grapes sweet. The sugar (carbohydrate) content of grapes averages 16%.

Raisins contain only 17% water; hence, many of the nutrients in grapes are more concentrated in raisins. Each 100 g of raisins contain a whopping 289 Calories (kcal), since the sugars (carbohydrate) comprise 77% of raisins. Additionally, raisins contain 2.1 mg of iron and 678 mg of potassium in each 100 g. Traditionally, raisins have been promoted as good sources of iron.

Food Composition Table F-21 provides more complete nutritional data on fresh grapes, canned grapes, and raisins.

GRAPEFRUIT *Citrus paradisi*

A large citrus fruit, popular as a breakfast or salad fruit. Grapefruit is misnamed, because it neither looks nor tastes like a grape. Like the other citrus fruits, it is a member of the rue family (*Rutaceae*).

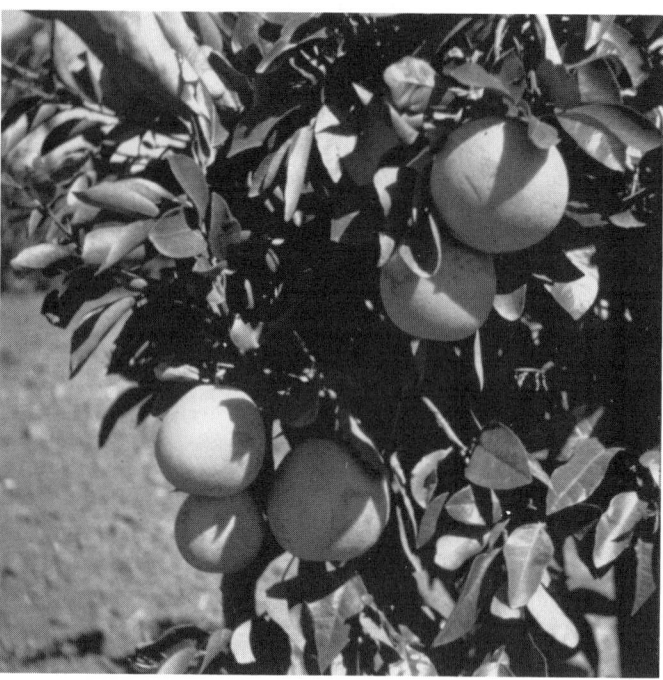

Fig. G-18. Grapefruit on tree. (Courtesy, USDA.)

ORIGIN AND HISTORY. The grapefruit originated in the West Indies, where it was first known about 1700. It is believed to be either a pomelo mutant or a hybrid resulting from crossing the pomelo with the sweet orange. The name grapefruit was first used in Jamaica in 1814.

WORLD AND U.S. PRODUCTION. The worldwide production of grapefruit totals about 4.3 million metric tons annually; and the leading grapefruit-producing countries, by rank, are: United States, Israel, Cuba, and China. The United States accounts for 41% of the world crop.[8]

Grapefruit ranks fourth among the fruit crops of the United States. The U.S. produces about 2.3 million short tons of grapefruit annually; and the leading states, by rank, are: Florida, California, and Arizona. Florida accounts for more than 72% of the U.S. grapefruit crop.[9]

PROCESSING. About 60% of the U.S. grapefruit crop is processed. Frozen grapefruit juice concentrate and grapefruit juice each account for about 42% of all processed grapefruit products. The remainder of processed products is made up of (1) chilled grapefruit juice in glass bottles, plastic bottles, and paperboard cartons; (2) canned grapefruit sections; and (3) chilled grapefruit sections in glass or plastic containers.

SELECTION. Fresh grapefruits of good quality are firm, but springy to the touch; not soft, wilted, or flabby. They are well-shaped, and heavy for their size. Fruits heavy for their size are usually thin-skinned and contain more juice than those that have a coarse skin or are puffy or spongy.

With a little practice, one can learn to prepare fresh grapefruit sections almost as rapidly as removing processed sections from a can or a jar. It pays to use fresh sections whenever feasible because (1) they usually cost less, and (2) the fresh fruit is likely to be richer in nutrients than the processed fruit.

Grapefruit uses are: appetizer, fruit dishes, fruit salads, and juices.

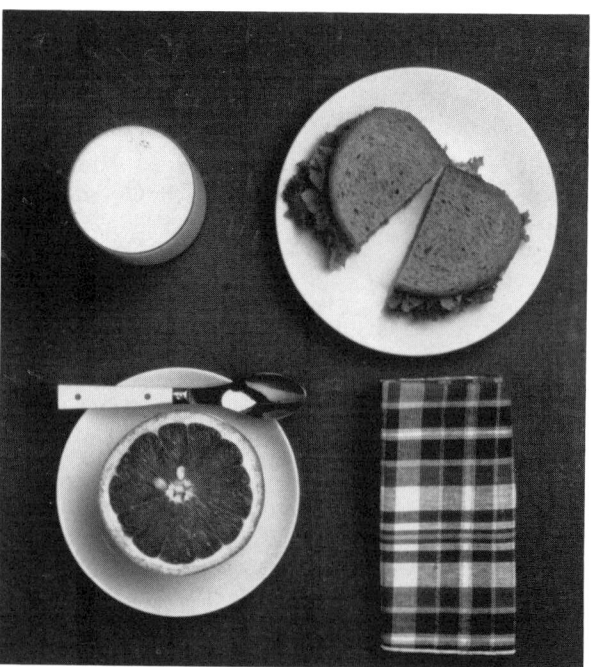

Fig. G-19. Half a grapefruit. (Courtesy, USDA.)

NUTRITIONAL VALUE. The nutrient compositions of various forms of grapefruit are given in Food Composition Table F-21.

---

[8]Data from *FAO Production Yearbook 1990*, FAO/UN, Rome, Italy, Vol. 44, p. 165, Table 72. **Note well:** Annual production fluctuates as a result of weather and profitability of the crop.

[9]Data from *Agricultural Statistics 1991*, USDA, p. 189, Table 278. **Note well:** Annual production fluctuates as a result of weather and profitability of the crop.

Some noteworthy observations regarding the nutrient composition of grapefruit follow:

1. Fresh grapefruit is low in calories (only 41 kcal per half of an average fruit), but it is a good source of fiber, pectin, potassium, vitamin C, inositol, and bioflavonoids (vitaminlike substances), a fair source of folic acid; and pink and red grapefruits contain moderate amounts of Vitamin A.

2. Frozen grapefruit juice concentrate is a rich source of the nutrients present in the fresh fruit.

3. Grapefruit drinks are low in all of the nutrients present in the fresh fruit, except for vitamin C, which is usually added during processing.

(Also see BIOFLAVONOIDS; and VITAMIN C.)

GRAPEFRUIT NARINGIN

The flavonoid naringin is the principal component of grapefruit which contributes to the bitter taste of the fruit.
(Also see BIOFLAVONOIDS.)

GRAPE JUICE

The fluid expressed from fully ripened grapes. Most of the grape juice produced in the United States is made from Concord and various other dark-colored varieties of grapes.

The nutrient compositions of various forms of grape juice are given in Food Composition Table F-21.

Some noteworthy observations regarding the nutrient composition of grape juice follow:

1. Bottled or canned grape juice is moderately high in calories (66 kcal per 100 g) and carbohydrates (17%).

2. The juice is an excellent source of chromium (a mineral that is part of the glucose tolerance factor, which acts along with insulin to promote the utilization of sugar), a good source of potassium, and a poor source of vitamin C—unless supplemental vitamin C has been added during processing.

(Also see CHROMIUM; and GRAPE[S].)

GRAPE SUGAR

Glucose occurs in a free form in grapes. Thus, in times past it was commonly called grape sugar.

GRAS (GENERALLY RECOGNIZED AS SAFE)

A designation of food additives that have been judged as safe by the Food and Drug Administration for human consumption by a panel of expert pharmacologists and toxicologists who consider available data, including experience of common use in food. The common use factor is often the major criterion on which judgment is based.

(Also see ADDITIVES.)

GREEN BEANS

(See BEAN, COMMON; and BEAN[S].)

GREEN REVOLUTION

This term refers to certain breakthroughs in wheat and rice farming which have the potential to double or triple the supplies of these grains for the developing countries of the world. Gaud, who was the Director of United States Aid for International Development (USAID), coined the term in a speech that he made in 1968. However, the father of the Green Revolution is considerd to be the American agricultural scientist *Norman Borlaug*, who was awarded the Nobel Peace Prize in 1970 for his breeding of new high-yielding varieties of wheat at the International Maize and Wheat

Improvement Center in Mexico. A related development was the similar production of special varieties of rice by scientists at the International Rice Research Institute (IRRI) in the Philippines. Dr. Borlaug's hybrid wheats were the results of crosses between varieties from the United States, Russia, Japan, and Mexico. This hybridization resulted in such favorable traits as (1) dwarfism, which prevents the plant from growing too tall and falling over (lodging) when extra water and fertilizer are applied; (2) an increase in the amount of grain per plant in response to increases in irrigation and fertilization; (3) resistance to diseases like rust; and (4) tolerance of a variety of climates and day lengths. (Certain strains of cereal crops require a fixed number of daylight hours in order to flower and set seed.)

The new varieties of wheat and rice are no panacea for the problems that the world now faces in feeding its people. Nevertheless, they have provided food for many who might otherwise have had none, and their success has encouraged similar efforts to improve other crops which are vital to mankind. Therefore, it is noteworthy that the Green Revolution did not occur as an isolated event, but that it is merely the latest victory in the never-ending struggle to obtain better yields from the major cereal crops.

(Also see WHEAT, section headed, "The Green Revolution.")

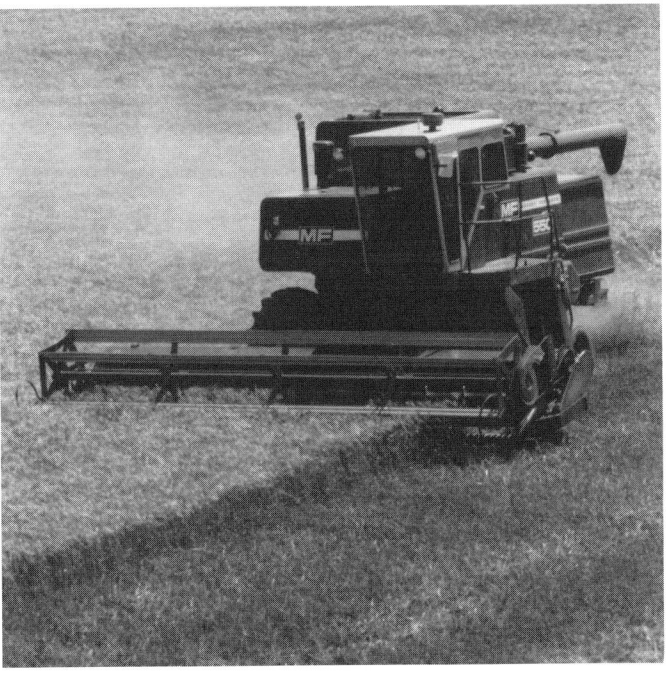

Fig. G-20. New high-yielding, *shorty* wheat, which along with improved varieties of maize and rice, spawned the Green Revolution. (Courtesy, Oklahoma State University, Stillwater, Okla.)

FUTURE IMPROVEMENT OF WORLD FOOD. Many agriculturalists believe that future increases in grain production will be less dramatic than those which have recently occurred under the Green Revolution. Hence, the provision of sufficient cereals for the peoples of the world will depend mainly upon reductions in human fertility rates in the developing countries, so that advances in agricultural production may be able to keep up with the demands for food. Also, our present varieties of grains are low in certain nutrients, so it will be necessary to (1) improve the nutritional qualities of the major cereal crops, and (2) produce sufficient amounts of the supplemental foods which supply the deficient nutrients in grains. Some approaches to these problems follow.

• **Breeding high-protein, high-lysine, and high-yielding cereals**—Agricultural scientists are currently attempting to breed varieties of cereals which have both high yields and high protein quality, since farmers are not utilizing fully the present types of high-lysine and high-protein grains because they have lower-than-average yields. The breakthrough that is most likely to occur in the near future is the development of a high-yielding, high-lysine corn because (1) corn may be crossbred much more readily than the other major grains, and (2) varieties which possess one or more of the desired traits are now under investigation by plant breeders.

• **Increasing the utilization of other important crops**— Although rice and wheat have long been the staple foods used by millions of people around the world, certain other crops such as potatoes, corn, and soybeans may yield more calories and/or protein per acre. Hence, the latter items should be more utilized. Fig. G-21 compares the yields of the five crops.

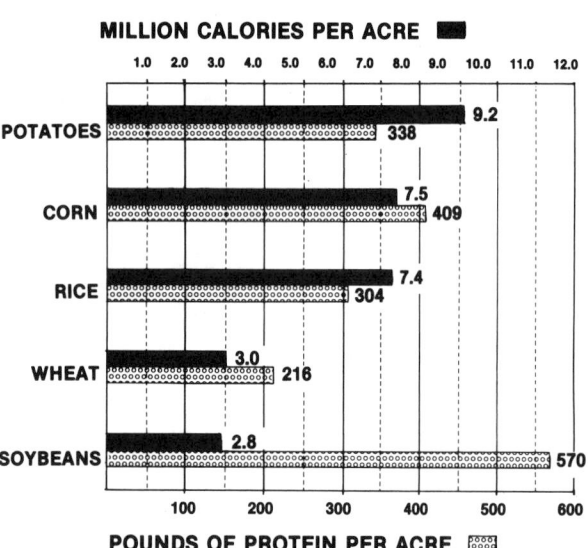

MILLION CALORIES PER ACRE ■

POTATOES — 9.2 — 338

CORN — 7.5 — 409

RICE — 7.4 — 304

WHEAT — 3.0 — 216

SOYBEANS — 2.8 — 570

POUNDS OF PROTEIN PER ACRE ▨

Fig. G-21. The yields of calories and protein from some leading food crops. (Values calculated from data in *A Hungry World: The Challenge to Agriculture,* University of California Food Task Force, pp. 37, 62, 206, Tables 2.12, 3.7, and 6.9)

It may be seen from Fig. G-21 that potatoes outstrip by far the caloric yields of the leading grains, whereas soybeans, corn, and potatoes each provide more protein per acre than either rice or wheat. Unfortunately, the merits of the potato are not appreciated fully by much of the world, as evidenced by the fact that most of this crop is grown in the region of Europe which extends from Ireland to the Soviet Union.

Corn appears to be more highly regarded than potatoes, since the peoples in most of Latin America and in parts of Africa use corn as their major food. Even countries like France and Italy have recently begun to use more of this grain. It is noteworthy that the American poultry, meat, and dairy industries owe their success in part to corn because

(1) the grain is the leading concentrate fed to swine, cattle and sheep in feedlots, and to dairy cattle; and (2) corn silage, which may be made from the leaves and stalks that might otherwise be wasted, is relished by and used extensively for both beef and dairy cattle.

Almost all of the efforts to increase man's supply of food have been directed towards improvement of the species which were domesticated thousands of years ago by primitive peoples. However, other lesser known plants might have even greater potential than the common crops used as staple foods around the world. For example, the native peoples of Latin America have long used the grainlike seeds of various species of *Amaranth* and *chenopodium,* each of which contain about 13% protein. Furthermore, it has been reported that cultivated strands of *Amaranth* yield a greater weight of seeds per acre than corn. At the present time the utilization of these plants is limited mainly to Latin America, although a few agriculturists in other parts of the world are studying their potential as alternative sources of food.

GRIND

To reduce to small segments or a powder by impact, shearing, or attrition (as in a mill).
(Also see CEREAL GRAINS; and FLOUR.)

GRISKIN

This is an English term for a pork chop, especially the lean part of it. It is also used when referring to lean bacon—better known in this part of the world as Canadian bacon.

GROUND BEEF (CHOPPED BEEF)

A product so labeled must be made with fresh and/or frozen beef, with or without seasoning, without the addition of fat as such, and shall contain no more than 30% fat.

GROUSE (CANADA SPRUCE GROUSE; PRAIRIE CHICKEN; AND RUFFED GROUSE)

This is an important game bird of the Northern Hemisphere. There are many species of grouse, all of which belong to the family, *Tetraonidae.* The ruffed grouse is genus *Bonasa,* species *B. umbellus.*

Grouse is a favorite with hunters of game birds, because its meat makes good eating. Young grouse is best roasted.

The prairie chicken (genus *Tympanuchus,* species *T. cupido*) is a member of the grouse family. It is an excellent game bird, esteemed for its delicate flesh.

GROWTH

The increase in size of bones, muscles, internal organs, and other parts of the body.

GRUEL

A food prepared by mixing ground ingredients with hot or cold water.

GUANINE

One of the nitrogenous bases in nucleic acids.

GUINEA CORN (SORGHUM)

The name given in West Africa to any of several grain sorghums, especially durra.
(Also see SORGHUM.)

GUINEA PIG

Domestic rodent of South American origin. Its flesh is edible, but in the United States it is used for laboratory experiments and as pets.

GUMS

As technically employed in industry, the term gum usually refers to polysaccharides (long chains of simple sugars) or their derivatives, which are dispersible in either hot or cold water to produce viscous mixtures. Gums also may include water-soluble derivatives of cellulose and modifications of other polysaccharides which in their natural form are insoluble. The original definition of gums applied only to the sticky gummy natural plant exudates.

Many of the plant gums originally used by man are still important today; for example, the dried exudates from trees and shrubs collected by hand in the hot, semiarid regions of the world. Also seed gums have been used for many centuries, and some ancient sources of gum include quince, psyllium, or flax seeds. Seaweeds provide another important source of gums.

Gums perform many food and nonfood functions. Since they are used in foods they are considered additives. In foods, gums serve as stabilizers and thickeners. They form viscous solutions which prevent aggregation of the small particles of the dispersed phase. In this way they aid in keeping solids dispersed in chocolate milk, air in whippping cream, and fats in salad dressing. Gum solutions also retard crystal growth in ice cream (ice crystals) and in confections (sugar crystals). Also, gums are employed to modify texture and increase moisture holding capacity; for example, as gelling agents in canned meats or fish, marshmallows, and jellied candies.

Table G-6 lists some of the common or potentially useful gums, their source and composition.

TABLE G-6
SOURCES OF GUMS AND THEIR COMPONENT CARBOHYDRATES

Gum	Source	Carbohydrates (sugars) Present[1]
Seaweeds		
Agar	Red algae (Gelidium group)	Galactose, 3,6-anhydro-L-galactose plus sulfate acid ester groups.
Algin	Brown algae (Macrocystis pyrifera)	Mannuronic acid, guluronic acid.
Carrageenan	Red algae (Chondrus crispus, Gigartina stellata)	Galactose, 3,6-anhydro-D-galactose plus sulfate acid ester groups.
Facoldan	Brown algae Fucus, and Laminaria groups)	Fucose plus sulfate acid ester groups.
Laminaran	Brown algae (Laminaria group)	Glucose and mannitol with branches.
Plant exudates		
Gum arabic	Acadia plants	Arabinose, galactose, rhamnose, glucuronic acid.
Ghatti	Anogeissus latifolia	Arabinose, xylose, galactose, mannose, glucuronic acid.
Karaya	Sterculia urens	Galactose, rhamnose, galacturonic acid.
Tragacanth	Astragalus plants	Galactose, xylose, glucuronic acid.
Plant extracts		
Pectin	Cell walls and intracellular spaces of all plants; commercial source, citrus waste.	Galacturonic acid, arabinose with galactose branches.
Larch gum	Western larch	Galactose, arabinose.
TI	Tubers of Cordyline terminalis	Fructose, glucose.
Plant seeds		
Corn-hull gum	Corn seed coat.	Xylose, arabinose, galactose, glucuronic acid.
Guar	Camposia teragonolobus endosperm.	Mannose, galactose with branches.
Locust bean	Carob tree (Ceratonia siliqua)	Mannose, galactose with branches.
Quince seed	Cydonia vulgaris	Arabinose, xylose, hexuronic acid, monomethyl hexuronic acid.
Psyllium seed	Plantago plants	Xylose, arabinose, galacturonic acid, rhamnose, galactose.
Flax seed	Linum usitatissimum	Galacturonic acid, xylose, rhamnose, arabinose, galactose, glucose.
Tamarine	Tamarindus indica	Glucose, galactose, xylose.
Wheat gum	Wheat	Xylose with arabinose branches.
Miscellaneous		
Cellulose derivates	Plant cell walls, wood pulp, and cotton.	Glucose
Starch and derivitives	Cereal grains and tubers.	Glucose with some branch points.
Dextran	Bacterial action on sucrose.	Glucose.
Xanthan	Bacterial action on glucose.	Glucose, mannose, glucuronic acid.
Chitin	Exoskeleton of insects.	Glucosamine

[1]The carbohydrates forming long chains which form gums are primarily sugars but some are carbohydrates or sugar derivatives such as guluronic acid, galacturonic acid, glucuronic acid and glucosamine.

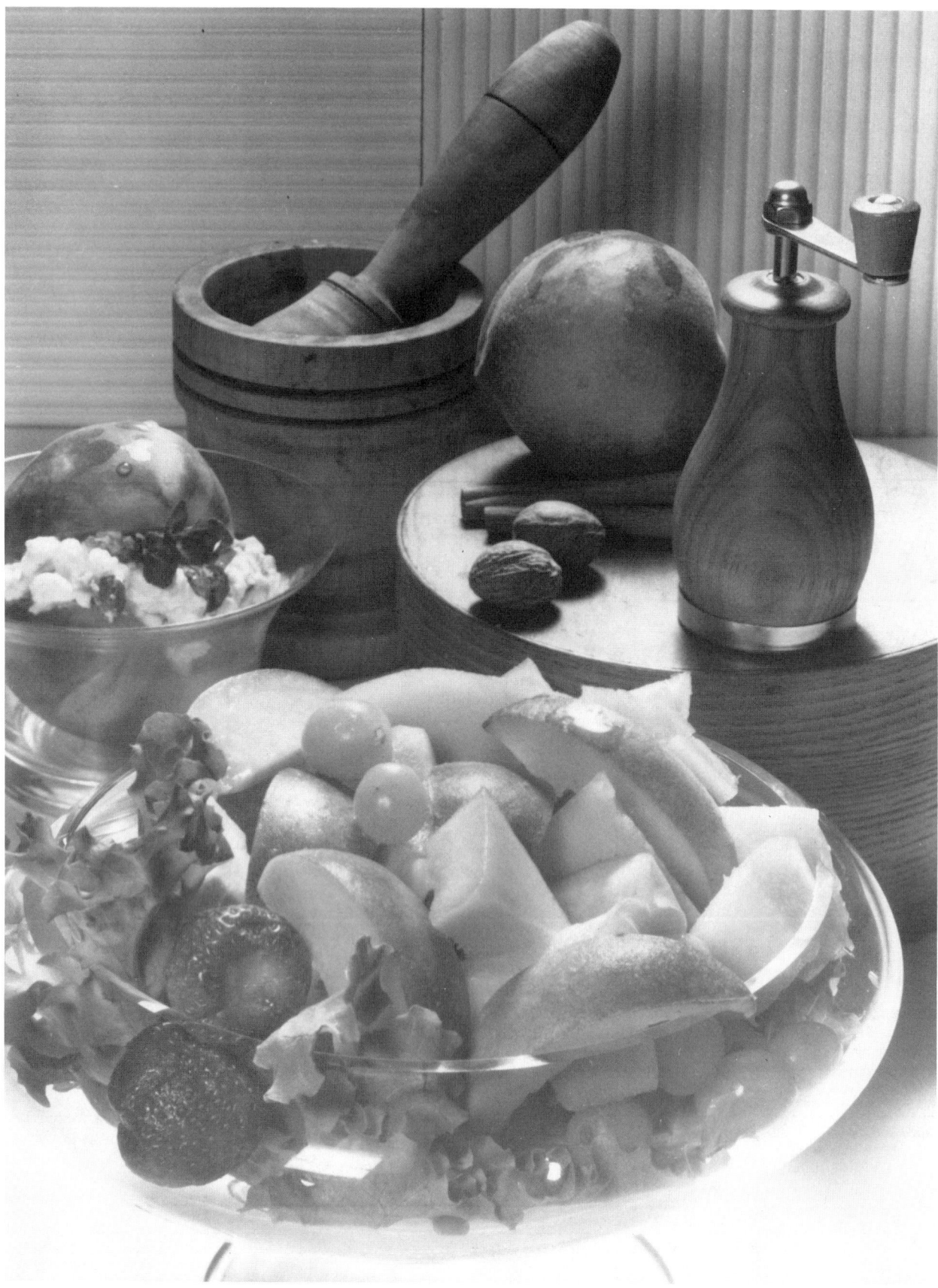

Fig. G-22. *Peaches 'N Spice 'N Everything Nice.* Fresh California peaches are delicious spiced up in a fruit compote and stuffed with cottage cheese. (Courtesy, The California Peach Commodity Committee, Sacramento, Calif.)

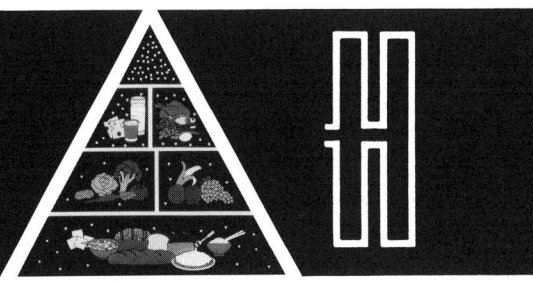

HACKBERRY (SUGARBERRY) *Cettia occidentalis*

Purple fruit of a small tree (of the family *Ulmaceae*) that is native to North America. It was much used as food by the American Indians.

HAFF DISEASE

This is a disease of humans characterized by the presence of hemoglobin in the urine (giving it a dark reddish color), muscular weakness, and pains in the limbs. Between World Wars I and II, it was rather prevalent among fishermen and their families around Haff in East Germany. Always on the day before an attack, fish (usually eel or burbot) had been eaten. The condition became known as Haff disease.

Haff disease appeared to be the human equivalent of Chastek paralysis, which affects mink and fox. Hence, it was concluded that it was caused by eating large quantities of inadequately cooked thiaminase-containing fish; with the enzyme thiaminase inactivating the thiamin molecule, resulting in a thiamin deficiency.

Some authorities now question that Haff disease is caused by thiaminase. Fortunately, whatever the cause, the malady is seldom reported nowadays.

HAGGIS

A favorite meat dish in Scotland, made of the heart, liver, and lungs of sheep or calves minced with suet, onions, oatmeal, and seasonings and boiled in the stomach of a sheep.

HAIR ANALYSIS

Minerals are deposited in hair as it grows; and, in theory, the hair reflects the mineral status of an individual at the time of hair growth. Scientific analytical methods, such as atomic absorption spectometry, neutron activation analysis, and x ray fluorescence spectometry, are sensitive enough to detect the levels of minerals in hair samples. Because hair samples are easily and painlessly obtainable, and because hair samples are stable and store easily, there is considerable interest in the use of hair as a diagnostic tool for mineral deficiencies and/or toxicities. However, like many other diagnostic tests, hair analysis is only a tool to complement other tests and observations. It is not a panacea. For the reasons which follow, an individual's nutritional status cannot be assessed solely on the basis of a hair analysis:

1. The relationship between the concentration of a mineral or of a vitamin in the hair and that in other body tissues is unknown.

2. Laboratory results depend upon the proper treatment of the hair sample. Hair samples must be washed properly to remove outside contamination from environmental sources, but washing leaches some of the deposited minerals out of the hair.

3. Sampling procedures vary. Mineral levels at the ends of hair may be different than that near the scalp, or mineral levels from hair at the nape of the neck may be different than that from the hair on the top of the head.

4. Factors other than diet influence the mineral content of hair. Such factors include sex, age, and hair color. For example, red hair contains more iron than other hair colors.

Clearly, some scientific findings demonstrate that if dietary intakes of certain minerals (chromium, copper, iron, manganese, and selenium) are extremely low, if the diet includes toxic minerals (arsenic, cadmium, lead, and mercury), hair analysis can detect these changes. Furthermore, some disorders such as anemia, hepatitis, hyperthyrosis and nephrocalcinosis are reported to change the mineral levels in the hair.

Hair analysis is a growing industry, and some laboratories encourage individuals to submit hair samples to assess their nutritional status by multiple mineral hair analysis. Some of these laboratories then prescribe minerals and vitamins to correct the "metabolic imbalances," or deficiencies, discovered by the analysis. Not surprisingly, some of these laboratories also sell minerals and vitamins.

In summary, while hair analysis has been used to detect certain types of heavy metal poisoning (e.g., lead, arsenic, mercury) in populations, its value on an individual basis remains to be established. There are a number of limitations to hair analysis both in terms of analytical procedures and in interpretation of results. For example, the relationship between hair concentration of a trace element or of a vitamin and the concentration of other body tissues is unknown. Basically, hair analysis is of limited value for assessing mineral status and questionable for assessing vitamin status.

(Also see DEFICIENCY DISEASES, Table D-2, Minor Dietary Deficiency Disorders; and MINERAL[S], section headed "Diagnosis of Mineral Deficiencies.")

HALF-LIFE

The time required to reduce a substance to one-half of its original amount, or to replace one-half of the original amount of a substance.

• **Physical**—In the field of radioactive isotopes, the half-life of radioactive carbon, carbon-14, is 5,568 years. In other words, if we start with 1 g of carbon-14, 5,568 years later only ½ g of carbon-14 will remain due to the radioactive decay. All radioactive isotopes have a specific half-life which may range from seconds to millions of years.

• **Biological**—In biology, chemicals in the body and tissues have half-lives. Follicle stimulating hormone has a half-life of 2 hours. That is, in 2 hours ½ of that secreted 2 hours earlier will have been eliminated from the circulation. One-half of the total protein in the body is replaced every 80 days. The radioactive element cesium-137 has a physical half-life of 28 years, while it has a biological half-life of about

140 days. That is, in 140 days, ½ of the initial cesium-137 will be excreted from the body.

(Also see RADIOACTIVE FALLOUT.)

HALIBUT LIVER OIL

Halibut liver oil is obtained from halibut livers. It is an excellent source of vitamins A and D and is frequently used as a primary material in making these vitamin products.

Although the livers of codfish are a good source of vitamins A and D, nature ordained that halibut livers be even richer for the following reason: Carotene is passed up through the food chain and concentrated as vitamin A in the livers of the higher level predators. Thus, codfish derive their vitamin A from the tiny vegetable plankton, upon which they feed, whereas halibut eat cod. It is noteworthy that at the top of the hierarchy is the polar bear, who eats the seal, who eats the halibut. Thus, the liver of the polar bear, which contains about 500,000 IU of vitamin A per gram, is toxic to man. A hungry explorer eating a 4-oz *(112 g)* serving of polar bear liver is in mortal danger, since he will have consumed 50,000,000 IU of vitamin A.

(Also see VITAMIN A.)

HALLUCINOGEN

A substance that induces hallucinations or false sensory perceptions.

HALVA

• A popular sweet in the lower Balkan area, made by crushing sesame seeds and mixing with honey or other syrup.

• In India, a halva is a pudding-like dessert that is always made from milk, but it is flavored with a variety of vegetables and fruits.

HAM

Cured and smoked hind leg of pork. Uncured hams should be labeled *fresh pork* or *pork ham*.

HAMBURGER

This is the best known and most popular American food. McDonald's, which features hamburgers, started with one fast-food restaurant at Des Plaines, Illinois, in 1955. Today, McDonald's competes with at least 15 other national chains, and the chains have more than 45,000 individual franchises. Different fast-food establishments feature different products, but the hamburger continues to be the mainstay of the industry.

The Code of Federal Regulation (CFR) defines *hamburger* as follows: chopped fresh or frozen beef, with or without added beef fat and/or seasonings. It shall not contain more than 30% fat, and it shall not contain added water, binders, or extenders. Beef cheek meat may be used up to 25% of the meat formulation. If hamburger contains extenders, it must be labeled as such.

(Also see CONVENIENCE AND FAST FOODS; FAST FOODS; and MEAT[S].)

HARD CIDER

Cider is usually the juice pressed out of apples. Before it is fermented, it may be referred to as sweet cider. However, after it is fermented and it contains alcohol, it is called hard cider. In some countries, the term cider alone refers to a fermented drink with an apple base. Fermenting cider is similar to the production of wine.

(Also see APPLE[S]; and WINE.)

HARDTACK (PILOT BREAD; SHIP'S BREAD)

A hard crackerlike bread which is similar to a soda cracker, but contains no salt. It was a staple on board the ships of old.

HARE

Wild rabbits with dark flesh, highly flavored and excellent for eating. The mountain hare is more delicate than the plains hare.

HASLET

• A piece of meat roasted on a spit.

• The edible viscera (as the heart, liver, or kidneys) of pork.

• A braised dish made of edible viscera.

HAWS (HAWTHORNE) *Crataegus* spp

The fruit of various species of hawthorne shrubs and trees (of the family *Rosaceae*) which grow wild throughout the New World and the Old World. *Haws* refers to the fruits, which resemble crab apples and are between ½ and 1 in. *(1 to 2.5 cm)* in diameter.

Haws are usually made into jams and jellies or brewed in herb tea.

A typical hawthorne fruit (in this case *C. pubescens* of Latin America) is moderately high in calories (89 kcal per 100 g) and carbohydrates (24%). It is a good source of fiber, iron, potassium, and vitamin C, and a fair source of vitamin A.

HAY DIET

The Hay Diet was first described by Dr. William Howard Hay in 1933 in his book, *Health Via Food*. Dr. Hay recommended that proteins and carbohydrates not be eaten at the same meal.

(Also see DIGESTION AND ABSORPTION.)

HEADCHEESE

A pork product made by skinning out a hog's head and removing the jaw bones, eyes, and ears; adding some hearts and tongues if desired; cooking the meat with the bones removed; grinding; adding enough broth to make a thick porridge; seasoning with salt, pepper, and marjoram to taste; and placing in crocks where the fat rises to the top. Usually, headcheese is eaten cold.

HEALTH

Contents	Page

Health is the state of complete physical, mental, and social well-being, and not merely the absence of disease or infir-

mity. The word *health* comes from the Old English *haeth,* meaning the condition or state of being hail—safe or sound.

The custom of drinking to the health of people is very old, probably derived from the ancient religious rite of drinking to the gods. Later, the Greeks drank to one another, and the Romans adopted the custom. By the beginning of the 17th century, health drinking had become a very ceremonious business in England; toasts were often drunk solemnly on bended knees. A Scots custom, still surviving, is to drink a toast with one foot on the table and the other on the chair. The French manner, when a health is drunk, is to bow to him that drank to you.

In 1992, the World Health Organization (WHO), the headquarters of which are located in Geneva, Switzerland, reported that at least 40% of the estimated 50 million annual deaths worldwide could be prevented by "improved health systems, drugs, and vaccines, and a healthier life-style and education."

SIGNS OF GOOD HEALTH. In order to know when disease strikes, people must first know the signs of good health, any departure from which constitutes a warning of trouble. Some of the signs of good health are:

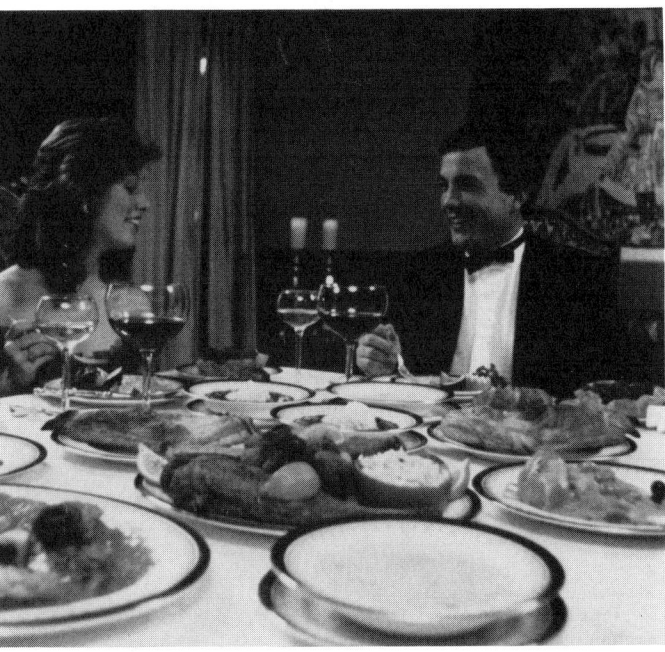

Fig. H-1. Signs of good health. (Courtesy, Mississippi Cooperative Extension Service, USDA)

1. **Seldom sick.** Healthy people are not susceptible to *every infection that comes along;* and they possess endurance and vigor.

2. **Good natured and full of life.** Healthy people are happy, contented, and full of *vim and vinegar.*

3. **Normal temperature, pulse rate, and breathing rate.** For the average person, this means: mouth temperature, 98.6°F *(37°C),* and rectal about 1 degree higher; pulse, 72 times a minute; breathing varies with age: in the baby it is about 45 times a minute; by age 6, it is down to about 25; between ages 15 and 25, it drops to about 18; and with advanced age, there is a tendency for it to increase.

Every family should have a thermometer, either oral or rectal type.

To take the pulse, place a finger on the radial artery at the wrist. The pulse is caused by the impact of the pressure of blood on the arteries as the heart beats.

Breathing rate can be determined by counting either the inhaling or exhaling of air.

4. **Average height for age, and average weight for height.** The body should not be undersized or poorly developed; and it should not be too thin (more than 10% underweight) or too fat and flabby (more than 10% overweight).

5. **Alertness.** Healthy people are alert; they are heads up.

6. **Good appetite.** In healthy people, the appetite is good and the food is eaten with relish; they're hungry when it's time to eat.

7. **Normal feces and urine.** The feces should be firm, and neither hard nor soft. The urine should be clear. Both the feces and urine should be passed without effort, and should be free from blood, mucus, or pus.

8. **Bright eyes and pink eye membranes.** In healthy people, the eyes are bright and clear; and the membranes—which can be seen when the lower lid is pulled down—are whitish pink in color and moist.

9. **Reddish pink tongue.** The tongue is reddish pink in color and not coated.

10. **Healthy gums and membranes of the mouth.** The gums should be firm, and the mucous membranes of the mouth should be reddish pink.

11. **Skin.** The skin is smooth, pliable, and elastic, and of a healthy color.

12. **Smooth, glossy hair.** The hair is lustrous (it has a gloss or shine) and firmly attached to the scalp (not easily pulled out).

13. **Firm, pink nails.** The nails are firm and pink, and not brittle or rigid.

SIGNS OF ILL HEALTH. Most sicknesses are ushered in by one or more departures from the signs of good health—by indicators that tell us that all is not well. If these signs exist and persist, you should see your doctor as soon as possible. Here are the most common signs of ill health:

1. **Loss of appetite; digestive disturbances.** Lack of appetite, nausea, indigestion, abdominal pain or cramps.

2. **Listless.** A tired run-down feeling—lack of energy.

3. **Abnormal feces.** Constipation, diarrhea, or passing blood.

4. **Abnormal urination or urine.** Difficulty in starting, stopping, dribbling, pain, or passing blood.

5. **Abnormal discharge from the nose, mouth, or eyes.** Pus or excess watering give reason for concern.

6. **Persistent cough or hoarseness.** When a cough or hoarseness lingers longer than normal, you should see a doctor.

7. **Lack of color of skin.** Paleness.

8. **Pale, dark red, or purple mucous membranes lining the eyes and gums.** Such signs give cause for concern.

9. **Sores on the skin, lips, or tongue.** If such sores fail to heal, there is reason for concern.

10. **Dull hair.** Lacking sheen; dry; and can be easily plucked.

11. **Nails.** Rigid, and brittle.

12. **Shortness of breath, or labored breathing.** This refers to shortness of breath when performing normal activities, and to labored breathing characterized by increased rate and depth.

13. **Chest pains.** Such pains may presage a heart attack.

14. **Persistent headaches.** The cause should be determined by your doctor.

15. **Prolonged aches in back, limbs, or joints.** See your doctor.

16. **Hard of hearing.** If hearing is worsening, see a specialist.

17. **Failing eyesight.** Dimming or fogging of vision should be checked by a specialist.

18. **Swelling of feet or ankles.** This may be serious. See your doctor.

19. **Sleeplessness.** Tendency to wake up during the night and difficulty in falling asleep again.

20. **Nervous, irritable, and depressed.** Such outward signs as crying spells, overwhelming sadness, worthlessness, and mental apathy may presage a nervous breakdown.

21. **Above normal body temperature.** If the temperature is more than 2° above normal.

22. **Sudden drop in weight or work.** Sudden loss of weight or work productivity should be checked.

23. **Malnutrition.** Malnutrition may result from a deficiency, excess, or imbalance of nutrients. This may include (a) undernutrition, which refers to a deficiency of calories and/or one or more essential nutrients; or (b) overnutrition, which is an excess of one or more nutrients and usually of calories.

24. **Noncontagious diseases.** Such noncontagious diseases as allergies, anemia, arthritis, diabetes, diverticulosis, and heart disease are signs of ill health, all of which may be influenced by diet.

Special for women:
25. **Vaginal bleeding at unexpected times.**
26. **Lump on breast.** This may be cancerous.

RULES OF GOOD HEALTH. It is within easy reach of every individual to attain a good state of health and to retain it to a ripe old age by following the rules of good health. It is established and accepted medical opinion that good health does not imply merely the absence of disease, but presumes a state of physical, mental, and social well-being. Observance of the following rules will make for good health.

1. **Eat an adequate and balanced diet.** Proper food provides energy, builds new tissue, repairs worn out tissue, and keeps the body working well. A balanced diet contains adequate proportions of carbohydrates, fats, and proteins, along with the recommended daily allowances of the essential minerals and vitamins.

2. **Exercise regularly.** Exercise builds muscles, helps the blood circulate, enhances appetite, and helps the body use food properly.

3. **Relax regularly.** Relaxation makes a person feel happier and more comfortable, prevents tenseness and nervousness, and enhances both work and play.

4. **Get enough sleep.** Sleep lets the body rid itself of poisons, repair worn tissue, and grow properly.

5. **Get plenty of fresh air.** People must breathe air to live. Fresh air is desired because it is rich in oxygen (O_2) and low in carbon dioxide (CO_2).

6. **Take care of teeth.** Teeth cut, tear, and grind food to make it ready for digestion; hence, they are important for good health. Also, germs from decaying teeth may spread disease throughout the body. Eating a balanced diet and brushing the teeth after eating help prevent tooth decay, or cavities.

7. **Visit your doctor and dentist regularly.** Doctors and dentists guard your health. Many diseases develop slowly and do not cause pain in early stages. Often, doctors and dentists can find hidden signs of illness, and can take steps to correct disorders that may cause trouble. So, have your doctor and your dentist examine you at least once a year.

8. **Personal hygiene.** Personal cleanliness—the care of your body, including cleanliness of the skin, the body cavities, and the eliminative organs—improves appearance and helps keep a person well.

9. **Sanitize your immediate environment.** Keep your immediate environment sanitary, including your home and place of employment—be it office, farm, factory, or coal mine.

10. **Dress comfortably.** Loose, light clothing lets a person move freely, and allows air to reach the body.

11. **Keep good posture.** Posture refers to the carriage of the body in walking, standing, or sitting. Women in some cultures maintain an erect posture by carrying a basket or pot on the head; and in the western world, fashion models are taught to do so by walking with a book on the head.

In standing, the ideal posture is erect with the abdomen and chin drawn in and the shoulders square and high. In sitting, the body is erect and the head is poised in a line with the hip bones.

12. **Work and play safely.** Many accidents can be prevented by following safety rules and avoiding hazardous situations.

13. **Enjoy your work.** Fortunate is the person for whom work is fun and fun is work. (I have never felt that I worked a day in my life. M.E.E.) Pleasure is important for mental and social health.

14. **Be at peace with the world and all humanity.** Think positive, healthful thoughts; it can help make life more pleasant and healthful. Religion and philosophy help develop peace of mind.

15. **Practice restraint in taking drugs, medicines, and alcoholic beverages.** Take drugs and medications on your own only for the most minor conditions, and seek medical advice if there is no improvement within a day or two. Those who drink an alcoholic beverage should imbibe intelligently and in moderation.

16. **Follow the golden rule.** Find ways to help others, and think less about yourself. Cultivate wholehearted consideration of and genuine affection for your family, friends, and your fellowmen.

17. **Never grow old.** Keep on keeping on.

HEALTH FOODS

Contents	Page

These are foods which are purported to improve health. The term "health food" encompasses both "natural" and "organic" foods, along with certain other foods. The two senior authors of this book patronize health food stores, especially for products that are not available in supermarkets.

Today, health food stores and health food sections in traditional supermarkets are doing a booming business—with retail sales of $3.3 billion in 1990. Their products may be extolled as "natural," "organically grown," "nothing artificial," "no preservatives," "no additives," "no chemicals," "anti-gray hair factors," or "dieters delight." Although most such claims are not supported by scientific evidence, it is difficult for the public to separate truth from fiction—particularly in regard to the use of the term *natural* for everything from whole grain flour to potato chips.

There is nothing wrong with the use of health foods. Most of them are beneficial. It is the exaggerated claims that some promoters make for them—the promise of better health through better eating—that needs to be questioned. However, it would be inaccurate to imply that all elements of the health food industry engage in questionable marketing practices. Also, not all items cost more; for example, at the time this section was written the senior author of this book checked the price of sesame seed at the local health food store and at the local supermarket. A 16 oz *(454 g)* package of sesame seed in the health food store cost $1.35 vs $9.09 for the similar product in the supermarket.

The labels and promotions of fad foods or diets usually do not make any direct claims that can be shown to be false. Instead, they refer to a book, a pamphlet, a speech, or a magazine article that has praised the product. Thus, the indirect promotions receive the protection of the First Amendment.

Other areas upon which health food promoters capitalize are beauty, eternal youth, retention of sexual potency, and long life. Such promotion may give hope to the users and improve their health and well-being by meeting their emotional needs. There is nothing wrong with these desires.

Health food can refer to natural and organic foods plus a wide range of other products. Such foods as alfalfa sprouts, blackstrap molasses, bone meal, ginseng, honey, kelp (seaweed), raw sugar, rose hips (seed pods of roses), seawater (bottled), sesame and sunflower seeds, wheat germ, whole grain flour, yeast, and yogurt have taken on a halo effect.

Science has found no magic or miracle foods. No one food is a preventive or cure-all for diseases. Foods are important because of their nutrient content; and no single food can serve as the source of all the essential nutrients. For example, wheat germ is considered a health food because it is a good source of vitamin E, the B vitamins, calories, essential fatty acids, protein, fiber, and most minerals. However, it lacks calcium, vitamin A, and vitamin C. So, the best way in which to ensure that nutritional requirements are met is to eat a variety of foods from each of the major food groups.

More and more health food stores are highly reputable. Some growers and distributors now supply affidavits or certificates of food grown and handled according to *organic* or *natural* precepts. Also, many health food operators are very knowledgeable about nutrition, and take pride in sharing helpful health information with their customers. Health food stores are coming of age!

HISTORICAL BACKGROUND AND CURRENT TRENDS.

Anthropologists, archaelogists, and other students of primitive peoples have found that beliefs in the superiority of certain foods were held by many ancient cultures. Some of the earliest concepts identified the organs of animals as beneficial to the analogous organs and functions in humans. For example, the American Indians and the Eskimos considered brains, eyes, and glands of birds and animals as special foods, good for health and vitality. Later studies have shown that these items are especially rich in minerals and vitamins. And bird eggs and fish eggs have long been thought to be promoters of fertility and the bearing of healthy children, as evidenced by the practice (by natives in the South Sea islands) of feeding roe to prospective parents. Unfortunately, many useful and reasonably accurate observations were often clouded by cultural biases, superstitions, and taboos.

Another set of factors that has tended to complicate matters in man's search for a more healthful diet has been those associated with the settlement of large populations within areas that could furnish only limited varieties of foods. This is best illustrated by the agricultural communities in which animal products were scarce and the people had to rely on only a few vegetable crops. Multiple nutritional deficiencies have often been found under these circumstances and it has often been surprising that the people have managed to propagate themselves. Any nutritious food that corrected even one of the severe deficiencies of these deprived people would have been regarded as a "health food". A contemporary example of this type is found among the natives in New Guinea who augment their predominately sweet potato diets with plant ashes (rich in essential minerals) and small amounts of pork and other animal foods.

During the Middle Ages, some people felt that the more unpalatable the food or its source, the greater its curative properties. This philosophy culminated in the development of such delectables as ground coffee beans blended with fat.

The development of the modern scientific approach to nutrition began with the French chemist Lavoisier's experiments in metabolism during the latter part of the 18th century. Nevertheless, ideas regarding nutrient requirements were grossly oversimplified until the dawn of the Vitamin Era in the early part of the 20th century. (Around the end of the 19th century, agricultural chemists limited their analyses of foods and feeds to carbohydrates, fats, proteins, fiber, a few minerals, and water. On that basis, they concluded that white corn was nutritionally equal to yellow corn. However, the farmers knew from experience that their animals did better on the latter grain, which was later found to be a much better source of Vitamin A.)

In 1773, Captain Cook fed sauerkraut to his sailors to prevent scurvy—the vitamin C deficiency disease; now, more than 200 years later, millions of Americans are taking vitamin C.

Meanwhile, the American health foods movement got underway in the early 1800s when the former Presbyterian preacher, the Reverend Sylvester Graham, toured the country giving lectures on the merits of eating coarse, whole grain breads and abstaining from fats and meat. He is immortalized by the graham cracker, which was named after him,

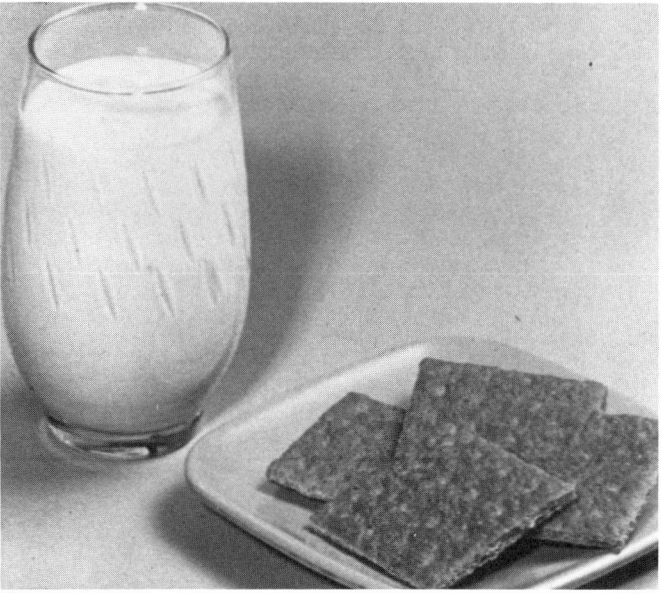

Fig. H-2. Graham crackers, immortalized by the health food crusader, the Reverend Sylvester Graham. (Courtesy, New Mexico State University, Las Cruces, New Mexico)

and which since his death has undergone an evolution to a soft modern product made from a mixture of graham flour and white flour. (A 100% whole wheat graham cracker is still sold in some health food stores.) Also, Graham's ideas were promoted by Sister Ellen White, one of the early leaders of the Seventh-day Adventist church, and a founder of the Western Health Reform Institute that was established in Battle Creek, Michigan in 1866. The institute was later operated by Dr. John Kellogg, who, with his brother Will, developed a dry, ready-to-eat breakfast cereal that marked the birth of the cereal industry in Battle Creek. It is noteworthy that (1) one of the patients of Dr. Kellogg was C. W. Post, who also started a cereal company in Battle Creek and invented a cereal substitute for coffee; and (2) the vegetarian dietary practices of the Seventh-day Adventists, who abstained from animal flesh, were the main reason for the development of the first meat analogs to be used in the United States. (However, the idea for making meatlike dishes from vegetable protein foods did not originate in America, but in Asia, where such dishes were prepared for many centuries.)

Health food stores became a notable part of the American scene in the 1920s and 1930s when shrewd businessmen capitalized on the news of the newly discovered vitamins and the foods from which they were obtained. An early mecca for these establishments was Hollywood, where actors and actresses stood in line to buy the five *wonder foods*—blackstrap molasses, brewers' yeast, powdered skim milk, yogurt, and wheat germ. In the eastern part of the United States, an interest in health, natural, and organically grown foods was sparked by the writings of Louis Bromfield, and later by Jerome Rodale, who moved from the dingy Lower East Side of New York City to the green meadows of Emmaus, Pennsylvania and started his own organic farming and gardening movement. (Rodale's entry into the field was financed by the successful electrical fixtures business which he operated with his brother. The continued success of the Rodale enterprises led to the founding of *Prevention* magazine in 1950.)

In its early days, the industry had its most ardent supporters among adults who were striving to retain or regain their youthful beauty, virility, and/or vitality. In the 1960s and 1970s, the health food industry received a very large boost from the ecology movement, when many young people, including the hippies, started to patronize health and natural food stores. Even the more conventional sector of the food industry has sought to capitalize on the evergrowing demand for *natural* foods, as evidenced by new products such as (1) many new types of yogurts; (2) natural whole-grain cereals with little or no added sweetener; (3) the substitution of carob powder for cocoa in many products (however, a major reason for this action was the high price of cocoa); (4) meat analogs made from soy protein; (5) natural coloring agents made from beets, marigolds, and turmeric; and (6) natural orange flavor, consisting of orange oil artificially extracted from natural oranges.

REASONS FOR POPULARITY OF HEALTH FOODS.
The public has been introduced to health foods through news media, magazines, books, and self-styled nutrition experts. The reasons for changing to health foods are numerous; among them, those that follow:

• **Affluence**—In today's affluent society, most people are assured of their basic needs for food and security. Consequently, they can devote both time and money to a wider range of interests, including health foods.

• **Arthritic treatment**— A study of a large population of arthritic patients revealed that half of them had followed dietary treatments at different times.

• **Athletic prowess**—Much nutritional fallacy goes with athletics. There isn't a health food (including royal jelly) known to man that is not advocated somewhere by a coach or athletic director to the boys or girls under his care.

• **Emotions**—For others, health foods serve as a symbol in meeting emotional needs. For them, food is a symbol of acceptance, friendliness, and socialization. So, to get *with it,* health foods are used.

• **Environment**—Others are concerned about the effect of chemical fertilizers and pesticides on the environment. Their concern causes them to buy health foods because they feel that less chemical fertilizer and pesticides have been used in their production.

• **Illness**—Some believe that particular foods have curative powers for certain diseases. At the same time they seek modern medical treatment, many persons look for something beyond what scientific medicine offers. This search is for a miracle drug, a secret formula, a special herb, or a wonder food.

• **Lifetime customer and advocate**—Once they're hooked, they usually become lifetime customers. It's virtually impossible to convince a true believer that his favorite health foods do not possess the purported magic. So, once they have concluded that health foods are their salvation from nutritional sins and the panacea and preventive for the world's mental and physical ills, they usually remain a lifetime health food customer and advocate.

• **Nature**—According to some health enthusiasts, nature cannot be improved upon; hence, it follows that natural, organic, or health foods are the best.

• **Nutrition experts**—Millions of people pose as self-styled nutrition *experts*. Some of these are content to ply their trade on themselves and their families. Others give their advice free to all who will listen. Still others are the modern counterpart of the medicine men of old—they sell their *expertise*. Television, newspapers and magazines, best-selling books—all feed us information and advice that's a mixture of scientific fact, half-truths, and just plain nonsense. (See FOOD MYTHS AND MISINFORMATION, section headed "The Medicine Man of Old.")

• **Nutritious and safe foods**—Some people are demanding health foods because they believe that they are getting more nutritious and safer foods. They associate their appearance and well-being with what they eat.

• **Obesity therapy**—Consumers are inundated with quick weight-loss plans; from megavitamin therapy to herbalism, from fasting to the wondrous grapefruit diet billed as follows:

"Lose 10 lbs (4.5 kg) in 10 days
on grapefruit diet"

Books abound, some of them assuring weight watchers that they can lose weight while eating all they want.

• **Personal attention**—Most health food store operators get to know their customers, much like the pop and mom corner grocery of old. By contrast, supermarkets seldom impart a personal touch.

• **Profit motive**—Many health food manufacturers and quack *doctors* have exploited the beliefs of some consumers at considerable profit to themselves.

• **Rebellion**—For some, health foods serve as a symbol against the establishment. Their reasoning: The food industry is linked with the establishment; therefore, foods normally found in supermarkets are undesirable.

• **Summary**—The movement toward a more primitive life-style has created a market as well as many gross untruths about health foods. Most health foods are very good—and good for you. For example, bread made with stoneground whole wheat flour may be enjoyed by all. Also, health food stores serve useful purposes by (1) focusing attention on certain foods that are more nutritious than others, (2) providing some items that are not found in other stores, and (3) stimulating beneficial innovation that might not otherwise occur in the food industry.

NOTE WELL: Some people have the impression that health food promoters—manufacturers; health food store operators; authors and publishers of books, pamphlets, leaflets, magazines, or newspapers; and health lecturers to live audiences, or over radio or TV—couldn't make the claims that they do if these claims were not proven and true. Nothing could be further from the truth. *The government can only regulate claims made on product labels and in product advertising.* The Food and Drug Administration (FDA) enforces proper labeling; and both the Post Office Department and the Federal Trade Commission are empowered to halt false advertising claims. Also, the American Medical Association maintains a Bureau of Investigation, which monitors the facts where there appears to be promotion and distribution of products that may be harmful to individuals. However, under the First Amendment (constitutional guarantees of a free press and free speech), purveyors of nutrition misinformation can (1) write, publish, and distribute books and other literature, or (2) lecture, proclaiming miraculous, but totally unfounded, benefits from foods.

COMMONLY CONSIDERED HEALTH FOODS.
The selling of certain items by health food stores and not by supermarkets is as much a matter of economics and marketing as it is a matter of providing items reputed to be of high nutritional value. (Both types of food stores sell a range of products that are designed to suit the preferences of their customers, and which differ widely in their nutritional values.) Furthermore, many health food stores carry more tablet forms of nutritional supplements than actual food items. Finally, quite a few products are merely combinations and/or variations of certain basic foods. Table H-1 is a summary of commonly considered health foods.

(Also see FOOD MYTHS AND MISINFORMATION; NATURAL FOODS; ORGANICALLY GROWN FOOD; PESTICIDES AS INCIDENTAL FOOD ADDITIVES; POISONS; PROCESSED FOODS, HIGHLY; VEGETARIAN DIETS; and ZEN MACROBIOTIC DIET.)

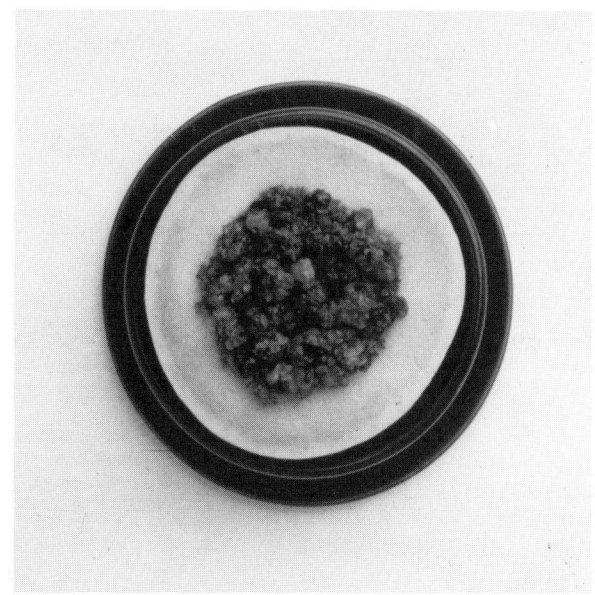

Fig. H-3. Granola cereal, a crunchy natural cereal mixture containing rolled oats, one or more sweeteners, oil, raisins, nuts, and/or flavorings. (Courtesy, USDA)

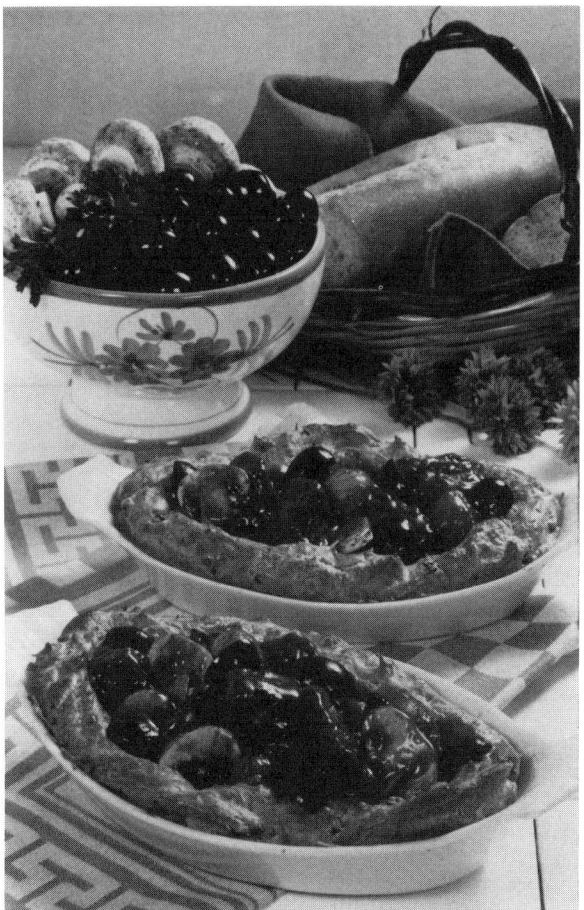

Fig. H-4. Mushrooms and olives with lean stew meat make for a healthy food. (Courtesy, Olive Administrative Committee, Fresno, Calif.)

TABLE H-1
COMMONLY CONSIDERED HEALTH FOODS

Name of Food	Type of Product(s)	Uses	Reputed Values and Claims	Comments
Acerola (Barbados cherry)	Tablets made from powdered, dried, acerola berries.	Vitamin C supplement.	Rich in vitamin C and bioflavonoids.	Acerola has the highest ascorbic acid (vitamin C) content of any known food.
Acidophilus	Bottled suspensions of *Lactobacillus acidophilus* bacteria, and powder and tablets made from the dried, but viable bacteria.	To promote the growth of this bacteria in the intestine.	The lactic acid produced by the bacteria may aid in the absorption of calcium and other minerals, while other substances it produces prevent the growth of less desirable bacteria.	The conditions that favor the growth of this bacteria are not known for certain.
Acidophilus milk	Fluid milk to which a culture of *Lactobacillus acidophilus* has been added.	To increase the *L. acidophilus* component of the gut microflora, thereby helping to maintain the balance of microorganisms in the intestinal tract. To regenerate intestinal flora after antibiotic treatment or other conditions that upset the microfloral balance in the gut.	Same as that for acidophilus, plus those values for milk.	The older types of products had a sour taste, but a sweet acidophilus milk is now available.
Adzuki bean	A small, dark red, dried bean that is popular in the Orient.	Cooked and eaten with brown rice, or ground into a powder that is used to make vegetarian milk substitute.	Good source of calories, carbohydrates, proteins, minerals (particularly phosphorus and iron), and the B vitamins.	Sweetened fillings and pastes may be made from the mashed cooked beans.
Agar-Agar (Japanese gelatin) (Also see Agar-Agar.)	A firm gumlike substance extracted from seaweed.	Emulsifier, gelling agent, and thickener in foods.	The calories and carbohydrates are not available, but iron, iodine, and other minerals may be utilized.	Sometimes used by vegetarians as a substitute for gelatin.
Alfalfa flour (powder)	A green, grassy-flavored flour made from the dried leaves of the alfalfa plant.	In baked goods, gravies, soups, and stews.	An excellent source of proteins, calcium, and trace minerals, carotene, vitamins E and K, and the unidentified factors. Used by some health food enthusiasts for treatment of diabetes.	Only small amounts should be used until one becomes accustomed to the color and flavor. There is no proof that alfalfa powder is effective as a treatment for diabetes.
Alfalfa seeds	Tiny seeds of the alfalfa plant.	Making an herb tea, and sprouting to obtain a raw salad vegetable.	The unsprouted seeds are not usually consumed.	The tea is reputed to ease aches and pains in the joints, but this is without experimental proof.
Alfalfa sprouts	Sprouts made from alfalfa seeds.	As a raw salad vegetable, sandwich fillings, and in soups.	Similar to alfalfa flour. Also, rich in vitamin C.	Fresh sprouts keep for only a few days in a refrigerator. There are cheaper sources of vitamin C.
Alfalfa tablets	Tablets made from alfalfa powder.	Nutritional supplement.	Same as alfalfa flour.	Some people are allergic to alfalfa powder.
Aloe vera	A gel made from the leaves of the aloe plant, a tropical & semitropical plant of the lily family, resembling a cactus.	Healing of burns, cuts, and ulcers.	Uncertain.	Should *not* be taken internally unless indicated on the product label.
Apricot kernels (Also see LAETRILE.)	The kernels from apricot pits.	As a source of highly controversial substance known as laetrile (also known as amygdalin).	Marketed as a dietary supplement as well as a drug for treatment of cancer, hepatitis, heart disease, alcoholism, allergies, and other conditions. Laetrile is not a nutrient.	Laetrile has no known value for humans. Anyone who consumes these kernels in excess runs the risk of cyanide poisoning.
Arrowroot starch	The powdered starch from the root of a tropical herb.	Ingredients of biscuits, gravies, sauces, and soups for infants and invalids.	Provides mainly calories and is easily digested.	Arrowroot cookies have long been given to teething infants.
Artichoke noodles	A pasta product made from the flour of Jerusalem artichoke tubers.	Dietetic pasta products for people who need to limit their consumption of calories and carbohydrates.	The major starchy constituent of the tubers is inulin, a carbohydrate that is not utilized by the body.	The actual calorie and carbohydrate contents of this product are rarely given on the label.
Avocado oil	Vegetable oil extracted from avocados.	In salad oils and cosmetics.	Source of essential fatty acids.	This oil is quite expensive.
Baking mixes, dietetic	Mixes for preparing baked goods that are suitable for people who have conditions that warrant the use of modified diets.	Preparation of special dietetic types of biscuits, breads, cakes, cookies, muffins, pancakes, rolls, etc.	Varies according to the type of mixture. May be deficient in the nutrients that are present in the ingredients which were replaced by substitutes.	Also see BREADS AND BAKING, Table B-8, Special Bakery Products.
Baking powder, low sodium	Chemical leavening agent in which potassium salts replace sodium salts.	Preparation of low sodium quick breads.	Rich in potassium, but contains little or no sodium.	Recipes may have to be modified to compensate for bitter taste of potassium salts.
Banana flakes	Flakes made from dried bananas.	Adding calories, flavor, and thickening to drinks and foods.	Rich in calories, magnesium and potassium; easily digested.	May be mixed in cereals, fruit drinks, or milk for infants or invalids.

(Continued)

Table H-1 *(Continued)*

Name of Food	Type of Product(s)	Uses	Reputed Values and Claims	Comments
Barbados molasses	Molasses residue from sugar refining.	As a flavoring in milk drinks, an ingredient or a spread for baked goods, and a laxative.	It is a variation of blackstrap molasses. Used by some enthusiasts as a general health food, and in the treatment of anemia.	Has a more pleasant flavor than blackstrap molasses, but rest of comments made for blackstrap molasses are applicable to Barbados molasses.
Barley flour	Flour milled from barley grains at various stages of refinement.	Preparation of baked goods for people with allergies to wheat.	Similar to wheat flours of equivalent degrees of refinement.	Contains gluten and is *not* useful for gluten-free diets.
Blackstrap molasses	Molasses residue from sugar refining.	As a flavoring in milk drinks, an ingredient or spread for baked goods, and a laxative.	Blackstrap molasses is purported to be a health-imparting food and a good source of iron; it is used by advocates as a cure for anemia and rheumatism.	There is no experimental proof that molasses improves health or cures anemia or rheumatism. Molasses is a fair, but unreliable source of iron. Molasses is eaten in such small amounts that it does not make an important contribution to the diet.
Bone meal	Tablets or powder made from ground sterilized bones of slaughter animals.	Nutritional supplement that provides calcium, phosphorus, and other minerals.	Rich source of calcium, phosphorus and other minerals.	The consumption of excessive amounts may reduce the absorption of certain trace minerals.
Bran	The seed coat of wheat and other grains. Available as flakes or in tablets.	May be added to cereals and baked goods to increase the fiber content.	Low in calories, but rich in fiber, protein, minerals, and B vitamins. Slightly laxative.	Should be eaten with plenty of fluid to prevent irritation of the g.i. tract.
Branch-chain amino acids	Individual amino acids in tablet or powder form.	As a dietary supplement—an alternative to anabolic steroids. To augment the protein in the regular diet.	Superior athletic performance.	Protein overloading may increase the amount of water the body loses and alter kidney function, and cause diarrhea and abdominal cramps. More creditable research on this product is needed.
Brewers' yeast (Also see YEAST.)	Dried food yeast derived from the brewing of beer and ale. Available in flake, powder, or tablet form.	Used primarily as a source of B vitamins and unidentified factors that may be taken with water or added to baked goods, drinks, puddings, soups, etc.	Rich source of B vitamins and unidentified factors. Also, an excellent source of protein of good quality.	The high nucleic acid content makes it unsuitable for people with gout or high blood levels of uric acid.
Buckwheat flour	Flour from dehulled buckwheat.	Preparation of buckwheat pancakes and blintzes (rolled thin pancakes filled or served with fish, fruit, meat, and/or sour cream).	Similar to that of wheat flour, except that amino acid patterns of the 2 flours are complementary. (Hence, mixtures of the flours are more nutritious than either one alone.)	This flour has a rich hearty flavor and produces baked goods that are a little heavier and moister than wheat flour items.
Buckwheat groats (kasha)	Dehulled and lightly milled pieces of buckwheat grains.	Cooked and served as a cereal, side dish, or stuffing for poultry.	Similar to that of buckwheat flour.	The groats add flavor when mixed with more bland cereal products.
Bulgur wheat	Grains of wheat that have been soaked, cooked, dried, lightly milled, and cracked.	The cooked grain is used as a cereal, stuffing for meats and poultry, or a substitute for rice.	Similar to that of whole wheat grains.	Cooks more quickly than whole wheat grains.
L-carnitine	This nonprotein amino acid is synthesized from two essential amino acids in the liver and kidneys.	As a dietary supplement—an alternative to anabolic steroids. Weight reduction. Endurance in athletic events.	Some endurance athletes feel that taking carnitine supplements helps them go the distance.	L-carnitine may have a sparing action of glycogen and improve fatty acid metabolism. More creditable research on this product is needed.
Carob powder (Also see LEGUMES, Table L-2.)	Chocolate colored, sweet powder made from deseeded carob pods.	A chocolate-like ingredient of cakes, candies, drinks, and puddings.	Lower in calories and fats than most chocolate products. Carob powder is low in sodium and high in potassium; hence, desirable for diets which restrict sodium and encourage potassium, such as those used in the treatment of congestive heart failure and hypertension.	
Carrageenan (Irish moss) (Also see CARRAGEENAN.)	A vegetable gum extracted from the Irish moss seaweed.	Emulsifier, gelling agent, and thickener for various types of food products.	Low in calories (most of the carbohydrate content is not utilizable), but rich in calcium, iodine, and other minerals.	Sometimes used by vegetarians as a substitute for gelatin.
Cheese, raw milk	Mild-flavored cheeses made from certified raw (unpasteurized) milk.	Same as for cheeses from pasteurized milk.	Similar to counterparts made from pasteurized milk.	Some people prefer not to use products made from pasteurized milk.
Chia seeds	Seeds from a wild sage that grows in Mexico and in southwestern U.S.	May be added as a thickener to cereals, doughs for baking, sauces, spreads, etc.	Data on the nutrient composition is not readily available.	These seeds become jellylike when soaked in a liquid.
Chickpeas (Also see LEGUMES, Table L-2.)	Salted roasted chickpeas or uncooked dried chickpeas.	Roasted peas—as a snack like peanuts. Boiled peas—as most other dried legumes.	Similar to that of most legumes.	Canned cooked chickpeas are sold in many American supermarkets.
Chicory root powder	Powder made from roasted roots of chickory.	As an extender of or a substitute for coffee, which it resembles in flavor.	The amounts that are generally used (1 tsp or 5 g) are too small to contribute much in the way of nutrients.	The practice of mixing chicory with coffee was brought to New Orleans by French settlers.

(Continued)

Table H-1 *(Continued)*

Name of Food	Type of Product(s)	Uses	Reputed Values and Claims	Comments
Chlorophyll	Green pigment extracted from the leaves of plants that is sold in liquid and tablet forms.	As a breath deodorizer and a "cleanser" of the digestive tract. For digestive disorders.	It is reputed to alleviate ulcers, but experimental proof is lacking.	May be obtained more economically by eating liberal amounts of fresh green leaves from edible plants.
Chromium picolinate	It is a natural compound of chromium and picolinic acid. Picolinic acid is a natural chelating agent that occurs normally in the human body to facilitate the assimilation of minerals.	As a dietary supplement—an alternative to anabolic steroids. Weight reduction and muscle building.	It is purported to speed fat loss while building muscle.	It works by enhancing insulin-dependent mechanisms that control hunger, stimulates metabolism, and conserves body protein.
Coffee substitutes	Powdered, toasted cereal preparations that may also contain chicory, figs, molasses and/or other ingredients.	For beverage use by people who may wish to avoid consuming caffeine.	The amounts consumed (1 tsp or 5 g) are too small to contribute much in the way of nutrients.	These products are now sold in many American supermarkets.
Cold-pressed oils	Vegetable oils that have been extracted from seeds heated to 200°F to 300°F *(94°C to 148°C)*.	By people who expect the oils to have higher nutritive values than those extracted by the conventional processes.	May be a little higher in vitamin E and tocopherol content than oils extracted by higher temperature processes.	Some of the vitamin E and related tocopherol content may be destroyed even by so-called "cold-pressing."
Corn, flaked	Flakes produced by rolling whole kernels of corn.	Whole grain cooked cereal.	Higher in protein, fiber, and certain trace minerals than ready-to-eat cornflakes.	Much more filling than the more commonly used breakfast cereal.
Corn flour, whole ground	Flour produced by milling whole kernels of corn.	Baked goods; breading for fish, meats, and poultry; soups; and stews.	Higher in calories, corn oil, and vitamin E than degerminated corn flours.	Should be kept refrigerated to prevent the development of rancidity.
Cornmeal, whole	Meal produced from whole kernels of corn.	Baked goods; cooked breakfast cereal; cornmeal mush, etc.	Higher in calories, corn oil, and vitamin E than degerminated cornmeal.	Yellow cornmeal is richer in vitamin A than white cornmeal.
Cottonseed flour	Flour made from ground cottonseed from which the oil has been extracted.	Mixed with cereal flours that are used to prepare baked products.	Richer in protein, calcium, phosphorus, iron and B vitamins than most cereal flours.	About 7% cottonseed flour may be used in a mixture with wheat flour.
Couscous	A semolina made from finely ground hard durum wheat.	As a side dish or an addition to soups and stews.	About the same as that for other products made from partly milled wheat.	Couscous is a staple food in North Africa and the Middle East.
Date syrup	A syrup made from ground fresh dates.	An ingredient or a topping for hot breads and desserts.	Provides mainly calories and carbohydrates.	Produces moist baked goods when used in place of some of the sugar.
Dolomite	Tablets or powdered, made from ground dolomitic limestone.	Nutritional supplement that provides calcium, magnesium, and other minerals.	Rich source of calcium, magnesium, and other minerals. May also be used as an antacid.	The consumption of excessive amounts may reduce the absorption of certain trace minerals.
Eggs, fertile	Fertile eggs, laid by hens mated to roosters.	Same as nonfertile eggs.	Advocates claim that fertile eggs are more nutritious and invigorating than nonfertile eggs.	Fertile eggs are no more nourishing than nonfertile eggs. Besides, they spoil more quickly due to the developing embryo.
Eggs, raw	Uncooked eggs.	Eaten raw, usually with salt and pepper added.	Faddists claim that raw eggs increase potency.	Raw eggs contain the antivitamin, avidin, which binds biotin and makes it unavailable.
Egg replacers	Egg-free mixtures made from various hypoallergenic vegetable gums and starches.	Baked preparations for people who cannot eat eggs (as in certain allergies.).	Provide mainly calories and carbohydrates.	These products are designed to provide binding for batter and doughs.
Egg white, dried	A powder prepared by drying separated egg white.	In baked goods and other foods prepared for people who wish to avoid egg yolks.	Moderately high in calories and very rich in high-quality protein.	1 lb *(454 g)* of dried egg white is equivalent to about 14 cups *(3,360 ml)* of liquid egg whites.
Fig syrup	Syrup made by evaporating a water extract of ground dried figs.	A flavoring for milk drinks, an ingredient or topping for baked items, and as a laxative.	Provides mainly calories and carbohydrates.	Whole dried figs are a more effective, but more irritating laxative.
Flaxseed	Whole or ground seeds from the flax plant.	Additions to cereals or porridges, for making a soothing tea, and as a laxative.	High in polyunsaturated fatty acids, protein, and fiber.	The seeds contain a mucilage that is extracted by steeping in hot water.
Fructose	Sugar obtained from certain fruits or from the chemical conversion of dextrose (glucose).	As a substitute for table sugar, because it is sweeter and less is needed.	Same caloric and carbohydrate values as most other pure sugars.	There is little evidence to support the use of fructose in treating blood sugar disorders.
Gamma oryzanol and other plant sterols	The chemical structure of this product is similar to cholesterol.	As a dietary supplement—and alternative to anabolic steroids. Users hope to obtain an increase in lean muscle mass.	Plant sterols are purported to increase testosterone production and stimulate human growth hormone release.	Gamma oryzanol is produced from rice bran oil. More creditable research on this product is needed.
Garlic	Pills.	Medicinal purposes.	May lower blood cholesterol levels.	By livening up the taste for food, garlic helps people reduce their consumption of salt.
Ginger root	Fresh root of the ginger plant.	Seasoning for various dishes, and for making spicy tea that is reputed by some to help open a clogged nose.	The amounts consumed (1 tsp or 5 g) are too small to contribute much in the way of nutrients.	The flavor of fresh ginger root is much more distinctive than that of powdered dried ginger.
Ginseng	Root of the ginseng plant which is sold in capsules, extract, instant powder, paste, tea, and whole root.	Claimed to be a general tonic for digestive trouble, impotence, and overall lack of vitality.	The amounts consumed (1 tsp or 5 g) are too small to contribute much in the way of nutrients.	Ginseng may raise the blood pressure of certain susceptible people.

(Continued)

Table H-1 *(Continued)*

Name of Food	Type of Product(s)	Uses	Reputed Values and Claims	Comments
Gluten flour	A high-protein, highly-elastic flour obtained by washing much of the starch from ordinary white flour.	Preparation of low-carbohydrate, high-protein breads and in baking mixtures with other flours or meals of low gluten.	Compared to ordinary wheat flour, it is lower in carbohydrates, higher in protein, and lower in minerals and vitamins.	Gluten flour strenthens and lightens doughs made with barley, corn, oat, potato, rice, rye, or soy flours.
Goat's milk	Fresh or evaporated goat's milk.	For people with an intolerance to cow's milk.	About the same as cow's milk.	Some infants digest goat's milk more readily than cow's milk.
Graham flour	Whole wheat flour made from winter wheat.	Baking of whole grain breads.	Similar to that of whole wheat flour.	Available in some supermarkets.
Granola cereal	A ready-to-eat toasted cereal mixture containing rolled oats, one or more sweeteners, oil, raisins, nuts, and/or flavorings.	Breakfast cereal or ingredient of bars, breads, muffins, pancakes, etc. Topping for other foods such as desserts.	Usually higher in calories and sometimes higher in fiber and certain minerals, but otherwise not much better than fortified breakfast cereals.	Granola mixtures vary considerably in their compositions and may contain several different sweeteners.
Guarana	Tablets or a bitter chocolatelike powder, made from the seeds of a Brazilian climbing shrub, that are mixed into drinks.	As a stimulant (see comments).	The amount used are too small to make any significant nutritional contributions.	Guarana contains 3 to 5 times as much caffeine as coffee or tea.
Honey	Produced by bees from the flower nectar of 1 or more plants such as alfalfa, buckwheat, clove, orange, sage, and tupelo.	Sweetener for baked goods, desserts, drinks, etc. Spread for breads, muffins, pancakes, etc. Some cultures claim that honey excites sexual desire. Unfounded medical claims have been ascribed to honey.	Due to its fructose content, honey is sweeter than table sugar; hence, less of it is needed.	Honey has no magical powers relative to either sexual desire or health. Breads and cakes that contain honey keep moist longer than those sweetened with sugar.
Honey and Vinegar	A mixture of honey and vinegar.	As a cure-all.	Honey and vinegar have been purported to cure an amazing array of ills, ranging from arthritis to the common cold and digestive disturbances.	Don't you believe it! The presence of honey makes the swallowing of vinegar more tolerable.
Kefir	Milk product similar to yogurt but produced by a double fermentation (bacterial and yeast).	Beverage, dessert, dressing, and ingredient of baked products.	The lactic acid content may increase the absorption of calcium and other minerals.	Kefir may be made by using granules.
Kelp	A seaweed that is rich in iodine. Available in tablet or powder form.	As an iodine supplement to prevent a deficiency of the mineral.	Very rich source of iodine.	Consumption should be limited to amounts which provide the RDA for iodine. (Too much iodine may be toxic.)
Lactobacillus	Bacteria (such as *L. acidophilus*) which ferment milk sugar (lactose) to lactic acid. Available as dried powder, liquid suspensions, and tablets.	Preparation of fermented milks. Colonization of the intestines by lactobacilli and elimination of undesirable intestinal microorganisms.	Dietary lactic acid may promote mineral absorption and the counteraction of ammonia accumulation in the intestine. (Excessive ammonia is toxic.)	There is still considerable uncertainty regarding the diet and other conditions which promote the colonization of the intestine by *Lactobacilli*.
Lecithin	Fatty substance that is obtained from egg yolks, unrefined soy bean oil and other oils.	Emulsifying agent (helps to keep constituents of mixtures from separating out). Certain therapeutic applications. Recent reports suggest that one of the constituents of lecithin, choline, may counter senile deterioration of the brain.	Some enthusiasts claim that added lecithin will prevent or cure arthritis, gallstones, heart disease, nervous disorders, and skin disorders.	Research has not backed up these claims. Supplements of lecithin contain little choline. Besides, more research is needed on senile deterioration of the brain.
Licorice root	Extracted from the root of an herb and used in the production of certain candies and drinks.	Chips from the root are used for brewing teas and making other home remedies.	Little nutritional value. May sooth minor colds and sore throats.	Licorice has a laxative effect for some people.
Liver powder	Powder or tablets made from defatted or undefatted dried liver.	Nutritional supplement for undernourished people.	Excellent source of protein, nucleic acids, phosphorus, iron, copper, and B vitamins.	Defatted liver powder is much more palatable than undefatted forms.
Maple sugar	Sugar obtained by evaporating maple syrup.	Ingredient of candies and other sweets.	Provides mainly calories and sugar.	Some products contain mixtures of maple and other sugars.
Maple syrup	The syrup obtained by boiling down the sap from maple trees.	Ingredient of baked goods, candies, pies, etc. Spread or topping for pancakes, waffles, etc.	Provides mainly calories and sugar.	Some products are only "maple-flavored" syrups, or blends of maple and other syrups.
Meat analogs	Vegetarian imitations of meat products that are made from cereal and legume derivatives such as gluten and soy protein.	Extenders or substitutes for fish, meats, and poultry. Vegetarian diets.	Values vary according to the ingredients. Usually the protein values approximate those of meat, but the levels of calories and other nutrients may be quite different.	Some products are much higher in sodium than fish, meats, or poultry.
Milk, raw	Unpasteurized milk, straight from the udder to the consumer.	For people who do not wish to use pasteurized milk.	Some supporters claim that raw milk is more nutritious than pasteurized milk—that pasteurization destroys vitamin C.	The amount of vitamin C in raw milk is so small that it makes no significant contribution of this vitamin to the diet. Raw milk can be a source of undulant fever (brucellosis) and tuberculosis—two dreaded diseases.

(Continued)

Table H-1 *(Continued)*

Name of Food	Type of Product(s)	Uses	Reputed Values and Claims	Comments
Milk substitutes	Milklike fluids that are usually made from soy derivatives and a sweetener.	Vegetarians who consume no animal foods. People who have an intolerance to milk.	Usually, amino acids, minerals, and vitamins are added to make these products nutritionally similar to milk.	Now available in pharmacies and supermarkets.
Millet	A tiny grain that is much more commonly used for food in Africa, the Middle East, and India than in the U.S. (It is used mainly for birdseed in America.)	Cooked breakfast cereal, side dish, or topping for other dishes. The ground grain may be added to flour mixtures used for breads, muffins, rolls, etc.	Millet is generally superior to wheat, rice, and corn in protein quality. However, like other grains, it is low or lacking in calcium and in vitamins A, D, C, and B-12.	Millet has a bland taste that is improved by browning or toasting it slightly before cooking.
Miso	A fermented food paste made from soybeans.	Ingredients of dips, dressings, salads, sandwich fillings, soups, and stews.	Varies considerably according to the way in which it is prepared. (However, it is a good source of calories and protein.)	Made with sea salt; hence, it has a high sodium content.
Mung bean sprouts	Small beans from India and other tropical countries that are used for sprouting.	Mung bean sprouts are good in salads, sandwiches, soups, and stir-fried dishes.	The sprouts are low in calories, but a good source of protein, fiber, and vitamin C.	The unsprouted beans are rarely used in the U.S.
Mushrooms, dried	Dried pieces of various species of mushrooms.	Salads, soups, and stews.	Varies according to the species. Proteins complement those of cereal grains.	The best flavored dried mushrooms are the wild species from Europe.
Oat flour	Flour made by milling dehulled and debranned oats.	Alone or with other cereal flours in baked products.	Slightly higher in protein than the other common cereal flours.	Oat flour produces a heavier and moister baked product than wheat flour.
Oats, steel cut	Oat grains cut into granules.	Cooked cereal, puddings, and soups.	Same as oat flour.	Also known as Scottish oats.
Papain	A protein-digesting enzyme extracted from papaya that is available in tablet and powder forms.	Meat tenderizer. Digestive aid for people lacking digestive secretions.	The amounts used are generally too small to contribute much in the way of nutrients.	Papain has also been used to heal festering sores.
Peanut butter, natural	Unhydrogenated peanut butter in which the oil separates and floats to the top of the jar.	Same as for hydrogenated peanut butter, except that in this case the oil may be skimmed off and used separately.	Similar to that of hydrogenated peanut butter, except that the natural oil is richer in essential fatty acids than the hydrogenated oil.	Natural peanut butter is now sold in many supermarkets.
Peanut flour	More of a meal than a true flour. It is made from finely ground peanuts.	In baked products (when mixed with wheat flour).	The proteins of peanut flour complement those of wheat flour.	The calorie and fat contents are variable. Flours may be low, medium, or high fat.
Pectin	A dry powder or a water solution of a carbohydrate gum used to make gels.	Preparation of jellies and other types of gels. In an antidiarrheal remedy.	Little or no nutritional value, but used medicinally to lower blood cholesterol.	Citrus pectin appears to be much more effective than apple pectin in lowering cholesterol.
Pollen	Male reproductive cells of flowering plants that are sold as granules or in tablets.	A nutritional supplement (according to some who promote its use).	Uncertain. However, it is said to be useful in desensitizing allergic people. Also, it is reported to be good for general health and vitality.	The claims for beneficial effects of pollen have *not* been confirmed in scientific tests.
Potato flour	Flour made from cooked, dried potatoes.	In baked goods, and as a thickener for gravies.	Good source of energy. Dried potato flour contains 8% protein, which is about the same as corn and rice; and potatoes supply lysine, the amino acid which is lacking in cereal grains. Potato flour may be substituted for wheat flour for those allergic to the latter.	Can be used to make instant mashed potatoes.
Protein supplements	Candylike bars, liquids, powders, and tablets made from high-protein derivatives of eggs, milk, and soybeans.	For protein-deficient people, muscle builders, and patients recovering from burns, cancer, injuries, and surgery.	High protein intakes during periods of great stress may help to prevent the loss of proteins from the body tissues.	An excessively high protein intake may lead to a large urinary loss of calcium and other undesirable effects.
Psyllium seeds	Ground refined or unrefined seeds of *Plantago ovata* in granule or powder form.	As a source of dietary fiber and a laxative.	Little or no nutritive value, but binds bile salts and lowers the blood cholesterol.	People with easily irritated bowels should use only the refined psyllium products.
Pumpkin seeds	Dried, salted or unsalted, toasted or raw seeds of pumpkins or squashes.	Snack food. Nutritional supplement.	Rich source of calories, fats, proteins, minerals, and vitamins.	The prehistoric Indians of the Americas grew pumpkins and squashes for the seeds.
Rice, brown	Grains of rice with the brown layer intact.	Cooked cereals, desserts, ingredient of entrees, soups, and stews.	A moderately good source of calories and protein, and a good source of minerals and B vitamins.	Asians have consumed brown rice for thousands of years.
Rice flours	Flours produced by milling grains of raw or parboiled brown, glutinous, or white rice.	Cookies, infant cereals, low-gluten baked goods. Thickener for sauces, soups, and stews.	The same as that of the type of rice used to make the flour.	Most infants, invalids, and sufferers from allergies tolerate rice flour well.
Rice, glutinous (sweet rice)	Grains or flour of a variety of rice that becomes sticky (glutinous) when cooked.	Desserts and fillings for pastries.	About the same as ordinary rice.	Available in Chinese markets and some food stores.
Rice polish	Tiny flakes of the inner bran layers of the rice grain that can be obtained by milling. Also available as an extract or syrup.	Ingredient of infant cereals, and special cakes (to which it imparts tenderness and moistness). Nutritional supplement.	Easily digested, low in fiber, rich in thiamin, and high in niacin.	This item is a well-documented "health-food" where thiamin is needed because it was first used to cure beriberi in Asia.

Table H-1 (Continued)

Name of Food	Type of Product(s)	Uses	Reputed Values and Claims	Comments
Rose hips	The bulb-shaped fleshy fruits that remain after the rose petals fall off. Available in dried pieces, powders, syrups, and tablets.	Preparation of fruit soups (a European dish), jams, jellies, syrups, and teas.	A very rich source of vitamin C and bioflavonoids.	Used as a source of vitamin C in Great Britain during World War II.
Royal jelly	Substance produced by worker bees for feeding the queen. (Available in capsules.)	Nutritional supplement. Ingredient of certain expensive cosmetics.	Very rich in certain B vitamins such as pantothenic acid. Some claim that royal jelly aids sexual rejuvenation.	An expensive item that has been promoted with many extravagant claims. The claim of sexual rejuvenation is an old wives' tale. Royal jelly should be left for the bees, for which it is intended.
Rye flours	Flours that vary from light to dark that are milled from rye grains at various stages of refinement.	Alone or in mixtures with other flours in baked products.	Dark rye flours are less refined and more nutritious than light rye flours.	Rye flours are low in gluten and produce heavier, moister breads than wheat flours.
Rye grain	Whole, cut, or rolled grains.	Cooked cereal, special breads for people allergic to wheat.	Similar to wheat, but a little higher in proteins, fiber, minerals, and B vitamins.	Rye has long been an important cereal in Northern Europe, where wheat grows poorly.
Safflower oil	Oil from the seeds of a hardy, thistlelike plant.	Same as other vegetable oils—frying, salads, shortenings, etc.	Rich in essential polyunsaturated fatty acids.	Excessive consumption of vegetable oils may promote the formation of gallstones.
Salt-free foods	Items made without added salt.	For people who are on low-sodium diets.	About the same as the salted counterparts.	Some items may contain sources of sodium other than salt. (Hence, labels should be read carefully.)
Sea salt	Salt produced by the evaporation of sea water.	Seasoning and source of certain trace minerals.	Contains more minerals than common salt.	The form of salt used by ancient peoples.
Seawater	Water from the sea.	As drinking water.	Good source of iodine and fluorine.	Seawater is abundant and cheap. Another great advantage, shared by few manufacturers: The raw material is also the finished product!
Sesame seeds	Tiny hulled or unhulled seeds of the sesame plant.	Baked products, candies (such as halvah), desserts, meat and poultry dishes, and salads.	Good source of calories, essential fatty acids, proteins, minerals, and B vitamins.	Taste best when lightly browned or toasted.
Sesame tahini	A creamy spread made by blending or grinding sesame seeds.	Alone or mixed with various sauces or spreads.	About the same as that for sesame seed, unless mixed with other items.	Should be kept refrigerated to prevent the development of rancidity.
Sorghum syrup	The syrup produced by evaporation of the sap expressed from sorghum stalks.	Same as other syrups or sweeteners. Sometimes, it is fermented to produce alcohol.	Rich in calories and sugar, and a good source of minerals.	Has a milder flavor than either balckstrap or Barbados molasses.
Soy flour	Flours made from heat treated soybean meals of varying fat contents.	Protein supplement, extender in meat products, and ingredient of baked products.	Caloric content depends upon fat content. Excellent source of protein, minerals, and vitamins.	Full-fat, medium-fat, low-fat, and *extra-lecithin* soy flours are available.
Soy milk powder	Finely ground soy powder of low to medium fat content.	Preparation of soy *milks* and *cheeses,* and fermented products.	Same as those of a soy flour having the same fat content.	Long used by the Chinese for the preparation of a milk substitute.
Soy protein powder	A concentrated source of protein (85 to 98%) produced by removal of most of the carbohydrates from a soybean flour or meal.	Protein supplement. Preparation of extenders or substitutes for fish, meat, milk, poultry, and seafood.	Very rich in protein. The levels of the other nutrients depend upon the extraction processes used.	The consumption of excessive amounts of protein may promote high urinary losses of calcium and other undesirable effects.
Spirullina	Powder or tablets made from a dried blue-green algae grown in Mexico and Africa.	Food and nutritional supplements, sold at very high prices in the U.S.	Good source of protein, fiber, minerals, and vitamins. (One of the few wholly vegetarian foods that contains vitamin B-12.)	Used for centuries by the African tribes around Lake Niger. Recently promoted as an aid to weight reduction.
Sprouts	Sprouted (germinated) seeds prepared by soaking them in water in the dark.	In salads, soups, stews, and stir-fried dishes.	Low in calories, but a fair to good source of proteins, fiber, minerals, and vitamins.	The exposure of newly emerged sprouts to sunlight develops the chlorphyll content.
Sugar, raw (Brown sugar)	A mixture of sugar crystals coated with a film of molasses.	Same as for white sugar, except that the taste of raw sugar is a little more appealing.	Closer in composition and nutritional value to white sugar than to molasses. Raw sugar is promoted on the basis of its mineral content, especially iron.	Raw sugar contains little iron now that it is processed in stainless steel and aluminum vessels. Besides, it is eaten in small servings. An adult woman would have to eat 2½ cups (600 ml) of brown sugar daily to meet her requirement for iron. So, brown sugar should be eaten for reason of taste, rather than for any health properties.

(Continued)

Table H-1 *(Continued)*

Name of Food	Type of Product(s)	Uses	Reputed Values and Claims	Comments
Tamari	A soy sauce made by water extraction of a fermented mixture of soybeans, grains, water, and salt.	As a flavoring for Oriental dishes such as chop suey, chow mein, sprouts, and stir-fried mixtures.	High in sodium content. Hence, only small amounts should be used, making the nutritional contribution small.	Some products contain added monosodium glutamate.
Tapioca	Starchy globules produced by heating a paste made from the cassava root.	Foods for infants and invalids, and starchy puddings.	Provides mainly calories and starch. Easily digested by infants and invalids.	In Latin America, the name tapioca is given to various cassava products.
Tapioca flour	Finely ground cassava root starch.	Same as those for other edible starches.	Same as for tapioca.	Hard to find in U.S.
Textured vegetable product (TVP)	Extracted soy protein that has been made into granules or spun into chewy pieces that have a texture like cooked animal tissues.	Extender or substitute for fish, meats, poultry, and seafood.	Moderately high in calories and high in protein. (The levels of the other nutrients vary with the type of product.)	Some products have a rather insipid taste and a dry crumbly texture. (They should be mixed with other more tasty and juicy ingredients.)
Tofu	A mild-flavored, cheeselike type of soybean curd.	As a cheese extender or substitute; and in salads, soups, and vegetarian dishes.	High in protein and B vitamins.	Now sold in the produce section of many supermarkets.
Torula yeast (Also see YEAST.)	Species of yeast grown specially for food use. (Available in powder or tablet form.)	Ingredient of fortified fruit or milk drinks, gravies, sauces, etc.; and nutritional supplement.	Contains from 50 to 62% protein, and is a good source of minerals and B vitamins.	More palatable than brewers' yeast. Some brands contain added nutrients.
Vegetable salt	Sea salt flavored with powdered dried vegetables.	Seasoning for various dishes.	Provides mainly salt and some trace minerals.	Excessive use of any form of salt may be detrimental to good health.
Vegetarian gelatin	Any of several vegetable gelling agents such as agar-agar and carrageenan.	In place of gelatin in the preparation of gelled desserts, salads, and soups.	Much of the carbohydrate in these items is not utilized but they furnish some essential minerals.	Used mainly by vegetarians who do not use animal gelatin.
Wheat, cracked	Cracked grains of wheat.	Baked products, cooked cereals, desserts, filler in meat and poultry dishes, salads, soups, and stews.	Good source of calories, carbohydrates, proteins, fiber, minerals, and B vitamins.	Cooks more rapidly than whole grains of wheat.
Wheat germ	The embryo of the wheat kernel.	As a ready-to-eat breakfast cereal; or in baked goods; breading for fish, meats, or poultry; casseroles; cooked cereals; desserts; salads; soups; and stews.	Good source of calories, essential fatty acids, proteins, fiber, minerals, vitamin E, and the B vitamins.	Should be kept refrigerated to prevent the development of rancidity. Light toasting improves the flavor.
Wheat germ flour	Finely ground wheat germ.	Preparation of baked products.	Same as for wheat germ.	Should be stored in a refrigerator.
Wheat germ oil	Oil extracted from wheat germ.	Salad oil, and nutritional supplement.	Primarily as a rich vitamin E supplement.	Heating (as in pan frying) may destroy some of the vitamin E.
Whey powder	A powder obtained by drying the whey from cheese production.	In baked goods, desserts, fruit or milk drinks, and soups; and a nutritional supplement.	Rich in milk sugar (lactose), protein; and a fair to good source of calcium, phosphorus, and B vitamins.	Much of the whey produced in the U.S. goes to waste because of lack of demand.
Whole wheat berries	Whole grains of wheat.	Cereals, desserts, puddings, and stuffings.	Good source of calories, carbohydrates, proteins, fiber, minerals, and B vitamins. Also a fair source of vitamin E.	The long cooking time may be shortened by using a pressure cooker.
Yeast, Instant (Also see YEAST.)	Powdered yeast treated to make it blend readily with various liquids.	Nutritionally fortified drinks for undernourished people.	Rich source of proteins, nucleic acids, and B vitamins.	Powdered yeast has long been used as a protein and vitamin supplement.
Yeast, Nutritional (Also see YEAST.)	Powdered or tableted yeast grown specially for use as a food.	Nutritional supplement or tonic for undernourished or debilitated people.	Very rich in proteins, nucleic acids, essential minerals, and B vitamins.	Has a milder flavor and a higher protein content than brewers' yeast.
Yogurt	Mildly fermented milk product (milk sugar converted to lactic acid by bacteria).	Dessert, entree, salad dressing, or snack. May be added to baked goods, in which it reacts with baking soda to leaven them.	Similar to milk, except that *Lactobacilli* (if alive) prevent the growth of certain undesirable microorganisms in the intestines.	A dairy food that has had a recent rapid growth in popularity. Although yogurt does not have any magical health-imparting properties, it is a nutritious food.

HEARTBURN

This condition is characterized by a burning and painful sensation under the sternum (breastbone), sometimes accompanied by a sour regurgitation (bringing up of gas and small bits of food from the stomach). The most common response to these symptoms is to take antacids to relieve what is thought to be hyperacidity. It is better, however, not to rely solely on these remedies, but to try to discover the cause(s) of these symptoms.

CAUSES OF HEARTBURN. Although the pain experienced in heartburn is sometimes due to a peptic ulcer, in many cases there is some type of irritation or spasm of the esophagus. Two of the most common esophageal disorders are: Esophageal Reflux and Hiatus Hernia.

(Also see ANTACIDS; HIATUS HERNIA; and ULCERS, PEPTIC.)

• **Esophageal reflux (esophagitis)**—This type of irritation, also known as esophagitis, results from regurgitation of stomach acid into the esophagus.

• **Hiatus hernia**—This refers to a slight protrusion of the upper part of the stomach through the opening (or hiatus) in the diaphragm, caused by intra-abdominal pressure.

TREATMENT AND PREVENTION OF HEARTBURN.
NOTE: Sufferers from chronic heartburn should consult a physician for diagnosis of the cause(s). They might then inquire as to the advisability of using antacids. (Indiscreet use of these compounds may result in other digestive disorders such as malabsorption.)

(Also see ANTACIDS; HIATUS HERNIA; and ULCERS, PEPTIC.)

HEART DISEASE

This term refers to a wide variety of disorders, ranging from congenital defects in the valves of the heart to degeneration of the heart muscle. However, the mass media and the public tend to identify heart disease with what is medically known as *coronary heart disease*—the various conditions that are associated with blockage of the coronary artery, which delivers blood to the heart muscle. Coronary heart disease is responsible for about 80% of the one million deaths from diseases of the heart and blood vessels (cardiovascular diseases) which occur in the United States each year.[1] Another name for coronary heart disease is *ischemic heart disease*. (The term *ischemia* means a drastic reduction in the flow of blood to a tissue.)

Lack of blood in the heart muscle may lead to a *heart attack*—an event usually characterized by the sudden onset of severe chest pain which may spread to nearby points of the body, although some people may suffer so-called *silent heart attacks*, which are not noticed at the time they occur, but which leave evidence of damage to the heart muscle. Some characteristic features of a heart attack are depicted in Fig. H-5.

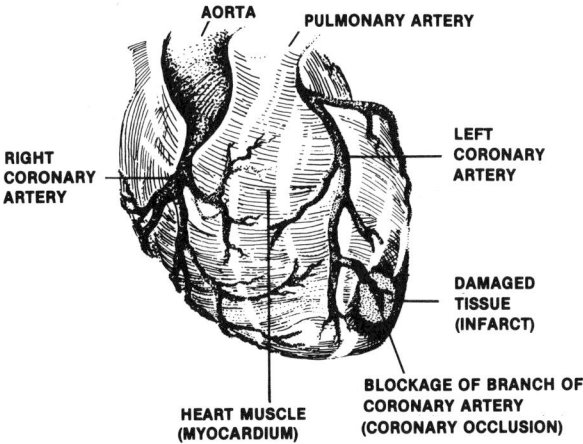

Fig. H-5. Some characteristic features of a heart attack. Interference with the flow of blood to the heart muscle is usually accompanied by such symptoms as (1) severe pain in the chest and surrounding areas, and (2) shortness of breath.

The three potentially modifiable heart disease risk factors of greatest concern are: cigarette smoking, high blood pressure, and high serum cholesterol.

HEART AND BLOOD VESSEL DISORDERS. Many of the ideas about heart disease which have been popularized by the mass media are limited to the dramatic aspects of blood clots, cardiac arrest, clogging of the blood vessels with plaques, excruciating pain, and sudden death. However, these aspects represent only the later stages of the disease. Detection and treatment of the early stages may forestall the later stages for a long time. Hence, it is worthwhile to consider the various aspects of the cardiovascular disorders that follow.

Angina Pectoris. This is the Latin term for an intense pain in the chest. It usually results from an insufficient flow of blood to the heart muscle for meeting the demands which are imposed. Often, the pain occurs during emotional excitement or exercise, and subsides when the stress factor is

[1]DeBakey, M., and A. Gotto, *The Living Heart,* David McKay Company, Inc., New York, N.Y., p. 219.

removed. However, similar pain felt in the chest may also originate from the upper part of the digestive tract in such disorders as gallstones, hiatal hernia, ulcers of the stomach or duodenum; or when the small intestine is distended with fluid, food, or gas.

Lying down may aggravate the pain from a diseased heart because (1) more blood than usual flows into the chambers of the heart, with the result that greater muscular force is needed to expel it; or (2) a full stomach may press up against the heart, cutting off some of its blood supply, therefore, the fastest relief from angina may usually be obtained by remaining still in either a sitting or standing position.

Angina may be a warning of an impending heart attack, so it should lead one to obtain prompt diagnosis and treatment.

Atherosclerosis.

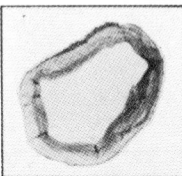 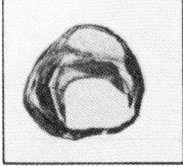 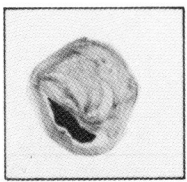

NORMAL ARTERY   FATTY DEPOSITS IN   PLUGGED ARTERY
                     VESSEL WALL   WITH FATTY DEPOSITS
                                             AND CLOT

**ACTUAL PHOTOGRAPH OF THE DEVELOPMENT OF
ATHEROSCLEROSIS**

Fig. H-6. The development of atherosclerosis in an artery. (Reprinted with permission, American Heart Association, Dallas, Tex.)

This degenerative disease, which is characterized by the buildup of abnormal patches (plaques) on the walls of arteries, is thought to be the main cause of heart attacks.

Coronary Occlusion (Coronary Thrombosis). If a coronary artery is partially blocked by a blood clot, it is commonly called a coronary thrombosis. If the blood clot completely blocks the blood flow, it is called a coronary occlusion.

Occlusion, or blocking, of the coronary circulation is usually caused by extensive atherosclerosis and/or a blood clot lodged in an artery. Occlusion is likely to occur in the coronary system before it does in other major arteries because, during the heartbeat, there is a moment when the blood literally "stands still" in these arteries. This condition occurs because each contraction of the heart muscle squeezes the coronary arteries and temporarily stops the forward flow of blood in them. The flow of blood in these arteries resumes when the muscle relaxes between contractions. Slowing of the movement of blood favors the development of such obstructions as atherosclerotic deposits and clots, when other conditions are also favorable for these developments.

Heart Failure. The heart may fail to pump sufficient blood to various tissues when there are conditions such as those which follow:

1. The heart muscle is weakened by chronic overwork, infectious disease, nutrient deficiencies, or a reduction in its blood supply.

2. There is damage to the heart valves which regulate the flow of blood.

3. The transmission of the heartbeat through the heart muscle is abnormal.

4. The beating of the heart muscle fibers is not coordinated in a regular rhythm.

5. The demands on the heart to pump blood are stepped up by such factors as emotional excitement, high blood pressure, strenuous exercise, an expansion of the volume of blood in circulation resulting from the enlargement (dilation) of small blood vessels, or a speeding up of metabolism such as occurs during a fever, or when the thyroid gland is overactive.

6. There is an increased resistance to the flow of blood because the openings in the blood vessels are narrowed or obstructed, the blood itself is thickened, or there is an accumulation of excessive fluid in various tissues.

Myocardial Infarction. When the coronary artery or one of its branches is obstructed (occluded), tissue may be damaged if there are areas of the heart muscle which do not receive sufficient blood. These damaged areas are called *infarcts*, and the coronary occlusion is simply called a *coronary*.

Irregular Heartbeats. Normally, the beating of the individual fibers in the heart muscle is coordinated so that the muscle contractions are regular and smooth. However, the normal rhythm of the heartbeat may be lost when the heart is sorely taxed and there may be a rapid and irregular twitching of the individual muscle fibers, which is called *fibrillation*. When this occurs in the muscle around the large chambers (ventricles) of the heart, the pumping action may stop, producing what is commonly called *cardiac arrest*. Death usually occurs within a few minutes, unless the fibrillation is corrected. Some people who have survived longer periods of fibrillation have had severe brain damage due to lack of blood. Disorders of heart rhythm are believed to be the main cause of sudden death due to cardiovascular disease in the United States.

FACTORS AFFECTING CARDIOVASCULAR DISEASES.

There have been countless studies of both animals and humans which were aimed at identifying the specific dietary and other factors responsible for cardiovascular diseases. Details follow.

Ethnic Groups. The first large-scale studies found that the countries with high rates of the disease were characterized by diets rich in butter, cheese, cream, and meat, and in highly refined sugars. Other researchers were quick to point out that certain peoples who eat plenty of animal fats have exceptionally low rates of heart disease, citing (1) the Masais of Africa, (2) the Georgians of the U.S.S.R., and (3) the Eskimos.

The Masai, a tribe of nomadic herdsmen in East Africa, have low death rates from cardiovascular diseases, even though their diet is rich in fat from blood, meat, and milk. (They regularly draw blood from the jugular veins of their cattle.)[2]

It is well known that the people in the Georgian region of the Soviet Union are among the most long-lived in the world, yet they consume plenty of dairy products, meats, and sweets—foods which are often blamed for the high rates of heart attacks in other societies.[3]

[2]Mann, G. V., et al., "Cardiovascular Disease in the Masai," *Journal of Atherosclerosis Research*, Vol. 4, 1964, p. 289.

[3]Leaf, A., "Search for the Oldest People," *National Geographic*, Vol. 143, 1973, p.93.

Finally, it has often been said that the Eskimos who still live under primitive conditions are an outstanding contradiction of the theory that animal fats cause heart disease, since their diet consists mainly of animal flesh and fish.

Findings from studies such as those cited above neither prove nor disprove that dietary fat is a cause of heart disease. Rather, they show that it is likely that this type of disease is the end result of many different dietary and nondietary conditions, which may not be obvious to those investigating only a few such conditions.

The Framingham Study Of Risk Factors.
This well-known study was conducted from 1949 to 1969 on over 5,000 men and women, aged 30 to 62, in Framingham, Massachusetts, which is about 20 miles southwest of Boston. The subjects were free of clinical signs of coronary heart disease at the beginning of the study, and they were examined once every other year for signs of the disorders which often accompany this disease. Data obtained in the study were used to estimate the risks for the development of heart disease by men and women who had certain characteristics. The factors which were found to add to the risk of heart disease follow.

• **Abnormal electrocardiograms (EKG) and/or enlargement of the heart**—While abnormalities in an EKG may not always indicate heart disease, the data from this study showed that EKG abnormalities usually indicated a high risk of heart disease.

• **Elevated blood cholesterol**—Even though the risk due to high blood cholesterol alone was small, a blood value of 335 mg per 100 ml of blood conferred about 3 times the risk of a value of 185.

• **Glucose intolerance**—The investigators in the Framingham Study defined this abnormality as one or more of the following: a blood sugar value of 120 or more, diabetes, or sugar in the urine. This condition, whether alone or accompanied by other risk factors, was always associated with a higher risk of heart disease.

• **High blood pressure**—The chances of developing heart disease markedly increased as the blood pressure rose. For example, when other factors were the same, people with a systolic blood pressure (the highest reading) of 180 had about twice the risk as those who had a blood pressure of 120.

• **Lack of exercise**—It was found that active persons had only from 1/3 to 1/2 the risk of angina pectoris, myocardial infarction, or sudden death, as sedentary persons.[4]

• **Obesity**—People who were 20% or more heavier than their ideal weights had about double the risk of angina pectoris, triple the risk of sudden death in a heart attack, and about an equal risk of myocardial infarction as persons whose weights were ideal.[5]

• **Sex of subject**—When all of the other risk factors were similar, 45-year-old men were about 3 times as likely to develop heart disease as 45-year-old women.

• **Smoking**—The risk of heart disease for smokers was consistently about 1 1/2 times as great as that for nonsmokers, when the other risk factors were the same for both groups.

Dietary Components and Heart Disease.
The American Heart Association has long asserted that most people in the United States might reduce their risk of developing cardiovascular diseases by (1) reducing their consumption of dietary sources of saturated fats and cholesterol such as beef, pork, eggs, butter, cheeses, and ice cream; and (2) substituting polyunsaturated vegetable oils for saturated animal fats. On the other hand, the opponents of these recommendations have argued that there has been a modest decline in heart disease mortality, even though the per capita consumption of beef and pork has recently reached an all-time high.

Some of the current, but controversial, ideas about individual foods and nutrients which contribute to heart disease follow.

ALCOHOLIC BEVERAGES. There have been many debates on the merits and demerits of the use of various alcoholic beverages by persons suffering from heart disease.

In moderation, alcoholic beverages, especially beer and wine, may have a beneficial effect by relaxing and calming jittery people. However, in people with healthy hearts, excessive alcohol can induce irregular heart beats, heart enlargement, and deterioration of heart function.[6]

(Also see ALCOHOLIC BEVERAGES; BEERS AND BREWING; DISTILLED LIQUOR; and WINE.)

CAFFEINE-CONTAINING BEVERAGES. Caffeine stimulates the heart directly. It causes the coronary arteries to dilate, thereby increasing the blood flow, the blood pressure, and the heart rate. Too much caffeine can cause irregular heart beats in heart patients.[7] Caffeine-containing beverages include coffee, cola beverages and certain other types of soft drinks, and tea.

(Also see CAFFEINE; COFFEE; SOFT DRINKS; and TEA.)

CARBOHYDRATES. Diabetes and other disorders of carbohydrate metabolism are frequently accompanied by various signs of heart disease. The most common of these disorders is high blood levels of triglycerides (hypertriglyceridemia) due to poor utilization of carbohydrates and fats. Many research studies on both animals and humans have produced evidence that high blood triglycerides may be associated with rapid clotting of the blood and angina pectoris.[8]

---

[4]Kannel, W. B., "The Disease of Living," Nutrition Today, Vol. 6, No. 3, 1971, pp. 2-11.

[5]Ibid.

[6]Rios, Jorge C., M.D., Chairman, Department of Medicine, George Washington University Medical Center; and a practicing cardiologist. From: Cardiac Alert, Mid-April, 1985, Vol. 7, No. 5, published by Phillips Publishing, Inc., 7315 Wisconsin Avenue, Suite 1200N, Bethesda, Maryland.

[7]Ibid.

[8]Scheig, R., "Diseases of Lipid Metabolism," in Duncan's Diseases of Metabolism, 7th ed., edited by P. K. Bondy and L. E. Rosenberg, W. B. Saunders Company, Philadelphia, Pa., 1974, p. 383.

It seems that the disorder(s) which result(s) in high triglycerides and poor carbohydrate utilization may be at least partly corrected in some people by the administration of glucose tolerance factor (GTF), a complex substance containing chromium, which increases the effectiveness of insulin.[9] The chronic consumption of table sugar (pure sucrose), white flour, and other highly refined sources of carbohydrates may deplete the body's stores of chromium because (1) the carbohydrates in the foods cause increased excretion of chromium, and (2) refining of these foods removes their naturally occurring chromium.

(Also see CARBOHYDRATE[S]; CHROMIUM; DIABETES MELLITUS; GLUCOSE TOLERANCE FACTOR.)

ENERGY. Consumption of more food energy (kilocalories) than is needed eventually leads to obesity and an increased risk of heart disease. Many studies have shown that the blood fats (cholesterol and triglycerides) which are believed to be involved in atherosclerosis rise in obesity and fall when the excess weight is lost. Also, it seems that cholesterol is synthesized, then stored in the body fat to a much greater extent in obese people compared to those who are lean.[10]

FATTY SUBSTANCES. The relationships between the various fatty substances in the diet, the blood levels of the substances, and the formation of clots and plaques in the major arteries are complex and not well understood. Nevertheless, some of the current ideas on the effects of the various fatty substances found in most diets are noteworthy.

Cholesterol. It appears that people differ considerably in their response to dietary cholesterol; so, many nutritionists question the wisdom of recommending that everyone cut down on cholesterol consumption when only a limited number of people have a tendency to develop high blood cholesterol from consuming foods high in cholesterol. Furthermore, other factors such as dietary energy, amount and type of fats, and fiber appear to affect the utilization of dietary cholesterol. However, the American Heart Association recommends a limit of 300 mg of cholesterol each day. **NOTE WELL:** There is evidence that total blood cholesterol is a poor indicator of a heart attack. Rather, the level of the lipoproteins which carry cholesterol in the blood, specifically high-density lipoproteins (HDL) and low-density lipoproteins (LDL) are better indicators. HDL has a protective role since it transports cholesterol back to the liver, while LDL seems to deposit cholesterol in cells, including blood vessels. Also, evidence indicates that high HDL decreases the risk of heart attack, while high LDL increases the risk.

(Also see CHOLESTEROL; and HYPERLIPOPROTEINEMIAS.)

Essential Fatty Acids. Certain polyunsaturated fatty acids (PUFA)—essential fatty acids (EFA)—are required in small amounts because they are not synthesized in the body. The most important of the essential fatty acids is linoleic acid because it has several vital functions in the body, one of which is to serve as raw material for the synthesis of other compounds. Although linoleic acid and other polyunsaturated fatty acids may lower blood cholesterol and retard the clotting of blood, it does not appear that the various cardiovascular disorders are due to deficiencies of these fatty acids, since they are abundantly supplied by most vegetable oils, fats from pork and poultry, and, in smaller amounts, by fats from beef and lamb.

Fats: Polyunsaturated vs Saturated. According to the American Heart Association, up to 30% of the total calorie intake may be from fat, but no more than one-third of this should be saturated fats. Sources of polyunsaturated fats are: canola (rapeseed), corn, cottonseed, olive, peanut, safflower, sesame, soybean, sunflower, and walnut oils.

(Also see FATS AND OTHER LIPIDS; OILS, VEGETABLE; and TRANS FATTY ACIDS.)

Lecithin and Other Phospholipids. These compounds act as bonds between fats and proteins in cell membranes, and in the special lipoproteins which carry cholesterol and fats (triglycerides) in the blood. They also promote the absorption of fatty substances in the intestine. For example, it is believed that the high rate of absorption of cholesterol from eggs is due in part to the lecithin which is present in the egg yolk.

The interest in lecithin as a protective factor against heart disease arose from the finding that high ratios of cholesterol to to phospholipids in the blood were correlated with the severity of atherosclerosis.[11] Furthermore, it is established that the phospholipids of the platelet plasma membrane play an important role in blood coagulation.[12]

It is thought that the body synthesizes the phospholipids that it requires as long as there is a sufficient body supply of methionine, magnesium, protein, polyunsaturated fatty acids, and vitamin B-6 (pyridoxine). However, this may not be the case when the feeding of diets rich in polyunsaturated fats causes a rise in the cholesterol content of bile, which may lead to gallstones. It has been reported that the feeding of lecithin raised the levels of phospholipid in the bile of patients afflicted with gallstones.[13]

(Also see LECITHIN; and PHOSPHOLIPIDS.)

FIBER. Adding soluble high-fiber foods to the diet may reduce blood cholesterol by as much as 13% to 22%. Soluble fiber (fiber which dissolves in water) slows down the stomach's digestive process. This affects cholesterol as follows: The liver uses cholesterol to form bile salts which digest food in the intestines. Slowing down the digestive process causes the body to excrete more bile salt, which, in turn, forces the liver to use up more of its stored cholesterol.

Good sources of soluble fiber are: root vegetables (such as carrots, parsnips, and potatoes); legumes (such as chickpeas, dried beans, green peas, and lentils; fruit (especially apples); oats; and sesame.

(Also see FIBER.)

---

[9]Doisy, R. J., et al., "Chromium Metabolism in Man and Biochemical Effects," *Trace Elements in Human Health and Disease,* Vol. II, edited by A. S. Prasad and D. Oberleas, Academic Press, New York, N.Y., 1976, pp. 91-96.

[10]Scheibman, P. H., "Diet and Plasma Lipids," in *Diet and Atherosclerosis,* edited by C. Sirtori, G. Ricci, and S. Gorini, Plenum Press, New York, N.Y., 1975, p. 159.

[11]Harper, H. A., *Review of Physiological Chemistry,* 15th ed., Lange Medical Publications, Los Altos, California, 1975, p. 320.

[12]Zwaal, R.F.A. and C.H. Hemker, "Blood Cell Membranes and Haemostasis," *Haemostasis,* Vol. 11, 1982, p. 12.

[13]Tompkins, R. K., et al., "Elevation of Phospholipid Concentrations in Human Bile by Feeding Lecithin," (Abstract), *Federation Proceedings,* Vol. 27, 1968, p. 573.

MACROMINERALS. Most of the mineral elements that are required in relatively large amounts (macrominerals) are supplied by diets containing a moderate variety of plant and animal foods. However, certain types of diets, which are low in such nutritious foods as dairy products, fish, fresh vegetables, lean meats, and unrefined grains, may furnish only marginal amounts of the essential macrominerals which, in addition to other functions, may protect against heart disease. Also, excesses of certain elements may aggravate deficiencies of others. Discussions of macrominerals associated with the functioning of the heart and blood vessels follow.

(Also see MINERAL[S].)

Calcium. Studies indicate that, in addition to building strong bones, calcium may lower blood pressure, which, in turn, will lessen the risk of heart attack. Good sources of calcium are milk and other dairy products, blackstrap molasses, green leafy vegetables, and fish eaten with bone (for example, sardines and salmon).

On the other hand, elevated blood levels of calcium (hypercalcemia) may promote irregular heartbeats, toxicity of cardiac drugs, and/or deposits of the mineral in the arteries and kidneys. Hypercalcemia is *not* usually due to dietary calcium, but to such factors as an excess of vitamin D or a deficiency of magnesium.

(Also see CALCIUM; and MINERAL[S].)

Magnesium. This element appears to provide at least partial protection against such cardiovascular disorders as arteriosclerosis, excessive clotting of the blood, high blood pressure, nonrhythmic heartbeats, and metabolic abnormalities in the heart muscle.[14] Magnesium also appears to protect arteries against the calcium deposits which occur with aging (arteriosclerosis).[15]

Although some nutritionists claim that the diets consumed by most Americans contain sufficient magnesium, others doubt whether this is true because (1) there has been a steady decline in the consumption of such sources of the element as green, leafy vegetables, legumes, and whole grains; and (2) the conditions of acidosis, alcoholism, chronic use of diuretic drugs, diabetes, and diarrhea tend to increase the loss of magnesium from the body.

(Also see MAGNESIUM; and MINERAL[S].)

Potassium. Adequate potassium may lower blood pressure, which, in turn, will lessen the risk of heart attack. Also, depletion of potassium from the heart muscle renders it more susceptible to nonrythmic beating, particularly when digitalis is used to treat heart failure.

Generally, a deficiency of potassium sufficient to impair the functioning of the heart does *not* result from a dietary shortage of the element since many foods are good sources. However, the supply of the mineral in the cells of the heart muscle may be low due to such factors as (1) excessive losses in the digestive tract (as diarrhea and vomiting), in sweat (particularly during hot and humid weather), or in urine (as a result of acidosis, diuretics, and various stress factors);

and/or lack of sufficient magnesium for the process which pumps potassium into the cells.

The best sources of potassium are dried fruits, wheat and rice bran, and meat.

An excess of potassium is dangerous and may cause cardiac arrest when kidney function is impaired because, when the latter condition exists, the body cannot get rid of an overload.

(Also see MINERAL[S]; and POTASSIUM.)

Sodium. This element is vital to life, so it is fortunate that the human body has remarkable ways of conserving it when dietary intakes are low. However, the ability to conserve short supplies, or to excrete excesses in the urine, varies considerably among different people, and the processes also vary according to the condition of health. For example, some of the people who consume moderate to large excesses of sodium may fail to excrete completely such excesses and, therefore, suffer such consequences as buildup of excessive fluid in the blood and tissues, damage to the kidneys, heart failure, and/or high blood pressure. There is evidence that susceptibility to these sodium-induced disorders may be a trait that runs in certain families.

At the other extreme are people who lose excessive amounts of sodium in their urine, due to such conditions as Addison's disease or kidney diseases. This may lead to excessive loss of water from the body, dangerous declines in the pressure and volume of the blood, and failure of the heart and blood vessels to deliver sufficient blood to the tissues. These circumstances may lead to the complete cutoff of blood flow to the kidneys, a condition which might cause kidney damage.

It is noteworthy that certain vegetarians may consume only small amounts of sodium because their diets are based mainly upon unprocessed, unsalted plant foods which contain only traces of the mineral. Animal foods and commercially processed plant foods usually contain sufficient sodium so that the adding of extra salt is not necessary. However, normally healthy people on low intakes of salt may suffer from sodium deficiency if they are exposed to hot environments, or if they engage in strenuous activities that provoke heavy losses of sweat.

(Also see MINERAL[S]; SODIUM.)

MICROMINERALS (Trace Elements). The importance of these essential elements may often be overlooked in investigations of the causes of heart disease, because only small quantities are required and deficiencies may develop only after long periods on poor diets. However, a variety of these elements is necessary for (1) various functions of the cardiovascular system, and (2) the regulation of metabolic processes which directly or indirectly affect the heart and blood vessels. Furthermore, they are often the nutrients most likely to be removed during the processing of such foods as whole grains, or to be rendered unavailable because they are bound by naturally occurring food constituents like oxalates and phytates, or by food additives like ethylenediaminetetraacetic acid (EDTA). (EDTA is added to foods so as to bind metals like copper and zinc which may cause discoloration of the products.) Therefore, a discussion of some trace elements and their functions follows.

Chromium and the Glucose Tolerance Factor. It was recently found that chromium in the form of glucose tolerance factor (GTF) may prevent disorders of carbohydrate metabolism which, in turn, could lead to heart disease.

[14]Seelig, M. S., and H. A. Heggtveit, "Magnesium Interrelationships in Ischemic Heart Disease: A Review," *The American Journal of Clinical Nutrition*, Vol. 27, 1974, p. 59.

[15]Szelenyi, I., "Magnesium and Its Significance in Cardiovascular and Gastro-Intestinal Disorders," *World Review of Nutrition and Dietetics*, Vol. 17, edited by G. H. Bourne, published by S. Karger, Basel, Switzerland, 1973, p. 195.

Evidence of a direct relationship between chromium deficiency and cardiovascular disorders in the United States consists of the findings that (1) chromium could not be detected in the aortas of people dying from heart disease, but it was found in those of people who died from accidents; (2) the levels of chromium in the hearts and aortas of people in the United States were only a fraction of the levels found in these tissues from people in most other parts of the world.[16]

(Also see CHROMIUM; GLUCOSE TOLERANCE FACTOR; and MINERAL[S].)

Copper. This mineral element is required for the production of red blood cells, the formation of connective tissue, and as a component of various enzymes. When rapidly growing young animals are given diets deficient in copper, they become susceptible to rupture of such major blood vessels as the aorta, enlargement of the heart, and degeneration of the heart muscle.[17] These findings suggest that similar disorders in man might be due in part to copper deficiencies during periods of rapid growth. It is noteworthy that high dietary levels of the minerals iron, molybdenum, and zinc may interfere with the utilization of copper.

(Also see COPPER; and MINERAL[S].)

Iodine. The sole function of iodine in the human body is as a component of the hormones secreted by the thyroid gland. A dietary deficiency of iodine may lead to low levels of these hormones (hypothyroidism), a condition which is often accompanied by high blood cholesterol, and in some cases, atherosclerosis. Studies in Finland have shown that, although the dietary levels of fat are similar throughout the country, there seem to be more cases of cardiovascular diseases in the areas where the rates of goiter (an enlargement of the thyroid due to iodine deficiency) are also high.[18]

(Also see IODINE; and MINERAL[S].)

Iron. It is well known that severe deficiencies of iron may cause the heart to race in order to pump enough oxygen-poor blood to the tissues. (The blood becomes oxygen-poor due to lack of red cells which require iron for their production.) Although these deficiencies are nowhere near as common in the developed countries as in the developing countries where iron-deficiency anemia may be a leading cause of disability or death, certain conditions such as heavy menstrual flow, hemorrhage, or pregnancy may lead to their occurrence in the developed countries.

(Also see IRON; and MINERAL[S].)

Manganese. This element is required for blood clotting, carbohydrate metabolism, and as a component of various enzymes. Studies have shown that animals deficient in manganese have abnormal metabolism of glucose (a simple sugar), a defect which is corrected by manganese supplementation.[19]

(Also see MANGANESE; and MINERAL[S].)

Selenium. It has been reported that the region of the United States where the crops have the highest content of this mineral (roughly, an area lying between the Mississippi River and the Rocky Mountains)[20] have the lowest incidence of deaths from heart disease.[21]

Other evidence of the protective effects of selenium against heart disease consists of (1) its action as part of the enzyme which breaks down toxic peroxides that may damage the heart muscle, particularly those formed from polyunsaturated fats;[22] and (2) its counteraction of the toxicity of cadmium, a common environmental pollutant which causes kidney abnormalities leading to high blood pressure.[23]

(Also see SELENIUM; and MINERAL[S].)

Silicon. A deficiency of this mineral might be a factor in the development of cardiovascular diseases, because the silicon content of human aortas decreases with aging and with the development of atherosclerosis.

Although silicon is one of the most abundant chemical elements on the face of the earth, its inorganic compounds are poorly utilized by man and the higher animals. Its more readily utilized organic forms are generally present in the connective tissues of animals and in the fibrous tissues of plants, two forms of food which are often spurned by people who prefer soft, highly refined items. For example, most of the silicon is removed during the production of table sugar from sugar cane, and in the milling of whole wheat to make flour.

(Also see MINERAL[S]; and SILICON.)

Zinc. Diabeticlike disorders of metabolism have been observed in zinc-deficient animals, but the basis for this abnormality is not understood.

Better known is the promotion of wound healing by zinc. This property appears to have been responsible for the marked improvement in the circulations of patients suffering from severe atherosclerosis.[24]

Finally, studies over the past 10 years or so have produced strong evidence that the counteraction of the toxic effects of cadmium by zinc may help to prevent various forms of cardiovascular diseases. For example, a study in North Carolina of the associations between cardiovascular disorders and the trace element levels in the organs of deceased people showed that low ratios of zinc to cadmium in the kidneys were associated with both atherosclerosis and high blood pressure.[25]

[16]Schroeder, H. A., "The Role of Chromium in Mammalian Nutrition," *The American Journal of Clinical Nutrition,* Vol. 21, 1968, p. 230.

[17]"Brain and Myocardial Lesions in Copper-Deficient Young Rats," *Nutrition Reviews,* Vol. 33, 1975, p. 306.

[18]Davidson, S., R. Passmore, and J. F. Brock, *Human Nutrition and Dietetics,* 5th ed., The Williams and Wilkins Company, Baltimore, Md., 1972, p. 323.

[19]Everson, G. J., and R. E. Shrader, "Abnormal Glucose Tolerance in Manganese Deficient Guinea Pigs," *The Journal of Nutrition,* Vol. 94, 1968, p. 89.

[20]Hodgson, J. F., W. H. Allaway, and R. B. Lockman, "Regional Plant Chemistry as a Reflection of Environment," *Environmental Geochemistry in Health and Disease,* edited by Helen L. Cannon and Howard C. Hopps, The Geographical Society of America, Boulder, Colo., *Memoir 123,* 1971, p.61, Fig. 2.

[21]Sauer, H. I., and F. R. Brand, "Geographic Patterns in the Risk of Dying," *Environmental Geochemistry in Health and Disease,* edited by Helen L. Cannon and Howard C. Hopps, The Geographical Society of America, Boulder, Colo., *Memoir 123,* 1971, p. 137.

[22]Hoekstra, W. G., "Biochemical role of Selenium," *Trace Element Metabolism in Animals-2,* edited by W. G. Hoekstra, et al., University Park Press, Baltimore, Md., 1974, p. 61.

[23]Underwood, E. J., *Trace Elements in Human and Animal Nutrition,* 4th ed., Academic Press, New York, N.Y., 1977, p. 253.

[24]Pories, W. J., W. H. Strain, and C. G. Rob, "Zinc Deficiency in Delayed Healing and Chronic Disease," *Environmental Geochemistry in Health and Disease,* edited by Helen L. Cannon and Howard C. Hopps, The Geographical Society of America, Boulder, Colo., *Memoir 123,* 1971, p. 90.

[25]Voors, A. W., M. S. Shuman, and P. N. Gallagher, "Atherosclerosis and Hypertension in Relation to Some Trace Elements in Tissues," *World Review of Nutrition and Dietetics,* edited by G. H. Bourne, published by S. Karger, Basel, Switzerland, 1975, Vol. 20, p. 299.

VITAMINS AND VITAMINLIKE FACTORS. Certain vitamins may be involved in processes associated with the cardiovascular system. Also, excesses of some vitamins may result in deficiencies of others. There is also evidence that the massive doses which may be used to treat deficiencies and other disorders may do more harm than good. Details follow.

Inositol. This vitaminlike substance is synthesized within the body. Nevertheless, under certain circumstances it may be like a vitamin in that a dietary supply is required for optimal health.

Like choline, which is part of the compounds which are commonly called lecithins, inositol is an important component of phospholipids which help to stabilize blood cholesterol and prevent its deposition on the walls of arteries. Sometimes, the administration of inositol has helped to reduce accumulations of fatty substances (lipids) in the blood and the liver. Hence, it is designated as an agent which aids in the utilization of lipids (a lipotropic factor). However, it appears that the actions of inositol are closely tied to those of such other nutrients as choline, essential fatty acids, phospholipids, niacin, and vitamin B-6 (pyridoxine). Finally, it is noteworthy that the heart muscle contains high levels of inositol, which suggests that it has an important cardiac function.

The body's requirements for inositol may exceed the rate of its synthesis when (1) the urinary excretion of this nutrient is high, such as in diabetes, or when there is copious urination resulting from the consumption of alcoholic beverages; or (2) there is an accumulation of fatty substances in the blood and/or the liver due to bad diets or various metabolic disorders.

(Also see INOSITOL; and VITAMIN[S].)

Vitamin A. Although various animal studies have shown that supplemental doses of this vitamin may help to heal atherosclerotic lesions and to lower blood cholesterol, similar studies in humans have yielded disappointing results. Hence, it is *not* certain at this time whether vitamin A supplements are beneficial for people with various cardiovascular disorders.

However, it is well established that vitamin A is involved in (1) the laying down of the connective tissue which lines the large blood vessels; (2) synthesis of various stress hormones; and (3) counteracting the effects of vitamin K in blood clotting (when large amounts of vitamin A are consumed). Therefore, it appears that adequate levels of vitamin A may help in maintaining the health of the cardiovascular system, but that excesses of the vitamin might be harmful.

(Also see VITAMIN[S]; and VITAMIN A.)

Thiamin (Vitamin B-1). It is well known that people suffering from severe thiamin deficiency, or beriberi, may die suddenly from heart failure. However, this severe deficiency is not often seen in the developed countries, except in certain alcoholics who eat poor diets. Also, hospital patients given only intravenous glucose (sugar) solutions without supplementary thiamin and other vitamins may develop severe thiamin deficiencies when such treatment lasts for prolonged periods of time (1 to 2 weeks).

(Also see THIAMIN; VITAMIN[S]; and VITAMIN B-COMPLEX.)

Niacin (Nicotinic Acid; Nicotinamide). Massive doses of this vitamin have been used to reduce elevated levels of blood fats. This practice may be dangerous because there is now evidence that it reduces the energy stores in the heart muscle.[26] (One of the effects of massive doses of niacin is the blocking of the release of free fatty acids from the fatty tissues, so the heart is forced to rely on its own stores of fat and glycogen.) However, the doses which have such effects are many times the amounts present in most diets.

(Also see NIACIN; VITAMIN[S]; and VITAMIN B-COMPLEX.)

Vitamin B-6 (Pyridoxine). Various studies conducted during the past 20 years or so have shown that monkeys fed a low-fat, vitamin B-6-deficient diet develop lesions of their blood vessels which are very similar to the atherosclerotic lesions in man. Hence, it has recently been suggested that perhaps some cases of atherosclerosis might be due to lack of this vitamin and/or excessive dietary amounts of the amino acid methionine, which requires pyridoxine for its metabolism.[27] Furthermore, the high-protein foods which are rich in cholesterol, such as dairy products, eggs, and meat, are also rich in methionine. Since the dietary requirement for pyridoxine depends to a large extent on the amount of protein eaten, the people who regularly consume large excesses of such foods might not receive sufficient amounts of this vitamin.

(Also see ATHEROSCLEROSIS; VITAMIN[S]; VITAMIN B-COMPLEX; and VITAMIN B-6.)

Vitamin B-12 (Cobalamin). Deficiencies of this vitamin are most likely to occur either among strict vegetarians who eat no animal foods, or among people over 40 who have various stomach disorders. Hence, some doctors inject large doses of this vitamin into people who show signs of the deficiency since it is generally thought that these doses may be beneficial, but never harmful. However, it has recently been found that massive doses have caused blood clots in certain people.[28] The explanation for this effect was that severe deficiency of the vitamin resulted in pernicious anemia, a condition where the formation of blood cells was impaired, and the time required for the blood to clot was prolonged. Repeated injections of large doses of the vitamin over short periods of time (1,000 mcg daily for 1 or 2 weeks) caused overcorrection of the abnormalities, so that the blood clotted more rapidly than normal.

(Also see VITAMIN[S]; VITAMIN B-COMPLEX; VITAMIN B-12.)

Vitamin C and the Bioflavonoids. Some recent reports have presented evidence of the beneficial effects of vitamin C (ascorbic acid) on heart disease, while others state that the vitamin failed to produce such effects.

Perhaps one reason for these contradictory reports is that many investigators have relied upon the reduction of blood cholesterol as an indicator of a beneficial effect in man,

---

[26]"Niacin and Myocardial Metabolism," *Nutrition Reviews,* Vol. 31, 1973, p. 80.

[27]"Study Questions Cholesterol Role," *Journal of the American Medical Association,* Vol. 212, 1970, p. 257.

[28]"A Qualitative Platelet Defect in Severe Vitamin B-12 Deficiency," *Nutrition Reviews,* Vol. 32, 1974, p. 202.

whereas in animal studies the arteries are usually examined for atherosclerotic lesions. For example, a series of studies of the effects of a mild lack of dietary vitamin C in guinea pigs (which, like man, need dietary ascorbic acid) has shown that a chronic deficiency led to (1) elevations in blood and liver cholesterol; (2) a reduced rate of conversion of cholesterol to bile salts (which may favor the buildup of cholesterol); and (3) atherosclerotic lesions, even when no cholesterol was given in the diet.[29]

Another reason for the variable results of vitamin C supplementation might be that certain people may need less of the vitamin than those who are exposed to chronic stresses and smoking. During stress, the ascorbic acid content of the adrenal glands drops markedly, while the synthesis of cholesterol in these tissues is greatly increased.

Finally many of the natural sources of vitamin C also contain substances called *bioflavonoids* which appear to have effects like those of the vitamin (such as strengthening capillary walls against breakage or leakage of fluid), and which may protect it against destruction.[30] Hence, the effects of a given amount of dietary vitamin C may vary according to the amounts of bioflavonoids which are present in the diet.

(Also see BIOFLAVONOIDS; VITAMIN[S]; and VITAMIN C.)

Vitamin D. It is well known that overdoses of this vitamin may promote the deposition of calcium in such soft tissues as the kidneys. Recently, it has been suggested that overdoses might also be responsible for various cardiovascular disorders. It seems that high intakes of the vitamin increase the requirement for magnesium, and that some of the damage might be prevented by equally high intakes of this mineral.

(Also see VITAMIN[S]; and VITAMIN D.)

Vitamin E. This vitamin has long been extolled as beneficial for both the prevention and treatment of heart disease. Certainly, it is necessary to consume greater amounts of vitamin E when extra polyunsaturated fats are taken, or when the dietary levels of selenium are low. (Vitamin E prevents the formation of toxic peroxides from polyunsaturated fats, while selenium is part of the enzyme which breaks down the peroxides once they are formed.)

Although the so-called anticlotting effect of large doses of vitamin E has often been described, the basis for the effect is not well understood. A recent report has attributed it to interference with the action of vitamin K, a factor which is required for the clotting of blood.[31] This report came from doctors who noted bleeding in the skin of a man treated with an anticlotting drug, who also took, without their advice, a daily dose of up to 1,200 IU of vitamin E per day. However, the anticlotting drug which was used also interfered with vitamin K activity, so it is not known whether vitamin E alone might have produced such a drastic effect. Nevertheless, this observation suggests that self-treatment

with large doses of vitamin E might be dangerous, particularly for people on anticlotting drugs, or for those who have high blood pressure.

(Also see VITAMIN[S]; and VITAMIN E.)

Vitamin K. Many people may not have to worry about whether they get sufficient amounts of this vitamin, if they regularly eat green leafy vegetables (the best of the food sources of the vitamin) or carry within their intestines bacteria such as *E. coli* which synthesize the vitamin (except when the bacteria are killed by medicines that are taken orally for various infectious diseases).

The traditional anticlotting therapy for victims of heart disease consists of drugs which block the action of vitamin K. However, people so treated have sometimes died from massive hemorrhages in the heart muscle, particularly in the days before the need for frequent checks on blood clotting times was recognized. A recent report suggests that the mineral manganese also must be present in adequate amounts in order for vitamin K to have its full effect on blood clotting.[32] Hence, people who are deficient in manganese may be extra susceptible to the effects of anticoagulant drugs.

(Also see VITAMIN K; and VITAMIN[S].)

Other Factors Associated with Heart Disease. The consequences of poor diet may be aggravated by various other factors. For example, a person with an inherited tendency to have high blood levels of various fats might be much more affected by a high-cholesterol, high-fat diet than a person who has no hereditary abnormality. Likewise, people with certain temperaments may be more susceptible to emotional stress factors.

In addition to the factors listed and discussed up to this point, the following additional risk factors may be associated with heart disease:

1. Advanced atherosclerosis and hardening of the arteries (Arteriosclerosis).
2. Allergic reactions.
3. Blood abnormalities other than high cholesterol, including—
   a. Acidosis and/or ketosis.
   b. Elevated blood sugar.
   c. Elevated free fatty acids.
   d. Excessive blood volume.
   e. High triglycerides.
   f. High uric acid levels.
   g. Imbalances between various ions (electrolyte imbalances).
   h. Thickening of the blood.
4. Body builds.
5. Chronic constipation.
6. Climate and weather, including—
   a. Cold weather.
   b. Warm weather.
   c. Dry weather.
   d. Humid weather.
7. Congenital defects.
8. Crash dieting.

[29]Ginter, L., "Vitamin C in Lipid Metabolism and Atherosclerosis," *Vitamin C*, edited by G. G. Birch and K. J. Parker, Applied Science Publishers, Ltd., Essex, England, 1974, p. 179.

[30]Kuhnau, J., "The Flavonoids. A Class of Semi-Essential Food Components: Their Role in Human Nutrition," *World Review of Nutrition and Dietetics*, Vol. 24, edited by G. H. Bourne, published by S. Karger, Basel, Switzerland, 1976, p. 175.

[31]"Hypervitaminosis E and Coagulation," *Nutrition Reviews*, Vol. 33, 1975, p. 269.

[32]Doisy, E. A., Jr., "Effects of Deficiency in Manganese Upon Plasma Levels of Clotting Proteins and Cholesterol in Man," *Trace Element Metabolism in Animals-2*, edited by W. G. Hoekstra, *et al.*, University Park Press, Baltimore, Md., 1974, p. 668.

9. Drugs, including—
   a. Antacids.
   b. Antibiotics.
   c. Antidepressants.
   d. Birth control pills.
   e. Cortisone.
   f. Digitalis.
   g. Insulin and oral antidiabetic drugs.
   h. Laxatives.
   i. Pep pills (or *uppers*).
   j. Rainbow pills for weight control.
   k. Thyroid hormones.
   l. Water pills.
10. Emotional stresses.
11. Glandular or hormonal disorders, including—
   a. Aldosterone and renin.
   b. Insulin.
   c. Stress hormones.
   d. Thyroid hormones.
12. Heavy meals.
13. Heredity.
14. Injuries to the blood vessels and/or the heart.
15. Kidney diseases.
16. Living in densely populated areas.
17. Medical treatments, including—
   a. Anesthesia.
   b. Dialysis of patients with kidney failure.
   c. Intravenous administration of glucose.
   d. Tube feeding of liquid formula diets.
18. Overly aggressive (Type A) behavior.
19. Physical stresses.
20. Soft drinking water.
21. Stickiness of blood platelets.
22. Toxic substances, including—
   a. Cadmium.
   b. Cobalt.
   c. Honey from poisonous plants.
   d. Lung irritants.
   e. Overheated fats.
   f. Pesticides.
   g. Poisonous potatoes.
   h. Tobacco smoke.

SIGNS AND SYMPTOMS OF HEART DISEASE.

Some of the characteristic features of heart disease may be so obvious that even lay people can recognize them. However, other more subtle signs may require special laboratory tests in order that experienced physicians may be certain of their diagnoses. Furthermore, the earlier that heart disease is detected, the better the outlook for the patient. Hence, it is worth noting the various ways in which heart disease may be diagnosed.

Easily Recognizable Abnormalities.

These conditions, which are readily recognizable by lay people, are often associated with major disorders of the heart although they may sometimes result from other types of medical problems. Therefore, it is wise to consider the possibility of heart disease whenever there are symptoms like those which follow:

1. **Pain in the chest (Angina pectoris).**
2. **Shortness of breath.**
3. **Fainting.**
4. **Fluid accumulation in various tissues.**
5. **Enlargement of the veins in the neck.**
6. **Chronic tiredness.**
7. **Palpitations.**

8. Coughing up blood.
9. Bluish coloring of the skin.
10. Arterial blockage in the legs.
11. Wheezing.

Detection Of Cardiovascular Disorders By Physical Examination.

Although it is usually preferable for a doctor to conduct a physical examination for heart problems, emergency situations may require that the examination be made by a nurse, paramedic, or even an untrained lay person. The common physical examination procedure is as follows:

1. Taking of the pulse.
2. Listening to the sounds of the heart.
3. Taking the blood pressure.
4. Examining the eyes.
5. Testing the functioning of the heart by exercising.

Special Diagnostic Procedures For Cardiovascular Problems.

Some of the characteristic features of heart disease are ambiguous in that they may sometimes be due to other causes. For example, severe pains in the chest may be due to a flare-up of gallstones, rather than a heart attack. Hence, the following clinical diagnostic procedures may be used:

1. Electrocardiogram (EKG).
2. Analysis of blood for certain enzymes.
3. X rays of the heart.
4. Analysis of blood for certain ions (electrically charged particles or electrolytes).
5. Measurement of hemoglobin in the blood.
6. Insertion of a catheter into the heart.
7. Analysis of blood for various fatty substances (lipids).

TREATMENT AND PREVENTION OF HEART DISEASE.

Many people with severe heart disease have lived full lives for long periods after the onset of their medical problems, thanks to well-designed therapies. Therefore, brief descriptions of a variety of helpful measures follow.

Emergency Care For Victims Of Heart Attacks.

While it is beyond the scope of this article to provide comprehensive descriptions of the various emergency measures for heart attacks, it is nevertheless appropriate to consider briefly what actions might be taken in certain critical situations, so that concerned people may take steps to prepare themselves for dealing with such emergencies. Hence, descriptions of both life-threatening emergencies and recommended countermeasures follow. (It is noteworthy that in many communities there are special courses in which lay persons are taught how to assist heart attack victims through severe crises.)

CARDIAC ARREST.

Stoppage of the pumping of blood by the heart is usually followed promptly by cessation of breathing. These are the most critical conditions which may accompany a heart attack because cells in the brain begin to die within a few minutes after the delivery of blood and oxygen is halted. Hence, *immediate* actions must be taken in order to (1) get the blood back into circulation, and (2) force air into the lungs.

Whether or not the heart is beating may be determined by feeling for a pulse in either one of the carotid arteries in the neck, or in the left or right femoral artery which runs along the inside of the thigh. The pulse in the wrist may be very difficult to detect when the heartbeat is weak. If a pulse appears to be absent in the patient, one should call for help and immediately begin the resuscitation procedure illustrated in Fig. H-7.

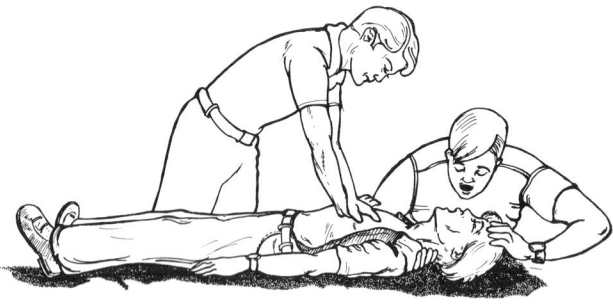

Fig. H-7. Revival of a person whose heart has stopped. This procedure is called *cardiopulmonary resuscitation (CPR)*. It involves (1) rhythmically pressing down the lower part of the breastbone against the heart 60 to 80 times per minute so as to pump blood to the tissues, and (2) mouth-to-mouth breathing 16 to 20 times per minute so as to force oxygenated air into the lungs of the victim. When resuscitation is attempted by only one person, every 15 chest compressions should be alternated with two respirations.

The procedure shown in Fig. H-7 should be continued until (1) the heart action and breathing of the victim resumes and remains steady, (2) help arrives with a defibrillator and a respirator, (3) at least 60 minutes have elapsed after cardiac arrest, when neither events (1) or (2) have occurred. Although *brain damage* may occur within a few minutes after cardiac arrest, the rhythmic compression of the chest and mouth-to-mouth breathing by the person(s) attempting resuscitation may provide a flow of blood to the brain which is sufficient to prevent such damage.

Another means of treating cardiac arrest is shown in Fig. H-8.

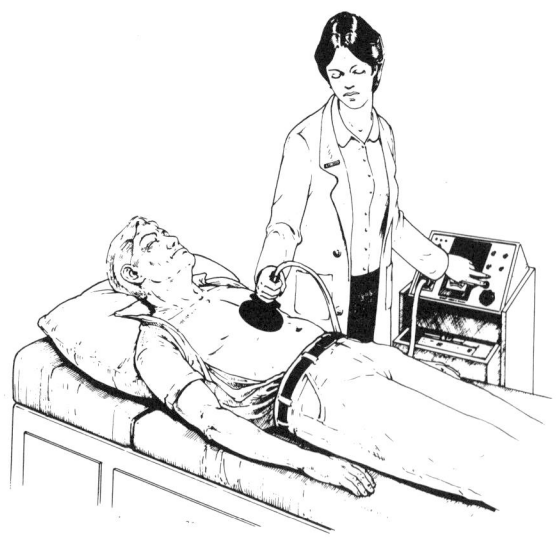

Fig. H-8. Using a defibrillator on a person in cardiac arrest. An electrical shock is applied to the chest of the victim in an attempt to induce the heart to resume its beating.

In addition to these emergency measures, doctors, nurses, or paramedics may inject one or more doses of adrenalin, atropine, digitalis, lidocaine, quinidine, or sodium bicarbonate so as to obtain the desired rhythm, speed, and force of the heartbeat.

If the attempts at reviving the patient have been successful, he or she is usually placed in the coronary care unit (CCU) of a hospital until it is fairly certain that the crisis has passed.

HEART ATTACK WITHOUT CARDIAC ARREST. A person might have the persistent chest pain of a heart attack, yet his or her heart rate and the blood pressure may remain normal. However, there is always the danger that the heartbeat will become highly irregular, or stop altogether, if the attack is not promptly and properly treated. Hence, some recommendations for handling this kind of emergency follow:

1. Send for assistance—a doctor, an ambulance, or a rescue squad. In some communities, paramedic teams may work with the firemen and police.

2. Make the patient as comfortable as possible by the loosening of tight clothing, helping him or her settle into a relaxed position on a soft surface, minimizing discomfort due to chilling or overheating, and generally going about things in a calm way so as to avoid exciting the patient.

3. Observe the patient carefully so that you might notice any turns for the worse, such as loss of consciousness and cardiac arrest. Be prepared to carry out promptly the revival measures outlined in the preceding section if such should be necessary.

ANGINA PECTORIS. This condition is characterized by pain similar to that which occurs in a heart attack, only it differs in that it is usually relieved in a few minutes by resting. However, it is noteworthy that the long-term survival rate for people with angina is only about as good as that for people who have had heart attacks. The outlook is disappointing because heart attacks may often strike those afflicted by one of the three dangerous types of angina which follow:

• **The first occurrence of angina pectoris**—It is difficult to predict the outcome when the patient has had no prior experience with this condition.

• **Angina which is not readily relieved by resting and nitroglycerine**—Pain which lasts after 15 to 20 minutes of resting and a moderate dose of nitroglycerine may indicate the onset of a heart attack.

• **Steadily worsening angina**—Sometimes, ever higher doses of nitroglycerine are needed to relieve the pain, the episodes of pain last longer, and they occur more frequently.

A doctor should be called for any of the three conditions described above.

• **Stable angina**—This refers to the type of angina which is predictably brought on by certain circumstances, and which is readily relieved by resting and/or moderate doses of nitroglycerine. The outlook for survival is much better in the case of stable angina than it is for any of the three dangerous types of the condition.

HEART FAILURE. The characteristics which differentiate heart failure from a heart attack are that the former (1) usually develops more slowly; (2) may occur without pain; (3)

is often accompanied by difficulty in breathing, weakness and chronic fatigue, fainting and/or dizziness, a rapid and feeble pulse, lack of appetite, swelling and tenderness of the liver, and fluid accumulation in the legs, lungs, and/or the abdomen.

However, the early stages of heart failure may be difficult for physicians to diagnose. Hence, the lay person is not likely to be in a position to make such a judgment. Therefore, anyone who suspects that a person they know has been stricken with heart failure should call a doctor. While awaiting medical assistance, someone should remain with the patient and be ready to carry out cardiopulmonary resuscitation, if necessary.

Long-Term Treatments.
There is good news for those who suffer from heart disease! Since 1975, there has been a reduction in deaths from heart disease in the United States. By following proper treatment, a heart patient can add many years to his or her life, and add life to the years. The sections that follow tell how this can be achieved.

BIOFEEDBACK.
This term refers to various techniques by which a limited amount of voluntary control is gained over certain body functions that were hitherto thought to be strictly automatic and therefore not subject to such control. It may be necessary for certain excitable people to learn how to exert control over their nerves so that they may prevent steep rises in blood pressure and/or racing of the heart when they become excited. Overreaction to emotional excitement, if habitual, could offset the benefits which accrue from the treatment of their disease. However, they may be taught how partially to control their blood pressure and heart rate by biofeedback, thereby countering the threat of various cardiovascular disorders.

Learning these techniques requires special exercises which are too detailed to describe here. However, briefly stated, the basic principles are: (1) the subject must have some means of measuring blood pressure, breathing, and heartbeat; (2) efforts are made to change the measurements by concentration, conjuring up various images, movements of certain muscles, and relaxation; and (3) the subject learns which of the various types of action were successful in altering certain functions. Hence, the *feedback* is the conscious *input* of the subject which alters the *output* of his or her body. For example, he or she watches for the tightening of the neck or shoulder muscles. Then, relaxation techniques are employed to loosen up the muscles.

Details of biofeedback may be obtained from recently published books on this subject, which are available in many public libraries.

CHANGING OF BEHAVIOR.
The effects of this type of therapy may augment or complement those obtained from biofeedback in that a patient learns how to avoid or minimize behaviors which may be self-destructive.

An important type of desirable behavior change is the development of certain attitudes which lessen stressful emotional reactions to common frustrations such as dealing with aggravatingly slow-paced people or driving in traffic jams. Also, the patient learns how to plan ahead so as to minimize the occurrence of stress-producing situations. Some suggestions for these behavior changes follow:

1. Try to anticipate slow traffic in bad weather, and allow extra time to get to work or to meet other commitments.

2. Drop unproductive, time-consuming activities such as participation in social affairs which fail to provide any tangible personal benefits.

3. Put in extra working hours, when necessary, on a regular basis so as to avoid *burning the midnight oil* on several consecutive nights prior to deadlines.

4. Beg off optional engagements which require staying up late on nights before working days.

5. Avoid excessive striving to win every argument, contest, or game engaged in with other people when the outcomes are not important.

6. Practice biofeedback, meditation, prayer, and/or other means of obtaining emotional peace without drinking, overeating, or taking drugs.

DIETARY MEASURES.
It is widely believed that many people might forestall the onset of cardiovascular disease by their adoption of more healthful diets. However, these diets should be planned on an individual basis so as to take into account the variable factors such as age, health status, heredity, level of activity, and sex. Not all people will need or benefit from drastic dietary changes.

Modified Diets for People Who May Be at Risk.
People who might be expected to have more than an average chance of developing heart disease are those who (1) have elevated blood levels of cholesterol (values over 240 mg per 100 ml of blood) and/or triglycerides (values over 150 mg per 100 ml of blood); (2) come from families with histories of premature heart disease; (3) show signs of angina pectoris or poor circulation of blood to various parts of the body; (4) have diabetic tendencies; or (5) who are obese (overweight by 20% or more). These people need to consult a physician in order to obtain the proper diagnosis and advice as to the dietary measures which might be most suitable for them.

One or more of the following types of diets may be recommended for people who may be at risk:

1. Low-cholesterol diet.
2. Low-energy diet.
3. Low-fat diet.
4. Low-salt (low sodium) diet.
5. Low-sugar diet.
6. Vegetarian diet.

Selection of Foods for Modified Diets.
Diets which are modified in order to avoid excessive intakes of cholesterol, energy, fats, and/or sugar may lead to nutritional deficiencies unless special efforts are made to select foods which have low levels of the restricted nutrients, but which have moderate to high levels of protein, minerals, and vitamins. These foods are generally called *protective foods* because the nutrients they contain help to maintain the health and strength of tissues against the onslaught of aging and various other stress factors. For example, a sound heart muscle might better withstand the effects of a *coronary* than one which has been weakened by deficiencies of various essential minerals and vitamins.

It would be desirable to rely as much as possible on obtaining nutrients from foods, and to resort to nutritional supplements only when certain nutrient-rich foods are not liked by the patient, or cannot be eaten because of medical problems. In order to plan diets containing optimal amounts of the required nutrients, it is necessary to (1) eat a wide variety of foods from both animal and plant sources, and

(2) select minimally refined foods whenever possible. This means that a typical diet might contain such items as those which follow:

1. Alcoholic beverages.
2. Beans and peas, eggs, fish, meats, nuts, oilseeds, and poultry.
3. Breads and cereal products.
4. Cocoa, coffee, and tea.
5. Dairy products.
6. Fruits and vegetables.
7. Herbs and spices.
8. Sweeteners.
9. Vegetable oils and margarines.

DONATIONS OF BLOOD.   In the not too distant past, the application of leeches to the skin of patients and bloodletting (the medical term is phlebotamy) were standard medical practices. Even today, doctors may periodically withdraw blood from people who have too many red cells (the condition called polycythemia) because an abnormally thickened blood clots too readily. Hence, it might be a good idea for those who have a high red cell count to make donations of their blood after first receiving assurance from their physicians that it is safe for them to do so.

DRUGS.   It may be tempting for people who have high blood levels of lipids and/or the earlier signs of cardiovascular disease to make only half-hearted attempts to adhere to stringent diets when they know that there are drugs which may be used to treat their disorders. However, more and more doctors are recommending that their patients make every effort to control their conditions by dieting, exercise, and healthy living habits because there are many dangers associated with most of the drugs which are commonly used. Nevertheless, there may be no choice other than drugs for people with hard-to-manage disorders; and, fortunately, many drugs—some old, some new—are available.

But the use of drugs in the prevention and treatment of heart disease should be only by prescription from an M.D.

EXERCISE.   Recently, there have been many reports describing how people with heart trouble so serious that they might in the past have been consigned to lives of semi-invalidism, have been given new leases on life by supervised programs of strenuous exercise. The reasons for such dramatic recoveries are still unclear, although it has long been suspected that exercise-induced enlargement of the small arteries of the heart, which are sometimes called the collateral circulation, has been a factor in this regard.

Now that it is known that recovered heart patients may safely tolerate a moderate amount of exercise stress, more and more health scientists are measuring various cardiovascular functions before and after periods of moderate to intensive physical training. One study showed that 6 weeks of training on an exercise bicycle, twice a day, 5 days per week enabled six middle-aged people who had suffered attacks to more than double the time that they could pedal vigorously before the onset of chest pain.[33] These patients were tested again 8 to 12 months later, and it was found that all of them had maintained their improved tolerance for exercise. However, one patient had suffered a nonfatal heart attack 3 months after the training period, which shows that

there is still a lot to be learned on this subject. For example, electrocardiograms which were taken of the participants in similar training programs have shown that damage to the heart muscle often remains for months or years, even though the ability to engage in strenuous activity may be greatly improved.

Furthermore, a few people have even had heart attacks while participating in exercise tests by physicians. Therefore, it is not wise for a customarily sedentary person to engage in vigorous exercise without first consulting a doctor who will make some type of evaluation of cardiovascular fitness before specifying the exercises which are most suitable.

Some exercising guidelines follow:

1. **Exercise regularly.** Exercise regularly—daily or every-other-day.

2. **Type of exercise.** There are many good exercises from which to choose, including walking, jogging, bicycling, swimming, tennis, or the use of a treadmill or an exercycle—all of them result in deep breathing and a speeding of the heart rate.

NOTE WELL: For some people, the stress which running places on the joints may do more harm than good.

3. **Warm-up; Cool-down.** Precede the exercise session with a warm-up period of at least 5 minutes. Following exercise, cool-down by doing more stretches and light exercises.

4. **Exercise sensibly.** Pay attention to warning signals—do not exercise when it becomes painful. Slow down if you're out-of-breath, fatigued, or mildly light-headed. Stop exercising immediately if you experience pain, tightness or pressure in your chest, irregular pulse, or dizziness. Do not exercise during the hottest part of the day.

5. **Avoid becoming dehydrated.** Strenuous activity tends to dehydrate, because of loss of fluid through perspiration. To compensate for this loss, drink a glass of water (*not* ice water) before and following exercising.

NOTE: It may be dangerous for people who have certain cardiovascular problems to perform isometric types of exercise (those which cause both the buildup of tension and the constriction of blood vessels in muscles) because these activities tend to raise the blood pressure. For example, pushups, knee bends, weight lifting, and similar activities have isometric components, whereas such activities as running and walking are basically nonisometric in nature.

SURGERY.   There have been remarkable advances in the surgical treatment of cardiovascular diseases since World War II. Hence, it is now possible, with certain limitations, to replace worn out or diseased parts of the heart and blood vessels with either those from human or animal donors, or with artificial analogs of human organs. Brief descriptions of some common types of surgery follow:

• **Bypass graft(s) of a piece of leg vein onto a coronary artery**—In this well-known operation, which is frequently called a *coronary bypass*, a piece of a leg vein is grafted onto a blocked coronary artery. The piece of vein is attached to the artery so that it allows the blood to flow from the heart side of the occluded artery, around the obstruction, and back into the artery on the other side of the occlusion. However, a few patients may develop atherosclerotic blockage of the vein graft within a year or so. The reason for this development is not known for certain, although it is suspected to be due to whatever factors might have been responsible for the original coronary occlusion.

---

[33]Redwood, D. R., D. R. Rosing, and S. E. Epstein, "Circulatory and Symptomatic Effects of Physical Training in Patients with Coronary-Artery Disease and Angina Pectoris," *The New England Journal of Medicine*, Vol. 286, 1972, p. 959.

• **Grafts of dacron patches of tubes onto blood vessels**
—This type of surgery uses dacron, rather than living tissue, to repair diseased blood vessels. For example, a dacron patch may be sewn into the wall of a blood vessel which has been surgically opened, because such a procedure allows for a larger opening in the vein or artery than might be obtained by merely stitching the cut edges together. Also, a knitted dacron tube may be used in lieu of a vein graft in a coronary bypass operation.

• **Heart transplantation**—In this procedure, the patient is connected to a heart-lung machine, then, his or her diseased heart is removed and replaced with a healthy heart from a donor. However, few medical centers now conduct this surgery because (1) there may be a rejection of the transplanted heart by the patient's body; and (2) treatments which decrease the likelihood of the transplant's rejection also render the patient more susceptible to infectious diseases.

• **Implantation of an artificial pacemaker**—Sometimes, it is necessary to provide artificial electrical stimulation of the heart for a patient who has what is commonly called a *heart block*. A heart block is a pathological condition in which there is some type of interference with the natural pacemaker action in the heart.

Certain types of heart blocks may be counteracted by an artificial electronic pacemaker which is surgically implanted in the body. The usual procedure is for the surgeon to insert the pacemaker's electrodes, which are connected by wires to the main body of the device, up through a vein and into the heart. Then, the main body of the pacemaker which contains the power supply and the electronic impulse generator is placed under the skin on the chest. It is usually necessary to replace the power source every 5 to 7 years.

Patients who are fitted with artificial pacemakers should discuss with their physicians the precautions which should be taken to avoid electronic interference from microwave ovens, x ray machines, and various types of electronic equipment.

• **Replacement of diseased heart valves with prosthetic ball valves**—The special flaps of tissue which serve as valves for the heart may become damaged or diseased, and require replacement. Most surgeons now use prosthetic valves as replacement parts rather than human or animal tissues because the artificial devices are better tolerated by the body. Hence, the type of valve which is implanted in the heart is likely to be a wear-resistant ball or disc that moves back and forth in a small wire cage in response to the ebb and flow of blood from the heart.

• **Removal of atherosclerotic plaques (endarterectomy)**—This operation consists of the removal of plaques from blood vessels, surgically or by rimming them out with a *balloon*.

• **Artificial heart**—Although artificial hearts are still in the experimental stage, they appear promising.

SUMMARY. The thought of suffering from some form of cardiovascular disease has led many people to become overly anxious about their hearts. Yet, it may be seen from this article that there has been a steady advance in the ability of physicians to detect and treat all stages and types of heart disease. However, people who wish to minimize their problems should read and heed what follows:

1. The earlier that heart disease is detected and treated, the safer the treatment(s), and the better the outcome.

2. Regular exercise and restraint in eating are about the best preventative measures for people whose hearts are still healthy.

3. Whole foods, which are richer in fiber, minerals, and vitamins than their refined counterparts, may provide the nutrition that the heart needs to withstand the emotional and physical stresses of a full life.

(NOTE WELL: For a more complete discussion of Heart Disease, see the two-volume *Foods & Nutrition Encyclopedia*, a work by the same authors as *Food For Health.)*

HEAT EXHAUSTION

The result of overtaxing the body's mechanisms for keeping cool, and for maintaining balance between body water and various mineral salts.

• **Water depletion heat exhaustion**—Inadequate water replacement during physical labor or exercise may result in water depletion heat exhaustion. It is characterized by thirst, fatigue, giddiness, fever, and decreased urine output (oliguria).

• **Salt depletion heat exhaustion**—During hard physical labor or exercise both sodium and water are lost in the sweat, especially in unacclimatized persons. Water may be replenished by drinking; however, a sodium deficit still remains. Inadequate sodium replacement leads to heat exhaustion characterized by fatigue, nausea, vomiting, and giddiness.

Water loss usually exceeds sodium loss. Hence, free access to water is essential whenever one expects significant sweat losses. Free access to water is especially important when additional sodium (salt) is provided.

(Also see DISEASES, section headed "Injuries from Physical Agents.")

HEAT LABILE

Unstable to heat.

HEAT OF COMBUSTION (GROSS ENERGY)

The heat of combustion, or gross energy, of a material is determined in a bomb calorimeter by the following procedure: An electric wire is attached to the material being tested, so that it can be ignited by remote control; 2,000 g of water are poured around the bomb; 25 to 30 atmospheres of oxygen are added to the bomb; the material is ignited; the heat given off from the burned materials warms the water; and a thermometer registers the change in temperature of the water. For example, if 1 g of material is burned and the temperature of the water is raised 1 °C, 2,000 Calories (kcal) are given off. Hence, the material contains 2,000 Calories (kcal) per gram. This value is known as the gross energy (GE) content of the material.

(Also see BOMB CALORIMETER; and CALORIC [ENERGY] EXPENDITURE.)

HEIGHT INCREMENTS

Human growth is composed of two periods of rapid growth: (1) the first year of life, and (2) during puberty or adolescence. As determined by height increments, the

first year of life, following which growth slows to 2 to 2¼ in. (5.1 to 5.6 cm) per year. Then, at puberty there is a growth spurt lasting about 4 years. This growth spurt usually begins earlier in females. During this time, height increments increase to about 2½ to 3 in. (6.4 to 7.6 cm) per year. In total, boys may grow 8 in. (20 cm) and gain 40 lb (18 kg) during this time. Girls grow slightly less during their growth spurt. Following this, the yearly height increments decline rapidly and by 17 or 18 years of age only slight height increments are noted. Understandably, during these growth spurts of adolescence, additional food requirements are indicated and usually met via increased food intake at mealtimes and between-meal snacks. Little actual information exists as to the nutritional requirements during this time.

HEM-, HEMA-, HEMO-

Prefixes referring to blood.

HEMAGGLUTININS (LECTINS OR PHYTOAGGLUTININS)

Naturally-occurring plant toxins capable of causing red blood cell agglutination—clumping—are proteins called hemagglutinins. These are found in soybeans and other legumes. Adequate cooking destroys hemagglutinins. Experimentally, these toxins induce weight loss and inhibit the growth of rats.

HEMATOCRIT

An instrument for separating the solid elements (largely red cells) of the blood from the plasma.

HEMATOPOIESIS (HEMOPOIESIS; HEMOPOIETIC)

The formation of blood or of blood cells within the body.

HEMATURIA

The presence of blood or blood cells in the urine.

HEMERALOPIA

A defect of vision characterized by reduced visual capacity in bright lights—also called day blindness.
(Also see NIGHT BLINDNESS.)

HEMIPLEGIA

The most common type of paralysis. It often involves the loss of strength in the arm, the leg, and sometimes the face on the same side of the body. In order of importance, hemiplegia may be caused by vascular diseases of the brain, trauma (injury), brain tumors, brain abcess, encephalitis, demyelination disease, and syphilis. Due to reduced activity, and the difficulties encountered in preparing and eating food, some dietary modification may be necessary.
(Also see MODIFIED DIETS.)

HEMODIALYSIS

Those individuals whose kidneys are completely nonfunctional—normal function continues when as little as two-thirds of one kidney remains—must have the waste products of metabolism removed from their blood. Without this, the concentrations of urea, uric acid, and creatinine increase. Also, acidosis or hyperkalemia (high blood potassium) and edema may develop. If not controlled, death results in 8 to

14 days. Hemodialysis, using an artificial kidney, provides a means of removing the waste products from the blood.

The blood leaves the body via an artery in the arm and flows through a dialyzer where a semipermeable cellophane membrane separates the blood and a dialyzing fluid. Metabolic waste products pass into the dialyzing fluid and are carried away. Blood proteins and red blood cells are too large to pass through the cellophane membrane. The refreshed blood is warmed to body temperature and then returned to the body via a vein in the arm. These connections, hookups, in the arm are usually permanent since dialysis must be repeated 2 or 3 times per week. Each treatment requires 4 to 12 hours depending upon the type of artificial kidney used. Blood is leaving and entering the body on a continuous basis until the process is complete. The treatments are expensive, but have saved many lives and allowed individuals to enjoy quite normal lives.

Persons using dialysis require restriction of sodium, potassium and water intake. Protein intake is also closely controlled and will vary from 30 to 60 g daily. The aim is to provide about ¾ of the protein allowance as protein of high biological value. Furthermore, to prevent high blood urea and potassium levels, it is especially important that adequate energy be supplied to prevent the catabolism of body protein. Dialysis patients also require vitamin supplementation in addition to the dietary controls.
(Also see KIDNEY DISEASES; METABOLISM; and MODIFIED DIETS.)

HEMOGLOBIN

The oxygen-carrying, red-pigmented protein of the red corpuscles.
(Also see ANEMIA; HEMOGLOBIN SYNTHESIS; and IRON.)

HEMOGLOBIN SYNTHESIS

The red oxygen-carrying pigment of the blood, hemoglobin, is comprised of two substances. The first substance, the red color, is the heme which is manufactured in the developing red blood cells from acetic acid, the amino acid glycine, and iron. Heme is rather an odd-shaped octagon with a hole in the center wherein the iron is found. Once the heme is manufactured, it combines with the second substance, globin, a protein classified as a globulin; forming hemoglobin. About 7 g of hemoglobin are formed every day. It constitutes 90% of the dry weight of the red blood cell. Iron is essential for the synthesis of hemoglobin. Copper, vitamin C, vitamin B-6 (pyridoxine), folic acid, and vitamin B-12 are also required. Each day, adult males normally lose about 1,000 mcg of iron; adult females may lose 1,500 mcg per day due to menstrual losses. If a deficiency of iron occurs, and is not corrected, iron deficiency anemia results. Liver, red meats, and dietary supplements are rich sources of iron.
(Also see ANEMIA; and IRON.)

HEMOLYSIS

Destruction of red blood cells.

HEMOLYTIC

Causing the separation of hemoglobin from the red blood cells.

HEMORRHAGE

Copious loss of blood through bleeding.

HEMORRHOIDS (PILES)

They are dilated and engorged veins of the anus and rectum which may be located either externally or internally. The veins in the area of the rectum and anus become stretched, dilated, and then knotted as the muscle fibers in the walls of the veins break down. Blood returning through these veins to the heart is slowed down and pooled thus distending a portion of the vein causing it to protrude and be covered by only the lining of the rectum (internal) or by the skin around the anus (external). Hemorrhoids are often noted during the following conditions: constipation, overweight, pregnancy, diarrhea, chronic liver disease, tumors, or incomplete evacuation of the feces. Likely, there is also a hereditary factor involved. The first signs of hemorrhoids is severe rectal pain and/or rectal bleeding. Most hemorrhoids respond to conservative therapy such as hot sitz baths, dietary changes to soften the stool and remove irritating roughages, and the proper use of local medication.

HEMOSIDERIN

The insoluble iron oxide-protein compound in which iron is stored in the liver and spleen if the amount of iron in the blood exceeds the storage capacity of ferritin. Such accumulation of excess iron occurs in diseases that are accompanied by rapid destruction of red blood cells (malaria, hemolytic anemia).

HEPARIN

A mucopolysaccharide that prevents clotting of blood by preventing the formation of fibrin.

HEPATITIS

The name hepatitis means *liver inflammation*. It can be caused by viruses, drugs, and chemicals (including alcohol), to name the most common offenders. In the minds of most people, however, it means a viral infection.

(Also see DISEASES.)

HEPATOMEGALY

Enlargement of the liver.

HERB

The word *herb* is usually applied to a plant or plant part valued for its savory, aromatic, or medicinal qualities.

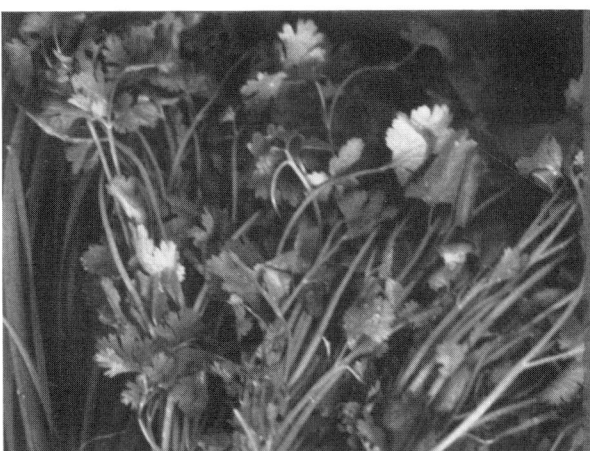

Fig H-9. Chinese parsley *(Cilantro)*, a common U. S. herb. (Courtesy, Dept. of Food Service and Human Nutrition, University of Hawaii.)

Some herbs are used in cooking—to flavor foods. Others give scent to perfumes; and still others are used for medicines. Some herbs, like balm and sage, are valued for their leaves. Saffron is picked for its buds and flowers. Fennel seeds are valued in relishes and seasoning. Ginseng is valued for its aromatic roots.

Some people grow herbs in their gardens. The plants do well with little care. When they are grown, the leaves, stems, or seeds are harvested and dried. Then, they are generally pounded to a fine powder, placed in airtight containers, and stored for later use.

Although herbs have little nutrient value, they make food tasty and more flavorful. Cooking with herbs is a culinary art, which adds great interest to menus.

(Also see FLAVORINGS AND SEASONINGS.)

HEXOSEMONOPHOSPHATE SHUNT PENTOSE SHUNT

An alternate mechanism for the breakdown of glucose. The function of this pathway is twofold: (1) the generation of energy through the use of NADPH, and (2) the production of pentoses—five carbon sugars—especially ribose which can be used in the synthesis of nucleic acids—DNA and RNA.

Also see METABOLISM.)

HIATUS HERNIA

Many persons have, under certain circumstances, a slight protrusion of the upper part of the stomach through the opening (or hiatus) in the diaphragm. Normally, the esophagus passes down through this opening and is attached to the stomach just below the hiatus. This disorder sometimes causes *heartburn* and sour regurgitation. These conditions may be wrongly attributed to heart disease or peptic ulcer. (It is difficult to diagnose the origin of pain in the region under the breastbone.) It is rare for more than a small portion of the stomach to protrude up into the chest cavity. Also, the amount of protrusion is usually variable with the hernia sliding up and down in response to the size of the hiatus, the amount of pressure on the stomach, and the length of the esophagus. (The esophagus may be shortened due to irritation or distention.) Serious consequences may result when there is chronic esophagitis caused by reflux of stomach acid (hiatus hernia makes this more likely to happen as it alters the action of the sphincter between the esophagus and the stomach), or under rare circumstances, where a large portion of the stomach protrudes into the chest cavity.

CAUSES OF HIATUS HERNIA. Some people appear to be more susceptible to this disorder than others. As in other hernias, an increased intra-abdominal pressure is the most common cause of herniation. Ways of avoiding such pressure are discussed in the section that follows.

TREATMENT AND PREVENTION OF HIATUS HERNIA. Although surgical reduction of the tendency for herniation might appear to be the best treatment most physicians are reluctant to advise such surgery, except when the hernia is very large. Therefore, the most common approach to the problem is to advise patients how to avoid large increases in intra-abdominal pressure. Preventive measures involve (1) reducing obesity; (2) avoiding straining at the stool, distention of the stomach with food and drink, chronic coughing and sneezing, and lying down soon after meals

(The stomach is held in a lower position by gravity when the patient is in an upright position.); and (3) sleeping with the head high and drinking water when there are signs of regurgitation coming on.

(Also see HEARTBURN.)

HIGH BLOOD PRESSURE (HYPERTENSION)

About 25% of Americans have some degree of high blood pressure. If not corrected, it is a risk factor for both heart disease and strokes. Each year about 300,000 people die from diseases linked to high blood pressure.

The force which the blood exerts against the wall of the blood vessels—blood pressure—is measured at two readings. The higher reading, which is called systolic blood pressure, occurs when the heart exerts its maximum force of contraction (systole). The lower reading, which is called the diastolic blood pressure, occurs when the heart rests between contractions (diastole). Normal blood pressure values for an adult between the ages of 18 and 45 center around readings of 120 systolic and 80 diastolic—when written as 120/80 and spoken as "120 over 80." High blood pressure, or at least the upper limits of normal, is considered as 160/95. However, the range for high blood pressure is from 140/90 to 165/95, and severe cases of high blood pressure may have readings as high as 200/115. Aside from the high extremes, a diagnosis of high blood pressure is based upon an individual's medical history, and the judgement of the physician.

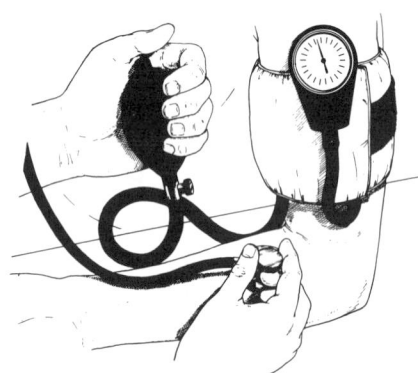

Fig. H-10. Taking blood pressure with a sphygmomanometer. The gauge is calibrated in millimeters of mercury. A stethoscope is placed over an artery in the arm to detect sounds characteristic of the systolic reading and the diastolic reading as the pressure is released from the cuff surrounding the arm.

The numbers used to express blood pressure are pressures in millimeters of mercury—the height that blood flow in an artery pushes a column of mercury in a glass tube—determined by an instrument known as a manometer. Normally, blood pressure is taken in the large artery of the upper arm. An inflatable pressure cuff connected to a mercury manometer (a sphygmomanometer) is wrapped around the upper arm. The pressure cuff is inflated until the wall of the artery collapses and blood flow ceases. Then a stethoscope is held below the inflated cuff, just over the artery. Next, pressure is gradually released from the cuff. Just at the instant when blood is heard to spurt through the artery—a tapping sound—the reading on the manometer is noted. This reading is the *systolic* pressure, since blood is being forced through the artery only when the heart contracts. Gradually more pressure is released from the cuff and the spurting sounds or vibration are still noted through the stethoscope. The reading noted on the manometer the moment the spurting sounds disappear is the *diastolic* pressure.

DANGERS. Untreated high blood pressure may, over a period of time, affect vital areas of the body, particularly the heart, brain, and kidneys.

High blood pressure causes the heart to pump harder than normal which in turn causes the heart to get larger but pump less effectively. Since the heart pumps less effectively, it dilates causing the signs and symptoms of heart failure to appear. High blood pressure may also speed up the process of atherosclerosis—a contributor to heart attacks.

High blood pressure increases the risk of a stroke due to the chance of accelerated blockage of an artery feeding the brain or hemorrhage (rupture) of a brain blood vessel. Both result in the destruction of brain tissue.

Aside from the brain, the other nervous tissue involved is the eye. High blood pressure may cause the tiny blood vessels in the back of the eyes to undergo atherosclerotic changes (narrowing), or hemorrhaging, resulting in blurred vision and even blindness. These small blood vessels of the eye can be examined directly by a physician, providing a means of following the effects of high blood pressure.

Oftentimes the blood vessels of the kidneys are the hardest hit by high blood pressure. Narrowing or rupturing of the small blood vessels of the kidneys eventually leads to the inability of the kidneys to perform their task of removing wastes from the blood—kidney failure.

(Also see HEART DISEASE.)

TYPES. High blood pressure is classified as (1) secondary hypertension, or (2) primary or essential hypertension. Most individuals suffer from primary or essential hypertension.

Secondary Hypertension. This is high blood pressure due to a clearly definable cause, primarily kidney disorders, endocrine malfunctions, pregnancy, and *the pill.*

In secondary hypertension, the underlying cause is dealt with first, thereby eliminating the high blood pressure.

Primary or Essential Hypertension. Unfortunately, relatively few individuals demonstrate a clear-cut cause of hypertension. Rather, about 90% of the people suffering from high blood pressure show no single, easily identifiable cause. This type of high blood pressure is called primary, or essential, or sometimes idiopathic hypertension.

POSSIBLE CAUSES. It is likely that primary hypertension is due to a variety of causes—some interrelated. The following list contains some of the most probable causes:

1. Advanced age.
2. Emotions.
3. Hormones.
4. Heredity.
5. High salt diet.
6. Smoking.
7. Obesity.

TREATMENT. Traditional treatment of high blood pressure depends upon dietary modifications, drugs, and life-style changes.

• **Dietary modifications**—Rigid, long-term sodium (salt) restriction can be successfully used to control, at least in part, high blood pressure.

Sodium and potassium are closely interrelated. Although sodium intake may be the most important dietary determinant of blood pressure, variations in the sodium:potassium ratio in the diet affect blood pressure under certain circumstances. In rats with high blood pressure due to a high intake of sodium, blood pressure may be lowered to a more normal level by increasing the potassium intake and lowering the sodium intake. It seems that a 1:1 ratio may be somewhat protective against the blood pressure-elevating effects of a given level of sodium. This ratio can be achieved by increasing the intake of potassium, or lowering the intake of sodium, or both.

Researchers in both Finland and Denmark report that, for people who do not eat fish regularly, fish oil may be helpful.

• **Drugs**—Individuals with blood pressure levels above 160/100 generally require drugs to lower their blood pressure. These drugs can be classified into three major groups: (1) diuretics which promote increased urinary excretion of sodium; (2) sympatholytics which block nerves controlling blood vessels, and allow blood vessels to dilate thus decreasing the pressure; and (3) vasodilators which act directly on blood vessels causing them to widen. The long-term use of diuretics leads to a potassium deficiency. Hence, dietary potassium supplementation is required.

• **Life-style changes**—These may be different for every individual suffering from hypertension. Life-style changes which appear to be beneficial include weight reduction, cessation of smoking, and regular exercise. Possibly an evaluation of the day-to-day events—coping with the stress of living—may point out the need for engaging is some relaxing activity. Biofeedback and meditation offer a means of relaxation and regaining control for some individuals. Perhaps just working out some personal problems will help.

PREVENTION. Most Americans who suffer from high blood pressure suffer from primary or essential hypertension—a condition without specific causes. Hence, preventive measures are difficult to designate. However, some suggestions can be made based on the current knowledge.

• **Diet**—Average Americans consume about 10 g of salt each day. This amount translates into 4,000 mg of sodium daily—considerably more than the upper limit of 500 mg currently recommended by the National Research Council. Furthermore, under ordinary circumstances the body requires only 115 mg of sodium daily and under conditions of profuse sweating only 780 mg daily. So, while no direct evidence links salt intake to the development of hypertension, there are no known benefits to the healthy person of excessive salt consumption. Moreover, it is reasonable to assume that a voluntary lowered salt intake will reduce the risk of developing high blood pressure in the 10 to 30% of all Americans born with a genetic predisposition to hypertension. In addition, a 1:1 ratio of sodium and potassium intake may be somewhat protective.

• **Exercise and weight control**—Many Americans suffer from too little exercise and too many calories. Since obesity is implicated with high blood pressure, the benefit of maintaining ideal weight appears obvious.

• **Smoking**—Give it up. Cigarette smoking is the principal preventable cause of chronic disease and death in the United States.

• **Periodic blood pressure checks**—Periodic screening is an invaluable preventative measure, so treatment can be started before damage occurs. Adults should have a screening exam for high blood pressure at least every 5 years, and every 2 or 3 years if over the age of 40, or if there is a family history of high blood pressure.

It is encouraging to note that death rates attributable to high blood pressure have been reduced by as much as 35% in the last 10 years due largely to earlier detection and effective treatment.

(Also see ENDOCRINE GLANDS; HEART DISEASE; MODIFIED DIETS; OBESITY; POTASSIUM; SALT; SODIUM; STRESS; and WATER AND ELECTROLYTES.)

HIGH DENSITY LIPOPROTEINS (HDL)

Also called alpha-lipoproteins.
(Also see ALPHA-LIPOPROTEINS; and LIPOPROTEINS.)

HIGH-NUTRIENT DENSITY

A high proportion of a specific nutrient to total kilocalories in a given amount of food.

HIGH RATIO FLOUR

Flour of very fine and uniform particle size, treated with chlorine to reduce the gluten strength, used for making cakes. It is possible to add up to 140 parts of sugar to 100 parts of this flour. The product can be classed as a *weak* flour which does not make good bread, but does make excellent cakes.

HISTIDINE

One of the essential amino acids.
(Also see AMINO ACID[S].)

HISTOLOGY

Microscopic anatomy; pertaining to minute structure, composition, and function of tissues.

HISTORY OF NUTRITION

In nutrition, more than in any other science, history is most important. In the final analysis, food and people are not only inseparable from history—they're part of it. Without them, there would be no history—no mankind.

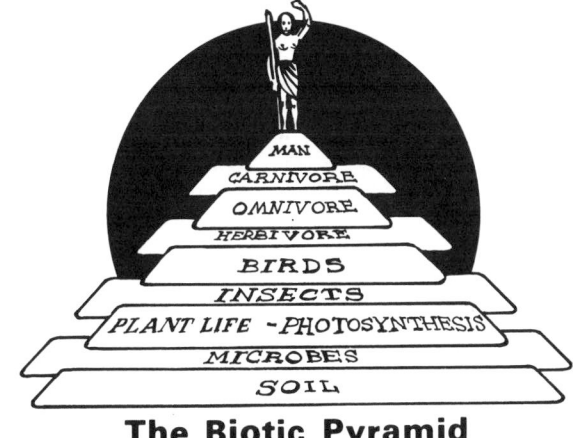

The Biotic Pyramid

Fig. H-11. The biotic pyramid.

For thousands of years, the quest for food has shaped the course of history. It dictated population growth, urban expansion, migration, and settlement of new lands. It profoundly influenced economic, social, and political theory. It promoted early sailing and the discovery of new worlds, widened the horizons of commerce, caused wars of dominion, and played no small role in the creation of empires.

Food has played an important role in many things. In religion, it helped to define the separateness of one creed from another by means of dietary taboos. In science, the prehistoric cook's discoveries of the effect of heat applied to raw materials laid the foundations on which much of early chemistry was based. In technology, the waterwheel, first used in the milling of grain, achieved immense industrial importance. In wars, battles were sometimes postponed until the harvest had been gathered in, and the well-fed armies usually defeated the hungry ones.

Although the ancient Greek philosophers were interested in science, logical reasoning—rather than experimentation—was the Greek way. Hippocrates (460 to 377 B.C.), known as the *father of medicine,* was the first great physician to indicate an interest in nutrition. Among his famous quotes were "Children produce more heat and need more food than adults"; and "Persons who are naturally very fat are apt to die earlier than those who are slender."

The naturalistic, or prescientific, era of nutrition was characterized by a fascinating maze of philosophy, taboos, bizarre superstitions, and religious precepts. During this period, little of truly scientific nature was accomplished in the field of nutrition. Then came the successful merger of the art and the science of food and nutrition, ushering in a new era. It stimulated increased research. Many maladies which had long plagued mankind were traced to dietary deficiencies, imbalances, and toxicities.

The great French chemist, Antoine Laurent Lavoisier (1743-1794), is credited with being the founder of the science of nutrition. He used guinea pigs to measure body heat, oxygen consumed, and carbon dioxide expired, and he concluded that the human body is like a little furnace using food to produce heat and energy. Further, he was able to show that heat production in the body is directly related to oxygen consumption.

Next came the Feeding Standard Era which held sway from 1810 to 1940, followed, in order, by the Vitamin-Biological Era of the early 1900s, the Amino Acid Era of the 1930s, and the Food Additive Era of the 1950s. Along the way, many researchers contributed richly to our knowledge of nutrition.

Today, we know that the chemical substances found in food materials can be used, and are necessary, for life itself. We know that the nutrient chemicals—more than 40 of them, including amino acids, minerals, and vitamins—reach the body cells and tissues and are utilized for growth, development, physical activity, reproduction, lactation, maintenance of health, and recovery from illness or injury.

Like other sciences, modern human nutrition does not stand alone. It draws heavily on the basic findings of chemistry, biochemistry, physics, microbiology, physiology, bacteriology, medicine, food technology, agricultural science, genetics, mathematics, endocrinology, behavior, cellular biology, and, most recently, genetic engineering.

Although the chasm between awareness and application is becoming smaller, there is still much to be learned about foods and nutrition. We need to know more about human nutritional requirements; we need to know more about food composition and availability; we need to know more about diet, disease causation, and food safety; we need to know more about food consumption and nutritional status.

We need to be able to distinguish between myths and facts. We are told that Americans are living happily against the odds. We are warned about cholesterol in our eggs, about nitrate in our bacon, and about caffeine in our coffee—all of which has taken the fun out of eating. But there is no escape! If we go on bread and water, just as soon as we begin to enjoy it, someone will tell us that it's bad for us.

So, despite the advances that typify nutrition, there are many unknowns. The search goes on!

NOTE WELL: For a chronological history of nutrition, see the two-volume *Foods & Nutrition Encyclopedia,* a work by the same authors as *Food For Health.*

HIVES

Small itchy swellings under or within the skin. They appear suddenly over large portions of the body and can be caused by food allergies.

(Also see ALLERGIES.)

HOME ECONOMISTS

Specialists in home economics. Home economists work to improve products, services, and practices that affect the comfort and well-being of the family. Some specialize in specific areas, such as child development and family relations, clothing and textiles, consumer economics, foods and nutrition, home furnishings and equipment, home management, and housing. Others have broad knowledge of the whole professional field.

Home economists are engaged in the following types of work: (1) teaching in colleges, high schools, and adult education programs; (2) research for the federal government, state agricultural experiment stations, colleges, and private organizations; (3) Cooperative Extension Service; (4) private business firms and trade associations; (5) social welfare programs conducted by federal, state, and local governments; (6) dietitians for hospitals, schools, group food services, and restaurants; and (7) health services.

About 350 U.S. colleges and universities offer a bachelor's degree in home economics.

The professional organization for home economists is: American Home Economics Association, 2010 Massachusetts Ave. N.W., Washington, D.C. 20036.

HOMEOSTASIS

A state of equilibrium of the body's internal environment; for example, the lungs provide oxygen as it is required by the cells; and the kidneys, through the processes of reabsorption and elimination, help to maintain normal blood composition.

HOMOGENIZATION

A process which creates small uniform particles in a mixture. Many substances are homogenized when a uniformity of particle size is desired.

(Also see MILK AND MILK PRODUCTS.)

HONEY

Honey originated with honeybees. They make honey to use as their food, and man exploits this trait.

Essentially, honey is an invert sugar—a mixture of glucose

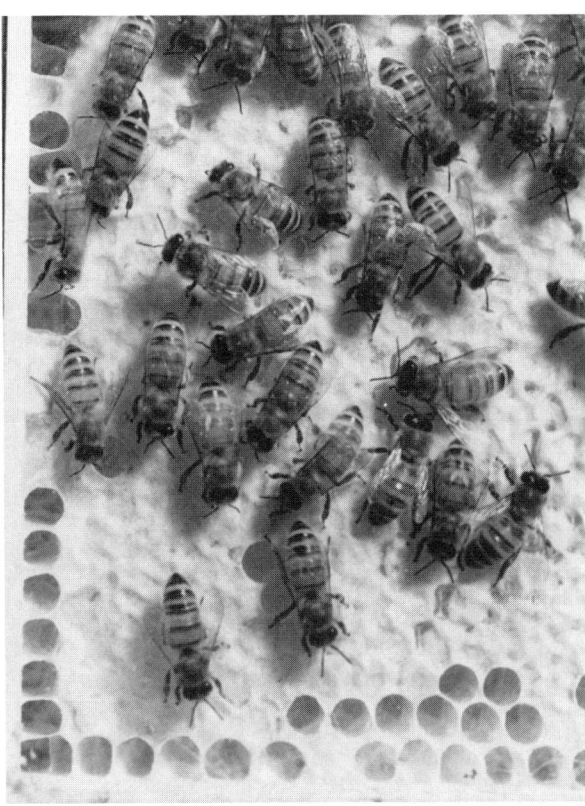

Fig. H-12. Bees on a honeycomb. (Photo by J. C. Allen & Son, West Lafayette, Ind.)

TABLE H-2
NUTRITIONAL VALUE OF HONEY[1]

Nutrient[2]	Unit	Amount	
		Per 100 g	Per Tbsp *(20 g)*
Energy	kcal	304.00	61.00
Protein	g	.30	.10
Carbohydrates	g	82.30	16.50
Calcium	mg	5.00	1.00
Phosphorus	mg	6.00	1.20
Sodium	mg	5.00	1.00
Magnesium	mg	3.00	.60
Potassium	mg	51.00	10.20
Iron	mg	.50	.10
Zinc	mg	.10	.02
Copper	mg	.20	.04
Vitamin C	mg	1.00	.20
Riboflavin	mg	.04	.008
Niacin	mg	.30	.06
Pantothenic acid	mg	.20	.04
Pyridoxine	mg	.02	.004
Folic acid	mcg	3.00	.60

[1]Values are from the Food Composition Table F-21 of this book.
[2]Nutrients not listed are not present.

The other major constituent of honey is water, about 14 to 20%. Hence, very little is left over for essential nutrients. Indeed, numerous other food sources provide more of the essential nutrients. One real advantage in using honey is that, due to the fructose content, it is sweeter than table

and fructose—dissolved in 14 to 20% water with minor amounts of organic acids, along with traces of minerals and vitamins. Honey is derived from the nectar of flowering plants which the honeybee collects. Nectar consists primarily of 10 to 50% sucrose, glucose, and fructose, and 50 to 90% water. Each worker bee has a special pouch, called a honey bag, inside its body. Here the bee stores the nectar that it collects. After collections, the bees (1) supply an invertase enzyme which converts the sucrose to glucose and fructose, (2) store it in honeycombs, and (3) reduce the water content. The color, flavor, and proportion of the sugars vary with the source of nectar. In the United States, most honey is produced from alfalfa and clover. These honeys are light colored and delicately flavored. Tupelo honey, from southern United States, contains about twice as much fructose and glucose; hence, it seldom granulates. Nectar from the flowers of goldenrod and aster yield a dark honey. Other common honeys include buckwheat from eastern United States, orange-blossom honey, and sage honey from California.

NUTRITIONAL VALUE AND USES.
Honey is pleasing to the senses—especially taste—so pleasing that some cultures have considered it an aphrodisiac (a product that excites sexual desire). Also, honey has acquired a special reputation as a nutritional food or medicine. Unfortunately, neither reputation is deserved. As Table H-2 shows, honey supplies substantial energy, since it is 75 to 80% fructose and glucose. But there are only traces of other nutrients. Despite its unimpressive chemical composition, honey continues to be appreciated by all who (1) can afford it and (2) enjoy its pleasant taste.

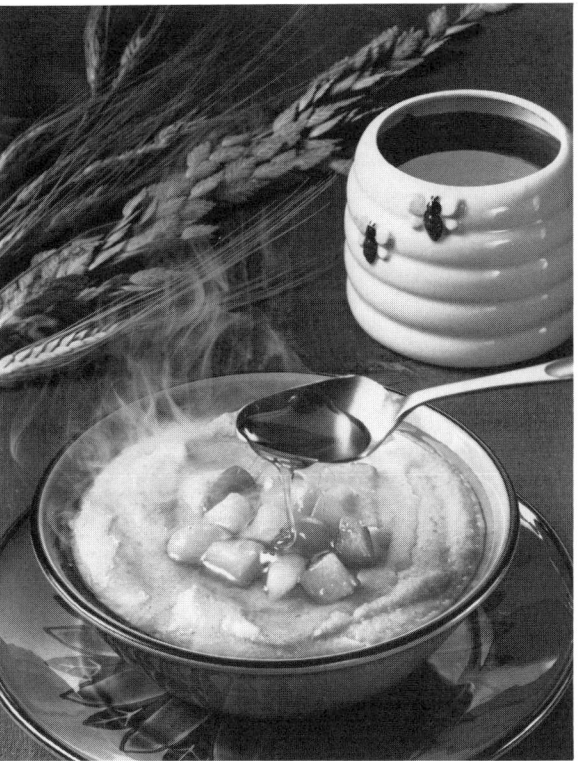

Fig. H-13. Honey over hot cereal. (Courtesy, California Honey Advisory Board, Whittier, Calif.)

sugar—sucrose—and less is needed; it has the same sweetness as invert sugar. As a sweetener, honey is used on breads, cereals, and desserts. About half the honey produced is used this way and the other half is used in the baking industry.

Because honey absorbs and retains moisture (it is hygroscopic), it is used by the baking industry to keep bread or cakes moist and fresh. Furthermore, the fructose in honey improves the browning quality. These same benefits of honey can be enjoyed in home baking. When honey is substituted for sugar, it is usually necessary to reduce the amount of liquid in the recipe by ¼ cup for each cup (240 ml) of honey. Many recipe books for cooking with honey are available. Honey may also be used in canned or frozen fruits, in jams and jellies, and in drinks. One popular drink in Viking and Elizabethan times was mead—fermented honey.

Honey has enjoyed some application in medicine for thousands of years. Any number of unfounded medical properties have been ascribed to it; among them, relief from nasal and bronchial pneumonia. And some really wild claims have been made for honey combined with vinegar; without doubt, the sweetness of the honey makes swallowing the vinegar tolerable, but not curative. Nowadays, honey is employed in some medicinal compounds just to cover up harsh bitter flavors and to prevent granulation.

It may not be wise to feed honey to infants under 1 year of age, since infant botulism—botulism resulting from the production of toxins after the ingestion of Colostridium botulinum—may result from the ingestion of raw agricultural products. Honey has been implicated as a source in a very few cases. This type of botulism does not occur in older children and adults.[34]

(Also see SWEETENING AGENTS.)

HORMONE

The word hormone comes from the Greek word hormon, which means to spur on, to set in motion, or to excite to action. These phrases are all very descriptive of a hormone. Released by the endocrine glands, hormones are chemical messengers which travel via the blood to specific organs or tissues and direct such processes as growth, reproduction, metabolism and behavior. In the blood they exist in extremely small quantities—millionths and billionths of a gram. Yet, their effects upon the body are profound, as demonstrated by diseased conditions where there is an over- or under-secretion of some hormone.

NOTE WELL: Hormone therapy for whatever reason, and whether oral or by injection, should always be under the direction of a physician.

(Also see ENDOCRINE GLANDS.)

HORSEMEAT

This refers to the flesh of the horse, which is used as a human food in most European countries, the U.S.S.R., and Japan. The leading horsemeat consumers are Belgium, Luxembourg, and France. Elsewhere in the Old World, horseflesh has been avoided by most Hindus, Buddhists, Jews, Moslems, and Christians, all of whom have followed closely the precepts of their religion or their cultural prejudices. Additionally, the notion that eating horseflesh is disreputable has persisted for a variety of reasons, not the least of which is man's attachment to the horse as a good friend and stout companion.

A variety of recipes for beef can be used in the preparation of horsemeat.

HOSPITAL DIET

Depending upon the needs of the patient it may be a regular, light, soft, or full liquid diet. Regular diets are for those persons who are ambulatory and require no therapeutic diet. Light diets are generally given during the early stages of convalescent periods, and differ from regular diets mainly in their mode of preparation. Rich pastries, fried foods, and most raw vegetables and fruit are avoided. The soft diet is an intermediate step between the light and liquid diet. Some hospitals, however, may omit the light diet. A soft diet consists mainly of liquids and semisolid foods; it is required in some gastrointestinal tract conditions, debilitated patients, and acute infections. Soft diets are low in residue and easily digested. They contain little or no spices and condiments, and are more restrictive in fruits, meats, and vegetables. The liquid diet is usually given postoperative, or to patients acutely ill with an infection, with gastrointestinal tract disturbances, or with myocardial infarction. It contains nothing but liquids such as fruit and vegetable juices, broth, milk, eggnogs (with powdered high-protein supplements added), junket, ice cream, etc.

(Also see MODIFIED DIETS.)

HOTHOUSE LAMBS

Considered by epicureans as the most delectable of the lamb age groups. They are very young lambs—usually less than 3 months of age at slaughter—which are born and marketed out of season. Such milk-fat lambs are usually marketed during the period from Christmas to the Easter holidays at weights ranging from 30 to 60 lb (14 to 27 kg). Hothouse lambs may consist of ewe, wether, or ram lambs.

(Also see LAMB.)

HOT POT

This dish, which originated in Lancashire, England, became popular as a national dish. It consists of layering sliced potatoes, lamb chops (trimmed), lamb kidneys, onions, and mushrooms in a baking dish. Water is added, and it is baked covered in the oven. Sometimes meats other than lamb are used.

HUCKLEBERRY Gaylussacia spp

The fruit of a bush that grows wild throughout the United States and southern Canada.

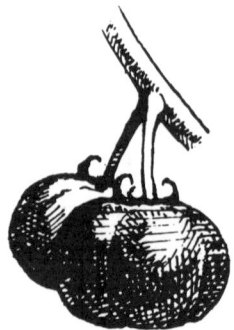

Fig. H-14. Huckleberry.

[34]The Harvard Medical School Letter, November, 1978, p. 5.

Huckleberries resemble blueberries, except that they are usually smaller, contain larger seeds, and are almost always gathered from wild bushes rather than from cultivated plants. They may be eaten fresh, or used to make jam, jelly, juice, pies, tarts, or wine.

(Also see FRUIT[S], Table F-23, Fruits of the World.)

HUCKLEBERRY, GARDEN (SUNBERRY; WONDERBERRY) *Solanum intrusum*

The fruit of a plant (of the family *Solanaceae*) that is believed to have originated in Africa. Garden huckleberries bear a close resemblance to the berries of the poisonous black nightshade, except that the former are a little larger.

Cultivated huckleberries are about ½ in. (*1.2 cm*) in diameter. The rather bland tasting fruit may be used in jams and pies.

HULLS

Outer covering of grain or other seed, especially when dry.

HUMBLE PIE

Originally, this was a meat pie made from the inferior parts of the carcass, usually eaten by the huntsman and the servants. Ironically, these variety meats were superior, nutritionally, to the more desired cuts.

HUMECTANT

A term for additives which prevent foods from drying out. Humectants keep marshmallows and shredded coconut soft. Glycerine (glycerol) and sorbitol are utilized for this purpose.

HUMULONE

One of the two resins of hops which imparts the traditional odor and bitter taste to beer.

(Also see BEERS AND BREWING.)

HUNGARIAN PARTRIDGE (CHUKAR; EUROPEAN PARTRIDGE; OR GRAY PARTRIDGE)

True partridges belong to the partridge family, *Phasianiidae*. There are about 150 kinds of these birds, the best known of which are: (1) the Hungarian (or gray partridge; European partridge), native to Europe, northern Africa, and Western Asia, which is genus *Perdix*, species *P. perdix*); and (2) the Chukar, native to Asia and Europe, which is *Alectoris chukar*.

The Hungarian, or gray partridge, was introduced into western United States as a game bird early in the 20th century. Today, most of these birds are found on the Canadian plains and in the North Central and Northwestern United States.

The chukar, which was also introduced into the United States, is an important game bird in northwestern United States.

HUNGER

Hunger is a physiological desire for food following a period of fasting . Appetite, on the other hand, is a learned or habitual response, which arises with the customary intervals of eating and may be influenced by numerous external and internal phenomena. Satiety is the opposite of hunger—a feeling of complete fulfillment of the desire for food.

(Also see APPETITE.)

HUNGER, WORLD

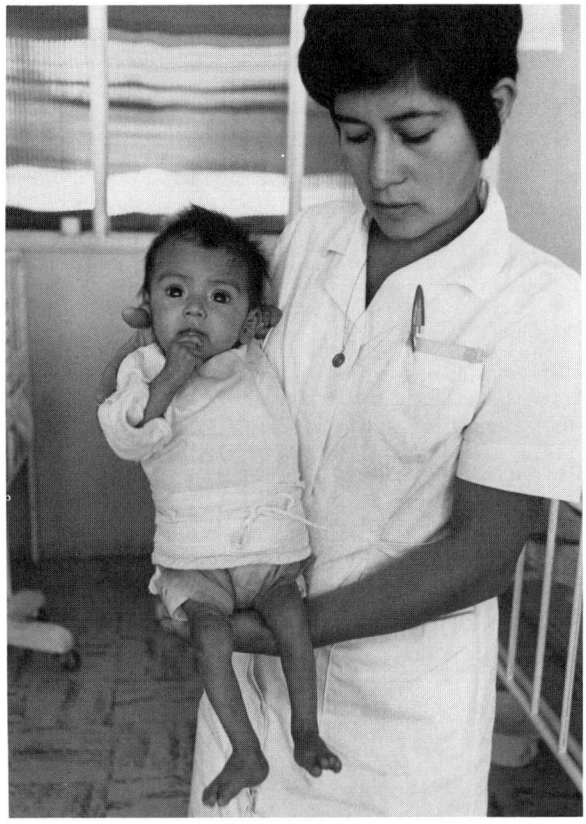

Fig. H-15. Hunger is a tragedy for millions of children and their families. Yet scenes like this can be avoided. (Courtesy, World Health Organization, Geneva, Switzerland.)

Many knowledgeable people subscribe to the view that the world is on the brink of being subjected to food shortages of unprecedented scale and urgency—a world broken by unshared bread.

The troubled 21st century will open with 1.3 billion malnourished people, up from one-half billion in 1986. Starvation will claim increasing numbers, and many of the surviving babies will grow up physically and mentally retarded. More disturbing yet, all nations and all people must realize that a hungry man is impelled only by his hunger and the right to survive, and that there can be no peace on an empty stomach.

The best way in which to lessen hunger and malnutrition in the developing countries is by a massive infusion of science, technology, and education—by self-help programs—so that they can produce more of their own food.

Improved genetics, along with improved feeding and management, have made for more meat, milk, and eggs in the United States, as shown in Fig. H-16. And similar achievements have been made in crops.

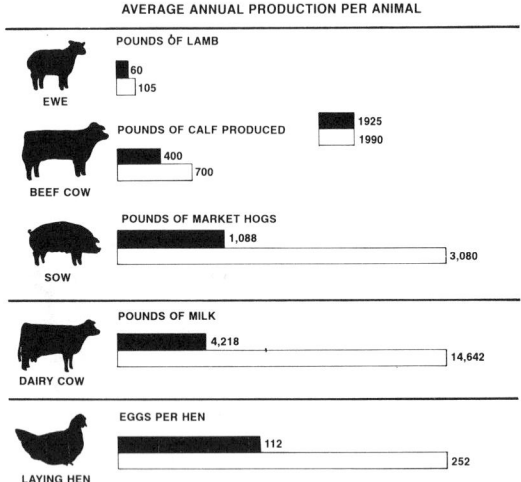

Fig. H-16. Improved efficiency in U.S. meat and milk animals from 1925 to 1990. The application of science and technology made the difference. *Sources:* Milk and egg statistics from USDA. Ewe, beef, cow, and sow statistics estimated by Dr. M. E. Ensminger.

The science and technology that have been so successful in the United States may be adapted to and applied by developing countries.

(Also see MALNUTRITION, PROTEIN-ENERGY; POPULATION, WORLD; PROTEIN, WORLD PER CAPITA; and WORLD FOOD.)

HUSKS

Leaves enveloping an ear of corn (maize).

HYDRAULIC PROCESS

A process for the mechanical extraction of oil from seeds, involving the use of a hydraulic press. Sometimes referred to as the old process.

(Also see SOYBEAN.)

HYDROCHLORIC ACID (HCL)

Formed by the chemical combination of hydrogen (H) and chlorine (Cl), it is important in the digestion of proteins. Hydrochloric acid secreted by the cells of the stomach breaks down some proteins, but, more importantly, it provides an environment conducive to the activity of the enzyme pepsin.

(Also see DIGESTION AND ABSORPTION; and HYPER-CHLORHYDRIA.)

HYDROCOOLING

To avoid loss of produce through decay and to preserve freshness, many fruits and vegetables are substantially cooled shortly after harvesting. In the past, packing produce with ice when loading for transport was the major practice. Now, many fruits and vegetables are cooled by spraying them continuously with cool water while they are in wholesale containers—hydrocooling. The water used is recirculated. It often contains salt to lower the freezing point and a fungicide or bacteriocide. There are portable hydrocoolers which cool fruits and vegetables as they are picked and before loading them into refrigerated trucks or railroad cars.

(Also see VACUUM COOLING.)

HYDROGENATION

The chemical addition of hydrogen to any unsaturated compound. However, the term is usually applied to the process for hardening vegetable oils.

(Also see OILS, VEGETABLE.)

HYDROLYSATE

The product of hydrolysis; for example, protein hydrolysate is a mixture of the constituent amino acids when the protein molecule is split by acids, alkalis, or enzymes.

HYDROLYSIS

The splitting of a substance into the smaller units by its chemical reaction with water.

(Also see DIGESTION AND ABSORPTION; and ENZYME.)

HYDROPONICS

Hydroponics is the growing of plants in chambers under conditions of controlled temperature and humidity with their roots immersed in an aqueous solution containing the essential mineral nutrient salts, instead of in soil. This means that food plants may be produced with water and chemicals, without soil.

HYDROSTATIC PRESSURE

The pressure exerted by a liquid on the surface of the walls that contain it, which is equal on all containing walls. In the body, hydrostatic pressure usually refers to the blood pressure; together with the plasma proteins, it maintains fluid circulation and volume in the blood vessels.

HYDROSTATIC STERILIZER

A type of continuous pressure cooker which is open to the atmosphere at the inlet and outlet. Steam pressure in the sterilizing chamber is balanced by tall columns of hot water in the inlet and cold water in the outlet. If the steam in the sterilizing chamber is 260°F (*127°C*), to balance the pressure developed the water columns would have to be 46 ft (*14 m*) high at the outlet and the inlet. The hydrostatic sterilizer is well suited for large scale production of canned goods. Canned goods on a conveyor transverse down the inlet column into the sterilizing chamber and then, after adequate time, leave via the outlet column.

HYDROXYLATION

The introduction of a hydroxy group (-OH) into an organic compound (a carbon-containing compound).

HYGROSCOPICITY

The degree of tendency to absorb and retain moisture. For example, nonfat dry milk (NDM) is hygroscopic in that it tends to absorb moisture.

HYPER–

A prefix meaning over, above, or beyond.

HYPERALIMENTATION, INTRAVENOUS

The term *hyperalimentation* alone literally means the provision of nutrients at levels considerably higher than those received in a normal diet, although in medical circles it is commonly used as a synonym for total parenteral nutrition (TPN). The latter procedure involves the provision of all nutrient requirements by intravenous means. However, the term *hyperalimentation* might also be used to indicate feeding by means of orally administered liquid diets which provide high levels of one or more nutrients. Furthermore, some patients on TPN are normal weight or overweight and will require only normal or somewhat subnormal levels of calories and nutrients such as carbohydrates and fats. Therefore, confusion about the nature of the various nutritional procedures may be avoided by using the terms *intravenous* and *parenteral* to denote feeding through the veins. (These subjects are covered in detail elsewhere in this book.)

(Also see INTRAVENOUS [PARENTERAL] NUTRITION, SUPPLEMENTARY; and TOTAL PARENTERAL [INTRAVENOUS] NUTRITION.)

HYPERCALCEMIA

An excessive quantity of calcium in the blood, above the normal level of 11 mg per 100 ml. Hypercalcemia may be caused by some cancers (especially lung cancer), overactivity of the parathyroid glands, chronic ingestion of large doses of vitamin D, and alkali and milk therapy for peptic ulcers. Affected persons demonstrate a loss of appetite, vomiting, flabby muscles, and possibly kidney stones.

(Also see CALCIUM.)

HYPERCALCIURIA

Excess calcium in the urine, as in hyperparathyroidism.

HYPERCHLORHYDRIA (HYPERACIDITY)

A term used to denote excess acidity of the gastric juice, most often hydrochloric acid, in the stomach. It is usually accompanied by burning pain after meals, heartburn, and acid indigestion. It is a common symptom of emotional upsets, duodenal ulcers, or inflammation of the gallbladder and is associated with hunger pains.

The distress may be relieved by antacids, including calcium carbonate, aluminum hydroxide gel, milk of magnesia, magnesium carbonate, and magnesium trisilicate.

(Also see ANTACIDS; GASTRITIS; HEARTBURN; INDIGESTION; and ULCERS, PEPTIC.)

HYPERCHOLESTEREMIA (HYPERCHOLESTEROLEMIA)

Excess of cholesterol in the blood.

HYPEREMIA

An excess of blood in any part of the body.

HYPERESTHESIA

Excess sensitivity to touch or pain.

HYPERGLYCEMIA

Excess of sugar in the blood.

HYPERKALEMIA

Excess potassium in the blood. Hyperkalemia is a serious complication of kidney failure, severe dehydration, or shock; it causes the heart to dilate, and the heart rate is slowed by weakened conditions.

HYPERLIPOPROTEINEMIAS (HYPERLIPIDEMIAS)

The term hyperlipoproteinemias refers to a group of disorders characterized by excessive concentrations of one or more of the lipoproteins in the blood.

Fats or lipids, which are not soluble in a water medium such as blood, are transported in the blood in the form of water-soluble, fat-protein complexes—lipoproteins. All of these lipoproteins contain phospholipids, triglycerides, and cholesterol, but in varying amounts.

The lipoproteins are classified as chylomicrons, very low density lipoproteins (VLDL), low density lipoproteins (LDL), or high density lipoproteins (HDL)—according to their density, from least dense to most dense. They are also named prebeta-lipoproteins (VLDL), beta-lipoproteins (LDL), and alpha-lipoproteins (HDL), based upon their migration on paper subjected to an electrical field—electrophoresis.

Levels of lipoproteins in the blood are controlled by diet, a number of hormones (anterior pituitary hormones, adrenal hormones, insulin, and thyroxine), age, weight change, emotions and stress, drugs, and illness. Abnormalities of blood lipid levels are best determined by measurement of the lipoproteins rather than the analyses of the blood lipid fractions alone. Thus disorders in blood lipid levels are classified according to the concentrations of the lipoproteins. The term hyperlipoproteinemias is used to describe a group of disorders characterized by excessive concentrations of one or more of the lipoproteins in the blood, the types of which follow:

Type I. Hyperchylomicronemia (normal or elevated cholesterol with markedly elevated triglyceride).
Type IIA. Hyperbeta-lipoproteinemia or hypercholesterolemia (increased LDL).
Type IIB. Hypercholesterolemia with hyperglyceridemia or combined hyperlipidemia (increased LDL and VLDL).
Type III. Broad-beta or floating beta (increased ILDL).
Type IV. Hyperpre-beta-lipoproteinemia (increased VLDL).
Type V. Mixed hyperlipidemia (increased chylomicrons and VLDL).

The specific causes of the hyperlipoproteinemias are not completely understood. In a broad sense, hyperlipoproteinemias occur for two reasons: (1) inadequate removal of the lipoprotein from the blood, and (2) increased production of lipoproteins. In turn this may be caused by secondary diseases such as diabetes, liver disease, and hypothyroidism. On the other hand, hyperlipoproteinemias may be the primary disorder, but their cause is not obvious. Many of the primary hyperlipoproteinemias indicate a genetic origin. They *run in families.*

Elevated lipoproteins are a major health concern due to their association with accelerated atherosclerosis—a basic pathologic process in coronary heart disease. Fortunately, the hyperlipoproteinemias generally respond to diet therapy and within a few weeks lipoproteins may be lowered. Both the American Heart Association and the National Heart and Lung Institute have published detailed diets for controlling the hyperlipoproteinemias. Overall, the therapeutic diet is palatable, selected from ordinary foods, and no more expensive than the usual diet.

If a personal medical history, family history, and physical examination suggest the existence of a hyperlipoproteinemia, the next step is to measure blood levels of cholesterol and triglycerides. These measurements are made on blood drawn after an overnight fast during a steady state period in an individual's habits and environment. Elevated levels of cholesterol and/or triglycerides, or the presence of a *creamy* layer on the top of plasma after overnight refrigeration indicates to a physician the type of hyperlipoproteinemia. The actual lipoproteins—chylomicrons, VLDL, LDL or HDL—which are involved may need to be determined by ultracentrifugal fractionation or electrophoretic analysis. However, both of these laboratory techniques are too time-consuming and complex for routine blood analyses.

(Also see DIGESTION AND ABSORPTION; ENDOCRINE GLANDS; FATS AND OTHER LIPIDS; HEART DISEASE; INBORN ERRORS OF METABOLISM; and METABOLISM.)

HYPERPHOSPHATEMIA

Excess phosphorus in the blood serum, which may result (1) when the kidneys do not excrete phosphorus adequately, or (2) from hypoparathyroidism, which causes an insufficient secretion of parathyroid hormone. When serum phosphorus rises, serum calcium falls, causing tetany.

HYPERPLASIA

Abnormal increase in number of normal cells.

HYPERTENSION

The medical term for high blood pressure. It is not a disease as such; rather, it is a sign of a variety of diseases differing in nature and significance. High blood pressure is indicated by a persistent elevation above normal limits. The normal: 120-150 systolic pressure (when the heart contracts), and 80-100 diastolic pressure (when the heart is at rest). Blood pressure is a measure of the pressure of the blood against the walls of the blood vessels produced by the beating of the heart.

(Also see HEART DISEASE; and HIGH BLOOD PRESSURE.)

HYPERTHYROIDISM

Overactivity of the thyroid gland.
(Also see GOITER.)

HYPERTONIC DEHYDRATION

Loss of water from cells as a result of hypertonicity (excess solutes [dissolved substances]; hence, greater osmotic pressure) of the surrounding extracellular fluid.

HYPERTRIGLYCERIDEMIA

Increased levels of triglycerides in the blood.

HYPERTROPHIED

Having increased in size beyond the normal growth.

HYPERURICEMIA

Excess of uric acid in the blood—a characteristic of gout.

HYPERVITAMINOSIS (VITAMIN OVERDOSES)

This refers to an excessive intake of certain vitamins. The best known vitamin toxicities are those which result from vitamin A (known as hypervitaminosis A) and vitamin D (known as hypervitaminosis D), because (1) these vitamins are fat-soluble, (2) small amounts of them have strong effects, and (3) they tend to accumulate in the liver. Toxic effects do not occur so readily with vitamins E and K, which are also fat-soluble, unless high potency supplements are taken. Excesses of water-soluble vitamins (vitamin C and the vitamin B complex) are not stored in the body to any great extent, so toxicities from food sources of these nutrients are rare. However, people who take very large doses (mega-

doses) of any vitamin in the form of supplements should be under the supervision of a physician or nutritionist.

(Also see DISEASES, section headed "Essential Nutrients"; and VITAMIN[S].)

HYPO-

Prefix meaning lack, or a deficiency.

HYPOALBUMINEMIA

Abnormally low albumin level of the blood.

HYPOCALCEMIA

A subnormal concentration of ionic calcium in blood resulting in convulsions, as in tetany. The most common cause of this problem in man is lack of parathormone, a secretion of the parathyroid glands.

(Also see CALCIUM.)

HYPOCHLOREMIC ALKALOSIS

An abnormal decrease of chlorides in the blood, with bicarbonate replacing the chloride ions, may lead to hypochloremic alkalosis. This condition may follow excessive loss of gastric secretion (hydrochloric acid) with the accompanying loss of chlorides. Excess vomiting may cause hypochloremic alkalosis unless the chloride is replaced promptly.

HYPOCHLORHYDRIA

Decreased secretion of hydrochloric acid by the cells of the stomach.

HYPOCHROMIC

An abnormal decrease in the hemoglobin content of the red blood cells, characterized by below normal color.

HYPOCUPREMIA

A deficiency in blood copper, which may be caused by urinary loss of ceruloplasmin (the copper binding protein of the plasma) in nephrosis (degeneration of the kidneys) or by malabsorption of copper in sprue.

HYPOGEUSIA

A diminished (or blunted) sense of taste.

HYPOGLYCEMIA (LOW BLOOD SUGAR)

This condition results when the level of glucose, the main

sugar found in the blood, is below normal. It may be accompanied by such irritating signs as anxiety, mental confusion, rapid pulse, and tiredness which is greater than might be expected under the circumstances. The diverse complaints accompanying hypoglycemia are due to the sensitivity of the brain and the nerves to deprivation of glucose, which is the major source of energy for these tissues. Some physicians believe the condition to be uncommon, while others suspect it to be regularly present in a fairly large group of people. Those doctors who subscribe to the latter thinking have, at various times, suggested that low blood sugar may be associated with such diverse disorders as alcoholism, excess coffee, allergies, behavior problems, brain damage in infants, depression, diabetes, drug addiction, fatigue, high blood pressure, impotency, obesity, ulcers, and under-achievement in school.

FACTORS WHICH RAISE OR LOWER THE BLOOD SUGAR IN HEALTHY PEOPLE.
The means by which people adapt to irregularities in the supply of dietary carbohydrates, and yet maintain normal functioning of their brain and nerves, is explored in the next two sections.

Control Of Blood Sugar After Meals.
The factors which affect the blood sugar after a meal are outlined in Fig. H-17.

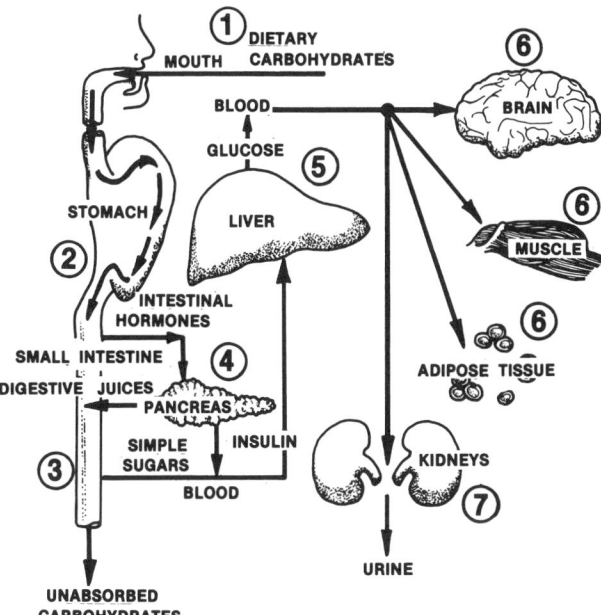

FACTORS WHICH AFFECT THE BLOOD SUGAR AFTER A MEAL

1. Size and nutrient composition of the meal
2. Rate at which the stomach empties into the small intestine
3. Efficiency of digestion and absorption
4. Rate of insulin secretion by the pancreas
5. Metabolism of sugars and insulin in the liver
6. Utilization of glucose by such tissues as brain, muscle, and adipose tissue
7. Spilling of sugar from the blood into the urine

Fig. H-17. Regulation of blood sugar after meals.

Control Of Blood Sugar During Fasting Or Starvation.
Many people are able to withstand considerable deprivation of food without experiencing signs of abnormalities in their mental and nervous functions. Others, not so

fortunate, may have symptoms of low blood sugar when they go too long between meals. The major factors which help to maintain the blood sugar during fasting or starvation are outlined in Fig. H-18.

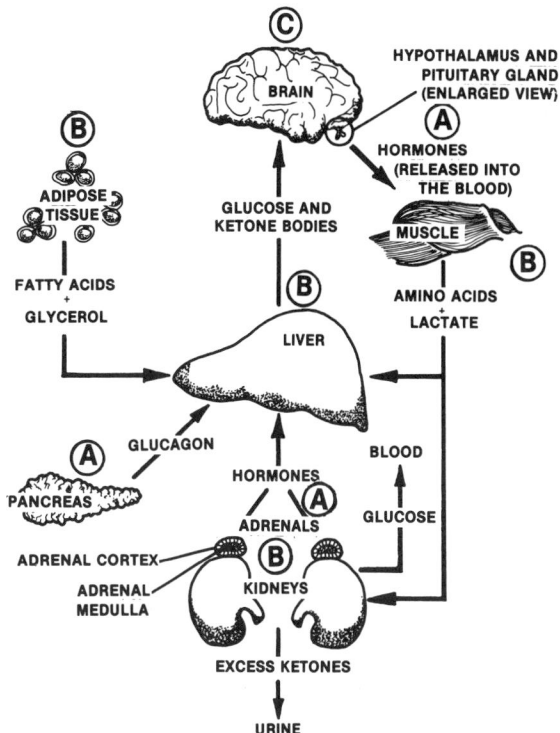

FACTORS WHICH HELP TO MAINTAIN THE BLOOD SUGAR DURING FASTING OR STARVATION

Ⓐ Release of hormones which trigger glucose-producing responses of tissues

Ⓑ Production of glucose from glycogen, fats, and amino acids

Ⓒ Reduced activity of satiety center in the brain, increased appetite for food

Fig. H-18. Regulation of blood sugar during fasting or starvation.

MAJOR CAUSES OF HYPOGLYCEMIA.
Low blood sugar is often nature's way of telling a person that he or she needs to eat some food; for if the blood sugar could be maintained at a normal level during fasting, one might go without eating and starve to death. Fortunately, there are also other factors, such as force of habit and rumblings of the stomach, which provoke us to eat. However, even persons who are well fed and apparently healthy may sometimes suffer from bouts of hypoglycemia. Furthermore, it would not be sensible to advise all persons with a tendency for low blood sugar to rely solely on eating when they have symptoms of this condition, since some might become obese, which could lead to even worse problems. Last, but not least, there is always the possibility that hypoglycemia might be due to a disorder requiring medical treatment. Therefore, it is important to note the causes of low blood sugar which follow:

1. Adrenal cortical exhaustion, or chronic insufficiency of the glands.
2. Alcoholism.
3. Caffeine consumption.
4. Children born to diabetic mothers.
5. Diabetes, adult onset type.
6. Dietary factors such as meals far apart or high in carbohydrates.
7. Drugs, especially insulin, tranquilizers, and aspirin.
8. Emotional stress.

9. Exercise.
10. Fasting or starvation.
11. Gastrointestinal problems.
12. Glucagon insufficiency.
13. Inborn errors of metabolism.
14. Insulin excess.
15. Kidney disease.
16. Liver disease.
17. Obesity.
18. Pituitary insufficiency.
19. Thyroid deficiency.
20. Tumors.
21. Women after childbirth.

OTHER DISORDERS WHICH MAY RESULT FROM HYPOGLYCEMIA. Just about everyone may have a mild hypoglycemic episode from time to time. Perfect regulation of the blood sugar in the face of all challenges is more than might be expected of a normal, healthy body. Experienced athletes and other people who strive hard to reach their goals learn that temporary weaknesses due to low blood sugar soon pass. However, severe forms of acute or chronic hypoglycemia pose some dangers, since upsetting the normal processes of the body may, along with other factors, produce harmful effects. Some possible effects of abnormally low levels of blood sugar follow:
1. Accident proneness.
2. Alcoholism.
3. Brain damage in infants.
4. Depression.
5. Diabetes.
6. Drug addiction.
7. Extra sensitivity to allergens.
8. Fatigue.
9. Glycogen depletion.
10. High blood pressure (hypertension).
11. Hunger for sweets.
12. Irritability.
13. Ketosis.
14. Liver damage.
15. Neurotic behavior.
16. Obesity.
17. Oversusceptibility to toxic agents.
18. Slackening of mental or physical performance.
19. Sleeplessness.
20. Ulcers.

DIAGNOSIS OF HYPOGLYCEMIA. A doctor should be relied upon to decide whether or not one has a tendency towards an abnormally low blood sugar level because a laboratory test on the blood is needed in order to be certain of the diagnosis. However, everyone should be able to recognize the major signs and symptoms of the condition so as to know when a physician should be consulted.

Signs And Symptoms. When hypoglycemia develops within a short period of time (such as from the oversecretion of insulin), the symptoms, which are mainly due to the adrenalin response, include rapid pulse, trembling, hunger, and a slight amount of mental confusion. However, hypoglycemia which has developed over many hours (such as when meals are skipped) is characterized by signs that the brain has undergone glucose deprivation, including headache, depression, blurred vision, incoherent speech, considerable mental confusion, and, occasionally, coma or convulsions. None of the above signs and symptoms can be attributed solely to hypoglycemia. There are similar syndromes

in drunkenness and in certain nutritional deficiencies. Therefore, a person suspected of having a tendency to low blood sugar should be given a glucose tolerance test.

Glucose Tolerance Test (GTT). The term *glucose tolerance* literally means the rate at which the cells of the body take up glucose from the blood. Factors which reduce glucose tolerance are those that slow the rate of glucose uptake by cells. Therefore, such factors tend to raise the blood sugar above the level considered normal under conditions of good health.

The test is administered in the morning, following an overnight fast. Sometimes, the doctor or dietitian tells the person who is to be tested to eat a diet moderately high in carbohydrates (250 to 300 g) for each of the 3 days preceding the test. The purpose of this so-called *carbohydrate-loading* is to stimulate the pancreas to its full capacity for secreting insulin. First, a sample of *fasting blood* is taken. Then, a test dose of glucose is given in the form of a water solution which the patient drinks. Blood samples are usually taken at hourly intervals for up to 6 hours. A diagnosis is made by comparing the hourly blood glucose levels of the patient to standard values. Depending upon the judgment of the physician and the laboratory methods used to measure glucose, a person is diagnosed as hypoglycemic when his or her blood sugar falls to values below 60 mg of glucose per 100 ml of blood. Fig. H-19 shows normal, hypoglycemic, and diabetic blood sugar curves. Explanations of these curves follow.

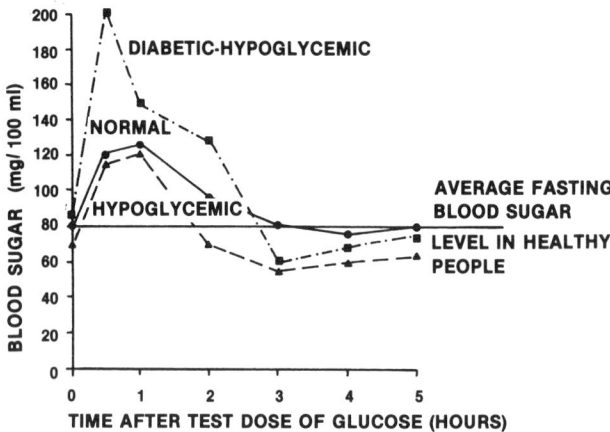

Fig. H-19. Glucose tolerance curves.

The normal blood sugar curve shows a moderate rise as the test dose of glucose is absorbed from the intestine and enters the blood. Soon after absorption, insulin secreted by the pancreas starts to promote the utilization of glucose by various tissues, thereby causing the blood sugar to drop back to the fasting level. A fasting blood sugar of around 80 mg per 100 ml of blood is considered to be normal.

A person with hypoglycemia may have a fasting blood sugar slightly below normal (70 instead of 80). However, the early response of such a person to a test dose of glucose will be very close to normal for the first hour or so of the test. Then, there is likely to be an abnormally sharp drop in the blood sugar due to an oversecretion of insulin. After about 3 hours, the blood glucose level of the hypoglycemic is likely to be below the normal fasting level. It may then start back up towards the normal level after the 4th or 5th hour. People whose blood sugar curve indicates hypoglycemia may be totally free of symptoms. For this reason, some doctors and health scientists think that a lowered blood sugar should not be considered hypoglycemic until it drops to 40. On the other hand, some people start to have symptoms while their blood sugar is on its way down, but is above 60.

Finally, many people with adult onset diabetes may have a blood sugar curve which typifies what at one time was called *dysinsulinism,* in which the insulin response is delayed and the blood sugar soars to a diabetic level. At this point, there is a heavy secretion of insulin which causes the blood sugar to plummet to a hypoglycemic level. Hence hypoglycemia is sometimes a prelude to, or an accompaniment of, diabetes.

(Also see DIABETES MELLITUS.)

Conditions Which May Mimic Hypoglycemia.
Many of the signs and symptoms of low blood sugar are similar to those which occur in other, unrelated disorders. Some of these conditions follow:
1. Reduced flow of blood to the brain and other tissues.
2. Depression.
3. Nutritional deficiencies.
4. Alkalosis.

TREATMENT AND PREVENTION OF HYPOGLYCEMIA.
It is important to treat severe hypoglycemia promptly, so as to avoid permanent damage to the brain and nervous system. After treatment has been given, measures should be taken to prevent such episodes in the future, since the victim might have another attack when alone or at night while sleeping. It makes one wonder how many times hypoglycemia might have been a contributing factor to deaths occurring in the early hours of the morning. Such thoughts give point and purpose to the recommendations which follow:

Emergency Treatment.
Every person known to have a tendency to diabetes or hypoglycemia should always have a source of sugar at hand, such as hard candy, fruit juice, or just plain packets of sugar. These items will pull a person out of the severe stage of hypoglycemia, but they may also render the victim more susceptible to a subsequent attack. Therefore, long-term measures to prevent future attacks need to be instituted at the first opportunity.

Diet Therapy.
The standard treatment for low blood sugar was formerly a low-carbohydrate, high-fat diet. However, many of those so treated developed adult onset diabetes. It is conjectured that the hypoglycemia of these patients was actually the first sign of diabetes. If that were the case, a high-fat diet did more harm than good, since it is well known that fat blocks the actions of insulin. This effect of fat was formerly thought to be desirable for hypoglycemics, because the therapy was aimed at countering what was thought to be the result of excessive insulin secretion. Recent research has shown that replacement of dietary carbohydrate with either fat or protein has undesirable effects on patients who develop low blood sugar after eating.[35] Therefore, the current dietary treatment for hypoglycemia is based upon the following considerations:
1. Insulin secretion should be regulated by avoiding excessive stimulation of the pancreas by either large meals or too much readily available carbohydrate.
2. Six small meals daily are preferable to three large ones. Reducing the intervals between meals from about 5 hours on a three-meal pattern to about 3 hours on a six-meal pattern helps to keep the blood sugar from dropping too low.
3. The dietary pattern should be essentially the same as that for adult onset diabetes.
4. Hard-to-manage cases may require nondietary treatments, rather than diets which are extremely low in carbohydrates.

Practical Hints for Controlling Blood Sugar.
People who have a tendency towards low blood sugar may often spare themselves from the agonies of this condition if they regularly eat a good diet and practice certain other health habits. Some beneficial practices follow:
1. Eat regular, well-balanced meals.
2. Avoid highly refined starches and sugars, especially between meals.
3. Avoid caffeine.
4. Exercise and avoid stress.

Nondietary Measures.
It may be necessary for a physician to resort to nondietary treatments to control hypoglycemia in some people. Discussions of some typical measures follow:

• **Adrenal cortical extract**—Some recent books and articles for the lay public have promoted injections of adrenal cortical extract as a remedy for low blood sugar. The American Medical Association is strongly opposed to such treatments on the grounds that (1) they are nowhere near as effective as injections of pure, steroid hormones; and (2) many people who have been given these injections do not need extra adrenal cortical hormones. A hypoglycemic glucose tolerance does *not* demonstrate the lack of sufficient adrenal cortical secretion. Special tests of the glands' function are necessary for such a diagnosis.

• **Antispasmodic (anticholinergic) drugs**—These drugs block some of the nerve impulses to the stomach and intestine, thereby slowing the rate of emptying of the stomach, and reducing the secretion of intestinal hormones which trigger the release of insulin. Such therapy has helped some highly nervous people who literally had jittery digestive systems.

• **Psychotherapy**—Although these treatments may be expensive and time-consuming, they may in the long run be well worth the cost, since continual emotional distress may ruin one's health. However, a thorough physical examination is often helpful in determining the extent to which hypoglycemia is mental and/or physical.

• **Steroid hormone treatments**—Sometimes, tests of adrenal cortical function reveal an insufficiency in the secretion of these glands. Then, it is necessary for the physician to inject regularly the hormones which are lacking.

• **Surgery**—Surgical removal of part of the pancreas may be necessary if it contains a tumor which is secreting a large excess of insulin.

(NOTE WELL: For a more complete discussion of Hypoglycemia, see the two-volume *Foods & Nutrition Encyclopedia,* a work by the same authors as *Food For Health.)*

---

[35]Anderson, J. W., and R. H. Herman, "Effect of Carbohydrate Restriction on Glucose Tolerance of Normal Men and Reactive Hypoglycemic Patients," *The American Journal of Clinical Nutrition*, Vol. 28, 1975, p. 748.

HYPOGLYCEMIC AGENTS

These agents are capable of lowering the sugar (glucose) content of the blood. The hormone insulin from the pancreas is the natural hypoglycemic agent. Some sulfa-type drugs (sulfonylureas) are used as hypoglycemic agents for some forms of diabetes. However, the action of these drugs is to stimulate the pancreas to release insulin.

(Also see DIABETES MELLITUS, section headed "Treatment and Prevention of Diabetes"; ENDOCRINE GLANDS; and HYPOGLYCEMIA.)

HYPOKALEMIA

Low potassium in the blood. Hypokalemia is a serious complication of severe diarrhea, in which large amounts of potassium are lost in intestinal secretions. Replacement therapy should involve added potassium.

HYPOMAGNESEMIA

An abnormally low level of magnesium in the blood. (Also see MAGNESIUM.)

HYPOPROTEINEMIA

An abnormally small amount of total protein in the blood plasma.

HYPOTHALAMUS

A group of nuclei at the base of the brain, including (1) centers of appetite control, and (2) cells that produce antidiuretic hormone.

HYPOTHYROIDISM

Under activity of the thyroid gland, of which there are two forms: (1) cretinism, a congenital defect, and (2) myxedema, subnormal secretion occurring anytime after birth.

(Also see ENDOCRINE GLANDS; GOITER, sections headed "Cretinism," "Myxedema," and "Prevention of Goiter and Related Disorders.")

HYPOTONE DEHYDRATION

Increase of water in cells (cellular edema) and decrease of extracellular fluid, as a result of hypotonicity (decreased solutes [dissolved substances]; hence, diminished osmotic pressure) of the extracellular fluid surrounding the cell.

HYPOVITAMINOSIS (AVITAMINOSIS)

A deficiency of one or more vitamins. Often the term is used in combination with a specific vitamin to identify the vitamin involved; for example, hypovitaminosis A.

HYSSOP

An herb whose natural camphoric characteristics are extracted and used to flavor liqueurs such as Benedictine and Chartreuse. It is a GRAS additive.

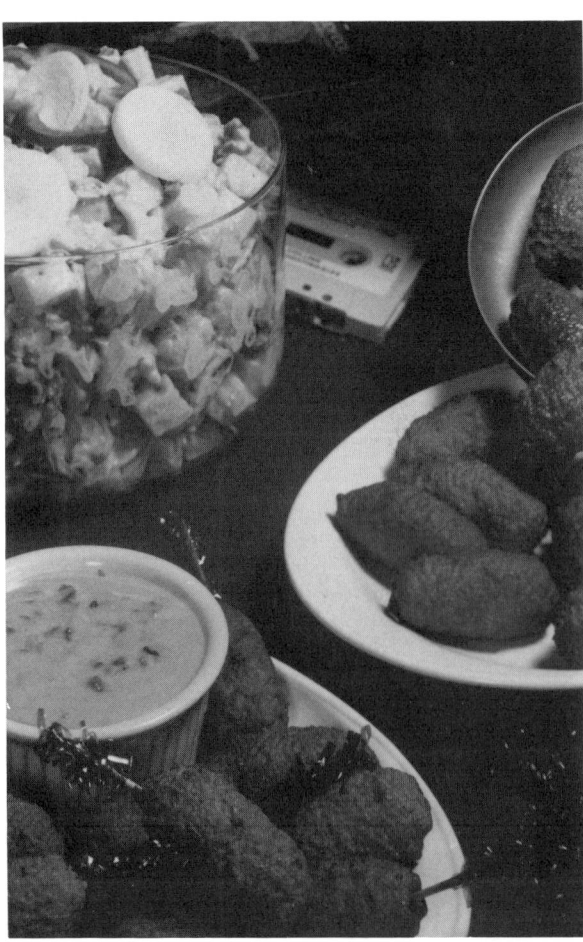

Fig. H-20. Corn dogs and potato salad. (Courtesy, Carnation, Los Angeles, Calif.)

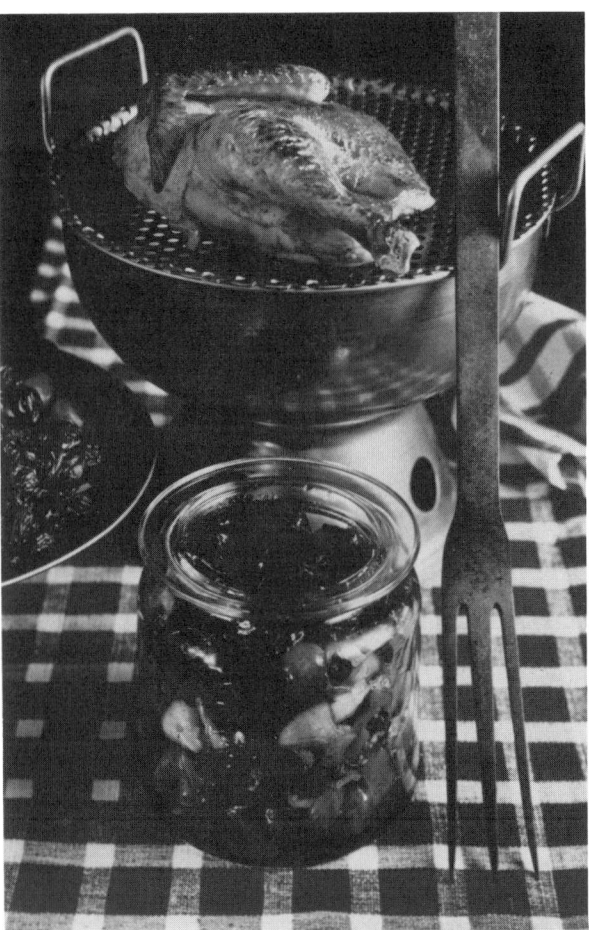

Fig. H-21. Chicken and chutney. Variety is the key to all successful diets. (Courtesy, Siegel/Ketchum, San Francisco, Calif.)

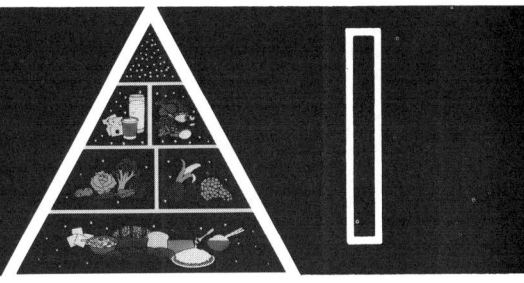

ICELAND MOSS *Cetraria*

This is a lichen, *Cetraria islandica*, which grows in all northern countries. Iceland, Norway, and Sweden export Iceland moss. When it is boiled with water it forms a jelly after cooling. Iceland moss is used like other gums—for foods, cosmetics, and textile sizing. The gum of Iceland moss is a polysaccharide containing uronic acid, galactose, mannose, and glucose.

(Also see GUMS.)

IDIOPATHIC

A condition of spontaneous origin; occurring without known cause.

ILEAL RESECTION

A surgical removal of part of the ileum section of the small intestine.

ILEITIS

Inflammation of the ileum, which is the last two-thirds of the small intestine before joining the large intestine. It may be caused by intestinal infections such as typhoid fever or dysentery, an obstruction, a chronic irritation, or a defect in the immune system. Also, like other gastrointestinal disorders, emotional upset seems to contribute to the cause. Sufferers experience loss of appetite, loss of weight, anemia, diarrhea, pain in the lower right of the abdomen, and soreness around the navel. Acute cases are usually self-limiting and respond to bed rest and a change in daily routine. More serious cases may require surgery and medication. Some dietary adjustments may also be necessary. Many persons respond to some degree of fiber restriction. Also vitamin and mineral supplementation are recommended.

(Also see DIGESTION AND ABSORPTION; and MODIFIED DIETS.)

ILEUM

The lower portion of the small intestine extending from the jejunum to the cecum.

(Also see DIGESTION AND ABSORPTION.)

ILEUS

Obstruction of the bowel.

ILLIPE BUTTER

This is oil pressed from the fruits of the *Bassia longifolia* plant, or ilpa, of the East Indies. People of India use it as a butter substitute.

IMMUNOGLOBULINS

A family of proteins found in body fluids which have the property of combining with antigens and, when the antigen is pathogenic, sometimes inactivating it and producing a state of immunity. They are also called antibodies. Colostrum is high in immunoglobulins. It is suspected that full protection against disease by these substances depends upon adequate protein nutrition.

(Also see PROTEIN[S].)

IMPERMEABLE

Not capable of being penetrated.

INBORN ERRORS OF METABOLISM

As often as the genetic code is correctly interpreted and reproduced, mistakes—mutations—do sometimes occur. Mutations result in genetically determined metabolic disorders due to specific defects, present at birth, though not always evident. Inborn errors of metabolism is a phrase coined by Archibald E. Garrod who described only four diseases of a hereditary nature, at the beginning of this century. These disorders may also be referred to as genetic diseases or hereditary molecular diseases. Outwardly, the infant appears normal at birth. However, once it begins to receive nutrition and/or interacts with other environmental factors, some dramatic changes may occur in mental and/or physical development due to abnormal utilization of nutrients by the body. Evidence of other genetic diseases does not appear until later in life. There are two main types of genetic disorders of metabolism: (1) the absence or severe reduction in the activity of an enzyme or enzymes, and (2) a defect in the transport of metabolites across cell membranes. Hence, both types may involve protein molecules whose synthesis is directed by the genetic material of the cells—the DNA. Detrimental effects of these metabolic errors are due to the accumulation of toxic levels of a biochemical and/or the reduced availability of an essential biochemical. Genetic defects vary widely, and may alter the metabolism of amino acids, carbohydrates, lipids, vitamins, and minerals. There are between 100 and 200 genetic disorders. Fortunately, many are extremely rare, while others are harmless and only represent biological variation.

Early diagnosis of inborn errors of metabolism is important so treatment may be initiated before irreversible mental and/or physical damage occurs. In general, some of the approaches to treatment of inborn errors include (1) environmental modification, (2) dietary restriction and/or supplementation, (3) product, enzyme, or cofactor replacement or enhancement, (4) depletion of toxic levels of stored substances, (5) drug avoidance, (6) surgical intervention, and (7) possibly in the future, genetic engineering. For some inborn errors no known therapy is available.

Tables I-1 to I-5 outline the specific defects, characteristic features, and treatment (particularly dietary management), of some of the more important inborn errors in the metabolism of amino acids, carbohydrates, lipids, nucleic acids, and miscellaneous inborn disorders of metabolism.

(Also see AMINO ACID[S]; CARBOHYDRATE[S]; DIGESTION AND ABSORPTION; DISEASES; ENZYME; FATS AND OTHER LIPIDS; and METABOLISM.)

TABLE I-1
INBORN ERRORS OF AMINO ACID METABOLISM

Disorder	Defect(s)	Characteristic Features	Treatment
Albinism	Insufficient levels of the enzyme tyrosinase.	Inability to form pigment melanin; lack of pigmentation of hair, skin, and eyes.	Protection from sunlight.
Alkaptonuria	Insufficient levels of the enzyme homogentisic acid oxidase.	Incomplete oxidation of tyrosine and phenylalanine; darkening of urine; pigmentation of connective tissue; inflammation of the vertebrae (spondylitis) and joint disease (arthropathy).	Once pigmentation of connective tissue is established, there is no effective treatment. Possible benefit if phenylalanine and tyrosine intake could be limited following early detection; ascorbic acid supplementation.
Argininosuccinic aciduria (Also see UREA CYCLE.)	Insufficient levels of the enzyme argininosuccinase.	Elevated arginosuccinic acid in blood, urine, and spinal fluid; ammonia intoxication; severe mental retardation; seizures; liver dysfunction.	Lowering protein intake to 0.5 to 1.0 g/kg body weight may be effective; frequent feedings.
Citrullinemia (Also see UREA CYCLE.)	Insufficient levels of the enzyme argininosuccinic acid synthetase.	Elevated blood ammonia after eating; nausea; vomiting; mental retardation; elevated blood level of citrulline.	Restriction of dietary protein to 0.5 to 1.0 g/kg per day.
Cystathioninuria (Also see VITAMIN B-6.)	Insufficient levels of the enzyme cystathionase.	Excessive levels of cystathionine in urine, blood, and spinal fluid; possibly mental deficiency; seizures.	Marked improvement with vitamin B-6 (pyridoxine) therapy.
Cystinuria	Defective membrane transport in kidney and small intestine.	Excessive urinary excretion of cystine, lysine, arginine, and ornithine; formation of cystine kidney stones.	Restriction of dietary methionine; high fluid intake; alkalinizing urine; possible penicillamine to increase solubility of cystine.
Fanconi's syndrome (Also see VITAMIN D.)	No specific enzyme; defect in kidney transport mechanism.	Loss of amino acids, glucose, phosphate, and bicarbonate in urine; often acidosis; rickets or osteomalacia.	Therapy aimed at replacing losses; control acidosis; infants require vitamin D therapy plus neutral phosphates.
Hartnup disease	Defective membrane transport in kidney and small intestine.	Excretion of the amino acids valine, leucine, isoleucine, threonine serine, tryptophan, and phenylalanine in urine; pellagra-like skin rash; mental retardation.	Skin and neurological features respond to nicotinamide therapy (50 to 200 mg/day). High protein diet recommended to counter loss in urine; avoidance of undue exposure to sunlight.
Histidinemia	Insufficient levels of the enzyme histidase.	Elevated blood and urine histidine levels; some mental retardation; speech and hearing disorders.	High protein diet in infancy avoided; no claims made for improvement by dietary treatment.
Homocystinuria (Also see AMINO ACID[S]; and PROTEIN.)	Insufficient levels of the enzyme cystathionine synthetase.	High blood levels of methionine and homocysteine; eye problems; bone deformities; mild mental deficiency; common circulatory disorders.	Some types respond to massive vitamin B-6 (pyridoxine); others require low methionine diet with supplemental cystine; soy and gelatin used as protein sources; supplemental synthetic amino acids, fruits, vegetables, breads, cereals, fats supply energy; folic acid supplementation.
Hydroxyprolinemia	Insufficient levels of the enzyme hydroxyproline oxidase.	Hydroxyproline elevated in urine and blood; severe mental retardation in some cases.	Little success with dietary treatment; some cases of hydroxyprolinemia not harmful.
Hyperammonemia	Insufficient levels of the enzyme ornithine transcarbamylase or carbamylphosphate synthetase.	Ammonia intoxication—high blood levels of NH_3; vomiting; lethargy; coma; mental retardation.	Dietary protein restricted to 0.5 to 1.0 g/kg per day.
Hyperlysinemia (lysine intolerance)	Insufficient levels of the enzyme lysine NAD oxidoreductase.	High blood levels of arginine and lysine and sometimes ammonia; vomiting; spasticity; coma; mental retardation.	Dietary protein restricted to 1.5 g/kg per day; no treatment necessary in some cases.
Hyperoxaluria	Insufficient levels of the enzyme 2-oxo-glutarate: glyoxylate carboligase or D-glyceric dehydrogenase.	Increased urinary oxalate, of which ⅓ to ½ originates from glycine, an amino acid; symptoms and signs of kidney stones and advancing kidney failure.	None satisfactory; some use of high phosphate diet; plenty of drinking water; some use of large doses of vitamin B-6 (pyridoxine) and folic acid; possibly restrict dietary sources of oxalate—rhubarb and spinach.
Hyperprolinemia	Insufficient levels of the enzyme proline oxidase, or pyrroline-5-carboxylatedehydrogenase.	Excess urinary excretion of proline, glycine, hydroxyproline, and possibly pyrroline-5-carboxylic acid; fever, diarrhea, convulsions, and possible mental retardation; one form is without signs or symptoms.	Proline is synthesized by the body. Dietary management probably is difficult. An intermediate restriction of proline (130 mg/kg per day) may be helpful; further study necessary.
Hypervalinemia	Insufficient levels of the enzyme valine transaminase.	Elevated urinary and blood valine; growth retardation; mental retardation; vomiting; involuntary rapid eye movements (nystagmus).	Formula diet low in valine.
Isovaleric acidemia	Insufficient levels of the enzyme isovaleryl-CoA dehydrogenase.	Elevated plasma isovaleric acid; incoordination; acidosis; stupor; coma, foul smelling breath.	Management of acidosis; control of acute catabolic stimuli; low protein diet; just sufficient to maintain growth and low in leucine.
Maple syrup urine disease (branched-chain ketoaciduria) (Also see AMINO ACID[S].)	Insufficient levels of the enzyme branched-chain keto acid decarboxylases.	High levels of leucine, isoleucine, valine, and their keto acids in the blood and urine; maple syrup odor of urine; mental retardation; spasticity; seizures; convulsions.	Necessary to begin diet therapy first week of life and run through lifetime; synthetic formula diet; small amounts of milk for growth requirements; some low protein foods identified by their leucine content, for example, low protein cereals, fruits, and vegetables; synthetic formula meets energy, protein, and all other nutrient requirements.

(Continued)

TABLE I-1 *(Continued)*

Disorder	Defect(s)	Characteristic Features	Treatment
Methionine malabsorption (Oasthouse urine disease)	No specific enzyme; defect in small intestine transport system.	Only a few cases; convulsions and mental retardation; foul odor to urine; large amounts of methionine in urine.	Methionine restriction.
Phenylketonuria (PKU)	Insufficient levels of the enzyme phenylalanine hydroxylase.	Plasma phenylalanine elevated; urinary phenylalanine, phenylpyruvate, phenyllactate, phenylacetate, and O-hydroxyphenylacetate elevated in urine; *mousy* odor to urine and skin; mental retardation; fair complexion; convulsions; tremors; eczema.	Early detection; *Diaper test,* controlled phenylalanine intake; use of commercial preparation, Lofenalac; other foods of known phenylalanine content used to meet requirements for phenylalanine; Lofenalac provides main source of protein and energy; continued adjustment of diet necessary; discontinue at 6 to 8 years of age except during pregnancy.
Tyrosinemia (neonatal tyrosinemia)	Insufficient levels of the enzyme hydroxyphenylpyruvic acid oxidase or tyrosine transaminase.	Transient condition of newborns; increased levels of tyrosine in blood and urine drop as infant matures; not associated with specific symtoms.	Tyrosine in blood and urine returns to normal as infant matures. Vitamin C helps reduce blood levels. Reduced protein intake beneficial; often occurs in premature babies.
Tyrosinosis	Insufficient levels of the enzyme parahydroxyphenylpyruvic acid oxidase.	Elevated thyroxin levels in plasma and urine; loss of the amino acids proline, serine, and threonine in urine; kidney damage; liver damage; mental retardation; rickets; may progress so rapidly that death results from liver damage.	Diet low in phenylalanine and tyrosine; casein hydrolysate possibly used as source of protein and calories; limited amounts of foods low in phenylalanine and tyrosine.

TABLE I-2
INBORN ERRORS OF CARBOHYDRATE METABOLISM

Disorder	Defect(s)	Characteristic Features	Treatment
Carbohydrate intolerance	Insufficient levels of the enzymes disaccharidases such as maltase, isomaltase, invertase, lactase, and trehalase.	Diarrhea most outstanding feature; abdominal cramps; flatulence.	Dietary elimination of the sugar that is not tolerated; for example, maltose, sucrose, or lactose.
Fructose intolerance (fructosemia)	Insufficient levels of the enzyme fructose-1-phosphate aldolase.	Release of glucose from liver blocked by accumulation of fructose-1-phosphate; vomiting; hypoglycemia; death if fructose source not removed from diet.	Exclusion of sucrose and fructose sources from diet; elimination of most fruits; no table sugar; no sorbitol; avoid sweets.
Galactosemia	Insufficient levels of the enzyme galactose-1-phosphate uridyl transferase.	Elevated blood and urine levels of galactose; vomiting; failure to thrive; enlarged liver; mental retardation; cataract formation.	Early diagnosis; complete exclusion of lactose and galactose from diet; use of synthetic milk; milk permanently excluded from diet; supplements of calcium and riboflavin.
Glycogen storage diseases (10 types): Type I (von Gierke's disease)	Insufficient levels of the enzyme glucose-6-phosphatase.	Large liver and kidneys; kidney stones; yellowing or orange growth on skin due to lipid deposits (xanthomas); hypoglycemia; convulsions; coma; retarded growth.	High protein diet promoting gluconeogenesis; feedings every 3 to 4 hours; carbohydrate in form of glucose or starch; no sucrose or lactose; feeding medium chain triglycerides for treatment of xanthomas.
Type II (Pompe's disease)	Insufficient levels of the enzyme lysosomal glucosidase.	Massive glycogen infiltration particularly of the heart; cardiac distress; heart failure.	Treatment is useless.
Type III (limit dextrinosis; Cori's disease; Forbes' disease)	Insufficient levels of the enzyme amylo-1, 6-glucosidase.	Accumulation of glycogen with abnormal chemical structure in liver and muscles; enlarged liver.	High protein, low fat diet; frequent feedings; prompt treatment of infections; prohibition of strenuous exercise.
Type IV (amylopectinosis; brancher glycogenosis; Anderson's disease)	Insufficient levels of the enzyme amylo-1, 4—►6-transglucosylase.	Abnormally formed glycogen; enlarged spleen; enlarged liver; cirrhosis; liver failure; cardiac failure.	Death before third year; supportive treatment only.
Type V (McArdle's disease)	Insufficient levels of the enzyme muscle phosphorylase.	Accumulation of muscle glycogen; weakness and cramping of muscles on exercise; no rise of blood lactate.	Intravenous glucose; limited exertion; no tight garments; plenty of carbohydrate.
Type VI (liver phosphorylase deficiency; Hers' disease)	Insufficient levels of the enzyme liver phosphorylase.	Liver glycogen accumulation; enlarged liver; cirrhosis.	Avoidance of prolonged fasting; high protein diet; frequent feedings.
Type VII	Insufficient levels of the enzyme phosphofructokinase and phosphoglucomutase.	Muscle pain and stiffness on exercise.	Experience with the value of dietary treatment is limited, due to rare occurrences of the disease.
Type VIII	Insufficient levels of the enzyme liver phosphorylase.	Glycogen accumulation in the liver; enlarged liver; brain degeneration.	
Type IX	Insufficent levels of the enzyme liver phosphorylase kinase.	Enlarged liver.	
Type X	Insufficient levels of the enzyme c-AMP-dependent phosphorylase kinase.	Enlarged liver.	

(Continued)

TABLE I-2 *(Continued)*

Disorder	Defect(s)	Characteristic Features	Treatment
Hemolytic anemia: I .... II .... III .... IV .... V	Insufficient levels of the following enzymes: Hexokinase Phosphohexose isomerase. Triosephosphate isomerase. Diphosphoglycerate kinase. Pyruvate kinase.	Enzyme deficiency in red blood cell energy yielding pathway reduces survival time of red blood cells, thus producing anemia. These 10 enzyme deficiencies (I through X) listed, are known to produce hemolytic anemia.	The relationship between abnormalities of the metabolism of glucose in red blood cells and their survival is not completely understood. Splenectomy may or may not be beneficial.
VI	Glucose-6-phosphate dehydrogenase.	Most common; requires inducing agent such as aspirin, antimalarial drugs, antibiotics, or fava beans.	Offending foods and chemicals avoided; transfusion may be necessary at times.
VII .... VIII .... IX .... X	6-Phosphoglucomate dehydrogenase. Glutothione reductase. Glutathione peroxidase. Glutathione synthetase.	Most hemolytic anemias due to these enzyme deficiencies are quite rare.	Transfusions may be necessary.
Leucine-induced hypoglycemia	Exact defect unknown.	Apparent 4th month of life; first sign may be convulsions; failure to thrive; possibly some delayed mental development; test dose of leucine produces profound lowering of blood glucose.	Diet low in leucine; diet furnishes minimum requirements of protein for growth; fruits and vegetables added; carbohydrate feeding (10 g) 30 to 40 min. after each meal; possible treatment with diazoxide; normal diet by age 5 to 6.
Pentosuria	Insufficient levels of the enzyme xylulose dehydrogenase.	Harmless; large amounts of zylulose—5-carbon sugar (pentose)—excreted in urine; almost exclusively found in Jews.	No treatment necessary.
Renal glycosuria	No specific enzyme; disorder in membrane transport in kidney.	Glucose excreted in urine while blood glucose at normal levels; storage and utilization of carbohydrates normal.	No treatment required providing diagnosis is correct.

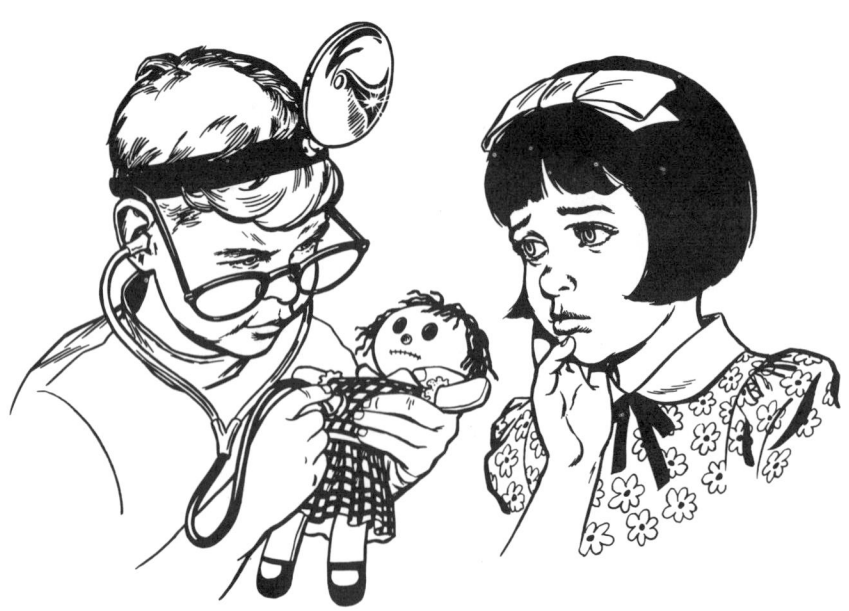

Fig. I-1. A serious case!

TABLE I-3
INBORN ERRORS OF LIPID METABOLISM

Disorder	Defect(s)	Characteristic Features	Treatment
Abetalipoproteinemia	No specific enzyme defect.	Absence of low density beta lipoprotein (LDL) in blood; steator-rhea (fatty diarrhea); malnutrition; growth retardation; nervous disorders; spiny or thorny shaped red blood cells.	Low fat diet with medium chain triglycerides (MCT) supplementation providing some fat intake; large doses fat-soluble vitamins particularly vitamins A, D, and E may be beneficial.
Angiokeratoma (Fabry's disease; glycolipid liposis)	Insufficient levels of the enzyme ceramide trihexosisidase.	Accumulation of glycolopids in tissues; joint pain; eye disorders; purplish papules on skin; males show progressive kidney failure; some nervous disorders.	Moderate quantities of the drug diphenyhydantion; no dietary therapy.
Familial high-density lipo-protein deficiency (Tangier disease)	No specific enzyme.	Absence of high-density or alpha lipoprotein (HDL); deposition of cholesterol in tonsils; enlarged orange tonsils; peripheral nerves may be affected.	Treatment may not be necessary; sometimes tonsillectomy and splenectomy; no definitive treatment.
Familial hyperlipoprotein-emias: Type I (hyperchylomicronemia) (Also see HYPERLIPO—PROTEINEMIAS.)	Insufficient levels of the enzyme lipoprotein lipase.	Elevated blood levels of chylomicrons; yellow papules with reddish base develop over skin and mucous membranes (xanthomas); enlarged spleen; enlarged liver; abdominal pain; possible pancreatitis.	Low fat (25–36 g/day); use of medium chain triglycerides; high energy, high protein diet; no alcohol.
Type II (hyperbetalipoprotein-emia or hypercholesterol-emia) (Also see ATHEROSCLERO-SIS; and HYPERLIPO-PROTEINEMIAS.)	No specific enzyme defect.	Increased blood levels of beta lipoprotein (LDL) and cholesterol; yellow lipid deposits in skin, tendons, and cornea; accelerated atherosclerosis.	Dietary saturated fat and cholesterol limited sharply; polyunsaturated fats increased; use of the drug cholestryamine.
Type III (broad-beta or float-ing beta disease) (Also see HEART DISEASE; and HYPERLIPOPROTEIN-EMIAS.)	No specific enzyme defect.	Elevated blood levels of abnormal prebetalipoproteins (VLDL), cholesterol, and triglycerides; and tendon xanthomas; creases in palm of hands show as yellow lines; accelerated athero-sclerosis of coronary and peripheral blood vessels; heart disease.	Low cholesterol intake; achieve ideal weight; no concentrated sweets; energy should be 20% from protein, 30% from fat, and 50% from carbohydrates; use of polyunsaturated fats; drug of choice clofibrate.
Type IV (hyperprebetalipo-proteinemia) (Also see HEART DISEASE; and HYPERLIPOPROTEIN-EMIAS.)	No specific enzyme defect.	High blood levels of prebetalipoprotein (VLDL) and triglycerides; cholesterol normal or elevated; accelerated heart disease; glucose intolerance.	Maintenance of ideal weight; controlled carbohydrate intake, about 50% of energy; moderate cholesterol restriction to 300 mg; polyunsaturated fats preferred; no concentrated sweets; drugs of choice clofibrate or nicotinic acid.
Type V (mixed hyperlipid-emia) (Also see FATS AND OTHER LIPIDS; and HYPERLIPO-PROTEINEMIAS.)	No specific enzyme defect.	Elevated blood levels of chylomicrons, prebetalipoproteins, cholesterol, and triglycerides; eruptive orange-yellow deposits of lipid on skin (xanthomas); abdominal pain; lipid in retina of eye; enlarged liver and spleen.	Fat restricted to 30% of energy; high protein diet; mainte-nance of ideal weight; 300 mg cholesterol daily; no concen-trated sweets; possible use of nicotinic acid; no alcohol.
Familial cholesterol ester deficiency	Insufficient levels of the enzyme lecithin: Cholesterol acyltrans-ferase (LCAT).	Proteinuria; anemia; corneal opacity; elevated blood levels of triglycerides, lecithin, and unesterified cholesterol.	Low fat diet under trial; none specific.
Glucosyl ceramide lipido-sis (Gaucher's disease) (Also see FATS AND OTHER LIPIDS.)	Insufficient levels of the enzyme glucocerebrosidase.	Accumulation of cerebroside in liver, spleen, and bone mar-row; enlarged spleen and liver; bone lesions.	Supportive therapy of vitamins and supplemental iron; splen-ectomy.
Niemann-Pick disease (sphingomyelin lipidosis) (Also see FATS AND OTHER LIPIDS.)	Insufficient levels of the enzyme sphingomyelinase.	Accumulation chiefly of sphingomyelin and lecithin in the liver, spleen, and central nervous system; enlarged liver and spleen; mental and physical retardation; cherry red spot on retina of eye.	None of value.
Refsum's disease (Phytanic acid storage disease)	Insufficient levels of the enzyme phytanic acid oxidase.	Accumulation of phytanic acid in blood and tissues; vision and hearing disorders; dry skin; bone deformities.	Phytanic acid restriction; diets exclude green vegetables, butter, and ruminant (cattle, sheep, goat) fat; all phytanic acid origin-ates in diet.
Tay-Sachs disease (ganglioside lipidosis)	Insufficient levels of the enzyme hexosaminidase A.	Abnormal glycosphingolipid metabolism; growth retardation; failure to develop coordinated muscular activity; listlessness, blindness with a cherry red spot on retina.	None of value.
Wolman's disease	Insufficient levels of the enzyme acid lipase.	Failure to thrive; vomiting; diarrhea; enlarged spleen and liver; accumulation of cholesterol and triglycerides in liver, lymph nodes, spleen, thymus, intestine, and bone marrow; adrenal calcification; death by 6 months of age.	None

TABLE I-4
INBORN ERRORS OF NUCLEIC ACID METABOLISM

Disorder	Defect(s)	Characteristic Features	Treatment
Gout[1] (Also see ARTHRITIS, section headed "Gout [Gouty arthritis]"; and PURINES.)	Insufficient levels of the enzyme hypoxanthine-guanine phosphoribosyltransferase (HPRT).	Uric acid secretion 5 to 6 times greater than normal; gout; severe neurological disorder called Lesch-Nyhan syndrome when there is a complete deficiency of the enzyme; transmitted on sex chromosomes; onset within first year of life; partial deficiency still produces some neurological disorders.	Valium (diazepam) for spasticity and self-mutilating behavior; allopuriol to reduce uric acid formation; adequate nutrition and secure environment beneficial; no treatment prevents neurological disorder.
	Insufficient levels of the enzyme glucose-6-phosphatase (glycogen storage disease, type I).	Over-production of uric acid and under-secretion of uric acid; gout; excessive deposition of glycogen in liver; yellowish or orange growth on skin due to lipid deposits (xanthomas); hypoglycemia; convulsions; coma; acidosis; stunted growth.	Colchicine, phenylbutazone, indomethacin, ACTH, or hydrocortisone for acute attacks; reduction to ideal weight; avoidance of high purine foods, high fluid intake; alkalinized urine.
	Insufficient levels of the enzyme phosphoribosylpyrophosphate synthetase.	Accelerated purine biosynthesis; high daily uric acid excretion; problems caused by excessive activity of the enzyme; kidney stones; gout.	
Orotic aciduria	Insufficient levels of the enzyme orotidylic pyrophosphorylase; orotidylic decarboxylase.	Very rare; appears first year or so of life; severe megoblastic anemia resistant to usual treatments; mental and physical retardation; excrete large quantities of ortic acid in urine; needle-shaped crystals in urine.	Dietary supplementation with large doses of uridine improves anemia and mental and physical development. Early diagnosis essential.
Xanthinuria	Insufficient levels of the enzyme xanthine oxidase.	Elevated blood and urine levels of xanthine and hypoxanthine and very low uric acid; a therapeutic xanthinuria accompanies use of allopurinol.	Most cases require no treatment; high fluid intake and restricted purine intake recommended.

[1]Gout that is associated with specific enzyme defects.

TABLE I-5
MISCELLANEOUS INBORN ERRORS OF METABOLISM

Disorder	Defect(s)	Characteristic Features	Treatment
Adrenal hyperplasia (Also see ENDROCRINE GLANDS.)	Insufficient levels of the enzyme 21-hydroxylase.	Most common; overproduction of testosterone; steroid excretion in urine elevated; virilization of the female; derangement of external female genitalia; growth of the penis within the first months of life; accelerated growth; early bone maturation; no sperm production; no ovarian function; sensitive to stress and infection; abnormal, excessive hair growth in unusual places especially in women (hireutism); possibly acne; one form demonstrates a salt-losing (sodium-losing) syndrome.	Daily administration of glucocorticoids; salt-losing form requires fluid replacement; therapy throughout life; prognosis excellent if noted first 2 years of life.
	Insufficient levels of the enzyme 11-hydroxylase.	Clinically indistinguishable from 21-hydroxylase deficit with exception of high blood pressure due to accumulation of 11-deoxycortisol, a steroid.	Daily administration of glucocorticoids; prognosis excellent.
	Insufficient levels of the enzyme 17-hydroxylase.	Accumulation of the steroids progesterone and pregnanediol; no virilization, however female fails to mature; sodium retention; potassium wasting; alkalosis; high blood pressure; males fail to mature or have ambiguous external genitalia.	Glucocorticoids correct high glood pressure; sex hormones necessary for sexual maturity.
Congenital lack of intrinsic factor	No intrinsic factor.	Megaloblastic anemia; onset early in life.	Vitamin B-12 therapy.
Congenital nonhemolytic jaundice: Type I (Crigler-Najjar syndrome)	Absence of the enzyme glucuronyl transferase.	Jaundice not due to red blood cell bursting; onset of jaundice at birth; serum bilirubin 18 to 50 mg/100 ml; severe neurologic defects; kernicterus (deposition of bile pigments in brain).	Death often in infancy; no response to phenobarbital; albumin infusions; phototherapy; prognosis poor.
Type II	Insufficient levels of the enzyme glucuronyl transferase.	Jaundice not due to red blood cell bursting; onset of jaundice usually at birth; serum bilirubin 6 to 22 mg/100 ml; no intellectual impairment.	Phenobarbital lowers bilirubin; phototherapy (blue light) lowers serum bilirubin.
Hemochromatosis (bronze diabetes or pigment cirrhosis)	Failure of the control mechanism for absorption of iron from the intestine.	Saturation of the plasma iron-binding protein, transferin; excessive deposits of iron in the tissues; enlarged liver; pigmentation of the skin; diabetes mellitus; frequently heart failure.	Once or twice weekly, blood-letting which removes 500 ml of blood and 250 mg of iron for about 2 years; once or twice yearly blood-letting thereafter; supportive treatment of damaged organs.
Hereditary spherocytosis (congenital hemolytic jaundice)	Defect in red blood cells due to excessive permeability to sodium.	Jaundice due to red blood cell bursting; enlarged spleen; increased fragility of red blood cells.	Blood transfusions necessary at times; splenectomy best treatment.

(Continued)

TABLE I-5 *(Continued)*

Disorder	Defect(s)	Characteristic Features	Treatment
Hypophosphatemia (Also see PHOSPHORUS; and VITAMIN D.)	Defect in kidney tubules.	Low blood phosphate; blood calcium level normal; rickets and dwarfism; transmitted on the sex chromosomes.	Large doses of vitamin D; oral phosphorus.
Mucopolysaccharidoses (11 types) (Also see CARBOHYDRATE[S].)	Deficiency in lysosomal enzyme important for mucopolysaccharide (complex polysaccharide) degradation.	Depending on the type, nervous disorders from mild to severe; stiff joints to severe bone changes; some forms transmitted on sex chromosomes.	No effective or practical treatment available.
Porphyria: Acute intermittent (Also see METABOLISM.)	Insufficient levels of the enzyme uroporphyrinogen I synthetase.	Disruption in porphyrin metabolism; urine changes to burgundy wine color on standing; intense abdominal colic with vomiting and nausea; neurotic or psychotic behavior; neuromuscular disturbances; actual lesions of the nerve; course of the disease variable; mortality rate high.	Unpredictable remission and expression of symptoms; no treatment uniformly successful; avoidance of estrogens and barbiturates; drugs for pain, and sedation; best prevention high carbohydrate intake; most effective treatment producing remission is glucose orally or intravenously.
Congenital erythropoietic	Insufficient levels of the enzyme uroporphyrinogen III cosynthetase.	Urinary excretion of large amounts of uroporphyrin I; mutilating skin lesions; photosensitivity; hemolytic (red blood cell bursting) anemia; pink or red urine; symptoms usually appear between birth and 5 years; teeth may turn red to reddish brown.	Avoidance of exposure to sunlight; possibly splenectomy or steroids.
Renal tubular acidosis	Disorder of membrane transport of hydrogen ion and bicarbonate by kidney tubules.	Inability of kidney to excrete an acid urine; persistent metabolic acidosis results; kidney stones; increased urinary calcium and phosphate; osteomalacia; potassium depletion.	Oral administration of sodium bicarbonate or citrate; supplemental potassium and/or calcium until body stores repleted; possibly vitamin D therapy.
Wilson's disease (hepatolenticular degeneration)	Deficient synthesis of ceruloplasmin, the copper-carrying protein of the blood.	Excess copper storage particularly in the liver, kidneys, brain, and cornea of the eye; eventually causing liver, kidney, and brain disorders and a characteristic rusty-brown ring in the cornea known as Kayser-Fleischer ring.	Early diagnosis; administration of the copper-chelating agent, D-penicillamine mobilizes copper in tissue and causes excretion in urine; sulfurated potash with meals prevents copper absorption.

INCAPARINA

A mixture of corn flour, cottonseed flour, torula yeast, minerals, and vitamins developed by the Institute of Nutrition of Central America and Panama (INCAP) with the aid of funds from Central American governments, the Kellogg Foundation, the Rockefeller Foundation, and several other foundations. It has a protein content of about 25%. Incaparina can be used as a cereal for weanling infants and young children. It was test marketed in Nicaragua, El Salvador, Guatemala, and Colombia for the treatment and prevention of protein-energy malnutrition.

(Also see CORN, Table C-23, Corn Products and Uses.)

INCOME, PROPORTION SPENT FOR FOOD

We tend to remember the *good ole days* when a loaf of bread was 25¢ and the Saturday afternoon show was 10¢, while forgetting that our yearly income was proportionately low for the same period. It is true that the price of many things has increased, but so has the average income. Therefore, to gain a better perspective, two important questions are: (1) how long must one labor to put food on the table, and (2) what portion of our income goes for food? The answers to both of these questions determines the money left over for the other necessities and the extras of life—prosperity.

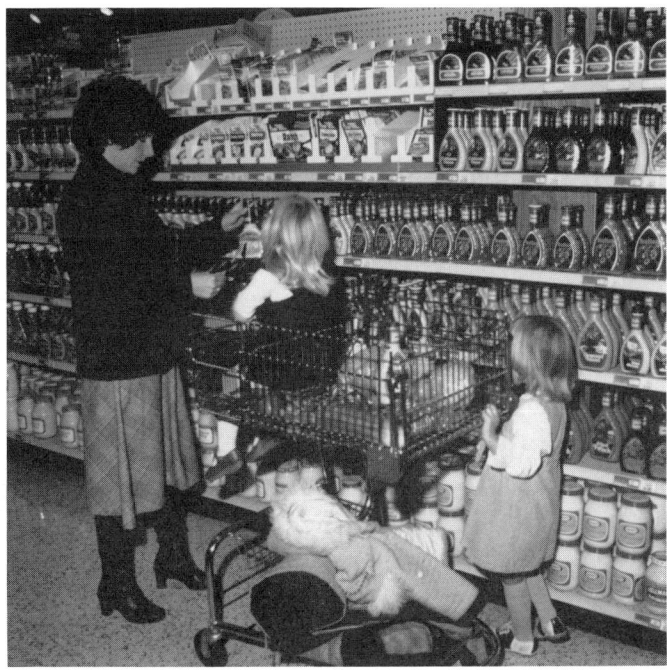

Fig. I-2. Food is a bargain in the United States and Canada, where consumers spend less than one-sixth of their income for food. (Courtesy, American Soybean Assn., St. Louis, Mo.)

Wage earners in various countries must work longer than their U.S. counterparts to purchase the same foods. Fig. I-3 shows that laborers of North America are in an enviable position. To buy 1 lb *(454 g)* of bread, bacon, steak, pork chops, chicken, tomatoes, and butter, along with 1 dozen oranges and 1 dozen eggs, Canadians and Americans needed to work slightly less than 1½ hours. Laborers of other countries toiled from nearly 2 hours in Australia to as long as 7½ hours in Japan.

As income rises, consumers spend a smaller proportion of their disposable income for food. Fig. I-4 demonstrates this general trend, worldwide.

In most low income countries, consumers spend ½ or more of their income for food, whereas in the higher income countries the proportion drops to about ⅕. The data contained in Fig. I-4 shows that consumers spent the following proportion of their income for food: United States, 10.3%; Canada, 11.3%; United Kingdom, 12.8%; Netherlands, 14.2%; Australia, 15.0%; Denmark, 15.7%; France, 16.4%; W. Germany, 16.6%; Sweden, 17.0%; Austria, 17.4%; Belgium, 17.7%; and Japan, 18.0%. Food is still a bargain in some countries, notably the United States and Canada. However, even in the United States, the level of income influences the proportion of income spent for food.

Worldwide, food preferences, or eating habits, change with income. The hierarchy of preferences, from lowest income to highest income, is: lowest for roots and tubers, a little higher for coarse grains (corn, sorghum, etc.) for human consumption, and progressively higher for other cereals (wheat and rice), pulses (the edible seeds of leguminous crops, like peas and beans), fruits and vegetables, and animal products.

Low-income consumers spend a high proportion of their budget for direct cereal grain consumption. High-income consumers spend less of their food budget for cereals and more of it for animal products.

(Also see MALNUTRITION, PROTEIN-ENERGY; MEAT[S], section on "Income—Proportion Spent for Food; Food—Kinds Bought"; and WORLD FOOD.)

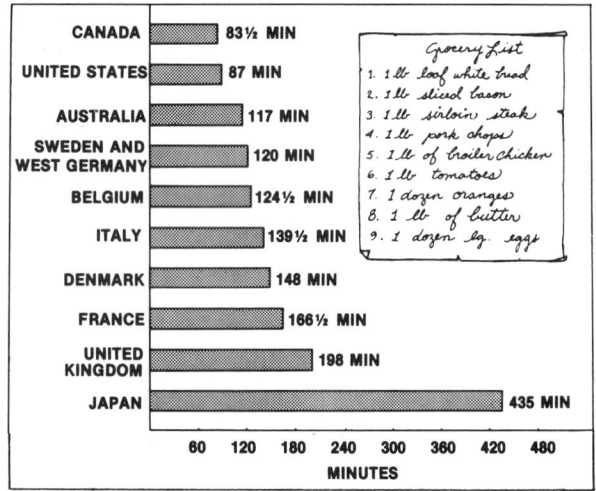

Fig. I-3. The amount of work required in various countries to earn the money necessary to purchase all of the items shown on the grocery list. *Note:* Food prices and wages of laborers in all countries change, but the work/food cost relationship remains about the same within each country.

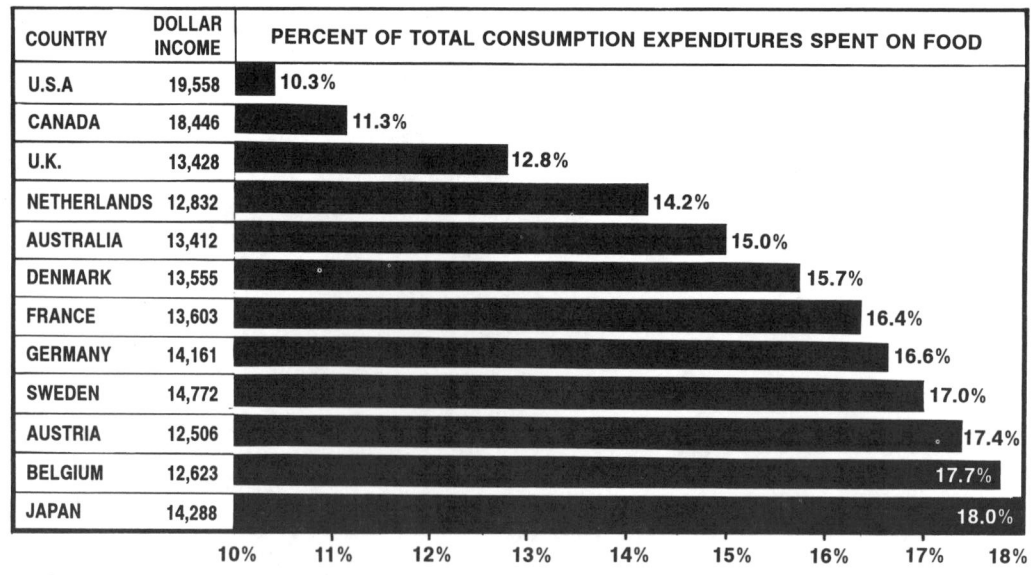

Fig. I-4. Proportion of income spent for food. As income rises, consumers spend a smaller proportion of their wages for food. (*Statistical Abstract of the United States 1991*, p. 843, Tables 1450, 1451)

INDIGESTION

The word is rather a catchall label for a variety of disorders associated with eating. Definitions vary between sufferers. Furthermore, a doctor will try to attach a more specific diagnosis to a patient's complaint of indigestion by determining

(1) the location and duration of discomfort; (2) occurrence of the discomfort in relationship to the time of eating; and (3) the relationship of the symptoms to certain food types. Among the disorders which may be referred to as indigestion are: peptic ulcer, gastritis, gastric hyperacidity, heartburn, flatulence (gas), stomach irritation (from corticosteroid

drugs, food intolerance, excessive smoking, or alcoholic stimulation), pylorospasm (spasm of the sphincter between the stomach and the small intestine), nervous dyspepsia, bleeding ulcers, colitis, hiccups, hypermotility, diverticulitis, and anxiety.

Where indigestion is caused by emotional or physiological problems rather than by organic or physical diseases or disorders, treatment often includes the following:

1. Eating meals at regular hours.

2. Eating small meals at frequent intervals, rather than large meals less frequently.

3. Eating slowly and in a relaxed atmosphere; avoiding gulping food.

4. Avoiding irritating stimulants, spicy foods, and greasy foods.

5. Drinking a glass of milk between meals.

(Also see ANTACIDS; GASTRITIS; HEARTBURN; and ULCERS, PEPTIC.)

INDISPENSABLE AMINO ACID

This phrase is synonymous to the phrase *essential amino acid*. Both phrases refer to an amino acid which the body cannot synthesize in sufficient amounts to carry out physiological functions and must, therefore, be supplied in the diet. The indispensable amino acids in the human diet are histidine, isoleucine, leucine, lysine, methionine (some used for the synthesis of cysteine), phenylalanine (some used for the synthesis of tyrosine), threonine, tryptophan, and valine.

NOTE WELL: Arginine is not regarded as indispensable for humans, whereas it is for animals; in contrast to human infants, most young mammals cannot synthesize it in sufficient amounts to meet their needs for growth.

(Also see AMINO ACID[S].)

INERT

Relatively inactive.

INFANT ALLERGY

In infants the prime concern is *food* allergies. Symptoms such as wheezing, coughing, running of the nose, colic, vomiting, diarrhea, constipation, rash, or eczema may suggest an allergy—an unusual or exaggerated response to a particular substance called an allergen. Major food offenders are milk, eggs, wheat, corn, legumes, nuts, and seafoods. The offending food, allergen, should be identified and eliminated from the diet. Dietary history, skin test, provocative food test, elimination diets, and pulse tests are all useful for identifying the causative food. Fortunately, children tend to outgrow food allergies. Foods known to have caused reactions in infancy may be tried months or years later when perhaps they can be taken with impunity.

(Also see ALLERGIES.)

INFANT ANEMIA

Anemia during infancy, a frequent occurrence, is closely related to the body iron stores at birth. Pregnant women may have an insufficient intake of iron; thus, the newborn infant may develop anemia early in the first year of life. Also, infants (1) born prematurely, (2) of low birth weight, (3) of multiple births, or (4) whose mothers have had several pregnancies are most likely to have inadequate iron reserves at birth. Furthermore, infants are apt to develop iron deficiency anemia because milk has a low iron content and babies are just not born with sufficient iron to meet their needs beyond 6 months. Infant anemia may also be caused by gastrointestinal bleeding due to the ingestion of homogenized milk, infections, diarrhea, or a hemolytic disease.

Clinical features of iron deficiency anemia are the impairment of general health and vitality, paleness of the skin and mucous membranes, and a hemoglobin concentration less than 11g/100 ml of blood.

Appropriate measures should be taken to insure that infants have a daily dietary iron intake of 6 mg from birth to 6 months of age, and of 10 mg from 6 to 12 months of age.

(Also see ANEMIA; and IRON.)

INFANT DIET AND NUTRITION

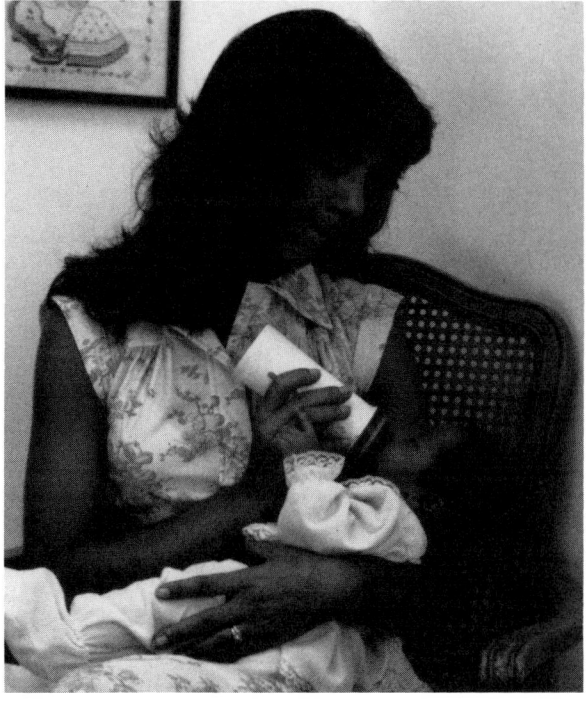

Fig. I-5. Infant being bottle fed. (Courtesy, Mead Johnson, Company, Evansville, Ind.)

The future of each society depends to some extent on how its infants are fed since subsequent repair of damage done by chronic malnutrition in the very young is difficult. Furthermore, there are ever increasing numbers of infants in the developing countries which have long had shortages of food. Therefore, economical and efficient infant feeding is a matter of worldwide concern.

HISTORY. It is not known for certain how the breast feeding of infants was supplemented in prehistoric times, since the remains of food found by archaeologists usually tell us what a group of people ate, but they do not always tell how it was allotted to individuals. What is known is that a wide variety of animal and plant foods were obtained by hunting, fishing, and gathering. Furthermore, modern day aborigines, whose modes of living are similar to those of prehistoric nomadic peoples, often eat a larger variety of foods than contemporary subsistence farmers in the developing countries. For example, Australian aborigines wean their babies on honey, turtle eggs, fish, meat, fruits, and vegetables.[1]

On the other hand, the peasants in the densely populated ancient agricultural societies depended mainly on cereal grains, starchy roots and tubers, legumes, vegetables, and only occasionally on some animal foods. Some of the ancient rural peoples may have benefited nutritionally from the raising of livestock, although it is difficult to determine the extent to which eggs, meat, milk, or poultry were used in the feeding of weanling infants. The contemporary counterparts of these early societies rely heavily on products made from cereal grains, such as watery gruels and doughy masses that are literally pushed down an infant's throat.

In ancient times the failure of a mother to have an adequate suppply of breast milk often meant death of her infant unless another lactating female was available as a wet nurse. Occasionally, attempts were made to have infants suckle asses, cows, goats, sheep, dogs, and other animals as evidenced by the story that Romulus and Remus (Romulus was the legendary first King of Rome) were nursed by a she wolf. Of course, the female animals may have been milked

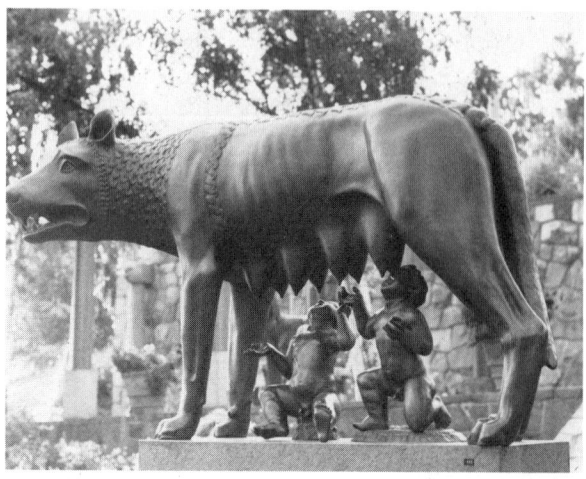

Fig. I-6. She wolf suckling Romulus and Remus. Bronze sculpture by Carl Milles, in Milles Garden, Stockholm, Sweden. (Photo by A. H. Ensminger)

and the milk given to babies, but the method of feeding was likely to have been accompanied by contamination with microorganisms that cause deadly diarrheal disease in infants. Furthermore, animal milks differ in composition from human milk. It is noteworthy, that of all the common species of livestock, mares have milk which is closest in characteristics to human milk. The Mongol tribes that roamed the steppes of Central Asia are known to have consumed mare's milk, but it is not known whether it was given to infants.

By the beginning of the 19th century, the search for ways to use animals' milks safely in infant feeding became almost desperate, because the practices of wet nurses in the urban societies endangered the health of the infants they fed. Contamination of cow's milk with harmful bacteria had been a problem for ages and the feeding devices (pitchers or pots with long spouts) left much to be desired. However, glass bottles fitted with Nipples made of cork or wood were also used. Another achievement of that era was the development of the first safe canning process by the Frenchman, Nicholas Appert, in 1810. Unfortunately, many years passed and countless infants died before these inventions were utilized in suitable feeding procedures. There were still great gaps in the knowledge of microbial growth, and of the significant differences in the chemical compositions and physical characteristics of human milk vs cow's milk.

The first major advances in the *humanization* of cow's milk were made around the middle of the 19th century by the great German chemist Justus von Liebig who showed by chemical analyses that cow's milk was considerably higher in protein and lower in carbohydrate than human milk. Shortly thereafter, he developed an infant formula that was a mixture of an extract of malt flour and liquid whole cow's milk. The main shortcoming of this product was that it spoiled readily. It is noteworthy that Nestle of Switzerland started the infant formula industry in 1867, when they produced a dried *milk food* mixture made from milk and malted wheat. Later, William Horlick, who had come to the United States from England, also utilized the principles of Liebig's formula in his invention of malted milk powder, which was patented in 1883.

Meanwhile, other developments for coping with the perishability of fresh milk were (1) the production of sweetened condensed milk, which was invented by Gail Borden in the 1850s; and (2) the pasteurization of milk, a process that had been first used in the 1870s by the French scientist Louis Pasteur to preserve wines from spoilage.

The prevention of the bacterial contamination of milk by pasteurization had its shortcomings in that the vitamin C content became almost negligible and infants developed scurvy. It was not until the late 1920s and early 1930s that the role of vitamin C in the prevention of scurvy was clarified. After that, mothers were told to supplement their infant's diet with orange juice. Rickets was also a common affliction of infants until cod-liver oil was given in the winter months.

Canning did not become an important means of preserving vegetables until the early 1900s, after researchers at the Massachusetts Institute of Technology devised means of killing heat-resistant bacteria. However, mothers who wished to prepare vegetables for infant feeding had to mash canned or home-cooked items through a pureeing cone or a sieve to remove the fibrous matter which had a laxative effect. Then, in 1928 Dan Gerber started the Gerber Baby Foods Division of the Fremont Canning Company (located in Fremont, Michigan) after his wife asked if canned pureed vegetables could be produced commercially. The birth of

[1]Robson, J. R. K., "Foods from the Past, Lessons for the Future," *The Professional Nutritionist*, Vol. 8, Spring 1976, pp. 13-15.

the baby food industry led eventually to the production of a wide variety of baked products, cereals, desserts, fruits, meats, and vegetables.

The ready availability of canned evaporated milk led to its extensive use in infant feeding. Usually, it was diluted with water and sweetened with corn syrup, lactose, and/or sugar. Preprepared mixtures, called *formulas,* came into widespread use in the 1920s, but many mothers found it more economical to prepare the feedings from evaporated milk and store them in nursing bottles in an ice box or a refrigerator. However, commercially prepared formulas became more popular in the 1940s when many mothers went to work to help the war effort.

During World War II, breads, cereals and milk were fortified with essential vitamins and minerals (mainly calcium, iron, vitamin A, vitamin D, thiamin, riboflavin, and niacin). British nutritionists noted that some children developed vitamin D toxicity, and advised the food technologists and government agencies to reduce the amount of vitamin D fortification after the war ended. However, there was a rise in the incidences of rickets in the large cities of northern England and Scotland during the 1950s, which attested to the dangers of inadequate consumption of the vitamin.

Aid to the needy nations of the world was a major part of American foreign policy in the 1950s, as exemplified by the Marshall Plan under President Truman and the Food for Peace program under President Eisenhower. Grains and nonfat dry milk were shipped to various parts of the world for the relief of impoverished people. Vegetable oils were generally used in skim milk formulas to provide the fat that would have been supplied by whole milk. When the cost of nonfat dry milk rose sharply during the 1960s and 1970s, nutritionists developed infant foods that were mixtures of cereal and legume flours fortified with essential minerals and vitamins.

Meanwhile, the cholesterol scare in the United States was one of the factors that led to the growing use of infant formulas containing nonfat dry milk and vegetable oils that were similar to those used in the developing countries. However, it was found that a few premature infants developed severe vitamin E deficiencies when fed the products that were rich in the polyunsaturated fatty acids present in certain oils. Hence, many formulas were fortified with vitamin E and other micronutrients deemed to be essential. Also, formulas based upon soybean substitutes for milk were developed for infants with milk allergies.

Today, there are a large variety of infant formulas that are considered to be nutritionally complete for infants up to age one, although American pediatricians generally recommend that the feeding of supplemental foods start between 3 and 6 months of age. Also, great progress has been made in the widespread application of nutritional and sanitary principles to infant feeding during the 20th century, as evidenced by the sharp drop in infant mortality shown in Fig. I-7.

GROWTH AND DEVELOPMENT OF INFANTS.
From a nutritional standpoint, a knowledge of normal infant growth and development is useful for gauging the adequacy of nutrient consumption. Growth that is too slow suggests (1) that the diet is nutritionally inadequate, or (2) that there is an impairment(s) in the utilization of food by the body. Excessively rapid growth may lead to obesity, which increases the likelihood of later development of cardiovascular diseases, diabetes, and high blood pressure. However, measurement of growth alone does not tell the whole story, since infants with normal growth may have abnormalities of certain functions due to nutritional deficiencies or

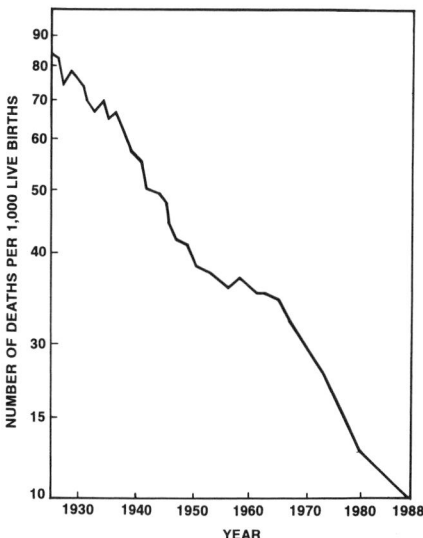

Fig. I-7. Infant mortality in the United States from 1925 to 1988. (Source: *Health, United States,* U.S. Department HEW, p. 345, Table CD II.1, and *Statistical Abstract of the United States,* 1991, U.S. Department of Commerce, p. 78, Table 114)

excesses, inherited tendencies, congenital defects, or certain illnesses. Some of the most commonly used means of assessing growth and development follow.

Measurement of Growth.   Although there are various procedures for determining the growth of bone, fatty tissue, and muscle, the measurement of height and weight is most readily accomplished as follows:

• **Height**—For infants, this measurement is the head to foot length of the subject in the recumbent position, as shown in Fig. I-8. Measurement of length should be made to the nearest ¼ in. (or *0.5 cm*).

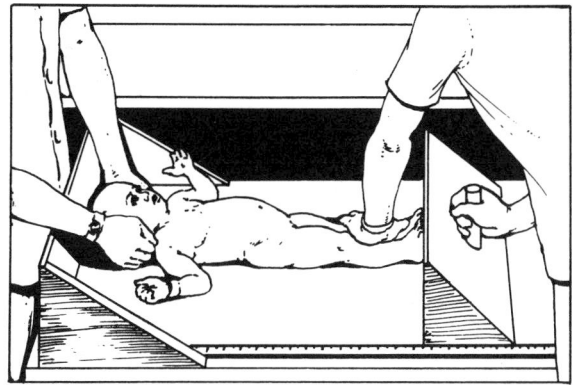

Fig. I-8. Measurement of an infant's length with the apparatus that is commonly used by pediatricians.

• **Weight**—Measurements of weight of infants are preferably made with the subjects unclothed. Weight should be recorded to the nearest ¼ lb (or *0.1 kg*).

The most recently published standard growth curves for infants are those from the National Center for Health

Statistics (NCHS)[2]. Data from plotting the curves was obtained in a study in which 867 children were measured from birth to 3 years of age. The curves are presented in Figs. I-9 through I-12.

To use the growth curves shown in Figs. I-9 through I-12, it is necessary to determine the percentile which corresponds most closely to the data from the infant that was measured. A simple procedure follows:

[2]*NCHS Growth Curves for Children, Birth–18 Years, United States,* U.S. Department HEW.

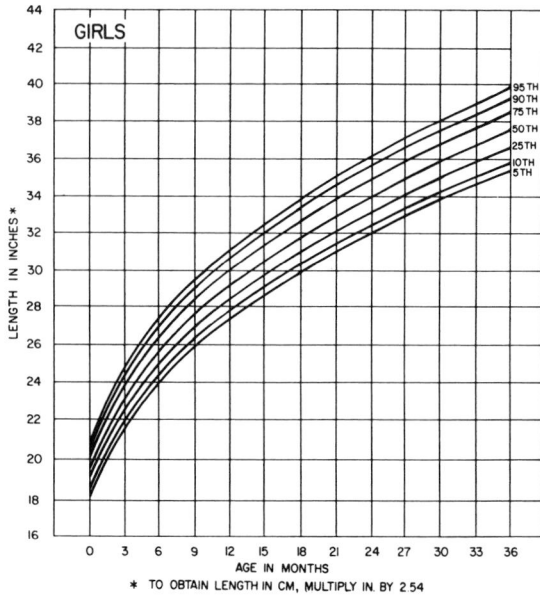

Fig. I-9. Lengths (heights) of girls by age percentiles from birth to 36 months. (Source: *NCHS Growth Curves for Children, Birth–18 Years, United States,* U.S. Department HEW)

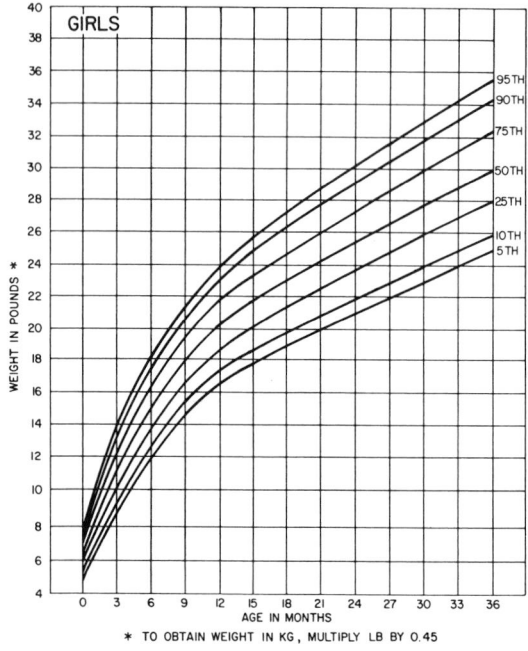

Fig. I-11. Weights of girls by age percentiles from birth to 36 months. (Source: *NCHS Growth Curves for Children, Birth–18 Years, United States,* U.S. Department HEW)

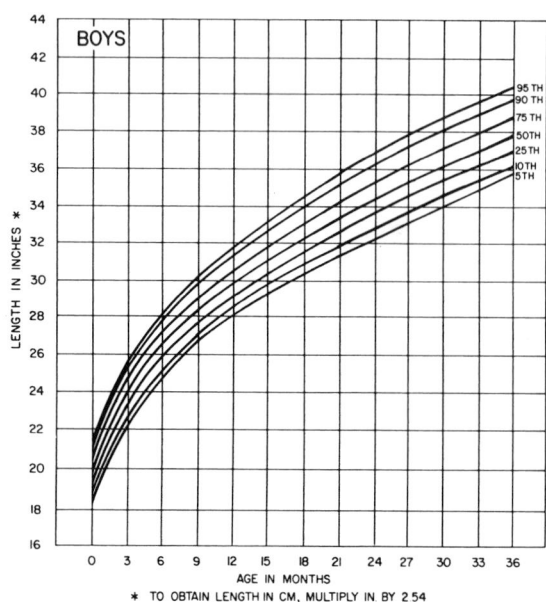

Fig. I-10. Lengths (heights) of boys by age percentiles from birth to 36 months. (Source: *NCHS Growth Curves for Children, Birth–18 Years, United States,* U.S. Department HEW)

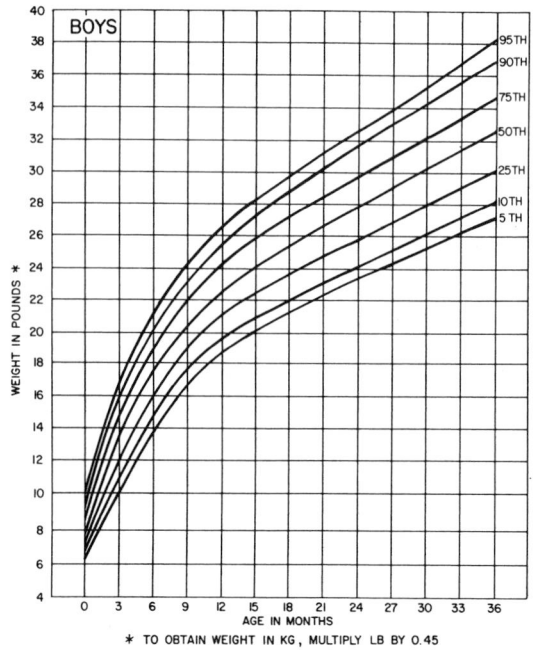

Fig. I-12. Weights of boys by age percentiles from birth to 36 months. (Source: *NCHS Growth Curves for Children, Birth–18 Years, United States,* U.S. Department HEW)

1. Locate and mark the height or weight of the infant on the vertical scale in the left margin of the appropriate chart. If the value of the measurement falls between the values marked on the scale, its placement should be estimated as accurately as possible.

2. With the aid of a ruler draw a light, horizontal line across the chart, starting from the marked value for height or weight.

3. Using a procedure similar to step 1 (above), locate and mark the age of the child on the horizontal scale at the bottom of the chart.

4. Draw a vertical line on the chart, starting from the marked value for age.

5. Circle the point at which the horizontal and vertical lines intersect on the chart and note the percentile curve which is closest to the intersection.

Values which fall between the 5th and 95th percentiles are considered to be within the normal range. However, there should not be a wide discrepancy between the percentiles for height and weight. Sometimes, a pediatrician will not diagnose and treat an otherwise healthy infant until a clear-cut trend of growth abnormality is indicated by measurements taken at 2 or more consecutive monthly or bimonthly visits.

Other Means of Assessing Infant Development and Nutritional Status. The measurement of growth is only part of the assessment of infant development. Pediatricians also look for signs of inherited or congenital disorders and nutritional deficiencies. For example, special attention is paid to general features such as pallor, apathy, and irritability. Similarly, the skin is examined carefully for signs of scurvy and the skeletal system for the signs of rickets.

Any potentially important abnormality that is detected by physical examination usually requires confirmation by laboratory tests, x ray, or other means such as (1) measurement of hemoglobin concentration or hematocrit when anemia is suspected, and (2) x rays of bones if signs of rickets are present.

NUTRIENT REQUIREMENTS. A growing infant usually triples its birth weight within the first year and has high nutrient needs in proportion to its size. Fortunately, much more is now known about infant requirements than was ever known before.

A complete presentation of nutrient allowances for different age groups, including infants, along with the nutrient functions and best food sources of each nutrient, is given in this book in the section on NUTRIENTS: REQUIREMENTS, ALLOWANCES, FUNCTIONS, SOURCES, and its accompanying Table N-3; hence, the reader is referred thereto.

It is not expected that mothers will use Table N-3 to make frequent checks on the nutrient compositions of their infants' diets, but rather that they will use it for guidance in selecting (1) fortified infant formulas and cereals, and (2) mineral and vitamin supplements.

FOODS AND FEEDING. Few subjects outside of politics and religion generate as much controversy as the selection of foods for infant feeding. Hence, the merits and demerits of the various alternatives are noteworthy.

Breast Feeding vs Bottle Feeding. About 350,000 babies are born around the world daily to face a very uncertain future while the partisans of these feeding systems argue over which one is best.[3] Few people on either side would deny that for the young infant up to age 6 months, breast feeding offers advantages such as (1) convenience for mothers who are able to remain near to their babies, (2) extension of the infertile period between births, (3) partial protection of the infant against diarrheal disease caused by microorganisms such as *Salmonella, Shigella,* and pathogenic strains of *E. coli,* and (4) physical and psychological bonding between the mother and infant. These and other benefits are detailed elsewhere.

(Also see BREAST FEEDING.)

INFANT FORMULAS. At this point it should be noted that modern infant formulas represent the latest in a long series of humanitarian efforts to save babies when breastfeeding is not feasible. Some anthropologists believe that in prehistoric nomadic societies, babies that failed to thrive on their mother's milk were allowed to die.[4] Perhaps it was in the early agricultural societies that the first attempts were made to develop substitutes for breast milk. For example, the Chinese have long used milklike products made from soybeans and a vegetable soup fortified with egg yolk, whereas in 16th-century England orphaned infants were strapped to the bellies of asses so they might suckle.[5]

Excellent results have been obtained with the modern types of mineral and vitamin fortified infant formulas when (1) the prices of the products are affordable by the customers, (2) feedings are prepared with safe water under sanitary conditions according to the manufacturer's instructions, and (3) unused portions of formula in opened cans are stored in a refrigerator. Unfortunately, these conditions are not met in certain *poverty pockets* within the developed countries, nor are they likely to be met in many of the Third World countries.

Although many families have fed their infants fresh pasteurized cow's milk, this practice may be harmful because (1) the protein in the milk may not be digested well, and (2) there is evidence that this type of milk often hastens the development of iron deficiency anemia because it has been found to induce the loss of blood from the gastrointestinal tract in about 50% of the infants who developed anemia. Boiling the milk renders the protein more digestible and reduces the likelihood of blood loss. However, it may be advisable to use either diluted evaporated milk or a commercial formula, rather than fresh homogenized milk, for infant feeding. This matter is still controversial. Therefore, the authors recommend that mothers consult their pediatricians for recommendations regarding the most suitable forms of milk or infant formulas.

Nutrient compositions of breast milk, cow's milk, and a typical commercial infant milk base formula are given in Table I-6.

³Edson, L., "Babies in Poverty—The Real Victims of the Breast/Bottle Controversy," *The Lactation Review,* Vol. IV, 1979, pp. 20-38.

⁴Raphael, D., "Of Mothers and Mothering—Remembrances by Margaret Mead," *The Lactation Review,* Vol. IV, 1979, pp. 5-18.

⁵Edson, L. "Babies in Poverty—The Real Victims of the Breast/Bottle Controversy," *The Lactation Review,* Vol. IV, 1979, pp. 20-38.

TABLE I-6
NUTRIENT ALLOWANCES VS. COMPOSITIONS
OF HUMAN, COW, AND FORMULA MILKS

Nutrient	Recommended Intakes for Infants Aged 0 to 6 mo.[1]	Nutrient Composition of Three Kinds of Infant Formula[2]		
		Human Milk[3]	Cow's Milk, Whole, Undiluted[3]	Milk Base Formula[4]
	(per day)	(per qt)	(per qt)	(per qt)
Calories ....kcal	650	833	824	645
Carbohydrates ....g	—	66	45	69
Fats ....g	—	36	36	34
Proteins ....g	13	11	31	15
Macrominerals:				
Calcium ....mg	400	322	1,192	484
Phosphorus ....mg	300	151	936	370
Sodium ....mg	120	142	548	208
Magnesium ....mg	40	38	123	39
Potassium ....mg	500	473	1,308	665
Microminerals:				
Copper ....mg	0.4–0.6	0.4	0.3	0.4
Iron ....mg	6	2	1.2	11
Zinc ....mg	5	6.2	3.3	5
Fat-Soluble Vitamins:				
Vitamin A ....mcg RE	375	537	291	711
Vitamin D ....mcg	7.5	0.5	0.3	9.5
Vitamin E .....mg α TE	3	1.7	0.4	14
Water-Soluble Vitamins:				
Biotin ....mcg	10	3.8	33	—
Folate ....mcg	25	2.1	2.7	47
Niacin ....mg	5	1.6	0.8	7
Pantothenic acid ....mg	2	1.9	3.3	3
Riboflavin ....mg	0.4	0.5	1.5	0.9
Thiamin ....mg	0.3	0.1	0.4	0.6
Vitamin B-6 ....mg	0.3	0.1	0.4	0.4
Vitamin B-12 ....mcg	0.3	0.3	3.8	1.4
Vitamin C ....mg	30	42	17	52

[1]*Recommended Dietary Allowances*, 10th rev. ed., 1989, NRC–National Academy of Sciences.
[2]To convert to amount per liter, multiply by 0.95.
[3]Based upon data in Toverud, K. U., *et al., Maternal Nutrition and Child Health, An Interpretive Review*, National Academy of Sciences.
[4]Based upon data from the manufacturers.

It may be noted from Table I-6 that both human milk and cow's milk are low in certain minerals and vitamins, whereas, the commercial infant formula provides levels of these nutrients that are close to the recommended intakes. Furthermore, cow's milk is exceptionally high in protein and mineral salts, and may stress the ability of the young infant's kidneys to rid the body of the waste products of metabolism. Nevertheless, undiluted cow's milk is a suitable food for infant feeding after supplemental foods have been introduced, provided that the infant receives sufficient water.

Usually, doctors recommend milk base formulas for infants. However, a few infants are allergic to cow's milk, as evidenced by the continuous or frequent occurrence of symptoms such as asthma, colds, colic, constipation, coughing, diarrhea, eczema, poor weight gain, runny nose, spitting up, and vomiting. In such cases, the pediatrician may put the baby on a soy base formula without conducting the usual tests for allergy, since elimination of the symptoms on the substituted formula confirm the diagnosis. Sometimes, babies are also allergic to soy base formulas and are given a meat base formula because the latter type of preparation is the least likely to provoke an allergic response.

Supplemental Foods. Some of the advocates of breast feeding have advised against the early introduction of supplemental foods on the grounds that it might tend to discourage the baby from nursing. Therefore, it is noteworthy that the noted anthropologist Margaret Mead observed nursing mothers who fed their infants a wide variety of supplemental foods soon after birth.[6] She thought that early supplementation (by about 3 months of age) was a good practice because (1) it alleviated some of the physical and emotional strain on the mother when the baby was growing rapidly and developing a large appetite, and (2) the mother was more likely to be able to continue breast-feeding when she was secure in the belief that her infant was contented and doing well. Furthermore, some supplementation is desirable because breast milk is low in protein, minerals, and vitamins.

The supplemental foods that are most commonly utilized in the United States are baby cereals; egg yolks; orange juice; and pureed fruits, meats, and vegetables. Guidelines for using these foods are given in the next section.

Guidelines for Infant Feeding. The liquids and solid foods fed to infants should be selected carefully in order to avoid giving them too much of some nutrients and too little of others. A typical feeding schedule is given in Table I-7.

MILK AND OTHER LIQUIDS. It is very important for mothers who are not breast feeding to recognize that undiluted cow's milk is not suitable for young infants because it contains too much protein and mineral salts and too little carbohydrate. (A calf has very high nutrient requirements because it grows so rapidly that it requires only 47 to 70 days to double its birth weight, whereas, a human infant grows much more slowly and requires about 150 days to double its birth weight.) Therefore, parents who wish to save money by preparing their infant's formula from evaporated milk instead of using a commercial preparation should consult with their pediatrician or local public health nurse or nutritionist for instructions regarding dilution and sweetening of the milk.

NOTE: Evaporated milk is low in iron, vitamin D (unless fortified with the nutrient), folacin, and vitamin C. Hence, babies fed evaporated milk formulas should be given the appropriate nutritional supplements and/or the supplemental beverages or foods that provide the deficient nutrients.

Preparation of Infant Formula. A typical set of instructions for preparing an infant formula follows:

1. The nursing bottles, caps, and nipples should be washed thoroughly with soap and hot water, then rinsed with boiling water to sterilize them and remove the last traces of soap, and allowed to dry while inverted on a sterilizer rack.

2. A commercially prepared infant formula is poured into clean nursing bottles for feeding, or an evaporated milk formula is prepared from carefully measured amounts of milk, sugar, and water. In the latter case, the filled bottles should be capped, placed on a rack in a sterilizer, and heated in gently boiling water for about 25 minutes. The sterilized bottles of formula should be stored in a refrigerator until used.

NOTE: Sterilized nipples should *not* be handled. Therefore, inserting them into the bottle caps prior to sterilization helps to avoid contamination. Bottles with

---

[6]Raphael, D., "Margaret Mead—A Tribute," *The Lactation Review*, Vol. IV, 1979, pp. 1-3.

TABLE I-7
SUGGESTED PLAN FOR FEEDING NORMAL, HEALTHY INFANTS DURING THE FIRST YEAR[1]

Time of the Day	1st Month	2nd & 3rd Months	4th & 5th Months	6th & 7th Months	8th & 9th Months	12 Months
2 a.m.	Breast milk or 3 to 4 oz (90 to 120 ml) of formula ──────────►	—	—	—		—
6 a.m.	Breast milk or 3 to 4 oz (90 to 120 ml) of formula ──────────►		5 to 6 oz (150 to 180 ml) formula[2]	7 to 8 oz (210 to 240 ml) formula[2]	1 cup (240 ml) of whole milk	—
8 a.m.	1 oz (30 ml) orange juice mixed with 3 oz (90 ml) of water. Mineral and vitamin supplement.[3] ──────────	2 oz (60 ml) orange juice mixed with 2 oz (60 ml) of water	3 to 4 oz (150 to 180 ml) orange juice or equivalent in vitamin C forti-fied strained fruit ──────────────────────────►			1 cup (240 ml) of whole milk (may be given later). ½ cup (120 ml) fruit or fruit juice. 1 to 2 oz (30 to 60 g) of iron and vitamin enriched bread, dry cereal, muffins, pancakes, toast, or waffles.
			2 to 4 oz (60 to 120 ml) of cooked boiled water ──────────►			
10 a.m.	Breast milk or 3 to 4 oz (90 to 120 ml) of formula ──────────►		5 to 6 oz (150 to 180 ml) formula.[2] ½ to 1 oz (15 to 30 g) infant cereal.	7 to 8 oz (210 to 240 ml) formula.[2] 1 to 2 oz (30 to 60 g) infant cereal, teething biscuits, or toast. ──────────►	1 cup (240 ml) of whole milk.	Milk, juice, water,[4] and/or bread or cereal (little or no food is needed if a hearty breakfast was eaten).
12 noon	—	1 to 4 oz (30 to 120 ml) of cooled boiled water (more may be needed in a hot environment) ──────────►			½ to 1 cup (120 to 240 ml) water	1 to 2 oz (30 to 60 g) of cottage cheese or yogurt, egg (whole), fish, meat, poultry, or mashed cooked beans or peas. 1 cup (240 ml) of whole milk (may be given later). 1 to 2 oz (30 to 60 g) fruit or vegetable.
2 p.m.	Breast milk or 3 to 4 oz (90 to 120 ml) of formula ──────────►		5 to 6 oz (150 to 180 ml) formula.[2] 1 to 2 oz (30 to 60 g) strained vegetable. ──────────►	7 to 8 oz (210 to 240 ml) formula.[2] 1 oz (30 g) of cottage cheese, or yogurt, egg yolk, meat, or poultry.	1 cup (240 ml) of whole milk.	Milk, juice, water,[4] and/or bread or cereal (little or no food is needed if a hearty lunch was eaten).
6 p.m.	Breast milk or 3 to 4 oz (90 to 120 ml) of formula ──────────►		5 to 6 oz (150 to 180 ml) formula.[2] ½ to 1 oz (15 to 30 g) infant cereal. 1 to 2 oz (30 to 60 g) strained fruit or vegetable. ──────────►	7 to 8 oz (210 to 240 ml) formula.[2] 1 to 2 oz (30 to 60 g) infant cereal, teething biscuits, or toast. ──────────►	1 cup (240 ml) of whole milk.	1 to 2 oz (30 to 60 g) of cottage cheese or yogurt, egg (whole), fish, meat, poultry, or mashed cooked beans or peas. 1 cup (240 ml) of whole milk (may be given later). 1 to 2 oz (30 to 60 g) of fruit or vegetable.
10 p.m.	Breast milk or 3 to 4 oz (90 to 120 ml) of formula ──────────►		5 to 6 oz (150 to 180 ml) of formula[2]	Some of the milk from the day's allowance may be given at bedtime (usually at about 8 p.m.) ►		

[1]This plan should be modified to meet the particular needs of individual infants. For example, underweight babies might be given more, and overweight ones less food.

[2]Or breast milk. Some mothers who go to work might breast-feed in the morning and evening, but have the sitter give the baby a formula at the other feeding times.

[3]May not be needed if diet contains adequate iron (formula and/or cereal), vitamin D (formula or fortified milk), vitamin C (formula, fruit juice, fruits, and vegetables), and folacin (formula, egg yolks, meats, and vegetables).

[4]Sufficient water should be given between meals so that the total daily intake of fluids is 6 cups (1,440 ml). Additional fluid may be needed in a hot environment.

tapered necks for nipples without caps should *not* be used because (a) the nipples cannot be put on without handling them, and (b) the nipples may come off while the infant is being fed.

3. Evaporated milk formulas should be changed as the infant grows older, according to a schedule such as outlined below.

    a. The formula for the first 2 months should be made from 1 oz of evaporated milk and 2 oz of water for *each pound* (65 ml evaporated milk + 130 ml water per kg) of body weight, plus 2 Tbsp (24 g) of corn syrup, sugar, or similar sweetener (but *not* honey, because it has been implicated as a source of infant botulism in a very few cases) in the total formula for the day.

    b. During the third, fourth, and fifth months, each day's feeding should consist of one 13 oz (385 ml) can of evaporated milk mixed with 19 oz (565 ml) of water plus 2 Tbsp (24 g) of sweetener.

    c. By the sixth month, the baby can be fed 16 oz (475 ml) of evaporated milk diluted with an equal amount of water and sweetened with 3 Tbsp (36 g) of sugar or syrup. The sweetener may be reduced or omitted if the infant is receiving supplemental foods and is growing

as might be expected.

NOTE: Parents should *not* attempt to force their infants to consume the total feeding for the day, since some infants do well on less than the recommended amounts of formula. Furthermore, obesity that develops at such an early age is difficult to correct later.

The health professional consulted by the parents may also recommend other liquids to supplement the milk formula.

• **Fruit juices**—Fruit juices are usually started between 2 and 4 weeks of age. Use citrus (especially orange and grapefruit) fruit juices that are high in vitamin C, or other fruit juices that have vitamin C added. Infants need vitamin C to help build strong healthy gums, strengthen the walls of blood vessels, and aid in healing scratches.

Fresh juice should be strained to remove the pulp. To prepare fruit juice, put a small amount of juice in a sterilized bottle and add cool boiled water. Each day decrease the amount of water and increase the juice until the baby is getting ¾ cup of pure juice daily. Give the infant cool fruit juice. Heating the juice destroys vitamin C. Do not add sugar to juices. This only adds energy (calories)—not nutrients, and it increases an infant's taste for sweets.

• **Water**—In addition to milk and fruit juice, an infant may be given cool, boiled water 2 to 3 times a day. Water is as important to a baby as food.

MINERAL AND VITAMIN SUPPLEMENTS. There is considerable controversy among nutritionists and pediatricians regarding the amounts and types of nutrient supplements that are required by infants, since breast-fed infants have long been given little or no supplementation. Furthermore, the need for supplementation depends upon a variety of factors such as (1) status of the infant at birth, since preterm or low birth weight infants have higher nutritional requirements to attain the rates of growth and development of normal infants; (2) type of milk or formula used; (3) affliction of the infant with diarrhea, fever, infection, and/or other stresses; and (4) age at which supplemental foods are introduced. It is noteworthy that even breast milk is low in iron, copper, fluoride, vitamins A, D, and E, and biotin, folacin, niacin, thiamin, and vitamin B-6. Furthermore, diluted evaporated milk is notably inferior to breast milk with respect to the contents of iron, zinc, vitamin A, vitamin E, and vitamin C. Therefore, the need for nutrient supplements should be evaluated by a health professional who is familiar with the diet and the overall health status of the infant.

SOLID FOODS. The time at which solid foods such as cereals, fruits, vegetables, and meats are added to the diet depends on the infant's (1) nutritional needs, (2) digestive tract ability to handle food other than milk, and (3) physical capacity to handle them. Usually, solid foods are introduced in the order which follows:

• **Cereals**—Nutrient-enriched cereals are usually started between 2½ and 3 months of age. Read the label to make certain that the product has been enriched or fortified with iron and other nutrients. Special baby cereal (in a box) is bound to contain the added nutrients, and many other ready-to-eat and cooked products are similarly enriched.

Use an enriched or fortified cereal each day. Cereal is usually offered at the morning and evening feedings. Try rice cereal first because there is less chance of an infant having an allergic reaction. Then try oat or barley cereals. Wheat cereals may then be added. Mixed cereals should not be started until all of the single-grain cereals have been accepted by the baby without any allergic reaction. Special baby cereals do not need cooking. Just add milk. An infant may be fed cereal cooked for the family, but it should be very soft. Do not add sugar, salt, or fat to cereals.

Begin with 1 tsp (5 ml) of cereal made *soupy* with milk. Gradually increase the amount of cereal and thicken it as the infant learns to swallow. Do not add cereal to a baby's bottle. Spoon feeding is important to the development of eating behavior.

• **Fruits**—These foods are usually started between 3 and 4 months. This is a new *sweet taste* for the baby. Fruits supply vitamins and minerals and provide bulk to prevent constipation.

Soft canned fruits such as applesauce, peaches, pears, and peeled apricots can be used if mashed thoroughly. Neither sugar nor syrup from the canned fruit should be used. Sugar only adds extra calories—not nutrients.

Begin with 1 tsp (5 ml) and gradually increase until the infant is getting 2 to 3 Tbsp (30 to 45 ml). Do not use raw fruit other than ripe bananas until the infant is older. If the baby's stools become soft and watery, stop the fruit for a

few days; then add a small amount gradually.

• **Vegetables**—Mashed, pureed, and/or strained vegetables are usually started between 3 and 4 months of age. They provide vitamins and minerals needed for growing. Dark yellow and leafy green vegetables provide vitamin A which helps keep the eyes and skin healthy. Bulk from vegetables helps to promote regular bowel movements.

Fresh, canned, or frozen vegetables may be used. Cook and mash vegetables thoroughly. At first, you may want to strain the vegetables. Do not add salt, spices, fats, or bacon to the vegetables. Commercial strained baby vegetables may also be used. Choose a pure vegetable rather than a creamed vegetable mixture or dinner. At first, offer the baby mild-tasting vegetables such as green beans, carrots, squash, green peas, and greens.

Begin with 1 tsp (5 ml) of vegetable. Gradually increase until the infant is getting 2 or 3 Tbsp (30 to 45 ml) a day. Offer the same vegetable for several days before trying a new one. This will give the infant a chance to learn to like the taste of the vegetable. It also gives the mother a chance to see if the baby is allergic to the vegetable. Potato may be added after the baby is eating other vegetables. White potatoes do not take the place of green or yellow vegetables.

Be sure to include a vegetable each day. Remember, that dark yellow and green vegetables are high in vitamin A.

• **Meats**—Easily digested forms of fish, legumes, meats, and poultry are usually started by 6 months of age. These foods supply protein needed to build and repair muscles and other body tissues. They also supply iron needed to prevent the baby from getting anemic and other nutrients needed to keep the body healthy.

Begin with 1 tsp (5 ml) of meat and gradually increase to 2 or 3 Tbsp (30 to 45 ml) daily. Start with one meat and feed it several days before adding a new flavor. This gives the infant a chance to learn to like the taste. It also gives the mother a chance to see if her baby is allergic to the meat.

Table meats such as ground beef, chicken, liver, and fish may be used. Ground beef should be boiled and mashed as it cooks. Fish, chicken, and liver should be finely mashed. Moisten the meat with broth or milk. Do not fry meat. Canned chicken or fish may be finely mashed and used. Remove all bones, fat, and skin.

Commercial strained baby meat may also be used. Use pure meat rather than dinners, meat mixtures, or soups. It takes five jars of meat-vegetable mixture to equal the protein content in one jar of pure meat such as strained chicken. Bacon, fat back, salt pork, broth, and gravy are *not* meat or protein—they are mainly fat.

Dried beans and peas, thoroughly cooked and mashed, may be used in place of part of the meat. Be sure to include milk or a small amount of meat with the beans. Cook beans without bacon, salt pork, lard, or other fats.

Vegetarian diets which contain no meat, eggs, or milk may be harmful for babies. These diets are likely to be lacking in several important nutrients that infants need to grow strong and healthy.

• **Egg yolks**—This food is usually started between 4 and 6 months of age. Egg yolks provide iron needed to make red blood. Begin with 1 tsp (5 ml) and gradually increase until the baby is getting one yolk each day. If a rash develops, see your doctor before giving egg yolk again.

NOTE: Egg whites should *not* be used until recommended by your doctor. They may cause the baby to have an allergic reaction.

Hard cooked egg yolk may be fed to a baby. Use a fresh, uncracked egg. Heat in water until it comes to a boil. Remove from heat. Let the egg set in water for 20 minutes. Crack the shell and remove the yolk. Add warm milk and mash the yolk. Boiling an egg makes it tough.

Special egg yolks in a jar may be used, but they are usually more expensive. Use pure egg yolks rather than egg mixtures such as cereal and egg or bacon-egg dinners.

SELF FEEDING.
At about 5 to 6 months of age, many babies will begin hand-to-mouth movements and chewing movements. These occur at about the same time they begin to cut teeth. It is important that an infant be given the opportunity to develop chewing and self-feeding skills at this time. Chewing strengthens a baby's throat muscles for the development of speech. Dry toast is a good food to develop chewing. To prepare, cut small strips of bread and put in low (200°F [94°C]) oven for 1 hour. Store this hard toast in an air-tight container.

When hand-to-mouth movements begin, the infant is ready to start drinking from a cup and using a spoon. Let the baby play with an empty cup; and teach it how to put the cup to its mouth. Then add a few drops of milk. Increase the amount of milk as he learns to handle the cup.

Choose *child-size* utensils for eating; small spoons with short handles; unbreakable broadmouth and broadbase small cups; dishes with rims that will help the baby push food onto the spoon.

Use of *finger foods* is an excellent way to teach the baby to self-feed. Offer bite-size pieces of meat, vegetables, and fruits that can be picked up with the fingers.

Remember that an infant will be messy while he is learning to feed himself. Don't get upset. Let him do it himself!

Common Problems Encountered in Feeding.
It is always best for parents to consult their pediatrician promptly when feeding problems arise, so that any serious conditions may be diagnosed and treated as soon as possible. However, many parents encounter minor problems that can be remedied by fairly simple measures, which may be recommended by a doctor in a telephone conversation. Therefore, some of the principles that may be applied to the most common problems are presented so that parents may have a better understanding of the physician's recommendations.

LOW BIRTH WEIGHT OR PREMATURITY.
Infants that are significntly smaller than average or premature at birth may be given formulas that are more concentrated than usual.

COLIC.
This condition, which is characterized by crying and tensing of the abdomen shortly after a feeding, is a painful cramping or spasm in the infant's digestive tract. Many infants have occasional bouts of colic during the first few months of life. However, frequent occurrences require the attention of a doctor.

DIARRHEA.
The passage of loose, watery bowel movements will occur occasionally in almost all infants. However, infant diarrhea should be treated promptly according to a pediatrician's recommendations so that dehydration does not occur.

CONSTIPATION.
This condition, which is characterized by the passage of dry, hard, small infrequent stools, is rarely as serious as diarrhea, unless there is considerable pain (indicated by crying of the baby) while having a bowel move-

ment. The doctor may recommend that a litte extra sugar be added to the formula, or that greater amounts of fruits and vegetables be fed. However, chronic constipation which persists in spite of feeding sufficient bulk may require a medical evaluation to rule out other more serious conditions.

UNDERWEIGHT.
Infants vary considerably in their caloric needs, so it is to be expected that some babies will be thinner than others. Nevertheless, a pediatrician will usually want to examine thoroughly any infant that fails to gain at the rate indicated by the growth curve for the 10th percentile of infants of the same age and sex. Some of the most common causes of the failure of infants to gain sufficient weight are (1) underfeeding; (2) frequent vomiting or diarrhea; (3) febrile disease(s); (4) refusal of some or all of the food that is offered; (5) expenditure of above average amounts of energy in crying, kicking, overexcitement, excessive neuromuscular tension, or functioning with various physical handicaps; and (6) digestive or metabolic abnormalities that interfere with the utilization of nutrients. Sometimes, the correction of one or more nutritional deficiencies brings about a normal rate of growth.

OVERWEIGHT AND/OR OBESITY.
The presence of excessive body fat (obesity) may be indicated by a weight that is excessive for an infant's age and height. However, overweight and obesity are *not* always equivalent, since a baby with a smaller than normal skeleton and musculature may be of normal weight but obese, whereas a large-boned and heavy-muscled baby may be overweight without being obese. Hence, a doctor or other health professional will most likely measure the thickness of skinfolds on either the triceps or below the shoulder blades, because these measurements are rough indicators of the body fat content. Once obesity has been diagnosed in an infant, the current mode of treatment is to reduce the caloric content of the diet just enough to restrict the rate of additional fat accumulation while allowing the full growth of lean body tissue. Attempts to reduce the amount of fat that is already present may retard the rate of growth for the bones, muscles, and vital organs. Hence, the dietary treatment of obese infants differs significantly from that used for older children or adults.

FOOD ALLERGY (Food Sensitivity).
This type of condition is not uncommon in children, especially during the first few months of life. Food allergy may be mild causing only a skin rash, or it may be more severe causing vomiting, diarrhea, and colic.

Cow's milk is a common cause of allergy. Infants with milk allergy can be given a milk-free formula made from soybean or meat. These formulas provide nutrients in amounts similar to those in milk.

Other foods to which infants may be allergic include egg (especially the white), wheat, nuts, chocolate, citrus fruit, tomatoes, strawberries, and fish. Since these foods increase the risk of young infants developing allergy, they are usually left out of the diet for the first few months.

Children tend to become less allergic to food as they grow older, providing that their exposure to the offending food(s) is limited. Food sensitivity is similar to immunity to various diseases in that repeated exposures to the sensitizing agent is like a *booster shot* that stimulates the defense reactions of the body.

(Also see ALLERGIES.)

ANEMIAS. The lack of sufficient red blood cells is considered to be a sign of anemia, although there is still controversy as to the hemoglobin levels that should be characterized as subnormal. Iron-deficiency anemia is the most common one found in infants, although this type of condition may also result from other nutritional deficiencies or certain nonnutritional causes such as slow, but prolonged internal bleeding. Fortunately, there are a variety of iron-fortified infant foods and formulas that may be used to treat mild cases of anemia, and certain forms of medicinal iron may be used in the more severe cases.

(Also see ANEMIA; and IRON.)

Modifications of Infant Diets. Major modifications of the nutrient composition of an infant's diet should be made only under the supervision of a physician or a nutritionist. For example, abnormalities in the metabolism of one or more nutrients may make it necessary to restrict the diet of an infant to special foods or formulas. These conditions are relatively rare and usually require special diagnostic tests for their detection. Thus, skim milk alone is not suitable for infant feeding, except when prescribed by a doctor for an infant that has an intolerance to dietary fat; normally, it should be used only in formulas or mixtures that contain added fats such as vegetable oils.

(Also see BABY FOODS; BREAST FEEDING; and NUTRIENTS: REQUIREMENTS, ALLOWANCES, FUNCTIONS, SOURCES.)

INFARCTION

Dead tissue caused by blockage of an artery, usually by a blood clot. Infarctions have specific names; for example, the term *myocardial infarction* is used when the area affected is a part of the heart muscle (it is usually the result of a blockage—occlusion—of a coronary artery).

(Also see HEART DISEASE; and MYOCARDIAL INFARCTION.)

INFECTION

A condition that occurs when the body is invaded by disease-producing germs or microorganisms.

(Also see DISEASES.)

INFLAMMATION

A reaction of the tissues of the body to an injury or ailment, characterized by redness , heat, swelling, and pain.

INGEST

To eat or take in through the mouth.

INORGANIC

Denotes substances not of organic origin (not produced by animal or vegetable organisms).

INOSITOL

Inositol, which has been known as a chemical compound since 1850, is widely distributed in foods and closely related to glucose. It was first commonly called muscle sugar and given the name inositol from two Greek roots: *inos,* meaning sinews; and *-ose,* the suffix for sugars.

Animal experiments conducted in the 1940s indicated that inositol was an essential nutritional factor and led many investigators to group it with the B vitamins. Today, there is no evidence that humans cannot synthesize all the inositol needed by the body, and its classification as a vitamin is disputed; more properly perhaps, it should be classified as an essential nutrient, rather than a vitamin, for certain species of bacteria and animals. Nevertheless, listing inositol among the B vitamins persists in some books, catalogs, and diet-ingredient lists, and on some labels.

HISTORY. In 1940, Woolley at the University of Wisconsin demonstrated that inositol could prevent alopecia (patchy-hair, or baldness, condition) in mice. Later studies demonstrated that rats on inositol-deficient diets developed a denuded area around the eyes that imparted a curious spectacled-eye appearance. Research has also indicated a need for dietary inositol for chicks, swine, hamsters, and guinea pigs.

CHEMISTRY, METABOLISM, PROPERTIES.

• **Chemistry**—Inositol is a cyclic 6-carbon compound with 6-hydroxy groups, closely related to glucose. It exists in nine forms, but only myo-inositol demonstrates any biological activity.

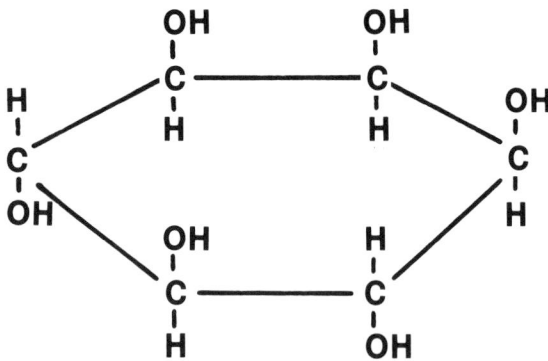

Fig. I-13. Structure of myo-inositol ($C_6H_{12}O_6$).

• **Metabolism**—In addition to food sources of inositol, it is synthesized within the cells. Myo-inositol is present in relatively large amounts in the cells of practically all animals and plants.

In animal cells, it occurs as a component of phospholipids, substances containing phosphorus, fatty acids, and nitrogenous bases. In plant cells, it is found as phytic acid, an organic acid that binds calcium, iron, and zinc in an insoluble complex and interferes with their absorption.

Inositol is stored largely in the brain, heart muscle, and skeletal muscle.

Small amounts of inositol are normally excreted in the urine. Diabetic patients excrete much larger amounts of inositol in their urine than nondiabetics.

• **Properties**—Inositol is a colorless, water-soluble, sweet-tasting crystalline material. It can withstand acids, alkalis, and heat.

MEASUREMENT/ASSAY. Inositol is measured in milligrams.

Formerly, myo-inositol analysis was by microbiological method only, based on growth of certain yeasts. Later, a time-consuming chemical method became available. Today, microbiologic and chemical assays are giving way to chromatographic methods and enzyme assays.

FUNCTIONS. The functions of inositol are not completely understood, but the following roles have been suggested:

1. It has a lipotropic effect (an affinity for fat, like choline). It promotes body production of lecithin; in turn, lecithin aids in moving fats from the liver to the cells. It follows that inositol aids in the metabolism of fats and helps reduce blood cholesterol.

2. In combination with choline, inositol prevents the fatty hardening of arteries and protects the heart.

3. It appears to be a precursor of the phosphoinosities, which are found in various body tissues, especially in the brain.

DEFICIENCY SYMPTOMS. Myo-inositol is a *growth factor* for certain yeasts and bacteria, and for several lower organisms up to and including several species of fish.

Earlier experiments indicated that a deficiency of inositol caused retarded growth and loss of hair in young mice (symptoms closely resembling deficiencies of vitamin B-6 or pantothenic acid), and loss of hair around the eyes in rats. But it is now known that these earlier studies were made with diets partially deficient in certain other vitamins; hence, in retrospect, the relationship of inositol to these symptoms is being questioned.

Large amounts of coffee (caffeine) may deplete the body's storage of inositol and result in deficiency symptoms.

RECOMMENDED DAILY ALLOWANCE OF INOSITOL. The inositol requirement of man is unknown for two reasons: (1) its role in human nutrition is undetermined, and (2) man and other higher animals appear capable of synthesizing all the inositol needed. So, no recommended daily allowances are given.

Myo-inositol appears to be required in the diet of the mouse, rat, hamster, guinea pig, duck, and pig, but there is still uncertainty as to whether (1) it is merely performing some of the functions of certain B vitamins, or (2) it is an essential metabolic requirement.

• **Inositol intake in average U.S. diet**—It is estimated that the average daily inositol consumption in the United States ranges from 300 to 1,000 mg per day.

TOXICITY. There is no known toxicity of inositol.

SOURCES OF INOSITOL. Inositol is abundantly present in nature. Sources are given in the section on VITAMIN(S), Table V-5, Vitamin Table.

Also, humans synthesize it within the cells. Perhaps it is also synthesized by intestinal bacteria, although this has not been proven.

(Also see VITAMIN[S], Table V-5.)

INSENSIBLE PERSPIRATION

Perspiration that evaporates before it is noticed as sweat on the skin.

INSIDIOUS

Denoting a disease which progresses with few or no symptoms to indicate its seriousness.

INSTITUTE OF FOOD TECHNOLOGY

This is the professional organization for food technologists. The address: Suite 2120, 221 North La Salle St., Chicago, Ill. 60601. The Institute issues two publications: (1) *Food Technology,* in which applied research articles and news of the society appear; and (2) *The Journal of Food Science,* which carries more fundamental research reports.

(Also see FOOD TECHNOLOGY.)

INTERESTERIFICATION

Fats are mixtures of triglycerides—various fatty acids esterified to glycerol. The process of interesterification is the migration of the various fatty acids between the glycerol molecules giving the fat different physical properties. Heating a fat will cause this process to occur. A major application of this process in the food industry is the production of mono- and diglycerides. In a mixture of triglycerides and glycerol heated to 400°F (*204°C*) in the presence of a sodium hydroxide catalyst, fatty acid molecules migrate from the triglyceride to the free glycerol molecules thus producing a mixture of mono- and diglycerides because there is an excess of glycerol molecules. Mono- and diglycerides have wide use in the food industry as emulsifiers.

(Also see ESTER; and TRIGLYCERIDES.)

INTERMEDIATE HYDROGEN CARRIER

The body utilizes a series of biological oxidations to form energy from foods. Oxidation refers to the loss of electrons—hydrogen—by a compound. For example, lactic acid is dehydrogenated to form pyruvic acid. This hydrogen is then passed to the intermediate hydrogen carriers, nicotinamide adenine dinucleotide (NAD) and flavin adenine dinucleotide (FAD), which, in turn, pass hydrogen to a system known as the electron transport chain, a series of intermediate hydrogen carriers. As the hydrogen is passed down this chain, energy is released. At the end of the chain, the hydrogen combines with the ultimate hydrogen carrier, oxygen, and water is formed.

(Also see METABOLIC WATER; and METABOLISM.)

INTERNATIONAL UNIT (IU)

A standard unit of potency of a biologic agent (e.g., a vitamin, hormone, antibiotic, antitoxin) as defined by the International Conference for Unification of Formulae. Potency is based on bioassay that produces a particular effect agreed on internationally. Also called a USP unit.

INTERSTITIAL (FLUID)

Situated in spaces between tissues.

INTESTINAL FLORA

Relating to the various bacterial and other microscopic forms of plant life in the intestinal contents.

INTESTINAL JUICE

A clear liquid secreted by glands in the wall of the small intestine. It contains the enzymes lactase, maltase, and sucrase, and several peptidases.

(Also see DIGESTION AND ABSORPTION.)

INTESTINE, LARGE

The tubelike part of the digestive tract lying between the small intestine and the anus. It is larger in diameter but shorter in length than the small intestine.
(Also see DIGESTION AND ABSORPTION.)

INTESTINE, SMALL

The long, tortuous, tubelike part of the digestive tract leading from the stomach to the cecum and large intestine. It is smaller in diameter but longer than the large intestine.
(Also see DIGESTION AND ABSORPTION.)

INTOLERANCE

Sensitivity or allergy of certain foods, drugs, or other substances.
(Also see ALLERGIES.)

INTRA-

Prefix meaning within.

INTRACELLULAR

Within the cell.

INTRAMURAL NERVE PLEXUS

A network of interwoven nerve fibers within a particular organ. The smooth muscle layers of the gastrointestinal wall are controlled by such a network of nerve fibers.

INTRAVENOUS FEEDING

At times it becomes necessary to correct acute losses of fluids, salts, vitamins, and other nutrients by application directly into the bloodstream. This process is intravenous feeding. Most times it is practiced on a short term basis. Often it is used to tide a patient over after injuries or operations involving the face, mouth, esophagus, stomach, and small intestine. Nutrient-containing fluids used for this purpose are dripped by gravity into a peripheral vein, often a vein in the arm. A bottle containing the fluid is suspended above the patient and connected to a needle in the vein via a small plastic tube. Long-term use of this procedure in patients who cannot be fed by mouth or a stomach tube is hazardous, expensive, and time consuming. It can, however, be accomplished if the plastic tube is inserted into one of the large central veins of the body. There are available a variety of solutions containing fats, amino acids, and glucose that can, if needed, provide complete nutrition for weeks and even years.
(Also see Fig. I-14.)

INTRAVENOUS (PARENTERAL) NUTRITION, SUPPLEMENTARY

Contents

This term refers to the temporary provision of supplementary nutrients in a solution that is infused into a vein. When a small vein on the surface of an arm, leg, or the scalp is

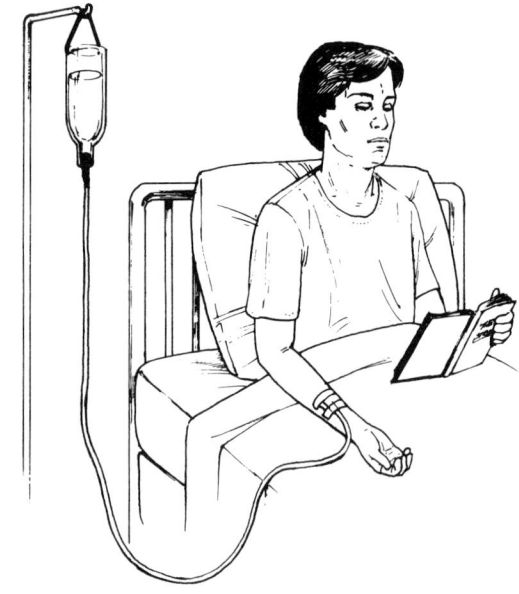

Fig. I-14. Intravenous feeding. This method of providing nutrients and/or medications has long been used to maintain patients when it is inadvisable to attempt to feed them via the mouth and the digestive tract.

used, it is called peripheral intravenous feeding, whereas the infusion of the nutrients into a large vein deep within the body is called central venous feeding. Furthermore, the amounts of nutrients which may be delivered to a peripheral vein is limited because concentrated solutions are likely to cause phlebitis and/or clots (thrombi). On the other hand, rather concentrated nutrient solutions may be infused by central veins because the blood flow is rapid enough to bring about a prompt dilution of the solution so that little irritation to the vein occurs.
(Also see TOTAL PARENTERAL [INTRAVENOUS] NUTRITION [TPN].)

HISTORY. The first experiments on feeding animals and people by intravenous means were conducted shortly after the English physician William Harvey discovered the circulation of the blood in 1616.

It appears that the modern era of intravenous nutrition began in 1843, when the renowned French physiologist Claude Bernard injected sugar solutions into a dog. By the end of the 19th century, the intravenous administration of dextrose (glucose) and saline solutions had become a regular practice.

Experiments on dogs in the 1950s suggested that higher levels of calories in intravenous feedings might be provided safely by the use of fat emulsions, which were much less irritating to veins than dextrose and amino acids. Unfortunately, the types of emulsions that were used then produced side effects such as asthma, chills, fever, liver disorders, low back pain, and various abnormalities of blood clotting. Better correlations between the effects of fat emulsions on dogs and on humans were obtained later by Dr. Arvid Wretlind and his co-workers in Sweden when the dogs used in the tests were given the fat emulsions on the basis of their metabolic rates rather than according to body weights. These studies led to the development of a safer fat emulsion in the early 1960s. This product has been used since then in Europe, but only recently in the United States.

The most recent major breakthrough in this field was the development of total parenteral nutrition (TPN) in the mid-1960s by Dr. Stanley Dudrick and his co-workers at the University of Pennsylvania School of Medicine. TPN involves the infusion of a complete and concentrated mixture of nutrients into the vena cava (a large vein that empties directly into the heart) by means of a catheter that is passed down through either the subclavian or jugular veins.

Supplementary parenteral nutrition continues to be used routinely, in spite of the development of TPN, because the latter is a serious surgical procedure, whereas, the former procedure is usually safer and easier to use.

INDICATIONS. Presently, there is a wide variety of intravenous solutions from which to choose and use for conditions such as acidosis, dehydration, diarrhea, elevated metabolic rate, fever, gastric suction, hemorrhage, malnutrition, N.P.O. (no nourishment may be taken orally), retention of excessive water in the tissues, severe burns, and vomiting.

The major reasons for correcting these conditions intravenously rather than orally are (1) oral treatment may be too slow and uncertain because of disorders of digestion and absorption, (2) inflammation, injury, or surgery of the digestive tract makes it inadvisable to use this route for therapy, (3) the patient may be comatose or paralyzed and subject to aspiration (sucking of material down the windpipe into the lungs) or choking on matter fed orally, and (4) it may not be possible to meet unusually high requirements by oral or tube feeding.

It is noteworthy that supplementary intravenous feeding is almost always a short-term procedure because it is difficult to meet all nutritional requirements by this means. Patients who require long-term intravenous feeding are usually given total parenteral (intravenous) feeding through a central vein.

Types Of Solutions Used In Peripheral Intravenous Feeding.
The selection of the proper solution for treatment of a particular condition may be a matter of life or death for a very ill patient. Descriptions and uses of the major types of intravenous solutions follow:

• **Amino acids and/or protein hydrolysates**—Whole proteins cannot be given intravenously because of the danger of a very strong antigenic reaction. (Blood transfusions are an exception because the proteins present are those which occur naturally in the blood.) Therefore, mixtures of purified amino acids or protein hydrolysates (proteins broken down to amino acids by means of acid, alkaline, and/or enzymatic hydrolysis) are used to meet protein requirements. However, newborn infants can be given only the amino acids, because protein hydrolysates contain more ammonia than their bodies can metabolize readily.

• **Carbohydrates**—Glucose is most commonly used at a concentration of 5 or 10%, although fructose is sometimes given to diabetics because it does not require insulin for its metabolism. The latter practice is falling into disfavor because the rapid administration of fructose may cause a buildup of lactate in the blood and a corresponding acidosis.

• **Fat (lipid) emulsions**—These preparations consist of very finely dispersed minute droplets of a vegetable oil in isotonic solutions that contain small amounts of lecithin which help to make the emulsions very stable.

Fat emulsions are used alone or in combination with other intravenous solutions to provide extra calories that often mean the difference between the sparing of body protein and the wasting of tissues.

• **Minerals and vitamins**—Generally, doctors are more likely to order the addition of supplementary minerals and vitamins to intravenous solutions infused into central veins (total parenteral feeding) than to those given peripherally (supplementary parenteral feeding) for short periods of time. However, doses of vitamin C as high as one or more grams per day have been utilized in the latter procedure because of the important role of this nutrient in healing.

It is not always necessary to give every essential mineral and vitamin intravenously, since some of these nutrients may be provided in intramuscular or subcutaneous injections made at regular intervals. The present trend appears to be leading in the direction of giving greater mineral and vitamin supplementation than was done in the past.

• **Plasma extenders such as dextran**—These substances are synthetic substances without nutritional value that are used in emergency situations to provide colloid that helps to maintain the water content of the blood. Normally, this function is served by the bloodborne proteins, but these constituents may be at critically subnormal levels when there has been hemorrhage, severe malnutrition, and other serious injuries or disorders.

• **Salt (sodium chloride) and/or other electrolytes**—The most commonly used solution in this category is 0.9% sodium choloride, which is also called *physiological saline* because it has the same solute strength (tonicity) as the body fluids. Some solutions also contain potassium and magnesium salts because these minerals are also highly essential in the maintenance of a variety of vital functions.

Solutions of electrolytes are administered when it is necessary to replace the mineral salts and water that have been lost under circumstances such as dehydration, diarrhea, gastric suction, hemorrhage, moderate to severe burns, and vomiting. For example, sodium bicarbonate is often given to correct acidosis, which occurs in diabetic coma. Also, magnesium sulfate is sometimes given intravenously to correct ventricular fibrillation.

BENEFITS. The leading benefits of intravenous solutions injected into a peripheral vein are as follows:

1. Solutions may be *tailor made* for the patient's needs.
2. Delivery of the required nutrients directly and rapidly into the bloodstream ensures that they get to where they are needed without being subjected to the uncertainties of a patient's appetite and the ingestion, digestion, and absorption of substances given via the digestive tract.
3. Infusion into a peripheral vein may be started by nurses and paramedics, whereas total parenteral feeding via a central vein is a procedure that requires a doctor.

HAZARDS AND PRECAUTION. The major hazards of supplementary intravenous feeding via a peripheral vein usually arise from attempting to supply too much, too rapidly, without considering the patient's condition carefully before proceeding.

CONTRAINDICATIONS. Intravenous feeding via a peripheral vein should not be used if (1) oral or tube feeding may meet all of the patient's requirements, (2) a long-term intravenous administration of all or most nutrients is required, and total parenteral nutrition is available, or (3) the risks (due to the instability of the patient's condition) outweigh the benefits gained. In the last case, intravenous feedings may be initiated as soon as the patient's condition has been stabilized.

SUMMARY. Supplementary intravenous feeding via a peripheral vein is best suited for meeting short-term needs of patients who are likely to fare poorly without it. It does not require the expertise needed to administer total parenteral nutrition (TPN), but it is more limited with respect to the amounts of nutrients which may be delivered intravenously. Therefore, it is being replaced by TPN in chronic care situations when the capability for administering the latter is present.

(Also see TOTAL PARENTERAL [INTRAVENOUS] NUTRITION.)

INTRINSIC FACTOR

A chemical substance secreted by the stomach which is necessary for the absorption of vitamin B-12. The exact chemical nature of intrinsic factor is not known, but it is thought to be a mucoprotein or mucopolysaccharide. A deficiency of this factor may lead to a deficiency of vitamin B-12, and, ultimately, to pernicious anemia.

(Also see ANEMIA, PERNICIOUS; DIGESTION AND ABSORPTION, section on "Stomach.")

INULIN

A polysaccharide found especially in Jerusalem artichokes which yields fructose upon hydrolysis.

INVERSION

The process of splitting table sugar (sucrose) into glucose and fructose—invert sugar. Inversion is carried out by invertase, an enzyme, or by acids. Invert sugar is sweeter than sucrose due to the fructose present. It is often incorporated in products to prevent drying out; thus, it is a humectant. Invert sugar is utilized in the confectionary and brewing industries.

(Also see SUGAR, section on "Consumption and Use of Sugar.")

INVERTASE (SACCHARASE; SUCRASE)

An enzyme produced by the cells of the small intestine and by yeast. It catalyzes the splitting of table sugar (sucrose) into glucose and fructose.

(Also see FOOD—BUYING, PREPARING, COOKING, AND SERVING, section on "Enzymes.")

INVERTASE (SUCRASE)-ISOMALTASE DEFICIENCY

This is a rare inborn error in the metabolism of carbohydrates. The most common symptom is diarrhea. In this disease the enzymes invertase and isomaltase are missing. Both enzymes are disaccharidases. Invertase splits sucrose (sugar) and isomaltase splits isomaltose, a product of starch digestion. Therefore, sources of sucrose and isomaltose—wheat and potatoes—should be omitted from the diet to control the disease.

(Also see INBORN ERRORS OF METABOLISM, Table I-2, Inborn Errors of Carbohydrate Metabolism, "Carbohydrate Intolerance.")

INVERT SUGAR

A sugar obtained by splitting sucrose—table sugar—into glucose and fructose. This process—inversion—may be carried out by the enzyme, invertase, or by acids. Invert sugar is sweeter than table sugar due to the presence of fructose.

It is a mixture of about 50% fructose and 50% glucose. It is used in foods and confections. In some foods it is used as a humectant to hold moisture and prevent drying. The brewing industry also uses invert sugar. Honey is mostly invert sugar.

(Also see SUGAR, section on "Consumption and Use of Sugar"; and SWEETENING AGENTS, Table S-18, Comparison of Some Sweet-Tasting Substances.)

IODINE (I)

Contents	Page

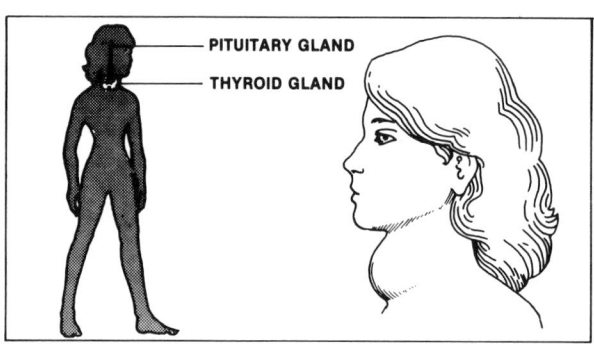

Fig. I - 15. When the hormone thyroxin must be made, the pituitary gland sends messages to the thyroid gland. When iodine is lacking in the diet, the thyroid works harder to build more thyroxin. This causes the thyroid to develop a goiter—an enlargement in the neck area.

Iodine is recognized as an essential nutrient for all animal species, including man. The human body contains about 25 mg of iodine, 10 mg of which is in the thyroid gland. It is an integral component of the thyroid hormones, thyroxin and triiodothyronine, both of which have important metabolic roles.

One of the factors affecting the output of thyroid hormones by the thyroid gland is iodine availability. In the absence of sufficient iodine, the gland attempts to compensate for the deficiency by increasing its secretory activity, and this causes the gland to enlarge. This condition is known as simple, or endemic, goiter. Females are consistently more affected than males, because goiter usually develops in periods when metabolic rate is high, such as during puberty and pregnancy. It should be noted that not all goiter is *simple goiter* due to lack of iodine. Another type of goiter, called *exophthalmic goiter (Graves' disease)*, is due to overactivity of the thyroid gland, which is usually—but not always—enlarged.

Iodine deficiencies are worldwide; wherever foods are grown on iodine-poor soil containing insufficient iodine to meet human needs. The highest incidence has been observed in the Alps, the Pyrenees, the Himalayas, the Thames Valley of England, certain regions of New Zealand, a number of Central and South American countries, and the Great Lakes and Pacific Northwest regions of the United States. Fig. I-16 shows the goiter areas of the world.

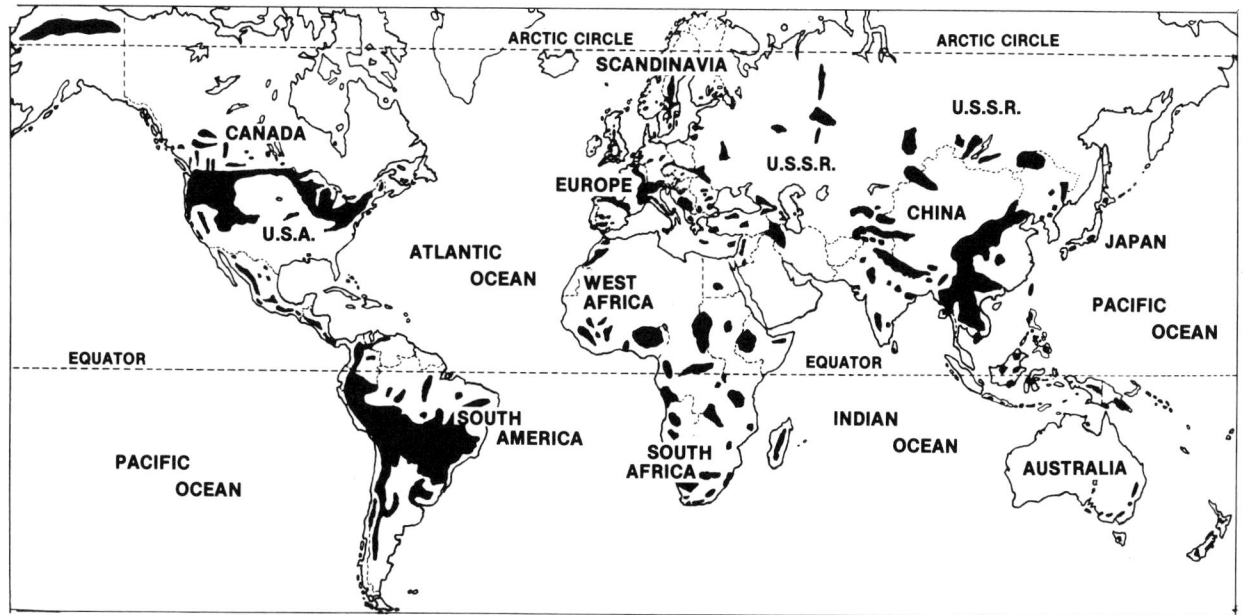

Fig. I-16. Goiter areas of the world. (Map prepared by the authors on the basis of information from the World Health Organization, Geneva, Switzerland)

The incidence of goiter in the United States fell sharply following the introduction of iodized table salt. Nevertheless, some *residual* goiter persists, probably not caused by insufficient iodine intakes, but strongly suggesting causes other than iodine deficiency—such as goitrogens (substances that can cause goiter).

HISTORY.
Iodine was the first nutrient to be recognized as essential for humans or animals. As early as 3000 B.C., the Chinese treated goiter by feeding seaweed and burnt sponge. Also, Hippocrates (460 to 370 B.C.), the Greek physician, used the same treatment for enlarged thyroid glands. The name *iodine* is derived from the Greek word *iodes*, meaning violet color, from the color of the fumes of iodine.

In 1811, Bernard Courtois, a French chemist, discovered iodine in seaweed and described some of its basic properties. Five years later, potassium hydriodate was introduced by Prout as a treatment for goiter. However, the widespread appearance of goiter continued in much of the world for many years.

In 1914, Kendall, at the Mayo Clinic, in Minnesota, reported the isolation of a crystalline compound containing 65% iodine from the thyroid gland and named it thyroxin. From this discovery and from other studies, the inclusion of iodine in the diets of man and animals led to a great reduction of goiter in the United States and other developed countries of the world. Kendall received the Nobel Prize for his work on thyroxin and other hormones.

ABSORPTION, METABOLISM, EXCRETION.
Most of the iodide present in food is iodine, in which form it is absorbed. Absorption takes place in the small intestine. Following absorption, iodine takes two main pathways within the body. Approximately 30% is removed by the thyroid gland and used for the synthesis of the thyroid hormones; most of the remainder is excreted in the urine, although small amounts are lost in the feces and sweat.

FUNCTIONS OF IODINE.
The sole function of iodine is for making the iodine-containing hormones secreted by the thyroid gland, which regulate the rate of oxidation within the cells; and in so doing influence physical and mental growth, the functioning of the nervous and muscle tissues, circulatory activity, and the metabolism of all nutrients.

DEFICIENCY SYMPTOMS.
Iodine deficiency is characterized by goiter (an enlargement of the thyroid gland at the base of the neck), coarse hair, obesity, and high blood cholesterol. Simple goiter is prevented by the addition of iodized salt to the diet. The most effective treatment is

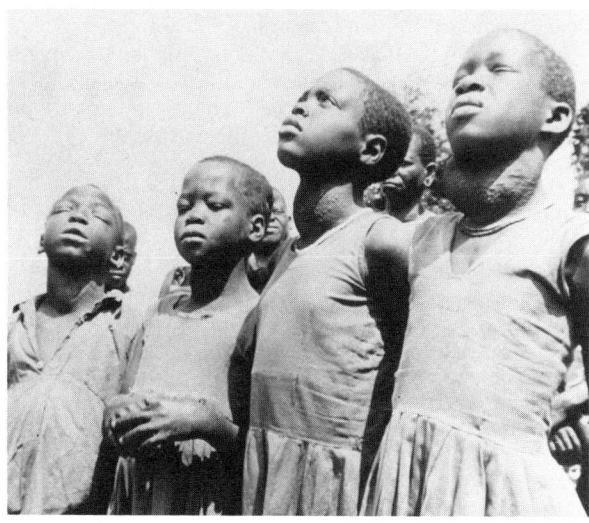

Fig. I-17. Goiter (big neck), caused by iodine deficiency. The enlarged thyroid gland (goiter) is nature's way of attempting to make sufficient thyroxin under conditions where a deficiency exists. (Courtesy, FAO/UN, Rome, Italy.)

thyroid hormone, obtained from the glands of animals and prescribed by the physician according to the patient's needs. Surgery may be necessary if the doctor suspects malignancy or to improve the victim's appearance.

Iodine-deficient mothers may give birth to infants with a type of dwarfism known as cretinism, a disorder characterized by malfunctioning of the thyroid gland, goiter, mental retardation, and stunted growth. Some of these effects may be prevented by diagnosis of the condition right after birth, followed by the administration of thyroid hormones. A similar disorder of the thyroid gland, known as myxedema, may develop in adults.

INTERRELATIONSHIPS. Certain foods (especially plants of the cabbage family—cabbage, kale, turnips, cauliflower, rapeseed, and mustard seed) contain goitrogens, which interfere with the use of thyroxin and may produce goiter. Fortunately, goitrogenic action is prevented by cooking, and an adequate supply of iodine inhibits or prevents it.

Jointly occurring deficiencies of iodine and vitamin A are likely to cause a more severe thyroid disorder than lack of iodine alone.

RECOMMENDED DAILY ALLOWANCE OF IODINE. The daily iodine requirement for prevention of goiter in adults is 50 to 75 mcg, or approximately 1 mcg/kg of body weight. In order to provide an extra margin of safety and to meet increased demands that may be imposed by natural goitrogens under certain conditions, the Food and Nutrition Board of the National Research Council (FNB-NRC) recommends an allowance of 150 mcg per day for adolescents and adults of both sexes, *plus* additional allowances of 25 and 50 mcg per day for pregnant and lactating women, respectively. The FNB-NRC recommended daily iodine allowances are given in the section on MINERAL(S), Table M-25, Mineral Table.

Iodine intake at the FNB-NRC recommended levels has no demonstrable adverse effects; in fact, an intake in adults between 50 and 1,000 mcg of iodine can be considered safe.

It is recommended that iodized salt be used in households in all noncoastal regions of the United States. In the coastal regions the need is not so great because of the higher iodine concentration in the environment.

It is suggested that all food products designed to provide complete nutrient maintenance of individuals (such as infant formulas and special medical diets) contain iodine in sufficient concentrations to provide their proportion of the recommended dietary allowance.

The FNB-NRC recommends that many added sources of iodine in the American food system, such as iodophors in the dairy industry, alginates, coloring dyes, and dough conditioners, be replaced wherever possible by compounds containing less or no iodine. This recommendation was prompted because the iodine consumed by human beings has increased in recent years, and there is evidence that the quantity of iodine presently consumed in the United States is well above the nutritional requirement. Although there is no direct evidence of an increased human iodine toxicity problem because of the increased intake, there is some concern that if this trend continues, the greater iodine concentration may contribute to an increase in thyroid disorders.

Because iodine content in milk has increased 300 to 500% since about 1965, the Kentucky Agricultural Experiment Station made a study of the factors contributing to this increase. They reported as follows:

Organic iodine additions to the feed supply have contributed large increases in iodine content in milk from some farms, and are considered the main factor contributing to the large increase in iodine content in milk values. Iodine teat dips and udder washes contribute to the increased iodine content of milk, but they generally do not result in increases of more than 150 mcg/liter. Iodine-sanitizing agents used on milking equipment or in milk transfer and storage equipment can contribute large amounts if improperly used, but the frequency of this problem is small. Iodine content in meat does increase with increased iodine intake, but the transfer of iodine to meat is relatively lower than it is in milk.[7]

• **Iodine intake in average U.S.diet**—Studies have estimated the average dietary iodine intake in the United States to range from 64 to 677 mcg per day. Higher intakes are likely in persons subjected to high levels of atmospheric iodine or in those consuming iodine-containing drugs.

TOXICITY. Long-term intake of large excesses of iodine may disturb the utilization of iodine by the thyroid gland and result in goiter. In Tasmania, goiter induced by high dietary iodine intake has been correlated with the introduction of bread fortified with iodine. Also, goiter induced by high iodine intake has been documented in Japan, where seaweeds rich in iodine are habitually consumed. It is unlikely that such adverse effects as those reported in Tasmania and Japan would result in a population with habitual iodine intakes of less than 300 mcg per day.

Therapeutic use of iodine or large intakes of kelp in the diet can be toxic. So, self-treatments with compounds of iodine or concentrates of iodine in dried seaweed over long periods can be hazardous.

It is noteworthy that people with iodine deficiencies have above average susceptibility to the toxic effects of I-131, an atmospheric contaminant produced during the open-air testing of nuclear weapons.

SOURCES OF IODINE. Of the various methods that have been proposed for assuring an adequate iodine intake, especially among populations in iodine-poor regions, the use of iodized salt has thus far proved to be the most successful, and therefore the most widely adopted method. In the United States, iodination is on a voluntary basis, nevertheless slightly more than half of the table salt consumed is iodized. Stabilized iodized salt contains 0.01% potassium iodide (0.0076% I), or 76 mcg of iodine per gram. Thus, the average use of 3.4 g of iodized salt per person per day adds approximately 260 mcg to the daily intake, more than three times the normal requirement.

Iodine may also be provided in bread. But the practice of using iodates (chemicals used as dough conditioners) in bread-making appears to be on the decline.

Among natural foods the best sources of iodine are kelp, seafoods, and vegetables grown on iodine-rich soils. Dairy products and eggs may be good sources if the producing animals have access to iodine-enriched rations. Most cereal grains, legumes, roots, and fruits have low iodine content.

[7]Hemkin, R. W., "Milk and Meat Iodine Content: Relation to Human Health," *Journal of the American Veterinary Medicine Association*, Vol. 176, No. 10, pp. 1119-1121.

So, for intakes of iodine, man is dependent upon food, soil, and water. The iodine content of foods varies widely, depending chiefly on (1) the iodine content of the soil, (2) the iodine content of the animal feeds (to which iodized salt is routinely added in most countries), and (3) the use of iodized salt in food processing operations. Iodine in drinking and cooking water varies widely in different regions; in some areas, such as near oceans, it is high enough to meet the daily requirement. For these reasons, iodine values in food composition tables should be accepted as indicative, but not precise.

Table I-8 gives the iodine content of some common foods. (Also see GOITER; and MINERAL[S], Table M-25.)

TABLE I-8
IODINE CONTENT OF SOME COMMON FOODS

Source	Iodine Content
	(mcg/100 g)
Dried kelp	62,400
Iodized salt	7,600
Saltwater fish (haddock, whiting, herring)	330
Blackstrap molasses	158
Catfish	118
Beans, dried	115
Seafoods	66
Spinach	56
Vegetables	30
Milk and products	14
Eggs	13
Whole grain wheat	9
Whole grain oats	9
Beef	8
Rice polish	7
Wheat bran	7
Rice bran	4
Whole grain barley	4
Rice	4
Fruits	3

IODINE DEFICIENCY (GOITER)

Failure of the body to obtain sufficient iodine from which the thyroid gland can form thyroxin, an iodine-containing compound.

(Also see GOITER; and IODINE.)

IODINE NUMBER

A number which denotes the degree of unsaturation of a fat or fatty acid. It is the amount of iodine in grams which can be taken up by 100 grams of fat.

(Also see FATS AND OTHER LIPIDS, section headed "Fatty Acids"; and OILS, VEGETABLE, section headed "Chemical and Physical Properties.")

IODINE 131

The radioactive form of iodine (I). It has a half-life of 8 days. Since its presence can be detected by a Geiger counter or similar instrument, iodine 131 has numerous uses in biology and medicine. Substances can be *tagged* with iodine 131 and then their metabolism, movement, or disappearance can be followed in the body. Medical diagnostic and therapeutic uses include: thyroid function, blood volume, location of brain tumors, cancer treatment, and hyperthyroid treatment.

(Also see RADIOACTIVE FALLOUT [CONTAMINATION].)

IODIZED SALT

Prevention of goiter is usually achieved in the developed countries by the use of iodized salt. For the purpose of iodizing, the FDA allows up to 0.01% of potassium iodide (KI) in table salt. Two grams of iodized table salt per day—most people use more—furnishes about 152 mcg of iodine or slightly more than the Recommended Dietary Allowance for adults.

(Also see GOITER; and IODINE, section headed "Sources.")

IODOPSIN

The main pigment found in the cones of the retina; it contains vitamin A.

(Also see VITAMIN A, section headed "Functions.")

ION

An atom or a group of atoms carrying an electric charge, either positive or negative. They are usually formed when salts, acids, or bases are dissolved in water.

IONIC IRON

Pertaining to an atom of iron, as Fe^{+++} or Fe^{++} (ferric and ferrous, respectively).

(Also see IRON.)

IONIZATION

The adding of one or more electrons to, or removing one or more electrons from, atoms or molecules, thereby creating ions.

IONIZED CALCIUM (Ca^{++})

This refers to the free, diffusible form of calcium in the blood and other body fluids, amounting to about 1% of the total body calcium. It exerts a profound effect on the function of bone, the heart, and the nervous system.

IRON (Fe)

The human body contains only about 0.004% iron, or only 3 to 4 g in an adult. About 70% of the iron is present in the hemoglobin, the pigment of the red blood cells. Most of the rest (about 30%) is present as a reserve store in the liver, spleen, and bone marrow. Despite the very small amount in the body, iron is one of the most important elements in nutrition and of fundamental importance to life. It is a component of hemoglobin, myoglobin (muscle hemoglobin), the cytochromes, catalase, and peroxidase. As part of these heme complexes and metalloenzymes, it serves important functions in oxygen transport and cellular respiration.

The red blood cells and the pigment within are broken down and replaced about every 120 days, but the liberated iron is not excreted; most of it is utilized to form new hemoglobin.

IRON, needed by the body to build red blood

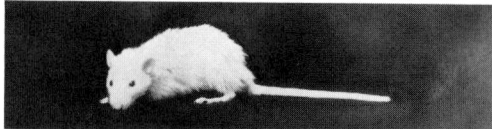

This rat did not have enough iron. It has pale ears and tail. Eight months old, it weighed only 109 g.

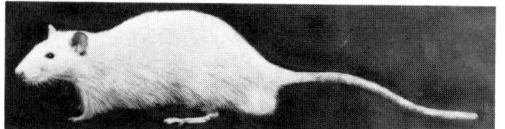

This rat had plenty of iron. Its fur is sleek and its blood has three times as much red coloring as the rat to the left. Though only about 5½ months old, it weighed 325 g.

TOP FOOD SOURCES

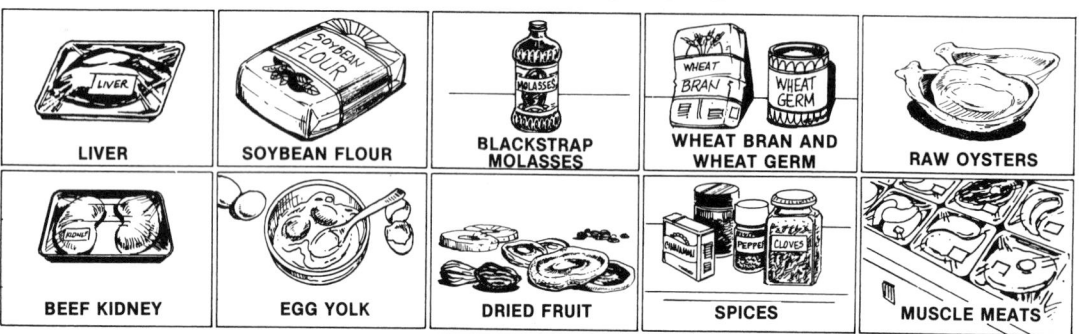

Fig. I-18. Iron made the difference! *Left*: Rat on iron-deficient diet. *Right*: Rat that received plenty of iron. Note, too, ten top sources of iron. (Adapted from USDA sources)

HISTORY. Elemental iron has been known since prehistoric times. Although how early humans first learned to extract the element from its ores is still debated, scientists are fairly certain that early, highly prized samples of iron were obtained from meteors. Several references to "the metal of heaven" (thought to be iron) have been found in ancient writings. By approximately 1200 B.C., iron was being obtained from its ores; this achievement marked the beginning of the *Iron Age*.

The early Greeks were aware of the health-imparting properties of iron. Ever since, it has been a favorite health tonic (for better or worse). As early as the 17th century in England, iron was found to be a specific treatment for anemia in man. In 1867, Boussingault, the French chemist, obtained experimental evidence of the essential nature of iron in nutrition.

Although the need for iron was discovered long ago, and although it is the most common and cheapest of all metals, more deficiencies of iron (chiefly in the form of anemia) exist in the United States and in most other developed countries than of any other nutrient. An estimated 10 to 25% of the population is affected. Lack of iron in the diet is attributed primarily to (1) the increased refining and processing of our food supply, and (2) the decreased use of cast-iron cookware.

ABSORPTION, METABOLISM, EXCRETION. The greatest absorption of iron occurs in the upper part of the small intestine—in the duodenum and jejunum, although a small amount of absorption takes place from the stomach and throughout the whole of the small intestine. Only 10% of the iron present in cereals, vegetables, and pulses, excluding soybeans, is absorbed. Absorption of iron from other foods is slightly higher—for example, 30% from meat, 20% from soybeans, and 15% from fish. For estimating the absorption of iron in diets, a value of 10% is usually taken as the percentage of iron absorbed from mixed foods.

It is noteworthy that there are two forms of food iron—heme (organic) and nonheme (inorganic). Of the two, heme is absorbed from food more efficiently than inorganic iron and is independent of vitamin C or iron-binding chelating agents. Although the proportion of heme iron in animal tissues varies, it amounts to about one-third of the total iron in all animal tissues—including meat, liver, poultry, and fish. The remaining two-thirds of the iron in animal tissues and all the iron of vegetable products are treated as nonheme iron.

Modern knowledge of the existence of two categories of iron-containing foods—heme and nonheme compounds—and of dietary factors influencing their absorption, now makes it possible to replace the estimate of an average 10% absorption of dietary iron by a more precise figure. This concept provides a means for the calculation of absorbable iron in any one meal and for increasing the availability of dietary iron through selection of appropriate food items. The application of this concept gives promise of improving the nutritional status of population groups in need of more iron, and of decreasing the exposure of individuals with excessive iron absorption.

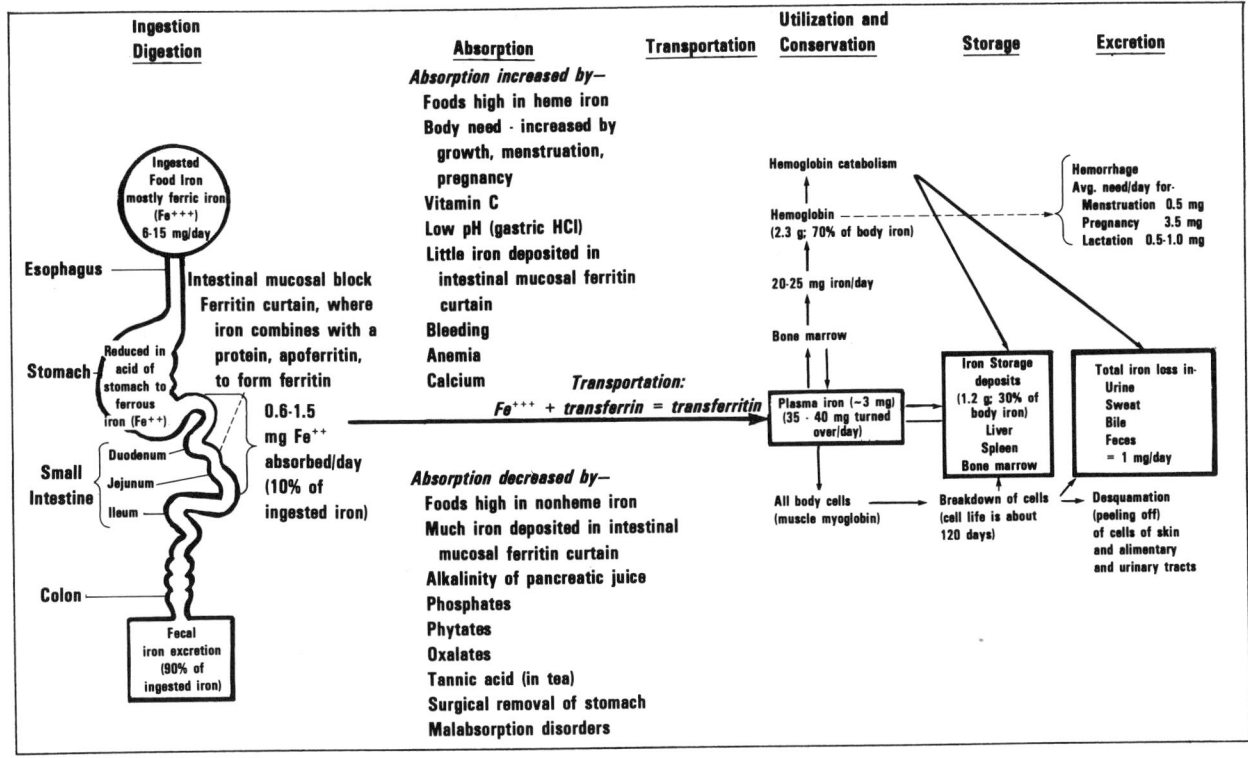

Fig. I-19. Iron absorption, metabolism, and excretion. Note that healthy adults absorb only about 10% of the iron in food, and that about 90% is excreted in the feces. Note, too, the factors that increase and decrease absorption.

Iron absorption is controlled by the intestinal mucosal block—the ferritin curtain, the exact mechanism of which is not known. It is increased (1) by foods high in heme iron; (2) by body needs—increased by growth, menstruation, and pregnancy; (3) by the presence of vitamin C (ascorbic acid) and gastric HCl, which convert the iron from the ferric (Fe + + +) to the ferrous (Fe + +) state; (4) when little iron is deposited in the intestinal mucosal ferritin curtain; (5) when there is increased *hemoglobin* synthesis—for example, following *hemorrhages* (bleeding), or as a result of anemia or *hemopoetic* abnormalities; and (6) by the presence of calcium. Iron absorption is impaired (1) by foods high in nonheme iron; (2) when much iron is deposited in the intestinal mucosal ferritin curtain; (3) by excess phosphates, phytates, oxalates, and tannic acid (in tea), all of which form insoluble compounds that are not readily absorbed—hence, excesses of such substances should be avoided in individuals suffering from severe nutritional anemia; and (4) following surgical removal of the stomach or when there are malabsorption disorders.

Mucosal ferritin delivers ferrous iron (Fe + +) to the portal blood system. Thence iron is converted back to the ferric (Fe + + +) state by oxidation. As ferric iron, it combines with protein (transferrin), forming a combination known as transferritin. In this form, iron is transported to the bone marrow where it may be incorporated into newly synthesized hemoglobin molecules; or, alternatively, it may be stored in the liver, spleen, and bone marrow, where it combines with a protein and is deposited as ferritin.

Absorbed iron is lost only by desquamation (shedding or peeling off of cells) from the alimentary, urinary, and respiratory tracts, and by skin and hair losses. The bulk of ingested iron (about 90%) is excreted in the feces. Only negligible amounts of iron are excreted in the urine. The body conserves and reuses iron once it has been absorbed. The combined losses of iron by all routes are of the order of about 1 mg per day for a healthy adult man, and about 1.5 mg per day for a woman during the reproductive period. Added losses of iron of importance occur from blood donation and pathological bleeding (hookworm infections, bleeding ulcers, etc.), and in cases of kidney diseases, particularly nephrosis.

FUNCTIONS OF IRON. Iron combines with protein to make hemoglobin for red blood cells. *Heme* means iron; *globin* means protein. A small amount of iron (heme) combines with a large protein (globin) to make hemoglobin, the iron-containing compound in red blood cells. So, iron is involved in transporting oxygen. It is also a component of enzymes which are involved in energy metabolism.

DEFICIENCY SYMPTOMS. A deficiency of iron may cause iron-deficiency (nutritional) anemia, clinically characterized by a decrease in the amount of hemoglobin and by small, pale-red blood cells, depleted iron stores, and a plasma iron content of less than 40 mg per 100 ml. The number of red blood cells may also be reduced, but not as markedly as the hemoglobin content. Iron-deficiency anemia is a medical and public health problem of primary importance, causing few deaths but contributing seriously to the weakness, ill health, and substandard performance of millions of people.

The symptoms of anemia are: paleness of skin and mucous membranes, fatigue, dizziness, sensitivity to cold, shortness of breath, rapid heartbeats, and tingling in the fingers and toes.

An inadequate dietary intake of iron by growing children, by adolescent girls, or by women—especially during pregnancy and in lactation, will produce nutritional anemia.

If a pregnant woman has an insufficient intake of iron, the newborn infant, in turn, will have a relatively low store of iron, causing anemia to develop early in the first year of life. Anemia during infancy, a frequent occurrence, is closely related to the body stores of iron at birth. It is especially common in premature infants and twins, because in such circumstances the body reserves of iron cannot be built up to desirable levels.

Many adolescent girls select a poor diet, to indulge the whims of a freakish appetite or to maintain ill-advised reduction regimens, with resultant anemia. Thus, it is necessary continually to emphasize to them that there is an accelerated demand for iron to satisfy their still-increasing blood volume as well as to compensate for losses through menstruation.

(Also see DEFICIENCY DISEASES, Table D-1, Major Dietary Deficiency Diseases—"Iron Deficiency Anemia.")

INTERRELATIONSHIPS. Iron is associated with hemoglobin and various enzymes. However, the production of hemoglobin in the body also requires protein, copper, vitamin C, vitamin B-6 (pyridoxine), folic acid, and vitamin B-12. An excess of iron in the diet can tie up phosphorus in an insoluble iron-phosphate complex, thereby creating a deficiency of phosphorus.

Free iron ions are very toxic. So, the iron molecule is always transported in combination with protein; 2 atoms of ferric iron are bound to 1 molecule of beta globulin protein called *transferrin*—and the combination forms *transferritin*. When the level of iron ions exceeds the binding capacity of the transferrin, iron toxemia occurs. Normally, the amount of iron in plasma is sufficient to bind only ⅓ of the transferrin—the remaining ⅔ represents the unbound reserve.

Iron overload may occur as a result of metabolic defects, such as idiopathic hemochromatosis—an inherited disease, or from high intakes of iron. The clinical signs and symptoms of iron overload may include hyperpigmentation of the skin, cirrhosis of the liver, diabetes, and myocardial failure. Dr. John R. K. Robson, M.D., one of the coauthors of this book, has observed excessive intakes of iron, characterized by hemosiderosis and cirrhosis of the liver, in the Bantu tribe of South Africa who cook their food in iron pots and ferment their beer in iron utensils—and who have iron intakes of up to 100 mg, or more, per day.

RECOMMENDED DAILY ALLOWANCE OF IRON. There are four situations in which iron intake is frequently inadequate in the United States: (1) in infancy, because of the low iron content of milk and because babies are not born with sufficient iron to meet their needs beyond 6 months; (2) during the periods of rapid growth in childhood and adolescence, because of the need to fill expanding iron stores; (3) during the female reproductive period, because of menstrual iron losses (at least 10% of menstruating women are iron deficient); and (4) in pregnancy, because of the expanding blood volume of the mother, the demands of the fetus and placenta, and blood losses in childbirth. In order to provide for the retention of 1 mg per day in adult males and postmenopausal females, and assuming an average availability of 10% of the food iron, an allowance of 10 mg per day is recommended. Higher recommended allowances are made during the critical periods; in infancy, in childhood and adolescence, during the female reproductive period, and in pregnancy and early lactation.

Recommended daily iron allowances are given in the section on MINERAL(S), Table M-25, Mineral Table.

• **Iron intake in average U.S. diet**—According to the U.S. Department of Agriculture, there is sufficient iron in foods available for consumption in the United States to provide an average intake of 17.1 mg per person per day. Of this total, the contribution of food groups is as follows: meat, poultry, and fish, 22.1%; flour and cereal products, 42.7%; other vegetables, including tomatoes, 6.9%; sugars and sweeteners, 2.3%; dry beans and peas, nuts, soya flour, and grits, 6.5%; eggs, 2.9%; potatoes, 4.7%; noncitrus fruits, 2.4%; dairy products, 2.4%; dark green and deep yellow vegetables, 1.7%; citrus fruits, 0.6%; and fats and oils, including butter, 0.1%.

Iron fortification of cereals, flour, and bread has added significantly to the total iron intake.

TOXICITY. Approximately 2,000 cases of iron poisoning occur each year in the United States, mainly in young children who ingest the medicinal iron supplements of their parents. The lethal dose of ferrous sulfate for a 2-year-old is about 3 g; for an adult it's between 200 and 250 mg/kg of body weight.

IRON LOSSES DURING PROCESSING AND COOKING. The size of the pieces, the amount of water used, the cooking method, and the length of cooking time affect the extent of mineral loss.

The use of cast-iron cookware increases the iron content of foods, especially those that have an acid reaction, such as applesauce and spaghetti sauce. However, it has not been established that the iron leached from iron cooking utensils is as available to the body as the naturally occurring iron in foods.

SOURCES OF IRON. Milk and milk products are poor sources of iron.

About 20% of the iron in the average U.S. diet comes from fortified products. Enrichment of flour (bread) and cereals with iron (along with thiamin, riboflavin, niacin, and with calcium enrichment optional), which was initiated in 1941, has been of special significance in improving the dietary level of iron in the United States. It is noteworthy that the major iron-enriched foods provide the following quantities of iron:

Food	Iron (mg/100 g)
Wheat flour, all-purpose or family enriched	2.9
Rice, white, enriched, raw	2.9
Cornmeal, degermed, enriched	2.9
Bread, white, enriched	2.5
Corn flakes, with added nutrients	2.4

Normal mixed human diets of good quality contain from 6 to 15 mg of iron per day, of which 0.6 to 1.5 mg is absorbed. This amount is adequate for adult males, but it is inadequate for adolescent girls or women on diets of less than 10% calorie content from animal foods; hence, the doctor may recommend iron supplementation for females. It is noteworthy, however, that diets consisting of highly refined foods, such as are common in the United States, contain only 6 to 7 mg of iron, a level that is not high enough to satisfy the requirements. The iron level of such refined food diets can be improved by fortification (through wheat flour and bakery products). The use of ferrous sulfate, one of the most available forms of iron, is recommended. Since too much iron can trigger the hereditary illness called hemochromatosis, iron-rich pills or tonics should be taken only on the advice of a physician or nutritionist.

The top iron sources are listed in Table I-9.

NOTE WELL: This table lists (1) the top sources without regard to the amount normally eaten (left column), and (2) the top food sources (right column); and the caloric (energy) content of each food.

For additional sources and more precise values of iron see Food Composition Table F-21 of this book.

(Also see MINERAL[S], Table M-25.)

TABLE I-9
TOP IRON SOURCES[1]

Top Sources[2]	Iron	Energy	Top Food Sources	Iron	Energy
	(mg/100 g)	(kcal/100 g)		(mg/100 g)	(kcal/100 g)
Thyme	123.6	276	Liver, hog, fried in margarine	29.1	241
Parsley, dried	97.9	276	Wheat-soy blend (WSB)/bulgur flour or straight grade wheat flour	21.0	365
Marjoram, dried	82.7	271	Molasses, cane, blackstrap	16.1	230
Cumin seed	66.4	375	Wheat bran, crude commercially milled	14.9	353
Fish flour from fillet waste	54.0	305	Liver, calf, fried	14.2	261
Celery seed	44.9	392	Kidneys, beef, braised	13.1	252
Dill weed, dried	44.8	253	Soybean flour, defatted	11.1	326
Oregano	44.0	306	Liver, chicken broiler/fryer, simmered	8.5	165
Bay leaves	43.0	313	Oyster, fried	8.1	239
Basil	42.8	251	Eggs, raw yolk, fresh	5.5	369
Coriander leaf, dried	42.5	279	Apricots, dehydrated, sulfured, uncooked	5.3	332
Turmeric	41.4	354	Sardines, Pacific, canned in brine or mustard, solids/liquid	5.2	186
Fish flour from whole fish	41.0	307	Prunes, dehydrated, uncooked	4.4	344
Cinnamon	38.1	261	Peaches, dried, sulfured, uncooked	3.9	340
Savory	37.8	272	Beef, all cuts[3]	3.8	300
Anise seed	38.0	337	Nuts, mixed, dry roasted	3.7	590
Fenugreek seed	33.5	323	Pork, all cuts[3]	3.2	325
Tea bag, orange pekoe	33.0	1	Beans, lima, mature, seeds, dry, cooked	3.1	138
Tarragon	32.3	295	Rice, white, enriched, raw	2.9	363
Curry powder	29.6	325	Wheat flour, all-purpose or family, enriched	2.9	365
			Raisins, natural, uncooked	2.8	289

[1]These listings are based on the data in Food Composition Table F-21. Some top or rich food sources may have been overlooked since some of the foods in Table F-21 lack values for iron.

Whenever possible, foods are on an *as used* basis, without regard to moisture content; hence, certain high-moisture foods may be disadvantaged when ranked on the basis of iron content per 100 g (approximately 3½ oz) without regard to moisture content.

[2]Listed without regard to the amount normally eaten.

[3]Values for different cuts range from 3.9 to 2.5 mg/100 g.

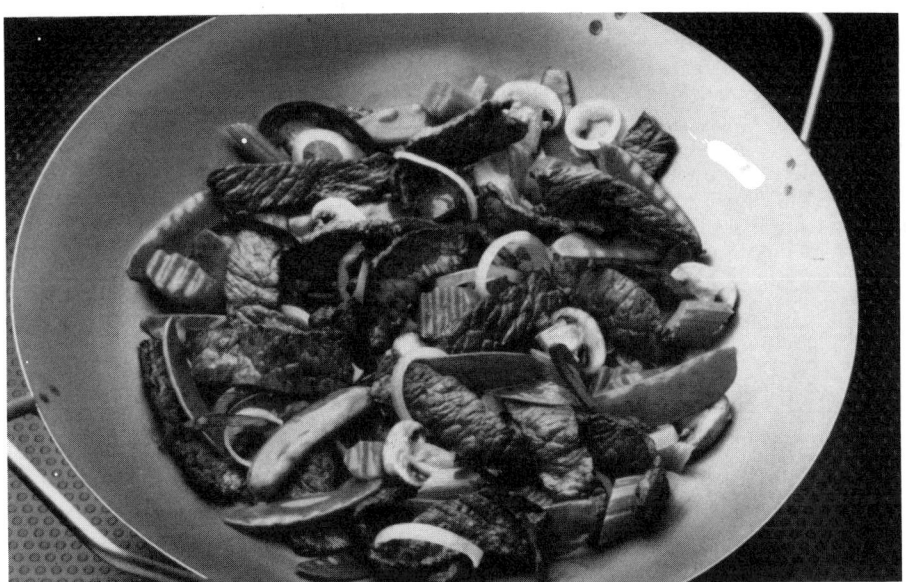

Fig. I-20. Beef strips, stir fried. Muscle meats are a top source of iron. (Courtesy, National Live Stock and Meat Board, Chicago, Ill.)

IRON-BINDING CAPACITY

The relative saturation of the iron-binding protein transferrin; the amount of transferrin bound to iron in relation to the amount remaining free to combine with iron determines the iron-binding capacity.

(Also see IRON.)

IRRADIATED YEAST

Yeast that has been irradiated. Yeast contains considerable ergosterol, which, when exposed to ultraviolet light, produces vitamin D.

(Also see VITAMIN D.)

IRRADIATION (FOOD)

This refers to the preservation of foods by radiation. It is sometimes referred to as *cold sterilization* because the microorganisms in the food are destroyed or inactivated by nuclear ionization rather than by heat or freezing.

(Also see PRESERVATION OF FOOD; and RADIATION PRESERVATION OF FOOD.)

ISCHEMIA

A local deficiency of blood, chiefly from narrowing of the arteries.

ISCHEMIC HEART DISEASE

A condition in which there is a deficiency of blood supply to the heart muscle due to obstruction or constriction of the coronary arteries.

(Also see HEART DISEASE.)

ISINGLASS

An extremely pure gelatin obtained from the swim bladders of certain species of fish. In the wine and beer industry it is used for clarification. It may also be used as an adhesive and as a lustering and stiffening agent in silks and other fabrics.

ISLETS OF LANGERHANS

The pancreas is a dual purpose organ. It secretes digestive juices to aid the process of digestion, and it secretes the hormones insulin and glucagon which regulate blood glucose levels. These hormones are secreted from the islets of Langerhans which are microscopic patches within the pancreas. In man there are 1 to 2 million islets. Actually, these patches or islands can be further divided into two types of cells: (1) beta cells secreting insulin, and (2) alpha cells secreting glucagon.

(Also see ENDOCRINE GLANDS, Table E-8, Hormones of the Endocrine Glands—Glucagon and Insulin.)

ISOASCORBIC ACID (ERYTHORBIC ACID)

A form of ascorbic acid, but it has only slight vitamin C activity. Isoascorbic acid is, however, a strong reducing agent and is used in food as an antioxidant and in cured meats to speed up color fixing.

(Also see VITAMIN C.)

ISOCALORIC

Containing an equal number of calories.

ISOENZYME

Proteins with the same enzymatic specificity but which can be made into different molecular forms by physiochemical techniques.

ISOLEUCINE

One of the essential amino acids.

ISOMALTOSE

Two molecules of glucose linked together, but linked between the first carbon of one glucose and the sixth carbon of the other instead of the first and fourth carbon linkage of maltose. Isomaltose and maltose are products of the breakdown of starch.

(Also see DIGESTION AND ABSORPTION, Table D-8, Enzymatic Digestion of Carbohydrates, Fats, and Proteins.)

ISOMER

Compounds having the same kind and number of atoms but differing in the atomic arrangements in the molecule.

ISOTONIC

Two solutions having the same total osmotic pressure; hence, if two isotonic solutions are separated by a semipermeable membrane, there is no net movement of solutions across the membranes.

ISOTOPE

An element of chemical character identical with that of another element occupying the same place in the periodic table (same atomic number) but differing from it in other characteristics, such as in radioactivity or in the mass of its atoms (atomic weight). Isotopes of the same element have the same number of protons in their nucleus but different numbers of neutrons. A *radioactive* isotope is one with radioactive properties. Such isotopes may be produced by bombarding the element in a cyclotron.

ISOTOPIC LABEL

The marking of a compound by introducing into it an isotope of one of its constituent elements; i.e., using a form of the element with a different atomic mass. For example, the atomic mass of carbon (C) is 12; an isotope of carbon has an atomic mass of 14, expressed as ^{14}C.

–ITIS

Suffix denoting inflammation; for example, colitis.

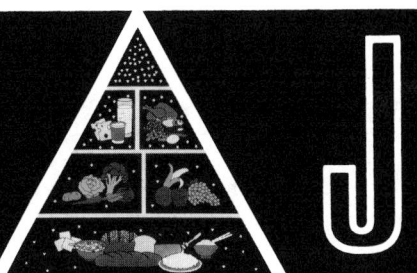

JABOTICABA *Myrciaria cauliflora*

The purple, grapelike fruit from an evergreen tree (of the family *Myrtaceae*) that grows in the tropics of Brazil. Individual fruits within the clusters are about ½ in. (*1.2 cm*) in diameter and contain a seedy pulp that may be eaten raw or made into jam, jelly, juice, or wine.

The fruit is fairly low in calories (46 kcal per 100 g) and carbohydrates (12.6%). Also, it is a fair to good source of vitamin C.

JAGGERY

Sap obtained from some palm trees contains 10 to 16% sucrose. In processing this sap, it is condensed by heating until the sucrose crystallizes. This product is poured into molds which form small sweet cakes, a product known as jaggery in some areas of the world.

(Also see SUGAR PALM.)

JAMBALAYA

This dish is most often found in the states bordering the Gulf of Mexico because it is usually made with crawfish which abound in the freshwater areas surrounding the gulf. It is made with rice, vegetables, herbs, and either ham, sausage, chicken, shrimp, oysters, or crawfish.

JAPANESE QUAIL (COTURNIX QUAIL, EASTERN QUAIL, PHAROAH'S QUAIL, AND STUBBLE QUAIL)

The Japanese quail (*Coturnix coturnix japonica*) has long been domesticated in Japan. The beginning of Japanese quail breeding can be traced back to 1595. Coturnix were first raised as pets and singing birds, but by 1900 they had become widely used for meat and egg production. Japanese quail develop 3½ times as fast as chickens; at 30 days of age they are almost fully grown. At 6 weeks of age, hens lay their first eggs; thereafter, they proceed, like machines, to lay an egg every 16 to 24 hours for 8 to 12 months.

Japanese quail are also game birds. The breast and legs are considered delicacies.

JAUNDICE

A symptom consisting of a yellow discoloration of both the bodily tissues and the body fluids with bile pigment (bilirubin) in which the skin and whites of the eyes are yellow.

JEJUNUM

The middle portion of the small intestine which extends from the duodenum to the ileum.

(Also see DIGESTION AND ABSORPTION.)

JELLY

A colloidal suspension which contains either gelatin, pectin, or agar. It can be flavored with fruit juice or synthetic flavors and colors. Some jellies are used as spreads on breads, others may be used as an accompaniment to meats.

JOULE

A proposed international unit (4.184j = 1 calorie) for expressing mechanical, chemical, or electrical energy, as well as the concept of heat. In the future, energy requirements and food values will likely be expressed by this unit.

(Also see WEIGHTS AND MEASURES.)

JUICE

The aqueous substance obtainable from animal or plant tissue by pressing or filtering, with or without the addition of water.

JUJUBE, INDIAN *Zizyphus mauritiana*

The orange-brown egg-shaped fruit of a tree that belongs to the *Rhamnaceae* family and is believed to have originated in India, but is now grown throughout the dry tropics of Asia and Africa. Usually, the fruits are almost 1 in. (*2 to 3 cm*) long and have a tart sweet flavor. They are eaten fresh, candied, dried, or the pulp is made into a refreshing beverage. The dried and fermented pulp may also be used in spice cakes.

Indian jujubes are moderately high in calories (97 kcal per 100 g) and carbohydrates (25%). They are also a good source of fiber and vitamin C. The dried fruit contains approximately 3 times the nutrient levels of the fresh fruit, except that much of the vitamin C is destroyed during drying.

JULEP (MINT JULEP)

• A drink usually consisting of sweet syrup, flavoring, and water.

• A tall drink made from gin, rum, or other alcoholic liquor and sometimes flavored with citrus juice.

• A tall drink consisting of bourbon, sugar, and mint served in a frosted tumbler filled with finely crushed ice—also called a mint julep.

JUNE BERRY (SERVICE BERRY; SUGAR PLUM) *Amelanchier canadensis*

Purplish-red fruits borne by a shrub or small tree (of the family *Rosaceae*) that is native to eastern North America.

June berries resemble blueberries and huckleberries and are used in many of the same ways (fresh, or in pies, puddings, and sauces).

JUNIPER BERRY *Juniperus communis*

The fruit of a shrub or small tree (of the family *Cupressaceae*) that grows wild around the world and is known as the common juniper.

Juniper berries are a little smaller than wild blueberries and have a blue-black color. They have long been used medicinally for digestive problems and to rid the body of excess water (diuretic action). It appears that they were first used in wine and then later to make gin. The berries are also used as a flavoring in herb teas, meat and vegetable dishes, sauces and soups, and in various confections and desserts.

JUNK FOODS

There is no agreement on the definition of a junk food. According to the U.S. Department of Agriculture, a 100-calorie portion of food that does not supply 5% or more of the required daily allowance of one of the eight specified nutrients (protein, vitamin A, ascorbic acid, niacin, riboflavin, thiamin, calcium, and iron) is classified as a food of "minimal nutritional value." However, most people attribute the following characteristics to junk food: high in sugar, fat, calories, salt and/or additives; bad for health; and limited in protein, minerals, and vitamins. But, regardless of definition, people eat junk food simply because they like it.

Despite parental concern, most fast foods are not junk foods. Indeed, many of them are very nutritious. Certainly, fast foods are not gourmet meals. Some of them have too few fresh fruits and vegetables. Others have an overabundance of fats and carbohydrates. But most people—whether they are age 6, 16, or 60—can eat today's fast foods that are good—and good for them.

(Also see CONVENIENCE AND FAST FOODS.)

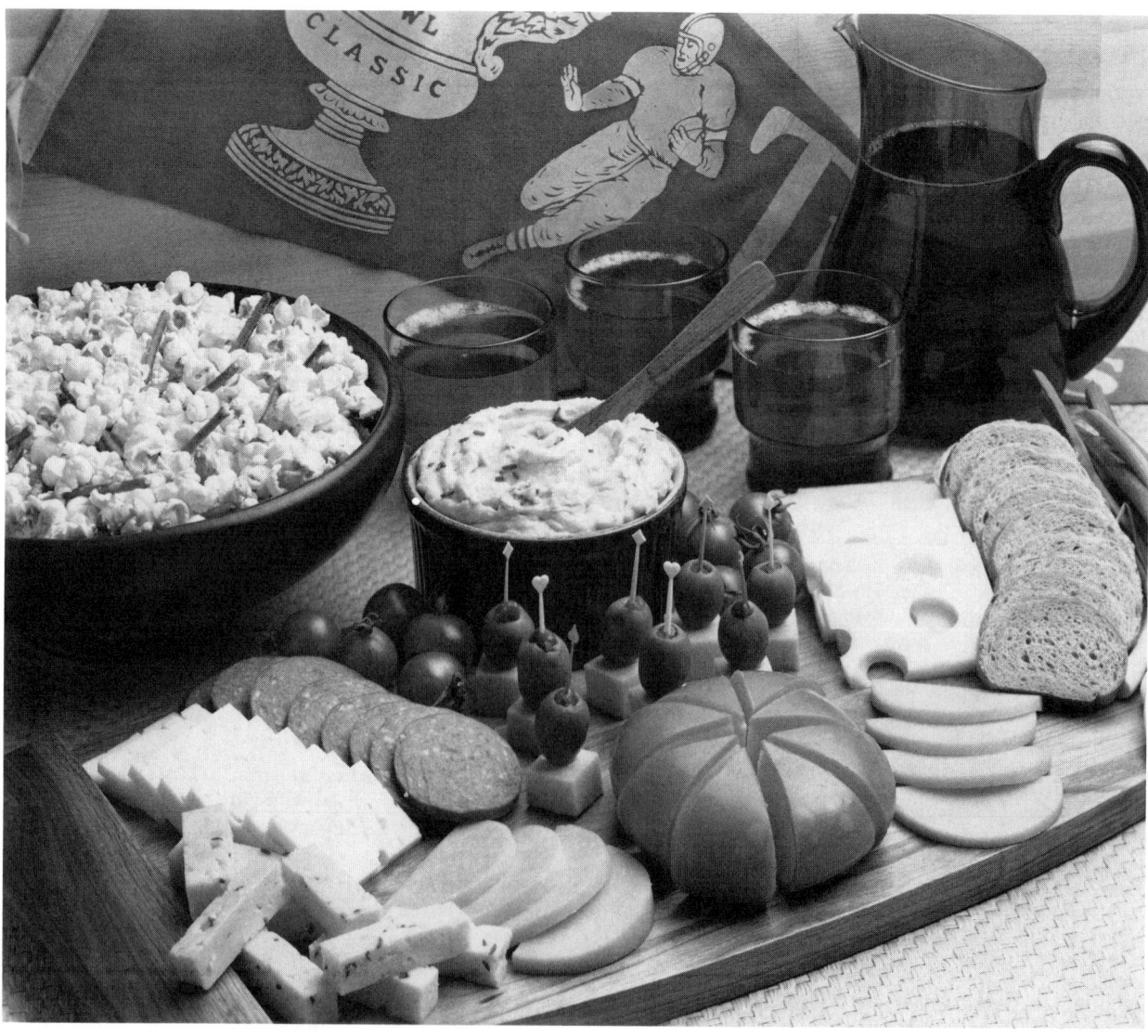

Fig. J-1. Junk foods are less attractive if there are plenty of interesting and nutritious snacks available. A bowl of seasoned popcorn, alone or with other goodies, is a favorite snack or fun food for armchair sports fans. (Courtesy, United Dairy Industry Assn., Rosemont, Ill.)

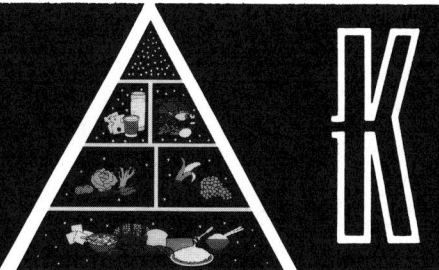

KANGAROO MEAT

Australian frontiersmen in remote areas boil or roast the legs of the kangaroo, which look something like ham, and which are especially good when spiked with bacon. Kangaroo tail is used as the base for a rich and heavy soup, which is considered quite a delicacy and is sold commercially. Fearing that the animal might become extinct, in 1973 the Australian Parliament passed a law banning the sale to other countries of live kangaroos or of kangaroo hides or meat.

KARELL DIET

A special diet for the early stage of victims of congestive heart failure or myocardial infarction. It is a low-calorie fluid diet consisting of only 27 oz (800 ml) of milk per day. The milk is given every four hours in 6½ oz (200 ml) servings. No other food and little additional fluid is offered for 2 to 3 days.

KCAL

The abbreviation for kilocalorie, a measure of food energy. (Also see KILOCALORIE.)

KEI-APPLE (UMKOKOLA) *Dovyalis caffra; Aberia caffra*

The fruit of a shrub (of the family *Bixaceae*) that is native to Africa, and is used locally to make jam.

KELP (SEAWEED)

One of the names by which seaweed is known. (Also see SEAWEED.)

KEMPNER DIET

Used in the treatment of high blood pressure, some kidney disorders, cirrhosis of the liver, and pregnancy toxemia, the Kempner diet is a rice-fruit diet. As such it is low in fat, protein, and sodium. Specifically, it is comprised of 10.5 oz (300 g) of raw rice cooked by boiling, or by steaming without milk, fat, or salt. With this, liberal amounts of canned or fresh fruit may be eaten. Daily fluid intake consists of 1 qt (700 to 1,000 ml) of fruit juice, but no additional water.

KERATIN

A sulfur-containing protein which is the primary component of epidermis, hair, wool, hoof, horn, and the organic matrix of the teeth. (Also see PROTEIN[S].)

KERATINIZATION

A condition occurring in a severe vitamin A deficiency, in which the epithelial cells either slough off or become dry and flattened, then gradually harden and form rough horny scales. The process may occur in the cornea the respiratory tract, the genitourinary tract, or the skin. (Also see VITAMIN A, section on "Deficiency Symptoms.")

KERNEL

The whole grain of a cereal. The meats of nuts and drupes (single-stoned fruits). (Also see CEREAL GRAINS.)

KETO–

A prefix denoting the presence of the carbonyl (CO) group.

KETO-ACID

The amino acid residue after deamination. The glycogenic keto-acids are used to form carbohydrates; the ketogenic keto-acids are used to form fats.

KETOGENESIS

The formation of ketones from fatty acids and some amino acids.

KETOGENIC

Capable of being converted into ketone bodies. The fatty acids and certain amino acids are the ketogenic substances in metabolism.

KETOGENIC AMINO ACID

The amino acids leucine, isoleucine, phenylalanine, tryptophan, and tyrosine are capable of undergoing a metabolic conversion to acetoacetate, a ketone body. Thus, they are said to be ketogenic. (Also see AMINO ACID[S]; KETOSIS; and METABOLISM.)

KETOGENIC DIET

Diets high in fat and low in carbohydrate are termed ketogenic since they cause the accumulation of ketone bodies in the tissues. These diets eliminate carbohydrate sources such as breads, cereals, fruits, desserts, sweets, and sugar-containing beverages while foods high in fat such as butter, cream, bacon, mayonnaise, and salad dressing are eaten in generous amounts. Ketones are produced from the breakdown (oxidation) of fats. When the ratio of fatty acids to available glucose in the diet exceeds 2:1, ketosis occurs.

A ketogenic diet is considered monotonous and unpalatable. In some cases a ketogenic diet may be prescribed to control epilepsy, if drugs prove ineffective. (Also see KETOSIS; METABOLISM; and MODIFIED DIETS.)

KETONE

Any compound containing a ketone (CO) grouping.

KETONE BODIES

Acetoacetic acid, acetone, and beta-hydroxybutyric acid.

KETONIC RANCIDITY

Decomposition of fats and oils results in the production of ketones. These ketones give fats or oils an off flavor or odor. The decomposition occurs slowly and spontaneously, however, certain molds of *Aspergillus* and *Penicillium* species may also be responsible.

KETOSIS

Shifting the metabolic machinery of the body to excessive utilization of fats instead of carbohydrates or a balance of fats and carbohydrates results in the buildup of ketone bodies—acetoacetate, beta-hydroxybutyrate, and acetone—in the blood and their appearance in the urine. This condition is referred to as ketosis, and outwardly noted by the sweetish, acetone odor of the breath. Three circumstances can cause ketosis: (1) high dietary intake of fat but low carbohydrate intake as in ketogenic diets; (2) diminished carbohydrate breakdown and high mobilization of fats as in starvation; or (3) disorders in carbohydrate metabolism as in diabetes mellitus. Unless ketosis goes unchecked and results in acidosis, it is a normal metabolic adjustment.

(Also see CARBOHYDRATE[S], section on "Regulation of Fat Metabolism"; FATS AND OTHER LIPIDS, section on "Recommended Fat Intake"; and METABOLISM.)

KIBBLED

Coarsely ground grain or meal.

KIDNEY DISEASES

Due to their importance, any disorder in the function or structure of the kidneys can have serious consequences, and often require some dietary adjustments. Glomerulonephritis (nephritis), nephrosis, nephroptosis, nephrosclerosis, renal (kidney) failure, kidney stones (nephrolithiasis), pyelitis, and pyelonephritis are all specific diseases which may in general be called kidney diseases.

Before there are any dietary adjustments, the extent of the kidney disease must be evaluated. It may be necessary to restrict sodium and potassium intake, and control the levels of protein and fluid intake. If protein intake is controlled, then it is important that sufficient high caloric but nonprotein food be eaten to meet the body's demand for energy, and to prevent the breakdown of the body's own protein for energy. Those proteins that are eaten should be proteins of high biological value—containing a large number of essential amino acids—like eggs, meat, milk, and milk products.

(Also see AMINO ACID[S]; GLOMERULONEPHRITIS; KIDNEY STONES; MODIFIED DIETS; NEPHROSCLEROSIS; NEPHROSIS; and PROTEIN[S].)

KIDNEYS

They are paired, bean-shaped organs located in the abdominal cavity at the level of the lower ribs next to the back with one on each side of the spine. The kidneys form urine and control the volume and the composition of the blood (extracellular fluid). Each day, the kidneys (1) filter about 50 gal *(190 liter)* of fluid, and (2) remove excesses of substances such as urea and uric acid while conserving needed substances such as water and glucose. Without their cleansing-filtering function, death results in 8 to 14 days. Kidneys also regulate red blood cell production, adrenal secretion of aldosterone, blood pressure, and calcium metabolism.

(Also see CALCIUM, section on "Excretion of Calcium"; GLOMERULONEPHRITIS; HEMODIALYSIS; and WATER BALANCE.)

KIDNEY STONES (NEPHROLITHIASIS; RENAL CALCULI; URINARY CALCULI; UROLITHIASIS)

Hard concentrations primarily composed of calcium oxalate or calcium phosphate which form within the kidney. They vary in size from very small gravel to very large stones. Apparently, a variety of factors may contribute to the formation of kidney stones, and to some extent they may be controlled by diet. Some common contributing factors are (1) a high phosphorus–low calcium diet; (2) a high potassium intake; (3) vitamin A deficiency; (4) high animal protein (meat, fish, poultry) intake; (5) renal infection; (6) urinary tract obstruction; (7) chronic dehydration; (8) long periods of immobilization; (9) hypercalcemia; or (10) heredity. Generally, a kidney stone goes unnoticed until it starts to move out of the kidney and down the ureter. When this occurs, there is excruciating pain until the stone is passed or removed surgically or nonsurgically.

Note: Currently, a German-built machine which uses high-energy shock waves to break up kidney stones from outside the body is being tested. The nonsurgical procedure is called extracorporeal shock wave lithotripsy, or stone exploding.

If at all possible the cause and type of kidney stones should be determined since a person forming a kidney stone once is apt to form them repeatedly.

Dietary modification depends on the type of stones formed. The formation of calcium phosphate stones may be lessened by a calcium- and phosphorus-restricted diet, and by aluminum gel which diminishes the absorption of phosphorus. Modification of the urine pH also prevents the formation of kidney stones. An acid urine helps prevent stones of calcium and magnesium phosphate and carbonates, while an alkaline urine helps prevent oxalate and uric acid stones. The diet should support therapy with alkalinizing or acidifying agents by supplying acid-producing or alkaline-producing foods. Also the formation of uric acid stones may be lessened by a purine-restricted diet.

Most importantly, a liberal intake of fluid—3 to 4 qt *(3 to 4 l)* or more depending upon the environment—is essential to prevent the formation of a concentrated urine which allows the stone-forming salts to precipitate.

(Also see CALCIUM, section headed "Calcium Related Diseases"; MODIFIED DIETS; and URIC ACID KIDNEY STONES.)

KILOCALORIE (kcal)

The amount of energy as heat required to raise the temperature of 1 kilogram of water 1°C (from 14.5 to 15.5°C). It is equivalent to 1,000 calories. In human nutrition, it may also be referred to as a kilogram calorie, k-calorie, kcal, or a *large Calorie.* The last designation is spelled with a capital C to distinguish it from the *small calorie.* However, in some of the literature, the word *calorie* is used, even though it is technically incorrect.

(Also see CALORIE.)

KILOGRAM

A metric measure of weight which is equal to 1000 g or about 2.2 lb.

(Also see WEIGHTS AND MEASURES.)

KILOJOULE (KJ)

A metric unit of energy, equivalent to 0.239 kcal.

KINETIC ENERGY (MECHANICAL ENERGY)

A body, an object, or a molecule in motion which is capable of performing work at once. It possesses kinetic energy, energy of motion.

KJELDAHL

Relating to a method of determining the amount of nitrogen in an organic compound. The quantity of nitrogen measured is then multiplied by 6.25 to calculate the protein content of the food or compound analyzed. The method was developed by the Danish chemist, J. G. C. Kjeldahl, in 1883.

(Also see ANALYSIS OF FOOD.)

KOHLRABI *Brassica oleracea,* variety *caulorapo*

The name of this vegetable, which belongs to the mustard family *(Cruciferae),* literally means "cabbage (kohl)-turnip (rabi)." It has both the wild cabbage *(B. oleracea)* and the wild turnip *(B. campestris,* species *rapifera)* as ancestors. Kohlrabi is unlike other cabbage vegetables in that it is comprised of stem tissue, while the rest of these vegetables are buds (sprouts), flowers, and leaves. Fig. K-1 shows a typical kohlrabi.

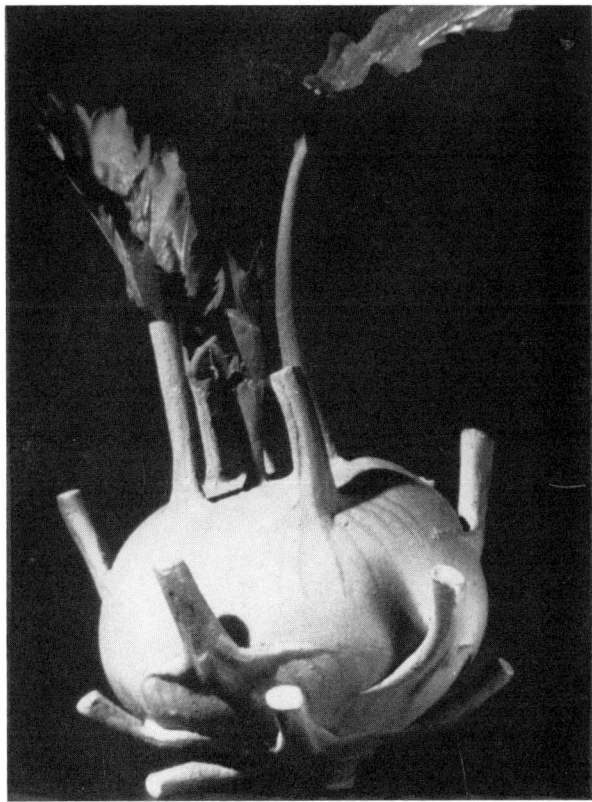

Fig. K-1. Kohlrabi, a vegetable derived from the wild cabbage and the wild turnip. (Courtesy, Field Museum of Natural History, Chicago, Ill.)

ORIGIN AND HISTORY. It is not known for certain when the kohlrabi was first developed, because a vegetable described in the writings of the Roman botanist, Pliny, (1st century, A.D.) had very similar characteristics. However, it is not mentioned in any other writings until after the Middle Ages, when it was a popular vegetable in the central and eastern parts of Europe. Since then, the utilization of kohlrabi has declined to the extent that it is difficult to find in vegetable markets. One of the reasons for the decline in popularity of the vegetable may have been the production of large, tough bulbs the size of softballs, rather than the more tender bulbs that are usually smaller than baseballs.

PRODUCTION. There is little commercial production of the kohlrabi in the United States; hence, statistics on the size of the crop are not available. But per capita consumption is low.

Kohlrabi seeds may be planted as soon as the soil can be cultivated in the spring. The vegetable may also be planted in the summer for harvesting in the fall. A rich soil is needed for high-quality kohlrabi. Therefore, it is often desirable to fertilize with nitrogen, phosphorus, and potassium.

The bulblike vegetables may be harvested when they are between 2 and 3 in. *(5 and 8 cm)* in diameter. It is not wise to let them grow any larger because the edible portion becomes fibrous and tough when it reaches full maturity. The edible portion is the bulbous enlargement of the stem, which like all stems, becomes very woody as it ages.

PROCESSING. It appears that most, or all, of the kohlrabi produced in the United States is marketed fresh, and that very little, if any, is processed.

SELECTION AND PREPARATION. Best quality kohlrabi is from 2 to 3 in. *(5 to 8 cm)* in diameter, and has fresh green tops and a tender rind. Bulbs that are overly large (over 3 in. in diameter), and that have blemishes or growth cracks, are likely to be of poor quality.

Raw kohlrabi may be sliced and added to relish trays and salads. The vegetable is usually cooked by steaming, although the people in the Central European countries may stuff and bake it after scooping out some of the center. Cooked kohlrabi is enhanced by a well-seasoned cheese sauce or cream sauce.

CAUTION: Kohlrabi and other vegetables of the mustard family *(Cruciferae)* contain small amounts of goiter-causing (goitrogenic) substances that may interfere with the utilization of iodine by the thyroid gland. In the quantities normally consumed, this is not a concern. Besides, this effect may be counteracted by the consumption of ample amounts of dietary iodine, a mineral that is abundantly present in iodized salt, ocean fish, seafood, and seaweeds such as kelp.

NUTRITIONAL VALUE. The nutrient composition of kohlrabi is given in Food Composition Table F-21.

Some noteworthy observations regarding the nutrient composition of kohlrabi follow:

1. Kohlrabi is high in water content (over 90%) and low in calories (only about 40 kcal per cup *[240 ml]*).
2. The levels of most nutrients are lower in kohlrabi than

in the other cabbage vegetables because it is comprises of tem tissue, whereas, the other vegetables are buds (sprouts), flowers, and leaves. However, kohlrabi is a good source of potassium and vitamin C.

3. Kohlrabi is most comparable to the potato and the other tuberous vegetables that are enlarged stems of plants. On this basis, kohlrabi has about the same amount of protein (2%) as the potato, but contains less then half as many calories, and more than three times as much vitamin C.

(Also see VEGETABLE[S], Table V-2 Vegetables of the World.)

KOJI

A yeast or other starter prepared in Japan from rice inoculated with the spores of the mold *Asperigillus oryzae* and permitted to develop a mycelium. Koji is used for making miso from soybeans, a popular fermented food in Japan.

KORSAKOFF'S SYNDROME (PSYCHOSIS)

A mental disease involving disintegration of the personality or escape from reality. Typical behavior includes confused thinking, making up stories to fill in gaps of memory (confabulation), irresponsibility, and the inability to learn new things. Eventually a stupefied state may result. These effects may be commonly found in chronic alcoholics, semistarved persons such as prisoners of war, and persons suffering from beriberi. Most evidence seems to indicate that the Korsakoff's Syndrome is due to a long-standing thiamin deficiency. Vitamin therapy restores responsiveness and alertness, but some irreversible structural damage to the nervous system may have occurred. Often the early symptoms of a thiamin deficiency—Wernicke's Syndrome—are noted prior to the mental disorders, and the physical and mental symptoms are together called the *Wernicke-Korsakoff Syndrome.*

(Also see ALCOHOLISM; and BERIBERI.)

KUBAN

A type of fermented milk.

KWASHIORKOR

Kwashiorkor is most common in the tropical areas of the world, where it afflicts children from weaning to age 4.

Kwashiorkor results from a severe protein deficiency, and is characterized by changes in pigmentation of the skin and hair, edema, skin lesions, anemia, and apathy. Kwashiorkor differs from marasmus in terms of the greater role of protein

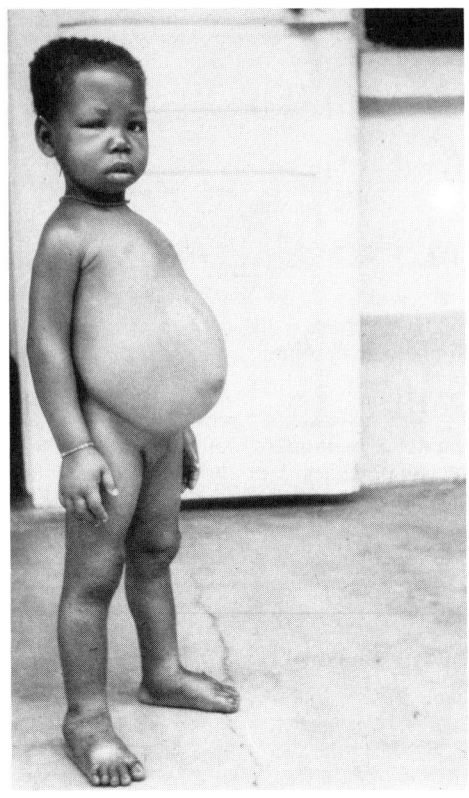

Fig. K-2. Kwashiorkor, a protein deficiency disease. Note characteristic bloated belly. Other usual symptoms are: stunted growth, diarrhea, brittle hair with an abnormal reddish color, and retarded mentality. (Courtesy, FAO, Rome, Italy)

deficiency in causing it.

The recommended treatment: Providing 1 to 2 g of high-quality protein per pound of body weight, along with sufficient energy. Cautious replacement of mineral salts may also be needed. In case of severe diarrhea, the protein intake should be temporarily restricted to 0.5 g per pound of body weight.

Prevention consists in feeding children an adequate amount of protein (particularly after weaning) from such sources as fish, legumes, meats, milk, and nuts. (Milk supplies 1 g of protein per oz [30 ml].)

(Also see MALNUTRITION, PROTEIN-ENERGY; and PROTEIN(S), section headed "Protein Malnutrition.")

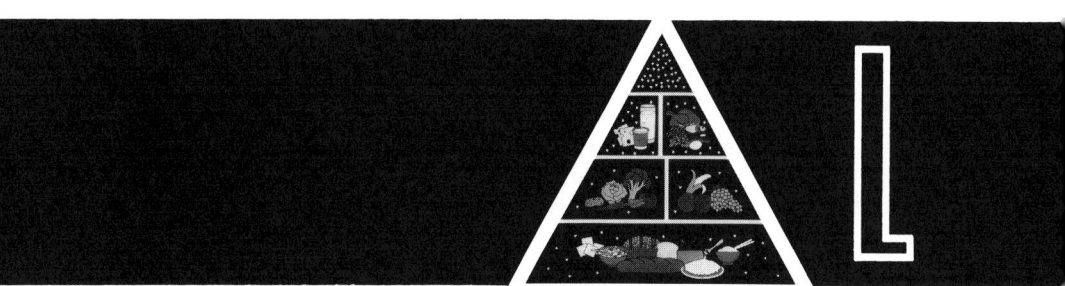

LABELS, FOOD

On November 8, 1990, President Bush signed into law *The Nutrition Labeling and Education Act of 1990*, the most significant revision of the U.S. food labeling law since 1938. The new labeling law requires that the majority of food products under FDA authority carry nutrition labeling, regulates the terms used on labels to describe a food's nutrient content, authorizes and regulates food health claims, and establishes national uniformity by federal preemption for many areas of food labeling other than safety warning statements. In 1992, FDA regulatory authority encompassed about 75% of all food consumed in this country. The remaining foods—mainly meat, poultry, and egg products—are largely under the U.S. Department of Agriculture regulatory authority.

The Nutrition Labeling and Education Act of 1990 (Public Law 101–538–Nov. 8, 1990) amends the Federal Food, Drug, and Cosmetic Act to require the following changes in food labels:

• **Nutrition labeling**—Nutrition labeling is required for all retail food products, including fresh produce, fish, and seafood. **NOTE WELL:** Subsequently President Bush ruled that the law would apply only to packaged foods.

• **Health claims on food**—The Nutrition Labeling and Education Act permits health claims on foods, provided (1) that such claims are based on scientific evidence (including evidence from well-designed experiments), and (2) that there is significant agreement among experts qualified by scientific training and experience.

• **Nutrient content claims**—The FDA is required to define the following nutrient terms as they relate to nutrient content: *free, reduced, low, less, light* or *lite*, and *high*.

Further, the Act prohibits a label claim for the absence of a nutrient (e.g., "sodium-free," "no cholesterol") where the nutrient is not normally present in the food.

• **Implementation of food labeling law**—On November 8, 1990, President George Bush signed into law The Nutrition Labeling and Education Act. However, implementation of the law was delayed due to disagreement between the U.S. Secretary of Agriculture and the U.S. Secretary of Health and Human Services relative to certain aspects of food labeling. Finally, on December 2, 1992, President Bush resolved the dispute between the two cabinet secretaries, made some changes in the application of the law, announced that the regulations will be final following their publication in the Federal Register, and ruled that all labels must be on packaged foods by May 1994.

Fig. L-1 shows the format and content of a new food label similar to the type that will be standard on all packaged foods in the future. The label on a carton of yogurt will look just like the label on a can of corn.

Pertinent new food labeling rules which were revealed on December 2, 1992, at the time of implementing the food labeling law, follow.

Nutrition facts

Serving size	½ cup (114 g)
Servings per container	4

Amount per serving

Calories 260	Calories from fat 120

		% Daily value*
Total fat	13 g	**20%**
Saturated fat	5 g	**25%**
Cholesterol	30 mg	**10%**
Sodium	660 mg	**28%**
Total carbohydrate	31 g	**11%**
Sugars	5 g	
Dietary fiber	0 g	**0%**
Protein	5 g	

Vitamin A 4% • Vitamin C 2% • Calcium 15% • Iron 4%

* Percents (%) of a Daily Value are based on a 2,000-calorie diet. Your Daily Values may vary higher or lower depending on your calorie needs:

Nutrient		2,000 calories	2,500 calories
Total fat	Less than	65 g	80 g
Saturated fat	Less than	20 g	25 g
Cholesterol	Less than	300 mg	300 mg
Sodium	Less than	2,400 mg	2,400 mg
Total carbohydrate		300 g	375 g
Fiber		25 g	30 g

1 g fat = 9 calories • 1 g carbohydrates = 4 calories • 1 g protein = 4 calories

Fig. L – 1. A new food label.

1. **All packaged foods must be labeled.** The regulations apply to all packaged foods, but not to fresh meat, poultry, fish, and produce.

2. **Percent Daily Value will be used.** Instead of Recommended Daily Allowance (RDA), the new labels will refer to percent of *Daily Value*.

3. **The nutritional value of a food can be compared with daily dietary needs.** The new labels will provide consumers with an opportunity to compare the nutritional value of a food with the daily dietary needs. Thus, the label will show how much fat is in a product, and how much of the daily quotient of fat the consumer will get from one serving of that product. Also, the label provides consumers a way in which to compare the nutrients found in their food with their total daily dietary needs, based on recommended diets of both 2,000 calories and 2,500 calories. Thus, from the label, consumers will be able to compare the percentage of the *Daily Value* of each nutrient contained in a particular product with a chart that shows the total amount of each nutrient they should be eating.

4. **Serving sizes and descriptive terms will be standardized.** Thus, the serving size in canned soups will be the same, no matter what the brand. Likewise, descriptive phrases like "low-fat" and "light" will be standardized.

5. **Labels must be rewritten and printed.** An estimated 257,000 labels must be rewritten and printed.

6. **Complete nutritional information will be required.** If manufacturers do not report complete nutritional information on their product labels, they will be required to have their products tested.

7. **Calorie information will be given.** The new labels will include information on how many calories are in a gram of fat, in a gram of carbohydrate, and in a gram of protein.

8. **Amounts of essential nutrients, along with the requirements, must be listed.** Every label must list total grams or milligrams, along with required amounts, of fat, saturated fat, cholesterol, sodium, total carbohydrates (sugar and dietary fiber), protein, and essential vitamins and minerals.

• **Basic label and other information to be continued**—In addition to requiring changes in nutrition labeling as detailed above, the following basic information will be continued on food nutrition labels: (1) the name of the product, (2) the net contents or net weight, and (3) the name and place of business of the manufacturer, packer, or distributor. Also, label information may include the following:

• **Grades**—Some food products carry a grade on the label, such as "U.S. Grade A." Grades are set by the U.S. Department of Agriculture, based on the quality levels inherent in a product—its taste, texture, and appearance. U.S. Department of Agriculture grades are not based on nutritional content.

Milk and milk products in most states carry a "Grade A" label. This grade is based on FDA recommended sanitary standards, for the production and processing of milk and milk products, which are regulated by the states.

• **Open dating**—To help consumers obtain food that is fresh and wholesome, many manufacturers date their product. Open dating, as this practice is often called, is not regulated by FDA. Four kinds of open dating are commonly used:

1. Pack date is the day the food was manufactured or processed or packaged. In other words, it tells how old the food is at the time of purchase. The importance of this information to consumers depends on how quickly the particular food normally spoils. Most canned and packaged foods have a long shelf life when stored under dry, cool conditions.

2. Pull or sell date is the last date the product should be sold, assuming it has been stored and handled properly. The pull date allows for some storage time in the home refrigerator. Cold cuts, ice cream, milk, and refrigerated fresh dough products are examples of foods with pull dates.

3. Expiration date is the last date the food should be eaten or used. Baby formula and yeast are examples of products that may carry expiration dates.

4. Freshness date is similar to the expiration date but may allow for normal home storage. Some bakery products that have a freshness date are sold at a reduced price for a short time after the expiration date.

• **Code dating**—Many companies use code dating on products that have a long *shelf life*. This is usually for the company's information, rather than for the consumer's benefit. The code gives the manufacturer and the store precise information about where and when the product was packaged, so if a recall should be required for any reason the product can be identified quickly and withdrawn from the market.

• **Universal product code**—Many food labels now include a small block of parallel lines of various widths, with accompanying numbers. This is the Universal Product Code (UPC). The code on a label is unique to that product. Some stores are equipped with computerized checkout equipment that can read the code and automatically ring up the sale. The UPC, when used in conjunction with a computer, also can function as an automated inventory system. The computer can tell management how much of a specific item is on hand, how fast it is being sold, and when and how much to order.

• **Symbols**—Food labels can possess a variety of symbols. The letter "R" on a label signifies that the trademark used on the label is registered with the U.S. Patent Office. The letter "C" indicates that the literary and artistic content of the label is protected against infringement under the copyright laws of the United States. Copies of such labels have been filed with the Copyright Office of the Library of Congress. The symbol which consists of the letter "U" inside the letter "O", is one whose use is authorized by the Union of Orthodox Jewish Congregations of America, more familiarly known as the Orthodox Union, for use of foods which comply with Jewish dietary laws. The symbol which consists of the letter "K" inside the letter "O" is used to indicate that the food is *kosher,* that is, it complies with the Jewish dietary laws, and its processing has been under the direction of a rabbi. None of these symbols is required by, nor under the authority of, any of the laws enforced by the FDA.

(Also see FOOD AND DRUG ADMINISTRATION; and U.S. DEPARTMENT OF AGRICULTURE.)

LABILE

Unstable. Easily destroyed.

LABILE PROTEIN

The reserve protein available in most tissues.

LABRADOR TEA

This term may refer to (1) any of a group of low evergreen shrubs growing in bogs and swamps of the arctic and sub-arctic regions, or (2) tea made from the leaves of these plants. Labrador tea was popular with miners, mountain-men, and American colonists during the Revolution.

LACTALBUMIN

It is one of the proteins of milk, sometimes called a *whey protein.* During the making of cheese, lactalbumin is not precipitated with the protein casein; and thus, it appears in the whey. One half, or more, of the protein in human milk is lactalbumin; the rest is casein.

(Also see MILK AND MILK PRODUCTS; and PROTEIN[S].)

LACTASE

An enzyme in intestinal juice which acts on lactose to produce glucose and galactose.

(Also see DIGESTION AND ABSORPTION.)

LACTATION

That process of milk formation common to all mammals for the purpose of nurturing their young. Milk formation occurs in the mammary gland following preparation during pregnancy, and it is initiated near the time of birth. Lactating mothers require more food and more nutritious food than non-lactating females.

(Also see BREAST FEEDING; INFANT DIET AND NUTRITION; and MILK AND MILK PRODUCTS.)

LACTIC ACID ($C_3H_6O_3$)

During strenuous exercise lactic acid is produced in the muscles of the body. Also, this important biochemical forms during some food processes. The fermentation of pickles, sauerkraut, cocoa, tobacco, and silage produces lactic acid. Lactic acid formed by *lactobacillus* bacteria in the fermentation of milk sugar (lactose) is responsible for the sour milk flavor, and for the formation of cottage cheese and yogurt. Furthermore, it is a food additive employed as an acidulant and antimicrobial in cheeses, beverages, and frozen desserts. In addition to the above, lactic acid has some nonfood uses in the tanning, plastic, and textile industries. Commercially, lactic acid is produced by the fermentation of whey, cornstarch, potatoes, or molasses.

(Also see METABOLISM; and MILK AND MILK PRODUCTS.)

LACTOBACILLUS ACIDOPHILUS

A lactic-acid forming organism, which occurs as rods sometimes united in short chains; found in intestinal contents of young infants.

LACTOFLAVIN

An obsolete name for riboflavin (vitamin B-2) which described the origin of the isolate in the early days of riboflavin research. Hence, riboflavin isolated from milk was called lactoflavin.

(Also see RIBOFLAVIN.)

LACTOSE (MILK SUGAR)

A disaccharide found in milk having the formula $C_{12}H_{22}O_{11}$. It hydrolyzes to glucose and galactose. Commonly known as milk sugar.

(Also see CARBOHYDRATE[S], and MILK AND MILK PRODUCTS, section headed "Carbohydrates in Milk.")

LAETRILE (VITAMIN B-17, AMYGDALIN, NITRILOSIDES)

Contents   Page

NOTE WELL: Laetrile (amygdalin, nitrilosides) has no known value for humans. The authors present this section relative to the controversial compound for informational purposes only. Further, it is listed with the vitaminlike substances because it is sometimes erroneously designated as vitamin B-17. Both the pros and cons relative to Laetrile are given, then the reader may make a judgment.

Laetrile, or amygdalin, is a natural substance obtained from apricot pits, which its advocates claim to have cancer preventive and controlling effects. Dr. Ernest Krebs, Sr., who was the first to use Laetrile therapeutically in this country, considered it to be an essential vitamin and called it vitamin B-17.

In the United States, Laetrile therapy is not approved by the Food and Drug Administration for treatment of cancer.

In a report before the American Society for Clinical Oncology (the society of cancer specialists) May 1, 1981, Dr. Charles G. Moertel of Mayo Clinic reported on the Laetrile treatment of 156 patients, all with cancers that either had not responded or were not likely to respond to other treatments. Nine months after the beginning of the study in July 1980, 102 of the patients were dead, and the other 54 had seriously *progressive cancer*, which did not respond to the Laetrile treatment. The results: Laetrile was not effective; the results were about the same as would be expected had the doctors given the patients either placebos (dummy pills, with no effectiveness), or no treatment at all.

NOTE WELL: This study pertained to the use of Laetrile as a treatment of patients "with cancers that either had not responded or were not likely to respond to other treatments"; and not as a preventive of cancer, or as a treatment of early cancers.

The following statement explains the position of the Soviet Union relative to Laetrile:

"The preparation has never been tested in the Soviet Union. And in our opinion, today there are no grounds to show any interest in it. Why? Because the Soviet medical profession feels that this chemical is a useless preparation. Laetrile does not possess those wonderful properties which are ascribed to it. Moreover, being toxic, Laetrile may actually harm a patient's health.

Soviet specialists in chemotherapy subscribe to the competent opinion of the American Cancer Society and the World Health Organization, who have conducted thorough tests of Laetrile and convincingly proved its quackish nature."[1]

Despite the above, the advocates of Laetrile advance the following arguments: There is usually a considerable time lag between the scientific validation of a medical treatment and its acceptance. Moreover, the bias against nutrition is frequently deep-seated when it comes to cancer. Then, they make the following statements in support of the use of Laetrile in the prevention and treatment of cancer:

1. It is harmless when not taken in excessive amounts all at once.

2. It is low cost.

3. The ancient Chinese got pretty good results using the same treatment (apricot kernels) for cancer.

4. Several distinguished doctors feel that it gives good results.

5. It is manufactured and used legally in about 20 countries throughout the world, including Belgium, Germany, Italy, Mexico, and the Philippines.

HISTORY. Laetrile was first extracted from apricot pits in the early 1900s, and first used as a therapy for cancer in the United States in the 1920s.

CHEMISTRY, METABOLISM, PROPERTIES.

• Chemistry—Laetrile or amygdalin is a nitriloside, a simple chemical compound consisting of two molecules of sugar (glucose), one molecule of benzaldehyde, and one molecule of hydrogen cyanide (HCN) (see Fig. L-2).

---

[1]Garbin, Avgust, Professor, Doctor of Science (Medicine), Deputy General, Director of the Oncological Research Center of the USSR Academy of Medical Sciences, "What is the Soviet Attitude Toward Laetrile?," *Soviet Life*, November 1980, p. 30.

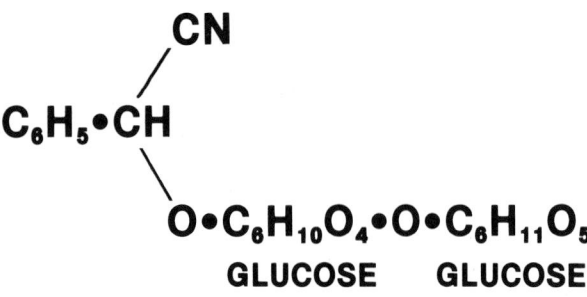

Fig. L-2. Structural formula of Laetrile ($C_{20}H_{27}NO_{11}$).

There are some 20 different nitrilosides occurring in at least 1,200 different plants, many of which were or are used as food, historically or at present. The natural cyanide in such foods, including apricot kernels or bitter almonds, is locked in a sugar molecule, and is released slowly in the digestive tract of man.

• **Metabolism**—Oral doses of Laetrile pass from the stomach into the small intestine, where the substance is acted upon by enzymes. The enzymes break down Laetrile into four components, which are then absorbed into the lymph and portal systems and circulated throughout the body.

• **Properties**—White crystals; bitter taste; soluble in water and alcohol; insoluble in ether.

MEASUREMENT. Laetrile is measured in grams.

FUNCTIONS. Nitrilosides, including apricot kernels and bitter almonds, supply the body a low, but steady, level of HCN. Man and other mammals have an enzyme, rhodanase, which converts the cyanide to thiocyanate.

There are at least three theories as to how the HCN interferes with tumor growth, but all theories relative to the action of nitrilosides recognize the steady low-level supply of HCN as the active agent. The simplest theory postulates that cancer cells do not have rhodanase; instead, they are surrounded by another enzyme, beta-glucuronidase, which releases the bound cyanide from the Laetrile at the site of the malignancy. So, Laetrile is believed to attack and destroy only the malignant cells.

The advocates claim that Laetrile is effective in preventing tumor cells from getting a foothold. In support of this thesis, the following epidemiological data has been cited by Dr. James Cason, Professor of Chemistry, University of California, Berkeley, an authority on carcinogenic hydrocarbons:[2]

1. In a 1958 publication, famed African physician Dr. Albert Schweitzer, stated that for *several decades* his hospital at Lamberene in Gabon did not see a single case of cancer among the cassava-eating tribes. This was attributed to the fact that the natives in the Lamberene area obtain 80 to 90% of their calories from cassava, the tubers of which contain about 0.5% of a nitriloside.

2. Studies by the Loma Linda Hospital and the U.S.C. Medical School on the incidence of cancer in the Los Angeles basin showed that the Seventh-day Adventists had only one-third the incidence of cancer suffered by the rest of the population. For religious reasons, the Adventists' diet is heavily vegetarian; hence, rich in nitrilosides. It is estimated that the Adventists consumed 6 to 8 mg of nitrilosides per person daily, in comparison with an estimated average daily consumption of less than 1 mg per capita by the U.S. population.

3. Among the Hunzakuts (natives of the Himalayan Kingdom of Hunza), it has been estimated that the average daily intake of nitrilosides per capita is more than 100 mg. In addition to being Moslems, a local twist to the religion calls for eating apricot kernels; with the priests seeing that the brethren keep that part of the faith. Moreover, a young woman is not regarded as properly marriageable unless she has at least seven apricot trees in her dowry. After doing a study of morbidity of the Hunzakuts covering 100 years, the World Health Organization reported that not a single death from cancer was recorded.

NOTE WELL: The three reports cited above pertain to the use of Laetrile as a preventive of cancer, and not as a treatment of cancer.

DEFICIENCY SYMPTOMS. The advocates claim that prolonged deficiency of Laetrile, or amygdalin, may lead to lowered resistance to malignancies.

DOSAGE. The usual dosage is 0.25 to 1.0 g taken at meals. Cumulative daily amounts of more than 3.0 g are sometimes taken, *but more than 1.0 g should never be taken at any one time*.

According to the advocates, 5 to 30 apricot kernels eaten through the day may be effective as a preventive of cancer, but they should not be eaten all at one time.

• **Laetrile intake in average U.S. diet**—It is estimated that the average daily consumption of nitrilosides by the U.S. population is less than 1 mg per person.

TOXICITY. Toxicity levels of Laetrile haven't been established, but one should exercise extreme caution in order to avoid ingesting excessive amounts. *More than 1.0 g should not be taken at any one time.*

SOURCES OF LAETRILE. A concentration of 2 to 3% Laetrile is found in the whole kernels of most fruits, including apricots, apples, cherries, peaches, plums, and nectarines.

SUMMARY. Regardless of the validity of the claims and counter claims pertaining to Laetrile, it is noteworthy that more and more medical authorities are accepting the nutrition approach in the prevention and treatment of cancer. Although the use of such nutrients as Laetrile, vitamin A (carotene), folic acid, and vitamin C, along with a general supplemental program of minerals and vitamins, is controversial as a cancer treatment, perhaps even more important in the long run is the apparent success of nutrients of many kinds in strengthening the body's immune system—as preventives.

There is evidence that a person's immune capability is enhanced by top physical and mental condition; in turn, physical and mental condition depend heavily on diet. Together, they impart the *fighting spirit* and the *will to live*, terms that are often heard in the medical profession.

(Also see VITAMIN[S], Table V-5.)

[2]Cason, James, "Ascorbic Acid, Amygdalin, and Carcinoma," *The Vortex*, June 1978, pp. 9-23.

FOOD PRODUCTION

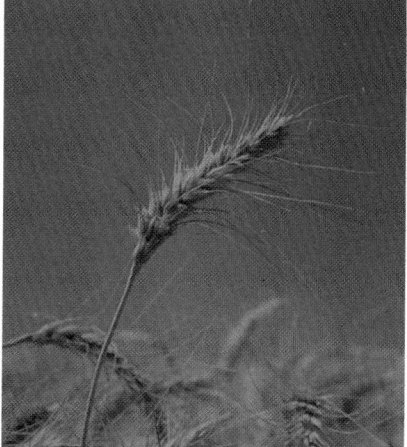

Plate 1. Wheat—the staff of life. It provides more nourishment for more people throughout the world than any other food. (Courtesy, USDA)

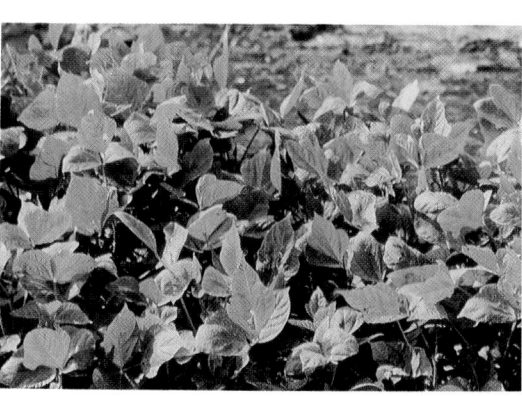

Plate 4. Adzuki beans, green and flowering. This legume ranks next to soybeans in the Orient. (Courtesy, University of Minnesota, St. Paul)

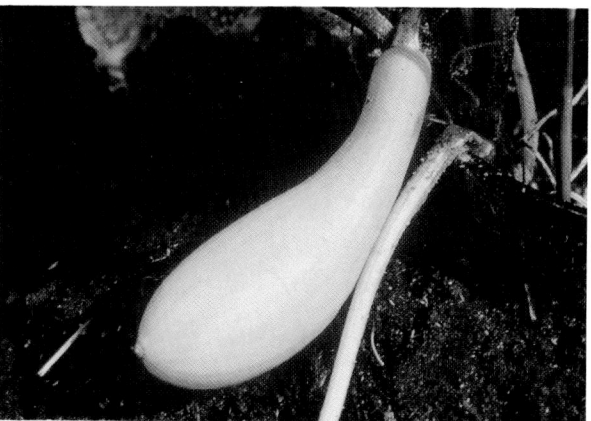

Plate 2. Summer squash. This shows a Yellow Crookneck Squash ready for harvest, when they are tender and before the rind has hardened. (Courtesy, USDA)

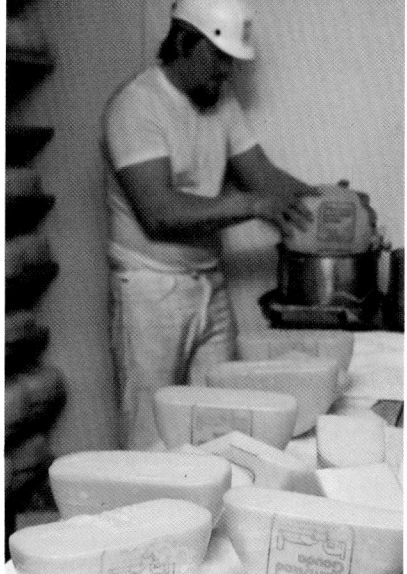

Plate 5. Cheese. This milk product is manufactured by (a) exposing milk to specific bacterial fermentation, and/or (b) treating with enzymes. (Courtesy, University of Minnesota, St. Paul)

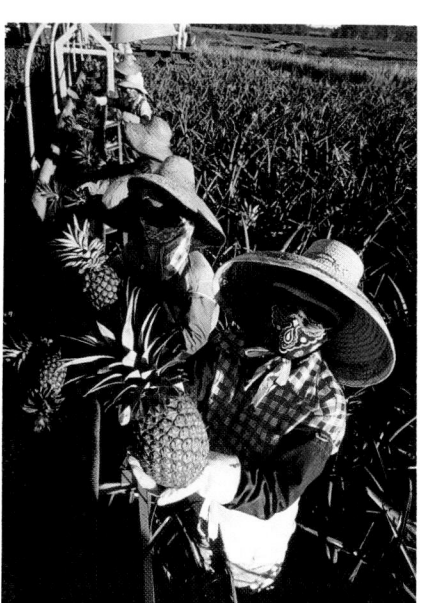

Plate 3. Pineapple. This shows ripe Hawaiian pineapple being hand-harvested and placed on a conveyor belt built into a long boom. (Courtesy, Castle & Cook, Inc.—Dole Pineapple)

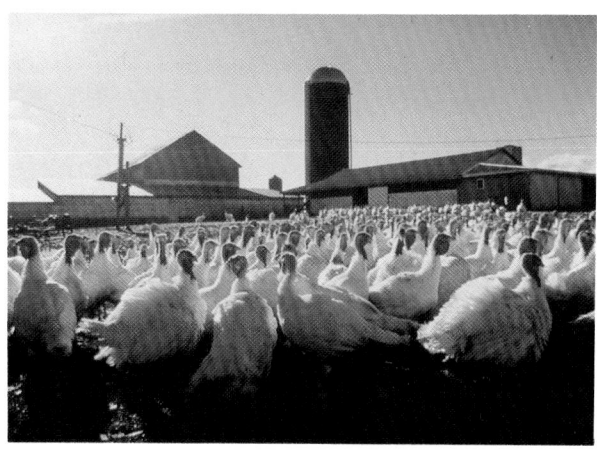

Plate 6. Turkeys. This shows Broad-Breasted White turkeys on the range. (Courtesy, USDA)

FOOD MARKETING

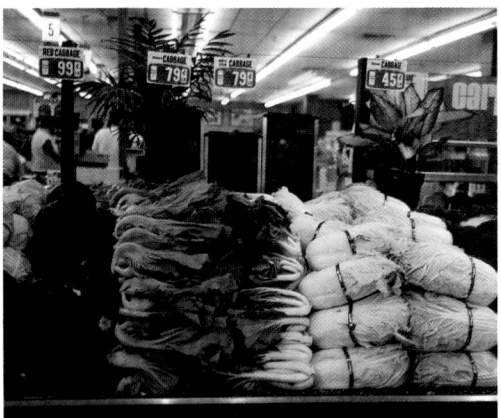

Plate 7. Cabbage. This shows several types of cabbage in a market, where it is sold by bundle and priced by weight. (Courtesy, University of Hawaii)

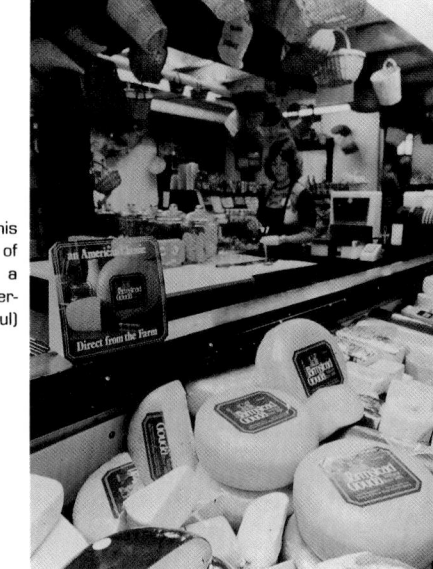

Plate 10. Cheese. This shows an assortment of cheeses on display in a market. (Courtesy, University of Minnesota, St. Paul)

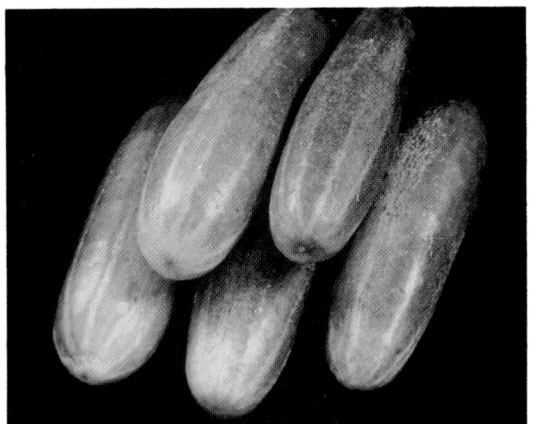

Plate 8. Cucumbers. Five long, slender cucumbers are shown on display in a market. (Courtesy, USDA)

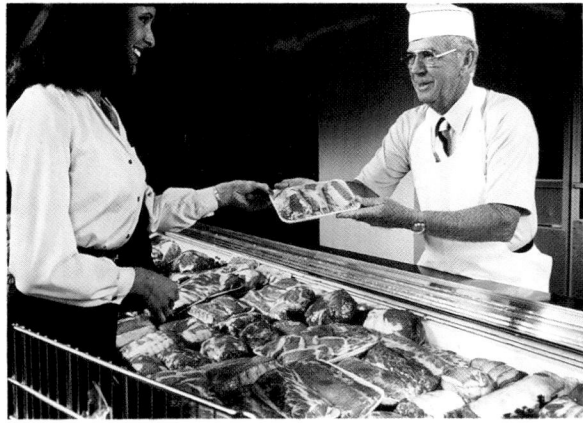

Plate 11. Meat. Customer being assisted at the supermarket. (Courtesy, National Live Stock & Meat Board, Chicago, Ill.)

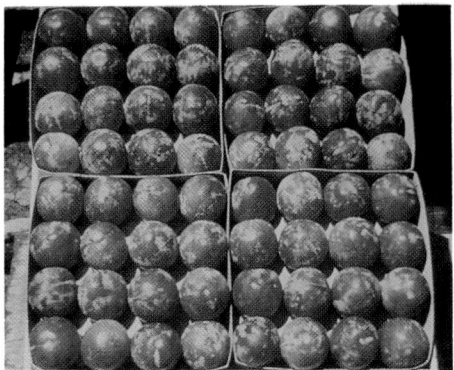

Plate 9. Plums. This shows plums on display in a market. (Courtesy, USDA)

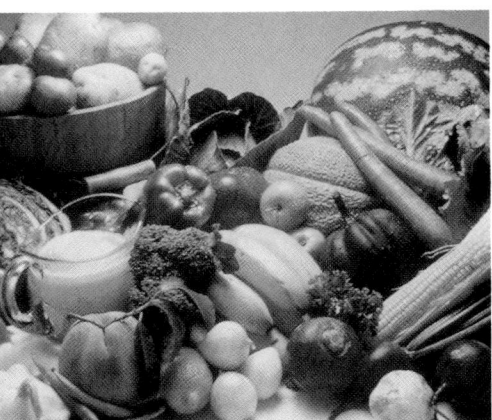

Plate 12. Vegetables and fruits. An assortment of vegetables and fruits on display in a market. (Courtesy, USDA)

BREAD, CEREAL, RICE, & PASTA GROUP

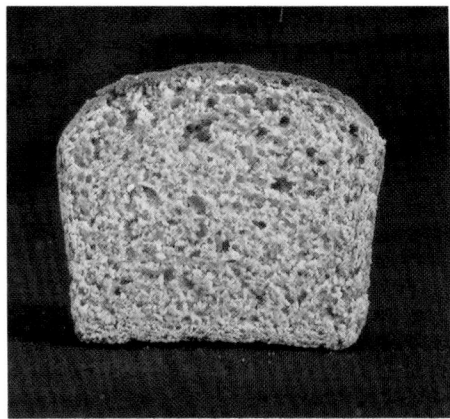

Plate 13. Bread—made from whole wheat. The Bread, Cereal, Rice, & Pasta Group forms the broad base of the *Food Guide Pyramid*, with 6-11 daily servings of this group recommended. (Courtesy, Washington State University, Pullman)

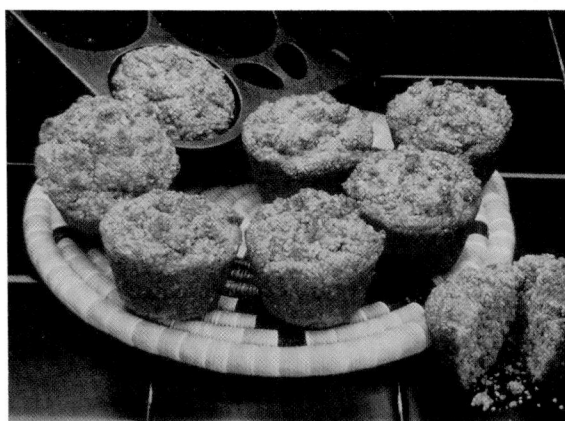

Plate 16. Bran muffins, made from the outer coat of wheat, are high in fiber (10 to 14%) and a good source of minerals and vitamins. (Courtesy, USDA)

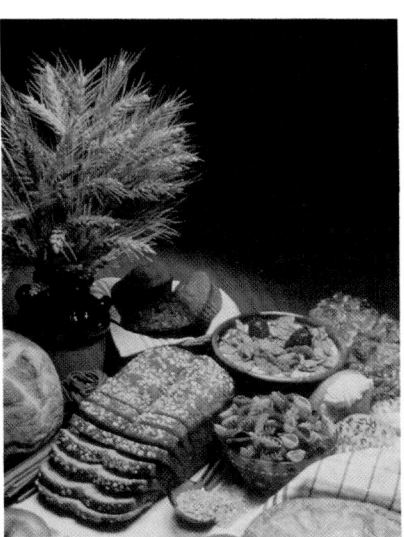

Plate 14. Wheat cereal grain products. Whole cereal products supply most of the essential nutrients. (Courtesy, USDA)

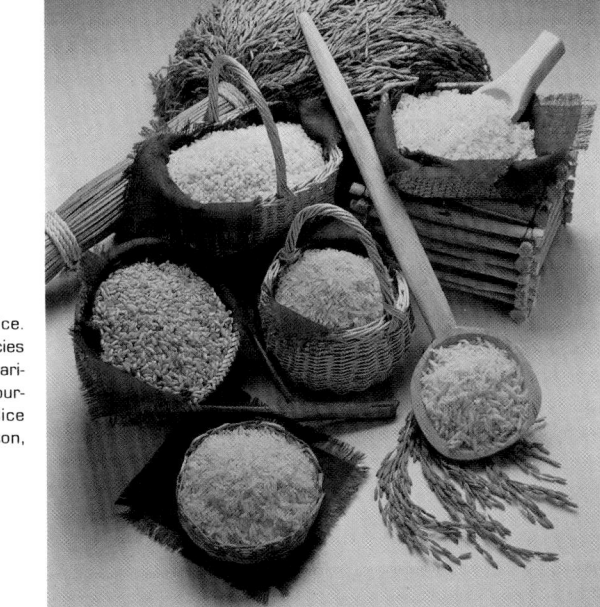

Plate 17. Rice. There are 25 species and thousands of varieties of rice. (Courtesy, USA Rice Council, Houston, Tex.)

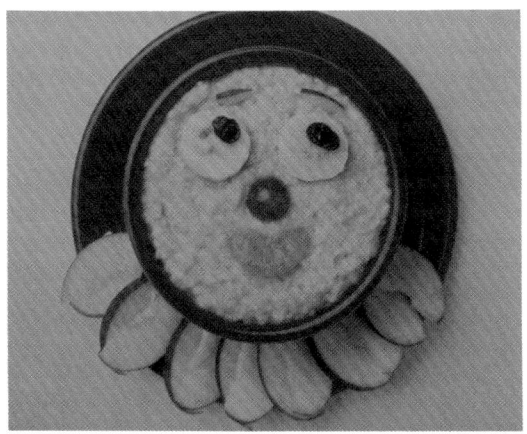

Plate 15. A bowl of cooked cereal decorated with a face made of assorted fruits, for a preschooler. (Courtesy, USDA)

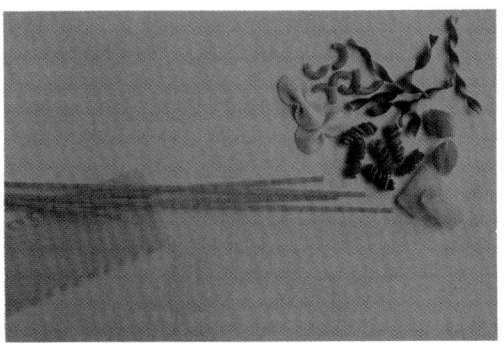

Plate 18. Pasta (macaroni), pieces of dough that have been formed into various shapes, then dried. Pasta contains sufficient calories and protein to be a major dietary source of these essentials. (Courtesy, USDA)

VEGETABLE GROUP

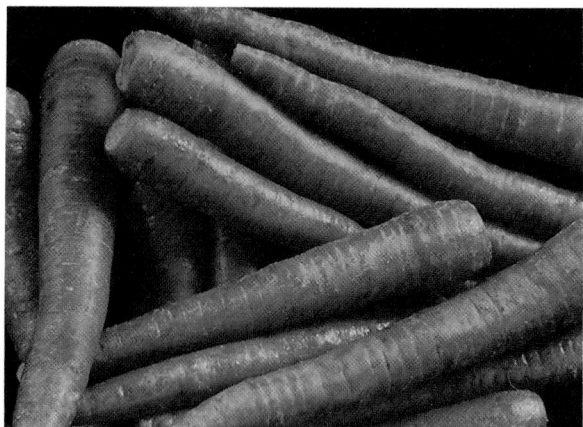

Plate 19. Carrots, the richest source of vitamin A among the common vegetables. The *Food Guide Pyramid* calls for 3-5 daily servings of the Vegetable Group. (Courtesy, USDA)

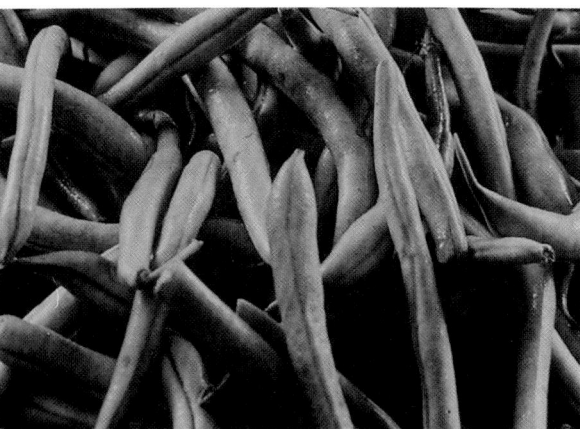

Plate 22. Green beans. They have higher nutritive value than most vegetables; they are a good source of protein, calcium, iron, and potassium. (Courtesy, USDA)

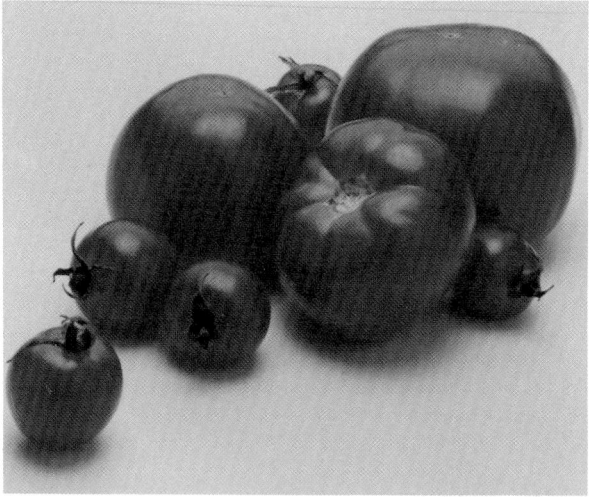

Plate 20. Tomatoes. Fresh tomatoes are high in water content (about 94%), low in calories, and a good source of vitamins A and C. (Courtesy, Shell Chemical Company, Houston, Tex.)

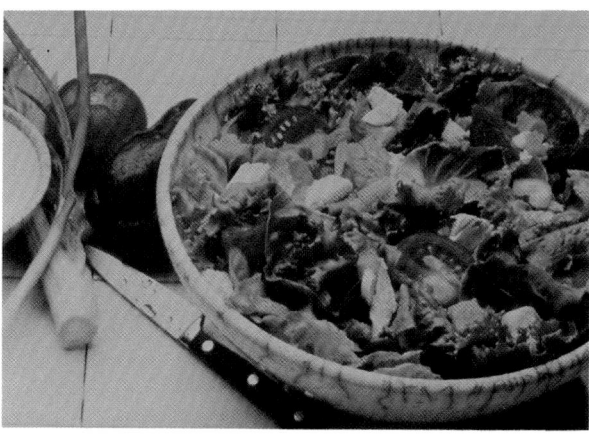

Plate 23. Chef's salad. The calories in such a salad may be minimized by using lowfat dressing, lowfat dairy products, and/or lean meat, poultry, or fish. (Courtesy, USDA)

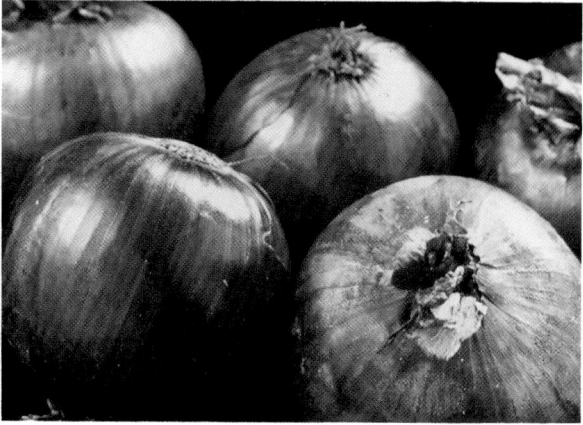

Plate 21. Onions. Dry mature onions are high in water content (89%) and low in calories. They are distinguished by their pungency when raw and the appetizing flavor that they impart when cooked with various other foods. (Courtesy, USDA)

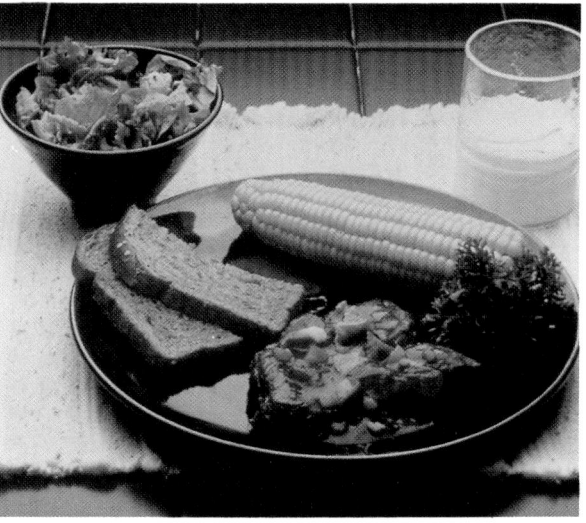

Plate 24. Corn-on-the-cob, a rich source of carbohydrates and fats, featured with the main meal. (Courtesy, USDA)

FRUIT GROUP

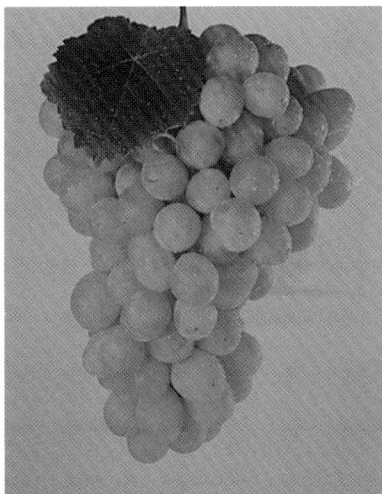

Plate 25. Grapes, one of the richest sources of chromium and a good source of potassium. The *Food Guide Pyramid* calls for 2-4 servings of the Fruit Group daily. (Courtesy, California Table Grape Commission)

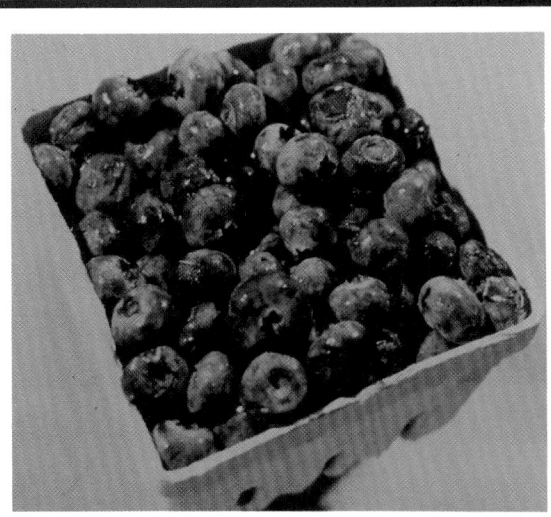

Plate 28. Blueberries. They are a good source of fiber, iron, and bioflavonoids, and fair sources of potassium and vitamin C. (Courtesy, USDA)

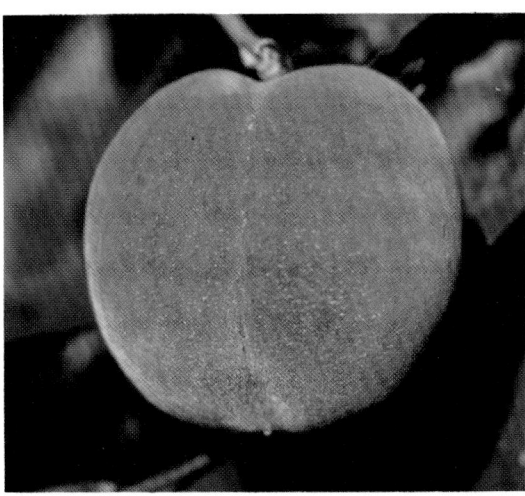

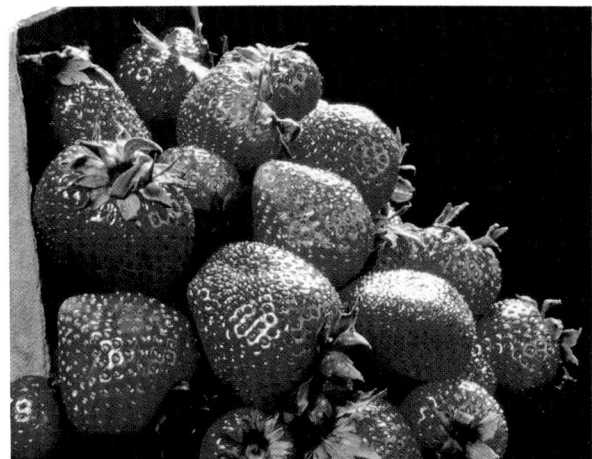

Plate 29. Strawberries, a good source of iron and potassium, and an excellent source of vitamin C. (Courtesy, USDA)

Plate 26. Peach, a good source of potassium and an excellent source of vitamin A. (Courtesy, National Film Board of Canada)

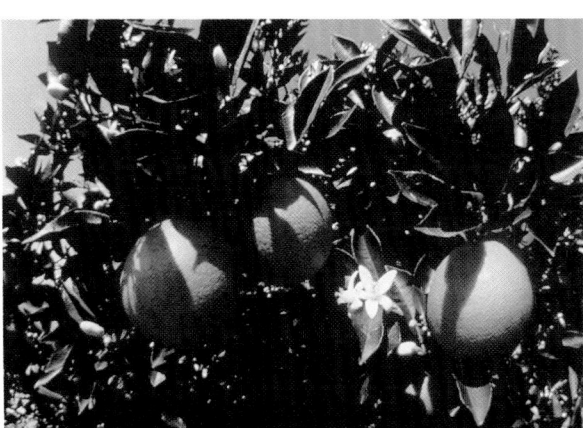

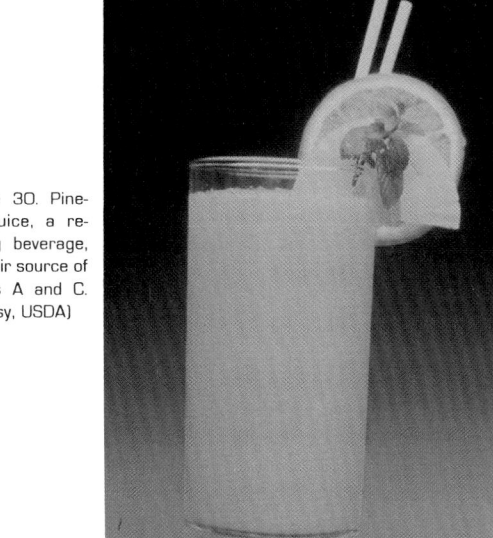

Plate 30. Pineapple juice, a refreshing beverage, and a fair source of vitamins A and C. (Courtesy, USDA)

Plate 27. Oranges. Note that ripe oranges and blossoms are on the same tree at the same time. Oranges are a good source of potassium and an excellent source of vitamin C. (Courtesy, USDA)

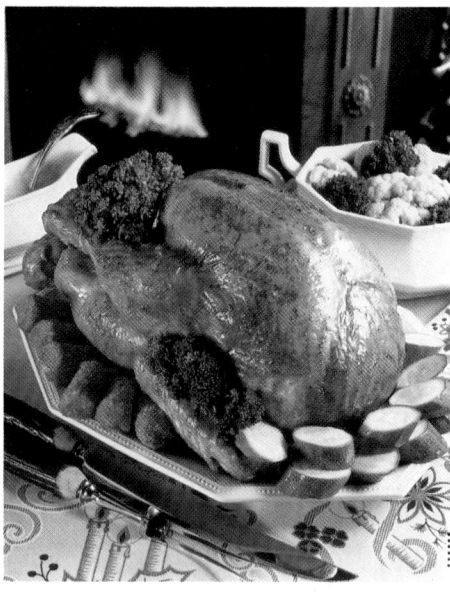

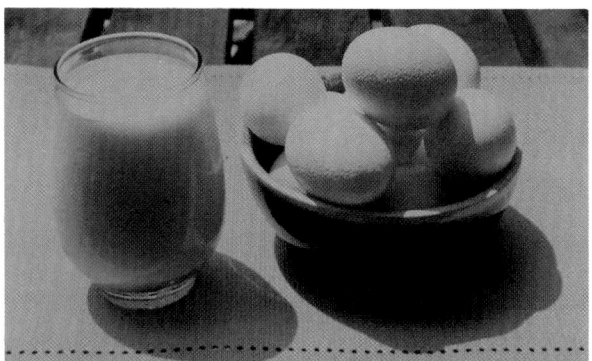

Plate 31. Beef burger, an excellent source of high-quality protein, iron, and the B-complex vitamins. Vitamin B-12 is found in all foods of animal origin, but not in plants. The *Food Guide Pyramid* calls for 2-3 daily servings of the Meat, Poultry, Fish, Dry Beans, Eggs, & Nuts Group. (Courtesy, National Live Stock and Meat Board, Chicago, Ill.)

Plate 34. Eggs and milk. Eggs contain an abundance of proteins, minerals, and vitamins. Also, egg protein is highly digestible and of high quality, having the highest biological value of any food. (Courtesy, USDA)

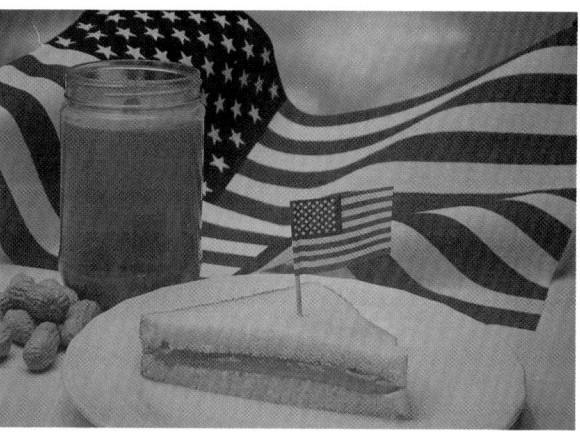

Plate 32. Roasted turkey, a Thanksgiving and Christmas tradition. Poultry meat is high in quality of protein and a rich source of all the amino acids. (Courtesy, Poultry International)

Plate 35. Peanut butter sandwich. Peanut butter is an excellent source of protein, contains no cholesterol, and the fat is mostly unsaturated. (Courtesy, Peanut Advisory Board, Atlanta, Ga.)

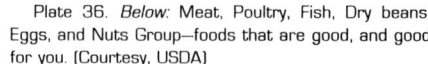

Plate 36. *Below:* Meat, Poultry, Fish, Dry beans, Eggs, and Nuts Group—foods that are good, and good for you. (Courtesy, USDA)

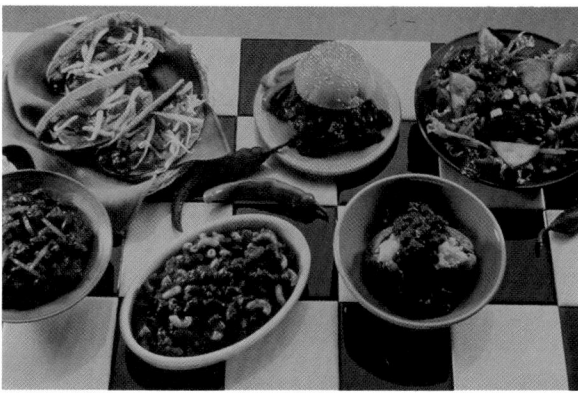

Plate 33. A variety of dishes made with beans and ground beef. Meat may be extended and lowered in cost by the use of beans. (Courtesy, USDA)

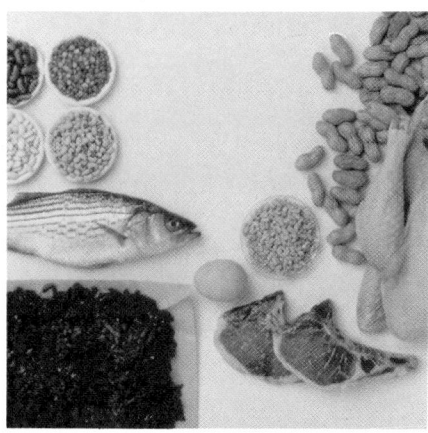

MILK, YOGURT, & CHEESE GROUP

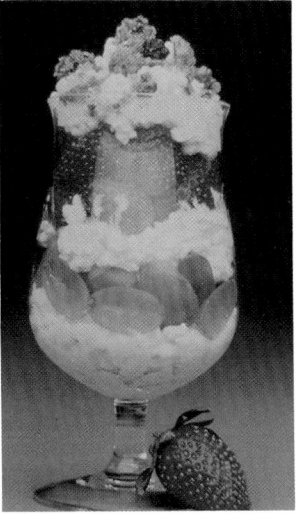

Plate 40. Cottage cheese-fruit parfait—cottage cheese layered with fruits. The most important cheese produced from skimmed milk is cottage cheese. (Courtesy, USDA)

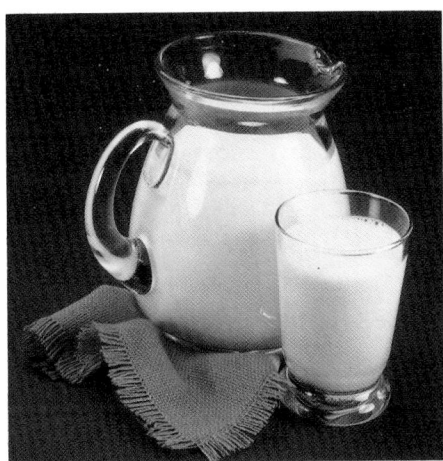

Plate 37. Milk, which Hippocrates, the father of medicine, described as "the most nearly perfect food." This must be so, for all newborn mammals rely almost entirely on their mother's milk for food. The *Food Guide Pyramid* calls for 2-3 servings daily of the Milk, Yogurt, & Cheese Group. (Courtesy, National Dairy Board, Arlington, Va.)

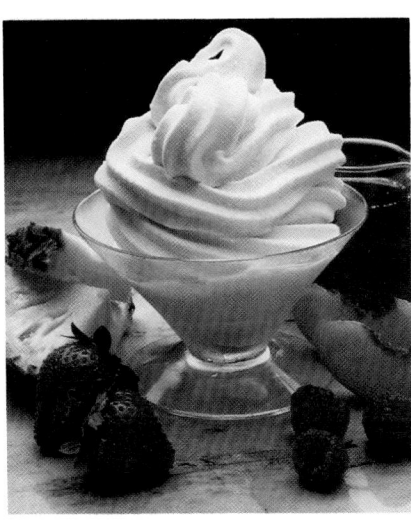

Plate 38. Yogurt, frozen. The increased consumption of yogurt in the U.S.A. in recent years is largely attributed to fruit-flavored and low-calorie yogurts. (Courtesy, American Dairy Assn., Rosemont, Ill.)

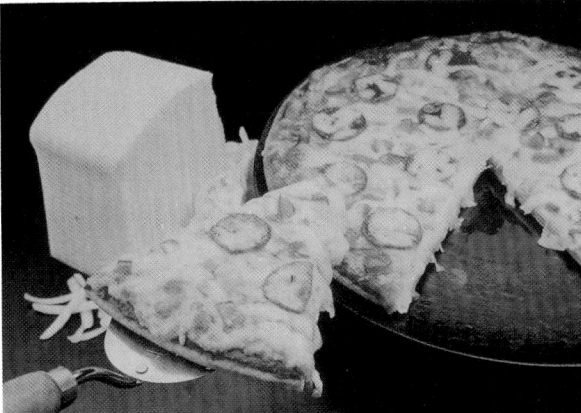

Plate 41. Pizza. This is an Italian word meaning pie, which a pizza resembles. Typically, pizzas contain mozzarella and parmesan cheeses, sausages, and other good things. (Courtesy, American Dairy Assn., Rosemont, Ill.)

Plate 42. *Below:* Assorted cheeses. There are more than 2,000 different named cheeses. Cheese is made by (a) exposing milk to specific bacterial fermentation, or (b) treating with enzymes, or both methods, to coagulate some of the proteins. More than 30% of all the milk used in manufactured dairy products in the U.S.A. is processed into cheese (exclusive of cottage cheese). (Courtesy, USDA)

Plate 39. *Below:* Ice cream. It consists primarily of milk fat, nonfat milk solids, sugar, flavoring, and stabilizers. (Courtesy, American Dairy Assn., Rosemont, Ill.)

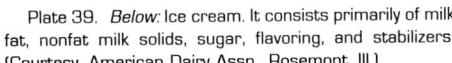

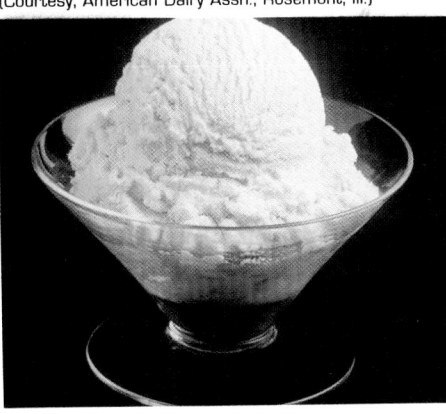

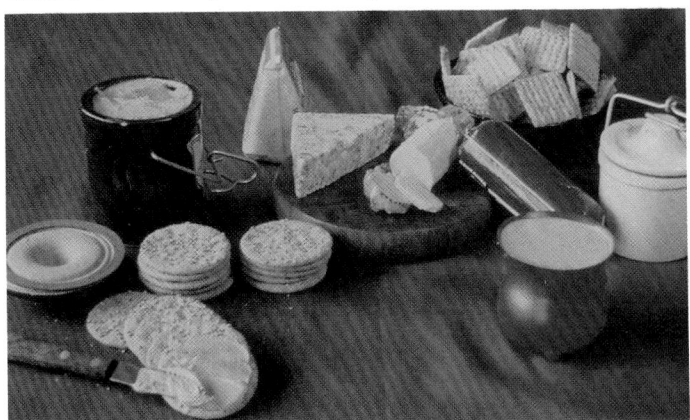

FATS, OILS, & SWEETS GROUP

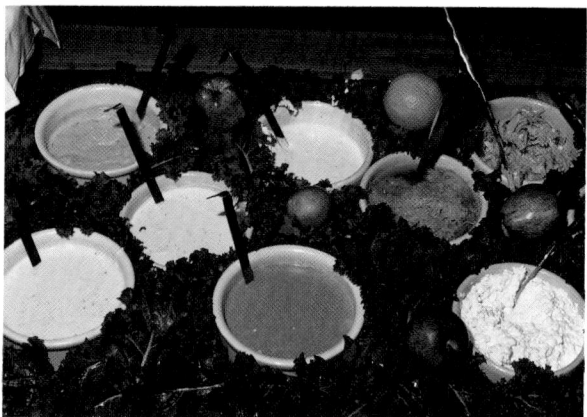

Plate 43. Salad dressings, many of which are high in fats and oils. **Caution:** The 1989 Recommended Dietary Allowances calls for maintaining total fat intake at or below 30% of the total caloric intake and saturated fatty acid intake of less than 10%. So, less fats and oils should be used in salad dressings.

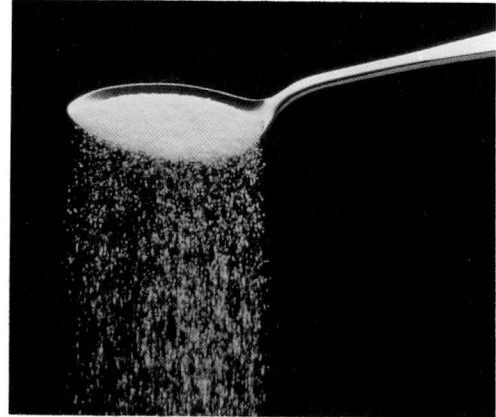

Plate 46. Sugar being poured from a spoon. **Caution:** The new *Food Guide Pyramid* admonishes that Fats, Oils, and Sweets should be *used sparingly.* (Courtesy, USDA)

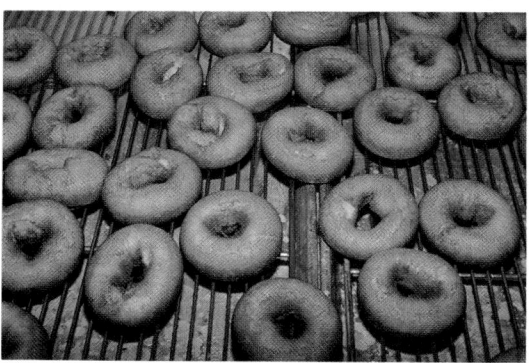

Plate 44. Doughnuts are generally high in oil because they are fried in deep oil. Thus, those who eat doughnuts will need to restrict the consumption of other foods high in fats/oils in order to restrict the total fat intake at or below the 30% of the total caloric intake as called for by the 1989 RDA. (Courtesy, American Soybean Assn., St. Louis, Mo.)

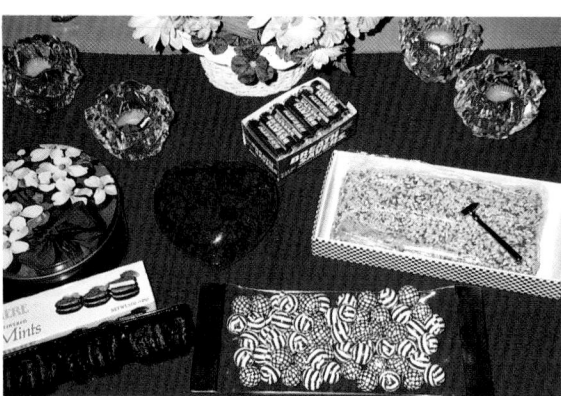

Plate 47. Candy. This shows candy on display. The story of candy is the story of sugar, because basically candymaking is simply the boiling of sugar. (Photo by A. H. Ensminger)

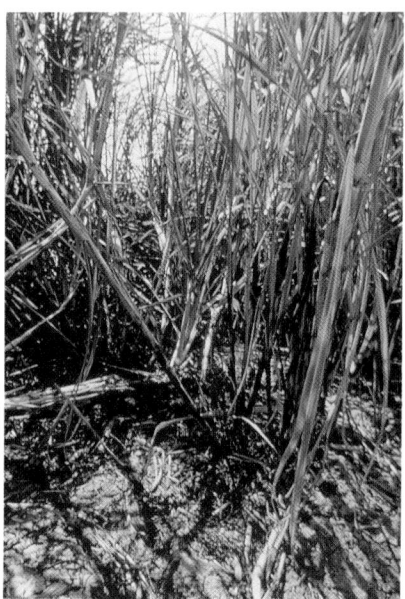

Plate 45. Sugarcane, source of 60 to 62% of the world's refined sugar. (Courtesy, USDA)

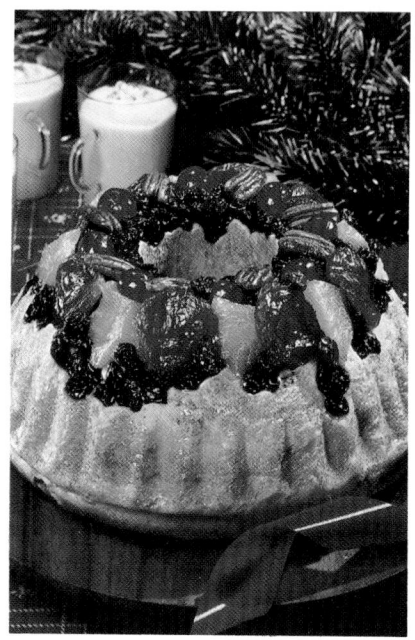

Plate 48. Coffee cake. Generally, coffee cake is low in fat, but high in sugar. So, remember the admonition of the *Food Guide Pyramid: Use sparingly.*

FOOD PRODUCTION

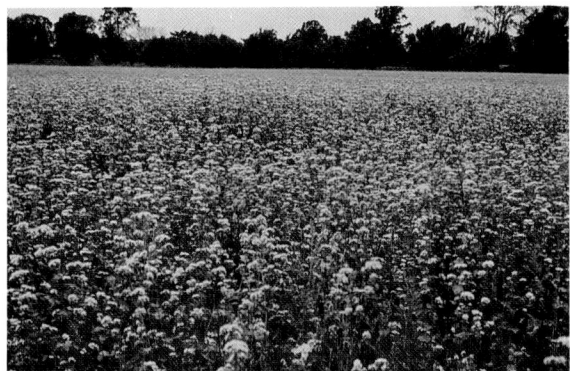

Plate 49. Buckwheat, in full bloom. Buckwheat is used for about the same purposes as the cereal grains, but it is not a cereal; it is related to rhubarb. (Courtesy, University of Minnesota, St. Paul)

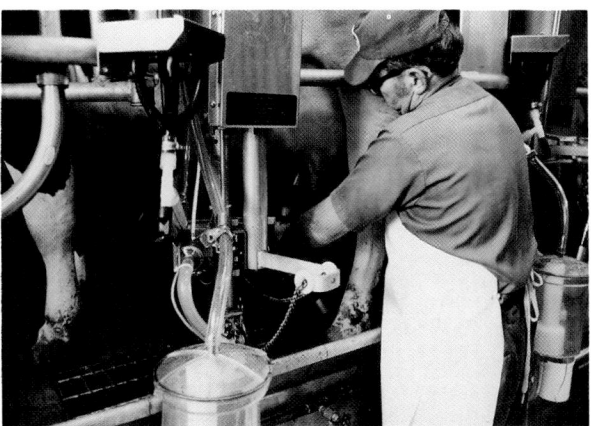

Plate 52. Milking. This shows dairy cows being milked by machine in a milking parlor. (Courtesy, University of Maryland, College Park)

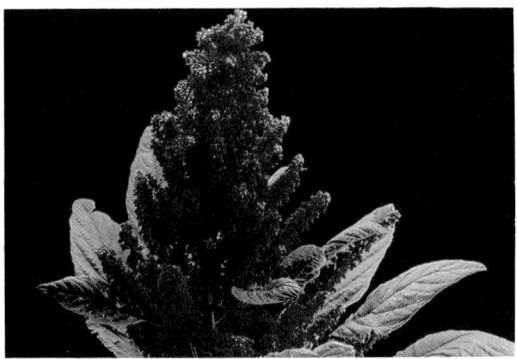

Plate 50. Amaranth. It is grown for the leaves as a green vegetable and for the seed as a grain. (Courtesy, University of Minnesota, St. Paul)

Plate 53. *Below:* Cowpeas. This shows a field of cowpeas in southeastern U.S.A. The plants have a trailing and bushy vine, but do not climb. (Courtesy, University of Minnesota, St. Paul)

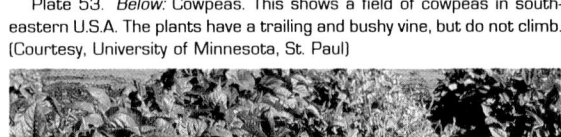
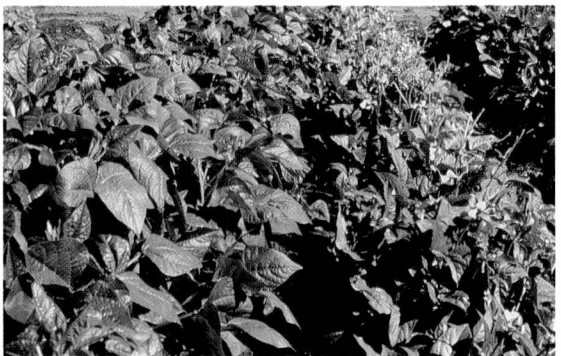

Plate 51. *Below:* Cherries. This shows a cluster of the fruit ready for harvest. (Courtesy, USDA)

Plate 54. Layers in cages. More than 90% of U.S. layers are in cages or on wire. (Courtesy, USDA)

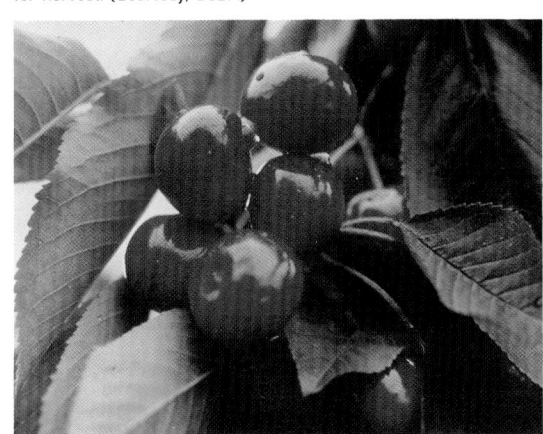

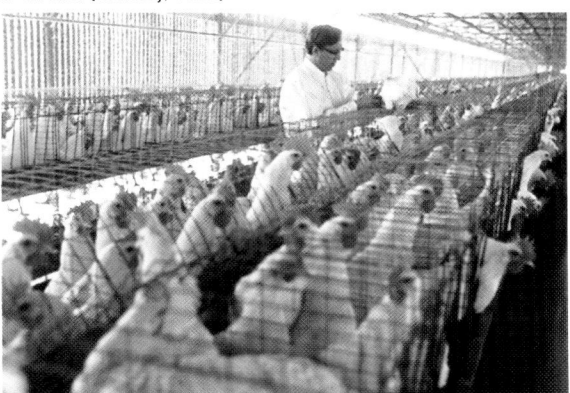

FOOD MARKETING

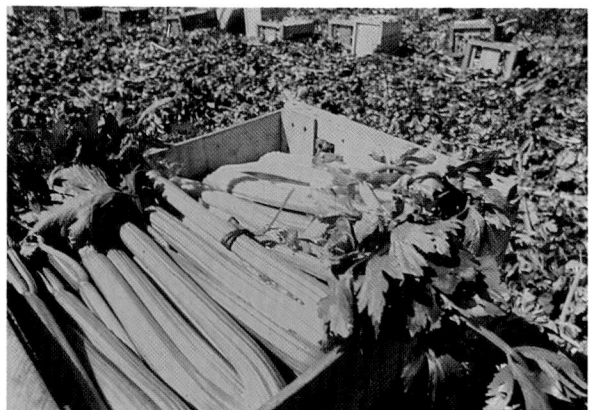

Plate 55. Celery. This shows harvested celery being packed in the field for shipment to market. (Courtesy, USDA)

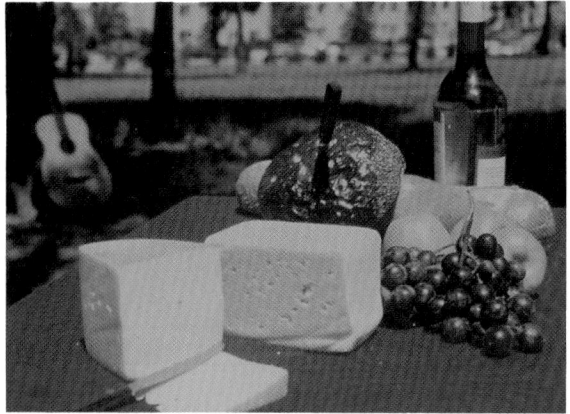

Plate 58. Cheese, bread, and wine—an attractive display. (Courtesy, USDA)

Plate 59. *Below:* Meat, showing customer selecting from a meat display in a supermarket. (Courtesy, USDA)

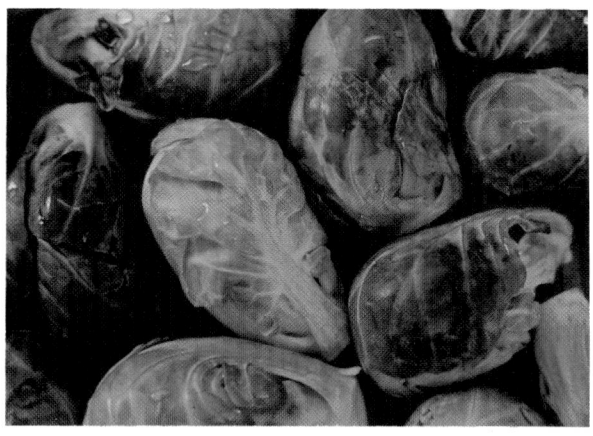

Plate 56. Brussel sprouts in a supermarket. (Courtesy, USDA)

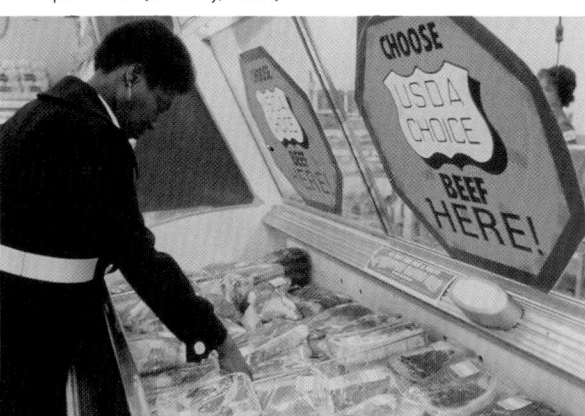

Plate 57. *Below:* Strawberries, fully ripe and glistening in a market. Strawberries are the world's leading berry-type fruit. (Courtesy, USDA)

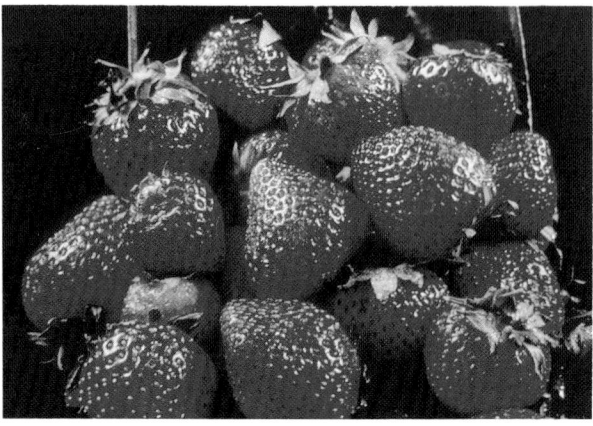

Plate 60. *Below:* Vegetables and fruits—an attractive display. (Courtesy, University of Florida, Gainesville)

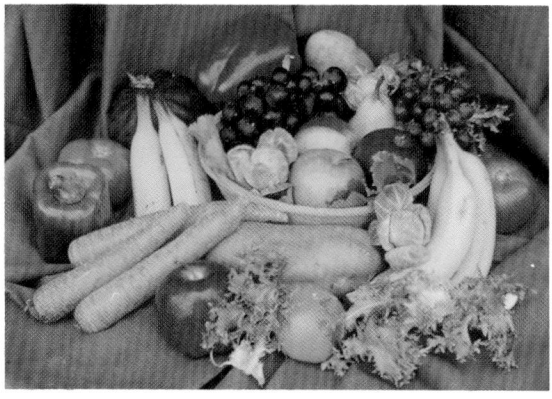

BREAD, CEREAL, RICE, & PASTA GROUP

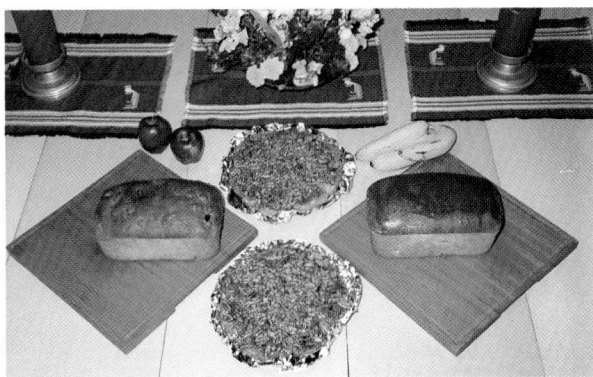

Plate 61. Whole wheat bread—a member of the Bread, Cereal, Rice, & Pasta Group, of which 6-11 daily servings are recommended in the *Food Guide Pyramid.* (Photo by A. H. Ensminger)

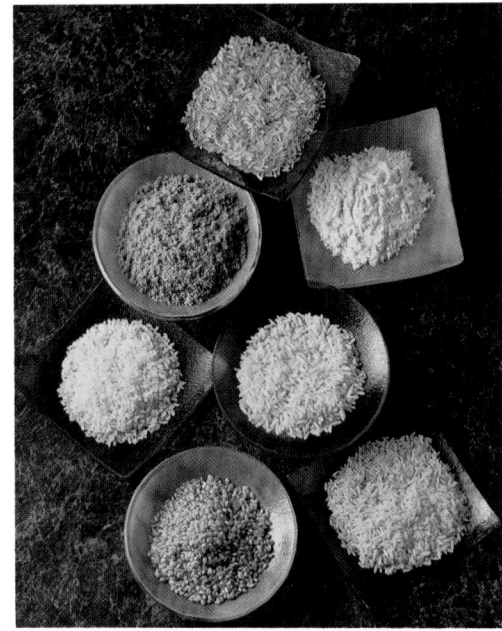

Plate 64. Rice, of which 7 kinds are displayed. Of the thousands of varieties, only about 25 are grown commercially in the U.S.A. (Courtesy, USA Rice Council, Houston, Tex.)

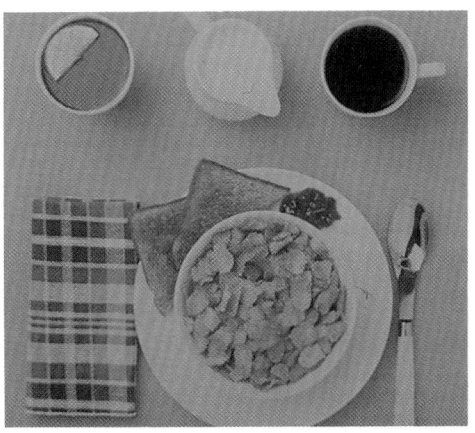

Plate 62. Corn flakes. This ready-to-eat breakfast cereal is manufactured from deskinned, degerminated kernels of soaked dried corn by flavoring, rolling, and toasting. (Courtesy, USDA)

Plate 65. A pita bread sandwich. (Courtesy, USDA)

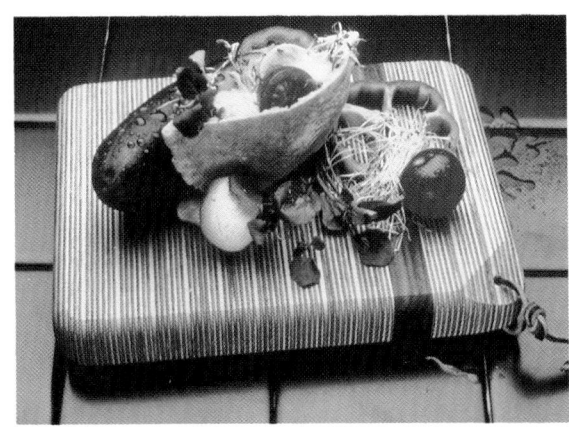

Plate 66. *Below:* Pasta (macaroni). This shows pasta used to extend meat—a high-quality protein. (Courtesy, National Live Stock and Meat Board, Chicago, Ill)

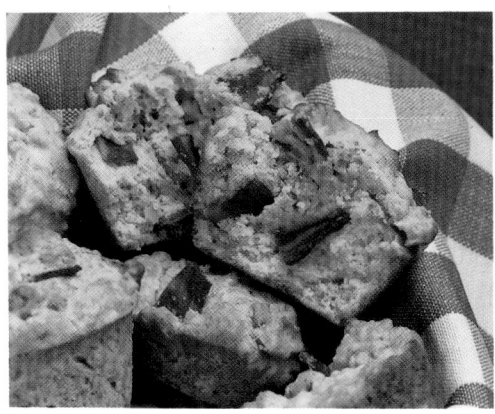

Plate 63. Muffins with turkey bacon. (Courtesy, Oscar Mayer Food Corp., Madison, Wisc.)

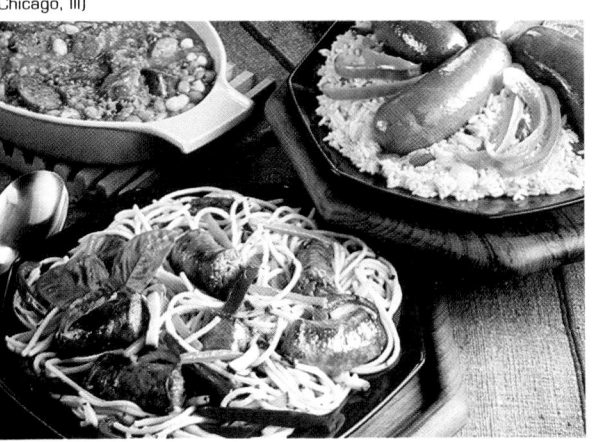

VEGETABLE GROUP

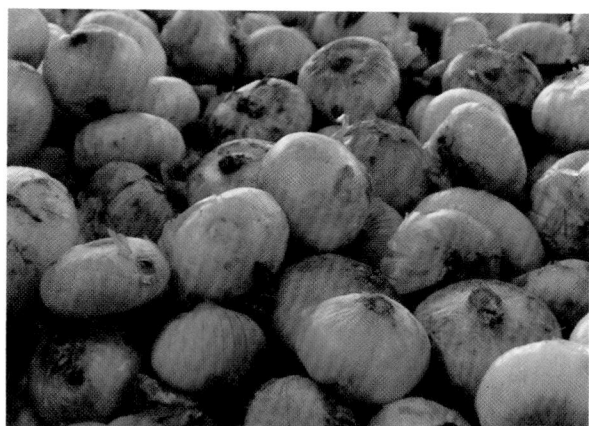

Plate 67. Onions. This vegetable is used primarily for its flavor and appetite appeal. The *Food Guide Pyramid* calls for 3-5 daily servings of the Vegetable Group. (Courtesy, USDA)

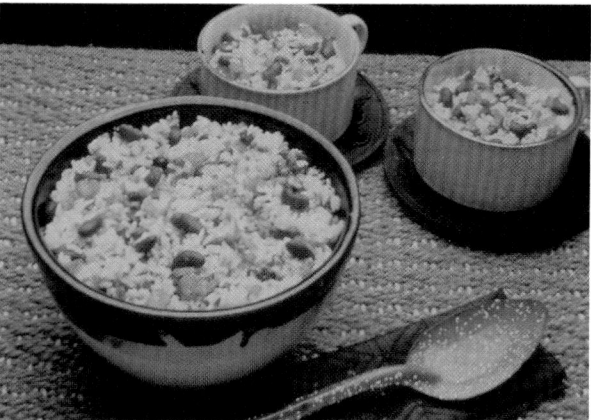

Plate 70. Red beans and rice. A mixture of 50% of each beans and rice has a protein quality that approaches meat, milk, and other animal proteins. (Courtesy, USDA)

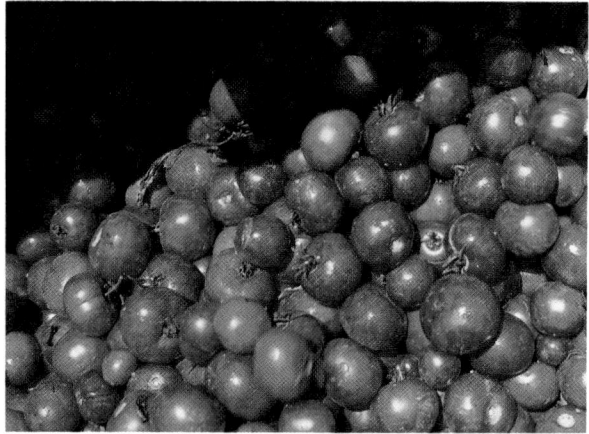

Plate 68. Tomatoes, a member of the nightshade family. Ripe (red) tomatoes are low in calories and a good source of vitamins A and C. (Courtesy, Rutgers University, New Brunswick, N.J.)

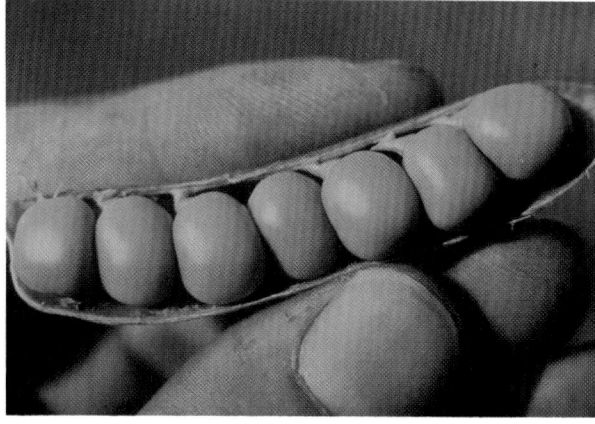

Plate 71. Peas in a pod. Peas are usually picked when immature. They are rich in protein, an excellent source of vitamin A, and a good source of vitamin C. (Courtesy, USDA)

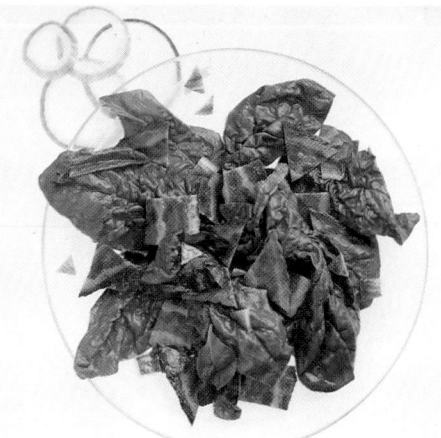

Plate 69. Spinach salad, with turkey and bacon. Spinach has a high water content (90 to 93%), is low in calories, and is an excellent source of magnesium, iron, potassium, and Vitamin A. (Courtesy, Oscar Mayer Food Corp., Madison, Wisc.)

Plate 72. *Below:* Corn-on-the-cob. Three ears of sweet corn-on-the-cob contain about 240 Calories (kcal). Yellow corn is also a fair source of vitamin A. (Courtesy, USDA)

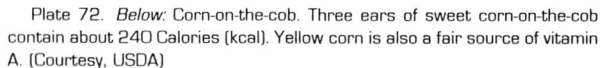

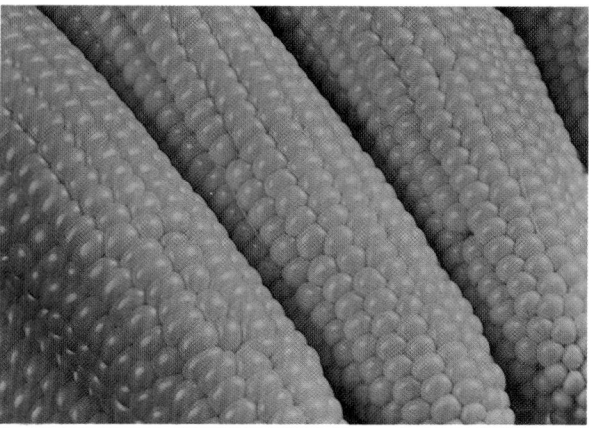

FRUIT GROUP

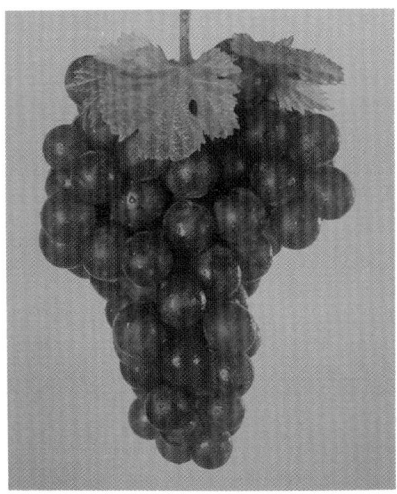

Plate 73. Grapes, the leading fruit crop of the world. Fresh table grapes are one of the richest sources of chromium and a good source of potassium. The *Food Guide Pyramid* calls for 2-4 servings of the Fruit Group daily. (Courtesy, California Table Grape Commission)

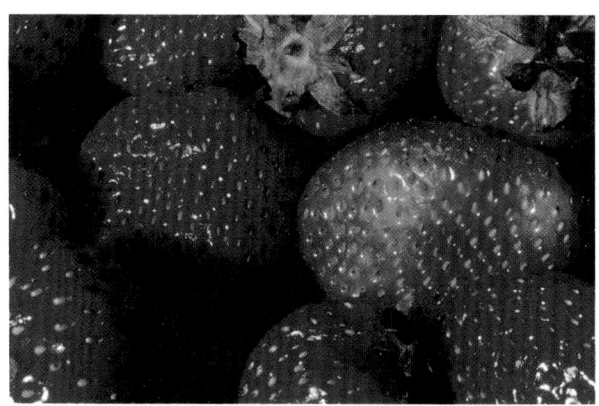

Plate 76. Strawberries, a good source of iron and potassium, and an excellent source of vitamin C. (Courtesy, National Film Board of Canada)

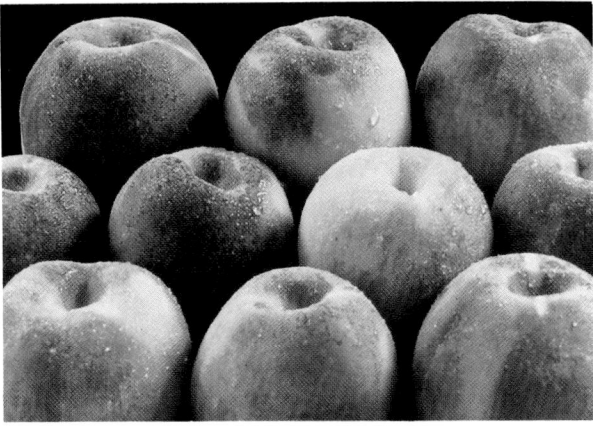

Plate 74. Peaches. Fresh peaches contain 89% water. Additionally, each 100 g (about 3 1/2 oz or I medium-sized peach) contain 38 Calories (kcal) of energy, 202 mg of potassium, 1,330 IU of vitamin A, and only I mg of sodium. (Courtesy, USDA)

Plate 77. *Below:* Fruits for snacks. Fruits provide fiber, few calories, no cholesterol, and little sodium or fat. (Courtesy, North Dakota State University, Fargo)

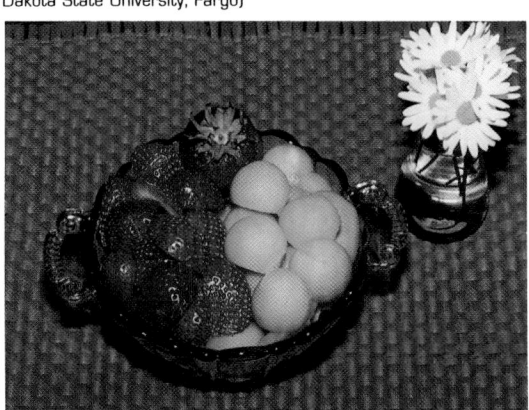

Plate 78. Lemonade, a refreshing beverage and a good source of vitamin C. (Courtesy, Sunkist, Van Nuys, Calif.)

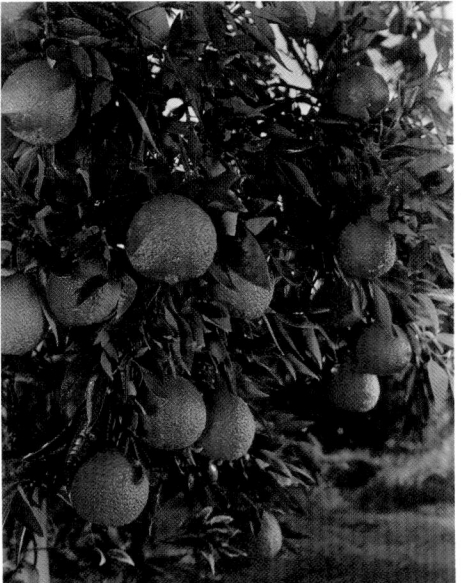

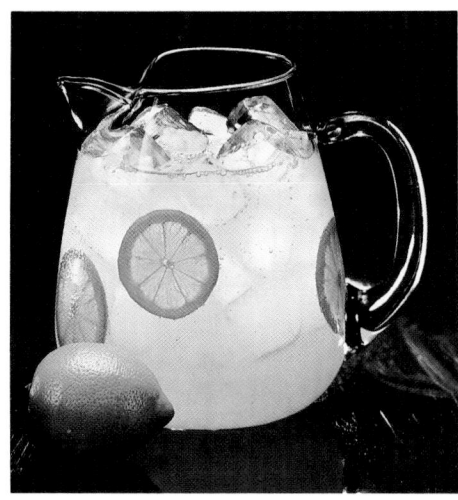

Plate 75. Oranges ready for harvest. Fresh oranges are low in calories (47 kcal per 100 g), but they are good sources of fiber, pectin, potassium, vitamin C, inositol, and bioflavonoids. (Courtesy, Sunkist, Van Nuys, Calif.)

MEAT, POULTRY, FISH, DRY BEANS, EGGS, & NUTS GROUP

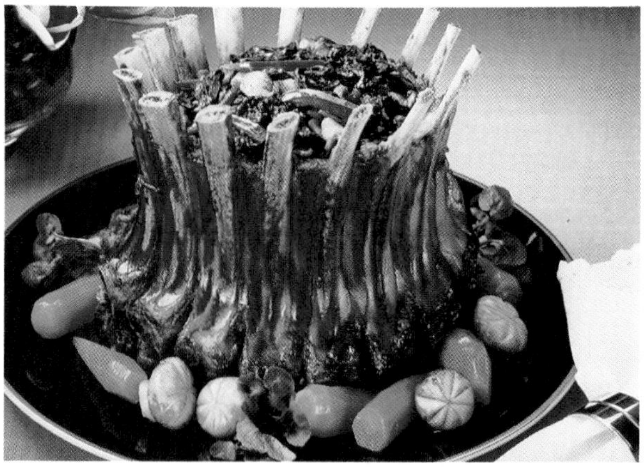

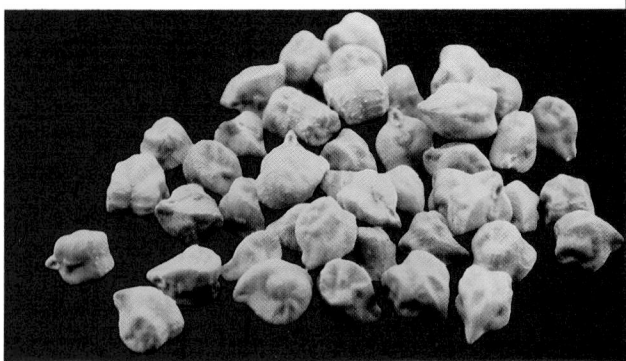

Plate 79. Crown roast of lamb—an elegant dish. Lamb is an excellent source of high-quality protein, a rich source of phosphorus and iron, and an excellent source of vitamins B-12, B-6, biotin, niacin, pantothenic acid, and thiamin. The *Food Guide Pyramid* calls for 2-3 daily servings of the Meat, Poultry, Fish, Dry Beans, Eggs, & Nuts Group. (Courtesy, National Live Stock and Meat Board, Chicago, Ill.)

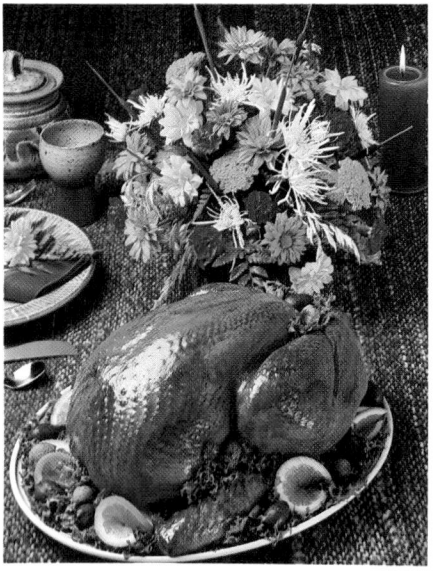

Plate 80. Roasted turkey. Poultry meat is a good source of phosphorus, iron, copper, and zinc; a rich source of vitamins B-12 and B-6; and a fair source of vitamins A, biotin, niacin, pantothenic acid, riboflavin, and thiamin. (Courtesy, Canadian Marketing Agency, Ontario, Canada)

Plate 82. Garbanzo beans (Chickpeas). Beans may be used (a) to upgrade the protein quantity and quality of diets based mainly on cereals and starchy foods, and (b) to extend and lower the cost of animal proteins. (Courtesy, University of Minnesota, St. Paul)

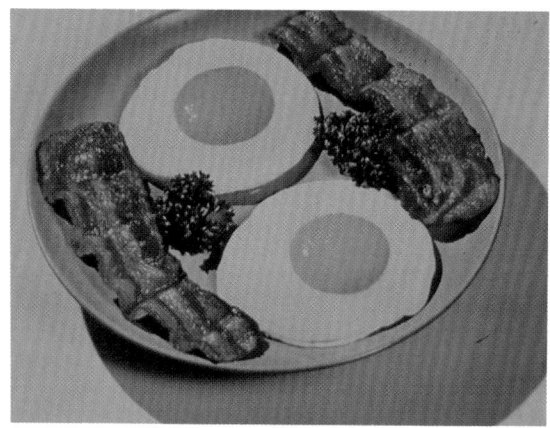

Plate 83. Bacon and eggs, the traditional American breakfast. Bacon contains all the essential amino acids, is rich in iron, and is high in the B-vitamins. Eggs contain an abundance of proteins, minerals, and vitamins. (Courtesy, USDA)

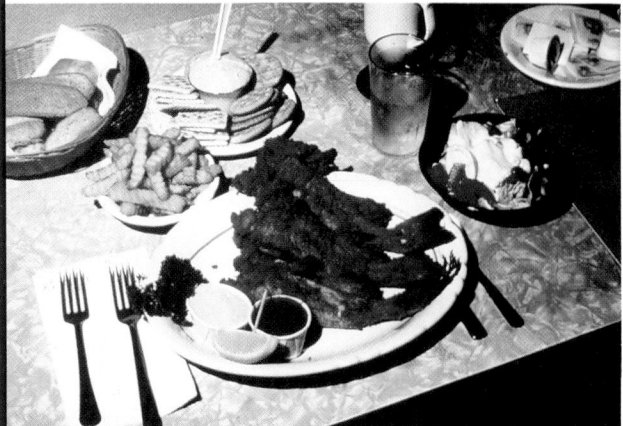

Plate 81. Seafood dinner. Fish and seafood are high in the essential amino acids, and rich in minerals and vitamins. Also, the fatty acids present are polyunsaturated; hence, they can play a major role in low-cholesterol diets. (Courtesy, U.S. Department of Interior)

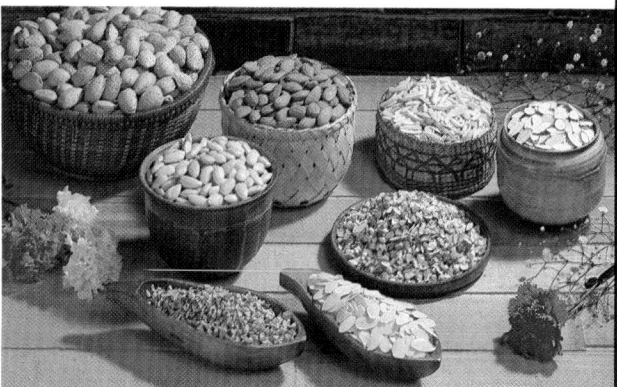

Plate 84. Almonds, which come in more forms than any other nut. Nuts are high in energy and protein; a good source of magnesium, zinc, and copper; and a good source of the B-vitamins. (Courtesy, Almond Board of California, Sacramento)

MILK, YOGURT, & CHEESE GROUP

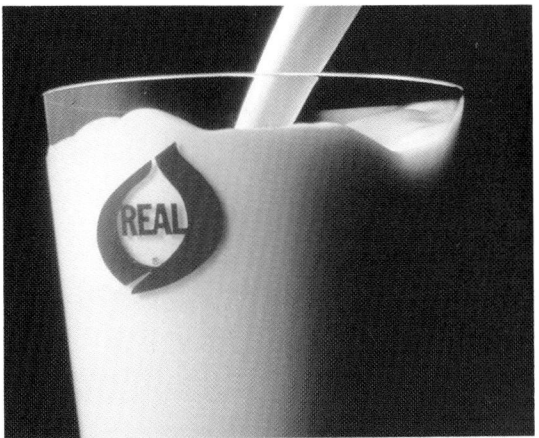

Plate 85. Milk, the major components of which are carbohydrates, fat, and protein. Milk is also a valuable source of certain minerals and vitamins. The *Food Guide Pyramid* calls for 2-3 servings daily of the Milk, Yogurt, & Cheese Group. (Courtesy, American Dairy Assn., Rosemont, Ill.)

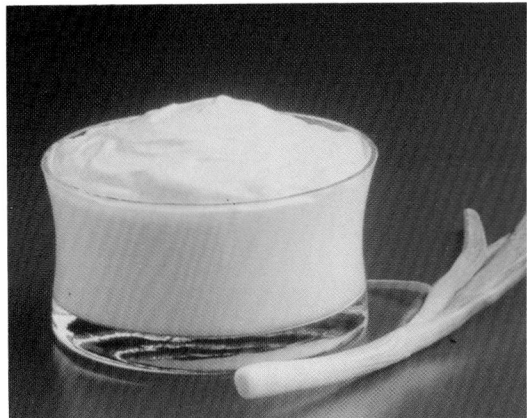

Plate 88. Sour cream. Today, most sour cream is cultured, much the same way as buttermilk. It is a uniformly textured, smooth product which is widely used for flavoring. (Courtesy, American Dairy Assn., Rosemont, Ill.)

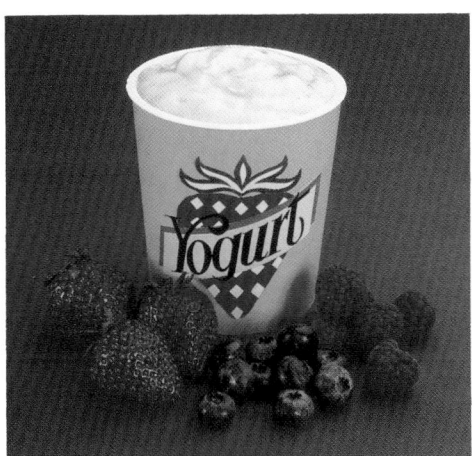

Plate 86. Yogurt, a fermented milk product prepared from lowfat milk, skim milk, or whole milk. (Courtesy, National Dairy Board, Arlington, Va.)

Plate 89. Pizzas. This Italian creation is a flat leavened bread topped with such good things as mozzarella and parmesan cheeses, sausages, anchovies, tomatoes, mushrooms, olives, herbs and spices. (Courtesy, USDA)

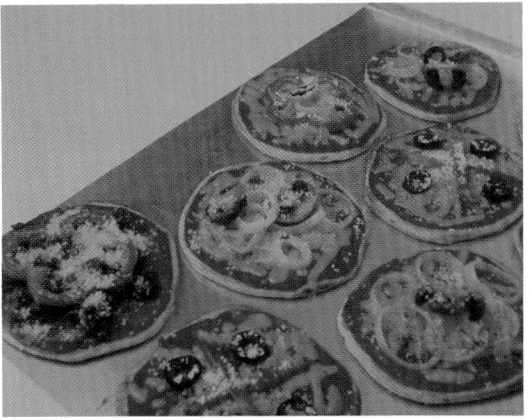

Plate 90. *Below:* Assorted cheeses. Milk can be, and is, processed into many different varieties of cheese. Some are made from whole milk, others from milk that has had part of the fat removed, and still others from skimmed milk. American types of cheese (Cheddar, Colby, Washed curd, Stirred curd, Monterey, and Jack) make up to 60% of the nation's cheese output. (Courtesy, American Dairy Assn., Rosemont, Ill.)

Plate 87. *Below:* Ice cream. Of all the frozen dairy desserts, ice cream contains the most milk solids (about 16 to 24%). (Courtesy, Carnation, Los Angeles, Calif.)

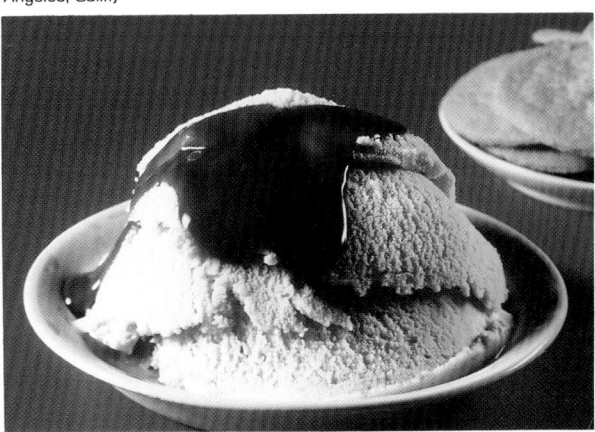

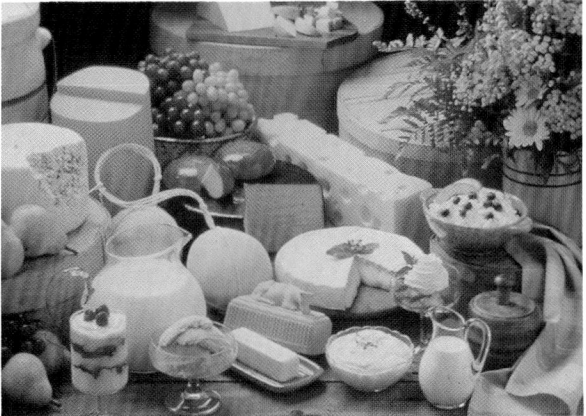

FATS, OILS, & SWEETS GROUP

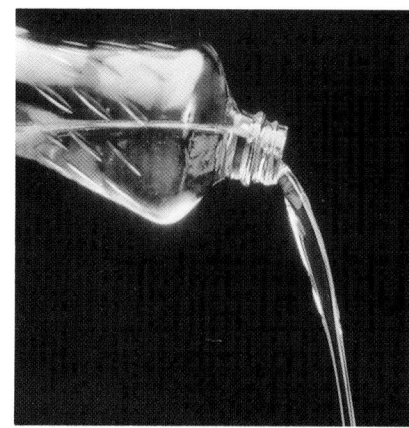

Plate 91. Cooking oil pouring out of a glass bottle. **Caution:** The new *Food Guide Pyramid*, released by the USDA in 1992, lists fats, oils, and sweets at the apex of the pyramid, where they are accorded the least space, along with the admonition to *use sparingly*. (Courtesy, USDA)

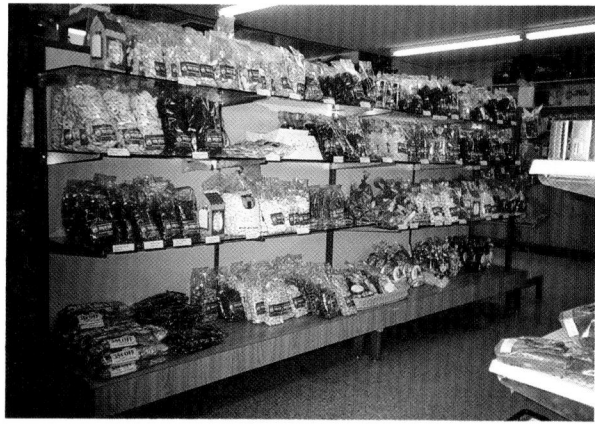

Plate 94. The Candy Store. An assortment of candy and chocolate covered nuts and raisins. **Note well:** The new *Food Guide Pyramid* admonishes that sweets should be *used sparingly*. (Photo by A. H. Ensminger)

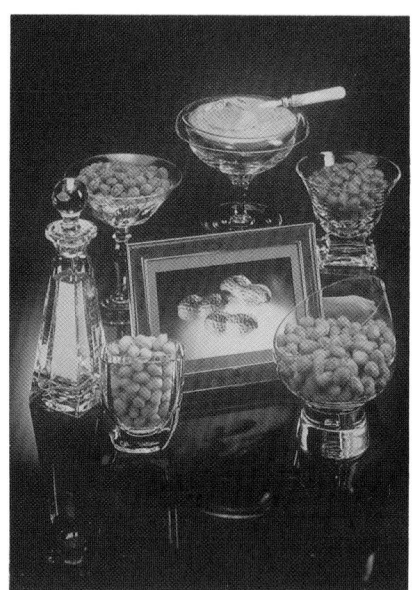

Plate 92. Peanut products. The nuts and skin yield about 47.5% oil. Peanuts supply about $\frac{1}{5}$ of the world's edible oil production. Peanut oil contains 76 to 82% unsaturated fatty acids. (Courtesy, Peanut Advisory Board, Atlanta, Ga.)

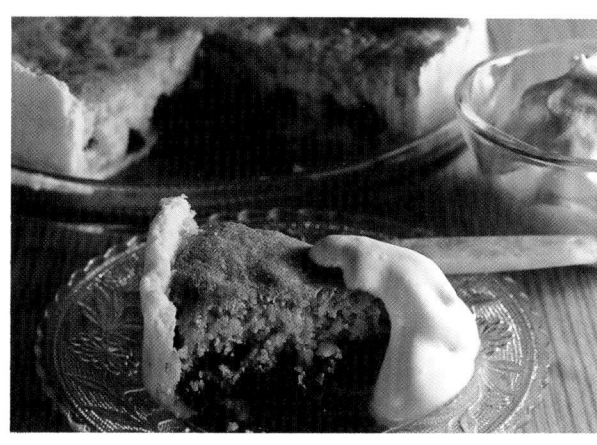

Plate 95. Raisin pie, which is moderately low in sugar, but moderately high in fat because of the crust. The calories in raisins are derived primarily from carbohydrates.

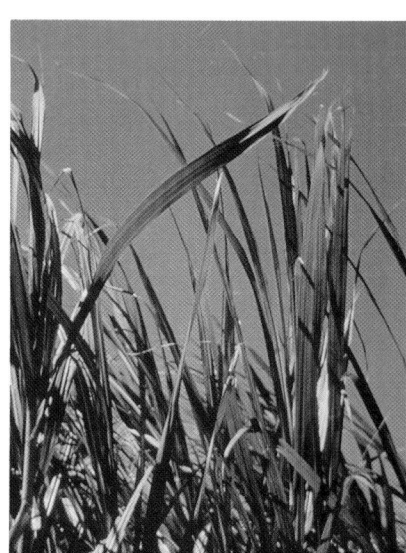

Plate 93. Sugarcane— a coarse grass of tropical and semitropical climates from which refined sugar is derived. (Courtesy, USDA)

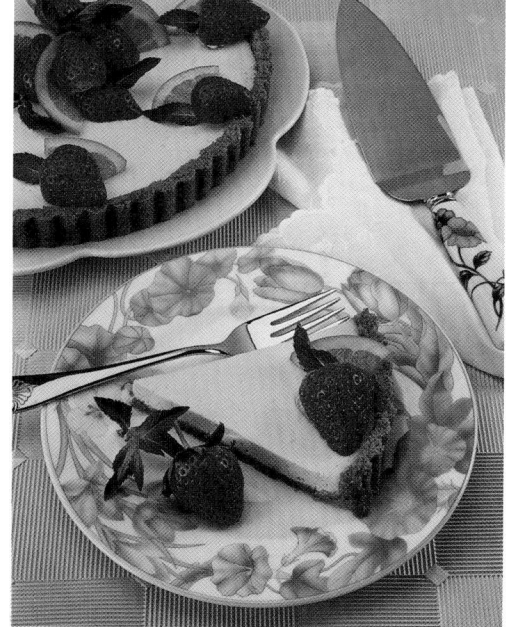

Plate 96. Yogurt cheese tart. Luscious desserts need not be high in fat. This creamy dessert made with lowfat yogurt has only 6 g of fat per serving. (Courtesy, National Dairy Board, Arlington, Va.)

LAMB AND MUTTON

Contents

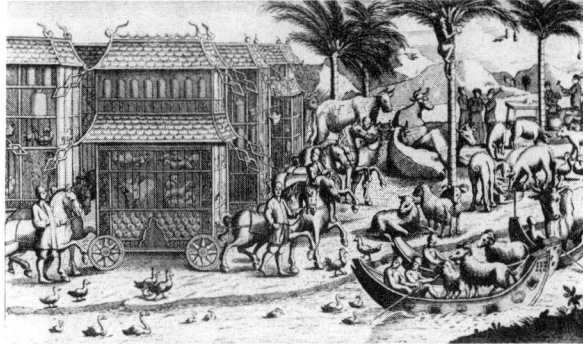

Fig. L-3. Live sheep and other animals sent to Persia and India with an Expeditionary Force in 1670. Until meat preservation was developed, live animals had to be taken along by the explorers. (Courtesy, the Bettmann Archive, Inc., New York, N.Y.)

Lamb is the flesh of young sheep; mutton is the flesh of mature sheep. Lamb differs from mutton in both tenderness and flavor.

QUALITIES IN LAMB DESIRED BY CONSUMERS.
Consumers desire the following qualities in lamb:

1. Palatability.
2. Attractiveness.
3. Maximum muscling; minimum fat.
4. Small cuts.
5. Ease of preparation.
6. Tenderness.
7. Repeatability.

FEDERAL GRADES OF LAMB AND MUTTON. The
quality grades of lambs, yearlings, and mutton may be defined as a measure of their degree of excellence based on conformation and quality, or eating characteristics of the meat; and the yield, or percent of retail cuts, is based on the thickness of fat over the ribeye. **Note:** 0.25 in. of fat over the ribeye is considered the line between desirable and somewhat overfat lambs.

The current federal grades, which became effective July 6, 1992, on a voluntary basis, call for both quality and yield grading after removal of most of the kidney and pelvic fat, although up to 1.0% of the carcass weight in kidney and pelvic fat is allowed in carcasses.

Federally graded meats are so stamped (with an edible vegetable dye) that the grade will appear on the retail cuts as well as on the carcass and wholesale cuts. The federal quality grades of lambs, yearlings, and mutton are:

Lambs and Yearlings	Mutton
Prime	Choice
Choice	Good
Good	Utility
Utility	Cull

In addition to the quality grades given, there are the following yield grades of lamb, yearling, and mutton carcasses: Yield Grade 1, Yield Grade 2, Yield Grade 3, Yield Grade 4, and Yield Grade 5. The new standards call for both quality and yield grades. Also, the new grades apply to both (1) lamb, yearling, and mutton carcasses; and (2) slaughter (live) lambs, yearlings, and mutton sheep.

The word *quality* infers superiority. It follows that quality grades indicate the relative superiority of carcasses or cuts in palatability characteristics. In turn, palatability is associated with tenderness, juiciness, and flavor. The major quality-indicating characteristics are (1) color and texture of bone, which indicates the age of the animal; (2) firmness; (3) texture; and (4) marbling—the intermixing of fat among the muscle fibers.

Yield grades indicate the *quantity* of meat—the amount of retail, consumer-ready, ready-to-cook, or edible meat that a carcass contains. Yield grade is not to be confused with dressing percent. Dressing percent refers to the amount of carcass from a live animal, whereas yield grade refers to the amount of edible product from the carcass.

The grades of lambs, yearlings, and mutton are based on separate evaluation of (1) the palatability indicating characteristics of the lean—the *quality grade;* and (2) the indicated percent of trimmed, boneless major retail cuts to be derived from the carcass—the *yield grade.*

LAMB CUTS AND HOW TO COOK THEM. Fig. L-5
illustrates the retail cuts of lamb, and gives the recommended method or methods of cooking each.

U.S. LAMB PRODUCTION. In 1990, 362,000,000 lb
(*165,000,000 kg*) of lamb and mutton were produced in the United States, which represented only 0.9% of the nation's total meat production. On January 1, 1991, there were 11,200,000 sheep and lambs in the United States.

PER CAPITA LAMB AND MUTTON CONSUMPTION. In 1990, the U.S. per capita consumption of lamb
and mutton (and most of it was lamb) was a mere 1.1 lb.

LAMB AND MUTTON AS FOODS.

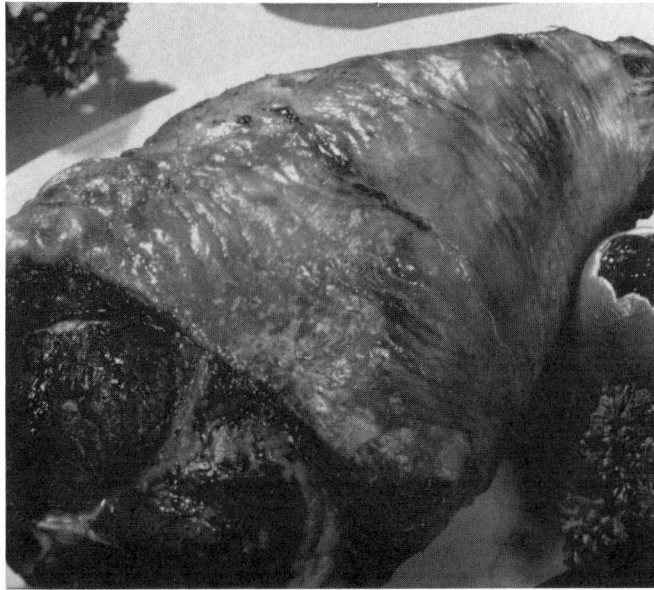

Fig. L-4. Roast leg of lamb. (Courtesy, National Live Stock and Meat Board, Chicago, Ill.)

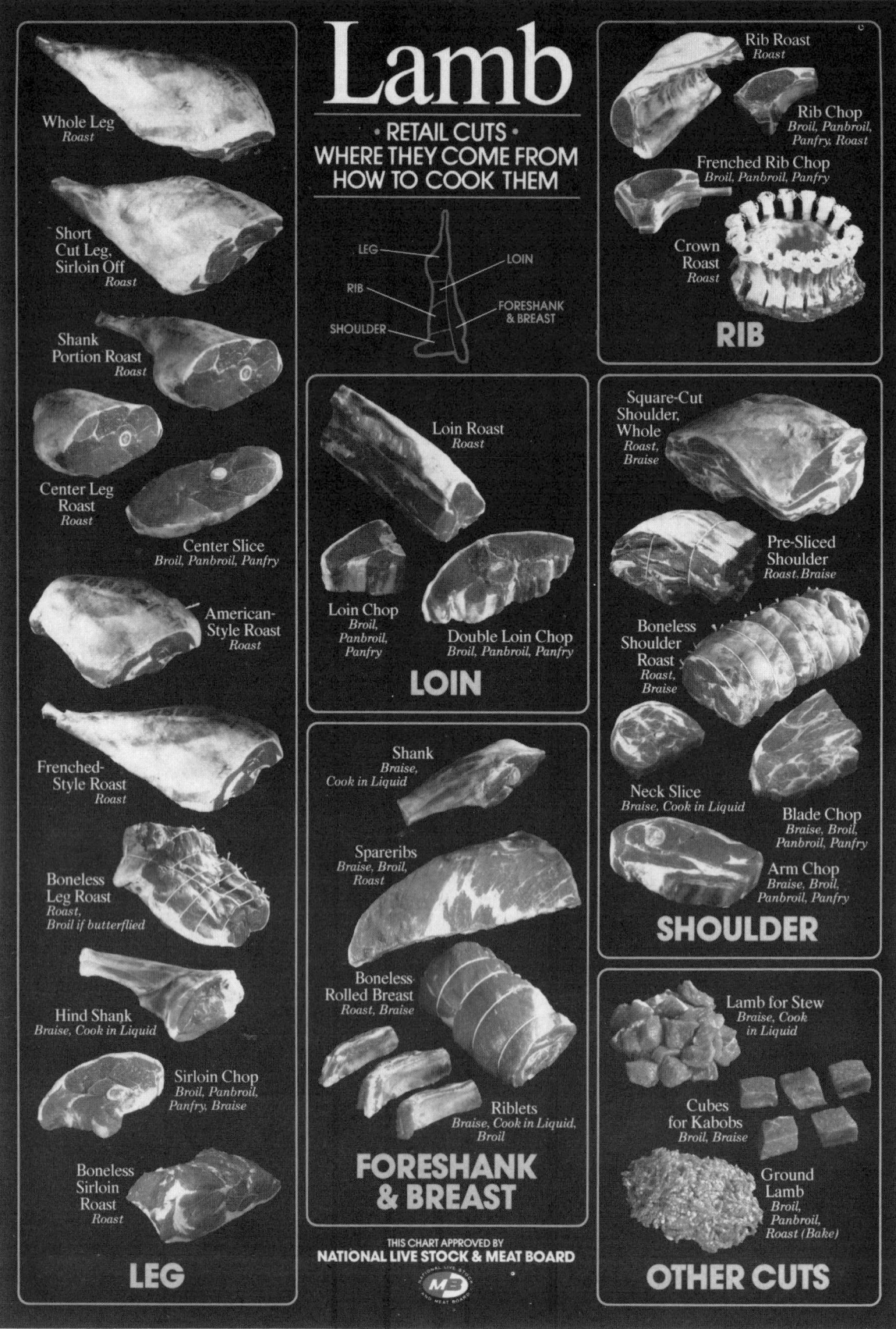

Fig. L-5. The retail cuts of lamb: where they come from, and how to cook them. (Courtesy, National Live Stock and Meat Board, Chicago, Ill.)

Lamb has long been noted for its delicate flavor and tenderness. In biblical times, frequent reference was made to the desirability of lamb meat. Today, it may be featured for gourmet dining at home and in hotels and restaurants.

Lamb is important in the diet, not for its appetite appeal alone, but for the essential food nutrients that it contains. It is an excellent source of high-quality protein for muscle building and body maintenance. In most cuts of lamb, the fat may be easily separated from the lean; hence, the calories can be adjusted to desired levels. Lamb is one of the best sources of iron, needed for hemoglobin formation; and it is rich in phosphorus, needed for bones and teeth. It is also an excellent source of vitamin B-12, vitamin B-6, biotin, niacin, pantothenic acid, and thiamin. Also, lamb muscle is easily digested, so it is included in the diet of both the young and aged.

In the past, lamb was often considered to be a seasonal meat—spring lamb. Today, it is available the year-round, primarily due to freezer storage and imported lamb. Since lamb will keep frozen for long periods (12 months), large volumes are now marketed as portion-cut, frozen, and ready-to-cook.

LARD

Lard is the fat rendered (melted out) from fresh, fatty pork tissue.

The proportion of live market weight made into lard varies with the type, weight, and finish of the hogs, and the relative price of lard and the cuts of meat. A market weight hog grading U.S. No. 1 yields about 8 lb of lard per 100 lb (3.6 kg/45 kg) liveweight, whereas the same weight hog grading U.S. No. 3 yields about 16 lb per cwt (7.3 kg/45 kg).

It is noteworthy, too, that lard consumption has steadily declined since 1950. The U.S. per capita consumption of lard in 1950 was 12.6 lb; in 1990, it was only 2.2 lb.

The three most important sources of lard obtained from a hog carcass are: (1) leaf fat, (2) fat trimmings, and (3) fat backs and plates. About 75% of the fat back is rendered for lard, the other 25% is marketed fresh, frozen, or cured.

LARDING

A method of adding fat to lean meat so that it does not dry out during cooking. Narrow strips of fat (as bacon fat) are inserted into the meat with a special larding needle—a large needle with a hollow split end. The strips of fat are called lardoons.

LARK (MEADOWLARK)

Singing and game birds of which there are numerous species, found mostly in Europe, Asia, and northern Africa. The lark has a very delicate flesh and is greatly esteemed by gastronomes.

LATHYRISM

A disease due to the toxicant found in the Lathyrus seed (*Lathyrus sativus*). The toxin produces an irreversible, gradual weakness, followed by paralysis of both legs (paraplegia). Outbreaks occur in Asia and North Africa mainly during years of poor wheat crops. In these areas, it is common practice to plant Lathyrus with the wheat. If rainfall is adequate, the wheat overgrows the Lathyrus. However, in a year when the rains fail, mainly Lathyrus seed is harvested and it becomes the main dietary energy source; and the symptoms

of Lathyrism begin appearing. The disease can affect horses and cattle, too.

(Also see Table L-2, Legumes of the World, Lathyrus Pea.)

LAXATIVE

A food or drug that will induce bowel movements and relieve constipation. Bran and other fibrous foods will soften the stool and encourage more rapid movement through the digestive tract. Numerous laxative drugs are sold, most of which act by increasing the water content of the stool, or by increasing the contraction of the bowel, or by lubricating the lining of the bowel. Persons seeking relief from constipation should exercise care in the choice and use of a laxative; and, when in doubt, consult a doctor.

(Also see CONSTIPATION.)

LEAD (Pb)

Lead poisoning has dogged man for centuries. It is even speculated that it may have caused the decline and fall of the Roman Empire. In recent years, lead poisoning has been reduced significantly with the use of lead-free paints.

(Also see MINERAL[S], section headed "Contamination of Drinking Water, Food, or Air with Toxic Minerals"; and POISONS, Table P-2, Some Potentially Poisonous [Toxic] Substances.)

LEAVEN

To make light by aerating (adding air) in any of three different methods: (1) by the fermentation of yeast, (2) by the action of baking powder, or (3) by beating air into egg whites.

(Also see BREADS AND BAKING.)

LEBEN

• A type of fermented milk in Egypt.

• A sour milk delicacy of biblical times, made from goat milk.

LEBKUCHEN

A Christmas cookie made with honey, brown sugar, almonds, candied fruit peel, and spices.

LECITHIN (PHOSPHATIDYL CHOLINE)

A versatile phospholipid found in all living organisms. It is a mixture of the diglycerides of the fatty acids stearic, palmitic, and oleic combined with the choline ester of phosphoric acid. The body is capable of synthesizing lecithin. In addition, lecithin is found in a wide variety of foods. *At this time, there is no evidence that lecithin has any nutritional significance.*

The commercial source of lecithin is predominately soybeans. It is an FDA approved food additive employed as a stabilizer and emulsifier in margarine, dressings, chocolate, frozen desserts, and baked goods. Furthermore, lecithin is also used in such products as paints, soaps, printing inks, and cosmetics, to name only a few.

(Also see ADDITIVES, Table A-3; CHOLINE, section on sources of Choline; and SOYBEAN, Table S-12, Soybean Products and Uses For Human Food.)

LEGUMES

Contents	Page

This very large family of plants contains about 13,000 species, most of which are distinguished by their seed-bearing pods. These species occur in such diverse forms as short, erect broad-leafed plants; climbing vines; and various types of trees. Legumes rank second only to cereals in supplying calories and protein for the world's population. They supply about the same number of calories per unit weight as the cereals, but they contain from 2 to 4 times more protein. Also, the amino acid patterns of legumes complement those of cereal grains so that combinations of the two foods provide dietary protein that is used much more efficiently by the human body than that from either food alone.

One or more types of edible legumes may be found almost everywhere in the world where the soil is arable and sufficient water is available, because these plants are endowed with certain characteristics which favor their growth and propagation. First, the roots of many legumes harbor bacteria which convert nitrogen gas from the air into nitrogen compounds that may be utilized by the plant. This process is called *nitrogen fixation*. Hence, these plants may grow on soils in which the fixed nitrogen has been exhausted by the growth of other plants such as cereal grains. Also, legumes release their nitrogen compounds upon decaying, so that grains may again grow well on soils that were once depleted. Second, wild legumes have pods that burst open when mature, and scatter their seeds in all directions.

HISTORY. Historians express wonderment at the apparent wisdom of primitive peoples who produced and utilized legumes and other foods in ways which have only recently received the endorsement of professional agriculturists and nutritionists. Therefore, the history of legumes merits special consideration.

It appears that the first cultivation of legumes occurred in Southeast Asia, rather than in the Middle East, as was originally thought. The recently discovered Spirit Cave near the border between Burma and Thailand contained seeds of beans, peas, and other plants that had been there since about 9750 B.C. (as estimated by radiocarbon dating), and which closely resembled the seeds of today's cultivated plants.

The next oldest sites of agriculture, which date to about 8000 B.C., are those in the Middle East, in the region commonly referred to as the Fertile Crescent, a broad arc of land

Fig. L-6. Soybeans, the leading legume of the world. (Courtesy, USDA)

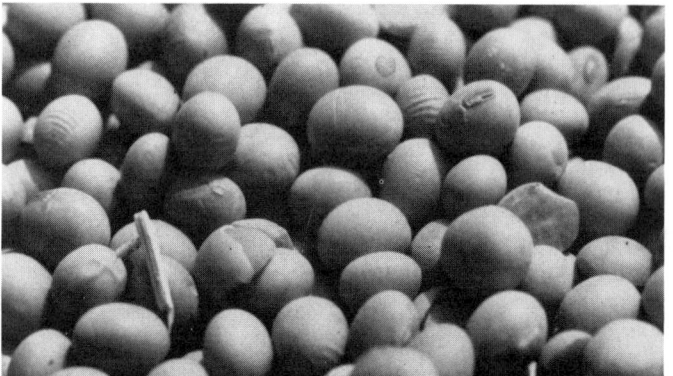

that curved northward and eastward from the Mediterranean coast of what is now Israel to the Zagros Mountains near the border between Iraq and Iran. This region was probably the place of origin of chickpeas, fava beans, and lentils.

The long dependence of China and India on almost wholly vegetarian diets led to (1) the development of soybean-based imitations of dairy products by the Chinese, and (2) the utilization of legumes for food in India; in a manner and to a degree that was unequaled elsewhere in the world.

Apparently, the first cultivation of legumes in the New World occurred around 4000 B.C. in both Peru and Mexico, but the practice gradually spread to other parts of North and South America. Hence, there was much similarity between the American Indian practices observed by the Spanish when they arrived in Latin America and those noted by the English settlers of New England. The Indians of both places planted beans among rows of corn so that the corn stalks might provide convenient supports for the climbing legume vines. This practice eliminated much of the necessity for weeding the crops.

The English colonists also learned from the Indians how to make succotash (a mixture of corn and beans). Boston baked beans were derived from the Indian method of soaking beans until they swelled, then baking them with deer fat and onions in clay pots surrounded by hot stones. The Pilgrims baked their beans on Saturday nights in order to avoid the performance of servile work on Sundays. Later, the custom changed as the strict observance of the sabbath abated, and baked beans were served on Saturday nights in New England.

During the great westward expansion in the 19th century, the settlers of the southwestern United States adopted many of the Mexican bean dishes such as frijoles (refried beans) and chili. It is believed that the original chili dish was invented by Mexican nuns.

At the present time, food technologists around the world are engaged in testing many new food products made from legumes in the hope that this approach might help to combat protein deficiency. Also, agricultural scientists are conducting experiments designed to (1) improve the per acre yields of legumes, and (2) increase the amount of nitrogen fixed by these plants.

WORLD AND U.S. PRODUCTION. The world production of major legumes totals about 186,503,000 metric tons annually. Fig. L-7 shows the leading legumes of the world, and the production of each. Fig. L-8 shows the contribution of each of the major legume crops to world production. It is noteworthy that soybeans account for 58% of the world's legumes.

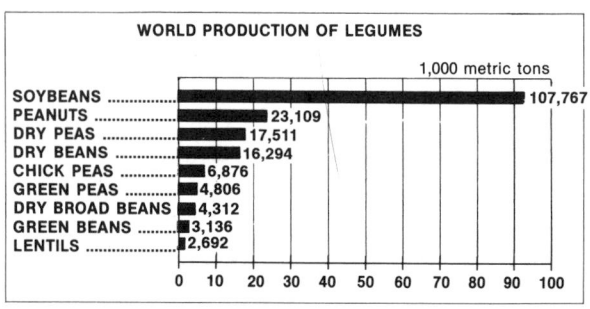

WORLD PRODUCTION OF LEGUMES

	1,000 metric tons
SOYBEANS	107,767
PEANUTS	23,109
DRY PEAS	17,511
DRY BEANS	16,294
CHICK PEAS	6,876
GREEN PEAS	4,806
DRY BROAD BEANS	4,312
GREEN BEANS	3,136
LENTILS	2,692

0 10 20 30 40 50 60 70 80 90 100

Fig. L-7. The leading legume crops of the world, and the annual production of each. Based on data from *FAO Production Yearbook 1990*, FAO/UN, Rome, Italy, Vol. 44. **Note well:** Annual production fluctuates as a result of weather and profitability of the crop.

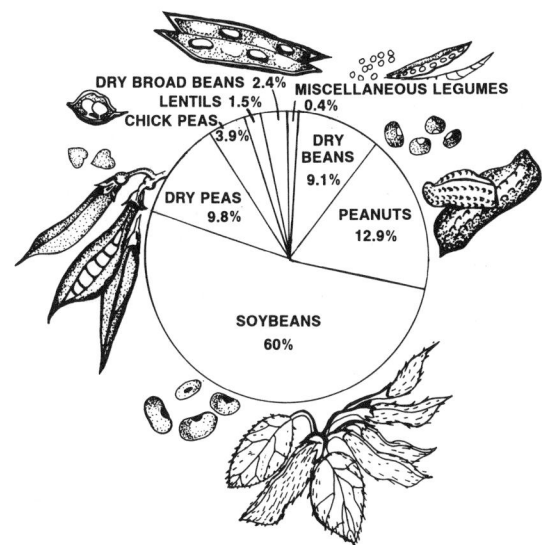

Fig. L-8. Contributions of the U.S. major legume crops to world production. (Based on data from *FAO Production Yearbook 1990*, FAO/UN, Rome, Italy, Vol. 44)

The U.S. production of major legumes totals about 60.4 million short tons annually. Soybeans and peanuts accounted for 92% and 3%, respectively, of the nation's legumes; hence, combined, these two legumes supplied an astounding 95% of U.S. legumes.

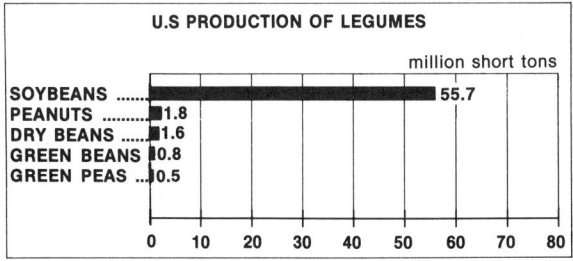

Fig. L-9. The leading legume crops of the U.S., and the annual production of each. Based on data from *Agricultural Statistics 1991*, USDA. **Note well:** Annual production fluctuates as a result of weather and profitability of the crop.

PREPARATION AND SERVING OF LEGUMES.

Today, many American homemakers work either part time or full time and have little time to boil beans for two or more hours, unless they wish to use a crock pot and start them cooking before they leave for work in the morning. However, long cooking uses a lot of electricity or gas, which are becoming more expensive. Therefore, the U.S. Department of Agriculture and various university departments have conducted research to find methods of simplifying the cooking and serving of legumes. Their findings have led to the suggestions which follow:

1. Soaking dry beans cuts cooking time considerably. However, the traditional overnight soaking is not needed if the beans are placed in water, heated to boiling and the boiling maintained for at least 2 minutes, then set aside to soak for at least an hour. The initial boiling rapidly softens the seed coats so that water may penetrate more readily.

2. If hard water is used in cooking, it will take much longer for the legumes to cook because the calcium and magnesium in hard water combine with pectin in the peas or beans and render them tough. The remedy is to add not more than ⅛ to ¼ teaspoon (*0.6 to 1.3 ml*) of baking soda per cup of legumes to the cooking water. Also, such acid ingredients as tomato sauce and vinegar should not be added until the peas or beans have become tender.

3. Most legumes can be made tender by pressure cooking for 10 to 15 minutes, if the pressure is allowed to fall without allowing the steam to escape. Pressure cooking has not usually been recommended because certain legumes generate considerable foam which may plug the vent on the cooker. However, the addition of about a teaspoon or so of oil or melted fat reduces foaming greatly.

4. Whenever feasible, at least small amounts (1 oz or more) of cheese, eggs, fish, meat, milk (1 glass per meal), or poultry should be served with cooked legumes since ½ cup (*120 ml*) or more of the latter are required to furnish an amount of protein equivalent to only 1 oz (*28 g*) of meat. (Adults require a minimum daily protein intake which is equivalent to that in 8 oz of meat.) Most legumes go well with most animal foods when appropriate seasoning is used.

5. Strict vegetarians who eat no animal products (vegans) need to keep track of their protein intake so as to be certain that they get enough, because most plant foods are low in protein. (However, legume flours are high in protein.) Therefore, vegans should eat from 1½ to 2 times as much legumes per meal as a person who eats some animal foods. For example, ¾ cup (*180 ml*) of cooked legumes furnishes about 11 to 13 g of protein. This would need to be supplemented with at least 1½ cups (*360 ml*) of cooked cereal product or 3 to 4 slices of bread to insure that the meal contained sufficient protein. Also, the breads used by vegans should either (1) contain plenty of nuts and/or soy flour; or (2) be eaten with peanut butter or mashed cooked bean spreads (homemade or commercial bean dips are suitable).

• **Sprouting legume seeds**—Using sprouted seed adds considerably to the dietary intake of vitamins with few added calories because much of the food energy stored in a seed is used up during the growth of the embryonic plant. Also, extra vitamins are synthesized by the seed when the embryo starts to grow. Therefore, it is noteworthy that a dormant seed usually starts sprouting when it has absorbed sufficient water to allow a stepping up of its metabolism. Directions for sprouting seeds follow.

1. Purchase seeds that are guaranteed to sprout. Most health food stores now carry alfalfa seeds for sprouting. Some also sell viable mung bean seeds and soybean seeds. It is not wise to use seeds intended for planting as food because they may have been treated with one or more chemical agents used to prevent fungus diseases.

2. Use only unbroken seeds, and soak them overnight in an amount of water at least four times as great as the seeds. After soaking, drain off water through a strainer. Place seeds in a special sprouter, or in a wide-mouthed jar or a tray. Cover with wet paper toweling. Rinse seeds in a strainer three or four times a day, and replace paper towels. Sprouts should be sufficiently developed for use after 3 to 4 days.

3. Fresh sprouts may be used in salads, sandwiches, soups, stews, casseroles, and baked goods. Generally, seeds yield six or more times their original weight in sprouts. Sprouts have only about ½ the solids content of cooked beans or peas. Hence, one has to eat from 1 to 1½ cups

(360 ml) of sprouts to obtain the amount of protein furnished by about ½ cup (120 ml) of cooked dried beans. However, the sprouts furnish fewer calories, but more vitamins per gram of protein.

CAUTION: Deleterious substances of various kinds are present in some legumes eaten by people; among them, the trypsin inhibitor, and the following toxins: cyanogenetic glucosides, saponins, alkaloids, goitrogenic factors, hemagglutinins (substances which agglutinate red cells and destroy them) and the unknown toxic factor which produces lathyrism. Further research on many of these substances is needed. And consumption of certain legumes should be limited to nontoxic species or to those where toxicity can be eliminated or reduced to safe limits by appropriate preparation and cooling. But present knowledge suggests that most of these substances are present only in raw grain and are eliminated by ordinary methods of preparation; e.g., adequate soaking and boiling. There is no existing evidence, for example, that poisoning by cyanogens has ever occurred in human beings as a result of eating cooked legumes, or that goitrogenic substances in legumes have caused goiter. Two toxic substances in certain legumes are, however, of special importance; namely, the factor in lathyrus pea (Lathrus sativus) which causes the disease lathyrism, and the hemolytic factor in broad bean (Vicia faba) associated with the disease favism.

Consumers should be aware of the potentially harmful substances present in certain legumes so that there will be proper preparation. To the latter end, the major antinutritional and toxic factors in certain legumes are presented in Table L-1.

TABLE L-1
ANTINUTRITIONAL AND/OR TOXIC FACTORS WHICH MAY BE PRESENT IN CERTAIN LEGUMES

Type of Factor(s)	Effect of Factor(s)	Method(s) of Counteracting Undesirable Factor(s)	Legumes Containing the Factor(s)
Antivitamin factors: Antivitamin A	Interfere with the actions of certain vitamins. Lipoxidase oxidizes and destroys carotene (provitamin A).	Roasting at 212°F (100°C) or higher.	Soybeans.
Antivitamin B-12	Increases requirement for vitamin B-12.	Heating.	Soybeans.
Antivitamin D	Causes rickets unless extra vitamin D is provided.	Autoclaving (pressure cooking).	Soybeans.
Antivitamin E	Damage to the liver and muscles.	Heat treatment (only partially effective).	Alfalfa, Common beans (Phaseolus vulgaris), Peas (Pisum sativum).
Cyanide-releasing glucosides	An enzyme in legumes causes the release of hydrocyanic acid (a cellular toxin) from the otherwise inert glucoside. The toxic factor may also be released by an enzyme in E. coli a normal inhabitant of the human intestine.	Soaking and cooking the beans releases much of the toxic factor. The E. coli population of the human intestine may be reduced by encouraging the growth of Lactobacilli species, which are present in fermented dairy products (sour milk, yogurt, etc.).	All legumes contain at least small amounts of these factors. However, certain varieties of lima beans (Phaseolus lunatus) may contain much larger amounts.
Favism factor	Causes the breakdown of red blood cells in susceptible individuals only (some of the people with ancestors from the Mediterranean, Taiwan, and various parts of Asia). Other people are not affected.	Avoidance of fava beans by people who are susceptible to this type of hemolytic anemia. Some of the more sensitive people are even affected by inhalation of the pollen from the bean flower.	Fava beans (Vicia faba)
Gas-generating carbohydrates	Certain indigestible carbohydrates are acted upon by gas-producing bacteria in the lower intestine.	Much of the indigestible carbohydrates may be broken down by (1) soaking and cooking (and discarding the water after each step); (2) acid treatment, followed by incubation; or (3) fermentation and sprouting.	Many species of mature dry legume seeds, but not peanuts. The immature (green) seeds contain much lower amounts.
Goitrogens	Interfere with the utilization of iodine by the thyroid gland. As a result, the thyroid gland may become enlarged (forms a goiter).	Heat treatment is partially effective. However it is a good idea to provide extra dietary iodine when large amounts of peanuts and/or soybeans are consumed.	Peanuts and Soybeans.
Inhibitors of trypsin	The inhibitor(s) binds with the digestive enzyme trypsin. As a result, the pancreas may become overworked as it attempts to produce additional enzyme. Normally, the secretion of adequate trypsin acts as a feedback to prevent excessive secretion of pancreatic enzymes.	Heat treatment (soaking, followed by steaming, pressure cooking, extrusion cooking); fermentation; or sprouting.	All legumes contain trypsin inhibitors to some extent.
Lathyrogenic neurotoxins	Consumption of the lathyrogenic legumes in large quantities (¼ or more of the total diet) for long periods (several months) results in severe neurological disorders.	Dehulling, then soaking overnight and steaming or roasting.	Lathyrus pea (L. sativus), which is grown mainly in India. Common vetch (Vicia sativa) may also be lathyrogenic.
Metal binders	These factors bind certain essential minerals (such as copper, iron, manganese, and zinc) so that they are not well utilized by the body.	Heat treatment.	Soybeans, Peas (Pisum sativum)
Red blood cell clumping agents (hemagglutinins)	The agents cause the red blood cells to clump together.	Soaking followed by heat treatment.	Occurs in all legumes to some extent.

It may be seen from Table L-1 that various types of heat treatment inactivate most of the antinutritional and toxic factors in legumes. However, heating has no effect on the favism-producing factor in fava beans. Hence, people troubled with favism should avoid eating the offending beans. Those who tolerate gassiness (flatulence) poorly would be better off eating only immature (green) beans or mature beans which have been specially treated.

The most effective detoxifying treatment for the home preparation of beans is soaking until the legumes begin to swell, discarding the water and covering with fresh water, then cooking them until tender. Also, some researchers have found that pressure cooking prior to grinding them into flour or meal inactivates most of the potentially harmful substances. Finally, it is noteworthy that various types of fermentation, which have been utilized by Asian peoples for centuries, are also means of detoxifying legumes.

NUTRITIONAL VALUE.

Seeds such as those of the common food legumes are good sources of certain nutrients, because they are storehouses of the carbohydrates, fats, proteins, minerals, and vitamins needed to sustain the embryonic plant until it has developed sufficiently to take care of its own needs. The nutritive composition of common legumes is given in Food Composition Table F-21.

Some noteworthy observations regarding the nutrient composition of legumes follow:

1. The items lowest in calories are those with the highest water content. Hence, weight watchers may eat their fill of cooked snap beans (92.4% water and 25 kcal per 100 g), but they should curtail their consumption of roasted, salted peanuts (1.6% water and 585 kcal per 100 g). However, it is noteworthy that the high caloric value of the latter item is also due to a high fat content, since defatted peanut flour is much lower in energy content (371 kcal per 100 g).

2. A 100 g portion (approximately ½ cup) of most types of cooked mature dry beans supplies between 100 and 130 Calories (kcal) and an average of about 7 g of protein, which is about the same as the amount of protein in 1 oz (28 g) of cooked lean meat. However, the quality of protein in legumes is somewhat lower than that of meat and other animal proteins.

3. Sprouted seeds supply more protein per calorie than unsprouted seeds because much of the stored carbohydrate is metabolized for energy during sprouting, whereas little protein is used for this purpose. For example, cooked sprouted soybeans contain 13.9 g of protein per 100 kcal, whereas cooked unsprouted soybeans contain only 8.4 g of protein per 100 kcal.

4. Defatted peanut flour and defatted soybean flour each contain almost 50% protein. Hence, small amounts of these products make major protein contributions when added to cereal flours, which contain only about 8 to 15% protein.

5. The various soybean flours are good sources of calcium and iron, although the beany flavor sometimes limits the amounts which may be used in certain foods.

6. All of the legumes are good to excellent sources of iron, potassium, thiamin, riboflavin, and niacin.

7. Immature cowpea (black-eyed pea) pods and seeds are the best legume sources of vitamins A and C, which are lacking in the mature dry seeds.

8. Cooked pigeon peas are high in fiber, which might be beneficial to people bothered with chronic constipation and certain other disorders. Some researchers have reported that the consumption of fibrous legumes lowers blood cholesterol significantly, even when substantial amounts of animal fats are consumed with the legumes.

Additional information on certain nutritional and antinutritional aspects of legumes are given in the sections which follow.

Protein Quantity and Quality. There is much current worldwide interest in the value of legumes as major sources of dietary protein because (1) the prices of meat and other animal products are rising rapidly, and (2) certain densely populated developing countries lack sufficient land to raise large numbers of animals for meat. Therefore, certain facts regarding protein quantity and quality of legumes are noteworthy:

1. Cooked legumes furnish less protein per gram, and per calorie than low and medium fat types of cheeses, eggs, fish, meats, and poultry. For example, 3½ oz (100 g) of cooked common beans supplying 118 Calories (kcal) are required to provide the protein in 1 oz (28 g) of cooked lean meat (55 kcal) or medium-fat meat (78 kcal). Also, the protein quality of the legumes is lower than that of the animal foods.

2. The proteins in legumes are moderately deficient in the sulfur-containing amino acids methionine and cystine. However, the importance of this problem has been exaggerated somewhat, because tests of protein quality are usually conducted with rats, which have a higher requirement for these amino acids than people. The feeding of a little extra protein from legumes usually insures that adequate amounts of the deficient amino acids are provided.

3. Mixtures of legumes and cereals have a protein quality which comes close to that of meat, milk, and other animal proteins. The highest protein quality is usually achieved in mixtures comprised of 50% legume protein and 50% cereal protein because the amino acid patterns of the two types of foods complement each other. Some examples of food combinations utilizing this principle are corn tortillas and refried beans, baked beans and brown bread, peanut butter sandwiches, and macaroni products fortified with soy protein.

4. Cooked legumes contain from 2 to 4 times the protein of most cooked cereals. For example, a cup of cooked dried legumes (approximately 200 g) supplies from 10 to 20 g of protein, whereas a cup of cooked cereal (150 g - 250 g) provides from 3 to 7 g of protein. Also, more calories (about 50% more) are supplied by the legumes.

5. Legumes may be used to upgrade the protein quantity and quality of diets based mainly on cereals and/or starchy foods such as bananas, cassava, and sweet potatoes. The latter foods are the mainstays of people in the developing tropical regions. For example, a protein-enriched flour or meal may contain about 15% defatted peanut or soybean flour or meal, and about 85% of cereal product made from corn, rice, or wheat. Highly starchy diets may be upgraded considerably by mixing 20% defatted legume flour with 80% starchy food. For example, one of the first attempts to rehabilitate African children suffering from protein-calorie malnutrition utilized a mixture of soybean flour and bananas.

6. Animal protein foods may be extended by the use of legumes. Some approximate *equations* of protein value follow:

a. 1 frankfurter + ½ cup cooked beans = 2 frankfurters

b. 10% legume flour + 5% skim milk powder + 85% cereal flour = 10% skim milk powder + 90% cereal flour

Both examples show that the requirement for expensive animal protein may be halved by the judicious use of legume products. However, it should be noted that the substitution of legumes for animal foods may raise the caloric value of the diet.

LEGUMES OF THE WORLD.

About a dozen species account for the greater part of the world's legume production. Additionally, many luguminous food plants with only minor roles in commercial food production at the present time have the potential to become important food crops. Also, most of these lesser known species thrive in subtropical and tropical areas where most of the world's impoverished people live. Table L-2 gives pertinent information relative to the legumes of the world. Additionally, the most important legumes are accorded narrative status, alphabetically, in this book.

NOTE WELL: Where production figures are given in Table L-2, Legumes of the World, in column 2 under "Importance," unless otherwise stated, they are based on 1990 data. Most world figures are from *FAO Production Yearbook 1990*, FAO/UN, Rome, Italy, Vol. 44. Most U.S. figures are from *Agricultural Statistics 1991*. Annual production fluctuates as a result of weather and profitability of the crop.

Although beans are often classed as vegetables, especially those that are used as immature green pods (snap beans, or green beans), all beans are legumes. So, in order to avoid double listing, the species of beans commonly used in the United States are listed and summarized in Table L-2, Legumes of the World.

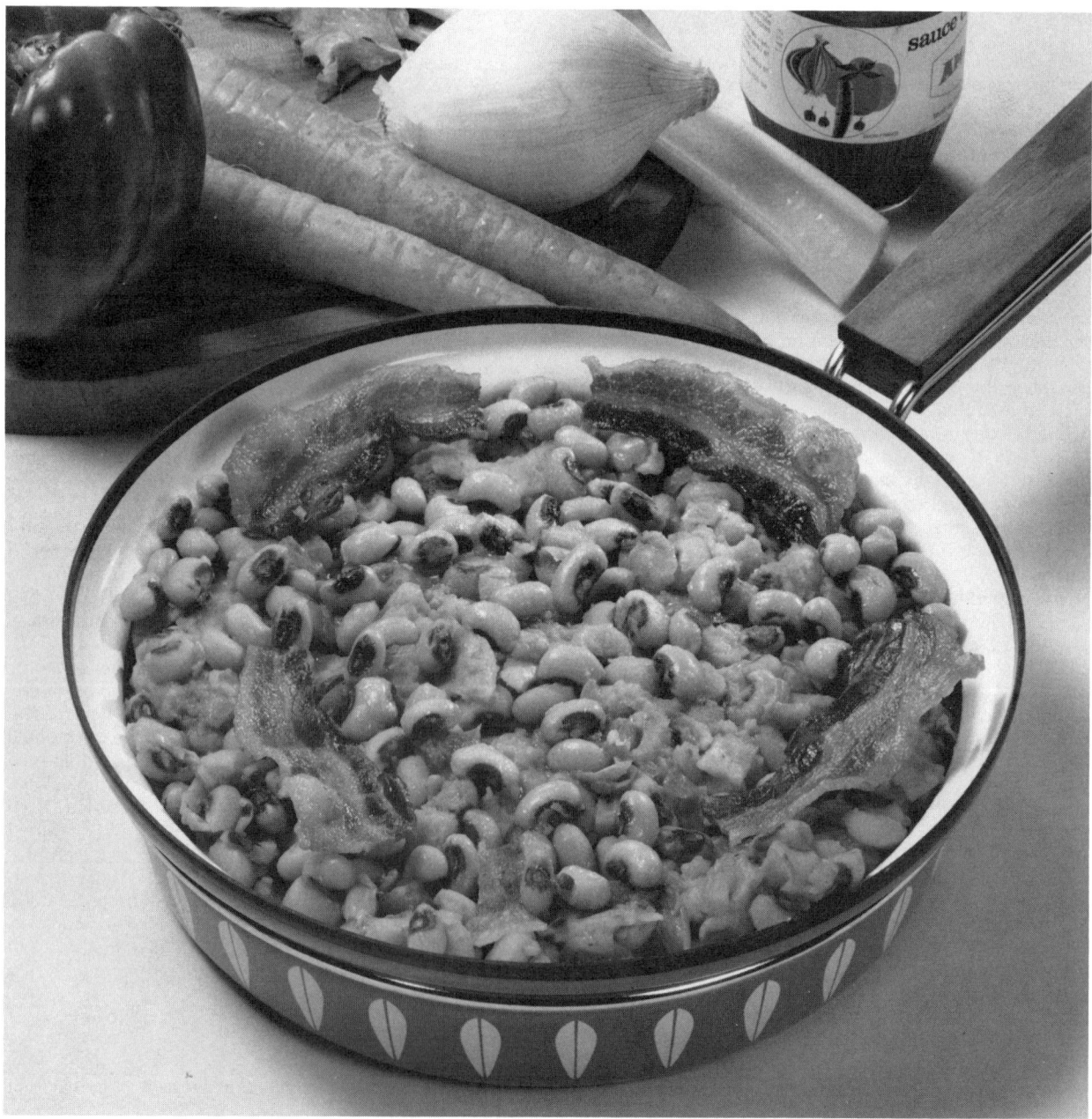

Fig. L-10. Cowpeas (black-eyed peas) used in an entree. Mixtures of legumes and cereals have a protein quality close to that of animal proteins. (Courtesy, California Dry Bean Advisory Board, Dinuba, Calif.)

TABLE L-2
LEGUMES OF THE WORLD

Popular and Scientific Name(s); Origin and History	Importance; Principal Areas; Growing Conditions	Processing; Preparation; Uses	Nutritional Value; Caution[1,2]
Adzuki Bean[3] *Phaseolus angularis* **Origin and History:** Originated in China and Japan, where it has been cultivated for centuries. (Also see BEAN[S]; BEANS, COMMON; and ZEN MACROBIOTIC DIETS.)	**Importance:** Ranks next to soybeans among the Chinese and Japanese. Recently, became known in the U.S. as a staple food in the Zen Macrobiotic Diets. **Principal Areas:** China, Japan, and Korea. **Growing Conditions:** Temperate climate with hot humid summers.	**Processing:** Usually, the beans are picked when mature. They may be left whole or pounded into a meal. **Preparation:** Whole beans boiled, then mashed; or used as a flour. **Uses:** Vegetable dish. Bean flour is used for cakes and various desserts and sweets, and as a substitute for milk, called *kokoh*.	**Nutritional Value:** 100 g of uncooked dried beans supply 324 kcal, 21.1 g protein, 1.0 g fat, 59.5 g carbohydrate, 3.9 g fiber, 82 mg calcium, and 6.4 mg iron. Adzuki beans are low in calcium, high in phosphorus, rich in iron and potassium, and almost totally lacking in vitamins A and C.
Alfalfa (Lucerne) *Medicago saliva* **Origin and History:** Alfalfa was seeded for livestock forage in southwestern Asia long before recorded history. The Persians took it to Greece when they invaded the country in 490 B.C. From Greece, it was taken to Italy in the first century A.D. from whence it spread to other parts of Europe.	**Importance:** The most valuable hay plant of the U.S., with an estimated annual production of 83 million short tons. **Principal Areas:** U.S., Argentina, Europe, and Asia. **Growing Conditions:** Temperate climate.	**Processing:** Mature seeds are sprouted. A flour made from the dried leaves, and a protein concentrate from the juice of the fresh leaves. **Preparation:** Sprouts may be cooked or left raw. **Uses:** Sprouts, in salads, and sandwiches. Flour may be added in small amounts to various cereal products. Protein concentrate is used mainly in livestock feeds.	**Nutritional Value:** 100 g of sprouted seeds contain 41 kcal, 5.1 g protein, 0.6 g fat, 1.7 g fiber, 28 mg calcium, and 1.4 mg iron. *CAUTION:* Usually, only the sprouts are eaten by people. Sprouting counteracts the potentially harmful agents.
Bambarra Groundnut[3] *Voandzeia subterranea* **Origin and History:** Native to tropical Africa. Taken to other parts of Africa, Brazil, and the Orient in the 17th century.	**Importance:** Its use in certain regions of Africa has been replaced to a large extent by the peanut. **Principal Areas:** District of Bambarra in Mali, Zambia, and Madagascar. (All are in Africa.) **Growing Conditions:** Tropical climate.	**Processing:** This plant, like peanuts, must be unearthed for harvesting of the seeds. The hard seeds require soaking and/or breaking up into pieces prior to cooking. **Preparation:** Dry seeds are roasted. Seeds in pods are boiled. **Uses:** Vegetable dish, source of calories and protein.	**Nutritional Value:** 100 g of uncooked dried seeds contain 370 kcal, 16.0 g protein, 6.0 g fat, 65.0 g carbohydrates, 4.8 g fiber, 62 mg calcium, and 12.2 mg iron.
Bean(s) (See BEAN[S].)			
Bean, common *Phaseolus vulgaris* (See BEAN, COMMON.)			
Broad Bean (Fava Bean) *Vicia faba* **Origin and History:** Believed to have originated in northern Africa and in the eastern Mediterranean region. The Chinese used broad beans as food 5,000 years ago. It has been cultivated in various parts of southern and northern Europe (particularly the British Isles) since the Iron Age (1000 B.C.). (Also see BEAN[S]; and BEAN, COMMON.)	**Importance:** Worldwide, about 4.3 million metric tons of dry broad beans are produced annually. Broad bean is one of the leading nonoilseed legumes grown in the temperate areas of the world. However, it is a minor crop in the U.S.A. **Principal Areas:** China, Ethiopia, Egypt, and Italy. **Growing Conditions:** Thrives under temperatures ranging from 50°F *(10°C)* to 86°F *(30°C)*, but is also planted in the British Isles in the autumn or early winter, for harvesting in June or in the late summer.	**Processing:** Immature pods and seeds may be picked, or mature seeds may be harvested, shelled, and dried. **Preparation:** May be boiled, cooked in casseroles, or steamed. Immature pods may be cooked whole or sliced. **Uses:** Vegetable dish, and in casseroles, soups, and stews.	**Nutritional Value:** Mature, uncooked, dried beans are rich in calories (328 kcal per 100 g), proteins (25%), and carbohydrates (56.9%), but low in fat (1.2%). Immature beans and cooked dried beans have a high water content and much lower levels of these nutrients. However, the immature beans are a fair source of vitamin C. *CAUTION:* Contains a hemolytic anemia factor[4] which triggers favism, but which affects *only* people who have an inherited susceptibility. Other potentially harmful constituents are rendered safe by soaking and cooking, sprouting, or fermentation.
Carob (Locust Bean, St. John's Bread) *Ceratona siliqua* **Origin and History:** Originated in the eastern Mediterranean region and introduced into tropical areas around the world.	**Importance:** Appears to be increasing in importance because the seeds yield a valuable gum, and the pods provide a substitute for expensive cocoa. **Principal Areas:** Subtropics and tropics. **Growing Conditions:** Thrives in hot, dry climate.	**Processing:** First, the pods with seeds are dried in the sun. Then, the pods are ground to a powder. Seeds are crushed, roasted, and boiled in water to extract the gum. **Preparation:** The pod powder may be mixed in hot or cold water or milk to make a drink. **Uses:** Powdered pods are a substitute for cocoa. The seed gum is a food additive.	**Nutritional Value:** 100 g of the dried pod powder supply 380 kcal, 3.8 g protein, 0.2 g fat, 90.6 g carbohydrate, 5.4 g fiber, and 290 mg of calcium per 100 g. *CAUTION:* The pods are not known to contain any harmful substances, and the seed gum is generally safe in the amounts used. Seeds are rarely prepared and eaten like other legumes.
Chickpea (Garbanzo Bean)[3] *Cicer arietinum* **Origin and History:** Most likely originated in the Near East. From there its cultivation spread eastward to India, and westward throughout the countries of north Africa and southern Europe. (Also see BEAN[S]; and BEAN, COMMON.)	**Importance:** Worldwide about 6.9 million metric tons are produced annually; and chickpeas rank fifth among the legume crops of the world. **Principal Areas:** Over 70% of the crop is produced in India. Most of the remainder is grown in Turkey, Pakistan, and Mexico. **Growing Conditions:** Grows best in areas where the temperature ranges from 36°F *(2°C)* to 86°F *(30°C)*. Hence, it may be grown during the warm season in northern India, and during the cool season in the dry tropics.	**Processing:** Dehulling, then drying. In India, the dried seeds are sometimes ground into flour. **Preparation:** Boil, fry, or roast. **Uses:** Snack, vegetable dish, and in soups, salads, and stews. In India, the flour is used to make various confections.	**Nutritional Value:** Similar to the various beans in nutritional value. Hence, chickpeas are a good source of calories and protein (100 g, or about ½ cup of cooked beans supplies about 10 g of protein). Also, they are a good source of phosphorus and iron.

Footnotes at end of table

(Continued)

TABLE L-2 *(Continued)*

Popular and Scientific Name(s); Origin and History	Importance; Principal Areas; Growing Conditions	Processing; Preparation; Uses	Nutritional Value; Caution[1,2]
Cowpea (Black-eyed Pea)[3,4] *Vigna sinensis; V. unguiculata* **Origin and History:** Originated in central Africa. Brought to the West Indies and to the southeastern U.S. by African slaves. Its cultivation also spread northward to the Mediterranean and eastward to China and India.	**Importance:** A valuable crop in the subtropical and tropical areas of the world. **Principal Areas:** Africa, India, China, West Indies, and southeastern U.S. **Growing Conditions:** 68°F *(20°C)* to 95°F *(35°C).* Hence, the growing season is not long enough in northern U.S. to produce mature beans. However, the immature pods and seeds may be produced in cool, temperate climates.	**Processing:** May be picked early for immature pods. Mature beans are dried, canned, and frozen. In Africa, the dried seed may be ground before cooking. **Preparation:** Mature dried beans may be boiled or baked. Immature pods and seeds may be chopped and stir-fried with meats and other foods. **Uses:** Vegetable dish, with or without cooked pork; and an ingredient of casseroles, salads, soups, and stews.	**Nutritional Value:** 3½ oz *(100 g,* or about ⅔ cup) of the cooked, mature beans supply 76 kcal and 5 g protein. Compared with cooked, mature beans, the cooked immature seeds contain more calories (108 kcal per 100 g), protein (8%), iron (50% more), and vitamins A and C.
Fenugreek *Trigonella foenum-graceum* **Origin and History:** Originated in the Mediterranean region.	**Importance:** Widely used spice. **Principal Areas:** Southern Europe, north Africa, Egypt, and India. **Growing Conditions:** Subtropical climate.	**Processing:** Dried seeds are often ground into flour. **Preparation:** Pods may be cooked. **Uses:** Pods as a vegetable. Powdered seeds as a condiment.	**Nutritional Value:** 100 g of uncooked dried seeds contain 323 kcal, 23 g protein,6.4 g fat, and 58.4 g carbohydrate, 10.1 mg fiber, 176 mg calcium, and 34 mg iron.
Guar (Cluster Bean) *Cyanopsis tetragonoloba* **Origin and History:** Originated in India. (Also see GUMS.)	**Importance:** Source of a valuable gum. **Principal Areas:** Southeast Asia, India, Indonesia, Burma, and the U.S. **Growing Conditions:** Subtropical climate.	**Processing:** In Asia, immature pods and seeds are picked. In the U.S., the mature seeds are harvested and the gum is extracted. **Preparation:** In Asia, pods are cooked for eating. **Uses:** As a food and livestock feed in Asia. As a source of a food additive in the U.S.	**Nutritional Value:** Data not available. Most likely the composition of the immature pods and seeds is similar to that of other legumes. *CAUTION:* The mature seeds[4] are used almost exclusively for extraction of the gum, which is a safe food additive. However, the residue from extraction requires detoxification.
Hyacinth Bean (Lablab Bean)[3] *Dolichos lablab* **Origin and History:** Originated in India. Cultivated for many centuries as a food plant, and lately as an ornamental plant. (Also see BEAN(S); and BEAN, COMMON.)	**Importance:** Its drought resistance makes it valuable in the developing countries, but it is little known in the developed countries. **Principal Areas:** Southern and eastern Asia and parts of Africa. It is an important crop of India. **Growing Conditions:** Dry, tropical climate.	**Processing:** Picked when immature or mature for human consumption. In India, the mature beans are dried, and sometimes split. **Preparation:** The whole beans or the split beans are cooked. The immature pods and seeds may be prepared as a green vegetable. **Uses:** The mature beans are used primarily as cooked whole beans or cooked split seeds. The immature pods and seeds may be used like snap beans. Because of its purple flowers and attractive purplish-red pods, the hyacinth bean is sometimes used for ornamental purposes.	**Nutritional Value:** 100 g of uncooked, dried whole mature seeds supply 338 kcal, 22.2 g protein, 1.5 g fat, 61 g carbohydrate, 6.9 g fiber, 73 mg calcium, and 5.1 mg iron. The seeds are low in calcium (they contain only ⅛ as much calcium as phosphorus); and the protein quality is inferior to animal proteins (the protein is low in the amino acids methionine and cystine).
Jack Bean (Horse Bean) *Canavalia ensiformis* **Origin and History:** Native to Mexico, Central America, and the West Indies. Known for 5,000 years in Mexico. (Also see BEAN(S); and BEAN, COMMON.)	**Importance:** A minor crop grown mainly for green manure or forage. However, the dried seeds and the immature pods and seeds are eaten at times of food scarcity. **Principal Areas:** Tropical regions around the world, including the southern U.S. **Growing Conditions:** Dry, tropical climate.	**Processing:** Immature pods or mature beans may be harvested. May also be plowed under as green manure. **Preparation:** Seeds require prolonged soaking and boiling with several changes of water to soften. Immature pods are cooked in water like snap beans. **Uses:** Human food, cattle fodder, green manure. During times of food scarcity, both the immature pods and seeds and the mature seeds are used for human food.	**Nutritional Value:** 100 g of uncooked dried beans contain 348 kcal, 21.0 g protein, 3.2 g fat, 61.0 g carbohydrate, 7.6 g fiber, 134 mg calcium, and 8.6 mg iron. The dried mature beans are deficient in calcium and in the amino acids cystine and methionine. The immature beans are similar in nutrient composition to snap beans, but they are poorer sources of vitamins A and C. *CAUTION:* They may contain more antinutritional factors than occur in most legumes. Hence, prolonged soaking and thorough cooking[5] are required.
Lathyrus Pea (Grass Pea) *Lathyrus sativus* **Origin and History:** Native to southern Europe and western Asia. Excessive consumption of the seeds, which occurs in time of famine, can cause a paralyzing disease known as lathyrism. (Also see LATHYRISM.)	**Importance:** An emergency food used by the impoverished and during famines because it grows well on poor soils and is drought resistant. **Principal Areas:** India, southern Europe, and South America. **Growing Conditions:** Semitropical climate.	**Processing:** Dehusked seeds may be soaked in water, dried in the sun, then ground into flour. Sometimes the seeds are steamed and/or roasted to remove a highly toxic constituent which causes the disease lathyrism. **Preparation:** Whole seeds cooked as other legumes. Flour made into thin, unleavened cakes (chapatis) and baked. **Uses:** Human food, livestock feed, green manure.	**Nutritional Value:** 100 g of uncooked, dried whole seeds supply 348 kcal, 27.4 g protein, 1.1 g fat, 59.8 g carbohydrate, 7.3 g fiber, 127 mg calcium, and 10.0 mg iron. *CAUTION:* Contains lathyrogens, in addition to factors found in other legumes. Toxicity is counteracted by overnight soaking and thorough cooking.[5] It is *not* sufficient to bake uncooked flour products.
Lentil *Lens esculenta* (See LENTIL.)			
Lima Bean (Butter Bean) *Phaseolus lunatus* (See LIMA BEAN.)			

Footnotes at end of table

(Continued)

TABLE L-2 *(Continued)*

Popular and Scientific Name(s); Origin and History	Importance; Principal Areas; Growing Conditions	Processing; Preparation; Uses	Nutritional Value; Caution[1,2]
Lupines *Lupinus* genus **Origin and History:** There are about 200 species of lupines, most of which are native to the U.S.	**Importance:** Mainly as an emergency food because the species grows in poor soils. **Principal Areas:** Southern Europe, northern Africa, and North and South America. **Growing Conditions:** Temperate to subtropical climate, depending upon species.	**Processing:** Seeds may be treated as most other legumes, or they may be roasted and ground to make a coffee substitute. **Preparation:** Seeds are soaked in water, then boiled. **Uses:** Vegetable dish, coffee substitute, livestock feed, green manure.	**Nutritional Value:** 100 g of uncooked dried seeds furnish 407 kcal, 44.3 g protein, 16.5 g fat, 28.2 g carbohydrate, 7.1 g fiber, 90 mg calcium, and 6.3 mg iron. *CAUTION:* Some varieties contain a toxic alkaloid which is removed by soaking in water. It might also be a good idea to rinse the beans after thorough cooking,[5] and to discard the cooking water.
Mesquite[3] *Prosopis* genus **Origin and History:** Most species probably originated in the tropical areas of the Americas, where they were long used by the Indians.	**Importance:** These wild plants are usually grazed by livestock, but occasionally serve as human food. Some species grow on poor soils and withstand severe droughts. **Principal Areas:** South, Central, and North America; Africa; and other subtropical areas. **Growing Conditions:** Subtropical to tropical climate.	**Processing:** Depending upon the species, either the pods and/or the seeds may be used. Sometimes, the dried seeds may be ground into a flour. **Preparation:** Pod and/or seeds may be boiled or steamed. **Uses:** Human food, livestock feed.	**Nutritional Value:** 100 g of uncooked dried seeds contain 347 kcal, 15.4 g protein, 1.6 g fat, 75.5 g carbohydrate, 7.3 g fiber, and 421 mg of calcium. *CAUTION:* The pods and pod pulp contain large amounts of indigestible carbohydrates (fiber) which may interfere with the utilization of various nutrients.
Mung Bean (Golden Gram; Green Gram)[3] *Phaseolus aureus* **Origin and History:** Probably originated in India. (Also see BEAN[S]; and BEAN, COMMON.)	**Importance:** Important food in India and Pakistan. Used mainly for sprouting in China and U.S. **Principal Areas:** India and Pakistan. **Growing Conditions:** Does well in temperatures between 68°F (20°C) and 113°F (45°C).	**Processing:** Picked when fully mature. In India and Pakistan, the beans are dried, debranned, and ground into flour, whereas in China and the U.S., the beans are usually allowed to sprout for about 4 days. **Preparation:** Boil, or sprout for eating raw or cooked. **Uses:** Cooked beans as a vegetable dish. Sprouts in salads, soups, sandwiches, etc. In Chinese cooking, the sprouts may be stir-fried with green onions and seasoned with soy sauce.	**Nutritional Value:** 3½ oz (100 g) of the raw, sprouted beans supply 53 kcal, 4.3 g of protein, and 16 mg of vitamin C.
Pea, Field *Pisum arvense* **Origin and History:** Thought to have originated in Central Asia and Europe, with possibly secondary developments in the Near East and north Africa, as evidenced by 9,000 year-old buried seeds found in archeological sites.	**Importance:** Less important for human food than garden peas (*Pisum sativum*), except in Africa, where it has long been used as human food. **Principal Areas:** Africa, Asia, and central and northern Europe. **Growing Conditions:** Grows best at temperatures between 50°F (10°C) and 86°F (30°C). However, they may also be grown in some parts of Africa and Europe as a cold season crop. Field peas are more hardy than garden peas.	**Processing:** Shelling, followed by drying. Entire plant may be plowed under as green manure, or used as forage. **Preparation:** Boil or bake, with or without meat. Field peas do not become soft like garden peas. **Uses:** Vegetable dish, livestock feed.	**Nutritional Value:** The nutrient composition of field peas is given in Food Composition Table F-21. A 3½ oz (100 g) serving (about ½ cup) of cooked field peas provides about 103 calories (kcal) and 7 g of protein. This is about double the caloric value and approximately equal to the protein value of 1 oz (28 g) of cooked lean meat. Field peas contain less than half as much calcium as phosphorus. Peas are a good source of iron and potassium. *CAUTION:* Antivitamin E factor (the diet should contain ample vitamin E and selenium). Metal-binding factor(s). Pressure cooking[4] is more certain to eliminate this problem than boiling at normal pressure.
Pea, Garden (English pea, Green pea) *Pisum sativum* (See PEA, GARDEN.)			
Peanut (Groundnut) *Archis hypogaea* (See PEANUT.)			
Pigeon Pea[3,4] *Cajanus cajan* **Origin and History:** Probably native to Africa; now widely grown in tropical and subtropical countries, paticularly India, equatorial Africa, the East Indies, and the West Indies. African slaves took it to the Caribbean.	**Importance:** A valuable drought-resistant tropical food crop. However, the tightly adhering seed coat has an acrid taste which reduces its acceptability in certain areas. **Principal Areas:** India, Africa, Burma, Dominicam Republic, Malawi. **Growing Conditions:** Tropical climate that is moderately dry.	**Processing:** Either immature pods with seeds or mature seeds may be harvested. The latter are canned in the West Indies. In India, the seed coats are removed before preparation. **Preparation:** Cooked as other legumes. **Uses:** Human food, forage plant.	**Nutritional Value:** 100 g of uncooked dried beans furnish 342 kcal, 20.4 g protein, 1.4 g fat, 63.7 g carbohydrate, 7.0 mg fiber, 129 mg calcium, and 8.0 mg iron.
Scarlet Runner Bean[3,4] *Phaseolus coccineus* **Origin and History:** Originated in Central America or Mexico. The Indians in Mexico used it as food 9,000 years ago. (Also see BEAN[S]; and BEAN, COMMON.)	**Importance:** Popular in U.K., Asia, and Africa, for its immature pods and seeds. Mature seeds used mainly in Central America. **Principal Areas:** Temperate climate areas of Europe, Asia, Africa, and Central America (grown in the Highlands). Commercial production is limited to Great Britain. **Growing Conditions:** Needs a mild climate.	**Processing:** Immature pods and seeds are picked and cut into string beans. May be sold fresh, cooked and canned, or frozen. **Preparation:** Cook briefly in water and serve with butter or margarine. Toss with hot oil and chopped garlic (Italian style). Dried seeds are prepared like kidney beans. **Uses:** Dried seeds are used like dried kidney beans. Immature pods and seeds are used like snap beans. Also, as an ornamental plant.	**Nutritional Value:** The immature pods and beans contain over 90% water. Hence, the nutrient levels are much lower than those for mature beans. The immature pods and seeds are fair to good sources of vitamins A and C. The dried seeds are deficient in the amino acids cystine and methionine, and deficient in calcium.

Footnotes at end of table

TABLE L-2 *(Continued)*

Popular and Scientific Name(s); Origin and History	Importance; Principal Areas; Growing Conditions	Processing; Preparation; Uses	Nutritional Value; Caution[1,2]
Soybean *Glycine max* (See SOYBEAN.)			
Tamarind Tree *Tamarindus indica* **Origin and History:** Native to eastern tropical Africa; spread to India long ago. 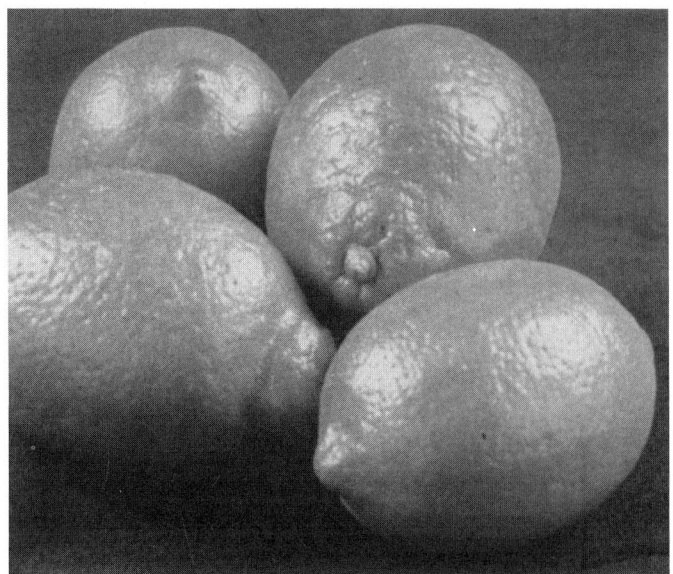	**Importance:** For a very long time, it was of limited local importance, but it may be increasing due to exporting of such products as tamarind juice. **Principal Areas:** India, Arabic countries, East Indies, and countries in the Caribbean. **Growing Conditions:** Tropical climate.	**Processing:** Pulp from ripened pods is made into juice, fruit paste, and other products. Seeds may be roasted or boiled, dehulled, and ground into a meal. **Preparation:** The pulp is usually mixed with other fruit products, because its strong flavor and acidity accentuate fruity tastes. **Uses:** Consumed fresh where produced, and exported in preserved forms (juices, pastes, etc.).	**Nutritional Value:** 100 g of dried pod pulp furnish 270 kcal, 5.0 g protein, 0.6 g fat, 70.7 g carbohydrate, 166 mg calcium, and 2.2 mg iron. *CAUTION:* The seeds should be soaked overnight and cooked thoroughly[5] like other mature legume seeds.
Tepary Bean[3] *Phaseolus acutifolius* **Origin and History:** Probably originated in Central Mexico, where it was cultivated by the Mexican Indians 5,000 years ago. It grows wild in Mexico and Arizona. (Also see BEAN[S]; and BEAN, COMMON.)	**Importance:** Not grown commercially, but still cultivated by various Indian tribes in U.S. and Mexico. It grows in areas of little rainfall. Less gas-forming than other beans. **Principal Areas:** Western Mexico and southwestern U.S. **Growing Conditions:** Hot, dry climate in tropical areas.	**Processing:** Shelling, drying. **Preparation:** Cook as other legumes. However, tepary beans absorb more water than other beans during soaking and require longer cooking time. **Uses:** Vegetable dish, in mixed meat and bean dishes.	**Nutritional Value:** 100 g of uncooked dried beans contain 353 kcal, 19.3 g protein, 1.2 g fat, 67.8 g carbohydrate, and 4.8 g fiber. *CAUTION:* Tepary beans contain less gas-forming carbohydrates than most other mature beans.
Yard-Long Bean; Asparagus Bean *Vigna unguiculata; Vigna sesquipedalis; Dolichos sesquipedalis* **Origin and History:** Thought to have originated somewhere in tropical Asia. However, the wild ancestors of cowpeas came from Central Africa over 5,000 years ago. (Also see BEAN[S]; and BEAN, COMMON.)	**Importance:** Mainly used as a food where grown. Green pods are much liked in Asia and the Americas. **Principal Areas:** Tropical parts of Asia. **Growing Conditions:** Semitropical climate.	**Processing:** Much of the crop is sold as a fresh vegetable, but some is also canned and frozen. **Preparation:** Brief cooking in water. **Uses:** Served in the same ways as snap beans.	**Nutritional Value:** The immature pods and seeds have a high water content (88.3%). Hence, a 100 g portion supplies only 37 kcal, 3.0 g protein, 0.2 g fat, 7.9 g carbohydrate, 44 mg calcium, and 0.7 mg iron. *CAUTION:* The mature seeds[4] should be treated the same as other mature beans.

[1]Refers to substances other than gas-generating carbohydrates, which are present in almost all types of mature legume seeds other than peanuts. The seeds are rendered less gassy by sprouting or fermentation.

[2]Additional details on specific antinutritional and/or toxic factors are given in the section of this article, *"CAUTION,"* and Table L-1.

[3]Much of the gassiness of these beans may be alleviated by (1) soaking and cooking (and by discarding the water after each step); (2) acid treatment, followed by incubation; or (3) fermentation and sprouting.

[4]Immature pods with seeds do not appear to contain the antinutritional factors found in the mature seeds of the same species. Hence, the green pods need only be cooked briefly.

[5]Time may be saved by pressure cooking. However, oil or melted fat should always be added to beans before cooking in a pressure cooker so that foaming is reduced. Foaming may result in the plugging of the safety valve and a buliding up of pressure which may cause the counterweight to be blown off.

LEMON *Citrus limon*

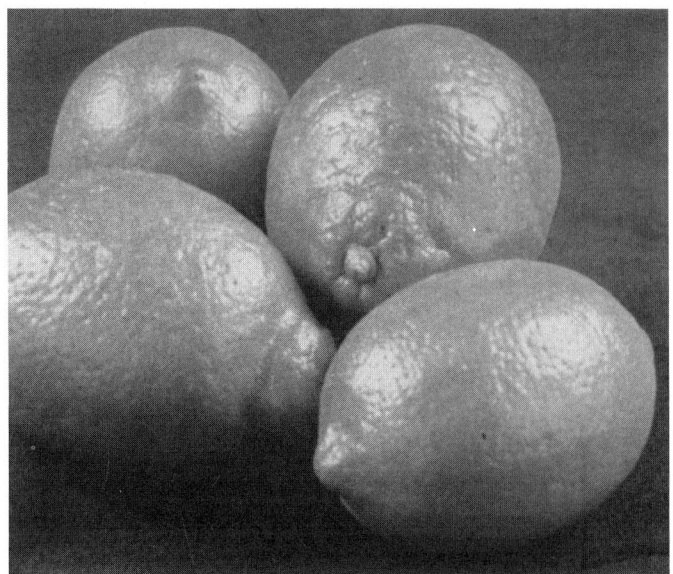

Fig. L-11. Lemons, a tangy-flavored fruit that is used to enhance the flavors of many beverages and foods. (Courtesy, USDA)

A small, yellow, oval-shaped citrus fruit. Although it is too sour to be eaten like other citrus fruits, it imparts an excellent flavor to a wide variety of beverages and other preparations. The lemon is a member of the rue family (*Rutaceae*).

ORIGIN AND HISTORY. The lemon tree is native to southeastern Asia. It was introduced in the Mediterranean area about l000 A.D. From the Mediterranean countries, it was taken to Europe, thence to the United States.

WORLD AND U.S. PRODUCTION. Worldwide, about 6.6 million metric tons of lemons and limes are produced annually; and the leading lemon-producing countries, by rank, are: United States, Mexico, Italy, Spain, India, Brazil, Iran, Argentina, Turkey, and Egypt.[3]

About 722,000 short tons of lemons are produced annually in the United States, with all the commercial production in California and Arizona. California produces 78% of the U.S. lemon crop.[4]

[3]Data from *FAO Production Yearbook 1990*, FAO/UN, Rome, Italy, Vol. 44, p. 163, Table 71. **Note well:** Annual production fluctuates as a result of weather and profitability of the crop.

[4]Data from *Agricultural Statistics 1991*, USDA, p. 189, Table 278. **Note well:** Annual production fluctuates as a result of weather and profitability of the crop.

PROCESSING. More than half of the U.S. lemon crop is processed. A major portion of the processed lemons are converted into lemon juice and related products such as frozen lemon juice concentrates, lemonade, frozen lemonade concentrates, and lemon flavored soft drinks. The peel, pulp, and seeds are used to make lemon oil, lemon essence, pectin, bioflavonoids (vitaminlike substances), and cattle feed ingredients.

SELECTION, PREPARATION, AND USES. Fresh lemons that have a fine-textured skin and are heavy for their size are generally of better quality than those that are coarse-skinned and light in weight. Deep-yellow-colored lemons are usually relatively mature and are not so acid as those of the lighter or greenish-yellow color; they are also generally thinner skinned and may have a relatively larger proportion of juice but they are not so desirable since lemons are wanted for their acid flavor.

Fresh lemons are available year long. Also they may be stored for much longer than other major citrus fruits. Lastly, lemon juice, peel, and pulp are strongly flavored so that small amounts of each of these items may be used to enhance relatively large amounts of food. Therefore, it would be worthwhile for most homemakers to use the fruit more often in their preparations. Some suggestions follow:

1. Lemon juice may be used instead of vinegar in salad dressings and sauces.

2. Squirt a little lemon juice on the cut surfaces of fresh fruits and vegetables in order to prevent them from darkening.

3. Mixtures of herbs and lemon juice may be substituted for oily, salty, and/or sugary dressings when certain types of restricted diets must be followed.

4. Lemon juice, peel, and pulp may be used to make homemade items such as candied peel, ice cream, ices, pie fillings, puddings, punches, and sherbets.

NUTRITIONAL VALUE. The nutrient compositions of various forms of lemons and lemon products are given in Food Composition Table F-21.

Some noteworthy observations regarding the nutrient composition of these items follow:

1. Fresh lemons are very low in calories (27 kcal per 100 g), and they are a good source of potassium, vitamin C, and bioflavonoids.

2. Bottled, canned, and fresh lemon juice are approximately equal to fresh lemons, except that the bioflavonoid levels may be much lower in the juices than in the fruit because most of the latter nutrient is found in the peel and the membranes of the fruit.

3. Frozen lemon juice concentrate has four times the caloric and nutrient levels of bottled, canned, or fresh lemon juice. Hence, it may make a significant nutritional contribution when added undiluted to drinks, salad dressings, and sauces. However, additional caloric or noncaloric sweetener may be needed because the pure juice concentrate is very tart.

4. Frozen lemonade concentrate contains considerable added sweetener and is 68% higher in calories (it contains 195 kcal per 100 g [3½oz]) than unsweetened frozen lemon juice concentrate. Furthermore, the lemonade concentrate contains much lower levels of potassium and vitamin C.

5. Candied lemon peel is high in calories (316 kcal per 100 g) and is low in almost all nutrients other than carbohydrates and fiber. However, it may contain significant amounts of bioflavonoids.

6. Lemon-flavored carbonated drinks consist primarily of water, sugar, and imitation or natural flavoring(s).

(Also see BIOFLAVONOIDS; CITRUS FRUITS; POTASSIUM; and VITAMIN C.)

LENHARTZ DIET

Initially, patients suffering from a bleeding peptic ulcer were sometimes offered this type of diet. It is mainly fluid; it consists of raw eggs or milk and vegetable purees fed frequently throughout the day.

(Also see MODIFIED DIETS; SIPPY DIET; and ULCERS, PEPTIC.)

LENTIL *Lens esculenta*

This appetizing legume is one of the oldest cultivated plants in the world. Fig. L-12 features both the plant and a closeup of the seed.

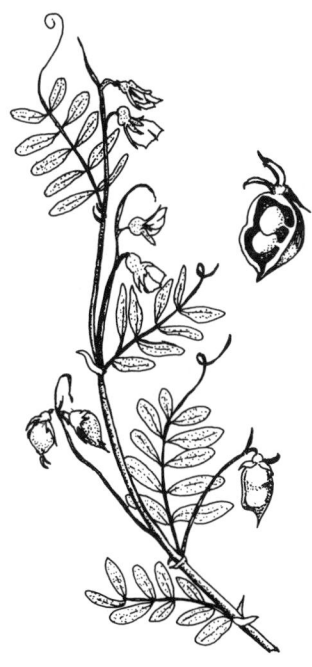

Fig. L-12. The lentil, an ancient food.

ORIGIN AND HISTORY. The lentil is indigenous to southwestern Asia, where it was cultivated 8,000 years ago. It was introduced into Greece and Egypt before Biblical times, and it was taken as far east as China. According to the Bible, Esau traded his inheritance to Jacob for some lentils.

WORLD AND U.S. PRODUCTION. Lentils rank ninth among the legume crops of the world. Worldwide, about 2.7 million metric tons of lentils are produced annually; and the leading producing countries of the world, by rank, are: Turkey, India, Canada, Bangladesh, and China. Turkey produces one-third of the world's crop of lentils.[5]

The United States produces about 40,000 metric tons of lentils annually, mostly in Washington and Idaho.[6]

---

[5]Data from *FAO Production Yearbook 1990*, FAO/UN, Rome, Italy, Vol. 44, p. 106, Table 36. **Note well:** Annual production fluctuates as a result of weather and profitability of the crop.

[6]*Ibid.*

PROCESSING.   Lentils may be marketed as whole dried seeds, split dried seeds, or as an ingredient of canned soups. Occasionally, the legume is ground into a flour and combined with cereal flour to make a protein supplement for children in the developing countries of North Africa and the Middle East.

SELECTION, PREPARATION, AND USES.   Lentils should be mature, plump, free from foreign matter, and dry.

Lentils may be boiled or stewed.

Cooked lentils go well with most other vegetables in casseroles, soups, and stews. Also, they may be used as substitutes for part or all of the more expensive animal foods such as cheeses, eggs, fish, meats, and poultry.

NUTRITIONAL VALUE.   The nutrient composition of lentils is given in Food Composition Table F-21.

Some noteworthy observations regarding the nutrient compositon of lentils follow:

1.   A 3½ oz (*100 g*) serving (about ½ cup) of cooked lentils is equivalent in protein value to 1 oz of cooked lean meat, but the legume supplies about twice as many calories.

2.   Lentils are a good source of iron, but they contain less than one-fourth as much calcium as phosphorus. Therefore, foods richer in calcium and lower in phosphorus (such as dairy products and green leafy vegetables) should be consumed to improve the dietary calcium to phosphorus ratio.

3. The substitution of lentils for animal protein foods on an equal protein basis usually results in an increase in the number of calories, whereas the replacement of cereal grains by lentils results in an increase in the amount of protein supplied per calorie.

4. The protein in lentils is quite deficient in the amino acids methionine and cystine, which are supplied amply by the protein in cereal grains. Furthermore, the grains are short of lysine, an amino acid that is present more abundantly in lentils. Therefore, the amino acid patterns of lentils and grains complement each other so that mixtures of the two foods contain higher quality protein than either one alone.

Protein Quantity and Quality.   Many of the people in India are vegetarians, so they rely heavily upon grains, lentils, and other legumes to supply much of their protein needs. (Milk and other dairy products may also be utilized, but the supply of these foods is limited.) Hence, the grams of protein per 100 Calories (kcal) provided by lentils compared to other selected foods are noteworthy:

Food	Grams of Protein per 100 Calories (kcal) (g)
Lentils	7.4
Cottage cheese	13.2
Lean meat	12.7
Eggs	8.6
Sweet corn	3.9
Brown rice	2.1

LETHARGY

Drowsiness and lack of energy.

LETTUCE *Lactuca sativa*

This vegetable is the major salad crop of the United States. Lettuce belongs to the Sunflower family (*Compositae*). Fig. L-13 shows a typical head of lettuce.

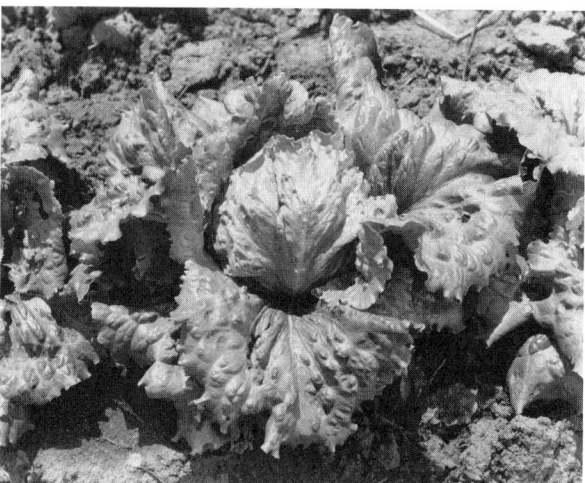

Fig. L-13. A head of the "New York" variety of lettuce. (Courtesy, J. C. Allen & Son, Inc., West Lafayette, Ind.)

ORIGIN AND HISTORY.   Lettuce is thought to have originated in Asia Minor from wild lettuce. It was popular with pre-Christian people, having appeared on the royal tables of Persian Kings as long ago as 550 B.C.

WORLD AND U.S. PRODUCTION.   Although lettuce is grown over a wide area, it is of lesser importance worldwide than many other vegetables.

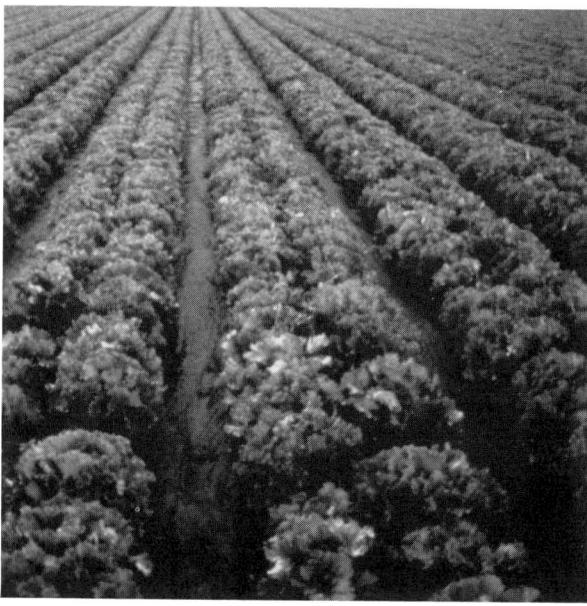

Fig. L-14. Field of mature Iceberg lettuce, ready for harvest. (Courtesy, California Iceberg Lettuce Commission, Monterey, Calif.)

Lettuce ranks fourth among the leading vegetable crops of the United States.

About 3.3 metric tons of lettuce are produced annually in the United States, 76% of which is produced in California.

The leading lettuce-producing states of the nation, by rank, are: California, Arizona, Florida, and Colorado.[7]

PROCESSING. Lettuce is processed to a very limited extent, since it cannot be frozen or heated without becom-

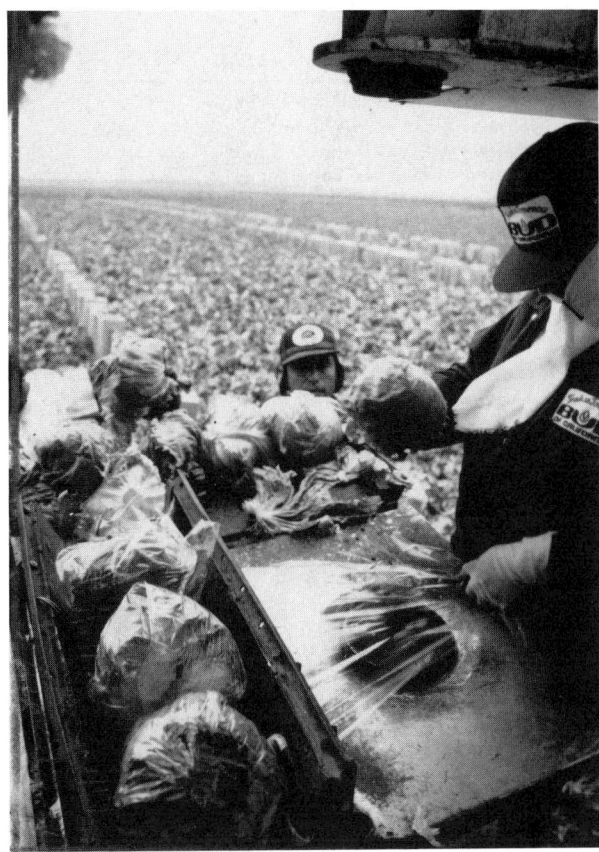

Fig. L-15. Harvested lettuce field—wrapped in a cello wrapper being packed in cardboard boxes, following which, it well be picked up and delivered to a centrally located vacuum-cooling unit. (Courtesy, California Iceberg Lettuce Commission, Monterey, Calif.)

ing limp and losing much of its appeal. However, the demand for ready-to-use shredded lettuce by many food service establishments has led to the production of prepacked shredded lettuce. This product is made from the freshly harvested vegetable by coring, shredding, cooling, and washing. The shredded lettuce is then packed in plastic bags that are shipped in styrofoam containers to prevent damage during transit.

SELECTION, PREPARATION, AND USES. Consumers are more likely to get the best buy if they know something about (1) the types of lettuce marketed in their locality, and (2) the indicators of quality.

Most of the varieties of lettuce sold in the United States fall into one of the types shown in Fig. L-16.

Good quality lettuce should be clean, crisp, and tender. The heads of crisp-head lettuce should be fairly firm to firm.

The enjoyment of lettuce dishes may be enhanced by keeping lettuce as fresh as possible until it is served.

[7]Data from *Agricultural Statistics 1991*, USDA, p. 155, Table 219. **Note well:** Annual production fluctuates as a result of weather and profitability of the crop.

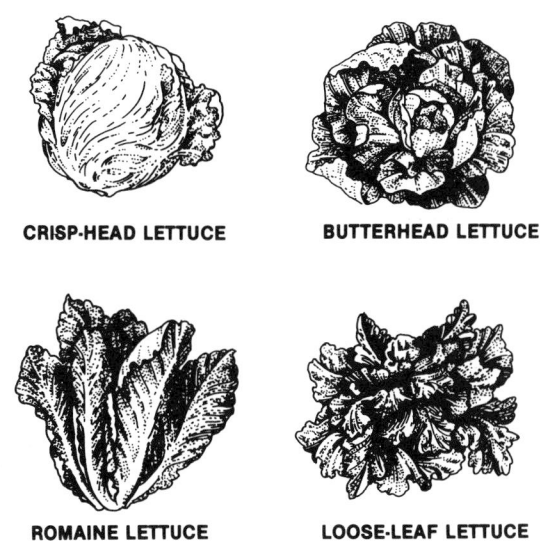

CRISP-HEAD LETTUCE   BUTTERHEAD LETTUCE

ROMAINE LETTUCE   LOOSE-LEAF LETTUCE

Fig. L-16. The four main types of lettuce grown in the United States.

Maximum meal pleasure and nutritional benefits may be obtained by utilizing the principles that (1) lettuce is a low-calorie food which goes well with cheese, eggs, fish and seafood, grains and cereal products, legumes, meats, nuts, poultry, and other vegetables; and (2) the larger the quantity of lettuce used, the more likely it will be that hunger will be satisfied and the digestive system stimulated to optimal functioning by the abundant water and gentle bulk provided by this vegetable. Fig. L-17 shows an appetizing and nutritious lettuce dish.

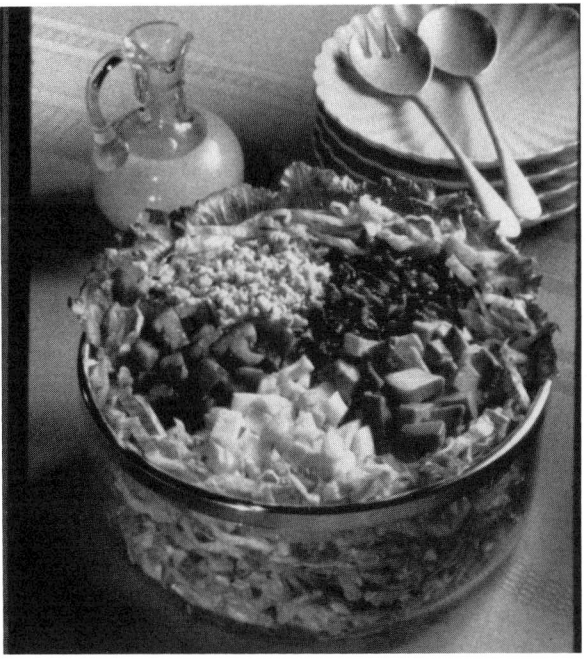

Fig. L-17. An appetizing and nutritious lettuce salad. (Courtesy, Iceberg Lettuce Commission, Monterey, Calif.)

Some appetizing ways of serving lettuce are: (1) as a salad, or as an ingredient of a salad (lettuce is by far the most commonly used salad green in the United States); (2) as a pocket bread sandwich; (3) as broiled prawns and cherry tomatoes on a lettuce raft; (4) as stir-fried; (5) as a wilted salad in which a hot dressing is poured over the raw vegetable, and (6) as cream of lettuce and minestrone soups.

NUTRITIONAL VALUE. The nutrient composition of the major types of lettuce are given in Food Composition Table F-21.

Some noteworthy observations regarding the nutrient composition of lettuce follow:

1. All types of lettuce have a high water content (94 to 96%) and are low in calories (13 to 18 kcal per 100 g). Therefore, a 1-lb (*454 g*) head of iceberg lettuce furnishes only about 56 Calories (kcal). Hence, people trying to cut their caloric intake in order to lose weight may assuage their hunger pangs by eating large quantities of this vegetable.

2. The darker the green color of lettuce, the richer it is likely to be in nutrients. For example, the butterhead, loose-leaf, and romaine types contain significantly more iron and vitamin A than the crisp-head type. Also, it is noteworthy that romaine lettuce contains about 10 times as much folic acid as the other types. Although each of the four types is only a fair source of vitamin C, lettuce may make a significant contribution of this vitamin to the diet if sufficiently large quantities are consumed.

LEUCINE

One of the essential amino acids.
(Also see AMINO ACID[S].)

LEUKEMIA

A malignant condition, a blood cancer, wherein there is uncontrolled production of abnormal white blood cells, leukocytes. These are produced in the bone marrow, spleen, and lymph tissues. Blood concentrations of leukocytes may increase a hundredfold. There are several forms of the disease, the exact causative factors of which are unknown. However, excessive radiation, certain chemicals, heredity, and hormonal abnormalities have been implicated. New techniques employed to combat leukemia have greatly increased a patient's chances of complete remission. During treatment, a supportive diet should be given which is higher than normal in energy and nutrient content and which is acceptable and appetizing.

(Also see CANCER.)

LEVULOSE

It is another name for fructose, fruit sugar. It is levoratatory (turning to the left) to polarized light; hence, the name levulose. Levulose, which is much sweeter than cane sugar, is found in honey, ripe fruits, and some vegetables.

(Also see CARBOHYDRATE[S]; and FRUCTOSE.)

LICORICE

Licorice is a herb, the root of which produces a flavoring that is used to flavor candy, chewing gum, and soft drinks.

Caution: Licorice raises the blood pressure of some people dangerously high, due to the retention of sodium.

LIEBERKUHN'S CRYPT

Tubular glands located in the mucous membrane of the small intestine, named after Johann Lieberkuhn, German anatomist, who first described them. Now they are simply called intestinal glands. They secrete intestinal juices.

(Also see DIGESTION AND ABSORPTION.)

LIFE EXPECTANCY AND NUTRITION

Contents   Page

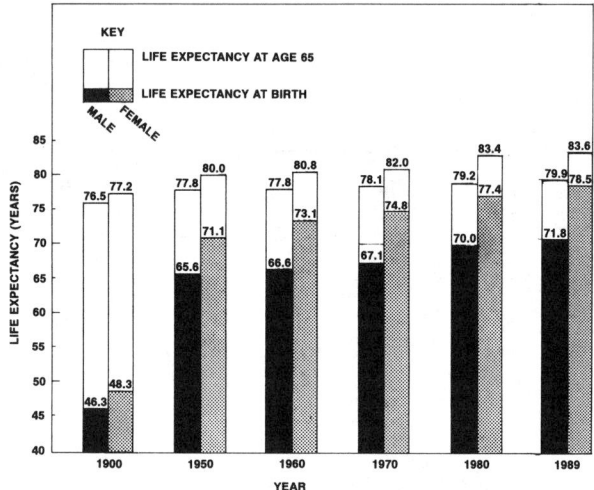

Fig. L-18. Life expectancies in the United States from 1900 to 1989. (Source: *Health, United States 1979*, U.S. Dept. HEW, p. 90, Table 9; and *Statistical Abstract of the United States 1991*, p. 73)

The great increase in life expectancy at birth has been due mainly to the control of many of the infectious diseases that formerly killed many infants and children. Therefore, researchers are now trying to identify the factors that may increase the life expectancies of older people by substantial amounts.

WELL-KNOWN STUDIES OF HEALTH AND LONGEVITY. Certain studies are referred to frequently in the popular and scientific literature on longevity. Hence, details of some of the better known observations follow.

Experiments with Laboratory Animals. In the early 1930s, Dr. Clive McKay of Cornell University succeeded in doubling the life expectancy of laboratory rats by drastically restricting their diets from after weaning to death. Furthermore, the incidence of tumors in the restricted rats was much lower than normal. However, the rats given the stringent diets failed to grow and develop at the normal rate and had an increaseed susceptbility to diseases and death early in their lifespan. These drawbacks make it unlikely that similar measures will be applied deliberately to people, although it has been suggested that very rigorous conditions of life in certain parts of the world have similar effects on human populations. That is, the more vulnerable people die young, while those with unusually strong constitutions live to ripe old ages.

Observations of Human Populations. The longest-lived peoples of the world are believed to be those that live in the geographic areas depicted in Fig. L-19. Descriptions of the people shown in Fig. L-19 follow:

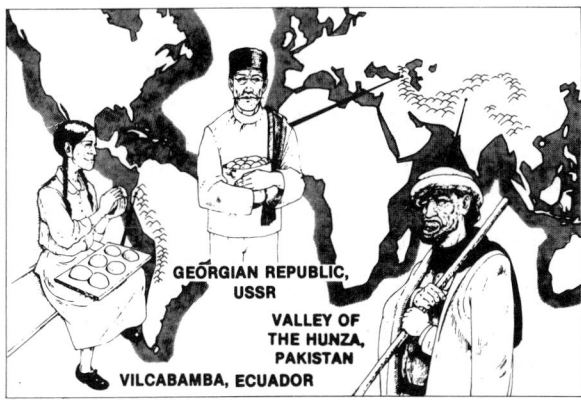

Fig. L-19. The locations where some people of apparently great longevity are found.

• **Ecuadorians of Vilcabamba**—These people live in a village that is located at an elevation of 4,600 ft (*1,400 m*) in the Andes mountains of southern Ecuador. They are reputed to live as long as 125 years, although this belief is now being questioned due to the fact that many people take the names of their parents and other close relatives. Hence, it is difficult to determine whether the names listed in the baptismal records of the local church are those for people that are now alive, or those that are deceased. Nevertheless, the older people in this village appear to be sufficiently vigorous and healthy to engage in a primitive type of farming. Furthermore, they have to contend with a mountainous terrain that makes getting about a test of physical fitness. Their caloric intake is low and they eat mainly vegetables because animal foods are scarce in their region. Most Vilcabambans drink moderate amounts of a rumlike alcoholic beverage called zuhmir, and they smoke.

• **Georgians of the Soviet Union**—Gerontologists have long thought that these people had the longest lives known to man, since some were once thought to be at least 150 years old. However, the Russian gerontologist Zhores Medvedev believes that the advanced ages may be gross exaggerations which started in the early 1900s as a means of avoiding military service under the Czars. Even if the reports of the advanced ages prove to be false, the fitness of the people and the scarcity of degenerative diseases in this region provide ample testimony to the benefits of a varied diet and strenuous exercise. The Georgians eat dairy products, meats, plenty of vegetables, and some sweets such as halvah. Many also drink and smoke. Apparently, the potential ill effects of the latter vices are offset by the heavy work on the farms.

• **Hunzas of Pakistan**—There are few American enthusiasts for health foods who have not heard of these people in the Karakorum Mountains (the western end of the Himalayas) in the northeastern part of Pakistan. Now, it appears that the reports of exceptional health and longevity of these people have been less than accurate, since a Japanese medical team found many cases of cancer, heart disease, and tuber-

culosis, and little evidence to confirm exceptional longevity.[8] Furthermore the death rates for the younger generations were quite high, since 30% of the children died before age 10, and 10% of the survivors died before 40. Therefore, it appears that the sprightly Hunza oldsters observed by the seekers of the secrets of longevity represented the hardiest of the group, who were endowed with exceptional ability to adapt to primitive conditions.

Even if it should be impossible to extend the human lifespan much beyond 100 years, it would still be a great achievement to cut the incidences of the major degenerative diseases drastically, so that more people might live healthier and longer lives. Hence, the groups of people who have lower-than-normal rates of these diseases are noteworthy.

• **Bulgarians**—In the early 1900s, the Russian microbiologist Elie Metchnikoff promoted the consumption of the yogurt bacteria *Lactobacillus bulgaricus* because he observed that the yogurt-consuming Bulgarians appeared to have healthier and more long-lived people than the other groups he studied. Furthermore, he theorized that the *Lactobacillus* organisms prevented the growth of undesirable toxin-producing species of bacteria in the intestine. Many other scientists of that era scoffed at Metchnikoff's ideas, but recent studies have yielded evidence that supports some of his concepts.[9] For example, the feeding of *Lactobacilli* has been beneficial to (1) infants afflicted with diarrhea induced by pathogenic microorganisms, and (2) people suffering from ammonia toxicity due to liver failure. In the latter case, intestinal bacteria convert urea that is present in digestive secretions to ammonia which is then absorbed into the blood. Normally, the liver converts excess ammonia to urea, but in liver failure the ammonia accumulates in toxic amounts. *Lactobacilli* reduce the buildup of ammonia.

• **Longshoremen in San Francisco**—A 22-year study (from 1951 to 1972) of 3,686 longshoremen revealed that those who performed heavy work (that requiring an average of 1,876 Calories [kcal] per day above the BMR) had a much lower risk of a fatal heart attack than those who performed light work which required an expenditure of about 1,066 Calories (kcal) per day over the BMR.[10]

• **Masai tribesmen of Africa**—The males of this tribe, who consume liberal amounts of cow's blood, milk, and meat, do not develop heart disease as they grow older even though atherosclerotic plaques form in their coronary arteries, because the exercise of walking about 11 miles (*18 km*) per day results in compensatory enlargement of the arteries.[11]

• **Mormons**—Various studies of these people have shown them to have a cancer death rate that is about ⅓ lower than the national average, and from ⅓ to ½ fewer deaths from

[8]Jarvis, W. T., "The Myth of the Healthy Savage," *Nutrition Today*, March-April 1981, pp. 14-22.

[9]"Interrelationships of Diet, Gut Microflora, Nutrition, and Health," *Dairy Council Digest*, July-August 1976, pp. 19-24.

[10]Paffenbarger, R.S., Jr., *et al.*, "Work-Energy Level, Personal Characteristics, and Fatal Heart Attack: A Birth-Cohort Effect," *American Journal of Epidemiology*, Vol. 105, 1977, pp. 200-213.

[11]Mann, G. V., Testimony in the hearings of the U.S. Senate Select Committee on Nutrition and Human Needs, March 24, 1977.

heart attacks.[12] Furthermore, many elderly Mormons stay active in businesses, farming, and church affairs well into their 80s and 90s. Their superior health and longevity is thought to result from factors such as (1) abstinence from alcoholic beverages, coffee and tea, habit-forming drugs, and smoking; (2) consumption of liberal amounts of whole grains, fruits and vegetables, and only moderate amounts of meat; (3) adequate physical activity and sufficient rest and recreation; (4) family unity; (5) extensive participation of the laity in church affairs; and (6) striving for high levels of occupational achievement.

• **Seventh-day Adventists**—Adventists men live an average of 6 years longer than other American men, and the women live 3 years longer than their counterparts.[13] Furthermore, the death rates of cancer, heart disease, and stroke for Adventists are only about 50 to 60% of that of other Americans. It appears that the reduced susceptibility of Adventists to degenerative diseases results from (1) abstinence from alcoholic drinks, caffeine-containing beverages, drugs, and smoking; (2) consumption of strict vegetarian (vegan) diets or lacto-ovo-vegetarian diets (those which contain milk and eggs, but no meat); (3) exercising on a regular basis; and (4) participation in the activities of their church.

PRACTICAL APPLICATIONS. The observations of the various groups of people who live full lives here and abroad provide some lessons regarding the types of health practices that promote longevity. First of all, the healthiest people usually eat a wide variety of fresh, minimally-processed foods such as meats and fish, dairy products, fruits and vegetables, and whole grain breads and cereals; and they may limit their consumption of potentially harmful items such as strong alcoholic drinks, caffeine-containing beverages, and refined fats, starches, and sugars. Furthermore, the quantities of foods consumed are sufficient to promote health and vitality, but not enough to bring on life-threatening obesity. Finally, the winners in the game of survival have harmonious relationships with their families and neighbors, and engage in moderate to vigorous levels of physical activity on a regular basis.

SELECTING FOODS. The food groups which comprise the framework of the daily food plan are: (1) bread, cereal, rice, and pasta group; (2) vegetable group; (3) fruit group; (4) milk, yogurt, and cheese group; (5) meat, poultry, fish, dry beans, eggs, and nuts group; and (6) fats, oils, and sweets. The minimum quantities indicated in the food groups form a foundation for an adequate diet, safeguarding the quantity and proportion of minerals, vitamins, and other nutrients. Many people will use more than the minimum number of servings suggested in each food group; and everyone will add some sugars, fats, and oils during food preparation and at the table. Perhaps a third to a half of the day's calories will come from such additions to the minimal number of servings. However, people who are overweight would be wise to limit their food selections to the basic foods in each group, and to restrict drastically their intake of sugars, fats, and oils.

PHYSICAL ACTIVITY. Regular physical activity helps to utilize dietary calories and prevent obesity, and imparts a good feeling. It is also useful in preventing degenerative

diseases and for rehabilitating people who contract them. For example, patients with heart disease have had their health and physical capacity improved by physical training.[14] Also, moderate to strenuous exercise performed on a regular basis helps to retard the loss of bone calcium that occurs with aging. The exercise is most effective in conjunction with adequate amounts of dietary calcium, phosphorus, and vitamin D.

CAUTION: It is wise to consult a doctor before starting strenuous activities that have not been performed recently.

LIGHT OFF-FLAVOR

In some foods, exposure to a light source creates an off-flavor. Light provides the energy for a chemical change which creates the undesirable odor. These chemical changes due to light are known to occur in fats, milk, and beer, and, depending upon the product, they may have a special name such as light-struck flavor in milk and sunlight off-flavor or skunky in beer.

LIGNIN

A practically indigestible compound which along with cellulose is a major component of the cell wall of certain plant foods, such as very mature vegetables.
(Also see FIBER.)

LIMA BEAN (BUTTER BEAN) *Phaseolus lunatus*

This bean is believed to have been named after Lima, Peru, the area where it was first cultivated. It belongs to the family *Leguminosae*. The beans may be picked while still immature and green for use as *baby* limas, or when fully mature. Fig. L-20 shows the beans at various stages of growth.

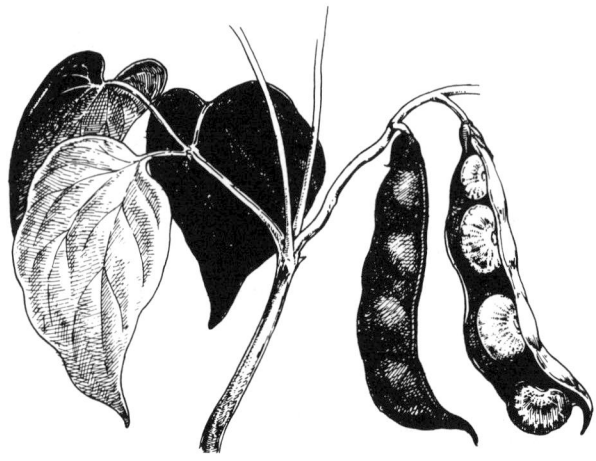

Fig. L-20. Lima beans, flowers and seeds.

ORIGIN AND HISTORY. The lima bean is native to Peru, where there is archeological evidence that it was first cultivated about 3800 B.C. It was spread throughout the Americas and the West Indies by the Indians; and it was taken to Europe by the Spanish explorers.

[12]Davidson, B., "What Can We Learn About Health from the Mormons?", *Family Circle,* July 1976.

[13]Walton, L. R., et al., *How You Can Live Six Extra Years,* Woodbridge Press Publishing Company, Santa Barbara, Calif., 1981, pp. 4-7.

[14]Redwood, D. R., et al., "Circulatory and Symptomatic Effects of Physical Training in Patients with Coronary-Artery Disease and Angina Pectoris," *The New England Journal of Medicine,* Vol. 286, May 4, 1972, pp. 959-965.

WORLD AND U.S. PRODUCTION.   Lima beans are grown in temperate and subtropical areas throughout the world, although production figures are not available.

About 140,000 short tons are produced annually in the United States, largely in the coastal area of California.

PROCESSING.   Only a very small part of the green lima beans grown in the United States is marketed fresh; most of the crop is processed. About 30% of the processed beans is canned and 70% is frozen.

Dried lima beans store well without refrigeration, as long as they are kept under dry conditions and protected from pests. Therefore, they are usually stored after harvesting and either marketed or sent to processors at the most profitable time. Most of the dried beans which are processed are cooked and canned, but small amounts are also ground into flour.

SELECTION, PREPARATION, AND USES.   Fresh green limas are often marketed in their pods. Hence, the suggestions which follow are noteworthy.

The pods of good quality unshelled lima beans are well filled, clean, bright, fresh, and dark green in color.

Shelled lima beans should be plump, have tender skins, and be green or greenish-white in color.

Green limas may be prepared and served in the same ways as green peas—in casseroles, salads, soups, and stews. Usually, they are made tender by 25 to 30 minutes of cooking.

Dry limas have a mild flavor which allows them to mix well with many other foods. Also, their ample protein content makes them nutritionally valuable for extending more expensive animal protein foods such as cheeses, eggs, fish, meats, and poultry.

• **Antinutritional and toxic factors**—Many foods contain components which may be harmful under certain circumstances, especially if they have not been improved through breeding, and/or if they are not processed properly; and lima beans are no exception.

Some varieties of lima beans, such as those that are native to the Caribbean region—and which are usually colored, contain harmful levels of cyanide-releasing glucosides. In such lima seeds, an enzyme in the legume causes the release of hydrocyanic acid (a cellular toxin) from the otherwise inert glucoside. The toxic factor may also be released by the enzyme in *E. coli* bacteria, a normal inhabitant of the human intestine. Fortunately, soaking and cooking the beans releases much of the toxic principle. Also, the *E. coli* population of the human intestine may be reduced by encouraging the growth of *Lactobacilli* species, which are present in fermented dairy products (sour milk, yogurt, etc.). Nevertheless, travelers in the Caribbean region should be wary of eating colored limas.

The varieties of limas grown in the United States contain only negligible amounts of cyanide. Besides, U.S. law prohibits the marketing of lima beans that contain harmful amounts of this toxic factor.

Lima beans also contain inhibitors of trypsin, which bind the digestive enzyme trypsin; and red blood cell clumping agents (hemagglutinins), which cause the red blood cells to clump together. Soaking followed by cooking (steaming, pressure cooking, extrusion cooking), fermentation, or sprouting greatly reduce the effects of trypsin inhibitors and blood cell clumping agents.

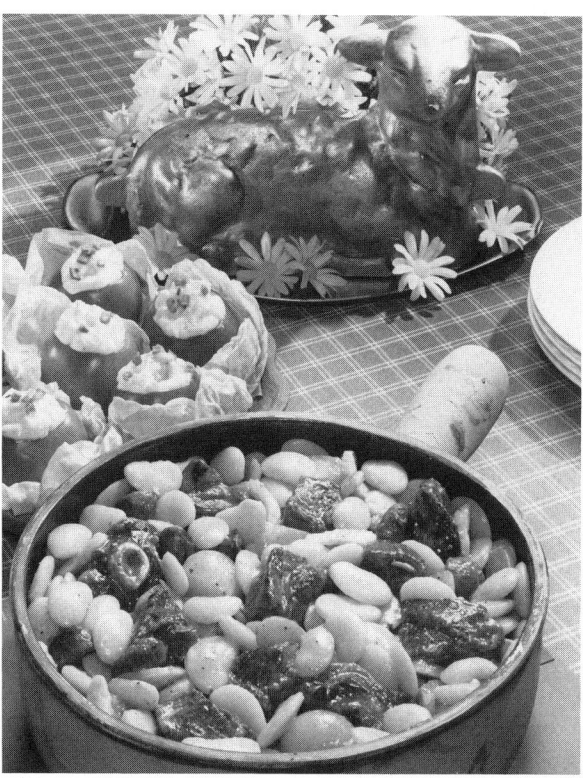

Fig. L-21. Golden limas and lamb. This casserole dish features large limas, lean lamb stew meat, celery, small white onions, carrots, fresh mushrooms, and a variety of delectable seasonings (butter or oil, garlic salt, chicken soup stock, onion salt, turmeric, white pepper, and a dash of brandy or Cognac). (Courtesy, The California Dry Bean Advisory Board, Dinuba, Calif.)

• **Gas-producing substances**—Lima beans, in common with most other mature beans, also contain gas-generating carbohydrates—certain indigestible carbohydrates which are acted upon by gas-producing bacteria in the lower intestine. Much of the indigestible carbohydrate may be broken down by incubation of the raw beans in a mildly acid solution for 1 to 2 days. However, people who are greatly troubled with gassiness (flatulence) are admonished not to eat lima beans.

NUTRITIONAL VALUE.   The nutrient composition of lima beans is given in Food Composition Table F-21.

Some noteworthy observations regarding the nutritive value of lima beans follow:

1. Cooked mature limas furnish considerably more calories, protein, carbohydrate, phosphorus, iron, and potassium than cooked immature beans (*green limas*). However, the latter are much higher in vitamins A and C. Both types of limas are low in fat.

2. One cup (*240 ml*) of cooked mature beans contains about the same amount of protein (*about 14 g*) as 2 oz (*57 g*) of lean meat, but the beans supply over three times as many calories (360 kcal vs 110 kcal).

3. Lima beans, like most other legume seeds, contain much less calcium than phosphorus. Hence, they should be eaten with foods such as milk and green leafy vegetables which have more favorable calcium to phosphorus ratios. An excessively low ratio of dietary calcium to phosphorus will result in poor utilization of calcium by the body.

4. Lima bean flour is a concentrated source of both calories and protein.

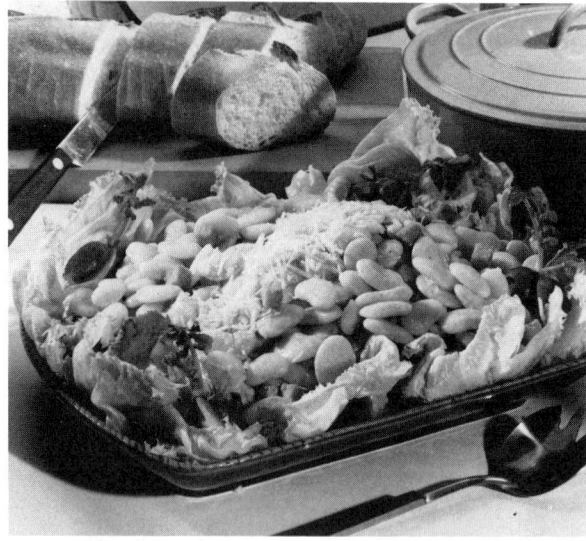

Fig. L-22. California potluck salad. An appetizing dish made from large limas, lettuce, celery, green pepper and pimiento strips, mayonnaise, pickle relish, mustard, dried dill weed, and fresh ground black pepper. (Courtesy, The California Dry Bean Advisory Board, Dinuba, Calif.)

Protein Quantity And Quality. Various types of beans are being used all over the world as protein supplements because many people consume only small amounts of animal protein. Lima beans are more acceptable in mixed dishes than many other beans because limas have a milder taste and a lighter color. Therefore, certain facts concerning the quantity and quality of protein in lima beans are noteworthy:

1. Cooked limas furnish less protein per gram of food, and per calorie than low and medium fat types of cheeses, eggs, fish, meats, milk, and poultry. For example, 3½ oz (*100 g*) of cooked green lima beans supplying 133 Calories (kcal) are required to provide the amount of protein (*about 8 g*) in 1¾ oz (*50 g*) of cottage cheese (45 kcal) or 1 large egg (82 kcal). It is noteworthy, too, that only 3 oz (*85 g*) of cooked mature limas are equivalent in calorie and protein values to 3½ oz (*100 g*) of cooked green limas.

2. Measure for measure, cooked lima beans contain from 2 to 3 times the protein of most cooked cereals. Similarly, lima bean flour provides twice as much protein per calorie as wheat flour.

3. The protein in lima beans is moderately deficient in the sulfur-containing amino acids methionine and cystine, but it contains ample amounts of lysine, which is deficient in cereal grains. Furthermore, the grains are good sources of methionine and cystine. Therefore, mixtures of the beans with cereal products have a higher quality of protein than either food alone. A good example of this type of mixture is succotash, a combination of lima beans and corn.

4. Bread made from 70% wheat flour and 30% lima bean flour contains about 40% more protein than bread made from wheat flour alone.

(Also see FLOURS, Table F-13, Special Flours.)

5. Expensive animal protein foods may be extended by replacing approximately half of the animal protein with an equivalent amount of protein from lima beans, without any significant reduction in the utilization of the dietary protein by the body. Some approximate *equations* of protein value follow:

    a. 1 frankfurter + ½ cup cooked beans = 2 frankfurters

    b. 10% lima bean flour + 5% skim milk powder + 85% cereal flour = 10% skim milk powder + 90% cereal flour.

However, the substitution of lima beans for protein rich animal foods usually results in the consumption of considerably more calories.

(Also see BEAN[S]; and BEAN, COMMON.)

LIME *Citrus aurantifolia*

A rounded fruit that is pointed at both ends and greener than the lemon. The juice of this fruit is used in various refreshing beverages. Limes, like the other citrus fruits, belong to the rue family (*Rutaceae*).

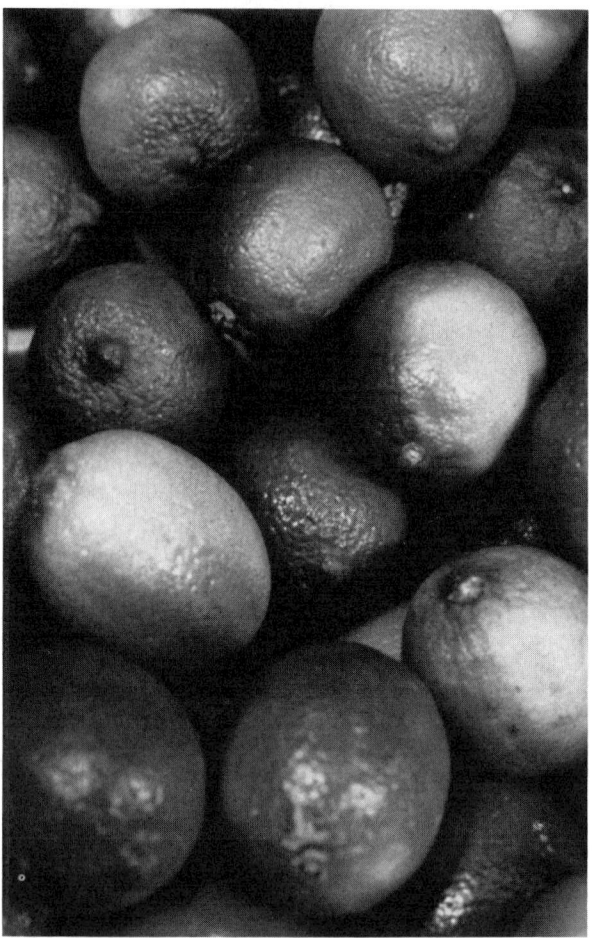

Fig. L-23. Limes, famed for protecting early-day sailors against scurvy. Because of this, British sailors were called limeys. (Courtesy, USDA)

ORIGIN AND HISTORY. The lime tree originated in India. The Arab traders first took the fruit to Arabia sometime before 900 A.D.; and about the same time, they introduced it to Egypt. Limes were taken to Spain in the 13th century. Columbus took lime seeds to Haiti during his second voyage to the New World in 1493.

WORLD AND U.S. PRODUCTION. FAO, United Nations, reports combined production figures for lemons and limes, without any breakdown between the two fruits. (See LEMONS.) However, it is estimated that annual world production of limes is about 360,000 metric tons. Most of the limes are grown in the warmer countries, especially in Mexico, Egypt, the West Indies, and in Florida.

The U.S. production of limes commercially is limited to Florida, where about 72,000 short tons are produced annually.[15]

SELECTION, PREPARATION, AND USES. Fresh limes that are green in color and heavy for their size are the most desirable. Many adult Americans have used alcoholic drinks made with lime juice. It is commonly used in the *coolers* served in hot weather. However, there are other good uses for fresh limes and lime juice. For example, the whole fruit makes excellent marmalade after slicing and removing the seeds. Also, the freshly squeezed juice imparts a superb flavor to fish and seafood dishes, fruits and fruit juices, meats, pie fillings, puddings, salad dressings, and sauces.

NUTRITIONAL VALUE. The nutrient compositions of various forms of limes are given in Food Composition Table F-21.

Some noteworthy observations regarding the nutrient composition of limes follow:

1. Fresh limes are low in calories (28 kcal per 100 g); and good sources of potassium, vitamin C, and bioflavonoids.

2. Fresh lime juice is similar to fresh limes in caloric and nutrient levels, except that the juice is likely to be much lower in bioflavonoids, which are found mainly in the peel and the membranes within the fruit.

3. Reconstituted frozen limeade concentrate contains about 50% more calories, but is much lower in nutrients than fresh lime juice.

4. Bottled lime juice contains only about two-thirds as much vitamin C as fresh lime juice.

(Also see BIOFLAVONOIDS; CITRUS FRUITS; POTASSIUM; and VITAMIN C.)

LIMITING AMINO ACID

The essential amino acid of a protein which shows the greatest percentage deficit in comparison with the amino acids contained in the same quantity of another protein selected as a standard.

(Also see AMINO ACID[S]; and PROTEIN.)

LIMONIN

The chemical responsible for the bitter principle of lemons. It is contained in the white spongy inner part of the rind. Too much limonin released into the juice during extraction produces bitter juice.

LINGONBERRY (COWBERRY)
Vacinnium vitis-idaea

The fruit of a vine (of the family *Ericaceae*) that grows wild throughout the cool, temperate regions of North America and Europe. Lingonberries, which are much esteemed in the Scandinavian countries, closely resemble their nearest

relative, the cranberry, and are about the same size. They are too tart to be eaten raw, but they make excellent jams and jellies.

LINOLEIC ACID

An 18-carbon unsaturated fatty acid having two double bonds. It is one of the essential fatty acids.
(Also see FATS AND OTHER LIPIDS.)

LINOLENIC ACID

An 18-carbon unsaturated fatty acid having three double bonds.
(Also see FATS AND OTHER LIPIDS.)

LIPASE

A fat-splitting enzyme, present in gastric juice and pancreatic juice. It acts on fats to produce fatty acids and glycerol.
(Also see DIGESTION AND ABSORPTION.)

LIP, CLEFT (HARELIP)

Usually infants born with a cleft palate (roof of the mouth) also have a cleft lip. These are congenital defects characterized by a gap in the palate and a gap in the upper lip. The condition may be bilateral—occurring on both sides of the face under each nostril. Infants with a cleft palate and/or lip have difficulty sucking, drinking, eating and swallowing. Hence, they require some special feeding techniques, depending upon the degree of the defect. Fortunately new plastic surgery methods have been developed and may be employed as early as the third month of life. Nevertheless, afflicted infants must build up their reserves for surgery; hence, the following suggestions will help to cope with feeding problems:

1. Sucking difficulties can be overcome by using a nipple with an enlarged opening, a medicine dropper, or a 10-20 cc syringe with a 2-in. (5 cm) piece of rubber tubing.

2. The tendency to choke should be countered by offering liquids slowly and in small amounts.

3. Frequent burpings are necessary as large amounts of air may be swallowed.

4. Irritating food such as spicy and acid foods should be avoided.

5. Foods such as peanut butter, nuts, leafy vegetables, and creamed dishes may adhere to the palate.

6. Pureed foods may be given from a bottle with a large nipple opening if diluted with milk, fruit juice, or broth.

7. Extra time should be allowed for feeding, and possibly five or six small meals may be better than three larger ones.

8. Supplementing the diet with the proper amounts of vitamins will insure optimal health and growth.

LIPIDS

An all-embracing term referring to any compound that is soluble in chloroform, benzene, petroleum, or ether. Included are fats, oils, waxes, sterols, and complex compounds such as phospholipids and sphingolipids. There are three basic types of lipids—simple lipids, compound lipids, and derived lipids. When fatty acids are esterified with alcohols, simple lipids result. If compounds such as choline or serine are esterified to alcohols in addition to fatty acids, compound lipids result. The third type of lipid, derived lipids, result from the hydrolysis of simple and compound lipids. The sterols and fatty acids are derived lipids.

---

[15]Data from *Agricultural Statistics 1991*, USDA, p. 177, Table 254. **Note well:** Annual production fluctuates as a result of weather and profitability of the crop.

(Also see FATS AND OTHER LIPIDS; and OILS, VEGETABLE.)

LIPOGENESIS

The formation of fat.

LIPOIC ACID

Lipoic acid is a fat-soluble, sulfur-containing substance. It is not a true vitamin because it can be synthesized in the body and is not necessary in the diet of animals. However, it functions in the same manner as many of the B-complex vitamins.

HISTORY. The continuing study of thiamin as a coenzyme in carbohydrate metabolism revealed that this metabolic system required other coenzyme factors in addition to thiamin. In work with lactic acid bacteria, Reed discovered, in 1951, that one of these factors is a fat-soluble acid which he named lipoic acid (after the Greek *lipos* for fat).

FUNCTIONS. Lipoic acid functions as a coenzyme. It is essential, together with the thiamin-containing enzyme, pyrophosphatase (TPP), for reactions in carbohydrate metabolism which convert pyruvic acid to acetyl-coenzyme A. Lipoic acid, which has two sulfur bonds of high-energy potential, combines with TPP to reduce pyruvate to active acetate, thereby sending it into the final energy cycle. It joins the intermediary products of protein and fat metabolism in the Krebs cycle in the reactions involved in producing energy from these nutrients. A metal ion (magnesium or calcium) is involved in this oxidative decarboxylation, along with lipoic acid and four vitamins: thiamin, pantothenic acid, niacin, and riboflavin. Thus, this underscores the concept of the interdependent relationships among the vitamins.

RECOMMENDED DIETARY ALLOWANCE OF LIPOIC ACID. Because the body can synthesize the needed lipoic acid, no dietary requirement for humans or animals has been established.

SOURCES OF LIPOIC ACID. Lipoic acid is found in many foods. Yeast and liver are rich sources.
(Also see VITAMIN[S], Table V-5.)

LIPOLYSIS

The hydrolysis of fats by enzymes, acids, alkalis, or other means to yield glycerol and fatty acids.

LIPOLYTIC RANCIDITY

Food spoilage that is caused by the enzymatic breakdown of fats by lipases. Lipases are produced by some microorganisms, and are present in tissues. Heating destroys the lipases, preventing this type of spoilage.
(Also see FATS AND OTHER LIPIDS; and RANCIDITY.)

LIPOPROTEIN

A lipid-protein complex that is water soluble. Hence, it is involved in the transport of lipids in the blood. Four types of lipoprotein circulate in the blood, all of which contain the lipids, triglycerides, cholesterol, and phospholipid in varying proportions. The four types of lipoprotein are (1) chylomicrons—lowest density; (2) very low density, VLDL; (3) low density, LDL; and (4) high density, HDL.

(Also see CHOLESTEROL; DIGESTION AND ABSORPTION, section on ''Lipids''; and FATS AND OTHER LIPIDS, section headed ''Other Lipids''.)

LIPOTROPIC (FACTOR)

A substance that prevents accumulation of fat in the liver. Choline is probably the most important of the lipotropic factors. So, any substance capable of contributing methyl groups for choline synthesis is lipotropic.
(Also see CHOLINE, section headed ''Functions.'')

LIQUID DIETS

This term covers a wide variety of dietary preparations that range from clear liquids which provide little in the way of nourishment to nearly complete diets in liquid form. For example, an infant formula is one type of liquid diet, whereas tube feedings are another.

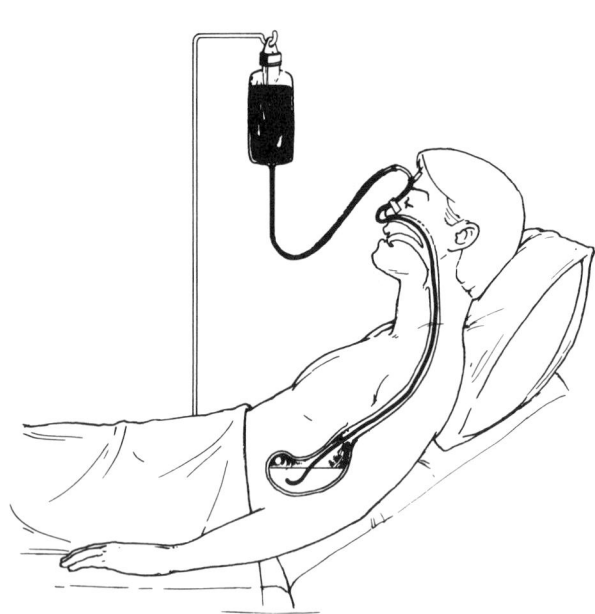

Fig. L-24. A hospital patient being tube fed a liquid diet. This type of feeding may be a lifesaver for people who are unable to eat in the normal way.

The use of liquid diets is growing rapidly, as evidenced by the various types of canned products that may be found in supermarkets and pharmacies. Some liquid diets are used for therapeutic purposes. Others are intended as replacements for, or supplements to, regular diets. Some department stores now have vending machines which dispense a liquid dietary formula in paper cups so that employees and shoppers may gulp their lunch down quickly and spend most of their lunch hour shopping.

TYPES OF LIQUID DIETS. The major types of liquid diets are described in Table L-3.

NOTE: Liquid diets should be used for therapeutic purposes only after consulting a doctor. *This caution also applies to liquid reducing diets.*

TABLE L-3
MAJOR TYPES OF LIQUID DIETS

Diet	Composition		Uses	Comments
	Foods[1] Included	Foods Excluded		
Clear Liquid	Only clear liquids such as tea; coffee; carbonated beverages; cereal beverages (coffee substitutes); flavored gelatin; ices made from strained fruit juices; fruit juices and drinks without pulp; fat-free fish, meat, and poultry broths; consomme; bouillon; sugar; clear syrups and honey.	All others.	To maintain the body's water balance when other foods and beverages cannot be taken by mouth, or when it is necessary to clear the colon of residue (in preparation for x rays; prior to, and following, surgery on the digestive track; during diarrheal disease; or as an initial oral feeding during the recovery of a critically ill patient).	This diet should be used for only a few days because it is deficient in almost all of the essential nutrients. Elemental diets serve most of the same purposes and are much more suitable for longterm use.
Elemental (semi-synthetic liquid diet) (Also see ELEMENTAL DIETS.)	Formula powders that are mixed with water and/or carbonated or noncarbonated fruit drinks that are free of fibrous residues, or bouillon. Essential nutrients are provided in the following forms: Carbohydrates as sugars and other well absorbed, rapidly utilized saccharides. Fat (usually only 0 to 10% of the diet) as a vegetable oil. (1) Amino acids as chemically pure crystalline powders; or (2) A protein hydrolysate such as digested casein; or (3) Egg albumin. Mineral salts and vitamins in chemically pure forms.	All others, unless allowed by a doctor, or a dietitian.	To promote ease of digestion and absorption and minimize food residue in the colon, while providing nearly all of the required nutrients, prior to and following surgery on the digestive tract; during diarrheal disease, infections, or inflammatory conditions; for the rehabilitation of severely injured and/or malnourished patients; minimizing nausea due to chemotherapy and/or radiation treatments; or as an initial oral feeding during the recovery of a critically ill patient. May also be used in tube feeding.	None of the products now available contain the essential trace minerals chromium and selenium, and only some brands contain vitamin K. Therefore, these nutrients must be provided by other means of nourishment for more than a few weeks. Patients have been maintained in good condition on elemental diets for as long as a year or more.

Full liquid diet (General liquid diet)
(See MODIFIED DIETS, Table M-28, Modified Diets—General liquid diet [Full liquid diet] for the composition and uses of Full liquid diet.)

Diet	Foods[1] Included	Foods Excluded	Uses	Comments
Infant formulas (Also see BABY FOODS; BREAST FEEDING; and INFANT DIET AND NUTRITION.)	Commercially produced infant formulas based mainly on milk or a milk substitute (usually soy protein isolates or pureed beef or lamb) that may contain added vegetable oil, sweetener, mineral salts, and/or vitamins. Homemade formulas prepared from diluted cow's milk with or without an added sweetener.	Homogenized cow's milk is not considered suitable for infants younger than 6 months, but evaporated milk is usually tolerated well.	In lieu of breast feeding young infants, and for older infants who do not tolerate cow's milk well. May be used by older children and adults who require liquid diets, when the latter is not available. Special modified types of infant formulas are available for children who have intolerances to certain foods and nutrients, but should be used only after consulting a doctor.	Some formulas furnish all the nutrients required by infants, whereas others should be supplemented by mineral and vitamin preparations. Infants aged 6 months and older should receive other foods besides a formula in order to develop good eating habits.
Special dietary products	Liquid or powdered (for mixing with water, milk, or other suitable liquid) dietary preparations that are designed to meet the special needs of patients placed on certain modified diets. Most of the products contain the appropriate types of carbohydrates, fats, amino acids or proteins, mineral salts and vitamins; but some furnish only supplementary nutrients for meeting unusual requirements.	Some products may contain little or no allergens, cholesterol, electrolytes, lactose, milk protein, protein in general, saturated fat, sodium, or other substances that are deemed to aggravate the patient's condition.	As a substitute for a normal diet that may be unsuitable in composition for the patient. Provision of calories and/or nutrients in addition to those in the normal diet where patients cannot or will not consume foods that supply the essential nutrients.	The use of these products alone may become very expensive and monotonous for the patient, who may benefit more by consuming homemade items prepared from common foods by modified recipes (when it is feasible for a lay person to prepare them).
Supplemental feedings	Dietary formulations designed to provide extra calories, proteins, and other nutrients in easily digested and readily absorbed forms when the patient is already receiving some, but not all, of his or her nutrient requirements from another source. Most products contain sugars, powdered milk or a substitute for milk protein, vegetable oils or their derivatives, added mineral salts and vitamins, and flavorings such as vanilla and chocolate.	Nutrients that are poorly digested or slowly absorbed, such as fiber, and long chain fatty acids.	Supplemenation of the normal or therapeutic diets of growing children athletes, underweight adults, people recovering from debilitating illnesses, injuries, burns, surgery, gastrointestinal disorders, anorexia, and various other conditions in which nutritional needs are likely to be in excess of the nourishment provided by the unsupplemented diets.	Some of the products in this category are called *nourishments* after the traditional dietary practice of providing certain patients with extra feedings between meals. In the past, these feedings often consisted of items such as cream, milk, milk drinks, puddings, custards, and other high-calorie foods.

Footnotes at end of table

(Continued)

TABLE L-3 *(Continued)*

Diet	Composition		Uses	Comments
	Foods¹ Included	**Foods Excluded**		
Tube feedings	Mixtures of liquids, dissolved powders, and/or pureed solid foods of sufficiently fluid consistencies to pass through feeding tubes without clogging them. Some typical ingredients of the common types of feedings are: commercial formulas; whole milk, evaporated milk, strained buttermilk, and/or ice cream; strained pureed meats, hard cooked yolk, fruits, and/or vegetables; fruit juices; sugar, syrup, and/or honey; added mineral salts and vitamins; and flavorings such as vanilla and chocolate.	Foods and nutrients that are poorly digested or slowly absorbed, such as fiber and long chain fatty acids. Substances that are likely to settle out and clog the tube are also excluded, such as pieces of foods, nuts, seeds, chocolate chips, milk curds, solidified fats, and powders that are difficult to dissolve.	Nutritional support of people who are unable to chew and/or swallow ordinary foods due to surgery on the face, oral cavity, neck, or throat; fractures of the jaw; esophageal strictures; injury, inflammation, or surgery affecting one or more parts of the upper digestive tract; partial paralysis, or unconsciousness. Sometimes, tube feedings are used for force feeding people who refuse to eat and become emaciated, such as those with anorexia nervosa or protesters on a *hunger strike.*² The tube for feeding may be inserted (1) up through the nose and down to the stomach (nasogastric feeding), (2) through the nose and down to the duodenum (nasoduodenal feeding), (3) into an opening on the abdomen leading to the stomach (gastrostomy feeding), or (4) into an opening on the abdomen leading to the jejunum (jejunostomy feeding).	Care has to be taken that tube feedings are not regurgitated and aspirated into the lungs. This may be prevented by giving the initial feeding at only ½ strength, keeping the rate of feeding slow; and by allowing the patient to rest in a sitting position after an intermittent feeding of a large volume of formula. It is noteworthy that some tube feeding formulas have a high concentration of dissolved materials (solutes) and may cause dehydration and/or diarrhea unless some additional water is given. Detailed instructions for tube feedings may be obtained from the manufacturers of the formulas and from nursing manuals.

¹Many liquid diets provide nutrients in highly purified forms rather than in the forms of ordinary foods.

²Long-term deliberate or unavoidable abstention from the consumption of adequate food may result in a loss of appetite and other abnormalities that often necessitate forced feeding to initiate recovery of the normal eating and digestive functions.

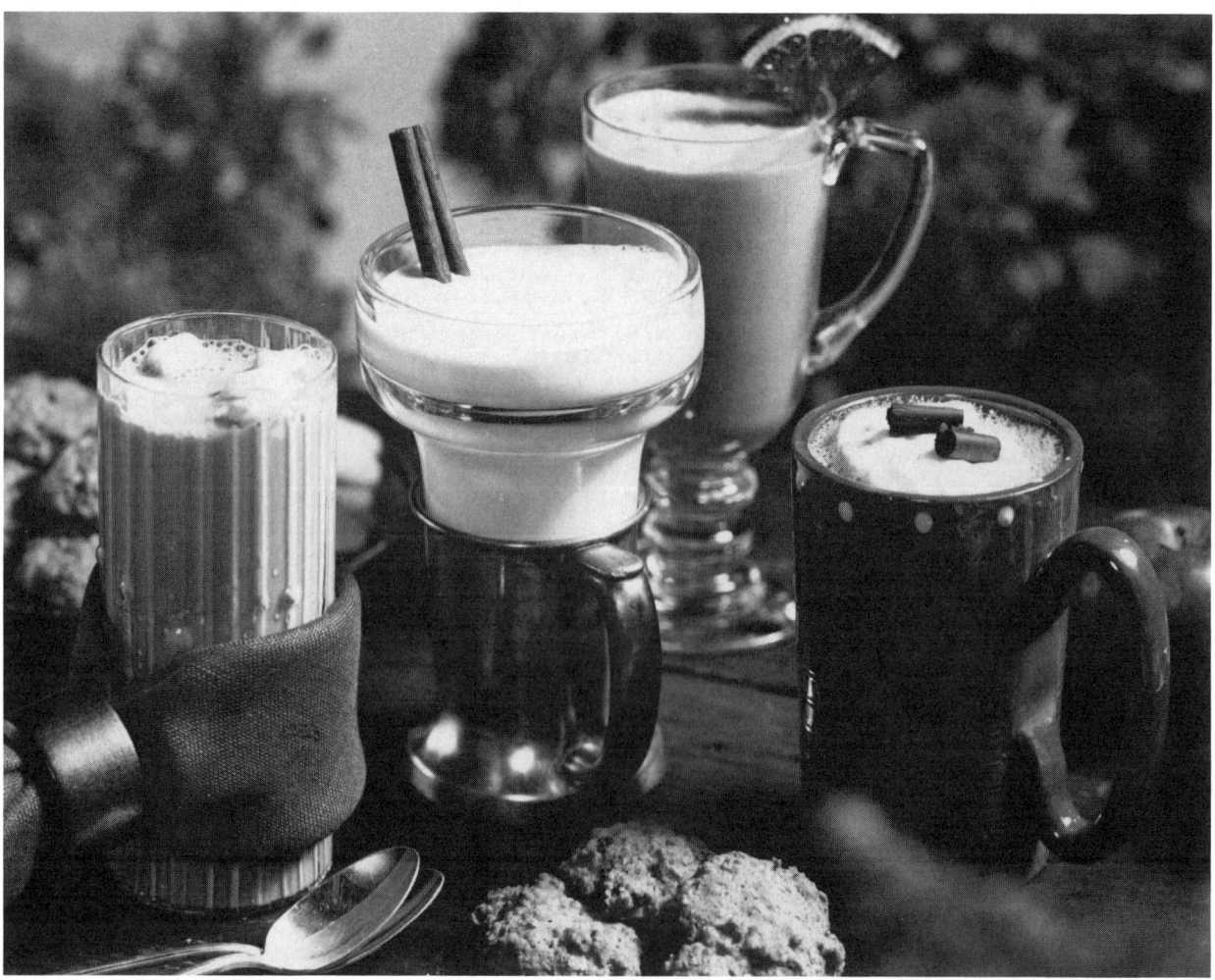

Fig. L-25. Liquid diets can be monotonous, so different tumblers and frills can *zip* them up. (Courtesy, American Dairy Assn., Chicago, Ill.)

SUMMARY. Providing most of a patient's nutrient needs by a liquid diet may be done successfully over long periods of time if this means of nourishment is carried out according to the recommendations of a doctor and/or a dietitian.

(Also see ELEMENTAL DIETS; and MODIFIED DIETS.)

LITHIASIS

The formation of calculi (stones) of any kind (as in the urinary tract and gallbladder).

LIVETINS

A collective term for the principal water-soluble proteins that are found in egg yolk—an albumin, a glycoprotein, and a globulin.

(Also see EGG.)

LOFENALAC

This term is the registered trademark of the commercially prepared protein formula sold by Mead Johnson & Company of Evansville, Indiana. Ninety-five percent of the amino acid phenylalanine is removed from Lofenalac. It provides the basis for dietary management of phenylketonuria (PKU), an inborn error of metabolism. Most proteins contain 4 to 6% phenylalanine and would be detrimental to an infant with PKU. Lofenalac is used to meet the infant's protein and energy needs while the requirement for phenylalanine, an essential amino acid, is just satisfied—no excess—with foods whose phenylalanine content is known.

(Also see INBORN ERRORS OF METABOLISM; and PHENYLKETONURIA.)

LOGANBERRY *Rubus loganbaccus*

A reddish-purple type of blackberry (fruit of the *Rosaceae* family) that was discovered growing in the garden of Judge Logan of Santa Cruz, California in 1881.

It is believed to have originated as a result of a natural crossbreeding (hybridization) between a western wild blackberry and a domesticated variety of red raspberry. The loganberry is grown mainly in the central coast region of California, the Willamette Valley of Oregon, and the southwestern part of British Columbia around Vancouver.

Only about 2% of the U.S. crop of loganberries is marketed fresh. The rest is canned, frozen, and made into jam, jelly, juice, and wine. It is noteworthy that the sharp tartness of the fresh berries is improved by cooking.

The nutrient compositions of various forms of loganberries are given in Food Composition Table F-21.

Some noteworthy observations regarding the nutrient composition of loganberries follow:

1. The raw fruit is moderately high in calories (62 kcal per 100 g) and carbohydrates (15%). It is an excellent source of fiber, a good source of potassium, iron, and vitamin C, and only a fair to poor source of vitamin A.

2. Canned loganberries contain about two-thirds of the nutrients of the fresh fruit, except that much of the vitamin C is destroyed during processing. Also, the products containing syrups may be rather high in caloric content.

LOGARITHMIC PHASE (EXPONENTIAL PHASE; LOG PHASE)

When pertaining to bacterial cultures in an adequate medium, it is the period of most rapid growth when numbers increase in geometric progression. On a rich medium bacteria can double in numbers every 20 minutes.

LONGAN *Euphoria longana; Nephelium longana*

The fruit of a tree (of the *Sapindaceae* family) that is native to the Asian tropics, and is now grown in some of the other tropical regions of the world. Longans are round, yellowish-brown fruits that contain a white, juicy pulp.

The nutrient compositions of raw and dried longans are given in Food Composition Table F-21.

Some noteworthy observations regarding the nutrient composition of longans follow:

1. The raw fruit is moderately high in calories (62 kcal per 100 g) and carbohydrates (14.9%). It is a good source of iron, but a poor source of vitamin C.

2. Dried longans contain about 5 times the nutrient levels of the fresh fruit. The vitamin C content is apparently retained completely during drying. Hence, the dried fruit is suitable for a nutritious high-calorie (286 kcal per 100 g) snack that contains almost 5% protein, 2% fiber, and is an excellent source of phosphorus and potassium, and a good source of vitamin C.

LONGEVITY

Long-lived.

LOW DENSITY LIPOPROTEIN (LDL)

A lipoprotein with a density of 1.006 to 1.063; composed of about 21% protein; high in cholesterol.

(Also see BETA-LIPOPROTEINS.)

LUCERNE (ALFALFA) *Medicago sativa*

The plant known as alfalfa (botanically *Medicago sativa*) in the United States is called lucerne in many parts of the world.

(See ALFALFA.)

LUPUS ERYTHEMATOSUS

Recent research indicates that systemic lupus erythematosus is primarily a disease of the immune system in which antigen-antibody complexes cause tissue damage. An early manifestation of the disease is the erosive inflammation of the skin typically in the form of a *butterfly rash* over the nose and cheeks. This rash gave the disease its original name—*lupus erythematosus* or *red wolf*. Besides the rash, other symptoms of lupus include an intermittent fever, severe joint pain, and periods of extreme fatigue. It afflicts about one woman in 500 in the United States, and about one-tenth as many men. Lupus affects not only the skin, but, at different times in different individuals, it may affect the joints, the blood vessels, the heart, the lungs, and the brain—and most significantly the kidneys. The disease probably arises from an interplay of genetics, drugs, hormones and viruses. Methods for early diagnosis have led to improved control of lupus, thereby preventing irreversible tissue damage, particularly to the kidneys.

Part of the treatment for lupus may involve cortisone or other steroids to control the inflammation; hence, a sodium-restricted diet may be necessary. Should the kidneys become involved, dietary changes similar to those for kidney diseases may be recommended.

(Also see MODIFIED DIETS.)

LYCOPENE

A chemical similar to carotene, but it has no vitamin A activity. It is the principal red pigment present in tomatoes, watermelon, pink grapefruit, paprika, rose hips, and palm oil.

LYMPH

The slightly yellow, transparent fluid occupying the lymphatic channels of the body. It is derived from the fluid between the cells—interstitial fluid. The chemical makeup of lymph is similar to that of blood plasma. Following a meal, some of the fat from the diet is absorbed into the lymph in the form of chylomicrons.

(Also see BODY FLUIDS; and DIGESTION AND ABSORPTION.)

LYMPHATIC SYSTEM

All the vessels and structures that carry lymph from the tissues to the blood.

LYOPHILIZATION (FREEZE DRYING)

A process of rapid freezing followed by drying under a vacuum. The ice sublimes off as water vapor without melting. Freeze drying results in the least damage to foods of all the commercial processes for drying. It can be applied to all foods, both raw and cooked, which can withstand freezing. Freeze drying yields a product that is dried without shrink, and which has a highly porous structure favoring rapid rehydration. After rehydration, freeze-dried foods are often indistinguishable from their commercially frozen counterparts.

(Also see PRESERVATION OF FOOD.)

LYSERGIC ACID

A chemical derived from the hydrolysis (breakdown) of the alkaloids of the fungus ergot. It is thought to be the active component of ergot. Lysergic acid can produce a state resembling psychosis. Also, its diethylamide derivative, LSD, is a potent hallucinogenic drug.

(Also see POISONS, Table P-2, Some Potentially Poisonous [Toxic] Substances—"Ergot.")

LYSINE

Contents   Page

Lysine is an essential amino acid. The body requires lysine but cannot synthesize it so it must be provided in the diet. High quality protein foods provide lysine. However, lysine is the limiting amino acid in most cereals—foods for much of the world. It is present in cereal grains, but at low levels. Inadequate lysine in the diet may create a negative nitrogen balance—protein being broken down and excreted. Chemically, lysine is unique among the essential amino acids since it possesses two amino groups (NH_2). This can further affect the availability of lysine when it is in short supply. All other essential amino acids possess one amino group. Since lysine, in the form of lysine monohydrochlorine, can be commercially produced at a reasonable cost, much consideration has been given to the supplementation of cereals with lysine in an effort to improve the nutrition of people who depend largely upon cereal grains.

INVOLVEMENT IN THE BODY. The requirement of lysine for growth is quite high, since tissue proteins contain a high proportion of lysine. Infants require 45 mg/lb (*99 mg/kg*) of body weight per day, and growing children require 20 mg/lb (*44 mg/kg*) of body weight per day, while adults require only 5.5 mg/lb (*12 mg/kg*) of body weight per day. Rats fed diets deficient in lysine grow very little while the addition of lysine to the same diet significantly increases growth. Since protein synthesis—growth of tissue—is an all-or-none phenomenon, it requires that all amino acids necessary for synthesis be present. Otherwise, synthesis will not proceed; hence, growth will be limited. The protein in most cereal grains is poorly utilized by infants and children due to its low lysine content.

SOURCES. Lysine may be obtained from both plant and animal dietary proteins. However, in terms of lysine content, plant proteins and animal proteins are not created equal. In general, plant proteins contain less lysine than animal proteins.

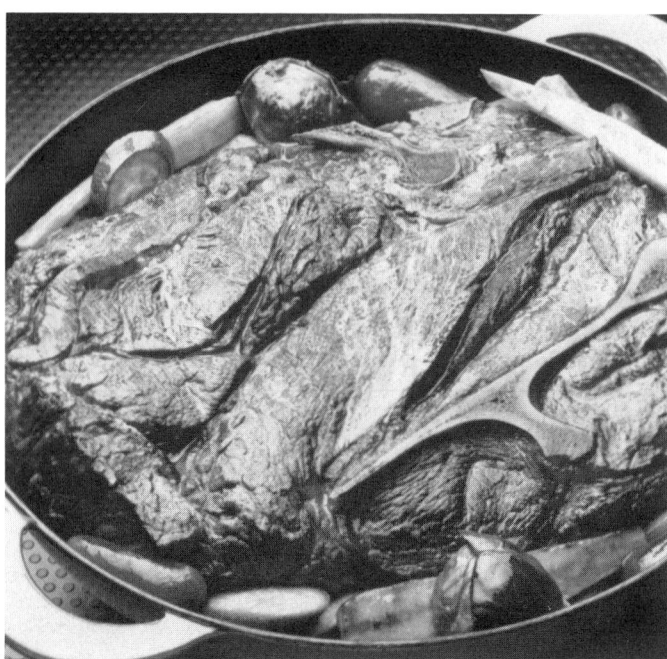

Fig. L-26. Lysine, an essential amino acid, is generally more abundant in animal proteins than in plant proteins. Beef is an especially rich source. (Courtesy, National Livestock & Meat Board, Chicago, Ill.)

Plant vs Animal. Protein is a part of all tissue—plant or animal. The seeds of many plants supply protein, hence lysine, to mankind; for example, wheat, corn, barley, lentils, peas, rice, and soybeans. Likewise, all animal foods—except pure fats—are good protein sources and, therefore, provide lysine. Table L-4 shows the comparative lysine content of some common protein sources.

TABLE L-4
LYSINE CONTENT OF SOME COMMON FOODS[1]

Food	Lysine	
	(mg/100 g)[2]	(mg/g protein)[3]
Beef steak, cooked	2,999	98
Chicken, cooked	1,830	86
Cheese, cheddar	2,072	83
Pork chop, cooked	2,044	83
Cod, cooked	2,421	83
Sardines, canned	1,552	83
Lamb leg, roasted	2,081	82
Milk, cow's (2% fat)	264	80
Soybeans, cooked	759	69
Eggs	820	68
Lentils, cooked	476	61
Peas, green, cooked	254	47
Peanuts, roasted	1,176	45
Rice, brown, cooked	99	40
Oatmeal, dry	521	37
Wheat, parboiled (bulgur)	217	35
Barley, pearled light, uncooked	279	34
Corn meal, cooked	29	26

[1]Data from Protein and Amino Acid Content of Selected Foods, Table P-16.

[2]One hundred grams is approximately equal to 3½ oz.

[3]Two grams per kilogram of body weight per day of a protein containing 51 mg of lysine per gram of protein would meet the lysine needs of the infant.

Cereal grains—barley, corn, oats, rice, and wheat—are low in lysine as Table L-4 shows, whereas the lysine content of legumes—lentils, peas, and soybeans—is better. The lysine content of animal products is highest.

It is a recognized fact that lysine is the limiting amino acid—the essential amino acid most deficient—of the cereal grain proteins. Since cereal grains provide much of the world's food, there have been attempts to increase their lysine content. Plant breeding programs have successfully increased the lysine content of barley, sorghum, and corn as shown in Table L-5. This brings the protein quality of the cereal grains closer to that of animal products.

TABLE L-5
LYSINE CONTENT OF CEREAL GRAINS

Grain	Lysine	
	(mg/100 g)	(mg/g protein)
Barley	435	34
High-lysine barley	1,089	56
Corn	290	29
High-lysine corn	491	45
Sorghum	297	27
High-lysine sorghum	611	33

These improved grains have been tested in animal and human trials with good results. However, farmers are reluc-

tant to grow the hybrid varieties because they yield 10 to 15% less grain per acre than the more common varieties.

(Also see CORN, section headed "High-Lysine Corn [Opaque 2, or O_2].")

Other Lysine Sources. Lysine itself may be produced by two processes: (1) the fermentation of carbohydrate materials; and (2) the Toray process, which converts cyclohexene, a by-product of nylon production, to lysine. Following purification procedures, lysine is available as a pure white powder, often as lysine monohydrochlorine. Currently, the cost of producing pure lysine is about $1.50 to $2.00 per pound ($3.30 to $4.40/kg).

FACTORS AFFECTING AVAILABILITY. Beside lysine being in short supply in cereal grains, the biological availability—availability to the body once ingested—may be adversely affected. As pointed out, lysine has an extra amino group (NH_2). This amino group can react with other compounds, primarily the aldehyde group of reducing sugars such as glucose or lactose. The reaction yields an amino-sugar complex that is no longer available for use in the body. Digestive enzymes cannot split the amino-sugar complex; hence, it is not absorbed. This reaction—the Maillard reaction—occurs due to extensive heating or prolonged storage. In protein sources such as the cereal grain products where lysine is already in short supply, the reaction can further reduce the lysine content of the diet.

LYSINE SUPPLEMENTATION. Since lysine is the limiting amino acid of cereal grains which make up the diets of a large portion of the world, some scientists propose the enrichment of these grains with pure lysine derived from processes described above. This practice would be similar to that in the United States wherein thiamin, niacin, riboflavin, and iron are added to many cereal products. Indeed, there have been experimental trials with animals and humans demonstrating the beneficial effects of adding lysine. Still, in countries where diets are extremely poor, more may be gained by increasing the food supply in general and providing other protein sources such as legumes which complement the protein of cereal grains. However, some countries have tried lysine supplemented foods. The Japanese school lunch programs fortified bread with lysine and vitamins. Government-controlled bakeries in India produced bread fortified with lysine, vitamins, and minerals. In Guatemala, Incaparina, a new product to increase the quality and quantity of protein, is fortified with lysine. In the United States, Pillsbury test marketed a flour containing added vitamins, minerals, and lysine.

Lysine enrichment is a debatable issue, depending on a variety of factors, primarily the continued availability of major sources of calories and protein. Supplementation is of little value if there is not enough food. But lysine supplementation is a potential tool.

(Also see AMINO ACID[S]; and PROTEIN[S].)

LYSINE AND HERPES INFECTIONS. The Herpes simplex viruses are responsible for cold sores, fever blisters, and genital herpes, while a close relative, Herpes zoster, is responsible for chickenpox, shingles, and *infectious mono.* In 1979, the Lilly Research Laboratories, a division of Eli Lilly and Company of Indianapolis, released research results showing that supplementary lysine speeded recovery and suppressed recurrences of herpes infections.

Tablets of lysine as the hydrochloride may be purchased at many general health food stores. Each tablet contains about 300 mg of lysine. A monograph from Lilly Research laboratories recommends the following:

1. When a clearly established herpes infection is present, two lysine tablets should be taken two to four times daily until the infection has cleared.

2. Those individuals who can predict an episode of herpes due to its association with such things as menstruation, exposure to sunlight, eating nuts, or any stressful situation, may take suppressive amounts of lysine—one, two, three, or four tablets daily depending upon the individual. Some individuals may prevent further infection with one tablet daily, while others may require two tablets twice a day.

3. Attacks may be completely aborted if lysine is taken in a dose of two tablets, three times per day for 3 to 5 days as soon as the signs of an attack are noted—a stinging and burning sensation followed by a little reddish nodule.

4. Some individuals can prevent herpes by avoiding known sources of another amino acid—arginine. These sources include: peanut butter, cashews, pecans, almonds, and chocolate. Tissue culture studies have shown that arginine enhances herpes growth.

Supplemental lysine does not produce any undesirable effect nor is it toxic. It is a normal constituent of protein. However, some individuals may not receive adequate amounts, and the needs from individual to individual may vary widely. Hence, to suppress herpes the dose of lysine must be varied.

Some recent work indicates that the continued use of lysine may antagonize (counteract) arginine, another amino acid. Also, drugs and vaccines raise the hope of suppressing the herpes virus. Thus, those who are persistently plagued with herpes are advised to confer with their physician.

LYSOSOMES

Structures of cell cytoplasm that contain digestive enzymes.

LYSOZYME

An enzyme that digests some gram-positive bacteria and certain high molecular weight carbohydrates; present in saliva, tears, and egg white.

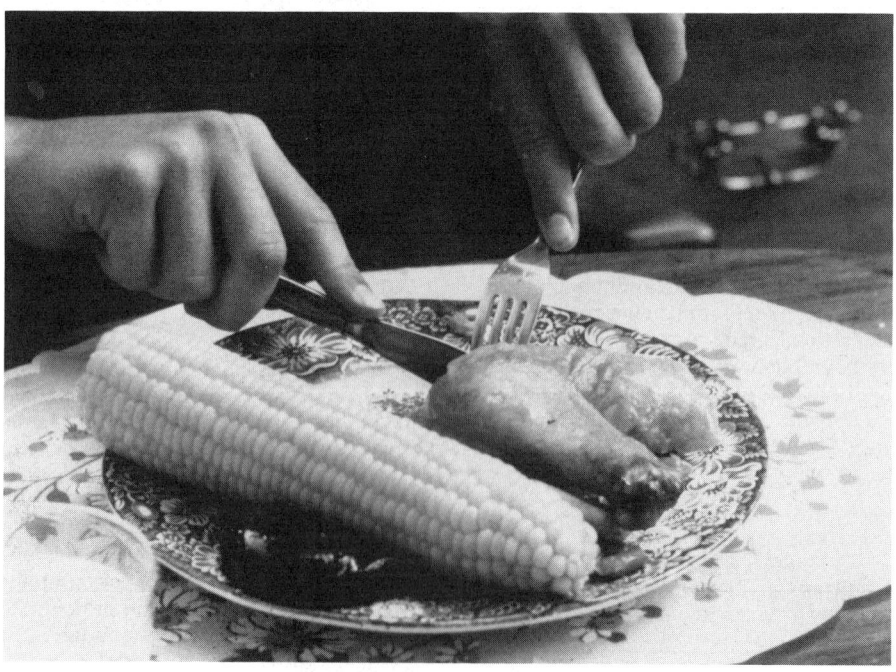

Fig. L-27. Balancing the lysine! Corn and other cereals are low in lysine, while chicken and other animal products are high in lysine. (Courtesy, USDA)

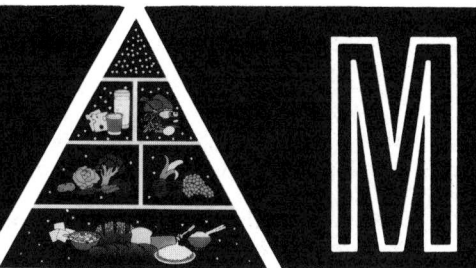

MACARONI AND NOODLE PRODUCTS

These items, which are also called pasta, are pieces of dough that have been formed into various shapes, then dried. In the United States, macaroni products may contain egg as an optional ingredient; but products labeled as noodles must contain a certain minimum amount of egg. The names *macaroni*, *spaghetti*, and *vermicelli* are applied to macaroni products that are cord-shaped and have certain diameters. *Macaroni* has the largest diameter of the macaroni products, while *vermicelli* has the smallest diameter.

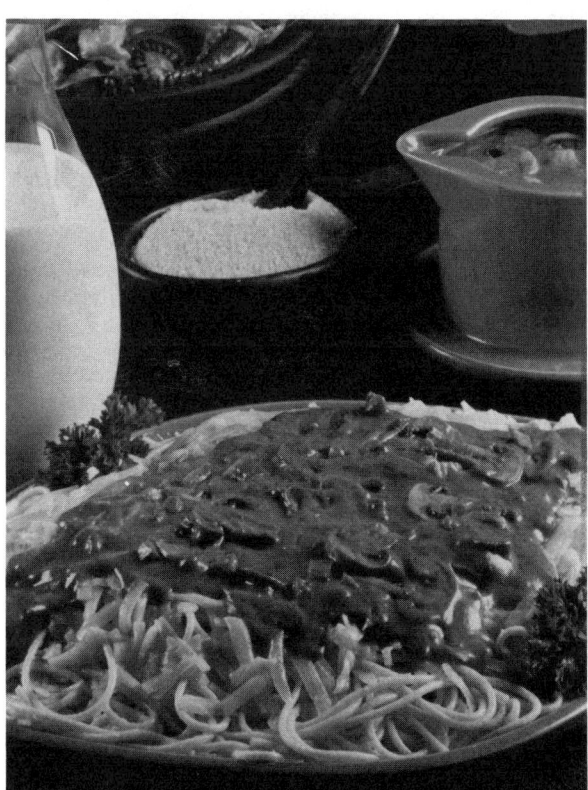

Fig. M-1. Spaghetti, a favorite pasta. (Courtesy, United Dairy Assoc., Rosemont, Ill.)

Macaroni and noodle products are important foods for many peoples around the world because they (1) are easy to make with simple equipment from ingredients that are available in most places, (2) keep well without refrigeration, (3) are bland flavored and mix well with most other foods, and (4) contain sufficient calories and protein to be major dietary sources of these nutrients.

HISTORY. Evidence suggests that forms of pasta were used by the ancient Etruscans (people who settled the upper western coast of the Italian peninsula around 700 B.C.). Some historians suspect that macaroni and noodle types of pasta were introduced into Italy during the Middle Ages by the Asian slaves who cooked for the affluent Italians, since threadlike noodles were then made in various places across Asia—from China to Arabia.

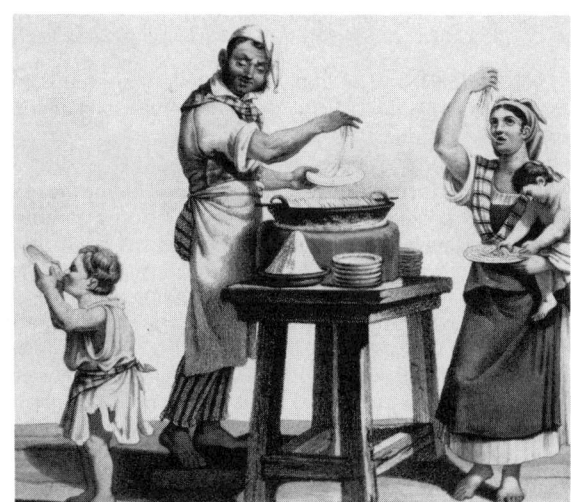

Fig. M-2. The macaroni seller, in Southern Italy. (After a colored lithograph by Muller. Courtesy, The Bettman Archive, Inc., New York, N.Y.)

Whatever the origin of pasta, the southern Italians became the masters of its production in Europe, because the northern Italians ate rice in their soups and with their sauces. Also, the warm, dry climate of southern Italy favored the drying of freshly made pasta in the sun. Finally, the southern Italians preferred their pasta firm (*aldente,* which means that it requires chewing), whereas the northern Italians cooked it until it was much more tender.

Pasta appears to have spread throughout Europe from Italy, although the peoples in the northern countries apparently preferred flat noodles to the rounded types (macaroni and spaghetti). It is believed that Thomas Jefferson brought pasta to America from France, where he had served as U.S. Ambassador. Later, immigrants from northern Europe brought their own noodle dishes. Still later, Italian immigrants came to America, and for a long time thereafter imported their pasta from Italy.

It is noteworthy that the production of good pasta (that which holds together in boiling water) requires hard wheats with a high gluten content. The Italians obtained most of their wheat from the U.S.S.R. until the Crimean War (1854-1856) cut off their supplies. Shortly thereafter, hard wheats were produced in Canada and the United States. Hence, North America soon became the major source of durum wheat for the pasta industry around the world. However, there was not much production of macaroni or spaghetti in the United States until World War I cut off the supply from Italy.

PRODUCTION.   The consumption of macaroni and noodle products in the United States has grown steadily since World War II, even though the total consumption of all types of wheat products declined. It is noteworthy that the production of macaroni utilizes most of the durum wheat grown in North Dakota. However, good macaroni may also be made from weaker flours if certain optional ingredients such as eggs are added.

Commercial Products.   The first machine powered pasta presses were developed around the mid-1800s. Prior thereto, most macaroni was produced in small shops which utilized hand operated equipment. Today, large machines make it possible to turn out large batches of these products. Details of commercial production follow.

INGREDIENTS.   The items which follow are the ingredients specified in the U.S. standards of identity for macaroni and noodle products:[1]

• **Semolina, durum flour, farina, flour**—One or more of these wheat products constitute(s) the major ingredient of pasta. Semolina is the coarsely milled endosperm of durum wheat, while durum flour is more finely milled. Farina is similar to semolina, but it is obtained from other than durum wheats, whereas flour is the more finely milled endosperm of nondurum wheats. Each of these four fractions may contain only minimal amounts of branny particles. Generally, pasta makers prefer to use semolina and/or farina since products made from these meals hold up better in cooking than those made from the flours.

• **Water**—This is the usual liquid for making a dough, although it may be replaced completely by fluid milk in certain products. Care is taken that the water is pure and free from undesirable flavors.

• **Eggs**—Egg whites (fresh, frozen, or dried) are optional ingredients for macaroni products, in which they help to strengthen the dough. On the other hand, noodles must contain at least 5½% egg solids from either whole egg or egg yolk. The latter is preferred for the color it imparts to noodles.

• **Disodium phosphate**—Small amounts (0.5 to 1.0%) of this optional additive make pasta cook more quickly.

• **Seasonings and spices**—Onions, celery, garlic, bay leaf, and salt are optional ingredients for macaroni and noodle products. When used, they must be listed on the label.

• **Gum gluten**—Sometimes, this product, which is made from wheat flour by washing out the starch, is added in small amounts to strengthen the dough.

• **Glyceryl monostearate**—Less than 2% of this additive (it is an emulsifying agent) may be used to prevent the formation of clumps of dough.

• **Minerals and vitamins**—Products labeled *enriched* must contain prescribed amounts of iron, thiamin, and riboflavin, which may be (1) added as chemically pure compounds, or (2) supplied by optional ingredients such as dried yeast, dried torula yeast, partly defatted wheat germ, enriched farina, or enriched flour. Certain specified amounts of calcium and vitamin D are optional.

• **Protein supplements**—The sources of extra protein are usually corn flour and soybean flour or meal, although other ingredients such as nonfat dry milk, fish flour, and derivatives of oilseeds (usually peanut, safflower seed, or sunflower seed) also may serve this purpose. These supplements raise both the quantity and quality of protein so that the macaroni and noodle products may be substituted for part of the dietary animal protein.

• **Milk products**—Whole fluid milk may replace completely the water used in making a dough, or the milk ingredient may be concentrated milk, evaporated milk, dried milk, a mixture of butter and skim milk, concentrated skim milk, evaporated skim milk, or nonfat dry milk. In the case of *Milk Macaroni Products,* the milk ingredient(s) must supply an amount of milk solids equal to 3.8% of the finished product. Also, the weight of nonfat milk solids cannot be more than 2.275 times the weight of milk fat. This regulation insures uniformity by making all products equivalent to those made with whole milk. It is *not* applicable to items designated as "Macaroni products made with nonfat milk."

• **Carrageenan or its salts**—This optional additive, which is a gum, is used to strengthen products containing greater than average amounts of nonfat dry milk, because the latter ingredient weakens doughs.

• **Vegetable products**—Colorful macaroni and noodle products are produced by the addition of red tomato, artichoke, beet, carrot, parsley, or spinach derivatives. The vegetable ingredient may be fresh, canned, dried, or in the form of a paste or a puree. However, the pasta product must contain at least 3% vegetable solids. Spinach is the most commonly used vegetable ingredient. It is noteworthy that 3% vegetable solids corresponds to a content of about 30% fresh vegetable matter since most fresh vegetables contain about 90% water.

MANUFACTURING PROCEDURES.   There must be careful control of each manufacturing stage in order to ensure that the product holds up well under (1) handling between the factory and the consumer, and (2) boiling in water. Therefore, the major processes that are utilized in manufacturing of pasta are noteworthy:

1. **Milling of the durum wheat into semolina.**   This milling procedure differs from that used to make flour in that a granular product is desired, with a minimum amount of flour. Hence, certain aspects of the flour milling procedure are altered in the production of semolina. The durum wheat is moistened before milling to toughen the outer layers of the wheat kernels so that they may be removed readily from

---

[1]*Code of Federal Regulations,* Title 21, Revised 4/1/78, Part 139, Sections 139.110 through 139.160.

the inner portion (endosperm) which yields the semolina. Then, the wheat is broken into coarse particles by corrugated rolls. Other rolls then crush the grain further and scrape the branny material from the pieces of endosperm. Finally, the particles of endosperm and bran are separated by sifting, and by a stream of air which lifts away the smaller flakes of bran.

2. **Preparation of the pasta dough.** The wheat ingredient may be semolina, durum flour, farina, nondurum flour, or various combinations of these items. About 31 parts of water (by weight) are mixed with about 69 parts of meal and/or flour to make a dough. Then, the dough is mixed well and a vacuum is applied to remove any air that might have been mixed into the dough, because air bubbles weaken the pasta.

3. **Shaping the products.** Macaroni products are given their shapes by a process called extrusion, in which the dough is forced through openings in a die made from bronze or Teflon. The shaped raw pasta which emerges from the die is cut to the proper length by either a rotating knife (in the case of short products), or by other means.

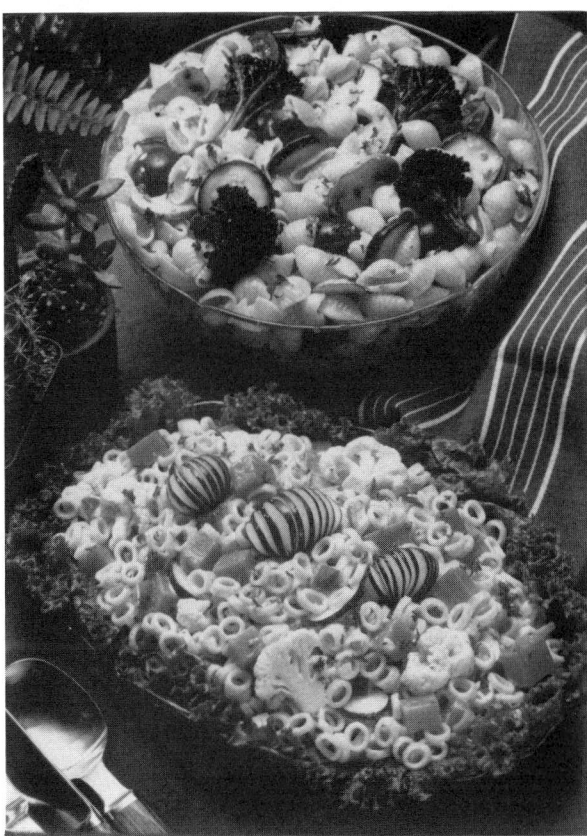

Fig. M-3. Two shapes of macaroni (Pasta)-shells and rings. (Courtesy, Hershey Foods Corp. Hershey, Pa.)

4. **Drying.** The newly shaped pieces of pasta are carefully dried under strictly controlled conditions to bring the moisture content down to between 12 and 13%.

5. **Packaging.** Most long, cordlike, or tubular macaroni products are packaged in boxes that protect the strands against breakage. However, noodle products are usually packed in plastic bags.

TYPES OF MACARONI AND NOODLES. Many new products have been developed recently by food technologists

for use in various parts of the world. However, it could be very confusing for the American consumer if each manufacturer were allowed to make products and label them in an arbitrary manner, since the ingredients and nutritive values might vary widely. Hence, the U.S. Food and Drug Administration, with the cooperation of American pasta manufacturers, has developed names and specifications (standards of identity) for each of the more common macaroni and noodle products. These follow:

1. Macaroni products.
2. Enriched macaroni products.
3. Enriched macaroni products with fortified protein.
4. Milk macaroni products.
5. Nonfat milk macaroni products.
6. Enriched nonfat milk macaroni products.
7. Vegetable macaroni products.
8. Enriched vegetable macaroni products.
9. Whole wheat macaroni products.
10. Wheat and soy macaroni products.
11. Noodle products.
12. Enriched noodle products.
13. Vegetable noodle products.
14. Enriched vegetable noodle products.
15. Wheat and soy noodle products.

NUTRITIVE VALUES OF MACARONI AND NOODLE PRODUCTS. People with low incomes have long relied on pasta dishes to supply most of their dietary calories and other nutrients. Furthermore, these dishes are served regularly in the school lunch programs around the United States. Therefore, it is noteworthy that the nutritive values of these foods vary widely, depending upon the type of macaroni or noodle product and the other items that might be served with them. The nutrient compositions of macaroni, noodles, pastinas, spaghetti, and some of the most common dishes prepared with these products are given in Food Composition Table F-21.

Some of the more noteworthy observations regarding the products listed in Food Composition Table F-21 are as follows:

1. A cup of a plain, tender cooked macaroni product contains about 5 oz (*140 g*) of food, 155 Calories (kcal), and 4.8 g of protein, whereas a cup of noodles supplies 5⅔ oz (*160 g*) of food, 200 Calories (kcal), and 6.6 g of protein. The superior nutritive values of the noodles are due mainly to the egg content.

2. Enriched macaroni and noodles supply fair amounts of iron, thiamin, riboflavin, and niacin, but only negligible amounts of calcium, phosphorus, vitamin A, and vitamin C.

3. The addition of cheese to macaroni provides considerable extra calories, protein, calcium, phosphorus, and vitamin A. Similarly, the addition of tomato sauce plus cheese or meat to spaghetti enhances the nutritive value of a pasta dish.

4. Chow mein noodles are a concentrated source of calories and protein because they contain almost no water. However, the ratio of protein to calories (2.7 g per 100 kcal) is less than those for either macaroni (3.1 g per 100 kcal) or noodles (3.3 g per 100 kcal), because the frying of the Chinese noodles raises the fat content without increasing the protein.

5. Another important observation regarding macaroni and noodles, which is not apparent from the data presented in Food Composition Table F-21, is that the protein in these products is deficient in the amino acid lysine, which is critical for the growth of infants and children. This defect is offset partly by the high quality of the protein in the eggs that are

added to noodles.

There is a great need for supplementing the nutritive contributions of pasta products when they are used as staple foods for infants and children. (Tiny egg noodles called pastina are used as a baby food in Italy.) Therefore, the current enrichment and fortification practices that are utilized in macaroni and noodle products merit some discussion.

Enrichment. The most common practice is to add the specified amounts of iron, thiamin, riboflavin, and niacin in chemically pure form. However, the restoration of iron and three vitamins replaces only a few of the two dozen or more essential nutrients that are removed in substantial amounts during the conversion of whole wheat kernels into semolina or flour.

Better, but more expensive, means of enrichment are permitted by the standards of identity for enriched macaroni products and enriched noodle products.[2] It consists of providing the specified amounts of iron and the B vitamins through the addition of the highly nutritive ingredients dried yeast, dried torula yeast, and/or partly defatted wheat germ. The use of these ingredients adds extra protein, minerals, and B vitamins that are not provided by the usual means of enrichment.

The federal standards of identity also provide for the optional calcium and vitamin D enrichment of both macaroni and noodles. These nutrients are rarely added, although they would be very beneficial for people who drink little milk or who receive limited amounts of sunshine.

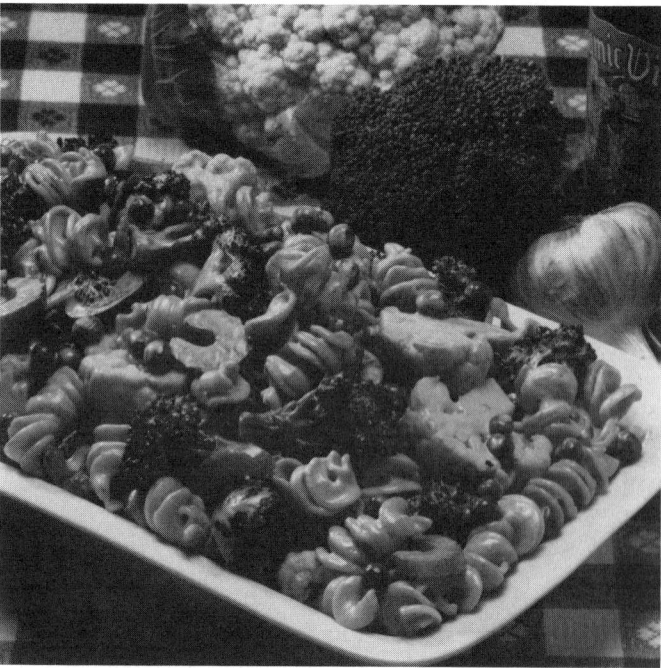

Fig. M-3a. Pasta salad. (Courtesy, Castle & Cooke, Inc.)

Fortification. The low quality of the wheat protein in macaroni and noodles is of considerable concern to nutritionists, because these foods are popular with children around the world. This concern led to the development of new products by food companies, which in turn led to the establishment of a standard of identity for "Enriched macaroni products with fortified protein."[3]

These products must contain at least 20% protein with a quality at least 95% that of casein (a major protein in cow's milk). The supplemental protein may be supplied by flours or meals made from nonwheat cereals or oilseeds such as soybeans, peanuts, sunflower seeds, and cottonseeds.

Similar protein fortified products are specified under the standards of identity for "Wheat and soy macaroni products" and for "Wheat and soy noodle products."[4] The quantities of protein in these items are at least 50% greater than those in similar items made from wheat flour alone. They are often sold in health food stores. However, products labeled "imitation soy macaroni" and "imitation soy noodles" may not contain as much protein because the word "imitation" denotes products which do not conform to a federal standard of identity.

Finally, "Nonfat milk macaroni products" contain between 12 and 25% nonfat milk solids.[5] These items contain from 36 to 75% more protein than is present in similar products made from wheat flour alone. A cup *(240 ml)* of cooked macaroni would also furnish from 89 to 175 mg of calcium and from 131 to 197 mg of phosphorus. Unfortunately, this type of fortified product does not appear to be available at the present time.

PREPARATION AND SERVING OF PASTA. Macaroni and noodle dishes may be utilized as main courses, appetizing side dishes, or as substitutes for starchy vegetables such as corn, potatoes, or rice.

MACEDOINE

A French word meaning a mixture of fruits or vegetables which are chopped and mixed with a dressing, or put into a gelatin. A macedoine can be served as a salad or as a dessert.

MACROBIOTICS, ZEN

This term encompasses both a diet and a philosophy of life. Zen refers to meditation, and macrobiotic suggests a tendency to prolong life.

(Also see ADZUKI BEAN, section on "Zen Macrobiotic Diets"; and ZEN MACROBIOTIC DIET.)

MACROCYTE

An exceptionally large red blood cell occurring chiefly in anemias.

MACRO (OR MAJOR) MINERALS

The major minerals—calcium, phosphorus, sodium, chlorine, magnesium, potassium, and sulfur.
(Also see MINERAL[S].)

MACRONUTRIENT

These are nutrients that are present in the body and required by the body in amounts ranging from a few tenths of a gram to one or more grams. Macronutrients include fat, water, protein, calcium, phosphorus, sodium, chlorine, magnesium, potassium, and sulfur.
(Also see MINERAL[S].)

MAGMA

• A suspension that is comprised of finely divided insoluble or nearly insoluble material in water; for example, magnesia magma (milk of magnesia).

---

[2]*Ibid.,* Sections 139.115 and 139.155.

[3]*Ibid.,* Section 139.117

---

[4]*Ibid.,* Sections 139.140 and 139.180

[5]*Ibid.,* Section 139.121.

• A crude organic mixture that is in the form of a paste; for example, the mixture of sugar syrup and sugar crystals produced during the refining process.

MAGNESIUM (Mg)

Contents	Page

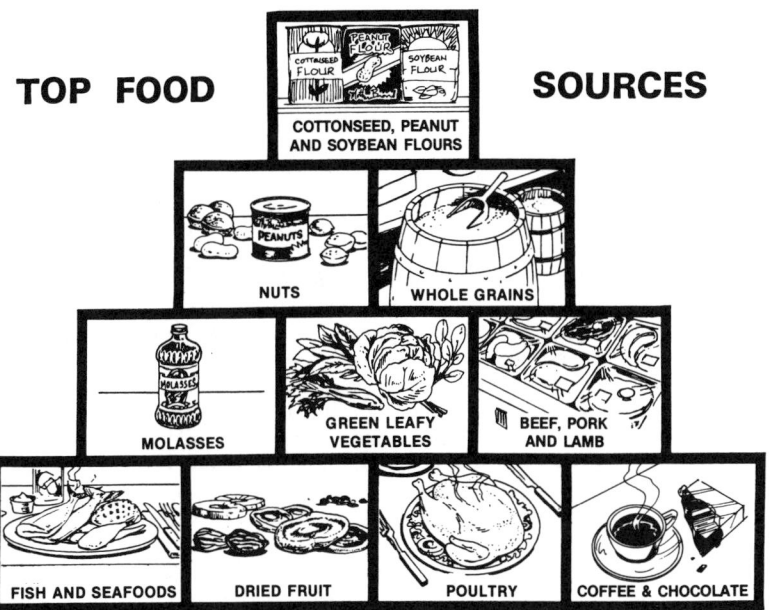

Fig. M-4. Top food sources of magnesium.

Magnesium is an essential mineral that accounts for about 0.05% of the body's total weight, or about 20 to 30 g. Nearly 60% of this is located in the bones in the form of phosphates and carbonates, while 28% of it is found in the soft tissues and 2% in the body fluids. The highest concentration in the soft tissues is in the liver and muscles. The red blood cells also contain magnesium. Blood serum contains 1 to 3 mg of magnesium per 100 ml, most of which is bound to proteins; the rest is in the form of ions.

HISTORY. Centuries ago, the ancient Romans claimed that *magnesia alba* (white magnesium salts from the district of Magnesia in Greece, from which the element was eventually named) cured many ailments. But, it was not until 1808 that Sir Humphrey Davy, the British chemist, announced that he had isolated the element, magnesium.

In 1926, LeRoy, in France, using mice, first proved that magnesium is an essential nutrient for animals. Subsequently, McCollum and co-workers described several magnesium deficiency signs in rats and dogs, including magnesium tetany, a form of convulsions in which the nerves and muscles are affected. Indications that magnesium is required by man followed during the period 1933-1944.

ABSORPTION, METABOLISM, EXCRETION. From 30 to 50% of the average daily intake of magnesium is absorbed in the small intestine. Almost all of the magnesium in the feces represents unabsorbed dietary magnesium. Its absorption is interfered with by high intake of calcium, phosphate, oxalic acid (spinach, rhubarb), phytate (whole grain cereals), and poorly digested fats (long chain saturated fatty acids). Its absorption is enhanced by protein, lactose (milk sugar), vitamin D, growth hormone, and antibiotics.

Magnesium is generally reabsorbed in the kidneys, thus minimizing the loss of body reserves.

The main route of excretion of magnesium is the urine. Aldosterone, a hormone secreted by the adrenal gland, helps regulate the rate of magnesium excretion through the kidneys. Losses tend to increase with the consumption of alcohol or the use of diuretics.

FUNCTIONS OF MAGNESIUM. Magnesium is involved in many functions. It is a constituent of bones and teeth; it is an essential element of cellular metabolism, often as an activator of enzymes involved in phosphorylated compounds and of the high energy phosphate transfer of ADP and ATP; and it is involved in activating certain peptidases in protein digestion. Magnesium relaxes nerve impulses and muscle contraction; functioning antagonistically to calcium which is stimulatory.

DEFICIENCY SYMPTOMS. A deficiency of magnesium is characterized by (1) muscle spasms (tremor, twitching) and rapid heartbeat; (2) confusion, hallucinations, and disorientation; and (3) lack of appetite, listlessness, nausea, and vomiting.

Magnesium deficiency has been observed in alcoholics, in severe kidney disease, in acute diarrhea, and in kwashiorkor.

Some scientists have cautiously theorized a magnesium-cancer link. In support of this thinking, it is noteworthy that fewer cases of leukemia (a form of blood cancer characterized by abnormal increase of white blood cells) have been reported in Poland in areas where magnesium is plentiful in the soil and drinking water than in areas where it is scarce. At this time the magnesium-cancer link theory is without adequate proof, but it merits further research.

INTERRELATIONSHIPS. When magnesium intake is extremely low, calcium is sometimes deposited in soft tissues forming calcified lesions.

An excess of magnesium upsets calcium and phosphorus metabolism. Also, with diets adequate in magnesium and other nutrients, increasing the calcium and/or phosphorus results in magnesium deficiency.

Magnesium activates many enzyme systems, particularly those concerned with transferring phosphate from ATP and ADP. Magnesium is also capable of inactivating certain enzymes, and is known to be a component of at least one enzyme.

Overuse of such substances as *milk of magnesia* (magnesium hydroxide, an antacid and laxative) or *Epsom salts* (magnesium sulfate, a laxative and tonic) may lead to deficiencies of other minerals, or even to toxicity.

RECOMMENDED DAILY ALLOWANCE OF MAGNESIUM. The Food and Nutrition Board (FNB) of

Allowances of magnesium are given in the section on MINERAL[S], Table M-25, Mineral Table.

● **Magnesium intake in average U.S. diet**—The U.S. Department of Agriculture reported that foods available for consumption in the United States in 1988 provided an average of 330 mg of magnesium per person per day, and that the leading sources were as follows: dairy products, 18.5%; flour and cereal products, 18.5%; meat, poultry, and fish, 15.4%; legumes, including dry beans and peas, nuts, soya flour, and grits, 12.7%; and vegetables, including tomatoes, 16.1%.

Surveys indicate that the magnesium content of the average American diet is about 120 mg per 1,000 Calories (kcal). Thus, a person consuming a varied diet of about 2,000 Calories (kcal) will get 240 mg of magnesium. However, a woman following diets limiting intake to 1,000 to 1,500 Calories (kcal) will likely have magnesium intakes below the recommended daily allowance.

TOXICITY. Magnesium toxicity may occur when the kidneys are unable to get rid of a large overload; characterized by slowed breathing, coma, and sometimes death. It is noteworthy that magnesium salts taken by pregnant mothers may affect their newborn babies.

SOURCES OF MAGNESIUM. Magnesium is relatively widespread in foods.

Human milk contains approximately 3 mg of magnesium per 100 g, while cow's milk contains about 13 mg/100 g. Processing grains causes them to lose most of their magnesium. Likewise, refined sugar, alcohol, fats, and oils do not contain magnesium. Excessive cooking of foods in large amounts of water can cause losses.

Groupings by rank of common food sources of magnesium are given in the section on MINERAL[S], Table M-25, Mineral Table.

For additional sources and more precise values of magnesium, see Food Composition Table F-21 of this book.

(Also see MINERAL[S], Table M-25, Mineral Table.)

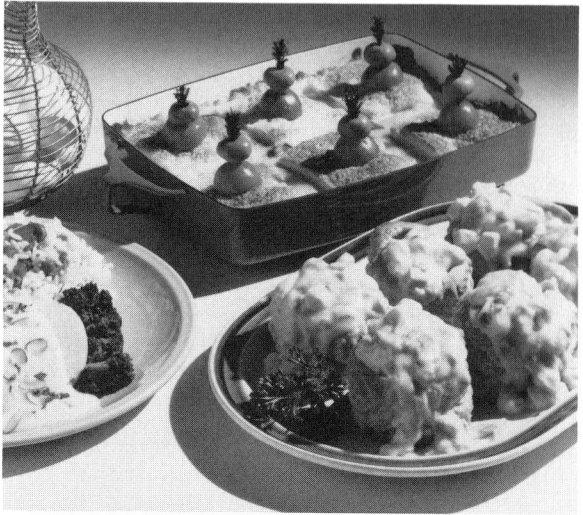

Fig. M-5. Soybean products, made from soybean flour—a top source of magnesium. (Courtesy, Worthington Foods, Worthington, Ohio)

MAILLARD REACTION

Nonenzymatic browning that takes place upon heating or prolonged storage of food is caused by this reaction. The responsible chemical reaction occurs between a sugar and a free amino group (NH_2) of an amino acid. Once the reaction occurs the amino acid is no longer biologically available, thus reducing the nutritive value of the food. Most Maillard reactions take place with the essential amino acid lysine, since it has a free amino group not involved in a peptide bond. Dr. L. C. Maillard, who first described the reaction, died in 1936 without ever receiving recognition for the importance of his pioneering work.

(Also see LYSINE.)

MALABSORPTION SYNDROME

This term is used to describe a number of symptoms and signs indicating a defect which limits or prevents absorption of one or more essential nutrient from the small intestine. Individuals suffering from a malabsorption syndrome display in varying degrees the following clinical manifestations: (1) diarrhea; (2) steatorrhea (fatty diarrhea) due to impaired fat absorption; (3) progressive weight loss and muscle wasting; (4) abdominal distention; and (5) evidence of vitamin and mineral deficiencies, such as macrocytic anemia due to inadequate folic acid and vitamin B-12 absorption, iron-deficiency anemia, hypocalcemic (low calcium) tetany, and inflammation of the tongue, mouth, and skin—glossitis, stomatitis, and dermatitis, respectively. The laboratory findings characteristic of malabsorption consist of decreases in the blood concentrations of electrolytes, albumin, and carotene, and increases in fecal fat and nitrogen (protein).

The causes of malabsorption syndrome are diverse, but they fall into seven general categories: (1) heart and blood vessel disorders, (2) endocrinal disorders, (3) inadequate absorptive surface, (4) inadequate digestion, (5) lymphatic obstruction, (6) defects in the absorption surface, and (7) reduced bile salts.

Diagnosis of a malabsorption syndrome is based on the results of absorption tests such as xylose absorption, fat absorption balance study, the Schilling test for vitamin B-12 absorption, and the folic acid test. Also gastrointestinal x ray studies, small intestine biopsy, prothrombin time, and serum levels of vitamin A are useful diagnostic tools.

Treatment is directed toward (1) eliminating, insofar as possible, the abnormality causing the malabsorption, (2) vitamin and mineral supplements, and (3) dietary modifications.

Dietary modification will differ due to the cause of the malabsorption syndrome. In general, the diet should be high in calories and protein, but some disorders require the elimination of certain carbohydrates, proteins, or amino acids. Persistent diarrhea may be dealt with by a soft or fiber-restricted diet. Furthermore, a modification of fat intake is beneficial; for example, the common practice of incorporating medium chain triglycerides (8- and 10-carbon chains) into the diet. Medium chain triglycerides substitution can reduce the steatorrhea and the losses of calcium, sodium, and potassium observed in many malabsorption syndromes.

MALAISE

A feeling of illness or depression.

MALARIA

Initially, there was some confusion over the cause-and-effect of this disease; hence, the name *malaria* which literally means *bad air.* Swamps do produce bad air but, more importantly, they also produce *Anopheles* mosquitoes which carry the malaria parasites. In the cycle of this parasite, man serves as an intermediate host, and the mosquito serves as a vector. Transmission of the disease requires at least two mosquito bites—one to pick up the malaria parasite, and another to infect the victim. Fig.M-6 illustrates the malaria cycle.

There are four types of *Plasmodium* which are responsible for three distinct forms of malaria. Each form of malaria can be distinguished by the length of time between the recurrent malaria attacks.

• **Tertian malaria**—Merozoites are released every other day—every 48 hours.

• **Quartan malaria**—Attacks occur every fourth day, or 72 hours apart; hence, the name quartan.

• **Falciparum malaria**—In this form of malaria there is no characteristic length of time between attacks since the mero-

zoites multiply in asynchronous cycles.

It is not possible to prevent infection, but while residing in an area where there is a risk of contracting malaria, drugs can be taken that suppress the symptoms.

Prevention can only come about through public health programs that eliminate the *Anopheles* mosquito.

From a nutritional standpoint, malaria is important for two reasons. First, malaria survives in areas where the mosquito and the infected human population remain above a critical density for each. This situation often occurs in time of famine when people congregate, following which rains come producing breeding grounds for mosquitoes. Malaria then spreads rapidly among the weakened survivors of the famine. Second, malaria attacks, chronic malaria, or repeated infections of malaria are taxing on the nutritional reserves of the body. Good nutrition is essential to recovery. A high calorie, high protein, high fluid intake with vitamin supplementation is recommended.

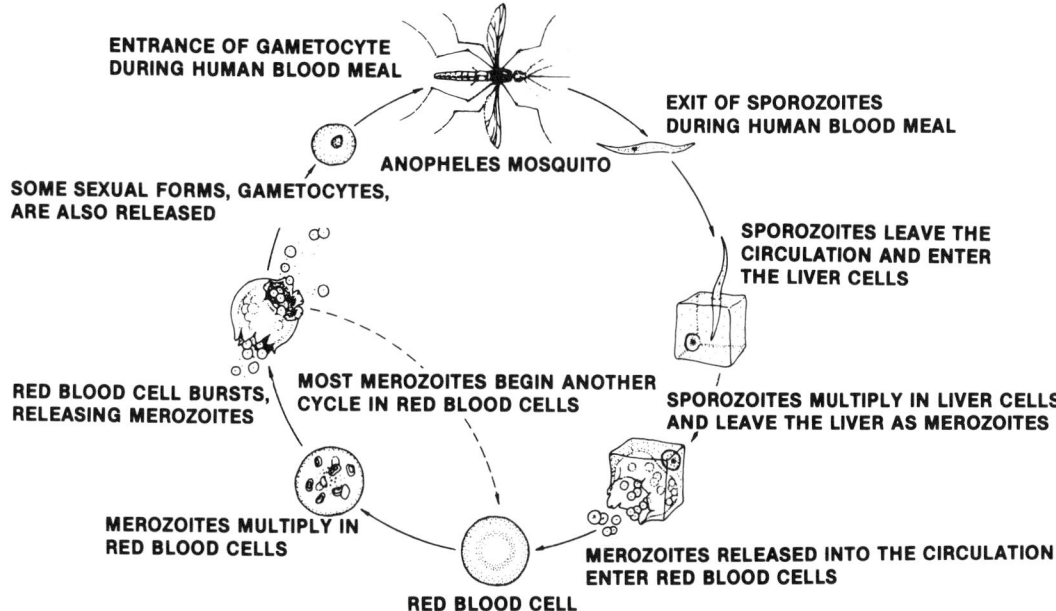

Fig. M-6. The malaria cycle.

MALAY APPLE (POMERAC) *Eugenia malaccensis*

The fruit of an evergreen tree (of a family *Myrtaceae*) that is native to Malaysia and is now grown throughout the tropics. Malay apples are reddish-pink, oblong or pear-shaped fruit that are about 3 in. (*8 cm*) long. They have a white flesh that surrounds the single large seed. The rather bland fruit may be eaten fresh or made into jam or jelly.

Malay apples have a high water content (91%) and are low in calories (32 kcal per 100 g) and carbohydrates (8%). They are a fair source of vitamin C.

MALFORMATION

Any abnormal development in the physical and physiological makeup of the body.

MALIGNANT

Cancerous growth, as distinguished from a benign growth. (Also see CANCER.)

MALNUTRITION

This term refers to an impairment of health resulting from a failure of the diet, or from a failure of the physiologic processes of the body itself, to provide to the tissues the correct proportions of nutrients. Thus, malnutrition may involve nutrient deficiencies, excesses of nutrients such as carbohydrates, or a combination of deficiencies and excesses.

(Also see DEFICIENCY DISEASES; and DISEASES.)

Disproportions or imbalances between the dietary supply and the tissue requirement for nutrients are responsible for severe deficiency diseases, like beriberi. Populations relying on dietary staples, such as commercially milled white rice, which is high in carbohydrates but low in the thiamin required for its metabolism, are very susceptible to beriberi. Other groups eating a similar diet may avoid the disease by using rice which has been parboiled prior to milling; parboiling rice drives the thiamin from the outside of the grain into the inner parts. As a result, less thiamin is lost when the outer layers of rice are removed during milling.

(Also see BERIBERI; and RICE, section headed "Nutritional Losses.")

Another example of a potential imbalance is the substitution of heat-processed polyunsaturated fats for saturated fats without the addition of vitamin E to the diet. The natural sources of these fats are plant seeds which usually contain ample amounts of vitamin E. But the vitamin E is easily destroyed in the extracted oils by exposure to heat, light, and oxygen. Although severe deficiencies of vitamin E are rare, marginal deficiencies may, over a long period, be responsible for cellular damage and premature senility. Both disorders may be caused by the peroxidation of polyunsaturated fatty acids, which is prevented by vitamin E.

(Also see VITAMIN E.)

Finally, there is evidence that high intake of dietary protein, such as 100 to 150 g/day, results in increased calcium excretion in the urine, thereby raising the requirement for dietary calcium to replace the extra loss from the body. Failure to provide the additional calcium in the diet may lead to the removal of calcium from bone, since the body maintains the level of the mineral in the blood by taking it from bone.

(Also see CALCIUM; and OSTEOPOROSIS.)

MALNUTRITION AROUND THE WORLD.

Many adverse physical conditions are brought about by prolonged periods of malnutrition, especially the absence of sufficient quantities of critical compounds in the diet. Rickets, scurvy, beriberi, pellagra, vitamin A deficiency (a major cause of blindness in many countries), anemia, iodine deficiency (which often leads to endemic goiter and cretinism), kwashiorkor, and marasmus are but a few of the many classical examples of nutritional deficiency diseases. When malnutrition begins at an early age and persists over a substantial period of time, a variety of defects may develop involving bone and body structures and mental condition, all of which may be irreversible. Unfortunately, in the developing countries, the basic problem is one of gross dietary inadequacies which may be compounded by specific vitamin or protein insufficiency.

The most malnutrition is found in the developing countries where 70% of the people in the world live, but where only 40% of the world's food is produced. Fig. M-7 shows the countries where the greatest deficits of protein and calories are found.

In Latin America, where protein-poor cereal grains are the imperfect staff of life, 82 out of every 1,000 children die before their first birthday; and another 12 die before they reach the age of 4. Even the survivors may envy the dead. Often brain damaged, they become the adults who are most in need of help and least able to help themselves.

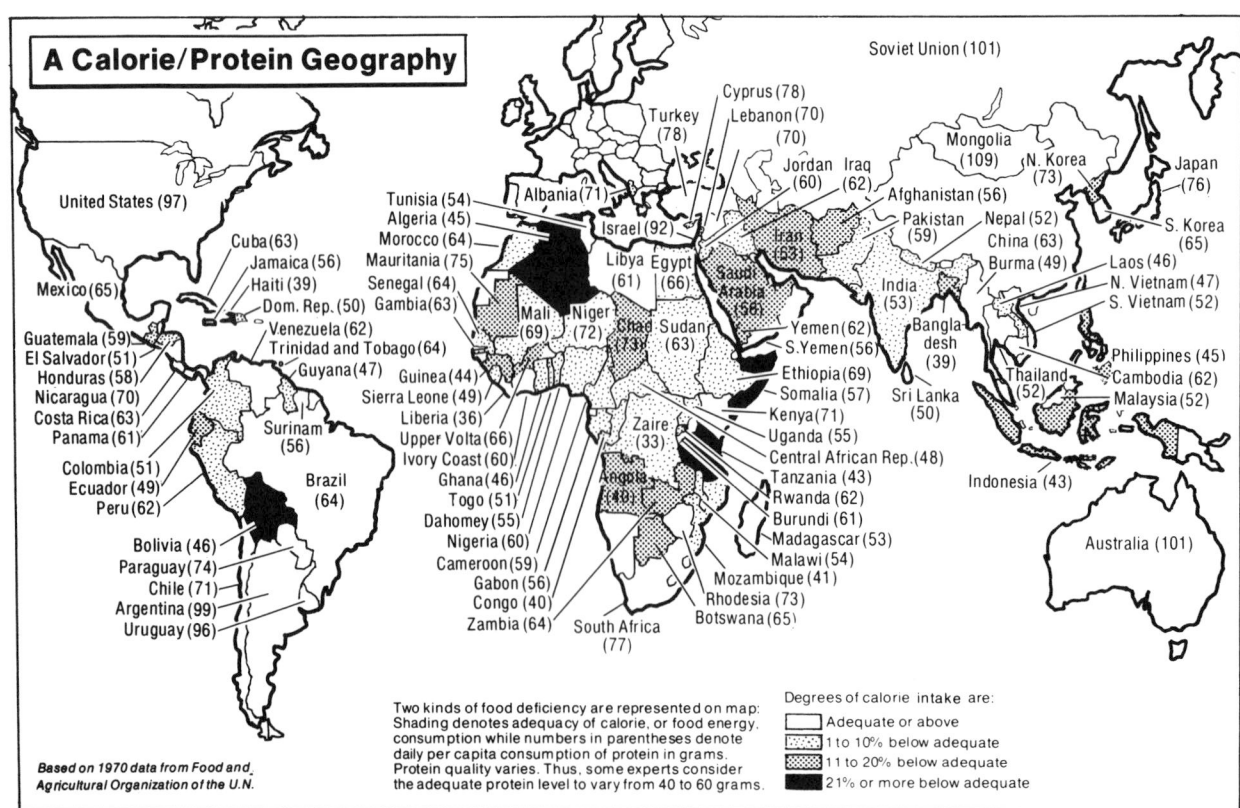

Fig. M-7. World geography of calories and proteins. (Courtesy, *The New York Times*)

In the Far East and Africa, 25 to 30% of the population is estimated to suffer from significant undernutrition. FAO estimates that (1) altogether in the developing world (exclusive of the Asian centrally planned economies for which insufficient information is available), malnutrition affects around 460 million people—that's nearly twice the population of the United States; and (2) one-half of the young children in the developing countries suffer in varying degrees from inadequate nutrition.[6]

According to the World Health Organization (WHO), 10 million children under the age of 5 are now chronically and severely malnourished, and 90 million more are moderately affected. While undernourished children may remain alive, they are extremely vulnerable to minor infectious diseases. WHO figures also show that of all the deaths in the poor countries, more than half occur among children under 5, and that the vast majority of these deaths, perhaps as many as 75%, are due to malnutrition complicated by infection.

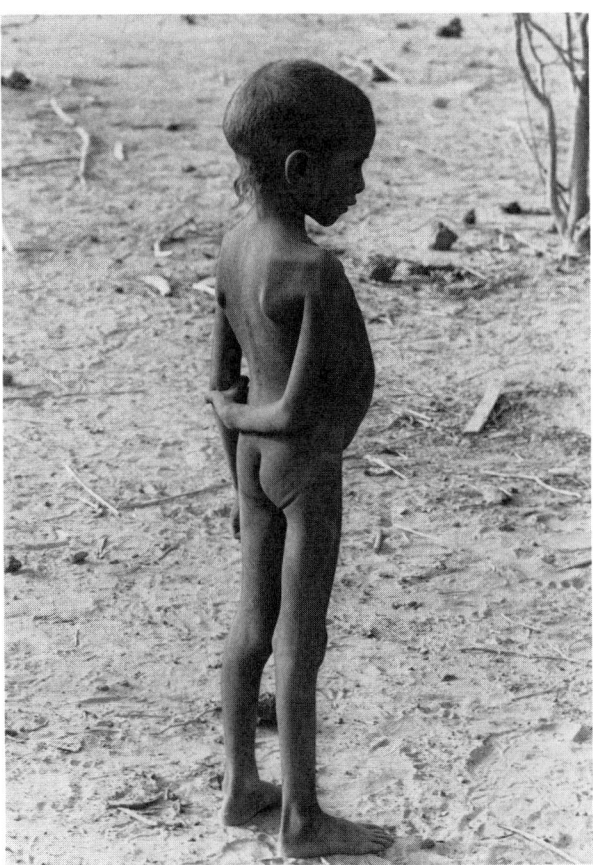

Fig. M-8. A malnourished youngster in the Sahel. Five years of drought caused human suffering and loss of cattle in the six countries along the southern edge of the Sahara. The Sahelian Zone includes Upper Volta, Mauritania, Niger, Senegal, Mali and Chad. (Courtesy, Agency for International Development)

CAUSES OF MALNUTRITION. Poor health due to malnourishment may be the result of one or more factors contributing to poor diets or reduced utilization of nutrients of the body. A listing of some of the more important causes of malnutrition follows:

1. Failure to cultivate available arable land.
2. Catastrophic events, including droughts, floods, earthquakes, wars, and civil disorders.
3. The population explosion.
4. Bad weather.
5. Inefficient food production due to lack of knowledge, skills, seeds, improved animals, feeds, fertilizer, pesticides, farming equipment, and irrigation.
6. Shortages of grains (a) forcing low-income people to resort to starchy plants, such as bananas, sweet potatoes, and cassava, for their staple foods, and (b) creating nutritional problems due to the low content of protein and other nutrients in these high-carbohydrate foods.
7. Lack of money.
8. High food costs.
9. Poor sanitation.
10. Poor nutritional knowledge and practices.
11. Disorders which hamper the utilization of nutrients, including uncontrolled diabetes, hyperthyroidism, hyperparathyroidism, diarrhea, vomiting, parasites, wasting diseases, infections, fevers, inborn errors of metabolism, and toxicants in food.
12. Medical treatments which interfere with nutritional processes; among them, the administration of antibiotics, laxatives, enemas, hormones, anticonvulsants, diuretics, and gastrointestinal surgery, and the severe restriction of diet.

(Also see DEFICIENCY DISEASES.)

CONSEQUENCES OF MALNUTRITION. The cost to the individual and to the society of illness, disability, and death from malnutrition far outweigh the expense of adequate nutrition. Some of these consequences are:

1. Impairment of physical and mental development.
2. Increased susceptibility to infectious diseases.
3. Increased susceptibility to metabolic disorders.
4. Reduced work capacity.

COMMON TYPES OF MALNUTRITION. About one billion cases of malnutrition around the world result mainly from lack of sufficient food.[7] However, hundreds of millions of people suffer from mild to severe nutritional deficiency diseases such as anemia, beriberi, blindness due to vitamin A deficiency (xerophthalmia), goiter, marasmus, pellagra, protein-energy malnutrition, rickets (children) or osteomalacia (adults), and scurvy.

Some of the more prevalent types of deficiencies are briefly described in the paragraphs which follow.

Energy-Protein Malnutrition. An insufficient intake of energy and/or protein needed to maintain the body functions—for activity, for growth, and for resistance to infectious diseases—may be manifested, in keeping with the severity of the deficiency, from the slight impairment of growth or thinness seen in mildly undernourished children to the gross alterations shown by persons suffering from kwashiorkor (protein deficiency) or marasmus (energy deficiency).

(Also see MALNUTRITION, PROTEIN-ENERGY; and STARVATION.)

Deficiencies of Minerals or Vitamins. The lack of sufficient quantities of critical vitamins or minerals may be the cause of many adverse conditions, even when the dietary

---

[6]*The World Food Situation and Prospects to 1985*, Foreign Ag. Econ. Report No. 98, Economic Research Service, USDA, p. 50.

[7]McLaren, D. S., "Hunger/Malnutrition: Some Misconceptions," *The Professional Nutritionist*, Fall 1978, p. 13.

amounts of protein and energy are adequate.

(Also see ANEMIA; BERIBERI; BLINDNESS DUE TO VITAMIN A DEFICIENCY; DEFICIENCY DISEASES; GOITER; PELLAGRA; RICKETS; and SCURVY.)

Disorders of Nutrient Utilization.

Malnutrition may result even when the diet contains adequate amounts of all of the nutrients which are known to be required. In these cases, disease may be caused by a failure of the body to utilize fully certain nutrients, by accumulation of excess amounts of nutrients and/or their metabolites, or by diet-induced changes of the normal environment in and around tissues so that these areas develop increased vulnerability to pathogenic agents and stress factors. However, there may also be nonnutritional causes of some of these disorders, since it has been difficult to explain why a given diet results in disease for some, and fairly good health for others.

(Also see HEART DISEASE; DENTAL CARIES; DIABETES MELLITUS; INBORN ERRORS OF METABOLISM; MALABSORPTION SYNDROME; OBESITY; OSTEOPOROSIS.)

SIGNS OF MALNUTRITION.

There are many signs which indicate moderate to severe malnutrition. Also, a number of laboratory tests are available for detection of tissue pathologies, metabolic imbalances, and deficiency diseases. It would be worthwhile, however, to be able to diagnose early stages of malnutrition, since prompt correction of dietary imbalances will, in the long run, be much less costly than later treatment of the more severe stages.

The incidence of malnutrition may be estimated for communities by examining hospital and autopsy records, and by interviewing the parents of deceased children. Also, some individual cases may be diagnosed by their features. Each of these types of assessment will be discussed under the items which follow.

Indicators of Malnutrition in Communities.

Although cases of malnutrition may be found among all socioeconomic classes, one is most likely to find this condition in areas where there are serious problems concerning the following factors: the production and distribution of food, unemployment and low incomes, environmental sanitation, public health and other community services, and unusual food preferences.

A survey of the living conditions in a community might, therefore, save time and money in assessing the nutritional status of its residents. The following types of data might be collected in such a survey: (1) population from latest census; (2) total food consumption by the population (which may be roughly estimated from figures showing local production and shipments of food into the area); (3) foods and nutrients available per capita, which may be calculated from (1) and (2) and a food composition table; (4) morbidity and mortality statistics, plus estimates of school attendance and absenteeism in local industry; (5) infant feeding practices, such as breast feeding, use of formulas, baby foods, table foods, etc.; (6) food preferences and customs of the ethnic and religious groups in the community; (7) employment and income status; (8) water quality and sanitary facilities for disposal of garbage and human and animal waste; (9) food, health, and financial services provided by public and voluntary agencies; and (10) the professional training and number of workers in the service agencies.

Analyses of the data should provide indications of the types of malnutrition and other health problems which are most likely to be present.

Signs of Malnutrition in Individuals.

Assessment of the nutritional status of individuals by laboratory tests is expensive, so it is necessary to have some screening procedures for identifying persons who are most likely to suffer from malnutrition. Such screenings may include medical histories of individuals and their families; heights, weights, and other growth data for children; dietary histories; and observations of the face, tongue, mouth, eyes, skin, muscular and skeletal development, and weight in proportion to height.

Also, the following are valuable adjuncts in screening: measurements of hemoglobin in finger prick samples of blood, testing of urine with pretreated tapes for sugar and ketone bodies, and examination for the presence of sediment in the urine. In adolescents, the stage of sexual development in relation to age may be determined by physicians or nurses, since maturation may be delayed in malnutrition.

Criteria for the diagnosis of specific nutritional disorders are given in this book under the separate entries for each disease. Physical signs often associated with malnutrition are shown in Table M-1.

(Also see DEFICIENCY DISEASES.)

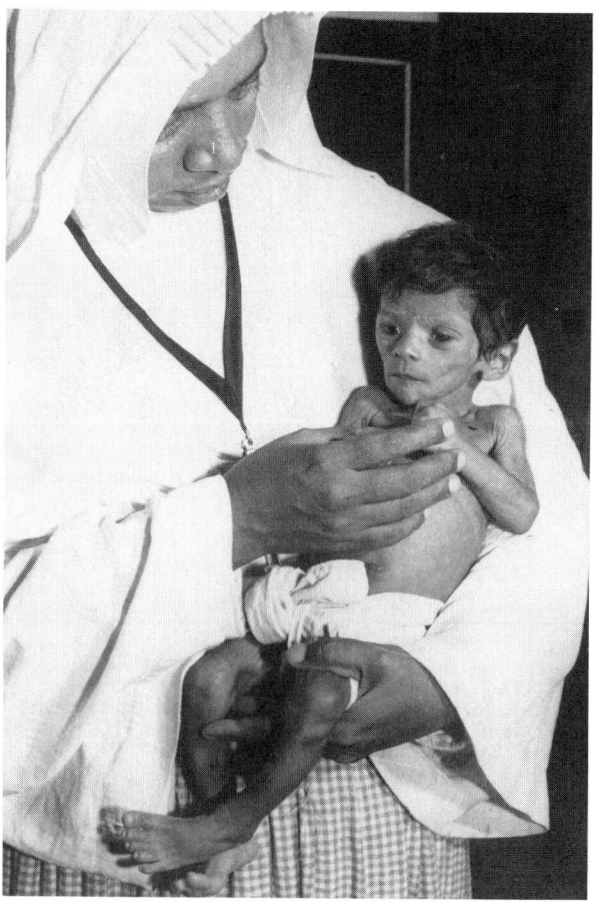

Fig. M-9. Malnutrition. (Courtesy, FAO, Rome, Italy)

TABLE M-1
PHYSICAL SIGNS WHICH ARE OFTEN ASSOCIATED WITH MALNUTRITION[1]

Area of Body Examined	Normal Appearance	Common Signs of Malnutrition	Differential Diagnoses (other causes of clinical signs)
Appearance in general	Normal weight for age, sex, and height. Alert and emotionally stable. No areas of edema.	Significant overweight or underweight. Apathetic or hyper-irritable. Loss or slowness of ankle or knee reflexes. Pitting edema.	Nonnutritional nervous or metabolic disorders. Endocrine diseases.
Eyes	Shiny and free from area of abnormal pigmentation, opacity, vascularization, and dryness.	Paleness, dryness, redness, or pigmentation of membranes (conjunctiva). Foamy patches on conjunctiva (Bitot's spots). Dullness, softness, or vascularization of the cornea. Redness or fissures on eyelids.	Exposure to environmental or chemical irritants. Tissue changes accompanying aging.
Face	Skin is clear and uniform in color, free of all except minor blemishes. Free of swollen or lumpy areas.	Skin is lighter (depigmentation) and darker (over cheeks and under eyes) areas. Greasy scales around nose and lips. Swollen or lumpy areas.	Poor hygiene. Addison's disease (moonface).
Glands	No swollen areas on face or neck.	Swelling of parotids (enlarged "jowls") or thyroid (front of neck near its base).	Mumps. Inflammation, tumor, or hyperfunction of the thyroid.
Gums	Red, free from bleeding or swelling.	Receded. *Spongy* and bleeding. Swelling of the gingiva.	Medication. Periodontal disease. Poor oral hygiene.
Hair	Shiny, firmly attached to scalp (not easily plucked without pain to patient).	Dullness, may be brittle and easily plucked without pain. Sometimes lighter in color than normal (depigmentation may be bandlike when hair is held up to a source of light).	Endocrine disorders.
Lips	Smooth, not chapped, cracked, or swollen.	Swollen, red, or cracked (cheilosis). Angular fissues and/or scars at the corners of the mouth.	Herpes (blisters). Exposure to strong sunshine, dry or cold climates.
Muscles	Muscles are firm and of normal size.	Wasting and flabbiness of muscle. Bleeding into muscle.	Wasting diseases. Trauma.
Nails	Firm, pink.	Spoon-shaped nails. Brittle and ridged nails.	Cardiopulmonary disease.
Organs, internal	Normal heart rate and rhythm. Normal blood pressure. Internal organs cannot be palpated (except liver in children).	Racing heartbeat (over 100 beats per minute). Abnormal rhythm of heart. High blood pressure. Palpable enlargement of liver or spleen.	Rheumatic fever. Nonnutritional diseases of the heart, liver, spleen, and kidneys.
Skeleton	Bones have normal sizes and shapes.	Softening, swelling, or distorted shapes of bones and joints.	Nonnutritional connective tissue disorders.
Skin	Smooth, free of rashes, swellings, and discoloration.	Roughness (follicular hyperkeratosis), dryness or flakiness. Irregular pigmentation, black and blue marks, *crazy pavement* lesions. Symmetrical, reddened lesions (like sunburn). Looseness of skin (lack of subcutaneous fat).	Secondary syphilis. Poor or improper hygiene (excessive washing with soap). Environmental irritants. Trauma. Anticoagulant therapy.
Teeth	Enamel is unbroken and unspotted. None or a few small cavities.	Caries. Mottled or darkened areas of enamel.	Developmental abnormalities. Stains from foods or cigarettes.
Tongue	Normal size of papillae (no atrophy or hypertrophy). Color is uniform and deep red. Sense of taste is without impairment.	Atrophy of papillae (the tongue is smooth) or hypertrophy of papillae. Irregularly shaped and distributed white patches. Swollen, scarlet, magenta (purple colored), or raw tongue.	Dietary irritants. Colors or dyes from food. Nonnutritional anemias. Antibiotics. Uremia. Malignancy.

[1]Adapted by the authors from *American Journal of Public Health*, Vol. 63, November 1973 Supplement, p. 19, Table 1.

TREATMENT AND PREVENTION OF MALNUTRITION.

The first step in the correction of a dietary imbalance is the use of a modified or supplemented diet, or when necessary, medical correction of a disorder which limits the utilization of nutrients.

(Also see MINERAL[S]; MINERAL SUPPLEMENTS; MODIFIED DIETS; NUTRITIONAL SUPPLEMENTS; and VITAMIN[S].)

Sometimes it is necessary to administer nutrients by tube feeding to hospitalized patients who can't eat, or by injection to persons who require a supplement such as vitamin B-12, which is stored in the body and needs only to be supplied once a month.

Overtreatment of malnutrition by administration of excessive amounts of nutrients in a short period of time may be dangerous, since the victim usually has a reduced ability to detoxify and excrete excess materials. The treatment may, therefore, produce effects worse than the disease. All treatments require supervision by health professionals who are able to recognize the clinical signs of deterioration in the patient.

It may be more expeditious at the community, state, or national levels to enrich and fortify foods of low nutrient quality with amino acids, minerals, and vitamins, than to try to supply foods which naturally contain the optimal quantities of nutrients. This is particularly applicable to situations where foods, which are rich in the desired nutrients, are rejected by the population to be fed. For example, there is a high rejection rate for broccoli, carrots, and other vegetable sources of vitamin A in the U.S. School Lunch Program. Therefore, food technologists have proposed the development of a snack food, like a potato chip, which would contain spinach powder and be fortified with minerals and vitamins.

Prevention of malnutrition requires correction of the factors leading to a poor diet. This calls for education of the consumer; instituting new patterns of food selection, preparation, and consumption; and insuring that supplies of the appropriate foods are available.

(Also see DEFICIENCY DISEASES; and ENRICHMENT [Fortification, Nutrification, Restoration].)

MALNUTRITION, PROTEIN-ENERGY

One of the most serious nutritional problems in the developing countries of the world is a group of disorders associated with inadequate or unbalanced intakes of protein and energy. It is often convenient to consider these disorders as various types of protein-energy malnutrition (PEM).

DIETARY PROTEIN AND ENERGY SUPPLIES AROUND THE WORLD. Although protein-energy malnutrition (PEM) may be found even in the developed countries, by far the greatest number of cases occur in the developing countries where food shortages limit the average consumption of protein and energy. Therefore, rough indicators of the incidence of PEM are the per capita deficits in protein and energy supplies of various countries. This means that there is the likelihood of there being a significant number of cases of PEM in countries where the per capita supplies of protein and/or energy fall below the recommended daily requirements defined by the Joint FAO/WHO Expert Committee on Energy and Protein Requirements.[8]

An assessment of the world situation, per capita protein and calories, by FAO/WHO, is summarized in Table M-2. It is noteworthy that, of the 127 countries included in Table M-2, 33 are classed as developed and 94 are classed as developing. Table M-2 also shows the per capita proteins and calories per day of countries in 2 groups: (1) developed countries, and (2) developing countries.

Additional facts pertinent to world per capita protein and energy in supplies follow:

1. In general, countries that are low in calories are also

TABLE M-2
PER CAPITA PROTEINS AND CALORIES PER DAY IN DEVELOPED COUNTRIES AND DEVELOPING COUNTRIES[1]

Year	Per Capita Protein/Day			Per Capita Calories/Day		
	World	Developed Countries	Developing Countries	World	Developed Countries	Developing Countries
	(g)	(g)	(g)	(kcal)	(kcal)	(kcal)
1970	69.0	96.4	57.4	2,480	3,150	2,200
1985	72.6	100.0	63.3	2,610	3,220	2,400

[1]United Nations data.

low in protein supplies; and countries that are low in total protein are also low in animal protein (which generally has a higher biological value than protein from plant sources).

2. A total of 65 countries—over half of all countries studied—fail to meet the recommended daily requirement of 2,385 Calories (kcal) per person.

3. All but two of the 127 countries studied meet or exceed the recommended daily requirement of 38.7 g of protein per person. But it should be noted that, on a worldwide basis, much protein is diverted to meet dietary energy deficits; it is estimated that 11% of the energy comes from protein. Remember, too, that many of the countries that are low in total protein depend to a large extent on protein from plant sources which is required in greater amounts than animal protein.

4. The developed countries average over 3,150 Calories (kcal) per capita per day in their energy supplies (23% above requirement), whereas the developing countries average only 2,200 Calories (kcal) per capita per day (see Table M-2). Similarly, the protein supply is over 96 g per capita per day in the developed countries vs less than 58 g in the developing regions; and much of the latter is vegetable protein rather than animal protein, and is diverted in an attempt to meet the energy deficits (see Table M-2).

5. Despite an apparently adequate supply of energy and protein, a country may have a considerable number of people who fail to have their requirements met due to the un-

equal distribution of food between the different socioeconomic classes. There may also be disproportionate distributions of food within households, with the male head receiving well over his needs while the wife and children receive less than their needs.[9]

TYPES OF PROTEIN-ENERGY MALNUTRITION. Depending upon the nature and extent of the deficiency, there is at one extreme *Kwashiorkor*, or severe deficiency of protein; and at the other, *marasmus*, or severe deficiency of energy. In between are the combination disorders such as *marasmic kwashiorkor* and *nutritional dwarfing*. More than likely, deficiencies of certain minerals and vitamins accompany all of these disorders, except that the problems due to severe deficiencies of protein or energy overshadow the other problems. A discussion of the characteristics of each type of PEM follows.

Kwashiorkor. Infants fed low-protein, starchy foods (such as bananas, yams, and cassava) after weaning may develop kwashiorkor. This imbalanced diet, which has a subnormal protein-to-calorie ratio for infants, prevents some

---

[8]Per capita requirements per day of 2,385 Calories (kcal) and 38.7 g of protein (as defined by the FAO/WHO Expert Committee in April 1971). From *Nutrition Newsletter*, Vol. 11, No. 4, FAO of the United Nations, October-December 1973, p. 4., Table 1.

[9]den Hartog, A. P., "Unequal Distribution of Food Within the Household," *Nutrition Newsletter*, Vol. 10, No. 4, FAO of the United Nations, October-December 1972, p. 8.

of the adaptive mechanisms of the body from operating the way that they do in the case of starvation or marasmus.

In kwashiorkor there is less breakdown of protein and release of amino acids from muscle than in marasmus since provision of adequate energy in the diet reduces the adrenal cortical response to starvation and, consequently, the flow of amino acids from muscle to viscera. The release of amino acids from muscle is, therefore, not sufficient to meet the needs of the internal organs.

Particularly critical is the loss of tissue cells from the gastrointestinal lining which leads to various types of malabsorption. Also, the severe shortage of protein results in a reduction in synthesis of digestive enzymes, normally secreted from the pancreas or present in the intestinal wall. Thus, there is likely to be diarrhea which may cause excessive loss of water or dehydration, loss of mineral salts, and an electrolyte imbalance.

There may also be glucose intolerance, and, in some cases, elevated levels of plasma growth hormones, although the particular role of this hormone in malnutrition is not fully understood. Also, there may be reductions in the secretions of the thyroid gland which could lead to failure of the body to maintain its temperature.

Liver function is greatly reduced due to lack of protein for the synthesis of enzymes. Also, there is likely to be fat accumulation in the liver due to its inability to package fat with protein for transport in the blood. Low blood levels of albumin, along with anemia, result from the scarcity of amino acids for protein synthesis; and edema is a consequence of the depletion of plasma proteins and electrolytes.

The production of antibodies is likely to be greatly reduced and the victim, therefore, will be prone to infectious diseases. In chronic cases, there is likely to be delayed eruption of teeth, poor enamel with many caries, and pale gums and mucous membranes due to anemia.

Marasmus. Starvation in adults has a counterpart in children called marasmus. It is a severe deficiency of energy usually found in infants and young children who are not getting enough food or who have suffered from bouts of infection and diarrhea which have depleted body reserves. Marasmus in infants and children is more severe than starvation in adults, who can survive for a long period (1 to 3 months) on their tissue stores of nutrients. An infant, or child, has very high requirements for nutrients in proportion to his size. His rate of metabolism is much higher than that of adults, and he has additional requirements for a rapid rate of growth.

Physiological adaptations in marasmus involve the breakdown of body tissues for energy which is stimulated by catabolic hormones, such as those from the adrenal cortex, and the reduction or cessation of protein synthesis and growth in many tissues. The specific effects of the adrenal cortical hormones are the breakdown of proteins to amino acids, and conversion of amino acids to glucose for use by the brain and nervous system.

Survival during extreme calorie deprivation is moderately enhanced by a large reduction in the utilization of nutrients for energy which is brought about by a diminished secretion of thyroid hormones and a reduced response of cells to insulin. Eventually, there may be dehydration and electrolyte imbalances due to depletion of sodium, potassium, magnesium, and chloride ions, which may in turn lead to disorders of the brain, heart, kidneys, and nerves. Therefore, these conditions can rapidly lead to death if not promptly corrected.

Marasmic Kwashiorkor. This condition is found in many situations where children are fed diluted gruels after weaning. It is characterized by a combination of disorders which accompany both marasmus and kwashiorkor. Today, the tendency is to use the generalized term, protein-energy malnutrition, to describe this condition.

Nutritional Dwarfing or Growth Failure. Nutritional dwarfing, or growth failure, while not always a severe handicap, is nonetheless an indicator of underlying protein-energy malnutrition, and may be the beginning of the development of kwashiorkor or marasmus.

Protein-Energy Malnutrition (PEM) in Adults. These disorders may occur in adults under the following circumstances: chronic illness or alcoholism; unemployment or retirement—which means living on very limited resources; or hospitalized and maintained on intravenous glucose solutions without any other nutrients. The latter situation is particularly dangerous in the case of postsurgical patients who need extra amounts of protein for the healing of their tissues. These patients may show signs like those of kwashiorkor since calories are provided without protein.

SIGNS OF PROTEIN-ENERGY MALNUTRITION.
Every effort should be made to detect PEM in its early stages, since the cost of treating a severe case of this disorder in a hospital may easily be several times that of the treatment of a mild case on an outpatient basis.[10]

Indicators of Protein-Energy Malnutrition in Communities. Even in the developed countries resources for health surveillance and follow-up care are limited. Therefore, it is necessary to identify communities where these services might yield maximum benefits. Regional health departments usually collect data which is helpful in locating areas where the needs for public health services are greatest. Statistics which suggest the possibility of finding PEM in a community are increased mortality and morbidity of preschool children, a high incidence of infectious diseases, and significant numbers of children who are below standard weights and heights for their ages. Unfortunately, it is not a common practice to obtain on a regular basis the heights and weights of preschool and school age children—not even in developed countries such as the United States.

Signs of Protein-Energy Malnutrition in Individuals. The extreme forms of PEM (kwashiorkor and marasmus) are not often found in the developed countries, unless there are provocative factors such as parental neglect of children, untreated diseases such as those that affect the gastrointestinal tract, and improper infant feeding. For example, a case of kwashiorkor was identified by a foreign-trained physician in Bronx, New York.[11] The circumstances of the case follow: An attending physician in a clinic told the mother of a child suspected of having an allergy to cow's milk to feed her child soy milk and rice. The mother misunderstood the physician and fed her child only the rice, and the child became very ill. Another physician who was foreign trained, later saw the child in the hospital and recognized kwashiorkor (by the depigmented hair). Fortunately, the child was brought

10Beghin, I. D., "Nutritional Rehabilitation Centers in Latin America: A Critical Assessment," *American Journal of Clinical Nutrition*, Vol. 23, 1970, p. 1412.

11Taitz, L. S., and L. Finberg, "Kwashiorkor in the Bronx," *American Journal of Diseases of Children*, Vol. 112, 1966, p. 76.

back to health. Thus, it is helpful for all health professionals to be able to recognize severe PEM. Some of the features of kwashiorkor and marasmus are given in Table M-3.

TABLE M-3
FEATURES OF KWASHIORKOR AND MARASMUS

Features[1]	Kwashiorkor	Marasmus
Albumin concentration in plasma[1]	Markedly low	Normal or slightly low
Anemia	Moderate	Moderate
Appetite	Depressed	Normal to increased
Dehydration	Sometimes	Often
Edema[1]	Often on the legs and feet	Sometimes
Electrolyte metabolism	Potassium depletion	Near to normal
Endocrine function:		
Adrenal cortex (glucocorticoids)	Normal to decreased secretion	Increased secretion
Pancreas (insulin)	Decreased secretion, impaired glucose tolerance	Normal to low secretion
Pituitary (growth hormone)	Increased secretion	Increased secretion
Thyroid	Decreased secretion	Decreased secretion
Essential/nonessential amino acids (blood)[1]	Subnormal ratio	Normal ratio
Gastrointestinal function	Decreased secretions, diarrhea	Atrophy of digestive tract
Growth failure[1]	Moderate	Severe
Hair	Depigmented in spots	Easily plucked
Liver[1]	Fatty (may be palpated)	Atrophied
Mouth	Smooth tongue	Normal
Muscle wasting[1]	Masked by edema	Noticeable
Psychological	Apathetic, miserable	Alert (early stages)
Skin[1]	Depigmentation, rashes	Dry and baggy
Weight (for age and height)[1]	Moderately subnormal	Severely subnormal

[1]Features which are commonly used to distinguish between marasmus and kwashiorkor.

It is also worthwhile to be able to distinguish between the types and degrees of PEM since in most cases the treatment should be directed towards correction of the causative factors and their resulting consequences. Distinguishing characteristics are discussed under the items which follow:

• **Kwashiorkor**—The specific features which distinguish this disorder from marasmus are (1) a significantly subnormal albumin concentration in plasma, (2) swollen parotid glands (just under and in front of the ears), (3) a depressed ratio of essential to nonessential amino acids in the blood plasma, (4) fatty liver (which often may be palpated), and (5) a moderate deficit in weight for height and age (the weight is usually 80% or more of normal).

Fig. M-10 shows a typical case of kwashiorkor.

• **Marasmus**—In contrast to kwashiorkor, this condition is distinguished by (1) severe growth failure where weight may be only 60 to 80% of normal, (2) noticeable muscle wasting, (3) dry and baggy skin (edema is not usually apparent), and (4) normal values for both the plasma albumin and the ratio of essential to nonessential amino acids.

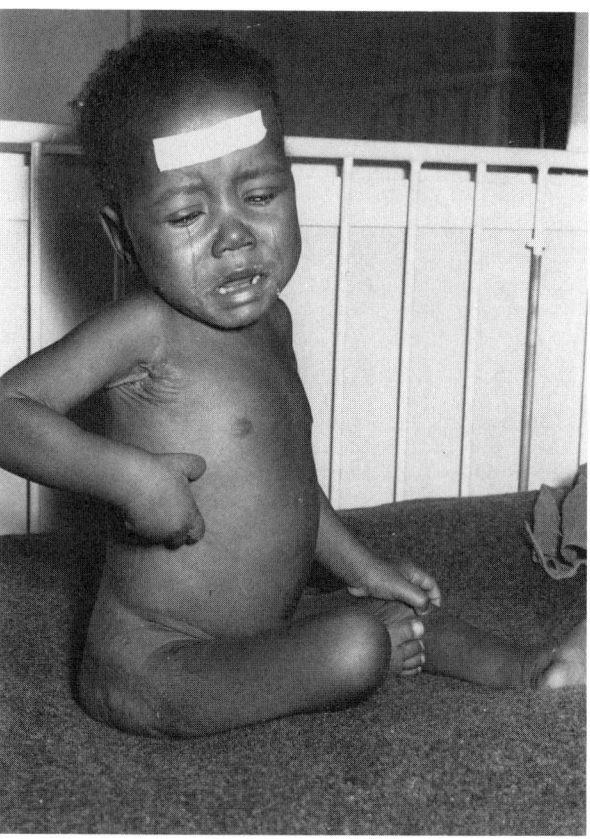

Fig. M-10. An African boy suffering from kwashiorkor. Note the misery reflected in his expression and the characteristic signs of swollen parotid glands and distended abdomen, flabby thigh muscles, flaky and roughened skin (on his right thigh). (Courtesy, FAO, Rome, Italy)

• **Marasmic kwashiorkor**—Patients who show features of both marasmus and kwashiorkor are usually given the general diagnosis of protein-energy malnutrition.

• **Nutritional dwarfing or growth failure**—One of the first effects of serious malnutrition in infants and children is growth retardation. Thus, it may often be possible to diagnose PEM in children who show none of the abnormal features other than growth deficits. New standard charts of growth curves are available for making comparisons.[12] These revised charts are now based on data from all contemporary U.S. children of the same age and sex, which is in contrast to the older standards based upon data from white, middle-class children living in Boston or Iowa 30 to 40 years ago.

Subnormal values for height and weight at a given age are considered to be those which are more than two standard deviations below the mean values (or below the curve representing the third percentile of values). Growth records should be kept over a period of time, since the child's placement on the chart for a single measurement is not as indicative of nutritional status as is the growth velocity, or increments of growth which occur between several measurements. For example, a child that was initially placed well up on a growth chart may subsequently experience protein-energy malnutrition and, as a result, drop down on the chart but still not fall below the curve representing the third per-

[12]National Center for Health Statistics, *NCHS Growth Charts*, 1976, Health Resources Administration, Monthly Vital Statistics Report, Vol. 25, No. 3, June 1976 Supplement.

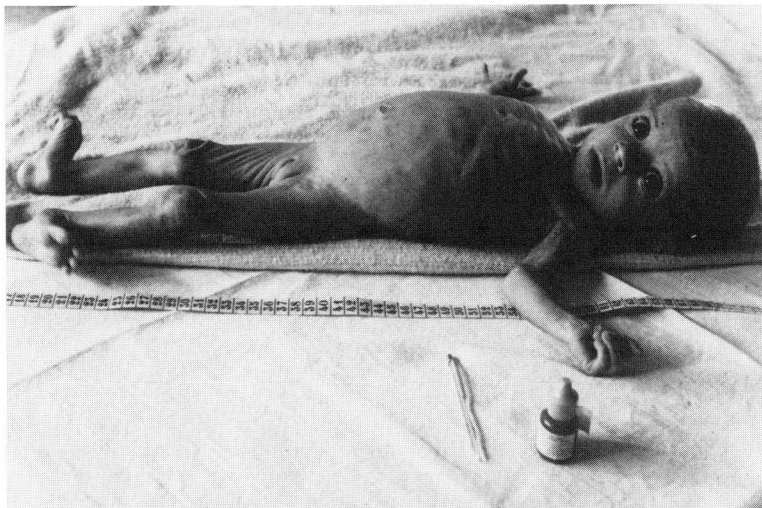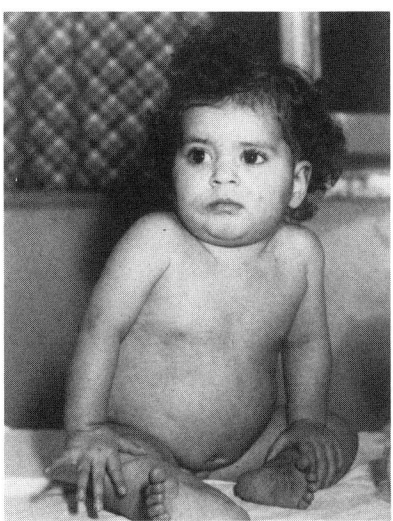

Fig. M-11. *Molok, a 4-month-old Iranian girl suffering from marasmus. Left:* When admitted to the demonstration foundling home in Teheran, she was 24 in. *(61 cm)* tall and weighed 7 lb *(3.2 kg). Right:* Following 10 months in the foundling home, Molok was 31 in. *(79 cm)* tall and weighed 16 lb *(7.3 kg).* She was restored to good health by a diet consisting of UNICEF milk powder, orange juice, green vegetables, potatoes, dried apricots, beef, liver, lentils, and bread. (Courtesy, FAO, Rome, Italy)

centile. When, however, the pattern of measurements is carefully examined, it can be seen that there has been a marked departure from the normal progress of growth.

• **Protein-energy malnutrition in adults**—Many of the signs observed in children suffering from PEM will be found in adult patients who have protein and/or energy deficiencies. However, in the case of adults, the ratio of weight to height has been found to be less sensitive than other indicators of PEM.[13] Better indicators of the severity of protein deficiency are serum albumin, triceps skinfold, and muscle circumference. These three measurements are distinctly subnormal in moderate to severe protein deficiencies.

TREATMENT AND PREVENTION OF PROTEIN-ENERGY MALNUTRITION.

Depending upon the severity of the disorder, the process of rehabilitation may require one or more levels of treatment. The main therapeutic levels follow.

Emergency Care of Severely Ill Patients. The severely malnourished person has usually adapted over a period of weeks or even months to greatly reduced amounts of food and drink. Therefore, a great deal of care has to be exercised during rehabilitation in order to avoid overloading the patient's imbalanced physiologic functions. Death has frequently resulted from overzealous administration of food, fluids, and mineral salts. The priorities for rehabilitation follow:

• **Correction of dehydration of electrolyte imbalances**—Intravenous administrations of fluid may be harmful to a patient with impaired kidney function resulting from malnutrition. This therapy should be undertaken only when it is certain that there is dehydration (it is not usually present in the malnourished unless there has been diarrhea and/or vomit-

ing). Signs of dehydration are dryness inside the mouth, and a rapid and weak pulse as a result of shrinkage of blood volume due to water loss, which, in turn, causes cardian insufficiency. If there is no vomiting, oral administration of an electrolyte solution for rehydration is preferable to intravenous administration. Half-strength Darrow's solution with 2.5% dextrose is suitable for either mode of administration (32 ml of solution per pound of body weight over a period of 24 hours). This procedure should be stopped when the pulse slows to normal.

Repletion with magesium should *not* be undertaken until rehydration has been accomplished. Dangerously high levels of this element may accumulate when there is dehydration. Magnesium should not be given intravenously, because it may cause a dangerous drop in blood pressure. Instead, it should be given either orally (as magnesium hydroxide) or intramuscularly (as 50% solution of magnesium sulfate).

The malnourished patient usually has an excess of body sodium, so intravenous sodium bicarbonate should be given only when there is severe acidosis.

• **Feeding by nasogastric tube**—Acutely ill infants and children may be very irritable, making it difficult to feed them by spoon or bottle. Also, the feeding of large quantities of food in a short period of time may aggravate diarrhea. Therefore, some rehabilitation centers usually begin the refeeding procedure with administration of milk-oil formula[14] by nasogastric drip. The compositon of the formula is as follows (percent by weight): dried skim milk, 9.3%; vegetable oil (medium-chain triglycerides, a special dietetic fat derived from coconut oil, have also been used successfully in rehabilitation), 6.8%; magnesium hydroxide, 0.12%; potassium chloride, 0.4%; and water, 83.4%. One-half cup of this formula provides approximately 4 g of protein and

[13]Blackburn, G. L., and B. Bistrian, "Report from Boston," *Nutrition Today,* Vol. 9, No. 3, May/June 1974, p. 30.

[14]Robson, J. R. K., and C. de joya-Agregado, "The Operation and Function of Malward in the Philippines," *The Journal of Tropical Pediatrics and Environmental Child Health,* March 1973, p. 43, Table IV.

115 Calories (kcal). The formula is usually diluted at the beginning of rehabilitation and fed at a rate of 0.5, 1.0, or 1.5 g of protein per pound (*1.1, 2.2, or 2.3 g/kg*) of body weight per day. The lower concentrations are used in the case of diarrhea, but the amounts of magnesium and potassium salts should be proportionately increased. Following 1 to 3 days the nasogastric feeding may be replaced with bottle, spoon, or cup feeding of the full-strength mixture at the rate of 2 g protein/pound/day.

There may initially be a loss of weight due to correction of edema by protein repletion. The excess water in the tissues is gradually excreted. Once weight gain is steady, the dried skim milk may be replaced by dried whole milk, or by an equivalent quantity of evaporated or pasteurized milk, provided suitable sanitary storage facilities are available for these products.

Treatment of Protein Depletion in Hospital Patients (With Trauma, Infection, Burns, or After Surgery). This has been most successfully accomplished by either (1) feeding meat, or (2) intravenous infusion of amino acids (compared to the lesser effect of intravenous glucose alone, or a combination of glucose and smaller amounts of amino acids).[15]

The rationale for not feeding patients who have had gastrointestinal surgery has been to prevent irritation or opening up of the surgical wounds. However, there are now available nutrient supplement powders which contain no indigestible residue, and which may be cautiously given to patients soon after surgery. These powders, generally called elemental diets, are marketed by several pharmaceutical companies.

Correction of Mild to Moderate Protein-Energy Malnutrition. The rehabilitation procedure in developing countries usually consists of cautiously feeding nonfat dry milk (dietary fat is restricted at the start of treatment to avoid aggravation of diarrhea) reconstituted with boiled water (to avoid bacterial contamination) until other foods are tolerated. Supplements of vitamins and minerals are given along with the food to prevent or correct deficiencies. Vitamin A deficiency frequently accompanies kwashiorkor, but may not be noticed until the protein deficiency has been corrected. As soon as possible, part of the milk should be replaced with low-cost, nutritious foods which are readily available in the local community. Sometimes the milk may be mixed with foods of high-energy content, such as butter, banana, cassava, beans, and mixtures of grains.

Part of the rehabilitation procedure should involve teaching the patient (or the mothers in the cases of infants and children) the principles of selecting a diet containing the correct proportions of nutrients. This is not achieved easily where food supplies are scarce, or cultural practices limit the use of certain foods.

Prevention of Protein-Energy Malnutrition. A high priority should be given to the identification of children who have been weaned early, or are being breast fed by mothers who cannot produce adequate amounts of milk. They should be fed a supplemental formula. When feeding formulas under primitive or unsanitary conditions, every effort must be made to prevent contamination of the food given to the baby. Lack of proper preparation of formulas is the most common cause of diarrhea; spoilage of the milk formula is another.

The diets of infants after weaning should be carefully planned to include a high-quality protein source, since infants and children require suitable patterns of amino acids in their diets. This means that if grains are a major dietary staple, there should be supplementation with animal proteins—such as milk, eggs, fish, or if these are unavailable, with legumes such as soybeans or peanuts (which may be in the form of a powder). None of the commonly used grains—corn, rice, wheat, and barley—are adequate as the major source of protein for growing children, unless the grain preparations have been supplemented with lysine and/or other deficient amino acids.

Adults are not as likely to suffer from protein deficiencies as are children because (1) their requirements for protein, in proportion to their body size, are much less; and (2) they do not require high-quality proteins—for example, adults have been adequately nourished when wheat flour constituted the sole source of protein. Lysine is not required by adults at as high a level as it is for growing infants and children.

Many cultures believe that males require the most animal protein. So, they tend to feed women less meat than men, and to feed children largely on cereals. These priorities should be reversed by feeding young children the highest quality protein, including animal protein whenever possible; by giving women more meat than men, in order to offset menstrual losses of blood and iron; and, when necessary, by providing mainly vegetarian diets for men. However, some animal proteins, such as egg and milk, are needed by men in order to provide vitamin B-12.

RECENT DEVELOPMENTS IN THE TREATMENT AND PREVENTION OF PROTEIN-ENERGY MALNUTRITION. A variety of new high-protein food products has been developed by large food concerns for distribution in developing countries. Many of these products are currently being test marketed in Latin American countries. For example, the protein quality of tortilla flour in Mexico has been enhanced by the mixing of soy flour with the traditional corn flour.

Another approach to meeting the protein needs of growing populations is the development of new, improved varieties of grains. Plant geneticists have recently produced high-lysine corn and both high-protein and high-yielding strains of wheat, rice, corn, barley, and sorghum; and they have crossed wheat and rye to obtain a nutritious new hybrid grain called *triticale*. Collectively, these developments, which are known as the *Green Revolution*, have made these much-used cereals more nearly the staff of life for growing children.

(Also see DEFICIENCY DISEASES; ENRICHMENT [Fortification, Nutrification, Restoration]; GREEN REVOLUTION; HUNGER, WORLD; POPULATION, WORLD; PROTEIN; and WORLD FOOD.)

MALT

Contents	Page

The term commonly applied to grains of barley which have been allowed to germinate under controlled condi-

---

[15]"Protein Sparing Produced by Protein and Amino Acids," *Nutrition Reviews*, Vol. 34, 1976, p. 174.

tions, then stripped of their sprouts and dried to prevent further sprouting or spoiling. However, the term malt may also refer to (1) the process of making malt; (2) germinated grains other than barley, such as wheat and rye; or (3) a water extract of the malted grain which may be either in the form of a dried powder or a concentrated syrup.

HISTORY OF MALTING.
It is known that the Chaldeans and Egyptians brewed beer on a regular basis as early as 5000 B.C. However, the ancient Egyptians became the first commercial malsters in 1300 B.C., when they produced malt for export by baking ground, malted barley into cakes which could be transported without spoilage. Beer was brewed from these malted cakes by soaking them in water until fermentation occurred.

The Greeks acquired these skills from the Egyptians around 700 B.C. About 300 years later, beer became a major beverage of the Roman legions when they learned about brewing from the Greeks. Shortly thereafter, all parts of the Roman Empire malted barley and brewed beer.

Although most of the malt which is produced today is used by brewers and distillers to make alcoholic beverages, some tasty, nonalcoholic foods are also made from malted grain.

MALT DERIVATIVES.
Malt retains most of its enzyme activity. Also, it contains maltose and other sugars which result from the breakdown of about 18% of the starch in the original grain. These properties lend themselves well to the production of the items which follow:

1. Beers.
2. Malt vinegar.
3. Distilled malt vinegar.
4. Whiskeys.
5. Malt flour.
6. Caramel malts.
7. Chocolate malts.
8. Malt extracts.
9. Malt bread.
10. Malted milk powder.

NUTRITIVE VALUES OF MALT PRODUCTS.
Table M-4 compares the nutrient content of the original barley grain, malt, and two of the products derived from it.

TABLE M-4
NUTRIENT COMPOSITION OF BARLEY AND MALT

	Unhulled Barley Grain	Dried Malt	Malt Extract Dried[1]	Malted Milk Powder[1]
	◄————(per 100 g portion)————►			
Food energy .... kcal	274	368	367	410
Carbohydrates .... g	66.6	77.4	89.2	72.9
Fat .... g	1.7	1.9	Trace	8.3
Protein .... g	12.2	13.7	6.0	13.1
Fiber .... g	5.3	3.3	Trace	.6
Calcium .... mg	40	60	48	266
Phosphorus .... mg	330	460	294	380
Sodium .... mg	30	80	80	440
Magnesium .... mg	140	180	140	93
Potassium .... mg	400	430	230	758
Iron .... mg	8	4	9	1
Niacin .... mg	8.5	5.7	9.9	.3
Riboflavin .... mg	.2	.3	.4	.5
Thiamin .... mg	.4	.4	.4	.3

[1]Data from Food Composition Table F-21.

Table M-4 shows that malt contains higher levels of energy and protein, but less fiber, than the grain from which it was derived. In general, the grain is rendered more digestible by malting as a result of enzymatic activity generated in this process.

Malt extract is composed mainly of carbohydrates in the form of sugars, since much of the protein in malt is insoluble, and, therefore, is not extracted by water. Also, there is only a negligible content of fiber in the extract. Thus, the malt extract is not as complete a food as the malted grain.

Malted milk powder is the most nutritious of the products listed in Table M-4 since the whole milk used in its preparation contributes extra energy, fat, protein, calcium, phosphorus, sodium, and potassium. It may be mixed with milk and used as a nearly complete food for convalescents, except that supplemental vitamins, minerals, and fiber should be provided if it is the exclusive food for a long period of time.

Additional nutritional information may be found on malt and malt products in Food Composition Table F-21.

COMMERCIAL USES OF MALT AND ITS DERIVATIVES.
Although malt products are almost exclusively consumed by man in the form of beverages and foods, producers of these items recover and sell the by-products from their processes for use as ingredients in livestock feeds. A brief summary of some of the commercial uses of malt and its derivatives follows.

Beverages and Foods.
The manufacturers of these products use malt because of (1) its enzymatic activity which helps to make foods more digestible, or more readily fermentable; (2) its content of sugars, such as maltose; and (3) its flavor. Examples of these applications follow:

1. Diastatic malts.
2. Malt-flavored beverages and foods.
3. Malt vinegars.

Feeds.
Even though malt has a higher nutritive value for feeding livestock than unmalted barley grain (see Table M-4), the higher cost of producing the malt makes such a use unprofitable. But, the by-products which are not consumed by man make good ingredients for animal feeds. Among them, diastatic malts, malt hulls, and sprouts, miller's screenings (from the production of malt flour), brewers' grains, brewers' yeast, distillers' grains, and distillers' solubles. These by-products are combined with various other ingredients to make up rations for both nonruminants like chickens and hogs, and for ruminants such as sheep and cattle.

USING MALT EXTRACTS IN HOME RECIPES.
Diastatic malts are sold mainly by wholesalers to bakers, brewers, and distillers. Therefore, consumers are not likely to be able to purchase such products in retail stores.

Malt extracts are available in powdered and syrup form, but they are rather expensive since they are sold mainly in drug stores as laxatives and tonics. However, a slightly less expensive diastatic malt is sold by some health food stores.

An inexpensive, hop-flavored, nondiastatic malt syrup is sold in some supermarkets. This syrup might be used to flavor beverages where a bit of bitterness (from the hops) is desired. It makes a good yeast food for bread baking because of its sugar content.

(Also see BEERS AND BREWING, section headed "Malting.")

MALTASE

An enzyme which acts on maltose to produce glucose. Salivary amylase is present in saliva, and intestinal maltase is present in intestinal juice.

(Also see DIGESTION AND ABSORPTION.)

MALTHUS

An English clergyman whose full name was Thomas Robert Malthus. In 1798, he prophesied that world population grows faster than man's ability to increase food production. He stated, "The power of population is infinitely greater than the power in the earth to provide subsistence for man." For almost 200 years, we proved Malthus wrong because, as the population increased, new land was brought under cultivation; and machinery, chemicals, new crops and varieties, and irrigation were added to step up the yields. Now, science has given us the miracle of better health and longer life; and world population is increasing at the rate of about 240,000 people a day, or 87.5 million per year; and it is predicted that world population will be 6.2 billion by the year 2000, and be doubled by the year 2045. To match population growth and feed people adequately, world food production needs to increase at an average rate of about 2.5% per year.

(Also see HUNGER, WORLD; POPULATION, WORLD; and WORLD FOOD.)

MALTOL

This substance is used both for its own flavor and for enhancing flavors of sweet, fruit-containing foods. It has a fragrant caramellike odor and a bittersweet taste.

FORMATION AND OCCURRENCE OF MALTOL. Chemists have demonstrated that maltol may be formed (1) by heating maltose at 375°F *(191°C)* for 1 hour (note the similarities of these conditions to those in baking), or (2) by heating mixtures of sugars, such as maltose and lactose, with amino acids, such as glycine (the latter procedure is known as nonenzymatic browning reaction of the Maillard type).

Maltol is found in roasted materials which have a moderate to high carbohydrate content, such as bread crusts, cocoa beans, cellulose, cereals, chicory, coffee beans, diastatic flour doughs (where some of the starch has been converted by enzyme action to maltose), malt products, soft woods, and soybeans. It is also found in heated products which contain moderate amounts of both sugars and amino acids, such as condensed and dried milks, dried whey, and soy sauce. Apparently heating is not always required for the production of maltol, since it also occurs in larch bark and the dry needles of cone-bearing evergreen trees.

USES OF MALTOL. When maltol flavor is desired in a food, it is often produced by careful attention to the conditions under which food is processed. For example, the roasting of cereal grains results in the production of maltol and other flavors which are similar to those in roasted cocoa and coffee. Thus, the distinctive flavors and aromas of many roasted foods are due to the different mixtures of the individual substances produced by the browning reactions.

The enhancement of fruit flavors in sweetened foods requires more precise control of the amounts of maltol in the food product than can be achieved by processing, since the flavor of maltol itself should not be evident in these foods. Thus, pure maltol is used in trace amounts ranging from 5 to 350 ppm (from about a teaspoon to 12 oz per ton of food)

in products such as cakes, fruit drinks, gelatin desserts, ice cream, jams, soft drinks, and sweet rolls which have fruit flavors (strawberry, raspberry, pineapple, black cherry, and orange). Maltol also enhances the sensation of sweetness in sweet, fruit-containing foods, but it is less effective for this purpose than for enhancing fruit flavor.

ETHYL MALTOL. The strength of maltol as an enhancer of fruit flavors and as a sweetener is increased by a factor of from 4 to 6 when the methyl group (CH_3) in the molecule is replaced by an ethyl group (CH_2CH_3). Also, water solutions of ethyl maltol at room temperature are 9 times more volatile, and, therefore, more aromatic than those of maltol. The use of ethyl maltol as an additive in foods allows the sugar content to be reduced by 15%.

MALTOSE (MALT SUGAR)

A disaccharide with the formula $C_{12}H_{22}O_{11}$; obtained from the partial hydrolysis of starch; yields 2 molecules of glucose on further hydrolysis.

MAMEY (MAMMEE APPLE) *Mammea americana*

The fruit of an evergreen tree (of the family *Guttiferae*) that is native to the West Indies, Central America, and South America.

The fruit is pear-shaped and from 3 to 6 in. (*7 to 14 cm*) in diameter with brown thick skin and an orange-colored flesh. It is eaten fresh, stewed and sweetened, or made into jam or jelly. Also, a liqueur is made from the flowers and a seasoning agent is made from the seeds of the fruit.

The fruit is fairly low in calories (59 kcal per 100 g) and carbohydrates (12%). It is a fair source of vitamin C.

MANATEE (MANATI; SEA COW)

A formerly common American herbivorous sea mammal of the West Indies and neighboring mainland coasts from Florida to Yucatan, now rare because of excessive killing. The manatee is about 10 ft long, nearly black, thick-skinned, and almost free from hair. The flesh of the manatee, which tastes something like pork, is much esteemed in the West Indies.

MANGANESE (Mn)

In industry, manganese is a metallic element used chiefly as an alloy in steel to give it toughness. In nutrition, it is an essential element for many animal species. Manganese is an activator of several enzyme systems involved in protein and energy metabolism and in the formation of mucopolysaccharides. The human body contains 12 to 20 mg of manganese. So, an essential function of the element must be assumed to exist in man.

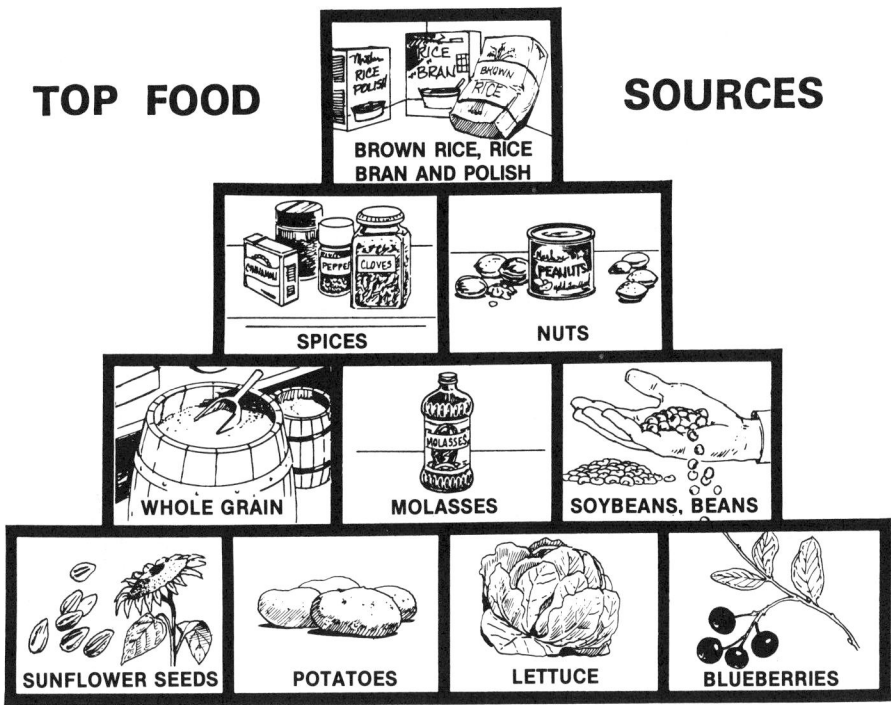

TOP FOOD SOURCES

BROWN RICE, RICE BRAN AND POLISH

SPICES

NUTS

WHOLE GRAIN

MOLASSES

SOYBEANS, BEANS

SUNFLOWER SEEDS

POTATOES

LETTUCE

BLUEBERRIES

Fig. M-12. Top food sources of manganese.

HISTORY. Manganese was first recognized as an element in 1774 by the famous Swedish chemist Carl W. Scheele. It was isolated in the same year by his co-worker, Johann G. Ghan. The name *manganese* is a corrupted form of the Latin word for a form of magnetic stone, *magnesia.*

About 95% of the world's annual production of manganese is used by the steel industry. Also, manganese is essential for plant growth, and it is found in trace amounts in higher animals, where it activates many of the enzymes involved in metabolic processes.

In 1931, University of Wisconsin researchers reported that manganese was a dietary essential for growth of rats. Later, it was shown to be essential for poultry (a deficiency results in slipped tendon; see Fig. M-13), swine, guinea pigs, cattle, and other animals. Undoubtedly, manganese is an essential nutrient for man, even though the deficiency symptoms have never been determined with certainty.

ABSORPTION, METABOLISM, EXCRETION. Manganese is rather poorly absorbed, primarily in the small intestine. In the average diet about 45% of the ingested manganese is absorbed, and 55% is excreted in the feces. Absorption can be depressed when excessive amounts of calcium, phosphorus, or iron are consumed.

Following absorption, manganese is loosely bound to a protein and transported as transmanganin. The bones, and to a lesser extent the liver, muscles, and skin, serve as storage sites.

Manganese is mainly eliminated from the body in the feces as a constituent of bile, but much of this is again reabsorbed, indicating an effective body conservation. Very little manganese is excreted in the urine.

The concentration of manganese in the various body tissues is quite stable under normal conditions, a phenomenon attributed to well controlled excretion rather than regulated absorption.

FUNCTIONS OF MANGANESE. Manganese is involved in the formation of bone and the growth of other connective tissues; in blood clotting; in insulin action; in cholesterol synthesis; and as an activator of various enzymes in the metabolism of carbohydrates, fats, proteins, and nucleic acids (DNA and RNA).

DEFICIENCY SYMPTOMS. Signs of deficiency in many animal species include poor reproductive performance, growth retardation, congenital malformations in the offspring, abnormal formation of bone and cartilage, and impaired glucose tolerance.

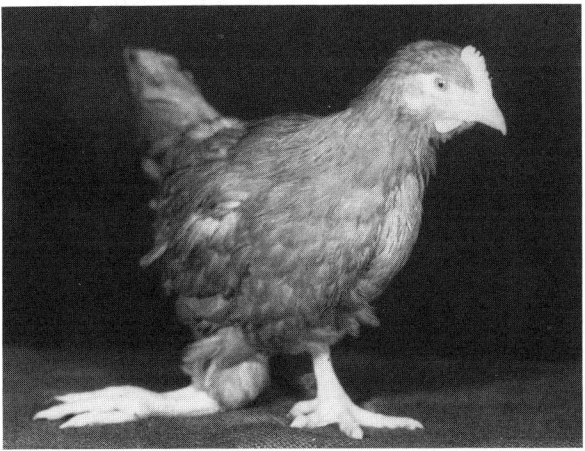

Fig. M-13. A bone disease known as perosis, or slipped tendon, in a chicken due to manganese deficiency. (Courtesy, Department of Poultry Science, Cornell University)

The only confirmed deficiency of manganese in man was in connection with a vitamin K deficiency, where administration of the vitamin did not correct the abnormality in blood clotting until supplemental manganese was provided.

Analyses of hair and blood samples for manganese content indicate that subclinical deficiencies of the mineral might aggravate such disorders as growth impairments, bone abnormalities, diabeticlike carbohydrate metabolism, lack of muscle coordination in the newborn, and abnormal metabolism of lipids (fatty acids, choline, and cholesterol).

In 1963, researchers at the University of California—Davis reported, in the *American Journal of Physiology,* on a study of convulsions in rats; they found that manganese levels helped determine the susceptibility to convulsions of rats subjected to electroshocks and a convulsive drug. In 1976, Yukio Tanaka, a clinical chemist at St. Mary's Hospital in Montreal, reported, before the American Chemical Society in Chicago, that about 30% of all children who have epileptic convulsions have low levels of manganese in their blood. These leads merit further study.

INTERRELATIONSHIPS. Manganese interacts with other nutrients. Excess calcium and phosphorus interfere with the absorption of manganese; the functions of manganese, copper, zinc, and iron may be interchangeable in certain enzyme systems; and manganese and vitamin K work together in the promotion of blood clotting.

RECOMMENDED DAILY ALLOWANCE OF MANGANESE. Extreme dietary habits can result in manganese intakes outside the limit suggested as safe, but the consumption of a varied diet, balanced with regard to bulk nutrients, can be relied on to furnish adequate and safe amounts.

Estimated safe and adequate intakes of manganese are given in the section on MINERAL(S), Table M-25, Mineral Table.

• **Manganese intake in average U.S. diet**—In the United States, the normal daily intake of manganese varies from 2 to 9 mg/day in adults, depending on the composition of the diet.

TOXICITY. Toxicity in man as a consequence of dietary intake has not been observed. However, it has occurred in workers exposed to high concentrations of manganese dust in the air (such as in mining ores rich in manganese, and in the production of dry-cell batteries where manganese dioxide is used). The excess accumulates in the liver and central nervous system. The symptoms resemble those found in Parkinson's and Wilson's diseases.

SOURCES OF MANGANESE. The manganese content of plants is dependent on soil content. It is noteworthy, however, that plants grown on alkaline soils may be abnormally low in manganese.

• **Rich sources**—Rice (brown), rice bran and polish, spices, walnuts, wheat bran, wheat germ.

• **Good sources**—Blackstrap molasses, blueberries, lettuce, lima beans (dry), navy beans (dry), peanuts, potatoes, soybean flour, soybeans (dry), sunflower seeds, torula yeast, wheat flour, whole grains (barley, oats, sorghum, wheat).

• **Fair sources**—Brewers' yeast, liver, most fruits and vegetables, orange pekoe tea, white enriched bread.

• **Negligible sources**—Fats and oils, fish, eggs, meats, milk, poultry, sugar.

• **Supplemental sources**—Alfalfa leaf meal, dried kelp, manganese gluconate.

For additional sources and more precise values of manganese, see Table M-5, Some Food Sources of Manganese, which follows:

TABLE M-5
SOME FOOD SOURCES OF MANGANESE

Food	Manganese	Food	Manganese
	(mg/100 g)		(mg/100 g)
Rice bran	34.7	Barley, whole grain	1.2
Cloves	30.3	Wheat flour	1.0
Rice polish	17.1	Lettuce	1.0
Ginger	17.8	Potato, raw	1.0
Walnuts	15.2	Blueberries, raw	1.0
Wheat germ	13.3	Spinach, raw	.8
Wheat bran	11.0	Beet, common red, raw	.7
Rice, whole grain	9.6	Yeast, brewers'	.6
Molasses, blackstrap	4.3	Corn, whole grain	.5
Wheat, whole grain	3.7	Bananas, raw	.5
Oats, whole grain	3.7	Carrot, raw	.4
Alfalfa leaf meal (powder), dehydrated	3.6	Turnip, raw	.4
		Cherries, raw	.4
Soybean flour	3.2	Green beans	.3
Soybeans, dry	3.0	Apple, raw	.3
Peanuts	2.5	Bread, enriched white	.3
Sunflower seeds	2.3	Sweet potato	.3
Beans, navy, dry	2.1	Cabbage, raw	.3
Beans, lima, dry	1.6	Strawberries, raw	.3
Sorghum, whole grain	1.6	Liver	.2
Yeast, torula	1.3	Orange pekoe tea	.2
		Rutabaga, raw	.1

MANGO *Mangifera indica*

The mango is a tropical evergreen tree of the cashew family, *Anacardiaceae,* which produces the mango fruit—a slightly sour juicy oval fruit with a thick yellowish-red rind.

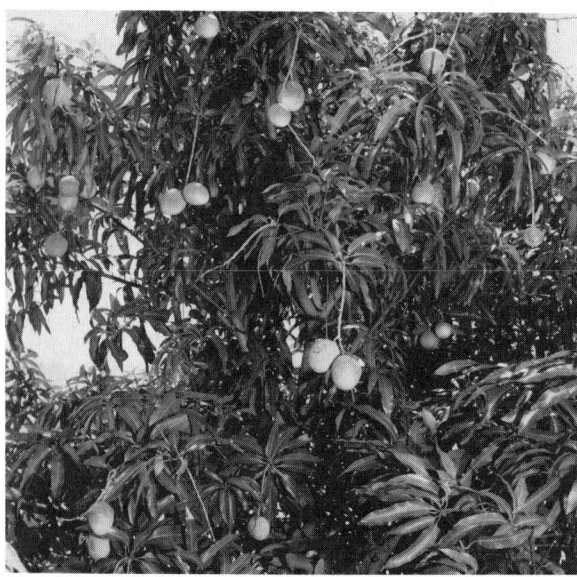

Fig. M-14. A fruiting mango tree. (Courtesy, USDA)

Although not very popular in the United States, it is an important fruit crop of tropical countries. Mangoes have a spicy taste. Centuries of selection have produced mangoes free of fiber and offensive flavors.

ORIGIN AND HISTORY. The mango tree originated in India, from the wild trees of the area. From here, it spread throughout the tropical regions of the world. Settlers brought it to America in the 1700s.

WORLD AND U.S. PRODUCTION. Worldwide, mangoes are the seventh leading fruit crop. About 15.7 million metric tons are produced annually; and the leading countries, by rank, are: India, Mexico, Pakistan, Thailand, China, Indonesia, Brazil, Philippines, Haiti, and Zaire.[16]

In the tropical countries, mangoes are more important than peaches and apples.

No production figures on mangoes for the United States are available. But it will grow in California, Florida, and Hawaii; and there is a limited amount of commercial production and sale in Florida and Hawaii.

PROCESSING. Virtually all of the mango crop is marketed fresh. However, small amounts are canned.

SELECTION, PREPARATION, AND USES. Mangoes should be nearly ripe, or ripe, firm, and free from bruises. Ripe fruits are eaten raw as a dessert, fruit dish, or used in juice, jams, jellies, or preserves. Small amounts are canned. Unripe mangoes are used in pickles and chutneys—a delicacy of India. Some are sun dried, and seasoned with turmeric to produce *amchur,* which may be ground and used in soups and chutneys.

NUTRITIONAL VALUE. Raw mangoes are about 82% water and contain 66 Calories (kcal) of energy per 100 g (about 3½ oz). Unripe fruits contain starch which changes to sugars during ripening. Also, mangoes are a good source of potassium, and an excellent source of vitamin A (4,800 IU/100 g), and a fair source of vitamin C (35mg/100 g). More complete information regarding the nutritional value of mangoes is presented in Food Composition Table F-21.

MANGO MELON *Cucumis melo*

This is a fairly uncommon variety (*Chito*) of muskmelon with fruit as small as lemons. The fruits are also called melon apples, orange melons, and vegetable oranges. They are used to make preserves.

MANGROVE *Rhizophera mangle*

The fruit of a tree (of the family *Rhizophoraceae*) which grows along the Atlantic coast from South Carolina to the American tropics. Mangrove fruit is sweet and edible if it is picked before it starts to develop roots. It is one of the rare fruits that sprouts while on the tree.

MANNA

The food provided by God to the Israelites during their 40 years of wandering in the wilderness as they left Egypt for Canaan—the Promised Land. Manna fell from the sky every day except the Sabbath, for which an extra portion was gathered the previous day. (Exodus 16; Numbers 11)

Some historians say that manna was a gluey sugar from the tamarisk tree.

MANNITOL ($C_6H_{14}O_6$)

Mannitol is a sugar alcohol. It tastes about 70% as sweet as sucrose—table sugar; hence, it is used as a sweetener in foods.

(Also see SWEETENING AGENTS.)

MANNOSE ($C_6H_{12}O_6$)

This is a hexose monosaccharide—a 6-carbon sugar. Mannose is not found free in foods, but it is derived from ivory nuts, orchid tubers, pine trees, yeast, molds, and bacteria. Although unimportant to human nutrition, it is a component of some glycoproteins and mucoproteins of the body. Its chemical structure is very similar to glucose.

(Also see CARBOHYDRATE[S]; and PROTEIN[S], Table P-11, "Classification Of Some Common Proteins.").

MAPLE SYRUP

A product unique to North America, made by boiling the sap of the sugar maple (*Acer saccharum*). Collection of the sap commences in the spring of the year, when warm days begin to follow cool nights, causing the sap of the sugar maple to flow. During the winter, some of the starch that the tree made the previous summer and stored in its roots is converted to sugar, primarily sucrose, and carried in the first sap of the spring. Spring sap contains 4 to 10% sugar. Collected sap is boiled to concentrate the sugar and produce the characteristic flavor. Maple syrup is esteemed for its sweet taste and *maple* flavor. Interestingly, the maple flavor of the syrup is not present in the sap, but develops during the boiling.

Although the United States produces more than one million gallons (*3.8 million liter*) of maple syrup yearly, this production is dwarfed by the Canadian province of Quebec which produces about 20 million gallons (*76 million liter*) of maple syrup yearly. Maple syrup produced in the United States is for both home and commercial use.

Fig. M-15. Fresh maple syrup pie is the first sign of spring. (Courtesy, Agriculture Canada, Ottawa, Ontario, Canada)

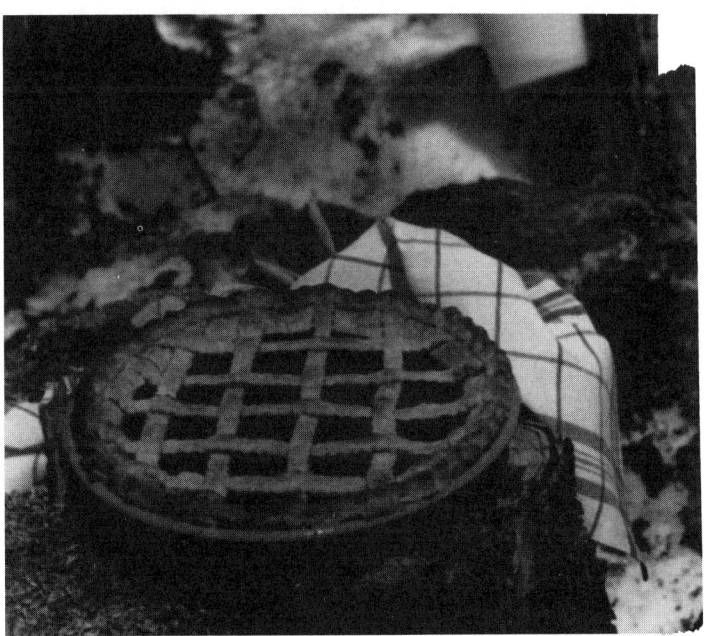

---

[16]Based on data from *FAO Production Yearbook 1990,* FAO/UN, Rome, Italy, Vol. 44, p. 167–168, Table 73. **Note well:** Annual production fluctuates as a result of weather and profitability of the crop.

Production of maple syrup begins with the spring tapping of maple trees. Although the sugar maple (*Acer saccharum*) is the major source of sap, the black maple (*Acer nigrum*) and the red maple (*Acer rubrum*) are also syrup sources. All of these types of maple trees are native to the eastern half of the North American continent. Their sap is harvested during a 4 to 6 week period before buds on the tree begin to open, usually between January and April.

Each day the accumulation of sap is collected from the pails, poured into a large tank, and hauled by sled or wagon to the sugarhouse.

PROCESSING. Processing occurs in the sugarhouse. It is here that the sap is strained and then placed in shallow pans—evaporators—over wood, oil, or gas fires. As the sap boils, the water evaporates. When the sugar concentration reaches 66.5%, it is drawn off, filtered, and bottled as maple syrup. During the boiling and evaporation, the characteristic maple flavor and color develop. Depending on the sugar content of the sap, 30 to 50 gal (*115 to 190 liter*) of sap are required to make one gallon (*3.8 liter*) of maple syrup. Maple sugar is produced by further boiling and evaporation of most of the water. One gallon of syrup yields about 8 lb of sugar. An old-fashioned treat enjoyed by those making maple sugar is called Jack wax—a taffylike confection formed by pouring the hot syrup onto the snow. The process of forming maple sugar is referred to as sugaring off. Often sugaring off gatherings are held at which people sample the maple syrup and sugar.

NUTRITIONAL VALUE AND USES. During colonial times, maple syrup and sugar were important and abundant, but nowadays these products are rather a treat and a luxury.

The composition of maple syrup is listed in Food Composition Table F-21 of this book. Nutritionally, maple syrup is primarily a source of energy; 1 Tbsp (*15 ml*) of maple syrup contains about 50 Calories (kcal) of energy, along with some calcium and potassium.

No doubt, maple syrup is esteemed more for its flavor than its nutritional value. Maple syrup on pancakes, French toast, or ice cream, is a real treat. The flavor can also be enjoyed in glazed hams, glazed carrots, and baked beans—all made with maple syrup. A delicious hot toast spread can be made by boiling two cups of syrup in a pot to 230°F (*110°C*), placing the hot pan in ice water without stirring, cooling to tepid but pliant state, and then beating until creamy.

U.S. Grade A Light syrup has a subtle flavor, while Grade A Medium and Dark syrups have a more robust flavor for cooking; besides, they cost less.

(Also see SUGAR, section headed "Other Sources of Sugar.")

MARASMUS

From the Greek *marasmos,* meaning a *dying away.* A progressive wasting and emaciation.

This disease is due to chronic protein-calorie malnutrition. It is found in infants and young children in many areas of the world, particularly in the developing and overpopulated countries, where protein-rich foods, especially those of animal origin, are practically unavailable to the poorer segments of the population. This is because (1) protein itself is deficient, and (2) total food consumption, and hence energy intake, is so inadequate that the protein eaten is not spared to function as an essential nutrient.

Physiological adaptations in marasmus involve the break-

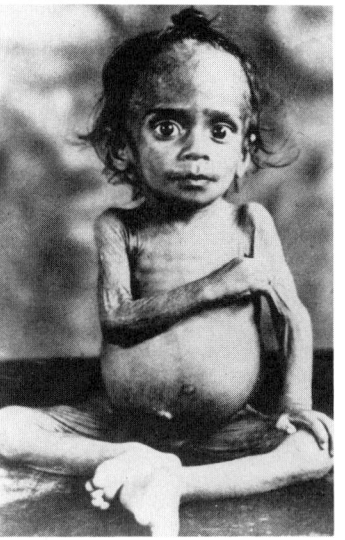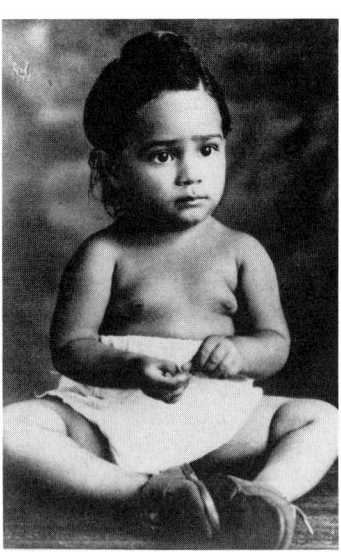

Fig. M-16. Marasmus, due to lack of energy foods. *Left:* A 2 year-old girl, weighing 11½ lbs. *Right:* Same little girl after 10 months of treatment. (Courtesy, FAO, Rome, Italy)

down of body tissues for energy which is stimulated by catabolic hormones from the adrenal cortex. Moreover, there is a reduction or cessation of protein synthesis and growth in many tissues. Outward signs and symptoms include wasting of muscle, loss of subcutaneous fat, dry baggy skin, general appearance of old age, low body weight (often less than 60% of weight expected for age and height), large sunken eyes, diarrhea, subnormal body temperature, and malabsorption. Survival during marasmus is moderately enhanced by a large reduction in the utilization of nutrients for energy which is brought about by a diminished secretion of the thyroid hormones, and a reduced response of the cells to insulin. Eventually, there may be dehydration and electrolyte imbalances due to depletion of sodium, potassium, magnesium, and chloride ions, which may in turn lead to disorders of the brain, heart, kidneys, and nerves. These conditions can rapidly lead to death if not promptly corrected. Treatment of marasmus consists of feeding an easily digested diet, such as milk and oil, which supplies at least 1.0 g of protein and 50 to 60 kcal per lb of body weight (2.2 g of protein, 110 to 132 kcal per kg of body weight).

Also see MALNUTRITION, PROTEIN-ENERGY.)

MARGARINE (OLEOMARGARINE)

This is an economical, nondairy product resembling butter in appearance, form, composition—and taste. Margarine contains about 80% fat as does butter, but the fat is generally entirely of plant origin—corn, soybean, safflower, and/or cottonseed, although a small amount of animal fat (not butterfat) is sometimes used by processors. Like many other products, margarine was developed in response to a need and an incentive.

ORIGIN AND HISTORY. Napoleon III, the ruler of France from 1852 to 1870, appealed to his people for an economical and nutritious butter substitute. Near the end of his rule, a chemist, Hippolyte Mege-Mouries, developed margarine, for which he was awarded a prize by the emperor. Mouries used oil obtained by pressing beef fat, oleo oil, salt, milk, and annatto for coloring. These ingredients were partially emulsified, then chilled rapidly with ice water to separate the solidified fatty granules from the excess water of the milk. This formed a solid emulsion which could be kneaded to the finished margarine. Even today, Mouries' method is the basis of margarine production. This first margarine had a pearly appearance and was called oleomargarine—a name derived from the oleo oil, and from the Greek word *margaron,* meaning pearl. In the United States, the name oleomargarine was required by law until 1952. Subsequently, the terms margarine and oleomargarine have been used interchangeably, but the term margarine is used most frequently.

Today, Americans consume much more margarine than butter, as Table M-6 shows. Most of the increased consumption of margarine can be explained by the price difference between butter and margarine; butter costs about 1¾ times more than margarine.

TABLE M-6
PER CAPITA CONSUMPTION OF BUTTER AND MARGARINE IN THE UNITED STATES SINCE 1950[1]

Year	Butter		Margarine	
	(lb)	(kg)	(lb)	(kg)
1950	10.7	4.9	6.1	2.8
1955	9.0	4.1	8.2	3.7
1960	7.5	3.4	9.4	4.3
1965	6.4	2.9	9.9	4.5
1970	5.3	2.4	11.0	5.0
1975	4.8	2.2	11.2	5.1
1980	4.5	2.0	11.4	5.2
1985	4.8	2.2	10.7	4.9
1990	4.3	2.0	10.9	5.0

[1]Data from *Agricultural Statistics,* USDA, 1965, p. 150, Table 220; 1980, p. 148, Table 208; and 1991, p. 139, Table 194.

PRODUCTION. Several types of plant oils may be used in the production of margarine. The most common is soybean oil, but corn, cottonseed, palm, peanut, and safflower oils may also be used by processors. Some of these oils may be hardened by hydrogenation. Also, some processors may employ a small amount of animal fat. Regardless of the oil source, the U.S. government stipulates that margarine must contain at least 80% fat.

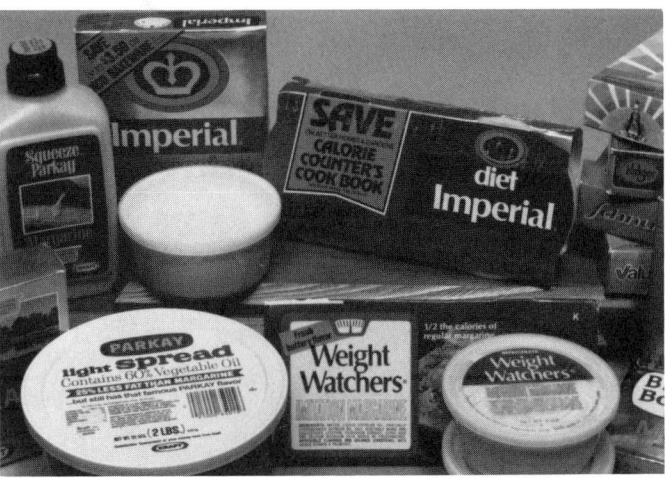

Fig. M-17. About 80% of all the margarines in the U.S. market contain soybean oil. (Courtesy, American Soybean Assoc., St. Louis, Mo.)

In 1990, about 2.8 billion lb *(1.3 billion kg)* of margarine were produced in the United States. Although most people consider margarine a household item, about 10 to 15% of the total production is used by the baking industry.

NUTRITIONAL VALUE. With the exception of the origin of the fat, the nutrient composition of margarine is very nearly the same as that of butter, as Table M-7 reveals.

TABLE M-7
COMPARISON OF THE NUTRIENT COMPOSITION OF BUTTER AND MARGARINE[1]

Nutrient		Butter	Margarine
		◄——(per 100 g)——►	
Food energy	kcal	717.0	718.7
Protein	g	0.9	0.9
Fats	g	81.1	80.5
Calcium	mg	24.0	29.9
Phosphorus	mg	23.0	22.9
Sodium	mg	826.0	943.4
Magnesium	mg	2.0	2.6
Potassium	mg	26.0	42.4
Iron	mg	0.2	—
Zinc	mg	0.1	—
Copper	mg	0.4	—
Vitamin A	IU	3,058.0	3,307.0[2]
Vitamin E	mg	1.6	15.0[3]
Thiamin	mcg	1.6	10.0
Riboflavin	mcg	34.0	37.0
Niacin	mcg	42.0	23.0
Vitamin B-6	mcg	3.0	9.0
Folic acid	mcg	3.0	1.2
Vitamin B-12	mcg	—	0.1

[1]Values from Food Composition Tale F-21.
[2]Vitamin A must be added to yield a finished margarine with not less than 15,000 IU per pound *(0.45 kg).*
[3]Varies depending on the type of oil used.

The major difference between margarine and butter—the fat—is expanded in Table M-8.

TABLE M-8
COMPARISON OF THE FATS OF BUTTER AND MARGARINE[1]

Fat	Butter	Margarine
	◄——(g/100 g)——►	
Total fat	81.1	81.1
Animal fat	81.1	—
Plant fat	—	81.1
Saturated fat	50.5	14.8
Polyunsaturated fat	3.0	—
Oleic acid	20.4	41.4
Linoleic acid	1.8	22.2
Cholesterol	.2	.0

[1]Values from Table F-4, Fats and Fatty Acids in Selected Foods.

Table M-8 indicates a difference that has been exploited as a selling point—no cholesterol in margarine. Furthermore, margarine contains significant amounts of the essential fatty acid, linoleic acid.

Despite attempts to stymie the growth of the margarine industry, it has become a success and is established as a high-quality, wholesome, nutritious food, with worldwide acceptance.

(Also see FATS AND OTHER LIPIDS; MILK AND MILK PRODUCTS; and OILS, VEGETABLE.)

MARGARINE, KOSHER

Made only from vegetable fats, and fortified only with carotene (derived from vegetable sources).

MARINADE

A mixture of liquids with herbs and spices which is used to steep meats and fish before cooking. By using pineapple juice, the marinade can be used to tenderize meats. The marinades containing oil and seasonings add oil and flavor to the fish or meat being cooked.

MARMITE

• A large metal or pottery soup kettle with a lid. Small individual ones are called *petite marmite*.

• Soup that is cooked in a marmite.

• A yeast product used for flavoring soups and meats; also as a spread or beverage.

MARRON

Chestnuts preserved in syrup flavored with vanilla.

MATÉ (BRAZILIAN TEA, PARAGUAY TEA, YERBA MATÉ)

This is a stimulating drink prepared from the dried leaves of maté or ilex plant (*Ilex paraguayensis*) of South America. It is prepared in much the same manner as tea. Boiling water is poured over maté leaves or powder and allowed to steep for about 10 minutes. Then the drink is strained and taken either hot or cold, with or without sugar. Maté is enjoyed throughout most of South America. It contains caffeine.

MATOKE *Musa paradisiaca* **var.** *sapientum*

The East African name for the local varieties of unripe bananas that are used mainly for cooking.
(Also see BANANA; and PLANTAINS.)

MATRIX

The ground work in which something is enclosed or embedded; for example, protein forms the bone matrix into which mineral salts are deposited.

MAY APPLE (INDIAN APPLE; MAYFLOWER)
Podophyllum peltatum

The small, yellow fruit of a wild herb (of the *Podophyllaceae* family) which is native to eastern North America from southern Canada to the Gulf of Mexico.

It is good fresh or when made into fruit drinks, jam, jelly, marmalade, pies, and wine. It is noteworthy that the unripe fruit, leaves, and roots of the plant are poisonous.

MAYONNAISE

This is an oil-in-water type of semisolid emulsion with egg yolk acting as the emulsifying agent. It consists of vegetable oil, egg yolk or whole egg, vinegar, lemon and/or lime juice, with one or more of the following: salt, a sweetener, mustard, paprika or other spice, monosodium glutamate, and other food seasonings. Vegetable oil comprises 65 to 80% of the composition. Thus, mayonnaise is high in calories. Each 3½ oz (*100 g*) contains 650 to 700 Calories (kcal). Vinegar and salt act as preservatives. A number of methods for manu-facturing mayonnaise are available, but all of them make use of high-speed beating or dispersing equipment in some stage of the process. Manufacturers employ machines and systems which allow the semicontinuous and continuous production of mayonnaise. Mayonnaise may be packaged in glass or plastic wide-mouth jars, tubes, sachets, or individual portion cups. It is used on salads, fish, vegetables, other foods, and in a variety of recipes.

MAYPOP *Passiflora incarnata*

The fruit of a wild species of passion fruit (family *Passifloraceae*) that grows in the southern United States. Maypop berries are yellow-colored, egg-shaped, and about 2 in. (*5 cm*) long. They may be eaten raw or made into jam, jelly, pies, and sauces.

The raw fruit is moderately high in calories (111 kcal per 100 g) and carbohydrates (21%). It is also high in fiber and a good source of iron.

MEAL

• A food ingredient having a particle size somewhat larger than flour.

• Mixtures of cereal foods, in which all of the ingredients are usually ground.
(Also see CEREAL GRAINS.)

MEAL PLANNING

Many factors enter into planning meals. Perhaps the most important one is nutritive value; but other things such as appearance, palatability, cost, and food preferences must be considered at the same time.

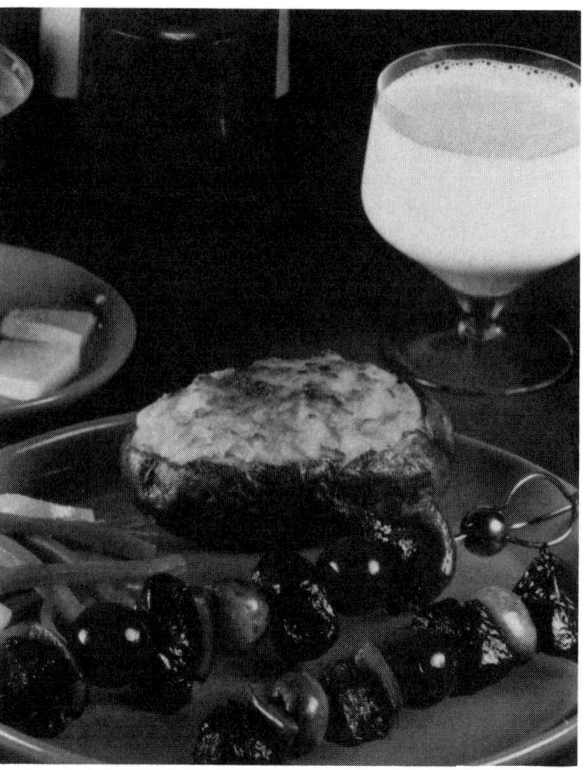

Fig. M-18. Meal planning should begin by using the food groups as a pattern. (Courtesy, American Dairy Assoc., Rosemont, Ill.)

The procedure should begin by using the food groups as a pattern. Choose the entree from the protein group, then add the milk group, follow with the vegetable and the fruit, and finish up with the cereal group. It is quite simple if every meal is planned this way.

There are some well-known food combinations which have stood the test of time, thus when combining foods it is best not to try unorthodox combinations. The public has demanded that restaurant meals be well balanced; thus, when in doubt, their menus can be used as patterns.

Table M-9 Meal Planning Guide, can be used for the purpose of planning the day's meals. It gives the number of servings of each food group, for the different ages. Thus, one menu can take care of every age, merely by varying the number of servings from each food group.

TABLE M-9
MEAL PLANNING GUIDE

Food Group and Serving Size[1]			Servings Per Person Per Day											
				Children			Adolescents		Adults (20–50 yrs)				Persons Older than 50 Yrs	
			Infants under 1 yr	1–3 yrs	4–7 yrs	8–11 yrs	12–19 yrs M	12–19 yrs F	M	Non-Preg. F	Preg-nant F	Lac-tating F	M	F
Low-Energy Foods	Medium-Energy Foods	High-Energy Foods												
MEATS, FISH OR SEAFOOD, EGGS, BEANS, PEAS, OR NUTS— each serving provides 12 to 20 g of protein			½	1	2	2	2	2	2	2	3	3	2	2
(50–150 kcal per serving)	(200–300 kcal per serving)	(350–500 kcal per serving)												
MILK PRODUCTS—each serving provides 250 to 300 mg of calcium and 8 g of protein			1½–2	3	3	3	4	4	3	3	4	4	3	3
(about 100 kcal per serving)	(150–200 kcal per serving)	(300–500 kcal per serving)												
BREADS AND CEREALS—should be whole-grain or enriched. Each serving provides 70 kcal and 2 g of protein			2	3	4	4	6	6	4	4	6	6	4	4
DARK-GREEN AND DEEP-YELLOW FRUITS AND VEGE-TABLES—each serving provides 3,000 or more IU of vitamin A			⅓	½	½	½	1	1	1	1	1½	1½	1	1
(less than 100 kcal per serving)		(100–200 kcal per serving)												
CITRUS FRUITS OR THEIR EQUIVALENTS—each serving provides 30 or more mg of vitamin C and less than 100 kcal			1	1	1	1	1	1	1	1	2	2	1	1
OTHER FRUITS AND VEGETABLES—sources of carbohydrates, fiber, minerals, and vitamins			½	1	3	3	3	3	3	3	4	4	4	4
(less than 100 kcal per serving)	(100–200 kcal per serving)	(200–350 kcal per serving)												
ESSENTIAL FATS—each serving provides approximately 1 g of essential fatty acids and 40–70 kcal			1	1½	2	2½	3	2½	3	2	2½	2½	2½	2
SUPPLEMENTAL SOURCES OF ENERGY—to bring the daily dietary energy up to the total allowance														
(Less than 100 kcal per serving)	(150–300 kcal per serving)	(350–500 kcal per serving)												
ENERGY ALLOWANCES (kcal per person per day)			50/lb	1,300	1,800	2,400	3,000	2,250	2,700	2,000	2,300	2,500	2,400	1,800

[1]Secure the foods according to the calories required for serving, from the Food Composition Table F-21.

Here is how to use Table M-9: Let us suppose that it is necessary to plan a daily meal pattern for a 25-year-old single, moderately active female, who is not overweight.

Step 1—Look down the column headed "Adults (20-50 years)" and subheaded "nonpregnant F." Note that the essential food groups and the number of servings are as follows:

Meat, Fish, or Seafood, etc. — 2
Milk Products — 3
Breads and Cereals — 4
Dark-Green Vegetables — 1
Citrus Fruits — 1
Other Fruits and Vegetables — 3
Essential Fats — 2

Optional items to make up a total of 2,000 Calories (kcal).

Step 2—Select items from the essential groups. Take care to balance their distribution between the meals and snacks, but avoid exceeding the total allowance for energy—2,000 Calories (kcal) per day. However, if the subject gains weight on 2,000 Calories (kcal) per day, then it will be necessary to choose servings from the *Low-Energy Foods*. On the other hand, if she wishes to gain weight, then choose servings from the *High-Energy Foods*. Optional items may be added from the group *Supplemental Sources of Energy* in order to bring the total energy up to the amount allowed. However, it would be better to obtain the supplemental sources of energy from among the essential groups. A typical day's selection might be as follows:

MEAL	FOOD	AMOUNT	CALORIES
Breakfast	Grapefruit	½	100
	Poached egg	1	74
	Whole wheat toast	2 slices	109
	w/butter	2 tsp	70
	Coffee w/evaporated milk	¼ c	50
	or Milk, 2%	1 c	122
Morning Snack	Yogurt, flavored	1 c	231
Lunch	Sandwich made w/		
	Cooked ham	2 oz	112
	Swiss cheese	½ oz	51
	Sliced tomato	4 slices	22
	Lettuce leaf		
	Mayonnaise	2 tsp	36
	Whole wheat bread	2 slices	109
	Milk, nonfat	1 c	83
Dinner	Roast beef	3 oz	300
	Tomato catsup	1 Tbsp	16
	Baked potato	1	93
	Mixed vegetables	½ c	64
	Biscuits made w/whole		
	wheat flour	2	204
	Butter	2 tsp	70
	Jam	1 Tbsp	54
Bedtime Snack	Apple	1	84
	Total		1932-2004

Step 3—After writing down the menu plan for the day, check the number of servings of each of the essential food groups and the total energy supplied as given in Table M-9.

Although Table M-9 is a useful guide in planning the day's diet, always remember the Golden Rule of Eating, which is—''The greater the variety of foods in the diet, the greater the chances of getting everything that the body requires.'' (Also see FOOD GROUPS.)

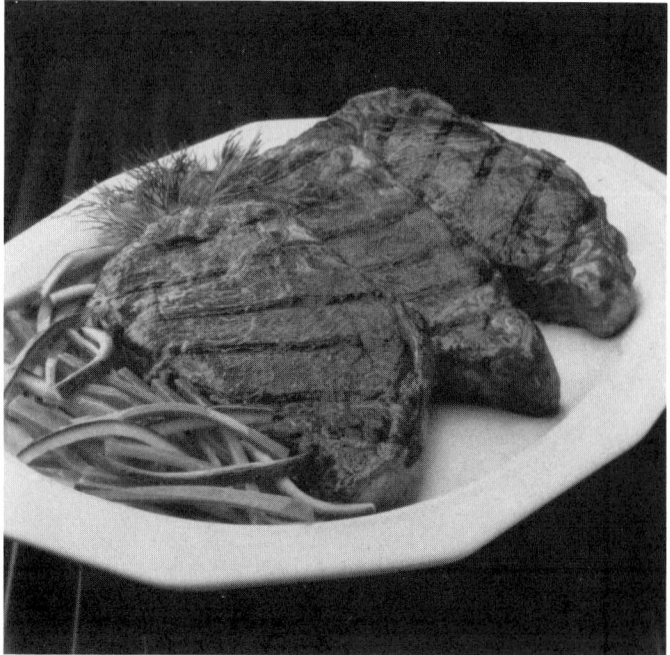

Fig. M-19. Rib eye steaks. People eat steaks because they're good, and good for them. (Courtesy, National Live Stock & Meat Board, Chicago, Ill.)

MEAT(S)

Contents   Page

For centuries, animals have made a major contribution to human welfare as sources of food, pharmaceuticals, clothing, transportation, power, soil fertility, fuel, and pleasure. The most important of these is food—meat and other animal products. This section contains information on the value of animal foods to humans, with particular emphasis on the meat and meat by-product supply.

Meat is the edible flesh, organs, and glands of animals used for food. Meat by-products include all products, both edible and inedible, other than the carcass meat. In a broad sense, the term meat may include the flesh of poultry, fish and other seafoods, and game. In this section, however, the discussion of meat will largely be limited to red meat and to by-products therewith—to beef, lamb, and pork. Poultry, fish and seafoods, game, and milk and milk products are treated in separate sections of this book.

That Americans enjoy eating meat is attested by the fact that, in 1990, the average American ate 112.3 lb of beef, veal, pork, and lamb. Of this total, beef accounted for 64 lb, pork for 46.3 lb, veal for 0.9 lb, and lamb for 1.1 lb.

Not only are meat and animal by-products good, but they are good for you. Foods from animals are the most nutritionally complete known. Today, they (meat, poultry, fish, and milk) supply to the U.S. diet an average of 95% of the vitamin B-12, 79% of the calcium (mostly from milk and milk products), 55% of the riboflavin, 63% of the protein, 64% of the phosphorus, 51% of the vitamin B-6, 46% of the niacin, 36% of the vitamin A, 33% of the thiamin, 25% of the iron (in a readily absorbed form), and 34% of the magnesium. Additionally, animal proteins provide the nine essential amino acids in the proportions needed for humans; hence, they are *high quality* proteins.

HISTORY OF MEAT.   The use of meat by man antedates recorded history. Primitive man recognized that a meat-rich diet was far more concentrated than leaves, shoots, and fruits. Thus, the adoption of the meat-eating habit allowed him, if he was lucky in his kill, more time for other pursuits and skills, such as devising new tools and learning the beginnings of pictorial art.

Until less than 10,000 years ago, man obtained his food by hunting, scavenging, or gathering from the animal and vegetable kingdoms in his environment. It is probable that taming, and then domestication, of animals occurred without people being aware of what was happening. Certainly, gatherers and hunters—the people who first domesticated animals—could not forsee any use for them other than those they knew already—for meat and skins. Only later, after a change from a nomadic to a more settled life-style, were animals used for such things as milk, wool, motive power, war, sport, and prestige.

It is recorded that pork was used as a food in Egypt, probably at certain feasts, as early as 3400 B.C., and in China beginning in 2900 B.C. Old Testament Laws, written about 1100 B.C., dictated what meats were considered wholesome and sanitary. In 1 Corinthians, 15:39, written about 54 A.D., the Bible tells us—"All flesh is not the same flesh, but there is one kind of flesh of men, another flesh of beasts, another of fishes, and another of birds."

FROM WHENCE MEAT COMES.   Animal agriculture is worldwide. Most of the livestock and poultry, along with 58% of the agricultural land, are found in Asia, Africa, and South America. Yet, North America, Europe, and Oceania, where scientific methods of production are most widely applied, produces 58% of the world's beef and veal, 62% of the milk, 41% of the lamb and mutton, 53% of the wool, 55% of the pork, 60% of the poultry meat, and 48% of the eggs.

Consumers—all—need to know from whence their meat comes; they need to know that meat on the table is the ultimate objective in producing cattle, sheep, and swine. Consumers need to know that only farmers produce foods—that neither governments nor supermarkets produce foods; and they need to know that people do those things that are most profitable for them—and that farmers are people.

HOW MEAT REACHES THE TABLE

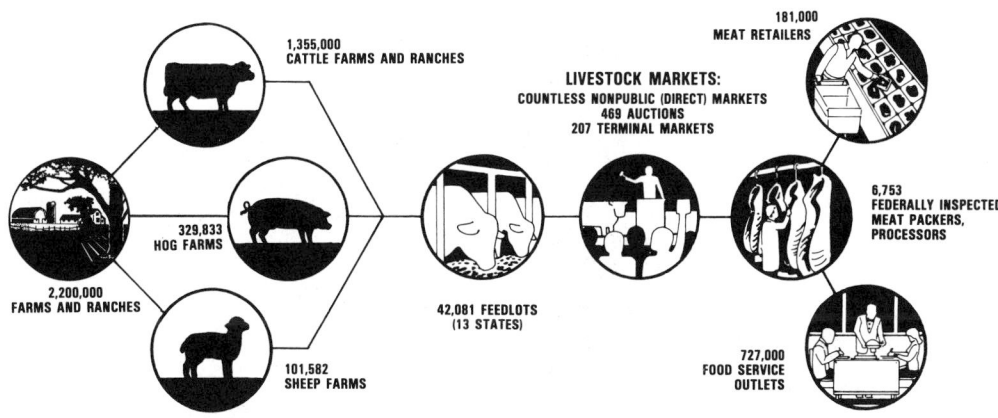

Fig. M-20. From whence meat comes. Back of the meat on the table are 2,200,000 farms, of which 1,355,000 are cattle farms and ranches, 329,833 are hog farms, and 101,582 are sheep farms. All statistics are from the USDA, and for 1988, except number of cattle farms, number of hog farms, and number of sheep farms are from 1982 Agricultural Census.

MEAT PACKING.   *Meat packing is the business of slaughtering cattle, hogs, and sheep, and of preparing the meat for transportation and sale.* It is an important industry in many countries; the United States ranks first in meat packing. In 1986, 6,753 U.S. establishments slaughtered 37.6 million cattle, 3.5 million calves, 5.8 million sheep and lambs, and 80 million hogs; and produced 39.3 billion pounds of red meat. Also, the meat packing industry employed 143,000 people.

Today, the name *packing* is a misnomer, for the barrelled or pickled pork from whence the name originated is only a mem-

ory. But modern meat slaughtering and processing developed slowly, and the original name was so well established that there has been no attempt to rename the industry.

Meat Tenderizing.   Consumers want tenderness, as well as flavor, in the meat they buy. The common methods of tenderizing are:

• **Aging, Natural (low temperature)**—Following slaughter, dressed carcasses are rapidly chilled in a room at 32°F (0°C), at a relative humidity of about 85% in order to reduce moisture loss. The chilled side or cuts may be held for aging.

Aging is accomplished by holding the beef carcass or cuts for 1 to 6 weeks at a temperature of 38 to 40°F (*3 to 4 °C*) and a relative humidity of 70 to 90%, with a gradual flow of air to provide a fresh atmosphere. These conditions permit selective enzymatic and bacterial action; the enzymes aid in the breakdown of various tissues, and the bacteria provide the nutlike flavor characteristic of aged beef. Today, very little beef is aged more than a week, because aging in carcass or wholesale cuts has become too costly in terms of shrinkage and cooler space.

Lamb carcasses are not aged.

• **Vegetable enzymes**—Three enzymes of vegetable origin which dissolve or degrade collagen and elastin are:

1. *Papain,* secured from the tropical American tree, *Carica papaya* (Also see PAPAYA.)

2. *Bromelin,* secured from the juice of the pineapple (Also see PINEAPPLE.)

3. *Ficin,* secured from figs (Also see FIG.)

The tenderizing action of enzymes does not occur until the meat is heated during cooking.

• **Mechanical tenderization (blade tenderization)**—Mechanical tenderizers, consisting of a machine that presses many sharp blades or needles through roasts and steaks, are being used by some segments of the meat trade. It is chiefly used on primal cuts (rib and loin) from lower quality grades and on the less tender cuts (chuck, round, shank) of higher grade carcasses. These machines have gained wide acceptance in the hotel, restaurant, and institutional trade in recent years. Research indicates that mechanical tenderization improves tenderness by 20 to 50%, without increasing cooking losses.

• **Electrical stimulation**—Electrical stimulation is a method of tenderizing meat with electricity. The passing of a current through the carcass causes the muscle fibers to loosen. Before rigor mortis sets in, the carcass is shocked until all the energy in the muscle that causes the fibers to contract is used up.

Electrical tenderizing is effective on beef, lamb, and goat carcasses, but not pork.

Meat Curing. In this country, meat curing is largely confined to pork, primarily because of the keeping qualities and palatability of cured pork products. Considerable beef is corned or dried, and some lamb and veal are cured, but none of these is of such magnitude as cured pork.

Meat is cured with salt, sugar, and certain curing adjuncts (ascorbate, erythorbate, etc.); with sodium nitrite or sodium nitrate (the latter is used only in certain products); and with smoke. Each of the most common curing additives will be discussed:

• **Salt**—Sodium chloride is added to processed meats for preservative and palatability reasons. The addition of salt makes it possible to distribute certain perishable meats through what are often lengthy and complicated distribution systems. Also, in products such as wieners, bologna, and canned ham, fat solubilizes myosin, the major meat protein, and causes the meat particles to hold together; the meat can then be sliced without falling apart.

(Also see SALT.)

• **Sodium nitrite ($NaNO_2$), sodium nitrate ($NaNO_3$), potassium nitrate or saltpeter (KNO_3)**—Nitrite and nitrate contribute to (1) the prevention of *Clostridium botulinum* spores in or on meat (*Clostridium botulinum* bacteria produce the botulin toxin that causes botulism, the most deadly form of food poisoning); (2) the development of the characteristic flavor and pink color of cured meats; (3) the prevention of *warmed-over flavor* in reheated products; and (4) the prevention of rancidity. Of all the effects of nitrite and nitrate, the antibotulinial effect is by far the most important. Nitrite is the essential ingredient for curing; the effectiveness of nitrate results from change of part of the nitrate to nitrite by reactions that occur during processing.

No entirely satisfactory substitute is known for nitrite in meat curing.

• **Smoking**—Smoking produces the distinctive smoked-meat flavor which consumers demand in certain meats.

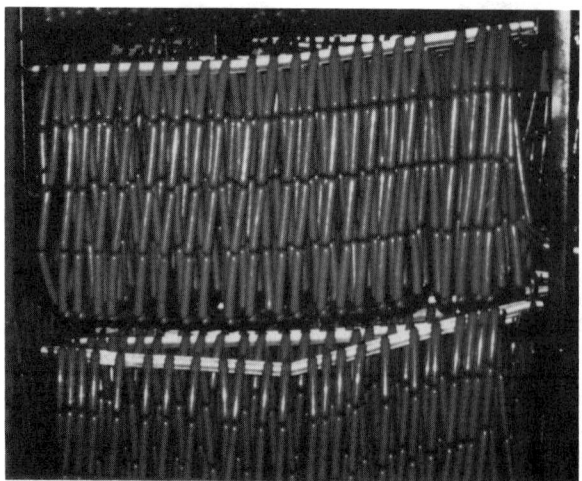

Fig. M-21. Hot dogs (Frankfurters, or wieners), the most popular sausage in America, processed by a large meat packing company. (Courtesy, University of Tennesse, Knoxville, Tenn.)

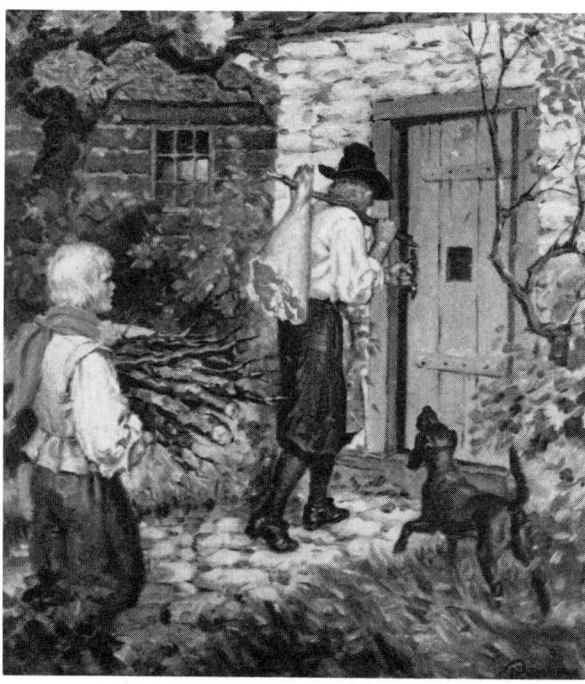

Fig. M-22. The Smoke House, in which meats were smoked in colonial days. This method of preserving meats is very old. Modern meat packers still smoke many of their products. (Courtesy, Swift and Company)

• **Phosphate (PO₄)**—Phosphate is added to increase the water-binding capacity of meat; its use increases yields up to 10%. Also, it enhances juiciness of the cooked product. Federal regulations restrict the amount of phosphates to: (1) not to exceed 0.5% in the finished product, and (2) not more than 5% in the pickle solution based on 10% pumping pickle. The addition of phosphate must be declared on the label.

Federal and State Meat Inspection. Most foods from animals are inspected by government officials to assure wholesomeness, proper labeling, and freedom from disease and adulteration. Federal inspection of animal products is the responsibility of the Food Safety and Quality Service of the U.S. Department of Agriculture. Imported meat and poultry are produced under USDA supervision in foreign countries where they originate, and samples are inspected by USDA upon arrival in the United States.

If meat passes federal inspection, an inspection stamp (Fig. M-23) is affixed to the wholesale cuts or package to assure the retailer and consumer that the products have been inspected. Products that do not pass inspection are denatured and rendered unusable for human consumption.

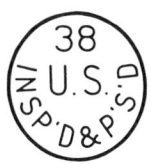

THIS IS THE STAMP USED ON MEAT CARCASSES. NOTE THAT IT ALSO BEARS THE OFFICIAL NUMBER ASSIGNED TO THE ESTABLISHMENT---IN THIS CASE NUMBER 38. THE STAMP IS USED ONLY ON THE MAJOR CUTS OF THE CARCASS; HENCE, IT MAY NOT APPEAR ON THE ROAST OR STEAK THE CONSUMER BUYS.

THIS MARK IS FOUND ON EVERY PREPACKAGED PROCESSED MEAT PRODUCT---SOUPS TO SPREADS--- THAT HAS BEEN FEDERALLY INSPECTED.

Fig. M-23. Federal inspection marks used on animal products.

Federal Grades of Meats. The grade of meat may be defined as a measure of its degree of excellence based on quality, or eating characteristics of the meat, and the yield, or total proportion, of primal cuts. Naturally, the attributes upon which the grades are based vary between species. Nevertheless, it is intended that the specifications for each grade shall be sufficiently definite to make for uniform grades throughout the country and from season to season, and that on-hook grades shall be correlated with on-foot grades.

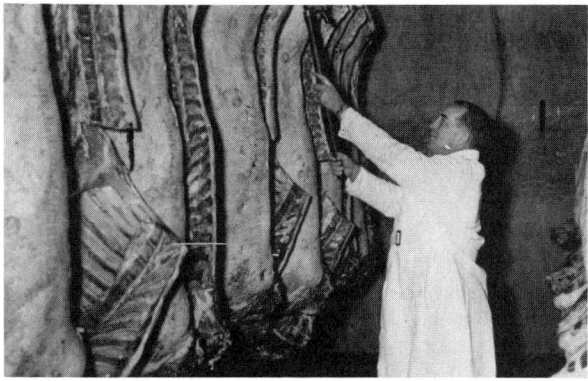

Fig. M-24. Federal grader shown rolling (grading or stamping) beef with an edible vegetable dye. (Courtesy, *Livestock Breeder Journal,* Macon, Ga.)

Government grading, unlike meat inspection, is not compulsory. Official graders are subject to the call of anyone who wishes their services, (packer, wholesaler, or retailer) with a charge per hour being made.

Consumers, especially the housewife who buys most of the meat, should know the federal grades of meats, because (1) in these days of self-service, prepackaged meats there is less opportunity to secure the counsel and advice of the meat cutter when making purchases, and (2) the average consumer is not the best judge of the quality of the various kinds of meats on display in the meat counter.

Federally graded meats are so stamped (with an edible vegetable dye) that the grade will appear on the retail cuts as well as on the carcass and wholesale cuts. These are summarized in Table M-10.

TABLE M-10
QUALITY GRADES OF MEATS BY CLASSES[1]

Beef[2]	Veal	Mutton and Lamb[2]	Pork
1. Prime[3]	1. Prime	1. Prime[4]	1. U.S. No. 1
2. Choice	2. Choice	2. Choice	2. U.S. No. 2
3. Select	3. Select	3. Select	3. U.S. No. 3
4. Standard	4. Standard	4. Utility	4. U.S. No. 4
5. Commercial	5. Utility	5. Cull[5]	5. U.S. Utility
6. Utility			
7. Cutter			
8. Canner			

[1]In rolling meat, the letters U.S. precede each federal grade name. This is important as only government-graded meat can be so marked. For convenience, however, the letters U.S. are not used in this table or in the discussion which follows.

[2]In addition to the quality grades given herein, there are the following yield grades of beef and lamb (and mutton) carcasses: Yield Grade 1, Yield Grade 2, Yield Grade 3, Yield Grade 4, and Yield Grade 5.

[3]Cow beef is not eligible for the Prime grade.

[4]Limited to lamb and yearling carcasses.

[5]Limited to mutton carcasses.

As would be expected, in order to make the top grade in the respective classes, the carcass or cut must possess a very high degree of the attributes upon which grades are based. The lower grades of meats are deficient in one or more of these grade-determining factors. Because each grade is determined on the basis of a composite evaluation of all factors, a carcass or cut may possess some characteristics that are common to another grade. It must also be recognized that all of the wholesale cuts produced from a carcass are not necessarily of the same grade as the carcass from which they are secured.

NOTE WELL: Federal grades of meats change from time to time, reflecting consumer preferences, technological developments in meat processing and marketing, and political expediency.

• **Proportion of U.S. meat federally graded**—In 1988, 93.6% of all lamb and mutton was quality graded, 56.4% of the beef was quality graded, but only negligible amounts of pork were quality graded.

Packer Brand Names. Practically all packers identify their higher grades of meats with alluring private brands so that the consumer as well as the retailer can recognize the quality of a particular cut.

A meat packer's reputation depends upon consistent standards of quality for all meats that carry his brand names. The brand names are also effectively used in advertising campaigns.

Kosher Meats.[17]—Meat for the Jewish trade—known as kosher meat—is slaughtered, washed, and salted according to ancient Biblical laws, called *Kashruth,* dating back to the days of Moses, more than 3,000 years ago. The Hebrew religion holds that God issued these instructions directly to Moses, who, in turn, transmitted them to the Jewish people while they were wandering in the wilderness near Mount Sinai.

The Hebrew word *kosher* means fit or proper, and this is the guiding principle in the handling of meats for the Jewish trade. Also, only those classes of animals considered clean—those that both chew the cud and have cloven hooves—are used. Thus, cattle, sheep, and goats—but not hogs—are koshered (Deuteronomy 14:4–5 and Leviticus 11:1–8).

Poultry is also koshered. Rabbinical law dictates that only cold water shall be used; hot or warm water cannot be used in defeathering or at any time in the processing of poultry products. Also, following picking and cleaning, kosher poultry must be washed, hung up to drip, hand-salted internally and externally, and rinsed; with constant inspection at all phases.

Both forequarters and hindquarters of kosher-slaughtered cattle, sheep, and goats may be used by Orthodox Jews. However, the Jewish trade usually confines itself to the forequarters. The hindquarters (that portion of beef carcass below the twelfth rib) are generally sold as nonkosher for the following reasons:

1. The Sinew of Jacob (*the sinew that shrank,* now known as the sciatic nerve), which is found in the hindquarters only, must be removed by reason of the Biblical story of Jacob's struggle with the Angel, in the course of which Jacob's thigh was injured and he was made to limp.

Actually, the sciatic nerve consists of two nerves; an inner long one located near the hip bone which spreads throughout the thigh, and an outer short one which lies near the flesh. Removal of the sinew (sciatic nerve) is very difficult.

The Biblical law of the sciatic nerve applies to cattle, sheep, and goats, but it does not apply to birds because they have no spoon-shaped hip (no hollow thigh).

2. The very considerable quantity of forbidden fat (Heleb) found in the hindquarters, especially around the loins, flanks, and kidneys, must be removed; and this is difficult and costly. Forbidden fat refers to fat (tallow) (a) that is not intermingled (marbled) with the flesh of the animal, but forms a separate solid layer; and (b) that is encrusted by a membrane which can be easily peeled off.

The Biblical law of the forbidden fat applies to cattle, sheep, and goats, but not birds and nondomesticated animals.

3. The blood vessels must be removed, because the consumption of blood is forbidden; and such removal is especially difficult in the hindquarters.

NOTE WELL: Forbidden fat and blood (the blood vessels) must be removed from both fore and hindquarters, but such removal is more difficult in the hindquarters than in the forequarters. However, the Sinew of Jacob (the sciatic nerve), which must also be removed, is found in the hindquarters only.

Because of the difficulties in processing, meat from the hindquarters is not eaten by Orthodox Jews in many countries, including England. However, the consumption of the hindquarters is permitted by the Rabbinic authorities where there is a special hardship involved in obtaining alternative supplies of meat; thus, in Israel the sinews are removed and the hindquarters are eaten.

Because the forequarters do not contain such choice cuts as the hinds, the kosher trade attempts to secure the best possible fores; thus, this trade is for high grade slaughter animals.

Kosher meat must be sold by the packer or the retailer within 72 hours after slaughter, or it must be washed (a treatment known as *begiss,* meaning to wash) and reinstated by a representative of the synagogue every subsequent 72 hours. At the expiration of 216 hours after the time of slaughter (after begissing three times), however, it is declared *trafeh,* meaning forbidden food, and is automatically rejected for kosher trade. It is then sold in the regular meat channels. Because of these regulations, kosher meat is moved out very soon after slaughter.

Kosher sausage and prepared meats are made from kosher meats which are soaked in water ½ hour, sprinkled with salt, allowed to stand for an hour, and washed thoroughly. This makes them kosher indefinitely.

The Jewish law also provides that before kosher meat is cooked, it must be soaked in water for ½ hour. After soaking, the meat is placed on a perforated board in order to drain off the excess moisture. It is then sprinkled liberally with salt. One hour later, it is thoroughly washed. Such meat is then considered to remain kosher as long as it is fresh and wholesome.

Meats and fowl are the only food items which require ritual slaughter, washing, and salting before they are rendered kosher.

As would be expected, the volume of kosher meat is greatest in those Eastern Seaboard cities where the Jewish population is most concentrated. New York City alone uses about one-fourth of all the beef koshered in the United States.

While only about half of the total of more than six million U.S. Jewish population is orthodox, most members of the faith are heavy users of kosher meats.

By-Products.   By-products include everything of value produced on the killing floor other than the dressed carcass; and they are classified as edible or inedible. The edible by-products include blood, brains, casings, fats, gelatin, hearts, kidneys, livers, oxtails, sweetbreads, tongues, and tripe. The inedible by-products include animal feeds, bone meal, bone products, brushes, cosmetics, feathers, fertilizer, glue, glycerin, hides and skins, lanolin, ligatures, lubricants, neat's foot oil, pluck (lungs, etc.), soap, and wool.

In addition to the edible (food) and nonfood (inedible) products, certain chemical substances useful as human drugs or pharmaceuticals are obtained as by-products. Among such drugs are ACTH, cholesterol, estrogen, epinephrine, heparin, insulin, rennet, thrombin, TSH, and thyroid extracts—all valuable pharmaceuticals which are routinely recovered from meat animals in the United States.

---

[17]Authoritative information relative to kosher meats was secured from: (1) Grunfeld, Dayton Dr. I., *The Jewish Dietary Laws,* The Soncino Press, London/Jerusalem/New York, 1975; (2) a personal letter to M. E. Ensminger dated December 22, 1981, from Rabbi Menachem Genack, Rabbinic Coordinator, Union of Orthodox Jewish Congregations of America, New York, N.Y.; and (3) John Ensminger, Lawyer, New York, N.Y.

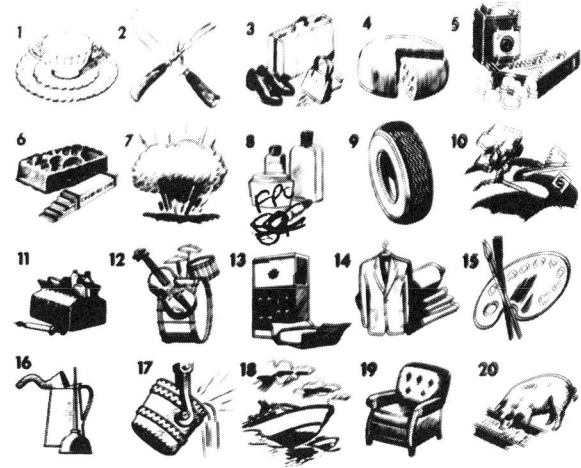

Fig. M-25. Some of the items for which by-products are used—items which contribute to the convenience, enjoyment, and health of people in all walks of life. (Courtesy, American Meat Institute, Washington, D.C.)

1. Bone for bone china
2. Horn and bone handles for carving sets
3. Hides and skins for leather goods
4. Rennet for cheese making
5. Gelatin for marshmallows, photographic film, printers' rollers
6. Stearin for making chewing gum and candies
7. Glycerin for explosives used in mining and blasting
8. Lanolin for cosmetics
9. Chemicals for tires that run cooler
10. Binders for asphalt paving
11. Medicines such as various hormones and glandular extracts, insulin, pepsin, epinephrine, ACTH, cortisone; and surgical sutures

12. Drumheads and violin strings
13. Animal fats for soaps
14. Wool for clothing
15. Camel's hair (actually from cattle ears for artists' brushes)
16. Cutting oils and other special industrial lubricants
17. Bone charcoal for high-grade steel such as ball bearings
18. Special glues for marine plywoods, paper, matches, window shades
19. Curled hair for upholstery. Leather for covering fine furniture
20. High-protein livestock feeds

KINDS OF MEAT.
The meat of cattle, hogs, sheep, and goats is known by several different names. These follow:

• **Beef**—This is the flesh of adult cattle. Good beef has white fat and bright cherry-red lean meat.

• **Veal**—This is the flesh of calves, usually 2 to 12 weeks old. Older calves are usually sold as *calves*. Veal is pink in color and has a fine texture.

• **Mutton**—This is the flesh of mature sheep. It is darker colored and stronger flavored than lamb.

• **Lamb**—This is the flesh of young sheep. The meat of a sheep becomes mutton when the animal is about a year old. Lamb has a light-pink color and white fat, and a much milder flavor than mutton.

• **Pork**—This is the flesh of hogs. It is known as pork no matter how old the animal from which it comes. The eating quality of pork does not change much with the animal's age.

• **Chevon (goat meat)**—This is goat meat. The meat from young goats (kids) is delicious. Chevon from older goats is likely to possess a strong flavor.

• **Variety meat**—The various organs of animals are called variety meats. The heart, liver, brains, kidneys, tongue, cheek meat, tail, feet, sweetbreads (thymus and pancreatic glands), and tripe (pickled rumen of cattle and sheep) are sold over the counter as variety meats or fancy meats.

• **Game meat**—The flesh of wild animals or birds used as food.

MEAT PRESERVATION.
Methods of preserving meat were well established before the dawn of recorded history. Meat was dried by the aborigines; smoking and salting techniques were well established long before Homer's time (about 1000 B.C.); preparation and spicing of some kinds of sausages were common practices in Europe and in the Mediterranean countries before the time of the Caesars.

Fundamentally, meat preservation is a matter of controlling putrefactive bacterial action. Various methods of preserving meats have been practiced through the ages, the most common of which (listed alphabetically), are: (1) acidity, (2) air exclusion, (3) canning, (4) drying, (5) freeze-drying, (6) radiation, (7) refrigeration and freezing, (8) salting, (9) dry sausage, (10) smoking, (11) spicing, and (12) sugar.

• **Acidity**—Commonly referred to as pickling or souring, an acid condition is unfavorable to bacteria. This method of preservation is used for pigs' feet, certain sausages, sauerkraut, pickles, and milk.

• **Air exclusion (vacuum packed)**—Vacuum packaging, or packaging with inert gas (e.g., N_2 or CO_2), are examples of the exclusion of air method. Elimination of oxygen from the package is the primary objective in vacuum and gas packaging. It extends the shelf life of fresh meats.

• **Canning**—*Canning is the temporary increasing of the heat content of a product that has been enclosed in an airtight container for the purpose of preventing the spoilage of the product being canned by the inactivation of particular organisms.* Two levels of heat may be applied in canning meat:

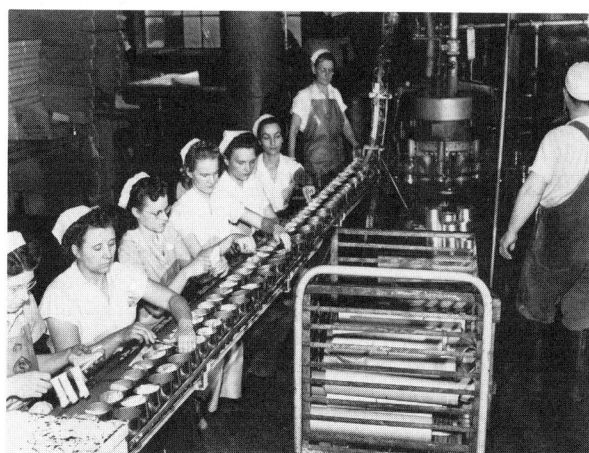

Fig. M-26. Canning meat, a method of meat preservation. (Courtesy, *Meat Magazine*)

1. **Pasteurization.** A low level of heat in the process of pasteurization, which is designed to kill all pathogenic organisms, but not all spoilage organisms. Since all spoilage organisms have not been destroyed, the product must still be stored under refrigeration. Most canned hams are pasteurized.

2. Sterilization. A high temperature in the process of sterilization. In this process, the canned meat is processed at a sufficiently high temperature and held there long enough to kill bacteria that cause spoilage, food poisoning, or infection. This calls for using a steam-pressure canner. By holding steam under pressure, one can get a temperature of 240°F (115.5°C) or more. Many luncheon meats are processed in this manner.

When canning, checking the sea level is important. More pressure in the canner is required at high altitudes than at low altitudes. A rule of thumb is: add 1 lb pressure for each 2,000 ft above sea level. Processing time depends on the container size.

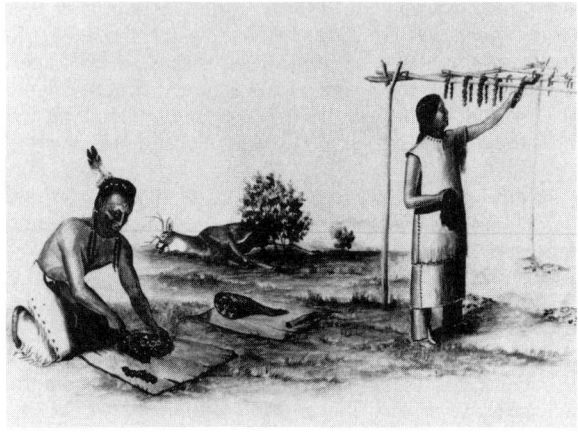

Fig. M-27. Indians drying and smoking venison. (Photo from a watercolor original by Ernest Smith. Owned by the Rochester Museum of Arts and Sciences)

Today, a limited amount of beef is cured and dried, in which form it is known as *beef jerky*. It has a tough, chewy consistency and may be smoked, unsmoked, or air- or oven-dried.

• **Freeze-drying**—This process involves the dehydration of meat by the freeze-drying process, which consists of subjecting frozen pieces of meat to heat under vacuum. Products retain their shape and form and do not shrink as with other methods of dehydration. Freeze-dried meat and poultry have a moisture content of 2% or less and will not support the growth of most microbes.

• **Radiation**—This is the newest development in meat preservation. Nonionizing and ionizing radiation are capable of deactivating microorganisms.

Ultraviolet light is an example of nonionizing radiation; however, it does not sterilize beneath the surface.

Ionizing radiation, in the form of soft x rays or gamma rays, is capable of destroying organisms in canned, packaged, or exposed meat products without raising the temperature appreciably (hence, it is known as *cold sterilization*). Some researchers report that radiation may result in slight odor, flavor, and color changes. Also, it is noted that small doses of radiation do not completely inactivate all the proteolytic enzymes in meat, with the result that there is danger of these enzymes causing serious changes in the product during storage. However, much research is in progress; hence, these deficiencies may soon be overcome.

In 1981, the control of the Mediterranean fruit fly in California caused the Food and Drug Administration to ease the ban on treating food with gamma rays. However, each food processed by radiation requires FDA's approval. Also, labels on foods that have been irradiated must so indicate.

Consumer reaction to radiation of foods will be watched closely. It has great potential, provided people are not squeamish about the *dangers*.

(Also see RADIATION PRESERVATION OF FOOD; and ULTRAVIOLET LIGHT.)

• **Refrigeration and freezing**—Meat is perishable, so proper care is essential to maintaining its keeping qualities.

Meat may be refrigerated for short-time storage, at a temperature of 36° to 40°F (2° - 4°C); or it may be frozen for longtime storage, at a temperature of 0°F or lower. Table M-11 gives recommended times for refrigerator and freezer storage. Additional pointers relative to refrigeration and freezing follow:

TABLE M-11
STORAGE TIME FOR REFRIGERATED AND FROZEN MEATS[1]
(Maximum storage time recommendations
for fresh, cooked, and processed meat)

Meat	Refrigerator	Freezer
	(36° to 40°F)[2]	(at 0°F or lower)
Beef (fresh)	2 to 4 days	6 to 12 months
Veal (fresh)	2 to 4 days	6 to 9 months
Pork (fresh)	2 to 4 days	3 to 6 months
Lamb (fresh)	2 to 4 days	6 to 9 months
Ground beef, veal and lamb	1 to 2 days	3 to 4 months
Ground pork	1 to 2 days	1 to 3 months
Variety meats	1 to 2 days	3 to 4 months
Luncheon meats	1 week	not recommended
Sausage, fresh pork	1 week	60 days
Sausage, smoked	3 to 7 days	—
Sausage, dry and semidry (unsliced)	2 to 3 weeks	—
Frankfurters	4 to 5 days	1 month
Bacon	5 to 7 days	1 month
Smoked ham, whole	1 week	60 days
Ham slices	3 to 4 days	60 days
Beef, corned	1 week	2 weeks
Leftover cooked meat	4 to 5 days	2 to 3 months
Frozen Combination Food		
Meat pies (cooked)	—	3 months
Swiss steak (cooked)	—	3 months
Stews (cooked)	—	3 to 4 months
Prepared meat dinners	—	2 to 6 months

[1]*Lessons on Meat*, published by the National Live Stock and Meat Board, Chicago, Ill., p. 60.
[2]The range in time reflects recommendations for maximum storage time from several authorities. For top quality, fresh meats should be used in 2 or 3 days, ground meat and variety meats should be used in 24 hours.

1. Storage of meat. Fresh meat which is not to be refrozen should be stored in the coldest part of the refrigerator or, when available, in the compartment designed for meat storage. Additional guides for storage of meats follow:

a. **Fresh meat, prepackaged by the meat retailer (self-service).** It may be stored in the refrigerator in the original wrapping for no more than 2 days, or it may be frozen without rewrapping and stored in the freezer 1 to 2 weeks. For longer freezer storage, the original package should be overwrapped with special freezer material.

b. **Fresh meat, not prepackaged.** It should be removed from the market wrapping paper, wrapped loosely in waxed paper or aluminum foil, and refrigerated for no more than 2 days.

c. **Variety meats and ground or chopped meats.** They are more perishable than other meats; so, they should be cooked in 1 or 2 days if not frozen.

d. **Cured, cured and smoked meats, sausages, and ready-to-serve meats.** These should be left in their original wrapping and stored in the refrigerator.

e. **Canned hams, picnics and other perishable canned meats.** These should be stored in the refrigerator unless the directions on the can read to the contrary. These meats should not be frozen.

f. **Frozen meat.** Meat that is frozen at the time of purchase should be placed in the freezer soon after purchase unless it is to be defrosted for immediate cooking. The temperature of the freezer should not go above 0°F (-18°C). Packages should be dated as they are put into the freezer, and the storage time should be limited as recommended in Table M-11.

g. **Cooked meats.** Leftover cooked meats should be cooled within 1 to 2 hours after cooking, then covered or wrapped to prevent drying, and stored in the refrigerator. Meats cooked in liquid for future serving should be cooled uncovered for 1 to 2 hours, then covered and stored in the refrigerator.

2. **Freezing of meat.** Most meats may be frozen satisfactorily if properly wrapped, frozen quickly, and kept at 0°F or below. The following guides will help ensure good quality in frozen meats:

a. **Freeze meat while it is fresh and in top condition.** Properly done, freezing will maintain quality, but what comes out of the freezer will be no better than what goes in.

b. **Select proper wrapping material.** Choose a moisture-vapor-proof wrap so that air will be sealed out and moisture locked in. When air penetrates the package, moisture is drawn from the surface of the meat and the condition known as *freezer burn* develops. Several good freezer wraps are on the market.

c. **Prepare meat for freezing before wrapping.** Trim off excess fat and remove bones when practical; wrap in family-sized packages; place double thickness of freezer wrap between chops, patties, or individual pieces of meat, for easier separation during thawing.

d. **Label properly.** This should include the kind and cut of meat enclosed, the number of possible servings (including weight if convenient), and the date of packaging.

e. **Freeze immediately.** Start freezing immediately following wrapping and labeling.

f. **Keep freezer temperature 0°F (– 18°C) or lower.** Higher temperatures and fluctuations above that temperature impair quality.

g. **Check freezer, Table M-11, for maximum storage times.** Frozen meat will be of best quality if not held longer than indicated.

h. **Avoid refreezing if possible.** Refreezing results in loss of juices when rethawed, thereby affecting juiciness and flavor.

• **Salting**—Dry salting of meats has been practiced since the 5th century B.C., and possibly longer. However, it was not until the latter part of the 18th century that salt curing of meat was done on a scientific basis.

The presence of salt has an effect on osmotic pressure. In addition, the action of chloride on microorganisms is detrimental.

Currently, salt curing is limited to a few specialized products, such as hams and bacon. Although there is no specified salt content for products labeled *salt cured,* most cured meats are acceptable at levels of 2.5 to 3% salt.

• **Dry sausages**—Dry sausages are often called summer sausages because of their keeping qualities. They can be held in a fairly cool room for a very long period of time. Dry salami is an example of a dry sausage.

• **Smoking**—This method of preserving meats is very old. The drying and smoking of meats was known to the Egyptians as well as to the ancient Sumerian civilization which preceded them. The advantage to this type of preservation lay in the fact that the smoke overcame objectionable flavors that developed if the drying did not proceed at a rapid rate. The favorite wood smoke in colonial America was produced by hickory or oak, although the Indians also used sage and various aromatic seeds and plants.

Smoking permits formaldehyde and phenolic compounds to accumulate on the surface of the meat. This, along with the surface drying, prevents microbial growth.

• **Spicing**—Many of the essential oils and other substances found in spices are effective bacteriostatic agents *provided* they are used at high levels. Mustard oil and allicin (allythio-sulfinic allyl ester) in garlic are examples of effective bacteriostatic substances. Contrary to historical and popular belief, in the concentrations generally employed in flavoring agents, spices cannot be depended upon to have any preservative action. Rather, it appears that they gained early popularity as a means of masking undesirable flavors resulting from microbial spoilage and other causes.

• **Sugar**—A high concentration of sugar exerts a high osmotic pressure and causes water to be withdrawn from microorganisms. However, the sugar concentrations normally employed in meat curing are far short of those needed to contribute to any preservative action. Mincemeat, of which only a minor proportion is meat, is an example of a meat-containing food which is preserved by a combination of sugar, acetic acid, and spices.

FABRICATED; PACKAGED MEAT. With the advent of the refrigerator car, meat was shipped in exposed halves, quarters, or wholesale cuts, and divided into retail cuts in the back rooms of meat markets. But this traditional procedure leaves much to be desired from the standpoints of efficiency, sanitation, shrink, spoilage, and discoloration. To improve this situation, more and more packers are fabricating and packaging (boxing) meat in their plants, thereby freeing the back rooms of 200,000 supermarkets.

After chilling, the carcass is subjected to a disassembly process, in which it is fabricated or broken into counter-ready cuts; vacuum-sealed; moved into storage by an automated system; loaded into refrigerated trailers; and shipped to retailers across the nation.

QUALITIES IN MEATS DESIRED BY CONSUMERS. Consumers desire the following qualities in meats:

1. Palatability
2. Attractiveness; eye appeal
3. Minimum amount of fat
4. Tenderness
5. Small cuts
6. Ease of preparation
7. Repeatability

If these qualities are not met by meats, other products will. Recognition of this fact is important, for competition is keen for space on the shelves of a modern retail food outlet.

MEAT BUYING. Meat buying is important because, (1) meat prices change, (2) one-fifth of the disposable personal income spent on food goes for red meats, and (3) buying food for a family may be a more intricate affair than its preparation at home. Hence, meat buying merits well informed buyers.

What Determines the Price of Meat? During those periods when meat is high in price, especially the choicest cuts, there is a tendency on the part of the consumer to blame either or all of the following: (1) the farmer or rancher, (2) the packer, (3) the meat retailer, or (4) the government. Such criticisms, which often have a way of becoming quite vicious, are not justified. Actually, meat prices are determined by the law of supply and demand; that is, the price of meat is largely dependent upon what the consumers as a group are able and willing to pay for the available supply.

• **The available supply of meat**—Because the vast majority of meats are marketed on a fresh basis rather than cured, and because meat is a perishable product, the supply of this food is dependent upon the number and weight of cattle, sheep, and hogs available for slaughter at a given time. In turn, the number of market animals is largely governed by the relative profitability of livestock enterprises in comparison with other agricultural pursuits. That is to say, farmers and ranchers—like any other good businessmen—generally do those things that are most profitable to them. Thus, a short supply of market animals at any given time usually reflects the unfavorable and unprofitable production factors that existed some months earlier and which caused curtailment of breeding and feeding operations.

• **The demand for meat**—The demand for meat is primarily determined by buying power and competition from other products. Stated in simple terms, demand is determined by the spending of money available and the competitive bidding of millions of housewives who are the chief home purchasers of meats. On a nationwide basis, a high buying power and great demand for meats exist when most people are employed and wages are high.

But the novice may wonder why these choice cuts are so scarce, even though people are able and willing to pay a premium for them. The answer is simple. Nature does not make many choice cuts or top grades, regardless of price. Moreover, a hog is born with two hams only, a lamb with two hind legs; and only two loins (a right and a left one) can be obtained from each carcass upon slaughter. In addition, not all weight on foot can be cut into meat. For example, the average steer weighing 1,050 lb *(477 kg)* on foot will only yield 448.8 lb *(204 kg)* of retail cuts (the balance consists of hide, internal organs, etc., see Fig. M-29, next page). Secondly, this 448.8 lb will cut out about 34.8 lb *(15.8 kg)* of porterhouse, T-bone, and top loin steaks. The balance of the cuts are equally wholesome and nutritious; and, although there are other steaks, many of the cuts are better adapted for use as roasts, stews, and soup bones. To make bad matters worse, not all cattle are of a quality suitable for the production of steaks. For example, the meat from most worn-out dairy animals and thin cattle of beef breeding is not sold over the block. Also, if the moneyed buyer insists on buying only the top grade of meat—namely U.S. Prime or its equivalent—it must be remembered that only a small proportion of slaughter cattle produce carcasses of this top grade. To be sure, the lower grades are equally wholesome, but they are simply graded down because the carcass is somewhat deficient in conformation, finish, and/or quality.

Thus, when the national income is exceedingly high, there is a demand for the choicest but limited cuts of meat from the very top but limited grades. This is certain to make for high prices, for the supply of such cuts is limited, but the demand is great. Under these conditions, if prices did not move up to balance the supply with demand, there would be a marked shortage of the desired cuts at the retail counter.

Where the Consumer's Food Dollar Goes. In recognition of the importance of food to the nation's economy and the welfare of its people, it is important to know (1) what percentage of the disposable income is spent for food, and (2) where the consumer's food dollar goes—the proportion of it that goes to the farmer, and the proportion that goes to the middleman.

Fig. M-28 reveals that of each food dollar, the farmer's share ranged from 7¢ (for white bread) to 62¢ (for eggs). For choice beef, the farmer's share was 52¢ in 1987; the rest—48¢—went for processing and retailing. This means that nearly one-half of today's meat dollar goes for meat packing and meat retailing.

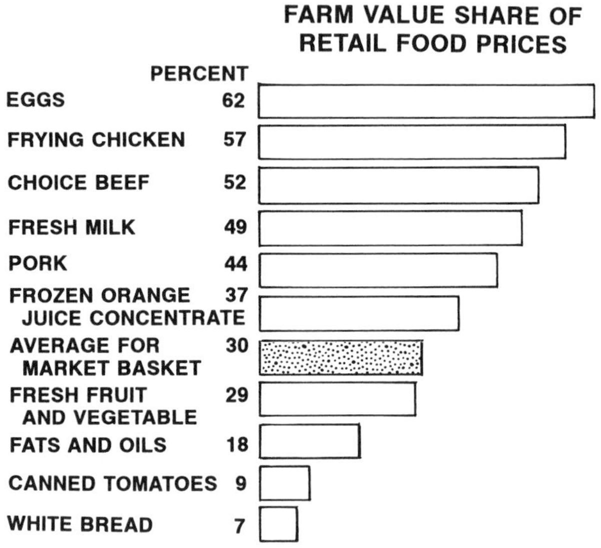

FARM VALUE SHARE OF RETAIL FOOD PRICES

	PERCENT
EGGS	62
FRYING CHICKEN	57
CHOICE BEEF	52
FRESH MILK	49
PORK	44
FROZEN ORANGE JUICE CONCENTRATE	37
AVERAGE FOR MARKET BASKET	30
FRESH FRUIT AND VEGETABLE	29
FATS AND OILS	18
CANNED TOMATOES	9
WHITE BREAD	7

Fig. M-28. Farm share of retail food prices. (From: *1989 Handbook of Agricultural Charts,* Agricultural Handbook No. 684, USDA, p. 61)

The farmer's share of the retail price of eggs, meat products, poultry, and beef is relatively high because processing is relatively simple, and transportation costs are low due to the concentrated nature of the products. On the other hand, the farmer's share of bakery and cereal products is low due to the high processing and container costs, and their bulky nature and costly transportation.

Among the reasons why farm prices of foods fail to go up, thereby giving the farmer a greater share of the consumer's food dollar, are: (1) rapid technological advances on the farm, making it possible for the farmer to stay in business despite small margins; (2) overproduction; and (3) the relative ease with which cost pressures within the marketing system can be passed backward rather than forward.

Over the years, processing and marketing costs have increased primarily because consumers have demanded, and gotten, more and more processing and packaging—more built-in services. For example, few consumers are interested in buying a live hog—or even a whole carcass. Instead, they want a pound of pork chops—all trimmed, packaged, and ready for cooking. Likewise, few housewives are interested in buying flour and baking bread. But consumers need to be reminded that, fine as these services are, they cost money—

A STEER IS NOT ALL STEAK!

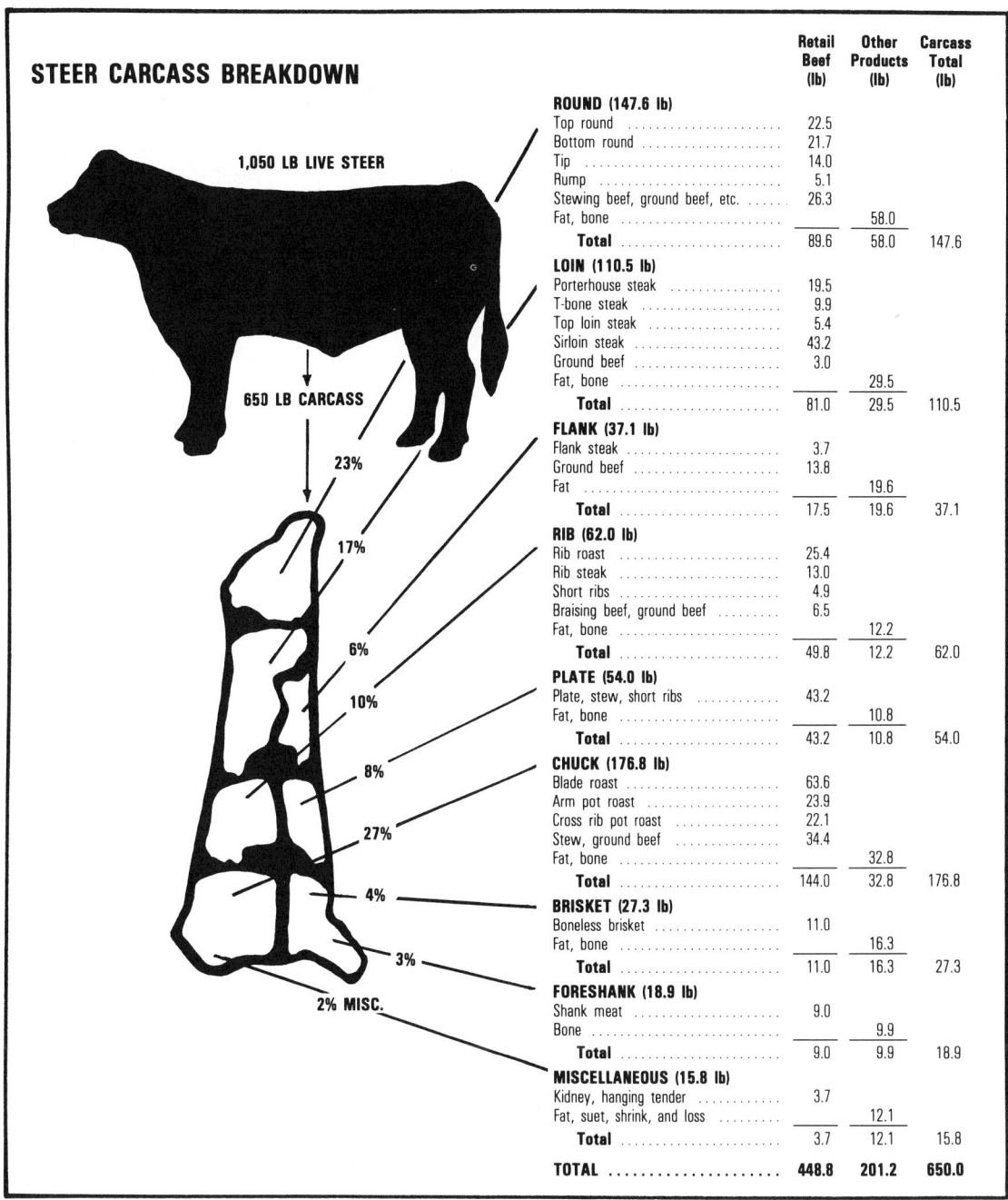

STEER CARCASS BREAKDOWN

1,050 LB LIVE STEER

650 LB CARCASS

23%

17%

6%

10%

8%

27%

4%

3%

2% MISC.

	Retail Beef (lb)	Other Products (lb)	Carcass Total (lb)
ROUND (147.6 lb)			
Top round	22.5		
Bottom round	21.7		
Tip	14.0		
Rump	5.1		
Stewing beef, ground beef, etc.	26.3		
Fat, bone		58.0	
Total	89.6	58.0	147.6
LOIN (110.5 lb)			
Porterhouse steak	19.5		
T-bone steak	9.9		
Top loin steak	5.4		
Sirloin steak	43.2		
Ground beef	3.0		
Fat, bone		29.5	
Total	81.0	29.5	110.5
FLANK (37.1 lb)			
Flank steak	3.7		
Ground beef	13.8		
Fat		19.6	
Total	17.5	19.6	37.1
RIB (62.0 lb)			
Rib roast	25.4		
Rib steak	13.0		
Short ribs	4.9		
Braising beef, ground beef	6.5		
Fat, bone		12.2	
Total	49.8	12.2	62.0
PLATE (54.0 lb)			
Plate, stew, short ribs	43.2		
Fat, bone		10.8	
Total	43.2	10.8	54.0
CHUCK (176.8 lb)			
Blade roast	63.6		
Arm pot roast	23.9		
Cross rib pot roast	22.1		
Stew, ground beef	34.4		
Fat, bone		32.8	
Total	144.0	32.8	176.8
BRISKET (27.3 lb)			
Boneless brisket	11.0		
Fat, bone		16.3	
Total	11.0	16.3	27.3
FORESHANK (18.9 lb)			
Shank meat	9.0		
Bone		9.9	
Total	9.0	9.9	18.9
MISCELLANEOUS (15.8 lb)			
Kidney, hanging tender	3.7		
Fat, suet, shrink, and loss		12.1	
Total	3.7	12.1	15.8
TOTAL	**448.8**	**201.2**	**650.0**

Fig. M-29. Cattle are not all beef, and beef is not all steak! This shows the approximate (a) percentage yield of carcass in relation to the weight of the animal on foot, and (b) the yield of differnet retail cuts. Note that a 1,050-lb live steer produces appoximately a 650-lb carcass, and ends up with only 448.9 lb of retail beef. Note, too, the small amount of steaks. (Source: Adapted by the authors from *Meat Facts,* published by the American Meat Institute, Washington, D.C. Data derived from USDA and industry figures.)

hence, they should be expected to pay for them. Without realizing it, American consumers have 18.2 million people working for them in the food and fiber sector after the products leave the nation's farms and ranches. Of these 18.2 million workers, 1.3 million are employed in food processing, 2.7 million in manufacturing, 6.6 million in transportation, trade and retailing, 3.7 million in eating establishments, and 3.9 million in other related work (1987 figures, latest available). They're the people who make it possible for the housewife to choose between quick-frozen, dry-frozen, quick-cooking, ready-to-heat, ready-to-eat, and many other conveniences. Hand in hand with this transition, and accentuating the demand for convenience foods, more women work outside the home; the proportion of the nation's labor force made up of women rose from 28% in 1947 to 52.2% in 1987. All this is fine, but it must be realized that these people engaged in food preparation must be paid, for they want to eat, too.

Income—Proportion Spent for Food; Food—Kinds Bought. U.S. consumers are among the most favored people in the world in terms of food costs and the variety of food products available. In 1988, only 14.5% of the U.S. disposable income was spent for food; 18.8% of this was spent for red meats, with 9.5% of the red meat share spent for beef and 1.8% of it spent for pork.

Food takes about ⅕ of the income in most other developed countries, and ½ or more of the income in most of the developing countries.

(Also see INCOME, PROPORTION SPENT FOR FOOD.)

Selecting the Meat Market.

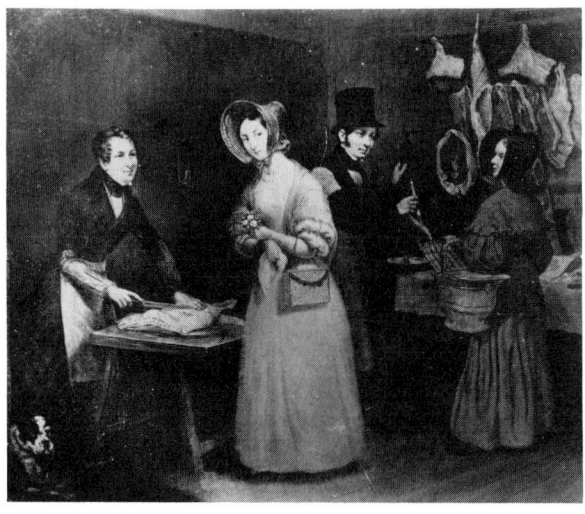

Fig. M-30. The way it used to be done. Early-day butcher shop, from a painting by W. S. Mount. There were neither wholesale cuts nor grades. (Courtesy, The Bettmann Archive)

Today's family may need help in meat buying. Meat is available in many places, in both supermarkets and meat specialty stores. Also, there is a selection from different species; and meat comes in many forms—fresh, cured, cured and smoked, frozen, freeze-dried, canned, and ready-to-serve. Then, there is the matter of deciding on which of the popular cuts to buy and serve on different occasions. All this leads most consumers to shop around until they find a retailer who provides the quality of meat and customer services desired, then remain loyal to that food store.

Selecting the Cut of Meat. The open refrigerated cases in a modern supermarket or meat specialty store present a sea of appetizing meats and meat products. Generally, meats are displayed wrapped in polyvinyl chloride (PVC) film that is sealed, on an affixed label on which is stamped the net weight, total price, price per pound, and the name of the cut.

The arrangement for displaying meats is rather standard. They are segregated as to kind (beef, veal, pork, lamb, poultry) and type of cut (steak, roast, ground beef, etc.). Smoked meats have separate display space as do fish, liver and other specialty items. Usually a clerk behind the display cases adds a personal touch and furnishes a source of information.

As the consumer pushes the cart along the refrigerated cases, selection is based primarily on preference, satiety, and nutritional value, along with the following practical considerations:

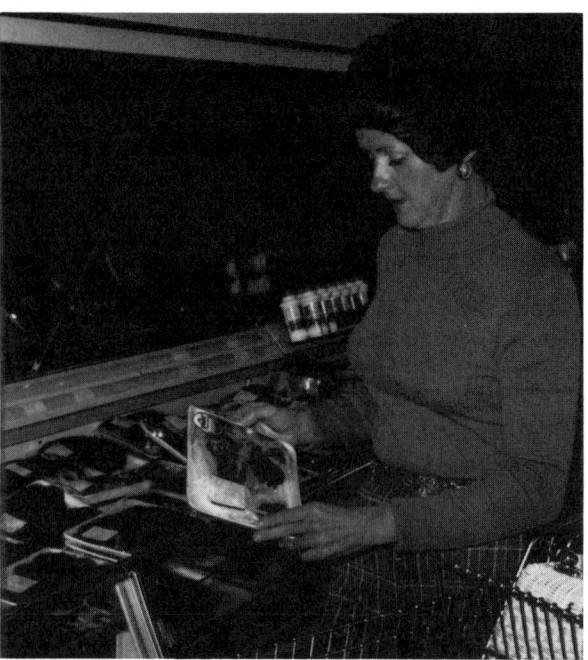

Fig. M-31. Consumer preference determines sales. (Courtesy, University of Tennessee, Knoxville, Tenn.)

1. The kind of meat that is best for the use planned. Skill in identifying cuts of meat and in cooking each of them properly is imperative.

2. The best buy on the basis of cost per serving. Except for such items as chopped meat and stew, the price per pound includes bone and fat, which are not eaten. Sometimes cuts like spareribs seem relatively inexpensive, but the amount of edible meat is small.

(Also see BEEF AND VEAL, section headed "Beef Cuts and How to Cook Them"; PORK, section headed "Pork Cuts and How to Cook Them"; and LAMB AND MUTTON, section headed "Lamb Cuts and How to Cook Them.")

Watching for Specials. Most meat retailers feature a good many meat specials. Experienced homemakers watch for these announcements and take advantage of them. When a home freezer is available, it may be possible to effect additional savings by buying extra large amounts of meat during special sales, then storing them.

Deciding How Much to Buy. Each meat shopper needs to be able to estimate how much meat, fish, or poultry to buy. Consideration should be given to the appetites and preferences of the members of the family. For example, active men and teen-agers generally have hearty appetites, and one child may like pork chops while another prefers hamburgers.

Other factors that should be considered in determining how much meat to buy are:

1. Time available for preparation.
2. The practicality of buying a particular cut for more than one meal.
3. Storage facilities.

MEAT COOKING—Every grade and cut of meat can be made tender and palatable provided it is cooked by the proper method. Also, it is important that meat be cooked at low temperature, usually between 300° and 350°F (*149 and 177°C*). At this temperature, it cooks slowly; and, as a result, it is juicier, shrinks less, and is better flavored than when cooked at high temperatures.

The method used in meat cookery depends on the nature of the cut to which it is applied. The common methods are:

1. **Dry-heat cooking**—Dry-heat cooking is used in preparing the more tender cuts; those that contain little connective tissue. The common methods of cooking by dry-heat are: (a) roasting, (b) broiling, and (c) panbroiling (see Fig. M-32).

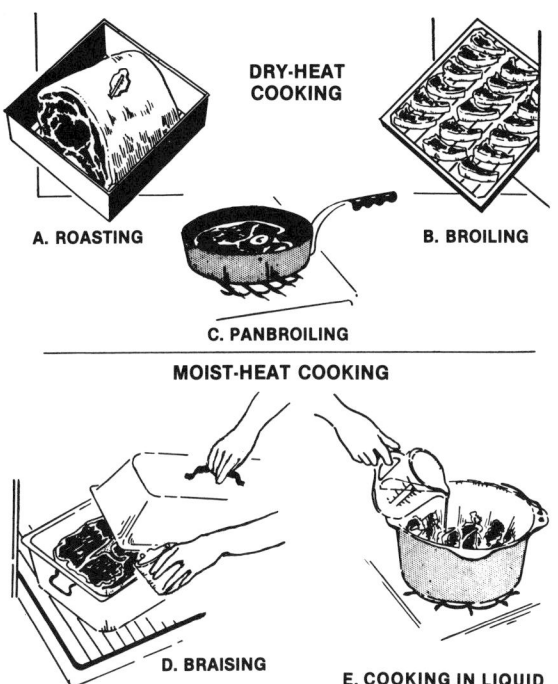

Fig. M-32. Common methods of meat cookery. *Dry-heat cooking:* A, roasting; B, broiling; and C, panbroiling. *Moist-heat cooking:* D, braising; and E, cooking in liquid.

a. **How to roast:**

(1) Season with salt and pepper, if desired.

(2) Place fat side up on rack in open roasting pan.

(3) Insert thermometer.

(4) Roast in oven at 300°to 350°F (*149 to 177°C*).

(5) Do not add water, nor cover, nor baste.

(6) Roast until the meat thermometer registers rare, medium, or well-done, as desired.

For best results, a meat thermometer should be used to test the doneness of roasts (and also for thick steaks and chops). It takes the guess work out of cooking. Allowing a certain number of minutes to the pound is not always accurate; for example, rolled roasts take longer to cook than ones with bones.

The thermometer is inserted into the cut of meat so that the bulb reaches the center of the largest muscle, and so that it is not in contact with fat or bone. Naturally, frozen roasts need to be partially thawed before the thermometer is inserted, or a metal skewer or ice pick will have to be employed in order to make a hole in frozen meat.

As the oven heat penetrates, the temperature at the center of the meat gradually rises and is registered on the thermometer. The meat can be cooked as desired—rare, medium, or well-done, except for pork which should always be cooked well-done (160° to 170°F [*71° to 77°C*] for cured pork; 185° [*85°C*] for fresh pork).

b. **How to broil:**

(1) Set the oven regulator for broiling.

(2) Place meat on the rack of the broiling pan and cook 2 to 5 inches from heat.

(3) Broil until the top of meat is brown.

(4) Season with salt and pepper.

(5) Turn the meat and brown the other side.

(6) Season and serve at once.

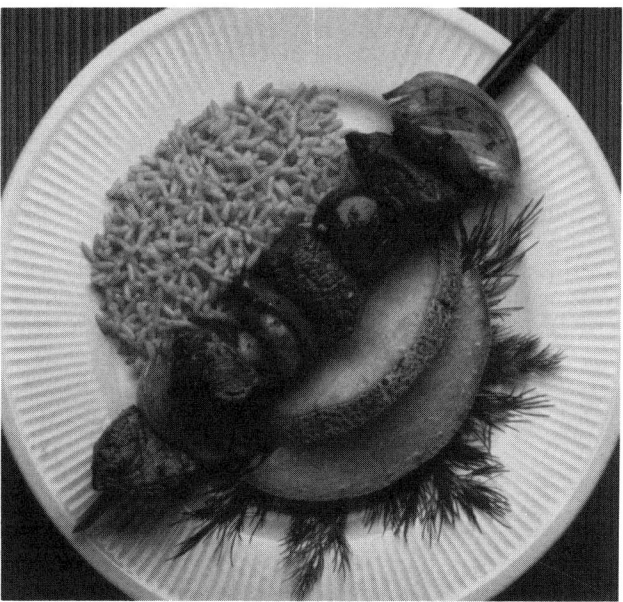

Fig. M-33. Beef Kabobs may be broiled or barbecued, forms of dry-heat cooking. (Courtesy, National Live Stock & Meat Board, Chicago, Ill.)

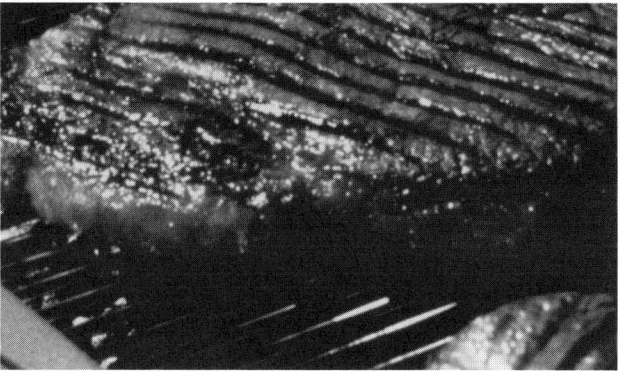

Fig. M-34. Barbecued steaks, a form of dry-heat cooking. (Courtesy, USDA)

c. **How to panbroil:**

(1) Place meat in a heavy, uncovered frying pan. Cook slowly.

(2) Do not add fat or water.

(3) Turn at intervals to ensure even cooking.

(4) As fat accumulates, pour it off.

(5) Brown meat on both sides.

(6) Do not overcook. Season.

2. **Moist-heat cooking**—Moist-heat cooking is generally used in preparing the less tender cuts, those containing more connective tissues that require moist heat to soften them and make them tender. In this type of cooking, the meat is surrounded by hot liquid or by steam. The common methods of moist-heat cooking are: (a) braising, and (b) cooking in liquid (see Fig. M-32).

a. **How to braise:**

(1) Brown the meat on all sides in a small amount of hot fat in a heavy utensil.

(2) Season with salt and pepper.

(3) Add small amount of liquid, if necessary.

(4) Cover tightly.

(5) Cook at simmering temperature, without boiling until tender.

b. **How to cook in liquid (large cuts and stews):**

(1) Brown on all sides in hot fat, if desired.

(2) Season with salt and pepper, if desired.

(3) Cover with water and cover kettle tightly.

(4) Cook slowly (simmer but not boil) until done.

(5) Add vegetables just long enough before serving to be cooked, if desired.

MEAT CARVING. *Carving is the art of cutting up meat, poultry, or game to serve at the table.*

Carving should be a proud accomplishment rather than drudgery. To master carving for the best presentation and maximum yield, the following simple rules should be observed:

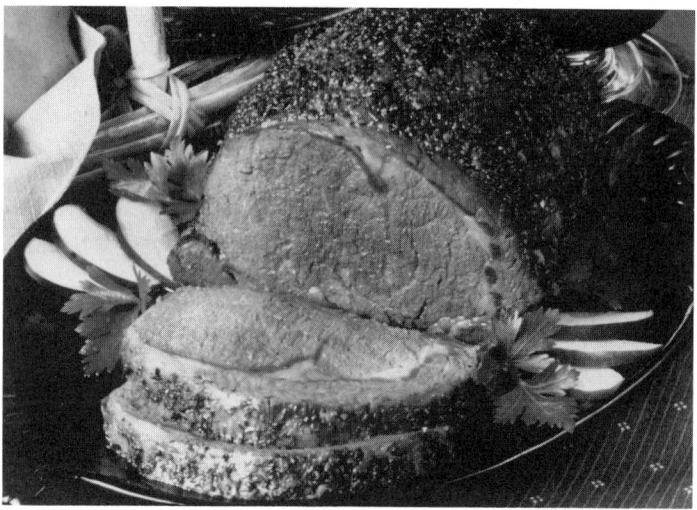

Fig. M-35. Roast beef on the table. (Courtesy, National Live Stock and Meat Board, Chicago, Ill.)

1. **Have proper tools.** Most carving needs can be met with a standard carving set and a steak set.

2. **Use sharp knife.** Always use a sharp carving knife (and never sharpen it at the table).

3. **Stand up if you prefer.** It is perfectly proper for the carver to stand if he prefers to do so.

4. **Know bone structure.** The carver should know something about anatomy; otherwise, the bones will get in his way.

5. **Know direction of muscle fiber and cut across the grain.** Except for steaks, meat should always be cut across the grain to avoid long meat fibers giving a stringy texture to the slices.

6. **Have a plan.** Start with a plan, cut with a plan, and make neat slices.

7. **Have ample platter or carving board.** The carving platter or board should be of ample size; large enough to accommodate slices.

8. **Have elbow room.** The carver must have plenty of elbow room.

9. **Use fork to hold cut.** The fork should be used for its intended purpose—to hold the cut; and not to dull the knife.

10. **Cut large and even slices.** The slices should be as large and even as possible.

11. **Be at ease.** The carver should always appear at ease. If the carver is nervous, the guests will be nervous, too.

U.S. MEAT PRODUCTION. U.S. production of red meat (total and by kinds) in 1990 follows:

	Million pounds
Total all meat	38,785
Beef	22,743
Pork, excluding lard	15,353
Veal	327
Lamb and mutton	362

U.S. PER CAPITA MEAT CONSUMPTION. Although comprising only 5.0% of the world's population, the people of the United States consume 10.5% of the total world production of meat. The amount of meat consumed in this country varies from year to year (see Fig. M-36).

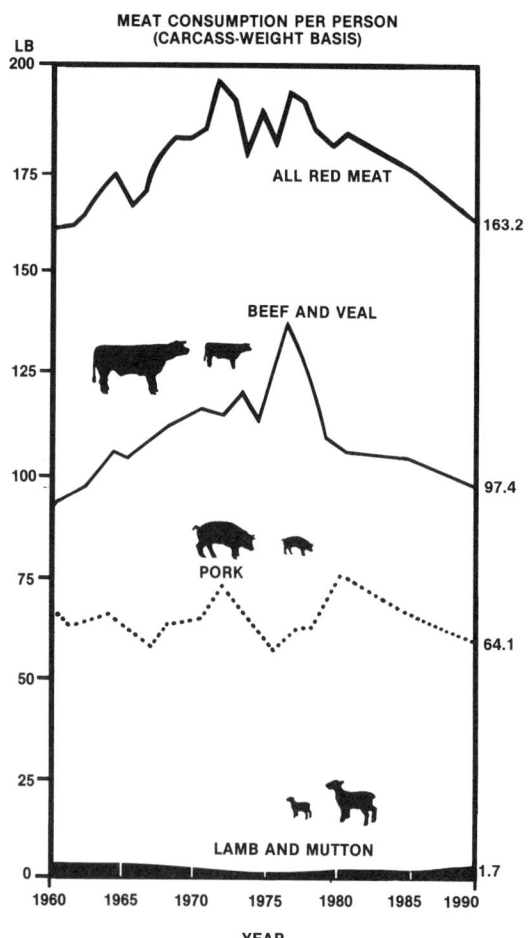

Fig. M-36. Per capita meat consumption in the United Sates, by kind of meat. As noted, the amount of meat consumed in this country varies from year to year. In recent years, the average American has consumed more beef than any other kind of meat. (Based on USDA figures)

In 1990 the average per capita red meat consumption was 163.2 lb, with distribution by types of meat as shown in Fig. M-36.

For the most part, meat consumption in this country is on a domestic basis, with only limited amounts being either imported or exported. Although cured meats furnish somewhat of a reserve supply—with more meats going into cure during times of meat surpluses—meat consumption generally is up when livestock production is high. Also, when good crops are produced and feed prices are favorable, market animals are fed to heavier weights. On the other hand, when feed-livestock ratios are unfavorable, breeding operations are curtailed, and animals are marketed at lighter weights. But during the latter periods, numbers are liquidated, thus tending to keep the meat supply fairly stable.

EATING HABIT TRENDS. Figs. M-37 and M-38, along with other data from the same source, clearly point up the following U.S. trends in eating habits in per capita consumption of meat and other foods by groups.

● The consumption of crop products is increasing, while the consumption of animal products is decreasing.

● Consumption of poultry and fish is on the increase; consumption of eggs continues to decrease; consumption of meat and dairy products has leveled off.

● Consumption of fruits stays about the same, vegetables show a slight increase, and cereal products continue to rise.

● Total consumption of sugars and sweeteners is rising again after a flat period during the 1970s. The consumption of sugar has dropped because it has been replaced by corn sweeteners, which are used primarily in soft drinks.

● Consumption of coffee, tea, and cocoa has declined rather sharply.

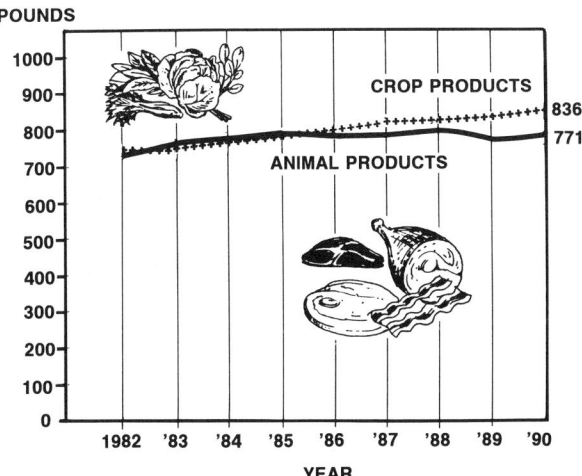

Fig. M-38. Per capita consumption of animal products vs crop products. (*Agricultural Statistics 1991*, USDA, p. 479, Table 672)

● Consumption of vegetable oils has increased, while consumption of animal fats has fallen.

The selection of food is based on taste preference, relative prices, dietary guidelines issued by government agencies and scientific groups, and myths.

WORLD MEAT PRODUCTION AND CONSUMPTION. In general, meat production and consumption are highest in those countries which have extensive grasslands, temperate climates, well-developed livestock industries, and sparse populations. In many of the older and more densely populated regions of the world, insufficient grain is produced to support the human population even when consumed directly. This lessens the possibility of keeping animals, except for consuming forages and other humanly inedible feeds. Certainly, when it is a choice between the luxury of meat and animal by-products or starvation, people will elect to accept a lower standard of living and go on a grain diet. In addition to the available meat supply, food habits and religious restrictions affect the kind and amount of meat produced and consumed.

Table M-12 shows the per capita consumption, by type, of the leading red meat-eating countries of the world.

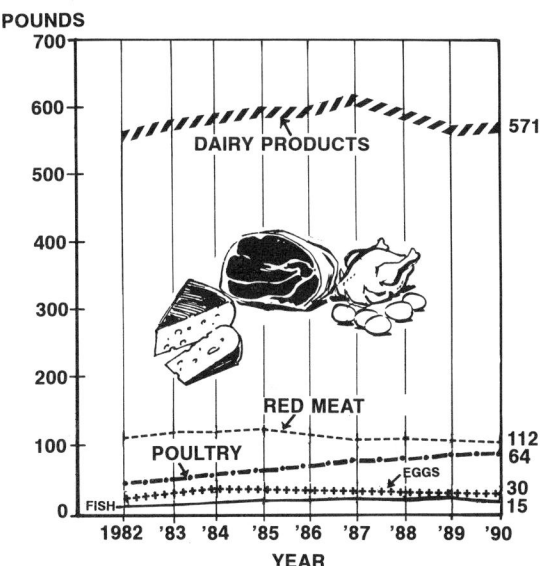

Fig. M-37. Per capita consumption of red meat, fish, poultry, eggs, and dairy products. (*Agricultural Statistics 1991*, USDA, p. 479, Table 672)

TABLE M-12
LEADING RED MEAT-EATING COUNTRIES OF THE WORLD[1]

	Beef and Veal		Pork	
Country	Quantity[2]	Country	Quantity[2]	
	(lb)		(lb)	
1. Argentina	143.3	1. Hungary	168.7	
2. Uruguay	127.0	2. Denmark	147.7	
3. U.S.A.	97.2	3. Czechoslovakia ...	130.3	
4. Australia	88.9	4. Austria	116.0	
5. Canada	86.2	5. Germany	115.8	

[1]*Statistical Abstract of the United States 1991*, U.S. Dept. of Commerce, p. 843, Table 1452.
[2]Pounds per capita. To convert to kilograms divide by 2.2.

As shown in Table M-12, in 1990 the United States with a per capita consumption of 97.2 lb *(44.2 kg)* ranked third in consumption of beef and veal, edging out the Australians who averaged 88.9 lb *(40.4 kg)*. But the United States was exceeded in per capita beef and veal consumption by Argentina, with 143.3 lb *(65.1 kg)*; and Uruguay, with 127 lb *(57.7 kg)*.

In per capita pork consumption, the five leading countries in 1990 were: Hungary, 168.7 lb *(76.7 kg)*; Denmark, 147.7 lb *(67 kg)*; Czechoslovakia, 130.3 lb *(59 kg)*; Austria, 116 lb *(52.7 kg)*; and Germany, 115.8 lb *(52.6 kg)*. The United States ranked twenty-fourth in per capita pork consumption.

The per capita red meat consumption of the leading meat-eating countries changes from time to time. Thus, from 1965 to 1968, New Zealand was the world's largest per capita consumer of red meat, followed closely by Australia. In 1969, Australia took the lead. In 1989, the leading countries in red meat consumption by rank were: East Germany, Uruguay, Czechoslovakia, New Zealand, Australia, and the United States.

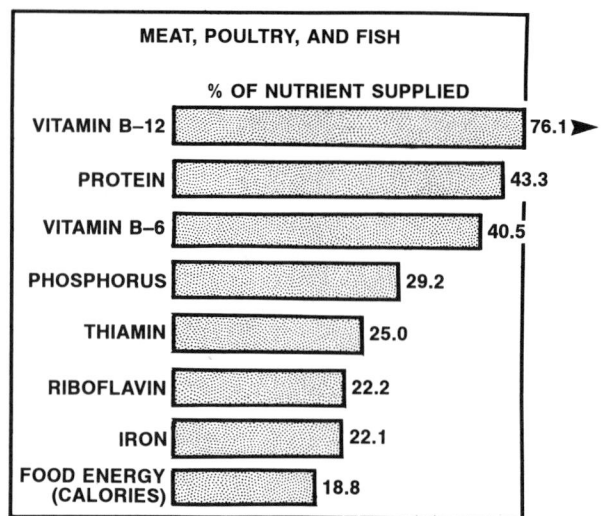

Fig. M-40. Contribution of meat, poultry, and fish combined, to the dietary intake in the United States. (*Agricultural Statistics 1991*, USDA, pp. 474-479)

NUTRITIVE COMPOSITION OF MEATS.

Meat is far more than just a very tempting and delicious food. From a nutritional standpoint, it contains the essentials of an adequate diet. This is important, for how we live and how long we live are determined in large part by our diet.

Meat is an excellent source of high-quality protein, of certain minerals, especially iron, and of the B-complex vitamins. It supplies phosphorus and nutrients which contribute significantly to the dietary balance of meals, and it is easily digested.

Although the RDAs are believed to be more than adequate to meet the requirements of most consumers, it is recognized that individuals vary greatly in their requirements. So, Fig. M-40 presents data showing the contribution of meat, poultry, and fish combined, toward the total dietary intake of each of the nutrients.

As shown in Fig. M-40, consumers obtain large proportions of their vitamin B-12, protein, Vitamin B-6, and iron from meat, poultry, and fish. Additionally, meat, poultry, and fish are fair sources of phosphorus, food energy, riboflavin, and thiamin.

The nutritive qualities of meats are detailed in the sections that follow.

Energy. The energy value of meat is largely dependent upon the amount of fat that it contains.

Today, meat-poultry-fish combined supply 18.8% of the dietary energy intake in the United States. Thus, meat is not a major contributor to excess energy intake.

(Also see CALORIC [ENERGY] EXPENDITURE; and ENERGY UTILIZATION BY THE BODY.)

Carbohydrate. Although the carbohydrates provide a major source of energy for man, they are found only in very limited amounts in meats and other animal products.

About half the carbohydrate is distributed through the muscles and in the bloodstream; the other half is stored in the liver in the form of glycogen (animal starch), where it constitutes 3 to 7% of the weight of that organ. Yet, most animal products contain little, if any, carbohydrate, for the reason that when an animal is slaughtered, the glycogen stored in the liver and muscles is rapidly broken down to lactic acid and pyruvic acid. Oysters and scallops contain some glycogen, but the amount is not significant to the diet. Milk, which contains the carbohydrate lactose or milk sugar, is the only animal food of importance as a carbohydrate source.

Only 0.4 g of carbohydrate comes from red meat daily, with most of it derived from the glycogen and reducing tissues naturally present in the tissues. Neither meat nor meat-poultry-fish make any significant contribution to total carbohydrate consumption; in each case they account for only 0.1%. A small amount of carbohydrate in the diet also

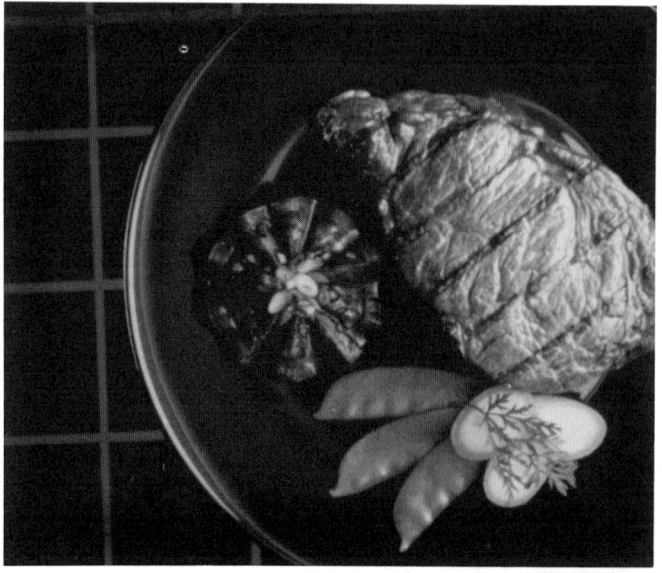

Fig. M-39. Rib eye steak. (Courtesy, National Live Stock and Meat Board, Chicago, Ill.)

comes from sugars and other carbohydrates added to sausages. The low level of carbohydrate in meat helps to keep its caloric contribution to a minimum. On the other hand, there is evidence that complex carbohydrates, i.e., fiber, contribute to bowel movement and the elimination of toxic substances from the digestive tract. Thus, it is recommended that fruit and vegetables be included in the diet to provide fiber.

(Also see CARBOHYDRATE[S].)

Fats. Energy is supplied by animal fats, which are highly digestible. Fats also supply needed fatty acids, transport fat-soluble vitamins (A, D, E, K), provide protection and insulation to the human body, and add palatability to lean meat. Highly unsaturated fats are soft and oily (as in soft pork). Generally, animal fats contain higher levels of saturated fat than vegetable oils.

The amount and composition of fats in the animal body are highly variable, depending upon the species, diet, and maturity. The species differences in the composition of fats are particularly noticeable between ruminants and nonruminants; ruminants (through rumen microorganisms) may alter the composition of the dietary fats, whereas nonruminants tend to deposit lipids in the form found in the diet. Australian researchers have developed a procedure for protecting dietary fats from the action of the rumen organisms by encapsulation of the fat, thus permitting alteration of the characteristics of fatty acid composition in both meat and milk.

The fats of the diet serve as a source of the essential fatty acids—arachidonic, linoleic, and linolenic acid, but only linoleic acid is required preformed in the diet. Although meats provide fat, the vegetable oils are generally richer sources of the essential fatty acids than animals fat; hence, no deficiency of fatty acids is likely to develop in a meatless diet unless there is impaired lipid absorption.

There is no RDA for fat consumption since there is seldom a deficiency. Rather, the main problem from fat consumption is its contribution to obesity.

Meat-poultry-fish combined contribute 53.3 g of fat per capita per day and account for 31.7% of the total consumption.

(Also see FATS AND OTHER LIPIDS.)

Protein. The need for protein in the diet is actually a need for amino acids, of which nine are essential for humans. (Ten are essential for animals; they require arginine, which is not required by humans.) But all proteins are not created equal! Some proteins of certain foods are low or completely devoid of certain essential amino acids. Hence, meeting the protein requirement demands quality as well as quantity. It is noteworthy that all the essential amino acids are present in muscle meats, heart, liver, and kidney. However, there is considerable variation in the protein content of meat, depending on the degree of fatness and the water content; the total protein content of animal bodies ranges from about 10% in very fat, mature animals to 20% in thin, young animals.

Because animal proteins are in short supply in the developing countries, it has been estimated that 20 to 30% of the children in these countries suffer severe protein-calorie malnutrition, and that it may contribute to as much as 50% of the mortality for this group. Kwashiorkor and marasmus are common manifestations of protein and protein-calorie deficiencies in infants and children. Also, the ability of the human body to produce antibodies (substances that attack specific foreign bodies) is dependent upon an adequate supply of amino acids in the diet. (The antibody molecule is actually a molecule of globulin—a class of protein.)

Fig. M-40 shows that meat-poultry-fish supply 43.3% of the dietary protein intake in the United States.

In spite of the high level of high-quality protein in the average American diet, there is evidence that some protein deficiencies occur in young children shortly after weaning. In these cases, it appears that protein intake is low due either to their economic status or a strict vegetarian diet. Regardless of the reason for the deficiency, inclusion of small amounts of meat or other animal protein would alleviate all signs of protein deficiency.

(Also see PROTEIN[S].)

Minerals. Meat is a rich source of several minerals, but it is an especially rich source of phosphorus and iron.

In the discussion that follows, minerals are divided into macrominerals or microminerals, based on the relative amounts needed in the diet.

(Also see MINERAL[S].)

MACROMINERALS. The macrominerals, or major minerals, are those that are needed in greatest abundance.

• **Calcium**—Meat is a poor source of calcium. However, it is noteworthy that mechanically deboned meat, which contains some bone, contains up to 0.75% calcium, and that it can make a considerable contribution to the calcium of the diet of man.

(Also see CALCIUM.)

• **Phosphorus**—Although meat is a poor source of calcium, it is usually a good source of phosphorus. Meat-poultry-fish combined contribute 56.2% of the RDA.

Meat Is A Good Source of Phosphorus

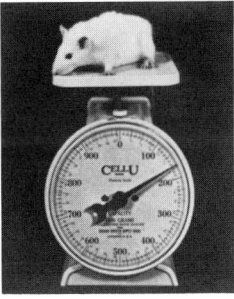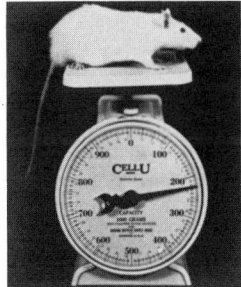

Low phosphorus diet
(no meat)
Wt. 168 grams

Same diet plus meat
Wt. 225 grams

Fig. M-41. This shows that meat is a rich source of phosphorus. Minerals are necessary in order to build and maintain the body skeleton and tissues and regulate body functions. Although meat is a good source of several minerals, it is especially rich as a source of phosphorus and iron. (Courtesy, National Live Stock and Meat Board and Rush Medical College)

Meat-poultry-fish combined provide 29.2% of the phosphorus intake in the United States (Fig. M-40).

(Also see PHOSPHORUS.)

• **Sodium**—Most of the sodium in the diet is in the form of salt (sodium chloride—NaCl). Deficiencies of sodium are rare because nearly all foods contain some sodium. However, excess dietary salt over a long period of time is believed to lead to high blood pressure in susceptible people. Also, excess salt may cause edema. So, a prudent diet should limit excess salt intake; this would call for limiting the intake of cured meats.

(Also see SODIUM.)

• **Chlorine**—Chlorine is provided by table salt (sodium chloride—NaCl) and by the foods that contain salt. Persons suffering from diseases of the heart, kidney, or liver, whose sodium intake is severely restricted by deleting table salt and such salty foods as cured meats, may need an alternative source of chloride; a number of chloride-containing salt substitutes are available for this purpose.

(Also see CHLORINE or CHLORIDE.)

• **Magnesium**—Meat, poultry, and fish are low in magnesium. Most of the magnesium in meat is found in the muscle and liver.

(Also see MAGNESIUM.)

• **Potassium**—Potassium is the third most abundant element in the body, after calcium and phosphorus; and it is present in twice the concentration of sodium.

Potassium is widely distributed in foods. Meat, poultry, fish, many fruits, whole grains, and vegetables are good sources. (Although meat, poultry, and fish are good sources of potassium, these items may be restricted when dietary sodium is restricted.)

(Also see POTASSIUM.)

• **Sulfur**—Meeting the sulfur needs of the body seems to be primarily a matter of providing sulfur for the sulfur-containing amino acids: methionine, cystine, and cysteine.

Inorganic sulfur is poorly utilized by man. Thus, meat, poultry, and fish, which are good sources of sulfur, serve an important function in supplying the body with its sulfur requirements.

(Also see SULFUR.)

MICROMINERALS. The microminerals, or trace or minor minerals, are those that are needed in least amounts.

• **Chromium**—Chromium, which has a number of important functions in the human body, is widely distributed in animal tissues and in animal products. In the section on Chromium, Table C-16, of this book, the chromium content of the following foods of animal origin, in mcg/100 g is reported: dried liver, 170; egg, 52; cheese, 51; fresh liver, 50; and beef, 32.

(Also see CHROMIUM.)

• **Cobalt**—This mineral, which is an integral part of vitamin B-12—an essential factor in the formation of red blood cells, must be ingested in the form of vitamin B-12 in order to be of value to man; hence, a table showing the cobalt content of human foods serves no useful purpose. The organ meats (liver, kidney) are excellent sources of vitamin B-12 (hence, of cobalt). The vitamin B-12 content, in mcg/100 g, of some rich animal food sources follows: beef liver, 111; clams, 98; lamb kidneys, 63; turkey liver, 48; and calf kidney, 25.

(Also see COBALT.)

• **Copper**—Organ meats (liver, kidney, brains) and shell fish are rich sources of copper.

(Also see COPPER.)

• **Fluorine**—Fluorine, which is necessary for sound bones and teeth, is widely, but unevenly, distributed in nature. Seafoods and tea are the richest dietary sources.

Because fluorine tends to concentrate in the bones and teeth and is toxic if used in excess, there has been some concern about fluorine levels in deboned meat. Yet, there seems to be little basis for such apprehension unless the bones come from animals suffering from fluorosis.

(Also see FLUORINE.)

• **Iodine**—Most of the iodine need of humans is met by iodized salt. Saltwater fish and most shellfish are rich sources of iodine. Dairy products and eggs may be good sources if the producing animals have access to iodine-enriched rations. Red meats and poultry are poor sources of iodine.

(Also see IODINE.)

• **Iron**—Liver is an excellent source of easily assimilated iron and is prescribed in the diet of anemia sufferers. Muscle meat, poultry, and fish are good sources of iron, but they contain less than half as much iron as liver.

There are two forms of food iron—heme (organic) and nonheme (inorganic). Of the two, heme is absorbed from food more efficiently than inorganic iron and is independent of vitamin C or iron binding chelating agents. Although the proportion of heme iron in animal tissue varies, it amounts to about ⅓ of the total iron in all animal tissues—including meat, liver, poultry, and fish. The remaining ⅔ of the iron in animal tissues and all the iron of vegetable products are treated as nonheme iron.

Meat also enhances the absorption of iron, as does vitamin C; it improves iron absorption by supplying what is referred to as the *meat factor*. It has been demonstrated that beef, veal, lamb, pork, liver, chicken, and fish all increase iron absorption by two to fourfold, while milk, cheese, and egg do not increase iron absorption.

Fig. M-40 shows that meat-poultry-fish combined provide 22.1% of the dietary iron intake in the United States.

There are four situations in life in which the iron requirement is increased (according to *Recommended Dietary Allowances*, NRC-National Academy of Sciences, 1980, p. 186): (1) in infancy; (2) during rapid growth and adolescence; (3) during the female reproductive period; and (4) in pregnancy. During these four stages in life, the iron status could be greatly improved by including meat, poultry, and fish in the diet on a regular basis.

(Also see IRON.)

• **Manganese**—Only a trace of manganese is found in muscle meat. Liver is a fair source.

(Also see MANGANESE.)

• **Molybdenum**—The organ meats (liver, kidney) are a good source of molybdenum.

(Also see MOLYBDENUM.)

• **Selenium**—Meat, poultry, and fish all contain small amounts of selenium, but liver and kidney are the best sources. The selenium content of animal products depends upon the content of the element in livestock feeds; for example, the Ohio Station reported that the addition of 0.1 ppm selenium to the animal's diet increased the selenium content of beef liver by 72%.[18]

---

[18]Moxon, A. L. and D. L. Palmquist, "Selenium Content of Foods Grown or Sold in Ohio," *Ohio Report*, Ohio State University, Columbus, Ohio, January-February 1980, pp. 13-14, Table 1.

Fortunately, foods eaten in the United States are generally varied in nature and origin; so, there does not appear to be any deficiency of selenium in man. However, a deficiency of selenium has been reported in a localized area in China where only locally produced foods are consumed.

(Also see SELENIUM.)

• **Silicon**—Meat, poultry, and fish all contribute silicon to the diet in appreciable quantities. However, the best sources of silicon are the fibrous parts of whole grains, followed by various organ meats (liver, kidney, brain), and connective tissues.

Because of the abundance of silicon in all but the most highly refined foods, it is of little concern in the human diet.

(Also see SILICON.)

• **Zinc**—Meat, poultry, fish, eggs, and dairy products are good sources of zinc. The animal proteins are generally much better sources of dietary zinc than plants because the phytate present in many plant sources complexes the zinc and makes it unavailable.

Since meat, poultry, fish, eggs, and dairy products are good sources of zinc, they should be included regularly in the diet. This recommendation is further reinforced by the fact that zinc deficiency is virtually unknown on a diet containing animal products.

(Also see ZINC.)

Vitamins. Many phenomena of vitamin nutrition are related to solubility—vitamins are soluble in either fat or water. This is a convenient way in which to discuss vitamins in meats; hence, they are grouped and treated as fat-soluble vitamins or water-soluble vitamins.

(Also see VITAMIN[S].)

FAT-SOLUBLE VITAMINS. The fat-soluble vitamins are stored in appreciable quantities in the animal body, whereas the water-soluble vitamins are not. Any of the fat-soluble vitamins can be stored wherever fat is deposited; and the greater the intake of the vitamin, the greater the storage. It follows that most meats, poultry, and fish are good sources of the fat-soluble vitamins.

• **Vitamin A**—Both vitamin A and the carotenes are found in the animal body associated with fats (lipids).

Cod and other fish liver oils are extremely high in vitamin A, sufficiently so that they are used as supplemental sources. Livers of all kinds are rich food sources of vitamin A, exceeding raw carrots.

(Also see VITAMIN A.)

• **Vitamin D**—Fish liver oils (from cod, halibut, or swordfish) are very high in vitamin D, sufficiently so that they are used as supplemental sources. Fatty fish and fish roe are rich food sources, while liver, egg yolk, cream, butter, and cheese are fair sources. Muscle meats and unfortified milk are negligible sources.

(Also see VITAMIN D.)

• **Vitamin E**—Meat and animal products are good to fair sources of vitamin E (the tocopherols); plant materials are much richer sources, especially vegetable oils, some grains, nuts, and green leafy vegetables.

The amount of vitamin E in animal tissues and products is influenced by the dietary consumption of tocopherols by the animal. Good animal sources are: beef and organ meats, butter, eggs, and seafoods. Cheese and chicken are fair sources.

(Also see VITAMIN E.)

• **Vitamin K**—Certain animal foods are good to fair sources of vitamin K, although they are far outranked by green tea, turnip greens, and broccoli. Beef liver is a rich source of vitamin K; bacon, cheese, butter, and pork liver are good sources; and beef fat, ham, eggs, pork tenderloin, ground beef, and chicken liver are fair sources.

(Also see VITAMIN K.)

WATER-SOLUBLE VITAMINS. The water-soluble vitamins are not stored in the animal body to any appreciable extent.

• **Biotin**—Biotin is widely distributed in foods of animal origin, with liver and kidney being rich sources, followed by eggs, sardines and salmon, cheese, chicken, oysters, and pork.

(Also see BIOTIN.)

• **Choline**—All animal tissues contain some choline, although it is more abundant in fatty than in lean tissues. Rich sources are: eggs, liver, and dried buttermilk.

(Also see CHOLINE.)

• **Folacin (folic acid)**—Folacin is widely distributed in animal foods, with liver and kidney being particularly rich sources. Eggs and fish are good sources, while cheese, cod, and halibut are fair sources. Chicken, milk, and most muscle meats are poor sources of folacin.

(Also see FOLACIN [FOLIC ACID].)

• **Niacin (nicotinic acid; nicotinamide)**—Generally speaking, niacin is found in animal tissue as nicotinamide. Animal foods are excellent dietary sources, with the richest sources being liver, kidney, lean meats, poultry, fish, and rabbit. Although low in niacin content, milk, cheese, and eggs are good sources because (1) of their tryptophan content (which may yield niacin), and (2) of their niacin being in available form.

The role of niacin-rich animal foods in eliminating pellagra, which was once a serious scourge in the United States, is generally recognized.

(Also see NIACIN.)

• **Pantothenic acid (vitamin B-3)**—Pantothenic acid is widely distributed in animal foods, with organ meats (liver, kidney, and heart) being particularly rich sources. Salmon, blue cheese, eggs, and lobster are good sources, while lean muscle and chicken are only fair sources.

(Also see PANTOTHENIC ACID.)

• **Riboflavin**—The organ meats (liver, kidney, heart) are rich sources of riboflavin; lean meat (beef, pork, lamb), cheese, eggs, and bacon are good sources; while chicken and fish are only fair sources.

Meat-poultry-fish combined supply 22.2% of the per capita daily consumption of riboflavin (Fig. M-40), and 31.3% of the RDA of riboflavin.

(Also see RIBOFLAVIN.)

• **Thiamin (vitamin B-1)**—Some thiamin is found in a large variety of animal products, but it is abundant in few.

Lean pork (fresh cured) is a rich source; kidney is a good source; while egg yolk, poultry, beef liver, luncheon meat, and fish are only fair sources. The thiamin content of pork

MEAT IS A GOOD SOURCE OF THIAMIN (VITAMIN B-1)

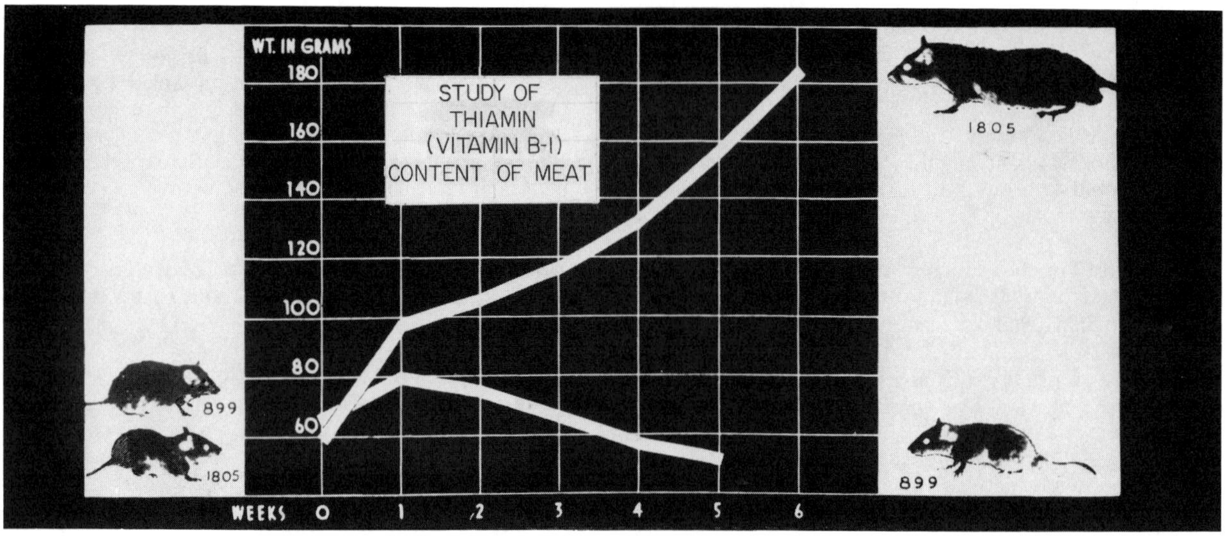

RAT NO. 899 RECEIVED ADEQUATE DIET EXCEPT FOR THIAMIN

RAT NO. 1805 RECEIVED SAME DIET + 2% DRIED PORK HAM WHICH IS RICH IN THIAMIN

Fig. M-42. Meat is a good source of thiamin (vitamin B-1). (Studies by the University of Wisconsin; supported by National Live Stock and Meat Board)

can be greatly altered by the thiamin level of the feed. Curing of meat causes only small losses.

Meat-poultry-fish combined contribute approximately 25% of the total thiamin intake (Fig. M-40).

(Also see THIAMIN.)

• **Vitamin B-6 (pyridoxine; pyridoxal; pyridoxamine)**—In animal tissues, vitamin B-6 occurs mainly as pyridoxal and pyridoxamine. Vitamin B-6 is widely distributed in foods of animal origin. Liver, kidney, lean meat, and poultry are good sources; eggs are a fair source; and fat, cheese, and milk are negligible sources.

Meat-poultry-fish combined contribute 40.5% of the total vitamin B-6 intake (Fig. M-40).

(Also see VITAMIN B-6.)

• **Vitamin B-12 (cobalamins)**—Vitamin B-12 is found in all foods of animal origin. Plants cannot manufacture vitamin B-12; hence, except for trace amounts absorbed from the soil (because of soil bacteria, soil is a good source of B-12) by the growing plant, very little is found in plant foods.

Liver and other organ meats—kidney, heart—are rich sources of vitamin B-12; muscle meats, fish, shellfish, eggs, and cheese are good sources; and milk, poultry, and yogurt are fair sources.

Fig. M-40 shows meat-poultry-fish contribute 76.1% of the consumption of vitamin B-12.

(Also see VITAMIN B-12.)

• **Vitamin C (ascorbic acid)**—Vitamin C is found only in small amounts in animal tissues, with the largest amounts being localized in the adrenal glands. Vitamin C is added to cured meats at a level of 550 ppm to reduce nitrosamine formation.

Summary. The unique contributions of meat, poultry, and fish to the nutritional needs of man have been presented in this section. In summary form, the major nutritive

contribution of foods of animal origin are:

1. They are an excellent source of protein, from the essential amino acids.

2. They are rich sources of phosphorus, iron, copper, and zinc.

3. They are the major dietary source of vitamin B-12 and vitamin B-6, and they supply appreciable amounts of vitamin A, biotin, niacin, pantothenic acid, riboflavin, and thiamin.

MEAT FACTS AND MYTHS. Much has been spoken and written linking the consumption of meat to certain health related problems in humans, including heart disease, cancer, high blood pressure (hypertension), and harmful residues. A summary of four incorrect statements, along with the correct facts, follows:

• **Fact or Myth: Meat fats cause coronary heart disease**—Coronary heart disease (CHD) is the leading cause of death in the United States, accounting for one-third of all deaths, according to *The Surgeon General's Report on Nutrition and Health* (1988, p. 4, Table 2). The major form of CHD results from atherosclerosis, a condition characterized by fatty deposits in the coronary arteries. These deposits are rich in cholesterol, a complex fatlike substance. Also, in general, serum cholesterol levels are relatively high among individuals with atherosclerosis.

Fact: Three major factors are associated with the risk of coronary heart disease; namely, elevated blood pressure, cigarette smoking, and elevated serum cholesterol. A serum cholesterol level in excess of 280 mg/dl is considered a major risk for heart disease. The concentration of cholesterol in the blood is strongly affected by the degree of saturation of the dietary fat.

Professional groups suggest that many people would benefit (1) if the amount of fat in the diet were reduced from the present level of 37% to less than 30% of the total calories; (2) if the amount of dietary cholesterol were restricted to less than 300 mg per day; (3) if polyunsaturated fats were substituted for some of the saturated fat in the diet so that the distribution among polyunsaturated, monounsaturated, and saturated fatty acids would be about equal; (4) if saturated fat were limited to 10% of the total caloric intake; and (5) if caloric intake were adjusted to maintain desired body weight.

The major dietary sources of fat in the American diet are meat, poultry, fish, dairy products, and fats and oils. Animal products tend to be higher in both total and saturated fats than most plant sources. Also, dietary cholesterol is found only in foods of animal origin.

The intake and types of fatty acids that made up an average American diet in 1956 is shown in Table M-13.

Since the 1956 report by the U.S. Department of Agriculture (Table M-13), health and dietary professionals have urged the American people to (1) reduce the consumption of total fat, especially saturated fat and cholesterol; (2) increase the intake of fruits, vegetables, and whole grain products and cereals; and (3) increase the consumption of fish, poultry prepared without skin, lean meats, and low-fat dairy products. Dietary changes have been made since 1956, but further improvements will lessen the risk of coronary heart disease.

(Also see HEART DISEASE.)

• **Fact or Myth: Meat causes bowel cancer**—This question has been prompted by the following reports: (1) that the age-adjusted incidence of colon cancer has been found to increase with the per capita consumption of meat in countries; (2) that, in a study done in Hawaii, the incidence of colon cancer in persons of Japanese ancestry was found to be greater among those who ate Western-style meals, especially those who ate beef; and (3) that an examination of (a) international food consumption patterns, and (b) food consumption survey data from the United States showed that a higher incidence of colon cancer occurred in areas with greater beef consumption.

Fact: A direct cause-effect relationship between diet and cancer has not been established. Such studies as the three cited provide valuable leads for researchers who are trying to determine the cause of a certain disease such as colon cancer, but they do not establish the cause. The reason is that the factor measured and found associated with the incidence of colon cancer or other condition is not the only difference among the population groups studied, and the factor measured in the study may be only associated in some way with the real cause.

(Also see CANCER.)

• **Fact or Myth: Meat causes high blood pressure (hypertension)**— Some have implicated meat as a cause of high blood pressure.

Fact: There is no evidence that meat per se has any major effect on high blood pressure. However, consumption of cured meat containing large amounts of salt should be minimized as should the amount of salt used as a condiment on meat and other foods. Other dietary factors that contribute to high blood pressure include obesity and excessive intake of alcohol.

(Also see HIGH BLOOD PRESSURE [HYPERTENSION].)

• **Fact or Myth: Meat contains harmful residues**—Do meats contain harmful toxic metals, pesticides, insecticides, animal drugs and additives?

Fact: If one pushed the argument of how safe is "safe" far enough, it would be necessary to forbid breast feeding as a source of food, because, from time to time, human milk has been found to contain DDT, antibiotics, thiobromine, caffeine, nicotine, and selenium.

The FDA requires drug withdrawal times on some of them, in order to protect consumers from residues. Additionally, federal agencies (USDA and/or FDA), as well as certain state and local regulatory groups, conduct continuous surveillance, sampling programs, and analyses of meats and other food products on their content of drugs and additives.

(Also see FOOD MYTHS AND MISINFORMATION; and POISONS.)

TABLE M–13
AVERAGE CONSUMPTION, IN GRAMS PER PERSON PER DAY, OF FATTY ACIDS FROM FOODS THAT
MADE UP AN AVERAGE AMERICAN DIET AS REPORTED BY THE U.S. DEPARTMENT OF AGRICULTURE IN 1956[1]

Commodity	Total Saturated Acids	Oleic Acid	Other Monounsaturated Acids	Linoleic Acid	Other Polyunsaturated Acids
Dairy products (milk, cheese, butter)	28.2	7.5	3.0	0.8	0.4
Fats, oils	10.0	18.9	0.4	9.5	0.4
Flour, cereal products	0.7	1.5	—	2.2	0.2
Bakery products, purchased	2.7	3.7	—	2.4	0.3
Meats, poultry, eggs	14.1	17.0	0.8	3.8	0.6
Sugar, sweets	1.1	1.0	—	0.4	—
Potatoes	0.4	0.3	—	0.3	0.2
Fruits, vegetables	0.3	0.6	—	0.4	0.1
Miscellaneous foods	0.9	2.2	—	0.7	—
Totals	58.4	52.7	4.2	20.5	2.2
% of Total	42.3	38.2	3.0	14.9	1.6

[1]From: *Diet and Health*, Council for Agricultural Science and Technology, Report No. 111, March 1987, p. 25. The per capita fat consumption represented 96.4% of the fat consumed.

MEAT ANALOGS

Food material usually prepared from vegetable protein to resemble specific meats in texture, color, and flavor.
(Also see SOYBEANS; and VEGETARIAN DIETS.)

MEAT EXTRACT

This is a boiled down and concentrated extract of beef, veal, poultry, or game. Meat extracts should be regarded as condiments which impart the same flavor as the meat stock from which they were obtained.

MEAT FACTOR

A factor in meat which enhances the absorption of iron in the body. It has been demonstrated that beef, veal, pork, liver, chicken, and fish all increase iron absorption by two-to fourfold, while milk, cheese, and egg do not increase iron absorption.

MECHANICALLY EXTRACTED

A method of extracting the fat content from oilseeds by the application of heat and mechanical pressure. The hydraulic and expeller processes are both methods of mechanical extraction.
(Also see OILS, VEGETABLE.)

MEDICINAL PLANTS

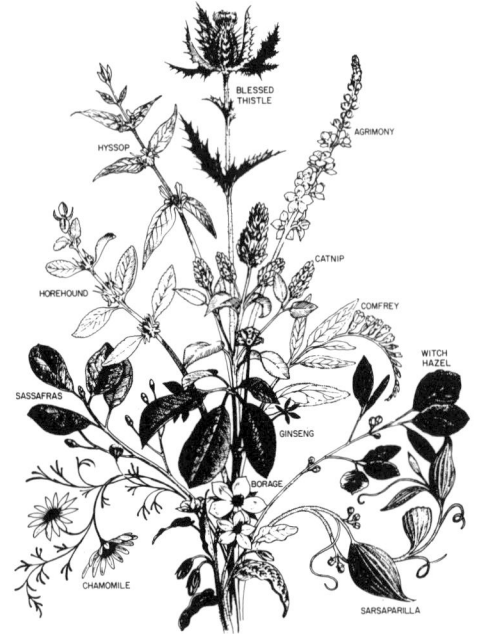

Fig. M-43. A bouquet of familiar medicinal herbs.

Through the ages various plants have been tried as medicine to see which ones helped cure certain ailments of mankind. Thus, by trial and error, people came to use thousands of plants as remedies for their ills. For example, many American Indian tribes used willow bark to treat pain, but how the Indians came to choose willow bark is not known. Willow bark contains salicin, a forerunner of aspirin. While not all plants actually cured or relieved ailments, many did. Prescribing and dispensing medicinal plants, was the pharmaceutical industry of the past. Then, as science advanced, those plants which demonstrated positive effects on certain ailments were extracted, chemically analyzed, and their active chemicals were discovered. Thus, some traditional medicinal plants became stepping stones for the development of modern day drugs as active chemicals were isolated from plants or synthesized in laboratories. Although drugs used in medicine today are composed of specific chemicals extracted or derived from plants or synthesized by other methods, the direct use of plants for medicine still survives. There are endless books available describing the medicinal plants, their combinations, and conditions which they prevent, relieve, or cure. Sometimes it is called folk medicine, or herbal medicine. Indeed, whole businesses have grown up around the uses of herbs or medicinal plants. This article deals specifically with plants used directly for medicinal purposes.

HISTORY. Almost every civilization has a history of medicinal plants. Perhaps, one of the oldest civilizations to record their use of plants for medicine is China. Books describing the use of plants as medicine are sometimes called herbals, and one of the earliest known herbals was supposedly written by the Chinese emperor Shen-Nung about 2700 B.C. About the time of the Chin and Han dynasties (202 B.C. to 220 A.D.), the first Chinese book on pharmacology was written. In it, 365 medicinal substances were recorded, with notes on the collection and preparation of the drugs. During the Tang dynasty, the government established a pharmacological institute which was called the Herbary. A total of 850 medicinal plants were grown on its 50 acres of fertile land. The cultivation, collection, and preparation of drugs were taught as basic subjects in this institute. In his *Magnum Opus*, Li Shih-chen (1518 to 1593 A.D.), the pharmacologist, recorded 1,892 drugs. In China today, there is an attempt to mesh traditional Chinese medical practices with Western medical practices. Chinese traditional medical prescriptions are the roots, stems, bark, leaves, flowers, and fruits of shrubs and trees. A small part comes from birds, animals, insects, fish, and minerals. About 70% of the prescriptions made out in the hospitals and in the rural areas are for herbal medicine.

In India, the oldest sacred writings of the Hindus, the four Vedas, refer to many healing plants.

Ancient Egyptian doctors practiced a combination of herbal medicine and faith healing. Carvings on tomb and temple walls indicate that people used plants for medicine around 3000 B.C., while a document written about 1500 B.C. described more than 800 remedies.

Hippocrates, the Father of Medicine, and other Greeks probably copied some of their plant lore from the Egyptians. About 370 B.C., Theophrastus, a pupil of Plato, wrote *An Enquiry Into Plants*, which contained a section on the medicinal properties of plants.

Dioscorides, a Greek surgeon in the Roman army, recorded the combined Egyptian, Greek, and Roman knowledge on the properties of plants. Much of the work of Dioscorides remained the basis of European medical practice for nearly 1500 years.

During the Middle Ages, Moslem pharmacists prepared herbal medicines for the disease-plagued Europeans. Men paid fantastic prices for these remedies since the Arabs controlled the drug and spice trade.

With the invention of printing, all knowledge became more widespread, and some of the first works printed following the *Bible* were books dealing with medicinal plants. In 1471, *De Agricultura* by Peter Crescentius, was published, containing complete, woodcut illustrated references to the useful and medicinal plants of southern Europe. More and more publications followed, and in 1597 *Gerard's Herbal* was published in England. Therefore, explorers of the New World must have been well versed in medicinal plants.

In the New World, Spanish explorers found the Incas and Aztecs using medicinal plants. The British and French explorers found the American Indians using still other plant remedies. As these plants were brought back to Europe, they were added to the European medicine chest and studied.

As the New World was settled, the herbal knowledge of the English soon meshed with that of the Indians who depended upon their medicine men. Benjamin Rush, a Philadelphia physician, investigated and wrote about the Indian cures. Soon, other compilers began to publish guides to Indian medicines during the early 1800s.

In the late 18th century and early 19th century, medicinal plants were primarily available to those who collected them in the wild. However, members of the Church of the United Society of Believers—the Shakers—were the first to mass produce herbs. By 1857, a Shaker settlement in New Lebanon, New York produced tons of medicinal plants which were shipped to every state and to England and Australia.

Gradually, as curiosity increased, scientists studied these medicinal plants handed down through the ages. They sought to discover the chemicals responsible for the healing properties of medicinal plants.

But herbal medicine still lives in this day and age of antibiotics, antibodies, vaccines, and synthetic chemicals! In fact, there seems to have been a revitalization of herbal medicine, with numerous new books printed and old books reproduced on the subject, and with increased sales of herbs and mixtures of herbs to cure, relieve, or prevent almost every ailment.

PLANT REMEDIES TO MODERN MEDICINE. As scientists studied the medicinal plants, they isolated the active chemicals, which could then be put into liquids or pills. Furthermore, once the active chemicals were discovered, the hope was that these chemicals could be synthesized in the laboratory, thus eliminating the need for collecting and extracting tons of plants to meet medicinal needs. Discovery of some active chemicals did lead to their laboratory synthesis, while some drugs still must come from plants. Examples of some important chemicals derived from plants include (1) the pain killer morphine from the opium poppy, (2) the tranquilizer reserpine from the snakeroot plant (rauwolfia), (3) the anesthetic cocaine from the coca plant, (4) the muscle relaxant and deadly poison curare from the curare vine, (5) the first malaria treatment, quinine from the bark of the cinchona tree, (6) the heart stimulant digitalis from the foxglove plant, and (7) the pupil-dilating drug atropine from the deadly nightshade. Thus, many medicinal plants handed down through the ages possess a chemical reason for their action. No doubt other important drugs will be discovered in plants as the search continues with more sophisticated techniques. Drug companies and government agencies are screening and testing thousands of plants yearly in an effort to find new and more effective cures for the ailments of mankind.

LANGUAGE OF PLANT REMEDIES. Along with the knowledge of the use of medicinal plants, a particular language has resulted which describes the method of use and/or the ailments for which plant remedies are employed. Some of the more important words commonly used follow:

• **Alteratives**—These are medicines that produce a gradual change for the better, and restore normal body function.

• **Anodyne**—Agents which relieve pain are called anodynes.

• **Astringent**—Substances which contract tissues and check the discharge of blood or mucus are termed astringents.

• **Carminative**—This is a substance that acts to reduce flatulence (gas).

• **Cathartics**—These are plant substances which relieve constipation by stimulating the secretions of the intestines.

• **Decoctions**—These are medicines made by simmering plant parts in water.

• **Demulcents**—These plant medicines are soothing to the intestinal tract and usually of an oily or mucilaginous nature.

• **Diaphoretic**—This type of substance has the ability to produce sweating.

• **Emollients**—These act similar to demulcents, but their soothing action is for the skin rather than the intestines.

• **Emmenagogues**—Plant remedies with this action are said to promote menstrual discharge.

• **Expectorants**—These are remedies which aid the patient in bringing up and spitting out excessive secretions of phlegm (mucus) from the lungs and windpipe.

• **Febrifuges**—These are the same as antipyretics—agents which help dissipate a fever.

• **Infusion**—This term applies to soaking of plant parts in water to extract their virtues. Infusions provide a quick and simple method for removing the medicinal principle from dried plant parts.

• **Nervines**—These substances are said to calm, soothe, and relax tensions caused by nervous excitement, strain, or fatigue.

• **Ointments and linaments**—The major difference between these is largely their consistency. An ointment is a semisolid in a fatty material, while a linament is a liquid or semiliquid preparation in a base of alcohol or oil.

• **Stimulants**—These are plant medicines which temporarily increase mental or physical activity.

• **Stomachics**—Plants with this property stimulate stomach secretions.

• **Tincture**—This refers to a solution of plant substances in alcohol. Tinctures contain those oils, resins, or waxes not soluble in water.

• **Tonic**—A tonic is said to be an agent which restores and invigorates the system and stimulates the appetite.

• **Vulneraries**—This word is often found in old herbals. It refers to medicines useful in healing wounds.

COMMON MEDICINAL PLANTS. Table M-14 groups some of the medicinal plants according to the language of herbal medicine.

TABLE M-14
SOME MEDICINAL PLANTS GROUPED ACCORDING TO THEIR REPORTED EFFECTS AND USES

Alterative	Anodyne	Appetite Stimulation	Astringent	Calmative
agrimony	birch bark	alfalfa	agrimony	catnip
black cohosh root	hops	anise	bayberry	chamomile
blue flag root	white willow bark	chamomile	blackberry	fennel seeds
burdock root	wintergreen	celery	valerian	linden flowers
dandelion		dandelion	witch hazel	
echinacea		ginseng		
ginseng		juniper		
goldenseal		mint		
red clover flowers		parsley		
sarsaparilla root		rosemary		
		sweet cicely		
		Virginia snakeroot		
		winter savory		
		wormwood		

Carminative	Cathartic	Demulcent	Diaphoretic	Diuretic
anise seed	barberry	borage	angelica root	alfalfa
capsicum	buckthorn bark	comfrey	borage	angelica
cardamom	chicory	marshmallow	catnip	bearberry leaves
catnip	colcynth		chamomile	buchu leaves
cumin	dandelion		ginger root	celery
fennel seed	senna		hyssop	chicory
ginger root			pennyroyal	cleaver's herb
goldenrod			senega root	corn silk
lovage root			serpentaria root	dandelion
nutmeg				elecampane root
peppermint				goldenrod
spearmint				horehound
valerian root				horse tail grass
				juniper berries
				parsley root
				wild carrot

Expectorant	Febrifuge	Nervine	Stimulant	Tonic
acacia	angelica	catnip	angelica	barberry root and bark
angelica	balm	chamomile	bayberry leaves	cascarilla bark
colt's foot	birch bark	hops	capsicum fruit	celery seed
garlic	borage	linden flower	cardamom	dandelion root
horehound	dandelion	passion flower	mayweed	gentian root
licorice root	eucalyptus	skullcap	Paraguay tea	ginseng
senega root	lobelia	valerian root	sarsaparilla root	goldenseal
	meadowsweet	yarrow	tansy	hops
	pennyroyal		vervain	mugwort
	senna		wintergreen	wormwood
	willow bark			

WORDS OF CAUTION. Herbal medicine, folk medicine, or whatever it is called, is back in vogue. It is appealing because most remedies are handy, inexpensive, and *natural*. Moreover, folk medicine gives people the feeling that they are taking care of themselves. With this return to folk medicine, there are numerous purveyors; hence, people should be wary. Many generalized and meaningless claims are employed to describe the action of certain plant remedies. For example, such claims include the following: purify the blood; strengthen the glands; establish a normal balance; strengthen the nerves; balance the female organism; encourage rejuvenation; and ease nerve pain. These claims could describe any number of symptoms or cures—or none at all. Moreover, some plant remedies are still recommended on the basis of the *doctrine of signatures*, which held that plant remedies could be identified by their resemblance to the afflicted part of the body. Names like liverwort and heartsease recall this belief.

As long as herbal medicine is not poisonous and does not replace traditional, professional medicine in serious ailments, no harm is likely. However, the individual subscribing to herbal medicine should be certain of the identity of the plants used, since some are poisonous and others may have serious side effects. Overall, herbal medicine is safe, fun, and some of it probably even helps ease minor ailments.

(Also see POISONOUS PLANTS; and WILD EDIBLE PLANTS.)

MEDIUM CHAIN TRIGLYCERIDES (MCT)

This is a special dietary product made from coconut oil by (1) steam and pressure hydrolysis of the oil into free fatty acids and glycerol, (2) separation of the resulting hydrolysate into medium-chain and long-chain fatty acids, and (3) recombination of the medium-chain fatty acids with glycerol to form MCT oil. It is composed of about ¾ caprylic acid, a saturated fatty acid containing 8 carbon atoms; and about ¼ capric acid, a saturated fatty acid containing 10 carbon atoms. The special nutritive values of this product are as follows:

1. It is much more readily digested, absorbed, and metabolized than either animal fats or vegetable oils which contain mainly long-chain triglycerides. The enzyme, pancreatic lipase, can easily break down MCT. Hence, MCT oil is valuable in the dietary treatment of fatty diarrhea and other digestive disorders in which the absorption of fat is impaired —malabsorption.

2. Medium-chain triglycerides, unlike other saturated fats, do *not* contribute to a rise in blood cholesterol. Therefore, they are used to treat some forms of hyperlipoproteinemia.

At the present time, MCT oil is used almost exclusively for special dietary formulations in the United States, but it is also available in various nonmedical consumer products in Europe.

(Also see HYPERLIPOPROTEINEMIAS; and MALABSORPTION SYNDROME.)

MEGADOSE

A very large dose; for example, taking 20 to 100 times the recommended allowance of vitamin C.

MEGAJOULE (MJ)

A metric unit of energy, equivalent to 240 kcal.

MEGALOBLAST

A large embryonic type of red blood cell with a large nucleus; present in the blood in cases of pernicious anemia, vitamin B-12 deficiency, and/or folacin deficiency.

MELANIN

Any of the various dark brown or black pigments of the skin, hair, and certain other tissues; derived from tyrosine metabolism.

MELBA TOAST

This is very thin bread which is toasted or baked until crisp and well browned. Thus, rusks, croutons, and melba toast all have one thing in common—all of them are made from bread which is baked until dry and crisp.

MELON(S)

The term *melon* is applied to the fruit of several closely related plants of the cucurbit family (*Cucurbitaceae*)—a family whose members include cucumbers, pumpkins, squashes, watermelons, and gourds.

Melons grow on plants that are either climbing or trailing vines with round, pointed or folded leaves, and small, yellow flowers. Melons are oblong to round. The surface of the melon is a skin called a rind which may be smooth, wrinkled, warty, netted, or ridged, and colored tan and yellow to light or dark green. The edible flesh—the pulp— may be green, white, yellow, pink, or red.

Melons include the summer melons, muskmelons, or cantaloupes; the winter melons, casaba, honeydew, crenshaw, and Persian melon; and watermelons. Descriptions of these melons follow:

• **Cantaloupe**—This is a variety of muskmelon, sometimes it is even called muskmelon. The netted-rind of the cantaloupe is yellow-green while the pulp is orange. Cantaloupes range in size from 4 to 7 in. *(10 to 17.5 cm)* in diameter. Although there are several varieties of cantaloupes which are grown in different climatic regions of the United States, California is by far the largest producer of the fruit. Usually, cantaloupes require about 3 months or so to reach maturity. Most of the crop is sold fresh, but some is canned or frozen in the form of melon balls.

• **Casaba**—The casaba is a golden-yellow, wrinkled-rind, round variety of muskmelon which has a white-colored flesh. Casabas range from 6 to 8 in. *(15 to 20 cm)* in diameter. This fruit requires a hot, dry climate and reaches maturity in about 3½ months. Most of the U.S. production is grown on irrigated fields in the southwestern and western states. All of the crop is marketed fresh right after harvesting or after a brief period of storage.

• **Honeydew**—This variety of melon has a white, smooth rind and light-green pulp. It is about 7 in. *(17.5 cm)* in diameter and 8 in. *(20 cm)* long. Honeydew melons grow best in hot, dry climates and require about 4 months to reach maturity. They are called winter melons because they ripen late in the season and are marketed during the winter. Most of the U.S. production comes from irrigated fields in the southwestern and western states. They are usually used fresh and as canned or frozen melon balls packed in syrup.

• **Crenshaw**—Crenshaw melons are oblong, with a yellow-tan, smooth rind. Their pulp is salmon-orange in color. Crenshaws are usually about 6 in. *(15 cm)* in diameter and about 7 in. *(17.5 cm)* long. These melons require a hot, dry climate and reach maturity in about 4 months. Most of the U.S. production is grown in irrigated fields in the southwestern and western states. All of this crop is marketed fresh.

• **Persian**—These melons are round with a dark green netted, rind and orange pulp. There are small Persian melons that are 4 to 5 in. *(10 to 12.5 cm)* in diameter and large types that are 7 to 10 in *(17.5 to 25 cm)* in diameter. Persian melons require a hot, dry climate and reach maturity in about 4 months. Most of the U.S. crop is grown in the southwestern states.

• **Watermelon**—All the melons listed above belong to the genus and species *Cucumis melo*, but the scientific name for watermelon is *Citrullus vulgaris*. Depending upon the variety, watermelons weight 5 to 85 lb *(2.3 to 38.3 kg)* and vary in shape from round to oval to oblong-cylindrical. The rind may be very light to very dark-green with stripes or mottling, while the pulp is red, pink, orange, yellow, or white. Watermelons are grown in tropical, semitropical, and temperate climates. In the United States commercial watermelon production occurs primarily in the southern states.

Nutritionally, melons are all quite similar containing only about 30 calories (kcal) per 100 g and being good sources of potassium, vitamin C, and vitamin A when the flesh is deep orange. Melons are all about 90% water.

(Also see CANTALOUPE; and WATERMELON.)

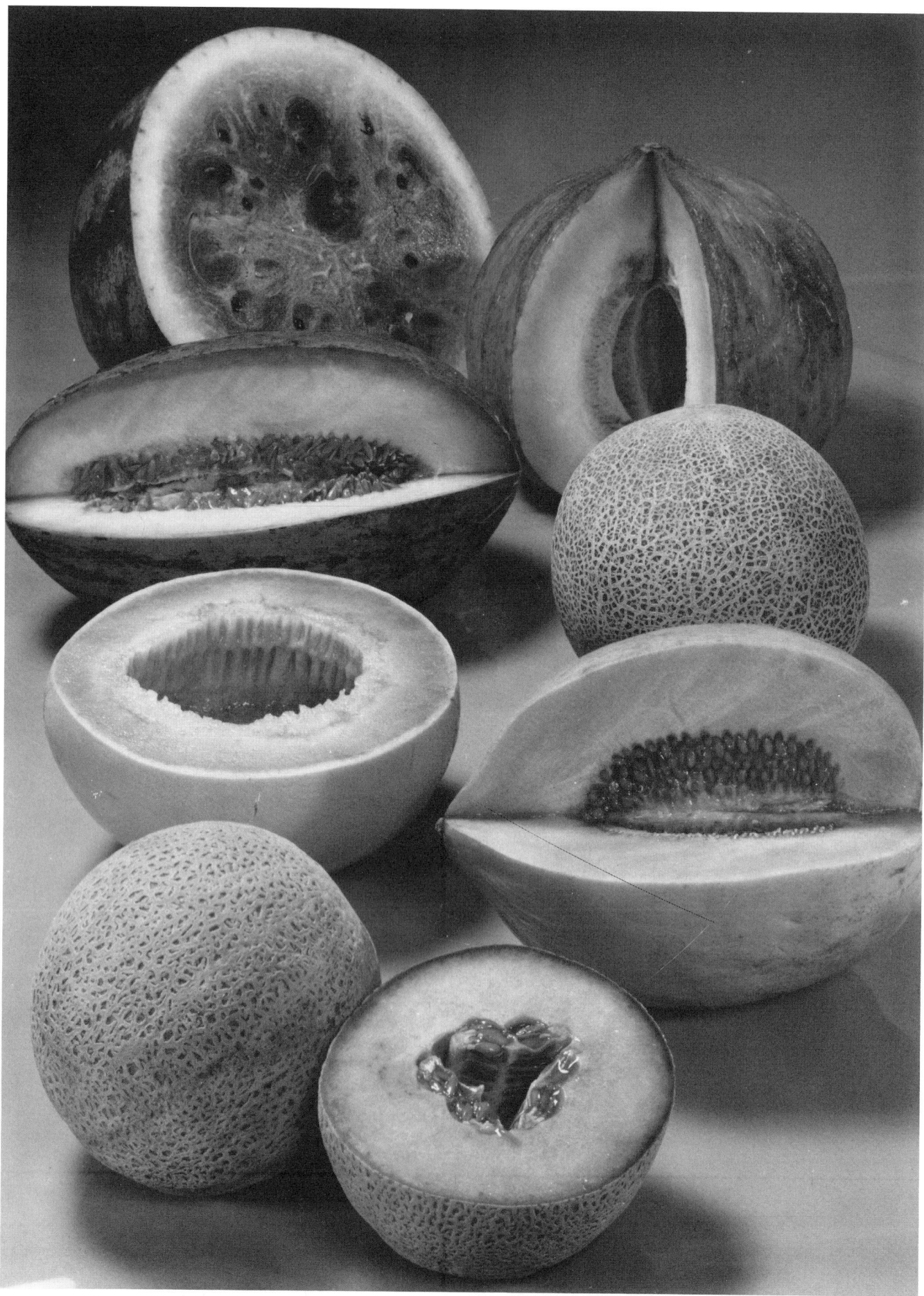

Fig. M-44. You can't get melancholy with melons. (Courtesy, United Fresh Fruit & Vegetable Assoc., Alexandria, Va.)

MELON PEAR (PEPINO) *Solanum muricatum*

The yellow and purple streaked fruit of a shrub (of the family *Solanaceae*) that is native to Peru, but is now grown in various parts of the American tropics. It is between 4 and 6 in. *(10 and 15 cm)* long, and has an aromatic pulp that is used to make drinks, jams, and jellies.

The pulp of the fruit is high in water content (92%) and low in calories (32 kcal per 100 g) and carbohydrates (6%). It is a good source of vitamin C.

MENIERE'S SYNDROME

Most common in the fifth decade of life, Meniere's syndrome denotes symptoms resulting from a disturbance of the inner ear due to fluid accumulation. The disease, whose symptoms were first collectively described by Prosper Meniere in 1861, is characterized by the sensation of whirling around in space—vertigo—fluctuating incidents of deafness, high pitch ringing or buzzing in the ear, nausea, vomiting, and headache. Many inner ear disorders can be traced to a variety of causes. However, the cause of Meniere's syndrome is difficult to pinpoint and it is rarely traceable to a disease or infection. Treatment, therefore, may proceed on a trial-and-error basis. Bed rest is an effective treatment since the sufferer can usually find a position in which vertigo is minimal. Other forms of treatment consist of diuretics and low salt diets to relieve the fluid accumulation in the inner ear and the use of sedatives and tranquil-izers. A preparation such as Dramamine may be given to relieve the vertigo. Should the condition become so annoying that normal activities are impossible, then surgery is often the only cure.

Some sufferers of Meniere's syndrome report obtaining relief from taking niacin (both oral and injections simultaneously) and other B-complex vitamins, and from adding yogurt or buttermilk to the diet. Also, a diet low in (1) saturated fats, (2) carbohydrates (especially sugar), and (3) salt has been found to be helpful.

(Also see MODIFIED DIETS.)

MENTAL DEVELOPMENT

Mental development is a complex, on-going process influenced by a multitude of factors. Furthermore, it is difficult to assess and compare due to various social, racial, and ethnic backgrounds. In general, mental development may be defined as the increased ability to function. It involves motor skills, social traits, behavioral traits and learning skills. Normal mental development is evidenced by the gradual development of certain skills—roll over, sit, creep, walk, coordination of eyes and hands, formation of words, formation of whole thoughts, and ability to relate to people. The overall desired outcome of mental development is the attainment of an individual's full genetic potential.

In humans, it is difficult to say whether nutrition *per se* contributes to mental development since the conditions of malnutrition and deprived social and environmental conditions coexist. However some animal models have been designed to separate the effects of nutrition and environment on mental development. Therefore, animal models and observations of human populations combine to form the following salient points in regards to nutrition and mental development:

1. The brain and spinal cord continue rapid growth during infancy.

2. Malnutrition during the early life of animals and humans alters the number of brain cells, brain cell size, and/or other biochemical parameters depending upon the time of onset and the duration of the malnutrition.

3. Malnourished animals demonstrate impaired learning abilities.

4. Teachers have observed that hungry, undernourished children are apathetic and lethargic.

5. Children suffering from kwashiorkor are apathetic, listless, withdrawn, and seldom resist examination or wander off when left alone.

6. Children who recover from marasmus have a reduced head circumference—brain size—even after five years of rehabilitation.

7. Numerous studies suggest that infants subjected to acute malnutrition during the first years of life develop irreversible gaps in mental development, and thus never attain their full genetic potential.

Nevertheless, no amount of food can compensate for the emotional and social deprivation, resulting primarily from the lack of fulfilling infant-parent interaction.

(Also see MALNUTRITION; and STARVATION.)

MENTAL ILLNESS

This is a catchall term referring to any alteration in the normal function of the mind, ranging from periods of brief depression to severe, long lasting, disabling personality disorders. Rather broadly, mental illnesses can be classified as (1) neuroses, (2) psychophysiologic disorders, (3) personality disorders, (4) psychoses, and (5) transient situational disturbances. It can be characterized by lack of control over emotions and actions plus anxiety and even the stimulation of various physical disorders; for example, a peptic ulcer. Mental illness may be inherited and/or induced by environmental factors—chemical, bacterial, viral, nutritional, psychological, and social. Indeed there are probably as many or more forms of mental illness as there are physical illnesses. It should also be noted that no sharp line exists between mental health and mental illness because every human is unique. What is normal or abnormal may be merely a matter of degree and the manner in which a person's behavior is interpreted by family, friends, and physicians. However, it is well documented that there are certain nutritional disorders which cause some modifications in normal nervous system function—mental illness. The following examples demonstrate that nutritional states modify nervous system function:

1. **Vitamins and minerals.** Dietary deficiencies of thiamin, riboflavin, niacin, pantothenic acid, vitamin B-6, and vitamin B-12 will modify sensory functions, motor ability, and personality. Deficiencies of minerals such as sodium and magnesium, and toxic intakes of minerals such as lead and mercury, produce mild to severe forms of mental disorders—hyperactivity, learning difficulties, hallucinations, confusion, and giddiness.

(Also see MINERAL[S]; and VITAMIN[S].)

2. **Hypoglycemia.** When hypoglycemia (low blood sugar) develops over a short period of time, the symptoms include rapid pulse, trembling, hunger, and a slight amount of mental confusion. However, hypoglycemia which has developed over many hours—meal skipping—is characterized by headache, depression, blurred vision, incoherent speech, and considerable mental confusion.

(Also see HYPOGLYCEMIA.)

3. **Starvation.** Short periods of starvation—4 days of water only—in healthy individuals decreases coordination and ability to concentrate. Semistarvation over long periods of time, such as existed in World War II concentration camps, decreased the ability to concentrate, lessened inter-

ests, decreased the ability of sustained mental effort, and created irritability, apathy, and sullenness.

(Also see STARVATION.)

4. **Beriberi.** Beriberi is a disease due to thiamin deficiency. Behavioral changes which have been noted include mental depression, loss of interest, diminution of the sense of humor, loss of ability to concentrate, and loss of patience with others. Rapid reversal of these symptoms depends upon restoration of thiamin to the diet.

(Also see BERIBERI.)

5. **Alcoholism.** Alcoholics make up about 10% of the first admissions to psychiatric wards. They possess some of the same symptoms noted in thiamin deficiency, and indeed respond to thiamin therapy. Often Korsakoff's syndrome—confusion, confabulation, fear, impaired learning, delirium—is associated with alcoholism. Vitamin therapy helps to restore the individual's attentiveness, alertness, and responsiveness.

(Also see ALCOHOLISM.)

(Also see ANOREXIA NERVOSA; DEFICIENCY DISEASES; INBORN ERRORS OF METABOLISM; MENTAL DEVELOPMENT; MENTAL RETARDATION; and STRESS.)

MENTAL RETARDATION

Various degrees of mental retardation occur, but all are characterized by faulty development or set-back in the mental processes which impairs an individual's ability to cope with and adapt to the demands of society. In the United States, there are about 6 million mentally retarded individuals. It is generally recognized that there are three classes of mental retardation: (1) high grade or educable; (2) middle grade or trainable; and (3) low grade. A physical injury to the brain; some childhood diseases; an infection such as rubella, syphilis, or meningitis during pregnancy; a genetic defect such as Down's syndrome; and inborn errors of metabolism such as phenylketonuria and galactosemia without dietary adjustments, can all cause mental retardation. Nutritionally, a low iodine intake by the mother during pregnancy may result in cretinism in the baby, and alcohol consumption during pregnancy may contribute to varying degrees of mental retardation in the infant. A poor diet by the mother during pregnancy, and/or a poor diet by the infant may contribute to abnormal mental development. In fact, a large number of cases of mild mental retardation, which are educable, are not related to any known physical or organic cause. In these cases, genetic, environmental, nutritional, or psychological factors, or a combination of factors, may be the cause. Depending upon the degree, a mentally retarded person can present some obvious feeding problems. Feeding may be messy and slow, and thus require frequent small feedings in an effort to provide adequate food. Mentally retarded individuals have food likes and dislikes, and, despite their mental differences, their nutritional requirements are like those of everyone else.

(Also see ALCOHOLISM; INBORN ERRORS OF METABOLISM; IODINE; and MENTAL DEVELOPMENT.)

MERCURY (Hg)

The element mercury is discharged into air and water from industrial operations and is used in herbicide and fungicide treatments. Although known cases of mercury poisoning have been limited, there is widespread concern over environmental pollution by this element.

(Also see MINERAL[S]; section on "Contamination of Drinking Water, Foods, or Air with Toxic Minerals"; and POISONS.)

METABOLIC POOL

The nutrients available at any given time for the metabolic activities of the body; e.g., the amino acid pool, the calcium pool.

METABOLIC RATE

Essentially all of the energy released from foods becomes heat. Therefore, the metabolic rate is a measure of the rate of heat production by the body. It is expressed in Calories (kcal) and can be determined by direct calorimetry which measures the heat given off by a person engaged in various activities. However, indirect calorimetry is more frequently used. This method determines the heat produced by measuring the oxygen consumed, since it is known that on the average for each liter of oxygen burned by the metabolic fires of the body 4.825 Calories (kcal) of energy are released. When a normal person is in a quiet resting state the metabolic rate is about 60 to 80 Calories (kcal) per hour. However, a variety of factors influence the metabolic rate. Many of these factors are interrelated and some are more important than others. Among the factors that affect the metabolic rate are: exercise, recent ingestion of food, envi-ronmental temperature, body surface area, sex, pregnancy, age, emotional state, state of nutrition, body temperature, and hormones.

(Also see CALORIC [ENERGY] EXPENDITURE, section headed "Special Circumstances that Affect Energy Requirements"; CALORIMETRY; and METABOLISM, section on "Factors Controlling Metabolism.")

METABOLIC REACTIONS

The chemical changes that occur in the body; some are synthetic (the formation of new compounds), others are degradative (the breaking down of compounds).

METABOLIC WATER

Water formed within the cells of the body during the combustion (breakdown) of nutrients for the release of energy. On the average 13 ml of metabolic water are formed for every 100 kcal of metabolizable energy in the typical diet of a human. It contributes to the daily intake of water, and must be accounted for in the maintenance of water balance. Table M-15 illustrates the oxygen requirement and the production of carbon dioxide, water, and energy for carbohydrates, proteins, and fats.

(Also see METABOLISM; and WATER BALANCE.)

TABLE M-15
OXYGEN REQUIREMENTS AND CARBON DIOXIDE, WATER, AND ENERGY PRODUCTION FOR THE BREAKDOWN OF EACH 100 GRAMS OF CARBOHYDRATE, PROTEIN, AND FAT

Nutrient	Oxygen Consumed	Carbon Dioxide Produced	Water Produced	Energy Released
	(liter)	(liter)	(ml)	(kcal)
Carbohydrate	82.9	82.9	60	410
Protein	96.6	78.2	40	410
Fat	201.9	142.7	110	930

METABOLISM

Contents Page

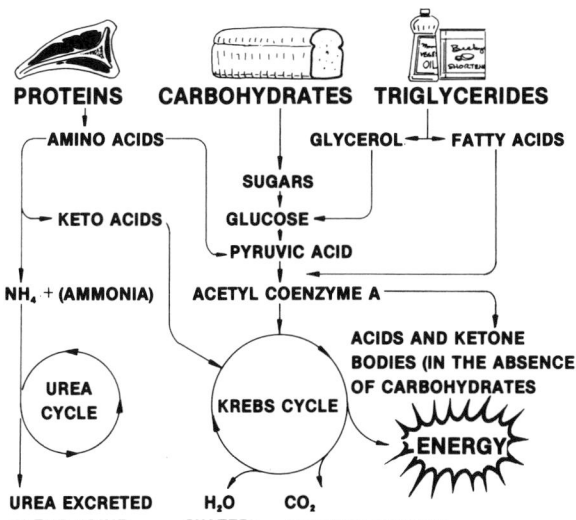

Fig. M-45. Metabolism of foods for the production of energy—the number one need.

Beefsteak, lettuce, tomatoes, and beans never get to the cells and tissues of our bodies, including our brains. But the nutrient chemicals—more than 40 of them, including amino acids, minerals, vitamins—do reach the body cells and tissues and are essential to their life. These are the ABCs of modern nutrition.

Once foods are eaten and digested, the nutrients are absorbed into the blood and distributed to the cells of the body. Still more chemical changes are required before the nutrients can be put to work in the body, by transforming them into energy or structural material. Thus, nutrients—carbohydrates, fats, proteins, minerals, vitamins, and water—are subjected to various chemical reactions. These chemical reactions occur on the cellular and subcellular level. The sum of all of these chemical reactions is termed metabolism. It has two phases: (1) catabolism, and (2) anabolism:

1. **Catabolism.** Catabolism is the oxidation—burning—of nutrients, liberating energy which is used to fulfill the body's immediate demands. When reactions liberate energy they are termed *exergonic reactions*.

2. **Anabolism.** Anabolism is the process by which nutrient molecules are used as building blocks for the synthesis of complex molecules. Anabolic reactions are endergonic—they require the input of energy into the system.

Basic to understanding the process of metabolism, is the realization that all of the reactions are catalyzed by enzymes —protein molecules which speed up biochemical reactions without being used up in the reactions. Furthermore, most all of the biochemical reactions of the metabolic processes are reversible. This is an important concept.

Life is a conquest for energy. Energy is required for practically all life processes—for the action of the heart, maintenance of blood pressure and muscle tone, transmission of nerve impulses, ion transport across membranes, reabsorption in the kidneys, protein and fat synthesis, the secretion of milk, and muscular contraction. A deficiency of energy is manifested by slow or stunted growth, body tissue losses, and/or weakness.

The diet contains carbohydrates, fats, and proteins. Although each of these has specific functions in maintaining a normal body, all of them can be used to provide the number one requirement—energy. Hence, the following discussion of their metabolism centers first, on their catabolism, and second, on their anabolism. Although they are not used for energy, minerals, vitamins, and water are essential to the metabolic processes.

In many ways, metabolism is similar to a factory. Like any manufacturing process, there are waste products with which to be dealt. Since the waste products of metabolism are toxic to the body at high levels, the body has developed reliable means for the removal of these wastes. Also, like any manufacturing process, there must be controls. Various factors control the rate and the direction of metabolism—anabolism or catabolism. Occasionally, a faulty piece of equipment hinders a manufacturing process. The body, too, can inherit faulty equipment for performing the metabolic processes.

CELLS—FUNCTIONAL UNITS. Every living thing is composed of cells and cell products. In an organism as complex as a human—with trillions of cells—the proper function of the body processes is dependent upon each individual cell carrying out its proper metabolic processes for the organ or tissue in which it is located. Just as the body has organs, the cells of the body contain organelles (little organs) which are involved in the metabolic processes.

A typical cell with the structures involved in metabolic processes is shown in Fig. M-46.

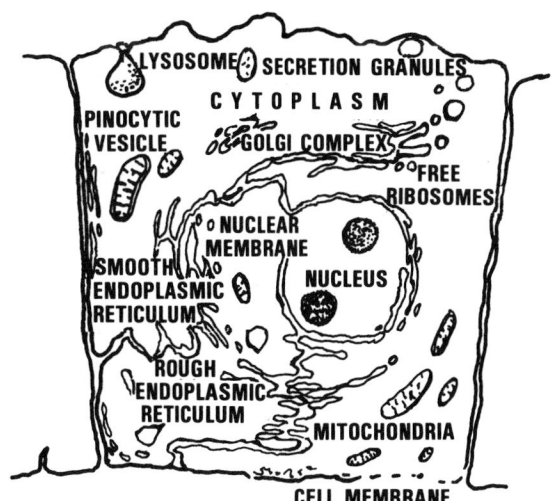

Fig. M-46. A typical cell showing some of the structural components most cells have in common, though cells of the body are variable in structure and function.

NUTRIENTS FOR METABOLISM.

NUTRIENTS FOR METABOLISM. From the standpoint of supplying the normal energy needs, carbohydrates are by far the most important, with fats second, and proteins third. Carbohydrates are usually more abundant and cheaper, and most of them are easily digested and absorbed. Moreover, excess carbohydrates can be transformed into body fat or into amino acids for protein synthesis.

Carbohydrates. The carbohydrates are organic compounds composed of carbon (C), hydrogen (H), and oxygen (O). They are formed in the plant by photosynthesis as follows: $6CO_2 + 6H_2O$ + energy from sun = $C_6H_{12}O_6$ (glucose) + $6O_2$. Carbohydrates form the woody framework of plants as well as the chief reserve food stored in seeds, roots, and tubers. As far as man is concerned, starch and sugars, primarily 6-carbon sugars, are the carbohydrates available for his use. Starch is composed of long chains of glucose which the digestive processes split into individual glucose molecules. Fructose (fruit sugar), glucose (grape sugar), sucrose (cane and beet sugar), and lactose (milk sugar) are the important dietary sugars. Other carbohydrates such as cellulose, hemicellulose, and pectin are not digestible; hence, they are unavailable for the metabolic processes. Sometimes these carbohydrates are called fiber or roughage. Ultimately, after being digested and absorbed, carbohydrates are converted to glucose.

No appreciable amount of carbohydrate is found in the body at any one time, but the blood supply of glucose is held rather constant at about 70 to 100 mg/100 ml. However, this small quantity of glucose in the blood, which is constantly replenished by changing the glycogen of the liver back to glucose, serves as the chief source of fuel with which to maintain the body temperature and to furnish the energy needed for all body processes. Maintenance of the blood glucose level is so important that at times amino acids and part of the fat molecule (glycerol) may be used to make glucose. The storage of glycogen (so-called animal starch) in the liver amounts to 3 to 7% of the weight of that organ. Glycogen is also stored in the muscles, but the latter is not available to raise blood glucose.

(Also see CARBOHYDRATE[S]; FIBER; HYPOGLYCEMIA; and STARCH.)

CATABOLISM. The primary use for carbohydrates is to produce energy. In the presence of oxygen, glucose will produce a maximum of 686 kcal/mole (*180.2 g*), as seen in the following equation:

$$C_6H_{12}O_6 + 6 O_2 \rightarrow 6 CO_2 + 6 H_2O$$
$$+ 686 \text{ kcal/mole (heat)}$$

The above reaction is a combustion or burning reaction. Hence, the expression of *burning off calories* can be understood.

No physiological system can approach 100% efficiency in the production of energy from the catabolism of a nutrient. Likewise, the body cannot produce 686 kcal from one mole (*180.2 g*) of glucose. Nevertheless, a great deal of energy is produced from the catabolism of glucose by a series of enzymatic reactions which permit the orderly transfer of energy from glucose to energy-rich compounds:

• **ATP—energy currency**—For metabolism to permit the orderly transfer of energy from foods to processes requiring energy, there must be a common carrier of energy— something cells can use to exchange goods for services. The energy currency—the primary mechanism by which energy is captured and stored—is a compound called adenosine triphosphate, often abbreviated ATP. Just as pennies are small units of a dollar, ATP is a small unit of energy.

ATP is a compound formed from the purine adenine, the 5-carbon sugar ribose, and three phosphate molecules as shown in Fig. M-47. Two of the phosphates are joined by high energy bonds.

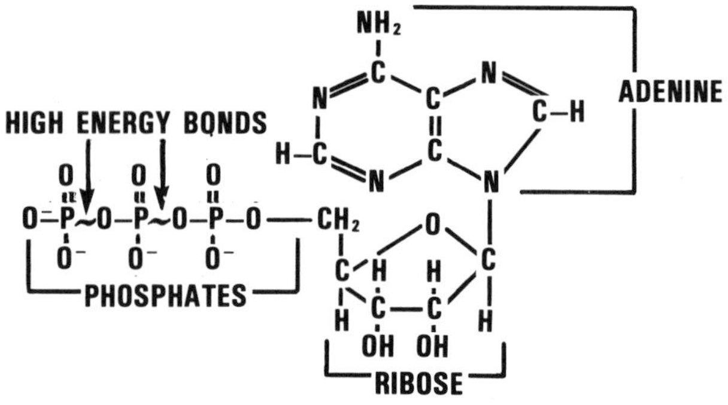

Fig. M-47. Structure of adenosine triphosphate.

When ATP is formed from ADP (adenosine diphosphate) by the addition of another phosphate, 8 kcal/mole must be put into the system—like a deposit in a bank account. The ATP then acts as a high-energy storage compound for the energy produced in the catabolism of various nutrients. When energy is required for body functions, ATP is broken down to ADP by releasing one phosphate and 8 kcal/mole of energy.

Releasing all of the energy contained in carbohydrates (fats and proteins, too) in one step would result in lost and wasted heat energy. Instead, energy is released in steps. The body utilizes a series of biological oxidations to form ATP. Oxidation refers to the loss of electrons (or hydrogen) by a compound. Conversely, reduction refers to the acceptance of electrons (or hydrogen) by a compound. Chemical energy is released as the lost electrons flow down energy gradients of an elevated state to the next lower hydrogen (electron) acceptor or carrier. Several coenzymes act as hydrogen (H^+) acceptors, many of which involve vitamins; for example, niacin and riboflavin. Compounds such as nicotinamide adenine dinucleotide (NAD^+), nicotinamide adenine dinucleotide phosphate ($NADP^+$), and flavin adenine dinucleotide (FAD) can accept and transfer hydrogen (or electrons) through a cytochrome system known as the electron transport system. Cytochromes are pigmented proteins similar to hemoglobin. In the electron transport system, electrons cascade from one intermediate carrier molecule—cytochrome—to the next lower in line, like water over a small waterfall. For every two electrons that tumble down the cytochrome system, enough energy is released to form three ATP molecules by adding a high energy phosphate to ADP. The ultimate hydrogen acceptor in the system is oxygen; hence, water (H_2O) is formed. This is metabolic water. Production of ATP through this system is known as oxidative phosphorylation. Oxygen is required. It should be noted that when oxidation is initiated and NAD^+ carries the hydrogen ($NADH + H^+$) there is a net production of three ATP molecules. Only two ATPs are yielded, however, when hydrogen is transferred by FAD ($FADH_2$).

Fig. M-48 illustrates the cytochrome system, and the formation of ATP as hydrogen drops to different energy levels.

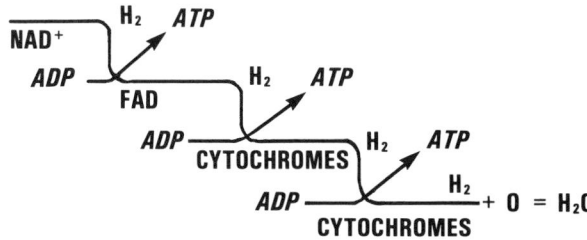

Fig. M-48. The formation of adenosine triphosphate (ATP) from adenosine diphosphate as hydrogen tumbles down a chain of hydrogen carriers—the electron transport system. NAD + stands for nicotinamide adenine dinucleotide, and FAD stands for flavin adenine dinucleotide—both hydrogen carriers similar to the cytochromes.

• **Glycolysis**—Before glucose can be used by the cells it must first enter from the blood. Entry into the cells depends upon the hormone insulin from the pancreas. Without insulin, glucose stays in the blood and creates the condition known as diabetes mellitus. Once inside the cell, the initial steps in the catabolism of glucose begin with a process called glycolysis—meaning glucose destruction. This pathway of chemical changes is referred to as the Embden-Meyerhof or glycolytic pathway. It is a series of reactions that are oxygen independent—no free or molecular oxygen needs to be involved; hence, these reactions are said to be anaerobic. The first reaction of glucose is that of providing activation energy—energy to get glucose *over a hump* before proceeding *downhill*. This is accomplished by a reaction in which ATP donates a high energy phosphate yielding a new compound called glucose-6-phosphate.

Next, glucose atoms are slightly rearranged to yield fructose-6-phosphate. Then another phosphate is added by a donation from ATP. The compound is now called fructose-1, 6-phosphate. Another enzyme splits this 6-carbon compound into two 3-carbon compounds each containing a phosphate. One compound is glyceraldehyde-3-phosphate and the other is dihydroxyacetone phosphate. Dihydroxyacetone phosphate can be converted to glyceraldehyde-3-phosphate which receives another phosphate after two hydrogen atoms are removed via NADH + H$^+$. When oxygen is present (aerobic), this hydrogen enters the electron transport system and yields three ATP. Next, the compound with two phosphates—1, 3, diphosphoglyceric acid—loses a phosphate thus forming ATP from ADP and converting the compound to 3-phosphoglyceric acid. Eventually, the other phosphate is lost to convert ADP to another ATP and pyruvic acid is formed. Since each glucose provides two 3-carbon compounds for glycolysis, the net gain in ATP to this point is two ATP. Two ATP were used to add phosphate to the 6-carbon compounds while two were gained for each 3-carbon compound converted to pyruvic acid.

Lactic acid is produced only under anaerobic conditions such as exercise, when oxygen cannot be delivered fast enough by the blood. Since the conversion of pyruvic acid to lactic acid requires the input of two hydrogen atoms, the NADH + H$^+$ generated earlier in glycolysis can be reconverted to NAD$^+$ thus allowing glycolysis to continue. Normally, NADH + H$^+$ would go to the electron transport system, but this requires oxygen. Lactic acid is a dead end. In order for the body to use it, it must be reconverted to pyruvic acid, and in some cases glucose.

The following items are important features of glycolysis:
1.   Two ATP are netted for each glucose.

2.   The system allows for the anaerobic breakdown of glucose.

3.   It provides a system whereby energy from glucose stored as glycogen can be made readily available in muscle even when oxygen is in short supply during exercise.

4.   Intermediates for the synthesis of other nutrients, such as glycerol and amino acids, are provided.

5.   In the step whereby glyceraldehyde-3-phosphate is converted to 1, 3-diphosphoglyceric acid, 2 moles of NADH + H$^+$ are produced which can subsequently be oxidized in the electron transport system under aerobic conditions to produce 6 additional ATP.

Through more chemical reactions, more energy can be derived from glucose which has reached the point of pyruvic acid. These additional reactions take place in a cellular structure appropriately called the powerhouse of the cell. These are the mitochondria.

• **Mitochondria**—These are watermelon-shaped microscopic structures within the cells of the body. The number and distribution of mitochondria within a cell depends upon the energy requirement of the cell. Those cells with large energy requirements possess a large number of mitochondria. The mitochondria contain the electron transport system. Moreover, they contain the enzymes necessary for the further metabolism of pyruvic acid, and other chemical transformations. It is their unique internal structure of cristae—a series of baffles—that allows for very efficient production of ATP.

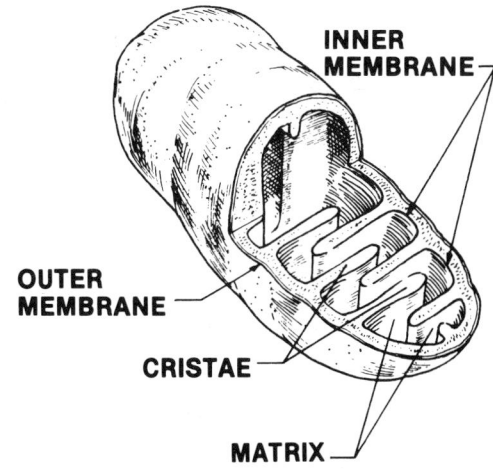

Fig. M-49. Microscopic view of a mitochondrion—powerhouse of the cell.

Pyruvic acid enters the mitochondria of the cell and begins another series of reactions variously referred to as the Krebs cycle, the tricarboxylic acid (TCA) cycle, or the citric acid cycle. First, pyruvic acid is converted to acetyl coenzyme A (acetyl CoA) by a loss of a carbon atom as carbon dioxide (CO_2) and two hydrogen atoms. This conversion yields 3 ATP, since the hydrogen atoms enter the electron transport system via NADH + H$^+$. Acetyl CoA is then condensed with oxaloacetic acid to form citric acid, thus initiating the Krebs cycle. As the cycle progresses, more electrons (hydrogens) are transferred to different coenzymes, which, in turn, enter the electron transport chain producing ATP. One complete turn of the cycle (1) produces 12 ATP and the loss of two carbons as carbon dioxides (CO_2) from citrate, and (2) the restoration of oxaloacetic acid; completing the cycle. Since 2 pyruvic acid molecules can be formed from 1 glucose molecule, 24 ATP are produced via the Krebs cycle. Thus, 38 ATP are produced from 1 molecule of glucose: 8 from glycolysis, 6 in the conversion of pyruvic acid to acetyl CoA, and 24 from the Krebs cycle. Each pass of the 2-carbon acetyl CoA through the Krebs cycle results in the formation of CO_2 (carbon dioxide) and H_2O (water), the end products of catabolism.

• **Energy efficiency**—One ATP molecule will yield about 8 Calories (kcal). Since 38 ATP are derived from the complete oxidation of glucose, 304 Calories (kcal) of energy are formed (38 × 8 = 304). Under ideal conditions, the oxidation of glucose yields 686 Calories (kcal). Hence, the human body is 44% efficient in converting glucose to energy (304 ÷ 686 × 100 = 44). Diesel engines have a maximum efficiency of about 40%, while many gasoline engines only convert about 25% of their fuel energy into work. The human body burns its fuel quite efficiently.

• **Hexosemonophosphate pathway (Pentose shunt)**—Not all glucose enters the glycolytic pathway. A small amount continually enters another pathway known as the pentose shunt or hexosemonophosphate (HMP) pathway. The functions of this pathway are twofold: (1) to provide some energy in the form of NADPH, another hydrogen carrier, which will function in the formation of fatty acids; and (2) to provide the 5-carbon sugar ribose for use in the nucleic acid DNA and RNA, or nucleotide coenzymes such as ATP. Products of this pathway eventually re-enter the glycolytic pathway.

ANABOLISM.   Two processes involved in carbohydrate metabolism may be considered anabolic in that they require energy: (1) storage of glucose as glycogen; and (2) the formation of glucose from noncarbohydrate sources, or gluconeogenesis.

• **Glycogen**—Upon absorption into the bloodstream, glucose travels to the liver where it is incorporated into glycogen. Glycogen is composed of numerous glucose molecules which are all chemically joined. Starch in plants is also composed of numerous glucose molecules joined together; hence, glycogen is sometimes referred to as animal starch. Each time a glucose molecule is linked with the glycogen already in the liver, two high-energy phosphate bonds are required. Then, as glucose is needed to maintain the blood glucose levels, glycogen is broken down to release glucose.

Some glycogen is manufactured and stored in the muscles. However, glucose derived from this glycogen is available only for use by the muscle and not the general circulation. Lactic acid may leave the muscle and be reconverted to glucose in the liver and released into the blood. This process requires six ATPs for each glucose molecule, and is referred to as the lactic acid cycle or Cori cycle. A husband and wife team, Carl and Gerty Cori, described it; and they were jointly awarded the Nobel Prize in 1947.

• **Gluconeogenesis**—Gluconeogenesis is the formation of glucose from nutrients other than carbohydrates. This pathway is extremely important when there is an insufficiency of dietary carbohydrates. The liver is the main site for gluconeogenesis. Amino acids are the primary precursors in gluconeogenesis. However, amino acids must first have their amino group (NH_2) removed by a process called deamination, following which the remaining carbon skeleton can enter the Krebs cycle and, essentially, be worked backwards through glycolysis to glucose. All of the amino acids except leucine are glycogenic—capable of forming

glucose. Production of glucose by this means is possible since most reactions catalyzed by enzymes are reversible. There is, however, one exception. Pyruvic acid in the mitochondria of cells cannot be directly converted to phosphoenolpyruvic acid. Rather, it is transformed into oxaloacetic acid and malic acid. Malic acid is then able to cross the mitochondrial membrane into the cytoplasm where it is reconverted to oxaloacetic acid. Oxaloacetic acid is then converted to phosphoenolpyruvic acid due to the presence of a specific enzyme in the cytoplasm. Once this is accomplished, the process closely resembles the reverse of the glycolytic pathway. The whole process requires an expenditure of energy.

Table M-16 indicates where each amino acid fits into the metabolic scheme following deamination.

TABLE M-16
GLUCONEOGENESIS FROM AMINO ACIDS

Amino Acid	Compounds Formed Following Deamination	Metabolic Fate[1]
Alanine	Pyruvic acid	Glycogenic
Arginine	Alpha-ketoglutaric acid	Glycogenic
Aspartate	Fumaric acid	Glycogenic
Cysteine	Pyruvic acid	Glycogenic
Glutamate	Alpha-ketoglutaric acid	Glycogenic
Glycine	Pyruvic acid	Glycogenic
Histidine	Alpha-ketoglutaric acid, beta-ketoglutaric acid	Glycogenic
Proline	Alpha-ketoglutaric acid	Glycogenic
Hydroxyproline	Alpha-ketoglutaric acid	Glycogenic
Methionine	Succinyl CoA	Glycogenic
Serine	Pyruvic acid	Glycogenic
Threonine	Succinyl CoA	Glycogenic
Valine	Succinyl CoA	Glycogenic
Isoleucine	Acetyl CoA, succinyl CoA	Glycogenic and ketogenic
Lysine	Alpha-ketoglutaric acid, acetyl CoA, acetoacetyl CoA	Glycogenic and ketogenic
Phenylalanine	Fumaric acid, acetyl CoA	Glycogenic and ketogenic
Tryptophan	Succinyl CoA, acetyl CoA	Glycogenic and ketogenic
Leucine	Acetyl CoA, acetoacetic acid	Ketogenic

[1]Glycogenic forms glucose while ketogenic forms ketone bodies—acetoacetic acid, beta-hydroxybutyric acid, and acetone.

Fats.   Fats are compounds composed of carbon, hydrogen, and oxygen—much like carbohydrates. However, because of the larger portion of carbon and hydrogen in their makeup, fats provide about 2.25 times as much energy as do the carbohydrates—more hydrogen atoms for the electron transport system. Dietary fats are primarily compounds composed of three fatty acid molecules linked to one glycerol molecule—a combination called triglycerides.

(Also see FATS AND OTHER LIPIDS.)

CATABOLISM.   When fats are hydrolyzed (water added), glycerol and fatty acids are released and subsequently catabolized separately. Glycerol is converted to glycerol-3-phosphate, then to dihydroxyacetone phosphate. Dihydroxyacetone phosphate can be readily converted to 3-phosphoglyceraldehyde which enters the last part of the glycolytic pathway and eventually enters into the Krebs cycle. Thus, it yields an amount of energy similar to that of one-half of the glucose molecule passing through glycolysis and the Krebs cycle.

The catabolism of fatty acids occurs in the mitochondria through a systematic process called beta-oxidation, whereby 2-carbon fragments are successively chopped from the fatty acid molecule to form acetyl CoA which then enters the Krebs cycle. The term lipolysis indicates mobilization of fats and their oxidation. Carnitine, a vitaminlike substance, facilitates the transport of fatty acids across the mitochondrial membrane. The first step in the beta-oxidation of a fatty acid is the addition of coenzyme A (CoA) to the end of the molecule. This requires energy, but not nearly as much energy as is subsequently generated. For example, the 16-carbon fatty acid palmitic acid can be oxidized seven times. Each time a 2-carbon fragment—acetyl CoA—is released from a fatty acid, 5 ATP are formed. However, 1 ATP is consumed in activating the fatty acid with CoA. Then, each acetyl CoA enters the Krebs cycle and produces 12 ATP. The energy balance sheet is as follows:

			ATP
Palmitic acid	→	Palmitoyl CoA............	− 1
Palmitoyl CoA	→	8 Acetyl CoA (7 × 5 ATP).	35
8 Acetyl CoA	→	H_2O + 18 CO_2 (8 × 12 ATP)	96
		Net....................................	130

Each mole of ATP contains about 8 Calories (kcal). Therefore, 1 mole of palmitic acid yields 1,040 Calories (kcal), which demonstrates that fats are high-energy compounds. Comparing this value to that obtained by burning fat in a laboratory bomb calorimeter, the efficiency of the biological burning of palmitic acid is about 42%—not bad for any machine.

Acetyl CoA is a common point—a crossroad— for many of the biochemical reactions of the body. It can be used for building other substances including (1) new fatty acids and cholesterol, (2) the formation of the ketone body, acetoacetic acid, and (3) the nerve transmitter substance, acetylcholine. It is formed during the catabolism of fatty acids, glucose, and amino acids; hence, excesses of these nutrients can be stored as fat. As already pointed out, acetyl CoA can enter the Krebs cycle. However, entry into this cycle is dependent upon continued availability of carbohydrates.

• **Ketosis**—Pyruvate, a product of carbohydrate catabolism, is needed to produce oxaloacetic acid. Oxaloacetic acid must then condense with acetyl CoA in order to produce citric acid. If there is insufficient oxaloacetic acid in the cell to keep the Krebs cycle functioning efficiently, the acetyl CoA is converted to acetoacetic acid, beta-hydroxybutyric acid, and acetone. These ketone bodies accumulate in the blood; and if the condition goes unchecked, acidosis will occur, often resulting in coma and death. Ketosis can be a complication of diabetes mellitus and starvation.

(Also see DIABETES MELLITUS; and STARVATION.)

ANABOLISM. Saturated fatty acids and monounsaturated fatty acids are rapidly and abundantly formed from acetyl CoA. Hence, any nutrient capable of yielding acetyl CoA during the metabolic processes can potentially contribute to fatty acid synthesis—a process called lipogenesis. While a limited amount of fat synthesis occurs in the mitochondria of the cell, most synthesis takes place outside the mitochondria via enzymes in the cytoplasm when supplemented with energy (ATP), carbon dioxide (CO_2), hydrogen, and the mineral magnesium (Mg +). The 2-carbon compound, acetyl CoA, is the primary building block. It is first carboxylated (organic acid group COOH added) to form malonyl CoA, and then it is transferred to a carrier protein—acyl-carrier protein (ACP). Malonyl-ACP then combines with acetyl CoA via acetyl ACP to form acetoacetyl-ACP which then has hydrogen added by NADPH generated in the pen-

tose shunt to convert to butyryl-ACP. More and more acetyl CoA and hydrogen are added to this molecule until the chain is 16 carbons long—palmitic acid. All fatty acids formed as described above are then transported back into the mitochondria where three fatty acids are joined—esterified—with one glycerol molecule, thus forming triglycerides. The glycerol is derived from the glycolytic pathway. Fatty acids may also be elon-gated in the mitochondria.

Acetyl CoA may also be used to synthesize cholesterol in many tissues, but the liver is the major site of synthesis.

(Also see CHOLESTEROL; and FATS AND OTHER LIPIDS.)

Proteins. Proteins are complex organic compounds made up chiefly of amino acids, which are present in characteristic proportions for each specific protein. This nutrient always contains carbon, hydrogen, oxygen, and nitrogen; and, in addition, it usually contains sulfur and frequently phosphorus. Proteins are essential in all plant and animal life as components of the active protoplasm of each living cell. The need for protein in the diet is actually a need for its constituents—the amino acids. For more than a century, the amino acids have been studied and recognized as important nutrients.

The dietary proteins are broken down into amino acids during digestion. They are then absorbed and distributed by the bloodstream to the body cells, which rebuild these amino acids into body proteins. Although the primary use of amino acids in the body is synthesis, amino acids can be catabolized as a source of energy.

CATABOLISM. Amino acids from the proteins are the primary sources of carbon skeletons utilized in gluconeogenesis—a process previously explained. In order that amino acids may enter energy metabolic pathways, they must first have their amino (NH_2) group removed—a process called oxidative deamination. This forms ammonia and a carbon skeleton that can be used for energy.

Following deamination, the carbon skeletons, depending upon their structure, can enter the Krebs cycle as pyruvic acid, alpha-ketoglutaric acid, succinic acid, fumaric acid, or oxaloacetic acid and be completely oxidized to carbon dioxide and water yielding the production of ATP (See Table M-16). Transamination—the transfer of an amino group (NH_2) to synthesize new amino acids—also forms carbon skeletons which can enter the Krebs cycle.

Most deaminated amino acids can be used to synthesize glucose by working backwards through glycolysis. This process is called gluconeogenesis, and amino acids capable of this are called gluconeogenic or glycogenic. Alanine is an important gluconeogenic amino acid. Alanine is formed in the muscles by transamination. When it is deaminated in the liver, it becomes pyruvic acid which the liver converts to glucose. Leucine is the only amino acid incapable of gluconeogenesis.

• **Urea**—The fate of the amino group (NH_2) split off from amino acids, presents a special metabolic problem. Fortunately, the body has developed the urea cycle for handling this substance. Most of the NH_2 is converted to urea in the liver for excretion by the kidneys. To facilitate elimination, 1 mole of ammonia (NH_3) combines with 1 mole of carbon dioxide (CO_2), another metabolic waste product. Phosphate is then added to this compound to produce carbamyl phosphate. Carbamyl phosphate then combines with ornithine to form citrulline—an intermediate in the urea cycle. The amino acid, aspartartic acid, contributes another amino group (NH_2), and citrulline is then converted to the amino acid arginine. Urea splits off from arginine forming ornithine, and the cycle is completed. The kidneys remove urea from the blood and excrete it in the urine.

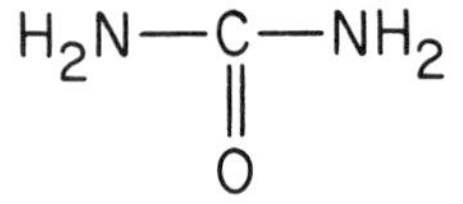

$$H_2N-\overset{\overset{\displaystyle O}{\|}}{C}-NH_2$$

Fig. M-50. The structure of urea—the means of eliminating amino groups from amino acids.

(Also see UREA CYCLE.)

ANABOLISM. The various amino acids are systematically joined together to form peptides and proteins. The amino portion (NH_2) of one amino acid will combine with the carboxyl (COOH) portion of another amino acid releasing water (H_2O) and forming a peptide linkage—like railroad cars joining to form a train. When numerous of these junctions occur, the resulting molecule is called a protein. The proteins of the body are the primary constituents of many structural and protective tissues—bones, ligaments, hair, fingernails, skin, organs, and muscles. Perhaps, most importantly enzymes are proteins, and they are responsible for most all of the catabolic and anabolic reactions.

Protein synthesis is not a random process whereby a number of amino acids are joined together; rather, it is a detailed predetermined procedure. Within the cell, DNA contains the coded information concerning the amino acid sequences of the various proteins to be synthesized in the cell. When DNA is decoded, amino acids are linked to form a specific protein which has its own particular physiological function.

Protein synthesis involves a series of reactions which are specific for *each* protein. A four step outline of this procedure follows:

1. Messenger RNA (ribonucleic acid) transcribes the sequence *message* from DNA to form a template (a pattern or guide) for protein synthesis. The sequences of the nucleotides in the DNA are the keys to the sequence pattern forming this template. This is possible because the nucleotides always pair off in the following manner: adenine (A) and thymine (T); adenine (A) and uracil (U); and guanine (G) and cytosine (C). Triplets of the purine (adenine and guanine) and pyrimidine (cytosine, thymine, and uracil) bases in the DNA form *codons* which correspond to specific amino acids and are signals which control protein synthesis. For example, the codon AGG (adenine, guanine, and guanine) signals the incorporation of arginine.

2. A specific transfer RNA (tRNA) combines with each respective amino acid to form an aminoacyl complex. This reaction requires the expenditure of energy. There is at least one specific tRNA for most of the 22 amino acids.

3. The initiation of protein synthesis occurs when the ribosome of the rough endoplasmic reticulum (site of protein synthesis) recognizes a codon specific for initiation. This first amino acid will be the amino (NH_2) terminal end of the protein. This amino acid is formulated to prevent the amino group of the amino acid from being incorporated in a peptide bond. Upon completion of the protein, the N-formyl group is cleaved from the protein.

4. Once synthesis has been initiated, the protein is elongated through a series of successive additions of amino acids as determined by the messenger RNA template. Each new amino acid is linked to the next by the formation of a peptide bond. Eventually the procedure will be terminated when a codon specific for terminating protein synthesis is reached. Thereupon, the protein splits off from the ribosomes.

Each sequence of amino acids is a different protein. Hence, different proteins are able to accomplish different functions in the body. With 22 amino acids, the different arrangements possible are endless, yielding a variety of proteins. For example, egg albumin, a small protein, contains approximately 288 amino acids. Thus, if one assumes that there are about 20 different amino acids in the albumin molecule, then mathematical calculations show that the possible arrangements of this number of amino acids are in excess of 10^{300}. (For comparison, one million is equal to 10^6.)

Since the DNA of each cell carries the master plan for forming proteins, genetic mutations often are manifested by disorders in protein metabolism. Many metabolic defects—inborn errors of metabolism—are the result of a missing or modified enzyme or other protein. The misplacement or omission of just one amino acid in a protein molecule can result in a nonfunctional protein. Therefore, when proteins are formed three requirements must be met: (1) the proper amino acids, (2) the proper number of amino acids, and (3) the proper order of the amino acid in the chain forming the protein. Meeting these requirements allows the formation of proteins which are very specific and which gives tissues their unique form, function and character.

(Also see INBORN ERRORS OF METABOLISM; and NUCLEIC ACIDS.)

Minerals And Vitamins. The metabolism of minerals and vitamins does not produce energy. However, minerals and vitamins are involved in many of the reactions in the body which comprise metabolism. The following table indicates some of the areas where minerals and vitamins are directly involved in metabolism. More information may be gained about minerals and vitamins under their separate entries.

(Also see MINERAL[S]; and VITAMIN[S].)

TABLE M-17
MINERAL AND VITAMIN FUNCTIONS IN METABOLISM

Mineral or Vitamin	Function
Minerals:	
Calcium	Cell wall permeability; enzyme activation; hormone secretion.
Phosphorus	Energy utilization (ATP formation); amino acid metabolism; protein formation; enzyme systems; formation of some fats (phospholipids).
Sodium	Acid-base balance of the body; absorption of sugars.
Chlorine	Acid-base balance; stomach acid; enzyme activitation.
Magnesium	Enzyme activation.
Potassium	Acid-base balance; enzyme reactions; nutrient transfer.
Sulfur	Component of the vitamins biotin and thiamin; component of coenzyme A (CoA).
Chromium	Component of the Glucose Transfer Factor; enzyme activation; stimulation of fatty acid synthesis.
Copper	Constituent of several enzyme systems.
Iodine	Constituent of thyroid hormones which act to regulate metabolism.
Iron	Component of cytochromes; component of hemoglobin which brings oxygen to the tissues.

(Continued)

TABLE M-17 *(Continued)*

Mineral or Vitamin	Function
Manganese	Enzyme activator.
Molybdenum	Component of enzyme systems.
Selenium	Enzyme component.
Zinc	Component of enzyme systems.
Vitamins:	
A	Synthesis of protein, some hormones, and glycogen.
D	Regulates calcium and phosphorus.
E	Regulator of DNA synthesis, and coenzyme Q, a hydrogen carrier.
Biotin	Coenzyme in decarboxylation (removal of carbon dioxide) and carboxylation (addition of carbon dioxide) reactions of carbohydrate, fat, and protein metabolism; for example, pyruvic acid to oxaloacetic acid, and acetyl CoA to malonyl CoA; formation of purines; formation of urea; deamination of amino acids.
Choline	Transport and metabolism of fats; source of methyl groups (CH_3).
Folacin	Formation of coenzymes for synthesis of DNA and RNA; amino acid synthesis.
Niacin	Constituent of the two coenzymes nicotinamide adenine dinucleotide (NAD) and nicotinamide adenine dinucleotide phosphate (NADP) which transport hydrogen during energy formation.
Pantothenic acid	Form part of coenzyme A (CoA) and the acyl carrier protein (ACP).
Riboflavin	Forms coenzymes like flavin adenine dinucleotide (FAD) which is responsible for transport of hydrogen ions.
Thiamin	A coenzyme in energy metabolism via decarboxylation of pyruvic acid and formation of acetyl CoA.
Vitamin B-6	As a coenzyme for: transamination, decarboxylation, deamination, transsulfuration, absorption of amino acids, conversion of glycogen to glucose, and fatty acid conversions.
Vitamin B-12	Coenzyme in protein synthesis.
Vitamin C	Makes iron available for hemoglobin synthesis, metabolism of the amino acid tyrosine and tryptophan.

Water.   Water is a vital nutrient. It is the solvent wherein the metabolic reactions of the body take place. Also, as a solvent, water carries (1) the nutrients which are subjected to cellular metabolism, and (2) the waste products of metabolism. Also, it serves to disperse the heat generated by the metabolic reactions. In many of the metabolic reactions water is either added or subtracted. Subtracted water is termed metabolic water. The addition of water is termed hydrolysis.

(Also see WATER; and WATER AND ELECTROLYTES.)

EXCRETION.   Products not used and products formed during metabolism must be continually removed from the body. The three major routes of removal are: (1) feces, (2) urine, and (3) lungs. The feces serve to remove materials that cannot be digested or absorbed. Urea, produced from the metabolism of amino acids is excreted by the kidneys into the urine, along with excess water, mineral salts, and some other compounds formed during metabolism. Carbon dioxide produced during metabolism is excreted from the body via the lungs. For every 2,100 Calories (kcal), about 327 liters of carbon dioxide are produced in the body.

FACTORS CONTROLLING METABOLISM.   The rate at which the body utilizes nutrients, and the direction of metabolism—anabolism or catabolism, are controlled by a variety of factors, but primarily the nervous system and endocrine systems. Many of these factors are interrelated and some are more important than others. Generally, metabolism is discussed in terms of energy, since energy to drive the machinery of the body is the first concern. The metabolic rate is the rate at which the body uses energy—calories—packaged in ATP. Some factors affecting metabolism follow:

• **Exercise**—Perhaps, muscular activity is the most powerful stimulus for increasing the metabolic rate. Short bursts of strenuous exercise can increase the metabolic rate to 40 times that of the resting state.

• **Recent ingestion of food**—Following a meal, the metabolic rate rises. This increase is dependent upon the type of food eaten. Carbohydrates and fats elevate the metabolic rate 4 to 15%, whereas proteins increase the rate 30 to 60%. This phenomenon is known as the specific dynamic action of foods (SDA).

• **Environmental temperature**—Increases or decreases in the environmental temperature increase the metabolic rate.

• **Body surface area**—Body surface area is a function of height and weight. A person weighing 200 lb (*91 kg*) has about 30% more surface area than a person weighing 100 lb (*45.5 kg*), when both are the same height. Hence, the larger person's metabolic rate is about 30% greater, not twice as great as is the weight.

• **Sex**—Females have a slightly lower metabolic rate than males throughout life.

• **Pregnancy and lactation**—The metabolic rate rises during pregnancy and lactation.

• **Age**—Metabolic rate gradually declines with age. During growth, energy is needed for the anabolic processes.

• **Emotional state**—Various emotional states—fear, anger, shock—stimulate the release of the hormones epinephrine and norepinephrine which can increase the metabolic rate 100% on a short term basis.

• **State of nutrition**—During prolonged undernutrition the body adapts by decreasing the metabolic rate by as much as 50%.

• **Body temperature**—For every one degree increase in body temperature during a fever, the metabolic rate increases 7%.

• **Hormones**—Many of the above changes in metabolism are ultimately due to some hormonal change. Most of the hormones direct the metabolic processes. The storage and release of glucose is hormone mediated. Protein synthesis is hormone mediated, as is the release of fatty acids from fats. The thyroid hormones can, on a long-term basis, raise the metabolic rate 100%. Conversely, undersecretion can cause the metabolic rate to fall 50% below normal. Other hormones control water and minerals, and still others control the digestive processes.

(Also see CALORIC [ENERGY] EXPENDITURE; ENDOCRINE GLANDS; and ENERGY UTILIZATION BY THE BODY.)

INBORN ERRORS OF METABOLISM.   At times the metabolism of the nutrients cannot proceed normally due to some defect in the genetic information that exists at birth or shortly thereafter. These defects can affect the metabolism of carbohydrates, proteins, and fats; hence, they are referred to as inborn errors of metabolism. Often they are due to production of a nonfunctional enzyme or complete lack of an enzyme involved in the metabolic scheme. Since enzymes are protein, their production relies upon correct genetic information. Many of these inborn errors have serious consequences, but fortunately most are rare. Familiar examples of errors in carbohydrate metabolism include lactose intolerance and galactosemia. Familiar examples of errors in protein metabolism include albinism, maple syrup urine disease, and phenylketonuria. The hyperlipoproteinemias are familiar examples of inborn errors of fat metabolism.

(Also see INBORN ERRORS OF METABOLISM.)

SUMMARY.   Although metabolism is discussed in parts —pathways, nutrients, and cycles—it is an interrelated, continuous process—the sum of all chemical changes in the body. While some organs have more important roles, metabolic processes occur in every cell of the body—from those in the big toe to brain cells. Energy production in the form of ATP is the first concern of metabolism, and water (H_2O), carbon dioxide (CO_2), and urea are the major waste products of metabolism.

METABOLITE

Any substance produced by metabolism or by a metabolic process.

METALLOENZYME

An enzyme of which a metal (ion) is an integral part of its active structure. Examples: carbonic anhydrase (zinc) and cytochromes (iron, copper).

METHIONINE

An essential amino acid which contains sulfur. Furthermore, methionine participates in a biochemical reaction in the body called transmethylation by donating a methyl group (CH_3).

(Also see AMINO ACID[S].)

METHYL ALCOHOL (WOOD ALCOHOL; CH₃OH METHANOL)

The simplest of the alcohols, but it is highly toxic when ingested. As little as 20 ml may cause (1) permanent blindness as a result of the formaldehyde formed by the metabolism of the methyl alcohol damaging the retina of the eye, or (2) death due to severe acidosis. Poisoning due to methyl alcohol is almost always a case of ingestion as a substitute for ethyl alcohol—the alcohol of liquors. Rather ironically, part of the treatment for methyl alcohol poisoning consists of administering ethyl alcohol. Aside from its adverse effects when ingested, methyl alcohol is an important industrial chemical utilized for numerous processes and products.

METHYLATED SPIRITS

Ethyl alcohol to which methyl alcohol has been added to render it unfit for consumption as a beverage. Often called denatured alcohol. The added methyl alcohol makes it highly poisonous.

(Also see METHYL ALCOHOL.)

MEULENGRACHT DIET

A diet for peptic ulcer patients first introduced by the Danish Physician Meulengracht in 1935. It is more liberal than the *Sippy Diet*, which was initiated in 1915 by the American Physician, Bertram Sippy. The Sippy Diet holds rather rigidly to a program of milk and cream feeding with slow additions of single soft food items over a prolonged period of time. To begin with, the Meulengracht Diet consists of milk, eggs, pureed fruits and vegetables, custard, ice cream, gelatin, plain pudding, crackers, bread and butter. Then, after 2 days, ground or minced meats and broiled, baked, or creamed fish are included. Taboo foods are coffee, tea, cocoa, soft drinks, alcoholic beverages, spices, nuts, and pastries.

(Also see MODIFIED DIETS; and ULCERS, PEPTIC.)

MEVALONIC ACID (C₆H₁₂O₄)

In the human body, mevalonic acid occurs as a precursor in the manufacture of cholesterol. In bacterial cultures, mevalonic acid can replace acetate as a growth promoting factor for *Lactobacillus acidophilus*, a bacterium producing lactic acid.

MICELLAR BILE-FAT COMPLEX

A micelle is a particle formed by an aggregate of molecules —a microscopic unit of protoplasm. In the micellar bile-fat complex, the particle is formed by the combination of bile salts with fat substances (fatty acids and glycerides) to facilitate the absorption of fat across the intestinal mucosa.

MICELLE

A microscopic particle of lipids and bile salts.

MICROCYTE

A small red blood cell.

MICROGRAM

A metric measure of weight which is equal to one millionth of a gram or one thousandth of a milligram. One ounce of a substance weighs over 28 million micrograms.

MICRONUTRIENTS

These are nutrients that are present in the body, and required by the body in minute quantities, ranging from millionths of a gram (microgram) to thousandths of a gram (milligram). Examples are vitamin B-12, pantothenic acid, chromium, cobalt, copper, fluorine, iodine, iron, manganese, molybdenum, selenium, silicon, and zinc. Their minuteness in no way diminishes their importance to human nutrition— many are known to be absolutely essential.

(Also see MINERAL[S]; TRACE ELEMENTS; and VITAMIN[S].)

MICROVILLI

Minute (visible only through an electron microscope) surface projections that cover the edge of each intestinal villus, called the brush border. The microvilli add a tremendous surface area for absorption.

MICROWAVE COOKING

Although microwave cooking has been available since the 1950s, it took 20 years for the microwave oven to become a common item on the market.

The magnetron tube is a vacuum tube which can convert electricity into electromagnetic energy radiation. In microwave cooking, food is cooked by the heat generated in the food itself.

The frequencies for microwave heating come under the rules of the Federal Communications Commission, which has designated four frequencies—915, 2450, 5800, and 22,125 mc/sec. The majority of the microwave ovens on the market today use 2450 megacycles.

It requires skill and experience to use the microwave oven successfully. Although it cooks foods in ½ to ⅓ the time of an electric oven, there are the following problems:

1. The microwave oven does not brown the food.

2. Frequently, microwaves do not penetrate a roast uniformly, with the result that there may be variations in doneness of meat. Thus, unless pork cooked in a microwave oven is subjected to a temperature of 170°F (77°C) *throughout* to destroy any organisms that might be present, *Trichinella spiralis* (the parasite that causes trichinosis) and food poisoning bacteria may not be destroyed.

(Also see FOOD—BUYING, PREPARING, COOKING, AND SERVING, section headed "Methods and Media of Cooking".)

MILK-ALKALI SYNDROME

A condition usually associated with sufferers of peptic ulcers wherein the sufferer consumes large amounts of milk and a readily absorbed alkali over a period of years resulting in hypercalcemia—high levels of calcium in the blood. Symptoms consist of vomiting, gastrointestinal bleeding, and increased blood pressure. Furthermore, kidney stones are common and calcium may be deposited in other soft tissues. The use of nonabsorbable antacids in peptic ulcer therapy seems to have lessened the prevalence of the milk-alkali syndrome.

(Also see ANTACIDS; and HYPERCALCEMIA.)

MILK AND MILK PRODUCTS

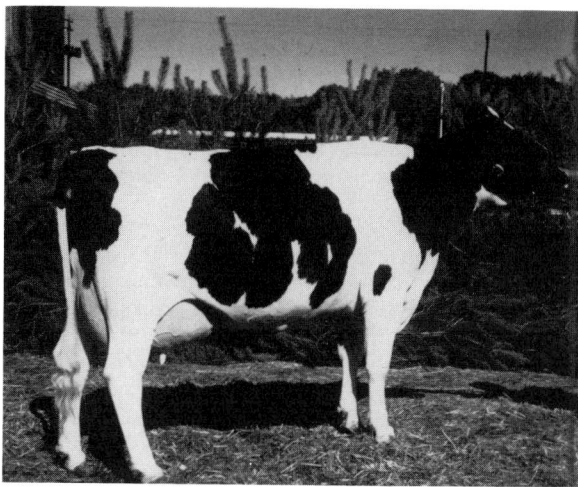

Fig. M-51. Foster mother of the human race. (Courtesy, Holstein-Friesian Assn. of America, Brattleboro, Vt.)

Milk is the fluid normally secreted by female mammals for the nourishment of their young.

Milk products include a diverse group of foods made from milk, including butter, cheese, dried nonfat milk, condensed and evaporated milk, yogurt, etc.

In different parts of the world, milk from various species of animals is used for food. In the United States, however, the cow furnishes virtually all of the available market milk. Therefore, unless otherwise stated, the terms *milk* and *milk products* as used in this section refer to cow's milk.

HISTORY AND DEVELOPMENT OF THE DAIRY INDUSTRY.

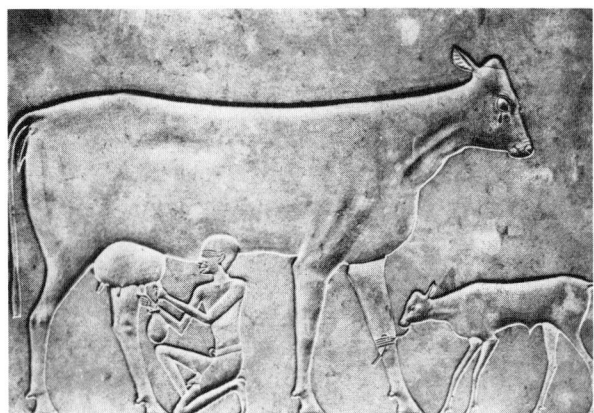

Fig. M-52. Dairy scene from ancient Egypt, from bas-relief found in the tomb of Princess Kewitt. Note man milking cow while calf is fastened to left foreleg. (Courtesy, The Bettmann Archive, Inc., New York, N.Y.)

Long before recorded history, the first food provided for mankind was from women's mammary glands. In remote times, when nature failed to bless the newborn child with a lactating mother, the baby suckled another mother, or suckled an animal, or died.

In due time, man found that milk was good—and good for him—with the result that he began domesticating milk-producing animals. However, under natural conditions, wild animals produce only enough milk for their offspring. So, man began selecting them for higher production for his own use. For the most part, this included the cow, the buffalo, and the goat—although the ewe, the mare, the sow, and other mammals have been used for producing milk for human consumption in different parts of the world. The importance of the cow in milk production is attested to by her well-earned designation as *the foster mother of the human race*.

As the cow population expanded throughout the world and as milk production became a specialized phase of agriculture, methods were developed for concentrating and preserving milk foods for future use, barter, and/or international trade. Dairying progressed from an art to a science—drawing upon genetics, chemistry, physics, bacteriology, heat, refrigeration, engineering, business, and other branches of knowledge, in order to improve dairy commodities, create new ones, and profitably distribute them in both domestic and world commerce.

Hand in hand with improvements and expansion in production and processing, recognition of the nutritional importance of milk and milk products increased. Following World War II, milk and milk foods were established as one of the groups of foods contributing the essentials of an adequate diet—first as one division of the Seven Food Groups, later in the Four Food Groups, and presently in the Six Food Groups (Food Guide Pyramid).

MILK FROM VARIOUS SPECIES.
Most of the world's milk is produced by cows. However, 8.6%—slightly less than one-twelfth—of the global milk supply comes from buffaloes, goats, and sheep. Yet, in 16 Asian countries for which data are available, only 51.5% of the milk is from cows, while water buffaloes, goats, and sheep produce 11.1, 15.2, and 22.2%, respectively. Mares are also used for producing milk for human consumption in different parts of the world.

A comparison of milks from various species, including humans, is given in Table M-18.

Goat Milk. Goats have played an important role in supplying milk for man since prehistoric times, and they still do in many areas. Approximately 400 million goats, including milk, mohair and meat goats, exist throughout the world, most of them in India, China, Turkey, Ethiopia, Iran, and Brazil. Although goats supply less than 3% of the worldwide milk supply for man, it is believed that more people consume goat milk than cow's milk, even though the per capita consumption may be small. This is because the highly populated countries of Asia and Africa have 70% of the world's goats.

Dairy goats commonly produce 3 to 4 qt (*2.9 to 3.8 liter*) of milk (6 to 8 lb) daily, although some yield 20 lb (*9.1 kg*) or more daily at the peak of lactation. Goat milk resembles cow's milk in composition (see Table M-18). However, the fat globules of goat milk are smaller and tend to remain suspended (little cream rises to the top); hence, homogenization is unnecessary. Also, goat milk is whiter in color than cow's milk, because the goat is essentially 100% efficient in converting carotene to vitamin A; it follows that butter made from goat milk is white, also. Goat milk produced under sanitary conditions is sweet, tasty, and free of off-flavors. Goat milk should be produced, handled, and processed much like cow's milk. The most important dairy goat products are milk and cheese, although goat milk can be manufactured into all the products made from cow's milk.

Since the time of Hippocrates, physicians have recommended goat milk for infants and invalids because it is easily digested. Also, those allergic to cow milk can usually drink goat milk without ill effects; and goat milk is widely used by persons afflicted with stomach ulcers.

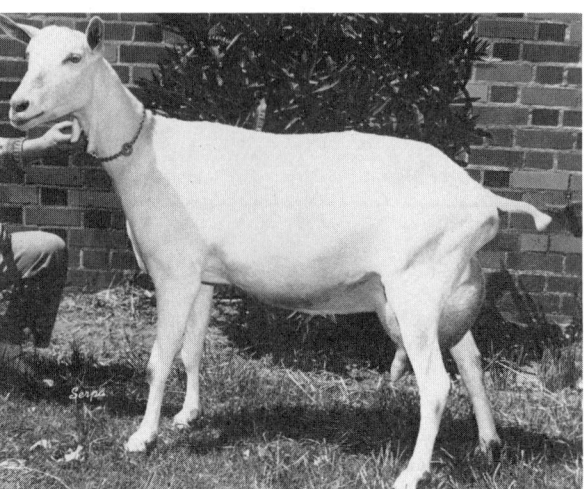

Fig. M-53. Saanen doe, Laurelwood Acres Merna, owned by Laurelwood Acres, Ripon, Calif. (Courtesy, *Dairy Goat Journal*)

TABLE M-18
COMPOSITION OF MILKS FROM DIFFERENT SPECIES[1]
(Amount in 100 g edible portion. Dashes denote lack of reliable data for a constituent believed to be present in measurable amounts.)

Nutrient	Species				
	Cow	Human	Buffalo	Goat	Sheep
Water .... (g)	87.99	87.50	83.39	87.03	80.70
Food energy .... (kcal)	61	70	97	69	108
.... (kj)	257	291	404	288	451
Carbohydrate, total .... (g)	4.66	6.89	5.18	4.45	5.36
Fat .... (g)	3.34	4.38	6.89	4.14	7.00
Cholesterol .... (mg)	14	14	19	11	—
Protein (N × 6.38) .... (g)	3.29	1.03	3.75	3.56	5.98
Fiber .... (g)	0	0	0	0	0
Ash .... (g)	.72	.20	.79	.82	.96
Macrominerals					
Calcium .... (mg)	119	32	169	134	193
Phosphorus .... (mg)	93	14	117	111	158
Sodium .... (mg)	49	17	52	50	44
Magnesium .... (mg)	13	3	31	14	18
Potassium .... (mg)	152	51	178	204	136
Microminerals					
Iron .... (mg)	.05	.03	.12	.05	.10
Zinc .... (mg)	.38	.17	.22	.30	—
Fat-soluble vitamins					
Vitamin A .... (RE)	31	64	53	56	42
.... (IU)	126	241	178	185	147
Water-soluble vitamins					
Folacin .... (mcg)	5	5	6	1	—
Niacin .... (mg)	.084	.177	.091	.277	.417
Pantothenic acid .... (mg)	.314	.223	.192	.310	.407
Riboflavin .... (mg)	.162	.036	.135	.138	.355
Thiamin .... (mg)	.038	.014	.052	.048	.065
Vitamin B-6 .... (mg)	.042	.011	.023	.046	—
Vitamin B-12 .... (mcg)	.357	.045	.363	.065	.711
Vitamin C (ascorbic acid)	.94	5.00	2.25	1.29	4.16

[1]*Newer Knowledge of Milk and Other Fluid Dairy Products,* National Dairy Council, Rosemont, Ill., 1979, p. 44, Table D.

MILK FROM COW TO TABLE. Fig. M-54 illustrates how milk gets from the cow to the table.

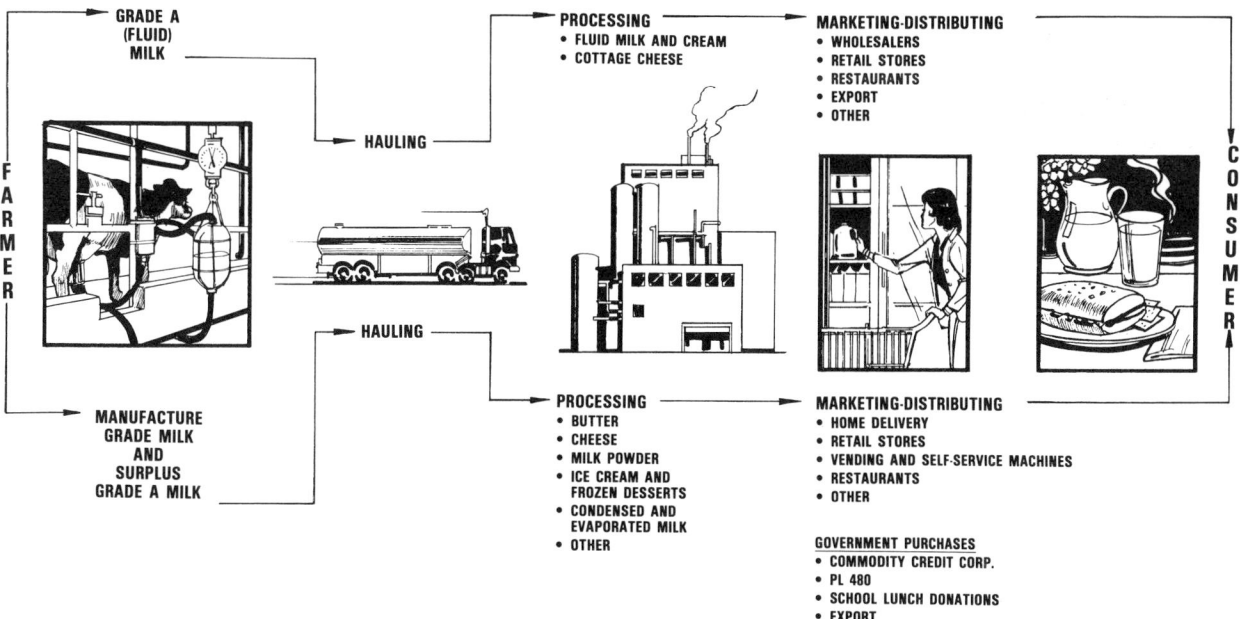

Fig. M-54. Steps and channels for getting milk from cows to table.

In summary form, the stages in getting milk from the cow to the table follow:

1. Milk is secreted by the mammary glands of a cow, beginning with the birth of a calf and continuing for about 305 days.

2. Milk is removed through the teats, generally by machine milking, although hand milking is still done.

3. Milk is cooled, usually in bulk tanks, to at least 50°F (preferably 40°F) as soon after milking as possible in order to inhibit bacterial growth.

4. Insulated trucks usually pick up milk from dairy farms daily and transport it to processing plants.

5. Processors (a) process and package fluid milk, or (b) manufacture milk into various products.

6. Milk and milk products are distributed through wholesale and retail channels to consumers.

NUTRIENTS OF MILK.[19] Although fluid whole milk is a liquid food (88% water), it contains an average of 12% solids (total solids include all the constituents of milk except water) and 8.6% solids-not-fat (includes carbohydrate, protein, minerals, and water-soluble vitamins).

More than 100 components have been identified in milk. Two glasses (1 pt) of whole milk provides approximately 23 g of carbohydrate (total), 16.3 g of fat, 16 g of protein, 3.5 g of minerals, plus fat-soluble and water-soluble vitamins. But the composition of milk varies in response to physiological factors (inherited or genetic) and environmental factors. Variations in composition occur among breeds, between milkings, and between milk taken from different sections of the udder. Also, the composition of milk is affected by the feed, the environment temperature, the season, and the age of the cow.

Milk plays an important role in the diet of the average American, as is shown in Table M-19 and Fig. M-55. The major nutrients provided by dairy products in the American diet are food energy (9.6%), fat (11.7%), protein (19.5%), calcium (75.1%), phosphorus (34.3%), vitamin A (15.8%), and riboflavin (32.6%).

TABLE M-19
FOOD NUTRIENTS: U.S. PERCENTAGE OF TOTAL CONTRIBUTED BY LIVESTOCK AND POULTRY PRODUCTS, 1988[1]

	Food Energy	Carbo-hydrates	Fat	Pro-tein	Cal-cium	Phos-phorus	Mag-nesium	Iron	Vitamin A Value	Niacin	Ribo-flavin	Thiamin	Vitamin B-6	Vitamin B-12
							(%)							
Dairy products, excluding butter	9.6	5.3	11.7	19.5	75.1	34.3	18.5	2.4	15.8	1.6	32.6	7.5	10.2	18.5
Meat, fish, and poultry ...	18.8	0.1	31.7	43.3	3.9	29.2	15.4	22.1	20.6	44.8	22.2	25.0	40.5	76.1
Eggs	1.4	0.1	2.0	4.0	1.9	3.9	1.0	2.9	4.0	0.1	7.2	0.9	2.2	3.7
Total	29.8	5.5	45.4	66.8	80.9	67.4	34.9	27.4	40.4	46.5	62.0	33.4	52.9	98.3

[1]*Agricultural Statistics 1991*, p. 478.

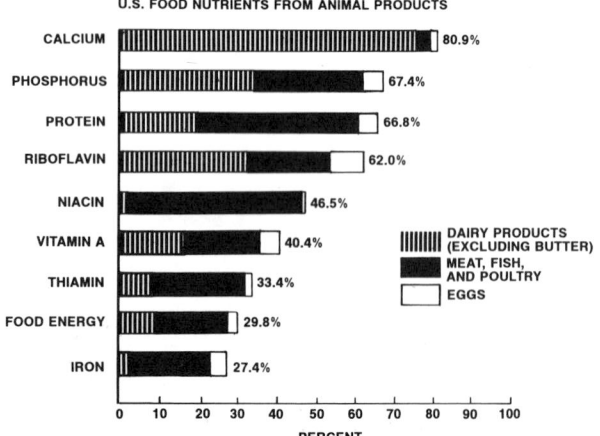

Fig. M-55. Percentage of food nutrients contributed by animal products of the total supply in the U.S.

The major components of milk—carbohydrate, fat, and protein—possess a wide range of nutritional and functional properties which lend themselves to application in a variety of food formulations. Milk is also a valuable source of certain minerals and vitamins.

Carbohydrates In Milk. Lactose is, by far, the most abundant sugar in milk, constituting about 4.9% of cow's milk and 7.0% of human milk. This disaccharide, consisting of glucose and galactose, is only one-sixth as sweet as sucrose (table sugar) and is less soluble in water. In the small intestine, lactose is cleaved to form its constituent monosaccharides. Glucose is readily absorbed, while galactose is slowly absorbed, thereby serving as a growth promotant for intestinal bacteria that synthesize the vitamins biotin, folacin, and riboflavin in the intestine. Lactose is also converted to lactic acid by intestinal bacteria. When lactic acid is produced in the intestines, growth of pathogenic bacteria is inhibited.

Lactose has been shown to facilitate the absorption of calcium. Also, there are reports that lactose enhances the absorption of barium, magnesium, phosphorus, radium, strontium, and zinc.

Glucose and galactose are the products of lactose hydrolysis by the enzyme lactase. Some individuals are unable to metabolize lactose because of reduced lactase levels, a condition termed lactose intolerance. Preparations of the enzyme lactase are now being marketed for commercial and consumer addition to milk. The resulting milk is sweeter tasting because the majority of the lactose is hydrolyzed to glucose and galactose.

Lactose has many food uses; among them, the following: as an anticaking ingredient in dry mixtures such as nondairy coffee whiteners; as a flavor enhancer in dusting powders to flavor potato chips, barbecue sauces, salad dressings, pie fillings, and puddings; in candies and confectionery products; and in the bakery industry.

(Also see subsequent section headed "Lactose Intolerance.")

---

[19]In the preparation of this section, the authors adapted material from the following publications by the National Dairy Council: *Newer Knowledge of Milk and Other Fluid Dairy Products*, and *Dairy Council Digest*, Vol. 48, No. 5; published by National Dairy Council, Rosemont, Ill.

Milk Fat. Milk fat, sometimes called butterfat, contributes about 48% of the calories of whole milk. Fat also gives milk its flavor.

Milk fat is highly emulsified, which facilitates its digestion. Since fats must be liquid or emulsified at body temperature to be digested and absorbed, and since milk fat has a melting point lower than body temperature, it is efficiently utilized—particularly by the young and the elderly.

Fat is the most variable constituent of milk, the amount being affected primarily by such factors as breed of cow and environmental temperature (a given cow will produce higher fat milk in cool weather than in hot weather). Minor factors affecting the amount of milk fat include the type and amount of feed and the stage of lactation. Feed also influences the fatty acid composition of the fat produced; for example, cows consuming succulent feed or pasture produce much more oleic acid than cows receiving dry roughage.

Milk fat consists of 12.5% glycerol and 87.5% fatty acids, by weight. The fatty acids combine with glycerol in units of three fatty acid molecules per glycerol molecule to form triglycerides which make up 95 to 96% of the total milk fat.

Milk fat contains a greater number of different fatty acids than any other food fat; approximately 500 different fatty acids and fatty acid derivatives have been identified in milk. Milk fat contains a relatively high proportion of short-chain fatty acids. These short-chain fatty acids (which are virtually absent in most vegetable oils) are water-soluble, are absorbed through the intestinal wall without being resynthesized to glycerides, and are transported in the portal vein directly to the liver where they are immediately converted to forms utilizable for energy. For this reason, they serve as a quick source of energy, which may be important—especially early in life.

Generally, the fatty acids are approximately 66% saturated (devoid of double bonds between the carbon atoms), 30% monounsaturated, and 4% polyunsaturated. The saturated fatty acids present in largest amounts in milk fat are myristic, palmitic, and stearic. The chief unsaturated (double-bond linkage between the carbon atoms) fatty acids are oleic, linoleic, and linolenic. Arachidonic acid, which has four double bonds, is present in trace amounts. Arachidonic acid and its precursor, linoleic acid, are essential fatty acids—they are not synthesized in the human body, or they are not synthesized fast enough; consequently, they must be supplied in the diet.

Milk fat is available in the food industry as conventional butter, anhydrous milk fat, or anhydrous butter oil.

Besides butter, fluid whole milk, cheeses, and ice cream are the main dairy foods in which milk fat is consumed in the United States. Milk fat is also used in the candy industry, in the baking industry; and, in the form of butter, in soups, and sauces for frozen and canned vegetables.

Cholesterol is the principal sterol in milk. An 8-oz (1 cup, or *240 ml*) serving of whole fluid milk (3.34% fat) contains 33 mg of cholesterol, whereas a similar serving of fluid skim milk (0.1% fat) contains 4 mg of cholesterol. In order to limit the consumption of cholesterol to 300 mg per day, as is recommended by most health professionals, low-fat dairy products may be used.

Protein In Milk. Fluid whole milk contains an average of 3.3% protein, mainly casein and whey proteins. Protein accounts for about 38% of the total solids-not-fat content of milk and for about 22% of the calories of whole milk. Dairy products (excluding butter) contributed 19.5% of the total protein in the U.S. diet in 1990.

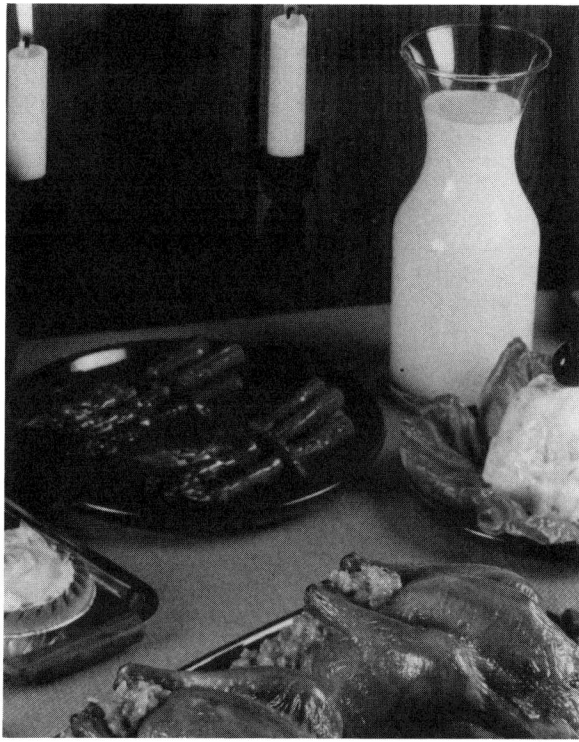

Fig. M-56. Dinner for two, includes, a carafe of milk. (Courtesy, American Dairy Assn., Rosemont, Ill.)

The proteins of milk are of very high quality, having a biological value of 85 as compared to 50 to 65 for the cereal proteins. They contain, in varying amounts, all of the amino acids required by man. Except for the sulfur-containing amino acids (methionine and cystine), 1 pt (*470 ml*) of milk supplies the recommended daily allowance of all the essential amino acids. Additionally, the protein to calorie ratio is very favorable in milk, assuring that the consumer is not ingesting *empty* calories.

It is also noteworthy that milk is rich in the amino acid tryptophan, a precursor of niacin; hence, milk is an excellent source of niacin equivalents. (One niacin equivalent is defined as 1 mg of niacin or 60 mg of tryptophan.) It is noteworthy, too, that the immunoglobulins in milk are a heterogeneous group of antibody proteins that serve as a source of passive immunity for the newborn, and that colostrum contains large quantities of globulins. A discussion of milk proteins follows:

• **Casein**—Comprising about 82% of the total protein content, casein is found only in milk, in which it is the principal protein. It gives milk its white color. Casein alone has a somewhat lower biological value than the whey proteins because of the limited quantity of the sulfur-containing amino acids. Commercial casein is made by either of two techniques: (1) precipitation by acid, or (2) coagulation by rennin. This procedure is followed by washing and drying the casein curd to a granular powder. The caseins and caseinates (sodium caseinate and calcium caseinate) are concentrated forms of proteins which have exceptional water-binding, fat-emulsifying and whipping capabilities.

Casein has been utilized as the main source of protein in the manufacture of meat analogs and as a protein supplement in some meat products. Also, it has found application in baked goods and as an ingredient of coffee whitener and whipped toppings.

Sodium caseinates are used in the meat industry as water-binding agents, as well as in the preparation of toppings, cream substitutes, and numerous desserts as whip-imparting agents.

Calcium caseinate, while significantly less soluble than the sodium salt, is used in various specialized dietary foods where low sodium intake is essential.

• **Whey protein**—A by-product of cheese and casein manufacture, whey is the liquid that remains after the removal of casein and fat from milk.

Like casein, whey protein is a complex mixture of a large number of protein fractions, with beta-lactoglobulin and alpha-lactalbumin being the principal ones of commercial interest. The whey proteins have a relative surplus of the sulfur-containing amino acids.

Recent advances have made the production of undenatured whey protein concentrates (WPC) a commercial reality. Among the uses made of WPC in food products are: in the fortification of acid fruit drinks and carbonated beverages; in cake flour; in dessert topping; and as a binder in the production of textured vegetable protein products. Also, the excellent binding, emulsifying, and gelling properties of WPC have been utilized in the formulation of meat products, soups, and sauces. In addition to the contributions that whey proteins make toward improved organoleptic characteristics in other foods, their nutritional contributions should not be underestimated.

• **Co-precipitates**—As the name implies, co-precipitates contain the total milk proteins that are precipitated from fresh milk. They are unique in that they contain both caseins and whey proteins, thus making them of high nutritional value. The low content of lactose also makes these coprecipitates useful in formulations where the use of dry milk powder may be unacceptable. Co-precipitates have found uses in baking, in dessert and confectionery products, and in meat analogs.

Minerals In Milk. Minerals are generally classified as macrominerals or microminerals, according to the amounts needed in the diet. These two groupings will be used in the discussion that follows:

• **Macrominerals**—Minerals that are needed at levels of 100 mg or more daily are generally classified as macrominerals.

1. **Calcium.** Of all the foods commonly eaten in the American diet, milk is one of the best and most commonly consumed sources of calcium. Dairy products (exclusive of butter) contributed 75.1% of the total calcium in the U.S. diet in 1990.

It is difficult to meet the RDA for calcium without including milk or milk products in the diet. Two 8-oz glasses (1 pt or *480 ml*) of milk daily will provide about 73% of the adult RDA for calcium. An additional allowance of 400 mg of calcium per day (a total of 1.2 g) during pregnancy and lactation will provide for the needs of the mother, the growing fetus, and the infant; a quart *(950 ml)* of milk will meet approximately 97% of this calcium allowance. For children 1 to 10 years of age, 800 mg of calcium daily are recommended, an allowance which is amply met by three 8-oz glasses of milk. During periods of rapid growth in preadolescence and puberty, 1.2 g of calcium per day are recommended, an amount supplied by 1 qt of milk.

2. **Phosphorus.** Dairy products (exclusive of butter) contributed 34.4% of the total phosphorus in the U.S. diet in 1990.

The RDA for phosphorus is the same as that for calcium after 1 year of age, thus two glasses *(480 ml)* of milk will supply the same percentage of the RDA for phosphorus as that for calcium.

3. **Magnesium.** Dairy products (exclusive of butter) contributed 18.5% of the total magnesium in the U.S. diet in 1990.

The RDA for magnesium is about 350 and 280 mg for adult males and females, respectively. Milk contains about 13 mg per 100 g; so, two 8-oz glasses (1 pt) furnish about 19% of the magnesium RDA for the adult male and 20.5% for the adult female.

• **Microminerals**—These are the minerals which are needed at levels of a few milligrams daily. Of the 103 known microminerals, 17 exhibit biological function in man and animals. The contribution which milk makes to the essential trace element intake is greatest with respect to zinc and possibly iodine.

The microminerals in milk are derived from the cow's feedstuffs, water, and environment. The concentrations are highly variable due to stage of lactation, season, milk yield, amount of the trace element in the cow's diet, handling of the milk following pasteurization, and storage conditions.

1. **Iodine.** Iodine is present in milk, but in variable amounts. As sea water is rich in iodine, milk from coastal agricultural areas contains more iodine than milk from inland areas. The iodine content of milk is highly dependent upon the composition of the animal's feed; it can be increased by as much as 200 times by adding iodine to the feed or by giving iodized salt blocks. Whole milk normally contains 13 to 37 mcg iodine per 100 g. So, two 8-oz glasses *(480 ml)* of milk supply about 25 to 69% of the iodine RDA for an adult man, 25 to 50 years of age.

2. **Iron.** Milk is a poor source of iron. The iron content of milk ranges from 10 to 90 mcg per 100 g. Feeding supplemental iron to cows does not increase the iron content of milk. However, milk is a very satisfactory food for iron fortification.

Two 8-oz glasses (1 pt) of milk provide about 1% of the iron recommended for women of childbearing age.

3. **Zinc.** This mineral occurs in many foods, including milk. The zinc content of milk varies from 0.3 to 0.6 mg per 100 g of milk, with an average of 0.38 mg. It may be slightly increased by feeding a zinc supplement to the cow. About 88% of zinc in milk is associated with casein; thus, the level of zinc in milk is mostly related to the milk protein content. It follows that the zinc content of lowfat and skim milk is virtually identical to that of whole milk.

Two 8-oz glasses (1 pt) of milk provide about 14% of the zinc RDA for adults.

(Also see MINERAL[S].)

Vitamins in Milk. For convenience, the vitamins in milk are grouped and discussed as fat-soluble vitamins and water-soluble vitamins in the discussion that follows:

• **Fat-soluble vitamins**—Vitamins A, D, E, and K are associated with the fat component of milk. Their quantities in milk, with the exception of vitamin K are dependent upon the dietary intake of the cow.

1. Vitamin A and its precursors, the carotenoids (principally beta-carotene), are present in high, but variable, quantities in milk. The carotenoids, which give milk its characteristic creamy color, constitute from 11 to 50% of the total vitamin A activity of milk. The carotenoid intake of the cow varies seasonally, generally being highest when the animals are on pasture.

One hundred grams of whole milk contain about 126 IU of vitamin A (31 RE); so, 1 qt *(960 ml)*, of whole milk will supply about 30% of the vitamin A recommended dietary allowance (RDA) of 5,000 IU (1,000 RE) for the adult male.

2. **Vitamin D.** Vitamin D (ergocalciferol and cholecalciferol), the ricket-preventing vitamin, is present in low concentrations in unfortified milk. However, approximately 98% of the fluid milk marketed in the United States is fortified with vitamin D to obtain standardized amounts of 400 IU (10 mcg cholecalciferol) per quart, the recommended intake for most persons.

The addition of vitamin D to fluid whole milk—thereby resulting in a widely used food providing calcium, phosphorus, and vitamin D—has been credited with the virtual eradication of rickets among children in the United States. The vitamin D fortification of milk to provide a concentration of 400 IU per quart has been endorsed by the Food and Nutrition Board, National Research Council–National Academy of Sciences; the American Academy of Pediatrics; and the American Medical Association.

3. **Vitamin E.** Vitamin E (principally alpha-tocopherol) is present in low concentrations in milk.

4. **Vitamin K.** Vitamin K is found only in trace amounts in milk. Also, there is some indication that part of the vitamin K of milk is destroyed by pasteurization.

• **Water-soluble vitamins**—All of the vitamins known to be essential for man have been detected in milk. The water-soluble vitamins are in the nonfat portion. The content of water-soluble vitamins in milk is relatively constant and not easily influenced by the vitamin content of the cow's ration.

1. **Biotin.** Milk is a fairly good source of biotin, generally providing about 3 mcg per 100 g. Two glasses of milk would provide between 7 and 23% of the average daily dietary intake of this vitamin. Less than 10% of biotin is destroyed by pasteurization.

2. **Folate (folic acid).** According to recent analyses, milk contains an average of 5 mcg of folate per 100 g. Two glasses *(480 ml)* of milk would supply about 12% of the 200 mcg RDA. Folate of milk is decreased by heat, but this can be minimized by excluding oxygen.

3. **Niacin.** The average niacin content of milk is only 0.08 mg per 100 g; so, two glasses of milk make little contribution (2 to 3%) to the 15 mg niacin RDA for adults. Nevertheless, milk and milk products are among the most effective pellagra-preventive foods because of (a) the complete availability of niacin in milk; and (b) the presence of the amino acid tryptophan (about 46 mg tryptophan per 100 g milk) in milk protein, which can be used for the synthesis of niacin in the body. (A dietary intake of 60 mg tryptophan is equivalent to 1 mg niacin.) Thus, the niacin value of milk is considerably greater than is reflected by its niacin concentration. Also, it is noteworthy that pasteurization does not destroy the niacin content of milk.

4. **Pantothenic acid (vitamin B-3).** Milk is a good source of pantothenic acid; it averages about 0.31 mg of pantothenic acid per 100 g. Pasteurization does not destroy the pantothenic acid in milk.

5. **Riboflavin (vitamin B-2).** Milk is an important source of this vitamin; dairy products (excluding butter) contributed 32.6% of the total riboflavin in the U.S. diet in 1990. The average riboflavin content of fluid whole milk is about 0.16 mg per 100 g. Two glasses *(480 ml)* of milk would supply between 45 and 60% of the 1.3 to 1.7 mg RDA for adults. Although riboflavin is not sensitive to heat, it can be destroyed by exposure to light. Riboflavin losses due to light can be minimized by protecting milk from exposure to strong light through utilizing opaque containers, transporting milk in special trucks, and storing milk in darkened refrigerators.

6. **Thiamin (vitamin B-1).** Significant quantities of this vitamin are found in milk—an average of 0.04 mg per 100 g. Since the RDA for thiamin is between 1.1 and 1.5 mg for the adult, two glasses of milk per day would supply about 13 to 18% of the RDA. Pasteurization results in the loss of about 10% of the thiamin.

7. **Vitamin B-6 (pyridoxine, pyridoxal, pyridoxamine).** An average of about 0.04 mg of vitamin B-6 are found in 100 g of milk; but there is considerable variation in the content of this vitamin in milk. Two glasses of milk furnish about 10% of the 2 mg RDA for adults. Pasteurization does not affect the vitamin B-6 content of milk.

8. **Vitamin B-12.** Milk is a good source of vitamin B-12; it contributed 18.5% of the total vitamin B-12 in the U.S. diet in 1990. Milk averages about 0.36 mcg of vitamin B-12 per 100 g. Two glasses of milk would furnish about 88% of the 2 mcg RDA for most adults. Pasteurization causes only minor destruction of the vitamin B-12 in milk.

9. **Vitamin C (ascorbic acid).** Fresh raw milk contains a small amount of ascorbic acid (about 0.94 mg per 100 g of milk), but processing and exposure to light and heat reduce the amount.

10. **Other vitamins.** Milk also contains choline, myoinositol, and para-aminobenzoic acid, the quantitative requirements of which have not been established.

(Also see VITAMIN[S].)

MILK AS A FOOD. Milk is often referred to as "the most nearly perfect food." It is consumed as a liquid and in the form of such products as butter, cheese, ice cream, and numerous other foods. Milk contains all the nutrients (food elements) needed for growth and good health.

The milk food group makes important contributions to the diet. Milk and milk products are the leading source of calcium and a good source of phosphorus. Also, they provide high-quality protein, the fat-soluble vitamins—A, D (when fortified), E, and K, and all the water-soluble vitamins. Lowfat or skim-milk products fortified with vitamins A and D have essentially the same nutrients as whole milk products, but with fewer calories.

No food has a wider acceptability or offers a greater variety of uses than milk. It is the first food of newborn babies, whether they are breast-fed or bottle-fed; and milk and milk products are important throughout life. For this reason, milk and dairy foods comprise a separate group in The Six Food Groups (Food Guide Pyramid).

(Also see FOOD GROUPS.)

Milk also fills a special role in meeting the nutrient needs of each of the following groups:

1. Pregnant and lactating women. (See PREGNANCY AND LACTATION NUTRITION.)

2. Infants. (See INFANT DIET AND NUTRITION.)

3. Children and adolescents. (See CHILDHOOD AND ADOLESCENT NUTRITION.)

4. Adults. (See ADULT NUTRITION.)

5. Elderly. (See GERONTOLOGY AND GERIATRIC NUTRITION.)

The recommended nutrient allowances (RDA) for each of the above groups are given in the section on Nutrients: Requirements, Allowances, Functions, Sources, Table N-3.

HEALTH ASPECTS OF MILK CONSUMPTION. Numerous advantages, along with some disadvantages, should be considered when incorporating milk in a nutrition program.

Health Benefits from Milk. The health, strength and vitality of people is dependent upon their getting an adequate supply of the right nutrients and foods. Milk, the most nearly perfect food, contributes richly to these needs. It bridges the gap all the way from the dependent fetus to independent old age.

The health imparting qualities of milk are indicated by the fact that daily consumption of a quart *(950 ml)* of cow's milk furnishes an average adult approximately all the fat, calcium, phosphorus, and riboflavin; ½ the protein; ⅓ of the vitamin A, ascorbic acid, and thiamin; ¼ of the calories; and, with the exception of iron, copper, manganese, and magnesium, all the minerals needed daily. These and other nutritional and health benefits of milk are detailed under two earlier headings of this section entitled "Nutrients of Milk" and "Milk as a Food"; hence, the reader is referred thereto.

Additional health benefits of milk are evidenced by its contribution to longevity, tranquilizing effect, ulcer therapy, symbolic meaning, and perhaps, lessening stomach cancer.

Health Problems from Milk. Several metabolic disorders are found in certain individuals when milk is introduced into the diet; among them, milk allergy, lactose intolerance, milk intolerance, galactose disease, milk anemia, or following gastric surgery.

MILK ALLERGY (MILK SENSITIVITY). Cow's milk is probably the most common food allergen in the United States, estimates of the incidence of which range from 0.3% to 3%. It tends to run in families; and an infant who has an allergy to milk may also be allergic to other foods, such as eggs.

When allergy to cow's milk exists, the following dietary alternatives are suggested:

1. Substitute goat's milk.
2. Change the form of the milk; that is, try boiled, powdered, acidulated, or evaporated milk.
3. Eliminate cow's milk and milk products from the diet, and substitute formulas in which the protein is derived from meat or soybeans.

(Also see ALLERGIES.)

LACTOSE INTOLERANCE. During digestion, nature ordained that lactose (milk sugar) be hydrolyzed (split) into its component monosaccharides, glucose and galactose, by the enzyme lactase. Sometimes this physiological process does not occur, and lactose intolerance results.

Lactose intolerance is the malabsorption of the milk sugar lactose due to a decrease in, or absence of, the enzyme lactase, which results in characteristic clinical symptoms (abdominal pain, diarrhea, bloating, flatulence). Three types of lactose intolerance are known:

1. Congenital lactose intolerance (often regarded as an inborn error of metabolism), a relatively rare condition, caused by an absence of lactase from birth.
2. Secondary lactose intolerance caused by damage by viruses, bacteria, allergens, etc. to the outer cell layer of the intestinal epithelium, possibly the brush border or the glycocalyx which surrounds the cell membrane, where the enzyme is confined.
3. Primary lactose intolerance due to an apparently normal development decrease in lactase activity.

The latter type—primary lactose intolerance—involving a normal decrease in the enzyme lactase after early childhood, is the most common type; hence, the discussion that follows pertains primarily thereto.

Normally, the enzyme lactase reaches maximum activity soon after birth, and its activity remains high throughout infancy (the suckling period). But, by late childhood, it decreases to a very low level in all but the Caucasian race.

Because of low intestinal lactase activity in a high proportion of non-Caucasian adults, their consumption of appreciable quantities of lactose can create considerable problems. In such cases, only a portion of the lactose is hydrolyzed; the excess passes down into the lower regions of the gastrointestinal tract, where it undergoes bacterial fermentation. As a consequence, large quantities of fluids are drawn into the lumen of the gut due to the osmotic effect of the uncleaved lactose molecule and its fermented by-products. A reaction follows, generally characterized by abdominal bloating, gaseousness, cramps, flatulence, and watery diarrhea. Initial symptoms are usually observed 30 to 90 minutes after the administration of the disaccharide; diarrhea usually occurs within 2 hours; and the symptoms disappear within 2 to 6 hours after the intake of lactose.

Lactose intolerance is of practical concern in developing countries, as well as in school lunch programs, where milk is commonly used in attempts to correct or avoid serious nutritional problems.

This metabolic disorder interests the anthropologist as well as the physiologist because certain populations throughout the world show extremely high rates of lactose intolerance. Less than 15% of Scandinavians and those of Western and Northern European extraction exhibit this affliction, while 60 to 80% of Greek Cypriots, American Indians, Arabs, Ashkenazi Jews, Mexican-Americans, and African Americans, and 90% of African Bantus and Orientals have been reported to be lactose intolerant. An estimated 30 to 50 million Americans are lactose intolerant. In general, populations in which dairying is traditional seem to tolerate lactose, whereas people from nondairying parts of the world do not; and the inability to utilize lactose in the latter groups persist in successive generations in spite of migration. The question posed by anthropologists is whether the intolerance to lactose evolved due to the inadequate consumption of milk over a period of generations or whether the low consumption of milk was a result of low gut lactase activity originally. That is, did these people once have the ability to digest lactose and eventually lose it, or have they always had this lactase insufficiency?

Fortunately, many people having lactose intolerance can digest most cheeses and other fermented dairy products, such as yogurt. Fortunately, too, lactase is now on the market. By adding it to milk, lactose is changed into two simple sugars, glucose and galactose. The resulting milk is four times sweeter than regular milk, but is otherwise unchanged. Another alternative is lactose-reduced lowfat milk currently available that contains 70% less lactose.

MILK INTOLERANCE. Milk intolerance is not the same as lactose intolerance. Rather, it refers to the development of significant symptoms similar to those described for lactose intolerance following the consumption of usual amounts of milk or milk-containing products. However, many persons with lactose intolerance (lactase deficiency) can consume milk in 1-cup quantities at meals without discomfort, and others can tolerate smaller quantities.

Suitable alternatives for milk-intolerant individuals should provide the same nutrients as does milk. Lactose hydrolyzed milk has been shown to be a suitable alternative in most cases. In addition, other dairy foods such as cheese and other fermented dairy products are well tolerated by the truly milk-intolerant individual.

On the basis of present evidence, it would appear inappropriate to discourage supplemental milk feeding programs targeted at children on the basis of primary lactose intolerance. Also, the use of milk should not be discouraged in feeding malnourished children—except when they have severe diarrhea.

GALACTOSE DISEASE (GALACTOSEMIA). Galactose disease, an inborn error of carbohydrate metabolism, inherited as an autosomal recessive trait, is caused by insufficient levels of the enzyme galactose-1-phosphate uridyl transferase, sometimes abbreviated P-Gal-transferase, which is needed in the liver for the conversion of galactose to glucose. Galactose is derived from the hydrolysis of lactose (milk sugar) in the intestine. (The enzyme lactase splits lactose into glucose and galactose.)

Where this genetic defect exists, galactose disease becomes apparent within a few days after birth by such symptoms as loss of appetite, vomiting, occasional diarrhea, drowsiness, jaundice, puffiness of the face, edema of the lower extremities, and weight loss. The spleen and liver enlarge. Mental retardation becomes evident very early in the course of the disease, and cataracts develop within the first year.

Dietary treatment consists of early diagnosis and the complete exclusion from the diet of milk, the only food that supplies lactose, along with all foods that contain milk. As a rule, the substitution of a nonmilk formula (usually a meat-base or a soy-base formula, supplemented with calcium gluconate or chloride, iron, and vitamins) leads to rapid improvement. All the symptoms disappear except the mental retardation which has already occurred and is not reversible.

Complete elimination of galactose is necessary for the young child, but breads and other prepared foods containing milk are usually permitted when the child enters school. Milk must be permanently excluded from the diet, however.

(Also see INBORN ERRORS OF METABOLISM, Table I-2, Inborn Errors of Carbohydrate Metabolism.)

MILK ANEMIA. *Milk anemia is the condition that results when infants and children drink milk over an extended period without iron supplementation by an iron salt or an iron-rich food(s).*

During growth, the demand for positive iron balance is imperative. At birth, a newborn infant has about 3 to 6 months' supply of iron, which was stored in the liver during fetal development. Since milk does not supply iron, supplementary iron-rich foods must be provided to prevent the classic milk anemia of young children fed cow's milk only after 6 months of age.

Iron is also needed for continued growth during the toddler stage (1 to 3 years). Sometimes excessive milk intake during this period, a habit carried over from infancy, may exclude some solid foods from the diet. As a result, the child may be lacking iron and develop a milk anemia.

AFTER GASTRIC SURGERY. The patient whose gastric or duodenal ulcer does not respond to medical treatment is the most common candidate for gastric surgery.

Immediately after gastric surgery, milk may or may not be included in the small frequent feedings, for the reason that the contents of the stomach may pass into the small intestine before it is in proper solution and cause distention of the jejunum. When this happens, the patient experiences nausea, cramps, diarrhea, light-headedness, and extreme weakness. This occurs 15 to 30 minutes after meals and is known as the *dumping syndrome.*

Also, some, but not all, individuals develop lactose intolerance following gastric surgery; therefore, some physicians regularly exclude milk after such surgery. However, other physicians exclude milk only after the patient has experienced distention and diarrhea that are relieved by the exclusion of milk.

Milk Myths: Some myths and incorrect statements related to health concerns appear to have acted as barriers to milk consumption; among them, the following:

Milk is toxic to nonwhite people.
Milk causes coronary heart disease.
Milk causes cancer.
Milk causes iron deficiency anemia.
Milk causes urinary calculi.
Milk causes acne.

U.S. PRODUCTION OF MILK. The United States ranks fourth in number of milk cows and third in production per cow, among the leading dairy countries of the world. The former U.S.S.R. holds a commanding lead in the number of milk cows; and Israel and Japan rank first and second, respectively, in average milk production per cow.

Milk is produced in every state of the Union. However, the greatest concentration of dairy cows is found in those areas with the densest human populations. This is as one would expect from the standpoint of the demand for, and the marketing of, fresh milk—a highly perishable product.

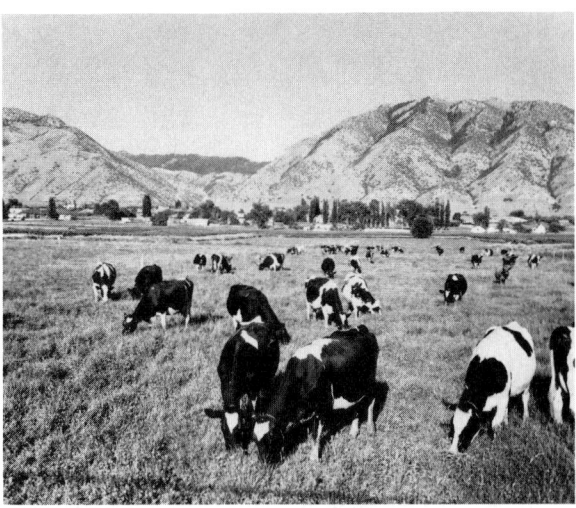

Fig. M-57. Cows convert the photosynthetic energy derived from solar energy and stored in grass into milk for humans. (Courtesy, Union Pacific Railroad, Omaha, Nebr.)

Dairy Producers. It is impossible to describe the *average* American dairy farm, for the dairyman can choose to tailor his operation in an infinite number of ways. Herd size, breeds, milking equipment, frequency of milking, and intensity of production all enter into the makeup of the dairy farm.

MILKING AND HANDLING MILK. Milk is secreted by the mammary glands of mammals. In the United States, cows furnish virtually all market milk.

Lactation begins at freshening, when a calf is born, and usually lasts 305 days. Milk is removed through the teats (the elongated nipples). Milking is carried out by either of two methods: (1) hand milking, or (2) machine milking.

The composition of milk depends mainly on the breed

of cows. The flavor and quality of milk vary according to how the cows are cared for, what they are fed, and how the milk is handled. Milk must be kept cool and clean from the moment it comes from the cows.

Milk possesses two characteristics which make it ideal for the development of bacteria: (1) It is a well-balanced food in which bacteria thrive; and (2) the temperature, as it comes from the cow, is ideal for bacterial growth. For these reasons, milk must be cooled to at least 50°F (preferably 40°F, or 4°C) as soon as possible in order to inhibit bacterial growth.

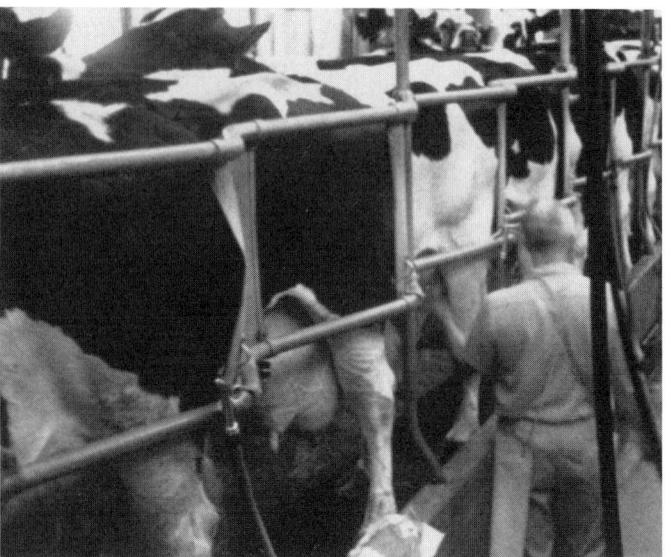

Fig. M-58. Cows being machine milked in a milking parlor. Note that the milk is piped directly into a refrigerated storage tank; without exposure—all very sanitary. (Courtesy, USDA)

Quality milk can be produced only when dairymen pay special attention to a number of factors; among them, herd health, clean cows, care of the milking equipment, cooling and storage of milk, and proper transportation of milk to market.

HAULING MILK.

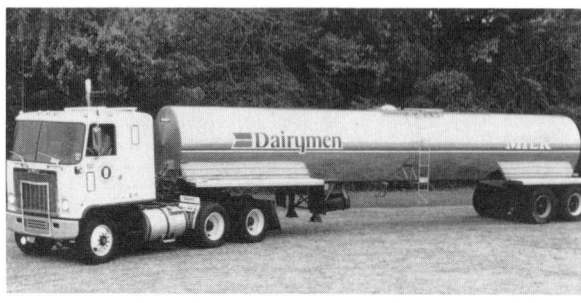

Fig. M-59. The bulk system of handling milk. This over-the-road transport is capable of moving 6,000 gal *(22,800 liter)* of milk. The insulated stainless steel tank holds milk within a few degrees of its original temperature. (Courtesy, Dairymen, Inc., Lexington, Ky.)

Practically all milk is now (1) placed in mechanically cooled bulk tanks on farms, and (2) transported to processing plants in bulk tank trucks with capacities ranging from 15,000 to 50,000 lb *(6,803 to 22,676 kg)*.

Because ownership changes at loading, this places responsibility on the truck operator to evaluate odor, flavor, and appearance of the milk, and to measure and sample the milk accurately and properly.

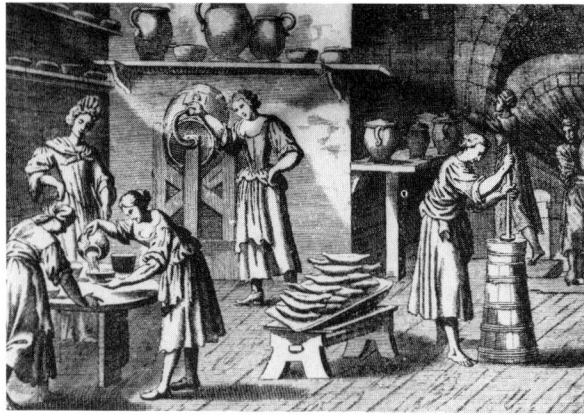

Fig. M-60. Seventeenth century dairy manufacturing plant. Note (1) division of labor among women workers; and (2) buttermaking, using two different types of churns: a barrellike churn with paddles inside (elevated in back of room and to the left), and a churn with a stirring stick called a *dasher* (right). (Courtesy, The Bettmann Archive, New York, N.Y.)

PROCESSING MILK. Upon arrival at the processing plant, trained laboratory technicians make many tests to ensure the quality and purity of milk, including temperature, flavor, odor, and appearance. They reject milk that does not meet the required high standards for quality.

Also milk is tested to determine its fat content; and different batches may be blended, in a process called standardization, to adjust the fat content.

Today, most milk is homogenized, pasteurized, and fortified (at least with vitamin D), the details of which follow:

• **Homogenization**—Most whole milk is homogenized to prevent formation of a cream layer. Homogenization is accomplished by passing hot milk under high pressure through a narrow constriction with a specially designed pump. In the process, fat globules are reduced in size so that they are no longer acted upon by force of gravity and remain evenly dispersed throughout the milk. The keeping quality and nutritive value of homogenized and nonhomogenized milk are similar. The main **advantages** of homogenizing are: (1) no separation of the cream—the product retains uniform consistency; and (2) a softer curd forms in the stomach, which aids digestion. The main **disadvantages**: (1) The protein is more readily coagulated by heat or acid so that care must be taken to avoid curdling; and (2) increased susceptibility of off-flavor induced by sun or fluorescent light.

• **Pasteurization**—*Pasteurization is the heating of raw milk in properly approved and operated equipment at a sufficiently high temperature for a specified length of time to destroy pathogenic bacteria.* Pasteurization is required by law for all Grade A fluid milk and milk products moved in interstate commerce for retail sale. This process was developed by and named after Louis Pasteur, the French scientist who in the early 1860s demonstrated that wine and beer could be preserved by heating above 135°F (57.2°C).

In addition to extending the shelf life of milk, pasteurization destroys pathogens that might be conveyed from infected cows to man.

Various time-temperature relationships are utilized in the pasteurization process. The first three that follow are most commonly used by milk processors. The fourth—sterilized or aseptic—milk is a relatively new development.

1. **Low temperature pasteurization.** Milk is heated to a minimum of 145°F (*63°C*) for at least 30 minutes.

2. **High temperature pasteurization.** Milk is heated to a minimum of 160.7°F (*71.5°C*) for at least 15 seconds, following which it is immediately cooled.

3. **Ultrapasteuriztion.** Milk is heated to 191.3°F (*88.5°C*) for 1 second. This method is common in Europe and is widely used for cream and eggnog in the United States.

4. **Sterilized milk (aseptic milk).** This refers to ultra-pasteurized milk products which are packaged aseptically. They can be stored at room temperature for several weeks.

• **Fortification**—Fortified milks are those that contain added minerals, vitamins, and/or milk solids-not-fat. Details follow:

1. **Fortification with vitamin D.** 400 IU of vitamin D per quart (*950 ml*) are added to most milk and lowfat milk. This has been common practice for many years. It has contributed significantly to a reduction in the incidence of rickets in infants. Milk provides the necessary calcium and phosphorus, but vitamin D must also be present for normal calcification of bones and teeth.

2. **Fortification of skim milk with vitamin A.** 2,000 to 4,000 IU of vitamin A per quart may be added to skim milk in most states, in addition to vitamin D.

3. **Multivitamin-mineral milk.** In addition to vitamins A and D, multivitamin-mineral milk typically has the following vitamins and minerals added per quart: thiamin (1 mg), riboflavin (2 mg), niacin (10 mg), iron (10 mg), and iodine (0.1 mg).

4. **Protein fortified lowfat and skim milks.** Federal standards for lowfat and skim milks provide for a protein fortified product containing a minimum of 10% milk-derived nonfat solids, with the stipulation that the product must be labeled *protein fortified* or *fortified with protein.* Fortification of milk with nonfat solids is desirable for two reasons: (1) The flavor of most milk is improved, and (2) the nutritive value is increased.

NOTE WELL: The Food and Drug Administration requires that fortified foods or foods that are labeled or advertised with a claim to their nutrition be labeled to show content, in terms of percent Recommended Daily Allowance, of protein, vitamin A, vitamin C, thiamin, riboflavin, niacin, calcium, and iron. Also, serving size and quantities per serving must be stated for calories, fat, protein, and carbohydrate.

State laws vary relative to fortification. In those states permitting such fortification, the levels are regulated by law.

Dairy Processing Plants. Dairy plants process fluid milk and/or manufacture dairy products from milk. Some of them produce several kinds of milk and milk products, others specialize—for example, they make cheese only, or they may condense and evaporate milk.

Fluid milk processors are located in and near population centers, where most fluid milk is consumed. The Great Lakes and Midwest regions of the United States are the primary centers for manufacturing grade milk. Thus, with the exception of ice cream production, the processing of manufactured dairy products—butter, nonfat dry milk, cheese, evaporated and condensed milk, and other products of minor importance—is concentrated near these areas of production. Other major production areas—California, New York, and Pennsylvania—produce substantial quantities of manufactured dairy products from excess Grade A milk.

Kinds And Uses Of Milk And Milk Products. Table M-20 shows the quantity of milk going into different uses, and Fig. M-61 shows the relative importance of each use.

TABLE M-20
HOW THE U.S. MILK SUPPLY IS USED[1]

Product	Milk Equivalent	
	(mil lb)	(mil kg)
Fluid milk and cream sales (25.8 billion quart)	55,370	25,168
Cheese	47,368	21,531
Creamery butter	25,043	11,383
Frozen dairy products[2]	12,307	5,594
Used on farms where produced	2,048	931
Evaporated and condensed milk	1,926	875
Other uses	4,413	2,006

[1]*1991 Milk Facts,* Milk Industry Foundation, Washington, D.C., p. 29.
[2]Plus 2,014 mil lb of milk equivalent in other manufactured dairy products used in production of frozen dairy products.

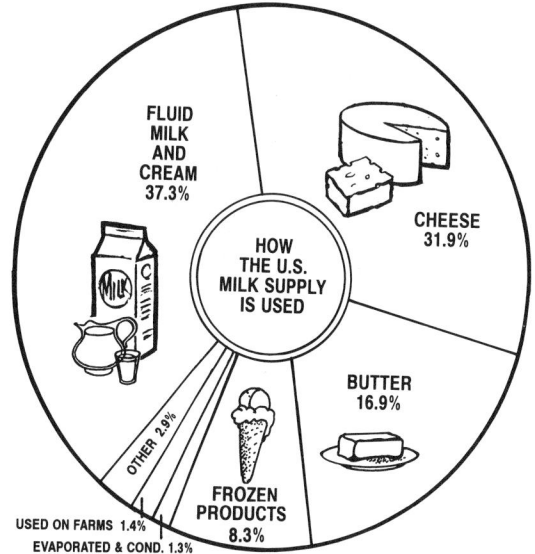

Fig. M-61. The uses of milk, in percentages. (From *1991 Milk Facts,* Milk Industry Foundation, p. 28)

Each of the branches of the dairy processing segment and each of the products will be listed and described briefly in the sections that follow.

FLUID MILK. This type of processing requires only a minimum of product alteration. Milk is usually homogenized, pasteurized, and fortified with vitamin D. The common forms of fluid milk follow:

• **Whole milk**—*Raw whole milk is defined as the lacteal secretion, practically free from colostrum, obtained by milking one or more cows.* Federal regulations require that whole milk as marketed contain not less than 3.25% milkfat and not less than 8.25% milk solids-not-fat. (Solids-not-fat include carbohydrate, protein, minerals, and water-soluble vitamins, whereas the total solids of milk includes all the constituents of milk except water.)

Various state standards provide that milkfat minimums may vary from 3.0 to 3.8% and solids-not-fat minimums from

8.0 to 8.7%. At the milk plant, the milk from different farms is pooled and *standardized* by removing excess milkfat or by adding cream, concentrated milk, dry whole milk, skim milk, concentrated skim milk, or nonfat dry milk to meet or exceed the minimum legal standards.

Whole fluid milk shipped in interstate commerce is usually pasteurized or ultrapasteurized; it must be pasteurized or ultrapasteurized before being sold for beverage use. Where milk is ultrapasteurized, it must be so indicated on the label.

The addition of vitamin A and/or vitamin D to fresh fluid milk is optional. If added, vitamin A must be present at a level not less than 2,000 IU per quart (*950 ml*) and vitamin D must be present at a level of 400 IU per quart. These amounts must be stated on the label. Milk is an excellent food for vitamin D fortification as it contains the proportion of calcium and phosphorus desirable for normal calcification of bones and teeth. Either vitamin D_2 or D_3 can be added to milk. Although vitamin D fortification of milk is optional, estimates indicate that approximately 98% of all homogenized milk contains vitamin D.

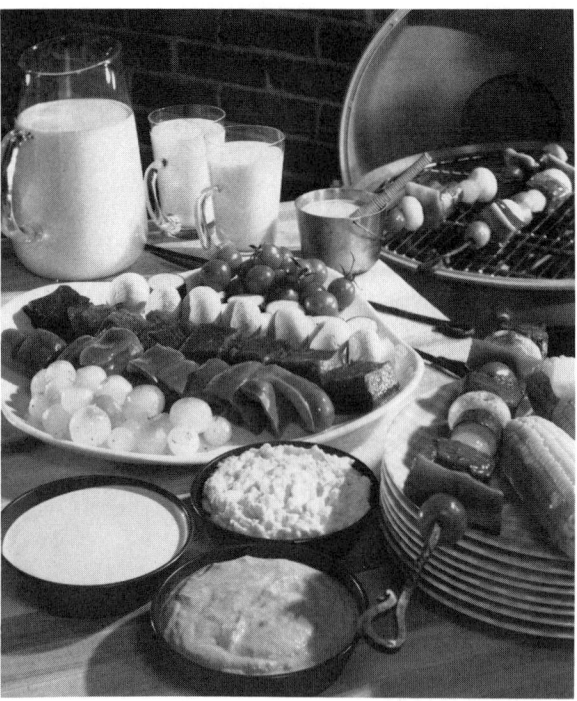

Fig. M-62. Fluid milk can be used in many forms and in many ways. This shows milk served with kabobs in outdoor cooking. (Courtesy, United Dairy Industry Assn., Rosemont, Ill.)

● **Lowfat milk**—Lowfat milk is milk from which sufficient milkfat has been removed to produce a food having one of the following milkfat contents: 0.5, 1.0, 1.5, or 2.0%; along with not less than 8.25% milk solids-not-fat. In 1987, for the first time ever, low-fat fluid milk consumption in the United States exceeded whole fluid milk consumption.

The addition of vitamin A to lowfat milk to a level of 2,000 IU per quart is mandatory. The addition of vitamin D is optional, but if added it must be present at a level of 400 IU per quart. If nonfat milk solids are added to reach the 10% solids-not-fat level, the product must be labeled *protein fortified* or *fortified with protein*.

● **Skim or nonfat milk**—This is milk from which as much fat as possible has been removed. But the milk solids-not-fat must be a minimum of 8.25%. The provisions for the addi-

tions of vitamins A and D and nonfat milk solids to skim or nonfat milk are identical to those described for lowfat milk.

● **Chocolate milk; other flavored milks**—Chocolate whole, lowfat, and skim milk are flavored with a chocolate syrup, cocoa, or a chocolate powder to give a final chocolate solids concentration of 1 to 1.5%. Additionally, a nutritive sweetener (about 5 to 7% sucrose) is added. Chocolate lowfat and skim milk must contain not less than 2,000 IU of vitamin A per quart. If vitamin D is added, it must be present in not less than 400 IU per quart.

Numerous other flavorings may also be added to milk; among them, strawberry, cherry, raspberry, pineapple, apple, orange, and banana. But chocolate is the most popular flavoring of milk.

SPECIAL MILKS. Certain fluid milks are sold under special labels. Among them are:

1. **Certified milk.** This is milk that is produced under special sanitary conditions prescribed by the American Association of Medical Commissioners. It is sold at a higher price than ordinary milk.

2. **Golden Guernsey milk.** Golden Guernsey milk is produced by owners of purebred Guernsey herds who comply with the regulations of the American Guernsey Cattle Club. Such milk is sold under the trade name "Golden Guernsey," at a premium price.

3. **All-Jersey milk.** This is produced by registered Jersey herds whose owners comply with the regulations of the American Jersey Cattle Club. It is sold at a premium price under the trademark of "All Jersey."

EVAPORATED AND CONDENSED MILK. The introduction of condensed milk in 1853 (patented in 1856) made available dairy products that expanded markets at home and abroad and significantly enhanced growth of the U.S. dairy industry. Today, candy manufacturers, bakers, and ice cream processors are large users of concentrated milk.

The primary products within this category are evaporated and concentrated (condensed) milk packed in cans for consumer use, and concentrated whole and skim milk shipped in bulk.

● **Evaporated milk**—Evaporated milk is made by preheating to stabilize proteins, concentrating in vacuum pans at 122°

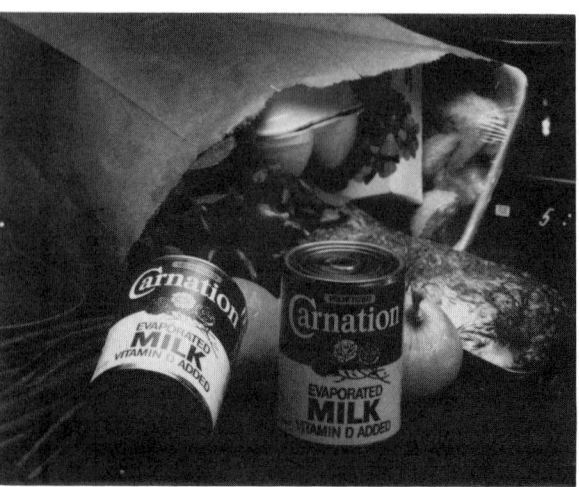

Fig. M-63. Evaporated milk. (Courtesy, Carnation Co., Los Angeles, Calif.)

to 131°F (50° to 55°C) to remove about 60% of the water, homogenizing (which is mandatory), standardizing to the required percentage of components, adding vitamins (vitamin D must be added to provide 400 IU per reconstituted quart), canning, and stabilizing (sealed in the container, then heat treated [240° to 245°F, or 115.5° to 118.5°C, for 15 minutes] to sterilize).

Federal standards require that the milkfat and total milk solids content of evaporated milk be not less than 7.5 and 25.5%, respectively. Evaporated skim milk is concentrated, fortified skim milk containing not less than 20% milk solids.

In recent years, per capita consumption of evaporated milk has declined, but bulk shipments of unsweetened concentrated milk to food and ice cream processors have increased.

• **Concentrated or condensed milk**—This is similar to evaporated milk because it is made by the partial removal of water from fluid milk; hence, the milkfat and total milk solids must not be less than 7.5 and 25.5%, respectively. Unlike evaporated milk, however, concentrated milk is usually not subjected to further heat treatment to prevent spoilage. The product is perishable and spoilage may occur rapidly at temperatures above 44.6°F (7°C).

• **Sweetened condensed milk**—This product is made by the removal of approximately 60% of the water from whole milk and the addition of a suitable sweetener such as sucrose. The amount of the sweetener (40 to 45% of the condensed milk) used is sufficient to prevent spoilage. Federal standards of identity require that sweetened condensed milk contain not less than 8.5% of milkfat and not less than 28% of total milk solids.

DRY MILK. Perishability and bulk of fluid milk have been a major drawback to transporting milk over long distances. However, the development of the dry milk industry made it possible to export milk abroad. Also, dry milk may be transported over relatively long distances domestically (1) to consumers who desire a less costly source of milk, and (2) to processors of other dairy products in areas where milk for manufacturing may not be readily available. The leading states producing dry milk are California, Wisconsin, and Minnesota. A discussion of each of the common dry milks follows:

• **Nonfat dry milk**—This product is prepared by removing water from pasteurized skim milk. Federal standards of identity require that it contain not more than 5% by weight of moisture and not more than 1.5% by weight of milkfat unless indicated. Except for small losses of ascorbic acid, thiamin, vitamin B-12, and biotin, the processing has no appreciable effect on the nutritive value of the milk. Due to its low moisture content, it can be kept for long periods.

• **Nonfat dry milk fortified with vitamins A and D**—This product is similar to nonfat dry milk except that it contains 2,000 IU of vitamin A and 400 IU of vitamin D per quart (950 ml) when reconstituted according to label directions. Almost all nonfat dry milk sold retail is fortified with vitamins A and D.

• **Dry whole milk**—This product is made from pasteurized whole milk from which water has been removed. Except for losses in ascorbic acid (20% for spray dried), vitamin B-6 (30% for spray dried), and thiamin (10% for spray dried, and 20% for roller dried), the processing has no appreciable

effect on the nutritive value of the product. The major deterioration of dry whole milk is oxidative changes in the fat. Stability of the product can be increased by special packaging, such as gas-pack (removal of air and replacement with inert gas such as nitrogen) or vacuum-pack containers.

CULTURED MILK AND OTHER PRODUCTS. Cultured milks are fluid products that result from the souring of milk or its products by bacteria that produce lactic acid, whereas acidified milks are obtained by the addition of food-grade acids to produce an acidity of not less than 0.20%, expressed as lactic acid. The word *cultured* is used because pure bacterial cultures are employed in commercial manufacture. It is proper also to use the words *fermented* or *sour* because lactic acid, which imparts sourness, is produced by fermentation of milk sugar (lactose). Kefir, koumiss, acidophilus milk, cultured buttermilk, sour cream, and yogurt are examples of lactic acid fermentations.

Sales of cultured products are increasing as consumers recognize their nutritional value and appreciate their flavors. Cultured products are also a practical means of introducing large numbers of particular organisms into the intestinal tract.

The body, flavor, and aroma developed in the finished product vary with the type of culture and milk, the concentration of milk solids-not-fat, the fermentation process, and the temperature. The vitamin concentration may be altered; the variation of specific vitamins depends on both the types of culture and the length of ripening. A discussion of each of the common cultured milk products follows:

• **Kefir and koumiss**—These are the two major types of cultured milks which have been subject to both acid and alcoholic fermentation.

Kefir, made from the milk of mares, goats, or cows, is popular in countries of southwestern Asia.

Koumiss, made from unheated mare's milk, is the typical fermented milk of the U.S.S.R. and western Asia.

• **Acidophilus milk**—Pasteurized milk, usually lowfat or skim, cultured with *Lactobacillus acidophilus* and incubated at 100.4°F (38°C) for at least 18 hours until a soft curd forms, is called acidophilus milk.

Today, there is increasing demand for health foods; and, frequently, acidophilus milk is promoted as such a food. Although much research is still needed, *L. acidophilus* is believed to be a normal bacterial component of the gut microflora that helps to maintain the balance of microorganisms in the intestinal tract. Cultures of products containing *L. acidophilus* are sometimes used to regenerate intestinal flora after antibiotic treatment or other conditions that upset the microfloral balance in the gut.

• **Cultured buttermilk; Bulgarian buttermilk**—The fluid remaining after churning cream to make butter is called buttermilk. Today, this product is used primarily by the baking industry; and most buttermilk for beverage purposes is a cultured product. Most of the cultured buttermilk marketed in the United States is made from fresh pasteurized skim or lowfat milk with added nonfat dry milk solids, cultured with *Streptococcus lactis*. However, cultured buttermilk can also be made from fluid whole milk, concentrated fluid forms, or reconstituted nonfat dry milk.

Bulgarian buttermilk is made with *Lactobacillus bulgaricus*.

• **Sour cream or cultured sour cream**—Pasteurized, homogenized cream cultured with *Streptococcus lactis* at 71.6°F (22°C) until the acidity is at least 0.5%, calculated as lactic acid, results in an acid gel product known as cultured sour cream. Federal standards of identity specify that cultured sour cream contain not less than 18% milkfat. If nutritive sweeteners or bulky flavoring ingredients are added, the product must not contain less than 14.4% milkfat.

Cultured sour cream is a uniformly textured, smooth product that is widely used for flavoring.

• **Acidified sour cream**—This product results from the souring of pasteurized cream with safe and suitable acidifiers, with or without the addition of lactic acid producing bacteria. Federal standards of identity call for not less than 18% milkfat and a titratable acidity of not less than 0.5% calculated as lactic acid. In the event nutritive sweeteners or bulky flavoring ingredients are added, the product may not contain less than 14.4% milkfat.

• **Sour half-and-half or cultured half-and-half**—The federal standards of identity state that this is the product of pasteurized half-and-half containing not less than 10.5% and not more than 18% milkfat and containing lactic acid producing bacteria.

• **Acidified sour half-and-half**—This product results from the souring of half-and-half with safe and suitable acidifiers, with or without the addition of lactic acid producing bacteria.

• **Sour cream dressing and sour half-and-half dressing**—The word dressing denotes a product in which other dairy ingredients such as butter have been substituted for cream and/or milk. Sour cream dressing is similar to sour cream and contains not less than 18% milkfat or not less than 14.4% milkfat if nutritive sweeteners or bulky ingredients are added. Sour half-and-half dressing is made in semblance of sour half-and-half and contains not less than 10.5% milkfat or not less than 8.4% if nutritive sweeteners or bulky ingredients are added.

• **Yogurt**—This product can be manufactured from fresh whole milk, lowfat milk, or skim milk. In the United States, yogurt usually is made from a mixture of fresh, partially skimmed milk and nonfat dry milk; and fermentation is generally accomplished by a one-to-one mixed culture of *Lactobacillus bulgaricus* and *Streptococcus thermophilus*, in a symbiotic relationship, with each microorganism metabolizing milk products which are subsequently used by the other.

The milk is pasteurized, homogenized, inoculated, incubated at 107.6° to 114.8°F (*42° to 46°C*) until the desired stage of acidity and flavor is reached, and chilled to 44.6°F (*7°C*) or lower to halt further fermentation. The usual milkfat levels of current products are: yogurt, at least 3.25% milkfat; lowfat yogurt, 0.5 to 2% milkfat; and nonfat yogurt, less than 0.5%. Milk solids-not-fat range from 9 to 16%, the higher amount reflecting the addition of solids. Today, three main types of yogurt are produced:
1. Flavored, containing no fruit.
2. Flavored, containing fruit.
3. Unflavored yogurt.

The rise in popularity of yogurt in the United States in recent years has been phenomenal. This increased consumption is largely attributed to development of fruit-flavored yogurts and the promotion of low-calorie, but highly nutritional, yogurts as diet foods.

• **Eggnog**—Eggnog is a mixture of milk, cream, sugar, milk solids, eggs, stabilizers, and spices that is pasteurized, homogenized, cooled, and packaged. Eggnog may refer to a product with 6.0 to 8.0% milkfat, 1.0% egg yolk solids, and 0.5% stabilizer. Also, eggnog-flavored milk is available; it contains a minimum milkfat level of 3.25%, minimum egg yolk solids of 0.5%, and a maximum stabilizer level of 0.5%.

SPECIALTY MILKS. Several specialty milks are on the market, including certified milk, low sodium milk, imitation milk, and filled milk. A discussion of each of these follows:

• **Certified milk**—The first certified milk was produced in 1893, in Essex County, New Jersey, before dairy sanitation had achieved the excellence that now exists in producing Grade A milk. Certified milk refers to raw or pasteurized milk produced and handled by dairies that operate according to the rules and sanitary regulations stated in the book *Methods and Standards for the Production of Certified Milk* issued and revised periodically by the American Association of Medical Milk Commissioners, Inc. Today, the quality of Grade A milk is so high that it has largely replaced certified milk—and at a lower cost, so certified milk is produced in only a few localities. The production of certified milk, conducted under the auspices of a Medical Milk Commission, involves the veterinary examination of cows, the sanitary inspection of the dairy farm and equipment, and the medical examination of employees who handle the milk.

• **Low sodium milk**—Ninety-five percent or more of the sodium that occurs naturally in milk can be removed by ion-exchange. Thus, the sodium content of whole milk generally can be reduced from a normal amount of about 49 mg to about 2.5 mg per 100 g of milk. Fresh whole milk is passed through an ion-exchange resin to replace the sodium in milk with potassium, following which the milk is pasteurized and homogenized.

Low sodium milk permits the inclusion of milk and milk-containing foods that might otherwise be limited in therapeutic diets because of their sodium content.

• **Imitation milk**—Imitation milks purport to substitute for and resemble milk. These products usually contain water, corn syrup solids, sugar, vegetable fat (coconut, soybean, cottonseed), and protein from soybean, fish, sodium caseinate, or other sources. Although imitation fluid milks do not contain dairy products as such, they may contain derivatives of milk such as casein, salts of casein, milk proteins other than casein, whey, and lactose. Sometimes vitamins A and/or D are added. Ingredient composition, and hence nutrient composition, vary widely. The American Academy of Pediatrics considers imitation milk products inappropriate for feeding infants and young children.

• **Filled milk**—These are milk products (milk, lowfat milk, half-and-half or cream, whether or not condensed, evaporated, concentrated, powdered, dried, or desiccated) from which all or part of the milkfat has been removed and to which any fat or oil other than milkfat has been added. The American Academy of Pediatrics does not recommend the use of filled milks for feeding infants and small children.

CREAM. Cream is the liquid milk product, high in fat, separated from milk, which may have been adjusted by the addition of milk, concentrated milk, dry whole milk, skim milk, concentrated skim milk, or nonfat dry milk. Federal standards of identity require that cream contain not less than 18% milkfat. The several cream products on the market are:

• **Half-and-half**—This is a mixture of milk and cream containing not less than 10.5% nor more than 18% milkfat. It is pasteurized or ultrapasteurized, and it may be homogenized.

• **Light cream (coffee cream, table cream)**—This product contains not less than 18% nor more than 30% milkfat. It is pasteurized or ultrapasteurized, and it may be homogenized.

• **Light whipping cream (whipping cream)**—This cream contains not less than 30% nor more than 36% milkfat. It is pasteurized, or ultrapasteurized, and it may be homogenized.

• **Heavy cream (heavy whipping cream)**—This cream contains not less than 36% milkfat. It is pasteurized or ultrapasteurized, and it may be homogenized.

ICE CREAM AND FROZEN DESSERTS.

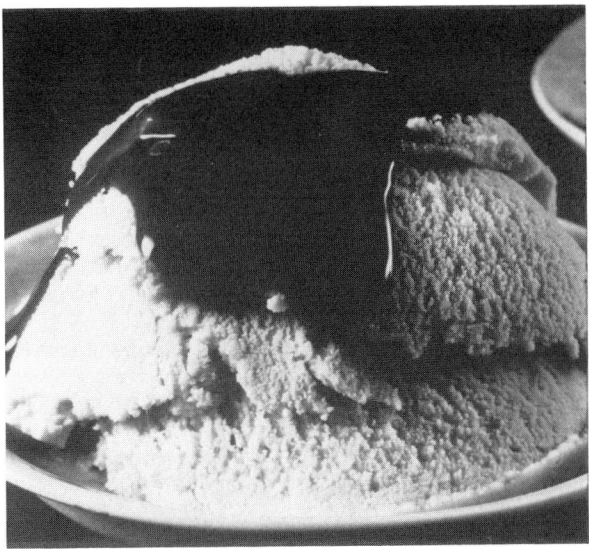

Fig. M-64. Homemade ice cream. (Courtesy, Carnation, Los Angeles, Calif.)

Today, the ice cream manufacturing industry is one of the largest in the realm of dairy processing. U.S. production of frozen dairy products increased from 936 million gallon *(3.5 billion liter)* in 1960 to 1.3 billion gallons *(4.9 billion liter)* in 1988.

Several products are classified under the category of frozen desserts. Some of these follow:

1. **Ice cream.** Of all the frozen dairy desserts, ice cream contains the most milk solids (about 16 to 24%). It consists primarily of milk fat, nonfat milk solids, sugar, flavoring, and stabilizers.

2. **Custards and French ice cream.** These products closely resemble ice cream except they must contain at least 1.4% egg yolk solids, additionally.

3. **Ice milk.** Ice milk contains less fat and less total solids than ice cream; hence, it contains fewer calories. It must contain at least 2%, but not more than 7%, milkfat.

4. **Mellorine.** Mellorine is essentially the same product as ice cream except that vegetable fat is used in place of milkfat.

5. **Sherbet.** Sherbet is a sweet, tart-flavored frozen dairy product that is low in total milk solids (about 3 to 5%). It can be made either by mixing water with ice cream or by

manufacturing from the raw ingredients. Since its melting point is lower than ice cream, it is softer than ice cream when the two products are stored at the same temperature.

BUTTER. Butter is made from cream. As marketed, it contains about 80 to 82% butterfat, 14 to 16% water, 0 to 4% salt, and 0.1 to 1.0% curd. *Sweet cream butter* is made from pasteurized sweet cream to which no starter has been added. *Ripened cream butter* is made by starter ripened cream. *Sweet butter* contains no salt. *Unsalted butter* is butter to which no salt has been added. *Salted butter* is butter to which salt has been added.

Butter is classed as Grade AA, A, B, or C based on flavor, body, color, and salt. Butter which does not meet the standards of Grade C cannot carry a USDA label.

Table M-21 shows the per capita consumption of butter and margarine for selected years from 1910 to 1990. Per capita consumption of margarine surpassed butter in 1957. In 1990, the per capita consumption of butter was 4.4 lb, as compared to 10.9 lb of margarine. Low prices and the controversy about cholesterol and heart disease are the primary reasons for the decrease in both butter and margarine consumption.

TABLE M-21
PER CAPITA CONSUMPTION OF BUTTER AND MARGARINE[1]

Year	Per Capita Consumption			
	Butter		Margarine	
	(lb)	(kg)	(lb)	(kg)
1910	18.3	8.3	1.6	0.7
1920	14.9	6.8	3.4	1.5
1930	17.6	8.0	2.6	1.2
1940	17.0	7.7	2.4	1.1
1950	10.7	4.9	6.1	2.8
1960	7.5	3.4	9.4	4.3
1970	5.3	2.4	11.0	5.0
1980	4.5	2.0	11.4	5.2
1990	4.4	2.0	10.9	4.5

[1]*Dairy Statistics Through 1960*, Stat. Bull No. 303, Supp. for 1963–64, Economic Research Service, USDA; *National Food Situation*, Economic Research Service, USDA, February 1966; *Agricultural Statistics 1980*, USDA, p. 148 and *1991*, p. 479.

CHEESE. *Cheese may be defined as the fresh or matured product obtained by draining after coagulation of milk, cream, skimmed or partly skimmed milk, buttermilk, or a combination of some or all of these products.*

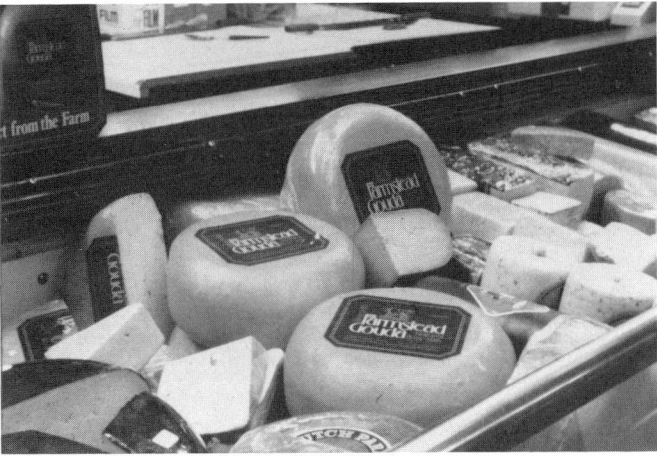

Fig. M-65. Assorted cheeses. (Courtesy, University of Minnesota, St. Paul, Minn.)

Cheese is manufactured by: (1) exposing milk to specific bacterial fermentation, and/or (2) treating with enzymes; to coagulate some of the protein. The first step in cheese making is to separate the casein and milk solids from the water in milk. The coagulated milk is then cut into small pieces and the water separated from the solids by a series of drainings and pressings. The characteristic flavor of the cheese is created by bacteria growth and subsequent acid production in the cheese during the cheese-making process and also by the bacteria and mold development during a period of curing.

Milk can be, and is, processed into many different varieties of cheese. In fact, there are over 2,000 different named cheeses. Some are made from whole milk, others from milk that has had part of the fat removed, and still others from skim milk. (The most important variety produced from skim milk is cottage cheese.) In 1990, American types of cheese accounted for 50% of the U.S. total cheese production, of which 96% was American Cheddar and 2.2% was other American types (Colby, washed curd, stirred curd, Monterey). Other important types of cheese are Italian (mostly soft varieties), Swiss, Muenster, cream, blue, and Neufchatel.

Fig. M-66 shows the kinds of cheese produced in 1990, exclusive of cottage cheese.

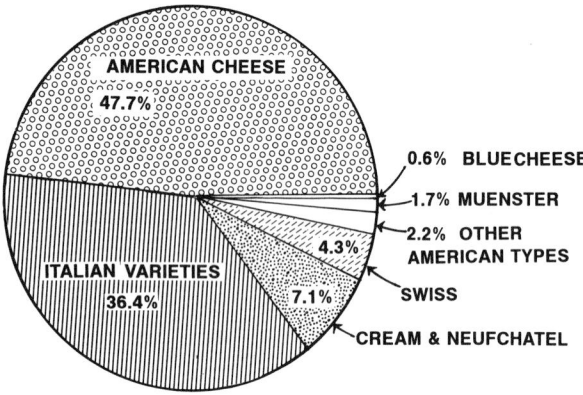

Fig. M-66. Relative importance of kinds of cheeses produced in the United States. (Source: USDA)

The U.S. per capita consumption of cheese has tripled since 1960, increasing from 8.3 lb in 1960 to 24.7 lb in 1990.

Hard cheese, such as Cheddar, is one of the most concentrated of common foods; 100 g (about 3.5 oz) supplies about 36% of the protein, 80% of the calcium, and 34% of the fat in the recommended daily allowance. Cheese is also a good source of some minerals and vitamins.

Cheese is a high-protein food, and the protein (principally casein) is partially digested. It is rich in the essential amino acids, calcium, phosphorus, certain other minerals, and vitamins, and has a high caloric value. Only a trace of the lactose present in milk remains in the cheese.

Cottage cheese (as made from skim milk) is low in fat and high in protein, but has only about one-eighth of the calcium content of American (Cheddar) cheese. Cream cheese differs from other soft cheeses in having more fat and less protein.

One ounce (about 28 g) of Cheddar-type cheese provides about the same nutritive value as a glass of milk. It is a particularly good food for children.

• **Processed cheese**—This product is formed by grinding, heating, and mixing hard-type cheeses. This type of cheese serves as an outlet to salvage defective cheeses as well as provide a uniform, widely marketable product.

• **Nutritive value of cheeses**—The composition and nutritive value of a number of varieties of cheeses is given in Food Composition Table F-21, in the section on "Milk and Products."

CASEINATES (COFFEE WHITENERS; WHIPPED TOPPINGS). *Caseinates are salts of casein.* They are classified as food chemicals derived from milk and are commonly used in (1) nondairy coffee whiteners (coffee whiteners are made from sodium caseinate) and (2) whipped toppings.

To produce caseinates, enough alkali, commonly called calcium hydroxide or sodium hydroxide, is added to acid coagulated casein to reach a pH of 6.7. The resulting suspension is pasteurized and spray dried.

WHEY. *Whey is the watery part of milk separated from the curd.* Whey is available as dried whey, condensed whey, dried whey solubles, condensed whey solubles, dried hydrolyzed whey, condensed hydrolyzed whey, condensed whey product, dried whey product, and condensed cultured whey.

Whey provides food processors with an inexpensive product that can be used as a source of lactose, milk solids, milk proteins, or total solids. Additionally, whey, which is relatively high in digestibility and nutritive value, is commonly used as a livestock feed.

MARKETING AND DISTRIBUTING MILK. Marketing milk is that all-important end of the line; it's that which gives point and purpose to all that has gone before.

Satisfactory milk marketing requires one basic ingredient—quality milk; and this begins with production on the farm.

The difference in price between Grade A milk and the lower grades is substantial. But it goes beyond this; quality influences consumer demand.

In our present system, the vast majority of the marketing of milk and dairy products is handled by specialists, usually under a myriad of complex regulations and controls. Both successful milk producers and enlightened consumers should be familiar with milk markets, regulations and controls, and pricing systems, along with the factors affecting them.

Milk Supply. In 1990, a total of 148 billion pounds (67 billion kilograms) of milk were marketed by U.S. dairy farmers for $20 billion delivered to plants. Of this amount, 37.3% was consumed in fluid form and 62.7% was processed into manufactured dairy products.

Fluid milk is retailed as pasteurized milk, homogenized milk, fortified milk (usually vitamin D), skim milk, and flavored milk. Of the milk used for manufacturing in 1990, 31.9% was used for making cheese (exclusive of creamed

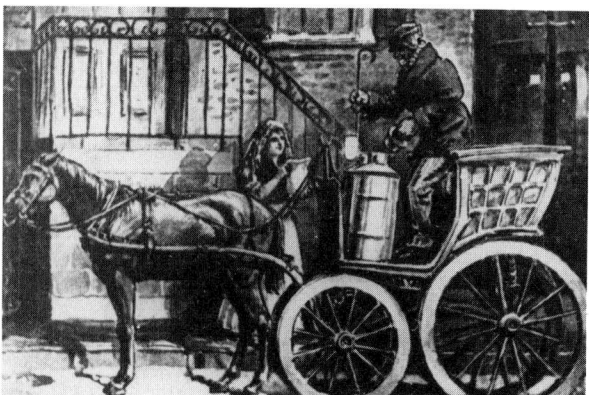

Fig. M-67. How it used to be done. Milkman transferring milk from can into customer's own pitcher, using a quart measure. (Courtesy, The Bettmann Archive, Inc., New York, N.Y.)

cottage cheese) and 16.9% was used for making butter.

Future milk supply will depend primarily on the profitability of dairy enterprises, for, like all other businesses, dairies are owned by people—and all people like to make a profit. In turn, profitability is determined by milk prices and cost of production. Also, dairy farmers will consider alternative farm and off-farm opportunities.

Milk Demand. There have been dramatic changes in the per capita consumption of milk and manufactured dairy products in recent years. Fig. M-68 clearly shows these changes.

PERCENT CHANGE IN PER CAPITA SALES
1977–87

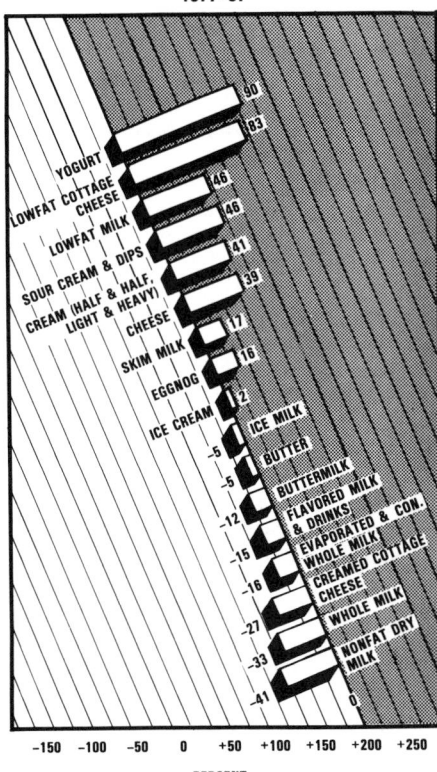

Fig. M-68. Change in U.S. per capita consumption of milk and dairy products 1977 to 1987, based on sales. Bars to the left of the vertical line represent decreases; bars to the right represent increases. (Source: *1988 Milk Facts*, Milk Industry Foundation, Washington, D.C., p. 16)

Because of increasing consumer infatuation with weight watching, low calorie diets, and cholesterol levels, it appears that present trends will continue—that there will be further increases in per capita consumption of low-fat and high-solids nonfat dairy products, and further decreases in per capita consumption of high-fat products.

Contrary to popular opinion, the United States ranks low among nations in per capita consumption of dairy products. Of the 18 major countries in per capita consumption of fluid milk, the United States ranks fifteenth in per capita consumption of fluid milk, last in consumption of butter, seventh in consumption of cheese, and twelfth in consumption of dry milk. Thus, based on (1) nutritive qualities, and (2) per capita consumption in those countries that exceed us, it would appear that there is a place and a need for increased consumption of milk and dairy products in the United States.

FACTORS INFLUENCING DEMAND. The demand for milk and milk products depends on a number of factors, chief of which are those which follow:

1. Price.
2. Availability and price of substitute products.
3. Consumer income.
4. Population growth.
5. Changes in consumer preference.
6. Age and sex.
7. Carbonated beverages.
8. Type and size of container.
9. Promotion of milk and dairy products.

Federal Milk Marketing Orders. Federal Milk Marketing Orders are established and administered by the Secretary of Agriculture under acts of Congress passed in 1933 and 1937. They are legal instruments, and they are very complex. However, stated in simple terms, they are designed to stabilize the marketing of fluid milk and to assist farmers in negotiating with distributors for the sale of their milk.

Federal Milk Orders (1) regulate only Grade A farm milk prices—they do not regulate Grade B milk prices, and (2) establish minimum, not maximum, farm milk prices. Prices paid to farmers are controlled, but there is no direct control of retail prices.

Federal orders are not concerned with sanitary regulations. These are administered by state and local health authorities.

State Milk Controls. Several of the states have milk control programs that also include some authority over milk prices.

In setting minimum farm prices, state control agencies often operate in a manner similar to Federal Milk Orders. They price only Grade A milk. State Orders price milk only within the particular state whereas Federal Orders can cover several states. Federal Milk Orders establish only farm milk prices, while State Orders establish prices at various stages along the way—farm, wholesale, retail, as well as regulating trade practices.

Some states set maximum prices at either wholesale or retail, or at both levels. Others set both minimum and maximum wholesale and retail milk prices. Still others require a minimum markup by retailers, while others require that milk prices be reported to the state. Most states specify Class I prices in their Orders.

All state control agencies have authority to require distributors to be licensed and to inspect and investigate operations of milk dealers and audit their records.

Other Regulatory Programs. Because of the essential nature of milk, plus the fact that it is easily contaminated and a favorable medium for bacterial growth, it is inevitable that numerous regulatory programs have evolved around it—federal, state, and local—some having been designed to control prices and assure a reasonably uniform flow of milk, and others for sanitary reasons.

SANITARY REGULATIONS. The sanitation of milk and dairy products is assured by the enforcement of sanitary regulations by federal, state, and local authorities.

All major cities and states have sanitary regulations governing the production, transportation, processing, and delivery of milk. Unfortunately, from area to area, there are a bewildering number of different regulations, with the result that milk going to more than one city market is often subjected to duplication and confusion in inspection. Also, sanitary and health regulations have sometimes been used as barriers to keep milk out of a certain area for competitive reasons.

In 1923, the U.S. Public Health Service (USPHS) established an Office of Milk Investigations; and, in 1924, the USPHS published its first Grade A pasteurized milk ordinance. Subsequently, this regulation has been revised several times.

Producers are issued permits allowing them to ship Grade A milk. The permit is revoked if either the bacteria count of raw milk exceeds 100,000 per milliliter or the cooling temperature exceeds 40°F in 3 of the last 5 samples.

The standard plate count of Grade A pasteurized milk may not exceed 20,000 per milliliter nor the coliform count 10 per milliliter in three of the last five samples or the processor's permit will be revoked.

A sample must be taken from each bulk tank at each farm every time the milk is collected.

The Food and Drug Administration (FDA) is charged with inspecting dairy products and processing plants for contamination and adulteration.

STANDARDS AND GRADES. Milk standards are established on the state and local levels and are patterned after the Pasteurized Milk Ordinance (PMO) formulated by the Food and Drug Administration (FDA). Essentially, the PMO is a set of recommendations for voluntary adoption by state and local regulatory agencies. Legal responsibility for the provision of quality milk rests mostly with state and local governments whose requirements are in some instances more stringent than the guidelines of the PMO.

The common grades are Grade A, manufacturing grade, or reject. In some areas, Grades A, B, and C are used.

Details relative to *Grade A Milk* and *Manufacture Grade Milk* follow, with a separate section devoted to each. For more specific regulations concerning the grading of milk in any particular area, the reader is advised to contact his local dairy extension agent.

Grade A Milk. *Grade A milk is milk that meets certain quality standards and is produced, processed, and handled in a stipulated manner in approved facilities and equipment.*

Grade A milk is produced and processed in accordance with the quality standards of the Pasteurized Milk Ordinance (PMO) formulated (and revised from time to time) by the Food and Drug Administration (FDA) for voluntary adoption by state and local milk regulatory agencies and the dairy industry. Federal specifications for the procurement of Grade A milk and milk products are based on the PMO, as are sanitary regulations for Grade A milk and milk products entering interstate commerce.

The Pasteurized Milk Ordinance is a very effective instrument for protecting milk quality. Strict compliance therewith is imposed so that the milk will be of high uniform quality. The sanitary dairy practices outlined by the PMO include:

1. Inspection and sanitary control of farms and milk plants.
2. Examination and testing of herds for the elimination of bovine diseases related to public health.
3. Regular instruction on desirable sanitary practices for persons engaged in production, processing, and distribution of milk.
4. Proper pasteurization or ultrapasteurization of milk.
5. Laboratory examination of milk.
6. Monitoring of milk supplies by federal, state, and local health officials to protect against unintentional chemical, physical, and microbiological adulterants.

Most rigid control is placed on the production and processing of Grade A market milk which is sold to consumers in its fluid state. Grade A pasteurized milk is obtained from dairy farms that conform with the sanitary requirements of the PMO or its equivalent as enforced by state or local authorities. The milk must be obtained from cows tested and found free of disease and disease-producing organisms. The raw milk is cooled immediately to the specified legal temperature and maintained at no higher temperature from the completion of milking until processing at a dairy plant that also conforms with state and local sanitation requirements.

At the processing plant, the milk is analyzed to be sure it contains not more than a specified bacterial count and is pasteurized according to the specified time-temperature relationships. Public health authorities advocate pasteurization since it is the only practical commercial process that destroys all disease-producing organisms that may be present in fluid milk. After processing, the milk is cooled again to the specified legal temperature and maintained at no higher temperature until sold. Today, practically all fluid market milk sold to consumers is Grade A pasteurized milk.

In order to become a producer of Grade A milk, the milking and milk storage facilities of the dairy must first pass the careful inspection of the state inspector. If approved by the inspector, the dairy is granted a permit for the shipment of Grade A milk. Once a permit is issued, the dairy operation is periodically inspected by a local health department official to ensure that adequate sanitation practices are maintained. The permit may be revoked if the bacteria count is too high, if the cooling temperature exceeds 40°F, and/or if the producer is found in repeated violation of other requirements of the ordinance.

Manufacture Grade Milk. As with Grade A milk, each state adopts and enforces its own regulations for the production, processing, and handling of Manufacture Grade milk, which is produced for, and processed into, ice cream, cheeses, etc. There is much less uniformity in the regulations governing Manufacture Grade milk than in Grade A milk, and the standards are not so high (although the trend is higher and more rigid).

Dairy farms producing Manufacture Grade milk must also conform to the sanitary requirements of state and local authorities, and the milk must come from cows tested and found free of disease and disease-producing organisms.

Processing plants manufacturing dairy products are subjected to general sanitation requirements similar to those for plants processing Grade A milk. Additionally, there are supplemental and specific requirements for plants that process dry milk products, butter, cheeses, and evaporated, condensed, or sterilized milk products.

Market Distribution of Fluid Milk. Once milk is processed, it must be marketed rather rapidly because of its highly perishable nature. When a consumer has a bad experience with milk, it is difficult to get him or her back into the habit of drinking milk. Hence, it is imperative that fluid milk be of high quality and possess desirable taste and packaging.

Milk is distributed in a number of ways: (1) home delivery, (2) retail stores, and (3) vending machines and self-service.

Dairy Imports and Exports. In order to protect the dairy industry from depressed prices caused by other countries dumping dairy products onto American markets, import quotas have been established. A number of dairy products, including several types of cheeses, butter, malted milk, butter oil, and dried milk are covered by specific import quotas. Although not formally restricted, certain other dairy products may be limited by agreement between the United States and the exporting country. Total imports on a milk equivalent basis have been very small. In 1988, imports of dairy products amounted to 2.4 million pounds *(1.1 mil kg)* when total milk production was more than 148 billion pounds *(67 bil kg)*. Hence, imports of dairy products were equivalent to only 0.002% of the total U.S. market milk.

As long as domestic prices are above world prices and world supplies are ample, exporting countries will look to the United States as a possible market. The four countries exporting the largest amount of dairy products are Italy, New Zealand, Denmark, and The Netherlands. As a result, import pressure will persist; yet, it is expected that imports of many commodities will continue to be limited by quotas.

As with imports, exports of dairy products by the United States are rather small. They fluctuate from year to year, but never amount to more than about 1% of the total milk supply.

Per Capita Milk Consumption of Milk and Milk Products. Milk is an important constituent of the American diet in terms of per capita consumption (Table M-22).

In 1990, the total milk equivalent consumption of all dairy products was 570. 6 lb *(259.4 kg)*, a 13% decline from 1960. But the growth in human population offset per capita decline, with the result that total consumption increased. From Table M-22, several trends are apparent: Americans have become weight conscious in recent years leading to a decreased per capita consumption of fluid whole milk and cream and an increased per capita consumption of low-fat milk. Per capita fluid whole milk consumption declined 67% from the period of 1960 to 1990, while per capita low-fat milk consumption increased 313%. Of the manufactured dairy products, per capita consumption of butter declined 41%, and evaporated milk 42%, in the period 1960 to 1990. Per capita total cheese consumption increased 34% in this same period. Per capita consumption of ice cream declined due to the increased popularity of frozen yogurt.

TABLE M-22
DAIRY PRODUCTS: U.S. PER CAPITA CIVILIAN CONSUMPTION, SELECTED YEARS 1960–88[1]

Year	Fluid Milk Products										Manufactured															
	Fluid Whole Milk		Cream		Low-fat Milk		Total Product		Whole Milk Equiv. of Butterfat		Butter		Total Cheese		Cottage Cheese		Ice Cream		Evap. & Cond. Milk		Nonfat Dry Milk		Yogurt		All Milk Equiv-alent	
	(lb)	(kg)	(lb)	(kg)	(lb)	(kg)	(lb)	(kg)	(lb)	(kg)	(lb)	(kg)	(lb)	(kg)	(lb)	(kg)	(lb)	(kg)	(lb)	(kg)	(lb)	(kg)	(lb)	(kg)	(lb)	(kg)
1960	276	125	9.1	4.1	23.8	10.8	309	140	309	140	7.5	3.4	8.3	3.8	4.8	2.2	18.3	8.3	13.7	6.2	6.2	2.8	0.3	0.1	653	296
1965	264	120	7.6	3.4	34.0	15.4	306	139	294	133	6.4	2.9	9.6	4.4	4.7	2.1	18.5	8.4	10.7	4.9	5.6	2.5	0.3	0.1	620	281
1970	229	104	5.6	2.5	57.5	26.1	292	132	260	118	5.3	2.4	11.5	5.2	5.1	2.3	17.7	8.0	7.1	3.2	5.4	2.4	0.9	0.4	561	254
1975	195	88	5.9	2.7	84.7	38.4	286	130	244	111	4.8	2.2	14.5	6.6	4.7	2.1	18.6	8.4	5.3	2.4	3.3	1.5	2.1	1.0	546	248
1980	148	67	5.7	2.6	97.8	44.5	251	114	231	105	4.1	1.9	17.1	7.8	4.6	2.1	17.6	8.0	7.2	3.3	3.0	1.3	2.5	1.1	554	252
1985	120	55	6.0	2.7	107.0	48.6	239	109	186	85	4.9	2.2	22.6	10.3	4.1	1.9	18.0	8.2	7.9	3.6	2.2	1.0	4.1	1.9	593	270
1988	100	45	6.0	2.7	132.0	60.0	238	108	184	84	4.4	2.0	23.6	10.7	3.8	1.7	17.8	8.1	7.9	3.6	2.7	1.2	4.7	2.1	585	266

[1]*1989 Dairy Producer Highlights*, National Milk Producers Federation, p. 17.

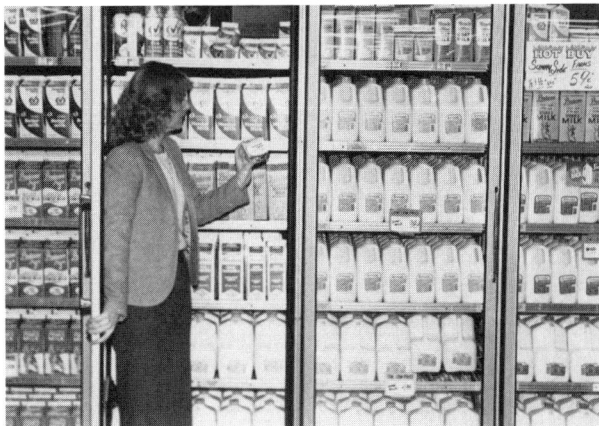

Fig. M-69. Milk and milk products in a modern retail store. (Photo by A. H. Ensminger)

Care of Milk in the Home.[20] The consumer also has responsibility for protecting the quality of milk. Proper handling of dairy products and open dating are designed to assure consumers of dairy products with a good shelf life, which is the length of time after processing that the product will retain its quality.

Open dating is the sometimes mandatory, often voluntary, inclusion of a date on milk containers to indicate when they should be withdrawn from retail sale. It is used by industry to reflect the age of individual packages. It does not indicate the shelf life of products. Generally, depending upon storage conditions and care in the home, a product will remain fresh and usable for a few days beyond this *pull date*, or *sell-by date*. Regulation of open dating varies among states and municipalities.

[20]This section and Table M-23 were adapted by the authors from *Newer Knowledge of Milk and Other Fluid Dairy Products*, National Dairy Council, Rosemont, Ill.

Dairy products are highly perishable, therefore, it is recommended that consumers observe the following practices to preserve quality:

1. Use proper containers to protect milk from exposure to sunlight, bright daylight, and strong fluorescent light to prevent the development of off-flavor and a reduction in riboflavin, ascorbic acid, and vitamin B-6 content.

2. Store milk at refrigerated temperatures 44.6°F (7°C) or below as soon as possible after purchase.

3. Keep milk containers closed to prevent absorption of other food flavors in the refrigerator. An absorbed flavor alters the taste, but the milk is still safe.

4. Use milk in the order purchased.

5. Serve milk cold.

6. Return milk container to the refrigerator immediately to prevent bacterial growth. Temperatures above 44.6°F (7°C) for fluid and cultured milk products for even a few minutes reduces shelf life. Never return unused milk to the original container.

7. Keep canned milk in a cool, dry place. Once opened it should be transferred to a clean opaque container and refrigerated.

8. Store dry milk in a cool, dry place and reseal the container after opening. Humidity causes dry milk to lump and may affect flavor and color changes. If such changes occur, the milk should not be consumed. Once reconstituted, dry milk should be treated like any other fluid milk: covered and stored in the refrigerator.

Guidelines on the storage life of various milk products at specific temperatures are shown in Table M-23. In this table, storage life refers to the approximate length of time after processing, not after purchasing, that the product will retain its quality.

TABLE M-23
APPROXIMATE STORAGE LIFE OF MILK PRODUCTS
AT SPECIFIC TEMPERATURES
(Storage life refers to the length of time after processing—not after purchasing—that the product will retain its quality.)

Product	Approximate Storage Life at Specific Temperatures		
	(Time)	(°F)	(°C)
Fresh fluid milk (whole, lowfat, skim, chocolate, and unfermented acidophilus)	8 to 20 days below ..	39.2	4
Sterilized whole milk	4 months at	69.8	21
	12 months at	39.2	4
Frozen whole milk	12 months at	-2.2	-23
Evaporated milk	1 month at	89.6	32
	12 to 24 months at ..	69.8	21
	24 months at	39.2	4
Concentrated milk	2 or more weeks at ..	34.7	1.5
Concentrated frozen milk	6 months at	-6.8	-26
Sweetened condensed milk	3 months at	89.6	32
	9 to 24 months at ...	69.8	21
	24 months at	39.2	4
Nonfat dry milk, extra grade	6 months at	89.6	32
(in moisture-proof pack)	16 to 24 months at ..	69.8	21
	24 months at	39.2	4
Dry whole milk, extra grade	6 months at	89.6	32
(gas pack: maximum oxygen 2%)	12 months at	69.8	21
	24 months at	39.2	4
Buttermilk	2 to 3 weeks at	39.2	4
Sour cream	3 to 4 weeks at	39.2	4
Yogurt	3 to 6 weeks at	39.2	4
Eggnog	1 to 2 weeks at	39.2	4
Ultrapasteurized cream	6 to 8 weeks at	39.2	4

Three to five days may elapse between processing and purchasing, so the shelf life from the point of purchasing would be correspondingly less.

Various dairy products such as fluid and concentrated milk may be preserved by freezing. Milk has a lower freezing point than water due to dissolved constituents such as lactose and salts. The average freezing point of milk is 31°F (-0.54°C).

A very low temperature is needed to freeze milk completely. About 75% of the milk will freeze at 14°F (-10°C). A temperature below 7.6°F (-18°C) is recommended for frozen storage.

Milk can be frozen and thawed in the refrigerator; however, it is not recommended. The quality of milk is impaired by freezing due to protein destabilization and settling of some milk solids. A watery wheylike liquid may collect on the top and curd particles may also appear. Mixing returns the product to its normal dispersion and subsequent separation does not occur. However, thawed milk may be susceptible to the development of an oxidized flavor. The homogenization of milk overcomes the problem of demulsification of fat, a result of freezing milk.

Cream can be frozen, as evidenced by the successful use of frozen cream by the ice cream industry for several decades. However, particles of fat are evident when frozen cream is thawed. Homogenization of high-fat products such as cream has little effect in preventing demulsification of fat which occurs during freezing. The addition of sugar and very rapid freezing tend to retard the fat coalescence. Generally, the home freezing of cream produces an unsatisfactory product. Similarly, sour cream does not freeze well, although some dishes prepared with sour cream can be frozen without adverse effects.

Freezing buttermilk is not advocated due to the separation of the watery portion from the solids. If inadvertently frozen, buttermilk can be thawed in the refrigerator, gently mixed and used in cooked products.

Freezing *per se* of milk, cream, and other dairy products does not influence their nutritional properties. However, ascorbic acid and thiamin levels in dairy products may decrease during frozen storage.

MILK, FERMENTED

Milk is fermented with selected bacteria, which convert some of the milk sugar, lactose, into lactic acid. In selected cases, some alcohol is formed additionally.

(Also see MILK AND MILK PRODUCTS, section headed "Cultured Milk and Other Products.")

MILK FREEZING POINT TEST

This test serves as an indicator of adulteration, especially the addition of water. Most milk samples freeze within the range of 31.01° to 31.05°F (-0.530° to -0.550°C). The addition of 1% of water to milk will raise the freezing point slightly more than 0.011°F (0.006°C). Thermistor cryoscopes are sensitive to changes in temperature of 0.002°F (0.001°C).

MILK, FROZEN OR FRESH FROZEN

This is milk that has been pasteurized, treated with an ultrasonic vibrator at 5 million cycles per second for 5 minutes, then frozen to 10°F (-12.2°C). It will keep for a year; when thawed, it is indistinguishable from the original milk.

MILK SHAKE

Milk and a flavored syrup sometimes with added ice cream either shaken up and down with a hand shaker or blended in an electric mixer.

MILK, TURBIDITY TEST

This is a test to distinguish sterilized milk from pasteurized milk. During sterilization, all the albumin is precipitated. So, in the test the filtrate from an ammonium sulfate precipitation should remain clear on heating, indicating that no albumin was present in solution and the milk had therefore been sterilized.

MILLET *Panicum miliaceum*

Millet is a rapid-growing, warm weather cereal grass of the family, *Gramineae*, genus *Panicum* and species *miliaceum*, whose small grains are used primarily for human food.

Millet provides the major part of the diet of millions of poor people living on the poor, dry lands of India, Africa, China, Russia, and elsewhere.

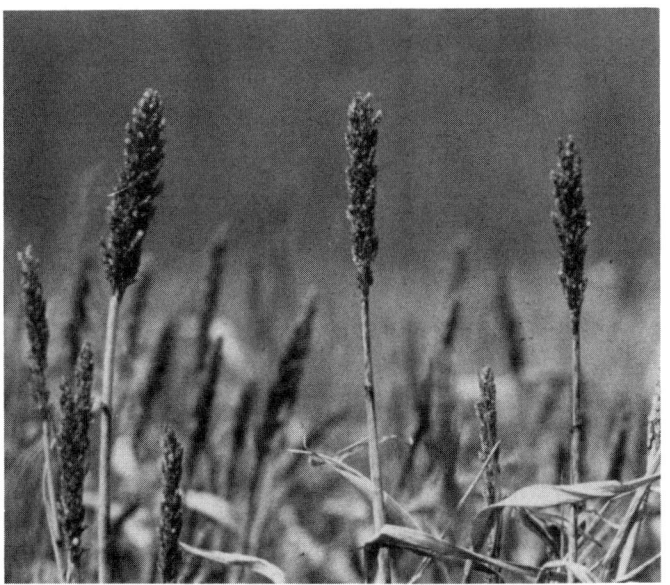

Fig. M-70. Millet the chief cereal grain of millions of people. (Courtesy, USDA)

ORIGIN AND HISTORY. Although millet has been grown in Asia and North Africa since prehistoric times, little is known of its origin. It probably came from Eastern and Central Asia. Millet was important in Europe during the Middle Ages, before corn and potatoes were known there. But it is of minor importance in Europe today.

WORLD AND U.S. PRODUCTION. The annual production of millet totals 30 million metric tons, grown on some 94 million acres *(38 million hectares),* more than 87% of which is produced in Asia and Africa. India alone produces 39% of the world's millet, followed by China and Nigeria, each produces 13% of the global total.[21]

Millet has never been of major agricultural importance in the United States. It is grown primarily as a substitute or emergency crop in the Great Plains and southeastern states.

NUTRITIONAL VALUE. Food Composition Table F-21 provides nutritional information regarding millet.

Some salient points concerning the nutritional value of millet follow:

1. Millet is high in starch—about 70%; hence, it serves as an energy food.

2. Like other grains, millet is low or lacking in calcium, vitamins A, D, C, and B-12.

3. The protein content varies greatly among various types, ranging from 5 to 20%, with an average of 10 to 12%.

MILLET PRODUCTS AND USES. Globally, about 85% of the millet crop is used for food. Millions of the poor in India, Africa, China, and parts of Eurasia depend on millet for 70% or more of their food calories.

Millet grain does not contain any gluten; hence, it is unsuited for making leavened breads. Millet meal and flour are used primarily for making flat breads and griddle-type cakes, and in boiled gruels. Ground millet is used in puddings, steamed meals, and deep-fried doughs, and is mixed with pulses (peas, beans, and lentils), vegetables, milk, cheese or dates. Whole grains are eaten with soups and stews or they are popped, roasted, sprouted, or malted.

Table M-24 presents, in summary form, the use of millet (1) in fortified foods, based on millet, for developing countries, and (2) in fermented beverages.

(Also see CEREAL GRAINS; and FLOURS, Table F-16, Special Flours.)

---

[21]Data from *FAO Production Yearbook 1990,* FAO/UN, Rome, Italy, Vol. 44, p. 83, Table 23. **Note well:** Annual production fluctuates as a result of weather and profitability of the crop.

TABLE M-24
MILLET PRODUCTS AND USES FOR HUMAN FOOD

Product	Description	Uses	Comments
FORTIFIED FOOD, BASED ON MILLET, FOR DEVELOPING COUNTRIES			
Ailment de Sevrage	Mixture of millet flour, peanut flour, skim milk powder, sugar, calcium, and vitamins A and D. It contains 20% protein.	High-protein infant food	Only the Senegal version of this food contains millet. The Algerian version contains wheat.
FERMENTED BEVERAGES			
Millet beers	Brewed beverages made from finger millet, a variety of millet, with or without corn (maize) and sorghum.	Alcoholic beverages	The beers are made by (1) sprouting millet by immersion in a stream, (2) drying and grinding the sprouted grain, (3) preparing a yeasty mixture from part of the sprouted grain by exposure to wild yeasts in the air, or on the surface of the brewing vessel, (4) mixing the freshly prepared yeast with a batch of sprouted grain, and pouring the mixture into gourds where fermentation occurs, (5) diluting the crude beer paste with hot water, and (6) allowing sediment to settle out prior to drinking.

MILLIEQUIVALENT (mEq)

An expression of concentration of a substance per liter of solution calculated by dividing the concentration in mg percent by the molecular weight.

MILLIGRAM

Metric unit of weight equal to 1/1,000 gram.

MINCE

To mince is to chop very finely. Sometimes the food is put through a food grinder to get it as fine as desired. In England, mince refers to ground beef or hamburger. Therefore, in England, rather than going for a hamburger, you would go for a mince.

MINCEMEAT

A special mixture used in pies, coffee cakes, and cookies. It is made with raisins, citron, apple, sugar and spices and usually contains some cooked beef and suet, which has been put through the food chopper along with the apple. The whole mixture is then simmered together. It can be used immediately, packed in sterilized jars, or put in the freezer.

MINERAL(S)

Contents

In nutrition, the term *mineral* denotes certain chemical elements which are found in the ash that remains after a food or a body tissue is burned. Some of these elements are essential to the proper functioning of the body—hence, they must be regularly supplied by the diet. Other elements are not known to be essential, yet they may get into the body by various means.

Each of the essential elements is considered to be either a macromineral or a micromineral, depending upon the quantity which is required in the diet.

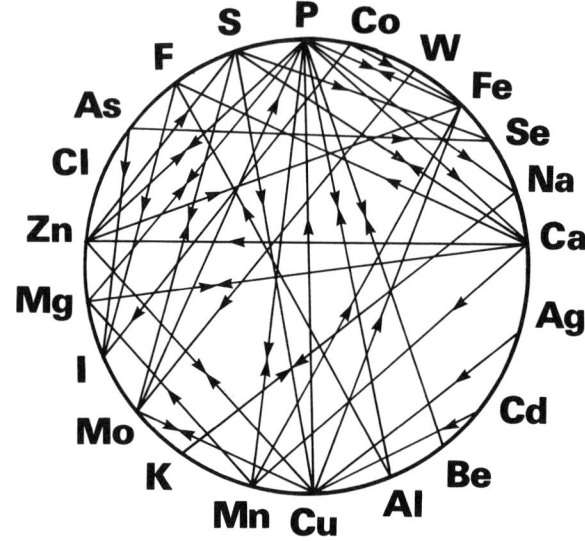

Fig. M-71. Mineral interaction chart, showing the interrelationship of minerals. The importance of such relationships is evidenced by the following:
1. A great excess of dietary calcium and/or phosphorus interferes with the absorption of both minerals, and increases the excretion of the lesser mineral.
2. Excess magnesium upsets calcium metabolism.
3. Excess zinc interferes with copper metabolism.
4. Copper is required for the proper utilization of iron, but excess copper can markedly depress iron absorption.
And there are others! The maze of connecting lines in this figure shows the relation of each mineral to other minerals.

• **Macrominerals**—These elements—which include calcium, phosphorus, sodium, chlorine, magnesium, potassium, and sulfur—are required in amounts ranging from a few tenths of a gram to one or more grams per day.

• **Microminerals (Trace elements)**—These elements are also known as *trace* elements because they are required in minute quantities, ranging from millionths of a gram (microgram) to thousandths of a gram (milligram) per day. As of this writing, the trace elements known to be essential for humans are chromium, cobalt, copper, fluorine, iodine, iron, manganese, molybdenum, selenium, silicon, and zinc. It seems likely that arsenic, vanadium, tin, and nickel may soon be added to this list.

HISTORICAL BACKGROUND. It is noteworthy that certain ancient peoples recognized and treated mineral deficiencies, although they did not understand the bases of their treatments. For example, a Chinese document dated about 3000 B.C. described goiter and recommended that the afflicted people eat seaweed and burnt sponge, which are good sources of the trace element iodine. Another deficiency disease, anemia, was treated in ancient Greece (around the time of Hippocrates, or about 4th century, B.C.) by giving the patient iron-containing water in which heated swords had been quenched. However, the effects of such treatments were often unpredictable, because there were no means of identifying or measuring the quantity of the active ingredients in the various medicinal substances.

The breakthroughs in our understanding of the functions of minerals in the body did not come for many centuries because laboratories for research were not developed until the Renaissance; although the medieval alchemists appear to have invented some of the techniques and tools of chemistry in their futile efforts to change base metals into gold.

The great French chemist Lavoisier, who is credited with being the founder of the science of nutrition, predicted in 1799 that such elements as sodium and potassium would soon be discovered because he believed that they were present in certain mineral compounds which were known as *earths*. Sure enough, within a few years the British chemist Davy discovered not only sodium and potassium, but also calcium, sulfur, magnesium, and chlorine. Davy's discoveries were so highly regarded by the French Academy that in 1806 they awarded him their new Volta medal, even though France and England were at war when the award was presented.

The pace of progress quickened as the noted Swedish chemist Berzelius added to our knowledge of minerals by (1) reporting his analysis of the calcium and phosphorus content of bone in 1801, and (2) concluding in 1838 that the iron in hemoglobin made it possible for the blood to absorb much oxygen. Similar contributions were made by the French chemist Boussingault, who (1) noted in 1822 that South American villagers who used salt containing iodine were protected from goiter which affected those who used plain salt; and (2) showed by means of animal feeding trials the necessity of providing dietary calcium and iron. Calcium studies were also conducted by Chossat, a physician in Switzerland, who won a prize in 1840 for his demonstration that the addition of calcium carbonate to a diet of wheat and water improved bone growth in pigeons.

Another half century elapsed before the value of iodine became widely accepted; thanks to (1) the discovery by the German biochemist Baumann in 1895 that the thyroid gland contained iodine, and (2) the demonstrations by the American medical scientist Marine and his co-workers between 1907 and 1918 that the administration of minute amounts of iodine prevented goiter in animals and in school children.

By the end of the 19th century only about 1/3 of the minerals now accepted as essential were known to be required in the diet. This state of affairs existed in spite of the many nutritional investigations which were conducted during that century because the need for vitamins had not yet been discovered. Hence, it was difficult to differentiate between the deficiency diseases due to lack of minerals and those due to lack of vitamins.

The first two decades of the 20th century were marked by a flurry of discoveries concerning the roles of various vitamins. Then, various minerals were found to be required by animals and man, as indicated by the dates of the discov-

eries which follow: phosphorus, 1918; copper, 1925; magnesium, manganese, and molybdenum, 1931; zinc, 1934; and cobalt, 1935. However, there was often uncertainty as to the metabolic roles of various minerals, even though they were known to be essential. For example, it was not until 1948 that it was established that cobalt functions as a component of vitamin B-12. Hence, the two decades between the 1930s and the 1950s were marked by feverish activity aimed at learning how each of the newly discovered essential elements acted in the body.

The most recent chapter in this story began when Schwarz, a medical scientist who had emigrated to the United States from Germany, and his co-workers discovered the essentiality of selenium in 1957, and of chromium in 1959. They then developed isolation equipment for shielding their animals and their ultrapure diets from contamination by minute amounts of elements in the environment. Their painstaking work paid off because in 1972 they were able to show that fluorine and silicon were also essential. It is ironic that only a short time ago each of these four trace elements was considered to be only an unwanted toxic contaminant of foods, water, and air.

Much work remains to be done in the areas of (1) testing whether other elements might be essential, (2) defining the limits of safe and toxic doses for those already known, and (3) determining how the various elements interact with each other in the human body.

MINERAL TABLE. The general functions of minerals are as follows:

1. Give rigidity and strength to the skeletal structure.
2. Serve as constituents of the organic compounds, such as protein and lipid, which make up the muscles, organs, blood cells, and other soft tissues of the body.
3. Activate enzyme systems.
4. Control fluid balance—osmotic pressure and excretion.
5. Regulate acid-base balance.
6. Exert characteristic effects on the irritability of muscles and nerves.
7. Act together with hormones, vitamins, and other metabolic regulators.

In addition to the general functions in which several minerals may be involved, each essential mineral has at least one specific role. Those which are present in large amounts, like calcium and phosphorus, are likely to have multiple and diverse roles. However, trace elements that are present at barely detectable levels, such as chromium and cobalt, appear to have highly specific functions centered around the organic molecules to which they are bound.

A summary of individual mineral functions, deficiency and toxicity symptoms, recommended daily allowance, and sources is given in Table M-25, Mineral Table. (Calcium, phosphorus, sodium, and chlorine are listed in this order, and first, under macrominerals, then the rest of the minerals are listed alphabetically under their respective categories—as macromineral or micromineral.)

Additionally, a separate presentation relative to each mineral appears alphabetically in this book under its respective name.

TABLE M-25
MINERAL TABLE

Functions	Deficiencies and Toxicity Symptoms	Recommended Daily Allowance			Sources	Comments
		Category	Age (Yrs)	Mineral		

MACROMINERALS:
Calcium (Ca)

The primary function of calcium is to build the bones and teeth, and to maintain the bones..
Other functions are:
1. Blood clotting.
2. Muscle contraction and relaxation, especially the heartbeat.
3. Nerve transmission.
4. Cell wall permeability.
5. Enzyme activation.
6. Secretion of a number of hormones and hormone-releasing factors.
(Also see CALCIUM.)

Deficiency symptoms—The most dramatic deficiency symptoms are manifested in the bones and teeth of the young, evidenced in—
1. Stunting of growth.
2. Poor quality bones and teeth.
3. Malformation of bones—rickets.
The clinical manifestations of calcium related diseases are—
1. Rickets in children.
2. Osteomalacia, the adult counterpart of rickets.
3. Osteoporosis, a condition of too little bone, resulting when bone resorption exceeds bone formation.
4. Hypercalcemia, characterized by high serum calcium.
5. Tetany, characterized by muscle spasms and muscle pain.
6. Kidney stones.
Toxicity—Normally, the small intestine prevents excess calcium from being absorbed. However, a breakdown of this control may raise the level of calcium in the blood and lead to calcification of the kidneys and other internal organs.
High calcium intake may cause excess secretion of calcitonin and such bone abnormalities as osteopetrosis (dense bone).
High calcium intakes have also been reported to cause kidney stones.

Calcium[1] (mg)

Category	Age (Yrs)	Mineral
Infants	0–0.5	400
	0.5–1.0	600
Children	1–3	800
	4–6	800
	7–10	800
Males	11–14	1,200
	15–18	1,200
	19–24	1,200
	25–50	800
	51+	800
Females	11–14	1,200
	15–18	1,200
	19–24	1,200
	25–50	800
	51+	800
Pregnant		1,200
Lactating		1,200

[1]*Recommended Dietary Allowances*, 10th ed., NRC–National Academy of Sciences, 1989, p. 285.

Rich sources—Cheeses, wheat-soy flour, blackstrap molasses.
Good sources—Almonds, Brazil nuts, caviar, cottonseed flour, dried figs, fish with soft edible bones, green leafy vegetables, hazel nuts, ice cream, milk, oysters, sour cream, soybean flour, yogurt.
Fair sources—Beans, bread, broccoli, cabbage, clams, cottage cheese crab, dehydrated apricots, dehydrated peaches, eggs, legumes, lettuce, lobster, okra, olives, oranges, parsnips, peanut butter, prunes, raisins, rhubarb, spinach, Swiss chard, turnips, wheat germ.
Negligible sources—Asparagus, beef, beets, Brussels sprouts, carrots cauliflower, corn and cornmeal and other grains and cereals, cucumbers, fats and oils, juices, kohlrabi, most fish, most fresh fruits, mushrooms, peas, pickles, popcorn, pork, potatoes, poultry, pumpkin, radishes, roe, squash, sugar, tomatoes, tuna.
Supplemental sources—Bone meal, calcium, carbonate, calcium gluconate, calcium lactate, dicalcium phosphate, dolomite, kelp. If calcium is taken as a pill, it should be in the form of some soluble salt, such as calcium lactate.

Calcium is the most abundant mineral in the body. It makes up about 2.0% of the body weight, or about 40% of the total mineral present; 99% of it is in the bones and teeth.
Normally, only 20 to 30% of the calcium in the average diet is absorbed from the intestinal tract and taken into the bloodstream. But growing children and pregnant-lactating women utilize calcium most efficiently—they absorb 40% or more of the calcium in their diets.
Calcium is involved in a number of relationships, which are detailed in the Calcium section of this book.
Generally, nutritionists recommend a calcium-phosphorus ratio of 1.5:1 in infancy, decreasing to 1:1 at 1 year of age and remaining at 1:1 throughout the rest of life; although they consider ratios between 2:1 and 1:2 as satisfactory.

Phosphorus (P)

Essential for bone formation and maintenance.
Important in the development of teeth.
Essential for normal milk secretion.
Important in building muscle tissue.
As a component of nucleic acids (RNA and DNA), which are important in genetic transmission and control of cellular metabolism.
Maintenance of osmotic and acid-base balance.
Important in many metabolic functions, especially—
1. Energy utilization.
2. Phospholipid formation.
3. Amino acid metabolism; protein formation.
4. Enzyme systems.
(Also see PHOSPHORUS.)

Deficiency symptoms—General weakness, loss of appetite, muscle weakness, bone pain, demineralization of bone, and loss of calcium.
Severe and prolonged deficiencies of phosphorus may be manifested by rickets, osteomalacia, and other phosphorus related diseases.
Toxicity—There is no known phosphorus toxicity *per se*. However, excess phosphate consumption may cause hypocalcemia (a deficiency of calcium in the blood).

Phosphorus[1] (mg)

Category	Age (Yrs)	Mineral
Infants	0–0.5	400
	0.5–1.0	600
Children	1–3	800
	4–6	800
	7–10	800
Males	11–14	1,200
	15–18	1,200
	19–24	1,200
	25–50	800
	51+	800
Females	11–14	1,200
	15–18	1,200
	19–24	1,200
	25–50	800
	51+	800
Pregnant		1,200
Lactating		1,200

[1]*Recommended Dietary Allowances*, 10th ed., NRC–National Academy of Sciences, 1989, p. 285.

Rich sources—Cocoa powder, cottonseed flour, fish flour, peanut flour, pumpkin and squash seeds, rice bran, rice polish, soybean flour, sunflower seeds, wheat bran.
Good sources—Beef, cheeses, fish and seafood, lamb, liver, nuts, peanut butter, pork, poultry, whole grain flours.
Fair sources—Breads and cereals, cottage cheese, dehydrated fruits, eggs, ice cream, kidneys, milk, molasses, most vegetables, mushrooms, sausages and luncheon meats, white flour, yogurt.
Negligible sources—Fats and oils, juices and beverages, raw and canned fruits, some vegetables (lettuce, celery, carrots, tomatoes), sugar.
Supplemental sources—Ammonium phosphate, bone meal, calcium phosphate, dicalcium phosphate, lecithin, monosodium phosphate, wheat germ (toasted), yeast (brewers', torula).

Phosphorus comprises about ¼ of the total mineral matter in the body.
Eighty percent of the phosphorus is in the bones and teeth in inorganic combination with calcium.
Normally, 70% of the ingested phosphorus is absorbed.
Generally, nutritionists recommend a calcium-phosphorus ratio of 1.5:1 in infancy, decreasing to 1:1 at 1 year of age, and remaining at 1:1 throughout the rest of life; although they consider ratios between 2:1 and 1:2 as satisfactory.

Sodium (Na)

Helps to maintain the balance of water, acids, and bases in the fluid outside the cells.
As a constituent of pancreatic juice, bile, sweat, and tears.
Associated with muscle contraction and nerve functions.
Plays a specific role in the absorption of carbohydrates.
(Also see SODIUM.)

Deficiency symptoms—Reduced growth, loss of body weight due to loss of water, reduced milk production of lactating mothers, muscle cramps, nausea, diarrhea, and headache.
Excess perspiration and salt depletion may be accompanied by heat exhaustion.
Toxicity—Salt may be toxic (1) when a high intake is accompanied by a restriction of water, (2) when the body is adapted to a chronic low salt diet, or (3) when it is fed to infants.

Sodium[1] (mg)

Category	Age (Yrs)	Mineral
Infants	0–0.5	120
	0.5–1.0	200
Children and adolescents	1	225
	2–5	300
	6–9	400
	10–18	500
Adults	18+	500

[1]**Note well:** The sodium values are "Estimated Minimum Requirements," from *Recommended Dietary Allowances*, 10th ed., NRC–National Academy of Sciences, 1989, p. 253, Table 11–1.

Generally speaking, the need is for low sodium diets, which calls for avoiding high sodium foods. Groupings of common food sources of sodium in descending order follow:
Rich sources—Anchovy paste, bacon, bologna, bran cereal, butter and margarine, Canadian bacon, corned beef, cornflakes cereal, cucumber pickles, cured ham, dehydrated cod, dried squid, frankfurters, green olives, luncheon meats, oat cereal, parmesan cheese, pasteurized process

Most of the salt in the diet is in the form of sodium chloride (NaCl).
Excess dietary salt, over a long period of time, is believed to lead to high blood pressure in susceptible people. Also, excess sodium may cause edema, evidenced by swelling of such areas as the legs and face. The simplest way to reduce sodium intake is to eliminate the use of table salt.
Deficiencies of sodium may occur from strict vegetarian diets without salt, or when there has been heavy,

(Continued)

TABLE M-25 *(Continued)*

Functions	Deficiencies and Toxicity Symptoms	Recommended Daily Allowance			Sources	Comments
		Category	Age (Yrs)	Mineral		
Sodium (Na) *(Continued)*	or others whose kidneys cannot excrete the excess in the urine.				cheese, potato chips, pretzels, sausages, seaweed, shrimp, smoked herring, soda crackers, soy sauce, tomato	prolonged sweating, diarrhea, vomiting, or adrenal cortical insufficiency. In such cases, extra salt should be taken.

catsup, wheat flakes cereal.

Good sources—Breads and cookies, canned vegetables, cheeses, condensed soups, many prepared foods and mixes, peanut butter, pickled foods, salad dressings, seafoods.

Fair sources—Beef, desserts and sweets, eggs, lamb, milk, pork, poultry, salt-loving vegetables (spinach, beets, chard, celery, carrots), some fish (cod, haddock, salmon, tuna) depending upon preparation, veal, yogurt.

Negligible sources—Lard, legumes, most fresh fruits and vegetables, rye flour, shortening, soybean flour, sugar, vegetable oils, wheat bran, wheat flour.

Supplemental sources—Salt (sodium chloride), baking soda, monosodium glutamate (MSG), sodium-containing baking powder.

Functions	Deficiencies and Toxicity Symptoms	Category	Age (Yrs)	Mineral	Sources	Comments
Chlorine or chloride (Cl) Plays a major role in the regulation of osmotic pressure, water balance, and acid-base balance. Required for the production of hydrochloric acid of the stomach; this acid is necessary for the proper absorption of vitamin B-12 and iron, for the activation of the enzyme that breaks down starch, and for suppressing the growth of microorganisms that enter the stomach with food and drink. (Also see CHLORINE or CHLORIDE.)	**Deficiency symptoms**—Severe deficiencies may result in alkalosis (an excess of alkali in the blood), characterized by slow and shallow breathing, listlessness, muscle cramps, loss of appetite, and occasionally, by convulsions. Deficiencies of chloride may develop from prolonged and severe vomiting, diarrhea, pumping of the stomach, injudicious use of diuretic drugs, or strict vegetarian diets without salt. **Toxicity**—An excess of chlorine ions is unlikely when the kidneys are functioning properly.			*Chlorine[1]* (mg)	Table salt (sodium chloride) and foods that contain salt. Persons whose sodium intake is severely restricted (owing to diseases of the heart, kidney, or liver) may need an alternative source of chloride; a number of chloride-containing salt substitutes are available for this purpose.	Chlorine is an essential mineral, with a special function in forming the hydrochloric acid (HCl) present in the gastric juice.
		Infants	0–0.5 / 0.5–1.0	180 / 300		
		Children and adolescents	1 / 2–5 / 6–9 / 10–18	350 / 500 / 600 / 750		
		Adults	18+	750		
		[1]**Note well:** The chloride values are "Estimated Minimum Requirements," from *Recommended Dietary Allowances*, 10th ed., NRC–National Academy of Sciences, 1989, p. 253, Table 11–1.				
Magnesium (Mg) Constituent of bones and teeth. Essential element of cellular metabolism, often as an activator of enzymes involved in phosphorylated compounds and of high energy phosphate transfer of ADP and ATP. Involved in activating certain peptidases in protein digestion. Relaxes nerve impulses, functioning antagonistically to calcium which is stimulatory. (Also see MAGNESIUM.)	**Deficiency symptoms**—A deficiency of magnesium is characterized by (1) muscle spasms (tremor, twitching) and rapid heartbeat; (2) confusion, hallucinations, and disorientation; and (3) lack of appetite, listlessness, nausea, and vomiting. **Toxicity**—Magnesium toxicity is characterized by slowed breathing, coma, and sometimes death.			*Magnesium[1]* (mg)	Groupings by rank of common food sources of magnesium follow: **Rich sources**—Coffee (instant), cocoa powder, cottonseed flour, peanut flour, sesame seeds, soybean flour; spices, wheat bran, wheat germ. **Good sources**—Blackstrap molasses, nuts, peanut butter, whole grains (oats, barley, wheat, buckwheat), whole wheat flour, yeast. **Fair sources**—Avocados, bananas, beef and veal, breads, cheese, chicken, corn, cornmeal, dates, dehydrated fruit, fish and seafoods, lamb, liver, olives, pork, raspberries, rice, turkey, most green leafy vegetables. **Negligible sources**—Cabbage, egg plant, eggs, fats and oils, ice cream, lettuce, milk, most fruits, mushrooms, rhubarb, rutabagas, sausages and luncheon meats, sugar, tomatoes. **Supplemental sources**—Dolomite, magnesium gluconate, magnesium oxide, wheat germ.	Overuse of such substances as "milk of magnesia" (magnesium hydroxide, an antacid and laxative) or "Epsom salts" (magnesium sulfate, a laxative and tonic) may lead to deficiencies of other minerals or even to toxicity.
		Infants	0–0.5 / 0.5–1.0	40 / 60		
		Children	1–3 / 4–6 / 7–10	80 / 120 / 170		
		Males	11–14 / 15–18 / 19–24 / 25–50 / 51+	270 / 400 / 350 / 350 / 350		
		Females	11–14 / 15–18 / 19–24 / 25–50 / 51+	280 / 300 / 280 / 280 / 280		
		Pregnant		320		
		Lactating		355		
		[1]*Recommended Dietary Allowances*, 10th ed., NRC–National Academy of Sciences, 1989, p. 285				
Potassium (K) Involved in the maintenance of proper acid-base balance and the transfer of nutrients in and out of individual cells. Relaxes the heart muscle—action opposite to that of calcium, which is stimulatory. Required for the secretion of insulin by the pancreas, in enzyme reactions involving the phosphorylation of creatine, in carbohydrate metabolism, in protein synthesis. (Also see POTASSIUM.)	**Deficiency symptoms**—Potassium deficiency may cause rapid and irregular heartbeats, and abnormal electrocardiograms; muscle weakness, irritability, and occasionally paralysis; and nausea, vomiting, diarrhea, and swollen abdomen. Extreme and prolonged deficiency of potassium may cause hypokalemia, culminating in the heart muscles stopping. **Toxicity**—Acute toxicity from potassium (known as hyperpotassemia or hyperkalemia) will result from sudden increases of potassium to levels of about 18 g per day for an adult,			*Potassium[1]* (mg)	**Rich sources**—Dehydrated fruits, molasses, potato flour, rice bran, seaweed, soybean flour, spices, sunflower seeds, wheat bran. **Good sources**—Avocado, beef, dates, guavas, most raw vegetables, nectarine, nuts, pork, poultry, sardines, veal. **Fair sources**—Breads, cereals, cheeses, cooked or canned vegetables, eggs, fruit juices, milk, raw, cooked, or canned fruits, shellfish, whole wheat flour, wine, yogurt. **Negligible sources**—Cooked rice, cornmeal, fats and oils, honey, olives,	Potassium is the third most abundant element in the body, after calcium and phosphorus; and it is present in twice the concentration of sodium. Sources of potassium other than foods, such as potassium chloride, should be taken only on the advice of a physician or nutritionist.
		Infants	0–0.5 / 0.5–1.0	500 / 700		
		Children and adolescents	1 / 2–5 / 6–9 / 10–18	1,000 / 1,400 / 1,600 / 2,000		
		Adults	18+	2,000		
		[1]**Note well:** The potassium values are "Estimated Minimum Requirements," from *Recommended Dietary Allowances*, 10th ed., NRC–National Academy of Sciences, 1989, p. 253, Table 11–1.				

(Continued)

TABLE M-25 (Continued)

Functions	Deficiencies and Toxicity Symptoms	Recommended Daily Allowance			Sources	Comments
		Category	Age (Yrs)	Mineral		

Potassium (K) (Continued)

	provided the kidneys are not functioning properly and there is not an immediate and sharply increased loss of potassium from the body. The condition may prove fatal due to cardiac arrest.		sugar. **Supplemental sources**—Potassium gluconate, potassium chloride, seaweed, yeast (brewers', torula), wheat germ.

Sulfur (S)

As a component of the sulfur-containing amino acids methionine, cystine, and cysteine.

As a component of biotin, sulfur is important in fat metabolism.

As a component of thiamin and insulin, it is important in carbohydrate metabolism.

Deficiency symptoms—Primarily retarded growth, because of sulfur's association with protein synthesis.

Toxicity—Except in rare, inborn errors of metabolism where the utilization of the sulfur-containing amino acids is abnormal, excess organic sulfur intake is essentially nonexistent. However, inorganic sulfur can be dangerous if ingested in large amounts.

There are no recommended allowances for sulfur because it is assumed that the sulfur requirements are met when the methionine and cystine intakes are adequate.

For the most part, the sulfur needs of the body are met from organic complexes, notably the amino acids of proteins, rather than from inorganic sources. Good food sources are: cheese, grains and grain products, eggs, fish, legumes, meat, nuts, and poultry.

Sulfur is found in every cell in the body and is essential for life itself. Approximately 10% of the mineral content of the body is sulfur.

As a component of coenzyme A, it is important in energy metabolism.

As a component of certain complex carbohydrates, it is important in various connective tissues.

As a component of insulin and glutathione, it regulates energy metabolism.

As a converter of toxic substances to nontoxic forms, it rids the body (via excretion) of such toxic substances as phenols and cresols.
(Also see SULFUR.)

MICROMINERALS OR TRACE ELEMENTS:

Chromium (Cr)

Component of the Glucose Tolerance Factor (GTF), which enhances the effect of insulin.

Activator of certain enzymes, most of which are involved in the production of energy from carbohydrates, fats, and proteins.

Stabilizer of nucleic acids (DNA and RNA).

Stimulation of synthesis of fatty acids and cholesterol in the liver.
(Also see CHROMIUM.)

Deficiency symptoms—Impaired glucose tolerance, which may be accompanied by high blood sugar and the spilling of sugar in the urine; seen especially in older persons, in maturity-onset diabetes, and in infants with protein-calorie malnutrition.

Disturbance in lipid and protein metabolism.
(Also see DIABETES.)

Toxicity—Chromium is seldom toxic because (1) only small amounts are present in most foods, (2) the body utilizes it poorly, and (3) there is a wide margin of safety between helpful and harmful doses.

Note well: Excesses of inorganic chromium are much more toxic than similar amounts of GTF-chromium.

Category	Age (Yrs)	Chromium[1,2] (mcg)
Infants	0–0.5	10–40
	0.5–1.0	20–60
Children and adolescents	1–3	20–80
	4–6	30–120
	7–10	50–200
	11+	50–200
Adults		50–200

[1]**Note well:** The chromium values are "Estimated Minimum Requirements."
[2]From *Recommended Dietary Allowances,* 10th ed., NRC–National Academy of Sciences, 1989, p. 284.

Groupings by rank of some common food sources of chromium follow:

Rich sources—Blackstrap molasses, cheese, eggs, liver.

Good sources—Apple peel, banana, beef, beer, bread, brown sugar, butter or margarine, chicken, cornflakes, cornmeal, flour, oysters, potatoes, vegetable oils, wheat bran, whole wheat.

Fair sources—Carrots, green beans, oranges, spinach, strawberries.

Negligible sources—Milk, most fruits and vegetables, sugar.

Supplemental sources—Brewers' yeast, dried liver.

Note well: The content and/or availability of chromium in foods may be affected by the following:
1. The chromium content of the soil.
2. The processing of grain.
3. The refining of molasses.
4. The type of cooking utensil.
5. Fermentation.
6. The alcohol-extractable fraction.
(Also see GLUCOSE TOLERANCE FACTOR.)

Further studies are needed to determine chromium's role in metabolism and its nutritional significance.

Chromium levels in the body decline with aging. Hence, it is suspected that some of the cases of adult-onset diabetes are due to lack of GTF-chromium.

Cobalt (Co)

The only known function of cobalt is that of an integral part of vitamin B-12, an essential factor in the formation of red blood cells.
(Also see COBALT; and VITAMIN B-12.)

A cobalt deficiency as such has never been produced in humans. The signs and symptoms that are sometimes attributed to cobalt deficiency are actually due to lack of vitamin B-12, characterized by pernicious anemia, poor growth, and occasionally neurological disorders.
(Also see ANEMIA, PERNICIOUS.)

There is no known human requirement for cobalt, except for that contained in vitamin B-12.

Cobalt is present in many foods. However, the element must be ingested in the form of vitamin B-12 in order to be of value to man; hence, a table showing the cobalt content of human foods serves no useful purpose. Instead, the need is for rich sources of vitamin B-12—liver, kidneys, fish, poultry, eggs, and tempeh.

Cobalt is an essential constituent of vitamin B-12 and must be ingested in the form of the vitamin molecule inasmuch as humans synthesize little of the vitamin. (A small amount of vitamin B-12 is synthesized in the human colon by *E. coli;* but absorption is very limited.

Copper (Cu)

Facilitating the absorption of iron from the intestinal tract and releasing it from storage in the liver and the reticuloendothelial system.

Essential for the formation of hemoglobin, although it is not a part of hemoglobin as such.

Constituent of several enzyme systems.

Development and maintenance of the vascular and skeletal structures (blood vessels, tendons, bones).

Deficiency symptoms—Deficiency is most apt to occur in malnourished children and in premature infants fed exclusively on modified cow's milk and in infants breast fed for an extended period of time.

Deficiency leads to a variety of abnormalities, including anemia, skeletal defects, demyelination and degeneration of the nervous system, defects in pigmentation and structure of the hair, reproductive failure, and pronounced cardiovascular lesions.

Toxicity—Copper is relatively non-

Category	Age (Yrs)	Copper[1] (mg)
Infants	0–0.5	0.4–0.6
	0.5–1.0	0.6–0.7
Children and adolescents	1–3	0.7–1.0
	4–6	1.0–1.5
	7–10	1.0–2.0
	11+	1.5–2.5
Adults		1.5–3.0

[1]**Note well:** The copper values are "Estimated Minimum Requirements," from *Recommended Dietary Allowances,* 10th ed., NRC–National Academy of Sciences, 1989, p. 284.

Groupings by rank of common food sources of copper follow:

Rich sources—Black pepper, blackstrap molasses, Brazil nuts, cocoa, liver, oysters (raw).

Good sources—Lobster, nuts and seeds, olives (green), soybean flour, wheat bran, wheat germ (toasted).

Fair sources—Avocado, banana, beans, beef, breads and cereals, butter, Cheddar cheese, coconut, dried fruits, eggs, fish, granola, green vegetables (turnip greens, collards, spinach), lamb, peanut butter, pork, poultry, turnip, yams.

Negligible sources—Fats and oils, milk, and most milk products (ice

Most cases of copper poisoning result from drinking water or beverages that have been stored in copper tanks and/or that pass through copper pipes.

Dietary excesses of calcium, iron, cadmium, zinc, lead, silver, and molybdenum plus sulfur reduce the utilization of copper.

(Continued)

TABLE M-25 *(Continued)*

Functions	Deficiencies and Toxicity Symptoms	Recommended Daily Allowance			Sources	Comments
		Category	Age (Yrs)	Mineral		

Copper (Cu) *(Continued)*
Structure and functioning of the central nervous system. Required for normal pigmentation of the hair. Component of important copper-containing proteins. Reproduction (fertility).
(Also see COPPER.)

toxic to monogastric species, including man. The recommended copper intake for adults is in the range of 2 to 3 mg/day. Daily intakes of more than 20 to 30 mg over extended periods would be expected to be unsafe.

cream, cottage cheese), other fruits and vegetables than listed above, sugar.
Supplemental sources—Alfalfa leaf meal, brewers' yeast, copper carbonate, copper sulfate.
Note well: Copper sulfate or copper carbonate should only be taken on the advice of a physician or nutritionist.

Fluorine (F)
Constitutes .02 to .05% of the bones and teeth. Necessary for sound bones and teeth. Assists in the prevention of dental caries.
(Also see FLUORINE.)

Deficiency symptoms—Excess dental caries. Also, there is indication that a deficiency of fluorine results in more osteoporosis in the aged. However, excesses of fluorine are of more concern than deficiencies.
Toxicity—Deformed teeth and bones, and softening, mottling, and irregular wear of the teeth.

Fluorine[1] (mg)

Category	Age (Yrs)	Mineral
Infants	0–0.5	0.1–0.5
	0.5–1.0	0.2–1.0
Children and adolescents	1–3	0.5–1.5
	4–6	1.0–2.5
	7–10	1.5–2.5
	11+	1.5–2.5
Adults		1.5–4.0

[1]**Note well:** The fluoride values are "Estimated Minimum Requirements," from *Recommended Dietary Allowances*, 10th ed., NRC–National Academy of Sciences, 1989, p. 284.

Fluorine is found in many foods, but seafoods and dry tea are the richest food sources. A few rich sources follow:

Source	Fluorine (F) (ppm)
Dried seaweed	326.0
Tea	32.0
Mackerel	19.0
Sardines	11.0
Salmon	6.8
Shrimp	4.5

Large amounts of dietary calcium, aluminum, and fat will lower the absorption of fluorine.
Fluoridation of water supplies (1 ppm) is the simplest and most effective method of providing added protection against dental caries.

Fluoridation of water supplies to bring the concentration of fluoride to 1 ppm.

Iodine (I)
The sole function of iodine is making the iodine-containing hormones secreted by the thyroid gland, which regulate the rate of oxidation within the cells; and in so doing influence physical and mental growth, the functioning of the nervous and muscle tissues, circulatory acitivity, and the metabolism of all nutrients.
(Also see IODINE.)

Deficiency symptoms—Iodine deficiency is characterized by goiter (an enlargement of the thyroid gland at the base of the neck), coarse hair, obesity, and high blood cholesterol.
Iodine-deficient mothers may give birth to infants with a type of dwarfism known as cretinism, a disorder characterized by malfunctioning of the thyroid gland, goiter, mental retardation, and stunted growth. A similar disorder of the thyroid gland, known as myxedima, may develop in adults.
Toxicity—Long-term intake of large excesses of iodine may disturb the utilization of iodine by the thyroid gland and result in goiter.
(Also see ENDOCRINE GLANDS; and GOITER.)

Iodine[1] (mcg)

Category	Age (Yrs)	Mineral
Infants	0–0.5	40
	0.5–1.0	50
Children	1–3	70
	4–6	90
	7–10	120
Males	11–14	150
	15–18	150
	19–24	150
	25–50	150
	51+	150
Females	11–14	150
	15–18	150
	19–24	150
	25–50	150
	51+	150
Pregnant		175
Lactating		200

[1]*Recommended Dietary Allowances*, 10th ed., NRC–National Academy of Sciences, 1989, p. 285.

Among natural foods the best sources of iodine are kelp, seafoods, and vegetables grown on iodine-rich soils. Dairy products and eggs may be good sources if the producing animals have access to iodine-enriched rations. Most cereal grains, legumes, roots, and fruits have low iodine content.
Of the various methods for assuring an adequate iodine intake, iodized salt has thus far proved to be most successful, and therefore the most widely adopted method. In the U.S., iodination is on a voluntary basis, nevertheless slightly more than half of the table salt consumed is iodized. Stabilized iodized salt contains 0.01% potassium iodide (0.0076% I), or 76 mcg of iodine per gram.
Iodine may also be provided in bread. But the practice of using iodates in bread making appears to be on the decline.

The enlargement of the thyroid gland (goiter) is nature's way of attempting to make sufficient thyroxine under conditions where a deficiency exists.
Certain foods (especially plants of the cabbage family) contain goitrogens, which interfere with the use of thyroxine and may produce goiter. Fortunately, goitrogenic action is prevented by cooking.
For intakes of iodine, man is dependent upon food, soil, and water. The iodine content of food varies widely, depending chiefly on (1) the iodine content of the soil, (2) the iodine content of the animal feeds (to which iodized salt is routinely added in most countries), and (3) the use of iodized salt in food processing operations. Iodine in drinking and cooking water varies widely in different regions; in some areas, such as near oceans, it is high enough to meet the daily requirement.

Iron (Fe)
Iron (heme) combines with protein (globin) to make hemoglobin, the iron-containing compound in red blood cells; so, iron is involved in transporting oxygen. Iron is also a component of enzymes which are involved in energy metabolism.
(Also see IRON.)

Deficiency symptoms—Iron-deficiency (nutritional) anemia, the symptoms of which are: paleness of skin and mucous membranes, fatigue, dizziness, sensitivity to cold, shortness of breath, rapid heartbeats, and tingling of the fingers and toes.
Toxicity—Approximately 2,000 cases of iron poisoning occur each year in the U.S., mainly in young children who ingest the medical iron supplements of their parents. The lethal dose of ferrous sulfate for a 2-year-old is about 3 g; for an adult it's between 200 and 250 mg/kg of body weight.
(Also see ANEMIA.)

Iron[1] (mg)

Category	Age (Yrs)	Mineral
Infants	0–0.5	6
	0.5–1.0	10
Children	1–3	10
	4–6	10
	7–10	10
Males	11–14	12
	15–18	12
	19–24	10
	25–50	10
	51+	10
Females	11–14	15
	15–18	15
	19–24	15
	25–50	15
	51+	10

Groupings by rank of common sources of iron follow:
Rich sources—Beef kidneys, blackstrap molasses, caviar, chicken giblets, cocoa powder, fish flour, liver, orange pekoe tea, oysters, potato flour, rice polish, soybean flour, spices, sunflower seed flour, wheat bran, wheat germ, wheat-soy blend flour.
Good sources—Beef, brown sugar, clams, dried fruits, egg yolk, heart, light or medium molasses, lima beans (cooked), nuts, pork, pork and lamb kidneys.
Fair sources—Asparagus, beans, chicken, dandelion greens, enriched bread, enriched cereals, enriched cornmeal, enriched flour, enriched rice,

About 70% of the iron is present in the hemoglobin, the pigment of the red blood cells. The other 30% is present as a reserve store in the liver, spleen, and bone marrow.
An excess of iron in the diet can tie up phosphorus in an insoluble iron-phosphate complex, thereby creating a deficiency of phosphorus.
Babies are not born with sufficient iron to meet their needs beyond 6 months.
Milk and milk products are poor sources of iron.
About 20% of the iron in the average U.S. diet comes from fortified products.
Ferrous sulfate is the supplemental

TABLE M-25 *(Continued)*

Functions	Deficiencies and Toxicity Symptoms	Recommended Daily Allowance			Sources	Comments
		Category	Age (Yrs)	Mineral		
		Pregnant[2]		30	fish, lamb, lentils, mustard greens, peanuts, peas, sausages and luncheon meats, spinach, Swiss chard, turkey, turnip greens, whole eggs. **Negligible sources**—Cheese, fats and oils, fresh and canned fruits, fruit juices and beverages, ice cream, milk, most fresh and canned vegetables, sour cream, sugar, yogurt. **Supplemental sources**—Dried liver, ferrous gluconate, ferrous succinate, ferrous sulfate, iron furmarate, iron peptonate, seaweed, yeast.	iron source of choice.
		Lactating		15		

[1]*Recommended Dietary Allowances*, 10th ed., NRC–National Academy of Sciences, 1989, p. 285.

[2]The increased requirement during pregnancy cannot be met by the iron content of habitual American diets nor by the existing iron stores of many women; therefore, the use of 30 to 60 mg of supplemental iron is recommended. Iron needs during lactation are not substantially different from those of nonpregnant women, but continued supplementation of the mother for 2 to 3 months after parturition is advisable in order to replenish stores depleted by pregnancy.

Manganese (Mn)

Functions	Deficiencies and Toxicity Symptoms	Category	Age (Yrs)	*Manganese*[1] (mg)	Sources	Comments
Formation of bone and the growth of other connective tissues. Blood clotting. Insulin action. Cholesterol synthesis. Activator of various enzymes in the metabolism of carbohydrates, fats, proteins, and nucleic acids (DNA and RNA). (Also see MANGANESE.)	**Deficiency symptoms**—The only confirmed deficiency of manganese in man was in connection with a vitamin K deficiency, where administration of the vitamin did not correct the abnormality in blood clotting until supplemental manganese was provided. Analysis of hair and blood samples for manganese content indicate that subclinical deficiencies of the mineral might aggravate such disorders as growth impairments, bone abnormalities, diabeticlike carbohydrate metabolism, lack of muscle coordination of the newborn, and abnormal metabolism of lipids (fatty acids, choline, and cholesterol).	Infants	0–0.5 0.5–1.0	0.3–0.6 0.6–1.0	Groupings by rank of common food sources of manganese follow: **Rich sources**—Rice (brown), rice bran and polish, spices, walnuts, wheat bran, wheat germ. **Good sources**—Blackstrap molasses, blueberries, lettuce, lima beans (dry), navy beans (dry), peanuts, potatoes, soybean flour, soybeans (dry), sunflower seeds, torula yeast, wheat flour, whole grains, (barley, oats, sorghum, wheat). **Fair sources**—Brewers' yeast, liver, most fruits and vegetables, orange pekoe tea, white enriched bread. **Negligible sources**—Fats and oils, eggs, fish, meats, milk, poultry, sugar. **Supplemental sources**—Alfalfa leaf meal, dried kelp, manganese gluconate.	In average diets, only about 45% of the ingested manganese is absorbed. The manganese content of plants is dependent on soil content. It is noteworthy, however, that plants grown on alkaline soils may be abnormally low in manganese.
		Children and adolescents	1–3 4–6 7–10 11+	1.0–1.5 1.5–2.0 2.0–3.0 2.0–5.0		
		Adults		2.0–5.0		

[1]**Note well:** The manganese values are "Estimated Minimum Requirements," from *Recommended Dietary Allowances*, 10th ed., NRC–National Academy of Sciences, 1989, p. 284.

Toxicity—Toxicity in man as a consequence of dietary intake has not been observed. However, it has occurred in workers (miners, and others) exposed to high concentrations of manganese dust in the air. The symptoms resemble those found in Parkinson's and Wilson's diseases.

Molybdenum (Mo)

Functions	Deficiencies and Toxicity Symptoms	Category	Age (Yrs)	*Molybdenum*[1] (mcg)	Sources	Comments
As a component of three different enzyme systems which are involved in the metabolism of carbohydrates, fats, proteins, sulfur-containing amino acids, nucleic acids (DNA and RNA), and iron. As a component of the enamel of teeth, where it appears to prevent or reduce the incidence of dental caries, although this function has not yet been proven conclusively. (Also see MOLYBDENUM.)	**Deficiency symptoms**—Naturally occurring deficiency in man is not known, *unless* utilization of the mineral is interfered with by excesses of copper and/or sulfate. Molybdenum-deficient animals are especially susceptible to the toxic effects of bisulfite, characterized by breathing difficulties and neurological disorders. Severe molybdenum toxicity in animals (molybdenosis), particularly cattle, occurs throughout the world wherever pastures are grown on high-	Infants	0–0.5 0.5–1.0	15–30 20–40	The concentration of molybdenum in food varies considerably, depending on the soil in which it is grown. Most of the dietary molybdenum intake is derived from organ meats, whole grains, leafy vegetables, legumes, and yeast.	The utilization of molybdenum is reduced by excess copper, sulfate, and tungsten. In cattle, a relationship exists between molybdenum, copper, and sulfur. Excess molybdenum will cause copper deficiency. However, when the sulfate content of the diet is increased, the symptoms of toxicity are avoided inasmuch as the excretion of molybdenum is increased.
		Children and adolescents	1–3 4–6 7–10 11+	25–50 30–75 50–150 75–250		
		Adults		75–250		

[1]**Note well:** The molybdenum values are "Estimated Minimum Requirements," from *Recommended Dietary Allowances*, 10th ed., NRC–National Academy of Sciences, 1989, p. 284.

molybdenum soils. The symptoms include diarrhea, loss of weight, decreased production, fading of hair color, and other symptoms of copper deficiency.

Toxicity—In the U.S.S.R., molybdenum toxicity in man is reported to have caused a high incidence of goutlike syndrome associated with elevated blood levels of molybdenum, uric acid, and xanthine oxidase.

Selenium (Se)

Functions	Deficiencies and Toxicity Symptoms	Category	Age (Yrs)	*Selenium*[1] (mcg)	Sources	Comments
Component of the enzyme glutathione peroxidase, the metabolic role of which is to protect against oxidation of polyunsaturated fatty acids and resultant tissue damage. Protecting tissues from certain poisonous substances, such as arsenic, cadmium, and mercury. Interrelation with vitamin E—they spare each other, and with the sulfur-containing amino acids. (Also see SELENIUM.)	**Deficiency symptoms**—There are no clear-cut deficiencies of selenium, because this mineral is so closely related to vitamin E that it is difficult to distinguish deficiency due to selenium alone. The selenium content of the blood, hair, and fingernails may be used as rough indicators of the selenium content of the rest of the body. **Toxicity**—Poisonous effects of selenium are manifested by (1) abnormalities of the hair, nails, and skin; (2) garlic odor on the breath; (3) intensification of selenium toxicity by arsenic or mercury; (4) higher than normal rates of dental caries.	Infants	0.0–0.5 0.5–1.0	10 15	The selenium content of plant and animal products is affected by the soil and animal feed, respectively. Nevertheless, such data are useful as they show which foods are likely to be good sources of the mineral. Groupings by rank of some common food sources of selenium follow: **Rich sources**—Brazil nuts, butter, fish flour, lobster, smelt. **Good sources**—Beer, blackstrap molasses, cider vinegar, clams, crab, eggs, lamb, mushrooms, oysters, pork kidneys, spices (garlic, cinnamon, chili powder, nutmeg), Swiss chard, turnips, wheat bran, whole grains (wheat, barley, rye, oats). **Fair sources**—Cabbage, carrots, cheese, corn, grape juice, most nuts, orange juice, whole milk. **Negligible sources**—Fruits and sugar. **Supplemental sources**—Wheat germ, yeast (brewers' and torula). **Note well:** Many drug stores and health food stores now carry special types of yeast which were grown on media rich in selenium; hence, they contain much greater amounts of this mineral than ordinary yeast. Tablets made from high-selenium yeast are also available.	The high selenium areas are in the Great Plains and the Rocky Mountain States—especially in parts of the Dakotas and Wyoming. The functions of selenium are closely related to those of vitamin E and the sulfur-containing amino acids. Selenium-rich supplements should be taken only on the advice of a physician or dietitian.
		Children	1–3 4–6 7–10	20 20 30		
		Males	11–14 15–18 19–24 25–50 51+	40 50 70 70 70		
		Females	11–14 15–18 19–24 25–50 51+	45 50 55 55 55		
		Pregnant		65		
		Lactating		75		

[1]**Note well:** The selenium values are "Estimated Minimum Requirements," from *Recommended Dietary Allowances*, 10th ed., NRC–National Academy of Sciences, 1989, p. 285.

TABLE M-25 *(Continued)*

Functions	Deficiencies and Toxicity Symptoms	Recommended Daily Allowance			Sources	Comments
		Category	Age (Yrs)	Mineral		
Silicon (Si) Necessary for normal growth and skeletal development of the chick and the rat. These findings suggest that it may also have essential functions in man. (Also see SILICON.)	**Deficiency symptoms**—Deficiencies in chicks and rats are characterized by growth retardation and skeletal alterations and deformities, especially of the skull. Deficiencies of silicon have not been produced in man. **Toxicity**—Silicon does not appear to be toxic in the levels usually found in foods.	A human requirement for silicon has not been established. The silicon intake in the average U.S. diet has been estimated at approximately 1 g per day.			The best sources of silicon are the fibrous parts of whole grains, followed by various organ meats (liver, lungs, kidneys, and brain) and connective tissues. Much of the silicon in whole grains is lost when they are milled into highly refined products.	A common nondietary form of silicon toxicity is a fibrosis of the lungs known as silicosis, due to inhalation of airborne silicon oxide dust.
Zinc (Zn) Needed for normal skin, bones, and hair. As a component of several different enzyme systems which are involved in digestion and respiration. Required for the transfer of carbon dioxide in red blood cells; for proper calcification of bones; for the synthesis and metabolism of proteins and nucleic acids; for the development and functioning of reproductive organs; for wound and burn healing; for the functioning of insulin; and for normal taste acuity. (Also see ZINC.)	**Deficiency symptoms**—Loss of appetite, stunted growth in children, skin changes, small sex glands in boys, loss of taste sensitivity, lightened pigment in hair, white spots on the fingernails, and delayed healing of wounds. In the Middle East, pronounced zinc deficiency in man has resulted in hypogonadism and dwarfism. In pregnant animals, experimental zinc deficiency has resulted in malformation and behavioral disturbances in offspring. **Toxicity**—Ingestion of excess soluble salts may cause nausea, vomiting, purging.	Infants Children Males Females Pregnant Lactating	0–0.5 0.5–1.0 1–3 4–6 7–10 11–14 15–18 19–24 25–50 51+ 11–14 15–18 19–24 25–50 51+	Zinc[1] (mg) 5 5 10 10 10 15 15 15 15 15 12 12 12 12 12 15 19	Groupings by rank of common food sources of zinc follows: **Rich sources**—Beef, liver, oysters, spices, wheat bran. **Good sources**—Cheddar cheese, crab, granola, lamb, peanut butter, peanuts, popcorn, pork, poultry. **Fair sources**—Beans, clams, eggs, fish, sausages and luncheon meats, turnip greens, wheat cereals, whole grain products (wheat, rye, oats, rice, barley). **Negligible sources**—Beverages, fats and oils, fruits and vegetables, milk, sugar, white bread. **Supplemental sources**—Wheat germ, yeast (torula), zinc carbonate, zinc gluconate, zinc sulfate. (Zinc carbonate or zinc sulfate are commonly used where zinc supplementation is necessary.)	The biological availability of zinc in different foods varies widely; meats and seafoods are much better sources of available zinc than vegetables. Zinc availability is adversely affected by phytates (found in whole grains and beans), high calcium, oxalates (in rhubarb and spinach), high fiber, copper (from drinking water conveyed in copper piping), and EDTA (an additive used in certain canned foods).

[1]*Recommended Dietary Allowances,* 10th ed., NRC–National Academy of Sciences, 1989, p. 284.

CAUSES OF MINERAL DEFICIENCIES AND/OR TOXICITIES. Recently, there has been much speculation as to whether many people in the United States might have subclinical deficiencies of certain minerals. It has also been speculated that mild, but chronic, toxicities, due to excesses of certain nutrients, might contribute to the development of such disorders as atherosclerosis, diabetes, heart failure, high blood pressure, and kidney stones. These concerns prompt conjecture that our distant ancestors were also prone to similar diet-related problems. Hence, it is revealing to review certain aspects of man's early existence and to compare dietary factors of the past with those of the present.

Our knowledge of prehistoric diets has been derived mainly from archaeological studies of charred food remains and dried fecal material found in caves and at the sites of ancient camps. Also, there have been many studies of the aborigines who are still engaged in stone age practices in such parts of the world as Africa, Australia, New Guinea, and the Philippines.

Some causes of mineral deficiencies and or toxicities are listed and discussed in the sections that follow.

Agricultural Practices Which May Be Harmful.
Plants use the energy of the sun, gases from the air, and water and minerals from the soil, to make the various substances which are essential for their life processes and for those of animals and man. Hence, the mineral composition of the soil is one of the major factors affecting the nutritive composition of the foods we eat. Agricultural practices affect the utilization of soil minerals by plants in ways which may, in turn, affect animals and people that eat the plants. However, the reader should note that the discussions which follow are not intended to be condemnations of certain practices; rather, they are designed to point out some pitfalls of carrying them to extremes. Consider:

• **Application of sewage sludge to soils**—Although organic wastes may be applied to the soil in order to improve its chemical and physical characteristics, sewage sludge may contain such toxic elements as cadmium, lead, and mercury—particularly when the sludge comes from highly industrialized areas.

• **Close grazing of seleniferous ranges**—This practice forces the grazing animals to eat plants which may contain extremely high levels of selenium. Some of these plants would not be eaten under conditions of light or moderate grazing.

• **Depletion of soil minerals by intensive single cropping**—Growing the same crop on the same area year after year may deplete the soil of certain minerals because they are removed more rapidly than they are replaced by the commonly used fertilizers.

• **Excessive use of copper-containing sprays**—Plants are sprayed with copper compounds in order to prevent certain fungus diseases. However, overspraying may cause the buildup of toxic levels of copper in the plants and/or the soil, which may interfere with the utilization of other minerals.

• **Feeding livestock unsupplemented feeds and forages which have been grown on mineral-deficient soils**—It is well known that products obtained from animals given such feedstuffs are likely to reflect the mineral deficiencies of the soils on which the feeds and/or forages were grown.

• **Overfertilization of soils with certain minerals**—The overapplication of such minerals as nitrogen, potash, potassium, lime, and sulfur to soils may (1) kill soil microorganisms which convert minerals to forms which are readily picked up by plants, and (2) change the chemical composition of the soil so that certain minerals form insoluble compounds which are not available to plants.

(Also see DEFICIENCY DISEASES, section headed "Eating Patterns Which Lead to Dietary Deficiencies.")

Contamination of Drinking Water, Foods, or Air with Toxic Minerals.
Toxic chemical elements—which include some of the essential trace minerals—may get into foods or drinking water from the environment, piping, commercial processing equipment, packaging, or utensils used in the home. In certain cases, such contamination might even be beneficial, if it results in the ingestion of essential minerals which are not supplied in adequate amounts by the foods or the drinking water. However, the margins between beneficial or harmless amounts and toxic levels are rather narrow for certain elements. Furthermore, excesses of certain elements may produce deficiencies of others that they counteract. Hence, it is important to consider how potentially toxic elements get into water, foods, or air so that appropriate measures might be taken to control the amounts which are ingested or inhaled. Consider:

• **Aluminum**—It is not certain whether it is safe to cook such highly acid foods as rhubarb and tomatoes in aluminum pots and pans, because aluminum is dissolved by acid solutions. Abnormally large intakes of aluminum have irritated the digestive tract. Also, unusual conditions have sometimes permitted the absorption of sufficient aluminum from antacids to cause brain damage.[22] Even if the amounts of aluminum leached from aluminum utensils by acid foods are not toxic, there is the possibility that insoluble complexes might be formed between the aluminum and some of the trace minerals, so that the absorption of these nutrients is blocked.

(Also see ANTACIDS; and POISONS, Table P-2, Some Potentially Poisonous [Toxic] Substances.)

• **Arsenic**—Although the public has long thought arsenic to be synonymous with poison, it may be less toxic than the essential trace element selenium, which it counteracts within the body. Also, recent studies on rats suggested that arsenic may be essential.

Minute amounts of arsenic are widely distributed in the common foods, in quantities that are more likely to be beneficial than toxic. However, poisoning may result from foods contaminated with excessive amounts of arsenic-containing sprays used as insecticides and weed killers.

(Also see POISONS, Table P-2, Some Potentially Poisonous [Toxic] Substances.)

• **Cadmium**—In the early 1970s there were many cases of cadmium toxicity in the Jinzu River basin near Toyama, Japan, which is about 160 miles northwest of Tokyo. The disease that resulted was known as itai-itai, or *ouch-ouch* disease, because of the pains the victims had in their bones. Eventually, the poisonings were traced to the chronic consumption of rice and soybeans containing about 3 ppm (parts per million) of cadmium, a nonessential trace mineral which came from the wastes of nearby mines and smelters. Therefore, it is noteworthy that cadmium levels of around 1 ppm have been found in soybeans grown in soil fertilized by sewage sludge, and that oysters taken from waters contaminated by industrial wastes contained about 3 ppm of cadmium.

Other sources of potential environmental contamination by cadmium are cigarette smoke, electroplating processes, paint pigments, the cadmium-nickel type of automobile storage battery, certain phosphate fertilizers, and some of the older types of galvanized water tanks.

While severe cadmium toxicity like that which occurred near Toyama has not been found elsewhere, it is suspected that mild to moderate types of chronic cadmium toxicity may cause disorders of the kidneys leading to high blood pressure. However, the milder forms of cadmium poisoning may be counteracted by such essential minerals as calcium, copper, iron, manganese, selenium, and zinc. Therefore, a few scientists believe that high ratios of cadmium to zinc in the diet and in the various tissues of the body are better indicators of potential cadmium toxicities than the dietary and tissue levels of this toxicant alone.

• **Chlorine**—This element may be ingested as essential chloride ions from inorganic salts, or as toxic organic compounds such as chlorinated hydrocarbons, which may cause liver damage, or even cancer.[23] The toxic chlorine compounds are formed when lake or river water containing nonchlorinated hydrocarbons is chlorinated prior to its use as drinking water. Chlorinated hydrocarbons have been found to be present at various levels in many of the drinking water supplies in the United States, but information is lacking as to the levels which pose either short-term or long-term hazards.

(Also see CHLORINE OR CHLORIDE.)

• **Copper**—Several groups of scientists have recently warned about the possibility of copper poisoning by acid and/or soft drinking water which has been conveyed through copper piping. The blue stains on the surface of sinks where the water drips from the faucet are an indication that drinking water may contain too much copper. About twice as much copper may be present in hot tap water as in cold tap water. Infants are particularly susceptible to the toxic effects of copper in tap water because (1) their water needs are high relative to their size, so they ingest more water in proportion to their body weights than adults; and (2) their diets are usually limited in variety, which means

---

[22]"Possible Aluminum Intoxication," *Nutrition Reviews,* Vol 34, 1976, pp. 166-167.

[23]Ibrahim, M.A., and R. F. Christman, "Drinking Water and Carcinogenesis: The Dilemmas," *American Journal of Public Health,* Vol. 67, 1977, p. 719.

that they may not receive much of the other mineral elements which counteract the effects of copper.

In view of the disorders associated with copper toxicity, it is heartening to note that many of these conditions may be counteracted by increasing the dietary levels of iron, molybdenum, sulfur, zinc, and vitamin C. However, in cases of severe poisoning, it is necessary to administer special metal-binding (chelating) agents which draw copper out of the body.

(Also see POISONS, Table P-2, Some Potentially Poisonous [Toxic] Substances.)

• **Fluorine**—This essential element, like chlorine, is beneficial when it is provided in ionic form (inorganic fluorides) at levels up to 1 ppm in drinking water. The major benefit obtained from such fluoridated water is the increased resistance to tooth decay which occurs when it is consumed by children whose teeth are developing. Higher levels of fluoride (3 to 10 ppm), such as may occur in certain naturally fluoridated waters, may cause mottling of the teeth in some of the children who drink it, although this does not occur if the initial exposure to excessive fluoride takes place after the teeth are fully developed. Furthermore, growing children appear to have greater resistance than adults to the other toxic effects of fluoride, like the development of brittleness in bones and the inhibition of certain enzymes, because growing bones apparently take up fairly large amounts of fluoride without harm.

In addition to fluoridated water, some other sources of significant amounts of fluoride are (1) the environments around aluminum refining plants; and (2) the consumption of tea, crude sea salt, bone meal, or fish (particularly, fish bones). However, the effects of excess fluoride may be reduced somewhat by diets rich in calcium and magnesium.

(Also see POISONS, Table P-2, Some Potentially Poisonous [Toxic] Substances.)

• **Iodine**—Only the radioactive isotope of this element—Iodine 131—is likely to be an environmental hazard, because it emits dangerous radiation. It is formed during the explosions of nuclear weapons; and it may get into foods.

When the contaminated foods are eaten, the radioactive iodine is utilized by the body as if it were normal, nonradioactive iodine. Most of it is picked up by the thyroid gland, which may be injured by the radioactivity that is emitted.

(Also see RADIOACTIVE FALLOUT.)

• **Iron**—The worldwide concern over iron-deficiency anemia has often obscured the fact that excesses of dietary iron might sometimes lead to such disorders as toxic accumulations of the mineral in the liver, spleen, pancreas, heart muscle, and kidneys. This overloading of the body with iron, called hemochromatosis, is most likely to occur in adult males who consume liberal amounts of alcohol. Females are less likely to have such an accumulation of iron because they regularly lose significant amounts of the mineral during their menstrual flow, or as a result of pregnancy and childbirth.

Moderate excesses of iron, which do *not* have direct toxic effects, may produce nutritional deficiencies by interfering with the absorption of copper, manganese, and zinc, and by destroying vitamins C and E.

Some of the sources of iron which may lead to overaccumulation of the mineral in the body are (1) acid foods which have been cooked in iron pots, (2) certain ciders and wines, and (3) occasionally, drinking water. Fortunately, diets containing abundant quantities of phosphorus, copper, manganese, and zinc tend to protect against excesses of iron, because these minerals interfere with its absorption.

• **Lead**—Apparently, lead poisoning has dogged man for a longer time than most people might suspect, because toxic levels of this nonessential mineral were found in the disinterred bones of ancient Romans. In fact, the use of lead for household utensils and wine containers by the Romans is suspected of having been responsible for widespread lead poisoning which, it is conjectured, may have led to weakness and infertility, and the eventual decline of the empire.

Today, there is great concern over acute lead poisoning in young children (ages 1 to 6) who live in urban slums where they may eat chips of lead-containing paints, peeled off from painted wood. The effects of such poisoning may be anemia, hyperactivity, learning difficulties, mental retardation, or even death.[24] There is also concern for older children and adults who might develop chronic lead poisoning from (1) exposure to such sources of the toxic mineral as automobile exhaust fumes, cigarette smoke, fumes from lead smelters, or smoke from coal fires; or (2) consumption of beer held in lead-containing pewter mugs, fruits from orchards sprayed with lead arsenate, fruits and vegetables grown near heavily traveled highways.

Children and pregnant women appear to be most susceptible to lead poisoning because (1) they are likely to have deficiencies of calcium and iron, minerals which protect against lead toxicity; (2) rapidly growing children absorb more lead and excrete less of this metal than other people, and (3) there is a rapid transfer of lead from the blood of pregnant women, through the placenta, to the fetus.

(Also see POISONS, Table P-2, Some Potentially Poisonous [Toxic] Substances.)

• **Mercury**—It is common knowledge that mercury fumes may be responsible for the mental deterioration encountered by some workers in the felt hat industry (often called *mad hatters*). Yet, widespread concern over environmental pollution by the mineral did not develop until the late 1950s when an epidemic of mercury poisonings occurred in Japan.

The mercury poisonings in Japan—which were characterized by losses of balance, hearing, speech, and vision; and by mental disorders—came to be known as "Minamata disease," because they first occurred in people who lived around Minamata Bay, about 50 miles (80 km) southeast of Nagasaki. However, another rash of poisonings occurred around the Agano River in Nugata, a region about 150 miles (240 km) north of Tokyo. Eventually, investigators identified more than 700 cases of mercury toxicity at Minamata, and more than 500 cases at Nugata.[25] The poisonings were traced to the consumption of large amounts of fish and shellfish which contained methylmercury, an organic compound of the element that is much more toxic than its inorganic compounds. It appears that the chain of events which led to the buildup of methylmercury in the fish was as follows:

1. Certain industries discharged their inorganic mercury wastes into Minamata Bay and the Agano River.

---

[24]King, B. G., A. F. Schaplowsky, and E. B. McCabe, "Occupational Health and Child Lead Poisoning: Mutual Interest and Special Problems," *American Journal of Public Health*, Vol. 62, 1972, pp. 1056-1058.

[25]*An Assessment of Mercury in the Environment*, National Academy of Sciences, 1978, p. 90.

2. The bay and the river contained abundant amounts of microscopic organisms which converted inorganic mercury into methylmercury. It also appears likely that the profuse growth of these organisms was promoted by the dumping of organic wastes into these waters.

3. The minute organisms which methylated and stored the mercury were eaten by larger forms of life, which in turn stored the methylmercury. Hence, the poisonous compound eventually became concentrated in the bodies of fish and shellfish.

Another recent outbreak of mercury poisonings occurred in Iraq, where more than 6,000 people were hospitalized after eating bread baked from wheat seed that had been treated with a methylmercury fungicide.[26] The poisonous seed grain had not been intended for human consumption; rather, it had been sent to Iraq for planting. Such fungicide-treated seed does not produce poisonous plants, because the methylmercury is detoxified in the soil.

Around the world, investigations were triggered by the reports of mercury poisonings. Only a few people were found to have unmistakable signs of mercury toxicity, even though some had abnormally high levels of the metal in their tissues. Recently, it has been found that the essential trace mineral selenium sometimes protects people against the toxic effects of mercury. Hence, a food which contains both mercury and selenium may not be as dangerous as one which contains mercury alone. Furthermore, the selenium in one food might also provide some protection against mercury in other foods.[27]

(Also see POISONS, Table P-2, Some Potentially Poisonous [Toxic] Substances.)

• **Selenium**—Although it is suspected that people living in areas with high levels of selenium in the soil may occasionally suffer from such effects of selenium toxicity as dental caries and dermatitis, poisoned livestock commonly develop severe deformities; or they may even die from eating excessive amounts of this essential mineral. It is not that people are immune to severe poisoning from selenium; rather, the grains eaten by people are relatively low in selenium compared to the forage plants eaten by grazing animals. Furthermore, high selenium soils alone will not yield wheat containing abnormally large amounts of the mineral unless it is in a form which is readily available to the growing wheat. Usually, this requires that *selenium converter plants*, such as *Astragulus racemosus*, be present to convert soil selenium to a form which is absorbable by wheat.

In the event that conditions in high-selenium areas should be conducive to the poisoning of people, it is noteworthy that selenium toxicity may be counteracted by arsenic and copper, which are less toxic.

(Also see SELENIUM.)

• **Strontium**—This nonessential element, which is normally nontoxic, has an artificial radioactive isotope—strontium 90—that is produced in man-made nuclear reactions, such as those occurring during the explosion of nuclear weapons or during the generation of nuclear energy. Strontium 90 is toxic because it is absorbed by the body and deposited in the bones, where it continuously emits radiation which may cause such disorders as bone cancer and leukemia.

Strontium is chemically similar to calcium, and is likely to be mixed with this element in foods such as milk, vegetables, and cereals. Hence, it follows that the foods which are most frequently fed to infants and young children are those most likely to be contaminated with radioactive strontium. However, diets high in noncontaminated calcium tend to reduce the absorption of strontium 90.

In the long run, the best protection against the buildup of radioactive strontium in the environment is the cessation of nuclear weapons tests conducted in the atmosphere.

(Also see RADIOACTIVE FALLOUT.)

• **Zinc**—It is not likely that people will receive toxic excesses of zinc from eating ordinary, unsupplemented diets unless some of the foods were stored in zinc-coated (galvanized) containers, because most of the common foods contain only small fractions of the levels of zinc which may be ingested safely. However, zinc toxicity due to contamination of food by galvanized containers or similar means may be accompanied by nausea, vomiting, stomachache, diarrhea, and fever.

Dietary and Medical Treatments. Various types of therapies may eventually lead to deficiencies or toxic excesses of certain essential minerals because they alter the ways in which the body absorbs, utilizes, retains, or excretes these nutrients. Often, countermeasures may be used to offset the undesirable effects of treatments, while retaining the desirable effects. Hence, the typical treatments and effects which follow are noteworthy:

• **Blood transfusions**—Sometimes, blood is given regularly, and over a period of time, to people with various diseases characterized by short-lived red cells. The danger of this practice is that it may lead to the overaccumulation of iron, since each pint of blood contains over 200 mg of the mineral, most of which is likely to be retained within the body.

• **Dialysis of patients with kidney failure**—Dialysis procedures, which are used to remove wastes from the blood of people whose kidney function is impaired, also remove essential minerals. Although certain procedures are designed to prevent the withdrawal of such major minerals as calcium, magnesium, potassium, and sodium, there is still the likelihood that various bloodborne trace elements will be reduced to deficient levels.

• **Dietary modifications**—Restriction or elimination of certain foods in order to produce diets which are low in carbohydrates, fats, or protein may lead to mineral deficiencies, unless great care is taken to provide other sources of the deleted elements. For example, it was found that some typical hospital diets tended to be deficient in copper, iron, magnesium, and manganese.[28]

Even more likely to lead to mineral deficiencies are the *crash diets* which cause rapid loss of weight primarily through loss of water, because there also may be excessive losses of minerals in the urine.

• **Intravenous administration of glucose and/or other nutrients**—Long-term maintenance of hospitalized patients on intravenous solutions may accentuate the effects of mild to moderate deficiencies of chromium, manganese, and zinc, because (1) each of these essential trace elements is involved, somehow, in the actions of insulin, and (2) increases in blood sugar add to the workload of the insulin-secreting system. Also, it is noteworthy that the solutions

---

[26]*Ibid.*, p. 91.

[27]"Mercury Toxicity Reduced by Selenium," *Nutrition Reviews*, Vol. 31, 1973, p. 25.

[28]Gormican, A., "Inorganic Elements in Foods Used in Hospital Menus," *Journal of the American Dietetic Association*, Vol. 56, 1970, p. 403.

commonly used for total parenteral nutrition may or may not contain manganese and zinc, and that most do not contain chromium.

- **Pumping the stomach**—Normally, the minerals which are abundantly present in the digestive juices secreted by the stomach are almost totally absorbed in the intestine so that only negligible amounts of these essential substances are lost in the stool. However, the pumping of gastric fluid from the stomach results in the removal of large quantities of chloride and potassium ions, so that deficiencies of these elements may result, unless measures are taken to replace them.

- **Tube feeding**—When concentrated liquid formulas are fed too rapidly to sick people by stomach tube, there may be diarrhea, dehydration, and losses of both the minerals which are present in the formulas and those which are secreted in the digestive juices. The causes of these undesirable effects are (1) reduction in the secretion of the digestive juices which would normally dilute the formula, due to the illness and the unnatural means of feeding; and (2) the drawing of water from the intestinal wall by the formula, so that a strong laxative effect is produced.

Drugs Which May Affect the Utilization of Minerals by the Body. Certain commonly used drugs affect the utilization of both essential and nonessential minerals by the body. Furthermore, many of these medicines may be used to treat chronic conditions over long periods of time. Therefore, brief descriptions of the effects of some of the most frequently used drugs are presented, so that appropriate measures may be taken to prevent mineral deficiencies or toxicities:

- **Antacids**—The nonabsorbable types of these compounds, such as aluminum hydroxide, may form insoluble complexes in the intestine, which reduce the absorption of phosphate, fluoride, and other essential minerals. Also, it recently became apparent that certain patients with kidney diseases who had been put on diets low in phosphate and who were given regular dialysis treatments absorbed considerable amounts of aluminum from antacids, because they developed toxic deposits of the metal in the brain and the bones.[29]

When consumed in excess, the absorbable antacids, which yield such absorbable ions as calcium, magnesium, sodium, and bicarbonate, may lead to toxic excesses of these ions in the body.
(Also see ANTACIDS.)

- **Antibiotics**—The tetracycline types of these drugs may form insoluble, unabsorbable complexes with such essential minerals as calcium, iron, and magnesium.

- **Anticonvulsants**—Epileptic patients given these drugs for the prevention of seizures have sometimes developed softening and distortion of their bones which may lead to rickets in children, or to softening of the bones (osteomalacia) in adults.[30] Apparently, the drugs produce their harmful effects on the bones by provoking increased rates of destruction of vitamin D and its active metabolites, so that the absorption and utilization of dietary calcium is reduced. Sometimes, their effects have been overcome by providing

extra vitamin D and/or additional exposure to sunlight.

- **Blood-cholesterol-lowering agents**—It is suspected that the types of these drugs which bind with cholesterol and bile salts in the intestine may similarly tie up calcium and other minerals so that their absorption is reduced.

- **Diuretics (*water pills*)**—Usually, these drugs are given to people with water accumulation in their tissues and/or high blood pressure. Some of them may promote excessive urinary losses of potassium and other essential minerals.

- **Hormones**—Although the administration of adrenocorticotropic hormone (ACTH) and cortisone has often provided great relief for those who suffer from allergies and from inflammatory diseases like arthritis, the long-term use of these hormones has sometimes caused loss of bone minerals to the extent that weakening of the bones (osteoporosis) and/or collapse of the spine have occurred.

- **Laxatives**—Habitual use of these drugs may result in mineral deficiencies because they reduce the intestinal absorption of (1) dietary minerals, and (2) minerals secreted in the various digestive juices.

- **Mineral supplements**—The consumption of excessive amounts of certain minerals in the form of pills or tonics may lead to the deficiencies of other minerals, because there are diverse interactions between the various essential elements. For example, high intakes of iron may interfere with the absorption of copper, phosphorus, and zinc.

- **Oral contraceptives (birth control pills)**—The full details are still uncertain, but it appears that these drugs alter the metabolic processes which involve calcium, magnesium, and phosphorus.

Food Additives. Many natural and synthetic substances are added to foods to improve their color, odor, texture, and taste. The U.S. Food and Drug Administration has established strict regulations governing food additives so that there is little likelihood of any direct toxic effects resulting from the proper use of such ingredients. However, some of these substances affect the utilization of certain minerals. Such effects may not be important to people who eat a little of everything, but they may be responsible in part for mineral deficiencies or toxicities in people whose diets are narrowly limited by choice, economic circumstances, or other factors. Therefore, some effects of various food additives on mineral metabolism follow:

- **Aluminum compounds**—The amounts of aluminum that most people consume in the form of food additives—mainly present in such items as baking powder, pickles, and processed cheeses—are probably less than that ingested by people who regularly take aluminum-containing antacids. For example, 3½ oz (*100 g*) of one brand of processed American cheese was found to contain 70 mg of aluminum,[31] which is about the amount present in a single tablet of a commonly used antacid. Nevertheless, even small amounts of aluminum may form nonabsorbable complexes with essential trace elements such as iron.

- **Bran**—This product of flour milling is sometimes added to breads and cereals to increase their fiber content.

[29]Alfrey, A. C., et al., "The Dialysis Encephalopathy Sydrome," *The New England Journal of Medicine*, Vol. 294, 1976, p. 184.

[30]"Anticonvulsant Drugs and Calcium Metabolism," *Nutrition Reviews*, Vol. 33, 1975, pp. 221-222.

[31]Gormican, A., "Inorganic Elements in Foods Used in Hosptial Menus," *Journal of the American Dietetic Association*, Vol. 56, 1970, p. 399, Table 1.

However, it is rich in phytates, phosphorus compounds that bind many of the essential minerals so that they are not readily absorbed. It is noteworthy that the leavening of breads with yeast overcomes much of the effects of phytates.[32]

• **Chelating agents**—These additives are used to bind metallic mineral elements like copper, iron, and zinc, because the unbound forms of the minerals may promote the deterioration and/or discoloration of foods.

The effects of added chelating agents may be beneficial, unfavorable, or uncertain with respect to mineral nutrition, because (1) foods may contain naturally occurring chelating agents which interact with the food additives; (2) some agents interfere with mineral absorption, while others enhance it; (3) sometimes, agents which enhance the absorption of metals also increase their urinary excretion; and (4) the overall mineral content of the diet often determines which of the various metals will be bound to the chelating agent(s), and which will remain free.

• **Gums**—These water-soluble mucilaginous materials may be added to a wide variety of processed foods to produce clarification (by binding with clouding agents), gelling, stabilization (prevention of the separation of various components), and thickening. Many of the gums used in foods are neither digested nor absorbed by man; hence, they may tie up essential minerals so that they are poorly absorbed. For example, sodium alginate—a seaweed derivative which is sometimes added to beers, cheeses, ice creams, salad dressings, sausages, whipped toppings, and wines—forms insoluble, nonabsorbable complexes with iron and copper.

• **Iodates**—Some nutritionists have expressed concern lest the use of these compounds as dough conditioners in the baking industry may lead to excessive consumption of iodine. Hence, it is noteworthy that the iodate fortification of bread for the prevention of goiter in Tasmania was accompanied by an increased incidence of iodine-induced overactivity of the thyroid gland (hyperthyroidism) in goiter-prone people.[33]

• **Iron**—In 1970, the American Bakers Association and the Millers' National Federation asked the U.S. Food and Drug Administration to triple the amount of iron permitted in the enrichment of flour and bread because there was widespread concern over iron-deficiency anemia in women and children.[34] However, it was strongly opposed by some of the leading blood specialists on the grounds that it might lead to toxic accumulations of iron in the tissues of susceptible people.

Finally, in late 1977, the FDA decided that there were too many unresolved questions regarding the safety of adding the proposed levels of iron to breads and flour, so they rejected the proposal by the bakers and the millers.

There is no evidence that the current amounts of iron which are added to foods pose any hazards.

• **Phosphates**—It has been estimated that the widespread use of phosphates as food additives may make the calcium to phosphorus ratio in the American diet as low as 1:4. This mineral imbalance may lead to poor absorption and utilization of dietary calcium, and perhaps even to certain bone disorders.

Sometimes, these effects may be prevented by extra dietary vitamin D, or by exposure to sunlight. However, newborn infants, whose kidneys do not excrete excess phosphate as well as those of older infants and children, may develop high blood levels of phosphate and have seizures when they are fed evaporated milk containing phosphate additives.[35] The seizures are attributed to the fact that cow's milk contains almost four times the calcium and over six times the phosphorus present in human breast milk.[36] Furthermore, extra phosphate is often added to evaporated milk to lengthen its shelf life. Hence, newborn babies fed evaporated milk (diluted with an equal volume of water) may receive between seven and eight times the phosphorus they would get from the same amount of human breast milk. An elevation of the blood level of phosphate causes a corresponding drop in the level of ionized calcium. The direct cause of the milk-induced seizures is the lack of sufficient ionized calcium in the blood.

Fortunately, such seizures have become much less of a problem in the United States, because (1) the use of commercial infant formulas which contain much less phosphate have essentially replaced the use of evaporated milk for feeding newborn infants; and (2) pediatricians generally advise mothers who neither breast feed nor use commercial formulas either to dilute fresh cow's milk or to use extra water in diluting evaporated milk.

Another problem which may result from high levels of dietary phosphate is the formation of nonabsorbable complexes with essential trace elements such as iron.

• **Sodium compounds**—It is suspected that high intakes of sodium may be one of the factors which lead to the development of high blood pressure in susceptible people. Natural, unprocessed foods contain only small amounts of sodium compared to most commercially processed foods. Furthermore, in addition to being present in foods in the form of common salt (sodium chloride), sodium may also be present in such additives as sodium bicarbonate, monosodium glutamate, and various types of phosphates. Therefore, the consumer who is on a low-sodium diet must read carefully the labels of food products because items which are low in salt may contain liberal amounts of other sodium compounds.

(Also see SODIUM.)

Food Processing. The development of food processing has enabled man to modify such undesirable qualities of natural foods as bulkiness, toughness, susceptibility to spoilage, and in some cases, even toxicity. However, certain processes may lessen the mineral values of foods, while others may enhance them. The favorable effects are given in the section of this article headed, "Production and Preparation of Foods to Maximize Their Mineral Values." The details which follow cover some of the detrimental effects:

• **Canning fruits and vegetables**—Some of the minerals in canned fruits and vegetables escape into the packing fluid,

---

[32]"Zinc Availability in Leavened and Unleavened Bread," *Nutrition Reviews,* Vol. 33, 1975, pp. 18-19.

[33]"Iodine Fortification and Thyrotoxicosis," *Nutrition Reviews,* Vol. 28, 1970, pp. 212-213.

[34]"Anatomy of a Decision,"*Nutrition Today,* Vol. 13, January/February, 1978, pp.6-7.

[35]Filer, L., Jr., "Excessive Intakes and Imbalance of Vitamins and Minerals," *Nutrients in Proposed Foods: Vitamins-Minerals,* (Papers from a symposium sponsored by the American Medical Association), Publishing Sciences Group, Inc., Acton, Mass., 1974, p. 27.

[36]Robson, et al., *Malnutrition: Its Causation and Control,* Gordon and Breach, Science Publishers, Inc., 1972, Vol. 1, p. 125, Table 12.

which may be discarded. The amount of mineral loss depends upon such factors as the type of processing, degree of acidity of the packing medium, and the length of storage.

• **Cheese making**—During this process, milk is clotted by either acid or rennet (an enzyme-containing substance derived from animal stomachs) so that it separates into cheese and whey. Usually, much more calcium and phosphorus are lost in the whey from acid-clotted items like cottage cheese than from the rennet-clotted cheeses like Cheddar and Swiss.

• **Milling grains**—The greater part of the mineral content of grains is lost during milling because these elements are usually concentrated in the outer layers of the seed. Hence, such by-products of milling as bran, hominy feed, and rice polishings are excellent sources of many essential minerals. Usually, these by-products are fed to livestock, although they are sometimes added to special breads and cereals.

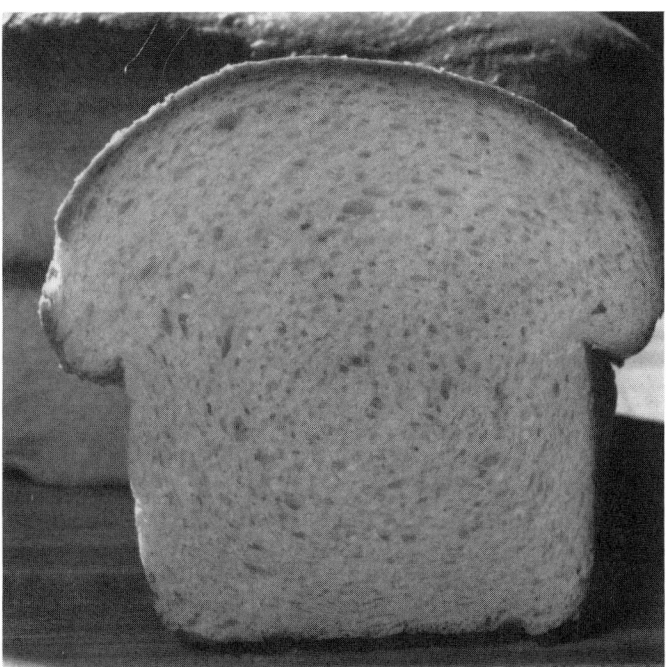

Fig. M-72. Milling wheat to produce white flour for the making of bread removes much of the mineral content because the minerals are concentrated in the outer layers of the seed. (Courtesy, University of Minnesota, St. Paul, Minn.)

• **Refining sugar**—Most of the minerals that are present in raw sugar made from either sugarcane or sugar beets are (1) removed as the sugar is refined, and (2) end up in the crude molasses, which is a by-product. Cane molasses may be marketed for human consumption as dark molasses, or *blackstrap* molasses, but because beet molasses is bitter, it is sold as a feed ingredient.

Metabolic Disorders Which May Alter Mineral Metabolism. Various disorders of metabolism may interfere with the ways in which the body normally absorbs, utilizes, and excretes essential minerals, so that deficiencies and/or toxicities may result. Sometimes, the disorders produce conditions so precarious that the maintenance of the proper blood levels of sodium, potassium, calcium, and magnesium may become a matter of life or death. Brief descriptions of some of these medical problems are given so that the reader may realize the importance of consulting a doctor before taking mineral supplements or making drastic dietary changes, since people differ widely in their susceptibility to these metabolic disorders. Metabolic disorders which may alter mineral metabolism follow:

• **Acidosis**—This condition is characterized by an excess of acid in the blood which may result from such diverse causes as diabetes; diarrhea; diets which are high in fat and protein, but low in carbohydrates; fever; kidney diseases; lung diseases; severe stress; starvation; or trauma. If prolonged, acidosis may lead to (1) excessive urinary loss of calcium and demineralization of the bones; (2) depletion of water, sodium, and potassium; and (3) retention of excessive amounts of phosphate and sulfate ions. The blood levels of potassium may be normal, even when the cells are low in the mineral. Hence, the feeding of injured, sick, or starved people must be done cautiously so as not to aggravate the imbalances in the body's mineral salts.

(Also see ACID-BASE BALANCE.)

• **Addison's disease**—Victims of this disorder have abnormally low secretions of adrenal cortical hormones, so they are unable to retain sufficient amounts of sodium and water in their bodies to counter such stresses as dehydration and low-sodium diets. However, they may retain excessive amounts of potassium in their blood, which may cause cardiac arrest.

(Also see ADDISON'S DISEASE; and ENDOCRINE GLANDS.)

• **Alkalosis**—The main causes of alkalosis, which is an excess of alkali in the blood, are: (1) the consumption of large amounts of such absorbable antacids as sodium bicarbonate, (2) the loss of large amounts of stomach acid through vomiting, (3) the depletion of the body's supply of chloride ions through vomiting or diarrhea, and (4) excessively deep breathing—due to nervousness or overdoses of aspirin—which eliminates too much carbon dioxide. Alkalosis may be accompanied by the development of a potassium deficiency, due to an excessive loss of the mineral in the urine; and a reduction in the blood level of calcium ions, so that muscle spasms may occur.

(Also see ACID-BASE BALANCE.)

• **Congestive heart failure**—Abnormalities such as the accumulation of fluid in the tissues, and an overtaxing of the heart muscle, make the patient with heart failure extra susceptible to the toxic effects of imbalances between the blood and tissue levels of such ions as sodium, potassium, calcium, and magnesium. Extra magnesium and potassium may be given to prevent irregular heartbeats when digitalis is used as a medication. However, too much potassium may cause cardiac arrest, if the kidneys are not able to excrete excesses of this mineral in the urine.

(Also see HEART DISEASE.)

• **Cushing's syndrome**—This disorder is characterized by oversecretion of adrenal cortical hormones which cause the breakdown and loss of protein from the bones and muscles. Potassium is lost along with muscle protein, and the bone minerals—mainly calcium and phosphorus—are lost when the protein structure of bone breaks down. People with Cushing's syndrome often have an accumulation of salt and water in their tissues, a condition which gives rise to a rounded body, *moon-face*, and high blood pressure.

(Also see CUSHING'S SYNDROME; and ENDOCRINE GLANDS.)

• **Diabetes**—Uncontrolled diabetes is frequently accompanied by acidosis and ketosis—conditions characterized by excesses of acid and ketones in the blood—which may lead to depletion of bone calcium and of muscle potassium. It is noteworthy that the treatment of diabetes with insulin results in the rapid uptake of bloodborne potassium by the tissues. Hence, there may be a dangerous drop in the blood level of this mineral, unless extra amounts are given.

(Also see DIABETES MELLITUS.)

• **Goiter**—People with goiter may be overly susceptible to the toxic effects of excess iodine because their thyroid glands have become extra efficient in the utilization of this mineral. Therefore, they may develop oversecretion of thyroid hormones (hyperthyroidism) when given extra iodine. This toxic condition may sometimes be accompanied by the loss of calcium from the bones, and of potassium from the muscles.

(Also see ENDOCRINE GLANDS; GOITER; and IODINE.)

• **Hemolytic anemia**—Several types of anemias are characterized by an overly rapid breakdown of red blood cells, which may be caused by genetic, nutritional, and/or toxic factors. Administration of extra iron or blood transfusions to people with these disorders may be dangerous because the iron which is released during the destruction of red cells may accumulate in various tissues where it may cause damage.

(Also see ANEMIA.)

• **High blood pressure**—Sometimes, this condition results from a failure of the kidneys to excrete excess sodium, which promotes the accumulation of water in the body. Certain people appear to be overly susceptible to the effects of only moderate excesses of dietary sodium, so they should restrict their salt intake in order to avoid high blood pressure.

(Also see HIGH BLOOD PRESSURE.)

• **Ketosis**—The most common causes of this condition—which is characterized by an excess of ketones in the blood—are (1) diabetes; (2) diets high in fat and protein, but low in carbohydrate; (3) fevers; and (4) starvation. A mild ketosis in normally healthy people is usually not dangerous, unless it occurs regularly over a long period of time. Then, it may lead to such problems as (1) excessive urinary loss of sodium and water; (2) acidosis which provokes the loss of calcium from bone, and potassium from muscle; and (3) the accumulation of uric acid (a waste product of protein metabolism) in the blood, and sometimes in the soft tissues where it causes damage and pain (the latter disorder is commonly called gout). Uric acid buildup is usually treated with alkalizers to prevent the formation of kidney stones. However, the alkalizers may cause other alterations in mineral metabolism.

It is noteworthy that two men who lived for 1 year on a ketogenic diet consisting only of beef, veal, lamb, pork, and chicken lost about 300 mg of calcium from their bodies each day.[37]

(Also see DIABETES MELLITUS; MODIFIED DIETS; and STARVATION.)

• **Kidney diseases**—These disorders are usually accompanied by excessive loss of certain minerals in the urine and/or excessive retention of others, depending upon the parts of the kidney which are diseased. Kidney function may also be impaired whenever the blood supply to the organs is reduced, such as occurs in heart failure and shock. Furthermore, certain kidney diseases impair the metabolism of vitamin D, so that the utilization of calcium and phosphorus may be greatly reduced.

(Also see KETOSIS; and KIDNEY DISEASES.)

• **Lack of stomach acid**—Older people may have a deficiency of stomach acid. This may contribute to mineral malnutrition because acid is needed to offset the alkalinity of bile and pancreatic juice which tends to reduce the absorption of certain minerals.

• **Oversecretion of parathyroid hormone (PTH)**—This condition may be due to (1) a tumorous growth of the parathyroid glands, or (2) enlargement of the glands due to prolonged stimulation by a chronically low blood level of calcium ions. The hormone raises the blood calcium by causing its withdrawal from the bones. Hence, the chronic oversecretion of PTH may lead to such troubles as demineralization of bones, excessive excretion of phosphorus so that muscle weaknesses result, and deposition of calcium in tissues such as the kidneys.

(Also see CALCIUM; ENDOCRINE GLANDS; and PHOSPHORUS.)

• **Rickets**—This disease of infancy and childhood, which is usually due to a deficiency of vitamin D, is characterized by poor utilization of dietary calcium and phosphorus for the mineralization of bones. A similar condition, which may occur in adults, is called *softening of the bones* or osteomalacia.

(Also see CALCIUM; PHOSPHORUS; RICKETS; and VITAMIN D.)

• **Starvation**—The extreme deprivation of food is increasingly being used as a means to achieve a rapid loss in body weight, even though there may be such harmful effects as severe depletion of water, sodium, and potassium. These effects have often led to serious disorders of the heart, and even death—in cases of both voluntary and involuntary starvation. Furthermore, there may be abnormal shifts of mineral salts and water between the tissues and the blood, so it may be difficult to decide how to rehabilitate starved people without aggravating their water and salt imbalances.

(Also see STARVATION.)

• **Vitamin D poisoning**—Overdoses of this vitamin may raise the blood calcium so high that the mineral forms harmful deposits in many of the soft tissues in the body. If this toxicity is prolonged, there may be demineralization of the bones since the high blood calcium is maintained at the expense of the bones. A similar, but milder type of poisoning may result from the overexposure of fair-skinned people to sunlight or other forms of ultraviolet light, such as sunlamps.

(Also see VITAMIN D.)

Mineral Composition of the Soil. There has been continuing controversy over how the mineral composition of the soil might affect the nutrient levels of the plants grown on it. The U.S. Food and Drug Administration has long maintained that (1) mineral deficiencies in soils may lead to reduced yields of plants rather than to plants containing sub-

---

[37]Randall, H. T., "Water, Electrolytes, and Acid-Base Balance," *Modern Nutrition in Health and Disease*, 5th ed., edited by R. S. Goodhart and M. E. Shils, Lea & Febiger, Philadelphia, Pa., 1973, p. 360.

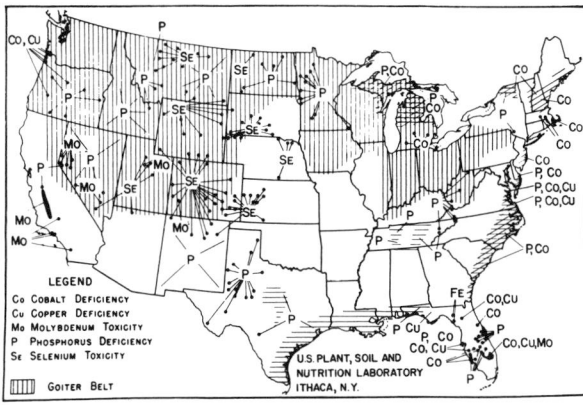

Fig. M-73. Known areas in the U.S. where mineral nutritional diseases of animals occur. The dots indicate approximate locations where troubles occur. The lines not terminating in dots indicate a generalized area or areas where specific locations have not been reported.

People need to be aware of any soil mineral dificiencies or of certain minerals that may cause toxicities because there is a direct and most important relationship between soil minerals and plant composition. (Courtesy, USDA)

normal levels of minerals; and (2) most people eat a wide variety of foods from different areas of the United States, so that variations in the mineral contents of foods tend to average out. On the other hand, certain proponents of organic farming may go so far as to assert that various human nutritional deficiencies may be due to the consumption of products grown on mineral-deficient soils. It is difficult to evaluate the information presented in support of each side of the controversy, because comparisons have often been made between different nutrients in different crops which have been grown on different soils.

Present research, together with practical observation, points to the fact that the mere evaluation of crop yields in terms of tons of forage or bushels of grain produced per acre is not enough. Neither does a standard food analysis (a proximate analysis) tell the whole story. Rather, there is a direct and most important relationship between the fertility of the soil and the composition of the plant.

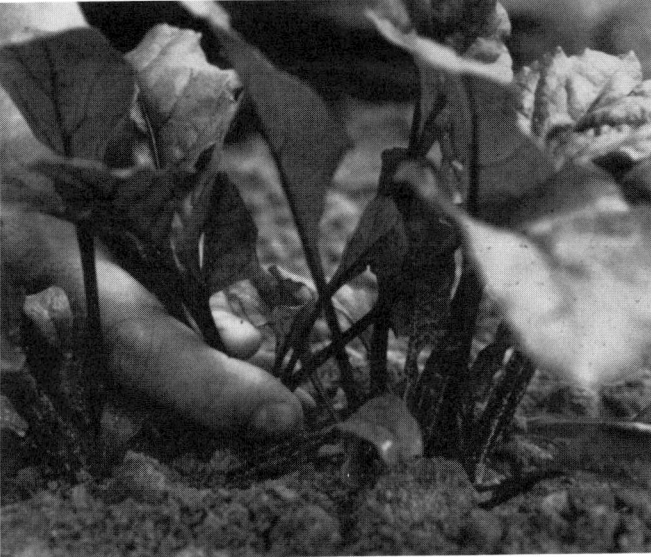

Fig. M-74. Mineral deficient soils may produce mineral deficient plants, which can cause mineral deficient people. (Courtesy, USDA)

The land surface of the earth is covered with many kinds of soil. Some of them naturally contain an abundant supply of most of the elements needed by both plants and animals. Other soils may have an abundant supply of most required elements and yet be deficient in one or more essential. For example, southwestern United States is known as a phosphorus-deficient area; northwestern United States and the Great Lakes region are iodine-deficient areas, and southeastern United States is a cobalt-deficient area.

At every step in the chain from soils to man, the essential mineral elements interact with other elements, and these interactions may profoundly affect the availability of essential elements or the amount of the essential element required for normal growth or metabolic function. For example, a high level of sulfate in the soil may depress the uptake of selenium by plants, and cause the people that eat the plants to suffer from selenium deficiency. The availability of zinc may be depressed if the diet is high in calcium. These and other interactions must be considered in assessing whether a given soil will supply plants with needed nutrients, and, in turn, whether plants will supply the people that consume them with needed nutrients.

Thus, the transfer of essential nutrient elements from soils to plants, thence to man, is a complicated process.

Naturally Occurring Mineral Antagonists in Foods. Although there has been much recent praise of the virtues of natural, unprocessed foods, certain naturally occurring substances present in foods may interfere with the absorption and utilization of minerals by the body. Sometimes, these interfering substances or antagonists may contribute to the development of mineral deficiencies, when diets are barely adequate with respect to these nutrients. Hence, it is important to identify the most common types of naturally occurring mineral antagonists, such as—

• **Fiber**—Plant foods that contain large amounts of indigestible carbohydrate (fiber) tend to stimulate more rapid movements of the intestine, so that the absorption of minerals and other nutrients may be reduced. Another way in which fiber may reduce mineral absorption is by enveloping certain mineral elements so that they pass into the stool with the indigestible matter.

• **Goitrogens**—Certain plants contain substances called goitrogens, which interfere with the utilization of iodine by the thyroid gland, so that the gland becomes enlarged. An enlarged thyroid gland is called a goiter. The most common food sources of goitrogens are Brussels sprouts, cabbage, kohlrabi, rutabaga, and turnip. Even the milk of cows which have been fed substantial amounts of these plants may be goitrogenic. Also, it is noteworthy that soybeans contain a goitrogen, which may be rendered less toxic by heating.[38]

(Also see DEFICIENCY DISEASES, section headed "Major Dietary Deficiency Diseases"; and GOITER.)

• **Interacting minerals**—Excesses of various essential or nonessential minerals may reduce the absorption and/or the activity in the body of other minerals. Such interferences are most likely to happen when large excesses of special mineral supplements are taken. However, they may occur to a lesser degree when (1) the diet lacks variety, and disproportionate amounts of phosphate are obtained from foods like fish, meats, nuts, and poultry; and (2) most of the

[38]Wills, J.H., Jr., "Goitrogens in Foods," *Toxicants Occurring Naturally in Foods,* National Academy of Sciences, 1966, p. 8.

foods have been produced in a particular area where the environment is heavily contaminated with such toxic elements as arsenic, cadmium, copper, lead, mercury, or selenium.

(Also see Table M-25 for additional details on mineral interrelationships.)

• **Naturally occurring chelating agents**—Many naturally occurring substances in foods—such as amino acids and other organic acids like citric, oxalic, salicylic, and tartaric—may bind with (chelate) metallic mineral elements in the digestive tract. The effects of such chelating agents may be either beneficial or detrimental, depending upon whether mineral absorption is enhanced or reduced. Also, the effects of chelating agents may be counteracted by dietary excesses of metal which are chemically similar, because such metals may compete for binding to the chelator. Therefore, it is not known at the present time whether these agents may have significant effects on mineral nutrition when ordinary, mixed diets are consumed.

• **Oxalates**—Nutritionists have long been concerned about whether oxalates, which are present in such foods as rhubarb and spinach, might bind with sufficient amounts of calcium and/or iron so as to produce deficiencies of these minerals. However, experiments have shown that such effects are not likely to occur in man unless (1) the mineral intake is marginal and (2) unusually large amounts of these foods are eaten, along with other sources of oxalates like almonds, beet greens, cashew nuts, cocoa, or tea.[39]

• **Phytates**—These poorly utilized compounds of phosphorus—which are present in the outer layers of grains—bind with such minerals as calcium, iron, and zinc and interfere with their absorption. Hence, mineral deficiencies may occur in people whose diets are composed mainly of whole grain breads. For example, diets based upon these breads were found to be the cause of combined zinc and protein deficiencies which led to stunting of growth and impaired sexual development of males in rural Iran.[40]

The interference of phytates with calcium absorption may be counteracted by supplemental vitamin D and/or exposure of the skin to ultraviolet light from the sun, or from an artificial source such as a sunlamp.[41]

Overconsumption of Alcohol. Alcoholics may suffer from deficiencies of minerals such as magnesium, potassium, and zinc, provoked in part by erratic eating habits and in part by an increased urinary loss of these minerals due to the effects of alcohol.

Alcoholism may also increase the toxicity of certain dietary minerals by causing alterations in the ways in which the body absorbs, utilizes, and excretes these substances. For example, iron deposits in organs such as the liver, pancreas, and spleen may sometimes result from the enhancement of iron absorption by alcohol. Similarly, a moderate to heavy consumption of alcohol appears to have contributed to the cobalt poisoning of certain beer drinkers, because the amounts of cobalt ingested by these people were less than the doses of the mineral which have been used medicinally without such ill effects.[42]

Poor Food Choices. Although a wide variety of foods rich in minerals is available in most supermarkets, people may eat only a few of them for reasons such as (1) lack of money to buy certain items, (2) dependence upon eating most meals away from home, (3) dislike of many types of nutritious foods, and (4) lack of knowledge of and/or the facilities for the preparation of various items. Even the consumption of a wide variety of foods may not guarantee the achievement of adequate mineral nutrition if most of the foods selected are high in fats and carbohydrates, but low in minerals.

Procedures Used in the Preparation of Meals. The preparation of meals may involve procedures which result in the loss of essential minerals. These losses may be great enough to make the difference between adequate and inadequate mineral nutrition. Hence, the food preparation procedures that follow are noteworthy:

1.   The thawing of frozen fish, meat, and poultry results in the loss of some of the juices, but data on their mineral content are scarce. Usually, the amount of fluid which is lost increases as the amount of cut surface increases. Thus, small cubes of beef for stewing will have greater losses than large pieces of meat. It may not always be safe to save the thaw juices from the food, because there may be considerable bacterial growth in the fluids during the period of thawing.

2.   Large amounts of peelings and trimmings may be removed from fruits and vegetables during meal preparation. Often, the material which is removed and discarded may be richer in certain minerals than the part which is retained for eating. For example, the outer green leaves of cabbage may contain from 1.5 to 3 times as much iron as the inner bleached leaves.

3.   Soaking vegetables in water prior to cooking tends to leach out some of the water-soluble minerals.

4.   Cooking fruits and vegetables in lots of water, then throwing away the cooking water, is a sure way to lose plenty of minerals. For example, in one study it was found that the boiling of cabbage led to the following losses of minerals: calcium, 72%; magnesium, 76%; phosphorus, 60%; and iron, 67%.[43] Boiling results in much greater losses of minerals than pressure cooking, baking, frying, steaming, or roasting. The greater the amount of cut surface, the greater the mineral losses. Hence, French cut green beans are subject to greater losses during cooking than cross cut beans.

Stress and Trauma. Many types of stresses and traumas (the term used for sudden shocks, injuries, or wounds to the body) may alter various aspects of mineral metabolism. The reactions of the body to various types of stresses and traumas are similar because (1) such stresses as the deprivation of food or water, extremes of heat or cold, or emotional upsets may damage the body tissues in ways which are similar to the effects of trauma; and (2) most traumas provoke substantial increases in the secretion of stress hormones by the pituitary and adrenal glands. The prolonged secretion of abnormally high levels of stress hormones may lead to excessive losses of potassium, phosphorus, calcium, magnesium, and zinc in the urine. Usually, such conditions are accompanied by greater than normal

[39]Fassett, D. W., "Oxalates," *Toxicants Occurring Naturally in Foods*, National Academy of Sciences, 1966, pp. 259-264.

[40]Prasad, A. S., "Nutritional Aspects of Zinc," *Dietetic Currents*, Vol. 4, September/October 1977, p. 27.

[41]"Phytates and Rickets," *Nutrition Reviews*, Vol. 31, 1973, pp. 238-239.

[42]"Synergism of Cobalt and Ethanol," *Nutrition Reviews*, Vol. 29, 1971, pp. 43-45.

[43]Lachance, P. A., "Effects of Food Preparation Procedures on Nutrient Retention with Emphasis upon Food Service Practices," *Nutritional Evaluation of Food Processing*, 2nd ed., edited by R. S. Harris and E. Karmas, The Avi Publishing Company, Inc., Westport, Conn., 1975, p. 476.

retention of sodium and water, so that fluid sometimes accumulates in tissues and the blood pressure may be raised.

Bad burns produce effects somewhat different from those due to other stresses and traumas because substantial amounts of body fluid and mineral salts may be lost. Hence, burn patients are often very thirsty and drink large amounts of water, which can be dangerous because there may be excessive dilution of the body fluids and the salts which remain. A severe deficiency of sodium might occur under such conditions. Therefore, considerable care must be taken to replenish the body with the proper mixture of mineral salts and water. It is noteworthy that attempts to replace the large losses of calcium and phosphorus rapidly have sometimes led to kidney stones, because the body was unable to use all of the minerals which were provided, so the excesses were filtered through the kidneys.

Another factor which causes increased mineral loss in the urine after an injury is the confinement of the patient to a bed and/or wheel chair. It seems that a certain amount of physical activity is required for the maintenance of optimal bone mineralization.

DIAGNOSIS OF MINERAL DEFICIENCIES.

There are various degrees of mineral deficiencies, ranging from a mild depletion of the body's stores of the mineral(s), to severe clinical disorders which may result in disability or even death. Hence, it may be possible to improve health and increase longevity if mineral malnutrition is detected early by means such as those which follow:

Dietary Histories.

Dietary patterns which might lead to mineral deficiencies may sometimes be discovered by (1) asking people to list the types and amounts of food that they usually eat; (2) calculating their mineral intakes with the help of food composition tables (see Food Composition Table F-21); and (3) comparing their mineral intakes with the mineral allowances which have been set by the Food and Nutrition Board of the National Research Council. These dietary histories may also reveal the presence of conditions that are known to interfere with the absorption and/or the utilization of certain minerals.

Table M-25, Mineral Table, gives the mineral allowances recommended by the Food and Nutrition Board, National Academy of Sciences. However, official allowances are given for only seven essential elements, while estimated safe and adequate ranges of intakes are given for five, and minimum requirements are given for three.

The Recommended Daily Allowances in Table M-25, Mineral Table, may be used for purposes of comparing the official mineral allowances with the actual mineral intakes of people who may be eating inadequate diets. However, a person who consumes a diet which lacks sufficient amounts of certain minerals may *not* necessarily have deficiencies of these minerals because (1) individual needs for minerals vary widely; (2) other dietary and nondietary factors affect the ways in which minerals are utilized; and (3) there may be stores of the minerals in that individual's body, which may be used to offset inadequacies of the diet. Nevertheless, the chances are that a markedly inadequate diet will eventually lead to nutritional deficiencies.

Calculating individual mineral intakes for large groups of people is an expensive and time-consuming procedure. Hence, a practical shortcut is to try to identify the most likely candidates for mineral deficiencies by scanning individual patterns of food selection. Some guidelines for identifying diets which may lead to certain mineral deficiencies follow:

1. **Calcium deficiency** may result from diets containing only small amounts of dairy products and/or green, leafy vegetables.

2. **Phosphorus deficiency** is likely only when the diet is low in protein foods.

3. **Iodine deficiency** usually occurs in areas where the soil is low in the mineral, unless iodized salt is used or there are such unsuspected sources of dietary iodine as (a) breads containing iodates as additives or (b) milk from cows which have been fed supplemental iodine, and/or which have had their udders washed with disinfectant solutions that contain iodine compounds.

4. **Iron deficiency** may often be due to lack of sufficient meat in the diet, because the forms of iron which are present in blood and muscle are utilized about three times as well as those in cereals, legumes, and vegetables; and about twice as well as those in fish.

5. **Magnesium deficiency** is not thought to be common in the United States, except among people whose diets consist mainly of highly milled grains and cereal products, and which are lacking in whole grains, leafy green vegetables, nuts, legumes, fish, and meats.

6. **Zinc deficiency** may occur in a mild form when the diet lacks meat, poultry, or fish.

Signs or Symptoms of Mineral Deficiencies.

Only a few clinical signs, such as a goiter which may result from an iodine deficiency, are specific indicators of certain mineral deficiencies. Other signs, like stunted growth, may be due to deficiencies of one or more minerals, vitamins, carbohydrates, fats, and/or proteins. (See Table M-25, Mineral Table, for a more complete coverage of the symptoms associated with various mineral deficiencies.) Hence, it is not wise to rely upon signs or symptoms for the early diagnosis of mineral deficiencies. Some other types of diagnostic measures are discussed in the next section.

Laboratory Tests for Mineral Deficiencies.

Tests for iron-deficiency anemia are widely used all over the world; but most of the tests for other mineral deficiencies are limited mainly to research studies, because there is a lack of information regarding normal values for such groups as infants, children, adults, and pregnant or nursing mothers. Nevertheless, a growing number of commercial laboratories offer analyses of hair and/or urine directly to customers. These laboratories may also sell mineral and vitamin supplements to the people who use their services.

It is not wise for lay people to attempt to interpret laboratory tests for mineral deficiencies without the aid of a doctor, because many factors other than the diet may raise or lower the levels of minerals in the body liquids and the tissues. Therefore, some of the better-known types of diagnostic tests are covered briefly, so that the reader may be knowledgable when discussing them with his or her physician. These follow:

• **Blood levels of various minerals**—Mild to moderate deficiencies of minerals may not be detected by analysis of the blood, because in mild deficiencies blood levels of essential elements are maintained at the expense of tissue supplies. Hence, subnormal blood values are likely to mean that the mineral reserves have been depleted. Unfortunately, there are only a few convenient procedures for measuring minerals in the tissues.

• **Bone marrow biopsies**—This procedure involves the sampling (by means of a needle) of a small amount of bone marrow for its iron content. It gives an indication of the amount of iron which is stored in the skeleton. However, it is used mainly in research studies.

• **Hair levels of minerals**—Hair is one of the last tissues of the body to be nourished and one of the first to show the effects of poor nutrition. Hence, there is much current interest in the use of hair as a test medium for various mineral deficiencies and/or toxicities. New analytical methods are now available for the rapid analysis of hair for more than a dozen minerals, so certain laboratories offer this service to the public. Some of the merits and demerits of these tests follow:

1. Abnormally high amounts of arsenic, lead, and mercury in hair usually indicate internal poisoning by these toxic elements.

2. Subnormal levels of such trace elements as chromium, manganese, and zinc are usually correlated with deficiencies of these essential minerals.

3. Sometimes, the minerals in hair originate from environmental contamination—from hair dyes, shampoos, and swimming pool water, rather than from the diet.

4. Standards for the mineral content of hair should take into consideration the color of the hair because certain minerals are constituents of hair pigments. For example, blonde hair has lower ratios of zinc to copper than dark shades of hair.[44] Also, red hair contains more iron than other colors, because iron is present in the red pigment. Also, age and sex can affect hair analyses.

5. The part of the body from which the hair sample is taken influences mineral content.

6. The rate of hair growth, which is influenced by several factors such as disease and season of the year, influences the concentration of minerals.

7. Genetic constitution, gender, and drugs may influence mineral content.

So, the results of hair analysis may be both inaccurate and misleading.

Many of the laboratories that analyze hair recommend supplements to correct deficiencies. It's no small coincidence, of course, that they just happen to sell the supplement that they are recommending.

(Also see HAIR ANALYSIS.)

• **Urinalysis**—Mineral deficiencies are likely to result in reductions in the amounts of the elements which are excreted in the urine, as the body attempts to conserve its dwindling supply of these essential nutrients. The trouble with urinalysis as a test for mineral nutrition status is that other factors, such as dehydration or stress, may raise or lower the rate of urinary excretion of minerals; hence, the effects of nutritional status alone cannot be readily measured.

• **X rays of bone**—X rays are used to diagnose demineralization of bones—which is usually due to deficiencies of calcium, phosphorus, and/or vitamin D—and the deposition of lead in the bones whch occurs in lead poisoning.

Often, tests such as those described are used in conjunction with tests of other metabolic functions, because the metabolic activities of certain minerals are not always correlated with the levels of the elements which are present in body fluids and tissues. For example, hair may be analyzed for its chromium content in order to determine whether a diabeticlike response to a glucose tolerance test is due to

a lack of chromium in the form of the glucose tolerance factor (GTF).

More details on the detection of specific mineral deficiencies will be found in the articles dealing with each of the individual minerals.

PREVENTION AND TREATMENT OF MINERAL DEFICIENCIES AND/OR TOXICITIES. The prevention and treatment of the various mineral deficiencies require the cautious use of mineral-rich foods or special supplements because (1) there is a narrow range between the safe levels and the toxic levels of such trace elements as iron, copper, fluorine, and selenium; (2) excesses of certain minerals are likely to reduce the absorption and utilization of others; and (3) large excesses of most minerals—except for potassium, sodium, and chloride—are not well absorbed, but are excreted in the stool. Therefore, lay persons should *not* dose themselves with *shotgun* amounts of mineral supplements; rather, they should limit themselves to more prudent measures, such as those which follow:

Selection of Foods Rich in Essential Minerals. Foods which comprise the most vital tissues of plants and animals are likely to be the richest in essential minerals, because mineral elements participate in the important life functions of these organisms. Hence, the animal products highest in mineral content are blood, bones, milk, and the vital organs, whereas leaves and seeds contain the highest levels of minerals found in the plant foods. Therefore, a mineral-rich diet may be assured by including a wide variety of such foods as dairy products; fish and other seafoods; meats and poultry (hearts, kidneys, and livers are much richer in minerals than the muscle meats); beans and peas; molasses; nuts; herbs; spices; tea; raw, unpeeled vegetables; and whole grain breads and cereal products.

Generally, foods which are only minimally refined contain the most minerals, because these elements are often present in the parts which are removed during processing. However, certain types of food processing may favorably alter the forms of the minerals present in foods so that these nutrients are better absorbed and utilized by the body. For example, yeast fermentation during the leavening of whole grain bread doughs is known to increase the availability of zinc and other minerals.

Production and Preparation of Foods to Maximize Their Mineral Values. Sometimes, animals and plants which have been produced *naturally*—with a minimum of interference from man—are not as nutritious as they might be. Correction of certain soil deficiencies and problems may enhance the mineral value of plants, and, likewise, the supplementation of natural animal feeds may improve the nutritive value of meat, milk, and eggs. Also, the procedures used in processing foods and in preparing meals may contribute to better mineral nutrition. Therefore, it is worth noting how the mineral values of various foods may be maximized through careful attention to certain details of food production and preparation.

BENEFICIAL PRACTICES IN AGRICULTURAL PRODUCTION. The profitable production of both animal and plant foods depends partly on the minerals which are provided by the farmers as supplements to the feedstuffs for livestock and as fertilizers for the soil. Although large excesses of certain elements will interfere with the utilization of other elements, it seems that small excesses—beyond the minimal amounts required for good production—may raise the levels

---

[44]Eads, E. A., and C. E. Lambdin, "A Survey of Trace Metals in Human Hair," *Environmental Research*, Vol. 6, 1973, p. 251.

of minerals present in the food products. However, this concept is highly controversial, so some of the evidence favoring liberal mineral supplementation for animals and plants follow:

1. Feeding livestock extra amounts of certain minerals like copper, iodine, manganese, selenium, and zinc tends to raise the levels of these elements in meat (including poultry) and eggs. But the amounts of mineral supplements which are required are considerably greater than the gains in mineral content of products achieved; hence, the method is inefficient.

2. Practices which encourage the growth of certain soil

SOME FOODS RICH IN ESSENTIAL MINERALS

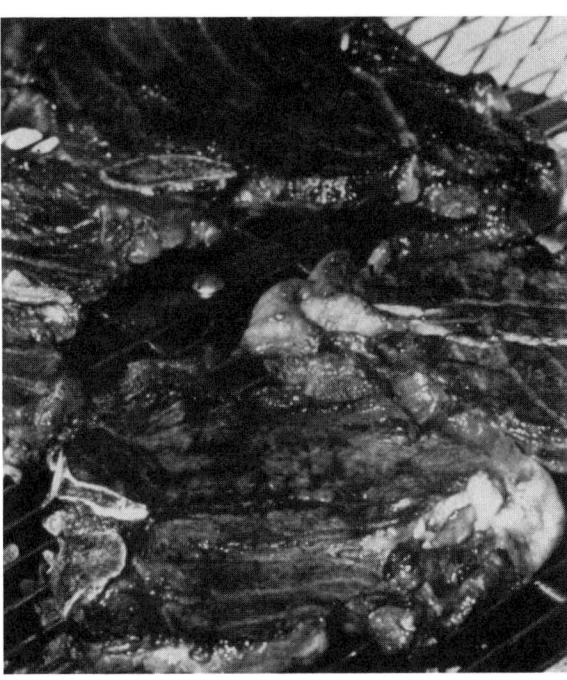

Fig. M-75. Barbecued steaks. (Courtesy, Agriculture Canada, Ottawa, Ontario)

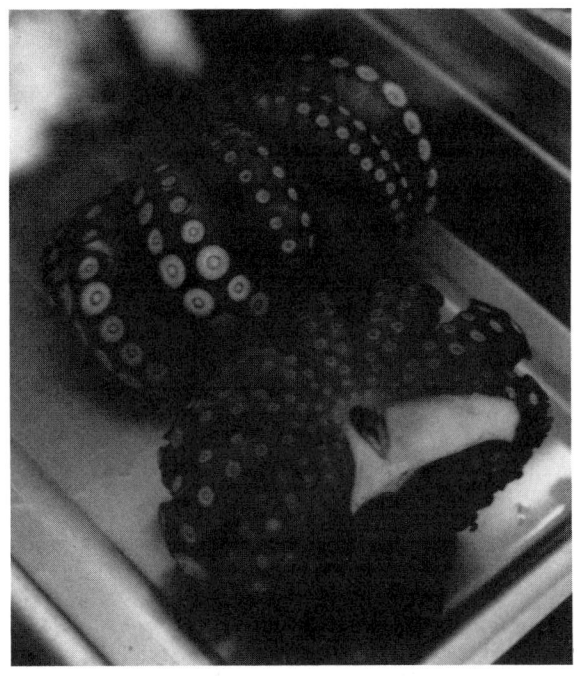

Fig. M-77. Octopus—a seafood. (Courtesy, Department of Food Science and Human Nutrition, University of Hawaii)

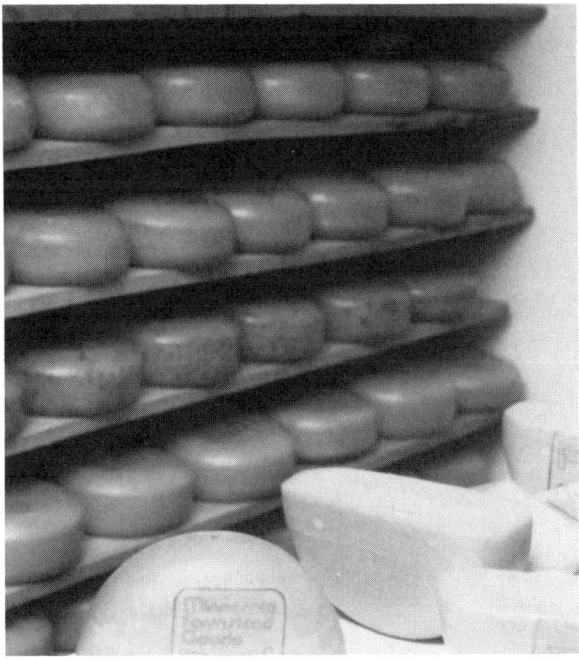

Fig. M-76. Cheeses. (Courtesy, University of Minnesota, St. Paul, Minn.)

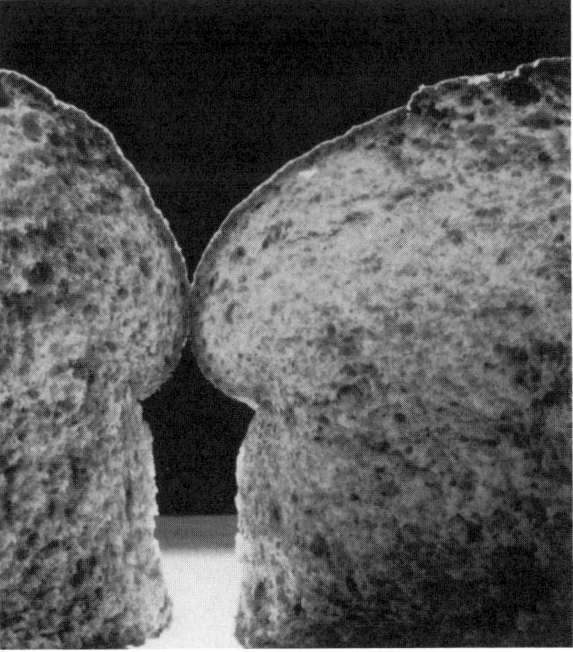

Fig. M-78. Whole grain breads. (Courtesy, University of Minnesota, St. Paul, Minn.)

microorganisms may also enhance the uptake of minerals by plants because the microorganisms convert insoluble mineral compounds to more soluble forms, which are more readily utilized by plants. The growth of beneficial microorganisms in the soil is favored by (a) organic matter which may be added as compost or manure; (b) the proper balance between acidity and alkalinity; and (c) minerals which are required by the microorganisms for growth and reproduction.

3. The improvement of mineral-depleted soils by balanced mineral fertilization has often resulted in both better overall crop yields and higher levels of certain minerals in individual plants. However, there are limits of the extent to which the mineral composition of plants may be improved by fertilization, because the utilization of minerals by plants is controlled mainly by genetic factors.

FOOD PROCESSING PROCEDURES WHICH RAISE THE MINERAL VALUES OF FOODS.

It is well known that certain types of food processing are detrimental to nutritive values. On the other hand, mention is seldom made of the types of food processing which either raise the level(s) of one or more minerals, or which alter foods in ways that make their minerals more available. Details follow:

1. The preparation of purees by homogenizing vegetables in water makes the iron in these items more available, because it breaks down the fibrous cell walls which enclose minerals and other nutrients.

2. Yeast fermentation which occurs during the leavening of whole grain breads breaks down the phytates (poorly utilized phosphorus compounds in the bran of the wheat grain) that interfere with mineral absorption.[45] Hence, there is better utilization of the minerals in such breads when yeast is used instead of baking powder.

3. The production of undistilled alcoholic beverages (beers and wines) from grains, grapes, and other plant materials appears to render minerals like iron more available for absorption. Alcoholic iron tonics have long been used to treat anemia. Also, alcoholic fermentation by yeast may convert the inorganic chromium which is present in various fermentable materials to the glucose tolerance factor (GTF)—an organically complexed form of chromium that augments the effects of insulin. (GTF has been found in beer and in yeast which has been grown on chromium-containing nutrient broths. Hence, it seems likely that yeast might similarly convert the chromium that is abundantly present in grape juice into GTF.)

(Also see BEERS AND BREWING; GLUCOSE TOLERANCE FACTOR; and WINE.)

4. Cheese making may raise or lower the amount of calcium in 100-Calorie (kcal) portions of the product compared to the original milk because variable amounts of calcium, phosphorus, protein, and lactose are lost in the whey, depending upon whether the milk is clotted with rennet, or with acid alone. Table M-26 shows how the contents of calories, calcium, and phosphorus vary between milk and several types of popular cheeses.

Dieters seeking to cut down their caloric intake while obtaining most of their calcium requirements from dairy products can use a few ounces of Swiss and/or Cheddar cheeses instead of cupfuls of whole milk or cottage cheese. However, each unit of calcium from Cheddar or Swiss cheese costs about 50% more than an equivalent amount from fresh whole milk.

---

[45]"Zinc Availability in Leavened and Unleavened Bread," *Nutrition Reviews*, Vol. 33, 1975, pp. 18-19.

TABLE M-26
SELECTED COMPONENTS OF MILK AND FOUR TYPES OF CHEESES[1]

Component	Milk[2]	Cheddar Cheese	Swiss Cheese	Cottage Cheese
Calories .... (kcal/100 g)	62	402	372	90
Calcium .... (mg/100 g)	119	718	961	68
Phosphorus .... (mg/100 g)	89	510	605	150
Calcium in 100 kcal portion of food .... (mg)	192	179	258	76
Calcium to phosphorus ratio	1.33:1	1.41:1	1.59:1	.45:1
Amount of product needed to supply 800 mg calcium .... (oz)	23.7	3.9	2.9	41.5
.... (g)	*672*	*111*	*83*	*1,176*
Amount of energy which must be consumed to obtain 800 mg calcium .... (kcal)	417	446	309	1,058

[1]The food composition data were obtained from Food Composition Table F-21 of this book.
[2]Milk which contains 3.5% fat.

5. The extraction of fat from soybean products prior to production of flour may raise the ratio of the mineral content (as represented by ash content) to the caloric content by more than 60%. This means that the consumer gets more minerals, but fewer calories, when defatted soybean products are selected.

6. Ascorbic acid (vitamin C) is a beneficial food additive because it converts oxidized iron to the reduced form, which is better absorbed. Also, the addition of sulfites (substances used to prevent discoloration and/or microbial growth) to foods may indirectly promote better utilization of iron, because these additives preserve ascorbic acid against oxidation.

7. The use of limewater (calcium hydroxide solution) in the production of tortillas (flat, thin cakes made of corn meal) adds about 100 mg of calcium per 100 g of product.

8. Heat treatment of soybeans improves the utilization of copper, iron, manganese, and zinc from this food because it inactivates a metal-binding constituent.

MEAL PREPARATION PRACTICES WHICH CONSERVE ESSENTIAL MINERALS.

It may not have been too important for prehistoric man to minimize the loss of mineral nutrients during cooking because the lack of laborsaving devices made it necessary to eat large amounts of food so as to provide for great expenditures of energy. Today, people expend much less energy and eat considerably less food; so, it is now necessary to use better methods of meal preparation. Some guidelines for conserving minerals follow:

1. Soaking spinach and rhubarb in water removes some of the oxalic acid from these items so that dietary minerals are better utilized. Oxalic acid forms insoluble, unabsorbable compounds with calcium, iron, and other minerals.

2. Cleaning fruits and vegetables with a stiff brush is preferable to peeling them, because the outer layers of many items are much richer in minerals than the inner parts. Hence, the mineral losses due to peeling may be disproportionately high for the amount of material that is removed.

3. It is better to purchase smaller amounts of fresh, leafy vegetables more frequently than to store large amounts in the refrigerator for long periods of time, because cutting down on storage time minimizes wilting and the need to discard the wilted outer leaves, which are the richest in minerals.

4. The loss of minerals during pressure cooking or steam cooking of vegetables is significantly less than that during boiling. Other ways of cooking which conserve minerals are baking and microwave heating. When other conditions are

the same, mineral losses may also be minimized by cooking vegetables in large pieces rather than small pieces, and by keeping the cooking time as short as possible.

5. There are considerable amounts of minerals in the packing fluids used in most canned foods, so the fluids should be saved and used whenever feasible.

6. The thawing of frozen foods results in losses of minerals with the juices which escape during thawing. Freezing food ruptures cell walls so that the cell contents escape readily during thawing. Although the thaw juices might be used in meal preparation, it may be dangerous to do so if there has been considerable time for the growth of microorganisms during thawing. Hence, it may be desirable to cook frozen foods without preliminary thawing so that the juices which escape may be used safely.

Microwave heating may be preferable to other ways of cooking unthawed frozen foods because when food is penetrated by the microwaves cooking proceeds uniformly throughout, whereas in other ways of cooking the heat acts mainly on the outside of the food, which may become overcooked, while the interior is undercooked.

ENRICHMENT AND FORTIFICATION OF FOODS WITH MINERALS.

Extra minerals may be added to foods so as (1) to restore those lost during processing (such restoration is called *enrichment*), or (2) to make certain popular foods richer in various nutrients than is natural for these items (this process is called *fortification*). For example, the level at which iron is added to white flour and other refined cereal products constitutes enrichment or restoration of the iron lost during milling, whereas the addition of iron to milk-based infant formulas is fortification, because milk is normally low in iron.

From such early beginnings as the iodine fortification of salt in the 1920s, and the enrichment of flour and bread with iron and vitamins in the 1930s, the addition of essential minerals has been extended to both traditional foods and new items which have been recently concocted by food technologists. Therefore, it is important to be knowledgeable relative to the following items that may be enriched or fortified with minerals:

• **Breakfast cereals**—Many of these items are made from highly milled grains, so they are often fortified with vitamins and iron, and sometimes with calcium. However, milling removes large amounts of other minerals like magnesium, chromium, manganese, copper, zinc, selenium, and molybdenum, which are not usually added during enrichment or fortification, unless the manufacturer does so indirectly by adding wheat germ, bran, or rice polish to his products. (The by-products of milling removed from the whole grains are rich sources of the minerals.) Hence, the consumer receives better overall mineral nutrition with whole grain cereals than with those made from refined grains which have been enriched or fortified with one or two minerals.

• **Complete diet formulas**—There are various types of powders and liquids, which usually contain skim milk or other sources of protein, that are fortified with minerals and vitamins so that they may be taken instead of regular meals. Nevertheless, they are not likely to contain adequate amounts of such newly discovered trace minerals as chromium, selenium, and silicon, because these elements are not usually added to the products. Hence, the formulas are best used as replacements for only one or two meals per day, so that the missing minerals may be obtained from regular foods.

• **Flour, grains, and bakery goods**—Usually, iron is the only mineral used to enrich these products when they are made from milled grains. It may be wise to avoid these items and select whole wheat or bran breads and muffins, and brown rice, unless the rest of the diet makes up for the mineral deficiencies in the highly refined products.

• **Imitation foods or analogs**—High prices for such staple foods as fruit juices, milk, ice cream, butter, meats, and poultry, along with the concern over the cholesterol and fat content of certain of these foods, have stimulated the development of imitation products or analogs. These products are made from lower-cost materials, like soybean derivatives, and they are usually fortified with minerals, vitamins, and amino acids so as to be nutritionally equivalent to the items which they are designed to replace in the diet.

Analogs are generally wholesome and nutritious for most healthy people. However, those who are prone to heart disorders and/or high blood pressure should note that (1) some of the soybean-based imitations of meats and poultry contain much more sodium than the authentic animal products, and (2) artificial fruitlike drinks may contain little or none of the potassium present in real fruit juices, which are often prescribed as sources of the mineral for therapeutic diets. Hence, there is a need for more extensive nutritional labeling on the packages of imitation foods.

• **Infant cereals**—These products generally provide better mineral nutrition than the breakfast cereals designed for older children and adults, because they are often fortified with calcium, iron, copper, and other minerals. Of course, whole grain cereals are also good, but the fiber they contain may have too much of a laxative effect on infants.

• **Infant formulas**—The manufacturers of these products have usually designed them to be nutritionally equivalent to human breast milk, perhaps with the following notable exceptions:

1. The calcium and phosphorus levels in the formulas may be considerably higher than those in human milk, but they are usually somewhat lower than those in fresh or evaporated cow's milk. Newborn infants may have seizures if they are fed excessive amounts of phosphorus. Hence, the formulas are safer than either undiluted, fresh cow's milk or evaporated milk diluted with only an equal volume of water.

2. The iron levels may be unusually high in certain formulas, because it is believed that the very low levels of this mineral in both human and cow's milk may sometimes be responsible for the development of anemia in infants and children.

• **Instant breakfast powders**—These powders, which are usually designed to be mixed with a glass of milk, are fortified with minerals and vitamins so as to supply at least one-fourth of the daily nutrient requirement for an adult. Probably they supply better balanced mineral nutrition than most people regularly receive from ordinary types of breakfast foods. However, they may not be suitable for people prone to constipation, unless the low fiber content of the formulas is offset by eating pulpy fruits or drinking unstrained juices.

• **Milk**—Minerals are not usually added to ordinary cow's milk, but vitamin D is usually added, so that the calcium and phosphorus which are present in the milk will be well utilized.

• **Nutrified** cakes, cookies, and food bars—The new term *nutrification,* which is derived from the words nutrient and fortification, was coined by food scientists to denote the providing of nutrients through fabricated, fortified foods such as snack cakes, cookies, food bars, and *chips* laced with minerals, vitamins, and amino acids. However, some of these products are too high in fats and/or sugars to be used by sedentary adults, who might easily eat too much of these concentrated sources of calories.

• **Salt**—Slightly more than half of the salt sold at the retail level is fortified with iodine for the purpose of preventing iodine-deficiency goiter.

Special Dietary Products. The use of special foods and mineral supplements may be justified when it appears that the diet is deficient in certain essential elements. Ordinary diets may not suffice to meet mineral needs under circumstances such as (1) pregnancy; (2) breast feeding of infants; (3) illnesses which depress the appetite; (4) types of malnutrition that require rapid restoration of the body's supply of certain minerals (*these conditions require the attention of physicians who are proficient in nutritional therapy*); (5) sharp restrictions in caloric intake in order to achieve rapid reduction in body weight; or (6) shortages of wholesome, nutritious foods.

The authors do *not* wish to suggest that any of the conditions listed are to be treated with special dietary products; rather, they wish to point out that certain products may be used to fill the gaps in mineral nutrition which may result from inadequate diets. Furthermore, the nutritional assessment of diets and the selection of products to provide minerals may be hazardous for a lay person to undertake without the assistance of a doctor or a dietitian. Unfortunately, this type of assistance is not always readily available.

Hence, some practical guidelines are presented with the hope that they may help to counteract the current tendency for many people to select nutritional products on the basis of questionable advertising claims.

SPECIALTY FOODS AND HIGHLY POTENT NUTRITIONAL SUPPLEMENTS. It is fortunate that most consumers are not able to purchase pure mineral salts and to mix them into their foods, because without special measuring equipment and experience in preparing such mixtures, it is very easy to add toxic excesses of trace elements like iodine and selenium to foods. However, even some of the products that are sold by health food stores may have undesirable, or even toxic effects, because they are very rich in certain minerals. The potentially hazardous products may be considered as *highly potent nutritional supplements,* in order to distinguish them from the less potent specialty foods, which are usually safe in the amounts consumed. Table M-27 shows the approximate amounts of these minerals that are provided by various specialty foods and nutritional supplements.

It may be seen from Table M-27 that it is safer to use specialty foods as sources of minerals than it is to use highly potent nutritional supplements because the former contain considerably lower levels of minerals than the latter, so the chance of receiving dangerous excesses of any of the elements is much less. For example, 3½ oz (*100 g*) of wheat germ contain about half of the daily allowance for copper, whereas an equal amount of liver powder contains seven times as much of the mineral. Furthermore, the contents of protein, vitamins, and other nutrients in the different products vary considerably. Hence, it is desirable to use a variety of these items, rather than a single one, to meet specific mineral needs. Some guidelines for using the various products follow.

Specialty Foods. The following items are good to excellent sources of energy, minerals, protein, and vitamins; so,

TABLE M-27
AMOUNTS OF SELECTED MINERALS IN SOME SPECIALTY FOODS AND NUTRITIONAL SUPPLEMENTS[1]

Product	Macrominerals					Microminerals					
	Calcium (Ca)	Phosphorus (P)	Potassium (K)	Sodium (Na)	Magnesium (Mg)	Iron (Fe)	Zinc (Zn)	Copper (Cu)	Selenium (Se)	Iodine (I)	Chromium (Cr)
	(mg/100 g)	(mg/100 g)	(mg/100 g)	(mg/100 g)	(mg/100 g)	(mg/100 g)	(mg/100 g)	(mg/100 g)	(mcg/100 g)	(mcg/100 g)	(mcg/100 g)
Specialty Food:											
Alfalfa (leaf) powder	1,640	230	2,070	60	350	36.0	1.6	1.0	28	—	—
Almonds, dried	234	504	773	4	293	4.7	3.1	1.2	—	—	—
Bran	119	1,276	1,121	9	598	11.0	10.4	1.3	63	6	40
Flaxseeds	271	462	1,460	30	400	9.0	—	—	—	—	—
Nonfat milk, dried, powder	1,308	1,016	1,794	532	144	.3	4.1	.5	—	—	12
Peanuts, roasted w/skins ..	72	407	701	5	175	2.2	3.0	.3	—	—	—
Rice polishings	69	1,106	714	100	650	16.1	2.6	.7	—	7	—
Sesame seeds	131	776	407	40	347	7.8	10.3	1.6	—	—	—
Soybean flour (low fat) ...	263	634	1,859	1	289	9.1	2.0	1.6	—	—	—
Sunflower seeds	120	837	920	30	38	7.1	4.6	1.8	—	—	—
Wheat germ, toasted	47	1,084	947	2	365	8.9	15.4	1.3	111	—	25
Nutritional Supplement:											
Blackstrap molasses	684	84	2,927	96	209	16.1	2.2	6.0	—	158	115
Bone meal	29,820	12,490	180	5,530	320	85.0	12.6	1.1	—	—	—
Brewers' yeast	210	1,753	1,894	121	231	17.3	3.9	3.3	125	—	118
Dolomite	22,080	40	360	—	9,870	76.0	—	—	—	—	—
Kelp	1,904	240	5,273	3,007	213	89.6	3.5	.6	43	62,400	Trace
Liver, dried, powder	40	830	930	450	—	20.0	—	9.0	180	—	170
Torula yeast	424	1,713	2,046	15	165	19.3	1.9	1.4	132	—	—

[1]A dash indicates a lack of authoritative data, *not* that the mineral is absent.

they may be used alone as foods, or they may be mixed with other items:

- **Alfalfa (leaf) powder or tablets**—Because of its grasslike taste, alfalfa powder should be mixed with other foods like baked goods (not more than a tablespoon per cup of flour), thick vegetable soups, or *green sauces* for pasta. It is noteworthy that the flavor of alfalfa blends well with mint or spices. Alfalfa is also available in the form of tablets that contain no other ingredient. Tablets avoid flavor problems because they may be swallowed whole. Alfalfa powder is an excellent source of calcium, iron, and magnesium.

- **Almonds, dried**—Although these nuts cost about twice as much as peanuts, they may be worth the price because (1) they are tasty without salt, and (2) their mineral content is higher than peanuts (three times the calcium, one and one-half times the magnesium, and two times the iron). Many people eat them plain, but they are also good in toppings, coatings (such as fish almondine), or in pastries and other desserts. Almonds, like other nuts, are also good sources of protein, polyunsaturated fats, and vitamins.

- **Bran**—This product has about nine times the overall mineral content of white flour. It may be (1) used alone as a cereal (a little goes a long way, because it soaks up liquid and is, therefore, very filling); (2) mixed with other cereals; (3) used as a breading for baked, broiled, or fried foods; or (4) mixed with chopped fish, meat, and poultry as a filler which aids in the retention of their juices. However, bran may have a laxative effect on some people, varying according to the amount eaten and individual susceptibilities. So, it should be added cautiously to the diet, in small amounts, until the level of tolerance is known. Also, plenty of liquid should be taken with bran, or it may cause irritation in the digestive tract. Bran is an excellent source of many of the essential minerals.

- **Flaxseeds**—These seeds, when ground, have long been used as the basis of various *natural* laxative preparations. They contain a mucilaginous material which thickens the porridge that is formed when they are cooked in water with other grains. Their bland taste makes it convenient to add them to various cereal products, where their ample supply of calcium, iron, and magnesium adds to the mineral values.

- **Nonfat milk powder**—This product, when mixed with water, yields a drink which is equal in mineral value to whole milk, but which is lower in calories. However, even greater mineral nutrition may be promoted by adding the dry powder to various foods, to which it contributes calcium and magnesium. For example, it blends well with the other ingredients in items such as cooked cereals, doughs, fudge-type candies, puddings, coffee, cocoa, and tea. Furthermore, milk sugar—lactose, which is abundantly present in nonfat milk powder, appears to promote the absorption of calcium and other essential elements.

- **Peanuts**—Peanuts and peanut butter are often used as meat substitutes, because of their protein content. However, they contain much more calcium, chromium, copper, magnesium, and calories than do muscle meats. They may be eaten alone, or in various combinations with other foods.

- **Rice polishings**—This product, like wheat bran, contains the minerals removed from whole grains (brown rice) during milling. It is an excellent source of iron, magnesium, and the vitamin B complex. The bland taste makes it a good additive for fortifying baked items, breading, and breakfast cereals.

- **Sesame seeds**—These seeds are often sprinkled over breads, cookies, crackers, and rolls. They are higher than muscle meats in content of several minerals and calories. Sesame seed butter (which resembles peanut butter) is sold in many health food stores.

- **Soy flour**—Usually soybeans have had most of their fat removed by crushing and extraction prior to being ground into flour. Hence, soy flour contains more minerals, but fewer calories, than most nuts and seeds. It is a good source of calcium and magnesium, as well as protein and certain vitamins. However, the use of this product is limited by (1) the beany flavor; and (2) its content of certain carbohydrates, which ferment in the digestive tract to form gas. Some ways of overcoming these disadvantages are: (1) adding soy flour to highly spiced foods like gingerbread cookies and ground sausage meat, so that the beany taste is disguised; and (2) using small amounts of soy flour at first, until the limit of one's tolerance to the gas-producing effects is determined.

- **Sunflower seeds**—Although many Americans formerly considered this chewy product to be best suited for feeding birds, it is now sold as a snack food. The seeds keep well without refrigeration, because of their protective outer covering. Their content of copper and iron, along with protein and vitamins, makes them a much better snack item than popcorn, potato chips, and sweets. Some health food stores carry sunflower seed butter and sunflower seed meal; but these items sometimes have a bitter taste, which may be due to rancidity that develops when the seed is crushed and the oil exposed to the air.

- **Wheat germ**—This by-product of wheat milling has about the same overall mineral content as bran, but it is better digested and it provides more protein, calories, and vitamins. Also, it ranks close to the vegetable oils as a source of vitamin E. It may be used alone as a breakfast cereal, or it may be added to various cereal products.

(Also see BREAKFAST CEREALS; and WHEAT.)

Highly Potent Nutritional Supplements. The following products should be used with caution so as to avoid over-doses of certain minerals or other potentially harmful substances:

- **Blackstrap molasses**—About two heaping tablespoons (40 g total) per day of this thick, sugary fluid will furnish liberal amounts of calcium, magnesium, chromium, copper, iodine, iron, and zinc. However, many people may find its licoricelike taste too strong for their liking when they attempt to take it alone, like a tonic. Also, it may be a strong laxative for some people. Hence, it might be mixed cautiously into other foods where its flavor may be either diluted or masked by other strong flavors. For example, it may be added to items like (1) a glass of milk, because the addition of 1 teaspoon (5 *ml*) of molasses per 1 or 2 teaspoons of carob powder makes a drink that is more nutritious than chocolate milk; (2) spice cakes or gingerbread cookies, which may also contain added soy flour; or (3) pumpernickel or other dark breads leavened with yeast, because the yeast may convert the inorganic chromium from the molasses into the glucose tolerance factor, an organic form of the mineral, which acts along with insulin in promoting the metabolism of carbohydrates.

(Also see MOLASSES, section headed "Food.")

• **Bone meal powder or tablets**—A little of this item goes a long way. A teaspoon of the powder provides over 1,000 mg of calcium, which appears to be more than enough for people other than pregnant or nursing mothers. Tablets may be more convenient than powder for most people, who usually lack scales for accurately measuring small quantities of powder. However, if the powder is to be mixed into such items as cereals, doughs, gravies, and sauces—*not* more than ¼ teaspoon per person per serving should be used. Careful trials should be conducted on a small scale, before adding the powder to recipes, because bone meal imparts a slightly gritty texture to foods.

• **Brewers' yeast powder or tablets**—This special product has long been used to prevent or treat malnutrition by providing extra protein and the vitamin B complex. However, it is also one of the richest sources of both chromium and selenium—minerals that are likely to be supplied inadequately by ordinary diets. Furthermore, the chromium is present in an organic form (glucose tolerance factor) which is much more beneficial to the body than the inorganic forms of the mineral.

Brewers' yeast is also rich in nucleic acids, which are substances that may cause certain susceptible people to develop high blood levels of uric acid (hyperuricemia) and/or gout. These disorders tend to run in certain families, so it may be wise to inquire whether any close relatives have had these disorders, before taking this supplement on a regular basis.

A suitable daily portion of the dried yeast—for people who are *not* prone to either hyperuricemia or gout—is 1 or 2 tablespoons (*15 or 30 ml*). It may be mixed in vegetable drinks like tomato juice, cooked cereals, flavored instant breakfast drinks, gravies, meat loaves, or various sauces. If there is a choice of product, one that is *debittered* should be selected. Tablets are also available for those who prefer a more convenient form of the product.

• **Dolomite tablets**—Usually, each tablet supplies about 130 mg of calcium, and about 60 mg of magnesium. Four such tablets daily should be an adequate supplement for most people, except for pregnant or nursing mothers, who may need as many as six tablets to fill the gap between intake and recommended allowances of these minerals. However, excesses of calcium and magnesium may interfere with the utilization of other essential minerals.

• **Kelp tablets**—Just about every brand of these tablets contains an amount of iodine equal to the U.S. RDAs for adults (150 mcg per day) in each tablet. It is not wise to exceed this amount because people who have tendencies to develop goiter are extra susceptible to iodine toxicity. Those who have suffered from dietary iodine deficiency may have thyroid glands which have adapted to low intakes of the mineral by becoming very efficient in the production of thyroid hormones. Thus, their glands may overproduce these hormones when the dietary level of iodine is raised.

CAUTION: Due to its high content of iodine, it is very easy to get an overdose of iodine from only small amounts of kelp powder.

(Also see ENDOCRINE GLANDS; and GOITER.)

• **Liver, dried, powder**—This excellent source of chromium, copper, iron, and selenium may also be rich in cholesterol and fat, unless it has been defatted. Also, the defatted types of liver powder have a more pleasant taste. However,

this supplement should *not* be used by people who might have tendencies to develop high blood levels of uric acid or gout because it is rich in nucleic acids, which are converted into uric acid in the body.

Two teaspoons (*10 ml*) of liver powder per day provide plenty of extra minerals for most people, when it is used on a regular basis. It may be added to gravies, meat loaves, or various sauces, provided sufficient seasonings are used to disguise the liver flavor.

MINERAL SUPPLEMENTS. Sometimes, it may be more convenient and economical to provide supplementary minerals in pill form than to attempt to meet all of one's mineral needs through ordinary foods and/or specialty products. However, mineral pills or tablets have certain disadvantages in that (1) people may neglect to take their pills regularly; and (2) small pills which contain large amounts of certain minerals may lead to overdosage by people who are impatient to obtain the expected beneficial effects, and to poisoning of small children who might be tempted to sample the pills. Nevertheless, there are circumstances under which it is necessary to take mineral pills in order to prevent nutritional deficiencies. Hence, some suggestions for using these products follow:

1. Whenever feasible, consult with a doctor or a dietitian before attempting to correct dietary inadequacies by means of special supplements.

2. Buy mineral pills which are labeled in accordance with the U.S. RDAs proposed by the Food and Drug Administration.

3. Use mineral supplements according to the directions on their lables.

4. Keep all types of pills out of the reach of infants and children.

5. Report any unusual signs or symptoms, such as changes in bowel habits, to a physician.

(Also see NUTRIENTS: REQUIREMENTS, ALLOWANCES, FUNCTIONS, SOURCES; NUTRITIONAL SUPPLEMENTS; and U.S. RECOMMENDED DAILY ALLOWANCES.)

MISCIBLE

Capable of being mixed easily with other substances.

MITOCHONDRIA

Minute spheres, rods, or filaments in the cytoplasm. Mitochondria are the sites of numerous biochemical reactions including amino acid and fatty acid catabolism, the oxidative reactions of the Krebs cycle, respiratory electron transport, and oxidative phosphorylation. As a result of these reactions, mitochondria are the major producers of the high energy compound adenosine triphosphate (ATP) in aerobically grown cells.

MODIFIED DIETS

This term refers to modifications of the ordinary American diet which are made for the purpose of providing nourishment when the consumption of a normal diet is inadvisable. (Strictly speaking, the term diet alone refers to whatever pattern of foods is consumed regularly, whether it conforms to a normal pattern or not.)

There is widespread current interest in various types of modified diets because many people are interested in increasing their productive years while minimizing the amounts spent on medical care. Also, an ever increasing number of nutritional supplements and special dietary products are marketed each year.

HISTORY. During most of human history, food patterns for most people have been based mainly upon whatever edible items could be obtained readily from nearby fields, forests, oceans, rivers, and streams, although some prehistoric peoples traveled long distances while hunting and gathering their foods. However, it appears that each of the preagricultural societies had some type of lore that attributed curative powers to certain special animal foods and druglike preparations from plants. For example, it was widely believed that eating the eyes of animals was the proper treatment for disorders of vision. (This idea was confirmed as valid in the 20th century, when it was found that eyes and other rich sources of vitamin A helped to cure visual problems due to deficiencies of this nutrient.)

The rise of agriculture made it possible for large numbers of people to dwell together in complex societies, but it also brought new health and nutritional problems because (1) infectious diseases spread rapidly through densely populated regions, and (2) the need to provide for large populations resulted in fewer types of foods being produced and consumed. The latter condition increased the likelihood of nutritional deficiencies because there were no means of identifying specific deficiencies and the nutrients that prevented them until a more scientific approach to nutrition was initiated by the great French chemist Antoine Lavoisier in the latter part of the 18th century. Nevertheless, the actual practice of dietetics began much earlier.

Dietetic concepts in the ancient civilizations of Babylon, China, Egypt, and India were based on various combinations of religious beliefs, superstitions, taboos, and trial-and-error observations. Even the last-named basis of judgment was clouded frequently by illness due to a contagious disease, contaminated water, or spoiled food. (The long-standing bias of some Greek and Roman physicians against the eating of fruit is believed to have been due to the fact that fruits were usually abundant in warm weather when diarrheal diseases were rampant because the conditions favored the rapid growth of microorganisms.) Another common type of prescientific concept was that (1) all matter was constituted of varying proportions of the elements air, earth, fire, and water (the Hindus believed that there were three elements, whereas the Chinese postulated five); and (2) the characteristic temperament of the patient (choleric, melancholic, phlegmatic, or sanguine) was due to the excess of one of the elements. Hence, it was considered desirable for an ill person to eat foods which counteracted the excess rather than those which augmented it. For example, a person with a fiery (choleric) temperament was usually told to eat only *cool* foods. In this case, coolness or hotness of foods referred to attributes other than temperature, which were deduced by rather convoluted reasoning. It is noteworthy that beliefs in cool and hot foods are still held by many poorly educated groups of people around the world.

Two major developments which contributed to the beginnings of modern dietetics in the 18th century were (1) the experiments on metabolism by Lavoisier whose career was literally cut short by the guillotine, and (2) founding of voluntary hospitals in England by private philanthropy. (The latter development helped to fill the gap created by the closing of the many hospitals operated by Catholic religious orders that occurred during the Reformation.) At first, the diet which was given to all patients was based mainly on beef, beer, and bread. Later, the diet was modified for (1) convalescent patients who were given *half diets* consisting of smaller quantities of meat that were augmented with light puddings, soups, broths, and vegetables; and (2) febrile patients who were fed *low diets* of gruels, milk, porridges, puddings, and small portions of cheese and/or meat. Use of these diets and variations of them persisted until the 20th century, because the nutritional science of the 19th century was dominated by the belief that adequate amounts of carbohydrates, fats, proteins, and minerals were all that were required to maintain good health. The need to prevent scurvy and other nutritional deficiencies by the provision of fruits and vegetables was not common knowledge until the latter part of the 19th century. Also, these items spoiled readily.

The major factors which accelerated the growth of modern dietetics in the first few decades of the 20th century were (1) the discoveries of the requirements for certain amino acids, trace minerals, and vitamins; (2) the founding of the American Dietetic Association in 1917 (this organization has contributed greatly to the standardization of the education and training of dietitians and the types of diets used for treating various disorders); and (3) the widespread recognition of the need for dietary modification in the treatment of certain conditions. (The designation *dietitian* originated in 1899 at the meeting of the National Home Economics Association at Lake Placid, New York.) It is noteworthy that the dramatic recoveries of some critically ill patients which resulted from the appropriate diet therapy led to a certain amount of unscrupulous promotion of nutritional supplements. These abuses inspired leading dietitians, doctors, and public health professionals to conduct vigorous educational campaigns against food faddism and nutritional hucksterism. The campaigns also emphasized that balancing diets with respect to all of the essential nutrients was much more important than relying on unusual dietary modifications or large quantities of a few minerals and vitamins to bring about the desired improvement of health.

Today, there are many types of modified diets that are used regularly in the treatment of a wide variety of abnormal conditions. However, there is a need for more accurate record keeping and monitoring of the patient's daily food intake so that the efficacy of these modifications may be judged with more certainty.

COMMON TYPES OF DIETARY MODIFICATIONS.
Two of the most important principles of dietary modification are (1) only necessary changes should be made in order to minimize the difficulty the patient will have in following the dietary prescription, and (2) every effort should be made to ensure that a modified diet is an adequate source of all essential nutrients, or if this is not feasible, appropriate nutritional supplementation should be recommended. The most common dietary modifications are given in Table M-28.

NOTE: This table lists only diets comprised of common foods and beverages that are taken orally. Special formulas and special means of administering nutrients are covered in the following articles: ELEMENTAL DIETS; INTRAVENOUS (PARENTERAL) NUTRITION, SUPPLEMENTARY; LIQUID DIETS; and TOTAL PARENTERAL (INTRAVENOUS) NUTRITION.

TABLE M-28
MODIFIED DIETS

Diet	Composition — Foods Included	Composition — Foods Excluded	Uses	Comments
General diet	The regular diet consumed by most Americans.	None	Patients who do not require any dietary modifications.	This is also called the house or full hospital diet and varies somewhat from one institution to another.

I. Modifications in texture and consistency

Diet	Composition — Foods Included	Composition — Foods Excluded	Uses	Comments
General diet, pureed	Same as general diet.	None	Toothless patients.	
General diet, liquid (Also see LIQUID DIETS.)	Finely homogenized and strained fish, meat, or poultry (visible fat should be removed before homogenization).	All other forms of fish, meat, or poultry.	For patients who are unable to chew and/or swallow foods due to circumstances such as surgery on the face, oral cavity, neck, or throat; fractures of the jaw; esophageal strictures; partial paralysis; or unconsciousness. As nutritional supplements for people who find it difficult to eat sufficient amounts of ordinary food. By athletes prior to, and/or during sporting events because liquids leave the stomach more rapidly than solid foods. Weight reduction when a low-calorie liquid diet is used at one or more daily meals in place of solid foods which contain more calories.	The daily allotment is usually divided into six feedings. Milk, milk drinks, and strained fruit or vegetable juices may be served between meals. Underweight patients may need supplemental feedings (commonly called "nourishments") that are rich in calories from foods such as melted butter or margarine (added to hot liquids), or honey, sugar, or syrups (added to fruit juices). Liquid diets are usually deficient in certain nutrients. Hence, the doctor or dietitian may recommend certain mineral and vitamin supplements if the diet is to be used for more than a week or so.
	Any type or kind of milk or cream.	None		
	Strained cottage cheese.	All other forms of cheese.		
	Eggs in cooked foods such as puddings and soft custards.	All other forms of eggs.		
	Strained fruit juices, pureed and strained fruits.	Berries with small seeds.		
	Strained vegetable juices, pureed and strained mild flavored vegetables such as asparagus, beans (green and wax), beets, carrots, peas, potatoes, spinach, squash, sweet potatoes, and tomatoes.	Strong flavored vegetables.		
	Cereal gruels made from enriched refined cooked cereals.	All prepared or dry cereals, and whole grain cooked cereals. All forms of bread.		
	Moderate amounts of butter, margarine, oil, or cream.	All other forms of fat.		
	Cream or broth-type soups made with pureed vegetables; strained fish, meats, or poultry; broth, bouillon, or consomme.	Highly seasoned soups or those containing pieces of vegetables, meats, or poultry.		
	Sugar, honey, syrups, jelly, and plain sugar candy.	Jams and marmalades.		
	Plain ice cream, sherbets, ices, puddings, junket preparations, soft custard, tapioca, and plain dessert gels.	Desserts that contain nuts, fruit, coconut, or other solids.		
	Carbonated beverages, cocoa, coffee, tea, and coffee substitutes.	All other beverages.		
	Salt, mild spices, and vanilla and other mild flavorings in moderate amounts.	All other types of condiments, flavorings, seasonings, and spices.		
Soft diet	Fresh, canned, or frozen fish; beef, lamb, liver, lean roast pork or ham, crisp bacon; or poultry meat. (These items should be cooked by baking, broiling, panbroiling, or roasting.)	Fried or deep fat fried fish, meats, or poultry; fish, meats, or poultry with small bones, gristle, or skin; fatty pork or ham, franks, corned beef; spiced or smoked items.	An intermediate diet that is given after a full liquid diet, and before a regular diet. Patients who are bedridden and likely to suffer from gas and other digestive problems when coarser foods are consumed. When difficulties in chewing and/or swallowing are present.	The compositions of soft diets vary somewhat between different hospitals. The diet may not furnish enough iron for women unless there is a liberal use of meats, enriched breads, and strained legumes. (The latter may be made into dips, soups, or spreads for bread.) Soft diets can be used for long periods of time, but they should not be used longer than necessary or the patient may lose his or her tolerance for coarser foods.
	Any type or kind of milk or cream.	None		
	Cottage and other mild-flavored varieties of cheeses.	Sharp or strong-flavored cheeses.		
	Eggs that are baked, hard or soft cooked, poached, or scrambled without fat (cooked in a nonstick fry pan).	Fried eggs or scrambled eggs cooked in fat.		
	All fruit juices; cooked and canned apples (without skin), applesauce, apricots, cherries, peaches, pears, plums, and prunes; and raw, ripe banana, grapefruit, and orange sections, ripe peeled peaches, and ripe peeled pears.	All fruits with small seeds or tough skins, unless these parts are removed completely. Dates, figs, and raisins.		
	All vegetable juices; cooked and canned asparagus, beets, carrots, eggplant, green beans, peas, pumpkin, spinach, squash, and tomatoes; corn and lima or navy beans that have been passed through a sieve; and raw lettuce.	Cooked broccoli, Brussels sprouts, cabbage, cauliflower, corn, cucumbers, kale, onions, parsnips, and whole lima or navy beans. All raw vegetables except lettuce.		
	Day old or toasted white bread; salted, soda, or graham crackers; refined cereals such as cornmeal, cream of wheat, oatmeal, or rice; dry cereals such as cornflakes.	All whole grain breads and cereals except oatmeal. Hot breads.		
	Sweet or white potatoes (without skins); macaroni, noodles, or spaghetti made with white flour; and white rice.	Spicy dressings or sauces on potatoes, pasta, or rice.		

(Continued)

| Diet | Composition | | Uses | Comments |
	Foods Included	Foods Excluded		
Soft diet (Continued)	Butter or margarine, cooking oils, cream, crisp bacon, mild-flavored salad dressings.	Fried foods and gravies.		
	Canned or homemade broths or soups made from items in this column.	Spicy soups or those containing large amounts of fat.		
	Sugar, syrups, honey, and clear jellies in moderation.	Jams and preserves which contain nuts, seeds, or skins.		
	Cakes (angel food, mild chocolate, plain white, sponge, yellow); cookies; custards; fruit whips; gelatin desserts with allowed fruits; ice cream or sherbet without fruit pulp or nuts; and puddings (bread, butterscotch, choclate, rice, tapioca, vanilla).	Pastries; pies; excessively sweet desserts; or those containing dates, fruits with small seeds, or raisins.		
	Carbonated beverages, coffee and coffee substitutes, and tea in moderation.	Alcoholic beverages, unless ordered by the doctor.		
	Salt, lemon juice, vanilla, cocoa, cinnamon, allspice, and ripe olives.	Spicy or fibrous condiments.		
Soft diet, pureed	Same foods as in the soft diet.	Same foods as in the soft diet.	Patients who have considerable difficulty in chewing and/or swallowing.	All solid foods are chopped fine, strained, or blended.
Bland diet	All of the foods in the soft diet, except those items excluded in the next column.	Those excluded from the soft diet *plus* chocolate, cocoa, coffee, decaffeinated coffee, cola beverages, tea; tomatoes, tomato juice, and citrus juices; and excessively fatty foods.	In some cases of chronic digestive disorders such as esophagitis, hiatus hernia, ulcers, colitis, diverticulitis, etc.	There is now some doubt as to whether the traditional types of bland diets promote healing any faster than regular diets which are free of strong irritants such as mustard and pepper. Pureed vegetables may also be used to make bland dressings and sauces. A vitamin C supplement is advisable.
Bland diet, low fiber	All the foods listed for the soft diet, except those items excluded in the next column.	Those excluded from the soft diet *plus* chocolate, coffee, decaffeinated coffee, cola beverages, tea; all fruit juices and fruits; all vegetables other than those pureed, strained, and prepared in cream soups; excessively fatty foods; and all spices other than salt.	In some cases of chronic digestive disorders such as esophagitis, hiatus hernia, ulcers, colitis, diverticulitis, etc.	The foods are usually distributed between 6 small meals per day. Additional feedings of milk and/or cream may be given between meals. A vitamin C supplement should be given. There is no reason for continuing this diet after the acute inflammatory stage of the disorder has subsided.
Milk and cream diet	A 1:1 mixture of whole milk and cream; or *coffee cream* with 12.5% butterfat; or if calories are to be reduced, only whole milk or skim milk.	All others	Acute stages of gastrointestinal disorders such as high gastric acidity, gastritis, ulcers, etc.	Generally, about 4 oz (*120 ml*) of the mixture are given every hour to keep some food in the stomach at all times. Mineral and vitamin supplements are needed.
Clear liquid diet (Also see LIQUID DIETS.)	Fat-free broth, bouillon, carbonated beverages, coffee, decaffeinated coffee, flavored gelatin, honey, popsicles, strained fruit juices, sugar, syrups (clear), and tea.	All others	Zero residue feeding used for (1) preparation for a barium enema and/or bowel surgery, (2) after surgery, (3) diarrhea, and (4) very weakened patients.	Supplies only a few calories (from the sugars in the allowed items) and some electrolytes (mainly sodium, chloride and potassium).
Tea and fat-free broth diet	Tea and fat-free broth (the doctor may allow the use of sugar).	All others	First feeding after surgery on the digestive tract.	Provides mainly water and little in the way of nutrients.
	*II. Modifications of caloric content*			
High-calorie diet (Also see UNDERWEIGHT.)	The regular American diet with an emphasis on eating greater-than-usual quantities of carbohydrate-rich items (breads, desserts, pasta products, and sweets); fat-rich items (bacon, butter, cream, margarine, mayonnaise, oils, peanut butter, salad dressings, and sour cream); and protein-rich items (cheeses, custards, eggs, eggnogs, fish, meats, poultry, and undiluted evaporated milk).	None, but low-calorie foods should be replaced in part by calorie-rich foods.	Providing the energy needs of (1) hypermetabolic patients (in cancer, hyperthyroidism, severe burns, and trauma), (2) underweight people, (3) victims of malnutrition and malabsorption syndromes, and (4) very active people such as athletes, explorers, laborers, miners, and soldiers.	Many of the people who have high energy needs also have high protein requirements. Hence, extra protein sources should be given. The metabolic status of the patient should be considered in determining whether the extra calories should be supplied by carbohydrates, fats, and/or protein.

(Continued)

Diet	Composition		Uses	Comments
	Foods Included	**Foods Excluded**		
Low-calorie diet (Also see OBESITY.)	Low-calorie items that are high in protein, fiber, minerals, and vitamins, such as eggs, fish, lean meats, poultry, low-fat cheeses and milk products, low-carbohydrate fruits and vegetables, and whole grain and bran types of breads and cereals. (The last named group of foods is not much lower in calories than those made from refined flour, but it contains very filling items that reduce the desire to overeat.)	Those which supply mainly calories, but little else in the way of nutrients (alcoholic beverages, cakes, cookies, desserts, highly refined fatty, starchy, and sugary foods, and many of the common snack foods).	Weight reduction for overweight people. (Loss of weight may also help to correct other undesirable conditions such as high blood pressure, an impaired utilization of sugars, and elevations in the blood levels of cholesterol and triglycerides.)	Drastic restrictions in dietary calories may lead to great reductions in certain energy-rich foods that are good sources of minerals and vitamins. Therefore, nutritional supplements may be needed in these cases. Vigorous exercise may offset some of the need for dietary restrictions. People attempting to lose considerable weight should be examined by a doctor before going on a very low calorie diet.

III. Modifications in the intakes of specific nutrients

Diet	Foods Included	Foods Excluded	Uses	Comments
Carbohydrate restricted diet (Also see DUMPING SYNDROME; HYPO-GLYCEMIA; and OBESITY.)	All types of cheeses, eggs, meats, and poultry; milk products without added sweetener; nuts; and peanut butter.	Sweetened milk products.	Treatment of the dumping syndrome in patients who have had all or part of their stomach removed. Correction of elevated blood levels of triglycerides when used with concurrent restrictions of alcohol, cholesterol, and saturated fats. Stabilization of the blood sugar in people with a tendency to low blood sugar (hypoglycemia). Weight reduction of patients who are obese due to an over-secretion of insulin in response to dietary sugars. Management of some types of juvenile diabetes in which it is difficult to adjust the dosages of insulin, or in the control of adult onset diabetes.	Some patients may also require the restriction of all milk products after they have had stomach surgery. This diet is high in cholesterol, saturated fats, and fats in general and should not be used without further modifications for patients with high blood levels of lipids (hyperlipo-proteinemias). The high protein content of this diet may be dangerous for people with certain kidney disorders. (Also see the ketogenic diet which is outlined in this table).
	Unsweetened fruit juices and fruits (limited to 3 exchanges a day).	Sweetened fruit juices and fruits.		
	Low-carbohydrate vegetables (limited to 2 exchanges per day).	Vegetables prepared with sweetener.		
	Unsweetened breads, cereals, pasta, and starchy vegetables (limited to 5 exchanges per day).	Breads and cereals with sugar, dates, or raisins (includes granola types).		
	Bacon, butter or margarine, cream (unsweetened), fats, French dressing, mayonnaise, shortenings, and vegetable oils.	Sweetened imitation cream toppings.		
	Soups made with allowed foods (starchy items limited as above).	Gravies thickened with cornstarch or flour.		
	Custards, gelatin desserts, and junket puddings made without a natural sweetener (an artificial sweetener may be used).	All desserts made with natural sweeteners.		
	Artificially sweetened carbonated beverages, coffee, herb teas, and tea (only artificial sweetener may be used in coffee and teas).	Alcoholic beverages, naturally sweetened carbonated beverages, sweetened coffee, imitation coffee creams, and sweetened ice tea.		
	Unsweetened condiments and spices.	Honey, jams, jellies, marmalade, molasses, sugar, and syrups.		
Carbohydrate, fiber, and fluid restricted diet	All of the foods listed for the soft diet, except the excluded items listed in the next column. Fluid intake should be restricted to 4 to 8 oz (*120 to 240 ml*) taken at each of 6 small meals per day. (The patient may be allowed to sip water or suck on cracked ice between meals.) Strained fruit juices should be diluted 1:1 with water. Only unsweetened cooked or canned fruits are allowed. The only allowed desserts are gelatin or baked custard made without added sugar (artificial sweeteners may be used).	Those excluded from the soft diet *plus* dried fruits, sweetened cooked or canned fruits, sweet potatoes, graham crackers, all types of sweetened desserts, all forms of sugar and sweets, all foods preserved with sugar or salt, and salt that is added at the table. (Some salt may be used in cooking.)	After gastrointestinal surgery when it is necessary to reduce the volume of fluids and foods in the stomach and intestines.	The amounts of food fluid served at each of the 6 daily meals should be increased cautiously in accordance with the patient's tolerance for food. Most nutrient requirements will be met if a variety of the allowed foods are consumed, and adequate amounts of food are eaten. However, a vitamin C supplement should be provided to compensate for the small amounts of fruits.
Fat restricted diet (Also see HYPERLIPO-PROTEIN-EMIAS.)	Canned fish (water pack), fresh or frozen fish (skin-less and unbreaded), lean meats, and poultry prepared by baking, or broiling (the pieces may be wrapped in foil to retain the juices), panbroiling (in a nonstick frying pan without added fat), and roasting.	Fish canned in oil, fresh or frozen salmon, fish cakes and frozen fish sticks, bacon, ham, pork, duck, goose, sandwich meats and sausages, canned and frozen meat dishes.	Patients who show signs of an impairment in the clearing of bloodborne fats such as chylomicrons and triglycerides from the blood within a normal period after a fat-containing meal. The major signs of this condition (Type I Hyperlipoproteinemia) are (1) a creamy upper layer that forms on a sample of blood plasma left overnight in a refrigerator, (2) abnormal pain after the consumption of fat, and (3) visible deposits of fat under the skin (eruptive xanthomas).	This diet imposes a drastic restriction on the dietary fats which form chylomicrons. However, the fat-soluble vitamins (vitamins A, D, E, and K) are absorbed and transported in the blood along with these fats. Hence, deficiencies of these vitamins may result from the diet unless supplements containing water-soluble forms of the vitamins are provided. Sometimes, patients are allowed to use specially prepared fats called medium chain triglycer-
	Evaporated skim milk, fat-free buttermilk, nonfat dry milk, and skim milk.	Chocolate milk, cultured buttermilk, whole milk, and yogurt.		
	Fat-free cottage cheese, pot cheese, and other skim-milk cheeses.	All other cheeses		
	Medium to hard cooked, poached, or scrambled egg (in a nonstick pan without added fat). Limit of 1 whole egg per day, but whites are not limited.	Eggs cooked with added fat or omelettes or souffles with fatty foods.		

(Continued)

Diet	Composition		Uses	Comments
	Foods Included	**Foods Excluded**		
Fat restricted diet *(Continued)*	All fruits and their juices, except avocado and coconut.	Avocado and coconut.	Other uses are in disorders of the biliary tract and/or the pancreas in which dietary fats are digested poorly and likely to cause a fatty diarrhea (steatorrhea).	ides (MCT) because they do not accumulate in the blood.
	All canned, fresh, or frozen vegetables prepared without a cream sauce, an oil, a fat, or a fatty food (such as a rich cheese).	Creamed vegetables or those prepared with a fat or an oil.		
	Breads and other baked goods made with little or no fat.	All other breads and baked goods.		
	All cooked and dry cereals (served with skim milk).	None		
	Baked, boiled, or mashed (with skim milk) potatoes served without any fat; hominy (corn), pasta, or rice without a fatty sauce; and unbuttered popcorn.	Escalloped, creamed, or fried potatoes; potato chips, ovenbrowned potatoes; buttered popcorn; and egg noodles.		
	Lowfat desserts such as cake (angel food), cookies (arrowroot, ladyfingers, and vanilla wafers), crackers (graham), fruit whips made with egg whites or gelatin, gelatin desserts, meringues, puddings (cornstarch, junket, rice, and tapioca) made with skim milk and egg whites, and water ices.	All cakes, cookies, ice cream, pastries, puddings, and other desserts made with eggs, egg yolks, fats, and whole milk.		
	Hard candy, fondant, jelly beans, honey, jams, and other lowfat sweets.	Candy made with fats or nuts, chocolate candy or chocolate syrup.		
	Carbonated beverages, coffee, grain beverages, and tea.	Alcoholic beverages, chocolate drinks.		
	Condiments, pickles, spices, white sauce made with skim milk.	Fat-containing gravies and sauces.		
Cholesterol and saturated fat restricted diet (Also see HEART DISEASE; and HYPERLIPO-PROTEIN-EMIAS.)	A modified regular diet that emphasizes foods containing little or no cholesterol and/or saturated fat (typical items are breads, cereals, eggs whites, fish, fruits, lean muscle meats, legumes [beans and peas], lowfat cheeses [such as cottage], margarines made from liquid vegetable oils other than coconut, nonfat milk products, oils, peanut butter [nonhydrogenated], poultry breast meats, salad dressings made from vegetable oils, and vegetables). Also, it is usually recommended that polyunsaturated vegetable oil products replace most of the eliminated saturated fats.	The foods that follow are *not* excluded, but should be eaten only in limited amounts: bacon, brains, butter, coconut oil, cream, creamy or fatty cheeses, chicken fat, egg yolks, kidneys, lard, liver, margarines made from animal fats, mayonnaise, meat fats, rich ice creams, sandwich meats and sausages, shellfish, sour cream, and whole milk products.	To prevent or treat certain hyperlipoproteinemias (high blood levels of cholesterol and/or triglycerides) in patients who (1) have a family history of early cardiovascular and/or cerebrovascular diseases (tendencies to have heart attacks and/or strokes), (2) are overweight and have high blood fats, or (3) have an abnormally rapid clotting of the blood.	The replacement of dietary saturated fats with polyunsaturated vegetable oils is considered by some doctors to be potentially hazardous because it may (1) increase the risk of cancer, (2) aggravate gallbladder disease, and (3) produce a deficiency of vitamin E, unless supplements of the latter are taken. It is not certain whether this diet is of any benefit to people other than those who tend to accumulate fats in the blood. Hyperlipemic patients should be given a glucose tolerance test before being put on this diet (to rule out the possibility that their condition is induced by dietary carbohydrates).
High fiber diet (Also see FIBER.)	A modification of the diet consumed by most Americans, with an emphasis on consuming greater-than-usual amounts of milk products, fruits, vegetables, whole-grain and bran-type breads and cereals, and nuts.	None, but some or all of the highly refined carbohydrate foods should be replaced by their unrefined equivalents.	Stimulation of larger, more frequent bowel movements to correct or prevent chronic constipation and its consequences (diverticulitis, hemorrhoids, and narrowing of the colon diameter).	Dietary fiber should be increased gradually for people accustomed to low fiber diets in order to prevent flatulence and looseness of the bowels. Should *not* be used when the bowel is inflamed.
Fiber-restricted diet	All the foods for the soft diet, except the excluded items listed in the next column. Milk intake should be restricted to 2 cups per day.	Those excluded from the soft diet *plus* all fruit and vegetable products other than strained fruit and vegetable juices and cooked white potatoes without skin; popcorn and potato chips, and prune juice (even when strained it has a laxative effect).	When gastrointestinal passages such as the esophagus or the intestines are narrowed by strictures and there is danger of blockage. Severe inflammation of the bowel in diverticulitis, infectious enterocolitis, or ulcerative colitis. As an intermediate diet that is used after a full liquid diet, and before a soft or regular diet.	A low fiber diet should not be used any longer than necessary because it produces small infrequent stools. This condition may encourage (1) excessive constriction of the colon, (2) narrowing of its diameter, (3) herniation of the colonic muscles and the production of pouches (diverticula), and (4) general aggravation of bowel problems.

(Continued)

Diet	Composition		Uses	Comments
	Foods Included	**Foods Excluded**		
Nonfiber, milk-free diet	All of the foods listed for the soft diet, except for the items listed in the next column.	Those excluded from the soft diet *plus* all milk products and cheeses, all fruit products other than strained fruit juices, all vegetable products other than strained tomato juice, potatoes, and all spices and condiments other than salt.	After intestinal surgery or trauma, when it is necessary to reduce bowel movements to a minimum.	This diet is usually given for only a few days until healing occurs because small, infrequent stools may result in (1) excessive con striction of the colon, (2) narrowing of its diameter, and (3) general aggravation of bowel problems. A calcium supplement should be given.
High protein, high calorie diet	The normal American dietary pattern supplemented by extra servings of protein-rich foods such as cheeses, eggs, fish, meats, milk products, peanut butter, poultry, and special proprietary formulas when necessary.	None, although certain filling low protein foods such as fruits and vegetables may be replaced in part by high protein foods.	Patients recovering from burns, cancer therapy, injuries, hepatitis, malnutrition, surgery, and ulcerative colitis and /or other inflammatory conditions of the gastrointestinal tract, and underweight.	High protein diets often increase the urinary losses of calcium so that a calcium supplement may be advisable. Should not be used when protein metabolism or nitrogen excretion is impaired.
Controlled protein, potassium, sodium, and water diet	A daily food pattern that provides 30 g of protein and about 800 mg each of potassium and sodium follows: 1½ oz (*28 g*) of unsalted eggs, fish, liver or muscle meat, or poultry.	Brains; kidneys; salted eggs; fish, meats, or poultry; sandwich meats; and sausages.	To provide as much nourishment as possible to patients with advanced kidney disease while preventing the accumulation in the body of excessive amounts of nitrogenous wastes and minerals salts. However, patients who are being treated regularly with hemodialysis or peritoneal dialysis may usually be given more liberal diets.	This type of diet should not be used until it is absolutely necessary, because if given prematurely, the patient may tire of it by the time it is needed the most. The diet may not supply sufficient calories for all patients and may need to be supplemented with intravenous feeding. Also, a mineral and vitamin supplement is required when a patient is given the diet for more than a few days.
	½ cup (*120 ml*) of unsalted cottage cheese or ½ oz (*14 g*) of unsalted American cheese.	All other forms of cheese and milk products.		
	½ cup (*120 ml*) of a canned, fresh, or frozen non-citrus-type of fruit.	Citrus fruits and dried fruits.		
	1 cup (*240 ml*) of cranberry juice or reconstituted frozen lemonade or limeade.	All other fruit juices.		
	1 cup (*240 ml*) of salt-free or unsalted cooked or raw cabbage, canned carrots, canned green beans, canned peas, canned wax beans, fresh cucumber, or lettuce.	All vegetables prepared with salt, and all others not listed.		
	3 slices of enriched white bread or 5 saltine crackers.	All other breads and baked goods.		
	½ cup (*120 ml*) of cooked cream of wheat, farina, or hominy grits served without milk.	All other cereals.		
	1 cup (*240 ml*) of cooked enriched pasta or enriched white rice that has been prepared without salt.	All forms of sweet and white potatoes, potato chips, and brown rice.		
	3 tsp (*15 ml*) of butter, cream cheese, margarine, mayonnaise, or salad dressing; and unresricted amounts of corn oil.	Cream gravies and all other fatty foods.		
	No soups.	All types of soups.		
	1 tsp (*5 ml*) of jam or jelly; moderate amounts of gum drops, hard candy, marshmallows, and sugar syrup (colorless-type).	All other types of sugars and sweets.		
	Moderate amounts of a homemade gelatin dessert prepared with sugar and artificial flavoring; dietetic gelatin; or lime ice.	Commercial gelatin desserts and all other types of desserts.		
	2 cups (*480 ml*) of ginger ale, or root beer.	All other beverages.		
	Unlimited amounts of cinnamon, mace, nutmeg, peppermint extract, vanilla, vinegar, and white pepper.	All other condiments, flavorings, herbs, and spices.		
Purine restricted diet	Cheeses; eggs; fishes and meats, except for those listed in the next column as excluded; and seafoods.	Brains, kidneys, liver, and sweetbreads; broths, extracts, gravies, sauces, and soups made from meats; fried meats; and anchovies, cavier, roe, and sardines.	Patients with high blood levels of uric acid (hyperuricemia), gout, and gouty arthritis.	A high fat diet may aggravate hyperuricemia. Hence, the amounts of dietary fats should be moderately restricted. The blood level of uric acid is also raised by the heavy consumption of alcoholic beverages and fasting. Vegetarian diets that are rich in microbically-fermented products, seeds, and yeast or yeast derivatives may furnish more
	All milk products, except that high fat products should be used in moderation.	None		
	All fruits and fruit juices.	None		
	Vegetables and vegetable juices as desired, except that cooked dried beans and peas should be limited to ½ cup (*120 ml*) per day.	None		

(Continued)

Diet	Composition		Uses	Comments
	Foods Included	**Foods Excluded**		
Purine restricted diet *(Continued)*	Most breads and cereals.	Wheat germ.		purines (uric-acid forming substances) per calorie than diets which contain fish, meats, and poultry.
	Most forms of sweet and white potatoes; and all pasta and rice products.	Fried potatoes and potato chips.		
	All types of fats when used in moderation.	None		
	Desserts that contain only small to moderate amounts of fats, such as custards made with skim milk, gelatin desserts, lowfat cakes, cookies, ice cream, and puddings.	High fat items such as rich cakes, cookies, ice cream, mince meat, pastries, and whipped cream or imitation whipped toppings.		
	Carbonated beverages and cereal beverages (coffee substitutes).	Alcoholic beverages, chocolate, cocoa, coffee, and tea.		
	Condiments, herbs, nuts, olives, peanut butter, pickles, popcorn, relishes, salt, spices, vinegar, and white sauce.	Fatty broths, extracts, gravies, sauces, and soups; and yeast.		
Ketogenic diet	This diet is very low in carbohydrates, high in fat content, and contains moderate amounts of protein. It is characterized by (1) the use of large and carefully calculated amounts of bacon, butter, cheese, cream, eggs, fish, meats, and poultry; (2) minimal amounts of low carbohydrate fruits and vegetables; and (3) exclusion of foods of moderate to high carbohydrate contents (such as those listed in the next column).	Beverages that contain sugar, breads and cereals, desserts other than small amounts of fruits with plenty of whipped cream, fruits and vegetables of moderate to high carbohydrate contents, milk products other than butter and cream, and all forms of sweets.	Prevention of seizures in epileptic children by inducing and maintaining a state of ketosis (the presence of ketone bodies in the blood and urine). Sometimes, this type of diet is used to induce a rapid loss of body weight in patients who find it difficult to reduce by other means. (The weight loss is largely made up of lost fluid.)	Some patients on this diet are prone to abdominal cramps, nausea, and vomiting. Small, frequent feedings are tolerated better than a few large meals per day. A special fat preparation called medium chain triglycerides is often given to patients on these diets.
Gluten-free diet	All types of cheeses, eggs, fish, meats, and poultry that are *not* breaded, creamed, extended, or served with a gravy made from barley, oats, rye, or wheat; sandwich meats and sausages if labeled as "pure meat."	Cheese, egg, fish, meat or poultry mixtures such as chili, croquettes, meat loaf, and canned products that are likely to contain flour.	The life-long diet of patients who have an intolerance to foods that contain the cereal protein gluten.	Sometimes, adults who have no previous history of gluten sensitivity have developed this condition after surgery on the digestive tract. (It has been suggested that any condition which allows incompletely digested gluten-containing proteins to be absorbed may lead to the development of a sensitivity.)
	Milk products that are not likely to contain cereal ingredients.	Chocolate and malted milk products that contain cereals or flours.		
	All fruit juices and fruits.	None		
	All vegetable juices, vegetables, except those listed in the next column as excluded.	Items prepared with bread, bread crumbs, or wheat flour.		
	Baked goods, breads and cereals made from corn, potato, rice, soybean, and/or tapioca flours or meals only.	Products containing barley, oat, rye, or wheat flour or meal.		
	Sweet or white potatoes other than those prepared by breading or flouring.	Macaroni, noodles, and spaghetti.		
	All types of fat except those listed in the next column as excluded.	All commercial salad dressings except pure mayonnaise.		
	Clear broths, consomme, and soups that contain no barley, oats, rye, or wheat; and cream soups that are thickened only with cornstarch or potato flour.	All canned soups other than clear broth; and all creamed soups that are thickened with the excluded grain products.		
	Gluten-free desserts such as custards, fruit products made without flour, gelatin desserts, homemade ice cream, ices, and sherbets, and junket, rice and other puddings thickened only with cornstarch, potato flour, or tapioca.	Cakes, cookies, ice cream containing a stabilizer made from wheat, ice cream cones, commercial baking mixes other than those labeled "gluten-free," and commercial puddings.		
	Corn syrup, honey, jams, and jellies, molasses, and brown and white sugars.	Commercial candies that contain the excluded grain products.		
Lactose-free diet	All types of eggs, fish, meats, nuts, and poultry without added lactose or milk.	Creamed or breaded preparations, sandwich meats and sausages unless labeled "all meat," and omelets and souffles made with cheeses or milk.	For people who cannot digest milk sugar (lactose) and suffer from unpleasant symptoms when lactose-containing foods are consumed.	It is believed that a large percentage of the world's people may have mild to severe symptoms of lactose intolerance (abdominal cramps,
	Nondairy creamers and similar lactose-free substitutes for milk.	All forms of milks, cheeses, ice creams, malted milks, etc.		

(Continued)

Diet	Composition		Uses	Comments
	Foods Included	**Foods Excluded**		
Lactose-free diet *(Continued)*	All fruits and vegetables and their juices that have been prepared without cheeses, cream sauces, lactose, or other milk products.	Fruit and vegetable products prepared with lactose or a milk product (such as breaded, buttered, or creamed items, corn curls, frozen french fries, and instant potatoes.)	In many cases the intolerance is congenital or hereditary, but it may also occur spontaneously in people who showed no prior indications of the condition. Usually, acquired lactose intolerance occurs as a result of injury to the intestinal lining in celiac disease (gluten intolerance), gastrointestinal milk protein allergy, irritable bowel syndrome, kwashiorkor, malnutrition, regional enteritis (Crohn's disease), ulcerative colitis, viral enteritis; and after some types of gastrointestinal surgery.	diarrhea, distention, gas, and malabsorption of nutrients) after the consumption of fairly small amounts of milk (as little as ¼ cup or *60 ml*). However, some types of fermented milks contain little or no unfermented lactose and do not produce the symptoms. (Many of the brands of yogurt sold in the U.S. contain added nonfermented skim milk solids.) Patients should be taught to scrutinize food labels for the presence of butter, casein, cheese, cream, lactose, milk, or whey. A commercial enzyme preparation that digests lactose in milk to harmless products is now available.
	Breads, cereals, and pasta made without lactose or milk.	Breads and other baked goods made from prepared mixes that contain lactose or milk products, cereals, and pasta made from milk.		
	Dressings, margarines, and shortenings made without any milk products; bacon; meats fats; nut butters that are lactose-free; oils, and certain brands of nondairy creamers and whipped toppings that contain no milk derivatives.	Dressings, margarines, certain nondairy creamers, peanut butter, and whipped toppings made with butter, cheese, cream lactose, or other milk products.		
	Broths, consomme, cream soups, and soups without milk products.	Items containing lactose or milk.		
	Candies, cakes, cookies, pies, and puddings made without milk.	Dessert items that contain milk.		
	Alcoholic and carbonated beverages, coffee, milk substitutes, tea.	Hot chocolate and some types of cocoa.		
	Condiments, jams, jellies, marmalades, spices, and sweeteners.	Artificial sweeteners that contain lactose.		
Calcium restricted diet	Most common foods, except those that are rich in calcium and are listed in the excluded list in the next column. However, meats are limited to 6 oz (*170 g*) per day, eggs to 1 per day, nonexcluded vegetables to 1 cup (*240 ml*) per day, and potatoes (prepared without milk) to 1 cup (*240 ml*) per day.	All milk products (except butter); canned mackerel, salmon, sardines, shellfish; foods that contain milk; baking powders and products made from them; green leafy vegetables; and molasses.	When the blood calcium of a patient is excessively high, and in certain tests of calcium metabolism. (Usually, only a few days of dietary calcium restriction will bring the blood calcium down to normal.)	This diet is *no* longer used to prevent the formation of calcium-containing kidney stones because keeping the urine acidic (by feeding cranberry juice or other means) works better.
Phosphorus restricted diet	3 oz (*85 g*) of cod, crab, haddock, lobster, and oysters; beef, bologna, corned beef, frankfurters, ham, heart, pork, tongue; and chicken, and duck.	Other fish and shellfish; bacon, brains, lamb. liver, turkey, and veal.	In hyperphosphatemia (excessively high blood levels of phosphate that occurs in hyperparathyroidism) and certain kidney diseases. Sometimes, a diet that is low in both phosphorus and calcium is given to prevent or treat calcium phosphate kidney stones.	When a rapid reduction in blood phosphate is essential to the patient's health, the diet is used in conjunction with the oral dosage of aluminum hydroxide antacids that bind with phosphate and prevent its absorption.
	½ cup (*120 ml*) of heavy cream (35% butterfat).	All other milk products		
	No cheeses	All cheeses		
	No eggs	All forms of eggs		
	3 cups (*720 ml*) of any canned, fresh, or frozen fruit or juice other than those listed as excluded in the next column.	Avocado, banana, blackberries; and all dried fruits.		
	1 ½ cups (*360 ml*) beets (roots are permitted, but not the leaves), cabbage, carrots, chicory, cucumbers, green bean, green peppers, lettuce, sauerkraut, spinach, squash, and tomatoes.	All dried beans and peas, and beet greens, broccoli, Brussels sprouts, and corn.		
	5 slices of enriched white bread or the equivalent in crackers made from enriched white flour.	Breads made from rye, or whole or cracked wheat, and all items made with baking powder.		
	½ cup (*120 ml*) of a dry or a cooked cereal made from refined grain.	All cereals made from whole or cracked (but not fully refined) grains.		
	½ cup (*120 ml*) of sweet or white potato; pasta made from refined white flour and white rice.	No milk products except the cream allowance may be used in dressings or sauces.		
	8 tsp (*120 ml*) of butter, margarine.	All other types of fats and salad dressings.		
	3 tsp (*15 g*) of white sugar, or 3 Tbsp (*45 ml*) of honey, jam, or jelly; and /or hard candy, drops, fondant, and mints as desired.	Candies that contain chocolate, cream or milk, dried fruits, or nuts; and all other desserts.		
	Unlimited coffee and tea	All other beverages		
	Unlimited olives and pickles	All other condiments and snacks		
High-potassium diet	A regular diet that emphasizes the consumption of potassium-rich foods such as those which follow: milk, citrus fruits and juices, apricots, bananas, cantaloupe, dates, figs, prunes, raisins, cooked dry beans and peas, green leafy vegetables, tomatoes and tomato juice, whole-grain and bran-type breads and cereals, nuts, catsup, chocolate, cocoa, herbs, spices, and sauces.	None. However, it would be wise to substitute the high-potassium foods in each food group (such as fruits and vegetables) for the low-potassium items in each group.	Patients who have become potassium depleted as a result of diarrhea, malnutrition, stresses, surgery, and treatment with certain diuretics.	When there is only mild to moderate potassium depletion it is generally safer to supply it in foods than as pure potassium salts which may cause gastrointestinal irritation. Potassium-containing salt substitutes should be used cautiously, and only after a doctor has authorized their use.

Diet	Composition		Uses	Comments
	Foods Included	**Foods Excluded**	**Uses**	**Comments**
Sodium restricted diet	The plan for a moderately restricted diet (800 to 1,000 mg of sodium per day) follows: 10 oz (*284 g*) of unsalted canned, fresh, or frozen fish, meats, or poultry; except the types listed as excluded in the next column. (Liver may be served only once every 2 weeks.)	All types of fish; cured meats such as bacon and ham; and poultry that contains added salt. (Also see Sodium, Table S-6.)	Patients with (1) fluid and sodium retention that is associated with congestive heart failure, liver disease such as cirrhosis, and certain types of kidney diseases; and (2) high blood pressure (hypertension).	Careful adherence to a moderately low salt diet may reduce or eliminate the need for some people to take diuretics and other medications. Many low salt foods are now available in health food stores, large supermarkets, and pharmacies. (A pharmacist can prepare a low sodium baking powder if a commercial product is not available.)
	3 cups (*720 ml*) of skim milk, unsalted buttermilk, and/or whole milk; or the equivalent in evaporated or nonfat dry milk.	Condensed milk, cultured buttermilk, and yogurt; all milk drinks containing chocolate syrup, ice cream, or a malt product.		
	1 oz (*28 g*) of unsalted American cheese, unsalted cottage cheese, or unsalted cream cheese.	All other cheeses		
	2 eggs, boiled, poached, scrambled, or fried in unsalted butter.	None		
	1½ cups (*360 ml*) of canned, fresh, or frozen fruit juice(s) and fruits, one of which should be citrus.	Candied fruits, dried figs, or raisins; tomato juice; all fruit drinks, juices, and other products to which sodium coloring, flavoring, or preservatives have been added.		
	1½ cups (*360 ml*) of salt-free canned, fresh, and frozen vegetables except those listed as excluded in the next column; dried lima beans, lentils, soybeans, and split peas, prepared without salt, salted pork, or a salty sauce.	Canned vegetables and vegetable juices that contain added salt; and frozen vegetables processed with salt.		
	6 slices of unsalted yeast bread, quick breads made with low sodium baking powder, and unsalted crackers. (Salt-containing yeast may be permitted, but not salt sticks.)	Products prepared with salt and/or baking soda that contains sodium.		
	½ cup (*120 ml*) of an unsalted, slow-cooking cereal such as barley, buckwheat groats (kasha), cornmeal, and hominy grits; unsalted dry cereals such as puffed rice and puffed wheat and some brands of shredded wheat (unsalted corn flakes are available in some health food stores).	Quick-cooking and enriched hot cereals; and dry cereals that contain salt.		
	1 cup (*240 ml*) of pasta, potatoes, and/or rice cooked without salt.	Potato chips and prepared potato products.		
	6 tsp (*30 ml*) of unsalted butter, cream, margarine, and homemade salt-free mayonnaise and salad dressings (commercial salt-free products are sold in some health food stores); cooking oils, salt-free shortenings and gravies.	Bacon, pork fat, salted butter and mayonnaise and salad dressings unless labeled "salt-free".		
	1 cup (*240 ml*) of unsalted broth, consomme, cream soup (made with part of the day's allowances for butter and milk), and other soups made from allowed foods listed in this column.	All canned, dehydrated, and frozen broths, bouillon cubes, consomme, extracts and soups that contain salt.		
	Moderate amounts of hard candy, honey, jams and jellies made without sodium benzoate, maple syrup, and brown and white types of sugar.	Chocolate syrups, commercial soft candies or syrups, molasses, and artificial sweeteners that contain sodium.		
	½ cup (*120 ml*) of unsalted desserts such as custards (made with part of the day's allowances for eggs and milk), fruit ices, gelatin desserts made with fresh fruit juices, ice cream and sherbets (commercial types must be deducted from the day's milk allowance), and salt-free puddings (cornstarch, rice, and tapioca).	All commercial cakes, cookies, gelatin desserts, chocolate junket desserts, pies, and puddings unless labeled "salt-free"; and all other desserts made with baking powder, soda, or salt.		
	Unlimited cocoa (milk deducted from day's allowance), coffee, decaffeinated coffee, fruit drinks without sodium benzoate or an artificial sweetener. Limit of 1 cup of carbonated drink.	Commercial chocolate drinks, diet soft drinks, ginger ale, and instant cocoa.		
	All seasonings, spices, and unsalted condiments except those excluded; unsalted nuts and popcorn; and low sodium catsup.	Salted condiments, seasonings, snacks, and spices; celery seed and dried celery leaves.		

Use of Exchange Lists in Planning Diets. Table M-28 shows that many types of modified diets are based upon the selection of certain allowed foods and the exclusion of others. However, it is often necessary to control the composition of diets quantitatively in regard to the levels of protein, carbohydrates, fats, and calories. In the early days of prescribing diets for diabetics this was done by stipulating the weights of the foods that were allowed. The preparation of meals for these patients was a tedious task for homemakers, who had to control their recipes carefully and weigh each portion of food that was served. This laborious task was simplified greatly in 1950, when the food exchange lists prepared by a joint committee of the American Dietetic Association, American Diabetes Association, and the U.S. Public Health Service were published. A revised version of this system is outlined in Table M-29.

TABLE M-29
FOOD EXCHANGE LISTS GROUPED ACCORDING TO CALORIC CONTENT AND SIZE OF PORTION[1]

Name and Description of Exchange	Low-Calorie Items	Medium-Calorie Items	High-Calorie Items
Meat and protein-rich meat substitutes 1 oz (28 g) of cooked fish, meat, or poultry; or the protein equivalent in cheese, eggs, cooked dried beans or peas, peanut butter, or a vegetable protein product.	***Lean meats and other protein-rich foods:*** 1 exchange furnishes about 7 g of protein, 3 g of fat, and 55 kcal. Baby beef, chipped beef, chuck, flank steak, tenderloin, plate ribs, plate skirt steak, round (bottom, top), all cuts rump, spare ribs, tripe 1 oz (28 g) Leg, rib, sirloin, loin, shank, shoulder of lamb .... 1 oz (28 g) Leg (whole rump, center shank) of pork, smoked ham (center slices) .... 1 oz (28 g) Leg, loin, rib, shank, shoulder, cutlets of veal .... 1 oz (28 g) Meat without skin of chicken, turkey, Cornish hen, guinea hen, pheasant .... 1 oz (28 g) Any fresh or frozen fish .... 1 oz (28 g) Canned crab, lobster, mackerel, salmon, and tuna .... 1 oz (28 g) Clams, oysters, scallops, shrimp 5 or 1 oz (28 g) Sardines, drained .... 3 Cheeses containing less than 5% fat . 1 oz (28 g) Cottage cheese, dry and 2% fat ... ¼ c (60 ml) Cooked dried peas and beans (omit 1 bread exchange) .... ½ c (120 ml)	***Medium fat meats and other protein-rich foods:*** 1 exchange furnishes about 7 g of protein, 5 g of fat, and 75 kcal (*omit ½ fat exchange*).[2] Canned beef, corned beef, ground (15% fat), ground round, rib eye .... 1 oz (28 g) Loin of pork (all cuts), tenderloin, shoulder arm shoulder blade (Boston butt), Canadian bacon, boiled ham, loin, picnic ham, shoulder 1 oz (28 g) Liver, heart, kidney, sweetbreads ... 1 oz (28 g) Cheese (farmer's, mozzarella, Neufchatel, ricotta) .... 1 oz (28 g) Cheese, Parmesan .... 3 Tbsp (45 ml) Egg .... 1 Peanut butter (omit 2 fat exchanges) . 2 Tbsp (30 ml)	***High fat meats and other protein-rich foods:*** 1 exchange furnishes about 7 g of protein, 8 g of fat, and 100 kcal (*omit 1 fat exchange*).[2] Brisket of beef, corned beef (brisket), ground beef (more than 20% fat), ground chuck, hamburger, rib roasts, club and rib steaks ..... 1 oz (28 g) Breast of lamb .... 1 oz (28 g) Ground pork loin (back ribs), spare ribs, country-style ham, deviled ham .... 1 oz (28 g) Breast of veal .... 1 oz (28 g) Capon, duck, goose .... 1 oz (28 g) Cheddar cheese and similar types .... 1 oz (28 g) Cold cuts—4½" (113 mm) diameter x ⅛" (3 mm) thick .... 1 slice Frankfurter 1
Milk and milk products 1 c (240 ml) or the equivalent in evaporated or nonfat dry milk.	***Nonfat items:*** 1 exchange furnishes about 8 g of protein, 12 g of carbohydrate, a trace of fat, and 80 kcal. Fluid nonfat or skim milk ..... 1 c (240 ml) Buttermilk made from skim milk ... 1 c (240 ml) Plain (unflavored) yogurt made with skim milk .... 1 c (240 ml) Canned evaporated skim milk .... ½ c (120 ml) Nonfat dry (powdered skim) milk .. ⅓ c (80 ml)	***Low fat items:*** 1 exchange furnishes about 8 g of protein, 12 g of carbohydrate, 5 g of fat, and 125 kcal (*omit 1 fat exchange*). Lowfat (2% fat) fluid milk .... 1 c (240 ml)	***Medium fat items:*** 1 exchange furnishes about 8 g of protein, 12 g of carbohydrate, 8.5 g of fat, and 160 kcal (*omit 2 fat exchanges*). Buttermilk made from whole milk ... 1 c (240 ml) Canned evaporated whole milk ..... ½ c (120 ml) Fluid whole milk .... 1 c (240 ml) Yogurt made from whole milk .. 1 c (240 ml)
Fruits and fruit juices Each of the designated portions furnishes 10 g of carbohydrate and 40 kcal.	***Large portions:*** 4½ to 7 oz (130 to 200 g) Cantaloupe, 6" (152 mm) diameter ...... ¼ Grapefruit, small .... ½ Honeydew melon 7" (178 mm) diameter .... ⅛ Raspberries .... ⅔ c (160 ml) Strawberries .... ¾ c (180 ml) Watermelon .... 1 c (240 ml)	***Medium portions:*** 2¼ to 4½ oz (65 to 129 g) Apple juice or apple cider .... ⅓ c (80 ml) Apple, 2" (51 mm) diameter .... 1 Applesauce, unsweetened .... ½ c (120 ml) Apricots, fresh, medium .... 2 Apricot nectar .... ⅓ c (80 ml) Blackberries .... ½ c (120 ml) Blueberries .... ½ c (120 ml) Fruit cocktail .... ½ c (120 ml) Grapefruit juice .... ½ c (120 ml) Grapes .... 12 Mango, small .... ½ Nectarine, small .... 1 Orange, small .... 1 Orange-apricot nectar .... ⅓ c (80 ml) Orange juice .... ½ c (120 ml) Papaya, medium .... ⅓ Peach, medium 1	***Small portions:*** ½ to 2¼ oz (15 to 64 g) Apricots, dried .... 4 halves Banana, small .... ½ Dates .... 2 Fig, dried, small .... 1 Fig, fresh, large .... 1 Grape juice .... ¼ c (60 ml) Prunes, dried, medium .... 2 Prune juice .... ¼ c (60 ml) Raisins .... 2 Tbsp (30 ml) Peach nectar .... ⅓ c (80 ml) Pear, small .... 1 Pear nectar .... ⅓ c (80 ml) Pineapple .... ½ c (120 ml) Pineapple juice .... ⅓ c (80 ml) Plums, medium .... 2 Tangerine, medium 1

Footnotes at end of table

(Continued)

TABLE M-29 *(Continued)*

Name and Description of Exchange	Low-Calorie Items	Medium-Calorie Items	High-Calorie Items
Vegetables and vegetable juices (The caloric contents of these items are dependent upon the carbohydrate contents. Hence, the low-calorie items are also low-carbohydrate items, and vice versa.)	***Free items to be used as desired when consumed raw:*** (If cooked, 1 c *(240 ml)* may be used without counting it, but the second cup of the cooked item should be counted as furnishing 2 g of protein, 5 g of carbohydrates, and 25 kcal.) Celery, Chicory, Chinese cabbage, Cucumbers, Endive, Escarole, Lettuce, Watercress / Asparagus, Bean Sprouts, Beets, Broccoli, Brussels sprouts, Cabbage, Carrots, Cauliflower, Eggplant, Green pepper	***Counted items:*** Each ½ c of the cooked or raw items (or their corresponding juices) that follow are to be counted as furnishing 2 g of protein, 5 g of carbohydrates, and 25 kcal. Greens: Beet, Chard, Collard, Dandelion, Kale, Mustard, Spinach, Turnip, Mushrooms, Okra, Onions, Radishes / Rhubarb, Rutabaga, Sauerkraut, String beans, green or wax, Summer squash, Tomatoes, Tomato juice, Turnips, Vegetable juice cocktail, Zucchini	***Starchy vegetables:*** 1 exchange furnishes 2 g of protein, 15 g of carbohydrates, and 70 kcal. Baked beans, no pork (canned) ..... ¼ c *(60 ml)*; Cooked dried beans, lentils, peas .... ½ c *(120 ml)*; Corn kernels, regular or cream-style .. ⅓ c *(80 ml)*; Lima beans .... ½ c *(120 ml)*; Parsnips .... ⅔ c *(160 ml)*; Peas, green (canned or frozen) .... ½ c *(120 ml)*; Potato, white, small .... 1; Pumpkin .... ¾ c *(180 ml)*; Winter squash, acorn or butternut ... ½ c *(120 ml)*; Yam or sweet potato .... ¼ c *(60 ml)*
Breads and cereals	***Low-fat items:*** 1 exchange furnishes 2 g of protein, 15 g of carbohydrate, and 70 kcal. Bread (French, Italian, pumpernickel, raisin, rye, white, whole wheat) .... 1 slice; Bread crumbs, dry .... 3 Tbsp *(45 ml)*; English muffin, small .... ½; Frankfurter roll .... ½; Hamburger bun .... ½; Pancake 5" *(127 mm)* diameter .... 1; Roll, plain, small .... 1; Tortilla 6" *(152 mm)* diameter .... 1; Waffle 5" *(127 mm)* square .... 1; Cooked cereals .... ½ c *(120 ml)*; Ready-to-eat cereals: Bran flakes .... ½ c *(120 ml)*; Others (unsweetened) .... ¾ c *(180 ml)*; Puffed grains .... 1 c *(240 ml)*; Pastas, cooked .... ½ c *(120 ml)*; Flour .... 2½ Tbsp *(38 ml)*; Wheat germ .... ¼ c *(60 ml)*	***Medium-fat items:*** 1 exchange furnishes 2 g of protein, 15 g of carbohydrate, 5 g of fat, and 115 kcal (*omit 1 fat exchange*). Biscuit, 2" *(51 mm)* diameter .... 1; Corn muffin, 2" *(51 mm)* diameter .... 1; Crackers, round butter-type .... 5; Muffin, plain, small .... 1; Potatoes, french fried, 2 to 3½" *(51 to 89 mm)* long .... 8; Crackers: Arrowroot .... 3; Graham 2½" *(64 mm)* square .... 2; Matzoh 4" x 6" *(102 x 152 mm)* ...... ½; Oyster .... 20; Pretzels 3⅛" *(80 mm)* long x ⅛" *(3 mm)* diameter .... 25; Rye wafers 2" *(51 mm)* x 3½" *(89 mm)* .... 3; Saltines .... 6; Soda 2½" *(64 mm)* square .... 4; Sponge cake, plain, 1½" *(38 mm)* cube .. 1; Vanilla wafers 5	***High-fat items:*** 1 exchange furnishes 2 g of protein, 15 g carbohydrate, 10 g of fat, and 160 kcal (*omit 2 fat exchanges*). Corn or potato chips .... 15; Ice cream .... ½ c *(120 ml)*
Fats Each of the designated portions furnishes 5 g of fat and 45 kcal.	***Least concentrated sources:*** 2 to 3 Tbsp *(30 to 45 g)*. Avocado 4" *(102 mm)* diameter .... ⅛; Cream, light, sweet or sour ...... 2 Tbsp *(30 ml)*; Half and half .... 3 Tbsp *(45 ml)*; Olives, green, medium 3	***Intermediate sources:*** 1 to 2 Tbsp *(15 to 30 g)*. Cream, heavy .... 1 Tbsp *(15 ml)*; Cream cheese .... 1 Tbsp *(15 ml)*; French dressing .... 1 Tbsp *(15 ml)*	***Most concentrated sources:*** 1 to 3 tsp *(5 to 15 g)*. Bacon, crisp .... 1 strip; Butter, lard, margarine, mayonnaise, meat fat (melted), oil, shortening ...... 1 tsp *(5 ml)*; Nuts, shelled, small .... 6; Salad dressing, mayonnaise type .... 2 tsp *(10 ml)*

[1]Adapted by the authors from *Exchange Lists for Meal Planning*, The American Dietetic Association and the American Diabetes Association, in cooperation with the National Institute of Arthritis, Metabolism and Digestive Diseases, and the National Heart, Blood and Lung Institute, Public Health Service, U.S. Dept. HEW, 1976.

[2]Most diets are based upon the use of lean meats and nonfat milk products. Hence, the use of items richer in fat must be compensated for by the deduction of fat exchanges from the total allowed.

The use of the food exchange lists presented in Table M-29 is illustrated by the sample calculations shown in Table M-30 and the typical menu in Table M-31.

The bases of the calculations shown in Table M-30 and the typical daily menu in Table M-31 are as follows:

1. A 48-year-old businessman who is 6 ft, 2 in. *(188 cm)* tall, is of medium build, and weighs 198 lb *(90 kg)*, has been diagnosed recently as an adult onset diabetic who does not require insulin injections but would benefit from a reduction of his body weight to one that is more desirable for his age, height, and condition.

2. The ideal weight of the patient is 176 lb, or *80 kg* (from a standard life insurance table) and the caloric intake for a sedentary person at that weight should be 176 lb x 13 Calories (kcal) per pound *(28.6 kcal/kg)*, or 2,288 kcal per day. (This allowance may be rounded to 2,300 kcal per day.)

3. It is decided that the weight reduction of the patient should be gradual (about 1 lb per week). Hence, his dietary prescription is for 1,800 kcal per day, distributed as follows: 20% from proteins, 45% from carbohydrates, and 35% from fats. (A caloric deficit of 500 kcal per day equals a weekly deficit of 3,500 kcal, or the amount needed to lose 1 lb [*0.45 kg*] of body weight.) The daily allowances (in grams) of proteins, carbohydrates, and fats are determined by dividing the caloric factors for nutrients (proteins, 4 kcal/g; carbohydrates, 4 kcal/g; and fats, 9 kcal/g) into the kcal contributed by each nutrient.

TABLE M-30
CALCULATION OF FOOD EXCHANGES FOR A PRESCRIBED DIET

Prescription: 1,800 kcal 20% protein (*90 g*), 45% carbohydrate (*202 g*), 35% fat (*70 g*)

Exchange	No. of Exchanges	Protein, g	Carbohydrate, g	Fat, g	Calories (kcal)
Meat, lean	3	(× 7) = 21	—	(× 3) = 9	(× 55) = 165
Meat, medium fat	3	(× 7) = 21	—	(× 5) = 15	(× 75) = 225
Running subtotal		(42)		(24)	(390)
Milk, lowfat	2	(× 8) = 16	(× 12) = 24	(× 5) = 10	(× 125) = 250
Milk, medium fat	1	(× 8) = 8	(× 12) = 12	(× 8.5) = 8.5	(× 160) = 160
Running subtotal		(66)	(36)	(42.5)	(800)
Fruit	3	—	(× 10) = 30	—	(× 40) = 120
Running subtotal		(66)	(66)	(42.5)	(920)
Vegetables, free items	unlimited	—	—	—	—
Vegetables, counted	2	(× 2) = 4	(× 5) = 10	—	(× 25) = 50
Vegetables, starchy	2	(× 2) = 4	(× 15) = 30	—	(× 70) = 140
Running subtotal		(74)	(106)	(42.5)	(1,110)
Bread, low fat	3	(× 2) = 6	(× 15) = 45	—	(× 70) = 210
Bread, medium fat	2	(× 2) = 4	(× 15) = 30	(× 5) = 10	(× 115) = 230
Bread, high fat	1	(× 2) = 2	(× 15) = 15	(× 10) = 10	(× 160) = 160
Running subtotal		(86)	(196)	(62.5)	(1,710)
Fats	2	—	—	(× 5) = 10	(× 45) = 90
Total		86	196	72.5	1,800
× calorie factor		× 4	× 4	× 9	
Calories		344	+ 784	+ 652.5 =	1,781

$$\text{Proteins} = \frac{1,800 \text{ kcal} \times 20\%}{4 \text{ kcal/g}} = 90 \text{ g}$$

$$\text{Carbohydrates} = \frac{1,800 \text{ kcal} \times 45\%}{4 \text{ kcal/g}} = 202 \text{ g}$$

$$\text{Fats} = \frac{1,800 \text{ kcal} \times 35\%}{9 \text{ kcal/g}} = 70 \text{ g}$$

4. The allowed food exchanges are worked out by (1) considering the meat and milk items to have the highest priorities, and (2) keeping a running count of the dietary content of proteins, carbohydrates, fats, and calories as the various exchanges are added to the diet. This calculation is simplified by the tabular format of Table M-30 in which the values shown in parentheses represent the nutrient values of the exchanges listed in the column on the left margin. The values shown after the equal signs were obtained by multiplying the nutrient values for the exchanges by the number of exchanges selected. It is noteworthy that the patient was allowed some medium fat exchanges for meat, milk, and bread products because he has to eat his lunch in a fast food restaurant.

5. After the bread exchanges were added to the diet, the running subtotal showed that only two separate fat exchanges could be added. Then, a check of the dietary totals of proteins, carbohydrates, fats, and calories showed that they were reasonably close to those in the dietary prescription.

6. The menu shows how the allowed exchanges may be used in meals. Although it may not always be possible to adhere perfectly to the plan, lapses on certain days should

be noted carefully in terms of the allowances that were exceeded and they should be compensated for in the days that follow the deviations. For example, extra fat taken on one day should be compensated for by an equivalent deduction the next day, such as the substitution of a lowfat exchange for an allowed medium fat exchange.

Special Dietetic Foods. Many types of special dietary products are now available for people who must limit their consumption of substances present in ordinary foods. For example, there are artificially sweetened jams, jellies, salad dressings, sauces, and soft drinks. The term *dietetic* does not always mean that the product contains an artificial sweetener. Rather, it may mean that considerably less than the normal amounts of natural sweetener were used in the recipe. It may also be used to designate lowfat varieties of items such as salad dressings. Also, both dry and liquid forms of low-cholesterol egg products are sold in most supermarkets. However, it is best for anyone who has been placed on a modified diet to consult his or her doctor or dietitian before using any special dietetic foods because use of the new product may result in a significant alteration in the nutritional value of the prescribed diet.

SUMMARY. The proper types of modified diets may be very useful in the treatment of people with various disorders or undesirable conditions such as overweight or underweight. Nevertheless, the combined expertise of a doctor and a dietitian are usually needed to determine the dietary patterns most suitable for individual patients.

TABLE M-31
A TYPICAL DAILY 1,800-CALORIE MENU
THAT WAS PLANNED FROM FOOD EXCHANGE LISTS[1]

Type of Food Exchange	No. of Exchanges	Typical Foods in Designated Exchange
Breakfast:		
Meat, medium fat ..	1	An egg, a 1 oz-slice of boiled ham, Canadian bacon, or 1 lamb kidney (cooked without fat, unless 1 of the allowed fat exchanges is used).
Milk, low fat (2%) ..	1	Taken as a beverage, in coffee or tea, and/or on cereal.
Fruit	1	Glass (4 oz, or *120 ml*) of fruit juice, or a serving of a fruit.
Bread, low fat	2	Bread and/or cereal.
Unrestricted items ..	—	Coffee, cereal beverage (coffee substitute), dietetic (artificially sweetened) soft drink, herb tea, or tea without a natural sweetener (unless ⅓ bread exchange is deducted for each tsp of sweetener used during the day).
Midmorning:		
Unrestricted items ..	—	Coffee, cereal beverage, dietetic soft drink, herb tea, etc. (See Breakfast.)
Bread, if *not* used at breakfast	1	Bread, cake, cookies, or crackers.
Milk, if *not* used at breakfast	1	Part of the allowed medium fat milk exchange (whole or evaporated milk) may be used in the unrestricted beverage.
Lunch:		
Meat, medium fat ..	2	2 slices (2 oz, or *56 g*) of broiled or roasted (not fried) meat.
Fruit	1	Glass (4 oz, or *120 ml*) of fruit juice, or a serving of a fruit.
Vegetable, free	—	Celery, cucumber, lettuce, etc. as desired.
Vegetable, counted .	1	Beets, carrots, green pepper, mushrooms, onions, tomatoes, etc.
Vegetable, starchy ..	1	Baked beans (without pork), cooked dried beans or peas, corn, green peas, sweet or white potato.
Bread, medium fat .	2	Allowance is intended to cover items such as a small serving of french fried potatoes, biscuits, or corn muffins. If 1 or more low fat items are used instead, 1 or more extra fat exchanges may be allowed.
Fat	1	Dressing for salad or vegetable, or spread for bread.
Unrestricted items ..	—	Coffee, cereal beverage, dietetic soft drink, herb tea, etc. (See Breakfast.)
Midafternoon:		
Unrestricted items ..	—	Coffee, cereal beverage, dietetic soft drink, herb tea, etc. (See Breakfast.)
Bread, if *not* used at breakfast or lunch .	1 to 2	Bread, cake, cookies, or crackers.
Milk, if *not* used as allowed at another meal	—	(See the note next to milk under Midmorning.)
Supper:		
Meat, lean	3	Fish, meat, poultry, or a meat substitute.
Fruit	1	Glass (4 oz, or *120 ml*) of fruit juice, or a serving of a fruit.
Vegetable, free	—	Celery, cucumber, lettuce, etc. as desired.
Vegetable, counted .	1	Beets, carrots, green pepper, mushrooms, onions, tomatoes, etc.
Vegetable, starchy ..	1	Baked beans (without pork), cooked dried beans or peas, corn, green peas, sweet or white potato.
Bread, low fat	1	Bread, roll, tortilla, etc.
Bread, high fat	1	Items such as 1 serving of ice cream or potato chips (if low or medium-fat bread is used instead, an extra fat exchange may be allowed).
Fat	1	Dressing for salad or vegetable, or spread for bread.
Unrestricted items ..	—	Coffee, cereal beverage, dietetic soft drink, herb tea, etc. (See Breakfast.)
Bedtime:		
Milk, low fat (2%) ..	1	
Bread, if the exchanges allowed at meals during the day are not all used . .	1 to 3	Bread, cake, cereal, cookies, or crackers.

[1]See Table M-30 and the accompanying text for the calculations used to determine the numbers of allowed food exchanges.

MOIETY

Any equal part.

MOISTURE

A term used to indicate the water contained in foods—expressed as a percentage.

MOISTURE-FREE (M-F, oven-dry, 100% dry matter)

This refers to any substance that has been dried in an oven at 221°F (*105°C*) until all the moisture has been removed. (Also see ANALYSIS OF FOODS.)

MOLASSES

Molasses is the thick brownish syrup by-product of the manufacture of cane or beet sugar from which part of the crystallizable sugar has been removed. However, molasses is also the by-product of several other industries. Citrus molasses is produced from the juice of citrus wastes. Wood molasses is a by-product of the manufacture of paper, fiberboard, and pure cellulose from wood; it is an extract from the more soluble carbohydrates and minerals of the wood material. Starch molasses, Hydrol, is a by-product of the manufacture of dextrose (glucose) from starch derived from corn or grain sorghums in which the starch is hydrolyzed by use of enzymes and/or acid. Cane molasses and beet molasses are, by far, the most extensively used types of molasses. The different types of molasses are available in both liquid and dehydrated forms.

Molasses contains sugar, which forms the basis of determining its quality. The sugar content is expressed as *Brix*. Brix is determined by measuring the specific gravity of molasses. After the specific gravity has been obtained, the value is applied to a conversion table from which the level of sucrose (or degrees Brix) can be determined. As sugar content increases, degrees Brix likewise increases. Since molasses also contains lipids, protein, inorganic salts, waxes, gums, and other material, the Brix classification can often be misleading, because each of these contaminants has an influence on the specific gravity of the solution. However, degrees Brix does give a relatively accurate indication of the sugar content of molasses and is, therefore, a good means of determining quality.

PRODUCTION. Molasses may be made by the open kettle method or by the vacuum pan method. In the open kettle method, the cane juice is boiled in a large open pan. Large sugar factories generally use the vacuum pan method, in which large, covered vacuum pans are used.

USES. Only a small portion of the molasses available in the United States is consumed by humans. Some molasses is used in industries for the production of yeast and organic fermentation chemicals. But the major utilization of molasses in the United States is in animal feeds, as blackstrap molasses—the molasses left after several boilings.

Food. The baking industry is the largest consumer of edible molasses. It imparts a pleasant flavor to breads, cakes, and cookies. Additionally, molasses serves as a humectant—helping to maintain the freshness of baked goods, and enhances the flavor of chocolate in baked goods or drinks.

In home cooking, molasses is employed for the same purposes as in the baking industry. Also, molasses is often incorporated in baked beans, and in glazes for sweet potatoes and meats such as hams. The flavor of toffees and caramel may be rounded out with molasses. Some table syrups contain molasses, and some individuals sweeten foods with molasses, while others mix a spoonful or two with hot water for a hot beverage. Many recipes have been developed which take advantage of the pleasant flavor and smell of molasses.

Generally, molasses is eaten in such small amounts it does not make an important contribution to the diet. The nutritional value of molasses is given in Food Composition Table F-21.

Molasses is (1) a good source of some minerals—especially calcium, magnesium, potassium, and iron; and (2) a concentrated energy source. Blackstrap molasses contains several of the minerals at higher levels than light or medium molasses. Vitamins are present only in low levels, or nonexistent.

Dark molasses (blackstrap molasses) is a fair, but variable and unreliable, source of iron. Today, there is less iron in molasses that is processed in stainless steel or aluminum vessels than in molasses processed in old-fashioned iron vats and pipes. Besides, molasses is generally eaten infrequently and/or in small servings. Some opinions to the contrary, molasses has no miraculous curative properties; rather, it should be eaten for reason of taste.

Rum is produced from the fermentation of molasses. After distillation, it is aged from 5 to 7 years. Rum gets its color from the oaken cask in which it is aged and from caramel added before aging. Some light rums are rapidly fermented with cultured yeast and aged from 1 to 4 years.

(Also see DISTILLED LIQUORS.)

MOLD INHIBITORS

Substances such as sodium and calcium propionate which are added to foods to prevent the growth of mold. Often, substances with this action are referred to as antimicrobials.

(Also see ADDITIVES, FOODS.)

MOLDS (FUNGI)

Fungi which are distinguished by the formation of mycelium (a network of filaments or threads), or by spore masses.

(Also see POISONS, Table P-2, Some Potentially Poisonous [Toxic] Substances—Mycotoxins; and SPOILAGE OF FOOD.)

MOLECULE

A chemical combination of two or more atoms.

MOLYBDENUM (Mo)

Although the essential role of molybdenum in plants is well known, the essentiality of this element in man is less well established. Evidence that molybdenum is an essential trace element is based on the facts that it is part of the molecular structure of two enzymes, xanthine oxidase (involved in the oxidation of xanthine to uric acid) and aldehyde oxidase (involved in the oxidation of aldehydes to carboxylic acids), and that diets low in molybdenum adversely affect growth in small animals. There is no evidence, however, that a low molybdenum intake produces deficiency signs and symptoms in man.

The adult human body contains only about 9 mg of molybdenum.

HISTORY. In 1778, Karl Scheele of Sweden recognized molybdenite as a distinct ore of a new element. Then, in 1782, P. J. Hjelm obtained the metal by reducing the oxide with carbon and called it molybdenum. The name molybdenum is derived from the Greek *molybdos*, meaning lead.

Molybdenum was long known as essential for the growth of all higher plants. Then, in 1953 it was found in the essential enzyme, xanthine dehydrogenase.

ABSORPTION, METABOLISM, EXCRETION. Molybdenum is readily absorbed as molybdate in the small intestine, although some absorption occurs throughout the intestinal tract. There is little retention of this element except in the liver, adrenals, kidneys, and bones. Molybdenum is excreted rapidly in the urine, and in limited amounts via the bile and feces.

FUNCTIONS OF MOLYBDENUM. Molybdenum is a component of three different enzyme systems which are involved in the metabolism of carbohydrates, fats, proteins, sulfur-containing amino acids, nucleic acids (DNA and RNA), and iron. Also, it is found in the enamel of teeth, where it appears to prevent or reduce the incidence of dental caries, although this function has not yet been proven conclusively.

DEFICIENCY SYMPTOMS. Naturally occurring deficiency of molybdenum in human subjects is not known, *unless* utilization of the mineral is interfered with by excesses of copper and/or sulfate.

Molybdenum-deficient animals are especially susceptible to the toxic effects of bisulfite, which is both a food additive and a product of the metabolism of sulfur-containing amino acids. Bisulfite toxicity is characterized by breathing difficulties and neurological disorders.

INTERRELATIONSHIPS. The utilization of molybdenum is reduced by excess copper, sulfate, and tungsten (an environmental contaminant). Also, even a moderate excess of molybdenum causes significant urinary loss of copper; and toxicity due to excess copper is counter-acted by molybdenum.

RECOMMENDED DAILY ALLOWANCE OF MOLYBDENUM. Man's requirement for molybdenum is so low that it is easily furnished by the diet.

The Food and Nutrition Board of the National Research Council (FNB-NRC) recommends that the molybdenum intake of an adult be within the range of 75 to 250 mcg/day.

Estimated safe and adequate intakes of molybdenum are given in the section on MINERAL(S), Table M-25, Mineral Table.

• **Molybdenum intake in average U.S. diet**—The daily intake from a mixed diet in the United States has been estimated at about 180 mcg/day.

TOXICITY. The greatest concern about molybdenum

is its toxicity. Adverse effects of high molybdenum concentrations in the environment have been reported in the human population living in a province of the U.S.S.R.[46] According to the U.S.S.R. report, an excessive dietary intake of 10 to 15 mg/day of molybdenum caused a high incidence of a goutlike syndrome associated with elevated blood levels of molybdenum, uric acid, and xanthine oxidase.

Potentially toxic levels of molybdenum are contained in some soils and herbage in parts of Florida, California, and Manitoba.

SOURCES OF MOLYBDENUM. The concentration of molybdenum in food varies considerably, depending on the soil in which it was grown. Most of the dietary molybdenum intake is derived from organ meats, whole grains, wheat germ, legumes, leafy vegetables, and yeast. Table M-32 gives the molybdenum content of some common foods. The molybdenum requirement should be met by most diets. Supplements of additional molybdenum are not recommended.

(Also see MINERAL[S], Table M-25.)

TABLE M-32
MOLYBDENUM CONTENT OF SOME COMMON FOODS

Food	Molybdenum
	(mg/100 g)
Lima beans, dry	.323
Wheat germ	.210
Liver	.150
Green beans	.067
Eggs	.050
Whole wheat flour	.048
Poultry	.040
White flours	.025
Spinach	.025
Cabbage	.017
Potato	.016
Cantaloupe	.016
Apricot	.011
Carrot	.010
Banana	.003
Milk	.003
Lettuce	.002
Celery	.002

MONOGLYCERIDE

An ester of glycerol with one fatty acid.

MONOPHAGIA

The habit of eating, or the desire to eat, only one type of food.
(Also see APPETITE.)

MONOSACCHARIDE

Any one of several simple, nonhydrolyzable sugars. Glucose, fructose, galactose, arabinose, xylose, and ribose are examples.
(Also see CARBOHYDRATE[S]; and SUGARS.)

MONOUNSATURATED

Having one double bond, as in a fatty acid; e.g., oleic acid.

---

[46]Kovalskiy, V. V., and G. A. Yarovaya, Molybdenum-infiltrated Biogeochemical Provinces, *Agrokhimiya*, Vol. 8, 1966, pp. 68-91.

MONOVALENT

Having a valence (the power of an atom to combine with another atom) of one. Example: sodium (Na+) has a valence of one; it combines with chloride (Cl–) to form sodium chloride (NaCl).

MORBIDITY

A state of sickness.

MORTADELLA

A dry or semidry sausage made of chopped pork and pork fat; seasoned with red pepper and garlic; stuffed in large casings; and cooked and smoked.

MOTILITY

The power of spontaneous movement.

MUCIN

A glycoprotein secreted by the secretory cells of the digestive tract. It functions to (1) facilitate the smooth movement of food through the digestive tract, and (2) provide a protective coating to the gastric and duodenal mucosa against the corrosive action of hydrochloric acid.
(Also see DIGESTION AND ABSORPTION; and ULCERS, PEPTIC.)

MUCOPOLYSACCHARIDE (GLYCOSAMINO-GLYCAN)

A group of polysaccharides which contains hexosamine (as glucosamine), which may or may not be combined with protein, and which, dispersed in water, form many of the mucins—thick gelatinous material that cements cells together and lubricates joints and bursas.

MUCOPROTEIN

Substances containing a polypeptide chain and disaccharides, found in mucous secretions of the digestive glands.

MUCOSA (MUCOUS MEMBRANE)

A membrane rich in mucous glands which lines the gastrointestinal, respiratory, and genitourinary tracts.

MUCOUS MEMBRANE

A membrane lining the cavities and canals of the body, kept moist by mucus.

MUCUS

A slimy liquid secreted by the mucous glands and membranes.

MULTIPLE SCLEROSIS (MS)

A strange and baffling disease of the nervous system of unknown origin whose victims are between the ages of 20 and 40. Some evidence suggests that it is caused by a slow-acting virus to which the body's immune system does not respond. Nerve tracts of the brain and spinal cord develop areas of faulty nerve transmission due to the development of areas of demyelination—loss of myelin, the insulation of nerves—which is thought to be the result of some alteration in lipid metabolism. These areas occur at random and may come and go. Symptoms signaling the onset of multiple sclerosis may be so minor that they are overlooked; for example, blurred or double vision. Once the initial symptoms disappear they may never recur, and a period of months or years may pass before other symptoms appear such as weakness of certain muscles, unusual tiring of a limb, minor interference with walking, muscle stiffness, dizziness, loss of bladder control and disturbances in the senses of touch, pain, and heat. Each symptom may appear and then disappear only to be followed by another. The disease continues to progress, and eventually the victim becomes crippled and even bedridden. However, the progression and remission of multiple sclerosis is different for every victim. Maintenance of good physical health, resistance to infection, and good mental health play a role in the severity of the symptoms. To this end a nutritionally adequate and appealing diet simply prepared is recommended. As the disease progresses, a pureed or liquefied diet may be necessary since victims have difficulty swallowing.

(Also see MODIFIED DIETS.)

MUSCLES

All physical functions of the body involve muscular contractions, which, in turn, require nutrients derived from the diet. Muscles conduct nervous impulses, contract in response to nervous impulses, and modify their activity according to the degree they are stretched. In the body, there are three types of muscles:

1. **Skeletal muscles.** These are attached to the 206 bones that make up the skeleton. Their coordinated contraction and relaxation results in the movement of body parts. Skeletal muscles are voluntarily controlled. They are also classified as striated muscles due to their microscopic appearance.

2. **Smooth muscles.** Most of the internal organs of the body contain smooth muscles. They are responsible for contractions of such organs as the intestines, blood vessels, and uterus. For the most part, smooth muscles are involuntarily controlled.

3. **Cardiac muscle.** Obviously, it is found only in the heart. Continually contracting and relaxing with a built-in rhythmicity until death, it pumps about 8,000 gallons (30,400 liters) of blood through 12,000 miles (19,200 km) of blood vessels each day.

Muscular contraction is a complicated process involving the actin and myosin filaments of the cell; requiring chemical energy and oxygen. It forms heat and a force capable of performing work.

(Also see ENERGY UTILIZATION OF THE BODY, section on ''Muscle Contraction'';METABOLISM; and MUSCULAR WORK.)

MUSCOVADO

Unrefined raw sugar obtained from the juice of sugarcane by evaporation and drawing off the molasses.

MUSCULAR DYSTROPHY (MD)

Any of the hereditary diseases of the skeletal muscles characterized by a progressive shrinking or wasting of the muscles. At the onset only certain muscles seem affected, but ultimately all muscles become involved. The exact cause is not known. The most common form of muscular dystrophy occurs almost entirely in males since its inheritance is sex linked—passed from mother to son on the X chromosome. There is no effective treatment. Physical therapy may delay the progression of the disease. Dietary adjustments due to limited mobility and feeding difficulties are necessary

as the disease advances.

(Also see MODIFIED DIETS.)

MUSCULAR WORK

Energy is the ability to do work. Mechanical work is accomplished when a force acts to move an object some distance. Muscles require chemical energy derived from the diet to contract and produce a force capable of performing work. Contraction of the heart produces a force which propels the blood through the blood vessels. Contracting limb muscles are capable of exerting a force to move an object from the floor to a table. Contracting limb muscles work to move the body—exercise. The amount of energy required is in direct relation to the intensity of the muscular work.

(Also see CALORIC [ENERGY] EXPENDITURE.)

MUSH

This is a dish made by boiling cornmeal in water, which is eaten as a hot cereal; or it can be put into a mold until cold, then sliced and fried in a little butter.

MUSHROOMS, CULTIVATED
Basidiomycetes, Ascomycetes

These much esteemed foods are the fleshy, fruiting bodies of higher fungi that grow in soil rich in organic matter, or on living trees or dead wood. From a strict botanical point of view, the term mushroom designates certain club fungi *(Basidiomycetes)*. However, many people extend the term to cover cup fungi *(Ascomycetes)* such as truffles.

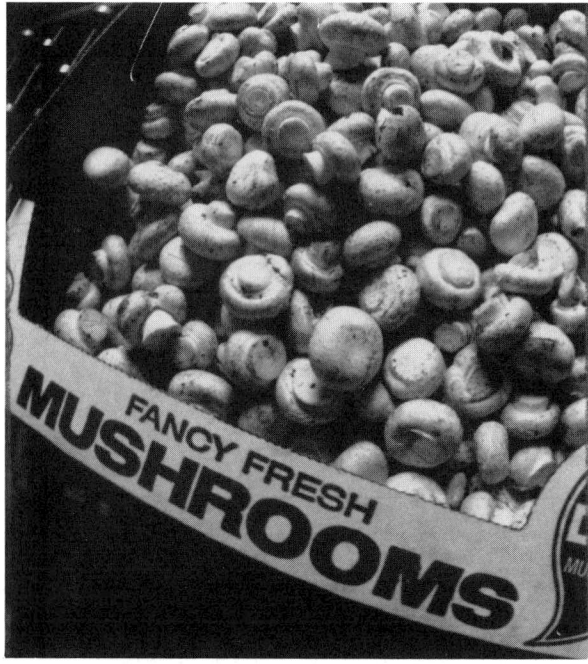

Fig. M-79. Mushrooms marketed in bulk. (Courtesy, Castle and Cooke, Inc.)

MAJOR TYPES. There are about 38,000 known species of mushrooms. Of course, it is impossible in this article to list or describe all the kinds of mushrooms. However, brief descriptions of the five most commonly cultivated mushrooms follow.

• **Common Cultivated Mushroom** *(Agaricus bisporus)*—This is the type that is best known to Americans. It is light colored and very mild flavored.

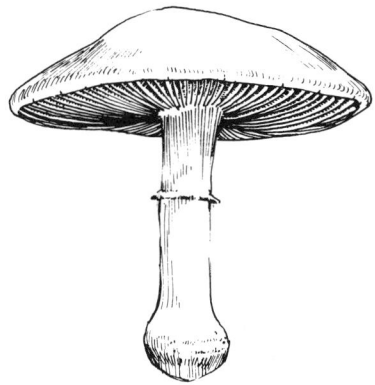

Fig. M-80. The common Cultivated Mushroom *(Agaricus bisporus)*.

• **Oyster Mushroom** *(Pleurotus ostreatus)*—The color and shape of this type are like those of an oyster. It is grown mainly in the Orient and Europe. The canned oyster mushrooms sold in the United States are usually imported from Taiwan.

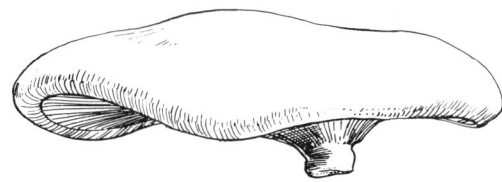

Fig. M-81. The Oyster Mushroom *(Pleurotus ostreatus)*.

• **Padi Straw Mushroom** *(Volvariella volvaceae)*—Most of this crop is produced in the Orient, where it is grown on rice (paddy) straw. These mushrooms are usually sold in the dried form.

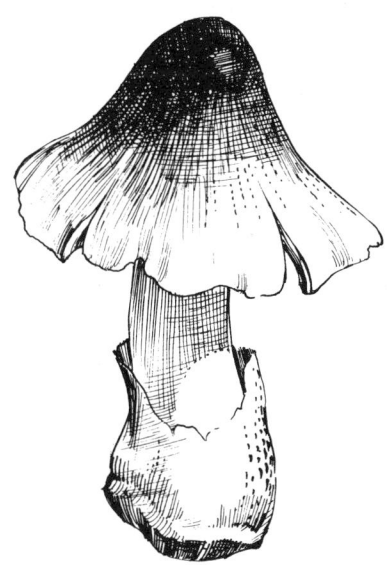

Fig. M-82. The Padi Straw Mushroom *(Volvariella volvaceae)*.

• **Shiitake** *(Lentinus edodes)*—This type is grown mainly in China and Japan, and is exported in canned, dried, and pickled forms.

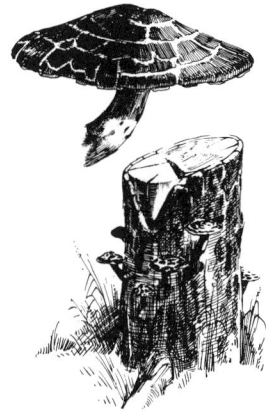

Fig. M-83. Shiitake *(Lentinus edodes)*, a mushroom which grows on hardwood logs.

• **Truffles** *(Tuber melanosporum; tuber magnatum)*—These are by far the most sought after and expensive of the mushrooms. Actually, they are cup fungi *(Ascomycetes)*, rather than mushrooms, and they grow underground in association with the roots of oak and beech trees. Most of the world's supply of this delicacy is produced in France and Italy. Terfezios are fungi that resemble truffles closely and are found mainly in the desert areas of North Africa and the Middle East.

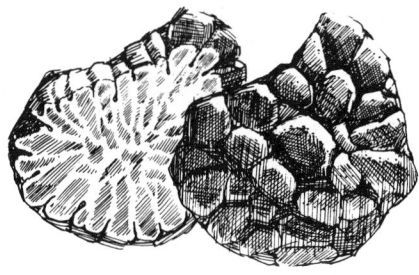

Fig. M-84. Truffles *(Tuber melanosporum)*, a gourmet fungus that is highly esteemed for its fragrant aroma.

NUTRITIONAL VALUE. The nutrient compositions of various forms of mushrooms are given in Food Composition Table F-21.

Mushrooms are high in water content (90%) and low in calories (28 to 35 kcal per 100 g). They contain about 20% more protein than potatoes, but they furnish less than half as many calories. Furthermore, they are very low in calcium, vitamin A, and vitamin C; moderately low in thiamin and riboflavin; and a good source of phosphorus, potassium, and niacin. However, many of the nutrients that are lacking in mushrooms may be provided by green leafy vegetables and milk products, which go well with the fungi.

(Also see VEGETABLE(S), Table V-2, Vegetables of the World.)

MUSKRAT *Ondatra zibethicus*

A small rodent found throughout the United States and Canada, and in parts of Europe, living in the holes in the banks of ponds and streams or in dome-shaped houses of rushes and mud. The muskrat is about the size of a small cat, has a long tail and webbed hind feet, is brown in color, and possesses small glands that give off a musky odor. Muskrat fur is sold as *Hudson seal.* Muskrat meat is tasty and is sold as *marsh rabbit.*

MUSTARD SEED *Sinapis alba; Brassica* spp

Mustard, which is made from the seeds of certain plants of the mustard family (*Cruciferae*), is the leading spice in worldwide usage. The four species of mustard seeds used for this purpose are: (1) white mustard (*Sinapis alba*), (2) brown mustard (*Brassica juncea*), (3) black mustard (*Brassica nigra*), and (4) Ethiopian mustard (*Brassica carinata*). It is noteworthy that brown mustard, which is also called Indian mustard, may also be grown for its green leaves rather than for its seeds.

PROCESSING. Mustard seed is usually marketed as a dry powder, or as a preparation with a pastelike consistency. Both of these forms are made by grinding the dry seed into a powder, then removing the seed hulls by milling, screening, and sifting. The dried mustard powder has no pungent odor because the ''hot'' components are present in a chemically inactive form. However, wetting the powder brings about an enzymatic action which liberates the pungent components.

Most prepared mustard is made by mixing the dried mustard powder with salt, vinegar, and other spices. Also, mustard is utilized in other products such as mayonnaise, salad dressings, and pickles.

SELECTION, PREPARATION, AND USES. Mustard powder, which is available in most supermarkets, may be added directly to casseroles (such as baked beans and pork), soups, stews, and other mixed dishes. However, it should be used cautiously, since the enzymatic action which releases the pungent components from the wetted powder requires a bit of time in which to develop the maximum flavor intensity. It is noteworthy that mixing the powder with very hot water, or with moderately strong acid such as lemon juice or vinegar, stabilizes the flavor intensity by stopping the enzyme action.

Prepared mustard may be used to spice up deviled eggs, fish, meats, and poultry. It also enhances the flavor of dressings and sauces.

NUTRITIONAL VALUE. Mustard seed is rich in nutrients (469 kcal per 100 g, 25% protein, and 29% fat), but it is not likely to contribute much to the diet, nutritionally, because the acrid components limit the amounts which may be consumed safely. (Mustard oil blisters the skin.) Nevertheless, the small amounts normally used are helpful in enhancing the taste of food and in stimulating the appetite. The nutrient composition of mustard powder is given in Food Composition Table F-21.

MUTAGENS

Any of a number of chemical compounds capable of inducing mutations (gene changes) in DNA and in living cells. The alkyl mustards, as well as dimethyl sulfate, diethyl sulfate, and ethylmethane sulfonate, comprise a group of alkylating agents, reacting with the nitrogen atoms of guanine (a purine base), a constituent of both RNA and DNA. This reaction affects the guanine molecule in such a way as ultimately to induce a mutation in DNA. Nitrous oxide can deaminate (remove the amino group from) both guanine and cytosine (a pyrimidine base).

Caffeine appears to be a weak mutagen in some nonmammalian systems. But its significance as a mutagen in humans is unknown. It is noteworthy, however, that studies of the caffeine intake of pregnant women have shown no association between caffeine and birth defects.

(Also see NUCLEIC ACIDS.)

MYASTHENIA GRAVIS

An autoimmune disease—failure of the body's immune system to recognize self—in which the body forms antibodies against its own muscle cell membranes. The antibodies attack the muscle cell membranes and destroy their responsiveness to nerve impulses. Nerve impulses fail to reach the muscle and contraction fails. Muscles unable to contract are paralyzed.

The cause of the disease is not known, but it is associated with an enlarged thymus. Myasthenia gravis is characterized by various groups of muscles which become easily fatigued and weakened. Respiratory, neck, tongue, trunk and shoulder muscles are affected. Some drugs are capable of improving muscular functions. Due to the muscles involved, there are some feeding difficulties as swallowing, and coughing; and grasping abilities are impaired.

MYELIN

The white, fatlike substance which forms a sheath around certain nerve fibers.

MYO–

Prefix meaning muscle.

MYOCARDIUM

The heart muscle.

MYOFIBRILS

The hundreds of small contractile units found in each muscle fiber. Myofibrils are composed of the muscle protein filaments, myosin and actin.

MYOGEN

A muscle protein, an albumin, that is found in the cytoplasm of the muscle cell. It is not a protein of the actin and myosin filaments.

MYOGLOBIN

A protein similar to hemoglobin in structure and function, found only in the muscles. Myoglobin receives oxygen from the blood and stores it for use by the muscle cells. It is responsible for the red color of meat.

(Also see HEMOGLOBIN.)

MYOSIN

One of two muscle cell proteins which play an important role in the contraction and elasticity of muscles. The other protein is actin.

(Also see MUSCLES.)

MYSORE FLOUR

This flour was developed in India and used for large-scale feeding trials as a partial substitute for cereals. It is a mixture of 75% tapioca flour and 25% peanut flour.

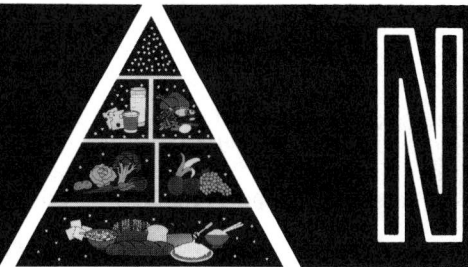

NAILS (FINGERNAILS)

Nails may be a sign of good health or of poor health. In good health, the nails are firm and pink. In poor health, the nails are rigid and brittle. In chronic iron deficiency anemia, the nails may be spoon-shaped (*koilonychia*). Severe protein deficiency may result in transverse white bands in the nails, occurring symmetrically on both hands. In other forms of malnutrition, the nails may be brittle, thickened, or lined on the surface either transversely or longitudinally; but these changes may also be seen in well-nourished people.

(Also see DEFICIENCY DISEASES, Table D-2, Minor Dietary Deficiency Disorders—Nails; and HEALTH, Sections headed ''Signs of Good Health'' and ''Signs of Ill Health.'')

NAPHTHOQUINONE

A derivative of quinone. Some of these derivatives have vitamin K activity.

NARANJILLA *Solanum quitoense*

The fruit of a very large herbaceous plant (of the family *Solanaceae*) that is 6 to 10 ft (*2 to 3 m*) tall and a native of the northern Andes.

Naranjilla fruits are orange-colored, fuzzy tomatolike fruits that have a sour green pulp. They are used mainly to make jam, jelly, juice, and pies.

The pulp of the fruit has a high water (92%) and a low content of calories (28 kcal per 100 g) and carbohydrates (7%). It is a good source of vitamin C.

NATAL PLUM *Carissa grandiflora*

Fruit of a shrub (of the family *Apocynaceae*) that is native to South Africa. Natal plums are pear-shaped and are up to 2 in. (*5 cm*) long. They have a reddish skin and reddish pulp with a white milky latex. The ripe fruits are used for making jellies and sauces. They may also be eaten fresh or stewed.

Natal plums are moderately high in calories (68 kcal per 10 g) and carbohydrates (16%). They are a good source of iron and ascorbic acid.

NATIONAL FLOUR

Presently, this is the name given to 85% extraction wheat flour in the United Kingdom.

NATIONAL RESEARCH COUNCIL (NRC)

A division of the National Academy of Sciences established in 1916 to promote the effective utilization of scientific and technical resources. Periodically, this private, nonprofit organization of scientists publishes bulletins giving nutrient requirements and allowances for man and animals, copies of which are available on a charge basis through the National Academy of Sciences, National Research Council, 2101 Constitution Avenue, N.W., Washington, D.C. 20418.

NATURAL FOODS

Natural foods are those that are grown naturally and subjected to little or no processing. But there is no official definition of a natural food. The Food and Drug Administration's policy on food labeling only prohibits a manufacturer from calling an entire food natural if it contains artificial colors or flavors or any synthetic ingredients.

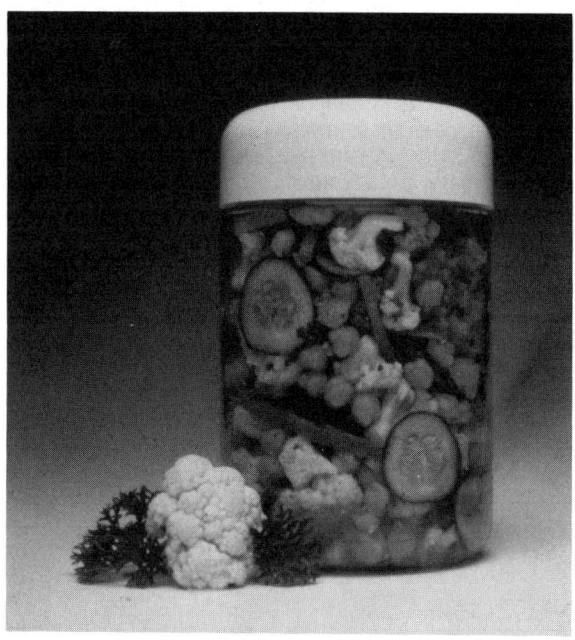

Fig. N-1. Natural foods—foods grown naturally and subjected to little or no processing. (Courtesy, USDA)

Natural food enthusiasts stress nature and the return to a more primitive way of life. Some of these advocates go so far as to suggest that something valuable has been removed from the traditional foods sold in the supermarket; that they are counterfeit, prefabricated, worthless, or devitalized. It is inferred that processing destroys the nutritive value of the food. Such notions have created doubts in the minds of some Americans about the integrity, purity, and nutritive content of the nation's food supply. It is true that modern food refining removes some valuable nutrients from such foods as white flour and wild rice. However, these foods, and many other processed foods, are enriched with minerals and vitamins to make them nutritious.

Usually, natural foods are grown with organic fertilizer and without chemical sprays in a garden, on a tree, or a farm, and just washed, possibly hulled and cracked, or cut before eating raw or cooked. And they contain no chemical additives, such as preservatives, emulsifiers, and antioxidants. Such foods include fresh fruits and vegetables, nuts, seeds, and stone-ground cereals. Honey, brown sugar, and fertile eggs are other foods which natural food enthusiasts consider to have superior power over their actual nutritive content.

The back-to-nature movement popularized granola, a *natural* food that had been around for years. Granola is a heavy, chewy, dry cereal made from such *healthy* ingredients as whole grains, nuts, seeds, raisins, and honey, and often (though not always) without chemical preservatives. The granola labels proclaim *all natural*. To its credit, granola does contain more protein, fiber, vitamins, and minerals than most popular cereals. However, its nutritious aspects may be offset by lots of fats (especially highly saturated coconut oil), and sugars (after all, honey is sugar, natural or not), and calories—four to six times as many calories as the same volume of more traditional cereals.

Some natural food advocates use raw milk, despite the hazard of brucellosis (undulant fever) and tuberculosis—disease-producing organisms that are destroyed by pasteurization. Others consider fish, chicken, and animal flesh as natural foods so long as the animals are grown without the use of commercial feeds, hormones, and antibiotics. Still, others imagine that natural vitamins are superior to synthetic vitamins; despite the fact that a vitamin is a vitamin whatever its source, and that a vitamin has a chemical formula and functions in a certain manner in the body whether it is natural or synthetic.

But the natural food movement has made for nutritional awareness and interest. In this respect, it has succeeded where mothers have failed. Many young people are now eating vegetables and a greater variety of other foods. Also, they are turning away from highly refined foods like candy, soft drinks, and other *empty calories*.

(Also see FOOD MYTHS AND MISINFORMATION; HEALTH FOODS; and ORGANICALLY GROWN FOODS.)

NAUSEA

Sickness at the stomach associated with an urge to vomit.

NECROSIS

Death of a part of the cells making up a living tissue.

NECTAR

The two major nutritional meanings of this term are as follows:

• A syrupy liquid produced by special glands of flowers that is collected by bees and converted by them into honey. The unique flavors of the honeys derived from the different nectars are due mainly to the essential oils and other aromatic substances produced by the flowers.
(Also see HONEY.)

• A pulpy fruit drink made from various combinations of ingredients such as water, fruit puree, fruit pulp, fruit juice, sweetener(s), citric acid, and vitamin C. The minimum amounts of fruit ingredient for each of the types of nectar are specified in the Standards Of Identity which have been established by the FDA. Some of the fruit nectars sold in the United States are apricot, guava, mango, papaya, peach, and pear.
(Also see the articles on the individual fruits for details regarding the various nectars.)

NEONATE

A newborn baby.

NEOPLASM (TUMOR)

A new and abnormal growth—a tumor, which serves no physiological purpose.

NEPHRITIS

Inflammation of the kidneys.
(Also see DISEASES.)

NEPHRON

The structural and functional unit of the kidneys consisting of a tuft of capillaries known as the glomerulus attached to the renal tubule. Urine is formed by filtration of blood in the glomerulus and by the selective reabsorption and secretion of solutes by cells that comprise the walls of the renal tubules. There are aproximately 1 million nephrons in each kidney.
(Also see GLOMERULONEPHRITIS [Nephritis].)

NEPHROSCLEROSIS

Hardening and narrowing of the arteries of the kidneys, a condition usually associated with high blood pressure and arteriosclerosis. Nephrosclerosis causes degeneration of the renal tubules, and fibrosis of the glomeruli, the points where filtration occurs. Its incidence increases with age but it often produces no outward symptoms. It may, however, account for the decrease in kidney reserve noted in the elderly. During its late stages some sodium and protein restrictions may be necessary.

NEPHROSIS

A degenerative kidney disease occurring without signs of inflammation. It may occur as a consequence of acute glomerulonephritis, lupus erythematosus, an allergic reaction, diabetes mellitus, or mercury poisoning. In children it appears for no apparent reason. Clinically, the patient exhibits massive losses of protein in the urine—proteinuria; low blood protein—hypoproteinemia; and water in the tissues of the body—edema. Treatment consists of replacing protein losses with a high protein diet, and controlling the edema with a restricted sodium intake. Possibly diuretics or steroids may also be involved in the treatment. Successful therapy is a long-term process. Full recovery seldom requires less than 2 years.
(Also see MODIFIED DIETS; GLOMERULONEPHRITIS; and LUPUS ERYTHEMATOSUS.)

NEROLI OIL

This is a fragrant essential oil obtained from certain flowers, especially the sour orange, which is used chiefly in perfumes, but which is also used in flavoring foods.
(Also see SEVILLE ORANGE.)

NERVOUS SYSTEM

The entire nerve apparatus of the body consisting of the brain and spinal cord, nerves, ganglia, and parts of the receptor organs that receive and interpret stimuli and transmit impulses to the effector organs.

NERVOUS SYSTEM DISORDERS

These may encompass everything from numbness in a limb to quadraplegia to mental illness, which in itself includes a multitude of disorders.

A variety of interrelationships exist between nutrition and nervous disorders. Among the nutritional factors which may cause or contribute to certain nervous system disorders are: energy, protein, lipid, minerals, and vitamins. Also many toxins have detrimental effects on the nervous system; for example, pesticides, ergot, mycotoxins, polybrominated biphenyls (PBBs), polychlorinated biphenyls (PCBs), neurotoxins, hallucinogens, and cholinesterase inhibitors.

Nutrition and nervous system disorders are further related since nervous disorders often require special dietary adjustments, and may present some feeding difficulties.

(Also see MODIFIED DIETS; MENTAL DEVELOPMENT; and MENTAL ILLNESS.)

NEURITIC

Of, relating to, or affected by neuritis.

NEURITIS

Inflammation of the peripheral nerves—the nerves which link the brain and spinal cord with the muscles, skin, organs, and other parts of the body.

NEUROPATHY

Disease of the nervous system, especially when involving degenerative changes.

NEUTROPENIA

The presence of neutrophile cells (white blood cells which do not stain readily) in abnormally small numbers in the peripheral bloodstream.

NIACIN (NICOTINIC ACID; NICOTINAMIDE)[1]

[1]Niacin has, along the way, been known as vitamin P-P, pellagra-preventive vitamin, vitamin G, vitamin B-3, vitamin B-4, and vitamin B-5.

NIACIN

IT'S ESSENTIAL FOR HUMANS TOO!

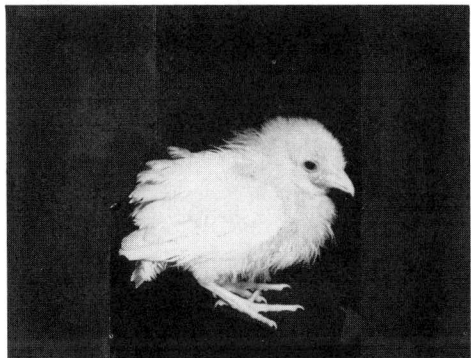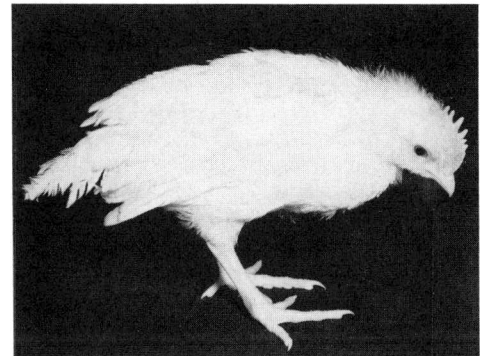

NIACIN MADE THE DIFFERENCE! LEFT: CHICK ON NIACIN-DEFICIENT DIET. NOTE POOR GROWTH AND ABNORMAL FEATHERING. RIGHT: CHICK THAT RECEIVED PLENTY OF NIACIN. (COURTESY,UNIVERSITY OF WISCONSIN)

TOP FOOD SOURCES

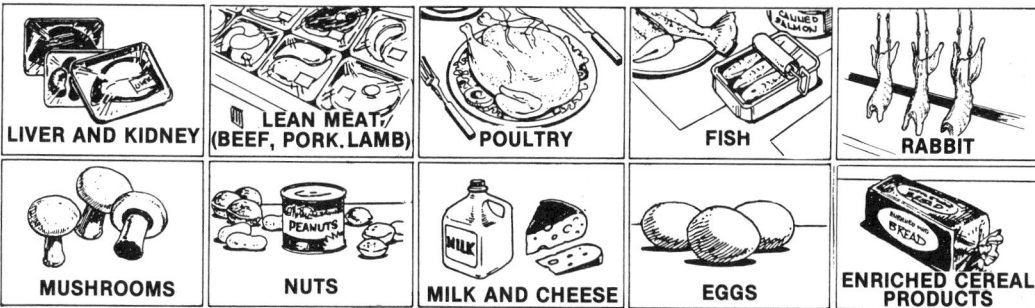

Fig. N-2. Niacin made the difference! *Left:* Chick on niacin-deficient diet. Note poor growth and abnormal feathering. *Right:* Chick that received plenty of niacin. (Courtesy, H.R. Bird, Department of Poultry Science, University of Wisconsin) Note, too, top ten food sources of niacin.

Niacin, a member of the B-complex, is a collective term which includes nicotinic acid and nicotinamide, both natural forms of the vitamin with equal niacin activity. In the body, they are active as nicotinamide adenine dinucleotide (NAD) and nicotinamide adenine dinucleotide phosphate (NADP) and serve as coenzymes, often in partnership with thiamin and riboflavin coenzymes, to produce energy within the cells, precisely when needed and in the amount necessary.

The discovery of the role of niacin as a vitamin of the B group was the result of man's age-old struggle against pellagra. The disease was first described by the physician Gaspar Casal in Spain in 1730, soon after the introduction of corn (maize) into Europe; and it was given the name pellagra (*pelle,* for skin; and *agra,* for sour) by physician Francesco Frapoli in Italy in 1771.

Pellagra spread with the spread and cultivation of corn. In the 19th century, it was common in almost all of the European and African countries bordering on the Mediterranean sea; and it later spread to other African countries. Pellagra had long been present in both North and South America, but it reached epidemic proportions in southern United States after the Civil War, which left poverty in its wake, as a result of which many of the poor subsisted almost entirely on corn. Outbreaks of the disease were so widespread and severe that most physicians considered the cause to be either an infectious agent or a toxic substance present in spoiled corn.

HISTORY. Nicotinic acid was first discovered and named in 1867, when Huber, a German chemist, prepared it from the nicotine of tobacco. But for the next 70 years it remained idle on the chemist's shelves because no one thought of it, even remotely, as a cure for pellagra. In the meantime, thousands of people died from the disease.

Subsequent to 1867, nicotinic acid was *rediscovered* many times as a compound present in foods and tissues. In 1912, Funk, in England, isolated nicotinic acid from rice polishings while attempting to isolate the antiberiberi vitamin; and, that same year, Suzuki, in Japan, isolated nicotinic acid from rice bran. But both researchers lost interest in the acid when they found it ineffective in curing beriberi.

In the early 1900s, pellagra reached epidemic proportions in southern United States, where the diet was based primarily on corn, which is extremely low in both available niacin and in tryptophan. In 1915, 10,000 people died of the disease; and, in 1917-18, there were 200,000 cases of pellagra in this country.

In 1914, the U.S. Public Health Service dispatched a team under the direction of Dr. Joseph Goldberger, a physician-researcher, to study the cause of, and hopefully find a cure for, pellagra. In a series of studies initiated in 1914 and continuing throughout the 1920s, Goldberger proved that the disease was caused by a dietary deficiency, and not an infection or toxin.

In 1925, Goldberger and Tanner classified common foods on the basis of their effectiveness in preventing or curing human pellagra. They studied the effects of supplementing a pellagra-producing diet with certain foods. From these results, (1) they concluded that there is a specific dietary factor of unknown nature present in certain foods, which is involved in preventing and curing pellagra; and (2) they rated foods on their content of this factor as follows: *abundant,* yeast; *good,* lean meat and milk; *fair,* peas and beans (and other vegetables).

In 1926, Goldberger and Wheeler showed that pellagra in man and blacktongue in dogs were similar. Goldberger and his associates observed that in towns where many people suffered from pellagra, a large percentage of the dogs had blacktongue, thereby noting the similarity between pellagra in man and blacktongue in dogs. Further, they confirmed that dogs with blacktongue could be cured by yeast. Goldberger and Wheeler designated this preventive and curative factor, present in certain foods, as P-P (pellagra-preventive); others designated it vitamin G for Goldberger.

In 1935, von Euler, Albers, and Schlenck studied the preparation of cozymase, the coenzyme which is necessary for the alcoholic fermentation of glucose by apozymase, shown later to be diphosphopyridine nucleotide (DPN). On hydrolysis, cozymase yielded nictotinic acid. This was the first evidence that nicotinic acid (in the form of its amide) formed a part of the structure of an enzyme, and placed it among the organic compounds of great importance in biological chemistry.

In 1936, two German scientists, Warburg and Christian, showed that nicotinamide was an essential component of the hydrogen transport system in the form of nicotinamide adenine dinucleotide (NAD).

In 1937, Dr. Conrad Elvehjem, and co-workers, at the University of Wisconsin, discovered that niacin (as either nicotinic acid or nicotinic acid amide, which he isolated from liver) cured blacktongue in dogs, a condition recognized as similar to pellaga in man. Shortly thereafter, several investigators found that niacin was effective in the prevention and treatment of pellagra in humans. Soon, the vitamin became recognized as a dietary essential for man, monkeys, pigs, chickens, and other species.

In 1945, Willard Krehl and his associates at the University of Wisconsin finally solved another mystery in the story of pellagra prevention when they discovered that tryptophan is a precursor of niacin, thereby explaining two things: (1) why milk, which is low in niacin but high in tryptophan, will prevent or cure pellagra; and (2) why, in earlier concepts, protein deficiency was often related to pellagra—for without protein, there could be no tryptophan (the precursor of niacin). Corn is low in tryptophan whereas meat contains both tryptophan and niacin.

In 1971, the name *niacin* was adopted by the American Institute of Nutrition and international agencies for all forms of the vitamin.

It is noteworthy that recent findings indicate that most persons suffering from pellagra have multiple deficiencies—that certain symptoms formerly associated with the disease are not relieved until thiamin and riboflavin are supplied along with niacin.

Today, pellagra is rare in the United States. Even in Latin America and Mexico, where many people eat large amounts of corn, pellagra is seldom seen. This is because of their common practice of soaking the corn in lime, which makes the niacin present in the corn in the bound form (niacytin) more available to the body. This probably explains why Mexicans who eat tortillas are relatively free of pellagra. In making tortillas, the pre-Columbian civilizations of Mexico (Aztec, Mayan, Toltec) devised a procedure to treat corn flour with lime water (alkali) before cooking in order to improve the plastic properties of the dough; and, presumably unbeknown to them, the lime water treatment also freed the niacin from the niacytin and made it fully available to the body tissues.

Africa is the only continent in which pellagra is still a public health problem.

CHEMISTRY, METABOLISM, PROPERTIES. The chemistry, metabolism, and properties of nicotinic acid and nicotinamide follow:

• **Chemistry**—The structure of nicotinic acid and nicotinamide are shown in Fig. N-3.

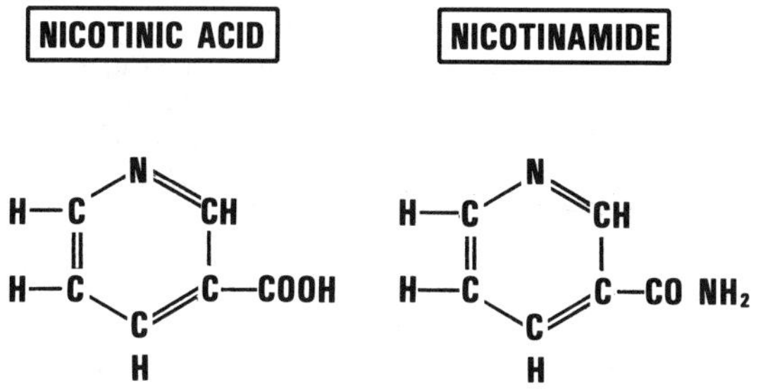

Fig. N-3. The formulas of nicotinic acid and nicotinamide reveal that the compounds are derivatives of pyrimidine.

• **Metabolism**—Niacin is readily absorbed from the small intestine into the portal blood circulation and taken to the liver. There it is converted to the coenzyme nicotinamide adenine dinucleotide (NAD). Also, some NAD is synthesized in the liver from tryptophan. NAD formed in the liver is broken down, releasing nicotinamide, which is excreted into the general circulation. This nicotinamide and the niacin that was not metabolized in the liver are carried in the blood to other body tissues, where they are utilized for the synthesis of niacin-containing coenzymes.

Niacin is found in the body tissues largely as part of two important coenzymes, nicotinamide adenine dinucleotide (NAD) and nicotinamide adenine dinucleotide phosphate (NADP); together, NAD and NADP are known as the pyridine nucleotides. The structure of NAD is given in Fig. N-4.

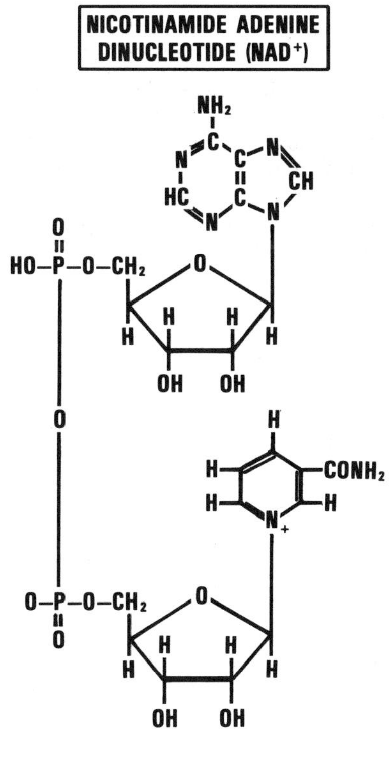

Fig. N-4. Structure of NAD.

NAD is composed of nicotinamide, adenine, two molecules of ribose, and two molecules of phosphate. NADP is similar in structure except it contains three phosphate groups.

Little niacin is stored in the body. Most of the excess is methylated and excreted in the urine, principally as N-methylnicotinamide and N-methyl pyridine (in about equal quantities). Also, small amounts of nicotinic acid and niacinamide are excreted in the urine. With a low niacin intake, there is a low level of metabolite excretion in any form.

• **Properties**—Nicotinic acid appears as colorless needle-like crystals with a bitter taste, whereas nicotinamide is a white powder when crystallized. Both are soluble in water (with the amide being more soluble than the acid form) and are not destroyed by acid, alkali, light, oxidation, or heat.

Nicotinic acid is easily converted to nicotinamide in the body. In large amounts, nicotinic acid acts as a mild vasodilator (as a mild dilator of blood vessels), causing flushing of the face, increased skin temperature, and dizziness. Since nicotinamide does not cause these unpleasant reactions, its use is preferred in therapeutic preparations.

MEASUREMENT/ASSAY. Niacin in foods and niacin requirements are expressed in milligrams of the pure chemical substance.

Chemical and microbiological methods for niacin assay are now generally used rather than animal assays.

The biological vitamin activity of new compounds can be assayed by the curative dog test (blacktongue disease) or by growth test with chicks and rats.

FUNCTIONS. The principal role of niacin is as a constituent of two important hydrogen-transferring coenzymes in the body: nicotinamide adenine dinucleotide (NAD) and nicotinamide adenine dinucleotide phosphate (NADP). These coenzymes function in many important enzyme systems that are necessary for cell respiration. They are involved in the release of energy from carbohydrates, fats, and protein. Along with the thiamin- and riboflavin-containing coenzymes, they serve as hydrogen acceptors and donors in a series of oxidation-reduction reactions that bring about the release of energy (see Fig. N-5).

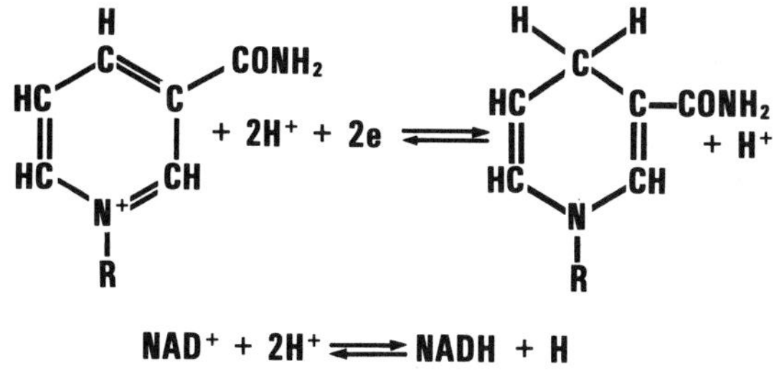

$$NAD^+ + 2H^+ \rightleftharpoons NADH + H$$

Fig. N-5. Hydrogen acceptor function of nicotinamide containing coenzymes. R = adenine dinucleotide (= NAD): = adenine dinucleotide phosphate (= NADP).

Also, NAD and NADP are involved in the synthesis of fatty acids, protein, and DNA. For many of these processes to proceed normally, other B-complex vitamins, including vitamin B-6, pantothenic acid, and biotin, are required.

Niacin also has other functions. It is thought to have a specific effect on growth. Also, there are reports that nicotinic acid (but not nicotinamide) reduces the levels of cholesterol; and that niacin in large doses is slightly beneficial in protecting to some degree against recurrent nonfatal myocardial infarction. However, because of possible undesirable effects, ingestion of large amounts (therapeutic doses) of niacin should be under the direction of a physician.

DEFICIENCY SYMPTOMS. In man, a deficiency of niacin results in pellagra, which generations of medical students have remembered as the disease of the three "Ds"—dermatitis, diarrhea, and dementia (insanity).

The typical features of pellagra are: dermatitis, particularly of areas of skin which are exposed to light or injury; inflammation of mucous membranes including the entire gastrointestinal tract, which results in a red, swollen, sore tongue and mouth, diarrhea, and rectal irritation; and psychic changes, such as irritability, anxiety, depression, and, in advanced cases, delirium, hallucinations, confusion, disorientation, and stupor.

Dogs develop a characteristic black tongue and lesions in the mouth, along with a skin rash, bloody diarrhea, and wasting; followed by eventual death.

(Also see PELLAGRA.)

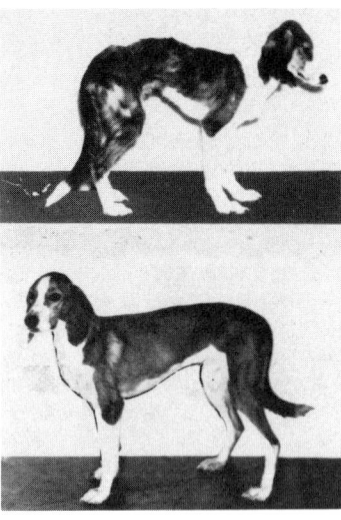

Fig. N-6. Niacin made the difference! *Top*: A dog that had been fed a diet extremely low in niacin. *Bottom*: The same dog after having been fed meat—a good source of niacin—for only 2 weeks. (Courtesy, University of Wisconsin)

RECOMMENDED DAILY ALLOWANCE OF NIACIN. Estimation of niacin requirements are complicated (1) by the fact that some tryptophan is converted to niacin in man, (2) by the paucity of people of different ages receiving diets varying in niacin and tryptophan content, and (3) by the possible unavailablity of niacin in some foods (such as corn).

The Food and Nutrition Board (FNB) of the National Research Council (NRC) recommended daily allowances of niacin are given in the section on VITAMIN(S), Table V-5, Vitamin Table, Niacin. Allowances for niacin are commonly related (1) to energy expenditure, based on the essential role of niacin in energy formation—the involvement of the coenzymes NAD and NADP in the functions of respiratory enzymes; and (2) to protein intake, because (a) a diet that fur-

nishes the recommended allowances of protein usually also provides enough niacin through the conversion of tryptophan to niacin, and (b) protein-rich foods are generally, except for milk, rich in preformed niacin. Hence, the section on VITAMIN(S), Table V-5, Vitamin Table, Niacin, gives niacin equivalent allowances in relation to both calories and protein.

Also in this same table, the recommended dietary allowances of niacin are presented as niacin equivalents (NE), recognizing that the contribution from tryptophan may be variable and unpredictable but may represent a substantial portion of the niacin activity of the diet. In estimating the amount of niacin available from foods, the average value of 60 mg of tryptophan should be considered equivalent to 1 mg of niacin. (See Fig. N-8.)

As with the other B-complex vitamins, the niacin requirements are increased whenever metabolism is accelerated as by fever or by the stress of injury or surgery.

Additional pertinent information relative to Table V-5, Vitamin Table, Niacin, follows:

• **Recommended allowance for infants, children, and adolescents**—Human milk contains approximately 0.17 mg of niacin and 22 mg of tryptophan per 100 ml or 70 Calories (kcal). Milk from a well-nourished mother appears to be adequate to meet the niacin needs of the infant. Therefore, the niacin allowance recommended for infants up to 6 months of age is 7.7 niacin equivalents per 1,000 Calories (kcal), about two-thirds of which will ordinarily come from tryptophan. The niacin allowance for children over 6 months of age and for adolescents is 7.1 niacin equivalents per 1,000 Calories (kcal).

• **Recommended allowance for adults**—The allowance recommended for adults, expressed as niacin equivalents, is 6.6 niacin equivalents per 1,000 Calories (kcal) and not less than 13 niacin equivalents at caloric intakes of less than 2,000 Calories (kcal). This amount provides an allowance for the differences in the contributions from tryptophan and the availability of niacin in diets.

• **Recommended allowances for pregnancy and lactation**—The recommended allowance provides an increase of 2 niacin equivalents daily during pregnancy, based on the recommended increase in energy intake of 300 Calories (kcal) daily.

With a recommended increase of 500 Calories (kcal) to support lactation, an additional intake of 3.3 niacin equivalents would be indicated; hence, a total additional intake of 5 niacin equivalents per day is recommended during lactation.

• **Pharmacological intakes of niacin**—Niacin in large doses has been found to be slightly beneficial in protecting to some degree against recurrent nonfatal myocardial infarction. However, ingestion of large amounts of nicotinic acid (3 g or more daily), *but not of the amide*, may produce vascular dilation, or *flushing*, along with other harmful side effects. So, it is recommended that great care and caution be exercised if this vitamin is to be used for the treatment of individuals with coronary heart disease. Megadoses of niacin should be taken under the supervision of a physician.

• **Niacin intake in average U.S. diet**—Average diets in the United States for women ages 19 to 50 supply 700 mg of tryptophan daily, and for men 19 to 50, 1,100 mg. The corresponding values for preformed niacin are 16 and 24 mg, respectively. Thus, the calculated intakes of total NEs are 27 mg for women and 41 mg for men. Proteins of animal origin (milk, eggs, and meat) contain approximately 1.4% tryptophan; most vegetable proteins contain about 1% tryptophan, whereas corn products contain only 0.6%. Some foodstuffs, such as corn, contain niacin-containing compounds from which the niacin may not be completely available. It has been estimated that the enrichment of cereal products adds about 20% more niacin to the food supply than would be provided if these products were not enriched.

The U.S. Department of Agriculture reports that there are sufficient available food sources in the United States to provide an average consumption of 26 mg of niacin per person per day; with 45% of the total contributed by meat, poultry, and fish, and 31% contributed by flour and cereal products.

TOXICITY.   Only large doses of niacin, sometimes given to an individual with a mental illness, are known to be toxic. However, the ingestion of large amounts of nicotinic acid (2 to 3 g per day) may result in vascular dilation, or *flushing* of the skin, itching, liver damage, elevated blood glucose, elevated blood enzymes, and/or peptic ulcer. So, high doses, which are sometimes prescribed for cardiovascular diseases and other clinical symptoms, should only be taken on the advice of a physician.

NIACIN LOSSES DURING PROCESSING, COOKING, AND STORAGE.
Niacin is the most stable of the B-complex vitamins. It can withstand reasonable periods of heating, cooking, and storage with little loss.

Canning, dehydration, or freezing result in little destruction of the vitamin.

Because niacin is water-soluble, some of it may be lost in cooking, but in a mixed diet usually such losses do not amount to more than 15 to 25%. Using a small amount of cooking water will minimize this loss.

Storage results in little loss. In a study of the niacin content of potatoes stored for 6 months at 40°F (4.4°C), only small losses of niacin were observed.

SOURCES OF NIACIN.
Generally speaking, niacin is found in animal tissues as nicotinamide and in plant tissues as nicotinic acid; both forms of which are of equal niacin activity and commercially available. For pharmaceutical use,

nicotinamide is usually used; for food nutrification (fortification), nicotinic acid is usually used.

As is true of other B vitamins, the niacin content of foods varies widely. A grouping and ranking of foods on the basis of normal niacin content is given in the section on VITAMIN(S), Table V-5, Vitamin Table, Niacin.

Food Composition Table F-21 gives the niacin content of foods. Proteins and Amino Acids in Selected Foods, Table P-16, gives the tryptophan content on a limited number of foods. In the absence of information on the tryptophan content of foods, the following thumb rules for estimating tryptophan content may be used: Proteins of animal origin (milk, eggs, and meat) contain about 1.4% tryptophan, those of vegetable origin about 1.0%, and corn products about 0.6%. An average mixed diet in the United States provides about 1% of protein as tryptophan. Thus, a diet supplying 60 g of protein contains about 600 mg of tryptophan, which will yield about 10 mg of niacin (on the average, 1 mg of niacin is derived from each 60 mg of dietary tryptophan). (See Fig. N-8.)

EXAMPLE OF CALCULATING NIACIN EQUIVALENTS

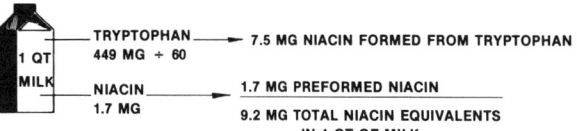

Fig. N-8. How to calculate the niacin equivalents in a quart of milk. A quart of milk containing 449 mg of tryptophan will form 7.5 mg of niacin (449 ÷ 60) from tryptophan. So, this is added to the 1.7 mg of niacin found as such in milk, bringing the total niacin equivalents of milk to 9.2.

Niacin may be present in foods in a *bound* form (i.e., niacytin in corn) which is not absorbable. This is particularly true of corn, wheat, oats, rice, and rye. Yet, pellagra occurs less frequently than one might expect in Mexico, where corn consumption is high. Born of centuries of experience, it is the custom in Mexico to treat corn with limewater before making tortillas, thereby liberating the nicotinic acid. Likewise, the Hopi Indians of Arizona roast sweetcorn in hot ashes, another traditional practice that liberates the nicotinic acid. But the ways of food preparation in Africa do not have this effect.

Coffee is a good source of niacin (a dark roast provides about 3 mg of niacin per cup). In certain areas of the world where the diet of the people is low in niacin and tryptophan, their high consumption of coffee may explain their low incidence of pellagra.

When considering sources of niacin, it should be noted that niacin can be, and is, synthesized by the intestinal flora. However, the amount produced is only of minor importance in the human. By contrast, as with thiamin and riboflavin, ruminants (cattle, sheep, etc.) have no dietary requirements for niacin because of bacterial synthesis in the rumen.

Niacin was one of the original vitamins, along with thiamin and riboflavin, first added to white flour in the United States in 1941; and later to other processed cereal products. Nicotinic acid is the form usually added to foods.

As with most other vitamins, the most inexpensive source of niacin is the synthetic source. Nicotinamide (niacinamide), the form usually taken as a vitamin supplement, is available in most food stores and pharmacies at a very reasonable cost.

Fig. N-7. Poultry, a rich source of niacin. (Courtesy, National Turkey Federation, Reston, Va.)

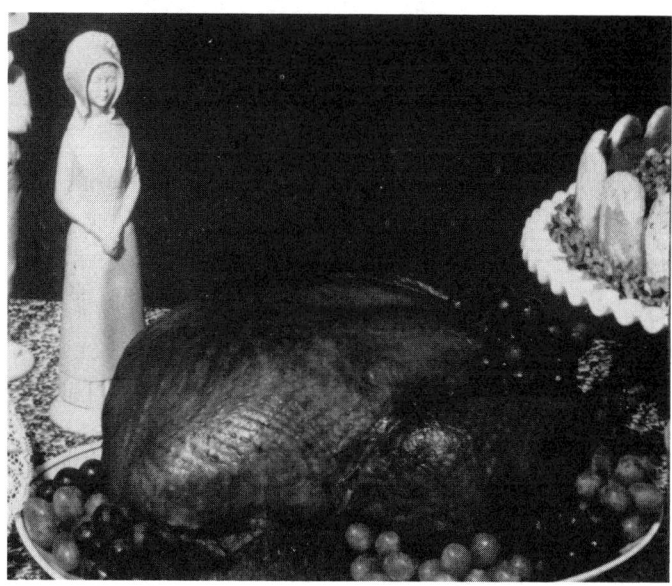

NOTE: When estimating the total amount of niacin suppled in the diet, the tryptophan content of the foods should be considered, also. Note, too, that most foods that are rich in animal protein are also rich in tryptophan.

(Also see VITAMIN[S], Table V-5.)

NIACINAMIDE

The biologically active form of niacin occurring in the tissues.

NIACIN EQUIVALENT (NE)

Because tryptophan is a precursor of niacin and thus an additional source, dietary requirements for niacin are usually given in terms of total niacin or niacin equivalents. Niacin equivalent is the total niacin available from the diet including (1) preformed niacin, plus (2) niacin derived from the metabolism of tryptophan (60 mg tryptophan = 1 mg niacin).

(Also see NIACIN; and VITAMIN(S).)

NICKEL (Ni)

This element, first discovered in 1751 by Cronstedt and named nickel after "Old Nick," a demon, is the same nickel that the U.S. five-cent piece is named after.

In 1970, F.H. Nielsen, of the U.S. Department of Agriculture, reported that chickens deficient in nickel (Ni) developed slightly enlarged hocks, thickened legs, bright orange leg color (instead of pale yellow-brown), a dermatitis, and a less friable liver; deficiency symptoms which were corrected by adding nickel at a level of 3 to 5 mg per kg of diet. Subsequently, deficiencies have also been reported in rats, pigs, and goats, and nickel has been found in a serum protein (called nickeloplasmin) in rabbits and humans.

NICOTINAMIDE

The amide of nicotinic acid. It has niacin (one of the B vitamins) activity as a constituent of two coenzymes.

(Also see NIACIN; and VITAMIN[S].)

NICOTINAMIDE ADENINE DINUCLEO-TIDE (NAD)

A coenzyme formed by the chemical combination of nicotinamide, adenine, ribose and phosphate. Its formation requires the vitamin niacin. In the body it is employed as a hydrogen (electron) acceptor during the oxidation (breakdown) of foods to form energy.

(Also see METABOLISM; and NIACIN.)

NICOTINAMIDE ADENINE DINUCLEO-TIDE PHOSPHATE (NADP)

A coenzyme of niacin with three high-energy phosphate bonds which facilitates oxidation within the cells.

NICOTINIC ACID

Another name for niacin.

(Also see NIACIN; and VITAMIN[S].)

NISIN

A naturally-occurring antibiotic, sometimes found in milk. Many countries use nisin as a food preservative. However, the direct addition of antibiotic to food is not permitted in the United States.

(Also see ANTIBIOTICS.)

NITRATES AND NITRITES

Nitrate refers to the chemical union of one nitrogen (N) and three oxygen (O) atoms, or NO_3, while nitrite refers to the chemical union of one nitrogen (N) and two oxygen (O) atoms, or NO_2. Of prime concern in foods are sodium nitrate (Chile saltpeter), potassium nitrate (saltpeter), sodium nitrite, and potassium nitrite.

OCCURRENCE AND EXPOSURE. Nitrates and nitrites are common chemicals in our environment whether they come from *natural* or *unnatural* sources.

Naturally Occurring. Most green vegetables contain nitrates. The level of nitrates in vegetables depends on (1) species, (2) variety, (3) plant part, (4) stage of plant maturity, (5) soil condition such as deficiencies of potassium, phosphorus, and calcium or excesses of soil nitrogen, and (6) environmental factors such as drought, high temperature, time of day, and shade. Regardless of the variation of nitrate content in plants, vegetables are the major source of nitrate ingestion as Table N-1 shows.

TABLE N-1
ESTIMATED AVERAGE DAILY INGESTION OF NITRATE AND NITRITE PER PERSON IN THE UNITED STATES[1]

Source	Nitrate (NO_3-)	Nitrite (NO_2-)
	(mg)	(mg)
Vegetables	86.1	.20
Cured meats	9.4	2.38
Bread	2.0	.02
Fruits, juices	1.4	.00
Water	.7	.00
Milk and products	.2	.00
Total	99.8	2.60
Saliva[2]	30.0	8.62

[1]*Nitrates: An Environmental Assessment*, 1978, National Academy of Sciences, p. 437, Table 9.1.

[2]Not included in the total since the amount of nitrite produced by bacteria in the mouth depends directly upon the amount of nitrate ingested.

Those vegetables which are most apt to contain high levels of nitrates include beets, spinach, radishes, and lettuce. Despite the shift from manure to chemical fertilizers over the years, the overall average concentration of nitrate in plants has remained unchanged. Other natural sources of nitrate are negligible.

Nitrite occurrence in foods is minimal. Interestingly, a naturally occurring source of nitrites appears to be the saliva.

Food Additives. Both nitrates and nitrites are used as food additives, mainly in meat and meat products, according to the guidelines presented in Table N-2. Their use in meat has been the subject of much publicity, though their use

TABLE N-2
FEDERAL NITRATE AND NITRITE ALLOWANCES IN MEAT

Meat Preparation	Level Allowed	
	Sodium or Potassium Nitrate	Sodium or Potassium Nitrite
Finished product . . .	200 ppm or 91 mg/lb (maximum)	200 ppm or 91 mg/lb (maximum)
Dry cure	3.5 oz/100 lb or 991 mg/lb	1.0 oz/100 lb or 283 mg/lb
Chopped meat	2.75 oz/100 lb or 778 mg/lb	0.25 oz/100 lb or 71 mg/lb

to cure meat is lost in antiquity. The role of nitrates in meats is not clear, though it is believed that they provide a reservoir source of nitrite since microorganisms convert nitrate to nitrite. It is the nitrite which decomposes to nitric oxide, NO, and reacts with heme pigments to form nitrosomyoglobin giving meats their red color. Furthermore, taste panel studies on bacon, ham, hot dogs, and other products have demonstrated that a definite preference is shown for the taste of those products containing nitrites. In addition, nitrites retard rancidity, but more importantly, nitrites inhibit microbial growth, especially *Clostridium botulinum*. Hence, cured meats provide a source of ingested nitrates and nitrites. However, as a source of nitrate, cured meats are minor compared to vegetables. The major dietary source of nitrites is cured meats, but this is small when compared to that produced by the bacteria in the mouth and swallowed with saliva. Currently, there is no other protection from botulism as effective as nitrites. So, for those wishing to eliminate nitrites, possible carcinogens, there is a Catch 22—eliminate the nitrites and increase botulism poisoning, a proven danger.

NOTE: Since 1990, 90% of the cured meat samples have contained less than 50 ppm nitrate; only 0.1% have contained more than 200 ppm.

Other Sources. Aside from very unusual circumstances, other sources of exposure to nitrates and nitrites are relatively minor. Nitrate concentrations in groundwater used for drinking range from several hundred micrograms per liter (1.06 qt) to a few milligrams per liter. Nitrates are generally higher in groundwater than surface water since plants remove nitrates from surface water.

DANGERS OF NITRATES AND NITRITES. Possibly these chemicals may present a hazard to man through two routes. First, under certain circumstances nitrates and nitrites can be directly toxic. Second, nitrates and nitrites contribute to the formation of cancer causing nitrosamine.

Toxicity. Our knowledge of the toxic effects of nitrates and nitrites is derived from its long use in medicine, accidental ingestion, and ingestion by animals. Overall, poisoning by nitrates is uncommon. An accidental ingestion of 8 to 15 g causes severe gastroenteritis, blood in the urine and stool, weakness, collapse, and possibly death. Fortunately, nitrate is rapidly excreted from the adult body in the urine, and the formation of methemoglobin generally is not part of the toxic action of nitrates.

Almost all cases of nitrate-induced methemoglobinemia in the United States have resulted from the ingestion of infant formula made with water from a private well containing an extremely high nitrate level. Overall, it is comforting to note that several hundred million pounds of beets and spinach—nitrate-containing vegetables—are eaten yearly without injury.

The Cancer Question. Without doubt, the greatest concern of people is the involvement of nitrates and nitrites in directly causing cancer, or in indirectly producing compounds known as nitrosamines. Since nitrosamines are definitely accepted as carcinogens in test animals, a majority of the furor around nitrates and nitrites stems from this fact.

It cannot be stated that any human cancer has been positively attributed to nitrosamines. However, some nitrosamines have caused cancer in every laboratory animal species tested.

EXPOSURE TO NITROSAMINES. When nitrosamines are mentioned, foods are the first items which come to mind. However, there are numerous other sources of nitrosamines. Furthermore, people are exposed to such nitrosamines as cosmetics, lotions, and shampoos containing N-nitrosodiethanolamine (NDELA), (the latter is carcinogenic in the rat). Other preformed nitrosamines have been found in tobacco and tobacco smoke. Hence, human exposure can result from breathing or eating preformed nitrosamines, or by applying them to the skin. Foods are not the only source of nitrosamines.

THE FDA AND THE DELANEY CLAUSE. To ban or not to ban the use of nitrates and nitrites in foods is the question. In the summer of 1978, this "fire" received more fuel when a study conducted for the FDA by Dr. Paul Newberne of Massachusetts Institute of Technology (MIT) reported that nitrite alone fed to rats increased the incidence of cancers of the lymphatic system. Immediately, and before the study was properly reviewed, the USDA and the FDA announced they would soon ban nitrites. Tempers flared and pork producers lost money due to the implication of bacon containing a cancer-causing substance. The MIT study has now been reviewed by an independent group, and the research has been shown to be in error. For the time being, the FDA and USDA have backed down from their earlier stand to ban nitrite; they now say that the evidence is insufficient to initiate any action to remove nitrite from foods. However, it is noteworthy that the U.S. Supreme Court has cleared the way for the USDA to approve no-nitrate labels in processed meats, should they wish to do so.

On an individual basis, after carefully considering the issue, it is the old question of benefit versus risk. The risk of botulism in cured meats in the absence of nitrite is both real and dangerous, while the risk of cancer from low levels of nitrosamines and/or nitrites remains uncertain. Thus, the risk of botulism is considered greater than the risk of nitrates, so their use is allowed. Furthermore, no acceptable alternative is as effective as nitrite in preventing botulism. Nevertheless, nitrite should be reduced in all products to the extent protection against botulism is not compromised.

(Also see ADDITIVES; and MEAT[S], section on "Meat Curing.")

NITROGEN (N)

A chemical element essential to life. All plant and animal tissues contain nitrogen. Animals and humans get it from protein foods; plants get it from the soil; and some bacteria get it directly from the air. Nitrogen forms about 80% of the air.

(Also see METABOLISM, section on "Proteins"; and PROTEIN[S].)

NITROGEN BALANCE (Nitrogen Equilibrium)

The nitrogen in the food intake minus the nitrogen in the feces, minus the nitrogen in the urine is the nitrogen balance. Normal adults are in nitrogen balance—intake equals output. Nitrogen is obtained from the proteins we eat.

• **Positive nitrogen balance**—When nitrogen intake exceeds nitrogen output a positive nitrogen balance exists. Such a condition is present in the following physiological states: pregnancy, lactation, recovery from a severe illness, growth, and following the administration of an anabolic steroid such as testosterone. A positive nitrogen balance indicates that new tissue is being built.

• **Negative nitrogen balance (Nitrogen deficit)**—This occurs when nitrogen intake is less than output. Starvation, diabetes mellitus, fever, surgery, burns or shock can all result in a negative nitrogen balance. This is an undesirable state since body protein is being broken down faster than it is being built up.

(Also see PROTEIN[S], section on "Quantity and Quality"; and BIOLOGICAL VALUE [BV] OF PROTEINS.)

NITROGEN-FREE EXTRACT (NFE)

It consists principally of the available carbohydrates—sugars, starches, pentoses, and nonnitrogenous organic acids in any given food. The percentage is determined by subtracting the sum of the percentages of moisture, crude protein, crude fat, crude fiber, and ash from 100. This fraction represents a catchall for the organic compounds for which there is no specific analysis when performing a proximate food analysis.

(Also see ANALYSIS OF FOODS.)

NITROGEN, METABOLIC

That nitrogen which is lost in the urine and feces due to the metabolic processes of the body and not due to that derived from the diet. Metabolic nitrogen consists of digestive enzymes, cells from the lining of the gastrointestinal tract and bacteria.

(Also see NITROGEN BALANCE.)

NITROSAMINES

A whole family of chemical compounds formed when chemicals containing nitrogen dioxide (NO_2)—so called nitrites—react with amine (NH_2) groups of other chemicals. Many nitrosamines are potent carcinogens when tested in animals. Because there are numerous chemicals capable of reacting with nitrite, nitrosamines have been found in the air, water, tobacco smoke, cured meats, cosmetics, pesticides, tanneries, alcoholic beverages, and tire manufacturing plants. It is even possible that they are formed in our body, though this process is not clearly demonstrated. Thus, human exposure may result from several routes. However, very few data are available to make estimates of levels of exposure by each route. Some epidemiological studies have associated increased incidence of human cancer with the presence of nitrosamines in the diet. Direct evidence that nitrosamines are carcinogenic for humans is lacking.

(Also see NITRATES AND NITRITES.)

NITROSOMYOGLOBIN

The chemical responsible for the red color of cured meat. It is formed by the decomposition of nitrites to nitric oxide

(NO) which reacts with the myoglobin of the muscle.

(Also see MEATS, section headed "Meat Curing"; MYOGLOBIN; and NITRATES AND NITRITES.)

NITROUS OXIDE (N_2O)

To most people it is better known as laughing gas, an inhalation anesthetic and analgesic. However, in the food industry it is approved by the FDA as a propellant and aerating agent in certain sprayed foods canned under pressure such as whipped cream or sprayed vegetable fats.

NOCTURIA

Excessive urination at night.

NONESTERIFIED FATTY ACIDS (NEFA)

Those fatty acids which are freed from triglycerides, and released into the blood. Often they are called free fatty acids (FFA).

(Also see FREE FATTY ACIDS; and TRIGLYCERIDES.)

NONHEME

Iron that is not a part of the hemoglobin molecule; a designation for iron in foods of plant origin.

(Also see IRON, section headed "Absorption, Metabolism, Excretion.")

NONPAREILS

Another name for colored sugar crystals used in decorating candies, cakes, or cookies.

NONPROTEIN NITROGEN (NPN)

Nitrogen which comes from other than a protein source but which under certain circumstances may be used by man in the building of body protein. NPN sources include compounds like urea and salts of ammonia. Persons on low protein diets make better use of NPN than those fed adequate or high levels of protein.

(Also see UREA.)

NONVEGAN

A nonvegetarian; a person who includes animal proteins in the diet.

NOURISH

To furnish or sustain with food or other substances necessary for life and growth.

NUCLEIC ACIDS

Nucleic acids were so named because they were originally isolated from cell nuclei. They are the carriers and mediators of genetic information, of which there are two types: *deoxy-*

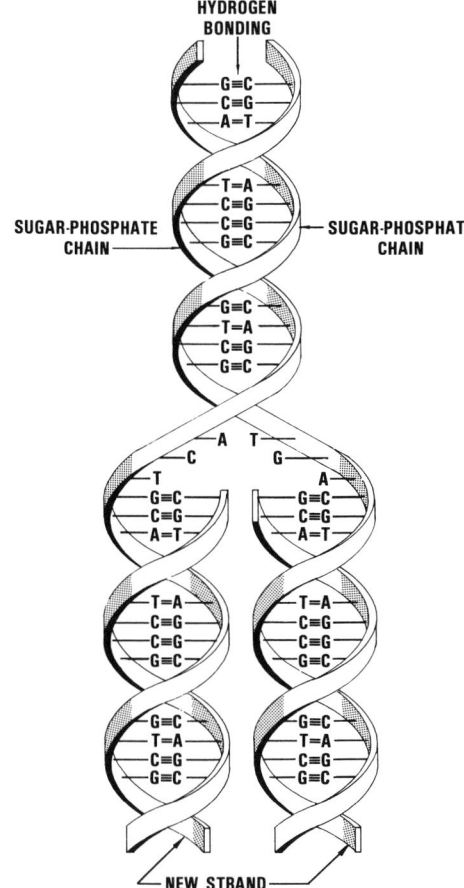

Fig. N-9. The spiral structure of deoxyribonucleic acid, or DNA—the basic building block of life on earth. It's a double helix (a double spiral structure), with the sugar (deoxyribose)-phosphate (phosphoric acid) *backbone* represented by the two spiral ribbons. Connecting the *backbone* are four nitrogenous bases (a base is the nonacid part of a salt): adenine (A) paired with thymine (T), and guanine (G) paired with cytosine (C); with the parallel spiral ribbons held together by hydrogen bonding between these base pairs. Adenine and guanine are purines, while thymine and cytosine are pyrimidines.

ribonucleic acid (DNA) and *ribonucleic acid (RNA)*. The two types of nucleic acids, DNA and RNA, differ in that DNA has one less oxygen molecule (carbon atom number 2) in its component sugar ribose, and is a double strand.

Every cell of the body contains the same amount of DNA with the exception of the sperm and egg cells. It is the DNA of the chromosomes in the nuclei of cells that carries the coded master plans for all of the inherited characteristics—size, shape, and orderly development from conception to birth to death. DNA is different for each species, and even for each individual within a species. These differences consist of minor rearrangements of sequences among the nitrogenous bases, which constitute a code containing all the information on the heritable characteristics of cells, tissues, organs, and individuals.

The messages carried by DNA are put into action in the cells by the other nucleic acid, RNA. To do this, DNA serves as a template (as the pattern or guide) for the formation of RNA. The genetic message is coded by the sequence of purine and pyrimidine bases attached to the *backbone* of the DNA structure—a long chain of the sugar deoxyribose and

phosphoric acid. Purine bases in DNA include adenine and guanine, while pyrimidine bases include cytosine and thymine. One molecule of DNA may contain 500 million bases. The *backbone* of RNA is also a sugar, the sugar ribose, plus phosphoric acid. However, in RNA the pyrimidine base thymine is replaced by uracil, another pyrimidine. RNA molecules are considerably smaller than DNA, containing from less than a hundred to hundreds of bases—not millions.

(Also see METABOLISM, section headed "Proteins.")

SYNTHESIS. Each time a cell divides, a new DNA is made, while within most cells RNA is continually being synthesized and broken down into its components. When the purines and pyrimidines are combined with the sugars ribose or deoxyribose, the resultant compound is referred to as a *nucleoside*. *Nucleotides* are nucleosides that are esterified (acid and alcohol combination) with phosphoric acid. When a series of nucleotides are joined together, nucleic acids are formed. The secret of the code is a process called base pairing.

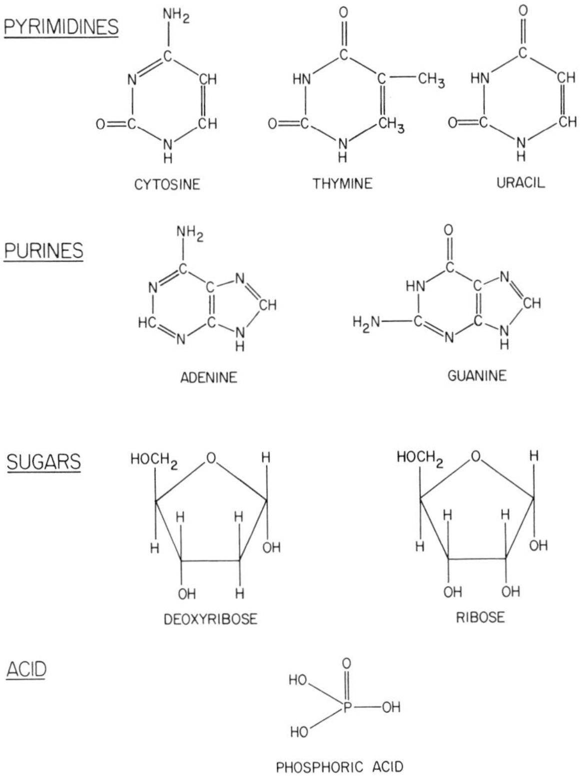

PYRIMIDINES

CYTOSINE   THYMINE   URACIL

PURINES

ADENINE   GUANINE

SUGARS

DEOXYRIBOSE   RIBOSE

ACID

PHOSPHORIC ACID

Fig. N-10. Components of nucleic acids.

During the formation of new DNA or RNA, the same bases always pair off—guanine with cytosine, adenine with thymine, and adenine with uracil in RNA. This ensures that the code is duplicated time and time again. During synthesis, the double helix splits, pulling the base pairs apart. New bases line up with the proper partner and form another sugar-phosphoric acid *backbone* (see Fig. N-9).

Purines, pyrimidines, ribose, and deoxyribose may be synthesized in the body from other compounds, or they may be recycled. Phosphorus, for the formation of phosphoric acid, is a required dietary mineral, and it is employed in a variety of other compounds besides DNA and RNA.

DIGESTION, ABSORPTION, AND METABOLISM.
The enzymes from the pancreas, called nucleases, split the nucleic acids into nucleotides. Then the nucleotides are split into nucleosides and phosphoric acid by other enzymes in the intestine. Finally, the nucleosides are split into their (1) constituent sugars (deoxyribose or ribose), (2) purine bases (adenine and guanine), and (3) pyrimidine bases (cytosine, thymine, and uracil). These bases are then absorbed into the blood via active transport. The sugars are absorbed slowly, and, as far as is known, there is no specific transport mechanism.

Once in the body, the purine and pyrimidine bases may be reused. They are not only used for DNA and RNA but also as components of a variety of coenzymes. If not used, pyrimidines are catabolized to beta-alanine, beta-aminoisobutyric acid, carbon dioxide (CO_2), and ammonia (NH_3), while the purines are converted to uric acid. Ammonia, uric acid, and beta-aminoisobutyric acid are excreted in the urine.

Ribose can be metabolized via the pentose shunt or hexosemonophosphate pathway—the same metabolic pathway that produces ribose.

(Also see METABOLISM.)

FUNCTIONS.
DNA is the component of the chromosomes that carries the blueprint for a species—the heritable characteristics of each cell in the body and its descendants. It functions in the egg and sperm cells to pass the blueprint along from parent to offspring. Messages are relayed from DNA in the nucleus of cells to the cytoplasm by RNA, whereupon the sequences of amino acids in protein synthesis are dictated by the order of the purine and pyrimidine bases transcribed from the DNA. Each cell of the body contains a full genetic blueprint, but only small parts of the genetic message are normally transcribed by RNA for cells to fulfill their role in whatever tissue they are located.

REQUIRED INTAKE.
There is no required level of intake of nucleic acids per se. A nutritious, well-balanced diet provides the precursors necessary for the synthesis of the purines, pyrimidines, and ribose sugar in the body. The only direct requirement is for the mineral phosphorus. Since it is a component of DNA and RNA, it is in every cell of the body. Children and adults require 800 to 1,200 mg daily.

SOURCES.
Since DNA and RNA are components of all cells, any food in which the cells are concentrated is a rich source of nucleic acids. Organ meats such as liver, kidneys, and pancreas are rich sources. Since these meats are rich sources of nucleic acids, it follows that they are rich sources of purines; hence, sufferers of gout are advised to avoid them. Other meats, poultry, and fish, the embryo or germ of grains and legumes, and the growing parts of young plants are good sources of nucleic acids. Butter and other fats, cheese, eggs, fruits, milk, nuts, starch, sugar, and vegetables are low in nucleic acids.

(Also see ARTHRITIS, section headed "Gout [Gouty Arthritis].")

GENETIC ENGINEERING.
The recent development of gene-splicing (also known as recombinant DNA) ushered in a new era of genetic engineering—with all its promise and possible peril. The scientific community is bitterly divided about the unknown risks of "tinkering with life." Proponents of research in DNA are convinced that it can help point the way to new scientific horizons—of understanding and perhaps curing cancer and such inherited diseases as diabetes and hemophilia; of a vastly improved knowledge of the genetics of all plants and animals, including eventually humans. The outcome being the potential of creating new or improved animals and plants, and correcting errors in human genetics. On May 23, 1977, scientists at the University of California-San Francisco reported a major breakthrough as a result of altering genes—turning ordinary bacteria into factories capable of producing insulin, a valuable hormone previously extracted at slaughter from pigs, sheep, and cattle, so essential to the survival of 1.8 million diabetics. The feat opened the door to further genetic engineering or splicing. Already, this genetic wizardry has been used in transplanting into bacteria (and recently into yeast cells) genes responsible for many critical biochemicals in addition to insulin.

Also, the advocates of DNA research argue, recombinant DNA techniques are of enormous help to scientists in mapping the positions of genes and learning their fundamental nature. They also point out that man has been intervening in the natural order for centuries—by breeding animals and hybrid plants, and more recently by the use of antibiotics. On the other hand, the opponents of tinkering with DNA raise the specter (1) of reengineered creatures proving dangerous, and ravaging the earth, and (2) of moral responsibility in removing nature's evolutionary barrier between species that do not mate.

Genetic manipulation to create new forms of life make biologists custodians of a great power. Despite different schools of thought, scare headlines, and political hearings, molecular biologists will continue recombinant DNA studies, with reasonable restraints, and work ceaselessly away at making the world a better place in which to live.

NUCLEOLUS

The nucleus usually contains a distinct body—the nucleolus, which is rich in RNA.

NUCLEOPROTEIN

A compound of one or more proteins and nucleic acid found in the nuclei of cells; found in large amounts in glandular tissue.

NUCLEOTIDES

Hydrolytic products of nucleic acid; they contain a sugar-phosphate component and a purine or pyrimidine base.

NUCLEUS

That part of the cell that contains the chromosomes; it's the control center of the cell, for both chemical reactions and reproduction; it contains large quantities of DNA.

NUTRIENTS: REQUIREMENTS, ALLOWANCES, FUNCTIONS, SOURCES

Nutrients are the chemical substances found in food that can be used, and are necessary for the maintenance, growth, and health of people. There are more than 40 nutrients,

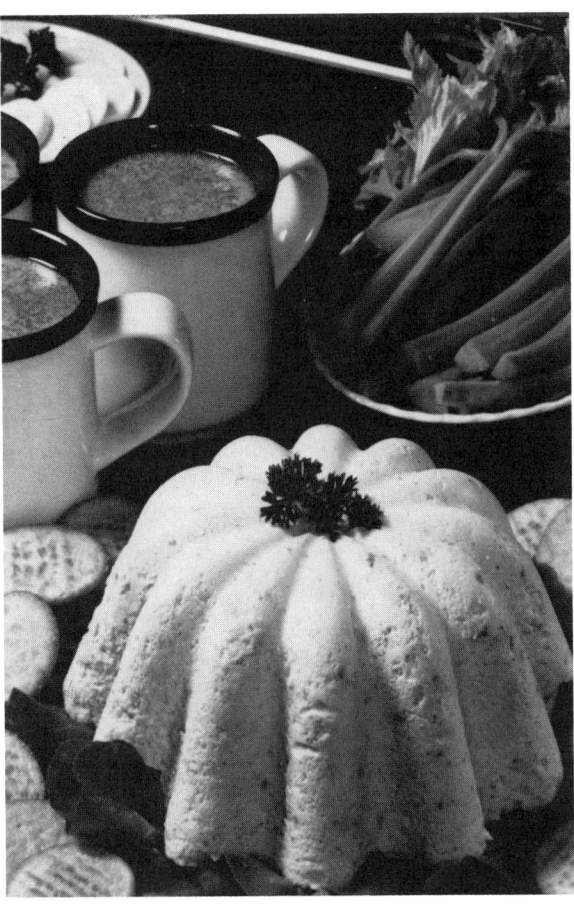

Fig. N-11. Soup in mugs, crackers with cheese spread, and celery sticks provide many nutrients for a luncheon. (Courtesy, Carnation Co., Los Angeles, Calif.)

including minerals, vitamins, and the amino acids from protein. Specific amounts of the nutrients are required, but their intake in the diet is expressed as allowances. Each nutrient from the various food sources reaches the cells of the body where it performs essential functions.

• **Requirements**—Nutrient requirements are the amount of nutrients necessary to meet an individual's minimum needs, without margins of safety, for maintenance, growth, pregnancy, and lactation. To meet nutrient requirements, individuals must receive sufficient food to furnish the necessary quantity of energy, protein, minerals, and vitamins. However, good nutrition is more than just meeting minimal needs.

• **Allowances**—To ensure good nutrition, allowances for the daily intake of nutrients are determined. These allowances provide reasonable margins of safety because of variations in such things as food composition, environment, stress, and individuality. Moreover, the nutritive needs vary according to age, sex, pregnancy, and lactation. Allowances must be determined; otherwise, imbalances may result, excesses may cause toxicity and needless expense, or deficiency diseases may develop. Recommended daily allowances of nutrients for humans are based on the *Recommended Dietary Allowances* compiled by the Committee on Dietary Allowances and the Food and Nutrition Board, National Research Council. The most recent edition

of the *Recommended Dietary Allowances* is the tenth revised edition, 1989, published by the National Research Council, National Academy of Sciences. (See Table N-3.)

• **Functions**—Nutrients perform a variety of specific functions in the body, from providing energy, to becoming tissue components, to acting as cofactors in enzymatic reactions. Altogether, the functions of these nutrients ensure good health as reflected in the general appearance, weight, posture, muscles, nerves, digestive system, heart, lungs, skin, hair, teeth, eyes, nails, and skeleton.

• **Sources**—However, nutrients are more than just chemicals. They are the components of foods, but nutrient distribution in foods is not equal. Some foods may contain virtually no nutrients, while others are good sources of several nutrients. Since there are thousands of foods from which to select, knowledge of foods providing good nutrition becomes very important.

Table N-3 provides summary information relative to the recommended daily allowance of each nutrient, its function in the body, and some of the best foods for obtaining the nutrient. More information about specific nutrients and their food sources may be obtained from individual articles on each nutrient. Also, Food Composition Table F-21 of this book lists complete nutrient composition data for a large number of foods.

(Also see RDA [Recommended Dietary Allowances]; and U.S. Recommended Daily Allowances [U.S.RDA].)

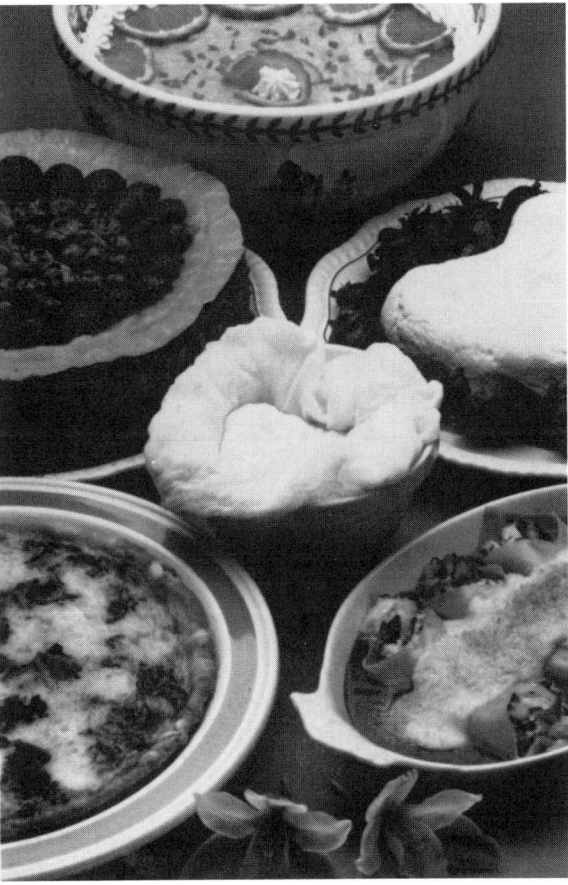

Fig. N-12. Nutrients are more than just chemicals, they are the components of foods. Shown: a variety of good foods. (Courtesy, National Film Board of Canada)

Nutrient	Recommended Daily Dietary Allowances By Age Group																
	Infants		Children			Males					Females						
Years	0–0.5	0.5–1	1–3	4–6	7–10	11–14	15–18	19–24	25–50	50+	11–14	15–18	19–24	25–50	50+	Preg-nant	Lacta-ting
Calories																	
REE ....kcal	320	500	740	950	1130	1440	1760	1780	1800	1530	1310	1370	1350	1380	1280	+300	+300
Energy allowance ....kcal/kg	108	98	102	90	70	55	45	40	37	30	47	40	38	36	30		
Total ....kcal	650	850	1300	1800	2000	2500	3000	2900	2900	2300	2200	2200	2200	2200	1900	2500	2700
Protein ....g	13	14	16	24	28	45	59	58	63	63	46	44	46	50	50	60	65
MACROMINERALS																	
Calcium ....mg	400	600	800	800	800	1200	1200	1200	800	800	1200	1200	1200	800	800	1200	1200
Phosphorus ....mg	300	500	800	800	800	1200	1200	1200	800	800	1200	1200	1200	800	800	1200	1200
Sodium [2] ....mg	120	200	225	300	400	500	500	500	500	500	500	500	500	500	500	500	500
Chloride ....mg	180	300	350	500	600	750	750	750	750	750	750	750	750	750	750	750	750
Magnesium ....mg	40	60	80	120	170	270	400	350	350	350	280	300	280	280	280	320	355
Potassium ....mg	500	700	1000	1400	1600	2000	2000	2000	2000	2000	2000	2000	2000	2000	2000	2000	2000
MICROMINERALS																	
Chromium [2] ....mcg	10–40	20–60	20–80	30–120	50–200	50–200	50–200	50–200	50–200	50–200	50–200	50–200	50–200	50–200	50–200	50–200	50–200
Copper [2] ....mg	.4–.6	.6–.7	.7–1.0	1.0–1.5	1.0–2.0	1.5–2.5	1.5–2.5	1.5–3.0	1.5–3.0	1.5–3.0	1.5–2.5	1.5–2.5	1.5–3.0	1.5–3.0	1.5–3.0	1.5–3.0	1.5–3.0
Fluoride [2] ....mg	.1–.5	.2–1.0	.5–1.5	1.0–2.5	1.5–2.5	1.5–2.5	1.5–2.5	1.5–4.0	1.5–4.0	1.5–4.0	1.5–2.5	1.5–2.5	1.5–4.0	1.5–4.0	1.5–4.0	1.5–4.0	1.5–4.0
Iodine ....mcg	40	50	70	90	120	150	150	150	150	150	150	150	150	150	150	175	200
Iron ....mg	6	10	10	10	12	12	10	10	10	15	15	15	15	15	10	30[3]	15[3]
Manganese [2] ....mg	.3–.6	.6–1	1–1.5	1.5–2	2–3	2–5	2–5	2–5	2–5	2–5	2–5	2–5	2–5	2–5	2–5	2–5	2–5
Molybdenum [2] ......mcg	15–30	20–40	25–50	30–75	50–150	75–250	75–250	75–250	75–250	75–250	75–250	75–250	75–250	75–250	75–250	75–250	75–250
Selenium ....mcg	10	15	20	20	30	40	50	70	70	70	45	50	55	55	55	65	75
Zinc ....mg	5	5	10	10	10	15	15	15	15	15	12	12	12	12	12	15	19
FAT-SOLUBLE VITAMINS																	
Vitamin A ....mcg RE	375	375	400	500	700	1000	1000	1000	1000	1000	800	800	800	800	800	1300	1200
Vitamin D ....mcg	7.5	10	10	10	10	10	10	10	5	5	10	10	10	5	5	10	10
Vitamin E ....mg alpha TE	3	4	6	7	7	10	10	10	10	10	8	8	8	8	8	10	12
Vitamin K ....mcg	5	10	15	20	30	45	65	70	80	80	45	55	60	65	65	65	65

Footnotes at end of table.

N–3
FUNCTIONS, SOURCES[1]

Nutrient	Major Function(s) in the Body	Best Food Source
Calories		
Carbohydrates	Supply food energy; in certain cases, fiber and bulk	Bread and cereal products made from whole grains, starchy vegetables, fruits, and sugars.
Fats	Provide food energy and the essential fatty acid; carrier of fat-soluble vitamins; body structure; and regulatory functions.	Vegetable oils, butter, whole milk and cream, margarine, lard, shortening, salad and cooking oils, nuts, and meat fat
Protein	Formation of new tissues; maintenance, regulatory functions; and provide energy.	Meats, fish, poultry, eggs, cheese, dried beans, soybeans, peas, lentils, nuts, and milk.
MACROMINERALS		
Calcium	Builds and maintains bones and teeth; blood clotting, muscles contraction and relaxation, cell wall permeability; enzyme activation; and nerve transmission.	Milk and milk products, most nuts, dried figs, fish with soft edible bones, and green leafy vegetables.
Phosphorus	Bone formation and maintenance, development of teeth, building muscles, genetic transmission and control of cellular metabolism, maintenance of osmotic and acid-base balance, and important in many metabolic functions.	Milk and milk products, rice bran, rice polish, wheat bran, sunflower seeds, beef, lamb, pork, poultry, liver, fish and seafoods, nuts, and whole grains.
Sodium	Helps maintain balance of water, acids, and bases in fluids outside of cells; a constituent of pancreatic juice, bile, sweat, and tears; associated with muscle contraction and nerve functions; involved in absorption of carbohydrates	Table salt, and most fresh or processed foods other than fresh fruits and vegetables. **NOTE WELL:** Generally, the need is for low-sodium diets, which calls for avoiding high-sodium foods.
Chlorine	Helps regulate osmotic pressure, water balance and acid-base balance; necessary for stomach acid formation and vitamin B-12 and iron absorption.	Table salt and foods containing table salt.
Magnesium	Constituent of bones and teeth; essential element of cellular metabolism; involved in protein metabolism; relaxes nerve impulses.	Nuts, sesame seeds, spices, wheat bran, wheat germ, whole grains, and molasses.
Potassium	Involved in acid-base balance and transfer of nutrients in and out of individual cells; relaxes heart muscle; required for secretion of insulin, phosphorylation of creatin, carbohydrate metabolism, and protein synthesis.	Fruits, molasses, rice bran, sunflower seeds, wheat bran, beef, most raw vegetables, nuts, pork, poultry, and sardines.
MICROMINERALS		
Chromium [2]	Component of the Glucose Tolerance Factor (GTF) which enhances the effect of insulin; enzyme activator; stabilizer of nucleic acids.	Apple peel, banana, beef, beer, blackstrap molasses, bread, brown sugar, butter or margarine, cheese, eggs, flour and whole wheat, liver, oysters, and potatoes.
Copper [2]	Facilitates iron absorption and release from storage; necessary for hemoglobin formation; hair pigmentation, component of important proteins.	Black pepper, blackstrap molasses, cocoa, green olives, liver, nuts and seeds, oysters, soybean flour, and wheat bran and germ.
Fluoride [2]	Necessary for sound bones and teeth.	Dry tea, fluoridated water, and seafoods.
Iodine	Essential component of hormones secreted by the thyroid gland.	Iodized table salt, kelp, seafoods, and vegetables grown on iodine-rich soils.
Iron	Iron (heme) combines with protein (globin) to make hemoglobin for red blood cells. Also, iron is a component of enzymes which are involved in energy metabolism.	Organ meats (liver, kidney, heart) blackstrap molasses, oysters, rice polish, wheat bran, beef, brown sugar, egg yolk, lima beans, nuts, pork, and iron-fortified products.
Manganese [2]	Formation of bone and growth of connective tissues; blood clotting; insulin action; enzyme activation.	Brown rice, legumes, rice bran and polish, spices, and whole grains.
Molybdenum [2]	Component of enzymes which metabolize carbohydrates, fats, proteins, and nucleic acids; component of tooth enamel.	Leafy vegetables, legumes, organ meats (liver, kidney, heart), whole grains, and yeast.
Selenium	Component of the enzyme glutathione peroxidase; interrelated with vitamin E as an antioxidant.	Beer, blackstrap molasses, Brazil nuts, butter, clams, crab, egg, lamb, lobster, mushrooms, oysters, smelt, Swiss chard, turnips, and whole grains
Zinc	Needed for normal skin, bones, and hair; component of many enzymes of energy metabolism and of protein synthesis.	Beef, lamb, liver, oysters, peanuts, pork, poultry, spices, and wheat bran.
FAT-SOLUBLE VITAMINS		
Vitamin A	Necessary for vision in dim light, the growth and repair of certain tissues, and resistance to infection.	Dark-green leafy vegetables, yellow vegetables, yellow fruits, crab, halibut, oysters, salmon, swordfish, butter, cheese, egg yolk, margarine (fortified), and whole milk.
Vitamin D	Essential for the absorption and utilization of calcium in the building of strong bones and teeth.	Fatty fish, liver, egg yolk, cream, butter, cheese, milk fortified with vitamin D. Exposure of the skin to sunlight results in the conversion of provitamin D (converted in the body to vitamin D).
Vitamin E	Serves along with selenium as an antioxidant; protects fatty acids from oxidative destruction.	Wheat germ, salad and cooking oils, margarine, nuts, sunflower seed kernels, beef and organ meats, butter, eggs, green leafy vegetables, oatmeal, and seafoods.
Vitamin K	Necessary for the clotting of the blood.	Green leafy vegetables, green tea, beef liver. Produced by microorganisms in the intestine.

(Continued)

Nutrient	Recommended Daily Dietary Allowances By Age Group																
	Infants		Children			Males					Females						
Years	0–0.5	0.5–1	1–3	4–6	7–10	11–14	15–18	19–24	25–50	50+	11–14	15–18	19–24	25–50	50+	Pregnant	Lactating
WATER-SOLUBLE VITAMINS																	
Biotin [2] ....mcg	10	15	20	25	30	30–100	30–100	30–100	30–100	30–100	30–100	30–100	30–100	30–100	30–100	30–100	30–100
Folate ....mcg	25	35	50	75	100	150	200	200	200	200	150	180	180	180	180	400	280
Niacin ....mg NE	5	6	9	12	13	17	20	19	19	15	15	15	15	15	13	17	20
Pantothenic acid [2] ...mg	2	3	3	3–4	4–5	4–7	4–7	4–7	4–7	4–7	4–7	4–7	4–7	4–7	4–7	4–7	4–7
Riboflavin (vitamin B-2) ....mg	.4	.5	.8	1.0	1.2	1.5	1.8	1.7	1.7	1.4	1.3	1.3	1.3	1.3	1.2	1.6	1.8
Thiamin (vitamin B-1) mg	.3	.4	.7	.9	1.0	1.3	1.5	1.5	1.5	1.2	1.1	1.1	1.1	1.1	1.0	1.5	1.6
Vitamin B-6 (pyridoxine) ....mg	.3	.6	1.0	1.1	1.4	1.7	2.0	2.0	2.0	2.0	1.4	1.5	1.6	1.6	1.6	2.2	2.1
Vitamin B-12 (cobalamins) ....mcg	.3	.5	.7	1.0	1.4	2	2	2	2	2	2	2	2	2	2	2.2	2.6
Vitamin C (ascorbic acid) .....mg	30	35	40	45	45	50	60	60	60	60	50	60	60	60	60	70	95

[1]Compiled from *Recommended Dietary Allowances*, 10th ed., National Academy of Sciences, 1989.

[2]These figures are given in the form of ranges of recommended intakes, since there is insufficient information to determine allowances.

[3]The increased requirement during pregnancy cannot be met by the iron content of habitual American diets nor by the existing iron stores of many women; therefore the use of 30–60 mg of supplemental iron is recommended. Iron needs during lactation are not substantially different from those of nonpregnant women, but continued supplementation of the mother for 2 to 3 months after parturition (birth) is advisable in order to replenish stores depleted by pregnancy.

NUTRITION

Nutrition can be defined as the science of food and its nutrients and their relation to health.

NUTRITIONAL DEFICIENCY DISEASES

Those disorders in normal structure and function of the body resulting from dietary shortages of one or more essential nutrients. They may be prevented or cured by the administration of the missing nutrient(s), except when there is irreparable damage to vital tissues of the body.

(Also see DEFICIENCY DISEASES.)

NUTRITIONAL STATUS

An evaluation or assessment of how well the needs of the body for essential nutrients are being met.

NUTRITIONAL SUPPLEMENTS

A nutritional supplement is any food(s) or nutrient(s), or a mixture of both, used to improve the nutritional value of the diet. Usually, a nutritional supplement consists of minerals, vitamins, and unidentified factor source(s), although it may include protein, one or more amino acids, and other substances.

Clearly, the above definition states that a nutritional supplement is "used to improve." It follows that if the diet is complete and balanced, and not in need of improvement, no supplementation is necessary. Certainly, nutritional supplementation is unnecessary for anyone who always eats a balanced diet consisting of such foods as fresh fruit, fresh vegetables, an animal protein (meat, milk, and/or eggs), whole grain breads and cereals, unroasted nuts, and honey—all produced on unleached, mineral-rich soils; the type of good eating that grandmother served up. But how many people eat such foods regularly today? Also, and most important, there is a wide difference between (1) the amount of a nutrient(s) required to prevent deficiency symptoms, and (2) the amount required for buoyant good health.

N–3 *(Continued)*

Nutrient	Major Function(s) in the Body	Best Food Source
WATER-SOLUBLE VITAMINS		
Biotin [2]	Essential for the metabolism of carbohydrates, fats, and proteins.	Cheese (processed), kidney, liver, most vegetables, eggs, nuts, sardines, salmon, and wheat bran. Also, considerable biotin is synthesized by the microorganisms in the digestive tract.
Folate	Important in metabolism, in cell division and reproduction, and in the formation of heme—the iron-containing protein in hemoglobin.	Liver and kidneys, beans, beets, eggs, fish, green leafy vegetables, nuts, oranges, and whole wheat products.
Niacin	Constituent of coenzymes that function in cell respiration and in the release of energy from carbohydrates, fats, and protein; involved in synthesis of fatty acids, protein, and DNA.	Liver, kidney, lean meats, poultry, fish, rabbit, cornflakes (enriched), nuts, milk, cheese, and eggs.
Pantothenic Acid[2]	Functions as part of two enzymes important in metabolism, nerve impulses, hemoglobin synthesis, synthesis of steroids, maintenance of normal blood sugar, and formation of antibodies.	Organ meats (liver, kidney, heart), wheat bran, rice bran, rice polish, nuts, salmon, eggs, brown rice, and sunflower seeds.
Riboflavin (vitamin B-2)	Essential for metabolism of amino acids, fatty acids, and carbohydrates, accompanied by release of energy; and necessary for formation of niacin from the amino acid tryptophan.	Organ meats (liver, kidney, heart), cheese, eggs, lean meat (beef, pork, lamb), enriched breads, turnip greens, wheat bran, and bacon.
Thiamin (vitamin B-1)	Energy metabolism—without thiamin there could be no energy; needed for conversion of glucose to fats, healthy nerves, normal appetite, muscle tone, and good mental attitude.	Rice bran, wheat germ, rice polish, lean pork, sunflower seeds, nuts, wheat bran, kidney, enriched breads, rye bread, whole wheat bread, and soybean sprouts.
Vitamin B-6 (pyridoxine)	In its coenzyme forms, involved in a number of physiologic functions, particularly (1) protein metabolism, (2) carbohydrate and fat metabolism, and (3) central nervous system disturbances.	Rice polish, rice bran, wheat bran, sunflower seeds, bananas, corn, fish, kidney, liver, lean meat, nuts, poultry, brown rice, and whole grains.
Vitamin B-12 (cobalamins)	Needed for red blood cell production, healthy nerves, and metabolism.	Organ meats, muscle meats, fish, shellfish, egg, cheese. Most plant foods contain little or none of this vitamin.
Vitamin C (ascorbic acid)	Formation and maintenance of collagen; involved in metabolism of amino acids tyrosine and tryptophan, absorption and movement of iron, metabolism of fats and lipids and cholesterol control; and makes for sound teeth and bones, and strong capillary walls and blood vessels.	Citrus fruits, guavas, peppers (green or hot), green leafy vegetables, cantaloupe, papaya, strawberries, and tomatoes.

NUTRITION EDUCATION

Nutrition education is concerned with (1) imparting sound knowledge of how food selection influences the health and well being of the individual, and (2) motivating the individual to use that information in daily living. Nutrition is, amongst other things, a behavioral science. It follows that nutrition education needs to be a practical program with a positive approach based on nutrition science and food composition, along with an understanding of human behavior. Additionally, cognizance should be taken that American consumers want freedom of choice in what they believe and in what they consume. This challenges nutrition educators to present scientifically based nutrition information in such a way that its authenticity is recognized and acted upon.

More people in the United States are malnourished because of nutritional ignorance and misinformation than because of poverty. The explanation is simple: In human folly, facts have never stood in the way of myths and misinformation. Faddism is costly, too. Americans spend more than $10 billion each year on magic to lose weight—more than is spent on research to discover the major causes of diseases that kill. Only a massive program of nutrition education can hope to have any overall effect in raising the quality of diets.

In the developing countries of the world where population growth is resulting in hunger and malnutrition, food production is the first requisite. Nutrition education has little effect where people have neither the food nor the money with which to buy food to quiet their hunger pangs.

NUTRITION EDUCATORS. All consumers, regardless of age, lifestyle, and cultural and socioeconomic background, need nutrition education. To reach everyone will require the enormous team approach of the following:
1. Government agencies.
2. Educational institutions.
3. Professional organizations.
4. Voluntary agencies.
5. Food industries.

Each of the above agencies or groups has its own special resources, facilities, programs, and opportunities to contribute to a national nutrition education program. Pertinent information about each of them follows:

Government Agencies. The golden rule is that "those who have the gold make the rules." It follows that government programs have the greatest impact of any agency or group on foods and nutrition.

The two government agencies having most to do with foods and nutrition issues are the U.S. Department of Agriculture (USDA) and the U.S. Department of Health and Human Services—notably two of its agencies, the Food and Drug Administration (FDA) and The National Institutes of Health (NIH).

The USDA is involved in massive food and nutrition programs, such as the School Lunch Program, the School Breakfast Program, and the Special Milk Program—all for children; the special supplemental food program for Women, Infants, and Children (WIC); and the Food Stamp Programs. These food programs cost more than $21.7 billion in 1990. Additionally, through its Cooperative Extension Programs, the USDA has a vast network of home economists who reach a large segment of the consuming public and have a tradition of success in consumer education programs.

The FDA is charged with protecting the safety of the food supply. Through its dietary guidelines for a variety of food products, and through its regulation of "standards of identity," the FDA can also influence the food supply in very significant ways. More recently, the FDA has become involved in nutrition education efforts through its nutrition labeling program, as a consequence of which more and more foods appearing on supermarket shelves are nutritionally labeled. This program, which represents the first effort in this country to provide nutrition information for consumers, should be augmented with adequate education efforts.

The National Institutes of Health supports nutrition and health research.

A host of other government agencies have an impact, in one way or another, upon the nation's food and nutrition. The Federal Trade Commission regulates food advertising and the application of anti-trust laws. The Office of Education supports educational research.

Also, Congress has become interested and involved in food and nutrition issues. Thus, there are more and more hearings dealing with nutrition topics. The dietary goals prepared by the Senate Select Committee on Nutrition and Human Needs indicate the tremendous impact which Congress can have on nutrition programs of this country.

All of the above comments indicate that the government recognizes that foods and nutrition are clearly linked to health and, as an important factor in the maintenance of health, demand government attention.

(Also see FOOD STAMP PROGRAM; GOVERNMENT FOOD PROGRAMS; HOME ECONOMISTS; SCHOOL LUNCH PROGRAM; U.S. DEPARTMENT OF AGRICUL-TURE; and U.S. DEPARTMENT OF HEALTH AND HUMAN SERVICES.)

Educational Institutions. Teachers (including physical education teachers and coaches, science teachers, and home economics teachers), doctors, nurses, dietitians, and social workers must receive adequate training in nutrition if they are to be competent educators in the area of health protection. Only through adequate training of these key personnel can sound nutrition education be imparted to students, patients, clients, and parents.

There is need for expanded nutrition instruction in higher education. For example, the professional preparation of most elementary school teachers does not include a single course in nutrition. It is noteworthy, however, that several American universities do have excellent postgraduate courses in nutrition.

In medical schools, some nutrition is taught as part of the undergraduate courses in biochemistry, physiology, pharmacology, pathology, internal medicine, pediatrics, obstetrics, surgery, and dentistry. However, there is a scientific core to nutrition which is unlikely to be covered except in one or more basic courses in nutrition. This includes such topics as the assessment of nutritional status, interactions of nutrients with one another and with diseases, recommended intakes of nutrients, food composition, food technology, world food problems, and psychological and sociological aspects of food habits.

Nurses should also have a sound elementary knowledge of nutrition and dietetics because of their responsibility in feeding patients.

Professional Organizations. Professional organizations engaged in human nutrition work need to be active in nutrition education. A number of these organizations are listed in the last section of this article, under the heading "Nutrition Education Sources."

Voluntary Agencies. Nutrition programs at the community level are greatly augmented by voluntary agencies; among them, parent-teachers associations, church organizations, the Salvation Army, children's camps, and day nurseries. Voluntary agencies are supported by private funds, such as the United Fund, foundations, and other means.

Food Industries. Government alone cannot meet the need for nutrition education, nor can a single agency, organization, institution or group accomplish what is needed. The demands are too great.

Some early leaders of our basic food industries perceived that their success depended both on quality of production and on consumers who were well informed about the nutritive value of their products and how to use them. Thus, in the 1920s, organizations came into being which were concerned with production, processing, distribution and household use of specific foodstuffs—organizations that were variously named councils, boards, institutes, or foundations. They were primarily concerned with kinds of food, rather than brand names. Earliest among these organizations were the National Live Stock and Meat Board and the National Dairy Council. Other food industries followed in the ensuing years. The Nutrition Foundation, an organization of many industries, was formed in 1941 and "dedicated to the advancement of nutrition knowledge and its effective application in improving the health and welfare of mankind."

NUTRITION EDUCATION CHANNELS.

NUTRITION EDUCATION CHANNELS. The solution lies in instituting and/or enlarging nutrition education programs through the following channels:

1. Elementary and secondary schools.
2. Doctors, nurses, dietitians, teachers, and social workers.
3. News media and community programs.
4. Food Industries.
5. Regulatory controls.
6. Food Assistance.
7. Books and news media.

Nutrition Education Sources.

Nutrition Education Sources. Sound nutrition information should be disseminated through good books and the news media.

All consumers, and all those who counsel with them—doctors, dentists, nutritionists, health experts, and others in allied fields—should have a book shelf on which good nutrition books are readily available.

Today's superstar M.D. will be tomorrow's mediocre M.D. without a continuing effort to keep abreast of medical progress. There are several ways to do this, but reading good books is one of the best. Look at the books in your doctor's office. Are they new editions, or are they dusty with disuse and tattered with age?

Sound nutrition information should also involve the news media—newspapers, radio, and television. Food advertising, particularly on the television, has a powerful influence on food choices. Many foods are promoted for their convenience and ease of preparation or for their taste, rather than for nutritional value. Although convenience and good taste are important considerations, a balanced presentation should also consider nutritional value.

In addition to good books and the news media, recommended sources of information about foods and nutrition follow:

• **County Agricultural Extension (Farm Advisor)**—Information can be secured from this office in each county.

• **State Universities**—A list of available bulletins and circulars, including information regarding foods and nutrition, can be obtained by writing to (1) the Foods and Nutrition Department, or (2) the Agricultural and Home Economics Extension Service at each State University.

• **U.S. Department of Agriculture, Washington, D.C. 20250**—The following USDA services can be contacted for information:

> Agricultural Research Service
> Consumer and Marketing Service
> Cooperative State Research Service
> Economic Research Service
> Federal Extension Service
> Foreign Agricultural Service
> International Agricultural Development Service
> Office of Communication

• **U.S. Department of Health and Human Services, F St. between 18th & 19th Streets N.W., Washington D.C. 20006**—The following USDHS services (agencies) can be contacted for information:

> Administration on Aging
> Children's Bureau
> Food and Drug Administration, 5600 Fishers Lane, Rockville, MD 20857
> Maternal and Child Health Services

> Office of Education
> Public Health Service
> National Institutes of Health, Bethesda, MD 20205

• **U.S. Department of State—**

Agency for International Development, U.S.A.I.D. Administration, 2401 E. St. N.W., Washington, DC 20523

• **Professional Societies and Voluntary Health Associations—**

American Academy of Pediatrics, P.O. Box 1034, Evanston, IL, 60204

American Council on Science and Health, 1995 Broadway, New York, NY 10023

American Dental Association, 211 E. Chicago Ave., Chicago, IL 60611

American Diabetes Association, 2 Park Ave., New York, NY 10016

American Dietetic Association, 430 North Michigan Ave., Chicago, IL 60611

American Heart Association, 7320 Greenville Ave., Dallas, TX 75231

American Home Economics Association, 2010 Massachusetts Ave. N.W., Washington, DC 20036

American Institute of Nutrition, 9650 Rockville Pike, Bethesda, MD 20814

American Medical Association, Council on Foods and Nutrition, 535 N. Dearborn St., Chicago, IL 60610

Council for Agricultural Science and Technology (CAST), 137 Lynn Ave., Ames, IA 50010–7197

Institute of Food Technologists, Suite 2120, 221 North LaSalle St., Chicago, IL 60601

National Academy of Sciences, National Research Council, 2101 Constitution Ave., Washington, DC 20418

Nutrition Today Society, 703 Giddings Ave., P.O. Box 1829, Annapolis, MD 21404

Society for Nutrition Education, 1736 Franklin St., Oakland, CA 94612

• **Foundations—**

Ford Foundation, 320 East 43rd St., New York, NY 10017–4801

Kellogg Foundation, 400 North Ave., Battle Creek, MI 49017–3398

Medical Education and Research Foundation, 1100 Waterway Blvd., Indianapolis, IN 46202

Vitamin Information Bureau, 612 N. Michigan Ave., Chicago, IL 60611

The Nutrition Foundation, 489 Fifth Ave., New York, NY 10017

Rockefeller Foundation, 1133 Avenue of the Americas, New York, NY 10036

• **Industry-Sponsored Groups—**

American Meat Institute (AMI), 1700 N. Moore St., Suite 1600, Arlington, VA 22209–1995

Cereal Institute, 1111 Plaza Drive, Schaumburg, IL 60195

National Dairy Council, 6300 North River Road, Rosemont, IL 60018

National Live Stock and Meat Board, 444 North Michigan Ave., Chicago, IL 60611

• **International Organizations—**

Food and Agriculture Organization (FAO) of the United Nations, Via delle Terme di Caracalla, 00100 Rome, Italy

League for International Food Education, 1126 Sixteenth St., N.W., Washington, DC 20036

United Nations Children's Fund (UNICEF), 331 East 38th St., New York, NY 10016

United Nations Scientific and Cultural Organization (UNESCO), 7, Place de Fontenoy, 75700 Paris, France

World Health Organization (WHO, Geneva, Switzerland), WHO Publication Centre, 49 Sheridan Ave., Albany, NY 12210

SUMMARY. Food choices are determined primarily by availability, personal and family likes and dislikes, marketing and advertising, and disposable income. There is need that the person who buys and prepares the food should give greater consideration to nutritional need.

Without sacrificing soundness and accuracy in the least, we need to emulate the purveyors of myths and misinformation when it comes to communicating effectively. Through whatever channel—books, news media, lecturers, schools, seminars, counselors—the chosen words and terms should always convey the intended meaning and concept. But a big word should not be used if it can be avoided. Choose words that are clear, specific, and simple, and that come alive. As an illustration, consider the words used by one of the masters of the English language, Sir Winston Churchill. During World War II, Churchill could never have rallied the British people to defend their country if he had called on them for "hemorrhage, perspiration, and lachrymation." Instead, he used the immortal words, "blood, sweat, and tears"—words that continue to live in history.

NUTRITION REVIEWS

This journal is published by the International Life Sciences Institute (formerly known as the Nutrition Foundation, Inc., which was formed in 1941 by the food and allied industries). The Institute's goal is to make essential contributions to the advancement of nutrition knowledge and its effective application, and thus serve the health and welfare of the public. *Nutrition Reviews* contains abstracts of current scientific literature in nutrition. Also, throughout the years, the Institute has published semipopular brochures on current topics in nutrition.

NUTRITIONIST

An individual who is trained in and able to apply a knowledge of foods and their relationship to growth, maintenance, and health. A nutritionist may apply his or her training and knowledge in clinics, consultation, medicine, public health, research, and teaching.

(Also see DIETITIAN and DIETETICS.)

NUTRITIVE RATIO (NR)

The ratio of digestible protein to other digestible nutrients in a food. It is the sum of the digestible protein, fat, and carbohydrate divided by the digestible protein.

NUTS

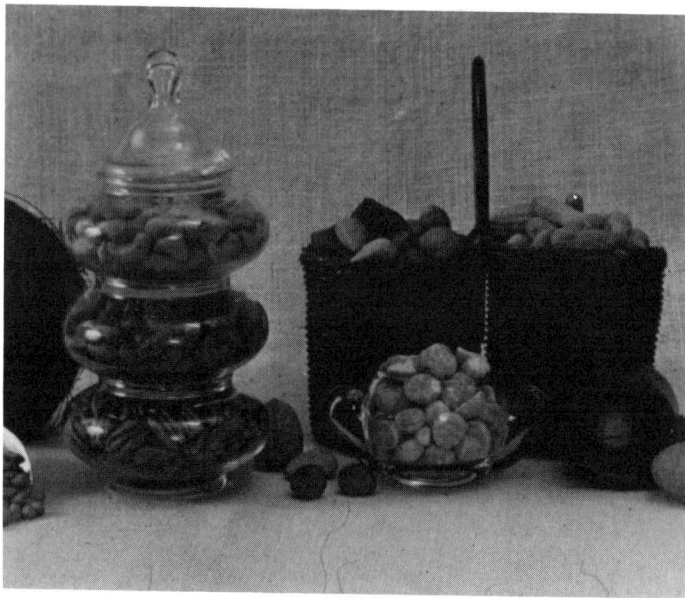

Fig. N-13. Assorted nuts—a good source of copper, zinc, magnesium, and the B-complex vitamins. (Courtesy, USDA)

This name is commonly given to the shell-encased seeds of nonleguminous trees, although various other seeds commonly called nuts may not grow on trees, and may even be legumes. (The peanut is the seed from a leguminous plant.)

ORIGIN AND HISTORY Archaeological evidence indicates that between 20,000 B.C. and 10,000 B.C. various nomadic peoples around the world began to form permanent settlements in certain areas where wild animals and plants were abundant. However, the numbers of large wild game species dwindled as the human populations grew. As a result, the settlers in the temperate regions came to depend upon small game and wild grains, legumes, and nuts to meet the greater part of their food requirements. Nuts could be handled and stored almost as well as cereal grains and legume seeds.

Soon after 10,000 B.C., some of the settlements began to cultivate the plants they favored. By Biblical times, almonds, pistachio nuts, and walnuts were grown in southwestern Asia; and cashew nuts and peanuts were grown in South America. The early agriculturalists experimented with various ways of processing nuts, which eventually resulted in the production of such items as *milks*, oils, and nut powders. The North American Indians made milks from hickory nuts and pecans; the southeastern Asians made milk from coconuts; and the Middle Eastern peoples made milks from almonds and walnuts. Similarly, oils were obtained from almonds, coconuts, and walnuts. Finally, the use of almond and pistachio nut powders in a variety of dishes appears to have been passed along by the Persians to the Arabs, who, in turn, spread the practice westward throughout the Mediterranean, and eastward to India. Today, food technologists are striving to perfect modern day counterparts of the nut products prepared by these ancient peoples.

The first Spanish explorers to reach the Americas found peanuts growing on some of the Carribean islands, to which they had apparently been brought by earlier migrations of South American Indians. These nuts were taken to Africa, where they soon became an important crop.

Through the years, several species of nuts have been improved by selection and breeding, and subjected to complex cultural systems. Today, most marketed nuts come from cultivated nut trees. But Brazil nuts are still produced only by wild trees, and wild trees contribute to the production of many other species, such as the pecan and filbert.

WORLD AND U.S. PRODUCTION. World nut production is small compared to grain, oilseed, and legume production.

Fig. N-14 shows the leading nut crops of the world, and the annual production of each. Fig. N-15 shows the leading nut crops of the United States, and the annual production of each.

WORLD NUT PRODUCTION

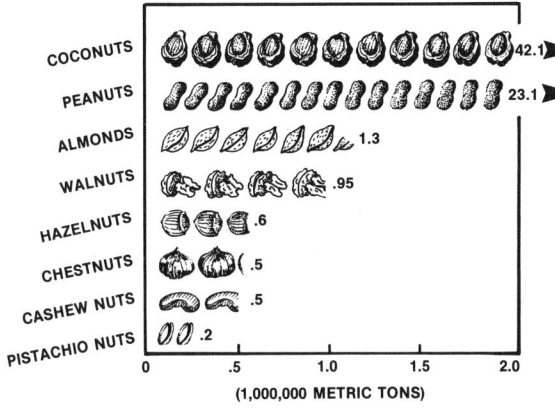

Fig. N-14. The world production of the leading nut crops. (Source: *FAO Production Yearbook 1990*, FAO/UN, Rome, Italy, Vol. 44)

Fig. N-14 shows that coconuts and peanuts are by far the most important nut crops of the world. Together, they account for about 94% of the world nut production. This situation prevails because coconut and peanut oils are among the leading ingredients of margarines and shortenings.

The production of nuts in the United States represents only a small fraction of the world production of these crops, except in the case of almonds, where the United States contributes almost one-fourth of the world's production.

U.S. NUT PRODUCTION

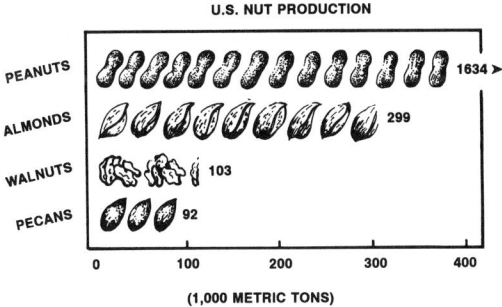

Fig. N-15. The U.S. production of nut crops. (Source: *FAO Production Yearbook 1990*, FAO/UN, Rome, Italy, Vol. 44, and *Agricultural Statistics 1991*, USDA, p. 221)

Fig. N-15 shows that the peanut crop accounts for most (about 68%) of the nut production in the United States. It is noteworthy that the per capita consumption of peanuts in the United States is the highest in the world.

PROCESSING. Following harvesting, nuts must be shelled. Also, green nuts contain 50% or more of water when harvested; hence, they must be cured or semidried for proper storage. Certain types of nut meats are often

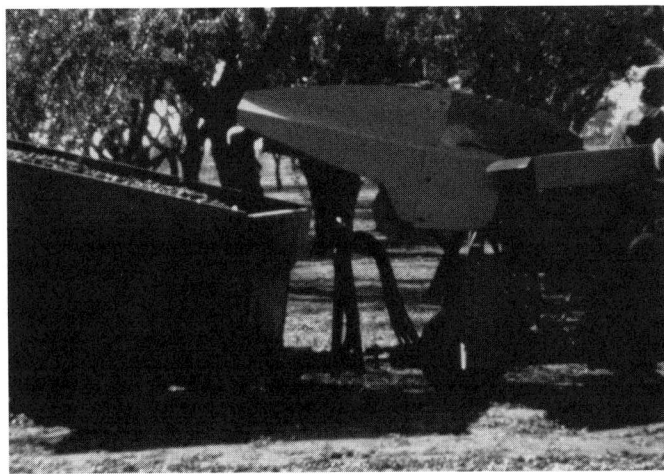

Fig. N-16. Harvesting almonds. (Courtesy, Anderson/Miller & Hubbard Consumer Services, San Francisco, Calif.)

roasted and salted, while others are packed without processing. The most common types of packaging are plastic bags, glass jars, and metal cans. However, some nuts are still sold unpacked or loose from bins or cannisters.

NUTRITIVE VALUES. The Food Composition Table F-21 gives the nutrient composition of some of the commonly used nuts and nut products.

A few pertinent points concerning the nutritive value of nuts follow:

1. Most nuts contain about 500 or more Calories (kcal) per 100 g portion (140 or more kcal per oz) due to their high fat content.

2. The protein content of nuts is about the same as that of legumes (close to 20%, on the average), except that the protein-to-calorie ratio for most nuts (about 4 g of protein per 100 kcal) is only two-thirds of that for legumes.

3. Defatted products, such as almond meal and peanut flour, are much better sources of protein (they contain 40% or more) and substantially lower in calories than nondefatted products.

4. Nuts contain only one-quarter to one-third as much carbohydrate as grains and legumes. Hence, nuts may be useful for low-carbohydrate diets.

5. Almonds, Brazil nuts, and filberts are moderately good sources of calcium (100 g furnish from ⅕ to ¼ of the Recommended Dietary Allowance [RDA] for adults). Almost all nuts furnish at least ⅓ of the RDA for phosphorus, and are fair to good sources of iron.

6. Nuts are also good sources of the B-complex vitamins, as indicated by the values for thiamin, riboflavin, and niacin. However, roasting destroys much of the thiamin. Nuts also furnish biotin, pantothenic acid, vitamin B-6, and vitamin E.

7. Nuts are good sources of (a) magnesium, a macromineral that activates enzymes and aids functioning of nerves and muscles, (b) zinc, a component of various enzymes, and (c) copper, the mineral that functions in enzyme actions, hair growth and pigmentation, connective tissue development, and red blood cell formation.

Details regarding some of the nutritive values not indicated in Food Composition Table F-21 are discussed in the sections that follow.

Fatty Acid Content. The fats in all of the common edible nuts, with the exception of coconuts, contain 77% or more of unsaturated fatty acids. Coconut fat contains over 90% saturated fatty acids. Table N-4 lists the unsaturated and polyunsaturated fatty acid content, as well as the content of the essential fatty acid linoleic acid, in some common nuts.

TABLE N-4
FATTY ACID CONTENT OF SOME COMMON NUTS[1]

Nut	Saturated Fatty Acids	Polyun-saturated Fatty Acids	Linoleic Acid
	(g/100 g)	(g/100 g)	(g/100 g)
Almond	4.3	10.5	9.9
Brazil nut	17.4	25.7	25.4
Cashew	9.2	7.7	7.3
Coconut	31.2	.8	.7
Filbert (hazelnut)	4.6	6.9	6.6
Hickory nut	6.0	12.7	12.0
Peanut	8.6	13.3	13.3
Pecan	6.1	18.3	17.0
Pistachio	7.4	7.3	6.8
Walnut, black	5.1	40.9	36.8
Walnut, English	6.9	42.0	34.9

[1]Data from Table F-4, Fats and Fatty Acids in Selected Foods.

All of the nuts in Table N-4, except almonds, cashews, coconuts, filberts, and pistachios contain liberal amounts of linoleic acid—the essential polyunsaturated fatty acid. One ounce (*28 g*) of peanuts, Brazil nuts, or English walnuts provides about 4, 7, and 10 g of linoleic acid, respectively. Therefore, it may be better to rely on nuts rather than vegetable oils to supply the essential fatty acid linoleic acid because the nuts also furnish protein, minerals, and certain vitamins that are not supplied by the oils. Shelled nuts, like vegetable oils, should be kept refrigerated to prevent them from becoming rancid.

(Also see FATS AND OTHER LIPIDS.)

Protein Quantity and Quality. Like legumes, nuts contain about twice as much protein as the common cereal grains, and have amino acid patterns that generally complement those of the cereals. However, nuts contain less of the amino acid lysine than legumes. Hence, the age-old practice of combining nut milks with cooked cereals made a lot of sense when animal protein was scarce. The American version of these complementary protein mixtures is peanut butter sandwiches, which children should eat with milk to offset the mild deficiency of lysine in the sandwich.

(Also see PROTEIN[S], section headed "Sources.")

Minerals and Vitamins. In addition to the minerals listed in Food Composition Table F-21, nuts are also good sources of (1) chromium, a micromineral which renders insulin more effective in promoting the passage of nutrients into cells; (2) manganese, an element required for growth of bones and other connective tissues, insulin action, blood clotting, and enzyme actions in many aspects of metabolism; and (3) selenium, which is present in an enzyme that detoxifies dangerous peroxides formed during metabolism. In general, nuts contain from 1 to 7 times the amounts of these minerals present in the other types of fresh, minimally processed natural foods.

Nuts also supply choline, a vitaminlike factor required for the transport of fats from the liver. Normally, the body synthesizes choline, but sometimes the amounts may be insufficient to meet its needs.

In general, the nutritive values of nuts are sufficient to enable people to live healthfully on them (provided that 12 to 16 oz [*340 to 454 g*] are consumed daily), plus some fruits and/or vegetables to supply the missing vitamin A and vitamin C. However, the prices of nuts have recently become so high that it is now more economical to eat dietary combinations of animal foods, cereals, and legumes instead of nuts. Also, the other foods are lower in calories. Therefore, it seems that with the exception of a few undeveloped areas blessed with an abundance of wild nut trees, most people of modest means will have to settle for using nuts as occasional snacks and garnishes for dishes based mainly upon other foods.

NUTS OF THE WORLD. Each type of nut tree (or vine in the case of peanuts) originated in an area with a particular climate and certain soil condition. Also, the growing conditions, harvesting, and processing for the market may vary for each species, as may the most important food uses.

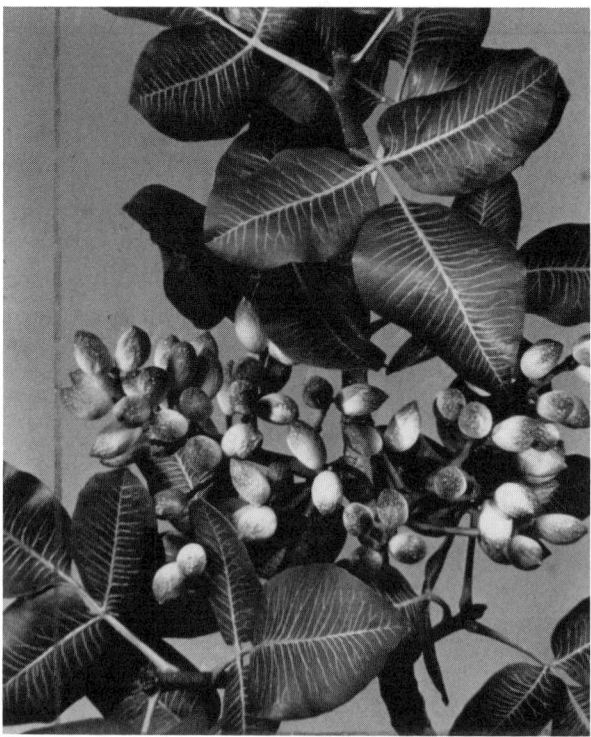

Fig. N-17. Pistachio nuts. (Courtesy, Field Museum of Natural History, Chicago, Ill.)

Finally, nutritive values vary over a spectrum ranging from fair to excellent with regard to the major nutrients. Information on these aspects is given in summary form in Table N-5. Additionally, the most important U.S. nuts—almonds, coconut, peanuts, pecans, and walnuts—are accorded narrative status in this book.

NOTE WELL: Where production figures are given in Table N-5, column 2 under "Importance," unless otherwise stated, they are based on 1990 data. Most world figures are from *FAO Production Yearbook 1990*, FAO/UN, Rome, Italy, Vol. 44. Most U.S. figures are from *Agricultural Statistics 1991*, USDA. Annual production fluctuates as a result of weather and profitability of the crop.

TABLE N-5
NUTS OF THE WORLD

Popular Name; Source; Scientific Name; Origin and History	Importance; Principal Areas; Growing Conditions	Processing; Preparation; Uses	Nutritive Value[1]
Almond (See ALMONDS.)			
Brazil Nut **Source:** The seed of the Brazil nut tree. **Scientific Name of the Brazil Nut Tree:** Family: *Lecythidaceae* Genus: *Bertholletia* Species: *B. excelsa* **Origin and History:** Originated in the Amazon valley in northern Brazil, the only region where it now grows.	**Importance:** An important native food in the areas where it is grown. Also, from 30,000 to 40,000 metric tons are exported to the U.S. and Europe. **Principal Areas:** The Amazon valley in Brazil. **Growing Conditions:** Grows wild in the forests of the Amazon valley. Little attempt is made to cultivate Brazil nut trees in their native area, and outside the Amazon valley they have survived poorly.	**Processing:** The nut-bearing fruits are allowed to fall to the ground when ripe. Then, the tough fruit capsules are cracked open and 15 to 30 nuts are removed. The hard shells may either be removed or left on the nuts prior to shipping and marketing. **Preparation:** No treatment is required for the shelled nuts. Sometimes, the kernels are crushed and oil is extracted. **Uses:** Snacks, ingredient of baked goods, confections, and nut mixtures. The oil may be used in salads.	Brazil nuts are similar in nutritive value to almonds, except that they contain more calories, essential fatty acids, phosphorus, and thiamin. Also, they contain less calcium, iron, magnesium, riboflavin, and niacin. The shelled nuts should be refrigerated or at least kept under cool conditions because their high oil content makes them very susceptible to rancidity. A 3½ oz (*100 g*) portion of Brazil nuts furnishes 715 kcal (204 kcal per oz).
Cashew Nut **Source:** The seed adhering to the cashew fruit. **Scientific Name of the Cashew Tree:** Family: *Anacardiaceae* Genus: *Anacardium* Species: *A. occidentale* **Origin and History:** Native to the West Indies and to Central and South America. Introduced into India and Africa by the Portuguese.	**Importance:** The fifth leading nut crop in the world, with an annual production of about 478,832 metric tons. **Principal Areas:** India, Brazil, Nigeria, Mozambique, and Tanzania. **Growing Conditions:** Dry, tropical climate. Well adapted to poor soils and sandy soils.	**Processing:** Nuts are allowed to fall to the ground. The shell around the nuts contains a caustic oil that blisters the hands. Hence, the shell oil is often extracted with solvents or by roasting or steaming after the nuts have been dried in the sun, cleaned, moistened, and allowed to stand in heaps. Then, the nuts are cracked and the kernels removed, after which the adhering skin is removed from the kernel. **Preparation:** Cashew nut kernels are usually consumed raw or after roasting and salting. **Uses:** Nut kernels are used as snacks, and as ingredients of baked goods and confections. Shell oil is used as a food and as a flavoring.	Cashew nuts are similar in nutritive value to almonds, except that they contain more thiamin. Also, they contain a little less energy (calories), protein, phosphorus, and iron; and much less essential fatty acids, calcium, riboflavin, and niacin. Oleic acid accounts for about 90% of the unsaturated fatty acids, and linoleic only 10%. Hence, cashew nuts are less likely to grow rancid than some of the other nuts which are much richer in linoleic acid. A 3½ oz (*100 g*) portion of cashew nuts contains 596 kcal (170 kcal per oz).
Chestnut **Source:** The seed of the chestnut tree. **Scientific Name of the Chestnut Tree:** Family: *Fagaceae* Genus: *Castanea* Species: *C. crenata* (Japanese), *C. dentala* (N. American), *C. mollissima* (Chinese), *C. sativa* (European) **Origin and History:** Different species native to each of 4 areas: Europe, Africa, Asia, and U.S.	**Importance:** The sixth leading nut crop in the world, with an annual production of about 488,161 metric tons. **Principal Areas:** China, South Korea, Italy, Japan, and Spain. **Growing Conditions:** Mild, temperate climate with few frosty nights. Does best on well drained soils. The N. American chestnut is the hardiest of the varieties, but it was practically wiped out by chestnut blight. Hence, hybrids of the American and Oriental chestnuts are now being grown.	**Processing:** The fallen burrs are gathered and the chestnuts removed. After roasting, the nuts may be left whole or ground into flour. **Preparation:** Roasting, boiling, making into a puree, grinding into a flour, preserving with sugar or syrup. **Uses:** Snacks; ingredients of confections, desserts, fritters, porridges, soups, stews, and stuffings.	Dried chestnuts differ greatly from all the other nuts in that they contain considerably more carbohydrate (3 to 4 times as much), and only fractions of the protein (about ⅓) and fat (about 1/15) content. Also, they furnish little more than ½ the calories of other nuts. The overall nutrient composition of chestnuts is quite close to that of dry cereal products made from corn or rice. A 3½ oz (*100 g*) portion of dried chestnuts contains 377 kcal (107 kcal per oz).
Coconut (coconut palm) (See COCONUT.)			
Hazelnuts (Filberts) **Source:** The seed of the hazel or filbert tree. **Scientific Names of the Filbert and Hazel Trees:** Family: *Betulaceae* Genus: *Corylus* Species: *C. maxima* (Filbert), *C. avellana* (Hazel) **Origin and History:** Various species are native to Europe, Asia, and N. America.	**Importance:** The seventh leading nut crop in the world, with an annual production of over 561,000 metric tons. **Principal Areas:** Turkey, Italy, and Spain. In the U.S., most commercial growing of filberts is in Oregon, Washington, and California. **Growing Conditions:** Moist, temperate climate. The filbert tree is usually larger and more hardy than the hazel tree.	**Processing:** Fallen nuts are gathered by hand and by mechanical sweepers. After shelling, the nuts may be dried and/or the oil extracted. **Preparation:** No treatment is required for shelled nuts. **Uses:** Snacks; ingredients of chocolates and other confections, and desserts. Filbert oil is used in the manufacture of cosmetics and perfumes.	Filberts are similar in nutritive value to almonds, except that they furnish more calories, fat, and thiamin; but less protein (only ⅔ as much), calcium, phosphorus, iron, and niacin. A 3½ oz (*100 g*) portion of filberts supplies 700 kcal (200 kcal per oz).

Footnote at end of table

(Continued)

TABLE N-5 *(Continued)*

Popular Name; Source; Scientific Name; Origin and History	Importance; Principal Areas; Growing Conditions	Processing; Preparation; Uses	Nutritive Value[1]
Macadamia Nut **Source:** The seed of the macadamia tree. **Scientific Name of the Macadamia Tree:** Family: *Proteaceae* Genus: *Macadamia* Species: *M. ternifolia* **Origin and History:** Native to Australia. Brought to Hawaii, where it has prospered.	**Importance:** One of the leading orchard crops of the Hawaiian Islands, where about 18,210 short tons are produced annually. **Principal Areas:** Australia and Hawaii. **Growing Conditions:** Moist semitropical climate. Does best on well-drained soils.	**Processing:** Fallen nuts are gathered and the outer husk is removed by a special machine. The unshelled nuts can be stored safely in a dry environment. Shelling is done by a cracking machine after the nuts have been air dried to a low moisture content. The shelled nuts are fried in deep fat, then salted and packaged. **Preparation:** No treatment is needed for packaged nuts. **Uses:** Snacks; ingredients of cakes, candy, and ice cream.	Macadamia nuts are very high in fat (75%), but low in protein (8%), calcium, phosphorus, iron, and the B vitamin complex. A 3½ oz (*100 g*) portion furnishes 776 kcal (259 kcal per oz).
Peanut (See LEGUMES, Table L-2, Legumes of the World; and PEANUTS.)			
Pecan (See PECAN.)			
Pine Nut (Pinon Nut) **Source:** The seeds of various species of pine trees. **Scientific Names of the Nut-bearing Pine Trees:** Family: *Pinaceae* Genus: *Pinus* Species: *P. cembra* (Swiss stone pine), *P. cembroides* (Mexican nut pine), *P. edulis* (pinon pine of southwestern U.S), and *P. pinea* (stone pine of the Mediterranean) **Origin and History:** Trees are native to the areas noted under Species.	**Importance:** Little of the crop enters the nut trade. The annual production in northern Mexico and southwestern U.S. averages 3,000 or more metric tons. **Principal Areas:** Northern Mexico, southwestern U.S., Europe, and Asia. **Growing Conditions:** Varies according to species. Generally, the nut-bearing species grow wild in the temperate zones of the Northern Hemisphere. The nut pines of N. America are adapted to an arid climate.	**Processing:** Most harvesting consists of picking the cones from the trees before the cone scales separate. Then, the cones are dried to free the nuts. Machines are used to shell the nuts. (American Indians gathered fallen nuts and cracked them with hand tools.) Some species require roasting to remove a turpentine flavor. **Preparation:** No further treatment is required for commercially processed nuts, but unprocessed items may require roasting. **Uses:** Snacks; ingredient of baked goods, confections, desserts, and vegetarian dishes.	The European types (generally called pignolias) are richer in protein (31%) but lower in carbohydrates (12%) than the American types (pinon nuts) which contain 13% protein and 20% carbohydrates. Compared to almonds, pinon nuts are richer in phosphorus, iron, and the vitamin B complex, but lower in calcium. All types of pine nuts contain fats that are highly susceptible to rancidity. Hence, they should be stored in a refrigerator. A 3½ oz (*100 g*) portion of pignolia nuts supplies 630 kcal (180 kcal per oz), whereas the same amount of pinon nuts furnishes 593 kcal (169 kcal per oz).
Pistachio Nut **Source:** The seed of the pistachio tree. **Scientific Name of the Pistachio Tree:** Family: *Anacardiaceae* Genus: *Pistacia* Species: *P. vera* **Origin and History:** Native to western Asia. Recently introduced to the central valley of California.	**Importance:** The eighth leading nut crop in the world, with an annual production of about 220,490 metric tons. **Principal Areas:** Iran, U.S., Turkey, Syria. **Growing Conditions:** Temperate to subtropical climate. Requires well-drained soils, and thrives on sandy loams. Tolerates drought well, and often grows wild on dry wastelands.	**Processing:** The nuts are harvested by picking the clusters or by beating them from the trees onto cloths. They may be husked immediately or after drying in the sun followed by soaking in water. Some of the nuts are roasted and salted in brine while in the shell, while others are cracked and the shells removed. **Preparation:** None required. **Uses:** Snacks; ingredient of confections, desserts, and ice cream.	Pistachio nuts are very similar in nutritional value to almonds, except that they are richer in iron and thiamin, and lower in calcium and niacin. A 3½ oz (*100 g*) portion contains 635 kcal (181 kcal per oz).
Walnut, English (See WALNUT.)			

[1]Additional details on the nutritive values are given in the Food Composition Table F-21, Table P-16 Proteins and Amino Acids in Selected Foods, and Table F-4, Fats and Fatty Acids in Selected Foods.

NYCTALOPIA

The medical term for night blindness.
(Also see NIGHT BLINDNESS.)

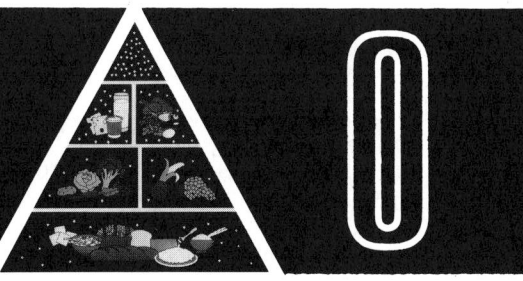

OATS *Avena sativa*

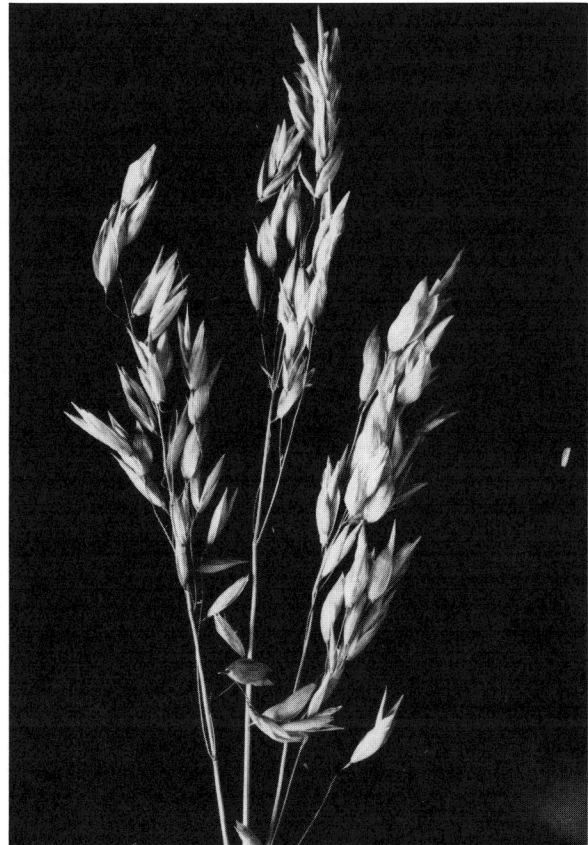

Fig. O-1. Oat panicles with many branches and spikelets. Note the loose-fitting hulls surrounding the grain, which are inedible by humans and must be removed when oats are processed for food. (Photo by J.C. Allen & Sons, West Lafayette, Ind.)

ORIGIN AND HISTORY. Oats, one of the most important food crops in the world, belong to the grass family, *Gramineae*, the same family as wheat, corn, rice, barley, and rye. Most cultivated oats have been developed from the genus *Avena*, species *A. sativa*.

Oats are grown in most temperate countries of the world for food for humans and livestock. They are believed to have developed from wild stocks that first grew in Asia. As a cultivated crop, oats were substantially later in origin than wheat. Not until about 2,000 years ago, at the beginning of the Christian era, are references to oats as a cultivated crop found in the literature. Early use of oats appears to have been medicinal, rather than as a food crop.

WORLD AND U.S. PRODUCTION. In 1990, 44 million metric tons of oats were produced in the world, almost exclusively in temperate North America and Europe. Oats rank sixth among the cereal grains, but account for only 2.2% of the total cereal grain produced globally. The ten leading oat-producing countries of the world by rank are: The Soviet Union, United States, Canada, Germany, Poland, Finland, Sweden, Australia, France, and Argentina.[1]

The United States produced 357,000,000 bushels of oats in 1990; and the ten leading oat-producing states, by rank, were: South Dakota, Minnesota, Wisconsin, Iowa, North Dakota, Ohio, Pennsylvania, Nebraska, Michigan, and Illinois.[2]

In the United States, oats rank fifth as a cereal crop in tonnage produced, being exceeded only by corn, wheat, grain sorghum, and barley.

PROCESSING OATS.

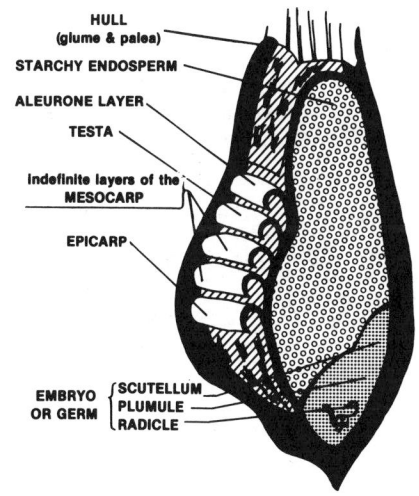

Fig. O-2. Covered kernel (caropsis) of oats.

---

[1]Based on data from *FAO Production Yearbook 1990*, FAO/UN, Rome, Italy, Vol. 44, p. 22. **Note well:** Annual production fluctuates as a result of weather and profitability of the crop.

[2]Based on data from *Agricultural Statistics 1991*, USDA, p. 41, Table, 51. **Note well:** Annual production fluctuates as a result of weather and profitability of the crop.

Only about 15% of the U.S. oat crop is processed for food.

The oat kernel has a fibrous hull, which is inedible by humans. So, the goal in milling oats is to obtain the maximum yield of clean, uniform, sound, whole oat kernels which are free from hulls, floury material, extraneous matter, and undesirable flavors. The hulls range from 21 to 43%, with an average of 25%.

The milling of oats involves the following steps:

1. **Cleaning.** Foreign material and oats not suitable for milling are first removed.

2. **Drying and roasting.** The grain is subjected to heat and the moisture is reduced to somewhere between 7 and 8½%. This process develops flavor, improves keeping quality, and facilitates the subsequent separation of the hull from the groats.

3. **Cooling.** After drying, the oats are cooled by air circulation.

4. **Hulling.** The hulling machine separates the groat kernel from the surrounding hull. The following products are obtained from the hullers: hulls, groats, broken groats and meal, flour, and unhulled oats. These materials are separated by air aspiration and screening. The choicest, plumpest groats are used to make package-grade rolled oats, while the less choice groats make either bulk or feed rolled oats. The broken kernels are used as livestock feed.

5. **Cutting.** The purpose of cutting is to convert groats to uniform granules.

6. **Flaking.** The granules are flaked between rolls to produce a quick-cooking breakfast cereal.

NUTRITIONAL VALUE OF OATS.
The nutrient composition of oats and oat products is given in Food Composition Table F-21.

A few salient points regarding the nutritional value of oats follow:

1. Oat cereals are palatable, rich in carbohydrates (starch), a good source of thiamin and vitamin E, but deficient in minerals, especially calcium.

2. Oat groats contain more protein than wheat. The protein is not of the glutenin type; hence, oat flour is not suitable as the sole flour for breads. However, it may be used for cakes, biscuits, and breakfast foods.

3. Oats lack protein quantity and quality. While dry oatmeal is about 14% protein, cooked oatmeal is only about 2% protein. Moreover, it is deficient in the essential amino acid lysine.

4. The oat grain very closely resembles a kernel of wheat in structure. Unlike wheat, however, the nutritious bran and germ are not removed in the normal processing because oats are not refined. The most important nutritional advantage of oats is the soluble fiber which helps to lower the cholesterol in the blood. Oat bran is a major source of this fiber.

When oats are processed, the hull is removed, leaving the whole grain. After further processing, the whole grain oat will become rolled, steelcut, or instant oats. The outer covering of the whole grain oat is bran. In the production of oat bran, however, the bran plus 3 to 4 layers of cells called aleurone layers are included in the final product.

(Also see CEREAL GRAINS and PROTEIN[S].)

OAT PRODUCTS AND USES.
The products from the milling of oats are: oat hulls, oat groats, steel-cut oats, oatmeal, rolled oats, oat flakes, oat flour, and the feed by-products.

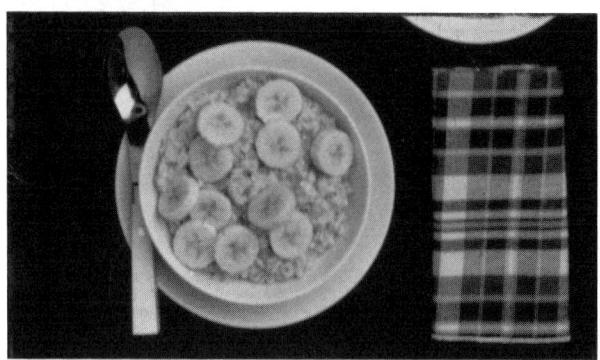

Fig. O-3. Many a school child has been raised on a breakfast of hot oatmeal porridge. (Courtesy, USDA)

Table O-1 presents in summary form the story of oat products and uses for human food.

(Also see BREAKFAST CEREAL[S]; CEREAL GRAINS; and FLOURS, Table F-13, Special Flours.)

TABLE O-1
OAT PRODUCTS AND USES FOR HUMAN FOOD

Product	Description	Uses	Comments
Oat flakes	The product made from the whole groats through (1) by-passing the cutting system, and (2) subjecting the whole kernel to steaming and flaking to a slightly greater thickness than regular rolled oats.	Porridge	This product is sometimes referred to as *old fashioned* or *5-minute* oat flakes.
Oat flour	The product produced by grinding and screening the oat flakes from the rolls.	As an antioxidant, as a constituent of baby foods, and in soaps and cosmetic preparations.	The antioxidant property of oat flour is due to the presence of caffeic acid derivatives which act as strong antioxidants. This explains why properly processed oatmeal is extremely stable and can be maintained in good quality in closed containers for many years.
Oatmeal	Uniform granules of a mealy texture, with a minimum of fine granules and flour.	Porridge	The decline in the consumption of oatmeal porridge is attributable to the greater convenience and speed of ready-cooked breakfast cereal. Oatmeal is made by subjecting groats to cutters, which convert them to uniform granules.
Rolled oats	The product resulting from rolling the groats after treating them with live steam, then passing the flakes through separators to remove all the fine material.	Breakfast foods, cookies, and breads. Granola (homemade or commercially prepared), eaten either— 1. As a ready-to-eat breakfast cereal; or 2. As a snack	Rolled oats and oatmeal contain about 1,850 calories (kcal) per lb (4,079 calories [kcal] per kg); hence, they are excellent food for the winter diet. Granola is a mixture of rolled oats, honey, vegetable oil, chopped nuts, shredded coconut, sunflower seeds, raisins, chopped dates, cinnamon, vanilla, and/or other ingredients. The raw granola is usually heated in an oven until crisp and slightly browned.

OATCAKES

These are thin, flat cakes made by mixing oatmeal with either water, milk, or sour milk, then cooked on a griddle.

OBESE

Overweight due to a surplus of body fat.
(Also see OBESITY.)

OBESITY

This term means an excess of body fat beyond that needed for optimal maintenance of body functions. Obesity is *not* synonymous with overweight because (1) a person may have an optimal body weight, yet have an excess of fat and less than the normal amount of lean (non-fat) tissue; or (2) some overweight people may have above average amounts of bone and muscle, but only normal amounts of body fat.

Some of our leading medical people consider obesity to be the most widespread nutritional disorder in the United States.[3] An estimated 100 million Americans are obese. In 1990, Americans spent an estimated $33 billion on diets and diet-related products. Statistics gathered by life insurance companies show that obese people are more likely to develop degenerative diseases and die early. However, these statistics have limited value when applied to the U.S. population at large because (1) they are based upon the characteristics of people who purchased life insurance policies; (2) the distinction between obesity and overweight is not made, since no measurements of fatness, other than body weight, are made; (3) the high sickness and death rates

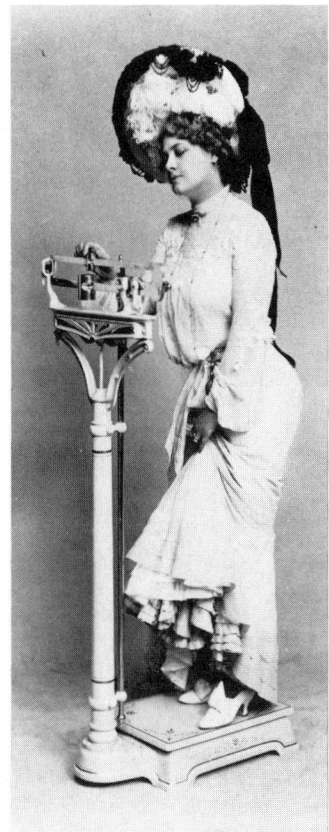

Fig. O-4. Down through the ages, people have been concerned with their weight. (Courtesy, The Bettmann Archive, Inc.)

of overweight people who have diseases that are aggravated by the gaining of weight, such as diabetes, heart disease, high blood fats, and high blood pressure, tend to distort the overall rates for overweight people who have none of these disorders, because unhealthy people are not considered separately from healthy people; and (4) the ranges of desirable weights for small, medium, and large frames were established arbitrarily, with no attempts to define criteria for assigning people to the appropriate categories.

In spite of the great uncertainty as to what constitutes the *ideal* weight for any particular person, the attainment of such a weight has long been promoted as a goal for those who wish to remain in good health. Some doctors devote their entire medical practice to the treatment of obesity. Also, great amounts of money are now being made by manufacturers of such items as dietetic foods, exercise devices, jogging attire, liquid and powdered formulas for losing weight, *rainbow* pills (mixtures of drugs for losing weight), and special suits which cause loss of weight by inducing a heavy loss of water as sweat.

TYPES OF OBESITY. Although all fat people may look alike to the untrained observer, there seems to be considerable variation in the physiological characteristics of obese people, judging from the many recent reports on this subject. Studies of the development of obesity in both animals and man have shown that there are two major types of obesity: early-onset and late-onset.[4] Descriptions follow:

[3]Sebrel, W. H., Jr., "Changing Concept of Malnutrition," *The American Journal of Clinical Nutrition*, Vol. 20, p. 653.

[4]Winick, M., "Childhood Obesity," *Nutrition Today*, Vol. 9, May/June 1974, p. 6.

• **Early-onset obesity**—This type is characterized by an abnormally large number of fat cells because it originates in childhood while the cells in the fatty tissues are still dividing. Early-onset obesity is often accompanied by extra nonfat tissue because the dietary, hereditary, and hormonal factors which spur the proliferation of fat cells also stimulate extra growth of bone and muscle.

• **Late-onset obesity**—This type, in contrast to early-onset type, is characterized by enlargement of normal numbers of fat cells because it usually begins after the division of cells in the tissues has ceased. Sometimes, adult obesity may be distinguished from that which began in childhood because the former is characterized by proportionately greater deposits of excess fat on the trunk of the body than on the arms and legs. Those who first became obese in adulthood are usually more successful in achieving long-term control of their body weight.

CAUSES OF OBESITY.   There are many different opinions as to the cause(s) of obesity. The simplest concept is that it is almost always due to a combination of overeating and underactivity. Hence, there tends to be an attitude of moral superiority in some people who flaunt their leanness at those who are obese. However, there may be many other reasons for obesity and leanness. Some of the current ideas on this subject follow:

Hereditary and Acquired Traits.   Each newborn baby has unique features which are determined mainly by heredity. However, the eventual development of the baby into a fat or lean adult depends upon a combination of both hereditary and environmental factors. Some well-known anthropologists, physicians, and psychologists believe that tendencies toward fatness or leanness may depend somewhat upon body build and other traits. Explanations follow.

BODY BUILDS (Somatotypes).   Dr. Sheldon, an American physical anthropologist, and his co-workers have described the temperaments they observed to be associated with each of three types of physique: ectomorph, mesomorph, and endomorph.[5] These types are shown in Fig. O-5.

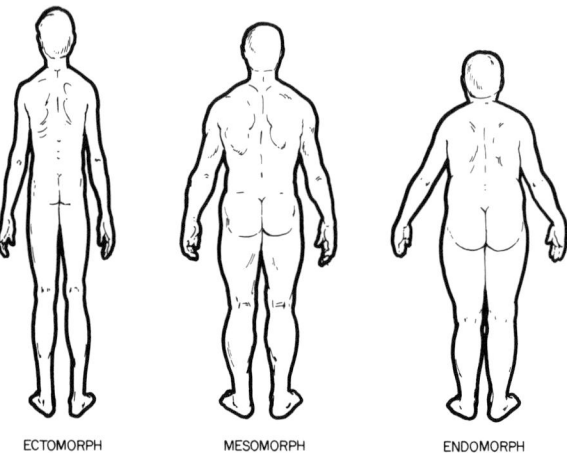

| ECTOMORPH | MESOMORPH | ENDOMORPH |

Fig. O-5. Sheldon's three extreme types of body build.

Details follow:

• **Ectomorph**—This type of physique is tall and slender with long arms and legs, but the trunk is short compared to the rest of the body. The personality of the person who has such a physique is generally of the introvert type. Most of the introvert's drive originates from within, so he or she works well alone, and with minimal supervision. Ectomorphs are often characterized by other people as ambitious and persevering, but also as somewhat inhibited and tense. Statistics which have been compiled by life insurance companies show that people with this physique live the longest. Hence, the tables of ideal weights for various heights tend to be closer to those of ectomorphs than to those of endomorphs or mesomorphs.

• **Mesomorph**—This body build has traditionally been viewed as the epitome of masculinity, although some women may also have this physique yet be truly feminine in every respect. It is characterized by an athletic build with good proportions between the arms, legs, and trunk. Usually, the chest is more prominent than the abdomen. Mesomorphs are rarely extreme extroverts or extreme introverts, but they are energetic and perform well in such team sports as football and hockey. Although life insurance statistics suggest that mesomorphs do not usually live as long as ectomorphs in sedentary, urban societies, it might be possible for people with this body build to live longer than expected by regularly engaging in strenuous physical activities. For example, a study of San Francisco longshoremen showed that those who consistently performed the heaviest work in loading cargo had only about ½ the death rate and ⅓ the sudden death rate as those who did lighter loading work.[6]

• **Endomorph**—People with this body build usually have large abdomens, long trunks, but short arms and legs. They are closest in personality to the extrovert type. In contrast to the introvert, the extrovert's drive depends mainly upon stimulation by such external factors as good food, interaction with other people, and a comfortable environment. Others often see endomorphs as good natured, pleasure loving, talkative, and on the lazy side. Extroverts sometimes have difficulty working alone. Many endomorphs may appear to be obese, but this designation may often be made without taking into consideration their marked differences in body build from the ectomorphic physique.

DIFFERENCES IN THE UTILIZATION OF FOOD ENERGY.
It has long been known that energy production by the body is stepped up after a meal has been consumed. The extra energy is usually lost from the body in the form of heat. *Hence, this effect of eating food is called thermo-genesis (heat production) or specific dynamic action (SDA).* Thermogenesis is taken into consideration in caloric allowances since they are usually increased by 10% after the energy costs of (1) basal metabolism, and (2) the daily activities have been estimated. However, the amount of extra heat production after meals varies considerably for different people, depending upon circumstances such as those which follow:

[5]Sheldon, W. H., and S. S. Stevens, *The Varieties of Temperament,* Harper and Row, New York, N.Y.

[6]Paffenbarger, R. S., Jr., and W. E. Hale, "Work Activity and Coronary Heart Mortality," *New England Journal of Medicine,* Vol. 292, 1975, p. 545.

• **Degree of fatness or leanness**—Certain obese patients had lower metabolic rates after eating, whereas thin patients had a rise in heat production in response to the test meal.[7] These results suggest there may be great differences in the efficiency with which various people utilize food energy, and that the obese may be able to maintain their body weights on below average caloric intakes.

• **Level of physical activity**—Subjects who exercised before and after a high calorie breakfast lost twice as much heat after eating as those who did not exercise.[8]

Hence, exercising before and after meals may result in a greater expenditure of calories than performance of the same amount of exercise at other times.

• **Prior level of dietary calories**—People who have long tried to lose weight by dieting sometimes find it difficult, if not impossible, to maintain a steady pattern of weight loss after having had some initial success in this regard. A study showed that about one-third of a group of women who had participated in weight control groups for 6 months or more could not lose weight on a diet containing 1,350 Calories (kcal).[9] Generally, the women who failed to lose weight had subnormal basal metabolic rates and low total energy expenditures. It was suspected that the low basal metabolism was an adaptation to the long use of low calorie diets.

• **Cellular metabolism**—Not all fat people are guilty of gluttony and sloth. On this point increasing physiological evidence agrees with the anguished testimony of overweight men and women. By and large, obese people do not eat more than thin people. As for sloth, it is noteworthy that physical activity accounts for only about 20% of most adults' energy expenditure. Why, then, do some people gain weight on a diet that allows others to remain slim, even at the same level of physical activity? It is not that the metabolic engine runs steadily at a lower energy cost in fat people than in thin people; it does not. Rather, it is because people with a tendency to obesity apparently are deficient in a particular cellular mechanism that in other people switches on automatically to burn off excess calories.

On being overfed, most people do not gain weight in proportion to the amount of overfeeding; they dispose of the extra energy by generating heat—through nonshivering thermogenesis (the production of heat in the body by oxidation). However, diet-induced thermogenesis is significantly reduced in obese and formerly obese individuals. This diminished thermogenesis may be due to a metabolic defect in brown fat, a particular tissue long known to be associated with heat production in young animals, and found mainly in the chest, upper back, and near the kidneys of adult animals. Brown fat is brown because it has more iron containing cytochrome molecules than white fat. The cytochromes are components of the membrane of the mitochondria; the cells of brown fat are packed with these organelles which carry out cellular respiration by oxidizing nutrient molecules. In the mitochondria of brown-fat cells, a proton leak bypasses the coupling of oxidation with adenosine triphosphate (ATP) pro-

duction. As a result, the mitochondria, oxidizing local stores of fat, generate heat instead of ATP.

Although more experimental work is needed, it does seem clear that there is diminished capacity in many obese people for thermogenesis induced by dietary fat. The defect seems to be associated with brown fat. It could be that the amount of tissue is inadequate, or that there is a difference in the proton-leakage pathway, or that there is a failure at some stage of the switching-on process.

Of course, not all fat people suffer from a metabolic defect; many people do eat too much. However, because of the possibility of a metabolic defect, a physician should not too readily condemn his fat patients for lack of willpower while he, unwittingly, enjoys a physiological system that allows him to stabilize his own weight with effortless ease.

HORMONAL INFLUENCES ON METABOLISM. The knowledge of the effects of the various hormones is at best a science in its infancy, since most of the major discoveries in this field have been made in the 20th century. When the early breakthroughs were first publicized, many doctors had high hopes of being able to treat obesity and other disorders with specific hormones which might produce immediate results like those seen in diabetics given insulin. The failure of these expectations to materialize led some doctors to abandon their interest in endocrinology. However, other doctors persist in the belief that hormones do exert a very considerable influence on metabolism. Some of those subscribing to the latter school of thought believe that a careful study of a patient's features (body build, distribution and type of hair, facial characteristics, head shape and size, skin, and trunk) will usually reveal which of three endocrine glands is most active: the adrenals, the pituitary, or the thyroid.

HORMONAL ABNORMALITIES IN THE OBESE. It is well known that patterns of endocrine secretion may be altered by such factors as the climate, diet, emotions, and the amount of body fat. For example, the development of obesity often results in increases in the secretion of insulin from the pancreas and of steroid hormones from the adrenal cortex; and by a decreased rate of secretion of growth hormones from the pituitary. However, this does not mean that such abnormalities are the causes of obesity, since they often disappear when the body weight is reduced to normal. Nevertheless, once the abnormalities are established, they may make it difficult to lose weight.

External Factors Which May Spur the Development of Obesity. Many of the lean people who believe that they have stronger character traits than the obese may not owe their success in staying lean to their own efforts; rather, they may owe them to complex physiological processes which regulate appetite. There is evidence for both the short-term and the long-term regulation of food intake in species of animals which are similar to man in their physiology.[10] Details of appetite regulation are given elsewhere in this book.

(Also see APPETITE.)

[7]Robson, J. R. K., et al., "Metabolic Response to Food," *The Lancet*, December 24 & 31, 1977, p. 1367.

[8]Miller, D. S., P. Mumford, and M. J. Stock, "Gluttony: 2. Thermogenesis in Overeating Man," *The American Journal of Clinical Nutrition*, Vol. 20, 1967, pp. 1228-1229.

[9]Miller, D. S., and S. Parsonage, "Resistance to Slimming: Adaptation or Illusion?," *The Lancet*, April 5, 1975, p. 773.

[10]Van Itallie, T. B., N. S. Smith, and D. Quartermain, "Short-Term and Long-Term Components in the Regulation of Food Intake: Evidence for a Modulatory Role of Carbohydrate Status," *American Journal of Clinical Nutrition*, Vol. 30, 1977, p. 742.

Animal experiments have also shown that under various circumstances, appetite control may be interfered with, or bypassed, so that the animals will eat sufficient food for fattening to occur. For example, it is well known that confining livestock in pens speeds up their gains in weight. Likewise, other procedures, such as changing the composition of rations and/or administering hormones, helps the farmer to fatten his animals. Therefore, it is reasonable to expect that similar factors may stimulate the development of human obesity.

The following external factors may spur the development of obesity:

1. **Birth-control pills (oral contraceptives).**—These agents may provoke elevated blood levels of insulin,[11] a condition which is known to favor the development of obesity.

2. **Climate.** Natives of tropical regions have about 10% lower basal metabolic rates than people living in cool regions, whereas people in cold environments expend extra energy to maintain their body temperature. Food consumption should be governed accordingly.

3. **Cultural factors.**—Obesity was, and still is, considered to be very desirable by various peoples; for example, in certain parts of Africa women are still being fattened up prior to marriage, and a man's worth may be partly based upon the total weight of his wives.

4. **Eating in response to external cues.**—This refers to such cues as the sight and smell of food, social gatherings, or while viewing movies or television. Hence, these people are likely to overeat and become obese if they are regularly exposed to these cues.

5. **Emotional stresses.**—With some people, overeating and obesity may stem from chronic emotional disturbances.[12]

6. **Excessive dietary carbohydrates.**—The overconsumption of such highly refined and easily utilized forms of carbohydrates as table sugar and white flour may be a major cause of obesity.

7. **Excessive dietary fats.**—The low bulk and high calories of fat may cause some people to consume too much fat before feeling satisfied.

8. **Excessive dietary proteins.**—Test feedings consisting only of lean meat have been found to be potent stimulators of the copious secretion of the growth hormone, an agent favoring the development of obesity in growing children.

9. **Fatigue.**—Eating when excessively tired may lead to a habit of eating when tired even when the tiredness is not due to lack of food and/or low blood sugar.

10. **Lack of exercise.**—Low levels of physical activity are usually accompanied by consumption of excess energy and a gaining of weight.

11. **Lack of fiber.**—There appears to be a minimum requirement for bulk in the diet so that distention of the small intestine may make for a feeling of satiety.

12. **Meal patterns.**—Eating two or three large meals per day is more likely to result in excessive fattening than five

or six smaller meals, even when the total consumption remains the same.[13]

13. **Nutritional deficiencies.**—Metabolic and nervous abnormalities may result from deficiencies of minerals and vitamins, so it seems reasonable to suspect that these nutritional deficiencies may lead to derangements in appetite control.

14. **Overfeeding of infants and children.**—Many bottle-fed babies are literally force fed, particularly when mothers enlarge the holes in the rubber nipples, then prop up the bottle so that the milk runs down the throats of their babies. Another practice is holding the infant and spooning in as much baby food as will be tolerated.

15. **Overseasoning of food.**—Heavy use of such seasoning agents as catsup, garlic, onions, mustard, pepper, and sugar may make food highly palatable, increase the flow of digestive juices, and generally promote overeating.

16. **Pregnancy.**—Many women gain weight after each pregnancy.

17. **Prenatal and early postnatal influences.**—Many recent research reports suggest that, if not genetic, the tendency towards lifelong obesity begins in a child at some time between the latter part of pregnancy and the end of the first year after birth.[14]

18. **Rapid eating.**—Rapid eating appears to lead to obesity, perhaps due to a delay in the operation of the various satiety mechanisms which allows rapid eaters to consume more than is required.

19. **Sexual and other frustrations.**—From time to time there are reports of studies which show that more obese than lean people complain of sexual frustrations.

20. **Social customs.**—Eating is often an important part of baptisms, bar mitzvahs or confirmations, business luncheons, funerals, professional meetings, and weddings. While these infrequent binges may seem to be unimportant, it may be difficult for some people to regain control of their eating.

21. **Types of food.**—Overeating is more likely to occur when the forms and types of food are high in calories, low in fiber, and do not require much chewing.

DISORDERS WHICH ARE OFTEN AGGRAVATED BY OBESITY.

Statistics from the Metropolitan Life Insurance Company show that obese people (those who are more than 20% overweight) have significantly higher death rates than the nonobese from such conditions as appendicitis, cancers of the gallbladder and liver, cirrhosis of the liver, diabetes, gallstones, heart disease, hernia and intestinal obstruction, kidney disease, stroke, and toxemia of pregnancy.

The statistical associations between obesity and various medical problems do not necessarily mean that the former is always the cause of the latter. For example, a tendency towards diabetes may make some people more susceptible to obesity and other problems, whereas similar problems may be absent in others who are obese. Furthermore, it is important to distinguish between those problems which are directly aggravated by obesity and those which are only indirectly affected, because the choice of the most effective

---

[11]Spellacy, W. N., K. L. Carlson, and S. A. Birk, "Carbohydrate Metabolic Studies after Six Cycles of Combined Type Oral Contraceptive Tablets. Measurement of Plasma Insulin and Blood Glucose Levels," *Diabetes*, Vol. 16, 1967, p. 590.

[12]Bruch, H., "Psychological Implications of Obesity," *Nutrition News*, Vol. 35, 1972, p. 9.

---

[13]Leveille, G. A., and D. R. Romsos, "Meal Eating and Obesity," *Nutrition Today*, Vol. 9, November/December 1974, p. 4.

[14]"Influence of Intrauterine Nutritional Status on the Development of Obesity in Later Life," *Nutrition Reviews*, Vol. 35, 1977, p. 100.

treatment for a disorder depends upon identification of the primary causative factor.

There is evidence that the following disorders are often aggravated by obesity:

1. Angina pectoris.
2. Breathing difficulties.
3. Coronary heart disease.
4. Diabetes.
5. Easy fatigability.
6. Enlargement of the heart.
7. Excessive numbers of red blood cells and abnormal clotting of the blood.
8. Gallstones.
9. Gout.
10. Hernia.
11. High blood pressure.
12. High levels of fats in the blood (hyperlipoproteinemias).
13. Increased sweating and susceptibility to heat exhaustion.
14. Infertility in men.
15. Kidney disease.
16. Low blood sugar (hypoglycemia).
17. Osteoarthritis.
18. Skin problems.
19. Sleepiness.
20. Stroke.
21. Sudden-unexpected death.
22. Surgical dangers.
23. Toxemia.
24. Troubles with the feet and legs.

WAYS OF DETECTING BORDERLINE OBESITY.
The standard practice of doctors and life insurance companies has been to consider their clients to be obese when their body weight is greater than their ideal weight (for their height and body build) by some arbitrary figure—commonly 20%. This arbitrary figure may be an unsatisfactory boundary between normal weight and obesity when (1) it is too low, as in the cases of people who have heavy bones and muscles; or (2) it is too high, as in the case of people with abnormally slender bones and muscles. Nevertheless, it is not wise to wait until someone is grossly obese before taking corrective measures, since the difficulty in achieving weight reduction increases with the degree of obesity. Therefore, it is worth noting the diagnostic standards which follow.

Formulas for Estimating Desirable Body Weights.
Doctors and dietitians commonly estimate desirable weights for (1) adult males by allowing 106 lb for the first 5 ft of height and 6 lb for each additional inch of height over 5 ft, and (2) adult females by allowing 100 lb for the first 5 ft of height and 5 lb for each additional inch. According to the formula for males, a man who is 6 ft 2 in. tall has a desirable weight of 106 lb + 14 × 6 lb (for each inch of height over 5 ft) = 190 lb.

Height-Weight Tables.
Different height-weight tables have been compiled, published, and used through the years. The first of these tables, one for men and the other for women, was compiled from data on people who purchased life insurance policies between 1885 and 1908. The Metropolitan Life Insurance Company introduced new tables in 1943. In 1959, data was published based on 26 life insurance companies in the United States and Canada pooling and analyzing their data on body weight and mortality which

had been compiled from records of several million policyholders over a period of 20 years.[15] Shortly thereafter, the Metropolitan Life Insurance Company issued new, revised tables of desirable weights, which were those found to be associated with the greatest longevity. These tables, like the ones which preceded them, give a range of weights for each of the three categories of build. It should be noted that the values for heights and weights which are presented in these tables represent those obtained from people wearing shoes and their usual indoor clothing. This means that the heights have been obtained from men wearing shoes with 1-in. heels, and from women wearing 2-in. heels; and that the total extra weight for clothing in the men was about 8 lb, while in women it was about 5 lb. Here again, it is necessary for the examiner to decide on a person's body build, since no directions are given for making such determinations. Even if body build were to be determined more precisely, there would still be considerable variation of the relative proportions of fat and lean tissues within each body build.

Therefore, desirable weights obtained from the life insurance tables, or from the formula given in the preceding section, give at best only rough indications of the most desirable body characteristics.

(Also see UNDERWEIGHT, section on "Body Weight for Height, Age, and Sex.")

An Index of Slenderness (Ponderal Index).
This derived quantity represents an attempt to express relative leanness as a function of height and weight. It is obtained through the use of the following formula:

$$\text{Ponderal Index (PI)} = \frac{\text{Height (in.)}}{\sqrt[3]{\text{Weight (lb)}}}$$

This quantity may also be calculated using metric units. However, the values so obtained cannot be compared with those obtained using English units because the ratios of the height to weight units differ between the two systems of measurement. The ponderal index has the applications that follow:

• **Prediction of the effect of body weight on health**—The higher the ponderal index, the greater the leanness and the lower the risk of cardiovascular disease since values under 12.0 are associated with higher rates of this type of disorder.[16] People who have ponderal indexes of 13 or more have very low risk for cardiovascular disease because they are more slender than average.

• **Estimation of trends towards fatness or leanness in growing children**—In this application, a ponderal index which increases with growth in height supposedly indicates a thinning out; while an index which decreases with growth indicates fattening. Although there has been little use of the ponderal index for this purpose, it has been suggested that

[15]*Build and Blood Pressure Study*, 1959, Society of Actuaries, Chicago, Ill., 1959.

[16]Seltzer, C. C., "Some Re-evaluations of the Build and Blood Pressure Study, 1959, as Related to Ponderal Index, Somatotype and Mortality," *New England Journal of Medicine*, Vol. 274, 1966, p. 254.

a value of less than 12.4 might indicate obesity in adolescent girls.[17]

Pinch Tests for Hidden Fat.

Skinfold measurements are more precise versions of the long used *pinch* tests for obesity. In a pinch test, one selects an area of the body where fat is likely to be deposited and grasps a double fold of skin between his thumb and forefinger. Excessive fat is present when the thickness of the double fat is an inch (*2.5 cm*) or more. Special calipers are available for accurately measuring skinfold thicknesses. The use of these calipers is shown in Fig. O-6.

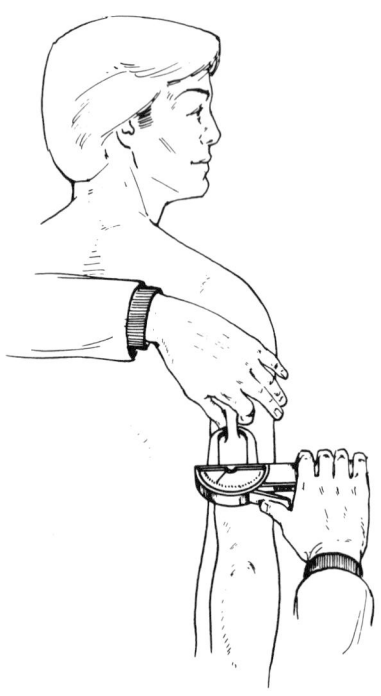

Fig. O-6. The use of skinfold calipers.

Weighing People Under Water.

Anyone observing obese people swimming can hardly fail to notice that their bodies float higher in the water than those of nonobese people. The reason for the greater buoyancy in the obese is that a given volume of fatty tissue weighs only about 90% as much as an equal volume of lean tissue. It follows that differences in the body fat content of people may be detected by weighing them while they're immersed in water.

Although measurement of body density is generally limited to research studies, it is a useful tool for evaluating other more convenient measurements such as skinfold thicknesses.

Detection of Early Signs of Obesity in Children.

Much might be done to prevent hard-to-manage obesity in adults if more efforts were made to detect and treat the early stages of fattening in children. However, children tend to grow at variable rates so many doctors are reluctant to advise

dietary restriction for heavier than average children for fear of slowing their rates of growth.

One means of detecting fattening in children is to pay close attention to the long-term pattern of growth in each child, rather than attempting to make a judgment on the basis of one-time measurements of height and weight. The pattern of growth is determined by plotting the monthly values of a child's height and weight on a standard growth chart. The standard charts usually have curved lines corresponding to growth rates for the 95th, 90th, 75th, 50th, 25th, 10th, and 5th percentiles of the population of children. There are separate charts for boys and girls.

For example, an infant, who at the age of 6 months had a height and weight corresponding to the 75th percentile of the population, would usually be judged to be growing at a normal rate, because the statistical range of normal values extends from the 5th to the 95th percentiles. However, if the same infant had from birth up to age 5 months followed the curves for the 25th percentile of heights and weights, then there would be reason to suspect that the child's growth might have been excessively rapid between 5 and 6 months of age, because of the progression from the 25th to the 75th percentiles in a month. This finding should lead the doctor or other examiner to question the parent as to the feeding of the infant, since overfeeding may force rapid growth and ultimately produce an obesity that is difficult to correct. Likewise, a body weight which is disproportionately high (for example, in the 75th percentile) for height (which might be in the 25th percentile) should lead an examiner to suspect excessive fattening.

(Also see CHILDHOOD AND ADOLESCENT NUTRITION, section on "Childhood Growth and Its Measurement"; and INFANT DIET AND NUTRITION, section on "Measurement of Growth.")

TREATMENT OF OBESITY.

While the prospects of developing any of the deadly disorders associated with obesity are enough to make anyone shudder, there are rarely good reasons for crash dieting, since extremely rapid rates of weight loss are metabolically equivalent to the eating of extraordinary quantities of dietary fat. Hence, the cure may be worse than the disease. Furthermore, many other metabolic abnormalities may accompany drastic changes in body weight. Therefore, the principles of weight control that follow are noteworthy.

Principles of Weight Reduction.

It is often said that all a person has to do to lose weight is to eat fewer calories than needed to meet his or her requirements. While this statement may be true over a long period of time, short-term changes in body weight often appear to defy these scientific principles. For example, a very lean person who skips supper one night might lose as much as 2 lb (*0.9 kg*) while a very obese person may go without food for two whole days and yet lose no weight. Furthermore, even very obese people might lose as much as 2 lb (*0.9 kg*) per day, when their daily diet is restricted to 400 Calories (kcal) from fat or protein alone, or from mixtures of these nutrients. The secret behind such seemingly contradictory observations is that weight losses may be due not only to loss of fat, but also to losses of variable amounts of water and protein from the lean tissues of the body.

Planning Diets and Selecting Foods.

Anyone with a tendency to become obese needs to plan a balanced diet

[17]Canning, H., and J. Mayer, "Obesity—Its Possible Effect on College Acceptance," *The New England Journal of Medicine*, Vol. 275, 1966, p. 1172.

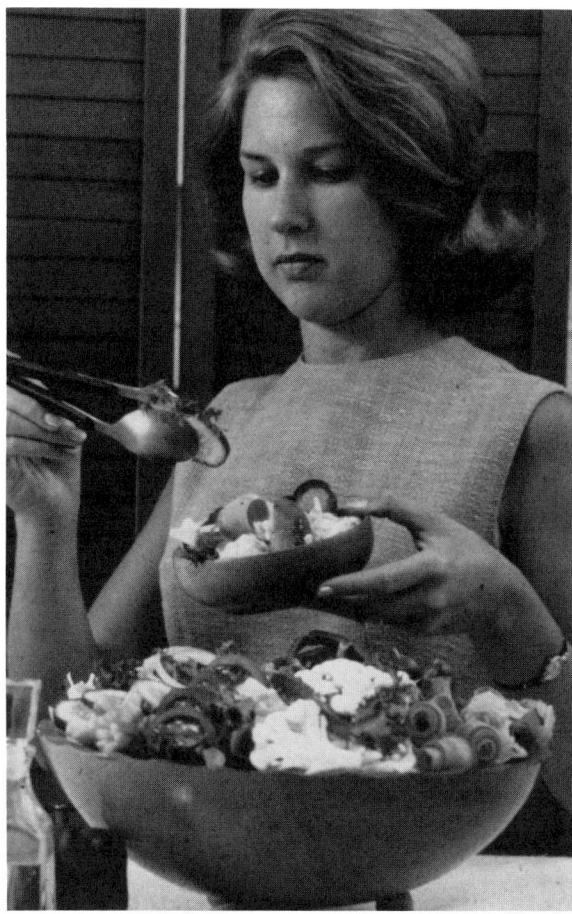

Fig. O-7. A low calorie salad. (Courtesy, USDA)

produce the appropriate caloric deficit. Descriptions of such calculations follow:

• **Estimating requirements for calories**—The equation for this calculation is: Calories (kcal) in modified diet equal caloric requirement minus caloric deficit for weight loss.

Most people require 15 Calories (kcal) or less per pound of desirable weight. (Desirable weights may be estimated by the means described in the section headed "Ways of Detecting Borderline Obesity.")

The caloric deficit is 500 Calories (kcal) per day to lose 1 lb (0.45 kg) per week, or 1,000 Calories (kcal) to lose 2 lb. People who wish to lose weight more rapidly should only do so under a doctor's supervision.

• **Selecting foods to make up a diet**—It is not wise to select foods solely on the basis of their calorie contents (a practice that is sometimes called *counting calories*) because it may lead to dietary deficiencies. Instead, one should select items

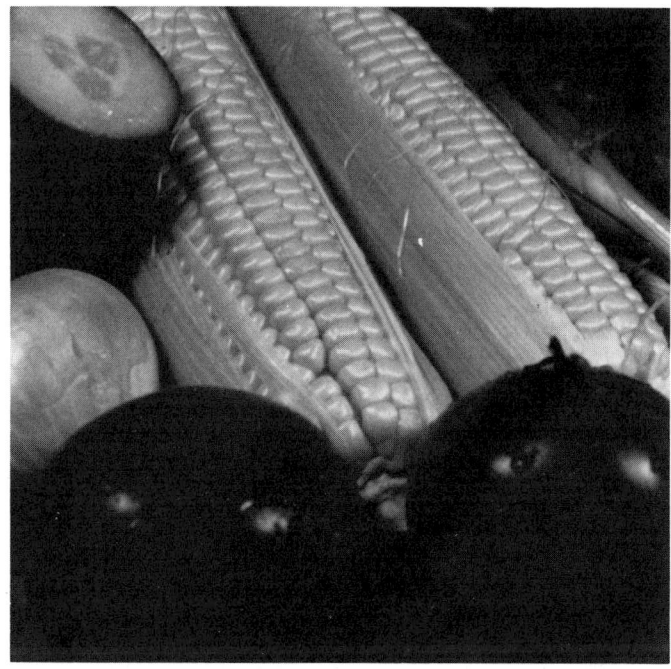

Fig. O-8. Slim cuisine calls for lots of vegetables. (Courtesy, National Film Board of Canada)

which provides the required nutrients, but which does not contain excess calories. It is easy to do such planning when one follows the procedures used by dietitians and others with expertise in planning such meals. Simplified versions of these procedures follow.

MODIFIED DIETS.   This term is now used instead of the older designation of *special diets* because nutritionists want to advance the idea that one should start with a basic diet which is suitable for most people, then modify it so as to achieve whatever composition may be desired. The modifications which are usually made for low-calorie diets involve reduction in the number of items high in carbohydrates and fats, but retention of those which are good sources of proteins, minerals, and vitamins. For example, it might be desirable to avoid candy, cookies, cakes, ice cream, butter or margarine, and table sugar, and to substitute in their place, whole grain breads, fruits, vegetables, and salad oils. Also, the leaner cuts of meat such as round steak might be used in place of short ribs, porterhouse steak, and luncheon meats (which tend to have higher fat contents).

However, such dietary modifications may not in themselves be sufficient to produce loss of weight, because excessive quantities of the low-calorie foods may be eaten. Therefore, it is often necessary to calculate caloric requirements so that the dietary calorie content may be low enough to

from each of the various food groups so as to obtain a nutritionally balanced diet. Even then, the diet may not furnish all of the required nutrients unless special effort is made to select foods which are good sources of these nutrients, such as dairy products, eggs, fish, fresh or frozen fruits and vegetables, meats, and whole grain cereal products. However, the amounts of these highly nutritious items must be limited in order to keep the energy content of the diet low enough for weight loss to occur. Hence, it is best to use the exchange system for planning diets. Table O-2 gives some typical diets planned by this system.

Table O-2 gives typical menus for diets which are (1) low in carbohydrates (thought to be useful for abnormally high levels of blood triglycerides), (2) moderately low in fat content (the basis of the most commonly used standard diets), and (3) high in carbohydrates and very low in fats (this type of diet may be helpful in preventing heart disease). However, it was noted earlier that when the dietary energy deficit is great enough to bring about the metabolism of large amounts of body fat, the mixture of nutrients metabolized by the body will have a much higher fat content than the diet. Hence, even low-fat diets may make it necessary for the body to burn considerable amounts of fat, which is mostly saturated because it is derived mainly from the fatty tissues. Therefore, one should avoid crash diets which result in the loss of more than 2 lb per week because the metabolic consequences of such programs are uncertain.

TABLE 0-2
TYPICAL MENUS FOR VARIOUS TYPES OF LOW-ENERGY DIETS

Types of Food Exchanges[1] (used for each meal or snack)	Number of Exchanges Per Meal (based upon daily energy requirements)					
	Low Carbohydrate Diet		Low-Fat Diet		High Carbohydrate Very Low-Fat Diet	
	1,200 kcal per day	1,500 kcal per day	1,200 kcal per day	1,500 kcal per day	1,200 kcal per day	1,500 kcal per day
Breakfast:						
Bread (or biscuits, cereals, crackers, muffins, pancakes, waffles, etc.)	1	1	1	1	1	2
Fat (bacon, butter, coffee whitener, margarine, mayonnaise, etc.)[2]	1	1	1	1	0	1
Fruit (or its equivalent in juice)	1	1	1	1	1	1
Lean meat (or low-fat cheese, fish, fowl, etc.)	1	1	1	1	0	0
Milk, nonfat[2]	0	0	0	0	1	1
Optional beverage: bouillon (fat free), clear broth, club soda, coffee, herb tea, tea, water	◄─────── Any amount, but limit sweetener[3] ───────►					
Mid-morning snack:						
Bread	0	0	1	1	1	1
Fat	0	1	0	0	0	0
Milk, nonfat	1	1	1	1	0	0
Optional beverage (see Breakfast)	◄─────── Any amount, but limit sweetener[3] ───────►					
Lunch:						
Bread	1	1	1	2	2	3
Fat	2	2	0	2	0	1
Fruit (or juice)	0	0	0	1	1	1
Meat, lean (see Breakfast)	3	3	3	3	2	2
Optional beverage (see Breakfast)	◄─────── Any amount, but limit sweetener[3] ───────►					
Raw vegetable, or salad without dressing	1	1	1	1	1	1
Mid-afternoon snack:						
Bread	0	0	1	1	0	1
Fat	0	1	0	0	0	0
Milk, nonfat	1	1	1	1	1	1
Optional beverage (see Breakfast)	◄─────── Any amount, but limit sweetener[3] ───────►					
Supper:						
Bread	1	1	1	2	2	2
Fat	3	3	1	2	0	1
Fruit	0	1	0	0	1	1
Meat, lean (see Breakfast)	3	4	3	3	3	3
Optional beverage (see Breakfast)	◄─────── Any amount, but limit sweetener[3] ───────►					
Nonstarchy vegetable, cooked	1	1	1	1	1	1
Raw vegetable, or salad without dressing	1	1	1	1	1	1
Late evening snack:						
Bread	0	1	0	0	1	1
Fat	0	1	0	0	1	0
Fruit (or juice)	0	0	1	1	0	0
Milk, nonfat	1	1	1	1	1	1

[1]Exchanges are portions of food which have been grouped together because they contain similar proportions of carbohydrates, fats, proteins, and calories. Portion sizes have been calculated so that the exchanges within each group may be substituted for one another because their nutritive values are approximately equal.
(Also see MODIFIED DIETS, section headed "Use of Exchange Lists in Planning Diets.")

[2]The distribution of fat at meals may have to be adjusted if the foods chosen from among the other groups of exchanges contain more or less fat than the amount which is typical for each of the groups. For example, two fat exchanges should be deducted from the amounts allowed each time that whole milk is used instead of the nonfat type, or one fat exchange deducted to compensate for the use of 2% milk or plain yogurt in lieu of nonfat milk. Similarly, one fat exchange should be deducted for each exchange of high-fat meat used instead of lean meat, or ½ fat exchange deducted for each exchange of medium-fat meat. Also, many doctors recommend that, wherever possible, the items used as fat exchanges be chosen from such sources of polyunsaturated fats as salad oils and soft margarines because ample amount of saturated fats are provided by the meat exchanges.

[3]These fluids contain few calories, so they may be taken as desired. However, the use of sugar and other sweeteners should be limited because 4 tsp (20 ml) of sugar furnish about the same amount of carbohydrates as one bread exchange, 1¾ fruit exchanges, one nonfat milk exchange, or three exchanges from the cooked vegetables.

The procedure for using the table follows:

1. Determine your desirable body weight by either referring to a standard height-weight table, or by using the appropriate formula given in the section headed "Formulas for Estimating Desirable Body Weights."

2. Calculate your caloric requirement for maintenance of weight by multiplying your ideal body weight by 15.

3. Choose a dietary calorie level by deducting a caloric deficit of either 500 Calories (kcal) (to lose 1 lb [0.45 kg] per week) or 1,000 Calories (kcal) (to lose 2 lb per week) from your caloric requirement calculated in step 2. Do not select a diet which furnishes less than 1,000 Calories (kcal) per day without consulting a physician.

4. Set up a daily menu by selecting exchanges from the food groups listed in Table O-2.

(Also see MODIFIED DIETS, section headed "Use of Exchange Lists in Planning Diets.")

EXAMPLE: An adult female who is 5 ft 4 in. (163 cm) tall and has a medium body build, weighs 140 lb (63 kg). She would like to get her weight down to normal as soon as possible. Her ideal body weight is 120 lb (54 kg) and her energy requirement for maintenance of this weight is 1,800 Calories (kcal) per day. It is not advisable for her to try to lose more than 1 lb (0.45 kg) per week because diets containing less than 1,200 Calories (kcal) per day are neither nutritious nor satisfying. Hence, it might take her about 17 weeks to reach her ideal weight if she sticks to her diet. (Her weight loss might be accelerated by extra activity.) Some typical meals and snacks for a 1,200 Calorie (kcal) low-fat diet are given in the column on the right. Generally, such low-fat, high-carbohydrate diets are more filling than low-carbohydrate, high-fat diets because the former contain more high-fiber foods like bread (if whole grain varieties are used) and fruits, while the latter are based upon foods where the calories are concentrated in a small amount of bulk.

(Also see FIBER.)

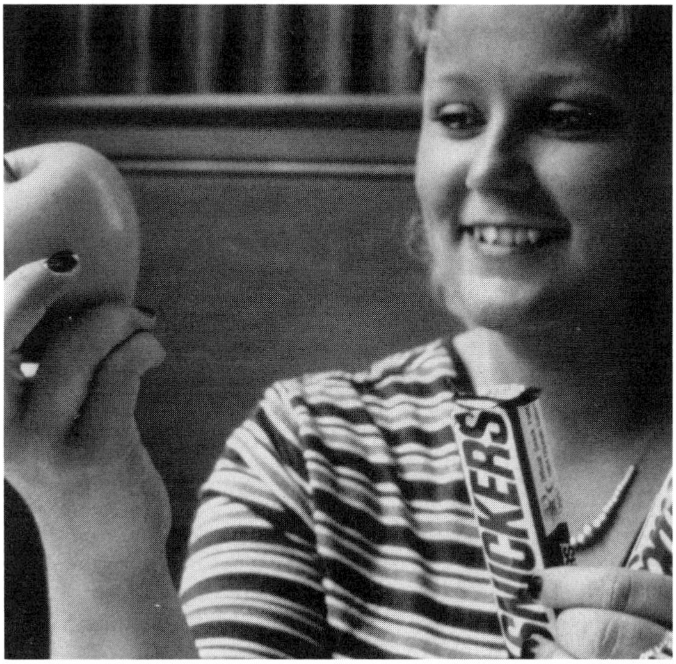

Fig. O-9. Weight watchers should snack on apples instead of candy bars. (Courtesy, Univ. of Tennessee, Knoxville, Tenn.)

Meal	Menu		Calorie (kcal)
Breakfast ..	Ready-to-eat cereal	¾ c ...	70
	with nonfat milk	¾ c ...	60
	and sliced fresh peaches .	1 whole peach	40
	Coffee	1 c	0
	Evaporated skim milk	2 Tbsp .	20
	Sugar	½ tsp ..	9
Mid-morning Snack ...	Graham crackers	two 2½ in. square	70
	Tea with lemon	1 c.....	0
Lunch	Sandwich made with whole-rye bread	2 slices	140
	boiled ham	2 slices	110
	lettuce, tomato, and mustard	no limit	0
	Clear, fat-free hot broth ...	1 c	0
	Apple	one 2 in. diameter ...	40
Mid-afternoon snack ...	Nonfat milk	1 c	80
Supper ...	Tossed salad made with chicory, chopped green peppers, mushroom slices, oregano (dried), and vinegar	no limit	0
	Flank steak	three 1 oz slices	165
	Horseradish sauce	2 tsp ..	0
	Mashed potato without butter or margarine	½ c ...	70
	Carrots, cooked	½ c ...	25
	Cantaloupe	¼ of 6 in. diameter fruit	40
	Whole-wheat bread	1 slice .	70
	Mint tea	1 c	0
Late-evening snack ...	Tortilla	one 6 in. diameter ..	70
	Low-fat yogurt, plain	1 c	125
Total food energy			1,204

SUGGESTIONS FOR PREPARING MEALS AT HOME. A good deal of study and planning is necessary in order for weight reduction to be achieved through dieting. One must learn (1) which foods are low in energy, yet are nutritious; (2) how to estimate correct portion sizes for various types of foods; and (3) ways of combining separate items in such dishes as casseroles, desserts, soups, and stews. Then, the necessary food ingredients must be purchased and kept available for meal preparation. In short, safe and successful weight reduction may require the expenditure of extra effort, money, and time.

EATING AWAY FROM HOME. Too many people who are frequently away from home may put on fat because they eat whatever is served to them. However, dieters should have a preplanned strategy for coping with the pitfalls of eating away from home. Suggestions follow:

• **Lunches Brought from Home**—It seems obvious that with careful planning it is possible both to stick to a diet and save money by bringing food from home for lunches, picnics, and short automobile trips.

• **Eating in Restaurants**—Although the staff in the better restaurants will usually make every effort to accommodate diners who are on diets, dieters must also be prepared to cope with much less flexibility in such places as fast food establishments where the foods and the cooking systems are designed for rapid turnover.

Changing Eating Behavior. This method of combating obesity, which is sometimes called *behavior mod* (mod is short for modification), differs from *crash* dieting in that it seeks permanent modification of the behavior that led to the obesity. Many people regain weight they lost by crash dieting because they failed to change their eating habits.

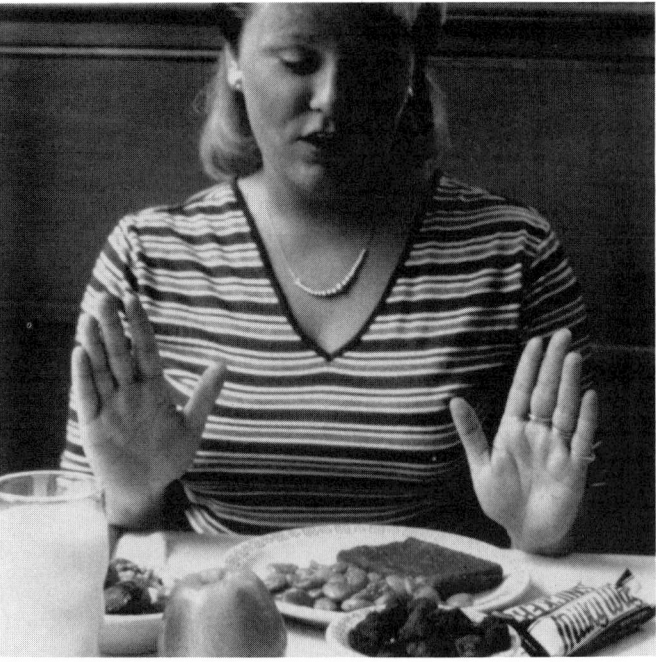

Fig. O-10. Changing eating behavior—say no to seconds. (Courtesy, Univ. of Tennessee, Knoxville, Tenn.)

However, before a person starts on such a program, it is a good idea to try and identify each of the factors which might be cues for his or her overeating. For example, some people habitually may eat, whether hungry or not, at such times and places as: (1) while engaged in such activities as conversation, reading, or watching television; or (2) in response to such emotions as anger, anxiety, boredom, excitement, frustration, happiness, or loneliness.[18] Hence, it might be necessary for a compulsive eater to keep a detailed diary for a week or so, noting both the circumstances (time, place, emotions, etc.) that prompt eating, and the amounts and types of foods which are eaten.

EATING BEHAVIOR AT HOME. Some do's and don'ts in changing eating behavior at home are:

1. Establish specific times and places for eating, then eat *only* under those circumstances. For example, this might mean that when one is home, eating is done only in the dining room at 7:30 a.m., 6:30 p.m., and 10:00 p.m.; and *never* while working in the kitchen or when people unexpectedly drop in between meals. Visitors may be served food,

but a dieter should learn to avoid eating just because others are doing so if the time is not in accordance with the new behavior pattern which is being established.

2. When eating, concentrate only on that activity. It might be necessary to ask other members of the family to cooperate by refraining from starting intense discussions at meals. One way to emphasize the importance of eating without distractions is to establish a regular etiquette for each meal and snack by using place settings and saying grace.

3. Do *not* put platters and bowls of food on the dining table so that diners may readily refill their plates; rather, put out only the servings of food needed for those present. It is rarely necessary to prepare more than one serving of foods per person, other than salads, since underweight members of the family would probably be better off eating extra food between meals; instead of eating more food at meals. However, the athletes or laborers in the family might go into the kitchen and serve themselves extra food, if such is absolutely necessary.

4. Put individual servings of all of the courses on the dining table before sitting down to eat. That way, everyone may see the total meal and thereby find it easier to avoid overeating the items which are normally served early in the meal. Using small dishes helps to emphasize the size of food portions.

5. Slow down your rate of eating by (a) breaking or cutting off only one small bite of food at a time, (b) chewing each bite of food thoroughly, and (c) swallowing each chewed bite before taking another. Development of a habit of chewing rather than bolting food may require the eating of such foods as dry breads, tough meats, and fibrous fruits and vegetables—all items which cannot be comfortably swallowed without thorough chewing.

6. The pace of eating may also be slowed by serving foods that require more time to eat like (a) fish or meat containing bones, (b) nuts with shells, and (c) fruits with rinds and seeds. Also, according to the rules of etiquette, one should *not* bring to the mouth a large piece of food, then chew off pieces; rather, he should use fingers (in the case of breads) or utensils to remove one bite size piece at a time.

7. When everyone has eaten, the leftovers should immediately be removed from the dining table and stored. Do *not* provide opportunities for nibbling after meals have been completed.

8. Allow sufficient time for meals and snacks each day so that food never has to be eaten on the run.

EATING BEHAVIOR AWAY FROM HOME. Some do's and don'ts in changing eating behavior away from home are:

1. Try to avoid conducting business or talking about work while eating, since emotionally disturbing discussions may (a) stimulate the flow of extra stomach acid and intensify movements of the digestive tract, two conditions which may increase the urge to eat more; (b) distract from the enjoyment of food so that the meal is completed without the usual satisfaction; and (c) provoke compulsive eating by susceptible people. There are very few people who cannot comfortably eat a moderate-sized meal in 30 minutes or less. Expenditure of this amount of time just for eating and small talk might in the long run prove to be a good investment, since a friendly relationship might be established at the meal so that unnecessary argumentation might be avoided when discussing business *after* the meal.

2. Planning in advance for uncertain eating conditions while traveling. For example, find out whether or not food will be served on an airline flight, so that one does not eat

---

[18]Leon, G. R., "A Behavioral Approach to Obesity," *The American Journal of Clinical Nutrition*, Vol. 30, 1977, p. 785.

both before and during the flight. Not all airline terminals have shops where nutritious, low-calorie snacks may be purchased. Some of those near large cities have various types of restaurants which serve a variety of salads, main dishes, and other items suitable for dieters. However, there are often long waits for service at the better restaurants, so at least an extra hour should be allowed for eating at airline terminals.

3.   Learn to be firm when coaxed by dining companions to have more food or drink. One may be gracious to hosts by praising them for their hospitality, rather than by trying to eat every morsel which is served. The old notion that guests should be filled almost to bursting is now considered passe.

Participation In Weight Control Groups.

It may be difficult for highly extroverted obese people to persist in dieting when the required sacrifices depend entirely upon their own initiative. Therefore, they might consider joining a dieting group which meets weekly to share experiences in the battle against the bulges. These groups differ in that (1) a few are affiliated with teaching hospitals whose doctors and dietitians provide guidance to members, (2) others operate as private, profit-making organizations which have paid nutrition consultants, and (3) still others are private, nonprofit clubs where there may be some voluntary participation by medical and/or nutrition professionals. It is desirable for weight control groups to have persons trained in food and nutrition as consultants because many members would benefit from professional evaluations of the new dietary concepts and the various dietetic foods which are promoted through the mass media.

Before joining a weight control group, a prospective member should obtain a thorough medical examination so as to rule out the possibility that a metabolic problem might be accompanying or contributing to his or her obesity. Then, the obese person might make certain that overeating is not a response to one or more emotional problems which are not related to foods. If the latter is the case, it might be necessary for the dieter to find some other means for coping with this situation. Finally, the prospective member should investigate the club to determine (1) whether the diet(s) recommended might be considered both safe and suitable by his or her doctor, and (2) if the techniques used by the group to modify behavior are compatible with the personality of the dieter. For example, some people might find it annoying to be chided, or even ridiculed, for dietary indiscretions, while others might find such tactics to be just what is needed to give a boost to their will power. However, certain members may so value the esteem of the group that a day or so prior to meetings they may resort to such drastic measures as depriving themselves of fluids and food, or taking enemas or strong laxatives. Hence, these groups might do well to advise against such practices.

People may find out about weight control groups in their local community by asking their doctor.

Drugs Which Affect Appetite and Metabolism.

Certain types of drugs, taken alone or in combination with others, may help to speed loss of weight when they (1) reduce appetite (these are called anorexic agents), (2) promote loss of water through urination (diuretics), and (3) increase the proportion of food energy lost as heat (thyroid hormones). In addition to these types of substances, other drugs might be used to counteract some of the undesirable side effects of those which promote the loss of weight.

NOTE: Each of the drugs which follow may have harmful side effects. Hence, their use in the treatment of obesity

should be done only under the close supervision of a physician. It would be much better to attempt to reduce the body weight by dieting and exercise, and to use drugs only as a last resort. Some reducing drugs follow:

• **Anorexic agents**—These drugs are appetite suppressants which are used as *part* of the treatment for obesity, augmenting the other part of the treatment consisting of a nutritious, calorie-restricted diet.

• **Atropine**—This antispasmodic drug slows excessive activity of the digestive tract, a condition sometimes resulting from the use of amphetamines. Hence, the two types of drugs may be combined in an antiobesity formulation.

• **Barbiturates**—These drugs, also known as *downers,* depress the activity of the central nervous system. Hence they may be combined with amphetamines.

• **Digitalis**—This substance slows the heart rate, so it may be used in combination with thyroid hormones, which speed up the heart rate. *The combination of these two types of drugs is considered to be both dangerous and unwarranted in the treatment of obesity.*[19]

• **Diuretics**—These agents increase the amounts of water lost from the body through urination. Some of the diuretic drugs also cause marked losses of potassium in the urine, a situation which might result in increased susceptibility of the heart muscle to the toxic effects of digitalis. Patients treated for congestive heart failure with combinations of these drugs are usually warned to obtain sufficient dietary potassium to compensate for urinary losses.

• **Hormones**—Thyroid hormones are often used to treat obesity because they increase the amount of food energy lost as heat so that the total energy metabolism of the body must be increased in order to meet the needs of the body tissues. However, the hormones may also cause palpitations of the heart. Therefore, many doctors believe that the use of these agents should be limited to people who have thyroid deficiencies.

• **Laxatives**—Drugs such as atropine and diuretics may make some people constipated, so laxatives may sometimes be added to such mixed medications. Some misinformed people also use excessive amounts of laxatives to cause weight loss which results in an increased loss of nutrients and water in the stool.

• **Rainbow pills**—These are multicolored pills which often contain mixtures of such drugs as amphetamines, barbiturates, digitalis, diuretics, laxatives, and thyroid hormones.

Exercise.

Although most people would not be able to exercise vigorously enough to lose weight by this method alone, more and more programs for weight control and physical fitness emphasize the need for frequent and brief periods of strenuous activity, e.g., bicycling, jogging, tennis, or swimming, all of which result in deep breathing and a speeding of the heart rate. These activities should be engaged in for at least 4 hours a week, and if possible, at least 1 hour every day. However, some people may be in such poor physical condition that they would be risking excessive strain on their hearts, joints, and muscles if they were suddenly to begin such exercises. Therefore anyone who

---

19"No End to the Rainbow," *Nutrition Today*, Vol. 3, June 1968, p. 24.

wishes to start an exercise program should first obtain a thorough physical examination, then ask his or her physician how much should be done. People unaccustomed to exercise might begin with walking at a moderate pace for an extra 30 minutes to 1 hour each day.

It is noteworthy that regular participation in vigorous activity might slow weight loss because the building up of muscles involves both protein and water. However, one might determine whether or not fat is being lost by periodically taking measurements of the skinfold thickness at various sites on the body.

Many of the dangerous tendencies which may accompany obesity may be reduced or eliminated by regular exercise, even when the rate of weight loss may be very slow. Therefore, some health benefits of exercise follow:

• **Appetite reduction**—It was mentioned earlier in this article that appetite decreases when sedentary people take up moderate physical activity. Hence, a good time for jogging or similar exercise would be after work, and just before supper.

• **Clearing of fats from the blood**—Many studies have shown that blood triglycerides often drop sharply when a person undertakes a daily program of exercise. This improvement in the levels of blood fats may occur even when the energy expended is compensated for by eating extra food.[20] There may also be gradual, but significant, declines in blood cholesterol.

• **Extra energy expenditure and loss of weight**—About the most weight which may be lost through extra exercise is 1 lb per week, when an additional 500 Calories (kcal) are expended each day, and no extra food is taken. However, it is not difficult at all to expend an extra 250 Calories (kcal) per day by jogging for half an hour, which will result in the loss of 13 lb (5.9 kg) over 6 months. Extra exercise might also help to rid the body of excess weight due to the buildup of water.

• **Firming up of muscles and improvement in appearance**— Men and women who lose weight without exercise may retain a protruding pot-belly or drooping breasts because flabby muscles allow these tissues to sag. Although most experts state that one cannot preferentially reduce certain fatty spots in the body without equally reducing all such deposits, the firming up of adjacent muscles helps to prevent unsightly sagging of flesh.

• **Improved tolerance for heat stress**—It was recently found that the tolerance of men for heat stress was improved when they underwent a 6-week training period where they engaged in such vigorous activities as basketball, handball, jogging, and running for 1 hour per day, 5 times a week.[21]

• **Increased flow of blood to vital organs and tissues**— Exercise speeds the heart rate and the flow of blood around the body. However, if the flow of blood in the muscles is greatly increased, as in strenuous exercise, there is likely to be a decreased flow to the visceral organs. Hence, it is *not* wise to do such exercises right after meals, since it may result in digestive problems.

• **Lowering of blood pressure**—Two conditions which may contribute to a drop in blood pressure during exercise are (1) the opening up of small blood vessels in the muscles, and (2) a similar dilation of blood vessels in the skin as part of the body's means of dissipating heat.

• **Lowering of elevated blood sugar**—It is well known that exercise lowers blood sugar, even in diabetics, since there appears to be an insulinlike effect of strenuous activity. Hence, diabetics who are required to take injections of insulin may often lower the dosage of this hormone when they take extra exercise.

• **Opening up of "emergency" blood vessels in the heart muscle**—Regular exercise may be one of the best forms of insurance against dying of a heart attack, since moderate working of the heart muscle causes enlargement of the branches of the coronary artery. Hence, if there is an obstruction to the flow of blood in one part of this system, the chances for survival are greatly enhanced when one has a highly functional system of alternative blood vessels for supplying the heart muscle.

• **Prevention of varicose veins**—Frequent exercising of the legs during the day helps to force the blood in the veins back up to the heart. It is believed that the enlargement of the leg veins is at least partly due to the pooling of blood in them when insufficient exercise is taken.

• **Reduction in the loss of calcium from bones**—Among the other benefits which accrue to older people from exercise is a dramatic decrease in the loss of calcium from their bones, which is considerable when people take little exercises.[22] (Also see OSTEOPOROSIS.)

• **Relaxation of tensions**—Getting out and exercising may help compulsive eaters since it helps to dissipate some of the tension which may build up from emotional stresses. Remember, that man's physiology is oriented towards "fight or flight" when confronted by various threats.

• **Slowing of the resting heart rate**—One of the signs that a person has achieved a high level of physical fitness is the slowing of his or her heart rate to as low as 60 beats per minute. A slower resting heart rate means that the organ has more time to rest between each beat.

• **Thinning of the blood**—Some obese, middle-aged men have excessive numbers of red blood cells (polycythemia) which increases the thickness (viscosity) of their blood along with its tendency to clot. It is believed that one cause of this condition may be a lack of oxygen in certain tissues, a condition which stimulates the production of extra red cells by the bone marrow. However, it has been found that vigorous exercise may cause a drop in the red cell count.[23] The lowering of the blood sugar by exercise might also help to prevent thickening of the blood since excess sugar produces excess glycoproteins, substances which contribute resistance to the flow of blood in the small blood vessels. (Also see DIABETES MELLITUS.)

[20]Gyntelberg, F., et al., "Plasma Triglyceride Lowering by Exercise Despite Increased Food Intake in Patients with Type IV Hyperlipoproteinemia," *The American Journal of Clinical Nutrition*, Vol. 30, 1977, p. 716.

[21]Gisolfi, C., and S. Robinson, "Relations between Physical Training, Acclimatization, and Heat Tolerance," *Journal of Applied Physiology*, Vol. 26, 1969, p. 530.

[22]Sidney, K. H., R. J. Shephard, and J. E. Harrison, "Endurance Training and Body Composition of the Elderly," *The American Journal of Clinical Nutrition*, Vol. 30, 1977, p. 326.

[23]Yoshimura, H., "Anemia during Physical Training (Sports Anemia)," *Nutrition Reviews*, Vol. 28, 1970, p. 251.

Surgery and Other Drastic Measures.

When all else fails to produce the desired loss in weight, drastic surgical measures may be taken. For example, one type of operation removes deposits of fat and some of the excess skin from the abdomen. Then, the wound is sewn together at the edges.

Another type of surgery is the removal of part of the small intestine so that the absorption of nutrients is greatly reduced. However, this operation may be followed by liver disorders, kidney stones, and other problems, and even death.[24] Hence, many doctors do not recommend it unless the risks of obesity are greater than those of the surgery.

Finally, a few people have had their jaws wired shut so that they might drink fluids, but could not take any solid foods. Dramatic losses of weight have occurred, but there has been no news as to whether these losses were sustained after the wires were removed.

SUMMARY.

No matter what the reason may be for obesity, it is not to be desired and should be avoided or treated promptly if it develops. The two most important points are:

1. Total caloric consumption must be reduced, and a new permanent pattern of eating established—otherwise, the weight will be regained eventually.
2. Exercise should be increased on a daily basis.

OBESITY DRUGS

Generally, this refers to anorexic agents—those drugs which suppress the appetite. Originally, amphetamines were used for this purpose but now a number of other drugs are available; among them, diuretics, hormones, barbiturates, and atropine, used alone or in combination. Drugs may be used as *part* of the treatment for obesity, with the other part of the treatment consisting of a nutritious calorie-restricted diet. But they should only be used as a last resort, and then only under the close supervision of a doctor.

(Also see OBESITY, section on "Drugs Which Affect Appetite and Metabolism.")

OCTACOSANOL ($C_{28}H_{58}O$)

This substance, which exists in nature as a constituent of many plant oils and waxes, including the oil of raw wheat germ, is reputed to be important in physical fitness. Based on a long series of human experiments on physical fitness conducted by Dr. Thomas Kirk Cureton of the University of Illinois Physical Fitness Institute, it appears that octacosanol is one of the factors responsible for the beneficial effects of unrefined, unheated wheat germ oil. Vitamin E alone was not effective.

Dr. Cureton's subjects were tested for pulse rates, breath-holding ability, basal metabolism, heart action, reaction time, agility, bicycling, strength, and many other physical activities. Improvements were noted in stamina, speed, reflexes, agility, and heart action.

Octacosanol, which has been concentrated from wheat germ oil, will be listed on any product that contains it.

NOTE WELL: More experimental work is needed relative to the importance of octacosanol as part of a nutritional pro-

gram for persons engaged in strenuous activities where agility, speed, and endurance are important. Also, persons eating plenty of whole grain cereals, unheated seeds and nuts, and other foods rich in this substance, do not need supplemental sources of octacosanol.

OFFAL

Formerly, the term offal, which literally means *off fall*, included all parts of the animal that fell off during slaughtering. As our knowledge of nutrition improved, the edible portions—liver, tongue, sweetbread, heart, kidney, brain, tripe, and oxtail—were upgraded and classed as *variety meats*. Hand in hand with this transition, the hide, wool, and tallow became known as by-products. Thus, in a modern packing plant, only the entrails and inedible trimmings are referred to as offal.

OIL

Although fats and oils have the same general structure and chemical properties, they have different physical characteristics. The melting points of oils are such that they are liquid at ordinary room temperatures.

(Also see FATS AND OTHER LIPIDS; and OILS, VEGETABLE.)

OIL CROPS

The main oil crops are soybeans, cottonseed, peanuts, and flaxseed. Sunflower, safflower, castor bean, and corn are also used for making oil.

OIL PALM *Elaeis guineensis*

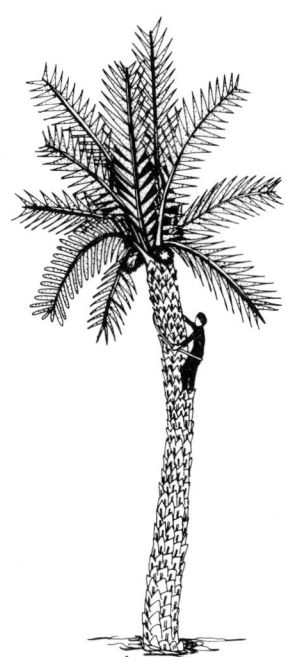

Fig. O-11. Oil palm of West Africa, showing climber ascending tree to harvest the fruit.

The oil palm is one of the world's most important sources of edible and soapmaking oil. It yields more per acre than can be obtained from any other vegetable oil; hence, its importance is not likely to decline.

[24]Bray, G. A., and J. R. Benfield, "Intestinal Bypass for Obesity: A Summary and Perspective," *The American Journal of Clinical Nutrition*, Vol. 30, 1977, p. 121.

ORIGIN AND HISTORY. The oil palm is indigenous to tropical Asia and/or Africa, where it grows wild in great numbers. A large proportion of the commercial palm oil comes from the fruits collected from wild palm groves. But plantations have also been established in the Congo, in Tanzania, along the Ivory Coast, and in Malaysia and Indonesia.

WORLD PRODUCTION. The world production of palm oil totals about 11,044,000 metric tons; and the world production of palm kernel oil totals about 3,468,186 metric tons.[25] The leading palm oil producing countries, by rank, are: Malaysia, Indonesia, Nigeria, Colombia, and Thailand.[26]

PROCESSING. The primitive method of processing, which is still used by many small farmers, consists of leaving the bunches of fruit to ferment for a few days (usually in holes in the ground); stripping off the fruits, then boiling and pounding them; and skimming off the oil from the surface of the water. The shells of the nuts are broken between two stones or in a hand-operated cracking machine. The kernels are usually sold for export, with their oil extracted by the importing country.

But modern oil processing factories are gradually replacing the primitive method, and recovering a larger percentage of oil from the fruits than can be secured by hand processing. The trend is toward steam distillation, followed by centrifuging and even hydraulic expression. In industrialized nations, the kernels are either expressed or solvent-treated.

PREPARING. Although liquid when first extracted, palm oil sets about as thick as butter at normal temperatures. It has a yellowish color (due to the carotene pigment), and a pleasant aroma.

NUTRITIONAL VALUE. Palm oils vary; in some cases resembling kernel oil, and in others olive oil. But they are always a rich source of vitamin A; they contain from 37,300 to 128,700 mcg of beta-carotene equivalent per 100 g. All kernel oils are very similar—they're high in lauric acid and high in saturation. Food Composition Table F-21 lists the nutrient composition of palm oil and palm kernel oil.

USES. The leading producing countries use palm oil locally as a food in all kinds of cookery, and export the surplus.

When exported, palm oil is used chiefly for soapmaking and industrial purposes; but with suitable treatment it may also be used in margarine. Palm kernel oil, which is white or pale yellow, is largely used for margarine. Following extraction, the oilcake is used as a protein supplement for livestock.

As with many other palms, wine may be prepared from the oil palm by tapping and fermenting the sugary sap, which contains a useful content of B vitamins.

OILSEED

Seeds from which oil is extracted for commercial use are termed oilseeds, including castor bean, cottonseed, flaxseed, peanut, safflower, sesame, soybean, and sunflower.

(Also see OILS, VEGETABLE, Table O-5.)

---

[25]Based on data from *Agricultural Statistics 1991*, USDA, p. 135, Table 189. **Note well:** Annual production fluctuates as a result of weather and profitability of the crop.

[26]Based on data from *FAO Production Yearbook 1990*, FAO/UN, Rome, Italy, Vol. 44, p. 124, Table 48.

OILS, VEGETABLE

Vegetable oils are obtained from the seeds and fruits of various plants. Many of their characteristics are similar to those of animal fats, which is fortunate because the per capita supply of the latter is ever dwindling as the human population grows larger. In fact, the past century has been marked by a continual effort to modify vegetable oils so that they may serve as replacements for butter, cream, and lard. Recently, there has been considerable controversy regarding the possible roles of the various fatty foods in the prevention or provocation of such disorders as atherosclerosis, cancer, heart disease, and obesity. Apparently, there are no simple answers to these questions, since dietitians, doctors, and nutritionists disagree on the relative merits and demerits of the different products. Therefore, some noteworthy background material on the vegetable oils is presented in the sections that follow.

HISTORY. The first fats produced by primitive peoples were those rendered from animal carcasses. Later, butter was obtained by churning the milk from domesticated animals. However, certain areas of the world became too densely populated to support a large population of wild or domesticated animals, and so the people in these places came to depend upon plants as sources of fats and oils.

It appears that olives may have been cultivated in various places around the eastern end of the Mediterranean Sea for at least 6,000 years. Similarly, the sesame plant has been grown for thousands of years in the tropical belt extending from Africa to India. Other sources of oil, such as coconut palm and the oil palm, have long grown wild in the tropics, where people gathered the nuts and extracted the oil. These oils (olive, sesame, coconut, and palm) keep better without refrigeration than most of the other vegetable oils. Hence, the stable oils have long been shipped to various parts of the world. Other, more perishable oils, such as safflower, were not articles of worldwide commerce until recently, when certain technological developments made it possible to reduce the potential for spoilage, or breakdown during frying.

PRODUCTION AND PROCESSING. At the present time, vegetable oils contribute the major share of the world production of fats and oils. Fig. O-12 shows the contribution of each of the important fats and oils.

The per capita utilization of the major fat and oil products in the United States is shown in Fig. O-13.

WORLD PRODUCTION OF FATS & OILS

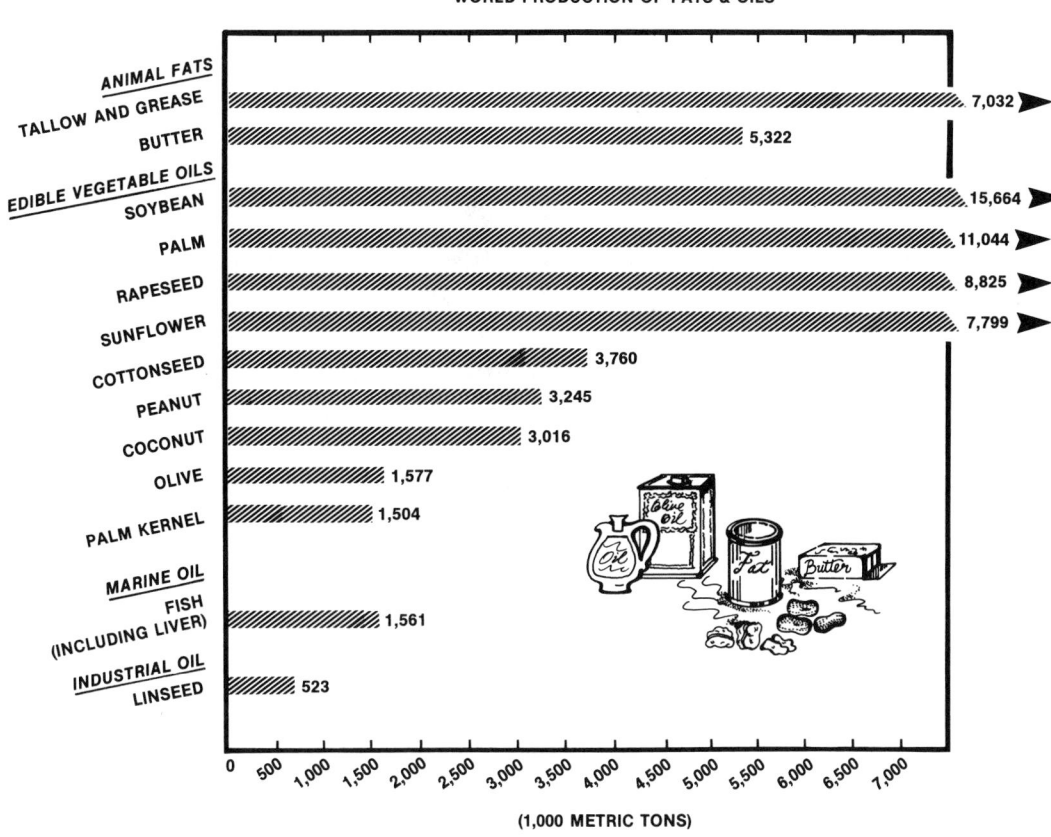

Fig. O-12. World production of fats and oils. (Source: *Agricultural Statistics 1991*, USDA, p. 135, Table 190)

U.S. PER CAPITA CONSUMPTION OF FATS AND OILS

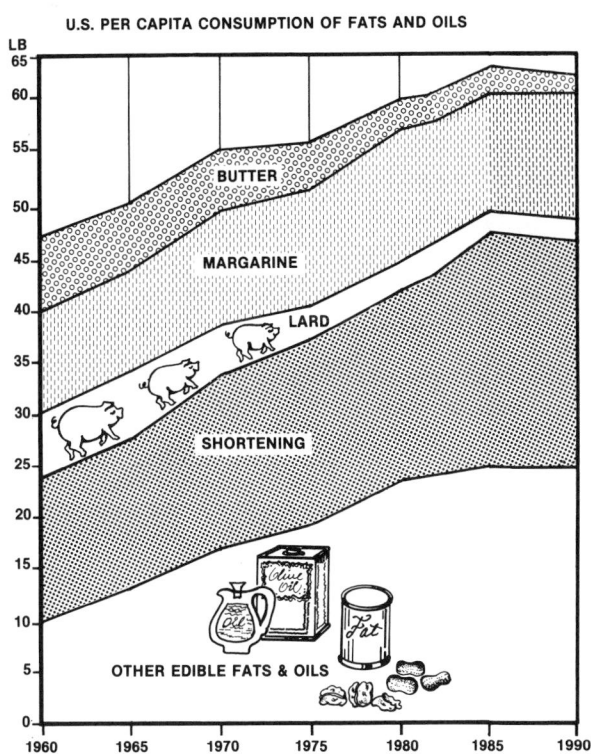

Fig. O-13. Per capita consumption of fats and oils in the United States between the years 1960 and 1990. (Source: *Statistical Abstract of the United States 1980*, p. 131, No. 211; and *Agricultural Statistics 1991*, USDA, p. 135, Table 190)

It may be seen from Fig. O-13 that the per capita consumption of both butter and lard has declined significantly in recent years, whereas the consumption of vegetable oil products has risen sharply. The categories of margarine, shortening, and other edible fats and oils represent mainly items made from vegetable oils.

Descriptions of the processes used in the production of vegetable oils and related products follow.

Extraction of Oils. Vegetable oils are enclosed within the cells of seeds or fruits. Hence, the plant tissues must be broken so that the oil may be extracted. Various processes have been developed to insure the maximum yield of oil because this product has generally brought considerably more profit than the extracted plant residue. Details of the more commonly used processes are noteworthy:

• **Cracking, crushing, flaking, or grinding of the oil-bearing tissue**—Depending upon the nature of the plant material, one or more of these processes are used to prepare the oil source for extraction; sometimes, the broken pieces are also cooked prior to extraction.

• **Pressing**—Various devices, ranging from small hand-operated presses to large mechanically driven expellers, are used to squeeze the oil from the pretreated pulverized plant tissue.

• **Solvent extraction**—Often, the residues from pressing are further treated with solvents such as ethylene dichloride or hexane to remove the remaining oil. Then, the oil and solvent mixture is heated to drive off the solvent.

(Also see SOYBEAN, Section headed "Extracting the Oil.")

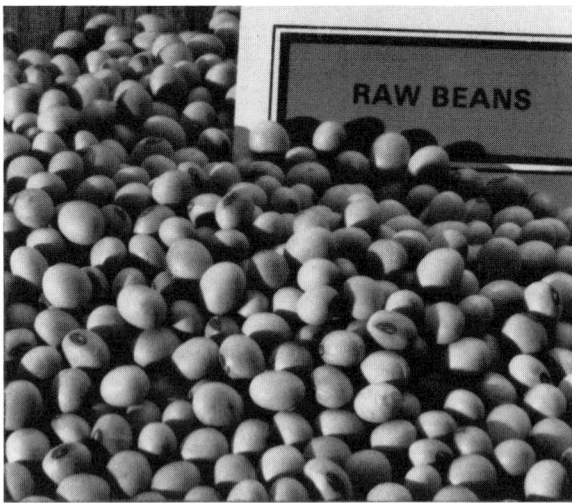

Fig. O-14. Soybeans, world's leading source of vegetable oil. (Courtesy, American Soybean Assn., St. Louis, Mo.)

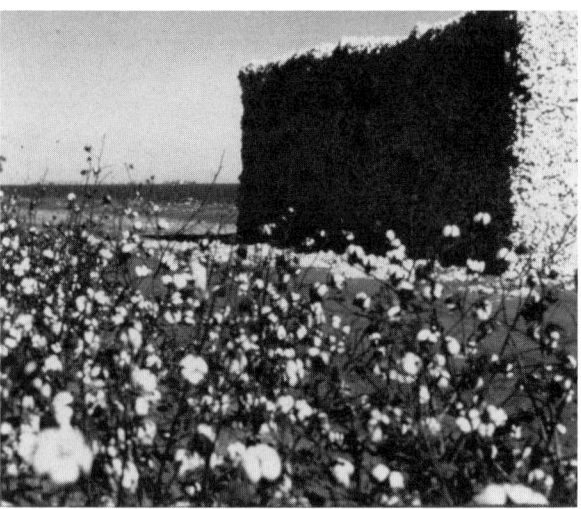

Fig. O-16. Cotton, the seed of which is the source of the fourth most consumed vegetable oil in the U.S. (Courtesy, USDA)

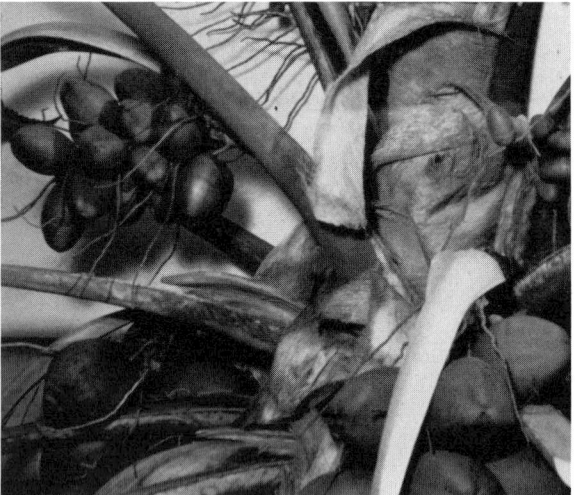

Fig. O-15. Coconuts, source of coconut oil, in demand by bakers and confectioners for use in coatings and fillings for baked goods and candy which may stand for a relatively long time between manufacture and consumption. (Courtesy, Field Museum of Natural History, Chicago, Ill.)

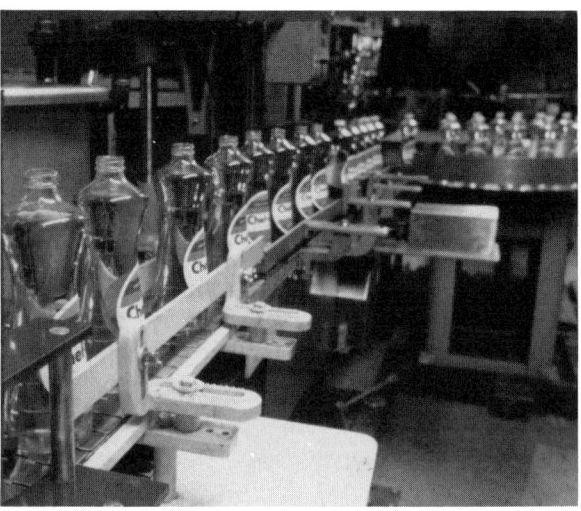

Fig. O-17. Soybean oil bottling line. (Courtesy, American Soybean Assn., St. Louis, Mo.)

Refining. Different processes may be used to refine each of the various oils, because the undesired constituents vary in each case:

• **Agitation with caustic soda**—The freshly extracted oil is stirred with alkali and heated in order to convert any free fatty acids to soaps. Then, centrifugation is used to remove the soaps, gums, sludge, and other undesirable materials. All traces of alkali are then removed by one or more washings with water, followed by centrifugation.

• **Bleaching (Decolorization)**—After alkali treatment, colored materials are removed from the oil by (1) the addition of fine particles of filtering clay and activated charcoal, and (2) passage of the mixture through a filter press to remove the colored materials absorbed into the clay and charcoal.

• **Deodorization**—Odoriferous materials are removed by the passage of steam through the heated oil in a vacuum chamber.

• **Winterization**—Certain oils contain fats which solidify (crystalize) at refrigerator temperatures and cause cloudiness. These harmless, but esthetically undesirable, components are removed by chilling the oil and filtering.

Hardening (Hydrogenation). This process is used to reduce the polyunsaturation of certain oils in order to (1) make them more solid at room temperature (for use in margarines and shortenings), and (2) increase their stability against deterioration when stored for long periods or when heated. It consists of (1) adding a trace amount of a nickel catalyst to the oil; (2) heating, and passing hydrogen gas through the oil in a converter kept under a vacuum; and (3) rebleaching, and removing the catalyst from the hydrogenated oil by filtration.

CHEMICAL COMPOSITION AND OTHER CHAR-ACTERISTICS. Both vegetable oils and animal fats are comprised mainly of mixtures of triglycerides, which are chemical compounds containing three molecules of fatty acids combined with one molecule of glycerol. Triglycerides differ from one another because their fatty acid content varies, while the glycerol in each triglyceride remains the same. Hence, the chemical and physical characteristics of vegetable oils depend ultimately on the types and amounts of chemically-combined fatty acids that they contain.

Fatty Acid Composition. Fatty acids are made up of hydrocarbon chains that contain an organic acid (COOH) grouping at one end. The backbone of the chain consists of carbon atoms connected by either single (saturated) or double (unsaturated) linkages (valence bonds). Saturated linkages are more stable than unsaturated linkages because the latter have the ability to combine readily with oxygen or other substances. Furthermore, fatty acids which contain two or more unsaturated bonds per molecule (polyunsaturated fatty acids or PUFA) are prone to rancidity (oxidative deterioration).

Another variable factor in the makeup of fatty acid molecules is the number of carbon atoms. Fatty acids are designated as having (1) short chains when the number of carbon atoms is 6 or less, (2) medium chains when there are 8 or 10 carbon atoms, and (3) long chains when the number of carbon atoms is 12 or more.

The properties of the various fatty acids depend mainly upon the combination of (1) the number of unsaturated bonds present, and (2) the length of the carbon chain. Table O-3 shows how these chemical characteristics affect melting points. Melting points of fats are very important in nutrition, because fats that remain solid in the digestive tract are utilized poorly.

It may be noted from Table O-3 that there is a steady rise in melting points as the chain lengths of fatty acids increase. However, for a given chain length, the melting points decrease as the degree of unsaturation increases. The latter principle is exemplified in the fatty acids with 18 carbon atoms by the high melting point for stearic acid (157°F, or 69°C), which is saturated; compared to those for monounsaturated oleic acid (56°F, or *13°C*) and polyunsaturated linolenic acid (12°F, or *-11°C*).

Although it is not shown in Table O-4, it is noteworthy that melting points of fats containing both low- and high-melting fatty acids are intermediate between the two extremes.

The relative amounts of saturated, monounsaturated, and polyunsaturated fats present in each of the commonly used vegetable oils are given in Table O-4.

TABLE O-4
FATTY ACID CONTENT OF 1-TBSP PORTIONS OF SELECTED VEGETABLE OILS[1]

Oil	Total Fat	Saturated	Mono-unsaturated	Poly-unsaturated	Other Minor Fats
	(g)	(g)	(g)	(g)	(g)
Coconut	13.6	11.8	0.8	0.2	0.8
Corn	13.6	1.7	3.3	8.0	0.6
Cottonseed	13.6	3.5	2.4	7.1	0.6
Olive	13.5	1.8	9.9	1.1	0.7
Peanut	13.5	2.3	6.2	4.3	0.7
Safflower	13.6	1.2	1.6	10.1	0.7
Sesame	13.6	1.9	5.4	5.7	0.6
Soybean	13.6	2.0	3.2	7.9	0.5
Sunflower, commercial	13.6	1.4	2.7	8.9	0.6
Sunflower, southern	13.6	1.4	6.2	5.5	0.5

[1]*Composition of Foods*, Ag. Hdbk. No. 8-4, USDA, 1979.

Chemical and Physical Properties. The wide variety of ways in which vegetable oils are utilized makes it necessary to have expeditious means for determining certain characteristics of these products. It is too expensive and time consuming for many commercial users of vegetable oils to assess the chemical and physical properties by the more comprehensive methods used in research studies. Some of the commonly conducted tests follow:

• **Iodine Number**—This test measures the degree of unsaturation of a fat. The higher the number, the greater the unsaturation. For example, the highly saturated coconut oil has an iodine value of only 9, whereas the highly unsaturated soybean oil has a value of 134. Susceptibility to oxidative rancidity increases, and the melting point decreases with the iodine value. It is noteworthy that this test is used to assess the amount of hydrogenation applied to vegetable oils. The value is usually given in the purchasing specifications for these products.

• **Saponification Value**—The name of this test is derived from the reaction (saponification) in which fats react with alkalis to form soaps, because the higher the value, the better the soap making potential. What is actually measured is the average length of the carbon chains in the fatty acids which constitute the fat. A high saponification value signifies a low melting point and a short chain length, and vice versa. For example, the value for coconut oil ranges between 250 and

TABLE O-3
CHEMISTRY OF FATTY ACIDS COMMONLY PRESENT IN VEGETABLE OILS

Name	Structure	Chain Length (no. C atoms)	Melting Point (°F)	Melting Point (°C)
Saturated:				
Caproic	$CH_3(CH_2)_4COOH$	6	18	*-8*
Caprylic	$CH_3(CH_2)_6COOH$	8	62	*16*
Capric	$CH_3(CH_2)_8COOH$	10	88	*31*
Lauric	$CH_3(CH_2)_{10}COOH$	12	112	*44*
Myristic	$CH_3(CH_2)_{12}COOH$	14	129	*54*
Palmitic	$CH_3(CH_2)_{14}COOH$	16	146	*63*
Stearic	$CH_3(CH_2)_{16}COOH$	18	157	*70*
Arachidic	$CH_3(CH_2)_{18}COOH$	20	170	*76*
Lignoceric	$CH_3(CH_2)_{22}COOH$	24	187	*86*
Mono-unsaturated:				
Palmitoleic	$CH_3(CH_2)_5CH = {}^1CH(CH_2)_7COOH$	16	31	*-1*
Oleic	$CH_3(CH_2)_7CH = CH(CH_2)_7COOH$	18	56	*13*
Poly-unsaturated:				
Linoleic	$CH_3(CH_2)_4CH = CHCH_2CH = CH(CH_2)_7COOH$	18	23	*-5*
Linolenic	$CH_3CH_2CH = CHCH_2CH = CHCH_2CH = CH(CH_2)_7COOH$	18	12	*-11*
Arachidonic	$CH_3(CH_2)_4CH = CHCH_2CH = CHCH_2CH = CHCH_2CH = CH(CH_2)_3COOH$	20	-57	*-50*

[1]The symbol = indicates a double valence (unsaturated) bond between adjacent carbon atoms.

264, because this product is rich in the fatty acids which contain 12 or fewer carbon atoms per molecule. On the other hand, the value for rapeseed oil ranges between 170 and 180, due to the high content of long-chain fatty acids.

• **Melting Point**—This is an important value for food processors because (1) consumers expect certain items to be solid at ordinary room temperatures, and others to be liquid; and (2) most shortenings should be at least semisolid at room temperature because flakiness of pastry depends upon the production of layers of solid fat. In common language, an item is called a fat if solid under ordinary conditions, or an oil if liquid. Ordinary conditions usually imply a temperature between 64°F (18°C) and 75°F (24°C). Products with a suitable melting point may be obtained by mixing high-melting items with low-melting ones.

NUTRITIVE VALUES. The nutrient compositions of the common vegetable oils are given in Food Composition Table F-21, and their fatty acid contents are given in Table F-4, Fats and Fatty Acids In Selected Foods.

Vegetable oils, like other highly edible fats, furnish about 9.3 Calories (kcal) per gram. Hence, 1 Tbsp (13.6 g) furnishes about 127 Calories (kcal). However, the most valuable nutritional assets of these products are the content of polyunsaturated fats and vitamin E. Nevertheless, the merits of the former may have been exaggerated somewhat over the past 3 decades, as exemplified by the growing doubts as to whether polyunsaturated fatty acids are efficacious in the prevention of heart disease. Also, the consumption of large amounts of vegetable oils might under certain conditions be hazardous to health. Therefore, some of the basic principles that bear on these and other controversial issues are noteworthy.

Essential Fatty Acids. The polyunsaturated fatty acid, linoleic acid, is required in the diet because it cannot be synthesized in the body. Linoleic appears to be needed in amounts of about 7.5 g per day.

Corn, cottonseed, safflower, soybean, and sunflower oils are excellent sources of linoleic acid, which comprises about one-half of the fatty acid content of these oils. Hence, about 1 Tbsp per day of any of them will provide the requirement for adults.

NOTE: The polyunsaturated fatty acid content of each of the oils listed in Table O-4 is mainly linoleic acid.

The essential fatty acids serve important functions in cell membranes, and as raw materials for the synthesis of hormonelike agents called prostaglandins. Deficiencies of these fatty acids result in skin disorders, reproductive difficulties, loss of hair, and perhaps even an increased susceptibility to high blood pressure. It is suspected that certain prostaglandins, that are synthesized from the essential fatty acids, help to control blood pressure.

(Also see FATS AND OTHER LIPIDS, section headed "Essential Fatty Acids.")

Polyunsaturated vs. Saturated Fats. Most vegetable oils, with the exception of cocoa butter, coconut oil, and the palm oils, are more unsaturated (they have higher iodine numbers) than most fats from animals. Marine animals and fish may also be rich in unsaturated fats. Also, vegetable oils are free of cholesterol, which is suspected of contributing to the development of atherosclerosis and heart disease, when excessive amounts of the sterol are consumed by susceptible people over long periods of time. Furthermore, the substitution of substantial amounts of vegetable oils for saturated animal fats such as butter, cream, lard, and meat drippings has sometimes led to (1) a modest (up to 20%) drop in blood cholesterol, and (2) a reduction in the tendency of the blood to form clots. However, arachidonic acid, a polyunsaturated fatty acid found mainly in peanut oil, promotes clotting.[27]

The effects of polyunsaturated fatty acids on the heart muscle are uncertain, since it has been found that the lifetime feeding of corn, cottonseed, or soybean oils produced more heart lesions in rats than beef fat, butter, chicken fat, or lard.[28]

Some of the other findings which call into question the wisdom of consuming large amounts of polyunsaturated vegetable oils have been summarized in a recent review.[29] They are as follows:

1. The drop in blood cholesterol may be due mainly to a shifting of the sterol from the blood to the tissues.
2. Polyunsaturated fats cause an increase in the amount of cholesterol secreted in the bile, a condition that sometimes leads to the formation of cholesterol gallstones.
3. Extra vitamin E is required to prevent the formation of toxic peroxides when the dietary level of polyunsaturated fats is raised. However, diets containing ample amounts of the essential trace mineral selenium (which is a part of the enzyme that breaks down the peroxides) may also help to offset this danger.

Medium-Chain Triglycerides (MCT Oil). This special dietary product is made from coconut oil by (1) steam and pressure hydrolysis of the oil into free fatty acids and glycerol, (2) fractionation of the resulting hydrolysate into medium-chain and long-chain fatty acids, and (3) recombination of the medium-chain fatty acids with glycerol to form MCT oil, which is made up of about ¾ caprylic acid (a saturated fatty acid containing 8 carbon atoms) and about ¼ capric acid (a saturated fatty acid containing 10 carbon atoms). The special nutritive values of this product are as follows:

1. It is much more readily digested, absorbed, and metabolized than either animal fats or vegetable oils which contain mainly long-chain triglycerides. Hence, MCT oil is valuable in the dietary treatment of fatty diarrhea and other digestive disorders in which the absorption of fat is impaired.
2. Medium-chain triglycerides, unlike other saturated fats, do *not* contribute to a rise in blood cholesterol.

At the present time, MCT oil is used almost exclusively for special dietary formulations in the United States, but it is also available in various nonmedical consumer products in Europe.

Vitamin E and Other Beneficial Substances. Vegetable oils and the seeds from which they are derived are the best food sources of vitamin E. For example, the amounts supplied by some typical oils (mg of vitamin E per 100 g [about 3½ oz] of oil) are as follows: wheat germ, 115; saf-

[27]"Dietary Essential Fatty Acids, Prostaglandin Formation and Platelet Aggregation," *Nutrition Reviews*, Vol. 34, 1976, p. 243.

[28]Kaunitz, H., and R. E. Johnson, "Influence of Dietary Fats on Disease and Longevity," *Proceedings of the Ninth International Congress of Nutrition (Mexico, 1972)*, Vol. 1, edited by A. Chavez, et al., published by S. Karger, Basel, Switzerland, 1975, p. 369, Table III.

[29]"The Biological Effects of Polyunsaturated Fatty Acids," *Dairy Council Digest*, Vol. 46, 1975, p. 31.

flower, 34; cottonseed, 32; peanut, 19; corn, 12; and soybean, 7.[30] It is noteworthy that these figures apply only to the amounts of alpha-tocopherol, which is the official standard for vitamin E activity. However, most vegetable oils also contain substantial quantities of related compounds (nonalpha-tocopherols) that have a reduced vitamin activity, but which, nevertheless, contribute to the total vitamin E value. Hence, some nutritionists have suggested that allowances also be made for the contributions of the other tocopherols.

Vegetable oils also contain plant sterols (phytosterols) that resemble cholesterol in structure, but which help to lower blood cholesterol by (1) interfering with its absorption, and (2) possibly accelerating its removal from the body.[31] It is noteworthy that vegetable oils which are very similar in fatty acid composition lower blood cholesterol by markedly different amounts. However, the anticholesterolemic effects of the oils are often in direct proportion to their content of plant sterols. For example, wheat germ oil, which contains approximately 5% phytosterols, has been shown to produce a much greater lowering of blood cholesterol than the other vegetable oils, which contain from 0.4% to about 1.0% phytosterols.[32] The higher plant sterol content of corn oil (about 1.0%) might also be the reason why this product is much more anticholesterolemic than soybean oil, which contains only about 0.4% phytosterols.

Antinutritional and/or Toxic Factors. Under certain conditions, small amounts of potentially harmful substances may be formed from polyunsaturated fatty acids. These substances present hazards only when large amounts of the affected oil products are consumed. This is *not* to suggest that these products be avoided, but rather that they should be used judiciously, while keeping in mind the possible consequences of misuse. Consider:

• **Peroxides**—The highly polyunsaturated fatty acids that are abundantly present in corn, cottonseed, safflower, soybean, and sunflower oils may be oxidized to toxic peroxides when exposed to air, heat, light, and metals such as copper and iron. Also, the long reuse of frying fats that have been overheated repeatedly is likely to result in the production of peroxides and other toxic substances.

Peroxides destroy vitamin E and help to speed the breakdown of polyunsaturated fatty acids in cell membranes. It is even suspected that these chemical reactions are responsible for some of the degenerative changes in the aging process because, upon autopsy, the brains of some senile people have been found to contain oxidized fats from cell membranes.

Some of the means by which the formation of peroxides in oils may be minimized are: (1) the addition of trace amounts of antioxidants; (2) storage of the oils in tightly capped, dark brown bottles in a refrigerator; (3) careful heating during frying so that smoking does not occur (a thermometer may be helpful to inexperienced cooks); and (4) straining of the oil

after frying to remove food particles, because they increase the tendency of the oil to smoke.

Peroxide formation and the breakdown of polyunsaturated fatty acids in the body may be prevented by vitamin E (synthetic antioxidants such as BHA and BHT do *not* act in the cells of the body). Also, the essential trace mineral selenium is part of the enzyme which breaks down peroxides once they have been formed. Therefore, adequate dietary intakes of both vitamin E and selenium are the best forms of insurance against toxicity from peroxides, when the handling of vegetable oils leaves much to be desired.

• **Trans Fatty Acids**—The hardening of vegetable oils by hydrogenation converts the naturally-occurring *cis* fatty acids to *trans* fatty acids which do *not* function as essential fatty acids. Also, some researchers have found that (1) the *trans* fatty acids were not as effective as their *cis* analogs in lowering blood cholesterol, and (2) fats rich in *trans* fatty acids appeared to promote atherosclerosis.[33]

The content of *trans* fatty acids generally increases with the extent to which a vegetable oil has been hardened by hydrogenation. For example, hard sticks of vegetable oil margarines may contain from 25 to 35% of *trans* fats, whereas lightly hydrogenated liquid oils usually contain 5% or less of these fats.

(Also see TRANS FATTY ACIDS.)

VEGETABLE OILS. Noteworthy information on each of the commonly used vegetable oils is given in Table O-5.

NOTE WELL: Where production figures are given in Table O-5, column 1 under "Importance," unless otherwise stated, they are based on 1990 data. Most world figures are from *FAO Production 1990*, FAO/UN, Rome, Italy, Vol. 44. Most U.S. figures are from *Agricultural Statistics 1991*, USDA. Annual production fluctuates as a result of weather and profitability of the crop.

[33]"Newer Concepts of Coronary Heart Disease," *Dairy Council Digest*, Vol. 45, 1974, p. 33.

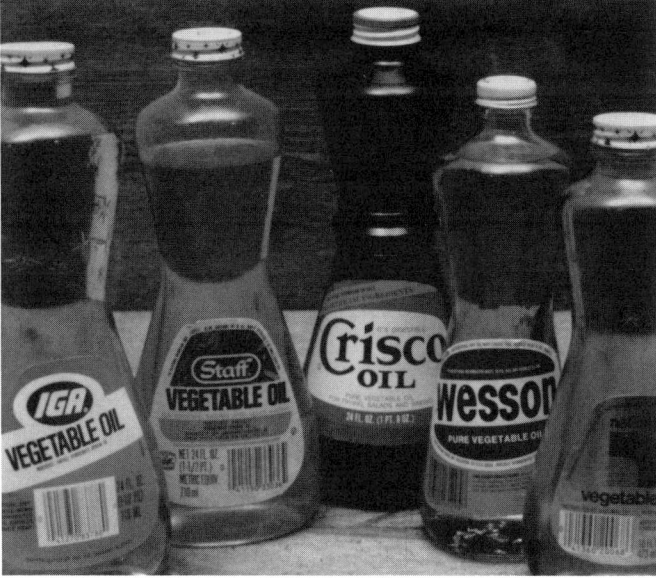

Fig. O-18. Several popular brands of vegetable oils. (Courtesy, American Soybean Assn., St. Louis, Mo.)

[30]Slover, H. T., et al., "Vitamin E in Foods: Determination of Tocols and Tocotrienols," *Journal of the American Oil Chemists' Society*, Vol. 46, 1969, p. 420, Table VII.

[31]Konlande, J. E., and H. Fisher, "Evidence for a Nonabsorptive Antihypercholestrolemic Action of Phytosterols in the Chicken," *The Journal of Nutrition*, Vol. 98, 1969, p. 435.

[32]Alfin-Slater, R. B., 1961, "Factors Affecting Essential Fatty Acid Utilization," *Drugs Affecting Lipid Metabolism*, edited by S. Garattini, and R. Paoletti, Elsevier Publishing Company, Amsterdam, Netherlands, 1961.

TABLE O-5
VEGETABLE OILS

Oil; Source; Scientific Name; Importance	Processing; Preparation; Uses	Nutritional Value[1]
COCONUT OIL **Source:** The nut (fruit) of the coconut palm tree, one of the world's most important crop trees. **Scientific name of coconut palm:** Family: *Palmae* Genus: *Cocos* Species: *C. nucifera* **Importance:** The world production of coconut oil totals about 9.6 million metric tons annually. (Also see COCONUT.)	**Processing:** Most coconut oil is obtained from copra by pressing in mechanical screw presses, sometimes followed by solvent extraction. In some areas, hydraulic cage and box presses are still used. **Preparation:** Crude coconut oil is refined and deodorized to remove free fatty acids and flavors. **Uses:** Because of the high percentage of lauric acid (45%), a saturated fatty acid, confectioners and bakers use coconut oil in coatings and fillings for baked goods and candy which may stand for a relatively long time between manufacture and consumption. Major uses of coconut oil are in shortening and oleomargarine, deep fat frying, detergents, laundry and toilet soaps. Minor uses are in filled milk, imitation milk, prepared flours, and cake mixes; lotions, rubbing creams, and in pressurized toppings. Recently, coconut oil has served as the raw material for producing medium chain triglycerides, which are very useful in the treatment of certain digestive disorders.	The fatty acids of coconut oil are: % Lauric .... 44 Myristic .... 18 Palmitic .... 11 Oleic .... 7 Caprylic .... 6 Capric .... 6 Stearic .... 6 Linoleic .... 2 Coconut oil has the highest percentage of saturated fatty acids of all common food oils; 86% vs 11% for corn oil. Hence, it is very stable, either alone or in products. Iodine value: 9 (This indicates the degree of unsaturation; It is the number of grams of iodine absorbed by 100 cm of fat. The higher the iodine value the greater the degree of unsaturation.) The high content of lauric, caprylic, and capric acids is a nutritional asset because these fatty acids are very useful in the dietary treatment of certain digestive disorders. However, the high degree of saturation of coconut oil may raise the blood cholesterol in some people, even though the oil itself contains no cholesterol.
CORN OIL **Source:** Corn (Maize) grain **Scientific name of corn:** Family: *Gramineae, the grass family* Genus: *Zea* Species: *Z. mays* **Importance:** Corn has always been important in North America. It accounts for 48% of the total world production of 475 million metric tons of corn grain; the United States alone produced 42% of the world total. (Also see CORN.)	**Processing:** Each year, about 6% of the U.S. corn crop is milled. Corn is wet milled for the production of starch, sweeteners, and oil; and corn is dry milled for the production of grits, flakes, meal, oil, and feeds. **Preparation:** Corn oil is further refined before using for food. **Uses:** Corn oil is used for salad dressings and cooking oil; and in such products as margarine and shortening. Also it is used in paints, varnishes, soaps, glycerine, and linoleum.	Corn oil is rich in essential fatty acid and contains moderate amounts of vitamin E. The chief fatty acids of corn oil are: % Linoleic .... 54 Oleic .... 29 Palmitic .... 13 Stearic .... 4 Iodine value: 127
COTTONSEED OIL **Source:** Derived from the seed of the cotton plant. **Scientific name of cotton:** Family: *Malvaceae* Genus: *Gossypium* Species: There are about 20 species, of which the following four are cultivated: *G. hirsutum,* American upland cotton; *G. barbadense,* Egyptian and Sea Island cottons; *G. herbaceum* and *G. arboreum,* the Asiatic cottons. **Importance:** Today, cottonseed oil is one of the most important food oils. It is the fourth most widely consumed vegetable oil in the United States, exceeded only by soybean oil, rapeseed oil, and sunflower oil. A ton of seed yields an average of 336 lb (152 kg) of oil. (Also see COTTONSEED.)	**Processing:** The oil is removed by three methods. The methods along with the proportion of the U.S. cottonseed production processed by each, follows: screwpressing, 40%; prepress solvent extraction, 28%; and direct solvent extraction, 32%. **Preparation:** The crude oil extracted from the seed is usually subjected to the following processes: (1) refined, (2) bleached, (3) deodorized, and (4) winterized. **Uses:** The principal use of cottonseed oil in the United States is in salad and cooking oils. It is also used in shortening, margarine, and mellorine—a frozen dessert that is comparable to ice cream in appearance and nutritive value. Cottonseed oil is also used in emulsifiers, pharmaceuticals, insecticides and fungicides, cosmetics, rubber, plastics, and finishes for leather, paper, and textiles.	Two major technological breakthroughs have largely eliminated gossypol as a barrier to cottonseed oil in food: (1) the separation of the pigment glands in processing; and (2) glandless cottonseed. Cottonseed oil is classified as a polyunsaturated vegetable oil. Linoleic acid, its principal fatty acid, comprises about 47 to 50% of the total fatty acids. Its unique crystalline properties result from the presence of about 26% palmitic acid. Its good flavor is generally attributed to the absence of linolenic acid. Cottonseed oil is preferred human food oil because of its flavor stability. Iodine value: 109

Footnote at end of table

(Continued)

TABLE O-5 *(Continued)*

Oil; Source; Scientific Name; Importance	Processing; Preparation; Uses	Nutritional Value[1]
OLIVE OIL **Source:** Derived from the olive, a fruit tree **Scientific name of olive tree:** Family: *Oleaceae* Genus: *Olea* Species: *O. europae* **Importance:** About 9.2 million metric tons of olives and 1.7 million metric tons of olive oil are produced annually in the world. In the United States, olive oil is a sideline. The major portion of the fruit is processed for eating. (Also see OLIVE.)	**Processing:** Olives are processed by crushing between stone or steel rollers. Then the crushed pulp is pressed, after which the oil is separated from the liquor. **Preparation:** Olive oil of good quality is ready to use following extracting, without refining. **Uses:** Olive oil is used chiefly in salad dressings and as a cooking oil. It is also used in soaps, perfumes, and medicines.	Olive oil is one of the most digestible of the edible oils. The fatty acid content of olive oil is: % Oleic .... 75 Palmitic .... 13 Linoleic .... 9 Stearic .... 2 Palmitoleic .... 1 Iodine value: 84 A medium size green olive averages about 5.8 Calories (kcal). Olives are a good source of calcium, iron, and vitamin A.

PALM OIL
Source: Derived from the oil palm tree.
Scientific name of oil palm:
Family: *Palmae*
Genus: *Elaeis*
Species: *E. guineensis*
Importance: Palm oil is one of the world's most important edible and soap-making oils. Moreover, the yield per acre is higher than can be obtained by any other vegetable oil. Annually, the world production of palm oil totals over 11 million metric tons, plus 3 million metric tons of palm kernel oil.
(Also see OIL PALM.)
	Processing: The traditional method of processing by farmers consists of (1) fermenting the fruits, followed by boiling, pounding, and skimming off the oil; and (2) cracking the nuts and exporting the kernels for processing.
	Modern factories process by steam distillation, followed by centrifuging or hydraulic expression. In industrialized nations, the kernels are either expressed or are solvent extracted.
	Correctly speaking, the fruits yield palm oil and the kernels yield palm kernel oil. But usually both are referred to as palm oil.
	Preparation: Palm oil of good quality is ready for certain uses following extracting, without refining. Although it is liquid when first extracted, it sets about as thick as butter at normal temperature.
	Uses: The leading producing countries use palm oil locally as food in all kinds of cookery, and export the surplus.
	When exported, palm oil is used chiefly for soap-making and industrial purposes. But, with suitable treatment, it may also be used in margarine.
	Palm kernel oil, which is white or pale yellow, is largely used for margarine.
		Palm oils vary; in some cases, they resemble kernel oil, and in others olive oil.
		The fatty acid profile of palm oil is:
		                            %
		Palmitic 48
		Oleic 38
		Linoleic 9
		Stearic 4
		Myristic 1
		The fatty acid profile of palm kernel oil is:
		                            %
		Lauric 51
		Myristic 17
		Oleic 13
		Palmitic 8
		Capric 4
		Caprylic 3
		Stearic 2
		Linoleic 2
		Iodine value of palm oil: 51
		Iodine value of palm kernel oil: 16

Footnote at end of table

(Continued)

TABLE O-5 *(Continued)*

Oil; Source; Scientific Name; Importance	Processing; Preparation; Uses	Nutritional Value[1]
PEANUT OIL **Source:** Derived from the peanut; a member of the pea family. **Scientific name of peanut:** Family: *Leguminosae* Genus: *Arachis* Species: *A. hypogaea* **Importance:** Peanuts, which contain 47 to 50% oil, are an important crop, especially in the warm regions of the world. Annual world production totals about: (1) peanuts in the shell, over 23 million metric tons; (2) peanut oil, 3.76 million metric tons. About ⅔ of the world's peanut crop is crushed for oil. Peanuts supply about 5% of the world's fats and oils. (Also see PEANUTS.)	**Processing:** The oil from peanuts is extracted by one of three methods: (1) hydraulic extraction, (2) expeller extraction, or (3) solvent extraction. **Preparation:** Following extraction, peanut oil is refined. The major portion of the characteristic peanut aroma and flavor is retained in the oil. **Uses:** In the United States, only a small proportion of the crop is processed for oil and protein concentrate. But in the rest of the world, peanuts are primarily processed for their separate constituents—oil and protein. Peanut oil is used primarily for food purposes; for frying foods, in salad oils, dressings, and margarine, and along with other vegetable shortenings. Also, peanut oil is used in soaps, face powders, shaving creams, shampoos, paints, as machinery oil, and in making nitroglycerin.	Peanut oil contains the following fatty acids: % Oleic .... 61 Linoleic .... 22 Palmitic .... 6 Stearic .... 5 Behenic .... 3 Arachidic .... 2 Lignoceric .... 1 Iodine value: 101 The major portion of the characteristic peanut aroma and flavor is imparted by the oil.
RAPESEED OIL **Source:** Derived from the rape plant, a member of the mustard family. **Scientific name of Rape:** Family: *Cruciferae* Genus: *Brassica* Species: *B. napus* and *B. camtestris* **Importance:** Rape oil is the only oil derived from an oilseed crop grown successfully in all parts of the world. Annually, world production of rapeseed totals about 24.5 million metric tons, and world production of rapeseed oil totals over 8.8 million metric tons. (Also see RAPE.)	**Processing:** The processing of rapeseed to obtain oil is similar to that of other oilseeds. There are three methods: (1) mechanical pressing, (2) straight solvent, or (3) prepress solvent-extraction. The latter is the method of choice. **Preparation:** The crude oil must still be refined. **Uses:** The primary use of rapeseed oil is for human food. It's relatively low linolenic acid content permits it to compete with other vegetable oils in shortenings, margarine, salad oils, and frying oils. Oils which are almost free of erucic acid will open up new uses of rapeseed oil.	In the past, rapeseed oil was high (it contained 40 to 45%) in the long-chain fatty acid, erucic acid. Since the nutritional studies indicate that this substance, along with glucosinolates which the meal formerly contained, can be detrimental to human and animal health if consumed in substantial quantities, plant breeders were stimulated to make genetic changes in the composition of rapeseed—to lower or eliminate erucic acid and glucosinolate. This change has proceeded at different rates in different countries, but is now nearly complete in Canada—one of the leading rapeseed producers of the world. Oil made from the new varieties of rape is almost free of the long-chain fatty acid, erucic acid, while the oleic acid content is significantly higher. Except for the presence of linolenic acid, the composition of the new oil greatly resembles olive oil. Canada renamed the changed plant; it is called *canola*.
SAFFLOWER OIL **Source:** Safflower, a relative of the thistle. **Scientific name of safflower:** Family: *Compositae* Genus: *Carthamus* Species: *C. tinctorius* **Importance:** The importance of safflower oil stems from its unique fatty acid composition, which places it highest in polyunsaturates and lowest in saturates of all commercial fats and oils. Annually, world safflower seed production totals about 922,000 tons. (Also see SAFFLOWER.)	**Processing:** In the United States, extraction of the oil is largely by the continuous screw-press solvent extraction method. **Preparation:** The oil must be refined. Due to the susceptibility of safflower oil to oxidation, care is taken to exclude air during storage, transport, and packaging. **Uses:** Safflower oil is used principally in the production of margarine, salad oils, mayonnaise, shortening, and other food products. The oil is also used as a drying agent in paints and varnishes.	Safflower oil is (1) extolled as a preventative of cholesterol build-up in the blood, and (2) recommended in the diets of persons suffering from heart disease and hypertension. The value of polyunsaturated fatty acids for such treatments, however, remains a matter of controversy. Safflower oil averages about 6.6% saturated acids and 93.4% unsaturated acids, with the latter consisting of 77.0% linoleic acid and 16.4% oleic acid. Linolenic acid is absent.

Footnote at end of table

TABLE O-5 *(Continued)*

Oil; Source; Scientific Name; Importance	Processing; Preparation; Uses	Nutritional Value[1]
SESAME OIL **Source:** Derived from the sesame plant, an annual herb. **Scientific name of sesame:** Family: *Pedaliaceae* Genus: *Sesamum* Species: *S. indicum* **Importance:** Annually, the world production of sesame seed now exceeds 2 million metric tons. (Also see SESAME.)	**Processing:** In those areas where sesame is primarily processed for its oil content, the seed is not dehulled; rather, the entire seed is crushed. **Preparation:** Sesame oil is natural salad oil requiring little or no winterization and is one of the few vegetable oils that can be used without refining. These are factors of increasing importance as energy costs escalate. **Uses:** Sesame oil is popular because of its pleasant, mild taste and remarkable stability—it is the most stable naturally-occurring liquid vegetable oil. Sesame oil is much sought because of the presence of a natural antioxidant, sesamol, and because of its high content of unsaturated fatty acids, 40% oleic and 44% linoleic. The oil is used as a substitute for olive oil—primarily as a salad and cooking oil and for margarine and soap. Also, a significant quantity of oil is used by the cosmetic industry for softening and soothing purposes and by the pharmaceutical industry as a carrier for medicines.	Due to the presence of natural antioxidants in the crude oil, sesame oil is the most stable naturally occurring liquid vegetable oil. It will keep for several years without turning rancid. The fatty acid composition of sesame oil is: **%** Linoleic .... 44 Oleic .... 40 Palmitic .... 9 Stearic .... 5 Linolenic .... 2 Sesame oil is classified as polyunsaturated. Iodine value: 114
SORGHUM OIL **Source:** Derived from the grain of the sorghum plant. **Scientific name of sorghum:** Family: *Gramineae* Genus: *Sorghum* Species: *S. bicolor* **Importance:** Sorghum is the staple food in parts of Asia and Africa. Sorghum is the fifth ranking cereal food crop of the world, being exceeded by wheat, corn, rice, and barley. Annually, the world sorghum crop totals over 58 million metric tons. (Also see SORGHUM.)	**Processing:** As with corn, sorghum may be either dry milled or wet milled. However, most sorghum is dry milled, simply because it is easier to accomplish. Sorghum oil is extracted from the germ of the grain. **Preparation:** For food use, sorghum oil must be refined, much like corn oil. **Uses:** Cooking oil; and in such products as margarine and shortenings.	The oil of sorghum is important nutritionally, and it influences flavor and acceptability of sorghum products. The fatty acid composition of sorghum germ oil is similar to corn oil (see CORN OIL). The ether extract of sorghum bran is composed mainly of long-chain alcohols and esters with some long-chain hydrocarbons.
SOYBEAN OIL **Source:** Soybean oil is derived from seeds produced by soybean plants. **Scientific name of soybean:** Family: *Leguminosae* Genus: *Glycine* Species: *G. max* **Importance:** Soybean oil is the leading vegetable oil for human food in the United States. In the Far East, soybean oil is consumed extensively as a food. Annually, world production of soybeans totals about 108 million metric tons, and world production of soybean oil is about 15.7 million metric tons. (Also see SOYBEANS.)	**Processing:** There are three basic processing methods of obtaining oil from soybeans: solvent extraction, hydraulic extraction, or expeller extraction. Today, almost all of the oil is extracted by the solvent process. **Preparation:** About 93% of soybean oil is used for food. To be suitable for human consumption, the extracted crude oil must undergo further processing, which is generally referred to as refining. **Uses:** Soybean oil is widely used throughout the world for human consumption as margarine, salad and cooking oils, and shortening. Also, soybean oil is used in paints, varnishes, enamels, soaps, linoleum, pharmaceuticals, cosmetics, core oil, synthetic rubber, and printing ink.	The fatty acid profile of soybean oil follows: **%** Linoleic .... 54 Oleic .... 24 Palmitic .... 12 Linolenic .... 8 Stearic .... 2 Soybean oil is low in saturated fat and free of cholesterol. Iodine value: 134

Footnote at end of table

(Continued)

TABLE O-5 *(Continued)*

Oil; Source; Scientific Name; Importance	Processing; Preparation; Uses	Nutritional Value[1]
SUNFLOWER OIL **Source:** Sunflowers **Scientific name of sunflower:** Family: *Compositeae* Genus: *Helianthus* Species: *H. annuus* **Origin and history:** The sunflower was first domesticated in the United States, although there is evidence that this honor should be shared with Peru and Mexico. **Importance:** Today, sunflower oil holds undisputed claim to third place among edible vegetable oils. Annually, world sunflower seed production totals about 22 million metric tons, and world sunflower oil production is about 7.8 million metric tons. Twenty-nine percent of the world's sunflower seed is produced in the U.S.S.R. Eighty percent of the vegetable oil produced in the Soviet Union comes from sunflowers. (Also see SUNFLOWERS.)	**Processing:** The separation of the oil from the seed may be acheived (1) by direct solvent-extraction, (2) by prepress solvent-extraction, or (3) by mechanical means (screwpressing). In the United States, sunflower oil is processed primarily by the prepress solvent-extraction method; and only small quantities of seed are dehulled prior to extraction. **Preparation:** Crude sunflower oil is stored in tanks following extraction until further processing. After refining, it has an attractive color and a pleasant, faintly nutty flavor. **Uses:** Cooking oil, salad oil, shortening, margarine, or for frying foods, making potato chips, producing modified butter with improved low temperature spreadability, and blending with other vegetable oils.	The fatty acid composition of sunflower oil makes it desirable as an edible oil. It follows: % Linoleic .... 66 Oleic .... 21 Palmitic .... 8 Stearic .... 5 As noted, sunflower oil is relatively low in the saturated fatty acids, palmitic and stearic. The high linoleic acid content and the high ratio of polyunsaturated to saturated fatty acid prompts some nutritionists to believe that sunflower oil might be useful in the prevention and treatment of high blood cholesterol and heart disease. Iodine value: 134

[1]Food Composition Table F-21 and Table F-4, Fats and Fatty Acids In Selected Foods contain additional information.

OLD PROCESS

Pertains to the extraction of oil from seeds. Same as hydraulic process.
(Also see SOYBEAN, section on ''Hydraulic Extraction.'')

OLEIC ACID

An 18-carbon unsaturated fatty acid (one double bond) which reacts with glycerol to form olein.
(Also see FATS AND OTHER LIPIDS.)

OLFACTORY

Pertaining to the sense of smell.

OLIGOSACCHARIDE

A complex carbohydrate which contains 2 to 10 molecules of monosaccharides combined through glycoside bonds.

OLIGURIA

Scanty urination.

OLIVE *Olea europaea*

Olives, which are classed as a fruit but used as a vegetable, belong to the olive family, *Oleaceae*.

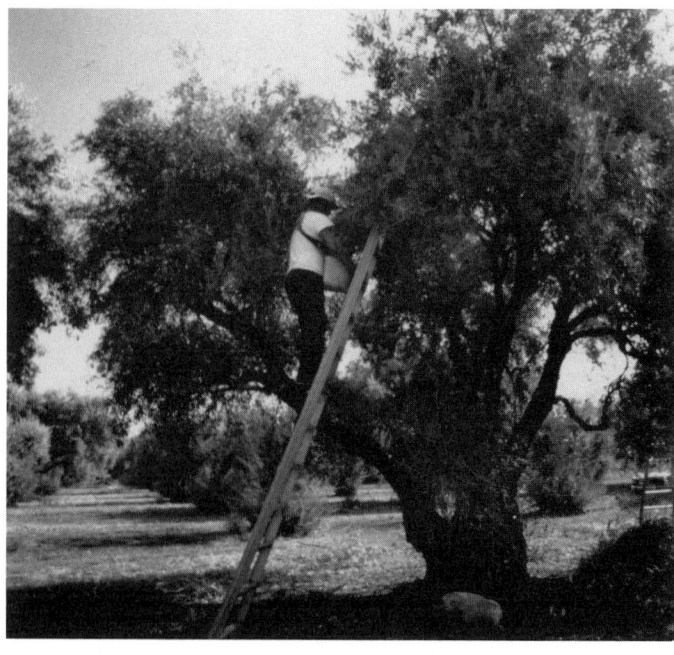

Fig. O-19. Olive tree showing olives being picked by hand—the way it is done. (Courtesy, California Olive Industry, Fresno, Calif.)

ORIGIN AND HISTORY.

It is not known when the wild olive was first brought under cultivation. But all indications are that the limestone hills of Attica, the Greek peninsula, was the seat of its first cultivation. The Spanish brought the olive to California in 1769.

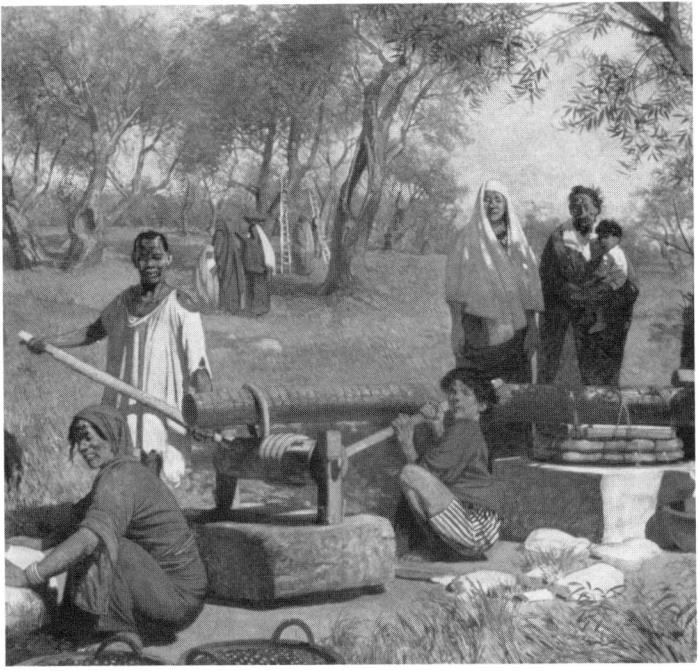

Fig. O-20. Primitive olive press. (Courtesy, Field Museum of Natural History, Chicago, Ill.)

WORLD AND U.S. PRODUCTION.

About 9 million metric tons of olives and 1.6 million metric tons of olive oil are produced in the world, annually. Most of the production is in the countries bordering the Mediterranean Sea. The leading olive-producers, by rank, are: Spain, Italy, Greece, and Turkey.[34] Spain and Italy produce 50% of the world's olives and 54% of the olive oil.

Olives rank fourteenth among the vegetable crops of the United States. About 131,000 short tons of olives are produced in the United States, annually.[35] California accounts for 99% of the olive production of the United States.

PROCESSING.

Olives were one of the first crops that man learned to adapt to his needs by developing special techniques for making the fruit edible and for extraction of the oil.

The methods of processing olives for the table vary widely. However, the three major commercial methods, known after the countries of their origin, are: (1) the Spanish method, in which unripe yellowish-green olives are fermented; (2) the American method, in which half-ripe, reddish fruit is used; and (3) the Greek method, in which the fully ripe, dark purple fruit is preserved. Additionally, there are numerous

local methods of processing, including pitting, stuffing, chopping, and spicing. In most processing methods, a weak solution of lye is applied for the purpose of neutralizing the bitter principle; the lye penetrates the olives and hydrolyzes the bitter phenolic glycoside, oleuropeen. The lye-treated olives are immediately rinsed and soaked in water with frequent changes in order to remove the lye. The washed olives are then placed in fermentation tanks and barrels and covered with brine.

Olive oil is produced by mechanical extraction of the ground fruit. Traditionally, this involves three steps: (1) crushing the fruit, (2) pressing (usually 2 to 4 times) the paste, and (3) separating the oil from the liquor. After the second pressing, the cake is usually solvent-extracted. Unlike most other vegetable oils, olive oil prepared from properly matured, harvested, and stored fruit is consumed without any refining treatment, thereby alleviating the need for added energy.

SELECTION, PREPARATION, AND USES.

Most table olives are prepared commercially in ready-to-serve form; hence, selection by the consumer is largely alleviated. Olives are commonly prepared commercially by one of the following methods:

1. **Canned or bottled green fermented olives (Spanish method).** This refers to green olives that are fermented, then put in jars or barrels. Increasingly, green olives are being pitted and the pit cavity stuffed with either pimientos, onions, almonds, anchovies, or other edibles.

2. **Canned ripe olives (American method).** The production of canned ripe olives is centered in California. The olives are picked when straw yellow to cherry red in color. In the curing process, the olives darken progressively due to the oxidation of the phenolic substances in a basic envi-

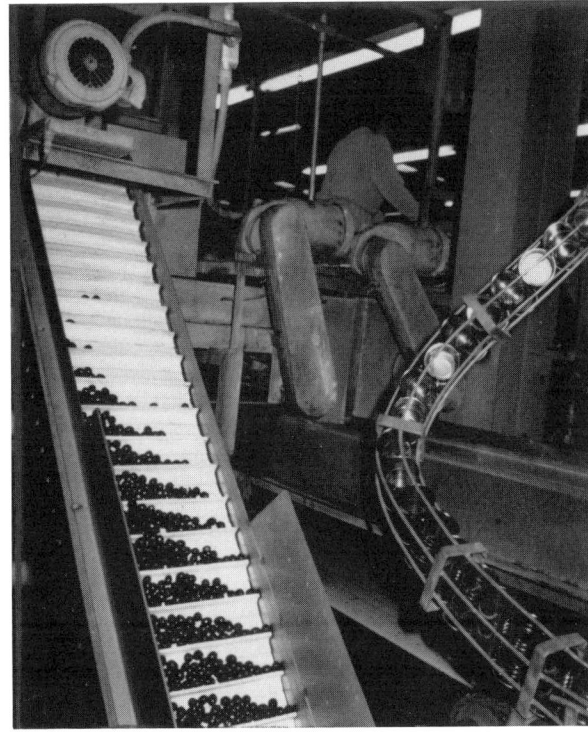

Fig. O-21. Ripe olives are canned in brine and heat sterilized. (Courtesy, California Olive Industry, Fresno, Calif.)

---

[34]Data from *FAO Production Yearbook 1990*, FAO/UN, Rome, Italy, Vol. 44, p. 120, Table 46. **Note well:** Annual production fluctuates as a result of weather and profitability of the crop.

[35]Data from *Agricultural Statistics 1991*, USDA, p. 371, Table 548. **Note well:** Annual production fluctuates as a result of weather and profitability of the crop.

ronment. The cured olives are packed in enamel-lined cans, covered with salt solution, sealed, and sterilized. More and more canned ripe olives are being pitted and stuffed.

3. **Black, naturally ripe olives (Greek method).** Olives to be prepared by this method are kept on the trees until they are fully matured and completely dark. The fruit is brined, with frequent changes of water in order to hasten the destruction of the bitter principle. Pretreatment with lye solution before brining, such as is used in the Spanish method, will hasten debittering and fermentation.

In addition to the above three major commercial procedures, a large number of different techniques for preparing olives for table use exist. Olives are often pitted, stuffed, chopped, and spiced, and put in fancy packs.

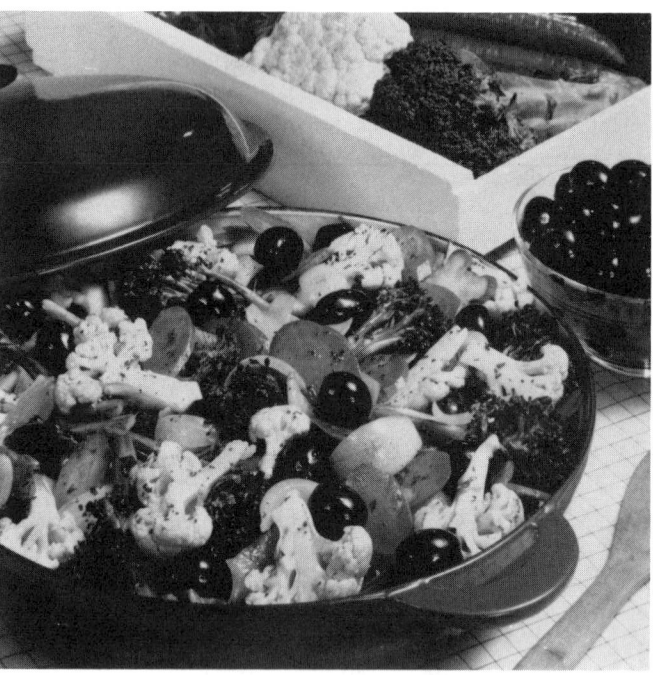

Fig. O-22. Olives enhance a vegetable dish. (Courtesy, Olive Administrative Committee, Fresno, Calif.)

Olives are used as a relish, and as an ingredient of salads and other mixed dishes such as pizza. Increasingly, table olives are becoming a luxury product in countries with high standards of living.

Olive oil of good quality needs no refining. The oil is highly esteemed by the gourmet. It is used chiefly in salad dressings, as a cooking oil, and for canning sardines.

NUTRITIONAL VALUE. The nutrient compositions of olives and olive oil are given in Food Composition Table F-21.

A few salient points regarding the nutritional value of olives follow:

1. At full maturity, the fruit meat (mesocarp) contains 15 to 35% oil. The pit, which accounts for 15 to 30% of the weight of the fruit, contains about 5% oil. The characteristic bitter glycoside, oleuropein, present in fresh olives, is concentrated close to the peel (exocarp).

2. Olives vary in calories according to size and oil content: On a per olive basis, they average about as follows:

Olive/Size and Kind	Calories/Olive
Medium, green	5.8
Medium, ripe	9.0

3. Olives contain fair amounts of iron and calcium and some vitamin A.

(Also see OILS, VEGETABLE, TABLE O-5.)

–OLOGY

Suffix meaning science of, or study of.

OMOPHAGIA

The practice of eating foods, particularly flesh, raw. The primitive diet of Eskimos consisted of raw meat and fish.

ONION *Allium cepa,* **variety** *cepa*

The onion, like the other related vegetables (*Allium* genus), has long been classified as a member of the Lily family (*Liliaceae*), but now some botanists place the onion and its close relatives in a new family called the *Alliaceae*. The common onion is classified as the variety *cepa* to distinguish it from other varieties of onions such as the shallot, which is the *aggregatum* variety. Fig. O-23 shows typical onion bulbs.

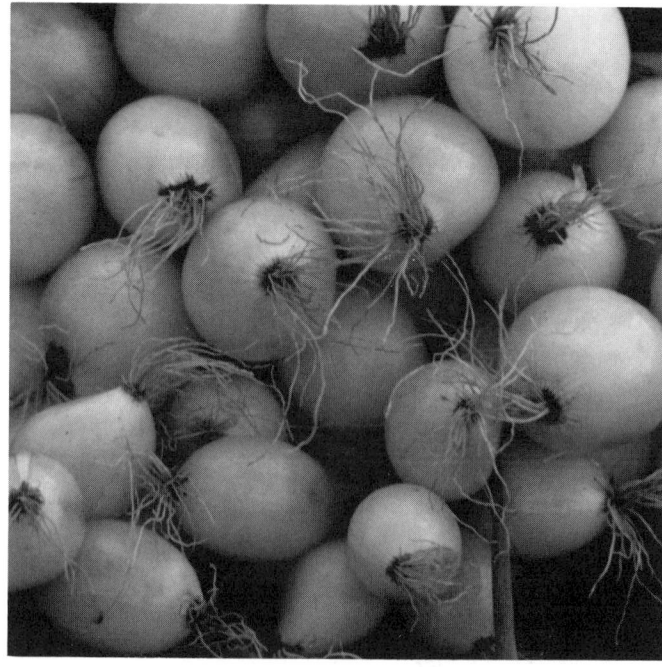

Fig. O-23. Onions, the sixth leading vegetable crop of the world. (Courtesy, University of Minnesota, St. Paul, Minn.)

The underground bulb of the onion plant is the sixth leading vegetable crop of the world. It is distinguished by its pungency when raw and the appetizing flavor it imparts when cooked with various other foods. The odor is due to an oil, which readily forms a vapor and escapes into the air when onions are peeled or cut. It affects nerves in the nose connected with the eyes, and makes tears flow.

ORIGIN AND HISTORY. Onions originated in the central part of Asia. Prehistoric man gathered and cooked wild onions. Some time after the dawn of agriculture in the Middle East, onions were grown in ancient Chaldea and Egypt. They were used as early as 5,000 years ago in the First Egyptian Dynasty.

WORLD AND U.S. PRODUCTION.

Onions rank sixth among the leading vegetable crops of the world, and fourth among the leading vegetable crops of the United States. About 27.9 million metric tons of onions are produced worldwide, annually. The leading onion-producing nations, by rank, are: China, India, United States, U.S.S.R., Turkey, Japan, and Spain.[36]

About 2.6 million short tons of onions are produced in the United States, annually. In descending order, the leading onion-producing states are: Texas, California, New Mexico, Georgia, Arizona, and Washington.[37]

PROCESSING.

The most common means of processing are:

• **Canning**—White-skinned onions, which are the most desirable ones for canning, are processed by removal of the papery skin, blanching, packing into cans, acidifying, and processing in a boiling water bath. Onions are also canned in prepared soups that require only heating.

• **Dehydration**—This procedure involves (1) burning off the onion skin and pieces of adhering roots, (2) washing with a high pressure stream of water to remove the charred pieces of skin, (3) slicing the deskinned onions thinly, (4) drying the slices with hot air, and (5) packaging the dehydrated pieces. Sometimes, dehydrated onion pieces are ground finely to make onion powder and onion salt.

• **Freezing**—Onions are commonly frozen in forms such as chopped raw onions, French fried onion rings, prepared soups, and TV dinners.

• **Pickling**—Small, immature onion bulbs are pickled by soaking in several changes of a salt solution (brine), boiling in fresh brine, and packing in a well-seasoned mixture of vinegar and sugar. Pickled onions are quite popular as an appetizer, and in certain cocktails.

SELECTION, PREPARATION, AND USES.

Professional chefs select types of onions according to how they will be utilized, since there are notable differences in flavor, pungency, and quality among the varieties commonly available in the United States. Hence, some guidelines for selecting and utilizing the various kinds of onions follow:

Dry Onions.

Pertinent information relative to the types, quality, and utilization of dry onions follow:

• **Types**—Two general classes of dry onions grown in the United States are found in retail markets: the mild flavored types, either large and elongated, or flat; and the usually stronger flavored types, generally globe shaped and medium in size. The former are *Spanish* or *Bermuda* types, and the latter are known as *globe* or *late crop* types.

• **Judging quality**—Bright, clean, hard, well-shaped, mature onions with dry skins are usually of good quality.

• **Utilization**—Onions are used as follows:

Chopped or sliced raw, which go well with roasted meats and poultry, and with other raw vegetables in relishes and salads.

Stewed, which may be served with butter, cheese sauce, or white sauce.

Broiled, which make a good accompaniment to broiled fish, fried liver, hamburger, and steak.

Stuffed with breadcrumbs, cooked kasha (buckwheat groats), fish, meat, poultry, and/or rice and baked like other stuffed vegetables. Stuffing requires large onions.

Dehydrated, and used in place of either raw or cooked fresh onions, provided that they are rehydrated sufficiently.

Powdered, or prepared as onion salt, which makes an excellent seasoning, but some of the flavor components of fresh onion are missing.

Finally, the various forms of onions may be added to a wide variety of casseroles, soups, and stews.

Green Onions.

These onions are usually early white or bulbless varieties that are harvested when the partially developed bulbs reach the desired size. Good quality green onions should have green, fresh tops, medium-sized necks well blanched for 2 or 3 in. (5 to 8 cm) from the root; and should be young, crisp, and tender.

Green onions may be served raw as an appetizer, or they may be chopped and added to cottage cheese, cream cheese, salads, and salad dressings. They are also good when pickled, stewed and served with a sauce, or when added to casseroles, soups, and stews.

NUTRITIONAL VALUE.

The nutrient compositions of various forms of onions are given in Food Composition Table F-21.

Some noteworthy observations regarding the nutrient composition of onions follow:

1. Dry, mature onions are high in water content (89%) and low in calories (38 kcal/100 g), protein (1.5%), and most other nutrients. They are a fair source of potassium, but they contain barely enough vitamin C to prevent scurvy (about 10 mg of vitamin C per 100 g).

2. Dehydrated onion flakes and onion powder contain almost ten times the solids content of fresh onions. Hence, the flakes and powder are much better sources of calories, protein, and other nutrients than the fresh bulbs.

3. The leafy tops of green onions are nutritionally superior to the green bulbs and to mature bulbs in that the tops are (a) a better source of potassium, (b) an excellent source of vitamin A, and (c) a good source of vitamin C. Hence, green onions should be eaten with the tops whenever feasible.

4. Europeans have long believed that onions have medicinal properties such as (a) prevention of colds, (b) loosening of phlegm, (c) correction of indigestion, (d) inducement of sleep, (e) stimulation of the appetite, (f) disinfectant in wounds, and (g) driving parasites from the digestive tract. Furthermore, they have often been added to food preparations to retard spoilage. So far, there has been only limited scientific documentation for these beliefs, consisting mainly of findings that onions (1) have a mild antibacterial effect, and (2) contain a substance (adenosine) which stimulates the breakdown of fibrinogen to fibrin, a protein in the blood which is involved in blood clotting.

---

[36]Data from *FAO Production Yearbook 1990*, FAO/UN, Rome, Italy, Vol. 44, p. 141, Table 58. **Note well:** Annual production fluctuates as a result of weather and profitability of the crop.

[37]Data from *Agricultural Statistics 1991*, USDA, p. 157, Table 222. **Note well:** Annual production fluctuates as a result of weather and profitability of the crop.

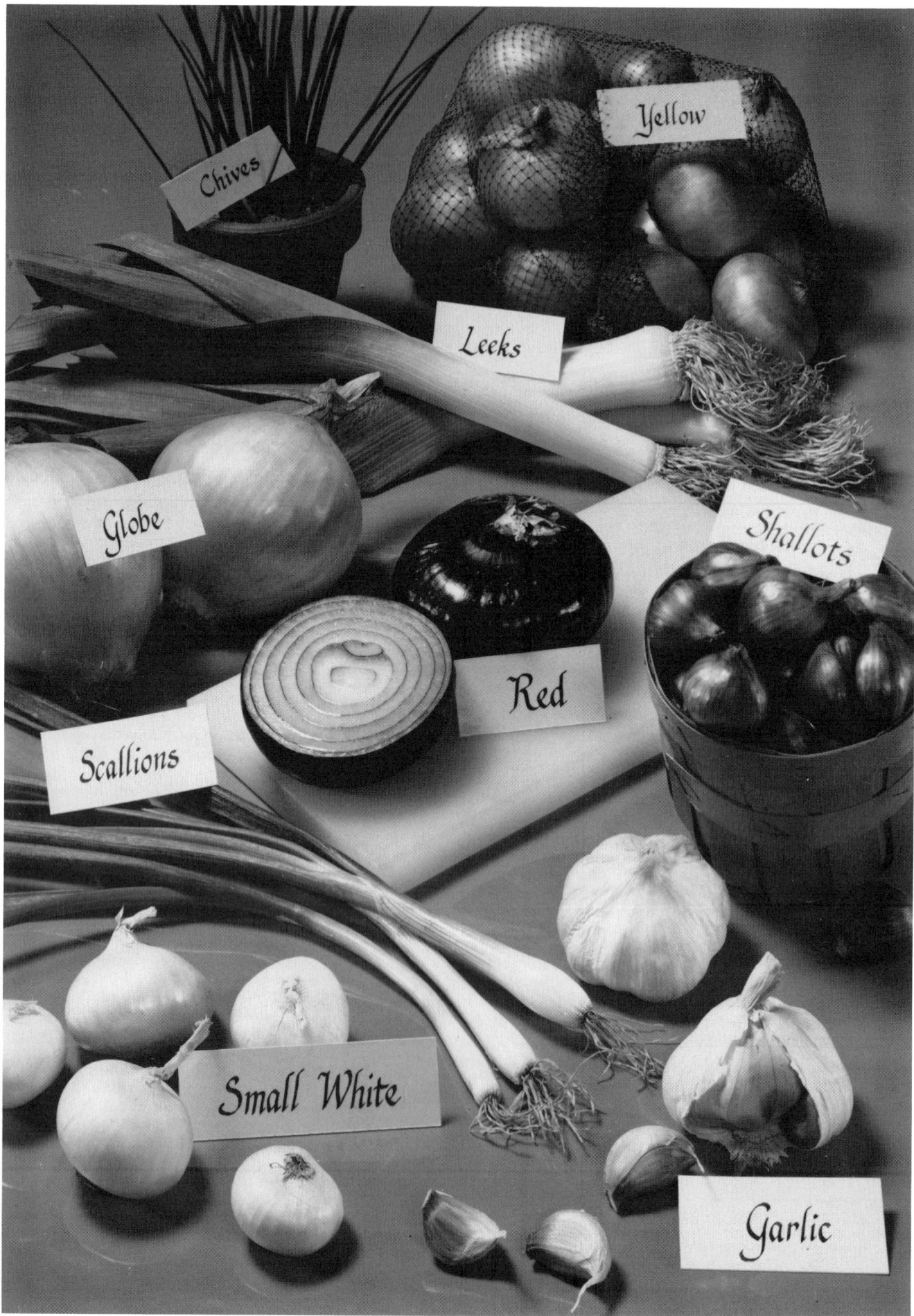

Fig. O-24. The onion and its close relatives. (Courtesy, United Fresh Fruit & Vegetable Assn., Alexandria, Va.)

ON-THE-HOOF

A term applied to a live animal; for example, the on-the-foot weight would be liveweight.

ON-THE-RAIL

A term applied to carcasses on the rail.

OPHTHALMIA

Severe inflammation of the conjunctiva (the membrane that lines the inner surface of the eyelids) or of the eyeball.

OPOSSUM

A marsupial, reaching the size of a rabbit, which abounds in certain regions of North America. The flesh is esteemed as a food in some sections and resembles that of rabbit.

OPSIN

A protein compound which combines retinal (vitamin A) to form rhodopsin (visual purple).
(Also see VITAMIN A, section headed "Functions".)

OPSOMANIA

Indicates a craving for special or certain foods—the pickles and ice cream appetite of pregnancy. In some cases, it may signal a deficiency of some essential element, for instance the periodic craving of chocolate may mean an insufficiency of chromium in the diet.
(Also see CISSA; and PICA.)

ORAL

Pertaining to the mouth.

ORANGE, BLOOD *Citrus sinensis*

Varieties of the sweet orange (a fruit of the *Rutaceae* family) in which the flesh of the fruit has a reddish tint due to the presence of anthocyanin pigments. It appears that the blood coloration develops only when the fruit is grown under hot, dry conditions such as those of the Mediterranean region. Hence, the major areas of production are Italy, Spain, Algeria, Morocco, and Tunisia. Blood oranges are usually consumed fresh, since the variability of the pigmentation presents difficulties in juice production and canning.
(Also see ORANGE, SWEET.)

ORANGE BUTTER

A mixture of butter or margarine, orange juice, grated orange peel, and/or other seasonings that is used as a sauce for dressing, cooked fish, meats, and poultry.

ORANGE JUICE

The fluid obtained from ripened oranges. Usually, it has been strained to remove excess pulp and seeds. Commercially canned orange juices may also contain juices from mandarin oranges (not more than 10%) and sour oranges (not more than 5%).

CAUTION: Some products may contain allergenic substances from the peel, but those made for infants contain little or none of these substances.

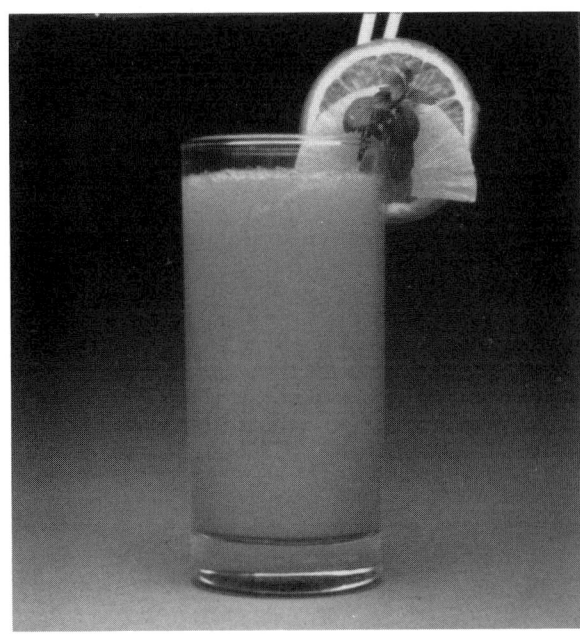

Fig. O-25. Orange juice, refreshing and high in vitamin C. (Courtesy, USDA)

The nutrient compositions of various forms of orange juice are given in Food Composition Table F-21.

Some noteworthy observations regarding the nutrient composition of orange juice follow:

1. A 1-cup (*240 ml*) serving of fresh orange juice provides 112 Calories (kcal) and 26 g of carbohydrates. It is an excellent source of potassium and vitamin C, and a fair to good source of vitamin A.

2. Canned, unsweetened orange juice is similar in composition to the fresh juice, except that it is about 20% lower in vitamin C.

3. Frozen orange juice concentrates contain over 3 times the nutrient level of the unconcentrated juice. Hence, it may make a significant nutritional contribution when added undiluted to sauces and toppings.
(Also see CITRUS FRUITS; and ORANGE, SWEET.)

ORANGE PEKOE

This refers to the grade of tea leaves from which a black tea is made. Orange pekoe leaves are the smallest grade of leaves, and they are generally from the tips of the branches of the tea plant.
(Also see TEA.)

ORANGE, SWEET *Citrus sinensis*

This citrus species is by far the leading fruit crop of the United States, and it is the second leading one of the world. (Grapes are first, and bananas, watermelons, and plantains follow in that order.)

There are two kinds of closely related oranges—the sweet orange, and the sour (Seville) orange. Both are members of the rue family, *Rutaceae*.

This article pertains to the sweet orange, which is the one commonly grown and eaten in the United States (for sour orange, see SEVILLE ORANGE).

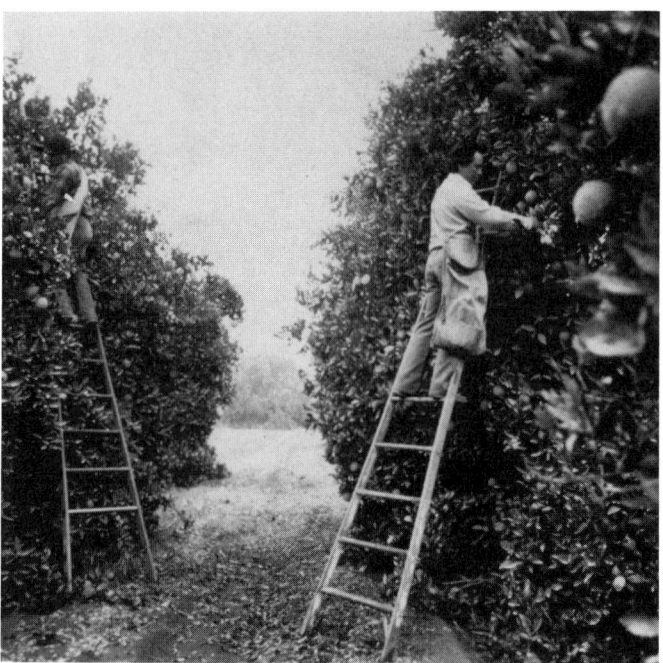

Fig. O-26. Orange trees, showing ripe oranges being hand-picked. (Courtesy, USDA)

Sweet oranges grow best in subtropical climates. Hence, commercial orange production in the United States is limited to Florida, Texas, Arizona, and California.

ORIGIN AND HISTORY. The sweet orange originated in southern China, but it was domesticated so long ago that it is no longer known in the wild. Oranges were not introduced to the Mediterranean region until about 1500 A.D. They were brought to America by the Spanish and Portugese in the 1500s.

WORLD AND U.S. PRODUCTION. Worldwide, over 52 million metric tons of oranges are produced annually; and the leading orange-producing countries, by rank, are: Brazil, United States, China, Spain, Mexico, India, Italy, Egypt, Iran, and Pakistan.[38]

Fourteen percent of the world's orange crop comes from the United States, where oranges are the number one fruit crop. About 7.8 million short tons of oranges are produced annually in the United States. Florida is the leading state by a wide margin; it accounts for more than 84% of the nation's orange crop. In descending order, the ranking of the other states are: California and Arizona.[39]

PROCESSING. About 84% of the U.S. orange crop is processed. The leading item is frozen orange juice concentrate, which utilizes almost 80% of the oranges that are grown for processing.

---

[38]Data from *FAO Production Yearbook 1990*, FAO/UN, Rome, Italy, Vol. 44, p. 163, Table 71. **Note well:** Annual production fluctuates as a result of weather and profitability of the crop.

[39]Data from *Agricultural Statistics 1991*, USDA, p. 189, Table 278. **Note well:** Annual production fluctuates as a result of weather and profitability of the crop.

An additional 15% of the orange crop is used to make chilled fresh orange juice that is packed in glass bottles, plastic bottles, and paperboard cartons; while the remainder is converted into canned orange juice and orange juice blends, canned orange sections, and chilled fresh orange sections packed in glass or plastic containers.

SELECTION, PREPARATION, AND USES. Fresh oranges of the best quality are firm, heavy, have a fine-textured skin for the variety, and are well-colored.

Preparation of fresh oranges is relatively simple. It consists of peeling, then serving fresh orange halves or sections alone or with other fruit.

Fresh orange sections and freshly squeezed orange juice have tangy flavors that may not be present in processed orange products because heating during processing drives off some of the aromatic constituents of the fruit. Furthermore, certain types of processing also reduce the content of vitamin C and bioflavonoids (vitaminlike substances). Therefore, some suggestions for using fresh fruit and juice follow:

1. Orange sections go well with other, more bland-flavored fruits such as apples, apricots, avocados, bananas, blueberries, cherries, figs, melons, peaches, and pears. It might also be a good idea to add some orange juice to the fruit mixtures to prevent cut pieces of certain fruits from darkening.

2. The flavor of oranges or orange juice also enhances such vegetables as beets, carrots, squash, and sweet potatoes. A little honey with butter or margarine helps to bring about the blending of the citrus and vegetable flavors.

3. Weight watchers may make a low calorie snack or a light meal by combining orange sections with lowfat cottage cheese or plain (unflavored) yogurt. The fruit also goes well with custard, ice cream, ices, puddings, and sherbets.

4. More nutritious gelatin desserts and salads may be prepared from fresh oranges, orange juice, and unflavored gelatin than from flavored gelatin dessert mixes.

5. The fruit sections may be added to sauces for fish, meats, poultry, and seafood, or to salads which contain these ingredients.

6. Orange juice may be mixed into thick jams and marmalades in order to (a) make them more spreadable and (b) raise their nutrient levels.

NUTRITIONAL VALUE. The nutrient compositions of various forms of oranges are given in Food Composition Table F-21.

Some noteworthy observations regarding the nutrient composition of oranges and orange products follow:

1. Fresh oranges are low in calories (49 kcal per 100 g), a good source of fiber, pectin, and potassium; an excellent source of vitamin C, inositol, and bioflavonoids (vitaminlike substances); and a fair source of folic acid.

2. Fresh orange juice contains about the same levels of most of the nutrients present in fresh oranges, except for fiber, pectin, and the bioflavonoids, which are present mainly in the peel and the membranes which surround the segments of fruit.

3. Higher quantities of vitamin C and folic acid are likely to be retained in chilled fresh orange juice packed in bottles or cartons than in canned orange juice which is heated strongly during canning, then stored at room temperature for an extended period of time.

4. Frozen orange juice concentrate contains from 3 to 4 times the levels of calories and nutrients of an equal amount of fresh orange juice. Hence, the concentrate may

make a significant nutritional contribution when it is added undiluted to various beverages, salad dressings, sauces, and toppings.

5. Dehydrated pure orange juice crystals contain over 8 times the levels of calories and nutrients of equal amounts of fresh orange juice. At the present time the crystals are sold mainly by institutional food service suppliers. (The dry mixes sold in retail groceries usually contain considerable amounts of added sugar.)

6. Orange and apricot drink (contains 40% fruit juices) supplies about 3 times the vitamin A of orange juice, but less than half as much potassium and vitamin C.

(Also see BIOFLAVONOIDS; CITRUS FRUITS; FIBER; and VITAMIN C.)

ORGANIC

Substances derived from living organisms. Carbon-containing compounds.

ORGANIC ACID

Any organic compound that contains a carboxyl group (COOH).

ORGANICALLY GROWN FOOD

This phrase and the phrases *organic food, organic gardening, natural foods,* and *health foods* are all related, carrying similar implications. Natural and health foods are often the products of organic farming or gardening methods.

At present, there is no national definition of *organic,* and no nationwide program to monitor produce labeled *organically grown.* However, 25 states have established their own definitions. Also, the Farm Bill of 1990 requires that by October 1993, plans for national certification be in effect.

Although the term organic traditionally refers to compounds of carbon, J. I. Rodale, the father of the organic farming and food movement in the United States, defined organic as meaning production of crops without using pesticides and chemical fertilizers. Recently, the USDA defined organic farming as follows:

"Organic farming is a production system which avoids or largely excludes the use of synthetically compounded fertilizers, pesticides, growth regulators, and livestock feed additives. To the maximum extent feasible, organic farming systems rely upon crop rotations, crop residues, animal manures, legumes, green manures, off-farm organic wastes, mechanical cultivation, mineral-bearing rocks, and aspects of biological pest control to maintain soil productivity and tilth, to supply plant nutrients, and to control insects, weeds, and other pests."[40]

Often, the meanings for *organic, natural,* and *health* which people imply or conjure up in their minds, are misleading, harmful, and tend to polarize people. The growing interest of consumers in the safety and nutritional quality of the American diet is a welcome development. Regrettably, however, much of this interest has been colored by those who state or imply that the American food supply is unsafe or somehow inadequate to meet our nutritional needs.

[40]*Report and Recommendations on Organic Farming,* USDA, 1980.

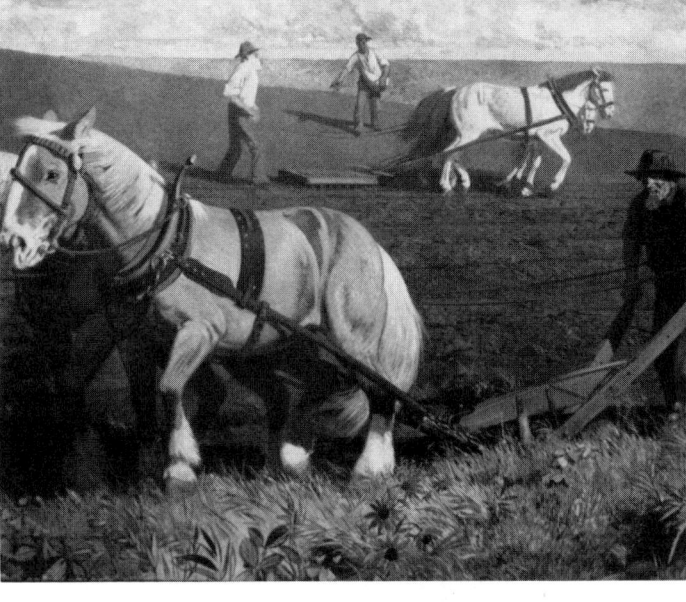

Fig. O-27. How it used to be done—organically grown. (Courtesy, Field Museum of Natural History, Chicago, Ill.)

The Food and Drug Administration (FDA) has taken no position on use of the terms *organic, natural,* and *health* in food labeling, since the terms are often used loosely and interchangeably. The Federal Trade Commission in its proposed Food Advertising Rule would prohibit use of the words *organic* and *natural* in food advertising because of concern about the ability of consumers to understand the terms in the conflicting and confusing ways they are used. FTC also proposes to prohibit the term *health food* in advertising because it is undefined and may fool consumers into thinking one particular food will provide good health.

Food Quality. Much of the promotion of organically grown food, natural and health foods included, comes from the idea that these foods are nutritionally superior to foods grown by conventional agricultural methods. Moreover, organically grown foods are promoted as containing no pesticides or additives, while conventionally grown foods are pictured as being poisoned with pesticides and additives. The truth is, that once organically grown and conventionally grown foods are removed from the field they cannot be identified as to their origin. Plants convert inorganic compounds to organic compounds. Therefore, it is relatively immaterial whether conventional methods or organic methods are followed. Inorganic ions—nitrates, potassium, iron, phosphate—are taken up by the plant roots and manufactured into new organic materials. The nutrient content of a crop—the amount of protein, carbohydrate, fat, vitamins, and most minerals—is largely determined by plant genetics, weather, and time of harvest. Scientific experiments at the Michigan Experiment Station for 10 years; at the United States Plant, Soil and Nutrition Laboratory in Ithaca, New York for 25 years; and as well as a 34-year investigation of organic and chemical agriculture on a British experimental farm failed to show a nutritional superiority of organically grown foods compared to conventionally grown foods.

Organically grown foods contain pesticide residues just as often as do conventional foods, although they may be present in smaller amounts. However, all residues are within Federal tolerance levels, which are set low enough to protect consumers. As for poisons in the food supply, many common foods contain naturally-occurring toxicants, but these are usually present in low levels and pose no health hazards. Poison is a matter of dosage. Further, a poisonous substance made by a plant is no different than the same substance made in a laboratory.

(Also see ADDITIVES; section on "Government Controls of Additives"; and POISONS.)

Food Quantity. The use of chemical fertilizers has been partly responsible for the abundance of food available. If all farmers were to adopt organic methods, there would be a decline in productivity as shown in Table O-6.

TABLE O-6
ESTIMATED NATIONAL AVERAGE CROP YIELDS
UNDER CONVENTIONAL AND ORGANIC FARMING[1]

Crop	Bushels per Acre	
	Conventional	Organic
Corn	98	49
Wheat	43	20
Soybeans	40	20
Other grains	57	17

[1]*Organic and Conventional Farming Compared,* Council for Agricultural Science and Technology (CAST), Report No. 84, October 1980, p. 24, Table 6.

Cost. One major difference between organically grown food and conventionally grown food is that it is often sold at relatively high prices to persons who are willing to tolerate imperfections in return for the suggestion that commercial fertilizers, pesticides, and additives have not been used. Numerous surveys have indicated that people will pay 30 to 100% more for organically produced foods than for their regular counterparts.

Individuals who desire organic foods—foods grown without the use of modern chemical technology—seem to be left with two choices: (1) purchase organic foods from a reputable dealer and pay the price; or (2) engage in organic gardening and grow their own.

Summary. Good farmers have always incorporated many of the so-called organic methods, and they have also incorporated new methods such as chemical fertilizer, pesticides, and the other chemical methods which ensure more food for all and at a reasonable price. Undoubtedly, world food production of the future will make use of a combination of both organic and inorganic fertilizers, with the nature and proportions of the combination for different farms and for different countries dependent on their access to fossil fuels, the availability and price of fertilizers, their

soils, their food production requirements, their environmental control problems, and many other factors. Regardless of the combination of organic and inorganic fertilizers used, feed and food plants of adequate nutritional quality can be produced.

Furthermore, to meet world food needs, pesticides and other chemical methods cannot be altogether abandoned. Even with the use of pesticides, about one-third of the food produced is lost to pests.

All foods are organic, and all edible foods, when properly selected for a balanced diet, are conducive to physiological and psychological health regardless of whether they are organically grown (as defined) or conventionally grown.

(Also see ADDITIVES, section on "Government Controls of Additives"; DELANEY CLAUSE; HEALTH FOODS; PESTICIDES; PESTICIDES AS INCIDENTAL FOOD ADDITIVES; and POISONS.)

ORGAN MEAT

Any edible part of a slaughter animal that consists of, or forms a part of, an internal organ, such as the liver, kidney, heart, or brain; distinguished from carcass meat.

ORGANOLEPTIC

It describes the employment of one or more of the special senses. Subjecting food to an organoleptic test employs the sensations of smell, taste, touch, and vision. We accept or reject food based on its organoleptic properties. The food industry sells food based on its organoleptic properties. First the consumer assesses the appearance (vision) and aroma (smell), but most important are the in-the-mouth properties—flavor, texture, and consistency.

(Also see TASTE.)

ORGEAT

• A nonalcoholic beverage prepared from the sweetened juice of almonds and other flavorings (such as orange blossom essence, or rose water), usually served cold.

• A sweet almond-flavored nonalcoholic syrup used as a cocktail ingredient or food flavoring.

ORNITHINE-ARGININE CYCLE (UREA CYCLE)

A cyclic sequence of biochemical reactions in protein metabolism in which citrulline is converted to arginine, thence urea splits off from arginine, producing ornithine.

(Also see UREA CYCLE.)

ORTANIQUE *Citrus reticulata X C. sinensis*

A citrus fruit (of the family *Rutaceae*) that was discovered growing in Jamaica, West Indies in 1920. It is believed to be the result of a natural crossbreeding (hybridization) between the mandarin orange (*C. reticulata*) and the sweet orange (*C. sinensis*). It is about the size of an average orange and it is flattened at both ends like certain tangerines. The fruit is quite juicy and its flavor is distinctive. Also, the rind adheres tightly, but is readily peelable.

OSMOPHILIC YEAST

Food preservation by high concentration of sugars or salts, such as in jams and pickles, takes advantage of the inability of most types of microorganisms to grow under this condition—high osmotic pressure. Some yeasts—osmophilic yeasts—are adapted. They thrive under the condition of high osmotic pressure.

(Also see PRESERVATION OF FOOD.)

OSMOSIS

The passage of a solvent such as water through a semipermeable membrane from the side of the membrane where the solution is dilute, to the side where the solution is more concentrated.

OSMOTIC PRESSURE

The force acting upon a semipermeable membrane placed between two solutions of differing concentrations.

OSSEIN

When the mineral salts of bone are dissolved by a dilute acid, the remaining organic material is called ossein.

(Also see PROTEIN[S].)

OSSIFICATION

The process of bone formation.

OSTEITIS

Inflammation of a bone.

OSTEO–

Prefix meaning bone.

OSTEOBLAST

Bone-forming cells.

OSTEODYSTROPHY (OSTEODYSTROPHIA)

Defective ossification of bone, usually associated with disturbed calcium and phosphorus metabolism and renal insufficiency.

OSTEOMALACIA

Osteomalacia is most prevalent in areas where either climate or clothing practices limit exposure of skin to sunlight, or where the diet does not supply correct proportions of calcium, phosphorus, and vitamin D.

Osteomalacia is an adult form of rickets caused by lack of vitamin D, inadequate intake of calcium or phosphorus, or an incorrect dietary ratio of calcium and phosphorus. It is characterized by a softening and deformity of bones, bone tenderness and pain, muscular weakness, and tetany.

The recommended treatment: administration of vitamin D (1,000 IU daily) and calcium (1-2 g per day). Care should be taken that vitamin D toxicity does not develop during treatment.

Prevention consists in exposure of skin to sunlight or sunlamps, fortification of milk with vitamin D, and provision of extra calcium when diets are high in oxalates or low in calcium (dietary phosphorus is usually adequate).

(Also see BONE, section on "Bone Disorders"; CALCIUM, section on "Calcium Related Diseases"; PHOSPHORUS, section on "Phosphorus Related Diseases"; VITAMIN D, section on "Deficiency Symptons"; and RICKETS.)

OSTEOPOROSIS

Contents   Page

A loss of bone mass which generally occurs with aging is called osteoporosis. When such loss is signficant (such as one-third of the original adult bone mass), bones will fracture easily and heal poorly. Recent research has shown that osteoporosis often occurs in the skeleton in the following order:[41]

1. The alveolar bone in the jaw.
2. The spinal column.
3. The long bones of the body.

CAUSES OF OSTEOPOROSIS. Many investigations conducted in man and animals have led to tentative explanations of why osteoporosis is a problem in the United States where, on the average, dietary calcium intakes are higher than elsewhere in the world. Some of the theories concerning this problem follow.

Dietary Deficiencies of Calcium. A dietary survey of the United States, made by the Department of Agriculture, showed that adult females had calcium intakes around two-thirds of their RDA (800 mg of calcium per day).[42]

Dietary Imbalances of Calcium and Phosphorus. Diets in the United States are believed to contain disproportionately high ratios of phosphorus to calcium (about 5 to 1), which have been shown in animal studies to result in significant loss of bone minerals.[43]

(Also see CALCIUM-PHOSPHORUS RATIO; and VITAMIN D.)

High Protein Intakes. Investigators at the University of Wisconsin found that the amounts of calcium needed to balance urinary and fecal losses in young adult males increased as their dietary protein levels were raised.[44] On the average, these young men required about 10 mg of calcium for every gram of protein.

Similar findings were obtained by researchers at the University of California at Berkeley, who also noted that the elevations in urinary calcium caused by high levels of dietary

---

[41]Lutwak, L., "Continuing Need for Dietary Calcium Throughout Life," *Geriatrics*, Vol. 29, 1974, p. 171.

[42]*Dietary Levels of Households in the United States, Spring, 1965*, Ag. Res. Serv. Bull. No. 62, 1968.

[43]Krook, L., et al., "Reversibility of Nutritional Osteoporosis: Physiochemical Data on Bones from an Experimental Study in Dogs," *Journal of Nutrition*, Vol. 101, 1971, p. 233.

[44]Linkswiler, H. M., C. L. Joyce, and C. R. Anand, "Calcium Retention of Young Adult Males as Affected by Level of Protein and of Calcium Intake," *Transactions of the New York Academy of Sciences*, Vol. 36, 1974, p. 333.

protein appeared to be independent of the levels of dietary calcium.[45] However, high protein intakes imply high phosphate intakes, because most of the nondairy sources of proteins contain liberal amounts of phosphate, but only small amounts of calcium. Thus, there is likely to be an imbalance in the ratios of phosphate to calcium in these diets.

Deficiencies of Vitamin D.

People who have moderate intakes of calcium, but who live in northern areas, seem to have more osteoporosis than people who eat diets low in calcium, but live in sunny, tropical areas. Furthermore, considerable effort is made in most countries to provide infants and children with adequate levels of the vitamin by either diet or exposure to sunlight, but there is often a lack of attention to the needs of adults, many of whom are kept indoors by either their occupations or the circumstances under which they live.

Stresses.

Many stresses—such as trauma, chilling, starvation, dehydration, surgery, and fear—are accompanied by great increases in the secretions of adrenal cortical hormones. The net effect of the hypersecretion of these hormones on bone is dissolution of both the mineral and protein components.

Lack of Sufficient Exercise.

There is some evidence that sedentary persons lose more calcium from their bones than active persons eating essentially the same diet. Also, it has been found that mechanical forces on bone, such as those which occur during exercise, produce a surface charge (a piezoelectric effect) which may stimulate the building up of bone.[46] Therefore, exercise may be an important factor in the development and maintenance of strong bones.

Postmenopausal Loss of Calcium.

Most cases of osteoporosis are diagnosed in women who are more than 50 years of age. Until recently, it has been assumed that the cessation of estrogen secretion after the menopause resulted in a loss of stimulation of bone remineralization. Now, it is not certain whether estrogen has more than a temporary effect in this regard.

The more rapid development of osteoporosis in women than in men might also be explained by the observation that women generally eat less calcium than men; therefore, they are more likely to have a chronic deficiency of the mineral, since the allowance is the same for both sexes. Both men and women consume, on the average, 30 mg of calcium per 100 Calories (kcal), but women consume far fewer calories.

Bone Loss—A Natural Accompaniment of Aging.

Some researchers have concluded that, irrespective of diet, bone loss is a general phenomenon which accompanies aging in man and may start as early as age 30.[47]

SIGNS OF OSTEOPOROSIS.

It has long been thought that the initial signs of this disorder are the occurrence of bone fractures when there has been little or no trauma. Since the long bones of the body do not readily lose bone mass until there has been loss in the jaw and the spinal column, it is difficult to detect early stages of osteoporosis by x rays of the long bones. However, research conducted at Cornell University showed that the early stages of this disorder might readily be observed in x rays of the jaw.[48] Thus, it would seem that dentists might be able to detect early stages of this disorder, particularly when patients seek treatment of periodontal disease caused by loss of bone in the jaw.

TREATMENT AND PREVENTION OF OSTEOPOROSIS.

A variety of therapeutic and prophylactic measures have been suggested, but each of them has its merits and demerits. Therefore, separate discussions of these measures follow:

• **Supplementation of dietary calcium**—It has been suggested that 1,000 mg of calcium per day might be an optimal intake for both the treatment of the early stages of the disease (when bone loss is detectable only in the jaw) and the prevention of the more severe stages.[49]

• **Combined therapy with fluoride, vitamin D, and calcium**—The supplementation of fluoride therapy with vitamin D and calcium apparently produced normal bone in patients with osteoporosis.[50]

• **Estrogen replacement therapy**—At one time it was thought that this therapy offered promise for the treatment of osteoporosis, but recent studies show that the beneficial effects of these hormones on bone may only be temporary.[51] Furthermore, physicians are cautious about the administration of estrogens for fear that long-term treatment with high doses of these hormones may lead to cancer in aging, estrogen-sensitive tissues.

Health Hints for Preventing Bone Fractures.

Every safe measure for the prevention of osteoporosis should be considered, because bone fractures are painful, incapacitating, and costly; and immobilization of the patient during recovery may result in other serious problems, such as further weakening of bones, formation of blood clots, and atrophy of muscles. Some practical recommendations for normal, healthy people follow:

1. Exercise regularly. This practice results in the improved utilization of calcium for bone remineralization.
2. Avoid exercises where sharp impacts are transmitted to bones and joints. For example, some joggers run in hard-soled shoes on hard pavement. It has been shown that this practice puts considerable force on the hip joints. Learn to be light on your feet and wear appropriate footwear.
3. Eat sufficient dairy foods and dark-green vegetables to obtain at least 800 mg of calcium per day (the amount in 3 cups [720 ml] of milk).

[45]Margen, S., et al., "Studies in Calcium Metabolism. 1. The Calciuretic Effect of Dietary Protein," *The American Journal of Clinical Nutrition*, Vol. 27, 1974, p. 584.

[46]Marino, A. A., and R. O. Becker, "Piezoelectric Effect and Growth Control in Bone," *Nature*, Vol. 228, 1970, p. 473.

[47]Garn, S. M., C. G. Rothman, and B. Wagner, "Bone Loss as a General Phenomenon in Man," *Federation Proceedings*, Vol. 26, 1967, p. 1729.

[48]Lutwak, L., et al., "Calcium Deficiency and Human Periodontal Disease," *Israel Journal of Medical Sciences*, Vol. 7, 1971, p. 504.

[49]Lutwak, L., "Dietary Calcium and the Reversal of Bone Demineralization," *Nutrition News*, Vol. 37, 1974, p. 1.

[50]Jowsey, J., et al., "Effect of Combined Therapy with Sodium Fluoride, Vitamin D and Calcium in Osteoporosis," *American Journal of Medicine*, Vol. 53, 1972, p. 43.

[51]Riggs, B. L., et al., "Short- and Long-Term Effects of Estrogen and Synthetic Anabolic Hormone in Postmenopausal Osteoporosis," *Journal of Clinical Investigation*, Vol. 51, 1972, p. 1659.

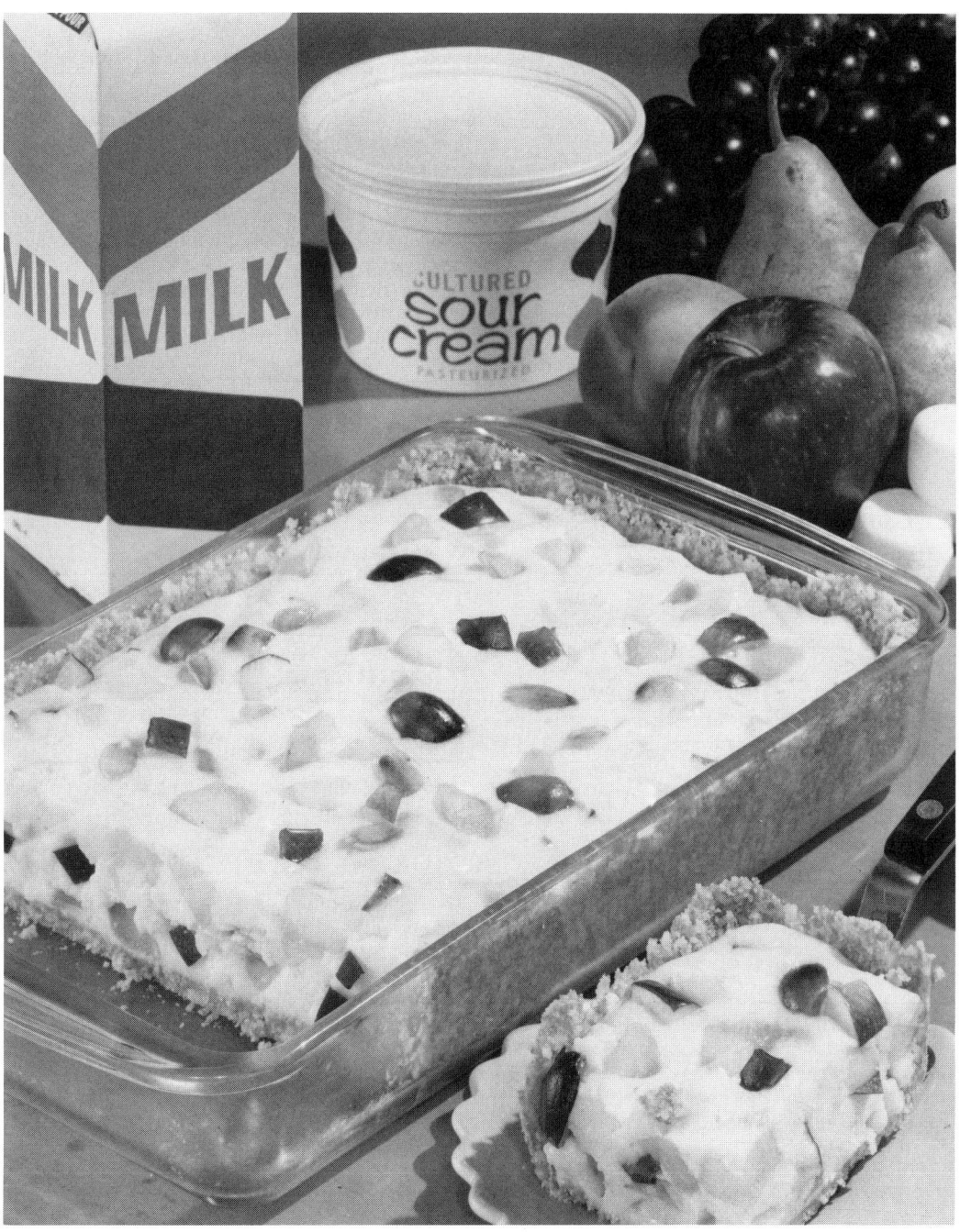

Fig. O-28. Dairy foods, important for prevention of osteoporosis, can be incorporated into many dishes. (Courtesy, United Dairy Industry Assn., Rosemont, Ill.)

4. Keep your protein intake down to around the RDA (63 g per day for males, and 50 g per day for females).

5. Add calcium supplements, such as dolomite, when either the protein intake is considerably higher than the RDA (like 90 g or more per day), or when circumstances prevent the consumption of adequate calcium in foods.
(Also see BONE MEAL; CALCIUM; and DOLOMITE.)

6. Obtain sufficient vitamin D by either diet or regular exposure to sunlight.
(Also see CALCIUM; MINERAL[S], Table M-25, Mineral Table, Calcium; and VITAMIN D.)

OTAHEITE APPLE (AMBARELLA)
Spondias cytherea.

The fruit of a tree (of the family *Anacardiaceae*) that is native to Polynesia. Otaheite is an old name for Tahiti. Otaheite apples are yellow, round fruits that range from 2 to 3 in. (*5 to 7 cm*) in diameter and contain a large stone. The fruit is usually eaten fresh, but is sometimes made into jam and jelly.

Otaheite apples are fairly low in calories (46 kcal per 100 g) and carbohydrates (12%). They are a good source of fiber and vitamin C.

OTAHEITE GOOSEBERRY (GOOSEBERRY TREE) *Phyllanthus acidus*

The fruit of a small tropical tree (of the family *Euphorbiaceae*) that is native to India and Madagascar.

Otaheite gooseberries are small, greenish, sour-tasting fruit about ¾ in. (*2 cm*) in diameter. They are usually eaten cooked with sugar and made into jam, jelly, pies, and tarts.

The fruit has a high water content (91%) and a low content of calories (37 kcal per 100 g) and carbohydrates (5%). It is an excellent source of iron, but only a fair source of vitamin C.

OVALBUMIN

This is egg albumin, the major protein of egg white representing 75% of the total egg white protein.
(Also see EGG[S].)

OVERWEIGHT

Persons who are 10 to 20% above the ideal weight for their height, age, build, and sex are said to be overweight. A person, especially an athlete, may be overweight without being obese since overweight does not imply fatness. Nevertheless, some use obesity and overweight interchangeably.
(Also see OBESITY.)

OVOMUCOID

A minor protein component of egg white containing large amounts of carbohydrate in its structure.
(Also see EGG[S].)

OXALIC ACID (OXALATE; $C_2H_2O_4$)

A naturally occurring toxicant present in such plants as beet leaves, cabbage, peas, potatoes, rhubarb, and spinach. There is some concern that oxalic acid may render calcium as well as some trace minerals less available for absorption from the gut. However, it is doubtful that oxalates pose a problem to man unless the intake of a mineral is marginal, and unusually large amounts of the oxalate-containing food are eaten. Poisoning could occur from the accidental ingestion of some cleaning compounds containing oxalic acid. Interestingly, oxalic acid is a normal constituent of urine derived from the metabolism of ascorbic acid (vitamin C) or glycine (an amino acid).
(Also see POISONOUS PLANTS.)

OXALOACETIC ACID

A 3-carbon ketodicarboxylic acid; an intermediate in the Krebs cycle.

OXALURIA

The presence of an excess of oxalic acid or of oxalates in the urine.

OXIDATION

Chemically, the increase of positive charges on an atom or the loss of negative charges or electrons. It also refers to the combining of oxygen with another element to form one or more new substances. Burning is one kind of oxidation.
(Also see METABOLISM.)

OXIDATIVE PHOSPHORYLATION

The principal function of the oxidation of carbohydrates and fatty acids is to make available to the cells the free energy released in the oxidation process, in a form physiologically usable for cellular energy processes, viz, ATP. This is accomplished by the process known as oxidative phosphorylation, whereby adenosine triphosphate (ATP) with three phosphate groups, two of which are held by high energy bonds, is formed from adenosine diphosphate (ADP) by the addition of phosphate.
(Also see METABOLISM, section headed "Carbohydrates, Catabolism, • ATP—energy currency.")

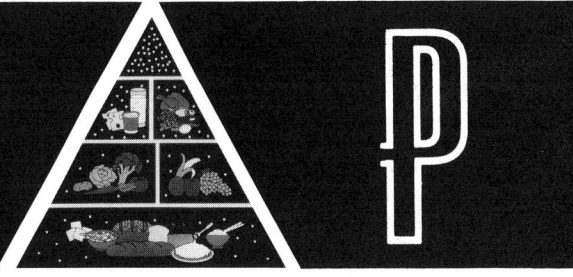

PALATABILITY

If they don't eat it, it won't do them any good. And that applies to all people.

The palatability of a food is the result of the following factors: taste, smell, texture, temperature, sound, and appearance. These factors are affected by the physical and chemical nature of foods.

(Also see FLAVORINGS AND SEASONINGS.)

PALM family *Palmae*

Palms are an ancient group of plants. Fossil (buried remains) palm leaves have been found that date from the age of dinosaurs.

The family *Palmae* embraces more than 2,600 kinds of palms, varying greatly in size and kind of flowers, leaves, and fruits they produce. They are of great economic importance; furnishing food, shelter, clothing, timber, fuel, building materials, sticks, fiber, paper, starch, sugar, oil, wax, wine, tannin, dyeing material, resin, and a host of other products, all of which render them most valuable to the natives and to tropical agriculture. Palms thrive in warm climates, especially in the tropics. They are most common in Southeast Asia, the Pacific Islands, and in tropical America. They grow wild along the coast of North Carolina, in Arizona, and in the deserts of southern California.

Most palms grow straight and tall, but a few do not. The trunks of some palms lie on the ground. Others have most of the trunk buried in the soil. Still others have slender, vinelike stems that are from 10 to 250 ft (*3 to 76 m*) long.

Because of their importance in food production, the following three palms are treated separately in this book:

Coconut (Coconut Palm) (*Cocos nucifera*)
Date(s) (*Phoenix dactylifera*)
Oil Palm (*Elaeis guineensis*)

PALMITIC ACID

A 16-carbon saturated fatty acid.
(Also see FATS AND OTHER LIPIDS.)

PANCREATIN

A commercially available preparation containing the enzymes of the pancreas of cattle or pigs. It is capable of breaking down starch, lipids, and proteins. Pancreatin may be used as an aid to digestion. However, the stomach environment destroys it; hence, coated pills are used to allow it to reach the small intestine.

PANCREATITIS

An acute or chronic inflammation of the pancreas whose cause is poorly understood. Cases may be mild to severe, and some may even cause death. Often its occurrence is associated with other diseases such as alcoholism, gallbladder disease, peptic ulcer, an infectious disease, or an acci-

dent. Symptoms of pancreatitis consist of a severe upper abdominal pain radiating into the back and stimulated by eating, tenderness above the stomach, distention, constipation, nausea, and vomiting. The basis of treatment is to limit pancreatic secretion to a minimum. Hence, during the first few days of treatment, intravenous feeding is employed, followed by a soft, bland, or low residue diet. When medical treatment is ineffective, surgery may be needed.

(Also see MODIFIED DIETS; DIGESTION AND ABSORPTION; and INTRAVENOUS FEEDING.)

PANDANUS FRUIT (SCREW-PINE FRUIT)
Pandanus adoratissimus

The fruit of a tree (of the family *Pandanaceae*) that grows throughout southeast Asia and the Pacific Islands. Pandanus fruits are usually yellow to red in color, round or pear-shaped, and range from 6 to 10 in. (*15 to 25 cm*) in diameter. The fleshy base of the fruit is usually the only part that is eaten. Some of the Polynesian peoples mix the fruit and coconut milk or grated coconut and bake the pasty mixture into flat cakes. The pandanus-coconut paste may also be made into a refreshing drink by diluting it with water.

Pandanus fruit is rich in calories (150 kcal per 100 g), carbohydrates (18%), fat (8%), protein (5%), and fiber (7%), but it is low in vitamin C.

PANGAMIC ACID (VITAMIN B-15)

The authors make this presentation for two primary purposes: (1) informational, and (2) stimulation of research.

The nutritional status and biological role(s) of pangamic acid await clarification. Its stimulation of such fundamental processes of transmethylation, cellular respiration, etc. may have physiological application. Certainly, there is sufficient indication of the value of pangamic acid as a therapeutic agent to warrant further study. In the meantime, pangamic acid should not be taken unless prescribed by a physician.

Pangamic acid (also known as vitamin B-15, calcium pangamate, and dimethylglycene) is a chemical substance of an organic nature. It is sometimes classed as a vitamin or vitaminlike substance. Obviously, however, pangamic acid does not meet the classical definition of a vitamin, which is: *A substance, organic in nature, necessary in the diet in small amounts to sustain life, in the absence of which a specific deficiency disease develops.* The proponents counter with the argument that: "It's not essential, strictly speaking, but it's helpful biologically under many circumstances."

The FDA classifies pangamic acid as a food additive, and, therefore, subject to the regulations requiring proof that it is nontoxic.

Pangamic acid has been widely studied and accepted in the U.S.S.R. as a necessary food factor with important physiological actions.

HISTORY. In 1951, Krebs *et al.* reported the presence of a water-soluble factor in apricot kernels, which they subsequently isolated in crystalline form from rice bran and polish. Later, it was extracted from brewers' yeast, cattle blood, and horse liver. The name *pangamic acid* (*pan*, meaning universal; *gamic*, meaning seed) was applied to the substance to connote its seeming universal presence in seeds; and it was assigned the fifteenth position in the vitamin B series by its discoverers.

The claim that pangamic acid is a B vitamin is based primarily on its presence in B-vitamin rich foods and on the broad spectrum of physiological functions attributed to it. However, it is not known whether man or other animals have the capacity to synthesize pangamic acid, and no specific disease can be attributed exclusively to a deficiency of the substance. Thus, the designation of pangamic acid as a vitamin is not accepted by most U.S. scientists.

CHEMISTRY, METABOLISM, PROPERTIES.

• **Chemistry**—The chemical structure of pangamic acid is given in Fig. P-1.

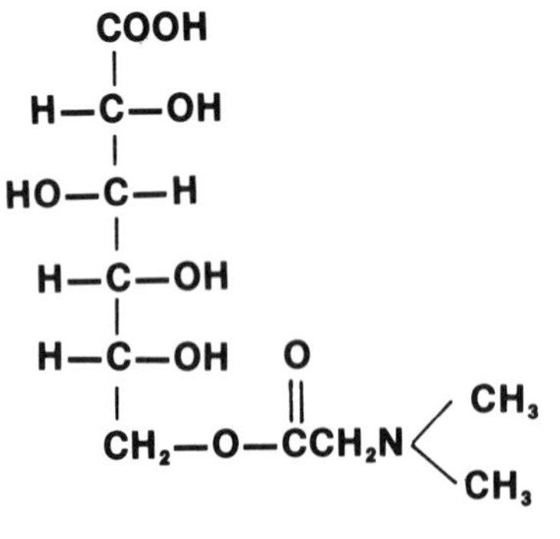

$$
\begin{array}{c}
COOH \\
|\\
H-C-OH \\
|\\
HO-C-H \\
|\\
H-C-OH \\
|\\
H-C-OH \qquad O\\
|\qquad\qquad \|\\
CH_2-O-CCH_2N \big\langle \begin{array}{c} CH_3 \\ CH_3 \end{array}
\end{array}
$$

Fig. P-1. Pangamic acid ($C_{10}H_{19}O_8N$).

But the chemical composition of pangamic acid varies from brand product to brand product, and even within the same brand. This, within itself, makes the substance controversial. Some products are a mixture of sodium (or sometimes calcium) gluconate, glycine, and diisopropylamine dichloroacetate. However, the Russians confine their product to pangamic acid, i.e., the form of vitamin B-15 in which it occurs in nature.

• **Metabolism**—Little is known about the metabolism of pangamic acid. Within 10 to 15 minutes after subcutaneous injection of the substance, it is found in the blood, brain, liver, heart, and kidney; the site of its highest concentration and longest duration in the body is the kidney, where it persists for at least 4 days.

Excessive amounts of pangamic acid are excreted in urine, feces, and perspiration.

• **Properties**—Pangamic acid is a white crystalline compound, very soluble in water.

MEASUREMENT/ASSAY. The content of pangamic acid is usually expressed in milligrams (mg).

Chromatographic and spectrophotometric techniques have been developed for the quantitative determination of pangamic acid in biological material.

FUNCTIONS. Numerous functions have been attributed to pangamic acid; among them, the following:

1. **Stimulation of transmethylation reactions.** Pangamic acid possesses methyl groups ($-CH_3$) which are capable of being transferred from one compound to another within the body, resulting in the stimulation of creatine synthesis in muscle and heart tissue. In turn, when ATP (adenosine triphosphate), a transitory form of energy, is in excess of immediate requirements, creatine forms phosphocreatine, a more permanent form of energy for storage in muscle. Then when the supply of ATP is insufficient to meet the demands for energy, more ATP is produced from phosphocreatine by the reverse reaction.

2. **Stimulation of oxygen uptake.** Pangamic acid stimulates tissue oxygen uptake, thereby helping to prevent the condition called *hypoxia*—an insufficient supply of oxygen in living tissue, especially in heart and other muscles. It does not add to the overall oxygen supply of the body; rather, it increases the efficiency with which the oxygen is delivered from the bloodstream to the cells.

3. **Inhibition of fatty liver formation.** Oral or injection of pangamic acid to rats and rabbits exerts a protective effect against fatty infiltration of the liver induced by starvation, protein-free diets, anesthetics, carbon tetrachloride, or cholesterol.

4. **Adaptation to increased physical activity.** Pangamic acid enables animals to adapt to increased exercise. After periods of enforced swimming, animals previously treated with pangamic acid demonstrate a better maintenance of oxidative metabolism and energy levels than untreated controls; moreover, these effects persist for several days.

Some horse trainers have been known to administer pangamic acid to racehorses because of its reputed, but undocumented, quality of enabling animals to run faster and tire less. Also, athletes have been taking it for years.

5. **Control of blood cholesterol levels.** In most cases, the administration of pangamic acid causes a fall in both cholesterol biosynthesis and blood levels.

DISORDERS TREATED WITH PANGAMIC ACID. Most treatments with pangamic acid have been conducted in the U.S.S.R., where the principal field of application of the drug has been in the treatment of cardiovascular disorders associated with insufficiency of oxidative metabolism. The Russians also report good results in treatment of liver disorders, a number of skin diseases, and some toxicoses. In the U.S.S.R. and/or elsewhere pangamic acid has been reported to be successful in treating the following disorders:

1. **Cardiovascular disease.** Pangamic acid is considered to be safe and effective in the treatment of—

a. **Arteriosclerosis (hardening of the arteries),** characterized by headaches, chest pains, shortness of breath, tension, and insomnia. In patients with arteriosclerosis, pangamic acid strengthens the action of the heart muscles.

 b. **Cardiopulmonary (heart-lung) insufficiency,** characterized by shortness of breath.

 c. **Angina pectoris,** characterized by chest pain, due to the arteries being incapable of supplying sufficient oxygen-rich blood to the heart muscle.

 d. **Congestive heart failure,** characterized by shortness of breath on slight exertion and dropsy (swelling around the ankles with pitting edema). This is a disease complex and group of symptoms caused by a failing heart, with congestion either in the lungs or the systemic circulation, or both. The chief causes are weakness of the heart muscles, high blood pressure, hardening of the arteries, and rheumatic or syphilitic disease of the heart valves. Treatment of patients suffering from congestive heart failure with pangamic acid increases diuresis (urination) and reduces high blood pressure and edema.

 e. **Patients recovering from serious heart attacks,** as an aid in speeding their recovery.

It is noteworthy, too, that pangamic acid increases the effectiveness of strophanthin (a heart tonic) on heart function of patients with congestive failure and reduces the incidence of side effects associated with digitalis therapy.

2. **Fatigue.** Pangamic acid is used to reduce fatigue and increase energy—to alleviate that tired feeling. According to the proponents, it accomplishes this by extracting more oxygen from the bloodstream for better metabolism in the cells. Some athletes, both professionals and amateurs, claim that it increases their physical endurance.

3. **Hypoxia.** Pangamic acid is effective in treating hypoxia, characterized by an insufficient supply of oxygen in tissues. It increases the efficiency with which oxygen is delivered from the bloodstream to the cells.

4. **High cholesterol.** Several workers have observed significant reductions in serum cholesterol levels as a result of daily treatment with pangamic acid for 10 to 30 days.

5. **Liver function.** As supportive treatment for infectious hepatitis in children, pangamic acid given orally for 10 to 20 days leads to a more marked and rapid decline in fever, liver size, jaundice, and serum transaminase levels and a 5 to 10 day shorter hospitalization period. Similar findings have been reported in adults with acute or chronic hepatitis treated with pangamic acid.

6. **Skin disorders.** It is claimed that pangamic acid is effective in the treatment of various skin diseases. It is reported that patients with scleroderma (*hidebound skin*), a chronic disease in which the skin and subcutaneous tissues become fibrous, rigid, and thickened, respond to daily treatment with pangamic acid for 45 days—relief is associated with softening of the affected skin and often with new hair growth. Also, a reduction of inflammation, edema, and itching has been reported in cases of eczema, psoriasis (a chronic skin disease that disfigures the face and body with recurrent red scaly patches), hives, and other skin disorders treated daily for 15 to 30 days with 100 to 150 mg of pangamic acid.

7. **Tumors.** Pangamic acid offers promise in the treatment of certain kinds of tumors. When given to rats with experimentally induced solid tumors, it did not interfere with the effectiveness of standard chemotherapeutic agents, but it significantly reduced the incidence and severity of the toxicity produced by certain drugs. Also, in preliminary work with rats, it has been reported that pangamic acid reduced both the incidence and latency of drug-induced mammary cancer. These limited studies await confirmation.

DEFICIENCY SYMPTOMS. There is indication that a deficiency of pangamic acid may cause fatigue (a tired feeling), hypoxia (an insufficient supply of oxygen in blood cells), heart disease, and glandular and nervous disorders.

DOSAGE. The usual dosage of pangamic acid is from 150 to 300 mg daily. But pangamic acid should not be taken unless prescribed by a physician.

TOXICITY. Despite initial caution regarding the use of pangamic acid in conditions of hypertension and glaucoma, "it is now regarded that the substance is without demonstrable toxicity in these or other disease states."[1] It is noteworthy, too, that, beginning in 1965, the U.S.S.R. Ministry of Health approved widespread manufacture and distribution of pangamic acid. One of the largest U.S. purveyors of pangamic acid—Da Vinci Laboratories, a subsidiary of Food Science Laboratories—cites several studies in which laboratory rats were fed quantities of B-15 equivalent to more than 100,000 times the recommended dosage for human consumption, without any ill effects.[2]

Perhaps the toxicity of pangamic acid depends on the particular formula. On the basis of available evidence, the so-called *Russian formula* appears to be relatively free of toxicity. Nevertheless, the U.S. Food and Drug Administration does not consider pangamic acid safe for human consumption.

Until the product is standardized (potency, quality, and chemical composition) and the question of toxicity is resolved, the authors recommend that pangamic acid be taken only under the direction of a physician.

SOURCES OF PANGAMIC ACID. The best natural sources of pangamic acid are sunflower seed, pumpkin seed, yeast, liver, rice, whole grain cereals, apricot kernels and other seeds. Evidence suggests its occurrence wherever B-complex vitamins are found in natural foods.

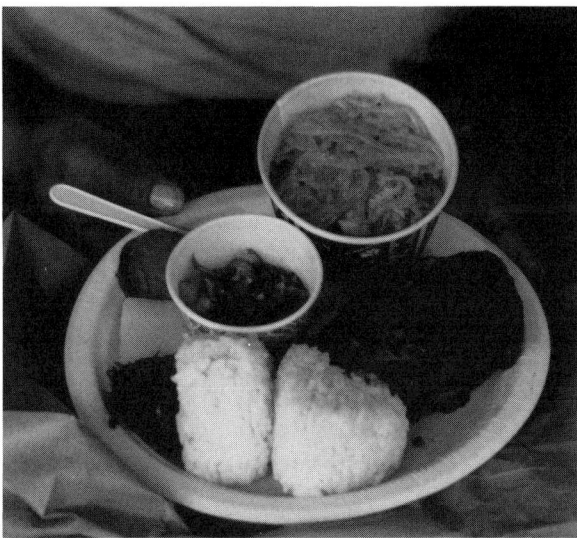

Fig. P-2. Rice is a rich source of pangamic acid. (Courtesy, Department of Food Science and Human Nutrition, University of Hawaii)

[1]Stacpoole, Peter W., "Pangamic Acid (Vitamin B-15)," *World Review of Nutrition and Dietetics—Some Aspects of Human Nutrition,* S. Karger, Basel, Munchen, 1977, p. 153.

[2]Grosswirth, Marvin, "B-15: Is it Superpill?," *Science Digest,* September 1978, p. 12.

CONCLUSION. Until more conclusive evidence on the role of pangamic acid is available, the authors subscribe to the view so well expressed by biochemist Richard A. Passwater, Ph.D., as follows:

"While the processes through which vitamin B-15 works are being elucidated, natural wisdom suggests that we take care to see that our diets are rich in vitamin B-15."[3]

(Also see VITAMINS[S], Table V-5.)

PANTOTHENIC ACID (VITAMIN B-3)

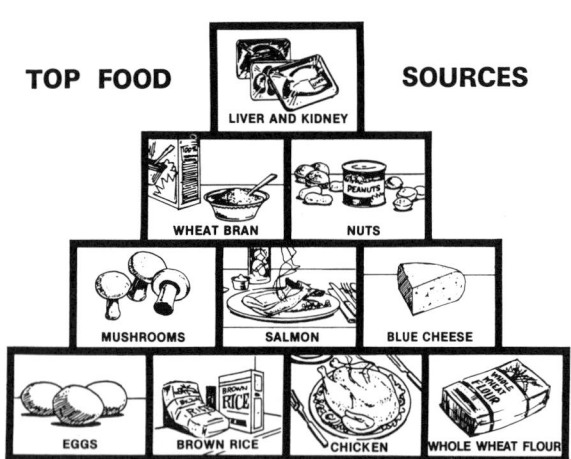

Fig. P-3. Top food sources of pantothenic acid.

Pantothenic acid, a member of the vitamin B complex, is a dietary essential for man and animals; and, as an important constituent of coenzyme A (CoA), it plays a key role in body metabolism.

In recognition of its wide distribution in foods, the name *pantothenic acid*, derived from the Greek word *pantothen*—meaning *everywhere*, was first given to it in 1933, by R. J. Williams, then of Oregon State, later at the University of Texas.

Before its structure was known, pantothenic acid was called by several other names, now obsolete, including: filtrate factor, chick antidermatitis factor, bios factor, the anti-gray hair factor, pantothen, factor H, factor 2, vitamin B-x, vitamin B-2, vitamin B-3.

HISTORY. The existence of pantothenic acid and its nutritive significance for the proliferation and fermentative activity of yeast cells first emerged from the studies of R. J.

Williams, beginning in 1919. In 1933, Williams fractionated this compound from yeast and called it pantothenic acid; and in 1939, he isolated pantothenic acid from liver. In 1939, Jukes concluded that the antidermatitis factor isolated from liver was one and the same thing as the factor found in yeast. In 1940, pantothenic acid was synthesized by Williams and two other laboratories, all working independently. Also, in 1940, pantothenic acid received widespread attention as a possible preventive for gray hair, since it had been observed that the black hair of a rat would turn gray when the animal was deprived of the vitamin; but subsequent studies did not reveal any such benefits to accrue to humans. In 1946, Lipmann and co-workers showed that coenzyme A is essential for acetylation reactions in the body; and in 1950 reports from the same laboratory showed pantothenic acid to be a constituent of coenzyme A.

CHEMISTRY, METABOLISM, PROPERTIES.

• **Chemistry**—Pantothenic acid is composed of pantoic acid and the amino acid beta-alanine, as shown in Fig. P-4.

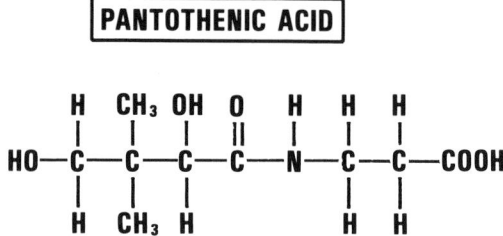

Fig. P-4. Structure of pantothenic acid.

• **Metabolism**—Pantothenic acid, like the other B vitamins, is readily absorbed through the mucosa of the small intestine and enters the portal circulation. Within the tissues, most of the panothenic acid is used in the synthesis of coenzyme A (CoA); but a significant amount found in the cells is bound to a protein in a compound known as acyl carrier protein (ACP).

Pantothenic acid is present in all living tissue, with high concentrations in the liver and kidney. (Large amounts of CoA are found in the liver, with lesser amounts in the adrenal glands.)

The vitamin is excreted from the body by way of the kidneys.

• **Properties**—In pure form, pantothenic acid is a viscous yellow oil, soluble in water, quite stable in neutral solutions, but destroyed by acid, alkali, and prolonged exposure to dry heat (2 to 6 days—far longer than the usual cooking or baking procedures). Calcium pantothenate, the form in which it is commercially available, is a white, odorless, bitter, crystalline substance, which is water-soluble and quite stable. (Pantothenic acid is also available as the sodium salt.)

MEASUREMENT/ASSAY. The activity of pantothenic acid is expressed in grams and milligrams of the chemically pure substance.

[3]Passwater, Richard A., Ph.D., "B-15—New Ally In The Fight Against Major Diseases," *The Health Quarterly*, Vol. 3, No. 5, 1979, p. 16.

Pantothenic acid content may be determined by chemical methods (including gas chromatography), microbiologic procedures, and the chick and rat bioassay.

FUNCTIONS. Pantothenic acid functions in the body as part of two enzymes—coenzyme A (CoA) and acyl carrier protein (ACP).

ACP is composed of a panthetheine linked through a phosphate group to protein. It, along with CoA, is required by the cells in the biosynthesis (the manufacture, or building up) of fatty acids (CoA, without ACP, is involved in their breakdown.)

Coenzyme A, meaning a coenzyme for acetylation, is one of the most important substances in body metabolism. It is a complex molecule containing the vitamin combined with adenosine 3-phosphate, pyrophosphate, and beta-mercaptoethylamine (a compound containing an -SH group), as shown in Fig. P-5.

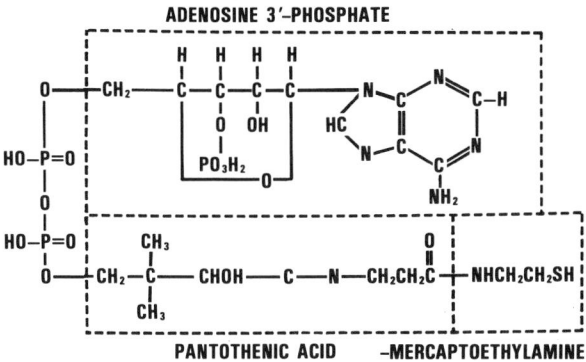

Fig. P-5. Structure of CoA.

The way in which pantothenic acid is incorporated in the molecule of coenzyme A is shown in Fig. P-5. The sulphydryl (-SH) group of the molecule is extremely active, but the other groups are also involved in some of the functions of coenzyme A.

CoA functions in any reaction in which an acetyl group (-CH$_3$CO) is formed or is transferred from one substance to another. In addition to acetyl, other acyl radicals require coenzyme A; it is required whenever succinyl, benzyl, or fatty acid radicals are formed or transferred.

Coenzyme A participates in several fundamental metabolic functions; these include the following:

1. **The synthesis (the building up) of fatty acids.** The most important function of coenzyme A (and, hence, of pantothenic acid) in metabolism is the transfer of radicals of acetic acid (or C$_2$) in the synthesis of fatty acids. During the process of digestion, the triglycerides which are present in the food are split by lipases of the pancreas and of the intestinal wall into glycerol, monoglycerides, and fatty acids which are simultaneously emulsified by the bile acids. The degree of absorption of the fatty acids through the wall of the small intestine depends on the length of the chain; the shorter the chain, the more complete the absorption. After passing through the intestinal wall, the short chain fatty acids are converted into longer chain fatty acids, the major step in the process being the combination of coenzyme A with acetic acid to form "activated acetic acid" or acetyl-coenzyme A.

Acetyl-coenzyme A is next converted to malonyl-coenzyme A (which contains one more carbon atom), a reaction which is catalyzed by an enzyme which contains biotin. Malonyl-

coenzyme A then reacts with another activated fatty acid (the chain of which has also become longer by one carbon atom) yielding a product which is a fatty acid with a chain which has been lengthened by two carbon atoms. In this manner, for example, stearic acid (C$_{18}$) is formed from palmitic acid (C$_{16}$) in the body.

2. **The degradation (the breaking down) of fatty acids.** In metabolism, both the synthesis and the degradation of fatty acids are required. Pantothenic acid, as a constituent of coenzyme A, participates in this breaking down process. The energy which is released in this process of degradation is gathered and transferred elsewhere by another system which is based on the (reversible) formation of adenosine triphosphate (ATP), which is high in energy, from two compounds having lower levels of energy, adenosine diphosphate (ADP) and monophosphate (AMP).

3. **The citric acid cycle.** A very large part of the energy required in metabolism is supplied by the citric acid cycle (or the *Krebs' cycle*), in which compounds high in energy (carbohydrates, fats, and proteins) are continually being converted into compounds which are lower in energy; the energy released is again contained in the form of ATP.

Pantothenic acid, as a constituent of coenzyme A, is involved in several of the steps of the citric acid cycle; these include the synthesis of citric acid from oxalacetic acid and its salts, and the oxidation by decarboxylation of a-keto-acids.

4. **The acetylation of choline.** Pantothenic acid is necessary for the formation of acetylcholine, the transmitter of nerve impulses.

5. **The synthesis of antibodies.** Pantothenic acid stimulates the synthesis of those antibodies which increase resistance to pathogens.

6. **The utilization of nutrients.** Coenzyme A is essential for the metabolism of fats, carbohydrates, and proteins; hence, a deficiency of pantothenic acid will necessarily impair the utilization of digestible nutrients. The function of coenzyme A is in the endogenous metabolism, not in the digestive tract. Hence, it cannot affect the digestible or metabolizable energy; only its utilization—the net productive energy which is most simply measured in terms of the retention of nutrients. This is true not only for those nutrients which supply energy, but also for those which supply protein.

7. **Other functions.** Pantothenic acid also affects the endocrine glands, and the hormones they produce. Thus, a deficiency of pantothenic acid in rats reduces not only the rate of gain in weight but also the rate of basal metabolism. Also, it has been postulated that the influence which pantothenic acid exerts on the fertility of various animals may be due to some relationship between pantothenic acid and the synthesis of steroid hormones.

Other functions attributed to pantothenic acid (or coenzyme A) are:

a. It is necessary in the synthesis of porphyrin, a precursor of heme, of importance in hemoglobin synthesis.

b. It is necessary for the maintenance of normal blood sugar levels.

c. It may facilitate the excretion of sulfonamide drugs.

d. It influences the metabolism of some of the minerals and trace elements.

e. It can be used for detoxification of drugs, including the sulphonamides.

DEFICIENCY SYMPTOMS. A deficiency of pantothenic acid has been associated with the "burning foot syndrome" that occurred in Japan and the Philippines among prisoners during World War II.

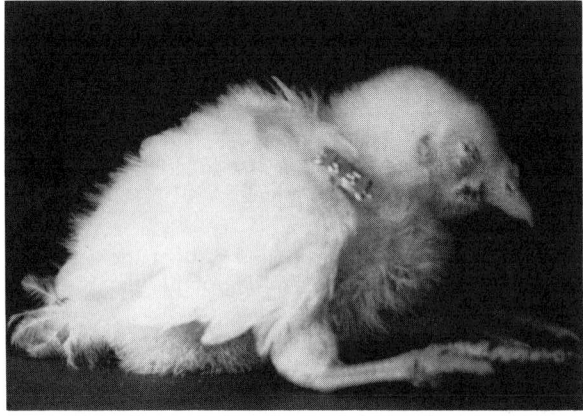

Fig. P-6. Pantothenic acid deficiency in chick. Note the lesions at the corners of the mouth and on the eyelids and feet. (Courtesy, Department of Poultry Science, Cornell University)

Pantothenic deficiency has been produced in human volunteers (1) by feeding them semisynthetic diets low in pantothenic acid for a period of 10 to 12 weeks; and (2) by feeding them diets to which the pantothenic acid antagonist omega-methylpantothenic acid was added. (A vitamin antagonist is a substance so similar in structure to the vitamin that the body accepts it in place of the vitamin, but the antagonist is unable to perform the functions of the true vitamin.) The subjects developed a wide variety of symptoms including: irritableness and restlessness; loss of appetite, indigestion, abdominal pain, nausea; headache; sullenness, mental depression; fatigue, weakness; numbness and tingling of hands and feet, muscle cramps in the arms and legs; burning sensations in the feet; insomnia; respiratory infections; rapid pulse; and a staggering gait. Also, in these subjects there was increased reaction to stress; increased sensitivity to insulin, resulting in low blood sugar levels; an increased sedimentation rate for erythrocytes; decreased gastric secretions; and marked decrease in antibody production. All symptoms were cured by the administration of pantothenic acid.

A lack of pantothenic acid results in premature graying of the hair in piebald rats, foxes, and dogs. But, neither pantothenic acid nor any other nutritional factor has been shown to be involved in the graying of hair in humans.

RECOMMENDED DAILY ALLOWANCE. The amount of pantothenic acid required by human beings has not been determined; so, a recommended daily allowance for pantothenic acid has not been made by the Food and Nutrition Board of the National Research Council. Nevertheless, they do give "estimated safe and adequate intakes" based on proportional energy needs (see section on VITAMIN(S), Table V-5, Vitamin Table). Further, they suggest that a higher intake may be needed during pregnancy and lactation.

NOTE WELL:

1. Processing of food can, in some instances, result in appreciable losses of pantothenic acid. Thus, it is possible that unrecognized marginal deficiencies may exist, along with deficiencies of other B-complex vitamins.

2. Deficiencies of pantothenic acid occur in farm animals (especially chickens and swine), fed *natural rations*. As a result, pantothenic acid is commonly added to commercial poultry and swine rations.

These two facts point up the need for more studies on the pantothenic requirement of humans, and perhaps the need for dietary supplementation for buoyant good health.

• **Pantothenic acid intake in average U.S. diet**—The average American diet provides 5 to 10 mg of pantothenic acid per day, with an average of 6 mg.

TOXICITY. Pantothenic acid is a relatively nontoxic substance. As much as 10 g of calcium pantothenate per day was given to young men for 6 weeks with no toxic symptoms; other studies indicate that daily doses of 10 to 20 g may result in occasional diarrhea and water retention.[4]

PANTOTHENIC ACID LOSSES DURING PROCESSING, COOKING, AND STORAGE. Losses up to 50%, and even more, of the pantothenic acid content of foods may occur from production to consumption. Here are some of them:

1. About 50% of the pantothenic content of grains is lost in milling.

2. Up to 50% of the pantothenic content of fruits and vegetables is lost in canning or freezing, and storage, of fruits and vegetables.

3. From 15 to 30% of the pantothenic acid content of meat is lost in cooking or canning.

4. Losses in pantothenic acid from dry processing of foods may exceed 50%.

Pantothenic acid is reasonably stable in natural foods during storage, provided that oxidation and high temperature are avoided. Cereal grains may be stored for periods up to a year without appreciable loss.

Henry A. Schroeder, M.D., of the Dartmouth Medical School, conducted an extensive survey of the pantothenic acid content in hundreds of common foods, and found that modern processing was causing massive losses of the vitamin. His studies showed pantothenic acid losses as follows: From milling wheat and making all-purpose flour, 57.7%; from canning vegetables, 56 to 79%; from freezing vegetables, 48 to 57%; from canning meat and poultry, 26.2%; and from canning seafood, 19.9%.[5]

SOURCES OF PANTOTHENIC ACID. Pantothenic acid is widely distributed in foods, with considerable variation in content according to food and processing. A grouping and ranking of foods according to pantothenic content is given in the section on VITAMIN(S), Table V-5, Vitamin Table.

---

[4]Committee on Dietary Allowances, Food and Nutrition Board, *Recommended Dietary Allowances,* 10th ed., 1989, National Research Council, National Academy of Sciences, Washington, D.C., p. 172.

[5]Schroeder, Henry A., M.D., "Losses of Vitamins and Trace Minerals Resulting From Processing and Preservation of Foods," *The American Journal of Chemical Nutrition,* Vol. 24, May 1971, pp. 562–573.

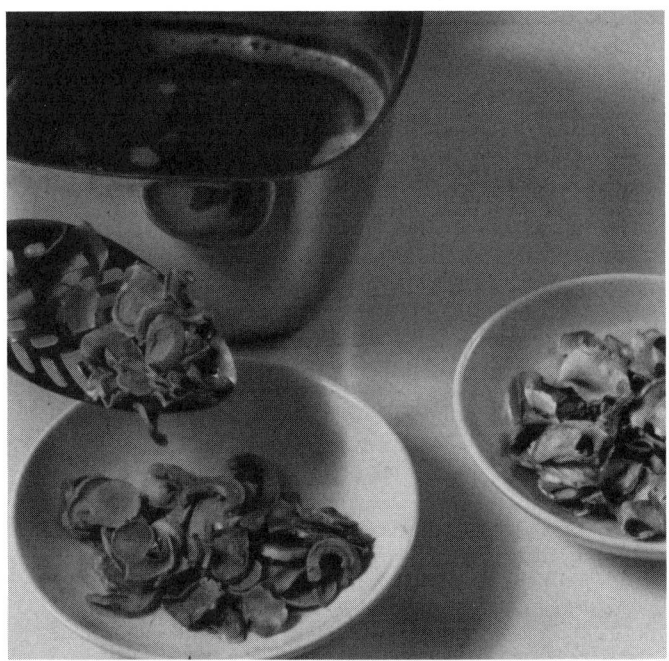

Fig. P-7. Mushrooms, a good source of pantothenic acid. (Courtesy, USDA)

Intestinal bacteria also synthesize pantothenic acid, but the amount produced and the availability of the vitamin from this source are unknown.

For additional sources and more precise values of pantothenic acid, see Food Composition Table F-21 of this book. (Also see VITAMIN[S], Table V-5.)

PAPAIN (VEGETABLE PEPSIN)

This is an enzyme obtained from the green fruit and leaves of the papaya. It is proteolytic; it breaks down proteins such as the digestive enzymes pepsin and trypsin. Papain can be employed to tenderize meats, clear beverages, prevent adhesions during wound healing, and aid digestion.

(Also see PAPAYA)

PAPAYA (MAMAO) Carica papaya

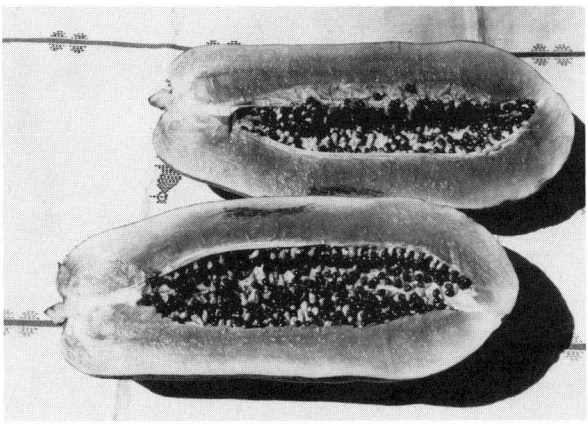

Fig. P-8. The papaya—fruit of a tropical tree that looks like a palm tree with a tuft of large leaves at the top. (Courtesy, USDA)

The papaya tree, a member of the family Caricaceae, is a fast-growing, short-lived tree native to tropical America. It is a soft wooded palmlike evergreen with palmate leaves clustered at the top. In tropical countries around the world, the papaya is cultivated for its edible melonlike fruit, the papaya, which is round to oblong and may weigh as much as 20 lb (9.1 kg).

ORIGIN AND HISTORY. The papaya is native to Central America. Since it grows readily from seed, the papaya was distributed quite early by man all over the tropical and subtropical areas of the world.

WORLD AND U.S. PRODUCTION. Papayas rank about nineteenth in quantity produced among the fruit crops of the world. Worldwide, about 4.4 million metric tons are produced annually; and the leading producing countries of the world, by rank, are: Brazil, Mexico, Thailand, Indonesia, India, Zaire, China, Philippines, Colombia, and Vietnam.[6]

The United States produces about 34,000 short tons annually. Most of the U.S. crop is grown in Hawaii.[7]

PROCESSING. Papayas are usually consumed fresh like a cantaloupe or in salads, pies, and sherbets. There is little processing involved. However, they can be squeezed for juice, pickled, candied, or made into jellies.

SELECTION, PREPARATION, AND USES. Papaya fruit ranges in shape from globose to long-ovid, in weight from 4 oz (113.4 g) to 20 lb (9.1 kg) or more, and in color from light yellow through deep yellow, orange, and pink to red. The fruit should be firm. Papaya is usually prepared by washing, peeling, and slicing ripe fruit, then serving with or without a little sugar. Unripe fruit may be cooked and used like a squash.

Papaya may be used as a fruit or vegetable dish, and in fruit salads, jams, jellies, juices, pickles, or sherbets. Also, papaya contain the enzyme papain which is used to tenderize meat.

NUTRITIONAL VALUE. Papayas are listed in Food Composition Table F-21. They contain about 89% water and only 39 Calories (kcal) per 100 g (about 3½ oz) or about 120 Calories (kcal) per medium-sized fruit. Papayas are rich in vitamin A and contain some vitamin C.

PARA-AMINOBENZOIC ACID (PABA)

Para-aminobenzoic acid (PABA) is a constituent of foods, which is sometimes listed with the B vitamins.

In addition to having activity as a growth factor for certain bacteria, PABA has considerable folacin activity when fed to deficient animals in which intestinal synthesis of folacin takes place. For example, for rats and mice, it can completely replace the need for a dietary source of folacin. This explains why para-aminobenzoic acid was once considered to be a vitamin in its own right.

For man and other higher animals, PABA is an essential part of the folacin molecule. But it has no vitamin activity in animals receiving ample folacin, and it is not required

---

[6]Data from *FAO Production Yearbook 1990*, FAO/UN, Rome, Italy, Vol. 44, p. 169, Table 74. **Note well:** Annual production fluctuates as a result of weather and profitability of the crop.

[7]Data from *Agricultural Statistics 1991*, USDA, p. 177, Table 254. **Note well:** Annual production fluctuates as a result of weather and profitability of the crop.

in the diet; hence, it can no longer be considered a vitamin, contrary to its listing in many vitamin preparations on the market.

HISTORY. PABA was first identified as an essential nutrient for certain microorganisms. Later, it was shown to act as an antigray hair factor in rats and mice (but not people) and as a growth-promoting factor in chicks.

CHEMISTRY, METABOLISM, PROPERTIES.

● **Chemistry**—The chemical structure of PABA is given in Fig. P-9.

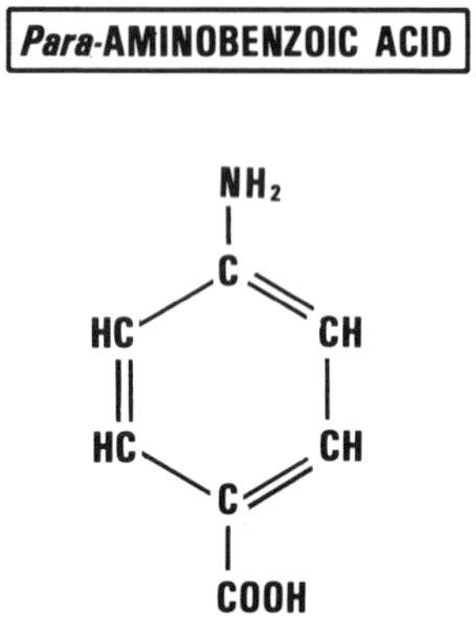

Para-AMINOBENZOIC ACID

Fig. P-9. Structure of *para*-aminobenzoic acid.

● **Metabolism**—The body manufactures its own PABA if conditions in the intestines are favorable.

● **Properties**—PABA is a yellow, crystalline, slightly water-soluble substance.

MEASUREMENT. The activity of PABA, and of its sodium and potassium salts, is ordinarily expressed in grams of chemically pure substances.

FUNCTIONS. For man and other higher animals, PABA functions as an essential part of the folacin molecule.

As a coenzyme, PABA functions in the breakdown and utilization of proteins and in the formation of blood cells, especially red blood cells.

● **Human pharmaceutical uses**—PABA is sometimes used as a human pharmaceutical, not as a vitamin, in the following: as an antirickettsial; to counteract the bacteriostatic action of sulfonamides; and as a protective agent against sunburn.

1. **Antirickettsial.** PABA is sometimes used in the treatment of certain rickettsial diseases—diseases in man and animals caused by microscopically small parasites of the genus *Rickettsia,* notably typhus and Rocky Mountain spotted fever.

The therapeutic use of PABA in the treatment of rickettsial diseases is based on the concept of metabolic antagonism. PABA acts as an antagonist to a material essential to these organisms, para-oxybenzoic acid; hence, the rickettsial organisms are killed because PABA blocks their essential metabolite.

2. **Sulfonamide antagonist.** PABA has the ability to reverse the bacteriostatic effects of sulfonamides, thereby counteracting their action. This is an antimetabolite action, explainable on the basis of similarity of structures (see Fig. P-10). According to this theory, sulfonamides suppress bacterial

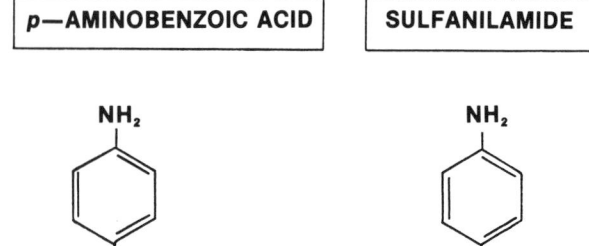

p—AMINOBENZOIC ACID   **SULFANILAMIDE**

Fig. P-10. The similarity of the structures of PABA and sulfanilamide is obvious.

growth by replacing their chemical analog PABA in bacterial enzyme systems; PABA in excess reverses the effect.

3. **Sunscreen agent.** PABA is used for protection against sunburn; usually about 5% PABA is incorporated in an ointment, to be applied over exposed parts of the body. Currently, some dermatologists are recommending other sunscreen lotions; so, for protection against sunburn, see your dermatologist.

DEFICIENCY SYMPTOMS. Sulfa drugs may induce a deficiency of not only PABA, but of folic acid as well. The symptoms: fatigue, irritability, depression, nervousness, headache, constipation, and other digestive disorders.

(Also see DISEASES, Table D-10, Food-Related Infectious and Parasitic Diseases; and MALARIA.)

RECOMMENDED DAILY ALLOWANCE OF PABA. The need for PABA has not been established; hence, it follows that there is no recommended daily allowance. The ordinary dose of PABA is 2 to 6 g, but even larger doses have been administered, in a variety of disorders.

TOXICITY. It has generally been considered that PABA is essentially nontoxic in man. But, continued high doses may be toxic, causing nausea and vomiting.

SOURCES OF PABA. Food composition tables do not list PABA, but the following foods are generally recognized as the richest sources: brewers' yeast, fish, soybeans, peanuts, beef liver, eggs, wheat germ, lecithin, and molasses.

(Also see FOLACIN; and VITAMIN[S], Table V-5.)

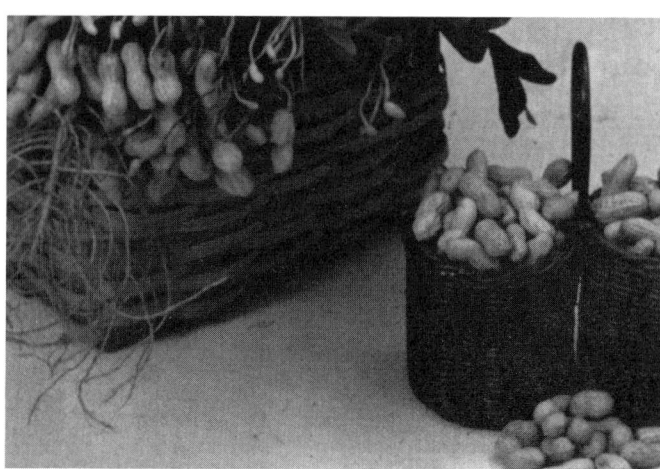

Fig. P-11. Peanuts, a rich source of para-aminobenzoic acid. (Courtesy, USDA)

PARABENS

This is a general term referring to the methyl, ethyl, propyl, or butyl esters (acid alcohol combination) of *p* hydroxybenzoic acid (parabens)—a group of antimicrobial agents used in foods, cosmetics, and drugs. Specifically, these compounds may be called methyl, ethyl, propyl, or butyl hydroxybenzoic acid, or methyl, ethyl, propyl, or butyl paraben.

PARAPLEGIA

Commonly found in spinal cord diseases, or accidents in which the spinal cord is severed in the lumbar region, it is the paralysis or weakness of both legs. Nutritionally, paraplegia is known to occur in humans who ingest Lathyrus seeds over a long period of time. Some dietary modification may be necessary due to reduced activity.

(Also see LATHYRISM; and MODIFIED DIETS.)

PARASITE INFECTIONS

People may harbor a wide variety of internal and external parasites (organisms that live in or on people). They include fungi, protozoa (unicellular animals), arthropods (insects, lice, ticks, and related forms), and helminths (worms). Some parasites require only one host—an animal or person serving as residence—while others need more in order to complete their life cycle.

While in residence, parasites usually seriously affect the host, but there are notable exceptions. Among the ways in which parasites may do harm are (1) absorbing food, (2) sucking blood or lymph, (3) feeding on the tissue of the host, (4) obstructing passages, (5) causing nodules or growths, (6) causing irritation, and (7) transmitting diseases. Two common infestations of man by parasites from undercooked meats are trichinosis and beef tapeworm.

(Also see DISEASES, Table D-10, Food-Related Infectious and Parasitic Diseases; and MALARIA.)

PARASITES

Broadly speaking, parasites are organisms living in, on, or at the expense of another living organism.

(Also see PARASITE INFECTIONS.)

PARATHYROID GLAND

As its name implies, the parathyroid is in the neck in close association with the thyroid gland. Both are endocrine glands. Normally, there are four very small (each weighs only 0.02 g) parathyroid glands lying behind the thyroid gland. They secrete the hormone parathormone, which controls blood calcium levels.

(Also see ENDOCRINE GLANDS.)

PARBOIL

Partial cooking which is sometimes done before finishing the cooking in the oven. Bagels are parboiled before baking in the oven. Some of the cereals that are partially cooked are parboiled.

PARENTERAL

Introduction of nutrients other than by mouth; it may be accomplished (1) subcutaneously (beneath the skin), (2) intramuscularly (into the muscle), or (3) intravenously (into the vein.)

PARESTHESIA

A sensation of burning, numbness, pricking, or tingling, usually associated with an injury or irritation of a sensory nerve or nerve root.

PARIETAL CELLS

The cells of the gastric glands of the stomach which secrete hydrochloric acid (HCl).

PARKIN

This is a popular cake in Scotland. It is made with oatmeal, butter, molasses, baking powder, and spiced with ginger.

PARTS PER BILLION (PPB)

It is an expression of extremely minute quantities. One part per billion equals 0.0000001%, 0.907 mg/ton, 1 mcg/kg, and 1 mcg/liter.

PARTS PER MILLION (PPM)

It is an expression of minute quantities. One part per million is equivalent to the following: 0.454 mg/lb; 0.907 g/ton; 0.0001%; 0.013 oz/gal; 1 mg/liter; and 1 mg/kg.

PARTURITION

Giving birth.

PASTA

Pasta consists of pieces of dough that have been formed in various shapes, then dried.

(Also see MACARONI AND NOODLE PRODUCTS.)

PASTEURIZATION

This is a method of processing food by destroying the microorganisms that cause disease and spoilage. The process was developed by and named for Louis Pasteur, the French scientist who in the early 1860s demonstrated that wine and beer could be preserved by heating above 135°F *(57.2°C)*. In the United States, milk, cheese, egg products, wine, beer, and fruit juice are pasteurized.

(Also see MILK AND MILK PRODUCTS, "Processing Milk"; PRESERVATION OF FOOD, Table P-10, Methods of Food Preservation; and ULTRAHIGH TEMPERATURE STERILIZATION.)

PÂTÉS

• The most common meaning for pâté is a meat or liver dish which has been finely minced and mixed with other ingredients to form a spread for crackers.

• A pastry filled with meat or fish.

PATH–, PATHO–, –PATHY

Each meaning disease; for example, pathological, apathy.

PATHOGENS

Those microorganisms responsible for producing disease. Many microorganisms are harmless.

(Also see DISEASES.)

PATHOLOGY

The science dealing with diseases; their essential nature, causes, and development, and the structural and functional changes produced by them.

PAVLOV POUCH

This is an experimental, surgical technique introduced by the famous Russian physiologist-psychologist, Ivan Petrovich Pavlov. A portion of the stomach is brought to the body wall and formed into a pouch from which samples may be taken. Secretions in the pouch are the same as those in the stomach.

PBI TEST

This test is a measure of thyroid activity by determining the amount of iodine that is bound to thyroxin and in transit in the plasma. The test is based upon the fact that the level of protein-bound iodine circulating in the blood is proportional to the degree of thyroid activity.

Since the hormone thyroxin constitutes the most important single factor influencing the rate of tissue oxidation, or basal metabolism, determination of the level of thyroid hormone in the bloodstream is used to detect the relative rate of basal metabolism. Good correlation with basal metabolism tests has been obtained by this method.

Thyroxin (tetraiodothyronine) is circulated in the blood in temporary union with blood proteins; hence, what the chemical test actually measures is the protein-bound iodine content of the blood, which, in turn, serves as an index of relative activity of the thyroid in releasing its hormone into the blood—hence, the approximate basal metabolic rate.

The PBI test has largely replaced the measurement of oxygen consumption by respiration apparatus (1) because it is much simpler for both patient and technician, and (2) because many doctors feel that it is better suited to clinical purposes. However, the basal metabolism test is still the method of choice for nutritional studies.

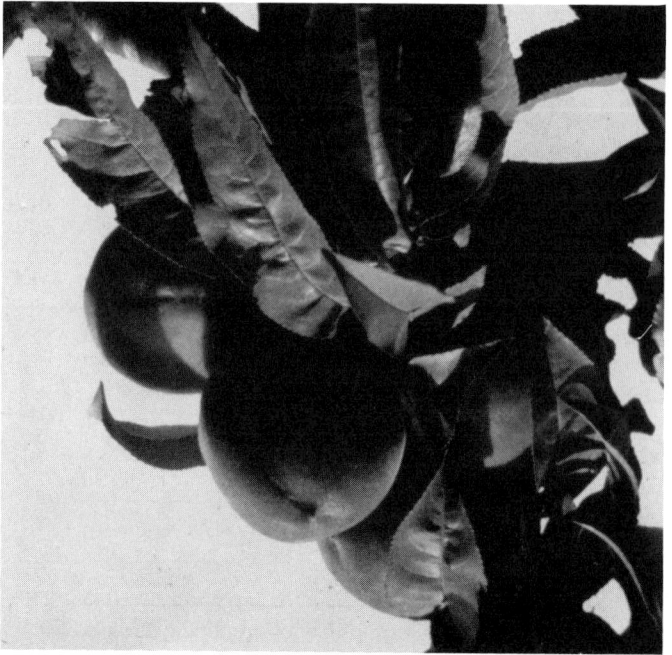

Fig. P-12. A cluster of peaches the juicy, but fuzzy fruit. (Courtesy, USDA)

PEACH AND NECTARINE *Prunus persica*

The peach is the fruit of a tree bearing the same name. Botanically, a peach is classified as a drupe—a fruit whose seed is contained in a hard pit or stone surrounded by soft, pulpy flesh with a thin skin. The peach tree belongs to the rose family, *Rosaceae*. As the genus name, *Prunus*, suggests, peaches are close relatives of the apricot, almond, cherry, and plum.

Peaches are round with yellow skin and edible flesh, though the skin may have areas of red. The edible flesh is either soft or quite firm. Peaches are classified as freestone or clingstone, according to how difficult it is to remove the pit from the fruit.

• **Nectarine**—The peach and the nectarine are essentially alike. Only the fuzz-free skin, the usually smaller size, greater aroma, and distinct flavor separate the two. The scientific name for nectarine is *Prunus persica*—the same as the peach. Nectarines have been called smooth-skin peaches. Herein, comments made regarding peaches also apply to nectarines, unless stated otherwise.

ORIGIN AND HISTORY. The peach is native to China, where it probably grew over 4,000 years ago. From China, it was taken to Persia (Iran), where it was known as the Persian apple. Thence, it spread to Europe, and from Europe to America.

WORLD AND U.S. PRODUCTION. Worldwide, about 8.7 million metric tons of peaches and nectarines are produced annually; and the leading producing countries, by rank, are: Italy, U.S.A., China, Greece, Spain, France, U.S.S.R., Turkey, Mexico, and Argentina. Italy and the United States are far in the lead; combined, they account for 34% of the world production.[8]

Peaches are the sixth leading fruit crop in the United States.

The U.S. produces about 1.3 million short tons of peaches annually; and the leading producing states, by rank, are: California, Georgia, South Carolina, Pennsylvania, Washington, New Jersey, Michigan, Texas, Arkansas, and Colorado. California accounts for almost 50% of the U.S. peach crop. In addition, the United States produces 211,000 short tons of nectarines.[9]

PROCESSING. Most of the U.S. peach crop is either marketed as fresh or canned produce. Sixty-seven percent is marketed as fresh fruit, while 28% is canned. The remaining 5% of the crop is distributed among the following processes: dried, 1%; frozen, 3%; and jams, preserves, brandy, and some other miscellaneous products, 1%. Nearly all nectarines are marketed as fresh fruit.

Before freezing or canning, peaches are inspected, graded, pitted, and peeled. Automatic pitters can remove pits from either freestone or clingstone varieties. Peaches are canned in water pack, juice pack, or in syrup from light to extra heavy. Frozen peaches are generally frozen in a syrup with a small amount of ascorbic acid to prevent browning.

Dried peaches are halved, pitted, peeled, sulfured, and then dried in the sun or in dehydrators. It takes 6 to 7 lb

---

[8]Data from *FAO Production Yearbook 1990*, FAO/UN, Rome, Italy, Vol. 44, p. 162, Table 70. **Note well:** Annual production fluctuates as a result of weather and profitability of the crop.

[9]Data from *Agricultural Statistics 1991*, USDA, p. 201, Table 303. **Note well:** Annual production fluctuates as a result of weather and profitability of the crop.

(2.7 to 3.2 kg) of fresh peaches to make 1 lb *(0.45 kg)* of dried fruit.

SELECTION, PREPARATION, AND USES. Fresh peaches should be fairly firm or becoming slightly soft. Peaches and nectarines can be enjoyed when eaten fresh out of the hand or they can be cooked in a variety of baked goods. Sliced fresh or canned peaches can be eaten alone as a dessert dish or in combination with other fruits in salads, or in fruit plates. Also, peaches are a component fruit of canned fruit cocktail. Dried fruit can be eaten as a snack or cooked. Additional uses of peaches include: baked goods, gelatin desserts, ice cream, jams, jellies, juices, pies, sherbets; and in the production of alcoholic beverages.

NUTRITIONAL VALUE. Fresh peaches contain 89% water. Additionally, each 100 g (about 3½ oz or one medium-sized peach) contain 38 Calories (kcal) of energy, 202 mg potassium, 1,330 IU vitamin A, and only 1 mg of sodium. The calories in fresh peaches are derived primarily from the natural sugars (carbohydrate) which give them their sweet taste. Canned peaches are slightly higher in calories due to the addition of syrup, and their vitamin A content is lower. Dried peaches contain only 33% water; hence, most of the nutrients are more concentrated, including calories. Each 100 g of dried peaches contain 237 Calories (kcal) of energy, 983 mg potassium, 3.9 mg of iron and 2,142 IU of vitamin A. Fresh nectarines are 82% water, and they contain 64 Calories (kcal) of energy, 294 mg potassium, 1,650 IU vitamin A, and 13 mg vitamin C in each 100 g (about two medium-size nectarines). More complete information regarding the nutritional value of fresh, canned, dried, and frozen peaches and fresh nectarines is presented in Food Composition Table F-21.

PEACH PALM (PEJIBAYE) *Guilielma gasipaes*

The fruit of a palm tree (of the family *Palmae*) that is native to Central America and northern South America, but is presently underutilized, considering that its production might be as profitable as that of the cereal grains in the temperate climates.

It is noteworthy that the egglike peach palm fruit develops a nutlike flavor when boiled in saltwater. The oily seeds of the fruit are also edible. They may also be made into flour or fermented into chicha (an alcoholic beverage made by allowing the previously chewed nuts to ferment).

The fruit is rich in calories (196 kcal per 100 g) and carbohydrates (42%). It also contains 2.6% protein (much more than most fruits), and is a good source of iron, vitamin A, and vitamin C.

PEACOCK (PEAFOWL)

This magnificent bird is prized for both its ornamental qualities and its gastronomical value.

In the Middle Ages, the peacock held sway at great state banquets. Its cooking called for all the skill of an experienced master-cook; and only the noblest at the feast had the right to carve it.

Peacocks are still regarded as a delicacy for special occasions. Culinary preparation is similar to pheasant.

PEA, GARDEN *Pisum sativum*

This legume is closely related to the field pea (*Pisum arvense*).

Fig. P-13 shows freshly harvested pods and seeds of the garden pea.

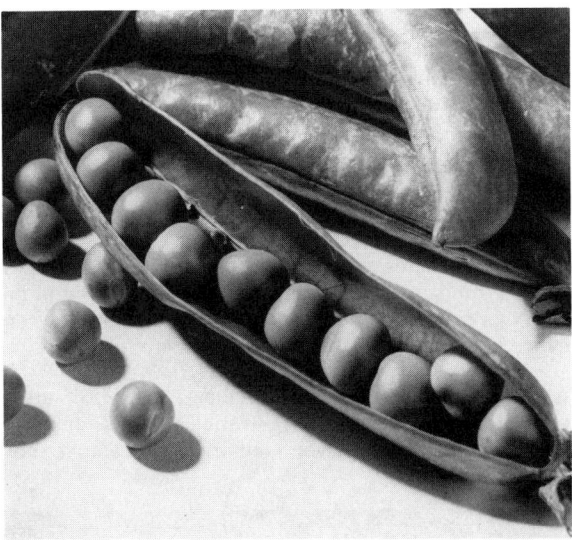

Fig. P-13. Close up of peas in a pod. (Photo by J. C. Allen & Son, Inc., West Lafayette, Ind.)

ORIGIN AND HISTORY. The garden pea appears to have been derived from the field pea by centuries of cultivation and selection for certain desired characteristics. Credence to this theory is lent by the fact that the garden pea is not found in the wild state, whereas the field pea grows wild in the Georgian Republic of the U.S.S.R.

The garden pea, like the field pea, is thought to have originated in Central Asia and Europe, with possibly secondary developments in the Near East and North Africa. Through the centuries, it spread westward and northward throughout Europe, southward into Africa, and eastward to India and China.

Peas were known to and used by the Chinese in 2000 B.C.; and the Bible mentions peas. Apparently, the Chinese were the first to use the green pods and seeds as food. (They also used other legumes similarly.) However, green peas did not appear on European menus until the 16th century, when they were popularized by French royalty. About this time, the agricultural writings began to distinguish between field peas and garden peas.

Peas appear to be the first crop that was scientifically bred to produce new varieties with more desirable characteristics. By the end of the 19th century, many cross breeding trials had been made, the most notable of which were those conducted by the Austrian monk Mendel.

The observations made by Mendel in his monastery garden at Brunn (now Brno, in Czechoslovakia) provided the foundation for the science of genetics.

Peas were brought to America about 1800.

WORLD AND U.S. PRODUCTION. Dry peas and green peas rank fourth and sixth, respectively, among the legumes of the world.

Worldwide, about 17.5 million metric tons of dry peas are produced annually; and the leading countries, by rank, are: U.S.S.R., France, China, Denmark, India, Hungary, Australia, U.K., Canada, and Czechoslovakia. The U.S.S.R. produces 49% of the world dry pea crop.[10]

---

[10]Data from *FAO Production Yearbook 1990*, FAO/UN, Rome, Italy, Vol. 44, p. 103, Table 34. **Note well:** Annual production fluctuates as a result of weather and profitability of the crop.

Worldwide, about 4.8 million metric tons of green peas are produced annually; and the leading countries, by rank, are: U.S.A., U.K., China, Hungary, India, U.S.S.R., Belgium/Luxembourg, France, Italy, and Romania.[11]

Green peas and dry peas rank fifth and sixth, respectively, among the legumes of the United States.

The United States produces about 528,150 short tons of green peas annually; and the leading states, by rank, are: Wisconsin, Minnesota, Washington, Oregon, New York, and Delaware.[12]

The United States produces about 108,000 metric tons of dry peas annually, virtually all of which is produced in the states of Washington and Idaho. It is noteworthy that dry peas represent only 20% of the U.S. pea crop.[13]

PROCESSING. Almost all of the U.S. crop of green peas is processed, since fresh peas spoil rapidly and there is little demand for them. Over half the crop is canned; most of the rest is frozen.

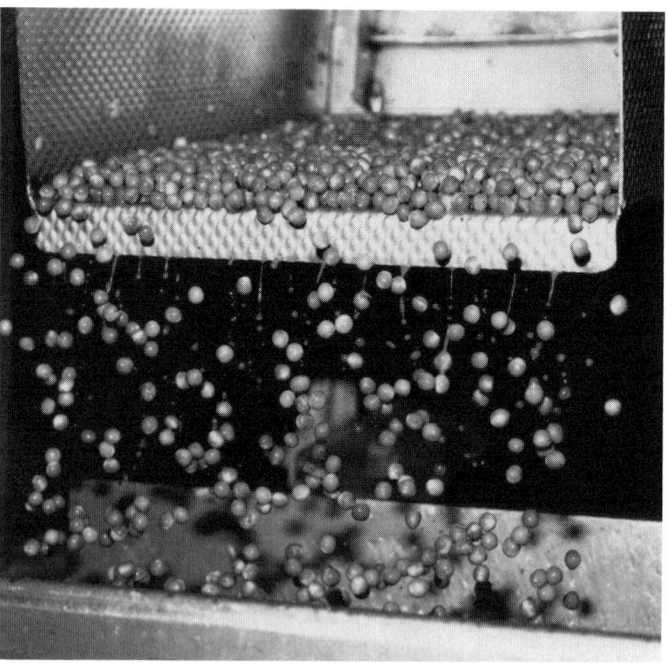

Fig. P-14. Processing peas. (Courtesy, University of Minnesota, St. Paul)

Dried peas may be utilized in the production of canned or dehydrated pea soups, or to a limited extent to make the following products: instant peas soup mixes, quick-cooking dried peas, pea flour, and pea protein concentrate.

SELECTION, PREPARATION, AND USES. Fresh peas of the best quality are young, tender, and sweet. The pods should be fresh, uniformly light-green in color, slightly velvety to the touch, and filled with well-developed peas.

Most homemakers use canned and/or frozen green peas (the leading frozen vegetable in the United States) in preparing meals for their families, since (1) the cooking of dried

---

[11]*Ibid,* p. 146, Table 61.

[12]Data from *Agricultural Statistics 1991,* USDA, p. 158, Table 225. **Note well:** Annual production fluctuates as a result of weather and profitability of the crop.

[13]Data from *FAO Production Yearbook 1990,* FAO/UN, Rome, Italy, Vol. 44, p. 103, Table 34.

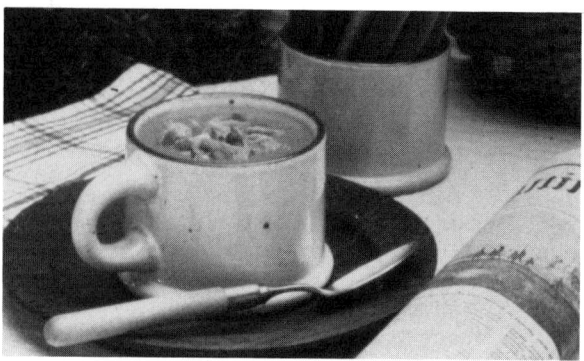

Fig. P-15. Split pea soup, made from dried peas. (Courtesy, USDA)

peas (the most economical form of this vegetable) at home has declined steadily over the past 3 decades, and (2) fresh green peas are sold in pods and require shelling. Some suggestions for preparing the different products follow:

1. Canned peas need no further cooking since they are already tender. Therefore, they might be added to cold salads, or to piping hot dishes that are ready to be served.

2. Frozen peas are usually sufficiently tender after thawing to be used without cooking, but most people enjoy them more after a very brief cooking, followed by the addition of butter or margarine. Only the minimal amount of water to prevent burning or sticking to the pan should be used in cooking.

3. Fresh green peas should be cooked from 10 to 15 minutes after the water comes to a boil. (About 1 lb [0.45 kg] of peas in pods yields a cup [240 ml] of shelled peas.)

4. Dried peas may be cooked much more quickly than dried beans, so it is necessary to use care not to convert the peas to a mushy consistency by overcooking them.

5. Each pound (about 2 cups, or 0.45 kg) of dried peas yields about 3 lb (6 cups, or 1.4 kg) of cooked peas. Usually, this form of peas is the most economical for use in preparing soups.

Peas go well with most other food items such as cereal products, cheeses and other dairy products, fish and seafood, meats, poultry, and vegetables. They may be used in casseroles, salads, soups, stews, and vegetable side dishes. The number and types of pea dishes need be limited only by the imagination of the cook and the ingredients on hand.

NUTRITIONAL VALUE. The nutrient composition of peas is given in Food Composition Table F-21.

Some noteworthy observations regarding the nutrient composition of garden peas follow:

1. Cooked dry (mature) peas provide about twice as much solids, calories, carbohydrates, and proteins as cooked green (immature) peas. However, the green peas are a good to excellent source of vitamin A, and a good source of vitamin C, whereas dried peas are a poor source of both vitamins.

2. A 3½ oz (100 g) portion (about ½ cup) of cooked dry peas or about 1 cup of cooked green peas provide an amount of protein (8 g) equivalent to 1 oz (28 g) of cooked lean meat. However, the peas provide about twice as many calories per gram of protein.

3. Peas are much lower in calcium and phosphorus than beans.

4. Both dry and green peas are good sources of iron and potassium.

Protein Quantity and Quality. The following facts regarding the quantity and quality of pea protein are noteworthy:

1. The grams of protein per 100 Calories (kcal) provided by green and dry peas compared to other selected foods follow:

Food	Grams of Protein per 100 Calories (kcal) (g)
Green peas	7.5
Dry peas	7.0
Cottage cheese	13.2
Lean meat	12.7
Eggs	8.6
Navy beans	6.6
Sweet corn	3.9
Brown rice	2.1

As noted, peas have almost as much protein as eggs. The above figures also show that the amount of protein per calorie in pea dishes may be increased by the addition of a high protein animal food. Similarly, peas may be used to raise the protein content of cereal dishes.

2. Pea protein is moderately deficient in the amino acids methionine and cystine, which are supplied in ample amounts by cereal proteins. However, the legume protein contains sufficient lysine to cover the deficiency of this amino acid in grain proteins. Hence, combinations of peas and cereal products supply higher quality protein than either food alone.

PEANUT (GROUNDNUT; EARTH NUT; GOOBER; GOOBER PEA; GROUNDPEA; PINDA; MONKEY NUT; CHINESE NUT) *Arachis hypogaea*

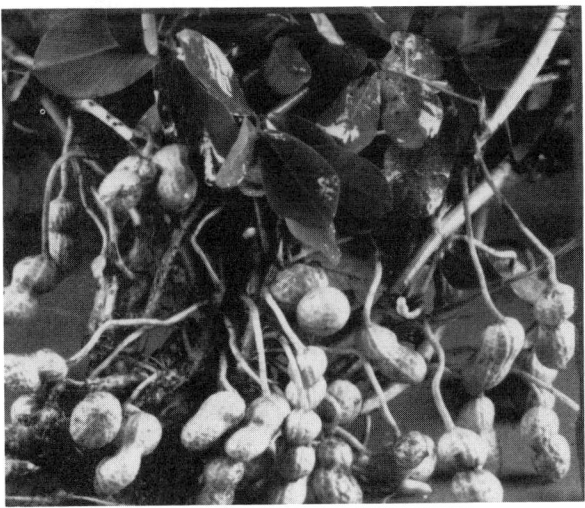

Fig. P-16. How peanuts grow. (Courtesy, National Peanut Council, Washington, D.C.)

The peanut is the strange fruit of the peanut plant. It begins as a fertilized flower above ground, but the pod and the seed mature in the ground; it's the plant with an aerial flower and subterranean fruit.

Unlike the soybean, peanuts are highly esteemed for human food in the United States; and they are standard fare at American sporting events, circuses, and cocktail parties; and, in the form of peanut butter, they have nourished millions of American youths.

ORIGIN AND HISTORY. Peanuts are native to South America. They were introduced to Africa by European explorers, and they reached North America with the slave trade. Early in the 19th century, the value of peanuts as a food crop was recognized. Today, the plant is cultivated on 6 continents in more than 40 countries.

WORLD AND U.S. PRODUCTION. Peanuts rank second among the legume crops of the world. World production in the shell totals about 23.1 million metric tons, annually; and the leading peanut-producing countries, by rank, are: India, China, United States, Nigeria, Indonesia, Senegal, Myanmar, Zaire, Argentina, and Vietnam. More than half of the world crop is produced by India and China.[14]

Peanuts also rank second as a legume crop of the United States; yet, the U.S. produces only 7% of the world's peanuts. About 1.8 million short tons of peanuts are produced annually in the United States; and the leading states, by rank, are: Georgia, Texas, North Carolina, Alabama, Virginia, Oklahoma, Florida, New Mexico, and South Carolina.[15]

PROCESSING PEANUTS. Following picking, peanuts are delivered to warehouses, where they remain until processed. Processing varies somewhat according to market use, with the following operations involved:

• **Cleaning**—The cleaning operation consists of removing sticks, stems, small rocks, and faulty nuts by a series of screens and blowers.

• **Storing**—Cleaned peanuts are either (1) stored unshelled in silos or warehouses for subsequent shelling and delivery to users; or (2) shelled, then stored in refrigerated warehouses at 32° to 36°F (0° to 2° C) and 65% relative humidity, so as to protect against insects and rancidity.

• **In the shell**—Large, unshelled peanuts may be cleaned, polished, whitened, then marketed in the shell.

Some peanuts are salted and roasted in the shell. This involves soaking in salt water under pressure, then drying and roasting.

• **Shelling**—This consists of breaking the shells by passing the nuts between a series of rollers. Then, the shells (along with small, immature pegs) are separated by screens and blowers; and the discolored kernels are removed by hand and by electric eye. Although varying according to variety, shelling reduces the weight of peanuts by 30 to 60%, the space occupied by 60 to 70%, and the shelf life by 60 to 75%.

---

[14]Data from *FAO Production Yearbook 1990*, FAO/UN, Rome, Italy, Vol. 44, p. 109, Table 38. **Note well:** Annual production fluctuates as a result of weather and profitability of the crop.

[15]Data from *Agricultural Statistics 1991*, USDA, p. 118, Table 160. **Note well:** Annual production fluctuates as a result of weather and profitability of the crop.

• **Blanching**—This consists of removing the skins or seed coats, (and usually the hearts) prior to use in peanut butter, bakery products, confections, and salted nuts.

Blanching may be done with heat or with water:

1. Blanching with heat consists of embrittling the skins by exposure to 259 to 293°F (126 to 145°C) heat for 5 to 20 minutes, followed by rubbing the kernels between soft surfaces and removing the skins by blowers and the hearts by screens.

2. Blanching with water is accomplished in different ways. The newest and most rapid method consists of wetting the nuts with 140°F (60°C) water and removing the skins by rapidly revolving spindles. The kernels are dried to 7% moisture prior to storage or conversion into peanut products.

• **Dry roasting**—Peanuts for use in peanut butter, confections, or bakery products are dry-roasted to develop desirable color, texture, or flavor. Dry roasting is accomplished by heating unblanched peanuts to 399°F (204°C) for 20 to 30 minutes, followed by cooling and blanching.

• **Oil roasting**—Peanuts for salting are first roasted in coconut oil or partly hydrogenated vegetable oil at 300°F (148.9°C) for 15 to 18 minutes.

• **Salting**—Either blanched or unblanched peanuts are roasted in oil and salted. Finely ground salt and an oil-base binder are mixed with freshly cooked nuts, which are then placed in flexible bags and canned under vacuum.

• **Extraction of oil**—The oil from peanuts is extracted by one of three methods: hydraulic extraction, expeller extraction, or solvent extraction.

One hundred pounds of peanuts in the shell will yield about 32 lb of crude oil, 45 lb of meal, and 25 lb of hulls.

NUTRITIONAL VALUE OF PEANUTS. The nutritive value of the different forms of peanuts and peanut products is given in Fig. P-17, and in Food Composition Table F-21.

Peanuts are a healthful food. The energy value in 1 lb (0.45 kg) of peanuts (containing about 2,558 Calories [kcal]) is about equal to any of the following: 14 oz (397 g) of cooked round steak, 15 oz (425 g) of natural Cheddar cheese, 3 qt (2.8 liter) of milk, or eight eggs.

Peanuts are also a good source of protein, containing about 26% and a fair balance of essential amino acids. They make a good complementary protein. (See Table P-16, Protein and Amino Acids in Selected Foods.)

Raw or processed peanuts are excellent sources of riboflavin and niacin, and peanut skins are high in the B vitamins.

PEANUT PRODUCTS AND USES. Peanuts have much to contribute to the world's food supply, whether the need be for calories, fats, proteins, or certain vitamins.

In the United States, peanuts are almost entirely a human food and not an oilseed crop as such, since so small a proportion of the crop is processed for oil and protein concentrate.

In the rest of the world, peanuts are primarily processed for their separate constituents—oil and protein. Fortunately, some of the highest peanut-producing countries are in greatest need of their food value. The biggest problem in these countries is to protect the peanuts from molds, rodents, insects, and rancidity. In such countries where there coexists protein deficiency and availability of peanuts, there is much interest in incorporating peanut protein concentrate in the diet of children (see Table P-1, section on "Fortified Foods, Based on Peanut Products, For Developing Countries"). The main deterrent to this program to date has been the cost of peanut protein.

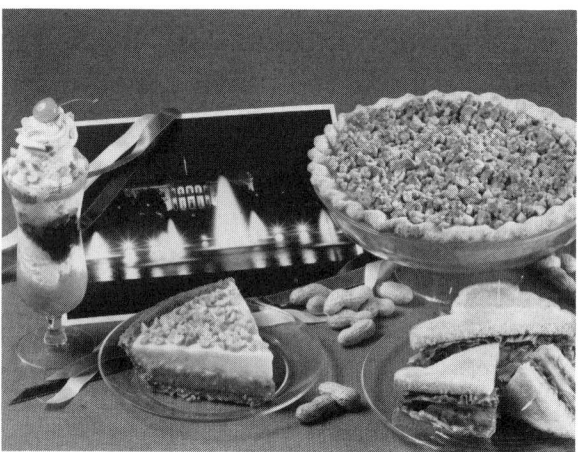

Fig. P-18. Here are three examples of peanut foods: (1) Presidential Peanut Pie; (2) peanut butter, lettuce and tomato sandwich; and (3) peanut butter parfait. (Courtesy, National Peanut Council, Washington, D.C.)

Table P-1 presents in summary form the story of peanut products and uses for human food. In addition to the products listed therein, the following human food products are among those that have not yet reached wide distribution: peanut protein, peanut milk, peanut cheese, boiled fresh peanuts, canned boiled peanuts—shelled and unshelled, frozen boiled peanuts, peanut bread, peanut cereals, and numerous products that may be developed from these.

(Also see FLOURS, Table F-13, Special Flours; and OILS, VEGETABLE, Table O-5.)

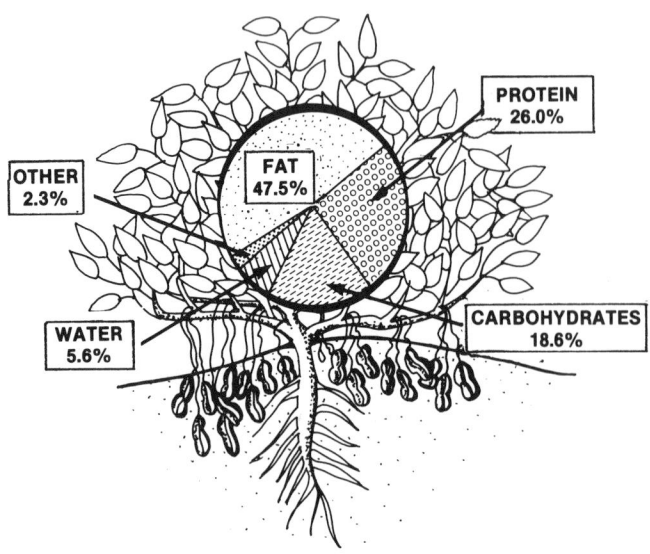

Fig. P-17. Food value of the peanut—the nut with skin.

TABLE P-1
PEANUT PRODUCTS AND USES FOR HUMAN FOOD

Product	Description	Uses	Comments
Whole, roasted-in-shell peanuts	Peanuts roasted inside the shells	Snacks	About ¼ of the peanuts marketed in the U.S. are in the form of roasted peanuts, primarily following shelling.
Defatted peanuts	This process removes 60 to 80% of the oil and ¾ of the calories, leaving intact a high-protein peanut with a flavor that is generally acceptable. Defatted peanuts are prepared as follows: shelled peanuts are reduced to a specific moisture content, then placed in a hydraulic press where most of the oil and calories are removed. Although the kernels are distorted due to the hydraulic pressure, they return to their original shape and size when soaked in water. Salt, sugar, spices and other flavors may be added during the reconstruction period. These low calorie nuts are then dried.	Defatted peanuts are consumed raw, roasted, or used in candy and confectionary products.	
Flour mix (In Congo)	A mixture of fish flour, millet, and peanut flour (50% protein). Made into biscuits.	For children ages 2 to 6 years	These biscuits, which have a good nutritive value and can be recommended for the prevention of malnutrition, are readily accepted by children.
Flour mix (In India)	A mixture of either (1) 25% roasted Bengal gram, 74% peanut flour (low fat), and 1% alfalfa (lucerne) powder; or (2) 25% roasted Bengal gram, 49% peanut flour, 25% low-fat sesame, and 1% alfalfa (lucerne) powder.	These mixtures are eaten with bread and jaggery (an unrefined brown sugar made especially from palm sap).	These vegetable protein diets are nearly as effective in controlling clinical manifestations of malnutrition as diets based on skim milk, but they are somewhat inferior to milk in restoring the level of blood protein (albumen) to normal.
Flour mix (In Senegal)	A mixture of 60% millet, 30% peanut flour, and 10% fish flour. Baked products.	Food for infants	This is a satisfactory food for infants.
Fresh peanuts	Fresh peanuts, not dried or roasted	As a vegetable	In tropical countries, peanuts are usually consumed in this form.
Granulated (chopped), artificially flavored peanuts	These are granulated, artificially flavored peanuts that have the identical flavor and taste of other nuts, especially black walnuts, almonds, and pecans.	Widely used for ice cream toppings, pies, cakes, and other confectionary products.	These artificially flavored nuts are now commercially available in many food stores.
High protein food (In India)	A mixture of equal parts of peanut protein isolate and skim milk powder	A high protein food suitable for treatment of protein malnutrition	
Peanut butter	A cohesive, finely ground product prepared from dry roasted, clean, sound, mature peanuts from which the seed coats and "hearts" are removed, and to which salt, hydrogenated fat, sugars (optional), antioxidants, and flavors have been added. About 90% of the peanut butter is stabilized with hydrogenated oil and antioxidants; 10% is unstabilized (and more flavorsome). Peanut butter contains about 50 to 52% fat, 28 to 29% protein, 2 to 5% carbohydrate, and 1 to 2% moisture.	Sandwiches, salads, desserts, ice cream, custards, confections, and in many baked goods	Peanut butter, consisting of shelled, ground, and parched peanuts, was first prepared as a kitchen product about 1890, as food for infants and invalids. Today, about half the peanuts consumed in the U.S. are made into peanut butter. By federal regulation, 90% of peanut butter must be peanuts in order to be labeled peanut butter. One lb (0.45 kg) of peanut butter has as much total food energy as any of the following: 1⅜ lb (0.6 kg) cheese, 2¼ lb (1 kg) of steak, 4 qt (3.8 liter) of milk, or 32 eggs. Peanut butter is an excellent source of protein (7.8 g per oz), contains no cholesterol and the fat (14.4 g per oz) is mostly unsaturated. An ounce of peanut butter contains 6.4 g of carbohydrate, making it acceptable for most diabetic diets. In a diabetic diet, 2 Tbsp (30 ml) of peanut butter is equivalent to one meat exchange, two fat exchanges, or one B vegetable exchange. However, as with any food, it should not be used indiscriminately.
Peanut flakes	After peanuts are blanched (skin removed) and cooked, they are ground to a slurry, then dehydrated. In the process of dehydration, most peanut flavor constituents volatize, leaving a "tasteless-faceless" peanut product.	Peanut flakes, which contain essentially the same nutritive value (protein and calories) as the peanut, offer virtually unlimited potential as a bland high protein extender for meat and bakery products without adversely affecting the flavor of the finished product.	The processing equipment for making peanut flakes is quite expensive. The worldwide demand for this new product is expected to increase substantially.
Peanut flour	In processing peanut flour, a high proportion of the oil is removed, leaving a product that contains about 60% protein, 22% carbohydrates, 5% minerals, and less than 1% fat.	When commecially available, it is expected that peanut flour will be widely used as a highly digestible protein extender in bakery and confectionary products.	Research has also demonstrated the possibility of using peanut protein fibers for manufacturing meat product substitutes.
Peanut oil	The oil obtained by crushing the nuts in hydraulic presses, or by using chemicals to dissolve the oil out of the nuts. The cold press method gives the lowest yield but the highest quality of edible oil.	Nearly 90% of the peanut oil used in the U.S is for food uses. For frying food. It smokes only	About ⅔ of the world's peanut crop is crushed for oil. Peanuts supply about 6% of the world's edible oil production. India produces 31% of the world's peanuts.

(Continued)

TABLE P-1 *(Continued)*

Product	Description	Uses	Comments
Peanut oil *(Continued)*		at high temperatures and does not absorb odors easily. In salad oils and dressings, margarine, and other vegetable shortenings	The large-podded, large-seeded varieties grown in the U.S. contain about 45% oil, and the small-podded, small-seeded kinds up to 50%. From the two types, a ton of nuts in the shell will yield about 480 lb and 580 lb*(218 and 263 kg)* of oil, respectively. Peanut oil contains at least 8 nutritionally essential fatty acids and 76 to 82% unsaturated fatty acids, of which 40 to 45% is unsaturated oleic acid and 30 to 35% polyunsaturated linoleic acid. The major portion of the characteristic peanut aroma and flavor is imparted by the oil.
Roasted peanuts (following shelling)	Whole nuts, following roasting and shelling. They are usually salted to improve their flavor, except where they go into peanut butter.	As snacks, eaten alone. In candies, salads, desserts, cookies, pies, and in other ways. In mixed, salted nuts. Peanut bread is made from ground peanuts.	There is a preference for the larger nuts for salted peanuts. About ¼ of all edible peanuts in the U.S. find their way into candies. Some of the most flavorsome, nutritious, and popular candies contain peanuts. Peanut candies are mostly bars and brittle.
FORTIFIED FOODS, BASED ON PEANUT PRODUCTS, FOR DEVELOPING COUNTRIES			
Biscuit (In Uganda)	A mixture of 41% peanuts, 26% corn meal, 12% sucrose, 6% cottonseed oil, and 15% dried skim milk. Baked into a biscuit containing 20% protein.	It can be mixed with water (1) into a gruel, or (2) into a drink (by adding more water).	When fed to infants and preschool children, it gives the same weight gain as a milk biscuit.

PEAR *Pyrus* spp

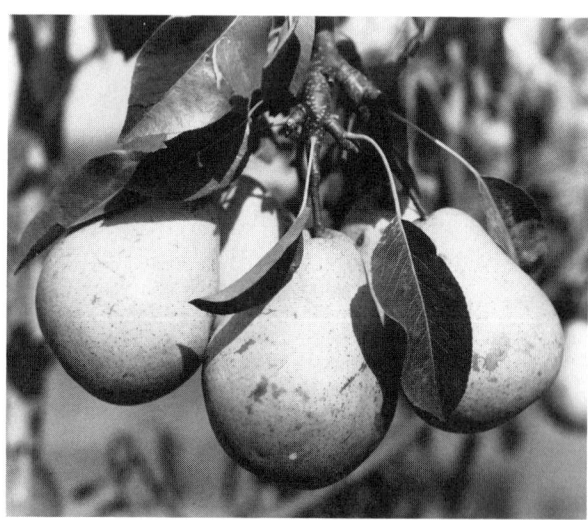

Fig. P-19. Pears—fruit of the ages and relative of the apple. Color may be yellow, russet, or red. (Photo by J. C. Allen & Son, Inc., West Lafayette, Ind.)

The pear which is a member of the rose family, *Rosaceae*, is classified as a pome fruit and is closely related to the apple and the quince. Generally pears are large and round at the bottom, tapering inward toward the stem. However, some are almost completely round and others are as small as a cherry. Pears are covered with a smooth thin skin that may be yellow, russet, or red when ripe. Its edible flesh is juicy, sweet, and mellow. The flesh of some pears has a sandy texture due to the presence of grit cells. Enclosed within the center of the fleshy portion is a core which contains as many as 10 seeds. There are hundreds of pear varieties. Depending upon variety, pears vary in shape, size, color, texture, flavor, aroma, time of ripening, and keeping qualities.

ORIGIN AND HISTORY. The pear is indigenous to western Asia; and it has long been cultivated there and in Europe. Pears were taken to America with some of the first colonists.

WORLD AND U.S. PRODUCTION. Worldwide, 9.8 million metric tons of pears are produced annually; and pears rank eighth among the fruit crops of the world. The leading pear-producing countries, by rank, are: China, Italy, United States, U.S.S.R., Japan, Spain, Turkey, Germany, France, and Argentina.[16]

About 963,800 tons of pears are produced annually in the United States; and the following states lead in production, by rank: Washington, California, and Oregon. These three states account for 97% of the U.S. pear crop.[17]

PROCESSING. About 48% of the pear crop is sold as fresh pears for consumption as fresh fruit and for home use. The remaining 52% is processed as canned or dried fruit. There are no recent estimates available as to the amounts canned or dried, though in past years, the amount dried has been less than 1% of the crop. Therefore, around 51% of the pear crop is probably canned.

---

[16]Data from *FAO Production Yearbook 1990*, FAO/UN, Rome, Italy, Vol. 44, p. 162, Table 70. **Note well:** Annual production fluctuates as a result of weather and profitability of the crop.

[17]Data from *Agricultural Statistics 1991*, USDA, p. 206, Table 313. **Note well:** Annual production fluctuates as a result of weather and profitability of the crop.

Preservation of pears by canning includes pears canned in water pack, juice pack, light syrup, heavy syrup or extra heavy syrup.

SELECTION, PREPARATION, AND USES. As pears ripen their skin color changes from green to the color characteristic for the variety. Bartlett pears turn yellow. Fresh pears are best when they yield to gentle palm pressure. If still green skinned when purchased, pears can be ripened at home by storing them at room temperature, preferably three or more together in a closed paper bag. When pears begin to turn colors and pass the palm pressure test they should be refrigerated. Bartlett pears can be held in the refrigerator for several days either before or after ripening.

Pears can be enjoyed by eating fresh out of the hand like an apple, or they may be used in salads, main dishes or desserts, limited only by the imagination. Canned pears are used alone as a dessert dish or in combination with other fruits and/or in gelatin dishes. Some pears are canned with other fruits in fruit cocktails. Dried pears are eaten as a snack or they may be cooked. Also, pears may be used in the production of alcoholic beverages.

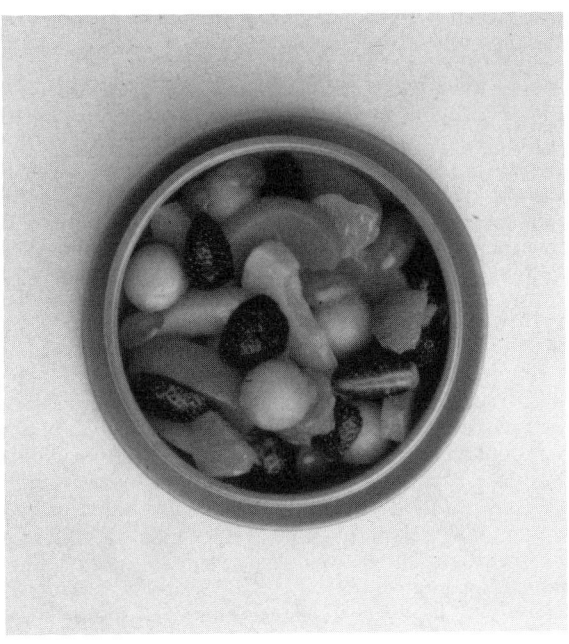

Fig. P-20. Pears are often used in fruit salad. (Courtesy, USDA)

NUTRITIONAL VALUE. Fresh pears contain 83% water. Additionally, each 100 g (about 3½ oz) provides 61 Calories (kcal) of energy, 130 mg of potassium, and only 2 mg of sodium. The calories in pears are derived primarily from the sugars (carbohydrate) which give pears a sweet taste. Pears canned in a syrup contain more calories due to the addition of sugar. Also, canning decreases the concentration of some minerals and vitamins. Dried pears contain only 26% water; hence, many of the nutrients, including calories, are more concentrated. More complete information regarding the nutritional value of fresh, canned, and dried pears is presented in Food Composition Table F-21.

PEARLED

Dehulled grains reduced to smaller smooth particles by machine brushing.

PECAN *Carya illinoensis*

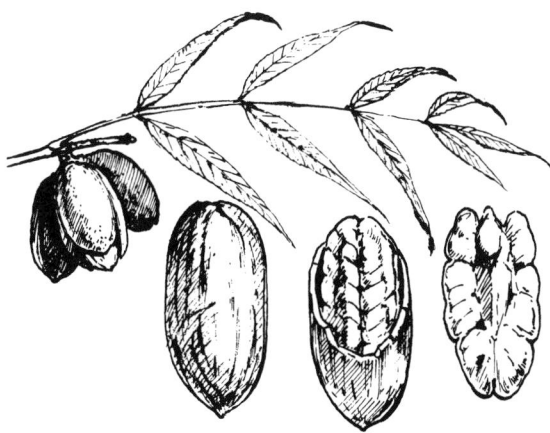

Fig. P-21. Pecans, an American crop requiring patience. Newly planted trees do not bear enough nuts to be profitable until they are about 11 years old.

The nut-bearing pecan tree is classified botanically as a hickory. The trees produce a popular U.S. nut—the delicately flavored, fat-rich pecan. The nut is the basis for pralines, pecan pie, and other foods originating in the South, where the tree grows and yields most abundantly.

ORIGIN AND HISTORY. Pecans are native to North America—to the middle southern United States, and to Mexico. Most pecans are still grown in the South, either as wild trees or as cultivars bred for thinness of shell.

WORLD AND U.S. PRODUCTION. Some wild pecan trees grow in Mexico; and some plantings of pecans have been made in Australia and South Africa. But no production figures for these countries are available.

Pecans are the fourth leading nut crop of the United States; outranked by peanuts, almonds, and walnuts. Most U.S. pecans are grown in the southern states. About 205,000 short tons of pecans are produced annually in the United States; and the leading states, by rank, are: Georgia, Texas, New Mexico, Louisiana, Alabama, Oklahoma, Florida, California, Mississippi, and Arkansas. Georgia alone produces 32% of the U.S. pecan crop. Wild, or native, trees produce 22% of the pecan crop, while improved varieties (cultivars), bred for thinness of shell, produce 78% of the crop.[18] The thin-shelled varieties are called *papershell*, because they can be cracked between the fingers.

PROCESSING. Following harvest, pecans are often dried or *cured* for a few weeks. At processing centers the nuts are cleaned, graded, and packaged. More than 90% of the pecans are marketed as shelled nuts. Pecans in the shell may be stored at 25°F (-4°C) or lower for 2 years or more.

Pecan processing equipment for shelled pecans can size, crack, and separate meats and shells. After separation from the shells, meats are dried to 3 to 4% moisture for better storage. Meats are graded by electric eye and by hand

---

[18]Data from *Agricultural Statistics 1991*, USDA, p. 221, Table 345. **Note well:** Annual production fluctuates as a result of weather and profitability of the crop.

whereupon they are packaged for distribution to bakeries, retail outlets, confectioners, and ice cream manufacturers. Some pecans are salted.

SELECTION, PREPARATION, AND USES.

Pecans in shells should be free from splits, cracks, stains, or holes. Moldy nuts may not be safe to eat. Nutmeat should be plump and fairly uniform in color and size. No further treatment following shelling is necessary. But pecans keep better if stored in tightly closed containers in the refrigerator or freezer.

Delicately flavored, sweet tasting pecans are eaten alone or in an array of dishes and products. It is estimated that there are 1,200 uses for pecans in prepared dishes.

Pecans are used to impart their qualities to such foods as baked goods, dairy products, confections, salads, desserts, fowl stuffings, puddings, souffles, meat combinations, cereals, and vegetable dishes. Pralines and pecan pie

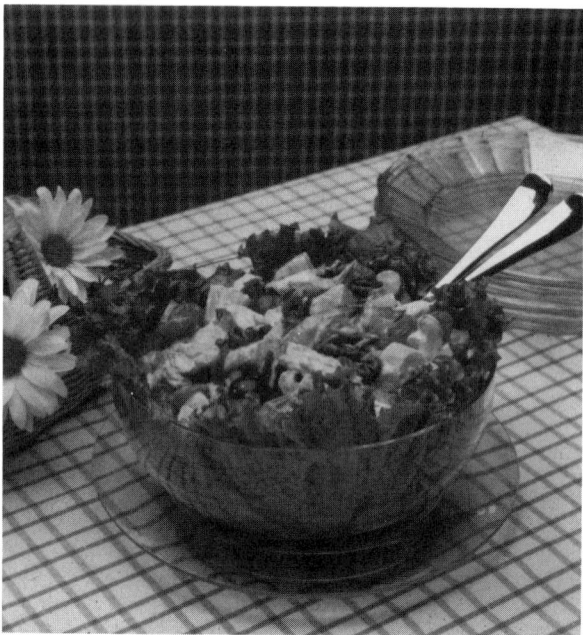

Fig. P-22. Pecans enhance many dishes, like the salad pictured here. (Courtesy, USDA)

originated in the South where most pecans grow. The flavor of pecans is compatible with that of most foods, so that they may be used natural, sweetened, salted, or spiced. The texture is such that they may be used as halves or pieces of any desired size. They may be eaten raw or toasted.

NUTRITIONAL VALUE.

Pecans are extremely nutritious. They contain only 3 to 4% water and they are loaded with energy. Each 100 g (about 3½ oz) of pecans contains 739 Calories (kcal), primarily due to their fat (oil) content of 71%. Additionally, each 100 g provides 9 g protein, 15 g carbohydrate, 2.4 mg of iron, and 4.1 mg of zinc. More complete information regarding the nutritional value of pecans is provided in Food Composition Table F-21.

PECTIN

Most plant tissue, fruits in particular, contain pectin—a polysaccharide which functions as a cementing material. Lemon or orange rind is one of the richest sources of pectin,

containing about 30% of this substance. Pectin, hemicellulose, and cellulose comprise a part of the diet which is often referred to as fiber or roughage. It is not digestible.

Chemically, pectin is a mixture of methyl esterified galacturonan—long chains of the uronic acid of galactose joined by methyl alcohol—plus some galactan and araban, depending upon the plant source. Hence, the complete breakdown of pectin into component parts yields galacturonic acid, methyl alcohol, and small amounts of the sugars arabinose and galactose.

In a pure form extracted from plant material, pectin is a powder, yellowish-white in color, almost odorless, and with a mucilaginous taste. Due to its ability to form gels in a water solution, pectin is an important commercial product used as a food additive by commercial and household food processors.

Many plant materials could be employed for the production of pectin, but apple pomace and citrus peel (lemon, lime, orange, and grapefruit) are the sources for the commercial extraction of pectin.

The type of pectin, hence, its uses in food, is governed by the amount of methyl alcohol joined to the galacturonic acid within the pectin molecule. Therefore, pectin is generally classified as high methoxyl pectin or low methoxyl pectin. Each type possesses different properties.

• **High methoxyl pectin**—When the degree of methylation is more than 50% for the high methoxyl pectin, half or more of the galacturonic molecules are associated with methyl alcohol. High methoxyl pectin requires 55 to 85% sugar and a pH of 2.5 to 3.8 (acid) to gel. This limits the use of high methoxyl pectin as a gelling agent in sweetened fruit products such as jams and jellies at a concentration of 0.1 to 1.5%.

• **Low methoxyl pectin**—Processing techniques can deesterify pectin (remove methyl alcohol) and create low-methoxyl pectin. This type of pectin requires no sugar or acid to gel. Therefore, low methoxyl pectin is used as a gelling agent in fruit products with a low sugar content or products containing no added sugar. The low methoxyl pectin has more and varied uses than high methoxyl pectin.

Pectin is a food additive, and since it is found naturally in plant material, and has always been part of man's diet, the Food and Drug Administration (FDA) accepts it as a generally recognized as safe (GRAS) additive. Moreover, pectin may be a beneficial constituent of the diet, even though it is not digested, since it has been shown to lower blood cholesterol levels.

(Also see FIBER, section on "Kinds of Fiber.")

PECTINASES

Like all living things, plants contain enzymes—protein molecules which catalyze chemical reactions. Pectinases are enzymes in plants or plant products which cause the chemical breakdown of the polysaccharide pectin, resulting in softening and viscosity changes in fruit products. Depending upon the food product, this may be desirable or undesirable. For example, pectins are desirable in tomato, orange, and apricot juices as they make the juice viscous and hold dispersed solids in solutions; hence, pectinase must be destroyed by heat during production. On the other hand, the fruit juices, such as apple and grape juice, a clear juice is desired so commercial pectinase is added. This ensures the production of a clear juice. Vinegar and jelly produced from depectinized juices are a brighter color. Pectinases are also used in making wines. Most commercial pectinases are

derived from *Aspergillus niger* fungi.
(Also see PECTIN.)

PEDIATRICS

Relating to the study and treatment of disease in children. A specialist in pediatrics is called a pediatrician. He is trained in both the medical and surgical diagnosis of the illnesses and disorders of infants and children.

PEKOE

This is a grade of tea leaves, from which a black tea is derived. Pekoe leaves are the middle-sized tea leaves, while orange pekoe leaves are the smallest.
(Also see TEA.)

PELLAGRA

Contents   Page
History of Pellagra...............................835
Causes of Pellagra..............................835
Signs of Pellagra...............................835
Treatment and Prevention of Pellagra................835

This dietary deficiency disease is due to lack of the vitamin niacin or of the amino acid tryptophan (which is converted in the body to nicotinic acid). It usually afflicts people whose dietary protein comes mainly from maize (corn) (which is deficient in both nicotinic acid and tryptophan). Also, it occurs in areas of India where the diet consists mainly of a millet called *jowar* (*Sorghum vulgare*) without any animal foods. Some alcoholics and persons with disorders of absorption have also been found to have the disease.

HISTORY OF PELLAGRA. There is no mention of pellagra in early medical writing in Europe. It appears that the first cases in Europe were observed after the cultivation of maize, taken there from the Americas. Casal first described the disorder in Spain in 1730; and by the end of the 18th century, the disease had spread through Europe, North Africa, and Egypt. Casal found that a milk diet cured the disease. Cerri demonstrated the dietary cure of Italian pellagra victims in 1795; and in the early 1800s Buniva showed, by inoculation of humans with material from diseased persons, that pellagra was not infectious. Most of the European investigators recognized the importance of diet in the prevention and treatment of the disease. In general, the dietary prescription was to eliminate corn from the diet and to replace it with foods of animal origin such as meat, milk, and eggs.

Pellagra, the age-old deficiency disease, killed thousands of people until Dr. Conrad Elvehjem, and co-workers, at the University of Wisconsin, discovered that the vitamin niacin cured blacktongue in dogs, a condition recognized as similar to pellagra in man. Shortly thereafter, several investigators found that niacin was effective in the prevention and treatment of pellagra in humans. Following closely in period of time, it was found that the amino acid tryptophan was a precursor of niacin; and that it would also prevent and cure pellagra.
(Also see NIACIN, section on "History.")

CAUSES OF PELLAGRA. Although pellagra was long associated with reliance on corn as a dietary staple, it took investigators over 200 years to identify the specific nutritional conditions which cause this disease. Today, it is known that pellagra may be caused by any one, or a combination, of the following nutritional conditions:

1. Deficiencies of niacin (nicotinic acid).
2. Deficiencies of tryptophan.
3. Amino acid imbalances which reduce the utilization of tryptophan.
4. Chronic alcoholism.

SIGNS OF PELLAGRA. Clinical signs of pellagra are the characteristic three D's—dermatitis, diarrhea, and dementia. The skin disorder is usually one of the first clear-cut signs of the development of the disease. There is reddening of the areas exposed to the sun or of those areas subjected to friction (such as the elbows). A characteristic dermatitis around the collarbone is called Casal's necklace after the man who first described the condition in Spain. Another very early sign in development of the disease is soreness of the tongue which is swollen, raw, and extra sensitive to hot or seasoned foods (apparently part of an irritation of the entire gastrointestinal tract). The diarrhea, which is not always present, may contain blood and mucus. The mental symptoms range from irritability, anxiety, and depression to psychosis. (In the days of endemic pellagra in the southeastern United States, there were many admissions of pellagra victims to mental hospitals.) A victim of pellagra is shown in Fig. P-23.

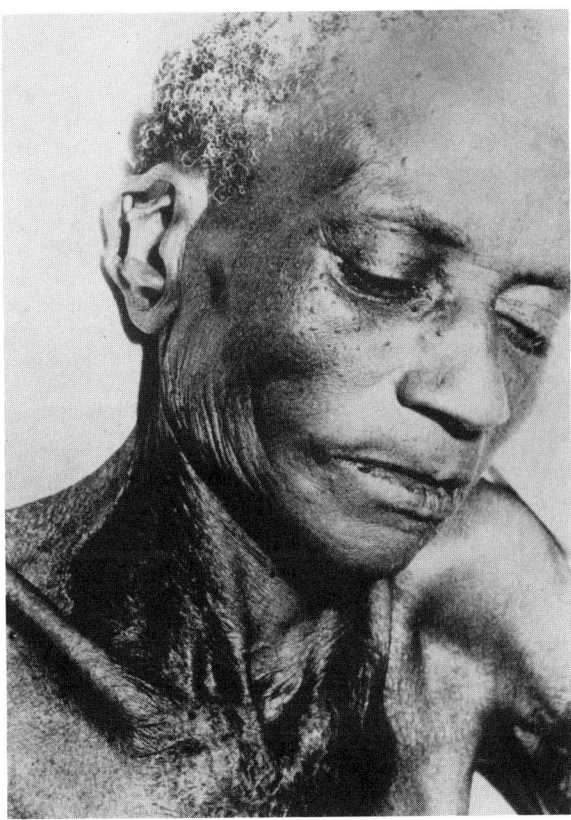

Fig. P-23. An East African victim of pellagra. Note the inflammation and darkening of the skin around his neck. (Courtesy, FAO, Rome, Italy)

TREATMENT AND PREVENTION OF PELLAGRA. Persons suffering from severe forms of the disease may be given either nicotinamide (a derivative of niacin) or nicotinic acid in oral doses as high as 100 mg every 4 hours. Such high doses of nicotinic acid often cause flushing, which does not result when similar doses of nicotinamide are given.

Niacin is well absorbed, even when gastrointestinal disorders are present. Often, a pellagra victim suffers from multiple vitamin and nutrient deficiencies, and, therefore, may require supplemental sources of the vitamin B complex and protein. Brewers' yeast has often been used as such a supplement.

Diets used for the treatment and prevention of pellagra should include abundant sources of animal protein such as meat, fish, eggs, and milk since these foods are good sources of both niacin and tryptophan. Vegetable protein sources high in tryptophan are peanuts, sesame seeds, sunflower seeds, and whole wheat. The refining of grains results in the loss of much of the niacin content, so it is wise to use either whole grain products or those which have been enriched. It should be noted that gelatin, and meats which are high in connective tissue (such as chitterlings, ham hocks, hog jowls, and maws), are very low in tryptophan. It is noteworthy, too, that these were the types of meats commonly used in the South in the years when pellagra was endemic.

(Also see NIACIN.)

PEPPERONI (PEPERONI)

A highly seasoned dry sausage made with beef, or with pork and beef. Also, poultry and turkey may be added to pepperoni provided it is properly labeled.

PEPPERS Capsicum spp

The species of peppers which are native to the Americas have been enthusiastically adopted as commercial crops around the world. These shrubby plants, which are called capsicums to distinguish from the viny pepper plants (*Piper* spp) of the Old World, are members of the nightshade family (*Solanaceae*). Hence, the capsicum peppers are close relatives of the eggplant, Irish potato, and tomato. Although many botanists believe that the different types of capsicums are simply different varieties of a single species, it is customary to classify most types as either (1) chilies (*C. frutescens*), which are usually very pungent; or (2) sweet peppers (*C. annuum*), which have milder flavored, larger fruits.

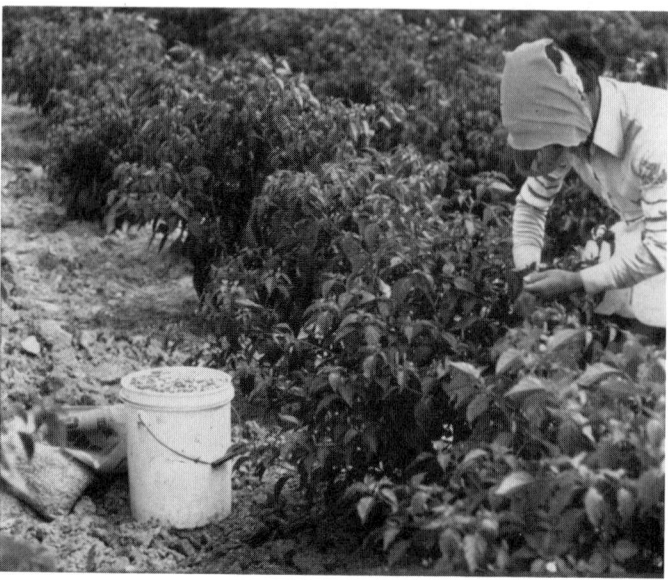

Fig. P-24. Harvesting hot peppers. (Courtesy, Louisiana Cooperative Extension Service, Louisiana State University, Baton Rouge, La.)

ORIGIN AND HISTORY. It seems likely that the prehistoric peoples of Latin America gathered wild peppers in much the same way as certain varieties are gathered today. Pepper seeds dating from more than 5000 B.C. were found by archaeologists at Techuacan, Mexico. It is believed that these seeds came from wild varieties of sweet peppers.

Chili peppers may also have been domesticated independently between 2000 and 1000 B.C. by the Indians living on the Peruvian coast.

The rapid spread of sweet and chili peppers around the world was due in large part to the Spanish and Portuguese explorers who introduced them wherever they went on their ocean voyages.

WORLD AND U.S. PRODUCTION. Peppers rank tenth among the leading vegetable crops of the world, and thirteenth among the leading vegetable crops of the United States.

About 9.1 million metric tons of chilies and sweet (green) peppers are produced worldwide, annually. The leading pepper-producing countries of the world, by rank, are: China, Turkey, Nigeria, Spain, Mexico, Romania, Indonesia, Yugoslavia, Italy, and Egypt.[19]

About 230,000 metric tons of chilies and sweet peppers are produced annually in the United States, with Florida and California ranking first and second, respectively. Most of the peppers produced in the United States are sweet peppers.[20]

PROCESSING. Much of the U.S. pepper crop is utilized as a fresh vegetable because refrigerated storage and transportation facilities make it possible for the vegetable to be marketed around the country with a minimum of spoilage. Most of the remainder is utilized in such items as (1) canned products—corn and peppers, pimientos, sauces, stuffed peppers, and tomatoes and peppers; (2) dehydrated or dried preparations for reconstitution with water, or for making condiments; (3) frozen items—chopped peppers, pizza, and stuffed peppers; and (4) pickles which utilize chilies or sweet peppers. Some are also used in the preparation of prepackaged salads and in making the stuffed peppers sold in the meat sections of certain supermarkets.

Good cooks often enliven their dishes with various condiments made from chilies and/or sweet peppers. Some of the more popular peppers are: Cayenne pepper, chili powder, chili sauce, dried chilies, paprika, pimiento, red pepper, and Tabasco sauce.

SELECTION, PREPARATION, AND USES. Good quality sweet peppers are fresh, firm, bright in appearance, thick fleshed, and have a fresh, green calyx.

The pungent or hot varieties are sold in either the green or red stage of maturity, and vary in size from the small chili peppers to nearly as large as the bell type. Red-colored pods are generally the most desired. The same quality characteristics noted for sweet peppers also apply to fresh hot peppers.

Many people remove the seeds from peppers, but some leave them in and eat them right along with the fleshy part of the vegetable.

Fresh, frozen, or pickled peppers may be (1) served without cooking in relishes, salads, and sandwiches; or (2) cooked in casseroles; Chinese stir-fried dishes; fried onion garnishes for fish, meats, and poultry; omelets; pizzas; soups;

[19]Data from *FAO Production Yearbook 1990*, FAO/UN, Rome, Italy, Vol. 44, p. 139, Table 57. **Note well:** Annual production fluctuates as a result of weather and profitability of the crop.

[20]*Ibid.*

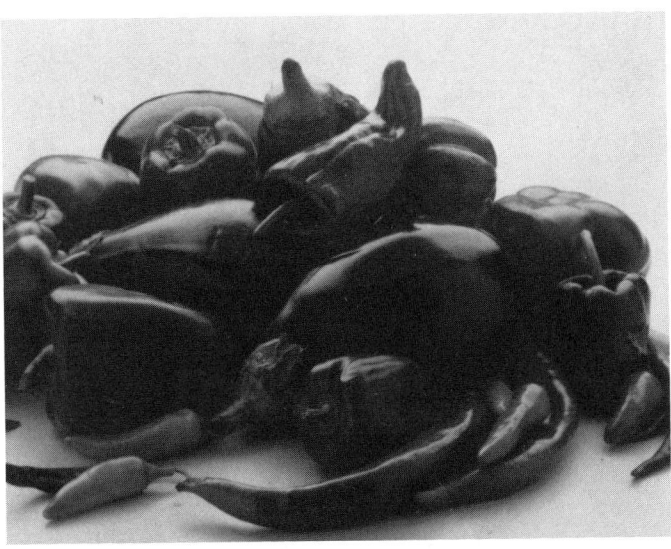

Fig. P-25. Several varieties of peppers. (Courtesy, Shell Chemical Company, Houston, Tex.)

and stews. Sweet peppers are also good when stuffed with bread crumbs, fish, meat, poultry, or rice, then baked. Chili peppers are used as seasoning, as an appetizer, or as a vegetable dish; and as an ingredient of casseroles, pizza, salads, sandwiches, soups, and stews. Chilies are suitable for making *rellenos* by stuffing them with cheese and either baking them in a sauce, or dipping them into an egg batter and deep-frying.

NUTRITIONAL VALUE. The nutrient compositions of various forms of peppers and pepper products are given in Food Composition Table F-21.

Some noteworthy observations regarding the nutrient composition of peppers and pepper products follow:

1. All types of raw peppers have a high water content (74 to 94%) which decreases with maturity, and a low caloric content which increases with maturity. These fresh vegetables are excellent sources of vitamin C and fair to excellent sources of vitamin A. The levels of both vitamins increase with the degree of ripeness. Red peppers have a significantly higher vitamin content than green peppers. Furthermore, chili peppers are richer in these vitamins than sweet peppers at comparable stages of ripeness. Canned, cooked, and dried peppers contain significantly less vitamin C, but approximately the same amount of vitamin A as raw peppers (on a moisture-free basis).

2. An average stuffed green pepper that weighs about 6½ oz (*185 g*) and is filled with a mixture of meat and bread crumbs is literally a nutritious meal in itself—supplying 314 kcal, 24 g protein, 78 mg calcium, 224 mg phosphorus, 477 mg potassium, 3.9 mg iron, 518 IU vitamin A, and 74 mg of vitamin C.

3. A 3½ oz (*100 g*) portion of canned pimientos contains 27 kcal, 2,300 IU of vitamin A, and 95 mg of vitamin C. Hence, this item makes an excellent addition to preparations based upon cereal products, cheeses, eggs, fish, meats, legumes, and poultry because it supplies the vitamins not furnished by the other foods.

4. The chili sauces made from chili peppers (the ones designated as "Hot chili sauces") usually contain only about one-fifth as many calories as the mild sauces made from tomato puree. Furthermore, the vitamin A content of the former preparations is usually several times that of the latter ones (about 1,630 IU vitamin A per Tbsp vs 238 IU vitamin A per Tbsp).

5. A teaspoon of paprika furnishes 1,212 IU of vitamin A, compared to the 800 to 900 IU provided by the same amount of chili powder or red pepper.

6. Although it is not shown in Food Composition Table F-21, it is noteworthy that peppers are excellent sources of bioflavonoids.

Certain types of hot chilies may contain potentially harmful amounts of a highly irritating substance called *capsaicin,* which can raise blisters on sensitive tissues or even cause ulceration. Also, peppers contain small amounts of solanine. (Also see SOLANINE.)

PEPSIN

The proteolytic enzyme present in the gastric juice. It acts on protein to form proteoses, peptones, and peptides.
(Also see DIGESTION AND ABSORPTION.)

PEPSINOGEN

The inactive precursor of pepsin, produced in the mucosa of the stomach wall and converted to pepsin by hydrochloric acid.
(Also see DIGESTION AND ABSORPTION.)

PEPTONE

An intermediate product of protein digestion.
(Also see DIGESTION AND ABSORPTION; and PROTEIN[S].)

PERINATAL

The period from just before to about 100 hours after birth.

PERISTALSIS

An advancing wave of circular constriction preceded by an area of relaxation in the wall of the gastrointestinal tract. This advancing wave propels the food from the esophagus to the anus. It is similar to the action obtained by wrapping one's fingers tightly around a plastic tube of shampoo and then sliding the fingers forward to expel the shampoo that is forced forward in front of the fingers.
(Also see DIGESTION AND ABSORPTION.)

PERNICIOUS

Denoting a severe disease that is usually fatal.

PERNICIOUS ANEMIA

(See ANEMIA, PERNICIOUS.)

PER ORAL

Administration through the mouth.

PER OS

Oral administration (by the mouth).

PEROXIDATION

Oxidation to the point of forming a peroxide—a compound (oxide) which contains an –0–0– group.

PEROXIDE VALUE

As fats decompose peroxides are formed. Chemically, peroxides are capable of causing the release of iodine from potassium iodide (KI). Therefore, the amount of iodine released from potassium iodide added to a fat is a rancidity test. The more peroxide present, the more iodine released; hence, the higher the peroxide value.

PERSIAN BERRY

The name given to the yellow to green dyes obtained from the native American fruits of the buckthorn family *Rhamnaceae*. Some of these berries are poisonous and have an extremely strong cathartic effect.

PESTICIDES

Some pesticides produce unplanned and undesirable side effects, particularly when they are not used properly. Among such effects are: reduction of beneficial species; drift; wildlife losses; honeybee and other pollinating insect losses; and pollution of air, soil, water, and vegetation. Farmers know that unless they follow federal and state regulations they risk having their products seized and condemned, or refused by food processors. It is, of course, essential that pesticide residues remaining on food following harvesting and processing be at levels that do not constitute a health hazard. Each pesticide is issued a tolerance for residues that may result from its use on food or feed crops. To this end, the Environmental Protection Agency (EPA) sets pesticide residue tolerances and the Food and Drug Administration (FDA) routinely monitors foods in an effort to enforce safe levels of pesticides on domestic food.

In recent years, several programs have evolved in both the public and private sectors to reduce the dependency on synthetic chemicals. These include: (1) breeding by both traditional and bio-engineered methods for crop resistance to pests; (2) integrated pest management, which stresses minimal use of pesticides; (3) organic production, which eliminates all synthetic chemical pesticides; (4) biological controls, which use either living organisms or toxic extracts from them; (5) low input sustainable agriculture, which applies integrated pest management principles to all areas of crop production.

No pest control system is perfect; and new pests keep evolving. So, research and development on a wide variety of fronts should be continued. We need to develop safer and more effective pesticides, both chemical and nonchemical. In the meantime, there is need for prudence and patience.

(Also see POISONS, Table P-2 Some Potentially Poisonous [Toxic] Substances.)

PETITGRAIN OIL

An essential oil extracted from the leaves and twigs of the bitter orange tree, the lemon tree, or the tangerine tree. Petitgrain oils are employed for flavoring purposes and are on the GRAS (generally recognized as safe) list of approved substances.

pH

A measure of the acidity or alkalinity of a solution. Values range from 0 (most acid) to 14 (most alkaline), with neutrality at pH 7.

(Also see ACID-BASE BALANCE.)

PHAGOCYTE

A cell capable of ingesting bacteria or other foreign material.

(Also see BACTERIA IN FOOD, section on "Bacterial Control Methods"; and BACTERIOPHAGE.)

PHAGOMANIA

An unusual or unreasonable fondness for eating. (Also see APPETITE.)

PHEASANT

The pheasant, which originated in the Orient, is classed as both a game bird and an ornamental bird. Connoisseurs of this savory bird prefer hen pheasants about 1 year of age. Pheasants are similar to chickens; so, they may be processed and cooked in a similar manner.

PHENOL OXIDASES (PHENOLASES)

A group of copper-containing enzymes responsible for the browning of the cut surfaces of certain fruits and vegetables. Browning reduces the acceptability of a food due to the off-color and off-flavor. Depending upon the intended use of a food, five different methods may be employed to prevent enzymatic browning by the action of phenol oxidases: (1) heat inactivation, blanching; (2) chemical inhibition with sulfur dioxide; (3) reducing agents such as ascorbic acid; (4) exclusion of oxygen during packaging; and (5) alteration of the phenol oxidase substrates by adding another enzyme.

(Also see PRESERVATION OF FOOD.)

PHENYLALANINE

One of the essential amino acids. (Also see AMINO ACID[S].)

PHENYLPYRUVIC ACID

An intermediate product in phenylalanine metabolism.

PHEOPHYTIN

A waxy, olive-brown pigment which results from the treatment of chlorophyll with an acid such as oxalic acid. The magnesium atom in the chlorophyll molecule is replaced by two hydrogen atoms. This accounts for the color change when green vegetables are cooked.

PHOSPHATE BOND, ENERGY RICH

Energy is required for practically all life processes—for the action of the heart, maintenance of blood pressure, muscle tone, transmission of nerve impulses, kidney function, protein synthesis, fat synthesis, secretion of milk, and muscular contraction. In the body, fats, proteins and carbohydrates represent potential energy sources. However, releasing all of the energy contained in these sources in one step would result in lost and wasted heat energy. Instead, energy is released in steps by a series of metabolic reactions. As the energy is released, it is captured and stored for use in the form of adenosine triphosphate (ATP). When this ATP is formed from ADP (adenosine diphosphate), 8 kcal/mole (molecular weight) must be put into the system. The ATP then acts as an energy rich storage compound. When energy is required for body functions, ATP is broken down to ADP and 8 kcal/mole of ATP are liberated.

(Also see METABOLISM.)

PHOSPHOLIPIDS

These are similar to triglycerides except one of the fatty acids attached to the glycerol molecule is replaced by phosphate and a nitrogen-containing compound. Lecithin, cephalin, phosphatidyl inositol, and phosphatidyl serine are all classified as phospholipids. Functionally, phospholipids are (1) structural components of membranes; (2) potential energy sources; (3) involved in the blood clotting mechanism; and (4) components of certain enzymes.

(Also see FATS AND OTHER LIPIDS.)

PHOSPHOPROTEIN

A conjugated protein that contains phosphorus; for example, casein found in milk.

PHOSPHORUS (P)

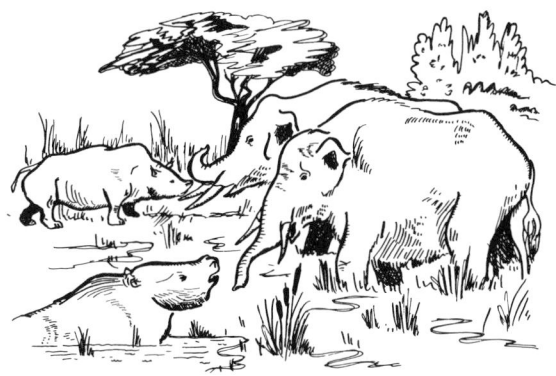

The era of phosphate formation

Fig. P-26. Primeval giants, such as rhinoceros (left) and mastodons (right) roamed Florida dulring the phosphate forming era.

Phosphorus is the Dr. Jekyll and Mr. Hyde of mineral elements—it can deal life or death. As white phosphorus, it's the flame of incendiary bombs; as red phosphorus, it's the heart of the common match; as organic phosphate, it's nerve gas and insecticides; and as organic combinations, it's a constituent of every cell and fluid of the body. Without phosphorus, no cell divides, no heart beats, and no baby grows.

Phosphorus is closely associated with calcium in human nutrition—to the extent that a deficiency or an overabundance of one may very likely interfere with the proper utilization of the other. Also, both calcium and phosphorus occur in the same major food source—milk; both function in the major task of building bones and teeth; both are related to vitamin D in the absorption process; both are regulated metabolically by the parathyroid hormone and calcitonin; both exist in the blood serum in a definite ratio to each other; and both, as the chief components of bone ash, were used in many ancient medieval remedies.

Phosphorus comprises about 1% or 1.4 lb (650 g) of the adult body weight. That's about ¼ the total mineral matter in the body. Eighty percent of the phosphorus is in the skeleton (including the teeth) in inorganic combination with calcium, where the proportion of calcium to phosphorus is about 2:1. The remaining 20% is distributed in the soft tissues, in organic combination, where the amount of phosphorus is much higher than calcium. In the soft tissues, it is found in every living cell, where it is involved as an essential component in interrelationships with proteins, lipids, and carbohydrates to produce energy, to build and repair tissues, and to act as a buffer. Whole blood contains 35 to 45 mg of phosphorus per 100 ml; of this, about ½ is in the red cells, and, in adults, 2.5 to 4.5 mg per 100 ml is in the serum. In children, the serum phosphorus level is somewhat higher, ranging from 4 to 7 mg per 100 ml; the higher level during the growth years reflecting its role in cell metabolism. Four to nine mg of the whole blood phosphorus is inorganic phosphorus, which is readily affected by dietary intake and is in constant exchange with the organic phosphate of the blood.

HISTORY. Phosphorus, a nonmetallic element, was first identified in urine by Hennig Brand, a German alchemist, in 1669. It created much interest because, in the unnatural free form, it glowed in the dark and took fire spontaneously upon exposure to the air. Eventually, the name phosphorus (from the Greek for *light-bringing*) was appropriated to this element. Fortunately, phosphorus exists in nature only in combined forms, usually with calcium, in such sources as bone and rock phosphates.

ABSORPTION OF PHOSPHORUS. Phosphorus is more efficiently absorbed than calcium; 70% of the ingested phosphorus is absorbed and 30% is excreted in the feces, whereas only 20 to 30% of the ingested calcium is absorbed and 70 to 80% is excreted in the feces.

Since much of the phosphorus in foods occurs as a phosphate compound, the first step (prior to absorption) is the splitting off of phosphorus for absorption as the free mineral. The phosphorus is then absorbed as inorganic salts.

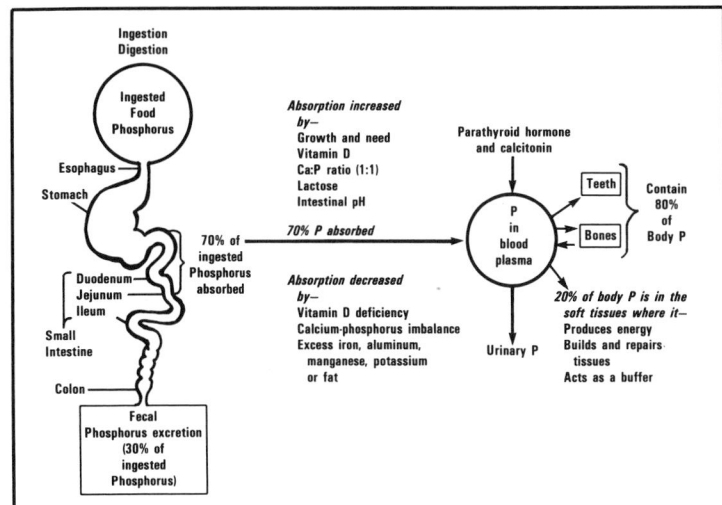

Fig. P-27. Phosphorus utilization. Note that healthy adults absorb 70% of the phosphorus in their food, and that 30% is excreted in the feces. Note, too, the factors that increase and decrease absorption.

Phosphorus is absorbed chiefly in the upper small intestine, the duodenum. The amount absorbed is dependent on several factors, such as source, calcium: phosphorus ratio, intestinal pH, lactose intake, and dietary levels of calcium, phosphorus, vitamin D, iron, aluminum, manganese, potassium, and fat. As is the case for most nutrients, the greater the need, the more efficient the absorption. Absorption increases, although not proportionally, with increased intake.

METABOLISM OF PHOSPHORUS. Phosphorus absorbed from the intestine is circulated through the body and is readily withdrawn from the blood for use by the bones and teeth during periods of growth. Some incorporation into the bones occurs at all ages. It may be withdrawn from bones to maintain normal blood plasma levels during periods of dietary deprivation.

The plasma phosphorus level (which generally falls within the range of 2.5 to 4.5 mg per 100 ml in adults—higher in children), along with calcium, is regulated by the parathyroid hormone and thyrocalcitonin (calcitonin) and is inversely related to the blood calcium level.

Phosphorus metabolism can be disturbed in many types of disease, notably those involving the kidneys and bone.

EXCRETION OF PHOSPHORUS. The kidneys provide the main excretory mechanization for regulation of the serum phosphorus level. All of the plasma inorganic phosphate is filtered through the renal glomeruli. If the serum phosphorus level falls, the renal tubules return more phosphorus to the blood; if the serum phosphorus level rises, the renal tubules excrete more. Also, when the diet lacks sufficient phosphorus, the renal tubules conserve phosphorus by returning it to the blood. On an average diet, an adult excretes from 0.6 to 1.0 g of phosphorus every 24 hours.

FUNCTIONS OF PHOSPHORUS. Among the mineral elements essential to life none plays a more central role than phosphorus. It is found throughout the body in every cell; and it is involved in almost all, if not all, metabolic reactions. The diverse and most important functions of phosphorus are given in the section on MINERAL(S), Table M-25, Mineral Table.

DEFICIENCY SYMPTOMS. Dietary deficiencies of phosphorus in man are unlikely, since this mineral is present in nearly all foods. However, deficiencies are seen in people in certain clinical conditions; in persons receiving excessive antacids over long periods, and in certain stress conditions such as bone fractures.

Vegetarian diets, especially those low in milk products, may be deficient in phosphorus as well as in other elements.

Severe and prolonged deficiencies of phosphorus may be manifested in rickets and phosphorus related diseases (see subsequent section headed "Phosphorus Related Diseases").

(Also see section on MINERAL[S], Table M-25, Mineral Table.)

INTERRELATIONSHIPS. Phosphorus is involved in certain relationships, the most important of which follow:

• **Calcium-phosphorus ratio and vitamin D**—Adequate phosphorus and calcium nutrition is dependent upon three factors: a sufficient supply of each element, a suitable ratio between them, and the presence of vitamin D. Generally, human nutritionists recommend a calcium-phosphorus ratio

of 1.5:1 in infancy, decreasing to 1:1 at 1 year of age, and remaining at 1:1 throughout the rest of life; although they consider ratios between 2:1 and 1:2 as satisfactory. With plenty of vitamin D, the ratio becomes of less importance, and more efficient utilization is made of the amounts of the element present.

• **Excess of calcium over phosphorus; excess of phosphorus over calcium**—If the diet contains an excess of calcium over phosphorus (that is, more calcium than can be absorbed in the first part of the small intestine) free calcium will be present at the points where phosphorus is absorbed. This excess calcium will combine with the phosphorus to form insoluble tricalcium phosphate, and thus interfere with the absorption of phosphorus.

An excess of dietary phosphorus over calcium will in the same way decrease the absorption of both calcium and phosphorus.

• **Excess intakes of iron, aluminum, and magnesium**—Large intakes of iron, aluminum, and magnesium may bind phosphorus in insoluble salts and inhibit its absorption.

• **Phosphorus present as phytin or phytic acid**—There is evidence that man utilizes phytin phosphorus poorly—that phytin is incompletely broken down in the digestive tract. As a result, the undigested phytate may depress the absorption of calcium and iron.

RECOMMENDED DAILY ALLOWANCE OF PHOSPHORUS. The National Research Council recommended daily dietary allowances, with provision for individual variation, of phosphorus are given in the section on MINERAL(S), Table M-25, Mineral Table.

Note that the recommended daily allowances for phosphorus range from 300 mg to 1,200 mg. Note, too, that the allowances vary according to age, and that provision is made for added allowances for pregnant and lactating females.

The recommended allowance of phosphorus in milligrams per day is the same as that for calcium, except for the young infant.

• **Phosphorus intake in average U.S. diet**—The intake of phosphorus in ordinary diets is usually higher than that of calcium and is thought to be adequate.

In recent years, the widespread use of phosphate food additives (mainly sodium salts of orthophosphates, pyrophosphates, and polyphosphates) as acidifiers, emulsifiers, chelators, leavening agents, and water-binders has significantly increased the phosphorus content of the food supply. Such additives currently appear to contribute an additional 0.5 to 1.0 g phosphorus per day to the diet of U.S. adults.

The average available phosphorus for consumption per capita per day in the United States is approximately 1,540 mg, the primary sources of which are: dairy products, 34.3%; meat, poultry, and fish, 29.2%; and flour and cereal products, 14.1%. Thus, except for unusual circumstances, a deficiency in man is unlikely.

TOXICITY. There is no known phosphorus toxicity *per se*. However, excess phosphate consumption may cause hypocalcemia (a deficiency of calcium in the blood) and result in enhanced neuroexcitability, tetany, and convulsions.

PHOSPHORUS RELATED DISEASES. Phosphorus is present in nearly all foods, with the result that a dietary deficiency is extremely unlikely to occur in man. Intake of this mineral is almost always, if not invariably, higher than that of calcium and is entirely adequate under most conditions. However, phosphorus deficiencies may occur (1) when there is excess intake of nonabsorbable antacids, (2) when infants are on cow's milk, and (3) when vegetarians are on high fiber diets produced on phosphorus-deficient soils. Phosphorus related diseases include rickets and osteomalacia.

(Also see RICKETS; and OSTEOMALACIA.)

• **Phosphorus depletion due to prolonged and excessive intake of nonabsorbable antacids**—The frequency of this syndrome is unknown. It is characterized by weakness, anorexia (reduced appetite), and pain in the bones. Treatment consists in discontinuing antacids and providing adequate dietary phosphorus.

• **Hypocalcemic tetany of infants**—Where infants are raised on cow's milk, the Ca:P ratio in cow's milk may contribute to the occurrence of hypocalcemic tetany during the first week of life. This postulation is based on the fact that the Ca:P ratio in cow's milk is approximately 1.2:1, compared with 2:1 in human milk. Because of this situation, the current recommendation is that in infancy the Ca:P ratio in the diet be 1.3:1, decreasing to 1:1 at 1 year of age.

• **Phosphorus deficiency of vegetarians on a high fiber diet produced on phosphorus-deficient soils**—Presently, this is without proof in humans, but there is abundant evidence that this condition occurs in animals.

At Washington State University, in a study with rabbits, the effect of soil phosphorus on plants, and, in turn, the effects of these plants on animals, was established.[21] Generation after generation, rabbits were fed on alfalfa, with one group receiving hay produced on low-phosphorus soils and the other group eating alfalfa grown on high-phosphorus soils. The rabbits in the low-phosphorus soil–alfalfa group (1) were retarded in growth—with 9.8% lower weaning weights, (2) required 12% more matings per conception, and (3) had a 47% lower breaking strength of bones than the rabbits on the high-phosphorus soil–alfalfa group. There is reason to believe that a phosphorus deficiency can affect people similarly, and that some people are consuming suboptimum levels of phosphorus—especially vegetarians on a high fiber diet produced on phosphorus-deficient soils.

In addition to the conditions noted above, a phosphorus deficiency may also interfere with the utilization of vitamin A and, in growing children, teeth as well as bones will be less dense and less completely mineralized.

• **Excess phosphorus syndrome**—Excess phosphorus may also create problems. For example, an inhibitory effect of excess dietary phosphorus on bone development in domestic animals has long been recognized. Chronic ingestion of high phosphate diets causes secondary hyperparathyroidism, bone resorption, and, in some cases, calcification of kidney and heart tissue. The level of dietary phosphate required to produce these effects is dependent upon the concentrations of calcium, magnesium, and other ingredients. Excess phosphate also causes the effects of magnesium deficiency to be more severe and increases the intake of calcium required to maintain normocalcemia.

The demonstration that adult animals fed high phospho-

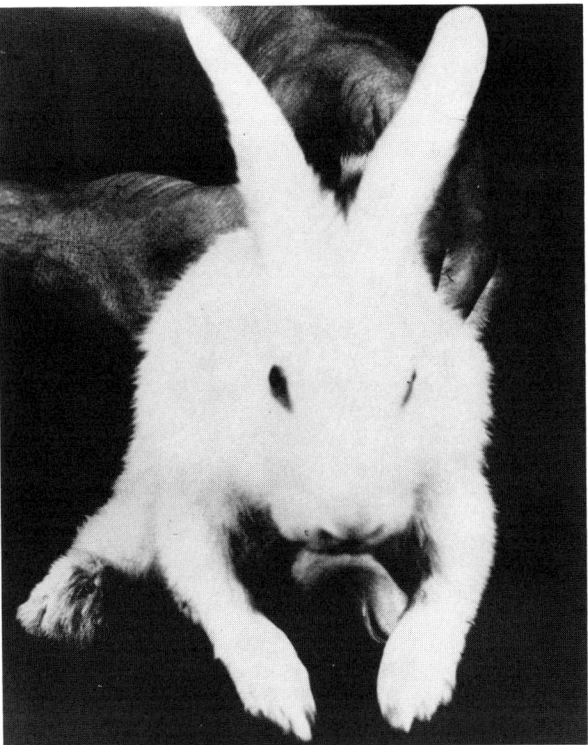

Fig. P-28. Rabbit with bowed legs and enlarged joints resulting from eating alfalfa produced on low-phosphorus soils. There is reason to believe that vegetarians on high fiber diets may suffer similar consequences. (Courtesy, Washington State University)

rus diets, even in the presence of normally adequate concentrations of calcium, undergo an enhanced rate of bone resorption and net loss of bone mass has raised the possibility that diets high in phosphorus, particularly those that are concomitantly low in calcium, may contribute to *aging bone loss* or of *osteoporosis* in man.

CALCIUM-PHOSPHORUS RATIO AND VITAMIN D. The proportional relation that exists between calcium and phosphorus is known as the calcium-phosphorus ratio. When considering the calcium and phosphorus requirements, it is important to realize that the proper utilization of these minerals by the body is dependent upon (1) a suitable calcium-phosphorus ratio (Ca:P), (2) an adequate supply of calcium and phosphorus in an available form, and (3) sufficient vitamin D to make possible the assimilation and utilization of the calcium and phosphorus. Generally speaking, a rather wide variation in Ca:P ratio in the diet is tolerated. However, nutritionists generally recommend a calcium-phosphorus ratio of 1.3:1 in infancy, decreasing to 1:1 at 1 year of age, and remaining at 1:1 throughout the rest of life; although they consider ratios between 2:1 and 1:2 as satisfactory. If plenty of vitamin D is present (provided either in the diet or by sunlight), the ratio of calcium to phosphorus becomes less critical. Likewise, less vitamin D is needed when there is a desirable calcium-phosphorus ratio.

It is noteworthy that there is much evidence indicating that calcium-phosphorus ratios of 1:1 to 2:1 for nonruminants (hogs and horses) and 1:1 to 7:1 for ruminants are satisfactory; but that ratios below 1:1 are often disastrous.

The dietary Ca:P ratio is particularly important during the critical periods of life—for children, and for women during the latter half of pregnancy and during lactation.

[21]Heinemann, W. W., M. E. Ensminger, W. E. Ham, and J. E. Oldfield, "Phosphate Fertilization of Alfalfa and Some Effects on the Animal Body," *Wash. Ag. Exp. Sta., Tech. Bull.* 24, June 1957.

SOURCES OF PHOSPHORUS. Good sources are meat, poultry, fish, eggs, cheese, nuts, legumes, and whole-grain foods. It is noteworthy, however, that much of the phosphorus in cereal grains occurs in phytic acid, which combines with calcium to form an insoluble salt that is not absorbed. Vegetables and fruits are generally low in phosphorus.

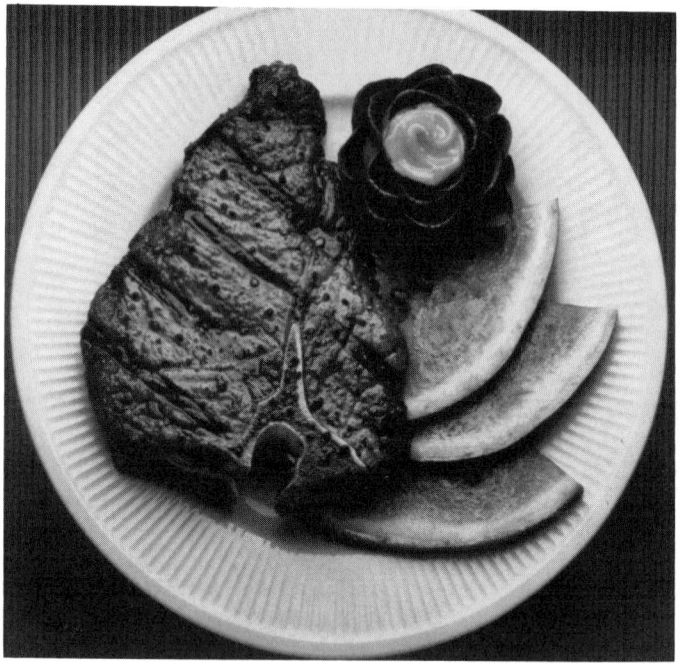

Fig. P-29. T-bone steak. Meat is a good source of phosphorus. (Courtesy National Live Stock & Meat Board, Chicago, Ill.)

Groupings, by rank, of common sources of phosphorus are given in the section on MINERAL(S), Table M-25, Mineral Table.

For additional and more precise values of phosphorus, see Food Composition Table F-21.

(Also see MINERAL[S], Table M-25, Mineral Table; and CALCIUM.)

PHOSPHORYLATE

To introduce a phosphate grouping into an organic compound; for example, glucose monophosphate produced by the action of phosphorylase.

PHOSPHORYLATION

The chemical reaction in which a phosphate group is introduced into an organic compound.

PHOTOSYNTHESIS

Life on earth is dependent upon photosynthesis. Without it, there would be no oxygen, no plants, no food, and no people.

As fossil fuels (coal, oil, shale, and petroleum)—the stored photosynthates of previous millennia—become exhausted, the biblical statement, "all flesh is grass" (Isaiah 40:6), comes alive again. The focus is on photosynthesis. Plants, using solar energy, are by far the most important, and the only renewable, energy-producing method; the only basic food-manufacturing process in the world; and the only major

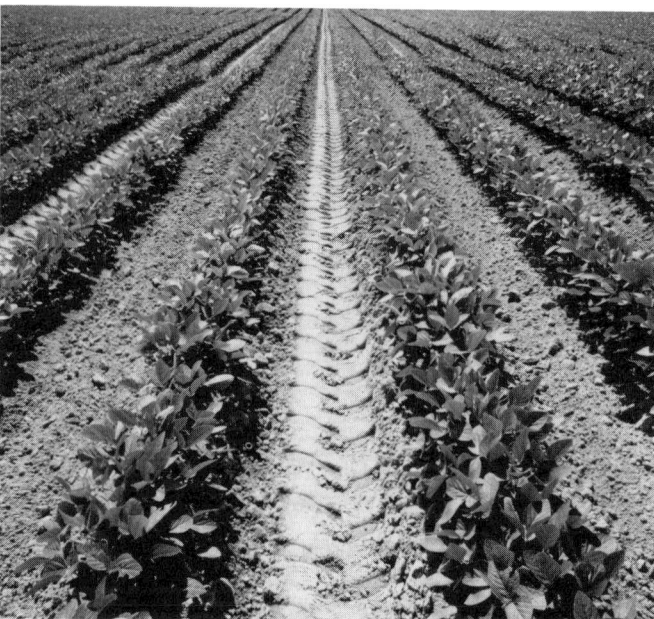

Fig. P-30. Photosynthesis. With their tops in the sun and their roots in the soil, plants are green factories producidng energy. (Courtesy, University of Maryland, College Park, Md.)

source of oxygen in the earth's atmosphere. Even the chemical and electrical energy used in the brain cells of man are the products of sunlight and the chlorophyll of green plants. Thus, in an era of world food shortages, it is inevitable that the entrapment of solar energy through photosynthesis will, in the long run, prove more valuable than all the underground fossil fuels—for when the latter are gone, they are gone forever. So, all food comes directly or indirectly from plants which have their tops in the sun and their roots in the soil. Hence, we have the nutrition cycle as a whole—from the sun and soil, through the plant, thence to animals and people, and back to the soil again. In summary form, the story is—

$$\text{Green factories} + \text{4-stomached animals} \xrightarrow[\text{(store)}]{\text{(convert)}} \text{energy}$$
(Plants)

Technically, green factories are known as photosynthetic plants, and 4-stomached animals are called ruminants; together, they convert and store energy in a form available to man. Not only that! They are relatively free from political control; they are universally available on a renewable basis; and, properly managed, they enhance the quality of the environment. Besides, they're free of cancer-laden carcinogens.

The energy required by every living creature, man included, is derived from the photosynthetic process occurring in green plants in which light energy from the sun is converted to chemical energy, then trapped in newly made sugar molecules.[22] Ultimately, all the energy in our food comes from this source.

---

[22]Certain types of microorganisms, termed chemoautotrophs, get their energy from inorganic compounds, but aside from this minor exception, the energy that runs the life support system of the biosphere comes from photosynthesis.

The word photosynthesis means putting together with light. More precisely, photosynthesis may be defined as *the process by which the chlorophyll-containing cells in green plants capture the energy of the sun and convert it into chemical energy; it's the action through which plants synthesize and store organic compounds, especially carbohydrates, from inorganic compounds—carbon dioxide, water, and minerals, with the simultaneous release of oxygen.*

Photosynthesis is dependent upon the presence of chlorophyll, a green pigment which develops in plants soon after they emerge from the soil. Chlorophyll is a chemical catalyst —it stimulates and makes possible certain chemical reactions without becoming involved in the reaction itself. By drawing upon the energy of the sun, it can convert inorganic molecules, carbon dioxide (CO_2) and water (H_2O), into an energy-rich organic molecule such as glucose ($C_6H_{12}O_6$), and at the same time release free oxygen (O_2). It transforms solar energy into a form that can be used by plants, animals, and man. Because of this capability, chlorophyll has been referred to as the link between nonliving and living matter, or the pathway through which nonliving elements may become part of living matter.

Through the photosynthetic process, it is estimated that more than a billion tons of carbon per day are converted from inorganic carbon dioxide (CO_2) to organic sugars ($C_6H_{12}O_6$—glucose), which can then be converted into carbohydrates, fats, and proteins—the three main groups of organic materials of living matter.

Photosynthesis is a series of many complex chemical reactions, involving the following two stages (see Fig. P-31):

Stage 1 —The water molecule (H_2O) is split into hydrogen (H) and oxygen (O); and oxygen is released into the atmosphere. Hydrogen is combined with certain organic compounds to keep it available for use in the second step of photosynthesis. Chlorophyll and light are involved in this stage.

Stage 2—Carbon dioxide (CO_2) combines with the released hydrogen to form the simple sugars and water. This reaction is energized (powered) by ATP (adenosine triphosphate), a stored source of energy. Neither chlorophyll nor light is involved in this stage.

The chemical reactions through which chlorophyll converts the energy of solar light to energy in organic compounds is one of nature's best-kept secrets. Man has not been able to unlock it, as he has so many of life's other processes. Moreover, photosynthesis is limited to plants; animals store energy in their products—meat, milk, and eggs—but they must depend upon plants to manufacture it.

Although photosynthesis is vital to life itself, it is very inefficient in capturing the potentially available energy. Of the energy that leaves the sun in a path toward the earth, only about half ever reaches the ground. The other half is absorbed or reflected in the atmosphere. Most of that which reaches the ground is dissipated immediately as heat or is used to evaporate water in another important process for making life possible. Only about 2% of the earthbound energy from the sun actually reaches green plants, and only half of this amount (1%) is transformed by photosynthesis to energy storage in organic compounds. Moreover, only 5% of this plant-captured energy is fixed in a form suitable as food for man.

With such a small portion of the potentially useful solar energy actually being used to form plant tissue, it would appear that some better understanding of the action of chlorophyll should make it possible to increase the effectiveness of the process. Three approaches are suggested: (1)

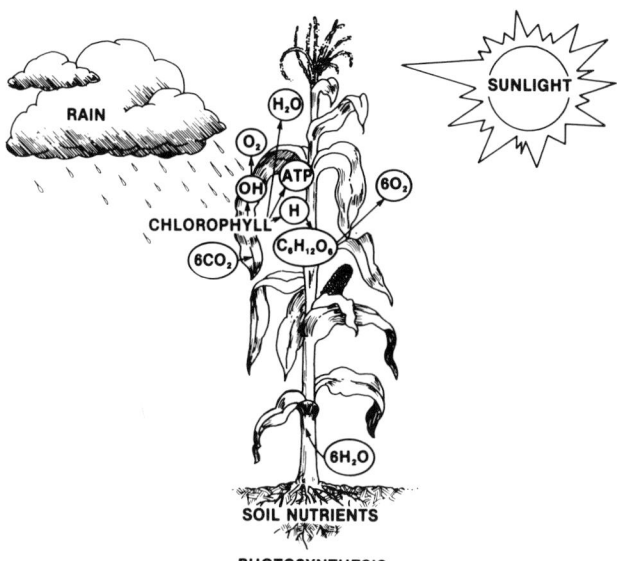

PHOTOSYNTHESIS

LIGHT REACTIONS:

WHERE: IN GREEN MESOPHYLL OF LEAVES.

REQUIRES: CHLOROPHYLL ENERGY FROM SUNLIGHT.

PRODUCES: ENERGY-RICH ATP.

DARK REACTIONS:

WHERE: IN STROMA OF CHLOROPLAST OF LEAVES.

REQUIRES: DOES NOT REQUIRE LIGHT OR CHLOROPHYLL, BUT REQUIRES ENERGY-RICH ATP.

PRODUCES: GLUCOSE-ENERGY-RICH CARBON COMPOUNDS.

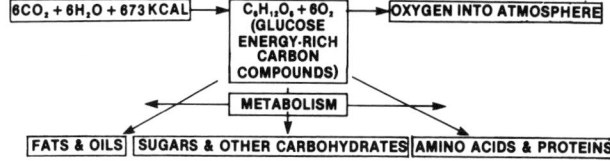

Fig. P-31. Photosynthesis fixes energy. Diagrammatic summary of (1) photosynthesis, and (2) the metabolic formation of organic compounds from the simple sugars. This diagram shows the following:

1. Carbon dioxide gas from the air enters the green mesophyll cells of plant leaves.

2. Plants take up oxygen from the air for some of their metabolic processes and release oxygen back to the air from other metabolic processes.

3. Plants take up water and essential elements from the soil.

4. The energy essential to photosynthesis is absorbed by chlorophyll and supplied by sunlight.

5. For a net input of 6 molecules of carbon dioxide and 6 molecules of water, there is a net output of 1 molecule of sugar and 6 molecules of oxygen.

6. The process is divided into light and dark reactions, with the light reactions building up the energy-rich ATP required for the dark reactions.

7. In the process, 673 Calories (kcal) of energy are used.

8. The sugar (glucose) manufactured in photosynthesis may be converted into fats and oils, sugars and other carbohydrates, and amino acids and proteins.

increasing the amount of photosynthesis on earth, (2) manipulating plants for increased efficiency of solar energy conversion, and (3) converting a greater percentage of total energy fixed as chemical energy in plants (the other 95%) into a form available to man. Ruminant (4-stomached) animals are the solution to the latter approach: they can convert energy from such humanly inedible plant materials as grains and other high-energy feeds and protein supplements, crop residues, pasture and range forages, and harvested forages into food for humans (see Fig. P-32). Also, it is noteworthy that animals do not require fuel to graze the land and recover the energy that is stored in the grass. Moreover, they are completely recyclable; they produce a new crop each year and perpetuate themselves through their offspring. It would appear, therefore, that there is more potential for solving the future food problems of the world by manipulating plants for increased solar energy conversion (*genetic engineering*) and by using ruminants to make more plant energy available to man than from all the genetic and cultural methods combined.

(Also see ENERGY REQUIRED FOR FOOD PRODUCTION.)

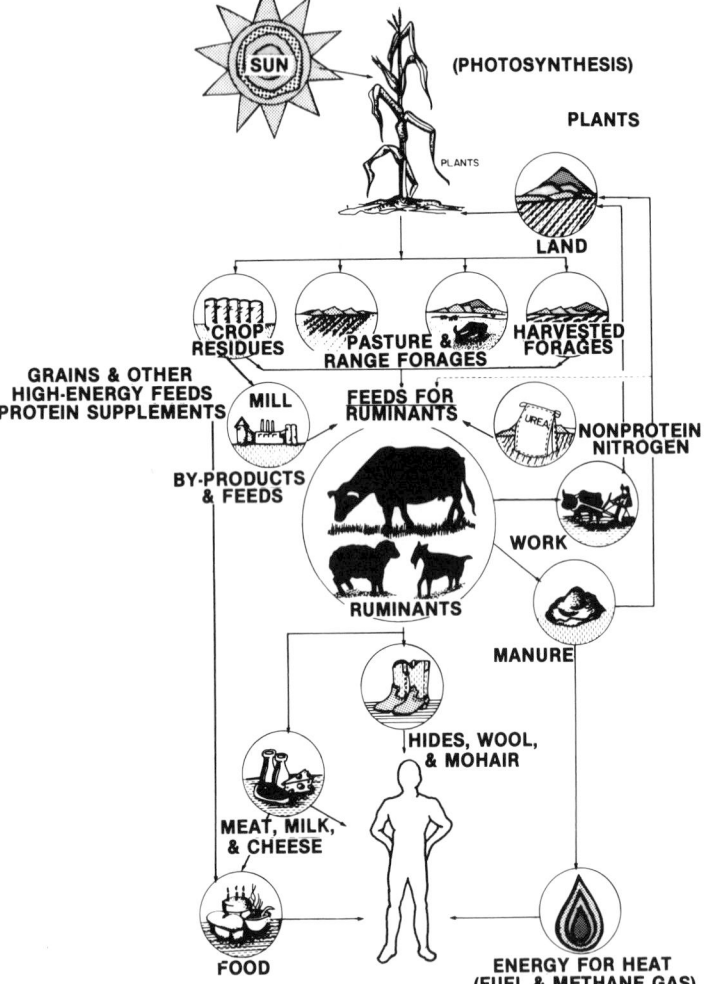

Fig. P-32. Ruminants step up energy. Their feed comes from plants which have their tops in the sun and their roots in the soil. Hence, we have the nutrition cycle as a whole—from the sun and soil, through the plant, thence to the ruminant (and man) and back to the soil again.

PHYLLOQUINONE

A form of vitamin K—K_1, which occurs in nature and is fat soluble.

(Also see VITAMIN K.)

PHYSICAL ACTIVITIES

The need for continuous, quick and strenuous movement of the body—physical activity—has declined over the years in our society. From youth to old age, we now spend most of our time engaged in moderate to very light activities. However, there has been a heightened interest in the need for physical activity coupled with sound nutrition as the two chief components of health.

The following major points indicate the need for physical activities:

1. Physical activity more than any other body process raises the body's energy requirements, and thus provides a means of weight maintenance and weight reduction.

2. Muscular tone and strength are increased by physical activity. This includes the heart and blood vessels.

3. A psychological benefit is derived from physical activities; it provides an outlet for tension and restlessness, and gives the individual a sense of well-being.

(Also see CALORIC [ENERGY] EXPENDITURE; and PHYSICAL FITNESS AND NUTRITION.)

PHYSICAL FITNESS AND NUTRITION

Many people equate fitness with the ability to perform either athletically or in feats of endurance and strength. However, health professionals consider it to be much broader in scope and to include functions such as (1) performance of work and other physical activities, (2) resistance to degenerative and infectious diseases, and (3) adaptation in beneficial ways to emotional and physical stresses.

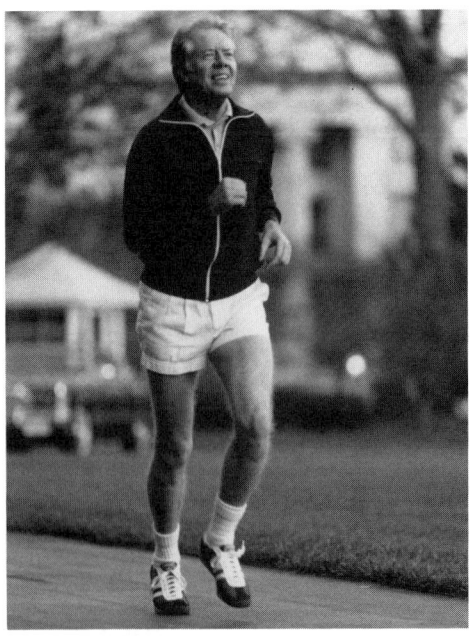

Fig. P-33. When he was president, Jimmy Carter kept fit by jogging. (Courtesy, Karl Schumacher of the Carter White House)

The treatment of nutrition as it relates to athletics is presented in the section on Athletics and Nutrition; hence, the reader is referred thereto.

PHYSICAL FITNESS AROUND THE WORLD.

Some well-known examples of exceptionally fit people, based on longevity and buoyant good health, in various parts of the world are:
1. The Ecuadorians of Vilcabamba.
2. The Georgians of the Soviet Union.
3. The Hunzas of Pakistan.
4. The Bulgarians.
5. The longshoremen in San Francisco.
6. The Masai tribesmen in Africa.
7. The Mormons.
8. The Seventh-Day Adventists.

Additional fit people, along with their cultural characteristics, follow:
1. **The Canadian Indians,** hunting and fishing tribes, in northern Canada near the Arctic Circle, whose physical fitness is attributed to a nutritious diet of meat and fish.
2. **The Eskimos of the Arctic,** who still live by hunting and fishing, are noted for a high aerobic capacity.
3. **The Polish farmers,** who live in the low mountains of southern Poland, enjoy a favorable climate, work hard, and are well fed, retain their fitness much longer than other Poles.
4. **The Swiss dairy farmers,** who consume considerable milk and cheese, are strong and healthy; many of the Pope's Swiss Guards come from this region.
5. **The Tarahumara Indians,** who live in the Madre mountains of northwestern Mexico, and whose diet is mainly vegetarian, are exceptionally good runners and have unusually high aerobic capacities.

Descriptions and life styles of each of the above groups are given in this book in the section on Life Expectancy and Nutrition; hence, the reader is referred thereto.

It is noteworthy that the health practices of some of the fittest groups of people around the world are characterized by (1) diets comprised of fresh, minimally processed foods, such as meats and fish, dairy products, fruits and vegetables, and whole grain breads and cereals; (2) limited consumptions of potentially harmful items such as strong alcoholic drinks, coffee and tea, and refined fats, starches, and sugars; and (3) engagement in moderate to vigorous physical activities.

IMPORTANT ASPECTS OF PHYSICAL FITNESS.

Although good overall fitness is to be desired by everyone, the particular circumstances that are unique to each person's life make it necessary to emphasize certain aspects, such as those which follow:

Ability to Perform Physical Work.

Certain types of jobs, such as construction work, firefighting, the harvesting of crops, military combat, and police work, require considerable physical exertion. Therefore, it is noteworthy that both the maximum rates of performing work and the times during which maximum performance may be sustained tend to decline with increasing age.

Athletic Prowess.

Many sports require agility, speed, and sufficient strength to make the required movements without excessive strain on the various organs and tissues. Therefore, the athletes who perform best owe their success to factors such as (1) development of the requisite neuro-

muscular coordination, (2) optimal cardiovascular functioning, (3) a high aerobic capacity, (4) well developed muscles, (5) a minimal accumulation of excess body fat, and (6) willpower to persevere.

It is generally believed that optimal nutrition somehow enhances these performance factors although hard data is often difficult to obtain since the effects of mediocre nutrition may not be evident in early adulthood.

(Also see ATHLETICS AND NUTRITION.)

Bearing of Healthy Children.

Even primitive tribes have long recognized the importance of the maternal diet to the successful outcome of pregnancy, as evidenced by the practices which follow:
1. Eskimos, Peruvian Indians, Polynesians, and other peoples living near the sea or inland lakes gave expectant mothers fish eggs and other aquatic foods.
2. Dairying tribes in Africa did not allow young women to marry until the season when the cattle were fed on lush, green pastures.
3. Papuans of New Guinea reserved special foods such as dried large snakes for their expectant mothers.

Fortunately, mothers-to-be may now skip the fish eggs and snakes since much is known about meeting the nutritional requirements with other types of foods.

(Also see PREGNANCY AND LACTATION NUTRITION.)

Emotional Well-Being.

For many people, peace of mind depends upon their feeling well, since symptoms of an illness may provoke anxiety, depression, and other distressful emotions. Recent research on the effects of diet on the nervous system has shown that mental depression may also arise from a subnormal brain content of the nerve transmitter, serotonin, which in turn may result from (1) lack of sufficient amounts of the amino acid tryptophan in the diet, or (2) excessively high levels of dietary fat and/or protein that interfere with the entry of tryptophan into the brain where it is converted to serotonin. Another factor which affects the emotional state and sense of well being is the level of blood sugar, since the brain requires a continuous supply of glucose for optimal functioning, and subnormal blood sugar makes many people feel poorly. Hence, erratic and imbalanced dietary patterns may be responsible for poor mental health.

In general, people who are physically fit appear to be more optimistic and more able to accomplish both mental and physical tasks. Hence, they may have a greater sense of self-sufficiency than those who have let themselves become weak, flabby, and overly dependent on others.

Sometimes, the emotional well-being and ability to work are also impaired by chronic disorders such as adrenal cortical insufficiency, allergies, anemia, depression, high or low blood pressure, hypochondriasis (an exaggerated sensitivity to minor discomfort that may be accompanied by unfounded fear of developing a deadly disease), insufficient flow of blood to the brain, nutritional deficiencies, and thyroid diseases. Therefore, a person who feels poorly much of the time should see a doctor to rule out the possibility of a chronic disease before resorting to the excessive use of stimulants such as caffeine and various mood elevating drugs.

Mental Acuity.

This type of fitness is closely related to overall physical fitness because the brain and nerves are very sensitive to changes in the blood chemistry. For example, the performance of tasks which require mental and sensory acuity is enhanced by meal patterns which maintain the blood sugar level at normal throughout the day. Skipping breakfast or having only coffee in the morning usually lowers the quality of work. Other dietary factors, particularly those relating to depression and emotional well being are also important.

Notable changes in a person's mental acuity may result from conditions or factors such as alcoholism, antihypertensive drugs, atherosclerosis, chronic stress, dehydration, depression, diabetes, fatigue, head injuries, insuffient blood flow to the brain, low blood pressure, low blood sugar (hypoglycemia), nutritional deficiencies, sedative or tranquilizer drugs, small strokes, and starvation. Sometimes these possibilities have been overlooked and the patient has been diagnosed as neurotic, psychotic, or senile and confined to an institution. However, some amazing improvements have resulted from the proper types of corrective measures.

Resistance to Infectious Diseases.

Both undernutrition and overnutrition impair the functioning of the body defenses against infection which are collectively called the immune system. Similarly, immunity may be reduced in disorders such as cancer and diabetes; and during severe emotional stress. Finally, some people fail to obtain the immunizations which are now available.

Scientists are now exploring the interactions between these and other factors that affect immunity. For example, there is evidence that the production of optimal immunity requires ample amounts of dietary selenium, zinc, vitamin A, and vitamin C; but only moderate amounts of dietary calories and proteins. Too little or too much of the latter nutrients may impair the functioning of the body's defense system. Hence, it should be possible in the near future to promote optimal functioning of the immune system by a balanced program of dietary measures, immunizations, medical treatment, and psychological counseling.

Slowing of the Physical Decline in Adulthood.

Mental and physical faculties must be used fully, but wisely, if they are to be kept operative at high levels of performance throughout adulthood. Furthermore, a vigorous life style helps to prevent obesity, which may hasten physical decline if not corrected soon enough. Finally, the progress of the various degenerative diseases that impair the faculties can be retarded by the proper diet and the use of corrective therapies when needed. This means that regular physical examinations and laboratory tests should be obtained to detect any early warning symptoms of degenerative diseases. It might also be a good idea to have tests of physical performance such as aerobic capacity and endurance.

Some of the symptoms that warrant dietary modification and/or other types of therapies are: diabetic glucose tolerance; high blood levels of cholesterol, triglycerides, and/or uric acid; low blood levels of hemoglobin, iron, red cells, and/or certain vitamins; and subnormal capacity for physical exertion, as evidenced by an electrocardiogram or stress testing on an exercise bicycle or a treadmill. Means of correcting these problems are described in the sections that follow.

DIETARY GUIDELINES.   In order to be certain of obtaining sufficient amounts of each of the required nutrients, one should consult a table showing the best food sources of these essential substances, such as the one given in Table N-3 of this encyclopedia.

Furthermore, meals can be planned with the aid of a food guide that groups commonly used items according to the nutrients which are furnished (see Food Groups).

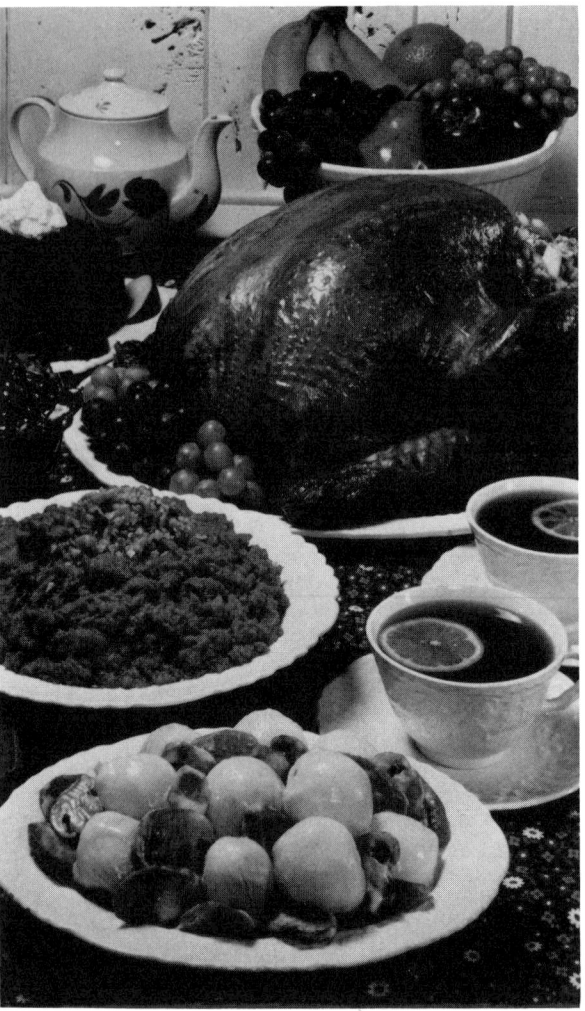

Fig. P-34. A wholesome diet, along with sufficient exercise, makes for physical fitness. (Courtesy, United Fresh Fruit & Vegetable Assn., Alexandria, Va.)

Finally, it appears that it would be beneficial to the fitness of many Americans to eat more food for breakfast and less at the evening meal. For example, breakfast should contain one or more sources of animal protein such as cheese, eggs, milk products, and meats, plus ample amounts of fresh fruit and whole grain breads or cereals. Lunch should also contain a good source of proteins, plus a milk product, one or more vegetables and whole grain bread. When two good meals have already been consumed, supper may consist of only small servings of protein foods with a bread or a cereal product, plus a large serving of vegetables in a salad or a freshly prepared soup. (Most canned soups have rather high salt contents, which may be harmful to people with tendencies to retain fluids and develop congestive heart failure or high blood pressure.)

(Also see FOOD GROUPS; NUTRIENTS: REQUIREMENTS, ALLOWANCES, FUNCTIONS, SOURCES; and RDA.)

Modified Diets and Nutritional Supplements.

The decision to make a radical change in one's dietary pattern should not be made without first consulting a doctor and/or a dietitian because many factors have to be considered before the appropriate changes can be made. For example, it may be dangerous for people with a family history of gout to lose weight rapidly.

PHYSICAL ACTIVITY AS AN ADJUNCT TO DIETARY PRACTICES. The need for following a carefully controlled diet is lessened somewhat by exercising enough to burn off at least 300 to 500 extra Calories (kcal) daily. Fig. P-35 shows that women who engaged in recreational physical activities were able to keep trim while consuming more calories than those whose activity levels were lower.

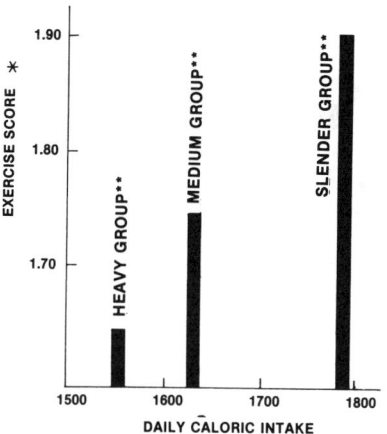

* AVERAGES OF REPORTED RECREATIONAL ACTIVITY
(LITTLE OR   NONE = 1, MODERATE = 2, MUCH = 3)

** ASSESSMENT OF BODY FATNESS FROM AVERAGE
MEASUREMENTS OF TRICEPS SKINFOLD
(13.5 MM = SLENDER, 20.8 MM = MEDIUM,
30.8 MM = HEAVY)

Fig. P-35. The effects of caloric intake and recreational exercise on a measure of body fatness in women. (Based on data from Habicht, J-P, testimony before the U.S. House of Representatives Committee on Science and Technology, July 28, 1977, p. 376, Fig. 2)

Physical activity is also valuable as a means of rehabilitation from various degenerative conditions. For example, the cardiovascular fitness of seven patients with heart disease was improved greatly by a 6-week program of intensive physical training that was supervised by doctors.[23]

(Also see CALORIC [ENERGY] EXPENDITURE; and ATHLETICS AND NUTRITION.)

SUMMARY. Studies around the world have shown that most people can remain fit well into middle age and beyond, providing that they consume a wholesome diet and engage in sufficient exercise. In fact, it is even possible to have a dramatic recovery from disabling heart disease when suitable measures are taken.

PHYSIOLOGICAL SALINE

A salt solution (0.9% NaCl) having the same osmotic pressure as the blood plasma.

PHYTIC ACID

It is a hexaphosphoric acid ester of inositol present mainly in cereal grains, nuts, and legumes.

(Also see MINERAL[S], section headed "Naturally Occurring Mineral Antagonists in Foods.")

[23]Redwood, D. R., et al., "Circulatory and Symptomatic Effects of Physical Training in Patients with Coronary Artery Disease and Angina Pectoris," *The New England Journal of Medicine,* Vol. 286, 1972, pp. 959-965.

PHYTOCHEMICALS

Phytochemical ("phyto" is derived from the Greek word for plant) is a new term embracing a host of plant chemicals which offer hope and help for the prevention of cancer. They are abundant in fruits and vegetables. In the mid-1990s, the race was on to find, isolate, and study them; hopefully, to find a magic pill that would go beyond vitamins.

Among the multitude of phytochemicals, their sources, and their claims, are the following:

• **Allylic sulfide**—Plentiful in onions and garlic, which detoxifies carcinogens.

• **Capsaicin**—Abundant in hot peppers, which keeps toxic molecules from attaching to DNA.

• **Ellagic acid**—Present in strawberries, grapes, and raspberries, which neutralizes carcinogens before they can invade DNA.

• **Flavonoids**—Present in berries, citrus, yams, and cucumbers, which keeps cancer-causing hormones from attaching to the surface of cells.

• **Genistein**—Abundant in soybeans, which prevents breast, prostate, and other lumps from growing and spreading.

• **Indole-3-carbinol**—Present in cauliflower and cabbage, seems to lessen breast cancer by acting on a precursor to the female hormone estrogen and producing a harmless form of estrogen rather than the form linked to breast cancer.

• **P-coumaric acid and chlorogenic acid**—Found in many fruits and vegetables, including tomatoes, green peppers, pineapples, strawberries, and carrots, which prevents the formation of cancer-causing nitrosamines from nitric acids and amines.

• **Phenethyl isothiocyanate (PEITC)**—Found in cabbage and turnips, which inhibits lung cancer.

• **Sulforaphane**—Found in broccoli, cauliflower, Brussels sprouts, turnips, and kale, which lessens breast cancer in animals.

But phytochemicals are not omnipotent! Remember, too, that lifelong vegetarians get cancer. Much more research is needed before the role of phytochemicals can be established. In the meantime, a balanced diet, including fruits and vegetables, is recommended for buoyant good health.

PICA

An abnormal craving of appetite for substances not usually considered as food—starch, clay, hair, dirt, chalk, and wood.

(Also see ALLOPRIOPHAGY; CISSA; and GEOPHAGIA.)

PIGMENTATION

This refers to melanin, the pigment which imparts color (1) to the skin, hair, and eyes, and (2) to bile and blood.

In sunburn, the skin darkens due to the ultraviolet rays of the sun. In albinos, melanin is absent. Certain skin diseases manifest excessive or unevenly distributed pigment, including freckles, liver spots, melanosis, vitiligo, and leukoderma.

Bile and blood color are due to melanin formed in the body. The two main bile pigments are bilirubin (red) and biliverdin (green). The red blood pigment is hemoglobin, from which the pigments hemosiderin, methemoglobin, bilirubin, and biliverdin are derived.

PIG SOUSE (PIG'S-FOOT JELL)

Made from pig's feet (free from hair and with toes removed), along with hearts, tongues, and shoulder hocks, by boiling in water until the meat separates from the bones;

removing the bones; cutting the meat into small chunks; placing the meat back in the broth in which it was cooked; seasoning to taste with salt, pepper, and vinegar; pouring into shallow pans and setting away to chill and jell.

PINEAPPLE *Ananas comosus*

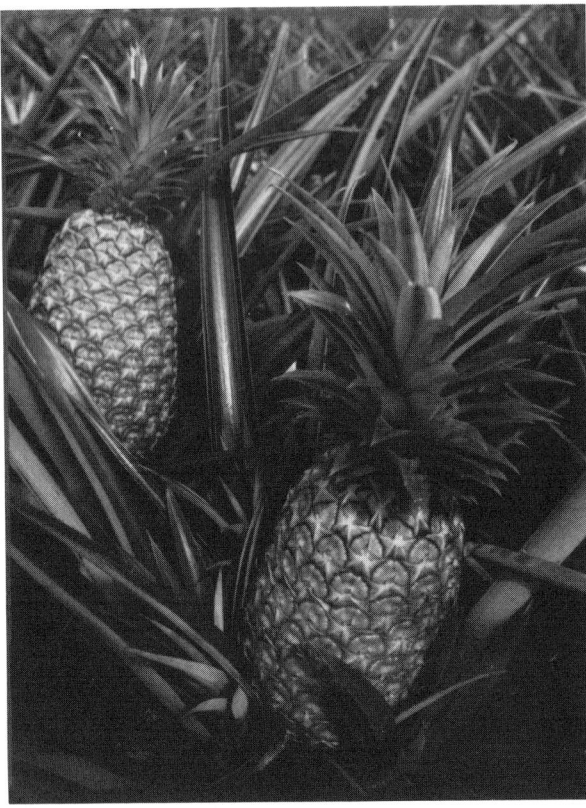

Fig. P-36. Pineapples ripening in the field. (Courtesy, Castle & Cooke, Inc.)

Pineapple is a tropical fruit plant, which grows from 2 to 3 ft (61 to 91 cm) tall, and produces a fruit weighing 4 to 8 lb (2 to 4 kg). It probably received its name because the fruit looks like a large pinecone. The pineapple is a member of the bromelaid family, *Bromeliaceae.*

The edible flesh of the pineapple is firm, pale yellow or white, and the flavor is a mixture of sweetness and tartness. Its flavor has been described as apple, strawberry, and peach mingled all at once.

ORIGIN AND HISTORY. The pineapple is native to South America, where it was domesticated by the Indians long before the coming of the white man to the New World.

WORLD AND U.S. PRODUCTION. Worldwide, about 9.7 million tons of pineapples are produced annually; and the leading pineapple-producing countries, by rank, are: Thailand, Philippines, China, Brazil, India, United States, Vietnam, Mexico, Indonesia, and South Africa.[24]

The United States ranks sixth among the leading pineapple-producing nations, with an annual production of

575,000 short tons. But pineapples are produced only in Hawaii.[25]

PROCESSING. A considerable amount of pineapple is consumed fresh. However, most exports are canned. Every part of a pineapple is used in the canning process. The flesh is canned as sliced, chunked or crushed pineapple. The juice is also canned.

At the cannery, pineapples are first washed and graded. Once graded, a machine called a *Ginaca* cuts the core from the fruit, removes the shell, and cuts off both ends. The flesh left on the shell is then scraped by machine so that it may be used for crushed pineapple and juice.

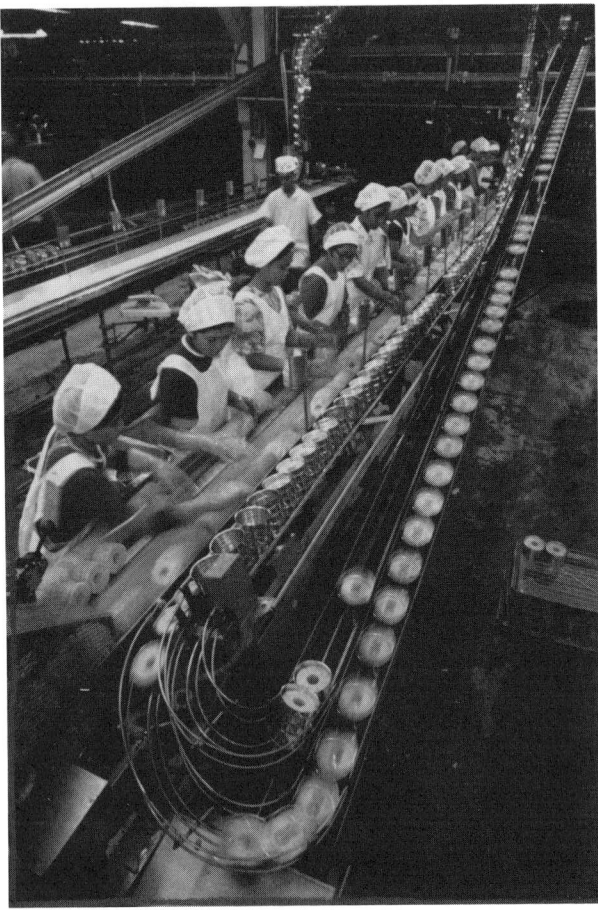

Fig. P-37. Processing pineapple, showing the fruit being sliced mechanically and placed in cans. (Courtesy, Castle & Cooke, Inc.)

The trimmed fruit is carefully inspected, sliced by machine, and placed in cans. Broken pieces are sent to the shredder to be crushed. The shells and other trimmings are shredded, pressed, and dried to make pineapple bran to feed livestock. Other by-products of the canning process are sugar, alcohol, and vinegar. Sugar is recovered by ion exchange purification of the juice pressed from the cannery waste. However, alcohol and vinegar, instead of sugar, may be produced from the by-product juice through fermentation.

---

[24]Data from *FAO Production Yearbook 1990*, FAO/UN, Rome, Italy, Vol. 44, p. 167, Table 73. **Note well:** Annual production fluctuates as a result of weather and profitability of the crop.

[25]Data from *Agricultural Statistics 1991*, USDA, p. 177, Table 254. **Note well:** Annual production fluctuates as a result of weather and profitability of the crop.

• **Bromelin**—Another by-product in some operations is the enzyme, bromelin, which is used to tenderize meat, to chill-proof beer, and to produce protein hydrolyzates. Bromelin is found in the stem and fruit of the pineapple.

(Also see MEAT, section headed "Meat Tenderizing."

SELECTION, PREPARATION AND USES. Pineapple varieties vary in color, but most are yellowish. Ripe pineapples have a fruity, fragrant aroma. Usually the heavier the fruit is for its size, the better the quality.

Pineapple may be served fresh or canned, by itself, or it may be used in pies, ice cream, puddings, baked goods, and salads, or with meats. The flavor blends well with other flavors. Cookbooks contain long lists of ideas for the uses

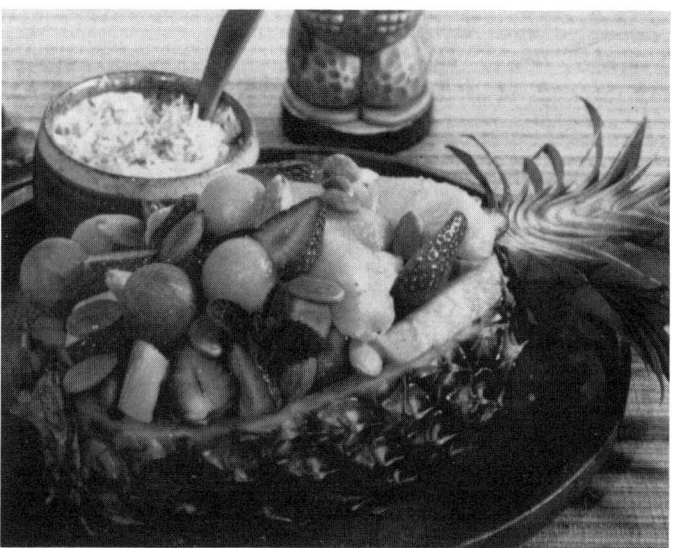

Fig. P-38. A fruit salad attractively served in a pineapple shell. (Courtesy, Anderson/Miller & Hubbard Consumer Services, San Francisco, Calif.)

of pineapple. The fresh fruit cannot be used in molded gelatin, because it contains the enzyme bromelin that digests and softens the gelatin. This enzyme is destroyed by heating; hence, canned pineapple can be used in gelatin dishes.

NUTRITIONAL VALUE. Fresh pineapple is 85% water and each 100 g (about 3½ oz) contains 58 Calories (kcal) as well as 70 IU of vitamin A and 17 mg of vitamin C. The calories in pineapples are derived primarily from the sugar (carbohydrate) present. They contain approximately 15% sugar. Canned and frozen pineapples are similar to fresh pineapples, but those canned in a heavy syrup contain more calories, and some vitamin A and C is lost during the processing. The nutrient composition of pineapple juice is very similar to the fresh fruit.

Further information regarding the nutritional value of fresh, canned, frozen, and candied pineapple, and pineapple juice is presented in Food Composition Table F-21.

PINEAPPLE GUAVA (FEIJOA) *Feijoa sellowiana*

The fruit of a small South American tree (of the family *Myrtaceae*) that is related to the common guava (*Psidium guajava*).

Feijoa is green outside and white inside, and has a tart sweet flavor somewhat like unsweetened pineapple. As a fresh fruit, it is good in fruit salads; or when made into jam.

PINEAPPLE JUICE

The fluid extracted from fresh pineapple by pressing the pulverized fruit pulp, filtering the juice, adding back some of the pulp, heat processing at 140-145°F (60-63°C), pressure homogenizing to keep the pulp suspended, filling into cans, and pasteurizing at 190°F (88°C).

The nutrient compositions of various forms of pineapple juice are given in Food Composition Table F-21.

Some noteworthy observations regarding the nutrient composition of pineapple juice follow:

1. A 1-cup (*180 g*) serving of canned pineapple juice supplies 138 Calories (kcal) and is a good source of potassium and a fair to good source of vitamin C. However, some pineapple drinks and juice products contain sufficient added vitamin C to make them much better sources of this vitamin.

2. Frozen pineapple juice concentrate contains over 3 times the caloric and nutrient contents of the single strength canned juice. Hence, it may make a significant nutritional contribution when added undiluted to dishes such as ice cream and sauces for ham and other meats.

(Also see PINEAPPLE.)

PINOCYTOSIS

The process by which liquid droplets are taken into the cell through invagination and subsequent dissolving of part of the cell membrane. This process enables cells to absorb certain lipids and dissolve proteins intact. As can be seen in Fig. P-39, the material to be engulfed comes into contact with the cell membrane. The membrane then invaginates to surround the material. Once the material has been completely surrounded, the membrane fuses, and the invaginated section of the membrane is dissolved by lysosomal enzymes. Absorptive cells in the small intestine are capable of using this mechanism during digestion.

(Also see DIGESTION AND ABSORPTION.)

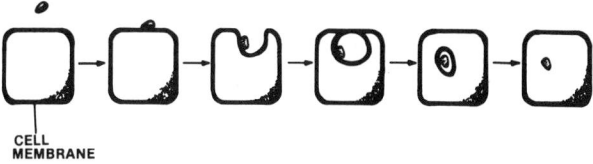

Fig. P-39. Pinocytosis involves the invagination of the cell membrane around the liquid to be engulfed. Once the liquid droplet has been completely engulfed, the membrane surrounding the material disintegrates and the material is incorporated into the cell.

PINTAIL (PINTAILED DUCK)

A river duck—a game bird.

PITH

In botany, this word has the following meanings:

• Soft white spongy material found in the center of certain plant stems. It is not usually consumed as a food.

• Another name for the albedo of citrus fruits, which is the white fibrous matter that lies between the fruit segments and the outer pigmented portion of the peel (flavedo). Citrus pith is rich in (1) bioflavonoids, and (2) pectin, a gelling agent and an ingredient in diarrhea remedies.

PITS

Stones or seeds of fruits such as cherries, plums, peaches, apricots, dates, or similar fruits.

PITUITARY GLAND

An endocrine gland, located at the base of the brain, which produces a number of hormones and regulates a large portion of the endocrine activity.

(Also see ENDOCRINE GLANDS.)

PIZZA

This is an Italian word meaning *pie,* which a pizza resembles. Pizza, the creation of which is credited to Naples, is flat leavened bread topped with a variety of such good things as tomatoes, mozzarella and parmesan cheeses,

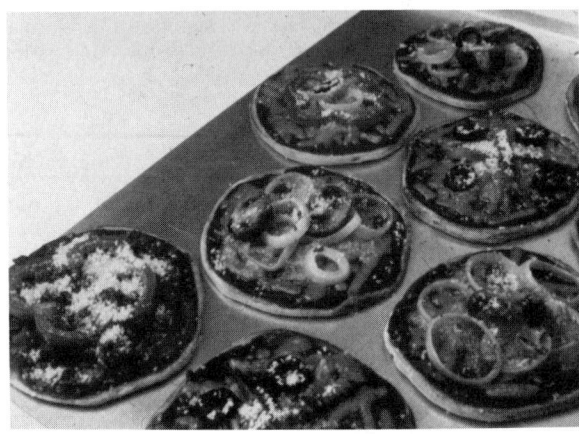

Fig. P-40. Pizza, a popular fast food in America. (Courtesy, USDA)

sausages, mushrooms, anchovies, olives, capers, and a profusion of herbs and spices. A pizza is actually an open sandwich.

Although pizza varies nutritionally according to the ingredients, typical pizza contains about 15% protein, 27% fat, and 58% carbohydrate; hence, it's a fairly well balanced food.

(Also see CONVENIENCE AND FAST FOODS; and FAST FOODS.)

PLACEBO

An inert preparation given for its psychological effect; especially (1) to satisfy the patient, or (2) to serve as a control in an experiment.

PLACENTA

The organ of communication between the fetus and the mother. It is the means by which the fetal blood receives oxygen and nourishment and gives up waste material; hence, the placenta performs the functions of respiration, nutrition, and excretion.

PLANTAIN *Musa paradisiaca*

Plantains belong to the banana family, *Musaceae,* which also includes bananas. The plantain is *M. paradisiaca,* while the common banana is *M. paradisiaca,* variety *sapientum.* Although plantains look like bananas, they have a higher starch content and a lower sugar content than bananas.

ORIGIN AND HISTORY. Plantains originated on the Malay Peninsula.

WORLD AND U.S. PRODUCTION. Statistically, plantains are never reliably distinguished from bananas. Nevertheless, they are an important fruit crop. World production totals 25,433 million metric tons; and the leading plantain-producing countries are: Uganda, Colombia, Rwanda, Zaire, Tanzania, Nigeria, Cameroon, and Cote Divoire.[26]

Plantain is not produced commercially in the United States.

PROCESSING. Plantains are processed much like bananas. However, they are not likely to be ripened after picking.

SELECTION, PREPARATION, AND USES. When purchased, plantains should be firm and free from bruises or other injury.

Because of their high starch content, it is necessary that plantains be cooked before eating. They are usually baked, boiled, fried, roasted, steamed, or made into a flour.

Plantains are generally used as a vegetable dish.

NUTRITIONAL VALUE. The nutrient composition of plantains is given in Food Composition Table F-21.

Plantains are high in carbohydrates (over 30%); and they contain more energy than bananas (more than 115 Calories [kcal] per 100 g versus 85 to 100 Calories [kcal] per 100 g for bananas). Also, they are an excellent source of potassium (385 mg/100 g), and a fair source of vitamin C.

(Also see BANANA.)

PLANT PROTEINS

Those proteins derived from plant sources. This consists of proteins from the seeds, nuts, fruits, vegetables, leaves, stalks, and roots. Common sources of plant proteins are the cereal grains and their products, and legumes, oil seeds, and green leafy vegetables. Plant proteins are less concentrated than animal proteins, and often lack some essential amino acids giving them a lower biological value.

(Also see PROTEIN[S].)

PLAQUE

Any patch; for example, atherosclerotic plaque refers to a deposit of lipid material in the blood vessel.

PLASMA

The colorless fluid portion of the blood in which corpuscles are suspended. It is often used as a basis for measurement of bloodborne nutrients and their metabolites.

PLATELETS

Small, colorless, round or rod-shaped bodies in the circulating blood of mammals.

PLUCK

• The organs that lie in the thoracic cavity, consisting of the heart, lungs, gullet, and windpipe.

• To remove the feathers of poultry before cleaning.

---

[26]Data from *FAO Production Yearbook 1990,* FAO/UN, Rome, Italy, Vol. 44, p. 169, Table 74. **Note well:** Annual production fluctuates as a result of weather and profitability of the crop.

PLUM AND PRUNE *Prunus* spp

The plum is the fruit of a tree bearing the same name. Botanically, a plum is classified as a drupe—a fruit whose seed is contained in a hard pit or stone surrounded by soft, pulpy flesh with a thin skin. Plums belong to the rose family, *Rosaceae*. As the genus name, *Prunus*, suggests, plums are close relatives of the apricot, almond, cherry, and peach.

Plums vary in size from those as small as a cherry to those as large as a small peach. Their shape may be round or oval, and their smooth skin may be colored green, yellow, red, blue, or purple. The edible flesh is thick, juicy, and sweet.

Plum trees range from low, shrubby type to trees 30 ft (9 m) high. Its white flowers blossom in the spring before the leaves appear. Since there are many species and hundreds of varieties, plums enjoy widespread distribution in different climates and soil conditions.

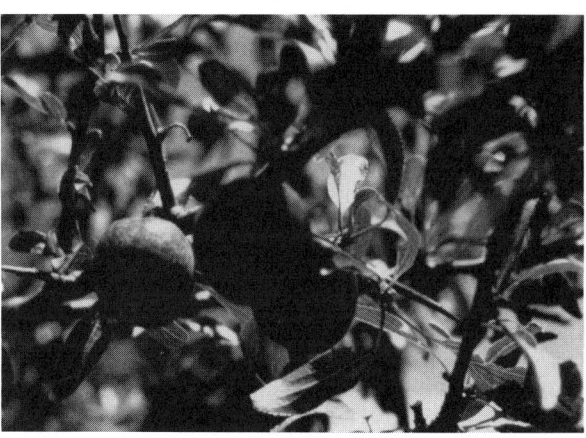

Fig. P-41. The fruiting branch of a plum tree. (Courtesy, USDA)

• **Prune**—A prune is a dried plum, but more than this a prune is a variety of plum that is satisfactory for drying without removing the pit. Growers use the term prune to refer to both the fruit in its fresh state and to the dried product. Also the following saying helps make the distinction between plum and prune: "The prune is always a plum—but a plum is not always a prune." Prune plums generally have firmer flesh and a higher sugar content. Popular varieties of the European plum, *Prunus domestica*, used for

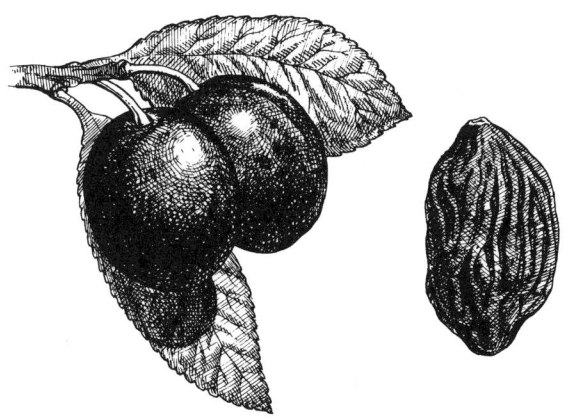

Fig. P-42. A prune (right) is a dried plum (left), but a plum is not always a prune.

prunes include: French or Agen (most popular), Imperial, Sugar, Robe de Sergeant, Burton, and Contes.

TYPES OF PLUMS. There are five main types of plums from which the important varieties are derived. These five types include the following: European, Japanese, American, damson, and ornamental.

• **European plum**—This plum is also called the garden or common plum. Its scientific name is *Prunus domestica*. Its fruits are blue or red and medium to large in size and may be eaten fresh or canned, though most are dried. European plums grown in the United States include: French or Agen, President, Tragedy, and Grand Duke.

• **Japanese plum**—This plum is also called the salicina plum. The fruits are yellow, crimson and purple, ranging in size from small to large. They are all very juicy and sweet, and they are eaten fresh, cooked, or canned—but never as prunes. The scientific name for the Japanese plum is *Prunus salicina,* and some common varieties include: Beauty, Burmosa, Santa Rosa, Wickson, Redheart, Duarte, Red Rosa, Kelsey, and Burbank.

• **American plum**—This group includes several species such as (1) the cold-resistant *Prunus americana* with amber skin and flesh; (2) the bushy and thorny Hortulan plum, *Prunus hortulana;* and (3) the sand cherry plum, *Prunus besseyi,* which grows in the Middle West and Canada. Some common names include De Soto, Pottawattomi, and Golden Beauty.

• **Damson plum**—These trees resemble the European type, but they are smaller and more cold resistant. Their fruits are tart and blue—favorites for jellies and jams. The scientific name for the damson plum is *Prunus insititia*. Several common varieties include Bullaces, St. Juliens, and Mirabelles.

• **Ornamental plum**—These trees produce red foliage and red fruit which is suitable for jams and jellies. The scientific name for the ornamental plum is *Prunus cerasifera* which is also the myrobalan plum. The major value of the myrobalan plum is its use as a rootstock for other stone fruits.

ORIGIN AND HISTORY. Over 2,000 varieties of plums are known. The most important species for commercial production in the United States is *Prunus domestica,* the common, or European, plum, which originated in Europe and was introduced to the United States by the Pilgrims. It produces most of the dessert plums and all of the prune plums in the United States. The Japanese plum, *Prunus salincina,* believed to be native to China, was introduced to the United States by way of Japan in 1870.

WORLD AND U.S. PRODUCTION. Worldwide, about 5.7 million metric tons of plums and prunes are produced annually; and the leading producing countries, by rank, are: U.S.S.R., China, Romania, U.S.A., Yugoslavia, Germany, Turkey, Hungary, France, and Italy.[27]

The United States produces 488,800 short tons of plums and prunes annually, on a fresh basis, with the following states leading in production, by rank: California, Oregon,

---

[27]Data from *FAO Production Yearbook 1990*, FAO/UN, Rome, Italy, Vol. 44, p. 162, Table 70. **Note well:** Annual production fluctuates as a result of weather and profitability of the crop.

Washington, Idaho, and Michigan. California produces 90% of the nation's plums and prunes.[28]

PROCESSING. Plums are marketed as fresh, dried (prunes), and canned or frozen fruit. Approximately 56.3% is marketed fresh, 20.6% dried, 22.2% is canned, and 0.9% frozen. In California, about 66% of the plum crop is dried for prunes, and the majority of the remaining crop is utilized fresh.

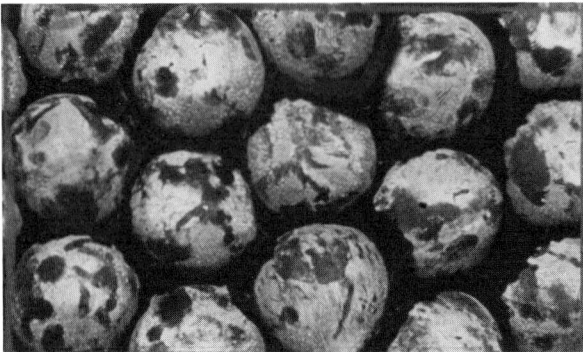

Fig. P-43. Plums. (Courtesy, USDA)

A few prunes are still sun dried, but most are dehydrated. Sun drying requires more than 1 week for completion, and may be hampered by bad weather. Prior to dehydration, plums are immersed in hot water for a few seconds to remove the natural wax, and then dipped in lye to prevent fermentation. Next, the plums (prunes) are placed in single layers on trays, and placed in the dehydrator where temperature, air movement, and humidity are controlled. In efficient operations drying in a dehydrator is completed in 3 to 4 days, when the fruit reaches 18 to 19% moisture. Some larger dehydrators may only require 12 to 24 hours. The drying ratio is approximately 2½ lb (1.13 kg) of fresh fruit to 1 lb (0.45 kg) of dried fruit.

Canned plums and prunes are canned in water pack, light syrup, heavy syrup, or extra heavy syrup. Prune juice is a by-product of prune dehydration. It is made by leaching prunes with hot water or by using pectic enzymes on a slurry of whole ground prunes. Prune juice is canned, and yearly production is about 7,000,000 cases of No. 2 cans. Plums are frozen primarily in large containers for remanufacture into jams and preserves at a later date.

SELECTION, PREPARATION, AND USES. With so many varieties which differ widely in appearance and flavor, it is best to buy a few of the fresh fruits and be certain that the taste and appearance is appealing. Fresh plums should be selected on the basis of their color characteristic for the type. Additionally, ripe plums are firm to slightly soft, and taste juicy and sweet. Slight softening at the tip is also a good sign of maturity.

If not quite ripe when purchased, keep plums at room temperature a day or so, but watch closely. Plums can turn overripe very quickly. Ripe plums should be refrigerated.

Plums can be eaten fresh out of the hand or prepared in a variety of fruit dishes. Plums make good jelly, preserves, plum butter, and jam. Canned prunes can be served alone

---

[28]Data from *Agricultural Statistics 1991*, USDA, pp. 207, 208, Tables 318, 319. **Note well:** Annual production fluctuates as a result of weather and profitability of the crop.

as a side dish or a dessert or in combination with other fruits, or in baked goods.

Prunes are used in baked goods, confections, desserts, salad, and meat dishes. Many prunes are served as a breakfast or dessert fruit, stewed and served with or without cream. Prunes are an excellent ready-to-eat snack.

NUTRITIONAL VALUE. Fresh plums contain 78 to 87% water, depending upon the variety. Additionally, each 100 g (about 3½ oz) provides 48 to 75 Calories (kcal) of energy, 170 to 299 mg potassium, 250 to 300 IU of vitamin A, and only 1 to 2 mg of sodium, depending upon the type of plum. The calories in plums are derived primarily from natural sugars (carbohydrates) which give them their sweet taste. Some canned plums contain more calories due to the addition of sugar, but some canned varieties are also excellent sources of vitamin A, containing 1,180 to 1,250 IU per 100 g. Dried plums (prunes) contain only 32% water; hence, many of the nutrients, including calories, are more concentrated. Prunes contain 239 Calories (kcal), 754 mg potassium, 2.5 mg iron, and 1,994 IU vitamin A in each 100 g. More complete information regarding the nutritional value of fresh plums, canned plums, prunes and cooked prunes is presented in Food Composition Table F-21.

POACH

A method of cooking eggs in a shallow amount of near-boiling water. A favorite method for cooking breakfast eggs.

POI

This is a Hawaiian food made from the root of the taro which is baked, pounded, moistened, and fermented. Poi tastes slightly sour; hence, some individuals trying poi for the first time find it unpleasant.

(Also see VEGETABLE[S], Table V-2, Vegetables of the World; and TARO.)

POISONING

The act of administering a substance which, in sufficient quantities and/or over a period of time, kills or harms living things. Many substances are poisonous in massive doses while other substances require only minute amounts to be lethal.

(Also see POISONS.)

POISONOUS PLANTS

Contents   Page

Herbal medicine enthusiasts and stalkers of the wild edible plants beware! Plants can be dangerous. But one does not have to be an herbal medicine enthusiast or stalker of the wild to encounter poisonous plants. Many poisonous plants grow in homes, gardens, and recreational areas. Some of the most prized cultivated ornamentals are extremely poisonous. However, this does not mean that poisonous plants should be destroyed, or that laws should be passed to ban their use. If this were done, many valuable plants, some of them edible plants, would require destruction or legislation. Rather, people should familiarize themselves with the hazards in their immediate environment, and develop a respectful attitude toward the potential hazards of unfamiliar plants.

Poisonous plants are those plants that contain substance(s) which in sufficient quantities and/or over a period of time kill or harm man or animals. Primarily, the effects of poisonous plants are noted when the poisonous plant parts are eaten. However, there are some plants whose poisons may be inhaled or contacted by the skin.

HISTORY.
Man's experience with plants over the ages has helped him to identify, use, and avoid poisonous plants. Primitive people obtained toxins from plants to use for hunting. African hunters tipped their arrows with ouabain from *Strophanthus gratus*—a poison powerful enough to stop an elephant. American Indians tipped blow gun darts with the powerful muscle relaxant curare from *Strychinos toxifera*.

Men used their knowledge of poisonous plants on other men. Plotters poisoned their enemies with deadly nightshade, *Atropa belladonna*. Some primitive tribes provided drinks from toxic plants to accused individuals as a trial—a survivor was held as innocent. Other cultures used poisonous plants to carry out death sentences. Socrates, about 400 B.C., was condemned to die by drinking a cup of poison hemlock.

The effects of some poisonous plants includes hallucinations. Through the ages men have used these plants for religious rites and to escape from everyday ills. The Aztecs revered a mushroom, *Psilocybe mexicana*, for its hallucinogenic properties, while the priests of India deified a toadstool, *Amanita muscaria,* for its intoxicating juices. Here in the United States, the Navajo Indians and other tribes employed the peyote cactus, *Lophophora williamsii,* to send users into a euphoric state.

No doubt, men watched their livestock get sick or die after eating certain plants. Stories of the Old West have made locoweeds famous because of their effects on animals. When eaten by dairy cows, White snakeroot transfers its poisonous alcohol, *tremetol,* to their milk. During the 19th century, this created the outbreaks of *milk sickness* in the Appalachians and the Midwest, and resulted in the loss of numerous lives.

Gradually, men learned to be cautious, to avoid and treat plant poisonings, and to identify poisonous plants.

PRECAUTIONS AND CAUTIONS.
Even in a modern society, that has to a large extent removed itself from the natural vegetation, poisonous plants may still be a hazard. Therefore, the following precautions and cautions will help avert the hazards of poisonous plants:

1. Become familiar with the poisonous plants in your home, garden, yard, and recreational areas; know them by sight and name.
2. Keep bright seeds, berries, and flowers out of the reach of small children, as they attract their curiosity.
3. Teach older children to keep unknown plants and plant parts out of their mouths; and instruct them as to the potential dangers of poisonous plants.
4. Know the plants that children use, or are apt to use, as play things.
5. Do not eat wild plants without *positive* identification.
6. Avoid all mushrooms and toadstools growing in the wild; their identification is too risky.
7. Never suppose a plant to be edible because it resembles a well-known edible plant.
8. Don't assume that a plant is safe for humans just because it is eaten by animals.
9. Be aware of the fact that some plants concentrate or confine the toxic substance to one part of the plant.

10. Be cognizant that in some cases cooking destroys or removes the poisonous substance, but that this is not the general rule.
11. Approach with caution the preparation of homemade herbal remedies from native or cultivated plants.
12. Remember that there are *no* absolute "tests" or "rules of thumb" which can be applied to distinguish edible from poisonous plants.

Fortunately, many poisonous plants must be eaten in relatively large amounts, and many are quite unpalatable and therefore will not be eaten in sufficient amounts to cause poisoning. Still, there are some plants that are very toxic and require only a bite or two, or a seed or two, to cause death. Also, some poisonous plants are not at all distasteful and may be eaten easily in large enough quantities to cause serious disturbances and even death.

AID FOR POISONED PERSONS.
Despite everything, people will be poisoned by plants. When this occurs, time is the most important factor. The toxic substance must be removed from the body before it is absorbed. When possible the first step should be to call a physician or the Poison Control Center immediately. The person calling should be able to (1) identify or describe the plant that was eaten, (2) tell when and how much was eaten, and (3) describe any observable symptoms. When the victim is transported, a sample of the plant should be taken for identification or verification. Also, it is important to keep parts of a plant that may be present in the stool or vomit, if there is a question about which plant part was eaten. Samples—fruits, flowers, and leaves—of the plants in the area should be quickly collected and taken with the victim.

When a physician is not available, first aid should be administered and the victim transported to a hospital. The first-aid treatment will be determined by the poison. If no other advice has been given by a doctor or a Poison Control Center, take the following emergency steps:

1. If the victim is unconscious, administer artificial respiration if necessary, and head for the hospital immediately.
2. If the swallowed poison is a noncaustic substance (not a strong alkali or strong acid), proceed as follows:

   a. Dilute the poison by getting the victim to drink lukewarm soapsuds, soda water made with common baking soda, or salt water (2 Tbsp of salt in a glass of warm water); but *beware of the danger of choking.* It may be necessary to give six or more glasses of the liquid. A poison diluted with a large amount of liquid is absorbed less quickly than a concentrate, and vomiting can be induced more easily when the stomach is filled.

   b. Induce vomiting by (1) using the fingers to stimulate gagging, (2) giving 1 tsp of syrup of ipecac (which should be in every medicine cabinet) every 5 minutes for 3 or 4 doses, or (3) giving either soda water made with baking soda, or salt water. When the victim vomits, lay him on his stomach with his head hanging over the edge of the bed or over your knees. If possible, catch any material thrown up in basin or bowl and save for laboratory analysis.

   c. After the stomach has been thoroughly emptied by vomiting, give an antidote (a substance to counteract the poison), such as an all-purpose product containing activated charcoal, magnesium hydroxide, or tannic acid.

3. If the poison is a strong alkali, a strong acid, or a petroleum distillate rather than a poisonous plant, *do not induce vomiting* because of the danger of perforating the stomach or esophagus and/or aspirating the corrosive fluid

into the lungs. Instead, neutralize and dilute with a weak acid such as dilute lemon juice or vinegar, or with an alkali, such as baking soda, lime water, milk of magnesia, or chalk, then give milk, olive oil, egg white, or an all-purpose antidote.

4. As soon as possible, transport the victim via private car, ambulance, police, or paramedics to the nearest hospital and/or physician. Be sure to take samples of the suspected poisonous plant.

(Also see POISONS.)

POISON CONTROL CENTERS.

Centers have been established in various parts of the country where doctors can obtain prompt and up-to-date information on treatment of poison cases, if desired. Poison Control Centers have information relative to thousands of poisonous substances, cross-indexed by brand name as well as generic or chemical name, and can give prompt, responsible advice about antidotes.

Local medical doctors have information relative to the Poison Contol Centers of their area, along with their telephone numbers. When the phone number is not known, simply ask the operator for the Poison Control Center. If this information cannot be obtained locally, call the U.S. Public Health Service at either Atlanta, Georgia, or Wenatchee, Washington.

SOME IMPORTANT POISONOUS PLANTS OF NORTH AMERICA.

A description of all plants that are potentially poisonous is not within the scope of this book. Almost all plants are poisonous if the wrong part is consumed or if too much is consumed. For example, the stalks of rhubarb are a wholesome and delicious food while the leaves contain poisonous levels of oxalic acid; or large quantities of apple seeds, peach pits, or apricot pits may cause cyanide poisoning.

The listing given herein includes some of the most important, and often the most common, poisonous plants in North America. It is presented for informational purposes and with the hope of stimulating reader interest in learning more about the poisonous plants in his particular environment. More can be learned through the advice of experts and by reading publications dealing with poisonous plants common to a specific area.

Listed alphabetically by common name, followed by the scientific name, some of the most important poisonous plants in North America follow:

Baneberry, *Actaea* spp
Buckeye; Horsechestnut, *Aesculus* spp
Buttercup, *Ranunculus* spp
Castor bean, *Ricinus communis*
Chinaberry, *Melia azedarach*
Death camas, *Zigadenus paniculatus*
Dogbane (Indian hemp), *Apocynum cannabinum*
Foxglove, *Digitalis purpurea*
Henbane, *Hyoscyamus niger*
Iris (Rocky Mountain Iris), *Iris missouriensis*
Jasmine, *Gelsemium sempervirens*
Jimmyweed (Rayless goldenrod), *Haplopappus heterophyllus*
Jimsonweed (Thornapple), *Datura stramonium*
Lantana (Red Sage), *Lantana camara*
Larkspur, *Delphinium* spp
Laurel (Mountain laurel), *Kalmia latifolia*
Locoweed (Crazyweed), *Oxytropis* spp
Lupine (Bluebonnet), *Lupinus* spp
Marijuana (hashish, Mary Jane, pot, grass), *Cannabis sativa*

Mescal bean (Frijolito), *Sophora secundiflora*
Mistletoes, *Phoradendron serotinum*
Monkshood (Wolfsbane), *Aconitum columbianum*
Mushroom (toadstools), *Amanita muscaria, Amantia verna, Chlorophyllum molybdites.*
Nightshade, *Solanum nigrum, Solanum elaeagnifolium*
Oleander, *Nerium oleander*
Peyote (Mescal buttons), *Lophophora williamsii*
Poison hemlock (poison parsley), *Conium maculatum*
Poison ivy, *Rhus radicans*
Poison oak, *Rhus toxicondendron*
Pokeweed (Pokeberry), *Phytolacca americana*
Poppy (common poppy), *Papaver somniferum*
Rhododendron; Azaleas, *Rhododendron* spp
Rosary pea (precatory pea), *Abrus precatorius*
Snow-on-the-mountain, *Euphorbia marginata*
Skunkcabbage, *Veratrum californicum*
Tansy, *Tancacetum vulgare*
Waterhemlock, *Cicuta* spp
White snakeroot, *Eupatorium rogosum*

(Also see MEDICINAL PLANTS; and WILD EDIBLE PLANTS. **NOTE WELL:** For a more complete discussion of poisonous plants, including a detailed summary relative to each of the poisonous plants, see the two-volume *Foods & Nutrition Encyclopedia,* a work by the same authors as *Food For Health.*)

POISONS

Contents	Page

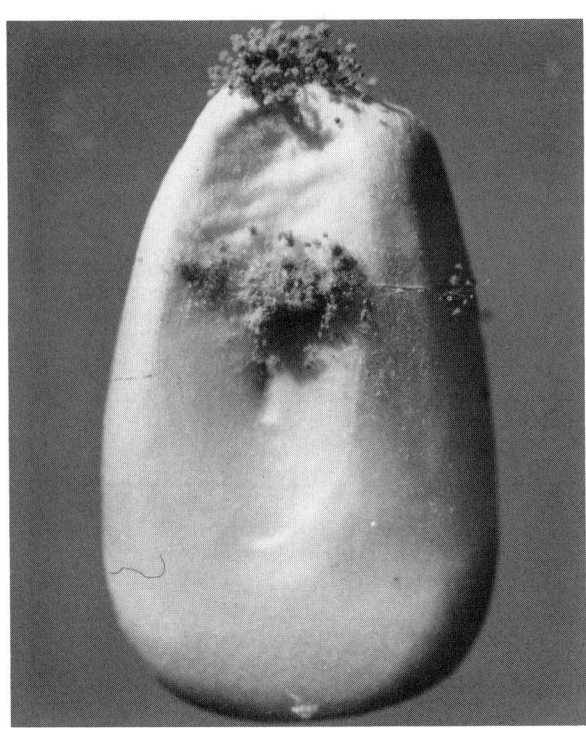

Fig. P-44. Sporulation of *Aspergillus flavus* on a kernel of corn. This fungus produces aflatoxin. Aflatoxin (1) is associated with a high indicence of liver cancer, and (2) may be involved in some types of acute poisoning of children. (Courtesy, C. W. Hesseltine, USDA, Agricultural Research, Peoria, Ill.)

Sola dosis facit venenum, means "only the dose makes the poison." Paracelsus, the noted German-born physician, said it in the 16th century. But it's just as true today as it was four centuries ago. For most food-related poisons, there is both a safe level and a poisonous level; and the severity of the effect depends upon (1) the amount taken, (2) the period of time over which the substance is taken (certain poisons are cumulative), and (3) the age and physical condition of the person.

Take potatoes, for example. They contain solanine, which can be toxic. In consuming an average of 119 lb (*54 kg*) of potatoes per year, the average American ingests 9,700 mg of solanine—enough to kill a horse. Yet it doesn't kill us because we don't eat it all at one time.

Or take lima beans! The average person eats about 1.85 lb (*0.84 kg*) of these tasty little morsels each year, not realizing that they contain hydrogen cyanide, a deadly poison. But they don't kill us simply because we can't eat enough at any one sitting to be deadly. Besides, most U.S. limas contain little hydrogen cyanide.

And so it goes, on and on through a long list of foods and drinks.

By definition, *a poison is a substance which in sufficient quantities and/or over a period of time kills or harms living things.* Many poisons are called toxins. The study of poisons is called *toxicology.* The discussion that follows and Table P-2 pertain primarily to food-related poisons that are eaten.

There are more than four million chemical compounds, of which more than 60,000 are commercially produced; and about 1,000 new ones are introduced each year. Some of these make their way into food and water. With the growth and use of chemicals, food supplies are subject to contamination from or treatment with chemicals in the course of growing, fertilizing, harvesting, processing, and storing.

Today, there are substantially fewer dangers than formerly from contamination of food and water by bacteria or from ingesting lead (now that paints are lead-free). Nevertheless, some two million ingestions of potentially dangerous substances occur in the United States each year; and there were 6,226 fatal poisonings in 1988.[29] Despite popular misconceptions, children are no longer the main victims of poisons. Today, only 1% of the deaths from poison involve children under 5 years of age; and poisoning now accounts for only 23% of the accidental deaths among children under age 5.[30] This decline is attributed primarily to the use of childproof safety caps in packaging poisonous agents; the storage of toxic substances separate and apart from other products and out of reach of children; and the banning of lead-containing paints, along with public health screening of children living in old housing areas in which lead-based paints may have been used years ago.

The general symptoms of poisoning are: nausea, vomiting, cramps, and stomach pains. If a corrosive poison (a strong alkali or a strong acid) has been taken, burns and stains may show on and around the mouth and tongue.

POISON PREVENTION AND TREATMENT. In
recent years, physicians, pharmacists, and Poison Control Center personnel have joined forces in advocating the following simple measures to avert poisoning and provide lifesaving aid when poisoning occurs:

---

[29]*Statistical Abstracts of the United States 1991,* U.S. Department of Commerce, Bureau of the Census, p. 85, Table 124.

[30]*Healthy People,* the Surgeon General's report on health promotion and disease prevention, U.S. Department of Health, Education, and Welfare, 1979, p. 70.

1. **Packaging and storing potential poisons with care.** The use of child-resistant containers (opened only with difficulty and know-how), strip packages (with pills and capsules sealed individually in a plastic strip), and safe storage have reduced the incidence of accidental poisoning, especially among children.

2. **Keeping a supply of syrup of ipecac on hand at all times.** As a reliable (and usually rapid) means of inducing vomiting, it is the best.

3. **Having an all-purpose antidote on hand.** Antidotes are usually listed on the labels of potentially poisonous products, but finding the ingredients and mixing them takes up valuable time. So, it is best to have an all-purpose antidote readily available. The main ingredients in all-purpose antidotes are powdered activated charcoal, which has a strong capacity to absorb many chemicals; a weak buffering alkali such as magnesium hydroxide to help neutralize an acid poison; and a weak buffering acid such as tannic acid to help neutralize any alkali present. This type of antidote is particularly useful in cases of poisoning in which it is best not to induce vomiting.

EMERGENCY MEASURES IN ACUTE POISONING.
In case of *acute* poisoning, it is important to act swiftly, calmly and knowledgeably. The following emergency measures, taken in the order listed, may save a life:

NOTE WELL: Although these measures were prepared especially for counteracting the poisons listed in Table P-2, they are applicable to all poisons, including those from drugs and household products.

1. **Call a doctor, the nearest Poison Control Center, or a hospital.** Describe over the phone exactly what the poison was (read off the label), provided it is known. If the victim is unable to give information, perhaps a nearby container or the symptoms will identify the poison. Based on this information, the doctor or Poison Control Center may be able to recommend emergency treatment, thereby saving precious time.

2. **Apply first-aid treatment.** The first-aid treatment will be determined by the poison. If no other advice has been given by a doctor or a Poison Control Center, take the following emergency steps:

   a. If the victim is unconscious, administer artificial respiration if necessary, and head for the hospital immediately.

   b. If the swallowed poison is a noncaustic substance (not a stong alkali or strong acid), proceed as follows:

      (1) Dilute the poison by getting the victim to drink lukewarm soapsuds, soda water made with common baking soda, or salt water (2 Tbsp of salt in a glass of warm water); but *beware of the danger of choking.* It may be necessary to give six or more glasses of the liquid. A poison diluted with a large amount of liquid is absorbed less quickly than a concentrate, and vomiting can be induced more easily when the stomach is filled.

      (2) Induce vomiting by (a) using the fingers to stimulate gagging, (b) giving 1 teaspoonful of syrup of ipecac (which should be in every medicine cabinet) every 5 minutes for 3 or 4 doses, or (c) giving either soda water made with baking soda, or salt water. When the victim vomits, lay him on his stomach with his head hanging over the edge of the bed or over your knees. If possible, catch any material thrown up in a basin or bowl and save for laboratory analysis.

(3) After the stomach has been thoroughly emptied by vomiting, give an antidote (a substance to counteract the poison), such as an all-purpose product containing activated charcoal, magnesium hydroxide, or tannic acid.

c. If the poison is a strong alkali or a strong acid, *do not induce vomiting* because of the danger of perforating the stomach or esophagus and/or aspirating the corrosive fluid into the lungs. Instead, proceed as follows:

(1) For alkali poisoning: (a) neutralize and dilute the alkali with a weak acid such as dilute lemon juice or vinegar, then give milk; or (b) give an all-purpose antidote.

(2) For acid poisoning: (a) neutralize and dilute the poison with an alkali, such as baking soda, lime water, milk of magnesia, or chalk, then (b) give milk, olive oil, egg white, or an all-purpose antidote.

3. **Control shock.** Keep the victim warm.

4. **See the doctor.** A physician should always see a victim of poisoning as soon as possible; with transportation provided by private car, an ambulance, the police, or paramedics (fire department). Also, take the poison container and label along.

POISON CONTROL CENTERS.
Centers have been established in various parts of the country where doctors can obtain prompt and up-to-date information on treatment of poison cases, if desired. Poison Control Centers have information relative to thousands of poisonous substances, cross-indexed by brand name as well as generic or chemical name, and can give prompt, responsible advice about antidotes.

Local medical doctors have information relative to the Poison Control Centers of their area, along with their telephone numbers. When the phone number is not known, simply ask the operator for the Poison Control Center. If this information cannot be obtained locally, call the U.S. Public Health Service at either Atlanta, Georgia, or Wenatchee, Washington.

ENVIRONMENTAL CONTAMINANTS IN FOOD.
Environmental contaminants include organic chemicals, metals and their derivatives, and radioactive substances that inadvertently enter the human food supply through agriculture, mining, industrial operations, or energy production. To regulate them under the law, the Food and Drug Administration (FDA) defines environmental contaminants as "added, poisonous, or deleterious substances that cannot be avoided by good manufacturing practices, and that may make food injurious to health."

Unlike food additives, environmental contaminants inadvertently find their way into the human food supply (including sports fish and game).

Four factors determine whether, and how seriously, the environmental contamination of food will affect human health: (1) toxicity of the contaminant, (2) the amount of the substance in the food, (3) the amount of the contaminated food eaten, and (4) the physiological vulnerability of the individual consuming the food.

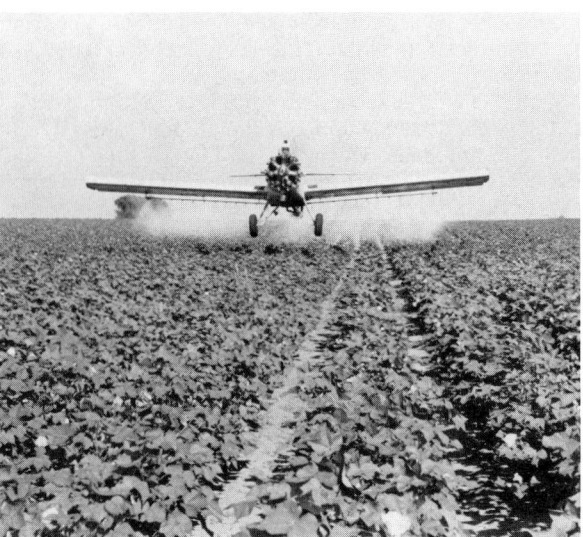

Fig. P-45. Pesticide being applied by airplane. When properly used, consumers benefit greatly from pesticides. It is important, however, to gauge the effect of each pesticide on the ecological food chain and human health.

Although the United States has escaped mass poisonings such as have occurred in most other industrialized nations, between 1968 and 1978, according to an Office of Technology Assessment (OTA) survey, 243 food-contamination incidents were reported in this country. During this same period (1968-1978), at least $282 million in food was lost to contamination—a conservative estimate that included only 30% of the known incidents and ignored such hidden costs as medical expenses and lost workdays.

The FDA sets permissible levels for all known contaminants. Then federal and state regulatory agencies monitor food to ensure that environmental contaminants do not exceed prescribed levels. Consequently, contamination involving an unregulated substance is rarely identified before it becomes a major problem. None of the major environmental contamination incidents in the United States—animal feeds in Michigan contaminated by polybrominated biphenyls (PBBs); the Hudson River contaminated by polychlorinated biphenyls (PCBs); Virginia's James River contaminated by kepone; and fat used to produce meat and bone meal feeds in a meat-packing plant in Billings, Montana, contaminated by PCBs from a damaged transformer—were initially discovered by ongoing monitoring programs. In each case, actual human or animal poisonings alerted authorities to the danger.

SOME POTENTIALLY POISONOUS (TOXIC) SUBSTANCES.
Table P-2 is a summary of some potentially poisonous (toxic) substances to people and animals.

(Also see POISONOUS PLANTS; and BACTERIA IN FOOD.)

NOTE WELL: For a more complete discussion of poisons, see the two-volume *Foods & Nutrition Encyclopedia*, a work by the same authors as *Food For Health*.

TABLE P-2
SOME POTENTIALLY POISONOUS (TOXIC) SUBSTANCES

Poison (Toxin)	Source	Symptoms and Signs	Distribution; Magnitude	Prevention; Treatment
Aflatoxins (See MYCOTOXINS in this table.)				
Aluminum (Al)	Food additives, mainly present in such items as baking powder, pickles, and processed cheeses. Aluminum-containing antacids. Aluminum cooking utensils.	Abnormally large intakes of aluminum irritate the digestive tract. Also, unusual conditions have sometimes resulted in the absorption of sufficient aluminum from antacids to cause brain damage. Aluminum may form nonabsorbable complexes with essential trace elements, thereby creating deficiencies of the trace elements.	**Distribution:** Aluminum is widely used throughout the world. **Magnitude:** The U.S. uses more aluminum than any other product except iron and steel. However, known cases of toxicity are rare.	**Prevention:** Based on the evidence presented herein, no preventative measures are recommended. **Treatment:** This should be left to the doctor.
Arsenic (As)	Consuming foods and beverages contaminated with excessive amounts of arsenic-containing sprays used as insecticides and weed killers. Arsenical insecticides used in vineyards exposing the workers (1) when spraying or (2) by inhaling contaminated dusts and plant debris. Arsenic in the air from three major sources: smelting of metals, burning of coal, and use of arsenical pesticides.	Burning pains in the throat or stomach, cardiac abnormalities, and the odor of garlic on the breath. Other symptoms may be diarrhea and extreme thirst along with a choking sensation. Small doses of arsenic taken into the body over a long period of time may produce hyperkeratosis (irregularities in pigmentation, especially on the trunk); arterial insufficiency; and cancer. There is strong evidence that inorganic arsenic is a skin and lung carcinogen in man.	**Distribution:** Arsenic is widely distributed, but the amount of the element consumed by man in food and water or breathed, is generally small and not harmful. **Magnitude:** Cases of arsenic toxicity in man are rather infrequent. Two noteworthy episodes occurred in Japan in 1955. One involved tainted powdered milk; the other, contaminated soy sauce. The toxic milk caused 12,131 cases of infant poisoning, with 130 deaths. The soy sauce poisoned 220 people. There are many scattered case reports of subacute to chronic arsenic poisoning.	**Prevention:** Avoid consuming (1) arsenic products, or (2) foods and beverages contaminated with excessive amounts of arsenic. **Treatment:** Induce vomiting and more vomiting, followed by an antidote of egg whites in water or milk. Afterward, give strong coffee or tea, followed by epsom salts in water or castor oil.
Chromium (Cr) (See CHROMIUM; and MINERAL[S].)				
Copper (Cu) (See COPPER; and MINERAL[S].)				
Ergot Although ergot is a small mycotoxin it is treated separately herein because it differs from the other mycotoxins in that it results from the consumption of a considerable amount of fungus tissue in which the toxin is found, whereas in the other mycotoxicoses the toxins are secreted into the substrate on or in which the fungus is growing, and very little fungus tissue as such is consumed. **Cause:** *Claviceps purpurea.* Ergotism is caused by overuse of ergot-containing foods or drugs.	Rye, wheat, barley, oats, and triticale. Ergot replaces the seed in the heads of cereal grains, in which it appears as a purplish-black, hard, banana-shaped, dense mass from ¼ to ¾ in. (*6 to 19 mm*) long.	When a large amount of ergot is consumed in a short period, convulsive ergotism is observed. The symptoms include itching, numbness, severe muscle cramps, sustained spasms and convulsions, and extreme pain. When smaller amounts of ergot are consumed over an extended period, ergotism is characterized by gangrene of the fingertips and toes, caused by blood vessel and muscle contraction stopping blood circulation in the extremities. These symptoms include cramps, swelling, inflammation, alternating burning and freezing sensations ("St. Anthony's fire") and numbness; eventually the hands and feet may turn black, shrink, and fall off. The amount of ergot in the food consumed determines how rapidly toxic effects will show. Ergotism is a cumulative poison, depending on the amount of ergot eaten and the length of time over which it is eaten.	**Distribution:** Ergot is found throughout the world, wherever rye, wheat, barley, oats, or triticale are grown. **Magnitude:** There is considerable ergot, especially in rye. But, normally, screening grains before processing alleviates ergotism in people.	**Prevention:** Consists of an ergot-free diet. Ergot in plants can not be controlled by treatment; and resistant varieties of cereal grains are not available. Control of ergot in cereal grains consists of using ergot-free seed, following a crop rotation, and using cultural practices which will reduce the incidence of ergot in plants and its spread to other crops. Ergot in food and feed grains may be removed by screening the grains before processing. In the U.S., wheat and rye containing more than 0.3% ergot are classed as *ergoty.* In Canada, government regulations prohibit more than 0.1% ergot in feeds. **Treatment:** An ergot-free diet; good nursing; treatment by a doctor.
Fluorine (F) (fluorosis) (See FLUORINE OR FLUORIDE; and MINERAL[S].)				

(Continued)

TABLE P-2 *(Continued)*

Poison (Toxin)	Source	Symptoms and Signs	Distribution; Magnitude	Prevention; Treatment
Lead (Pb)	Consuming food or medicinal products (including health food products) contaminated with lead. Inhaling the poison as a dust by workers in such industries as painting, lead mining, and refining. Inhaling airborne lead discharged into the air from auto exhaust fumes. Consuming food crops contaminated by lead being deposited on the leaves and other exposed portions of the plant by direct fallout. Consuming food or water contaminated by contact with lead pipes or utensils. Old houses in which the interiors were painted with leaded paints prior to 1945, with the chipped wall paint eaten by children. Such miscellaneous sources as illicitly distilled whiskey, improperly lead-glazed earthenware, old battery casings used as fuel, and toys containing lead.	Symptoms develop rapidly in young children, but slowly in mature people. **Symptoms of acute lead poisoning:** Colic, cramps, diarrhea or constipation, leg cramps, and drowsiness. The most severe form of lead poisoning, encountered in infants and in heavy drinkers of illicitly distilled liquor, is characterized by profound disturbances of the central nervous system, and permanent damage to the brain; damage to the kidneys; and shortened life span of the erythrocytes. **Symptoms of chronic lead poisoning:** Colic, constipation, lead palsy especially in the forearm and fingers, the symptoms of chronic nephritis, and sometimes mental depression, convulsions, and a blue line at the edge of the gums.	**Distribution:** Predominantly among children in poverty-stricken neighborhoods, living in dilapidated housing built before 1945, where they may eat chips of lead-containing paints, peeled off from painted wood. Leaded paints are no longer used on the interior surface of houses. **Magnitude:** The Center for Disease Control, Atlanta, Georgia, estimates that (1) lead poisoning claims the lives of 200 children each year, and (2) 400,000 to 600,000 children have elevated lead levels in the blood. Lead poisoning has been reduced significantly with the use of lead-free paint.	**Prevention:** Avoid inhaling or consuming lead. Workers in industries where lead poisoning is an occupational hazard should follow the safety regulations that have been established. **Treatment:** **Acute lead poisoning:** An emetic (induce vomiting), followed by drinking plenty of milk and ½ oz (*14 g*) of epsom salts in a glass of water. **Chronic lead poisoning:** Remove the source of lead. Sometimes treated by administration of magnesium or lead sulphate solution as a laxative and antidote on the lead in the digestive system, followed by potassium iodide which cleanses the tracts. Currently, treatment of lead poisoning makes use of chemicals that bind the metal in the body and help in its removal.
Mercury (Hg)	Mercury is discharged into the air and water from industrial operations and is used in herbicide and fungicide treatments. Mercury poisoning has occurred where mercury from industrial plants has been discharged into water and has then accumulated as methylmercury in fish and shellfish. Accidental consumption of seed grains treated with fungicides that contain mercury, used for the control of fungus diseases of oats, wheat, barley, and flax.	The toxic effects of organic and inorganic compounds of mercury are dissimilar. The organic compounds of mercury, such as the various fungicides, (1) affect the central nervous system, and (2) are not corrosive. The inorganic compounds of mercury include mainly mercuric chloride, a disinfectant; mercurous chloride (calomel), a cathartic; and elemental mercury. Commonly the toxic symptoms are: corrosive gastrointestinal effects, such as vomiting, bloody diarrhea, and necrosis of the alimentary mucosa.	**Distribution:** Wherever mercury is produced in industrial operations or used in herbicide or fungicide treatments. **Magnitude:** Limited. But about 1,200 cases of mercury poisoning identified in Japan in the 1950s were traced to the consumption of fish and shellfish from Japan's Minamata Bay contaminated with methylmercury. Some of the offspring of exposed mothers were born with birth defects, and many victims suffered central nervous system damage. Still another outbreak of mercury toxicity occurred in Iraq, where more than 6,000 people were hospitalized after eating bread made from wheat that had been treated with methylmercury.	**Prevention:** Do not consume seed grains treated with a mercury-containing fungicide. Surplus of treated grain should be burned and the ash buried deep in the ground. Control mercury pollution from industrial operations. **Treatment:** This should be left to a medical doctor.
Mycotoxins ("myco", prefix from the Greek word *mykes*, meaning fungus), which may produce the toxicity syndromes referred to as mycotoxicoses. There are an estimated 800 species of fungi (yeasts and molds), but fortunately not all fungi produce metabolites that are toxic. Some mycotoxins are carcinogens—capable of causing malignant tumors (cancers). **Cause:** Toxin-producing molds: e.g. *Aspergillus flavus, Aspergillus parasiticus, Penicillium cyclopium, P. islandicum, P. palitans, Fusarium roseum, F. tricinctum.* The aflatoxins constitute a family of 14 naturally-occurring toxins. (Also see ERGOT which is presented alphabetically in this table.)	Contaminated foods. Mycotoxins can produce toxic compounds on virtually any food (even synthetic) that will support growth. It is important to know that mycotoxins remain in food long after the organism that produced them has died; thus, they can be present in food that is not visibly moldy. Moreover, many kinds of mycotoxins are relatively stable substances that survive the usual methods of processing and cooking. The possibility of mycotoxicoses resulting from the ingestion of previously contaminated meat and eggs remains uncertain, unless the intake level is extremely high. But there is abundant evidence that lactating cows and lactating mothers consuming diets containing more than 20 ppb of aflatoxin on a dry matter basis will produce milk which contains aflatoxin residues. High levels of phytic acid in soybeans prevents aflatoxin synthesis.	In animals, liver damage is the most charcteristic symptom. It is reasonable to assume that man would respond similarly and that liver disease, particularly liver cancer, would be associated with aflatoxin exposure. Studies conducted in Uganda, Thailand, and Kenya have shown that high incidence of liver cancer is associated with high aflatoxin intake. Practically nothing is known about the acute effects of aflatoxins in humans. However, evidence is accumulating that suggests that aflatoxins and mycotoxins may be involved in some types of acute poisoning in children. In the Thailand study mentioned above, it was found that the liver, brain, and other tissues of children dying of a form of acute encephalitis, characterized by degeneration of the liver and other visceral organs (known as Reye's syndrome), contained far higher amounts and frequencies of aflatoxin B₁ than the tissues from children from the same region dying of other causes.	**Distribution:** Mycotoxins are widely distributed throughout the world. It has been known for a long time that liver cancer, which is relatively uncommon in the U.S. and Europe, occurs at much higher frequency in central and southern Africa and Asia. This prompted several field studies which confirmed that elevated liver cancer incidence is associated with aflatoxin exposure. **Magnitude:** Mass poisoning of human population by mycotoxins occurred in the U.S.S.R. during World War II. (See column headed "History.") Also, there has long been a high incidence of aflatoxin toxicity in Uganda, Thailand, and Kenya. In contrast to the limited numbers of documented mycotoxicoses in humans, there have been hundreds of reports of toxicity symptoms in livestock.	**Prevention:** The best way to control aflatoxins is to control their production. This calls for the maintenance of food and feed quality during growth, harvest, transportation, processing, and storage. The most important means of controlling mold growth and subsequent aflatoxin production is preventing damage to crops during harvest and reducing post harvest moisture levels below those required for fungal growth. Moisture levels below 18.5% in cereal grains, below 9% in such oilseeds as peanuts, sunflower, and safflower, and below 6% in copra. Organic acids (acetic acidpropionic acid mixture or propionic acid alone) may be applied to inhibit the growth of molds. The high aflatoxin risk crops are: peanuts, cottonseed, and copra. Aflatoxin in cottonseed may be inactivated by treating with anhydrous ammonia. Ultraviolet irradiation will also reduce the toxicity of aflatoxin. Certain spices, i.e. pepper.

TABLE P-2 *(Continued)*

Poison (Toxin)	Source	Symptoms and Signs	Distribution; Magnitude	Prevention; Treatment
Pesticides are chemicals used to destroy, prevent, or control pests. Pesticides also include (1) chemicals used to attract or repel pests, and (2) chemicals used to regulate plant growth or remove or coat leaves. Pests can be classified into six main groups: 1. Insects (plus mites, ticks, and spiders) 2. Snails and slugs 3. Vertebrates, including rats, mice, and certain birds (starling, linnets, English sparrows, crows, and blackbirds) 4. Weeds 5. Plant disease 6. Nematodes (Also see PESTICIDES AS INCIDENTAL FOOD ADDITIVES.)	Pesticides are chemicals. When properly used, they are beneficial; when improperly used, they may be hazards. Pesticide poisoning may be caused by either (1) sudden exposure to lethal quantities, or (2) as a result of repeated exposure to nonlethal quantities (chronic poisoning) during a protracted period of time. Farmers know that unless they follow state and federal regulations they risk having their products seized and condemned, or refused by processsors. Nevertheless, economics dictate that new products be used as soon as they prove useful. On the other hand, food faddists may feel that they are being poisoned; wildlife conservationists may be concerned over possible damage to songbirds and other animals; beekeepers may become unhappy if insectants kill honeybees; and public health officials may be concerned about contamination of soil and food supplies.	Knowing something of the toxicity and symptoms or signs of poisoning of each type of pesticide may result in getting medical advice quickly and in saving a life. The leading chemical groups, along with the toxicity symptoms of each follow: **Chemical Group:** Organophosphates—most toxic; they injure the nervous system. Carbamates—safer than the organo-phosphates. Fumigants—make a person seem drunk. Plant-derived pesticides—some are very toxic.	**Distribution:** In every pursuit of modern agriculture, more and more pesticides are being used. They are the first line of defense against pests that affect human health and well-being and attack crops, livestock, pets, and structures. **Magnitude:** Pesticides are used to control many of the estimated 10,000 species of harmful insects; more than 160 bacteria, 250 viruses, and 8,000 fungi known to cause plant diseases; 2,000 species of weeds and brush; and 150 million rats. **Symptoms or signs of toxicity:** *Mild poisoning:* Fatigue, dizziness, sweating, vomiting. *Moderate poisoning:* Inability to walk, constriction of pupil of eye. *Severe poisoning:* Unconsciousness, tremors, convulsions. They produce the same symptoms and signs as the organophosphates, but they respond more easily to treatment. Poor coordination, slurring words, confusion, sleepiness. Technical pyrethrum may cause allergic reaction. Some rotenone dusts irritate the respiratory tract. Nicotine is fast-acting nerve poison.	**Prevention:** The first and most important precaution to observe when using any pesticide is to read and heed the directions on the label. In the event of an accident, the label becomes extremely important in remedial measures. For public protection, all chemicals are rigidly controlled by federal laws. Each one is required to be registered by the Environmental Protection Agency before it can be sold in the United States, and each one is issued a tolerance for residues that may result from its use on food or feed crops. **Treatment:** Each label contains a "Statement of Practical Treatment." Read it before handling a pesticide. First aid procedures follow: **Happenstance: What to do:** Pesticide skin Wash with soap contact or detergent and plenty of water. Pesticide inhalation Get to fresh air right away. Pesticide in eyes Flush eyes and face thoroughly with water. Pesticide in mouth Rinse mouth with or stomach water. Do not induce vomiting. Go to physician immediately. *CAUTION:* Take the pesticide label to the physician; it will help him treat the problem.
Polybrominated biphenyls (PBBs), a fire retardant which may cause cancer when taken into the food supply.	All of the 1973 Michigan toxicity problem was traced to livestock feed which became contaminated with PBB when the fire retardant was shipped by mistake to a feed manufacturer.	People exposed to PBB in Michigan reported suffering from neurological symptoms such as loss of memory, muscular weakness, coordination problems, headaches, painful swollen joints, acne, abdominal pain, and diarrhea.	In 1973, the accidental contamination of animal feeds exposed many people in Michigan to PBB in dairy products and other foods. The Michigan incident eventually led to the slaughter and burial of nearly 25,000 cattle, 3,500 hogs, and 1.5 million chickens; and the disposal of about 5 million eggs and tons of milk, butter, cheese, and feed.	**Prevention:** Avoid human error such as substituting PBB for a livestock feed supplement. Avoid harmfully contaminated food. **Treatment:** Follow the prescribed treatment of a medical doctor.
Polychlorinated biphenyls (PCBs), industrial chemicals; they're chlorinated hydrocarbons which may cause cancer when taken into the food supply.	Sources of contamination to man include: 1. Contaminated foods. 2. Mammals or birds that have fed on contaminated food or fish. 3. Residues on foods that have been wrapped in papers and plastics containing PCBs. 4. Milk from cows that have been fed silage from silos coated with PCB-containing paint; and eggs from layers fed feeds contaminated with PCBs. 5. Absorption by humans beings of PCBs through the lungs, the gastrointestinal tract, and the skin.	The clinical effects on people are: an eruption of the skin resembling acne, visual disturbances, jaundice, numbness, and spasms. Newborn infants from mothers who have been poisoned show discoloration of the skin which regresses after 2 to 5 months.	**Distribution:** PCBs are widespread. They have, directly and indirectly, found their way into animal feeds and animal food products through water, paints, sealants used on the interior of silos, heat transfer fluids, and plastic and cardboard food-packaging materials.	**Prevention:** Comply with the law; do not use PCBs. Avoid harmfully contaminated food. **Treatment:** People afflicted with PCB should follow the prescribed treatment of their doctor.

Magnitude: PCB constitutes the first example of a widespread environmental hazard from an industrial chemical not classed as a pesticide. The wide usage and persistence indicate that PCB will be of considerable concern for many years.

In 1968, the accidental contamination of edible rice-bran oil by PCBs led to a poisoning epidemic among the Japanese families who consumed the oil. The disease, which afflicted 1,291 people, became known as Yusho or rice-oil disease—a condition marked by chloracne (a severe form of acne), eye discharges, skin discoloration, headaches, fatigue, abdominal pains, and liver and menstrual disturbances. In 1972, Japan banned the manufacture of PCB.

(Continued)

TABLE P-2 *(Continued)*

Poison (Toxin)	Source	Symptoms and Signs	Distribution; Magnitude	Prevention; Treatment
Polychlorinated biphenyls (PCBs) *(Continued)*		The following U.S. incidents dramatically illustrate the potential health hazard and economic harm that can be caused by PCBs: (1) the discharging of PCBs into the Hudson River with waste water from capacitor plants from 1946 to 1976, and the contamination of Hudson River fish; (2) in 1977, a fire in an animal-feed warehouse in Puerto Rico contaminated fish meal, which was subsequently fed to poultry and resulted in the desruction of 400,000 chickens and millions of eggs in the U.S.; and (3) in 1979, the fat used to produce meat and bone meal feeds in meat-packing plant in Billings, Montana, contaminated by PCBs from a damaged transformer, resulted (to October 1979) in the destruction of 600,000 to 700,000 chickens, several hundred thousand eggs, and 16,000 lb of fresh pork. In 1980, the EPA estimated that 91% of Americans carry a measurable quantity of PCB in their fatty tissues.		
Salt (NaCl—sodium chloride) poisoning (Also see MINERAL[S]; and SALT.)	Table salt (sodium chloride) and foods containing salt.	Excess dietary salt over a prolonged period of time is believed to lead to high blood pressure in susceptible people. Salt may be toxic (1) when it is fed to infants or others whose kidneys cannot excrete the excess in the urine, or (2) when the body is adapted to a chronic low-salt diet.	**Distribution:** Salt is used all over the world. Hence, the potential for salt poisoning exists everywhere. **Magnitude:** Salt poisoning is relatively rare.	**Prevention:** Do not deplete the body of salt such as can occur (1) when on a strict vegetarian diet without salt, or (2) when there has been heavy and prolonged sweating; followed by gorging on salt. The best preventative against salt poisoning is to provide plenty of water. **Treatment:** Drink large quantities of water.
Selenium poisoning (See MINERAL[S]; and SELENIUM.)				
Tin (Sn)	From acid fruits and vegetables canned in tin cans. The acids in such foods as citrus fruits and tomato products can leach tin from the inside of the can. Then the tin is ingested with the canned food. In the digestive tract tin goes through a methylation process in which nontoxic tin is converted to methylated tin, which is toxic.	Methylated tin is a neurotoxin—a toxin that attacks the central nervous system, the symptoms of which are numbness of the fingers and lips followed by a loss of speech and hearing. Eventually, the afflicted person becomes spastic, then coma and death follow.	**Distribution:** Tin cans are widely used throughout the world. **Magnitude:** The use of tin in advanced industrial societies has increased 14-fold over the last 10 years.	**Prevention:** Many tin cans are coated on the inside with enamel or other materials. Perhaps such coating should be a requisite when canning acidic fruits and vegetables. **Treatment:** This should be left to the medical doctor.

POISONS, CHEMICAL

The issue of chemical poisons is complicated, and sometimes emotional. We should remember that no chemical is totally safe, all the time, everywhere. Many chemicals, however, help make life more livable; hence, rather than banishing all chemicals, or discouraging the production of new ones, the obvious hazards must be eliminated. Then, our challenge for those chemicals with unknown hazards is their prudent and proper use and disposal coupled with monitoring their levels in food, water, and the environment. If we are able to do this, then we can reap the benefits derived from chemicals without suffering from their misuse.

(Also see PESTICIDES; and POISONS.)

POLLUTION CONTROL

Today, there is worldwide awakening to the problem of pollution of the environment (air, water, and soil) and its effects on human health and on other forms of life. Much of this concern stems from the sudden increase of animals in confinement.

We must be mindful that life, beauty, wealth, and progress depend upon how wisely man uses nature's gifts—the soil, the water, the air, the minerals, and the plant and animal life.

Certainly, there have been abuses of the environment (and it hasn't been limited to agriculture). There is no argument that such neglect should be rectified in a sound, orderly manner. But it should be done with a minimum disruption of the economy and lowering of the standard of living.

(Also see PESTICIDES; and POISONS.)

POLY-

Prefix meaning much or many.

POLYARTERITIS NODOSA (KASSMAULMAIER DISEASE)

A usually fatal disease affecting the connective tissue in the arteries of the kidneys, heart, lungs, liver, gastrointestinal tract, eyes, and joints. Diseased arteries allow blood to clot, become inflamed, and deteriorate. This causes functional impairment of the organs and tissues supplied by the affected arteries. Outward symptoms of the sufferer include fever, weight loss, abdominal and muscular pains, skin disturbances, and high blood pressure. The disease usually occurs in middle age, and affects three times as many men as women. The cause of polyarteritis is unknown, but it belongs to a class of diseases called collagen diseases. If detected early enough, steroids may provide temporary relief and slow the progess of the disease. During steroid therapy, dietary sodium may have to be restricted since many steroid preparations promote sodium retention.

POLYCYTHEMIA

Excess blood cells that contain a high concentration of hemoglobin. One type of polycythemia may be caused by an excess of cobalt in the diet of humans, resulting in stimulation of bone marrow accompanied by excessive production of red corpuscles and higher than normal hemoglobin.

POLYDIPSIA

An abnormal or excessive thirst due to the loss of body fluids, as observed in diabetes mellitus.

POLYNEURITIS

Neuritis of several peripheral nerves at the same time,

caused by metallic and other poisons, infectious disease, or vitamin deficiency. In man, alcoholism is also a major cause of polyneuritis.

POLYNEUROPATHY

A disease which causes the noninflammatory degeneration of many of the peripheral nerves. It may result from: (1) certain deficiency diseases, (2) metabolic diseases, (3) chemical poisoning, (4) some infective diseases, (5) a carcinoma, or (6) some rare genetic diseases. Symptoms consist of cramps, numbness, weakness, loss of reflexes, loss of positional senses, and partial paralysis. Usually the legs are affected first, and then the arms. Those deficiency diseases exhibiting polyneuropathy are beriberi, pellagra, chronic alcoholism, burning feet syndrome, and pyridoxine or pantothenic acid deficiency.

POLYPEPTIDES

Ten to one hundred amino acids chemically joined by a peptide bond are termed polypeptides. In the body, polypeptides occur as a result of protein digestion or protein synthesis.
(Also see PROTEIN[S].)

POLYPHAGIA

Continuous eating or excessive appetite.
(Also see APPETITE.)

POLYPHOSPHATES

The ability of the phosphates (PO_4) to chemically link up with each other and form long chains gives rise to a variety of phosphate compounds called polyphosphates. They have numerous uses in the food industry as nutrient and/or dietary supplements, sequestrants (chelating agents), flavor improvers in processed meats, and chemical aids to curing meats. The FDA considers most polyphosphates and their sodium, calcium, potassium and ammonium salts as GRAS (generally recognized as safe) additives.

POLYURIA

A medical term indicating excessive formation and discharge of urine. It is a sign of disease. For example, polyuria is noted in diabetics.

POMACE

The residue of a fruit pulp that remains after the fruit has been pressed to extract the juice. Large amounts of apple, citrus, and grape pomace are produced in the United States during the manufacturing of the respective juices. The apple and citrus pomaces are the raw materials used in the production of pectin, a gelling agent and an ingredient in diarrhea remedies. All three types of pomace are used as animal feed ingredients.

POME

A type of fruit that contains many seeds enclosed within a central cartilagenous core which, in turn, is surrounded by the fleshy portion and skin of the fruit. The best known pome fruits are apples, pears, and quinces.
(Also see FRUIT[S].)

POPULATION, WORLD

Population growth is the major determinant of demand for food.

It took from the dawn of man until 1,600 years after the birth of Christ for the number of people in the world to reach one-half billion. The population of the world first topped 1 billion in 1830. And it took another 100 years—until 1930—for the population to reach 2 billion. In 1960, it was 3 billion; in 1975, it was 4 billion; and in 1982, it was 4.5 billion. Even more frightening in the people-numbers game is the estimation of population experts for the years ahead. By the year 2000, it's predicted that the world will have 6.2 billion mouths to feed; and that by the year 2045, world population will be doubled. (See Fig. P-46.)

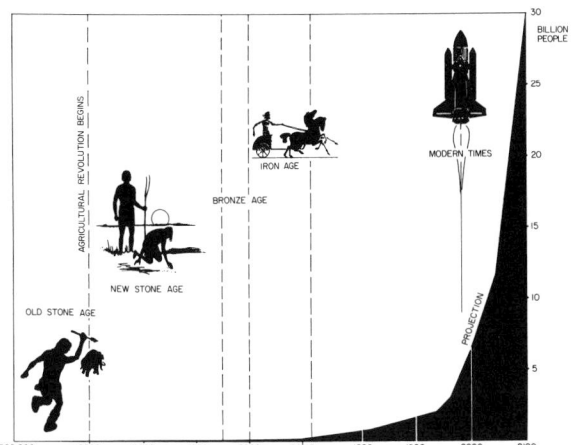

Fig. P-46. Human population growth over the past 1.5 million years, with projections to 2100 A.D.
NOTE: If the Old Stone Age were in scale, its base line would extend 8 feet to the left.

Assuming 6.2 billion (the estimated population in the year 2000) people standing shoulder to shoulder and occupying an average width of 2 ft, 6.2 billion people would circle the world 97 times, or reach to the moon and back (477,750 mi) 5 times. Today's one-year-old baby will likely see the world's population reach 12 billion—three times present numbers—within his or her lifetime.

Do these population figures foretell the fulfillment of the doomsday prophecy of Thomas Malthus, made in 1798, that world population grows faster than man's ability to increase food production? For almost 200 years, we proved Malthus wrong. Disease had a major role in holding population down; and as population increased, new land was brought under cultivation; and machinery, chemicals, new crops and varieties, and irrigation were added to step up the yields. Now science has given us the miracle of better health and longer life. Malthus was right!

The ominous challenge of our children is that the demand for food will triple in their lifetime. And that's not all! Seventy-five percent of the people of the world live in the developing countries where only 40% of the world's food is produced. Also, this is where most of the world's increase in population is occurring; population in the developing countries is now growing more than 2.1% annually compared to just under 0.6% in the developed countries. The developing countries now account for 89% of the world's annual population increase. More disturbing yet, rate of increased food production per capita in the developing countries is only two-thirds of that in the developed countries. So, people in some of the developing countries will starve to death because of population growth outrunning food production. Increased agricultural production in the developing countries requires more scientific knowledge than the older methods.

(Also see HUNGER, WORLD; MALNUTRITION, PROTEIN-ENERGY; MALTHUS; PROTEIN, WORLD PER CAPITA; and WORLD FOOD.)

PORK

Contents   *Page*

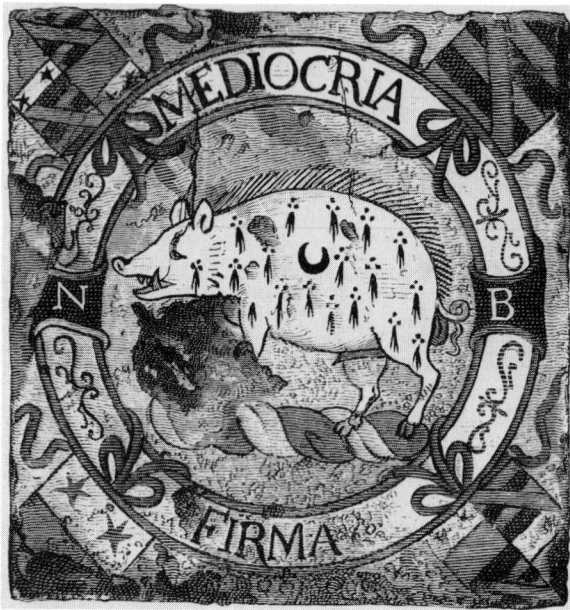

Fig. P-47. The crest of Lord Bacon (1561–1626)—noted English Viscount, lawyer, statesman, politician. According to some authorities, the word "bacon" was derived from Lord Bacon. (Courtesy, Picture Post Library, London, England)

Pork is the flesh of hogs, which are usually slaughtered at about 240 lb liveweight. About 70% of the pork carcass becomes salable retail cuts; the remaining 30% consists of fat trim, sausage trimmings, and feet, tail, and neckbones.

Only about 1/3 of the pork processed in the United States is sold as fresh product, the other 2/3 is cured and smoked. Originally, pork was cured to preserve it, but, today, pork is cured primarily to enhance flavor and provide variety and convenience.

QUALITIES IN PORK DESIRED BY CONSUMERS.
Consumers desire the following qualities in pork:

1. **Quality.** The quality of the lean is based on firmness, texture, marbling, and color.

2. **Firmness.** Pork muscle should be firm so as to display attractively. Firmness is affected by the kind and amount of fat. For example, pigs that are fed liberally on peanuts produce soft pork. Also, pork with small quantities of fat will contain more moisture and tend to be soft.

3. **Texture.** Pork lean that has a fine-grained texture and porous pinkish bones is preferred. Coarse-textured lean is generally indicative of greater animal maturity and less tender meat.

4. **Marbling.** This characteristic contributes to buyer appeal. Feathering (flecks of fat) between the ribs and within the muscles is indicative of marbling.

5. **Color.** Most consumers prefer pork with a white fat on the exterior and a greyish pink lean marbled with flecks of fat.

6. **Maximum muscling; moderate fat.** Maximum thickness of muscling influences materially the acceptability by the consumer. Also, consumers prefer a uniform cover of not to exceed 1/4 in. (6 mm) of firm, white fat on the exterior.

7. **Repeatability.** The housewife wants to be able to secure a standardized product; pork of the same eating qualities as her previous purchase.

If these seven qualities are not met by pork, other products will meet them. Recognition of this fact is important, for competition is keen for space on the shelves of a modern retail food outlet.

FEDERAL GRADES OF PORK.
Grades of barrow and gilt carcasses are based on quality-indicating characteristics of the lean and expected yields of the four lean cuts (ham, loin, picnic shoulder, and Boston butt). Quality and yield are combined in one set of grades and are not kept separate, in contrast to the system used with beef and lamb.

From the standpoint of quality, two general levels are recognized—*acceptable* and *unacceptable*. Acceptability is determined by direct observation of the cut surface and is based on considerations of firmness, marbling, and color, along with the use of such indirect indicators as firmness of fat and lean, feathering between the ribs, and color. The degree of external fatness is not considered in evaluating the quality of the lean. Suitability of the belly for bacon (in terms of thickness) is also considered in quality evaluation, as is the softness and oiliness of the carcass. Carcasses which have unacceptable quality lean, and/or bellies that are too thin, and/or carcasses which are soft and oily are graded U.S. Utility.

If a carcass qualifies as acceptable in quality of lean and in belly thickness, and is not soft and oily, it is graded U.S. No. 1, 2, 3, or 4, based entirely on projected carcass yields of the four lean cuts; carcasses not qualifying for these four grades are graded U.S. Utility. The expected yields of each of the grades in the four lean cuts, based on using the U.S. Department of Agriculture standard cutting and trimming methods, are as given in Table P-3.

TABLE P-3
EXPECTED YIELDS OF THE FOUR LEAN CUTS
BASED ON CHILLED CARCASS WEIGHT, BY GRADE

Grade	Yield
U.S. No. 1	60.4% and over
U.S. No. 2	57.4% to 60.3%
U.S. No. 3	54.4% to 57.3%
U.S. No. 4	Less than 54.4%

Carcasses vary in their yields of the four lean cuts because of variations in their degree of fatness and in their degree of muscling (thickness of muscling in relation to skeletal size).

PORK CUTS AND HOW TO COOK THEM.
The method of cutting pork is practically the same in all sections of the United States. Fig. P-48 illustrates the common retail cuts of pork, and gives the recommended method or methods for cooking each. This informative figure may be

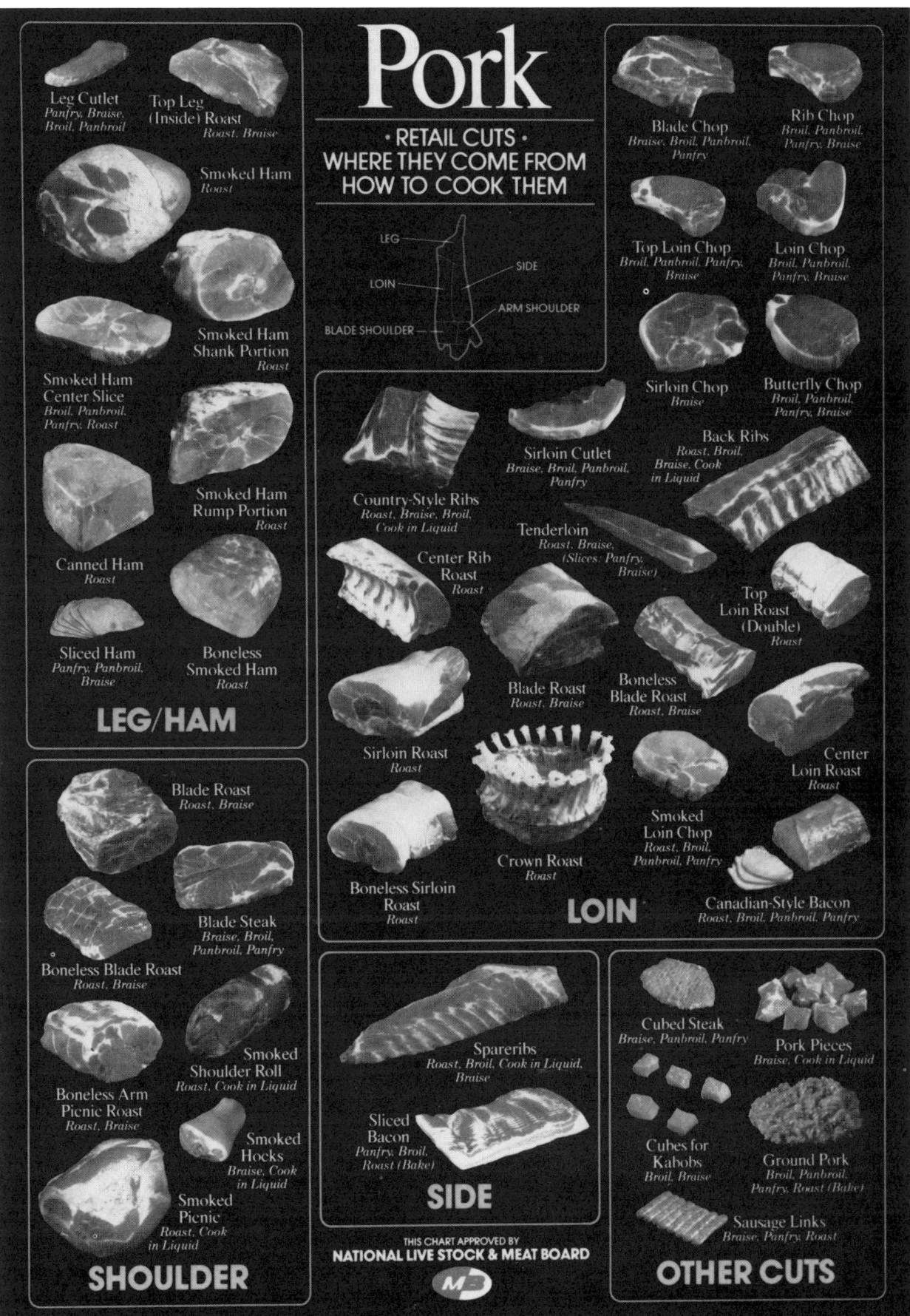

Fig. P-48. Pork Retail Cuts and how to cook them. (Courtesy, National Live Stock and Meat Board, Chicago, Ill.)

used as a guide to wise buying, in dividing the pork carcass into the greatest number of desirable cuts, in becoming familiar with the types of cuts, and in preparing each type of cut by the proper method of cookery.

U.S. PORK PRODUCTION.
On December 1, 1990, there were 54,562,000 hogs in the United States; and 15.3 billion pounds *(7 bil kg)* of pork were produced in the calendar year 1990. In 1990, pork production accounted for 40% of all red meats produced in the United States, while beef accounted for 59%.

PER CAPITA PORK CONSUMPTION.
In 1990, U.S. per capita consumption of pork, carcass basis, was 46.3 lb *(21 kg)*. That same year, U.S. per capita beef consumption was 112.3 lb *(51 kg)*.

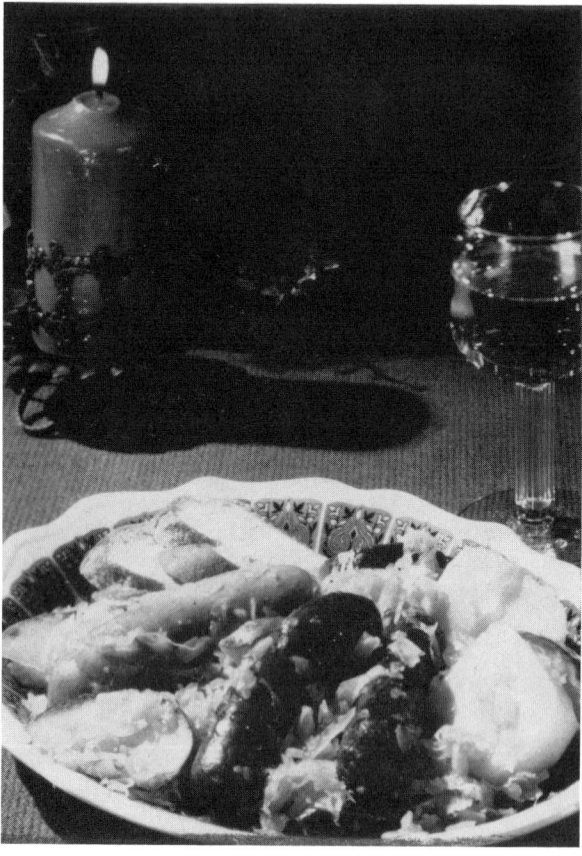

Fig. P-49. Pork sausage, rich in essential nutrients. (Courtesy, National Live Stock & Meat Board, Chicago, Ill)

Although comprising less than 5% of the world's human population and having only 6.3% of its hogs, the people of the United States eat 10% of the total world production of pork.

In general, pork consumption (and production) is highest in the temperate zones of the world, and in those areas where the human population is relatively dense. In many countries, such as China, pigs are primarily scavengers; in others, hog numbers are closely related to corn, barley, potato, and dairy production. As would be expected, the per capita consumption of pork in different countries of the world varies directly with its production and availability. Food habits and religious restrictions also affect the amount of pork consumed.

PORK AS A FOOD.
Pork is an important food and a rich source of many essential nutrients. An average 3.5 oz *(99.4 g)* serving of cooked pork ham provides 37 g of protein (that's ⅔ of the recommended daily allowance of protein) and 8.8 g of fat, along with being an excellent source of minerals and vitamins. Its high-quality protein contains all the essential amino acids needed to build, maintain, and repair body tissues. Pork is rich in iron, and the iron is readily used in the formation and maintenance of red blood cells. Also, pork is a major dietary source of the B vitamins, especially thiamin, riboflavin, and niacin. Also pork is about 98% digestible.

Because of its high concentration of several key nutrients, many physicians and nutritionists regard pork as a desirable part of many special diets, such as those for peptic ulcer, diabetes, diseases of the liver, and in geriatric and pediatric conditions where it is important to maintain a good supply of high-quality protein and other body-building and restorative nutrients which patients need. The lean cuts of fresh and cured pork are excellent foods, which afford appetizing variety for the patient.

(Also see MEAT[S].)

PORPHYRIN

A derivative of porphin. Porphyrin is present in hemoglobin; heme is ferroprotoporphyrin, a porphyrin combined with iron (ferro- for Fe^{++}).

PORTAL

An entrance. When applied to blood, it may refer to—

• **Portal blood**—The blood in the portal vein passing from the gastrointestinal tract to the liver.

• **Portal circulation**—The circulation within the liver; blood is taken into the liver by the portal vein and carried out by the hepatic vein.

• **Portal system**—The portal vein and its branches through which the portal circulation takes place; the portal system begins and ends in capillaries.

• **Portal vein**—A vein carrying blood from the digestive organs and spleen to the liver where the nutrients are altered by liver cells before passing into the systemic circulation.

POSTOPERATIVE NUTRITION

Major surgery results in a generalized loss of tissue—a catabolic phase—placing the patient in a negative nitrogen balance state. This is in part due to the changes brought about by the neuroendocrine system stimulating the secretion of adrenal cortical hormones. However, the nutritional concerns for most patients immediately following surgery are fluids, electrolytes, and energy. Depending upon the type of surgery these can be given (1) orally, (2) by a nasogastric tube, (3) by a tube placed directly in the small intestine or stomach, or (4) intravenously. As soon as possible the patient should be returned to an adequate oral intake of energy and protein to support a positive nitrogen balance during the time new tissues are being synthesized—the anabolic phase. As normal convalescence proceeds, and if there are no complications, the patient's appetite provides a reliable guide to requirements.

Specific information regarding postoperative situations requiring specialized methods is explained in detail elsewhere.

(Also see MODIFIED DIETS; INTRAVENOUS [Parenteral] NUTRITION, SUPPLEMENTARY; LIQUID DIETS; and TOTAL PARENTERAL [Intravenous] NUTRITION.)

POTASSIUM (K)

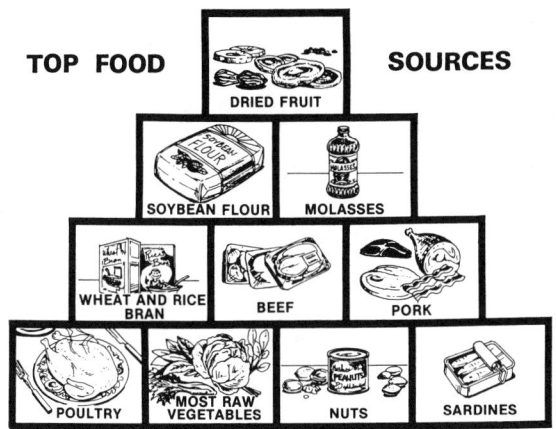

Fig. P-50. Top food sources of potassium.

Potassium is a silver-white metallic element. It is never found as a pure metal—it is always combined with other substances.

Potassium is the third most abundant element in the body, after calcium and phosphorus; and it is present in twice the concentration of sodium.

Potassium constitutes about 5% of the mineral content of the body. It is the primary cation of intracellular (within the cells) fluids. Approximately 98% of the total body potassium is located intracellularly, where its concentration is 30 or more times that of the extracellular (between cells) fluid. The concentration of sodium in blood plasma is much higher than potassium. On the other hand, the potassium concentration in muscle tissue and milk is many times higher than sodium.

HISTORY. The history of potassium is closely linked to that of sodium. Materials containing their compounds, particularly carbonates and nitrates, were known to some of the earliest civilizations. Records show that they were used in Mesopotamia in the 17th century B.C. and in Egypt in the 16th century B.C. However, the ancient technicians and artisans who used these materials, having no knowledge of the chemical and physical methods of analysis and identification, did not distinguish between them. This problem was finally solved in 1807 by the brilliant young English chemist Sir Humphry Davy, who isolated the metal which he named potassium, and gave it the chemical symbol K, from *Kalium,* the Latinized version of the Arabic word for *alkali.* However, more than 100 years elapsed following discovery before McCollum, in 1938—using the rat, obtained positive proof that potassium is an essential nutrient, although this had been suggested earlier.

ABSORPTION, METABOLISM, EXCRETION. Absorption of dietary potassium is very efficient; more than 90% of ingested potassium is absorbed. Most of the absorption occurs in the small intestine.

Although the digestive juices contain relatively large amounts of potassium, most of it is reabsorbed and the loss in the feces is small.

The kidneys provide the major regulatory mechanism for maintaining potassium balance; and relatively wide variations in intake are not reflected in fluctuations in plasma concentration. Aldosterone, an adrenal hormone, stimulates potassium excretion. Also, alcohol, coffee, and excess sugar increase the urinary excretion of potassium.

Excessive potassium buildup may result from kidney failure or from severe lack of fluid.

FUNCTIONS. Potassium and sodium are closely interrelated in the maintenance of proper osmotic pressure within cells. Both minerals are involved in the maintenance of proper acid-base balance and the transfer of nutrients in and out of individual cells. The potassium ion relaxes muscle; hence, a high concentration in the heart relaxes the heart—action opposite to that of calcium, which is stimulatory.

Potassium is also required for the secretion of insulin by the pancreas, in enzyme reactions involving the phosphorylation of creatine, in carbohydrate metabolism, and in protein synthesis.

DEFICIENCY SYMPTOMS. A potassium deficiency may cause rapid and irregular heartbeats, and abnormal electrocardiograms; muscle weakness, irritability, and occasionally paralysis; and nausea, vomiting, diarrhea, and swollen abdomen.

Hypokalemia (decreased serum potassium) of dangerous degree may be caused by a prolonged wasting disease with tissue destruction and malnutrition; by prolonged gastro-intestinal loss of potassium as in diarrhea, vomiting, or gastric suction; or by continuous use of diuretic drugs. Finally, the heart muscle may stop.

It should be noted that deficiencies of potassium rarely result from dietary lack of the mineral; rather, they result from crash diets, diarrhea, diabetic acidosis, vomiting, intense and prolonged sweating, body burns, and heavy urine losses induced by diuretic drugs (also known as "water pills").

INTERRELATIONSHIPS. A magnesium deficiency results in failure to retain potassium; hence, it may lead to a potassium deficiency.

Excessive levels of potassium interfere with magnesium absorption. Also, large excesses of potassium may slow the heart to a standstill when the kidneys are unable to excrete the surplus in the urine.

Because sodium and potassium must be in balance, excessive use of salt depletes the body's potassium supply. Although sodium intake may be the most important dietary determinant of blood pressure, variations in the sodium:potassium ratio in the diet affect blood pressure under certain circumstances.

Potassium is almost a constant component of lean body tissue, so much so that one method of estimating the amount of lean tissue in a person is by measuring the amount of potassium present. (This is accomplished by determining the amount of radioactive potassium that is naturally present in a constant ratio to ordinary potassium.) The need for potassium is increased when there is growth or deposition of lean tissue; and potassium is lost whenever muscle is broken down owing to starvation, protein deficiency, or injury.

Potassium is often prescribed for people with high blood pressure who are required to take diuretics to reduce excess water in the body because of the belief that diuretics deplete the body of potassium. However, newer knowledge indicates that diuretics do not seriously deplete natural potassium levels of the great majority of patients taking these drugs for high blood pressure. Since high blood potassium concentration can cause cardiac arrest (a heart attack) and death, potassium supplements should be taken with caution and only on the advice of a physician.

RECOMMENDED DAILY ALLOWANCE OF POTASSIUM.
The exact potassium requirements are unknown. But it is known that the daily intake on typical diets far exceeds the requirements.

Growth (increase in lean body mass) and fecal losses are the major determinants of potassium needs during the early years of life. The Food and Nutrition Board of the National Research Council (FNB-NRC) estimated minimal potassium requirements for the infant and young child are 65 mg per day (*Recommended Dietary Allowances*, 10th ed., 1989, p. 257). Human milk contains 500 mg of potassium per liter, whereas commonly used commercial formulas contain slightly more and cow's milk contains about 1,364 mg per liter. Average intakes of potassium during the first year of life range from about 780 mg per day at age 2 months to about 1,600 mg per day at the end of the first year; hence, normal diets of infants and young children provide a surplus of potassium.

Under ordinary circumstances, the healthy adult can maintain potassium balance with an intake of 1,600 to 2,000 mg per day.

Estimated safe and adequate intakes of potassium are given in the section on MINERAL(S), Table M-25, Mineral Table. The levels of potassium suggested in this table were calculated from the sodium intakes in order to achieve equivalent amounts of potassium on a molar basis. Older individuals need relatively less potassium than the rapidly growing infant, but an equivalent intake of potassium appears to be somewhat protective against the blood pressure-elevating effects of a given level of sodium.

• **Potassium intake in average U.S. diet**—The normal adult dietary intake of potassium is about 2,500 mg per day, which is more than adequate.

TOXICITY. Acute toxicity from potassium (known as *hyperpotassemia* or *hyperkalemia*) will result from sudden increases of potassium to levels of about 18 g per day for an adult, provided the kidneys are not functioning properly and there is not an immediate and sharply increased loss of potassium from the body. Although no significant increase in intracellular potassium content or in total body potassium occurs in this condition, hyperkalemia may prove fatal due to cardiac arrest.

SOURCES OF POTASSIUM. Potassium is widely distributed in foods. Meat, poultry, fish, many fruits, whole grains, and vegetables are good sources. (Although meat, poultry, and fish are good sources of potassium, these items may be restricted when dietary sodium is restricted.)

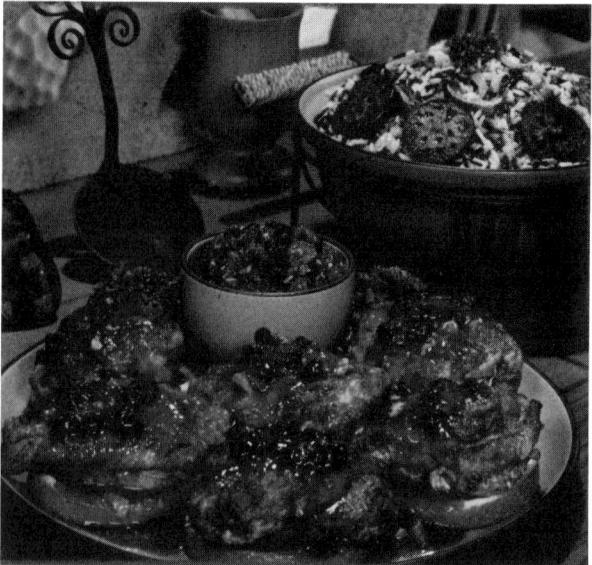

Fig. P-51. Chicken Valencia, with raisins. Chicken and raisins are good sources of potassium. (Courtesy, P. Sigel/Ketchum, San Francisco, Calif.)

Groupings by rank of common food sources of potassium are given in the section on MINERAL(S), Table M-25, Mineral Table.

NOTE WELL: Sources of potassium other than foods, such as potassium chloride, should be taken only on the advice of a physician or nutritionist.

For additional sources and more precise values of potassium, see Food Composition Table F-21 of this book.

(Also see MINERAL[S], Table M-25.)

POTATO (IRISH POTATO) *Solanum tuberosum*

This vegetable, commonly known as Irish or white potato, is grown around the world and ranks after the major grains (wheat, rice, and corn) in importance as a food. It is a member of the nightshade family of plants (*Solanaceae*), which includes the tomato, red pepper, tobacco plant, and eggplant. However, it is not related to the sweet potato or the yam. The scientific name *Solanum* is derived from the Latin word *solamen*, which means soothing.

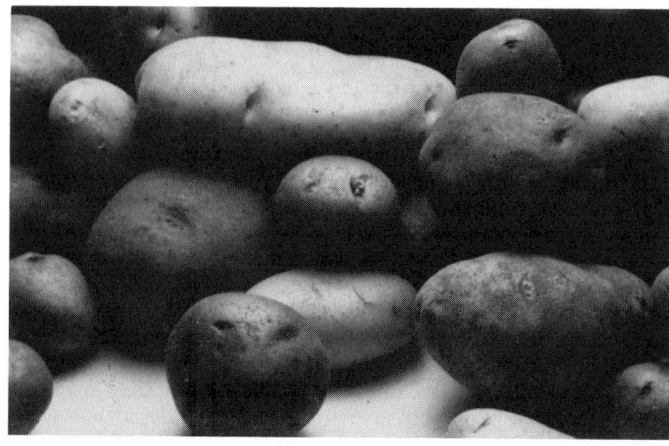

Fig. P-52. Potatoes, a vegetable which feeds millions of people around the world. (Courtesy, Shell Chemical Co., Houston, Tex.)

The edible part of the potato plant is the tuber, which grows in the ground. Tubers are not part of the roots of the plant, but are formed from underground stems. The tubers of the modern types of potatoes range in size from as small as a pea to so large that they can hardly be lifted by a strong man.

ORIGIN AND HISTORY.
Native to the Andes mountains of Peru and Bolivia, the potato was first cultivated between 4,000 and 7,000 years ago. It, along with corn (maize), was a staple of the Inca Indian diet. Spanish explorers took potatoes to Europe in the 16th century.

WORLD AND U.S. PRODUCTION.
The potato is the leading vegetable crop of the world, by a wide margin. About 270 million metric tons are produced worldwide, annually. The leading potato-producers, by rank, are: U.S.S.R., Poland, China, United States, India, Germany, U.K., Netherlands, France, and Spain.[31]

The potato is also the leading vegetable crop of the United States. The United States produces about 20 million short tons annually. By rank, the leading states are: Idaho, Washington, Colorado, Wisconsin, Oregon, Maine, California, North Dakota, Minnesota, and Michigan. Idaho alone accounts for 27% of the nation's potatoes.[32]

PROCESSING.
The consumption of fresh potatoes has declined steadily since World War II, while the use of various forms of processed potatoes has risen to the point where over half the crop is processed. Over 97% of the processed products is represented by chips and shoestring potatoes, dehydrated items (mainly instant mashed potatoes), and frozen french fries and other frozen products.

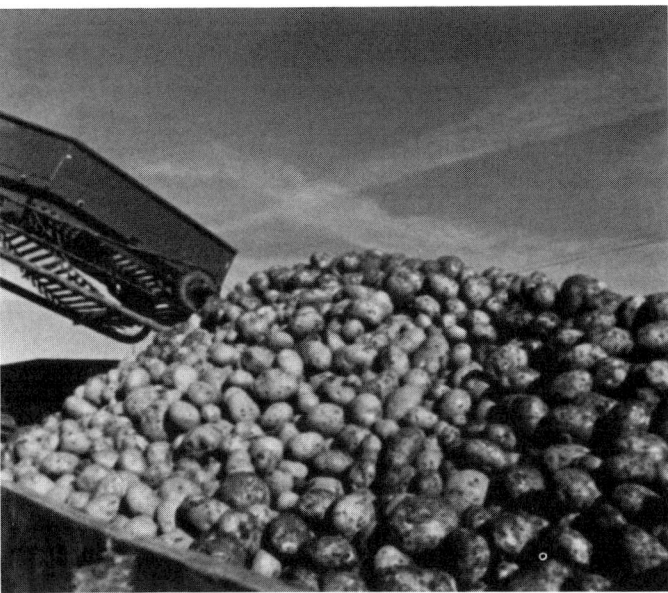

Fig. P-53. Newly harvested potatoes. (Courtesy, USDA)

---

[31]Data from *FAO Production Yearbook 1990*, FAO/UN, Rome, Italy, Vol. 44, p. 90, Table 26. **Note well:** Annual production fluctuates as a result of weather and profitability of the crop.

[32]Data from *Agricultural Statistics 1991*, USDA, p. 159, Table 228. **Note well:** Annual production fluctuates as a result of weather and profitability of the crop.

SELECTION, PREPARATION, AND USES.
Good quality potatoes are sound, firm, relatively smooth, and well shaped.

Several hundred varieties of potatoes are grown in the world. They differ in time of maturity, appearance, skin colors, resistance to insects and diseases, yield, and cooking and marketing qualities. A variety that thrives in one area may do poorly in another area.

Most supermarkets carry many types of canned, dehydrated, or frozen products that enable homemakers to prepare potato dishes with a minimum expenditure of time. Fig. P-54 shows a dish made from fresh potatoes.

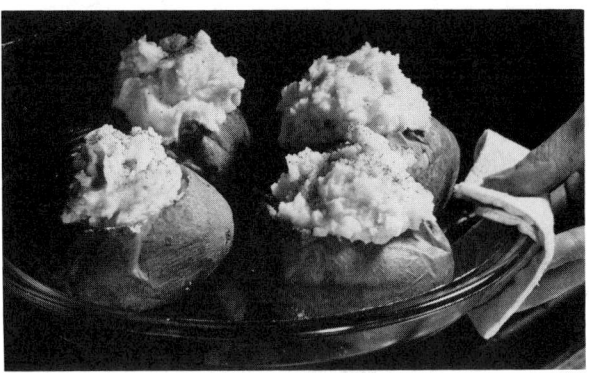

Fig. P-54. Baked and stuffed potatoes being browned in an oven. (Photo by J. C. Allen & Son, Inc., West Lafayette, Ind.)

Some suggestions for preparing various potato dishes follow:

1. There is no need to peel potatoes unless dirt is ground into the skins. The outer layer of the tuber is richer in nutrients than the inner layers. However, the skins should be cleaned thoroughly with a vegetable brush.

2. Microwave heating of baked potatoes is much faster than baking them in an ordinary oven. Also, the use of a microwave oven is a more efficient use of energy because it does not give off heat to the room in which it is located.

3. Cooking potatoes in a pressure cooker requires only a fraction of the time needed for boiling them in an open saucepan.

4. The oil or fat used to fry potatoes should *not* be heated to the smoking point because it may break down into bitter tasting and harmful products that are likely to be absorbed by the potatoes.

5. It is better to cook frozen french fries without any additional fat by placing them in an oven or under a broiler than it is to refry them because the second frying often gives the pieces a tough, poorly digested "skin" that contains more fat than most people need.

6. The fat content of homemade french fries may be kept low by tossing the raw pieces of potato in a little heated fat or oil (about 1 Tbsp per cup of potatoes), then baking them in an oven.

7. Yogurt or cottage cheese that has been blended or whipped until smooth may be substituted for butter, cheese, mayonnaise, or sour cream as a dressing for potatoes. The substitution works best when liberal amounts of seasonings such as chives, dried horseradish, mustard powder, oregano, pepper, and/or thyme are used.

NUTRITIONAL VALUE.
The nutrient composition of various forms of potatoes is given in Food Composition Table F-21.

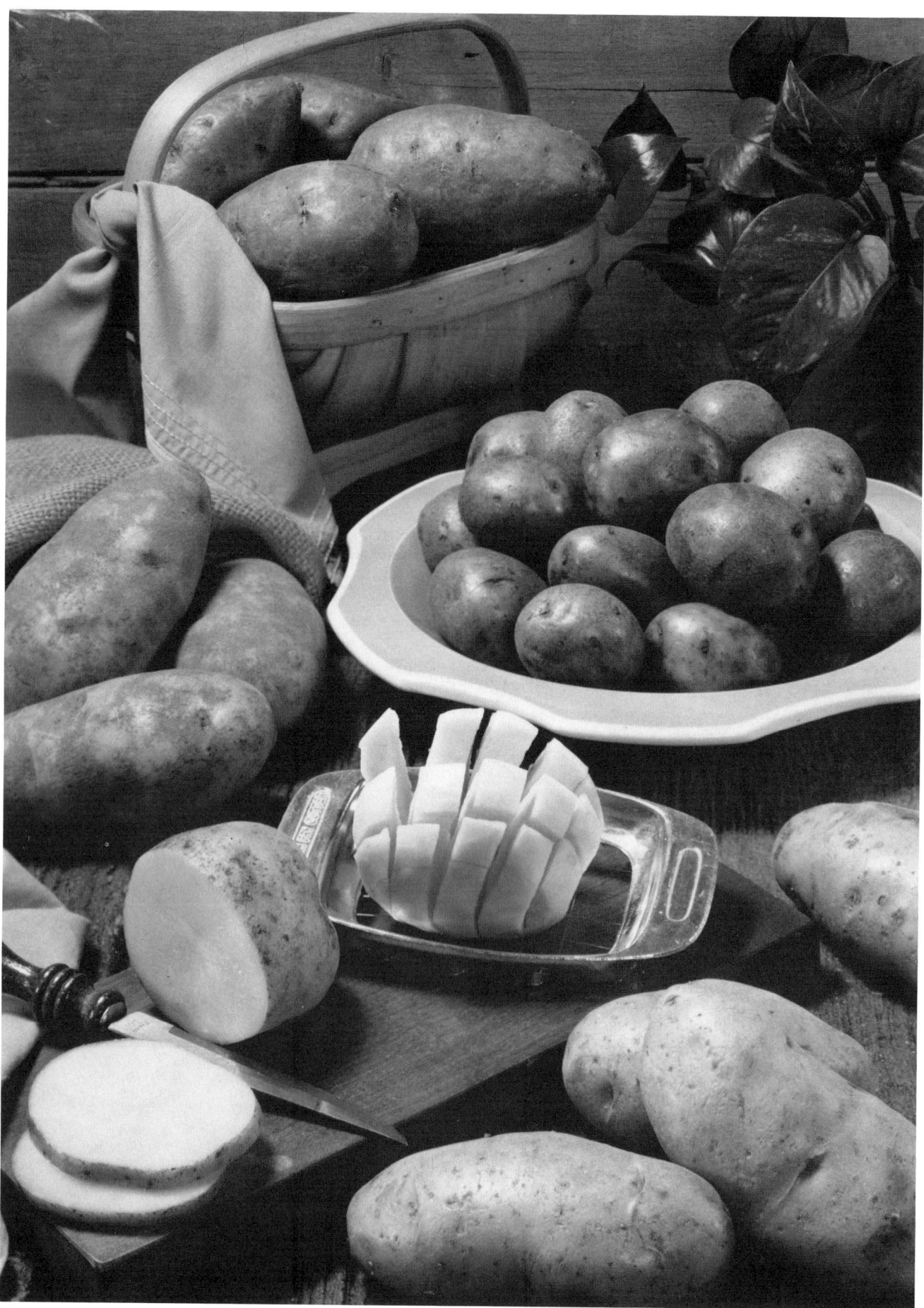

Fig. P-55. Versatile, everyway potatoes. (Courtesy, United Fresh Fruit & Vegetable Assn., Alexandria, Va.)

Some noteworthy observations regarding the nutrient composition of potatoes follow:

1. An average size raw potato (7 oz or *200 g*) contains about 115 Calories (kcal), 3.2 g of protein, 80 mg of phosphorus, 1 mg of iron, and 30 mg of vitamin C (about the amount in one-half of an average size orange), but only small amounts of calcium and vitamin A. Boiled potatoes have a similar nutrient composition, except that some of the vitamin C is destroyed by cooking.

2. Baked potatoes contain about 25% more solids and proportionately higher levels of all nutrients than raw or boiled potatoes. Also, an average size baked potato is equivalent in nutritional value to a cup of mashed potatoes, and contains about 4 g of protein, or the amount present in about a cup of cooked cereal such as cornmeal or rice.

3. French frying reduces the water content of potatoes to the extent that the cooked product contains over twice the solids, 3 to 4 times the calories, and double the protein content of baked or boiled potatoes. Furthermore, each ounce (*28 g*) of french fries contains almost 1 tsp (*5 ml*) of fat.

4. Potato chips and shoestring potatoes are high in calories because of their very low water content (2%) and high fat content (40%). Therefore, they are concentrated sources of calories (2,400 to 2,600 kcal per lb, or *0.45 kg*), protein (24 to 29 g per lb), and salt (up to 5,000 mg of sodium per lb). However, salt-free potato chips are sold in many health food stores.

5. Dried potato products, such as instant mashed potato granules and potato flour, are similar in composition to cereal flours. Therefore, they may be used in breads, pancakes, waffles, and similar baked products. Moist forms of potatoes may be used to make these items if the liquid called for in the recipes is reduced somewhat. The Irish have long made potato breads with mashed potatoes.

6. A 1-cup (*240 ml*) serving of au gratin potatoes made with cheese contains slightly more calcium and protein than a cup of milk, and about twice as many calories.

7. Potato salads are usually high in calories due to the liberal use of fat-rich mayonnaise or salad dressing in their preparation. Nevertheless, 1 cup of potato salad made with chopped egg usually provides about twice as much protein as a cup of cooked cereal.

Potatoes that are green on the surface (due to exposure to light), spoiled, or sprouted may contain harmful amounts of solanine. (See SOLANINE.)

• **The use of potatoes as a staple food**—People living in certain regions where grains do not grow well have long depended upon potatoes as a staple food. Nevertheless, there is a widely held belief that the potato-dominated diets of the Peruvian Indians and the Irish were likely to have led to multiple nutritional deficiencies. Therefore, Fig. P-56 is presented to help dispel such a belief.

It may be seen from Fig. P-56 that the yield from 1 acre (*0.4 ha*) of potatoes meets both the energy and protein requirements for over ten people, whereas, the other major life-sustaining crops are not as balanced in these nutrients. The requirements for most of the other nutrients may be met if sufficient quantities of potatoes are consumed together with other foods that supply calcium and vitamin A. The Peruvian Indians obtained these supplemental nutrients from the leaves of amaranth (pigweed) and chenopodium (lambsquarters), but, it is likely that the Irish received them from Irish moss (a seaweed) and other plants.

• **Protein Quantity And Quality**—Potatoes, which contain only 2% protein on a fresh basis, are being tested in

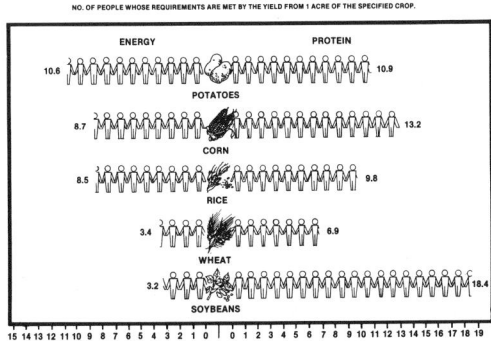

Fig. P-56. Number of people whose requirements are met by the yield from 1 acre of the specified crop.

Peru and in other countries for use as a protein supplement. Some of the reasons for this interest in the tubers are: (1) dried potato contains 8% protein; (2) the protein-to-calorie ratio of potatoes is 2.3 g per 100 Calories (kcal), which is about the same as that for corn and rice; and (3) potato protein supplies ample lysine, the amino acid that is lacking in cereal grains. Hence, mixtures of potato and cereal proteins contain higher quality protein than either type of food alone.

(Also see FLOURS, Table F-13, Special Flours.)

POTATO SYRUP

A clear, viscous, syrup produced by the hydrolysis—splitting—of potato starch with heat and acids, or enzymes. It contains dextrins, maltotetrose, maltotriose, maltose, and dextrose (glucose). The amount of each depends upon the conditions and duration of the hydrolysis. Corn syrup, derived in the same manner from corn starch, is more common in the United States.

POULTRY

The term *poultry* applies to a rather wide variety of birds of several species, and it refers to them whether they are alive or dressed. Poultry appears more frequently in the diet of people throughout the world than any other type of meat.

KINDS OF POULTRY. The most common kinds of poultry used for meat follow (the respective names of each kind of poultry also refer to the flesh of each of them used for food):

• **Chicken**—The common domestic fowl (*Gallus gallus*).

• **Turkey**—The large American bird (*Meleagris gallopavo*) derived primarily from a Mexican variety of the wild turkey and raised chiefly for their flesh.

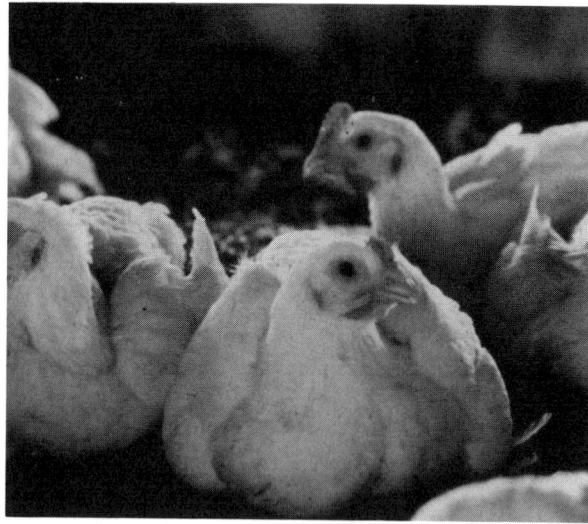

Fig. P-57. Chickens, the most common type of poultry. (Courtesy, USDA)

• **Ducks**—Swimming birds of the family *Anatidae,* characterized by short neck and legs, a broad, flat bill, the sexes differing from each other in plumage, and smaller in size than swans and geese.

• **Geese**—Swimming birds of a distinct subfamily of *Anatidae,* characterized by a high somewhat compressed bill, legs of moderate length, and longer necks and larger size than ducks.

• **Guinea fowl**—A West African bird of the subfamily *Phasianidae* (now usually classed as a separate family, *Numididae*), characterized by a bare neck and head.

• **Pigeon**—A bird of the widely distributed family *Columbidae,* characterized by a stout body with rather short legs, a bill that is horny at the tip but soft at the base, and smooth, compact plumage.

WORLD POULTRY NUMBERS, PRODUCTION, AND CONSUMPTION.
Through the ages, poultry meat and eggs have been basic foods throughout the world. In the future, they will become increasingly important for feeding the hungry for the following reasons:

1. Poultry convert feed to food efficiently.

2. The poultry industry can adjust rapidly to a variety of economic factors, e.g., feed availability, demand for animal products, cost, etc.

3. Poultry feeds are not commonly used for human consumption.

4. Layers provide a continuous source of food.

5. Most vegetarians eat eggs.

6. Poultry products are inexpensive.

7. Poultry manure can be used as a fertilizer or as a feed.

• **World poultry numbers**—The production of poultry is worldwide. Figs. P-58, P-59, and P-60 show the leading poultry-producing countries of the world.

China holds a commanding lead in chicken numbers, followed by the United States and the U.S.S.R., respectively.

The United States ranks first in turkey production with the U.S.S.R. second, and France third.

China ranks first in duck numbers, followed by Bangladesh, Indonesia, Vietnam, Thailand, and France, respectively. The duck numbers given in Fig. P-60 are, as shown, from the *FAO Production Yearbook 1991,* United Nations.

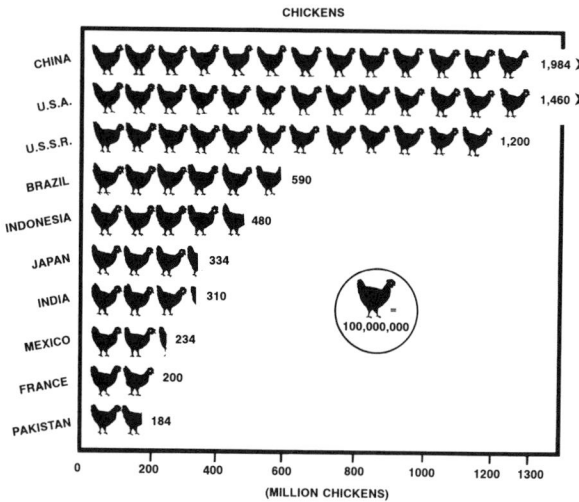

Fig. P-58. Leading chicken producers of the world. (Data from *FAO Production Yearbook 1990,* FAO/UN, Rome, Italy, Vol. 44, p. 197)

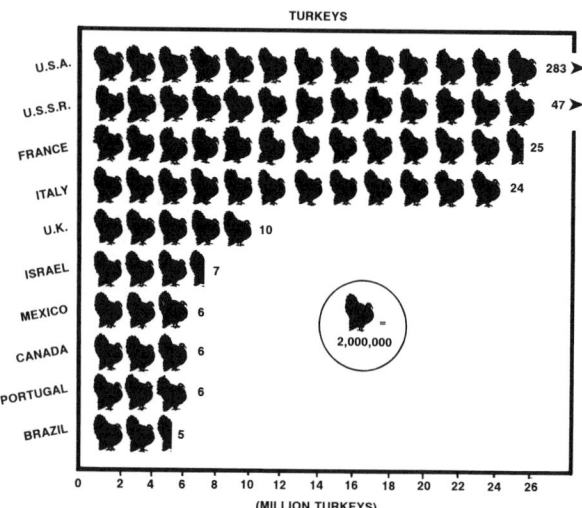

Fig. P-59. Leading turkey producers of the world. (Except for U.S. turkeys raised, data from *FAO Production Yearbook 1990,* FAO/UN, Rome, Italy, Vol. 44, p. 197. U.S. turkey data, showing turkeys raised, from *Agricultural Statistics 1991,* USDA, p. 347, Table 516)

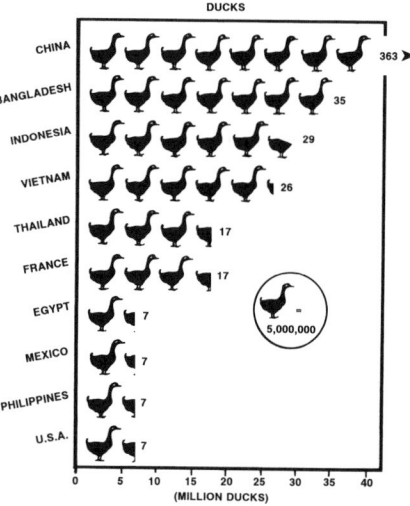

Fig. P-60. Leading duck producers of the world. (Data from *FAO Production Yearbook 1990,* FAO/UN, Rome, Italy, Vol. 44, p. 198, Table 91)

Although not shown in the FAO report, it is noteworthy that the annual production of ducks in the United States is approximately 20 million.

• **World poultry meat production**—Table P-4 shows the poultry meat production of the ten leading countries of the world in 1990. With a production of 10,851 metric tons, the United States ranks first in total poultry meat production; that is 27% of the world total.

TABLE P-4
POULTRY MEAT PRODUCTION IN
TEN LEADING COUNTRIES OF THE WORLD[1]

Country (leading countries, by rank, of all poultry meats)	Total Poultry Meat Production 1990
	(1,000 MT)
U.S.A.	10,851
China	3,295
U.S.S.R.	3,280
Brazil	2,417
Japan	1,487
France	1,384
Italy	1,104
United Kingdom	981
Spain	825
Canada	699
World Total	39,862

[1]*FAO Production Yearbook*, Vol. 44, 1990, p. 212.

• **World poultry meat consumption**—United States, with a per capita consumption of 91.9 lb *(41.8 kg)*, is the leading poultry meat consumer, followed by Singapore with 81.8 lb *(37.2 kg)*.

Table P-5 shows the leading poultry eaters of the world.

TABLE P-5
LEADING POULTRY MEAT-EATING
COUNTRIES OF THE WORLD 1990[1]

Country (leading countries by rank)	Per Capita Consumption, Dressed Weight Basis	
	(lb)	(kg)
U.S.A.	91.9	41.8
Singapore	81.8	37.2
Israel	77.6	35.3
Hong Kong	70.8	32.2
Canada	61.5	28.0
Saudi Arabia	56.0	25.5
Australia	54.0	24.5
Taiwan	53.8	24.5
Hungary	51.2	23.3
Spain	50.3	22.9

[1]*Statistical Abstract of the United States 1991*, U.S. Dept. of Commerce, p. 843, Table 1452 (with bone in). Per capita consumption is on ready-to-cook basis.

MARKETING POULTRY. It is estimated that 100% of the broilers and 90% of the turkeys are produced under some kind of integrated or contract arrangement. This means that a limited number of big firms are organized in such manner as to control every level of production—all the way from producing broilers and turkeys, through the processing, and finally, the ultimate promotion and marketing of the finished product.

Processing, Inspecting, Classifying, and Grading.
The slaughter and processing of broilers and turkeys is an assembly line operation conducted under sanitary conditions. Inspecting, classifying, and grading are a part of the processing operation.

FEDERAL INSPECTION. The Poultry Products Inspection Act was enacted on August 28, 1957, and became fully effective January 1, 1959. It requires inspection of poultry and poultry products by the U.S. Department of Agriculture. Birds are inspected twice: (1) live (antemortem); and (2) after slaughter (postmortem), when the carcasses and entrails are examined. Inspection assures U.S. consumers that the retail meat supply has been inspected to assure wholesomeness; sanitary preparation and handling; and freedom from disease, adulteration, and misbranding.

MARKET CLASSES OF POULTRY. The U.S. Department of Agriculture has established specifications for different kinds, classes, and grades of poultry. *"Kind" refers to the different species of poultry, such as chickens, turkey, ducks, geese, guineas, and pigeons. "Class" refers to kinds of poultry by groups which are essentially of the same physical characteristics, such as fryers or hens. These physical characteristics are associated with age and sex.* The kinds and classes of live, dressed, and ready-to-cook poultry listed in the U.S. classes, standards, and grades are in general use in all segments of the poultry industry.

MARKET GRADES OF POULTRY. Dressed and ready-to-cook poultry are graded for class, condition, and quality. These are most important since they are the grades used at the retail level. These grades are:

U.S. Grade A
U.S. Grade B
U.S. Grade C

These grades apply to dressed and ready-to-cook chickens, turkeys, ducks, geese, guineas, and pigeons.

Additionally, there are U.S. Procurement Grades, which are designed primarily for institutional use. These grades are: U.S. Procurement Grade 1 and U.S. Procurement Grade 2. In procurement grades, more emphasis is placed on meat yield than on appearance.

The factors determining the grade of carcass, or ready-to-cook poultry parts therefrom are: conformation, fleshing, fat covering, pinfeathers, exposed flesh, discoloration, disjointed bones, broken bones, missing parts, and freezing defects.

Retailing Poultry. Most of the poultry meat marketed consists of broilers and turkeys, although ducks, geese, guineas, and pigeons are also marketed.

• **Broilers**—In 1989, processors sold 18.3% of their broilers as whole carcasses, 50.4% as cut-up parts, 6.3% as further processed, and 25% in other forms. In 1992, approximately 40% of the broilers were further processed.

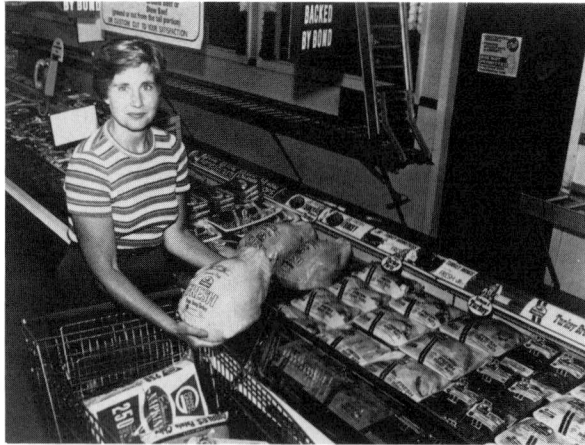

Fig. P-61. Fresh dressed turkey in the supermarket fresh meat case. (Courtesy, Cryovac Division, W. R. Grace & Co., Duncan, S.C.)

● **Turkeys**—About 80% of the turkey meat produced today is cut-up or used as further processed product. Whole bird processed turkeys, such as self-basting turkeys, comprise about 20% of the total.

Most turkeys marketed whole are Grade A. To the extent possible, Grades B and C and lower-priced parts are utilized in further processing.

More and more further processed and whole bird turkeys are being marketed directly to retail outlets and institutional outlets.

HOW TO BUY POULTRY. When buying any kind of poultry—chicken, turkey, duck, goose, guinea, or squab—in addition to price, the buyer should look for and select on the bases of the following:

1. **Look for the inspection mark.** Poultry must be officially inspected for wholesomeness before it can be graded for quality. Often the inspection mark and the grade shield are displayed together, as shown in Fig. P-62.

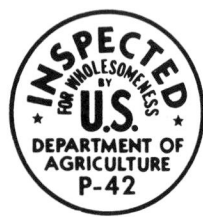 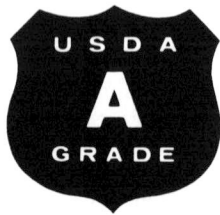

Fig. P-62. *Left:* the mark of wholesomeness. *Right:* the mark of quality.

2. **Select by grade (quality).** Look for the USDA shield, which certifies that the poultry has been graded for quality by a technically trained government grader and is the buyer's assurance of quality (see Fig. P-62, *right*).

The highest quality is Grade A. Grade A birds are—

● fully fleshed and meaty.

● well finished.

● attractive in appearance.

Grade B birds may be less attractive in finish and appearance and slightly lacking in meatiness.

3. **Select by class.** The grade of poultry does not indicate tenderness—the age (class) of the bird determines tenderness. Young birds are more tender than older one.

4. **Select to suit the occasion.** Poultry can be selected to fill every need.

● Chilled or frozen ready-to-cook poultry may be purchased in various sizes and forms to suit every occasion.

● Most kinds of ready-to-cook poultry are available as parts and in whole, halved, and quartered form. Some kinds are also available as boneless roasts and rolls.

HOW TO STORE POULTRY. All poultry is perishable. So, it is important that it be properly stored. To this end, the following pointers will be helpful.

For Refrigeration:

● Store poultry in the refrigerator only if you are going to use it within a few days. Temperatures between 35° and 40°F *(2° and 4°C)* should be maintained for refrigerator storage. Keep it in the coldest part of the refrigerator, which is usually near the ice cube compartment or in a special meat keeper.

● Wrap poultry properly for refrigeration. The special wrap on prepackaged poultry is designed to control moisture loss in the refrigerator. Raw poultry wrapped in paper should be unwrapped, placed on a platter, and then covered for refrigeration. Wrap and store giblets separately.

● Use fresh-chilled poultry within 1 to 2 days.

● Follow Table P-6, Poultry Storage Time Chart, relative to refrigerating poultry.

For Freezing:

● Keep frozen poultry at 0°F *(–18°C).*

● Keep frozen poultry hard-frozen until time to thaw, then cook promptly after thawing.

● Refreeze poultry only if it still contains ice crystals or if it is still cold and has not been held at refrigerator temperature for more than 1 to 2 days. Remember that refreezing may reduce the quality of a product.

● Follow Table P-6, Poultry Storage Time Chart, relative to freezing poultry.

TABLE P-6
POULTRY STORAGE TIME CHART

Product	Refrigerator 35°–0°F (2°–4°C)	Freezer 0°F (–18°C)
	(days)	(months)
Fresh Poultry:		
Chicken and turkey (whole)	1 to 2	12
Chicken (pieces)	1 to 2	6
Turkey (pieces)	1 to 2	6
Duck and goose (whole)	1 to 2	6
Giblets	1 to 2	3
Cooked Poultry:		
Pieces (covered with broth)	1 to 2	6
Pieces (not covered)	1 to 2	1
Cooked poultry dishes	1 to 2	6
Fried chicken	1 to 2	4

HOW TO HANDLE AND COOK POULTRY. Care and cleanliness should be used in the preparation , cooking, and serving of poultry products. The following pointers will be helpful:

• Wash poultry before preparing it for cooking.

• Wash your hands often when preparing poultry.

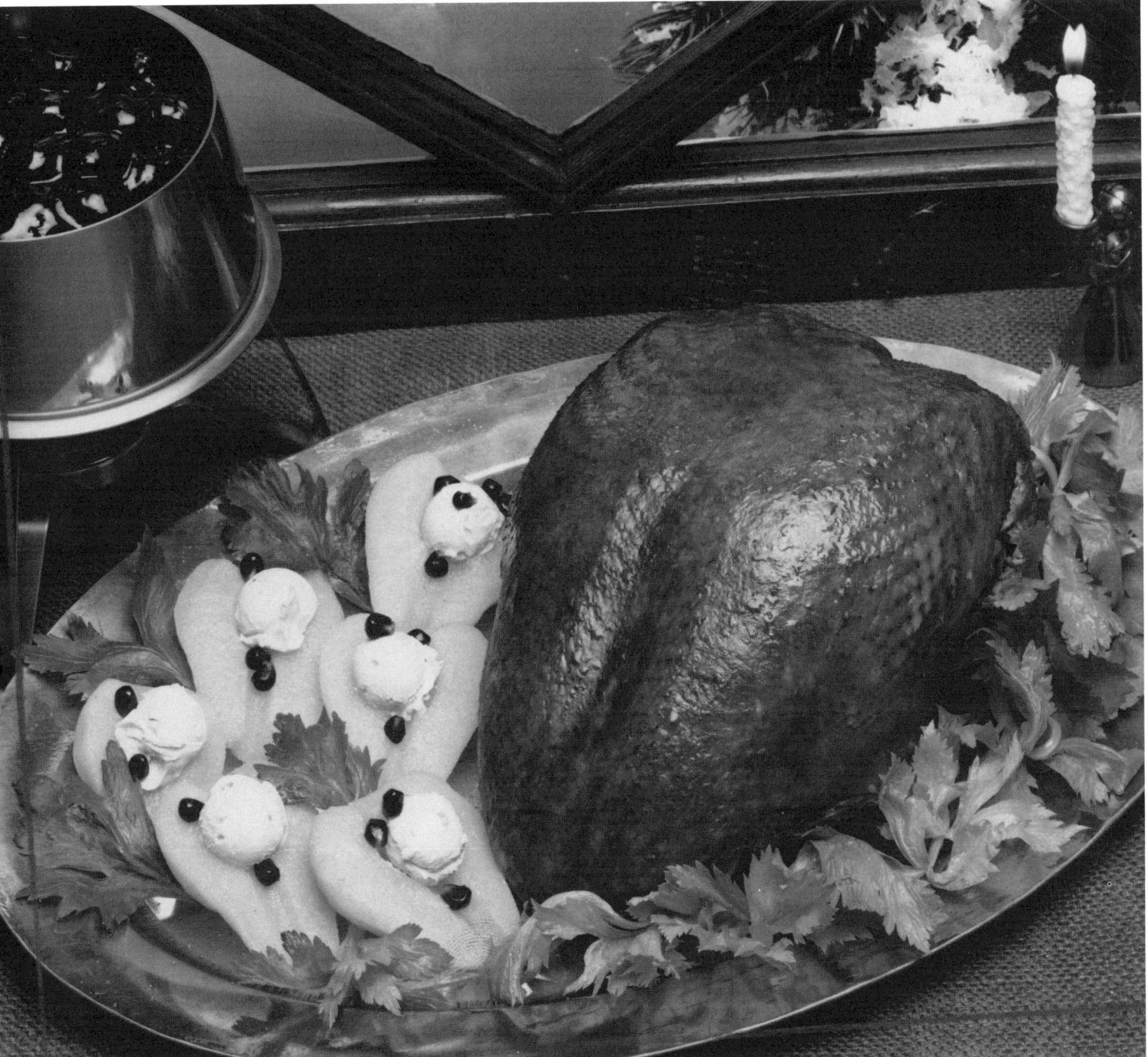

Fig. P-63. Roast turkey. Turkeys produce a higher proportion of edible meat to liveweight than any other species, and compare favorably with other meats as a source of amino acids. (Courtesy, National Turkey Federation, Reston, Va.)

• Completely cook poultry at one time. Never partially cook, then store, and finish cooking at a later date.

• It is safest to cook dressing outside the bird, but if you want to stuff it, do so right before roasting; don't stuff raw poultry and then refrigerate or freeze it. Commercially stuffed poultry should always be cooked without thawing.

• Left-over cooked poultry, broth, stuffing, and gravy should be separated, covered, and refrigerated. Use within 1 to 2 days. Freeze for longer storage.

U.S. PER CAPITA CONSUMPTION OF POULTRY MEAT.
Poultry meat is supplied chiefly by chickens and turkeys, although ducks, geese, guinea fowl, squabs (pigeon), and other fowl contribute thereto. Poultry meat is economical, and quick and easy to prepare and serve.

Fig. P-64 shows the U.S. per capita consumption of ready-to-cook poultry since 1965. Note that most of the increase occurred with broilers. In 1990, poultry meat consumption on boneless trimmed weight, or edible weight, totaled 63.8 lb *(29 kg)*.

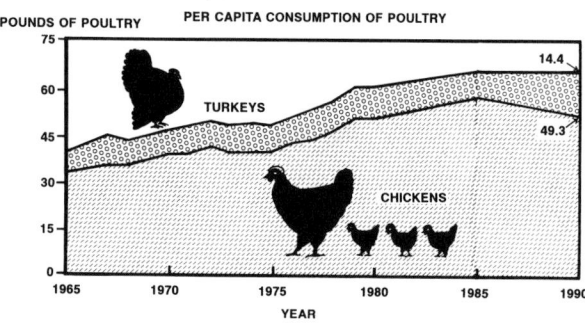

Fig. P-64. Per capita consumption of poultry—boneless, trimmed weight, or edible weight. (From: USDA)

Fig. P-65 shows how the consumption of poultry meat is fast catching up to beef and pork. From 1960 to 1990, the per capita consumption of poultry almost doubled. During this same period of time, beef and pork consumption both dropped 39%. If the recent trends shown in Fig. P-65 con-

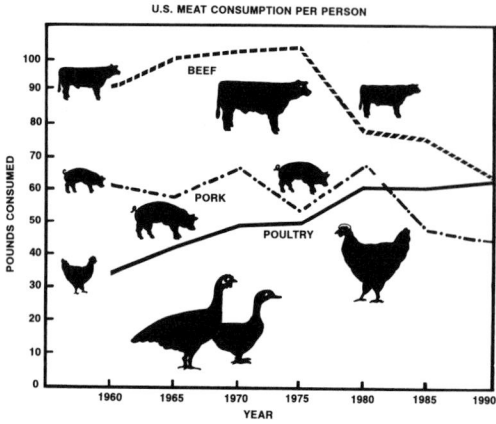

Fig. P-65. U.S. consumption of poultry, pork, and beef.

tinue, soon Americans will be eating more pounds of poultry meat than of beef or pork.

NUTRITIVE QUALITIES OF POULTRY MEAT.
Poultry meat has a number of desirable nutritional properties. Chicken and turkey meat is higher in quality protein and lower in fat than beef and pork. Additionally, the protein is a rich source of all the essential amino acids. The close resemblance of the amino acid content of poultry meat to the amino acid profiles of milk and eggs serves to emphasize the latter point.

Poultry meat is also a good source of phosphorus, iron, copper, and zinc. Additionally, it is a rich dietary source of vitamin B-12 and vitamin B-6, and it supplies appreciable amounts of vitamin A, biotin, niacin, pantothenic acid, riboflavin, and thiamin.

Poultry is a good, low-fat source of protein. However, poultry skin contains 32.35% saturated fat. Removing the skin reduces the amount of fat by approximately 5 grams per 2.5 oz breast. Because consumers are turning to foods that are lower in cholesterol and saturated fats, beginning in the early 1990s almost all U.S. restaurants included low fat, skinless chicken on their menus.

Although the RDAs are believed to be more than adequate to meet the requirements of most consumers, it is recognized that individuals vary greatly in their requirements—by as much as twofold. So, Table P-7 presents data showing the contribution of meat-poultry-fish combined, toward the total dietary intake of each of the nutrients.

TABLE P-7
CONTRIBUTIONS OF MEAT-POULTRY-FISH COMBINED, TO THE DIETARY INTAKE IN THE UNITED STATES[1,2]

Nutrition	Average Per Capita Consumption Per Day	Total Consumption Contributed by Meat-Poultry-Fish Combined
		(%)
Energy	3,600 kcal	18.8
Carbohydrate	425 g	0.1
Fat	168 g	31.7
Protein	105 g	43.3
Calcium	890 mg	3.9
Phosphorus	1,540 mg	29.2
Magnesium	339 mg	15.4
Copper	1.7 mg	17.5
Iron	17.1 mg	22.1
Zinc	12.7 mg	47.2
Vitamin A (R.E.)	1,630 mcg	20.6
Folate	284 mcg	9.8
Niacin	26 mg	44.8
Riboflavin	2.4 mg	22.2
Thiamin	2.2 mg	25.0
Vitamin B-6	2.2 mg	40.5
Vitamin B-12	9.1 mcg	76.1
Vitamin C	118 mg	2.2

[1]*Agricultural Statistics 1991*, USDA, pp. 474–479.

[2]The average yearly per capita consumption (carcass basis) amounted to 112.3 lb of red meat, 63.8 lb of poultry, and 15.4 lb of fish that was consumed in 1990.

PRECURSOR

A compound that can be used by the body to form another compound; for example, carotene is a precursor of vitamin A.

(Also see VITAMIN A.)

PREGNANCY AND LACTATION NUTRITION

Women who consume a good diet before conception and during pregnancy and lactation greatly improve their chances of successful reproduction, including (1) absence of complications during pregnancy, (2) birth of a healthy full-term baby, and (3) having little or no trouble in meeting the nutritional needs of their infants, whether they are breast-fed or formula-fed. Although even poorly fed mothers may have healthy babies, this result is sometimes achieved at the expense of the mother's tissues and health. Therefore, proper prenatal care is a means of promoting optimal health in both the baby and the mother.

HISTORY. Many ancient cultures appear to have been concerned about the successful result of pregnancy, judging by the many depictions of this condition on the artifacts found at various archaeological sites. Furthermore, students of contemporary primitives, whose practices have changed little over the centuries, have often discovered that the diets which are culturally prescribed for pregnant women have higher nutritional values than some of the food consumption patterns of people in the developed countries.

It appears that primitive diets have often deteriorated in both quantity and quality as a result of factors such as (1) rapid growth of the population as a result of which the per capita supply of food decreased greatly; (2) people changing their diets from a wide variety of native foods to a few highly refined imported foods such as flour, lard, and sugar; and (3) migration of the people to new areas where the foods are unfamiliar and likely to have been rejected because of cultural biases. Nevertheless, some groups apparently made a gradual and healthful transition from nomads to settled agriculturalists, as demonstrated by the outstanding physiques of the Swiss dairy farmers in isolated high Alpine valleys.

A new era in nutrition was ushered in during the early 1900s when the first discoveries of the vitamins were made. Before that time it was assumed that diets were adequate if sufficient amounts of carbohydrates, fats, and proteins were provided. Nevertheless, the application of sound nutritional principles to pregnancy and lactation diets lagged behind the many advances in nutritional science which were made during the first half of the 20th century.

In the 1920s, many doctors believed that a calorie-restricted diet protected pregnant women against toxemia because there was a reduction in the incidence of this condition in Austria, Hungary, and Germany during World War I when scarcities of fats and meats led to smaller weight gains during pregnancy. However, few systematically planned observations were made of (1) the weights of the women before pregnancy, and (2) the effects of dietary restrictions on the health and survival of infants. Evidence concerning the dangers of inadequate diets during pregnancy was provided by studies conducted in the 1930s which showed that toxemia might result from low protein intakes, because subnormal levels of blood proteins sometimes allowed fluid from the blood to accumulate in the tissues.

After World War II, there was considerable interest in (1) the wartime experiences of pregnant women, and (2) studies which had been conducted in the United States and England during the 1940s. Most of the studies provided evidence that fetal and neonatal deaths, low-birth-weight infants, and congenital malformations were linked to dietary deficiencies during pregnancy. However, interest in the subject waned during the 1950s after other studies failed to find significant relationships between diet and the outcome of pregnancy. One of the main reasons for the contradictory findings in the various studies may have been the failure to obtain information on the eating patterns of the subjects prior to conception. Previously, well-fed women would have had more tissue reserves to carry them through their pregnancies.

Throughout the 1950s and 1960s many American doctors told pregnant women not to gain more than 15 to 20 lb (7 to 9 kg) because they believed that excessive weight gain rendered the women more susceptible to complications such as toxemia. Furthermore, salt was often restricted and diuretics were administered to prevent the buildup of fluids in the tissues. However, this period was also characterized by a growing trend towards prescribing mineral and vitamin supplements for pregnant women. Hence, the latter practice may have offset some of the consequences of dietary restriction.

In the decade following the National Academy of Science (NAS) report, infant mortality in the United States decreased by an average of about 5% annually, thanks to the efforts of an ever-growing number of dedicated doctors, educators, medical researchers, nurses, nutritionists, and public health workers who have applied nutritional principles for the benefit of pregnant and lactating women.

CHANGES IN THE FEMALE BODY DURING PREGNANCY AND LACTATION.

Few people are aware of the amount of tissue growth that occurs in women during their reproductive years. For example, a woman who bears no children has to produce blood and repair uterine lining tissue to cover the loss of menstruation. This task alone is equivalent to the production of about 110 lb (*50 kg*) of body tissue between ages 15 and 45. However, a woman who bears 6 children and nurses each one for 9 months builds the equivalent of about 220 lb (*100 kg*)of body tissue during her reproductive years.[33]

A depiction of the tissue growth during pregnancy is given in Fig. P-66.

Details of the changes during pregnancy and lactation are given in Table P-8.

[33]Toverud, K. U., et al., *Maternal Nutrition and Child Health, An Interpretive Review,* National Academy of Sciences, 1950, p. 116.

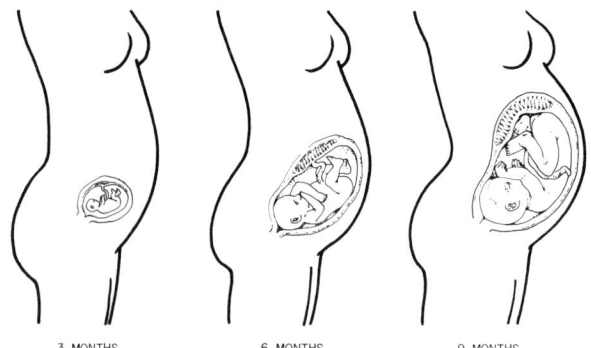

3 MONTHS   6 MONTHS   9 MONTHS

Fig. P-66. The growing fetus depends on its mother for nutrients and removal of wastes. The mother's heart pumps blood through the uterine arteries into the placenta; nutrients and oxygen diffuse through the placental membranes into the fetal bloodstream by way of the umbilical cord; and wastes pass in the reverse direction to the maternal bloodstream through the uterine veins.

TABLE P-8
MAJOR CHANGES IN THE FEMALE BODY DURING PREGNANCY AND LACTATION

Part of the Body	Changes[1]	Biological Significance	Comments
Body Composition Protein	Gain of over 2 lb (*0.9 kg*), which is equal to about 8 lb (*3.6 kg*) of lean body tissue.	Used for enlargement of maternal tissues, production of additional blood plasma and blood cells, and growth of the placenta and fetus.	About ⅓ of the additional protein is converted to fetal tissue. The rest is used for the various "support systems."
Fat	Gain of almost 10 lb (*4.5 kg*), which is equivalent to 47,500 kcal.	Provides energy for both the mother and the fetus, and subsequent lactation.	A woman may build up considerable fat in several pregnancies, unless it is lost between pregnancies.
Water	Gain of about 15 lb (*7 kg*), or about 60% of the weight gained in pregnancy.	All newly synthesized body tissues in pregnancy contain considerable fluid. A reserve of fluid against blood loss in childbirth.	Over 40% of all pregnant women have some degree of excess fluid retention in their tissues, but it is usually harmless.
Circulatory System Heart	Volume of blood pumped per minute increases by ⅓. Heart rate increases by 40% (from 70 to 85 beats per minute).	The heart has to work harder to pump the extra blood formed during pregnancy to the enlarged body mass of the mother.	Sometimes, there is a temporary enlargement of the heart during pregnancy.
Total blood volume	Increases by about 30% (from 4,000 to 5,250 ml).	Extra blood is needed to serve the tissues added during pregnancy.	The increased flow of blood to the skin causes it to feel warm and moist.
Plasma	Plasma volume increases by about 40%.	Plasma is the vehicle for transporting nutrients and other substances within the body.	This increase ocurrs early in pregnancy. Hence, the blood is temporarily diluted.
Red blood cells	Increased by about 18%.	These cells carry oxygen to the tissues.	The ratio of red cells to total blood volume is usually about 10% subnormal in pregnancy.
Digestive System Stomach	Sphincter between the esophagus and stomach is relaxed and emptying of the stomach is slowed.	Food is more thoroughly mixed with gastric juice.	Sometimes, the stomach contents pass up into the esophagus, causing heartburn.[2]
Intestines	Motion is slowed. Towards the end of pregnancy, the fetus presses against the lower bowel.	The slower passage of food results in better digestion and absorption.	Pregnant women tend to be constipated unless the diet is rich in fiber and water.
Endocrine Glands[3] Adrenals	Increased secretion of the adrenal cortical hormone aldosterone.	Promotes sodium and water retention by the body, thereby meeting the special needs of pregnancy.	Progesterone from the placenta prevents the development of excessive fluid retention and high blood pressure.
Kidneys	Increased production of renin, which acts to increase the secretion of aldosterone.	Initiates the chain of events which leads to sodium and water retention by the body.	The renin-initiated reactions may induce high blood pressure in some pregnant women.
Ovary	At the beginning of pregnancy, hormones from the placenta induce the corpus luteum in the ovary to (1) survive much longer than it does in nonpregnant women, and (2) secrete hormones such as the estrogens and progesterone.	The estrogens and progesterone from the ovary help to maintain pregnancy and prevent spontaneous abortion during the first 8 weeks.	After the first 8 weeks of pregnancy, the placenta has usually developed sufficiently to provide the hormones that were secreted by the corpus luteum.
Pancreas	Insulin secretion is usually higher than normal in the second half of pregnancy because the placenta hormone HCS[4] antagonizes the effects of insulin and causes an elevation in the blood sugar.	Resistance to the effects of insulin in normal pregnant women results in (1) higher than normal maternal blood levels of nutrients, and (2) a continuously available supply of nutrients for the fetus.	The insulin-secreting capacity of some diabetic women may be overtaxed to the extent that both the mother and fetus are harmed.

Footnotes at end of table

(Continued)

TABLE P-8 *(Continued)*

Part of the Body	Changes[1]	Biological Significance	Comments
Pituitary	Secretion of prolactin increases throughout pregnancy. Increased secretion of MSH.[4] Increased secretion of TSH.[4]	Brings about milk production by the mammary glands. Causes pigmentation in various areas of the body. Stimulates the growth of the thyroid so that it becomes more efficient in the use of iodine.	There is competition between the maternal and fetal thyroids for the supply of iodine. The placenta efficiently takes up iodine and transfers it to the fetus.
Placenta	Secretion of HCG[4] at the onset of pregnancy. Secretion of HCS[4], estrogens, and progesterone throughout pregnancy. (The amounts of the latter hormones increase as the placenta grows larger along with the fetus.)	HCG maintains the functions of the corpus luteum so that pregnancy is maintained during the first 8 weeks. HCS acts as a growth hormone and stimulates development of functioning mammary glands. Estrogens and progesterone promote many of the maternal adaptations to pregnancy. (After the first 8 weeks, the major source of estrogens and progesterone is the placenta. Hence, poor development and growth of the placenta may lead to a poor outcome of pregnancy.)	
Thyroid	May become a little enlarged.	Enlargement allows the thyroid to use iodine more efficiently.	The formation of a goiter is a sign that the dietary supply of iodine is inadequate.
Fetus	Growth proceeds slowly until about 3 months after conception. The weight of the fetus is tripled during the third trimester (final 13 to 14 weeks).	Optimal growth of the fetus and accompanying placenta are best ensured by a good diet and a maternal weight gain of about 1 lb *(0.5 kg)* per week in the latter half of pregnancy.	Restriction of the maternal diet may jeopardize the growth of the fetus and placenta.
Kidneys	Secrete greater amounts of renin, usually without causing an increase in maternal blood pressure. The flow of blood to the kidneys is increased by about 40%, and the glomerular filtration rate by about 60%.	Renin initiates actions that bring about greater retention of sodium and water in the mother. Waste products are removed with high efficiency so that the fetus is protected against toxic accumulations of substances.	Extra sodium and water is required in the maternal body during pregnancy. The high rate of urination in early pregnancy decreases somewhat in the latter half of this period.
Lungs	Although the rate of breathing remains at the nonpregnancy level, the amount of air inspired and expired with each breath increases by more than 40%.	Abundant oxygen is provided for the increased metabolism of pregnancy. However, the blood levels of carbon dioxide become subnormal.	Resting pregnant women may feel lightheaded and have other symptoms that disappear when they increase their activity. (The symptoms are due to the subnormal blood levels of carbon dioxide.)
Mammary Glands	Preparation for lactation is stimulated during pregnancy by hormones from ovaries, adrenal glands, pituitary, and the placenta. After childbirth, the hormone prolactin from the pituitary stimulates milk production. Then, sucking by the infant brings about the letdown and release of milk through the action of the hormone oxytocin from the pituitary.	Little is wasted in human lactation because (1) milk production is delayed until after childbirth, (2) sucking stimulates continuation of production, and (3) lactation ceases when mothers either fail to nurse or stop nursing after having done it for a while.	

[1]Adapted by the authors from *Maternal Nutrition and the Course of Pregnancy*, National Academy of Sciences, 1970; and *Laboratory Indices of Nutritional Status in Pregnancy*, National Academy of Sciences, 1978.
[2]Also see HEARTBURN; and HIATUS HERNIA.
[3]Only the well established endocrine changes are presented. It seems likely that other glandular changes occur in pregnancy, but firm evidence of them is lacking.
[4]HCS is human chorionic somatomammotropin; MSH is melanocyte stimulating hormone; TSH is thyroid stimulating hormone, and HCG is human chorionic gonadotropin.

NUTRIENT ALLOWANCES. Although the nutrition of the fetus is aided by the metabolic alterations that take place in the mother's body during pregnancy, adequate levels of nutrients must be provided in the mother's diet to ensure that (1) the fetus is nourished adequately without depletion of maternal tissues, and (2) maternal reserves for childbirth and lactation are accumulated. Some examples of how certain metabolic changes affect dietary needs follow:

• **Calories**—The requirement for food energy is high during the latter half of pregnancy because the fetus is accumulating a reserve supply of fat for the period after childbirth and the mother is putting on fat in order to be able to supply the necessary food energy in her breast milk. Although some women have given birth to apparently healthy babies after having gained little or no weight during pregnancy, it is likely that there was some withdrawal of fat, protein, and other nutrients from the mother's tissues. Hormones secreted during pregnancy maintain high levels of sugar (glucose), amino acids, and fatty acids in the maternal blood by (1) slowing the rate of nutrient utilization by the maternal tissues, and (2) bringing about the withdrawal of these substances from the maternal tissues when the blood levels decline. However, overweight women should *not* try to lose weight by restricting their diets during pregnancy because harmful conditions such as ketoacidosis may result.

• **Protein**—Most of the growth of the fetus takes place in the latter half of pregnancy, when the rate of protein synthesis is high, as indicated by Fig. P-67.

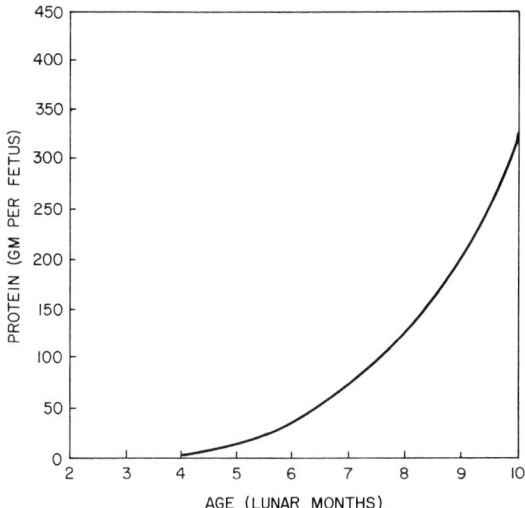

Fig. P-67. Protein accumulation in the fetus during pregnancy. (Adapted by the authors from Toverud, K. U., *et al.*, *Maternal Nutrition and Child Health, An Interpretive Review*, National Academy of Sciences, 1950, p. 36, Fig. 3)

It is noteworthy that the placenta can extract amino acids from the maternal blood so efficiently that the fetal blood levels of these nutrients are usually considerably greater than those of the mother. However, the mother herself has higher than normal needs for protein which is used to enlarge her uterus, mammary glands, and the other tissues that grow to support pregnancy and lactation. Hence, the maternal blood levels of proteins such as plasma albumin may drop to subnormal levels. This condition may be dangerous to both the mother and the fetus because lack of sufficient blood protein may allow fluid from the blood to accumulate in the maternal tissues, causing waterlogging and/or an elevated blood pressure. There appears to be an association between subnormal levels of blood protein and the tendency to develop toxemia of pregnancy.

• **Calcium and phosphorus**—Fetal bone growth proceeds on the same schedule as the growth of the lean body soft tissues, except that the rate of calcium accumulation in the bones literally skyrockets during the last 2 months of pregnancy, as is shown in Fig. P-68.

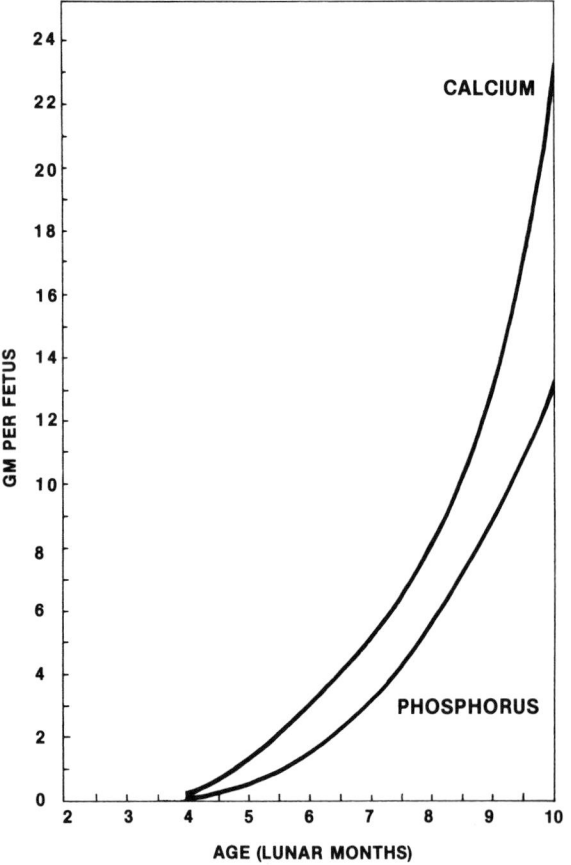

Fig. P-68. Calcium and phosphorus accumulation in the fetus during pregnancy. (Adapted by the authors from Toverud, K. U., et al., *Maternal Nutrition and Child Health, An Interpretive Review*, National Academy of Sciences, 1950, p. 55, Fig. 4)

It is noteworthy that the mother's diet should contain extra calcium from the beginning of pregnancy until the end of lactation, because the early accumulation of the mineral in the maternal tissues provides a reserve for later use, when it becomes almost impossible to consume enough to meet the needs. There is evidence to indicate that (1) dietary

calcium is about twice as well absorbed by pregnant women compared to nonpregnant women, and (2) adequate vitamin D during pregnancy enhances calcium utilization. The extra phosphorus that is required is usually provided in diets that contain sufficient protein. Infants that have received adequate calcium while in their mother's womb are less likely to develop rickets.

(Also see MINERAL[S]; CALCIUM; and PHOSPHORUS.)

• **Iodine**—The placenta extracts this essential mineral from the mother's blood so efficiently that fetal blood levels of iodine are usually several times those of the mother. However, the mother may develop a goiter when the supply of the mineral is inadequate to meet her needs. Enlargement of the maternal thyroid gland makes it more efficient in using iodine for the synthesis of thyroid hormones. Goitrous mothers have an increased risk of giving birth to infants that are cretins. Cretinism is a severe form of thyroid hormone deficiency in infants that is characterized by (1) failure of the fetal thyroid to develop, (2) mental retardation, (3) poor mineralization of the bones, and (4) dwarfism. Infants that are born with little or no functioning of the thyroid gland cannot be cured of this condition. Rather, they require the administration of thyroid hormone preparation for the rest of their lives.

(Also see MINERAL[S]; and IODINE.).

• **Vitamin E**—This vitamin does *not* readily pass across the placenta into the fetus. Hence, infants are born with low levels of vitamin E in their tissues. However, the consumption of adequate amounts of this vitamin by the pregnant mother is likely to be reflected in the amounts provided in her breast milk.

(Also see VITAMIN[S]; and VITAMIN E.)

• **Vitamin B-6**—Some pregnant women have developed a diabeticlike condition while consuming diets moderately high in protein, but low in vitamin B-6. Most of them were brought back to normal by giving them a supplement containing the vitamin.[34] It is noteworthy that the placenta concentrates the vitamin in the fetus, which may be a factor in the production of subnormal maternal blood levels of vitamin B-6 during pregnancy. Furthermore, women who have long used oral contraceptives prior to becoming pregnant may need extra amounts of this vitamin.

(Also see VITAMIN[S]; and VITAMIN B-6.)

Many other nutrients are required in greater amounts by pregnant and lactating women than by nonpregnant women. So, the Food and Nutrition Board of the National Academy of Sciences has established the allowances that are given in the section on Nutrient: Requirements, Allowances, Functions, Sources, Table N-3; hence, the reader is referred thereto.

Many other nutrients are required in greater amounts by pregnant and lactating women than by nonpregnant women. Hence, the Food and Nutrition Board of the National Academy of Sciences has established the allowances that are given in Table P-9.

---

[34]Coelingh Bennenk, H. T. J., and W. H. P. Schreurs, "Improvement of Oral Glucose Tolerance in Gestational Diabetes by Pyridoxine," *British Medical Journal*, July 5, 1975, pp. 13-15.

TABLE P–9

AVERAGE HEIGHTS, WEIGHTS, AND RECOMMENDED DAILY NUTRIENT INTAKES FOR PREGNANT OR LACTATING WOMEN OF VARIOUS AGES[1]

Category	Pregnant Age				Lactating Age			
	11–14 years	15–18 years	19–24 years	25–50 years	11–14 years	15–18 years	19–24 years	25–50 years
Weight[2] ....lb (kg)	101 (46)	120 (55)	128 (58)	138 (63)	101 (46)	120 (55)	128 (58)	138 (63)
Height ....in. (cm)	62 (157)	64 (163)	65 (164)	64 (163)	62 (157)	64 (163)	65 (164)	64 (163)
Energy ....kcal	2,500	2,500	2,500	2,500	2,700	2,700	2,700	2,700
Protein.........................g	76	76	74	74	66	66	64	64
MINERALS								
Calcium ....mg	1,200	1,200	1,200	1,200	1,200	1,200	1,200	1,200
Phosphorus ....mg	1,200	1,200	1,200	1,200	1,200	1,200	1,200	1,200
Sodium[3,4] ....mg	500	500	500	500	500	500	500	500
Chloride[4] ....mg	750	750	750	750	750	750	750	750
Magnesium ....mg	320	320	320	320	355	355	355	355
Potassium[4] ....mg	2,000	2,000	2,000	2,000	2,000	2,000	2,000	2,000
Chromium[4,5] ....mcg	50–200	50–200	50–200	50–200	50–200	50–200	50–200	50–200
Copper[4,5] ....mg	1.5–3.0	1.5–3.0	1.5–3.0	1.5–3.0	1.5–3.0	1.5–3.0	1.5–3.0	1.5–3.0
Fluoride[4] ....mg	1.5–2.5	1.5–2.5	1.5–4.0	1.5–4.0	1.2–2.5	1.5–2.5	1.5–4.0	1.5–4.0
Iodine ....mcg	175	175	175	175	200	200	200	200
Iron[6] ....mg	30	30	30	30	15	15	15	15
Manganese[4,5] ....mg	2.0–5.0	2.0–5.0	2.0–5.0	2.0–5.0	2.0–5.0	2.0–5.0	2.0–5.0	2.0–5.0
Molybdenum[4,5] ....mcg	75–250	75–250	75–250	75–250	75–250	75–250	75–250	75–250
Selenium[4,5] ....mcg	65	65	65	65	75	75	75	75
Zinc[8] ....mg	15	15	15	15	19–16	19–16	19–16	19–16
VITAMINS, FAT-SOLUBLE								
Vitamin A ....mcg RE	800	800	800	800	1,300	1,300	1,300	1,300
Vitamin D ....mcg	10	10	10	10	10	10	10	10
Vitamin E ....mgαTE	10	10	10	10	12	12	12	12
Vitamin K[4] ....mcg	65	65	65	65	65	65	65	65
VITAMINS, WATER SOLUBLE								
Biotin[4] ....mcg	30–100	30–100	30–100	30–100	30–100	30–100	30–100	30–100
Folate[7] ....mcg	400	400	400	400	280	280	280	280
Niacin ....mg	17	17	17	17	20	20	20	20
Pantothenic acid[4] ....mg	4–7	4–7	4–7	4–7	4–7	4–7	4–7	4–7
Riboflavin ....mg	1.6	1.6	1.6	1.6	1.8	1.8	1.8	1.8
Thiamin ....mg	1.5	1.5	1.5	1.5	1.6	1.6	1.6	1.6
Vitamin B-6 ....mg	2.2	2.2	2.2	2.2	2.1	2.1	2.1	2.1
Vitamin B-12 ....mcg	2.2	2.2	2.2	2.2	2.6	2.6	2.6	2.6
Vitamin C ....mg	70	70	70	70	95	95	95	95

[1]Adapted by the authors from *Recommended Dietary Allowances*, 10th ed., National Academy of Sciences, 1989.

[2]Average weight of nonpregnant, nonlactating women in each age group.

[3]There is no justification for the restriction of sodium in the diets of healthy women during pregnancy. Hence, the recommended intakes are those for nonpregnant women.

[4]These figures are given in the form of ranges of recommended intakes, because there is insufficient information to determine allowances.

[5]Since the toxic levels for many trace elements may be only several times average intakes, the upper values of the intakes should not be habitually exceeded.

[6]The increased requirement during pregnancy cannot be met by the iron content of habitual American diets nor by the existing iron stores of many women. Therefore, the use of 30 to 60 mg of supplemental iron is recommended. Iron needs during lactation are not substantially different from those of nonpregnant women, but continued supplementation of the mother for 2 to 3 months after childbirth is advisable in order to replenish stores depleted by pregnancy.

[7]The use of a folacin supplement appears to be desirable during pregnancy in order to maintain maternal stores and keep pace with the increased folacin turnover.

[8]For the first 6 mo. of lactation, the recommended allowance is 19 mg; and for the second 6 mo., it is 16 mg.

DIETARY GUIDELINES. If the mother does not have good nutrition during pregnancy, there is a greater chance of having a premature infant or one of low birth weight. There is also a greater chance of problems during

pregnancy and delivery, infant death, infant defects, and failure of the infant to grow and develop normally. The benefits of eating well during pregnancy are illustrated in Fig. P-69.

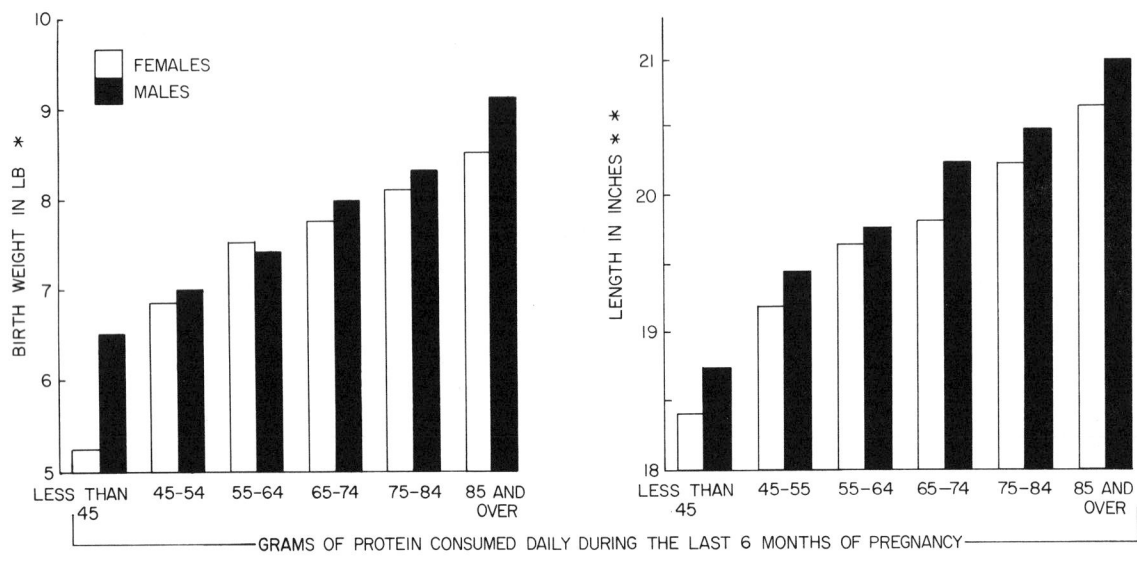

* DIVIDE BY 2.2 TO CONVERT TO KG   * * MULTIPLY BY 2.54 TO CONVERT TO CM

Fig. P-69. The effect of dietary protein during pregnancy on the weights and heights of newborn infants. (Based upon data from Toverud, K. U., *et al., Maternal Nutrition and Child Health, An Interpretive Review,* National Academy of Sciences)

The rate at which the pregnant woman gains weight is also important. Weight should be gained slowly over the entire pregnancy. A good rate of weight gain is 1½ to 3 lb *(0.7 to 1.4 kg)* the first trimester (first 3 months), and then about ¾ lb *(0.3 kg)* a week until the end of pregnancy. Gaining too much weight too quickly may be harmful to mother and baby. Excess weight gain is often due to extra fluid which causes swelling (edema) of the mother's feet, hands, and face.

Excessive weight gain during pregnancy may cause complications or problems for the mother and baby. It also places a strain on the back and leg muscles that may cause pain and fatigue. Too much weight gain will make it difficult to get back to normal size and figure after the baby is born.

Weight reduction is not generally recommended during pregnancy. And crash diets or fad diets should never be used during pregnancy. They may be harmful to mother and baby because essential nutrients may be provided in limited amounts. Low calorie diets should usually be restricted to before pregnancy or following pregnancy.

The mother is eating for two—but that's not two adults! A slight increase of 300 Calories (kcal) per day the last half of pregnancy is recommended for the woman whose activity is light. This is for the growth of the fetus, the placenta, and other maternal tissue. The pregnant woman who is working at a job requiring physical activity or at home with small children may need more than 300 additional calories per day.

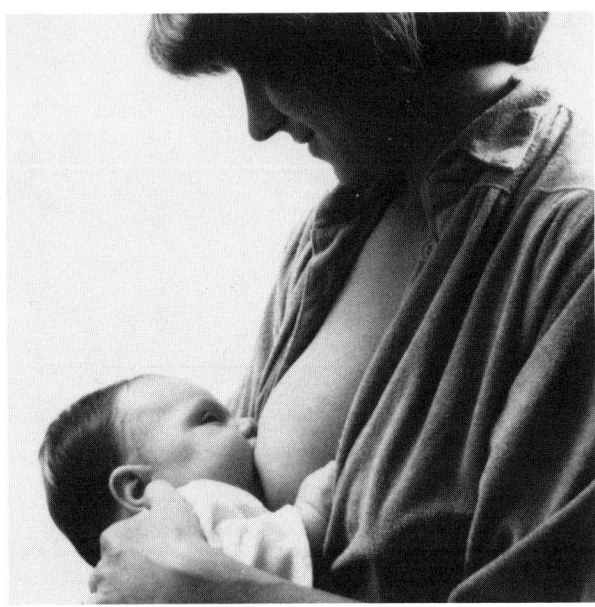

Fig. P-70. Mother and baby. (Courtesy, Gerber Products Co.)

COMMON NUTRITION-RELATED PROBLEMS OF PREGNANCY.

The physiological changes that occur in the maternal body as a result of conception may bring on or aggravate certain conditions that tend to make pregnancy burdensome to the mother. However, there are nutritional ways of coping with these problems so that the well being of the mother and fetus is promoted.

Anemia. This condition is characterized by a subnormal blood level of hemoglobin and/or red blood cells. It is usually the result of a chronic dietary deficiency of iron, although it may also result from (1) deficiencies of other nutrients such as protein, copper, folacin, vitamin B-6, vitamin B-12, and vitamin C; or (2) losses of blood that have not been replaced fully.

The need for iron during pregnancy is quite high because it is used to (1) maintain the hemoglobin level of the mother, (2) maintain the mother's store of iron, (3) promote fetal development, and (4) provide a reserve in the infant for blood formation during early infancy before iron-rich foods are added to the diet. Furthermore, the iron stores in women of childbearing age are apt to be inadequate for pregnancy because of (1) loss of blood during menstruation, and (2) failure to consume sufficient amounts of iron-rich foods. Therefore, the Committee on Maternal Nutrition of the National Academy of Sciences has recommended that pregnant women take a daily supplement that contains from 30 to 60 mg of iron.[35]

(Also see IRON.)

One of the benefits of iron supplementation during pregnancy is shown in Fig. P-71.

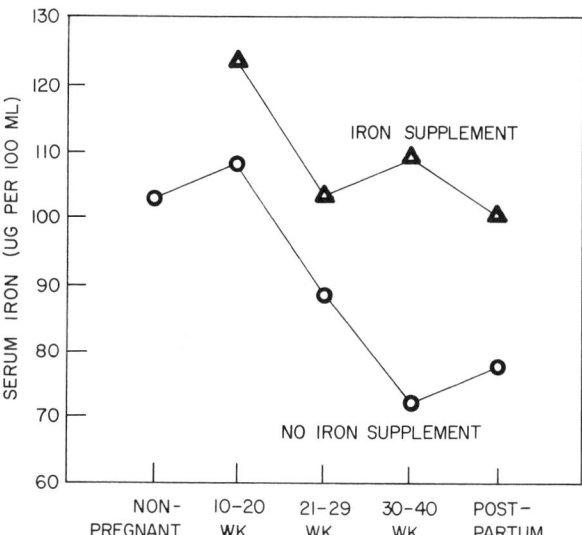

Fig. P-71. The effects of iron supplementation on the serum iron of the mother during and after pregnancy. (The points on the graphs represent averages of the different values given in *Laboratory Indices of Nutritional Status in Pregnancy,* National Academy of Sciences, 1978, p. 161, Table 7–1)

It may be noted from Fig. P-71 that the women who received the iron supplement maintained significantly higher levels of serum iron than the women who did not receive the supplement.

(Also see ANEMIA.)

Constipation. This condition may occur in late pregnancy. It may be due to pressure of the growing fetus on the digestive tract and to a decrease in the firmness (tone) of the muscles in the abdomen which slows down digestion. Thus, nutrients remain longer in contact with the walls of the intestines and nutrient absorption is increased.

Constipation may be prevented by drinking plenty of water and eating foods that add bulk to the diet such as fruits and vegetables (preferably raw) and whole grain cereals such as oatmeal, cracked wheat, all bran, etc.

(Also see CONSTIPATION.)

Cravings for Unusual Foods and Nonfood Items (Pica). Pregnant women sometimes have cravings for unusual items such as starch, clay, plaster, or chalk. The appetite for nonfoods is called pica. Eating of these substances should be discouraged because the practice may result in (1) filling of the digestive tract and reduction of the appetite for nutritious foods, (2) and poisoning by contaminants in the nonfoods. (Some types of plaster contain lead.)

Recently, evidence has been found that pica may be associated with iron deficiency anemia.[36] The abnormal cravings have often been reduced by treatment of the iron deficiency of pregnancy.

It is noteworthy that the craving for pastrami, pickles, or pizza in the wee hours of the morning is not pica and may be satisfied without harm, providing that pregnant women do not overindulge in these foods.

(Also see PICA.)

Diabetes. Diabetes poses a great risk to the developing fetus. The hormones of pregnancy (estrogen, human chorionic gonadotropin, and human placental lactogen) act to antagonize (counteract) the action of insulin in the body. Because of this antiinsulin activity, women are more prone to display diabetes when they are pregnant. To counteract this situation, the physician may prescribe increased insulin doses and put the mother on a special diet.

Problems with a fetus in a diabetic pregnancy include unexplained stillbirth, placental malfunction, and a large infant (macrosomia).

(Also see DIABETES MELLITUS.)

Excessive Gain in Weight. Weight, *per se,* is no indication of nutritional status. Food selections of some pregnant women who have gained weight too rapidly are likely to emphasize foods high in fats or carbohydrates and calories, yet be low in protein, minerals, or vitamins. Diets of other heavy women may be low in many nutrients, including calories. For the expectant mother with poor food practices, the prenatal period provides an opportunity to learn better food practices under medical supervision. There is little room in prenatal menus for foods that contribute mainly calories.

The *minimal caloric level recommended for the obese expectant mother is 1,500 Calories (kcal) per day.* It is very difficult to provide the needed nutrients below this caloric level. If insufficient calories are taken, protein may be used for the mother's energy needs instead of for building new tissue. Even though vitamin and mineral supplements may be given, these supplements do not furnish protein. Major efforts toward weight loss should not be attempted. Weight

[35]*Maternal Nutrition and the Course of Pregnancy,* National Academy of Sciences, 1970, p. 189.

[36]Gibbs, C. E., and J. Seitchik, "Nutrition in Pregnancy," *Modern Nutrition in Health and Disease,* 6th ed., edited by R. S. Goodhart and M. E. Shils, Lea & Febiger, Philadelphia, Pa., p. 748.

reduction in pregnancy has been associated with neuro-psychological abnormalities in the infant.

Guidelines released by the Institute of Medicine in 1990 indicate that weight gain of 25 to 35 lb during pregnancy is satisfactory.

Fluid Retention (Preeclampsia, Eclampsia). Many pregnant women accumulate a little fluid in their legs, which in itself is not usually harmful unless it is accompanied by (1) notable fluid retention in other parts of the body, (2) high blood pressure, and (3) passage of protein in the urine. These three conditions are signs of toxemia (preeclampsia) which may pose a threat to mother and fetus. However, it is noteworthy that salt restriction and the administration of diuretics may be hazardous in pregnancy and not advisable unless there is a clear cut threat of toxemia. Some doctors advise pregnant women who have some fluid retention and a moderate elevation in blood pressure to lie down for 30 to 45 minutes several times a day so that an increased amount of fluid is passed in the urine. Furthermore, they may allow the continued use of small amounts of salty foods, but it would be wise to avoid highly salted items such as pizza, potato chips, and other similar snacks.

The incidence of toxemia in American women has declined steadily in recent years, thanks to better diets and earlier prenatal care. Also, the condition is more severe when it develops in women who are markedly underweight at conception and who fail to gain weight normally during the early part of pregnancy.

Heartburn. This condition sometimes occurs when stomach contents are forced back into the esophagus. It usually happens during the latter part of pregnancy when the growing fetus puts pressure on the stomach. As with morning sickness, small, frequent meals may help. It is best to avoid greasy, fried foods and other foods that have previously caused digestive problems.

(Also see HEARTBURN; and HIATUS HERNIA.)

High Blood Pressure (Hypertension). Two forms of high blood pressure may be recognized during pregnancy: (1) chronic hypertension, which may cause fetal death and placental malfunction; or (2) acute hypertension, particularly in the last 12 weeks of pregnancy, which is indicative of toxemia. Toxemia can cause stroke, as well as blood-clotting difficulties in the mother, and lead to placental malfunction, separation of the placenta from the uterine wall, and stillbirth.

High blood pressure always warrants the attention of a physician. The blood pressure of the mother before pregnancy is an important factor to be considered in the diagnosis because many teenage girls have low blood pressure when not pregnant so that the rise which occurs may be much greater than suspected. Hence, high blood pressure is declared to be present when (1) the systolic blood pressure is 140 or greater, or the diastolic blood pressure is 90 or greater; or (2) the systolic reading has risen by 30 points or the diastolic reading has risen by 15 points.

Some moderately hypertensive pregnant women benefit by (1) staying off their feet as much as possible and/or (2) lying down for 30 to 45 minutes several times during the day. Many doctors refrain from restricting salt or giving diuretics to pregnant women for fear of creating an even greater problem. However, it would be wise for even a moderately hypertensive woman to avoid eating very salty foods.

(Also see HIGH BLOOD PRESSURE.)

Insufficient Gain in Weight. Recent studies of pregnant women show that markedly underweight expectant mothers have a greater than average incidence of toxemia

and a strikingly increased incidence of prematurity of the infant. In subsequent pregnancies, these same expectant mothers on an adequate diet had a great reduction in the incidence of prematurity over an untreated control group.

This does not mean that the women benefited from an overabundance of calories, but rather that mothers who had various nutritional deficiencies profited from a correction of these shortcomings during pregnancy.

Morning Sickness. Nausea and vomiting, symptoms often called morning sickness, may occur in early pregnancy. This is usually due to changes taking place in the body. It may also be due to tension or anxiety. Morning sickness usually ends about the third or fourth month.

Morning sickness may be relieved by eating small, frequent meals rather than three large meals. Foods that are fairly dry and easily digested such as toast or crackers may be eaten by the mother before getting out of bed in the morning. Liquids should be taken between meals instead of with food.

THE DECLINE OF TOXEMIA (PREECLAMPSIA, ECLAMPSIA) AS A PROBLEM DURING PREGNANCY.

Fortunately, the rate of maternal deaths from toxemia dropped by 88% between 1940 and 1965 (from a rate of 52.2 to 6.2 per 100,000 live births).[37] Nevertheless, many pregnant women may have a fear of becoming toxemic as a result of horror stories told by older female relatives. Therefore, some background on this increasingly uncommon condition follows.

First of all, the term *toxemia* is a misnomer in that there does not appear to be any toxic agent involved in the conditions it designates. Therefore, the Working Group on Nutrition and the Toxemias of Pregnancy (of the National Academy of Sciences Committee on Maternal Nutrition) has suggested that this term be replaced by preeclampsia and eclampsia. They also suggest (1) that the term preeclampsia be used only when the three abnormalities of fluid retention are present—(a) fluid retention throughout the body, not just in the legs, (b) high blood pressure, and (c) passage of protein in the urine; and (2) that the term eclampsia be used to designate the convulsive disorder that sometimes accompanies or follows the development of preeclampsia. These highly specific criteria for diagnosis are designed to prevent the overreporting of toxemia as a complication of pregnancy. (In the past, women were sometimes diagnosed as toxemic on the basis of a single abnormality such as fluid retention or high blood pressure.)

At one time, toxemia was thought to have resulted from the gain of excessive weight during pregnancy, but recent epidemiological studies have shown that it is much more likely to be associated with the conditions that follow:

1. Underweight at the time of conception, followed by failure to gain sufficient weight by the latter part of pregnancy.

2. Dietary deficiencies of calories and/or protein that produce a marked decrease in the blood level of protein.

3. High blood pressure that was present prior to conception.

4. Little or no prenatal care or counseling prior to the latter part of pregnancy.

5. First pregnancy, or a pregnancy following a multiple birth.

---

[37]*Maternal Nutrition and the Course of Pregnancy*, National Academy of Sciences, 1970, p. 177.

6. Inadequate consumption of calcium during pregnancy.

BREAST-FEEDING (Lactation). Lactation is the period after childbirth when a woman breast-feeds her baby. This is an important time for both the mother and her infant. Maternal nutrition plays a significant role during this time. A good diet is necessary for maternal tissue maintenance and replenishment of nutrient stores. In addition, a high-quality diet helps produce breast milk that is an excellent and natural source of nutrients for growth and development of the infant.

Inadequacies in the maternal diet during lactation may have severe consequences. The woman's health status may deteriorate as a result of large withdrawals of nutrients from her tissues. A poor maternal diet will also result in a decreased volume of breast milk. Also, there will be a reduction in vitamin levels. As a result, the infant may be short-changed with regard to calories and essential nutrients.

Since human milk has unique properties not found in other milks, it is the best initial food for infants. The use of breast milk will reduce the possibility of allergic reactions to protein or other components of cow's milk formulas. In addition, breast milk contains a smaller amount of casein, and therefore forms smaller and softer curds in the stomach. This makes it easier to digest by the infant whose digestive processes are not fully developed.

Another advantage of breast milk is that it contains antibodies against infectious microorganisms. This helps the infant resist infections during the first few months of life. In addition, breast milk has the advantage of being sterile. Hence, there is no problem with the type of contamination that can occur during formula preparation.

Breast-feeding is an excellent way to prevent overeating during infancy because the breast-fed baby usually consumes fewer calories than the infant who is bottle fed. The lactating woman simply allows her baby to feed at her breast until satisfied. On the other hand, a mother who bottle feeds her infant tends to see that the baby consumes the entire content of the bottle. Excessive caloric intake during infancy can lead to a permanently increased number of fat cells in the body. This can increase the chance of obesity in later life.

Besides its physiological advantages, breast-feeding has a psychological benefit for both mother and infant. Both experience close attachment. This is a natural situation for the mother to provide a soothing and loving atmosphere; it helps the infant develop desirable emotional characteristics. (Also see BREAST FEEDING.)

Maternal Diet During Lactation. In order to ensure adequate infant nutrition, the maternal diet must meet the nutrient requirements for lactation. (See Table P-9.) Ethnic, social, and economic factors may influence what the mother eats. The health professional should consider these in counseling.

Contrary to a prevalent belief, the diet of a lactating woman must contain an even higher number of calories than during pregnancy. These additional calories are necessary for milk production. Furthermore, the mother should consume the equivalent of 2 to 3 qt (*1.9 to 2.8 liter*) of liquids daily. This fluid is essential to provide the liquid volume for the breast milk and to meet the other needs of the mother. (Also see BREAST FEEDING.)

Nutritional Supplementation. During lactation, there is a need to supplement the maternal diet with certain nutrients. As in pregnancy, 30 to 60 mg of elemental iron should be taken daily by all women. This supplement should be continued for at least 2 or 3 months after childbirth. Iron supplementation during this period is necessary to replenish maternal iron stores depleted by pregnancy. Doctors may recommend other mineral and vitamin supplements for some patients.

Since breast milk does not contain an adequate amount of vitamin D, it is advisable to give the infant an oral supplement of 7.5 mcg daily.

The fluoride content of breast milk varies with the fluoride concentration of the community's water supply. If the fluoride content of the water exceeds 1.1 ppm, the infant will receive sufficient fluoride through breast milk. However, an oral supplement of 0.5 mg fluoride daily should be given to the infant if the water supply has less than 1.1 ppm fluoride. (Also see BREAST FEEDING.)

Use of Drugs by the Lactating Mother. If oral contraceptives are taken sooner than 6 weeks after childbirth, the amount of breast milk a woman produces may be diminished. (Hormones such as estrogen and progesterone in these pills reduce milk production.) Clinical experience shows that the majority of women will not have difficulty producing an adequate amount of milk if they do not use oral contraceptives for 6 weeks after delivery. Hence, they should substitute another form of birth control.

In addition to oral contraceptives, other drugs such as barbiturates (sleeping pills), laxatives, and salicylates (aspirin and similar substances) can be transmitted through breast milk. The taking of any drug during lactation should be done only under a doctor's supervision. (Also see BREAST FEEDING; and INFANT DIET AND NUTRITION.)

FACTORS THAT MAY WARRANT SPECIAL COUNSELING OF PREGNANT WOMEN. Experience has shown that even an affluent and educated woman can have nutritional problems throughout her pregnancy. Sufficient money to buy food is not a guarantee that the mother's diet will be nutritionally adequate. In some cases, her diet may consist of a limited variety of foods due to misinformation or adherence to unsound weight reduction diets. For example, the pregnant woman may not drink milk for fear that it will cause leg cramps, or she may eat only low-calorie foods to lose weight. Meals may be infrequent or eliminated with the result that the mother may be vulnerable to nutritional deficiencies. This type of deprivation may have harmful effects on the outcome of her pregnancy. Furthermore, certain factors related to the mother's status may classify her as a higher-than-average risk. These factors may be physiological, socioeconomic, and/or psychological. A high risk pregnant woman needs continuous nutritional assessment and in depth nutritional counseling. Some of the more common risk factors follow.

Adolescence. Girls younger than 17 years, who are pregnant before completion of their own growth, have greater nutritional requirements than adult women. For these patients, pregnancy creates a dual growth demand—that of the fetus, and of the patient herself. Compounding this, many adolescent girls may restrict their caloric intake in order to lose weight or may have poor dietary habits. Adolescent pregnancies have been associated with low birth weight, premature births, and a high death rate of newborn infants. Fig. P-72 shows how the mother's age is associated with infant death rates.

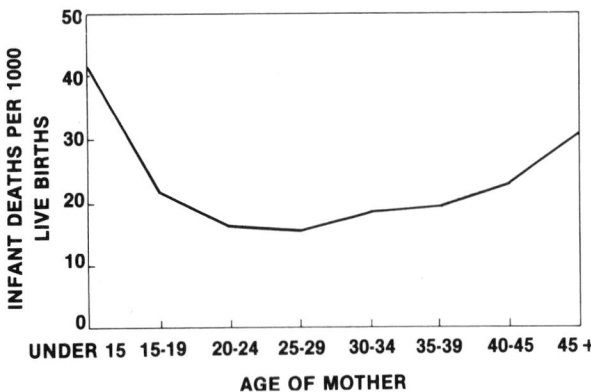

Fig. P-72. Infant mortality rates by age of mother. (Based upon data from *Maternal Nutrition and the Course of Pregnancy*, National Academy of Sciences, p. 144, Table 3)

Ethnic and/or Language Differences.

The U.S. population is composed of many national, cultural, and regional groups. These groups have a variety of dietary practices, many of which are excellent, that are part of their cultural traditions. However, some families may be unfamiliar with compositions and nutritional values of many foods available in local markets. Unfortunately they frequently adopt poor food practices and replace nutritious foods with ones that contain large amounts of fats, starch, and sugars, but few other nutrients. For example, substituting soft drinks for fruit juice or potato chips for potatoes increases the calories consumed and reduces the intake of essential minerals and vitamins.

For certain individuals, English is not a familiar language. This may present a problem, if the woman is not able to read or understand information about the foods commonly eaten in this country. In many cases, ethnic and/or language differences have been associated with anemia and inadequate or sporadic weight gain during pregnancy.

Habituation to Alcohol, Drugs, and/or Smoking.

Some of the current ideas on each of these harmful habits follow:

• **Alcohol**—Dr. David Smith of the University of Washington in Seattle, medical researcher who discovered that alcoholic mothers gave birth to infants with various defects, states that there is no *safe dose* of alcohol for a pregnant woman.[38] It is suspected that the consumption of alcohol during pregnancy may be the greatest single cause of birth defects and the most common cause of mental retardation in infants. Dr. Smith has named the complex of abnormalities the *fetal alcohol syndrome*.

Therefore, anyone who has a role in the counseling of pregnant women should strongly advise against the consumption of alcoholic beverages and help alcoholic mothers find the appropriate therapy means for breaking the habit.

• **Drugs**—The use of addictive drugs such as heroin and morphine by pregnant women has been reported to have neurological effects on their newborn infants. Sometimes, the infants are addicted at birth and have characteristic symptoms of withdrawal such as irritability, sleeplessness, and lack of interest in eating. The symptoms may occur as late as 7 days after delivery.

It is noteworthy that the identification and treatment of drug-addicted mothers early in pregnancy has resulted in great reduction in the harmful effects of the addiction on infants.

• **Smoking**—Women who smoke during pregnancy may give birth to a low-birth-weight infant. The reduction of weight in the fetus is due to the interference of carbon monoxide (from the smoke) with its oxygen supply. Therefore, women of childbearing age or younger should be discouraged from starting to smoke or given assistance in breaking the habit once it is established.

History of Obstetrical Complications.

Previous obstetrical complications reflect potential problems which may recur in subsequent pregnancies. Nutrition related factors in the obstetrical history include inadequate weight gain, preeclampsia and/or toxemia, anemia, diabetes, bleeding prior to delivery, multiple pregnancy, premature or small-birth-weight infant, and fetal or neonatal death.

Low Income.

Women from low-income families may find it difficult to obtain sufficient food and to consume adequate diets during pregnancy. Furthermore, the likelihood of prematurity rises sharply with a decrease in nutritional status. The lowest birth weights and the largest number of deaths in the neonatal period occur among the infants born to the most poorly nourished mothers.

In order to help improve the nutritional quality of the diet, the low-income person should be encouraged to participate in food programs such as Food Stamps and WIC (Special Supplemental Feeding Program for Women, Infants, and Children). These programs increase the buying power or provide specific high-quality foods.

Nutrition education and counseling are important to maximize the benefits from the limited resources available to low-income individuals. Information on food buying, storage, and preparation can be extremely useful. In many cases, existing community resources may help provide this support. It is important and valuable to coordinate these efforts.

Psychological Conditions.

Depression, anorexia nervosa, and other mental problems may affect the course and outcome of a patient's pregnancy. These conditions may result in reduced caloric and nutrient intake, which is associated with poor weight gain of the fetus, low-birth-weight infants, and a high death rate of newborn babies.

RH Factor Incompatibility.

This problem, which is also known as erythroblastosis fetalis, has little to do with nutrition, but it is presented here so that it will not be overlooked by prospective parents. (All obstetricians are well aware of this problem and the appropriate preventive measures, but some American women may have their babies with little or no prenatal advice from a doctor.)

The medical name of this condition is actually a description of the effects of the Rh incompatibility on the fetus. During pregnancy, a mother whose blood is Rh negative (from 12 to 15% of Americans have this type of blood) may develop antibodies against a fetus that is Rh positive. Some of the maternal antibodies may cross the placenta into the fetus, where they may destroy some of the red blood cells (this effect is called erythroblastosis). Pigment released from the blood cells may poison the infant's brain before or after birth. It is noteworthy that this condition was the cause of death in 1 of every 400 births at the Chicago Lying-In

[38]Iber, F. L., "Fetal Alcohol Syndrome," *Nutrition Today*, September/October 1980, pp. 4-11.

Hospital in the early 1940s (most of the deaths occurred within the first few days of life). Since then, the cause of the problem was studied intensively and appropriate preventative measures were developed. Fig. P-73 shows the most common combinations of parental Rh blood types that occur.

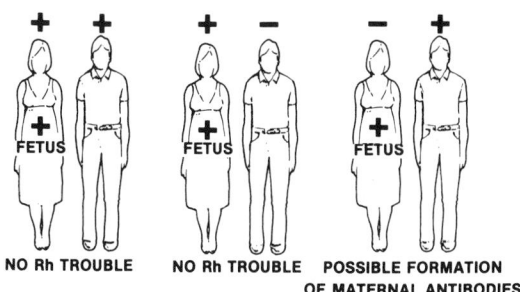

NO Rh TROUBLE   **NO Rh TROUBLE**   **POSSIBLE FORMATION OF MATERNAL ANTIBODIES**

Fig. P-73. Combinations of parental Rh blood types and the possibility of Rh factor incompatibility.

It may be seen from Fig. P-73 that only the combination of an Rh-negative mother and an Rh-positive father may lead to incompatibility. Even in these cases, the problem does not occur very often. Nevertheless, all couples should have their blood types checked to rule out the possibility of trouble. (A vaccine may be administered to prevent the formation of maternal antibodies if the potential for incompatibility is discovered early enough.)

Several Previous Pregnancies. Expectant mothers who have had many pregnancies in rapid succession are often in a depleted nutritional state. For example, if there is not enough time between pregnancies, the losses of iron and other nutrients will not be restored. Careful attention should be given to these dietary needs.

Use of an Oral Contraceptive. An estimated 10 to 11 million American women use oral contraceptives. Some have used them for many years prior to discontinuing their use in order to have a child. Researchers have found that these agents change the nutritional needs of some women. The levels of several vitamins and minerals in the blood are known to be, or suspected to be, influenced by *the pill.* As a result, some oral contraceptive users need increased amounts of certain nutrients in their diets to maintain normal blood levels (a sign of adequate nutrition). Folacin, a B vitamin, is of particular concern since many oral contraceptive users may need a supplement of folacin. In addition, adequate amounts of vitamin C (ascorbic acid), vitamin B-2 (riboflavin), vitamin B-6 (pyridoxine), vitamin B-12, and zinc are needed.

Therefore, pregnant women who previously used an oral contraceptive should ask their doctor whether they should take a mineral and vitamin supplement during pregnancy.

Vegetarianism. The types of diets used by people who abstain from eating meat vary widely in terms of the other foods that are used or not used.

Lacto-vegetarians do not consume meat, poultry, fish, or eggs. However, they do use milk, cheese, and other dairy products. The pure vegetarian (vegan) abstains from all animal protein foods and milk and milk products.

The fruitarian, unlike the majority of vegetarians, eats a more restricted diet of raw or dried fruits, nuts, honey, and oil. Even more restrictive is the macrobiotic diet. This

regimen consists of ten diets, ranging from the lowest level which includes cereals, fruits, vegetables, and some animal products, to the highest level made up entirely of brown rice. At all levels, fluids are avoided as much as possible. Individuals who continue to follow the higher levels of this diet are in serious danger of developing nutritional deficiencies.

A vegetarian who eats a wide variety of grains, legumes, nuts, fruits, vegetables, and milk and milk products can have a nutritionally sound diet. However, the vegan and fruitarian diets do not contain any significant amount of vitamin B-12. Lacto-ovo vegetarians will obtain the Recommended Dietary Allowance for this vitamin by consuming the equivalent of four glasses of cow's milk daily. Soybean and goat's milk contain less vitamin B-12 than cow's milk. Therefore, both vegans and vegetarians who do not drink cow's milk will need to take a vitamin B-12 supplement. A deficiency of vitamin B-12 causes an anemia and eventually results in spinal cord degeneration. A high intake of folacin will mask this anemia and thus vitamin B-12 deficiency may go undiagnosed. The irreversible neurological changes will then be the first indication of a deficiency.

The omission of cow's milk or goat's milk from a strict vegetarian diet is also likely to lead to deficiencies of calcium and vitamin D since few other foods contain adequate quantities of these nutrients in forms that are utilized readily. Hence, supplements containing them should be taken.

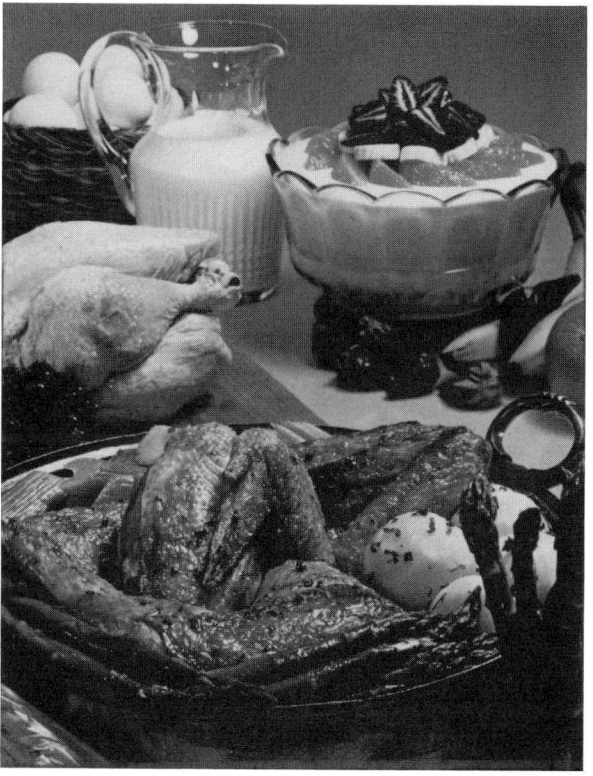

Fig. P-74. Pregnancy and lactation can be great opportunities for the mother to give her child a good start in life, providing a wide variety of nutritious foods are consumed before and during these periods. (Courtesy, United Fresh Fruit & Vegetable Assn., Alexandria, Va.)

(Also see NUTRIENTS: REQUIREMENTS, ALLOWANCES, FUNCTIONS, SOURCES.)

PREGNANCY ANEMIAS

The total iron requirements of pregnancy are considerable; hence, it is not uncommon to detect an iron deficiency anemia during pregnancy because the iron content of habitual U.S. diets is not sufficient. Such an iron deficiency anemia has three contributing factors: (1) low iron storage which may result from iron loss during a previous pregnancy; (2) low dietary iron intake; and (3) greatly increased demand for iron for maternal and fetal hemoglobin synthesis. Iron deficiency anemia during pregnancy can be corrected, and even more important it can be prevented, by appropriate iron supplementation. A daily supplement of 15 mg of iron, averaged over the entire pregnancy, should satisfy the needs of most women. Also, pregnant women should eat foods rich in iron. Liver contains far more iron than any other food. Other meats, dried beans, dried fruit, green vegetables, eggs, and enriched cereals are good sources of iron.

Although not very common in the United States, megaloblastic anemia due to a folate deficiency does occur during pregnancy. In most cases it appears to be the result of long term use of an oral contraceptive, a marginal diet, vomiting, and increased demands of the developing fetus. Pregnant women have double the requirement of other persons for folic acid. The administration of folic acid causes prompt reversal of the symptoms. If not treated during pregnancy, the baby may show symptoms of megaloblastic anemia and require folic acid supplementation.

(Also see ANEMIA, section headed "Groups of Persons Susceptible to Nutritional Anemias"; ANEMIA, MEGALOBLASTIC; FOLIC ACID; INFANT ANEMIA; IRON; and PREGNANCY AND LACTATION NUTRITION.)

PRENATAL

Before birth.

PRESERVATION OF FOOD

Since the beginning of time, man has searched for ways to protect himself from hunger—for ways to save food in times of plenty for times of scarcity. No doubt, man learned that he could often collect more food than he could eat, but that it soon spoiled and became unfit for consumption—or even poisonous.

There are no records to indicate when some of the first methods of preservation were discovered. Like other discoveries, some of the preservation methods were based on a series of enlightening observations which led to the development of a process. The methods of preservation became refined and more effective as men like Anton van Leeuwenhoek, Lazaro Spallanzani, and Louis Pasteur contributed to the understanding of spoilage of food. Until men learned some of the modern methods of preservation, large cities could not develop. Nearby farms were required to feed the city people, since food spoilage was a major problem.

Spoilage of food is caused by growth of microorganisms, enzyme action, oxidation (chemical reactions), extremes in physical surroundings, and/or pests. Insofar as possible, the aim of preservation is to reduce, eliminate, and/or control the causes of spoilage. With the modern methods of preservation, seasonal harvests can be enjoyed year round, and food specifically grown in one area can be shipped across the country or even worldwide. Still, scientists continue to search for better methods of preservation that yield a nutritious, flavorful, and desirable product, with minimal long-term requirements.

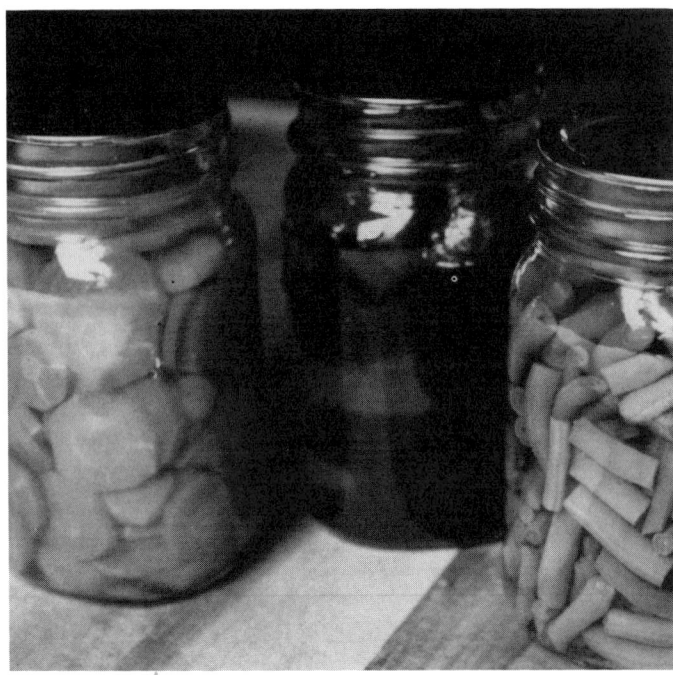

Fig. P-75. Home-canned foods. (Courtesy, University of Minnesota, St. Paul)

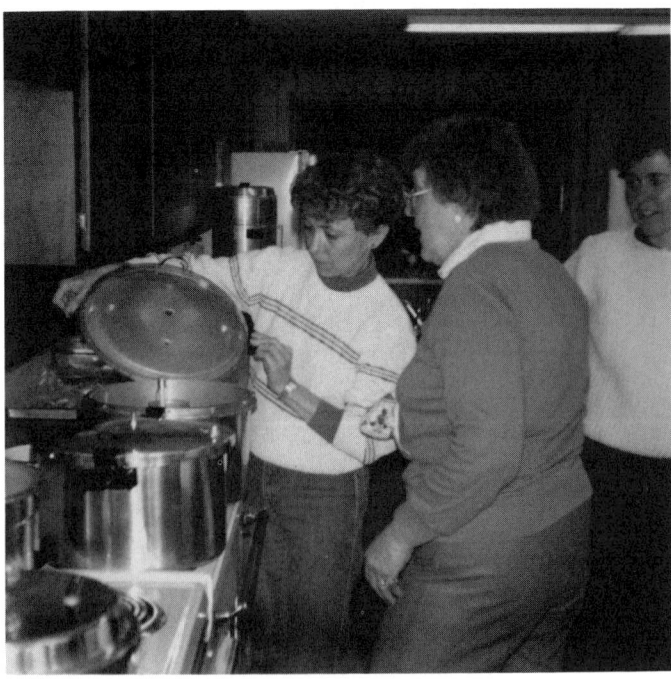

Fig. P-76. Pressure processing low-acid home canned foods is essential for food safety. (Courtesy, North Dakota State Cooperative Extension Service)

Table P-10, which follows, summarizes in a general way the methods of preservation which are applied to food. Often more details concerning the preservation of a food item may be found in the articles dealing specifically with that food. Foods are often preserved by a combination of the methods listed in Table P-10.

(Also see BACTERIA IN FOOD; FRUIT[S]; MEAT[S]; MILK AND MILK PRODUCTS; SPOILAGE OF FOOD; and VEGETABLE[S].)

TABLE P-10
METHODS OF FOOD PRESERVATION

Method(s); History	Description and Principle; Food Application	Length of Storage; Changes in Quality	Remarks
CANNING **History:** A Frenchman, Nicholas Appert, invented canning in response to a prize offered in 1795 by the French government for a food preservation method that would not seriously impair the natural flavor of fresh food. After 14 years of experimenting, Appert won the prize in 1809. His method involved heating foods in glass flasks sealed with corks. Pasteur later explained why the metod worked. An Englishman, Peter Durand, conceived the idea of using cans, and by 1839 tin-coated steel containers were widely used.	**Description and Principle:** Properly prepared foods are placed in the glass or can containers and sealed. Then depending upon the type of food (primarily the acidity [pH]), the cans or bottles are heated to a known temperature and then held at that temperature for a specified time. Low acid foods such as meats and vegetables are heated to 240° to 265°F (116° to 129° C) while acidic foods such as fruits are heated to about 212°F (100°C). The principle of canning is twofold: (1) to destroy spoilage, and disease-causing microorganisms, and (2) to keep air away from the food. **Food Application:** Meat, fish, poultry, vegetables, fruits, soups, orange juice, tomato paste, jams, jellies, and other manufactured foods.	**Length of Storage:** Most canned foods keep well for more than 1 year when properly canned. Commercially canned items are dated. **Changes in Quality:** This varies with the food and the process, but some general statements can be made; (1) color and texture often differ from fresh products; (2) no practical effect on protein, carbohydrates, and fats; (3) no effect on vitamins A, D, and riboflavin if protected from oxygen; (4) vitamin C destroyed by heat and exposure to oxygen; and (5) thiamin destruction dependent upon heat treatment and acidity of food.	The chief canning processes are: (1) the conventional retort method for most vegetables, fruits, fish and meat products; (2) preheating and hot filling for very acid foods like orange juice, tomato paste, jams and jellies; and (3) fast canning for foods such as baby foods, sauces, potted meats, and cream-style corn. Fast canning uses high temperatures of 250° to 280°F (121° to 138°C) for short periods of time. The major concern is proper processing to ensure the destruction of the spores of *Clostridium botulinum*—a toxin-producing bacterium. Commercially canned foods have been free of the botulism hazard for over 30 years.
CHEMICAL ADDITIVES **History:** Man's first uses of salt to preserve foods are lost in antiquity. Sugar has also enjoyed a long-time usage as a preservative. More recently, other chemicals have been tested and used in minute amounts to prevent spoilage and the growth of microorganisms. The uses of chemicals (food additives) in foods for preservative purposes are controlled by the government under the Food Additive Amendment of 1958. (Also see ADDITIVES; and NITRATES AND NITRITES.)	**Description and Principle:** A variety of chemicals will destroy microorganisms. Other than salt and sugar, chemicals used for this purpose must act at low levels. Some common chemical preservatives include ethyl formate, sodium benzoate, sodium and calcium propionate, sodium nitrate or nitrite, sorbic acid, and sulfur dioxide. Some chemicals act by preventing the growth of microorganisms, while others prevent oxidation or enzymatic deterioration of quality during manufacture and distribution. **Food Application:** Depends on the chemical and processing method; ranges from fruits and vegetables to meats to soft drinks; common examples include: BHA (butylated hydroxyanisole) and BHT (butylated hydroxytoluene) in beverages, cereals, chewing gum, and oil; calcium propionate in baked goods; and sodium nitrite in meats.	**Length of Storage:** This varies widely depending upon the chemical(s) used and the food product. Some chemical additives merely increase the shelf life a few days or weeks while others may increase storage time to an indefinite period. **Changes in Quality:** The prime reason for the addition of many chemicals is to maintain the quality of the food. Some chemicals actually increase the value of a food; for example, vitamin C (ascorbic acid) may be added to fruits to prevent browning.	Chemicals may be added to foods for reasons other than preservation. They are also added to enrich, or to improve a food. New chemicals added to food, regardless of the purpose, must undergo rigorous testing for safety.
DRYING AND DEHYDRATION **History:** Drying is one of the oldest methods of preserving food and is still a common practice in the world today. Prehistoric man probably dried foods in the sun or near fires. There is evidence that drying foods by the fire was an ancient practice in both the New and Old Worlds. Artificial drying (dehydration) via hot air was develpoed in France in 1795, where it was used to dry thin slices of vegetables. Technology gained during World War II resulted in the dehydration of more foods.	**Description and Principle:** Drying is accomplished via the sun in hot, dry areas of the world or via dehydrators which produce heat at certain temperatures, maintain humidity, and produce a flow of air. Whatever the method, the heated air carries away the moisture. Depending on the food, drying or dehydration may reduce foods to 2% moisture. Drying or dehydrating is effective because microorganisms require water to grow and many enzymatic and nonenzymatic reactions require water to proceed. **Food Application:** Eggs, milk and milk products, fruits, vegetables, juices, meats, spices, soups, coffee, tea, gelatin dessert mixes, and macaroni.	**Length of Storage:** This varies with the product, storage conditions, and the final moisture content. Some very dry items can be stored indefinitely if protected from moisture. Molds can grow on foods with as little as 5 to 16% moisture. Bacteria and yeast usually require a moisture content greater than 30%. **Changes in Quality:** Drying concentrates the nutrients. Protein, fat, and carbohydrate are present in larger amounts per unit weight. Often the reconstituted or rehydrated food is comparable to the fresh foods. However, the vitamin content of dried meat is much less than that of fresh meat.	Many foods dry as part of the natural process in their production on the plant; for example, legumes, nuts, and grains. Vacuum driers may be used for foods that are especially sensitive to heat. Besides the preservative action of drying, it also reduces the size and weight of foods making them easier to transport and store. There are many methods of drying (dehydrating) foods that are especially adapted to certain food products. Occasionally some toxin-producing bacteria may survive the process and cause poisoning when water is added.
FREEZE DRYING (Lyophilization) **History:** First application of freeze drying to a biological sample was reported in 1890 by the German histologist, Altmann. During the 1930s, the technology was applied to blood plasma. World War II stimulated the development of the technology to a commercial basis.	**Description and Principle:** The process removes water from food while the food is still frozen. After cooling food to about −20°F (−29°C), it is placed on trays in a vacuum chamber and heat is carefully applied. Water is evaporated without melting since it goes from the frozen-ice state to the gaseous state without passing through the liquid state—sublimation. The food is not exposed to high temperature until most of the water is removed. Without water, microorganisms cannot grow, and most enzymatic and nonenzymatic reactions cannot proceed. **Food Application:** Any food, raw or cooked, which can withstand freezing.	**Length of Storage:** Freeze-dried foods are often packaged in an inert gas such as nitrogen and they must be packaged in moisture-proof containers. When properly packaged, most products are acceptable after 1 year of storage at 100°F (38°C)—a temperature much higher than normal storage. Longer storage times can be expected at lower temperatures. **Changes in Quality:** Upon rehydration (adding water), freeze-dried foods are equal in acceptability to their frozen counterparts. There is a substantial retention of nutrients, color, flavor, and texture.	Freeze drying usually produces higher quality foods than the other drying methods, but it costs more. The first significant commercial application of freeze drying was in the production of an improved instant coffee.

(Continued)

TABLE P-10 *(Continued)*

Method(s); History	Description and Principle; Food Application	Length of Storage; Changes in Quality	Remarks
FREEZING **History:** Since early times, farmers, fishermen, and trappers, living in regions with cold winters, have preserved their meat and fish by freezing and storage in unheated buildings. About 1880, ammonia refrigeration machines were introduced for use in freezing fish. Clarence Birdseye stimulated the development of the business of packaging frozen foods by forming a company that began quick freezing foods in 1924. The frozen food business boomed when home freezers became available after World War II.	**Description and Principle:** Foods are subjected to temperatures below 32° to 25°F (0° to -3°C) where the water in the food turns to ice. Foods are best if rapidly frozen. Freezing methods may employ direct immersion in a cooling medium, contact with refrigerated plates in a freezing chamber, freezing with liquid air or nitrogen, or dry ice. Freezing does not kill microorganisms or destroy enzymes, it merely arrests or slows spoilage changes. **Food Application:** Most kinds of fruits and vegetables, meat, fish, poultry, and some dairy products; a variety of precooked foods (convenience foods) from french fries to complete dinners. Some foods such as tomatoes, cabbages, bananas, avocados, pears, and some shellfish are not well suited for freezing.	**Length of Storage:** Each food has its own recommended storage period, after which time undesirable off-flavors slowly develop. **Changes in Quality:** Many foods are pre-treated further to ensure quality during frozen storage. In general, freezing promotes the retention of nutrients and does not destroy nutrients. However, some destruction of vitamins may occur during the processing that preceeds freezing.	Frozen foods must be kept frozen since partial thawing and refreezing lowers the quality. Freezing and canning are the two most widely used methods of food preservation. Frozen foods must be protected from dehydration and freezer burn during storage.
FERMENTATION **History:** Some of the earliest writings describe the fermentation of grapes and other fruits. Most cultures devised some type of fermented beverage. Fermentation of milk has been known for ages; it is mentioned in the Old Testament. Nomadic tribes fermented milk. Sauerkraut is fermented cabbage—a product of ancient China. (Also see BEERS AND BREWING; MEAT[S], section headed "Meat Processing"; MILK AND MILK PRODUCTS; and WINE.)	**Description and Principle:** In fermentation, the growth of certain bacteria and yeasts which synthesize chemicals that aid in preservation of the food is encouraged. These products of fermentation are primarily lactic acid and ethyl alcohol. Lactic acid is important in the fermentation of cucumbers, olives, cabbage, meats, and milk. Ethyl alcohol is produced by the fermentation of fruits and cereals. **Food Application:** Fruits, vegetables, cereals, meats, and milk.	**Length of Storage:** Fermented products are often subjected to other preservation methods to increase storage time. Milk products are refrigerated while wines are pasteurized. **Changes in Quality:** Fermentation changes the quality of both plant and animal products to a marked degree. Some foods are made more edible, others are made more nutritious, and still others are made more flavorful.	Some fermented products require that individuals acquire a taste for their distinctive flavor. Fermentations create wine, beer, rum, hard liquor, breads, cheeses, pickles, salami sausage, olives, Sajur asin (vegetables and rice), poi (taro), yogurt, buttermilk, and acidophilus. Fermentations producing lactic acid are encouraged by the level of salt in the product.
PASTEURIZATION **History:** The process is named for Louis Pasteur, who, in the 1860s, found that heating liquids, especially wines, to a temperature of 140°F (60°C) improved their keeping qualities.	**Description and Principle:** This process is the application of mild heat for a specified time to a liquid, food, or beverage. Pasteurization destroys molds, yeasts, and the non-spore forming bacteria. The lower the temperature, the longer the application time, and vice versa. For example, milk can be pasteurized at 143°F (62°C) for 30 min. or 162°F (72°C) for 15 seconds. Time and temperature vary with the type of food. Foods are rapidly cooled following the treatment. **Food Application:** Milk, cheese, wine, beer, and other beverages such as fruit juices.	**Length of Storage:** This depends upon the type of storage following the pasteurization and upon the type of food. **Changes in Quality:** Since heat is less than boiling temperature and for a short time, the quality of the food is maintained. Foods which are pasteurized include those whose flavor and appearance may be adversely affected by high temperatures.	For milk, the times and temperatures employed are based upon the heat tolerance of *Mycobacterium tuberculosis*, one of the most heat resistant of the nonspore-forming pathogens (disease causing).
PICKLING **History:** Pickling of plant and animal foods is an ancient practice. Sauerkraut was manufactured in ancient China. In the 18th century, scientists recognized that vinegar (acetic acid) was good for preserving biological specimens. The pickling industry has grown rapidly since the 1930s.	**Description and Principle:** Preserving foods in vinegar and salt is called pickling. Vinegar is an acid, and microorganisms are sensitive to acids. Moreover, acids increase the lethality of heat on microorganisms. There are two methods of pickling: (1) fresh pack pickling, and (2) fermentation pickling. Both rely on brine and vinegar as the primary preservatives. The vinegar needs an acetic acid content of 4 to 6%, and either cider vinegar or white vinegar is acceptable. The addition of spices is a common practice. **Food Application:** Vegetables, fruits, meats, eggs, and nuts; most common include cucumbers, pears, peaches, plums, cured meats, cabbage, mushrooms, cauliflower, onions, tomatoes, beets, peppers, and watermelon.	**Length of Storage:** Pickling alone is not sufficient for long-term storage. Pickled products should be heat treated (canned) unless they are consumed soon after pickling. Even vinegar is often pasteurized for a longer shelf life. **Changes in Quality:** Pickling not only increases the keeping quality of a food, it adds an appealing flavor to the food. The nutritional quality depends on other preservative processes employed on the food.	Pickled foods are not likely to be suspect in a food poisoning incident—at least where sufficient vinegar is used. Vinegar is a chemical preservative used in other foods such as mayonnaise and salad dressing. Cucumbers are the most commonly pickled vegetable. Near perfect produce should be used for pickling.

(Continued)

TABLE P-10 *(Continued)*

Method(s); History	Description and Principle; Food Application	Length of Storage; Changes in Quality	Remarks
RADIATION **History:** The first patent related to the radiation treatment of food was taken out in France in 1930. Serious investigations in the U.S. were conducted during the 1950s. Radiation preservation of foods was considered to be in the experimental stages until 1981, when the ban on treating food with gamma rays was eased by the FDA. (Also see RADIATION PRESERVATION OF FOOD.)	**Description and Principle:** Ionizing radiation— moving subatomic particle or energetic electromagnetic waves— is used to treat foods. The radiation prevents the proliferation of microorganisms, insects, and parasites, and inactivates enzymes. The source of radiation may be cobalt-60, or cerium-137 or X rays. This process does *not* make the food radioactive. **Food Application:** Very adaptable; considered for use on fruits, vegetables, meats, fish, poultry, eggs, cereals, flours, and dried fruits; many potential foods tested.	**Length of Storage:** Radiation significantly increases the storage of any food in comparison to its preservation by conventional methods. **Changes in Quality:** Only minimal changes in texture, flavor, color, and odor are experienced; and nutrient destruction is no greater than that which occurs when food is preserved by more conventional methods.	At low levels of radiation, the process is comparable to pasteurization; at high levels, it is equivalent to sterilization. Some doses inhibit sprouting and delay ripening in foods. The process has great potential since irradiated foods can be stored for long periods without refrigeration. Also, it is very flexible, adapting to various sizes and shapes of food.
REFRIGERATION (Cold Storage) **History:** In ancient Rome, snow from the mountains was used to pack prawns and other perishables. Root cellars were constructed by many settlers to keep foods cool. The use of ice for refrigeration was introduced toward the beginning of the 19th century. It was not until 1890 that mechanical refrigeration came into use on a large scale.	**Description and Principle:** Refrigeration temperatures may range from 29° to 60°F (−1.6° *to 15.5°C).* Commercial and household refrigerators run at about 40° to 45°F *(4.5° to 7.2°C).* Refrigeration retards deterioration by slowing the growth of microorganisms and decreasing the rate of chemical reactions that deteriorate foods. **Food Application:** Meats, poultry, fish, eggs, fruits, vegetables, and all in different stages of processing—cooked, fresh, etc.; baked goods.	**Length of Storage:** The amount of time foods can be stored depends on the type of food and its age. At 40°F *(4.5°C),* meats, fish, and poultry keep for 2 to 10 days depending upon their stage of processing, while some fruits and vegetables keep for weeks or months. **Changes in Quality:** Gradual changes in quality and nutrient composition continue during storage.	Large cold storage warehouses keep huge quantities of apples, apricots, pears, butter, cheese, and eggs for periods of 6 to 10 months. Some fruits and vegetables are harvested at full size, but unripe. These are shipped in refrigerated transports, and allowed to ripen or held in cold storage to ripen.
SALT CURING (Brining) **History:** Salting is an ancient method of food preservation. Dry salting and the pickling of meats and fish in brine were practiced before 2000 B.C. (Also see CABBAGE; CUCUMBER AND GHERKIN; MEAT[S], section headed "Meat Processing"; and OLIVE.)	**Description and Principle:** There are 4 basic methods of salt curing: dry salting, brining, low-salt fermentation, and pickling. Dry salting and brining require concentrated amounts of salt. When a food is impregnated with salt, water is drawn out of the cells of the microorganisms and their growth is inhibited. Microorganisms vary in their sensitivity to salt, but usually 15 to 20% dissolved in the water phase of a food is highly preservative. **Food Application:** Meat, fish, poultry, and almost any fruit or vegetable by one or more of the salt curing methods.	**Length of Storage:** Most produce will remain fit for consumption 3 weeks to several months when stored at 38°F *(3.3°C),* though the actual salt-curing process may take several weeks. For longer periods of storage the food needs to be subjected to some other type of preservative process such as canning, drying, or smoking. **Changes in Quality:** Dry salt and brining require the greatest concentrations of salt, and generally the more salt used the better the food is preserved, but the greater the loss in food value. Heavily salted food must be soaked and rinsed to make it palatable—a process which further depletes vitamins and minerals.	Nowadays most people use a salt curing method for the distinctive flavor it imparts to foods such as cucumber pickles, sauerkraut, green olives, and sausage. Low-salt fermentation and pickling ensure that the proper microorganisms develop and suppress the development of undesirable microbial activity.
SUGAR **History:** Early man used some sugar for preserving. However, sugar (sucrose) availability in the world began increasing after the mid-1750s; hence, more sugar continued to be used in the preservation of foods.	**Description and Principle:** Concentrated sugar solutions draw water out of the microorganisms and bind water, thereby preventing their growth. Microorganisms differ in their sensitivity to sugar, but around 70% sucrose (sugar) is highly preservative. **Food Application:** Preservation of fruits in jellies, jams, conserves, marmalades, preserves, fruit butters, and candied and glaced fruits.	**Length of Storage:** After the addition of sugar, many fruits require further heat processing. When properly bottled or stored, these fruits may be stored a year or more. Some may be stored without hermetic sealing, though such protection is useful to control mold growth, moisture loss, and oxidation. **Changes in Quality:** Due to the addition of sugar, these foods contain more calories than fresh fruit. Also, some of the processing may leach minerals and destroy vitamins. However, some unpalatable fruits may be given a pleasing taste with this method.	Flavoring, coloring agents, and additional pectin may be added to overcome any deficiencies in the fruit. Most fruits contain significant amounts of sugars, and dried fruits are preserved in part by the increased concentration of natural sugars. Sugar is added to meat in some curing processes.
SMOKING **History:** Early settlers relied on curing and smoking of meats for their preservation. The old smokehouse was a common sight on many early farms. This old method led to the development of sausages, hams, and bacon, which are still popular. (Also see MEAT[S], section headed "Meat Processing.")	**Description and Principle:** Chemicals contained in smoke help prevent the growth of microorganisms, but, smoking is combined with other preservation methods which cure the product. Curing may be accomplished with salt alone, but generally herbs, spices, and sugar are also added. Cured meats are stored in rooms which can be filled with smoke, derived from burning hard woods. The amount of smoke, the temperature, and time of smoking depend upon the desired product. **Food Application:** Meat and fish, and some meat and fish products.	**Length of Storage:** Smoking by itself, as a cool smoke, contributes little to the preservation of meats and fish. In times past, the addition of smoke was associated with heat and drying of the product. Thoroughly cured and smoked meats such as Smithfield hams are reported to keep for years. **Changes in Quality:** The primary use of smoking today is to give the food a desirable smoked taste—an improvement in quality.	Modern refrigeration has opened the way for mild, sweet cures in which the smoked flavor is more important than the long-term preservation by smoke. Many people cure and smoke their game catches.

PRESSED

Compacted or molded by pressure; having fat, oil, or juice extracted under pressure.
(Also see OILS, VEGETABLE.)

PRESSURE COOKING

A pressure cooker is a heavy pan with a tight lid which can be clamped down, a safety valve, and an instrument for measuring the pressure. As the pressure increases, so does the boiling point of water, which means that the food cooks at a higher temperature, thus shortening the length of time required. The pressure cooker is also used for processing canned meats and vegetables.

PRETZELS

The name came from the German word, *brezel*, which originally came from the Latin word, *brachiatus*, meaning *having branches like arms*. Pretzels are brittle, glazed and salted crackers made of ropes of dough typically twisted into forms resembling the letter "B." The dough consists of a mixture of flour, salt, yeast, vegetable shortening, water, and malt. In the final step of their production, they are dipped into a tank of coconut oil maintained at a temperature of about 225°F (107°C), which seals the pretzel and extends its shelf life by 300%. Pretzels are a commercial product, difficult to duplicate in the home kitchen. They are used mainly as a snack food.

PRICKLY PEAR (INDIAN FIG; TUNA)
Opuntia ficus-indica

The fruit of a cactus (of the family *Cactaceae*) which is native to Mexico and now grows throughout the dry, subtropical areas in the northern and southern hemispheres.

Prickly pears are a little larger than large plums, but they have a prickly outer skin and a sweet inner pulp. They may be eaten fresh, stewed, or made into jams.

The nutrient composition of the prickly pear (Indian fig) is given in Food Composition Table F-21.

Some noteworthy observations regarding the nutrient composition of the prickly pear follow:

1. The fresh fruit is moderately high in calories (67 kcal per 100 g) and carbohydrates (17%).

2. Prickly pears are a good source of fiber and iron, and a fair source of calcium and vitamin C.

PROCESSED FOODS, HIGHLY

Many species of animals collect and store food, but only *Homo sapiens* processes it. *Processing refers to all the physical and/or chemical operations that are applied to foodstuffs.* Food processing influences the nutritional value of foodstuffs—enhancing some, lowering others.

The term "highly processed foods" designates foods that have been altered significantly in appearance, culinary characteristics, nutritional value, structure, and/or texture as a result of a considerable amount of processing. Some of the reasons why foods are highly processed are: (1) to prevent

spoilage; (2) to render them more storable and transportable, by reducing their bulk and water content; (3) to meet special dietary requirements; and (4) to produce concentrated sources of certain nutrients. Often, processing increases the levels of certain nutrients while reducing the levels of others. Hence, selected nutritional and economic aspects of highly processed foods are discussed in the sections which follow.

CURRENT TRENDS. Some of the most commonly employed types of processing tend to concentrate solids, carbohydrates, fats, and/or proteins at the expense of fiber, certain essential minerals, and certain vitamins. Examples of some highly processed items follow.

Cereal Products. The processing of grains has traditionally yielded products that are higher in starch than the original grains, but lower in most other nutrients. Enrichment of the products results in the restoration of only four of the more than 2 dozen essential nutrients that are depleted significantly by processing. Furthermore, many cereal products are made with substantial amounts of added fats and sugars. However, there has been a recent trend to restore some of the bran and wheat germ that was removed during processing.

Dairy Products And Eggs. These foods were once considered to be ideal for nourishing growing children and hard-working adolescents and adults. Now, many of the traditional items are being modified by (1) replacement of the animal fats with vegetable oil derivatives, (2) removal of much of the fat content without replacement, and (3) extension of certain expensive dairy and egg products with air, emulsifying agents, fillers, gummy binders, water, and less expensive animal or plant products that may possess analogous characteristics. Some noteworthy examples of these trends are cream substitutes (often called *nondairy blends*), filled milks, imitation cheeses, imitation eggs, imitation ice cream, imitation milk (this type of product may contain a soybean derivative plus vegetable oil), margarines, process cheeses, and sour cream substitutes. Producers often capitalize on the current concern over the alleged dangers of animal fats and cholesterol in promoting the modified items as being more beneficial to health than the traditional products.

Fish, Meats, Poultry, And Seafood. These items are steadily becoming more expensive, which makes it increasingly profitable to extend or even replace them with various plant products such as soybean derivatives or wheat gluten.

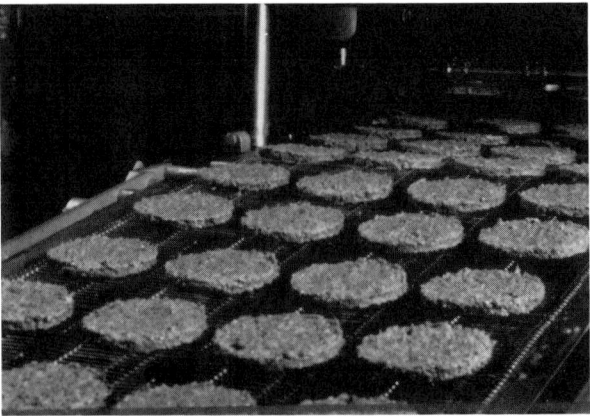

Fig. P-77. A hamburgerlike vegetetable protein product made from soybeans. (Courtesy, Worthington Foods, Inc.)

Fruits And Vegetables. Here again, binders and fillers come to the rescue of food processors beset with rising production costs. *Simulated* pieces of fruits or vegetables may be made from mixtures of fruit or vegetable pulp, vegetable gums, mineral salts, starch, sugar, artificial or natural coloring and flavorings, and water.

Meal Replacements. These products, which are often in the form of beverage powders or sweetened bars, are designed to be consumed with milk, water, or other beverage in lieu of the various mixtures of foods which usually constitute a meal. Federal regulations require that a typical serving of an item designated as a "meal replacement" provide at least 25% of the Recommended Daily Allowance (RDA) for certain specific nutrients. The macronutrients in these products are provided by various combinations of sugar, nonfat dry milk, soybean derivatives, and peanut butter and/or flour, whereas the required levels of micronutrients are usually met by fortification with selected minerals and vitamins. However, these products usually contain little or no fiber.

Limitations Of Enrichment and Fortification. In theory, it should be possible to add pure forms of the nutrients present in minimally processed foods to highly processed foods in order to obtain nutritional equivalency. However, the U.S. Food and Drug Administration specifies enrichment and fortification levels for only some of the nutrients known to be essential. There are no specified levels for other essential nutrients such as chromium, selenium, and vitamin K. It might even be illegal to add the purified forms of these nutrients to foods.

Secondly, foodborne nutrients may in certain cases be present in combinations which work together. For example, the metabolic activities of the members of the vitamin B complex are interrelated. Hence, the failure to provide sufficient dietary quantities of one or more of these vitamins may impair the functions of other B vitamins in the diet.

(Also see NUTRITIONAL SUPPLEMENTS; and PROCESSING OF FOOD.)

PROCESSING OF FOOD

Many foods are altered before they reach the table. Grains are ground into flour and other cereal foods. Milk is pasteurized, homogenized, or used in making cottage cheese, butter, or yogurt. Meat animals such as cattle and pigs are slaughtered, graded and cut into steaks, ground to hamburger, salted, dried, corned, or cured and smoked. Fruits and vegetables are sold fresh, canned, or frozen. All of these represent some stage or some portion of processing —treatment, preparation, or handling by some special method.

Processing starts on the whole raw material of whatever the food may be. Then, for some foods the whole raw material may be broken into parts which are futher processed, or the parts may be mixed with other components and used to form new products. The final stages of processing includes preservation so that the foods may be stored without spoiling. Finally processing includes some form of packing for shipment, storage, and consumer appeal.

(Also see NUTRITIONAL SUPPLEMENTS; and PROCESSED FOODS, HIGHLY.)

PROENZYME (ZYMOGEN)

Inactive form of an enzyme; e.g., pepsinogen.

PROGNOSIS

Prediction of the outcome of an illness based on the person's condition and on scientific knowledge concerning the usual course and results of such illnesses, together with the presence of certain symptoms and signs that indicate the expected outcome.

PROPHYLAXIS

Preventive treatment against disease.

PROPYL GALLATE (PG)

An FDA approved food additive which acts as an antioxidant in foods, fats, oils, and waxes. It is often used in combination with butylated hydroxyanisole (BHA) and butylated hydroxytoluene (BHT).

PROSTAGLANDINS

These are a class of hormonelike compounds, made in various tissues of the body from arachidonic acid (and other derivatives of linoleic acid), which are important in the regulation of such diverse reactions as gastric secretion, pancreatic functions, release of pituitary hormones, smooth muscle metabolism, and control of blood pressure. Some 16 prostaglandins have been identified.

PROSTHETIC GROUP

A protein conjugated with a nonamino acid substance; for example, hemoglobin is a conjugated (joined together) protein—each chain in the protein moiety, globin, is combined with a heme group to form the biologically functional molecule. Proteins are often described in terms of their prosthetic group; thus, hemoglobin is a *hemeprotein*, and proteins containing lipid, carbohydrate, or metals are called *lipoproteins*, *glycoproteins*, and *metalloproteins*, respectively.

PROTEASE

An enzyme that digests protein.

PROTEIN(S)

Chemically, proteins are complex organic compounds made up chiefly of amino acids. For each different protein there are specific amino acids and a specific number of amino acids which are joined in a specific order. Since amino acids always contain carbon, hydrogen, oxygen, and nitrogen, so do proteins. Moreover, the presence of nitrogen provides a tool for chemically estimating the amount of protein in a tissue, food, or some other substance. Crude protein is routinely determined by finding the nitrogen content and

PROTEIN is needed for growth

THREE RATS FROM THE SAME LITTER, 11 WEEKS OLD

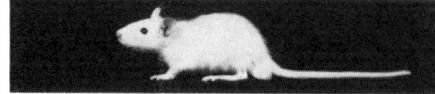

THIS RAT ATE FOODS THAT FURNISHED GOOD QUALITY
PROTEIN, BUT NOT ENOUGH. IT WEIGHED ONLY 70 GRAMS.

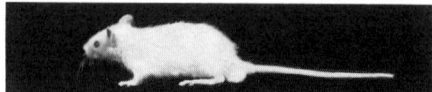

THIS RAT ATE FOODS THAT FURNISHED PLENTY OF PROTEIN,
BUT NOT THE RIGHT COMBINATION TO GIVE GOOD QUALITY.
IT WEIGHED ONLY 65 GRAMS.

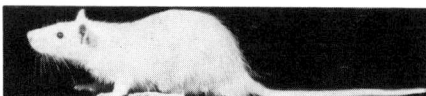

THIS RAT HAD PLENTY OF GOOD QUALITY PROTEIN FROM A
VARIETY OF FOODS. IT HAD GOOD FUR, A WELL-SHAPED
BODY, AND WEIGHED 193 GRAMS.

TOP FOOD SOURCES

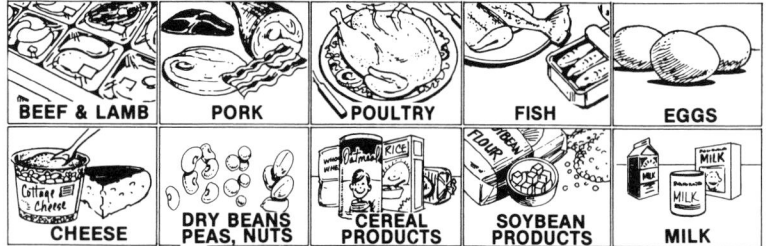

Fig. P-78. Protein quantity and quality made the difference! The top rat ate too little of a good quality protein. The middle rat ate plenty of poor quality protein, while the bottom rat ate plenty of a good quality protein. (Adapted from USDA sources)

multiplying the result by 6.25 since the nitrogen content of all protein averages about 16% (100 ÷ 16 = 6.25). In addition, proteins usually contain sulfur and frequently phosphorus. Proteins are essential in all plant and animal life as components of the active protoplasm of each living cell.

In plants, the protein is largely concentrated in the actively growing portions, especially the leaves and seeds. Plants also have the ability to synthesize their own proteins from such relatively simple soil and air compounds as carbon dioxide, water, nitrates, and sulfates, using energy from the sun. Thus, plants, together with some bacteria which are able to synthesize these products, are the original sources of all proteins.

In animals, proteins are much more widely distributed than in plants. Thus, the proteins of the body are primary constituents of many structural and protective tissues—such as bones, ligaments, hair, fingernails, skin, and the soft tissues which include the organs and muscles. The total protein content of animal bodies ranges from about 10% in very fat, mature animals to 20% in thin, young animals. By way of further contrast, it is also interesting to note that, except for the bacterial action in the rumen of ruminants—cows, sheep, and goats—animals, humans included, lack the ability of the plant to synthesize proteins from simple materials. They must depend upon plants or other animals as a source of dietary protein. Hence, humans must have certain amino acids or more complete protein compounds in the diet.

Animals of all ages and kinds require adequate amounts of protein of suitable quality. The protein requirements for growth, reproduction, and lactation are the greatest and most critical.

The need for protein in the diet is actually a need for amino acids. Proteins in the food are broken down into amino acids by digestion. They are then absorbed and distributed by the bloodstream to the body cells, which rebuild these amino acids into body proteins.

The various amino acids are then systematically joined together to form peptides and proteins. The amino portion of one amino acid will combine with the carboxyl (acid) portion of another amino acid to form a peptide linkage. When several of these junctions occur, the resulting molecule is called a polypeptide. Generally polypeptide chains contain 50 to 1,000 amino acids.

HISTORY. In 1838, the Dutch chemist Geradus Johannes Mulder applied the name *proteins* to a group of complex organic compounds found in both plant and animal materials. It was because of their recognized importance to the structure and function of living matter that proteins were so named from the Greek word *proteios,* meaning *of first quality.*

In 1841, Justus von Liebig, a German scientist, published a paper on the analysis of proteins. Liebig thought that the protein values of different foods could be assessed on the basis of nitrogen content. Then, in 1881, while studying the changes in protein content in grain during germination and fermentation, Johan Kjeldahl found his progress blocked by lack of an accurate method for determining nitrogen. Kjeldahl concentrated all his efforts on developing an analytical method for determining nitrogen; hence, protein content of substances. The Kjeldahl method is still routinely used today.

Gradually, the constituents of proteins—the amino acids—were discovered. In 1902, Emil Fischer, determined the chemical structure of amino acids, the building blocks of protein; and he determined the nature of the chemical bond—the peptide bond—holding the amino acids together.

One of the first recommendations as to protein intake was made by Carl von Voit, a student of Liebig. He suggested in 1881 that 118 g of protein daily was desirable. In 1902, a student of Voit and an American, W. O. Atwater, recommended 125 g per day. However, in 1904, R. H. Chittenden of Yale University recommended only 44 to 53 g of protein per day. Then, between 1909 and 1921, T. B. Osborne and L. B. Mendel conducted numerous experiments on rats which involved protein quantity and quality. Between 1935 and 1955, W. C. Rose conducted experiments in humans to determine how much of each amino acid was needed.

Further studies of actual proteins increased scientists' knowledge of exactly how proteins function in the body. In about 1927, James B. Sumner demonstrated that an enzyme was a protein. Then, during the 1950s, Frederick Sanger made a major discovery when he described the actual amino acid sequence of the protein hormone insulin.

Other studies pointed to the relationships between DNA (deoxyribonucleic acid) and RNA (ribonucleic acid) and protein. In 1953, Francis Crick and James Watson described the structure of the DNA molecule, and gradually scientists have unraveled how cells manufacture specific proteins with specific amino acid sequences.

(Also see NUCLEIC ACIDS.)

SYNTHESIS. The basic structural components of protein are amino acids. Many of the amino acids can be synthesized within the body. These are called nonessential amino acids or dispensable amino acids. If the body cannot synthesize sufficient amounts of certain amino acids to carry out physiological functions, they must be provided in the diet; hence, they are referred to as essential or indispensable amino acids. Actually, it is not entirely correct to say that all indispensable amino acids need to be provided in the diet; rather, the requirement is for the preformed carbon skeleton of the indispensable amino acids, except in the case of lysine and threonine.

According to our present knowledge, the following division of amino acids as essential and nonessential seems proper for humans:

Essential (indispensable)	Nonessential (dispensable)
Histidine	Alanine
Isoleucine	Arginine
Leucine	Asparagine
Lysine	Aspartic acid
Methionine (some	Cysteine
used for the synthe-	Cystine
sis of cysteine)	Glutamic acid
Phenylalanine (some	Glutamine
used for the synthe-	Glucine
sis of tyrosine)	Hydroxyproline
Threonine	Proline
Tryptophan	Serine
Valine	Tyrosine

NOTE WELL: Arginine is not regarded as essential for humans, whereas it is for animals; in contrast to human infants, most young mammals cannot synthesize it in sufficient amounts to meet their needs for growth.

(Also see AMINO ACID[S].)

In order for a protein to be synthesized, all of its constituent amino acids must be available. If one amino acid is missing, the synthesis procedure is halted. When a particular amino acid is deficient, it is referred to as a limiting amino acid because it limits the synthesis of protein. This is why protein quality is so important in human nutrition. Upon digestion, high-quality proteins provide balanced supplies of the various amino acids which can subsequently be absorbed as precursors for protein synthesis. Plant foods often contain insufficient quantities of lysine, methionine and cystine, tryptophan, and/or threonine. Lysine is the limiting amino acid of many cereals, while methionine is the limiting amino acid of beans (legumes). In general, the proteins of animal origin—eggs, dairy products, and meats—provide mixtures of amino acids that are well suited for human requirements of maintenance and growth.

Protein synthesis is not a random process whereby a number of amino acids are joined together; rather, it is a detailed predetermined procedure. When proteins are formed three requirements must be met: (1) the proper amino acids, (2) the proper number of amino acids, and (3) the proper order of the amino acid in the chain forming the protein. Meeting these requirements allows the formation of proteins which are very specific and which give tissues

their unique form, function, and character.

Protein synthesis involves a series of reactions which are specific for each protein. The directions for manufacturing protein are received in coded form from the genetic material of the cell—the DNA (deoxyribonucleic acid).

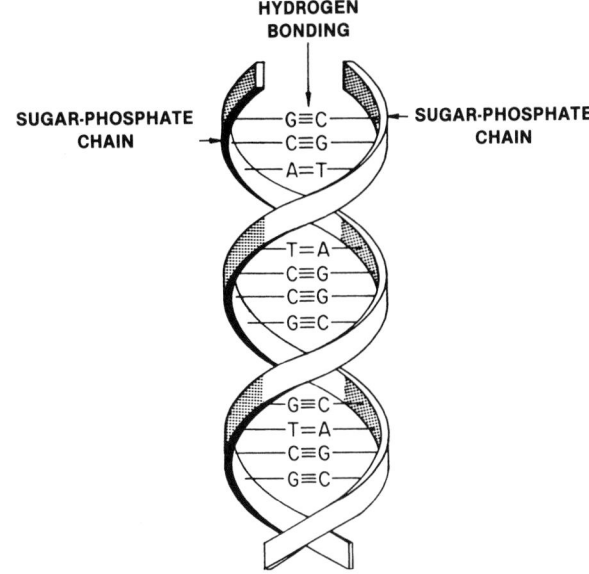

Fig. P-79. Deoxyribonucleic acid or DNA—the code of life. It's a double helix (a double spiral structure), with the sugar (deoxyribose)-phosphate *backbone* represented by the two spiral ribbons. Connecting the *backbone* are four nitrogenous bases (a base is the nonacid part of a salt): adenine (A) paired with thymine (T), and guanine (G) paired with cytosine (C); with the parallel spiral ribbons held together by bonding between these base pairs. The sequence of the bases codes for the synthesis of every protein in the body.

The code of the DNA is put into action by ribonucleic acid (RNA). There are three forms of RNA, each one with a special function. Messenger RNA (mRNA) transcribes the information from the DNA and transports it to the cytoplasm of the cell as a single strand. Transfer RNA (tRNA) are small molecules which act as carriers for the specific amino acids. The third type of RNA, ribosomal RNA (rRNA), is a major component of the ribosomes within the cytoplasm of the cell. The site of protein synthesis is ribosomes bound to mRNA. Ribosomes bound to the mRNA translate (decode) the genetic code. As the message from DNA is translated, tRNA supplies the proper amino acid. These amino acids are then linked by peptide bonds. The amino portion (NH_2) of one amino acid will combine with the carboxyl (COOH) portion of another amino acid releasing water (H_2O) and forming a peptide linkage—like railroad cars joining to form a train. When numerous of these junctions occur, the resulting molecule is called a protein.

Each sequence of amino acids is a different protein. Hence, different proteins are able to accomplish different functions in the body. With 22 amino acids, the different arrangements possible are endless, yielding a variety of proteins.

Since the DNA of each cell carries the master plan for forming proteins, genetic mutations often are manifested by disorders in protein metabolism. Many metabolic defects—inborn errors of metabolism—are the result of a missing or modified enzyme or other protein. The misplacement or omission of just one amino acid in a protein molecule can result in a nonfunctional protein. The disease called sickle-cell anemia results because the blood cells of afflicted individuals contains a faulty protein, with the result that the blood cells often collapse, causing anemia.

(Also see INBORN ERRORS OF METABOLISM; METABOLISM, section headed "Proteins"; and NUCLEIC ACIDS.)

CLASSIFICATION. Proteins occur in nature in a number of forms, each one possessing unique chemical properties. Based on chemical composition, proteins may be divided into two main categories: (1) simple and (2) conjugated. Simple proteins consist of only amino acids or their derivatives, while conjugated proteins are joined to various nonprotein substances. Then, these two main categories are further subdivided. Table P-11 lists the various categories of proteins along with their distinguishing characteristics.

Possibly a third category—*derived proteins* may be added

to the two above. Essentially derived proteins are the product of digestion. They are fragments of various sizes. From largest to smallest, in terms of the number of amino acids, derived proteins are proteoses, peptones, polypeptides, and peptides.

Proteins may also be classified according to their structure which is very important to their function in the body. Some proteins are round to ellipsoidal and are called *globular proteins*. These include *enzymes, protein hormones, hemoglobin,* and *globulins.* Other proteins form long chains bound together in a parallel fashion, and are called *fibrous proteins.* These include *collagen, elastin,* and *keratin*—the proteins of connective tissue, elastic tissue, and hair. Many of the fibrous proteins are not very digestible, and if they are, they are poor-quality proteins.

TABLE P-11
CLASSIFICATION OF SOME COMMON PROTEINS

Type	Chemical Properties	General Comments
SIMPLE PROTEINS		
Albuminoids (scleroproteins)	Insoluble in water; highly resistant to enzymatic digestion; some become gelatinous upon boiling in water or dilute acids and bases.	Includes collagen, elastin, and keratin; common in supporting tissues; sometimes referred to as fibrous protein.
Albumins	Readily soluble in water; coagulate upon heating.	Present in egg, milk, and serum.
Globulins	Low solubility in water; solubility increases with the addition of neutral salts; coagulates upon heating.	Abundant in nature; examples are serum globulins, muscle globulins, and numerous plant globulins.
Glutelins	Insoluble in water; soluble in dilute acids or bases.	Abundant in cereal grains; an example is wheat gluten.
Prolamins	Insoluble in water, absolute alcohol or neutral solvents; soluble in 80% ethanol.	Zein in corn and gliadin in wheat are prolamins.
CONJUGATED PROTEINS		
Chromoproteins	Combination of a protein and a pigmented (colored) substance.	Common example is hemoglobin—hematin and protein.
Lecithoproteins	Combination of protein and lecithin.	Found in fiber of clotted blood and vitellin of egg.
Lipoproteins	Water soluble combination of fat and protein.	A vehicle for the transport of fat in the blood; all contain triglycerides, cholesterol, and phospholipids in varying proportions.
Metalloproteins	Proteins that are complexed with metals.	One example is transferrin, a metalloprotein that can bind copper, iron, and zinc. Various enzymes contain minerals.
Mucoproteins or glycoproteins	Contain carbohydrates such as mannose or galactose.	Examples are mucin from the mucus secretion, and some hormones such as that in human pregnancy urine.
Nucleoproteins	Combination of proteins and nucleic acids.	Present in germs of seeds and glandular tissue.
Phosphoproteins	Compounds containing protein and phosphorus in a form other than phospholipid or nucleic acid.	Casein in milk and ovovitellin in eggs, are examples.

DIGESTION, ABSORPTION, AND METABOLISM. Protein digestion—the breakdown into smaller units—begins in the stomach and continues to completion in the small intestine. Enzymes from the pancreas and the small intestine eventually split dietary protein into individual amino acids. These amino acids are absorbed from the intestine by the process of active transport whereupon they are distributed to the cells of the body via the blood. In the body, amino acids may be used for primarily protein synthesis or energy production, depending upon the (1) protein quality, (2) caloric level of the diet, (3) stage of development, including growth, pregnancy, and lactation, (4) prior nutritional status, and (5) stress factors such as fever, injury, and immobilization.

Occasionally, individuals are born with very specific disorders related to the metabolism of protein or amino acids. These are often referred to as inborn errors of metabolism. Albinism, maple syrup urine disease, and phenylketonuria are examples of some of the more familiar types.

(Also see DIGESTION AND ABSORPTION; INBORN

ERRORS OF METABOLISM, Table I-1, Inborn Errors of Amino Acid Metabolism; and METABOLISM.)

FUNCTIONS. Each specific protein performs a specific function in the body. One protein cannot and will not substitute for another. Rather broadly, proteins may be classified as performing the following five functions:

1. The formation of new tissues from infancy to adulthood—*anabolism.*

2. Maintenance of body tissues—a process called *protein turnover.* Protein maintenance involves replacing blood cells every 120 days, replacing the cells that line the intestine every 1½ days, and replacing the protein lost from the body in the perspiration, hair, fingernails, skin, urine, and feces.

3. *Regulatory.* The protein in the cells and body fluids provide regulatory functions. Thus, hemoglobin, an iron-bearing protein, carries oxygen to the tissues; The protein of the blood plasma regulates water balance and osmotic pressure; the proteins act as buffers controlling the acid-base balance of the body; many of the hormones which regulate body processes are proteins; enzymes, the catalysts for most

all chemical reactions of the body, are proteins; antibodies, which protect the body from infectious diseases are proteins; the blood clotting mechanism of the body is dependent upon proteins; and certain amino acids derived from dietary protein or synthesized in the body also perform important regulatory functions.

4. *Milk production.* Each liter of human milk contains about 12 g of protein.

5. *The production of energy*—the catabolism (breakdown) of amino acids yields energy.

REQUIRED PROTEIN INTAKE. The minimum protein requirement of humans (other animals, too) may be determined by nitrogen balance studies. Nitrogen is obtained from the consumption of protein. As indicated previously, each 100 g of protein contains approximately 16 g of nitrogen. Nitrogen is lost from the body each day in the feces, urine, skin, hair, nails, perspiration and other secretions. Dietary protein (nitrogen) must be sufficient to cover the daily losses. Normal, healthy adults should be in a state of nitrogen equilibrium—intake approximately equals output. When nitrogen intake exceeds nitrogen output, a positive nitrogen balance exists. Such a condition is present in the following physiological states: pregnancy, lactation, recovery from a severe illness, muscular buildup, growth, and following the administration of an anabolic steroid such as testosterone. A positive nitrogen balance indicates that new tissue is being formed. A negative nitrogen balance occurs when nitrogen intake is less than output. Starvation, diabetes mellitus, fever, surgery, burns or shock can all result in a negative nitrogen balance. This is an undesirable state since body protein is being broken down faster than it is being built up.

Protein Allowance. Using nitrogen balance, the recommended daily dietary allowance for protein may be derived as follows:

1. Obligatory urinary nitrogen losses of young adults amount to about 37 mg/kg of body weight.

2. Fecal nitrogen losses average 12 mg/kg of body weight.

3. Amounts of nitrogen lost in the perspiration, hair, fingernails, and sloughed skin are estimated at 3 mg/kg of body weight.

4. Minor routes of nitrogen loss such as saliva, menstruation, and seminal ejaculation are estimated at 2 mg/kg of body weight.

5. The total obligatory nitrogen lost—that which must be replaced daily—amounts to 54 mg/kg, or in terms of protein lost this is 0.34 g/kg.

6. To account for individual variation the daily loss is increased by 30%, or 70 mg/kg. In terms of protein, this is 0.45 g/kg of body weight.

7. This protein loss is further increased by 30%, to 0.6 g/kg of body weight, to account for the loss of efficiency when consuming even a high quality protein such as egg.

8. The final adjustment is to correct for the 75% efficiency of utilization of protein in the mixed diet of Americans. Thus, the daily recommended allowances for protein becomes 0.8 g/kg of body weight for normal healthy adult males and females, or 63 g of protein per day for a 174-lb *(79 kg)* man and 50 g per day for a 138-lb *(63 kg)* woman.

Growth, pregnancy, and lactation, and possibly work and stress, require an additional intake of protein. Aging may present some special considerations.

The Food and Nutrition Board (FNB) of the National Re-

search Council (NRC) recommended daily allowance of protein are given in Table P-12.

TABLE P-12
RECOMMENDED DAILY PROTEIN ALLOWANCES[1]

Group	Age	Weight		Height		RDA
	(years)	(lb)	(kg)	(in.)	(cm)	(g)
Infants	0.0–0.5	13	6	24	60	13
	0.5–1.0	20	9	28	71	14
Children	1–3	29	13	35	90	16
	4–6	44	20	44	112	24
	7–10	62	28	52	132	28
Males	11–14	99	45	62	157	45
	15–18	145	66	69	176	59
	19–24	160	72	70	177	58
	25–50	174	79	70	178	63
	51+	170	77	68	173	63
Females	11–14	101	46	62	157	46
	15–18	120	55	64	163	44
	19–24	128	58	65	164	46
	25–50	138	63	64	163	50
	51+	143	65	63	160	50
Pregnant						60
Lactating						65

[1]*Recommended Dietary Allowances*, 10th ed., 1989, NRC-National Academy of Sciences, p. 284.

Table P-13 presents the recommended protein allowance for the elderly on the basis of their energy intake.

TABLE P-13
RECOMMENDED DAILY PROTEIN ALLOWANCES FOR THE ELDERLY[1]

Group	Age	Weight		Height		Energy Needs	Protein
	(years)	(lb)	(kg)	(in.)	(cm)	(kcal)	(g)
Males	51+	170	77	68	173	2,300	63
Females	51+	143	65	63	160	1,900	50

[1]Based on 12% of the energy intake in the form of protein. Age, weight, height, and energy needs are from *Recommended Dietary Allowances*, 10th ed., 1989, NRC-National Academy of Sciences, p. 284.

Both dietary protein and energy supplies are adequate in the United States. Individuals in the United States derive about 14 to 18% of their calories from protein. Average consumption levels of proteins are quite generous: about 50 g/day in preschool children; 70 to 85 g in older children; 90 to 110 g in male, and 65 to 70 g in female adolescents and adults; and 75 to 80 g in men and 55 to 65 g in women over age 65.

Amino Acid Requirement. The requirement for protein carries a restriction. Protein must supply individuals with amounts of the essential amino acids at levels sufficient to meet the protein synthesizing needs of the body. Based on a number of studies on infants, children, and adults, some estimated daily requirements for the essential amino acids have been made; and these are listed in Table P-14.

TABLE P-14
ESTIMATED AMINO ACID REQUIREMENTS OF MAN[1]

Amino Acid	Requirement, mg/kg Body Weight/Day			
	Infants	Children		Adults
	(3–4 mo.)	(2 yr)	(10–12 yr)	
Histidine	16	19	19	11
Isoleucine	40	28	28	13
Leucine	93	66	44	19
Lysine	60	58	44	16
Total S-containing amino acids (methionine and cystine)	33	25	22	17
Total aromatic amino acids (phenylalanine and tyrosine)	72	63	22	19
Threonine	50	34	28	9
Tryptophan	10	11	(9)	5
Valine	54	35	25	13

[1]*Recommended Dietary Allowances*, 10th ed., 1989, NRC-National Academy of Sciences, p. 67.

These requirements are adequate only when the diet provides enough nitrogen for the synthesis of the nonessential amino acids so that the essential amino acids will not be used to supply amino groups for the nonessential amino acids via the process of transamination. Even in infants the essential amino acids make up only about 35% of the total need for protein. In adults, essential amino acids account for less than 20% of the total protein requirement. Most proteins contain plenty of dispensable amino acids; usually the concern is to meet the essential amino acid needs, particularly of infants and children.

SOURCES. The protein content of numerous foods is given in Food Composition Table F-21.

Unfortunately, meeting the protein requirement is more involved than just choosing foods which provide the daily amount of protein. As previously indicated, the requirement for protein is primarily a requirement for essential amino acids. In terms of amino acid composition, all proteins are not created equal. Some proteins of certain foods are low or completely devoid of some essential amino acids. Hence, meeting the protein requirement demands quality as well as quantity.

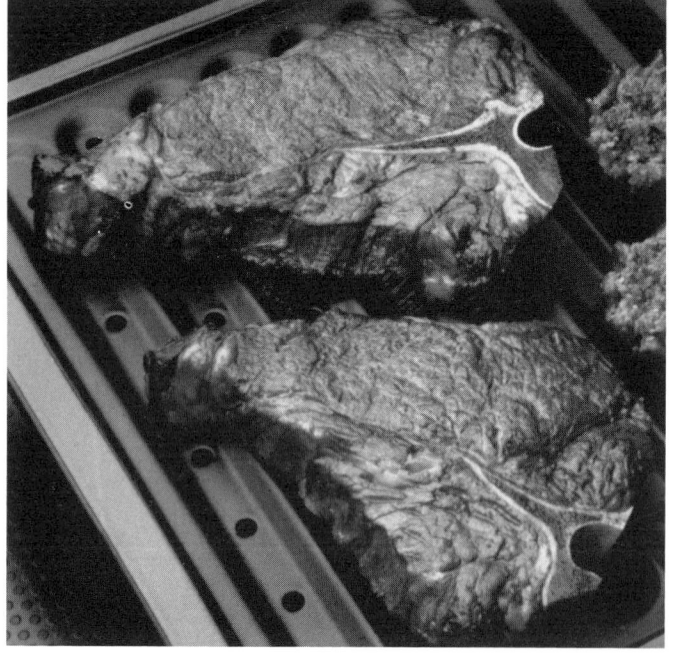
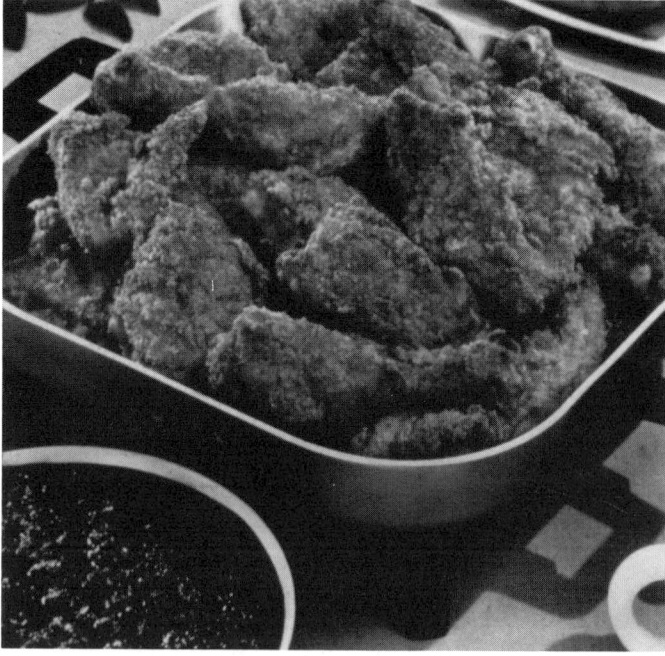

Fig. P-80. All proteins are not created equal. Animal proteins generally have a higher biological value than plant proteins. Shown: (left) T-bone steak, (Courtesy, National Live Stock & Meat Board, Chicago, Ill.); and (right) fried chicken. (Courtesy, USDA)

Quantity and Quality. Protein values such as those in Food Composition Table F-21 are crude protein values derived by the Kjeldahl method, which determines the nitrogen content of a substance and then assumes that each gram of nitrogen represents 6.25 g of protein. This procedure estimates protein quantity; and quantity is important. For example, boiled potatoes contain 1.9 g of protein per 3½ oz (100 g). To obtain just the extra 30 g of protein daily during pregnancy, a woman would have to consume about 3½ lb (1.6 kg) of potatoes, while only 3½ to 4 oz (100 to 113 g) of beef, fish, or poultry would supply the extra 30 g of protein. Still, crude protein values may be misleading. For example, gelatin ranks second among the top protein sources; yet, gelatin contains virtually no tryptophan and very low levels of other essential amino acids. Used as a protein source, gelatin will not support growth or life. Hence, some evaluation of protein quality is necessary.

In 1911, T. B. Osborne, of the Connecticut Agricultural Experiment Station, and L. B. Mendel, of Yale University, formed a brilliant partnership and pioneered in studies of protein quality. Their early work on the quality of protein resulted in proteins being classified as complete, partially incomplete, and incomplete. Complete proteins contain all of the essential amino acids in sufficient amounts to maintain life and support growth. Partially incomplete proteins can maintain life, but cannot support growth. Incomplete proteins cannot maintain life or support growth. Following the work of Osborne

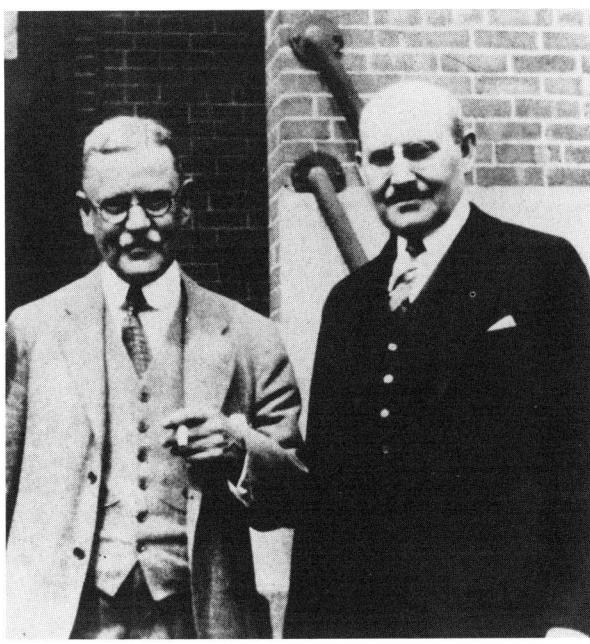

Fig. P-81. Thomas B. Osborne (left) and Lafayette B. Mendel (right), who prioneered in studies of protein quality. (Courtesy, The Connecticut Agricultural Experiment Station, New Haven, Conn.)

and Mendel, there was a quest for some method of evaluating proteins in terms of their ability to meet the needs of the body. The following are descriptions of some of these methods:

• **Biological value**—This method assumes that the retained nitrogen—ingested nitrogen not recovered in the urine or feces—represents a perfect assortment of amino acids utilized by the body. Biological value is a measure of the efficiency of utilization of absorbed nitrogen, and it depends primarily on the amino acid composition of the dietary protein. Needless to say, determining the quality of protein in the diet by this means is time-consuming, and hence, not often used. Moreover, few animals other than rats will consume protein-free diets long enough to complete the trial. However, biological value is often used to describe protein quality.

(Also see BIOLOGICAL VALUE [BV] OF PROTEINS.)

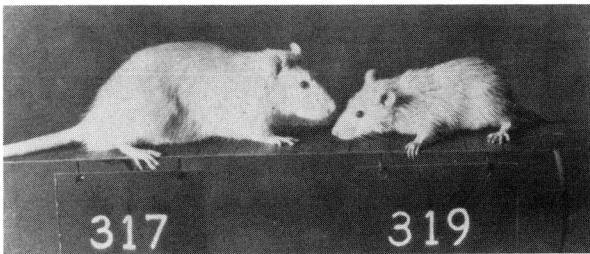

Fig. P-82. High protein vs. low protein diets! The rat on the left had a diet with 18% casein. The other rat's diet consisted of 4% casein. This experiment was conducted by Thomas B. Osborne, of the Connecticut Agricultural Experiment Station, and Lafayette B. Mendel, of Yale University, who in 1911, formed a brilliant partnership and pioneered in studies of protein quality. (Courtesy, The Connecticut Agricultural Experiment Station, New Haven, Conn.)

• **Net protein utilization (NPU)**—Digestibility is estimated from the quantity ingested that is subsequently not recovered in the feces, expressed as a percentage of the intake. The multiplication of the biological value and the digestibility gives the net protein utilization, a measure of the efficiency of overall utilization of the ingested nitrogen. For proteins that are completely digested, net protein utilization and biological value are the same. For less digestible proteins or for foods containing large amounts of fiber, the biological value does not provide a measure of efficiency of utilization of the protein consumed—only the efficiency of utilization of that absorbed.

• **Protein efficiency ratio (PER)**—This is the simplest test of protein quality, and the one used widely in comparing the nutritive value of proteins in individual foods. The PER is defined as the weight gain of a growing animal divided by its protein intake over the period studied, often 10 days. Although simple in application, it does not provide protein evaluations that are directly proportional to quality, because no account is taken of loss of weight when animals are given no protein in the diet. It assumes that all protein is used for growth and no allowance for maintenance is made.

• **Net protein ratio (NPR)**—This method attempts to correct the fault of the PER by making some allowance for maintenance. The NPR accomplishes this by the inclusion of a control group of animals receiving no dietary protein. Thus, the NPR is the weight gain of a group of animals (rats) fed the test diet plus the weight loss of a similar group fed a protein-free diet, and the total divided by the weight of the protein consumed by the animals on the test diet.

• **Nitrogen balance index**—This method is similar to the biological value but there is no period of feeding a protein-free diet. It is simply the nitrogen in the food minus that in the urine and feces. Nitrogen balance has been used as a means of evaluating protein foods in the human diet and determining the amino acid requirements of humans. When proteins (amino acids) are adequate in the diet, the nitrogen balance is positive. W. C. Rose, using a diet consisting of sugar, starch, fat, and a mixed solution of purified amino acids in known amounts, was the first to determine the amount of each essential amino acid needed for young men. One at a time, the amino acids were left out of the solution and nitrogen balance was noted. When the omitted amino acid was essential, a negative nitrogen balance resulted. The method used for determining the nutritive value of proteins for humans is an extension of nitrogen balance and is termed a nitrogen balance index. The food to be evaluated is fed at several intakes below and slightly above nitrogen equilibrium. Then, values for nitrogen balance versus nitrogen absorbed or nitrogen intake are plotted on a graph, and a straight line connects these points and the slope of the line is determined. When nitrogen intake is used in place of nitrogen absorbed, the values obtained are equivalent to net protein utilization (NPU).

• **Slope ratio method**—This is a modification of the nitrogen balance index wherein various levels of protein are fed *adlibitum* to growing animals. Then growth rate and protein intake are plotted on a graph, and the slope of this line is taken as the measure of protein quality.

• **Chemical score (CS)**—By chemically examining the essential amino acid content of a food, some idea of its nutritive value may be gained. To determine the chemical score one must first have a reference pattern of amino acid concentrations with which to compare the dietary protein. Table P-15 indicates what type of amino acid pattern a high-quality protein should possess in order to meet the body's needs. This amino acid pattern is based on the essential amino acid requirements of children 10 to 12 years of age. Also, Table P-15 shows how the essential amino acid patterns of human milk and eggs compare to that of the requirement of children 10 to 12 years of age. Human milk and eggs are frequently used

TABLE P-15
AMINO ACID REQUIREMENT OF CHILDREN 10–12 YEARS COMPARED TO THE AMINO ACID PROFILES OF HUMAN MILK AND EGGS

Amino Acid	Amino Acid Requirement for Children 10–12 Years[1]	Human Milk[2]	Whole Egg[2]
	(mg/g protein)		
Histidine	19	26	22
Isoleucine	28	46	54
Leucine	44	93	86
Lysine	44	66	70
Methionine and cystine	22	42	57
Phenylalanine and tyrosine	22	72	93
Threonine	28	43	47
Tryptophan	9	17	17
Valine	25	55	66

[1]Recommended Dietary Allowances, 10th ed., 1989, National Academy of Sciences, p. 67, Table 6–5.
[2]Values for the protein and amino acid content are from Proteins and Amino Acids in Selected Foods Table p. 37.

as standards due to their amino acid patterns. The reference or standard pattern is assigned a value of 100, and the percentage by which each essential amino acid in the food or dietary protein differs from the value of the standard is calculated. The essential amino acid showing the greatest deficit is considered to be the amino acid limiting utilization of the protein. The amount of this amino acid present, expressed as a percentage of that in the standard, provides the chemical score. This score usually shows good agreement with biological evaluation of protein quality but tends to overestimate quality for proteins that are not well digested.

The following equation may be used to calculate the chemical score of each essential amino acid:

$$CS = \frac{mg \text{ of amino acid per g test protein} \times 100}{mg \text{ of amino acid per g reference protein}}$$

Often, only the chemical scores for lysine, methionine and cystine, and tryptophan are calculated as one of these is commonly the limiting amino acid. The following is an example for potatoes:
1. Consider the reference pattern of whole eggs:
    Methionine and cystine .... 56 mg/g
    Lysine .... 68 mg/g
    Tryptophan .... 16 mg/g
2. List the amount of the same amino acids in the protein of potatoes:
    Methionine and cystine .... 27 mg/g
    Lysine .... 127 mg/g
    Tryptophan .... 35 mg/g
3. Calculate the chemical score for these amino acids as indicated by the above formula:
    Methionine and cystine 48
    Lysine 187
    Tryptophan 219

Obviously, the amino acids methionine and cystine—the sulfur-containing amino acids—are limiting in potatoes.

• **Net dietary protein calories percent (NDₚCal%)**—This method of evaluating protein considers the percentage of the calories from protein in the food which is adjusted according to the net protein utilization (NPU) or quality. The following formula describes $ND_pCal\%$:

$$ND_pCal\% = \frac{g \text{ of protein} \times 4 \text{ kcal} \times 100}{total \text{ kcal in food or diet}} \times NPU$$

One must bear in mind that each method for evaluating protein quality is only a tool to aid in identifying foods capable of meeting the protein—amino acid—needs of the body. These protein quality measurements are useful for comparing the nutritive value of different lots of a single protein, such as an infant formula, a processed food, or a uniform diet for man or animals. However, measurements made on individual foodstuffs do not give useful information about the protein quality of complex human diets. The only meaningful measure of the protein quality of a diet is one made on the total diet as consumed. To this end, there are some steps which can be taken to ensure that the total diet provides the needed amino acids.

Complementary Proteins. Fortunately, the amino acid deficiencies in a protein can usually be improved by combining it with another, and the mixture of the two proteins will often have a higher food value than either one alone. In other words proteins having opposite strengths and weaknesses complement each other. For example, many cereals are low in lysine, but high in methionine and cystine. On the other hand, soybeans, lima beans, and kidney beans are high in lysine but low in methionine and cystine. When

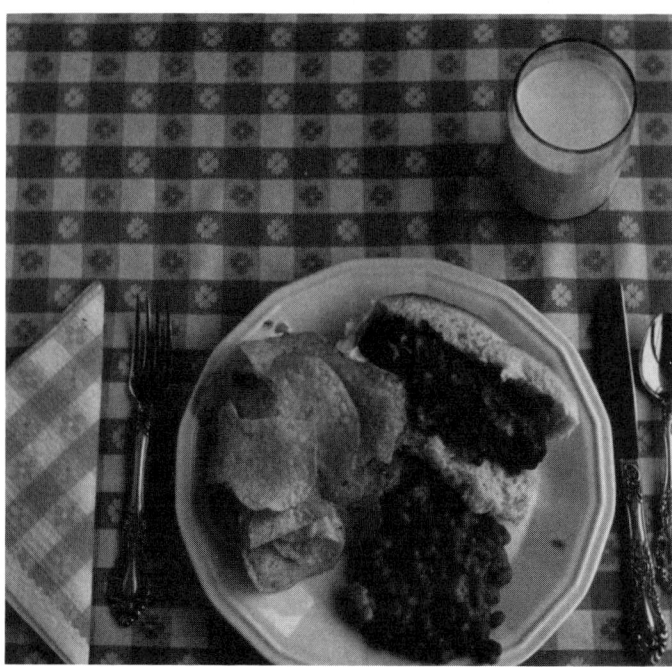

Fig. P-83. Complementary proteins of bun (low in lysine, but high in methionine and cystine) and beans (high in lysine, but low in methionine and cystine). (Courtesy, University of Minnesota, St. Paul)

eaten together, the deficiencies are corrected. Complementary protein combinations are found in almost all cultures. In the Middle East, bread and cheese are eaten together. Mexicans eat beans and corn (tortillas). Indians eat wheat and pulses (legumes). Americans eat breakfast cereals with milk. This kind of supplementation works only when the deficient and complementary proteins are ingested together or within a few hours of each other.

Other examples of complementary food proteins may include: (1) rice and black-eyed peas; (2) whole wheat or bulgur, soybeans, and sesame seeds; (3) cornmeal and kidney beans; and (4) soybeans, peanuts, brown rice, and bulgur wheat.

Factors Affecting Amino Acid Utilization. The presence of amino acids in a protein does not assure their utilization. So, in addition to the amino acid content of a food(s), the following related factors must be considered:

• **Digestibility**—The amino acids of most animal proteins are efficiently absorbed, but this is not necessarily so for many proteins of plant origin. Animal proteins are about 90 to 95% digestible, but the digestibility of some plant proteins may be as low as 73%.

• **Energy**—Protein is used inefficiently when the energy intake is grossly inadequate. When the energy intake is below a certain level, the nutritive value of the protein to the consumer diminishes. For example, an increase in the protein supply to undernourished subjects will not be fully effective if the energy content of the diet is restricted. This principle also applies to replenishment of body protein following malnutrition and during convalescence after injury or disease; full utilization of dietary protein for replenishment is best assured by an adequate calorie intake.

The influence of calorie intake on protein metabolism is shown by the rapid development of a negative nitrogen balance when the energy content of the diet is reduced below requirements—an unfavorable effect which persists if the sub-maintenance diet continues to be fed. From this, it can be concluded that an inadequate intake of energy will, by itself, cause a loss of protein from the body and will consequently aggravate protein deficiency in the diet. Hence, carbohydrates are said to have a protein-sparing effect. A daily intake of 50 to 100 g of digestible carbohydrates is required for protein-sparing.

• **Vitamins and minerals**—Any essential mineral or vitamin whose presence is needed for normal growth and metabolism can be presumed to affect utilization of dietary protein, in so far as deficiency of the vitamin or mineral leads to loss of body substance. For this reason, tests of protein quality are normally performed with diets containing adequate amounts of vitamins and minerals.

In treating persons with protein deficiency, the supply of some vitamins and minerals appears to be more critical than that of others. In particular enough niacin, potassium, and phosphorus should be given to ensure that they are not limiting factors in protein replenishment. Thus, in a niacin deficiency, not only is tryptophan converted to niacin when present in excess but there is evidence that some conversion may occur even when there is insufficient tryptophan for protein synthesis.

(Also see MINERAL[S]; and VITAMIN[S].)

• **Amino acid imbalances**—One type of amino acid imbalance arises when the addition of a single amino acid or mixture of amino acids to a diet reduces the utilization of the dietary protein. Even a small increase in the concentrations of certain amino acids can increase the needs for others when the total protein intake is low.

Utilization of one dietary amino acid may also be depressed by addition to the diet of another structurally related to it. The two best-known examples are the interference of an excess of leucine with the utilization of isoleucine and valine, and the interference of lysine with the utilization of arginine. Large amounts of single amino acids added to experimental diets may induce various toxic reactions, including depression of growth. The most toxic amino acids are methionine, tyrosine, and histidine, and their effect is most serious when the diet is low in protein.

Not enough is presently known about the practical bearing these observations may have in relation to human diets but they must be taken into account in studies of the biological effectiveness of essential amino acid patterns. Circumstances in which amino acid imbalances would occur are unlikely in individuals at normal levels of dietary protein.

• **Nonessential amino acid nitrogen**—The proportion of nonessential amino acid nitrogen has an influence on the essential amino acid requirements. If the ratio of essential amino acids to the total nitrogen in a food is too high, essential amino acids will be used as a source of nitrogen for the nonessential amino acids which, in spite of their being so designated, are necessary parts of the protein molecule and needed for protein synthesis. When the nonessential amino acids are in short supply, some of the essential amino acids furnish nitrogen (NH_2) more readily than others for the synthesis of the nonessential amino acids.

• **Food processing**—Heat and chemicals used during processing can affect amino acid availability. For example, loss of available lysine can occur from mild heat treatment in the presence of reducing sugars such as glucose or lactose.

Heating can also have favorable effects. Heating soybean flour improves the utilization of protein by making the amino acid methionine more available, and heating raw soybeans destroys the inhibitor of the protein digestive enzyme trypsin. Cooking eggs destroys the trypsin inhibitor ovomucoid in the white.

PROTEIN MALNUTRITION. Protein deficiency is common worldwide. This is primarily because in many underdeveloped areas of the world protein intake is marginal, but energy intake is so low that the protein eaten is not spared for its essential functions. The name, protein-energy (calorie) malnutrition is applied to a whole spectrum of protein and energy deficiencies. At one end of the spectrum is kwashiorkor—a severe clinical syndrome caused by a deficiency of protein. Pertinent protein malnutrition information follows:

• **Kwashiorkor**—Infants fed low-protein, starchy foods such as banànas, yams, and cassava after weaning may develop kwashiorkor. This imbalanced diet, which has a subnormal protein-to-calorie ratio for infants, prevents some of the adaptive mechanisms of the body from operating the way that they do in the case of starvation or marasmus—a wasting condition due to lack of food.

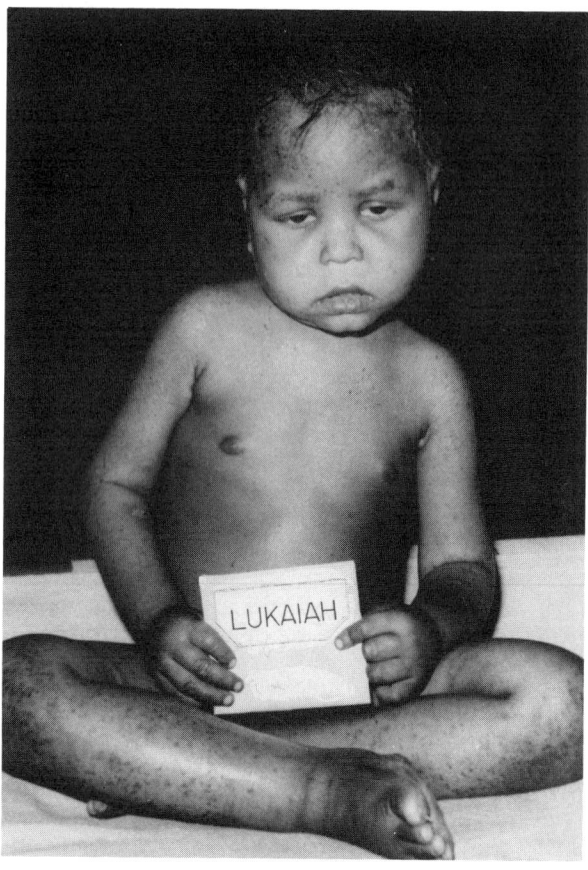

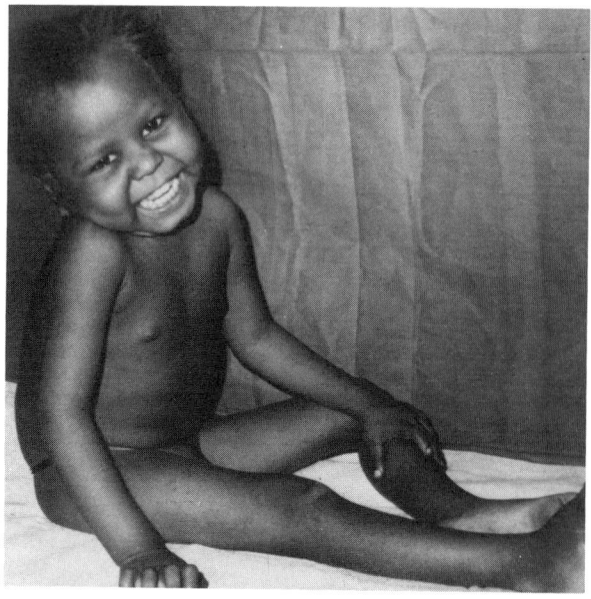

Fig. P-84. A 4½-year-old child from South India suffering from kwashiorkor. *Top:* Lukaiah before rehabilitation weighed 21½ lb (9.8 kg) and was in a state of severe kwashiorkor showing edema, hair and skin changes, and misery. *Bottom:* After 1 month of rehabilitation, Lukaiah weighed almost 24 lb (10.9 kg). The edema disappeared; the skin was normal, and the hair was recovering. Furthermore, Lukaiah was happy and full of mischief—like any child. (Courtesy, WHO, Geneva, Switzerland)

In kwashiorkor there is less breakdown of protein and release of amino acids from muscle than in marasmus since provision of adequate energy in the diet reduces the adrenal gland response and, consequently, the flow of amino acids from muscle is not sufficient to meet the synthesizing needs of the internal organs. Particularly critical is the loss of tissue cells from the gastrointestinal lining which leads to various types of malabsorption. Also, the severe shortage of protein results in a reduction in synthesis of digestive enzymes, normally secreted from the pancreas or present in the intestinal wall. Thus, there is likely to be diarrhea which may cause excessive loss of water or dehydration, loss of minerals salts, and an electrolyte imbalance.

Liver function is greatly reduced due to lack of protein for the synthesis of enzymes. Also, there is likely to be fat accumulation in the liver due to its inability to package fat with protein for transport in the blood. Low blood levels of albumin, along with anemia, result from the scarcity of amino acids for protein synthesis. Edema—swelling—is a consequence of the depletion of plasma proteins and electrolytes.

The production of antibodies is likely to be greatly reduced and the victim, therefore, will be prone to infectious diseases. In chronic cases, there is likely to be delayed eruption of teeth, poor enamel with many caries, and pale gums and mucous membranes due to anemia.

Besides the physical changes in kwashiorkor, there are also some mental changes such as general indifference, irritability, and apathy.

(Also see KWASHIORKOR; and MALNUTRITION, Protein-Energy.)

• **Ill and elderly**—Once protein is ingested, an individual's condition may preclude proper digestion or absorption of the intact protein source. Problems may include various types of inflammatory bowel disease, such as pancreatitis or enteritis, or a gastrointestinal fistula or bowel resection, or just the stress of an infection or surgery. Elderly individuals with low incomes, poor health, and poor appetites may not secure food with high-quality protein. In both the ill and the aged, the protein deficiency may be manifested by delayed convalescence or poor wound healing.

(Also see GERONTOLOGY AND GERIATRIC NUTRITION.)

• **Infants**—The diets of infants after weaning should be carefully planned to include a high-quality protein source since infants and children require suitable patterns of amino acids in their diets. This means that if grains are a major dietary staple, there should be supplementation with animal proteins—such as milk, eggs, fish, or if these are unavailable, with such legumes as soybean or peanuts (which may be in the form of a powder). None of the commonly used grains—corn, rice, wheat, and barley—are adequate as the major source of protein for growing children. Mental function disturbances may follow a severe protein deficiency occurring in infancy.

(Also see INFANT DIET AND NUTRITION.)

• **Pregnancy**—Many uncertainties exist concerning the storage and efficiency of protein utilization during pregnancy, but inadequate protein may have adverse effects on the mother and fetus. Pregnant adolescents and women from low-income groups ignorant of the essentials of a good diet may be particularly susceptible.

(Also see PREGNANCY AND LACTATION NUTRITION.)

• **Vegetarians**—Strict vegetarian diets which offer little variety such as the Zen macrobiotic diet can be dangerous. Some individuals on the Zen diet plan eat only brown rice, which fails to provide many essential nutrients. Fruitarians, who eat only raw or dried fruits, nuts, honey, and olive oil may also suffer from an inadequacy of essential nutrients. Although many adults may get along through well-planned vegetarian diets, the protein needs of infants and growing children may not be met. Indeed, children of some vegetarian cults have demonstrated retarded growth and poor nutrition.

(Also see VEGETARIAN DIETS; and ZEN MACROBIOTIC DIET.)

PROTEIN FOR THE WORLD. While there is adequate protein and energy available in the United Sates and other developed countries, many countries are low in calories and low in protein supplies. Moreover, countries low in total protein are also low in animal protein, which generally has a higher biological value than plant protein. Several approaches have been and are being taken to develop and supply good-quality proteins to undeveloped countries. The aim is to provide acceptable, nutritious, and inexpensive products from the foods available. Some of the approaches to feeding the world include the following:

1. **Food combinations.** Using foods common to an area, various nutritious food combinations have been developed and tried by agencies and governments throughout the world. Some examples of these include: (a) Incaparina, a mixture of whole grain corn, whole grain sorghum, cottonseed flour, torula yeast, calcium carbonate,

and vitamin A developed for use in central America; (b) L' aubina, developed in Lebanon and containing chick peas, parboiled wheat, some dried skim milk, and bone ash; (c) corn-soy-milk (CSM) fortified with minerals and vitamins; and (d) whey soy drink mix (WSDM)—a mixture of sweet whey, full-fat soy flour, soybean oil, corn syrup solids, and a vitamin and mineral premix.

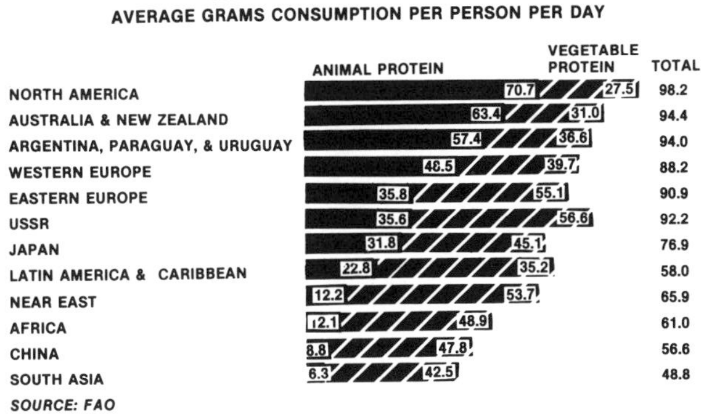

2. **Genetic improvement of grains.** Scientists at Purdue University developed a special corn called Opaque-2 in which the incomplete protein, zein, is reduced to one-half the normal amount, while the complete protein glutelin is doubled. Moreover, lysine and tryptophan concentrations are increased about 50%, and leucine and isoleucine are in a better balance. Feeding trials on both animals and humans have demonstrated the increased value of Opaque-2. Breeding programs have also developed (a) high lysine sorghum and barley, (b) high protein rice and wheat, and (c) a cross between wheat and rye, called triticale. These genetic improvements bring plant protein quality closer to that of the animal proteins, and are very promising.

(Also see CEREAL GRAINS; and CORN, section headed "High-Lysine Corn.")

3. **Protein concentrates.** Protein concentrates from oilseeds, nuts, and leaves provide another method of increasing the supply of quality protein.

Isolating protein from plant leaves may provide a protein source which could be used as a complementary protein in countries where it is too rainy to dry seed crops. Green leaves are among the best sources of protein. By pressing the leaves, a protein-containing juice can be obtained which may be coagulated and dried forming a product that is 50% protein. This product is called leaf protein concentrate (LPC).

(Also see COTTONSEED; PEANUTS; and SOYBEANS, Table S-12, Soybean Products and Uses, Soybean Protein Isolates, and Textured Soybean Proteins.)

4. **Single-cell protein.** This refers to protein obtained from single-cell organisms or simple multicellular organisms such as yeast, bacteria, algae, and fungi. The most popular and most familiar of these are brewers' yeast and torula yeast, both of which are marketed. The potential for producing single-cell protein (SCP) is tremendous. Furthermore, many of the industrial by-products with little or no economic value may be used as a growing media. Some of these by-products include petroleum products, methane, alcohols, sulfite waste liquor, starch, molasses, cellulose, and animal waste. Still with all its potential, problems such as (a) safety, (b) acceptability, (c) palatability, (d) digestibility, (e) nutrient content, and (f) economics of production need to be solved.

(Also see ALGAE; and SINGLE-CELL PROTEIN.)

5. **Amino acid supplementation.** Since lysine is the limiting amino acid in wheat and other grains, the addition of limited amounts of lysine to cereal diets improves their protein quality. Indeed, studies in Peru and Guatemala demonstrated that growing children benefited by this addition. However, in most countries there is more to be gained by focusing on increasing the food supply in general.

(Also see LYSINE.)

PROTEINS AND AMINO ACIDS IN SELECTED FOODS. Table P-16, Proteins and Amino Acids in Selected Foods, provides information on a number of foods. This information can be used to select foods and plan diets which yield a high-quality protein.

(Also see MALNUTRITION; MALNUTRITION PROTEIN-ENERGY; and VEGETARIAN DIETS.)

THERE IS PROTEIN AND PROTEIN!
AVERAGE GRAMS CONSUMPTION PER PERSON PER DAY

	ANIMAL PROTEIN	VEGETABLE PROTEIN	TOTAL
NORTH AMERICA	70.7	27.5	98.2
AUSTRALIA & NEW ZEALAND	63.4	31.0	94.4
ARGENTINA, PARAGUAY, & URUGUAY	57.4	36.6	94.0
WESTERN EUROPE	48.5	39.7	88.2
EASTERN EUROPE	35.8	55.1	90.9
USSR	35.6	56.6	92.2
JAPAN	31.8	45.1	76.9
LATIN AMERICA & CARIBBEAN	22.8	35.2	58.0
NEAR EAST	12.2	53.7	65.9
AFRICA	12.1	48.9	61.0
CHINA	8.8	47.8	56.6
SOUTH ASIA	6.3	42.5	48.8

SOURCE: FAO

Fig. P-85. Average grams protein consumption per person per day, with a breakdown into animal and vegetable protein, by geographic areas and countries. (From: *Ceres*, FAO/UN, Vol. 8, No. 3)

TABLE P-16
PROTEINS AND AMINO ACIDS IN SELECTED FOODS[1]

FOOD NAME— 100 Gram (3.5 oz) Portion	Water	Food Energy Calories	Total Protein	Animal Protein	Plant Protein	Amino Acids										
						Cystine	Histidine	Iso-leucine	Leucine	Lysine	Methi-onine	Phenyl-alanine	Threo-nine	Trypto-phan	Tyrosine	Valine
	(g)	(kcal)	(g)	(g)	(g)	(mg)	(mg)	(mg)	(mg)	(mg)	(mg)	(mg)	(mg)	(mg)	(mg)	(mg)
BAKERY PRODUCTS																
BREADS																
CRACKED WHEAT BREAD	34.9	263	8.7	0	8.7	—	—	373	582	234	130	426	252	104	—	400
FRENCH BREAD	30.6	290	9.1	0	9.1	—	—	255	695	205	115	495	260	110	—	385
RAISIN BREAD	35.3	262	6.6	Trace	6.6	—	—	278	434	173	95	321	130	78	—	300
RYE BREAD, DARK (pumpernickel)	34.0	246	9.1	0	9.1	—	—	390	606	371	143	425	334	100	—	471
RYE BREAD, LIGHT	35.5	243	9.1	0	9.1	—	—	391	613	291	139	439	291	100	—	473
WHITE BREAD, enriched	35.6	270	8.7	0.2	8.5	—	—	417	691	260	126	469	269	104	—	400
WHOLE WHEAT BREAD	36.4	243	10.5	—	—	—	—	460	721	308	160	508	313	126	—	491
CAKES																
ANGEL FOOD CAKE	34.0	259	5.7	4.4	1.3	—	—	262	439	131	74	314	165	68	—	245
DOUGHNUTS																
DOUGHNUT, cake type, plain	23.7	391	4.6	1.5	3.1	—	—	240	381	165	81	256	159	59	—	237
DOUGHNUT, raised type, plain	28.3	414	6.3	2.1	4.2	—	—	323	513	223	106	346	216	80	—	320
LEAVENINGS																
YEAST, DRY (active), baker's	5.0	282	36.9	0	36.9			2280	3970	3160	844	2090	2270	440	—	2900
MUFFINS																
BLUEBERRY	39.0	281	7.3	3.1	4.2	—	—	388	608	305	133	393	265	95	—	393
PLAIN, enriched	38.0	294	7.8	3.3	4.5	—	—	415	650	328	143	420	283	103	—	420
QUICK BREADS																
BAKING POWDER BISCUIT	27.4	369	7.4	0.2	7.3	—	—	342	571	171	97	408	214	88	—	320
BOSTON BROWN BREAD, canned	45.0	211	5.5	1.6	3.9	—	—	257	480	225	97	265	200	57	—	302
CORNBREAD OR JOHNNYCAKE	37.9	267	8.7	—	—	—	—	400	1130	260	160	400	350	52	—	440
POPOVER, home recipe	54.9	224	8.8	4.8	4.0	—	—	514	766	468	200	478	366	124	—	542
ROLLS																
CINNAMON BUN, w/raisins	32.0	275	6.9	1.6	5.3	—	—	315	527	157	88	377	198	82	—	293
DANISH PASTRY, plain w/o fruit or nuts	22.0	422	7.4	—	—	—	—	366	586	220	120	411	240	94	—	357
DINNER TYPE (pan), enriched	31.4	289	8.2	0.2	8.0	—	—	403	655	268	124	437	268	100	—	392
HARD ROLL, enriched	25.4	312	9.8	0.3	9.5	—	—	480	780	320	149	520	320	120	—	469
SWEET ROLL	31.5	316	8.5	2.0	6.5	—	—	436	698	309	142	464	291	109	—	431
CEREALS & FLOURS																
CEREALS																
BARLEY, pearled light, uncooked	11.1	349	8.2	0	8.2	—	—	343	568	279	114	429	279	100	—	411
BULGUR (parboiled wheat) canned, unseasoned	56.0	168	6.2	0	6.2	—	—	—	—	217	148	—	—	347	—	—
CORN GRITS, degermed, enriched, cooked	87.1	51	1.2	0	1.2	—	—	55	155	34	22	54	47	7	—	60
CORN MEAL, white or yellow, degermed, enriched, cooked	87.7	50	1.1	0	1.1	—	—	46	131	29	19	45	40	5	—	51
FARINA, quick cooking, enriched, cooked	89.0	43	1.3	0	1.3	—	—	489	689	200	121	521	279	—	—	439
MACARONI, any shape, enriched, cooked	72.0	111	3.4	0	3.4	—	—	171	226	110	51	179	134	41	—	196
NOODLES, EGG, cooked	70.4	125	4.1	2.6	1.5	—	—	202	273	137	70	198	173	46	—	243
OATMEAL, dry	8.3	390	14.2	0	14.2	309	261	733	1065	521	209	758	470	183	524	845
RICE, BROWN, long grain, cooked	70.3	119	2.5	0	2.5	—	—	119	218	99	45	127	99	28	—	177
RICE, WHITE, enriched, long grain, cooked	72.6	109	2.0	0	2.0	—	—	96	172	78	36	100	78	22	—	140
SPAGHETTI, enriched, cooked	72.0	111	3.4	0	3.4	—	—	170	225	109	51	177	133	41	—	194
WHEAT GERM, dry	11.5	363	26.6	0	26.6	—	—	1270	1840	1650	430	970	1430	270	—	1460
BREAKFAST CEREALS																
SHREDDED WHEAT	6.6	354	9.9	0	9.9	204	236	449	684	331	139	481	405	85	236	577
FLOURS																
FLOUR, WHITE, all purpose, enriched	12.0	364	10.5	0	10.5	210	210	483	809	239	138	577	302	129	359	453
DESSERTS & SWEETS																
GELATIN, unsweetened, dry powder	13.0	335	85.6	85.6	0	77	771	1357	2930	4226	787	2036	1912	6	401	2421
GELATIN, sweetened, dry powder	1.6	371	9.4	9.4	0	—	—	94	207	301	56	150	141	—	—	169
TOPPINGS, DESSERT																
non-dairy powdered	1.5	577	4.9	4.9	0	21	145	301	484	394	149	263	207	68	280	351
non-dairy pressurized	60.4	264	1.0	1.0	0	4	29	60	97	79	30	53	41	14	56	70
non-dairy frozen, semisolid	50.2	318	1.3	1.3	0	5	37	77	123	101	38	67	53	17	72	89
EGGS AND SUBSTITUTES																
EGG, WHOLE, fresh & frozen, raw	74.6	158	12.1	12.1	0	289	293	759	1066	820	392	686	596	194	505	874
EGG WHITE, fresh & frozen, raw	88.1	49	10.1	10.1	0	251	230	618	883	625	394	638	451	156	407	759
EGG YOLK, fresh, raw	48.8	369	16.4	16.4	0	291	394	939	1396	1110	417	714	890	241	706	1000
EGG OMELET, made w/butter and milk	76.3	148	9.3	9.3	0	208	227	581	883	641	294	519	453	147	394	666
EGG, WHOLE, POACHED	74.3	157	12.1	12.1	0	288	292	756	1062	816	391	683	594	193	503	870
EGG, WHOLE, DRIED	4.1	594	45.8	45.8	0	1093	1107	2876	4026	3094	1481	2588	2251	733	1907	3300
EGGNOG	74.4	135	3.8	3.8	0	38	95	230	369	298	87	182	175	54	182	253
DUCK EGG, whole fresh, raw	70.8	185	12.8	12.8	0	285	320	598	1097	951	576	840	736	260	613	885

Footnote at end of table

(Continued)

TABLE P-16 *(Continued)*

FOOD NAME— 100 Gram (3.5 oz) Portion	Water	Food Energy Calories	Total Protein	Animal Protein	Plant Protein	Amino Acids Cystine	Histidine	Iso-leucine	Leucine	Lysine	Methi-onine	Phenyl-alanine	Threo-nine	Trypto-phan	Tyrosine	Valine
	(g)	(kcal)	(g)	(g)	(g)	(mg)	(mg)	(mg)	(mg)	(mg)	(mg)	(mg)	(mg)	(mg)	(mg)	(mg)
FATS & OILS																
MARGARINE, regular, soft, whipped, or low sodium	15.5	720	0.6	0	0.6	—	—	50	70	60	20	40	40	10	—	50
FISH & SEAFOODS																
ANCHOVY, pickled, canned	58.6	176	19.2	19.2	0	—	—	1067	1590	1840	607	772	900	209	—	1109
CAVIAR, sturgeon, granular	46.0	262	26.9	26.9	0	—	—	1510	2210	1920	700	1190	1620	240	—	1650
COD, cooked	64.6	129	28.5	28.5	0	—	—	1400	2084	2421	800	1010	1210	273	—	1463
FLOUNDER, baked	58.1	140	30.0	30.0	0	—	—	1530	2250	2640	870	1110	1290	300	—	1590
HADDOCK, cooked	66.3	90	19.6	19.6	0	—	—	1000	1491	1725	568	725	843	196	—	1039
HALIBUT, cooked	66.6	130	25.2	25.2	0	—	—	1285	1915	2218	731	933	1083	252	—	1336
HERRING, pickled	59.4	223	20.4	20.4	0	—	—	1040	1530	1775	592	755	877	204	—	1081
HERRING, w/tomato sauce, canned	66.7	176	15.8	14.8	1.0	—	—	806	1185	1375	458	585	679	158	—	837
LOBSTER, whole, cooked	76.8	95	18.7	18.7	0	—	—	742	1558	1721	580	852	798	164	—	815
SALMON, broiled or baked	63.4	182	27.0	27.0	0	—	—	1350	2025	2349	783	999	1161	270	—	1431
SALMON, canned, Sockeye (red)	67.2	171	20.2	20.3	0	271	—	1025	1526	1771	588	750	876	200	546	1076
SARDINE, Pacific canned, w/mustard	64.1	196	18.8	18.8	0	238	—	898	1337	1552	515	657	767	176	479	943
SHRIMP, canned	70.4	116	24.2	24.2	0	—	—	1234	1839	2130	702	895	1041	242	—	1283
SWORDFISH, broiled	64.6	174	28.0	28.0	0	—	—	1428	2100	2464	812	1036	1204	280	—	1484
TUNA, canned w/oil or water	60.6	197	28.8	28.8	0	—	—	1469	2160	2534	835	1066	1238	288	—	1526
WHITEFISH, lake, cooked	63.2	125	13.7	13.7	0	—	—	775	1140	1338	441	562	654	152	—	806
WHITEFISH, smoked	68.2	155	20.9	20.9	0	—	—	1066	1568	1839	606	773	899	209	—	1108
FLAVORINGS & SEASONINGS																
BASIL, ground	6.4	251	14.4	0	14.4	159	287	588	1078	618	202	733	588	221	432	717
DILL SEED	7.7	305	16.0	0	16.0	—	320	767	925	1038	143	670	575	—	—	1120
FENNEL SEED	8.8	345	15.8	0	15.8	222	331	695	996	758	301	647	602	253	410	915
FENUGREEK SEED	8.8	323	23.0	0	23.0	369	668	1241	1757	1684	338	1089	898	391	764	1102
GARLIC POWDER	6.4	332	18.6	0	16.8	172	309	648	1027	578	336	484	468	215	215	712
GINGER, ground	9.4	347	9.1	0	9.1	42	158	266	387	299	67	236	187	63	102	382
MUSTARD SEED, YELLOW	6.9	469	24.9	0	24.9	582	762	1081	1783	1519	480	1067	1095	526	744	1325
ONION POWDER	5.0	347	10.1	0	10.1	181	136	293	327	467	86	249	199	120	232	238
POPPY SEED	6.8	533	18.0	0	18.0	453	528	905	1484	1099	470	882	905	255	681	1287
SESAME SEEDS, decorticated	4.8	588	26.4	0	26.4	523	677	1289	2150	831	896	1528	1180	473	1125	1478
THYME, ground	7.8	276	9.1	0	9.1	274	—	468	430	207	274	482	252	186	482	502
FRUITS																
APPLE, w/skin, raw	84.4	58	0.2	0	0.2	—	—	—	—	—	—	6	—	—	3	—
APRICOTS, raw	85.3	51	1.0	0	1.0	—	—	—	—	—	—	24	—	—	—	—
AVOCADO, raw	74.0	167	2.1	0	2.1	—	—	—	—	74	12	—	—	14	—	—
BANANA, raw	75.7	85	1.1	0	1.1	—	—	—	—	55	11	34	—	18	33	—
CANTALOUPE, cubed, raw	91.2	30	0.7	0	0.7	—	—	—	—	15	2	21	—	1	—	—
DATES, moisturized or hydrated	22.5	274	2.2	0	2.2	—	49	74	77	65	27	61	61	61	17	94
FIGS, dried, uncooked	23.0	274	4.3	0	4.3	—	—	—	—	—	—	107	—	—	179	—
GRAPEFRUIT, sections, all varieties, raw	88.4	41	0.5	0	0.5	—	—	—	—	6	0	—	—	1	—	—
GRAPES, GREEN, seedless raw, Thompson	81.4	67	0.6	0	0.6	11	25	6	14	15	23	18	19	3	11	19
HONEYDEW MELON	90.6	33	0.8	0	0.8	—	—	—	—	15	2	—	—	1	—	—
LIME, acid type	89.3	28	0.7	0	0.7	—	—	—	—	15	2	—	—	3	—	—
MANGO, raw	81.7	66	0.7	0	0.7	—	—	—	—	93	8	—	—	14	—	—
NECTARINES, raw	81.8	64	0.6	0	0.6	—	—	—	—	—	—	19	—	—	—	—
ORANGE, raw	86.0	49	1.0	0	1.0	—	—	—	—	24	3	12	—	3	21	—
PEACH, raw	89.1	38	0.6	0	0.6	9	17	13	29	30	31	12	27	4	15	40
PEAR, canned, water pack	91.1	32	0.2	0	0.2	—	—	—	—	—	—	6	—	—	10	—
PEAR, canned, heavy syrup	79.8	76	0.2	0	0.2	—	—	—	—	—	—	6	—	—	10	—
PINEAPPLE, raw	85.3	52	0.4	0	0.4	—	—	—	—	9	1	8	—	5	8	—
PINEAPPLE, canned, water pack	89.1	39	0.3	0	0.3	—	—	—	—	7	1	8	—	4	8	—
PRUNES, dried, uncooked	28.0	255	2.1	0	2.1	—	—	—	—	—	—	88	—	—	—	—
RAISINS, uncooked	18.0	289	2.5	0	2.5	—	—	—	—	—	—	36	—	—	—	—
STRAWBERRIES, fresh	89.9	37	0.7	0	0.7	7	16	18	42	32	1	17	25	9	26	23
TANGERINE, raw	87.0	46	0.8	0	0.8	—	—	—	—	28	4	—	—	5	—	—
WATERMELON, raw	92.6	26	0.5	0	0.5	—	—	—	—	—	—	12	—	—	12	—
JUICES																
GRAPEFRUIT, canned, unsweetened	90.0	39	0.5	0	0.5	—	—	—	—	6	0	11	—	1	6	—
ORANGE, canned, unsweetened	87.4	48	0.8	0	0.8	—	—	—	—	21	2	—	—	3	—	—
PINEAPPLE, canned, unsweetened	85.6	55	0.4	0	0.4	—	—	—	—	9	1	—	—	5	—	—
TOMATO, canned or bottled	93.6	19	0.9	0	0.9	—	—	26	37	38	6	25	30	8	—	25
MEAT																
BEEF																
dried, chipped, uncooked	47.7	203	34.3	34.3	0	—	—	1795	2809	2996	850	1410	1515	401	—	1903
flank steak, braised	61.4	196	30.5	30.5	0	—	—	1793	2808	2999	851	1409	1513	401	—	1904
hamburger (ground beef), cooked	54.2	286	24.2	24.2	0	—	—	1342	2101	224̈	636	1055	1132	300	—	1424
kidney, braised	53.0	252	33.0	33.0	0	—	—	942	1678	1402	396	911	858	285	—	1130
liver, fried	—	229	26.4	26.3	0.1	—	—	1246	2197	1781	560	1200	1130	357	—	1495
stew w/vegetables, canned	82.5	79	5.8	—	—	—	—	282	427	459	126	235	241	67	—	308
tongue, braised	60.8	244	21.5	21.5	0	—	—	792	1286	1364	356	661	708	196	—	840

Footnote at end of table

TABLE P-16 *(Continued)*

FOOD NAME— 100 Gram (3.5 oz) Portion	Water	Food Energy Calories	Total Protein	Animal Protein	Plant Protein	Amino Acids										
						Cystine	Histidine	Iso-leucine	Leucine	Lysine	Methi-onine	Phenyl-alanine	Threo-nine	Trypto-phan	Tyrosine	Valine
	(g)	(kcal)	(g)	(g)	(g)	(mg)	(mg)	(mg)	(mg)	(mg)	(mg)	(mg)	(mg)	(mg)	(mg)	(mg)
MEAT *(Continued)*																
CHICKEN																
chicken, canned	65.2	198	21.7	21.7	0	—	—	1100	1507	1830	543	820	887	253	—	1023
liver, simmered	65.0	165	26.5	26.5	0	—	—	1533	2707	2197	690	1480	1393	440	—	1847
LAMB																
ground, cooked	54.0	279	25.3	25.3	0	—	—	1332	1990	2081	617	1045	1176	332	—	1267
leg roast, roasted	54.0	279	25.3	25.3	0	—	—	1332	1990	2081	617	1045	1176	332	—	1267
LUNCHEON MEATS																
BRAUNSCHWEIGER (smoked liver sausage)	52.6	319	15.4	15.4	0	187	458	754	1291	1200	320	700	668	172	471	956
CORNED BEEF, canned	59.3	216	25.3	25.3	0	—	—	1185	1857	1982	560	932	1000	264	—	1260
HEAD CHEESE	58.8	268	15.5	15.5	0	209	278	509	946	907	250	569	418	79	569	617
LIVERWURST	53.9	307	16.2	16.2	0	203	497	818	1400	1301	347	759	724	187	510	1037
POLISH SAUSAGE (kolbassi), cooked	53.7	304	15.7	15.7	0	—	—	1420	1580	1717	507	800	890	147	—	1080
SALAMI, beef	29.8	450	23.8	23.8	0	298	642	1159	1713	1923	505	872	979	203	776	1201
SPICED LUNCHEON MEATS, pork/ham type	54.9	294	15.0	15.0	0	241	479	741	1151	1252	362	570	610	143	575	775
VIENNA SAUSAGE	63.0	240	14.0	14.0	0	197	425	766	1133	1272	334	576	647	134	513	794
PORK																
Canadian bacon, cooked	49.9	277	27.6	27.6	0	—	—	1471	2281	2481	719	1129	1210	286	—	1538
Loin roast or chops, cooked	45.8	362	24.5	24.5	0	—	—	1279	1833	2044	621	980	1155	323	—	1295
VEAL																
cutlet, braised or broiled	60.4	216	27.1	27.1	0	—	—	1751	2429	2769	758	1346	1438	435	—	1714
loin roast or chop, cooked	58.9	234	26.4	26.4	0	—	—	1189	1657	1889	517	919	981	297	—	1169
TURKEY, canned	64.9	202	20.9	20.9	0	—	—	1109	1611	1904	586	837	900	—	—	1046
MILK & PRODUCTS																
BUTTER, regular or unsalted	15.9	717	0.9	0.9	0	8	23	51	83	67	21	41	38	12	41	57
CHEESE																
AMERICAN, pasteurized process	39.2	375	22.1	22.1	0	142	903	1024	1958	2198	573	1125	719	323	1212	1326
AMERICAN, spread, pasteurized process	47.7	290	16.4	16.4	0	—	509	833	1780	1507	538	931	628	—	890	1366
BLUE	42.4	353	21.4	21.4	0	108	759	1126	1922	1855	585	1089	786	313	1297	1559
BRICK	41.1	371	23.2	23.2	0	131	823	1137	2244	2124	565	1231	882	324	1115	1472
BRIE	48.4	334	28.8	20.8	0	114	716	1015	1929	1851	592	1158	751	322	1200	1340
CAMEMBERT	51.8	300	19.8	19.8	0	109	683	968	1840	1766	565	1105	717	307	1145	1279
CHEDDAR, shredded	36.8	403	24.9	24.9	0	125	874	1546	2385	2072	652	1311	886	320	1202	1663
COLBY	38.2	394	23.8	23.8	0	119	834	1475	2275	1978	622	1251	845	305	1147	1586
COTTAGE,creamed	79.0	103	12.5	12.5	0	116	415	734	1284	1010	376	673	554	139	666	773
COTTAGE, lowfat, 2% fat	79.3	90	13.7	13.7	0	127	457	808	1413	1111	413	741	609	153	732	851
CREAM	53.8	349	7.6	7.6	0	66	271	399	731	676	181	419	321	67	360	443
EDAM	41.6	357	25.0	25.0	0	—	1034	1308	2570	2660	721	1434	932	—	1457	1810
GOUDA	41.5	356	24.9	24.9	0	—	1032	1306	2564	2654	719	1431	930	—	1454	1806
GRUYERE	33.2	413	29.8	29.8	0	304	117	1612	3102	2710	822	1743	1089	421	1776	2243
LIMBURGER	48.4	327	20.0	20.0	0	—	578	1219	2093	1675	619	1116	739	289	1197	1439
MONTEREY	41.0	373	24.5	24.5	0	123	859	1519	2344	2037	641	1289	871	315	1182	1635
MOZZARELLA	54.1	281	19.4	19.4	0	116	731	931	1893	1972	542	1014	740	—	1123	1215
MUENSTER	41.8	368	23.4	23.4	0	132	829	1145	2260	2139	569	1240	888	327	1123	1482
PARMESAN, grated	17.7	456	41.6	41.6	0	274	1609	2202	4013	3843	1114	2234	1531	560	2319	2853
PIMIENTO, pasteurized process	39.1	375	22.1	—	—	142	902	1023	1956	2196	572	1124	718	323	1211	1325
PORT DU SALUT	45.5	352	23.8	23.8	0	—	686	1446	2482	1987	734	1323	876	343	1420	1707
PROVOLONE	41.0	351	25.6	25.6	0	116	1115	1091	2297	2646	686	1287	982	—	1520	1640
RICOTTA, made w/whole milk	71.7	174	11.3	11.3	0	99	459	589	1221	1338	281	556	517	—	589	692
RICOTTA, made w/part skim milk	74.4	138	11.4	11.4	0	100	464	596	1235	1353	284	562	523	—	596	700
SWISS	37.2	376	28.4	28.4	0	290	1065	1537	2959	2585	784	1662	1038	401	1693	2139
CREAM																
half & half (milk & cream, fluid)	80.6	130	3.0	3.0	0	27	80	179	290	235	74	143	134	42	143	198
heavy whipping	57.7	345	2.0	2.0	0	19	56	124	201	163	51	99	93	29	99	137
CREAM SUBSTITUTES																
non-dairy liquid, w/hydrogenated vegetable oil & soy protein	77.3	136	1.0	0	1.0	18	28	56	85	68	15	55	43	15	37	56
non-dairy, powdered	2.2	546	4.8	4.8	0	21	142	294	473	385	145	257	203	.66	274	343
ICE CREAM																
French vanilla ice cream, soft serve	59.8	218	4.1	4.1	0	42	109	244	393	317	102	195	188	58	194	269
vanilla ice cream, regular (10% fat) hardened	60.8	202	3.6	3.6	0	33	98	218	354	286	91	174	163	51	174	242
vanilla ice milk, hardened	68.6	140	3.9	3.9	0	36	107	238	386	312	99	190	178	56	190	264
orange sherbet	66.1	140	1.1	1.1	0	10	30	68	110	89	28	54	51	16	54	75
MILK, COW'S																
whole milk, 3.7% fat	87.7	64	3.3	3.3	0	30	89	198	321	260	82	158	148	46	158	220
lowfat milk, 2% fat	89.2	50	3.3	3.3	0	31	90	201	326	264	84	161	150	47	161	223

Footnote at end of table

TABLE P-16 (Continued)

FOOD NAME— 100 Gram (3.5 oz) Portion	Water (g)	Food Energy Calories (kcal)	Total Protein (g)	Animal Protein (g)	Plant Protein (g)	Cystine (mg)	Histidine (mg)	Iso-leucine (mg)	Leucine (mg)	Lysine (mg)	Methi-onine (mg)	Phenyl-alanine (mg)	Threo-nine (mg)	Trypto-phan (mg)	Tyrosine (mg)	Valine (mg)
MILK & PRODUCTS *(Continued)*																
MILK, COW'S *(Continued)*																
skim milk	90.8	35	3.4	3.4	0	32	92	206	334	270	86	165	154	48	165	228
chocolate milk, whole, 3.3% fat	82.3	83	3.2	3.2	0	29	86	192	311	251	79	153	143	45	153	212
chocolate milk, 2% fat	83.6	72	3.2	3.2	0	30	87	194	314	255	81	155	145	45	155	215
buttermilk, cultured	90.1	40	3.3	3.3	0	31	95	204	329	277	81	174	158	36	139	243
whole milk, evaporated, canned	74.0	134	6.8	6.8	0	63	185	412	667	540	171	329	307	96	329	456
sweetened condensed milk, canned	27.2	321	7.9	7.9	0	73	214	479	775	627	198	382	357	112	382	529
nonfat dry milk powder, instantized	4.0	358	35.1	35.1	0	325	952	2124	3438	2784	880	1694	1584	495	1694	2349
hot cocoa, homemade w/whole milk	81.6	87	3.6	3.6	0	34	99	220	357	289	91	176	164	51	176	244
malted milk powder, natural flavor	2.6	411	13.1	—	—	261	261	391	749	356	180	439	335	140	362	445
malted milk beverage, chocolate flavor	81.2	88	3.5	—	—	11	28	61	100	79	26	51	47	14	50	71
milkshake, vanilla flavor, thick type	74.4	112	3.9	—	—	36	105	234	378	306	97	186	174	54	186	258
milkshake, chocolate flavor, thick type	72.2	119	3.0	—	—	28	83	185	299	242	76	147	138	43	147	204
MILK, GOAT'S, whole	87.0	69	3.6	3.6	0	46	89	207	314	290	80	155	163	44	179	240
MILK, HUMAN, whole	87.5	70	1.0	1.0	0	19	23	56	95	68	21	46	46	17	53	63
YOGURT																
plain	87.9	61	3.5	3.5	0	—	86	189	350	311	102	189	142	20	175	287
plain, lowfat	85.1	63	5.3	5.3	0	—	130	286	529	471	155	286	216	30	265	434
coffee & vanilla varieties, lowfat	79.0	85	4.9	4.9	0	—	122	269	497	442	145	269	202	28	249	408
fruit varieties, lowfat (10 g protein/8 oz)	74.5	102	4.4	—	—	—	108	238	440	392	129	238	179	25	221	362
NUTS & SEEDS																
ALMONDS	4.7	598	18.6	0	18.6	377	517	873	1454	582	259	1146	610	176	618	1124
BRAZIL NUTS	4.6	654	14.3	0	14.3	—	—	593	1129	443	941	617	422	187	—	832
CASHEW NUTS	5.2	561	17.2	0	17.2	—	—	1135	1410	740	327	877	688	430	—	1479
COCONUT, fresh	50.9	346	3.4	0	3.4	62	69	180	269	152	71	174	129	33	101	212
COCONUT, dried, shredded, sweetened	3.3	548	3.6	0	3.6	—	—	190	284	162	75	183	136	35	—	223
FILBERTS OR HAZELNUTS	5.8	634	12.7	0	12.7	165	288	853	939	417	139	537	415	211	434	934
PEANUTS, roasted, Spanish or Virginia	1.6	585	26.0	0	26.0	—	—	1355	2003	1176	290	1666	886	364	—	1639
PEANUT BUTTER	1.8	581	26.1	0	26.1	449	727	1228	1816	1066	263	1510	803	330	1071	1487
PECANS	3.4	687	9.4	0	9.4	216	273	553	773	435	153	564	389	138	316	525
PISTACHIO NUTS	5.3	594	18.9	0	18.9	385	471	881	1523	1080	367	1088	613	—	667	1344
PUMPKIN OR SQUASH SEEDS	4.4	553	29.0	0	29.0	—	—	1624	2291	1334	551	1624	870	522	—	1566
SUNFLOWER SEED KERNELS, hulled	4.8	560	23.0	0	23.0	464	586	1276	1736	868	443	1220	911	343	647	1354
WALNUTS, ENGLISH	3.5	651	15.0	0	15.0	320	405	767	1228	441	306	767	589	175	583	974
PICKLES & RELISHES																
BREAD & BUTTER PICKLES	78.7	73	0.9	0	0.9	—	—	28	39	40	9	21	24	6	—	31
DILL PICKLE, whole	93.3	11	0.7	0	0.7	—	—	22	30	31	7	16	19	5	—	24
OLIVE, ripe	73.0	184	1.2	0	1.2	—	24	53	79	15	17	45	40	—	38	60
PEPPER, HOT CHILI, green, canned	92.5	25	0.9	0	0.9	—	—	34	34	38	12	42	38	6	—	25
PICKLE, SWEET	60.7	146	0.7	0	0.7	—	—	22	30	31	7	16	19	5	—	24
PIMIENTOS, canned	92.4	27	0.9	0	0.9	—	22	37	60	48	6	45	43	—	22	49
SALADS																
COLESLAW, w/salad dressing	82.9	99	1.2	0	1.2	—	—	47	48	56	11	25	34	10	—	36
SNACK FOODS																
POPCORN, plain	4.0	386	12.7	0	12.7	—	—	593	1671	371	243	579	514	79	—	657
POPCORN, popped in coconut oil w/salt	3.1	456	9.8	0	9.8	—	—	461	1300	289	189	450	400	61	—	511
POTATO CHIPS	1.8	568	5.3	0	5.3	—	—	233	265	281	64	233	217	53	—	281
SOUPS & CHOWDERS																
BEEF BROTH, bouillon, consomme, canned, diluted w/water	5.8	13	2.1	2.1	0	—	—	27	70	76	14	47	79	1	—	58
BEEF NOODLE, canned, diluted w/water	92.8	29	1.6	—	—	—	—	80	65	156	56	65	75	14	—	77
CHICKEN NOODLE, canned, diluted w/water	93.1	27	1.5	—	—	—	—	80	75	180	43	75	65	13	—	55
CHICKEN W/RICE, canned, diluted w/water	94.7	22	1.3	—	—	—	—	60	65	176	47	52	50	11	—	40
CHICKEN VEGETABLE, canned, diluted w/water	92.3	30	1.7	—	—	—	—	62	92	87	21	47	53	18	—	56
CREAM OF ASPARAGUS, canned, diluted w/milk	85.2	69	2.7	—	—	—	—	159	254	181	57	119	155	28	—	173
CREAM OF CHICKEN, canned, diluted w/water	92.2	38	1.4	—	—	—	—	60	60	115	42	53	50	11	—	47
CREAM OF MUSHROOM, canned, diluted w/milk	83.4	92	2.6	—	—	—	—	151	213	227	85	124	109	31	—	152
CREAM OF SHRIMP, frozen, made w/milk	81.8	100	3.8	—	—	—	—	194	316	265	84	165	242	38	—	209
MINESTRONE, canned, diluted w/water	91.2	36	1.6	0	1.6	—	—	68	98	78	16	56	54	17	—	71
ONION, canned, diluted w/water	94.5	24	1.5	—	—	—	—	39	85	86	15	47	99	6	—	58
PEA, green, canned, diluted w/water	85.1	58	3.5	1.1	2.3	—	—	135	167	359	43	141	104	22	—	42
TURKEY NOODLE, canned, diluted w/water	92.7	32	1.6	—	—	—	—	92	108	81	23	53	58	16	—	70
TOMATO, canned, diluted w/water	90.5	36	0.8	0	0.8	—	—	33	28	75	32	37	27	6	—	25
VEGETABLE BEEF, canned, diluted w/water	91.9	33	2.1	—	—	—	—	71	170	234	36	92	94	21	—	124

Footnote at end of table

(Continued)

TABLE P-16 *(Continued)*

FOOD NAME—100 Gram (3.5 oz) Portion	Water	Food Energy Calories	Total Protein	Animal Protein	Plant Protein	Amino Acids										
						Cystine	Histidine	Iso-leucine	Leucine	Lysine	Methionine	Phenyl-alanine	Threonine	Trypto-phan	Tyrosine	Valine
	(g)	(kcal)	(g)	(g)	(g)	(mg)	(mg)	(mg)	(mg)	(mg)	(mg)	(mg)	(mg)	(mg)	(mg)	(mg)
VEGETABLES																
ASPARAGUS, green, cooked	93.6	20	2.2	0	2.2	—	—	79	97	103	33	68	66	26	—	106
white, canned	92.3	22	2.1	0	2.1	—	—	56	68	73	14	48	46	19	—	75
BEANS, common, red (kidney), unsalted, cooked	69.0	118	7.8	0	7.8	—	—	437	671	577	78	429	335	70	—	468
common, white, canned w/pork & sweet sauce	66.4	150	6.2	Trace	6.2	—	—	355	536	462	62	343	269	56	—	381
green, cut or french style, boiled	92.4	25	1.6	0	1.6	—	—	72	92	83	24	38	60	21	—	76
lima, frozen, cooked	73.5	99	6.0	0	6.0	—	—	429	614	496	118	437	348	67	—	466
sprouts (mung beans), cooked	91.0	28	3.2	0	3.2	—	—	179	291	218	35	154	99	22	—	189
BEET GREENS, cooked	93.6	18	1.7	0	1.7	—	—	71	109	92	29	99	65	20	—	85
BEETS, red, whole, cooked	90.0	32	1.1	0	1.1	—	—	34	37	59	4	18	22	9	—	33
BROCCOLI, raw	89.1	32	3.6	0	3.6	—	—	137	176	158	54	131	133	40	124	184
BRUSSELS SPROUTS, cooked	88.2	36	4.2	0	4.2	—	—	176	185	189	42	151	147	42	86	185
CABBAGE, raw	92.4	24	1.3	0	1.3	28	25	40	57	66	13	32	39	11	27	43
CABBAGE, RED, raw	90.2	31	2.0	0	2.0	-	—	78	80	94	18	50	56	16	41	60
CARROT, raw	88.2	42	1.1	0	1.1	29	17	46	65	52	10	36	43	10	17	56
CAULIFLOWER, raw, whole flowers	91.0	27	2.7	0	2.7	—	—	116	181	151	54	84	113	35	—	162
cooked	92.8	22	2.3	0	2.3	—	—	99	154	129	46	71	97	30	—	138
CELERY, raw	94.1	17	0.9	0	0.9	—	1	19	22	25	2	15	16	—	7	26
CHICORY GREENS, raw	92.8	20	1.8	0	1.8	6	24	—	—	52	16	—	—	24	40	—
COLLARDS, leaves & stems, cooked	90.8	29	2.7	0	2.7	—	—	84	151	140	32	86	78	38	—	135
CORN, sweet, cooked, cut off cob before cooking	76.5	83	3.2	0	3.2	—	—	—	—	—	—	—	—	—	—	—
sweet, cooked on cob, white/yellow	74.1	91	3.3	0	3.3	—	—	122	363	122	63	185	135	20	88	208
CUCUMBER, raw, pared	95.7	14	0.6	0	0.6	—	—	18	26	26	6	14	16	4	—	20
DANDELION GREENS, cooked	89.8	33	2.0	0	2.0	—	—	—	—	—	—	—	—	—	—	—
ENDIVE, curly, & escarole, raw	93.1	20	1.7	0	1.7	13	31	72	123	78	22	78	71	—	54	81
KOHLRABI, cooked	92.2	24	1.7	0	1.7	—	—	—	—	—	—	43	—	—	—	—
LENTILS, whole seeds, cooked	72.0	106	7.8	0	7.8	—	—	413	554	476	55	359	273	70	—	421
LETTUCE, Bibb or Boston, raw	95.1	14	1.2	0	1.2	—	—	—	—	70	4	—	—	12	—	—
MUSHROOMS, raw, *Agaricus campestris*	90.4	28	2.7	0	2.7	—	—	597	316	—	189	—	—	8	—	424
MUSTARD GREENS, leaves w/o stems & midribs, boiled	92.6	23	2.2	0	2.2	—	—	73	59	108	22	70	57	35	—	103
OKRA PODS, cooked	91.1	29	2.0	0	2.0	—	—	78	112	84	24	72	74	20	—	100
ONION, raw	89.1	38	1.5	0	1.5	—	14	21	37	64	13	38	22	21	42	31
PARSLEY, raw	85.1	44	3.6	0	3.6	—	—	—	—	230	18	—	72	—	—	—
PEAS, green, immature, raw	78.0	84	6.3	0	6.3	—	—	290	397	296	44	223	101	50	161	258
PEPPERS, green, sweet, raw	93.4	22	1.2	0	1.2	—	14	46	46	51	16	55	50	9	—	33
POTATO, baked in skin	75.1	93	2.6	0	2.6	—	101	463	486	330	70	295	225	90	84	420
pared, boiled	82.8	65	1.9	0	1.9	—	—	84	95	101	23	84	78	19	—	101
french fried	44.7	274	4.3	0	4.3	—	—	184	210	222	50	184	172	42	—	222
RADISHES, raw	94.5	17	1.0	0	1.0	—	—	—	—	34	2	—	59	5	—	30
SOYBEANS, mature seeds, cooked	71.0	130	11.0	0	11.0	—	—	649	935	759	165	594	423	165	—	638
SPINACH, raw	90.7	26	3.2	0	3.2	—	—	150	246	198	54	145	141	51	116	176
SQUASH, summer, cooked	95.5	14	0.9	0	0.9	—	—	29	41	34	12	24	21	7	—	33
winter, baked	81.4	63	1.8	0	1.8	—	—	58	81	68	23	49	41	14	—	66
SWEET POTATO, baked in skin	63.7	141	2.1	0	2.1	—	—	101	120	99	38	104	99	36	61	157
TOMATO, raw	93.5	22	1.1	0	1.1	—	15	29	41	42	7	28	33	9	24	28
TOMATO, GREEN, raw	93.0	24	1.2	0	1.2	—	15	29	41	42	7	28	33	9	14	28
TOMATO PASTE, canned, w/o salt	75.0	82	3.4	0	3.4	—	58	70	95	98	18	72	78	—	45	78
TOMATO PUREE, canned	87.0	39	1.7	0	1.7	—	—	49	70	71	12	48	56	15	—	48
TURNIP GREENS, frozen, chopped, cooked	92.7	23	2.5	0	2.5	—	—	81	156	99	40	100	95	35	71	112
TURNIP, cooked	93.6	23	0.8	0	0.8	—	—	14	—	42	9	17	—	—	21	—
WATER CRESS or GARDEN CRESS, raw	89.4	32	2.6	0	2.6	—	—	140	230	160	20	110	150	50	—	150

[1]The authors gratefully acknowledge that these food compositions were obtained from the HVH-CWRU Data Base developed by the Division of Nutrition, Highland View Hospital, and the Departments of Biometry and Nutrition, School of Medicine, Case Western Reserve University, Cleveland, Ohio.

PROTEIN, ANIMAL

Generally high quality protein derived from meat, milk, poultry, fish, and eggs, and their products.

(Also see PROTEIN[S].)

PROTEIN AS ENERGY SOURCE

In the body, protein functions in the (1) building of new tissues, (2) upkeep of tissues, (3) regulation of water and acid base balance, (4) production of enzymes, antibodies, hormones, and vitamins, (5) formation of milk, and (6) provision of energy. When more protein is eaten than is needed for the first five functions listed above, the excess protein is metabolized for energy. In addition, protein of the diet, along with tissue proteins, is burned for energy when the diet contains insufficient carbohydrates and fats. When this occurs, the building or repair processes of the body suffer. However, energy needs of the body have a higher priority. As a source of energy, protein yields about 4 kcal/g.

(Also see METABOLISM; PROTEIN[S]; and BIOLOGICAL VALUE [BV] OF PROTEINS.)

PROTEIN-BOUND IODINE (PBI)

The iodine that is bound to thyroxin and in transit in the plasma is known as protein-bound iodine. In the normal individual, PBI values range from 4 to 8 micrograms/100 milliliters of plasma.

PROTEIN, COMPLETE

Casein and egg albumin are examples of complete proteins. They contain all of the essential amino acids in sufficient amounts to maintain life and support growth.

(Also see PROTEIN[S], Table P-16.)

PROTEIN, CRUDE

This refers to all the nitrogenous compounds in a food. It is determined by finding the nitrogen content, as determined by the Kjeldahl process, and multiplying the result by 6.25. The nitrogen content of protein averages about 16% ($100 \div 16 = 6.25$).

(Also see PROTEIN[S].)

PROTEIN EFFICIENCY RATIO (PER)

By definition, *it is the weight gain of a young growing animal expressed in grams divided by the grams of protein eaten over a 4-week period, or some other predetermined time.* It provides a biological means for evaluating protein quantity. Casein and egg albumin yield the maximum values, while proteins like gliadin will not even support growth.

(Also see PROTEIN[S] section on Quantity and Quality; and BIOLOGICAL VALUE [BV] OF PROTEINS.)

PROTEIN FACTOR

A number used to convert the Kjeldahl nitrogen content of food to protein, since most of the nitrogen measured by the Kjeldahl method is derived from the protein contained in the food. On the average, protein contains about 16% nitrogen (16 g of nitrogen for every 100 g of protein); however, this can range from 15 to 18%. For most foods, to determine the crude protein content, the Kjeldahl nitrogen value is multiplied by 6.25 ($100 \div 16$). Where greater accuracy is desired, the specific factor for converting nitrogen to protein may be used. For example, the factor for most nuts is 5.30 while for milk and cheese it is 6.38.

(Also see KJELDAHL; and PROTEIN[S].)

PROTEIN HYDROLYSATE

A solution containing the amino acids derived from an artificially digested protein, usually milk or beef protein. Used extensively in medicine and surgery. Usually administered by a stomach tube or intravenous injection.

PROTEIN, INCOMPLETE

A protein that cannot maintain life or support growth is classified as incomplete; for example, zein (corn protein) and gelatin.

(Also see PROTEIN[S].)

PROTEIN MALNUTRITION

When the diet fails to meet the body's needs for protein quality and quantity, impaired function, growth and/or development result. The extreme case of protein malnutrition is kwashiorkor, which develops in infants consuming a deficiency of protein and marginal to adequate amounts of energy. Often there is an inadequate or imbalance of both protein and energy; hence, it is convenient to class the resulting disorders as various types of protein-energy malnutrition (PEM).

(Also see DEFICIENCY DISEASES, Table D-1, Major Dietary Deficiency Diseases—"Protein-energy malnutrition"; MALNUTRITION; and MALNUTRITION, PROTEIN-ENERGY.)

PROTEIN, MILK

When the term milk refers to cow or human milk, the proteins involved are casein and lactalbumin, both high quality proteins. In cow milk, casein is the predominate protein. In human milk, casein and lactalbumin are present in about equal amounts. However, human milk contains only about one third as much protein as cow milk.

(Also see MILK AND MILK PRODUCTS; and PROTEIN[S].)

PROTEIN, PARTIALLY COMPLETE

Gliadin, a protein found in wheat, is an example of a partially complete protein. It can maintain life, but it cannot support growth.

(Also see PROTEIN[S].)

PROTEIN SCORE (CHEMICAL SCORE)

A chemical means of evaluating a protein on the basis of its amino acid content. More often this is called the chemical score or amino acid score.

(Also see PROTEIN[S], section headed "Quantity and Quality.")

PROTEIN, SINGLE-CELL

Protein obtained from single-cell organisms, such as yeast, bacteria, and algae, and grown on specially prepared growth media. Dried brewers' yeast is one of the most familiar examples.

(Also see PROTEIN[S], section headed "Protein of the World.")

PROTEIN, VEGETABLE

Protein derived from plants. Most vegetable protein supplements, although not all, are the by-products that remain after extracting oil from soybeans, cottonseed, linseed, peanuts, safflower, sunflower, rapeseed, and coconut. Soybean is by far the most widely used vegetable protein.

(Also see PROTEIN[S].)

PROTEINURIA

Presence of protein in the urine.

PROTEIN UTILIZATION (NET PROTEIN UTILIZATION; NPU)

A procedure employed to determine protein quality. It is the proportion of the nitrogen in the food that is retained by the tissues of the body. In other words, it is the amount of nitrogen contained in the food consumed, minus the amount lost in the urine and feces, divided by the amount of nitrogen in the food.

(Also see PROTEIN[S], section headed "Quantity and Quality.")

PROTEIN, WORLD PER CAPITA

Worldwide, there are about 69 g of protein available each day for every individual—an amount which should be more than adequate. However, each individual does not receive this amount and the following must be considered: (1) distribution of protein, (2) the source of protein, and (3) the calories available.

(Also see HUNGER, WORLD; INCOME, PROPORTION SPENT FOR FOOD; MALNUTRITION; POPULATION, WORLD; PROTEIN[S]; and WORLD FOOD.)

PROTEOLYSIS

The breakdown of proteins or peptides into smaller units—polypeptides tripeptides, dipeptides and amino acids. Digestion of proteins entails proteolysis.

(Also see DIGESTION AND ABSORPTION; and PROTEIN[S].)

PROTEOSE

A derivative of protein formed during digestion.

PROTHROMBIN

One of four blood clotting proteins synthesized by the liver, the manufacture of which is regulated by vitamin K, present in the blood plasma, essential to clotting of blood.

(Also see VITAMIN K.)

PROTHROMBIN ACTIVATOR

A complex substance that splits prothrombin to form thrombin, an essential step in the blood clotting process.

PROTON

A particle of the nucleus of an atom that has a charge of plus one. A proton is a positive hydrogen ion (H^+).

PROTOPLASM

The living matter in all cells.

PROTOPORPHYRIN

The precursor of heme.

PROVITAMIN A

Carotene.
(Also see VITAMIN A.)

PROXIMAL

Next to or nearest the point of attachment or origin.

PRUNE Prunus spp

A type of plum that may be dried satisfactorily without removal of the pith. Only a few of the many cultivated varieties of plums can be so dried. Usually, the prune types of plums have a higher than average sugar content.

(Also see PLUM AND PRUNE; and PRUNE JUICE.)

PRUNE JUICE

A water extract of dried prunes that is produced by (1) pulverizing the prunes (this may be done with the aid of enzymes that break down the pectin which binds the fruit tissue), and (2) leaching the prune pulp with hot water. The resulting prune juice may be either (1) sweetened, or (2) left unsweetened, because the natural sugar content of prunes is generally high.

The nutrient composition of prune juice is given in Food Composition Table F-21.

Some noteworthy observations regarding the nutrient composition of prune juice follow:

1. A ½-cup serving (*125 g*) of unsweetened prune juice is moderately high in calories (96 kcal) and carbohydrates (24 g).

2. Prune juice is an excellent source of iron and potassium, but it is a poor source of vitamins A and C.

3. Many people find that the consumption of prune juice helps to promote regularity of bowel movement. However, the amounts required to produce this effect vary considerably among different people, from as little as a small glass to as much as a pint or more.

(Also see PLUM AND PRUNE; and PRUNE.)

PSORIASIS

A condition of the skin wherein red, itchy patches frequently appear on the scalp, knees, elbows, chest, abdomen, palms, and soles of the feet. These red patches tend to grow and join together creating extensive, unsightly and uncomfortable areas. However, psoriasis seldom causes long-term physical harm. Its cause is obscure but there is evidence to suggest it runs in families. No single treatment exists which will completely clear up the disease. Some treatments providing relief include ointments containing coal tar derivatives or mercury compounds, cortisone pills or ointment, x rays, and sunbathing. In the past, low taurine—a product of cysteine metabolism and normal constituent of animal protein—diets were designed, and recommended for sufferers of psoriasis.

PSYCHROPHILIC BACTERIA

These bacteria are "cold lovers," but despite their name they actually tolerate cold rather than prefer it. Most bacteria, mesophiles, have optimal growth at 97-111°F (*37-44°C*). Psychrophiles grow and reproduce at the usual refrigeration temperatures. In fact, some types can substantially multiply at 32°F (*0°C*). These bacteria are important as they are responsible for most of the fresh food spoilage that occurs. Low temperatures should not be relied on to destroy bacteria. Even in frozen foods some bacteria survive; hence, after thawing, frozen foods should not be allowed to stand at room temperature.

(Also see BACTERIA IN FOOD.)

PSYLLIUM Plantago psyllium

An annual herb grown in southern Europe and India. It bears a seed that has laxative qualities and is used in medicines. When the seed is moistened, it looks like gelatin.

PTOMAINES

The word ptomaine comes from the Greek word *ptoma*, meaning *dead body*. It refers to a group of extremely poisonous organic compounds formed during the microbial or enzymatic decomposition of animal proteins. Ptomaines are easily detected by the deteriorated appearance of the material (almost to a liquid state) and the putrid odor. Such food is hardly human fare!

Food poisoning by bacterial toxins, such as salmonellosis or staphylococcal intoxication, is sometimes called *ptomaine poisoning,* which is incorrect.

(Also see BACTERIA IN FOOD.)

PUBERTY

The age at which the sex organs begin to function and at which sexual features begin to appear. The average age of puberty in boys is from 13 to 16, in girls from 11 to 14.

PUERPERIUM

The period from delivery of the infant to the time when the uterus regains its normal size, usually about 6 weeks.

PULP

The solid residue remaining after extraction of juices from fruits, roots, or stems.

PULSES

Pulses are the seeds of leguminous plants. The following pulses are commonly used for human food: beans, chickpeas, cowpeas, field peas, peanuts, pigeonpeas, and soybeans.

PUMMELO (POMELO; SHADDOCK)
Citrus grandis

This fruit is the largest of the citrus fruits (which belong to the family *Rutaceae*) ranging in size between 4 and 12 in. *(10 and 30 cm)* in diameter.

The pummelo was brought from its native home of Malaysia to Barbados in the 17th century by Captain Shaddock of the British East India Company. The grapefruit (*C. paradisi*), which was discovered in Barbados in 1750, is believed to have arisen as either a mutation or a natural hybrid of this fruit.

Pummelos are low in calories (34 kcal per 100 g) and carbohydrates (8.5%). However, they are also a good source of vitamin C.

(Also see GRAPEFRUIT.)

PUMPERNICKEL BREAD

This is a sourdough bread made from unbolted (unsifted) rye flour.

PUMPKINS *Cucurbita* spp

The fruits of these plants provide both edible flesh and edible seeds. Also, the flowers are edible. Pumpkins belong

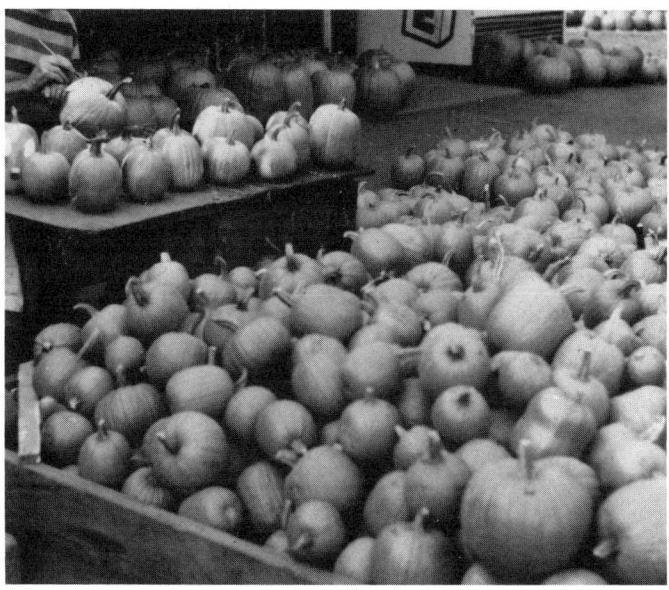

Fig. P-86. Pumpkins, a sign of autumn in North America. (Courtesy, New Jersey Department of Agriculture)

to the gourd or melon family (*Cucurbitaceae*), which also includes squashes and cucumbers. The different species of pumpkins are *C. maxima, C. mixta, C. moschata,* and *C. pepo.* Certain varieties of fruits within each of these species are squashes rather than pumpkins. Although there is some confusion between the terms *pumpkin* and *squash,* pumpkins are generally considered to be the large, orange fruits that have a coarse, strongly flavored flesh. They are not usually served as table vegetables, but are used mainly for (1) pies, and (2) decorations during the holidays in the fall.

ORIGIN AND HISTORY. The pumpkin descended from wild ancestors in Mexico and Guatemala, where it is reasonable to conclude that it has been under cultivation for at least 9,000 years. Most likely, the modern varieties with abundant sweet flesh arose when the Indians selected mutant varieties for cultivation.

WORLD AND U.S. PRODUCTION. Statistics on the world production of pumpkins are not available. *The FAO Production Yearbook* groups pumpkins, squash, and gourds together. Since squashes are much more widely grown and utilized than pumpkins, the combined data reflects mainly the production of squashes (See SQUASHES). Likewise, U.S. production figures on pumpkins are not available.

PROCESSING. Pumpkins are processed by removal of the rind and seeds, followed by cooking of the pulp prior to canning, freezing, or baking into cakes, custards, or pies.

Other noteworthy, but less common, pumpkin products are (1) dehydrated pumpkin flakes that are made by drum-drying cooked pumpkin puree which has been mixed with starch and sugar; (2) dehydrated pumpkin pie mix which contains dehydrated pumpkin flakes, dried milk powder, dried egg, sugar, corn syrup solids, starch, flavorings, and a vegetable gum; (3) pumpkin pickles made from pumpkin cubes that have been cooked briefly, then mixed with sugar, vinegar, water, and spices, and canned in glass jars; and (4) pumpkin seeds that are sold raw or roasted and salted.

SELECTION, PREPARATION, AND USES. The rind of a pumpkin should be hard. However, slight variations in the color of the skin do not affect the quality.

For the most part, pumpkins are either cooked or baked.

Some suggestions for utilizing the various parts of the pumpkin plant follow:

• **Pumpkin flesh**—The fruits should be cut into halves or small sections, the rind, fibrous matter, and seeds removed, and the remaining flesh cut into smaller pieces. Usually, a half hour to an hour of boiling is required to tenderize the flesh, but only 15 minutes of cooking in a pressure cooker is sufficient. Then, the cooked pumpkin may be mashed or pureed in a blender. The puree may require straining to remove residual fibers. Cooked pumpkin is usually made into custards, pies, and puddings. Canned, cooked pumpkin serves these purposes very well. However, Latin Americans utilize pumpkin mainly in soups and stews.

• **Pumpkin flowers**—These should be picked when open so that no bees will be trapped within the blossoms. The flowers are good when dipped in a batter and fried in deep fat.

• **Pumpkin seeds**—The seeds of pumpkins may be dried for a few days, after which any adhering tissue should be removed. Then, they may be roasted or fried in oil. Some people boil the seeds briefly in salted water before roasting or frying.

NUTRITIONAL VALUE. The nutrient compositions of various forms of pumpkin are given in Food Composition Table F-21.

Some noteworthy observations regarding the nutrient composition of pumpkin follow:

1. Fresh and canned pumpkin contains over 90% water and is low in calories (about 33 kcal per 100 g). However, it is an excellent source of vitamin A.

2. A 4 oz (*114 g*) serving of pumpkin pie plus an 8 oz (*244 g*) glass of milk constitute a nutritious meal for a growing child, except that insufficient iron is provided unless dark molasses is used as the sweetener in the pie. The pie supplies ample calories and vitamin A, a moderate amount of protein, and fair amounts of calcium and phosphorus; whereas the milk is rich in protein, calcium, phosphorus, and the vitamin B complex.

3. Pumpkin flowers contain 95% water and are low in calories (16 kcal per 100 g) and most other nutrients, except that they provide fair amounts of phosphorus, iron, vitamin A, and vitamin C. It is suggested that calorie-conscious people eat pumpkin flowers in a salad, soup, or stew.

4. The seeds from pumpkins are very rich in calories (553 kcal per 100 g), protein (29%), iron (11.2 mg per 100 g), and phosphorus (1,144 mg per 100 g). Hence, the consumption of as little as 1 oz (*28 g*) of the seeds per day will make a significant nutritional contribution to the diet.

PURGATIVE

A strong laxative.
(Also see LAXATIVE.)

PURINES

These are nitrogen-containing substances with a ring structure. They are widely distributed in nature, and are components of the nucleic acids. Important purines are adenine, guanine, xanthine, and uric acid, which is the excretory form of the purines in humans. Another common purine is the stimulant caffeine. Persons suffering from gout or uric acid kidney stones should limit their dietary sources of purines. Some of the richest food sources of purines are anchovies, asparagus, brains, kidney, liver, mincemeats, mushrooms, sardines, and sweetbreads. Foods with a low purine content include breads, cereals, fats, cheese, eggs, fruits, milk, nuts, sweets, and most vegetables.

(Also see ARTHRITIS, section headed "Gout [gouty arthritis]"; CAFFEINE; and NUCLEIC ACIDS.)

PURIS

A puri is a very light, fried wheat cake which originated in India. Butter is the preferred fat in which to fry it. Because it is an expensive dish, it is usually reserved for festive occasions.

PUROTHIONIN

A small, easily digested protein of wheat. It has antibacterial properties, and in excess it may interfere with the rising of dough.
(Also see WHEAT.)

PUTREFACTION

The decomposition of proteins by microorganisms under anaerobic conditions.

PUTRESCINE

A foul-smelling chemical which arises in the bacterial fermentation of animal protein. It can be formed from ornithine or the amino acid arginine.

PYRIMIDINE

The parent substance of several nitrogenous compounds found in nucleic acids. The principal pyrimidines found in RNA are uracil and cytosine; in DNA they are thymine and cytosine.
(Also see NUCLEIC ACIDS.)

PYRUVIC ACID (PYRUVATE; $CH_3COCOOH$)

An organic 3-carbon acid that is a key intermediate in carbohydrate, fat, and protein metabolism. It can participate in several metabolic pathways in the body. These pathways include (1) complete oxidation to water and carbon dioxide in the tricarboxylic acid (Krebs) cycle, (2) formation of fatty acid, (3) reversible conversion to lactic acid, (4) conversion to the amino acid alanine, and (5) formation of glucose by reversal of the enzymatic sequence which normally breaks down glucose.
(Also see METABOLISM.)

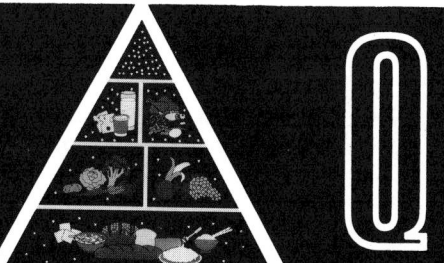

QUADRIPLEGIA

Paralysis of both arms and both legs. It can be caused by disease—poliomyelitis, Landry's acute ascending paralysis (due to an acute infection of the spinal cord), diptheria, leprosy—or injury which severs the spinal cord at the fifth or sixth cervical vertebra. Quadriplegics require some special dietary considerations due to reduced activity and difficulties encountered in preparing and eating food.

(Also see MODIFIED DIETS; and DISEASES.)

QUAIL (CALIFORNIA QUAIL, GAMBEL'S QUAIL, MEARN'S QUAIL, MOUNTAIN QUAIL, SCALED QUAIL)

Quail is the name given to several different kinds of birds. In Europe, it refers to several kinds of game birds of the pheasant family. Americans use the name for the bobwhite.

The bobwhite quail and the Japanese quail are listed in separate sections of this book. Other kinds of American quail are the California quail, Gambel's quail, Mearn's quail, mountain quail, and scaled quail. These birds live in western and southwestern United States.

All of the different quails are highly prized game birds and furnish good eating.

QUICK BREADS

Contents   Page

This term is usually applied to batters or doughs that are baked (in some cases, boiled, fried, grilled, or steamed) right after mixing, rather than being allowed to rise before baking. Hence, quick breads are not made with yeast. Instead, they are unleavened, or leavened with air, baking powder, a sourdough starter, or steam.

The elimination of the need for yeast leavening allows the use of a wide variety of flours that may contain little or no gluten—the elastic protein in wheat flour that helps to trap the leavening gas. Weaker flours may be used for quick breads because rising takes place in the oven, as the proteins in the dough are gradually made firm by baking. Furthermore, egg white has a greater strengthening effect on doughs that are baked right after mixing.

HISTORY. There is archaeological evidence that the first breads baked by primitive peoples were crude, unleavened forms of quick breads similar to those used today. These breads were made by mixing flours or meals with water and baking the dough on hot stones. Fig. Q-1 depicts the making of an early type of quick bread.

Thin, unleavened pancake-type breads became popular

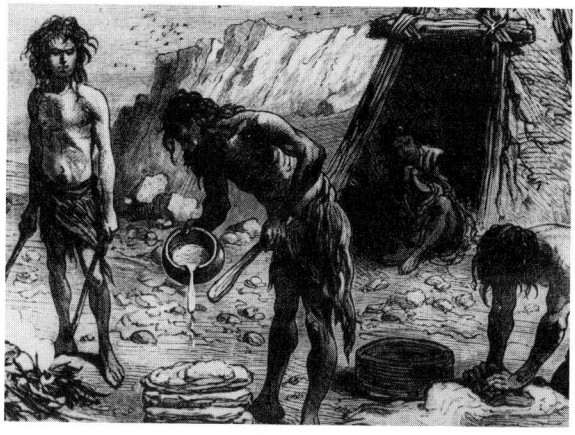

Fig. Q-1. History's first pancake-maker: prehistoric man pouring dough on heated stones. At the right side, a boy is preparing the dough. On the left side, another boy is heating the baking stones. Stones were piled, one upon the other, until sufficient pancakes were made for the whole family. (Courtesy, The Bettmann Archive, Inc.)

in many places around the world, because they could be prepared more rapidly, and they were more palatable after baking. The thicker types of unleavened breads were likely to remain soggy inside even though the outside had been baked until brown, or burned. Some of the thin breads which have remained popular to the present day are: (1) Chinese unleavened pancakes (egg roll wrappers); (2) chapaties made from whole wheat flour in India; (3) tortillas made from corn in Mexico; (4) crepes, usually made from wheat, in France; (5) the crackerlike matzo—the only form of bread eaten by orthodox Jews during Passover; (6) Swedish crispbreads made by mixing rye meal with snow or powdered ice; and (7) bannocks made from oats and/or barley in Scotland. Even the American pioneers made an unleavened corn bread called a *hoe cake,* which was baked on the blade of a hoe placed over hot coals. Wheat was scarce in North America until the Great Plains were settled and hardy Northern European wheats were planted.

The first type of baking powder appears to have been pearl ash, a crude form of potassium carbonate derived from wood ashes, which was invented in America in the 1790s. (Carbonates react with acids and give off carbon dioxide gas, the most commonly used leavener. Sometimes, heating is required to bring about the leavening reaction.) However, pearl ash left an unpleasant taste that had to be masked with sugars and other ingredients. Later, in 1835, a mixture of cream of tartar (obtained from the residue in wine vats) and baking soda was developed. Shortly thereafter, the mixture was utilized in commercial baking powders. Also, a self-rising flour (one that contains baking powder) was developed in England in 1849. The marketing of these quick acting leavening agents soon led to the development of many new types of baked goods, such as baking powder biscuits, layer cakes, quick muffins, and soda bread. By the early 1900s, many home-makers were using self-rising flour and preleavened pancake mixes. Other preleavened baking mixes, which contained all required ingredients except a liquid, did not become popular until the 1940s, when new products were developed for the use of the military services.

At the present time, most people use preleavened baking mixes for preparing quick breads, cakes, and similar items. (Also see BAKING POWDER AND BAKING SODA.)

MAJOR TYPES OF QUICK BREADS.   Fig. Q-2 shows some of the more popular items.

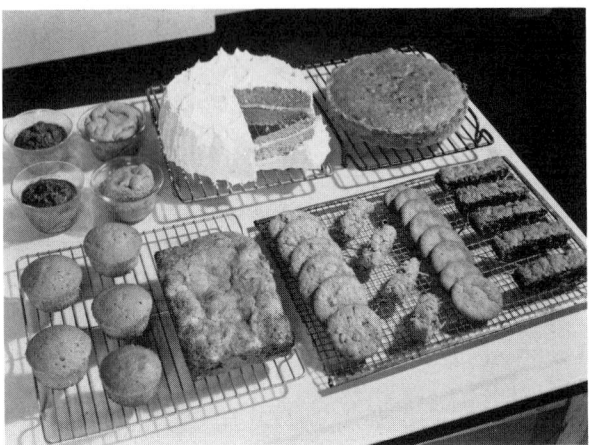

Fig. Q-2. Cakes, cookies, muffins, and other highly desirable quick breads. (Courtesy, J. C. Allen & Son, West Lafayette, Ind.)

The basic ingredients used in all quick breads are flour, liquid, and a leavening agent. Many also contain shortening, eggs, sugar, salt, flavorings, and other ingredients. However, the characteristics of each baked product are determined mainly by the proportions of the ingredients, and the ways in which they are mixed. Some of the more common types of quick breads are: biscuits, cakes (angel food, chiffon, plain, pound, sponge), coating batter, cookies, cornbread, crackers (soda, hard tack, pilot bread), doughnuts, dumplings, gingerbread, muffins, pancakes, pastry (pie crust, puff), popovers, scones, soda bread, and waffles.

(Also see BREADS AND BAKING, sections headed "Quick Breads Made With Baking Powder or Baking Soda," and "Products Leavened With Air or Steam.")

NUTRITIVE VALUES.   Most quick breads are higher in calories than most yeast-leavened breads because they are usually made with more sugar and fat. Since many people have to control their caloric intake in order to avoid becoming obese, careful selection of dietary breads is necessary if one is to obtain the optimal nutritional benefits from these products without putting on excess weight. It is noteworthy that both the American Diabetes Association and the American Dietetic Association have advised dieters not to include cakes, cookies, and pies in their meal plans without the permission of a diet counselor.[1] However, certain dessert items such as custard pie may equal or exceed the nutritive values of many plain breads (in terms of nutrients per calorie). What is most important is that portion sizes of high caloric items be chosen within appropriate limits.

The Food Composition Table F-21 presents the nutritive values for many of the most popular baked goods—biscuits, cakes, cupcakes, cookies, crackers, doughnuts, muffins, pancakes, pies, waffles, and wafers.

In general, the information in Food Composition Table F-21 shows that there are wide variations in the values for calories and other nutrients supplied by the various quick breads. However, a dieter should not judge the merits of an item solely by its caloric content because sometimes a rich but nutritious item might be substituted for one or more of the nonbread foods in the diet. For example, two popovers have the protein content of 1 oz (28.4 g) of meat. This type of substitution should not be carried too far, because popovers supply from 2 to 3 times as many calories as the lean types of meat.

A convenient way of assessing the protein contribution of quick breads is to consider items containing less than 2.0 g of protein per 100 Calories (kcal) as poor sources of protein, those supplying from 2.0 g to 2.9 g as fair sources, and those containing 3.0 g or more of protein per 100 Calories (kcal) as good sources. Therefore, some poor choices for dieters are most cakes with icing and/or filling, cookies, doughnuts, gingerbread, and pies. Fair choices are biscuits, uniced angelfood cake, peanut cookies, cheese crackers, muffins, coconut custard and custard pies, and waffles. Some good choices are the items made with plenty of eggs and milk, but with only small amounts of fat and sugar. The best examples of the latter types of products are pancakes and popovers. Dieters might also select whole rye wafers, which contain more than 3 g of protein per 100 Calories (kcal). However, the protein quality of items containing only cereal protein (rye wafers) is lower than those containing a mixture of cereal with eggs and milk (pancakes).

Most quick breads are low in minerals and vitamins because they are made from white flour. Even the use of enriched flour does little to correct these deficiencies because only iron, thiamin, riboflavin, and niacin are restored; whereas more than 2 dozen essential minerals and vitamins are removed during the production of white flour.

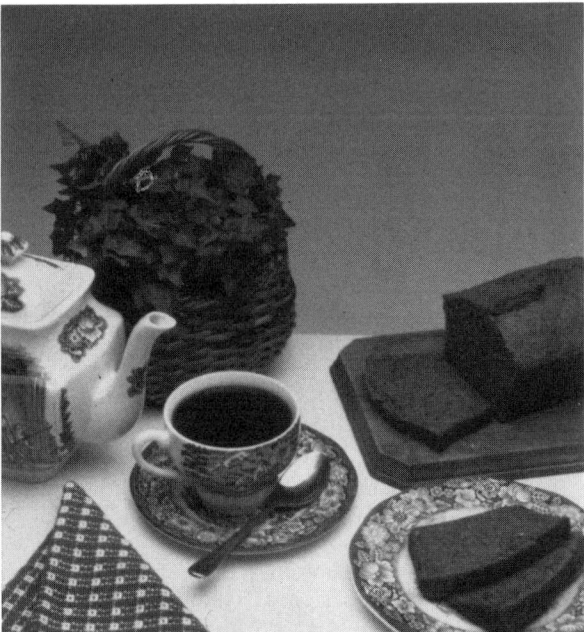

Fig. Q-3. Quick bread, made with baking powder and baked right after mixing. (Courtesy, USDA)

---

[1]*Exchange Lists for Meal Planning*, American Diabetes Association, Inc., and The American Dietetic Association, 1976, p. 4.

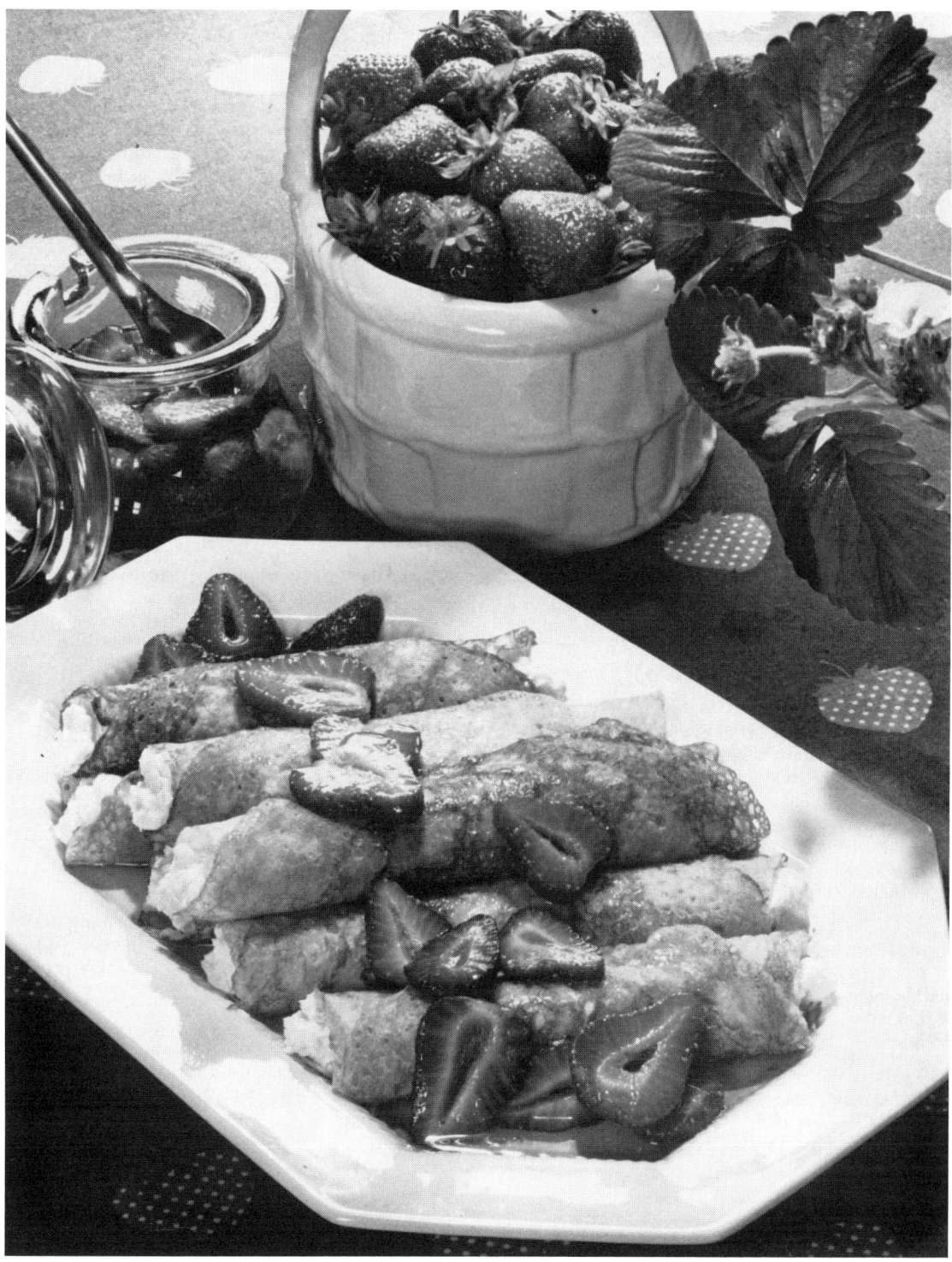

Fig. Q-4. A delectable *quick bread* dessert—Strawberry crepes—which is easier to prepare than it looks. (Courtesy, California Strawberry Advisory Board)

Improving The Nutritive Values Of Homemade Quick Breads. Most baked goods supply too many calories and too few other nutrients. Hence, it is necessary for modern homemakers to revise recipes for quick breads by (1) reducing fat and sugar content, and (2) adding other ingredients that are low in calories and rich in more essential nutrients. Some suggestions for modifying recipes follow:

1. Muffins and pancakes lend themselves readily to experimentation because (a) wide ranges of consistencies and textures are acceptable in these products, and (b) small amounts may be prepared so that wastage of food is minimized if an experiment is unsuccessful.

2. Low-calorie, high-protein items may be prepared from mixtures of whole wheat flour, nonfat dry milk, beaten egg white, and water.

3. The use of a nonstick frying pan or griddle for making pancakes eliminates the need for oiling the cooking surface.

4. About ⅓ cup of grated cheese may be added for each cup (240 ml) of flour. This addition raises the content of protein, calcium, and phosphorus.

5. Sprouted seeds (usually those of beans or grains) add protein, fiber, minerals, and vitamins (about ⅓ cup per cup of flour).

6. Extra eggs may be added to most baked products, providing that a soft flour is used. Too many eggs toughen doughs.

7. About ⅛ cup of soy flour or nonfat dry milk may be substituted for a cup of wheat flour.

8. The caloric content of dessert items may be reduced by mixing one part of cake or cookie mix with one part of biscuit mix.

RECENT TRENDS IN QUICK BREAD TECHNOLOGY.

The continuing rise in the employment of mothers has been accompanied by a reduction in the amount of time available for baking at home. Furthermore, the growing trends of eating out and of buying baked goods from bakeries have brought about a shortage of experienced bakers in certain areas. Hence, food technologists have recently developed some almost foolproof, time-saving products, such as those which follow:

• **Emulsified shortenings for packaged cake mixes**—The need to cream fats has been eliminated by the specially emulsified shortenings used in prepared cake mixes. Air bubbles are trapped by the special shortenings during mixing.

• **Frozen batters**—After thawing, these products may be poured right from the package (which is usually a short, squat cardboard container like those used for cream or milk) onto a pancake griddle or a waffle iron.

• **Frozen quick breads**—These items are available in the forms of unbaked doughs and frozen baked products. The state of the art is such that few people can tell the difference between frozen and unfrozen products once they have been heated.

• **Fruit pie fillings**—Thickened fillings containing pieces of fruit have long been available in grocery stores. Now, a new line of pie fillings is made from gums, starches, sugar, and fruit purees. The new types of fillings make more efficient use of available fruit, so, hopefully, the cost of these products may be lower than those of the former types of fillings.

• **Gums**—These ingredients are often added to commercial baked goods and to packaged mixes because they strengthen weak flours without causing excessive toughening. Some other functions of these additives are: (1) thickening pie fillings and jellied ingredients, and (2) reducing the fat absorption of fried doughnuts.

Prebaked items—Most prebaked products require only a little warming and/or browning in an oven prior to serving. Hence, they are being utilized increasingly by both homemakers and commercial and institutional food service establishments.

Prepackaged items for microwave baking—Certain items packaged in cardboard trays may be heated in microwave ovens, but *not* those that are sold in metal foil pans. Metal foil may cause damage to microwave ovens.

• **Refrigerated doughs**—Most of these products require only (1) their placement in a suitable pan, and (2) baking. Cookie doughs also require slicing. The most popular items in this line are ready-to-bake biscuits, pastry, and rolls.

• **Separation of flours into high-protein and low-protein fractions**—In the past, high-protein hard wheats were used to make flours suitable for yeast-leavened doughs and low-protein soft wheats yielded flours for quick breads. Now, either type of wheat may be milled and separated into high-protein and low-protein fractions by swirling streams of air in a process called air classification. This procedure enables millers to produce flours to meet customers' requirements.

QUILLAJA (SOAP BARK)

This is the inner dried bark of *Quillaja saponaria*, which grows in Peru and Chile. It contains quillaic acid, quillajasaponin, sucrose, and tannin. Soap bark is used to manufacture saponin, and to produce foams in various products. It is also approved as a natural flavor which can be used in foods.

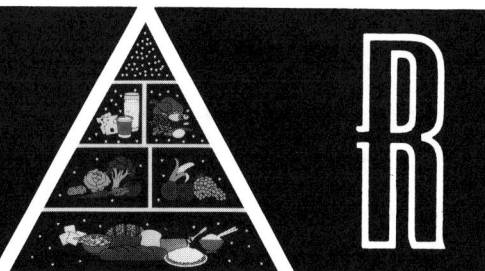

RABBIT

A small grayish brown mammal, native to southern Europe and northern Africa, which has been introduced into various other regions where it is often a pest because of its rapid reproduction. Under domestication, many breeds have been developed, with special adaptation for meat, fur, or show.

Ready-to-cook domestic rabbit is classed as either (1) fryer or young rabbit, or (2) roaster or mature rabbit. Fryers weigh from 1 ½ to 3 ½ lb (0.7 to 1.6 kg) and are usually less than 12 weeks of age; and the flesh is fine grained, tender, and a bright pearly pink color. Roasters usually weigh more than 4 lb (1.8 kg) and are 8 months of age or older; and the flesh is more coarse grained, slightly darker, less tender, and the fat more creamy in color than fryers.

RACCOON (RACOON)

A small wild animal, with longish grey fur, living in the forests of America. It is edible and cooked like wild rabbit.

RAD

In relation to radiation, it is a unit for measuring the radiation energy absorbed by a substance. One rad equals the absorption of 100 ergs of energy per gram.

(Also see RADIATION PRESERVATION OF FOOD.)

RADIATION (IRRADIATION)

The emission and propagation of energy in the form of waves or particles through space or matter.

• **In food**—It refers to ionizing radiation which kills off various microorganisms—so-called cold sterilization.

• **In health and disease**—It refers to the process in which any one or a combination of rays—sunshine, radioactive particles, x rays, for example—are used for diagnostic or therapeutic purposes.

RADIATION PRESERVATION OF FOOD (COLD STERILIZATION; IRRADIATION; RAD APPERTIZATION; RADICIDATION; RADURIZATION)

Ionizing radiation—fast moving subatomic particles or energetic electromagnetic waves which are strong enough to strip electrons from atoms or molecules—provides the basis for a new method of food preservation. By subjecting foods to ionizing radiation a number of desirable storage characteristics—sprouting inhibition, slowed ripening, pasteurization, and complete sterilization—may be induced, depending upon the dose of radiation. Since the radiaton must not make the food radioactive, the sources of radiation are limited to the isotopes cobalt-60 and cesium-137, and to x rays. The doses of ionizing radiation to which these sources subject foods are expressed by a unit called the rad—the energy absorption of 100 ergs per gram. Since one million rads only increases the temperature of food by about 2°C, radiation processing of foods is sometimes called cold sterilization. Table R-1 indicates some of the potential uses of this process.

Despite the fact that some people are somewhat squeamish about accepting irradiated products, irradiation under approved processes does not make food radioactive; hence, it poses no danger to consumers.

The possible use of radiation preservation is especially important in tropical and subtropical countries, where the temperature is high and the humidity is often excessive. In India, for example, 10 to 50% of the food production is often lost because of spoilage.

(Also see PRESERVATION OF FOOD, Table P-10, Methods of Food Preservation; RADIATION.)

TABLE R-1
POTENTIAL APPLICATIONS OF RADIATION TO FOOD PROCESSING

Use	Foods	Action of Radiation	Rads of Exposure
Extension of storage life	Potatoes, onions, and other tubers and bulbs	Inhibits sprouting	Less than 20,000
	Fruits and some vegetables	Delays ripening and reduces the yeast and mold population	100,000 to 500,000
	Meat, fish, poultry, and other highly perishable foods	Reduces the population of microorganisms capable of growth below 37°F (3°C)	50,000 to 1 million
	Cereals, flours, dried fruits, and any other food prone to insect infestations	Kills or sexually sterilizes the insects preventing loss during storage or spread of the pests	10,000 to 50,000
	Meat, fish, poultry, and other highly perishable foods	Complete sterilization, destruction of any organism capable of causing spoilage thus preparing food for long-term storage when properly packaged	4 to 6 million
Prevention of *Salmonella* food poisoning	Frozen meat, eggs, poultry, and other foods liable to contamination	Destroys *Salmonella* bacteria	300,000 to 1 million
Prevention of parasitic diseases	Meat or any other parasite-carrying food	Destroys parasites such as *Trichinella spiralis* and *Taenia sagnata*	10,000 to 30,000

RADIATION THERAPY

The therapeutic use of x rays or radioactive substances such as radium and radioactive cobalt-60 isotope in the treatment of disease, primarily of a malignant nature.

RADIOACTIVE FALLOUT (CONTAMINATION)

As a safeguard to our health, the Food and Drug Administration (FDA), the U.S. Department of Agriculture (USDA), the U.S. Public Health Service (USPHS) and the Federal Radiation Council (FRC), are among the groups that periodically monitor the level of radioactivity in the food supply. The FRC has stipulated the lower levels of radioactive contamination of foods. Should the level exceed these limits, the Agency will recommend actions which should be taken.

RADIOACTIVE ISOTOPES

An isotope is an element which has the same atomic number as another element but a different atomic weight. A radioactive isotope is one that decomposes spontaneously, emitting alpha or beta particles or gamma rays through the disintegration of its atomic nuclei. Usually, when fed or injected, its course and concentration can be traced and tagged by use of a special instrument, a Geiger counter. More than 150 radioactive isotopes are used (some experimentally) in the treatment of various diseases; among them, radioactive iodine (sodium iodide I-131)—used in the treatment of hyperthyroidism and other ailments, radioactive gold, radioactive phosphorus, and radioactive iron.

RADIOACTIVE I131 TEST

This is a test of thyroid function by using a radioactive isotope of iodine, I131. After administering the test dose, the uptake and utilization of iodine by the thyroid gland is measured by tracing the I131.

RAFFINOSE

A trisaccharide containing the three hexoses, glucose, fructose, and galactose. Raffinose is found in molasses, cottonseed meal, and Australian manna.
(Also see CARBOHYDRATE[S].)

RAGOÛT

This dish is essentially the same as a stove-top stew. The meat is browned, then the onion, garlic, parsley, stock, and vinegar are added along with seasonings, and the mixture is simmered until the meat is tender. Duck, chicken, rabbit, hare, lamb, or young partridge maybe prepared in this way. The gravy is usually thickened at the end. The name comes from the French word *ragoûter*, which means *to awaken the senses*.

RAISIN(S)

These are the dried fruit produced from certain varieties of grapes. The word raisin comes from the Latin *racemus*, which means *a cluster of grapes or berries*. All of the U.S. production, and nearly half of the world's supply of raisins comes from the San Joaquin Valley in California. Other raisin-producing countries include Turkey, Australia, Greece, Iran, South Africa, and Spain.

Many varieties of grapes are produced in California, but only four principal varieties have been found suitable for drying into raisins. These four varieties are the Thompson Seedless, Muscat, Sultana, and Zante Currant, and they are either sun-dried or mechanically dehydrated.

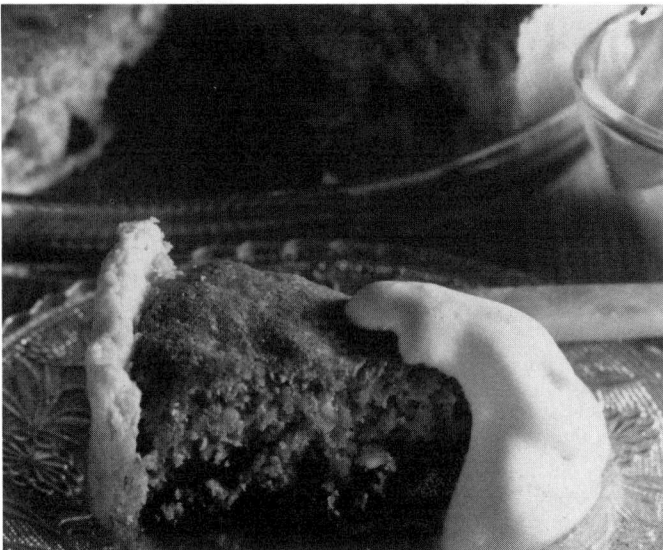

Fig. R-1. Raisin pie. (Courtesy, Phil Seagle/Ketchum, San Francisco, Calif.)

Raisins contain only 17% water whereas grapes contain about 80% water. Therefore, many of the nutrients in grapes are more concentrated in raisins. Each 100 g (about 3 ½ oz) of raisins provides 289 Calories (kcal) of energy, 2.8 mg of iron, and 678 mg of potassium. The calories in raisins are derived primarily from the naturally occurring sugars (carbohydrates). More complete information regarding the nutritional value of raisins is presented in Food Composition Table F-21.
(Also see GRAPE [RAISINS].)

RAISINE

A preserve made with either pears or grapes plus quinces, and cooked slowly in sweet wine or cider.

RAISIN OIL

The oil that is extracted from the seeds of muscat grapes before they are dried to make raisins. It gets its name from its use as a coating on raisins to prevent them from (1) sticking together, (2) becoming excessively dried out, and (3) being attacked by insects.

RAMP (WILD LEEK) *Allium tricoccum*

The ramp is a wild leek that is native to North America. An onionlike odor is emitted by the leaves, which are often eaten with the bulbs.

Data on the nutrient composition of ramp is not readily available. However, it is believed that they are a fair to good source of vitamin C, and that the green leaves may supply valuable amounts of vitamin A.

RAMPION *L. rapa*

This now-neglected vegetable is of the same family as the turnip. It has an edible root which can be eaten raw in salads and tastes like a walnut. The leaves are used raw in salads, or cooked like spinach.

RANCID

A term used to describe fats that have undergone partial decomposition.
(Also see FATS AND OTHER LIPIDS.)

RANGPUR (RANGPUR LIME; MANDARIN LIME)
Citrus limonia

A highly-acid citrus fruit (of the family *Rutaceae*) that is native to India and which (1) resembles the mandarin orange (*C. reticulata*) and (2) is highly acid. It is *not* related to the lime (*C. aurantifolia*). Rather, it is thought to be a sour mutant of the mandarin orange. The rangpur is used mainly as an ornamental plant and a rootstock for bearing the grafts of other citrus fruit trees.

RAPE (CANOLA) Brassica napus; B. campestris

Rape is a general term applied to members of the *Cruciferae* family. It ranks number two among the edible vegetable oils globally; and it is the only oilseed grown successfully in all parts of the world.

Development of new varieties of rape which contain little or no erucic acid and glucosinolate, two antinutritional factors, has made for expanded production and utilization of rapeseed, a cool climate oilseed. This has had a significant impact on producer countries, lessening their dependence on soybeans, sunflowers, peanuts, or cottonseed.

• **Canola**—The name "canola" is registered by the Western Canadian Oilseed Crushers Association; it stands for CANadian Oil Low Acid. To qualify as canola, rapeseed must yield oil with less than 2% erucic acid and meal with less than 30 micromoles of glucosinolate per gram.

ORIGIN AND HISTORY. It is probable that the primary types of rape came from Asia, the Mediterranean, and western Europe. It has a long history, with earliest references found in Indian Sanskrit writings of 2000 to 1500 B.C.

WORLD AND U.S. PRODUCTION. World production of rapeseed totals about 24.5 million metric tons annually; and the leading producing countries, by rank, are: China, India, Canada, Germany, and France.[1]

U.S. production of rapeseed in 1990 totaled 67,000 metric tons. The Food and Agricultural Organization of the United Nations reports that a mere 1,000 metric tons of seed are produced in the United States, annually.

PROCESSING RAPESEED. The processing of rapeseed to obtain oil and meal is similar to that of other oilseeds. There are three methods: (1) mechanical pressing, (2) straight solvent, or (3) prepress solvent extraction. The latter is the method of choice. In the prepress solvent extraction method, a large portion of the oils is removed from the seeds by mechanical presses (expellers), then the remaining oil is extracted by using the organic solvent n-hexane. After discharging from the extractor, the meal, which contains about 1% oil, is dried to about 10% moisture, cooled, and placed in storage. The crude oil must still be refined.

NUTRITIONAL VALUE OF RAPE. The seeds contain 40 to 45% oil and 25% protein. When processed, rapeseed yields about 40% oil and 50% oil meal which ranges from 32 to 40% protein.

[1]Based on data from *FAO Production Yearbook 1990*, FAO/UN, Rome, Italy, Vol. 44, p. 113, Table 41. **Note well:** Annual production fluctuates as a result of weather and profitability of the crop.

High glucosinolate rapeseed meal can cause goiter—an enlargement of the thyroid gland. Here again the best solution to the problem is to lower or eliminate the causative substance from the seed. This has been accomplished.

Plant breeders in Canada and northern Europe have been highly successful in changing rapeseed species to meet consumer needs. Today, these new products are being promoted as canola products, rather than rapeseed products.

It is noteworthy that the reduction or elimination of glucosinolates from rapeseed meal also results in more effective use of the favorable amino acid balance of rapeseed protein.

Oil made from the new varieties of rape is almost free of the long chain fatty acid, erucic acid, while the oleic acid content is significantly higher. Except for the presence of linolenic acid, the composition of the new oil greatly resembles olive oil.

Rapeseed meal, the residue remaining after removal of oil from the seed, contains 35 to 40% protein, 20 to 25% carbohydrate, 12 to 16% crude fiber, and 5 to 7% ash. Due to its high content of lysine, methionine, and cysteine, rapeseed protein has a higher nutritive value than any other known vegetable protein. Based on growth studies with rats and on a nitrogen balance study on student volunteers, the nutritive value of rape protein is as high as that of good animal protein. With the exception of a negative effect on the zinc balance in rats, which can be compensated, no negative findings have been recorded.

RAPESEED PRODUCTS AND USES. The primary use of rapeseed oil is for human food. Its relatively low linolenic acid content permits it to compete with other vegetable oils in shortenings, margarines, salad oils, and frying oils. Oils which are almost free of erucic acid will open up new uses of rapeseed oil.

Until now, rapeseed meal has been used almost solely as a protein supplement for animals. With the development of glucosinolate-free rapeseed meal, it is expected that rapeseed protein will join soybean protein as an ingredient in meat analogs, meat extenders, dairy products, bakery goods, and other processed foods.

(Also see CANOLA [RAPE]; and OIL, VEGETABLE, Table O-5.)

RASHER

A portion, usually 2 or 3 slices, of bacon.

RATAFIA

A liqueur made by infusing and usually not distilled, flavored with plum, peach, and apricot kernels and bitter almonds, and supplied with a base of brandy and fruit juices. There are many different ratafias in different countries; obviously, they are of great potential value to cooks.

RAVIOLI

This is a favorite pasta dish of Italy, and Italians around the world. It is made by rolling out the pasta dough and dropping a spoonful of special cheese filling on each 2-inch square (*13 cm²*) of pasta. This is covered with another sheet of pasta, sealed, and cut with a ravioli cutter. These little squares are cooked in rapidly boiling water and served with or without a tomato sauce, grated Parmesan cheese, or butter.

(Also see MACARONI AND NOODLE PRODUCTS.)

RAW SUGAR

This is the stage in cane sugar manufacturing at which

sugar is transferred from the sugar mills to the refineries. Raw sugar is about 96 to 98% sucrose covered with molasses, but containing extraneous materials which prevent its use without further refining. FDA regulations prohibit the sale of raw sugar unless impurities such as dirt and insect fragments are removed.

(Also see SUGAR, section on "Processing.")

RDA (RECOMMENDED DIETARY ALLOWANCES)

The first edition of *Recommended Dietary Allowances* (RDA) was published in 1943. The current RDA was published in 1989.

Ideally, these allowances should be determined through experimentation on humans. However, for a number of reasons—some quite obvious—this is not always possible. Therefore, estimates of nutrient requirements are determined by the following six methods, some rather indirect: (1) determination of nutrient intake in apparently normal, healthy people; (2) biochemical studies; (3) studies of clinical cases of nutrient deficiencies; (4) balance studies that determine nutrition status in relation to nutrient intake; (5) experiments that maintain individuals on diets low or deficient in a nutrient followed by correction of the deficiency; and (6) animal studies.

The RDAs are estimates, not standards, and should be employed as a goal—not ideal nor optimal, but acceptable—for meeting the nutritional needs of a group of people. If nutrients are consumed at the level of the RDA, the needs of nearly all healthy members of the group will be satisfied, since the RDAs are not averages (except energy), but calculated for individuals with the highest requirements. How-

ever, the RDAs do not allow for the special needs of inherited metabolic disorders, infections, and chronic diseases. Furthermore, the RDAs are not intended for use to evaluate individual nutritional status.

In the 1989 edition of *Recommended Dietary Allowances,* compiled by the Committee on Dietary Allowances and the Food and Nutrition Board, nutrient allowances are given by age, weight, height, sex, pregnancy, and lactation.

• **Dietary recommendations for Americans**—The National Academy of Sciences has also called on the American public to make the following changes in its eating habits:

1. Reduce total fat consumption to 30% or less of total daily calorie intake.

2. Reduce cholesterol intake to less than 300 mg a day.

3. Increase the amount of starches and other complex carbohydrates in the daily diet.

4. Increase the amount of fiber in the diet.

5. Increase the amount of fruits and vegetables eaten daily.

6. Avoid drinking alcohol, especially during pregnancy. If abstaining is impossible, drink in moderation.

7. Reduce daily intake of sodium to 6 g or less.

8. Maintain desirable body weight through prudent diet and regular exercise.

NOTE WELL: Table N-3 in section headed "Nutrients: Requirements, Allowances, Functions, Sources" of this encyclopedia gives the United States Recommended Daily Allowances (RDA) of each nutrient, *plus* its major function(s) in the body and best food sources; hence, the reader is referred thereto. A comparison of United States RDAs with the recommended daily dietary guidelines of selected countries and FAO follows.

TABLE R–2
COMPARATIVE DAILY DIETARY GUIDELINES FOR ADULTS IN SELECTED COUNTRIES AND FAO[1]

Country	Sex	Age	Weight		Activity[2]	Calories	Protein	Calcium	Iron	Vitamin A (retinol eq.)	Thiamin	Ribo-flavin	Niacin eq.	Vitamin C
		(yr)	(lb)	(kg)			(g)	(g)	(mg)	(mcg)	(mg)	(mg)	(mg)	(mg)
United States	M	25–50	174	79	MA	2,900	63	0.8	10	1,000	1.5	1.7	19	60
(1989)	F	25–50	138	63	MA	2,200	50	0.8	15	800	1.1	1.3	15	60
Canada	M	19–35	154	70	MA	3,000	56	0.8	10	1,000	1.5	1.8	20	30
	F	19–35	123	56	MA	2,100	41	0.7	14	800	1.1	1.3	14	30
United Kingdom	M	18–34	143	65	MA	2,900	63	0.5	10	750	1.0	1.6	18	30
	F	18–34	120	55	MA	2,150	54	0.5	12	750	0.9	1.3	15	30
FAO	M	25	143	65	MA	3,000	37[3]	0.4–0.5	5–9	750	1.2	1.8	19.8	30
	F	25	120	55	MA	2,200	29[3]	0.4–0.5	14–28	750	0.9	1.3	14.5	30

[1]Daily dietary guidelines for Canada, United Kingdom, and FAO provided by Z. I. Sabry, Director, Food Policy and Nutrition Division, Food and Agriculture Organization of the United Nations, Rome, Italy.
[2]Moderate activity.
[3]Expressed in reference protein.

RECOMMENDED DAILY DIETARY GUIDELINES OF SELECTED COUNTRIES AND FAO.

Table R-2 gives a comparison of the daily dietary guidelines for adults in selected countries and in all countries as made by the Food and Agriculture Organization (FAO) of the United Nations. The FAO dietary guidelines are intended to apply to people in all countries when translated in terms of local foods.

1. They are set for population groups that live under different environmental conditions (climate, occupation, and activity) and that have different dietary practices.

2. Those who prepare the standards give varied interpretations to scientific data; differences which have narrowed with increased research and knowledge of the nutrient needs of human beings.

All the standards include recommended intakes of only those nutrients for which the requirements for human beings have been established. In order to assure that the nutrients that are known to be essential, but for which the requirements are as yet unknown, will be included in the diet, the selected diet should include as much variety of foods as practical, acceptable, and palatable.

(Also see NUTRIENTS: REQUIREMENTS, ALLOWANCES, FUNCTIONS, SOURCES.)

RECTUM

The last 6 in. *(15 cm)* of the large intestine (colon) before ending at the anal opening.

(Also see DIGESTION AND ABSORPTION.)

RED MEAT

Meat that is red when raw. Red meats include beef, veal, pork, mutton, and lamb.

(Also see MEAT[S].)

REDUCING DIETS

The principle is to decrease the calorie intake. However, a good reducing diet must still provide the required nutrients. At the same time it should be acceptable and palatable, offer a variety, be economically feasible, and promote a sense of well-being.

Basically, the modifications which are usually made in low-calorie diets involve reduction in the number of items high in carbohydrates and fats, but retention of those which are good sources of minerals and vitamins. However, it is often necesary to calculate caloric requirements so that the dietary calorie content may be low enough to produce the appropriate caloric deficit. Generally a weight loss of 1 to 2 lb (0.45 to 0.91 kg) per week is ideal. This requires a caloric deficit of 500 to 1,000 Calories (kcal) per day.

(Also see FOOD GROUPS; and OBESITY, section headed "Treatment of Obesity.")

REFERENCE MAN

A healthy man of specified age, weight, environmental temperature, and physical activity permitting the formulation of standard calorie allowances. In the 1989 *Recommended Dietary Allowances*, the average mature male used for the basis of energy recommendation is engaged in light activity, is presumed to live in an area where the mean environmental temperature is 68°F (20°C), and has the desirable weight of 174 lb (79 kg). The energy requirements for the average mature male are given for two age groups: (1) 25 to 50 years of age; and (2) 51 years and over.

REFERENCE PROTEIN (CHEMICAL SCORE)

Proteins differ in nutritive value mainly due to their amino acid composition. A reference protein provides all of the essential amino acids in sufficient quantities and balances so as to meet the body's requirements without an excess.

A hypothetical reference pattern of amino acids expressed as milligrams per gram of protein, along with the amino acid patterns of human milk and eggs, is given under Protein, section on "Quantity and Quality," Table P-15; hence, the reader is referred thereto.

(Also see AMINO ACID[S]; and PROTEIN[S].)

REFERENCE WOMAN

A healthy woman of specified age, weight, environmental temperature, and physical activity permitting the formulation of standard calorie allowances. In the 1989 *Recommended Dietary Allowances,* the average mature female used for the basis of energy recommendation is engaged in light activity, is presumed to live in a climate where the mean environmental temperature is 68°F (20°C), and has a desirable weight of 138 lb (63 kg). Her energy requirements are given for two age groups: (1) 25 to 50 years of age, and (2) 51 years and over.

REGURGITATION

The return of food from the stomach, gullet, or duodenum (first portion of the small intestine) after eating, without vomiting. Patients with this affliction can usually lessen regurgitation (1) by sleeping with the head and chest higher than the rest of the body, and (2) by drinking lots of water.

REINDEER

The flesh of the reindeer provides venison, which, however, is inferior to that of the roebuck or deer. The venison from reindeer is prepared in the same way as venison from roebuck or deer. The meat of young reindeer is delicate; the meat from old reindeer is less tender and needs marinating.

RELAPSE

The return of the symptoms of a disease after convalescence has begun.

RELIGIONS AND DIETS

Religion and food have always played an important role in the lives of men. Often, food was the most precious and scarce of man's possessions. Not surprisingly, religious rituals or customs became associated with food. Religions have (1) decreed what foods man could or could not eat, (2) prescribed the preparation of foods, (3) indicated what food may or may not be eaten on certain days or certain occasions, and (4) symbolized foods and drink, and their ingestion. Furthermore, the religious idea of defiling or polluting objects influenced food choices. Since food is taken into the body, many religions held beliefs that certain foods and drinks were polluting or defiling.

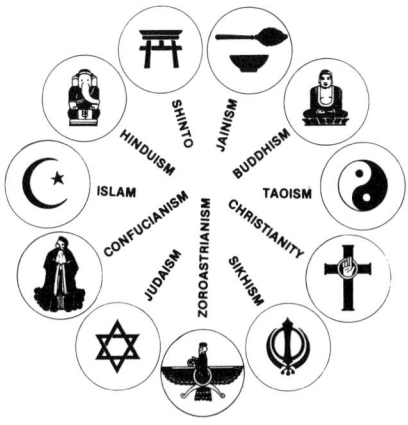

Fig. R-2. Symbolic representation of man's religions.

Through the ages, man has had many different religions, 11 of which have survived. While there are countless religious groups in the world, the broad groupings of these 11 living religions represents the wellspring of religious thought.

These religions developed from various areas of the world and then spread. Hinduism, Buddhism, and Jainism originated in India. Confucianism and Taoism originated in China. Shintoism started in Japan. Christianity, Islam, Judaism, and Zoroastrianism arose from the Middle East. Sikhism is a hybrid of Islam and Hinduism from India. Some of these religions prescribe very specific dietary practices while others do not appear to do so. Nevertheless, the philosophy of a religion may have subtle influences over food selection. For this reason, Table R-3 presents the basic tenets of the 11 living religions as well as foods or drinks which are specifically taboo or encouraged by the religion.

TABLE R-3
LIVING RELIGIONS OF THE WORLD, AND THE DIET PRESCIBED BY EACH

Religion; Origin; Adherents	Chief Scripture(s); Basic Tenets	Food Taboos	Foods Encouraged by Beliefs
BUDDHISM **Origin:** More than 2,500 years ago in India with the teachings of Prince Siddhartha Guatama, the Buddha. **Adherents:** About 245 million, primarily in Asia. About 60,000 in the United States.	**Chief Scriptures:** The *Pali Canon* **Basic Tenets:** The way beyond sorrow and suffering is a middle path between striving and spiritual contemplation. Buddhists believe in the rebirth of persons through transmigration of the soul. Also, Buddhists abstain from killing or injuring any living being.	Strict Buddhists are vegetarians. They will not eat the flesh of any animal and many will not eat milk and eggs. Part of rite action includes a vow to abstain from intoxicating beverages.	Buddhist monks do not eat after midday, but they are allowed to drink tea and coconut milk. Every morning Buddhist monks make the rounds in the village with their beggar's bowls and receive the very best of the rice, curry, or fruit available. Abstaining from taking life limits the use of livestock, but encourages the growing of rice and the introduction of new food crops. Eating fish is not viewed as killing but simply removing the fish from water.
CHRISTIANITY **Origin:** Began with the birth of Jesus Christ about 2,000 years ago. **Adherents:** About 1 billion throughout the world, of which about 135 million are in the United States.	**Chief Scriptures:** The *Bible* (Old and New Testament) **Basic Tenets:** Jesus Christ—the Savior—was the Son of God. He suffered for man's sins. He was crucified and then resurrected. Jesus Christ will return. Teachings and life of Christ are contained in the New Testament of the Bible. Christ taught love of God and love of fellow men.	Overall, Christianity does not teach that any specific foods are taboo, but several of the major Christian religions prohibit some foods: • **Greek Orthodox**—On Fridays and Wednesdays, the use of meat, fish, poultry, eggs, and dairy products is restricted. These foods are also restricted during the first and last weeks of the Greek Orthodox Lent. Devout members may abstain from olive oil. • **Mormons (Latter-day Saints)**—The Mormons prohibit the use of alcoholic beverages, tea, coffee, and tobacco, and encourage the sparing use of meat. • **Roman Catholic**—Historically, the most notable dietary law in Christianity was the Roman Catholic ban on eating meat on Friday. During the reign of Pope John XXIII, this ban was lifted. • **Seventh-day Adventists**—Adventists are taught to avoid meat, fish, poultry, alcohol, tea, coffee, ripened cheese, excess sugar, and excess refined grains, as well as irritating spices and too much salt.	Several of the major Christian religions encourage certain types of foods or diets: • **Greek Orthodox**—Dietary laws have been interpreted more liberally in recent years. On fast days—days meat and dairy products are restricted—shell fish may be eaten. Koliva, a boiled whole wheat dish, is important in memorial services for the dead. • **Mormons (Latter-day Saints)**—The Mormon "Word of Wisdom" encourages the use of grains, fruits, and vegetables. • **Roman Catholic**—Local customs vary with regard to foods allowed on fast days and days of abstinence. • **Seventh-day Adventists**—In general, Adventists are ovolactovegetarians, and allow the use of eggs and milk. Furthermore, they encourage the use of nuts, legumes, and whole grains. The Adventists have encouraged the development of meat analogs such as the soy protein products.
CONFUCIANISM **Origin:** Developed around the philosophy of Confucius (K'ung Fu-tzu) who lived in China from 551 to 479 B.C. **Adherents:** About 276 million, primarily in China and Taiwan.	**Chief Scriptures:** The *Analects* (Conversations or sayings) **Basic Tenets:** Confucianism is primarily a group of ethics or proper conduct: kindness, righteousness, decorous behavior, wisdom, and uprightness. The chief ethic is benevolence. Confucianism encourages ancestor worship.	Confucianism does not seem to have any specific food taboos.	Confucianism does not seem to encourage the use of any certain foods, other than those that may be part of ancestor worship.
HINDUISM **Origin:** No founder, but developed gradually over 5,000 years. **Adherents:** Over 500 million in India and in Indian communities throughout the world.	**Chief Scriptures:** The *Vedas* which includes the *Rig Veda*, the *Upanishads*, the *Bhagavad-Gita*, and many other writings **Basic Tenets:** Hinduism does not have a common creed or one doctrine to bind Hindus together. Membership in an Indian caste is encouraged by Hinduism. Brahman is the unifying spirit, and Hindus may worship many gods. Hindus believe in reincarnation or rebirth. They will not injure or kill an animal.	Some Hindus reject pork because of the value they place on life and because of the filth of pigs. Hindus view the cow as sacred; hence, beef is not a food, though there are numerous cows in India. Both eggs and poultry are rejected by the Hindus. Strict Hindu will not eat the flesh of any animal. Strict Hindus also avoid onions, garlic, turnips, and mushrooms, and for some, the association of blood with the color of some lentils and tomatoes has made these vegetables unacceptable.	Strict Hindus are vegetarians. Ghee (clarified butter) and milk from the cow are sacred foods. The coconut is also considered sacred. To insure success, new enterprises may be started by breaking a coconut. Following a fast, which may be either a complete fast or at least abstaining from cooked foods, a Brahman—high priest of Hinduism—can be fed ghee, coconuts, fruits, or some uncooked food.
ISLAM **Origin:** Founded by Mohammed, who was born in Mecca (now Saudi Arabia) and who lived from about 570 to 632 A.D. **Adherents:** About 700 million worldwide, with about 1 million in the United States.	**Chief Scriptures:** The *Koran*, A compilation of revelations Mohammed received from Allah. **Basic Tenets:** The simple article of faith of Islam is that they worship one God (Allah) and Mohammed was his messenger. Moslems believe that good deeds will be rewarded in paradise and evil deeds will be punished in hell. Duties of Islam include: 5 daily prayers, observance of Ramadan, giving of alms, and a pilgrimage to Mecca at least once in a lifetime.	Eating pork and drinking intoxicating beverages is forbidden. The observance of the month of Ramadan involves fasting during the daylight hours. With the exception of fish and locusts, no animal food is considered lawful unless it has been slaughtered according to the proper ritual. At the instant of slaughter, the person killing the animal must repeat, "In the name of God, God is great."	During the month of Ramadan, nights are often spent in feasting, possibly beginning with an appetizer like dates and a sherbetlike drink. Then following Ramadan there may be a feast lasting up to 3 days. This is called Eid-al-Fitr, where chicken or veal sauteed with eggplant and onions and simmered in pomegranate juice and spices may be served. But the highlight is a whole lamb stuffed with a rich dressing of dried fruits, cracked wheat, pine nuts, almonds, onions, and spices. The feast is concluded with rich pastries and candies, some of which are taken home and used over a period of time as reminders of the festival.

(Continued)

TABLE R-3 *(Continued)*

Religion; Origin; Adherents	Chief Scripture(s); Basic Tenets	Food Taboos	Foods Encouraged by Beliefs
JAINISM **Origin:** Founded in the 6th century B.C. in India by Prince Vardhamana who later became known as Mahavira or "the Great Hero." **Adherents:** About 2¼ million, mostly in the western part of India.	**Chief Scriptures:** None **Basic Tenets:** Jainism stresses nonviolence to all living creatures, a doctrine called *ahismsa*. Jains also believe in reincarnation or transmigration of the soul. Jainism does not recognize a supreme diety.	Since Jainism stresses nonviolence to all living creatures, any food that requires the taking of life is forbidden. Also, Jains refrain from eating certain fruits, honey, wine, and root vegetables which carry organisms on their skin.	Jains are vegetarians. A Jain monk carries a broom representing the sacredness of a life and a bowl for begging. The broom is used to sweep insects from his path so he will not step on them, and the bowl for begging represents the asceticism or self denial.
JUDAISM **Origin:** From the time of Abraham in about 1800 B.C. **Adherents:** Worldwide, about 15 million; in the United States about 6 million.	**Chief Scriptures:** The *Torah*, containing the first 5 books of the *Old Testament*, and the *Talmud*. **Basic Tenets:** The Jews believe in one God. Their life is guided by the commandments contained in the *Torah*. Judaism teaches that man is responsible for his actions and that he has a choice between right and wrong. The Jewish Sabbath is from sunset Friday to sunset Saturday. Judaism is a way of life, which assumes that life is significant, has value, and that the individual is important. Jews look forward to the coming of the Messiah—Savior.	Eating unclean animals is forbidden. The *Torah* provides the distinction between animals considered as clean and those which are unclean (see Leviticus Chap. 11 and Deuteronomy Chap. 14). Unclean foods include pork, camel, horse, most winged insects, reptiles, creeping animals such as the mouse, and birds of prey. All shellfish and eels are eliminated from the diet. Blood is taboo for human consumption, as is the internal fat from an animal. Meat and dairy foods can't be eaten in the same meal. Trefah is the term used to indicate an unclean food or a food not correctly prepared.	Clean foods which are permitted to be eaten include cow, sheep and goat, and fish (see Leviticus Chapter 11 and Deuteronomy Chapter 14). Dietary laws are further expanded in the *Talmud* which contains the Laws of Kashrut. Kosher foods are those which are permitted according to the *Torah (Bible)* and foods which have been processed in a prescribed manner. A rabbi must supervise the killing of all animals which is performed by a trained person called a shohet. A swift deep slash at the throat renders the animal unconscious and allows the blood to drain from the animal. Then truly kosher meat is soaked in cold water, drained, sprinkled with salt, washed in cold water, and cooked.

The *Talmud* forbids Jews to eat certain sinews of the hindquarters which presents some problems since the sinews are difficult and costly to remove. Many of the processed foods contain the symbols U or K on the label which refers to the Union of Orthodox Jewish Congregations and O.K. Laboratories, respectively. These symbols indicate that the food is kosher.

Food plays a major role in the symbolism of the Jewish holidays and festivals. Familiar foods during these times include honey, honey cake, carrot tzimmes, holishkes, strudel, potato latkes, potato krugel, St. John's Bread, fruit, nuts, raisins, pastry, wine, cheese blintzes, cheese kreplach, egg and unleavened wheat bread (matzo).

(Also see MEAT, section headed, "Kosher Meats.")

Religion; Origin; Adherents	Chief Scripture(s); Basic Tenets	Food Taboos	Foods Encouraged by Beliefs
SHINTO **Origin:** Originated in ancient times with the beginnings of the Japanese culture. **Adherents:** About 63 million Japanese.	**Chief Scriptures:** None **Basic Tenets:** The word *shin-to* or in Japanese Kami-no-michi means "the way of the gods." The gods and goddesses that are worshipped are the forces of nature which may reside in rivers, trees, rocks, mountains, certain animals, and particularly in the sun and moon. Today, Shinto sects stress world peace and brotherhood but no universal prophetic message.	No foods seem to be forbidden by the Shinto religion.	The only foods that may be considered as encouraged are those associated with ceremonies dealing with abundant harvest or good health. Gifts of cakes are offered at some public shrines. In traditional villages, the diet tends to be largely vegetarian with an occasional fish or chicken. These food habits may be the influence of Shinto and/or other religions which entered Japan over the years.
SIKHISM **Origin:** Founded by Guru Nanak about 1500 A.D. **Adherents:** About a million worldwide, primarily in India. Sikhs are easily identified by their turbans.	**Chief Scriptures:** *Granth Sahib* **Basic Tenets:** Sikhism combines the beliefs of Islam and Hinduism. Nanak taught that there is one God, and opposed the caste system, uniting his followers into one class.	Sikhs vow not to smoke or to drink alcoholic beverages.	No foods seem to be encouraged by the Sikh beliefs. There are certainly some traditional foods which may in part reflect the Hindu and Moslem influence.
TAOISM **Origin:** Founded about 2,600 years ago by Lao-tzu. **Adherents:** About 30 million worldwide. In China a person may be a Confucian, a Taoist, and a Buddhist all at the same time.	**Chief Scriptures:** *Tao te ching* **Basic Tenets:** In Chinese, the word "tao" means way or path. Taoism stresses quiet contemplation, and the elimination of all striving and strong passions which allows a man to live in harmony with the principles that underlie and govern the universe. Taoism divided all reality into male and female principles of *yang* and *yin*, respectively. Taoism developed beliefs of an afterlife with a heaven and hell.	No specific food taboos seem to be taught.	Yang and yin philosophy may have some influence in the food choices, as may the philosophy of living close to nature. Some Taoist groups have included special diets as part of their search for immortality. Early Taoists practiced alchemy—mixing elixirs designed to ensure immortality.
ZOROASTRIANISM **Origin:** Founded in the 6th century B.C. by Zoroaster, a religious teacher and prophet of Persia (now Iran). **Adherents:** Only about 200,000, primarily in limited areas of Asia.	**Chief Scriptures:** The *Avesta* or *Zend-Avesta* **Basic Tenets:** Zoroaster taught monotheism—the belief in one god. Also, this religion teaches that the world is ruled by two forces—good and evil. A lie is a great evil in Zoroastrianism.	No specific foods are limited by the teachings of Zoroastrianism.	Zoroastrians have a ritual drink called hoama. There are traditional foods which are associated with religious festivals. Zoroaster encouraged people to till the soil, raise grain, grow fruits, irrigate and weed crops, reclaim wasteland, and to treat animals kindly.

RELISH, CHUTNEY, PICCALILLI

All three of these words mean essentially the same thing: a mixture of chopped vegetables, with a blend of spices and vinegar.

REMISSION

An interval in the course of a disease in which the symptoms subside or abate.

RENAL GLUCOSURIA

A term which implies the excretion of glucose (sugar) in the urine while blood glucose remains within the limits of normal concentrations. It is caused by a disorder in kidney (renal) function and is sometimes called renal diabetes. Glucosuria or the excretion of sugar in the urine is often, but not always, associated with diabetes mellitus. However, in diabetes mellitus the blood sugar is elevated far beyond normal concentrations.

(Also see INBORN ERRORS OF CARBOHYDRATE METABOLISM, Table I-2.)

RENAL THRESHOLD

The level of concentration of a substance in the blood beyond which it is excreted in the urine. For example, the renal threshold of glucose is about 180 mg per 100 ml; diabetics excrete glucose because this level is exceeded.

RENDERING

• The process of liberating the fat from the fat cells, as in the production of lard and tallow.

• The processing of inedible animals and meats into livestock feeds, industrial fats and oils, and fertilizers.

RENNET

An extract of the stomach of certain mammals, which contains the enzyme rennin. It is used in making most cheeses and junkets.

RENNET, VEGETABLE

The name given to proteolytic enzymes derived from plants, such as bromelin (from the pineapple) and ficin (from the fig).

RENNIN (CHYMOSIN)

The milk-coagulating enzyme found in the gastric juice of the fourth stomach compartment of certain mammals.

REPLETION

To fill up; the act of overeating or the state of being overfed.

RESECTION

Removal of part of an organ.

RESERPINE

An active alkaloid that is extracted from the root of shrubs of the genus *Rauwolfia*, and used as a tranquilizer or sedative. It is also used as an antihypertensive drug, in the treatment of high blood pressure, various mental diseases, and tension.

RESIDUE

Left over, remaining; dietary residue refers to the content remaining in the intestinal tract after digestion of food—including fiber and other unabsorbed products.

RESORPTION

A loss of substance; for example, the withdrawal of calcium from bone.

RESPIRATION (BREATHING)

Commonly used to mean the taking in of oxygen and the throwing off of carbon dioxide and water vapor through the lungs, but it also includes the metabolism of the cells.

RESPIRATORY CHAIN (ELECTRON TRANSPORT SYSTEM)

The series of chemical reactions in the oxidation system of the cell that transfer hydrogen ions or electrons to produce ATP (high-energy phosphate compounds.)

(Also see METABOLISM, section on "Catabolism, • ATP—energy currency.")

RESPIRATORY SYSTEM

The body's apparatus for inhaling oxygen and exhaling carbon dioxide and water vapor; it consists mainly of the lungs and bronchial tubes, and its movements are activated by the midriff and the muscles between the ribs.

RESTAURANT

The word *restaurant* is a French word meaning *restorative*. It was originally applied to establishments that served soups. The soups, with their variety of ingredients, were thought to be restorative of one's health. In 16th-century France, one enterprising person advertised his soup establishment as a *restaurant*. Soon others copied him, and the name eventually became popular around the world.

In America, changing life-styles have contributed to the popularity of eating out, whether it be at a restaurant serving haute cuisine, or a fast-food chain. According to the National Restaurant Association, the average American family spent 39.5% of its food dollar in restaurants in 1983.

RETICULOCYTE

A young red blood cell.

RETICULOENDOTHELIAL SYSTEM

Groups of cells, except leukocytes, with phagocytic properties, functioning to rid the body of debris.

RETINAL

Retinal (or retinene) is the aldehyde form of retinol (formerly called vitamin A); it is one of the three biologically active forms of retinol (retinol is also active as an alcohol and as an acid).

(Also see VITAMIN[S], Table V-5; and VITAMIN A.)

RETINOIC ACID

Retinol (formerly called vitamin A) is biologically active as an alcohol, as an aldehyde, and as an acid. The acid form is usually referred to as retinoic acid. Retinoic acid can partially replace retinol in the rat diet; it promotes growth of bone and soft tissues and sperm production, but it cannot be used in the visual process and will not permit maturation of embryos. Retinoic acid is converted by the rat to an unknown form that is several times as active as the parent compound in the usual vitamin A nutritional assays.

(Also see VITAMIN[S], Table V-5; and VITAMIN A.)

RETINOL

One of the two forms of vitamin A as such; the other form is dehydroretinol. Retinol (formerly called vitamin A), which is found as an ester (retinyl palmitate) in ocean fish oils and fats, and in liver, butterfat, and egg yolk, is biologically active as an alcohol, as an aldehyde, and as an acid. The alcohol, the most common form, is usually referred to as retinol, the aldehyde as retinal or retinene, and the acid as retinoic acid.

(Also see VITAMIN[S], Table V-5; and VITAMIN A.)

RETINOPATHY

Degenerative disease of the retina.

RETROGRADATION

Starch is insoluble in cold water, but in a heated suspension the granules swell and form a paste or gel. However, upon aging or freezing, the amylose portion of starch aggregates, forming an insoluble substance and reducing the water-holding ability of the starch. This process, which is termed retrogradation, is undesirable in foods. In the food industry, monoglycerides are added to starch to reduce the tendency of retrogradation.

RHAMNOSE

A hexose monosaccharide found combined in the form of plant glycosides. It occurs in free form in poison sumac.

RHEUMATIC FEVER

A childhood disease that is always preceded by an infection of *Streptococcus* bacteria or scarlet fever. It occurs in acute and chronic forms, and it is one of the leading causes of chronic illness in children. Rheumatic fever belongs to a class of diseases termed collagen diseases.

(Also see MODIFIED DIETS.)

RHODOPSIN (VISUAL PURPLE)

The pigment in the rods of the retina that contains vitamin A. When light strikes the normal retina, this pigment is bleached to another pigment known as retinaldehyde (visual yellow). As a result of this change, images are transmitted to the brain through the optic nerve. Vitamin A is required for regeneration of rhodopsin.

(Also see VITAMIN A, section headed "Functions • **Vision**.")

RHUBARB (PIEPLANT) *Rheum rhaponticum*

Rhubarb is believed to be a native of Asia minor. It is a perennial plant which forms large fleshy rhizomes and large leaves with long, thick petioles. It is one of the few vegetables in which the petiole is the part consumed. The leaf portion contains a toxic substance. Rhubarb's popularity in preserves, pies, and desserts causes many people to think of it as a fruit; however, it is a vegetable.

RIBOFLAVIN (B-2)

RIBOFLAVIN
PROMOTES HEALTH BY HELPING BODY CELLS USE OXYGEN TO RELEASE ENERGY FROM AMINO ACIDS, FATTY ACIDS, AND CARBOHYDRATES.

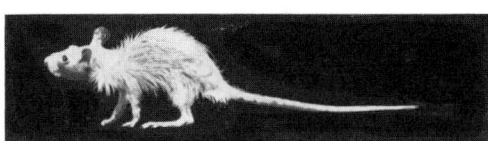 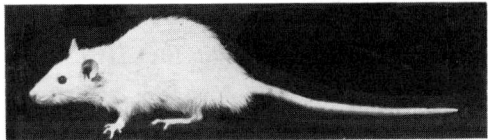

RIBOFLAVIN MADE THE DIFFERENCE! SAME RAT BEFORE (LEFT) AND AFTER (RIGHT). LEFT: THIS RAT 28 WEEKS OLD, HAD NO RIBOFLAVIN. IT SOON BECAME SICK, AND LOST HAIR, ESPECIALLY ABOUT THE HEAD. IT WEIGHED ONLY 63 g. RIGHT: THE SAME RAT 6 WEEKS LATER, AFTER RECEIVING FOOD RICH IN RIBOFLAVIN. IT RECOVERED ITS FINE FUR AND WEIGHED 169 g. (COURTESY, USDA.)

TOP FOOD SOURCES

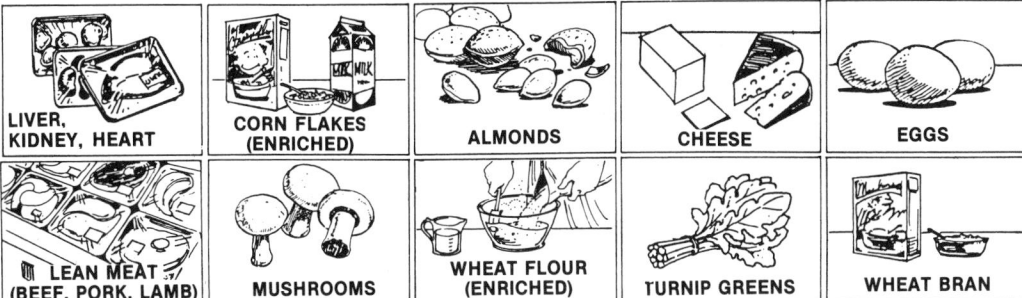

Fig. R-3. The riboflavin story.

Riboflavin is present in virtually all living cells; and, like niacin, it has an essential role in the oxidative mechanisms in the cells.

As early as 1879, the existence of a yellow-green fluorescent pigment in milk whey was recognized. Subsequently, other workers found this pigment in such widely varying sources as liver, heart, and egg white. This pigment, which possessed fluorescent properties, was called *flavin*. But, at the time, the biological significance of the pigment was not understood.

By 1928, it became evident that what had been called vitamin B was not a single vitamin. Numerous investigators found that a growth-promoting substance remained after heat had destroyed the beriberi-preventive factor (thiamin, or vitamin B-1) in yeast. This unknown substance was called *vitamin G* by U.S. research workers and *vitamin B-2* by British scientists. At the time, it was thought to be only one vitamin; later, it was found that the heat-stable fraction was composed of several vitamins.

HISTORY. The first serious attempts to isolate the long-known and widely-distributed fluorescent pigment was undertaken by workers in Germany and Switzerland in the early 1930s. In 1932, two German scientists, Warburg and Christian, isolated the *yellow enzyme,* part of which was later identified as flavin mononucleotide (FMN)—riboflavin phosphate. In the following year (1933), Kuhn, working at the University of Heidelberg, isolated pure riboflavin from milk; and, in 1935, he elucidated the structure and synthesized the vitamin. Independently, Swiss researchers, Karrer and co-workers, accomplished the same feat that year (in 1935). Karrer[2] named it riboflavin, because it was found to have a pentose side chain—ribitol (similar to the sugar, ribose)—attached to a flavinlike compound; and, in 1952, the name was adopted by the Commission on Biochemical Nomenclature.

Riboflavin is widely distributed in both plant and animal tissues. It is formed by all higher plants, chiefly in the green leaves. Also, the bacteria in the intestinal tract may be a considerable, but variable, source of it for man and other animals, just as with thiamin. So, higher animals must rely on food for their riboflavin.

CHEMISTRY, METABOLISM, PROPERTIES.

• **Chemistry**—Chemically, riboflavin is composed of an

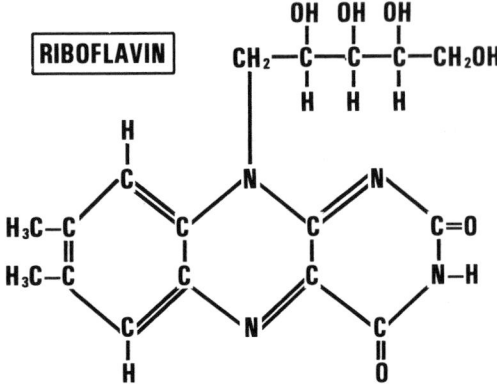

Fig. R-4. Structure of riboflavin.

[2]Karrer, who died in 1971, was also the first to synthesize carotene. In 1937, he was awarded the Nobel Prize for his important discoveries in nutrition.

alloxine ring linked to an alcohol derived from the pentose sugar ribose (see Fig. R-4)

• **Metabolism**—Riboflavin is absorbed in the upper part of the small intestine by passive diffusion, which controls the amount of the vitamin taken up by the cells of the intestinal mucosa. It is phosphorylated in the intestinal wall and carried by the blood to the tissue where it may occur as the phosphate or as a flavoprotein.

The body has limited capacity for storing riboflavin, although higher concentrations are found in the liver and kidneys than in other tissues. So, day-to-day tissue needs must be supplied by the diet. Excretion is primarily via the urine, with the amount excreted related to uptake. When the intake is high, urinary excretion is high; when the intake is low, excretion is low. Some riboflavin is excreted in the feces. All mammals secrete riboflavin in their milk.

• **Properties**—In pure form, riboflavin exists as fine orange-yellow crystals, which are bitter tasting and practically odorless. In water solutions, it imparts a greenish-yellow fluorescence. It is sparingly soluble in water. (It is much less soluble in water than thiamin.) It is heat-stable in neutral or acid solutions, but it may be destroyed by heating in alkaline solutions. It is easily destroyed by light, especially ultraviolet light; for example, it may be destroyed by sunlight striking milk kept in glass bottles. (Milk in cartons is protected against such losses.) Synthetic riboflavin should always be kept in dark bottles. Because of its heat stability and limited water solubility, very little riboflavin is lost in processing and cooking foods.

MEASUREMENT/ASSAY. Riboflavin is measured in terms of the metric weight of pure riboflavin; human requirements are expressed in milligrams, and food content in milligrams or micrograms.

Although the growth of rats and chicks may occasionally be used to assay riboflavin in mixed diets, the biologic method of assay has been generally superseded by microbiological and chemical methods.

The assessment of riboflavin nutriture in man is determined by urinary excretion or by blood analysis.

FUNCTIONS. Riboflavin functions as part of a group of enzymes called flavoproteins. *Flavin mononucleotide (FMN)* and *flavin adenine dinucleotide (FAD)* operate at vital reaction points in the respiratory chains of cellular metabolism. The structure of these two compounds is shown in Fig. R-5.

FMN and FAD function as coenzymes in a number of different flavoprotein systems. They play a major role with thiamin- and niacin-containing enzymes in a long chain of oxidation-reduction reactions by which energy is released. In the process, hydrogen is transferred from one compound to another until it finally combines with oxygen to form water. Thus, riboflavin functions in the metabolism of amino acids, fatty acids, and carbohydrates. During this process, energy is released gradually and made available to the cell. In addition, riboflavin, through its role in activating pyridoxine (vitamin B-6), is necessary for the formation of niacin from the amino acid tryptophan. Also, riboflavin is thought to be (1) a component of the retinal pigment of the eye; (2) involved in the functioning of the adrenal gland; and (3) required for the production of corticosteroids in the adrenal cortex.

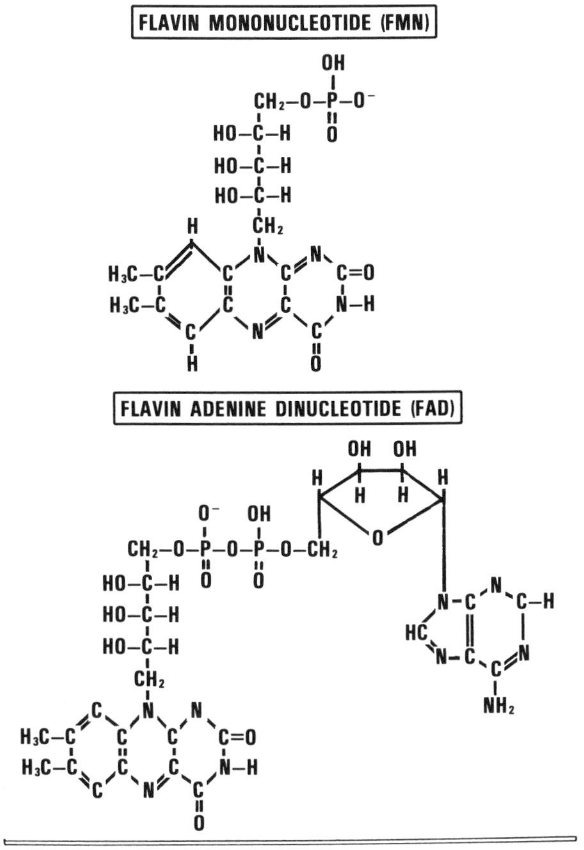

FLAVIN MONONUCLEOTIDE (FMN)

FLAVIN ADENINE DINUCLEOTIDE (FAD)

Fig. R-5. The structure of FMN and FAD.

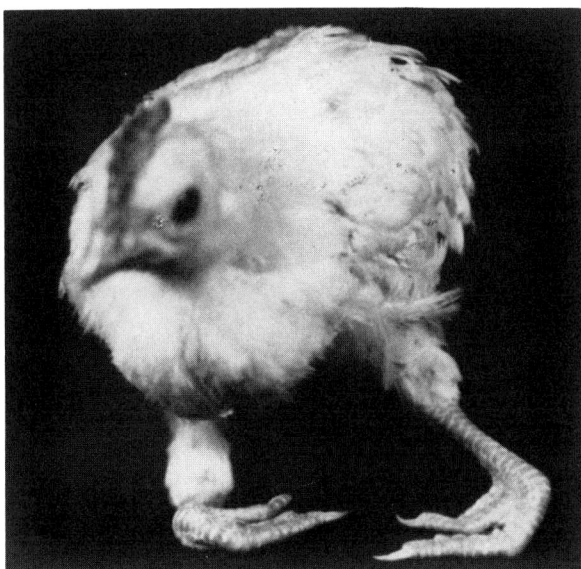

Fig. R-6. Riboflavin deficiency in a young chick. Note the curled toes and the tendency to squat on the hocks; this condition known as *curled toe paralysis,* is caused by degenerated nerves. (Courtesy, Department of Poultry Science, Cornell University)

DEFICIENCY SYMPTOMS. Unlike some of the other vitamins, riboflavin deficiency does not cause any serious disease in human beings; nevertheless, clinical signs associated with riboflavin deficiencies are found among persons of all ages in developing countries.

Manifestations of riboflavin deficiency center around the following symptoms:

1. **Fatigue.** The most important of the nonspecific symptoms is fatigue and inability to work.

2. **Wound healing.** Even minor wounds become aggravated and do not heal easily.

3. **Mouth.** Cheilosis (sores around the mouth) develops. The lips become swollen, reddened, and chapped, and characteristic cracks develop at the corners of the mouth (angular stoma).

4. **Nose.** Cracks and irritation develop at nasal angles.

5. **Tongue.** Glossitis (inflammation of the tongue) develops. The tongue becomes swollen, reddened, fissured, and painful.

6. **Eyes.** Extra blood vessels develop in the cornea (the eyes become bloodshot—a condition known as corneal vascularization), and the eyes become sensitive to light and easily fatigued. There is also blurring of the vision, and the eyes burn, itch, and tear. Cataracts have been observed in rats, mice, chickens, pigs, and monkeys after prolonged deficiency of riboflavin.

7. **Skin.** Seborrheic dermatitis (oily crusts and scales) may develop. The skin may become scaly, and greasy eruptions may develop—especially in the skin folds, around the nose, and on the scrotum in males.

8. **Anemia.** Anemia has been produced experimentally in human subjects given galactoflavin, a riboflavin antagonist. The anemia, along with other symptoms, responded rapidly to riboflavin therapy.

9. **Pregnancy.** Deficiency of riboflavin during pregnancy leads to skeletal abnormalities of the fetus, including shortened bones; deformed growth between ribs, toes, and fingers; and short fingers with fewer joints.

All of the above conditions are common, especially in children in the developing countries where the supply of meat, milk, and eggs is poor. The same conditions are sometimes seen among the elderly in well-fed countries.

Also, it is noteworthy that riboflavin deficiencies seldom occur alone. Instead, they are apt to be found along with deficiency diseases of the other members of the B complex.

RECOMMENDED DAILY ALLOWANCE OF RIBOFLAVIN. Prior to 1980, the Recommended Dietary Allowances of the Food and Nutrition Board (FNB), National Research Council-National Academy of Sciences, related the allowances for riboflavin to (1) protein allowances (1958), (2) energy intake (1964), and (3) metabolic body size (1968). In the ninth edition, 1980, the FNB concluded that the information available does not support strongly any one of these over another. In the tenth edition, 1989, the FNB listed the following factors as being known to affect the riboflavin requirements: nitrogen balance, energy (work) expenditure, and pregnancy–lactation.

The current FNB Recommended Daily Allowances are given in the section on VITAMIN(S), Table V-5, Vitamin Table.

• **Adults and children**—The riboflavin allowances in Table V-5 have been computed on the basis of 0.6 mg/1,000 Calories (kcal) for people of all ages. However, for elderly people and others whose calorie intake may be less than 2,000 Calories (kcal), a minimum intake of 1.2 mg/day is recommended.

• **Pregnancy**—The recommended allowances call for an additional 0.3 mg/day of riboflavin during pregnancy.

• **Lactation**—An additional daily intake of approximately 0.5 mg is recommended during lactation.

• **Riboflavin intake in average U.S. diet**—According to the U.S. Department of Agriculture, the riboflavin available for civilian consumption in the United States was 2.4 mg per person per day. Further, 79.5% of the riboflavin in the U.S. diet is supplied by three food groups: (1) meat, fish, and poultry; (2) milk and dairy products; and (3) flour and cereal products.

A U.S. enrichment program for white flour (with standards for riboflavin, thiamin, niacin, and iron) was initiated in 1941. Subsequently, several other products have been designated for enrichment, and the levels of added nutrients have been changed.

Currently, the riboflavin supplementation of flour and cereal products from synthetic and/or fermentation sources contributes an average of 0.33 mg of riboflavin per person per day, which is about one-fifth of the requirement of an adult male—a very significant amount. However, not all states require an enrichment program; hence, where products are not involved in interstate commerce, they need not be enriched. Besides, average consumption figures do nothing for those persons whose consumptions are below the recommended allowances, or who have higher than normal requirements. Chronic or borderline riboflavin deficiencies are most likely to occur to a variable extent in persons with inadequate intake of animal proteins (especially among those not consuming adequate milk) and enriched foods, in alcoholics, in the aged, in women taking oral contraceptives or who are pregnant or lactating. Also, it is recognized that riboflavin deficiencies, usually along with deficiencies of vitamin A, folacin, calcium, iron, and sometimes vitamin D, are commonplace in many other countries.

TOXICITY.   There is no known toxicity of riboflavin.

RIBOFLAVIN LOSSES DURING PROCESSING, COOKING, AND STORAGE.

The two properties of riboflavin that may account for major losses are (1) that it is destroyed by light, and (2) that it is destroyed by heat in alkaline solution. The following facts relative to riboflavin losses during processing, cooking, and storage are noteworthy:

• **Milk**—As much as 20% of the riboflavin content of fluid milk is destroyed in pasteurization, evaporation, or drying. Also, one-half or more of the riboflavin in milk may be lost in 2 hours if it is exposed to light; as happened prior to 1960 when clear glass bottles of milk were delivered on the doorsteps of U.S. homes—a practice still common in many countries. The use of opaque cartons or dark bottles for the distribution of milk markedly reduces the loss of riboflavin.

• **Blanching**—In the blanching processes used prior to canning or freezing certain foods, losses of 5 to 20% of riboflavin occur.

• **Drying**—Dehydration and freeze-drying processes have little effect on the vitamin content of foods. However, the practice of sun-drying of foods, such as fish and vegetables in tropical countries, results in considerable destruction of riboflavin.

• **Cooking**—Because riboflavin is heat stable and only slightly soluble in water, little of it is lost in home cooking or commercial canning. Average losses of riboflavin in cooking are 15 to 20% in meats, 10 to 20% in vegetables, and 10% in baking bread.

• **Alkali**—Riboflavin may be destroyed by heating in alkaline solutions; hence, sodium bicarbonate should not be used in the cooking of vegetables.

SOURCES OF RIBOFLAVIN.

Riboflavin is widely distributed in most foods. However, there is wide variation in levels, due primarily to source, harvesting, processing, enrichment, and storage. For example, whole cereal grains contain useful amounts, but much of this is removed in milling; hence, highly milled cereals and breads contain very little riboflavin unless they are enriched. Riboflavin is the only vitamin present in significant amounts in beer; beer drinkers may find consolation in knowing that 1 liter (1.06 qt) of beer daily almost meets the recommended intake. Green leafy vegetables vary greatly, but some are fair sources of riboflavin. Fruits, roots and tubers, with few exceptions, contain relatively small amounts of riboflavin. Pure sugars and fats are entirely lacking in riboflavin.

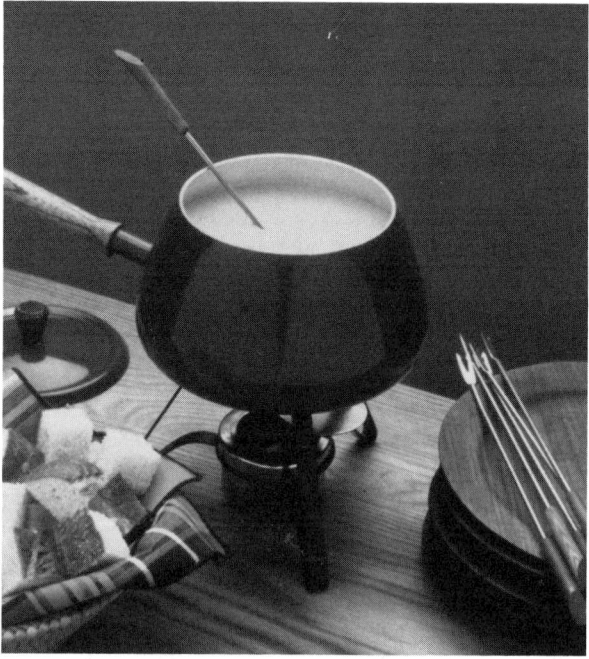

Fig. R-7. Cheese fondue, cheese is a good source of riboflavin. (Courtesy, USDA)

A grouping and ranking of foods according to normal riboflavin content is given in the section on VITAMIN(S), Table V-5, Vitamin Table.

The average person is not apt to get an optimum amount of riboflavin unless he/she consumes a generous amount of milk. Each quart (950 ml) of milk contains 1.66 mg of riboflavin, which just meets the recommended daily allowance of adult males. Of course, the addition of riboflavin in the enrichment of flour, bread, and certain other products has helped to raise the average intake.

For additional sources and more precise values of riboflavin (B-2), see Food Composition Table F-21 of this book.

(Also see VITAMINS, Table V-5.)

RIBONUCLEIC ACID (RNA)

Molecules in cell cytoplasm which serve for the transfer of the amino acid code from nuclei and the synthesis of protein.

(Also see METABOLISM; and NUCLEIC ACIDS.)

RIBOSE

A 5-carbon sugar—a pentose—synthesized by the body in all animals, including man. Hence, it is not essential in the diet, but in the body ribose plays an important role. When it is joined with pyrimidines—cytosine, thymine, and uracil; and purines—adenine and guanine—nucleosides are formed. When phosphoric acid is esterified with the nucleosides, nucleotides are formed. These compounds are then used in the formation of ribonucleic acid (RNA) and deoxyribonucleic acid (DNA). The nucleotides of adenosine monophosphate (AMP), adenosine diphosphate (ADP), and adenosine triphosphate (ATP) are compounds that are essential to cellular metabolism. Ribose is also a constituent of the vitamin riboflavin.

(Also see CARBOHYDRATE[S]; and METABOLISM.)

RIBOSOMES

The site of protein synthesis in the cell.
(Also see METABOLISM.)

RICE *Oryza sativa*

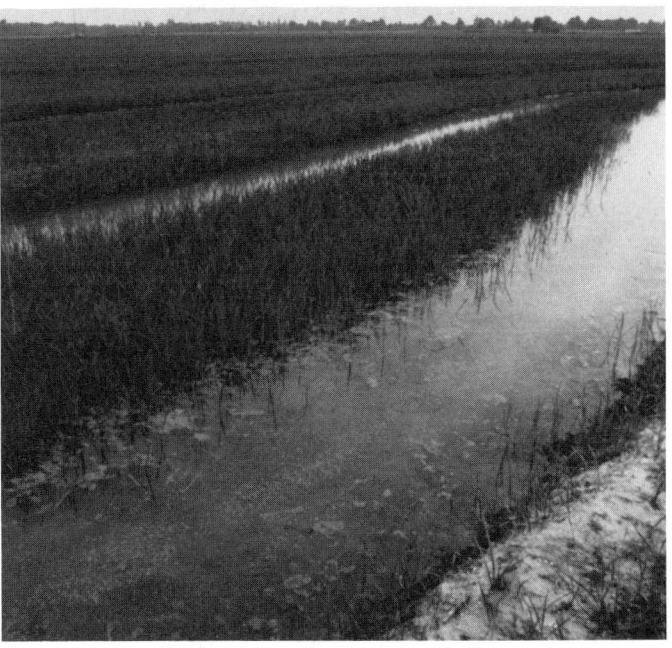

Fig. R-8. Rice. Yields of flooded rice are higher than those of upland rice. (Courtesy, USDA)

Rice is an annual grass of the family *Gramineae*, genus *Oryza*. Species *O. sativa* is the kind most commonly cultivated for food.

Rice is one of the most important cereal grains of the world. It provides most of the food for over half the human population of the earth, most of them living in the Orient. In some countries of the Orient, the per capita consumption of rice is 200 to 400 lb (90 to 180 kg) per year; by contrast, the yearly per capita consumption of rice in the United States is less than 8 lb (3.6 kg). In several national languages and local dialects, the word *eat* means *to eat rice*. American children associate rice with chopsticks.

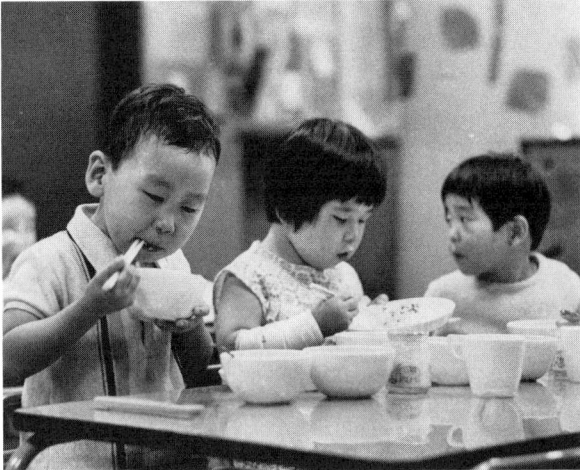

Fig. R-9. Japanese children eating rice, precious grain of the Orient. (Courtesy, *Sankei Kawashima*—newspaper, Tokyo, Japan.)

Rice is the only major cereal that is largely consumed by man directly as harvested (after hulling, and usually polishing). Wheat is usually milled to flour, then baked; and corn (maize) is largely fed to animals for the production of meat, milk, and eggs.

(Also see CEREAL GRAINS.)

ORIGIN AND HISTORY. Rice originated from wild species indigenous to southeastern Asia, where wild types still persist, although there is some evidence of an African center of domestication. Primitive man collected wild rice. Eventually, he cultivated it and selected mutant types with larger nonshattering grains. Hybridization with various wild species followed, contributing to great variability in the plant.

WORLD AND U.S. PRODUCTION. Rice is the third ranking cereal grain of the world. It is a cheap and abundant crop, easy to grow on little land, and well adapted to the climatic conditions of the East Indies and the Asian Coast from India to Japan. Asia produces 92.3% of the world's rice crop.

World production of rice totals about 518.5 million metric tons annually; and the ten leading rice-producing countries of the world are: China, India, Indonesia, Bangladesh, Thailand, Vietnam, Myanmar, Japan, Philippines, and Korea.[3]

The United States, which produces less than 1% of the world crop, usually accounts for a third of the world rice trade. Over half of the U.S. crop of about 7.7 million short tons annually is exported, largely to the Asian countries.

---

[3]Data from *FAO Production Yearbook 1990*, FAO/UN, Rome, Italy, Vol. 44, p. 72, Table 17. **Note well:** Annual production fluctuates as a result of weather and profitability of the crop.

The leading rice-producing states of the United States, by rank, are: Arkansas, California, Louisiana, Texas, Mississippi, and Missouri.[4]

PROCESSING RICE.   The main parts of the rice grain are the hull (husk, lemma), the seed coat (pericarp), the embryo (germ), and the endosperm (starchy endosperm).

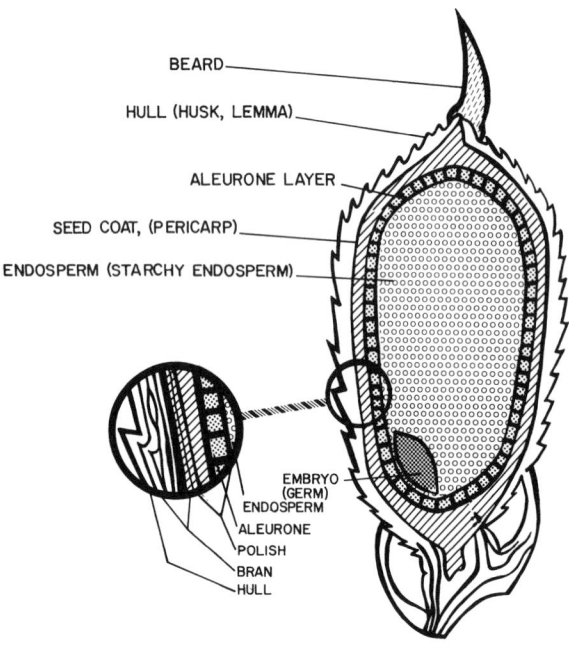

Fig. R-10. Structure of the rice grain.

The seed coat consists of six layers of differentiated types of cells, the innermost one of which is the aleurone layer.

Table R-4 shows that, together, the pericarp, aleurone, and scutellum (which is part of the germ) contain 79% of the

---

[4]Data from *Agricultural Statistics 1991*, USDA, p. 22, Table 28. **Note well:** Annual production fluctuates as a result of weather and profitability of the crop.

TABLE R-4
THIAMIN CONTENT OF FRACTIONS OF THE RICE GRAIN[1]

Part of Grain	Proportion of Grain	Thiamin Content	Proportion of the Total Thiamin of the Grain
	(%)	(mcg)	(%)
Pericarp and aleurone . . .	5.95	31	} 35.2
Covering to germ	.20	12	
Epiblast	.27	78	3.9
Coleorhiza	.20	94	3.5
Plumule	.31	46	2.7
Radicle	.17	62	2.0
Scutellum	1.25	189	43.9
Outer endosperm	18.80	1.3	} 8.8
Inner endosperm	73.10	.3	

[1]Davidson, Sir Stanley, *et al.*, *Human Nutrition and Dietetics*, 7th ed., The Williams and Wilkins Company, Baltimore, Md., 1979, p. 173, Table 17.5.

---

total thiamin present in the grain, although constituting only 6.2% of the weight. By contrast, the endosperm, which represents 92% of the grain by weight, contains only 8.8% of the thiamin.

• **Rice milling**—The purpose of milling rice is to separate the outer portions from the inner endosperm with a minimum of breakage. In modern mills, the rough rice passes through several processes in the mill: cleaning (usually parboiling), hulling, pearling, polishing, and grading.

Dramatic changes of immense health importance occur when rice is milled, the most important of which is the loss of much of the thiamin. Fig. R-11 shows the thiamin content of rice at different stages of milling. As noted, highly milled rice is almost devoid of thiamin. This loss has been responsible for much beriberi among people whose diet consists almost entirely of white rice.

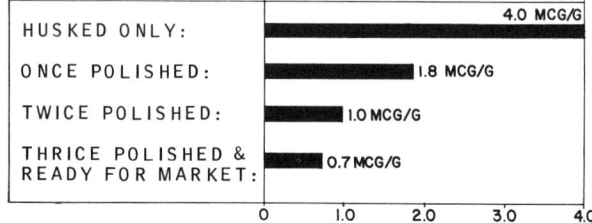

Fig. R-11. Thiamin content of rice at different stages of milling.

In the United States, most rice undergoes a polishing process, during which the outer, colored, protein-rich parts (12%) become livestock feed, and the starchy white endosperm alone is left for human consumption. Polished rice is approximately 92% carbohydrates and has only 2% additional materials of nutritional value.

Dried rice that still has its hull is referred to as *rough* or *paddy* rice. Following the removal of foreign material by means of vibrating sieves and air currents, the rough rice passes into an awning machine where the awns are removed from the grain. The grain then passes through a series of shellers, and the hulled grain is separated from the unhulled in the paddy machine—a complex sifter. At this stage, the hulled rice, which represents approximately 79% of the weight of rough rice, is referred to as *brown rice*.

In the next milling step, the brown rice is conveyed to the hullers, which scour off the outer bran coats and germ from the rice kernels. The term *hullers* is a misnomer because these machines remove the bran, not hulls, from the rice kernel. Loosened bran and smaller pieces of kernel pass through the huller screen and are later separated by aspiration and screening. The rice bran is sold as a by-product for livestock feed.

Thence, the undermilled rice is passed through the brushing machine (polisher) which removes most of the inner bran coat or polish, producing a by-product known as rice polishings; which is sold for animal feeds, and sometimes as an ingredient of baby foods. The rice resulting from this operation is termed *polished rice*, which consists of the white, starchy endosperm, together with fragments of the aleurone layer.

Rice may be sold either as (1) polished or uncoated rice, or (2) coated with talc and glucose, an inert, harmless coating used to give it a high gloss or sheen, which is desired by the Puerto Rican market.

Throughout the entire milling process, a number of kernels are unavoidably broken. So, a series of machines classify the different size kernels as head rice (whole and ¾ kernels), second heads (¾ to ⅓ size grains), screenings (⅓ to ¼ length grains), or brewers' rice (under ¼ length fragments).

In the United States, there are the following grades of rice: U.S. No. 1, U.S. No. 2, U.S. No. 3, U.S. No. 4, U.S. No. 5, U.S. No. 6, and U.S. Sample grade. The grades are determined by size of kernels, number of heat-damaged kernels and objectionable seeds, percent of red rice and damaged kernels, percent of chalky kernels, percent of broken kernels, and color.

• **Parboiled rice**—In southern Asia, rice is parboiled before milling. Approximately 20% of the world's rice is treated in this manner. Essentially, the process consists of soaking dry rough or paddy rice (in the hull) in warm water, steaming under pressure, and drying before milling.

In the United States, there are several patented methods of parboiling. When parboiled, the rice retains more minerals and vitamins (some of the minerals and vitamins present in the bran and embryo move into the grain proper), breaks less in subsequent processing, and stores better.

After parboiling, rice is milled in the conventional manner. It requires a longer cooking period (25 min) than regular rice (20 min). Because parboiling eliminates the surface starch common to regular rice, it ensures a separateness of grain that's especially desirable for kitchens preparing rice in large quantities.

NUTRITIONAL VALUE. Rice without hulls contains about 80% starch, 8% protein, and 12% water.

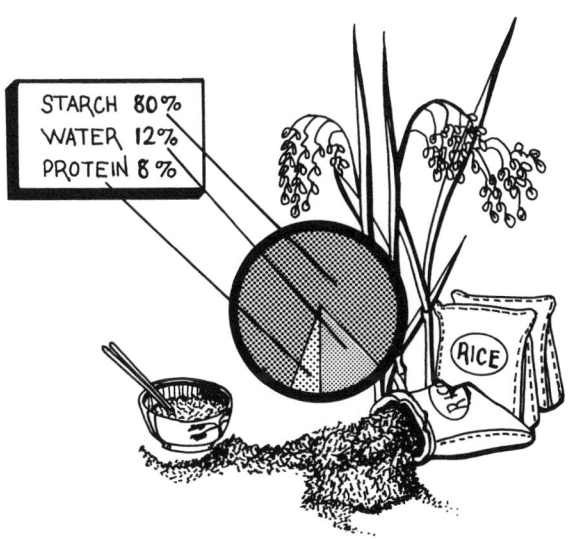

Fig. R-12. Food value of rice.

Because rice is such a predominant food in the diets of Oriental people, its nutrient composition is relatively more important than the nutritional composition of wheat in Western countries. In most wheat-eating countries, the cereals contribute only 30 to 40% of the average food-caloric consumption, whereas in the rice-eating nations some 60 to 80% of the calories come from rice. Thus, at best, the Oriental diet includes only 20 to 40% vegetables, meats, fish, fruits, and all other foods that could furnish the missing vitamins and minerals. Under such dietary conditions, it is easy to understand how the nutrient composition of rice determines the health of those who subsist largely on it.

In its natural state, rice has good nutritional values, comparing favorably with those of the other major cereals used as food staples around the world. It is better than corn and approximately as good as wheat. Brown rice—rice freed only of its chafflike hulls—has about the same caloric content, vitamins, and minerals as whole wheat; somewhat less proteins, but better quality proteins; and more fats and carbohydrates. Compared with corn, it has the advantage of carrying liberal amounts of the antipellagra vitamin, niacin. White rice—brown rice that has been milled and polished to remove the bran and germ—loses a portion of its best protein and most of its fat, vitamins, and minerals, especially if it is cooked in an excess of water which is discarded. Thus, where white rice is the main food, growth retardation, kwashiorkor, marasmus, vitamin A deficiency, and beriberi (thiamin deficiency) are commonplace.

Nutritional Losses.   In most of the rice-eating areas of the world, there is chronic undernourishment, malnutrition, low vitality, impairment of general health and physical development, and a high incidence of diseases resulting from insufficient and improper diet. Ranking high among these diseases as a killer of mankind is beriberi.

(Also see BERIBERI.)

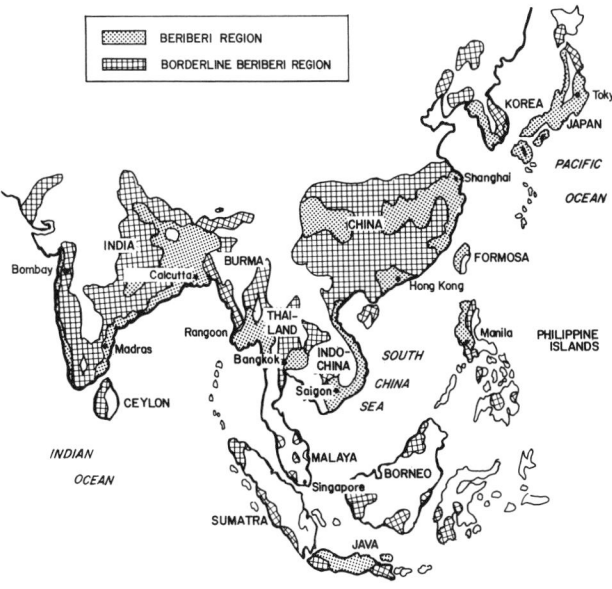

Fig. R-13. Probable beriberi regions of the world. The field for action in the fight against beriberi is most of the rice-growing and rice-eating area of the Orient. Although health statistics are largely lacking, there are probably high death rates from beriberi in all the regions where ordinary white rice is the chief food.

High beriberi death rates and high consumption of rice, occurring in the same areas, are not the result of coincidence. The kind of rice most of the people prefer is white—the kind that deprives them of the natural food substances that would prevent or cure beriberi.

The rice grown by these people has many of the vitamins and minerals they need, but by the time it is milled and polished, then washed and cooked, it has lost most of them. The taste of cooked white rice appeals to their palates; the bulk appeases their hunger; the protein, carbohydrate, and calorie content give them the strength to live and work; but the grain, robbed of many of its health-giving elements and reinforced with little other food, brings disease and death.

As early as 1897, Eijkman, working in Java, showed that beriberi was due to the continued consumption of polished rice. Thus, it might seem that the rice-eating nations of the world have been either negligent or indifferent. This is not the case, however, for many of the nations have made intensive studies of the problem. Some have attempted to reform milling practices or to bring about wider consumption of other foods, only to find that these solutions could not be effected because of very real economic or human factors. Important among these is the cost of other and more varied foods. Even more important is the extraordinary resistance of the people to changes in their established dietary habits and food practices.

Washing and cooking practices in many Asian countries are also obstacles to better rice. In general, the more water used in cooking, and the more water thrown away, the more vitamins and minerals lost—whether from brown, parboiled, white, or enriched rice. However, somewhat more thiamin, riboflavin, niacin, and iron are retained in all improved forms of rice, even with the worst cooking practices. Fortunately, the Filipinos, Cantonese, and Malays customarily cook rice with relatively small amounts of water which is fully absorbed by the swelling of the grains. Elsewhere, it is to be hoped that education may in time improve cooking methods so that the vitamin-laden water will not be thrown away.

Enrichment.
Enrichment is another possible solution for the rice-eating peoples who insist on the pure white product. Enrichment of white rice is a process in which selected vitamins and minerals are sprayed on rice grains. The treated rice is then coated with a film of edible substances, which protects the added elements against deterioration and reduces losses of vitamins during washing prior to cooking. The *premix* thus produced is as white as the untreated milled grain. When it is mixed with white rice in the proportion of one part of the premix to 200 parts of ordinarily milled rice, the resulting enriched rice contains approximately the same amounts of thiamin, niacin, and iron as brown rice.

While the addition of riboflavin, another vitamin lost in milling, is perfectly feasible, it is presently being omitted because it colors the premix grains. Confirmed white-rice eaters would undoubtedly be suspicious of these yellow grains, and sort them out and throw them away. However, in those rice-eating countries where it is desirable, riboflavin or other nutrients can be included. With proper public education, the occasional yellow grain might become the hallmark of enrichment.

Table R-5 shows the enrichment levels for rice in the United States.

TABLE R-5
ENRICHMENT LEVELS FOR MILLED RICE

Nutrient	Level	
	(mg/lb)	**(mg/100 g)**
Thiamin	2.0–4.0	.44–.88
Riboflavin[1]	1.2–2.4	.26–.53
Niacin	16–32	3.53–7.05
Iron	13–26	2.87–5.73
Calcium[2]	500–1,000	110–220

[1]The addition of riboflavin is feasible but the practice was stopped many years ago since its addition colors the rice yellow; hence, rice may or may not be enriched with riboflavin.

[2]The addition of calcium is optional.

Protein Quality.
Table R-6 presents a comparison between the essential amino acid content of brown rice, white rice, and milk—a high quality protein. Like the other cereal

TABLE R-6
PROFILE OF THE ESSENTIAL AMINO ACIDS OF BROWN RICE AND WHITE RICE COMPARED TO MILK—A HIGH-QUALITY PROTEIN[1]

Amino Acid	Brown Rice	White Rice	Cow's Milk
	(mg/g protein)		
Histidine	26	25	27
Isoleucine	40	46	47
Leucine	86	89	95
Lysine	40	39	78
Methionine and cystine	36	40	33
Phenylalanine and tyrosine	91	87	102
Threonine	41	36	44
Tryptophan	13	13	14
Valine	57	63	64

[1]*Recommended Dietary Allowances*, 10th ed., 1989, NRC-National Academy of Sciences, p. 67, Table 6–5. The essential amino acid requirement of infants can be met by supplying 0.79 g of high-quality protein per pound of body weight (1.7 g/kg of body weight per day).

grains, rice—brown and white—is deficient in the amino acid lysine; hence, lysine is the limiting amino acid. Infants and small children in particular need their essential amino acid requirement fulfilled. Therefore, due to the amino acid deficiency, and other vitamin and mineral deficiencies, brown or white rice alone is not a diet on which children will thrive or survive.

(Also see PROTEIN[S], section headed "Sources.")

The nutritive value of 1 cup *(240 ml)* of each of the different forms of rice is given in Food Composition Table F-21. Of the whole rice forms, brown rice ranks highest and unenriched white rice lowest. Of course, enriched rice can be fortified to any desired level. As shown, rice polish is a rich source of thiamin, which explains why it will prevent and cure beriberi.

BETTER RICE FOR MILLIONS.
While the dramatic results of the Bataan experiment (See ENRICHMENT, section headed "The Bataan Experiment")—a full-scale enrichment program which reduced beriberi among a rice-eating population—gave world health authorities another means for bringing better rice and better health to millions of people, the difficulties of actually adopting this measure should not be underestimated. Most of these are the obstacles which have stood in the way of adopting undermilling and parboiling, the earlier known measures. Principal among them have been the lack of popular understanding of the need for better rice (as portrayed in Fig. R-14), inadequately financed governments, authorities too busy with other problems to enforce the necessary inspection systems, and an inadequate supply of technically trained and administratively effective personnel to perform required services for the protection of the masses.

Enrichment avoids one additional barrier that has hindered adoption of undermilling and parboiling—the distaste of many people for any but white forms of rice. This is an enormous gain, but the money shortage may be a serious deterrent to importing vitamins for fortification.

Perhaps the greatest significance of the Bataan project was to point up the possibility of doing something about beriberi immediately. The ready and rapid introduction of enrichment in the Philippines produced far more striking evidence than could be cited for any measure which by its nature requires slow introduction, bit by bit, over a period of years. This success furnishes a basis for reconsidering the merits of all the possible measures.

Where the difficulties of undermilling or parboiling appear insurmountable, rice enrichment may be the answer, as was demonstrated in the Philippines.

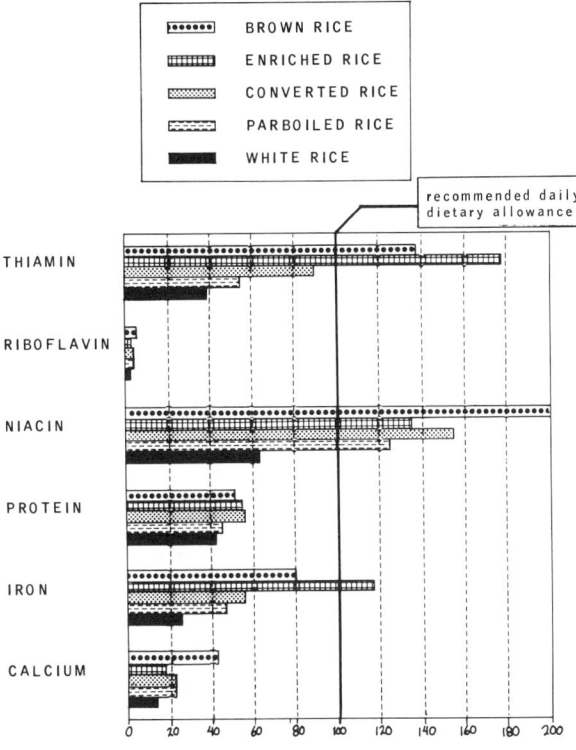

Fig. R-14. Nutritional values of rices. One pound per day of any of the rices shown here will yield these proportions of recommended daily dietary allowances. Of the "natural" forms, brown rice ranks highest, milled white rice lowest, with undermilled rice (not shown) ranging between the direct proportion to the degree of undermilling. The enriched rice is of the strength used in the Philippines, but the formula is adjustable to any level. "Converted" rice is a patented method of parboiling in the United States; it is highly milled, polished rice of greatly improved nutritive value.

RICE PRODUCTS AND USES. The whole grain of rice, with the hulls on, is known as rough rice or paddy rice. Milled rice (raw or parboiled), consisting of the kernels, is the major rice product. But rice milling produces a number of other products (see Table R-7).

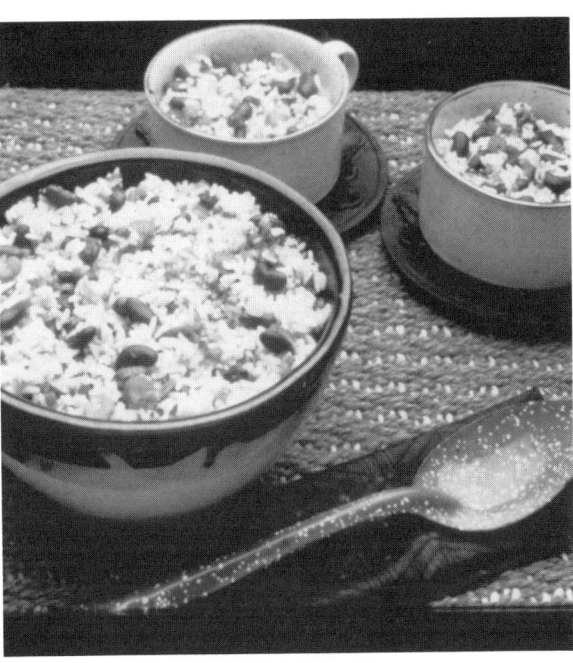

Fig. R-15. Rice is used in many dishes, from soup to dessert. (Courtesy, USDA)

Milled rice is used mainly for human food; it may be sold as raw, quick-cooking, or canned rice. Rice is also used extensively as breakfast food—as puffed rice, rice flakes, or rice crispies. Broken rice is used as food or in the manufacture of alcoholic beverages. Rice flour is used in various mixes. Hulls are used as fuel, insulation, and certain manufactured products. The bran is used mainly as livestock feed. The products and uses of rice for human food are summarized in Table R-7.

TABLE R-7
RICE PRODUCTS AND USES FOR HUMAN FOOD

Product	Description	Uses	Comments
Brown rice	Rice with the hulls removed, but with the bran left on.	To provide more protein and more of the antipellagra vitamin, thiamin, than can be obtained from white rice.	Because of its color and relatively long cooking period (45–60 min.), this highly nutritious rice is a specialty food in the U.S. It is available in many health food stores and in some supermarkets.
Milled rice	The kernels, after the milling is completed and the hulls, bran layers, and germ are removed.	Cooking, mostly by boiling.	The U.S. per capita consumption of milled rice averages about 7.5 lb (3.4 kg). Milled rice with the hulls removed, either polished or parboiled, is the major rice product.
Polished rice	Kernels from which the outer bran coats and germ have been removed, followed by polishing. Polished rice consists of the white, starchy endosperm, with fragments of the aleurone layer.	Cooking, mostly by boiling. Quick-cooking rice (instant rice), a convenience food, some types of which can be cooked in 5 minutes. Canned rice.	For the Puerto Rican market, polished rice is coated with talc and glucose, an inert, harmless coating to give it a high gloss or sheen. There are many approaches to making raw milled rice into a quick-cooking product. Essentially, the process consists of selecting premium grade rice, and, under carefully controlled conditions, soaking, cooking, cooling, and drying it. The canning process consists of (1) soaking the rice to a moisture of 30 to 35%; (2) cooking in excess water for 4 to 5 min.; (3) draining and packing the rice in cans; and (4) vacuum sealing and retorting. "Clumping" of the kernels and difficulty in emptying the contents of the can have been overcome by using surface-active agents to produce a free-flowing product, or freeze-processing, with the processed rice frozen in the can, then thawed prior to labeling.

(Continued)

TABLE R-7 *(Continued)*

Product	Description	Uses	Comments
Parboiled rice	Rough or paddy rice (in the hull) soaked in warm water, steamed under pressure and dried before milling.	Parboiled rice is used in cooking much the same as polished rice. Parboiling retains higher portions of the vitamins and lessens beriberi among people eating it.	In the United States, there are several patented methods of parboiling.
Enriched rice	Polished or parboiled rice enriched by spraying with a watery solution of vitamins (usually thiamin and niacin, and sometimes riboflavin) and sometimes iron and other minerals.	In rice-eating areas to prevent beriberi and other nutritional diseases.	See Table R-5 for the federal standard for enriched rice.
Ang-khak	A product prepared in China by culturing a red pigment-producing fungus *(Monascus purpureus)* on whole rice kernels until they are thoroughly permeated with mycelia which produce the color. They are then dried and powdered.	Used as a food coloring agent in China, Taiwan, and the Philippines, for coloring cheese, fish, red wine, and other foods.	The Chinese are very secretive about the method of preparation of ang-khak Apparently the amount of water used in producing ang-khak is quite critical; the secret of success is to have the rice grains just moist enough to permit the fungus to grow.
Bran	Rice bran is the layer beneath the hull, containing outer bran layers and parts of the germ.	As a water-soluble fiber, similar to oat bran. Cholesterol responds to water-soluble fibers, which combine with bile acids and decrease the body's absorption of fat. Rice bran is also used as a livestock feed.	In addition to being high in water-soluble fiber, rice bran is rich in protein and B-vitamins. Rice oil is extracted from rice bran.
Breakfast foods: Puffed rice Rice crispies Rice flakes	Made from quality milled rice, usually of the short-grain type, which is generally precooked, dried, flaked, foamed and/or puffed or expanded, then toasted.	Ready-to-eat breakfast cereals.	Preparations of different products vary in cooking time, steam pressure, temperature, and the addition of malt and nutrients.
Brewers' rice (Chipped rice, broken rice)	Small, broken rice segments, separated out in the grading process.	Much of it is mixed back with whole grain rice and sold as low-grade rice. As the raw material for rice flour.	Brewers' rice has the same chemical composition as polished rice.
Flour, of which there are two types: 1. Flour made from regular rice, raw or parboiled	Fine, powdery, white particles.	Primarily as a thickening agent in gravies and sauces.	Because rice protein does not contain gluten, its use for confectionery and baking purposes is limited.
2. Waxy rice flour. (Also see FLOURS, Table F-12, Major Flours.)	Waxy rice flour is made from waxy glutinous rice. It has little starch or amylose; it is essentially amylopectin.	As a thickening agent for white sauces, gravies, and puddings—preventing liquid separation (syneresis) when these products are frozen, stored, and subsequently thawed.	Both types of rice flour are available commercially in the United States.
Rice baby foods	Flaked rice.	Baby foods.	Most rice baby foods are prepared by cooking ground, broken rice kernels and rice polishings; adding nutrients; and drum drying the rice slurry.
Rice oil	A high-grade oil extracted from rice bran, followed by refining and bleaching.	Rice oil is used in margarine, salad oil, and cooking oil.	Rice bran contains 14 to 18% oil. When refined, bleached, and deodorized, rice oil has greater stability than other vegetable oils.
Rice polishings	Inner white bran, protein-rich aleurone layers, and starchy endosperm; obtained in the milling operation by brushing the grain to polish the kernel.	In many baby foods. To prevent and cure beriberi.	Rice polishings are easily digested, low in fiber, rich in thiamin, and high in niacin.
Wild rice (Also see WILD RICE.)	The kernels are slender, round, purplish-black, and starchy. It's high in protein and low in fat.	Highly esteemed for its unique taste.	Normally, wild rice sells at 2 to 3 times the price of regular white rice.
FORTIFIED FOOD, BASED ON RICE PRODUCTS, FOR DEVELOPING COUNTRIES			
Protex	Defatted mixture of rice bran, germ, and polish. Contains between 17% and 21% protein, plus minerals and vitamins present in the outer layers of the rice grain.	Acceptable at levels of 5%, 10%, and 15% in yeast-leavened and quick breads. Base for breakfast cereals, pasta, and milklike beverages.	The process for producing Protex commercially was developed by Riviana Foods, Inc. at their Abbeville, Louisiana plant.
BEVERAGES (Also see BEERS AND BREWING; DISTILLED LIQUORS)			
Brewers' rice (Chipped rice, broken rice)	Small, broken rice segments, separated out in the grading process.	Used by the brewing industry, where it is mixed with barley. Used for the production of arrak in the Orient, a liquor of high alcoholic content distilled from a fermented mash of rice and molasses.	
Polished rice	Cooked, whole grains of white rice.	Japanese rice beer (sake), which has an alcohol content of 14 to 16%. (It is sometimes called *rice wine.*)	Sake is prepared by (1) conversion of the starch in cooked rice to sugar by the fungus *Aspergillus oryzae;* (2) a multistage conversion of the rice sugar to alcohol; (3) filtration, settling, heating, and aging; and (4) bottling for distribution. It is usually warmed before serving.

RICE PAPER

A thin delicate material resembling paper made by cutting the pith of the rice-paper tree into one roll or sheet and flattening under pressure. It is edible; so, macaroons and similar biscuits are baked on it and the paper can be eaten with the biscuit.

RICE, WHITE (POLISHED RICE)

Brown rice from which the outer bran layers up to the endosperm and germ have been removed.
(Also see RICE.)

RICKETS; OSTEOMALACIA

The most common disorder of bone formation in growing children is rickets. It is characterized by softening and deformation of the bones. The adult counterpart of rickets is called *osteomalacia*. Both of these conditions result from subnormal mineralization of the protein structure of bone, which is also called the bone matrix.

(Also see OSTEOMALACIA.)

A third bone disorder, *osteoporosis*, differs from rickets and osteomalacia in that it is characterized by a normal amount of mineralization of the bone matrix, but there is a reduction in the total bone mass and a tendency for fractures rather than deformation of bone.

(Also see OSTEOPOROSIS.)

HISTORY. In 1924, Steenbock and Black, of the Wisconsin Experiment Station, discovered that irradiation of liver and a rickets-producing diet with ultraviolet light transformed these materials into cures for rickets. In 1936, the German chemist, Windaus, demonstrated that provitamin D (7-dehydrocholesterol) is found in the skin, and that it is converted into vitamin D (calciferol) by the action of sunlight. The demonstration of Windaus led to an argument as to whether vitamin D might better be considered a hormone, rather than a vitamin, since its effect on bone is like that of a hormone. There are present in the body some related hormones, such as parathormone and calcitonin, which act on bones; and these hormones, together with vitamin D, regulate the net flow of calcium in and out of bones. It might also be argued that vitamin D is not actually a vitamin since it can be made in the body when the skin is exposed to ultraviolet light. In the absence of sufficient sunlight, however, it is necessary to provide an adequate source of vitamin D in the diet.

CAUSES OF RICKETS AND OSTEOMALACIA. These disorders may result from dietary deficiencies and/or poor utilization of calcium, phosphorus, and/or vitamin D; or from an incorrect ratio of the two minerals. However, different circumstances may be responsible for the development of each disorder. Also, rickets is a disease of children, while osteomalacia occurs in adults. Therefore, separate discussions of these disorders follow.

Rickets. This disease is most commonly caused by lack of vitamin D since it is usually found in children whose skin has had only a limited exposure to sunlight. The ultraviolet rays in sunlight convert provitamin D on the surface of the skin to vitamin D. Even children living in tropical areas may not have sufficient exposure to sunlight if clothing covers most of their skin, or they are kept indoors by their parents. In some areas, it is desirable to have a light-colored skin, so parents try to protect their children from the skin-darkening effects of sunlight.

Recently, it has been found that even when sufficient vitamin D may be obtained from the diet and/or its synthesis in the body, some persons may be unable to convert efficiently the vitamin to its physiologically active forms.[5] Vitamin D is converted to its 25-hydroxy derivative in the liver; then, the derivative is carried through the blood to the kidneys, where it is converted to 1, 25-dihydroxy-vitamin D. Sometimes rickets occurs in conditions such as uremia where the kidney fails to synthesize the 1, 25-dihydroxy form of the vitamin.

Exposure to sunlight or oral administration of the vitamin may fail to be effective in preventing or curing the disease when there are great reductions in the amount of calcium absorption from the gastrointestinal tract (either as a result of severe dietary deficiencies of the mineral, or due to malabsorption). For example, diets consisting mainly of whole grain cereals which contain phytates (phosphorus compounds found in the bran) may result in reduced absorption of dietary calcium, due to the binding of calcium by the phytates.

Osteomalacia. This disease is more likely to be found in women than men because (1) women usually wear more clothing than men, with the result that they have less synthesis of vitamin D in their skin; (2) pregnancy and lactation greatly increase the requirements of women for calcium (it is mobilized from their bones when it is not provided in adequate amounts in the diet); and (3) the average bone mass of an adult woman is about one-third less than that of an adult man, so women have a lower margin of safety against deformation of bone due to physical stresses.

Like rickets, osteomalacia may also be caused by interference with calcium absorption by phytates in cereals, disorders of absorption, excessive excretion of calcium and/or phosphate in the urine, and subnormal synthesis of the physiologically active form of vitamin D.

SIGNS AND SYMPTOMS OF RICKETS AND OSTEOMALACIA. Although these two disorders have essentially the same causes, the features of the two diseases differ somewhat because rickets occurs while the bones are still growing, while osteomalacia develops after growth of the

---

[5]"Recent Developments in Vitamin D," *Dairy Council Digest*, Vol. 47, No. 3, May-June 1976, p. 13.

long bones has ceased. Therefore, the signs and symptoms of these conditions will be considered separately.

Rickets. The characteristic signs of rickets are protruding abdomen, beaded ribs or *rachitic rosary,* bowed legs, knock knees, cranial bossing (thickening of parts of the skull), pigeon chest (the breastbone or sternum is pushed backwards as it descends, forming a depression between the ribs), and enlargement of the epiphyses.

The epiphyses are the regions at the ends of the long bones which are separated from the shaft of bone or diaphysis by a layer of cartilage called the epiphyseal plate. These regions are mineralized during growth and eventually become part of the shaft of bone.

Teeth may erupt in an abnormal manner and the enamel may be defective. Malformed pelvic bones in women cause serious difficulties in childbirth. Permanent crippling results if severe cases are not treated. Other abnormalities associated with rickets are weak and flabby muscles, and muscle spasms (in severe cases). The deformities of rickets (curving and twisting of the bones from their normal shapes) are likely to be found in the bones that bear the most weight or stress, such as the legs.

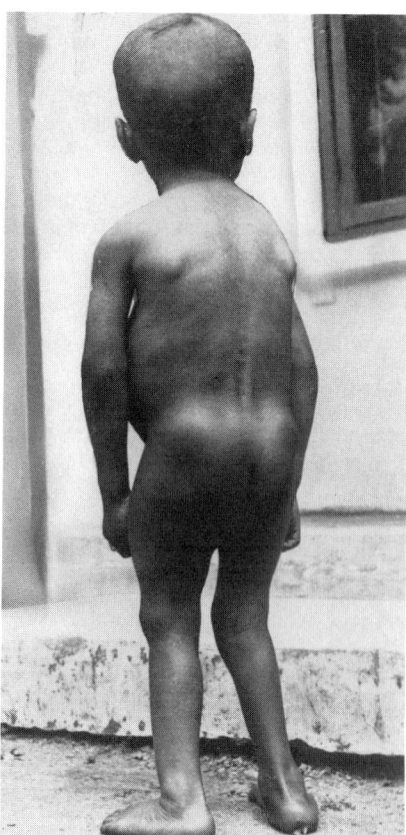

Fig. R-16. An Indian boy suffering from rickets. Note the protruding abdomen, knock knees, enlarged skull, and enlarged wrists. (Courtesy, FAO, Rome, Italy.)

Osteomalacia. One of the worst features of this disorder in a woman is the deformation of the pelvic bones so that she has great difficulty in childbirth. Another common feature of this disorder is a curvature of the spine (kyphosis) which gives the person a bent or hump-backed shape. Other features are pains in the bones, muscle weakness, a waddling gait, and muscle spasms (a mild form of tetany due to a subnormal level of serum calcium).

TREATMENT AND PREVENTION OF RICKETS AND OSTEOMALACIA. Treatment of these disorders is based upon the administration of therapeutic doses of vitamin D (1,000 to 5,000 IU per day) together with the provision of adequate levels of dietary calcium (ranging from 800 mg [milligrams] per day for infants and children, to 2,400 mg per day for adults suffering from severe osteomalacia). Periodic x-rays may be used to determine whether healing is taking place as expected. There may be cases of either rickets or osteomalacia that are resistant to therapeutic doses of vitamin D. It has sometimes been necessary to administer massive doses of the vitamin (50,000 to 100,000 IU per day). However, prolonged administration of such large doses of the vitamin may result in toxic effects.

Prevention of rickets and osteomalacia is usually achieved by the provision of adequate dietary calcium (a daily amount equivalent to that in 1½ pints [720 ml] of milk) and making certain that vitamin D is obtained from the diet or from the effect of sunlight on the skin. There is usually sufficient phosphorus present in the diets of people that a deficiency occurs only when there is an abnormally high level of urinary excretion of this element. Therefore, there have been worldwide efforts to promote the fortification of all milk with 400 IU of vitamin D per quart (950 ml). Should this prophylactic measure be unfeasible in some instances, calcium and vitamin D might be administered in the form of a mineral and vitamin supplement. It is noteworthy that in some areas of the Middle East, infants are fitted with miniature goggles (to protect their eyes) and placed out in the sun in bassinets.

(Also see BONE, section on "Bone Disorders"; CALCIUM, section on "Calcium Related Diseases"; OSTEOMALACIA; PHOSPHORUS, section on "Phosphorus Related Disease"; and VITAMIN D, section on "Deficiency Symptoms.")

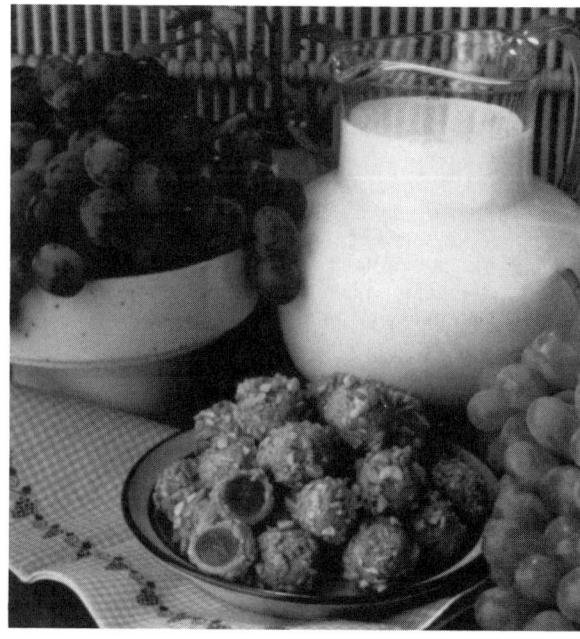

Fig. R-17. Prevention of rickets and osteomalacia is usually achieved by using fortified milk, a good source of both calcium and vitamin D. (Courtesy, California Grape Commission, Fresno, Calif.)

RIGOR MORTIS

Within a few hours after death the muscles become stiff and rigid. Since the blood no longer delivers oxygen to the tissues, anaerobic metabolism produces lactic acid which lowers the pH. As the ATP (adenosine triphosphate) is depleted, the muscles harden—contract.

RISSOLES

• These are like little turnovers, filled with a highly seasoned mixture of chopped chicken, ham, or other tender meat moistened with a little sauce, dropped onto pastry, which is sealed, then fried in deep fat.

• A patty of ground meat or fish, rolled in crumbs and dipped in egg, and more crumbs, then fried. The English name for the American croquette.

ROASTED GRAIN DRINKS (CEREAL COFFEE, CEREAL BEVERAGE, COFFEE SUBSTITUTE)

By roasting certain grains and grain products in combination with other flavor sources, a product may be obtained which can be mixed with hot water yielding an aromatic beverage similar to coffee. These cereal beverages are commercially available or they may be homemade. One popular product, developed over 75 years ago by C.W. Post, helped form the foundation for the General Foods Corporation.

Grains and grain products in the commercially prepared products are generally barley, wheat, rye, malt, and bran, while additional flavor is contributed by molasses, chicory, carob, cassia bark, allspice, and star anise, depending upon the manufacturer. A homemade roasted grain drink can be prepared by baking a combination of wheat bran, eggs, cornmeal, and molasses. There are even those cereal beverages which can be percolated like coffee.

Roasted grain drinks are caffeine-free. With the recent publicity involving the health effects of coffee and caffeine, these cereal grain beverages have gained in popularity.

ROASTERS (ROASTING PIGS)

Roasters are fat, plump, suckling pigs, weighing 30 to 60 lb (14 to 27 kg) on foot. They are dressed shipper style (with the head on), and are not split at the breast or between the hams. When properly roasted and attractively served with the traditional apple in the mouth, roast pig is considered a great delicacy for the holiday season.

ROCAMBOLE *Allium scorodoprasum*

European leek, usually cultivated like the shallot and used in the same way.

ROLLS

These can be defined as yeast-leavened miniature loaves of bread. There are as many kinds of rolls as the cook can devise. Some are the same basic recipe, but formed into different shapes. Others have slight variations in the proportion of fat or sugar to flour; and eggs may or may not be added. And the choices of added ingredients such as raisins, other fruits, spices, nuts, and poppy, sesame, or caraway seeds give added dimensions. A good basic roll recipe is like a good basic suit in the wardrobe—it can be used for all occasions. Any bread recipe can be used for rolls. Some of the more familiar rolls are: bagels, bread sticks, brioche, butterflake, cinnamon, clover-leaf, crescents (butterhorns),

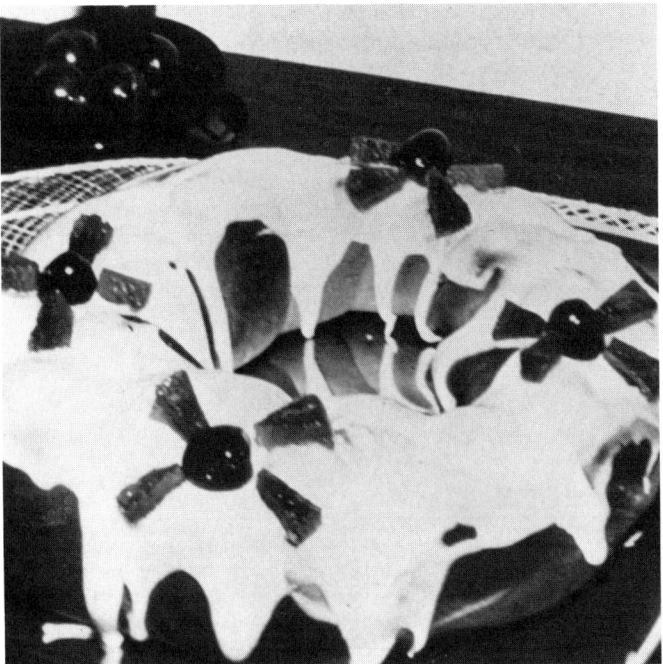

Fig. R-18. Christmas bread roll. (Courtesy, New Mexico State Univ., Las Cruces, N.M.)

croissants, English muffins (crumpets), hamburger buns, hot cross buns, Parker House (pocket rolls), pecan, submarine, twists, and wiener buns.

Rolls are as nutritious as the ingredients in them. See Table F-21, Food Composition Table, under "Bakery Products," for the nutritive qualities of rolls.

(Also see BREADS AND BAKING.)

ROPE

A condition in breads caused by *Bacillus mesentericus* or *Bacillus subtilis*. Spores of these bacteria can survive baking and then germinate under proper moisture and temperature surroundings. The bread develops sticky yellow patches that can be pulled into ropelike threads; hence, the name rope. Obviously, the bread is inedible. Food additives such as calcium acetate, calcium propionate, and sodium diacetate retard this bacterial growth.

(Also see ADDITIVES.)

ROSE APPLE (POMARROSA) *Eugenia jambos*

The fruit of a small tree (of the family *Myrtaceae*) that is native to the Indo-Malaysian region, and which was introduced into the New World tropics where it now grows wild. The rose-centered fruits are egg-shaped, about 1½ in. (4 cm) in diameter, yellowish-white or pink with a yellow flesh and one or two seeds. The fruit is eaten fresh or made into jam or pies.

The nutrient composition of rose apples is given in Food Composition Table F-21.

Some noteworthy observations regarding the nutrient composition of rose apples follow:

1. The raw fruit is low to moderately high in calories (56 kcal per 100 g) and carbohydrates (14%).

2. Rose apples are a good source of iron and a fair to good source of vitamin C.

ROSE HIPS *Rosa* spp

The fleshy fruit at the base of the rose bloom of plants of the family *Rosaceae*.

Rose hips are not eaten as such; rather, they are concentrated as a powder, made into jams, jellies, and syrups, or brewed as a tea. Rose hips are used as an ingredient of many vitamin C products, often in combination with ascorbic acid.

(Also see VITAMIN C, section on "Sources of Vitamin C.")

ROSELLE

An East Indian herb, cultivated for its fleshy calyxes, which are used to make tarts and jellies, and a very acid drink.

ROUX

A mixture of fat and flour which is used as a base for thickened sauces. It is prepared by melting the butter or other fat, adding the flour, and stirring until it is browned. This produces some dextrin which gives the sauce an enjoyable flavor, that gourmet cooks feel is superior to other methods of making white or other sauces.

ROWE ELIMINATION DIETS

Widely used elimination diets formulated by Dr. Albert H. Rowe. These diets are used to determine food allergies by removing certain types of foods from the diet. In general, elimination diets are tedious and time-consuming and should be employed only when dietary history, skin tests, and provocative food tests fail to detect the causative food. Rowe diets are organized on the basis of food items that have proven the least likely to produce an allergic response.

(Also see ALLERGIES, section on "Elimination Diets; Rowe Elimination Diets.")

ROYAL JELLY

This is the milky white food that is prepared exclusively for the queen bee in a beehive. Royal jelly, which is available as a supplement in capsule form, is a rich source of the B-complex vitamins, along with 20 amino acids. But about 3% of this substance made by bees still defies analysis.

Queen bees look different from worker bees: they are about twice the size; they live up to 8 years—fully 40 times longer than the normal lifespan of worker bees; and they lay about 2,000 eggs per day, whereas female worker bees are infertile. What makes queen bees so different? All the eggs start out the same, fed on a rich protein diet secreted from the glands of the worker bees. After 2 days, the eggs that are to become worker bees are changed to a diet of honey. Meanwhile, the egg that is to become the queen is fed royal bee jelly throughout her growth stage. Royal jelly makes the difference!

The implication of the promotors of royal jelly is that it will do as much for humans as for queen bees; that it will increase size, longevity, and fertility.

No effect has been demonstrated in humans, except a tendency to produce wakefulness. Royal jelly is judged to be of no practical value in human nutrition because of the very large amounts required for any definite effect.

RUMEN (PAUNCH)

The large first compartment of the stomach of a ruminant from which the food is regurgitated for cud-chewing and in which cellulose is broken down by bacterial and protozoan symbionts.

RUSKS (ZWIEBACK)

Zwieback is the German word meaning *twice-baked*. Originally, rusks were developed to take on ships for long voyages. They are made from either plain or sweet bread which is baked, then sliced and baked again to produce a hard crisp product. Rusks are a favorite food on which the infant can chew. They are also good for taking on camping or fishing trips, instead of trying to keep fresh bread on hand.

RYE *Secale cereale*

Contents   Page

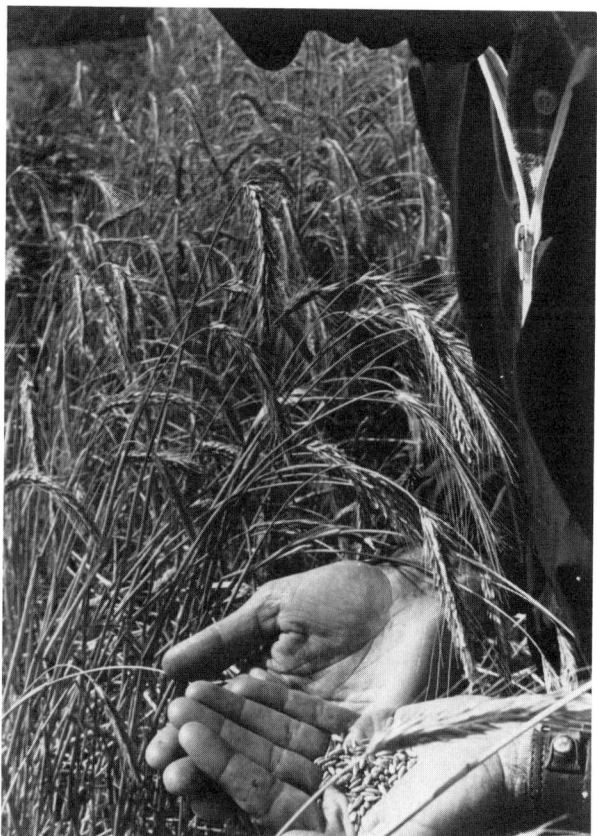

Fig. R-19. Rye, ripe and ready to harvest. (Courtesy, North Dakota State University, Fargo, N.D.)

The cereal grain, rye, *Secale cereale* of the grass family, *Gramineae*, is closely related to wheat and is grown as a bread grain, for distillation into grain alcohol spirits, and as a livestock feed. The most winter-hardy of the cereals, rye is the main bread grain of the Scandinavian and eastern European countries. Although nutritious, and palatable to some people, rye bread is not comparable to wheat bread in crumb quality and bold appearance of the loaf. As living standards rise, the consumption of rye bread falls, and the consumption of wheat bread rises.

(Also see CEREAL GRAINS.)

ORIGIN AND HISTORY. Rye was domesticated relatively recently, about the 4th century B.C., in Germany, and later in southern Europe. According to N. I. Vavilov, the Rus sian plant scientist, cultivated rye originated from wild species that occurred as weeds in wheat and barley crops, and rye was introduced into cultivation simultaneously and independently at many localities in central Asia or Asia Minor.

During the Middle Ages, the poorer people of England ate bread made from rye, or from a mixture of rye and wheat, known as *maslin*.

WORLD AND U.S. PRODUCTION. World production of rye is about 37 million metric tons, only about 6% of the world production of wheat, and only 2% of the world production of cereals.[6] Rye is more important in Europe and Asia than in the western hemisphere. The Soviet Union is the leading world producer, followed by Poland, Germany, China, Canada, Czechoslovakia, Denmark, Austria, Sweden, and Spain.[7]

Rye production in the United States has steadily declined since World War I. Annually, about 245 thousand metric tons are harvested from about 373,000 acres, with an average yield of 27.1 bu per acre. The U.S. wheat crop averages 36.7 bu per acre (*2,069 kg/ha*). The leading rye-producing states, by rank, are: South Dakota, Georgia, Minnesota, North Dakota, Nebraska, South Carolina, Michigan, Wisconsin, and North Carolina.[8]

---

[6]Data from *FAO Production Yearbook 1990*, FAO/UN, Rome, Italy, Vol. 44, p. 81, Table 21. **Note well:** Annual production fluctuates as a result of weather and profitability of the crop.

[7]*Ibid.*

[8]Data from *Agricultural Statistics 1991*, USDA, p. 16, Table 19. **Note well:** Annual production fluctuates as a result of weather and profitability of the crop.

PROCESSING. The processing of rye involves cleaning, conditioning, and milling.

The cleaning principles and machinery are similar to those used in wheat cleaning, complicated by two primary differences: (1) The grain is more variable in size; and (2) the grain is more subject to ergot (a poisonous fungus), which should be separated out before it is broken up and rendered difficult to remove (see ERGOT).

Conditioning, or tempering, consists of bringing the grain to a moisture content of about 14.5%.

The milling process resembles wheat flour milling, but it deviates from the latter because of two important differences between the grains; (1) the endosperm of rye breaks up into flour fineness more readily than the endosperm of wheat, and (2) the separation of the endosperm from the bran of rye is more difficult.

NUTRITIONAL VALUE. Food Composition Table F-21 gives the nutrient compositions of rye grain and rye products.

The food value of rye is similar to wheat. It is a good source of starch (carbohydrates) and a fair source of protein. However, the protein, in terms of essential amino acids, falls short in lysine compared to high-quality proteins. Therefore, like wheat and the other cereal grains, lysine is the limiting amino acid. Of the vitamins, rye is devoid of vitamins A, C, and B-12.

PRODUCTS AND USES. Rye is used for human food, fermented products, livestock feed, and for certain other purposes.

The uses of rye and rye products are summarized in Table R-8.

(Also see CEREAL GRAINS, and BREADS AND BAKING.)

TABLE R-8
RYE PRODUCTS AND USES FOR HUMAN FOOD

Product	Description	Uses	Comments
Rye	Whole grain, unground	Hot breakfast cereal. Served with main dish.	The whole grains may be cooked like rice by (1) soaking overnight in water (2-3 c of water per c [*240 ml*] of rye) then boiling until tender; or (2) cooking in a pressure cooker, using a standard recipe for rice.
Rye	Ground, dry whole rye grain. Rye meal, consisting of any extraction rate less than 100%.	Rye crisp Rye crisp	Rye crisp is a popular bread served with most meals in Sweden. Traditionally, rye crisp bread in Sweden is made by mixing rye meal with snow or powdered ice, then the expansion of the small air bubbles in the ice cold foam raises the dough when it is placed in the oven.
Rye flakes	Rolled whole rye	Hot breakfast cereal	
Rye flour (Also see FLOURS, Table F-12, Major Flours.)	Produced by milling rye, much like milling wheat. It does not contain as much gluten as wheat flour.	Bread. In the U.S., rye bread is usually made from a combination of rye flour and wheat flour. Biscuits and crackers (usually made from mixtures of about 10% rye flour and 90% wheat flour). Rye pancakes. Filler for sauces, soups, and custard powders.	In most countries, rye is used as a bread grain—for human food. Yeast does not raise rye dough as easily as wheat dough, because of lack of gluten in rye flour. When bread is made from straight rye flour, it is black, soggy, and rather bitter. For centuries, a large portion of the population of Europe lived mainly on schwarzbrot, made from rye flour, which is still rather common in rural Germany, Poland, and the U.S.S.R. Whole rye and mixed rye-wheat breads have a longer shelf life than wheat bread. Rye contains more pentosans than other cereals; hence, it is used in reducing diets because: (1) the pentosans gelantinize and swell in the stomach, imparting a feeling of satisfaction; and (2) digestion of the polysaccharides is slow, with the result that the blood sugar level rises slowly but is maintained for 5 to 6 hours, thereby controlling appetite.
		FERMENTED BEVERAGES	
Rye grain	Cleaned whole grain	Rye whiskey. Industrial alcohol.	Rye whiskey is made from a fermented mash containing a minimum of 51% rye.
Rye bread	Brown rye bread	Russian rye bread beer (kvass or quass)	A mash made by pressure cooking the bread is treated with rye malt, then fermented by a mixture of yeast and *Bacillus lactis*. The beer, which contains only about 0.7% alcohol, is usually dispensed cold from tank trucks.

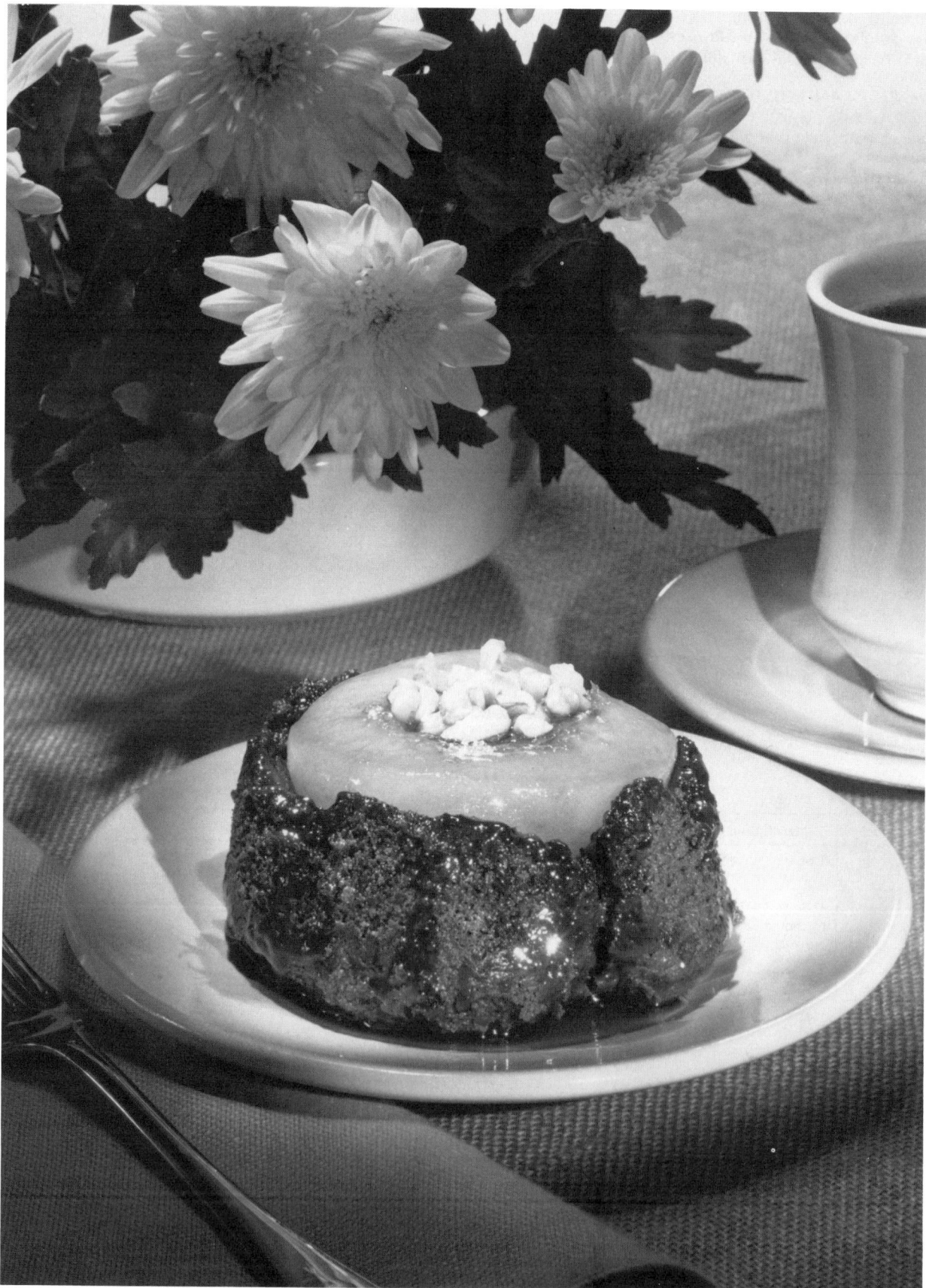

Fig. R-20. Besides using rye flour for rye bread, and pumpernickel, rye flour can be substituted for some of the wheat flour in such quickbreads as steamed brown bread, muffins, and gingerbread (as above). (Courtesy, California Foods Research Institute for Cling Peach Advisory Board, San Francisco, Calif.)

SACCHARIMETER

An apparatus for determining the concentration of sugar in a solution, based on the optical activity of the sugar; especially a polarimeter adapted for distinguishing different kinds of sugar in a solution.

SACCHARIN

A nonnutritive, noncaloric synthetic sweetener which is 300 to 500 times sweeter than table sugar. It was on the first GRAS (generally recognized as safe) list published in 1959. However, in 1972, following the ban on cyclamates, saccharin was removed from the GRAS list and given a provisional food additive status.

Today, saccharin is still being used on a limited basis.

(Also see ADDITIVES, Table A-3 Common Food Additives; ARTIFICIAL SWEETENERS; CANCER; and DELANEY CLAUSE.)

SACCHAROMETER

A floating apparatus, a special hydrometer, used to determine the specific gravity of sugar solutions. It can be graduated to read directly the percentage of sugar in solution. It is distinct from a saccharimeter.

SAFETY OF FOOD

Food safety involves a number of concerns, the most important of which are: (1) pesticides, and (2) harmful bacteria.

1. Pesticide residues in and on foods are the public's number one food safety fear. Because pesticides cannot be seen or smelled, consumers feel that they have little control over their level of exposure. So, we need to develop safer and more effective pesticides, and to use less pesticides on fruits and vegetables.

(Also see PESTICIDES AND INCIDENTAL FOOD ADDITIVES; and POISONS.)

2. Without bacteria in food there would be no yogurt, no blue cheese, and no sourdough bread. However, other bacteria left to grow unchecked can cause spoilage and even food-related illness. Making sure that this does not happen is the job of producers, workers, supervisors, and quality control specialists from farm to food counter, and finally to the consumer. Despite some concerns and scares from time to time, America's cornucopia of foods remains the envy of the world, both in quantity and quality.

(Also see DISEASES, sections on "Sanitary Measures Which Help to Prevent the Spread of Diseases" and "Health and Nutrition Functions of Government Agencies"; FOOD—BUYING, PREPARING, COOKING, AND SERVING; BACTERIA IN FOOD; and FOOD POISONING.)

SAFFLOWER Carthamus tinctorius

The safflower is a relative of the thistle. Its scientific identity: family, *Compositae*; genus, *Carthamus*, species, *C. tinctorius*.

The seed, which resembles a small sunflower seed, is com-

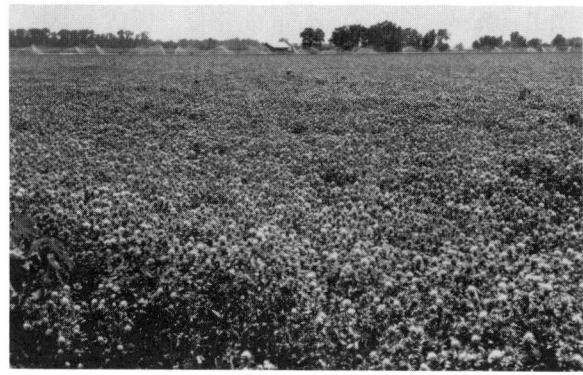

Fig. S-1. Field of safflowers in bloom in the Sacramento Valley of California. The safflower is a relative of the thistle family. (Courtesy, Pacific Oilseeds Incorporated, Woodland, Calif.)

posed of a thick fibrous white hull encasing a yellow kernel.

In the 1950s, interest in safflower oil as a food ingredient skyrocketed as a result of studies relating saturated fats in the diet to atherosclerotic heart disease. Safflower's unique fatty acid composition places it highest in polyunsaturates and lowest in saturates of all commercial fats and oils.

ORIGIN AND HISTORY. Safflower is native to Southeastern Asia, but it has long been cultivated in India, Egypt, China, and Northern Africa.

WORLD AND U.S. PRODUCTION. The world production of safflower seed totals 922,000 metric tons annually. India is far in the lead globally with a production of about 491,000 metric tons—over half of the world production. The United States with 170,000 metric tons ranks second, and Mexico with a production of about 159,000 metric tons ranks third. Lesser quantities are produced in Spain.[1]

Total U.S. seed production reached a high of 350,000 metric tons in 1967, but has since declined to around 170,000 metric tons.

PROCESSING SAFFLOWER SEED. Normally, the steps in processing consist of: (1) cleaning the seed by screening and aspiration; (2) grinding the seed; (3) cooking under steam pressure; (4) extracting the oil by the continuous screw press-solvent extraction method; (5) grinding and screening the cake to produce meal; and (6) refining the oil.

NUTRITIONAL VALUE OF SAFFLOWER SEED. The commercial varieties of safflower grown in the United States average 35 to 40% hull and yield 39 to 40% oil and 15% protein. However, varieties with up to 50% oil content have been developed.

The oil is extremely variable, perhaps reflecting its mixed heredity. California studies on safflower procured from many parts of the world showed great variation in the content of

[1]Data from *FAO Production Yearbook 1990*, FAO/UN, Rome, Italy, Vol. 44, p. 117, Table 44. **Note well:** Annual production fluctuates as a result of weather and profitability of the crop.

polyunsaturated fats, with iodine numbers ranging from 87 to 149. It averages about 6.6% saturated acids and 93.4% unsaturated acids, with the latter consisting of 77.0% linoleic acid and 16.4% oleic acid (The high linoleic acid content makes the oil susceptible to rancidity). Linolenic acid is absent. Genetically modified varieties of safflower with greater resistance to rancidity have been introduced that contain 80% oleic, 15% linoleic, and 5% saturated fatty acids. Safflower oil is listed in Food Composition Table F-21 and Table F-4, Fats and Fatty Acids in Selected Foods.

The extracted cake is ground to yield a 20 to 42% protein meal, with the higher protein content obtained from decorticated (dehulled) seed. Meal produced by the solvent method contains about 1% fat vs 5% when the expeller process is used. Safflower meal is of good quality, although somewhat deficient in lysine and methionine.

SAFFLOWER PRODUCTS AND USES. Safflower oil is a bland, almost colorless product. Due to its susceptibility to oxidation, care is taken to exclude air during storage, transport, and packaging. Interest in the oil as a food ingredient stems largely from its high percentage of unsaturated (polyunsaturated) fatty acids.

Safflower oil is used principally in the production of margarine, salad oils, mayonnaise, shortening, and other food products. The oil is also used as a drying agent in varnishes and paints.

High protein content safflower meal, made from dehulled seed and containing about 42% protein, is now considered a protein source for human consumption. However, most safflower meal is used as a protein supplement for livestock. The meal is not very palatable when used alone.

(Also see OILS, VEGETABLE, Table O-5.)

SAINT ANTHONY'S FIRE

A thousand years ago, this name was given to the condition known now as ergotism—a poisoning due to the consumption of foods containing the fungus ergot. Symptoms of ergotism include alternating burning and freezing sensations; hence, the name Saint Anthony's Fire.

(Also see POISONS, Table P-2, Some Potentially Poisonous [Toxic] Substances, "Ergot.")

SALAMI

A highly seasoned sausage made of pork and beef in various proportions; either (1) air-dried, hard, and of good keeping qualities, or (2) fresh, soft, and requiring refrigeration until consumed.

SALEP

A starchy foodstuff from the Middle East which consists of the dried tubers of various orchids. It is easily digested and highly esteemed in the East.

SALINE

It refers to anything containing or consisting of salt. Physiological saline is a solution containing 0.9% NaCl (salt). Since it is compatible with the blood, it is sometimes administered intravenously.

SALIVA

A clear, somewhat viscid solution secreted into the mouth by three pairs of salivary glands—the parotid, the sublingual, and the submaxillary.

The functions of saliva are manyfold including the follow-ing: lubrication, enzymatic activity, buffering capacity, taste, and moistening the membranes of the mouth and providing some antibacterial action.

Secretion of saliva is stimulated by the sight, the smell, and even the mere thought of food.

(Also see DIGESTION AND ABSORPTION, section on "Mouth.")

SALLY LUNN

This bread came to America from Bath, England, the home of Sally Lunn. It is baked in a tube-center pan, and it should have a porous, cakelike texture.

SALMONELLA

A genus of bacteria responsible for one of the most common foodborne infections in the United States—salmonellosis. *Salmonella* bacteria grow rapidly in cooked foods such as meats, eggs, custards, and salads which have been left unrefrigerated for several hours. It may also be transmitted by sewage-polluted water.

(Also see BACTERIA IN FOOD, Table B-2, Food Infections [Bacterial], "Salmonellosis.")

SALT (SODIUM CHLORIDE; NaCl)

Salt is created by the combination of the soft silvery-white metal sodium (Na), and the yellow poisonous gas chlorine (Cl). Sodium and chlorine are vital elements found in the fluids and soft tissues of the body. Salt also improves the appetite, promotes growth, helps regulate the body pH, and is essential for hydrochloric acid formation in the stomach.

HISTORICAL IMPORTANCE OF SALT. Throughout history, salt has occupied a unique position. Wars have been fought over it, empires have been founded on it and have collapsed without it, and civilizations have grown up around it.

Mosaic law prescribed the use of salt with offerings made to Jehovah; and there are frequent Biblical references to the purifying and flavoring effects of salt. The Greeks used salt as the medium of exchange in buying and selling slaves; a good slave was said to be *worth his weight in salt*. The word salary is derived from the Latin *salarium*, referring to the salt which was part of a Roman soldier's pay. In medieval England, royal banquet halls had imposing salt cellars; and the seating arrangement in relation thereto served as a status symbol. Important persons were invited to *sit above the salt*, where they could use the salt on their food freely; those of lesser importance were seated *below the salt*. In some parts of Africa, gold was once evaluated in terms of how much salt it would buy—rather than the reverse. Salt caravans, part of the ancient lore of Africa, still ply certain desert areas to this day. By common use, the expression *salt of the earth* refers to a really good person. These and other salt lore give ample evidence that in olden times salt was a valuable and relatively scarce commodity.

FUNCTIONS OF SALT.
Most people think of salt as a seasoning, but it is probably used in greater quantities and for more applications than any other chemical. In fact, it is estimated that over 14,000 uses are made of salt.

Physiological.
Sodium (Na) and chlorine (Cl) are essential parts of the human diet. (Salt as such isn't essential, since other sources of Na and Cl are satisfactory; for example, Na_2CO_3 and KCl.)

In body solution, salt dissociates into two ions—sodium and chloride, both of which are normal and necessary constituents.

(Also see CHLORINE OR CHLORIDE [Cl]; and SODIUM [Na].)

SALT DEFICIENCY.
Salt deficiency is rarely a problem since most Americans consume many times more salt than is recommended. Fortunately, the body adjusts.

If there is a low intake, the excretion rate is low. Deficiencies may occur from strict vegetarian diets without salt, or when there has been heavy, prolonged sweating, diarrhea, vomiting, or adrenal cortical insufficiency—Addison's disease.

A deficiency of salt (sodium) may cause reduced growth, loss of appetite, loss of body weight due to loss of body water, reduced milk production of lactating mothers, muscle cramps, nausea, diarrhea, and headache. In cases of prolonged or severe vomiting, or indiscreet use of diuretics, chloride losses may exceed that of sodium—resulting in a state of metabolic alkalosis. To restore the acid-base balance of the body, adequate chloride must be provided.

SALT TOXICITY.
Excess dietary salt, over a long period of time, is believed to contribute to the development of high blood pressure in susceptible individuals.

In addition, salt may be toxic (1) when ingested in large quantities, especially with a low water intake; (2) when the body has been depleted by a salt-free vegetarian diet or excess sweating, followed by gorging on salt; (3) when large amounts are fed to infants or others afflicted with kidney diseases, whose kidneys cannot excrete the excess in the urine; or (4) when the body is adapted to a chronic low-salt diet, followed by ingesting large amounts.

(Also see HIGH BLOOD PRESSURE; MINERAL[S]; POISONS, Table P-2, Some Potentially Poisonous, [Toxic] Substances; and SODIUM.)

Commercial Uses.
The majority of the millions of tons of salt produced each year is used by a variety of industries and businesses; it's used commercially.

FOOD INDUSTRY.
Its first uses in foods are lost in antiquity. Thus, not surprisingly, salt is on the FDA list of GRAS (generally recognized as safe) food additives. In foods, salt performs three primary functions: (1) as a flavor enhancer or seasoner; (2) as a preservative; and (3) as a solubilizing agent.

CHEMICAL INDUSTRY.
Much of the salt is utilized in the manufacture of other chemicals. By passing an electric current through salt—electrolysis—it can be broken up into sodium metal and chlorine gas. The sodium can be used as a catalyst, or it can combine with other elements to form new chemicals such as sodium carbonate, sodium bicarbonate, and lye (sodium hydroxide). The chlorine formed by electrolysis can also be used to make other chemicals, or it can be employed in bleaching paper and textiles, or in

disinfecting water supplies. Many of the chemicals derived from salt find their way into numerous other industries.

OTHER INDUSTRIES AND BUSINESSES.
Salt is important to a number of other industries and businesses. The leather industry uses salt for the preservation of hides. Salt can be employed to soften water. Railroads use salt to keep their switches from icing up. Highway departments use salt on icy roads, and on secondary roads to stabilize the soil and control the dust. Farmers feed salt to livestock. It is also employed in heat-treating, smelting, and refining metals. The list of uses seems endless for this basic chemical.

EXCESS SALT; LABELING.
For years, the subject of salt and its relation to hypertension has been debated by consumers, federal officials, and food industry representatives. Finally, in 1981, for the first time, the food industry was asked by the Food and Drug Administration to lower the salt content in foods, voluntarily and not by regulation. In support of the request, Richard S. Schweiker, Secretary of Health and Human Service, had the following to say:

"Sixty million Americans suffer from hypertension, which can lead to strokes and heart attacks. Hypertension can be significantly controlled."

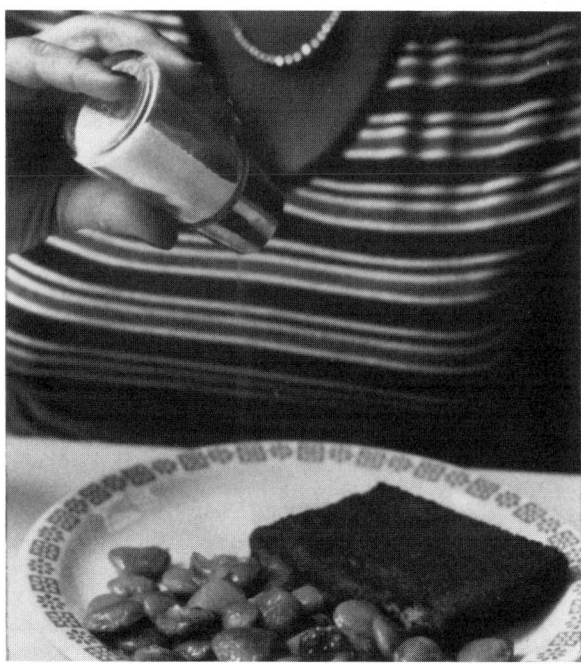

Fig. S-2. Use salt sparingly. (Courtesy, University of Tennessee, Knoxville, Tenn.)

At about the same time, a bill was introduced in the U.S. Congress that would *require* food processors and manufacturers to disclose, through a label, the salt content of their products if the salt is above a certain level. Also, it was revealed that the FDA had drafted a regulation that would *require* sodium labeling, but it would have to be approved by the Office of Management and Budget before it could be instituted.

The FDA, which has jurisdiction over about 80% of all processed foods, indicated that labeling would apply to both natural and added salt in a product.

Simultaneously, the U.S. Department of Agriculture announced that the department plans to encourage sodium disclosure for meat products under its jurisdiction through similar action to that of the FDA.

(Also see SODIUM, section headed "Recommended Daily Allowances of Sodium.")

SOURCES OF SALT. The United States is by far the leading salt-producing country. The states of Louisiana, Texas, New York, and Ohio produce 88% of U.S. salt. In 1985, 39.5 million short tons of salt, worth $741.8 million, were taken from the seas, mines, and wells in the United States.

(Also see ADDITIVES; CHLORINE OR CHLORIDE; MINERAL[S]; and SODIUM.)

SALT DIET, LOW

Low salt diet is a rather misleading term. Since table salt is by far the most important source of sodium in the diet, most sodium-restricted diets begin with the elimination or at least restricted use of table salt on food. Hence, sodium-restricted diets are sometimes called low salt diets. A mild sodium restriction which is used as a maintenance diet in cardiac and renal diseases limits daily sodium intake to 2,000 to 3,000 mg. This means no salty foods and no salt used at the table. Other sodium-restricted diets include moderate sodium restriction (1,000 to 1,500 mg daily), strict sodium restriction (500 mg), and severe sodium restriction (250 mg). All of these diets require limited or no use of salt at all stages of food preparation. The strict and severe sodium restriction necessitates careful selection of foods for all sources of sodium, not just salt.

(Also see MODIFIED DIETS, Table 28, Modified Diets, "Sodium restricted diet"; and SODIUM.).)

SALT FOODS, LOW

Table salt—sodium chloride—is the most important source of sodium in the diet. Salt may be added to foods during processing, during cooking, and at the table by the consumer. When an individual requires the restriction of daily sodium intake, the first step involves limiting the intake of salt. Depending upon the level of sodium restriction, foods may need to be carefully selected in regards to the amount of salt used in processing. However, salt is not the only source of sodium in foods, so if a strict or severe restriction of sodium is needed, all sources of sodium in foods must be considered. Other sodium sources include baking soda, baking powder, sodium benzoate, sodium citrate, monosodium glutamate (MSG), sodium propionate, and sodium alginate. When selecting foods for sodium restricted diets, labels should be noted for the words *salt* and *sodium*. Furthermore, some foods possess a naturally high level of sodium and must be used in measured amounts in sodium restricted diets.

(Also see MODIFIED DIETS; SALT, section on "Excess Salt; Labeling"; and SODIUM.)

SALT-FREE DIETS

A more accurate description of these diets is sodium restricted or low sodium. Since much of the sodium added to foods comes from table salt—sodium chloride—the first step in a sodium-restricted diet is the elimination of table salt. Hence, these diets are commonly called salt-free.

Sodium-restricted diets, varying in the amount of sodium restriction, are prescribed for the elimination, control, and prevention of edema—water accumulation in the tissues—which accompanies such things as congestive heart failure, cirrhosis, kidney disorders, and corticosteroid therapy.

Sodium restriction is also helpful in control of some cases of high blood pressure.

For persons on sodium restricted diets, a 1:1 mixture of table salt (NaCl) and potassium chloride (KCl) for salting foods will lessen the sodium intake without a change in taste. However, excessive use of dietary potassium should be avoided due to toxic effects at high levels.

(Also see MODIFIED DIETS; HIGH BLOOD PRESSURE; and SODIUM.)

SALTINE

This is a thin crisp cracker covered with salt. All saltines are soda crackers, but not all soda crackers are saltines.

SALTPETER

A name sometimes applied to potassium nitrate; sodium nitrate is called Chile saltpeter.

(Also see NITRATES.)

SAMBAL

A condiment common to Indonesia and Malaya, eaten with curry and rice. Typically, it contains peppers, pickles, grated coconut, salt fish, or fish roe.

SAMP

Coarse hominy or a boiled cereal made from it.

SAPONIFICATION

The formation of soap and glycerol from the reaction of fat with alkali.

SAPONINS

A group of heart-stimulating glycosides derived from plants such as foxglove, squill, and legumes. They can be broken down into a sugar and a steroid. All saponins foam when shaken with water, and all are surface-active agents. When injected into the bloodstream they are capable of bursting (hemolyzing) red blood cells. Saponins are used as an emulsification agent for fats and oils, as a soap or detergent, and as a subject of research on steroid sex hormones.

SARCOMA

A tumor of fleshy consistency—often highly malignant.

SATIETY

Full satisfaction of desire; may refer to satisfaction of appetite.

(Also see APPETITE.)

SATURATED

A state in which a substance holds the most of another substance that it can hold.

SATURATED FAT

A completely hydrogenated fat—each carbon atom is associated with the maximum number of hydrogens; there are no double bonds.

(Also see FATS AND OTHER LIPIDS.)

SAUCES

The word *sauce* comes from the Latin word *salsa* meaning *salted*. A *sauce can be defined as a liquid food, which*

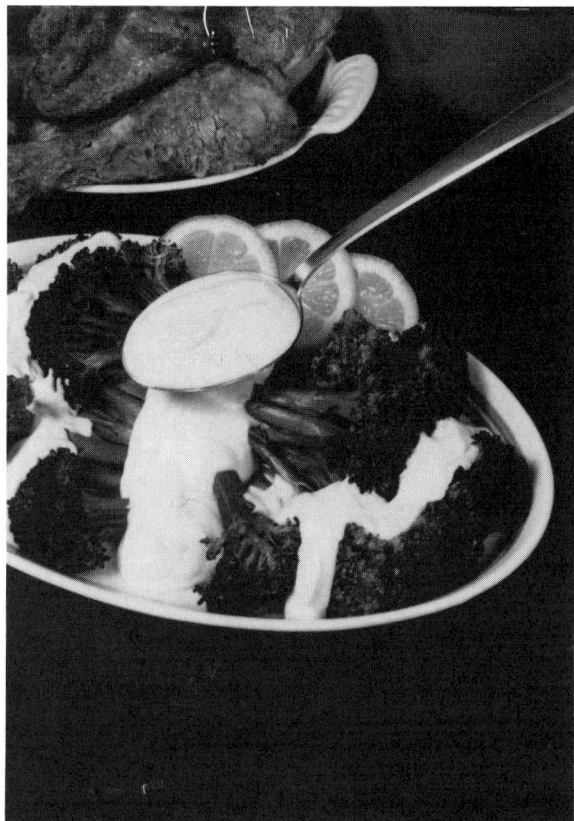

Fig. S-3. Sauce—the crowning touch. (Courtesy, Carnation Co., Los Angeles, Calif.)

is poured over a solid food. It can appear on the menu from appetizer to dessert. It can range from liquid to very thick; from no seasoning to highly seasoned; from cold to piping hot; from sour to extremely sweet; from simple to complicated and rich; and from the same every time to never the same way twice.

Sauces do not take any great amount of time to make. Nevertheless, they should not be a neglected art, for, in the final analysis, the sauce often lifts up the dish: it glamorizes the simplest food; it gives the recipe distinction; it increases the appetite appeal; it is the crowning touch.

There are so many kinds of sauces that it is difficult to organize them into any kind of order; for instance, a white sauce can be used either for fish or for dessert, depending on the added flavorings and seasonings.

Some of the basic sauces are:

• **For hors d'oeuvres and salads**—French dressing, mayonnaise, and salad dressings.

• **For main dishes**—Barbecue sauce, butter sauce, cheese sauce, fruit sauce, gravies, hollandaise sauce, tartar sauce, tomato sauce and ketchup, and white sauce.

• **For desserts**—Chocolate sauce, custard sauce, fruit sauces, hard sauce, and white sauce.

SAUERKRAUT

This is salted sliced cabbage that has undergone fermentation by lactic acid bacteria. In the fermentation process, the sugars of the cabbage are converted primarily to lactic and acetic acids, ethyl alcohol, and carbon dioxide.

The first description of sauerkraut manufacture, comparable to the methods used commercially today, was given by James Lind in 1772, in his treatise on scurvy. Barrels, kegs, and stone crocks were the common containers. Wooden vats were introduced in the United States about 1885. Recently, reinforced concrete with plastic coatings and glazed tile vats have been introduced.

In most modern kraut factories, salt is weighed and applied at a 2.25% level to the shredded cabbage. Ordinarily, sauerkraut is left in the vats until completely fermented.

Very little kraut is retailed in bulk today. Most of it is canned, although the use of plastic and glass containers is increasing.

Sauerkraut is often eaten as an adjunct to other foods, thereby making them more appetizing and digestible. It is generally recognized that when sauerkraut is cooked with other foods, particularly meats, it enhances their palatability.

(Also see CABBAGE.)

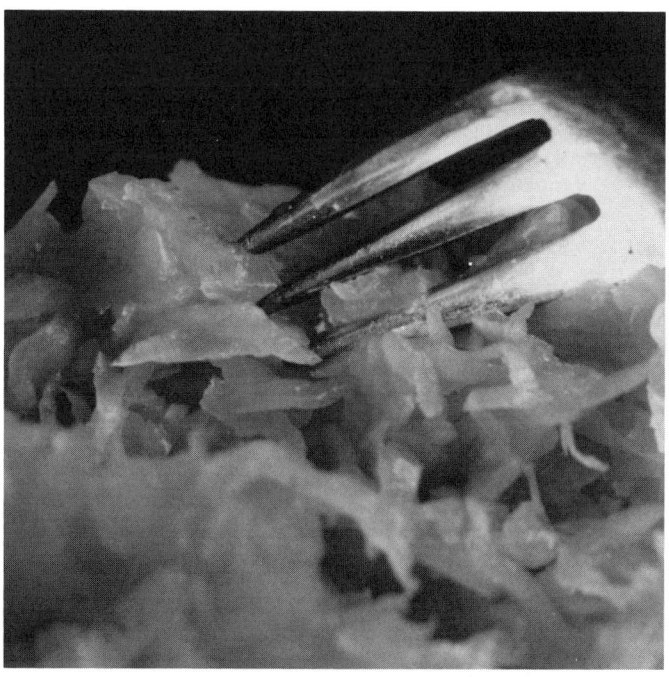

Fig. S-4. Sauerkraut—fermented cabbage—is often eaten as an appetizing adjunct to other foods. (Courtesy, University of Minnesota, St. Paul, Minn.)

SAUSAGE

Highly seasoned finely ground meat (usually pork or beef, but other meats may be used), most of which is stuffed in casings, used either fresh or cured.

SAUSAGE CASINGS

Natural casings are made from the middle wall of the small and large intestines of cattle, hogs, sheep, and goats. Also, the lung, bladder, and (in the case of hogs) the stomach are used as containers for special sausages.

Additionally, there are: cellulose casings, made from cotton linters; collagen casings, made from a collagen source, such as the corium layer of beef hide; and plastic netting made of polyethylene threads.

SCHOOL LUNCH PROGRAM

The National School Lunch Program, which is administered by the U.S. Department of Agriculture (USDA), was established for the purposes of (1) safeguarding the health and well-being of American children, and (2) encouraging the consumption of nutritious agricultural commodities and other foods. It operates by assisting the states, through grants-in-aid and other means, in the establishment, maintenance, conduct, and expansion of nonprofit school lunch programs. Hence, the costs of providing lunches are shared by the USDA, state and local government, and the recipients of the meals.

A good understanding of the school lunch program is important to parents and teachers who influence the child's eating habits.

HISTORY. United States surplus agricultural commodities were distributed on a limited basis for free lunches as early as 1932. In 1935, the U.S. Department of Agriculture was authorized by law to purchase and distribute the commodities on a much larger scale. In 1942, surplus foods were used to feed 6.2 million children.

By 1948, however, the supplies of surplus agricultural commodities were greatly reduced as a result of wartime demands. Hence, the USDA started a cash reimbursement program to pay schools for a part of the food purchased locally. But, the participating schools were required to (1) meet certain nutritional standards in the lunches served, (2) provide free meals for the children unable to pay, and (3) operate their lunch programs on a nonprofit basis. These provisions formed much of the basis for the National School Lunch Act of 1946, which placed the basic responsibility for the administration of school lunch programs in the hands of state education agencies. Since then, the provisions of the original act have been modified several times by new laws that were enacted to bring about the serving of greater numbers of free and reduced-price lunches to needy children. Participating schools are provided (1) cash assistance, (2) donation of surplus food commodities, and (3) technical assistance in the purchase and use of foods and in the equipping and managing of the school lunchroom.

During the 1970s, authorizations and regulations were established for a Nutrition Education and Training Program (NET) that had the objectives of (1) teaching students about the relationships between food, nutrition, and health, (2) training food service personnel in the principles and skills of food service management, and (3) instructing teachers in sound principles of nutrition education.

On a typical day in 1990, lunches were served to 24.6 million children and adolescents. That year, the federal cost of school lunches was $3.2 billion.

PROVISIONS OF THE NATIONAL SCHOOL LUNCH ACT.

The enactment of the National School Lunch Act of 1946 placed the school lunch program of the USDA on a firm foundation.

Eligibility for participation in the National School Lunch Program is contingent upon (1) operating the program on a nonprofit basis, (2) providing free or reduced-price lunches

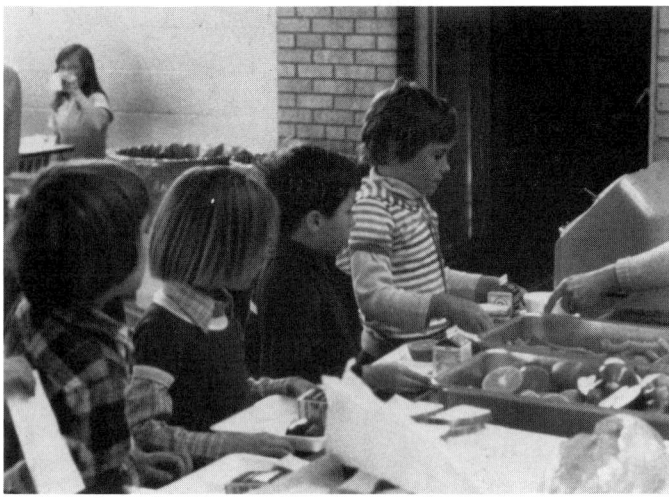

Fig. S-5. School Lunch Program. (Courtesy, University of Minnesota, St. Paul, Minn.)

to needy children, (3) making lunches available without regard to race, color, or national origin, (4) providing kitchen and dining facilities, (5) avoiding public identification or segregation of needy children, and (6) serving nutritious lunches that conform to USDA guidelines.

BENEFITS OF THE SCHOOL LUNCH.

Some of the main benefits of the National School Lunch Program follow:

1. Since the 1940s most of the children attending public and private schools in all 50 states, the District of Columbia, Puerto Rico, the Virgin Islands, and Guam have had the opportunity to obtain a school lunch.

2. Many needy children have been served nutritious lunches which they would not likely have received through other means. Fig. S-6 shows that the numbers of children receiving free or reduced-price lunches increased steadily throughout the 1980s.

3. About 50% of the families with children receiving lunches free or at reduced prices had incomes below $10,000.

Children In the National School Lunch Program

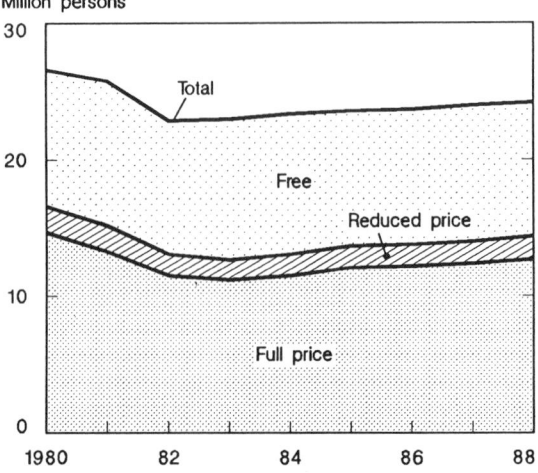

Fig. S-6. The number of children in the National School Lunch Program during the 1980s. (Source: *1989 Agricultural Chartbook*, USDA Ag. Hdbk. No. 684, p. 70)

4. School lunches have provided about one-third of the Recommended Dietary Allowances for school children on a daily basis.

5. Recent modifications in the food patterns have provided pupils with experiences in (1) eating foods used mainly by minority ethnic groups (items such as bulgur wheat and corn grits), and (2) new types of food preparations (such as meat dishes extended with soy protein).

6. Teachers have been motivated by students' comments on their lunches to spend more time discussing foods, health, and nutrition subjects.

7. Children, parents, teachers, and community groups have had opportunities to contribute viewpoints regarding the types of foods served. Some of these groups have been successful in making significant improvements in their local programs. For example, whole wheat pizza, sprouts, yogurt, and other highly nutritious foods are now served in certain local schools.

8. Poorly equipped and staffed schools have received both financial and technical assistance in developing better cooking and serving facilities and in upgrading the education and training of their personnel.

9. Surplus commodities have been utilized profitably and have helped to keep the prices of the lunches within the means of the students.

10. Local food suppliers have benefited from the purchases made for the program.

11. States have been induced to contribute some of their revenues to the program. At first, the state contributions came mainly from the payments of school children for the lunches.

SCHOOL LUNCH GUIDELINES.
Published U.S. Department of Agriculture school lunch guidelines are given in Table S-1.

GOAL OF THE SCHOOL LUNCH PROGRAM.
The goal of the school lunch program should be twofold:

1. The lunches offered to children should be nutritionally adequate and designed to develop and encourage the child's liking for a wide variety of the protective foods which frequently are not included in home diets.

2. The meals should be closely linked to the school's education program for better health.

These objectives merit further implementation. They need to be carried out by informed food service managers, cooks, and helpers in thousands of participating schools in every section of the country.

In addition to school lunches, it is noteworthy that, today, more and more children eat at least one meal outside the home—in day nurseries, child-care centers, day-care centers, or nursery schools. Usually, the noon meal is provided.

TABLE S-1
SCHOOL LUNCH GUIDELINES[1]
(Minimum amounts of foods listed by food components to serve students of various age/grade groups)

Food Component and Description	Preschool Children		Elementary School Students		Secondary School Students
	Group I (1 and 2 years of age)	Group II (3 and 4 years of age)	Group III (5-8 years of age; or Grades 1 to 3)	Group IV (9-11 years of age; or Grades 4 to 6)	Group V (12 years of age and over; or Grades 7 to 12)
	(amount per day)	(amount per day)	(amount per day)	(amount per day)	(amount per day)
Meat and meat alternates[2] Meat—a serving (edible portion) of cooked lean meat, poultry, or fish. Alternates: The following meat alternates may be used alone or in combination to meet the meat/meat alternate requirement:[3] Cheese (1 oz = 1 oz of meat), eggs (1 large egg = 1 oz of meat), cooked dry beans or peas (½ cup [120 ml] = 1 oz of meat),[4] peanut butter (2 Tbsp [30 ml] = 1 oz of meat)	1 oz (28 g)	1½ oz (43 g)	1½ oz (43 g)	2 oz (57 g)	3 oz (85 g)
Vegetables and fruits 2 or more servings consisting of vegetables or fruits or both. (A serving of full strength vegetable or fruit juice can be counted to meet not more than ½ of the total requirement.)	½ cup (120 ml)	½ cup (120 ml)	½ cup (120 ml)	¾ cup (180 ml)	¾ cup (180 ml)
Bread and bread alternates[5] 1 serving (1 slice) of enriched or whole-grain bread, or a serving of biscuits, rolls, muffins, etc. made with whole-grain or enriched meal or flour, or a serving (½ cup [120 ml]) of cooked enriched or whole-grain rice, macaroni, noodles, and other pasta products.[6]	5 servings per week	8 servings per week	8 servings per week	8 servings per week	10 servings per week
Milk, fluid[7] Unflavored fluid, lowfat milk, skim milk, or buttermilk must be offered as a beverage. If a school serves whole or flavored milk, it must offer unflavored fluid lowfat milk, skim milk, or buttermilk as a beverage choice.	¾ cup (180 ml)	¾ cup (180 ml)	½ pint (240 ml)	½ pint (240 ml)	½ pint (240 ml)

[1]Adapted by the authors from *Code of Federal Regulations*, Title 7, Revised January 1, 1980, Part 210, Sec. 210.19b.

[2]It is recommended that in schools not offering a choice of meat/meat alternate each day, no one form of meat (ground, sliced, pieces, etc.) or meat alternate be served more than three times per week. Meat and meat alternates must be served in a main dish, or in a main dish and one other menu item.

[3]When it is determined that the serving size of a meat alternate is excessive, the particular meat alternate shall be reduced and supplemented with an additional meat/meat alternate to meet the full requirement.

[4]Cooked dry beans or peas may be used as the meat alternate or as part of the vegetable/fruit component, but not as both food components in the same meal.

[5]One-half or more slices of bread or an equivalent amount of bread alternate must be served with each lunch with the total requirement being served during a 5-day period. Schools serving lunch 6 or 7 days per week should increase the quantity specified for a 5-day week by approximately 20% for each additional day.

[6]Enriched macaroni products with fortified protein may be used as part of a meat alternate or a bread alternate, but not as both food components in the same meal.

[7]One-half pint of milk may be used for all age/grade groups if the lesser specified amounts are determined by the school authority to be impractical.

A sound school lunch program can help to improve the diets and food habits of children, and, thus, eventually lead to better diets and food habits for the population as a whole. This goal merits the support of federal, state, and local governments, and of parents and school officials.

(Also see CHILDHOOD AND ADOLESCENT NUTRITION, section on "School Lunch and Breakfast Programs"; and GOVERNMENT FOOD PROGRAMS.)

SCLERODERMA

One of the first signs of scleroderma is tight, firm skin, and eventually a diffuse thickening and rigidity of the skin and subcutaneous tissue. These changes in the skin are reflected in the name of this disease, which means *hard skin*. Sometimes the disease is called *hidebound skin*. As the disease progresses, it involves the internal organs, specifically the intestinal tract, the heart, and the kidneys.

The cause of scleroderma is unknown. It belongs to a larger group of diseases sometimes classed as collagen diseases. In scleroderma, the changes in the skin and internal organs seem to be due to the overproduction of collagen—connective tissue.

There is no specific treatment for scleroderma. Corticosteroid therapy may slow the disease, or produce improvement in the early stages. This may require a sodium-restricted diet to prevent sodium retention during corticosteroid therapy. As the disease progresses, swallowing difficulties and a malabsorption syndrome may be encountered, which require some dietary adjustments.

SCRAPPLE

Made from head meat, feet, hearts, tongues, shoulder, spare ribs, fresh picnic shoulders, or any pork trimmings that contain some fat. Liver may be used if desired. Twenty percent of the meat may consist of beef or veal, but all pork is preferable.

Cook the meat in sufficient water to keep it covered; drain off the liquid when the meat separates readily from the bones. Remove the bones, then grind the meat. Place the ground meat and the liquor in which it was cooked together in a kettle and bring it to a boil.

Mix meal or flour (cornmeal, oatmeal, buckwheat flour, or soybean flour) with some water or some of the meat juice, add slowly and work the cereal to avoid lumps. Pour the diluted meal or flour into the cooked meat, season with condiments and herbs, and cook for another 30 minutes. Pour into a mold to cool, and serve sliced and fried.

SCREENED

A ground material that has been separated into various-sized particles by passing over or through screens.

SCREENINGS

By-products obtained from screening grains and other seeds.

SCURVY

Contents   Page

A severe deficiency of ascorbic acid (vitamin C) results in a specific disease called scurvy. The major lesions of scurvy are believed to be due to an impairment in the formation of connective tissue which requires ascorbic acid for its synthesis and repair. This impairment leads to pathologies of bone, teeth, skin, muscle, joints, adrenal glands, and blood vessels. Also, scurvy may be accompanied by hemorrhages of the adrenal glands and a gross impairment of adrenal function. If scurvy is not promptly treated, internal hemorrhages of increasing severity occur and death may follow.

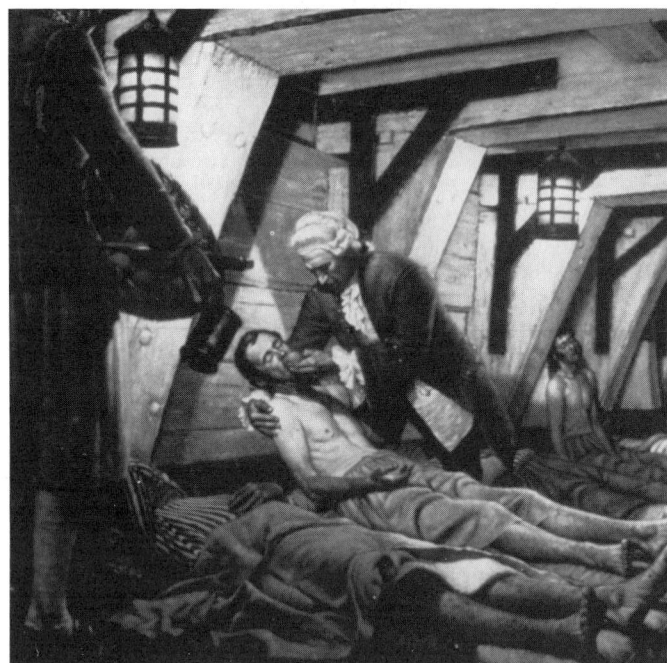

Fig. S-7. This shows British Sailors who ate little except salt meat and biscuits when on long voyages 200 years ago, collapsing and dying of scurvy. (Reproduction with permission of *Nutrition Today*, P.O. Box 1829, Annapolis Maryland, 21404, 1979)

HISTORY OF SCURVY. Although disorders resembling scurvy were described in ancient medical writings (such as *Papyrus Ebers* in Egypt about 1550 B.C., and in Greek and Roman writings), the causative agent was frequently attributed to a plague or other infectious diseases. Perhaps this happened because scurvy may be accompanied by lesions that resemble those associated with certain contagious diseases.

Most long sea voyages suffered large losses of men from scurvy. The greatest number of outbreaks occurred, however, after the change from oar-driven vessels which traveled only short distances from land, to sail-powered ships which traversed the high seas. There was not enough time during short voyages for depletion of the vitamin C stored in the tissues. Fresh fruits were not generally carried aboard such ships, since it was feared that they might spoil, and thereby cause diarrhea.

The first production of scurvy in an experimental animal was accomplished in 1907 by Holst and Frolich. These Norwegian investigators showed that it was necessary to supplement a ration of oats, rye, and rice, with vegetables and fruits, in order to protect guinea pigs against scurvy. This was a landmark experiment because only guinea pigs, monkeys, and man require vitamin C in their diets; other species are able to synthesize this substance in their livers.

These investigators also found that substances which did not normally protect against scurvy (dried grains and legumes—such as oats, barley, peas, beans, and lentils) developed the ability to protect against scurvy when they were germinated into sprouts.

The concept of vitamins was born in 1912 when Hopkins, in England, showed that animals apparently required in their diet small amounts of what he called *accessory food factors.* At the same time, Funk, a Polish scientist working in London, developed the concept of special organic compounds called *vitamines* (later changed to vitamins). In 1928, Szent-Gyorgyi, a Hungarian biochemist, working in Hopkins's laboratory, isolated "hexuronic acid" from orange and cabbage juices and adrenal glands of animals. That same year, King, at the University of Pittsburgh, showed that hexuronic acid was vitamin C. In 1933, the British chemist, Haworth, determined the structure of ascorbic acid and Reichstein, of Switzerland, synthesized ascorbic acid. These investigations made possible the development of a commercial synthesis of vitamin C from glucose. As a result, vitamin C can now be made in very large quantities and at a low cost.

(Also see VITAMIN C, section on "History.")

CAUSES OF SCURVY.
Scurvy is caused by a severe deficiency of vitamin C.

In recent times, very few persons are known to have died from scurvy, except, perhaps, prisoners of war and malnourished infants. However, mild cases of scurvy may occur in infants, especially when they're raised on cow's milk; in adults who eat few vegetables or fruits; and in older persons who live on reduced incomes and under stress.

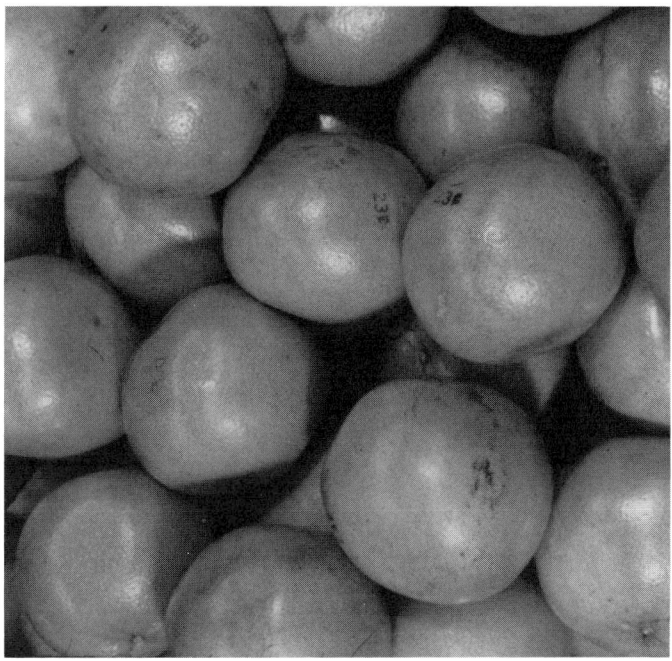

Fig. S-8. Scurvy can be prevented by a daily serving of citrus fruit or juice-grapefruit (shown above) oranges, lemons or limes. (Courtesy, USDA)

SIGNS AND SYMPTOMS OF SCURVY.
Prior to the appearance of specific signs of the disease, the victim may feel feeble and listless, be short of breath, and have slow healing of wounds. Next, there develops the characteristic feature of swollen, bleeding gums (gingivitis), which may become at least slightly infected and impart a foul odor to the breath. Sometimes, there is loosening or loss of teeth. Another early sign of scurvy is the minute hemorrhages (petechiae) which appear around the hair follicles on the abdomen, buttocks, arms, and legs. As the disease progresses, these petechiae merge into larger hemorrhagic areas or bruises, which are unusual in that they occur in the absence of trauma. At this stage of the disease, the victim usually experiences severe pain in his or her bones, joints, and muscles.

Fig. S-9 depicts the afflictions which often accompany scurvy.

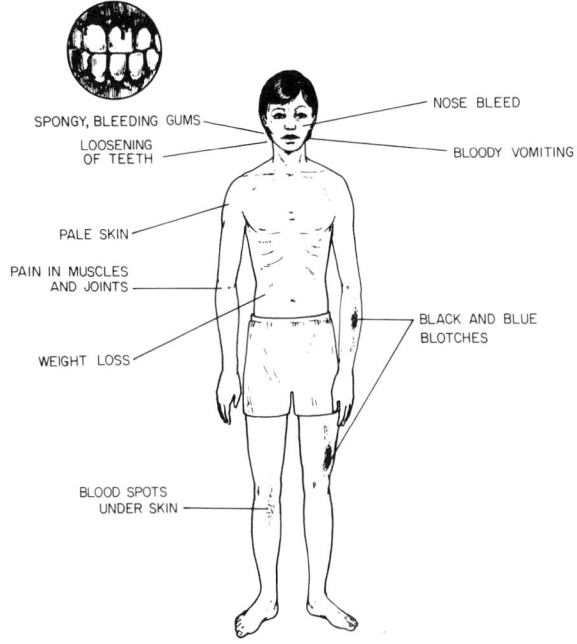

SPONGY, BLEEDING GUMS
LOOSENING OF TEETH
PALE SKIN
PAIN IN MUSCLES AND JOINTS
WEIGHT LOSS
BLOOD SPOTS UNDER SKIN
NOSE BLEED
BLOODY VOMITING
BLACK AND BLUE BLOTCHES

Fig. S-9. Signs and symptoms of scurvy.

Special Features of Scurvy In Infants. The first signs and symptoms of scurvy in infants differ from those in adults because the infant has special requirements for ascorbic acid to sustain growth and development. Thus, early features of infant scurvy may be retarded growth, irritability, lack of appetite, and shrinking from the touch of others in anticipation of pain. Soon, the infant may assume the *frog-legs* position (lying on its back, with the thighs spread widely apart and the legs flexed at the knees). There may also be bone malformations such as *bayonet chest* (a condition in which the breastbone or sternum gradually slopes out from the collarbone, then is indented sharply at its tip due to the sinking of the chest wall just above the belly) and beading of the ribs like that which occurs in rickets. Sometimes, there may be bloody stools or urine and discoloration of the eyelids.

TREATMENT AND PREVENTION OF SCURVY.
Sudden death sometimes occurs in severe scurvy, so prompt and aggressive treatment is necessary. The usual treatment consists of ascorbic acid in doses as high as 250 mg each, four times a day, for a week. The purpose of such high levels is to achieve rapid saturation of the body fluids with ascorbic acid so as to hasten the healing of diseased tissues. Excesses of the vitamin are excreted in the urine, so there is little

danger of large doses over a *short* period of time. The long-term effects of such dosage may be hazardous. When the crisis has passed, sufficient amounts of the vitamin may be provided by diets which contain one or more servings per day of fresh fruits or vegetables. Vitamin tablets may need to be provided for persons who do not eat such foods.

Although it has been estimated that as little as 10 mg per day of ascorbic acid will prevent scurvy, such a low intake is not likely to provide a reserve against such unexpected stresses as disease, trauma, and chilling. The Recommended Dietary Allowances (RDAs)[2] are 60 mg per day of ascorbic acid for adult males and for females who are neither pregnant nor lactating.

Infants should receive 30 mg of vitamin C from birth to 6 months of age, and 35 mg from 6 to 12 months of age. Therefore, at least one rich source of ascorbic acid (such as orange juice) should be given to a baby each day. In the event that citrus juices are not tolerated well, there are vitamin C drops which may be put in the drinking water.

(Also see DEFICIENCY DISEASES, Table D-1 Major Dietary Deficiency Diseases; and VITAMIN C.)

SEAFOOD

This refers to marine fish and shellfish used as food. A great variety of food is prepared from many species of fish and shellfish. Seafood products are preserved by refrigerating, freezing, canning, salting, smoking, pickling, dehydrating, or by combinations of these processes. In many countries, seafoods serve as a principle source of protein and an important source of fat, minerals, and vitamins in the diet.

(Also see FISH AND SEAFOOD[S].)

SEA KALE *Crambe maritiima*

This is a European perennial herb that has a fleshy branching rootstalk and is sometimes cultivated for its large ovate long-stalked leaves which are used as a potherb.

SEAWEED (KELP)

Any plant that grows in the sea is a seaweed. Botanically, seaweeds are algae.

For centuries, seaweed has been used as a food for humans and animals; prized for its minerals and vitamins.

• **Many names and varieties of seaweed**—One of the most confusing things about seaweed is the various names by which it is known; among them, seaweed, agar-agar, algae, carrageenan, dulse, Iceland moss, Irish moss, kelp, laver, rockweed, and sea lettuce. It has been estimated that there are some 2,500 varieties of marine plants; so, seaweed embraces a great variety of plants of many hues, shapes, and sizes. It is noteworthy, too, that seaweed is one of the few members of plant life that has remained unchanged for centuries, since its cultivation and growth is still controlled by the elements—not man.

Seaweeds are algae, of which there are four principal groups:

Brown algae
Red algae
Green algae
Blue-green algae

When the botanist speaks of seaweed, he usually means one of the larger brown or red algae. The seaweeds of cold waters are chiefly brown algae; those of the tropics are mainly red algae.

• **Composition of seaweed**—The Norwegian Seaweed Institute reports the following proximate analysis of seaweed:

Component	Percent
Protein	5.7
Fat	2.6
Fiber	7.0
Nitrogen-free extract	58.6
Ash	15.4
Moisture	10.7
	100.0

Contrary to claims that are sometimes made, seaweeds are low in protein, and the protein is of very low biological value.

The Norwegian Seaweed Institute has found an assortment of 60 different mineral elements in seaweed, all harnessed from the sea. Additionally, seaweed contains carotene, vitamin D, vitamin K, and most of the water-soluble vitamins, including vitamin B-12.

CAUTION: Dried kelp (seaweed) is so rich in iodine that consumption of a large amount for a prolonged period may be harmful; hence, it should be taken according to directions.

(Also see IODINE, section headed "Toxicity.")

• **Uses**—Seaweed has many important uses. Mention has already been made of seaweed as a staple food for humans and animals. For human food, kelp can be used in a variety of ways. In powdered form, it can be added to soups, salads, cottage cheese, tomato juice, fruit juices, or sprinkled on baked potatoes. Some persons use it as a salt substitute. Also, it is made into tablets and sold as a mineral-vitamin supplement in health food stores. About 25% of all food consumed in Japan consists of one form or another of seaweed (sea-vegetable), prepared and served in many forms.

Seaweed has many important uses, in addition to food. It has long been harvested and made into fertilizers. During World War I, giant kelp was harvested and made into explosives. Chemists extract large amounts of iodine and algin from seaweeds. Algin has many commercial uses because it can hold several different liquids together. In ice cream, it keeps the water in the milk from forming crystals. In the food and bakery industry, it is used for thickening, gelling, or binding products. It is also used in salad dressings, chocolate milk, aspirin, and in other foods and drugs.

Seaweed is sometimes promoted for its therapeutic properties in alleviating constipation, gastric catarrh, mucous colitis, and other disorders. But these claims need to be substantiated by more properly conducted and controlled experiments.

Some years ago, scientists became interested in the longevity of the population of Hizato situated in the Nagano province of Japan. Nearly 10% of the villagers were over 70 years of age; and a survey showed that there were 250% more 70-year-olds than in any other Japanese village. After extensive study, the conclusion was reached that the diet of the inhabitants of Hizato was a contributing factor to their longevity. The food consumed by these villagers consisted of all kinds of vegetables, including dried seaweed.

• **Sea farming and world food shortage**—There exist almost unlimited opportunities for increased sea farming. The water area of the world is many times greater than the land space; and phenomenal yields of seaweed are obtained

[2]*Recommended Dietary Allowances,* 10th rev. ed., Food and Nutrition Board, NRC-National Academy of Sciences, 1989.

—as much as 60 tons per acre. Not only that, seaweed farming does not suffer from drought or loss of crop through pests and disease; and seaweed requires no planting, weeding, or fertilizing. Some scientists predict that by the turn of the century the world's sea crops will have to be farmed to ensure the survival of our teeming population.

With one of the world's densest populations and a long coastline, the Japanese already have great expertise in the art of sea farming. Teams of girls, all expert swimmers and skin divers, play a part in this form of cropping, which is also known as aqua-culture. These underwater laborers are specially trained and equipped to carry out the cutting of seaweed from cultivated beds off the seashores.

(Also see ALGAE; and CARRAGEENAN.)

SEEDS

Lots of seeds are eaten for human nutrition. A seed is the primary reason for which whole plants exist. It is the next generation of plants, since it contains a new plant in the form of an embryo plus stored food to nourish the embryo as it develops. Since the plant embryo requires proper nutrition from the stored food, seeds are good sources of protein, carbohydrate, fat (oil), minerals, and vitamins.

Seed types are as diverse as the plant kingdom. Seeds come in all shapes and all sizes, from the dustlike seeds of the orchid to the large seed contained in the coconut.

Man has learned to use a variety of seeds for the food stored in them.

Specific information about seeds consumed by humans can be located under individual articles or in Food Composition Table F-21.

SELECTIVE PERMEABILITY

When only certain substances are permitted to pass through the membrane, and others are rejected.

SELENIFEROUS

Areas in which the soil is high in the mineral selenium. (Also see SELENIUM.)

SELENIUM (Se)

This comparatively rare, nonmetallic element, which makes up less than 0.0001% of the earth's crust, has recently been found to be essential. Fortunately, it is needed only in minute amounts, because (1) only traces are present in most foods, and (2) poisoning may result when the dietary level of this element is 0.0003% or greater. However, it seems that adequate dietary selenium is one of the keys to the maintenance of health under stressful conditions such as (1) prematurity at birth, (2) protein-energy malnutrition, and (3) the tissue disorders which accompany aging.

HISTORY. This element also occurs as a trace contaminant of substances which contain sulfur, because the chemical properties of the two elements are similar. Therefore, it is noteworthy that in 1817 the Swedish chemist Berzelius discovered the element selenium while testing the residue which remained after sulfur had been burned to make sulfuric acid.

In the 1950s, indirect evidence of the beneficial effects of dietary selenium accumulated slowly, but steadily. During the 1940s, German scientists had tested the European type of brewers' yeast for use as a protein supplement and found that it sometimes produced a liver disease in rats which was prevented by feeding wheat germ or other sources of vitamin E. Then, in 1951, the German medical researcher Schwarz, who at the time was a visiting scientist at the National Institutes of Health (NIH), discovered that the American type of brewers' yeast contained an unidentified *Factor 3* which apparently acted along with vitamin E and sulfur-containing amino acids in protecting the liver against damage due to certain types of diets. Schwarz stayed in the United States to continue his research, and, in 1957, he and a co-worker, Foltz, reported that Factor 3 contained selenium.

Other studies by the group at NIH, and by Scott and his co-workers in the Department of Poultry Husbandry at Cornell, showed that the addition of selenium salts to the diets of chicks prevented certain disorders which resulted from vitamin E deficiencies. The pace of discovery quickened as other investigators showed that selenium protected calves and lambs against white muscle disease (nutritional muscular dystrophy). Finally, in 1973, Rotruck and his co-workers at the University of Wisconsin reported that selenium acted as a co-factor for a recently-discovered enzyme (glutathione peroxidase) which breaks down toxic peroxides, most of which are formed from the oxidation of polyunsaturated fats. Hence, the link between selenium and vitamin E was shown; with selenium participating in the breaking down of these highly toxic compounds, and with vitamin E preventing their formation. Nevertheless, it may be that new chapters will be added to the story on selenium, as recent research suggests that there are other roles for this essential element.

SELENIUM IN SOILS. In large areas of the United States, the soils contain little available selenium. Plants produced in these areas are low in this element, and selenium deficiency in livestock (and perhaps in people) is a serious problem. It would appear, therefore, that if foodstuffs grown in these areas are to exert their maximum benefit, some means of combatting their selenium deficiency must be achieved, and this must be accomplished without hazard.

In the Great Plains and Rocky Mountain States (especially in parts of the Dakotas and Wyoming), however, some of the soils are so rich in available selenium that the plants produced thereon are so high in selenium that they are poisonous to animals that eat them.

Fig. S-10 is a map showing areas of the United States where forages and grains have been found (1) low, (2) variable, and (3) adequate or high in selenium. As noted, deficient and high regions are scattered around the country, and some states contain two or more levels of concentration.

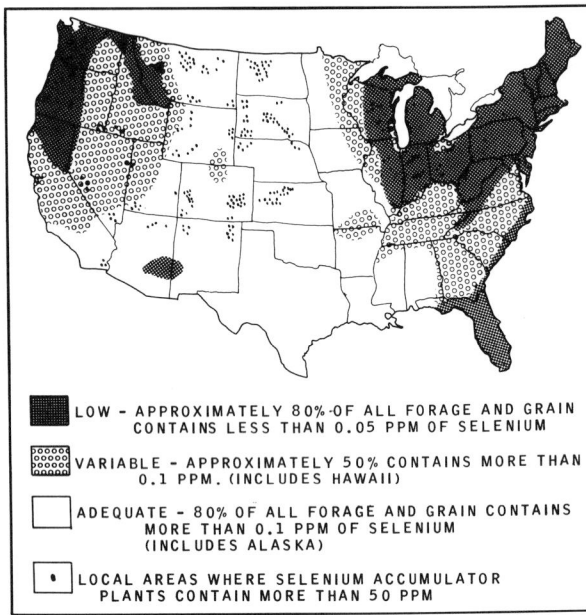

LOW - APPROXIMATELY 80%-OF ALL FORAGE AND GRAIN CONTAINS LESS THAN 0.05 PPM OF SELENIUM

VARIABLE - APPROXIMATELY 50% CONTAINS MORE THAN 0.1 PPM. (INCLUDES HAWAII)

ADEQUATE - 80% OF ALL FORAGE AND GRAIN CONTAINS MORE THAN 0.1 PPM OF SELENIUM (INCLUDES ALASKA)

LOCAL AREAS WHERE SELENIUM ACCUMULATOR PLANTS CONTAIN MORE THAN 50 PPM

Fig. S-10. Geographic distribution of low, variable and adequate or high selenium areas in the United States. (Source: Kubota, J. and W. H. Allaway, "Geographic Distribution of Trace Element Problems," *Micronutrients in Agriculture*, Soil Science Society of America, 1072.)

Regional Differences in the Selenium Content of Foods.

The average selenium content of the crops used for human foods and livestock feeds is highest in the region of the United States which lies west of the Mississippi River and east of the Rocky Mountains. On the other hand, the areas which yield the crops that are very low in selenium are (1) the northern states between the Atlantic Ocean and the Mississippi River; (2) the southeastern coastal plain, including most of the state of Florida; and (3) the western sections of Washington, Oregon, and northern California. Hence, it is noteworthy how these regional differences affect the selenium content of grains and meats, which are the main sources of the mineral in the American diet.

ABSORPTION, METABOLISM, EXCRETION.

Ingested selenium is absorbed in the intestine, mainly in the duodenum. Thence, it is bound to a protein and transported in the blood to the tissues, where it is incorporated into tissue protein as selenocysteine and selenomethionine; in the latter process, selenium replaces the sulfur in the amino acids cysteine and methionine. Excretion of selenium is largely by way of the kidneys, although small amounts are excreted in the feces and in sweat.

Many factors may affect dietary selenium; some enhancing it, others reducing it. These factors are elucidated in the section that follows:

Factors Which May Affect Dietary Selenium.

It is not surprising that deficiencies of selenium are sometimes hard to detect, because vitamin E and the sulfur-containing amino acids (cysteine and methionine) may act as partial substitutes for the mineral in some of its functions. Other nutrients, such as fat and protein, may also affect the body's need for selenium. Therefore, some of the major factors which influence selenium nutrition follow:

• **Biological availability of selenium from various foods** —All of the selenium in wheat appears to be biologically available whereas only about ⅓ of that in herring and tuna is available.[3] It might be that the selenium in certain species of ocean fish—which contain more of this element than most other foods—has a reduced availability because some of it is chemically bound to mercury. This idea is supported by the following evidence: (1) Many ocean fish contain small amounts of methylmercury; (2) selenium compounds have been shown to bind tightly with methylmercury; and (3) the toxicity of the methylmercury in tuna appears to be reduced greatly by the presence of selenium.[4]

• **Dietary protein**—Increasing the dietary protein intake reduces the chances of selenium poisoning when foods containing potentially hazardous amounts of the mineral are consumed. (High-selenium foods are produced only in the areas of the United States around the Rocky Mountains and in the Upper Missouri River Valley of the Dakotas.) However, most people are more likely to consume too little selenium rather than too much; so, protein foods are also valuable in this regard, because they are generally the best sources of selenium.

• **Form and source of the mineral**—Although seafood has a high selenium content, its value as a dietary source is reduced because of the poor availability of its selenium. For example, the selenium in tuna is only 33 to 50% available, possibly because it tends to bind to heavy metals such as mercury.

The selenium content of plant foods reflects the content of the soil in which they are grown. The soil content also influences the amount of selenium in muscle, eggs, or milk of animals raised on crops grown in the soil. Organ meats, muscle meats, cereals, and dairy products rank in descending order as good sources of selenium. The amount of selenium present in food tends to parallel the protein content of the food. Selenium is reduced in the milling process and is lost as vegetables are boiled.

Inorganic salts of selenium, called selenites, should be taken only under the direction of a medical doctor.

• **Intestinal microorganisms**—*E. coli, Streptococcus faecalis* and certain species of *Clostridia* and *Salmonella* metabolize selenium by (1) incorporating it into their enzymes, (2) utilizing selenium amino acids instead of sulfur amino acids, and/or (3) converting soluble forms of selenium into insoluble forms. The insoluble selenium is not likely to be absorbed, if it is produced in the intestines of people who harbor these microorganisms. Therefore, the dietary allowances for selenium should take into account the possibility that intestinal bacteria might somehow interfere with the utilization of selenium by animals and man.

• **Iron-deficiency anemia**—This disorder may be accompanied by a reduction in the activity of a selenium enzyme (glutathione peroxidase) in human red blood cells. Supplementation of the diet with iron sometimes restores the enzyme activity to normal, providing that the dietary supply of selenium is adequate. Hence, the optimal utilization of selenium may depend upon adequate iron nutrition.

• **Malnutrition**—Certain malnourished children who were given therapeutic formulas based upon skim milk powder did not respond well and had (1) subnormal blood levels of selenium, (2) a persistent anemia, and (3) very poor

---

[3]*Selenium and Interrelationships in Animal Nutrition*, Hoffman-La Roche, Inc., Nutley, N.J., 1974, p. 4.

[4]*An Assessment of Mercury in the Environment*, National Academy of Sciences, 1978, pp. 84-86.

growth; all of which were corrected by giving them a selenium supplement.[5] However, one of the children required extra vitamin E to bring about the restoration of red blood cells. These findings show the need for (1) administering selenium supplements when rehabilitation diets contain only minimal amounts of this mineral; and (2) providing sufficient vitamin E, which enhances some of the effects of selenium.

- **Polyunsaturated fats from vegetable oils**—A diet rich in polyunsaturated fatty acids (PUFA) but poor in vitamin E might raise the requirement for selenium because (1) PUFA may be readily converted to toxic peroxides by various metabolic processes unless there is sufficient vitamin E to prevent this conversion, and (2) selenium is needed to activate the enzyme (gluthathione peroxidase) which destroys the peroxides.

- **Processing and preparation of foods**—The losses of selenium during the milling of grains into flours are smaller than those for the other essential minerals, because selenium is distributed throughout the kernel, whereas the other minerals are concentrated in the outer layers of the grain which are removed during milling.

Most cooking procedures have been found to cause little loss of selenium from most foods, except that the boiling of asparagus and mushrooms resulted in significant losses of the mineral (29% and 44%, respectively).[6]

- **Stresses**—Pigs which had been subjected to social and environmental stresses such as crowding, chilling, and overheating developed the severe disorders associated with selenium deficiency much sooner than unstressed animals.[7] Hence, it seems likely that highly stressed people might have above average requirements for selenium, since pigs and people are very similar in the ways that their bodies respond to various stresses.

- **Sulfur-containing amino acids**—Certain disorders which result from selenium-deficient diets are prevented in part by the sulfur-containing amino acids methionine and cysteine because they are converted in the body to glutathione, a substance that has a limited ability to carry out some of the functions of the selenium enzyme glutathione peroxidase. Hence, the need of the human body for selenium is greater when the dietary levels of the sulfur-containing amino acids are low. It is noteworthy that vegetarian diets may be low in the amino acids and low in selenium, unless large amounts of high-selenium wheat are consumed.

- **Vitamin E**—The metabolic roles of selenium and vitamin E overlap, so that each nutrient may replace the other to a limited extent in preventing certain types of disorders. However, there are also unique functions for each nutrient, so each must be supplied in the diet to ensure good nutrition. Furthermore, the experimental supplementation of animal feed with vitamin E resulted in an improvement in selenium absorption, and a doubling of the amount of the mineral which accumulated in the liver.[8]

[5]Hopkins, L. L., Jr., and A. S. Majaj, "Selenium in Human Nutrition," *Selenium in Biomedicine*, edited by O. H. Muth, The Avi Publishing Company, Inc., Westport, Conn., 1967, pp. 205-206.

[6]Higgs, D. J., V. C. Morris, and O. A. Levander, "Effect of Cooking on Selenium Content of Foods," *Journal of Agricultural and Food Chemistry*, Vol. 20, 1972, p. 678.

[7]Ullrey, D. E., "The Selenium-Deficiency Problem in Animal Agriculture," *Trace Element Metabolism in Animals-2*, edited by W. G. Hoekstra, *et al.*, University Park Press, Baltimore, Md., 1974, pp. 276-277.

[8]Combs, G. F., Jr., "Influences of Vitamin A and Other Reducing Compounds on the Selenium-Vitamin E Nutrition of the Chicken,"*Proceedings of the 31st Distillers' Feed Conference*, 1976, p. 44, Table VIII.

FUNCTIONS OF SELENIUM. The essential functions of selenium have been proven conclusively in many species.

The best known biochemical function of the element is its role as part of the enzyme glutathione peroxidase, which protects vital components of the cell against oxidative damage. Selenium also functions as a protective agent against toxic substances. It appears that inorganic forms of selenium somehow bind with toxic minerals such as arsenic, cadmium, and mercury—and render them less harmful. However, the detoxification of these poisonous elements might tie up some of the selenium which would ordinarily be utilized by the body. This effect may be desirable when dietary selenium is excessive, but undesirable when it is marginal or deficient. Additionally, selenium functions in an interrelationship with vitamin E. Details relative to the selenium-vitamin E relationship follow.

Interrelationship of Selenium and Vitamin E. During the 1950s, an interrelationship between selenium and vitamin E was established. It was found that selenium prevented exudative diathesis in vitamin E-deficient chicks and liver necrosis in vitamin E-deficient rats. Subsequent research demonstrated that both selenium and vitamin E protect the cell from the detrimental effects of peroxidation, but each takes a distinctly different approach to the problem. Selenium functions throughout the cytoplasm to destroy peroxides, while vitamin E is present in the membrane components of the cell and prevents peroxide formation. This explains why the biological need for each nutrient can be offset, at least partially although not totally, by the other.

DEFICIENCY SYMPTOMS. There are no clear-cut signs or symptoms which indicate when people are mildly to moderately deficient in selenium. However, many tests on diverse species of animals and man have shown that blood and tissue levels of selenium are in most cases accurate reflections of the selenium nutritional status. But the interpretation of laboratory findings and the diagnosis of selenium deficiency are strictly jobs for health professionals, even though certain laboratories may analyze specimens for lay persons. Hence, the information which follows is presented so that the patient and his or her doctor might consider whether such tests are advisable.

- **Blood tests**—The selenium content of red blood cells is higher than the levels in either whole blood or plasma, because more of the selenium enzyme glutathione peroxidase is present in the red cells than in the other fractions of blood. The selenium concentration in the red blood cells of normal vs sick children is about as follows: healthy children, 0.4 mcg/ml; malnourished children, 0.2 mcg/ml.

- **Analysis of hair and fingernails**—The selenium contents of the hair and fingernails appear to be rough indicators of the selenium content of the rest of the body, so clippings of these materials might be a painless way of testing people for their nutritional status. However, the tests may be invalid if the patient has recently used a shampoo or a medication which contains selenium. Selenium is the active ingredient in preparations used to treat dandruff and fungus infections of the skin.

Evidence of Selenium Deficiencies. There is no hard evidence of human selenium deficiency in the United States. Nevertheless, a growing number of nutrition researchers believe that the well-documented and severe disorders which occur in all species of selenium-deficient farm animals show the need for closer examination of the circumstantial evidence for human deficiencies. Also, it is noteworthy that several studies have shown that there are low levels of selenium in the diet and/or in the blood of severely malnourished children in developing countries.

Associations Between Certain Diseases And Selenium.

Studies of the geographical distribution of certain diseases have shown that the disease rates are lower in areas where the selenium content of crops is higher than average. Such findings do not necessarily prove that selenium prevents the diseases, or that high rates of the diseases indicate selenium deficiencies; although they give reason to probe further into the association between certain diseases and selenium.

According to the National Research Council, National Academy of Sciences, "One could reasonably suppose that selenium is involved in such human medical problems as cancer, cataracts, diseases of the liver, cardiovascular or muscular diseases, and the aging process."[9] Additional health problems which appear to result from a selenium deficiency are discussed in this section, also.

Selenium participates in some of the important metabolic processes which take place in many of the body's tissues. Therefore, the disruption of these processes by deficiencies of selenium might be expected to result in various disorders if the deficiencies are not corrected promptly.

NOTE: This is *not* to say that selenium deficiency is the one and only cause of the disorders which follow, but rather that the possibility of such a deficiency ought to be taken into account in the planning of measures to prevent or to treat these conditions.

• **Cancer**—Certain forms of this disease might result from both the effects of potent carcinogens and the weakening of the body's defenses by deficiencies of nutrients such as selenium.

Some human population data and laboratory experiments indicate that selenium may have anticancer properties. An increased incidence of cancer in human beings has been correlated with decreased levels of selenium in the blood. Also, selenium has been found to have some inhibitory effect on the development of tumors in rodents given certain carcinogens.

The cancer rates are generally higher in the states which have low levels of selenium in their crops.[10] In many cases, however, the states which have high cancer rates have other potentially health-threatening conditions such as (1) heavy industrialization, (2) mining and ore processing, and/or (3) large populations.

Shamberger and Frost reported that human cancer mortality might bear an inverse relationship to selenium distribution.[11] Also, controlled animal studies conducted by Shamberger at the same time showed an inhibitory effect of selenium on cancer.[12]

Other studies showed that (1) certain male cancer patients had subnormal blood levels of selenium; and (2) administration of supplemental selenium slowed the growth of tumors

which were induced in animals by various carcinogens.[13]

One of the current theories regarding the prevention of cancer by selenium postulates that this element acts by (1) counteracting poisonous substances which may cause cells to mutate; and (2) stimulating the defenses of the body that act against abnormal cells.

Professor Gerhard N. Schrauzer of the University of California, San Diego, considers selenium to be a promising candidate for human cancer protection. He has been studying the effects of selenium in animals for 15 years. Using mice infected with viral particles which cause breast cancer, he showed that only 10% of the animals given nontoxic amounts of selenium in the drinking water or the diet developed breast cancer as compared to 80-90% in the controls.[14] His work was confirmed by Dr. Daniel Medina,[15] Baylor College of Medicine, in Houston.

Currently research on the cancer-protecting effects of selenium is being conducted in laboratories all over the world.

• **Heart disease and selenium**—A review of the effects of selenium deficiency reveals a repetitious undercurrent of vascular-type lesions suggesting a heart involvement in selenium disorders. Sudden death associated with selenium deficiency in newborn or rapidly growing lambs and calves apparently results from weakening of the heart muscle, commonly called white muscle disease. Selenium-deficient monkeys also have heart lesions. This disorder is characterized by white streaks in muscles, and in some cases, by abnormal electrocardiograms. Often, the animals affected with this disease die suddenly when they are subjected to moderate stresses.

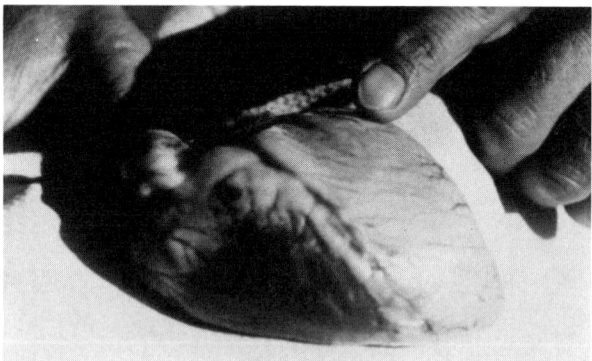

Fig. S-11. Heart of a 6-week-old calf afflicted with white muscle disease. Note abnormal white areas in the heart muscles. (Courtesy, Oregon Agricultural Experiment Station, Corvallis, Ore.)

Some researchers have suggested that combined deficiencies of selenium and vitamin E might contribute to heart disease in man because these nutrients help maintain adequate levels of coenzyme Q in the heart muscle. *(Coenzyme Q is a vital cofactor in energy metabolism.)* If this cofactor is lacking, the production of energy in the heart and in other muscles may fall off to the extent that these tissues can no longer carry their workloads. This hypothesis is supported by the finding that biopsy samples from the hearts of people with heart disease had subnormal levels of coenzyme Q. Hence, it is noteworthy that the administration of selenium to farm animals raised the levels of coenzyme Q in their hearts.

[9]*Selenium*, Subcommittee on Selenium, National Research Council, National Academy of Sciences, Washington, D.C., 1976, p. 152.

[10]Schrauzer, G. N., "Trace Elements, Nutrition and Cancer: Perspectives of Prevention," *Inorganic and Nutritional Aspects of Cancer*, edited by G. N. Schrauzer, Plenum Press, New York, N.Y., 1978, p. 326, Fig. 1.

[11]Shamberger, R. J., and D. V. Frost, "Possible Protective Effect of Selenium Against Human Cancer," *Canadian Medical Association Journal*, Vol. 100, 1969, p. 682.

[12]Shamberger, R. J., "Relation of Selenium to Cancer. 1. Inhibitory Effect of Selenium on Carcinogenesis," *Journal of National Cancer Institute*, Vol. 44, 1970, pp. 931-936.

[13]"Selenium and Cancer," *Nutrition Reviews*, Vol. 28, 1970, pp. 75-80.

[14]Schrauzer, G. N., "Trace Elements, Nutrition and Cancer: Perspectives of Prevention," *Inorganic and Nutritional Aspects of Cancer*, edited by G. N. Schrauzer, Plenum Press, New York, N.Y., 1978, p. 330, Scheme 1.

[15]Medina, D. and F. Shepherd, *Cancer Lett.* 8, 241-245, 1980.

A sure sign of a dietary deficiency of selenium and/or of vitamin E in poultry and pigs is damaged blood vessels that leak into the surrounding tissues.[16] It is believed that this disorder is prevented by (1) selenium which circulates in the blood as part of the enzyme glutathione peroxidase, and (2) vitamin E which protects the membranes in the cells lining the blood vessels. While it does not appear that people develop the acute disorder which occurs in farm animals, it may be that the development of atherosclerosis is hastened by selenium deficiency, because the selenium-containing enzyme has been found to break down the cholesterol complexes that build up in lesions within the walls of arteries.

The following studies indicate that selenium is likely involved in heart disease:

1. The death rates from heart disease have consistently been highest in the low-selenium states.[17] However, these states are also the most densely populated and heavily industrialized states—so this evidence is open to other interpretations.

2. A comparison of the maps of early heart mortality and cardiovascular-related deaths of different areas of the United States revealed an inverse relationship between selenium levels and the mortality pattern.[18]

3. It has been hypothesized that selenium deficiency (rather than manganese deficiency as was first thought), which is prevalent all over Finland, may contribute to the unusually high death rates from heart disease and cancer in Finland.[19]

4. Lesions of selenium deficiency in rats have been associated with vascular abnormalities.[20]

5. Selenium is required by the enzyme that breaks down toxic peroxides which may damage the heart muscle.[21]

6. In May 1980, in a report before the Second International Symposium in Biology and Medicine, held at Texas Tech University, Lubbock, Texas, Dr. G. R. Yang, Chinese Academy of Medical Sciences, Peking, reported that selenium was effective in preventing heart muscle disease in certain parts of China. The malady, known as keshan, is common to certain areas of China where the soil is low in selenium. In a study involving 45,000 Chinese—the most massive study ever done on selenium deficiency in people—supplementation with selenium wiped out a heart disorder affecting 40 out of every 1,000 children in certain areas of China. Although there is no question that selenium was a pivotal factor in the Chinese study, Dr. Yang hastened to add that it is unlikely that it is the only factor.

• **Cloudiness in the lens of the eye (cataracts)**—Normally, the selenium content of the lens of the eye increases steadily from birth to death, but it has been found that lenses with cataracts may contain less than one-sixth of the normal amounts of this element.[22] It is suspected that lack of selenium to activate the enzyme glutathione peroxidase impedes the destruction of peroxides in the lens of the eye, and that the peroxides may then accumulate in amounts sufficient to damage the lens.

It is noteworthy, too, that cataracts are one of the selenium deficiency symptoms noted in rats.[23] Many other injurious agents and nutrient deficiencies might also be associated with the formation of cataracts, so it is uncertain whether selenium deficiency is a frequent cause of this disorder.

• **Growth failure during the rehabilitation of malnourished children**—So far, no evidence has been found to indicate that any normal, apparently healthy children suffer from a deficiency of selenium. However, several groups of children who were suffering from protein-energy malnutrition were found to have very low blood levels of selenium.[24] Selenium and protein are found together in both the diet and the body, so it is not surprising that children who lacked protein were also deficient in selenium. The standard rehabilitation procedures —which are based upon providing a good source of protein such as skim milk, extra fat and/or sugar, and certain vitamins and minerals—produced only limited improvement until selenium supplements were given.

• **Hemolytic anemia of newborn infants**—Newborn infants are more prone than other people to have abnormally short-lived red blood cells because blood levels of vitamin E—which together with selenium protects the membranes of red cells from premature disintegration—are often subnormal at birth. Hence, it is suspected that selenium deficiency might tend to aggravate this condition, since the selenium enzyme glutathione peroxidase protects against this disorder. It is noteworthy, therefore, that cow's milk contains only half as much selenium as human milk, and that both types of milk are relatively poor sources of the mineral.

• **Increased susceptibility to infections**—The germ-eating (phagocytic) white blood cells constitute one of the body's major defenses against infectious disease, because their formidable cells ingest living microorganisms, enclose them in killing chambers (phagocytic vacuoles) and kill them with blasts of highly potent forms of oxygen. The selenium enzyme glutathione peroxidase might extend the lifespan of these white blood cells by breaking down the toxic peroxides which may escape from the "killing chambers" into the more vulnerable parts of the cells. It is noteworthy that phagocytic white cells from selenium-deficient rats had a reduced ability to kill yeast cells, even though they had no difficulty ingesting the yeast.

So far, it has been difficult to confirm that selenium deficiency might be responsible for chronic susceptibility to infections in people, because many other factors affect this condition.

• **Infertility**—Studies on various species of farm animals and laboratory animals have shown that selenium deficiency causes infertility which is characterized in the male by fluid accumulation in the testicles, and feeble and broken sperm cells; and in the female by death of the fetus during early embryonic development. Although no similar investigations have been made in man, it is well known that people are subject to most of the disorders of fertility which have been observed in selenium-deficient animals.

[16]*Selenium*, National Academy of Sciences, 1976, pp. 84-88.

[17]Sauer, H. I., and F. R. Brand, "Geographic Patterns in the Risk of Dying," *Environmental Geochemistry in Health and Disease*, edited by H. L. Cannon and H. C. Hopps, The Geological Society of America, Inc., Boulder, Colo., Memoir 123, 1971, p. 137.

[18]Frost, D. V., "Selenium Has Great Nutritional Significance for Man; Should Be Cleared for Feed," *Feedstuffs*, Vol. 44 (8), 1972, pp. 58-59.

[19]Marjanen, H., and S. Soini, "Possible Causal Relationship Between Nutritional Imbalances, Especially Manganese Deficiency and Susceptibility to Cancer, in Finland," *Ann. Agric. Fenn*, Vol. 11, 1972, pp. 391-406.

[20]Sprinker, L. H., et al., "Selenium Deficiency Lesions in Rats Fed Vitamin E Supplemented Rations," *Nutr. Rep. Int.*, Vol. 4, 1971, pp. 335-340.

[21]Hoekstra, W. G., "Biochemical Role of Selenium," *Trace Element Metabolism in Animals-2*, edited by W. G. Hoekstra, et al., University Park Press, Baltimore, Md., 1974, p. 61.

[22]Ganther, H. E., et al., "Selenium and Glutathione Peroxidase in Health and Disease—A Review," *Trace Elements in Human Health and Disease*, edited by A. S. Prasad and D. Oberleas, Academic Press, Inc., New York, N.Y., 1976, p. 205.

[23]*Selenium*, Subcommittee on Selenium, National Research Council, National Academy of Sciences, 1976, p. 143.

[24]Hopkins, L. L., Jr., and A. S. Majaj, "Selenium in Human Nutrition," *Selenium in Biomedicine*, edited by O. H. Muth, The Avi Publishing Company, Inc., Westport, Conn., 1967, pp. 203-214.

• **Liver disease**—The liver is vulnerable to damage by the toxic peroxides generated during fat metabolism, unless it is supplied with sufficient amounts of selenium, vitamin E, and/or sulfur-containing amino acids (methionine and cysteine) to prevent the buildup of peroxides.

• **Pancreatic disease**—The reason for the degeneration of the pancreas in selenium-deficient animals is not clear. It does *not* appear to be related to the level of activity of the selenium enzyme glutathione peroxidase. Furthermore, an abundant dietary supply of vitamin E does not protect the pancreas when selenium is lacking. Eventually, deficiencies of vitamin E and other fatborne nutrients may develop, when the damage to the pancreas is great enough to interfere with the secretion of enzymes which digest the fatty components of foods.

• **Poisoning by normally harmless amounts of toxic substances**—In addition to the counteraction of the toxic effects of arsenic, cadmium, and methylmercury by inorganic selenium, selenium in the enzyme glutathione peroxidase may protect against the effects of poisonous organic compounds such as carbon tetrachloride (a common dry-cleaning agent) and certain drugs.

• **Sudden infant death syndrome (crib or cot death)**—Infants that are fed cows milk receive only ½ as much selenium and 1/10 as much vitamin E as infants that are breast fed. It follows that several researchers have advanced the hypothesis that combined deficiencies of selenium and vitamin E in cow's milk may be contributory to *crib death*, where an infant that had appeared to be healthy is found to have died suddenly in its bed.[25]

However, the tentative explanation of crib deaths which is entertained by many doctors is that (1) an infant may develop antibodies (become sensitized) to cow's milk after bringing up part of a feeding and inhaling it into its bronchial tubes (the air passages which lead from the windpipe into the lungs), and (2) repetitions of these episodes lead to such a severe allergy to cow's milk that eventually one such event leads to a fatal allergic shock. Other doctors believe that the severe allergic shock may be triggered by a variety of allergens, or perhaps even by a virus.

The explanations are all compatible because severe allergic reactions are accompanied by (1) a marked enlargement (dilation) of the blood vessels, and a great drop in the blood pressure; and (2) a speeding up of the heart rate as the heart attempts to maintain the normal circulation of blood. Deficiencies of selenium and vitamin E may weaken the heart muscle so that it cannot cope with the increased workload brought about by a state of allergic shock.

TREATMENT AND PREVENTION OF SELENIUM DEFICIENCY.
As a result of extensive animal experiments, in 1974 the Food and Drug Administration (FDA) approved the use of selenium for livestock, with certain restrictions.[25]

In 1989, for the first time ever, the Food and Nutrition Board (FNB), National Research Council (NRC), included selenium in its *Recommended Dietary Allowances*, 10th Edition.

INTERRELATIONSHIPS.
The major selenium relationships are:

1. The functions of selenium are closely related to those of vitamin E and the sulfur-containing amino acids.

2. Selenium protects against the toxic effects of arsenic, cadmium, copper, mercury, and silver. Likewise, these elements counteract the toxic effects of selenium.

3. A diet high in protein or high in sulfate provides some protection against selenium poisoning.

4. The optimal utilization of selenium may depend upon adequate iron nutrition.

5. Diets rich in polyunsaturated fatty acids but poor in vitamin E may raise the requirements for selenium.

RECOMMENDED DAILY ALLOWANCE OF SELENIUM.
Tables S-1a and M-25 give selenium intakes that the FNB–NRC deems to be appropriate for various age groups.

TABLE S–1A
RECOMMENDED SAFE AND ADEQUATE
DAILY DIETARY INTAKES OF SELENIUM[1]

Group	Age	Selenium Intake
	(years)	(mcg)
Infants	0.0–0.5	10
	0.5–1.0	15
Children	1–3	20
	4–6	20
Adolescents	7–10	30
	11+	40
Adults		55–70

[1]Adapted by the authors from *Recommended Dietary Allowances*, 10th ed., 1989, NRC-National Academy of Sciences, p. 285.

Certain researchers, such as Dr. Schrauzer and his co-workers at the University of California at San Diego, believe that many cases of cancer might be prevented by selenium intakes that are approximately double the level recommended by the Food and Nutrition Board.[26]

• **Selenium intake in average U.S. diet**—Analyses of national food composites in the United States indicate that the overall adult mean dietary selenium intake was 108 mcg/day between 1974 and 1982. The daily mean for each year ranged from 83 to 129 mcg.

TOXICITY.
Confirmed cases of selenium poisoning in man are not often found because (1) the foods and beverages which are consumed by people are not likely to contain toxic excesses of the element, and (2) well-nourished people are protected by metabolic processes that convert selenium into harmless substances which are excreted in the urine, or in the breath. Nevertheless, a few cases of poisoning sometimes occur under unusual circumstances such as (1) very high levels of the element in drinking water, or (2) the presence of malnutrition, parasitic infestation, or other factors which may make people highly susceptible to selenium toxicity. Therefore, descriptions of some poisonous effects of selenium follow:

• **Abnormalities of the hair, nails, and skin**—It appears that some of the toxic effects of selenium might be due to its interference with the normal structures and functions of proteins rich in sulfur-containing amino acids. Hence,

[25]*Selenium*, National Academy of Sciences, 1976, pp. 93–94.

[26]Schrauzer, G. N., "Trace Elements, Nutrition and Cancer: Perspectives of Prevention," *Inorganic and Nutritional Aspects of Cancer*, edited by G. N. Schrauzer, Plenum Press, New York, N.Y., 1978, pp. 330-331.

poisoning by this element is characterized by abnormalities in the hair, nails, and skin; tissues which are rich in sulfurous proteins. For example, a group of children living in a high-selenium area of Venezuela had loss of hair, discolored skin, and chronic digestive disturbances.[27] However, most of the children were infested with intestinal parasites, which might have weakened them so that they had increased susceptibility to the toxic effects of selenium.

• **Garlic odor on the breath**—Normally, people who have consumed large excesses of selenium excrete it as trimethyl selenide in the urine, and/or as dimethyl selenide on the breath. The latter substance has an odor resembling garlic.

• **Intensification of selenium toxicity by arsenic or mercury**—Usually, the toxicity of selenium is reduced by the presence of either arsenic or mercury. However, the methyl derivatives of selenium—which are formed when animals or people are chronically exposed to excessive amounts of the mineral—may become highly toxic when they react in the body with arsenic or mercury. So far, these reactions have been observed only in animals in laboratory experiments. Hence, it is not certain whether there are circumstances under which they might occur in man.

• **Promotion of tooth decay**—Various studies have shown the rates of tooth decay to be slightly higher in high-selenium areas than in low-selenium areas. Research on laboratory animals has produced evidence that excesses of selenium interfere with the formation of the protective tooth enamel. However, this research has usually been conducted with much higher levels of the mineral than are likely to be encountered by man.

SOURCES OF SELENIUM. The selenium content of plant products varies according to the amounts and availability of the mineral in the soil. Likewise, the selenium content of animal products depends upon the content of the element in livestock feeds; for example, the Ohio Station reported that the addition of 0.1 ppm selenium to the animal's diet increased the selenium content of beef liver by 72%.[28] Also, there are cooking losses in some cases, although these are minor for most foods. Hence, the data regarding the amounts of the mineral supplied by various foods *cannot* be taken to indicate a constant content of selenium for any particular food. Nevertheless, such data are useful in that they show which foods are likely to be good sources of the mineral.

Fortunately, food eaten in the United States is generally varied in nature and origin. Nevertheless, it appears likely that most diets barely meet minimal requirements; hence, many diets are bound to be deficient.

Groupings by rank of some common food sources of selenium are given in the section on MINERAL(S), Table M-25, Mineral Table.

For additional sources and more precise values of selenium, see Table S-2, Selenium Content of Some Foods, which follows.

SUMMARY. It might be desirable for people who live in low-selenium areas of the United States—which are generally located east of the Mississippi River and west of

TABLE S-2
SELENIUM CONTENT OF SOME FOODS

Food	Selenium
	(mcg/100 g)
Fish flour	193
Butter	146
Eulachon (smelt)	123
Torula yeast	123
Wheat germ	111
Lobster	104
Brazil nuts	103
Brewers' yeast	91
Cider vinegar	89
Pork kidneys	64
Wheat, whole grain	63
Wheat bran	63
Clams	55
Whole wheat flour	53
Crab	51
Oysters	49
Pork	42
Rye, whole grain	37
Kidney beans	36
Lamb	30
Soybean flour	30
Turnips	27
Swiss chard	26
Blackstrap molasses	26
Garlic	25
Oats, whole grain	21
Beer	19
Barley, whole grain	18
Eggs	16
Skim milk (dehy)	13
Mushrooms	13
Soybeans	11
Cheese	8
Corn	7
Orange juice	6
Grape juice	4
Cow's milk, whole 3.7% fat	3
Pecans	3
Filberts (hazelnuts)	2
Almonds	2
Carrots	2
Cabbage	2

the Rocky Mountains—to make certain that they get enough selenium by eating ample amounts of foods rich or good in selenium. However, undesirable effects or toxicities might result from consuming too much selenium, so one should consult with a doctor or a dietitian before taking special, selenium-rich supplements.

(Also see MINERAL[S], Table M-25; and POISONS, Table P-2, Some Potentially Poisonous [Toxic] Substances.)

SEMIDISPENSABLE AMINO ACID

An amino acid which is essential only under certain circumstances or which may replace part of one of the essential amino acids. Arginine, cystine, and tyrosine fall into this group.

(Also see AMINO ACID[S].)

SEMIPERMEABLE MEMBRANE

A membrane that is permeable to some small molecules (like water and inorganic salts) but bars the passage of larger particles (like protein molecules).

SEPTICEMIA

A diseased condition resulting from the presence of pathogenic bacteria and their associated poisons in the blood.

[27]Burk, R. F., "Selenium in Man," *Trace Elements in Health and Disease,* edited by A. S. Prasad and D. Oberleas, Academic Press, Inc., New York, N.Y., 1976, p. 121.

[28]Moxon, A. L. and D. L. Palmquist, "Selenium Content of Foods Grown or Sold in Ohio," *Ohio Report,* Ohio State University, Columbus, Ohio, January-February 1980, pp. 13-14, Table 1.

SERENDIPITY BERRY
Dioscoreophyllum cumminsii

A very sweet tasting berry that is native to West Africa. The substance which is responsible for the sweet taste has been isolated and named monellin.

SEROTONIN

A derivative of the essential amino acid tryptophan which plays a role in brain and nerve function.

SERUM

The colorless fluid portion of blood remaining after clotting and removal of corpuscles. It differs from plasma in that the fibrinogen has been removed.

SERUM CHOLESTEROL

The level of the sterol cholesterol in the blood.

SERUM TRIGLYCERIDE

The level of fat in the blood.

SESAME *Sesamum indicum*

The sesame plant belongs to the family *Pedaliaceae;* genus *Sesamum;* species, *S. indicum.*

Sesame has been grown in tropical countries since time immemorial, primarily to obtain seed for use on bakery goods and food delicacies and for edible oil production. It appears to be the earliest condiment used and the oldest crop grown for edible oil. The magic words *open sesame* found in the Arabian Nights are thought to have been inspired by the characteristic bursting open of the sesame pods when the grain is ripe, a nettlesome trait that has necessitated hand harvesting of the crop.

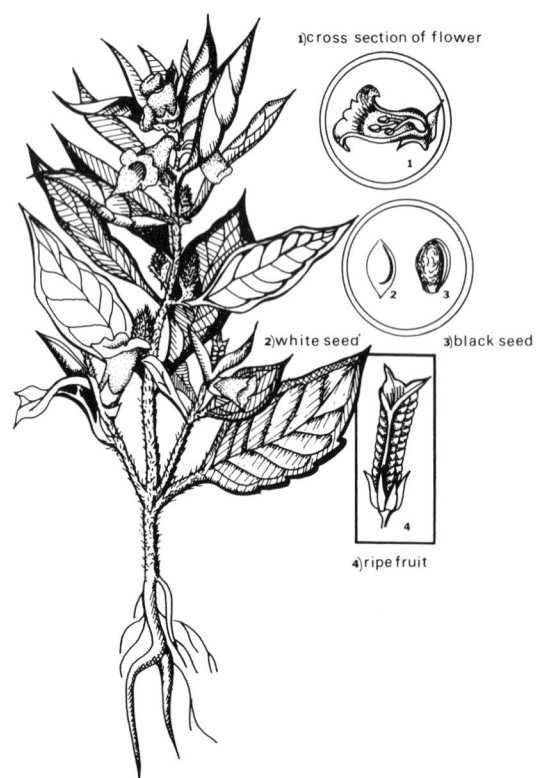

Fig. S-12. Sesame plant.

Production of sesame is limited to countries where labor is plentiful and inexpensive, and will so remain until and unless nonshattering varieties with satisfactory yields and/or improved mechanical harvesting techniques are developed. Intense breeding and engineering research programs to alleviate these problems are in progress.

ORIGIN AND HISTORY. Although sesame has not been identified in the wild state, it is believed to have originated in the Indian archipelago. Archeological evidence indicates that sesame was cultivated in Palestine and Syria around 3000 B.C., and by the civilization of Babylonia in 1750 B.C. An Egyptian tomb bears a 4,000-year-old drawing of a baker adding sesame to bread dough. In 1298, Marco Polo observed the Persians using sesame oil for cooking, body massage, medicinal purposes, illumination, cosmetics, and lubricating primitive machinery.

WORLD AND U.S. PRODUCTION. World production of sesame seed totals about 2,000,000 metric tons annually; and the six leading nations, by rank, are: India, China, Myanmar, Mexico, Nigeria, and Sudan.[29]

The United States produces only about 1,000 metric tons annually. However, this country is a large importer of sesame seed; the U.S. imports close to 43,000 metric tons each year.

NUTRITIONAL VALUE OF SESAME. Sesame seed averages about 50% oil, which is highly resistant to oxidation, and 25% protein, which has a unique balance of amino acids. Dehulled, defatted meal contains 50 to 60% protein and is bland. Food Composition Table F-21 gives the nutrient composition of sesame seeds and sesame oil.

The unique quality of sesame protein is the presence of a high level of the sulfur-containing amino acids, methionine and cystine. The limiting amino acid of sesame protein is lysine (Table S-3). It is also noteworthy that sesame does not contain some of the objectionable characteristics found in soy protein, particularly with regard to the trypsin inhibiting factor.

[29]Data from *FAO Production Yearbook 1990,* FAO/UN, Rome, Italy, Vol. 44, p. 114, Table 42. **Note well:** Annual production fluctuates as a result of weather and profitability of the crop.

TABLE S-3
PROFILE OF ESSENTIAL AMINO ACIDS IN DEHULLED SESAME PRODUCTS COMPARED TO MILK—A HIGH-QUALITY PROTEIN[1]

Amino Acid	Meal	Isolate	Cow's Milk[2]
	(mg/g protein)		
Histidine	24	21	27
Isoleucine	47	36	47
Leucine	74	66	95
Lysine	35	21	78
Methionine and cystine	56	37	33
Phenylalanine and tyrosine	106	79	102
Threonine	39	33	44
Tryptophan	19	18	14
Valine	46	46	64

[1]Adapted from Johnson, L.A., T. M. Suleiman, and E. W. Lusas, "Sesame Protein: A Review and Prospectus," *Journal of the American Oil Chemists' Society,* Vol. 56, No. 3, March 1979, p. 465, Table 3.
[2]*Recommended Dietary Allowances,* 10th ed., 1989, National Academy of Sciences, p. 67, Table 6–5. The essential amino acid requirements of infants can be met by supplying 0.79 g of a high-quality protein per pound of body weight (*1.7 g/kg body weight*) per day.

PROCESSING SESAME SEED. In those areas where sesame is primarily processed for its oil content, the seed is not dehulled; rather, the entire seed is crushed. However, in areas such as India, where the meal is an important food, dehulling is necessary.

Table S-4 shows the average analysis of crude sesame oil. Due to the presence of natural antioxidants in the crude oil, sesame oil is the most stable naturally-occurring liquid vegetable oil. It will keep for several years without turning rancid. Sesame oil is classified as polyunsaturated; it contains approximately 44% of the essential fatty acid, linoleic acid, and 40% oleic acid.

(Also see FATS AND OTHER LIPIDS; and OILS, VEGETABLE, Table O-5.)

TABLE S-4
ANALYSIS OF CRUDE SESAME OIL (AVERAGE)[1]

Free fatty acid (as oleic)	1.3%
Color	35y/1.2r
Iodine Value	110
Peroxide Value	13
AOM	24 hr
Percent unsaponifiable	2.3%
Smoke point	330°F
Specific gravity @ 25°C	.918
Saponification Value	185.8
Fatty acids (natural oil)	**(%)**
Oleic	40
Linoleic	44
Other unsaturates	1
Palmitic	9
Stearic	5

[1]Source: USDA Southern Regional Laboratories.

SESAME PRODUCTS AND USES. Sesame in many forms is now offered to the food industry for human consumption; among them, the following:

> Dry, cleaned, unhulled sesame seed
> White, hulled sesame seed
> Toasted sesame seed
> Toasted, flaked sesame seed
> Partially defatted sesame flour
> Solvent extracted sesame flour
> Sesame butter made from toasted sesame
>   seed

In the United States, sesame is used primarily in the bakery industry, where whole, hulled sesame seed is used as a decoration and flavoring agent on specialty breads, rolls, buns, candies, and other delicacies. Sesame is also used in high-protein snack foods and granola.

The protein (meal) of sesame has become increasingly important for human food due to the following unique properties: (1) the presence of a high level of the sulfur-containing amino acids, methionine and cystine; (2) its freedom from the trypsin inhibiting factor, an objectionable characteristic of soy protein; and (3) its pleasant flavor. The meal is very palatable to humans. In India, it is used extensively in human foods; and in India and Java, it is sometimes fermented for food.

Sesame oil (also known as gingili, benne, or til) is straw-colored, with a pleasant, mild taste and remarkable stability. It is a natural salad oil requiring little or no winterization and is one of the few vegetable oils that can be used without refining. These are factors of increasing importance as energy costs escalate. It is popular because of the presence of a natural antioxidant, sesamol, and because of its high content

of polyunsaturated fatty acids, 43% oleic and 43% linoleic. The oil is used as a substitute for olive oil—primarily as a salad and cooking oil and for margarine and soap. Also, a significant quantity of oil is used by the cosmetic industry for softening and soothing purposes, and by the pharmaceutical industry as a carrier for medicines.

In addition to the uses listed above, sesame is being used to enhance the flavor of fried or baked snacks, high-protein beverages, cereals, seasoning blends; and as a garnish for vegetables, high-protein breads, and pies.

Blends of peanut/chickpea, wheat/chickpea, rice/chickpea, peanut/soybean, sunflower/maize, and cowpea/rice have all shown improved nutritional qualities with supplementation of sesame meal. Even more significant, however, is the finding that a simple blend of one part sesame and one part soy protein has about the same protein nutritive value as casein, the main protein of milk. The high-lysine and low-methionine content of soy protein is complementary to sesame protein.

(Also see OILS, VEGETABLE, Table O-5, Vegetable Oils.)

SEVEN FOODS PLAN (BASIC 7 FOODS PLAN)

The different types of foods are sometimes divided into the following seven groups: *Group 1*—Green and yellow vegetables; *Group 2*—Oranges, tomatoes, grapefruit, or raw cabbage or salad greens; *Group 3*—Potatoes and other vegetables, and fruits; *Group 4*—Milk and milk products; *Group 5*—Meat, poultry, fish, or eggs, or dried beans, peas, nuts, peanut butter; *Group 6*— Bread, flour, and cereals; and *Group 7*—Butter and fortified margarine. A well-balanced diet should include food from each group every day. A more common plan is the selection of foods from the basic four food groups—(1) the meat, poultry, fish, and beans group; (2) the milk and cheese group; (3) the vegetable and fruit group; and (4) the bread and cereal group.

(Also see FOOD GROUPS.)

SEVILLE ORANGE (SOUR OR BITTER ORANGE) *Citrus aurantium*

This citrus fruit is rarely seen in the fresh form in the United States because it is grown mainly in Seville, Spain, for making marmalade. The Seville orange, like the other citrus fruits, belongs to the rue family (*Rutaceae*). It is distinguished from the Sweet orange (*C. sinensis*) by its much rougher skin and very sour taste.

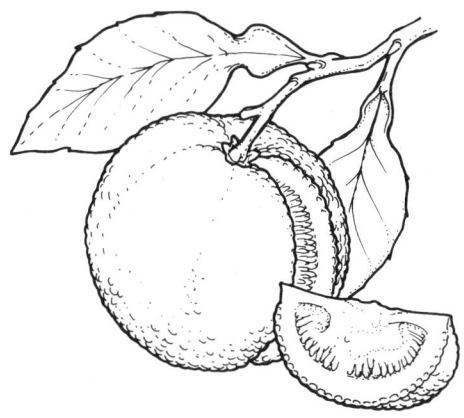

Fig. S-13. The Seville orange, a sour-flavored fruit which is used mainly for making marmalade and flavorings.

ORIGIN AND HISTORY. The sour orange originated in Indonesia and was brought to India in ancient times. The first orchards were planted on the Arabian peninsula in the beginning of the 10th century. Later, the trees were planted in Mesopotamia and Syria. The spread of Islam and Arabic culture across North Africa and into Spain led to the introduction of the sour orange into Seville, Spain, in the 11th century.

WORLD AND U.S. PRODUCTION. Most of the world's crop of sour oranges is produced in the area around Seville, Spain, although production figures are not available.

PROCESSING. Most of the sour orange crop is processed because the fruit is too sour to eat raw. Large quantities of the oranges are exported to Great Britain, where they are used to make a marmalade that has a strong distinctive flavor that is not found in similar products made from sweet oranges.

In Spain, the peel is scraped from the oranges and pressed to yield an oil that is much used as a flavoring agent. The clarified juice is used to impart a strong orangy flavor to highly diluted beverages such as orangeades and other fruit drinks. The U.S. Standards of Identity permit the use of up to 5% sour orange juice in the production of frozen orange juice concentrate.

SELECTION, PREPARATION, AND USES. One is not likely to see fresh sour oranges in the United States except in a few orchards in Florida. However, sour oranges are grown rather extensively in the Mediterranean region, especially Spain. Bitter orange marmalade and flavorings are made from it. Also, bitter oranges are grown for two additional purposes: (1) they are used as rootstock seedlings on which to bud-graft sweet oranges and other citrus fruits; and (2) in France, the flowers of the bitter orange are distilled for their perfume—eau de cologne is made from it.

NUTRITIONAL VALUE. The fruit and juice of the sour orange are rarely consumed alone, but are usually mixed with other citrus products. Hence, data on the nutrient composition of this fruit are not readily available. However, it might be expected to be similar to the sweet orange in its content of potassium, vitamin C, and bioflavonoids.

Citrus peel contains citral, an aldehyde which antagonizes the effects of vitamin A. Hence, people should not consume large amounts of peel-rich products such as candied peel and marmalade without making certain that their dietary supply of this vitamin is adequate.

(Also see CITRUS FRUITS.)

SHEA BUTTER

This is a fat obtained from the kernel of the fruit of the African tree, *Butyrospermum parkii*, also called butter tree or shea tree. Natives use the fat as a substitute for butter.

SHORTENING

Fat substances given this name are used to *shorten foods*. Their function is accomplished by forming films or clumps of fat throughout the food thereby preventing the protein and carbohydrate from cooking into one continuous hard mass. Thus, shortenings tenderize foods. Also, cake batters and icings often contain tiny air bubbles trapped in shortening that help to develop a fine delicate structure. It is the plastic consistency of shortenings that helps hold air in the

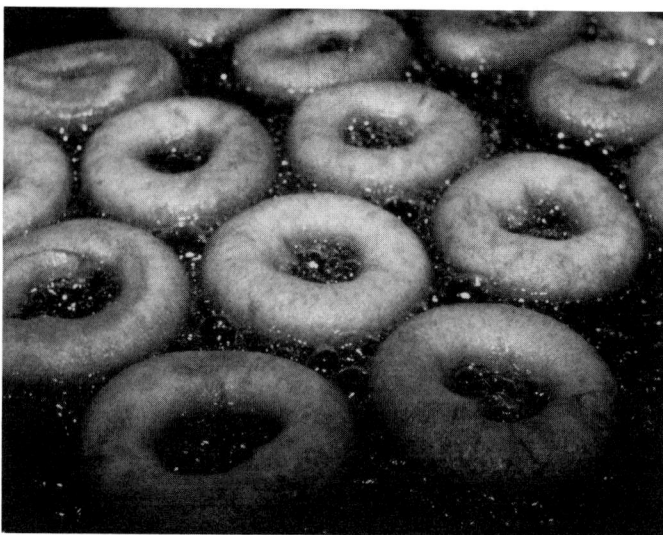

Fig. S-14. Frying doughnuts in shortening. (Courtesy, American Soybean Assn., St. Louis, Mo.)

food. The amount of shortening varies according to the product. Breads and rolls contain 1 to 2%, cakes 10 to 20%, and piecrusts contain over 30%. When shortenings are used in frying they serve for heat transfer and as antisticking agents, and provide some tenderness and richness of flavor.

Rendered animal fats and butter are shortening agents, but the term generally refers to fats which have been especially processed. For a number of years, lard or beef tallow were the main shortenings. Then with the development of hydrogenated vegetable oils came the increased use and acceptance of vegetable shortenings. Hydrogenation—adding hydrogen to the unsaturated fatty acids—can convert naturally liquid fats to semisolids. These shortenings may be prepared in all degrees of stiffness, from liquid to solid, depending upon their melting point. Melting point is determined by their degree of saturation. Then, in order to achieve specific physical, chemical, and biological properties, it is common to blend three or more different fats. Vegetable oils used include corn oil, cottonseed oil, soybean oil, olive oil, palm oil, peanut oil, safflower oil, and sesame oil. Thus, there are several general types of shortening meeting different needs.

• **General purpose**—These shortenings meet a variety of uses and are the household shortenings sold in grocery stores in metal containers. General purpose shortenings are semisolids when temperatures range from 60 to 90°F (16 to 32°C). They may be employed by the home cook in biscuits, cookies, pie crusts, breads and rolls, pancakes, and pan frying. Also, these shortenings usually contain monoglycerides (glycerol molecules with only one fatty acid) so they may also be employed in cakes, icings, frostings, and other recipes wherein relatively large amounts of fat and water must be mixed without danger of separation. Monoglycerides act as emulsifiers.

• **Frying**—Shortenings used in frying must resist oxidation at high temperatures. Oxidation causes fat to darken, become thicker, foam during frying, and develop unpleasant flavors and odors. To resist oxidation at high temperatures, frying fats are composed of saturated fatty acids—low iodine value, and cannot contain mono- or diglycerides as these produce smoke at high frying temperatures. Moreover, fats whose fatty acids are short chain such as coconut oil are not suitable for deep fat frying because they break down and foam. Frying fats generally contain some antioxidants and antifoaming agents.

• **Special emulsifying**—These shortenings contain at least four emulsifying agents which complement each other and provide some particular characteristic. They provide the special properties necessary in prepared baking mixes, whipped toppings, icings, fillings, and the like.

• **Liquid oils**—Vegetable oils are required in mayonnaise and salad dressings, and may be used as a shortening agent in rolls, breads, and other baked goods. They are a notable convenience in many kitchens. Also, the vegetable oils are the basis of margarine which may also be a shortening agent.

(Also see FATS AND OTHER LIPIDS; LARD; MARGARINE; and OILS, VEGETABLE.)

SHREDDED

Cut into long, narrow pieces.

SIFTED

Materials that have been passed through wire sieves to separate particles of different sizes. The common connotation is the separation of finer material than would be done by screening.

(Also see FLOURS.)

SILICON (Si)

Silicon is one of the most abundant elements on earth—present in large amounts in soils and plants. The highest concentrations in animal tissue are found in the skin and its appendages; for example, the ash of feathers is more than 70% silicon.

HISTORY. Although the early chemists considered silica (SiO_2) an elementary substance, Antoine Lavoisier, founder of quantitative chemistry, suspected in 1787 that it was an oxide of an undiscovered element. In 1823, Jons J. Berzelius, the Swedish chemist, discovered the element. The name *silicon* is derived from the Latin *silex* or *silicis*, meaning flint—appropriately indicating its hardness.

In 1972, Dr. E. Carlisle, nutritionist at the University of California, Los Angeles, reported that the trace element silicon (Si) is needed in microgram amounts for normal growth and skeletal development of chicks and rats.

The free element silicon is not found in nature, but it occurs either as the oxide silica (SiO_2) in such forms as sand and quartz, or as silicates in such materials as granite. Silicon is important in plant and animal life; it is present in the ashes of plants and in human skeletons.

ABSORPTION, METABOLISM, EXCRETION. Silicon is absorbed readily. Even over a wide range of intake, the concentration in the blood remains relatively constant—not more than 1 mg per 100 ml. It is excreted easily—via both the feces and urine.

FUNCTIONS OF SILICON. Silicon appears to be essential for chicks and rats; its absence from the diet impedes normal growth and skeletal development. These findings suggest that it may also have essential functions in man.

DEFICIENCY SYMPTOMS. The production of deficiencies in chicks and rats, characterized by growth retardation and skeletal alterations and deformities, especially of the skull, depends on strict control of dietary and environmental contamination; this suggests a low requirement that is easily met by the amount in the environment.

Deficiencies of silicon have not been produced in man. However, it has been found that the silicon content of the aorta, skin, and thymus decrease significantly with age; this is probably related to the fact that the mucopolysaccharide (the substance that binds with water to form the thick gelatinous material which cements cells together and lubricates joints and bursas) content of body tissues also declines with aging.

INTERRELATIONSHIPS. Silicon appears to take part in the synthesis of mucopolysaccharides and is a component of the mucopolysaccharide-protein complexes of connective tissue.

Normally, urinary silicon is eliminated efficiently. However, high levels of silicon in the diet of farm animals may be detrimental. In a manner not yet fully understood, part of it is sometimes deposited in the kidney, bladder, and urethra to form calculi (stones).

A common nondietary form of silicon toxicity is a lung condition known as silicosis, due to inhalation of airborne silicon oxide dust. The amount of silicon in the blood and urine increases in silicosis.

RECOMMENDED DAILY ALLOWANCE OF SILICON. A human requirement of silicon cannot be established on the basis of available knowledge.

• **Silicon intake in average U.S. diet**—Human intake of silicon has been estimated at approximately 1 g per day.

TOXICITY. Silicon does not appear to be toxic in the levels usually found in foods.

SOURCES OF SILICON. Because of the abundance of silicon in all but the most highly purified foods, it is of little concern in human diets.

The best sources of silicon are the fibrous parts of whole grains, followed by various organ meats (liver, lungs, kidneys, and brain) and connective tissues. Much of the silicon in whole grains is lost when they are milled into highly refined products.

(Also see MINERAL[S], Table M-25.)

SIMPLE SUGARS

The *monosaccharides*. The most important simple sugars are *fructose, galactose, glucose,* and *mannose.*

(Also see CARBOHYDRATES, section on "Monosaccharides.")

SINGLE-CELL PROTEIN (SCP)

This refers to protein obtained from single-cell organisms, such as yeast, bacteria, and algae, that have been grown on specially prepared media. Production of this type of protein can be attained through the fermentation of petroleum derivatives or organic waste, or through the culturing of photosynthetic organisms in special illuminated ponds.

CURRENT PROBLEMS ASSOCIATED WITH SINGLE-CELL PROTEIN. Although single-cell protein appears to be an excellent alternative or supplemental source of protein, several problems must be overcome before it becomes a widely used food; among them, palatability, digestibility, nucleic acid content, toxins, protein quality, and economics.

As the world's human population increases, there will be an increasing demand for cheap protein. This demand could dry up the sources of traditional protein, thereby opening the way for intensive development of alternative sources of proteins.

(Also see PROTEIN, section on "Protein For The World.")

SIPPY DIET

A type of diet offered to bleeding peptic ulcer patients, originated by an American physician, Bertram Sippy, in 1915. It broke the previous practice of initial starvation treatment and established the beginning principles of continuous control of gastric acidity through diet and alkaline medication. To start with, the Sippy Diet consists of hourly feedings of 3 oz (150 ml) of whole milk, skim milk, or equal parts of cream and milk. After 2 or 3 days, up to 3 oz (85 g) of soft eggs, or strained cereals are added to the milk. Bland, easily digested foods may be occasionally added to break the monotony. Never does the total bulk of one feeding exceed 6 oz (300 ml).

(Also see LENHARTZ DIET; MODIFIED DIETS; and ULCERS, PEPTIC.)

SKIMMED

Material from which floating solid material has been removed. It is also applied to milk from which fat has been removed by centrifuging.

SKIN

• Outer coverings of fruits or seeds, as the rinds, husks, or peels.

• Dermal tissue of man and animals.

SLOE (BLACKTHORN) *Prunus spinosa*

A small, wild European plum (of the family *Rosaceae*) that is blackish purple with a very sour, green-colored flesh.

The sloe plum is used mainly in the production of sloe gin, jam, and a highly esteemed liqueur. Few people care to eat it raw.

SNACK FOODS

Snacks are those small portions of food eaten between meals; hence, no certain food is really a snack food. Individuality and need determine snack foods.

Snacking can be good or bad, depending upon the snack food and the frequency of snacking. Unfortunately, many people choose foods loaded with sugar and fat—calories—but low in protein, vitamins, and minerals. In keeping with the objective of good nutrition for good health, it just makes sense to eat nutritious snacks; for example, an orange, an apple, peanut butter and crackers, milk, nuts, raw vegetables, juice, etc. However, the type of snack depends on age and activity. Small children often fail to consume the amount of food in regular meals that will add up to their nutritional needs. A slice of cheese, a wheat cracker, or a banana at various times helps supply the added energy they need. The active growing bodies of teenagers need nutritious snacks which provide extra protein, vitamins, minerals, and energy; for example, nuts, yogurt, milk, fruit salads, and left-

overs. Senior citizens often have chewing or digestion problems which interfere with regular eating habits. Here again nutritious snacks are helpful to meet daily needs.

Nutritious snacks are, however, no excuse for overindulgence. A calorie is still a calorie, and lots of little snacks add up. If more energy is consumed than used, the excess is stored as fat. Dieters should choose nutritious, but filling, snacks such as fresh fruits and raw vegetables.

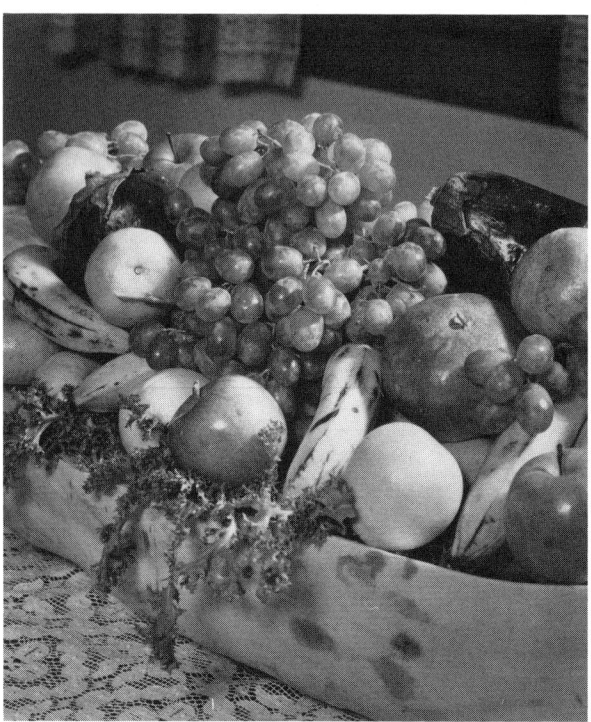

Fig. S-15. America is blessed with a distribution system that provides a wide variety of fresh fruits and vegetables the year round. (Photo by J. C. Allen and Son, West Lafayette, Ind.)

The best way to ensure nutritious snacking is to keep the nutritious snacks on hand and available. Ideas for nutritious snacks are endless, and may be chosen by evaluating foods in terms of energy, protein, mineral and vitamin content as given in Food Composition Table F-21 of this book.

(Also see CONVENIENCE AND FAST FOODS; and FAST FOODS.)

SNIPE

Any of several game birds (genus *Capella*) that are widely distributed in the New and Old Worlds, especially in marshy areas. The snipe is best prepared by roasting.

SOAP

Chemically, soap is the alkali salt of fatty acids. It is formed by a process called saponification. Specifically, soap is a mixture of the sodium salts of the following fatty acids: stearic acid ($C_{17}H_{35}COOH$); palmitic acid ($C_{15}H_{31}COOH$); and oleic acid ($C_{17}H_{33}COOH$). Soft soaps are the potassium salts of these fatty acids. Hence, saponification is accomplished with either sodium hydroxide or potassium hydroxide. Glycerin or glycerol is a by-product of saponification, since the fatty acids are triglycerides—three fatty acids joined to glycerol. Saponification releases the fatty acids from glycerol. During World War II, housewives saved used cooking fats to be used in making soap, and more importantly glycerin for explosives. In a broad sense, soap is any salt of long-chain fatty acids. In the body, fatty acids which leave via the feces are almost entirely soaps.

(Also see FATS AND OTHER LIPIDS.)

SODA WATER

Water charged with carbon dioxide is termed soda water. It bubbles and fizzes as the gas is released. Soda water is added to syrups in soft drinks and to mixed alcoholic drinks. It does not possess any medicinal properties.

(Also see SOFT DRINKS [Carbonated Beverages].)

SODIUM (Na)

Most of the sodium in the diet is in the form of sodium chloride (NaCl), a white granular substance used to season and preserve food. It is created by combining the elements sodium (Na), a soft silvery-white metal, and chlorine (Cl), a poisonous, yellow gas; neither of which is desirable for use alone.

The need for sodium in the diet has been recognized since the classic experiment of Osborne and Mendel, reported in 1918.[30]

The body contains about 0.2% sodium, or about 100 g in a 154-lb (70 kg) person. About 50% of the sodium is in the extracellular (between cell) fluids, 40% is in the skeleton, and only about 10% is within the cells. In the blood, most of the sodium is in the plasma, which contains 320 mg per 100 ml.

HISTORY. Compounds of sodium were known and used extensively during ancient times, but the element was not isolated until 1807, when Sir Humphrey Davy, the English chemist, used electricity (in a process called electrolysis) to extract the pure metal from sodium hydroxide. Although sodium had long been believed to be a dietary essential, final proof was not obtained until 1918 when Osborne and Mendel conducted laboratory animal experiments.

ABSORPTION, METABOLISM, EXCRETION. Virtually all sodium ingested in the diet is readily absorbed from the gut, following which it is carried by the blood to the kidneys, where it is filtered out and returned to the blood in amounts needed to maintain the levels required by the body.

Excess sodium, which usually amounts to 90 to 95% of ingested sodium, is, for the most part, excreted by the kidneys as chloride and phosphate and controlled by aldosterone, a hormone of the adrenal cortex. A deficiency of aldosterone, known as Addison's disease, leads to excessive losses of sodium in the urine.

The levels of sodium in the urine reflect the dietary intake; if there is high intake of sodium the rate of excretion is high, if there is low intake the excretion rate is low.

In hot weather, sodium excretion through the skin is important because each liter of sweat contains 0.5 to 3.0 g of sodium.

FUNCTIONS OF SODIUM. Sodium is the major positively charged ion in the fluid outside the cells, where it helps to maintain the balance of water, acids, and bases. Also, it is a constituent of pancreatic juice, bile, sweat, and tears.

Sodium is associated with muscle contraction and nerve functions. Sodium also plays a specific role in the absorption of carbohydrates.

(Also see section on MINERAL[S], Table M-25, Mineral Table.)

DEFICIENCY SYMPTOMS. Deficiencies of sodium are rare because nearly all foods contain some sodium. However, deficiencies may occur from strict vegetarian diets without salt, or when there has been heavy prolonged sweating, diarrhea, vomiting, or adrenal cortical insufficiency.

Excess perspiration and salt depletion may be accompanied by heat exhaustion. Salt tablets taken with a liberal amount of water may be advised under these conditions.

(Also see section on MINERAL[S], Table M-25, Mineral Table.)

INTERRELATIONSHIPS. Sodium, potassium, and chlorine are closely related metabolically. They serve a vital function in controlling osmotic pressures and acid-base equilibrium; and they play important roles in water metabolism. Both sodium and potassium ions occur in the body chiefly in close association with the chloride ion; therefore, a sodium or potassium deficiency is rarely found in the absence of a chlorine deficiency.

Excess dietary salt, over a long period of time, is believed to lead to high blood pressure in susceptible people. Also, excess sodium may cause edema, evidenced by swelling of such areas as the legs and face. The simplest way to reduce sodium intake is to eliminate the use of table salt.

RECOMMENDED DAILY ALLOWANCES OF SODIUM. The salt requirements of the infant and young child are estimated to be about 120–300 mg per day. Human milk contains 161 mg of sodium per liter, whereas commonly used bottle formulas contains between 161 and 391 mg per liter, and cow's milk contains about 483 mg per liter. Average intake of sodium during the first year of life ranges from about 300 mg per day at 2 months of age to about 1,400 mg per day at 12 months—far in excess of needs.

The healthy adult can maintain sodium balance with an intake of little more than the minimum requirements of the infant. When doing hard physical labor in high ambient temperatures, an adult may lose 8.0 g of sodium per day in sweat. Whenever more than 3 liter of water per day are required to replace sweat losses, extra salt (NaCl) should be provided; somewhere between 2 and 7 g of sodium chloride per liter of extra water loss, depending on the severity of losses and the degree of acclimatization. For those with a family history of high blood pressure, the food intake of salt should be limited to 500 mcg per day.

Pregnancy increases the sodium requirement, by an estimated 69 mg of sodium per day.

Estimated safe and adequate intakes of sodium are given in the section on MINERAL[S], Table M-25, Mineral Table.

• **Sodium intake in average U.S. diet**—The average daily American intake of salt is 10 to 15 g, or about 5 g of sodium (salt is approximately 40% sodium and 60% chlorine by weight).

---

[30]Osborne, T., and L. Mendel, "Inorganic Elements in Nutrition," *Journal of Biological Chemistry*, Vol. 34, 1918, p. 131.

• **Salt intake and high blood pressure**—There is strong evidence linking too much salt to high blood pressure, which affects 20 million Americans. Also, there is evidence that high salt intake increases the incidence of hypertension among various societies and cultures of the world (Altschal, A. M. and J. K. Grommet, "Sodium Intake and Sodium Sensitivity," *Nutrition Reviews*, Vol. 38, December 1980, No. 12, pp. 393-402).

Under ordinary circumstances, children and adults require no more than 0.2 g—about 1/10 tsp—of salt per day. With strenuous exercise or labor accompanied by profuse sweating, only 2 g—just under 1 tsp— is necessary. Normally, therefore, an allowance of 1 g of salt per day is sufficient. Yet, studies reveal that the average American consumes about 10 g of salt per day—ten times more than the recommended allowance.

People with high blood pressure should drastically curtail their salt intake. Fortunately, salt appetite can be readily revised downward, for there are no withdrawal pains from giving up salt. This can be accomplished by using the salt shaker sparingly, both in the kitchen and in the dining room; and by avoiding salty foods, such as olives, popcorn, potato chips, french fries, and sauerkraut.

It is noteworthy that cultural factors appear to determine the salt consumption. For example, the Japanese commonly consume 25 to 50 g of salt per day, whereas the Eskimos, Lapps, Australian aborigines, numerous tribes of New Guinea, South America and Africa, and many midwestern American Indian tribes consume from a few hundred milligrams to no more than 5 g of salt per day.

(Also see SALT.)

TOXICITY. Salt may be toxic when (1) a high intake is accompanied by a restriction of water, (2) when the body is adapted to a chronic low salt diet, or (3) when it is fed to infants or others whose kidneys cannot excrete the excess in the urine.

SOURCES OF SODIUM. In addition to salt (sodium chloride) used in cooking, processing, and seasoning, sodium is present in all foods in varying amounts. Generally more sodium is present in protein foods than in vegetables and grains. Fruits contain little or no sodium. The salt added to these foods in preparation may be many times that found naturally in foods. Also, the sodium content of the water

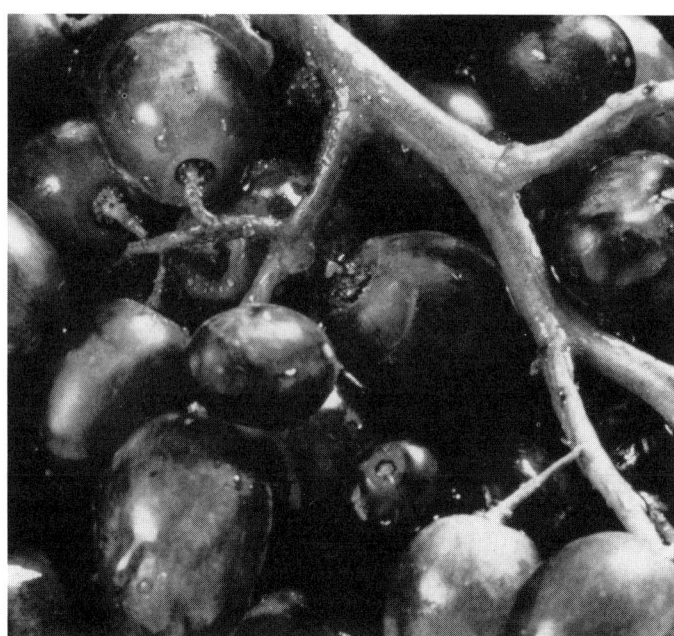

Fig. S-16. Grapes and other fruits contain little or no sodium. (Courtesy, USDA)

supply varies considerably; in some areas of the country, the amount of sodium in the water is of sufficient quantity to be of significance in the total daily intake.

Generally speaking, the need is for low sodium diets, rather than high sodium diets; especially by people with high blood pressure. Table S-5 has been prepared to meet this need.

TABLE S-5
GROUPINGS OF SOME LOW SODIUM FOODS

SODIUM LEVEL					
0-5 mg/100 g		**5-10 mg/100 g**	**10-20 mg/100 g**	**20-40 mg/100 g**	**40-60 mg/100 g**
Almonds	Oranges	Apples, dried	Avocados	Artichokes	Arrowroot
Apples	Peaches	Apricots, dried	Broccoli	Brown sugar	Black pepper
Asparagus	Pears	Chestnuts	Brussels sprouts	Chinese cabbage	Beef
Apricots	Pineapples	Cucumbers	Cabbage	Coconut	Carrots
Bananas	Potatoes	Dock	Cantaloupe	Cream	Chicken giblets
Blackberries	Raspberries	Green onions	Cauliflower	Hot chili peppers	Dandelion greens, cooked
Cherries	Rhubarb	Honey	Collards	Passion fruit	Egg yolks
Currants	Rye flour	Kohlrabi	Dried figs	Potato flour	Kale
Dates	Shortening	Lettuce	Endive	Red cabbage	Milk
Eggplants	Soybean flour	Nectarine	Garden cress	Sunflower seeds	Parsley
Figs	Squash	Parsnips	Garlic	Turnips	Pork pancreas
Fresh fruit juices	Strawberries	Peaches, dried	Mangoes		Rabbit meat
Grapefruit	Sugar	Peanut flour	Mature onions		Red beets, boiled
Grapes	Sweet corn	Peanuts	Molasses		Sablefish
Green beans	Tomatoes	Pears, dried	Mushrooms		Sole
Green peas	Walnuts	Persimmons	Mustard greens		Sunflower seed flour
Guavas	Watermelon	Pigeonpeas	Pecans		Tamarinds
Lard	Wax beans	Waxgourd	Prunes		Tuna
Lima beans	Wheat flour	Wheat bran	Radishes		Turkey
Oils	Wheat germ		Raisins		Walleye pike
Okra	Whole wheat flour		Split peas		Watercress
			Sweet potatoes		Yogurt, whole milk
			Turnip greens		
			Yeast		

NOTE WELL: Many processed foods contain high levels of sodium due to the addition of salt and other sodium-containing additives; among them, sodium alginate, sodium aluminum sulfate, sodium benzoate, sodium citrate, sodium diacetate, sodium erythorbate, sodium nitrate, sodium nitrite, sodium propionate, and sodium sorbate.

For additional sources and more precise values of sodium, see Food Composition Table F-21.

HIGH SODIUM SOURCES. In order that consumers may intelligently cut back on sodium intake, it is important that they know which foods are high in sodium. Table S-6 lists some of the high sodium foods and gives the precise sodium content of each.

(Also see MINERAL[S], Table M-25; and SALT.)

TABLE S-6
SOME HIGH SODIUM FOODS[1]

Food	Sodium
	(mg/100 g)
Canadian bacon	2,555
Olives, green	2,400
Shrimp, canned	2,300
Caviar	2,200
Corned beef	1,740
Pretzels	1,680
Parmesan cheese	1,602
Pasteurized process cheese	1,430
Cucumber pickles	1,428
Bologna	1,300
Oat cereal	1,267
Luncheon meat	1,200
Soda crackers	1,100
Cured ham	1,100
Frankfurters	1,084
Wheat flakes cereal	1,032
Bacon	1,021
Bran cereal	1,012
Corn flakes cereal	1,005
Potato chips	1,000
Rice flakes cereal	987
Sausage	958

[1]Data from the Food Composition Table F-21.

SODIUM BICARBONATE (NaHCO₃)

A chemical compound which is known to function as a buffer and pH agent, maintaining sufficient alkaline reserves (buffering capacity) in the body fluids to ensure normal physiological and metabolic functions.

(Also see ACID-BASE BALANCE; and ANTACIDS.)

SODIUM DIACETATE

An antimicrobial food additive which controls both rope (bacterial action) and mold in breads. The FDA allows flour used in bakery goods to contain 0.4% sodium diacetate.

SODIUM PHYTATE

A chelating agent that is formed from phytic acid. In the past, it has been employed as part of a treatment for calcium phosphate kidney stones.

(Also see PHYTIC ACID.)

SODIUM-POTASSIUM RATIO

Sodium and potassium are closely interrelated. Although sodium intake may be the most important dietary determi-nant of blood pressure, variations in the sodium: potassium ratio in the diet affect blood pressure under certain circum-stances. In rats with high blood pressure due to a high intake of sodium, blood pressure may be lowered to a more normal level by increasing the potassium intake and lowering the sodium intake. It seems that a 1:1 ratio may be somewhat protective against the blood pressure-elevating effects of a given level of sodium. This ratio can be achieved by increas-ing the intake of potassium, or lowering the intake of sodium, or both. Good dietary sources of potassium include meats, milk, dried dates, bananas, cantaloupe, apricots, tomato juice, and the dark green leafy vegetables.

(Also see HIGH BLOOD PRESSURE; POTASSIUM; and SODIUM.)

SOFT DRINKS (CARBONATED BEVERAGES)

This name is given to the familiar American beverages, often called *soda pop* or *pop*. The name *soft* is used to distinguish these beverages from *hard* or alcoholic beverages. Soft drinks are generally, but not always, car-bonated, and contain a sweetening agent, edible acids, and natural or artifical flavors. Today, everywhere people work or play, soft drinks are available and their yearly consump-tion reflects their availability—and the advertising budget of the major producers.

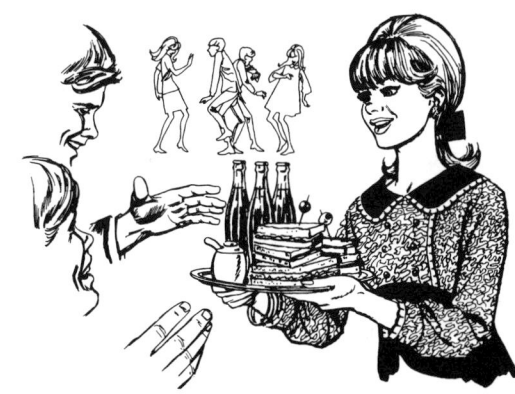

Fig. S-17. In moderation, the occasional soft drink at a party can be part of the fun.

HISTORY. In 1772, the Englishman, Joseph Priestley, described a pleasant-tasting, sparkling water which he pro-duced by introducing carbon dioxide (CO₂) into the water. Thus, carbonated beverages were born; however, Priestley is better known for his discovery of oxygen.

In 1806, the real business of selling soft drinks was started by Benjamin Silliman, a chemistry professor at Yale College in Connecticut. In New Haven, he bottled and sold soda water—water charged with carbon dioxide. Sometime after 1830, flavored soda water became popular, and by 1860, the census reported 123 plants producing carbonated drinks. In 1886, a druggist and former Confederate soldier named John Styth Pemberton created a drink which is still favored. He added an extract from the African kola nut to an extract from cocoa. Another enterprising pharmacist named Hires, introduced bottled root beer in 1893. Currently, the popular flavors are cola, lemon-lime, orange, ginger ale, root beer, and grape, but every conceivable type of flavor has been produced. Cola drinks are the most popular.

CONSUMPTION. In 1850, the United States per capita consumption of soft drinks was only about 1 pt (*470*

year. In 1990, the per capita consumption was about 47.5 gal—more than 3.5 times the consumption in 1960 (see Fig. S-18). But that's not all! Ponder these figures:

• In 1990, the average man, woman, and child in the United States drank 760 8-oz soft drinks (in comparison to only 25.4 gal of milk)—that's an average of 1½ 12-oz cans per day.

• Soda pop now provides about 8% of the calories consumed daily by the average person, with virtually all these calories coming from sugar.

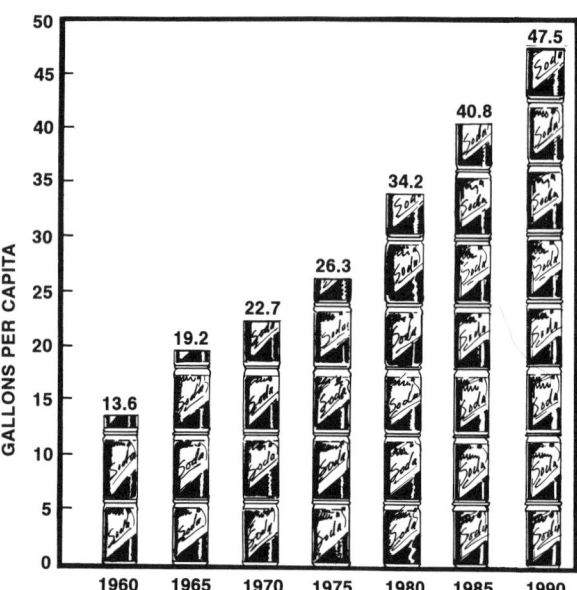

Fig. S-18. The rise in soft drink—carbonated beverage—consumption. (Sources: USDA; J. C. Maxwell, *Beverage Industry*, February 1991)

Yearly, consumption of soft drinks surpasses milk, beer, or coffee. This popularity is probably due to their availability and the tremendous advertising efforts of the major companies. The ad expenditures of the soft drink companies total over $200 million each year—all for convincing people to drink "the real thing," "the uncola," or to join a certain "generation" or to become a "pepper."

INGREDIENTS. The precise formulaton of most soft drinks is not well known. However, certain aspects of soft drinks are governed by standards of identity enforced by the Food and Drug Administration (FDA).

• **Soda water**—According to the standards of identity, soda water is the class of beverages made by absorbing carbon dioxide in potable water. The amount of carbon dioxide used is not less than that which will be absorbed by the beverage at a pressure of one atmosphere and at a temperature of 60°F *(15.5°C)*. It either contains no alcohol or only such alcohol as is contributed by the flavoring ingredient used, but not in excess of 0.5% by weight of the finished beverage.

• *Cola or pepper*—Soda water designated by any name which includes the word *cola* or *pepper* shall contain caffeine from kola nut extract and/or other natural caffeine-containing extracts. Also, caffeine may be added to any soda water. The total caffeine content in the finished food shall not exceed 0.02% by weight.

Soda water may contain any safe and suitable optional ingredient, except that vitamins, minerals, and proteins added for nutritional purposes and artificial sweeteners are

not suitable for food encompassed by this standard.

The optional ingredients include: sweetening agents, acids, flavors, colors, preservatives, emulsifying, stabilizing or viscosity-producing agents, and foaming agents. Sweetening agents may consist of the following nutritive sweeteners (calorie-containing): dry or liquid sugar (sucrose), invert sugar, dextrose, fructose, corn syrup, glucose syrups, or sorbitol, singly or in combination.

With the sudden popularity of diet soft drinks in the early 1960s, low-calorie sweeteners, once used primarily by diabetics and other individuals with special dietary restrictions, came into vogue. Since that time, consumer demand for reduced-calorie beverages has increased greatly, with a corresponding increase in the use of low-calorie sweetening agents, chiefly aspartame. The present status of each of three well-known low-calorie sweeteners follows:

• **Saccharin**—Used as a sweetener by diabetics. Also used in some cosmetics, toothpastes, and cough syrups.

• **Cyclamate**—Cyclamate was taken off the U.S. market completely in 1970.

• **Aspartame**—In the United States, both aspartame alone and aspartame-saccharine mixtures are used as sweeteners in diet sodas. In Canada, aspartame is the only sweetener used in soft drinks. In 1991, aspartame had 75% of the U.S. sweetener market.

(Also see SWEETENING AGENTS.)

Flavoring agents in a carrier of ethyl alcohol, glycerin, or propylene glycol may include fruit juices, including concentrates and natural flavoring derived from fruits, vegetables, bark, roots, leaves, and similar plant materials. Artificial flavoring may also be used, as well as natural or artificial color. The edible acids which may be used singly or in combination are acetic, adipic, citric, fumaric, gluconic, lactic, malic, tartaric, and phosphoric acids. Table S-7 shows how some of these ingredients make up the familiar soft drinks.

TABLE S-7
SOFT DRINK INGREDIENTS

Soft Drink	Flavors	Color	Sugar (%)	Edible Acid	Carbon Dioxide (CO_2) (volume of gas)[1]
Cola	Extract of kola nut, lime oil, spice oils, caffeine.	Caramel	11–13	Phosphoric	3.5
Orange	Oil of orange and orange juice.	Sunset yellow FCF with some Tartrazine.	12–14	Citric	1.5–2.5
Ginger Ale	Ginger root, oil of ginger, and lime oil.	Caramel	7–11	Citric	4.0-4.5
Root beer	Oil of wintergreen, vanilla, nutmeg, cloves or anise.	Caramel	11–13	Citric	3
Grape	Methyl anthranilate and oil of cognac, sometimes grape juice.	Amarinth and Brilliant Blue FCF.	11–13	Tartaric	1.0-2.5

[1]A volume of gas is equivalent to 15 lb per square inch at sea level and 60°F *(15.5°C)*. Correct carbonation results in pungent taste.

Soft drink plants are subject to state and federal laws and regulations which are designed to protect the consumer and to serve as an operational guide for the manufacturer.

NUTRITIONAL VALUE. Probably the best thing that can be said about soft drinks is that their flavor encourages people to drink water. Soft drinks containing nutritive sweeteners contribute empty calories to the diet. Each 12-oz (*360 ml*) can supplies about 147 Calories (kcal); hence, excessive usage may contribute to tooth decay and overweight. Diet soft drinks, which became popular during the 1960s, are essentially flavored water. Also, sparkling water (club soda) is carbonated water without sugar (calories), and sometimes with added sodium bicarbonate or sodium sulfate in an effort to simulate natural mineral water. Despite the nutritional shortcomings of carbonated beverages, many people indulge primarily because they enjoy the taste, the tingling sensation of the carbonation, and the mildly stimulating effects. Food Composition Table F-21 compares some of the common soft drinks.

Considering the alternatives, water costs less and quenches the thirst, and milk provides a few more calories but better nutrition. Moreover, 12 oz of milk costs less than 12 oz of a soft drink. Fruit juices are also viable alternatives providing substantially more nutrition at a cost comparable to soft drinks.

SOLANINE

A naturally occurring toxicant found in the nightshade family, which includes such useful plants as the potato, tomato, ground cherry, red pepper, and eggplant. In large enough doses it acts on the nervous system since it is an inhibitor of acetylcholinesterase, an enzyme involved in the transmission of nervous impulses. Also, the feeling persists (without research proof) that consumption of vegetables in the nightshade family may aggravate arthritis in susceptible people. Potatoes contain the highest levels of solanine. However, a person would have to eat, at one sitting, 4.5 lb (*2.0 kg*) of potatoes containing 200 mg (100 ppm) of solanine to produce the initial effects of poisoning—drowsiness and itchiness behind the neck.

CAUTION: When potatoes are exposed to light, or when they sprout, their solanine content increases; it's concentrated chiefly in the sprouts and to a lesser extent in the skin. Thus, potatoes that are green, spoiled, or sprouted may contain harmful amounts of solanine.

(Also see POISONOUS PLANTS; and POTATO, section headed "Selection.")

SOLIDS, MILK

The solids, or total solids, of milk includes all the constituents of milk except water. Milk contains an average of 12% total solids.

SOLIDS-NOT-FAT, MILK

This includes the carbohydrate, protein, minerals, and water-soluble vitamins of milk—it excludes the fat. Milk contains an average of 8.6% solids-not-fat.

SOLUTES

Particles in solution in body water. Three types of solutes influence internal shifts and balances of body water: (1) electrolytes, (2) plasma proteins, and (3) organic compounds of small molecular size.

SOLVENT-EXTRACTED

Fat or oil removed from materials (such as oilseeds) by organic solvents. Also called *new process.*

(Also see OILS, VEGETABLE, section on "Extraction of Oils"; and SOYBEAN, section headed "Extracting the Oil.")

SORBIC ACID (SORBATE; $C_6H_8O_2$)

A food additive possessing antimicrobial activity especially toward yeast and molds. It is commonly used in the form of *sodium sorbate* and *potassium sorbate.* In the body, all evidence indicates that sorbate is metabolized like other fatty acids. It is on the GRAS (generally recognized as safe) list of approved food additives. Food applications of sorbic acid are numerous, among them, baked goods, beverages, cheese and cheese products, dried fruits, fish, fruit juices, jams, jellies, meats, pickled products, salads, and wines.

SORGHUM (GUINEA CORN; KAFFIR; MILO)
Sorghum bicolor

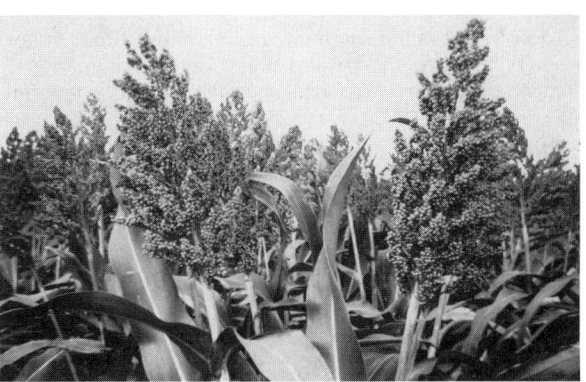

Fig. S-19. Hybrid grain sorghum, headed out and nearing harvest. (Courtesy, National Grain Sorghum Producers Assn., Abernathy, Tex.)

Sorghum, a member of the grass family, *Gramineae,* is of great importance in dry and arid lands. The genus *Sorgum* embraces hundreds of varieties and many hybrids which are commonly lumped as the many-faceted species, *Sorghum bicolor.* Different varieties are grown for different uses—grain, syrup, forage, and broom fiber.

ORIGIN AND HISTORY. Sorghum has been cultivated in Africa and Asia for 4,000 years. It is said to have been a principal item in the diet of the ancient city of Ninevah on the Tigris.

WORLD AND U.S. PRODUCTION. Sorghum is the fifth ranking cereal crop of the world, being exceeded by wheat, corn, rice, and barley. The world sorghum crop averages 58 million metric tons. Ten leading producing countries, by rank, are: United States, India, Mexico, China, Nigeria, Argentina, Sudan, Ethiopia, Australia, and Burkino Faso.[31]

---

[31]Data from *FAO Production Yearbook 1990,* FAO/UN, Rome, Italy, Vol. 44, p. 85, Table 24. **Note well:** Annual production fluctuates as a result of weather and profitability of the crop.

The United States produces about 25% of the world's sorghum grain. The U.S. *sorghum belt* is the Southern Great Plains. The ten leading states, by rank, are: Kansas, Texas, Nebraska, Missouri, Arkansas, Oklahoma, Illinois, South Dakota, Colorado, and Louisiana. Kansas and Texas account for 56% of the nation's production.

KINDS. The cultivated sorghums can be classified into the following four broad classifications according to use:

1. **Grain sorghums.** These sorghums are bred specially for grain production. Most types in the United States are less than 5 ft tall. Common grain varieties include kaffir, milo, feterita, Durra, shallu, koaliang, and hegari.

2. **Sweet sorghums (sorgos).** These have tall, sweet, juicy stalks that are used for forage, syrup, and sugar production.

3. **Grass sorghums.** These have thin stems, narrow leaves, and numerous tillers—characteristics which make them useful for hay or grazing by animals. Sudangrass and Johnsongrass belong to this group.

4. **Broomcorn sorghums.** These have panicle branches which are suitable for making brooms.

Today, most of the sorghums grown in the United States are hybrids, developed by crossing varieties. For grain production, crosses involving kaffir and milo are most common.

PROCESSING. As with corn, sorghum may be either dry milled or wet milled. However, most sorghum is dry milled, simply because it is easier to accomplish.

• **Dry milling**—The objective in dry milling of sorghum grain is to separate the endosperm, germ, and bran from each other.

The endosperm is processed into grits and flour. The other products of dry milling are bran, germ, and hominy feed. Sorghum grits from dry milling are used for brewing and industrial purposes.

(Also see CORN, section headed "Dry Milling.")

• **Wet milling**—The wet milling of sorghum closely resembles the wet milling of corn. However, sorghum is more difficult to wet mill than corn because (1) it is difficult to separate the starch and protein, (2) it is difficult to extract the sorghum germ from the kernel, (3) pigments discolor the starch and must be removed by bleaching, and (4) recovery of starch is lower than with corn. It is noteworthy, however, that new hybrids with improved wet milling qualities have been developed.

(Also see CORN, section headed "Wet Milling.")

NUTRITIONAL VALUE. Generally speaking, sorghum and corn are interchangeable in the diet; with corn preferred and grown where adapted, and sorghum grown in hot, dry regions where corn cannot be grown successfully. So, both the nutritionist and the consumer need to com-

pare the two foods. Table S-8 gives a comparison of selected nutrients of sorghum grain and corn. Also, Food Composition Table F-21 gives the nutrient compositions of corn and sorghum, and their products.

TABLE S-8
COMPARISON OF SELECTED NUTRIENTS IN SORGHUM GRAIN AND CORN

Nutrient		Sorghum Grain	Corn
		◄--- (per 100 g) ---►	
Calories	kcal	366.0	348.0
Carbohydrates	g	73.0	71.1
Fat	g	3.3	3.9
Protein	g	11.0	9.6
Calcium	mg	28.0	30.0
Phosphorus	mg	287.0	270.0
Iron	mg	4.4	2.0
Niacin	mg	3.9	3.0
Riboflavin	mg	.15	.13
Thiamin	mg	.38	.21

It is recognized that compositional data provide only an approximate comparison because the influence of environment is very striking, affecting both the physical and chemical properties of both sorghum and corn. Nevertheless, the following comparisons of the two grains appear to be justified: sorghum grain is higher in protein but lower in fat than corn.

The amino acid composition of sorghum grain and corn is strikingly similar. The most limiting amino acid is lysine —a feature common to all grains.

Although not shown in Table S-8, cognizance is taken of the following additional differences between sorghum and corn: yellow corn contains more carotene (vitamin A) than sorghum; sorghum has slightly more starch than corn; sorghum contains 0.1 to 0.3% waxes, which is 50 times the quantity of waxes in corn; tannins are present in the pericarp and testa of sorghums, especially in bird-resistant varieties, but absent in corn; and high yields of sorghum are generally inversely related to the protein content of the grain.

Other than the differences noted above, the nutrient composition of sorghum grain and corn are similar.

PRODUCTS AND USES. Sorghum is used for food, fermentation products, feed, and industrial purposes.

The sweet stalks of sorghum are chewed by the natives in various countries; and sorghum is the staple food and basis of beverages in much of Asia and Africa. It is usually consumed as a porridge or stiff paste prepared by adding pounded flour to hot water. Sometimes a flat cake is prepared. Also, the grain may be parched, popped, or boiled whole.

In the United States, the vast majority of grain sorghum is used as livestock feed; hence, in this country sorghum enters the human diet primarily as meat, milk, and eggs. Some sorghum is also used for industrial products.

Table S-9 presents in summary form the use of sorghum products for human food.

(Also see BEERS AND BREWING; BREADS AND BAKING; CEREAL GRAINS; and OILS, VEGETABLE, Table O-5.)

---

[32]Data from *Agricultural Statistics 1991*, USDA, p. 52, Table 67. **Note well:** Annual production fluctuates as a result of weather and profitability of the crop.

TABLE S-9
SORGHUM PRODUCTS AND USES FOR HUMAN FOOD

Country/Product	Description	Uses	Comments
In the United States: Sorghum flour—wheat flour, blended	An off-white flour	Muffins, bread, and griddle cakes	Only about 1.3% of U.S. sorghum grain is used for food, alcohol, and seed; The rest is used for livestock feed. Nevertheless, sorghum has many potential uses in food products.
Sorghum oil	Oil extracted from the germ of the grain	Cooking oil; and in such products as margarines and shortening	
Sorghum starch	An off-white powdery material (varieties with dark colored outer layers may stain the starch)	Thicken puddings	
Sorghum syrup	A distinctly flavored, mild, sweet, light amber-colored syrup. Sorghum syrup is a good source of carbohydrates, calcium, potassium, and iron.	A speciality product, especially in southeastern U.S. As a carbohydrate source, it is about equal to maple syrup and molasses.	The technology for satisfactorily converting sweet sorghum beyond the syrup stage—into sugar— is known. Thus, when the price is right, sweet sorghum can serve as a supplementary crop for the sugar cane and sugar beet industries.
Africa and Asia: East Africa	Pounded sorghum flour	Porridge, made by adding pounded sorghum flour to hot water	
Ethiopia and Sudan	Sorghum flour. Sorghum grain, whole.	Flat cakes. Parched, popped, or boiled white.	
India	Sorghum grain, ground or cracked	Prepared into a dough and baked as flat, unleavened bread (called *rotti*), or cooked like rice.	White, pearly grains are preferred for bread.
	Sorghum grain	Whole grain is parched or "fried" in a hot pan, then ground and mixed with salt, buttermilk, or molasses. Special sorghums for popping or roasting are grown in small quantities.	
Nigeria	Sorghum flour	A food called *tuwo*, prepared by stirring flour in hot water, then allowing the thick paste to cool and gel.	Pieces of the cooled gel are eaten with soup.
	Immature sorghum heads Sorghum (special varieties)	Roasted, much like sweet-corn in the U.S. Popped, similar to popcorn.	
Uganda	Sorghum grain, whole	The grain is malted and sprouted, the radicle (root portion) removed, and the grain dried.	Some of the pigment and the bitter principle are removed. The sugars produced make the porridge sweet.
West Africa	Sorghum flour	Porridge or stiff paste made from stirring flour in hot water. These may be allowed to cool and gel, or the paste may be fried to make pancakes.	

FERMENTATION PRODUCTS

Country and beverage: United States Alcohol	The whole grain is ground, cooked, hydrolyzed by enzymes or acid, fermented by yeast, and the alcohol distilled off. Beverage alcohol production is similar, except malt enzymes are preferred for hydrolysis.	1. Ethyl alcohol for beverages. 2. Denatured alcohol for industrial purposes. 3. Gasohol (10% anhydrous ethanol/90% gasoline)—a motor fuel.	In the U.S., the use of sorghum depends on its price relative to other grains.
Sorghum grits Sorghum starch	The starchy portion of the endosperm. An off-white powdery material.	Brewing and distilling, making industrial alcohol Brewing and distilling, making industrial alcohol	
Africa (Bantu tribe or family)	Sorghum beer	Beer, made by malting and brewing sorghum (preferably red grains)	It differs from beer made from barley malt in that it is an opaque reddish-colored liquor, contains 5 to 6% solids, has a yeasty sour taste, has a low alcohol content, and is high in nutritional value.
Central Africa; tribes in Zambia, Zaire, and the Central African Republic	Homemade sorghum beer; made from sorghum alone, or from a mixture of sorghum with maize (corn) and/or millet.	As a nutritious beer	The grain is soaked in water, sprouted, dried, ground, mixed with water, and allowed to ferment in clay pots. The crude beer may or may not be filtered prior to consumption. Sprouting and fermentation of sorghum results in a more nutritious product than the original grain because additional amounts of the vitamin B complex are produced during the processes.
China Mao-tai	About a 53% alcoholic beverage made from grain sorghum.	At Chinese banquets, Mao-tai is used for toasts.	The Chinese claim that "it's easy on the throat, and it doesn't go to the head." But *first timers* are admonished to approach it with caution. It's potent! (As a result of experiencing the traditional Chinese toasts on 5 different visits to China, two of the authors of this book, the Ensmingers, concluded that the only reason Mao-tai is not used for airplane fuel is that it is readily combustible.)

SOUPS

Probably the first dish ever cooked in a kettle over the open fire was a soup, and because this method of cooking was the only one for countless years, soups were standard fare.

In France, the evening meal is called *la soupe*; and in English, our word *supper* came from the word *soup*.

Each nation has its own special soups, rich in meat, chicken, or fish; health-giving vegetables; and nourishing barley, rice, or macaroni. At one time, soups were thought to be restorative of one's health, and in 16th-century France, one enterprising person advertised his soup establishment as a *restaurant*—alluding to its reputed health-restoring properties. Soon others copied him. Eventually, the name *restaurant* came to be used for all establishments that serve any kind of food.

The purpose of soup in the meal is twofold: (1) to improve digestion and stimulate appetite; and (2) to increase the variety of foods served at the meal. The clear, stock soups serve the first purpose, and the cream soups serve the latter. A heavy meal such as steak or roast, should be preceded by a clear soup, but a light meal of fish, eggs, or salad, is best with a heartier soup.

The number of good soup recipes would, literally speaking, stretch around the world. Usually the soup is named after the ingredients, but there are some world-famous soups with which everyone should become acquainted, unless they are already old friends. Some of these, the recipes for which can be found in the local cookbook library, follow:

• **Bird's nest soup (Chinese)**—The Asian swiftlets coat their nests with a translucent gelatinous material (their saliva), which is high in protein (11.9 g/100 g). It is packaged and available in Chinese specialty shops. First, the nest is soaked, then simmered in chicken stock. "Chicken velvet" is added and it is served garnished with ham. The chicken velvet is made by finely mincing the chicken and mixing it with cornstarch and beaten egg whites. When added to soup, this becomes light and frothy. Bird's nest soup is considered a delicacy.

• **Bisque**—A cream soup made from fish.

• **Borsch (Russian)**—This soup, of which there are several different recipes, is popular in both the U.S.S.R. and in Poland. Basically, it is a beet soup which is thickened with cornstarch. It may or may not have added vegetables and meats.

• **Bouillabaisse (French)**—This is a fish soup with a hot pepper sauce.

• **Bouillon**—Meat and/or meat scraps are simmered slowly to produce the stock or bouillon. It is usually served clear, but it can also be served with added vegetables and pieces of meat.

• **Chowder**—This word comes from the French word, *chaudiere*, meaning *caldron*. The chowder of today has not changed much from the chowder of yesterday. It consists of pieces of different vegetables, or of fish and potatoes, with seasonings, all cooked in milk, and with crackers added just before serving.

• **Cock-a-leekie**—This soup is made by boiling chicken and leeks together.

• **Consomme**—From the French word meaning *to boil down*. Basically, there is little difference between consomme and bouillon. But bouillon is usually thought of as strictly beef stock, whereas consomme may be beef, veal, and/or chicken stock.

• **Cream soups**—A thin white sauce is combined with any desired vegetables or meats. When vegetables or meats are pureed to make a soup, this can be classified as a cream soup, also.

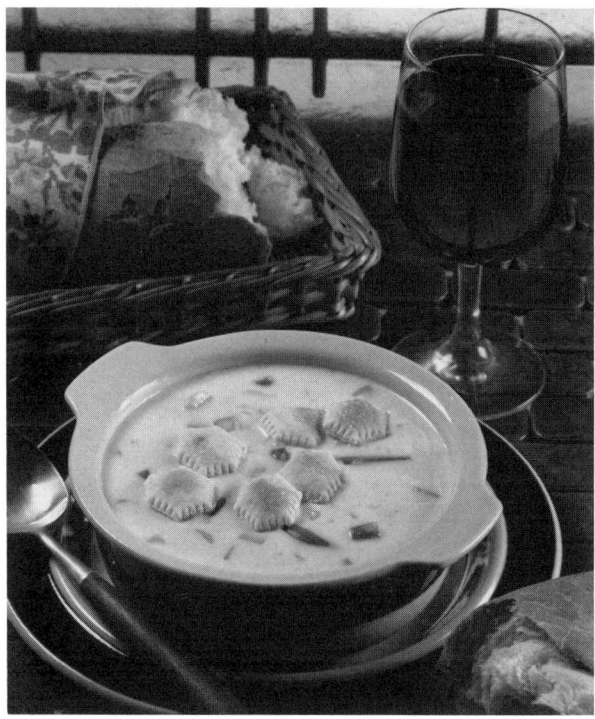

Fig. S-20. Plain and fancy—creamy vegetable soup is welcome at any meal. (Courtesy, Pet Incorporated, St. Louis, Mo.)

• **Egg drop soup (Chinese)**—A clear stock soup, into which is dropped a slightly beaten egg. The egg is cooked in the soup the same way that a poached egg is cooked.

• **Gazpacho (Spain)**—This soup, which originated in Spain, and is popular in Mexico and the southwestern United States, is a highly-seasoned tomato soup with added vegetables, which is served chilled. It may also be jellied.

• **Minestrone (Italy)**—A mixed vegetable soup with beans and macaroni.

• **Mulligatawny (East Indies)**—Chicken, carrots, green pepper and apple are cooked together. The vegetables and apple are pureed and returned to the pot, seasonings, including curry, cloves, and mace, are added.

• **Printanier soup**—This name comes from the French word *printemps*, meaning *spring*. The soup is made from fresh spring vegetables.

• **Vichyssoise (French)**—Potatoes and leeks are cooked together in a chicken broth, then blended, or put through a sieve. Thick cream is added and the mixture is served chilled with a garnish of chopped chives.

Soups can be served with inumerable garnishes, plus a raft of soup accessories. All good cookbooks will furnish the recipes for these.

The nutritive value of soups depends on the ingredients. See Table F-21, Food Composition Table, under the section, "Soups and Chowders" for the analysis of some of the more popular soups.

SOYBEAN *Glycine max*

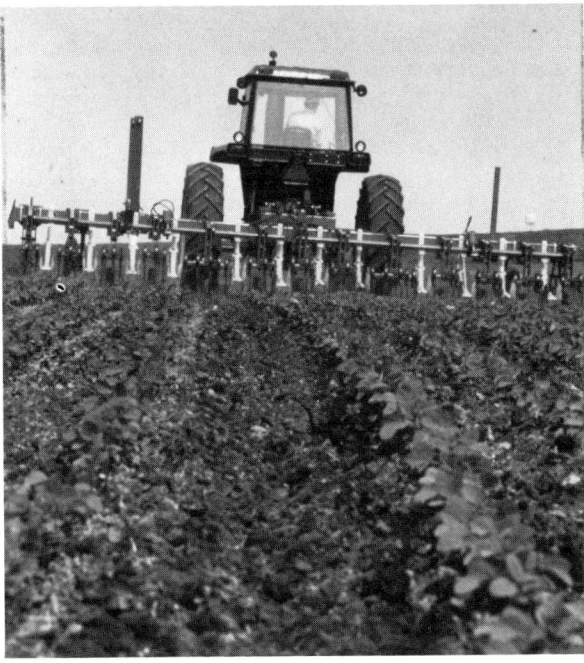

Fig. S-21. Cultivating soybeans. (Courtesy, Deere & Co., Moline, Ill.)

Soybeans belong to the pea family, *Leguminosae*. It is classed as genus *Glycine*, species *G. max*.

Soybeans were cultivated in China long before written history. The ancient Chinese used the soybean as food and made medicines from it.

Today, U.S. soybeans supply food for human beings, feed for animals, and many raw materials for industry.

ORIGIN AND HISTORY. The soybean plant is native to China, where it emerged as a cultivated crop in the 11th century B.C. Records of methods of culture, varieties for different purposes, and numerous usages indicate that the soybean was among the first crops grown by man. The ancient Chinese considered the soybean their most important crop, and one of the five sacred grains necessary for living. Soybeans were taken from China to Japan in the 7th century.

Soybeans were taken to Europe in the 17th century. They were introduced into the United States in 1804. However, scant attention was given to soybeans in North America until the 1930s. At that time, the U.S. Department of Agriculture and the agricultural experiment stations of the states and the Canadian provinces cooperated in developing improved soybean varieties through hybridization and selection.

WORLD AND U.S. PRODUCTION. Soybeans are the leading legume crop of the world, and the leading legume crop of the United States.

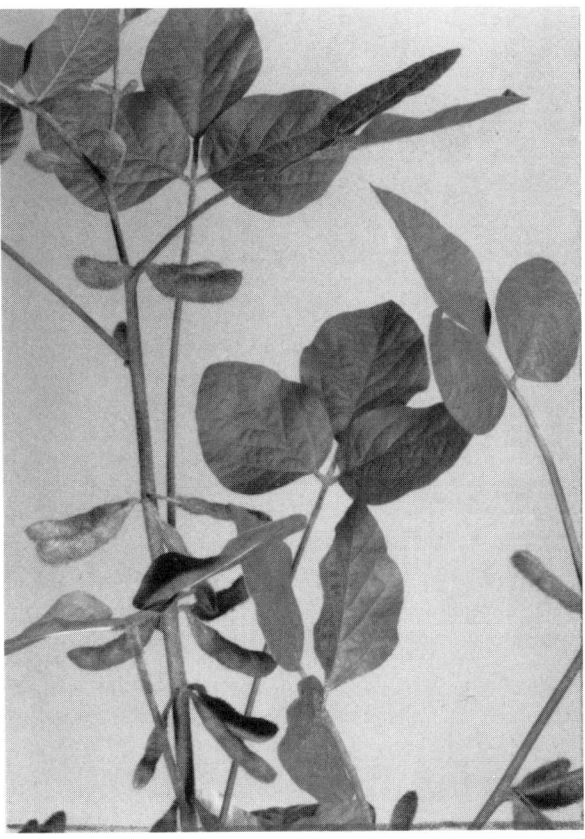

Fig. S-22. A soybean plant. Soybeans are the leading legume crop in the world. (Courtesy, Field Museum of Natural History, Chicago, Ill.)

World production of soybeans totals about 107,767,000 metric tons annually; and the ten leading soybean-producing countries of the world, by rank, are: United States, Brazil, China, Argentina, India, Italy, Paraguay, Indonesia, Canada, and U.S.S.R.[33] The United States is, by far, the leading soybean-producing country, producing more than 49% of the world's soybeans.

The United States produces about 1.9 billion bu of soybeans annually; and the ten leading states, by rank, are: Illinois, Iowa, Minnesota, Indiana, Ohio, Missouri, Arkansas, Nebraska, South Dakota, and Kansas.[34]

[33]Data from *FAO Production Yearbook 1990*, FAO/UN, Rome, Italy, Vol. 44, p. 107, Table 37. **Note well:** Annual production fluctuates as a result of weather and profitability of the crop.

[34]Data from *Agricultural Statistics 1991*, USDA, p. 123, Table 169. **Note well:** Annual production fluctuates as a result of weather and profitability of the crop.

PROCESSING SOYBEANS.

About 59% of the soybeans produced in the United States are crushed and processed domestically, 35% are exported as whole beans, 5% are used for seed, and 1% have miscellaneous uses.

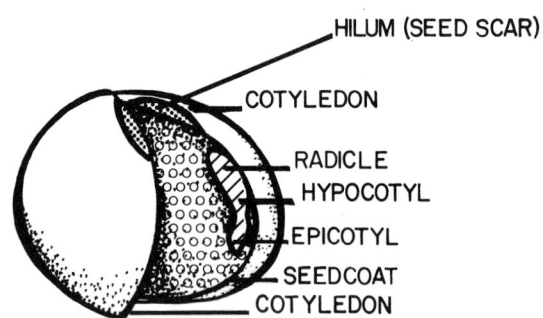

Fig. S-23. The soybean seed. There are three basic parts: (1) the seedcoat, which protects the embryo from fungi and bacteria before and after planting; (2) the embryo, consisting of (a) the radicle (which becomes the primary root), (b) the hypocotyl (which is the main stem and growing point); and (3) the cotyledons, which account for most of the bulk and weight of the seed and contain nearly all the oil and protein.

The processing of soybeans into oil and meal began in the Orient. The oil was used primarily for human food, while the meal was used for animal feed.

In the United States, soybeans are processed primarily to obtain (1) oil for use in shortenings, margarines, and salad dressings; (2) soybean protein products for direct human consumption; and (3) soybean meal for use as a protein supplement for livestock.

Extracting the Oil.

Oil, primarily for human food, is extracted from several rich oil-bearing seeds; among them, soybeans, coconuts, cottonseed, linseed, peanuts, rapeseed, safflower seed, sesame seed, and sunflower seed. The oil is extracted from these seeds by one of the following basic processes or modifications thereof: solvent extraction, hydraulic extraction, or expeller extraction. For purposes of illustration, all three processes are discussed relative to soybeans, since soybeans are the most widely used oilseed in the United States, and since the principles involved in processing all oilseeds are essentially the same. However, it should be noted that little of the U. S. soybean crop is processed via hydraulic or expeller extraction.

SOLVENT EXTRACTION.

In this method, the soybeans are first cracked, then heated to 140°F (60°C) for about 10 minutes. After the cracked seeds are heated, they proceed through a series of grinding rollers where they are flaked. The flakes are allowed to cool to about 113°F (45°C) and are then moved to the extraction equipment where the oil is removed by a petroleum solvent—usually hexane.

The extracted flakes then proceed to driers where the solvent is completely volatilized. From the drier, the flakes are conveyed to a toaster, thence they are cooled and ground.

The normal processing yields are: crude oil, 17 to 19.3%; and meal and feed products, 80.7 to 83%. One bushel (60 lb) of soybeans gives approximately 48 lb (22 kg) of meal and 11 lb (5 kg) of oil. The maximum yield of crude oil is always sought. Generally, less than 2% oil remains in the meal after solvent extraction. The hulls, accounting for about 5% of the beans, are ground and may be added back to the meal for the production of meal of a specific protein content.

HYDRAULIC EXTRACTION.

In the hydraulic extraction procedure, raw soybeans are cracked, ground, and flaked. The flakes (called meats) are then transported to cookers where they are exposed to both dry and steam heat. The cooking stage takes about 90 minutes.

After cooking, the meats are formed into cakes and wrapped in heavy cloth whereupon they are placed in hydraulic presses for the mechanical extraction of the oil. This procedure takes about 1 hour. Following extraction, the cakes are ground. Hydraulic press cake may have 5 to 8% residual oil.

Since this form of extraction is labor intensive and inefficient in the removal of oil, very few soybeans are processed by this method today.

EXPELLER EXTRACTION.

In this type of extraction, raw soybeans are initially cracked and dried to about 2% moisture. The dried soybeans are then transported hot to a steam-jacketed tempering apparatus which is directly above the expeller apparatus. The tempering apparatus stirs the cracked soybeans for about 10 to 15 minutes so that the seeds are heated uniformly.

From the tempering bin, the soybeans are fed into the expeller barrel (screw presses). A central revolving worm shaft creates pressure within the expeller barrel thereupon extracting the oil from the ground soybeans. The extracted soybeans leave the expeller in the form of flakes, which are subsequently ground.

The expeller process tends to extract less oil than the solvent process; consequently, it is used less frequently. Generally, expeller-extracted soybean meal contains 4 to 5% oil while solvent-extracted soybean meal contains less than 1%.

Refining Soybean Oil.

About 93% of soybean oil is used for food. To be suitable for human consumption, the extracted crude oil must undergo further processing, which is generally referred to as refining.

The steps in processing are:

1. **Degumming.** This consists in the removal of the soybean phospholipids, which are dried and sold as soybean lecithin. The crude lecithin, which is dark colored, may be bleached with hydrogen peroxide to produce a light, straw-colored product. Fatty acids may be added to make a fluid product, or the lecithin may be treated with ammonia to form a firm, plastic consistency. More refined grades (pharmaceutical lecithins) are produced by acetone extraction of the entrained soybean oil.

2. **Alkali refining.** The degummed soybean oil is next alkali-refined (treated with caustic soda, soda ash, or a combination of the two) to neutralize the free fatty acids. The neutralized free fatty acids, known as soap stock, may be removed from the oil and sold to soap manufacturers, fatty acid industries, or feed manufacturers in either (a) the alkaline form, or (b) the acidulated form after treatment with acid.

3. **Bleaching (decolorizing).** Bleaching agents (activated earth or carbon) are used to remove the pigments present in the oil.

4. **Hydrogenating.** Hydrogenation is achieved by treating the oil with hydrogen gas at an elevated temperature and pressure in the presence of a catalyst.

5. **Winterizing.** Hydrogenated soybean oil that is to be used as a salad oil must remain clear at refrigerator temperatures. This is accomplished by winterization—cooling the oil and filtering off the cloudy haze that forms.

6. **Deodorizing.** Undesirable flavors and odors are removed under high temperature and vacuum, with steam injected to assist volatization of the undesirable components.

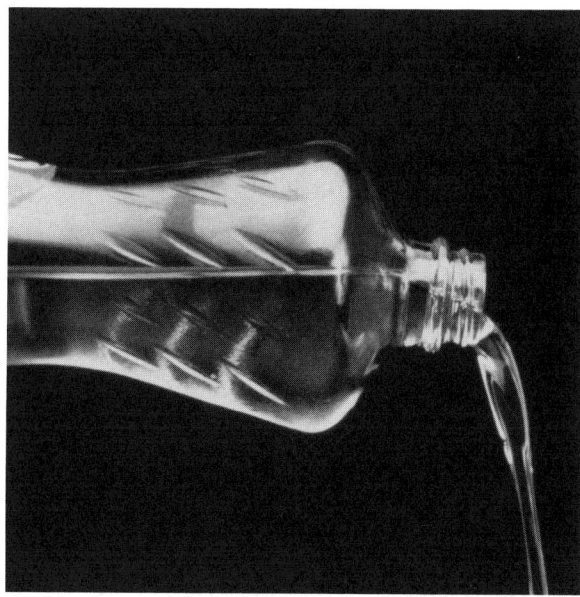

Fig. S-24. Soybean oil, widely used throughout the world for human consumption, as margarine, salad and cooking oils, and shortening. (Courtesy, USDA)

NUTRITIONAL VALUE.
The nutritive value of different forms of soybeans and soybean products is given in Food Composition Table F-21.

The soybean seed is 13 to 25% oil, 30 to 50% protein, and 14 to 24% carbohydrate. The fatty acid composition of the oil is: linoleic acid, 55%; oleic acid, 21%; palmitic acid, 9%; stearic acid, 6%; and other fatty acids, 9%. The ratio of polyunsaturated to saturated fatty acids (P/S ratio) is 82:18, which is conducive to lowering blood cholesterol. The soybean contains more protein than beef, more calcium than milk, and more lecithin than eggs. Also, it is rich in minerals, vitamins, and amino acids.

In terms of essential amino acids—those not produced by the body, and which must be eaten—soybeans are an excellent source as shown in Table S-10. Indeed soybeans and soybean products are good complementary protein sources when the diet consists largely of cereal grains.

TABLE S-10
PROFILE OF ESSENTIAL AMINO ACIDS IN SOYBEANS
COMPARED TO MILK—A HIGH-QUALITY PROTEIN

Amino Acid	Soybeans	Cow's Milk[1]
	(mg/g protein)	
Histidine	28	27
Isoleucine	50	47
Leucine	85	95
Lysine	70	78
Methionine and cystine	28	33
Phenylalanine and tyrosine	88	102
Threonine	42	44
Tryptophan	14	14
Valine	53	64

[1]Recommended Dietary Allowances, 10th ed., 1989, NRC–National Academy of Sciences, p. 67, Table 6–5. The essential amino acid requirements of infants can be met by supplying 0.79 g of a high-quality protein per pound of body weight (1.7 g/kg body weight) per day.

Fig. S-25 compares the levels of essential amino acids of soybeans and certain other foods.

V. R. Young and N. S. Scrimshaw, Clinical Research Center and Department of Nutrition and Food Science, Massachusetts Institute of Technology, make the following authoritative statement relative to the nutritional value of processed soy protein in human nutrition:

> When well-processed soy products serve as the major or sole source of protein intake, their protein value approaches or equals that of foods of animal origin, and they are fully capable of meeting the long term essential amino acid and protein needs of children and adults...For feeding of the newborn, the limited data available suggest that supplementation of soy-based formulas with methionine may be beneficial.[35]

---

[35]Young, V. R., and N.S. Scrimshaw, "Soybean Protein in Human Nutrition: An Overview," Journal of the American Oil Chemists' Society, Vol. 56, No. 3, March 1979, p. 110.

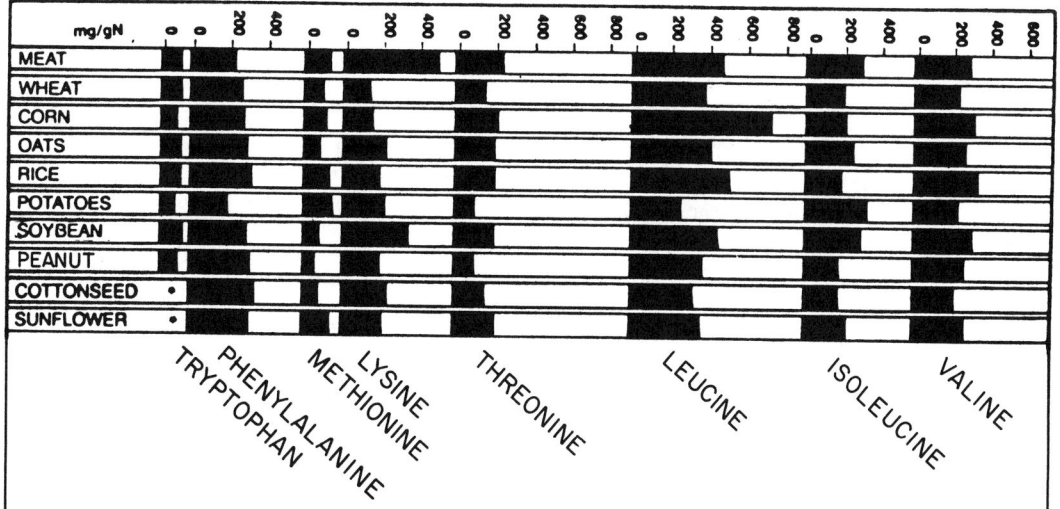

Fig. S-25. Comparative levels of essential amino acids (in mg/g of nitrogen) of soybeans and other foods. (Source: Vegetable Protein: Products and the Future, Food Protein Council, Washington, D.C.)

Perhaps more important than the individual nutritional strength of soy protein is its ability to complement the biological quality of other protein sources. For example, corn meal, which is the basis of many human diets around the world, is of low protein quality when used alone because of certain amino acid deficiencies. But, when blended with soy flour, the resulting nutritive value is comparable to milk protein (casein). This is accomplished because the low lysine content of corn meal is offset by the naturally high lysine content of soy protein. Conversely, the limited methionine content in soy products is offset by the excess of methionine in corn products. The results, when the two are combined at levels that do not inhibit palatability, is a combined meal nutritionally superior to corn meal alone. This same complementary relationship occurs when soy products are used with wheat and other foods (see Fig. S-25).

The cereals and meals based on corn and wheat are a vital basis of diets in the less developed countries. But these grains do not provide adequate nutrition. If combined with soybeans, however, these grains can boost the general nutritional value of the foods eaten in the less developed countries.

Different nutritional needs prevail in industrialized economies. For the affluent, meat analogs made from textured soy protein are largely free of cholesterol and high in polyunsaturates. For example, one kind of sausage made from textured soy protein contains 40% more polyunsaturated fats than saturated fats, while traditional pork sausage contains 400% more saturated than polyunsaturated fats.[36]

Evidence relative to the effectiveness of a soy protein diet in reducing serum cholesterol concentrations was dramatically corroborated by an Italian research team, whose work was reported in *The Lancet*, a respected British journal of medicine. A group of patients found to have high blood serum cholesterol levels was put consecutively on two kinds of diets: (1) a low-fat animal protein diet, and (2) a predominantly soy protein diet. The study showed that the soy protein reduced serum cholesterol concentrations in the patients by about 20%.[37]

It is noteworthy, too, that among the leading users of soy protein products are mass feeding institutions, including schools, hospitals, and military units, where nutritional standards must be maintained in the face of cost restrictions. The Federal Government's National School Lunch Program is the largest consumer of soy protein for food served in institutional settings. Hydrated soy protein may constitute up to 30% by weight of meat products served in that program. Over 50 million lb of soy protein are used each year in the school lunch program.

• **Savings in protein costs**—Savings realized by food service operators and feeding institutions explain why the applications of soy protein continue to expand and diversify. Also, the individual consumer is becoming increasingly aware of these savings. (See Table S-11.)

To determine relative protein costs from Table S-11, multiply the cost of a product by its cost multiplying factor. *Example:* Soy flour at 20¢ per pound has a protein cost of 40¢ per pound (20¢ x 2); whereas beef at 80¢ per pound has a protein cost of $4.80 per pound (80¢ x 6).

TABLE S-11
RELATIVE COST INDICATORS FOR LEADING PROTEIN FOODS

	Approximate Percent Protein	Cost Multiplying Factor
Soy isolates	90.	1
Sodium caseinate	90	1
Soy concentrates	65	1.5
Soy flour	50	2
Dried skimmed milk	36	3·
Cheese (Cheddar)	25	4
Dried beans	22	5.5
Fish/chicken	20	5.5
Beef (chuck—35% fat)	16	6
Dried whey	13	8
Wheat flour	12	8.5
Corn meal (whole)	9	11
Rice	7	15
Whole milk	3.5	28.5

• **Improved nutritive value of infant products**—Soy protein-based infant formulae are a universal staple for babies who are (1) allergic to milk protein, or (2) unable to utilize lactose. Soy protein infant products provide the same order of growth and weight gain as cow's milk. Also, soy protein is used in baby cereal blends and canned baby foods to improve nutritive value.

• **Improved nutritive value of breakfast cereals and pastas**—New emphasis on nutrition in breakfast cereals has meant more use of soy protein to increase their protein quantity and value. Today, soy proteins are used extensively as additives to hot cereal mixes, and as components of granola bars and compound breakfast bars. Also, U.S. standards of identity for pasta products permit fortification with soy protein.

SOYBEAN PRODUCTS AND USES FOR HUMAN FOOD.

In the People's Republic of China, Taiwan, Japan, Korea, and Indonesia, soybeans are a regular part of the diet and a major source of protein and oil. Soybean milk, soybean curd, soy sauce, fermented soybean paste, soybean sprouts, immature green seed, and deep-fried mature seed are common foods in the Orient.

Soybean oil is widely used throughout the world for human consumption as margarine, salad and cooking oils, and shortening.

In the United States, about 30% of the soybean production is used for food and industrial products, and soybean products are the leading protein supplements for livestock. In addition to the use of soybean oil, soy protein is revolutionizing the modern food system; its use as an ingredient, extender, and analog has spread to products in every category of food available to the public—in home and away from home.

Soy protein is available to the food industry in a multitude of forms, most of which may be classified according to protein content as: (1) soy flour and grits, containing 40 to 50% protein; (2) soy protein concentrates, with about 70% protein; (3) soy protein isolates, with 90 to 95% protein; and (4) textured soy protein, which is made from one or more of the other three types. Fig. S-26 shows an attractive meat-substitute dish.

---

[36]*Vegetable Protein: Products For the Future*, Food Protein Council, Washington, D.C.
[37]*Ibid.*

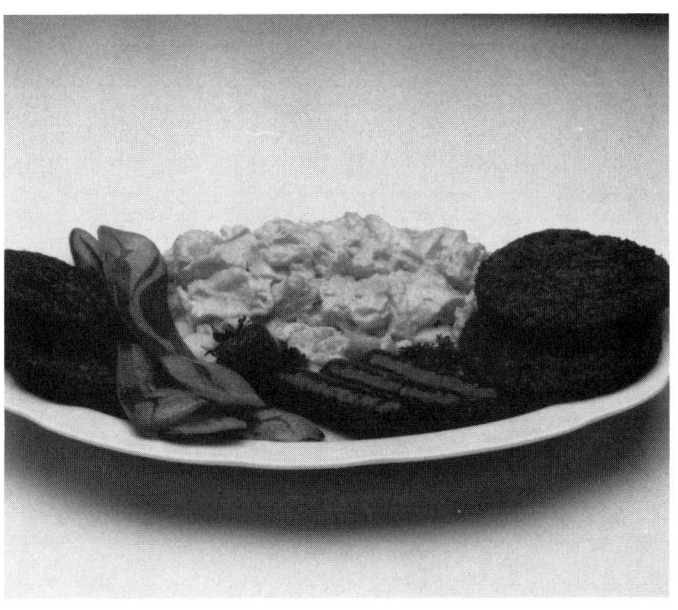

Fig. S-26. Textured soybean hamburger made from spun soy fiber. (Courtesy, Worthington Foods, Worthington, Ohio)

• **Soy proteins in foreign-feeding programs**—Soy flour is included in many commodities used in foreign-feeding programs, such as soy-fortified bulgur, soy-fortified bread flour, corn-soy milk, corn-soy blend, and wheat-soy blend. In particular, soy protein fortification improves the amino acid composition of the foods to which it is added.

Low cost, good nutrition, and functional versatility account for the ever-increasing quantities of soy proteins in food programs in the less-developed countries. Soy flour is the major ingredient in blended foods with flour and grits added to corn, sorghum, and oat products distributed overseas. Whey-soy drink mix is a new product recently added to the list of commodities available for distribution in feeding programs. It was developed as a replacement for dry milk. The finished product—41.4% sweet whey, 36.5% full fat soybean flour, 12.1% soybean oil, and 9.5% corn sugar—when mixed with water at 15% solids, provides a drink with nearly the same energy and protein content as whole milk.

Table S-12 presents in summary form the story of soybean products and uses for human food.

(Also see FLOURS, Table F-13, Special Flours; LEGUMES, Table L-2, Legumes of the World; OILS, VEGETABLE, Table O-5; and VEGETABLE[S], Table V-2, Vegetables of the World.)

TABLE S-12
SOYBEAN PRODUCTS AND USES FOR HUMAN FOOD

Product	Description	Uses	Comments
Soybeans	Whole soybeans	As mature, dry soybeans are used (1) in recipes like other dry beans, or (2) as roasted soybeans—a snack food. As immature, green seed served hot as a vegetable, like peas or corn.	In the Orient, soybeans (including whole soybeans) are the principal source of protein in the diet. Soybeans are also rich in minerals, vitamins, and amino acids. Direct food usage of soybeans is expected to increase dramatically around the world due to population pressure on the food supply.
Chee-fan	A type of sufu made by salting small cubes of soybean curd, innoculating with a species of *Mucor*, and allowing them to ferment for about 7 days. After fermentation, allowed to age in yellow wine for a year.	Consumed much like cheese is eaten in the western world.	
Fermented soybeans	Prepared from black soybeans in China, using a species of *Mucor* as the fermentation organism. After fermentation, they are aged for 6 months or longer in sealed earthenware jars, then seasoned with salt, spices, and wine or whiskey.	As an appetizer	
Hamanatto (A similar product called Meitanza or tu su is prepared in China. In the Philippines, it is known as taosi)	A liquid, fermented soybean product prepared from whole soybeans by using a starter (koji) made from roasted wheat or barley treated with spores of the mold *Aspergillus oryzae*.	For flavoring many foods	Hamanatto is expensive and very dark in color. Nagoya University, in Japan, reported the following analyses of hamanatto: water, 38%; protein, 25%; carbohydrate, 25%; salt and calcium, 12%.
Ketjap	A type of soy sauce made from black soybeans in Indonesia	As a flavoring agent for many foods	
Metlauza	A product prepared from the insoluble protein and other materials which are separated out from the soybean milk in the preparation of tofu. These residual solids are pressed into cakes; fermented with *Actinomucor elegans* for 10 to 15 days; then sun dried.		
Miso	A fermented food paste; made by inoculating trays of rice with *Aspergillus oryzae*, and leaving it to mold abundantly. Then a ground preparation of cooked soybeans and salt is mixed in, and the mass is allowed to ferment and age for several days before being ground into the paste of the consistency of peanut butter.	As a food in Japan. It is used primarily as flavoring material, added to soups and vegetables. Miso is also spread thinly on cucumbers or substituted for meat sauce on spaghetti.	Miso originated in China. A Japanese missionary who was sent to China in the 7th century learned how it was made and modified it into a product suited to the Japanese taste. The entire process of making miso requires from 10 to 40 days, varying according to the temperature at which the yeast fermentation is conducted. The qualities and proportions of amino acids in miso compare quite favorably with those of casein and soybean meal.

(Continued)

TABLE S-12 *(Continued)*

Product	Description	Uses	Comments
Natto	A fermented whole protein food, fermented by *Bacillus natto*. In this product, the shape of cooked whole soybeans is retained.	Natto is served with soy sauce (shoyu) and mustard.	Natto originated in Japan. In 1087, a ruler in the northern part of Japan discovered natto to be part of the local farmers' diets.
Soybean flour	An extremely fine powdered product, containing 40 to 50% protein, the particles of which are 100 or finer mesh size (U.S. standard screen)	Bakery products: breads, rolls, and buns; doughnuts; sweet goods; cakes and cakes mixes; pancake and waffle mixes; specialty crackers and cookies. Meat products: sausages, luncheon loaves, patties, canned meats in sauces. Breakfast cereals. Infant and junior foods. Confectionery items. Dietary foods.	Soybean flour is produced like soybean meal, except that the hulls are carefully removed before extraction. Flours are differentiated from grits on the basis of particle size. In Israel, 10% soybean flour is included with wheat flour in baking bread.
Soybean grits	A granular product containing 40 to 50% protein, the particles of which range from 10 to 80 mesh size (U.S. standard screen)	Same as for soybean flour	Soybean grits are produced like soybean meal, except that the hulls are carefully removed before extraction.
Soybean lecithin	The phospholipids which are removed from the crude oil during the degumming process	Baked goods, cake mixes, instant foods, candies, and drugs. As an antioxidant, emulsifier, and softener in food manufacturing.	Crude soybean oil contains 1 to 3% lecithin.
Soybean milk	The product obtained by soaking beans in water, grinding the soaked beans, and filtering the insoluble pieces out.	Consumed primarily by the Chinese. As the starting material for the preparation of a soybean curd, probably the most important and popular soybean food in the Orient. In soybean-milk-based infant formulas.	The soft cheeselike curd, known as "toufu," "tofu," "tubu," and other local names, contains about 53% protein, 26% fat, 17% carbohydrate, and 4% fiber, minerals, and vitamins. Curd has a bland taste and can be flavored with seasoning or blended with other foods. It is made into a variety of products by frying, dehydrating, or freezing and is consumed daily in the same manner as high-protein foods in the U.S.
Soybean oil	The crude oil which is extracted from soybeans, then refined.	Margarine, shortening (cooking oil), and salad oil. The hydrogenated oil finds much use in restaurant chains and institutions for deep fat frying of foods. In the Far East, oil is consumed extensively as a food.	About ⅕ of the bean is oil. More than 90% of the oil is refined and used for food—for margarine, shortening, and salad oil. All edible oils are deodorized. Hydrogenation varies, depending upon the final use of the oil.
Soybean protein concentrates	Soybean protein products containing 70% protein. They are prepared from defatted flakes or flours by removing water soluble sugars, ash, and other minor constituents.	Bakery products: bread, biscuits, and buns; cakes and cake mixes. Meat products: sausages, luncheon loaves, poultry rolls, patties, meat loaves, canned meats in sauces. Breakfast cereals. Infant foods. Dietary foods.	
Soybean protein hydroslysates	Soybean proteins that are partially hydrolyzed by a number of agents such as enzymes, acids, alkalis, or steam, or by yeasts, molds, or bacteria. Hydrolysates are soluble in water over the entire pH scale.	Soy sauce and other flavorings, foaming agents, and whipping agents	
Soybean protein isolates (Also see "textured soybean proteins")	Soybean protein isolates, which contain 90 to 95% protein, are the purest form of soybean protein marketed. They are produced by (1) washing out the proteins from dehulled, defatted soybean flakes, (2) precipitating the protein out of the liquid solution with a mild alkali, and (3) drying by a spray process.	As the basic ingredient of spun fiber types of meat analogs. Meat products: sausages, luncheon loaves, poultry rolls. Dairy-type foods: whipped toppings, coffee whiteners, frozen desserts, beverage powders. Infant foods. Dietary foods.	Soybean protein isolates are required for spinning.
Soybean sprouts	Sprouts of soybeans about 4 in. *(10 cm)* long. Prepared by germinating whole soybeans under optimum moisture conditions at a temperature of 72-86°F *(22-30°C)* for 4 to 7 days.	As a fresh vegetable, or in soup	Soybean sprouts are a rich source of vitamin C. On a moisture-free basis, soybean sprouts run about 50% protein content.
Soy sauce (shoyu in Japan, chiang-yu in China)	A salty brown sauce made by fermenting soybeans—a liquid food. The *starter* (koji) for making soy sauce is prepared from rice inoculated with the spores of the molds of either *Aspergillus oryzae* or *Aspergillus soyae*. In Japan, about equal quantities of soybeans and wheat are used in making soy sauce. In China, more soybeans and less wheat is used.	As a flavoring agent for many foods—especially in Chinese and Japanese cooking	Soy sauce originated in China some 2,500 years ago and was introduced in Japan in the 7th century by Buddhist priests. The average annual per capita consumption in Japan is about 3 gal. *(11.4 liters)*. Good soy sauce contains large amounts of amino acids, especially glutamic acid.
Tao-cho	Prepared from light colored soybeans. They are soaked, dehulled, and boiled, then mixed with rice flour and roasted. Next, they are inoculated with *Aspergillus*, then fermented for 3 days and sun-dried. The cakes are dipped in brine, arenga sugar and a paste of glutinous rice, following which they are exposed to the sun for a month or more.	As an appetizer	

TABLE S-12 *(Continued)*

Product	Description	Uses	Comments
Tao-si	A soybean product, made from unhulled soybeans. Soybeans are soaked and boiled; wheat flour is added; the mix is inoculated with *Aspergillus oryzae* and incubated for 2 to 3 days; thence placed in earthenware jars and salt brine is added; and the product is finished in about 2 months.	As an appetizer	
Taotjo	A soybean product of the East Indies. Boiled soybeans are mixed with roasted wheat meal or glutinous rice; inoculated with *Aspergillus oryzae* for 2 to 3 days; then placed in brine for several weeks, with palm sugar added at intervals.	As a condiment	
Tempeh	An Indonesian food made entirely from soybeans; prepared by using a phycomycete, *Rhizopus oligosporus*.	Tempeh is used as a main dish, rather than as a flavoring agent for other foods. Raw tempeh is sliced and then fried or baked.	A similar product called *tempeh bongkrek* is sometimes made from coconut meat. Tempeh made from coconut meat may become poisonous, but tempeh made from soybeans never does. The *Rhizopus* mold synthesizes vitamin B-12; hence, tempeh is one of the few vegetable products that contain significant amounts of this vitamin.
Textured soybean proteins (analogs) (Also see "soybean protein concentrates" and "soybean protein isolates.")	Further processing of the basic forms—flours and grits, concentrates, and isolates— is now practiced to give soybean proteins a texture that resembles specific types of meat; these items range from extenders to be used with ground meats to complete meat analogs. Two basic types of textured soybean protein products are now available: 1. *Extruded*, made by cooking soybean flour and other ingredients and forcing the mixture through small holes into a chamber of lower temperature and pressure. Granules of these expanded materials are available in both colored and uncolored and flavored and unflavored forms.	Ground meat extenders. Meat analogs (baconlike bits, etc.)	Textured items, mainly of the extruded type, are the fastest growing segment of the edible soy protein business. Production of meat analogs either by extruding soybean flour or by spinning protein isolate into fibers results in products that look and taste like beef, pork, and other kinds of meat. Soy protein can augment whole fish, improve the texture and eating characteristics of finished consumer fish products, and replace the functional fish protein. It can, for example, build the visual content of processed shellfish without altering the distinctive flavor and mouthfeel of such products. Soy protein seems assured of increased use in dairy product analogs made for people who have special health or religious diet requirements. The extruded soy process is patented and licensing is required.
	2. *Spun*, made by spinning the fibers and then flavoring, coloring, and forming them in shapes which resemble pieces of meat, poultry, and fish.	Meat analogs: baconlike bits, simulated sausages, simulated ham chunks, simulated chicken chunks, simulated bacon slices. Meat extenders.	The basic patent for spun protein isolates has expired, but companies now engaged in this business hold patents on improved methods for converting the fiber into meat analogs.
Tofu and Sufu (soybean cheese)	In producing sufu, a product called tofu, the Oriental equivalent of curdled milk, is produced. It is made by soaking, grinding, and straining soybeans to produce soybean milk; then boiling to coagulate the proteins and pressing to remove water. At this stage, which is prior to inoculation with fungi, it is called tofu; hence, tofu is not fermented. Sufu, a fermented soybean product, is often referred to as Chinese cheese, because it closely resembles cheese of the western world. At least 5 species of fungi have been isolated from sufu, but *Actinomucor elegans* appears to be the organism of choice.	Both tofu and sufu are sliced and eaten much like cheese is consumed in the western world.	Tofu has been one of the most important foods in the Orient for centuries. Sufu, which originated in China in the 5th century, is widely used in China today.

BEVERAGES			
Soy protein shake	A beverage containing soy protein	As shakes at fast food outlets	Shakes with soy protein have been widely marketed.
Whey-soy drink	A beverage containing whey and soy protein. The base product (41.4% sweet whey, 36.5% full fat soybean flour, 12.1% soybean oil, and 9.5% corn sugar) is mixed with water at 15% solids.	As a drink with nearly the same energy and protein content as whole milk	This is a new product available for distribution in the developing countries.

SPANISH GOAT

The primary meat-type goat, represents a cross of many dairy goat breeds. The meat from this type of goat is known as *cabrito*, meaning little goat in Spanish.

SPANISH LIME (MANONICILLO)

Melicocca bijuga

The fruit of a tropical American tree (of the family *Sapindaceae*) that is related to the litchi of Asia. Spanish limes, which are not related to the citrus fruits, are greenish plumlike fruits that have a tart sweet flesh and a large pith. They may be eaten fresh or when made into preserves.

The fruit is moderately high in calories (59 kcal per 100 g) and carbohydrates (20%). It is a poor source of vitamin C.

SPECIFIC DYNAMIC ACTION (SDA)

The increased production of heat by the body as a result of a stimulus to metabolic activity caused by ingesting food.

SPECIFIC GRAVITY

The ratio of the weight of a body to the weight of an equal volume of water.

SPECIFIC HEAT

- The heat-absorbing capacity of a substance in relation to that of water.
- The heat expressed in calories required to raise the temperature of 1 g of a substance 1°C.

SPHINCTER

A muscle surrounding a bodily opening or channel, which is able to contract and close it.

SPHINGOMYELIN

A lipid composed of a fatty acid such as stearic or palmitic, phosphate, choline, and the amino alcohol, sphingosine. It is found primarily in nervous tissue.

SPICES

The word *spice* is of French origin, meaning *fruits of the earth*. *Spice is the name given to food seasonings made from plants.* They have a sharp taste and odor—they're more pungent than herbs. Some spices are valued for their taste, others for their smell. Common spices include pepper, nutmeg, cloves, ginger, allspice, mace, mustard, and cinnamon.

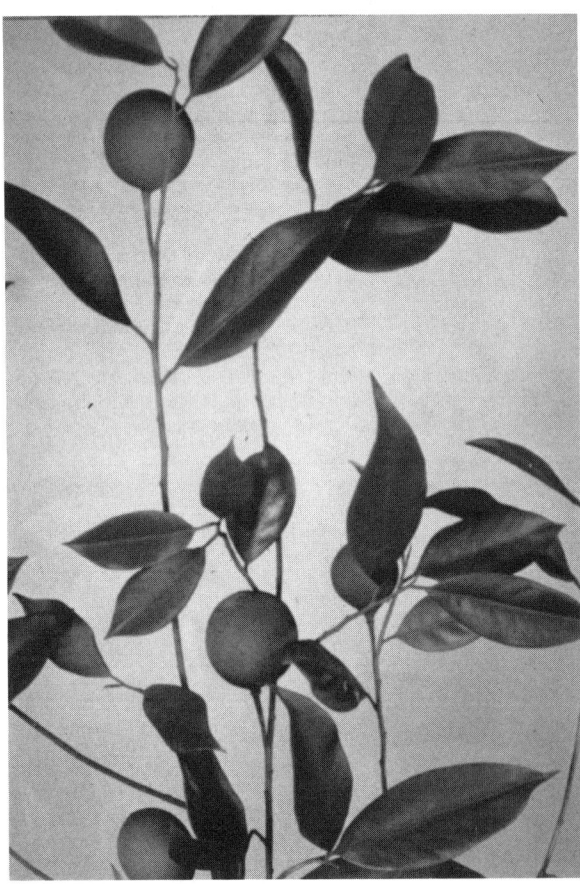

Fig. S-27. Fruiting nutmeg branch. Nutmeg is a common spice. (Courtesy, Field Museum of Natural History, Chicago, Ill.)

Spices have little in common except for their use. They usually come from tropical plants; and different parts of various spice plants may be used. For example, cloves come from the bud, cinnamon comes from the bark, pepper comes from the fruit, ginger and horseradish come from the root, and mustard comes from the seed.

Some people grow spice plants such as sage, marjoram, thyme, and others in their gardens; others grow them in pots in sunny windows. They then dry the plants for later use.

Spices have little food value, but they do increase the appetite and stimulate the organs of digestion. Before foods were canned or refrigerated, spices were used to make tainted foods taste better.

(Also see FLAVORINGS AND SEASONINGS.)

SPOILAGE OF FOOD

Although food spoilage is often thought of as something caused by bacteria, molds, or yeast, it is actually any change which renders a food unfit for human consumption. Here a distinction should be drawn between unfit and undesirable. Food may be undesirable due to the dislikes of an individual, but this does not mean it is unfit for everyone. Furthermore, food spoilage cannot be equated to danger to the consumer. Spoilage results in abnormal colors, flavors, odors, texture, or other unacceptable changes. The causes of food spoilage can be grouped into five broad categories: (1) microbial spoilage, (2) enzymatic spoilage, (3) chemical spoilage, (4) physical spoilage, and (5) pest spoilage.

The aim of modern food production, processing, and preservation is to, so far as is possible, reduce and/or eliminate all sources of food spoilage. By the time a food reaches the consumer, proper heat and/or chill treatments, canning, drying, freezing, sanitation, and food additives may all play a role in eliminating spoilage. Then the control of spoilage is passed on to the consumer who must exercise proper storage and preparation methods.

(Also see ADDITIVES; BACTERIA IN FOODS; POISONS; and PRESERVATION OF FOOD.)

SPORE

A resting reproductive form of certain microorganisms.

SPRAY-DEHYDRATED

Material which has been dried by spraying onto the surface of a heated drum. It is recovered by scraping it from the drum.

SPRUCE BEER

This is a fermented drink made from an extract of spruce needles and twigs boiled with molasses or sugar. At one time it was used as a diuretic and antiscorbutic.

SPRUE

A collective term for a group of nutritional deficiency diseases characterized by impaired absorption of nutrients from the small intestine, especially fats, glucose, and vitamins. Although all sprues exhibit the same general clinical manifestations of intestinal malabsorption and steatorrhea (fatty diarrhea), the following three etiologic classifications are presented in this book:

1. **Celiac disease,** a rare metabolic disorder of children, which results from a sensitivity to gluten.
2. **Nontropical sprue,** the term commonly applied to adults exhibiting a sensitivity to gluten.
3. **Tropical sprue,** caused by a deficiency of folic acid and vitamin B-12.

(Also see CELIAC DISEASE; SPRUE, NONTROPICAL; and SPRUE, TROPICAL.)

SPRUE, NONTROPICAL (CELIAC-SPRUE)

The term nontropical sprue is commonly applied to adults exhibiting a sensitivity to gluten. It is due to an intolerance to wheat gluten, a main constituent of wheat flour, which is also present to a small extent in rye, barley, and oats, but not in rice. Symptoms are provoked by the ingestion of any of the numerous foods containing wheat gluten. Characteristic symptoms of sprue include steatorrhea (fatty diarrhea), weight loss, and lesions of the small intestine. As the disease progresses, a multitude of other symptoms may appear due to the loss of fat and other nutrients in the stool.

Treatment consists of a gluten-free diet. This means the exclusion of all cereal grains except corn and rice and the use of potato and soy flours.

(Also see ALLERGIES, section headed "Wheat Allergy"; MODIFIED DIETS—GLUTEN-FREE DIET; and SPRUE.)

SPRUE, TROPICAL

A malabsorption syndrome affecting mainly individuals living in the West Indies, Central America, and the Far East. Even individuals from temperate climates visiting these countries may develop tropical sprue during or after their visit. Although somewhat similar to nontropical sprue, tropical sprue responds to different therapy. Both types of sprue are characterized by the typical flat mucosa of the small intestine, secondary enzyme deficiencies in the intestinal mucosa, and steatorrhea. However, in tropical sprue, a macrocytic anemia occurs as a manifestation of folic acid and vitamin B-12 deficiencies. Indeed, marked improvement of the sufferer is noted following the administration of folic acid and vitamin B-12. Diet therapy consists of a diet high in calories and protein. Substitution of fat with medium-chain triglycerides has alleviated the steatorrhea (fatty diarrhea), and weight gain. Unlike nontropical sprue, response to a gluten-free diet is minimal. Although no infective agent has been demonstrated, broad-spectrum antibiotics have proven beneficial.

(Also see MODIFIED DIETS; FOLACIN; and SPRUE.)

SQUAB

A young pigeon that is about 4 weeks old and weighs 1 lb. Squabs should be slaughtered just before leaving the nest. They are processed and cooked much like any other poultry.

SQUASHES *Cucurbita* spp

The fruits of these plants provide both edible flesh and edible seeds. Also, the flowers are edible. Squashes belong to the gourd or melon family (*Cucurbitaceae*), which also includes pumpkins and cucumbers. Most summer squashes are classified as *C. pepo* and bear relatively small fruits that are eaten while immature. Winter squashes are *C. maxima* and *C. moschata*. Winter squashes are eaten when mature and tend to be more nutritious than summer squashes.

ORIGIN AND HISTORY. The wild ancestors of the squashes appear to have originated in the vicinity of the border between Mexico and Guatemala. The first use of these vegetables as food appears to have occurred around 8000 B.C. At that time the Indians gathered the wild plants mainly for the seeds because the fruits contained only small amounts of bitter-tasting flesh. From Mexico and Central America, squashes spread throughout North and South America.

WORLD AND U.S. PRODUCTION. Production figures on squashes alone are not available. However, the worldwide production of pumpkins, squashes, and gourds totals about 6.8 million metric tons annually; and the leading producing countries, by rank, are: China, Romania, Egypt, Argentina, Turkey, Japan, Italy, Spain, Indonesia, and Thailand. Pumpkins, squashes, and gourds rank eleventh among the leading vegetables of the world.[38]

The United States produces a mere 1,000 tons of pumpkins, squashes, and gourds annually.[39] Without doubt, the actual production is higher than this figure would indicate, but this does show that they are produced primarily in home gardens rather than for commercial purposes.

PROCESSING. Summer squashes are often sliced and cooked briefly in preparation for canning or freezing, whereas winter squashes are usually cooked much longer before being similarly processed.

SELECTION, PREPARATION, AND USES. The culinary characteristics of summer squash and of winter squash, and of the varieties within each group, vary considerably. Hence, the cook should know the differences between them.

Types of Squashes. Descriptions follow:

• **Summer squash**—A bush-type cucurbit that produces many fruit which are usually harvested in the summer, while they are immature (the rind is still quite soft) and very watery.

The most common white or creamy-white variety of this type is the White Bush Scallop which is disk-shaped and smooth with scalloped edges. It is also called Cymling and Patty Pan.

[38]Data from *FAO Production Yearbook 1990*, FAO/UN, Rome, Italy, Vol. 44, p. 134, Table 54. **Note well:** Annual production fluctuates as a result of weather and profitability of the crop.
[39]*Ibid.*

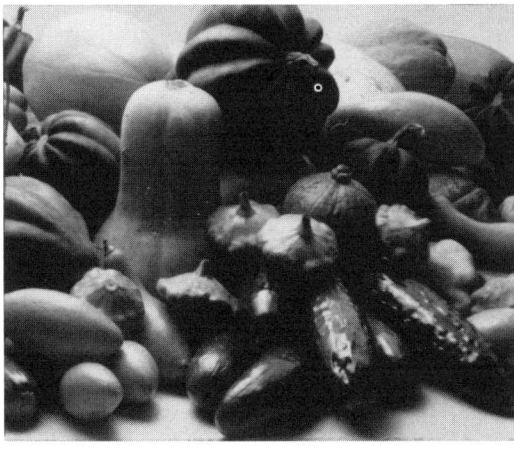

Fig. S-28. Squashes for all seasons, including the pumpkin, a favorite at Thanksgiving and Christmas. (Courtesy, Shell Chemical Co., Houston, Tex.)

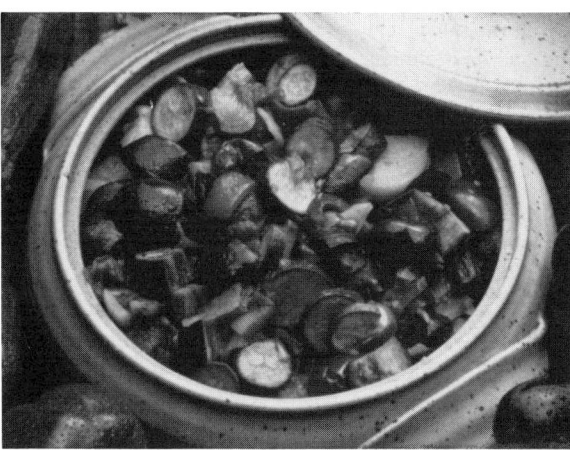

Fig. S-29. Summer squash featured in a vegetable dish. (Courtesy, National Film Board of Canada)

Most yellow summer varieties are elongated-bulbous in shape with a rough warty rind and are designated as either Straight or Crookneck.

Green, green-black or green-striped varieties, such as Zucchini and Italian Marrow, are elongated-cylindrical in shape.

• **Winter squash**—A bush-type, semivining, or vining cucurbit that is harvested in the fall when fully mature. The flesh of these squashes is usually less coarse and less fibrous, darker in color, milder flavored, and sweeter than that of pumpkins. They are often used in baked vegetable dishes and are sometimes used instead of pumpkin in making custards and pies.

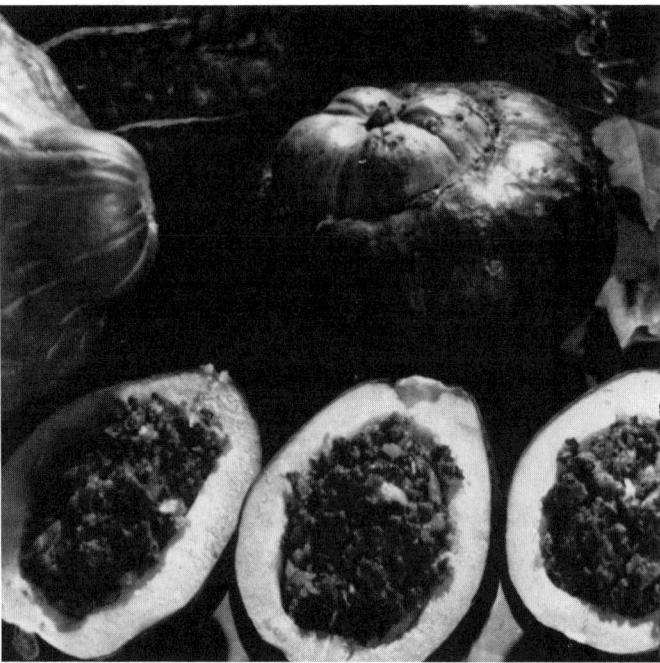

Fig. S-30. Winter squash stuffed with ground meat. (Courtesy, Agriculture Canada, Ottawa, Canada)

Common fall and early winter varieties are the green-colored corrugated Des Moines, Acorn, or Danish, the buff-colored Butternut, and the green or golden Delicious.

Vegetable spaghetti is an unusual variety of winter squash that has a large cylindrical fruit which contains a spaghetti-like pulp.

Most of the late winter squash varieties are relatively large and may have either a light-green, dark-green, bluish-green, or orange-colored rind.

Indicators of Quality. Summer squash should be fresh, fairly heavy in relation to size, free from cuts or noticeable bruises, crisp, and tender. The rind of winter squash should be hard.

Some suggestions for utilizing the various forms of squashes follow:

• **Squash flowers**—These should be picked when open so that no bees will be trapped within the blossoms. The flowers are good when dipped in a batter and fried in deep fat.

• **Squash seeds**—The seeds of winter squashes may be dried for a few days, after which any adhering tissue should be removed. Then, they may be roasted or fried in oil. Some

people boil the seeds briefly in salted water before roasting or frying.

• **Summer squash**—Usually these fruits are left unpeeled and cooked whole, sliced, cubed, or grated. The cooked item may be served with butter, margarine, or a special sauce. Some other ways in which summer squash may be prepared are (1) stuffed with ingredients such as bread crumbs, cheese, chopped eggs, ground meat, nuts, seasonings, and/or sour cream, and then baked; (2) peeled, grated, mixed with eggs, flour, baking powder, salt, and seasonings, shaped into patties, and fried on a griddle or baked in a bread; (3) sliced, dipped in batter, and fried in deep fat; (4) cooked, pureed, and used as a soup stock; or (5) sliced and baked in casseroles with cheese and other ingredients.

• **Vegetable spaghetti**—This special type of winter squash is usually baked or boiled whole until the rind softens, then it is cut open lengthwise, and the spaghettilike strands removed for serving alone with butter or margarine as a substitute for spaghetti, or it may be added to sauces or soups.

• **Winter squash**—These fruits should be cut in half and the fibrous matter and seeds removed. Then, they may be baked, broiled, or steamed and served with butter, margarine, and/or seasonings. Most varieties are equal or superior to pumpkin in recipes calling for the latter. The mashed, cooked vegetable is also good when it is (1) used to make breads, cakes, muffins, and pancakes, or (2) added to soups and stews near the end of the cooking periods to give them more body and to enhance their nutritional values.

NUTRITIONAL VALUE. The nutrient compositions of various forms of squashes are given in Food Composition Table F-21.

Some noteworthy observations regarding the nutrient composition of squashes follow:

1. Squash flowers contain 95% water and are low in calories (16 kcal per 100 g) and most other nutrients, except that they provide fair amounts of phosphorus, iron, vitamin A, and vitamin C. It is suggested that calorie-conscious people eat squash flowers in a salad, soup, or stew.

2. Boiled summer squashes contain more than 95% water and are very low in calories (14 kcal per 100 g) and most other nutrients. However, they are fair sources of potassium, vitamin A, and vitamin C. (The yellow and dark green varieties are generally richer in vitamin A than the white and pale green varieties.)

3. Baked winter squashes have a lower water content (81%) than most other cooked vegetables. They contain more than 4 times the calories, twice the potassium, and 10 times the vitamin A content of summer squashes. Although all winter squashes are excellent sources of vitamin A, the content is greatest in the varieties with deeply-colored yellow-orange flesh.

4. The seeds from winter squashes are very rich in calories (553 kcal per 100 g), protein (29%), iron (11.2 mg per 100 g), and phosphorus (1,144 mg per 100 g). Hence, the consumption of as little as 1 oz (*28 g*) of the seeds per day will make a significant nutritional contribution to the diet.

SQUIRREL

A rodent of the family *Sciuridae*, characterized by a bushy tail and long strong hind limbs. In some countries, squirrel is highly esteemed as game. It is cooked in the same way as rabbit.

STABILIZED

Made more resistant to chemical change by the addition of a particular substance.

STABILIZER

Any substance which tends to make a compound, mixture, or solution resistant to changes in form or chemical nature. In the food industry stabilizers are used to thicken, to keep pigments and other components in emulsion form, and to prevent the particles in colloidal suspensions from precipitating. Algin, methyl cellulose, carrageenan, and propylene glycol alginate are but a few of the stabilizers utilized.

(Also see ADDITIVES; and EMULSIFYING AGENTS.)

STACHYOSE

A tetrasaccharide composed of two molecules of galactose and one molecule of fructose and glucose. It occurs in many beans, beets, peas, soybeans, and tubers. Since the intestinal tract does not produce enzymes able to split stachyose, bacteria in the intestine act on it—forming gas. Hence, it is believed to be responsible for the gas-producing properties of beans.

(Also see BEAN[S], COMMON, section headed "Dried Beans.")

STALING

This term generally relates to bakery products where it is characterized in breads by (1) a firming of the crumb due to loss of water, (2) loss of flavor, and (3) loss of crispness in the crust resulting in leatheriness. The staling of breads is a complex combination of changes. Methods have been developed to detect these changes. However, the method most commonly employed to study staling is the detection of changes in the compressibility of a loaf of bread, since consumers associate softness with freshness. Softness of a bread may be increased by the inclusion of monoglycerides (emulsifiers), but this does not necessarily retard staling. Storing bread at refrigerator temperature increases the rate of staling while freezing bread arrests staling. Furthermore, staling can be reversed by heat; hence, stale bread makes good toast. No bakery products stale as fast as bread, but even rich cakes stale if kept long enough. Also, dry bakery goods like crackers stale, but they stale because they pick up moisture from the air.

STAR-APPLE (CAINITO) *Chrysophyllum cainito*

The fruit of a tree (of the family *Sapotaceae*) that is native to the West Indies and Central America. The fruit is apple-like, purple, round, up to 4 in. (*10 cm*) in diameter, with a white, sweet, edible pulp. The pulp is usually eaten fresh after removal of the skin.

The ripe fruit pulp is moderately high in calories (68 kcal per 100 g) and carbohydrates (14.5%). It is a fair source of vitamin C.

STARCH

Contents   Page

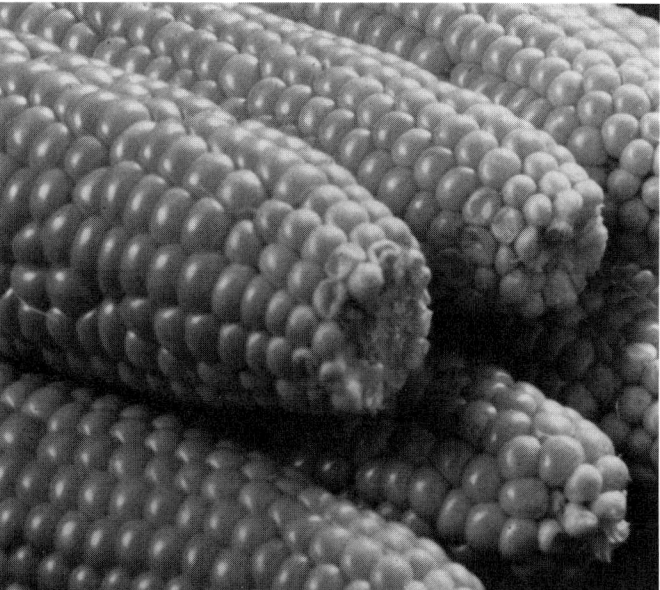

Fig. S-31. Corn, a major source of starch. (Courtesy, USDA)

Starch is a polysaccharide—long chains of the simple sugar, glucose—formed by the process of photosynthesis. It is the storage carbohydrate, stored as granules in seeds, roots, tubers, or stems of the higher plants. The chemical formula of starch is $(C_6H_{10}O_5)_n$. The "n" outside of the parentheses indicates an indefinite number of repeating glucose molecules. Furthermore, these glucose units may be linked in either of two patterns: (1) a straight-chained pattern called amylose; or (2) a highly branched pattern called amylopectin. The amount of amylose and amylopectin in starch depends on the source, but on the average starch is about 27% amylose and 73% amylopectin. Fig. S-32 illustrates the structures of amylose and amylopectin.

Unlike cellulose, which is also a long chain of glucose molecules, starch can be split by the digestive enzymes of the body. When either amylose or amylopectin are split, dextrins are formed. Dextrins may vary in length from five or more glucose molecules, and the final product of enzymatic splitting of starch is glucose.

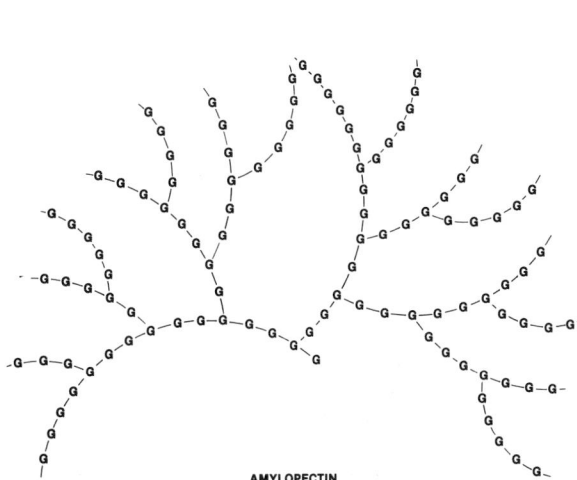

Fig. S-32. The structure of amylose and amylopectin of starch. Each "G" represents a glucose molecule.

IN THE DIET.   Since starch is a product of photosynthesis, many foods contain starch. It is the primary digestible carbohydrate in foods. Furthermore, starch and starch products are employed in many foods to facilitate processing or to give foods specific properties. Hence, starch and starch products are food additives.

Natural Starch.   Very little of the available carbohydrate occurring naturally in foods occurs as the disaccharides sucrose, lactose, or maltose or as the monosaccharides glucose or fructose. Cereal grains, roots, tubers, legumes, nuts, and some fruits and vegetables provide carbohydrate to the diet mainly as starch. The major sources of starch are the seeds of corn, rice, rye, sorghum, and wheat. Potatoes,

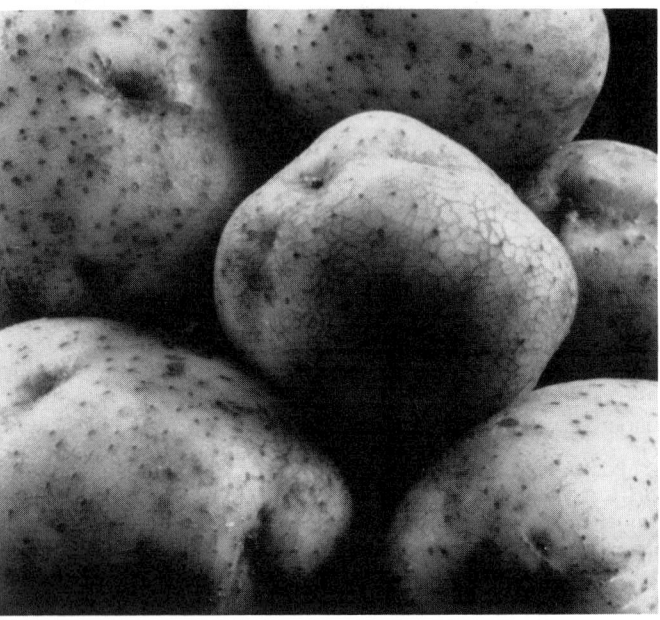

Fig. S-33. Potatoes, a good source of starch. (Courtesy, USDA)

which are tubers, are also a good source of starch. Dry mature beans and peas also contain starch, while fresh beans and peas contain starch but at much lower levels. Carbohydrate values given in Food Composition Table F-21 for the cereal grains, roots, tubers, nuts, dried beans, and peas can be considered as approximating the starch content of these foods.

Worldwide, natural starch is an important energy food. The staple food of a country provides the primary source of starch; for example, corn in Mexico; roots, tubers, and sorghum in parts of Africa; and rice in India, China and Indonesia. Starch is an economical food; hence, it contributes a large portion to the diets where income is low. As income increases, the amount of starch in the diet decreases while consumption of fat, animal protein, and sugar increase.

Aside from the starch which is natural in many foods, starch is an important commercial product, and it is extracted from several plant sources which produce it in sufficient quantities.

Commercial Starch.   Commercially extracted starch, due to some unique chemical and physical properties, low cost, and availability, may be added to foods during processing—as a food additive. While many plants produce starch, only a few produce it in quantities to make extraction feasible.

PRODUCTION.   Corn is the major source of commercial starch in the United States, followed by sorghum, wheat, and rice. Other sources include oats, barley, rye, potato, sago, arrowroot, and tapioca (cassava).

Starch production from corn is achieved by the wet milling process. Corn kernels are soaked in warm water containing sulfur dioxide until they become soft. Then, the kernels are cracked and the germ is removed. Next, the kernel fragments are ground and screened down to starch granules and gluten. The gluten is removed, and the starch is filtered, washed, dried, and packaged.

A newer process for obtaining wheat starch involves the milling of wheat into flour, followed by preparing a flour and water dough. Starch granules are then washed from the dough.

Starch is obtained from rice by soaking the grain in an alkaline chemical which dissolves the gluten, leaving the starch.

Starch from roots and tubers such as potato, arrowroot, and cassava is prepared by grinding the root or tuber to free the starch granule, screening to remove the fiber and skins, soaking, and separating the starch from other water-soluble material by settling or centrifugation. Starch granules are insoluble in cold water.

(Also see CEREAL GRAINS; CORN; POTATO; SORGHUM; and WHEAT.)

CHARACTERISTICS.   Although starch is a white powder to the unaided eye, it appears as granules or grains under the microscope, which vary in size and shape depending upon the plant source. Furthermore, the content of amylose and amylopectin vary depending upon the source. These characteristics of the starches affect their gelatinization, modification, and uses.

Gelatinization.   Starch gelatinizes, when mixed with water and heated beyond 133° to 167°F (56° to 75°C)—the critical temperature. This temperature differs depending upon the type of starch. As starch is heated, the chemical bonds (hydrogen bonds) holding the granules together start to weaken. This permits the water to penetrate the granules causing them to swell to many times their original size—a change referred to as gelatinization. As gelatinization occurs the clarity and the viscosity (thickness) of the solution increases, and the starch granules lose their unique microscopic shape by rupturing and releasing amylose and amylopectin.

The characteristics of these cooked viscous solutions vary from starch to starch. After cooling to room temperature, the starch from roots are clearer and more fluid, while starch from the cereal grains yield a cloudy less fluid paste that tends to be jellylike. These characteristics are dependent upon the amylose and amylopectin content of the starch and upon the size of the amylose and amylopectin molecule. Some hybrids—waxy hybrids—of corn and sorghum have been developed which yield starch that is almost entirely amylopectin, while other hybrids have a high amylose content. Overall, the tendency to thicken or gel upon cooling, and to become opaque is caused by the presence of amylose.

Modifications.   Besides the property of gelatinization, starch may be modified to yield some unique and useful properties which are used advantageously by the food industry and others; syrups and sugars are well-known products of modification.

• **Syrups and sugars**—Starch from any starch source—rice, corn, or other grains, or potatoes—may be broken down into its component sugar either enzymatically or with dilute acids. The most familiar example in the United States is corn syrup (Karo). Complete hydrolysis of starch yields glucose—dextrose.

Corn syrup is the product of the incomplete hydrolysis of starch. It is a viscous liquid containing dextrose, maltose, and dextrins. Unlike sugar, it has a distinct flavor other than sweetness. The degree of conversion is expressed by the *dextrose equivalent* (D.E.) which is, in effect, the measure of sweetness in the syrup, or in other words the amount of starch converted to glucose. Even high conversion syrups are substantially less sweet than sugar. A special corn syrup on the market is a *high fructose corn syrup* (HFCS) which is made by treating high conversion corn syrup with enzymes. The enzymes convert some of the glucose to fructose, which is much sweeter than glucose.

Corn sugar is glucose (dextrose) recovered by crystallization from hydrolyzed starch. Two types of refined dextrose are commercially available: dextrose hydrate, containing 9% by weight of water of crystallization, and anhydrous dextrose, containing less than 0.5% of water. Dextrose hydrate is most often used by food processors.

USES. Starch and modified starches are considered food additives, and they are employed in a wide variety of foods. As additives they contribute calories to foods, but starch and modified starches are primarily used in foods to facilitate processing or impart specific properties to foods. The following are some examples of the uses of starch in its various forms:

• **Dry granular starch**—One pound of cornstarch granules has a surface area of about 3,500 sq ft (*315 m²*). Dried starch or modified starch serve as moisture absorbing agents in many products. Starch is added to baking powder to absorb moisture and keep the ingredients from losing their activity. Confectioners sugar is protected from lumping during storage by the addition of cornstarch. Aside from food, the absorbing capacity of starch is sometimes employed on the human body as a substitute for powder, including baby diapers.

Candy and gum molds are formed from powdered cornstarch or modified starch.

Dry starch derivatives are used in foods to maintain their flow properties.

Starch powders are used as bulking or diluting agents in enzyme preparations or flavorings so that a larger unit of measurement may be used.

• **Starch pastes**—Most of the uses of starch as a food additive are for thickening and gelling. The proper starch or modified starch is chosen which yields the desirable properties. In the canning industry starches are used in baby foods, soups, sauces, pie fillings, gravies, vegetables in sauces, chow mein, chili, spaghetti, stews, and cream style corn. In the baking industry, starch, cross-linked starch and pregelatinized starches are employed in flour, fruit pie fillings, imitation jellies, whipped topping stabilizers, icing stabilizers, cream fillings, custards, salad dressings, candies, and gums.

• **Starch films**—The ability of starch to form films is utilized in covering foods with decorative and protective coatings, binding foods and providing a matrix to carry food substances. Starches are used as binders in meat products, and pet food, while modified starches are used as a matrix to carry flavor oils. Futhermore, starch coatings are oil resistant and can be used on nut and chocolate confections to prevent the migration of oil.

Starch coatings are found on chewing gums or other confections with hard sugar coatings.

• **Starch syrups and sugar**—Since corn syrups can (1) control crystallization, (2) retain moisture, (3) ferment, (4) produce a high osmotic pressure solution for preservation, and (5) aid browning; they are employed in many food products including the following: baby foods, bakery products, canned fruits, carbonated beverages, confections, dry bakery mixes, fountain syrups and toppings, frozen fruits, fruit juice drinks, ice cream and frozen desserts, jams, jellies and preserves, meat products, pickles and condiments, and table syrups (Karo syrup).

Due to its browning, fermentability, flavor enhancement, osmotic pressure, sweetness, humectancy (prevention of drying), hygroscopicity (moisture absorption), viscosity, and reactivity properties, starch sugar—dextrose—is utilized in many food products. The major uses of dextose are the confection, wine, and canning industries.

In medicine, various concentrations of glucose (dextrose) are utilized for intravenous administration.

NUTRITIONAL VALUE. Starch contributes energy—calories—to the diet. On the average, each gram of starch supplies 4 Calories (kcal) of energy. Upon ingestion, enzymes in the saliva begin breaking starch down to its component sugar, glucose. This process continues in the small intestine where the glucose is absorbed into the bloodstream and used by the cells of the body for energy production, stored as glycogen, or converted to chemicals used in the synthesis of fatty acids. Raw starch, as it occurs naturally in food, is contained in granules, and cooking of starch softens and ruptures these granules making the starch-containing food more palatable and more digestible.

Over the past 70 years, the value of starch in American nutrition has been decreasing. As shown in Fig. S-34, starch now supplies about 21% of the calories in the American diet. The decreased intake of starch has been countered by an increase in fat intake, particularly unsaturated fats.

(Also see ADDITIVES; CARBOHYDRATE[S]; CEREAL GRAINS; DIGESTION AND ABSORPTION; and METABOLISM.)

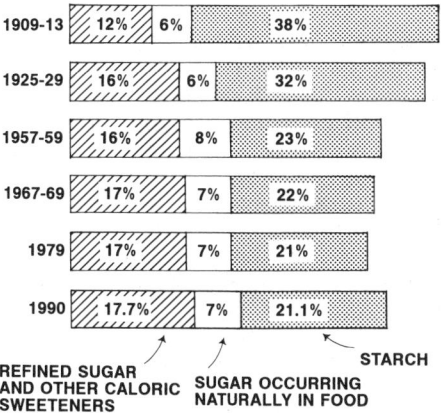

Fig. S-34. Changes in the percentage of calories in the American food supply derived from sugars and starch. (Courtesy, USDA)

STARCHES, WAXY

Properties of starch are influenced by the ratio of amylose (linear chains of glucose molecules) to amylopectin (branched chains of glucose molecules). Common starches contain 17 to 27% amylose, and 73 to 83% amylopectin. Waxy starches contain nearly 100% amylopectin. These do not form gels except at high concentrations; they remain as relatively clear solutions. Waxy starches can be derived from corn, grain sorghum, and rice.

(Also see STARCH.)

STARCH, PREGELATINIZED

None of the raw starches will form a paste with cold water unless they are precooked and then rolled or spray-dried. Therefore, pregelatinized starch is starch which has been cooked and dried. It can then be used in instant puddings, fillings, imitation jellies, whipped toppings, etc.

(Also see STARCH.)

STARVATION

This condition usually results from the prolonged and drastic deprivation of food. It is characterized by wasting of tissues and other alterations of normal physiology. If continued sufficiently long, there may be disability, or even death. Situations where large numbers of people starve are called *famines*.

Failure of children to get sufficient food results in growth failure, marasmus, and other serious disorders developing much sooner than in adults because children have proportionately higher requirements for nutrients to support their rapid rate of growth.

(Also see MALNUTRITION, PROTEIN-ENERGY.)

CAUSES OF STARVATION. The ultimate effect of starvation is the deprivation of the cells of the body of their essential nutrients. Although lack of food is the main cause of this condition, other factors may produce starvation at the cellular level.

The main causes of starvation are:

1. Unavailability of food.

2. Restriction of food intake due to such things as surgery or deprivation of food imposed for coercion or punishment.

3. Self-denial of food for purposes of weight reduction, protest, or religious fasting.

4. Failure to eat due to lack of appetite because of physiological or psychological reasons, including anorexia (lack of appetite), acidosis or ketosis, uremic poisoning in kidney failure, or emotional aversions to food such as in *anorexia nervosa*.

5. Disorders of the digestive tract due to reduced nutrient absorption in conditions such as diarrhea, malabsorption, vomiting, or surgical removal of part of the digestive tract.

6. Metabolic abnormalities caused by such conditions as fever, diabetes, hyperthroidism, Cushings' syndrome, extreme stress, or wasting diseases such as cancer.

ADAPTATION TO STARVATION. Persons, who are otherwise healthy, can adapt to deprivation of nutrients for short periods of time by means of various physiological processes which have helped the human race to survive many famines.

Prolonged dietary deficiency of energy results in an eventual reduction in voluntary activities and in the metabolic rate, so that it is possible to survive on about one-half of the energy which had been the normal intake in the diet. It is thought that the reduction in metabolic rate may be due in part to a shortage of energy-yielding nutrients and in part to subnormal blood levels of thyroid hormones. Likewise, body temperatures of starved persons are often subnormal.

Energy is supplied first from stored fat, then from body protein. Stored fat, in the form of triglycerides, is split into fatty acids and glycerol by hormone-sensitive lipase enzymes in adipose tissue. The fatty acids are then released into the blood where they immediately form complexes with plasma albumin, while the glycerol travels free in the blood to the liver where it may be converted to glucose or recombined into triglycerides. Many tissues, such as muscles, are able to utilize fatty acids as their sole sources of energy, although the metabolism of carbohydrates when they are available, requires about 10% less oxygen to produce the same amount of energy.

Blood glucose (critical for the brain and nervous system) is maintained at close to a normal level by the breakdown of protein in muscle to amino acids which travel through the blood to the liver where they are converted to glucose. The breakdown of body protein is limited, however, and so it is fortunate that the brain can adapt to the utilization of ketone bodies which are formed from fat in the liver when glucose becomes scarce.

Catabolism of body tissue for energy results in rapid weight loss, particularly when fat stores have been exhausted, since each pound of protein loss results in a corresponding loss of 3 lb of water which are eliminated from the body.

Starved persons vary in their susceptibility to low blood sugar and ketosis. Some become weak and feel dizzy after only a day of starvation, while others feel few effects after weeks of total fasting; hence, the use of starvation to obtain weight reduction should be done only under the supervision of a physician.

If fluids are limited, the kidneys set into play a mechanism which conserves water. They secrete renin, an enzyme which initiates the conversion of a bloodborne protein (an alpha-globulin) to angiotension II, a hormonelike substance. The latter substance stimulates the adrenal cortex to secrete aldosterone—a hormone which causes the retention of water and sodium by the kidney and a reduction in the amount of urine volume.

The edema of starvation results from a flow of water from the blood to the tissues because the ability of blood to retain water is reduced when proteins in the blood are depleted.

Diarrhea results from the loss of absorptive cells in the intestine which occurs as part of the wholesale catabolism of body tissues in severe starvation.

Minerals—such as potassium, magnesium, and phosphate ions—are released into the blood from the catabolism of tissues, thereby delaying the appearance of clinical deficiencies of these essential nutrients. However, there are likely to be deficiencies of nutrients which are not stored in the body and need to be provided on a regular basis in the diet, such as water-soluble vitamins, chloride, and other ions. Also, the absorption of vitamins and minerals is increased and their urinary excretion is decreased. Thus, there is more efficient utilization of vitamins and minerals by the body in starvation.

(Also see FASTING.)

EFFECTS OF STARVATION. The effects of food deprivation are dependent upon the severity and length of the deprivation, and the status of the victim prior to starvation. Thus, one cannot draw up an exact timetable of survival. There have been reports of survival after 8 months of total fasting, but the survivors were obese adult women at the beginning of starvation.

Death results from the loss of function of vital organs such as the digestive tract, which may become almost transparent and nonfunctional due to wasting, and the heart, where muscle wasting often results in circulatory failure.

Some crude generalizations about survival from starvation are as follows: Young adults may survive much longer than chidren (due to the proportionately higher nutrient requirements of the latter) or older persons; women survive longer than men because of their greater proportions of body fat to lean tissue which results from the action of female hormones; and the obese survive longer than lean persons. Thus, the now frowned-upon practice of trying to fatten children had a basis in the more precarious times of our ancestors.

Some of the specific effects of starvation follow:

1. **Physical defects.** Low birth-weight babies from food-deprived mothers are unlikely to show any long-term physical defects as a result of maternal starvation, *unless* the mother was subjected to both insufficient food and malnutrition.

2. **Impaired mental development.** Nutritional deprivation will most likely have a lasting effect on children if it occurs during the first year of life. Studies on the brains of infants who died from starvation at less than 1 year of age showed a significant reduction (15 to 20%) in the number of brain cells.[40] Smaller head circumferences of children who suffer from marasmus early in life are indicative of proportionate reductions in brain size. Itelligence tests have shown that such children do not seem to catch up in mental development by 6 years of age. However, when starvation occurs after 2 or 3 years of age, the effect on learning is temporary, since brain tissue is not affected once complete development of the brain has occurred.

3. **Stunted growth.** Children subjected to acute or chronic deprivation of water, calories, and protein in fetal life, or in the years between birth and school age, may show permanent retardation in growth and development or even disability and death.

4. **Increased susceptibility to disease.** Both children and adults who have been starved are more susceptible to, and suffer more severely from, diseases such as diarrhea, measles, plague, influenza, tuberculosis, and cholera. This is due to the exhaustion of nutrient reserves and concomitant reduced immunity.

5. **Abnormal behavior.** In the beginning stages of starvation, the victims become preoccupied with food and are increasingly restless, irritable, undisciplined, and nervous. Eventually there is increasing apathy, depression, and decreasing sociability until the victims become totally withdrawn and inactive. During rehabilitation from severe starvation, the patients go through a rebellious period that may last until recovery.

6. **Reduced work capacity.** Studies of worker produc-

tivity in the coal mines and steel mills of Germany showed that the average output per worker declined in proportion to the decrease in food energy which occurred as a result of decreasing food supplies during the course of war.[41] The work output returned to the original levels when it became possible for the workers to consume additional food.

SIGNS OF STARVATION. Signs of this disorder are weight loss, wasting of tissue, loose skin, ketone breath, ketones in urine, dehydration, low blood sugar, weakness, diarrhea, low blood pressure, edema, irritability, and anti-social behavior. It is usually easier to detect starvation in children than in adults, since one can readily observe in the former the great reduction in activity, smaller body weight for height and age, and other signs of malnutrition.

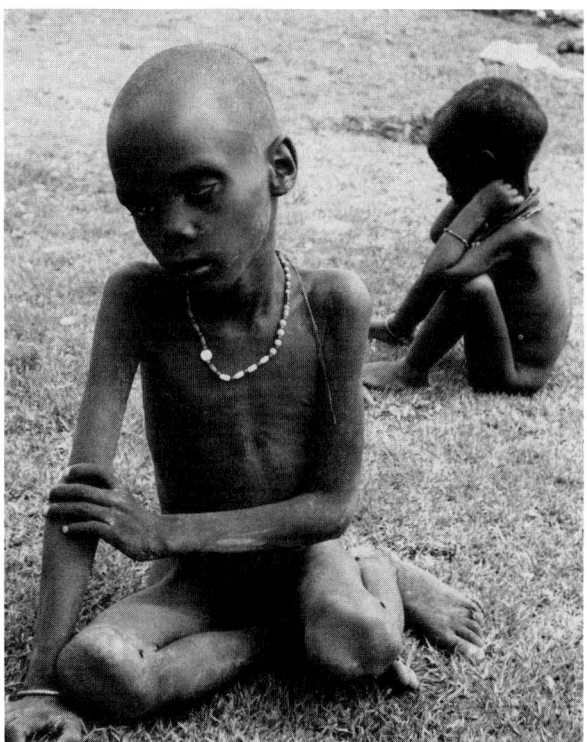

Fig. S-35. African children suffering from starvation. (Courtesy, FAO, Rome, Italy)

TREATMENT AND PREVENTION OF STARVATION. Although many victims of starvation are ravenously hungry, their digestive functions may be severely impaired. Therefore, care must be taken not to feed foods known to cause or aggravate diarrhea (fats, fried foods, beans, and high-fiber foods), which is one of the main causes of death from starvation. It may be necessary to provide small, but frequent feedings of skim milk. Supplements of vitamins and minerals may need to be provided when there is likely to have been depletion of nutrients. Vitamins A and C are needed for optimal healing of tissues, while mineral elements such as potassium, sodium, and magnesium are critical for cardiac function and electrolyte balance. Persons who cannot eat normally by mouth may have to be fed intravenously or by tube feedings.

(Also see INTRAVENOUS FEEDING; and TUBE FEEDING.)

[40]Keller, W.D., and H.A. Kraut, "Work and Nutrition," *World Review of Nutrition and Dietetics*, G.H. Bourne, Editor, S. Karager Ag, Basel, Switzerland, Vol. 3, 1959, p. 69.

[41]Keller, W. D., and H. A. Kraut, "Work and Nutrition," *World Review of Nutrition and Dietetics*, G. H. Bourne, Editor, S. Karager Ag, Basel, Switzerland, Vol. 3, 1959, p. 69.

Programs For The Prevention Of Starvation follow:

• **Distribution of food**—Although this is the most direct approach, it may well be the least satisfactory means of long-term assistance for chronically underfed populations, since these people may come to depend upon free or low-cost food from outside sources, rather than developing their own food supply. However, increasing food production takes time; in the meantime, it may be necessary to provide food for such vulnerable groups as infants and children, pregnant mothers, handicapped persons, and the aged.

• **Provision of money or scrip to buy food**—When a local supply of food is available, its sale through commercial channels may help to encourage local enterprises such as farming and marketing. However, the money or scrip may be used to purchase items other than food, as evidenced by abuses of the food stamp program in the United States (for example, their use to purchase liquor followed by their illicit redistribution at discounts). Furthermore, such doles to the able-bodied unemployed may lead to their rejection of employment when it is available.

• **Price controls**—The government may attempt to control food prices in order to prevent those with more money from buying large quantities of food for resale at higher prices. When controls are stringent, this type of policy sometimes makes food production and distribution unprofitable in the private sector, thereby creating more problems than it solves. Also, just about every attempt at price control or rationing has been accompanied by diversion of foods into *black market* channels. Thus, there must be adequate provision for enforcement of price controls.

• **Planning for the relief of famines**—Famines are often presaged by such events as bad weather during the planting, growing, and harvesting of crops; outbreaks of plant or animal diseases; steady increases in unemployment and reduction of food production; and political unrest. Failure to heed such warnings has frequently resulted in considerable wasted effort and materials as public and private groups have rushed aid to famine-stricken areas.

(Also see DEFICIENCY DISEASES; HUNGER, WORLD; and WORLD FOOD.)

STASIS

A slowing or stoppage of the normal flow of fluid or semifluid material in an organ or vessel in the body, as (1) slowing the flow of blood in arteries and veins, or (2) reduced motility of the intestines accompanied by retention of feces.

STEARIC ACID

An 18-carbon saturated fatty acid which occurs in tallow and other animal fats, and in cocoa butter and other hard vegetable fats, and which reacts with glycerol to form stearin.
(Also see FATS AND OTHER LIPIDS.)

STEATORRHEA

Describes a greasy or fatty bowel movement (stool), a characteristic of many malabsorption syndromes such as celiac disease and sprue.
(Also see CELIAC DISEASE; MALABSORPTION SYNDROMES; and SPRUE.)

STENOSIS

A constriction or narrowing of a channel.

STERILIZATION

A process used to destroy all living microorganisms. (Also see PRESERVATION OF FOOD.)

STEROIDS

Any of a group of fat-related organic compounds. They include cholesterol, numerous hormones, precursors of certain vitamins, bile acids, alcohols (sterols), and certain natural drugs and poisons (such as the digitalis derivatives).

STEROL

One of a class of complex, fatlike subtances widely distributed in nature.

STILLAGE

The mash from fermentation of grains after removal of alcohol by distillation.

STOMATITIS

Inflammation of the mucous membrane of the mouth due to a variety of causes, including a riboflavin deficiency.

STOOL

Fecal material; that which is evacuated from the digestive tract following the digestive process.

STRAWBERRY *Fragaria* spp

This fruit is borne by a small herbaceous plant (of the family *Rosaceae*) that grows close to the ground; embracing both *Fragaria virginiana,* the wild strawberry, and *Fragaria chiloensis,* from which most common cultivated strawberries descend.

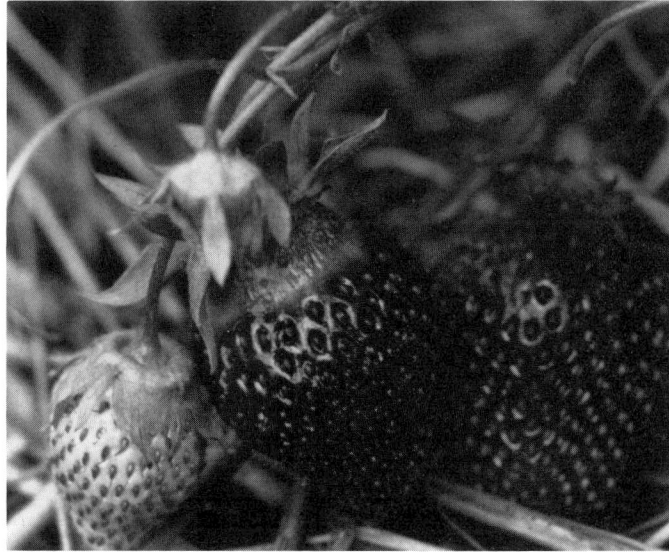

Fig. S-36. Strawberries are often grown with a straw mulch or plastic sheeting between the rows, both of which keep the berries clean. (Courtesy, University of Minnesota, St. Paul, Minn.)

Strawberries are the world's leading berry-type fruit, although they are not true berries from a strict botanical point of view because the tiny seeds are carried on the outside of the fleshy part of the fruit, whereas, true berries have seeds enclosed within the flesh.

ORIGIN AND HISTORY.   Strawberries are indigenous over a very wide area—to Chile; to North America from California to Alaska; and to the U.S.S.R. Cultivation of the strawberry as a garden plant began in the 13th century in France.

Most of the great advances in strawberry culture occurred after certain New World varieties of the fruit were introduced into Europe by the returning explorers. In the latter part of the 16th century, the explorer Cartier brought Canadian strawberries back to France, and Sir Francis Drake brought the Virginia strawberry to England. Both types are believed to have been varieties of *Fragaria virginiana.*

Strawberries remained a luxury during the first part of the 19th century and only the most affluent could enjoy them. The problem was that they spoiled readily and could not be shipped very far by the means of transport then available. By the middle of the century, this problem had been solved in the United States by the initiation of railway shipment, followed in short order by the development of a high-yielding variety of the hybrid strawberry. Today, fresh strawberries are carried thousands of miles in refrigerated railcars and trucks.

WORLD AND U.S. PRODUCTION.   Worldwide, about 2.4 million metric tons of strawberries are produced annually; and the leading producing countries, by rank, are: United States, Poland, Japan, and Spain. These four countries produce more than 52% of the strawberries of the world.[42]

The United States produces about 570,300 metric tons of strawberries, annually; and the three leading strawberry states, by rank, are: California, Florida, and Oregon. California alone produces more than 78% of the U.S. strawberry crop.[43]

---

[42]Data from *FAO Production Yearbook 1990*, FAO/UN, Rome, Italy, Vol. 44, p. 171, Table 75. **Note well:** Annual production fluctuates as a result of weather and profitability of the crop.

[43]Data from *Agricultural Statistics 1991*, USDA, p. 210, Table 323. **Note well:** Annual production fluctuates as a result of weather and profitability of the crop.

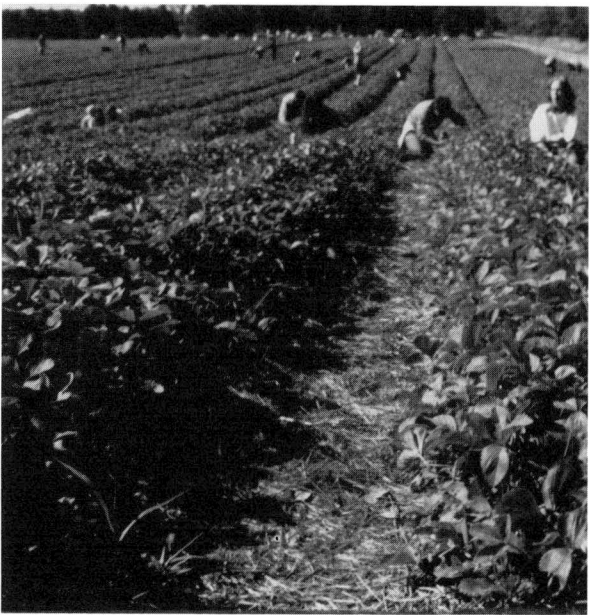

Fig. S-37. Picking strawberries. (Courtesy, University of Minnesota, St. Paul, Minn.)

Strawberries that are to be sold fresh in distant markets are often picked before they are fully ripe in order to minimize spoilage during shipment, but the fruit intended for nearby markets or processing plants may be allowed to attain optimal ripeness.

Much of the crop is still picked by hand, although the labor requirement has been reduced somewhat in recent years by the development of mechanical pickers and other harvesting aids. The fruit keeps best during shipment if it is precooled within 2 hours of picking, followed by shipment or storage at a temperature below 40°F (4°C).

PROCESSING.   Over ⅓ of the U.S. strawberry crop is processed. About 95% of processed fruit is frozen and most of the rest is made into preserves. However, it is noteworthy that sometimes freezing merely serves as a means of pre-serving the highly perishable berries until they can be utilized by the manufacturers of baked goods, ice cream, jams and jellies, and other items.

The most common ways in which frozen strawberries are packed for retail sales are (1) sliced and packed with sugar at a ratio of 80% by weight of fruit to 20% sugar, and (2) frozen whole berries without added sugar.

Frozen strawberries that are destined for manufacturing into various processed food products are usually packed with sugar at the ratio of 80% fruit to 20% sugar.

SELECTION, PREPARATION, AND USES.   Fresh strawberries should be bright red, plump, medium size, free from dirt, and well rounded with attached stems and caps. Unripe berries will not ripen after picking. Excessively large berries may have an overly bland flavor, while small, misshapen berries may be bitter.

Some preparation tips follow:

1. Fresh strawberries may be kept in a refrigerator for several days if they are removed from their store containers and placed in a single layer in a shallow container.

2. The berries should not be washed until just before using. Then, they should be rinsed with caps and stems intact under a gentle stream of cold water.

3. After washing, the caps and stems may be removed and the berries patted dry with paper towels.

4. Fresh strawberries are good in dishes such as breakfast cereals, cheesecake, compotes, cottage cheese salads, crepes, custards, French toast, gelatin salads, ice cream, milk shakes, pancakes, pies, puddings, sherbets, sundaes, and waffles. Thawed frozen strawberries may also be used in many of these dishes.

5. The syrup from thawed, sweetened frozen strawberries may be mixed with unflavored carbonated water, or plain water flavored with a little lemon juice, to make a refreshing drink.

6. Some of the flavorings which enhance strawberry dishes are almond extract, brandy, cinnamon, citrus juices (particularly when diluted and sweetened a little), fruit-flavored liqueurs, and vanilla extract.

In summary, the main uses of strawberries are: desserts, fruit dishes, baked goods, gelatin desserts, ice cream, ices, jams, jellies, pies, sherbets, soft drinks, and syrups; and in the production of liqueurs and wines.

NUTRITIONAL VALUE.   The nutrient compositions of various strawberry products are given in Food Composition Table F-21.

Some noteworthy observations regarding the nutrient

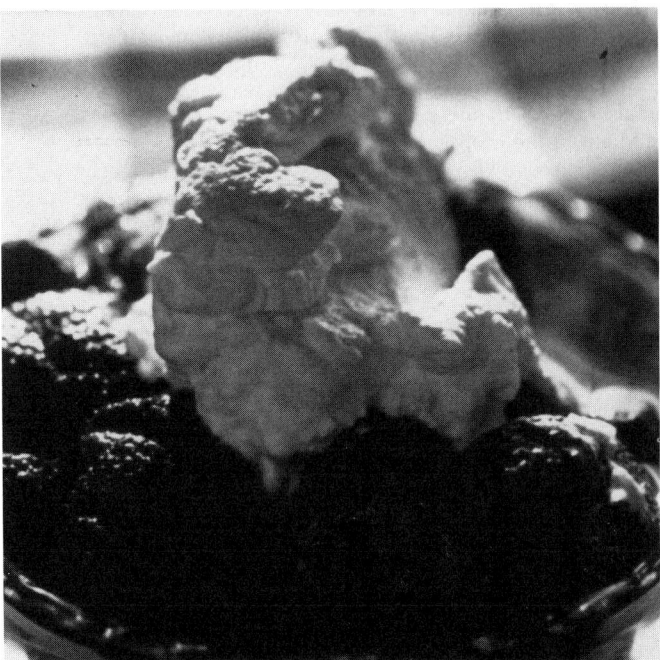

Fig. S-38. Strawberries and cream an all-time favorite. (Courtesy, USDA)

composition of the more common strawberry products follow:

1. The raw fruit and the frozen unsweetened berries are fairly low in calories (37 kcal per 100 g) and carbohydrates (8%). They are good sources of fiber, potassium, and iron; and an excellent source of vitamin C, and bioflavonoids.

2. Frozen sweetened strawberries contain about 3 times the caloric and carbohydrate levels of the raw fruit and the frozen unsweetened fruit, but the levels of the other nutrients are similar to those of the unsweetened products.

3. Strawberry ice cream is rich in calories (188 kcal per 100 g) and carbohydrates (24%). It is a good source of calcium, phosphorus, and potassium, and a fair to good source of vitamin A.

4. Pie made from strawberries is rich in calories (198 kcal per 100 g) and carbohydrates (31%). It is a fair to good source of potassium and vitamin C.

5. The red color of strawberries is due mainly to the anthocyanin pigment pelargonidin 3-monoglucoside (which belongs to the large family of substances called bioflavonoids).

STRAWBERRY GUAVA *Psidium cattleianum.*

A specie of guava, sometimes planted in the West Indies.

The nutrient composition of the strawberry guava is given in Food Composition Table F-21.

(Also see FRUIT[S], Table F-23, Fruits of the World—"Guava.")

STRAWBERRY PEAR *Hylocereus undatus*

The red egg-shaped fruit of a cactus that is native to the West Indies. It is fairly low in calories (54 kcal per 100 g) and carbohydrates (13%), and is a good source of iron, but only a fair source of vitamin C.

STRAWBERRY TOMATO (TOMATILLO)
Physalis pubescens

A member of the husk tomato fruits (*Physalis* species of

the family *Solanaceae*) which is native to Mexico and is related closely to the Cape Gooseberry and the ground cherry.

It is noteworthy that the Indians of Mexico used this plant for food long before they used the related plant that was developed into the common tomato *(Lycopersicum esculentum)*. Some botanists suspect that the latter was eventually domesticated because it resembled the strawberry tomato.

The strawberry tomato is low in calories (40 kcal per 100 g) and carbohydrates (9%). It contains much less vitamin A and vitamin C than the common tomato.

(Also see CAPE GOOSEBERRY; and TOMATO.)

STREPTOCOCCAL INFECTIONS, FOOD-BORNE

Streptococcus pyogenes may get into foods from infected handlers since they are carried on airborne droplets from the respiratory tract of infected people who may sneeze or cough on food. The disease caused by this bacteria is commonly called strep throat. Other *Streptococcal* bacteria can get into the food and cause scarlet fever. However, this is uncommon in the United States today. These diseases are characterized by fever, vomiting, and sore throat. To prevent their spread, food should be protected from contamination by infected handlers. Once contracted, the disease responds to penicillin and other antibiotics. Occasionally streptococcal infections produce complications such as rheumatic fever and glomerulonephritis.

(Also see DISEASES, Table D-10, Food-Related Infections and Parasitic Diseases—"Strep Throat" and "Scarlet Fever.")

STRESS

Stress is one of those words often used and assumed to be understood—until one is required to become precise about its meaning. Then stress becomes different things to different people. Stated simply, stress is a strain, a force, or a great pressure acting on an individual resulting from physical factors—illness, injury, and environment—or psychological factors—prolonged fear, anger, and anxiety.

Stresses of many kinds affect people; among such external forces are previous nutrition, abrupt diet changes, a large number of people crowded together, changing houses or offices, irregularity, travel, excitement, presence of strangers, fatigue, previous illness, temperature, and abrupt weather changes.

Due to our individuality, what stresses one person may have no effect on another. Physiologically, stress is characterized by increased blood pressure, increased muscle tension, rapid heart rate, rapid breathing, and altered endocrine gland function. In the whole scheme, the nervous system and the endocrine system are intimately involved in the response to stress and the effects of stress. In turn, changes produced by these two systems—collectively the neuroendocrine system—can alter nutritional processes and increase the needs of tissues for nutrients. Moreover, stress and nutrition interact since (1) malnutrition itself may produce a

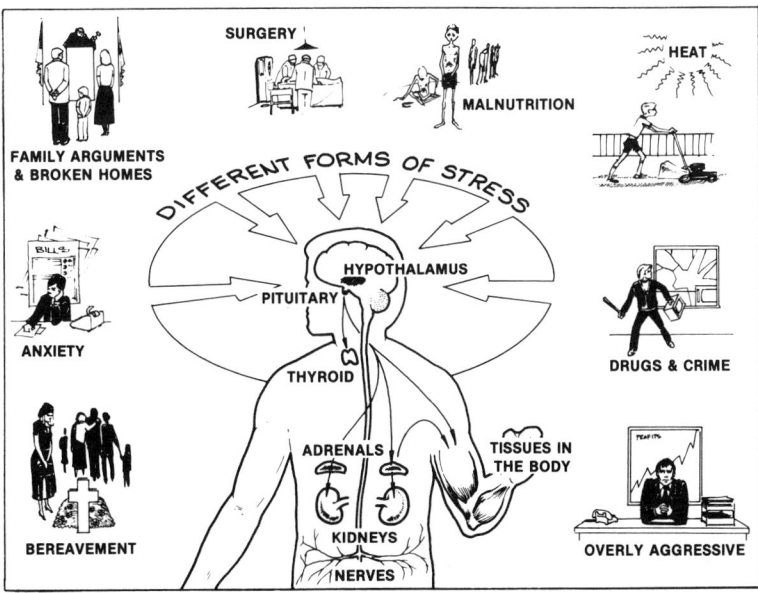

Fig. S-39. The different forms of stress and the action of stress on the body.

energy, and the body may fall victim to other disorders.

NUTRITIONAL DEMANDS OF STRESS. Nutrient requirements of the stressed individual are affected by the previous nutritional status, and the type and duration of the stress. The 1989 edition of *Recommended Dietary Allowances* (RDAs), compiled by the Committee on Dietary Allowances and the Food and Nutrition Board, provides for the nutrient needs of healthy people living under usual environmental stresses. (See Table N-3.) The RDAs do not allow for the special needs of infections and chronic diseases—both forms of stress. Due to the individuality of the response to stress, persons under severe stress must be individually identified. Stress severe enough to increase the body's needs for essential nutrients may come from physical factors, or from psychological or emotional factors.

Physical Stress. Stress due to physical, tangible, and specific events is well understood, and results in some definite nutritional recommendations.

INJURIES AND INFECTIONS. Injuries, surgery, burns, and infections result in increased energy expenditure via the neuroendocrine system. The magnitude of the changes elicited depends upon (1) the prestress nutritional status of the individual, (2) age of the individual, (3) the severity and duration of the stressing event.

Energy and protein requirements of physical stresses have been the prime concern. Little information exists concerning vitamins, minerals, and electrolytes.

• **Energy**—Stress associated with minor surgery increases the energy requirements of the body by less than 10%, while multiple bone fractures may increase energy expenditure by 10 to 30%. Some infections increase the basal metabolic rate (BMR); hence, energy expenditure, by 20 to 50%. The largest energy drain on the body is incurred by third degree burns, where the need for energy increases by 40%. When burns are complicated by infection, the requirement for energy is further increased. Some patients may require 4,000 to 8,000 kcal/day.

Often, individuals subjected to injuries, surgery, and/or infections have a depressed food intake which may complicate the nutritive requirements. Once carbohydrate stores of energy (muscle and liver glycogen) are depleted—usually within 24 hours—energy must be provided by fat and protein stores. Amino acids from the catabolism—breakdown—of skeletal muscle are an important energy source. If prolonged, this results in massive tissue wasting.

Energy replacement in some cases may be accomplished by oral feeding, tube feeding, or intravenous feeding, thus preventing or lessening tissue catabolism.

• **Protein**—As indicated, protein and energy metabolism are closely related. Injury, burns, surgery, and infection all induce protein breakdown via glucocorticoid secretion. Protein catabolism results in a negative nitrogen balance—the hallmark of stress which stimulates the catabolic mechanism. Adequate protein, with a high biological value, is necessary to prevent tissue wasting during a stressful illness, and to encourage convalescence following diminution of the stress.

stress response, (2) response to stress is determined by the nutritional state of an individual, and (3) stress can produce nutritional deficiencies or aggravate already existing deficiencies. Ultimately, through the neuroendocrine system, the nutrition and stress interactions are mediated via hormones released or inhibited by the body's response to stress.

THE STRESS RESPONSE. Normally, the secretion of the hormones is not viewed as a single event, but as a concert. As one hormone comes into play, another may fade out; or one hormone may cause the secretion of another, or the action of one may complement the action of another. Furthermore, the brain or nervous system in many cases acts as the conductor by signaling the proper time for increased or decreased secretion of a hormone. In particular, the hypothalamus acts like a "switchboard" by "plugging in" the proper hormone in response to a variety of nervous stimuli received by the brain. Thus, such things as stress, nutritional status, emotions, nursing, time of day, season of the year, etc. may manifest themselves as disruptions in bodily function.

The hormones involved in the stress response alter the metabolic reactions of the body, and hence, increase the nutritional needs of the body, possibly for protein, energy, fat, carbohydrates, minerals, and vitamins.

The response to stress is characterized as occurring in three stages, even when the cause is nonspecific:

1. **Alarm.** The body recognizes a stress and prepares for flight or fight. This preparation occurs via the release of hormones from the endocrine glands, primarily the adrenal medulla. These hormones cause increased heart rate, respiration, blood sugar, perspiration, dilated pupils, and slowed digestion. During the alarm stage, the burst of energy or alertness may be used for flight or fight. However, resistance is down.

2. **Resistance.** During this stage the body adapts to, and the body reaches, a heightened level of resistance or preparedness. The body attempts to repair any damage caused by the stress. The resistance stage cannot be maintained indefinitely; if the stress is not removed, then the body plunges into the third stage.

3. **Exhaustion.** Continued stress depletes the body's

• **Vitamins, minerals, and electrolytes**—Studies have shown that during moderate to severe stresses, more zinc, copper, magnesium, and calcium are lost in the urine. Furthermore, stress results in altered blood levels of vitamins A and C, and of zinc and iron. Also, part of the response to stress includes water and sodium retention, via vasopressin and aldosterone secretion. As for the water-soluble vitamins—thiamin, riboflavin, niacin, pyridoxine (B-6), pantothenic acid, folic acid, and vitamin C—stress increases their requirement. However, no dietary recommendations are made for these nutrients for individuals under stressful situations. Still, it seems wise to supply some supplementation before deficiency symptoms appear.

ENVIRONMENTAL EXTREMES. Overall, man has learned to protect himself from extreme heat or cold. However, nutrient requirements are increased during adaptation to environmental temperatures above 97°F (37°C). Protein, energy, and water needs are elevated while losses of minerals and electrolytes (calcium, iron, sodium, and potassium) may be anticipated, all depending upon the amount of physical work performed. Also, vitamin C requirements may be increased by stress of a hot environment. Exposure to a cold environment increases the metabolic rate, and hence, the energy requirement of unprotected individuals. Warm clothing and dwellings have minimized the effects of cold on man.

Psychological or Emotional Stress. Day-to-day psychological or emotional stress is normal, and it is inevitable—a part of life. In our society, stressful situations may include family arguments, death of a loved one, drug addiction, crime, unemployment, broken homes, and executive positions requiring aggressive personalities. The degree each individual is stressed depends on how the individual perceives day-to-day situations. Some individuals react excessively, causing hormonal and metabolic responses which tax the body's protective mechanisms. Indeed, some studies indicate a relationship between emotional stress and diseases such as cardiovascular disease, high blood pressure, peptic ulcers, cancer, and streptococcal throat infections, which in turn may increase or alter nutritional requirements.

Nutritionally, emotional stress may have a variety of effects. Prolonged fear, anxiety, anger, and tension all may stimulate hormonal and metabolic responses thus depleting energy, and increasing the need for energy, protein, vitamins, and/or minerals. Overeating, extreme undereating (anorexia nervosa), and eating binges with self-induced vomiting—bulimarexia—may be the result of psychological stress.

Without question, more research is needed in this area—especially in a society such as ours—so that stressed individuals may be identified and specific recommendations made. It seems reasonable to assume that persons experiencing emotional stresses need nutrient adjustments similar to those of individuals experiencing physical stresses. Most of the hormones altering the metabolism are influenced by either emotional or physical stimuli. Ultimately the brain determines the body's response to any stimuli.

COPING WITH STRESS OR DISTRESS. Stress is unavoidable. Therefore, the best protection comes from recognizing it, and coping with it. Recognizing stress requires individual evaluation. Stress is different for every individual. Coping with stress involves relaxation, regular exercises, and periodic evaluation of priorities. Moreover, one should recognize that stress may be turned into a positive force since it can stimulate some form of favorable action on the part of an individual. Therefore, people should differentiate between stress and distress in their lives. Thus, distress—not being able to adapt—is responsible for the harmful effects. Health professionals are beginning to recognize stress as a legitimate health concern, which may produce damaging or predisposing responses in the body, though clear cut connections between stress and disease are difficult to establish.

Diet-Stress Connection. It is noteworthy that most people have certain foods that they instinctively turn to when under stress—foods that create a feeling of security. The most common security food is milk, perhaps as a symbol of the more protected days of childhood and a desire to return to them. But the food or foods that comfort one person may trigger anxiety in another. So, individuals are best advised to study their own responses to stress, and to evaluate the effectiveness of their coping strategies, possibly by keeping a diary. If eating custard makes one feel better able to cope, then custard it should be. But because a certain approach works for one person it should not necessarily be urged upon the entire population. A moderate, well-balanced diet with emphasis on the stress-related nutrients and regular but not excessive meals is one approach that can be recommended for all.

(Also see ANOREXIA NERVOSA; BULIMAREXIA; DISEASES; ENDOCRINE GLANDS; HEART DISEASE; HIGH BLOOD PRESSURE; METABOLISM; and ULCERS, PEPTIC.)

STROKE (APOPLEXY)

An interruption in the normal circulation of the blood through the brain leading to a sudden loss of consciousness and some degree of paralysis, which may be temporary or permanent depending on the severity of the oxygen deprivation of the brain cells. Most strokes can be traced to previously existing conditions of atherosclerosis, hypertension, or arterial aneurysm.

The three immediate causes of stroke are:

1. **Cerebral thrombosis**, in which normal blood circulation through the brain is cut off from a part of it by a clot in an atherosclerotic artery.

2. **Cerebral embolism**, in which a traveling blood clot, fat, or an embolus of air (a bubble of air) settles in one of the cerebral arteries and chokes off the circulation.

3. **Cerebral hemorrhage**, in which there is a rupture of a blood vessel within the brain, usually an artery with a thin spot (aneurysm) in its wall. The latter type of stroke may be triggered by overexertion, overeating, great stress, or a violent coughing fit.

The most effective prevention of stroke consists in having a complete physical checkup once a year, following the doctor's instructions, and eliminating emotional stress and pressure.

STRONTIUM (Sr)

This is a soft, silvery metal with physical and chemical properties similar to those of calcium. There is no evidence as yet that strontium plays an essential role in man and other higher animals; so, it must be considered as a nonessential element at this time. It is noteworthy, however, that it has been reported that the omission of this element from the diet of rats and guinea pigs on a purified diet resulted in (1) growth depression, an impairment of the calcification of bones and teeth (but this report has been neither confirmed nor invalidated); and (2) a higher incidence of carious teeth.

The strontium content of bone has attracted particular interest because of the affinity of this tissue for strontium and, therefore, its relevance to the problem of strontium retention from radioactive fallout.

SUB–

Prefix denoting beneath, or less than normal.

SUBCUTANEOUS

Situated or occurring beneath the skin.

SUBSTRATE

The base on which an organism lives; a substance upon which an enzyme acts; a source of reactive material.

SUCCINIC ACID

An intermediate product in the Krebs cycle.

SUCCOTASH

A mixture of corn and beans with some milk and butter added. The beans may be either string, butter, or lima. It makes a good combination of cereal and beans together, and a more complete protein.

SUCRASE

An enzyme present in intestinal lining cells which acts on sucrose to produce glucose and fructose.

(Also see DIGESTION AND ABSORPTION, Table D-8.)

SUCROSE

A disaccharide having the formula $C_{12}H_{22}O_{11}$. It is hydrolyzed to glucose and fructose. Commonly known as cane, beet, or table sugar.

(Also see ADDITIVES; CARBOHYDRATE[S]; and SUGAR.)

SUCROSE ESTERS

Sucrose, table sugar, can form esters with fatty acids like lauric acid and stearic acid. These esters are surface active agents—surfactants, used as additives. An example is sucrose monostearate.

SUGAR

Contents   Page

To most people, sugar is sucrose, the white granular sweetener, obtained from cane and beets, and sold in 1, 5, 10, and 25 lb bags at the supermarket. It contributes virtually pure energy to the diet—16 Calories (kcal) per teaspoonful. To the chemist, sugar includes many carbohydrates such as ribose, glucose, fructose, galactose, lactose, maltose, and sucrose—the chemical combination of the two sugars glucose and fructose. Since sugar is usually recognized as sucrose, the following discussion deals specifically with sucrose; hence, the terms *sugar* and *sucrose* are used inter-changeably. Other sugars, when mentioned, are specified.

SOURCES. Although sucrose is widely distributed in nature in green plants, it is obtained commercially in large quantities from the sugarcane and sugar beet plants.

In 1990, world production of cane and beet sugar totaled over 109 million metric tons; and the 10 leading producing countries, by rank, were: India, U.S.S.R., Cuba, Brazil, China, United States, France, Germany, Thailand, and Australia.[44] That year, these 10 countries produced 60% of the world's cane and beet sugar. The United States produces more than 5.9 million metric tons of sugar annually, it imports 1.8 million metric tons and exports 463,000 metric tons.

In 1990, the United States per capita consumption of refined sugar totaled 64.2 lb *(29.2 kg).*[45]

Sugarcane. Sixty to sixty-two percent of the world's refined sugar is derived from sugarcane—a coarse grass of tropical and semitropical climates. Sugarcane produces stalks 7 to 20 feet *(2 to 7 m)* high and about 2 in. *(5 cm)* in diameter which contain a sugary juice. Most of the cultivated cane today is probably an ancestor of *Saccharum officinarum*, a native of New Guinea.

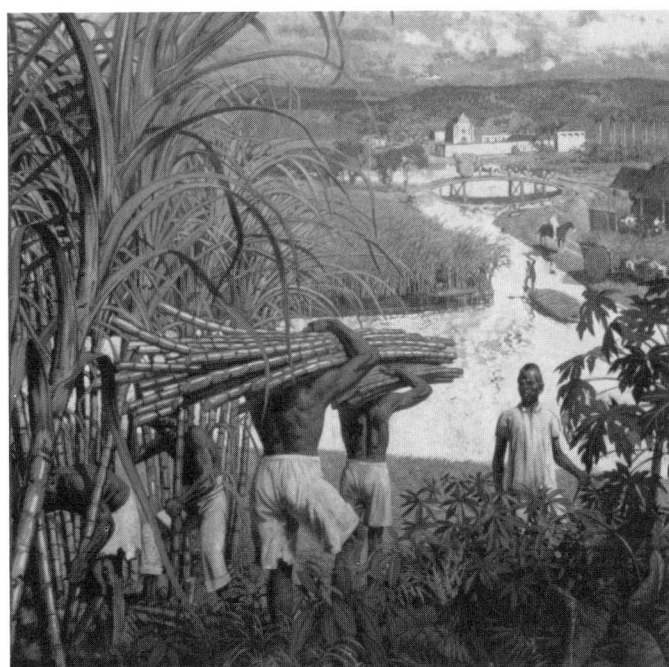

Fig. S-40. Sugar plantation in Brazil. (Courtesy, Field Museum of Natural History, Chicago, Ill.)

ORIGIN AND HISTORY. It is believed that sugarcane culture began in New Guinea. From there, it eventually spread throughout the islands of the South Pacific, and then to Indonesia, Asia, China, and the Philippines. On the second voyage of Christopher Columbus to the New World, he carried sugarcane. However, his transplants failed. But, other explorers who soon followed were able to introduce success-

[44]Data from *FAO Production Yearbook 1990*, FAO/UN, Rome, Italy, Vol. 44, p. 160, Table 69. **Note well:** Annual production fluctuates as a result of weather and profitability of the crop.

[45]*Agricultural Statistics 1991*, USDA, p. 479, Table 672.

fully sugarcane to the West Indies, Brazil, and Mexico. The first sugar mill in the New World was built in 1508 near Santo Domingo. Soon tropical America became the world's greatest sugar producing area. In 1751, Jesuit missionaries brought sugarcane from Haiti to New Orleans, Louisiana. By 1791, the commercial production of sugar had begun in a mill set up by Antonio Mendez. Then in 1795, Etienne de Bore produced the first granulated sugar in what was soon to become part of the United States. With the increased planting and processing of sugarcane in the New World and the development of the sugar beet industry, sugar became accessible to everyone.

WORLD AND U.S. PRODUCTION. In 1990, the worldwide production of sugarcane totaled over one billion metric tons. In the United States, all of the sugarcane is grown in four states—Florida, Hawaii, Louisiana, and Texas—where the yield per acre is about 34 tons on about 791,200 acres (320,324 ha).

PROCESSING. At the sugar mill the cane is washed, shredded, crushed, and passed through a series of heavy rollers (mills) under great pressure to extract the cane juice.

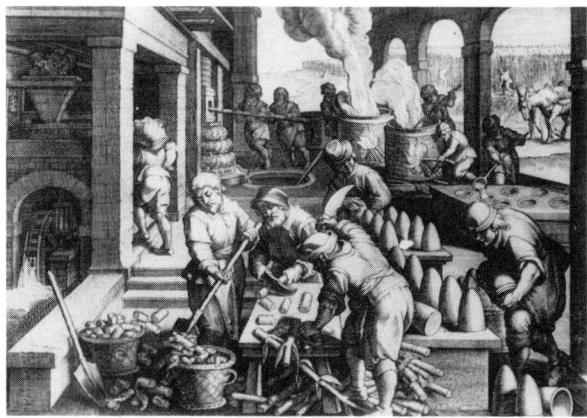

Fig. S-41. An early *sugar factory* where sugar was made from sugarcane and poured into molds. (Courtesy, The Bettmann Archive, Inc., New York, N.Y.)

Each set of rollers (mills) crushes the mat of cane stalks a little harder, pressing out more juice. At the end of the series of rollers, nothing remains but the fibrous part of the cane, termed bagasse. This is used to fuel the mill furnaces or to produce other by-products. Next, the juice is strained, and then pumped to large tanks for clarification by the addition of lime which precipitates impurities. After clarification, the juice is filtered and then transferred through a series of evaporators which remove water. The resulting syrup is then transferred to heated vacuum pans where it is reduced to a mixture of sugar crystals and molasses—massecuite. After the vacuum pans, the thick syrup is cooled and further crystallization occurs. Next this mass is moved to centrifugals which spin at high speeds and separate the sugar and molasses. The sugar is dried, cooled, weighed, and then readied for shipment as raw sugar, about 96% sucrose. The molasses is collected and reworked until no more sugar can be profitably extracted. At this point, usually the third extraction, the molasses—blackstrap molasses—becomes a by-product of the sugarcane industry.

Some raw sugar, in which part of the natural molasses remains in the crystals, is marketed and consumed as raw sugar. But most of it is further refined to produce granulated white sugar.

Raw sugar is an economical form in which to ship sugar in bulk to refineries where it is washed to remove the molasses, and dissolved in water. This syrup is then filtered, decolorized, crystallized in vacuum pans, and centrifuged to remove the sugar crystals which are then dried, screened, and packaged as the familiar granulated white sugar. The crystallization process is repeated as long as extractable sugar remains in the syrup. Brown sugar consists of the sugar crystals in the molasses syrup remaining after the granulated white sugar has been removed, although some commercial brown sugar is prepared by adding molasses back to the refined white sugar. Brown sugar is actually a mass of fine crystals covered with a film of brown, highly refined, molasses-flavored syrup. Brown sugar is not usually made from sugar beets due to the strong flavor of sugar beet molasses.

BY-PRODUCTS. The principal by-products of sugarcane processing are bagasse and molasses. Bagasse is used as a fuel for the sugar mill furnaces, and for the manufacture of paper products and building boards. In some areas, bagasse is ammoniated and used as cattle feed. Also, bagasse has been used effectively as a carrier of molasses for cattle feed. Molasses may contain up to 50% sugar. It is used either for livestock feed, for alcohol production, or for yeast production, which is subsequently manufactured into food for humans and livestock. Also, some molasses is sold for human consumption, and some is used to make rum. Cane wax and aconitic acid are also recovered during the processing of sugarcane. Cane wax is used in the manufacture of polishes, cosmetics, and paper coatings, while a derivative of aconitic acid is used in the manufacture of plastics.

(Also see MOLASSES; and SINGLE-CELL PROTEIN.)

Sugar Beet. Sugar beets rank second to sugarcane as a source of sugar. The sugar beet is a biennial plant. During the first year, it produces the fleshy root which contains 13 to 22% sugar. Hence, sugar beets are harvested and the sugar extracted following the first growing season. The scientific name for the sugar beet is *Beta vulgaris*, a newcomer as a world sugar source.

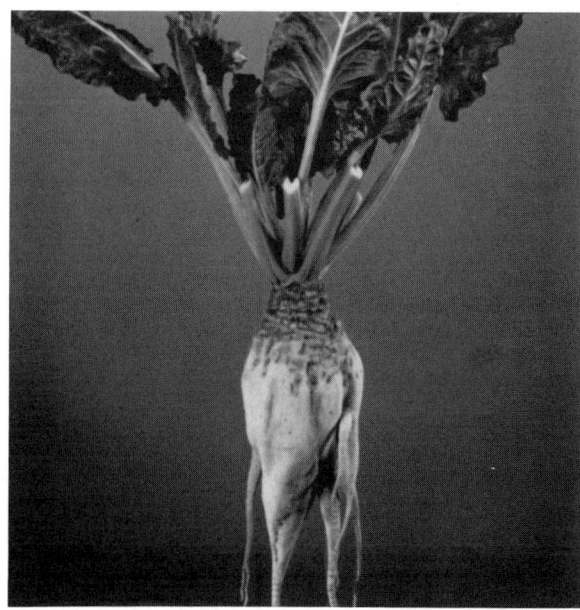

Fig. S-42. The sugar plant. (Courtesy, Field Museum of Natural History, Chicago, Ill.)

ORIGIN AND HISTORY. The sugar beet was cultivated in ancient times in southern Europe and North Africa. During the middle of the 18th century, a practical method for extracting sugar from beets was developed. Following this discovery, sugar beet culture spread into France, Austria, Hungary, and Russia. The world's first sugar beet factory was built in Germany in 1803.

During the middle of the 19th century, the sugar beet was brought to the United States, where the first successful beet sugar processing plant was built in 1870 at Alvarado, California, by E. H. Dyer. Today, sugar beets are grown in 17 states where the soil and climate are favorable.

WORLD AND U.S. PRODUCTION. In 1990, the worldwide production of sugar beets totaled 305.9 million metric tons, of which the United States accounted for only 25 million metric tons, or 8%. The leading U.S. sugar beet-producing states, by rank, are: Minnesota, Idaho, California, Michigan, and North Dakota.

PROCESSING. The major difference between processing sugarcane and sugar beets is that sugar beet processing is a single, continuous process. Upon arrival at a sugar factory, the beets are thoroughly washed and then shredded. The shreds are soaked in tanks of circulating hot water. This allows the diffusion of about 97% of the soluble sugar into the water. Next the shreds are pressed to squeeze out all of the sugary water. The squeezed shreds are called pulp, which is a by-product of the sugar beet industry. The sugar solution or *raw juice* contains about 10 to 15% sugar and many nonsugar substances. Clarification of the sugar solution is accomplished by the application of lime, carbon dioxide, and eventually sulfur dioxide. The sugar solution is filtered several times to remove sediments. Next the juice is concentrated by boiling, which promotes crystallization of the sucrose. Centrifuges separate the sugar crystals from the liquid portion or molasses. The molasses is subjected to additional crystallizations, but eventually it becomes a by-product. The sugar at this point is raw sugar and it is subjected to further refining which involves repeated washings and recrystallizations and decolorization until it is pure white and nearly 100% sucrose. At this stage, beet sugar and cane sugar are identical. However, for years beet sugar was considered inferior, and sold at a price disadvantage.

BY-PRODUCTS. All of the by-products of the sugar beet industry can be used as livestock feeds. The resulting beet pulp can be fed wet, or it can be ensiled or dried. Molasses is often added to beet pulp to increase the energy content. Furthermore, beet tops and crowns—very top portion of the beet—are relished by livestock. These can be fed fresh, dried, or ensiled.

NUTRITIONAL VALUE OF SUGAR. During digestion, sugar—sucrose—is split by the digestive enzyme, sucrase, into its two single sugars, glucose and fructose. Both of these sugars are easily used by the body for the production of energy since fructose is eventually converted to glucose. One ounce (28 g) of refined granulated sugar provides the body with 109 Calories (kcal) of energy and little else. Refined sugar is a concentrated form of energy. One ounce of brown sugar also provides nearly as much energy (106 kcal/oz) and small amounts of calcium, phosphorus, sodium, magnesium, potassium, and iron—hardly enough to contribute to our requirements.

Assuming our yearly consumption of sugar to be about 64.5 lb (29.3 kg), then each day we supply approximately 306 Calories (kcal) of our daily energy requirement from refined sugar—sucrose. For an average man, that is 10.5% of the recommended daily intake; for an average woman, it is 14%.

OTHER SOURCES OF SUGAR. Production and consumption of beet and cane sugar are so enormous that other sources are dwarfed, but several other important sugar sources or sweetening agents do exist. Other sugar sources are: maple sugar, palm sugar, sorghum, honey and plant nectar, and starch hydrolysis. A discussion of each of these follows:

• **Maple Sugar**—Making sugar from the sugar maple, *Acer saccharum*, was practiced by the American Indians long before there were any settlers. Early in the spring, the Northeast Indians tapped the hard maple trees by gashing them with their tomahawks, and then collecting the sap in a birch bark dish. By continually adding heated rocks, they evaporated the sap down to a thick, dark syrup. It was a rather crude, but effective, process. Upon arriving in the New World, the early settlers soon learned the skill from the Indians, and improved upon the Indian system by using iron drill bits to tap the tree and copper or iron kettles to evaporate the sap to syrup and sugar.

Even today, in the late winter or early spring when the sap flow begins, sugar maple trees—a common forest tree of the northeastern United States—are tapped. Large stands of maple trees are called *sugar bushes.* The sap of the sugar maple is about 95% water, and 15 to 20 gal (57 to 76 liter) of sap yields about 2 qt (1.9 liter) of maple syrup. Sugar in the sap is mainly sucrose. During the winter, some of the starch that the tree made the previous summer and stored in its roots is converted to sugar. When the sap begins to rise in the spring, the sugar is carried along. Sap flows for an average of 34 days when warm sunny days are fol-lowed by cool crisp nights.

Although collecting and processing sap have changed some since colonial days, gathering sugar from the maple is picturesque and truly American. Today, power drills are used to bore holes 2 to 3 in. (4.1 to 7.6 cm) deep in the trunk of the maple about 3 ft (1 m) above the ground. The number of holes varies with the size of the tree. Large trees, over 2 ft (0.6 m) in diameter, can be tapped in four or more locations. These holes usually heal by midsummer. Once the hole is drilled a spike is inserted and a pail hung below it. Sometimes the rate of flow is better than one drop per second. Collection of sap is a daily operation by hand using a sap-yoke with pails hung from its ends, by sleds, by wagons, or by gravity piping using plastic pipes connected to the hole in the tree and transporting to a single collection point.

The final stages of processing occur in the sugarhouse. Immediately after the sap is collected, it is strained. Then it is boiled in shallow aluminum evaporating pans which are 20 to 30 ft (6.2 to 9.2 m) long. The sap is boiled down to a specific thickness for maple syrup. Still more boiling produces maple sugar. A good tree yields up to 40 gal (152 liter) of sap in a season, but 30 to 50 gal (114 to 190 liter) of sap are required to make 1 gal (3.8 liter) of syrup, depending upon the quality of the sap. It is the boiling which gives maple syrup its characteristic flavor.

Nowadays, maple sugar and syrup are rather a treat and a luxury, but for the Indians and colonists they were important and abundant. Production of maple sugar increased in the colonies until about 1860, when cane sugar began to take its place. But, even today, about 1 million gal (3.8 million liters) of maple syrup, plus 1 million lb (0.45 million kg) of maple sugar are produced in the United States every year—some for home use and some for commercial use—almost entirely from wild trees.

The composition of maple sugar and maple syrup are given in Food Composition Table F-21. Maple sugar contains about 98 Calories (kcal) of energy per ounce and several macrominerals, while maple syrup contains about 71 Calories (kcal) of energy per ounce and several macrominerals. Both are slightly less concentrated sources of sugar than refined sugar.

(Also see MAPLE SYRUP.)

• **Palm sugar**—In tropical regions of the world, obtaining sugar from several species of palm is an important village industry. Collecting the sap from the sugar palm is an old practice in India and in the eastern tropics. The sap is collected from the stalk of the male flower rather than from a hole in the trunk as practiced with maple trees. At the time of collection, the sap is 10 to 16% sucrose. To process the sap, it is evaporated much the same way as maple sap until it becomes a thick syrup containing sucrose crystals. It may be crudely centrifuged or poured into molds to form small cakes, a product known as *jaggery*.

• **Sorghum**—Generally, sorghum is considered a grain, forage, or silage crop, but some sorghum is sweet. Sweet sorghum, or sorgo, has a tall, sweet, juicy stalk that can be used for syrup and sugar production. In some countries, the sweet stalks of sorghum are chewed by the natives. The juice contains about 12% sugar. In the United States, sorghum syrup is a distinctly flavored, mild, sweet, light amber-colored syrup. It is a specialty product of the southeastern United States. Although seldom carried beyond the syrup stage, the technology exists for converting sweet sorghum to sugar. Thus, sweet sorghum could serve as a supplementary crop for the sugarcane and sugar beet industries.

The composition of sorghum syrup is given in Food Composition Table F-21. It contains about 73 Calories (kcal) of energy per ounce, several of the macrominerals, and some iron.

(Also see SORGHUM.)

• **Honey and plant nectars**—Honey is essentially an invert sugar, a mixture of equal portions of the monosaccharides, glucose, and fructose. Bees collect plant nectar which contains sucrose, contribute an enzyme to invert the sucrose, and evaporate the water to produce the honey they store in combs. Man has learned to exploit this instinct of the honeybees.

Nutritionally, honey provides energy—about 86 Calories (kcal) per ounce—plus traces of minerals and vitamins, and 14 to 19% water. The composition of honey is given in Food Composition Table F-21.

(Also see HONEY.)

• **Starch hydrolysis**—Starch from any starch source—rice, corn, and other grains, and potatoes—may be broken down into its component sugar, either enzymatically or with dilute acids. The most familiar example in the United States is corn syrup (Karo). Complete hydrolysis of starch yields glucose or dextrose. Corn syrup and dextrose (corn sugar) are widely used in food products. Crystallized dextrose is pure energy. One ounce supplies 120 Calories (kcal) of energy. Each year, the foods we eat contain about 71.9 lb (32.7 kg) of corn sugar and 22 lb (10 kg) of corn starch.

(Also see CORN MILLING, WET MILLING AND DRY MILLING; STARCH; and SYRUPS.)

• **Naturally occurring**—Of course, all sugar occurs naturally in some form or another before being processed. Many raw fruits and some vegetables contain sugar—sucrose, fructose, and glucose.

Also, one other sugar—a nonplant sugar—is derived from an important food source. Milk sugar or lactose is present as 4.5% of whole cow's milk and 7.5% of human breast milk.

(Also see CARBOHYDRATE[S]; and MILK AND MILK PRODUCTS, section on "Carbohydrates in Milk.")

CONSUMPTION AND USE OF SUGAR. Sugar comes from a variety of sources, and the overall consumption of sugar from all sources is about 137.5 lb (63 kg) per person per year. Of this total, about 64.2 lb (29 kg) comes from sucrose or table sugar and 73 lb (33 kg) from corn syrup, honey, and other sweeteners. That translates into a per capita consumption of 658 empty Calories per day!

Most homes maintain a supply of sugar for use in baking, cooking, and sweetening, but a large share of the sugar consumed is derived from food products. Sugar is classified as a food additive, and on the basis of intake it is the number one food additive. Sugar—glucose, fructose, sucrose, corn syrup, and invert sugar—is employed as a food additive to make the aroma or taste of a food more agreeable or pleasurable. Sugar of one kind or another is commonly used in the following: cereals, baked goods, candies, processed meats, processed foods, and soft drinks. Table S-13 shows the level of sugar contained in some common foods.

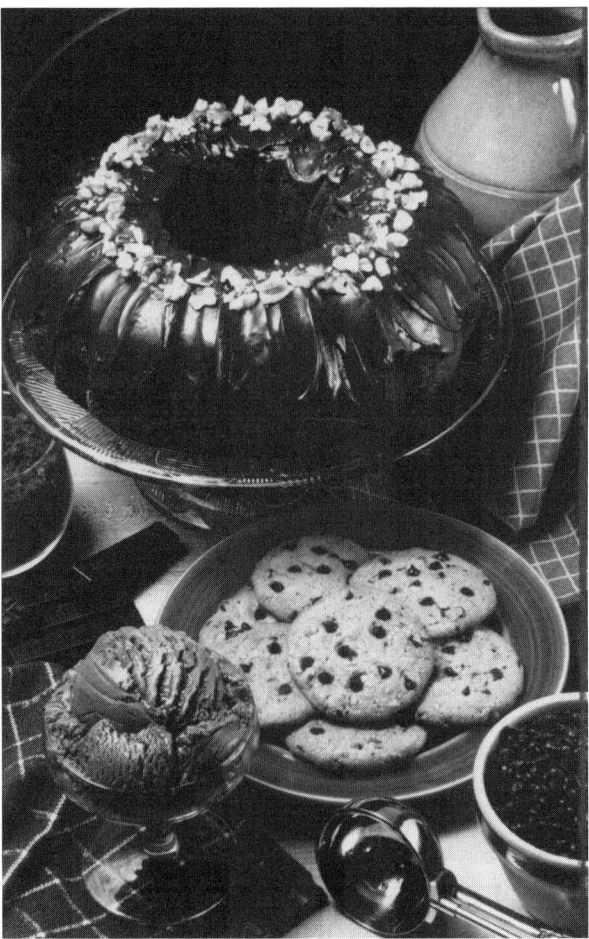

Fig. S-43. Some uses of sugar. (Courtesy, Hershey Food Corp., Hershey, Pa.)

TABLE S-13
SUGAR CONTENT OF
SOME CANNED OR PACKAGED FOODS[1]

Food	Sugar
	(%)
Nondairy creamer	57-65
Ready-to-eat cereals[2]	1-56
Milk chocolate candy	44-51
Brownies	50
Chocolate cake	36
Salad dressings	7-30
Ketchup	29
Ice cream	21
Peaches, canned	7-18
Yogurt	14
Crackers	12
Fruit juice drink	12
Corn, canned	11
Cola-type beverages	9-10
Peanut butter	9

[1]Values from *CNI Weekly Report,* Vol. 4, May 2, 1974, and *Consumer Reports,* March 1978, pp. 136-141.

[2]For more information also see BREAKFAST CEREALS, section headed "The Sugared-Breakfast-Cereal Binge."

Today, the use of sugar in households is less than one-half of what it was at the beginning of this century, but the use of sugar by industry in processing foods and beverages is three times greater. Industry uses about 70% of the refined sugar.

Sugar is available in a variety of forms the more common of which follow:

• **Granulated sugar**—The white, refined sugar used in the home and in commerce comes from sugarcane and sugar beets. It is 99.9% pure, and keeps indefinitely. Granulated sugar is classified according to crystal size as fine, or ultrafine. Three other forms of granulated sugar are produced mainly for industrial use: very fine, medium-coarse, and coarse.

• **Powdered sugars**—Powdered sugars are a form of sucrose made by grinding the sugar crystals. They are used for icings, frostings, uncooked candies, and for dusting on finished products. Confectioners' sugars are usually packed with small amounts of cornstarch to prevent caking.

• **Raw sugar**—This is the tan to brown product obtained from the evaporation of sugarcane juice. FDA regulations prohibit the sale of raw sugar unless the impurities—dirt, insect fragments, etc.—are removed.

• **Turbinado sugars**—A partially refined sugar which is similar in appearance to raw sugar. Turbinado sugar is sold for consumption without further refining.

• **Brown sugar**—So called *soft* sugar or brown sugar is a mass of fine crystals covered with a film of highly-refined, colored, molasses-flavored syrup. It is valued primarily for flavor and color. Four grades are commonly available for food manufacturing—Numbers 6, 8, 10, and 13. The higher numbers are darker and more flavorful. Brown sugar contains 91 to 96% sucrose.

• **Invert sugar**—When a solution of sugar is heated in the presence of an acid or treated with enzymes, the sugar breaks up into the two sugars of simpler chemical structure that characterize sucrose as a disaccharide. One is glucose, commercially called dextrose. The other is fructose, commercially called levulose. This mixture of dextrose and levulose in equal weights, is known as invert sugar.

Invert sugar is sold only in liquid form and is sweeter than sucrose. It helps prolong the freshness of baked goods and confections and is useful in preventing food shrinkage.

• **Liquid sugars**—Sugar syrups or liquid sugars are clear solutions that contain a highly purified sugar, of which there are many grades.

• **Levulose**—Fructose, or levulose as it is known commercially, is one of the two components of invert sugar. It is intensely sweet and highly soluble, and is produced in small quantities mainly for pharmaceutical applications.

• **Dextrose (Glucose)**—Dextrose is the commercial name for glucose, the second component of invert sugar. Dextrose is also called corn sugar. It is made commercially from starch by the action of heat and acids, or enzymes. Two types of refined dextrose are available commercially: dextrose hydrate, containing 9% by weight of water of crystallization; and anhydrous dextrose, containing less than 0.5% of water. Dextrose hydrate is most often used by food processors. It is 74% as sweet as sugar.

• **Lactose**—Milk sugar, or lactose, is generally made from whey and skim milk. Compared to sugar, it is only slightly sweet and markedly less soluble in water. It is used primarily in pharmaceuticals.

• **Maltose**—Malt sugar is formed from starch by the action of yeast. Maltose is much less sweet than sugar. Preparations containing maltose, often in mixture with dextrose, are used in bread-baking and in infant foods.

• **Corn syrup**—This is a viscous liquid containing maltose, dextrin, dextrose, and other polysaccharides—glucose chains of various lengths. Unlike sugar, it has a distinct flavor other than sweetness. Corn syrup is the product of the incomplete hydrolysis of starch; it is usually obtained by heating cornstarch with a dilute acid or by enzymatic action. The degree of conversion is expressed by the *dextrose equivalent* (D.E.) which is, in effect, the measure of sweetness in the syrup. Even high conversion syrups are substantially less sweet than sugar. Corn syrup can control crystallization in candy-making, and has moisture-containing properties. A special corn syrup on the market is a *high fructose corn syrup* (HFCS) which is made by treating high conversion corn syrup with enzymes. The enzymes convert some of the glucose to fructose.

• **Molasses**—Molasses consists of concentrates extracted from sugar-bearing plants, such as the thick liquid produced in the refining of sugar. It contains other substances that occur naturally in the plants as well as sugar. The highest grade is edible molasses. It is most often seen as a table syrup or as an ingredient in a blend of table syrups. It is suitable for use in gingerbread, spice and fruit cakes, rye and whole wheat breads, cookies, baked beans, and certain candies. Edible molasses provides nutrition in the form of sugar and certain minerals—primarily iron. Blackstrap molasses is the final molasses in the sugar manufacturing process.

(Also see MOLASSES.)

• **Honey**—Honey is essentially an invert sugar, but it contains a slight excess of fructose. It is used in food products where its distinctive flavor is desired.

• **Maple sugar and syrup**—Both are products of the condensation of the sap of the maple tree. However, their characteristic flavor is not manifested until the sap has been boiled. Maple sugar and syrup are also used in food products for their distinctive taste and aroma.

Whether sugar is utilized in the home or in the food industry, its properties have made it (1) the world's most widely used sweetener, and (2) one of the most versatile ingredients in food preparation. Six of sugar's qualities are particularly important; namely—

1. Sweetening.
2. Moistening—sugar absorbs and holds moisture.
3. Solubility—sugar is completely soluble in water.
4. Coloring (caramelization)—sugar turns dark brown when heated and thus adds to the browning of baked goods.
5. Preservation—a concentrated sugar solution acts as a preservative; it inactivates microorganisms.
6. Crystallization.

(Also see ADDITIVES; and CARBOHYDRATE[S].)

SUGAR AS A FACTOR IN HUMAN DISEASES.

Recently, charges have been leveled at sugar as a causative factor in some human diseases. Some studies have claimed that sugar intake is related to the development of coronary heart disease, diabetes mellitus, obesity, and dental caries. To date, however, any causative role of sugar in coronary heart disease is far from certain, and as for diabetes mellitus no proven direct links exist. As for obesity, any time the amount of energy flowing into our body exceeds the amount flowing out, the remainder is deposited as triglycerides in adipose tissue—fat. Excess energy derived from fats, carbohyrates, and proteins may all contribute to the deposition of fat. No reliable evidence exists that implicates any specific nutrient as contributing excess energy—rather, excessive intake creates the problem. Dental caries—tooth decay—is influenced by such factors as structural resistance of the teeth, oral hygiene, oral microflora, salivary flow, and composition of the diet. Nevertheless, indirect proof has been obtained implicating sugar. In China and Ethiopia, where the consumption of sugar is low, the incidence of tooth decay is also very low, while in Australia, Hawaii, and French Polynesia where sugar consumption is high, so is the incidence of dental caries. A number of studies have shown a firm link between sugar exposure and tooth decay. However, the manner of exposure and dental hygiene make a large contribution to the development and prevention of dental caries. Frequent exposure to a solid and/or sticky form of sugar between meals has resulted in a high incidence of dental caries, while taking sugar with meals, followed by quick brushing or rinsing, prevents the accumulation of bacteria and plaque, and removes the substrates for acid production by bacteria.

(Also see DENTAL HEALTH, NUTRITION, AND DIET; DIABETES MELLITUS; HEART DISEASE; and OBESITY.)

Until more definitive evidence can be gained, the real danger of sugar seems to be its attractiveness to the human taste buds—its palatability. Hence, excesses are often eaten, displacing more nutritious foods from the diet and possibly creating a diet low in other essential nutrients.

(Also see CARBOHYDRATE[S].)

SUGAR DOCTOR

Sucrose crystallizes. Since many foods, especially confectionery products like creams, fondants, and fudge, are dependent upon a balance between sugar crystals and sugar syrup for their texture characteristics, a sugar doctor helps prevent, or helps control, the degree of sucrose crystalliza-

tion, thus extending the shelf-life by maintaining the desired consistency of the product. Often invert sugar is employed as a sugar doctor. Invert sugar may be added during the candy making process or developed from sucrose during the candy making process. Invert sugar "doctors" because it crystallizes more slowly and forms smaller crystals than sucrose. Glycerine, sorbitol, and the polyhydric alcohols also are used to control crystal formation.

(Also see INVERT SUGAR; and SUGAR, section on "Consumption and Use of Sugar.")

SUGAR, ICING

Icing for cakes is made from a grade of sugar termed powdered sugar or confectioners' sugar; hence, the name icing sugar.

(Also see DESSERTS; and SUGAR, section on "Consumption and Use of Sugar.")

SUGARING OF DRIED FRUITS

The whitish deposits of sugar that are sometimes seen on the surface of dried fruits are formed during drying when water containing dissolved sugars flows from the inside of the fruit to the surface. Hot air at the surface of the fruit causes the water to evaporate, leaving behind the sugars in the form of tiny crystals.

SUGARING OFF

The process of making maple sugar by boiling off the water from the maple sap. The early spring of the year, when warm days follow cool nights, is the sugaring off season in the northeastern and north central states and eastern Canada. During this time of year, the sap begins to flow and maple trees are tapped for collection. Traditionally, sugaring off gatherings where held at the sugarhouse—the shed where the sap is boiled—there neighbors helped in the making and sampling of the maple sugar. For the production of 1 gal (*3.8 liter*) of maple syrup, 30 to 50 gal (*114 to 190 liter*) of maple sap are required; and 1 gal of maple syrup yields about 8 lb (*3.6 kg*) of maple sugar.

(Also see MAPLE SYRUP.)

SULFA DRUGS (SULFONAMIDE DRUGS)

Any of a group of compounds characterized by the presence of both sulfur and nitrogen, with high specificity for certain bacteria. Among the best known are sulfanilamide, sulfadiazine, sulfapyridine, sulfamerazine, and sulfasoxazole.

SULFHYDRYL GROUP

The -SH radical that forms high-energy bonds in chemical compounds, which are similar to the high-energy bonds formed by phosphates in compounds such as ATP.

SULFUR

Sulfur is a nonmetallic element that occurs widely in nature; it is found in every cell of the body and is essential for life itself, mostly as a component of three important amino acids—cystine, cysteine, and methionine. Also, it is a part of two vitamins—thiamin and biotin, and it is present in saliva and bile, and in the hormone, insulin. Approximately 0.25% of the body weight (or 175 g in the adult male) and 10% of the mineral content of the body are sulfur. It is sometimes referred to as nature's *beauty mineral*, because it is reputed to keep the hair glossy and the complexion clear and youthful.

HISTORY. The name is derived from the Latin word *sulphurum*. Sulfur has been used since ancient times. It was often called brimstone (burning stone); and ignited sulfur is mentioned in the earlier records of many countries as having been used in religious ceremonies and for purifying (fumigating) buildings. The early medical books of Dioscorides of Greece and Pliny the Elder mention sulfur; and the Romans used it in medicine and in warfare. Alchemists recognized sulfur as a mineral substance that could be melted and burned. It was first classified by Antoine Lavoisier in 1777.

ABSORPTION, METABOLISM, AND EXCRETION. The small intestine is the major site of sulfur absorption.

During digestion, the sulfur-containing amino acids are split off from protein and taken into the portal circulation. Sulfur is stored in every cell of the body, with the highest concentration found in the hair, skin, and nails.

Excess sulfur is excreted in the urine and in the feces. About 85 to 90% of the sulfur excreted in the urine is in the organic form, derived almost entirely from the metabolism of the sulfur amino acids. Since inorganic sulfates are poorly absorbed, it follows that the fecal excretion of sulfur is about equal to the inorganic sulfur content of the diet.

FUNCTIONS OF SULFUR. Sulfur has an important relationship with protein. It is a necessary component of the sulfur-containing amino acids methionine, cystine, and cysteine. Sulfur is present in keratin, the tough protein substance in the skin, nails, and hair; and it appears to be necessary for the synthesis of collagen.

As a component of biotin, sulfur is important in fat metabolism; as a component of thiamin and insulin, it is important in carbohydrate metabolism; as a component of coenzyme A, it is important in energy metabolism; as a component of certain complex carbohydrates, it is important in various connective tissues. Insulin and glutathione, regulators of energy metabolism, contain sulfur. Also, sulfur compounds combine with toxic substances such as phenols and cresols and convert them to a nontoxic form, following which they are excreted in the urine.

DEFICIENCY SYMPTOMS. Sulfur deficiencies are manifested primarily in retarded growth because of sulfur's association with protein synthesis.

INTERRELATIONSHIPS. Sulfur is related to the amino acids methionine, cystine, and cysteine, and to biotin, thiamin, insulin, coenzyme A, certain complex carbohydrates, insulin, and glutathione.

RECOMMENDED DAILY ALLOWANCE OF SULFUR. Sulfur requirements are primarily those involving amino acid nutrition.

There are no recommended allowances for sulfur because it is assumed that the sulfur requirements are met when the methionine and cystine intakes are adequate.

TOXICITY. Except in rare, inborn errors of metabolism where the utilization of the sulfur-containing amino acids is abnormal, excess organic sulfur intake is essentially nonexistent. However, inorganic sulfur can be dangerous if ingested in large amounts.

SOURCES OF SULFUR. Inorganic sulfur is poorly utilized by man and other monogastrics. So, the sulfur needs of the body are largely met from organic complexes, notably the amino acids of proteins, rather than from inorganic sources. The sulfur content of protein foods varies from 0.4 to 1.6%, depending on the quality of the protein. The

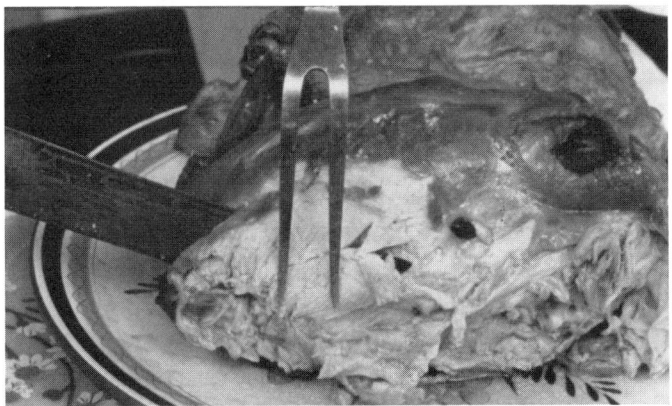

Fig. S-44. Poultry—a good source of sulfur. (Courtesy, USDA)

average mixed diet contains about 1% sulfur. Good food sources of sulfur are: cheese, eggs, fish, grains and grain products, legumes, meat, nuts, and poultry.

Unfortunately, few foods have been analyzed for sulfur, with the result that sulfur content is not given in Food Composition Table F-21. So, a special table, Table S-14, was prepared for this book; this gives some good sources of sulfur.

(Also see MINERAL[S], Table M-25.)

TABLE S-14
SOME FOOD SOURCES OF SULFUR AND THEIR CALORIC CONTENT

Food	Sulfur	Energy
	(mg/100g)	(kcal/100 g)
Soybean flour	410	386
Brewers' yeast	380	283
Peanuts, roasted, salted	380	582
Molasses, blackstrap	350	230
Pork chops, lean, roasted	300	254
Brazil nuts	290	715
Turkey, light or dark meat, roasted	290	190
Sardines, canned in oil, drained solids	310	246
Beef, variety of lean cuts	270	220
Chicken, light or dark meat, fried	255	210
Lamb, shoulder roast, lean	240	205
Wheat germ	240	391
Navy beans, dry	230	340
Cheese, natural cheddar	230	402
Soybeans, dry	220	405
Wheat bran	220	353
Salmon, canned	220	124
Oats, whole grain	210	283
Beans, lima, dry	200	359
Wheat flour	190	345
Rice bran	180	276
Rice polish	170	265
Wheat, whole grain	160	360
Barley, whole grain	150	305
Almonds	150	598
Sorghum, whole grain	150	339
Eggs, chicken	140	157
Corn, whole grain	120	348
Cabbage, raw	110	24
Buttermilk, dehydrated	80	387
Alfalfa leaf meal, dehydrated	60	215
Peas, raw	50	84
Rice, whole grain	50	363
Sweet potato	40	82
Turnip greens, raw	40	28
Turnip, raw	40	28
Milk, skim	30	34
Rutabaga, raw	30	46
Beet, common, red, raw	20	43
Carrot, raw	20	42
Potato, raw	20	76
Apple, raw	10	58

SULFUR AMINO ACIDS

The two amino acids, cystine and methionine, contain sulfur in their chemical structure. Methionine is an essential amino acid; cystine is not.

(Also see AMINO ACID[S]; and PROTEIN[S].)

SULFUR DIOXIDE (SO₂)

A colorless, nonflammable gas derived from burning sulfur. Its odor is pungent and suffocating. The ancient Egyptians and Romans used the fumes of burning sulfur in their wine making. Thus, they were utilizing the antimicrobial properties of sulfur dioxide. It also prevents enzymatic and nonenzymatic decolorization of some foods. In the food industry, sulfur dioxide is applied to dehydrated fruits and vegetables; to increase storage life, preserve color and flavor, and aid in the retention of ascorbic acid and carotene. In wine making, it is employed first to sanitize the equipment, then at several stages as an antioxidant, and finally during bulk storage to prevent bacterial spoilage.

SULTANAS

This term is used differently in the United States and Europe. Hence, the two major meanings follow:

• In the United States, the term designates the raisins produced *without* sulfuring from sultana grapes. They are used mainly by commercial food manufacturers and food service establishments.

• In Europe, this term refers to golden seedless raisins which are produced from Thompson Seedless grapes or a related variety of grape by (1) washing the freshly harvested fruit, (2) dipping it in a solution to crack the skin, (3) sulfuring the grapes by exposure to the fumes of burning sulfur, and (4) drying the sulfured fruit in heating chambers. In the Mediterranean region, a delicate white wine is also made from sultana grapes.

SUN-CURED

Material dried by exposure in open air to the direct rays of the sun.

SUNFLOWER *Helianthus annuus*

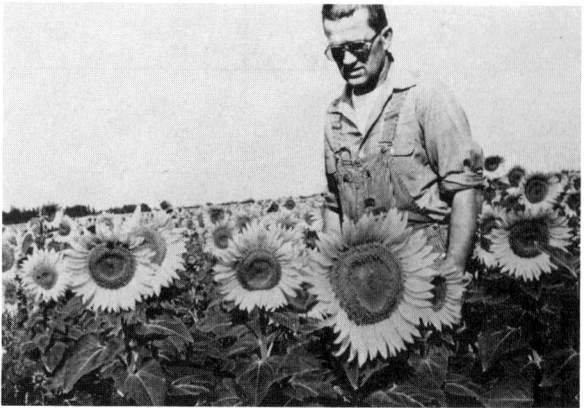

Fig. S-45. Sunflowers at bloom stage. (Courtesy, Sunflower Association of America, Fargo, N.D.)

Sunflowers belong to the composite family *Compositae*. The common annual is genus *Helianthus*, species *H. annuus*.

United States sunflower production has spiraled in recent years largely because of two breakthroughs which vastly improved oil production: (1) the development in the 1960s of sunflower varieties with an oil content of more than 40%—a ⅓ increase over earlier varieties; and (2) the development of hybrid sunflowers in the 1970s, which boosted yields another 25%.

Sunflower oil is higher in polyunsaturates than corn oil and is much more stable than safflower oil. Thus, it has an edge over these two competitors for use in premium grade margarine and in cooking and salad oils.

ORIGIN AND HISTORY. The sunflower is one of the few annual cultivated plants which was first domesticated in the United States, although there is evidence that this honor should go to, or be shared with, Peru and Mexico. Its culture for food by the Indians was at an advanced state when the colonists came to America.

In the Soviet Union, superior varieties were selected, and in the 1830s a method was developed for obtaining oil from the seed. The present-day interest in sunflowers in Europe, and elsewhere, stems primarily from the work of the Russian scientist, Dr. V. S. Pustovoit, at the Sunflower Research Institute, near Krasnodar, U.S.S.R. Today, some of the newer varieties in the Soviet Union produce up to 60% oil, and 95% of the nation's sunflower seed averages 50% oil content. Eighty percent of the vegetable oil produced in the Soviet Union comes from sunflowers.

Although U.S. production of sunflowers for oil started in the 1940s, present-day interest in sunflowers began in 1962 when new high-oil varieties were introduced.

WORLD AND U.S. PRODUCTION. The global growth in the 1960s of sunflower seed production and of the sunflower seed and oil trade is the most impressive of any in the fat and oil industry. In 1990, sunflowers ranked third in the world among sources of edible vegetable oils, exceeded only by soybean oil and rape oil.

World production of sunflower seed totals about 22 million metric tons annually; and the 10 leading sunflower-producing countries, by rank, are: U.S.S.R., Argentina, France, China, Spain, United States, Turkey, Hungary, South Africa, and Romania. The U.S.S.R. accounts for ⅓ of the world's sunflower production.[46]

In addition to being the world's leading producer of sunflower seed, the U.S.S.R. is the world's largest exporter of sunflower oil. Sunflowers are grown throughout a wide geographical area of the country, and generally occupy about 11.4 million acres (4.6 mil ha).

The United States produces about one million metric tons of sunflower seed annually; and the four leading sunflower-producing states, by rank, are: North Dakota, South Dakota, Minnesota, and Kansas.[47]

PROCESSING SUNFLOWER SEED. The sunflower seed is a four-sided, flattened fruit or achene. It has a dry, brittle hull which ranges in color from white, white and grey

[46]Data from *FAO Production Yearbook 1990*, FAO/UN, Rome, Italy, Vol. 44, p. 112, Table 40. **Note well:** Annual production fluctuates as a result of weather and profitability of the crop.

[47]Data from *Agricultural Statistics 1991*, USDA, p. 129, Table 179. **Note well:** Annual production fluctuates as a result of weather and profitability of the crop.

striped, white and black striped, to black. The hull encloses a whitish kernel which has a thin, translucent skin covering or coat.

High-oil-type sunflower seeds are processed to obtain the oil and meal. The separation of the oil may be achieved (1) by direct solvent extraction, (2) by prepress solvent extraction, or (3) by mechanical means (screw pressing).

The steps in processing are: (1) cleaning, (2) dehulling, (3) rolling and cooking, and (4) extracting the oil.

NUTRITIONAL VALUE OF SUNFLOWER SEED.
Composition data on sunflower seed kernels, flour, and oil are given in the Food Composition Table F-21.

A few salient features of the nutritional value of sunflower products follow:

• **Composition of nonoil sunflower seeds for human food**—The seeds are a concentrated source of many nutrients. The oil is desirable in the human diet due to the high linoleic fatty acid content, the essential fatty acid. Their protein content is sufficient to recommend them as a meat substitute; and the nonoil varieties are substantially higher in lysine, an essential amino acid, than the high-oil varieties. Sunflower seeds contain 31% more iron than raisins—a popular source of iron; and they are a good source of the vitamins thiamin and niacin.

• **Composition of the hulls**—The fibrous hulls have only a small percentage of oil and crude protein and contain about 50% crude fiber. Chemically, the hulls are largely lignin, pentosans, and cellulosic constituents.

• **Composition of sunflower meal (sun meal)**—The composition of defatted sunflower meal varies considerably, depending primarily on the method of processing. A typical commercial sunflower meal contains approximately 9.0% water, 45% protein, 3.5% fat, 9.5% fiber, 7.0% ash (mineral), and 26% carbohydrate.

Sunflower meal compares favorably with other oilseed meals as a source of calcium and phosphorus; it runs about 0.46% calcium and 1.47% phosphorus.

The meal is superior to other oilseed meals in vitamin content. It is richer in B-complex vitamins than soybean meal; it is equal in nicotinic acid content to peanut meal, which is rated as an outstanding source; the pantothenic content is similar to soybean meal; and it is a rich source of vitamin A. Sunflower flour is similar to sunflower meal.

The toxic compounds present in several vegetable proteins have not been found in sunflower meal. Also, sunflower meal products cause considerably less flatus (gases) in the digestive tract than soybean meal products.

• **Protein quality**—Table S-15 shows the essential amino acid composition of the protein of sunflower seed kernels and of a typical sunflower meal. Kernels and meal are deficient in lysine, but adequate in the other essential amino acids. It is noteworthy, however, that the amino acids of sunflowers vary with varieties and planting locations.

The main disadvantage of sunflower meal as a source of high-protein human food is that it turns off-color (generally to green or brown) during processing. These off-colors are caused by the reaction of chlorogenic acid at high pH values.

The commercial use of sunflower flour for human food is dependent on the development of low chlorogenic acid varieties and hybrids and efficient procedures for dehulling them.

• **Composition of sunflower oil (sun oil)**—The fatty acid

TABLE S-15
PROFILE OF ESSENTIAL AMINO ACIDS IN SUNFLOWER SEEDS COMPARED TO MILK—A HIGH-QUALITY PROTEIN

Amino Acid	Sunflower Seeds		Cow's Milk[1]
	Kernels	Meal	
	◄──── (mg/g protein) ────►		
Histidine	25	17	27
Isoleucine	55	52	47
Leucine	75	62	95
Lysine	38	38	78
Methionine and cystine	39	34	33
Phenylalanine and tyrosine	81	80	102
Threonine	40	40	44
Tryptophan	15	13	14
Valine	59	52	64

[1]*Recommended Dietary Allowances*, 10th ed., 1989, NRC–National Academy of Sciences, p. 67, Table 6–5. The essential amino acid requirements of infants can be met by supplying 0.79 g of a high-quality protein per pound of body weight (1.7 g/kg body weight) per day.

composition of sunflower oil makes it desirable as an edible oil. Of all oils produced in the United States, sunflower oil strikes the most ideal compromise between the amount of polyunsaturated fatty acids and stability. Its polyunsaturated fatty acid composition is superior to all oils except safflower oil; hence, it offers a popular approach to the prevention and/or cure of cardiovascular diseases. It contains only trace amounts of linolenic acids, which makes it a fairly stable oil. The stability imparts the capacity of the oil to maintain its flavor (not go rancid) and to resist change in viscosity (not congeal or leave deposits on cooking vessels) after prolonged periods of high temperature. The latter characteristic is particularly important to the rapidly growing fast food and snack industries where deep fat frying is used. Oils which can be reused without flavor deterioration and which allow maximum shelf life of products are desired.

TABLE S-16
COMPOSITION OF COMMERCIAL SUNFLOWER OIL

Nutrient		Amount	
		100 g	Tablespoon (13.6 g)
Calories	kcal	884	120
Vitamin E	mg	44.9	6.1
Palmitic acid[1]	g	5.9	.8
Stearic acid[1]	g	4.5	.6
Oleic acid[2]	g	19.5	2.7
Linoleic acid[3]	g	65.7	8.9

[1]Saturated fatty acid.
[2]Monounsaturated fatty acid.
[3]Polyunsaturated fatty acid and the essential fatty acid.

As shown in Table S-16 sunflower oil is relatively low in the saturated fatty acids, palmitic and stearic, but it is rich in the unsaturated fatty acids, oleic and linoleic. The lack of linolenic acid is primarily responsible for its good storage qualities. The oleic and linoleic acid contents of sunflower oil are quite variable, ranging from 13.9 to 60.0% for oleic and from 29.9 to 76.4% for linoleic acid. Seeds grown in cold climates (such as those in central U.S.S.R., Canada, and northern U.S.) contain less oleic acid and more linoleic acid than those grown in warmer areas (such as southern U.S.).

The high linoleic acid content and the high ratio of polyunsaturated to saturated fatty acids suggest that sunflower oil may be useful in the prevention of high blood cholesterol and heart disease. It is noteworthy, however, that the degree of unsaturation of sunflower oil is affected by plant location, climatic conditions during the growing season, and genetics.

SUNFLOWER PRODUCTS AND USES FOR HUMAN FOOD.
Table S-17 presents in summary form the story of sunflower products and uses.

(Also see FLOURS, Table F-13, Special Flours; and OILS, VEGETABLE, Table O-5.)

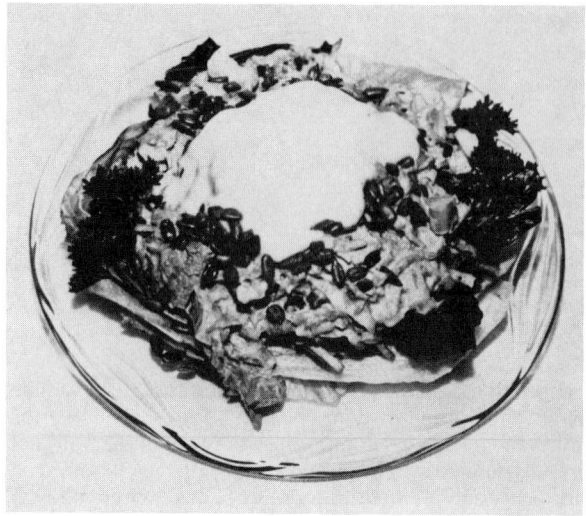

Fig. S-46. Sunflower kernels used in salad. (Courtesy, Sunflower Assn. of America, Fargo, N.D.)

SUPERGLYCINERATED FATS

These are mono- and diglycerides which are the products of interesterification. They are employed as emulsifiers by the food industry.

(Also see INTERESTERIFICATION.)

SUPEROXIDE DISMUTASE (SOD)

An enzyme contained in most cells of the body and in most organisms. It catalyzes the breakdown of superoxide free radicals—oxygen joined by an extra electron—to oxygen and hydrogen peroxide. This protects cells from the toxic effects of oxygen, since these superoxide radicals damage DNA, and age and destroy cells. Deactivation of these superoxide radicals is called dismutation; hence, the name superoxide dismutase. Some chemicals, poor nutrition, shock, and radiation therapy may increase the formation of superoxide radicals. Scientists feel that gaining an understanding of this enzyme may unlock secrets which (1) control the rate of human aging, (2) block tumor formation, and (3) maintain the body's immune system. As an injectable drug, SOD could be used to fight inflammatory diseases. Currently, the FDA has approved SOD for use by veterinarians. Human use is for investigational purposes only. Several European nations permit its use for rheumatoid arthritis, osteoarthritis, urological disorders, and the side effects of radiation treatment. In the United States, claims are sometimes made that SOD will reverse aging and degeneration. However, no firm evidence demonstrates that taking SOD will increase the life span.

TABLE S-17
SUNFLOWER PRODUCTS AND USES FOR HUMAN FOOD

Product	Description	Uses	Comments

Whole seed, with hulls	Whole seed may be:
	1. Dehulled with fingernails or teeth and eaten raw.
	2. Roasted by heating (a) in an oven for 15 min. at 350°F (177°C) or (b) in a frying pan while stirring.
	3. Salted by—
	  a. Soaking the whole seed overnight in salt brine (2 Tbsp salt to 1 cup water), boiled for a few minutes then dried with heat;
	  b. boiling in brine for at least 20 minutes; or
	  c. frying the salted whole seed in edible oil.
		Snack food	Consumers prefer a large seed and kernel with a loose hull to facilitate cracking. Also, they like uniformity, and bright black and white stripes.
			Roasted seeds have a relatively short shelf life because of high oil content and high proportion of polyunsaturated fatty acids.
			Many snack foods contribute little to the diet except calories. Raw or roasted sunflower kernels, with or without salt, are nutritious. They are a valuable source of unsaturated fat, quality protein, and some vitamins and minerals.
			Roasted seeds are very popular in the U.S.S.R.

Whole seed, hulled	Seed dehulled commercially in an impact dehuller, following which the mixed hulls and meats are separated by screening and aspiration. Then the dehulled seed is either— 1. Marketed raw as dehulled sunflower kernels, 2. roasted in sunflower or other vegetable oil, or 3. dry roasted, salted, and vacuum packed.	Considerable attention has been given to the use of hulled seed in candies, salads, cereals, bakery goods, and health foods. As a nut substitute in a number of confectionery and bakery formulas.	Dehulled kernels must be stored under refrigeration.
Sunflower meal and flour	Sunflower meal is the product obtained by grinding the residue that remains after extraction of most of the oil from the seed. Sunflower flour is similar to sunflower meal, except that it is finer and more of the hulls have been removed. Sunflower flour has high protein content, bland flavor, and contains no antinutritive factors.	Sunflower meals and flours have not been used commercially as a protein source for human nutrition in the U.S. Experimentally, sunflower flour has been added to wheat flour at 3 to 20% levels to make breads, griddle cakes, cupcakes, pies, dips, rolls, and candies; without loss in attractiveness, volume, or acceptance, and enhanced by a pleasant distinctive, nutty flavor.	Sunflower proteins are deficient in lysine and isoleucine, but they contain adequate levels of the other essential amino acids for humans. The vitamin B-complex content of defatted sunflower seed flour is superior to the products prepared from wheat germ, corn germ, and soya. A major problem in using sunflower meal in human foods is the presence of hulls and chlorogenic acid in the meal, both of which may cause undesirable discoloration. Hulls also cause excessive bulk and fiber in a food product.
Sunflower oil	Oil of an attractive color and pleasant, faintly nutty flavor	1. Cooking and salad oil. 2. In Europe, it is used extensively in shortening and margarine. 3. For frying foods, popping corn, and other culinary processes that require a liquid oil with a high smoke point. 4. For blending with other vegetable oils. 5. As a cooking fat for potato chip frying. 6. For producing a modified butter with improved low temperature spreadability.	Sunflower oil is a high-quality edible oil, high in the polyunsaturated acid linoleic acid. The oil is considered equal to olive oil and almond oil for table use. Oil from sunflowers produced in the South has a lower linoleic acid content than oil from sunflowers produced in the North; hence, it is more stable. Because of the high ratio of polyunsaturated to saturated fatty acids, sunflower oil possesses serum cholesterol-lowering abilities.

SUPPLEMENTS

Food supplements are foodstuffs used to improve the value of basal foods.

(Also see NUTRITIONAL SUPPLEMENTS.)

SURFACE AREA

The area covered by the exterior of cubes, spheres and cylinders is fairly easy to calculate. However, the area covered by the exterior of the body is not quite as easy to figure due to the variety of body shapes, heights, and weights. Charts and mathematical formulas are available for determining body surface area in relationship to height and weight. It is the body surface area which determines heat loss from the body; therefore, basal metabolism is correlated to surface area.

(Also see BASAL METABOLIC RATE; BODY SURFACE; and METABOLIC RATE.)

SURFACTANT (SURFACE ACTIVE AGENT)

Surface tension is that inward force acting on the surface of a liquid. It is an effect of the forces of attraction existing between the molecules below the surface. Water has a high surface tension compared to alcohol, and mercury has the highest surface tension of any known liquid. The surface tension of a liquid is related to (1) the tendency of a liquid to spread or wet a solid surface, and (2) the ability of a liquid to blend with other liquids. Hence, surface tension plays a role in a variety of processes; for example, emulsification, bubble formation, fabric cleaning, foams, and adhesives. Surface active agents or surfactants reduce the surface tension of a liquid, thereby increasing the wetting or blending ability. There are three categories of surfactants: (1) detergents, (2) wetting agents, and (3) emulsifiers. A variety of surfactants are employed as food additives by the food industry.

SWEETBREADS (THYMUS GLAND)

The sweetbreads, which are considered to be the most delicate of the variety meats, are located in the neck area of young bovines (veal); as the animal matures, they disappear.

SWEET CORN Zea mays saccharata

Varieties of corn grown chiefly for human food and harvested at an immature stage.

(Also see CORN.)

SWEETENING AGENTS

Sweet is a taste sensation—a pleasurable sensation for which man relies upon for his food selection. To satisfy his desire to stimulate the sweet taste sensation, man discovered and learned to keep honey bees. Later, he cultivated sugarcane and sugar beets. But the search for sweet tasting substances continues; primarily, for low-calorie or no-calorie substances which satisfy the taste sensation and are safe to eat.

There are over 200 chemicals known to taste sweet, but many sweet-tasting chemicals present problems such as bitter aftertaste, lack of stability, and toxicity.

Many people desire, or need, to limit their intake of sugar—and not just table sugar (sucrose) alone. Diabetics and individuals cutting down on calories also need to control their intake of monosaccharides such as glucose and fructose.

Any new sweetener should (1) possess a flavor that is clean and without aftertaste, (2) be made for a price competitive with sugar (sucrose) on a cost-per-sweetness basis, (3) be adequately soluble and stable, and (4) be subjected to and pass the lenthy and costly program of rigorous safety testing required by the U.S. Food and Drug Administration. Very few meet all of these requirements.

Table S-18 gives a comparison of the common sweet-tasting substances, ranked in descending order of sweetness. Note that sucrose is used as the standard; hence, it is given a sweetness rating of 1.0 and all other products are compared to it. Note, too, that Table S-18 gives the following information relative to each substance: (1) the caloric value, where available, and (2) the identity.

TABLE S-18
COMPARISONS OF SOME SWEET-TASTING SUBSTANCES

Substance	Sweetness[1]		Substance Identification
	(Calories)	(kcal/g)	
Neohesperidin dihydrochalone	1,500	0	Nonnutritive; artificial
Saccharin	500	0	Artificial sweetener
Aspartame (Nutrasweet)	180	4	Two amino acids
Cyclamate	100	100	Artificial sweetener
Tryptophan	30	0	Amino acid
Fructose (levulose)	1.7	4	Monosaccharide
Invert sugar[2]	1.3	0	Monosaccharide
Sucrose	1.0	4	Disaccharide
Maltitol	0.9	0	Sugar alcohol
Xylitol	0.9	4	Sugar alcohol
Glycine	0.8	4	Amino acid
Glucose (dextrose)	0.7	4	Monosaccharide
Mannitol	0.7	2	Sugar alcohol
Sorbitol	0.6	0	Sugar alcohol
Inositol	0.5	0	Sugar alcohol
Maltose	0.4	0	Disaccharide
Galactose	0.3	0	Monosaccharide
Lactose	0.2	0	Disaccharide
Raffinose	0.2	0	Trisaccharide
Starch	0	0	Polysaccharide

[1]The sweetness of sucrose taken as the standard.

[2]Invert sugar is formed by the splitting of sucrose. Thus, it is a mixture of half glucose and half fructose. Honey has the same sweetness as invert sugar.

Additional pertinent information relative to each of the sweeteners listed in Table S-18 follows, with the products listed in the same order as in Table S-18.

• **Neohesperidin dihydrochalone**—This is a new sweetener derived from citrus peel. It is slow to elicit the taste sensation, but it has a lingering licoricelike aftertaste. Potential uses include chewing gum, mouthwash, and toothpaste.

• **Saccharin**—Saccharin was discovered in 1879. Initially, FDA recognized it as safe (GRAS). But in 1972, saccharin was removed from the GRAS list. Presently, saccharin-containing foods and beverages are available under a Congressional moratorium requiring warning labels on packages.

No food energy is derived from saccharin, so its calorie count is zero. It is valuable in managing diabetes and obesity.

There is no evidence to indicate that, at conventional levels of use, it causes cancer in humans, or any other disease.

(Also see SACCHARIN.)

- **Aspartame (Nutrasweet)**—Discovered in 1965, Aspartame was introduced in the United States in 1981 as a low-calorie sweetener. Aspartame consists of three substances: two amino acids (phenylalanine and aspartic acid), and methanol (methyl alcohol). Aspartame's greatest virtue is its taste, which is very similar to sugar, and there is no unpleasant aftertaste.

Because aspartame contains phenylalanine, it can be consumed only in carefully controlled amounts by people with certain medical problems such as phenylketonuria; hence, labeling is required indicating that phenylalanine is present in aspartame-sweetened foods and beverages. Aspartame is unstable if subjected to prolonged heating, so it is not suitable for use in cooking or baking. Also, it gradually breaks down in beverages, but it can be used successfully in soft drinks if distribution and storage conditions are well controlled.

- **Cyclamate**—This noncalorie substance was discovered in 1937 and used as a dietetic sweetener in a variety of foods and drinks in the early 1950s. In 1969, in response to scientific evidence implicating cyclamate as a possible cancer-causing agent in rats, FDA removed the sweetener from the GRAS list; and in 1970, it was taken off the U.S. market completely. Presently cyclamate is being reevaluated by FDA, based on evidence that it may not pose a cancer hazard.

- **Tryptophan**—A sweet-tasting essential amino acid.
  (Also see AMINO ACID[S].)

- **Fructose (levulose)**—This is a carbohydrate—a monosacchride. It is found naturally in fruits, and it makes up about 50% of the sugar in honey. Commercially, it is found in high-fructose syrups and invert sugars. It is used in beverages, baking, and canned goods—wherever invert sugar or honey may be used.
  (Also see FRUCTOSE.)

- **Invert sugar**—This is a mixture of glucose (dextrose) and fructose (levulose). Invert sugar resists crystallization and has moisture-retention properties. It prolongs the freshness of baked goods and confectionery.
  (Also see INVERT SUGAR; and SUGAR, section on "Consumption and Use of Sugar.")

- **Sucrose (sugar)**—This is the standard with which other sweet substances are compared; hence, in Table S-18 it is given a sweetness rating of 1.0. Sucrose is widely used in many beverages and processed foods, and in homes. It is one of the oldest, most popular, and most available sweetening agents.
  (Also see SUGAR.)

- **Maltitol**—A sugar alcohol, used to add sweetness to *sugarless* chewing gum and some dietetic foods.

- **Xylitol**—This is a sugar alcohol or polyhydric alcohol (polyol). It occurs naturally in some fruits and vegetables. Commercially, it is produced from plant parts containing xylans—oat hulls, corncobs, and birch wood chips. Xylitol is used in *sugarless* chewing gums and dietetic foods.
  (Also see XYLITOL.)

- **Glycine**—This is a sweet-tasting nonessential amino acid. It is used to modify the taste of some foods.
  (Also see AMINO ACID[S].)

- **Glucose (dextrose)**—It is commercially produced from the conversion of starch (corn starch) by the action of heat and acids, or enzymes. Primarily, glucose is used in the confection, wine, and canning industries; and in intravenous solutions.
  (Also see GLUCOSE; and SUGAR, section on "Consumption and Use of Sugar.")

- **Mannitol**—This is a sugar alcohol or polyhydric alcohol (polyol). Mannitol occurs naturally in pineapples, asparagus, carrots, and olives. Commercially, it is prepared by the hydrogenation of mannose or glucose. Mannitol is used in candies, chewing gums, confections, and baked goods. Also, it is used in dietetic foods and in medicine—as a diuretic and to test kidney function.

- **Sorbitol**—This is a sugar alcohol or polyhydric alcohol (polyol). Sorbitol occurs naturally in many fruits. Commercially, it is prepared by the hydrogenation of glucose. It is used in chewing gum, dairy products, meat products, icings, toppings, and beverages.

- **Inositol**—Inositol is widely distributed in many foods and is closely related to glucose.

- **Maltose**—Malt sugar is formed from starch by the action of yeast. It is much less sweet than sugar. Preparations containing maltose, often in mixtures with dextrose, are used in bread-baking and in infant foods.
  (Also see MALTOSE.)

- **Galactose**—This is a hexose sugar (a monosaccharide) obtained along with glucose from lactose, found in milk.
  (Also see GALACTOSE.)

- **Lactose**—This disaccharide is composed of one molecule of galactose and one molecule of glucose. It is the only sugar not found in plants. It is found in milk; hence it is called milk sugar.
  (Also see LACTOSE.)

- **Raffinose**—This is a trisaccharide containing the three hexoses—glucose, fructose, and galactose. Raffinose is found in molasses, cottonseed meal, and Australian manna.
  (Also see RAFFINOSE.)

- **Starch**—Starch (as such) is tasteless (not sweet). But starch from any starch source—cereal grains or potatoes—may be broken down into its component sugar, either enzymatically or with dilute acids. The most familiar example in the United States is corn syrup (Karo). Complete hydrolysis of starch yields glucose (dextrose), which is sweet.
  (Also see STARCH.)

(Also see SUGAR.)

SWEET POTATO *Ipomoea batatas*

This tropical plant, which forms nutritious tubers, is a member of the morningglory family (*Convolvulaceae*).

ORIGIN AND HISTORY. The sweet potato is native to the American tropics. It was once an important component of the Aztec diet. Remains of sweet potatoes estimated to be between 10,000 to 20,000 years old were found in a cave in Peru. However, it is not certain whether the

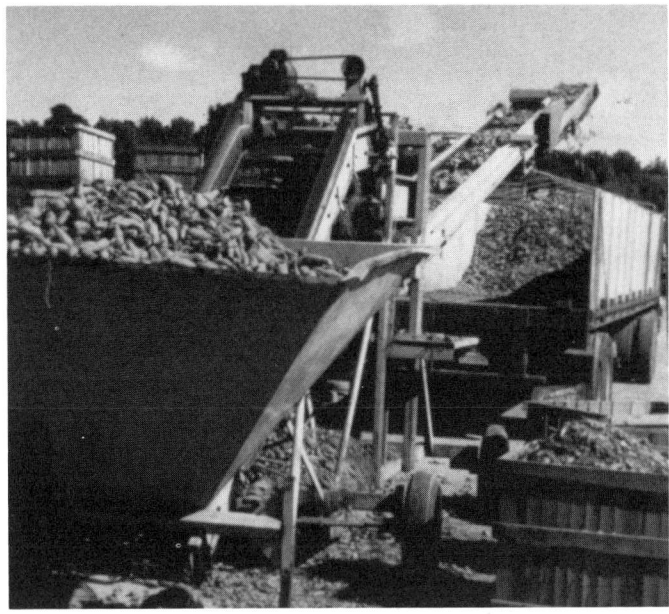

Fig. S-47. Loading sweet potatoes in the field. (Courtesy, Louisiana Cooperative Extension Services, Louisiana State University, Baton Rouge, La.)

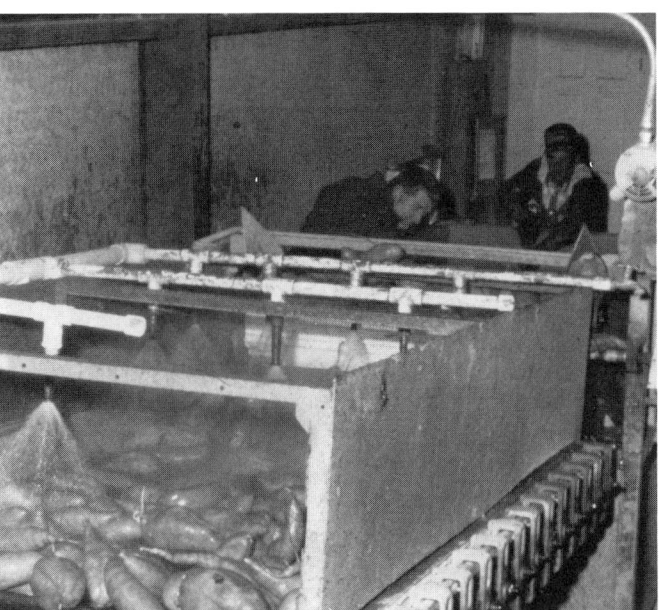

Fig. S-48. Washing sweet potatoes. (Courtesy, Louisiana Cooperative Extension Services, Louisiana State University, Baton Rough, La.)

ancient tubers had grown wild or been cultivated. Europeans introduced the plant to their continent in the 16th century, and it later spread to Asia.

WORLD AND U.S. PRODUCTION. Sweet potatoes rank second among the leading vegetables of the world, and tenth among the vegetables of the United States.

Worldwide, about 132 million metric tons of sweet potatoes are produced annually; and the leading sweet potato-producing nations in descending order are: China, Indonesia, Vietnam, Uganda, Japan, India, Rwanda, Brazil, Philippines, and Kenya.[48]

The United States produces about 651,000 short tons of sweet potatoes annually; and the leading sweet potato-producing states in descending order are: North Carolina, Louisiana, California, Georgia, Alabama, Mississippi, South Carolina, Texas, New Jersey, and Virginia.[49]

PROCESSING. Tubers which are to be stored keep better if they are cured after harvesting. Curing consists of holding the sweet potatoes in a facility where the temperature is about 85°F *(30°C)* and the relative humidity is about 85%. These conditions promote the healing of small wounds in the tubers.

Various means of processing have been developed, the two most common of which follow:

• **Canning**—This process is used mainly for small whole tubers or cut pieces of larger tubers, which are first cooked, then packed in syrup. Only small amounts of canned sweet potato puree are produced, most of which is packed in glass jars by baby food manufacturers.

• **Dehydration**—The sun-drying of raw sweet potato chips

or slices has long been one of the major means of preservation utilized in the developing countries of the tropics. However, dehydration in the United States usually involves the drum drying of a puree made from the cooked tubers. The retail market for this type of product is limited because most people use either fresh or canned sweet potatoes. Nevertheless, the dried powder is used by the armed forces, in school lunch programs, and by bakers who produce sweet potato cakes and pies.

SELECTION, PREPARATION, AND USES. There are two general types of sweet potatoes. One type has soft, moist flesh when cooked and a high sugar content (sweet potatoes of this type are commonly, but incorrectly, called yams). The second type, when cooked, has a firm, dry, somewhat mealy flesh, which is usually light yellow or pale orange in color, as contrasted to the usually deeper yellow or distinctly orange-red colored flesh of the moist type. The skin of the dry type is usually light yellowish-tan or fawn colored, while the skin of the moist-fleshed varieties may vary in color from whitish-tan to brownish-red. Varieties of each type vary considerably in shape, but most moist-fleshed varieties are usually more plump in shape than most dry-fleshed varieties. A mixture of types or a mixture of varieties within types is undesirable because of lack of uniformity in cooking, as well as differences in flavor and color of flesh.

Best quality sweet potatoes are clean, smooth, well-shaped, firm, and bright in appearance.

Many people like sweet potatoes prepared with a sweetener such as honey, molasses, sugar, or a syrup. However, the yam type of tuber provides much of its own sweetening when it is cooked slowly, because it contains an enzyme (beta-amylase) that converts starch to maltose and dextrins. Heating the tuber activates the enzyme, which is eventually inactivated when the internal temperature becomes too high. Prior to cooking, the tubers should be scrubbed well with a vegetable brush so that they may be cooked with the skins intact. Removal of the skin before cooking may result in darkening of the flesh. Also, the skins loosen and are easier to remove after cooking.

---

[48]Data from *FAO Production Yearbook 1990*, FAO/UN, Rome, Italy, Vol. 44, p. 92, Table 27. **Note well:** Annual production fluctuates as a result of weather and profitability of the crop.

[49]Data from *Agricultural Statistics 1991*, USDA, p. 164, Table 237. **Note well:** Annual production fluctuates as a result of weather and profitability of the crop.

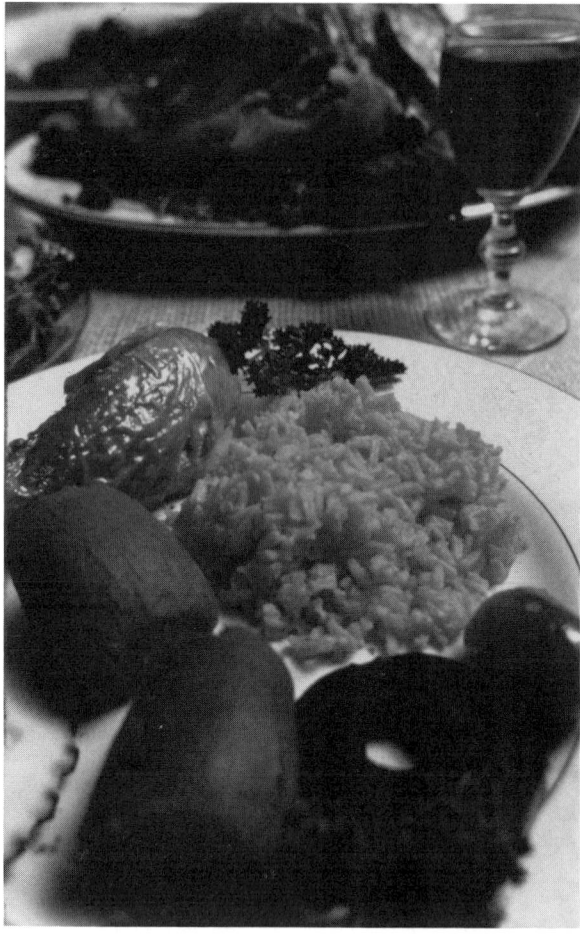

Fig. S-49. Sweet potatoes enhance the meal. (Courtesy, USDA)

Sweet potatoes may be cooked in much the same ways as Irish potatoes, but they require only about half as much cooking time. In addition, they are good in casseroles when accompanied by apple slices or pineapple rings and seasoned with spices such as allspice and cinnamon. Finally, mashed cooked sweet potato may be used to make biscuits, breads, cakes, cookies, custards, muffins, and pies.

NUTRITIONAL VALUE. The nutrient compositions of various forms of sweet potatoes are given in Food Composition Table F-21.

Some noteworthy observations regarding the nutrient composition of sweet potatoes follow:

1. Compared to cooked Irish potatoes, cooked sweet potatoes contain about an equal number of calories, less protein and vitamin C, and much more vitamin A—they are one of the leading plant sources of the latter vitamin.

2. A 1-cup serving (*about 9 oz or 225 g*) of mashed cooked sweet potatoes provides 275 Calories (kcal) and 5 g of protein, which is almost double the calories and about equal to the protein furnished by a cup of a cooked cereal such as corn or rice.

3. Candied sweet potatoes supply almost 50% more calories than the unsweetened cooked tubers.

4. The quantity and quality of protein is barely adequate to meet the needs of adults, and is inadequate for the needs of children. Fortunately, many tropical peoples supplement their diets with small amounts of protein-rich foods such as fish, legumes, and wild game.

SWEETSOP (SUGAR APPLE) *Annona squamosa*

The fruit of a small tree (of the family *Annonaceae*) that is native to the American tropics. The yellowish-green heart-shaped fruit are 3 to 4 in. (*8 to 10 cm*) in diameter, white, and have a sweet granular custardlike pulp. They are used as a dessert fruit, and are closely related to the other *Annona* species of fruit (the most common ones are the cherimoya, custard apple, and soursop). Their flavor is best when fully ripe, a stage at which the fruit is very perishable.

The nutrient composition of sweetsop (sugar apple) is given in Food Composition Table F-21.

Some noteworthy observations regarding the nutrient composition of sweetsop follow:

1. The raw fruit is moderately high in calories (94 kcal per 100 g) and carbohydrates (24%).

2. Sugar apples are a good source of fiber, potassium, and vitamin C, and a fair source of iron.

SYMPTOM

A complaint by patients which may lead them to seek medical advice.

SYN–

Prefix meaning with, or together.

SYNDROME

A combination of symptoms occurring together.

SYNERGISM

The joint action of agents in which their combined effect is greater than the sum of their separate actions; each agent enhances the action of the other.

SYNTHESIS

The process of building up a chemical compound by a reaction or a series of reactions.

SYNTHETIC

An artificially produced product that may be similar to the natural product.

SYRUPS

Although there is a large variety of syrups, they all contain sugar and water. There are those syrups which come from sources used to manufacture sugar and glucose, such as corn syrup, maple syrup, molasses, and sorghum syrup. Specialty syrups can be created from sugar, water, and a variety of flavors such as almond, cherry, chocolate, currant, orange, strawberry, and other fruit flavors. Plain sugar and water syrups are used for canning fruits. Also, syrup serves as a carrier of medicines as in cough syrup.

(Also see CARBOHYDRATE[S], section headed "Sources"; MAPLE SYRUP; MOLASSES; SORGHUM; and SUGAR.)

SYSTEMIC

Pertaining to the body as a whole, as distinguished from local.

TACHYCARDIA

An abnormally rapid heart beat, faster than 100 beats per minute. It occurs during exercise, in fevers, in certain heart conditions, and in a number of diseases.

TALLOW

The fat extracted from adipose tissue of cattle and sheep. (Also see FATS AND OTHER LIPIDS.)

TANGERINE (MANDARIN ORANGE)
Citrus reticulata

The names *tangerine* and *mandarin* are now used interchangeably in the United States. The tangerine, or mandarin, refers to citrus fruit which resembles the sweet orange (*C. sinesis*), but which are orange-red and have loose skins that peel easily. Tangerines, like the other citrus fruits, belong to the rue family (*Rutaceae*).

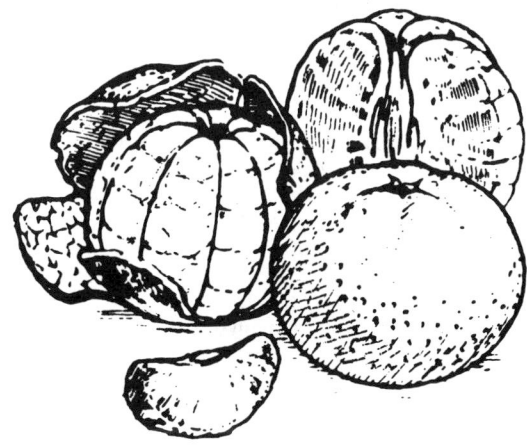

Fig.T-1. The tangerine, a species of citrus fruit that has a loose, easily peeled skin and a distinctive sweet flavor.

Of the many tangerine hybrids, the most widely produced in the United States are the tangelo, the tangor, and the temple orange. Details follow.

• **Tangelo**—This term designates the hybrids of the grapefruit and the tangerine. Usually, the fruits have the loose skin and sweetness of the latter parent, but they tend to have a distinctive flavor of their own.

• **Tangor**—Most lay people are unfamiliar with this name, which refers to hybrids of the tangerine or the sweet orange.

• **Temple orange**—This naturally occurring tangor (a hybrid of tangerine and grapefruit) was discovered in Jamaica. It is by far the most important hybrid of the mandarin.

ORIGIN AND HISTORY. Tangerines are native to China, where they were grown for 3,000 years. They did not reach Europe and the Americas until the 1800s. Today, tangerines and their hybrids are grown in most of subtropical and tropical areas of the world. As they spread throughout the world, many new varieties developed as a result of (1) mutations, and (2) accidental or intentional crossbreeding (hybridization) with the local varieties.

WORLD AND U.S. PRODUCTION. Worldwide, about 8.8 million metric tons of tangerines (and their hybrids) are produced annually; and the leading producing countries, by rank, are: Japan, Spain, Brazil, Korea, Italy, and Pakistan. Japan alone accounts for approximately 23% of the world tangerine production.[1]

The United States produces about 359,000 short tons of tangerines (and their hybrids) annually. Most of the U.S. crop (79% of it) is produced in Florida; California and Arizona rank second and third, respectively.[2]

PROCESSING. A little over half of the U.S. crop of tangerines is processed into single-strength juices and frozen concentrates. Much of the fruit juice is blended into orange juice and frozen orange concentrates because the tangerines contribute a deep orange color. However, U.S. regulations limit the amount of tangerine juice in orange juice blends to 10%. Greater amounts impart off-flavors to the orange juice products.

Some of the tangerine crop is made into single-strength tangerine juice and frozen tangerine juice concentrate. The latter product is by far the major one, because it is much more stable during storage.

Small amounts of tangerine segments are used in prepared citrus salads and gelatin desserts. It is noteworthy that almost all of the canned tangerine segments used in the United States are imported from the Orient.

SELECTION, PREPARATION, AND USES. Fresh tangerines are thin-skinned, and are usually oblate or decidedly flattened at the ends. The skin is easily removed; there is little coarse fibrous substance between the skin and the flesh, and the segments of the fruit separate readily. The flavor is distinctive; the aroma is pungent and pleasant. Because of the looseness of the skin these oranges are likely to feel puffy; therefore, judgment as to quality should be based mainly on weight for size and deep yellow or orange color of the skin.

Tangerines are at their best when served fresh in appetizers, desserts, or toppings for frozen desserts and puddings.

---

[1]Data from *FAO Production Yearbook 1990*, FAO/UN, Rome, Italy, Vol. 44, p. 163, Table 71. **Note well:** Annual production fluctuates as a result of weather and profitability of the crop.

[2]Data from *Agricultural Statistics 1991*, USDA, p. 189, Table 278. **Note well:** Annual production fluctuates as a result of weather and profitability of the crop.

However, their juice and/or their peel may be used to flavor ice cream, ices, sherbets, and sauces.

NUTRITIONAL VALUE. The nutrient compositions of various types of tangerine products are given in Food Composition Table F-21.

Some noteworthy observations regarding the nutrient composition of tangerines follow:

1. Fresh tangerines, fresh tangerine juice, and canned tangerine segments have similar nutritional values in that they are (a) moderately low in calories; (b) good sources of potassium and vitamin C; and (c) fair sources of vitamin A. Also, they all contain the vitaminlike bioflavonoids.

2. Frozen tangerine juice concentrate contains about 4 times the nutrient levels of the fresh, unconcentrated juice. Hence, the concentrate may make a significant nutritional contribution when it is added undiluted to drinks, sauces, and other preparations.

3. Canned tangerine juice has a nutritional value comparable to fresh juice, except that the canned product contains only two-thirds as much vitamin C.

4. Raw tangelos contain only half as much vitamin C as tangerines, but they supply about the same amount of potassium.

TANNIA (YAUTIA; MALANGA; COCOYAM)
Xanthosoma sagittifolium

This plant of the aroid family (*Araceae*) yields edible leaves and tubers. However, it is sometimes confused with taro (another aroid plant) because of certain similar characteristics.

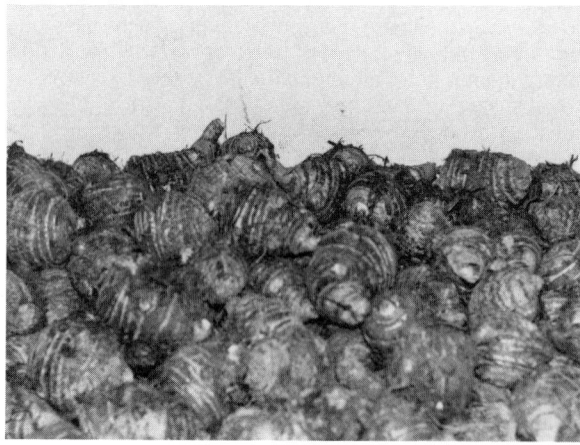

Fig. T-2. Tannia (malanga) tubers in a Cuban market. (Photo by Audrey Ensminger)

The various names given to the plant are also responsible for cases of mistaken identity. Therefore, some definitions of the more common names follow:

• **Tannia and Yautia**—These common names designate all varieties of the species *X. sagittifolium*.

• **Malanga**—This Latin American name is often applied to tannia, but it may also refer to similar tuberous plants of different species.

• **Cocoyam**—Some people give this general name to various tuberous plants grown alongside cocoa (*Theobroma cacao*) to provide shade for the young plants. Africans

distinguish between tannia and taro by calling the former the *new* cocoyam, and the latter the *old* cocoyam.

Only the name tannia will be used in the remainder of this article.

PREPARATION. In West Africa, tannia is used to prepare *fufu*, a pasty dough made by mashing boiled peeled tubers. People in other tropical areas of the world use the plant in much the same ways as they have long used cassava, taro, and yams. For example, the tubers may be baked, boiled, fried, or roasted; and the cooked young leaves may be used as a green vegetable.

CAUTION: Neither tannia roots nor tannia leaves should be consumed without cooking them thoroughly because some varieties contain high levels of calcium oxalate crystals, which are very irritating to the digestive system. The latter possibility may be alleviated by boiling the roots or leaves for about 15 minutes in water containing a small amount of baking soda (sodium bicarbonate), discarding the used water, rinsing the vegetable thoroughly, and boiling again in clear water.

NUTRITIONAL VALUE. The nutrient compositions of various forms of tannia are given in Food Composition Table F-21. Note that—

1. Compared to Irish potatoes, tannia tubers furnish about twice as many calories, the same amount of protein, and less than half as much vitamin C. The protein to calorie ratio (1.6 g per 100 kcal) of the tubers is barely high enough to meet the protein requirements of adults. So, children fed a tannia-rich diet are likely to develop protein-energy malnutrition unless they are given supplemental protein foods in their diets. Finally, tannia tubers are deficient in many vitamins and minerals.

2. Tannia leaves are nutritionally superior to the tubers with respect to protein, calcium, phosphorus, iron, vitamin A, and vitamin C. They are an excellent source of vitamin A. Hence, they compensate for most of the nutritional deficiencies of the tuber. However, the leaves may contain much higher levels of highly irritating calcium oxalate crystals than the tubers. Therefore, the leaves should not be consumed raw by people or livestock, unless it is certain that they contain little or no oxalates. The leaves may be rendered safe by boiling.

TANNINS

This refers to a complex group of chemicals found naturally in many plants. They are responsible for the astringent taste of coffee and tea. Tannic acid, a commercial tannin, is used widely in industry.

TAPIOCA

This is a starch derived from the roots of the tropical cassava plant. It is extracted by washing, peeling, and grinding the roots to fine pulp which is passed over a series of screens to remove root fibers. In some processes it may be further refined in settling basins or centrifuges. The moist starchy mass is dried; and, during the drying process, it forms small, uneven milky white balls known as pearl tapioca. High grade tapioca has a brilliant white color.

Tapioca is used like starch from other sources. It swells and thickens the liquid in which it is cooked. It is used in its natural state, as well as in modified and pregelatinized versions like other starches. The most familiar use of tapioca is the popular pudding which contains small lumps or granules. Special cooking, grinding, and screening methods produce this type of tapioca. Pearl tapioca requires prior soaking and yields larger lumps in puddings.

(Also see CASSAVA; and FLOURS, Table F-13, Special Flours)

TAPIOCA-MACARONI

A product developed in India. It may be a mixture (1) of 80 to 90 parts of tapioca flour and 10 to 20 parts peanut flour; or (2) of 60 parts of tapioca, 15 parts peanut, and 25 parts semolina. It is baked into shapes resembling rice grains or macaroni.

TARTAR

• A mineral deposit on the teeth, mainly calcium phosphate.

• A substance consisting basically of cream of tartar found in the juice of grapes, and often deposited in wine casks during the production of wine.

TARTAR EMETIC

This is another name for the chemical antimony potassium tartrate. Under hospital supervision, its slow intravenous administration is a dangerous but effective treatment used to eliminate certain parasites from the body.

TARTARIC ACID (HOOC[CHOH]₂–COOH)

A strong dicarboxylic acid. It is widely found in plants—especially fruits—both free and combined with salts.

TARTAZINE

This is an alternate name for the yellow color, FD & C Yellow no. 5, which is approved for use in food, drugs, and cosmetics. It may also be employed to dye wool and silk.

(Also see COLORING OF FOODS, Table C-19, Synthetic Color Additives Approved for Food Use.)

TASTE

This is a chemical sense detected by receptors—the taste buds—in the mouth, primarily on the tongue. Upon entering the mouth, certain dissolved chemicals create nervous impulses in the taste buds. These impulses travel to the brain where they are interpreted as (1) salty, (2) sweet, (3) bitter, or (4) sour. Humans have about 12,000 taste buds, and each taste bud possesses a greater degree of sensitivity to 1 or 2 of the taste sensations. In general, the tip of the tongue is the most sensitive to sweet, the sides to sour, the back to bitter, while salt sensitivity is distributed over most of the tongue.

Taste plays a major role in the acceptance or rejection of foods. Most of the time, salty foods are considered pleasant, but very salty foods will be rejected. Sweet is, of course, considered pleasant, and is associated with the sugar content of a food. However, much effort has been directed toward finding substances such as saccharin, which will *fool* the sweet taste buds, without contributing to calories as do the sugars. Foods with a bitter taste are generally rejected. This may have been a protective mechanism for early man, since many poisonous wild plants taste bitter due to alkaloid compounds. The sour taste may be considered as pleasing or objectionable. For example, foods containing dilute vinegar solutions are very palatable, while extremely sour foods are rejected. Sourness is a measure of the degree of acidity—

hydrogen ion concentration—of foods. Although, taste is important in food acceptance, most of the pleasurable experience associated with food is known as flavor. The flavor of foods results from the interaction of taste and smell—another chemical sense. Humans can detect as many as 10,000 different smells. Much of what is called taste is actually smell. This is emphasized during a cold when foods seem to lose their *taste*.

(Also see SUGAR; and SWEETENING AGENTS.)

TASTE BUDS

The sense organs for taste located in the epiglottis, palate, pharynx, and tongue. Taste buds are excited by chemical substances in the food we eat. We can detect four types of taste: (1) salty, (2) sweet, (3) bitter, and (4) sour. Taste sensations from these taste buds help regulate the diet. Much of what we usually call taste is actually smell.

(Also see TASTE.)

TAURINE (C₂H₇NO₃S)

This chemical is present in bile, combined with cholic acid.

TEA

The word *tea* refers to (1) a common drink made by pouring boiling water over the dried and prepared leaves of an oriental evergreen tree, (2) the dried and prepared leaves from which the drink is made, or (3) the tree upon which these leaves grow. Tea may also mean (1) a brew made from kinds of leaves other than tea, (2) an afternoon or early evening meal in Britain, or (3) a large reception at which tea is served. Herein, the word tea will refer to the dried leaves of the plant and the drink made from them. Tea is the most popular beverage in the world.

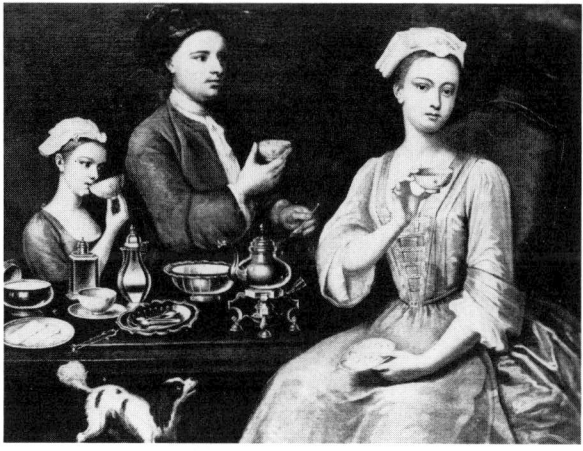

Fig. T-3. Tea for two, or three, or four—the pause that refreshes. (Painting by an unknown master, English. Courtesy, The Bettmann Archive, New York, N.Y.)

ORIGIN AND HISTORY. It is believed that the tea plant originated in a region encompassing Tibet, western China, and northern India. The exact origin of tea culture and brewing tea leaves into a drink is obscure. But, according to an ancient Chinese legend, tea was discovered by the Chinese emperor, Shen-Nung, in 2737 B.C. Leaves from a wild tea bush accidentally fell into the water that he was boiling; and he discovered that the drink was good. However, the earliest mention of tea in Chinese literature appeared about 350 A.D. Then, in 780 A.D. Lu Yu's *The Classic of Tea*, published in China, described the cultivation, processing, and use of tea. By the 9th century A.D., tea was growing in Japan after being introduced by Chinese Buddhist monks. Eventually, tea culture spread to Java, the Dutch East Indies, and other tropical and subtropical areas. Traders from Europe sailing to and from the Far East in the 16th century began to introduce Europeans to the unusual oriental beverage called tea, a word derived from the Chinese local Amoy dialect word *t'e,* pronounced *tay.* By the 18th century, tea had become the national beverage of England. Tea also was popular in the American colonies, but in 1767 the British government placed a tax on the tea used by the colonists. The rest of the story Americans know as the Boston Tea Party of 1773—a contributing factor to the Revolutionary War.

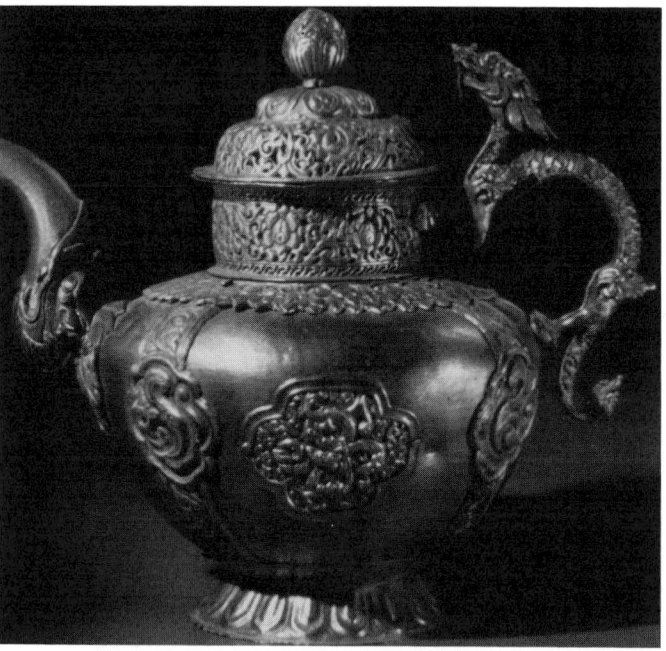

Fig. T-4. Teapot from Tibet. (Courtesy, Field Museum of Natural History, Chicago, Ill.)

WORLD AND U.S. PRODUCTION.
No longer is it "all the tea in China," since India ranks as the number one producer of tea. Sri Lanka (previously Ceylon) is, however, the major supplier of tea to the United States. Worldwide, about 2.5 million metric tons of tea are produced annually; and the leading tea-producing countries, ranked in descending order, are: India, China, Sri Lanka, Kenya, Indonesia, Turkey, U.S.S.R., Japan, Iran, and Bangladesh.[3]

Propagation and Growing.
The tea plant is an evergreen tree with the botanical name of *Camellia sinensis*. In the wild, the tree may grow to a height of 30 ft (10 m), but on tea plantations, or so-called gardens or estates, the tea plants are constantly pruned to keep their height at about 3 ft (1 m) to encourage new growth and to keep at a convenient picking height.

Tea plants grow best in warm climates where the rainfall averages 90 to 200 in. (220 to 500 cm) yearly, and the plants

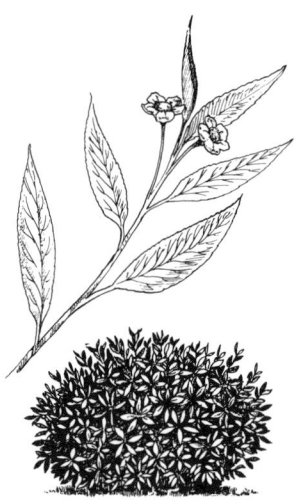

Fig. T-5. A pruned tea plant with abundant foliage, and a twig showing the camellialike flowers. It is the two leaves at the end of the twig which are plucked for tea.

grow at altitudes from sea level to 7,000 ft (2,200 m). The best teas are produced at the higher altitudes where plants grow more slowly in the cooler air and their leaves yield a better flavor.

Tea plants may be started from cuttings or seeds. The tea seedlings or small plants are placed in the soil about 3 to 5 ft (1.0 to 1.5 m) apart, and then, depending upon the altitude, 2½ to 5 years are required before the tea plants produce leaves for commercial production. Young plants are often shaded to protect them from the heat of the sun. Once in production a plant may produce for almost a century.

Harvesting.
Tea plants produce abundant foliage, a camellialike flower, and berries containing one to three seeds. However, it is the smallest and youngest leaves that are plucked for tea. Two leaves and a bud at the top of each young shoot are picked. A growth of new shoots is termed a flush. At lower altitudes a new flush may grow every week, while at higher altitudes more time is required. Flushes are picked off the tea plant by hand by workers called *tea pluckers.* Good pluckers harvest about 40 lb (18 kg) per day, or enough to make 10 lb (4.5 kg) of manufactured tea.

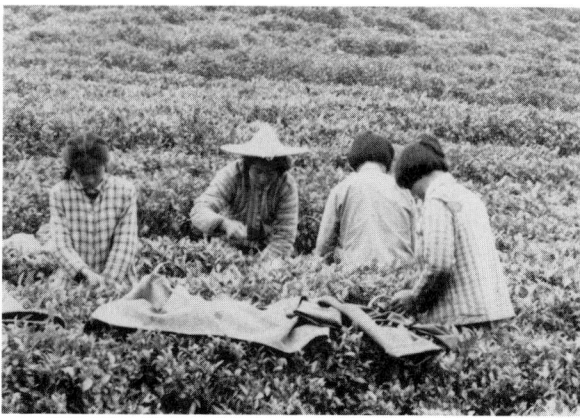

Fig. T-6. Picking tea in Hangchow, China. (Photo by Audrey Ensminger)

---

[3]Data from *FAO Production Yearbook 1990*, FAO/UN, Rome, Italy, Vol. 44, p. 177, Table 80. **Note well:** Annual production fluctuates as a result of weather and profitability of the crop.

PROCESSING. Although the kind and quality of leaves vary somewhat according to the local conditions and particular strains, the real difference in color, aroma, and flavor is caused by the way in which the leaves are processed. There are three different types of tea: black, green, and oolong. Most green and oolong tea comes from China, Japan, and Taiwan, while all tea-producing countries manufacture black tea.

• **Black tea**—First the leaves are transported from the plantation to the factory as rapidly as possible. The leaves are spread on withering racks and air is blown over the leaves to remove excess moisture. This removes about one-third of the moisture, and the leaves become soft and pliable. After this they are rolled to break the cells and release the juices, which are essential for the fermenting process. Then the leaves are spread out and kept under high humidity to promote fermentation, which develops the rich flavor of black tea, and the leaves become a coppery color. Finally, the leaves are hot-air dried (fired) until the moisture is removed, leaving the leaves brownish black.

• **Green tea**—In making green tea, the plucked leaves are steamed as quickly as possible. Steaming prevents the leaves from changing color and prevents fermentation. After steaming, the leaves are rolled and dried in the same way as black tea until they are crisp.

• **Oolong tea**—Oolong tea is somewhat like both green tea and black tea. It is semifermented. Fermentation is stopped before the process is complete. This produces a greenish-brown leaf with a flavor richer than that of green tea but more delicate than that of black tea.

GRADES OF TEA AND BLENDING. Tea is graded according to the size of the leaf, which has nothing to do with the quality of the tea. Large and small, broken and unbroken leaves are sorted by passing them across screens with different size holes. The largest leaves, classified in order of size, are orange pekoe, pekoe, and pekoe souchong. These large leaves are generally packaged as loose tea. The smaller or broken leaves are classified as broken orange pekoe, broken orange pekoe fannings, and fannings. These smaller grades of tea are generally used in tea bags.

Since tea grown in different countries, or even different parts of the same country, varies in taste, flavor, and quality, tea companies employ a tea taster. The tea taster selects the tea to purchase so that a company can sell tea with the flavor for which it is known. To achieve a particular flavor, teas are often blended. Nevertheless, some unblended varieties are popular.

BREWING TEA. A cup of tea is brewed by pouring fresh, boiling water over l tsp (*5 ml*) of loose tea or one tea bag. The best flavor is obtained by allowing the tea to steep (soak) for 3 to 5 minutes before being served. If tea is steeped too long, it will have a bitter taste from the excess tannins that are released. Also, the longer steeping times yield tea with a higher caffeine content.

Iced tea is made with 50% more tea leaves, to allow for the melting ice. The tea is poured into tall glasses that are two-thirds full of ice. Sliced lemons are served with it, and each person sweetens the tea to his taste. Flavorings of cloves, grated orange peel, or mint are sometimes added.

• **Instant tea**—Instant tea is an innovation developed in the United States. A strong brew of tea is made in large vats, and then the water is removed by a drying process. Consumers can make hot or cold tea by merely adding water to the powder which remains after the drying process.

NUTRITIONAL VALUE. Without sugar, cream, or other additions, tea provides little nutrition other than a few calories, and trace amounts of some minerals as indicated in Food Composition Table F-21. Green tea is, however, an excellent source of vitamin K.

Caffeine in tea accounts for its mildly stimulating properties, while the tannins contribute pungency, slight astringency, and color to tea. An essential oil contributes the flavor. The amount of caffeine in a cup of tea depends upon the steeping time.

(Also see CAFFEINE.)

TEASEED OIL

This is a vegetable oil extracted from *Camellia sinensis*, the tea-oil plant, and cultivated in China. Teaseed oil is used for salad oil and frying. It is claimed to be similar to olive oil.

TEFF *Eragrostis abyssinica*

This is an important cereal food of Ethiopia and the eastern African highlands. It is a leafy, quick-maturing annual plant that grows up to 4 ft in height. Teff is adapted to dry areas with a short rainy season.

The teff of Africa is grown by primitive methods. Fields are cultivated by crude plows drawn by oxen, followed by hand sowing and another tilling to cover the seed. When ripe, the grain is harvested by small hand sickles and threshed by treading with animals.

Women grind the white or black grain (grain color depends on variety) on flat stones to make a flour, which is baked into large, flat pancakes called injara.

Nutritional data on teff grains and meal are listed in the Food Composition Table F-21.

Teff is used as an annual grass hay as well as a food grain. Following threshing, the straw may be mixed with mud for constructing huts.

Table T-1 tells about *faffa*, a special fortified food based on teff.

TABLE T-1
A FORTIFIED FOOD BASED ON TEFF

Product	Description	Uses	Comments
Faffa	A finely ground mixture of teff, chickpeas, skim milk powder, sugar, salt, and vitamins. Contains from 14% to 15% protein.	May be mixed with water to make a porridge for infants. Leavened or unleavened breads. Mixed with the false banana (*Ensete ventricosum*).	The Ethiopian and Swedish governments established the Children's Nutrition Unit in Addis Ababa to conduct the development, production, and test marketing of Faffa. Sufficient vitamins are added to the product to ensure that 3½ oz (*100 g*) supplies the daily allowances for all of the essential vitamins. A large scale feeding trial with children aged 6 months to 10 years produced dramatic decreases in the incidence and severity of goiter, rickets, and skin infections; and a noticeable increase in muscle mass. However, the cereal did not cure anemia as rapidly as it did the other deficiency diseases.

TEMPLATE

A mold, pattern, or guide.

TENDERLOIN

The most tender muscle of the carcass (beef, lamb, and pork), located inside the loin and running nearly the entire length of the loin.

TERRAMYCIN AS PRESERVATIVE

Terramycin is a brand name for the broad-spectrum antibiotic oxytetracycline. Although low levels of antibiotics such as Terramycin effectively extend the shelf life of food, the direct addition of antibiotics to foods is not permitted in the United States. After some initial studies and limited usage of antibiotics as food preservatives, the FDA withdrew their approval because of concern that repeated exposure of the consumer to low concentrations of antibiotics could lead to the development of antibiotic-resistant strains of bacteria. Furthermore, there was wariness lest antibiotics provide a substitute for good sanitary practices.

(Also see BACTERIA IN FOOD, section headed "Bacterial Control Methods"; and ANTIBIOTICS, section headed "Antibiotics in Foods.")

TETANY

Spontaneous muscular spasms in the wrists and ankles, resulting when the parathyroid secretion is deficient, causing the amount of calcium in the blood to drop and the phosphorus to increase.

TEXTURE

Food is accepted or rejected on the basis of its chemical and physical properties as perceived by the senses—sight, sound, touch, smell, and taste. Therefore, the texture of a food is important. Texture is a physical quality of food perceived by the sense of touch in the mouth—mouth feel. It is described by such adjectives as chewy, tacky, stringy, hard, soft, rough, smooth, gritty, firm, crisp, coarse, etc. Through experience, people learn the customary texture of foods in their diet, and when the texture is different than expected, the food is judged to be of lower quality. Often, unacceptable foods feel slimy, stringy, and greasy, or they contain unchewable parts, grit, or foreign particles.

THEINE

This is an alternative name for caffeine.

THERAPEUTIC

Pertaining to the medical treatment of disease.

THERAPEUTIC DIETS

Diets designed to treat a disease or metabolic disorder. They are diets adapted or modified to meet special needs of specific diseases. Some common examples of diseases requiring therapeutic or modified diets are diabetes mellitus, phenylketonuria, kidney diseases, and galactosemia. Depending upon the disorder, these diets may be modified in energy content, in consistency or bulk, or in the kinds and amounts of nutrients such as vitamins, minerals, fats, proteins, or fluids. Despite the modification, the therapeutic diet should remain nutritionally adequate.

(Also see MODIFIED DIETS.)

THERAPY

The medical treatment of disease.

THERMAL

Refers to heat.

THERMODURIC

A term used to describe microorganisms (bacteria) that are heat tolerant. Thermodurics survive for short periods of time at high temperatures, but they do not grow at high temperatures. For example, thermodurics survive pasteurization of milk for short periods of time.

THERMOGENESIS

The production of heat, especially within the body.

THERMOPHILES

Bacteria that are *heat lovers*. These bacteria grow at temperatures of 131°F (55°C) to as high as 167°F (75°C). They are somewhat of a curiosity, since many of the proteins of other organisms would coagulate at these high temperatures. Thermophiles are commonly found in hot springs and compost heaps, and do not pose any real health problems. However, thermophiles are responsible for the *flat sour* which occurs in some home-canned food.

(Also see FLAT SOURS.)

THI– (THIO–)

Prefix meaning sulfur-containing.

THIAMIN (VITAMIN B-1)

Thiamin (vitamin B-1)—the antiberiberi, or antineuritic, or antipolyneuritis vitamin—was the first of the B complex vitamins to be obtained in pure form; hence, the name B-1, a name proposed by the British in 1927. Various other names were used for short periods along the way, including antineuritic factor, antiberiberi factor, water-soluble B, aneurin, and simply vitamin B.

The mystery of beriberi, an ancient disease among rice-eating peoples in the East, was eventually unraveled as a deficiency disease caused by a lack of thiamin.

Thiamin is required by all species of animals. They must have a dietary source, unless it is synthesized for them by microorganisms in the digestive tract, as in the case of ruminants.

A patient with wet beriberi—lying in bed breathless, waterlogged, and apparently dying—may recover in 1 or 2 hours after being given an injection of thiamin; this is perhaps the most dramatic cure in medicine.

THIAMIN (vitamin B-1) HELPS THE BODY CELLS CONVERT CARBOHYDRATES (STARCHES AND SUGARS) OF FOOD TO ENERGY, AND KEEPS THE NERVOUS SYSTEM, APPETITE, MUSCLE TONE AND ATTITUDE BUOYANT.

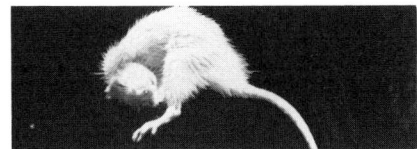 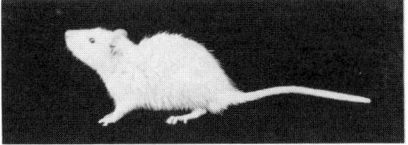

ONE OF THE MOST DRAMATIC CURES IN MEDICINE! SAME RAT BEFORE (LEFT) AND AFTER (RIGHT). LEFT: THIS RAT, 24 WEEKS OLD, HAD PRACTICALLY NO THIAMIN. IT LOST THE ABILITY TO COORDINATE ITS MUSCLES. RIGHT: THE SAME RAT 24 HOURS LATER, AFTER RECEIVING FOOD RICH IN THIAMIN—FULLY RECOVERED. (COURTESY, USDA)

TOP FOOD SOURCES

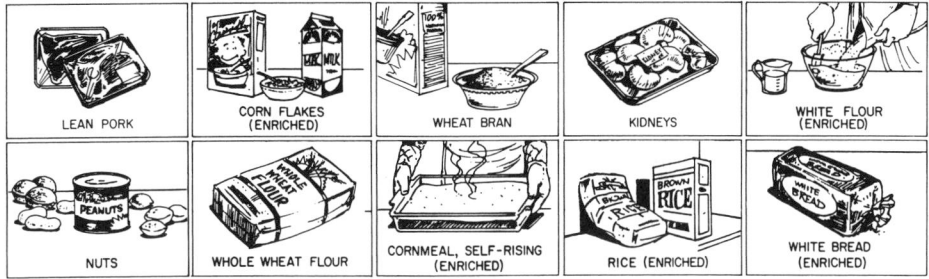

LEAN PORK | CORN FLAKES (ENRICHED) | WHEAT BRAN | KIDNEYS | WHITE FLOUR (ENRICHED)

NUTS | WHOLE WHEAT FLOUR | CORNMEAL, SELF-RISING (ENRICHED) | RICE (ENRICHED) | WHITE BREAD (ENRICHED)

Fig. T-7. The thiamin (vitamin B-1) story.

HISTORY. The history of thiamin begins with a study of the age-old disease beriberi.

Beriberi, which affects the nervous system, was known to the Chinese as early as 2600 B.C. The word *beriberi* means *I cannot,* referring to the fact that persons with the disease cannot move easily. But the cause of beriberi in man, and of polyneuritis—the counterpart in poultry—remained elusive for centuries.

Recognition of the cause of beriberi, and its possible cure by better diet, is a landmark in the history of nutrition, a chronological record of which follows:

In 1873, Van Lent was the first to conclude that the type of diet had something to do with the origin of beriberi, based on reducing the ration of rice in the diet of sailors in the Dutch navy.

In 1882, Kanehiro Takaki, a Japanese medical officer, cured beriberi in sailors of the Japanese navy by giving them less rice and more meat and milk.

In 1897, Christiaan Eijkman, a Dutch physician, working in a military hospital in the East Indies, produced polyneuritis, a condition resembling beriberi, in chickens, pigeons, and ducks by feeding polished rice; which he wrongfully attributed to too much starch.

In 1901, G. Grijns, another Dutch physician, who continued the work of Eijkman at the same hospital, concluded that beriberi in birds and man resulted from lack in the diet of an essential nutrient.

In 1912, Casimir Funk, working at the Lister Institute in London, coined the term *vitamine* and applied it to the anti-beriberi substance.

In 1916, Elmer V. McCollum of the University of Wisconsin, designated the concentrate that cured beriberi as *water-soluble B.*

In 1926, B. C. P. Jansen and W. P. Donath, in Holland, isolated the antiberiberi vitamin, which, at first, was called

aneurin because of its specific action on the nervous system.

In 1936, Robert R. Williams, an American, determined the structure, synthesized it, and gave it the name *thiamine* because it contains sulfur (from *thio,* meaning sulfur-containing) and an amine group. Subsequently, the "e" was dropped and the spelling *thiamin* came to be preferred.

CHEMISTRY, METABOLISM, PROPERTIES.

• **Chemistry**—Thiamin is made up of carbon, hydrogen, oxygen, nitrogen, and sulfur (see Fig. T-8). It consists of a molecule of pyrimidine and a molecule of thiazole linked by a methylene bridge.

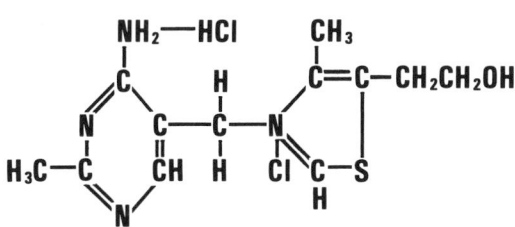

PYRIMIDINE RING   THIAZOLE RING

Fig. T-8. Structure of thiamin hydrochloride, the white, crystalline, stable form in which thiamin is usually marketed.

• **Metabolism**—The thiamin ingested in food is available (1) in the free form, or (2) bound as thiamin pyrophosphate (also called thiamin diphosphate), or (3) in a protein-phosphate complex. The bound forms are split in the digestive tract, following which absorption takes place principally in the upper part of the small intestine where the reaction is acid. It is noteworthy, however, that the absorption of thiamin is impaired in alcoholics with folate deficiency.

Following absorption, thiamin is transported to the liver where it is phosphorylated under the action of ATP to form the coenzyme thiamin diphosphate (formerly called thiamin pyrophosphate or cocarboxylase), (see Fig. T-9); although this phosphorylation occurs rapidly in the liver, it is noteworthy that all nucleated cells appear to be capable of bringing about this conversion.

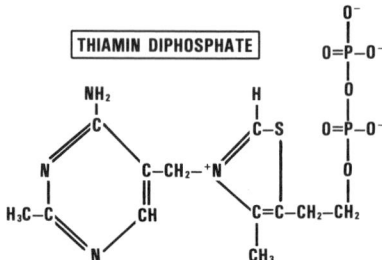

Fig. T-9. Structure of thiamin diphosphate.

Thiamin is the least stored of all the vitamins. The adult human body contains approximately 30 mg. Of the thiamin stored in the body, about 80% is thiamin pyrophosphate, about 10% is thiamin triphosphate, and the remainder is thiamin monophosphate. The liver, kidneys, heart, brain, and skeletal muscles have somewhat higher concentrations than the blood. If the diet is deficient, tissues are depleted of their normal content of the vitamin in 1 to 2 weeks, so fresh supplies are needed regularly to provide for maintenance of tissue levels. Body tissues take up only as much thiamin as they need; with the need increased by metabolic demand (fever, increased muscular activity, pregnancy, and lactation) or by composition of the diet (carbohydrate increases the need for thiamin, while fat and protein spare thiamin). Because thiamin is water soluble, most of the vitamin not required for day-to-day use is excreted in the urine. This means that the body needs a regular supply, and that unneeded intakes are wasted. With a well-balanced diet, approximately 0.1 mg is normally excreted every 24 hours. However, the amount excreted in the urine decreases as the intake becomes inadequate and increases as the intake exceeds body needs; because of this, the most widely used biochemical method to assess thiamin status in individuals is the measurement of the vitamin in the urine.

• **Properties**—Synthetic thiamin is usually marketed as thiamin hydrochloride, which is more stable than the free vitamin. It is a crystalline white powder, with a faint yeastlike odor and a salty nutlike taste. It is stable when dry but readily soluble in water, slightly soluble in alcohol, and insoluble in fat solvents. Heating in solutions at 248°F (120°C) in an acid medium (pH 5.0 or less) has little destructive effect. But cooking foods in neutral or alkaline reaction is very destructive. Also, autoclaving and ultraviolet light destroy thiamin.

Thiamin mononitrate is more stable in heat than thiamin hydrochloride; for which reason it is often used for the thiamin fortification of cereal products that have to be cooked. Derivatives of thiamin, thiamin propyl disulfide and thiamin tetrahydrofurfural disulfide, have been synthesized. These products are recommended for oral administration when there is evidence of thiamin deficiency, because they are absorbed more rapidly than thiamin hydrochloride.

MEASUREMENT/ASSAY. The thiamin content of foods is expressed in milligrams or micrograms. It is usually determined by rapid chemical or microbiological methods, which have largely replaced the older bioassay methods in which pigeons, rats, and chicks were used.

FUNCTIONS. Thiamin is essential as a coenzyme (or cofactor) in energy metabolism, as a coenzyme in the conversion of glucose to fat, in the functioning of the peripheral nerves, and in such indirect functions as appetite, muscle tone, and a healthy mental attitude. A discussion of each of these functions follows:

• **As a coenzyme in energy metabolism**—Without thiamin, there could be no energy.

The major functioning form of thiamin is as thiamin diphosphate (formerly called thiamin pyrophosphate or cocarboxylase)—thiamin combined with two phosphate groups, in which it serves as a coenzyme in a number of enzyme systems.

In the metabolism of carbohydrates, thiamin diphosphate is needed in the conversion of pyruvic acid and the subsequent formation of acetyl coenzyme A, which in turn enters the Krebs cycle and produces vital energy. This is one of the most complex and important reactions in carbohydrate metabolism. In addition to thiamin diphosphate, it also requires the following cofactors: coenzyme A, which contains pantothenic acid, nicotinamide adenine dinucleotide (NAD), which contains niacin; magnesium ions; and lipoic acid.

Oxidative decarboxylation (removal of CO_2) in carbohydrate metabolism is also involved in the Krebs cycle in the conversion of alpha-ketoglutaric acid to succinic acid. Because fats and amino acids, as well as carbohydrates, can contribute to alpha-ketoglutaric acid, it follows that thiamin is involved in the metabolism of all three energy producing units.

In thiamin deficiency, pyruvic and alpha-ketoglutaric acids tend to accumulate in the body; sometimes they are measured as a means of determining thiamin status.

• **As a coenzyme in the conversion of glucose to fats—the process called transketolation (keto-carrying)**—Thiamin diphosphate is also a coenzyme with the enzyme transketolase in the important reaction which provides active glyceraldehyde through the pentose shunt. This is a key link providing activated glycerol for lipogenesis for the conversion of glucose to fat. Thiamin diphosphate is the key activator which provides the high energy phosphate bond. Ionized magnesium (Mg^{++}) is another cofactor present.

• **In the functioning of peripheral nerves**—Thiamin is involved in the functioning of the peripheral nerves. In this role, it has value in the treatment of alcoholic neuritis, the neuritis of pregnancy, and beriberi.

• **In indirect functions**—Because of its primary role in carbohydrate metabolism, thiamin appears to have several indirect functions in the body; among them, the maintenance of normal appetite, the tone of the muscles, and a healthy mental attitude.

DEFICIENCY SYMPTOMS.   The numerous symptoms of thiamin deficiency vary with the severity and duration of the deprivation of the vitamin.

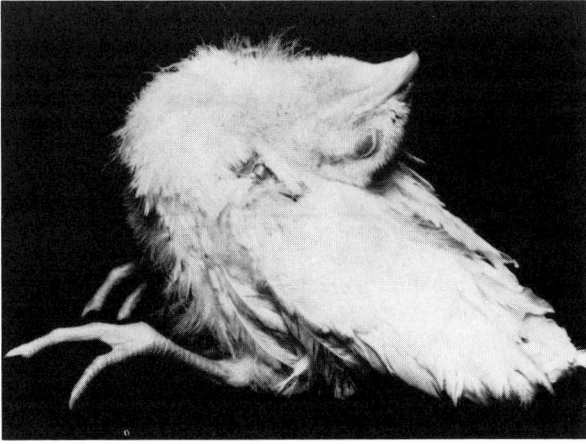

Fig. T-10. Polyneuritis (inflamation of the nerves) in the chick, the counterpart of beriberi in man, caused by thiamin (B-1) deficiency. Note the characteristic head retraction. (Courtesy, H. R. Bird, Department of Poultry Science, University of Wisconsin)

Moderate symptoms may be caused by poor diet, liver damage, or alcoholism. (In many cases, the latter is due to impaired absorption of thiamin caused in part by a deficiency of folacin.) Other persons at risk are kidney patients who are undergoing long-term dialysis treatment, patients fed intravenously for long periods of time, and patients with chronic febrile infections. Individuals consuming large amounts of tea, which contains a thiamin antagonist, or large amounts of raw fish, which contains thiaminase, an enzyme which inactivates the thiamin molecule by splitting it into two parts, may also run increased risk of developing a deficiency.

Symptoms of moderate thiamin deficiency include fatigue; apathy (lack of interest in affairs); loss of appetite; nausea; moodiness; irritability; depression; retarded growth; a sensation of numbness in the legs; and abnormalities of the electrocardiogram.

Clinical Effects of Thiamin Deficiency.   If a deficiency of thiamin is not corrected (if thiamin is not present in sufficient amounts to provide the key energizing coenzyme factor in the cells), the clinical effects will be reflected in the gastrointestinal system, the nervous system, and the cardiovascular system. Severe thiamin deficiency of long duration will culminate in beriberi, the symptoms of which are polyneuritis (inflammation of the nerves), emaciation and/or edema, and disturbances of heart function.

• **Gastrointestinal system symptoms**—The gastrointestinal symptoms of a thiamin deficiency are loss of appetite, indigestion, severe constipation, gastric atony (lack of tone), and decreased hydrochloric acid secretion. These manifestations likely result from insufficient energy from glucose being available for the smooth muscles and the glands of the intestinal tract to do their work of digestion.

• **Nervous system symptoms**—The central nervous system depends solely upon glucose for its energy. So, without thiamin to provide this need, neuronal activity is impaired, alertness and reflex responses are diminished, and fatigue and apathy (lack of interest) follow. If thiamin deficiency

persists, degeneration of myelin sheaths of nerve fibers in the central nervous system and the peripheral nerves occurs, resulting in nerve irritation, which produces pain and prickly or deadening sensations. Unchecked progressive degeneration of the nervous system may cause paralysis and muscle atrophy (wasting).

• **Cardiovascular system symptoms**—If the thiamin deficiency persists, the heart muscles weaken and heart failure may result. Also, the smooth muscles of the vascular system may be involved, causing peripheral vasodilation. As a result of cardiac failure, peripheral edema may be observed in the extremeties.

• **Beriberi**—The various forms and symptoms of beriberi follow:

1. **Dry beriberi (wasting of tissues).** In humans, this form is characterized by numbness or tingling in the feet and toes, stiffness of ankles, soreness in and wasting (atrophy) of the muscles of the legs, a decrease in the reflex of the knee, a drop in the muscles that support the toes and foot, and difficulty in walking. As the disorder advances, the arms and the other parts of the body are affected because there is nerve degeneration and lack of muscle coordination.

2. **Wet beriberi (collection of fluid in the tissues).** The presence of edema, especially of the legs, distinguishes this form from dry beriberi. Other symptoms are loss of appetite, breathlessness, and disorders of the heart.

3. **Infantile beriberi.** This acute disorder is common between the second and fifth months of life in children who are being suckled by mothers subsisting on beriberi-producing diets. Symptoms of the disease are weakness of voice during bawling (complete lack of sound in severe cases), lack of appetite, vomiting, diarrhea, rapid pulse, cyanosis (dark blue coloration of the skin and mucous membrane), and sudden death.

(Also see BERIBERI.)

• **Other clinical symptoms of thiamin deficiency**—Additional symptoms of thiamin deficiency include: low excretion of thiamin in the urine; electrocardiogram changes; reduced transketolase activity of the red blood cells; and an increase of pyruvic acid in the blood.

RECOMMENDED DAILY ALLOWANCE OF THIAMIN.   The Food and Nutrition Board (FNB) of the National Research Council (NRC) recommended daily allowances of thiamin are given in the section on VITAMIN(S), Table V-5, Vitamin Table.

In general, the recommended allowances are based (1) on assessments of the effects of varying levels of dietary thiamin on the occurrence of clinical signs of deficiency, (2) on the excretion of thiamin or its metabolites, and (3) on erythrocyte transketolase activity. Most studies have been conducted on subjects fed diets with ratios of carbohydrate and fat similar to those commonly consumed in the United States. There is evidence that dietary fat *spares* thiamin to some extent.

Because thiamin is essential for key reactions in energy metabolism, particularly carbohydrate metabolism, the requirement for thiamin has usually been related to energy intake.

• **Allowances for infants, children, and adolescents**—As shown in Table V-5, during the growth periods of infancy, childhood, and especially adolescence, thiamin needs are increased.

• **Allowances for adults**—The National Research Council recommended thiamin allowances for adults is 1.5 mg/day for males and 1.1 mg/day for females. Because there is some evidence that older persons use thiamin less efficiently, it is recommended that they maintain a minimum intake of 1 mg/day even if they consume fewer than 2,000 Calories (kcal) daily.

• **Allowance for pregnant and lactating women**—Increased thiamin needs accompany gestation and pregnancy. An allowance of 0.9 mg of thiamin per 1,000 Calories (kcal) is recommended throughout pregnancy, or about an additional 0.4 mg/day. To account for both the thiamin loss in milk and the increased energy consumption during lactation, an allowance of 1.0 mg/1,000 Calories (kcal) is recommended, amounting to an additional 0.5 mg/day.

Increased thiamin needs exist (1) during times of stress, fevers, infections, chronic illness, or surgery; (2) in old age; (3) with increased muscular work; and (4) in chronic alcoholism (due to high intake of energy in the form of alcohol and to reduced thiamin absorption).

• **Thiamin intake in average U.S. diet**—According to the U.S. Department of Agriculture, there is sufficient thiamin in foods available for consumption in the United States to provide an average intake of 2.2 mg per person per day. Of this total, the contribution of food groups is as follows: meats, poultry and fish, 25%; dairy products, 7.5%; and flour and cereal products, 43.3%.

TOXICITY.   There are no known toxic effects from thiamin.

THIAMIN LOSSES DURING PROCESSING, COOKING, AND STORAGE.   The thiamin content of foods is influenced by the practices employed in harvesting, handling, processing, cooking, and storing. Factors contributing to thiamin losses are pH, heat, oxidation, inorganic bases, enzymes, metal complexes, and radiation. The bond between the pyrimidine and thiazole rings is weak with the result that the vitamin is easily destroyed, particularly in an alkaline medium or by heat in the presence of moisture. Thiamin is sensitive to both oxidation and reduction. Sulfur dioxide, sulfites, etc., easily break the bond and vitamin activity is lost.

Pertinent facts about thiamin processing and cooking losses follow:

• **Parboiled (*converted*) rice**—Rice that is soaked and parboiled (*converted*) contains much more thiamin than rice that is milled from the raw state. The parboiling causes the thiamin and other water soluble nutrients to move from the outer layers to the inner layers of the rice kernel. As a result, fewer of them are removed in the milling process.

(Also see RICE.)

• **Processing losses**—Canning causes thiamin losses because of the solubility of the vitamin in the canning fluid; hence, the more canning fluid drained away, the greater the loss.

Drying (dehydrating) food, except fruit, results in only small losses. Thiamin is destroyed rapidly by sulfite, a fact which may explain the loss of thiamin in dried fruits, such as apricots and peaches, treated with sulfur.

Fresh frozen vegetables maintain in storage the thiamin content that is present following blanching to destroy the enzyme activity.

Irradiation destroys thiamin. Thus, the thiamin content of

pork is virtually depleted by irradiation in food preservation.

• **Normal cooking losses**—Normal cooking of an ordinary mixed diet results in the loss of about 25% of the thiamin.

• **Moist heat**—Boiling for not more than an hour causes little destruction of this vitamin. But, because thiamin is soluble in water, as much as one-third of the original thiamin content may be lost if cooking water is liberal and is discarded.

• **Dry heating**—High dry-heat temperatures, as in toasting bread, can cause considerable loss.

• **Cooking breakfast cereals**—Little thiamin is lost in the cooking of breakfast cereals since they are cooked at moderate temperatures and the cooking water is absorbed.

• **Alkali medium**—Thiamin is readily destroyed in an alkali medium. Hence, the practice of adding baking soda (an alkali) to cooking water to preserve the color of green vegetables is not recommended.

• **Meat losses**—Generally, the thiamin losses in cooking meats are greater than in cooking other foods, ranging from 30 to 50% of the raw value; with the least loss occurring in frying.

• **Bread baking losses**—In baking bread, 15 to 20% of the original thiamin content is lost.

• **The same principles apply to both ascorbic acid and thiamin**—When the principles for the retention of ascorbic acid are observed in food processing and cooking, the maximum thiamin content will be preserved, also.

There is little destruction of thiamin from exposure to air at ordinary temperatures. Hence, storage losses of thiamin in foods are minimal.

ANTITHIAMIN FACTORS IN FOOD.   Certain raw fish and seafood—particularly carp, herring, clams, and shrimp—contain the enzyme thiaminase, which inactivates the thiamin molecule by splitting it into two parts. This effect has been seen in mink and fox fed 10 to 25% levels of certain raw fish, giving rise to a thiamin deficiency disease known as Chastek paralysis. This action can be prevented by cooking the fish prior to feeding, thereby destroying the thiaminase. Of course, humans seldom eat sufficient thiaminase-containing raw fish or seafood to produce a thiamin deficiency.

Other agents known to affect thiamin levels in the body are: a large amount of live yeast in the diet of man, which reduces the amount of thiamin absorbed from the intestine; drinking large amounts of tea or chewing fermented tea leaves, a common practice in some parts of Asia; or imbibing alcohol in excess, which contains an antithiamin substance. Also, it is noteworthy that thiamin-splitting bacteria have been found in the intestinal tract of some Japanese with symptoms of beriberi, but the significance of this is not known at present.

SOURCES OF THIAMIN.   Some thiamin is found in a large variety of animal and vegetable products but is abundant in few. Therefore, a deficiency of thiamin is a distinct possibility in the average diet, especially when calories are curtailed.

In addition to food sources, synthetic thiamin is also available; mostly as thiamin hydrochloride, although thiamin mononitrate is often used for the thiamin fortification of cereal products that have to be cooked.

The thiamin content of sources varies according to food and may be affected by harvesting, processing, enrichment, and storage. A grouping and ranking of foods according to normal thiamin content is given in the section on VITAMIN(S), Table V-5, Vitamin Table.

For additional sources and more precise values of thiamin, see Food Composition Table F-21.

Whole grains and enriched grain products are the best daily sources of thiamin. A quart of milk each day contributes 0.29 mg of the thiamin intake.

Foods lacking in thiamin are man-made—refined rice and cereal flours (from which almost all the natural store of the vitamin has been removed by the millers), refined sugar, separated animal and vegetable oils and fats, and alcoholic beverages. None of the thiamin in yeast used for fermentation is present in beers, wines, and spirits that enter normal commerce, although home-brewed beers and country wines may contain significant amounts. Indeed, there are communities in Africa and Latin America which derive the major part of their thiamin from native beers.

Enrichment of flour (bread) and cereals, with thiamin, riboflavin, niacin, and iron (with calcium enrichment optional), which was initiated in 1941, has been of special significance in improving the dietary level in the United States. On the basis of the average per capita consumption of flour and bread in the United States, slightly more than 40% of the daily thiamin requirement is now supplied by these foods.

Rice enrichment has been practiced for years in some of the rice-eating countries; for example, much of the rice used in Japan is enriched.

NOTE WELL: The thiamin requirements are usually met if the diet does not contain disproportionate amounts of the following:
1. Refined, unfortified cereal
2. White sugar
3. Alcohol

Since these three foods are usually matters of personal choice, nutrition education is important.

(Also see RICE; WHEAT, section on "Enriched Flour"; and VITAMIN[S], Table V-5, Vitamin Table.)

THIAMIN DIPHOSPHATE (TDP)

The activating coenzyme necessary for the transketolation reaction in the hexose monophosphate shunt (glucose oxidation) by which active glyceraldehyde is formed for synthesis of fats.

THIRST

Thirst (in humans) is the conscious desire for water. It is the primary means of regulating water intake, and generally, the thirst sensation ensures that water intake meets or exceeds the body's requirement for water. The sensation of thirst is caused by nerve centers in the hypothalamus of the brain which monitor the concentration of sodium (osmolarity) in the blood. When the sodium concentration of the blood increases above the normal 310 to 340 mg/100 ml (*136 to 145 mEq/1*), cells in the thirst center shrink. This shrinking causes more nervous impulses to be generated in the thirst center, thereby creating the sensation of thirst.

An increase of only 1% in the osmolarity of the blood is sufficient to evoke the sensation of thirst. Increased osmolarity of the blood is primarily associated with water loss from the extracellular fluid—blood—through low cardiac output, hemorrhage, or intracellular dehydration may stimulate the thirst sensation. As water is lost, the sodium concentration of the remaining fluid increases. When the individual drinks, the sensation disappears.

Increased osmolarity of the blood simultaneously stimulates other nerve centers in the hypothalamus causing the release of antidiuretic hormone (ADH) from the posterior pituitary. ADH release results in the formation of less urine by the kidneys; hence, conserving body water. Thus, drinking water and excreting water are controlled by centers in the hypothalamus which maintains the water balance of the body within narrow limits.

Constant thirst is a classical symptom of diabetes mellitus.

(Also see ENDOCRINE GLANDS; WATER; and WATER AND ELECTROLYTES.)

THREONINE

One of the essential amino acids.
(Also see AMINO ACID[S].)

THROMBIN

An enzyme that facilitates the clotting of blood by promoting the conversion of fibrinogen to fibrin.

THROMBOSIS

The obstruction of a blood vessel by the formation of a blood clot.

(Also see HEART DISEASE, section headed "Coronary Occlusion [Coronary Thrombosis]".)

THYMINE

One of the four nitrogenous bases in nucleic acid.
(Also see NUCLEIC ACID.)

THYROCALCITONIN

Another name for calcitonin, the hormone secreted by the thyroid gland which acts to lower blood calcium levels.
(Also see CALCITONIN; and ENDOCRINE GLANDS.)

THYROID GLAND

An endocrine gland which is located in the neck on top of the windpipe. It secretes the iodine-containing hormones thyroxine (T_4) and triiodothyronine (T_3), and the calcium regulating hormone calcitonin. The thyroid gland may grow to enormous proportions in the condition of goiter.

(Also see ENDOCRINE GLANDS; GOITER; and IODINE.)

THYROIDITIS

Inflammation of the thyroid gland.

THYROID-STIMULATING HORMONE (TSH)

A hormone secreted by the anterior pituitary gland that regulates uptake of iodine and synthesis of thyroxin by the thyroid gland.

THYROTOXICOSIS

Overactivity of the thyroid gland, causing exophthalmic goiter, which is characterized by nervousness, rapid pulse, bulging eyes, high basal metabolism, and loss of weight.

THYROXIN (T₄)

One of the two iodine-containing hormones secreted by the thyroid gland. It contains four iodine atoms per molecule. Hence, it is often called T_4. Thyroxin is less active than its counterpart triiodothyronine. Thyroxin's actions include increased metabolic rate, increased nervous system activity, stimulated protein synthesis, and increased motility and secretion of the gastrointestinal tract.

(Also see ENDOCRINE GLANDS.)

TIMBALE

• A creamy mixture of chicken, lobster, cheese, or fish cooked in individual molds or cups.

• A small pastry shell fried with a timbale iron and filled with a cooked timbale mixture, or served with fruit sauce, or dusted with powdered sugar.

TISSUE

A collection of cells, usually of a particular kind which form a definite structure, such as connective tissue, epithelium, muscle, and nerve.

(Also see BODY TISSUE.)

TISSUES OF THE BODY

Tissues are an aggregate of similar cells together with their intercellular substances. In turn tissues combine to form the organs of the body. The major tissues of the body are (1) nervous tissue, (2) muscles, (3) skin, (4) blood cells, (5) fat or adipose, and (6) bone.

TOASTED

Brown, dried, or parched by exposure to a fire, or to a gas or electric heat.

TOCOPHEROL

Any of four different forms of an alcohol. Also known as vitamin E.

(Also see VITAMIN E.)

TOCOTERIENOL

Compounds found in nature that have vitamin E activity, but which are less potent than alpha-tocopherol.

(Also see VITAMIN E.)

TOLBUTAMIDE

An oral drug, a derivative of sulfonylurea, capable of lowering blood glucose (sugar) when a functioning pancreas is still present. Since it acts by stimulating the release of insulin, it may be used in the treatment of diabetes when there is still some residual function of the pancreas.

(Also see DIABETES MELLITUS, section headed "Sulfatype Drugs [Sulfonylureas].")

TOMATO *Lycopersicon esculentum*

The tomato is a member of the Nightshade family (*Solanaceae*), which also claims as members capsicum peppers, eggplant, and Irish potatoes.

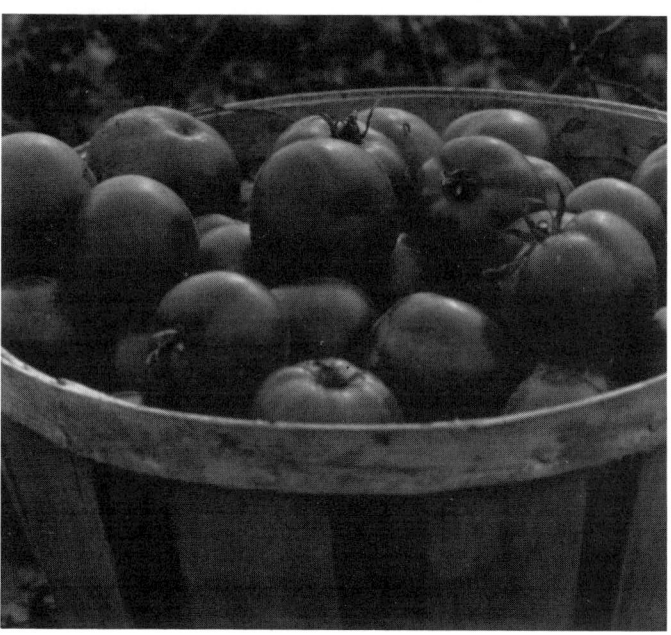

Fig. T-11. Tomatoes, the second leading vegetable of the U.S. (Courtesy, National Film Board of Canada)

ORIGIN AND HISTORY. The modern tomato descended from a wild ancestor, the cherry tomato, native to Peru and Ecuador. It was first domesticated by the Indians in Central America. But it had spread to both North and South America long before Columbus arrived.

WORLD AND U.S. PRODUCTION. Tomatoes rank fourth among the leading vegetables of the world. Worldwide, about 69 million metric tons of tomatoes are produced annually; and the leading tomato-producing countries, ranked by descending order, are: United States, U.S.S.R., Turkey, China, Italy, Egypt, Spain, Romania, Brazil, and Greece.[4]

Tomatoes rank second among the leading vegetables of the United States, with a production of about 16.8 million short tons annually; and the leading tomato-producing states are: Florida, California, and South Carolina. Florida alone produces 43% of the U.S. tomato crop.[5]

PROCESSING. About 75% of the U.S. tomato crop is processed; still, the demand for tomato products can hardly be met, as evidenced by the various tomato extenders that are used in certain products. Among the popular tomato products are the following: canned tomatoes, catsup (ketchup), chili sauce, juice, juice crystals, paste, powder, puree, salad dressings, sauces, soups, and vegetable juice cocktails.

---

[4]Data from *FAO Production Yearbook 1990*, FAO/UN, Rome, Italy, Vol. 44, p. 131, Table 52. **Note well:** Annual production fluctuates as a result of weather and profitability of the crop.

[5]Data from *Agricultural Statistics 1991*, USDA, p. 165, Table 240. **Note well:** Annual production fluctuates as a result of weather and profitability of the crop.

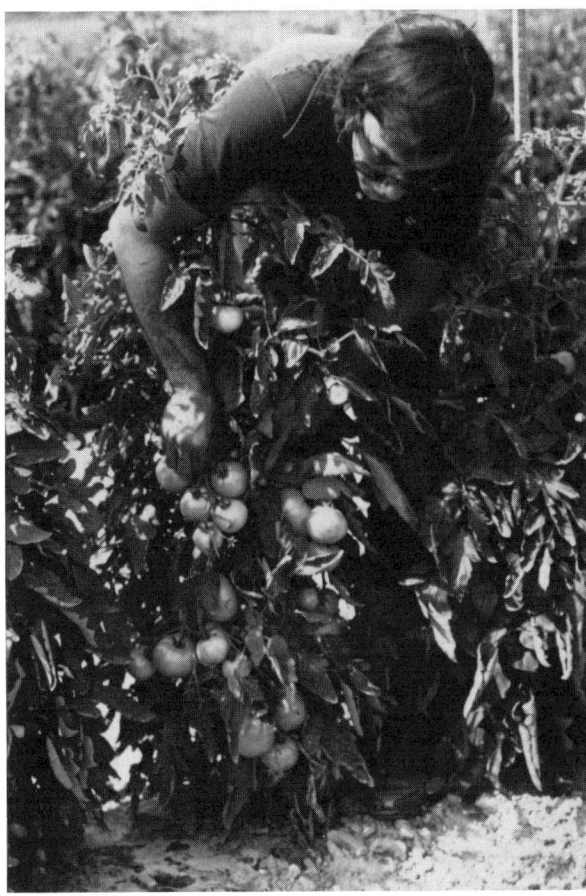

Fig. T-12. Closeup of a tomato plant. (Courtesy, Louisiana State University, Baton Rouge)

SELECTION, PREPARATION, AND USES. Good quality tomatoes are well formed and plump, of uniform red color, free from bruise marks, and not overripe or soft.

Fresh tomatoes and canned tomato products are very convenient foods for the busy homemaker because (1) the raw vegetable lends itself well to cold soups, relishes, and salads; (2) only a few minutes of simmering is needed to cook the raw vegetable; (3) canned tomato juice may be used to make a wide variety of molded gelatin salads, (4) canned tomato paste or puree may be used when concentrated sauces are desired, and (5) the flavor and color of the tomato blends well with those of many other ingredients. Some examples of easy-to-prepare tomato dishes and a few gourmet-type preparations follow:

• **Aspic**—This type of appetizer or side dish is usually made from tomato juice, flavored or unflavored gelatin, and seasonings such as lemon juice, sugar, salt, pepper, and Worcestershire sauce.

• **Chinese stir-fried dishes**—Tomatoes may be added near the end of the cooking period to stir-fried dishes

• **Eastern European tomato salad**—In Serbia (a region of Yugoslavia) this type of salad is made from tomatoes, raw onions, chili peppers, goat cheese, and baked sweet peppers.

• **Gazpacho soup**—This chilled tomato soup, which originated in Spain, contains small pieces of peeled and seeded tomatoes, other vegetables that have been finely chopped or pureed, olive oil, wine vinegar, and various seasonings.

• **Green tomato pie**—Although this dessert is very similar to apple pie with respect to ingredients and preparation, it differs in that deskinned, green tomato wedges are substituted for sliced apples.

• **Guacamole**—Deskinned, deseeded, chopped tomatoes are mixed with mashed avocado pulp, chopped onions, hot green chili peppers, coriander leaves or parsley, and a pinch of salt to make this popular Mexican sauce.

• **Italian pasta dishes**—Many of these items are served with a rich tomato sauce that is easily prepared if one starts with a canned tomato product such as tomato paste or tomato sauce.

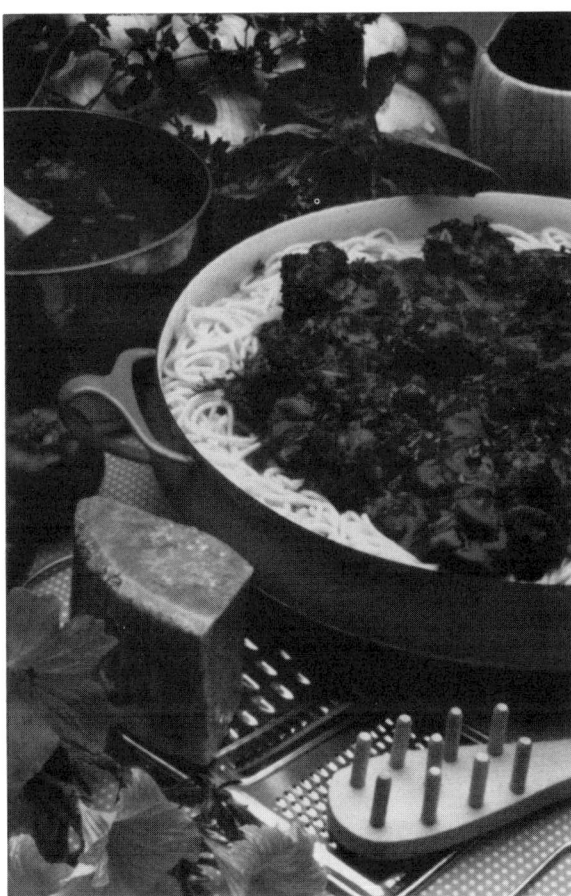

Fig. T-13. Tomatoes in a casserole. (Courtesy, National Film Board of Canada)

• **Lobster with tomato sauce**—Peeled and chopped tomatoes are simmered with white wine, fish stock, brandy, butter, chopped shallots, crushed garlic, parsley, Cayenne pepper, salt, and black pepper to make a delectable French sauce for lobster.

• **Piccalilli**—This popular relish is commonly made from green tomatoes, green peppers, red chili peppers, vinegar, sugar, salt, horseradish, ground mustard, cinnamon, and ginger.

• **Spanish rice**—Quick-cooking types of rice and canned tomato sauce make it possible to prepare this dish in less than one-half hour. Other ingredients are ground beef, chopped onion, chopped green pepper, chili sauce, butter or margarine, salt, Worchestershire sauce, and black pepper.

• **Stuffed tomato**—Fillings such as bread crumbs, cheese, chopped egg, crumbled bacon, fish or seafood, legumes, meats, nuts, poultry, and/or cooked rice may be used to stuff tomatoes. However, the fillings should be cooked first, so that the stuffed tomato shells will require only a few minutes of simmering in a sauce.

• **Tomato chutney**—Chutneys are condiments or relishes that appear to have spread to the rest of the world from India and Indonesia. A typical tomato chutney may contain chopped peeled tomatoes plus chili pepper, chopped dried fruit, vegetable oil, salt, and other seasonings.

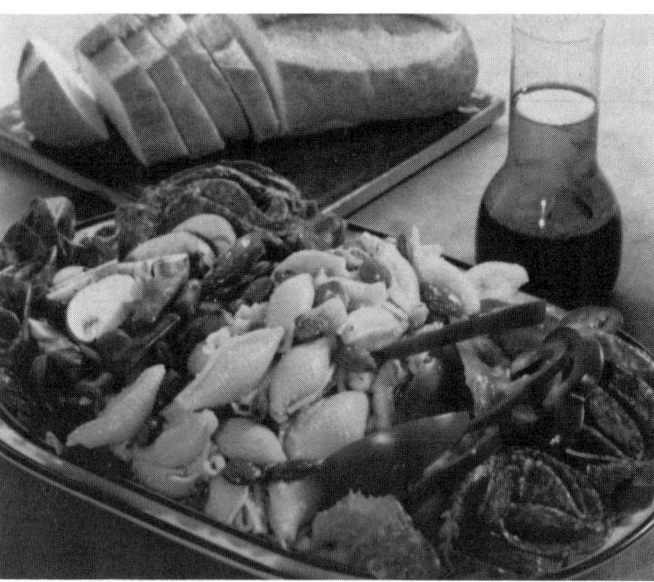

Fig. T-14. Tomatoes in a salad. (Courtesy, Anderson/Miller & Hubbard Consumer Services, San Francisco, Calif.)

NUTRITIONAL VALUE. The nutrient compositions of various forms of tomatoes are given in Food Composition Table F-21.

Some noteworthy observations regarding the nutrient composition of tomatoes follow:

1. Fresh tomatoes and tomato juice are high in water content (about 94%) and low in calories. Both items are good sources of vitamins A and C, except that the unfortified juice has only about two-thirds the vitamin C content of raw, ripe tomatoes. However, tomato juice may be fortified to bring the level of the vitamin up to 10 milligrams per fluid ounce (*30 ml*).

2. Ripe (red) tomatoes contain from 3 to 4 times as much vitamin A as mature green tomatoes. Otherwise, green and red tomatoes are about equal in nutritional value.

3. Canned tomatoes contain only about three-fourths the vitamin C content of fresh ripe tomatoes.

4. Tomato puree and plain types of tomato sauce (those without added ingredients such as cheese, meat, mushrooms, etc.) have about twice the solids content and about double the nutritional value of fresh tomatoes and tomato juice.

5. Tomato paste, which has about four times the solids content of fresh tomatoes, is a concentrated source of nutrients. Table T-2 compares the composition of this product with canned corn.

TABLE T-2
NUTRIENT COMPOSITIONS OF TOMATO PASTE AND CANNED CORN[1]

Nutrient or Other Constituent		Tomato Paste	Canned Corn[2]
Water content	(%)	75	76
Calories	(kcal)	82	83
Protein	(g)	3.4	2.5
Phosphorus	(mg)	70	73
Potassium	(mg)	888	97
Iron	(mg)	3.5	0.5
Vitamin A	(IU)	3,300	350
Vitamin C	(mg)	49	5
Thiamin	(mg)	0.20	0.03
Riboflavin	(mg)	0.12	0.06
Niacin	(mg)	3.10	1.10

[1]Nutrients per 3½ oz (*100 g*) portion.
[2]Yellow sweet corn, vacuum packed, solids and liquid.

Table T-2 shows that tomato paste provides considerably greater amounts of nutrients per calorie than canned corn. A similar nutritional superiority is noted when the paste is compared to other grains and cereal products. Therefore, this product may make a valuable contribution when it is used in the preparation of pastas, pizzas, and other dishes.

6. Catsup and chili sauce are about equal in nutritional value, since each item is made with similar ingredients and contains about 32% solids (about 5 times the content of fresh tomatoes and tomato juice). However, the nutrients provided per calorie by these products are significantly less than those furnished by tomato paste, because the solid contents and caloric values of the two condiments are boosted by added salt and sugar.

Tomatoes contain small amounts of solanine. (See SOLANINE.)

(Also see VEGETABLE[S], Table V-2, Vegetables of the World.)

TOMATO JUICE

The juice extracted from tomatoes that is produced by chopping fresh fruit which may or may not have been preheated, pressing the fruit pulp through a series of screens, adding back some of the pulp to the screened juice, canning, and pasteurization.

The nutrient composition of various forms of tomato juice is given in Food Composition Table F-21.

Some noteworthy observations regarding the nutrient composition of tomato juice follow:

1. 1-cup (*250 g*) of bottled or canned tomato juice provides only 38 Calories (kcal), and is a good source of potassium, iron, vitamin A, and vitamin C. Most juice products often contain added sodium (about 400 mg per cup), but low sodium products are also available.

2. Frozen tomato juice concentrate contains about 4 times the caloric and nutrient contents of the single strength canned juice. Hence, it will make a significant nutritional contribution when added undiluted to dishes such as sauces and soups.

(Also see TOMATO.)

-TOMY

Suffix meaning to cut into; e.g., gastrectomy.

TONIC

- A drug or agent said to improve the health or vigor of an organ, or of the body.

- When referring to muscles, it can mean the state of muscular tension or continuous muscular contraction.

- A bottled quinine water used to make the drink "Gin & Tonic." This drink originated in the tropics where it was used to alleviate fevers, either real or imagined.

TOPHUS

Sodium urate deposits in the fibrous tissues near the joints or in the cartilage of the external ear; present in gout.

TORULARODIN

Carotenoid pigment in *Torula ruba* and *Rhodotorula mucilaginosa* yeasts, with vitamin A activity.

TORULA YEAST

Torula yeast (*Torulopsis utilis*) is a hardy type of yeast that can be propagated on a variety of substrates, such as press liquor obtained during the manufacture of dried citrus pulp, molasses, sulphite waste liquor from the paper industry, saccharified wood (both hexoses and pentoses can be used), and fruit wastes such as coffee beans, apples, etc. While brewers' yeast is truly a by-product food, torula yeast is cultured specifically as a foodstuff for man and animals.

Dried torula yeast is an excellent source of high-quality protein (50 to 62% crude protein), minerals, B vitamins (including vitamin B-12), unidentified factors, and of vitamin D if irradiated. Unlike the bitter-tasting brewers' yeast, torula yeast is tasteless, thereby facilitating its use as a palatable foodstuff.

Torula yeast is available in powder and tablets.

TOTAL CRUDE PROTEIN

The equivalent amounts of crude protein in the food represented by the total nitrogen present.
(Also see ANALYSIS OF FOODS.)

TOTAL MILK SOLIDS

Primarily milk fat, proteins, lactose, and minerals.
(Also see MILK AND MILK PRODUCTS.)

TOTAL PARENTERAL (INTRAVENOUS) NUTRITION (TPN) (CENTRAL INTRAVENOUS NUTRITION)

This nutritional procedure can provide all or most of a patient's nutrient requirements by intravenous means. Total parenteral nutrition is used when the patient cannot be fed through the gastrointestinal tract because of the danger of aggravating an abnormal condition, or because some part of the tract is functioning poorly. Usually, it involves infusion of nutrients by means of a catheter that is passed through a large vein into the vena cava, as is shown in Fig. T-15.

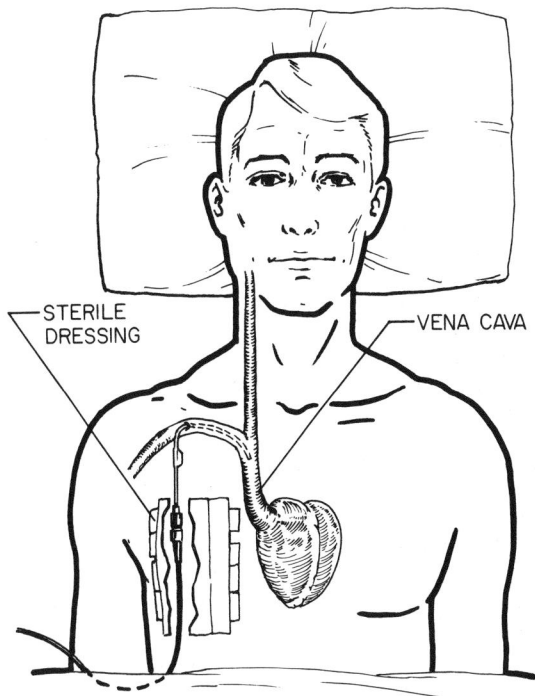

Fig. T-15. Total parenteral (intravenous) nutrition. The concentrated solution of nutrients flows through a sterile tubing attached to a catheter passed through the subclavian vein into the vena cava. This procedure results in rapid mixing of the nutrients with blood returning to the heart, which then pumps the nutrient-rich blood throughout the body.

It is noteworthy that the solutions used in total parenteral nutrition have much higher solute contents than those used in ordinary intravenous feedings (about 30% solute in TPN vs 5% solute in an IV) because (1) nutrient needs cannot be met completely by the latter, and (2) the means by which the former is administered (into a large central vein where rapid mixing with the blood occurs) is sufficiently safe, whereas concentrated (hypertonic) solutions cannot be infused safely into the peripheral veins. Phlebitis and clots are more likely to result from the injection of hypertonic solutions into peripheral veins because the flow of blood in them is slow. Therefore, TPN is sometimes referred to as *central intravenous nutrition* in order to distinguish it from peripheral IVs.

INDICATIONS FOR TPN.   The foremost types of conditions requiring total parenteral nutrition are those in which the patient's nutritive needs are high, and cannot be met by more commonly used procedures such as oral, tube, or peripheral intravenous feeding. However, it may also be indicated even when some food can be taken orally or through a nasogastric tube because the nutritional requirements may be so high that they cannot be met via the digestive tract alone. Some of the most common indications for TPN follow:

1. Burns over large areas of the body.
2. Cancer.
3. Chronic diarrhea.
4. Fistulas of the digestive tract.
5. Inflammatory bowel disease.
6. Kidney failure.
7. Liver failure.
8. Refusal to eat.
9. Surgery on the digestive tract.
10. Undernourished and very-low-birth-weight infants.

Use of TPN at Home.   The success of TPN in hospital settings led to the development of techniques and equipment that could be used at home so that patients requiring this therapy would not have to be kept in a hospital. Generally, the most likely candidates for home TPN are patients with reasonable chances of benefiting from it because their major nutritional problems are due to gastrointestinal disorders such as (1) a loss of considerable amounts of small intestine, (2) inflammatory bowel disease, and (3) digestive disorders resulting from chemotherapy and/or radiation treatments.

Home TPN is rather expensive because it requires a special pump or a gas pressure device, sterile tubing, special valves, and the nutrient solutions. It is noteworthy that the valves permit patients to be disconnected from the apparatus for 8 to 14 hours so that many normal acitivities may be carried out. Hundreds of patients have been placed on home TPN, and some have received this therapy for 5 years or more. It is expected that the cost will be reduced as the number of people on home TPN increases. At any rate, it is usually less expensive than receiving care in an institution.

Composition of Infusions.   The TPN solutions that were first used on an experimental basis by Dr. Dudrick and his co-workers at the University of Pennsylvania School of Medicine contained approximately 20% dextrose (glucose), 5% protein, and 5% minerals and vitamins. Hence, the total solute concentration was about 6 times that of an ordinary 5% dextrose (glucose) intravenous feeding. Since then, many modifications of Dudrick's original TPN solutions have been made to accommodate the particular needs of individual patients. However, the commercial TPN preparations that are available in the United States do not always contain essential fatty acids. Therefore, it is noteworthy that deficiencies of these nutrients have been observed in patients receiving parenteral nutrition. This risk is reduced to zero if fat emulsions are infused on a regular basis (1 to 2 times per week). No doubt there are other essential nutrients that should be provided by supplemental means when patients are on TPN for long periods of time.

BENEFITS.   Some of the recoveries that were brought about by TPN have been so remarkable that one eminent physician has ranked the development of this procedure on a par with other great medical innovations such as anesthesia, antiseptics, and antibiotics. What TPN has done is to demonstrate very dramatically the pivotal role played by nutrition in healing. Typical benefits of TPN follow:

1.   The need to search all over the body for intact veins through which to make peripheral intravenous infusions is eliminated by TPN because an indwelling catheter may remain in place for long periods of time when the proper safeguards are observed.

2.   Wasting of tissues after burns, injury, surgery, or other extremely stressful occurrences is minimized by TPN, which provides the high levels of nutrients needed for healing.

3.   Bypassing of the digestive tract does away with the needs to cope with diarrhea, flatulence, nausea, vomiting, and other gastrointestinal reactions that interfere with nourishment. Hence, the tract may be rested and allowed to heal without disturbance.

4.   Nutrient patterns may be tailormade to suit the needs of the patient because the infusions are made directly into a major blood vessel for delivery to the tissues of the body by the pumping of the heart.

HAZARDS AND PRECAUTIONS.   TPN is not a routine nutritional procedure because special precautions must be taken in its administration to prevent undesirable consequences. The main hazards and precautions of TPN are:

• **Aggravation of disorders of metabolism**—When people obtain their nourishment via the digestive tract the absorbed nutrients are conveyed by the portal system of blood vessels to the liver, where excess sugars are converted into fats and glycogen (a complex carbohydrate that is stored in the liver and muscles), fats are combined with proteins for safe transport in the blood, and amino acids are converted into proteins and waste products such as urea.

However, in TPN the regulation of the blood levels of nutrients by the liver is bypassed to a great extent because the infused substances flow to the heart, where they are pumped through the arteries to the body tissues. The latter situation may be dangerous to diabetics because they utilize nutrients more slowly than normal people. Hence, they may develop excessively high blood levels of nutrients, which can lead to (1) loss of excessive amounts of nutrients and water through urination (osmotic diuresis), (2) dehydration (due to excessive loss of water), and/or (3) coma. On the other hand, people with some types of kidney disease may fail to excrete a normal amount of water and consequently become waterlogged (overhydrated) to the point of developing congestive heart failure.

Finally, some people who have been on TPN for 5 months or longer have developed bone demineralization and bone pain. Therefore, patients receiving TPN for the first time should be monitored carefully by blood chemistries, blood gas analyses, urine collection and analyses, and other laboratory tests for metabolism so that the appropriate therapies may be administered for any abnormal conditions that may develop.

• **Injuries resulting from the procedure**—The experts who have used TPN on a regular basis consider the placement of the catheter to be a serious surgical procedure and proceed accordingly. Failure to observe certain precautions may result in mishaps such as puncturing of the vein and passage of the catheter into neighboring blood vessels or organs such as the heart and lungs, and consequences such as bleeding, production of irregular heartbeats, the introduction of air or fluids into the lungs, or inflammation of the catheterized vein so that a spasm occurs or a clot is formed. Therefore, it is best to place the patient in an inclined position with the head downward (15% Trendelenburg position) so that the subclavian vein sticks out and is more easily entered. Also, an x ray should be taken after the catheter has been placed and before it is used to make certain that its location is correct for the patient. It is noteworthy that complications are rare when these precautions are observed strictly.

• **Microbiological contamination**—Infectious microorganisms may get into the body via (1) the point where the vein is punctured, (2) the surface of the catheter, (3) the inside of the tubing and/or the catheter. Also, inside the vena cava the tip of the catheter may serve as a place for bloodborne bacteria to lodge and multiply, then detach themselves and spread through the bloodstream to susceptible body tissues. Therefore, a sudden unexplainable rise in the body temperature of a patient should lead the attending doctors and nurses to suspect a catheter-induced infection, and/or any of the other sources of infection that are likely under the circumstances.

Some of the antiseptic precautions that are commonly used to prevent a catheter-induced infection of the patient consist of (1) shaving the hair from the chest and defatting of the skin with ether or acetone; (2) washing of the shaved and defatted area with sterile gauze sponges wetted with iodine solution; (3) handling of the catheterization assembly with sterile gloves while making sure that it does not come into contact with nonsterile items; (4) application of an antibiotic ointment and a sterile dressing on the area of catheterization, followed by the application of tincture of benzoin around the dressing; (5) periodic changing of the dressing and inspection of the catheter site for redness, infection, leakage, or other problems (ideally, the same nurse should perform this function so that she will readily recognize any changes); and (6) taking care that the solutions are changed under strictly aseptic conditions. These measures ensure a continued sterility of the catheter for months, or even years. The longevity of the preparation is important because there are only four sites (right and left subclavian veins, and right and left jugular veins) that are highly suited for this procedure as it is normally carried out. (Other means of central venous infusion are more complicated and dangerous.)

- **Nutritional deficiencies**—Recent reports in the medical literature have indicated that certain nutritional deficiencies may result from the long-term use of some proprietary brands of TPN infusions, unless the nutrients not present in the solutions are provided by other means. The deficiencies reported up to now have been those of essential fatty acids, the essential minerals chromium and selenium, and the vitamin biotin. Normally, biotin is synthesized by intestinal bacteria, but the administration of broad spectrum antibiotics in the case reported eliminated that source of the vitamin.

It is the responsibility of the doctor who orders the TPN procedure to make certain that all of the essential nutrients are provided to the patient. This may be done readily by adding the required substances to the TPN infusion.

- **Psychological impact**—Many patients may be quite apprehensive of being put on TPN because (1) they may not have known anyone else who received this type of therapy, (2) the providing of nutrients parenterally for more than a few weeks may cause concern over whether normal eating will ever be resumed, and (3) their lives may depend upon the apparatus functioning properly. Therefore, it may be necessary for the doctor, nurse, a knowledgeable member of the family, or a trusted friend to give the patient repeated assurances about the efficacy of the procedure and the possibility of eventually resuming many normal activities, even though it should be necessary to continue TPN for a long time at home.

The expression of anger, disbelief, grief, and/or depression is common for patients dependent upon complex treatments delivered by the medical care team, who may sometimes deliberately or inadvertently create a mystique about their procedures. Some type of psychiatric consultation may be required to help the patient cope with the situation and cooperate in the healing process.

CONTRAINDICATIONS. TPN carries some risks, and should not be used when (1) it is possible to meet all or most of a patient's nutritional needs by oral or tube feeding (some supplementation may be given by peripheral intravenous feeding); (2) the patient is moderately healthy and will be required to abstain from eating for only a few days; (3) there is little hope for improvement of the patient; and (4) certain disorders (cardiovascular, metabolic, or organ disfunctions) are present that are likely to be aggravated by TPN. In the latter cases, it may be possible to use TPN after the patient's condition has been stabilized.

SUMMARY. Total parenteral nutrition is a recently developed procedure that carries some risks, but may help to get seriously ill patients back on their feet, provided that the proper precautions are observed.

TOX-

Prefix meaning poison.

TOXEMIA

A condition produced by the presence of poisons (toxins) in the blood.

TOXEMIA OF PREGNANCY (PREECLAMPSIA AND ECLAMPSIA)

A cardinal indication of toxemia of pregnancy is a sudden weight gain sometime during the last trimester. It is a serious disorder of uncertain origin involving decreased kidney function. Numerous factors including endocrine, metabolic, and nutritional may be responsible for the disorder, and not a toxic substance as the name implies. Other features of the condition consist of high blood pressure, blurred vision, protein in the urine, and puffy neck, ankles, and face—edema. It is most often observed in (1) first pregnancies before the age of 30 years; (2) twin pregnancies; (3) economically underprivileged segments of the population—the malnourished; and (4) women with prior kidney or vascular disease. Preeclampsia and eclampsia are two stages of toxemia of pregnancy. Preeclampsia is characterized by those items mentioned above, while eclampsia indicates that the symptoms have intensified—circulatory failure, convulsions, and coma—possibly resulting in the death of the mother and the baby.

The most effective treatment is delivery of the baby. However, during the course of pregnancy, routine urine analysis and blood pressure checks by a doctor indicate the onset of toxemia. Once the onset of toxemia is noted, control measures such as sodium restriction, diuretics, sedatives, and bed rest may be initiated. Nevertheless, toxemia becomes increasingly difficult to manage the last month of pregnancy, and delivery may be induced slightly before term to prevent harmful effects to both the mother and the child.

Although the involvement of dietary factors in the development of toxemia is not clear, three points deserve mention. First, a vitamin B-6 deficiency during pregnancy may have a role in the development of toxemia. Second, while sodium restriction and diuretics are traditional approaches to the control of toxemia, there is also an increased demand for sodium during pregnancy; moreover, the Committee on Maternal Nutrition discourages the routine use of salt restriction and diuretics during pregnancy. Third, well-balanced diets provide the best protection against the development of complications during the course of pregnancy.

(Also see PREGNANCY AND LACTATION NUTRITION, section on "Fluid Retention.")

TOXINS

The poisons produced by certain microorganisms. They are products of cell metabolism. The symptoms of bacterial diseases, such as diptheria, tetanus, botulism, and staphylococcal food poisoning, are caused by toxins.

(Also see FOODBORNE DISEASE; and POISONS.)

TOXINS, BACTERIAL, FOODBORNE

Food poisoning is caused by the ingestion of bacterial toxins that have been produced in the food by the growth of specific kinds of bacteria before the food is eaten. The powerful toxins are ingested directly, and the symptoms of food poisoning develop rapidly, usually within 1 to 6 hours after the food is eaten. Two common bacteria that produce toxins in food are *Clostridium botulinum* (botulism) and *Staphylococcus aureus* (staphylococcus food poisoning). Each type is quite different in growth habits and in the symptoms of poisoning.

(Also see BACTERIA IN FOOD, Table B-3, Food Poisonings [Bacterial Toxins]; and POISONS.)

TRANSAMINATION

A metabolic process involving the transfer of an amino group (NH_2) from one compound to another. This is one process which makes possible the synthesis of a limited number of amino acids—nonessential amino acids. Carbon skeletons for this process are produced through various intermediates of carbohydrate metabolism. A new amino acid can be produced when an amino group (NH_2) is transferred from an amino acid to the carbon skeleton. The deaminated molecule—past amino acid—can be used as an energy source.

(Also see METABOLISM; section on "Proteins-Catabolism;" and PROTEIN[S].)

TRANS FATTY ACIDS

The hardening of vegetable oils by hydrogenation (the chemical addition of hydrogen) converts the naturally-occurring *cis* fatty acids to *trans* fatty acids. Generally speaking, it follows that the more an oil has been hardened, the higher the content of trans fatty acids.

(Also see FATS AND OTHER LIPIDS, section headed "Fatty Acids"; and OILS, VEGETABLE, section headed "Antinutritional and/or Toxic Factors.")

TRANSFERASE

Any of various enzymes that promote a transfer reaction; for example, transaminase.

TRANSFERRIN (SIDEROPHILIN)

Iron-binding protein for transport of iron in the blood. (Also see IRON.)

TRANSKETOLASE

The enzyme is a transketolase and the process is called transketolation (keto-carrying). Transketolase uses thiamin diphosphate as a coenzyme to bring about the transfer of a 2-carbon unit from one sugar (a 2-keto sugar) to aldoses (monosaccharides with the characteristic aldehyde group [-CHO]).

TRAUMA

• A wound or injury.

• A psychological or emotional stress.

TREE TOMATO *Cyphomandra betacea*

The fruit of a small tree (of the family *Solanaceae*) that is native to Peru and is now grown throughout the tropics.

Tree tomatoes resemble the plum type of common tomato (*Lycopersicum esculentum*) in many respects in that they are usually yellow to red in color, 2 to 3 in. (*5 to 7.5 cm*) long, and contain many seeds. They may be eaten raw, stewed, or when made into jam, jelly, or juice.

The fruit ranges from low to moderately high in calories (50 kcal per 100 g) and carbohydrates (10%). It is a good source of fiber and vitamin C, and a fair source of iron.

TRIGLYCERIDES

Chemical compounds which contain three (tri-) molecules of fatty acid combined with one molecule of glycerol. Triglycerides differ from each other because the types of fatty acids linked to the glycerol vary. Fig. T-16 illustrates the formation of a triglyceride. The R in Fig. T-16 indicates a carbon chain which varies according to the fatty acid, while the COOH in Fig. T-16 is the acid portion of the fatty acid. When fatty acids combine with glycerol, water (H_2O) is formed.

(Also see FATS AND OTHER LIPIDS; and OILS, VEGETABLE.)

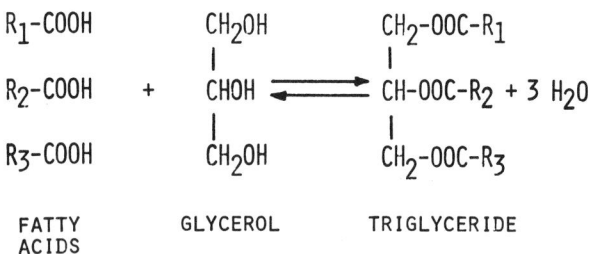

Fig. T-16. The formation of a triglyceride.

TRIPE

Most tripe is made from the first and second (rumen and reticulum) stomachs of cattle by: washing thoroughly; removing the stomach lining by scalding and scraping; and either (1) pickling in a 60°F (*16°C*) salt brine, or (2) cooking and pickling in a weak salt and vinegar brine.

TRIPEPTIDES

These are three amino acids chemically joined together by peptide bonds. They may be a step in the synthesis of new protein, or a step in the breakdown of dietary protein.

(Also see DIGESTION AND ABSORPTION; and PROTEIN[S].)

TRISTEARIN

A triglyceride of stearic acid.

TRITICALE *Triticum X Secale*

This is a hybrid cereal derived from a cross between wheat (*Triticum*) and rye (*Secale*), followed by doubling the chromosomes in the hybrid. The objective of the cross: to combine the grain quality, productivity, and disease resistance of wheat with the vigor and hardiness of rye. The first such crosses were made in 1875 when the Scottish botanist Stephen Wilson dusted pollen from a rye plant onto the stigma of a wheat plant. Only a few seeds developed and germinated; and the hybrids were found to be sterile. In 1937, the French botanist Pierre Givaudon produced some fertile wheat-rye hybrids with the ability to reproduce. Intensive experimental work to improve triticale was undertaken at the University of Manitoba, beginning in 1954.

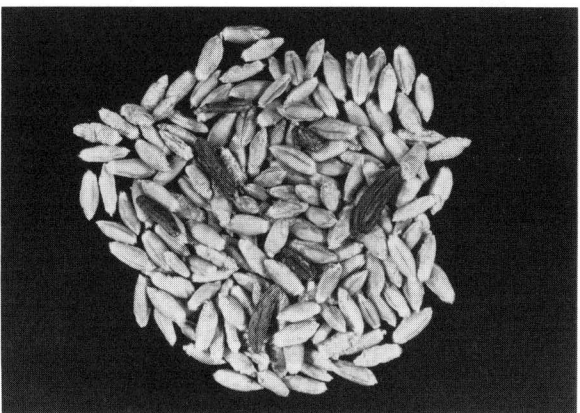

Fig. T-17. Triticale grains. (Photo by International Development Research Center, Ottawa, Canada)

In comparison with wheat, triticale (1) has a larger grain, but there are fewer of them in each head (spike), (2) has a higher protein content, with a slightly better balanced amino acid composition and more lysine, and (3) is more winter hardy. Nutritional information on triticale flour is presented in the Food Composition Table F-21.

Earlier varieties of triticale did not offer much promise for milling and baking; they resembled their rye parent more than their wheat parent. However, bread of good quality has been made from more recent triticale selections. So far, the main use for triticale has been as a feed grain, pasture, green chop, and silage crop for animals.

(Also see CEREAL GRAINS.)

TRUFFLE *Tuber* spp

The truffle is a pungent wild fungus that grows underground, which is highly prized as a food. The fungus is believed to have a symbiotic relationship with the roots of oak and beech trees, near which it is usually found. Agronomists have not been successful in cultivating truffles. Depending on the species, they vary from white to brown or black in color. They range from ¼ to 4 in. (0.6 to 10 cm) in diameter; and they grow in clusters 3 to 12 in. (7.7 to 30 cm) below the ground. They resemble an acorn, a walnut, or a potato in shape. Most culinary truffles are found in western Europe. *Tuber melanosporum* is the famed black truffle of France, while *Tuber magnatum* is the more pungent and odoriferous white truffle that grows in the Italian Piedmont. Also, North Africa produces a truffle (*Terfezios*) in some quantity and they are occasionally found along the Pacific Coast in the United States. Trained dogs or pigs are usually used to sniff out the location of truffles (See Fig. T-18). From 300 to 500 tons are harvested annually.

(Also see MUSHROOMS.)

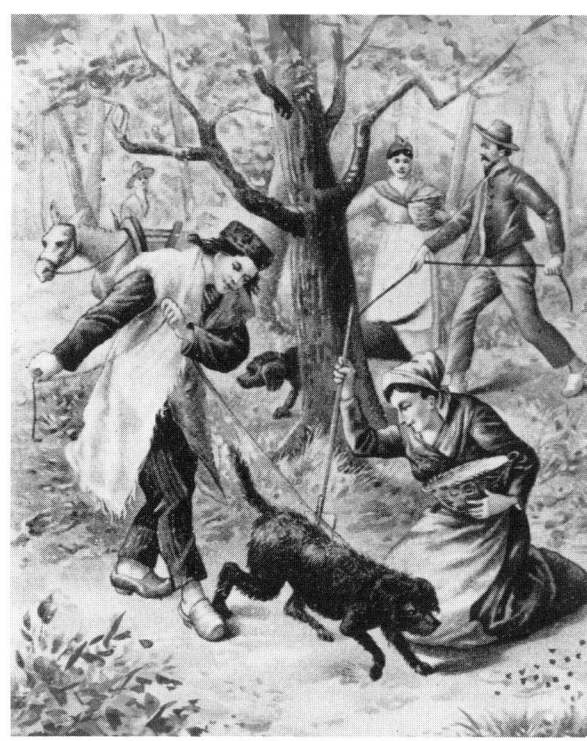

Fig. T-18. Hunting for truffles in France. (Courtesy, The Bettmann Archive)

TRYPSIN

A digestive enzyme formed in the small intestine when another enzyme, enterokinase, acts on trypsinogen, an inactive secretion of the pancreas. Trypsin cleaves polypeptides or proteins at peptide bonds adjacent to the amino acids arginine or lysine.

(Also see DIGESTION AND ABSORPTION.)

TRYPSINOGEN

Inactive form of trypsin.

TRYPTOPHAN

One of the essential amino acids, isolated and described by E. G. Hopkins of Cambridge University, England.

(Also see AMINO ACID[S].)

TUBE FEEDING

Among the circumstances which may necessitate tube feeding are surgery of the head and neck, esophageal obstruction, severe burns, gastrointestinal surgery, anorexia nervosa, and coma. Three types of tube feeding may be employed depending upon the situation: (1) a nasogastric tube (from the nose to the stomach) or a nasoduodenal tube (from the nose to the duodenum); (2) a surgically formed opening (stoma) in the stomach; or (3) a surgically formed opening (stoma) in the small intestine. Obviously, the nasogastric tube or the nasoduodenal tube is the method of choice but instances may arise when it is impossible to pass a tube from the nose to the stomach or the duodenum, or when there is gross disease of the stomach or the duodenum. All three types of tube placements are capable of supplying all types of adequate nutrients in a liquid form.

Since the nasogastric tube or the nasoduodenal tube is the most common, it will serve to illustrate the principles of tube feeding.

As the name implies, the tube is passed down the nose through the esophagus, and then to the stomach or duodenum. Extreme caution must be exercised in ensuring that the tube is in the stomach or duodenum, and not in the lungs. Also, in precoma or in comatose patients, the danger of aspiration pneumonia as a result of regurgitation of digestive juices must be kept in mind. Because there is less hazard of aspiration from nasoduodenal tube feeding than from nasogastric tube feeding, it is the method of choice of most physicians.

In order for tube feeding to be effective, it must meet several criteria. It must be: (1) nutritionally adequate; (2) easily digested without reactions such as diarrhea or constipation; (3) simply prepared; (4) well tolerated without inducing vomiting; and (5) low cost. There are three tube feedings which meet these criteria and are commonly used: (1) milk-base; (2) milk-base with suspended solids from strained or blenderized foods; and (3) synthetic low-residue formulas. Recipes are available for home preparation of these types of tube feedings. Commercial preparations are also available. All tube feedings generally contain ½ to 1½ kcal/ml.

Foods introduced into the tube are generally warmed to body temperature, and flow into the tube by gravity, or by the use of a food pump. The first tube feedings should be frequent and in small volumes, then if tolerated the volume of feedings may be gradually increased. Two liters per day is a common volume.

Several potential hazards of tube feedings are apparent: (1) tube feeding is dangerous when the patient is vomiting; (2) contaminated food leads to gastrointestinal infections; (3) concentrated feeding (high sodium or high protein) may lead to diarrhea, dehydration, and elevated blood urea; and (4) high concentrations of sugar, particularly lactose, are apt to produce diarrhea.

TUBER

A short, thickened, fleshy stem, or terminal portion of a stem or rhizome that is usually formed underground, bears minute leaves each with a bud capable under suitable conditions of developing into a new plant, and constitutes the resting stage of various plants such as the potato and Jerusalem artichoke.

(Also see VEGETABLE[S].)

TUBERIN

A globulin constituting the principal protein of the potato tuber.

TUN

Liquids, especially wine, ale, or beer, may be stored in a large cask or barrel called a *tun*. At one time, wine, liquor, and some other liquids were measured in terms of a tun, which equals 252 gallons (*958 liters*).

TURBINADO SUGAR

Sometimes this sugar is viewed erroneously as a raw sugar (sucrose), but turbinado sugar goes through a refining process to remove impurities and most of the molasses. It is produced by separating raw sugar crystals and washing them with steam. If produced under proper conditions, it is edible.

(Also see RAW SUGAR; and SUGAR.)

TURTLE

Reptiles with bodies encased in a bony shell. Both land turtles and water turtles are eaten, but it is the water turtle that is made into the famous turtle soup. The English hold turtle soup in high esteem; it is often served at their great diplomatic dinners and ceremonial repasts.

TWADDELL

This is a hydrometer used for measuring density (specific gravity) of industrial liquids which are greater than one. Measures of specific gravity between 1 and 2 are divided into 200 equal parts, and each division is 1 degree. The specific gravity of a solution equals the number of degrees on the Twaddell scale multiplied by 5 and divided by 1,000. The Twaddell is named for its inventor.

TYRAMINE

A pressor amine that has action similar to epinephrine; found in mistletoe, certain cheeses, some wines, and ergot, and also obtained from tyrosine by strong heating or by bacterial action.

TYROSINASE

A copper-containing enzyme responsible for the conversion of tyrosine to the dark pigment, melanin. Skin color depends, in part, upon the concentration of melanin. A genetic absence of tyrosinase results in albinism. Tyrosinase is also the enzyme responsible for the browning of cut surfaces of certain fruits and vegetables; as such, it is described by the generic term phenolase.

(Also see PHENOL OXIDASES.)

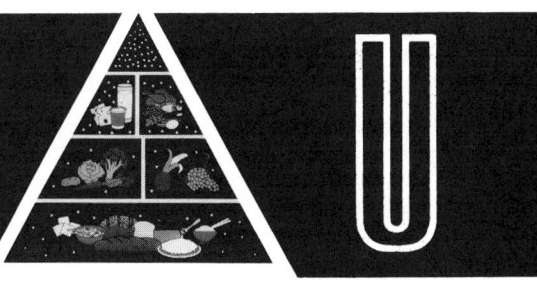

UDO

A Japanese plant grown for its tender young shoots which are eaten as a vegetable and in salads.

ULCERS, PEPTIC

An ulcer is any open sore, other than a wound. Peptic ulcers are open sores or erosions of the surface lining of the digestive tract, usually in the stomach or duodenum. Their appearance is roughly comparable to that of canker sores of the mouth—for those unfortunate sufferers familiar with the appearance of canker sores. The term peptic ulcer is employed since it appears that these ulcers develop from the lessened ability of the lining of the digestive tract to withstand the digestive action of pepsin and hydrochloric acid (HCl). Ulcers can occur in any area of the digestive tract which is exposed to the action of these two substances. However, a vast majority of ulcers occur in two locations: (1) the first part of the small intestine, or duodenum, before the point of entry of the alkaline secretions of the pancreas; and (2) the stomach or gastric portion of the digestive tract, usually along the lesser curvature near the pylorus—opening from the stomach into the duodenum.

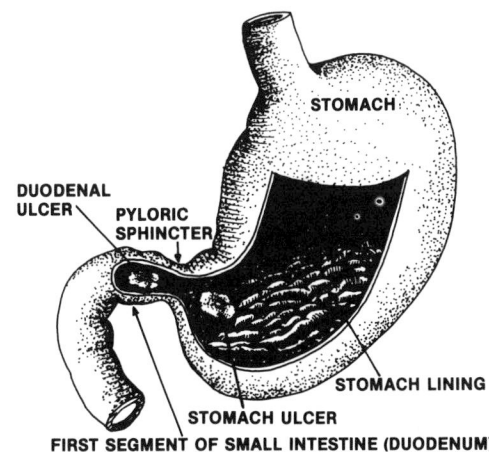

Fig. U-1. The major sites where peptic ulcers occur.

OCCURRENCE. Overall, peptic ulcers occur in about 10% of all Americans at some time of their lives. Between the two locations, duodenal ulcers are far more common than gastric ulcers. Unfortunately, both are characterized by high recurrence rates.

Duodenal. About 80% of all peptic ulcers are duodenal ulcers. These occur most often in men between the ages of 20 and 50. Thus, after puberty and before menopause the ratio of affected males to females varies from 3:1 to 10:1. For some unexplained reasons, duodenal ulcers are now less common than they were 20 years ago.

Gastric. Again, more males than females are affected by a ratio of about 3.5:1, and, as indicated, gastric ulcers occur less frequently than duodenal ulcers—the ratio being about 1:4. Interestingly, about 20% of the gastric ulcers occur in individuals who have, or who had, a duodenal ulcer.

CAUSES. The basic causes of peptic ulcers remain obscure. It is known that physiologically there is a disturbance in the acid-pepsin secretion and the tissue resistance of the digestive tract lining. Other factors, such as chemicals, heredity, and emotions also seem involved in some cases. Hence, peptic ulcers are likely to be caused by multiple factors.

SYMPTOMS. The hallmark of peptic ulcers is the sequence of pain-food-relief—the upper abdominal pain associated with ulcers when the stomach is empty, which is relieved by ingesting food or bland liquids. Thus, pain usually relates to eating patterns, and usually occurs several hours after eating and between midnight and 2:00 a.m. Interestingly, this pain is not present before breakfast. Occurrence of the pain relative to eating habits is an important point of differential diagnosis, as persons suffering from gallbladder diseases experience pain that is triggered by eating, rather than relieved. The pain experienced by ulcer sufferers is described as a steady, gnawing, burning, aching, or hungerlike discomfort. However, some victims have no pain even before serious complications develop, and, in some cases, gastric ulcer symptoms may be worsened by eating. A good rule is to have any persistent abdominal pain checked by a physician.

Ulcers that bleed slowly cause the stool to be black and may produce anemia. Other ulcers may bleed more profusely and lead to vomiting of dark brown blood.

DIAGNOSIS. Once a physician suspects an ulcer, x rays are taken after barium is swallowed. These x rays outline the stomach and small intestine and will clearly demonstrate a crater in most ulcer victims. This x ray procedure is commonly called an upper GI series. In most duodenal ulcers, an upper GI series is all that is required. Gastric ulcers, however, require some further tests since a small percentage of gastric ulcers are cancers that look like ulcers by x ray. Hence, gastric ulcer patients will probably be subjected to gastroscopy in an effort to rule out malignant disease. This involves passing a flexible lighted tube into the stomach for the direct visual inspection of the ulcer.

TREATMENT. Treatment, of course, varies with each individual; however, there are some general practices and recommendations which deserve mention. The facets of treatment involve tangible or physical approaches and intangible or psychological approaches.

Physical. Since psychological factors such as emotions and personality can have a large role in development of ulcers, treatment should stress individualized attention to the whole person and not just the ulcer. Nevertheless, some physical manipulations have proven helpful in the treatment of ulcers. These include diet, drugs, and surgery.

Psychological. Many ulcer patients improve within 24 to 48 hours with a change in environment; hence, the psychological side of treatment cannot be ignored. Both physical and psychological rest promote the healing of peptic ulcers. To this end sedatives may be prescribed. Often victims are urged to curtail their business and social responsibilities. Furthermore, those treating peptic ulcer patients need to demonstrate support and reassurance.

DIET. Table U-1 provides some general guidelines from which various diet plans may be derived for each individual during convalescence from a peptic ulcer.

PREVENTION. Peptic ulcers tend to recur. Those that recur and do not respond to treatment, or that recur frequently, may require surgery. Of course, at the first inkling of recurrent symptoms active therapy should be initiated.

A peptic ulcer provides one more reason for giving up smoking, since it appears to aggravate and contribute.

Being able to relax—although difficult to determine for each individual—would seem to offer some prevention due to the implication of emotions and personality type in the development of peptic ulcers. Each individual should determine the best form of relaxation based on needs and experiences.

(Also see ANTACIDS; MODIFIED DIETS; SIPPY DIET; and STRESS.)

TABLE U-1
GUIDELINES FOR SELECTING FOODS FOR PERSONS WITH PEPTIC ULCERS

Food Category[1]	Foods to Use	Foods to Avoid
Bakery products	Enriched white bread; toast; soda crackers; zwieback; melba toast; hard rolls; sponge cakes; other plain cakes; sugar cookies.	Whole wheat and other grain breads; hot bread; graham or coarse crackers; cakes and pastries containing dried fruit or nuts; spice cakes.
Beverages	Postum; decaffeinated coffee.	Alcohol; carbonated drinks; coffee; tea; chocolate.
Cereals and flours	Refined cereals; all ready-to-eat cereals; rice; oatmeal; macaroni; spaghetti; noodles.	Whole grain cereals; cereals containing bran; shredded wheat.
Desserts and sweets	Plain custard; rennet; plain puddings; gelatin desserts; clear plain jelly; honey; moderate amounts of sugar.	Excesses or concentrated sources like candy.
Eggs and substitutes	Boiled; poached; coddled; or scrambled; plain omelets.	Fried eggs.
Fats and oils	Margarine	All fried foods.
Fish and seafoods	Fresh or frozen; boiled; broiled; or baked; scalded canned tuna or salmon; oysters fresh or canned.	Smoked, preserved or pickled fish, crab, lobster, or sardines; other salted fish or fatty fish such as herring or mackerel.
Flavorings and seasonings	Salt	Most all, such as pepper, horseradish, catsup, mustard, vinegar, spices.
Fruits	Applesauce, baked apples without peel; ripe bananas; papayas; stewed or canned pears, peaches, apricots—all without peel.	Dried fruits, skins and peel of all fruits; raisins.
Gravies and sauces	Creamed sauces.	Gravies made from meat extracts.
Juices	Most all, but dilute half and half with water or drink after eating other foods.	
Meats	Tender cuts of beef, lamb, and veal; sliced chicken; liver; crisp bacon.	Fried, smoked, pickled, or cured meats; fat; sausages; ham; salami; wieners.
Milk and Milk products	Buttermilk; cream; milk; plain ice cream; plain milk shakes; cottage cheese; mild cheeses; butter; sour cream; yogurt.	Chocolate; strong cheeses.
Nuts and seeds		All nuts and seeds.
Pickles and relishes		All pickles and relishes.
Soups and chowders	Cream soups using such vegetables as asparagus, beets, carrots, peas, green beans, potatoes, tomatoes, and spinach.	All meat soups, soups from any other vegetables; all canned soups; dehydrated soups; broths; bouillon.
Vegetables	Raw cabbage, well-cooked or canned asparagus, carrots, peas, beets, peeled tomatoes, squash, spinach, green beans, mashed or baked potatoes without skins; sweet potatoes without skins; mushrooms.	All gas-forming vegetables which include cauliflower, Brussels sprouts, broccoli, cucumbers, onions, radishes, turnips; salad, coleslaw.

[1]Food categories are those listed in the Food Composition Table F-21 of this book.

ULTRAHIGH TEMPERATURE STERILIZATION (UHT STERILIZATION)

Rapid heating of a food to temperatures in the range of 205° to 307°F (96° to 153°C), then holding at these temperatures for three seconds or less. In combination with aseptic packaging, this process is designed for the manufacture of products with improved keeping qualities.

(Also see PRESERVATION OF FOOD.)

ULTRASONIC HOMOGENIZER

The use of high-frequency—over 20,000 vibrations per second—pressure waves of the same nature as sound waves to disintegrate fat globules or break up particles. This process is employed in a variety of food emulsifications, such as fruit and vegetable purees, milk homogenization, and peanut butter.

ULTRAVIOLET LIGHT (ULTRAVIOLET RADIATION)[1]

Light is a form of radiant energy. It travels in vibrations or waves. Each color of light vibrates with a different wavelength and carries a specific amount of energy.

The range of these wavelengths is measured in nanometers (nm), a unit of length equal to:

$$\frac{1}{100,000,000} \text{ mm}$$

The range of electromagnetic waves of some radiations follows:

Radiation	Approximate Wavelength (nanometer [nm])
X ray	50
Ultraviolet	300
Visible light	600
Infrared rays	1000

All radiations are important, but the discussion that follows will be limited to ultraviolet light because of its importance in human health and nutrition.

Ultraviolet light is generally divided into the near (400 to 300 nm), the far (300 to 200 nm), and the vacuum (200 to 4 nm) ultraviolet regions. The last wavelengths, which are particularly harmful to life, are strongly absorbed by the earth's atmosphere.

Ultraviolet light is created by the same processes that generate visible light—transitions in atoms in which an electron in high-energy state returns to a less energetic state.

USES OF ULTRAVIOLET LIGHT. Ultraviolet light serves mankind in numerous ways; among them, the following:

1. **Manufacture of vitamin D in the skin.** If the skin is exposed to the sun or to a sunlamp, the ultraviolet rays act on the provitamin 7-dehydrocholesterol in the skin and transform it into vitamin D_3.

(Also see VITAMIN D.)

2. **Formation of vitamin D in plant foods.** If ergosterol (the provitamin found in plants) is irradiated with ultraviolet light, vitamin D_2 is produced. This is the well-known Steenbock Irradiation Process, which was patented by Dr. Harry Steenbock of the University of Wisconsin.

3. **Sterilization.** Certain ranges of ultraviolet rays can kill bacteria. This property is used in sterilizing water, milk and other foodstuffs, and medicinal facilities and equipment. Also, modern food and drug plants often use germicidal lamps to disinfect their products and the containers.

4. **Industrial uses.** Ultraviolet rays have many important industrial uses, including use in fluorescent lamps and sun lamps, in testing materials, in identifying ores in mining, and

in lighting the instrument panels of aircraft. Scholars use the fluorescent effect of ultraviolet rays to examine old documents.

Ultraviolet rays, within moderation, are believed to have an invigorating effect upon the human body. But excessive exposure may be harmful, especially to the eyes and skin. Fair skinned people and those who sunburn easily and do not tan are especially susceptible to ultraviolet light-induced cancer of the skin.

NOTE WELL: Currently, there are many sunscreen lotions available. Some contain para-aminobenzoic acid (PABA). However, some dermatologists are recommending other sunscreen lotions; so, for protection against sunburn, see your dermatologist.

(Also see PARA-AMINOBENZOIC ACID.)

UMBLES

The entrails of an animal used as a food.

UNDERWEIGHT

This term means different things to different people. To some, it refers to mere slenderness, whereas to others it signifies undernourishment to the extent that a risk to health may be present. This article considers underweight to be a body weight that is notably low for a person's age, height, sex, and other personal characteristics. It is also considered to be an indication that the body contents of fat and lean tissue may be too low to ensure optimal responses to stresses such as chilling, diseases, fasting, injuries, prolonged and/or strenuous physical activities, and surgery.

EFFECTS ON HEALTH. The desirable or undesirable effects of underweight on the health of different people depend somewhat upon factors such as their life-styles (active or sedentary), their overall states of physical fitness, and the presence or absence of certain other health conditions. This means that some people are likely to be healthiest when they are moderately underweight, whereas others might be fittest for the important activities of their lives when they are average weight, or a little overweight. Therefore, the various effects of underweight are noteworthy.

Beneficial Effects. The people who may benefit the most from being moderately underweight are those who engage in predominantly intellectual work (artists, office workers, students, teachers, writers, etc.) and live otherwise sedentary lives because it is generally believed that slender people are less likely to become sleepy and tired when physical activity is limited. Runners and other athletes whose sports require the ability to maintain a rapid pace may also benefit from being a little underweight. Finally, people living in tropical climates or those troubled with one or more of the following conditions may be better off underweight than overweight: adult onset diabetes, angina pectoris, athero-

[1]This section was authoritatively reviewed by, and helpful suggestions were received from, Stephen A. Book, Ph.D., California Environmental Protection Agency, State of California, Sacramento.

sclerosis, breathing difficulties, chronic tiredness, congestive heart failure, coronary heart disease, enlargement of the heart, excessive numbers of red blood cells (polycythemia), gallstones, and troubles with the legs and feet.

Potentially Harmful Effects. In the early 1900s, underweight people were charged higher life insurance premiums than other policy holders because they were more susceptible to tuberculosis, which at that time was often fatal. Today, tuberculosis is rare, except in certain poverty-stricken areas, and leanness is extolled as a virtue. (Now, some obese policyholders may be charged higher premiums.) Nevertheless, there are certain other potentially harmful effects of a pronounced underweight, which may sometimes be the result of chronic undernutrition. Some of the more common undesirable effects are:

1. Cessation or irregularity of menstrual periods in females.
2. Growth retardation in growing infants and children.
3. Increased susceptibility to chilling and infections.
4. Lack of vigor, endurance, and sexual drive.
5. Low resistance to certain stresses.
6. Slow healing of injuries and surgical wounds.
7. Tendencies to be apathetic, irritable, listless, mentally depressed, nervous, restless, and sleepless.
8. Weak muscles.

FACTORS THAT MAY BE RESPONSIBLE FOR UNDERWEIGHT.

Lack of sufficient dietary calories is only one of the causes of underweight. Hence, attempts to bring about a gain in weight by merely increasing the caloric content of the diet may fail when there are other contributing factors that are unrecognized. Therefore, some of the major causes of underweight are noteworthy.

Dietary Practices. Many people would like to be able to eat more food without gaining weight, yet there are some who appear to have difficulty eating enough to maintain a normal body weight. Furthermore, the problem of consuming sufficient calories is more common in infancy, childhood, and adolescence than it is in adulthood because much more food energy per pound of body weight is required during growth.

Other reasons why some people may find it difficult to consume sufficient calories follow:

1. The diet may contain too much fibrous vegetable matter, which is very filling. Distention of the small intestine with bulky food curbs the appetite in many people. It is noteworthy that, on the average, vegetarians tend to be more slender than meat eaters.
2. Excessive amounts of fluids may be taken with meals. Hence, filling occurs before sufficient solid food is consumed. A similar effect occurs when the foods themselves are very high in water content, as in the cases of gelatin desserts or salads, thin soups and stews, and various vegetable dishes.
3. Oversalted foods may cause feelings of fullness in some people because the salt draws fluid from the intestinal wall into the intestinal contents, thereby producing a bulking effect.
4. Too much fat may be consumed. Fatty foods delay the emptying of the stomach and may make some people lose their appetites.

Finally, the diets of some underweight people may be lacking in the minerals and vitamins that promote hearty appetites. For example, a deficiency of the essential trace mineral zinc leads to loss of taste, and, an insufficient amount of the vitamin thiamin can lead to loss of appetite.

Other Factors. Even when adequate amounts of calories are consumed, various factors that alter the normal utilization of food by the body may prevent the gaining of weight; among them, the following:

1. Digestive disturbances.
2. Febrile illnesses.
3. Glandular disorders.
4. Parasitic infestations.
5. Excessive physical activity.

ASSESSMENT OF WEIGHT STATUS.

It may not always be easy to determine when a person is sufficiently underweight to require that remedial measures be taken because there is considerable variation in body weights among people of equal heights and the same sex.

Body Weight for Height, Age, and Sex. One procedure for assessing the weights of adults is to consider that the ranges of normal weights for males or females extend from the 10th to the 90th percentiles of the average weights for selected heights of persons aged 25 to 34. The young adult group is taken as a standard because it is widely believed that weight gained after the attainment of maturity is a detriment rather than a benefit to health. These data are given in Table U-2.

The problem with the data in Table U-2 is that there is no specification of body build. Hence, an adult with a large frame might be underweight with a weight falling between the 10th percentile and the average weight. Therefore, some other measures of the *fleshiness* of a person are needed.

NOTE: Weight norms for infants, children, and adolescents are given in the sections on CHILDHOOD AND ADOLESCENT NUTRITION; and INFANT DIET AND NUTRITION.

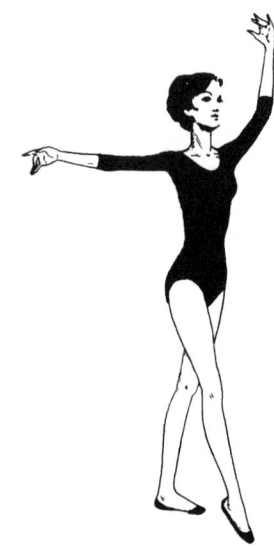

Fig. U-2. Slenderness is considered attractive, but being too thin may be hazardous to health.

TABLE U-2
AVERAGE WEIGHTS (without clothing) FOR PERSONS AGED 25 TO 35 YEARS[1,2]

Height (without shoes)			Men						Women					
			Light[3] (10th percentile)		Average		Heavy[4] (90th percentile)		Light[3] (10th percentile)		Average		Heavy[4] (90th percentile)	
(ft)	(in.)	(cm)	(lb)	(kg)	(lb)	(kg)	(lb)	(kg)	(lb)	(kg)	(lb)	(kg)	(lb)	(kg)
4	10	147	—	—	—	—	—	—	97	44	119	54	147	67
4	11	150	—	—	—	—	—	—	97	44	126	57	151	69
5	0	152	—	—	—	—	—	—	97	44	125	57	171	78
5	1	155	—	—	—	—	—	—	103	47	130	59	172	78
5	2	157	—	—	—	—	—	—	107	49	135	62	172	78
5	3	160	110	50	151	69	196	89	109	50	138	63	178	81
5	4	163	126	57	151	69	195	89	110	50	141	64	188	86
5	5	165	128	58	155	71	194	88	115	52	143	65	187	85
5	6	167	134	61	160	73	191	87	118	54	146	67	190	86
5	7	170	136	62	168	77	199	91	123	56	153	70	191	87
5	8	173	140	64	166	76	196	89	129	59	162	74	217	99
5	9	175	148	68	176	80	225	102	124	56	153	70	177	81
5	10	178	148	68	185	84	215	98	—	—	—	—	—	—
5	11	180	142	65	178	81	212	96	—	—	—	—	—	—
6	0	183	157	72	190	86	224	102	—	—	—	—	—	—
6	1	185	165	75	195	89	224	102	—	—	—	—	—	—
6	2	188	158	72	191	87	226	103	—	—	—	—	—	—

[1]Adapted by the authors from *Weight by Height and Age for Adults 18-74 Years: United States 1971-74*, U.S. Dept. of Health, Education, and Welfare, 1979, pp. 18, 21, Tables 2 and 3.
[2]**Note:** These weights are not what are commonly called "ideal" or "desirable" weights because recent studies have cast doubt upon the basis for the latter.
[3]Most people who weigh less than this amount are likely to be underweight.
[4]Most people who weigh more than this amount are likely to be obese.

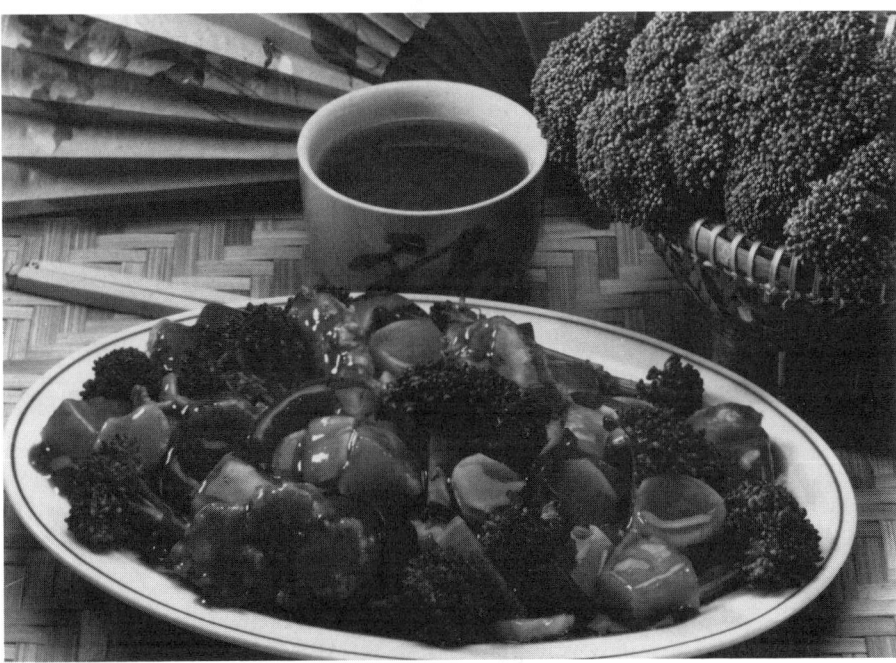

Fig. U-3. Underweight people don't need to worry about eating too many calories. Sweet and Sour Broccoli Chicken.
(Courtesy, Castle & Cooke, Inc.—Bud of California Fresh Vegetables.)

Skinfold Thicknesses. About one-half of the body fat content is distributed under the skin. Therefore, the thicknesses of various skinfolds are measures of body fatness. For example, it is generally considered that a triceps skinfold (which is usually measured at a point about halfway between the shoulder and the elbow) smaller than ½ in. *(12.5 mm)* for men or less than ⅝ in. *(16 mm)* for women is indicative of insufficient subcutaneous fat or underweight condition.

Midarm Muscle Circumference. This calculated value gives an approximate estimate of the muscle mass, which is useful in determining whether an underweight person is lacking fat alone (measured by skinfold thickness) or is short on both fat and muscle. The value for the midarm muscle circumference (MAMC) is derived from measurements of the triceps skinfold (TSF) and the midarm circumference (MAC) by the following formula:

$$MAMC = MAC - (3.14 \times TSF)$$

For example, a man who has a midarm circumference (measured by placing a tape measure around the upper arm where the triceps skinfold is measured) of 11 in. *(279 mm)*, and a skinfold thickness of ½ in. *(12.5 mm)* would have a midarm muscle circumference of 9 ⁹⁄₁₆ in. *(240 mm)*. These measurements would indicate that while he has just enough subcutaneous fat, he is lacking some muscle since the standard values for muscle circumferences are 10 in. *(254 mm)* for males and 9 in. *(232 mm)* for females.

MEASURES FOR GAINING WEIGHT. The selection of the measures to be used for gaining weight should take into account whether additional fat alone is needed, or a combination of extra muscle and fat is required. A diet high in calories will be suitable for the former objective, but the latter objective requires a diet that is high in both calories and protein.

Some suggestions for using high-calorie foods to gain weight are given in MODIFIED DIETS, Table M-28, Modified Diets/High-calorie diet.

Suggestions for using high-protein foods as sources of additional calories and protein are given in MODIFIED DIETS, Table M-28, Modified Diets—High protein, high calorie diet.

SUMMARY. Ideal body weights for different people vary according to age, sex, body build, life-style, and other factors. Hence, some feel better when slender, whereas others may benefit from a little extra weight. Therefore, a doctor should be consulted before one attempts to gain or lose a considerable amount of weight.

UNESCO

United Nations Educational, Scientific, and Cultural Organization, with headquarters in Paris, France.

UNIDENTIFIED FACTORS

In addition to the vitamins as such, certain unidentified or unknown factors are important in nutrition. They are referred to as *unidentified* or *unknown* because they have not yet been isolated or synthesized in the laboratory. Nevertheless, rich sources of these factors and their effects have been well established. A diet that supplies the specific levels of all the known nutrients but which does not supply the unidentified factors may be inadequate for best performance. There is evidence that these factors exist in dried whey, marine and animal products, distillers' solubles, antibiotic fermentation residues, yeasts, alfalfa meal, and certain green leafy vegetables.

UNSATURATED FAT

A fat having one or more double bonds; not completely hydrogenated.
(Also see FATS AND OTHER LIPIDS.)

UNSATURATED FATTY ACID

Any one of several fatty acids containing one or more double bonds, such as oleic, linoleic, linolenic, and arachidonic acids.
(Also see FATS AND OTHER LIPIDS.)

UREA (NH_2CONH_2)

Before amino acids (protein) can enter energy metabolic pathways, the amino group (NH_2) must first be removed. This is accomplished by a process called deamination which produces a carbon skeleton that can be used for energy, and ammonia (NH_3). To facilitate elimination from the body, this ammonia is converted to urea in the urea cycle in the liver. Urea circulates in the blood, and is removed from the blood by the kidneys. It is the main nitrogenous constituent of urine. Normally 20 to 35 g of urea are excreted in the urine every 24 hours.
(Also see METABOLISM; PROTEIN[S]; and UREA CYCLE.)

UREA CYCLE (KREBS-HENSELEIT CYCLE)

Most of the ammonia (NH_3) produced through deamination—removal of amino groups (NH_2) from amino acids—is converted to urea in the liver for excretion by the kidneys. To facilitate elimination, 1 mole of ammonia (NH_3) combines with 1 mole of carbon dioxide (CO_2), another metabolic waste product. This compound is then phosphorylated to produce carbamyl phosphate. Carbamyl phosphate then combines with ornithine to form citrulline—an intermediate in the urea cycle. The amino acid, aspartic acid, contributes another amino group (NH_2), and citrulline is then converted to the amino acid arginine. Urea splits off from arginine forming ornithine, and the cycle is completed. Fig. U-4 illustrates the urea cycle.
(Also see METABOLISM; PROTEIN[S]; and UREA.)

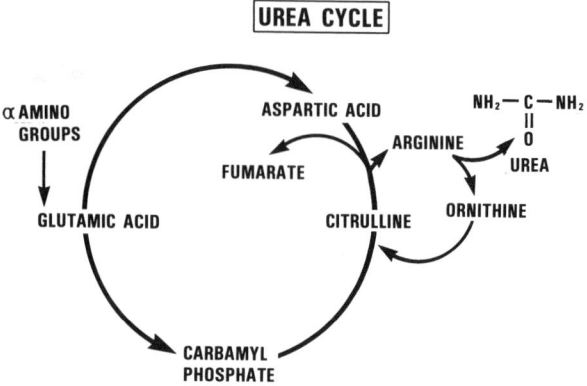

Fig. U-4. Urea cycle (nitrogen excretion).

UREASE

An enzyme which acts on urea to produce carbon dioxide and ammonia. It is found in the human digestive tract where it acts on the urea in the digestive secretions.

UREMIA

A toxic accumulation of urinary constituents in the blood.

URIC ACID

The main end product of purine—adenine, guanine and xanthine—metabolism in birds, reptiles, and man, which is excreted in the urine. Uric acid is formed from purines consumed in the diet, and from body purines derived from the breakdown of nucleic acids. Mammals other than man further metabolize uric acid to allantoin, which is excreted in the urine. However, man lacks the enzyme, urate oxidase, necessary for this conversion. Therefore, about 0.5 to 1.0 g of uric acid is lost in the urine each day. A high level of uric acid in the blood is associated with the development of gout. In addition, uric acid may form kidney stones, especially in individuals suffering from gout.

(Also see ARTHRITIS, section headed "Gout [gouty arthritis]"; PURINES; and URIC ACID KIDNEY STONES.)

URIC ACID KIDNEY STONES

Kidney stones formed from uric acid—the excretory product of purines in humans. Stones develop when (1) blood levels of uric acid are elevated, (2) urinary uric acid excretion is high, and (3) an acid urine is produced. Individuals suffering from gout are a thousand fold more likely to develop uric acid kidney stones than the general population. Formation of uric acid kidney stones may be minimized by keeping the urine alkaline, increasing the fluid intake, and reducing the purine intake. Most fruits and vegetables contribute to the formation of an alkaline urine, while meat, fish, and poultry contribute to the formation of an acid urine. A purine-restricted diet begins with the elimination of foods with high purine content such as anchovies, asparagus, brains, kidneys, liver, meat extracts, mincemeat, sardines, and sweetbreads.

(Also see ARTHRITIS, section headed "Gout [gouty arthritis]"; MODIFIED DIETS; and KIDNEY STONES.)

URICASE (URATE OXIDASE)

A copper-containing enzyme which all mammals possess with the exception of man and other primates. It is responsible for the conversion of uric acid to allantoin.

(Also see URIC ACID.)

URINARY CALCULI (WATER BELLY, KIDNEY STONES, UROLITHIASIS)

Mineral deposits which occur in the urinary tract. These deposits may block the flow of urine, followed by rupture of the urinary bladder and death. In severe cases of some duration, watery swellings (edema) of the lower abdomen may develop.

(Also see KIDNEY STONES; and URIC ACID KIDNEY STONES.)

URINARY SYSTEM

The organs engaged in the excretion of urine. They consist of the kidneys, the ureters, the bladder, and the urethra.

URINE

Liquid or semisolid matter produced in the kidneys and discharged through the urinary organs. Normally, it is a clear, transparent, amber-colored, slightly acid fluid.

(Also see KIDNEYS; UREA; and UREA CYCLE.)

USDA

The abbreviation commonly used for the United States Department of Agriculture.

(Also see U.S. DEPARTMENT OF AGRICULTURE.)

U.S. DEPARTMENT OF AGRICULTURE (USDA)

In 1796, President George Washington recommended the creation of a national board of agriculture, which eventually developed into the United States Department of Agriculture. The USDA and the FDA (Food and Drug Administration) share the responsibility for assuring the safety of the nation's food supply. Meat and meat products, and poultry and poultry products are the main food concerns of the USDA, operating under the authority of the Federal Meat Inspection Act (FMIA) and the Poultry Products Inspection Act (PPIA). Also, the USDA is involved in research, educational, nutritional, and health programs. The following eight divisions of the USDA have primary responsibilities in the areas of human health and nutrition: (1) the Agriculture Research Service; (2) the Animal and Plant Health Inspection Service; (3) the Consumer and Marketing Service; (4) the Cooperative State Research Service; (5) the Federal Extension Service; (6) the Food and Nutrition Service; (7) the Labeling and Registration Section; and (8) the Veterinary Services Division.

(Also see DISEASES, section headed "U.S. Department of Agriculture.")

U.S. DEPARTMENT OF HEALTH AND HUMAN SERVICES (FORMERLY, HEALTH, EDUCATION, AND WELFARE)

An agency of the federal government with responsibility for public health in its broadest aspects. This agency is under the jurisdiction of the U.S. Public Health Service (USPHS) and includes the following: (1) Alcohol, Drug Abuse and Mental Health Administration; (2) Center for Disease Control (CDC); (3) Food and Drug Administration (FDA); (4) Health Resources Administration; (5) Health Services Administration; and (6) National Institutes of Health (NIH).

(Also see DISEASES, section headed "U.S. Department of Health and Human Services.")

USP (UNITED STATES PHARMACOPIA)

A unit of measurement or potency of biologicals that usually coincides with an international unit. (Also see IU.)

U.S. PUBLIC HEALTH SERVICE (USPHS)

This service is in the U.S. Department of Health and Human Services and is concerned with the prevention and treatment of disease. It works in the areas of vector control, pollution control, and control of communicable diseases of man. In addition to its own research program, the USPHS provides grants for health-related research at many universities and research institutes in the United States.

A part of this important complex is the National Institutes of Health (NIH), which was formed in 1930, and is composed of the following nine sister institutes:

    The National Cancer Institute
    The National Heart Institute
    The National Institute of Allergy and Infectious Diseases
    The National Institute of Arthritis and Metabolic Diseases
    The National Institute of Dental Research
    The National Institute of Mental Health
    The National Institute of Neurological Diseases and Blindness (including multiple sclerosis, epilepsy, cerebral palsy, and blindness)
    The National Institute of Child Health and Human Development
    The National Institute of General Medical Science

U.S. RECOMMENDED DAILY ALLOWANCES (U.S. RDA)

These allowances are guides to the amounts of vitamins and minerals an individual needs each day to stay healthy. They were set by the Food and Drug Administration (FDA) as nutritional standards for labeling purposes. The U.S. RDAs are *based* on the Recommended Dietary Allowances established by the Food and Nutrition Research Council, and they replace the Minimum Daily Requirements (MDR) which were used for years as guidelines for labeling products. For practical purposes, the many categories of dietary allowances for males and females of different ages were condensed to as few as nutritionally possible for labeling. Generally, the highest values for the ages combined in a U.S. RDA were used. For example, the U.S. RDAs for adults and children over 4 years are representative, generally, of the dietary allowances recommended for a teenage boy.

There are four groupings of the U.S. RDAs, shown in Table U-3. The best known, and the one that will be used on most nutrition information panels and most vitamin and mineral supplements, is for adults and children over 4 years of age. The second is for infants up to 1 year, and the third is for children under 4 years. The latter two are to be used on infant formulas, baby foods, and other foods appropriate for these ages, as well as vitamin-mineral supplements intended for their use. The fourth is for pregnant women or women who are nursing their babies.

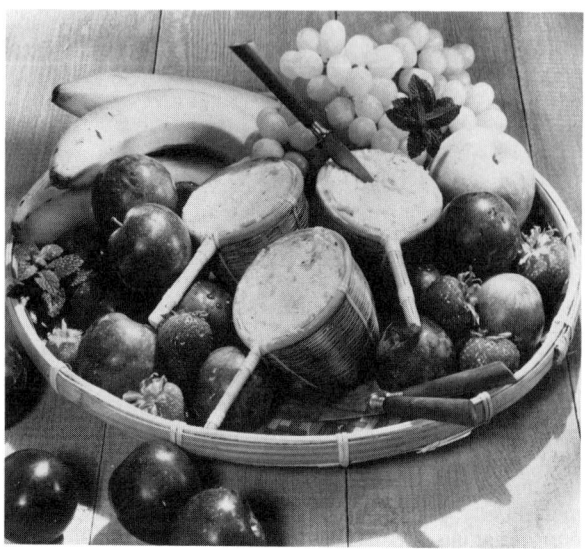

Fig. U-5. Fruit and cheese—common contributors to RDAs. (Courtesy, The California Plum Commodity Committee, Sacramento, Calif.)

TABLE U-3
U.S. RECOMMENDED DAILY ALLOWANCES (U.S. RDA)[1]

Nutrient	Adults and Children 4 Years or Older	Infants from Birth to 1 Year	Children Under 4 Years	Pregnant or Lactating Women
Required on labels:				
Protein ....g	50–63	13–14	16	60/65
Vitamin A ...mcg RE	500–1000	375	400	800/1,300
Vitamin C ....mg	60	30–35	40	70/95
Thiamin ....mg	1.5	0.3–0.4	0.7	1.5/1.6
Riboflavin ....mg	1.7	0.4	0.8	1.8
Niacin ....mg NE	20	5–6	9	17–20
Calcium ....mg	1,200	600	800	1,200
Iron ....mg	15	6–10	10	30/15
Optional on labels:				
Vitamin D ......mcg	10	7.5–10	10	10
Vitamin E ....IU	30	3–4	6	10–12
Vitamin B-6 .....mg	2	0.3–0.6	1	2.2
Folate ....mcg	200	25–35	50	400/280
Vitamin B-12 .mcg	2	0.3–0.5	0.7	2.2/2.6
Phosphorus .....mg	1,200	400–600	800	1,200
Iodine ....mcg	150	40–50	70	175/200
Magnesium .....mg	350	40–60	80	320/355
Zinc ....mg	15	5	10	15/19
Copper ....mg	2	0.6	1	2
Biotin ....mcg	30–100	10–15	20	30/100
Pantothenic acid mg	4–7	2–3	3	4–7

[1]*Recommended Dietary Allowances*, NRC, 1989, pp. 284–285.

• **Labels and U.S. RDA**—Whenever a food product is labeled "enriched," or a product has added nutrients, or a nutritional claim is made for a product, the FDA requires that the nutritional content be listed on the label. In addition, many manufacturers put nutrition information on products when not required to do so. The lower part of the nutrition label must give the percentages of the U.S. Recommended Daily Allowances (U.S. RDA) of protein and of seven vitamins and minerals in a serving of the product, in the following order: protein, vitamin A, vitamin C, thiamin, riboflavin, niacin, calcium, and iron. As shown in Table U-3, listing is optional relative to the percentage of 12 other vitamins and minerals. Likewise, listing of cholesterol, fatty acid, and sodium content is optional—for now. Nutrients present at levels less than 2% of the U.S. RDA may be indicated by a zero or an asterisk which refers to the statement, "contains less than 2% of the U.S. RDA of these nutrients." Nutrition labels also list how many calories and how much protein, carbohydrate, and fat are in a serving of the product.

Unfortunately, some confusion has arisen since the National Research Council's *Recommended Dietary Allowances* have for years been called the RDAs; hence, U.S. RDA should always refer to the U.S. Recommended *Daily* Allowances used for labeling purposes.

(Also see ENRICHMENT [Fortification, Nutrification, Restoration]; LABELS, FOOD; NUTRIENTS: REQUIREMENTS, ALLOWANCES, FUNCTIONS, SOURCES; and RDA [Recommended Dietary Allowances].)

UTERUS (WOMB)

The organ that receives the fertilized egg from the fallopian tube and holds it during the 9 months of its growth until the infant is expelled at childbirth. It is situated deep in the pelvic cavity between the bladder and the rectum.

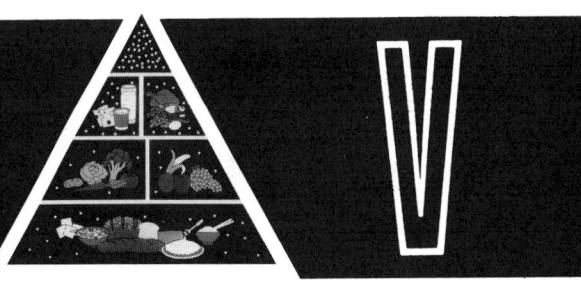

VACUUM COOLING

A means of rapidly cooling fruits and vegetables to prevent deterioration. Produce is sprayed with water, then while still wet it is subjected to a vacuum which causes the water to evaporate; thereby rapidly chilling the produce. Some vacuum coolers are railroad car size.
(Also see HYDROCOOLING.)

VACUUM-DEHYDRATED

Freed of moisture after removal of surrounding air while in an airtight enclosure.

VACUUMIZATION (VACREATION)

In milk processing, the subjection of heated milk to vacuum for the purpose of removing volatile off-flavors and odors and/or moisture.
(Also see DEAERATION.)

VALENCE

The power of an element or radical to combine with (or to replace) other elements or radicals. The valence number of an element is the number of atoms of hydrogen with which one atom of the element can combine.

VALINE

One of the essential amino acids.
(Also see AMINO ACID[S].)

VANADIUM (V)

Vanadium was first identified in 1831 by Sefstrom, of Sweden, who named it after the Norse goddess of beauty, Vanadis (because of the beautiful color of its compounds). However, it was not obtained in pure form until 1927. It has many industrial uses, especially in Vanadium steel.

In 1970, Dr. Klaus Schwarz demonstrated that the trace element Vanadium (V) is needed by higher animals. Vanadium-deficient diets resulted in retarded growth, impaired reproduction, increased packed blood cell volume and iron in the blood and bone of rats, and increased hematocrit in chicks.

VANASPATI

This is a term applied in India to hydrogenated fat made from vegetable oils. It is a butter substitute, like margarine in the United States.

VASCULAR

Pertaining to the blood vessels of the body.

VEGANS

A vegan is an individual who is a strict vegetarian. All foods of animal origin—meat, poultry, fish, eggs, and dairy products—are excluded from the diet of vegans. In addition, vegans share a philosophy and life-style.
(Also see VEGETARIAN DIETS.)

VEGETABLE(S)

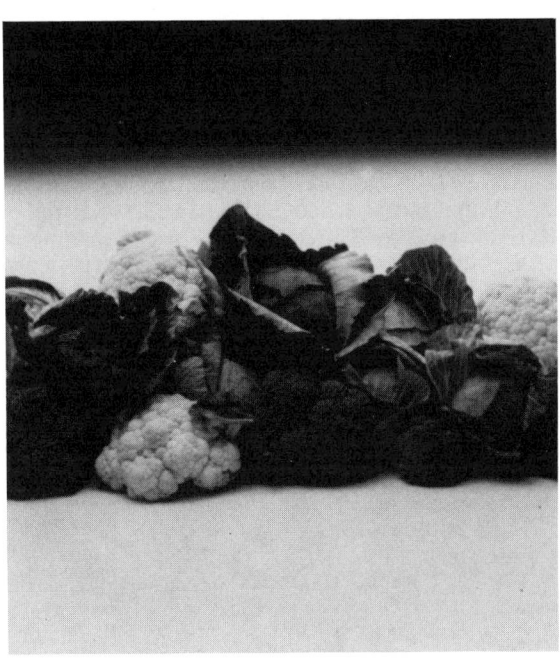

Fig. V-1. Common vegetables. (Courtesy, Shell Chemical Co., Houston, Texas)

In the phrase the vegetable kingdom, the word vegetable refers to the entire world of plants. In an 1893 decision, the U.S. Supreme Court held, in effect, that a plant or plant part generally eaten as part of the main course of the meal is a vegetable, while a plant part which is generally eaten as an appetizer, as a dessert, or out of hand is a fruit. As used herein, the term refers to the edible part of a plant that is consumed in raw or cooked form with the main course of a meal. Some typical parts of plants used as vegetables are: bulbs (garlic, onions), flowers (broccoli, cauliflower), fruits (pumpkins, squashes, tomatoes), leaves (lettuce, spinach), roots (beets, carrots), seeds (beans, corn, peas), stalks (celery), stems (asparagus), and tubers (Irish potatoes, yams). Although green land plants provide most of the vegetables for human diets, certain fungi and algae may also be used for vegetables. The different types of vegetables are shown in Fig. V-2.

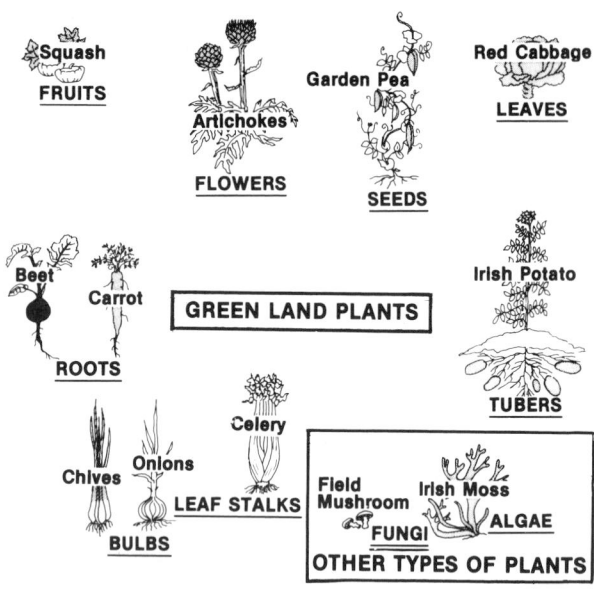

Fig. V-2. Common types of vegetables.

HISTORY. It has been difficult for archaeologists, botanists, geographers, and other researchers to trace the history of all of the vegetables people have used through the ages because (1) few remains of the more succulent parts of plants have been found at archaeological excavations since these parts decay very readily; (2) most of the identifiable plant fragments have been found in relatively dry areas, while evidence of vegetables used in the humid tropics is scarce; and (3) some of the vegetables that were once consumed by man may have become extinct, and others may have evolved into forms that bear little resemblance to the ancestral species. Nevertheless, enough evidence has been found to support some tentative conclusions about the first cultivation of the important vegetable crops.

Long before the development of the first agricultural societies some 10,000 to 12,000 years ago, most people lived in nomadic bands that obtained their food by fishing, hunting, and gathering wild plants. This period of human history lasted approximately 2 million years. It is not known why some of the nomads eventually settled in certain areas, but this change appears to have been accompanied by (1) the herding of animals and (2) a regular pattern of harvesting wild plants. The first cultivation of local plants appears to have occurred in the regions where systematic gathering had long been practiced. In many cases, the first long-term settlements were made in places where diverse geographical features such as mountains, foothills, valleys, and rivers were in close proximity. Hence, the varied habitats favored the growth of numerous plant species. A wide variety of plant foods would have been needed to form a nutritious diet when fish and game became scarce, or the early settlers would have succumbed to malnutrition. Fig. V-3 shows the locations of the regions where many of the important vegetables were first cultivated.

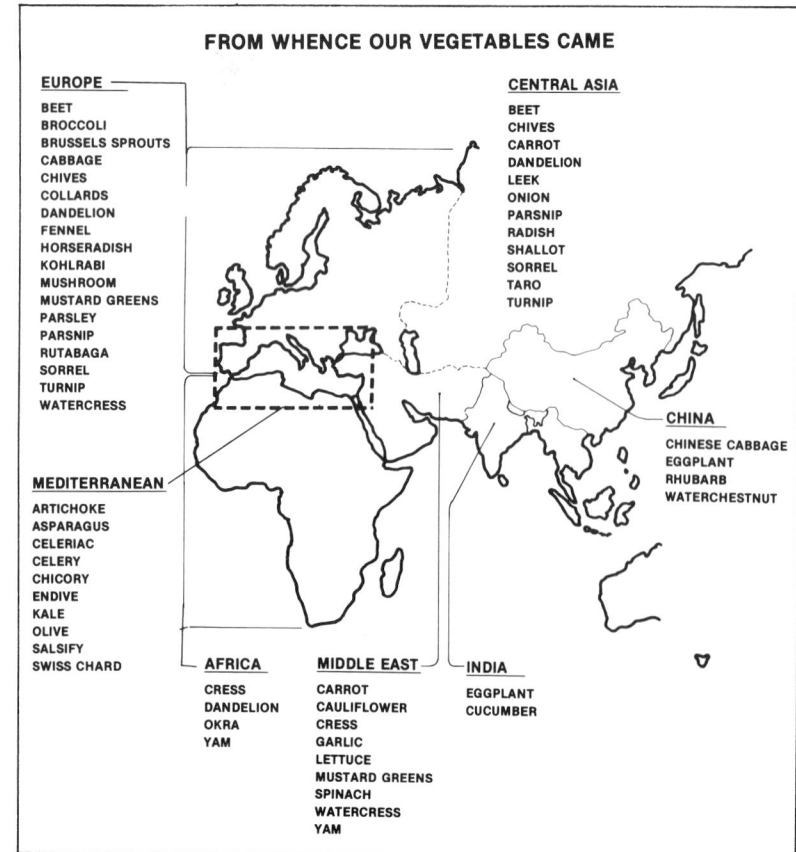

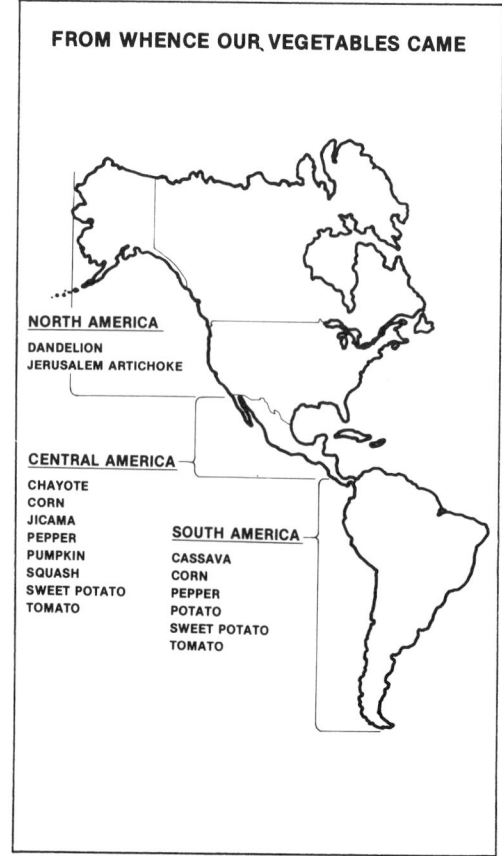

Fig. V-3. Places of origin and/or domestication of vegetables in the Old World (left) and in the New World (right).

Details on the history of individual vegetables are given in Table V-2 of this article, and in the separate articles covering each of the leading vegetable crops.

WORLD AND U.S. PRODUCTION.

The production of vegetables is an important part of the American agricultural scene. Market gardeners live near centers of population. Truck farmers live farther away; they grow vegetables and ship them in refrigerated trucks or cars to all parts of the nation. Home gardeners are everywhere; their vegetables provide (1) healthful exercise, and (2) cheap food and the maximum freshness and nourishment from crops that lose some of their goodness after harvesting.

Fig. V-4 shows the leading vegetable crops of the world, and the annual production of each. Fig. V-5 shows the leading vegetable crops of the United States, and the annual production of each.

Fig. V-4 shows that starchy roots and tubers (Irish potatoes, cassava, and sweet potatoes) are by far the leading vegetable crops of the world.

Fig. V-5 shows that the five leading U.S. vegetable crops, by rank, are: tomatoes, sweet corn, lettuce, onions, and Irish potatoes.

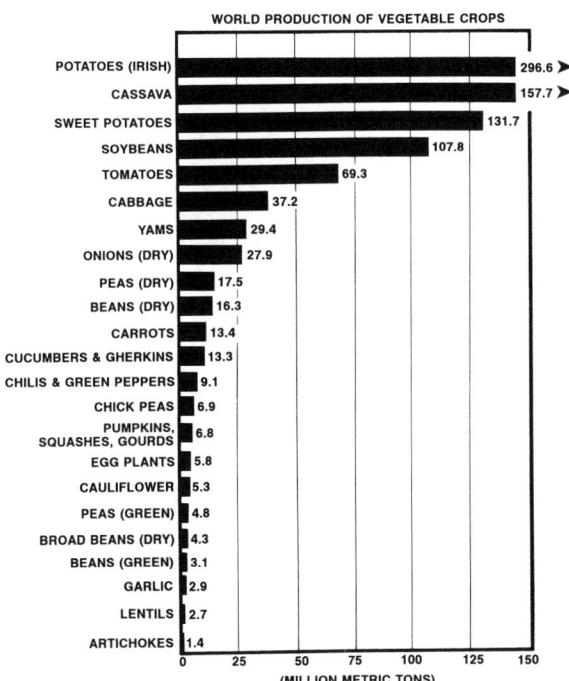
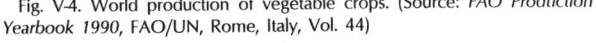

Fig. V-4. World production of vegetable crops. (Source: *FAO Production Yearbook 1990*, FAO/UN, Rome, Italy, Vol. 44)

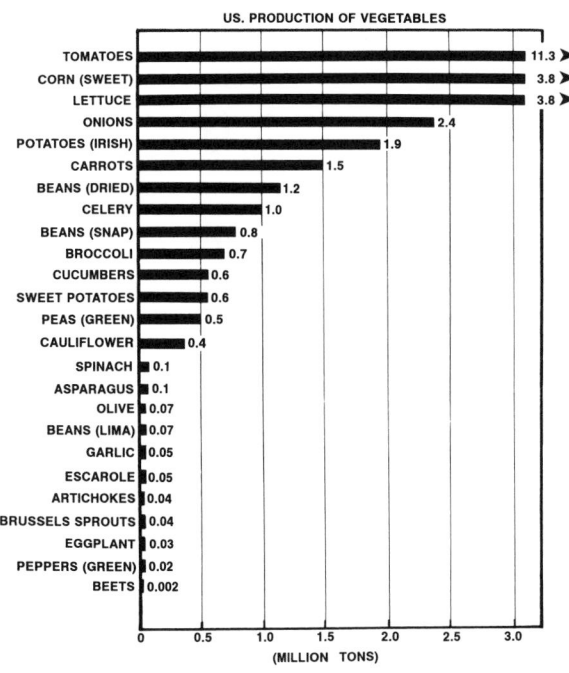

Fig. V-5. U.S. production of vegetable crops. (Source: *Statistical Abstract of the United States*, U. S. Dept. of Commerce, 1991, p. 669, Table 1167, and *Agricultural Statistics 1991*)

NUTRITIVE VALUES.

"Eat your vegetables" is the admonition of mothers and doctors alike; and with reason. They know that vegetables are good—and good for you. They give bulk to the diet, which aids the digestive process; and they are rich sources of certain essential minerals and vitamins.

Vegetables are high in water content; hence, they are considerably lower in calories and proteins than most of the grains and legumes. However, most vegetables are fair to excellent sources of fiber (poorly digested carbohydrate which stimulates movements of the digestive tract), various essential macrominerals and microminerals, vitamins, and vitaminlike factors. The nutrient composition of the commonly used vegetables is given in Food Composition Table F-21. Table V-1 groups vegetables according to the amounts of vitamins A and C that they supply.

TABLE V-1
AMOUNTS OF VITAMIN A, VITAMIN C, AND CALORIES FURNISHED BY 100 G OF SELECTED VEGETABLES[1,2]

Nutritional Group	Vegetable	Vitamin Content A	Vitamin Content C	Food Energy
		(IU)	(mg)	(kcal)
High in vitamins A and C	Parsley (raw)	8,500	172	44
	Spinach	8,100	28	23
	Collards	7,800	76	33
	Kale	7,400	62	28
	Turnip Greens	6,300	69	20
	Mustard Greens	5,800	48	23
	Cantaloupes	3,400	33	30
	Broccoli	2,500	90	26
High in vitamin A	Carrots (raw)	11,000	8	42
	Carrots (cooked)	10,500	6	31
	Sweet Potatoes	8,100	22	141
	Swiss Chard	5,400	16	18
	Winter Squash	4,200	13	63
	Green Onions	2,000	32	36
High in vitamin C	Peppers (immature green)	420	128	22
	Brussels Sprouts	520	87	36
	Cauliflower	60	55	22
	Kohlrabi	20	43	24
	Cabbage	130	33	20
	Chinese Cabbage	150	25	14
	Asparagus	900	26	20
	Rutabaga	550	26	35
	Radishes (raw)	322	26	17
	Tomatoes (ripe, raw)	900	23	22
	Tomatoes (ripe, cooked)	1,000	24	26
Other green vegetables	Beans, green	540	12	25
	Celery	540	9	17
	Lettuce (leaf)	1,900	18	18
	Lettuce	330	6	13
	Okra	490	20	29
	Peas (garden)	540	20	71
	Beans (lima)	280	17	111
Starchy vegetables	Corn, sweet (yellow)	400	9	91
	Onions (dry)	40	10	38
	Peas (field, southern)	350	17	108
	Potatoes (baked in skin)	Trace	20	93
Other vegetables	Beets	20	6	32
	Cucumbers	250	11	15
	Eggplants	10	3	19
	Pumpkins	1,600	9	26
	Rhubarb	80	6	141
	Summer Squash	440	11	15
	Turnips (roots)	Trace	22	23

[1]Data from Food Composition Table F-21.

[2]Figures are for amounts of vitamins and calories per 100 g sample of cooked vegetables (unless normally eaten raw). 100 g are equal to about ½ cup. Vitamin C values are generally higher if the vegetable is eaten raw; for example, 100 g of cabbage contains 33 mg of vitamin C when cooked, but 47 mg when raw.

Effects of Processing and Preparation. The maximum amounts of essential nutrients are supplied by raw, fresh vegetables that are harvested at just the right stage of maturity. However, many people find some vegetables unappealing when raw, and it is not practical to use only fresh vegetables, which are available only at certain times of the year. Furthermore, raw vegetables contain more undigestible carbohydrates (fiber) than cooked vegetables, and might have a strong laxative effect on people unaccustomed to so much fiber. Therefore, the effects of the various processing and preparation procedures should to be taken into account when planning menus that furnish all of the required nutrients.

NOTE: The information which follows is based on relatively few studies and may not be valid in all cases because (1) different vegetables are affected in different ways; (2) the effects depend partly upon the condition of the vegetables—whether immature or mature, fresh or taken from long storage, whole or in pieces, and untreated or treated; and (3) information is lacking on some of the effects of commonly used procedures. Nevertheless, pertinent information pertaining to nutrient losses in processing and preparation follow:

• **Artificial ripening**—Most commercially grown tomatoes are picked before full maturity in order to avoid excessive softness and oversusceptibility to damage and spoilage. However, one study showed that tomatoes ripened on the vine contained up to one-third more ascorbic acid than those allowed to ripen after picking.[1]

• **Baking**—Various studies of baked Irish potatoes and baked sweet potatoes have shown that baking results in vitamin losses as follows: carotene (provitamin A), 24%; thiamin, 24%; riboflavin, 11%; niacin, 18%; pantothenic acid, 23%; pyridoxine (vitamin B-6), 20%; and ascorbic acid (vitamin C), 20%.[2] Much lower losses of these vitamins were observed when the potatoes were boiled instead of baked.

• **Blanching**—This procedure is used to stop enzyme action in vegetables prior to canning, drying, or freezing. There are considerable losses (up to 80%) of water soluble minerals and vitamins when the vegetables are blanched in boiling water, then cooled by immersion in cold water.[3] Apparently, the nutrients are leached out into the water. These losses may be reduced greatly by (1) blanching with steam instead of boiling water, (2) cooking with air instead of water, or (3) blanching with microwaves. It is noteworthy that the vitamin losses from unblanched vegetables during frozen storage are from 2 to 3 times as great as those from blanched vegetables.

• **Boiling**—The losses of minerals and water-soluble vitamins increase as the amount of cooking water increases. Hence, greater mineral and vitamin retention results in steaming and waterless cooking.

[1]Pantos, C. E., and P. Markakis, "Ascorbic Acid Content of Artificially Ripened Tomatoes," *Journal of Food Science*, Vol. 38, 1973, p. 550.

[2]Lachance, P. A., "Effects of Food Preparation Procedures on Nutrient Retention with Emphasis on Food Service Practices," *Nutritional Evaluation of Food Processing*, 2nd ed., edited by R. S. Harris and E. Karmas, The Avi Publishing Company, Inc., Westport, Conn., 1975, pp. 508-509.

[3]Fennema, O., "Effects of Freeze-Preservation on Nutrients," *Nutritional Evaluation of Food Processing*, 2nd ed., edited by R. S. Harris and E. Karmas, The Avi Publishing Company, Inc., Westport, Conn., 1975, pp. 246-247.

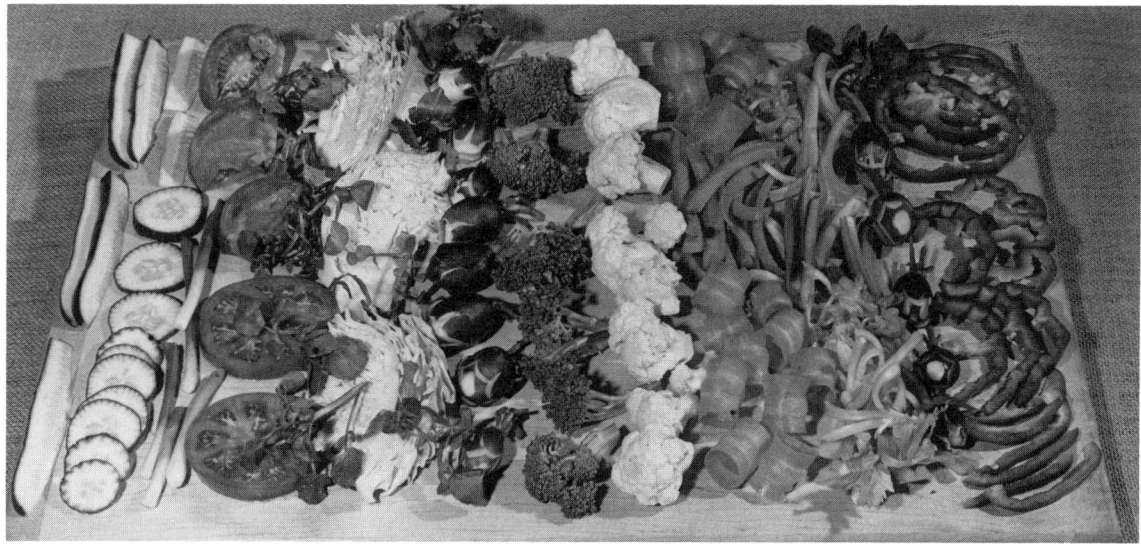

Fig. V-6. Raw, fresh vegetables ready-to-eat. Shown here are cucumbers, green onions, tomatoes, watercress, cabbage, radishes, broccoli, cauliflower, carrots, celery, and green peppers—ideal finger foods when cut and served in interesting shapes like these. (Courtesy, U.S. Department of Agriculture)

• **Canning**—Blanching, plus the strong heat treatments applied to nonacid vegetables, appears to be responsible for the large vitamin losses in canning, because much less loss occurs in the more mildly processed tomato products. The nutrient losses may be reduced or offset by (1) utilization of newer procedures, such as microwave blanching, and (2) restoration of nutrients lost during processing (enrichment or fortification).

• **Chopping, dicing, grating, mashing, mincing, or slicing**—Any process which breaks many vegetable cells is likely to be responsible for significant losses of certain vitamins. The longer the broken pieces of vegetables are held, the greater the losses. Therefore, vitamins may be conserved by (1) cutting up vegetables just prior to serving, and (2) using a plastic knife for cutting, because metals speed up the destruction of vitamin C.

• **Drying**—Moderate amounts of carotene (provitamin A) and vitamin C may be destroyed in the process, unless the vegetables are sulfured before drying. However, sulfuring destroys most of the thiamin content. Vitamin losses are greater during slow processes, such as sun drying, than they are for more rapid processes like freeze drying.

• **Fermenting and/or pickling**—Pickles, olives, and sauerkraut are the only fermented and pickled vegetables used to any extent in the United States. Vitamin losses in these products may vary widely as a result of factors such as heat developed during fermentation, volume of pickling solution, and temperatures under which the pickles are canned and stored.

• **Freezing**—Most of the losses of vitamins in frozen vegetables occur during blanching, since freezing itself is responsible for only small losses. The vitamin losses during frozen storage may be considerably greater when blanching is omitted prior to freezing. The use of less drastic blanching procedures may help to prevent vitamin losses in frozen vegetables.

• **Frying**—Vitamin losses during the frying of vegetables vary greatly as a result of factors such as (1) time and temperature of frying, (2) type of frying (shallow fat, deep fat, or stir frying), and (3) fat or oil that is used (those which break down during frying may increase the rate of vitamin destruction).

• **Holding on a steam table**—Losses of vitamin C, thiamin, and riboflavin appear to increase with the length of time that vegetables are kept warm on a steam table.

• **Microwave cooking**—The vitamin losses during this procedure are small, and are comparable to those which occur when vegetables are cooked with little or no water.

• **Peeling, scraping, and/or trimming**—Removal of the outer leaves, peels, and/or skins of certain vegetables may result in disproportionately high losses of nutrients because the outer layers are often richer in minerals and vitamins than the inner layers. Therefore, these measures, which are often performed mainly for cosmetic reasons, should be used only to the extent that is absolutely necessary.

• **Pressure cooking**—This method of cooking vegetables results in a greater retention of minerals and vitamins than boiling in a saucepan. However, best results are obtained when the vegetables are placed on a rack above the water so that they are cooked only by steam.

• **Steaming**—Vegetables cooked with steam, but not in contact with water, have better nutrient retention than those cooked in boiling water.

• **Sulfuring**—This process, which consists of either exposing vegetables to fumes from burning sulfur, or dipping them in a sulfite solution, is used to prevent discoloration and spoilage. It is generally utilized before vegetables are to be dried. Sulfuring helps to prevent the losses of both carotene (provitamin A) and vitamin C, but it destroys thiamin. Fortunately, vegetables are utilized more as sources of the first two vitamins, than as a source of thiamin.

VEGETABLES OF THE WORLD. A relatively few species of vegetable plants account for most of the world's vegetable production.

Most of the better-known vegetables of the world are listed in Table V-2, Vegetables of the World. The *most important* (those produced in greatest quantity), worldwide and/or in the United States, are accorded detailed narrative coverage, alphabetically, whereas vegetables of lesser importance are presented in summary form only in Table V-2, Vegetables of the World.

TABLE V-2
VEGETABLES OF THE WORLD

Popular and Scientific Name(s); Origin and History	Importance; Principal Areas; Growing Conditions	Processing; Preparation; Uses	Calories; Nutritive Value[1]
Artichoke, Globe (See ARTICHOKE, GLOBE)			
Asparagus *Asparagus officinalis* **Origin and History:** Originated around the eastern Mediterranean. The ancient Egyptians cultivated asparagus. First used as a medicinal plant.	**Importance:** The U.S. produces much of the world's asparagus—about 110,000 tons annually. **Principal Areas:** U.S., Europe, Mexico, and Taiwan. **Growing Conditions:** Temperate climate and well-drained soil. Propagated by suckers from the root crown of the parent plant, which may have originally grown from seed.	**Processing:** The freshly cut spears are washed, bunched, and packed. About ⅔ of the U.S. asparagus crop is processed, with about twice as much canned as frozen. **Preparation:** Poached in water. Usually served with butter, sauce, or in an omelet. Slices may be stir-fried. **Uses:** Vegetable dish, entree (when served with a sauce and chopped hard boiled eggs on toast), soups, and salads.	High in water (92%), low in calories (26 kcal per 100 g), and a good source of vitamin A. Also, it is a fair source of thiamin, riboflavin, and niacin. Herbal lore has it that asparagus juice eases the discomforts of arthritis, neuritis, and rheumatism.[2]
Beets *Beta vulgaris* **Origin and History:** One of the vegetables derived in pre-Christian times from the wild beet that is native to Europe and Asia.	**Importance:** Beets are a minor commercial vegetable crop. **Prinicpal Areas:** U.S. and European countries. **Growing Conditions:** Temperate climate.	**Processing:** When ripe, they are pulled from the ground by hand or by machine, and the tops are removed. About 95% of the beet roots are canned or pickled, while the greens are sold fresh. **Preparation:** Beets are peeled by steaming, following which the skins are washed away with high velocity jets of water. The peeled roots may be canned whole, sliced, or cut in narrow strips; or the root may be pickled in vinegar. Tops may be eaten raw. **Uses:** Roots—vegetable dish, pickles, baby foods, beet soup (Borsch). Greens—ingredient of salads and soups.	Boiled beets are high in water content (91%) and low in calories (32 kcal per 100 g). Beet greens are much richer in calcium, iron, and vitamins A and C than beet roots. The heavy consumption of beets may lead to the passage of red-colored urine (beeturia), a condition generally regarded as harmless. Beets and beet juice have long been used as herbal remedies for a wide variety of ailments.[2]
Broccoli (See BROCCOLI)			
Brussels Sprouts *Brassica oleracea* It is closely related to cabbage, which it resembles; and is a member of the mustard family. **Origin and History:** Believed to have first been developed from wild cabbage sometime around the 15th century in the area that is now Belgium.	**Importance:** A minor U.S. vegetable crop. **Principal Areas:** U.S. and European countries. **Growing Conditions:** Mild, temperate climate. Benefits from nitrogenous fertilizers.	**Processing:** The lower sprouts are usually picked first. Some of the crop is sold fresh, while the rest is frozen. **Preparation:** Boiled briefly until tender, but crisp. May be served with butter or a special sauce. **Uses:** Vegetable dish.	High in water (88%), low in calories (36 kcal per 100 g), a good source of vitamin C and a fair source of vitamin A. Brussels sprouts contain small amounts of goitrogens. (See GOITROGENS)
Cabbage (See CABBAGE)			
Carrot (See CARROT)			
Cassava (manioc, yucca) (See CASSAVA)			
Cauliflower (See CAULIFLOWER)			
Celeriac (turnip rooted celery) *Apium graveolens* Celerica, which is closely related to celery, is a member of the parsley family, *Umbelliferae.* **Origin and History:** Native to the Mediterranean region.	**Importance:** A minor vegetable that is popular in certain European countries. Little used elsewhere. **Principal Areas:** European countries. **Growing conditions:** Moist, temperate climate. Plants are started from seed in greenhouses or hotbeds, then transplanted when the weather is suitable for growth in a field.	**Processing:** The plant is harvested by pulling it up when mature. The root is the edible portion. **Preparation:** Steamed, then served whole, diced, or pureed (Europeans often mix it with hot, mashed potatoes and serve it with butter or a cream sauce.) **Uses:** Vegetable dish; ingredients of salads, soups, and stews.	Low in calories (40 kcal per 100 g) due to its high water content (88%). Also contains about twice as much protein (1.8%) and fiber (1.3%) as ordinary celery. Herbalists have long claimed that celeriac is a cure for dropsy because it is thought to increase the flow of urine.[2]
Celery (See CELERY)			

Footnotes at end of table

(Continued)

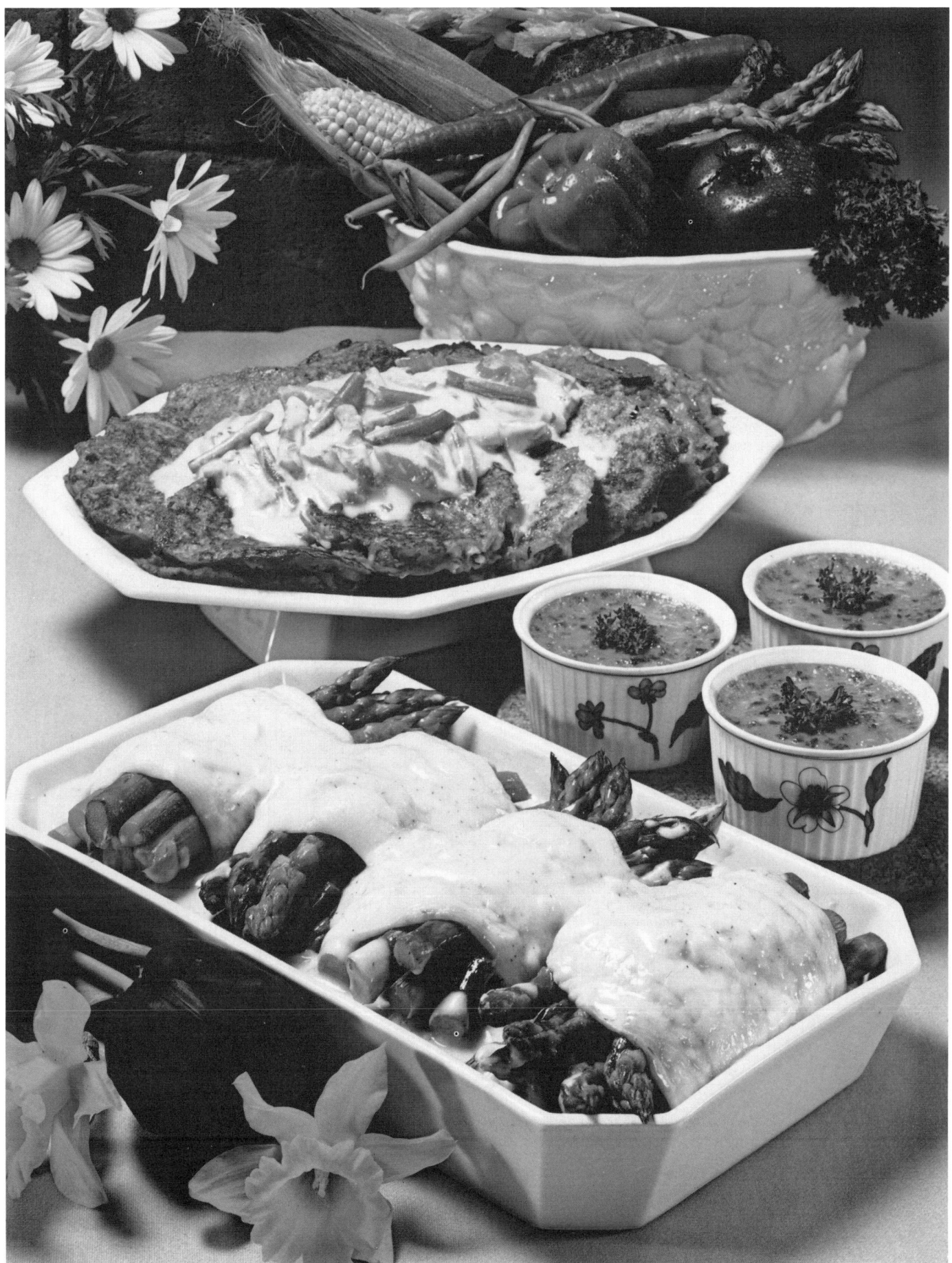

Fig. V-7. Fresh vegetables in dishes that speak of springtime. (Courtesy, United Fresh Fruit and Vegetable Assn.)

TABLE V-2 *(Continued)*

Popular and Scientific Name(s); Origin and History	Importance; Principal Areas; Growing Conditions	Processing; Preparation; Uses	Calories; Nutritive Value[1]
Chayote *Sechium edule* Chayote is a member of the gourd and melon family, *Cucurbitaceae*. **Origin and History:** Native to southern Mexico and Central America. Spread throughout Caribbean by local Indians.	**Importance:** A minor, but popular, vegetable in the tropical areas of the New World. **Principal Areas:** Mexico, Central America, and West Indies. **Growing Conditions:** Subtropical or tropical climate (freezing kills the plant); requires large amounts of water.	**Processing:** Usually, the fruits are picked when ripe and used immediately. Some of the fruit may be preserved by pickling. The large tuberous roots may also be harvested for food use. **Preparation:** Boiled, steamed, baked (after stuffing), or dipped in batter or fried. **Uses:** Vegetable dish (served with butter or cream sauce), ingredient in salads, and relish (when pickled).	Chayote fruit resembles squash in water content (92%) and caloric value (28 kcal per 100 g). However, the mineral and vitamin content of this vegetable is low. (It is a fair source of potassium and vitamin C).
Chicory *Chicorium intybus* Chicory belongs to the composite family *Compositae*. **Origin and History:** Thought to have originated in the Mediterranean region. Certain varieties have been developed as green leafy vegetables, while others have been selected mainly for their roots.	**Importance:** A minor, but popular, vegetable in Italy, France, Belgium, and Holland. **Principal Areas:** It grows wild in Europe, Asia, and North America. Chicory is cultivated in the U.S. and southern Canada. **Growing Conditions:** Temperate climate. It is often grown in greenhouses or in heated beds in cellars. (Growing in the dark produces light colored leaves).	**Processing:** Blanching (the production of light colored leaves) may be done in the field by tying the outer leaves together around the head of each plant so that light is excluded. The darker outer leaves may be removed after harvesting. Roots may be chopped, roasted until brown, and ground into a finely ground coffee. **Preparation:** Greens—served raw or boiled briefly. Roots—roasted or boiled. **Uses:** Greens—vegetable dish, ingredient of salads, soups, and stews. Roots—vegetable dish; extender or substitute for coffee, when roasted.	The leaves are high in water (93%) and low in calories (20 kcal per 100 g). Unblanched (green) chicory is an excellent source of potassium and vitamin A, but the blanched forms contain only traces of vitamin A. Sometimes used as a tonic for the digestive system, and to treat disorders of the skin. In the skin treatment, the juice of the leaves is mixed with a little vinegar and applied externally.[2]
Chinese Cabbage *Brassica chinensis* and *Brassica pekinensis* Chinese cabbage belongs to the mustard family, *Cruciferae*. It decends from the wild turnip and rape. **Origin and History:** Thought to have originated in Asia Minor and to have been brought to China, where it was developed over thousands of years.	**Importance:** Major vegetable crop in eastern Asia, where about one-half of the world's crop of various cabbages is produced. **Principal Areas:** China and Japan. **Growing Conditions:** Cool temperate climate. It is usually grown in southern China during the winter, and elsewhere in China during the fall.	**Processing:** In China, the mature heads are harvested when winter approaches. After removal of loose outer leaves, the heads are stored in a cold cellar. Some of the crop is preserved by pickling. **Preparation:** Boiled briefly, or minced and stir fried with other vegetables, meats, poultry, and/or seafoods. **Uses:** Vegetable dish; ingredient of salads, soups, and various Chinese dishes.	Very high in water (95%) and low in calories (14 kcal per 100 g). Green types are good to excellent sources of calcium, potassium, and vitamin A, and fair sources of iron and vitamin C. Chinese cabbage contains small amounts of goitrogens. (See GOITROGENS.)
Chives *Allium schoenoprasum* A member of the amaryllis family, *Amaryllidaceae*, closely related to the onion. **Origin and History:** Native to the temperate zones of Asia and Europe.	**Importance:** Commercial production is limited to that utilized by a few processors. Very popular among home gardeners. **Principal Areas:** Temperate zones of Asia, Europe, and North America. **Growing Conditions:** Cool temperate climate. Propagated by bulbs or by seeds.	**Processing:** Common ways of processing are: (1) chopping and flash freezing; (2) chopping and blending into cottage cheese, cream cheese, or salad dressings; or (3) drying. **Preparation:** Chopped and added to various dishes. **Uses:** Decorative flavoring or garnish for cottage cheese, cream cheese, omelets, salads, sandwich fillings, and soups.	Low in calories (28 kcal per 100 g) due to high water content. A fair source of calcium; and a good source of iron and potassium. An excellent source of vitamin A and a fair source of vitamin C.
Collards *Brassica oleracea acephala* Collards belong to the mustard family, *Cruciferae*, and are closely related to cabbage. **Origin and History:** Developed from the primitive leafy, nonheading cabbage of Europe. (Collards and kale are very closely related.)	**Importance:** A minor vegetable crop. **Principal Areas:** Southeastern U.S. **Growing Conditions:** Temperate climate. One of the hardiest of the cabbage vegetables, in that it is quite resistant to cold and heat.	**Processing:** Small, young heads or large, mature heads may be harvested. Much of the crop is chopped and frozen; some is canned. **Preparation:** Boiled with salt pork; stir fried chopped greens with bits of bacon and chopped onions. **Uses:** Vegetable dish; ingredient of casseroles, salads, soups, and stews.	The cooked leaves with stems are like other greens—they're high in water content (91%) and low in caloric content (29 kcal per 100 g), but they contain about twice as much protein (about 3.4%). Also a good source of calcium and iron, and an excellent source of potassium; and excellent source of vitamin A, and a very good source of vitamin C. Collards contain small amounts of goitrogens. (See GOITROGENS.)

Footnotes at end of table

(Continued)

TABLE V-2 *(Continued)*

Popular and Scientific Name(s); Origin and History	Importance; Principal Areas; Growing Conditions	Processing; Preparation; Uses	Calories; Nutritive Value[1]
Corn, Sweet *Zea mays saccharata* **Origin and History:** Probably developed from older varieties of corn indigenous to Mexico and South America. (Also see CORN, section on "Kinds of Corn," "Sweet Corn.")	**Importance:** The second ranking vegetable crop in the U.S., which produces about 4.0 million short tons annually. The leading states, by rank, are: Wisconsin, Minnesota, Washington, and Oregon. **Principal Areas:** U.S., Mexico, and Canada. **Growing Conditions:** Mild temperate climate with a hot, humid summer. Usually requires the application of fertilizers containing nitrogen, phosphorus, and potassium.	**Processing:** Once sweet corn reaches its flavor peak, it must be harvested, husked, and processed rapidly to avoid excessive loss of its sweetness. Hence, the fresh ears cannot be stored for long. Much of the crop is canned and frozen. **Preparation:** Boiled, steamed with husk on but with silk removed, or roasted. **Uses:** Vegetable dish; ingredient of casseroles, fritters, salads, soups, stews, and succotash.	Fresh corn cooked on the cob has a high water content (74%) and a fairly high caloric content (91 kcal per 100 g) and protein content (3.3%). Yellow corn is a fair source of vitamin A.
Cress *Lepidium sativum* Cress belongs to the mustard family, *Cruciferae*. **Origin and History:** Appears to have originated in Western Asia and/or Ethiopia. Cultivated for many centuries in various European countries.	**Importance:** A minor vegetable crop that is grown mainly by home gardeners. **Principal Areas:** All over the world. **Growing Conditions:** Cool, temperate climate. Seeds germinate quickly when exposed to light.	**Processing:** May be harvested within a few weeks after sowing, and should be picked before the arrival of hot weather, when it quickly goes to seed. **Preparation:** No cooking is required, but it may be added to various hot dishes. **Uses:** Ingredient of salads, sandwiches, and soups.	High in water (89%) and low in calories (32 kcal per 100 g). The raw vegetable is an excellent source of vitamin A and a good source of vitamin C. Cress contains small amounts of Goitrogens. (See GOITROGENS.)
Cucumber (See CUCUMBER and GHERKINS)			
Dandelion *Taraxacum officinale* The dandelion is a member of the daisy family, *Compositae*. **Origin and History:** There are many related species native to various parts of the world, including Europe, North Africa, Central Asia, and North America.	**Importance:** A very common wild plant or weed that is cultivated on a small scale. **Principal Areas:** U.S. and European countries. **Growing Conditions:** Temperate climate.	**Processing:** The leaves should be picked while they are still young and tender (before flowers appear). Roots are harvested by digging up the entire plant. **Preparation:** The leaves need not be cooked, but the roots should be boiled or roasted. Roasted roots may be ground to make an extender or substitute for coffee. **Uses:** Greens—vegetable dish, ingredient of salads and soups. Roots—vegetable dish and coffee substitute.	Boiled dandelions are high in water (90%) and low in calories (33 kcal per 100 g). Dandelions are an excellent source of iron and potassium, and a good source of calcium; and an excellent source of vitamin A, and a good source of vitamin C. Through the years, dandelion greens have been used by some advocates as a laxative, as a tonic to aid digestion, or as a help to rid the body of excessive water.[2]
Eggplant (aubergine) (See EGGPLANT)			
Endive (escarole) *Cichorium endivia* This lettucelike vegetable is a member of the sunflower family, *Compositae*. **Origin and History:** Native to the eastern Mediterranean region.	**Importance:** Most of the winter crop is grown in Florida, and most of the summer crop is grown in New Jersey and Ohio. **Principal Areas:** Italy produces about half of the world's crop, while France contributes one-quarter. **Growing Conditions:** Mild temperate climate. May be started from seed in a hotbed or a greenhouse, then transplanted when there is no danger of frost.	**Processing:** The leaves are harvested by cutting them off near the surface of the soil. Endive is not processed—it is marketed exclusively as a fresh vegetable. **Preparation:** May be served raw, stuffed, baked, or tossed in hot bacon drippings or melted butter. **Uses:** Vegetable dish, ingredient of salads and sandwiches, and added to soups and stews.	Similar to other greens in high water content (93%), and low caloric content (20 kcal per 100 g). Endive is a good source of calcium, phosphorus, iron, and potassium; an excellent source of vitamin A, and a fair source of vitamin C. The bitter flavor is believed to stimulate the flow of digestive juices.[2]

Footnotes at end of table

(Continued)

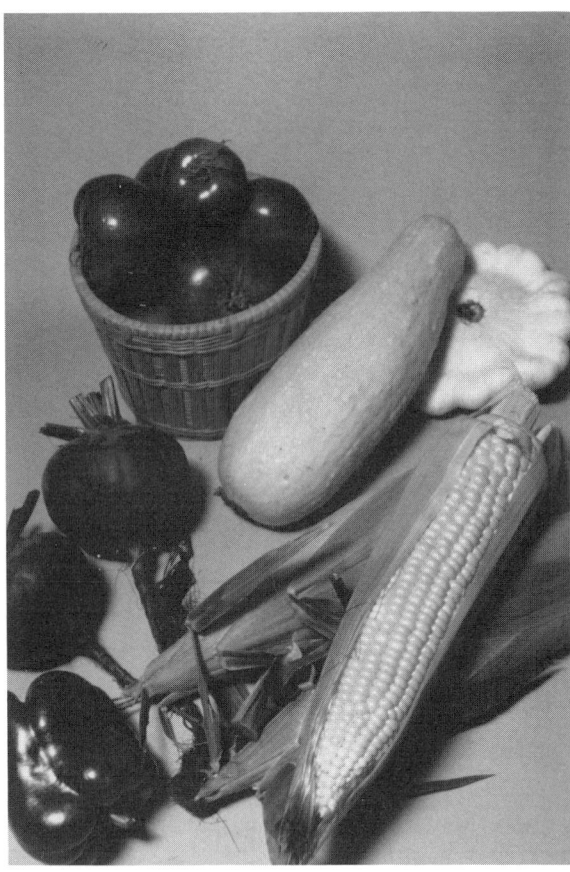

Fig. V-8. Vegetables; sweet peppers, beets, tomatoes, summer squashes, and corn. Vegetables are rich sources of certain essential minerals and vitamins. (Courtesy, University of Minnesota, St. Paul, Minn.)

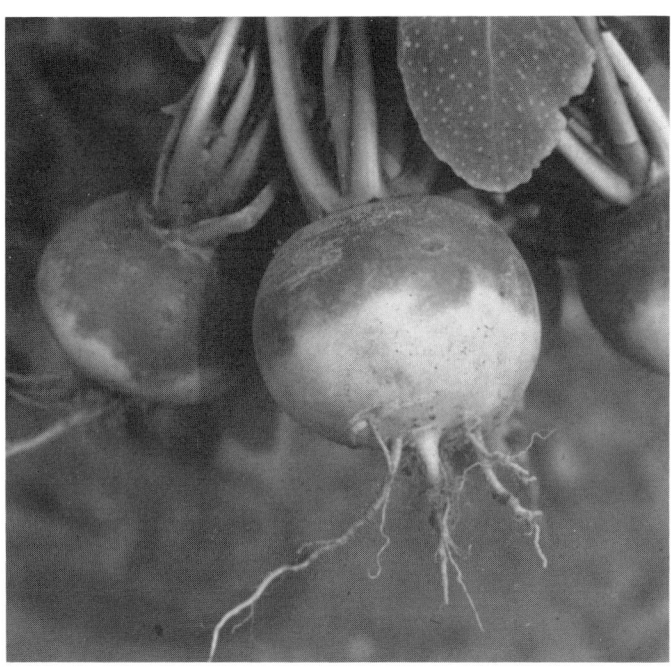

Fig. V-10. Turnips may be boiled and mashed or cooked with other items in mixed dishes. (Courtesy, USDA)

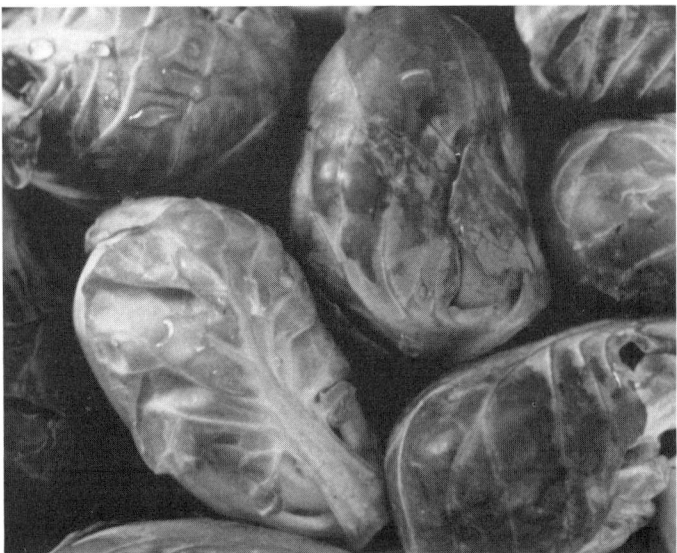

Fig. V-9. Brussels sprouts, used as a vegetable dish. A good source of vitamin C. (Courtesy, USDA)

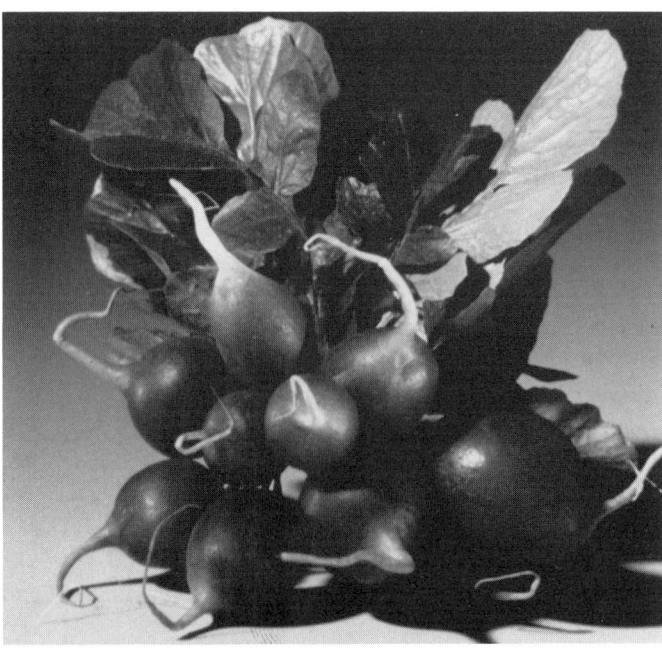

Fig. V-11. Radishes, used as an appetizer, ingredient of mixed vegetable dishes, relishes, and salads. (Courtesy, Field Museum of Natural History, Chicago, Ill.)

TABLE V-2 *(Continued)*

Popular and Scientific Name(s); Origin and History	Importance; Principal Areas; Growing Conditions	Processing; Preparation; Uses	Calories; Nutritive Value[1]
Fennel (Florence Fennel) *Foeniculum vulgare* Fennel belongs to the parsley family, *Umbelliferae.* **Origin and History:** Originated in southern Europe. The variety with the fleshy leaf stalks (Florence fennel) was developed in Italy.	**Importance:** A minor vegetable used mainly as a flavoring agent and a medicinal plant. **Principal Areas:** European countries and U.S. **Growing Conditions:** Mild, temperate climate. It is often planted in the summer for harvesting in the fall.	**Processing:** The plant should be pulled from the ground when the leaf stalks are between 3 and 6 in. *(8 to 15 cm)* long. Both the thickened leafstem bases and the leaves are used. **Preparation:** Leaves and stalks may be served raw, boiled, or parboiled with butter, cheese, and seasonings. **Uses:** Leaves and stalks—vegetable dish; ingredient of casseroles, salads, soups, and stews. Oil is extracted from the seeds and used as a flavoring agent.	The stalks are high in water (90%) and low in calories (28 kcal per 100 g). The green stalks contain a fair amount of vitamin A. The leaves are a good source of calcium, and an excellent source of iron and potassium; and an excellent source of vitamin A, and a good source of vitamin C. Long used as a medicinal plant since it is believed to stimulate the digestive processes.[2] The ancient Greeks believed that it increased the fitness in their athletes.[2]
Garlic (See GARLIC)			
Horseradish *Amoracia rusticana* It is a member of the mustard family, *Cruciferae.* **Origin and History:** Horseradish is a native of Europe, where it is commonly cultivated. It was domesticated about the time of Christ.	**Importance:** A minor vegetable crop used mainly as a seasoning agent. **Principal Areas:** Temperate regions around the world. **Growing Conditions:** Temperate climate, and a rich, deep, moist, fertile soil. Propagated by root cuttings (usually those that are trimmed from the sides of the main root).	**Processing:** The highest quality horseradish is obtained by stripping the smaller side roots from the main root during the growing period. When the roots are harvested, the leaves and side roots are trimmed off. Fresh horseradish should be grated as soon as possible. **Preparation:** Grated horseradish is usually mixed with vinegar or beet juice, but it may also be mixed with sweet or sour cream. Also powdered horseradish is sold in grocery stores and served in restaurants. **Uses:** Condiment.(One of the 5 bitter herbs of the Jewish Passover).	The raw root has a moderately high water content and caloric content (87 kcal per 100 g). Also it is a good source of potassium and vitamin C. However, the pungent flavor limits the amount which may be eaten. It may make a valuable nutritional contribution by stimulating the appetite and enhancing the enjoyment of food. When eaten, the pungency is thought to help clear out congested breathing passages.[2] Used externally as a counter-irritant.
Jerusalem Artichoke *Helianthus tuberosis* This tuber-bearing plant is a member of the daisy family, *Compositae,* and is closely related to the sunflower. **Origin and History:** Native to North America; it was cultivated by the Indians.	**Importance:** It is a minor crop. **Principal Areas:** Europe, Asia, and the Americas. **Growing Conditions:** Adapted to a wide variety of conditions in temperate climates. Propagated by pieces of tubers.	**Processing:** The long, woody stems must be cut off before the tubers can be harvested. The most common type of processing consists of drying and grinding the tubers into flour. **Preparation:** The flour may be used to make dietetic baked goods and pastas. Also, it may be served unpeeled and raw, cooked with other vegetables, pureed and served like mashed potatoes, or fried, (after dipping the cooked vegetable in a batter). **Uses:** Baked products, and vegetable dishes and substitute for Irish potatoes. It can be used in the diet of diabetics.	Composed mainly of water (80%) and carbohydrates (17%). Most of the latter consists of inulin, a substance not utilized by the body. Hence, the caloric value of the fresh vegetable is negligible. However, the inulin is slowly converted to fructose (fruit sugar) when the tubers are left in the ground. This conversion tends to raise the caloric value. Jerusalem artichoke tubers are deficient in calories, minerals, and vitamins.
Jicama (Yam bean) *Exogonium bracteatum* It is a member of the morning glory family, *Convolvulaceae,* and is related to the sweet potato. **Origin and History:** Originated in Mexico.	**Importance:** A minor vegetable crop that is much appreciated where it is available. **Principal Areas:** Mexico and California. **Growing Conditions:** Subtropical climate. Requires rich, moist soil. Propagated by tubers.	**Processing:** After the vine has flowered, the tubers are harvested by digging around the base of the vine. There is little processing. However, they may be canned, dried, or frozen like potatoes. **Preparation:** Peeled and served raw, or pan fried like potatoes. **Uses:** Appetizer, ingredient of raw salads, or as a substitute for waterchestnuts in various Oriental dishes.	Raw jicama is high in water content (88%) and low in calories (55 kcal per 100 g) and protein (1.4%).

Footnotes at end of table

(Continued)

TABLE V-2 *(Continued)*

Popular and Scientific Name(s); Origin and History	Importance; Principal Areas; Growing Conditions	Processing; Preparation; Uses	Calories; Nutritive Value[1]
Kale *Brassica oleracea acephala* Kale, which belongs to the mustard family, is similar to collards, except that it has leaves with curly edges and is less tolerant to hot weather. **Origin and History:** Believed to have been developed from the wild cabbage that is native to the Mediterranean region. 	**Importance:** A minor vegetable crop. **Principal Areas:** U.S. and European countries. **Growing Conditions:** Cool, temperate climate (Kale differs from collards, in that it does not tolerate hot weather.) Requires well-drained fertile soil.	**Processing:** In commercial production, the leaves are harvested by cutting the plant off at soil level with a large knife. Much of the crop is frozen, but some is canned. **Preparation:** Boiled briefly, or stir fried (in preparation of Chinese dishes). Often served with butter or a cheese sauce. **Uses:** Vegetable dish, ingredient of various mixed dishes, or in soups.	Kale is high in water (88%), low in calories (39 kcal per 100 g), high in protein (4.5%), high in calcium, iron, and potassium, but low in phosphorus; and very high in vitamin A, and moderately good in vitamin C. The eating of moderately large quantities of this vegetable may give some people gas pains. Kale contains small amounts of goitrogens. (See GOITROGENS.)
Kohlrabi *Brassica oleracea caulorapo* Kohlrabi is closely related to cabbage. It is a member of the mustard family, *Cruciferae*. **Origin and History:** Kohlrabi is native to Europe. Selections from a cabbage-like ancestral form were made near the end of the Middle Ages. 	**Importance:** A minor vegetable crop which is more appreciated in Eurnpe (especially Germany) than in the U.S. **Principal Areas:** European countries and U.S. **Growing Conditions:** Cool temperate climate. Requires a rich soil, or one to which fertilizer has been added.	**Processing:** Kohlrabi is usually harvested when the swollen stem is 2 to 3 in. (*5 to 8 cm*) in diameter. The root is cut off after harvesting. Kohlrabi is marketed fresh. **Preparation:** May be eaten raw, or after steaming. Eastern European cooks scoop out the center and stuff the hollow with various mixtures of bread crumbs, meat, seasonings, etc. **Uses:** Vegetable dish; ingredient of salads, soups, and stews.	Similar to the other vegetables of the cabbage species in water content (92%), caloric value (24 kcal per 100 g), protein content (l.7%), and potassium and vitamin C content (a good source). Kohlrabi contains small amounts of goitrogens. (See GOITROGENS.)
Leek *Allium porrum* This onion relative differs from onion in having flat leaves instead of tubular and relatively little bulb development. **Origin and History:** Native to southern Asia. 	**Importance:** Grown to a much greater extent in Europe market gardens than in U.S. The leek is also the national flower of Wales. **Principal Areas:** Northwestern European countries. **Growing Conditions:** Temperate climate. May be transplanted from greenhouse or hot-bed.	**Processing:** Often blanched (lightened in color) during growth by the banking of soil around the plants. (Some growers wrap the stems with cardboard before piling up the soil.) There is little processing of leeks other than canning or drying small amounts of soup preparations. **Preparation:** Boiled, braised, cooked in mixed dishes similar to those which utilize asparagus, or used raw as relishes. **Uses:** Appetizer; ingredient of quiches, salads, soups, and stews.	Like most other vegetables in water content (85%), caloric value (52 kcal per 100 g), and protein content (2.2%). Leeks are a good source of vitamin C.
Lettuce (See LETTUCE)			
Mushroom, Cultivated *Basidiomycetes (club fungi)* *Ascomycetes (truffles)* Mushrooms are fungi. There are 38,000 known species of mushrooms. **Origin and History:** Wild mushrooms were consumed by primitive peoples long before the dawn of agriculture. However, it appears that the common mushroom was first grown commercially in France around 1700. 	**Importance:** Commercial mushroom production is important in Asia and the United States. In 1981, the U.S. produced about 337,000 metric tons. **Principal Areas:** U.S., and European countries. **Growing Conditions:** Commercial production usually involves the planting of specially grown spores in a bed of compost inside a growing shed where the temperature and humidity may be controlled.	**Processing:** Young mushrooms are usually plucked from the bed shortly after they have emerged and while they are still in the button stage. Much of the crop is canned, but some is frozen, dried, or sold fresh. **Preparation:** May be sliced and served raw, stuffed and baked, fried or stewed alone or with other items, or cooked in sauces. **Uses:** Vegetable dish; ingredient of casseroles, quiches, salads, soups, and stews.	High in water content (over 90%) and low in caloric value (around 28 to 35 kcal per 100 g). Contains between 2 and 3% protein. Mushrooms are a good source of phosphorus and potassium, but low in calcium; and they're a good source of niacin, moderately low in thiamin and riboflavin, and very low in vitamins A and C. People who have gout and/or high blood pressure are usually advised to avoid eating mushrooms and other foods that are rich in nucleic acids.

Footnotes at end of table

TABLE V-2 *(Continued)*

Popular and Scientific Name(s); Origin and History	Importance; Principal Areas; Growing Conditions	Processing; Preparation; Uses	Calories; Nutritive Value[1]
Mustard Greens (Indian Mustard) *Brassica juncea* Mustard is a member of the family *Cruciferae*. It is grown for its pungent seed, and for its leaves, which are eaten as greens. **Origin and History:** Native to southern Europe and southwestern Asia. Cultivated since ancient times.	**Importance:** A minor vegetable crop that is much appreciated in the southeastern U.S. **Principal Areas:** Southeastern U.S., central and southern Europe, North Africa, and western Asia. **Growing Conditions:** Temperate climate. Must be planted at the beginning of spring, or in the fall, because high temperatures make the crop go to seed.	**Processing:** Leaves may be harvested anytime from the time they emerge to just before the seedstalks develop. Much of the crop is sold fresh, although mustard greens are frozen. **Preparation:** Steamed, boiled with salt pork, or stir-fried chopped greens with bits of bacon and chopped onions. **Uses:** Vegetable dish; ingredient of casseroles, salads, soups, and stews.	Boiled mustard has a nutritional value like that of most greens (92% water; 23 kcal per 100 g; and 2 to 3% protein). Mustard greens are high in calcium, iron, and potassium; and an excellent source of vitamins A and C. Mustard greens contain small amount of goitrogens. (See GOITROGENS.)
Okra *Hibiscus esculentus* Okra is a member of the mallow family, which includes cotton. **Origin and History:** Thought to be native to Ethiopia. Used in Egypt for many centuries. Brought to Louisiana from France.	**Importance:** A minor vegetable crop. **Principal Areas:** Southern U.S., Europe, Africa, and Asia. **Growing Conditions:** Warm temperate climate. The fruit develops during the summer.	**Processing:** Continuous harvesting of the young pods insures maximum yield. (Old pods are virtually inedible.) A large part of the crop is frozen, while much of the remainder is canned. **Preparation:** May be dipped in egg and cornmeal, then fried; boiled or stewed, alone or with other items. **Uses:** Vegetable dish; ingredient of soups and stews. The Creole cuisine of New Orleans includes various *gumbos*, or okra-containing stews.	Boiled okra contains about 90% water and around 30 kcal per 100 g. Okra is a fair to good source of calcium, potassium, vitamin A, and vitamin C. The mucilaginous material from cooked okra has been used to soothe irritations of the digestive tract.[2]
Olive (See OLIVE)			
Onion (See ONION)			
Parsley *Petroselinum crispum* It is a member of the parsley family, *Umbelliferae*. **Origin and History:** Parsely is native to southern Europe.	**Importance:** A minor vegetable crop. **Principal Areas:** European countries and U.S. **Growing Conditions:** Cool, temperate climate. However, the seeds need warmth to germinate. Hence, it is often transplanted from greenhouses and hotbeds.	**Processing:** Usually, the outer leaves of the plant are harvested when large enough. Some of the crop is dried or frozen, and some is sold fresh. **Preparation:** Served raw, stir fried with other items, or boiled briefly in mixed dishes. **Uses:** For garnishing and flavoring. Ingredient of casseroles, quiches, relishes, salads, soups and stews. It is essential to French cooking.	It is lower in water (85%) and higher in calories (44 kcal per 100 g) than most other leafy vegetables. Also, it is very rich in protein, calcium, iron, potassium, and vitamins A and C.
Parsnip *Pastinaca sativa* Parsnips belong to the parsley family *Umbelliferae*, which also includes carrots, celery, and other vegetables. **Origin and History:** It is native to Eurasia and was cultivated by the Greeks and Romans.	**Importance:** A minor vegetable crop. **Principal Areas:** European countries and U.S. **Growing Conditions:** Requires a rich, moist soil, that does not pack down too readily. Usually planted in the early spring.	**Processing:** Harvested in the late fall by digging, and/or loosening the roots by plowing the ground around them. Eating quality is improved by storage at 34°F (1°C) for 2 weeks. Parsnip roots are generally processed as cooked food. However, they are also used for making parsnip wine. **Preparation:** Parboiled or steamed. Cooked parsnips may be mashed, formed into cakes, and fried. **Uses:** Vegetable dish; ingredient of soups and stews.	A typical root vegetable in water content (80%), and caloric value (76 kcal per 100 g). Parsnips are a good source of potassium, but only a fair source of vitamin C.
Pepper, Chili (See PEPPERS)			
Pepper, Sweet (See PEPPERS)			
Potato (Irish Potato) (See POTATO)			
Pumpkin (See PUMPKIN)			

Footnotes at end of table

(Continued)

TABLE V-2 (Continued)

Popular and Scientific Name(s); Origin and History	Importance; Principal Areas; Growing Conditions	Processing; Preparation; Uses	Calories; Nutritive Value[1]
Radish *Raphanus sativus* The radish is a member of the mustard family, *Cruciferae,* grown for its edible root. **Origin and History:** The radish was developed from a wild plant in the cooler areas of Asia. From here, it spread to the Mediterranean region before the Greek era, thence to the New World early in the 16th century.	**Importance:** A minor, but popular, vegetable. Often grown in home gardens and kept for family use. **Principal Areas:** Temperate and sub-tropical areas of the world. **Growing Conditions:** Requires warm, light, well-drained soils that are highly fertile.	**Processing:** The roots are harvested when they reach marketable size. There is little or no processing except in the Orient, where they may be made into fermented and pickled preparations. **Preparation:** Served raw in salads, or steamed with other ingredients and seasonings. **Uses:** Appetizer; ingredient of mixed vegetable dishes, relishes, and salads.	High in water (94%) and low in calories (17 to 19 kcal per 100 g) and protein (1%). Oriental radishes, which have a milder flavor and can be eaten in larger quantities than common radishes, are lower in potassium and higher in vitamin C than common radishes. Long used to stimulate digestive processes and to help rid the body of excessive water.[2]
Rhubarb (Pieplant) *Rheum rhabarbarum* The rhubarb is a member of the buckwheat family, *Polygonaceae.* **Origin and History:** Originated in Mongolia; used as a medicine in China in 2700 B.C.; introduced into U.S. in late 1700s.	**Importance:** A minor vegetable crop, grown chiefly in home gardens. **Principal Areas:** In Zurich, where it seems to be more appreciated than elsewhere, every small family vegetable garden displays at least one large rhubarb plant. **Growing Conditions:** Adapted to cool, moist climates and cold winters.	**Processing:** Rhubarb is frozen and canned, but many people prefer to cook the fresh stalks. **Preparation:** The thick stalks may be either stewed or baked. **Uses:** Rhubarb is classed as a vegetable, but used as a fruit in America. It is used as a side-dish or as a dessert—often in pie fillings and sauces. In France, it is used in jams and compotes.	The nutrient composition of rhubarb is given in Food Composition Table F-21. Rhubarb contains some vitamin C, and has laxative properties. The leafy portions and the roots contain toxic substances, including oxalic acid, and should not be eaten. (See OXALIC ACID [OXALATE]).
Rutabaga (Swede) *Brassica napobrassica* Rutabagas belong to the mustard family, *Cruciferae.* **Origin and History:** A hybrid of the turnip and cabbage, which originated in Europe in the Middle Ages.	**Importance:** A minor vegetable for human consumption, but an important feed and forage crop for livestock. **Principal Areas:** Europe and North America. **Growing Conditions:** Cool, temperate climate.	**Processing:** Usually, the roots are harvested in the fall. Then some of the crop is stored in a cold, damp environment. The roots keep better if they are covered with a thin layer of wax before storage. **Preparation:** Boiled and mashed, or cooked with other items in mixed dishes. **Uses:** Vegetable dish; ingredient of soups and stews; and feed for livestock.	Similar in nutritive value to other root vegetables (90% water, 35 kcal per 100 g, and 1% protein). It is noteworthy that a mashed mixture of rutabaga and potatoes is lower in calories than mashed potatoes alone. Rutabagas are a good source of vitamins A and C. Rutabagas contain small amounts of goitrogens. (See GOITROGENS.)
Salsify (Oysterplant) *Tragopogon porrifolius* Salsify is a member of the sunflower family, *Compositae.* **Origin and History:** Native to the Mediterranean countries.	**Importance:** A minor vegetable crop. **Principal Areas:** Soviet Union and other European countries. **Growing Conditions:** Temperate climate. Requires a well-drained crumbly soil.	**Processing:** There is little or no processing of salsify. Some of the crop is usually stored. **Preparation:** Boiled; sauteed (after breading), served raw; or roasted to make a coffee substitute. **Uses:** Vegetable dish; ingredient of salads, soups, and stews; and low-carbohydrate substitute for starchy vegetables. (Most of the carbohydrate in salsify is inulin, which is not metabolized by the body.)	Very similar to the Jerusalem artichoke in water content (78%) and carbohydrates (18%). Most of the latter consists of inulin, a substance not utilized by the body. Hence, the caloric value of the fresh vegetable is negligible. However, the caloric value increases when some of the inulin is converted into fructose after long storage of the roots in the ground. Salsify roots are a good source of iron and potassium, a fair source of calcium and phosphorus; a fair source of vitamin C, but a poor source of vitamin A.

TABLE V-2 *(Continued)*

Popular and Scientific Name(s); Origin and History	Importance; Principal Areas; Growing Conditions	Processing; Preparation; Uses	Calories; Nutritive Value[1]
Shallot *Allium cepa* Like the onion, which it resembles, the shallot belongs to the *Alliaceae* family. **Origin and History:** Believed to have originated in Central Asia as a modification of the ordinary type of onion. Onions produce larger and fewer bulbs.	**Importance:** Of little commercial importance. Grown mainly in home gardens. **Principal Areas:** European countries and the U.S. **Growing Conditions:** Temperate climate. Grown in the winter for green onions, and in the summer for dry, mature onions.	**Processing:** The *green onions* are trimmed and skinned, whereas, the dry bulbs are treated like ordinary onions. There is little or no processing of shallots because most of the crop is marketed as a fresh vegetable. **Preparation:** Chopped and served raw; sauteed; or boiled. **Uses:** Appetizer; ingredient of relishes, salads, soups, and stews.	Like other members of the onion family in water content (80%) and caloric value (72 kcal per 100 g). Shallot bulbs are similar in nutrient composition to the Irish potato. However, only small amounts of shallots are usually consumed.
Sorrel (Dock) *Rumex acetosa* Sorrel belongs to the buckwheat family, *Polygonaceae.* **Origin and History:** Native to Asia and Europe. Cultivated in France and Italy since the 14th century.	**Importance:** A minor vegetable crop. **Principal Areas:** Popular in Europe. **Growing Conditions:** Temperate climate. Requires rich, moist soil and abundant sunshine.	**Processing:** Almost all of the sorrel is consumed fresh. Sometimes the leaves are dried for storage. **Preparation:** Served raw, or boiled briefly. **Uses:** Seasoning; and an ingredient of casseroles, salads, soups, and other mixed dishes.	Similar in nutritional value to other green leafy vegetables (91% water, 28 kcal per 100 g, 2% protein); a good source of iron and potassium, and a fair source of calcium and phosphorus; and an excellent source of vitamins A and C. Sorrel is rich in oxalates. (See OXALIC ACID [OXALATE]).
Spinach *Spinacia oleracea* Spinach is a member of the goosefoot family, *Chenopodiaceae.* **Origin and History:** Native to Southwestern Asia (believed to have orginated in Persia).	**Importance:** Spinach is a popular garden vegetable, which is widely cultivated throughout the world. **Principal Areas:** The U.S., the Netherlands, and the Scandinavian countries are the major producers. **Growing Conditions:** Cool, temperate climate (goes to seed readily in hot weather.)	**Processing:** Leaves may be harvested as soon as they are large enough. Some spinach is consumed fresh, but ¾ of the crop is processed—mostly by canning or freezing. **Preparation:** Cooked briefly in as little water as possible; served raw in salads; baked in casseroles and quiches. **Uses:** Vegetable dish; main dish (when served with chopped eggs and/or a cheese sauce on toast); and an ingredient of casseroles, quiches, salads, and soups. Small quantities are used to 'make baby foods, spinach noodles, and other special items.	Like other greens in water content (91%), caloric value (26 kcal per 100 g) and protein content (3%). Spinach is an excellent source of magnesium, iron, and potassium, and a good source of calcium; and an excellent source of vitamin A, and a good source of vitamin C. Spinach is rich in oxalates. (See OXALIC ACID [OXALATE]).
Squash, Summer (See SQUASHES)			
Squash, Winter (See SQUASHES)			
Sweet Potato (See SWEET POTATO)			
Swiss Chard (seakale beet) *Beta vulgaris* Swiss chard belongs to the goosefoot family, *Chenopodiaceae.* **Origin and History:** One of the vegetables derived in pre-Christian times from the wild beet that is native to the shores of the Mediterranean.	**Importance:** A minor, but popular vegetable in Europe and the U.S. **Principal Areas:** Swiss chard is grown more widely in Europe than in U.S. **Growing Conditions:** Temperate climate. May be started from seed in a greenhouse or a hotbed, then transplanted when the danger of hard frost is over.	**Processing:** Leaves may be picked from the plants until fall frost occurs. Little chard is processed. It is used mainly as a fresh vegetable. However, it may be canned or frozen like spinach. **Preparation:** Served raw as greens, or leaves and stems cooked (usually boiled or fried) separately, since the stems require longer cooking. **Uses:** Vegetable dish; entree (with cheese sauce and hard boiled eggs on toast); ingredient of salads, soups, and mixed dishes (such as chard fried with meat and onions or garlic).	Very high in water (91%) and low in calories (25 kcal per 100 g). A good source of iron and vitamin C, and an excellent source of vitamin A. The protein-to-calorie ratio of Swiss chard (9.6 g per 100 kcal) is about equal to that of skim milk. Hence, significant amounts of dietary protein may be supplied by this vegetable, if sufficiently large amounts are consumed. Has a high oxalic acid content which may reduce utilization of calcium, iron, and other essential minerals.

Footnotes at end of table

(Continued)

TABLE V-2 *(Continued)*

Popular and Scientific Name(s); Origin and History	Importance; Principal Areas; Growing Conditions	Processing; Preparation; Uses	Calories; Nutritive Value[1]
Taro (Cocyam, Dasheen, Eddoe) *Colocasia esculenta* Taro is a tropical plant of the Arum family, *Aracea.* **Origin and History:** Native to southeastern Asia, where it was first cultivated 4,000 to 7,000 years ago. Spread throughout the Pacific Basin by the ancestors of the Polynesians.	**Importance:** Among the leading tuberous plants grown and consumed in Africa. **Principal Areas:** Moist, tropical areas around the world. **Growing Conditions:** Warm, moist climate. Requires a highly fertile soil.	**Processing:** Small tubers may be stored more successfully than large ones. Only small amounts of taro are processed commercially; most of the crop is consumed where it is produced. **Preparation:** Baked, boiled, or fried (like potato chips). **Uses:** Starchy vegetable; used to make *poi,* a fermented starchy paste, in Hawaii.	Boiled taro tubers are similar in nutritional value to other root and tuber vegetables (67% water, 124 kcal per 100 g, and 1.9% protein). The nutritional value of taro tubers is similar to that of potatoes, except that the taro is much lower in vitamin C. The leaves are more nutritious than the tubers. Neither the roots nor the leaves of taro should be consumed raw, because some varieties contain potentially harmful amounts of calcium oxalate crystals.
Tomato (See TOMATO)			
Turnip *Brassica rapa* The turnip belongs to the mustard family, *Cruciferae.* **Origin and History:** One type is native to Europe, while another is native to central Asia. Turnips were first cultivated 4,000 years ago in the Near East.	**Importance:** A minor vegetable crop that is more important in Europe than in the U.S. **Principal Areas:** European countries. Most of the U.S. crop is produced in the southern states. **Growing Conditions:** Cool, temperate climate. Grows best during spring and early fall since it does not do well in hot weather.	**Processing:** Although fresh greens and roots are still marketed, much of the crop is now frozen. **Preparation:** Turnip roots are boiled and mashed, or cooked with other items in mixed dishes. Southern cooks prepare turnip greens as a hot vegetable, often mixed with bacon or pork. **Uses:** Vegetable dish; ingredient of salads, soups, and stews.	Boiled turnip roots have a high water content (94%) and are low in calories (23 kcal per 100 g) and protein (0.8%). They are a fair source of vitamin C. Compared to the roots, the cooked greens contain about the same amounts of water and calories, but twice as much protein, iron, and vitamin C, and many times as much vitamin A (of which they are an excellent source). Turnips contain small amounts of goitrogens. (See GOITROGENS.)
Waterchestnut, Chinese (Ma-tai, Pi-tsi) *Elocharis tuberosa,* and *Elocharis dulcis* The Chinese waterchestnut is not related to the waterchestnut *(Tropanatans).* It is a member of the sedge family, *Cyperaceae.* **Origin and History:** Native to southern China.	**Importance:** Minor, but much appreciated vegetable. **Principal Areas:** China, Japan, and East Indies. **Growing Conditions:** Temperate climate. Grows wild in shallow water near the shores of lakes, and in marshes. Cultivated in China (grown in rice paddies).	**Processing:** The corms are dug from the mud by hand after the rice paddies have been drained. Much of the Chinese crop is canned for export. Sometimes starch is extracted by washing grated raw tubers on a fine screen. **Preparation:** Boiled briefly (after peeling). **Uses:** Ingredient of mixed Oriental dishes, salads, and soups.	Has a nutritional value like that of the other tuberous vegetables. Compared to Irish potatoes, Chinese waterchestnuts contain about the same calories, but only 2/3 the protein, and 1/6 the vitamin C.
Watercress *Nasturtium officinale* Watercress is a member of the mustard family, *Cruciferae.* **Origin and History:** Watercress is a native of Europe, but it has become naturalized wherever there is clear, cold, shallow water.	**Importance:** Minor crop, which also grows wild. **Principal Areas:** Germany, France, and the United Kingdom. **Growing Conditions:** Temperate climate. Requires an abundant supply of running water which is alkaline and contains nitrates.	**Processing:** None of the crop is processed; all of it is sold fresh. **Preparation:** Served raw in salads and sandwiches, or cooked with other vegetables to add flavor. **Uses:** Ingredient of salads, sandwiches, and soups.	Very similar to other greens in nutrient composition (93% water, 19 kcal per 100 g, and 2.2% protein). Watercress is high in calcium and iron, and an excellent source of vitamins A and C. Herbal remedy for minor disorders (lack of appetite, mild depression, and waterlogging).[2] Watercress contain small amounts of goitrogens. (See GOITROGENS.)

Footnotes at end of table

(Continued)

TABLE V-2 *(Continued)*

Popular and Scientific Name(s); Origin and History	Importance; Principal Areas; Growing Conditions	Processing; Preparation; Uses	Calories; Nutritive Value[1]
Yam (Asiatic Yam) *Dioscorea alata* Yams belong to the family, *Dioscoreaceae.* Although the starchy tubers resemble sweet potatoes, the two plants are not even distantly related. **Origin and History:** Originated in Africa, where they were cultivated 11,000 years ago; and in southeast Asia, where they were cultivated 10,000 years ago.	**Importance:** Among the leading tuberous plants grown and consumed in the tropics. Worldwide, production of yams is about 29.4 million metric tons per year. **Principal Areas:** Moist, tropical areas of Africa, Asia, and the Americas. About half of the yams of the world are grown in western Africa. **Growing Conditions:** Warm, moist climate. Do not grow well below 68°F *(20°C).* Require fertile soils and at least 40 in. *(250 cm)* of rainfall during the 8 months growing season.	**Processing:** Toxic varieties must be soaked or boiled in water to remove the harmful substances. Some of the crop is made into flour, which stores better than the whole tubers. **Preparation:** Baked; boiled and mashed; or fried (after slicing). **Uses:** Staple food, starchy vegetable, and ingredient of soups and stews.	Somewhat like the potato in nutritional value, but yam tubers contain 50% more calories, and about the same amount of protein. Yams are a fair to good source of calcium, phosphorus, and iron; and a fair source of vitamin C, but they contain little carotene.

[1]See Food Composition Table F-21 for additional details.

[2]No medical claims are made for any of the vegetables listed in this table. The various beliefs regarding the beneficial effects of certain items are presented (1) for historical and informational purposes, and/or (2) to stimulate further investigation of the claimed merits.

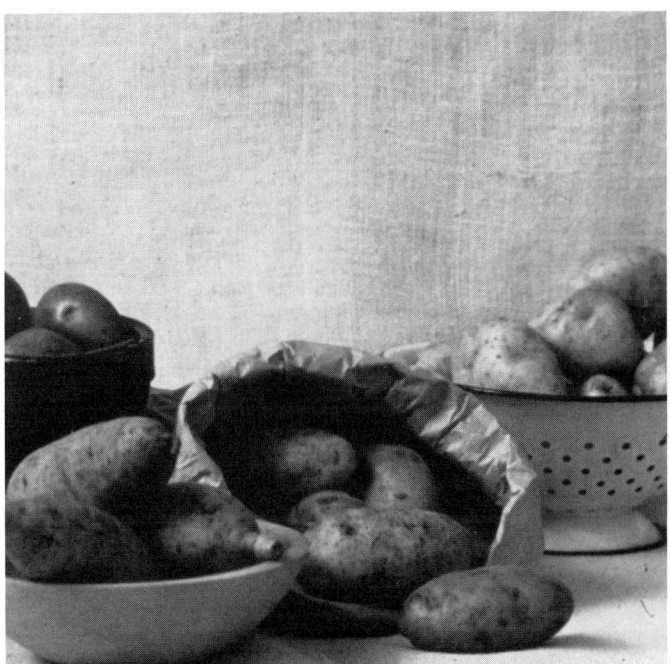

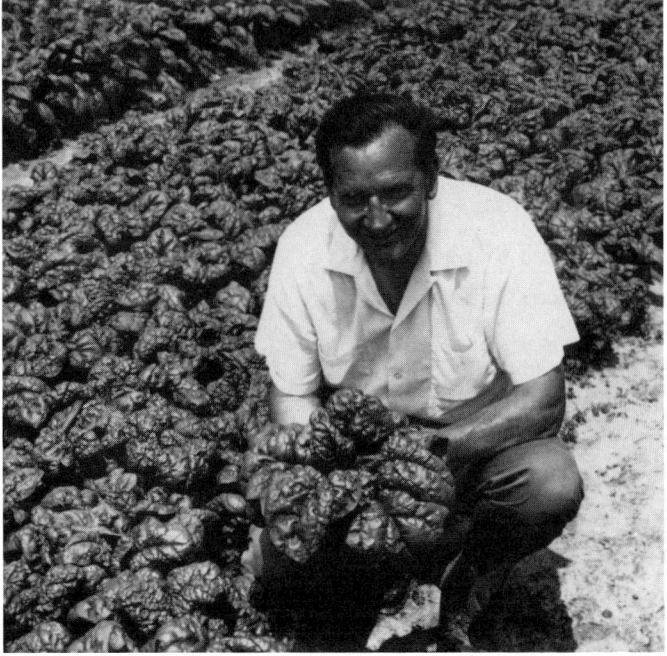

Fig. V-12. Potatoes, the leading vegetable crop of the world and of the U.S. (Courtesy, USDA)

Fig. V-13. Swiss chard, used as a vegetable dish, entree, and ingredient of salads, soups, and mixed dishes. (Courtesy, New Jersey Department of Agriculture)

NOTE WELL: Where production figures are given in Table V-2, column 2 under "Importance," unless otherwise stated, they are based on 1990 data. Most world figures are from *FAO Production Yearbook 1990,* FAO/UN, Rome, Italy, Vol. 44. Most U.S. figures are from *Agricultural Statistics 1991.* Annual production fluctuates as a result of weather and profitability of the crop.

Although beans are often classed as vegetables, especially those that are used as immature green pods (snap beans or green beans), all beans are legumes. So, in order to avoid double listing, the species of beans commonly used in the United States are listed and summarized in Table L-2, Legumes of the World.

VEGETABLE BUTTERS

Due to their fatty acid composition, the lipids extracted from some plants are solids—fats—at room temperature and, hence, exhibit the consistency of butter and even the yellow color. Most lipids extracted from plants are liquids—oils—at room temperature. Two familiar vegetable butters are cocoa butter and coconut butter.

• **Cocoa butter**—The fat pressed from the roasted cacao bean is known as cocoa butter. It is yellow and possesses a slight chocolate smell and flavor. Cocoa butter is mainly used in drugs and cosmetics. As a food it is pleasant to the taste and easily digestible.

• **Coconut butter**—This is derived by pressing the dried coconut meats or copra, and then after bleaching and various other processes the oil is transformed into a product of firm consistency that looks like butter. Coconut butter is common in France.

Other less known vegetable butters include Shea butter from the African plant *Butyrospermum parkii*, Mowrah fat or illipe butter from the Indian plant *Bassia longifolia*, and nutmeg butter. By broadening the definition of butter to include foods that are spread like butter, peanut butter, hazelnut butter, and walnut butter are included as vegetable butters.

VEGETABLE OILS

These oils are pressed or extracted from a variety of plant seeds. Of primary importance as sources of edible oil on a world basis are soybeans, cottonseed, peanuts, corn germ, olives, coconut, rapeseed (canola), sesame, sunflower, safflower, cocoa beans, and various oil palms.

(Also see OILS, VEGETABLE; and FATS AND OTHER LIPIDS, section headed "Animal and Vegetable.")

VEGETARIAN DIETS

In its purest form, a vegetarian diet consists of only foods of plant origin—no meat, fish, or other animal products are allowed. Most vegetarian diets allow vegetables, fruits, cereals and breads (often whole grain), yeast, dry beans, peas and lentils, nuts and peanut butter, seeds, vegetable oils, sugars and syrups, and possibly some rather unusual foods. Often a vegetarian diet is assumed to mean only no meat in the diet. For some types of vegetarianism this may be true.

TYPES OF VEGETARIANS.   Persons following vegetarian patterns fall into one of the four basic types of vegetarianism.

1. *Ovolactovegetarians.* These individuals consume a diet of plant origin supplemented with milk, milk products, and eggs.
2. *Lactovegetarians.* These individuals eat a diet of plant origin supplemented with milk and milk products only.
3. *Pure vegetarians or vegans.* These individuals eat all foods of plant origin, and no animal-originating foods, dairy products, or eggs. In addition, the term vegan may embody

a philosophy which discourages the use of anything that even indirectly requires the taking of animal life.

4. *Fruitarians.* These individuals consume diets consisting of raw or dried fruits, nuts, honey, and olive oil. Some may supplement with grains and legumes.

Each type of vegetarianism may run some risk of dietary inadequacy—some more than others.

PREVALENCE OF VEGETARIANISM.   The practice of vegetarianism is not new. Throughout history there have been various individuals, groups or cults that have subscribed to a vegetarian diet. Of the five major religions of the world—Christianity, Judaism, Islam, Hinduism, and Buddhism—all place restrictions on some food of animal origin. Because of the belief in the transmigration of souls, the preservation of animal life is a basic tenet of Hinduism, Brahmanism, Buddhism, and Jainism.

Organized vegetarianism was brought to the United States by the Reverend William Metcalfe and 41 members of his church, who landed in Philadelphia in 1817. Their numbers grew, and their cause was furthered by the influence of several prominent men who became convinced of the advantages of the fleshless diet. Among these were Reuben D. Mussey (1780-1866), fourth president of the American Medical Association and Edward Hitchcock (1793-1864), professor of Science and then president of Amherst College, whose "Lectures on Diet, Regimen, and Employment" were published in 1831. Also, contributing to the vegetarian movement in 1829 was Sylvester Graham, a young Presbyterian who believed he had regained his health on a vegetarian diet, and who began writing and speaking on moderation in eating. Graham is best remembered for advocating the use of unbolted *graham* flour and the *graham* cracker. In 1858, Dr. James Caleb Jackson opened Our Home Hygienic Institute in Danville, New York, which emphasized, among other things, the Graham-type diet. Mother Ellen Harmon White, spiritual leader of the Seventh-day Adventist Church, founded the Western Health Reform Institute at Battle Creek, Michigan, in 1866. Later, Dr. John Harvey Kellogg was hired as superintendent, and the name was changed to the Battle Creek Sanitarium or "San" where, in an effort to provide a wholesome, palatable nonflesh diet for the sanitarium patrons, Dr. Kellogg and his brother, W. K. Kellogg, developed cereal foods. From this vegetarian movement sprang two breakfast cereal businesses—Kelloggs of Battle Creek and General Foods Corporation. C. W. Post, the founder of General Foods, had been a patient-guest at the "San."

While the history of vegetarian movements can be traced, it is important to remember that in much of the world, adherence to a vegetarian diet is not by choice but by economics and availability. For centuries large populations of the world have survived on vegetarian diets of one type or another out of necessity.

Vegetarianism has more or less always existed. However, in the United States, there is a renewed movement toward vegetarianism—some for religious convictions, and some for personal convictions as an attitude of the future. In recent years, various religious cults such as Zen Buddhism, Hare Krishnas, and some yogic groups, which promote vegetarianism, have gained popularity in the United States. As a movement of the future, vegetarianism seems to have roots in various other movements; for example, ecology, counterculture, environmental pollution, and population studies suggesting increased heart disease, cancer, and various other ills with increased meat consumption. Many animal products have been promoted as unhealthy due to additives, preservatives, cholesterol, fat, and lack of fiber. Hardest hit have been eggs, cured meats, and red meats. Moreover, proponents of animal rights make animal production methods seem inhumane; hence, eating animal products becomes an inhumane activity. Still other individuals say cereal grains could be better used to feed the hungry world than to feed cattle and pigs. So, much of the move toward vegetarianism may actually be a move toward what many feel is a more healthful diet—at least based upon popularized theories, or a move toward some feeling of a right action.

PROBLEMS OF VEGETARIANISM. Whatever the reason for choosing a vegetarian life-style, some nutritional problems are inherent unless the person practicing possesses a sound knowledge of nutrition. Furthermore, the level of vegetarianism is important. Those at the greatest risk are the vegans or pure vegetarians and fruitarians, and among these individuals their dietary practices are the most hazardous to pregnant or lactating women, infants, growing children, adolescents, and people who are ill or recovering from disease. Dietary concerns for fruitarians and vegans include energy, protein, calcium, iron, zinc, vitamin D, riboflavin, and vitamin B-12.

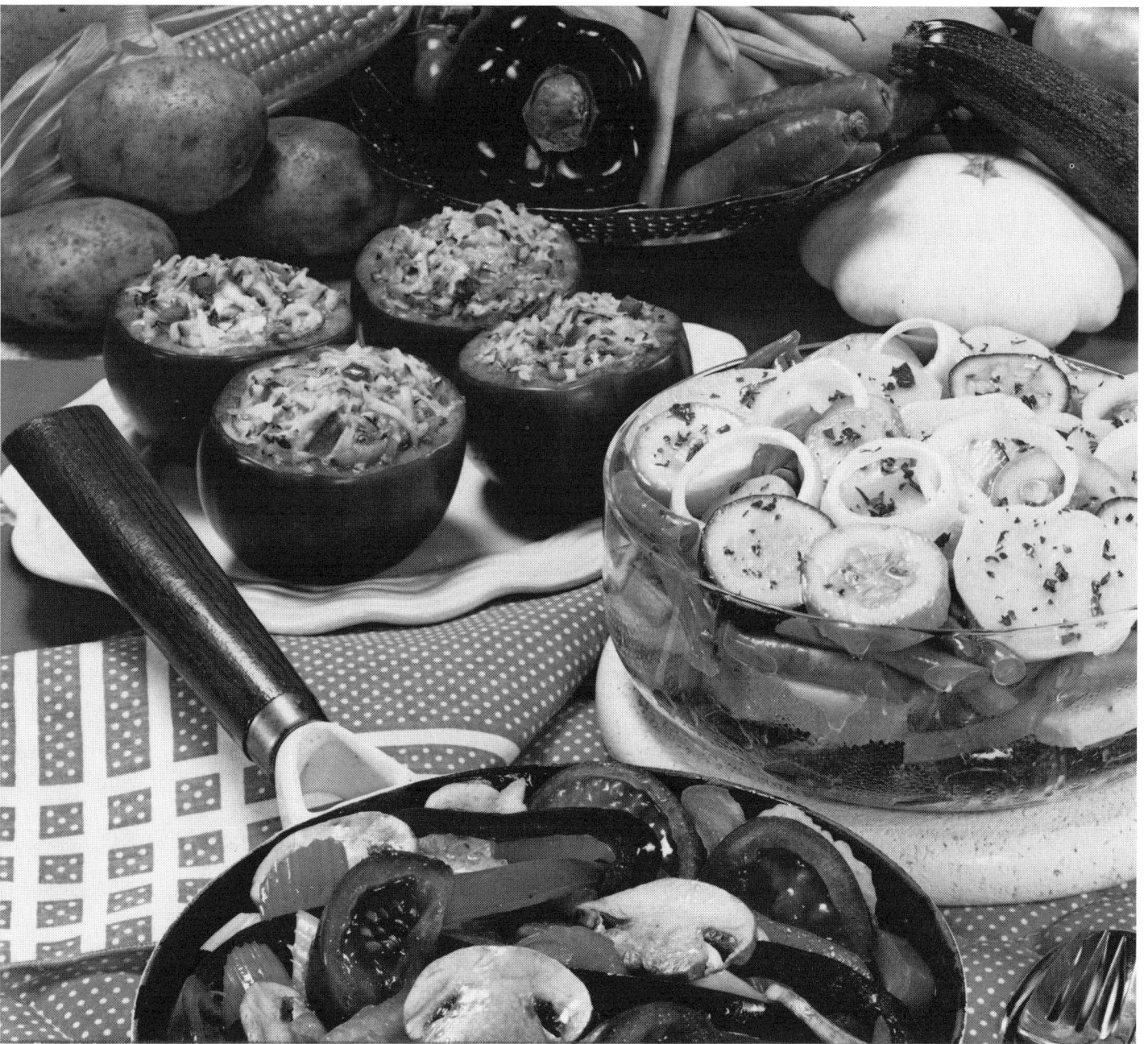

Fig. V-14. A wide variety of vegetables provides adventures in good eating and rich sources of certain essential minerals and vitamins. (Courtesy, United Fresh Fruit and Vegetable Assn.)

HEALTHFUL VEGETARIAN DIETS. Planning nutritious total vegetarian diets requires care and knowledge of the strengths and weaknesses of the various foods. By combining the information contained in Table V-3 and using the following guidelines, healthful vegetarian diets may be planned:

1. Reduce substantially all high calorie, low nutrient density foods (empty-calories). Instead, use unrefined foods as far as practical, which, on a caloric basis, supply their share of nutrients.

2. Replace meat by the protein-rich group of legumes, seeds, and nuts.

3. Increase intake of whole grain breads and cereals, legumes, nuts, and seeds to maintain energy intake.

4. Use a variety of legumes and whole grains, with some seeds and/or nuts, in meals each day to achieve good protein complementation; for example, beans with corn or rice, cereals with legumes and green, leafy vegetables, and peanuts with wheat.

5. Use a variety of fruits and vegetables, but be sure to include food high in ascorbic acid *in each meal* to enhance iron absorption.

6. Replace the nutrients lost by deleting milk and dairy products by (a) taking a modest amount of nutritional yeast (brewers' or torula), (b) eating dried fruits, (c) providing supplemental vitamin D by daily exposure to the sun, and (d) providing supplemental vitamin B-12.

7. Secure added food energy (calories) from such foods as sweeteners (sugar and syrups), margarine, oils, and shortenings; used either as ingredients in recipes, or at the table.

8. Eat sufficient amounts to maintain ideal weight for age and height. Larger servings and additional foods such as nuts or margarine may be necessary.

9. Consult the Food Composition Table F-21 when planning vegetarian diets to ensure the selection of nutritious foods.

TABLE V-3
THE VEGETARIAN FOUR FOOD GROUPS—THE BASIC FOUR[1]

Group	Foods Included	Amount Recommended	Contribution to the Diet	Comments
Protein rich	Dry beans, dry peas, soybeans, lentils, nuts, including peanuts and peanut butter; meat analogs.	Choose five servings every day. Count as a serving: ½ c. of cooked dry beans, dry peas, soybeans, or lentils; 2 Tbsp peanut butter; ¼ to ½ c. nuts, sesame, or sunflower seeds. Count one serving as equivalent to 1 oz of lean meat, poultry, or fish.	Foods in this group are valued for their protein. They also provide iron, thiamin, riboflavin, niacin, and phosphorus.	Commercially prepared plant protein products are not essential for a well-balanced diet. However, when changing from a nonvegetarian to a vegetarian diet, meat analogs are helpful because they replace the accustomed entree without further changes in the menu being necessary. They are convenience-type foods. Labels should be checked for nutritional data. Nuts are concentrated foods contributing flavor and unsaturated fat to the diet.
Milk and cheeses	Fortified soy milk and soy cheese (tofu).	Some milk every day for everyone. Recommended amounts are given below in terms of 8-oz cups: (8-oz cup) **Children under 9** . . . . 2 to 3 **Children 9 to 12** . . . . 3 or more **Teenagers** . . . . 4 or more **Adults** . . . . 2 or more **Pregnant women** . . . . 3 or more **Nursing mothers** . . . . 4 or more	Provides calcium, and vitamin B-12.	Children, in particular, need fortified soybean milk. Large servings of greens like collards, kale, mustard greens, turnip greens, and dandelion greens contribute to meeting the calcium requirement. Vitamin D normally obtained from milk should be supplemented by daily exposure to sunlight. Vitamin B-12 must be provided in fortified foods such as soy milk or yeast grown on B-12 enriched media; or provided as a supplement. Nursing mothers need supplemental vitamin D and B-12.
Vegetables and fruits	All vegetables and fruits including dried fruits; with emphasis on those that are valuable sources of vitamin C and vitamin A.	Choose 4 or more servings every day, including: 1 serving of a good source of vitamin C or 2 servings of a fair source; 1 serving, at least every other day, of a good source of vitamin A. If the food chosen for vitamin C is also a good source of vitamin A, the additional serving of a vitamin A food may be omitted. The remaining 1 to 3 or more servings may be of any vegetable or fruit, including those that are valuable for vitamin C and vitamin A. Count as one serving: ½ c. of vegetable or fruit; or a portion as ordinarily served, such as 1 medium apple, banana, orange, or potato, ½ a medium grapefruit or cantaloupe or the juice of 1 lemon.	Fruits and vegetables are valuable chiefly because of the vitamins and minerals they contain. In this plan, this group is counted on to supply nearly all the vitamin C needed and over ½ of the vitamin A. In addition, some members of this group supply fiber. Dark-green and deep-yellow vegetables are good sources of vitamin A. Most dark-green vegetables, if not overcooked, are also reliable sources of vitamin C, as are citrus fruits. Dark-green vegetables are valued for riboflavin, folacin, iron, and magnesium as well. Nearly all vegetables and fruits are low in fat, and none contain cholesterol. Unpeeled fruits and vegetables and those with edible seeds supply fiber. Dried fruits are good sources of iron.	A food high in vitamin C (ascorbic acid) at each meal enhances iron absorption. For sweetening cereals use raisins, dates, or sliced bananas. Avocados supply some fat. Dried fruits concentrate the mineral content.
Breads and cereals	All breads and cereals should be whole-grain or enriched products; whole grains include: wheat, oats, corn, rye, millet, barley, rice, wild rice.	Choose 5 or more servings daily; or if no cereals are chosen, have an extra serving of breads or baked goods, which will make at least 5 servings from this group daily. Count as 1 serving: 1 slice of bread; 1 oz ready-to-eat cereal; ½ to ¾ c. cooked cereal, cornmeal, grits, macaroni, noodles, rice, spaghetti, etc.	Foods in this group furnish worthwhile amounts of protein, iron, several of the B vitamins, and food energy. Whole-grain products also contribute magnesium, folacin, and fiber. Yeast fermentation of whole-grain flours, such as in breadmaking, lowers the phytates and significantly increases the availability of zinc.	Includes all products made with whole-grains or enriched flour, or meal. Example: bread, biscuits, muffins, waffles, pancakes, cooked or ready-to-eat cereals, cornmeal, flour, grits, macaroni and spaghetti, noodles, rice, rolled oats, barley, and bulgur. Most breakfast cereals are fortified at nutrient levels higher than those occurring in the natural grain. Use whole grains to complement the protein-rich group.

[1]In ovolactovegetarian or lactovegetarian diets, eggs and/or milk and milk products are used in place of some of the servings of food from the protein-rich group. Milk recommendations follow those set forth in the milk and cheese group. To convert to metric, see WEIGHTS AND MEASURES.

10. Make use of a number of good vegetarian cookbooks for preparing tasty and nutritious dishes.

NOTE WELL: Pure vegetarian diets are not recommended for infants and small children. Also, pure vegetarian diets for pregnant or lactating women should be planned with great care.

(Also see INFANT DIET AND NUTRITION; and PREGNANCY AND LACTATION NUTRITION.)

MEAT SUBSTITUTES. Vegetarians can have their meat and eat it too! There is a whole line of products developed primarily from plant proteins that look like meat and taste like meat. Similar to the vegetarian movement of the late 1800s which spawned the development of Kelloggs and

General Foods, the vegetarian movement of the late 1900s has created a market for meat analogs or substitutes. These are manufactured by two companies, primarily—Loma Linda Foods and Worthington Foods. Although these products are not necessary for a well-balanced vegetarian diet, they do help when an individual is shifting from a nonvegetarian diet to a vegetarian diet. Furthermore, meat analogs add variety to a vegetarian diet. They can be produced to simulate the appearance, texture, and flavor of meat, poultry, and fish; and they can be made to meet the known nutrients in animal sources. Individuals purchasing these meat analogs should realize that they are convenience foods. Also, nutritional information on the labels must be checked to determine their adequacy.

(Also see MEAT[S], section headed "Meat Substitutes.")

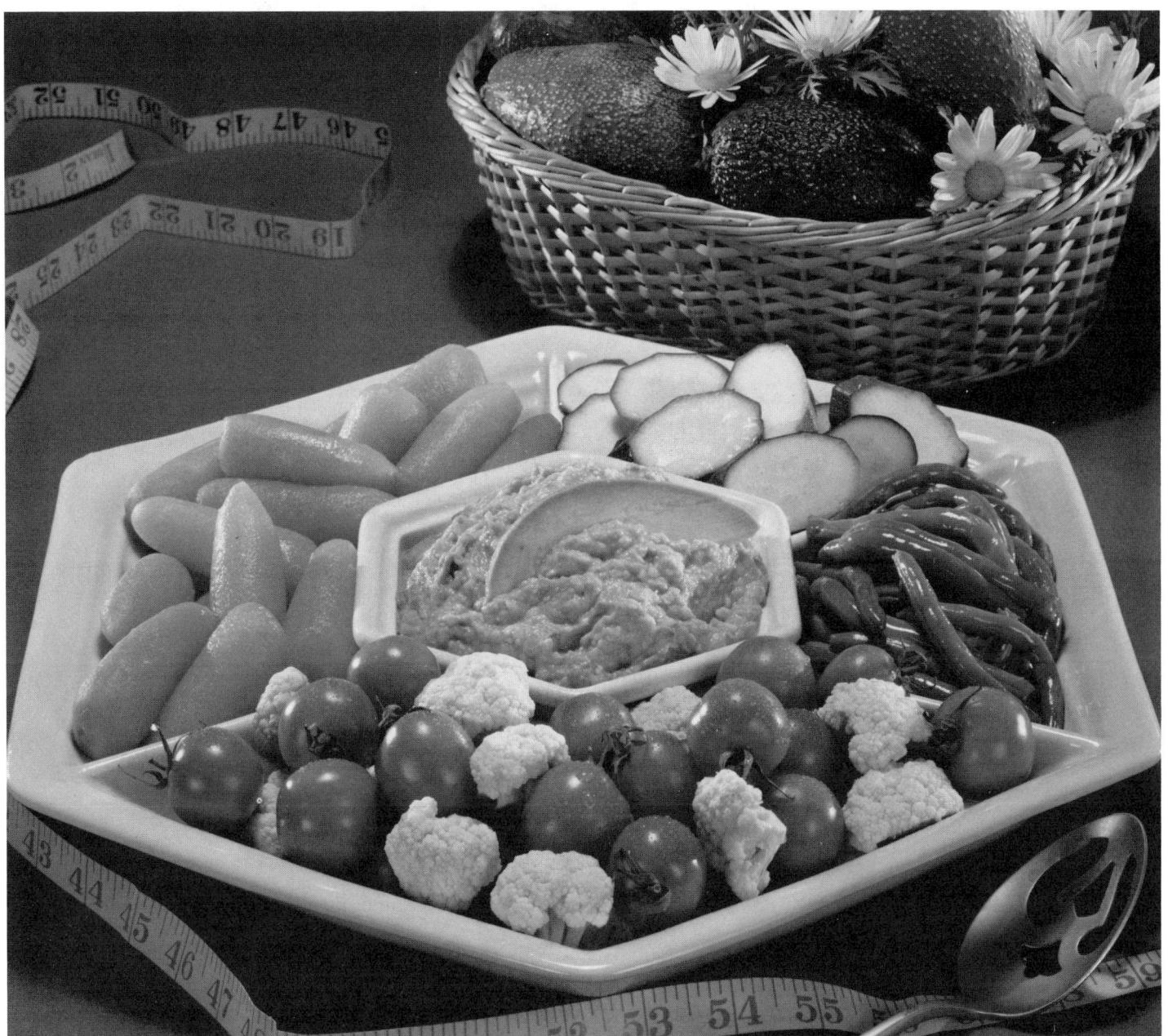

Fig. V-15. Vegetables measure up to *good nutrition.* (Courtesy, Harshe-Rotman & Druke, Inc., Public Relations, Los Angeles, Calif.)

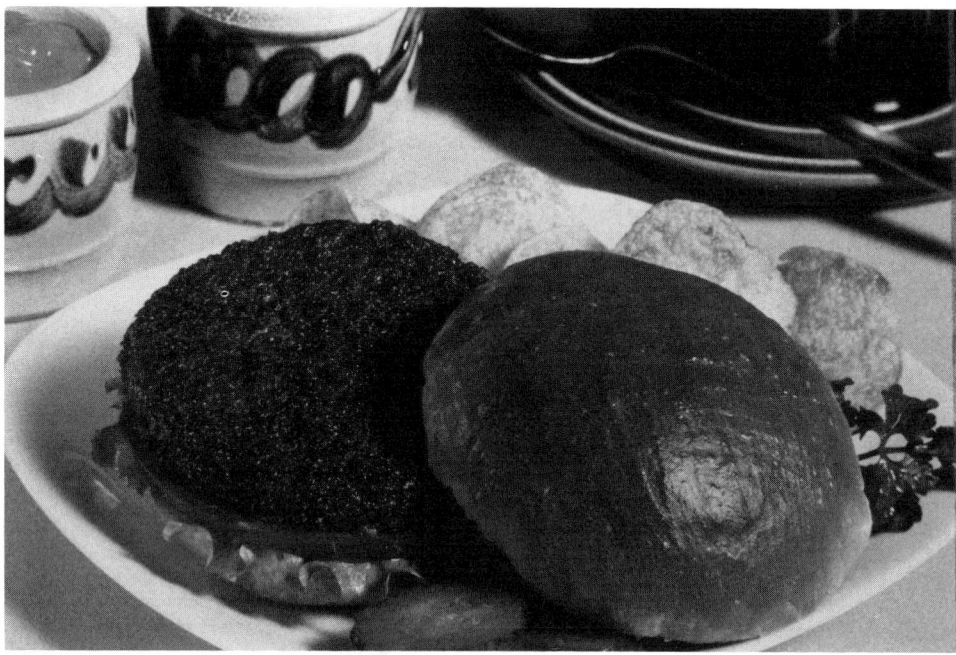

Fig. V-16. A textured vegetable protein patty which can be fried, baked, or grilled to taste like a hamburger. (Courtesy, Worthington Foods, Worthington, Ohio)

POSSIBLE HEALTH BENEFITS OF VEGETARIAN-ISM. Vegetarianism has been credited with minimizing a variety of diseases including obesity, cancer, coronary heart disease, dental caries, diabetes, and diverticular disease of the colon. However, in many cases, lack of complete data prohibits sound conclusions.

(Also see CHOLESTEROL; FIBER; FOOD GROUPS; MEATS; WORLD FOOD; and ZEN MACROBIOTIC DIET.)

VENISON

The name venison comes from the Latin *venatio*, meaning *game* or *hunting*. Presently, the term connotes the flesh of any antlered animal.

Venison should be aged before eating or freezing. This may be accomplished by hanging the carcass in a walk-in cooler at 34° to 36°F (1° to 2°C); aging young deer for 1 week, and older deer for 2 to 3 weeks.

Venison lends itself well to corning (corned venison); to curing, drying, and smoking (dried venison); to sausage making, when mixed with 50% or more of fat pork trimmings, and prepared as summer or smoked sausage; and to freezing. The most widely used method of preservation is by freezing at 0°F (-18°C) or lower. Ground meat may be stored in the freezer for 2 to 3 months, and roasts and steaks for 8 to 12 months.

Venison may be cooked like beef—steaks and chops broiled or sauteed, legs roasted, and the less tender cuts pot-roasted. The best tenderizer for game is a tasty marinade. Any fat should be cut off and replaced with other fat, such as bacon or salt pork. Salt pork is excellent for larding large pieces of meat; smaller pieces may be wrapped in bacon. Venison, like beef, may be served rare, medium, or well done.

VERJUICE

The two different meanings of this term are as follows:

• The juice extracted from either unripe apples or unripe grapes, which was once used to make various drinks, but is now used mainly to impart a tart flavor to various sauces in European cuisine.

• Any tart juice, such as that expressed from cress, crab-apples, gooseberries, or sorrel, which may be either fermented or unfermented.

VERMICELLI

This refers to a pasta that is much like spaghetti—only thinner.

(Also see MACARONI AND NOODLE PRODUCTS.)

VERMOUTH

A white wine flavored with wormwood or other herbs such as anise, cinnamon, bitter orange peel, cloves, and elderberries. There are two types: (1) a dark or reddish, richly flavored (sweet) Italian variety; and (2) a pale yellow or light, dry French variety. Vermouth can be used as a liqueur or in cocktails.

(Also see WINE.)

VETCH

The name applied to several different legumes (pulses) some of which are used for food. The starchy root of the tuber-vetch is roasted, while the chick-vetch is prepared in the same manner as chick peas.

VICILIN

A globulin (simple protein) associated with a legume, such as peas, lentils, and broad beans.

VIENNA BREAD

A bread that is eaten in France mainly as toast or croutons, or in sandwiches. It has a very thin crust; and it is baked in square pans.
(Also see BREADS AND BAKING.)

VILLI

Small threadlike projections attached to the interior side of the wall of the small intestine.
(Also see DIGESTION AND ABSORPTION.)

VINEGAR

The word vinegar is derived from the French word *vinaigre*, literally meaning sour wine. Indeed, sour wine was the original source of vinegar. Vinegar was a by-product of wine makers and brewers until about the 17th century when vinegar making became a separate industry in France.

By definition, vinegar is a sour liquid containing 4 to 12% acetic acid. Any product that will yield alcoholic fermentation—apples, grapes, pears, peaches, plums, figs, oranges, berries, honey, sugar, syrups, hydrolyzed starchy materials, beers and wines—is acceptable for the production of vinegar. However, wine and cider are the best raw materials for vinegar production. In addition to the acetic acid, other organic acids and esters are present in vinegar giving it a flavor and aroma characteristic of the material from which it was derived. Thus, there are a variety of vinegars: wine vinegar, apple-cider vinegar, beer vinegar, and malt vinegar.

In 1864, Louis Pasteur demonstrated that bacteria caused the conversion of alcohol to acetic acid. Hence, vinegar making is dependent upon the action of yeast and bacteria on the raw product. Fig. V-17 illustrates the chemical reactions involved in the production of vinegar. Cider and wine

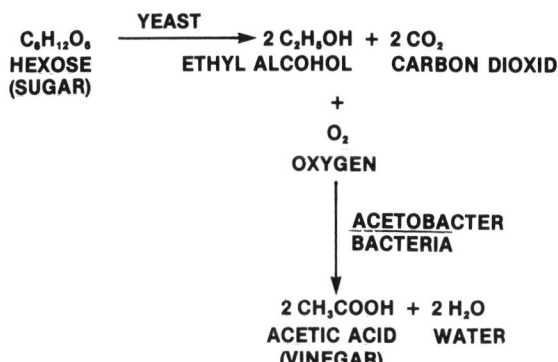

Fig. V-17. Biochemical changes of vinegar making.

are the best raw materials for vinegar production. In the United States, cider is most frequently used. Basically, apples are mechanically crushed and pressed, and adjusted to contain not less than 8%, and not more than 20%, fermentable sugar. Following fermentation by yeast, the sugar content should preferably be below 0.3%. Next, this alcohol-containing substrate is subjected to the action of acetobacter organisms until the alcohol is converted to acetic acid, following which the vinegar is usually clarified, possibly pasteurized, then bottled.

USES OF VINEGAR. In the home, vinegar is used for baking, candies, pickling, production of sour milk, salad dressings, and sweet-and-sour sauces.

Commercially, vinegar is used for mayonnaise, mustard, pickled foods, salad dressings, and tomato products.
(Also see PRESERVATION OF FOODS, Table P-10, Pickling.)

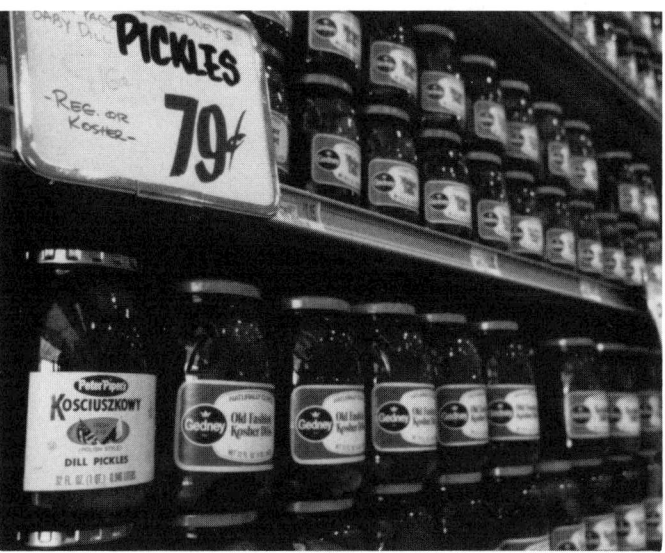

Fig. V-18. Pickles (cucumbers) preserved in vinegar. (Courtesy, University of Minnesota, St. Paul, Minn.)

VIRAL INFECTIONS, FOODBORNE

Infectious hepatitis is the most common foodborne viral disease. The virus is found in excreted stools and blood of infected persons. It may be spread by poorly handled food or seafood taken from sewage contaminated water. In addition to hepatitis, there is some suggestion that the viruses responsible for epidemic diarrhea of the newborn, intestinal flu, and poliomyelitis may be transmitted in contaminated foods.
(Also see DISEASES, section on "Food-Related Infectious and Parasitic Diseases.")

VIRUS

A disease-producing agent that (1) is so small that it cannot be seen through an ordinary microscope (it can be seen by using an electron microscope), (2) is capable of passing through the pores of special filters which retain ordinary bacteria, and (3) propagates only in living tissues.

VISCOSITY

A term which indicates the condition or the property of being thick like syrup or glue. Viscous fluids resist flow or motion.

VISUAL PURPLE (RHODOPSIN)

Photosensitive vitamin A-containing pigment found in the rods of the retina.
(Also see VITAMIN A, section headed "Functions.")

VITAMERS

A substance structurally related to a certain vitamin, which possesses some biological activity—although usually less than the true vitamin, and which may relieve a particular vitamin deficiency.

VITAMIN(S)

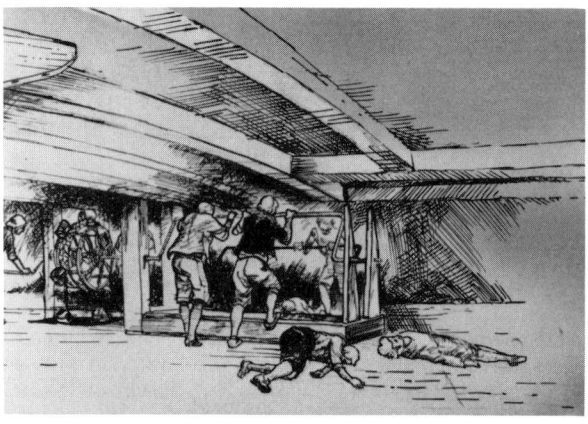

Fig. V-19. This shows an artist's dramatic impression of how British sailors, who ate little except salt meat and biscuits when on long voyages 200 years ago, suddenly collapsed and died of scurvy. (Reproduced with permission of *Nutrition Today*, P.O. Box 1829, Annapolis, MD 21404, ©, 1979)

For proper physiological function, the human body requires some 40 to 50 dietary essentials, of which 14 are vitamins.

Throughout history, vitamin deficiencies have been a major cause of disease, morbidity, and death. Pellagra, scurvy, and beriberi decimated armies, ships' crews, and nations; they even reshaped the course of history. The importance of dietary factors in the genesis of diseases became recognized in the 18th century. But the significance of these observations was not fully understood until early in the 20th century, when scientists found it desirable in many types of investigations to use the biological approach—the use of laboratory animals (largely white, albino rats and mice; guinea pigs; and chicks) fed on purified diets using pure protein such as casein or albumen, pure fat such as lard, and pure carbohydrate such as dextrin, plus minerals to supplement chemical analyses in measuring the value of food. These diets were made up of relatively pure nutrients (proteins, carbohydrates, fats, and minerals) from which the unidentified factors were largely excluded. With these purified diets, all researchers shared a common experience—the animals not only failed to thrive, but they even failed to survive if the investigations were continued for any length of time. At first, many investigators explained such failures on the basis of unpalatability and monotony of diets. Finally, it was realized that these purified diets were lacking in certain factors, minute in amounts, the identities of which were unknown to science. These factors were essential for the efficient utilization of the main ingredients of the food and for the maintenance of health and life itself. The discovery, synthesis, and commercial production of vitamins followed. With these developments, the vitamin era of science was ushered in and the modern approach to nutrition was born.

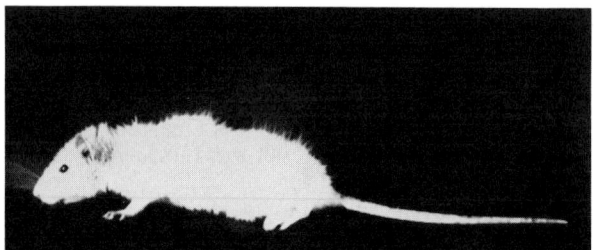

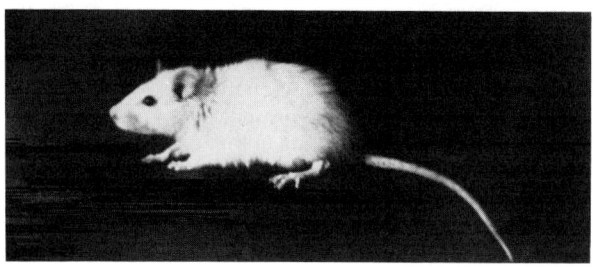

Fig. V-20. The belief that certain factors in very minute amounts are needed by people and animals was difficult to conceive and hold in the early 1900s. Like many episodes of science, it was a mystery story. Yet, finally it was solved by the biological approach—the use of laboratory animals in controlled feeding experiments.

In 1909, Thomas B. Osborne and Lafayette B. Mendel of the Connecticut Agricultural Experiment Station (New Haven), began investigations with purified foodstuffs. (Although different mixtures were used, the basic ingredients of their purified diets were: casein, starch, sugar, and lard.)

The two white rats pictured above were the result of pioneering vitamin studies conducted by Osborne and Mendel during the years 1913 to 1917. *Top*: Rat on a diet deficient in B vitamins; note the rough, scraggly coat, and the emaciation. *Bottom*: The same rat after 12 days on a diet that included B vitamins; note the marked changes in the coat. (Courtesy, The Connecticut Agricultural Experiment Station, New Haven, Conn.)

HISTORY/DISCOVERY OF VITAMINS.
Until the early 1900s, if a diet contained proteins, fats, carbohydrates, minerals, and water, it was considered to be a complete diet. True enough, the disease known as beriberi made its appearance in the rice-eating districts of the Orient when milling machinery was introduced from the West, having been known to the Chinese as early as 2600 B.C.; and scurvy was long known to occur among sailors fed on salt meat and biscuits. However, for centuries these diseases were thought to be due to toxic substances in the digestive tract caused by pathogenic organisms, rather than food deficiencies; and more time elapsed before the discovery of vitamins.

Largely through the trial-and-error method, it was discovered that specific foods were helpful in the treatment of certain of these maladies. Hippocrates (460-377 B.C.), the Greek, known as the father of medicine, advocated liver as a cure for night blindness 400 years before the birth of Christ. At a very early date, the Chinese also used a concoction rich in vitamin A as a remedy for night blindness; and cod-liver oil was used in treating or preventing rickets long before anything was known about the cause of the disease. In 1747, James Lind, a British naval surgeon, in a study involving 12 sailors with scurvy on board the "Salisbury," showed that the juice of citrus fruits was a cure for the disease. Nicholas Lunin, as early as 1881, while a student of von Bunge at the University of Dorpat, had come to the conclusion that certain foods, such as milk, contain, beside the principal ingredients, small quantities of unknown substances essential to life. In 1882, Kanehiro Takaki, Director-General of the Japanese Navy, greatly reduced the number of beriberi cases among naval crews by adding meat and evaporated milk to their diet of rice. In 1897, Christiaan Eijkman, a Dutch medical officer, working in Java, had satisfied himself that the disease beriberi was due to the continued consumption of a diet of polished rice.

In 1912, Dr. Casimir Funk, a 28-year-old Polish biochemist working in London, coined the word *vitamine*. Funk postulated, as others had before him, that beriberi, scurvy, pellagra, and possibly rickets, were caused by a lack in the diet of "special substances which are of the nature of organic bases, which we will call vitamines." Presumably, the name vitamines alluded to the fact that they were vital to life, and that they were chemically of the nature of amines (nitrogen-containing). The name caught the popular fancy and persisted, despite the fact that the chemical assumption was later proved incorrect, with the result that the "e" was dropped in 1920; hence, the word *vitamin*. In 1922, Funk's book entitled *The Vitamins* was published.

A chronological summary of the discovery/isolation and synthesis of the various vitamins is given in Table V-4.

The actual existence of vitamins, therefore, has been known only since 1912, and it was much later before it was possible to see or touch any of them in a pure form. Previously, they were merely mysterious invisible *little things* known only by their effects. In fact, most of the present fundamental knowledge relative to the vitamin content of both human foods and animal feeds was obtained through measuring their potency in promoting growth or in curing certain disease conditions in animals—a most difficult and tedious method. For the most part, small laboratory animals were used, especially rats, guinea pigs, pigeons, and chicks.

Today, there are 14 known vitamins. Additionally, there are at least nine other vitaminlike substances that have been proposed as a result of various experiments, but it is unlikely that all of them are distinct essentials. Yet, the probability that there are still undiscovered vitamins is recognized. Each of the vitamins and vitaminlike substances is alphabetically listed and discussed in a separate section of this book

DEFINITION. *Vitamins are organic substances that are essential in small amounts for the health, growth, reproduction, and maintenance of one or more animal species, which must be included in the diet since they either cannot be synthesized at all or in sufficient quantities in the body.*

Each vitamin performs a specific function; hence, one cannot replace, or act for, another. In general, the human body cannot synthesize them, at least in large enough amounts to meet its needs. However, vitamin D is an exception; when a person is exposed to ultraviolet rays, the vitamin is synthesized from its precursor, which is found in the skin.

TABLE V-4
CHRONOLOGY OF THE
DISCOVERY/ISOLATION AND SYNTHESIS OF VITAMINS

Year	Discovery/Isolation	Synthesis
1849[1]	Choline	
1866–67		Choline
1913	Vitamin A[2]	
1926	Thiamin (B-1)	
1929	Vitamin K[3]	
1931	Vitamin A[2]	
1932	Vitamin C (Ascorbic Acid) Vitamin D₂	
1933	Riboflavin (B-2)	Vitamin C (Ascorbic Acid)
1935		Riboflavin (B-2)
1936	Biotin Vitamin E	Thiamin (B-1)
1937	Niacin (Nicotinic acid)	
1938	Vitamin B-6 (pyridoxine)	Vitamin E
1939	Pantothenic acid (B-3) Vitamin K[3]	Vitamin B-6 (pyridoxine) Vitamin K[3]
1940		Pantothenic acid (B-3)
1943		Biotin
1945	Folacin (Folic acid)	Folacin (Folic acid)
1947		Vitamin A[2]
1948	Vitamin B-12	
1952		Vitamin D₃
1955		Vitamin B-12

[1]In 1844 and 1846, Gobley isolated a substance from egg yolk, which he called lecithin. In 1849, Strecker isolated a compound from hog bile, to which he subsequently (in 1862) applied the name choline.

[2]A more detailed chronology of vitamin A is: in 1913, it was discovered, independently, by McCollum and Davis of the University of Wisconsin, and Osborne and Mendel of the Connecticut Experiment Station; in 1931, its chemical formula was determined by P. Karrer, a Swiss researcher; and, in 1947, it was synthesized by Isler, working in Switzerland.

[3]Vitamin K was discovered in 1929, isolated in 1939, and synthesized in 1939.

NOMENCLATURE AND CLASSIFICATION. There is no universal agreement on the nomenclature of the vitamins. But the modern tendency is to use the chemical name, particularly in describing members of the B complex. In this book, the most common designations are used.

Today, vitamins are generally classed as (1) fat-soluble vs water-soluble vitamins, (2) vitamin B complex, and (3) vitaminlike substances.

Fat-Soluble vs Water-Soluble Vitamins. Many phenomena of vitamin nutrition are related to solubility—vitamins are soluble in either fat or water. Consequently, it is important that both nutritionists and consumers be well informed about solubility differences in vitamins and make use of such differences in programs and practices. Based on solubility, vitamins may be grouped as follows:

The Fat-Soluble Vitamins	The Water-Soluble Vitamins
Vitamin **A**	Biotin
Vitamin **D**	Choline
Vitamin **E**	Folacin (folic acid)
Vitamin **K**	Niacin (nicotinic acid; nicotinamide)
	Pantothenic acid (vitamin B-3)
	Riboflavin (B-2)
	Thiamin (vitamin B-1)
	Vitamin B-6 (pyridoxine; pyridoxal; pyridoxamine)
	Vitamin B-12 (cobalamins)
	Vitamin C (ascorbic acid; dehydroascorbic acid)

It is noteworthy that vitamin C is the only member of the water-soluble group that is not a member of the B family.

The two groups of vitamins exhibit the following several differences that distinguish them both chemically and biologically:

• **Chemical composition**—The fat-soluble vitamins contain only carbon, hydrogen, and oxygen, whereas the water-soluble B vitamins contain these three elements plus nitrogen.

• **Occurrence**—Vitamins originate primarily in plant tissues; with the exceptions of vitamins C and D, they are present in animal tissues only if an animal consumes foods containing them or harbors microorganisms that synthesize them. Fat-soluble vitamins can occur in plant tissue in the form of a provitamin (or precursor of a vitamin), which can be converted into a vitamin in the animal body. But no provitamins are known for any water-soluble vitamin. Also, the B vitamins are universally distributed in all living tissues, whereas the fat-soluble vitamins are completely absent from some.

• **Absorption**—Fat-soluble vitamins are absorbed from the intestinal tract in the presence of fat. It follows that any factor that increases the absorption of fat, such as small particle size or the presence of bile, will also increase the absorption of fat-soluble vitamins. Generally speaking, the absorption of the water-soluble vitamins is a simpler process because there is constant absorption of water from the intestine into the bloodstream.

• **Storage**—The fat-soluble vitamins are stored in appreciable quantities in the body, whereas the water-soluble vitamins are not. Any of the fat-soluble vitamins can be stored wherever fat is deposited; and the greater the intake, the greater the storage. By contrast, the water-soluble B vitamins are not stored in any appreciable amount. Moreover, the large amounts of water which pass through the body daily tend to carry out the water-soluble vitamins, thereby depleting the supply. Hence, they should be supplied in the diet on a daily basis. However, because all living cells contain all the B vitamins, and because the body conserves nutrients that are in short supply by using them only in vital reactions, deficiency symptoms do not appear immediately following their removal from the diet.

• **Excretion**—The fat-soluble vitamins are excreted exclusively in the feces via the bile. The water-soluble vitamins are excreted primarily in the urine, although limited amounts may be present in the feces. This difference in pathway of excretion reflects the difference in solubility.

• **Physiological action**—The fat-soluble vitamins are required for the regulation of the metabolism of structural units, and each vitamin appears to have one or more specific roles. Collectively, the water-soluble B vitamins are primarily concerned with the transfer of energy.

• **Deficiency symptoms**—The absence of one or more vitamins in the diet may lead to failure in growth or reproduction, or to characteristic disorders known as deficiency diseases. In severe cases, death may follow.

The sign of a fat-soluble vitamin deficiency can sometimes be related to the function of the vitamin. For example, vitamin D is required for calcium metabolism and a deficiency results in bone abnormalities. On the other hand, the signs of a B-vitamin deficiency are much less specific

and are difficult to relate to function in most cases. Most B-vitamin deficiencies result in dermatitis, rough hair, and poor growth. Deficiencies of some produce loss of pigment in the hair, whereas deficiencies of others cause anemia. It is noteworthy, too, that not all animals suffer from the same deficiency diseases. Thus, man, the monkey, and the guinea pig get scurvy on diets that provide no vitamin C in the diet, whereas rats, fowl, and ruminants make this vitamin in their bodies and do not need it in their food.

The short supply of a vitamin may be more serious than a short supply of food. However, such vitamin deficiencies are less widespread throughout the world than hunger itself, for starvation has always stalked across much of the world, being referred to as famine only when the numbers dying approach the millions.

• **Toxicity**—Excesses of fat-soluble vitamins A and D can cause serious problems, whereas the water-soluble vitamins are relatively nontoxic.

Vitamin B Complex. With the exception of vitamin C, all of the water-soluble vitamins can be grouped together under the vitamin B complex, of which there are the following nine:

Biotin
Choline
Folacin (folic acid)
Niacin (nicotinic acid; nicotinamide)
Pantothenic acid (vitamin B-3)
Riboflavin (vitamin B-2)
Thiamin (vitamin B-1)
Vitamin B-6 (pyridoxine; pyridoxal; pyridoxamine)
Vitamin B-12 (cobalamins)
(Also see VITAMIN B COMPLEX.)

Vitaminlike Substances. Certain substances, although not considered true vitamins, closely resemble vitamins in their activity, and are sometimes classed with the B-complex vitamins. They're commonly refered to as *vitaminlike substances.* When listed in vitamin preparations, usually the names of these substances are followed by an asterisk, which is tied in with another asterisk at the bottom of the label reading: "Need in human nutrition has not been established."

The nutritional status and biological role(s) of each of the vitaminlike substances require further clarification; indeed, some of them are very controversial. In the meantime, the authors discuss each of them for two primary purposes: (1) historical and informational, and (2) stimulation of research. Additionally, cognizance is taken of the fact that there is usually a considerable time lag between the scientific validation and the acceptance of a vitamin, essential nutrient, and/or medical treatment. A list of the vitaminlike substances follows:

Bioflavonoids
Carnitine (vitamin B-T)
Coenzyme Q (ubiquinone)
Inositol
Laetrile (vitamin B-17), amygdalin, nitrilosides)
Lipoic acid
Pangamic acid (vitamin B-15)
Para-aminobenzoic acid (PABA)
Vitamin B-13 (orotic acid)

Each of these vitaminlike substances is alphabetically listed and discussed in this book.

DETERMINATION OF THE VITAMINS IN FOOD.
The potency, or vitamin content, of foods may be determined by biological, microbiological, chemical, physical methods, and/or human assay.

Biological (Animal) Assay. Before the chemical nature of vitamins was known, their potency could be measured by their ability to promote growth or cure a deficiency when test doses were fed to experimental animals—usually rats, mice, guinea pigs, pigeons, or chicks. Such measurement is known as *biological assay* or *bioassay* and is expressed in terms of units. Vitamins A, D, and E are still measured in international units (IU). (Also, vitamin A values are given in RE [mcg retinol equivalent]; vitamin D is given in micrograms of cholecalciferol; and vitamin E is given in milligrams of alpha-tocopherol equivalents.)

In most common methods of bioassay, laboratory animals are first depleted of the particular vitamin being studied by being fed a diet lacking in it. Then some of the depleted animals are divided into different groups and fed graded doses of the known vitamin, with each group receiving one of the doses in the series. The response of the animals to the intake, in growth and/or other appropriate criteria, is measured and recorded in a standard response curve. Simultaneously, a second set of depleted animals is divided into different groups, with each group fed increasing amounts of the food being assayed; and the responses of each of these groups is recorded. Then, the vitamin potency of the product being tested is estimated by comparing the responses of the second set of animals with the standard response curve of the first group.

Biological assays are laborious, time-consuming, and costly. Large numbers of samples are needed to produce statistically reliable results; the animals should be of approximately the same age, sex, and weight; it takes time to produce nutrient-deficient animals; and quite often the data obtained are highly variable. In addition, data from one species are not always relevant to another species.

The fundamental value of the biological assay is that it gives positive proof of biological activity. It is still the basis of comparison or standardization for newer microbiological or chemical methods.

Microbiological Assay. This assay is a measure of the ability of a vitamin to promote the growth of a microorganism. A microorganism is selected that is known to require the vitamin, or other nutrient, in question. Therefore, if the vitamin is not present, the selected microorganism will not grow. Actually, the procedure is the same as the biological assay; the only difference is that some suitable microorganism is used in place of rats or other animals. Growth media is prepared so that it is nutritionally complete except for the vitamin to be tested. Graded levels of the vitamin are then added to the media and a growth response curve is prepared. Then, the sample to be assayed can be tested and compared to the growth response curve to determine the concentration of the nutrient. The B vitamins may be assayed in this manner.

The microbiological assay requires less time than the biological assay. Its main disadvantage is that the vitamin being tested must first be extracted from the foodstuff before being added to the growth medium used for the microorganism.

Chemical Assay. Today, foods may be analyzed by highly sophisticated chemical procedures, with the vitamin content expressed in units of weight—milligrams (mg) or micrograms (mcg).

Chemical assays are much faster than biological assays, but, at intervals, they must be compared with bioassays in order to rule out the possibility of assaying as a vitamin some substance that does not function as a vitamin in the body.

Physical Assay. Each of the vitamins may now be determined by physical methods—measurement of absorption spectra, chromatography, fluorescence, turbidity, etc.

Human Assay. Actually, this is a special biological type of assay designed for humans. Experiments with people are very costly and difficult to control. Besides, it is necessary to protect the health and rights of the subjects, and to avoid psychic factors in interpreting the results. The use (1) of *placebos* as controls (pills that, unknown to the subject, contain an inactive substance such as sugar), and (2) of double blind tests (in which none of the participants—the subjects, the investigator, the person giving the diets or supplements, and the diagnostician—know the composition of the dietary variables) is standard procedure in human nutrition studies. In such studies, a code may be used for various test groups, the disclosure of which is not revealed until all tests are completed.

FACTORS INFLUENCING THE UTILIZATION OF VITAMINS.
Vitamin deficiency is usually caused by an insufficiency of the nutrient in the diet being consumed. However, the utilization of vitamins may be influenced by availability, antivitamins, provitamins, synthesis in the gut, and interactions of nutrients.

Availability. Not all the vitamins in foods are in absorbable form. For example, (1) niacin in many cereals is bound to a protein and cannot be absorbed through the intestinal wall, unless the food is treated with an alkali to release the vitamin from the inaccessible complex; (2) fat-soluble vitamins may fail to be absorbed if the digestion of fat is impaired; and (3) vitamin B-12 requires a factor produced in the stomach (the intrinsic factor) for its absorption.

Antivitamins (Vitamin Antagonists, or Pseudovitamins). Antivitamins, which are present in some natural foods, are compounds that do not function as vitamins even though they are chemically related to them. As a result, they may cause vitamin deficiencies if the body (1) is unable to distinguish between them and true vitamins, and (2) incorporates them into essential body compounds.

Provitamins. These are nonvitamin substances that occur in foods which can be converted into vitamins in the body. Well-known examples of provitamins are: (1) beta-carotene, which is converted to vitamin A in the intestinal wall; (2) 7-dehydrocholesterol in the skin, which is converted to vitamin D_3 by ultraviolet light (sunlight); (3) ergosterol of plants, which is converted to vitamin D_2 by ultraviolet light; and (4) the amino acid tryptophan, which can be converted to niacin. (Because of the poor efficiency—60 mg of tryptophan is required to produce 1 mg of niacin—tryptophan is not utilized for its provitamin value.)

Synthesis In The Gut. Although some species of bacteria can synthesize vitamins, other species compete with the host for the vitamins ingested in food and retain them until they are excreted in the feces.

In health, the small intestine of man is usually sterile. The large intestine carries a heavy load of bacteria, but usually absorption from the large intestine is limited to water and salts. It is unlikely, therefore, that bacterial synthesis in the gut affects the amounts of most vitamins available to the healthy human body.

When an intestinal disorder is present, especially if there is diarrhea, the small intestine may harbor large numbers of bacteria. These are likely to reduce, rather than increase, the amounts of available vitamins.

Interaction Of Nutrients. Several vitamins are closely linked to other nutrients. For example, (1) if the diet is rich in carbohydrates or alcohol, more thiamin is needed for metabolism; and (2) if the intake of polyunsaturated fats is high, more vitamin E is required. There are several other similar interactions. For this reason, the nutritive value of a diet in respect to a given vitamin may differ from the chemical analysis of its vitamin content. For this reason, too, the diet should supply a well-balanced mixture of all the nutrients, including the vitamins, such as is provided by eating a wide variety of traditional foods—meat, milk, eggs, fruits (including citrus fruits), vegetables (including green leafy vegetables), whole grain cereals and bread, and butter or fortified margarine.

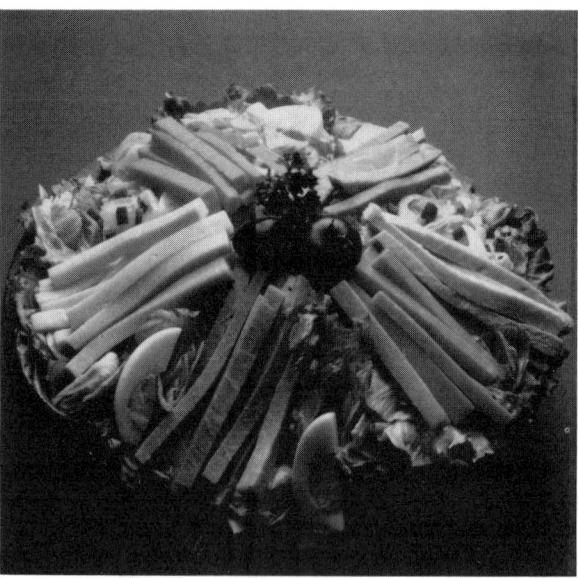

Fig. V-21. Vitamin-rich salad. (Courtesy, California Iceberg Lettuce Commission, Monterey, Calif.)

VITAMIN CONTENT OF FOODS. The vitamin content of foods is given in Food Composition Table F-21. However, in selecting foods to furnish vitamins in the diet, it is well to keep in mind the following:

1. The vitamin losses of vegetables due to storage tend to parallel the degree of wilting. Such losses are progressive in the long storage of fresh vegetables and fruits.

2. The effects of processing and preparation of foods on vitamin retention must be clearly understood. For example, the fat-soluble vitamins (A, D, E, and K) are not easily lost by ordinary cooking methods, and they do not dissolve out in the cooking water. On the other hand, the water-soluble vitamins (B complex and C) are dissolved easily in cooking water, and a portion of the vitamins may be destroyed by heating; therefore, cooking food only until tender and in as little water as possible is, in general, the best procedure.

3. It is important to determine (a) how often any given food will be included in the diet, and (b) the size serving that will normally be eaten.

4. Economic factors such as availability and cost must be considered.

VITAMIN SUPPLEMENTATION OF THE DIET. Ideally, there should be enough of all the vitamins in the natural diet selected on the basis of the Six Food Groups to prevent disease and promote health. When we get our vitamins from such a diet, we usually also obtain the various other nutrients essential to health. Also, when vitamins are consumed in ordinary foods, they are never at a toxic level. The rule, therefore, is: Eat *enough* of *proper* foods *consistently* and chances are you'll get your full complement of needed vitamins. But for many Americans these three words—*enough, proper,* and *consistently*—are the catch. In the first place, lots of folks don't know what constitutes a good diet; and, worse yet, altogether too many people neglect or ignore the rules even if they know them. In either case, the net result is always the same: We shortchange ourselves on the right amounts of good, nutritious food, including vitamins. As a result, more and more doctors and nutritionists are recommending vitamin preparations as supplements. Additional arguments advanced in favor of judicious vitamin supplementation are:

1. **The vitamin content of animal and plant species and parts differ.** The vitamin content of foods varies widely; it's affected by species (for example, pork, is higher in thiamin than beef), and by parts (leaf, stalk, and seed of plants; and organ meats vs muscle meats of animals).

2. **Vitamin losses occur in processing, cooking, and storing.** Unfortunately, many of the vitamins naturally present in foods are destroyed by sunlight, oxidation, mold growth, and heat, to which they are subjected in processing, cooking, and storing. So, by the time they reach the table, much of their vitamin value has disappeared. By contrast, during olden times, for the most part man ate whole or natural foods which were subjected to little processing except for field preparation prior to consumption. Then came the food processing and refinement era, followed by the convenience, fabricated, and fast-food era.

Although it is apparent that raw foods supply adequate amounts of vitamins and other micronutrients, it's unlikely that today's processed, cooked, and stored foods provide adequate amounts of certain vitamins and other trace nutrients, especially for certain critical periods of life, unless they are enriched or supplemented.

One authoritative study revealed the following losses of vitamins from the processing and preservation of foods:[4]

a. The losses in seven vitamins from milling wheat and making flour ranged from 50 to 86.3%. Half of the pantothenic acid, 71.8% of the vitamin B-6, 86.3% of the alpha-tocopherol, and 66% of the folacin were removed.

b. The average losses by food groups in vitamin B-6 and pantothenic acid from canning and freezing were as follows:

Food Group	Frozen		Canned	
	Vitamin B-6	Pantothenic Acid	Vitamin B-6	Pantothenic Acid
	(% loss)	(% loss)	(% loss)	(% loss)
Fish and seafood	17.3	20.8	48.9	19.9
Meat and poultry		70.2	42.6	26.2
Vegetables, roots		36.8	63.1	46.1
Vegetables, legumes	55.6	57.1	77.4	77.8
Vegetables, green	36.7	48.2	57.1	56.4
Fruit and fruit juices	15.4	7.2	37.6	50.5

[4]Schroeder, Henry A., M.D., "Losses of Vitamins and Trace Minerals Resulting From Processing and Preservation of Foods", *The American Journal of Chemical Nutrition*, Vol. 24, May 1971, pp. 562-573.

The appalling processing and preservation losses revealed above underscore the dietary need for whole grains and unprocessed foods of many varieties. They also suggest that the vitamin enrichment and/or supplementation of certain refined and processed foods may be necessary in order to meet the recommended allowances of certain vitamins.

3. **Poor eating habits are commonplace.** Although there is an abundance of good food available, strange as it may seem many folks have fallen into poor eating habits.

But for the millions of Americans with poor eating habits supplemental vitamins are in the nature of *diet insurance* —they're a way of making sure that they are getting enough vitamins each day. That's the reason many of today's doctors and nutritionists recommend vitamin supplementation of the food we eat.

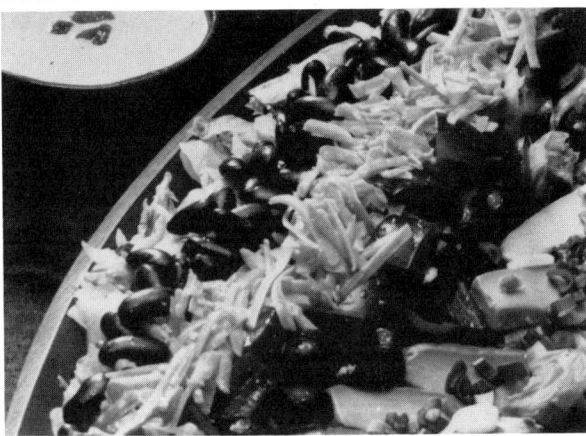

Fig. V-22. People who eat a variety of the proper foods consistently, generally get their full complement of vitamins. (Courtesy, Castle and Cooke, Inc.— Bud of California Fresh Vegetables)

4. **Several vitamins are not stored.** Several of the vitamins cannot be accumulated and stored in the body for any considerable period of time; they are used up quickly and therefore must be constantly replaced or renewed with a continuing supply from the outside.

5. **Fewer calories usually mean fewer vitamins.** With increased mechanization and decreased manual labor, fewer calories are consumed—and with it fewer vitamins.

6. **More vitamins required for growth, pregnancy, and lactation.** Vitamin intakes need to be increased during the critical periods of growth, pregnancy, and lactation. Babies are given supplemental vitamins from the time they are born until they are at least a year old and sometimes longer. Also, vitamin intakes are usually increased during pregnancy and lactation.

7. **Increased vitamins may be needed for therapeutic reasons.** Vitamin supplementation may be needed when a person is unable to consume an adequate diet due to illness, allergies, or emotional upsets. Likewise, vitamin supplementation may be prescribed when a serious dietary deficiency has occurred because of ignorance or poor eating habits; however, such supplementation should never replace the correction of factors leading to the dietary inadequacy. At such times, vitamin supplementation should be taken on the recommendation of physicians to help control particular conditions diagnosed by them.

8. **More vitamins needed during stress.** There are times when vitamin intakes may need to be increased, such as during infections; chronic disease; heavy drinking and/or smoking; regular use of birth control pills; restrictive dieting; environmental stress; and regular use of drugs which interfere with vitamin function. In these situations, professional advice should be sought relative to the given need, and

proper adjustment should be made in the dietary pattern or the diet should be supplemented with a vitamin or a vitamin-mineral preparation.

9. **Lack of vitamins not easily recognizable.** *Too much* or *too little* of some food nutrients may soon show up on the bathroom scale as a pound or two gained or lost. But a lack of a vitamin(s) isn't so immediately recognizable.

Initially, it was thought that each vitamin was primarily a protective substance, which prevented a specific disease. While it is true that a specific disease can result from lack of a specific vitamin, specific deficiencies of a single vitamin are comparatively rare today. Instead, it is recognized that vitamins are interdependent of each other and on other nutrients for buoyant good health; hence, people are likely to have a deficiency of a group of vitamins, some consequences of which may be: a tired, run-down feeling; not quite up to par; insomnia; easily irritated; or lowered resistance to minor infection. Such signs and illnesses do not necessarily indicate vitamin deficiency, but, of course, the physician should be consulted. Also, everyone should understand the essential role of vitamins in maintaining health.

10. **Vitamin needs vary with individuals.** Vitamin needs vary according to age, kind of work, and general physical condition. Moreover, different individuals have different needs for different vitamins.

11. **We can learn from animals.** Much of the research on vitamins has been done with laboratory animals—rats, mice, guinea pigs, chicks, monkeys, dogs, etc. This makes sense when one realizes that many generations of white mice, for example, can be studied over a period of a few months or years, whereas if such clinical research were limited to humans, it would take 50 years or longer to make comparable tests with successive generations. Therefore, many conclusions concerning the role of vitamins in nutrition have been reached through basic research with animals.

So, today, more and more physicians and nutritionists rely on vitamin supplements, which in many cases are chemically pure sources that need to be taken only in very minute amounts, and which cost only a small fraction of the total food bill. Also, informed physicians and nutritionists no longer prescribe vitamins merely to prevent deficiency symptoms, or to meet minimum requirements, but, rather, to impart buoyant good health.

Undoubtedly, the use of vitamin supplements far exceeds the need for them in many cases. The potency of preparations on the market varies widely, and the number of nutrients present differs from one product to another. Moreover, the consumer may be unable to interpret the label information in terms of his/her own requirements.

Although water-soluble vitamins in excess of body needs will be excreted in the urine—with no harm done, except to the pocketbook, excessive intakes of vitamins A and D may be toxic. So, large amounts of vitamins should be taken under the direction of a physician or nutritionist.

VITAMIN TABLE. Table V-5 is a summary of each of the 14 known vitamins and of the 9 vitaminlike substances, totaling 23. Note that the 23 factors are divided into 3 appropriate groups—(1) fat-soluble vitamins, (2) water-soluble vitamins, and (3) vitaminlike substances—with the members within each group listed alphabetically. Note, too, that information relative to each of the 23 substances is given under the following headings: functions; deficiency and toxicity symptoms; recommended daily allowances; sources; and comments.

Additionally, a separate and more complete presentation relative to each vitamin and vitaminlike substance appears alphabetically in the book under its respective name.

TABLE V-5
VITAMIN TABLE

Functions	Deficiency and Toxicity Symptoms	Recommended Daily Allowance				Sources	Comments
		Age Group	Years	Vitamin			

FAT-SOLUBLE VITAMINS:
Vitamin A

Helps maintain normal vision in dim light—prevents night blindness.

Prevents xerophthalmia, an eye condition which may lead to blindness in extreme vitamin A deficiency.

Essential for body growth.

Necessary for normal bone growth.

Necessary for normal tooth development.

Helps keep the epithelial tissues of the skin, and of the lining of the nose, throat, respiratory and digestive systems, and genitourinary tract, healthy and free of infection.

May help prevent miscarriage of women during the first three months of pregnancy.

New information suggests that vitamin A (1) acts in a coenzyme role, as for instance in the form of intermediates in glycoprotein synthesis; and (2) functions like steroid hormones, with a role in the cell nuclei, leading to tissue differentiation.

Other functions of vitamin A: necessary for (1) thyroxine formation and prevention of goiter; (2) protein synthesis; and (3) synthesis of corticosterone from cholesterol, and the normal synthesis of glycogen.
(Also see VITAMIN A.)

Deficiency symptoms—Night blindness (nyctalopia), xerosis, and xerophthalmia.

Stunted growth of children.

Slowed bone growth, abnormal bone shape, and paralysis.

Unsound teeth, characterized by abnormal enamel, pits, and decay.

Rough, dry, scaly skin—a condition known as follicular hyperkeratosis (it looks like "gooseflesh"); increased sinus, sore throat, and abscesses in ears, mouth, or salivary glands; increased diarrhea and kidney and bladder stones.

Reproductive disorders, including poor conception, abnormal embryonic growth, placental injury, and death of the fetus.

Toxicity—Toxicity of vitamin A is characterized by loss of appetite, headache, blurred vision, excessive irritability, loss of hair, dryness and flaking of the skin (with itching), swelling over the long bones, drowsiness, diarrhea, nausea, and enlargement of the liver and spleen.

Vitamin A[1]

Age Group	Years	(mcg RE)	(IU)
Infants	0.0–0.5	375	1,250
	0.5–1.0	375	1,250
Children	1–3	400	1,333
	4–6	500	1,667
	7–10	700	2,333
Males	11–14	1,000	3,333
	15–18	1,000	3,333
	19–24	1,000	3,333
	25–50	1,000	3,333
	51+	1,000	3,333
Females	11–14	800	2,667
	15–18	800	2,667
	19–24	800	2,667
	25–50	800	2,667
	51+	800	2,667
Pregnant		800	2,667
Lactating		1,200	4,000

[1]*Recommended Dietary Allowances*, 10th ed., NRC–National Academy of Sciences, 1989, p. 285.

The recommended daily allowances (RDA) are given in both International Units (IU) and Retinol Equivalents (RE). An International Unit (IU) of Vitamin A is defined on the basis of rat studies as equal to 0.344 mcg of crystalline retinylacetate (which is equivalent to 0.3 mcg of retinol, or to 0.6 mcg of beta-carotene). These standards are based on experiments which show that in rats only about 50% of the beta-carotene is converted to vitamin A.

Rich sources—Liver and carrots.
Good sources—Dark-green leafy vegetables; beet greens, collards, dandelion greens, kale, mustard greens, spinach, Swiss chard, turnip greens. Yellow vegetables: pumpkins, sweet potatoes, squash (winter). Yellow fruits: apricots, peaches. Some seafoods: crab, halibut, oysters, salmon, swordfish, whale meat.
Fair sources—Butter (regular salted), cantaloupe, cheese, cream, egg yolk, lettuce, margarine (fortified), tomatoes, whole milk.
Negligible sources—Breads and cereals (except yellow corn), chicken, cottage cheese (not creamed), dry beans, muscle meats, potatoes, skim milk.
Supplemental sources—Synthetic vitamin A, cod and other fish liver oils.
For additional sources and more precise values of vitamin A, see Food Composition Table F-21.

The forms of vitamin A are: alcohol (retinol), ester (retinyl palmitate), aldehyde (retinal or retinene), and acid (retinoic acid).

Retinol, retinyl palmitate, and retinal are readily converted from one form to another, but retinoic acid cannot be converted to other forms. Retinoic acid fulfills some of the functions of vitamin A, but it does not function in the visual cycle.

Vitamin D

Increases calcium absorption from the small intestine.

Promotes growth and mineralization of the bones.

Promotes sound teeth.

Increases absorption of phosphorus through the intestinal wall, and increases resorption of phosphates from the kidney tubules.

Maintains normal level of citrate in the blood.

Protects against the loss of amino acids through the kidneys.
(Also see VITAMIN D.)

Deficiency symptoms—Rickets in infants and children, characterized by enlarged joints, bowed legs, knocked knees, outward projection of the sternum (pigeon breast), a row of beadlike projections on each side of the chest at the juncture of the rib bones and joining (costal) cartilage (called rachitic rosary), bulging forehead, pot belly, and delayed eruption of temporary teeth and unsound permanent teeth.

Osteomalacia in adults, in which the bones soften, become distorted, and fracture easily.

Tetany, characterized by muscle twitching, convulsions, and low serum calcium.

Toxicity—Excessive vitamin D may cause hypercalcemia (increased intestinal absorption, leading to elevated blood calcium levels), characterized by loss of appetite, excessive thirst, nausea, vomiting, irritability, weakness, constipation alternating with bouts of diarrhea, retarded growth in infants and children, and weight loss in adults.

Vitamin D[1]

Age Group	Years	(mcg)	(IU)
Infants	0.0–0.5	7.5	300
	0.5–1.0	10	400
Children	1–3	10	400
	4–6	10	400
	7–10	10	400
Males	11–14	10	400
	15–18	10	400
	19–24	10	400
	25–50	5	200
	51+	5	200
Females	11–14	10	400
	15–18	10	400
	19–24	10	400
	25–50	5	200
	51+	5	200
Pregnant		10	400
Lactating		10	400

[1]*Recommended Dietary Allowances*, 10th ed., NRC–National Academy of Sciences, 1989, p. 285.
400 IU of vitamin D = 10 mcg cholecalciferol.

Vitamin D is more sparse in foods than any other vitamin.
Rich sources—Fatty fish (bloater, herring, kipper, mackerel, pilchard, salmon, sardines, tuna) and fish roe.
Fair sources—Liver, egg yolk, cream, butter, cheese.
Negligible sources—Muscle meats, milk (unfortified), fruits, nuts, vegetables, grains.
D-fortified foods—Milk (400 IU/qt) and infant formulas. Other foods to which vitamin D is often added include: breakfast and infant cereals, breads, margarines, milk flavorings, fruit and chocolate beverages, and cocoa.
Supplemental sources—Fish liver oils (from cod, halibut, or swordfish); irradiated ergosterol or 7-dehydrocholesterol such as viosterol.
Exposure to sunlight or sunlamp—Manufacture in the skin.
For additional sources and more precise values of vitamin D, see Food Composition Table F-21.

Vitamin D includes both—D_2 (ergocalciferol, calciferol, or viosterol) and D_3 (cholecalciferol).

Vitamin D is unique among vitamins in three respects: (1) it occurs naturally in only a few common foods (mainly in fish oils and a little in eggs and milk), (2) it can be formed in the body and in certain foods by exposure to ultraviolet rays, and (3) the active compound of vitamin D (1, 25-[OH]$_2$-D$_3$) functions as a hormone.

Vitamin E (Tocopherols)

As an antioxidant which (a) retards rancidification of fats in plant sources and in the digestive tracts of animals, and (b) protects body cells from toxic substances formed from the oxidation of unsaturated

Deficiency symptoms—Innumerable vitamin E deficiency symptoms have been demonstrated in animals; and they are highly variable from species to species. But vitamin E deficiency symptoms as such rarely

Vitamin E[1]

Age Group	Years	(mg αTE)	(IU)
Infants	0.0–0.5	3	4.47
	0.5–1.0	4	5.96
Children	1–3	6	8.94
	4–6	7	10.43
	7–10	7	10.43

Rich sources—Salad and cooking oils (except coconut oil), alfalfa seeds, margarine, nuts (almonds, Brazil nuts, filberts, peanuts, pecans), sunflower seed kernels.
Good sources—Asparagus, avo-

There are 8 tocopherols and tocotrienols, of which alphatocopherol has the greatest vitamin E activity.

(Continued)

TABLE V-5 *(Continued)*

Functions	Deficiency and Toxicity Symptoms	Recommended Daily Allowance			Sources	Comments
		Age Group	Years	Vitamin		

Vitamin E *(Continued)*

fatty acids. As a powerful antioxidant, vitamin E readily oxidizes itself (it combines with oxygen), thereby minimizing the destruction by oxidation of unsaturated fatty acids and vitamin A in the intestinal tract and in the tissues.

As an essential factor for the integrity of red blood cells.

As an agent essential to cellular respiration, primarily in heart and skeletal muscle tissues.

As a regulator in the synthesis of DNA, vitamin C, and coenzyme Q.

As a protector of lung tissue from air pollution (smog).

As a sometimes replacement for selenium.

(Also see VITAMIN E.)

Deficiency — occur in humans.

Newborn infants (especially the premature), suffering from a deficiency of vitamin E (caused by shortened life span of red blood cells), characterized by edema, skin lesions, and blood abnormalities.

Patients unable to absorb fat (like those suffering from sprue or from fibrocystic disease of the pancreas) have low blood and tissue tocopherol levels, increased red blood fragility and shortened red blood cell life span, and increased urinary excretion of creatine.

Toxicity — Vitamin E is relatively nontoxic. Some persons consuming daily doses of more than 300 IU of vitamin E have complained of nausea and intestinal distress. Excess intake of vitamin E appears to be excreted in the feces.

Age Group	Years	Vitamin	
Males	11–14	10	14.90
	15–18	10	14.90
	19–24	10	14.90
	25–50	10	14.90
	51+	10	14.90
Females	11–14	8	11.92
	15–18	8	11.92
	19–24	8	11.92
	25–50	8	11.92
	51+	8	11.92
Pregnant		10	14.90
Lactating		12	16.39

[1]*Recommended Dietary Allowances*, 10th ed., NRC–National Academy of Sciences, 1989, p. 285.

The recommended daily allowances (RDA) are given in both International Units (IU) and alpha-tocopherol equivalents. 1 mg d-tocopherol = 1 alpha-TE. See section on Vitamin E. (tocopherols) for variation in allowances and calculation of vitamin E activity of the diet as alpha-tocopherol equivalents.

Sources: cados, beef and organ meats, blackberries, butter, eggs, green-leafy vegetables, oatmeal, potato chips, rye, seafoods (lobster, salmon, shrimp, tuna), tomatoes.

Fair sources — Apples, beans, carrots, celery, cheese, chicken, liver, peas.

Negligible sources — Most fruits, sugar, white bread.

Supplemental sources — Synthetic dl-alphatocopherol acetate, wheat germ, wheat germ oil. Most of the commercial vitamin E is synthetic dl-alphatocopherol acetate. It is the least expensive source of the vitamin, but, unlike natural food sources, it provides no other essential nutrient.

For additional sources and more precise values of vitamin E (alphatocopherol), see Food Composition Table F-21.

Vitamin K

Vitamin K controls blood coagulation; recent research suggests that it acts in some way to convert precursor proteins to the active blood clotting factors.

Vitamin K is essential for the synthesis in the liver of four blood clotting proteins:
1. Factor II, prothrombin.
2. Factor VII, proconvertin.
3. Factor IX, Christmas factor.
4. Factor X, Stuart-Power.
(Also see VITAMIN K.)

Deficiency symptoms —
1. Delayed blood clotting.
2. Hemorrhagic disease of newborn.

Vitamin K deficiency symptoms are likely in —
1. Newborn infants, especially if premature and breast-fed.
2. Infants born to mothers receiving anticoagulants.
3. Obstructive jaundice (lack of bile).
4. Fat absorption defects (celiac disease, sprue).
5. Anticoagulant therapy or toxicity.

Toxicity — The natural forms of vitamin K_1 and K_2 have not produced toxicity even when given in large amounts. However, synthetic menadione and its various derivatives have produced some toxic symptoms in rats and jaundice in human infants when given in amounts of more than 5 mg daily.

Age Group	Years	Vitamin K[1] (mcg)
Infants	0.0–0.5	5
	0.5–1.0	10
Children	1–3	15
	4–6	20
	7–10	30
Males	11–14	45
	15–18	65
	19–24	70
	25–50	80
	51+	80
Females	11–14	45
	15–18	55
	19–24	60
	25–50	65
	51+	65
Pregnant		65
Lactating		65

[1]Estimated Safe and Adequate Daily Intake from *Recommended Dietary Allowances* 10th ed., NRC-NAS, 1989, p. 285

Vitamin K is fairly widely distributed in foods and is available synthetically.

Rich sources — Tea (green), turnip greens, broccoli, lettuce, cabbage, beef liver, spinach.

Good sources — Asparagus, watercress, bacon, coffee, cheese, butter, pork, liver, oats.

Fair sources — Peas (green), wheat (whole), beef fat, ham, beans (green), eggs, pork tenderloin, peaches, ground beef, chicken, liver, raisins.

Negligible sources — Applesauce, bananas, bread, cola, corn, corn oil, milk (cow's), oranges, potatoes, pumpkin, tomatoes, wheat flour.

Supplemental sources — Chiefly synthetic menadione.

The vitamin K values of some common foods is given in Table V-7.

There are 2 naturally occurring forms of vitamin K: K_1 (phylloquinone, or phytylmenaquinone), and K_2 (menaquinones), multiprenyl-menaquinones. Vitamin K_1 occurs only in green plants. Vitamin K_2 is synthesized by many microorganisms, including bacteria in the intestinal tracts of human beings and other species.

There are several synthetic compounds, the best known of which is menadione, formerly known as K_3.

The intake for young infants is based on 1 mcg/kg, assuming no intestinal synthesis. Thus, the amount provided by current formulas of 4 mcg/100 kcal should be ample for normal infants. The suggested intake of 10 mcg/day is also in the range supplied by breast milk (15 mg/liter).

WATER-SOLUBLE VITAMINS:

Biotin

Biotin is required for many reactions in the metabolism of carbohydrates, fats, and proteins. It functions as a coenzyme mainly in decarboxylation-carboxylation and in deamination.

Biotin serves as a coenzyme for transferring CO_2 from one compound to another (for decarboxylation—the removal of carbon dioxide; and for carboxylation—the addition of carbon dioxide).

Numerous decarboxylation and carboxylation reactions are involved in carbohydrate, fat, and protein metabolism; among them, the following:

Deficiency symptoms — The deficiency symptoms in man include: a dry scaly dermatitis, loss of appetite, nausea, vomiting, muscle pains, glossitis (inflammation of the tongue), pallor of skin, mental depression, a decrease in hemoglobin and red blood cells, a high cholesterol level, and a low excretion of biotin; all of which respond to biotin administration.

There is now substantial evidence that seborrheic dermatitis (an abnormally oily skin, which results in chronic scaly inflammation) of infants under 6 months of age is due to nutritional biotin deficiency.

Toxicity — There are no known toxic effects.

Age Group	Years	Biotin[1] (mcg)
Infants	0.0–0.5	10
	0.5–1.0	15
Children and adolescents	1–3	20
	4–6	25
	7–10	30
	11+	30–100
Adults		30–100

[1]**NOTE WELL:** the biotin values are "Estimated Safe and Adequate Daily Intakes," and *not* RDA; from *Recommended Dietary Allowances*, 10th ed., NRC–National Academy of Sciences, 1989, p. 284.

Rich sources — Cheese (processed), kidney, liver, soybean flour.

Good sources — Cauliflower, chocolate, eggs, mushrooms, nuts, peanut butter, sardines and salmon, wheat bran.

Fair sources — Cheese (natural), chicken, oysters, pork, spinach, sweet corn, whole wheat flour.

Negligible sources — Refined cereal products; most fruits and root crops.

Supplemental sources — Synthetic biotin, yeast (brewers', torula), alfalfa leaf meal (dehydrated).

Considerable biotin is synthesized by the microorganisms in the intestinal tract, and much of it is absorbed, as evidenced by the fact that 3 to 6 times more biotin is excreted in the urine and feces than is ingested. For additional sources and more precise values of biotin, see Food Composition Table F-21.

Biotin is closely related metabolically to folacin, pantothenic acid, and vitamin B-12.

It is noteworthy that the amount of avidin in raw egg white exceeds the amount of biotin in the whole egg. But, since avidin is destroyed by cooking, the usual diet includes little of the biotin-interfering substance.

TABLE V-5 *(Continued)*

Functions	Deficiency and Toxicity Symptoms	Recommended Daily Allowance			Sources	Comments
		Age Group	Years	Vitamin		

Biotin *(Continued)*

1. Interconversion of pyruvate and oxaloacetate. The formation of oxaloacetate is important because it is the starting point of of the tricarboxylic acid cycle (TCA), known as the Krebs cycle, in which the potential energy of nutrients (ATP) is released for use by the body.
2. Interconversion of succinate and propionate.
3. Conversion of malate to pyruvate.
4. Conversion of acetyl CoA to malonyl CoA, the first step in the formation of long chain fatty acids.
5. Formation of purines, essential part of DNA and RNA, and for protein synthesis.
6. Conversion of ornithine to citrulline, an important reaction in the formation of urea.

Biotin also serves as a coenzyme for deamination (removal of -NH_2) reactions that are necessary for the production of energy from certain amino acids (at least aspartic acid, serine, threonine); for amino acids to be used as a source of energy, they must first be deaminated—the amino group must split off.
(Also see BIOTIN.)

Choline

Choline has several important functions; it is vital for the prevention of fatty livers, the transmitting of nerve impulses, and the metabolism of fat.

1. It prevents fatty livers through the transport and metabolism of fats. Without choline, fatty deposits build up inside the liver, blocking its function and throwing the whole body into a state of ill health.

2. It is needed for nerve transmission. Choline combines with acetate to form acetylcholine, a substance which is needed to jump the gap between nerve cells so that impulses can be transmitted.

3. By a phenomenon known as transmethylation, it serves as a source of labile methyl groups, which facilitate metabolism.
(Also see CHOLINE.)

Deficiency symptoms—Poor growth and fatty livers are the deficiency symptoms in most species except chickens and turkeys. Chickens and turkeys develop slipped tendons (perosis). In young rats, choline deficiency produces hemorrhagic lesions in the kidneys and other organs.

Toxicity—No toxic effects have been observed.

The Food and Nutrition Board of the National Research Council does not recommend any human allowance for choline because of lack of evidence of need.

The Committee of the American Academy of Pediatrics recommends that choline be added to infant formulas in amounts equivalent to breast milk. Human milk contains about 145 mg of choline per liter, nearly 0.1% of total solids. It is estimated that the average mixed diet for adults in the U.S. contains 400 to 900 mg per day of choline and betaine, or about 0.1 to 0.18% of the diet.

Rich sources—Egg yolk, eggs, liver (beef, pork, lamb).

Good sources—Soybeans, potatoes (dehydrated), cabbage, wheat bran, navy beans, alfalfa leaf meal, dried buttermilk and dried skimmed milk, rice polish, rice bran, whole grains (barley, corn, oats, rice, sorghum, wheat), hominy, turnips, wheat flour, blackstrap molasses.

Negligible sources—Fruit, fruit juices, milk, vegetables.

Supplemental sources—Yeast (brewers', torula), wheat germ, soybean lecithin, egg yolk lecithin, and synthetic choline and choline derivatives.

Also, the body manufactures choline from methionine, with the aid of B-12. So, the needs for choline are supplied in two ways: (1) by dietary choline, and/or (2) by body synthesis through transmethylation.

It is noteworthy that choline has been known for a very long time. It was isolated in 1849, named in 1862, and synthesized in 1866-67. But the compound did not attract the attention of nutrition investigators at the time.

The classification of choline as a vitamin is debated because it does not meet all the criteria for vitamins, especially those of the B vitamins.

Folacin (Folic Acid)

In the body, folic acid is changed to at least five active enzyme forms, the parent form of which is tetrahydrofolic acid. Folacin coenzymes are responsible for the following important functions:

1. The formation of purines and pyrimidines which, in turn, are needed for the synthesis of the nucleic acids DNA and RNA, vital to all cell nuclei. This explains the important role of folacin in cell division and reproduction.

2. The formation of heme, the iron-containing protein in hemoglobin.

3. The interconversion of the three-carbon amino acid serine from the two-carbon amino acid glycine.

4. The formation of amino acids tyrosine from phenylalanine and glutamic acid from histidine.

5. The formation of amino acid methionine from homocysteine.

6. The synthesis of choline from ethanolamine.

7. The conversion of nicotinamide to N-methylnicotinamide, one of the metabolites of niacin that is excreted in the urine.
(Also see FOLACIN.)

Deficiency symptoms—Megaloblastic anemia (of infancy), also called macrocytic anemia (of pregnancy), in which the red blood cells are larger and fewer than normal, and also immature. The anemia is due to inadequate formation of nucleoproteins, causing failure of the megaloblasts (young red blood cells) in the bone marrow to mature. The hemoglobin level is low because of the reduced number of red blood cells. Also, the white blood cell, blood platelet, and serum folate levels are low.

Other symptoms include a sore, red, smooth tongue (glossitis), disturbances of the digestive tract (diarrhea), and poor growth.

Toxicity—Normally, no toxicity.

Age Group	Years	Folate[1] (mcg)
Infants	0.0–0.5	25
	0.5–1.0	35
Children	1–3	50
	4–6	75
	7–10	100
Males	11–14	150
	15–18	200
	19–24	200
	25–50	200
	51+	200
Females	11–14	150
	15–18	180
	19–24	180
	25–50	180
	51+	180
Pregnant		400
Lactating		280

[1]*Recommended Dietary Allowances*, 10th ed., NRC–National Academy of Sciences, 1989, p. 285.
The RDA are expressed in terms of "total" folacin; that is, the amount of folic acid activity available from all food folates.

Rich sources—Liver and kidney.

Good sources—Avocados, beans, beets, celery, chickpeas, eggs, fish, green leafy vegetables (such as asparagus, broccoli, Brussels sprouts, cabbage, cauliflower, endive, lettuce, parsley, spinach, turnip greens), nuts, oranges, orange juice, soybeans, and whole wheat products.

Fair sources—Bananas, brown rice, carrots, cheese (Cheddar), cod, halibut, rice, and sweet potatoes.

Poor sources—Chicken, dried milk, milk, most fruits, muscle meats (beef, pork, lamb), products made from highly refined cereals (including white flour), and most root vegetables (including Irish potatoes).

No folacin—Fats and oils, and sugar supply no folacin.

Supplemental sources—Yeast, wheat germ, and commercially synthesized folic acid (pteroylglutamic acid, or PGA).

Intestinal bacterial synthesis of folacin may be important in man, but the amount produced has not been determined.

For additional sources and more precise values of folacin (folic acid), see Food Composition Table F-21.

There is no single vitamin compound with the name *folacin*; rather, the term folacin is used to designate folic acid and a group of closely related substances which are essential for all vertebrates, including man.

Ascorbic acid, vitamin B-12, and vitamin B-6 are essential for the activity of the folacin coenzymes in many of their metabolic processes; again and again pointing up to interdependence of various vitamins.

Folacin deficiencies are thought to be a health problem in the U.S. and throughout the world. Infants, adolescents, and pregnant women are particularly vulnerable.

The folacin requirement is increased by tropical sprue, certain genetic disturbances, cancer, parasitic infection, alcoholism, and oral contraceptives.

Raw vegetables stored at room temperature for 2 to 3 days lose as much as 50 to 70% of their folate content.

Between 50 and 95% of food folate is destroyed in cooking.

(Continued)

TABLE V-5 *(Continued)*

Functions	Deficiency and Toxicity Symptoms	Recommended Daily Allowance					Sources	Comments
		Age Group	Years	Calories	Protein	Niacin[1]		
				(kcal)	(g)	(mg NE)		

Niacin (Nicotinic acid; nicotin-amide)

The principal role of niacin is as a constituent of two important coenzymes in the body: nicotina-mide adenine dinucleotide (NAD) and nicotinamide adenine dinu-cleotide phosphate (NADP). These coenzymes function in many important enzyme systems that are necessary for cell respiration. They are involved in the release of energy from carbohydrates, fats, and protein.

NAD and NADP are also involved in the synthesis of fatty acids, protein, and DNA.

Also, niacin is thought to (1) have a specific effect on growth, (2) reduce the levels of cholesterol, and (3) protect to some degree against nonfatal myocardial infarction. However, because of possible undesirable side effects, massive doses should be under the direction of a physician.

(Also see NIACIN.)

Deficiency symptoms—A deficiency of niacin results in pellagra, the symptoms of which are: dermatitis, particularly of areas of the skin which are ex-posed to light or injury; inflam-mation of mucous membranes, including the entire gastrointes-tinal tract, which results in a red, swollen, sore tongue and mouth, diarrhea, and rectal irritation; and psychic changes, such as irritability, anxiety, depression, and in advanced cases, delirium, hallucinations, confusion, disorientation, and stupor.

Toxicity—Only large doses of niacin, sometimes given to an individual with mental illness, are known to be toxic. However, ingestion of large amounts may result in vascular dilation, and *flushing* of the skin, itching, liver damage, elevated blood glucose, elevated blood enzymes, and/or peptic ulcer.

Age Group	Years	Calories (kcal)	Protein (g)	Niacin[1] (mg NE)
Infants	0–.5	650	13	5
	.5–1	850	14	6
Children	1–3	1,300	16	9
	4–6	1,800	24	12
	7–10	2,000	28	13
Males	11–14	2,500	45	17
	15–18	3,000	59	20
	19–24	2,900	58	19
	25–50	2,900	63	19
	51+	2,300	63	15
Females	11–14	2,200	46	15
	15–18	2,200	44	15
	19–24	2,200	46	15
	25–50	2,200	50	15
	51+	1,900	50	13
Pregnant		+300	60	17
Lactating		+500	65	20

[1]*Recommended Dietary Allowances*, 10th ed., NRC–National Academy of Sciences, 1989, p. 285. Calorie values from p. 33, Table 3–5 of the same report.
On the average, 1 mg of niacin is derived from each 60 mg of dietary tryptophan.

Sources:

Generally speaking, niacin is found in animal tissues as nico-tinamide and in plant tissues as nicotinic acid. Both forms are of equal niacin activity.

Rich sources—The best food sources of niacin are liver, kid-ney, lean meats, poultry, fish, rabbit, corn flakes (enriched), nuts, peanut butter.

Good sources—Milk, cheese, and eggs, although low in niacin content, are good anti-pellagra foods, because of their high tryptophan content, and because their niacin is in avail-able form. Other good sources are: bran flakes, sesame seed, sunflower seed.

Also, enriched cereal flours and products are good sources of niacin.

Negligible sources—Cereals (corn, wheat, oats, rice, rye) tend to be low in niacin. Moreover, 80 to 90% of the niacin is in the bran layer (outer seed coat) and removed in milling; and the niacin may be present in bound form (i.e. niacytin) and unavailable.

Fruits, roots, vegetables (other than mushrooms and legumes), butter, and sugar (white) are insignificant sources of niacin.

Supplemental sources—Both synthetic nicotinamide and nicotinic acid are com-mercially available. For pharmaceutical use, nicotinamide is usually used; for food nutrification, nicotinic acid is usually used. Also, yeast is a rich natural source of niacin.

For additional sources and more precise values of niacin, see Food Composition Table F-21.

Comments:

Although nicotinic acid was prepared and named in 1867, it took another 70 years before it was known that it would cure blacktongue in dogs and pellagra in humans.

An average mixed diet in the U.S. provides about 1% protein as tryptophan. Thus, a diet sup-plying 60 g of protein contains about 600 mg of tryptophan, which will yield about 10 mg of niacin (on the average, 1 mg of niacin is derived from each 60 mg of dietary tryptophan).

Niacin is the most stable of the B-complex vitamins. Cooking losses of a mixed diet usually do not amount to more than 15 to 25%.

Born of centuries of experience, (1) in Mexico, corn has long been treated with lime water before making tortillas; and (2) the Hopi Indians of Arizona have long roasted sweet corn in hot ashes. Both practices liberate the nico-tinic acid in corn.

Functions	Deficiency and Toxicity Symptoms	Recommended Daily Allowance			Sources	Comments
		Age Group	Years	Vitamin		
				Pantothenic Acid[1] (mg)		

Pantothenic Acid (Vitamin B-3)

Pantothenic acid functions in the body as part of two enzymes—coenzyme A (CoA) and acyl carrier protein (ACP).

CoA functions in the following important reactions:

1. The metabolic processes by which carbohydrates, fats, and proteins are broken down and energy is released.

2. The formation of acetyl-choline, a substance of importance in transmitting nerve impulses.

3. The synthesis of porphyrin, a precursor of heme, of importance in hemoglobin synthesis.

4. The synthesis of cholesterol and other sterols.

5. The steroid hormones formed by the adrenal and sex glands.

6. The maintenance of normal blood sugar, and the formation of antibodies.

7. The excretion of sulfonamide drugs.

ACP, along with CoA, required by the cells in the biosynthesis (the building up) of fatty acids. (CoA, without ACP, is involved in the breakdown of fatty acids.)

(Also see PANTOTHENIC ACID.)

Deficiency symptoms—Panto-thenic acid deficiency has been pro-duced in human volunteers by either (1) feeding semi-synthetic diets low in pantothenic acid, or (2) adding a pan-tothenic antagonist to the diet. The symptoms are: irritableness and restless-ness; loss of appetite, indigestion, abdominal pains, nausea; headache; sullenness; mental depression; fatigue, weakness; numbness and tingling of hands and feet, muscle cramps in the arms and legs; burning sensation in the feet; insomnia; respiratory infections; rapid pulse; and a staggering gait. Also, in these subjects there was increased reaction to stress; increased sensitivity to insulin, resulting in low blood sugar levels; increased sedimentation rate for erythro-cytes; decreased gastric secretions; and marked decrease in antibody production.

Toxicity—Pantothenic acid is relatively nontoxic. However, doses of 10 to 20 g per day may result in occasional diarrhea and water retention.

Age Group	Years	Pantothenic Acid[1] (mg)
Infants	.0-0.5	2
	.5-1.0	3
Children and Adolescents	1-3	3
	4-6	3-4
	7-10	4-5
	11+	4-7
Adults		4-7

[1]**NOTE WELL:** The pantothenic acid values are "Estimated Safe and Adequate Daily Intakes," and *not* RDA; from *Recommended Dietary Allowances*, 10th ed., NRC–National Academy of Sciences, 1989, p. 284.

Sources:

Rich sources—Organ meat (liver, kidney, and heart), cottonseed flour, wheat bran, rice bran, rice polish.

Good sources—Nuts, mush-rooms, soybean flour, salmon, blue cheese, eggs, buckwheat flour, brown rice, lobster, sunflower seeds.

Fair sources—Chicken, broccoli, sweet peppers, whole wheat flour, avocados.

Negligible sources—Butter, corn flakes, white flour, fats and oils, margarine, precooked rice, sugar.

Supplemental sources—Syn-thetic calcium pantothenate is widely used as a vitamin supplement. Yeast is a rich natural supplement.

Intestinal bacteria synthesize pan-tothenic acid, but the amount and availability is unknown.

For additional sources and more precise values of pantothenic acid, see Food Composition Table F-21.

Comments:

Coenzyme A, of which panto-thenic acid is a part, is one of the most important substances in body metabolism. The following two facts indicate that there may be need for dietary supplementa-tion of pantothenic acid for buoyant good health:

1. Losses of up to 50%, and even more, of the pantothenic content of foods may occur from production to consumption.

2. Deficiencies of pantothenic acid occur in farm animals fed natural rations (which are much less refined than human foods); hence, pantothenic acid is commonly added to commercial poultry and swine rations.

(Continued)

TABLE V-5 *(Continued)*

Functions	Deficiency and Toxicity Symptoms	Recommended Daily Allowance				Sources	Comments
		Age Group	Years	Vitamin			

Riboflavin (Vitamin B-2)

Riboflavin has an essential role in the oxidative reductions in all body cells by which energy is released. Thus, riboflavin functions in the metabolism of amino acids, fatty acids, and carbohydrates.

Riboflavin, through its role in activating pyridoxine (vitamin B-6), is necessary for the formation of niacin from the amino acid tryptophan.

Riboflavin is thought to be (1) a component of the retinal pigment of the eye; (2) involved in the functioning of the adrenal gland; and (3) required for the production of corticosteroids in the adrenal cortex.

(Also see RIBOFLAVIN.)

Deficiency symptoms—Unlike all the other vitamins, riboflavin deficiency is not the cause of any severe or major disease of man. Rather, riboflavin often contributes to other disorders and disabilities such as beriberi, pellagra, scurvy, keratomalacia, and nutritional megaloblastic anemia.

Riboflavin deficiency symptoms are: sores at the angle of the mouth (angular stomatitis); sore, swollen, and chapped lips (cheilosis); swollen, fissured, and painful tongue (glossitis); redness and congestion of the cornea of the eye; and oily, crusty, scaly skin (seborrheic dermatitis).

Toxicity—There is no known toxicity of riboflavin.

Riboflavin[1] (mg)

Age Group	Years	Riboflavin[1] (mg)
Infants	0.0–0.5	0.4
	0.5–1.0	0.5
Children	1–3	0.8
	4–6	1.1
	7–10	1.2
Males	11–14	1.5
	15–18	1.8
	19–24	1.7
	25–50	1.7
	51+	1.4
Females	11–14	1.3
	15–18	1.3
	19–24	1.3
	25–50	1.3
	51+	1.2
Pregnant		1.6
Lactating		1.8

[1]*Recommended Dietary Allowances*, 10th ed., NRC–National Academy of Sciences, 1989, p. 285.

Rich sources—Organ meats (liver, kidney, heart).

Good sources—Corn flakes (enriched), almonds, cheese, eggs, lean meat (beef, pork, lamb), mushrooms (raw), wheat flour (enriched), turnip greens, wheat bran, soybean flour, bacon, cornmeal (enriched).

Fair sources—Chicken (dark meat), white bread (enriched), rye flour, milk, mackerel and sardines, green leafy vegetables, beer.

Negligible sources—Fruits (raw), roots and tubers, white sugar, fats and oils (butter, margarine, salad oil, shortening).

Supplemental sources—Yeast (brewers', torula).

Riboflavin is the only vitamin present in significant amounts in beer.

For additional sources and more precise values of riboflavin (B-2), see Food Composition Table F-21.

Body storage of riboflavin is very limited; so, day-to-day needs must be supplied in the diet.

Two properties of riboflavin may account for major losses: (1) it is destroyed by light; and (2) it is destroyed by heat in an alkaline solution.

Because riboflavin is heat stable in neutral or acid solutions and only slightly soluble in water, little of it is lost in home cooking or commercial canning.

Thiamin (Vitamin B-1)

As a coenzyme in energy metabolism. Without thiamin, there could be no energy. As a coenzyme in the conversion of glucose to fats—the process called transketolation (Keto-carrying).

In the functioning of the peripheral nerves. In this role, it has value in the treatment of alcoholic neuritis, the neuritis of pregnancy, and beriberi.

In the direct functions in the body, including (1) maintenance of normal appetite, (2) the tone of the muscles, and (3) a healthy mental attitude.

(Also see THIAMIN.)

Deficiency symptoms—Moderate thiamin deficiency symptoms include fatigue, apathy (lack of interest); loss of appetite; nausea; moodiness; irritability; depression; retarded growth; a sensation of numbness in the legs; and abnormalities of the electrocardiogram.

More advanced thiamin deficiency is reflected in the gastrointestinal system, the nervous system, and the cardiovascular system.

Severe thiamin deficiency of long duration culminates in beriberi, the symptoms of which are polyneuritis (inflammation of the nerves), emaciation and/or edema, and disturbances of heart function.

Additional symptoms of thiamin deficiency include low excretion of thiamin in the urine; electrocardiogram measurement; reduced transketolase activity of the red blood cells; and increase of pyruvic acid in the blood.

Toxicity—None, for there are no known toxic effects from thiamin.

Age Group	Years	Calories (kcal)	Thiamin[1] (mg)
Infants	0.0–0.5	650	0.3
	0.5–1.0	850	0.4
Children	1–3	1,300	0.7
	4–6	1,800	0.9
	7–10	2,000	1.0
Males	11–14	2,500	1.3
	15–18	3,000	1.5
	19–24	2,900	1.5
	25–50	2,900	1.5
	51+	2,300	1.2
Females	11–14	2,200	1.1
	15–18	2,200	1.1
	19–24	2,200	1.1
	25–50	2,200	1.1
	51+	1,900	1.0
Pregnant		+300	1.5
Lactating		+500	1.6

[1]*Recommended Dietary Allowances*, 10th ed., NRC–National Academy of Sciences, 1989, p. 285.

1 kcal = 4.184 kj (kilojoules)
1,000 kj = 1 mj (megajoules)
Because the principal functions of thiamin are concerned in energy metabolism, its requirement by the body bears a direct relation to the energy intake.

Thiamin is found in a large variety of animal and vegetable products but is abundant in few.

Rich sources—Lean pork (fresh and cured), sunflower seeds, corn flakes (enriched), peanuts, cottonseed flour, safflower flour, soybean flour.

Good sources—Wheat bran, kidney, wheat flour (enriched), rye flour, nuts (except peanuts, which are a rich source), whole wheat flour, cornmeal (enriched), rice (enriched), white bread (enriched), soybean sprouts.

Fair sources—Egg yolk, peas, turkey (hamloaf), beef liver, luncheon meat, crab mackerel (fried), salmon steak (broiled), roe (cod, herring), lima beans, refried beans, lentils.

Negligible sources—Most fruits, most vegetables, polished rice, white sugar, animal and vegetable fats and oils, milk, butter, margarine, eggs, alcoholic beverages.

Supplemental sources—Thiamin hydrochloride, thiamin mononitrate, yeast (brewers', torula), rice bran, wheat germ, and rice polish.

Enriched flour (bread) and cereal, which was initiated in 1941, has been of special significance in improving the dietary level of thiamin in the U.S.

For additional sources and more precise values of thiamin, see Food Composition Table F-21.

A patient with wet beriberi—lying in bed breathless, waterlogged, and apparently dying—may recover in one to two hours after being given an injection of thiamin. This is perhaps the most dramatic cure in medicine.

Synthetic thiamin is usually marketed as thiamin hydrochloride or thiamin mononitrate.

Antithiamin factors are present in certain raw fish and seafood, live yeast, tea and fermented tea leaves, and alcohol.

Vitamin B-6 (Pyridoxine; pyridoxal; pyridoxamine)

Vitamin B-6, in its coenzyme forms, usually as pyridoxal phosphate but sometimes as pyridoxamine phosphate, is involved in a large number of physiologic functions, particularly:

1. In protein (nitrogen) metabolism, including—
   a. Transamination
   b. Decarboxylation
   c. Deamination

Deficiency symptoms—In adults, the deficiency symptoms are: greasy scaliness (seborrheic dermatitis) in the skin around the eyes, nose, and mouth, which subsequently spread to other parts of the body; a smooth, red tongue; loss of weight; muscular weakness; irritability; mental depression.

In infants, the deficiency symptoms are: irritability, muscular twitchings, and convulsions.

Age Group	Years	Vitamin B-6[1] (mg)
Infants	0.0–0.5	0.3
	0.5–1.0	0.6
Children	1–3	1.0
	4–6	1.1
	7–10	1.4
Males	11–14	1.7
	15–18	2.0
	19–24	2.0
	25–50	2.0
	51+	2.0

Rich sources—Rice bran, wheat bran, sunflower seed.

Good sources—Avocados, bananas, corn, fish, kidney, lean meat, liver, nuts, poultry, rice (brown), soybeans, whole grain.

Fair sources—Eggs, fruits (except bananas and avocados, which are good sources), milk, vegetables.

Negligible sources—Cheese (Cheddar, cottage), fat, milk,

In rats, the three forms of vitamin B-6 have equal activity; and it is assumed that the same applies to man.

Processing or cooking foods may destroy up to 50% of the B-6.

Because vitamin B-6 is limited in many foods, supplemental B-6 with synthetic pyridoxine hydrochloride may be indicated, especially for infants and during preg-

(Continued)

TABLE V-5 (Continued)

Functions	Deficiency and Toxicity Symptoms	Recommended Daily Allowance			Sources	Comments
		Age Group	Years	Vitamin		
Vitamin B-6 (Continued)	**Toxicity**—B-6 is relatively non-toxic. But large doses may result in sleepiness and be habit-forming when taken over an extended period.	Females	11–14	1.4	sugar, white bread.	nancy and lactation.
d. Transsulfuration			15–18	1.5	**Supplemental sources**—Pyridoxine hydrochloride is the most	
e. Tryptophan conversion to nicotinic acid.			19–24	1.6	commonly available synthetic form;	
f. Hemoglobin formation.			25–50	1.6	and yeast (brewers', torula), rice	
g. Absorption of amino acids.			51+	1.6	polish, and wheat germ are used as	
2. In carbohydrate and fat		Pregnant		2.2	natural source supplements.	
metabolism, including—		Lactating		2.1	**F**or additional sources and more	
a. The conversion of glycogen to glucose-1-phosphate.		[1]*Recommended Dietary Allowances*, 10th ed., NRC–National Academy of Sciences, 1989, p. 285.			precise values of vitamin B-6 (pyridoxine), see Food Composition Table F-21.	

Vitamin B-6 functions continued (left column):

b. The conversion of linoleic acid to arachidonic acid.
3. In clinical problems, including—
a. Central nervous system disturbances.
b. Autism, a mental and emotional affliction in children.
c. Anemia that is iron-resistant.
d. Kidney stones.
e. Tuberculosis, in countering the antagonistic drug isonicotinic acid used in its treatment.
f. Physiologic demands in pregnancy.
g. Oral contraceptives.
(Also see VITAMIN B-6.)

Functions	Deficiency and Toxicity Symptoms	Age Group	Years	Vitamin	Sources	Comments
Vitamin B-12 (Cobalamins)	**Deficiency symptoms**—Vitamin B-12 deficiency in man may occur as a result of (1) dietary lack, which sometimes occurs among vegetarians who consume no animal food; or (2) deficiency of intrinsic factor due to pernicious anemia, total removal of the stomach by surgery, or infestation with parasites such as the fish tapeworm.			**Vitamin B-12**[1] (mcg)	**Rich sources**—Liver and other organ meats—kidney, heart.	**P**lants cannot manufacture vitamin B-12. Hence, little is found in vegetables, grains, legumes, and fruits.
In the body, vitamin B-12 functions in two coenzyme forms: coenzyme B-12, and methyl B-12.		Infants	0.0–0.5	0.3[2]	**Good sources**—Muscle meats, fish, shellfish, eggs, and cheese.	**V**itamin B-12, like so many other members of the B-complex,
Vitamin B-12 coenzymes perform the following physiological roles at the cellular level, especially in the cells of the bone marrow, nervous tissue, and gastrointestinal tract:			0.5–1.0	0.5	**Fair sources**—Milk, poultry, yogurt.	is not a single substance; rather, it consists of several closely related
		Children	1–3	0.7	**Negligible sources**—Bread (both whole wheat and white),	compounds with similar activity.
			4–6	1.0	cereal grains, fruits, legumes,	**V**itamin B-12 is the largest and
1. Red blood cell formation and control of pernicious anemia.			7–10	1.4	vegetables.	the most complex of all vitamin molecules.
2. Maintenance of nerve tissue.	The common symptoms of a dietary deficiency of vitamin B-12 are: sore tongue, weakness, loss of weight, back pains, tingling of the extremities, apathy, and mental and other nervous abnormalities. Anemia is rarely seen in dietary deficiency of B-12.	Males	11–14	2.0	**Supplemental sources**—Cobalamin, of which there are at least	**I**t is noteworthy (1) that vitamin B-12 is the only vitamin that
3. Carbohydrate, fat, and protein metabolism.			15–18	2.0	three active forms, produced by	requires a gastrointestinal tract
4. Synthesis or transfer of single carbon units.			19–24	2.0	microbial growth; available at the corner drugstore.	secretion for its absorption (intrinsic factor); and (2) that the
5. Biosynthesis of methyl groups (-CH₃), and in reduction reactions such as the conversion of disulfide (S-S) to the sulfhydryl group (-SH).			25–50	2.0	**S**ome B-12 is synthesized in the intestinal tract of human beings.	absorption of vitamin B-12 in the small intestine requires about 3
			51+	2.0	However, little of it may be absorbed.	hours (compared to seconds for most of the other water-soluble
In the following therapeutic uses:	In pernicious anemia, the characteristic symptoms are: abnormally large red blood cells, lemon-yellow pallor, anorexia, dypsnea, prolonged bleeding time, abdominal discomfort, loss of weight, glossitis, and unsteady gait, and neurological disturbances, including stiffness of the limbs, irritability, and mental depression. Without treatment, death follows.	Females	11–14	2.0	**F**or additional sources and more precise values of vitamin B-12, see Food Composition Table F-21.	vitamins).
1. The control of pernicious anemia.			15–18	2.0		
2. In the treatment of sprue. (Also see VITAMIN B-12.)			19–24	2.0		
			25–50	2.0		
			51+	2.0		
		Pregnant		2.2		
	Toxicity—No toxic effects of vitamin B-12 are known.	Lactating		2.6		

[1]*Recommended Dietary Allowances*, 10th ed., NRC–National Academy of Sciences, 1989, p. 285.
[2]The recommended dietary allowance for vitamin B-12 in infants is based on average concentration of the vitamin in human milk. The allowances after weaning are based on energy intake (as recommended by the American Academy of Pediatrics) and consideration of other factors, such as intestinal absorption.

Functions	Deficiency and Toxicity Symptoms	Age Group	Years	Vitamin	Sources	Comments
Vitamin C (Ascorbic acid)	**Deficiency symptoms**—Early symptoms, called latent scurvy: loss in weight, listlessness, fatigue, fleeting pains in the joints and muscles, irritability, shortness of breath, sore and bleeding gums, small hemorrhages under the skin, bones that fracture easily, and poor wound healing.			**Vitamin C**[1] (mg)	**N**atural sources of vitamin C occur primarily in foods of plant origin—fruits (especially citrus fruits) and leafy vegetables.	**A**ctually, several compounds have vitamin C activity. So, the term vitamin C is a combined name for all of them. The terms
Formation and maintenance of collagen, the substance that binds body cells together. So, vitamin C makes for more rapid and sound healing of wounds and burns.		Infants	0.0–0.5	30	**Richest natural sources**—acerola cherry, *camu-camu*, and rose hips.	ascorbic acid and dehydroascorbic acid should be used when specific reference is made
			0.5–1.0	35	**Excellent sources**—Raw,	to them.
Metabolism of the amino acids tyrosine and tryptophan.		Children	1–3	40	frozen, or canned citrus fruit or juice: oranges, grapefruit, lemons, and	**A**ll animal species appear to require vitamin C, but dietary need
Absorption and movement of iron.			4–6	45	limes. Guavas, peppers (green, hot),	is limited to humans, guinea pigs,
			7–10	45	black currants, parsley, turnip greens,	monkeys, fruit-eating bats, red-
Metabolism of fats and lipids, and cholesterol control.		Males	11–14	50	poke greens, and mustard greens.	vented bulbul birds, certain fish,
Sound teeth and bones.	**Scurvy**: swollen, bleeding, and ulcerated gums; loose teeth; malformed and weak bones, fragility of the capillaries with resulting hemor-		15–18	60		
Strong capillary walls and			19–24	60		
			25–50	60		
			51+	60		
		Females	11–14	50		
			15–18	60		

TABLE V-5 *(Continued)*

Functions	Deficiency and Toxicity Symptoms	Recommended Daily Allowance			Sources	Comments
		Age Group	Years	Vitamin		

Vitamin C *(Continued)*
healthy blood vessels.
  Metabolism of folic acid. (Also see VITAMIN C.)

rhages throughout the body; large bruises; big joints, such as the knees and hips, due to bleeding into the joint cavity; anemia; degeneration of muscle fibers; including those of the heart; and tendency of old wounds to become red and break open. Sudden death from severe internal hemorrhage and heart failure is always a danger.
  Toxicity—Adverse effects reported of intakes in excess of 8 g per day (more than 100 times the recommended allowance) include: nausea, abdominal cramps, and diarrhea; absorption of excessive amounts of iron; destruction of red blood cells; increased mobilization of bone minerals; interference with anticoagulant therapy; formation of kidney and bladder stones; inactivation of vitamin B-12; rise in plasma cholesterol; and possible dependence upon large doses of vitamin C.

		19–24	60
		25–50	60
		51+	60
Pregnant		70
Lactating		95

¹*Recommended Dietary Allowances*, 10th ed., NRC–National Academy of Sciences, 1989, p. 285.
  0.05 mg of ascorbic acid = 1 IU of vitamin C.

Good sources—Green leafy vegetables: broccoli, Brussels sprouts, cabbage (red), cauliflower, collards, kale, lamb's-quarter, spinach, Swiss chard, and watercress. Also, cantaloupe, papaya, strawberries, and tomatoes and tomato juice (fresh or canned.)
  Fair sources—Apples, asparagus, bananas, blackberries, blueberries, Irish potatoes, lima beans, liver, peaches, pears, sweet potatoes.
  Negligible sources—Cereal grains and their by-products, cow's milk, eggs, fats, fish, meat, nuts, poultry, sugar.
  Supplemental sources—Vitamin C (ascorbic acid) is available wherever vitamins are sold. For additional sources and more precise values of vitamin C, see Food Composition Table F-21.

and perhaps certain reptiles.
  Of all the vitamins, ascorbic acid is the most unstable. It is easily destroyed during storage, processing, and cooking; it is water-soluble, easily oxidized, and attacked by enzymes.

VITAMINLIKE SUBSTANCES:
Bioflavonids (Vitamin P)
  Bioflavonoids function as follows:
  1. They influence capillary fragility and permeability, perhaps together with vitamin C; increasing the strength of the capillaries and regulating their permeability. These actions help prevent hemorrhages and ruptures in the capillaries and connective tissues and build a protective barrier against infection.
  2. They are active antioxidant compounds in food, ranking second only to fat-soluble tocopherols in this regard.
  3. They possess metal-chelating capacity; and they affect the activity of the enzymes and membranes.
  4. They have a synergistic effect on ascorbic acid, and they appear to stabilize ascorbic acid in human tissues.
  5. They possess a bacteriostatic and/or antibiotic effect, which is sufficiently high to account for measurable anti-infectious properties of normal daily food.
  6. They possess anticarcinogenic activity in two ways; a cytostatic effect against malignant cells and a biochemical protection of the cell from damage by carcinogenic substances.
  (Also see BIOFLAVONOIDS.)

Deficiency symptoms—The symptoms of bioflavonoid deficiency are closely related to those of a vitamin C deficiency. The tendency to bleed (hemorrhage) or bruise easily are especially noted.
  Toxicity—Bioflavonoids are nontoxic.

There are no NRC-National Academy of Sciences recommended daily allowances (RDA) of bioflavonoids.
  The average daily intake of flavonoids in the American diet amounts to about 1 g, of which one-half (0.5 g) is absorbed from the gut.
  The label on a rather typical vitamin C-bioflavonoid supplement reads as follows:

Each tablet contains:	**(mg)**
Rose hip powder	500
Vitamin C	500
Lemon bioflavonoid	500
Rutin (buckwheat)	50

NOTE: Need in human nutrition not established.

Rich sources—Citrus peel (especially orange and lemon peel), white pulp of citrus fruits, tangerine juice, rose hips, buckwheat leaves.
  Good sources—Onions with colored skins, leafy vegetables, fruit, coffee, tea, cocoa, red wine, beer.
  Poor sources—Frozen orange juice, most root vegetables.

Bioflavonoids are a group of natural pigments in vegetables, fruits, flowers, and grains. They appear as companions of vitamin C, but they are not present in synthetic vitamin C.
  Bioflavonoids do not fill the two prerequisites of a vitamin; they are not essential food constituents, and deficiency symptoms which can be cured by their administration are unknown.
  NOTE: At this time, no evidence exists that bioflavonoids serve any useful role in human nutrition or in the prevention or treatment of disease in humans; hence, this presentation is for two purposes (1) informational, and (2) stimulation of research.

Carnitine (Vitamin B$_T$)
  Carnitine plays an important role in fat metabolism and energy production in mammals. It functions as follows:
  1. *Transport and oxidation of fatty acids.* Carnitine plays an important role in the oxidation of fatty acids by facilitating their transport across the mitochondrial membrane. Carnitine is part of the shuttle mechanism whereby long-chain fatty acids are made into acyl carnitine derivatives and transported across the mitochondrial membrane, which is impermeable to long-chain fatty acids *per se* and to their coenzyme A esters. Once across the membrane, the acyl carnitines are reconverted to their fatty acid CoA form and undergo B-oxidation to liberate energy.
  2. *Fat synthesis.* Although this role is controversial, carnitine appears to be involved in transporting acetyl groups back to the cytoplasm for fatty acid synthesis.
  3. *Ketone body utilization.* Carnitine stimulates acetoacetate oxidation; thus, it may play a role in ketone body utilization.
  (Also see CARNITINE.)

Deficiency symptoms—If the body's supply of carnitine is low, the cells cannot get the fatty acids they need for energy production and growth. This is rare, but life-threatening. The symptoms of carnitine deficiency include muscle weakness, failure to thrive, poor growth, recurrent infections, cardiomyopathy, and hypoglycemia.
  Toxicity—Not known.

Under normal conditions, there is no dietary requirement for carnitine. However, where a metabolic abnormality exists which inhibits synthesis, interferes with use, or increases catabolism of carnitine, illness may follow, which is sometimes relieved by a dietary supplement. There is need for further research on the role of carnitine in human health and disease.

Generally speaking, carnitine is high in animal foods and low in plant foods. Few foods have been assayed for carnitine, but based on available data, the following evaluation of dietary sources of carnitine may be helpful.
  Rich sources—Muscle meat, liver, heart, yeast (torula and brewers'), chicken, rabbit, milk, whey.
  Good sources—Avocado, casein, wheat germ.
  Poor sources—Cabbage, cauliflower, peanuts, wheat.
  Negligible sources—Barley, corn, egg, orange juice, spinach. likely deficient in the essential amino acids, lysine and methionine, precursors of carnitine. Thus, a vegetarian diet will likely be low in carnitine, in both preformed carnitine and the amino acid precursors of carnitine.

Carnitine, a vital coenzyme in animal tissues and involved in fat metabolism, is another vitaminlike substance that has received much attention recently. It is similar to a vitamin with the exception that under normal conditions higher animals synthesize their total needs within their bodies; hence, no need appears to exist to supply this substance in food on a daily basis.
  The lower level of carnitine in plant foods in comparison with animal foods is explainable on the basis that plant materials are most

---

Coenzyme Q (Ubiquinone)
  Coenzyme Q functions in the respiratory chain in which energy is released from the energy-yielding nutrients as ATP.
  There is evidence that specific ubiquinones function in the remission (prevention) of some of the symptoms of vitamin E deficiency.
  (Also see COENZYME Q.)

Deficiency symptoms—Nonspecific.
  Toxicity—Unknown.

Coenzyme Q is synthesized in the body. So, dietary allowance seems unimportant.

synthesized in the body, they cannot be considered a true vitamin.
  The entire series of ubiquinones has been prepared synthetically.

Quinones occur widely in aerobic organisms, from bacteria to higher plants and animals. Because they are

Coenzyme Q, or ubiquinone, is a collective name for a number of ubiquinones—lipidlike compounds that are chemically somewhat similar to vitamin E.
  The importance of coenzyme Q as a catalyst for respiration im-

parts status as an essential metabolite. It may have other significant roles. For man and other higher animals a simple precursor substance with an aromatic ring may have vitaminlike status, but dietary ubiquinone seems, on the whole, to be unimportant unless it provides the aromatic nucleus for endogenous (body) synthesis.

(Continued)

TABLE V-5 *(Continued)*

Functions	Deficiency and Toxicity Symptoms	Recommended Daily Allowance	Sources	Comments
Inositol The functions of inositol are not completely understood, but the following roles have been suggested: 1. It has a lipotropic effect (an affinity for fat, like choline). In this role, inositol aids in the metabolism of fats and helps reduce blood cholesterol. 2. In combination with choline, inositol prevents the fatty hardening of arteries and protects the heart.	**Deficiency symptoms**—Myoinositol is a *growth factor* for certain yeasts and bacteria, and several species of fish. Earlier experiments indicated that a deficiency of inositol caused retarded growth and loss of hair in young mice, and loss of hair around the eyes (spectacled-eyes) in rats. But these	**N**eed for inositol in human nutrition has not been established. So, no recommended daily allowance is given. **M**ost authorities feel that people should consume about the same amount of inositol as choline. **T**herapeutic doses, which should be under the supervision of a physician, range from 500 to 1,000 mg daily.	**I**nositol is abundantly present in nature. **Rich sources**—Kidney, brain, liver, yeast, heart, wheat germ, citrus fruits, and blackstrap molasses. **Good sources**—Muscle meat, fruits, whole grains, bran of cereal grains, nuts, legumes, milk, and vegetables.	**T**here is no evidence that human beings cannot synthesize all the inositol needed by the body. So, its classification as a vitamin is disputed. More properly perhaps, it should be classified as an essential nutrient, rather than a vitamin, for certain species of bacteria and animals.

symptoms are now being questioned because the experimental diets used were partially deficient in certain other vitamins.   **In** animal cells, inositol occurs as a component of phospholipids. In plant cells, it is found as phytic acid, an organic acid that binds calcium, iron, and zinc in an insoluble complex and interferes with their absorption.

Toxicity—There is no known toxicity of inositol.

3. It appears to be a precursor of the phosphoinosities, which are found in various body tissues, especially in the brain.
(Also see INOSITOL.)

Functions	Deficiency and Toxicity Symptoms	Recommended Daily Allowance	Sources	Comments
Laetrile (Vitamin B-17, amygdalin, nitrilosides) **A**ccording to its advocates, Laetrile, or amygdalin, is a highly selective substance that attacks only cancerous cells. They explain this phenomenon as follows: Upon being absorbed by normal body cells, the enzyme rhodanese detoxifies the cyanide, which is	**Deficiency symptoms**—The advocates claim that prolonged deficiency of amygdalin may lead to lowered resistance to malignancies. **Toxicity**—None reported. But not more than 1.0 g should be taken at one time because of the hazard of hydrogen cyanide poisoning.	**T**he usual dosage is 0.25 to 1.0 g taken at meals. Cumulative daily amounts of more than 3.0 g are sometimes taken, *but more than 1.0 g should never be taken at any one time.* **A**ccording to the advocates, 5 to 30 apricot kernels eaten through the day may be effective as a preventive of cancer, but should not be eaten all at one time.	**A** concentration of 2 to 3% Laetrile is found in the whole kernels of most fruits, including apricots, apples, cherries, peaches, plums, and nectarines.	**NOTE WELL**; Laetrile has no known value for humans. The authors present this section relative to the controversial compound for informational purposes only. Further, it is listed with the vitaminlike substances because it is sometimes erroneously designated

then excreted through the urine. But cancer cells are completely deficient in rhodinese; instead, they are surrounded by another enzyme, beta-glucosidase, which releases the bound cyanide from the Laetrile at the site of the malignancy. So, Laetrile is believed to attack only the malignant cells.   as vitamin B-17. Both the pros and cons relative to Laetrile are given, then the reader may make a judgement.

Those who oppose Laetrile submit evidence that it is not effective as a treatment.   **R**egardless of the validity of the claims and counter claims pertaining to Laetrile, it is noteworthy

Those who support the use of Laetrile do so primarily on the basis that it is a preventive of cancer, rather than as a treatment of cancer.
(Also see LAETRILE.)   that more and more medical authorities are accepting the nutrition approach in the prevention and treatment of cancer. Although the results of such nutrients as Laetrile, vitamin A (carotene), folic acid, and vitamin C, along with a general supplemental program of minerals and vitamins are significant for cancer treatment, perhaps even more important in the long run is the apparent success of nutrients of many kinds in strengthening the body's immune system.

Functions	Deficiency and Toxicity Symptoms	Recommended Daily Allowance	Sources	Comments
Lipoic acid **L**ipoic acid functions as a coenzyme. It is essential, together with the thiamin-containing enzyme, pyrophosphatase (TPP), for reactions in carbohydrate metabolism which convert pyruvic acid to	**Deficiency symptoms**—No characteristc deficiency symptoms have been produced. **Toxicity**—Not known.	**B**ecause the body can synthesize the needed lipoic acid, no dietary requirement for humans and animals has been established.	**Y**east and liver.	**L**ipoic acid is not a true vitamin because it can be synthesized in the body and is not necessary in the diet of animals. However, it functions in the same manner as many of the B-complex vitamins.

aceytl-coenzyme A. Lipoic acid, which has two sulfur bonds of high-energy potential, combines with TPP to reduce pyruvate to active acetate, thereby sending it into the final energy cycle. It joins the intermediary products of protein and fat metabolism in the Krebs cycle in the reactions involved in producing energy from these nutrients. A metal ion (magnesium or calcium) is involved in this oxidative decarboxylation, along with lipoic acid and four vitamins: thiamin, pantothenic acid, niacin, and riboflavin.
(Also see LIPOIC ACID.)

Functions	Deficiency and Toxicity Symptoms	Recommended Daily Allowance	Sources	Comments
Pangamic acid (Vitamin B-15) **N**umerous functions have been attributed to pangamic acid; among them, the following: 1. Stimulation of transmethylation reactions. 2. Stimulation of oxygen intake. 3. Inhibition of fatty liver formation. 4. Adaptation to increased physical activity. 5. Control of blood cholesterol levels. (Also see PANGAMIC ACID.)	**Deficiency symptoms**—There is indication that a deficiency of pangamic acid may cause fatigue (a tired feeling), hypoxia (an insufficient supply of oxygen in blood cells), heart disease, and glandular and nervous disorders. **Toxicity**—The so-called *Russian formula* appears to be relatively free of toxicity.	**N**o NRC-National Academy of Sciences recommended daily allowances (RDA) have been established. But the usual dosage of pangamic acid is from 150 to 300 mg daily.	**Rich sources**—All cereals and cereal products, with corn and rice particularly rich. Also, apricot kernels and brewers' yeast. **Good sources**—Wherever B-complex vitamins are found in natural foods.	**NOTE:** The authors make this presentation for two primary purposes: (1) informational, and (2) stimulation of research. The nutritional status and biological role(s) of pangamic acid await clarification. Its stimulation of such fundamental processes as transmethylation, cellular respiration, etc. may have physiological application. Certainly, there is sufficient indication of the value of pangamic acid as a therpeutic agent to war-

rant further study. In the meantime, pangamic acid should not be taken unless prescribed by a physician.

Pangamic acid is a vitaminlike substance, rather than a vitamin.

FDA classifies it as a food additive.

It has been widely studied and accepted in the U.S.S.R. as a necessary food factor (with important physiological actions). The Russians have used pangamic acid in treating cardiovascular disorders associated with insufficiency of oxidative metabolism, and in the treatment of liver disorders, a number of skin diseases, and some toxicoses.

(Continued)

TABLE V-5 *(Continued)*

Functions	Deficiency and Toxicity Symptoms	Recommended Daily Allowance	Sources	Comments
Para-aminobenzoic acid (PABA) **F**or man and other higher animals, PABA functions as an essential part of the folacin molecule. **Human pharmaceutical uses**— PABA is sometimes used as a human pharmaceutical, not as a vitamin, in the following: as an antirickettsial; to counteract the bacteriostatic action of sulfonamides; and as a protective agent against sunburn.	**Deficiency symptoms**—Sulfa drugs may induce a deficiency of not only PABA, but of folic acid as well. The symptoms: fatigue, irritability, depression, nervousness, headache, constipation, and other digestive disorders. **Toxicity**—PABA is not known to be toxic to man. But continued high doses may result in nausea and vomiting.	The need for PABA has not been established; hence, it follows that there is no recommended daily allowance.	**F**ood composition tables do not list PABA, but the following foods are generally recognized as the richest sources: brewers' yeast, fish, soybeans, peanuts, beef liver, eggs, wheat germ, lecithin, molasses.	**I**n addition to having activity as a growth factor for certain bacteria, PABA has considerable folacin activity when fed to deficient animals in which intestinal synthesis of folacin takes place. For example, in rats and mice, it can completely replace the dietary source of folacin. This explains why para-aminobenzoic acid was once considered to be a vitamin in its own right. **F**or man and other higher animals, PABA has no vitamin activity in animals receiving ample folacin, and it is not required in the diet; hence, it can no longer be considered a vitamin.

1. **Antirickettsial**. PABA is sometimes used in the treatment of certain rickettsial diseases—diseases in man and animals caused by microscopically small parasites of the genus *Rickettsia*, notably typhus and Rocky Mountain spotted fever.

2. **Sulfonamide antagonist**. PABA has the ability to reverse the bacteriostatic effects of sulfonamides, thereby counteracting their action. This is an antimetabolite action, explainable on the basis of similarity of structures. According to this theory, sulfonamides suppress bacterial growth by replacing their chemical analog PABA in bacterial enzyme systems; PABA in excess reverses the effect.

3. **Sunscreen agent**. PABA is used for protection against sunburn; usually about 5% PABA is incorporated in an ointment, to be applied over exposed parts of the body.

(Also see FOLACIN; and PARA-AMINOBENZOIC ACID.)

Functions	Deficiency and Toxicity Symptoms	Recommended Daily Allowance	Sources	Comments
Vitamin B-13 (Orotic acid) **V**itamin B-13 has been found to stimulate the growth of rats, chicks, and pigs under certain conditions. **O**rotic acid is utilized by the body in the metabolism of folic acid and vitamin B-12. Also, it appears to aid the replacement or restoration of some cells. **T**here is indication that vitamin B-13 may be helpful in the treatment of multiple sclerosis. (Also see VITAMIN B-13.)	**Deficiency symptoms**—Deficiency symptoms have not been proven. But it is believed that a deficiency may lead to liver disorders, cell degeneration, and premature aging; and to degenerative symptoms in multiple sclerosis victims. **Toxicity**—Not reported.	**D**ietary requirements are not known.	**V**itamin B-13 is found in such natural sources as distillers' solubles, whey, sour or curdled milk, and root vegetables. Also, this nutrient is available in supplemental form as calcium orotate.	**I**t is highly possible that the so-called vitamin B-13 is a growth promotant and a preventive of certain disorders. At this time, however, it is not known whether it plays an essential role in an otherwise adequate diet.

VITAMIN A (CAROTENE)

Contents

Vitamin A is probably the most important of all vitamins, if any vitamin can be singled out and ranked. More than any other vitamin, deficiencies of vitamin A are still widespread throughout most developing countries of the world and involve millions of people, especially children.

Vitamin A is required by man and all other animals. It is strictly a product of animal metabolism—present in all species of mammals, birds, and fish, no vitamin A being found in plants. The counterpart in plants is known as carotene, which is the precursor of vitamin A. Because the animal body can transform carotene into vitamin A, this compound is often spoken of as *provitamin A*.

Carotene, which derives its name from the carrot, from which it was first isolated over 100 years ago, is the yellow-colored, fat-soluble substance that gives the characteristic color to carrots and many other vegetables and to several fruits.

Thus, the ultimate source of all vitamin A is the carotenes which are synthesized by plants. Man and other animals convert a considerable proportion of the foods they eat into vitamin A.

HISTORY. At a very early date, the Chinese used a concoction rich in vitamin A as a remedy for night blindness; and, in ancient Greece, Hippocrates prescribed various forms of liver, a good source of preformed vitamin A, as a treatment for night blindness. But it remained for laboratory experiments conducted in the early 1900s to identify vitamin A as a distinct nutrient.

In 1913, vitamin A was discovered by Elmer V. McCollum and Marguerite Davis of the University of Wisconsin, and by Thomas B. Osborne and Lafayette B. Mendel of the Connecticut Experiment Station. Working independently, each research team demonstrated the presence of an essential dietary substance in fatty foods. McCollum and Davis found it in butterfat and egg yolks; Osborne and Mendel discovered it in cod-liver oil. These researchers believed that only one factor, which they called fat-soluble A, was needed to supplement purified diets. They described the condition as the "type of nutritive deficiency exemplified in the form of an infectious eye disease prevalent in animals inappropriately fed." In 1915, McCollum and Davis also noted that a deficiency of fat-soluble A caused night blindness. (It is noteworthy that Miss Marguerite Davis, a young biologist who had just obtained her bachelor's degree from the University of California, volunteered to do the rat work for McCollum without salary.)

VITAMIN A . . .
needed for growth, healthy eyes, skin and other tissues

TWO RATS FROM SAME LITTER, 11 WEEKS OLD

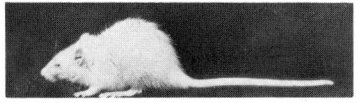

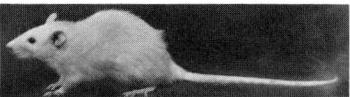

THIS RAT HAD NO VITAMIN A. NOTE THE INFECTED EYE, ROUGH FUR, AND SICK APPEARANCE. IT WEIGHED ONLY 53 g.

THIS RAT HAD PLENTY OF VITAMIN A. IT HAS BRIGHT EYES, SLEEK FUR, AND APPEARS ALERT AND VIGOROUS. IT WEIGHED 123 g.

TOP FOOD SOURCES

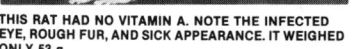

LIVER | CARROTS | DARK-GREEN LEAFY VEGETABLES | SWEET POTATOES | SQUASH (WINTER)

PEACHES AND APRICOTS | BUTTER AND MARGARINE (FORTIFIED) | EGG YOLK | CHEESE | TOMATOES

Fig. V-23. Vitamin A made the difference! *Left*: Rat on vitamin A-deficient diet. *Right*: Rat that received plenty of vitamin A. (Adapted from USDA sources.) Note, too, top ten sources of vitamin A.

In 1919, Steenbock and co-workers at the University of Wisconsin noted that an unknown substance, present in sweet potatoes, carrots, and corn, later to be identified as carotene, would support normal growth and reproduction.

In 1920, the English scientist Drummond proposed that this compound be called vitamin A.

In 1930, Moore, of England, demonstrated that this provitamin A activity was beta-carotene.

In 1931, P. Karrer, a Swiss researcher, isolated the active substance in halibut-liver oil and determined the chemical formula for vitamin A—the first vitamin to have its chemical structure determined. For this, and for his work with riboflavin, he received the Nobel Prize. However, vitamin A was not produced (by Karrer) in crystalline form from fish liver oils until 1937, and it did not become available in synthetic form (by Isler working in Switzerland) until 1947. Today, pure, inexpensive synthetic forms of vitamin A are readily available.

CHEMISTRY, METABOLISM, PROPERTIES.

• **Chemistry**—*Vitamin A* may be a misleading term because it sounds as if only one chemical compound has vitamin A activity. Actually, several forms of vitamin A exist, with each possessing different degrees of activity.

There are two forms of vitamin A as such, retinol and dehydroretinol. Retinol (formerly called vitamin A), which is found as an ester (retinyl palmitate) in ocean fish oils and fats, and in liver, butterfat, and egg yolk, is biologically active as an alcohol, an aldehyde, and an acid. The alcohol, the most common form (see Fig. V-24 for formula), is usually referred to as retinol, the aldehyde as retinal or retinene, and the acid as retinoic acid.

Dehydroretinol, or vitamin A_2, differs from retinol in that (1) it has an extra double bond, and (2) it has about 40% the biological value (activity). It is found only in freshwater fish and in birds that eat these fish; hence, it is of limited interest.

Today, the general term *vitamin A* is used for both *retinol* and *dehydroretinol*.

In addition to the actual forms of vitamin A, related compounds, known as *carotenes*, are found in several fruits and vegetables. Carotene is also called (1) provitamin A, because it can be converted to vitamin A in the body; and (2) precursor of vitamin A, because it precedes vitamin A. At least 10 of the carotenoids found in plants can be converted with varying efficiencies into vitamin A. Four of these carotenoids—alpha-carotene, beta-carotene, gamma-carotene, and cryptoxanthine (the main carotenoid of corn)—are of particular importance due to their provitamin A activity. Of the four, *beta-carotene* (see Fig. V-25) has the highest vitamin A activity and provides about two-thirds of the vitamin A necessary for human nutrition.

VITAMIN A

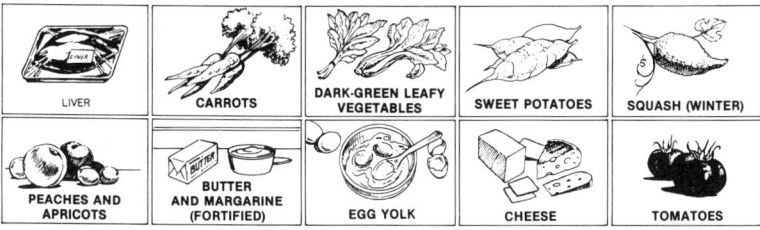

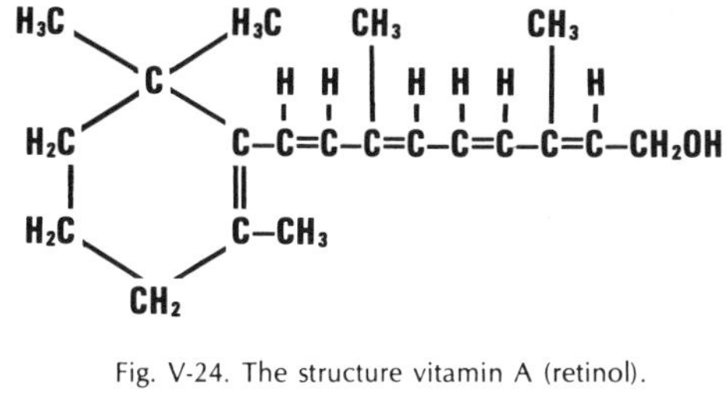

Fig. V-24. The structure vitamin A (retinol).

β-CAROTENE

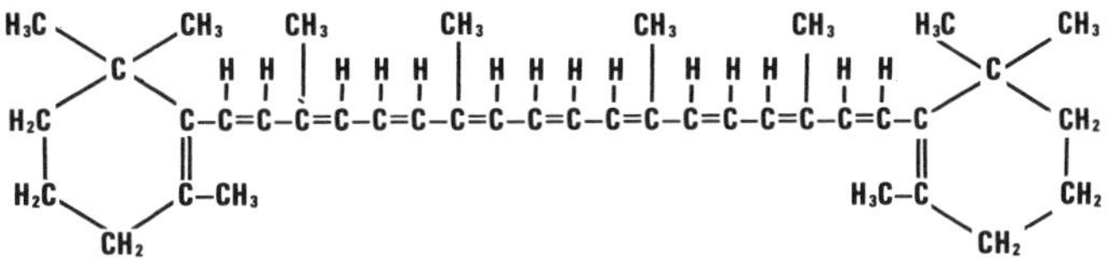

Fig. V-25. The structure of beta-carotene.

• **Metabolism**—Foods supply vitamin A in the form of vitamin A, vitamin A esters, and carotenes. Almost no absorption of vitamin A occurs in the stomach. In the small intestine, vitamin A and beta-carotene are emulsified with bile salts and products of fat digestion and absorbed in the intestinal mucosa. Here, much of the conversion of beta-carotene to vitamin A (retinol) takes place. There are wide differences in species and individuals as to how well they utilize the carotenoids. Their absorption is affected by several factors, including the presence in the small intestine of bile, dietary fat, and antioxidants. Bile aids emulsification; fat must be absorbed simultaneously; and antioxidants, such as alpha-tocopherol and lecithin, decrease the oxidation of carotene. Also, the presence of enough protein of good quality enhances the conversion of carotene to vitamin A—a matter of great importance in developing countries where protein is limited in both quantity and quality.

The absorption of vitamin A is adversely affected by the presence of mineral oil in the intestinal tract. Since mineral oil is not absorbed, and since it holds carotene and vitamin A in solution, carotene and vitamin A are lost through excretion. Therefore, mineral oil should never be used as a substitute for regular fats in food preparation (for example, as a salad dressing); neither should it be taken at mealtime when it is used as a laxative. It is noteworthy, too, that intestinal parasites adversely affect the absorption of vitamin A and carotene and the conversion of carotene to vitamin A—a factor of importance in tropical regions where intestinal parasite infections are common.

In the blood, vitamin A esters are transported in association with a retinol-binding protein, whereas the carotenoids are associated with the lipid-bearing protein. Storage of vitamin A is largely in the liver, but small amounts are also stored in the lungs, body fat, and kidneys. The amount of body storage of vitamin A tends to increase with age, but of course this depends on the quantity in the diet and the amount absorbed. It is estimated that a normal adult may store sufficient vitamin A in his/her liver to meet the needs for 4 to 12 months. Infants and children do not build up such reserves; hence, they are much more susceptible to deficiencies.

From the liver, vitamin A enters the bloodstream as a free alcohol, whereupon it travels to the tissues for use.

No vitamin A is excreted in the urine because it is not water-soluble, but considerable unabsorbed carotene is normally found in the feces.

• **Properties**—Vitamin A (retinol) is an almost colorless (pale yellow) fat-soluble substance. It is insoluble in water; hence, there is no loss by extraction from cooking. Although the esters of vitamin A are relatively stable compounds, the alcohol, aldehyde, and acid forms are rapidly destroyed by oxidation when they are exposed to air and light. Since vitamin A occurs in the stable form (the ester) in most foods, normal preparation procedures do not destroy much vitamin A activity. However, fats that undergo oxidative rancidity, can lose their vitamin A rapidly. We depend mainly on storage in a cool, dark place (refrigeration) and on added antioxidants, such as vitamin E, to protect fats and oils from vitamin A loss.

The carotenoid pigments (which are referred to as carotene in this discussion) are deep red color, but in solution they are bright yellow or orange yellow. They impart the color to many fruits and vegetables, including apricots, peaches, carrots, sweet potatoes, squash, pumpkins, and yellow corn. As a general rule of thumb, the more intense the pigmentation in these foods, the higher the provitamin A content. Green vegetables, particularly dark green and leafy ones, are also rich in provitamin A. They contain carotenoids, although their color is masked by that of the green pigment, chlorophyll. The properties of solubility and stability of carotene and carotenoid pigments are similar to those of vitamin A.

The yellow color of beta-carotene is so intense that it is widely used as a coloring agent by the food industry. For such purposes, beta-carotene is valued more for its aesthetic contribution than its nutritive value, although the potential vitamin A value of the food it colors is also increased.

MEASUREMENT/ASSAY. The assay of vitamin A is accomplished by two basic methods: biological, or chemical. The bioassay procedure is based on a biological response such as growth of rats or chicks deficient in vitamin A. It measures the total vitamin A, including provitamin A, present. But, because of the difficulties and time factor in bioassays, chemical assays are usually used.

Until recently, dietary allowances of vitamin A were stated in terms of either International Units (IU) or United States Pharmacopeia (USP) units, which are equal. An International Unit (IU) of vitamin A is defined on the basis of rat studies as equal to 0.344 mcg of crystalline retinylacetate (which is equivalent to 0.300 mcg of retinol, or to 0.60 mcg of beta-carotene). These standards were based on experiments that showed that in rats only about 50% of the beta-carotene is converted to vitamin A. In man, however, beta-carotene is not as available as in the rat, due to poorer absorption in the intestines and other factors, with the result that various factors have been used to compensate for this when vitamin A activity of foods and diets have been expressed in IU.

In order to quantify vitamin A values for humans within the metric system, therefore, international agencies have now introduced the biological equivalent of 1 microgram (1 mcg) of retinol as the standard. In 1967, the FAO/WHO proposed that vitamin A allowances be expressed as the equivalent weight of retinol, and that the use of IU be discontinued. The United Kingdom adopted this change and coined the term *Retinol Equivalent* (RE). The U.S. Food and Nutrition Board (National Academy of Science, National Research Council) and Canada followed suit. The RE system of measurement takes into account the amount of absorption of the carotenes as well as the degree of conversion to vitamin A; hence, it is more precise than the IU system.

In terms of International Units, beta-carotene (by weight) is ½ as active, and the other provitamin A carotenoids are ¼ as active, as retinol. Also, retinol is completely absorbed by the intestine, but only about ⅓ of the intake of provitamin A carotenoids is absorbed. Of the absorbed carotenoids, only ½ of the beta-carotene and ¼ of the other provitamin A carotenoids are converted to retinol. It follows that beta-carotene is only ⅙ as active, and the other carotenoids ¹⁄₁₂ as active, as retinol.

The vitamin A values in the food composition tables of this book are in International Units.[5]

But the recommended daily dietary allowances (RDA) are expressed in both IU and RE.

Functions. Vitamin A is essential for a number of physiological processes: among them, (1) vision, (2) growth, (3) bone development, (4) tooth development, (5), maintenance of body epithelial tissues, (6) protective effect

---

[5]Both the FAO/WHO and the FNB recommend that, in the future, foods be analyzed separately for (1) retinol, (2) beta-carotene, and (3) other provitamin A carotenoids, for inclusion in food composition tables, and that (4) total RE, as micrograms, also be listed in the tables. Until this information is available, we will primarily employ the still widely used IU values.

against cancer, (7) reproduction, and (8) coenzyme and hormone roles.

It is noteworthy that the basic physiological functions of vitamin A are, in general, common to man and all other animals. These follow:

• **Vision**—The best understood function of vitamin A is related to the maintenance of normal vision in dim light — the prevention of night blindness. The retina of the eye — the light-sensitive inside layer at the back of the eye which may be likened to the film of a camera—contains two kinds of light receptors: the rods for vision in dim light, and the cones for vision in bright light and color vision. (The terms *rods* and *cones* are derived from the shape of the cells.) *Rhodopsin* (*visual purple*) is the pigment in the rods that contains vitamin A; iodopsin is the main pigment in the cones that contains vitamin A. All of the pigments are composed of the same vitamin A fraction (retinol) but of different proteins. Opsin is the protein of rhodopsin.

The visual cycle proceeds as follows: When light strikes the normal retina, this pigment—called rhodopsin (visual purple)—is bleached to another pigment known as retinaldehyde (visual yellow). As a result of this change, images are transmitted to the brain through the optic nerve. Rhodopsin is rebuilt in the dark, but some vitamin A is lost in the reactions, and rod vision is impaired unless sufficient vitamin A is supplied by the blood from the diet or body stores to replace it. The ability of the eyes to adjust to changes from bright light to dim light is reduced. This condition is known as *night blindness*, or nyctalopia. Fig. V-26 shows, in simplified form, the role of vitamin A in vision.

The cones are not as sensitive to changes in the amount of vitamin A as the rods. Thus, vision in bright light and color vision are not affected to any extent in the early stages of vitamin A deficiency.

Night blindness is the earliest symptom of vitamin A deficiency in humans. It first manifests itself as a slow, dark adaptation, thence it progresses to total night blindness. In man, the *dark adaptation test,* which measures the eyes' ability to recover visual activity in dim light, is used as a means of determining vitamin A status. However, night blindness or dark adaptation tests are not always reliable in diagnosing a deficiency. Measurements of serum vitamin A and carotene values in comparison with known standards are most useful. Serum levels of 10 to 19 mcg of vitamin A, or of 20 to 39 mcg of carotene, per 100 ml are considered low.

Night blindness can usually be cured in a half hour or so by the injection of vitamin A. It is noteworthy that both retinol and retinaldehyde are effective in the visual process, but retinoic acid has no visual function; if retinoic acid is the only form of vitamin A fed to experimental animals, blindness results.

In 1967, the Nobel Prize in Medicine was awarded to Dr. George Wald of Harvard University, who clarified the role of vitamin A in vision, which, to that time, had been an extremely complicated picture.

Night blindness has a long medical history, associated with diet. It is common in Newfoundland among fishermen working in open boats in bright sunshine with their eyes exposed to the glare on the water. There, it is said that if a man cannot see at night his vision will be restored by the next night if he eats the liver of a codfish or of a sea gull.

Vision can also be impaired because of *xerophthalmia* (from the *Latin* words for *dry* and *eye*), another manifestation of a vitamin A deficiency. In this condition, the conjunctiva (the covering of the eye) dries out, the cornea becomes inflamed, and the eyes become ulcerated. It may progress to blindness in extreme deficiency of vitamin A. Xerophthalmia is a very common disease in infants and undernourished children in those parts of the world where the deficiency is prevalent; but it may be prevented by including in the diet a good source of vitamin A.

• **Growth**—Vitamin A aids in the building and growth of body cells; hence, it is essential for body growth. Because of this, prior to the time that vitamin A was isolated and its chemical formula determined, its potency in food was measured by growth rate. Since animals on a vitamin A-free diet stop growing when their bodies are depleted of its stores, foods to be assessed were fed to these animals in

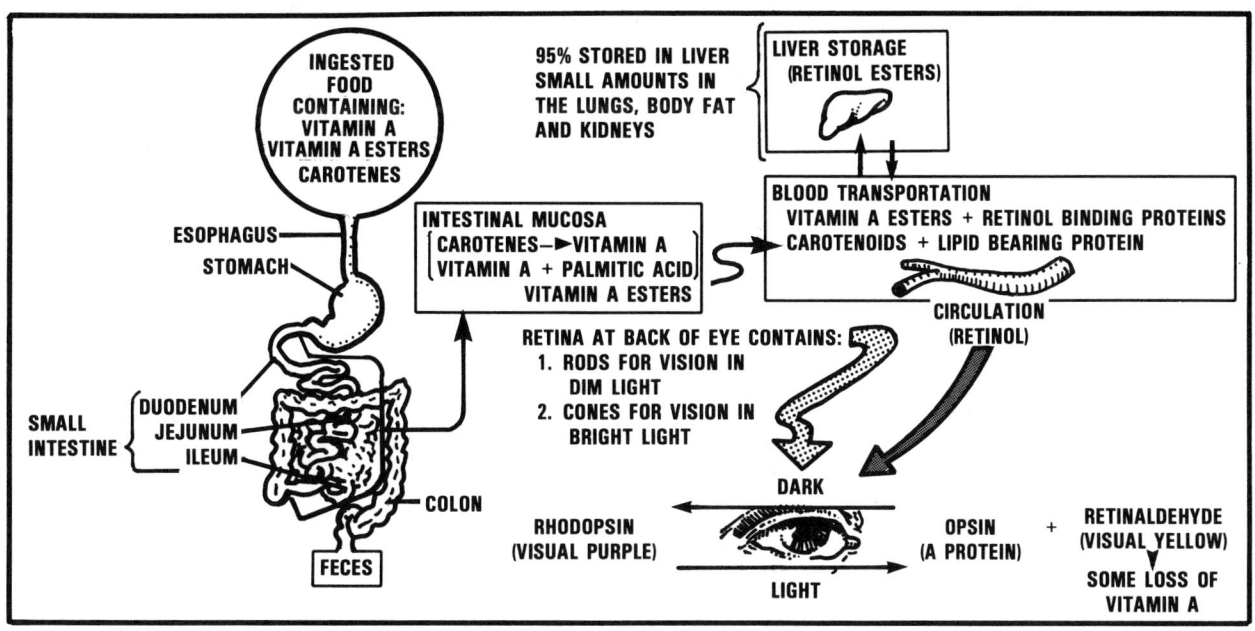

Fig. V-26. Metabolism of vitamin A and its role in vision in dim light.

known amounts for a prescribed period of time and their growth response noted. Better growth meant a higher vitamin A content in the food. Also, it has long been known that vitamin A is essential for the growth of children and for the normal development of babies before birth.

Although the relationship of vitamin A to growth was the first function studied, its role in the growth process is poorly understood. Experimental animals on vitamin A-deficient diets lose their appetites and fail to grow. The loss of appetite is attributed to the loss of the sense of taste because of keratinization (drying out) of the taste buds. When supplements of retinol or of retinoic acid are given in amounts to bring about growth, sense of taste returns to normal.

• **Bone development**—Vitamin A is especially needed for bone growth. If the intake is not sufficient, the bones will stop growth before the soft tissues are affected. Thus, if the brain and spinal cord grow too fast for the stunted skull and spinal column, injury of brain and nerves may occur and paralysis and various other neurological signs may result. In some cases, there is a constriction of the bone canal through which the optic nerve passes, thereby resulting in blindness. It is noteworthy, however, that a deficiency of vitamin A may cause degeneration of the nervous tissue without causing bone malformation.

• **Tooth development**—Vitamin A is essential for normal tooth development. Like other epithelia, the enamel-forming cells are affected by lack of vitamin A; instead of an even protective layer of enamel, fissures and pits will be present and the teeth will tend to decay. Also, when there is a shortage of vitamin A, the odontoblasts which form dentine become atrophied.

• **Maintenance of healthy epithelial tissues**—Epithelial tissues are of two kinds: (1) those that cover the outer surface of the body—the resistant, protective skin (epidermis); and (2) those that line all the tubular system—the secretory mucous membranes. Without vitamin A, the epithelial cells become dry and flat, and gradually harden to form scales that slough off. This process is known as keratinization. The skin may become rough, dry and scaly; and the membranes lining the nose, throat, and other air passages, and the gastrointestinal and genitourinary tracts, may become keratinized. Whenever these tissue changes occur, the natural mechanism for protection against bacterial invasion is impaired and the tissue may become infected easily. It follows that vitamin A deficiency commonly manifests itself in those parts that are particularly susceptible to infections. Vitamin A is also necessary for the health of the membranes lining the stomach and intestinal wall, and for the health of the sex glands, uterus, and the membranes that line the bladder and urinary passages. Renal calculi (kidney stones) may be related to the keratinization of the urinary tract.

Although adequate vitamin A is necessary to maintain healthy epithelial tissues, excessive intakes will not increase resistance to infections which enter through the epithelium.

• **Protective effects against cancer**—Vitamin A, either as retinol or carotene, appears to play an important nutritional role in keeping the body free of certain kinds of cancer, especially cancers of epithelial tissue (the skin and various membranes that line the mouth, internal passages, and hollow organs). This does not call for megadoses of vitamin A; rather, it indicates that getting sufficient vitamin A in the daily diet is likely a very important anticancer measure.

• **Reproduction**—In most animals, the absence of vitamin A in the diet will dramatically reduce reproductive ability. In the male rat, spermatogenesis stops; in the female, there may be an abnormal estrus cycle, fetal resorption, or congenital malformations. In rabbits, there is a reduction in fertility and an increase of abortion in pregnant does. Hatchability is significantly reduced when hens are fed a vitamin A-deficient ration. Lack of vitamin A in the diet of pregnant women during the first trimester (the first 3 months) may cause miscarriage.

Quite often, retinoic acid, the acid form of vitamin A, is used to study the effects of vitamin A deficiency on reproduction, because it can be substituted freely for retinol and retinaldehyde (the aldehyde form of vitamin A) for all physiological functions except reproduction and vision.

• **Coenzyme and hormone roles**—New information suggests that vitamin A (1) acts in a coenzyme role, as for instance in the form of intermediates in glycoprotein synthesis; and (2) functions like steroid hormones, with a role in the cell nuclei, leading to tissue differentiation.

• **Other functions of vitamin A**—Studies have indicated that vitamin A deficiency reduces the rate of thyroxine formation and increases the incidence of goiter in people. Also, protein synthesis is adversely affected by vitamin A deficiency. Animal studies indicate that vitamin A functions in the synthesis of corticosterone from cholesterol, resulting in a decrease in the body's capacity to synthesize glycogen.

DEFICIENCY SYMPTOMS.   A deficiency of vitamin A may be due to a dietary lack of vitamin A and/or provitamin A, or to poor absorption. A diet that contains an insufficiency of vitamin A activity will, in due time, cause night blindness, xerosis, or xerophthalmia; stunted growth; slowed bone growth; unsound teeth; rough, dry, scaly skin; increased sinus trouble, sore throat, and abscesses in the ears, mouth, or salivary glands; and increased diarrhea and kidney and bladder stones.

It is noteworthy that vitamin A deficiency symptoms, and their prominence, vary from one species to another, as is true for other vitamins. Common deficiency symptoms follow:

• **Night blindness, xerosis, and xerophthalmia**—The earliest symptom of a vitamin A deficiency is the inability to see in dim light—the condition known as night blindness (nyctalopia). Night driving—facing the bright lights of oncoming vehicles—is difficult, and even dangerous, for persons whose eyes are slow to adjust.

The next symptom (following night blindness) to appear is usually xerosis (dryness) of the conjunctiva (the delicate membrane that lines the eyelids and covers the exposed surface of the eyeball), in which there may be (1) wrinkling, pigmentation, and accumulation of debris, and (2) loss of transparency.

When associated with generalized xerosis in children, Bitot's spots (named for the French physician who first discovered them)—which appear as small plaques of silvery gray, usually with a foamy surface, on the conjunctiva—are usually caused by a deficiency of vitamin A. However, in adults these spots may have another cause.

Extreme vitamin A deficiency over a long period of time may cause xerophthalmia, characterized by the following stages: (1) the cornea (the transparent membrane that coats the outer surface of the eye) becomes dry, then inflamed and edematous; (2) the eyes become cloudy and infected, which leads to ulceration; and (3) keratomalacia, a softening and keratinizing of the cornea, culminating in permanent blindness if the disease is not arrested. Xerophthalmia occurs most frequently in undernourished infants and children in India, the Middle East, Southeast Asia, and parts of Africa and South America. It has been estimated that throughout the world (exclusive of China) about 80,000 children become blind each year from vitamin A deficiency, and that about one-half of these die.

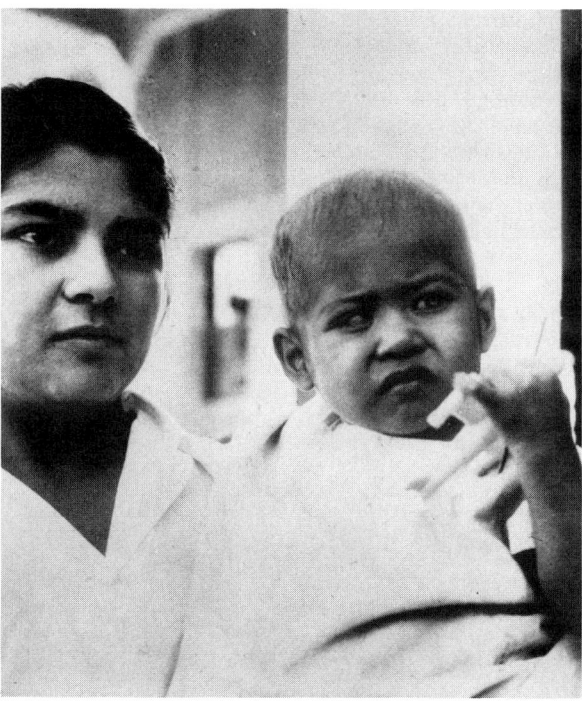

Fig. V-27. Keratomalacia, characterized by softening and ulceration of the cornea of the eye, due to a vitamin A deficiency. Unless vitamin A or carotene is provided, blindness may follow. (Courtesy, FAO, Rome, Italy)

• **Stunted growth**—A deficiency of vitamin A results in stunted growth of children.

• **Slowed bone growth**—When young animals are deprived of vitamin A, the bones fail to lengthen, and the remodeling processes necessary for the formation of compact bone cease to operate. Abnormalities in bone shape result. Bone growth in the cranium and spine slows, while nerve tissue continues to grow; sometimes this results in overcrowding of the skull and spine, and mechanical compression damage to nerve tissue with paralysis and degeneration.

• **Unsound teeth**—If a child gets too little vitamin A when his teeth are developing, the enamel forming cells become abnormal and pits are formed. Such pits may harbor food deposits, which may ferment and form acids that etch the enamel and lead to decay.

• **Rough, dry, scaly skin; increased sinus trouble, sore throat, and abscesses in ears, mouth, or salivary gland; increased diarrhea and kidney and bladder stones**—A deficiency of vitamin A injures the epithelial tissues throughout the body, and leads to a peculiar type of horny degeneration called keratinization. The epithelial cells form the outer layer of the skin and the mucous membranes that line the mouth and digestive, respiratory, and genitourinary tracts. Instead of being soft and moist, they become hard and dry. As a result, (1) the skin, especially in the areas of the arms, legs, shoulders, and lower abdomen, may become rough, dry, and scaly—a condition known as follicular hyperkeratosis or phrynoderma (it looks like *gooseflesh*); and (2) bacteria have easy access to the mucous membranes, with the result that there is increased susceptibility to infections such as sinus trouble, sore throat, and abscesses in the ears, mouth, or salivary glands. Also, certain other troubles, noninfective in character, increase as a result of the damaged epithelium, including diarrhea and the formation of kidney and bladder stones.

• **Reproductive disorders**—Deficient animals of all species studied—rat, fowl, pig, cow, sheep, dog, guinea pig, and others—show the following reproductive disorders: poor conception, abnormal embryonic growth, placental injury; and, in severe deficiency, death of the fetus. The same deficiency symptoms have been described in humans.

RECOMMENDED DAILY ALLOWANCE OF VITAMIN A.
The Food and Nutrition Board (FNB) of the National Research Council (NRC) recommended daily allowances of vitamin A are given in the section on VITAMIN(S), Table V-5, Vitamin Table.

• **Infants and children**—The daily allowance for infants from birth to 6 months is based on the average retinol content of human milk, which is about 49 mcg per 100 ml. Thus, an infant consuming 850 ml of breast milk would receive approximately 420 mcg of retinol (RE). The allowance for infants from 6 months to 1 year of age, who are fed solid foods in addition to milk, is reduced to 375 RE (280 as retinol, 95 as beta-carotene).

• **Adults**—The FNB-NRC recommended daily allowance of vitamin A for adult men is set at 1,000 mcg RE (3,333 IU). The allowance is based on the assumption that the average American diet provides half the total vitamin A activity as retinol and half as provitamin A carotenoids. In terms of Retinol Equivalents (RE), this is 750 mcg retinol (1 RE = 3.33 IU retinol) and 250 Retinol Equivalents as beta-carotene (1 RE = 10 IU beta-carotene) for a total of 1,000 RE.

Because the body size of women is usually smaller than that of men, the RDA of vitamin A for adult women is set at 80% of that of men, or 800 mcg RE (2,667 IU).

• **Pregnancy and lactation**—During pregnancy, the RDA remains the same as for adult women, but during lactation, the RDA is increased to 1,200 mcg RE (4,000 IU) to compensate for the vitamin A secreted in breast milk.

• **Therapeutic uses**—Retinol is valuable in the treatment of night blindness and xerophthalmia, malabsorption syndrome or obstructive jaundice, and malnourished people who show Bitot's spots or follicular keratosis.

For the prevention of blindness in vitamin A-deficient children, massive doses of vitamin A (200,000 IU) by mouth at 6-month intervals have been effective.

• **Vitamin A intake in average U.S. diet**—The vitamin A value of foods available in the United States amounts to about 1,630 RE per person per day: 44.3% of which is from fruits and vegetables; 31.7% from fats, oils, and dairy products; 24.6% from meat, fish, and eggs; and 4% from miscellaneous foods. This does not account for subsequent losses in processing, cooking, and storage.

Vegetarians will need to increase their intake of provitamin A carotenoids in order to meet the recommended allowances.

Vitamin A is efficiently stored in the liver, and well-nourished persons have several months' supply that the body can utilize.

TOXICITY (Hypervitaminosis A). Excessive intake of preformed vitamin A, called hypervitaminosis A, may cause serious injury to health. However, massive intakes of carotene are not harmful because they are not converted to vitamin A rapidly enough to cause toxicity. The excess carotene will merely produce a yellow coloration of the skin, which disappears when the intake is reduced.

Symptoms of vitamin A toxicity are: loss of appetite, headache, blurred vision, excessive irritability, loss of hair, drying and flaking of the skin (with itching), swelling over the long bones, drowsiness, diarrhea, nausea, and enlargement of the liver and spleen. The most direct and positive diagnosis of hypervitaminosis A is the determination of the vitamin A concentration in the plasma or serum from a fasting blood sample. Values higher than 100 mcg per 100 ml (normal 20 to 60 mcg/100 ml) can be considered suspect, whereas values greater than this indicate toxicity.

Poisoning of men and dogs from eating polar bear liver has been reported in the Arctic since 1596. Polar bear liver contains 13,000 to 18,000 IU of vitamin A per gram. It is estimated that a hungry Arctic explorer may eat about 500 g of liver per day, containing about 9,000,000 IU of vitamin A.

Chronic toxic symptoms (hypervitaminosis A) may occur in adults who receive doses of vitamin A in excess of 50,000 IU daily over a prolonged period. Lesser doses will produce symptoms in children; infants who receive 18,500 IU daily may show signs of toxicity within 12 weeks. Acute toxicity occurs in adults who are given massive doses of 2 to 5 million IU daily, and in infants from doses as low as 75,000 to 300,000 IU daily. Vitamin C can help prevent the harmful effects of vitamin A toxicity. When excess intake of vitamin A is discontinued, recovery is usually rapid and complete; in some cases, the toxicity symptoms disappear within 72 hours.

On the basis of the evidence presently available, prolonged daily doses of vitamin A to adults in excess of 50,000 IU, and to infants in excess of 18,500 IU, should be under the supervision of a qualified physician or nutritionist.

VITAMIN A LOSSES DURING PROCESSING, COOKING, AND STORAGE. The carotene losses of vegetables following harvest tend to parallel the degree of wilting. In order to conserve their maximum carotene value, they should be stored at low temperatures or be quick frozen.

Freezing and freeze-drying causes little loss. But drying of eggs, vegetables or fruits, with exposure to air, sunlight, or high temperatures, may cause serious loss of vitamin A value.

Because vitamin A and the carotenes are insoluble in water and stable to heat at ordinary cooking temperatures, it was once thought that little vitamin A activity was lost from foods in cooking and processing, *unless* they were exposed to air. However, cooking or canning vegetables produces a rearrangement of atoms in the carotene molecule, resulting in carotenes of substantially lower vitamin A value. It is estimated that, on the average, the vitamin A value of cooked green vegetables is decreased by 15 to 20% and the value of yellow vegetables by 30 to 35%.

Both vitamin A and the carotenoids are easily oxidized and rapidly destroyed on exposure to ultraviolet light, with the rate of destruction influenced by the associated substances and the temperature and moisture conditions. Butter exposed in thin layers in air at 122°F (*50°C*) loses all of its vitamin A potency in 6 hours, but in the absence of air there is little destruction at 248°F (*120°C*) over the same period. Yellow corn has been reported to lose as much as 60% of its carotene in 7 months' storage.

Animal fats should be kept in a cold, dark place; and fish liver oils should be protected from light by being kept in dark bottles. Rancid fat destroys both vitamin A and carotene. Also, minerals such as iron oxide, charcoal, sulfur, ground limestone, bone meal, manganese, and iodine, contribute to the destruction of vitamin A in foods.

SOURCES OF VITAMIN A. Grouping by rank of common sources of vitamin A is given in the section on VITAMIN(S), Table V-5, Vitamin Table.

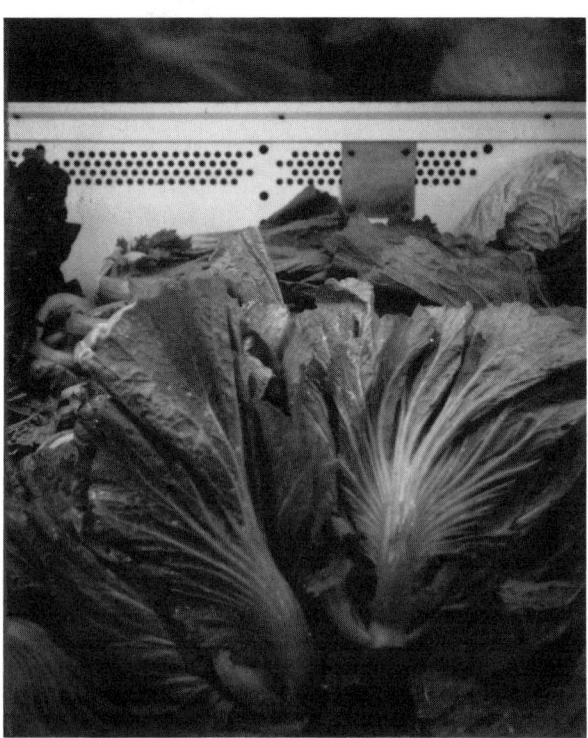

Fig. V-28. Green mustard cabbage. Dark green leafy vegetables are a good source of vitamin A. (Courtesy, Department of Food Science and Human Nutrition, University of Hawaii)

For additional sources and more precise values of vitamin A, see Food Composition Table F-21.

Only animal foods contain vitamin A as such. Although they are usually classed as food supplements rather than foods, the fish liver oils are the richest natural sources. Fish eat smaller fish or crustaceans, which, in turn, have fed on marine plants that contain provitamins A. Herbivorous animals eat green plants and convert these substances into the vitamin itself in their bodies. Carnivorous animals get the vitamin from feeding on plant-eating animals. The cow and the hen are efficient in converting the provitamins A in plant foods into the vitamin A in milk fat and eggs, respectively; and into the vitamin A in their body tissues. But some provitamin A in the diet escapes their conversion, with the result that milk fat, egg yolk, and other animal products contain a mixture of vitamin A and its plant precursors. The proportion of each depends partly on the animal species, or even the breed, and partly on the feed consumed. For example, the *golden* color of Guernsey milk is due to the high content of provitamin A, while whiter Holstein milk contains a higher proportion of vitamin A. But both milks have about the same amount of total vitamin A activity.

Also, the vitamin A value of animal foods varies widely according to the vitamin A value of the feed of the animals that produced them. For example, livers from older animals and from animals on green grass are higher in vitamin A than the livers of younger animals on dry, bleached feeds; and the butterfat in milk is usually yellower and of higher vitamin A value when the cows are grazing on green pastures than when they are confined to a corral.

The principal source of vitamin A in the diet is likely to be from the carotenes, which are widespread in those plant foods that have high green or yellow colorings. There is a direct correlation between the greenness of a leaf and its carotene content; dark-green leaves, such as beet greens, collards, dandelion greens, kale, mustard greens, spinach, Swiss chard, and turnip greens, are rich in carotene, but pale leaves, like cabbage and lettuce, are insignificant sources. The yellow vegetables and fruits, such as carrots, apricots, cantaloupe, peaches, pumpkins, squash (winter), sweet potatoes, and yellow corn, are rich in provitamin A carotenoids.

• **Synthetic vitamin A**—Today, synthetic forms of vitamin A are the most potent and inexpensive sources. They are just as effective and safe as the natural forms, but it must be remembered that they contain no other nutrients.

(Also see VITAMIN[S], Table V-5.)

VITAMIN A DEFICIENCY

This refers to an insufficiency of vitamin A, which may be due to either (1) a dietary lack of vitamin A and/or provitamin A, or (2) poor absorption.

(Also see VITAMIN A, sections headed "Deficiency Symptoms;" and "Blindness Due to Vitamin A Deficiency.")

VITAMIN ANTAGONIST

A substance so similar in structure to the vitamin that the body accepts it in place of the vitamin is known as a vitamin antagonist. But the antagonist is unable to perform the functions of the true vitamin.

VITAMIN B-6 (PYRIDOXINE; PYRIDOXAL; PYRIDOXAMINE)

VITAMIN B-6

PROMOTES GROWTH AND FEATHERING IN CHICKS.
IT'S ESSENTIAL FOR HUMANS, TOO.

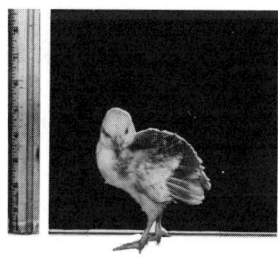
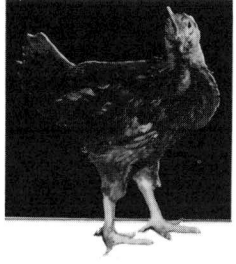

VITAMIN B-6 MADE THE DIFFERENCE! LEFT: CHICK SHOWS RETARDED GROWTH AND ABNORMAL FEATHERING DUE TO VITAMIN B-6 DEFICIENCY. RIGHT: NORMAL, CONTROL CHICK. (COURTESY, G.F. COMBS, UNIVERSITY OF GEORGIA)

TOP FOOD SOURCES

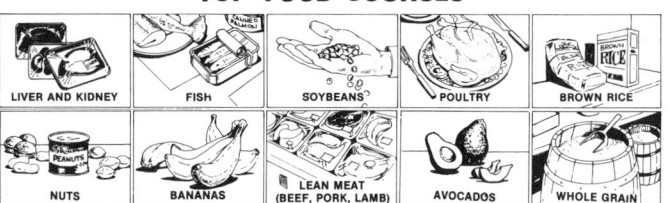

Fig. V-29. The vitamin B-6 story.

By official action of the Society of Biological Chemists and the American Institute of Nutrition, vitamin B-6 is now the approved collective name for three closely related naturally occurring compounds with potential vitamin B-6 activity: pyridoxine, pyridoxal, and pyridoxamine. Pyridoxine is found largely in vegetable products, whereas the pyridoxal and pyridoxamine forms occur primarily in animal products. There is no information on the relative biological activity of the three compounds in man, but in rats they are equally active if given parenterally (injected intramuscularly or intravenously).

The need for vitamin B-6 was first demonstrated in rats, but it is now established that it is also a dietary essential for the human, pig, chick, dog, and other species, including microorganisms.

HISTORY.

In 1926, Goldberger and Lillie conducted an experiment designed to produce pellagra in rats. A severe dermatitis resulted, which was believed to be analogous to pellagra. In 1934, the Hungarian scientist, Gyorgy, produced a cure for this condition with an extract from yeast; but the curative compound of the extract was neither thiamin, niacin, nor riboflavin, but a substance which he called *vitamin B-6*. In 1938, five different laboratories, working independently, isolated the vitamin in crystalline form, but credit for obtaining the first crystals is generally given to Lepkovsky of the University of California. In 1939, Stiller *et al.*, of Merck and Co., established the chemical structure of the vitamin; and Harris and Folkers, of Merck, along with Kuhn, the German scientist, synthesized the compound.

When the vitamin was first isolated, the German biochemists gave it the name of adermin, while American researchers called it pyridoxine. Because the compound has a pyridine ring (five carbon and one nitrogen) and three hydroxy groups, Gyorgy, the Hungarian, expressed preference for the name pyridoxine, which became widely adopted.

In 1942, Snell discovered the vitamin B-6 activity of two closely related substances in natural products, which he named pyridoxal and pyridoxamine. Umbreit followed in 1945 with a report of the coenzyme functions of the vitamin in phosphate forms.

CHEMISTRY, METABOLISM, PROPERTIES.

• **Chemistry**—Vitamin B-6 is found in foods in three forms which are readily interconvertible—pyridoxine, pyridoxal, and pyridoxamine. Also vitamin B-6 is found in physiological systems in the forms of pyridoxal phosphate and pyridoxamine phosphate. The structural formulas of the three naturally occurring free forms of these compounds are given in Fig. V-30.

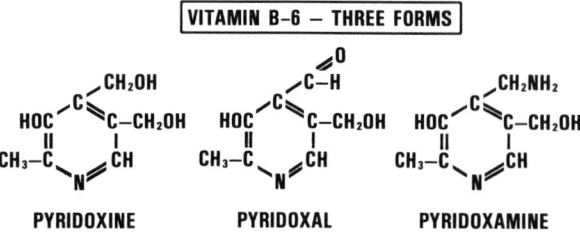

Fig. V-30. Structure of pyridoxine, pyridoxal, and pyridoxamine.

• **Metabolism**—In the free form, vitamin B-6 is absorbed rapidly from the upper part of the small intestine, thence it enters the body by the portal vein. It is present in most body tissues, with a high concentration in the liver. It is secreted into milk and excreted primarily via the urine. Measurement of B-6 in the urine is the assay method used in nutrition surveys.

• **Properties**—Vitamin B-6 is readily soluble in water, quite stable to heat and acid, but easily destroyed by oxidation and exposure to alkali and ultraviolet light. All three forms are white crystalline substances.

Of the three forms, pyridoxine is more resistant to food processing and storage conditions and probably represents the principal form in food products.

MEASUREMENT/ASSAY.

No international standard or unit system of vitamin B-6 is in current usage. Analytical results are expressed in weight units of pyridoxine hydrochloride. One milligram of pyridoxine hydrochloride is equivalent to 0.82 mg pyridoxine or 0.81 mg pyridoxal, or 0.82 mg pyridoxamine.

The vitamin B-6 content in foods and tissues is determined by microbiological assay, chemical methods, and animal bioassays. The animal bioassays, using either the rat or chick, are time consuming, expensive, and variable; therefore, they have been generally replaced by microbiological and chemical methods.

FUNCTIONS.

Vitamin B-6, in its coenzyme forms, usually as pyridoxal phosphate but sometimes as pyridoxamine phosphate, is involved in a large number of physiologic functions, particularly in protein (nitrogen) metabolism, and to a lesser extent in carbohydrate and fat metabolism. Also, it appears to hold a key role in a number of chemical problems. Discussion follows:

• **Vitamin B-6 in protein metabolism**—Vitamin B-6 in its phosphorylated forms is active metabolically in the following types of reactions in amino acid metabolism:

1. **Transamination.** It is involved in shifting an amino group (NH_2) from a donor amino acid to an acceptor acid to form another amino acid. This reaction is important in the formation of nonessential amino acids. Transamination is illustrated in Fig. V-31.

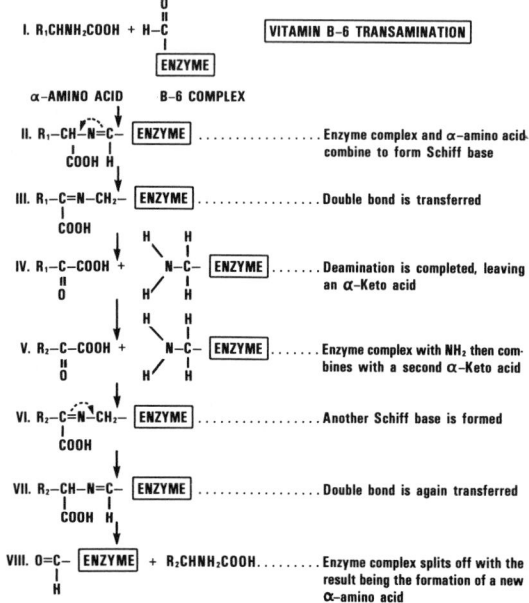

Fig. V-31. Vitamin B-6 in transamination.

2. **Decarboxylation.** It is active in the removal of the carboxyl groups (COOH) from certain amino acids to form another compound. Decarboxylation is necessary for the synthesis of serotonin, norepinephrine, and histamine from tryptophan, tyrosine, and histidine, respectively.

3. **Deamination.** It aids in deamination. By removing amino groups (NH_2) from amino acids not needed for growth, it helps to render carbon residues available for energy.

4. **Transulfuration.** It aids in the transfer of sulfhydryl-group (HS) from the amino acid methionine to another amino acid (serine) to form the amino acid cysteine.

5. **Tryptophan conversion to niacin (nicotinic acid).** It assists in forming niacin (nicotinic acid) from tryptophan, thereby playing a role in the niacin supply.

6. **Hemoglobin formation.** It is necessary for the formation of a precursor of porphyrin compounds which is part of the hemoglobin molecule.

7. **Absorption of amino acids.** Vitamin B-6 is believed to play a role in the absorption of amino acids from the intestine.

• **Vitamin B-6 in carbohydrate and fat metabolism**—Vitamin B-6 in its phosphorylated forms also plays a role in carbohydrate and fat metabolism, although this role is less important than protein metabolism:

1. **Catabolism of glycogen.** It is an essential part of phosphorylase, the enzyme that brings about the conversion of glycogen to glucose-1-phosphate in muscle and liver.

2. **Fatty acid metabolism.** It takes part in fat metabolism, although the exact mode of action is unknown; for example, it is believed to be involved in the conversion of the essential unsaturated fatty acid, linoleic acid, to another fatty acid, arachidonic acid.

• **Clinical problems of pyridoxine deficiency**—It seems apparent that vitamin B-6 is also involved in a number of clinical problems; among them, the following:

1. **Central nervous system disturbances.** It assists in energy transformation in brain and nerve tissue; hence, the functioning of the central nervous system. When vitamin B-6 is lacking, convulsive seizures occur in both human infants and experimental animals.

2. **Autism.** This is a severe disturbance of mental and emotional development in young children, characterized chiefly by withdrawal from reality and lack of responsiveness or interest in other people in the normal activities of childhood. Although more experimental work is needed, nine studies reported in the world literature show that megadoses of vitamin B-6 are helpful in treating autism.[6]

3. **Anemia.** In studies on human subjects, vitamin B-6 has been effective in treating anemia that does not respond to iron—so-called iron-resistant anemia.

4. **Kidney stones.** It has been reported that a deficiency of vitamin B-6 causes increased urinary excretion of oxalates; thus, a lack of the vitamin may result in the formation of kidney stones.

5. **Tuberculosis.** The drug isoniazid (isonicotinic acid hydrazide, INH), which is used as a chemotherapeutic agent in treating tuberculosis, has been shown to be an antagonist to pyridoxine, causing a side effect of neuritis in some patients. Treatment with large doses (50 to 100 mg daily) of pyridoxine prevents this effect.

6. **Physiologic demands in pregnancy.** Pyridoxine defi-

ciencies during pregnancy have been demonstrated and subsequently corrected by supplementation with vitamin B-6.

7. **Oral contraceptives.** Some women on estrogen-progesterone oral contraceptives appear to require additional vitamin B-6.

• **Other functions**—It appears from experimental studies that vitamin B-6 is involved in—

1. Antibody formation, for protection against infectious diseases, although this role is unproved.
2. Messenger RNA synthesis.
3. Nucleic acid metabolism.
4. Endocrine gland functions.
5. Biosynthesis of coenzyme A.

DEFICIENCY SYMPTOMS. It is difficult to produce a dietary deficiency of vitamin B-6 in human beings because it is so widely distributed in foods. The characteristic symptoms are: skin lesions—especially at the tip of the nose, anemia, convulsive seizures, and reduced antibody production. In adults, there may also be depression and confusion. If the vitamin B-6 deficiency is prolonged, the symptoms may include dizziness, nausea, vomiting, and kidney stones.

Experimentally, vitamin B-6 deficiency in adults has been produced by using a low vitamin B-6 diet along with one of the antagonists of the vitamin—desoxypyridoxine. After 2 to 3 weeks, the following symptoms were noted: greasy scaliness (seborrheic dermatitis) in the skin around the eyes, nose, and mouth, which subsequently spread to other parts of the body; a smooth, red tongue; loss of weight; muscular weakness; irritability; and mental depression. Administration of as little as 5 mg of pyridoxine, pyridoxal, or pyridoxamine daily corrected all the abnormalities in a few days.

The effects of vitamin B-6 deprivation appear to be more dramatic in infants than in adults.

RECOMMENDED DAILY ALLOWANCE OF VITAMIN B-6. The Food and Nutrition Board (FNB) of the National Research Council (NRC) recommended daily allowances of vitamin B-6 are given in the sections on VITAMIN(S), Table V-5, Vitamin Table.

The establishment of allowances for vitamin B-6 is complicated by the following facts: (1) the requirement varies with dietary protein intake—there is increased need for vitamin B-6 with increased intakes of protein; (2) the uncertainty of the availability of the vitamin in the diet; and (3) the uncertainty as to the extent of intestinal bacterial synthesis of the vitamin, and the degree to which it is utilized by the body. Also, there is evidence of increased need of the vitamin in pregnancy and lactation, in the elderly, and in various pathologic and genetic disturbances. Nevertheless, the NRC has set recommended allowances to assure a safety margin and to make a deficiency unlikely under most circumstances. Discussion follows:

• **Recommended allowance for infants**—Although based on limited information, a recommended dietary allowance of 0.3 mg of vitamin B-6 per day is considered adequate for the young infant. For older infants (0.5 to 1.0 year of age) consuming a mixed diet, a daily allowance of 0.6 mg of vitamin B-6 is recommended.

• **Recommended allowance for children and adolescents**—The recommended allowances for children range from 1.0 mg to 1.4 mg per day, depending on age.

• **Recommended allowance for adults**—For males 11–14 years = 1.7 mg; 15 years and over = 2.0 mg. Females 11–14 years = 1.4 mg; 15–18 years = 1.5 mg; 19 and over = 1.6 mg.

[6]Rimland, Bernard, Ph.D., Letters (to the editor), *Science News*, Vol. 119, No. 16, April 18, 1981, p. 243.

• **Recommended allowance for pregnancy**—Theoretically, several factors imply an increased need for vitamin B-6 in pregnancy: (1) because vitamin B-6 requirements increase with increasing protein in the diet, the extra protein allowance for the pregnant woman necessitates a modest increase in intake of the vitamin; (2) all forms of vitamin B-6 cross the placenta readily and are concentrated in the fetal blood; and (3) estrogens apparently increase tryptophan oxygenase activity, which will result in need for additional vitamin B-6.

An additional allowance of 0.6 mg of vitamin B-6 per day (for a total allowance of 2.2 mg/day) is recommended during gestation.

• **Recommended allowance for lactation**—The content of vitamin B-6 in milk appears to reflect the nutritional state of the mother with respect to the vitamin.

An additional allowance of 0.5 mg of vitamin B-6/day (for a total allowance of 2.1 mg/day) is recommended during lactation.

• **Vitamin B-6 and oral contraceptive agents**—Recent studies indicate that the vitamin B-6 requirement for most oral contraceptive users is approximately the same as that for nonusers; thus, the current evidence does not appear to justify the routine supplementation of the dietary vitamin B-6 with pyridoxine. However, some women report that depression occurs when they are taking oral contraceptives, probably as a result of the failure to convert tryptophan to serotonin, a neurotransmitter in the brain. When this problem occurs, the physician may suggest higher levels of vitamin B-6 (about 30 mg daily) in order to normalize tryptophan metabolism.

• **Vitamin B-6 intake in average U.S. diets**—According to the U.S. Department of Agriculture, the overall average per capita availability of vitamin B-6 per day in the United States is 2.2 mg, not including waste or cooking losses. Also, it is noteworthy that 40.5% of the available vitamin B-6 is provided by meat, poultry, and fish.

TOXICITY. Although vitamin B-6 is relatively nontoxic, side effects, such as sleepiness, may follow injection of large doses. Also, it may be habit-forming when taken in large doses over an extended period; a vitamin B-6 dependency has been induced in normal human adults given a supplement of 200 mg of pyridoxine daily for 33 days while on a normal diet.

VITAMIN LOSSES DURING PROCESSING, COOKING, AND STORAGE. More than 75% of the vitamin B-6 content of wheat is lost in milling white flour. Although vitamin B-6 is not added in white flour enrichment programs, perhaps it should be.

Canning and freezing result in considerable losses of vitamin B-6 with the losses being smaller in frozen foods. Freeze-dehydration and subsequent storage appear to have no adverse effect on the vitamin B-6 content of meat and poultry.

Considerable losses of vitamin B-6 occur during cooking. Beef loses 25 to 50% of its raw vitamin B-6 content in cooking, with the losses higher from oven braising than from oven roasting. Home cooking of fruits and vegetables results in a loss of about 50% of the vitamin B-6.

Storage losses appear to be minimal. Studies have shown that the storage of potatoes for as long as 6 months at 40°F (4.4°C) results in no loss of the vitamin.

Henry A. Schroeder, M.D., of the Dartmouth Medical School, conducted an extensive survey of the B-6 content in hundreds of common foods, and found that modern processing was causing massive losses of the vitamin. His studies showed B-6 losses as follows: From milling wheat and making all-purpose flour, 82.3%; from canning vegetables, 57 to 77%; from freezing vegetables, 37 to 56%; from canning meat and poultry, 42.6%; and from canning seafood, 48.9%.[7]

SOURCES OF VITAMIN B-6. In animal tissues and yeast, vitamin B-6 occurs mainly as pyridoxal and pyridoxamine. In plants, all three members of the vitamin are found, but pyridoxine predominates. The occurrence of vitamin B-6 in various forms has complicated the task of determining the content of the vitamin in foods.

Although vitamin B-6 is widely distributed in foods, many sources provide very small amounts. Thus, there is concern, as well as ever-increasing evidence, that in more than a few instances normal diets may be borderline or low in this vitamin.

Groupings by rank of common food sources of vitamin B-6 are given in the section on VITAMIN(S), Table V-5, Vitamin Table.

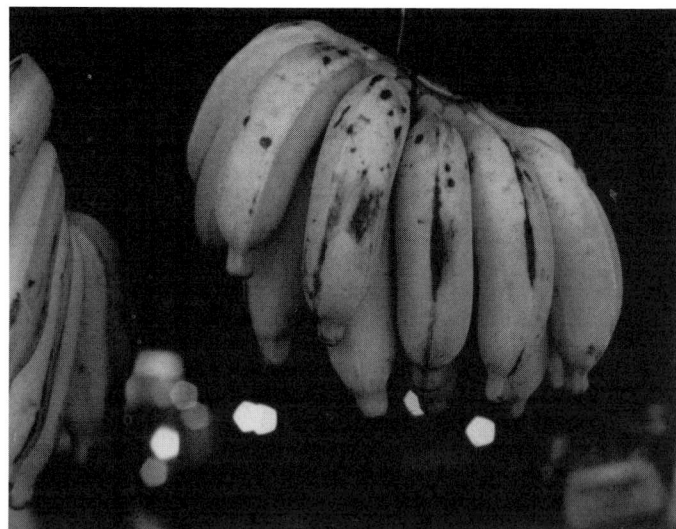

Fig. V-32. Bananas, a good source of vitamin B-6. (Courtesy, Department of Food Science and Human Nutrition, University of Hawaii)

For additional sources and more precise values of vitamin B-6 (pyridoxine), see Food Composition Table F-21.

Fat and sugar, which supply over ⅓ of the energy intake of the average American, are devoid of vitamin B-6. Generally speaking, processed or refined foods are much lower in vitamin B-6 than the original food; thus, white bread, rice, noodles, macaroni, and spaghetti are all quite low in vitamin B-6.

There is evidence that intestinal bacteria produce vitamin B-6. But the extent of this source, and the degree to which the bacterial-synthesized vitamin is utilized by the body, are undetermined.

Because vitamin B-6 is important for buoyant good health, and because it is limited in many foods, supplemental vitamin B-6 may be indicated, especially for infants and during pregnancy and lactation.

(Also see VITAMIN[S], Table V-5.)

[7]Schroeder, Henry A., M.D., "Losses of Vitamins and Trace Minerals Resulting From Processing and Preservation of Foods," *The American Journal of Chemical Nutrition*, Vol. 24, May 1971, pp. 562-573.

VITAMIN B-12 (COBALAMINS)

Vitamin B-12, like so many other members of the B complex, is not a single substance; rather, it consists of several closely related compounds with similar activity. The term *cobalamins* is applied to this group of substances because all of them contain cobalt. Vitamin B-12, which is the most active member, is cyanocobalamin, named after the cyanide ion in the molecule. Other chemically related compounds known to have vitamin B-12 activity include hydroxocobalamin, nitritocobalamin, and thiocyanate cobalamin.

The most distinguishing characteristics of vitamin B-12 are: (1) unlike any other vitamin, the inability of higher plants to synthesize it (although it can be synthesized by animals); and (2) its most important deficiency state—Addisonian pernicious anemia, named after Thomas Addison, a physician working in London, who first described the malady in 1849. The anemia progressed slowly and ended with the death of the patient in 2 to 5 years. So feared and fatal was its course that it became known as pernicious anemia.

HISTORY. For 77 years (from 1849 to 1926) following the description of pernicious anemia by Thomas Addison of England, there was no hope for victims of the disease. Finally, step by step, scientists evolved with the treatment for Addisonian pernicious anemia and the discovery of vitamin B-12, a chronological record of which follows:

1. In 1925, George Hoyt Whipple, the Dean of the School of Medicine and Dentistry, University of Rochester, from 1921 to 1953, showed that liver was a great benefit in blood regeneration in dogs rendered anemic by bleeding.

2. In 1926, Minot and Murphy of the Harvard Medical School reported that feeding large amounts of raw liver (¼ to ½ lb per day) restored the normal level of red blood cells in cases of pernicious anemia. For this discovery, they shared a Nobel Prize with Whipple.

Following the report of Minot and Murphy, liver concentrates were developed, alleviating the necessity of eating large quantities of this food; and biochemists began a long series of studies to isolate the active component present in liver, which, at the time, was called the *antipernicious anemia factor*.

3. In 1929, W. B. Castle of Harvard showed that pernicious anemia could be controlled by feeding patients beef muscle incubated in normal gastric juice, although neither beef muscle nor gastric juice was effective alone. This finding

VITAMIN B-12
IT'S ESSENTIAL FOR HUMANS, TOO!

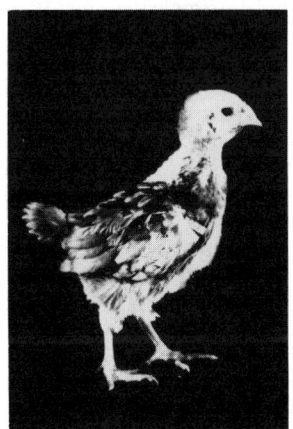 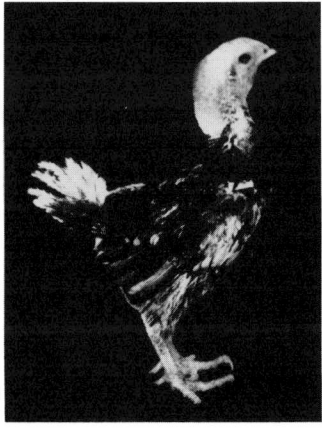

VITAMIN B-12 MADE THE DIFFERENCE! THE BIGGER CHICK AT THE RIGHT AND HIS SMALLER COMPANION ARE BOTH 3½ WEEKS OLD. LEFT: THE SMALL CHICK, FED A RATION DEFICIENT IN VITAMIN B-12, WEIGHED 157 g. RIGHT: THE LARGER CHICK, FED THE SAME RATION PLUS VITAMIN B-12, WEIGHED 280 g. (COURTESY, MERCK AND COMPANY, RAHWAY, N.J.)

TOP FOOD SOURCES

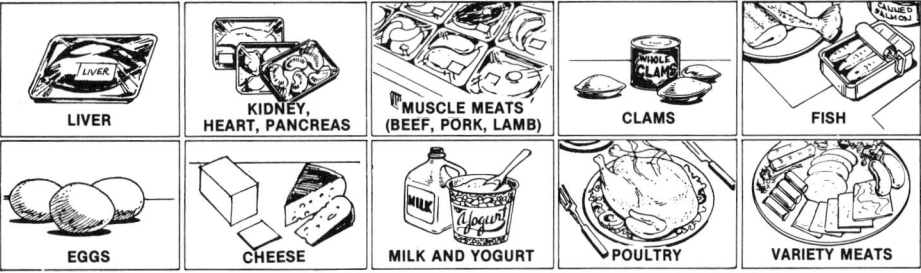

Fig. V-33. The vitamin B-12 (cobalamins) story.

led him to postulate that two factors were involved: one an *extrinsic factor* in food, and the other an *intrinsic factor* in normal gastric secretion; which, given together, caused red blood cell formation in pernicious anemia.

4.   In 1948, two groups of researchers working independently, Rickes and co-workers of Merck and Co., Inc. of New Jersey, and Smith and Parker of England, isolated from a liver concentrate a crystalline, red pigment, which they called vitamin B-12.

5.   In 1948, R. West, of Columbia University, New York, showed that injections of vitamin B-12 induced a dramatic beneficial response in patients with pernicious anemia.

6.   In 1955, the structure of vitamin B-12 (cyanocobalamin) was determined by Dorothy Hodgkin and co-workers, at Oxford. Later (1964), Hodgkin was awarded the Nobel Prize.

7.   In 1955, Woodward's group at Harvard synthesized vitamin B-12 using a very complicated and expensive procedure. Fortunately, soon thereafter, it was found that highly active vitamin B-12 concentrates can be produced from cultures of certain bacteria and fungi grown in large tanks containing special media; and this remains the main method of commercial production.

CHEMISTRY, METABOLISM, PROPERTIES.

• **Chemistry**—Vitamin B-12 is the largest and the most complex of all vitamin molecules. The main part of the molecule consists of a porphyrin ring containing cobalt as the central element. A cyanide (-CN) group may be attached to the cobalt, in which case the compound is called cyanocobalamin (or vitamin B-12); the commercially available form of the vitamin, little of which occurs naturally. The cyanide group attachment to the cobalt can be replaced by a hydroxy group (-OH), giving hydroxocobalamin, the common naturally occurring form of the vitamin; or it can be replaced by a nitrite group ($-NO_2$), giving nitritocobalamin, a form found in certain bacteria.

A coenzyme form of vitamin B-12 contains an adenosine (a nucleoside, which consists of a purine [adenine] combined with a pentose sugar, ribose) molecule in place of the cyanide and is thought to be the most common form in foods. Methylcobalamin is another form of the vitamin with a coenzyme role. All these forms have approximately equal vitamin B-12 activity in the diet.

The structure of vitamin B-12 ($C_{63} H_{90} O_{14} N_{14} PCo$) is shown in Fig. V-34.

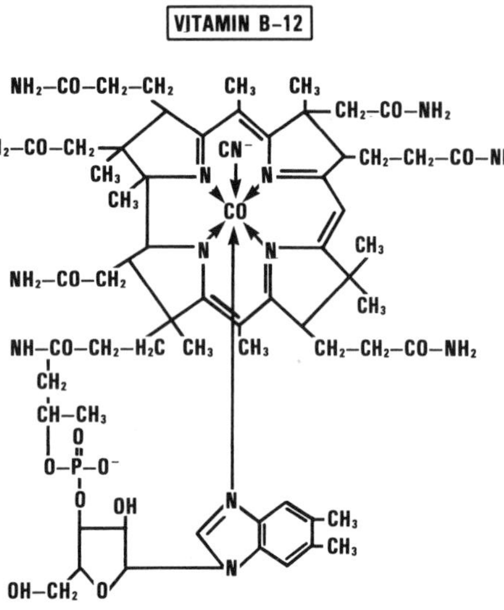

Fig. V-34. Structure of vitamin B-12.

Vitamin B-12 occurs as a protein complex in animal proteins. The ultimate source, however, is the microorganisms in the gastrointestinal tract of herbivorous animals. Such microorganisms are found in large amounts in the rumen (the first stomach) of cows and sheep. Apparently, some synthesis occurs in the intestinal bacteria of man, also; but the amount supplied from this source is small and unknown.

• **Metabolism**—It is noteworthy (1) that vitamin B-12 is the only vitamin that requires a specific gastrointestinal tract secretion for its absorption (*intrinsic factor*); and (2) that the absorption of vitamin B-12 in the small intestine requires about 3 hours (compared to seconds for most other water-soluble vitamins). The absorption of vitamin B-12 involves the following five steps:

1.   First, vitamin B-12 is released from the protein (the peptide bonds) to which it is linked in foods by the action of hydrochloric acid and intestinal enzymes.

2.   Next, vitamin B-12 is bound to a highly specific glycoprotein, Castle's intrinsic factor, which is secreted in the stomach.

3.   The vitamin B-12 intrinsic factor forms a complex with calcium and passes through the upper part of the small intestine to receptor sites in the ileum through which absorption of vitamin B-12 takes place.

4.   In crossing the intestinal mucosa, vitamin B-12 is freed from the complex (the B-12-intrinsic-factor-calcium complex).

5.   In the intestinal cells, vitamin B-12 is transferred to a plasma transport protein known as transcobalamin II, for transport in the blood circulation.

In normal persons, from 30 to 70% of the vitamin B-12 is absorbed as outlined above, in comparison with 1 to 3% absorbed by simple diffusion. Pernicious anemia results from a complete failure to absorb the vitamin, a condition caused by gastric abnormality (usually lack of intrinsic factor). Hence, therapeutic doses of B-12 given to pernicious anemia patients usually must be administered intramuscularly.

Intrinsic factor regulates the amount of absorption of vitamin B-12 to about 1.5 to 3.0 mcg daily. Absorption decreases with age (it drops to about 5% in the elderly), and with iron and vitamin B-6 deficiencies; and it increases with pregnancy. Infant levels are approximately twice that of the mother. Also, absorption is greater if the vitamin is provided in three meals than if all of it is provided in a single meal.

The liver is the principal site of storage of vitamin B-12; normally, it contains 2,000 to 5,000 mcg, sufficient to take care of the body needs for 3 to 5 years. Small amounts of vitamin B-12 are stored in the kidneys, muscle, lungs, and spleen. Storage in the bone marrow is limited, amounting to only 1 to 2% of that in the liver.

Vitamin B-12 is excreted by way of the kidneys and in the bile.

The most useful measurement for the detection of a vitamin B-12 deficiency is the serum vitamin B-12 level. Normal serum levels of vitamin B-12 range from 200 to 700 picograms (1 pg = 10^{-12} g per milliliter).

• **Properties**—The deep-red needlelike crystals are slightly soluble in water, stable to heat, but destroyed by light and by strong acid or alkaline solutions. There is little loss (only about 30%) of the vitamin by ordinary cooking procedures.

Vitamin B-12 is remarkably potent. It has a biologic activity 11,000 times that of the standard liver concentrate formerly used in the treatment of pernicious anemia.

MEASUREMENT/ASSAY.   No International Units have been defined for the biological activity of vitamin B-12.

However, pure cobalamin can be used as a standard substance. Vitamin B-12 is measured in micrograms or picograms (pg, micromicrograms).

High potency preparations of vitamin B-12 are usually assayed by spectrophotometry. Also, vitamin B-12 may be assayed colorimetrically or fluorometrically. Some assays involve measurement of cobalt. However, food sources are usually assayed for vitamin B-12 by either (1) the microbiological method, or (2) the biological method, using chicks or rats.

FUNCTIONS.   In the human body, vitamin B-12 is converted to a coenzyme form, if it is not already in such form. There are two active coenzyme forms: Coenzyme B-12 (adenosylcobalamin), and methyl B-12 (methylcobalamin). Coenzyme B-12 has an adenosine ribonucleoside attached to the cobalt atom in the vitamin B-12 molecule in place of the cyanide group, whereas methyl B-12 contains a methyl group in place of the cyanide group. The conversion of vitamin B-12 to coenzyme forms requires many nutrients, including riboflavin, niacin, and magnesium.

Vitamin B-12 coenzymes perform the following physiological roles at the cellular level, especially in the cells of the bone marrow, nervous tissue, and gastrointestinal tract:

1. **Red blood cell formation and control of pernicious anemia.** Vitamin B-12 is essential for the blood-forming organs of the bone marrow to function properly. Without sufficient B-12 coenzymes, the red blood cells do not mature normally, with the result that large, immature cells (megaloblasts) form and are released into the blood, causing megaloblastic anemia.

2. **Maintenance of nerve tissue.** Vitamin B-12 is essential to the health of the nervous system. Vitamin B-12 coenzymes are necessary for the synthesis of myelin, a lipoprotein, in the nervous tissue; but it is not known whether the vitamin is involved in the synthesis of the lipid of the protein part of myelin.

3. **Carbohydrate, fat, and protein metabolism.** Since coenzyme B-12 is necessary for the conversion of methylmalonate to succinate, it is required for normal carbohydrate and fat metabolism. It is also involved in protein metabolism, since the requirement for B-12 increases as protein intake increases.

4. **Synthesis or transfer of single carbon units.** Vitamin B-12 is thought to be required for the synthesis of single carbon units, whereas folacin participates in their transfer. It follows that B-12 takes part in most of the same reactions as folacin, including—
    a. The interconversion of serine and glycine
    b. The formation of methionine from homocysteine
    c. The formation of choline from ethanolamine

5. **Other functions.** Vitamin B-12 also serves as a coenzyme in the biosynthesis of methyl groups ($-CH_3$), and in reduction reactions such as the conversion of disulfide (S-S) to the sulfhydryl group (-SH).

• **Therapeutic uses of vitamin B-12**—Vitamin B-12 is being used in the treatment of the following maladies:

1. **Pernicious anemia.** The discovery that B-12 would control pernicious anemia was a great clinical breakthrough. Now a patient can be given intramuscular injections of 15 to 30 mcg of B-12 daily during a relapse, then maintained afterward by an injection of about 30 mcg every 30 days.

2. **Sprue.** Vitamin B-12 is effective in the treatment of sprue, especially if used in conjunction with folic acid. Actually, the role of B-12 may be indirect—to facilitate the action of folic acid.

DEFICIENCY SYMPTOMS.   Vitamin B-12 deficiency in man may occur as a result of (1) dietary lack, which sometimes occurs among vegetarians who consume no animal foods; or (2) deficiency of intrinsic factor, due to pernicious anemia, total or partial removal of the stomach by surgery, or infestation with parasites such as the fish tapeworm.

The common symptoms of a dietary deficiency of vitamin B-12 are: sore tongue, weakness, loss of weight, back pains, tingling of the extremities, apathy, and mental and other nervous abnormalities. Anemia is rarely seen in dietary deficiency of B-12.

In pernicious anemia, the characteristic symptoms are: abnormally large red blood cells (macrocytes), lemon-yellow pallor, anorexia, dyspnea (short of breath), prolonged bleeding time, abdominal discomfort, loss of weight, glossitis (inflammation of the tongue), an unsteady gait, and neurological disturbances, including stiffness of the limbs, irritability, and mental depression. Without treatment, death follows. Only injections of vitamin B-12 can alleviate efficiently the symptoms of pernicious anemia.

• **Dietary deficiencies**—Dietary deficiencies of vitamin B-12 may occur under the following circumstances:

1. **Among vegans and ovolactovegans.** People who live exclusively on plant foods (vegans) may be seriously deficient in vitamin B-12. Vegetarianism is, for religious reasons, common among Hindus in India and elsewhere, but most of them are ovolactovegetarians. (They consume animal products other than flesh foods.) Yet, for large numbers of Hindus, the intake of animal foods, and therefore of vitamin B-12, falls far short of the recommended allowances.

2. **In some developing countries.** Vitamin B-12 deficiencies are not uncommon in developing countries where foods of plant origin predominate, especially among pregnant and lactating women. For example, very low intakes of the vitamin have been reported in Peru and in parts of Africa.

3. **Where consumption of animal products by mothers is low.** In areas of the world where intakes of animal products by mothers is low, vitamin B-12 deficiency in infants may occur.

When and where animal foods are in short supply, vitamin B-12 now makes it possible to rectify the above situations, and to use plant and cereal foods much more wisely in the human diet.

RECOMMENDED DAILY ALLOWANCE OF VITAMIN B-12.   The Food and Nutrition Board (FNB) of the National Research Council (NRC) recommended daily allowances (RDA) of vitamin B-12 are given in the section on VITAMIN(S), Table V-5, Vitamin Table.

These recommended daily allowances provide for a margin of safety to cover variance in individual needs, absorption, and body stores. However, in using this table as a nutritional guide, the following facts should be noted: (1) exact daily human requirements of vitamin B-12 cannot be given because it is synthesized by intestinal flora; (2) in the absence of intrinsic factor (e.g., pernicious anemia), the vitamin is not absorbed; and (3) it is assumed that at least 50% of the vitamin B-12 in food is absorbed.

• **Infants and children**—The recommended allowance for infants up to 6 months of age is 0.3 mcg per day. This is based on the average concentration of the vitamin in human milk. For infants receiving commercial formulas, the Committee of Nutrition of the American Academy of Pediatrics recommends a daily vitamin B-12 intake of 0.15 mcg/100 kcal; thus, a 1-year-old child weighing 10 kg and receiving 1,000 kcal should receive 1.5 mcg of vitamin B-12 per day. The recommended daily allowances given in Table V-5 for older infants and preadolescent children have been calculated on the basis of average energy intakes by using the latter formula.

• **Adults**—The recommended daily allowance for both males and females over 10 years of age is 2.0 mcg of vitamin B-12. This value will maintain adequate vitamin B-12 nutrition and a substantial reserve body pool in most normal persons.

• **Pregnancy and lactation**—The recommended dietary allowance for pregnant women is 2.2 mcg/day; and for lactating women it is 2.6 mcg/day.

Only the effects of gross deficiency of vitamin B-12 are known; hence, it is possible that a minor degree of deficiency, especially if of long duration, may prevent buoyant good health, even in well-fed populations.

• **Vitamin B-12 intake in average U.S. diet**—According to the U.S. Department of Agriculture, the amount of vitamin B-12 in the U.S. food supply averages 9.1 mg per person per day. (But the intake may range from a low of 1 to a high of 100 mg per day.) Meat, fish, and poultry contribute 76.1% of the 9.1 mg of vitamin B-12 available in the typical U.S. daily diet; dairy products contribute 18.5%; eggs, 3.7%; and 1.7% comes from other sources.

TOXICITY.   No toxic effects of vitamin B-12 are known.

VITAMIN B-12 LOSSES DURING PROCESSING, COOKING, AND STORAGE.
About 30% of the vitamin B-12 activity of foods is lost during ordinary cooking.

Although only about 10% of the vitamin B-12 activity in milk is lost by pasteurization, from 40 to 90% of the B-12 is destroyed by evaporating milk.

It is noteworthy that in the presence of ascorbic acid vitamin B-12 withstands less heat.

Vitamin B-12 is destroyed by light.

SOURCES OF VITAMIN B-12.
The sole source of vitamin B-12 in nature is synthesis by microorganisms. It is synthesized by the many microorganisms in the rumen and intestine of herbivorous animals. The vitamin B-12 bound to a protein in animal foods results from such synthesis. This explains why vitamin B-12 is found in all foods of animal origin.

Plants cannot manufacture vitamin B-12; hence, except for trace amounts absorbed from the soil (because of the bacteria, soil is a good source of B-12) by the growing plant, very little is found in plant foods—in vegetables, grains, legumes, fruits, etc.

A classification of the B-12 content of food sources is given in the section on VITAMIN(S), Table V-5, Vitamin Table.

For additional sources and more precise values of vitamin B-12, see Food Composition Table F-21.

Some vitamin B-12 is formed by microorganisms in the intestinal tract of human beings. However, the synthesis is so far down in the colon that little of it may be absorbed.

The story of vitamin B-12 lends support to all developing country programs designed to improve animal production and to increase the supply and consumption of animal protein. Also, it is recognized that vitamin B-12 deficiency is not an uncommon consequence of many diseases and of

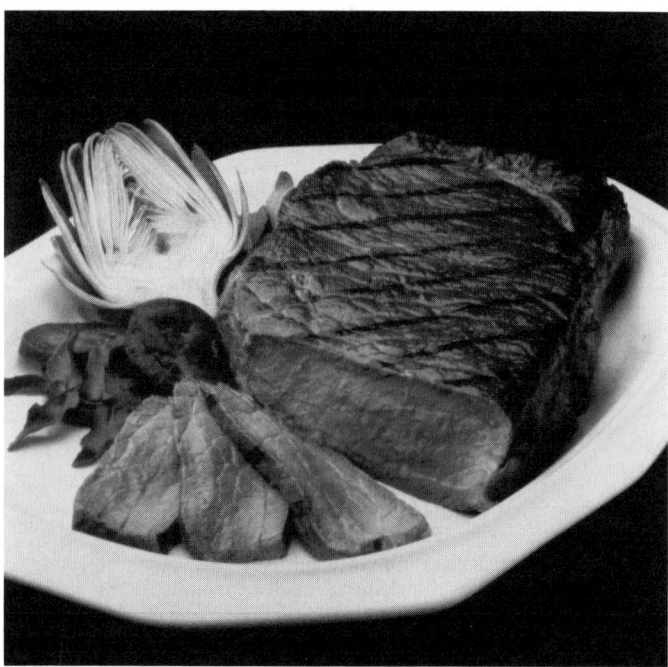

Fig. V-35. Slices of top round steak. Muscle meats are a good source of vitamin B-12. (Courtesy, National Live Stock and Meat Board, Chicago, Ill.)

surgical operations on the stomach and small intestine.
(Also see VITAMIN[S], Table V-5.)

VITAMIN B-13 (OROTIC ACID)

It is highly possible that the so-called vitamin B-13 is a growth promotant and a preventative of certain disorders. At this time, however, it is not known whether it plays an essential role in an otherwise adequate diet; hence, this presentation is for two purposes; (1) informational, and (2) stimulation of research.

HISTORY.   This compound, called B-13, was first obtained from distillers' solubles. Subsequently, one of its constituents, orotic acid, has been synthesized in Europe and used to treat multiple sclerosis.

CHEMISTRY.   Vitamin B-13 is a compound of unknown structure which appears either to contain orotic acid or to yield it on decomposition (see Fig. V-36).

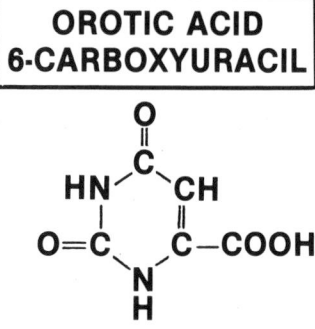

Fig. V-36. Orotic acid.

FUNCTIONS. Vitamin B-13 has been found to stimulate the growth of rats, chicks, and pigs under certain conditions.

Orotic acid is utilized by the body in the metabolism of folic acid and vitamin B-12. Also, it appears to aid the replacement or restoration of some cells.

There is indication that vitamin B-13 may be helpful in the treatment of multiple sclerosis.

DEFICIENCY SYMPTOMS. Deficiency symptoms have not been proved. But it is believed that a deficiency may lead to liver disorders, cell degeneration, and premature aging; and to degenerative symptoms in multiple sclerosis victims.

RECOMMENDED DAILY ALLOWANCE OF VITAMIN B-13. Dietary requirements are not known.

SOURCES OF VITAMIN B-13. Vitamin B-13 is found in such natural sources as distillers' solubles, whey, soured or curdled milk, and root vegetables. Also, this nutrient is available in supplemental form as calcium orotate.

(Also see VITAMIN[S], Table V-5.)

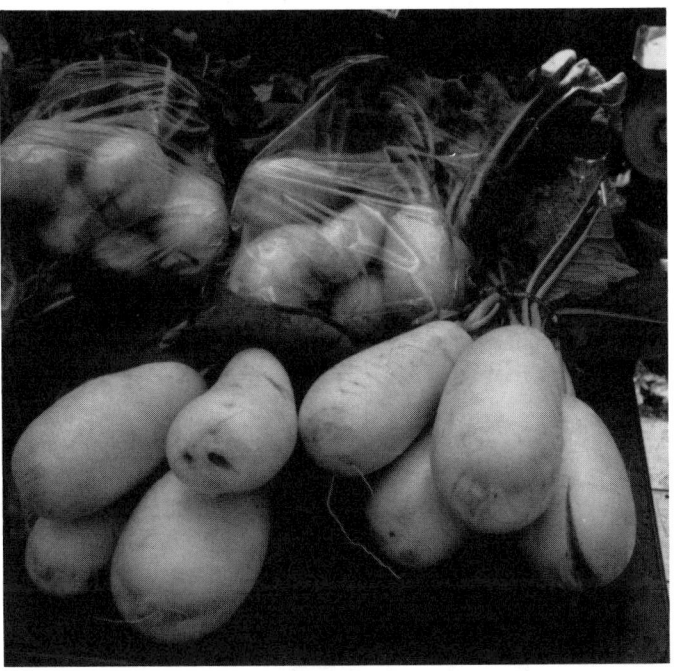

Fig. V-37. White turnips. Root vegetables are a good source of vitamin B-13. (Courtesy, Dept. of Food Service and Human Nutrition, University of Hawaii)

VITAMIN B COMPLEX

With the exception of vitamin C, all of the water-soluble vitamins can be grouped together under the vitamin B complex.

The story of the B vitamins begins with the study of the age-old disease beriberi.

In 1873, Van Lent was apparently the first to conclude that the type of diet had something to do with the origin of beriberi. By reducing the ration of rice in the diet of the sailors in the Dutch navy, he was able to eradicate beriberi almost entirely.

In 1882, Kanehiro Takaki, a Japanese Naval medical officer, reported that he had cured beriberi in sailors of the Japanese Navy by giving them less rice and more meat, milk, and vegetables. Takaki attributed the cure to the protein content of the diet.

Fifteen years later (1897), Christiaan Eijkman, a Dutch physician assigned to a prison hospital in the East Indies, observed beriberi among the inmates and sought the answer through experiments with chickens. To save money, he fed the birds scraps—mostly polished rice—from the patients' meals. The chickens unexpectedly developed a bad nerve ailment, which resulted in paralysis.

Later, the unsympathetic director of the hospital withheld permission to use scraps, and Dr. Eijkman had to buy natural (unmilled) rice for the chickens he used in his experiment. The ailing birds improved after they began eating the natural rice.

Dr. Eijkman then began a series of experiments that led to the first clear concept of disease due to nutritional deficiency. He fed polished white rice to chickens, pigeons, and ducks. They developed the paralysis that he had observed previously, then recovered when he fed them natural (unmilled) rice. Birds fed whole rice remained well.

Eijkman noted that the disease in birds which resulted from a polished rice diet resembled beriberi in man. He theorized that rice contained too much starch, which poisoned nerve cells, and that the outer layers, removed from the grain in milling, were an antidote.

Another Dutch physician, Dr. G. Grijns, continued the work of Eijkman. But he interpreted Eijkman's findings differently. In 1901, he concluded that beriberi in birds and man was due to a deficiency or absence of an essential nutrient from the diet.

From then on, chemists in many countries tried to concentrate the substance in rice that prevented beriberi in order to obtain it in pure form. Among them was Casimir Funk, of the Lister Institute, London, who, in 1912, coined the term *vitamine* and applied it to the antiberiberi substance.

In 1916, Dr. Elmer V. McCollum of the University of Wisconsin designated the concentrate that cured beriberi as *water-soluble B*, to distinguish it from the antinightblindness factor (called vitamin A) which had been found in carrots and butterfat of milk. At that time, McCollum thought that the antiberiberi substance was one factor only.

In 1926, B. C. P. Jansen and W. P. Donath, in Holland, isolated the antiberiberi vitamin, and in 1936 Robert R. Williams, an American, determined the structure and synthesized it.

As research continued (1919-1922), it was found that vitamin B was not a single substance, that it actually consisted of several factors. Collectively, they came to be known as the *vitamin B complex*, but each factor was given a separate designation. Some members of the group came to be referred to by subscript numbers as vitamins B_1, B_2, etc.; others became known by their chemical names; still others received both a number and a chemical designation. These vitamins differ in both chemical structure and specific functions. Yet, there are similarities. All of them are water-soluble; all of them are abundant in liver and yeast, and they often occur together in the same foodstuffs; each of them contains carbon, hydrogen, oxygen, and nitrogen; some of them contain mineral elements in their molecules (thiamin and biotin contain sulfur, and vitamin B-12 contains cobalt and phosphorus); most of them are part of a coenzyme molecule concerned with the breakdown of carbohydrate, protein, and fat in the body; the actions of many of them are interrelated; few of them are stored in large amounts in the body, so they must be provided daily; certain organs, particularly the liver, contain higher concentrations of them than others; and they are excreted from the body by way of the kidneys.

excreted from the body by way of the kidneys.

Another noteworthy characteristic of the B vitamins is that they are synthesized by microbial fermentation in the digestive tract, especially by ruminants (cattle and sheep) and herbivorous nonruminants (horse and rabbit). Some animals eat their own feces (coprophagy), thus recycling the vitamins synthesized in the microbial fermentation in the large intestine and cecum; rabbits, in particular, are known to do this on a routine basis. Unlike ruminants and herbivorous nonruminants, however, man, pigs, and poultry have only one stomach and no large cecum like the horse and rabbit. As a result, they do not synthesize enough of most B vitamins. Consequently, for man and other monogastrics, the B vitamins must be provided regularly in the diet in adequate amounts if deficiencies are to be averted.

At the present time, 9 fractions of the vitamin B complex are generally recognized, and others are postulated. Those discussed in this book (alphabetically under their name designations) are: biotin, choline, folacin (folic acid), niacin (nicotinic acid; nicotinamide), pantothenic acid (vitamin B-3), riboflavin (vitamin B-2), thiamin (vitamin B-1), vitamin B-6 (pyridoxine, pyridoxal; pyridoxamine), and vitamin B-12 (cobalamins).

A lack of B-complex vitamins is one of the forms of malnutrition that occur often throughout the world. Because the B vitamins are usually found in the same foodstuffs, a deficiency of several factors is usually observed rather than a deficiency of a single factor.

Many physiologic and pathologic stresses influence the need for the B vitamins. Larger amounts are needed during growth and in pregnancy and lactation than in maintenance of health in adult life. The requirement may be increased by diseases that elevate metabolism and by conditions associated with poor absorption, improper utilization, or increased excretion. Administration of antibiotics may lead to vitamin deficiency in some circumstances; in others, antibiotics spare vitamin requirements.

(Also see BERIBERI; and VITAMIN[S].)

VITAMIN C (ASCORBIC ACID; DEHYDROASCORBIC ACID)

Vitamin C—also called *ascorbic acid, dehydroascorbic acid, hexuronic acid,* and the *antiscorbutic vitamin*—is the very important substance, first found in citrus fruits, which prevents scurvy, one of the oldest scourges of mankind. All animal species appear to require vitamin C, but a *dietary need* is limited to humans, guinea pigs, monkeys, bats, certain fish, and perhaps certain reptiles. These species lack the enzyme L-gulonolactone oxidase which is necessary for vitamin C synthesis from 6-carbon sugars.

HISTORY. Scurvy, now known to be caused by a severe deficiency of vitamin C, has been a dread disease since ancient times. It was once common among sailors who ate little except bread and salt meat while on long voyages.

The historical incidence and conquest of scurvy constitute one of the most thrilling chapters in the development of nutrition as a science. A chronological summary of the saga of scurvy and vitamin C follows:

As early as 1550 B.C., scurvy was described by the Egyptians on medical papyrus rolls (man's first writing paper, made by the Egyptians from the papyrus plant as early as 2400 B.C.), discovered in Thebes by George Moritz Ebers,

VITAMIN C
helps to build healthy gums, teeth, and bones
TWO GUINEA PIGS OF SAME AGE

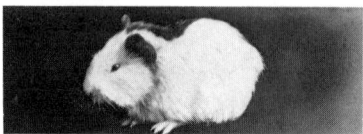

THIS GUINEA PIG HAD NO ASCORBIC ACID AND DEVELOPED SCURVY. NOTE CROUCHED POSITION DUE TO SORE JOINTS.

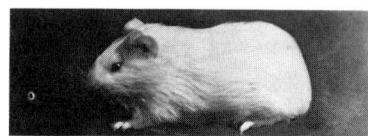

THIS GUINEA PIG HAD PLENTY OF ASCORBIC ACID. IT IS HEALTHY AND ALERT; ITS FUR IS SLEEK AND FINE.

TOP FOOD SOURCES

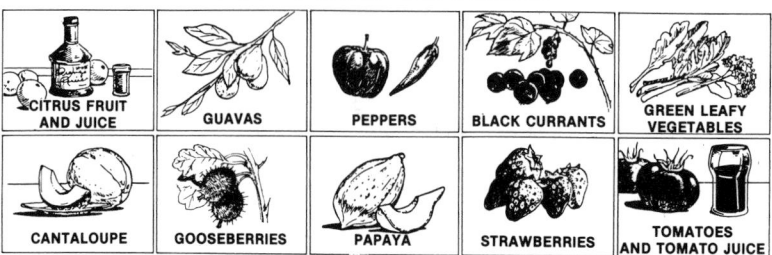

CITRUS FRUIT AND JUICE | GUAVAS | PEPPERS | BLACK CURRANTS | GREEN LEAFY VEGETABLES

CANTALOUPE | GOOSEBERRIES | PAPAYA | STRAWBERRIES | TOMATOES AND TOMATO JUICE

Fig. V-38. Vitamin C (ascorbic acid) made the difference! *Left:* Guinea pig on vitamin C-deficient diet. *Right:* Guinea pig that received plenty of vitamin C. Note, too, top sources of vitamin C. (Adapted from USDA sources.)

a German Egyptologist and novelist, who, in 1874, edited it in a romantic historical novel on medicine which he titled *Papyrus Ebers*).

In the Old Testament (which was written over a long period of time, thought to be from 1100 B.C. to 500 B.C.), reference is made to this disease.

About 450 B.C., Hippocrates, the Greek *father of medicine* described the symptoms of the malady—gangrene of the gums, loss of teeth, and painful legs in soldiers.

In 1248-54, Jean Sire de Joinville, the French chronicler, accompanied Louis IX of France to Cyprus and Egypt. In 1309, he completed in final form the *History of Saint Louis*, an account of the Crusade, in which he told of a disease (scurvy) "which attacked the mouth and the legs."

In 1497, when Vasco da Gama, Portuguese navigator, sailed around the Cape of Good Hope and established the first European trading colony on the coast of Malabar in India, 100 of his crew of 160 men perished from scurvy on the voyage.

During the winter of 1535 in Canada, Jacques Cartier, the daring explorer who laid claim to Canada for France, recorded in his log that the lives of many of his men dying of scurvy were saved "almost overnight," when they learned from the Indians that drinking a brew made from the growing tips of pine or spruce trees cured and prevented the malady. (It is now known that the *brew* contained vitamin C.)

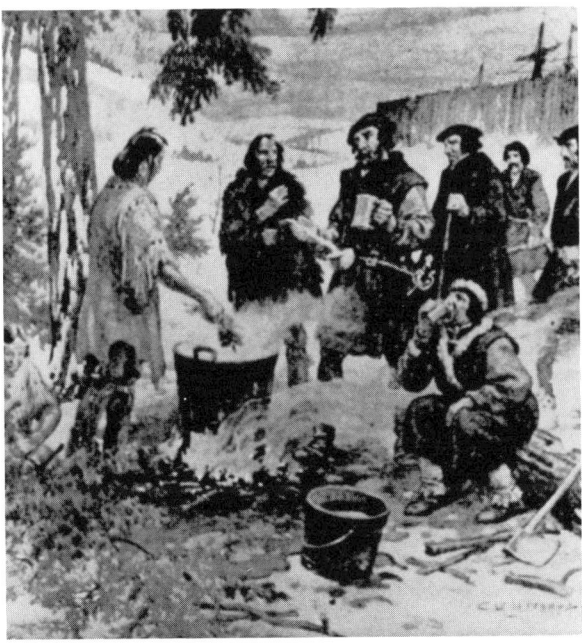

Fig. V-39. Friendly Huron-Iroquois Indians shown in Quebec in 1535, (1) making a broth from pine branches, and (2) serving it to Jacques Cartier and his men to cure scurvy. (Reproduced with permission of *Nutrition Today*, P.O. Box 1829, Annapolis, MD, 21404, © 1979)

In the 15th and 16th centuries, scurvy was a scourge throughout Europe, so much so that medical men wondered if all diseases might stem from it. It was particularly prevalent and severe on long voyages of sailing ships, in cities, and in times of crop failures. During this period, there was also a tendency to associate scurvy and venereal disease; some authorities of the day believed that both diseases were brought from abroad by sailors. Mercury was sometimes used as a treatment, with disastrous results.

In 1600-1603, Captain James Lancaster, English navigator, recorded that on the long voyage to the East Indies he kept his crew hearty merely by the addition of a mandatory "three spoonfuls of lemon juice every morning."

In 1747, James Lind, an English naval surgeon, tested six remedies on 12 sailors who had scurvy and found that oranges and lemons were curative. His classical studies, the results of which were published in 1753, are generally credited as being the first experiments to show that an essential food element can prevent a deficiency disease. But another 50 years elapsed before the British Navy required rations of lemons or limes on sailing vessels.

On two historic voyages, each of three-years duration, from 1768 to 1771 and from 1772 to 1775, British Captain James Cook, avoided scurvy—hitherto the scourge of long sea voyages. He had his ship stocked with concentrated slabs of thick brown vegetable soup and barrels of sauerkraut. Of the sauerkraut he said: "It is not only a wholesome vegetable food, but, in my judgment, highly antiscorbutic, and spoils not by keeping." In addition, he sent seamen ashore at every port visited to gather all sorts of fresh fruits and green vegetables (including grasses), which the crew prepared, served, and ate. As a result, not one of the crew died from scurvy.

In 1795 (one year after Lind's death), by Admiralty Order, the British Royal Navy began providing 1 oz of lime juice daily in every sailor's food ration; from this date forward, British sailors were stuck with the nickname *limeys*.

In 1907, Holst and Frolich, of Norway, produced scurvy experimentally in guinea pigs by feeding them a diet deficient in foods containing ascorbic acid.

In 1928, Szent-Gyorgy, a Hungarian scientist, working in Hopkins' laboratory at Cambridge University, in England, isolated a substance from the ox adrenal glands, oranges, and cabbage leaves, which he called hexuronic acid; but he did not test it for antiscorbutic effect.

In 1932, Charles Glen King and W. A. Waugh, at the University of Pittsburgh, isolated from lemon juice a crystalline material that possessed antiscorbutic activity in guinea pigs; this marked the discovery of *vitamin C*, a deficiency of which caused the centuries-old scourge of scurvy.

In 1933, vitamin C was synthesized by Reichstein, a Swiss scientist.

In 1938, *ascorbic acid* was officially accepted as the chemical name for vitamin C.

CHEMISTRY, METABOLISM, PROPERTIES.

• **Chemistry**—Ascorbic acid is a compound of relatively simple structure, closely related to the monosaccharide sugars. It is synthesized from glucose and other simple sugars by plants and by most animal species (see Fig. V-40).

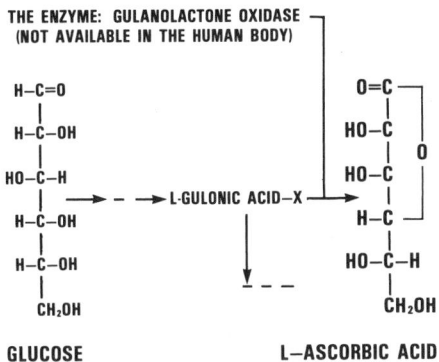

Fig. V-40. Metabolic relation of glucose to ascorbic acid. In man, the absence of oxidase prevents this reaction, making the intake of preformed ascorbic acid in food necessary.

Man, monkeys, guinea pigs, fruit-eating bats, and red-vented bulbul birds (the latter two are native to India), cannot make the conversion from glucose to ascorbic acid, because these species lack the necessary enzyme (oxidase). Scurvy, then, in man can really be classed as a disease of distant genetic origin—an inherited metabolic error; a defect in carbohydrate metabolism due to the lack of an enzyme, which, in turn, results from the lack of a specific gene.

Two forms of vitamin C occur in nature: ascorbic acid (the reduced form), and dehydroascorbic acid (the oxidized form).[8] Their structural formulas are shown in Fig. V-41.

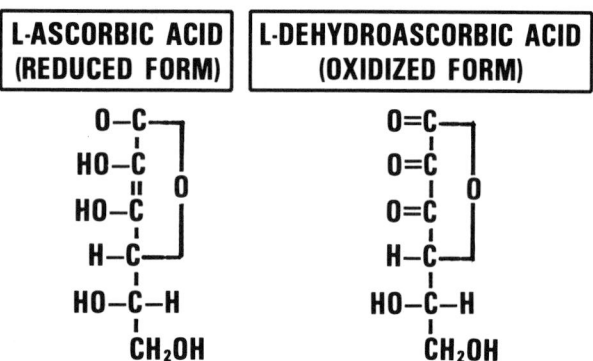

Fig. V-41. Structural formulas of vitamin C.

Although most of the vitamin C exists as ascorbic acid, both forms appear to be utilized similarly by the human. Also, the body efficiently utilizes either synthetic L-ascorbic acid or the vitamin in its natural form as in orange juice.

Ascorbic acid is easily oxidized to dehydroascorbic acid, which is just as easily reduced back to ascorbic acid. However, dehydroascorbic acid may be irreversibly oxidized, particularly in the presence of alkali, to diketogulonic acid, which has no antiscorbutic activity (see Fig. V-42.)

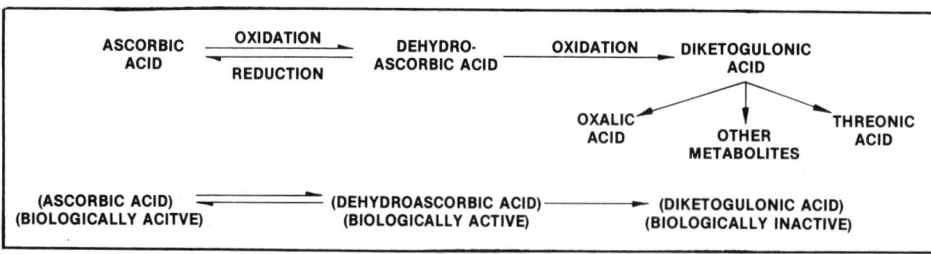

Fig. V-42. Relationship of ascorbic, dehydroascorbic, and diketogulonic acids.

Certain derivatives of vitamin C (for example, erythrobic acid and ascorbyl palmitate) are used as antioxidants in food products to prevent rancidity, to prevent browning of fruit, and to cure meat. Erythrobic acid (D-araboascorbic acid) is poorly absorbed and has little antiscorbutic activity.

• **Metabolism**—Pertinent facts about the absorption, storage, and excretion of vitamin C follow:

1. **Absorption.** Vitamin C is readily and rapidly absorbed from the upper part of the small intestine into the circulatory system. Thence, it is taken up unevenly by the tissues; the adrenal gland and the retina of the eye contain an especially high concentration of vitamin C, but the liver, spleen, intestine, bone marrow, pancreas, thymus, pituitary, brain, and kidney also contain appreciable amounts. Blood cells contain more than blood serum.

2. **Storage.** Unlike the majority of the water-soluble vitamins, limited stores of vitamin C are held in the body. Thus, the signs of scurvy do not appear for some weeks in humans receiving no vitamin C.

3. **Excretion.** Vitamin C is largely excreted in the urine, with the amount excreted controlled by the kidney tubules. When the tissues are saturated, a large amount is excreted; but when the tissue reserves are depleted, only a small amount is excreted. Some vitamin C is always excreted by the kidneys even when the tissues are severely depleted.

• **Properties**—Ascorbic acid is a white, odorless crystalline powder, which is quite stable when dry.

Of all the vitamins, ascorbic acid is the most unstable when in solution. It is highly soluble in water, but not in fat. The oxidation (destruction) of ascorbic acid is accelerated by air, heat, light, alkalies, oxidative enzymes, and traces of copper and iron. It is markedly destroyed by cooking, particularly where the pH is alkaline. Cooking losses also result because of its solubility. The destruction of ascorbic acid is slowed down by foods that are acidic, by refrigeration, and by protection from exposure to air.

MEASUREMENT/ASSAY. The concentration of ascorbic acid in tissues and foods is expressed in milligrams. One IU is the activity of 0.05 mg of ascorbic acid.

Ascorbic acid is generally determined by chemical assay, accomplished by taking advantage of its reducing properties.

For bioassay work, guinea pigs are the preferred experimental animals because of their susceptibility to a deficiency of vitamin C. Thus, they are still used for demonstration of deficiency of the vitamin and to make comparative assays.

FUNCTIONS. The specific biochemical functions of vitamin C are not clearly understood. Nevertheless, it is established as a very important substance for body welfare because of being implicated in the following roles: (1) formation and maintenance of collagen, which makes for more rapid and sound healing of wounds and burns; (2) metabolism of the amino acids tyrosine and tryptophan; (3) absorption and movement of iron; (4) metabolism of fats and lipids, and cholesterol control; (5) as an antioxidant in the protection of vitamins A and E and the polyunsaturated fatty acids; (6) sound teeth and bones; (7) strong capillary walls and healthy blood vessels; (8) metabolism of folic acid; and perhaps in a number of other roles. Details follow:

• **Collagen formation**—The most clearly established functional role of vitamin C is the formation and maintenance of collagen, the substance that binds body cells together in much the same manner as mortar binds bricks.

Collagen is a fibrous protein that contains large amounts

---

[8]Actually, several chemical compounds have vitamin C activity. So, it is now recommended that the term *vitamin C* be used as the combined name of all compounds having the biological activity of ascorbic acid, and that the terms *ascorbic acid* and *dehydroascorbic acid* be used only when specific reference to them is made.

of the amino acids proline and hydroxyproline. Postulation is that vitamin C is essential for making hydroxyproline in the body as follows: Vitamin C activates the enzyme prolyl hydroxylase, which, in turn, effects the conversion of proline (by the addition of an "OH" group) to hydroxyproline in the formation of collagen.

Vitamin C is also required for the conversion of lysine to hydroxylysine, another amino acid that is an essential part of collagen. The reaction is brought about by the enzyme lysine hydroxylase. The role of vitamin C in the formation of hydroxylysine is thought to be similar to its role in the formation of hydroxyproline.

Both of the above reactions require vitamin C, and both are essential for collagen formation. In turn, failure to synthesize collagen results in delayed healing of wounds and burns. So, the administration of vitamin C makes for more rapid and sound healing of wounds.

- **Metabolism of tyrosine and tryptophan**—Vitamin C is necessary in the metabolism of the amino acids tyrosine and tryptophan.

In the metabolism of tyrosine, a deficiency of vitamin C will result in the build-up and excretion of the intermediary product, P-hydroxyphenylpyruvate, as a result of inactivating the enzyme P-hydroxyphenylpyruvic acid oxidase. When large amounts of tyrosine are being metabolized, vitamin C protects the enzyme P-hydroxyphenylpyruvic acid oxidase from inactivation (rather than activates as was formerly thought), and enhances the synthesis of norepinephrine, a neurotransmitter, from tyrosine.

Also, vitamin C is required for the conversion of tryptophan to 5-hydroxytryptophan, the first step in the formation of the serotonin, a compound that raises blood pressure through vasoconstrictor action.

- **Iron utilization**—When the two nutrients are ingested simultaneously, dietary vitamin C increases the absorption of iron by converting ferric iron to the more readily absorbed ferrous form. Vitamin C is also necessary for the movement of transferritin (a combination of ferric iron and the protein transferrin) to the liver, and for the formation of the iron-protein compound ferritin for storage in the liver, spleen, and bone marrow.

(Also see IRON.)

- **Metabolism of fats and lipids**—There is some evidence that vitamin C affects fat and lipid metabolism as follows:

1. Vitamin C serves as a cofactor, along with ATP and magnesium ions, in the inactivation of the enzyme *adipose tissue lipase*, the enzyme that mobilizes the free fatty acids from adipose tissue to meet the energy demands of the body. When the body's energy needs have been met, vitamin C (along with the other two controlling agents—ATP and magnesium ions) inactivates the adipose tissue lipase.

2. Vitamin C may have a role in the metabolism of cholesterol. The levels of cholesterol in the liver and blood serum appear to rise during a deficiency of the vitamin, and to fall with the administration of the vitamin. The increased accumulation of cholesterol appears to be due to a decrease in the rate of conversion of cholesterol to bile acids when vitamin C intake is inadequate.

Vitamin C also appears to be involved in the metabolism of cholesterol in another way. Through its sulfated metabolite, *ascorbic acid sulfate*, it appears to bring about the formation of cholesterol sulfate, a water-soluble compound that is excreted in the urine. By this means, cholesterol may be mobilized from the body tissues, with the result that there is a lowering of blood cholesterol levels.

- **Antioxidant in the protection of vitamins A and E and the polyunsaturated fatty acids**—Ascorbic acid is an important antioxidant; thus, it has a role in the protection of vitamins A and E and the polyunsaturated fatty acids from excessive oxidation.

- **Sound teeth and bones**—Vitamin C is required for the normal development of odontoblasts, a layer of cells that forms dentin in teeth. It follows that a deficiency of vitamin C may cause defects in tooth dentin, especially during the critical period of tooth formation.

Also, vitamin C is necessary for the proper calcification and soundness of bone.

- **Strength of capillary walls and blood vessels**—Vitamin C is necessary for maintaining strength of capillary walls, especially of the small blood vessels. Shortages of the vitamin result in weakened and inelastic capillary walls, which may rupture and hemorrhage, evidenced by easy bruising, pinpoint peripheral hemorrhages, bone and joint hemorrhages, easy bone fracture, fragile bleeding gums with loosened teeth, and poor wound healing.

- **Metabolism of folic acid (folacin)**—Vitamin C is required for the conversion of the inactive form of the vitamin, folic acid (folacin), to its active form, folinic acid. When there is an insufficiency of vitamin C in the diet, the metabolism of folic acid (folacin) is impaired and the megaloblastic anemia that occurs in scurvy, and sometimes in infancy, may result.

In addition to the above functions of vitamin C, investigators have suggested a number of other roles for vitamin C. Although the evidence for most of these functions is not conclusive, a brief summary of each of them follows in the hope that it will stimulate further research:

- **Synthesis or release of the steroid hormones; stress**—It has been observed (1) that the normally high concentration of ascorbic acid in the adrenal glands is depleted with the synthesis of steroid hormones, and (2) that there is an increased requirement of vitamin C in all forms of stress—extremely high or low temperature, shock, fatigue, injury, burns, surgery, cigarette smoking, toxic levels of heavy metals (such as lead, mercury, and cadmium, etc.). Hence, it has been theorized that vitamin C is involved with either the synthesis or release of the steroid hormones by the adrenal glands; and that the greater the stress, the higher the vitamin C requirement.

Dr. James Cason, Professor of Chemistry, University of California, Berkeley, cites the following item in support of the role of ascorbic acid in resisting stress: A 150-lb goat makes about 13 g of ascorbic acid daily under ordinary circumstances, but if a goat is put under stress it will produce up to twice this amount.[9] It seems reasonable, therefore, that ascorbic acid would help man to resist stress, too.

- **Protection in infection and fever**—There are decreased tissue and blood levels of ascorbic acid during infections and fever, indicating either increased need for this vitamin or increased destruction of it. Thus, higher than normal intakes of vitamin C may be needed to provide maximum protection against infections and fevers.

- **Prevention and cure of colds and flu**—There is much controversy concerning the effectiveness of massive doses of vitamin C in the prevention and cure of the common cold and flu. Linus Pauling, a respected chemist with the rare

---

[9]Cason, James, "Ascorbic Acid, Amygdalin and Carcinoma," *The Vortex*, June 1978, pp. 9-23.

distinction of receiving two Nobel Prizes—one for science and the other for peace, is the most enthusiastic advocate of using vitamin C as a drug. His book *Vitamin C and the Common Cold and the Flu*, published in 1970, has had great influence. As a result of his advocacy, many people throughout the world began taking tablets of ascorbic acid. Nevertheless, as a result of studies on thousands of people, the only reasonable conclusion that can be drawn is that vitamin C has no effect on the number of colds people get, but in some people it lessens the severity of cold symptoms.

There should be an awareness that large doses of vitamin C are known to increase (1) the urinary output of oxalic acid and uric acid, and (2) the intestinal absorption of iron. Thus, massive doses of vitamin C may be hazardous to those with a liability to kidney stones or iron-storage disease.

• **Phagocyte activity and formation of antibodies—** Ascorbic acid may have a stimulating effect on the phagocytic activity, and on the formation of antibodies.

• **Reducing the requirements for certain vitamins—** Ascorbic acid (the reduced form of vitamin C) lessens animal requirements for thiamin, riboflavin, pantothenic acid, folacin, vitamin A, and vitamin E; likely, it has a similar role in man.

• **Smoking—**Recent research confirms the long-time claim that smoking lowers the blood level of vitamin C, although it is not known whether this is due to actual destruction or reduced availability of ascorbic acid. But there is no evidence that heavy smokers need more vitamin C than that supplied by the recommended dietary allowances.

• **Cancer—**Dr. Linus Pauling declares that vitamin C is beneficial to cancer victims, according to Dr. James Cason, Professor of Chemistry, University of California, Berkeley, who reported on the following cancer-vitamin C study in which Dr. Pauling was involved.[10]

In 1976, Cameron and Pauling published the results of an ongoing investigation of cancer therapy with vitamin C at a hospital in Scotland, where Dr. Cameron is physician in residence. The study involved 1,100 cancer victims who had been diagnosed as *terminal*. One hundred of these (matched for sex, age, and type of cancer for comparison with a control group) were given massive doses of 10 g/day of vitamin C in double blind placebo procedure, and the remaining 1,000 were the comparison group. The vitamin C-treated patients lived an average of four times longer than the comparison group. At the time of publication in 1976, all the comparison group were dead, while 16 of the 100 who received vitamin C were alive. Moreover, 1 year after publishing the results, Dr. Pauling reported, "13 of these 'hopeless' patients are still alive, some as long as 5 years after having been pronounced untreatable, and most of them are in such good apparent health as to suggest that they now have normal life expectancy."

But a controlled study by Dr. Edward T. Creagan, Mayo Clinic, showed no anticancer effect or improved survival as a result of megadoses of vitamin C. Likewise, Drs. J. Roberto Moran and Henry L. Greene, researchers at Vanderbilt University School of Medicine

concluded from a study of the benefits and risks of vitamin C megadoses that "at present no strong evidence can be found to support the routine prophylactic (preventive) use of ascorbic acid in well-nourished people."

• **Removal of ammonia in the deamination of proteins and peptides—**Vitamin C appears to accelerate the deamination of proteins and peptides and the conversion of ammonia (NH_3) to urea for excretion. Some have even conjectured that these processes (the oxidative deamination and the urea cycle) affect aging and longevity.

• **Antihistamine—**Ascorbic acid is an antihistamine; hence, it may be effective in treating respiratory infections due to a histamine.

• **Detoxifying drugs—**Vitamin C appears to be involved in a set of biochemical reactions responsible for detoxifying drugs, and for eliminating them from the body. Specifically, the vitamin may facilitate steps in which iron is introduced into the heme groups that subsequently become part of the proteins that carry out the detoxification reactions.

• **Longevity—**In 1992, the UCLA School of Public Health reported in the *Journal of Epidemiology* that (1) daily intake of 300 mg of vitamin C from food and supplements may increase life expectancy in men by 6 years, and (2) daily intake of 150 mg vitamin C from food, without supplements, may increase life expectancy in men by 2 years. The study focused on 11,000 adults, 25 to 74 years of age.

DETERMINING VITAMIN C STATUS. Vitamin C status in people may be determined by clinical signs and by blood levels of the vitamin. Evidence of capillary bleeding in the skin (perifolliculosis) and in the gums are clinical signs that may indicate a vitamin C deficiency.

Different investigators have employed a variety of tests for estimating the vitamin C nutrition of man and animals. The simplest of these is measurement of the L-ascorbic acid content of serum or plasma. Approximate values of L-ascorbic acid of man which may be used for guide purposes follow:

Nutritional Status	Serum or Plasma Concentration (mg/100 ml)
Well nourished	over 0.60
Adequate	0.40–0.59
Low	0.10–0.39
Deficient	under 0.10

In a study of the ascorbic acid level per 100 ml of blood plasma of 48 women and 41 men, the senior author of this book, Audrey H. Ensminger, found 14 subjects, or 15.7%, at the scurvy level.

DEFICIENCY SYMPTOMS. When deprived of a dietary source of vitamin C for a sufficient length of time, man, along with other primates and several other species, develops scurvy, a potentially fatal disease.

• **Early symptoms, called latent scurvy—**Early symptoms of vitamin C deficiency, called latent scurvy, include: loss of weight, listlessness, fatigue, fleeting pains in the joints and muscles, irritability, shortness of breath, sore and/or bleeding gums, small hemorrhages under the skin, bones that fracture easily, and poor wound healing.

---

[10]Cason, James, "Ascorbic Acid, Amygdalin and Carcinoma, " The *Vortex*, June 1978, pp. 9-23.

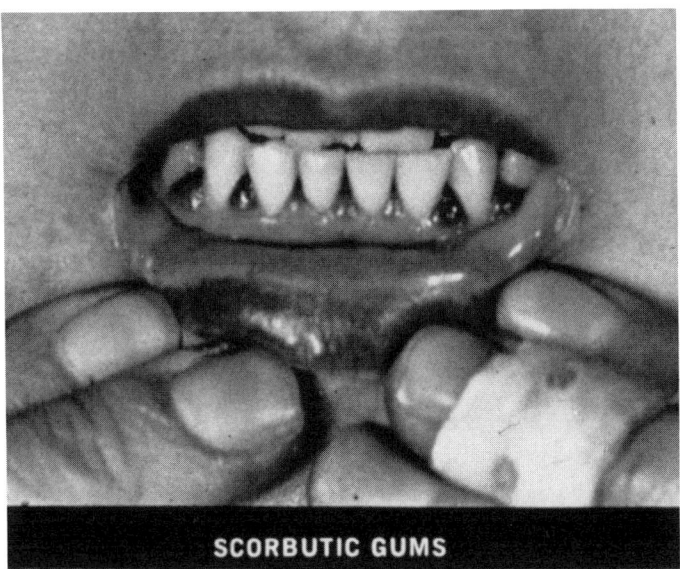

Fig. V-43. Scorbutic gums. (Reproduced with permission of *Nutrition Today*, P.O. Box 1829, Annapolis, MD, 21404, ©, 1979)

• **Scurvy**—A severe deficiency of vitamin C results in acute scurvy, characterized by: swollen, bleeding, and ulcerated gums; loose teeth; malformed and weak bones; fragility of the capillaries with resulting hemorrhages throughout the body; large bruises; big joints, such as the knee and hip, due to bleeding into the joint cavity; anemia; degeneration of muscle fibers, including those of the heart; and tendency of old wounds to become red and break open. Sudden death from severe internal hemorrhage and heart failure is always a danger.

RECOMMENDED DAILY ALLOWANCE OF VITAMIN C.

Many studies have been conducted to determine the human vitamin C requirements. Consideration has been given to the effect of age, environment, physical exertion, infections, and fevers. Also, various measurements for determining the adequacy of vitamin C have been devised, including: (1) the daily intake of vitamin C necessary to prevent the symptoms of scurvy; (2) the amount of vitamin C required to saturate whole blood, blood plasma, white blood cells, or body tissue; and (3) the intake of vitamin C necessary to maintain blood and urinary ascorbic acid levels within normal range. The results of these studies vary widely.

A daily intake of 10 mg of ascorbic acid will prevent scurvy. But this should be regarded as a minimum level. In order to provide for individual differences and margins of safety, the Food and Nutrition Board of the National Academy of Sciences recommends the following allowances: 30–35 mg for infants, 40–45 mg for children, 60 mg for males and females over 14 years, 70 mg for pregnancy, and 95 mg for lactation. (See the section on VITAMIN[S], Table V-5, Vitamin Table.)

It is noteworthy that the joint FAO/WHO Expert Committee makes somewhat lower recommendations than those given in Table V-5: 20 mg for infants and children up to 13 years of age, 30 mg for adults (males and females over 13 years), and 50 mg during pregnancy and lactation.

It is recognized, however, that these allowances are not necessarily adequate to meet the additional requirements of persons depleted by disease, traumatic stress, or prior dietary inadequacies. Also, the recommended levels given in Table V-5 may not be sufficient to assure vigorous good health.

• **Recommended allowances for infants, children, and adolescents**—A dietary allowance of 30 mg per day is recommended from birth to six months, and 35 mg per day from six months to twelve months. This is based on the fact that (1) human milk contains 30 to 55 mg/liter of vitamin C, although it varies with the mother's dietary intake of the vitamin; and (2) the breast-fed infant receives approximately 850 ml of milk per day. However, newborn infants, especially if they are premature, may have an increased requirement for the metabolism of tyrosine during the first week of life.

For children 1 to 3 years, an allowance of 40 mg/day is recommended; up to the age of 11 years, an allowance of 45 mg/day of vitamin C is recommended. For older children, an allowance of 50 mg/day is recommended as adequate to meet individual needs and to provide a margin of safety.

• **Recommended allowance for adults**—A dietary allowance of 60 mg of vitamin C per day is recommended for adults of both sexes. This will maintain an ascorbate body pool of 1,500 mg—a body pool of sufficient magnitude to protect against signs of scurvy in the adult male for a period of 30 to 45 days, and allow for an ascorbate catabolism rate of 3 to 4% and an average ascorbate absorption efficiency of approximately 85%.

• **Recommended allowances for pregnancy and lactation**—During pregnancy, plasma vitamin C levels fall. It is not known whether this is due to a physiological response to pregnancy and/or to increased demands of pregnancy. It is known that the placenta normally transmits sufficient ascorbic acid from mother to fetus to result in fetal levels 50% greater than maternal levels at birth. To provide for this fetal need, an additional allowance of 10 mg of ascorbic acid per day is recommended for pregnant women, particularly during the second and third trimester of pregnancy.

Human milk from well-nourished women is relatively high in ascorbic acid, but it varies with the mother's dietary intake of the nutrient. During lactation, a daily loss of 25 to 45 mg of vitamin C may occur in the secretion of 850 ml of milk. So, for lactating women, an additional allowance of 35 mg/day of vitamin C is recommended for the first six months in order to assure a satisfactory level of the vitamin in breast milk.

• **Massive doses of ascorbic acid**—Intakes of ascorbic acid in excess of 1,000 mg/day (1 g/day) or more have been reported to have some effect in reducing the frequency and severity of symptoms of colds and flu. To date, the results of research work have generally shown that the benefits of large doses of vitamin C are too small to justify recommending routine intake of large amounts. But further studies are needed.

Large doses of ascorbic acid have been reported to lower serum cholesterol in some hypercholesterolemic subjects, but not in others.

Ascorbic acid supplements can prevent the reduced platelet and plasma concentrations of ascorbic acid observed in aspirin-treated rheumatoid-arthritis patients.

The use of massive doses of vitamin C to improve the performance of athletes has long been a controversial issue. Present findings indicate that the vitamin is ineffective for this purpose, and that large doses may have a negative effect on athletic performance by disturbing the equilibrium between oxygen transport and oxygen utilization.

Large doses of ascorbic acid have generally been considered nontoxic, except for gastrointestinal symptoms experienced by some people. However, a number of adverse effects of excessive intakes of ascorbic acid have been reported, such as acid-induced uricosuria, absorption of excessive amounts of food iron, and impaired bactericidal activity of leucocytes.

Since many of the claims of significant beneficial effects of large intakes of ascorbic acid have not been sufficiently substantiated, and since excessive intakes may have some adverse effects, routine consumption of large intakes of ascorbic acid is not recommended without medical advice.

• **Vitamin C intake in average U.S. diet**—According to the U.S. Department of Agriculture, the foods available for civilian consumption in the United States provide 120 mg of vitamin C per person per day. Of this amount, fruits (especially citrus fruits) and vegetables provide 91% of the total.

TOXICITY.   Doses of up to 2 g per day (which is more than 30 times the recommended daily allowance) of ascorbic acid are nontoxic to adults. However, in amounts of 2 to 8 g per day, caution should be exercised; and there is clear evidence that intakes in excess of 8 g per day (more than 100 times the recommended daily allowance) may be distinctly harmful.

A number of adverse effects of excessive intakes of vitamin C have been reported, such as: nausea; abdominal cramps and diarrhea; absorption of excessive amounts of food iron; destruction of red blood cells; increased mobilization of bone minerals; interference with anticoagulant therapy; formation of kidney and bladder stones; the inactivation of vitamin B-12; a rise in plasma cholesterol; and possible dependence upon large doses of vitamin C (small doses no longer meet nutritional needs). It is also noteworthy that undesirable side effects may be greater in certain physiological states (e.g. pregnancy).

Since excessive intakes of vitamin C may be hazardous, routine consumption of large amounts (above 2 g daily by adults) of the vitamin is not recommended without medical advice.

LOSSES OF VITAMIN C DURING PROCESSING, COOKING, AND STORAGE.   Of all the vitamins, ascorbic acid is the most unstable. It is easily destroyed during harvesting, processing, cooking, and storage, because it is water-soluble, easily oxidized, and attacked by enzymes. Thus, a warm environment, exposure to air, solubility in water, heat, alkalinity, and dehydration are detrimental to the retention of ascorbic acid in foods. Also, cutting of vegetables releases an enzyme and increases the leaching by water. Hence, foods may lose much of their original vitamin C content from the time they are harvested until they are eaten. Details follow:

• **Processing losses**—The method of preparing fruits and vegetables affects the amount of the vitamin. Much vitamin C is lost when the products are washed slowly, cut up into small pieces, and soaked after peeling. In preparing foods for quick freezing, canning, or drying, a brief blanching with steam favors retention of vitamin C, because this process destroys the enzymes that hasten destruction of the vitamin in raw foods. The least loss of vitamin C occurs when foods are preserved by quick freezing; the most loss occurs when foods are preserved by drying, especially if they are exposed to sunlight. Losses of vitamin C from drying may be lessened by sulfuring before drying and by rapid dehydration (away from sunlight). Manufacturers of canned and frozen fruits

and vegetables should take special care to use products of high quality, then process them quickly. If this precaution is taken—if the products reach the cannery fresh from nearby fields and are heated quickly in vacuum-sealed cans—commercially canned fruits and vegetables may compare favorably in vitamin C content with home-cooked products. The vitamin C content of canned fruit juices varies considerably, unless they are specially protected in processing or fortified with vitamin C.

• **Cooking losses**—There is a great deal of variation in the amount of vitamin C lost in home cooking, depending on the nature of the food, the reaction (acid or alkaline), the length of time and the degree of heating, and the extent to which the food is exposed to water and air in the cooking process.

To retain a maximum of the ascorbic acid, frozen fruits should be used promptly, and frozen vegetables should be plunged directly into boiling water for immediate cooking.

Losses may be minimized by cooking with peel left on or with the product in large pieces, by cooking with as much exclusion of air as possible (e.g., using a tightly covered vessel or pressure cooker); by boiling the cooking water for a minute before adding the food; by shortening the boiling time; by using a small amount of water; and by consuming the cooking water.

Increased cooking losses of vitamin C result from cooking in copper or iron utensils (the ions of which inactivate the vitamin); from adding baking soda to vegetables to retain the green color (as an alkaline medium facilitates oxidation); from mashing the food and leaving it in a hot place or exposed to air; or from holding cooked foods warm for prolonged periods of time, such as on hot plates or on steam tables in cafeterias.

• **Storage losses**—Losses of vitamin C occur during prolonged storage, whether at home or in a market, especially if the product is damaged or is in a warm place. New potatoes, which contain about 30 mg/100 g of ascorbic acid, may lose 75% of the vitamin during 9 months of storage. Leafy vegetables (with large surface areas) lose more vitamin C in storage than do roots and tubers. Refrigeration during storage reduces losses. In markets, more of the vitamins of vegetables are retained when they are kept in crushed ice than when they are kept in a refrigerator.

Citrus fruit juices stored in the refrigerator lose negligible amounts of the vitamin; the acid content of the juice helps preserve vitamin C.

HOW TO CONSERVE VITAMIN C IN FOODS IN THE HOME.   Since vitamin C is essential for health, its maximum value should be conserved in foods. Losses may be minimized by keeping in mind that vitamin C is water-soluble and easily destroyed by oxidation, and that heat, alkalinity, and exposure to air hasten its destruction.

Practical suggestions for conserving vitamin C in foods in the home follow:

• Buy fresh fruits and vegetables in small quantities so that they will be used promptly. Store them in the refrigerator.

• Prepare foods immediately before they are to be served raw or cooked; do a minimum of chopping and cutting, and cook with the skins left on when possible; and do not allow foods to be exposed to air or stand in water before cooking.

• Use frozen foods promptly.

• Do not thaw frozen vegetables before cooking; keep them in the refrigerator until ready to cook, then, in their frozen state, plunge them directly into a limited amount of boiling water for immediate cooking.

• Cook in a small quantity of water, for as short a period of time as feasible, in a tightly covered cooking vessel; cook by steaming or broiling (instead of boiling).

• Never cook in copper or iron pans, and do not add soda in cooking; copper, iron, and soda hasten vitamin C destruction.

• Serve vegetables as soon after cooking as possible.

• Prepare fresh fruit juices immediately before serving. It is noteworthy, however, that acid juices (orange, grapefruit, tomato) may be left in a covered glass container in the refrigerator for several days with little loss in vitamin C.

SOURCES OF VITAMIN C.
Vitamin C occurs primarily in foods of plant origin—fruits (especially citrus fruits) and vegetables; those that may be eaten fresh, uncooked, or previously frozen are the best sources.

Contrary to common opinion, it takes 3 times as much tomato juice as citrus juice to supply the same amount of vitamin C.

If the mother's diet has contained sufficient vitamin C, human milk will contain 4 to 6 times as much ascorbic acid as cow's milk and will protect the infant from scurvy.

It is noteworthy that the vitamin content of plant foods varies greatly, depending on such factors as variety, climate, amount of sunshine, stage of maturity, part of plant (little is found in dry seeds), and length of storage. In general, the more sunshine to which a plant is exposed, the higher the vitamin C content; and the more mature the plant, the lower the vitamin C content.

A good rule to follow in order to assure sufficient vitamin C in the diet is to include a daily serving of citrus fruit or juice.

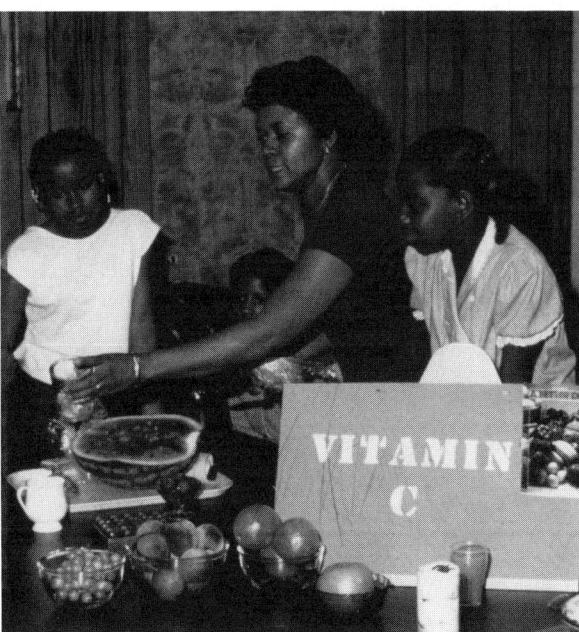

Fig. V-44. Rich, natural sources of vitamin C. (Courtesy, Louisiana Cooperative Extension Service, Louisiana State University, Baton Rouge, La.)

• **Richest natural sources**—The richest natural sources of vitamin C are the acerola cherry, *camu-camu*, and rose hips. Rose hips, which form the base of the rose bloom, are not eaten as such; rather, they are either made into a syrup (or extract) or brewed as a tea. During World War II food rationing in England, rose hip syrup was issued by the British Ministry of Food to help fortify the vitamin C intake of the English people. The acerola cherry, commonly called the Barbados cherry or West Indian cherry, which is grown in Florida, Hawaii, and Puerto Rico, has the highest ascorbic acid content of any known food. The *camu-camu* is native to the jungles of Peru. Also, pine needles, which are rich in vitamin C, have long been extracted (brewed) and used to prevent scurvy by the Indians of Canada and the northern Russians.

• **Synthetic ascorbic acid**—Pure ascorbic acid is available wherever vitamins are sold, at a cost of as little as ½¢ or less per 100 mg (which is more than the recommended daily allowance). It is less expensive than an equivalent amount in natural foods, but natural foods also supply a variety of minerals and other vitamins; hence, vitamin C supplements should be used to augment, rather than replace, natural food sources. Also, the satiety derived from eating fresh strawberries is not experienced when swallowing a tablet or a capsule. Nevertheless, the body utilizes synthetic vitamin C as effectively as it does the vitamin C in foods.

Groupings by rank of foods according to vitamin C values are given in the section on VITAMIN(S), Table V-5, Vitamin Table.

For additional sources and more precise values of vitamin C, see Food Composition Table F-21.

(Also see VITAMIN[S], Table V-5.)

VITAMIN D

Contents	Page
History	1092
Chemistry, Metabolism, Properties	1093
Measurement/Assay	1094
Functions	1094
Deficiency Symptoms	1095
Recommended Daily Allowance of Vitamin D	1096
Toxicity (Hypervitaminosis D)	1096
Vitamin D Losses During Processing, Cooking, and Storage	1097
Sources of Vitamin D	1097

The importance of vitamin D—the sunshine vitamin—in human nutrition lies in the role of regulating calcium and phosphorus metabolism. Vitamin D promotes intestinal absorption of calcium and phosphorus and influences the process of bone mineralization. In the absence of vitamin D, mineralization of bone matrix is impaired, resulting in rickets in children and osteomalacia in adults. Although rickets is rare in the United States, it is still prevalent in many countries.

A bone disorder, which we now call rickets, has been known since 500 B.C. But the disease was first properly described in London about 300 years ago. The word *rickets* is derived from the Old English word *wrikken*, meaning to bend or twist.

Vitamin D is unique among the vitamins in two respects: (1) it occurs naturally in only a few common foods (mainly in fish oils, and a little in liver, eggs, and milk), and (2) it can be formed in the body by exposure of the skin to ultraviolet rays of the sun—light of short wavelength and high frequency; hence, it is known as the *sunshine vitamin*.

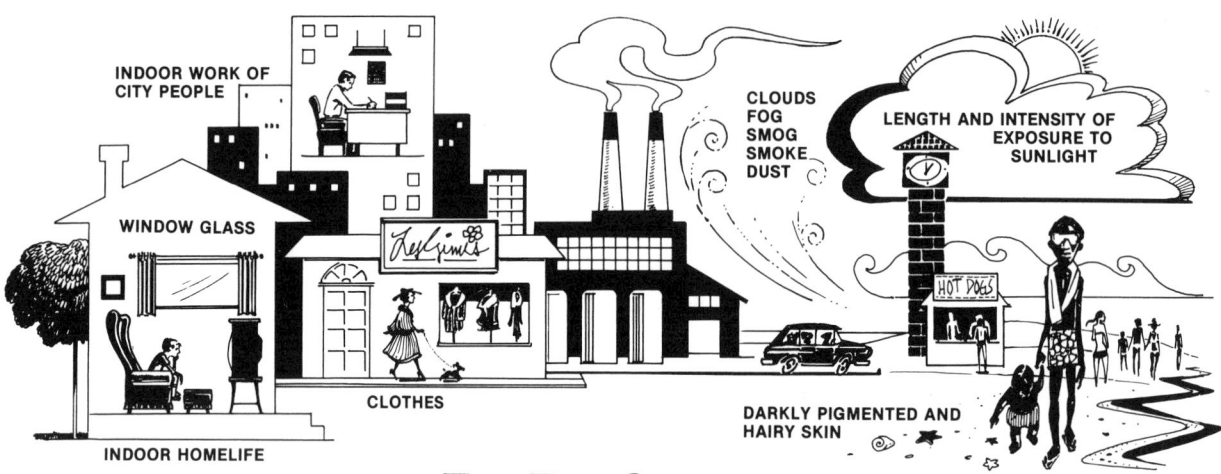

Ten Top Sources

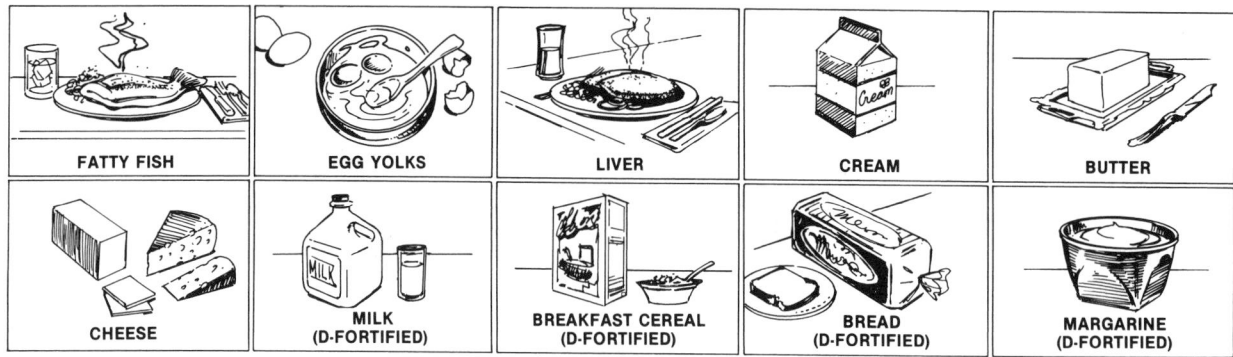

Fig. V-45. Factors that inhibit the sunshine vitamin—that screen out light and prevent the formation of vitamin D. Note, too, top food sources of vitamin D.

HISTORY. The history of rickets as a deficiency disease is much older than our knowledge of how to prevent it. During the Industrial Revolution in England in the 1600s, the disease became very prevalent in children in the crowded slums. Industrial smoke and high tenement buildings shut out the sunlight; so, as industrial cities grew, rickets spread. But no one blamed lack of sunshine (vitamin D) for the crippling disease. Instead, it was attributed to bad home environment and hygiene, and it became known as "a disease of poverty and darkness."

In 1824, cod-liver oil, long known as a folk medicine, was found to be important in the treatment of rickets. But the remedy lost favor with the medical profession because physicians could not explain its action.

As early as 1890, Palm, an English physician, observed that where sunshine was abundant, rickets was rare, but where the sun seldom shone, rickets was common.

In 1918, Sir Edward Mellanby of England demonstrated that rickets was a nutritional deficiency disease. He produced rickets in puppies, then cured it by giving them cod-liver oil. But Mellanby incorrectly attributed the cure to the newly discovered fat-soluble vitamin A.

In 1922, McCollum at Johns Hopkins University found that, after destruction of all the vitamin A in cod-liver oil, (oxidation, by passing heated air through cod-liver oil) it still retained its ricket-preventing potency. This proved the existence of a second fat-soluble vitamin, carried in liver oils

and certain other fats, which he called *calcium-depositing vitamin*. It is of interest to note that, though McCollum discovered the existence of vitamin D, he did not call it by this name until after this designation was in common use by others.

In 1924, the mystery of how sunlight could prevent rickets was partially solved. Dr. Harry Steenbock of the University of Wisconsin and Dr. A. Hess of Columbia University, working independently, showed that the antirachitic activity could be produced in foods and in animals by ultraviolet light. The process, known as the Steenbock Irradiation Process was patented by Steenbock, with the royalties assigned to the Wisconsin Alumni Research Foundation of the University of Wisconsin. Subsequent research disclosed that it was certain sterols in foods and animal tissues that acquired antirachitic activity upon being irradiated. Before irradiation, the sterols were not protective against rickets.

By the late 1920s, it had been established that rickets could be prevented and cured by exposure to direct sunlight (ever since, vitamin D has been popularly called *the sunshine vitamin*), by irradiation with ultraviolet light, by feeding irradiated food, or by feeding cod-liver oil. Later, the natural vitamin D of fish liver oils was identified as the same substance that is produced in the skin by irradiation.

In 1932, crystals of pure vitamin D_2 (ergocalciferol) were isolated from irradiated ergosterol by Windaus of Germany and Askew of England; and in 1936, crystals of pure vitamin

D_3 (cholecalciferol) were isolated from tuna liver oil by Brockmann of Germany.

In 1952, the first total synthesis of a form of vitamin D (in this case vitamin D_3) was accomplished by R. B. Woodward of Harvard. He was awarded the Nobel Prize in Chemistry in 1965 for this and other similar achievements.

CHEMISTRY, METABOLISM, PROPERTIES.

Although about 10 sterol compounds with vitamin D activity have been identified, only two of these, known as provitamins D or precursors, are of practical importance today from the standpoint of their occurrence in foods—ergocalciferol (vitamin D_2, calciferol, or viosterol) and cholecalciferol (vitamin D_3); the name cholecalciferol of the latter is a reflection of its cholesterol precursor. Because these substances are closely related chemically, the term vitamin D is used collectively to indicate the group of substances that show this vitamin activity.

• **Chemistry**—Fig. V-46 shows the structures of vitamins D_2 and D_3.

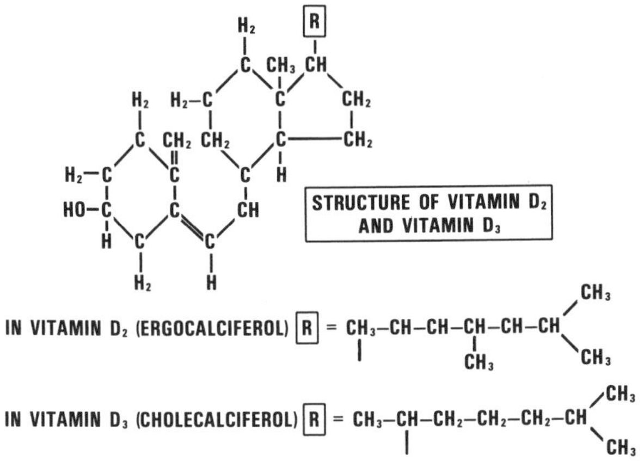

STRUCTURE OF VITAMIN D_2 AND VITAMIN D_3

IN VITAMIN D_2 (ERGOCALCIFEROL) R = CH_3–CH–CH–CH–CH–CH with CH_3 and CH_3/CH_3

IN VITAMIN D_3 (CHOLECALCIFEROL) R = CH_3–CH–CH_2–CH_2–CH_2–CH with CH_3/CH_3

Fig. V-46. Structure of vitamin D_2 and vitamin D_3.

Ultraviolet irradiation of the two provitamins—ergosterol and 7-dehydrocholesterol—will produce vitamins D_2 and D_3, respectively. Ergosterol is found in plants (in yeasts and fungi), whereas 7-dehydrocholesterol is found in fish liver oils and in the skin of man and other animals. Therefore, people or animals that are exposed to sunlight for extended periods of time do not need dietary supplementation of vitamin D. Both forms of vitamin D, D_2 and D_3, have equal activity for people and most other mammalian species. But chickens, turkeys, and other birds are exceptions—they utilize vitamin D_3 more efficiently than vitamin D_2.

• **Metabolism**—Vitamin D is unique in that man and animals normally obtain it from two sources; formation in the skin, and by mouth. The steps involved in the metabolism of vitamin D follow:

1. **Formation of vitamin D_3 in the skin and its movement into the circulation.** The unique mechanism for the synthesis, storage, and slow, steady release of vitamin D_3 from the skin into the circulation is shown in Fig. V-47.

When the skin is exposed to the ultraviolet radiation of sunlight, part of the store of 7-dehydrocholesterol undergoes a photochemical reaction in the epidermis and the dermis and forms previtamin D_3. Once previtamin D_3 is formed in the skin, it undergoes a slow temperature-dependent transformation to vitamin D_3, which takes at least 3 days to complete. Then, the vitamin D-binding protein transports D_3 from the skin into the circulation.

2. **Absorption.** Vitamin D taken by mouth is absorbed with fats from the small intestine (from the jejunum and ileum), with the aid of bile. Vitamin D formed in the skin by irradiation of the provitamin present there is absorbed directly into the circulatory system.

3. **Utilization.** Cholecalciferol—obtained either from the diet or from the irradiation of the skin—is transported by a specific vitamin D carrier protein (a globulin) to the liver where it is converted to 25-hydroxycholecalciferol (25-OH-

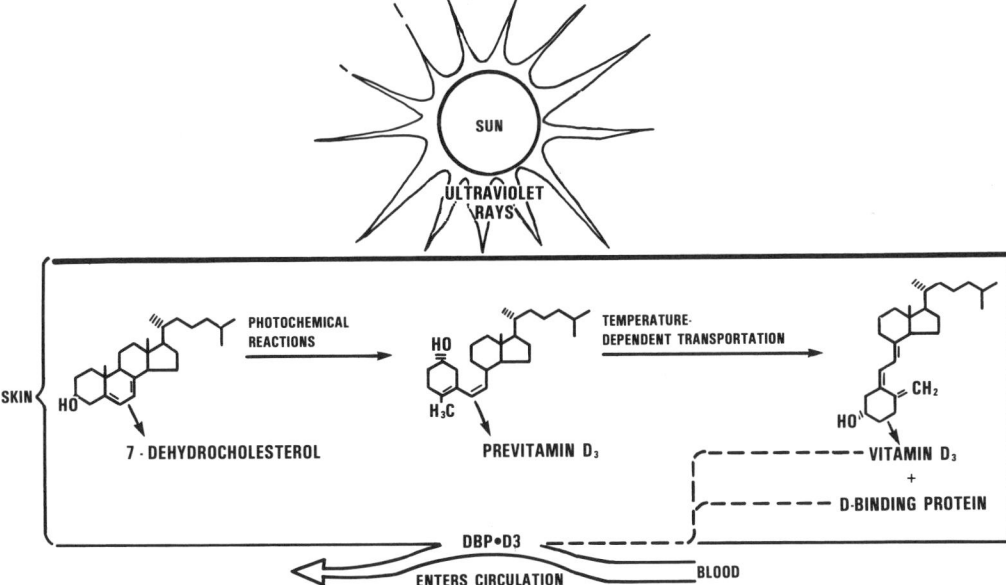

Fig. V-47. Diagram showing the sequence of steps in the formation of vitamin D_3 in the skin and its transport into the circulation.

D_3).[11] From the liver $25\text{-}OH\text{-}D_3$ is transported to the kidneys where it is converted to $1,25\text{-}(OH)_2\text{-}D_3$, the most active form of vitamin D in increasing calcium absorption, bone calcium mobilization, and increased intestinal phosphate absorption. The active compound $1,25\text{-}(OH)_2\text{-}D_3$ functions as a hormone, since it is a vital substance made in the body tissues (the kidneys) and transported in the blood to cells within target tissues. This physiological active form of vitamin D_3 is then either transported to its various sites of action or converted to its metabolite forms of 24,25-dihydroxycholecalciferol or 1,24,25-trihydroxycholecalciferol (see Fig. V-48).

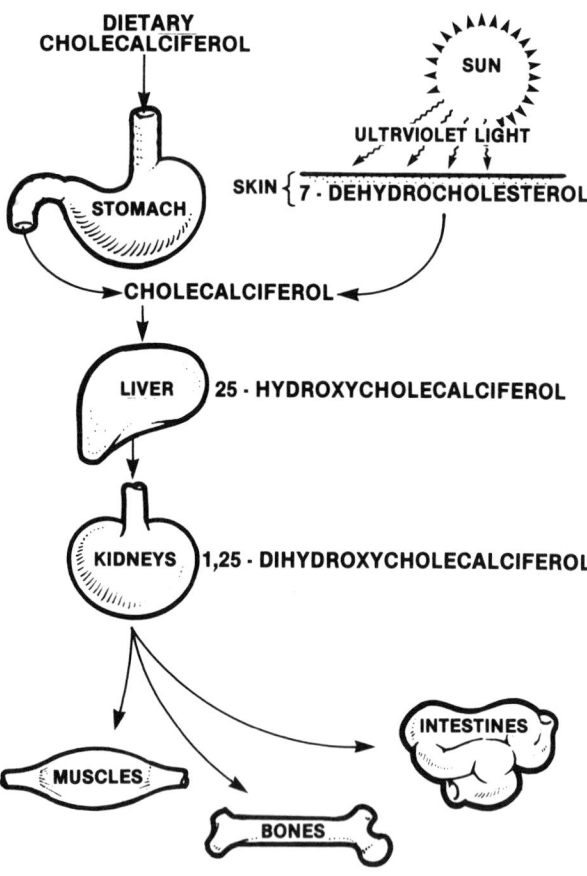

Fig. V-48. Fate of cholecalciferol in the body.

Although most of the research on vitamin D metabolism has been conducted on cholecalciferol, studies by DeLuca on ergocalciferol indicate that it is metabolized similarly to cholecalciferol; that it is changed to a similar active metabolite in the liver—25-hydroxyergocalciferol ($25\text{-}OH\text{-}D_2$).

4. **Storage.** The major storage sites of vitamin D are the fatty tissues and skeletal muscle. Some of it is also found in the liver, brain, lungs, spleen, bones, and skin. But body storage of vitamin D is much more limited than the storage of vitamin A.

5. **Excretion.** The main pathway of excretion of vitamin D is by way of the bile into the small intestine, thence the feces. Less than 4% of the intake is excreted in the urine.

---

[11]Identified by DeLuca and co-workers of the University of Wisconsin. First reported in *Proc. Nat. Acad. Sci.*, 61:1503, 1968.

• **Properties**—Pure D vitamins are white, crystalline, odorless substances that are soluble in both fats and fat solvents (such as ether, chloroform, acetone, and alcohol). They are insoluble in water, and they are resistant to heat, oxidation, acid, and alkali.

Although the precursors are activated by ultraviolet light, excessive irradiation results in the formation of slightly toxic compounds that have no antirachitic activity.

MEASUREMENT/ASSAY. Vitamin D potency is expressed in International Units (IU) and United States Pharmacopeia Units (USP), which are equal. One IU, or one USP, of vitamin D is defined as the activity of 0.025 mcg of pure crystalline vitamin D_3 (cholecalciferol).

The ultraviolet light absorption property of vitamin D may be used for the assay of pure preparations free of irrelevant absorption. But it does not distinguish between vitamin D_2 and D_3.

Both vitamin D_2 and D_3 give a yellow-orange color with antimony trichloride. This color reaction forms the basis of the USP XVIII method for vitamin D. Since color reactions are subject to interferences from many sources, they should be limited to high potency pharmaceutical preparations or fortified foods. Combinations of column and thin-layer chromatographic purification steps with the antimony trichloride reaction have been successfully used.

Gas-liquid chromatography provides a means of combining qualitative and quantitative assays.

Food and feed samples, which contain vitamin D in very low concentrations, are not usually assayed by chemical methods. For these substances, bioassays are the only means available for the assessment of vitamin D activity. Rats and chicks are used as test animals; rats respond equally well to D_2 and D_3, whereas chicks respond only to D_3. The assays measure the alleviation (curative test) or the development (prophylactic test) of vitamin D deficiency in terms of the degree of rickets produced.

A bioassay method, known as the *line test*, uses stained longitudinal sections of the distal end of radius bones to evaluate calcification. Usually the test animal is the rat, although the chick must be used if the vitamin D activity of a sample intended for poultry nutrition is to be determined. Young rats from mothers having a deficient supply of vitamin D are kept on a rachitogenic diet so that no calcification occurs in the ends of the long bones. When a test material is fed to these vitamin D-deficient rats, its value as a source of vitamin D is measured by the amount that must be fed for 7 to 10 days to produce a good calcium line (line test) in the ends of the long bones. Standard cod-liver oil is fed to a similar group of animals and is used as a basis of comparison.

FUNCTIONS. Vitamin D is primarily associated with calcium and phosphorus. It influences the absorption of these minerals and their deposit in bone tissue. Research is continuing to unfold the relationship of vitamin D to calcium and phosphorus metabolism. Although there are many gaps in our knowledge relative to the exact mechanism by which vitamin D carries out its various physiological functions, the current thinking is as follows:

• **Calcium absorption**—It has been clearly established that vitamin D increases calcium absorption from the small intestine, and that a vitamin D deficiency produces large calcium losses in the feces.

• **Phosphate level**—Adequate vitamin D enhances the levels of phosphates in the body, because of (1) improved absorption of phosphorus through the intestinal wall, independent of calcium absorption; and (2) increased resorption of phosphates from the kidney tubules. When sufficient vitamin D is not available, urinary excretion of phosphate increases and the blood level drops.

Maintenance of a satisfactory phosphate level, and of the vital balance between calcium and phosphorus in the blood, is essential (1) to the process of bone calcification and (2) to the prevention of tetany.

• **Bone and teeth metabolism**—The growth and proper mineralization of the bones and teeth require vitamin D.

Lack of vitamin D or lack of exposure to sunlight of children results in weak bones and overgrowth of the softer tissues (cartilage) at the ends of the bones. The joints enlarge, and bowed legs, knock knees, beaded ribs, and skull deformities may result. Lack of vitamin D in adults may result in osteomalacia, in which changes occur in the shafts of bones and bone structure softens. Adequate vitamin D is also important during reproduction and lactation. Extreme deficiencies may result in congenital malformations of the newborn and injury to the skeleton of the mother.

With lack of vitamin D, the enamel and the dentin of the teeth, which are composed almost entirely of calcium and phosphorus, may not develop normally. Thus the teeth of rachitic children and animals have thin, poorly calcified enamel, with pits and fissures, and are especially prone to decay.

The withdrawal of calcium and phosphorus storage from bone (resorption) is stimulated by the action of vitamin D. In this way, vitamin D helps to maintain the blood levels of the two minerals.

• **Citrate metabolism**—The level of citrate in the blood decreases in a vitamin D deficiency. Citrate is an important organic acid involved in many metabolic functions, including mobilization of minerals from bone tissue and removal of calcium from the blood.

The effect on citrate metabolism is thought to be due to changes in mineral metabolism brought about by the absence or presence of vitamin D rather than to a direct action of the vitamin on the formation of citrate.

• **Amino acid levels in the blood**—Vitamin D is involved in the amino acid levels in the blood, by protecting against the loss of amino acids through the kidneys. When there is a deficiency of vitamin D, the excretion of amino acids in the urine is increased.

DEFICIENCY SYMPTOMS. A deficiency of vitamin D leads to inadequate absorption of calcium and phosphorus from the intestinal tract and to faulty mineralization of the bones and teeth, followed by skeletal malformations. The major deficiency symptoms follow:

• **Rickets**—Lack of vitamin D will cause rickets in infants and children, even though the diet is adequate in calcium and phosphorus. (Rickets may also be caused by lack of either calcium or phosphorus, or an incorrect ratio of the two minerals.) This disease is caused from failure of the bones to calcify normally (meaning that the deposition of calcium and phosphorus salts is not normal). As a result, they are soft and pliable and become deformed. The weight of the body causes the ends of the long bones of the legs

to flatten and mushroom outward, giving the appearance of enlarged knee and ankle joints. Other bone changes occurring in rickets include enlarged wrist joints; bowed legs; knocked knees; outward projection of the sternum (*pigeon breast*); a row of beadlike projections on each side of the chest at the juncture of the rib bones and joining (costal) cartilage (called *rachitic rosary*); delayed closure of the fontanel of the skull, causing a bulging of the forehead; narrowing of the pelvis so as to make childbirth difficult in subsequent years; and spinal curvature.

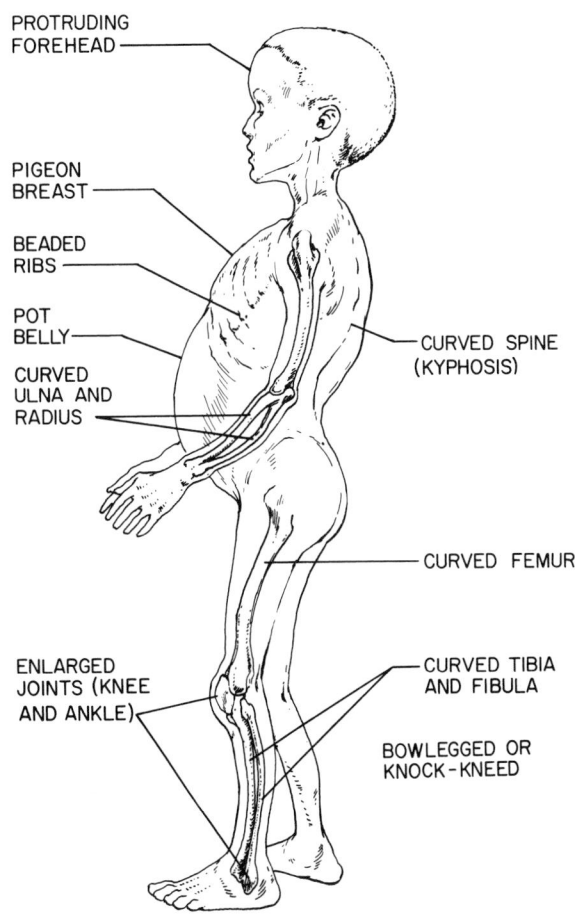

PROTRUDING FOREHEAD

PIGEON BREAST

BEADED RIBS

POT BELLY

CURVED ULNA AND RADIUS

CURVED SPINE (KYPHOSIS)

CURVED FEMUR

ENLARGED JOINTS (KNEE AND ANKLE)

CURVED TIBIA AND FIBULA

BOWLEGGED OR KNOCK-KNEED

Fig. V-49. Symptoms of severe rickets.

Sometimes muscles are poorly developed. Often rickets is associated with protrusion of the abdomen, or *pot belly*, due to weakness of the abdominal muscles.

Eruption of the temporary teeth is delayed; and the permanent teeth may be thin, pitted, and grooved, with the result that they decay easily.

Since the 1930s, the incidence of rickets in the United States has declined, largely because of the addition of vitamin D supplements to breast-fed infants and of the fortification of infant formulas and fluid and evaporated milk with vitamin D. Since 1968, nonfat dry milk for use in various food programs has also been fortified with vitamin D (and vitamin A).

The best protection against rickets and the most favorable bone growth are secured when calcium and phosphorus are supplied in approximately equal amounts (as in milk) and when liberal quantities of vitamin D are available.

When preventive measures are not taken, rickets occurs in northern regions, especially in dark, crowded cities during the winter months, where the ultraviolet rays of sunshine cannot penetrate through the fog, smoke, and soot. Dark-skinned children are more susceptible to rickets than those of the white race; and premature infants are more susceptible than full-term infants, because of the additional demands for vitamin D imposed by increased growth rate and calcification of the bones.

Rickets is still a serious problem in many tropical and semitropical countries and among the poor in overcrowded sections of large cities. In Africa, rickets may be caused by the custom of not exposing babies to sunlight, little vitamin D or calcium in the diet, intestinal parasites, and recurrent diarrhea.

• **Tetany**—A deficiency of vitamin D may cause tetany, though it is not the only cause. Tetany may also result from insufficient absorption of calcium or from a disturbance of the parathyroid gland. Tetany is characterized by muscle twitching, cramps, convulsions, and low serum calcium—less than 7 mg per 100 ml.

• **Osteomalacia**—This is the adult form of rickets, caused by depletion of the bone stores of calcium and phosphorus, as a result of a lack of vitamin D or exposure to sunlight, or lack of either calcium or phosphorus. It is most common during pregnancy, lactation, and old age. Since longitudinal bone growth has stopped in adults, only the shafts on long and flat bones, such as the pelvis, are affected. The bones soften, become distorted, and fracture easily. Also, osteomalacia generally causes rheumatic-type pain in the bones of the legs and lower back.

RECOMMENDED DAILY ALLOWANCE OF VITAMIN D.

The minimum vitamin D requirements are not known, mainly because information on the amount of cholecalciferol formed by the action of sunlight on the skin is not available. The amount formed varies with the length and intensity of exposure to sunlight; the color of skin (dark-pigmented skins can prevent as much as 95% of the sun's ultraviolet light from penetrating into the skin and forming cholecalciferol); the amount of window glass and clothing, which prevent ultraviolet rays from reaching the skin; the season (sunlight is usually scarce during the winter months, when there are cloudy and foggy days); and the amount of atmospheric pollution (*smog*, smoke, dust).

The Food and Nutrition Board (FNB) of the National Research Council (NRC) recommended dietary allowances of vitamin D are given in the section on VITAMIN(S), Table V-5, Vitamin Table.

• **Infants and children**—The vitamin D content of human milk has long been regarded as inadequate for infant needs. Thus, an allowance of 7.5 to 10 mcg should be provided to both breast-fed and bottle-fed infants, either as an oral supplement or included in the formula, particularly since exposure to sunlight of infants is often inadequate.

• **Adults**—Young adults, ages 19–24, may still be growing, therefore their requirements remain at 10 mcg. With the cessation of skeletal growth, calcium needs decrease, and with it, the need for vitamin D. So, the recommended allowance for vitamin D is reduced to 5 mcg after the age of 25 years. Actually, the requirements for the normal adult can usually be met by adequate exposure to sunlight. However, solar radiation may be inadequate under certain climatic conditions or because of chronic air pollution, under which circumstances a dietary source may be necessary.

• **Pregnancy and lactation**—Calcium needs increase during gestation. Moreover, vitamin D and its active metabolites cross the placenta readily. The recommended allowance for both pregnancy and lactation is 10 mcg.

Because vitamin D is a potentially toxic substance, and because there is a lack of evidence that amounts above the recommended allowance confer health benefits, intakes should closely approximate the recommended allowances. Only individuals with diseases affecting vitamin D absorption or metabolism should take vitamin D in excess of the recommended allowances; even then, such treatment should be on the recommendation, and under the supervision, of a physician or a nutritionist.

• **Vitamin D intake in the United States**—It is difficult to estimate the average daily intake of vitamin D per person in the United States because there is no way in which to determine the amount manufactured in the body by the action of sunlight. However, because of the widespread use of fortified milk and other foods, intakes of at least 10 mcg daily per person appear probable.

TOXICITY (HYPERVITAMINOSIS D).

There is wide individual difference in the tolerance to vitamin D; hence, it is impossible to give the level at which vitamin D intake becomes toxic. But, generally speaking, the intake of vitamin D should not exceed a total of 400 IU per day. Excessive amounts of vitamin D (above 2,000 IU/day) can lead to hypercalcemia (toxicity caused by elevated blood levels of calcium) as a result of increased intestinal absorption of calcium. Symptoms of mild toxicity include loss of appetite, excessive thirst, nausea, vomiting, irritability, weakness, constipation (which may alternate with bouts of diarrhea), retarded growth in infants and children, and weight loss in adults. Chronic hypercalcemia results in abnormal deposition of calcium in the soft tissues (including the heart, blood vessels, lungs, and tubules of the kidneys), with particular damage to the kidneys. If massive doses of vitamin D are continued, widespread calcification of the soft tissues may ultimately prove fatal.

Excessive intakes of vitamin D during pregnancy and early infancy may cause idiopathic hypercalcemia, or the hypercalcemic syndrome, a condition characterized by narrowing of the aortic valve of the heart, a peculiar facial appearance, and mental retardation.

The ingestion of excess vitamin D is due mainly to the use of dietary supplements that contain large amounts of the vitamin. Because of the vitamin D added to milk and infant formulas, as well as the vitamin D produced by exposure to sunlight, parents should consider all these sources before giving their children vitamin D supplements.

Adults should also be warned about taking massive doses of vitamin D (as well as about taking massive doses of vitamin A) over a long period of time *unless* it is under the supervision of a physician or nutritionist. Even moderate overdosage of vitamin D is not wise for the elderly.

The concurrent administration of large quantities of vitamin A with potentially toxic levels of vitamin D will reduce the toxicity of the latter.

VITAMIN D LOSSES DURING PROCESSING, COOKING, AND STORAGE.

Vitamin D in foods and food supplements is remarkably stable. Processing does not affect its activity; and because vitamin D is stable to heat and insoluble in water, there is little loss in cooking foods. Foods containing vitamin D can be stored for long periods of time with little deterioration.

The commercial forms of vitamin D_2 and D_3 supplements, which come in either oily solutions or powders, are destroyed relatively rapidly by light, oxygen, and acids. Therefore, they must be stored in opaque, hermetically-sealed containers from which the air is displaced by an inert gas, such as nitrogen. The crystalline compounds are relatively stable to heat.

SOURCES OF VITAMIN D.

Vitamin D is found in foods more sparsely than any other vitamin. But, fortunately, nature ordained that man could generate some of his supply of vitamin D by sunlight.

Groupings by rank of common sources of vitamin D are given in the section on VITAMIN(S), Table V-5, Vitamin Table.

For additional sources and more precise values of vitamin D, see Food Composition Table F-21. However, few vitamin D values are available, because foods do not lend themselves well to chemical analysis for this vitamin. For foods, costly and time-consuming bioassays with rats or chicks are the only means available for the assessment of vitamin D activity.

Among animal foods, fatty fish are rich sources of vitamin D. They obtain the vitamin by feeding on plankton which live near the surface of the sea exposed to sunlight. Liver, egg yolk, and butter contain useful amounts of vitamin D, but the potency of these foods varies widely according to the extent to which the animals have been exposed to sun-

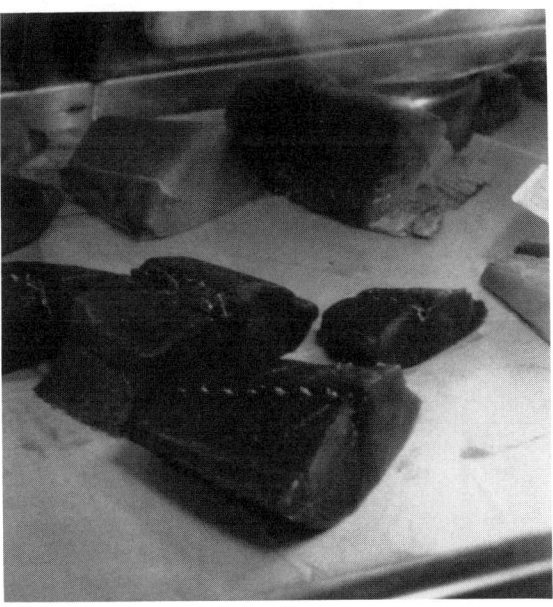

Fig. V-50. Tuna fish, a rich source of vitamin D. (Courtesy, Department of Food Service and Human Nutrition, University of Hawaii)

light or ultraviolet light and to the feeds given them. Muscle meats contain only traces. Both human milk and cow milk are a poor source of vitamin D.

Vegetables, grains and their products, and fruits have little or no vitamin D activity. Although it is usually assumed that living plants do not contain vitamin D activity, an important exception is certain tropical and subtropical shrubs and plants of the *Solanum* family,[12] native to the West Indies, recently found to contain such large amounts of the vitamin D hormone as to be extremely toxic to animals and cause extensive economic losses.

Vitamin D is added to most commercial milk and infant formulas. These two foods are considered most suitable for vitamin D fortification because of their calcium and phosphorus content and the role of vitamin D in the absorption and utilization of the two minerals. Also, milk is consumed in large quantities by the young, who especially need vitamin D for skeletal development.

Practically all whole, low-fat, and nonfat fluid milks on the market today are fortified with 400 IU of vitamin D per quart. Either vitamin D_2 (ergosterol) or D_3 (irradiated cholecalciferol) is added, with the form of the added vitamin listed on the label. Evaporated milk is required by federal law to be fortified with sufficient vitamin D to provide 400 IU per quart when it is reconstituted. Although the fortification of nonfat dry milk is optional, most of it is fortified at a level that supplies 400 IU per reconstituted quart.

Although milk is the only food for which vitamin D fortification is recommended by the Food and Nutrition Board of the National Research Council and the Council of Foods and Nutrition of the American Medical Association, other foods to which vitamin D is added include breakfast cereals, infant cereals, breads, margarine, milk flavorings, fruit and chocolate beverages, and cocoa. Concern has been expressed about the possibility of overconsumption of vitamin D as a result of widespread fortification of foods with the vitamin. Obviously, when vitamin D-enriched milk is used in the amount of 1 qt daily, no other source of vitamin D is required.

All fish liver oils (cod-liver, halibut, and swordfish liver oils) are rich sources of vitamin D, but they are not part of the usual American diet. Preparations containing them are available for use as supplementary sources of vitamin D, particularly for infants. Other vitamin D concentrates are made by irradiating pure ergosterol or 7-dehydrocholesterol; these are available in liquid and tablet form. Viosterol, which is a solution of irradiated ergosterol dissolved in neutral oil, is an example. Such preparations are labeled with the units per dose or tablet and are prescribed accordingly.

The alternative to oral sources of vitamin D is its manufacture in the skin. The vitamin can be produced in the skin if it is exposed to the short wavelengths of the sun's rays (or to a sunlamp), the ultraviolet rays, which act on the provitamin 7-dehydrocholesterol in the skin and transform it into vitamin D_3. But the amount of these rays that act on the skin is affected by atmospheric clouds, smoke, fog, dust, window glass, clothing, skin pigmentation, and season; hence, it is highly variable and cannot either be determined or relied upon. So, some other source of vitamin D is usually needed.

(Also see VITAMIN[S], Table V-5.)

---

[12]Potatoes and eggplant belong to the *Solanum* family, but they are not known to be a source of vitamin D activity. The *Solanum*-toxic plant known as day-blooming jessamine, wild jessamine, or King-of-the-Day has been introduced into the United States and cultivated for ornamental purposes.

VITAMIN E (TOCOPHEROLS)

For many years, vitamin E was known as the *antisterility* vitamin, a name taken from early work with rats, in which species a dramatic improvement in fertility was observed when vitamin E was added to a diet deficient in the substance.

Today, vitamin E is recognized as an essential nutrient for higher animals, including man. In humans, however, sexual potency has never been linked with vitamin E.

HISTORY. In 1922, Evans and Bishop, of the University of California, discovered that a fat-soluble dietary factor (then called *factor X*) in lettuce and wheat germ was essential for successful reproduction in rats. In 1924, Sure, of the University of Arkansas, named the factor vitamin E. In 1936, Evans and co-workers isolated crystalline vitamin E from wheat germ oil and named it tocopherol, from the Greek words *tokos* (offspring) and *pherein* (to bear), meaning *to bear offspring*. In 1938, the vitamin was first synthesized by the Swiss chemist, Karrer.

CHEMISTRY, METABOLISM, PROPERTIES.

• **Chemistry**—Eight tocopherols and tocotrienols with vita-

min E activity, collectively called vitamin E, have been identified. Differing from each other in the number and position of the methyl (CH₃) groups around the ring of the molecule, they are: alpha- (see Fig. V-51), beta-, gamma-, and delta-tocopherol; and alpha-, beta-, gamma-, and delta- tocotrienol. Alpha-tocopherol has by far the greatest vitamin E activity; the other tocopherols have biological activities ranging from 1 to 50% that of alpha-tocopherol. Nevertheless, the nonalpha-tocopherol compounds in foods normally consumed contribute vitamin E activity equivalent to about 20% of the indicated alpha-tocopherol content of a mixed diet.

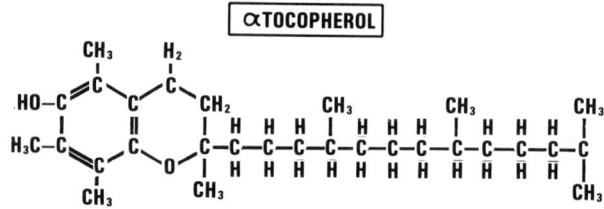

Fig. V-51. Structure of alpha-tocopherol.

• **Metabolism**—A discussion of the absorption, transportation, storage, and excretion of vitamin E follows.

1. **Absorption.** As with other fat-soluble vitamins, the presence of both bile and fat are required for the proper absorption of vitamin E. Absorption takes place in the small intestine, where 20 to 30% of the intake passes through the intestinal wall into the lymph.

2. **Transportation.** Once absorbed, vitamin E is transported attached to the beta-lipoprotein fraction of the blood. In normal adults in the United States, the total tocopherol content of the plasma ranges from 0.5 to 1.2 mg/100 ml.

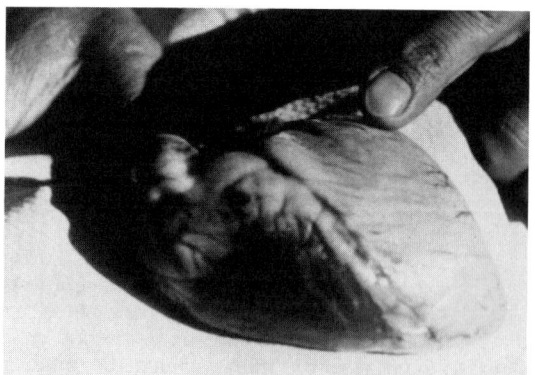

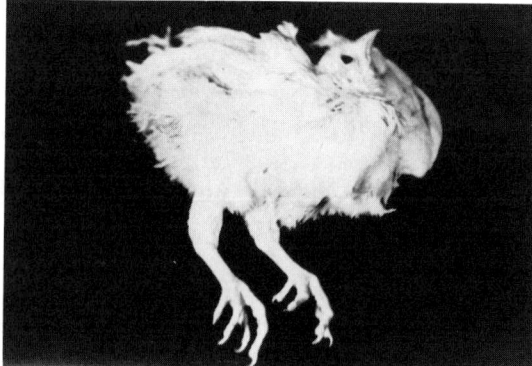

TOP FOOD SOURCES

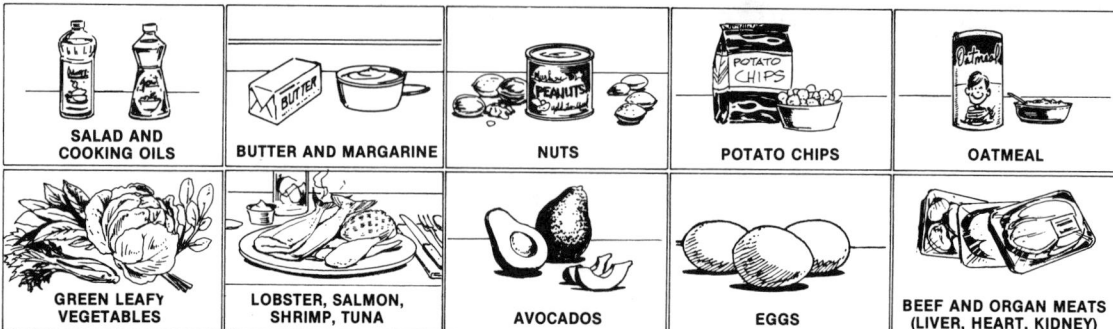

SALAD AND COOKING OILS | BUTTER AND MARGARINE | NUTS | POTATO CHIPS | OATMEAL

GREEN LEAFY VEGETABLES | LOBSTER, SALMON, SHRIMP, TUNA | AVOCADOS | EGGS | BEEF AND ORGAN MEATS (LIVER, HEART, KIDNEY)

Fig. V-52. *Left:* White muscle disease in a lamb, showing characteristic whitish areas or streaks in the heart. (Courtesy, Oregon State University) *Right:* A chick with nutritional encephalomalacia (crazy chick disease), due to a lack of vitamin E. Note head retraction and loss of control of legs. (Courtesy, Department of Poultry Science, Cornell University) Note, too, top food sources of vitamin E.

A level below 0.5 mg is considered undesirable. The ratio of total tocopherol to the total lipids in the plasma appears to be more important than the actual tocopherol level; a ratio of 0.8 mg of total tocopherol to 1 g of total lipids in the plasma is accepted as an indication of adequate vitamin E nutritional status. The predominant form of vitamin E in both the plasma and red cells is alpha-tocopherol, which accounts for 83% of the total tocopherol; gamma-tocopherol accounts for most of the remainder.

3. **Storage.** Adipose (fatty) tissue, liver, and muscle are the major storage sites, although small amounts of vitamin E are stored in most body tissues. Relatively high amounts are found in the adrenal and pituitary glands, heart, lungs, testes, and uterus. Vitamin E is deposited in the fat of tissues and is mobilized from them with fat.

There is little transfer of vitamin E across the placenta to the fetus; hence, newborn infants have low tissue stores.

4. **Excretion.** The major pathway of excretion of vitamin E is by way of the feces, although a small amount is excreted in the urine.

• **Properties**—The tocopherols and tocotrienols are light yellow, viscous oils, soluble in alcohol and fat solvents, but insoluble in water. They are stable to acids and heat, but they are destroyed upon exposure to oxygen, ultraviolet light, alkali, and iron and lead salts. Their ability to take up oxygen gives them important antioxidant properties. Vitamin E is not destroyed to any great extent by normal cooking temperatures, but there are appreciable losses of vitamin E activity in oils heated long periods of time at high temperature, such as in deep-fat frying, because rancidity develops.

Currently, the bulk of commercial vitamin E is synthetic di-alpha-tocopherol acetate, an ester of alpha-tocopherol, a form more stable to heat and oxidation than the free alcohol form, but with the same vitamin E activity. This stable form of alpha-tocopherol is added to vitamin preparations, various medicinal products, foods, and animals feeds.

MEASUREMENT/ASSAY. By agreement of international committees, it is now preferred to use "milligrams of alpha-tocopherol equivalents" as a summation term for all vitamin E activity. In this book, however, both International Units (IU) and alpha-tocopherol equivalents will be used because (1) food composition tables generally give values in IU, and (2) IU is still used for labeling most food products. Table V-6 shows the relationship between milligrams of alpha-tocopherol equivalents and IU.

For purposes of calculating the total vitamin E activity of mixed diets, the milligrams of beta-tocopherol should be multiplied by 0.5, those of gamma-tocopherol by 0.1, and those of alpha-tocotrienol by 0.3. (These are the only vitamins with significant activity that may be present in U. S. diets.) When these are added to the milligrams of alpha-tocopherol, the sum is the total milligrams of alphatocopherol equivalents. If only alpha-tocopoherol in a mixed diet is reported, the value in milligrams should be increased by 20% (multiply by 1.2) to account for the other tocopherols that are present, thus giving an approximation of the total vitamin E activity as milligrams of alpha-tocopherol equivalents.

A colorimetric method is the most commonly used assay method for estimating vitamin E activity. Additionally, spectrofluorometric and gas-liquid chromatographic methods are sometimes used. Animal tests are available, but are now rarely used.

TABLE V-6
RELATIONSHIP BETWEEN ALPHA-TOCOPHEROL EQUIVALENTS AND INTERNATIONAL UNITS (IU)

Compound (1 mg)	Alpha-tocopherol Equivalents in 1 mg	IU Activity in 1 mg
	(mg)	(IU)
d-alpha-tocopherol[1]	1.0	1.49
d-alpha-tocopheryl acetate	0.91	1.36
d-alpha-tocopheryl acid succinate	0.81	1.21
dl-alpha-tocopherol	0.74	1.10
dl-alpha-tocopheryl acetate[2]	0.67	1.00
d-gamma-tocopherol[3]	0.10	0.15

[1]The natural form in foods and the standard for *alpha-tocopherol equivalents*, usually just called alpha-tocopherol.

[2]The common commercial form of vitamin E—a synthetic and stable form. Naturally occurring di-alpha-tocopheryl acetate is considered to have the same potency as the synthetic product. This is the standard for International Units.

[3]The most abundant form in food oils.

FUNCTIONS. The primary function of vitamin E (tocopherols) is to help protect the integrity of cellular and intracellular structures and to prevent destruction of certain enzymes and intracellular components. But there is much controversy as to how this function is carried out.

The authors of this book are of the opinion that vitamin E is more important in human nutrition than is now known; based on current evidence, they subscribe to the following thinking relative to the functions of vitamin E:

1. **As an antioxidant which (a) retards the rancidification of fats in foods and in the digestive tract, and (b) protects cells from toxic substances formed from the oxidation of unsaturated fatty acids.** As a powerful antioxidant, vitamin E readily oxidizes itself (it combines with oxygen), thereby minimizing the destruction by oxidation of unsaturated fatty acids and vitamin A in the intestinal tract and in the tissues.

As an antioxidant, vitamin E prevents rancidity of fats in plant sources and in the animal's digestive tract. But the primary biological role of vitamin E is as an antioxidant inhibiting the oxidation of polyunsaturated fatty acids in tissue membranes, especially at the cellular level—in the membranes that surround the cells, the subcellular particles, and the erythrocytes. It stabilizes the lipid (fat) parts of cells and protects them from damage from toxic free radicals formed from the oxidation of polyunsaturated fatty acids; it reacts with the peroxides, converting them to forms that are not harmful to the cells. By functioning as a natural inhibitor of the destruction of cells, and by protecting tissue from breaking down, vitamin E may have a role in preventing a number of degenerative disorders—including aging.

In its antioxidant role, vitamin E also protects vitamin A (and carotene), vitamin C, sulfur-containing enzymes, and ATP from being oxidized, thereby enabling these essential nutrients to perform their specific functions in the body.

It is noteworthy that when fat is added to the diet it will destroy the vitamin E in both the diet and the digestive tract if rancidity occurs. For this reason, the quantitative relationship between vitamin E and the amount and kind of dietary fat is of practical importance; the higher the consumption of polyunsaturated fats, the higher the vitamin E requirement.

2. **As an essential factor for the integrity of red blood cells.** Evidence has been accumulating that vitamin E functions in the body in maintaining the integrity of the red blood cells. Thus, it is noteworthy that hemolytic anemia, an abnormality of the red blood cells in premature babies, may be corrected with vitamin E. Also, full-term babies with this same abnormality make a more rapid and complete recovery when fed with human milk (rather than cow's milk); and laboratory tests show that human milk contains from 2 to 4 times as much vitamin E as cow's milk.

3. **As an agent essential to cellular respiration.** Alpha-tocopherol appears to be necessary in cellular respiration, primarily in heart and skeletal muscle tissues. Thus, muscular dystrophy has been produced experimentally in various animals on E-deficient rations; however, vitamin E supplements have not been effective in treating people with muscular dystrophy.

4. **As a regulator in the synthesis of body compounds.** The tocopherols appear to be involved in the biosynthesis of DNA, probably by regulating the incorporation of pyrimidines into the nucleic acid structures.

Vitamin E also appears to act as a cofactor in the synthesis of vitamin C, and in the synthesis of coenzyme Q—a factor that is essential in the respiratory mechanism of cells that releases energy from carbohydrates and fats.

5. **As a protector of lung tissue from air pollution.** Recent studies on rats have shown that vitamin E may protect lung tissue from smog—from damage by such oxidant components of air pollution as nitrogen dioxide (NO_2) and ozone. At the present time, it is not known whether or not vitamin E protects human lungs from damage by air pollution.

6. **As a sometimes replacement for selenium.** Both vitamin E and selenium are antioxidants, although each takes a different approach. Nevertheless, vitamin E has a sparing or replacement effect on selenium.

The belief among some people that vitamin E is *the sex vitamin* and will reduce sterility and increase potency in man is not based on scientific fact; it is one of the falsities of nutrition information which is given wide publicity.

INTERRELATIONSHIP OF VITAMIN E AND SELENIUM.

During the 1950s, an interrelationship between vitamin E and the element selenium was established. It was found that selenium prevented exudative diathesis (a hemorrhagic disease) in vitamin E-deficient chicks and liver necrosis in vitamin E-deficient rats. Subsequent research demonstrated that both selenium and vitamin E protect the cell from the detrimental effects of peroxidation, but each takes a distinctly different approach to the problem. Vitamin E is present in the membrane components of the cell and prevents free-radical formation, while selenium functions throughout the cytoplasm to destroy peroxides. This explains why selenium will correct some deficiency symptoms of vitamin E, but not others.

There is also some indication that vitamin E and selenium work together to protect cell membranes, cell nuclei, and chromosomes from carcinogens—substances that can cause cancer. But much more experimental work is needed on this subject.

DEFICIENCY SYMPTOMS.

Many dietary factors seem to contribute to the development of vitamin E deficiency symptoms; among them, total fat, unsaturated fats, cod-liver oil (which is high in unsaturated acids), amount of protein, choline, cystine, inositol, cholesterol, vitamin A, and minerals have been implicated, at one time or another, as causing or aggravating deficiency symptoms.

Vitamin E deficiency symptoms as such rarely occur in humans because vitamin E (1) is widely distributed in foods, (2) is stored in almost all body tissues, and (3) is retained in the body for relatively long periods. However, clinical evidence of deficiency has been observed in infants, especially those born prematurely and formula-fed. Also, vitamin E deficiency occurs in individuals suffering from kwashiorkor (a protein deficiency), and in children and adults who have impaired fat absorption.

Newborn infants (especially the premature) have low plasma levels of vitamin E (the vitamin E concentration in full-term newborn infants is about one-third that of adults, and that of premature infants is even lower), because transfer of vitamin through the placenta to the fetus is limited. As a result, hemolytic anemia (caused by shortened life span of red cells) may occur in the early weeks of life. In this condition, the membranes of the red blood cells are weakened by the action on them of the products of peroxidation of polyunsaturated fats and the cells rupture easily, producing a condition characterized by edema, skin lesions, and blood abnormalities. Supplements of vitamin E bring about increases in blood levels of the vitamin, decreases in red blood cell hemolysis, and a return to normal hemoglobin levels.

Individuals suffering from kwashiorkor, due to a severe protein deficiency, have very little tocopherol in their serum; the fragility of their red blood cells is greater than normal, and they frequently suffer from an accompanying anemia.

The symptoms of vitamin E deficiency produced by artificial diets high in unsaturated fatty acids or observed in patients unable to absorb fat (sprue, fibrocystic disease of the pancreas) include low blood and tissue tocopherol levels, increased red blood cell fragility and shortened red blood cell life-span, and increased urinary excretion of creatine (the latter is indicative of muscle damage). Marked improvement in these conditions is noted following administration of alpha-tocopherol.

RECOMMENDED DAILY ALLOWANCE OF VITAMIN E.

The Food and Nutrition Board (FNB) of the National Research Council (NRC) recommended daily allowances of vitamin E are given in the section on VITAMIN(S), Table V-5, Vitamin Table.

The requirements of vitamin E for humans is known to vary with other ingredients in the diet; for example, the presence of large amounts of polyunsaturated fatty acids (PUFA), such as linoleic acid, markedly increases the requirement. This is important in today's diets, in which large amounts of vegetable oils are used. So, individuals consuming diets high in PUFA need more vitamin E than the amounts listed in Table V-5, Vitamin Table; those whose diets are low in PUFA need less. Also, the presence of rancid fats, oxidizing substances, and selenium modify the requirements for vitamin E.

• **Infants**—The vitamin E content of human milk, 2 to 5 IU (1.3 to 3.3 mg d-alpha-tocopherol equivalent) per liter (1.06 qt), is considered to be adequate for full-term infants. Table V-5 lists the daily allowances in mg d-alpha-TE of infants, as follows: birth to 6 months, 3 mg; from 6 months to 1 year of age, 4 mg.

Cow's milk differs from human milk in two ways: (1) it contains only 1/10 to 1/2 as much vitamin E, varying with the feed consumed by the cow; and (2) it is much lower in polyunsaturated fats, containing about 1/2 as much.

Increased vitamin E is required for both premature and full-term infants fed commercial formulas made from vegetable oils that are high in polyunsaturated fats, like linoleic acid. According to the Committee on Nutrition of the Academy of Pediatrics, full-term infants require at least 0.7 IU (about 0.47 mg) of vitamin E per gram of linoleic acid in a formula preparation.

• **Children**—Table V-5 lists the daily allowances in mg d-alpha-TE of children as follows: from 1 to 3 years of age, 6 mg; from 4 to 10 years of age, 7 mg.

• **Adults**—Table V-5 lists the daily allowances in mg d-alpha-TE of adults as follows: males, 10 mg; females, 8 mg.

• **Pregnancy and lactation**—During pregnancy and lactation, the Food and Nutrition Board recommends that the daily allowance of vitamin E be increased to compensate for the amount deposited in the fetus and secreted in the milk; that the RDA be 10 mg α TE during pregnancy, and 12 mg α TE during lactation.

• **Vitamin E intake in average U.S. diet**—Limited reports on the vitamin E intake in the U.S. diet show a daily intake of 16.7 mg α tocopherol. To this must be added the additional forms of vitamin E other than alpha-tocopherol, particularly gamma-tocopherol from soybean oil, which provide significant amounts of vitamin E activity in usual diets in the United States. Generally, nonalpha-tocopherol forms of vitamin E in a mixed diet are considered to supply about 20% of the total vitamin E activity. For the latter reason, calculations based only on alpha-tocopherol underestimate the amount of dietary vitamin E activity.

TOXICITY. Compared with vitamins A and D, vitamin E is relatively nontoxic. Excess intakes of vitamin E are excreted in the feces.

VITAMIN E LOSSES DURING PROCESSING, COOKING, AND STORAGE.

Food processing, storage, and packaging cause considerable loss of vitamin E. The tocopherols are subject to destruction by oxygen; and oxidation is accelerated by exposure to light, heat, alkali, and the presence of certain trace minerals such as iron (Fe^{+++}) and copper (Cu^{++}).

The milling of grains removes about 80% of the vitamin E; for example, in converting whole wheat to white flour, and in processing corn, oats, and rice.

Various methods of processing cause considerable destruction of vitamin E. Dehydration causes 36 to 45% loss of alpha-tocopherol in chicken and beef, but little or none in pork. Canning causes losses of 41 to 65% of the alpha-tocopherol content of meats and vegetables. An 80% destruction occurs during the roasting of nuts.

Deep-fat frying of foods causes vitamin E losses of 32 to 75%. However, normal home baking or cooking in water do not involve large losses of tocopherol. Also, being insoluble in water, tocopherols are not drained off with water.

There is a great loss of tocopherol in the storage of potato chips and french fried potatoes. One study showed after-manufacture losses of tocopherol in potato chips stored at 73°F (23°C) of 71% in 1 month and 77% in 2 months. When the chips were frozen at 10°F (–12°C), the losses were 63% in 1 month and 68% in 2 months. The after-manufacture losses of french fries stored at 10°F (–12°C) were 68% in 1 month and 74% in 2 months.

SOURCES OF VITAMIN E. Vitamin E (the tocopherols) occurs mainly in a variety of plant materials, especially oil seed crops (vegetable oils), some grains, nuts, and green leafy vegetables. The amount in plant foods is affected by species, variety, stage of maturity, season, time and manner of harvesting, processing procedures, and storage time. Animal tissues and animal products are usually low to poor sources of vitamin E and are influenced by the dietary consumption of tocopherols by the animal.

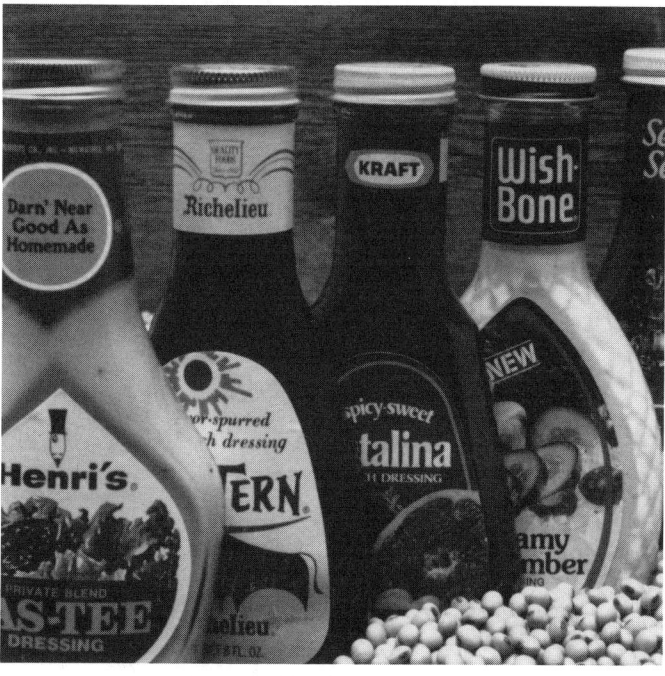

Fig. V-53. Salad dressings, a rich source of vitamin E. (Courtesy, American Soybean Assn., St. Louis, Mo.)

Groupings by rank of common food sources of vitamin E are given in the section on VITAMIN(S), Table V-5, Vitamin Table.

For additional sources and more precise values of vitamin E (alpha-tocopherol), see Food Composition Table F-21.

Wheat germ and wheat germ oil, which are used as supplements, are the richest natural sources of vitamin E, followed by the vegetable oils (almond, corn, cottonseed, olive, palm, peanut, rapeseed, safflower, soybean, and sunflower—coconut oil is a poor source of vitamin E). It follows that margarine and cooking and salad oils are major sources in the diet; fortunately, the hydrogenation process used in their manufacture has little, if any, effect on the vitamin E content.

Refined grain products contain little vitamin E—most of the vitamin is removed in the milling process.

Human milk contains 2 to 4 times as much vitamin E as cow's milk.

(Also see VITAMIN[S], Table V-5.)

VITAMIN K

Vitamin K, known as the *antihemorrhagic vitamin*, is necessary for the synthesis of prothrombin and other blood clotting factors in the liver. Presently, the term vitamin K is used to describe a chemical group of quinone compounds, rather than a single entity, which have characteristic antihemorrhagic effects.

Defective blood coagulation is the only well-established symptom of vitamin K deficiency. Deficiencies are rare in humans, but considerable use is made of synthetic substances that act as antagonists of vitamin K (such as dicoumarol, an anticoagulant) to prevent clotting of blood in patients with certain circulatory disorders.

HISTORY. In 1929, Professor Carl Peter Hendrik Dam, biochemist at the University of Copenhagen, Denmark, observed that certain experimental diets produced fatal hemorrhages in chicks. Bleeding could be prevented by giving a variety of foodstuffs, especially alfalfa (lucerne) and fishmeal. Further, it was found that the active principle in these materials could be extracted with ether; thus, a new fat-soluble factor was discovered. In 1935, Dam named it the Koagulation vitamin (the Danish word for coagulation), from which the shortened term vitamin K (from the first letter of Koagulation) was derived. In 1939, Dam and Karrer isolated vitamin K in pure form; and, that same year, Almquist and Klose synthesized vitamin K. In 1943, Dam received the Nobel Prize in physiology and medicine for his brilliant work.

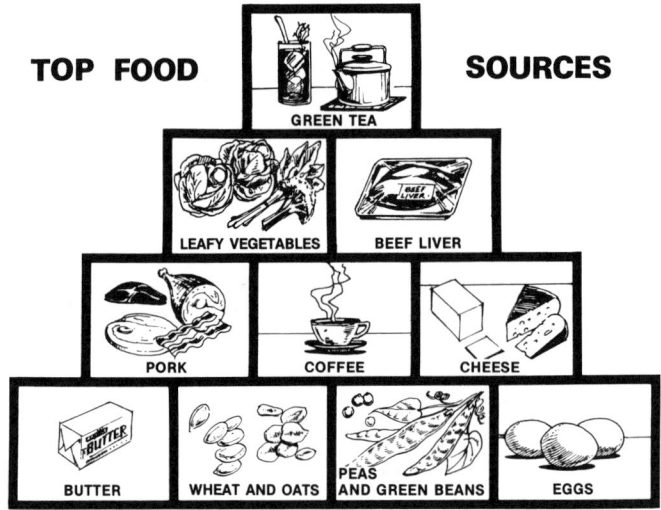

Fig. V-54. Top sources of vitamin K for common foods.

In 1941, Link and co-workers at the University of Wisconsin discovered dicoumarol—an antimetabolite of vitamin K.

CHEMISTRY, METABOLISM, PROPERTIES.

• **Chemistry**—A number of chemical compounds possessing vitamin K activity have been isolated or synthesized. There are two naturally occurring forms of vitamin K; vitamin K_1 (phylloquinone or phytylmenaquinone) which occurs only in green plants, and K_2 (menaquinones or multiprenylmenaquinones), which is synthesized by many microorganisms, including bacteria in the intestinal tracts of human beings and other species. Additionally, several synthetic compounds have been prepared that possess vitamin K activity, the best known of which is menadione (2-methyl, 1, 4-naphthoquinone), formerly known as K_3. Menadione,

CHEMISTRY. METABOLISM. PROPERTIES.

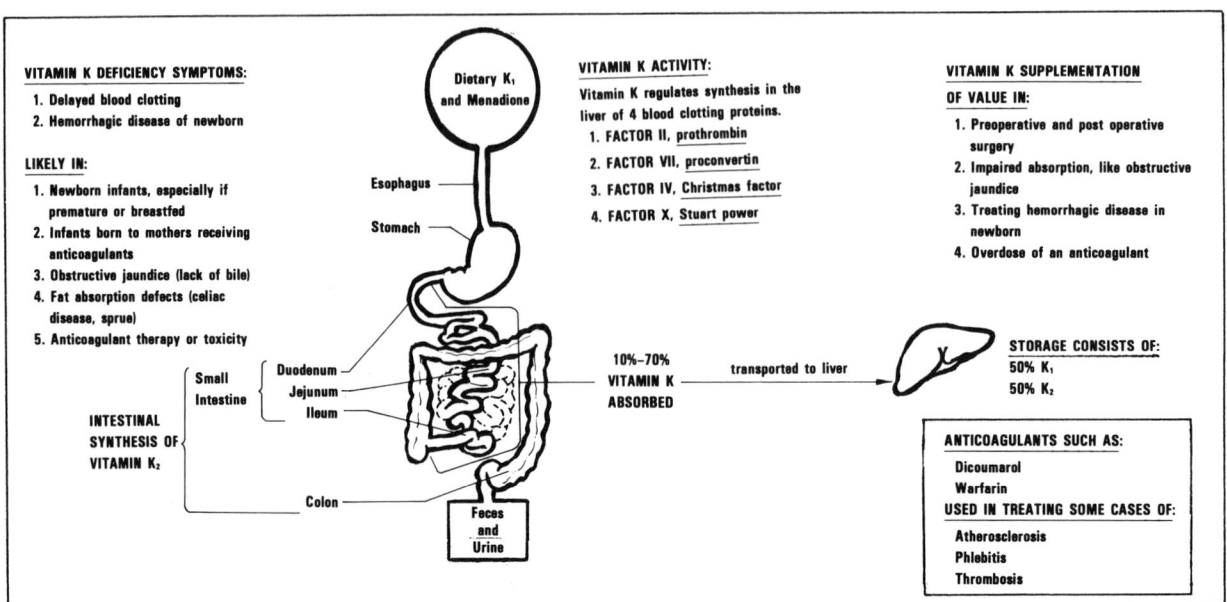

Fig. V-55. Vitamin K utilization.

which is converted to vitamin K_2 in the body, is 2 to 3 times as potent as K_1 and K_2. The structural formulas of K_1, K_2, and menadione, all of which are called vitamin K, are shown in Fig. V-56.

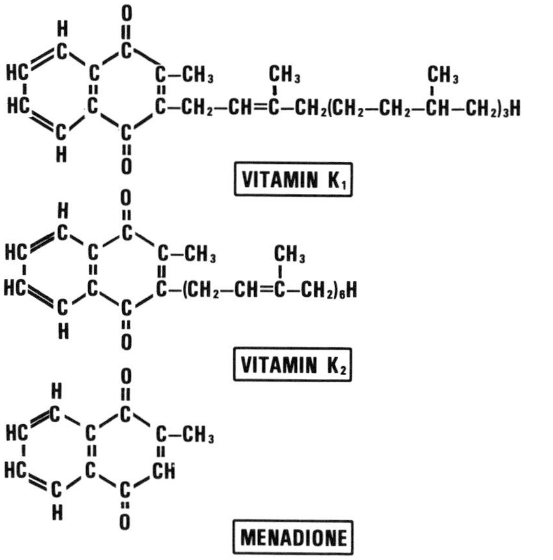

Fig. V-56. Structures of vitamin K, vitamin K_2, and menadione.

• **Metabolism**—Normally, vitamin K_1 is taken into the body in the diet, vitamin K_2 is synthesized in the intestine, and menadione is taken as a vitamin supplement.

1. **Intestinal synthesis.** Vitamin K_2 is synthesized by the normal bacteria in the small intestine and the colon; hence, an adequate supply is generally present. Since the intestine of a newborn infant is sterile at birth, however, the supply of vitamin K is inadequate until normal bacterial flora of the intestine develops on about the third or fourth day of life.

The intestinal synthesis of vitamin K reduces the food dietary requirements for the vitamin in man and other mammals (but not birds; birds have such a short intestinal tract and harbor so few microorganisms that they require a dietary source of vitamin K), although it appears that little of the vitamin K produced in the lower gut is absorbed. It is noteworthy, however, that animals that practice coprophagy, such as the rabbit, can utilize much of the vitamin K that is eliminated in the feces.

2. **Absorption.** Since the natural vitamins K (K_1 and K_2) are fat soluble, they require bile and pancreatic juice in the intestine for maximum absorption. Thus, anything that interferes with the normal absorption of fat, interferes with the absorption of natural vitamin Ks. By contrast, some of the synthetic vitamin K compounds are water soluble and more easily absorbed. Absorption takes place mainly in the upper part of the small intestine. Normally, 10 to 70% of the vitamin K in the intestines is absorbed. However, there is uncertainty as to how much of the vitamin K_2 that is synthesized in the colon is absorbed, based on the fact that absorption of nutrients in general from the large intestine appears to be limited because of the nature of the epithelial lining.

3. **Transportation.** Vitamin K passes unchanged from the small intestine into the lymph system. Thence, it is carried to the thoracic duct, where it enters the bloodstream. In the blood, it is attached to beta-lipoproteins and transported to the liver and other tissues.

4. **Metabolism.** Whether the vitamin Ks' functions are unchanged or are transformed to other metabolically active forms has not been determined. It is known that menadione must be converted to K_2 in the bodies of both animals and humans for it to be biologically active.

5. **Storage.** Vitamin K is stored only in small amounts. Modest amounts are stored in the liver, with the skin and muscle following in concentration. About 50% of the vitamin K found in the human liver is K_1 from the diet; the other 50% is K_2 from bacterial synthesis in the intestine.

6. **Excretion.** Excess vitamin K is excreted in the feces and urine.

• **Properties**—The naturally occurring forms of vitamin K are yellow oils; the synthetic forms are yellow crystalline powders. All K vitamins are resistant to heat and moisture, but they are destroyed on exposure to acid, alkali, oxidizing agents, and light—particularly ultraviolet light. Since natural vitamin K is stable to heat and not water soluble, little of it is lost in normal cooking processes. However, some of the synthetic forms of vitamin K are soluble in water.

MEASUREMENT/ASSAY. Vitamin K can be measured in micrograms of the pure synthetic compound (menadione), and the vitamin K activity of other substances can be expressed in similar terms.

The potency of low concentration samples, such as occurs in most foods, is commonly determined by bioassay, using young chicks, and is based on the minimum dose that will maintain the normal coagulation of the blood at the end of 1 month. In pure solutions, vitamin K may be assayed by U.V. spectrophotometry or colorimetric methods. Other accepted techniques are the oxidimetric assay after catalytic reduction to the hydroquinone and the polarographic determination.

FUNCTIONS. Vitamin K is essential for the synthesis by the liver of four blood clotting proteins—factor II, or prothrombin; factor VII, or proconvertin; factor IX, Christmas factor; and factor X, Stuart-Power factor. The exact way in which vitamin K functions in the synthesis of these proteins is unknown. Recent research suggests that vitamin K acts in some way to convert precursor proteins to the active blood clotting factors. Without vitamin K, or when an antagonist is given, the level of the blood clotting proteins in the blood is reduced and clotting time is prolonged.

At this time, there is no evidence that vitamin K has any functions in humans or animals other than in the blood coagulation process, although vitamin K-dependent proteins have been identified in the bone, kidney, and liver.

VITAMIN K ANTAGONISTS (ANTICOAGULANTS). The discovery of vitamin K antagonists stemmed primarily from investigations into a disorder in cattle known as *sweet clover disease,* in which there is a loss of clotting power of the blood. The causative agent of *sweet clover disease* was identified by Campbell, et al., (1941) of the University of Wisconsin, as dicoumarol, an oxidative product of coumarin, found in sweet clover hay that had undergone spoilage during harvesting or storage.

The discovery of the cause of *sweet clover disease* opened up an entirely new field. The synthesis of several dicoumarol derivatives followed. These antivitamins, or antagonists, decrease the ability of the blood to clot by inhibiting the synthesis of prothrombin and the other K-dependent blood clotting factors. They are used medically to reduce clotting of the blood in patients with certain circulatory disorders, especially some forms of atherosclerosis, phlebitis, and thrombosis.

DEFICIENCY SYMPTOMS.   The symptoms of vitamin K deficiency are increased clotting times and hemorrhaging. Two laboratory tests are commonly used to assess vitamin K status: (1) the *prothrombin time*—the measurement in a plasma sample of the speed of conversion of prothrombin to thrombin; and (2) the *blood clotting time*—the placing of freshly drawn blood in a clean test tube, tilting it once each minute, and determining the time required for the clot to form (for normal blood the clotting time is about 10 minutes).

Fowl are very susceptible to vitamin K deficiency. When vitamin K is absent, they develop delayed blood clotting, causing hemorrhages under the skin and serious internal bleeding, followed by death if not corrected. Deficiencies have also been produced in cattle, pigs, rats, dogs, and all other species studied.

Although a hemorrhagic syndrome, due to a vitamin K deficiency, is rare in adult humans, it can be caused by the following:

1.   Some defect in the absorption as in obstructive jaundice, or in malabsorption due to celiac disease or sprue.
2.   Sterilization of the bowels by an antibiotic or a sulfa drug, thereby reducing the synthesis of vitamin K.
3.   Anticoagulant therapy for certain circulatory disorders.

Hemorrhagic disease, due to a vitamin K deficiency, may occur in newborn babies—particularly those born prematurely and breast fed, those on unfortified soy formulas, or those whose mothers have been taking anticoagulants—between the second and fifth days of life; causing bleeding either in the skin, nervous system, peritoneal cavity, or alimentary tract. Because human milk provides less vitamin K than cow's milk, vitamin K deficiency is more common in breast-fed than in formula-fed babies. Hemorrhagic disease due to a vitamin K deficiency can be prevented by giving a dose of 1 mg of vitamin K_1 intramuscularly immediately after birth. It is noteworthy, however, that vitamin K deficiency is not always the cause of hemorrhagic disease; injury at birth is undoubtedly responsible in some cases.

Vitamin K has proved ineffective in treating hemophilia, an inherited condition causing abnormal hemorrhaging in man.

RECOMMENDED DAILY ALLOWANCE OF VITAMIN K.   Because of the synthesis of vitamin K by intestinal bacteria in healthy individuals (except newborn babies), no specific recommended allowance is made for this vitamin by the Food and Nutrition Board of the NRC–National Academy of Sciences. However, because the adequacy of the intestinal synthesis over a long period is uncertain, NRC does give an estimated adequate dietary intake of vitamin K. (See section on VITAMIN[S], Table V-5, Vitamin Table.)

The Table V-5 estimated safe and adequate daily intakes of vitamin K, in mcg, are as follows: Infants birth to 6 months, 5 mcg; infants 6 months to 1 year, 10 mcg; children 1 to 3 years, 15 mcg; children 4 to 6 years, 20 mcg; children 7 to 10 years, 30 mcg; males 25 to 50 years, 80 mcg; females 25 to 50 years, 65 mcg, with no increase in pregnancy or lactation.

In 1989, the Committee on Nutrition of the American Academy of Pediatrics recommended that infant formulas include a minimum of 4 mcg per 100 kcal of vitamin K for milkbase formulas and 8 mcg per 100 kcal for soy isolate and other milk substitute formulas. Vitamin K hypoprothrombinemia (due to K deficiency) occurs in infants fed certain soy protein isolates, meat base formula, or formula containing hydrolyzed casein. Such diets may be low in vitamin K.

The intake suggested for young infants is based on 2 mcg/kg, assuming no intestinal synthesis. Therefore, the amount provided by current formulas of 4 mcg/100 kcal should be ample for normal infants. The suggested intake of 12 mcg/day is also in the range supplied by breast milk (15 mcg/liter).

• **Vitamin K intake in average U.S. diet**—The average mixed diet in the United States supplies 300 to 500 mcg of vitamin K per day; hence, there is little danger of insufficiency under normal conditions.

TOXICITY (HYPERVITAMINOSIS K).   The natural forms of vitamins K_1 and K_2 have not produced toxicity even when given in large amounts. However, synthetic menadione and its various derivatives (formerly called K_3) have produced toxic symptoms in rats and jaundice in human infants when given in amounts of more than 5 mg daily. Consequently, the U.S. Food and Drug Administration does not allow any menadione in any food supplements, including prenatal vitamin capsules.

Vitamin K_1 preparations are preferred for the treatment of such medical conditions as liver disease, severe malabsorption syndromes, and anticoagulant overdosage.

VITAMIN K LOSSES DURING PROCESSING, COOKING, AND STORAGE.   For maximum vitamin K, food should be fresh. Frozen foods tend to be deficient in vitamin K. Ordinary cooking processes destroy very little natural vitamin K, since the vitamin is stable to heat and not water soluble. However, some of the synthetic compounds are soluble in water and subject to greater loss in cooking. Sunlight destroys vitamin K_1; and all vitamin K compounds tend to be unstable to alkali.

SOURCES OF VITAMIN K.   Vitamin K is fairly widely distributed in foods.

Also, synthesis in the intestine is an important source of vitamin K_2; and vitamin K supplements (chiefly the synthetic menadione) are available.

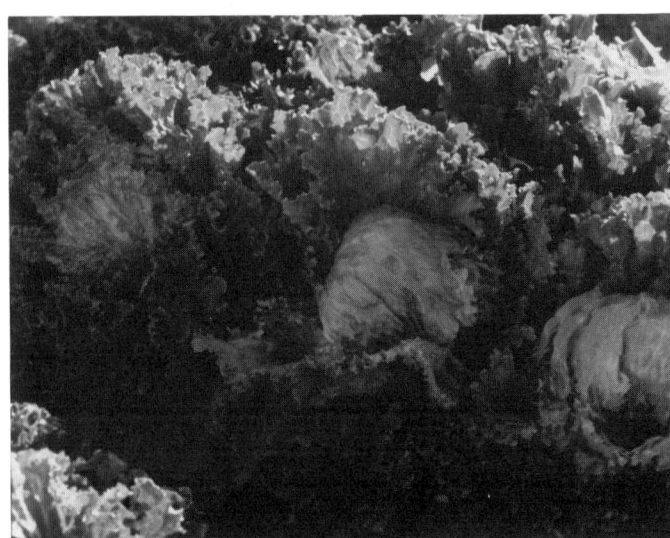

Fig. V-57. Lettuce, a good source of Vitamin K. (Courtesy, California Iceberg Lettuce Commission, Monterey, Calif.)

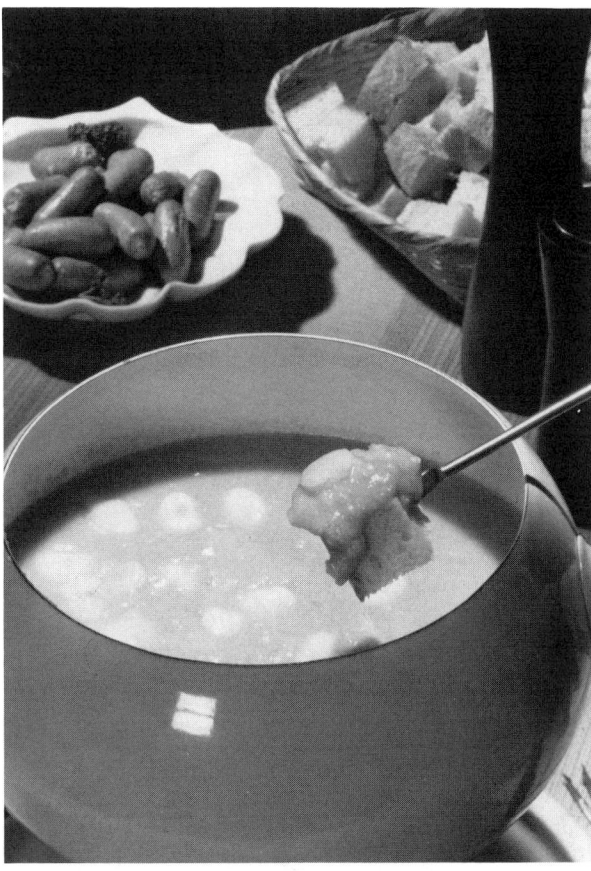

Fig. V-58. Cheese fondue, a good source of vitamin K. (Courtesy, California Dry Bean Advisory Board, Dinuba, Calif.)

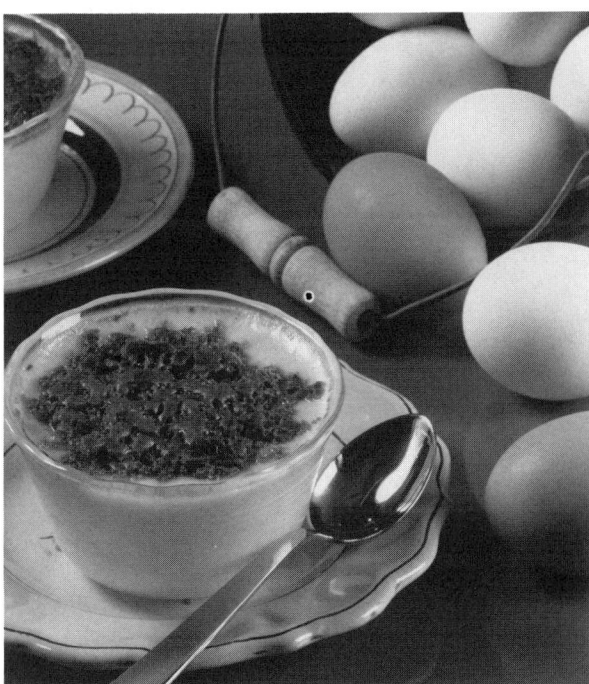

Fig. V-59. Egg custard is another good source of vitamin K. (Courtesy, American Egg Board, Park Ridge, Ill.)

Groupings by rank of common sources of vitamin K are given in the section on VITAMIN(S), Table V-5, Vitamin Table.

No vitamin K values are listed in Food Composition Table F-21, for the reason that few foods have been assayed for this vitamin.

The vitamin K content of some common foods is given in Table V-7.

(Also see VITAMIN[S], Table V-5.)

TABLE V-7
VITAMIN K AND CALORIE CONTENT OF SOME COMMON FOODS[1]

Food	Vitamin K	Energy
	(mcg/100 g)	(kcal/100 g)
Tea, green	712	1
Turnip greens	650	28
Broccoli	200	26
Lettuce	129	15
Cabbage	125	24
Beef liver	92	222
Spinach	89	26
Asparagus	57	20
Watercress	57	19
Bacon	46	300
Coffee	38	3
Cheese	35	402
Butter	30	717
Pork liver	25	241
Oats	20	390
Peas, green	19	71
Wheat, whole	17	357
Beef fat	15	902
Ham	15	350
Beans, green	14	24
Eggs	11	157
Pork tenderloin	11	254
Peaches, raw	8	38
Ground beef	7	301
Chicken liver	7	165
Raisins	6	289

[1]Adapted from Goodhart, Robert S. and Maurice E. Shils, *Modern Nutrition in Health and Disease*, 6th ed., Lea & Febiger, 1980, p. 172, Table 6C-1; data taken from the studies of Dam and Glavind, Richardson, Doisy and Matschiner and Doisy.

VITAMIN L

Factors L_1 and L_2, which are found in yeast, are said to be necessary for lactation. However, they have not become established as vitamins; hence, there is no such thing as vitamin L at this time.

VITAMIN SUPPLEMENTS

Rich synthetic or natural food sources of one or more of the complex organic compounds, called vitamins, that are required in minute amounts by people and animals for normal growth, production, reproduction, and/or health.

(Also see VITAMIN[S].)

VOLATILE OILS

These are obtained from flowers, stems, leaves, and often the entire plant, and they are used for perfumery and flavorings. Often these are called essential oils. They vaporize quickly.

(Also see ESSENTIAL OILS.)

VOMITING

The forcible expulsion of the contents of the stomach through the mouth.

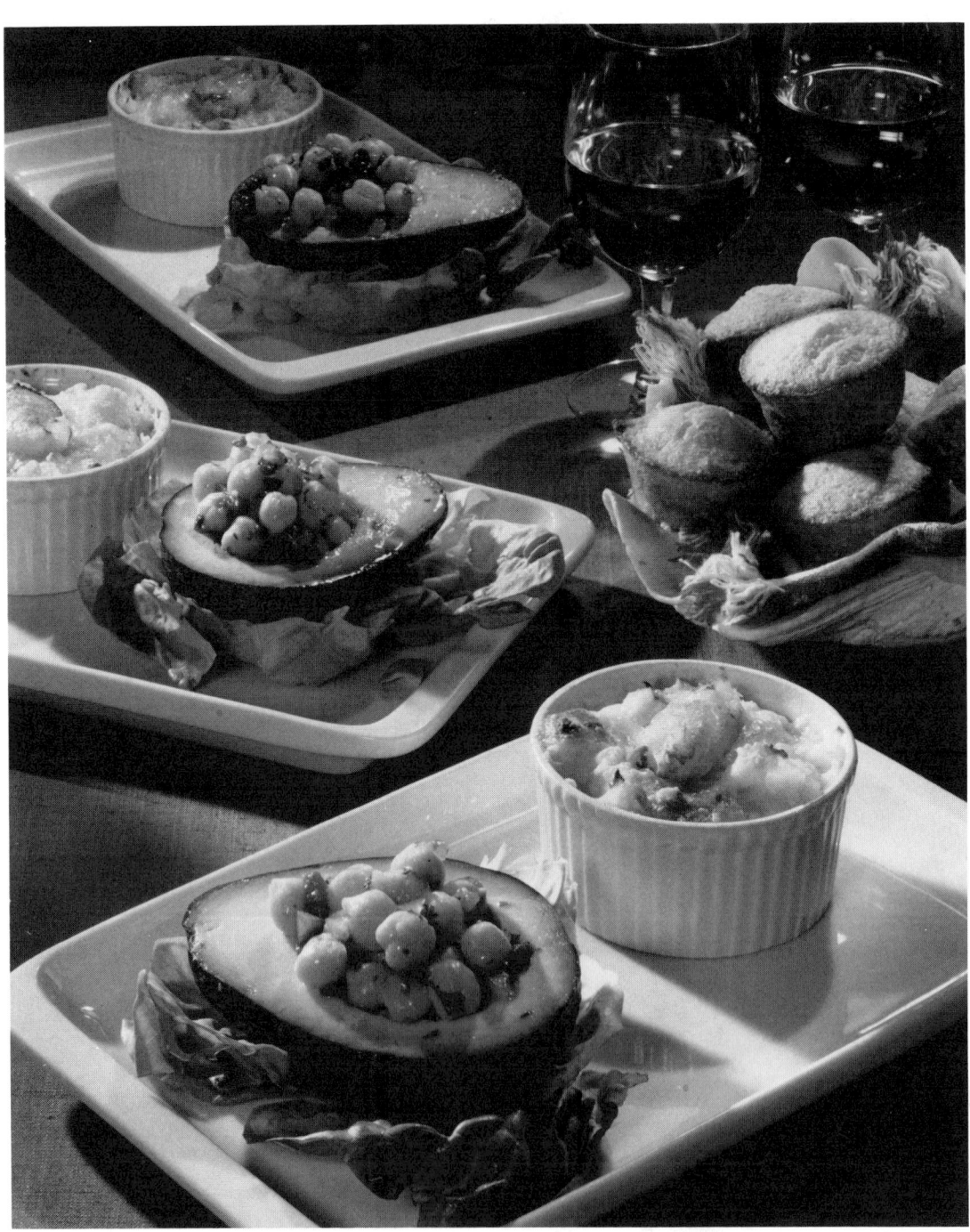

Fig. V-60. Most vitamins originate in plants; and they come in many different shapes, sizes, and colors. (Courtesy, California Dry Bean Advisory Board, Dinuba, Calif.)

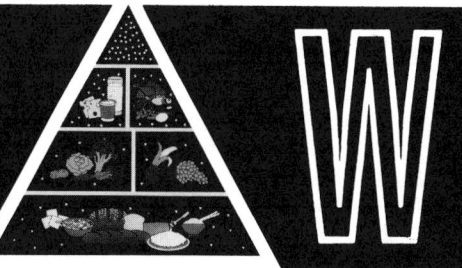

WALNUT (BLACK WALNUT; ENGLISH WALNUT)
Juglans spp

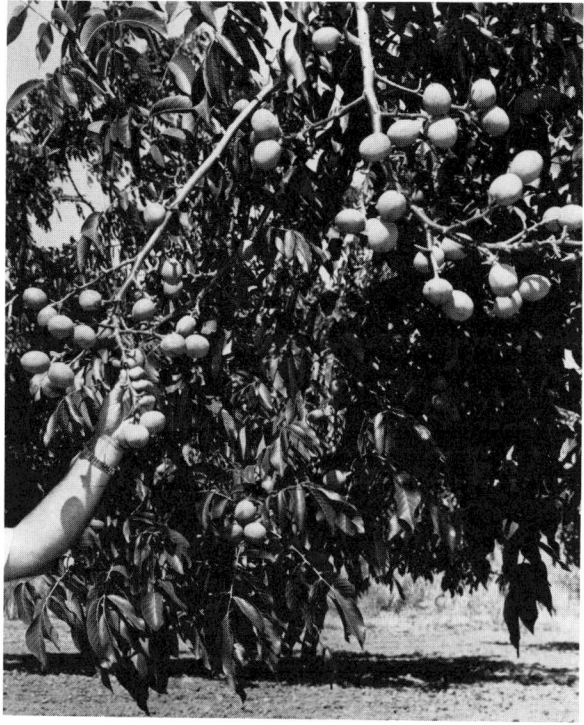

Fig. W-1. English walnuts approaching maturity. (Courtesy, Sun-Diamond Growers of California, Stockton, Calif.)

The term walnut refers to several varieties of nuts. Two are of importance: (1) the English walnut (Persian walnut), *Juglans regia*; and (2) the black walnut, *Juglans nigra*. Of these two, the English walnut tree bears walnuts that are the most valuable commercially.

ORIGIN AND HISTORY.
English, or Persian walnuts, as they are also called, are a native of southeastern Europe and western Asia—not England as the name suggests. Perhaps, it gained the name English walnut because it was brought to America on English ships. English walnuts are commercially produced in orchards.

Black walnuts are native to the Central Mississippi Valley and the Appalachian region of North America. However, they have been planted beyond their natural range and they grow over a wide area on good agricultural soils. Black walnuts were an important source of food for the American Indians and early settlers.

Black walnut production is limited to trees in forests and farmsteads. In some areas, they are collected, shelled, and sold.

WORLD AND U.S. PRODUCTION.
Worldwide, about 946,626 metric tons of English walnuts are produced annually; and the leading producing countries, by rank, are: United States, Turkey, China, Romania, Iran, France, and Yugoslavia. The U.S. produces 21% of the world walnut crop.[1]

The entire U.S. commercial crop of English walnuts is produced in California, where about 210,000 metric tons are produced annually.[2]

No reliable production figures on the production of black walnuts are available.

PROCESSING.
At packing houses, those English walnuts to be marketed in the shells (about 40%) are sized, bleached, and bagged for shipment. Others are machine-shelled, and the kernels are graded for color and size, and packaged for the retail trade. Some of the poorer grades may be used to make walnut oil and shell flour.

It is difficult to remove the hulls of black walnuts, so they are usually allowed to rot away. The nutmeats are sold in broken pieces because it is difficult to remove whole nuts from the shell of black walnuts.

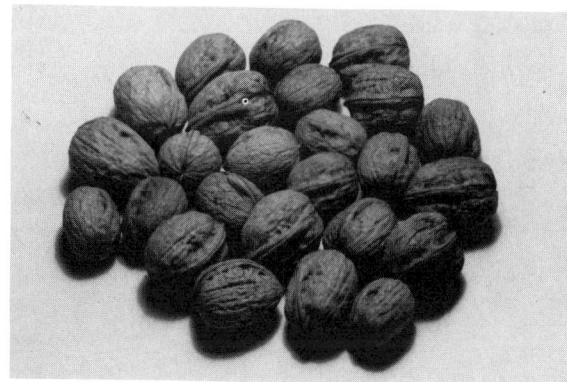

Fig. W-2. English walnuts with their husks removed are ready for selling or cracking. (Courtesy, Sun-Diamond Growers of California, Stockton, Calif.)

SELECTION, PREPARATION, AND USES.
Walnuts in shells should be free from splits, cracks, stains, or holes. Nutmeats should be plump and fairly uniform in color and size.

The dried nuts will store for at least a year under fairly variable conditions, up to 2 years if the storage temperature is kept below 40°F (4.8°C).

No preparation of walnut meats is required.

[1]Data from *FAO Production Yearbook 1990*, FAO/UN, Rome, Italy, Vol. 44, p. 173, Table 77. **Note well:** Annual production fluctuates as a result of weather and profitability of the crop.

[2]Data from *Agricultural Statistics 1991*, USDA, p. 219, Table 339. **Note well:** Annual production fluctuates as a result of weather and profitability of the crop.

Walnuts (kernels) are eaten alone as a snack, or they are used in endless ways in baking and confectionery.

The few black walnuts that are available can be used in baked goods, candy, and ice cream.

NUTRITIONAL VALUE. Walnuts—English and black—are extremely nutritious. They contain only 3 to 4% water and they are *supercharged* with energy. A 3½ oz (*100 g*) portion of black walnuts supplies 678 kcal (194 kcal per oz), whereas the same amount of English walnuts supplies 694 kcal (198 kcal per oz). Walnuts are high in calories, primarily because they are about 60% fat (oil). Additionally, each 100 g also provides 15 to 20 g of protein, 3 mg of iron and zinc, and only 2 mg of sodium.

Among the leading nuts, walnuts are the richest source of essential polyunsaturated fatty acids. Hence, they should be kept refrigerated to prevent rancidity.

More complete information regarding the nutritional value of walnuts is provided in Food Composition Table F-21.

WARBURG'S YELLOW ENZYME

A protein isolated in 1932 by two German scientists, Warburg and Christian. It played a role in the discovery of the vitamin riboflavin.

(Also see RIBOFLAVIN.)

WATER (H₂O)

Contents	Page
Importance of Water to Life	1108
Water Balance	1108
Requirement for Water	1109
Water Sources	1109
Drinking Water	1109
Foods	1109
Metabolic Water	1110

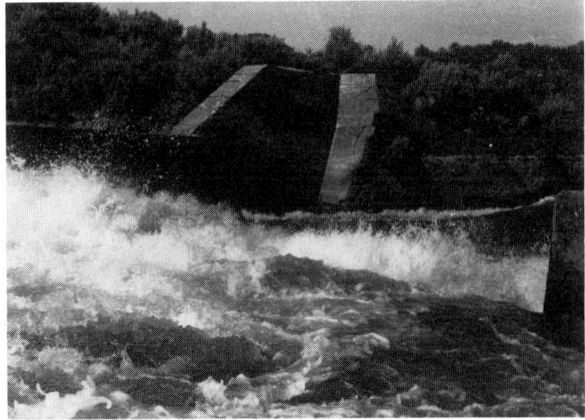

Fig. W-3. Plenty of cool, fresh, clean water, Lake Walcott canal, Minidoka County, Idaho. (Photo by Jayne Parker)

Chemically, water is the combination of two gases—hydrogen (H) and oxygen (O)—which are joined in the ratio of two hydrogen atoms to one oxygen. Thus, the chemical formula for water is H_2O. It is the most abundant chemical, and it performs endless functions in one of its three forms—liquid, solid, gas.

IMPORTANCE OF WATER TO LIFE. Water is a nutrient. It is one of the most vital of all nutrients. In fact, water is the only substance necessary to all life. Many organisms can live without air, but none can live without water. Humans and animals can survive for a longer period without food than without water. Only oxygen is more important to human life. Fortunately, water is usually provided in abundance and at little cost. In most U.S. cities it can be delivered to the kitchen for about 15¢ per ton.

Water is the most abundant body constituent. The younger the individual the more water the body contains. It accounts for about 98% of the embryo, for about 75% of infants, and for about 50 to 65% of the body weight of adults. In general, as the fat content of the body increases, the water content decreases.

In the body, water performs the following important functions:

1. It is necessary to the life and shape of every cell, and a constituent of every body fluid.

2. It acts as a carrier for various substances, serving as a medium in which nourishment is carried to the cells and waste products are removed therefrom.

3. It assists with temperature regulation in the body, cooling the individual by evaporation from the skin as perspiration.

4. It is necessary for many important chemical reactions of digestion and metabolism.

5. It lubricates the joints, as a constituent of the synovial fluid; it acts as a water cushion for the nervous system, in the cerebrospinal fluid; it transports sound, in the perilymph in the ear; and it is concerned with sight and provides a lubricant for the eye.

6. It acts as a solvent for a number of chemicals which can subsequently be detected by taste buds.

7. It aids in gas exchange in respiration by keeping the alveoli of the lungs moist.

The total body water involved in all of these functions is contained in two major compartments in the body: (1) the extracellular or water outside the cells (about 20% of the body weight), and (2) the intracellular or the water inside each cell (about 45% of the body weight).

Deficits or excesses of more than a few percent of the total body water are incompatible with health; large deficits, of about 20% of the body weight lead to death. Under normal circumstances, thirst ensures that water intake meets or exceeds the requirement for water. Surplus water is excreted from the body, principally in the urine, and to a lesser extent in the perspiration, feces, and water vapor from the lungs.

Water Balance. In healthy individuals, total body water remains reasonably constant. An increase or decrease in water intake brings about an appropriate increase or decrease in water output to maintain the balance. Water enters the body as a liquid, and as a component of the food—including metabolic water derived from the breakdown of food. Water is lost from the body (1) by the skin as perspiration, (2) by the lungs as water vapor in expired air, (3) by the kidneys as urine, and (4) by the intestines as feces. Therefore, under normal conditions the intake of water from the various sources is approximately equal to output of water by the various routes. For example, if a large volume of water is drunk, then the volume of urine excreted increases, or if water drinking is severely limited then the volume of urine formed is drastically reduced.

Water intake for a normal adult during a 24-hour period averages about 2.1 to 2.9 qt (*2 to 2.7 liter*) and water output via all four routes averages the same, assuming light activity and no visible perspiring, as Table W-1 shows.

TABLE W-1
DAILY WATER LEDGER

Water In		Water Out	
Source	Amount	Source	Amount
	(ml)		(ml)
Fluids	1,500	Skin	700
Water in foods	850	Lungs	350
Metabolic water	250	Kidneys	1,400
		Feces	150
Total	2,600	Total	2,600

The body is equipped with a number of mechanisms for regulating body water within narrow limits. Important among these mechanisms are nerve centers in the hypothalamus of the brain which control the sensation of thirst and water output by the kidneys. Stimulation of the thirst center in the hypothalamus results when water loss amounts to about 1% of the body weight, and creates the conscious desire for water. If water is not drunk, discomfort increases—heart rate increases, body temperature rises, and working and thinking abilities deteriorate. Heat exhaustion is certain if physical work is attempted when water loss is 10% of the body weight. Stimulation of other nerve centers in the hypothalamus causes the release of antidiuretic hormone (ADH) from the posterior pituitary. Release of ADH results in the formation of less urine, thereby conserving body water. The urine formed appears more concentrated, dark, and cloudy than when water intake is adequate. Despite the controls to maintain water balance, several factors can influence water balance and the requirement for water.

Requirement for Water. The requirement for water to maintain the water balance can be influenced by age, physical activity, heat, diet, illness, and injury. In general, the requirement for water can best be taken care of by allowing free access to plenty of clean, fresh water at all times. A discussion of each of the factors influencing the requirement for water follows:

• **Age**—Water needs for infants and children are proportionately higher than those for adults. The normal turnover rate of water per day is about 6% of the total body water in the adult and about 15% in the young infant.

Under ordinary circumstances, a reasonable allowance is 1 ml/kcal for adults and 1.5 ml/kcal for infants. Table W-2 presents daily water allowances in terms of the recommended dietary allowances for energy.

TABLE W-2
DAILY WATER ALLOWANCE FOR INFANTS AND ADULTS[1]

Category	Age	Weight		Energy Needs	Water Needs		
	(years)	(lb)	(kg)	(kcal)	(ml/kcal)	(ml)	(8 oz cups)
Infants	0.0–0.5	13	6	650	1.5	975	4.1
	0.5–1.0	20	9	850	1.5	1,275	5.4
Males	25–50	174	79	2,900	1.0	2,900	12.3
Females	25–50	138	63	2,200	1.0	2,200	9.4
Pregnancy				2,500	+30 ml	2,530	10.8
Lactating				2,700	+750 ml	3,450	14.7

[1]Based on *Recommended Dietary Allowances*, 10th ed., 1989, National Academy of Sciences–National Research Council, pp. 247–250.

• **Physical activity**—Even in a comfortable environment, physical activity increases the loss of water from the body through perspiration and water vapor from the lungs. Al-though considerable amounts of sodium are lost in the perspiration, the loss of water significantly exceeds that of sodium. Hence, water depletion is the major problem. If water loss is not replenished then physical performance begins to deteriorate when the water deficit exceeds 3% of the body weight. Despite this fact, extremely ill-advised practices—withholding water, wearing rubberized apparel, and inducing vomiting—are sometimes used to meet weight ranges in competitive sports such as wrestling.

• **Heat**—The combination of high temperature and increased physical activity may increase water losses from the skin and lungs threefold to tenfold. These increased water losses must be covered by increased intake, and free access to water is essential. Water needs for individuals living in hot dry climates are increased as losses from the lungs and skin are elevated 50 to 100%. Failure to replace water losses arising from prolonged sweating may result in heat exhaustion. Furthermore, providing salt (sodium chloride) without free access to water may lead to the development of significant hypernatremia—elevated blood sodium. Symptoms of acute water lack during hard work in a hot environment appear rapidly, and recovery following water ingestion is even more rapid.

(Also see HEAT EXHAUSTION.)

• **Diet**—High-protein diets require extra water for excretion of urea. Special attention must be given to the water needs of infants on high-protein formulas, since the concentrating ability of the infant's kidneys is not well developed.

• **Illness**—In persistent vomiting large amounts of water are lost. Prolonged diarrhea also results in excessive loss of water. Fever accelerates the loss of body water though increased perspiration and the excretion of body waste. Illnesses in which a fever, vomiting, and/or diarrhea are present, can rapidly result in dehydration especially in infants, children, and older individuals.

In the opposite direction, some conditions are associated with excessive retention of water or edema. Often edema is noted in the following diseases: congestive heart failure, cirrhosis of the liver, nephritis, and nephrosis. In all of these diseases there is a reduction in sodium excretion which promotes the retention of water.

• **Injury**—During the postoperative period adequate fluid is essential since large fluid losses may occur due to vomiting, hemorrhage, exudates, diuresis, or fever. Abnormal loss of water also occurs from burns.

Water Sources. The water required to replace body losses is available from three sources: (1) drinking water and other beverages, (2) water contained in solid foods, and (3) metabolic water resulting from the breakdown (catabolism) of fats, carbohydrates, and proteins.

DRINKING WATER. Nearly three-fourths of the earth's surface is covered with water, but only 3% of this is *fresh* water—fit drinking water. Today, our drinking water comes from underground wells and reservoirs. Some is transported through miles of pipelines in huge quantities to places where the demand is great.

FOODS. Many solid foods contain a high water content, and contribute to meeting our water requirement. Even such *dry* foods as crackers, ready-to-eat cereals, and nuts provide some water, while some fruits and vegetables contain over 90% water. Table W-3 illustrates, over a wide range, the water content of foods.

TABLE W-3
WATER CONTENT OF FOODS[1]

Foods	Water
	(%)
Fruits and vegetables	70-95
Milk	87
Cooked cereals	80-88
Fish and shellfish	60-86
Cheese, cottage	79
Meat and poultry	40-75
Eggs	74
Cooked beans	69
Cheese, Cheddar	39
Bread	36
Butter	16
Crackers	2-6
Nuts	2-5

[1]Approximate values from Food Composition Table F-21.

METABOLIC WATER. Metabolic water is produced from the catabolism—breakdown—of nutrients. When 100 g of carbohydrates are oxidized, 60 g of water are produced. The oxidation of proteins yields 42 g of water for every 100 g of protein. Fats can be said to be "wetter than water." For every 100 g of fats that are oxidized, close to 110 g of water are produced. However, there are some losses of water in the oxidation of both proteins and fats. Water must be used to excrete nitrogen in the deamination process of protein—thus lowering the net availability of water. In fact, it requires more water to excrete nitrogen as urea than is formed in the deamination process. The oxidation of fats requires increased respiration. Water is lost from the lungs during this increased respiration, and the net yield of water produced from fat is less than that from the oxidation of carbohydrates.

On the average, 13 g of metabolic water are formed for every 100 Calories (kcal) of metabolizable energy in the typical human diet.

(Also see MINERAL[S], section on "Contamination of Drinking Water, Foods, or Air with Toxic Minerals"; THIRST; WATER ELECTROLYTES; and WATER BALANCE.)

WATER, AERATED

Municipal water works may aerate water by spraying into the air to remove disagreeable tastes and odors. Also, well water can be improved by aeration, particularly if it contains carbon dioxide, hydrogen sulfide, or iron. The term aerated water is synonymous to mineral water in British usage. However, mineral water in Britian is water that has been aerated or charged with carbon dioxide—soda water, or soft drink.

WATER AND ELECTROLYTES

Thoughts of constant, never ending motion are almost inseparable from thoughts of water—the water of the sea, of the rivers, and even household water. The water of our bodies is no different. It is constantly in motion—entering the body, leaving the body, and moving in and around the cells of the body. Life depends upon the movement of water and substances dissolved in the water which bathes the cells. Water is one of a few inorganic chemicals which exists as a liquid at the temperature of life processes. It is the chemical of life. Among the many important properties of water is its ability to act as a solvent for a variety of organic and inorganic chemicals. Of the inorganic chemicals, some of these—for example, acids, alkalis, and salts—will separate into ions when dissolved in water. Ions are atoms or molecules that carry an electrical charge—positive or negative. Such compounds which separate into positive and negative ions in solutions are called electrolytes. Those with a positive charge are cations, while those with a negative charge are anions.

Table W-4 lists ions which are found dissolved in the water of the body. Sodium, potassium, and chloride are the primary electrolytes which are most often discussed due to their important relationships in body fluids.

TABLE W-4
IMPORTANT IONS OF THE BODY

Cations			Anions		
Name	Formula	Charge	Name	Formula	Charge
Sodium	Na^+	+1	Chloride	Cl^-	−1
Potassium	K^+	+1	Bicarbonate	HCO_3^-	−1
Calcium	Ca^{++}	+2	Phosphate	$HPO_4^=$	−1
Magnesium	Mg^{++}	+2	Sulfate	$SO_4^=$	−2

Hence, electrolytes become chemical compounds such as sodium chloride (table salt), potassium chloride, calcium phosphate, magnesium sulfate, sodium bicarbonate, and so on.

Electrolytes may be dissolved in water at different concentrations. This introduces another concept. Electrolytes are measured according to the total number of particles in solution, not their total weight. Thus, the unit of measure for electrolytes is milliequivalents, which is abbreviated as mEq. It refers to the number of ions—cations and anions—in solution in a given volume, generally one liter. Hence, milliequivalents are expressed as mEq/liter. The concentration of electrolytes in the compartments of the body determines the flow of water within the body.

BODY FLUID COMPARTMENTS. Fluids—water, electrolytes, and other dissolved substances—are contained in two major compartments within the body. In order to gain this concept of body compartments, all the cells of the body must be thought of as a whole. Then, all fluid outside of the cells is termed extracellular fluid, while all fluid within the cells is termed intracellular fluid. Fluids in each compartment differ in composition.

(Also see WATER BALANCE, Fig. W-4.)

REGULATION OF WATER AND ELECTROLYTE BALANCE. Basically, water (1) enters the body via the digestive tract as liquid or food, (2) moves into the blood and tissue, and (3) leaves via the kidneys, skin, lungs, or feces. Water entering and leaving the body is under rigid control, and under normal conditions water leaving the body equals the water entering the body—a condition of water balance. Moreover, the shifts of water between various body compartments and water balance are controlled by the concentration and distribution of the electrolytes.

Movement of Water and Electrolytes.
In the body, water and electrolytes are moved across cell membranes by one or more of five processes: (1) osmosis, (2) diffusion, (3) active transport, (4) filtration, and (5) pinocytosis.

Putting these five processes into perspective requires the realization that the body is a dynamic system. Adjustments are constantly taking place. Water and electrolyte balance is no different. Water enters the body as a liquid, and as a component of the food—including metabolic water derived from the breakdown of food. In the digestive tract water and the many substances dissolved in water—including electrolytes—are transported across the membrane lining the digestive tract into the blood. Then the blood plasma—a water solution—transports nutrients and other substances to the cells, and picks up the waste products from the cells. The kidneys act to regulate the composition of the body fluids by conserving some substances and excreting others into the urine. Furthermore, the kidneys regulate water loss from the body. Additional water is lost from the body by the skin, the lungs, and the feces. As water and the substances dissolved in it move through the body, some or all five of these processes—osmosis, diffusion, active transport, filtration, and pinocytosis—are at work maintaining balance within the body. In order to maintain the composition of the extracellular fluid and the intracellular fluid, the volume of water intake is very nearly equal to the volume of water lost. Whenever body fluids become too concentrated, water moves into this area and dilutes the body fluid. However, a number of factors act to regulate the movement of water.

(Also see DIGESTION AND ABSORPTION, section on "Water.")

Factors Regulating Movement.
The body requires water. To ensure that this requirement is fulfilled, the sensation of thirst creates a conscious desire for water. The sensation of thirst is caused by nerve centers in the hypothalamus of the brain which monitors the concentration primarily of sodium in the blood. When the sodium concentration, and hence the osmolarity of the blood, increases above the normal 310 to 340 mg/100 ml (136 to 145 mEq/liter), cells in the thirst center shrink. They shrink because the increased osmotic pressure of the blood pulls water out of their cytoplasm. This shrinking causes more nervous impulses to be generated in the thirst center, thus creating the sensation of thirst. Increased osmolarity of the blood is primarily associated with water loss from the extracellular fluid. As water is lost the sodium concentration of the remaining fluid increases. When water is drunk, it moves across the membrane lining the gut into the blood thereby decreasing the sodium concentration—osmolarity—of the blood. In turn, the cells of the hypothalamus take on water and return to their normal size. This time water moves back into these cells via osmosis in the opposite direction.

Increased osmolarity of the blood simultaneously stimulates other nerve centers in the hypothalamus causing the release of antidiuretic hormone (ADH) from the posterior pituitary. This hormone makes a portion of the kidney permeable to water. Thus, water originally destined to be urine moves, by osmosis, back into circulation. ADH release results in the formation of less urine by the kidneys; hence, conserving body water and helping dilute the body fluids and decrease the sodium ion concentration. Thus, drinking water and excreting water are controlled by centers in the brain which help maintain body water within appropriate ranges, and in turn control the extracellular sodium ion concentration. While many changes in the body fluids are compensated for by shifting water, electrolytes are also regulated to some degree.

Sodium and potassium, the major electrolytes of the extracellular and intracellular fluid, respectively, are controlled by the hormone aldosterone which comes from the cortex (outside layer) of the adrenal gland. Of prime importance is the regulation of the potassium ion in the extracellular fluid since both nerve and muscle function are dependent on its close regulation. Aldosterone also acts to conserve sodium. Secretion of the hormone aldosterone is controlled by a chain of events called the renin-angiotensin system. Briefly, renin is released from the kidney in response to (1) changes in blood pressure, (2) blood levels of potassium, or (3) nervous stimulation. It then converts angiotensinogen, a protein in the blood, to angiotensin which stimulates the secretion of aldosterone. Aldosterone causes the reabsorption of sodium from the urine and the loss of potassium in the urine. Potassium is exchanged for sodium. This conservation also causes water to be reabsorbed via osmosis. Under some stressful situations such as surgery, the release of adrenocorticotropin hormone (ACTH) from the anterior pituitary may cause the secretion of aldosterone.

It is evident that a marvelous organ, the kidney, is largely responsible for regulating the water and electrolyte balance of the body. Each kidney contains about one million minute functional units called nephrons. As the blood passes through these nephrons, they select, reject, conserve, and eliminate water, electrolytes, and other substances in order to maintain the volume and the composition of the extracellular fluid. Each day they rejuvenate about 50 gal (190 liter) of blood. Moreover, they function to regulate red blood cell production, aldosterone secretion, blood pressure, and calcium metabolism. So important is their function that without it death results in 8 to 14 days.

IMBALANCES OF WATER AND ELECTROLYTES.
When the day-to-day and individual-to-individual variations in water and electrolyte intake are considered, maintaining the consistent water and electrolyte levels of the body is truly an amazing feat. However, there are times when the controlling mechanisms are disrupted and excesses or deficiencies result. Of prime concern are water and the major electrolytes, sodium, potassium, and chlorine. So intimate are the relationships between water and the major electrolytes that separation is often difficult.

Water Depletion.
Life without water is short. When water is unavailable, or when water is lost faster than it can be replaced, events occur in the following order:
1. Sensation of thirst, when water loss amounts to about 1% of body weight.
2. Thirst accompanied by vague discomfort and loss of appetite.
3. Tingling and numbness in arms and hands.

4. Increase in pulse rate, respiratory rate, and body temperature.

5. Weakness, spastic muscles, and mental confusion.

6. Increase in concentration of the blood (hemoconcentration), decreased blood volume, and difficult circulation.

7. Cracked skin and cessation of urine formation.

8. Death when dehydration weight loss becomes greater than 20% of the initial weight.

Various stages of the above may occur when losses of water are incurred by (1) evaporation, (2) vomiting and diarrhea, (3) hemorrhage, or (4) burns.

Water Excess. Sometimes excessive water accumulates in the tissues, specifically the interstitial compartment. Outwardly, this condition is noted as swelling and it may occur in any area of the body. It is called *edema*, though some may still call it *dropsy*. In general, there are four causes of edema: (1) elevated fluid pressure in the capillaries as in heart failure; (2) low osmotic pressure in the blood due to decreased blood protein in such conditions as liver cirrhosis, kidney disease, severe burns, and starvation; (3) blockage of the lymph vessels as caused by the parasitic worm, filariae, in the disease ˙elephantiasis; or (4) increased capillary permeability due to the release of histamine in allergic reactions. Edema may require the restriction of dietary sodium and/or diuretics.

• **Diuretics**—These are drugs which act to increase the output of sodium and water in the urine, and are often used to treat disorders of the heart, kidneys, or liver which cause edema. A majority of the diuretics act upon the kidneys by depressing the sodium reabsorbed. Thus, sodium remaining in the urine carries more water out of the body with it. Diuretics include thiazides, furosemide, and ethacrynic acid. Xanthine diuretics are mild diuretics but they are used by many people—perhaps unknowingly —since they are the caffeine, theophylline, and theobromine present in tea, coffee, cola and other soft drinks, cocoa, and many over-the-counter pain relievers. Moreover, water and ethyl alcohol (alcoholic beverages) can act as diuretics by inhibiting the release of ADH.

• **Water intoxication**—When water intake is more rapid than urine formation, the extracellular compartment fluid is diluted and water moves into the cells—cellular edema. Swelling of the cells of the brain causes drowsiness and weakness, convulsions, and coma. Water intoxication may be observed in (1) patients given excessive amounts of intravenous glucose and water, (2) individuals who absorb water from the colon during enemas or colon irrigations, (3) individuals who absorb water from wounds or burns treated with wet dressings, or (4) individuals who have impaired antidiuretic hormone.

Sodium Depletion. Sodium is the major positively charged ion—cation—in the extracellular fluid. Depletion is rare. Urinary output reflects the dietary intake. However, strict vegetarian diets without salt, heavy prolonged sweating, diarrhea, and vomiting or adrenal cortical insufficiency —lack of aldosterone—may result in sodium depletion. Continued depletion results in loss of appetite, muscle cramps, mental apathy, loss of body water, headache, and reduced milk production in lactating mothers. Sodium depletion/heat exhaustion occurs most frequently in persons unacclimatized to working in a hot environment who replace water losses but fail to replace electrolyte losses. It is characterized by fatigue, nausea, giddiness, vomiting, and exhaustion. The blood volume decreases, kidney blood flow is impaired, and cellular edema occurs.

Sodium Excess. Most of the sodium ingested is excessive, and for the most part it is excreted by the kidneys in combination with bicarbonate or phosphate. However, under some circumstances sodium accumulates in the extracellular fluid and causes edema since the retention of sodium is accompanied by water retention. Such conditions include (1) cardiac or renal failure, (2) adrenal tumors which secrete excessive cortical hormones, and (3) adrenocorticotropic hormone (ACTH) or steroid hormone therapy. In these conditions, individuals benefit from sodium-restricted diets.

Excessive sodium may be harmful (1) when ingested in large quantities, especially with a low water intake; (2) when the body has been depleted by a salt-free vegetarian diet or excess sweating, followed by gorging on salt; (3) when large amounts are fed to infants or individuals afflicted with kidney diseases, whose kidneys cannot excrete the excess in the urine; or (4) when the body is adapted to a chronic low-salt diet, followed by ingesting large amounts of salt. A dramatic example of excessive sodium (salt) is provided by imagining a sailor lost at sea who decides to drink sea water. The sea water is a much more concentrated salt solution than the extracellular fluids. Drinking sea water would only worsen a stranded sailor's condition.

(Also see SALT; and SODIUM.)

Potassium Depletion. Deficiencies of potassium rarely result from dietary lack of the mineral. Potassium is lost whenever muscle is broken down owing to starvation, malnutrition, or injury since it is tied to protein inside cells. Crash diets, diarrhea, vomiting, gastric suction, diabetic acidosis, and burns also induce potassium loss from the body. Also lean tissue growth increases the need for potassium. A potassium-depleted individual may display irregular heart function, muscle weakness, irritability, paralysis, nausea, vomiting, diarrhea, and swollen abdomen.

(Also see MALNUTRITION, PROTEIN-ENERGY; and STARVATION.)

Potassium Excess. The kidneys provide the major regulatory mechanism for maintaining potassium balance. Hence, a potassium buildup in the blood—hyperkalemia—is the frequent complication of kidney failure. Other causes of potassium excess include adrenal insufficiency, severe dehydration, or shock after injury wherein the potassium in the cells leaks into the blood. Symptoms of an excess are muscular weakness, mental apathy, and irregular heart action. Both an excess and depletion of potassium affect the heart muscle. Indeed, if either becomes severe enough the heart will stop. Although, it would be nearly impossible to ingest enough potassium-containing foods to create an excess, ill advised individuals who take a supplemental source such as potassium chloride run the risk of increasing potassium to dangerous levels.

(Also see POTASSIUM.)

Chloride. Excess chlorine in the diet is excreted via the urine accompanied by excess sodium or potassium and sometimes ammonia. Loss of chloride generally parallels that of sodium. However, deficiencies of chloride may develop from vomiting, diarrhea, stomach pumping, injudicious use of diuretic drugs, or strict vegetarian diets used without salt. A deficiency of chloride causes an increase in the pH of the body. This condition is called alkalosis and it is characterized by slow and shallow breathing, listlessness, muscle cramps, lack of appetite, and sometimes convulsions.

(Also see CHLORINE OR CHLORIDE.)

ACID-BASE BALANCE. Aside from their involvement in body fluid distribution, water and electrolytes are involved in the acid-base balance of the body. This is important since the body tolerates only very minor shifts in this balance which refers to the hydrogen ion concentration of the body fluids. An acid is a chemical that can release hydrogen ions, whereas a base, or alkali, is a chemical that can accept hydrogen ions. The degree of acidity is expressed in terms of pH. A pH of 7 is the neutral point between an acid and alkaline (base). Substances with a lower pH than 7 are acid, while substances with a pH above 7 are alkaline. The normal pH of the extracellular fluids of the body is 7.4, with a range of 7.35 to 7.45. Maintenance of the pH within this narrow range is necessary to sustain the life of cells. The extremes between which life is possible are 7.0 to 7.8. To help maintain this narrow range the body has other chemicals called buffers. A buffer protects the acid-base balance of a solution by rapidly offsetting changes in its ionized hydrogen concentration—a chemical sponge. It protects against added acid or base. The three most important chemical buffers are the bicarbonate buffer, phosphate buffers, and hemoglobin and protein buffers.

The lungs and kidneys also have an important role in maintaining the acid-base balance. The extent to which they are involved depends upon the amount of adjustment necessary.

WATER BALANCE

Water is the major constituent of the body; it accounts for 50 to 75% of the body weight. Next to oxygen, it is the most important constituent for life itself. A person can live for several weeks without food but for only a few days without water. Dehydration (water loss) will kill far quicker than starvation.

Large deficits or excesses in the body water are reason for concern. In healthy individuals, the total amount of body water remains reasonably constant. Therefore, an increase or decrease in water intake brings about an appropriate increase or decrease in water output to maintain the balance. Fig. W-4 illustrates the intake of water, the routes of water output, and the movement of fluid between the compartments of the body. Water enters the body as a liquid, and as a component of the food—including metabolic water derived from the breakdown of food. Water is lost from the body by (1) the skin as perspiration, (2) the lungs as water vapor in expired air, (3) the kidneys as urine, and (4) the intestines in the feces. As Fig. W-4 shows, under normal conditions total water intake is approximately equal to total water output by the various routes.

The body is equipped with a number of mechanisms for regulating body water within narrow limits. Important among these mechanisms are nerve centers in the hypothalamus which control the sensation of thirst and water output by the kidneys. Stimulation of the thirst center in the hypothalamus creates the desire for water, while stimulation of other nerve centers in the hypothalamus causes the release of antidiuretic hormone (ADH) from the posterior pituitary. Release of ADH results in the formation of less urine; hence, conserving the body water. Water needs of the body are disrupted by fever, high protein diets, dry hot climates, high altitudes, vomiting, diarrhea, and injury.

(Also see BODY FLUIDS; ENDOCRINE GLANDS; METABOLISM; METABOLIC WATER; and WATER AND ELECTROLYTES.)

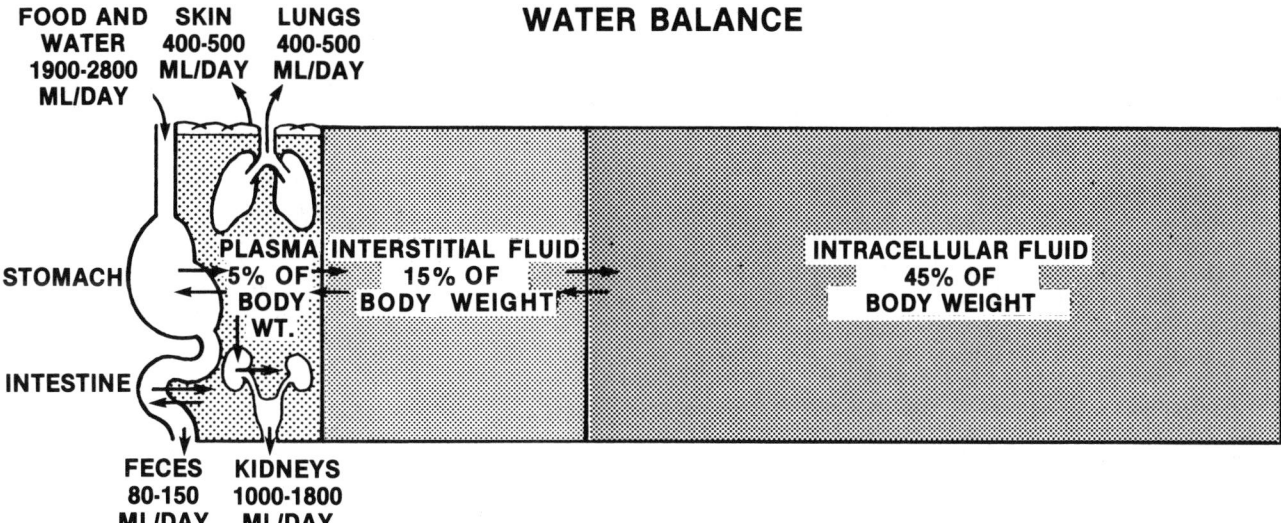

Fig. W-4. Water balance in humans showing the daily amount of water input and output by the various routes, and the compartments of the body which contain water. Arrows represent fluid movement.

WATERBORNE DISEASES

Many of the same diseases that are transmitted by contaminated food may also be transmitted by contaminated water. Important among these diseases are amebic dysentery, bacillary dysentery, cholera, intestinal flu, infectious hepatitis, poliomyelitis, salmonellosis, and typhoid fever. In addition, certain parasitic diseases, including beef tapeworms, fish tapeworms, liver flukes, and round worms, may be spread to man, either directly or indirectly, through contaminated water.

Because of the importance of water to the normal function of the body, it is imperative that our water supplies be safeguarded. Large cities sterilize water by the addition of chlorine, while questionable water in the home may be boiled vigorously for 1 to 3 minutes. However, chlorine or boiling does not eliminate toxic levels of industrial chemicals or metals that find their way into water supplies.

(Also see DISEASES, Table D-10, Infectious and Parasitic Diseases Which May Be Transmitted By Contaminated Foods and Water; and WATER.)

WATER, DEMINERALIZED (DEIONIZED WATER)

By passing water through two ion exchange resins, all mineral salts can be removed—both anions (negatively charged elements) and cations (positively charged elements). This is demineralized water. It is as pure as water can be. Frequently, demineralized water is utilized in scientific investigation to prevent the introduction of interfering substances during sensitive analyses of minute quantities.

(Also see WATER.)

WATER, EXTRACELLULAR

That water in the body which is found outside of the cells of the body. The blood plasma and interstitial fluid make up the extracellular water.

(Also see BODY FLUIDS; and WATER BALANCE.)

WATER GLASS

This is a common term for the chemical, *sodium silicate,* a solution of which may be used to preserve eggs by sealing the pores in the shell. Other uses include fireproofing of fabrics, waterproofing, a detergent in soaps, and adhesives.

WATER HARDNESS

Hard water contains the bicarbonate (HCO_3) and sulfate (SO_4) salts principally of calcium (Ca) and magnesium (Mg) leeched from mineral deposits in the earth, though aluminum and iron salts are sometimes involved. Water hardness due to calcium and magnesium bicarbonate is known as temporary or bicarbonate hardness since boiling the water results in the decompositon of the bicarbonates and the precipitation of calcium and magnesium carbonate (CO_3) or hydroxide (OH). Boiling produces no change in water containing calcium and magnesium sulfate. Hence, the hardness caused by sulfates is known as permanent or noncarbonate hardness.

Following a chemical analysis, water hardness is expressed in parts per million (ppm) of an equivalent amount of calcium carbonate. This method is used for expressing the amount of magnesium as well as the amount of calcium, and for expressing the noncarbonate as well as the carbonate hardness. Total hardness of water varies with locality and source. A water with a total hardness of less than 100 ppm of calcium carbonate is generally considered soft, while a water with a total hardness about 300 ppm is considered very hard.

Hard water requires more soap because of the formation of insoluble salts of calcium and magnesium with soap. Furthermore, hard water leaves deposits in pipes and appliances. Some municipal water supplies have reported 2,000 ppm and some are known to be as high as 4,400 ppm.

(Also see WATER.)

WATER, INTRACELLULAR

That water in the body which is contained within the cells of the body. It represents about 45% of the body weight.

(Also see BODY FLUIDS; and WATER BALANCE.)

WATER LEMON (YELLOW GRANADILLA)
Passiflora laurifolio

This type of passion fruit (of the family *Passifloraceae*) grows wild in the hot, humid lowlands of the West Indies and northeastern South America. The fruits of this vine have an orange-yellow peel and a seedy, white pulp. They may be eaten fresh or made into confections, ice cream, ices, jams, jellies, juices, and sherbets. Its excellent flavor has made it popular throughout the tropical areas of the world.

(Also see FRUIT[S], Table F-23, Fruits of the World—"Passion Fruit.")

WATERMELON *Citrullus vulgaris*

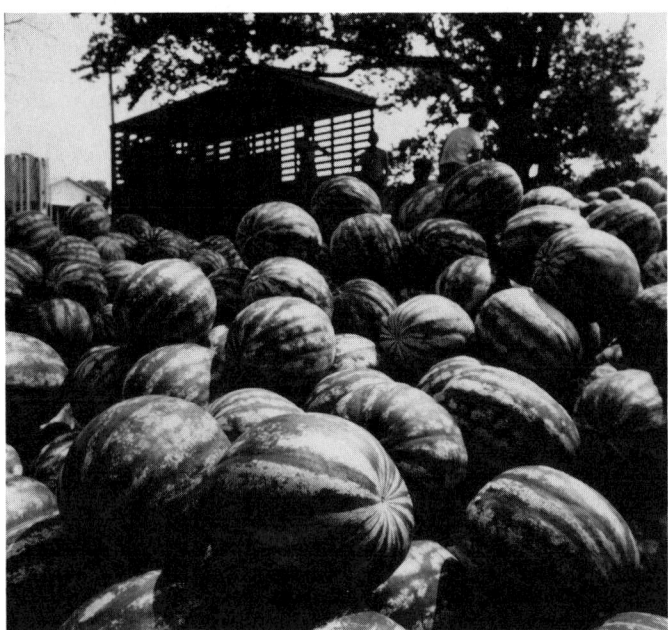

Fig. W-5. Watermelons. (Courtesy, University of Maryland, College Park, Md.)

Watermelons are the fruit of an annual prostrate vine with multiple stems, branching out 12 to 15 ft (*4 to 5 m*). They may weigh 5 to 85 lb (*2.3 to 38.3 kg*), and vary in shape from round to oval to oblong-cylindrical. On the outside the hard rind of watermelons may be very light to very dark green with stripes or mottling, while the inside edible flesh (pulp) is red, pink, orange, yellow, or white. Red is the most familiar color in the United States. Most watermelons contain white, brown, or black seeds, but there are seedless watermelons.

The pumpkin, squash, muskmelon, and cucumber are relatives of the watermelon and all are members of the cucumber family, *Cucurbitaceae*.

ORIGIN AND HISTORY. Watermelons originated in Africa, where they still occur in the wild, and where they have been cultivated for 4,000 years. From Africa, they spread to Asia, thence throughout the world. They were introduced in America soon after its discovery.

WORLD AND U.S. PRODUCTION. Watermelons rank fifth among the leading fruit crops of the world.

Worldwide, about 28.9 million metric tons of watermelons are produced annually; and the leading producing countries, by rank, are: China, U.S.S.R., Turkey, Egypt, and United States.[3]

The United States produces about 1.3 million short tons of watermelons each year. Florida and Texas are the leading producers.[4]

PROCESSING. Almost all of the watermelon crop is consumed fresh after being chilled. Only small amounts are used to make processed fruit products.

SELECTION, PREPARATION, AND USES. Judging the quality of a watermelon is very difficult unless it is cut in half or quartered. When cut, indicators of a good watermelon include firm, juicy flesh with good red color, free from white streaks, and seeds which are dark brown or black.

When selecting an uncut watermelon, a few appearance factors are helpful, though not totally reliable. The watermelon surface should be relatively smooth; the rind should have a slight dullness (neither shiny nor dull); the ends of the melon should be filled out and rounded; and the underside, or *belly,* of the melon should have a creamy color.

Preparation is simple; after being chilled, watermelons are generally sliced and served with a fork or spoon. Some people prefer a little salt to enhance the sweetness. Also, the seeds can be removed from fresh watermelon, following which it can then be used in fruit dishes and desserts.

Sometimes, the rinds of watermelons are pickled or candied. In the U.S.S.R., a fermented drink is made from the juice. Sometimes, Orientals preserve chunks of watermelon in brine.

In some countries of the Middle East and in China, the seeds are also eaten. They are roasted and eaten like popcorn, or preserved in salt.

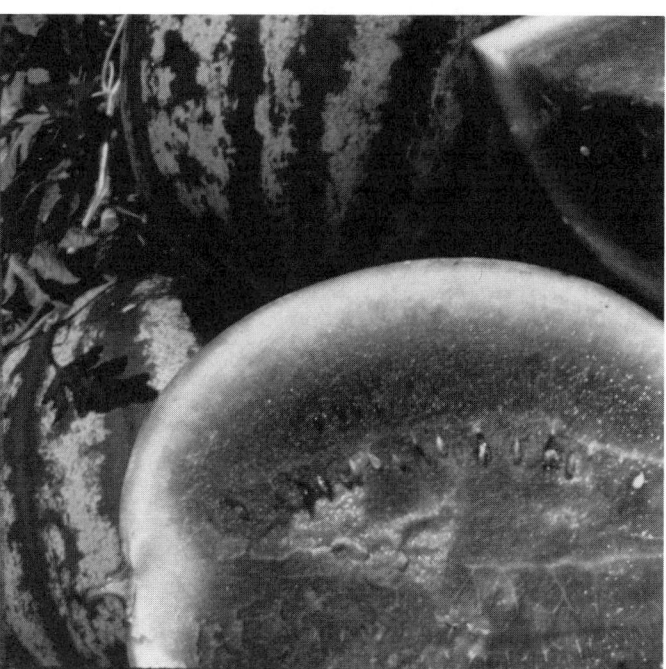

Fig. W-6. Sliced watermelon; simple preparation; significant amount of vitamin A. (Courtesy, USDA)

---

[3]Data from *FAO Production Yearbook 1990,* FAO/UN, Rome, Italy, Vol. 44, p. 149, Table 63. **Note well:** Annual production fluctuates as a result of weather and profitability of the crop.

[4]*Ibid.*

NUTRITIONAL VALUE. The nutritional values of fresh watermelon and watermelon seeds are listed in Food Composition Table F-21.

Fresh watermelon is true to its name. It contains about 93% water, and only 26 Calories (kcal) per 100 g (about 3 1/2 oz). The calories are primarily derived from the naturally-occurring sugar which gives watermelon its sweetness. Watermelons contain 6 to 12% sugar (carbohydrate) depending upon the variety and growing conditions. Vitamin A is present in significant amounts—about 590 IU/100 g.

The nutritional composition of watermelon seeds is typical of many other seeds and nuts—high in protein, fat, carbohydrates, and calories. Each 100 g of seeds contains about 23 g protein, 40 g of fat, and 27 g of carbohydrate for a whopping 536 Calories (kcal) per 100 g.

WATER-SOLUBLE VITAMINS

The large amounts of water which pass through most animals daily tend to carry out the water-soluble vitamins of the body, thereby depleting the supply. Thus, they must be supplied in the diet on a day-to-day basis. The water-soluble vitamins are: vitamin C (ascorbic acid), B-1 (thiamin), B-2 (riboflavin), B-6 (pyridoxine), niacin (nicotinic acid), pantothenic acid, biotin, folic acid (folacin), choline, B-12, and inositol.

(Also see VITAMIN[S].)

WAX, APPLE

The waxy material present in apple skin which is sometimes removed by dewaxing with hot isopropyl alcohol vapor in order to reduce the amount of peel lost during the processing of apples into canned slices or juice. Dewaxing of apples makes it possible to remove the peel with a lye solution.

(Also see APPLE.)

WAX GOURD (CHINESE PRESERVING MELON)
Benincasa hispida

The fruit of a vine (of the family *Cucurbitaceae*) that is native to Malaysia, but is now grown throughout the tropics of Asia.

Wax gourds are large, heavy, oblong fruits that range from 6 to 8 in. (*15 to 20 cm*) in diameter, and from 8 to 14 in. (*20 to 35 cm*) long. The fruits may be boiled or candied, and the seeds fried. Also, the young leaves and flower buds are eaten as vegetables.

The nutrient composition of the wax gourd is given in Food Composition Table F-21.

Some noteworthy observations regarding the nutrient composition of the wax gourd follow:

1. The raw fruit has a very high water content (96%) and is very low in calories (13 kcal per 100 g) and carbohydrates (3%).

2. Wax gourds are a fair to good source of potassium and vitamin C.

(Also see GOURDS.)

WEIGHT AND HEIGHT-AGE PERCENTILE STANDARDS

Charts or tables used to determine deviations in growth patterns—weight and height—from normal growth patterns. They are based on careful measurements of selected populations of children over a period of years, and they are expressed in percentiles—distribution of ranked values for weight and height divided into hundreths. Thus, the 50th percentile on the table or chart represents the median, or in other words the central tendency of all children. These weight and height-age percentile standards or growth charts may be used to spot undernutrition or overnutrition in children or adolescents.

(Also see CHILDHOOD AND ADOLESCENT NUTRITION, Section on "Childhood Growth and It's Measurement"; and INFANT DIET AND NUTRITION, section on "Measurement of Growth.")

WEIGHTS AND MEASURES

Weights and measures are the standard employed in arriving at weights, quantities, and volumes. Even among primitive people, such standards were necessary; and with the growing complexity of life, they became of greater and greater importance.

COMMON FOOD WEIGHTS AND MEASURES.

In preparing foods, it is often more convenient for the cook to measure the ingredients, rather than weigh them. Table W-5, Common Food Weights and Measures, will serve as a useful guide when preparing foods by measure.

TABLE W-5
COMMON FOOD WEIGHTS AND MEASURES
(All measurements are level)

ABBREVIATIONS COMMONLY USED

tsp	= teaspoon	oz	=	ounce or ounces
Tbsp	= tablespoon	lb	=	pound or pounds
c	= cup	sq	=	square
pt	= pint	min	=	minute or minutes
qt	= quart	hr	=	hour or hours
gal	= gallon	mod.	=	moderate or moderately
pk	= peck	doz	=	dozen
bu	= bushel			

MEASUREMENTS

3 tsp	= 1 Tbsp	1 c	=	½ pt
4 Tbsp	= ¼ c	2 c	=	1 lb
5⅓ Tbsp	= ⅓ c	2 c	=	1 pt
8 Tbsp	= ½ c	2 pt (4 c)	=	1 qt
16 Tbsp	= 1 c	4 qt (liquid)	=	1 gal
1 oz	= 2 Tbsp	8 qt (solid)	=	1 pk
1 gill	= ½ c	4 pk	=	1 bu
8 oz	= 1 c			
16 oz	= 1 lb			

BUTTER OR MARGARINE

2 Tbsp = 1 oz
½ c = ¼ lb = 1 stick
2 c = 1 lb

CEREALS

Rice	1 c	=	½ lb
Rice	1 c raw precooked	=	2 c cooked
Rice	1 c raw converted	=	3 to 4 c cooked
Rice	1 c raw long-grain	=	4 c cooked
Noodles	1 c	=	1¼ c cooked
Macaroni	1 c	=	2¼ c cooked

COFFEE, GROUND

1 lb = 80 Tbsp or 5 c
= ½ c makes 10 c beverage

EGGS

5 eggs = about 1 c
8 to 10 egg whites = 1 c
12 to 15 egg yolks = 1 c

FLOUR

All-purpose	4 c sifted	=	1 lb
Cake	1 c sifted	=	1 c all-purpose flour less 2 Tbsp
Cornmeal	3 c	=	1 lb
Potato flour (for thickening)	1 Tbsp	=	2 Tbsp flour
Cornstarch (for thickening)	1 Tbsp	=	2 Tbsp flour
Arrowroot (for thickening)	2 tsp	=	5 tsp flour

FRUITS

Apples	1 lb	=	3 med. or 3 c sliced
Candied fruit	1 lb	=	1½ c
Lemon (whole)	1	=	2 to 3 Tbsp juice
Lemon (grated rind)	1	=	about 1½ to 2 tsp
Orange (whole)	1	=	6 to 8 Tbsp or ⅓ to ½ c juice
Orange (grated rind)	1	=	about 1 Tbsp
Raisins	1 lb	=	3 c

MARSHMALLOWS

¼ lb = 16

MILK AND CHEESE

Milk	1 c	=	½ c evaporated milk + ½ c water
Milk	1 c	=	4 Tbsp powdered whole milk + 1 c water
Cream	1 c	=	2 c whipped cream
Cheese (grated)	4 to 5 c	=	1 lb
Cottage cheese	1 c	=	½ lb
Cream cheese	3-oz package	=	7 Tbsp

NUTS

Unshelled	1 lb	=	2 c nut meats
Shelled	1 lb	=	3 to 4 c nut meats

SUGAR

Granulated	1 lb	=	2 c
Brown	1 lb	=	2¼ c
Confectioners	1 lb	=	3½ c
Powdered	1 lb	=	2⅓ c

CONTENTS OF CANS

Size (No.)	Weight	Measure (c)
¼	4 to 4.5 oz	½
½	7.5 to 8 oz	1
Picnic		1¼
No. 1 short or No. 300	10 to 13 oz	1¾
No. 1 tall or No. 303	1 lb	2
No. 2	1 lb 4 oz	2½
No. 2½	1lb 14 oz to 15 oz	3½
No. 3	2 lb to 2 lb 1 oz	4
No. 10	6 lb 8 oz to 8 lb 12 oz	12 to 13

TEMPERATURES

	Fahrenheit (°F)	Centigrade (°C)
Simmering point	180	82
Boiling point of water at sea level	212	100
Ovens		
Very slow	200 - 250	93 - 121
Slow	300	149
Moderately slow	325	163
Moderate	350	177
Moderately hot	375	191
Hot	400	204
Very hot	450 - 500	232 - 260
Extremely hot	over 500	260

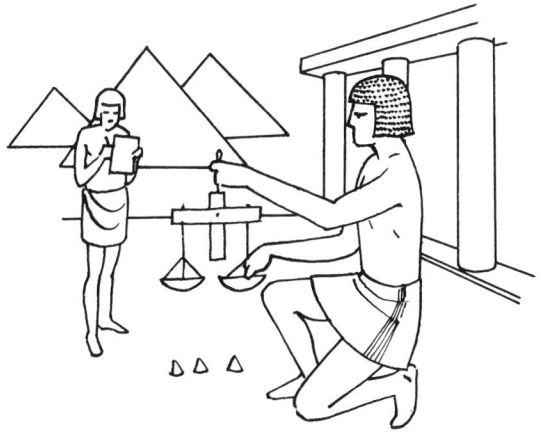

Fig. W-7. Scales were developed by the ancient Egyptians to weigh grains.

ENGLISH SYSTEM.

In about 1300, London merchants adopted a weight system called *avoirdupois* (from the old French term, *aveir-de-peis*), meaning *goods of weight*. This system, which was used to weigh bulky goods, is based on a pound of 7,000 grains or 16 oz. It is still used in many English-speaking countries.

U.S. CUSTOMARY SYSTEM.

On May 29, 1830, the Senate passed a resolution directing the Secretary of the Treasury to make a comparison of the weights and measures in use in the principal customhouses. The study was made, followed by real progress toward the unification of weights and measures in the United States through the subsequent distribution of uniform standards to the customhouses based on the following: (1) the yard of 36 in.; (2) the avoirdupois pound of 7,000 grains; (3) the wine gallon of 231 cu. in.; and (4) the Winchester bushel of 2,150.42 cu.in. These units are still in use in the United States.

METRIC SYSTEM.

The Metric System is a decimal system based on multiples of ten.

The basic metric units are the *meter* (length/distance), the *gram* (weight), and the *liter* (capacity). The units are then expanded in multiples of 10 or made smaller by $\frac{1}{10}$. The prefixes, which are used in the same way with all basic metric units, follow:

"milli-"	=	1/1,000
"centi-"	=	1/100
"deci-"	=	1/10
"deca-"	=	10
"hecto-"	=	100
"kilo-"	=	1,000

CONVERSIONS OF U.S. CUSTOMARY AND METRIC.

A comparison of U.S. Customary and Metric Systems is shown in Figs. W-9 and W-10.

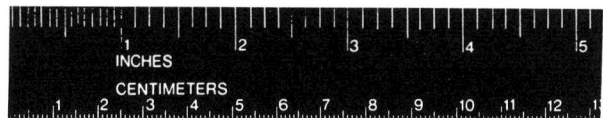

Fig. W-9. Inches-centimeter scale for direct conversion and reading.

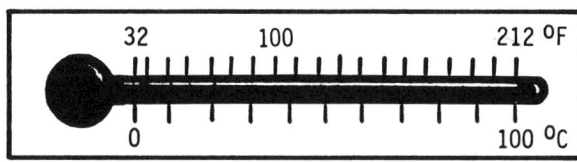

Fig. W-10. Farenheit-Celsius (Centigrade) scale for direct conversion and reading.

The following tables will facilitate conversion from U.S. Customary to Metric units, and vice versa:

TABLE W-6
WEIGHT EQUIVALENTS

1 lb	= 453.6 g = .4536 kg = 16 oz
1 oz	= 28.35 g
1 kg	= 1,000 g = 2.2046 lb
1 g	= 1,000 mg
1 mg	= 1,000 mcg = .001 g
1 mcg	= .001 mg = .000001 g
1 mcg per g or 1 mg per kg is the same as ppm	

TABLE W-7
WEIGHT-UNIT CONVERSION FACTORS

Units Given	Units Wanted	For Conversion Multiply By	Units Given	Units Wanted	For Conversion Multiply By
lb	g	453.6	kcal/kg	kcal/lb	0.4536
lb	kg	0.4536	kcal/lb	kcal/kg	2.2046
oz	g	28.35			
kg	lb	2.2046	ppm	mcg/g	1.
kg	mg	1,000,000.	ppm	mg/kg	1.
kg	g	1,000.	ppm	mg/lb	0.4536
g	mg	1,000.	mg/kg	%	0.0001
g	mcg	1,000,000.	ppm	%	0.0001
mg	mcg	1,000.	mg/g	%	0.1
			g/kg	%	0.1
mg/g	mg/lb	453.6			
mg/kg	mg/lb	0.4536			
mcg/kg	mcg/lb	0.4536			
Mcal	kcal	1,000.			

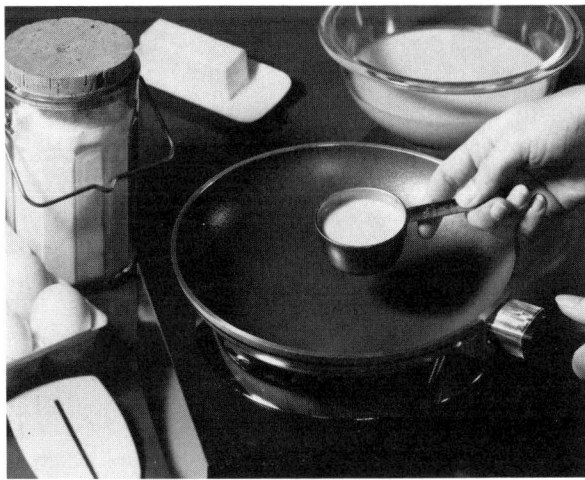

Fig. W-8. Accurate measurements make for a successful cook. (Courtesy, American Egg Board, Park Ridge, Ill.)

TABLE W-8
CONVERSION FACTORS
U.S. CUSTOMARY TO METRIC

Symbol	When You Know	Multiply By	To Find	Symbol
U.S. Customary			*Metric*	
LENGTH				
in.	inches	**2.5**	*centimeters*	*cm*
ft	feet	**30.**	*centimeters*	*cm*
yd	yards	**0.9**	*meters*	*m*
mi	miles	**1.6**	*kilometers*	*km*
AREA				
in.²	square inches	**6.5**	*square centimeters*	*cm²*
ft²	square feet	**0.09**	*square meters*	*m²*
yd²	square yards	**0.8**	*square meters*	*m²*
mi²	square miles	**2.6**	*square kilometers*	*km²*
	acres	**0.4**	*hectares*	*ha*
MASS (weight)				
oz	ounces	**28.**	*grams*	*g*
lb	pounds	**0.45**	*kilograms*	*kg*
	short tons (2000 lb)	**0.9**	*metric ton*	*t*
VOLUME				
tsp	teaspoons	**5.**	*milliliters*	*ml*
Tbsp	tablespoons	**15.**	*milliliters*	*ml*
in.³	cubic inches	**16.**	*milliliters*	*ml*
fl oz	fluid ounces	**30.**	*milliliters*	*ml*
c	cups	**0.24**	*liters*	*liter*
pt	pints	**0.47**	*liters*	*liter*
qt	quarts	**0.95**	*liters*	*liter*
gal	gallons	**3.8**	*liters*	*liter*
ft³	cubic feet	**0.03**	*cubic meters*	*m³*
yd³	cubic yards	**0.76**	*cubic meters*	*m³*
TEMPERATURE (exact)				
°F	degrees Fahrenheit	**5/9 (after subtracting 32)**	*degrees Celsius*	*°C (Centigrade)*

TABLE W-9
CONVERSION FACTORS
METRIC TO U.S. CUSTOMARY

Symbol	When You know	Multiply By	To Find	Symbol
Metric			*U.S. Customary*	
LENGTH				
mm	*millimeters*	**0.04**	inches	in.
cm	*centimeters*	**0.4**	inches	in.
m	*meters*	**3.3**	feet	ft
m	*meters*	**1.1**	yards	yd
km	*kilometers*	**0.6**	miles	mi
AREA				
cm²	*square centimeters*	**0.16**	square inches	in.²
m²	*square meters*	**1.2**	square yard	yd²
km²	*square kilometers*	**0.4**	square miles	mi²
ha	*hectares (10,000 m²)*	**2.5**	acres	
MASS (weight)				
g	*grams*	**0.035**	ounces	oz
kg	*kilograms*	**2.2**	pounds	lb
t	*metric ton (1000 kg)*	**1.1**	short tons	

VOLUME				
ml	*milliliters*	**0.03**	fluid ounces	fl oz
ml	*milliliters*	**0.06**	cubic inches	in.³
liter	*liters*	**2.1**	pints	pt
liter	*liters*	**1.06**	quarts	qt
liter	*liters*	**0.26**	gallons	gal
m³	*cubic meters*	**35**	cubic feet	ft³
m³	*cubic meters*	**1.3**	cubic yards	yd³
TEMPERATURE (exact)				
°C	*degrees Celsius (Centigrade)*	**9/5 (then add 32)**	*degrees Fahrenheit*	*°F*

WHALE OIL

A yellowish-brown oil made by (1) boiling the blubber of whales, and (2) skimming off the oil. After hardening by hydrogenation some of it is used for making margarine and soap.

WHEAT, family *Gramineae;* genus *Triticum*

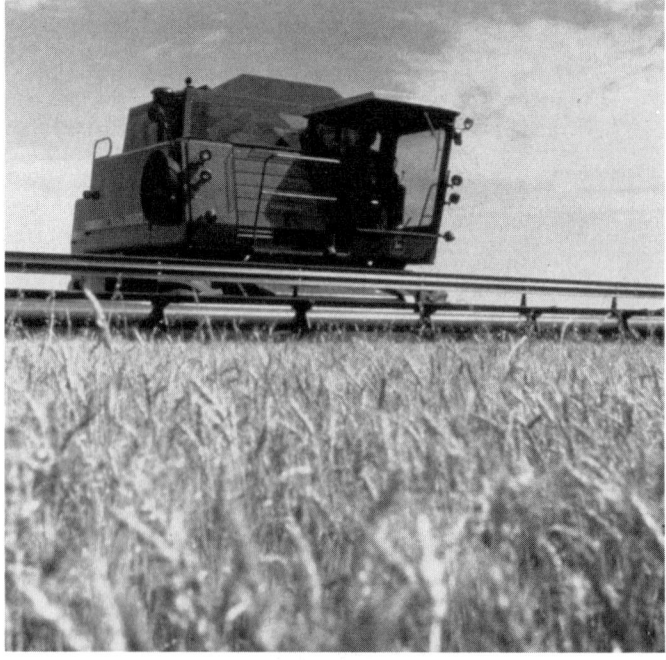

Fig. W-11. Harvesting wheat. (Courtesy, Deere & Co., Moline, Ill.)

Wheat, the world's most important grain crop, is a member of the grass family, *Gramineae,* and of the genus *Triticum.*

Wheat provides more nourishment for more people throughout the world than any other food; indeed, it is the staff of life. While rice is the common food in the Orient, wheat is basic to the diet of Europe, Africa, North and South

America, Australia, and a large part of Asia. One-third of the world's poplulation depends on wheat as its main staple. Total world production of wheat is about 250 g per day per person, enough to supply 800 Calories (kcal) and 30 g of protein daily if it were evenly distributed and unrefined. In many developing countries, wheat supplies 40 to 60% of the available energy and protein.

Wheaten foods provide generously of carbohydrates, protein, and certain minerals and vitamins. Of all the cereals, wheat alone could meet minimum protein requirements if used as the sole cereal product, with the exception of infants and young growing children (who need supplemental lysine when fed wheat-based diets) and possibly pregnant and lactating females. A diet with large amounts of wheat and only small amounts of protein from animal sources provides adequate quantity and quality protein.

(Also see CEREAL GRAINS.)

ORIGIN AND HISTORY. The development and progress of civilization can be linked to the history of wheat. Prior to recorded history, man cultivated wheat.

No one knows where the wheat plant originated, although it was cultivated where modern man is supposed to have first appeared—in southwestern Asia. The common ancestor of all wheats is believed to be a species called *wild einkorn* (meaning *one seed*), found in excavated ruins in the upper reaches of the Tigris-Euphrates basin in Southwestern Asia—called the "Fertile Crescent," the presumed birthplace of our civilization. The 14- and 21-chromosome species of wheats are believed to have developed as natural hybrids of the original einkorn.

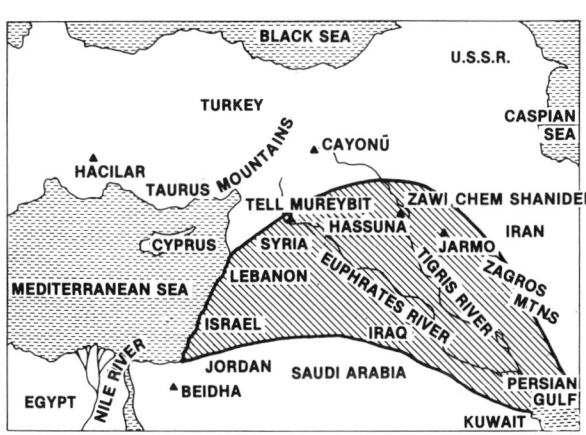

Fig. W-12. The fertile crescent.

Man probably used wheat as food 10,000 to 15,000 years before Christ. In 1948, archaeologists from the University of Chicago found kernels of wheat, believed to be about 6,700 years old, preserved in the ruins of an ancient village in Iraq.

The first wheat food was probably the grain itself, stripped of its husk, or glumes, and chewed, a way in which it is still eaten in many parts of the world. But a form of bread was found in the remains of a Stone Age village of Swiss lake dwellers.

The reverence in which people held wheat and bread through the ages still lives in the Lord's Prayer: "Give us this day, our daily bread." In the Hebrew faith, the eating of unleavened matzoh during the Passover also marks the significance of bread in religion. In Europe, bread is commonly referred to as "the staff of life."

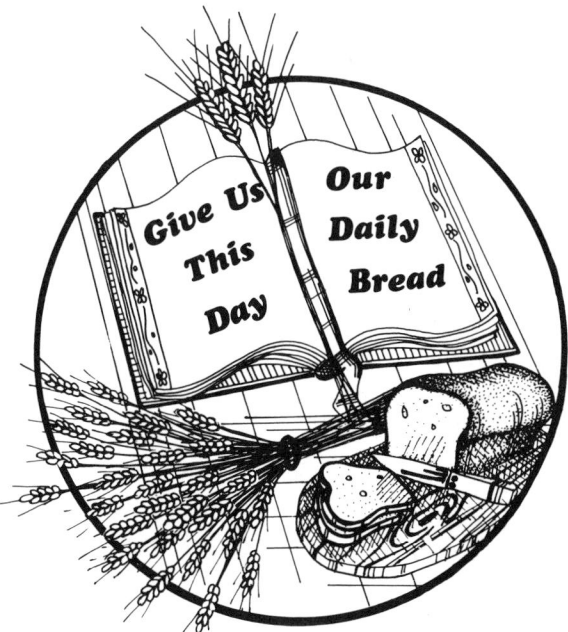

Fig. W-13. Throughout the ages, wheat and bread have lived in the Lord's Prayer.

WORLD AND U.S. PRODUCTION. Wheat is the leading cereal grain of the world. Farmers of the world grow approximately 595 million metric tons of wheat each year.[5] The Soviet Union, which produces about 18% of the world crop, is the leading wheat-producing nation of the world. But the U.S.S.R. does not grow enough wheat for its own needs.

The United States ranks third among the wheat-producing countries of the world. The ten leading wheat-producing countries of the globe are: U.S.S.R., China, United States, India, France, Canada, Turkey, Australia, Germany, and Pakistan.[6]

In the United States, wheat ranks second only to corn among the cereal grains in total acreage and production. Wheat is grown in every state of continental United States, although production in New England is minor. The greatest acreage is in the Central Plains and north central states.

The United States produces 74.5 million metric tons of wheat annually; and the ten leading wheat-producing states of the United States, by rank, are: Kansas, Oklahoma, Washington, Texas, North Dakota, Montana, Illinois, Nebraska, Colorado, and Ohio.[7]

KINDS OF WHEAT. Wheat is classified according to climatic adaptation, color of kernel, relative hardness of kernel, species, and varieties.

• **Winter wheat vs spring wheat**—There are two broad kinds of wheat, winter wheat and spring wheat.

Winter wheats, which are adapted to the Middle Great Plains, are planted in the fall and harvested in the following June and July.

---

[5]Data from *FAO Production Yearbook 1990*, FAO/UN, Rome, Italy, Vol. 44, p. 70, Table 16. **Note well:** Annual production fluctuates as a result of weather and profitability of the crop.

[6]*Ibid.*

[7]Data from *Agricultural Statistics 1991*, USDA, p. 6, Table 8. **Note well:** Annual production fluctuates as a result of weather and profitability of the crop.

Spring wheats are planted in the spring after the threat of frost is over and the ground is dry enough to work, and they ripen in the summer of the same year, usually a few weeks after winter wheat. Each group includes varieties of both hard and soft wheat.

• **Color of kernel**—Both winter and spring wheat produce grain that is red or white, with various shades of yellows or amber.

• **Texture of the ripened grain**—Wheat is classed as hard or soft. Hard wheats tend to be higher in protein content than soft wheats, and are primarily used in bread flour. Durham wheats are also hard wheats, used for macaroni production. Softer wheats are lower in protein and are chiefly milled into flour for cakes, cookies, pastries, and crackers.

• **Species of wheat**—All the wheats grown throughout the world belong to one of 14 species.

Of the 14 species, only three—common, club, and durum—account for 90% of all wheat grown in the world today.

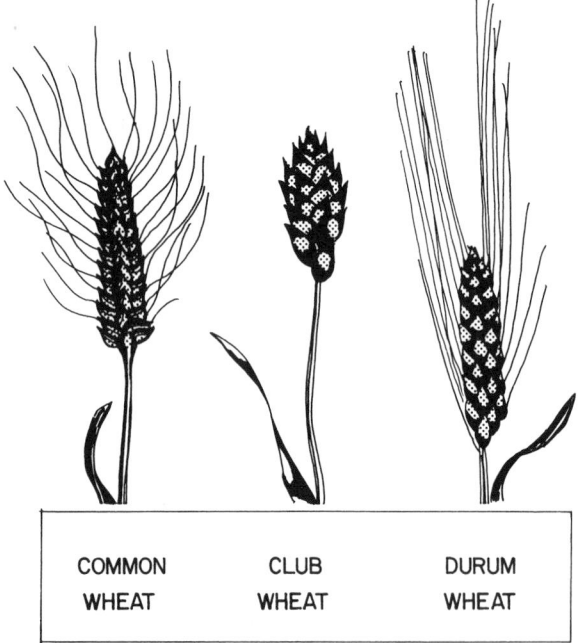

Fig. W-14. Heads of three most common types of wheat.

Common wheat is bread wheat. It probably originated in Turkey and southern U.S.S.R. Over 200 varieties of common wheat have been described, of which about 100 are now cultivated. They may be either red or white, hard or soft, and spring or winter type.

Club wheat is grown primarily for flour, in the Pacific Northwest. It may be either winter or spring type.

Durum wheat is grown for spaghetti, macaroni, and noodles. The kernels are white or red. The varieties of this species grown in North America are all spring wheats, grown in North Dakota, South Dakota, Montana, Minnesota, and parts of Canada.

MILLING WHEAT. The main parts of the wheat grain are:

1. **The endosperm**, which constitutes about 83% of the kernel and is the source of white flour.

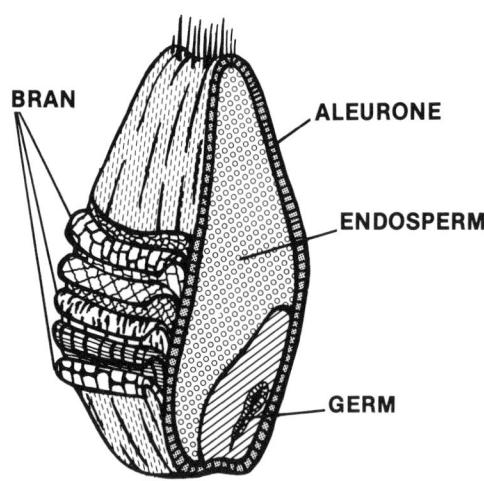

Fig. W-15. Structure of the wheat grain.

2. **The coat** (bran or coarse bran; and aleurone or fine bran), which constitutes about 14.5% of the kernel and is the source of bran, used primarily for animal feed.

3. **The germ**, which constitutes 2.5% of the kernel and is the source of wheat meal and wheat germ oil, used for human food or animal feed.

On threshing, the husk is removed and the grain is made naked. The wheat endosperm is covered with two kinds of fibrous coatings; the coarsest outer layer is called bran, and the less fibrous layer is the aleurone. At the base of the kernel is the germ. The objective of milling is to separate the starchy endosperm from the other parts of the grain. Whole wheat yields about 72% white flour, and 28% by-products, consisting of bran and germ. (By contrast, in China, by official ruling, the minimum extraction rate permissible for wheat flour is 81%; hence, the wheat flour of China is less refined than in the United States.) Since an average bushel of wheat weighs 60 lb (*27 kg*), this means that approximately 2.3 bu of wheat are required to produce 100 lb (*45 kg*) of flour and 38 lb (*17 kg*) of millfeed.

Whole wheat flour, as the name would indicate, contains the finely ground endosperm, bran, and germ. In comparison with products made from white flour, whole wheat products have a distinctive flavor and a coarser texture, and, because of the higher fat content of the germ, they are more difficult to keep and sometimes become rancid.

Since prehistoric times, the goal of milling has been the separation of the bran and germ from the endosperm, to make white flour.

• **Modern milling**—In modern milling, wheat passes through about 2 dozen processes before it is made into table flour. Fig. W-16 is a simplified diagram showing what happens in milling.

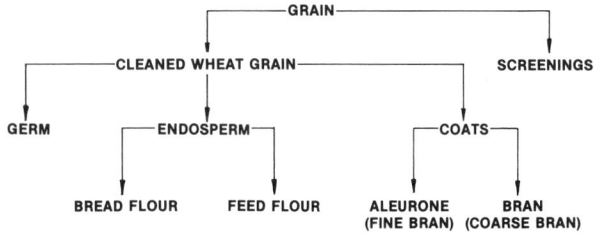

Fig. W-16. A simplified flow diagram of wheat milling.

Flour. Different grades and kinds of wheat are required for milling into the several grades and kinds of flours.

GRADES OF FLOUR; TEST BAKING.

The highest quality flour is known as *patent flour.*

The percentage of protein in a flour generally serves as one standard of quality. The protein of wheat and flour is composed of *gliadin* and *glutenin*, which, when mixed with liquid, form *gluten.* The elastic gluten developed by kneading the dough entraps the carbon dioxide formed by the fermentation of sugar and starches by yeast, or released by chemical leavening or air beaten into the mixture. The result is the unique *rising* or expansion characteristics of wheat flour doughs.

The mineral or ash content of flour is also used as an index of flour quality or grade; the lower the ash, or the less residue, the whiter or more refined the flour.

Small quantities of wheat are usually milled for test baking. Various flours are checked by different baking procedures according to end use. For hard wheat, test loaves are baked to determine the mixing time and tolerance of doughs, the degree to which the flour will absorb liquid, potential loaf volume, texture, crumb, color, and flavor. For soft wheat, similar determinations are made with test cakes, cookies, or crackers.

KINDS OF FLOURS.

There are many kinds of flours, each designed and best suited for a specific purpose, the main ones of which are discussed in the sections that follow:

• **Bakery flour**—Bakery bread wheat doughs are usually processed by machinery; therefore, the dough must have machine tolerance, or strength, in order to withstand the beating action of mechanical kneading and handling. This calls for *stronger* wheat—higher in the proteins, gliadin and glutenin, which form gluten—resulting in stronger doughs.

• **Family flour**—The decreasing production and sale of family flour reflects the decline in home baking.

Bread doughs worked by hand require strong arms, somewhat limiting the market to flour made from mellow gluten wheats that produce doughs that can be hand manipulated. There has been a trend away from the use of very strong wheats because the average homemaker does not have the strength or the patience to knead the dough long enough to develop the strong gluten.

The problems of the family flour requirements were partially solved with the making of *all-purpose* flours—mixed flours suited for both (1) good cakes, biscuits, and pastries, and (2) good bread.

Another innovation of family flour developed in the early 1960s was a granular or more dispersible type of flour. From the standpoint of the family, this flour offers the following advantages in comparison with regular flour: free-pouring—like salt; dust-free; alleviating the need for sifting; and dispersing in cold liquid, rather than balling or lumping.

Special soft wheat cake flours, and whole wheat flours are also available to homemakers. Graham flour is a whole wheat product made from 11.5% protein hard red winter wheat.

• **Specialty flours**—For the bakery trade, millers make a wide variety of different flours designed for different products, such as Italian and French breads and rolls.

Small retail shops keep a supply of several different kinds of flour, including: hard wheat flour for breads; soft wheat or cake flour for cookies, cakes, doughnuts, and cakelike products; and in-between flour for certain rolls, coffee cakes, and other pastries.

Special soft wheat flours are milled for cookie, cracker, and pretzel bakers; and other special flours are prepared for canners who make soups, gravies, desserts requiring thickening, and flour-based sauces.

• **Durum wheat flour**—The milling of durum wheat flour for making macaroni requires additional purifiers to separate the branny material from the desired semolina, a coarse granulation of the endosperm. By federal definition, semolina cannot contain more than 3% flour.

Durum millers also make *granulars,* or a coarse product with greater amounts of flour; or they grind the wheat into flour for special use in macaroni products, particularly in noodles.

• **Bleached flour**—At one time, it was necessary to age flour by storing it in a warehouse for a considerable time and turning it so as to expose it to the oxidizing action of the air. The stored flour lost some of its creamy color and baked better. But the process necessitated storage facilities, took time, and required labor; and the results were variable. Today, the same end result is achieved, more quickly and better, by the use of additives. In either case, the proteins are slightly oxidized. In storage, they're oxidized from the air; in bleaching, they're oxidized from the maturing agent. The oxidation of flour makes gluten stronger, or more elastic, and produces better baking results. Some oxidizing agents, such as those in which a calcium or phosphorus compound is used as a carrier, also improve the nutritive value of the flour. Only cookie, pie crust, and cracker flours are more satisfactory without bleach.

Today, flour must be plainly marked "bleached" if one of several government approved oxidizing-maturing agents has been added.

• **Phosphated flour**—Phosphated flour is popular in certain areas, particularly where biscuits are commonly made with sour milk and buttermilk. Since the acid content of sour milk varies, phosphated flour provides a greater assurance of leavening action from baking soda. The amount of calcium phosphate permitted in the flour is very small, not less than 0.25% and not more than 0.75%. Nevertheless, this low level of phosphation constitutes a significant nutritional enhancement, because a cup *(115 g)* of sifted phosphated flour supplies from 68 mg to 165 mg of calcium, and from 176 to 328 mg of phosphorus—compared to only 18 mg of calcium and 100 mg of phosphorus in unphosphated flour.

• **Self-rising flour**—Calcium phosphate is an ingredient of baking powder as well as in the leavening agents of self-rising flour, which also contains salt and soda. A typical self-rising flour contains 305 mg of calcium and 536 mg of phosphorus per cup *(115 g).*

In chemically-leavened flour, in the presence of liquid, the acid of the phosphate reacts with baking soda to produce a leavening gas, carbon dioxide—the same as the yeast organisms produce in yeast-raised products. Additionally, the calcium and phosphorus improve the nutritive qualities of the flour.

• **Whole wheat, cracked wheat, farina**—Whole wheat (or graham flour) is made from the entire wheat kernel.

Cracked or crushed wheat refers to wheat that has been broken into fragments.

Farina is purified middlings; it is the glandular endosperm that contains no bran and no more than 3% flour. Farina is most commonly used as a cooked breakfast cereal.

(Also see FLOUR, Table F-12, Major Flours.)

Enriched Flour. Since 1941, millers and bakers have followed the practice of enriching their products. Earlier surveys had indicated that the levels of certain nutrients were inadequate in the national diet; among them, the B vitamins, iron, iodine, and vitamin D. Since public need was demonstrated, the American Medical Association, leading nutritionists, government agencies, millers, and bakers worked together to develop an enrichment program with widely used, available, and inexpensive foods, like bread, to serve as carriers.

Originally, the FDA differentiated between enrichment and fortification, but now the two programs are used interchangeably. Nevertheless, the following vocabulary for and definition of food improvement persist:

• **Enriched**[8]—Refers to the addition of specific nutrients to a food *as established in a federal standard of identity and quality* (for example: enriched bread). The amounts added generally are moderate and include those commonly present at even lower levels.

• **Fortified**[9]—Refers to the addition to foods of specific nutrients. The amounts added are usually in excess of those normally found in the food because of the importance of providing additional amounts of the nutrients to the diet. Some foods are selected for fortification because they are an appropriate carrier for the nutrient. *Example:* Milk is frequently fortified with vitamin D.

---

[8]"Nutrition Labeling—Terms You Should Know," *FDA Consumer Memo,* DHEW Publication No. 74-2010, 1974, pp. 2-3.
[9]*Ibid.*

• **Restored**—The replacement of nutrients lost in processing food.

Although the principle followed with white flour is basically enrichment, rather than restoration, and although the quantity of the nutrients in the enrichment formula were established on the basis of dietary need, they also happen to restore to white flour the approximate amounts of those same nutrients as were present in whole wheat (see Table W-10).

Tables W-11, W-12, W-13, and W-14 show the standards for enriching flour, self-rising flour, macaroni products, and enriched bread, buns, and rolls. Calcium and vitamin D are permitted as optional additions to flour and bread, in the amounts specified. At about the same time that the flour enrichment program got underway (1941), iodine was added to table salt to prevent goiter, and vitamin D was added to milk to prevent rickets (Since most milk is now fortified with vitamin D, it is seldom added to bakery foods).

Since the start of the enrichment program in 1941, the available supplies of the B vitamins—thiamin, riboflavin, and niacin—and of iron in the national diet have increased. The enrichment program has played a significant role in the practical elimination of the vitamin deficiency diseases ariboflavinosis, beriberi, and pellagra, and of simple iron-deficiency anemia.

Today, enrichment is required in 34 states and Puerto Rico. In practice, however, all family flour is enriched, and about 90% of all commercially baked standard white bread is enriched.

TABLE W-10
COMPARISON OF NUTRIENTS IN WHEAT FLOUR AND WHEAT BREAD[1]
(Minimum and maximum enrichment levels for the three B vitamins—thiamin, riboflavin, and niacin—and iron are given in the table below)

One pound[2]	Protein	Fat	Calcium	Iron	Thiamin	Riboflavin	Niacin
	(g)	(g)	(mg)	(mg)	(mg)	(mg)	(mg)
Flour							
Whole Wheat	60.3	9.1	186	15.0	2.49	.54	19.7
Unenriched (all purpose)	47.6	4.5	73	3.6	.28	.21	4.1
Enriched (all purpose)	47.6	4.5	73-960[3]	13-16.5[3]	2.90[3]	1.80[3]	24.0[3]
Bread							
Whole Wheat (2% nonfat dry milk)	47.6	13.6	449	10.4	1.17	.56	12.9
Unenriched (white), (3 to 4% nonfat dry milk)	39.5	14.5	381	3.2	.31	.39	5.0
Enriched (white), (3 to 4% nonfat dry milk)	39.5	14.5	381-600[4]	8-12.5[4]	1.80[4]	1.10[4]	15.04[4]

[1]The source of this data is *From Wheat to Flour,* published by Wheat Flour Institute, Chicago, Ill., 1976, p. 68, except where noted otherwise.
[2]Multiply by 2.2 to obtain the amount per kg.
[3]*Code of Federal Regulations,* Title 21, Revised 4/1/78, Section 137.165 provides that enriched flour must contain the specified amounts of iron, thiamin, riboflavin, and niacin; but that the addition of calcium is optional. However, no claim for calcium on the label may be made if the flour contains less than 960 mg per lb.
[4]*Code of Federal Regulations,* Title 21, Revised 4/1/78, Section 136.115 provides that enriched bread, buns, and rolls must contain the specified amounts of iron, thiamin, riboflavin, and niacin; but that the addition of calcium is optional. However, no claim for calcium on the label may be made if the bread contains less than 600 mg per lb.

TABLE W-11
STANDARD FOR ENRICHED FLOUR[1]

Required Ingredients per Pound of Flour[2]	
Thiamin	2.9 mg
Riboflavin	1.8 mg
Niacin	24.0 mg
Iron	13.0-16.5 mg
Optional Ingredient	
Calcium	960 mg

[1]*Code of Federal Regulations,* Title 21, Revised 4/1/78, Section 137.165.
[2]Multiply by 2.2 to obtain the amount per kg.

TABLE W-12
STANDARD FOR ENRICHED SELF-RISING FLOUR[1]

Required Ingredients per Pound of Flour[2]	
Thiamin	2.9 mg
Riboflavin	1.8 mg
Niacin	24.0 mg
Iron	13.0-16.5 mg
Optional Ingredient	
Calcium	960 mg

[1]*Code of Federal Regulations,* Title 21, Revised 4/1/78, Section 137.185.
[2]Multiply by 2.2 to obtain the amount per kg.

TABLE W-13
STANDARD FOR
ENRICHED MACARONI PRODUCTS[1]

Required Ingredients per Pound of Flour[2]		
	(minimum)	(maximum)
Thiamin	4.0 mg	5.0 mg
Riboflavin	1.7 mg	2.2 mg
Niacin	27.0 mg	34.0 mg
Iron	13.0 mg	16.5 mg
Optional Ingredient		
Calcium	500.0 mg	625.0 mg
Vitamin D	250 U.S.P. units	1000 U.S.P. units

[1]*Code of Federal Regulations*, Title 21, Revised 4/1/78, Section 139.115.

[2]Multiply by 2.2 to obtain the amount per kg.

TABLE W-14
STANDARD FOR
ENRICHED BREAD, BUNS, AND ROLLS[1]

Required Ingredients per Pound of Flour[2]	
Thiamin	1.8 mg
Riboflavin	1.1 mg
Niacin	15.0 mg
Iron	8.0-12.5 mg
Optional Ingredient	
Calcium	600.0 mg

[1]*Code of Federal Regulations,* Revised 4/1/78, Section 136.115.

[2]Multiply by 2.2 to obtain the amount per kg.

It is noteworthy that England, Canada, and a few other countries have enrichment programs somewhat similar to the United States, but that France forbids enrichment.

NUTRITIONAL VALUE OF WHEAT. Whole wheat flour is made by grinding the entire kernel of wheat. Thus, it contains nutrients found in all three parts—the bran, endosperm, and germ. To produce white flour which has better keeping qualities than whole wheat flour, millers remove the bran and germ and use only the endosperm. Some of the B vitamins, calcium, and iron are lost. The processing of white flour removes additional nutrients.

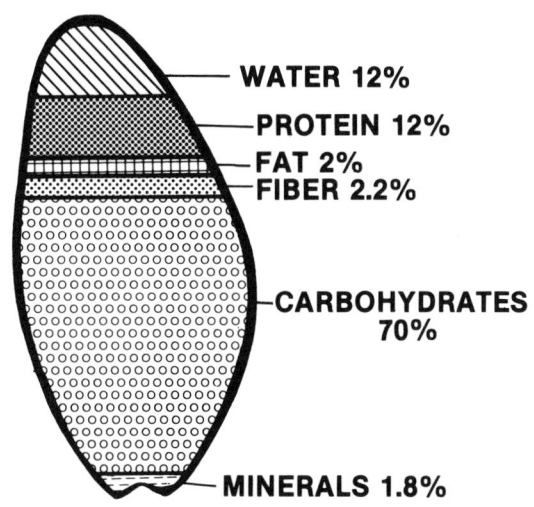

Fig. W-17. Proximate analysis of whole wheat.

Wheat is high in carbohydrates; hence, it is a high energy source. Its contribution to the available food energy of the following countries is noteworthy: Israel, 35%; France, 30%; Australia, 25%; England, 20%; and United States, Canada, and West Germany, 18%. As a source of energy in the United States, wheat ranks on a par with three other major sources of energy: meats, processed fats, and processed sugar. Together, these four foods comprise three-fourths of the food energy available in the United States.

Wheat has the highest protein value of any of the cereals. Still, the protein is of poor quality. Table W-15 compares the essential amino acids in whole wheat, white flour, and wheat germ to a high quality protein product—cow's milk. Like rice and corn and their products, wheat is particularly deficient in lysine; hence, it should be eaten with a complementary protein source such as a legume. Although not indicated in Table W-15, wheat germ contains about 23% protein, whole wheat contains about 12% protein, and white flour contains about 11% protein. Interestingly, the protein in wheat germ is extra rich in lysine, the amino acid that is deficient in the rest of the wheat grain.

TABLE W-15
PROFILE OF ESSENTIAL AMINO ACIDS IN
WHOLE WHEAT, WHITE FLOUR, AND WHEAT GERM
COMPARED TO MILK—A HIGH-QUALITY PROTEIN[1,2]

Amino Acid	Whole Wheat	White Flour	Wheat Germ	Cow's Milk
	(mg/g protein)			
Histidine	19	20	27	27
Isoleucine	32	46	36	47
Leucine	58	77	64	95
Lysine	25	22	63	78
Methionine and cystine	33	33	37	33
Phenylalanine and tyrosine	68	89	68	102
Threonine	26	29	40	44
Tryptophan	11	12	12	14
Valine	38	43	48	64

[1]Additional information about the essential amino acid content of wheat and flour products may be found in Table P-16, Proteins and Amino Acids in Selected Foods.

[2]*Recommended Dietary Allowances*, 10th ed., 1989, National Academy of Sciences, p. 67, Table 6–5. The essential amino acid requirements of infants can be met by supplying 0.79 g of a high-quality protein per pound of body weight (1.73 g/kg body weight) per day.

The nutritive value of the many different forms of wheat and wheat products is given in Food Composition Table F-21.

(Also see BREADS AND BAKING, sections headed "Nutritive Values of Breads and Related Items," and "Improving the Nutritive Values of Breads and Baked Goods"; MINERAL[S]; PROTEIN[S]; and VITAMIN[S].)

For some individuals, the consumption of wheat creates health problems. If supplementary foods are inadequate, excessive amounts of wheat products can lead to kwashiorkor or beriberi. However, persons to whom wheat products are available are usually able to obtain a wider variety of foods, and deficiency diseases have not been directly attributed to overdependence on wheat products. Celiac disease, however, is apparently due to a genetically-determined intolerance to wheat gluten or an acquired defect in the intestinal lining. Also, the use of refined flour in wheat products, especially those of a sticky nature such as biscuits, is believed to be a major factor predisposing to dental caries.

WHEAT PRODUCTS AND USES.

The most common use of wheat is for food made from flour. Breakfast foods and beer or other alcoholic fermentations also take considerable quantities of wheat.

Breads date back thousands of years, in war and in peace, in famine and in plenty, to the discovery of wheat, the invention of milling, and the development of baking.

Wheat is not normally fed to animals because of its high cost and greater value for human food. However, surplus or damaged wheat and the by-products of milling find important use as livestock feeds and, eventually, enter the human diet as meat, milk, and eggs. Some wheat products are also used for industrial purposes.

Table W-16 presents in summary form the story of wheat products and uses for human food.

(Also see BREADS AND BAKING; CEREAL GRAINS; and BREAKFAST CEREALS.)

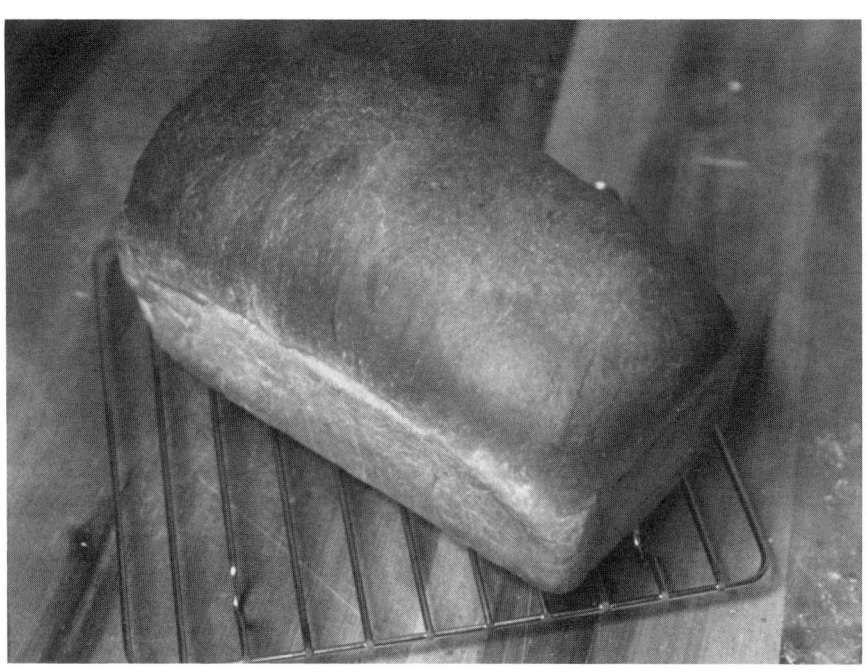
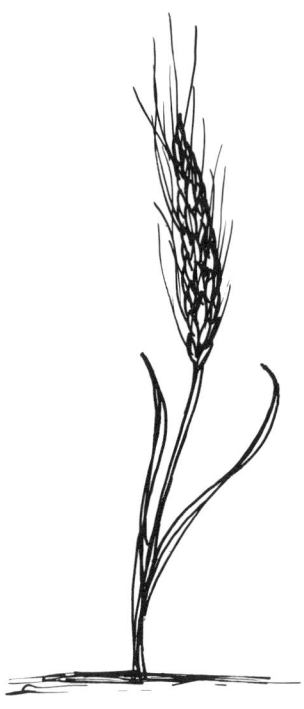

Fig. W-18. Home-made wheat bread. (Courtesy, University of Minnesota, St. Paul, Minn.)

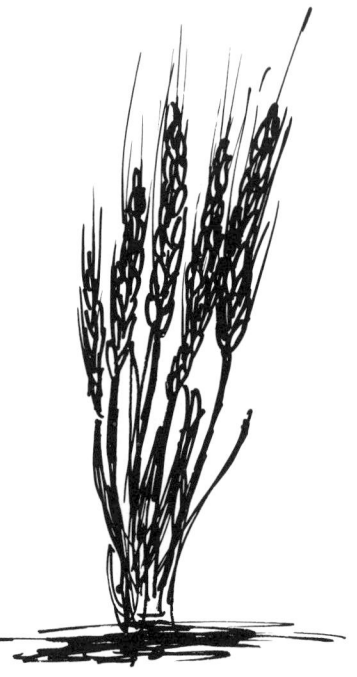
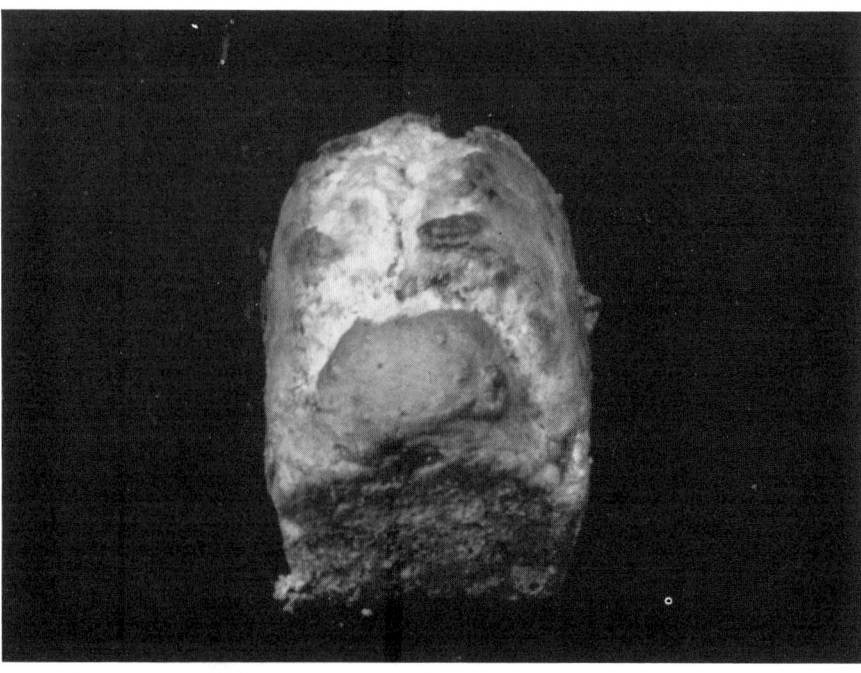

Fig. W-19. There are an unlimited number of recipes for wheat flour production. (Courtesy, Washington State University, Pullman, Wash.)

TABLE W-16
WHEAT PRODUCTS AND USES FOR HUMAN FOOD

Product	Description	Uses	Comments
Flour	White flour is finely ground endosperm of wheat. Whole wheat flour contains the finely ground endosperm, bran, and germ.	Wheat flours are used for many purposes, such as bread, pastries, cakes, cookies, crackers, macaroni, puddings, and soups. (Also see BREADS AND BAKING, section headed "Types of Breads and Baked Doughs.")	For each purpose, a flour of particular properties is required. Additives, such as maturing agents, bleaching agents, and self-rising ingredients, are frequently blended into wheat flours at the mill. Family flour is enriched at the mill, while flour being shipped to the baker is enriched at the bakery.
Bulgur	A partly debranned, parboiled wheat product, used either whole or cracked.	Bulgur is used as a substitute for rice; e.g., in pilaf, an eastern European dish consisting of wheat, meat, oil, and herbs cooked together.	Bulgur is exported in large quantities, especially to the Far East. Bulgur provides a cheap food that is acceptable to rice-eating people because it can be cooked in the same way as rice, and it resembles rice superficially.
Fermented minchin	A product made by putting wheat gluten in a tightly covered container for 2 to 3 weeks and allowing it to be overgrown with both molds and bacteria. Then 10% salt is added and the mixture allowed to age for 2 weeks.	Aged fermented minchin is cut into thin strips and used as a condiment with other foods.	
Wheat germ	The germ is the embryo or sprouting part of the wheat seed.	As an ingredient of speciality breads.	Wheat germ is available for human food, but is usually added to animal feeds.
Wheat gluten	Wheat gluten is a mixture of two proteins, gliadin and glutenin. When mixed with water, they impart the characteristic stickiness to dough.	For making monosodium glutamate which imparts a meatlike flavor to foods. For adding to white flour to make a high-gluten bread.	Some people may develop an intolerance to gluten.
Wheat starch	A white, odorless, tasteless granular or powdery material.	Wheat starch is used as a thickener in soup where its lower gelatinization temperature and shorter gel temperature range is an advantage. Syrup and sugar.	
Wheat tempeh	Fermented cake of cooked wheat grains.	Vegetarian main dish when sliced and baked or fried, and/or an ingredient of salads, sandwiches, soups, sauces, casseroles, and spreads.	An experimental food developed by USDA scientists who utilized the mold *Rhizopus oligosporus* in a procedure similar to that used by Asians to make soybean tempeh. The nutritional value of the original grain is enhanced by the mold fermentation in that (1) proteins are partially digested, and (2) certain B vitamins are synthesized. It is noteworthy that the mold synthesizes vitamin B-12, which makes tempeh one of the few vegetable foods that contain the vitamin.
Breakfast foods, ready-to-eat: Bran flakes	Tan colored, paper thin flakes.	Ready-to-eat breakfast food	
Puffed wheat	Whole wheat depericarped (the outer covering removed), cooked, puffed by extruding through a machine, then dried-toasted.	Ready-to-eat breakfast food	(Also see BREAKFAST CEREALS.)
Shredded wheat	Whole wheat is cooked with water to gelatinize starch, cooled, shredded by machine, cut to shape, baked, then dried and cooled.	Ready-to-eat breakfast food	Shredded wheat has a protein content considerably lower than puffed wheat.
Wheat flakes	Whole wheat, that has been rolled, cooked, flavored, then dried.	Ready-to-eat breakfast food	
Breakfast foods, to be cooked: Whole wheat grains	Unground whole wheat	Cooked cereals, starchy vegetable, puddings such as frumenty.	Cook 40-50 minutes in an open pot or a pressure cooker after soaking overnight in water. Frumenty is cooked grains which have been reheated with milk and served with cream, butter, sugar, and/or jam.
Cracked wheat	Whole grains broken into small pieces	Cooked cereals, breads, soups, casseroles.	Cracked wheat has a nutlike flavor and texture, and cooks much faster than whole kernels of the grain. Only limited amounts can be used in breads because the sharp edges on the particles cut the strands of gluten which make the dough elastic.

(Continued)

TABLE W-16 (Continued)

Product	Description	Uses	Comments
Farina (Cream of Wheat)	This is granulated endosperm that contains no bran and no more than 3% flour; it's similar to semolina except that the wheat is not a durum variety.	A hot breakfast cereal.	Encriched farina is popularly known as *Cream of Wheat,* a product made famous by Nabisco.
Malted cereals	Cracked wheat and malted barley, mixed	Cooked cereals, baked items	May also be used to make muffins and other quick breads.
Rolled wheat	Whole grains rolled into flat pieces (flakes) after steaming	Cooked cereals, cookies, filler in meatloaf	Can be substituted for rolled oats in most recipes.
Wheat meal	Ground wheat from which the bran has been removed	Cooked wheat breakfast foods	
Fortifled foods for developing countries: Bal Ahar	Coarsely ground mixture of bulgur wheat, peanut flour, skim milk powder, minerals, and vitamins. Contains 22% protein.	Infant cereal, suitable for mixing with water	Produced by the government of India. The protein quality is on a par with that of milk.
Bread fortified with low-fat cottonseed flour	Bread made from a mixture of 90% wheat flour and 10% cottonseed flour	High protein bread	Developed at Universidad Agraria La Molina in Lima, Peru. The special cottonseed flour (Protal) raises the protein level of wheat bread from 9% to 11%.
Cereal products fortified with fish protein concentrate (FPC)	Products made from wheat flour fortified with dried, defatted, whole fish powder	Breads, crackers, and noodles	Developed at Universidad Agraria La Molina in Lima, Peru.
Fortified atta	Whole wheat flour mixed with peanut flour, minerals, and vitamins	Baked goods commonly used by people in India	Produced by flour mills that are subsidized by the Indian government. Breads resemble unleavened breads in consistency, and contain about 13.5% protein.
Fortified couscous	Coarsely ground wheat mixed with high protein wheat fractions.	Cereals, casseroles, soups, and other traditional dishes prepared by people in Algeria and neighboring countries.	Developed by International Milling for U.S. Agency for International Development (AID). High protein wheat fractions are obtained by special milling procedures. Fortified couscous has higher quantity and quality of protein than ordinary couscous.
Laubina	Finely ground mixture of cooked bulgur wheat, cooked chickpeas, skim milk powder, sugar, minerals and vitamins.	Infant cereal	Developed at the American University of Beirut in Lebanon. Promoted prompt recovery of hospitalized infants suffering from severe protein-energy malnutrition, but was not effective in curing anemia.
Leche alim	Mixture of toasted wheat flour, fish protein concentrate (FPC), sunflower meal, and skim milk powder. Contains 27% protein.	High protein infant cereal suitable for mixing with water.	Produced by the Pediatrics Laboratory of the University of Chile in Santiago.
Rolled wheat and soy flake mixture	Mixture of 85% rolled wheat and 15% soy flakes.	Cereal	Developed by USDA and test marketed by AID.
Superamine	Finely ground mixture of wheat flour, chickpea flour, lentil flour, skim milk powder, sugar, minerals, vitamins, and flavoring. Contains 21% protein.	High protein powder which may be mixed with water and cooked briefly (2 to 4 minutes)	Developed as a cooperative project between FAO, WHO, UNICEF, and the Algerian government.
Vitalia macaroni	Pasta made from semolina, wheat, soy, corn, and rice derivitives. Contains 18% protein.	High protein macaroni product	Produced by Instituto de Investigaciones Tecnoligicas, in Bogota, Colombia.
Wheat protein beverage powder	A finely ground mixture of wheat protein concentrate, skim milk powder, sugar, vegetable oil, minerals, vitamins, and flavoring	Powder suitable for mixing with water to make a high protein beverage	Experimental products developed by USDA scientists, who devised means of producing a partially digested, low starch, high protein concentrate from wheat flour. Protein quality is intermediate between milk and egg proteins.
Fermented beverages: Wheat grain	Cleaned, whole wheat	Canadian whiskey	Canadian whiskey is produced from any one of the cereal grains; hence, corn, rye, or barley may also be used.
Wheat starch	Malt converts wheat starch to sugar, which is fermented by yeast to ethyl alcohol and carbon dioxide.	1. Ethyl alcohol, used largely for alcoholic beverages. 2. Denatured alcohol for industrial purposes. 3. Gasohol (10% anhydrous ethanol, 90% gasoline)—a motor fuel.	(Also see CORN, section headed "Distilling and Fermentation.")

WHEAT GERM

Wheat germ is the embryo or sprouting part of the wheat seed. A kernel of wheat is composed of three principal parts: The starchy endosperm, which constitutes about 83% of the kernel and is the source of white flour; the coat, which constitutes about 14.5% of the kernel and is the source of bran; and the germ, which constitutes 2.5% of the kernel and is the source of wheat germ meal and wheat germ oil. Wheat germ meal is used chiefly as a livestock feed, although some of it is now used as a human nutritional supplement. Wheat germ oil is used primarily as a rich vitamin E supplement for man and animals.

Wheat germ meal consists chiefly of wheat germ together with some bran and middlings or shorts. It is low in fiber, good in protein (minimum 25% crude protein), high in fat (7%), and rich in vitamin E. Defatted wheat germ meal is the product that remains after removal of part of the oil or fat from wheat germ meal. It must not contain less than 30% crude protein; and it is much lower than wheat germ meal in vitamin E.

Flour millers use the endosperm to make white flour and discard the bran and germ. In discarding the bran and germ, they are losing 77% of the thiamin, 80% of the riboflavin, 81% of the niacin, 72% of the vitamin B-6, 50% of the pantothenic acid, 67% of the folacin, 86% of the alpha-tocopherol, and 29% of the choline.[10]

Thus, wheat germ is a rich source of the nutrients that are discarded from the flour in milling. However, the oil of wheat germ decomposes readily after the germ is removed from the kernel, causing short shelf life and problems in marketing raw wheat germ. Thus, the product is usually defatted when offered for sale. The label will show whether the germ is defatted.

Wheat germ is added to many kinds of foods, such as bread, cookies, cereals, and milkshakes. Wheat germ oil may be taken to restore nutrients lost in defatting the germs.

(Also see WHEAT.)

WHEATMEAL, NATIONAL

The name given to 85% extraction wheat flour when introduced into the United Kingdom in 1941 (as distinct from whole wheat meal, which is 100% extraction). Later, the name was changed to *national flour.*

WHIPPLE'S DISEASE (INTESTINAL LIPODYSTROPHY)

A relatively rare, and previously considered fatal, disease of predominantly middle-age men. It is characterized by adominal pain, diarrhea progressing to steatorrhea (fatty diarrhea), marked weight loss, anemia, arthritis, fever, and impaired intestinal absorption—a malabsorption syndrome. Whipple's disease produces structural changes in the lymphatics and intestinal mucosa which seem responsible for the malabsorption. Usually there is evidence of the malabsorption of fat with the loss of fat-soluble vitamins, vitamin B-12, and xylose. Furthermore, the victim demonstrates low blood levels of calcium, magnésium, and potassium—hypocalcemia, hypomagnesemia, and hypokalemia, respectively. Excessive loss of albumin into the intestine results in low circulating levels of albumin in the blood—hypoalbuminemia. Evidence from intestinal biopsies suggests that it is due to a microorganism. Moreover, antibiotic therapy brings

about dramatic improvement, but it is required on a long-term (10 to 12 months) basis.

Diet and replacement therapy are based on the nutritional deficiencies evident, on-going needs, and specific absorptive defects.

(Also see MODIFIED DIETS; and MALABSORPTION SYNDROME.)

WHITE BLOOD CELLS (LEUKOCYTES)

The colorless blood cells, generally called white blood cells or corpuscles.

WHOLE WHEAT MEAL

Meal that is made by grinding the entire wheat kernel.

WILD EDIBLE PLANTS

In the beginning, all plants were wild. Then, through the ages man collected, selected, and cultivated those plants which fitted his needs, while the others remained in the wild. As man started to travel more widely, he carried plants with him to introduce to new locations. Occasionally, these would escape his cultivation and fare so well in their new environment that they eventually became a wild plant—sometimes a weed. Still others came as weeds, but they came from other countries with crop seeds or on animals or birds.

Often what is called a wild plant, and an unfamiliar food source to most, was however, very familiar to the natives of a land. When colonists arrived in the New World, very few Indians had gardens or cultivated crops. Instead, most of them supplemented their diets by collecting edible wild plants with which they were familiar. Instead of the potatoes, carrots, radishes, parsnips, beets, and turnips known today, Indians relied on wild roots and tubers. They also collected various nuts, fruits, greens, and seeds. In some areas, natives still depend upon edible wild plants for food, and at times a distinction between wild and domesticated is difficult.

Perhaps, the future of edible wild plants lies ahead, as some wild plants may represent forgotten or undiscovered food sources. Wild edible indigenous plants, if exploited, could offer alternative food sources in some areas of the world. In addition, there are other plants which could be exploited for fiber, energy, and medicine.

TYPES OF WILD FOODS AVAILABLE. In the wild, a knowledgeable person may find the selection of foods as varied as that in the supermarket. Wild greens for use in salads or for cooking as a potherb include dandelions, chickweed, clover, chicory, miner's lettuce, mint, purslane, lamb's quarter, and watercress. Roots and tubers, or potato-like wild foods include the arrowhead, bulrush, cattail, and water lily. Shoots and stems that can be used as a vegetable include asparagus, burdock, bracken fern, and thistle. There is an endless array of wild nuts and berries available. Many plants produce seeds which can be ground and used like meal or flour. Nature even provides substitutes for coffee and tea. Many leaves can be brewed green or dried for tealike beverages; for example, wintergreen, catnip, colt's foot, Labrador tea, and cassina (holly). Caffeineless coffee substitutes can be made from roasted roots of chicory, chufa, dandelions, or salsify. Such examples of edible wild plants continue on and on.

[10]Schroeder, Henry A., M.D., "Losses of Vitamins and Trace Minerals Resulting from Processing and Preserving Foods," *The American Journal of Clinical Nutrition,* Vol. 24, May 1971, pp. 562-573, Table 3.

STALKING WILD EDIBLE PLANTS. In the United States, people just buy their plants in the supermarkets in cans, or frozen, or fresh, so why should anyone be interested in what grows wild and what may have an unfamiliar flavor? There are several reasons:

• **Outdoor groups**—Groups such as the Boy Scouts, Girl Scouts, garden clubs, nature study groups, and campers and hikers always have a natural curiosity about the plants they observe, and often wish to know or need to know the identity of edible plants.

• **Hobby**—For many people, identifying and collecting wild edible plants represents a satisfying hobby. By starting with a few familiar plants, they gradually branch out to identifying more and more plants as they acquire new knowledge and sharpen their techniques of identification. To these individuals, the *weeds* in the garden, in the lawn, and along the roads take on new meaning. Collecting and eating wild greens, potherbs, berries, nuts, roots, and tubers, is an enjoyable adventure. Also, foods of the wild are tasty and can be preserved for future use by drying, freezing, canning, or use in jams. It is doubtful, however, that collecting wild edible plants would ever result in saving money. Gathering wild plants requires much time and often travel, and some must be hulled, or soaked, or prepared in some time-consuming way.

• **Survival**—Some individuals have experienced a time when life depended on being able to identify wild edible plants. Experienced outdoorsmen have stated: "If you starve to death in the wilderness it is because you are just plain tired of living." Indeed, manuals for training members of the United States Armed Forces contain sections on the identification, collection, and preparation of edible wild plants in areas throughout the world. Each year, campers, fishermen, and hunters become lost and many suffer needlessly because of their lack of knowledge of edible wild plants.

There are many more examples of the role of wild plants in the survival of people. When the Forty-Niners stampeded California's streams, deserts, and mountains in search of gold, the scarcity of fresh food brought scurvy to the camps. The Indians and Spanish introduced the Forty-Niners to what is now called miner's lettuce. To combat scurvy in the northern portions of this continent, frontiersmen, explorers, and gold diggers learned to identify and use a plant now called scurvy grass. When rations were low on the Lewis and Clark expedition, the sweet yellow fruit of the papaw was eaten. During World War II, the people of England and Scandinavia collected vitamin C-rich rose hips from wild roses.

While stalking the wild plants can spell fun, adventure, and survival, it may also spell danger. Before eating a wild plant it should be positively identified. For most plants, this requires knowledge, skill, and experience. Some poisonous plants are easily confused with edible plants. Some edible plants are poisonous at certain stages of development, or certain parts of the plant are poisonous. However, in times of *survival emergencies* the following advice is often given:

1. Never eat large quantities of a strange plant food without first testing it. (A disagreeable taste in a food item, which is otherise safe to eat, may sometimes be removed. If cooking is possible, boiling in one or more changes of water may remove the unpleasant taste.)

2. Take a teaspoonful of the plant food, prepared in the way it will be used (raw, boiled, baked, etc.), hold it in your mouth for about 5 minutes. If, by this time no burning sensation, or other unpleasant effect, has occurred, swallow it.

3. Wait 8 hours. If no ill effects such as nausea, cramps, or diarrhea occur, eat a handful and wait 8 hours. If no ill effects are noted at the end of this time, the plant may be considered edible.

4. If serious ill effects develop, induce vomiting.

5. Even foods deemed safe should be eaten with restraint until you become used to them.

6. Remember that olives are bitter and grapefruit is sour, so an unpleasant taste does not, in itself, mean poison. But a burning, nauseating, or bitter taste is a warning of danger. A small quantity of even poisonous food is not likely to prove fatal or even dangerous, whereas a large quantity may be. This, however, does not apply to mushrooms, which are best avoided in any case.

7. In general, it is safe to try foods that you observe being eaten by birds and mammals, but there are some exceptions.

Enthusiasts who are unable to escape completely into the wilds, and must do their foraging near civilization, should be somewhat cautious. Vacant lots and roadsides where wild plants may be found may get sprayed with herbicides. Also, plants along busy roads have been known to contain high levels of lead, due to the lead in some gasolines burned in cars. Plants should be gathered at least 100 ft (*31 m*) away from a busy road.

EDIBLE WILD PLANTS OF NORTH AMERICA. In North America, there are hundreds of edible wild plants, and worldwide there are hundreds more.

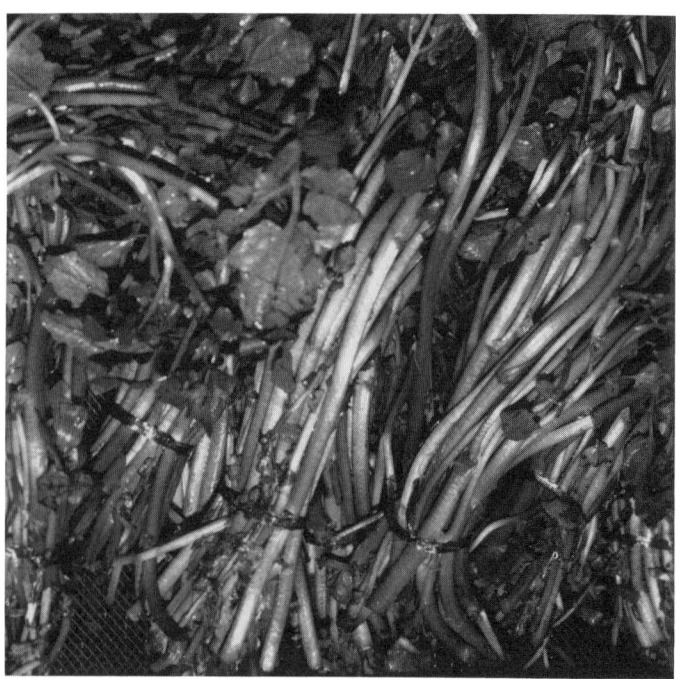

Fig. W-20. Watercress, which requires an abundance of water, often grows wild. (Courtesy, Dept. of Food Science and Human Nutrition, University of Hawaii)

Foragers of wild plants should completely familiarize themselves with the identification of edible and poisonous wild plants in an area. Moreover, beginners would do well to take lessons from persons with experience in stalking the wild life. An alphabetical listing of a few of the edible wild plants of North America follows:

Acorn (oak), *Quercus* spp
Amaranth (pigweed, redroot, wild beet), *Amaranthus* spp
Arrowhead (wapatoo), *Sagittaria latifolia*
Asparagus, *Asparagus officinalis*
Beechnuts (American beech), *Fagus grandiflora*
Bitterroot, *Lewisia rediviva*
Bulrush, *Scirpus* spp
Burdock, *Arctium minus* and *Arctium lappa*
Cattail, *Typha* spp
Chokecherry, *Prunus virginiana*
Chufa (earth almond, nut grass, zula nuts), *Cyperus esculentus* and *Cyperus rotundus*
Chickweed, *Stellaria media*
Cranberry, *Vaccinium* spp
Currants and Gooseberries, *Ribes* spp
Dandelion, *Taraxacum officinale*
Dock, *Rumex* spp
Elderberry, *Sambusus* spp
Evening primrose, *Oenothera* spp
Glasswort (Samphire), *Salicornia* spp
Ground Cherry, *Physalis* spp
Groundnut (Indian Potatoes), *Apios americana*
Hazelnut (filbert), *Corylus* spp
Hickory, *Carya* spp
Jerusalem Artichoke, *Helianthus tuberosus*
Jojoba, *Simmondsia chinensis*
Kinnikinic, *Arctostaphylos* spp
Lamb's Quarter (Goosefoot), *Chenopodium* spp
Maple (Sugar maple), *Acer saccharum*
Miner's Lettuce, *Montia* spp
Mountain Sorrell (Scurvy grass), *Oxyria digyna*
Mulberry (Red Mulberry), *Morus rubra*
Nettles (Stinging Nettle), *Urtica* spp
Pinon Pine, *Pinus monophylla* and *Pinus edulis*
Plantain, *Plantago* spp
Pokeweed (Poke), *Phytolacca* spp
Poplar, *Populus* spp
Prairie Turnip (Bread root), *Psoralea* spp
Prickly Pear (Indian fig), *Opunita* spp
Purslane, *Portulaca oleracea*
Salsify (Oyster plant), *Tragopogon* spp
Tepary Bean, *Phaseolus acutifolius*
Thistle, *Cirsium* spp
Water Cress, *Nasturtium officianale*
Water Lily (Yellow water lily), *Nuphar* spp
Wild Rose, *Rosa* spp

NOTE WELL: For a more complete summary of edible wild plants of North America including their description, geographical distribution, and preparation and uses, see the two-volume *Foods & Nutrition Encyclopedia,* a work by the same authors as *Food For Health.*

WILD RICE *Zizania aquatica*

Wild rice (*Indian rice, water oats*), which is native to the Great Lakes Region—especially in what is now Minnesota, Wisconsin, and Manitoba, is the only native cereal crop to be domesticated in the United States; all other cereal grains were cultivated elsewhere and brought to America. Wild rice is not closely related to true rice, *Oryza*; it belongs to a different genera and even a different tribe of the grass family.

Taming wild rice was not easy. It ripened at different stages, and, as it ripened, the grain fell off the stalk, making harvest difficult. As a result, it was formerly harvested by Indians by *ricing,* which to the Indians meant harvesting from canoes by bending the stems over the boat and beating the heads with a stick. Following harvesting, the moist seeds were dried by parching in a heat-rotated drum or in an open kettle with constant stirring to prevent burning. However, in the 1960s, the University of Minnesota developed an improved variety of wild rice that ripened more uniformly without shattering, adapted to harvest with combines—just like wheat or barley. Today, 75% of the annual U.S. wild rice crop of 3 to 4 million lb (*1.4 to 1.8 mil kg*) is grown in the marshy areas of northern Minnesota (the remaining 25% of the supply comes from Canada, Wisconsin, Michigan, and California); and, today, 90% of Minnesota's wild rice is grown in paddies and harvested by combine, and only 10% is grown in lakes and harvested by canoes.

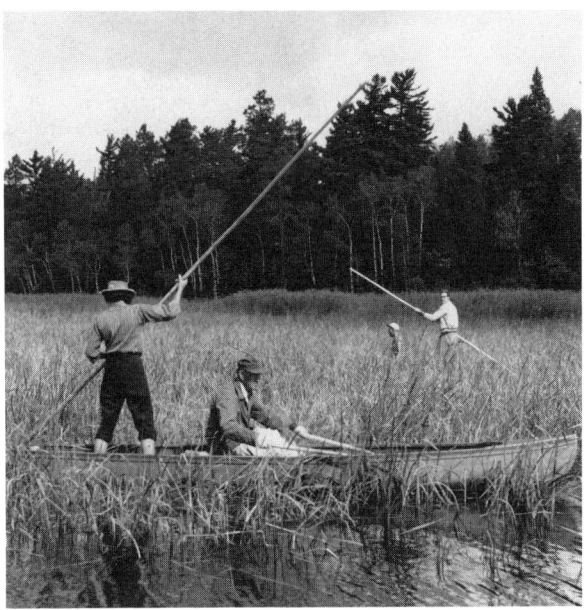

Fig. W-21. Harvesting wild rice in the Chippewa National Forest, Minnesota. One person *poles* the boat, and the other person harvests the rice by means of two sticks—he pulls a batch of ripe rice stalks over the boat with one stick, then knocks the rice into the bottom of the boat with the other stick. (Courtesy, USDA)

Wild rice can be cooked by the same methods as regular rice. Cooking times vary, depending on the size, color, and processing; generally, the larger the kernel and the darker the color, the longer it takes to cook. When properly cooked, the slender, round, purplish black, starchy grain is excellent food, highly esteemed by gourmets and others familiar with the taste. Wild rice is usually high in protein content and low in fat compared to other cereals. (For the composition of wild rice, see Food Composition Table F-21.) Normally, it sells at 2 to 3 times the price of cultivated rice.

(Also see CEREAL GRAINS; and RICE, section headed "Wild Rice.")

WINDBERRY (BILBERRY) *Vaccinium myrtillus*

A fruit of a low shrub (of the family *Ericaceae*) that is native to Europe and northern Asia. It is closely related to blueberries and huckleberries. Windberries are used fresh or in confections, jams, and pies.

(Also see FRUIT[S], Table F-23, Fruits Of The World—"Blueberry.")

WINE

Contents   Page

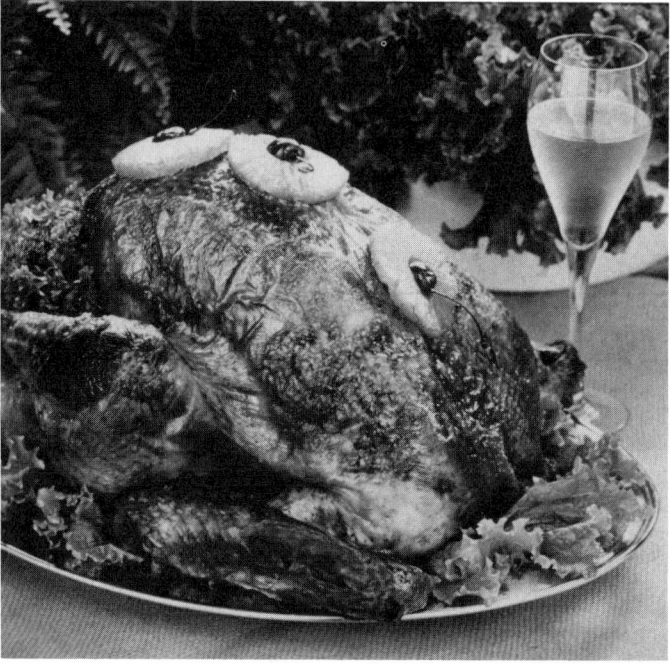

Fig. W-22. Wine enhances a meal. (Courtesy, Cryovac Divison, W. R. Grace & Co.)

The term *wine* refers to the fermented juice of the grape. If other fruit juices are used to make wine, the name of the fruit must precede the word *wine*. Wine is believed to have been one of the oldest medicines in the world and has long been used as a base for many tonics. However, most people drink wine for enjoyment. Recently, Americans increased their consumption of this beverage at the expense of other alcoholic drinks, as evidenced by the fact that the per capita sales of all types of wine in the United States doubled in the period between 1956 and 1976.[11] Since 1976, the per capita consumption of wine has not changed much; it has gone from 2.7 gal to 3.0 gal.

By comparison, the per capita wine consumption in Portugal is 23 gal; in Italy, 21 gal; and in France, 20 gal.

HISTORY OF WINE MAKING. Some historians suspect that certain cave dwelling, primitive peoples of the Eurasian continent may have enjoyed fermented juices from spoiled wild fruit long before grapes were first cultivated some 7,000 years ago in the region around the Caspian Sea. (Grapes naturally contain the vital ingredients for fermentation because they are rich in sugar and have a waxy outer coating that collects wild airborne yeast cells.)

---

[11]Folwell, R. J., and J. L. Baritelle, *The U.S. Wine Market*, Agri. Economic Report No. 417, USDA, 1978.

Archaeologists have found 6,000 to 7,000 year old pottery wine jars that suggest that the first wines were made in the Middle East from grapes, figs, and dates. Apparently the art of grape growing (viticulture) was spread westward by migratory peoples, such as the Jews, since the *Bible* mentions that Noah raised grapes and made wine (Genesis 9:20-21). It is noteworthy that Egyptian accounts of wine making date back to about 2500 B.C. They also stored jars of wine in special wine cellars dug out of the earth, because they apparently realized that this highly esteemed drink kept better when it was stored in a cool environment. The ancient Minoan, Greek, and Etruscan civilizations also produced wine for their own use and trading, as evidenced by the airtight clay pots they used as containers. Later, the Greeks originated symposiums, which were gatherings of people who drank wine together, engaged in intellectual discussions, and played simple games. (The symposia may have represented a refinement of the earlier dionysian orgies that often ended in drunkenness and violence.)

Roman wine festivals, or bacchanalia (named after Bacchus, the god of wine), were characterized by drinking to intoxication and resembled the dionysian orgies, except that the Romans did not allow women to drink wine. The Romans were the first to retard the spoilage of wine by storing it in their smoke houses. They also became experts in vine growing and helped to spread this art throughout their European colonies.

By the early Christian era, the Gauls in France rivaled the Romans in their wine-making skills. When Rome fell, each region of Europe made its own types of wines from the fruits of the vineyards that were planted by the Romans. Because wine was used sacramentally in the celebration of the Mass, the monasteries developed special recipes for making local wines. Later, some groups of monks (such as the Benedictines) took winemaking a step further and made special distilled liqueurs by processes that were kept secret to insure their livelihood.

The European colonists of North America found fields of wild grapes when they arrived. However, the first wines made from the American species (*Vitis labrusca*) were inferior to those made from Old World grapes (*V. vinifera*). Nevertheless, the wild species were much hardier in the climate

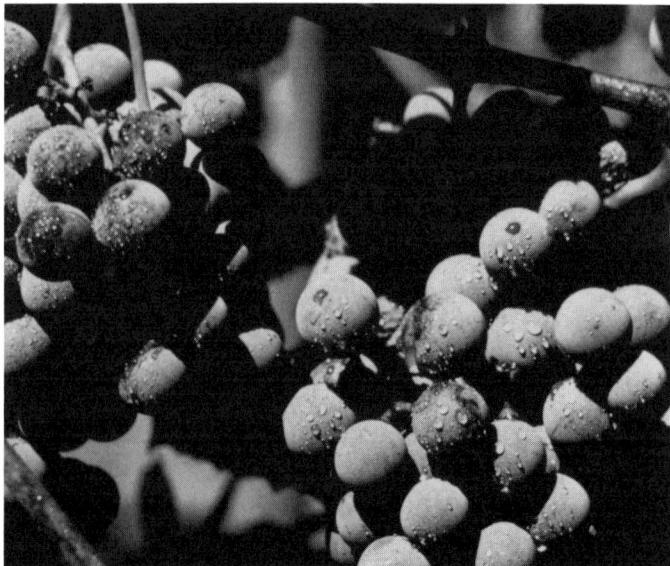

Fig. W-23. Wine grapes. (Courtesy, USDA)

of eastern N. America than the Old World species. (There is some evidence that the Vikings who landed in eastern Canada found grapes there, also). Finally, in 1769 the Old World varieties were successfully introduced into California by the Spanish priest Father Junipero Serra who founded a string of missions with vineyards.

By the 19th century, many European varieties of wine grapes were brought to western United States, where they grew well in the mild climate. A better native American grape was developed after the Concord grape was first grown by E. W. Bull of Concord, Massachusetts in 1852. The hardiness of the American vines led to their introduction into European vineyards to which they carried the plant louse, *phylloxera*. This parasite caused massive destruction of vines throughout Europe until it was found that resistant vineyards could be produced by grafting European vines onto the louse-resistant American rootstocks. Eventually, most of the vineyards of Europe were reestablished, but many years were required for the production of the mature vines that yield the best wine grapes. Another important development of the 19th century was the discovery by the French microbiologist Pasteur that the heating of wines destroyed the undesirable bacteria that caused spoilage.

The growth of the American wine industry during the 20th century was interrupted by Prohibition, which lasted from 1919 to 1933. However, the consumption of wine has risen steadily since 1933; and there have been many innovations and improvements in the production of wines as a result of research programs in viticulture and enology. What were formerly the trade secrets jealously guarded by a few winemakers have now been formulated into scientific practices of the entire industry. As a result, many high quality American wines are available at very reasonable prices.

BASIC PRINCIPLES OF WINE PRODUCTION.
Actual production practices vary somewhat from winery to winery, since the grapes used and the wines produced are distinctively different for each growing region. For example, the high acid and low to moderate alcoholic content of the European-type table wines are produced from the grapes grown in the cooler areas of northern California, Oregon, and Washington, whereas the dessert wines are made from the high sugar content grapes grown in the hot Central Valley of California. (A long, hot growing season is needed to produce grapes that are very rich in sugars.) Only the basic principles that are utilized in most wineries will be presented here.

Fermentation. The juice from the crushed grapes is usually fermented by pure cultures of certain strains of yeasts, by processing steps like those that follow:

1. **Preparation of the must.** The must, or juice, to be fermented is extracted by passing the fresh grapes through a *stemmer-crusher*, after which the juice is treated with sulfur dioxide to kill any undesirable wild yeasts. **NOTE WELL:** Because sulfites trigger severe reactions among some people, since June 1978, the Bureau of Alcohol, Tobacco, and Firearms has required that all wines containing more than 10 parts per million of sulfites carry the phrase "Contains sulfites" on the neck, back, or side panels of containers.

2. **Fermentation.** A culture of the most suitable strain of yeast is added to the must in fermentation tanks. In most cases, the juice contains sufficient sugar to produce the desirable alcoholic content. However, some of the grapes grown in cool climates are too low in sugar and require additional sugar for complete fermentation. Large fermenta-

tion tanks may be equipped with cooling coils to prevent the temperature from rising too high, since the yeast cells may be killed by too much heat. The dark-colored wines are produced by fermenting the grape pulp with the skins present, whereas the lighter-colored wines are fermented with only minimal contact with the skins.

Clarification. Newly fermented wines contain considerable sediment which is usually removed by (1) fining, in which an agent such as gelatin or egg white is added to bring certain materials out of solution or suspension; (2) settling out of suspended materials; (3) filtration of the wine through special filter pads; and (4) centrifugation, when the wines are not fully clarified by the preceding processes.

Aging. Some wines are intended for consumption right after their production but others must be mellowed by aging for a few years to remove the harsh flavors and allow the more desirable ones to develop. This process has long been carried out in wooden barrels that contribute flavors of their own, while absorbing some of the astringent constituents. However, many of the less expensive wines are held in redwood, concrete, or lined wine tanks for periods ranging from a few months to 2 years or so.

After aging, the wines are filtered, treated with sulfur dioxide to prevent spoilage; and bottled.

A little more aging may occur in the bottle, as the sulfur dioxide content decreases gradually. Corked bottles of wine are stored with the cork end inclined downward so that the cork is kept wet and the admission of air is prevented. **NOTE WELL:** In 1991, the Food and Drug Administration issued a temporary standard for wine prohibiting the sale of wine with more than 300 parts per billion of lead as a temporary measure until a permanent standard can be set. Also, FDA has said that it will soon propose a ban on lead foil wrappers to cover corks in wine bottles.

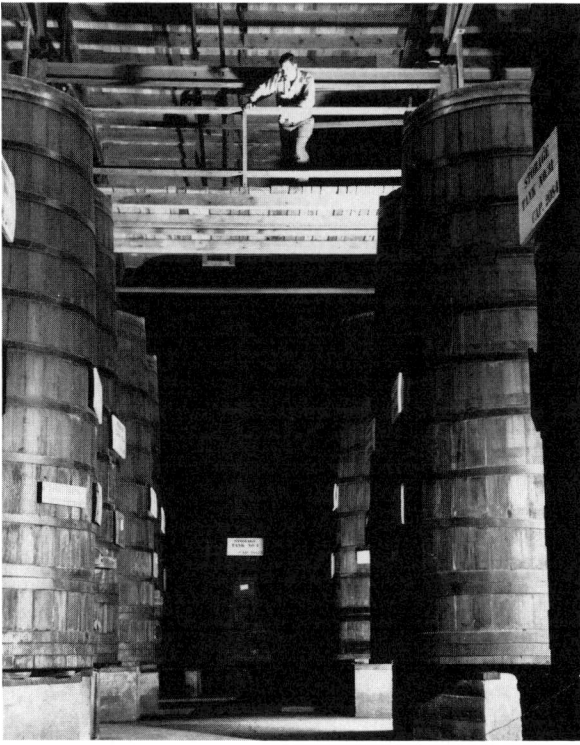

Fig. W-24. These great wooden tanks, filled with aging wines, are in a cool winery in a California valley. (Courtesy, Wine Institute, San Francisco, Calif.)

TYPES OF WINES AND RELATED PRODUCTS.
The names listed on the labels of European wines are confusing to all but the experts in the field because they give vineyards and regions of production that are unfamiliar to most consumers. Furthermore, the quality of these wines varies from year to year because the climates of the grape producing regions are quite variable. Therefore, high class restaurants allow the customers to taste imported wines before they are served.

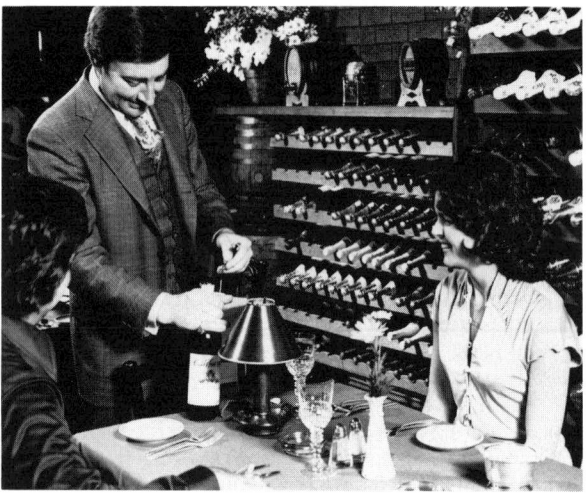

Fig. W-25. The opening and tasting of a bottle of wine is a pleasant ritual that is performed in many high class restaurants. (Courtesy, Wine Institute, San Franciso, Calif.)

The years in which good wines were produced in a region are called *vintage years*. However, wines produced in the more predictable climate of California vary little from year to year. Some of the common types of wines, along with brief descriptions, follow:

Apple wine (hard cider). Apple cider or juice that has been allowed to ferment.

Aromatic wine. A fortified wine flavored with one or more aromatic plant parts such as bark, flowers, leaves, roots, etc.

Bordeaux. A wine produced in the Bordeaux region of France. May be red, white, or rose.

Brandy. Distillate from a wine (Hence, the characteristics of each product stem from those of the original wine, the type of distillation, and the aging process).

Burgundy. A wine produced in the Burgundy region of France. May be red, white, or sparkling.

Cabernet. Wine made from the Cabernet Sauvignon grape, which was brought from Bordeaux, France to California.

Chablis. An excellent dry white wine (with a green-gold tint) from the French town of Chablis. However, the name is sometimes applied to similar dry, white wines made elsewhere.

Champagne. A sparkling wine that is made by allowing wine from Pinot grapes to undergo a second fermentation after a small amount of sugar has been added to the bottle.

Chianti. Red wine from the Tuscany region of Italy that is often sold in a round-bottom flask placed in a straw basket. However, the best wine comes in tall bottles that can be binned for aging.

Claret. A dry, red Bordeaux wine made from Cabernet Sauvignon grapes.

Cognac. Brandy that is double distilled from wine made in the Charente district of France.

Cold Duck. A sparkling wine that is similar to champagne.

Concord wine. A strong-flavored, dark red wine made from Concord grapes (a native American variety).

Crackling wines. Wines that are less carbonated than sparkling wines.

Cream sherry. A heavy, dark-colored, sweetened sherry that is made by a process similar to the one developed in Jerez de la Frontera, Spain.

Dessert wines. Fortified (with additional alcohol in the form of brandy), wine that contains from 15 to 20% alcohol by volume.

Dry wines. A wine that is *not* sweet or sweetened. (In other words, all or most of the natural sugar content has been converted to alcohol.)

Fortified wines. Wines that have had their natural alcohol content increased by the addition of a brandy.

Honey wine (mead). An ancient type of wine that was made from fermented honey flavored with herbs.

Light wines. A wine that has a low alcoholic content.

Madeira. One of the wines made on the island of Madeira, which is located 500 mi (800 km) southeast of the coast of Portugal. (The wines range from light and dry to heavy and rich.)

May wine. A light, white Rhine wine that is flavored with the herb woodruff.

Moselle wines. Light wines (the alcohol content is usually about 10% or less) made in the valley of the Moselle River in Germany which lies to the west of the Rhine.

Mulled wine. Heated, sweetened, spiced wine served in a cup.

Muscatel. A sweet fortified wine made from Muscat grapes.

Perry (pear wine). Light wine made from pear juice.

Pinot. Wine made from Pinot grapes.

Port. The type of fortified wine that originated in the town of Oporto in Portugal.

Pulque. Fermented juice of the agave plant that grows in Mexico and in southwestern United States.

Red wines. Wines produced from dark-colored grapes that are fermented together with their skins (which contains most of the color pigments).

Resinated (Greek) wines. Greek wines that contain a resin which imparts a pinelike flavor.

Rice wine (sake). A Japanese wine made from fermented white rice.

Riesling. White wine made from the Riesling grape, which is considered to be the finest wine grape grown in Germany.

Rhine wines. Wines from grapes grown in the Rhine River Valley of Germany. (The wines range from dry and light to rich and sweet.)

Rose wines. Rose-colored wines produced by fermenting dark-colored grapes without the skins present, or from lighter grapes in the presence of their skins.

Sauternes. Wines made in the Sauternes district of Bordeaux, France from grapes withered somewhat by a *Botrytis* mold that is also called *noble rot*.

Sherry. A fortified wine made by a process similar to the one developed in Jerez de la Frontera, Spain. (Sherries range from pale-colored dry wines to rich, sweet ones.)

Sparkling wines. Wines that are bubbly with carbon dioxide gas by virtue of having undergone a second fermentation initiated by the addition of a small amount of sugar.

Sweet wines. Fortified wines that contain considerable amounts of unfermented sugars. The addition of extra alcohol prevents the fermentation of the sugars which are present.

Table wines. Unfortified wines of low to moderate alcoholic content. (They usually contain 14% or less of alcohol.)

Tokay. A rich white dessert wine made in Hungary that comes in dry and sweet varieties.

Vermouth. A fortified wine that is flavored with a variety of aromatic herbs and comes in dry and sweet varieties.

White wines. Made by fermenting grapes separated from their skins in order to keep the content of colored pigments low.

Zinfandel. A red wine made from Zinfandel grapes grown in California.

NOTE WELL: For a more complete summary of types of wines and related products, including their uses, see the two-volume *Foods & Nutrition Encyclopedia,* a work by the same authors as *Food For Health.*

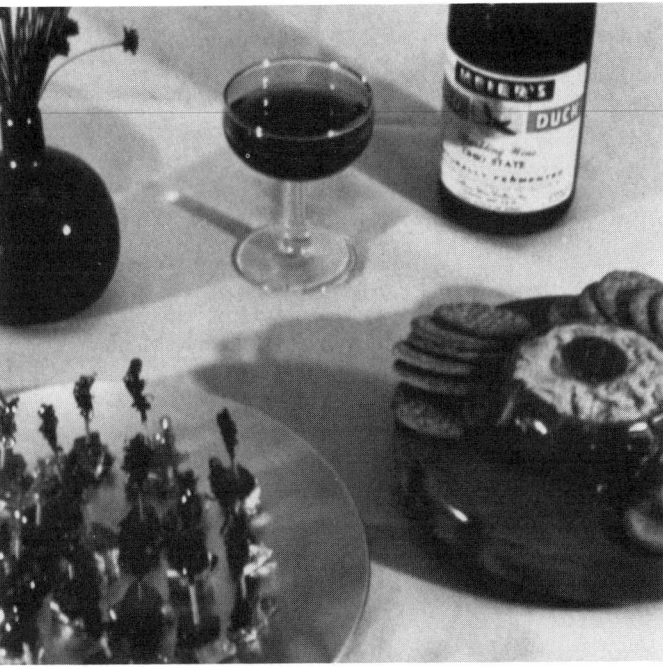

Fig. W-26. Wine and hors d'oeuvres are a favorite pre-dinner snack. (Courtesy, New Mexico State University, Las Cruces, N.M.)

MEDICINAL AND NUTRITIONAL EFFECTS. Many curative powers have been attributed to wine, since it has been used medicinally from the time of the ancient Greek physician, (460 to 370 B.C.) Hippocrates. However, the observations made in the early days of medicine were often clouded by unidentified factors that may have helped to alleviate or worsen diseases. Therefore, some of the beneficial effects ascribed to wine in a recent article are noteworthy:[12]

1. Wine contains many constituents other than alcohol that tend to slow the rate at which the alcoholic content is absorbed. (Earlier studies showed that wine consumed with a meal produced a peak blood alcohol level that was only about one-quarter of that resulting from the same amount of alcohol taken in the form of gin or vodka.) Hence, intoxication is less likely to occur when moderate amounts of wine are consumed.

2. The anthocyanins (colored pigments) and tannins (astringent substances) in wines have greater antiviral effects than unfermented grape juice. However, these experiments were conducted in laboratory vessels, rather than in animal or human subjects.

3. Two 4 oz (120 ml) glasses of wine taken daily alter the blood patterns of cholesterol and other fats so that the likelihood of atherosclerotic heart disease is reduced by a small, but significant, amount.

4. Wine has a relaxing effect that may be due in part to ingredients other than alcohol.

5. The aroma and taste of good wines stimulate the appetite.

6. Substances present in both normal wine and dealcoholized wine promote better absorption of the essential minerals calcium, phosphorus, magnesium, and zinc than pure alcohol or deionized water. (It has long been thought that the absorption of iron is improved by wine. Hence, an old time remedy for iron deficiency anemia was "beef, iron, and wine.")

DANGERS OF DRINKING TOO MUCH WINE.
Intoxication and other serious threats to health may result from the overconsumption of any of the alcoholic beverages. Experiments have shown that the body of a medium size man can metabolize about ½ oz (15 ml) of pure alcohol per hour. This is equivalent to the amount of alcohol present in a 4 oz (120 ml) glass of most table wines. It is noteworthy that four 8 oz (250 ml) portions of California Zinfandel wine were consumed with meals at 4 hour intervals (between 9 A.M. and 9 P.M.) by young male volunteers who showed no signs of intoxication.[13] However, the consumption of similar amounts of wine without food has been shown to produce blood alcohol levels that are twice as high as those resulting from the consumption of wine with food. Therefore, it seems best to restrict the consumption of table wines to not more than 1 pt (480 ml) per day in order to allow for differences in the rates of alcohol absorption under various conditions of drinking.

(Also see ALCOHOLISM.)

WINEBERRY *Rubus phoenicolasius*

The fruit of an oriental type of raspberry (fruit of the family *Rosaceae*).

Wineberries are orange-colored and originated in northern China and Japan. They may be eaten fresh or made into jam, jelly, juice, pies, and wine.

(Also see FRUIT[S], Table F-23, Fruits Of The World—"Raspberry".)

WINTERIZATION

Some oils solidify or crystallize and become cloudy at refrigerator temperatures, due to the presence of triglycerides containing saturated fatty acids which have a higher melting point. The process of winterization filters out these triglycerides from a chilled oil thus improving consumer acceptability by providing an oil that remains clear. The higher melting triglycerides removed from the oil may be used in margarines and shortening.

(Also see OILS, VEGETABLE, section on "Refining.")

---

[12]McDonald, J. B., "Not by Alcohol Alone," *Nutrition Today,* Vol. 14, January/February, 1979, pp. 14-19.

[13]*Ibid,* p. 18.

WITCHES' MILK

Secretion from the mammary glands of the newborn of both sexes thought to be due to placental permeability to the lactation-producing hormones of the mother.

WOOD ALCOHOL (METHANOL; METHYL ALCOHOL; CH₃OH)

Originally, this product was obtained from the destructive distillation of wood; hence, it was termed wood alcohol. It is extremely poisonous (causes blindness). Poisoning due to methyl alcohol is almost always a case of ingestion as a substitute for ethyl alcohol—the alcohol of liquors. Rather ironically, part of the treatment for methyl alcohol poisoning consists of administering ethyl alcohol. Aside from its adverse effects when ingested, methyl alcohol is an important industrial chemical utilized for numerous processes and products.

(Also see METHYL ALCOHOL.)

WOODCOCK

Many hunters consider the woodcock to be the best winged game bird; and many gourmets consider it one of the most succulent morsels. It is full of glory when roasted and served to the hunter who shot it.

WORK, MUSCULAR; ENERGY REQUIREMENTS

Work is accomplished when a force acts to move an object some distance. Muscles are capable of creating a force and of performing work. However, for muscles to create a force they require chemical energy. Thus, any time muscular work is performed the energy demands of the body increase. In fact, muscular activity is the most powerful stimulus for increasing the metabolic rate—the rate at which the body utilizes energy. Short bursts of strenuous exercise can increase the metabolic rate forty times that of the resting state. From day to day, a person engaged in sedentary work may require only 2,500 Calories (kcal) or less per day, while a person doing hard manual labor may require 5,000 Calories (kcal) or more per day.

(Also see CALORIC [ENERGY] EXPENDITURE; and METABOLIC RATE.)

WORLD FOOD

In 1798, an English clergyman named Thomas Robert Malthus predicted part of the world food problem. He stated, ''The power of population is infinitely greater than the power in the earth to provide subsistence for man.'' Malthus, however, failed to see the many changes of the future. For almost 200 years, we proved Malthus wrong because, as the population increased, new land was brought under cultivation; and machinery, chemicals, new crops and varieties, and irrigation were added to step up the yields.

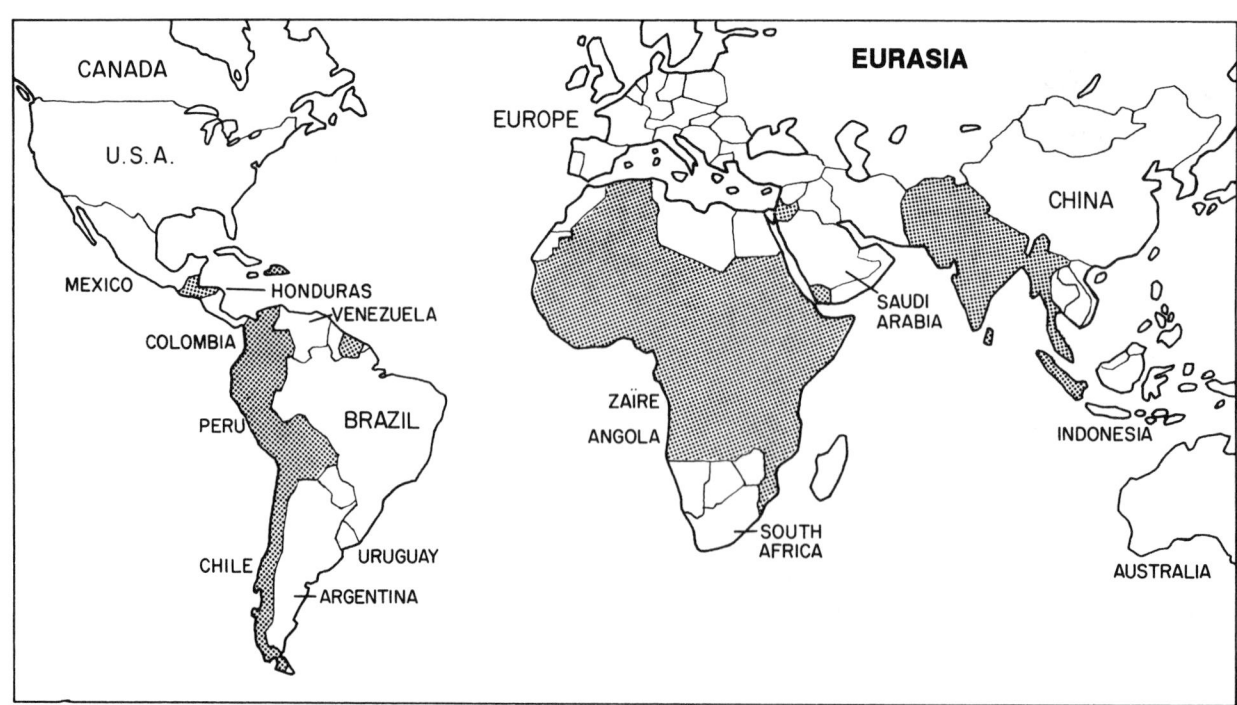

Fig. W-27. The geography of world food problems. The darkened areas are countries where the undernourished population exceeded 15%.

Now, science has given us the miracle of better health and longer life; and world population is increasing at the rate of about 240,000 people a day. At this rate, world population will double by the year 2045. To meet the needs of a more sophisticated and demanding world population of this size, world food production needs to increase at an average rate of about 2.5% per year.

World food problems are more complex than just too many people and too little food. Thus, during the 25-year period 1961–63 to 1983–85, people as a whole were better fed than previously. On the average, the food available per capita rose from 2,320 calories to 2,660 calories. But the exceptions were many! In the low income countries as a group, apart from China and India, per capita food supplies in 1983–85 were no higher than 15 years earlier. More

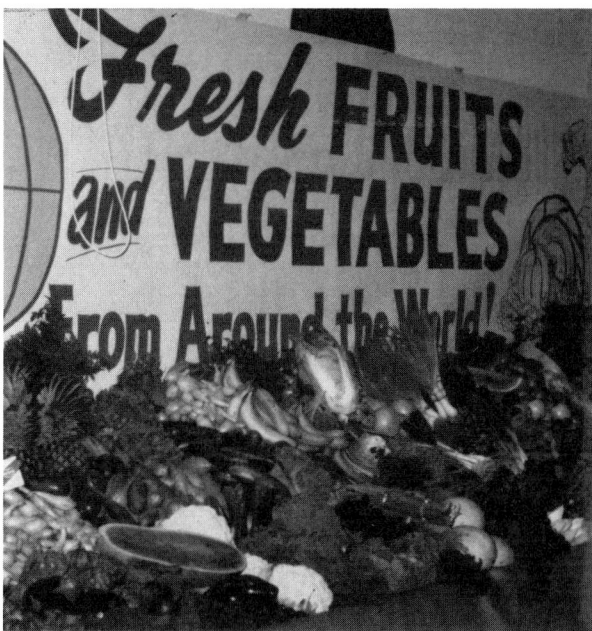

Fig. W-28. Fresh fruits and vegetables from around the world. (Courtesy, University of Tennessee, Knoxville)

disturbing yet, about 75% of the people in the world live in the developing countries where only 40% of the world's food is produced. Also, this is where most of the world's increase in population is occurring. Their rapid population growth causes severe economic strains on food production, processing and distribution. Finally, there is the problem of money. Countries able to produce sufficient food for their needs could supply food to the developing countries where production does not meet the needs. However, these developing countries generally lack the money necessary to purchase food from other countries. Therefore, the world food problems are related to (1) population, (2) production and distribution, and (3) wealth.

(Also see MALTHUS.)

POPULATION, PRODUCTION, AND WEALTH AROUND THE WORLD.
Around the world, population, food production, and wealth are unequally distributed, and will remain so in the future.

• **Population**—The world population is about 5.3 billion and by the year 2000 it will be 6.2 billion. Assuming all 6.2 billion people stood shoulder to shoulder and occupied an average width of 2 ft, 6.2 billion people would circle the world 91 times, or reach to the moon and back nearly five times!

Numbers are, however, only part of the problem. As Table W-17 shows, there is and will be dramatic unequal distribution of the people of the world. Only 21% of the population will be in developed regions of the world by the year 2000. Africa, Asia, and Oceania, will have 70% of the population. Among the individual nations the United States will have only 4% of the world's population, compared to 21% in the People's Republic of China, or 16% in India.

TABLE W-17
POPULATION PROJECTIONS FOR WORLD
MAJOR REGIONS, AND SELECTED COUNTRIES[1]

Area	Year 1975	Year 2000	Percent of World Population in 2000
	(millions)	(millions)	(%)
World	4,090	6,351	100
More developed regions	1,131	1,323	21
Less developed regions	2,959	5,028	79
Major regions			
Africa	399	814	13
Asia and Oceania	2,274	3,630	57
Latin America	325	637	10
U.S.S.R. and Eastern Europe	384	460	7
North America, Western Europe, Japan, Australia, and New Zealand	708	809	13
Selected countries and regions			
People's Republic of China	935	1,329	21
India	618	1,021	16
Indonesia	135	226	4
Bangladesh	79	159	2
Pakistan	71	149	2
Philippines	43	73	1
Thailand	42	75	1
South Korea	37	57	1
Egypt	37	65	1
Nigeria	63	135	2
Brazil	109	226	4
Mexico	60	131	2
United States	214	248	4
U.S.S.R.	254	309	5
Japan	112	133	2
Eastern Europe	130	152	2
Western Europe	344	378	6

[1]*Global 2000 Report to the President, Entering the Twenty-First Century*, p. 9, Table 1.

• **Production**—Food production depends upon a number of factors, among which are (1) the availability and use of land, (2) farming methods, (3) soil fertility, (4) water, (5) weather and climatic conditions, (6) civil order, and (7) incentives to producers. Therefore, the ability of countries to produce sufficient food for their need varies as shown in Table W-18.

TABLE W-18
PER CAPITA GRAIN PRODUCTION, CONSUMPTION, AND TRADE, ACTUAL AND PROJECTED, AND PERCENT INCREASE IN PER CAPITA TOTAL FOOD PRODUCTION AND CONSUMPTION[1]

Area	Grain			Food (Percent increase over the 1970-2000 period)
	1969-71	1973-75	2000	
	(kilograms per capita)			(%)
United States				
Production	1,018.6	1,079.3	1,640.3	51.1
Consumption	824.9	748.0	1,111.5	28.3
Trade[2]	+194.7	+344.0	+528.8	
Western Europe				
Production	364.9	388.4	394.0	1.0
Consumption	432.4	443.3	548.8	15.5
Trade	-65.4	-57.6	-154.8	
Japan				
Production	121.7	108.5	135.4	6.1
Consumption	267.5	274.4	452.3	54.2
Trade	-138.1	-175.9	-316.7	
U.S.S.R.				
Production	697.6	711.2	903.2	28.1
Consumption	663.1	796.1	949.9	41.4
Trade	+16.1	-42.0	-46.7	
People's Republic of China				
Production	216.3	217.6	259.0	17.4
Consumption	220.2	222.4	267.8	19.1
Trade	-4.0	-4.8	-8.8	
Latin America				
Production	236.1	241.0	311.4	33.7
Consumption	226.5	238.3	278.1	25.1
Trade	+11.8	+2.7	+33.3	
North Africa/Middle East				
Production	217.1	214.6	222.5	1.8
Consumption	276.2	273.8	292.8	2.2
Trade	-50.8	-69.8	-70.3	
South Asia				
Production	161.6	162.4	170.0	4.6
Consumption	170.0	171.8	181.0	5.8
Trade	-8.4	-11.8	-11.0	
Southeast Asia				
Production	244.7	214.5	316.5	35.9
Consumption	207.2	182.6	228.5	14.6
Trade	+37.5	+31.9	+87.5	
East Asia				
Production	137.3	136.0	163.5	22.8
Consumption	176.2	171.5	217.3	27.3
Trade	-40.4	-38.8	-53.8	

[1]*Global 2000 Report to the President, Entering the Twenty-First Century*, pp. 20 and 21, Table 6.
[2]In trade figures, a plus indicates export, while a minus sign indicates import.

Several important observations can be made from Table W-18. As far as past and future grain production is concerned, only three areas listed produce more grain than is consumed; thus leaving grain for export to other countries. Of the three—United States, Latin America, and Southeast Asia—the United States has the greatest excess for export. In terms of the percent increase in production and consumption of food between now and the year 2000, only the United States, Latin America, and Southeast Asia will significantly increase the percentage of food produced over

that consumed. Most areas of the world will consume more food than they produce.

• **Wealth**—Living standards have risen during the 20th century, but wealth remains unequally distributed. In many countries the economic development lags; hence, they are unable to purchase food or apply technology to increase food production within their country. By comparing the per capita income, some idea may be gained of the economic well-being of the countries and of the citizens' ability to purchase a nutritious diet. Table W-19 presents some of the countries with the highest incomes, and some of the lowest incomes.

TABLE W-19
PER CAPITA INCOME FOR SELECTED COUNTRIES[1]

Country	Per Capita Income
Highest:	(U.S. $)
Qatar	27,000
Switzerland	26,309
Iceland	21,660
Denmark and West Germany	19,750
U.S.A.	16,490
Japan	15,030
Australia	14,458
Norway	13,790
Luxumbourg	13,380
United Kingdom	13,329
Netherlands	13,065
France	13,046
Austria	12,521
United Arab Emirates and Finland	11,900
Lowest:	
Niger	310
Zambia	304
India	300
Somalia	290
Zimbabwe	275
Tanzania and China	258
Togo	240
Uganda and Afghanistan	220
Myanmar (Burma)	210
Vietnam	180
Nepal	160
Ethiopia	121
Bangladesh	113

[1]*The World Almanac and Book of Facts 1991*, pp. 684–771.

Several crucial observations can be made from the information in Table W-19. There is a wide gap between the highest per capita income countries and the lowest per capita income countries, and the gap will widen by 2000. In general, areas with the greatest population have the lowest per capita income.

In most low income countries, consumers spend ½ or more of their income for food; whereas, in the higher income countries, the proportion drops to less than ⅕. For example, consumers in different countries spend the following proportion of their income for food: U.S.A., 10.3%; Canada, 11.3%; United Kingdom, 12.8%; Netherlands, 14.2%; Australia, 15%; Denmark, 15.7%; France, 16.4%; West Germany, 16.6%; Sweden, 17%; and Austria, 17.4%. Moreover, among the people of all countries, food takes a larger chunk of the income of the poor than it does of the rich, e.g., India where they spend 53% on food; the Philippines, 51%; and South Korea, 36%. The great disparities of wealth within countries can also be expected to widen by the year 2000. (Also see INCOME, PROPORTION SPENT FOR FOOD.)

TYPE OF DIET. A country's staple food is its primary source of carbohydrate, and for much of the poor population it must also serve as the principle source of protein. The degree to which this generally low-quality protein is supplemented by a more valuable or complementary source of protein (animal or legume protein) depends on income. The developing countries where wheat and rice are the principal crops have been the most successful in meeting food demand. In countries where corn is the chief crop, about 15% of the population is undernourished. In countries where the people subsist on millet and sorghum or root and tubers (much of Africa), some degree of malnutrition is virtually universal.

OUTLOOK AND OPTIONS RELATIVE TO WORLD FOOD.

Increasingly, the charge will be made that much of the world goes hungry because of the substitution of meat, milk, and eggs for direct grain consumption. The goal is to feed the world a nutritious diet by the most efficient methods. Before deciding, individuals in both camps—(1) feed the grain to people, or (2) feed the grain to animals—should possess a sound knowledge of the options rather than moral indignation. When this is done, the outlook for the future may be brighter. To this end the important sections that follow are presented.

Who Shall Eat? Cereal grain is the most important single component of the world's food supply, accounting for between 30 and 70% of the food produced in all world regions. It is the major, and sometimes almost exclusive, source of food for many of the world's poorest people, supplying 60 to 75% of the total calories many of them consume. However, in many developed countries, more grain is fed to animals than is consumed directly by humans. Under such circumstances, sporadic food shortages and famine in different parts of the world give rise to the following recurring questions:

1. Who should eat grain—people or animals? Shall we have food or feed?

2. Can we have both food and feed?

FAVORING BREAD ALONE. Among the arguments sometimes advanced by those who favor bread alone—the direct human consumption of grain—are the following:

1. **More people can be fed.** About 2,000 lb (*907 kg*) of grain must be supplied to livestock in order to produce enough meat and other livestock products to support a man for a year, whereas 400 lb (*181 kg*) of grain (corn, wheat, rice, soybeans, etc.) eaten directly will support a man for the same period of time. Thus, a given quantity of grain eaten directly will feed five times as many people as it will if it is first fed to livestock and then is eaten indirectly by humans in the form of livestock products. This is precisely the reason why the people of the Orient have become vegetarians.

2. **On a feed, calorie, or protein conversion basis, it is not efficient to feed grain to animals and then to consume the livestock products.** This fact is pointed up in Figs. W-29 through W-31.

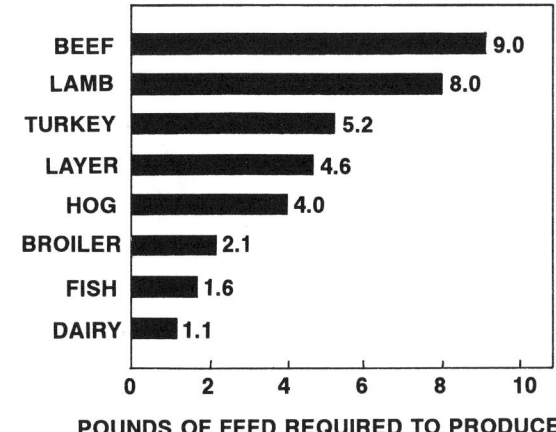

POUNDS OF FEED REQUIRED TO PRODUCE ONE POUND OF PRODUCT

Fig. W-29. Pounds of feed required to produce 1 lb of product. This shows that it takes 9 lb of feed to produce 1 lb of on-foot beef, whereas it takes only 1.1 lb of feed to produce 1 lb of milk. (One lb equals *0.45 kg*.)

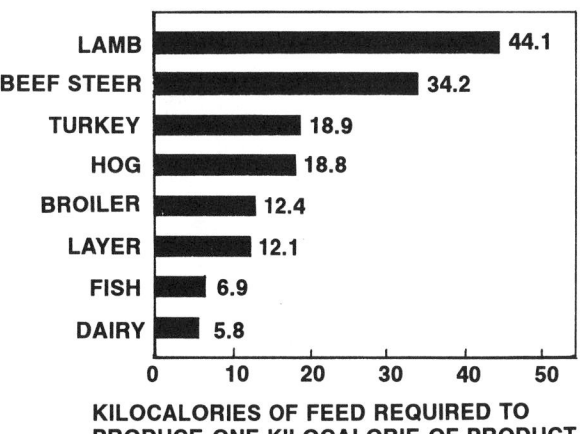

KILOCALORIES OF FEED REQUIRED TO PRODUCE ONE KILOCALORIE OF PRODUCT

Fig. W-30. Kilocalories in feed required to produce 1 kcal of product. This shows that it takes 44.1 kcal in feed to produce 1 kcal in lamb, whereas only 5.8 kcal in feed will produce 1 kcal in milk.

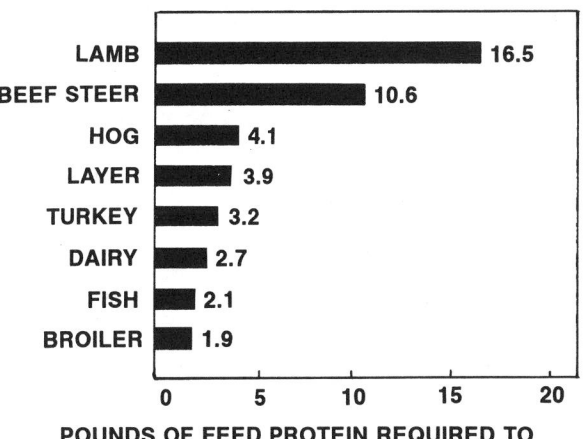

POUNDS OF FEED PROTEIN REQUIRED TO PRODUCE ONE POUND OF PRODUCT PROTEIN

Fig. W-31. Pounds of feed protein required to produce 1.0 lb of product protein. This shows that it takes 16.5 lb of feed protein to produce 1 lb of lamb protein, whereas only 1.9 lb of feed protein will produce 1 lb of broiler protein. (One lb equals *0.45 kg*.)

Thus, in the developing countries, where the population explosion is greatest, virtually all grain is eaten directly by people; precious little of it is converted to animal products.

As people become more affluent, they actually use more grain, but most of it is converted into animal products, for they consume more meat, milk, and eggs. It is noteworthy, too, that no nation appears to have reached such a level of affluency that its per capita grain requirement has stopped rising.

FAVORING ANIMALS. Practicality dictates that a hungry world should consider the following facts in favor of sharing grain with animals, then consuming the animal products:

1. **Animals provide needed power.** In the developing nations, cattle, water buffalo, donkeys, and horses still provide much of the agricultural power. Such draft animals are a part of the agricultural scene of Asia, Africa, the Near East, Latin America, and parts of Europe; areas characterized by small farms, low incomes, abundance of manpower, and lack of capital. They can be fueled on roughages to produce power, a most important consideration in times of energy shortage; and both cattle and water buffalo may be used for work, milk, and meat.

Although the general trend in the world is toward more and more mechanization, animals will continue to provide most of the agricultural power for the small farm food/crop agriculture in many of the developing countries.

If the entire world were suddenly to adopt American farming and food processing methods, increasing the diets of all people to the American level, the energy consumed would exhaust the world's known petroleum reserves in 13 years.

Modern mechanized feed and food production requires an extra input of fuel, which is mostly of fossil origin. This auxiliary energy is expended in endless ways to improve agricultural productivity; it is used for drainage and irrigation, clearing of forest land, seedbed preparation, weed and pest control, fertilization, and efficient harvesting. In addition to production as such, there are two other important steps in the feed-food line as it moves from the producer to the consumer; namely, processing and marketing, both of which require higher energy inputs than to produce the food on the farm. In 1990, U.S. farms expended an average of 2.8 Calories (kcal) on the farm per calorie of food grown. By contrast, the Chinese wet rice peasant, using animal power (water buffalo), expends only 1 Calorie (kcal) of energy to produce each 50 Calories (kcal) of food.

(Also see ENERGY REQUIRED FOR FOOD PRODUCTION.)

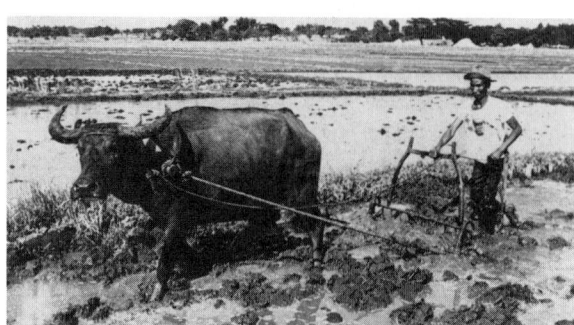

Fig. W-32. An Oriental wet rice peasant, using animal power (water buffalo), expends only 1 Calorie (kcal) of energy to produce each 50 calories (kcal) of food. By comparison, the average U.S. farmer, using mechanical power (tractors), expends 2.5 Calories (kcal) of fuel energy to produce 1 Calorie (kcal) of food. (Courtesy, International Bank for Reconstruction and Development, Washington, D.C.)

2. **Animals provide needed nutrients.** Animal products provide all the essential amino acids (including lysine and methionine in which vegetable sources are deficient), plus minerals and vitamins, along with palatability and digestibility.

Foods of animal origin (meat, milk, and their various by-products) are especially important in the American diet; they provide ⅔ of the total protein, about ⅓ of the total energy, ⅘ of the calcium, ⅔ of the phosphorus, and significant amounts of the other minerals and vitamins needed in the human diet.

In addition, meat, dairy products, and eggs are a rich source of vitamin B-12, which does not occur in plant foods—only in animal sources and fermentation products. Also, it is noteworthy that the availability of iron in beef is twice as high as in plants.

About ⅔ of the world's protein supply is provided from plant sources, ⅓ from animal sources. Since the Food and Agriculture Organization of the United Nations reports that the world's diet needs animal protein in amounts equivalent to ⅓ of the total protein requirements, there should be ample animal protein, *provided* it were equally distributed. But it isn't. The people in the developed countries have five times as much high-quality animal protein per person as the people living in the developing countries (Table W-20). The gap between total protein (animal and plant combined) is not as wide (106.2 g vs 58.3 g per person per day in the developed and developing countries, respectively).

TABLE W-20
WORLD PROTEIN PER PERSON PER DAY
IN GEOGRAPHIC AREAS OR COUNTRY[1]

Area or Country	Total Protein	Source	
		Animal	Plant
	←	(g/day)	→
U.S.S.R.	106.2	56.1	50.1
Europe	102.0	59.6	42.4
North-Central America	95.6	56.7	38.9
Oceania	88.9	56.8	32.1
South America	65.0	29.5	35.5
Asia	61.0	13.2	47.8
Africa	58.3	12.5	45.8
World Total	70.4	24.7	45.7

[1]*FAO Production Yearbook 1991*, FAO/UN, Rome, Italy, p. 239.

The most important role of animal protein is to correct the amino acid deficiencies of the cereal proteins, which supply about two-thirds of the total protein intake, and which are notably deficient in the amino acid, lysine. The latter deficiency can also be filled by soybean meal, fish, protein concentrates and isolates, synthetic lysine, or high-lysine corn. But such products have neither the natural balance in amino acids nor the appetite appeal of animal protein.

(Also see PROTEIN[S], section headed "Protein for the World.")

3. **Much of the world's land is not cultivated.** Vast acreages throughout the world—including arid and semiarid grazing lands; and brush, forest, cutover, and swamplands—are unsuited to the production of bread grains or any other type of farming; their highest and best use is, and will remain, for grazing and forest.

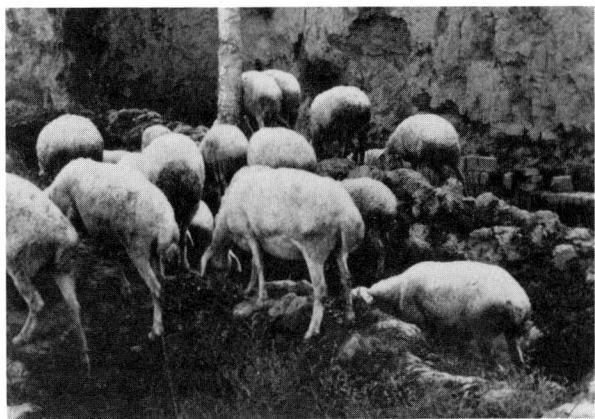

Fig. W-33. Vast areas throughout the world, such as this rough terrain, are not suited to cultivation. Hence, their only use is for grazing or forest.

In the United States, only 21% of the land area of the 50 states is cultivated. About 900 million acres, or 46.8%, of the land area, exclusive of Alaska and Hawaii, is pasture and grazing land.

In China, only 10% of the land is cultivated. North of China's Great Wall, life centers on pastoral areas; large flocks and herds of cattle, sheep, and horses roam these vast grasslands.

4. **Forages provide most of the feed for livestock.** Pastures and other roughages—feeds not suitable for human consumption—provide most of the feed for livestock, especially for ruminants (four-stomached animals such as cattle, sheep, goats, buffalo, and certain wild species including deer, antelope, and elk), throughout the world. Fortunately, the uniqueness of the ruminant's stomach permits it to consume forages, and, through bacterial synthesis, to convert such inedible (to humans) roughages into high-quality proteins—meat and milk. Hence, cattle and sheep manufacture human food from nonedible forage crops. Additionally, they serve as the primary means of storing (on the hoof, without refrigeration) such forage from one season to the next.

Despite grains being relatively plentiful in the United States, forages provide the bulk of animal feeds; pastures and other roughages account for 94% of the total feed of sheep, 85% of the feed of beef cattle, 59% of the feed of dairy cattle, and 62% of the feed of all livestock.

5. **Food and feed grains are not synonymous.** Animals do not compete to any appreciable extent with the hungry people of the world for food grains, such as rice or wheat. Instead, they eat feed grains and by-product feeds—like field corn, grain sorghum, barley, oats, milling by-products, distillery wastes, and fruit and vegetable wastes—for which there is little or no demand for human use in most countries, plus forages and grasses—fibrous stuff that people cannot eat. For example, in the United States only 3% of the corn—the major animal feed grain—is used for human food. Also, it is noteworthy that the feed grains which the United States ships overseas are used almost entirely for livestock and poultry production abroad.

6. **Ruminants utilize low-quality roughages.** Cattle, sheep, and goats efficiently utilize large quantities of coarse, high-cellulose roughages, including crop residues, straw,

and coarse low-grade hays. Such products are indigestible to humans, but from 30 to 80% of the cellulose material is digested by ruminants.

Of all U.S. crop residues, the residue of corn (cornstalks and husklage) is produced in the greatest abundance and offers the greatest potential for expansion in cow numbers. In 1990, 66,952,000 acres of corn, yielding 118.5 bushels per acre, were harvested in this country.

Normally, over and above the grain, corn produces over 200 million tons of corn residue each year. That's more than 200 million tons of potential cow feed, enough to winter more than 150 million pregnant cows. Mature cows are physiologically well adapted to utilizing such roughage. Moreover, when corn residue is used to the maximum as cow feed, acreage which would otherwise be used to pasture the herd is liberated to produce more corn and other crops. Also, there are many other crop residues which, if properly utilized, could increase the 150 million head figure given above.

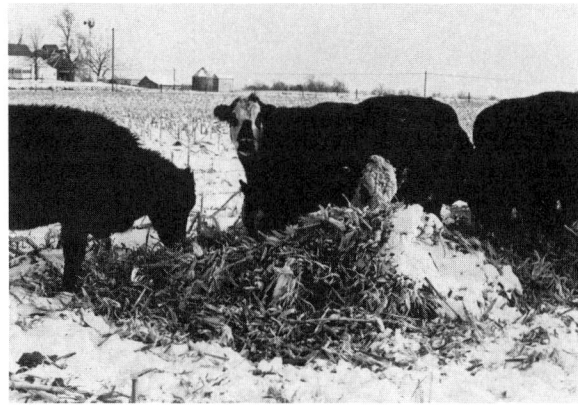

Fig. W-34. Cattle can utilize efficiently large quantities of coarse, humanly inedible roughages, like cornstalks. This shows cows feeding on corn residue which had been harvested by mechanical means. (Courtesy, Iowa State University)

7. **Animals utilize by-products.** Animals provide a practical outlet for a host of by-product feeds derived from plants and animals, which are not suited for human consumption. Some of these residues (or wastes) have been used for animal feeds for so long, and so extensively, that they are commonly classed as feed ingredients, along with such things as the cereal grains, without reference to their by-product origin. Most of these processing residues have little or no value as a source of nutrients for human consumption. Among such by-products are corncobs, cottonseed hulls, gin trash, oilseed meals, beet pulp, citrus pulp, molasses (cane, beet, citrus, and wood), wood by-products, rice bran and hulls, wheat milling by-products, and fruit, nut, and vegetable refuse. It is estimated that each year ruminants convert more than 9 million tons of by-products into human food.

8. **Animals provide elasticity and stability to grain production.** Livestock feeding provides a large and flexible outlet for the year-to-year changes in grain supplies. When there is a large production of grain, more can be fed to livestock, with the animals carried to heavier weights and higher finish. On the other hand, when grain supplies are low, herds and flocks can be maintained by reducing the grain that is fed and by increasing the grasses and roughages

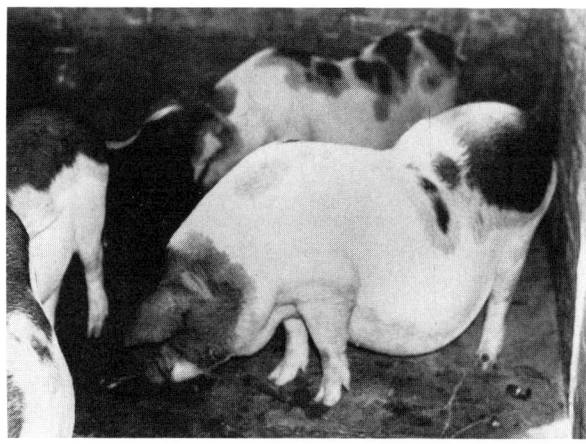

Fig. W-35. Chinese hogs in Kwang Tung Province, China. Their ration consisted of two by-products—rice millfeed and bagasse (the pith of sugarcane), along with water hyacinth—all of which the pigs ate with relish. In China, swine utilize millions of tons of otherwise wasted crop residues and by-products. (Photo by A. H. Ensminger)

in the ration. Thus, when grains are in short supply, fewer slaughter cattle are grain fed—more are grass finished. In the years ahead, depending on future grain supplies and prices, it is predicted that less than two-thirds of the U.S. domestic beef supply will come from feedlot cattle, in comparison with the 77% of U.S. slaughter cattle that were grain fed in 1973. Also, during periods of high-priced grains, heavier feeder cattle will go into feedlots, and they will be fed for a shorter period on less grain and more roughage than when grains are more abundant and cheaper.

In the future, animals will increasingly be *roughage burners,* with the proportion of grain to roughage determined by grain supplies and prices.

Beef cattlemen, dairymen, and sheepmen will more and more rely upon the ability of the ruminant to convert coarse forage, grass, and by-product feeds, along with a minimum of grain, into palatable and nutritious food for human consumption, thereby competing less for humanly edible grains. The longtime trend in animal feeding will be back to roughages; increasingly, all flesh will be grass.

9. **Animals step up the protein content and quality of foods.** Grains, such as corn, are much lower in protein content in cereal form than after conversion into meat, milk, or eggs. On a dry basis, the protein contents of selected products are corn, 10.45%; beef (Choice grade, total edible, trimmed to retail level, raw), 30.7%; milk, 26.4%; and eggs, 47.0%. Also, animals increase the quality (e.g., biological value) of the protein—a higher proportion of the protein is assimilated by the body.

(Also see PROTEIN[S].)

10. **Ruminants convert nonprotein nitrogen to protein.** Ruminant animals (cattle, sheep, and goats) can use non-protein nitrogen, like urea, to produce protein for humans in the form of meat and milk.

11. **Animals provide medicinal and other products.** Animals are not processed for meat alone. They are the source of hundreds of important by-products, including some 100 medicines such as insulin, epinephrine, and heparin, without which the lifestyle and health of people would be altered.

Besides medicines, many familiar products are derived

from animals, including leather, shoe polish, photographic film, soap, lubricants, candles, glue, buttons, and bone china, to name a few.

12. **Animals maintain soil fertility.** Animals provide manure for the fields, a fact which was often forgotten during the era when chemical fertilizers were relatively abundant and cheap. One ton *(907 kg)* of average manure contains 18 lb *(8.2 kg)* of nitrogen, 9 lb *(4.1 kg)* of phosphorus, and 13 lb *(5.9 kg)* of potassium.

The energy crisis prompted concern that farmers would not have sufficient chemical fertilizers at reasonable prices in the years ahead. Since nitrogenous fertilizers are oil- and petroleum-based, there is cause for concern. As a result, a growing number of American farmers are returning to organic farming; they are using more manure—the unwanted barnyard centerpiece of the past, and they are discovering that they are just as good reapers of the land and far better stewards of the soil.

(Also see ORGANICALLY GROWN FOOD.)

Meeting the Feeds Vs Foods Dilemma. Life on earth is dependent upon *photosynthesis.* Without it, there would be no oxygen, no plants, no feed, no food, no animals, and no people.

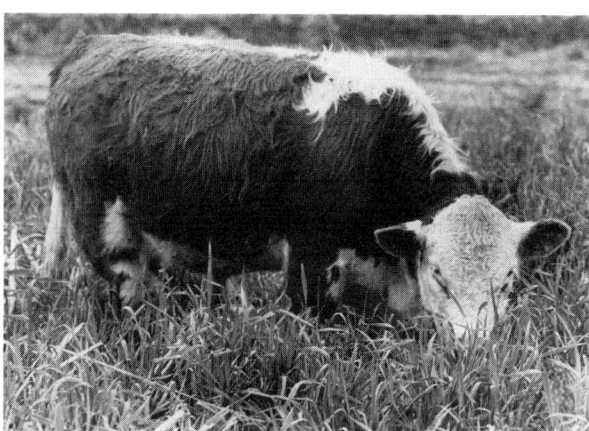

Fig. W-36. Ruminants—cattle, sheep, and goats—convert the photosynthetic energy derived from solar energy and stored in grass into food for humans. (Courtesy, *The Progressive Farmer,* Birmingham, Ala.)

As fossil fuels (coal, oil, shale, and petroleum)—the stored photosynthates of previous millennia—become exhausted, the biblical statement, "all flesh is grass" (Isaiah 40:6), comes alive again. The focus is on photosynthesis. Plants, using solar energy, are by far the most important, and the only renewable, energy-producing method; the only basic food-manufacturing process in the world; and the only major source of oxygen in the earth's atmosphere. Even the chemical and electrical energy used in the brain cells of man is the product of sunlight and the chlorophyll of green plants. Thus, in an era of world food shortages, it is inevitable that the entrapment of solar energy through photosynthesis will, in the long run, prove more valuable than all the underground fossil fuels—for when the latter are gone, they are gone forever.

(Also see PHOTOSYNTHESIS.)

Practicality dictates that a hungry world should, and will, proceed in about the following order in meeting the feeds vs foods dilemma:

1. Consume a higher proportion of humanly edible grains and seeds, and their by-products, directly—without putting them through animals, simply because approximately five times more people can be fed by doing it this way.

2. Utilize a higher proportion of roughages to concentrates in animal rations as increasing quantities of cereal grains are needed for human consumption.

3. Retain more of those species that can utilize a maximum of humanly inedible feeds and a minimum of products suitable for human consumption. This would favor cows, sheep, and goats, provided they are fed a maximum of pasture and other roughages. Both poultry and swine may compete with man for grains. Nevertheless, it is expected that further increases in poultry will come, primarily because of their efficiency as converters of protein from feed to food, and their adaptability to small-scale production. Also, it is expected that there will be further increases in swine, especially in China, where pigs are scavengers and manure producers par excellence.

4. Propagate the most efficient feed to food species converters (see Figs. W-29, W-30, and W-31). This means dairy cows, fish, and poultry. Because beef cattle and sheep are at the bottom of the totem pole when it comes to feed efficiency, the pressure will be to eliminate them, except as roughage consumers. Although not mentioned yet, rabbits are also efficient converters of feed to food, and can utilize roughages to some extent. Moreover, rabbits are easily adapted to small-scale agriculture.

5. Increase the within-species efficiency of all animals and eliminate the inefficient ones. This calls for more careful selection and more rigid culling than ever before.

6. Improve pastures and ranges. Good pasture will produce 200 to 400 lb (91 to 181 kg) of beef or lamb per acre annually (in weight of young weaned, or in added weight of older animals); superior pastures will do much better.

Improving The World Food Situation. The world food situation can be improved provided major problems are solved, many of which are not self-correcting. Among the most pressing are curbing population growth, transferring food from the developed food-exporting countries to the developing food-deficit countries, providing for emergency disaster and famine relief, achieving an acceptable degree of stability of world food prices, and finding the proper combination of techniques and policies to bring about a substantial improvement in food production in developing countries. On a longtime basis, the world food situation can best be improved by a massive infusion of education, science, and technology—by self-help programs —so that they can produce more of their own food.

• **Population control**—Members of the animal kingdom other than man have their numbers held in check by the many factors encompassed in the term *balance of nature*. Man is different! His strong propensity is to overpopulate the earth and to create conditions which threaten his very existence—his food supply, the water he drinks, the environment in which he lives, and the very air he breathes.

Without doubt, people will continue to live longer. Hence, curbing population growth will be required to maintain the balance between production and demand for food. It will be necessary to bring the number of people and their supply of food into proper balance. Alternate methods of population control are starvation, disease, and/or war.

• **Fair prices and profits**—People do those things which

are most profitable to them; and farmers are people. The American farmer, and farmers in certain other countries of the world, can produce more, but higher prices than have existed in the past will be necessary to assure this.

Farmers, like any businessmen, have always demonstrated their willingness to respond to incentives—prices and profits.

• **Increase cultivable land**—Ever since man stopped living a nomadic life, he has been hunting for arable (cultivable) land. Fortunately, there is still much of it to be had. Studies show that about twice as much of the world's land is suitable for crops as is presently used. More than half of the potential, but presently unused, arable land is in the tropics, and about a sixth of it is in the humid tropics—the largest areas being in Africa and South America.

• **More irrigation**—The value of irrigation for increasing crop yields is generally known. Yet, a study of the world's 20 major irrigating countries, in areas irrigated, showed that only 15% of their total cultivated area is irrigated. Thus, the potential to increase crop yields through irrigation is very great.

• **Improve crop yields**—While the amount of land that could be brought into production is perhaps double that currently used, all recent studies of world food production conclude that, outside of Africa and Latin America, yield-increasing techniques—irrigation, fertilizer, new seeds, and improved technology—will be the primary source of future food increases.

In addition to irrigation, fertilizer is a key factor in yield increases, although it must be combined with improved varieties of seeds and improved cultural practices if it is to have much impact on yields. As evidence of the soundness of the fertilizer approach, it is noteworthy that almost half of the 50% gain in crop output per acre in the United States since 1940 is attributed to the increased use of fertilizers. From this, it may be concluded that increased use of fertilizer could increase world food output by 50% in the years ahead.

• **Full use of pastures and ranges**—Some sparsely populated areas of the world, such as Australia, New Zealand, Argentina's pampas area, and the western range areas of the United States and Canada, are now important sources of livestock products. But there are still vast areas of sparsely settled grasslands where the production of livestock products is small; among them, large portions of Africa, the highlands of central Asia, some portions of the Andean area of South America, and the nomadic grazing areas of the Near East. In these areas, subsistence is the goal and animal numbers are generally regarded as being more important than the yield of salable products. Nevertheless, the potential for increased production in these areas is considerable. Also, and most important, the only practical way of harvesting human food from many of these areas is through livestock. So, grass—the world's largest crop—should no longer be taken for granted. In an era of world food shortages, the contribution of properly managed grazing lands in terms of food and fiber production needs to be pursued. No other program offers so much potential to increase the world's food production capacity quickly and at so little cost; this is especially true of the grasslands in the tropics and subtropics.

• **Produce leaner beef**—Leaner beef is higher in protein content than fat beef. On a carcass basis, trimmed to retail level, Standard grade runs 19.4% protein vs 17.4% for Choice grade—that's 2% higher. Besides, leaner beef can be produced with much less grain.

Consumer preferences and costs of production underlie

the relative prices of fat and lean beef, but changes in U.S. grading standards help consumers adjust their consumption patterns. For this reason, when grain prices are high, producers exert pressure to have the beef-grading system changed so as to reduce the amount of grain fed.

• **Select efficient animals**—Improved genetics, along with improved feeding and management, have made for more meat, milk, and eggs. Yet, further improvements are possible and needed, especially in the developing countries. Although 60% of the animals of the world are raised in the developing countries, primarily in Africa and Asia, these nations produce less than 30% of the world's meat, milk, and eggs. This low productivity is largely due to the failure to utilize the scientific principles of husbandry and disease control.

• **Feed roughage and by-products**—In the future, cattle and sheep will increasingly be *roughage burners.* Stockmen will rely upon the ability of the ruminant to convert coarse forage, grass, and by-product feeds, along with a minimum of concentrate, into palatable and nutritious food for human consumption, thereby competing less for humanly edible grains.

Ruminants can make the transition to more roughage with ease. For them, it is merely a *return to nature,* for they evolved as consumers of forage.

• **Control disease and parasites**—Diseases in farm animals reduce the supply of meat and other products by a large quantity, and add substantially to the cost of food and fiber. The cost of animal diseases, parasites, and pests of livestock and poultry to U.S. producers and consumers is estimated to aggregate $10 to $12 billion.

Deaths of animals take a tremendous toll. Even greater economic losses—hidden losses—result from failure to reproduce living young, and from losses due to retarded growth and poor feed efficiency, carcass condemnations and decreases in meat quality, and labor and drug costs. Also, considerable cost is involved in keeping out diseases that do not exist in a country, such as keeping foot-and-mouth disease out of the United States. Quarantine of a diseased area may cause depreciation of land values or even restrict whole agricultural programs. Additionally, and most importantly, it is recognized that some 200 different types of infectious and parasitic diseases can be transmitted from animals to human beings; among them, such dreaded diseases as brucellosis (undulant fever), leptospirosis, anthrax, Q fever, rabies, trichinosis, tuberculosis, and tularemia. Thus, rigid meat and milk inspection is necessary for the protection of human health. This is added expense which the producer, processor, and consumer must share.

Thus, the potential throughout the world of providing more food through animal disease and parasite control is very great. The level of animal health attained in the advanced countries shows that tremendous scope exists for improvement in most developing areas. It is estimated that if the tsetse fly of the high rainfall belt of tropical Africa were brought under control, the savannah pastures could carry a cattle population of 120 million head, equal to the total cattle population of the United States.

• **Create new and improved protein sources**—It is generally recognized that diet customs are somewhat emotional in character—that many people will put synthetic clothes on their backs long before they will put synthetic food in their stomachs. Yet, when people are hungry or suffering from malnutrition, they are not finicky about the *pedigree* of their food.

Researchers are attempting to bolster traditional protein sources and to develop entirely new proteins, with their efforts centered around the following approaches and protein sources: (1) improvement of traditional sources through genetic manipulation, (2) fortification with synthetic nutrients, or addition of protein concentrates from fish, oilseeds, and other foods, (3) use of the versatile soybean, and (4) development of single cell protein technology.

(Also see SINGLE-CELL PROTEIN; and SOYBEAN.)

• **Improve small-scale farming methods**—The United States and other developed countries are well known for agriculture that is large in scale and high in capital investments, substituting machinery for human labor. Although it has made the United States the world's largest exporter of food, the technology for large-scale agriculture has been difficult to implement abroad.

Subsistence farming is the principal agricultural practice internationally, especially in the developing countries. Unlike the large U.S. operations, subsistence farms are small in scale and low in capital investments, requiring intensive labor of the approximately one billion farmers who operate them. About 40% of the world's farmers have fewer than 11 acres (4.5 ha) of land; 35% have fewer than 2.5 acres (1 ha). These farms feed a majority of the world population. To provide effective technical assistance to these farmers, scientists must understand the problems of small-scale agriculture.

Although leading scientists have recently identified small-scale agriculture as a priority for research and several international agricultural research centers have initiated mixed cropping and homestead farming studies, research is still lacking on integrated small-scale agriculture, including crop production, methodology, vegetable crops, small animal production, and energy generation.

History shows that world food production has never been immune from shortfalls. These food shortages become more likely as world population increases. As food prices increase because of higher energy costs, the needy will depend on diets made up of the cheapest, most-accessible food without regard for nutrition.

One way to increase the food base and income is for farmers in densely populated agrarian regions to increase the agricultural production on their small land holdings. These farmers would then have the incentive to remain on the farm, avoiding the social problems that result when farmers migrate to the city. Appropriate small-scale agriculture could integrate crops and small animals (poultry, rabbits, milking goats, and sheep) into a system that would meet the nutritional requirements of the family, improving the quality as well as the quantity of food. This integrated approach could make a significant contribution to national health, wealth, and stability.

• **Farm the sea**—The ocean, which covers 70.73% of the earth's surface and, therefore, receives a proportionate amount of all the solar energy reaching this planet, is one of the most promising potentials for providing added food for the world's spiraling human population. It is an immense reservoir of food which man has only lightly tapped. Hence, there is growing interest in the sea as a source of food supply, including both fish and vegetables.

• **Eliminate waste**—Waste of food supplies will increasingly nag the consciences and pocketbooks of all people—producers and consumers alike.

Pests cause an estimated 30% annual loss in the worldwide potential production of crops, livestock, and forests.

Every part of our food, feed, and fiber supply—including marine life, wild and domestic animals, field crops, horticultural crops, and wild plants—is vulnerable to pest attack. Obviously, if these losses could be prevented, or reduced, world food supplies would be increased by nearly one-third. The problems are complex, but the stakes are high.

This worldwide annual loss of 30% potential food productivity occurs despite the use of advanced farming technology and mechanized agriculture. Furthermore, in many of the developing countries losses greatly exceed this figure.

Pests of many kinds attack plants during all stages of their growth, and they attack food and food products after harvest—in storage, during transportation to market, in warehouses, in elevators, in ships, in supermarkets, and in homes after purchase. A few notable pest losses include: plant diseases, insects, weeds, rats, and birds.

• **Increase scientific and cultural exchange between countries**—There will always be international boundaries. But scientists and agriculturalists the world over can, and will, work together through the *tie that binds*—their desire to help mankind. Since no nation has a corner on all the brains, scientific and cultural exchange between countries offers our best hope for survival.

• **Increase teaching, research, and extension**—The best long-run solution to the problem of world food and nutrition shortages is to develop teaching, research, and extension programs that provide farmers in the developing countries with the necessary tools and techniques to increase their production, augmented by fortification of foods and education of consumers.

Each of the developing countries needs: (1) an agricultural teaching-research-extension program patterned after the Land Grant Colleges of America, but adapted to their respective countries; (2) seminars and agricultural short courses for adults; and (3) to send more of their best and brightest students abroad for graduate training. These programs need to be implemented by imaginative and bold approaches because, on a longtime basis, they afford the most logical way in which to provide adequate food and clothing for the world's expanding population.

Why Be Your Brother's Keeper? Famine and starvation are not new to the people of the world, but what is new are the electronic means of communication which are shrinking the size of the world and increasing our awareness. People can sit in their living rooms and watch others starve in some other area, or people in a remote village can become aware that there is another world where people have enough of life's essentials. There are numerous reasons to worry enough to take action, but the three major ones follow:

1. **Humanitarian.** Developing countries need help and many developed countries have the knowledge and resources to help. The challenge of a difficult task and the moral uplift that comes only from doing for others can serve to temper and balance the affluence of American life as exemplified in the late Albert Schweitzer's dictum: ''It is only giving that stimulates.''

2. **Security.** By the year 2000, there will be four times as many people in the developing countries as in the developed countries. Developed countries cannot afford to be too little and too late with their assistance. The idea that security is more than military might is not new. Seneca, nearly 2,000 years ago, warned the Roman Senate: ''A

hungry people listens not to reason nor is its demand turned aside by prayers.''

The expectations of the poor are demanding fulfillment. Hopefully, some measure of their ambitions can be realized by peaceful means.

3. **Economic.** An important way to expand our own economy in the future will be the creation of additional markets for U.S. goods and products. This aim is not entirely self-serving, because achievement of sustained economic growth by the hungry countries will depend upon their participation in world markets on a competitive basis.

While people of the world do not share a common history, they do share a common future. By sharing and applying know-how, the whole world will have a brighter tomorrow. Dreams will come true—faster and more abundantly, with more food and animals in the future.

(Also see CEREAL GRAINS, sections headed ''Feeds for Livestock'' and ''Future Prospects for the Cereal Grains''; ENERGY REQUIRED FOR FOOD PRODUCTION; GREEN REVOLUTION; HUNGER, WORLD; MALNUTRITION, PROTEIN-ENERGY; MALTHUS; NUCLEIC ACIDS, section headed ''Genetic Engineering''; PHOTOSYNTHESIS; POPULATION, WORLD; and PROTEIN, WORLD PER CAPITA.)

WORLD HEALTH ORGANIZATION (WHO)

A specialized agency of the United Nations founded in 1948 to further international cooperation for improved health conditions—physical, mental, and social well-being. The main offices are located in Geneva, Switzerland; and there are six regional offices around the world. Primarily, member governments, on the basis of their relative ability, finance the WHO with yearly contributions. About 130 countries are members. The World Health Assembly, the policy-making body; the Executive Board, a board of health specialists; and the Secretariat, the regional offices and field staff, are the principle organs through which the WHO operates.

The WHO is involved in three distinct health-related areas:

1. It provides a research service and sets standards of international sanitary regulations. The WHO keeps member countries informed on the most recent developments in the use of vaccines, control of drug addiction, nutritional discoveries, cancer research, and health hazards of nuclear radiation. It also standardizes quarantine measures with minimal interference of international trade and air travel.

2. It encourages member nations to enlarge and strengthen their health programs. To do this, the WHO, on request, provides (a) technical advice to governments, (b) sends out international teams of experts, (c) helps set up health centers, and (d) offers aid for the training of medical and nursing personnel.

3. It helps control epidemic and endemic diseases by promoting mass campaigns involving nationwide vaccination programs, clinics for early diagnosis and prevention of diseases, pure water supplies, good sanitation systems, health education, and antibiotic and insecticide use. It has been effective with campaigns against tuberculosis, malaria, and smallpox.

Besides its own programs, the WHO often works closely with the FAO (Food and Agriculture Organization).

(Also see FOOD AND AGRICULTURE ORGANIZATION OF THE UNITED NATIONS; and DISEASES, section headed ''International and Voluntary Organizations Engaged in Health and/or Nutrition Activities.'')

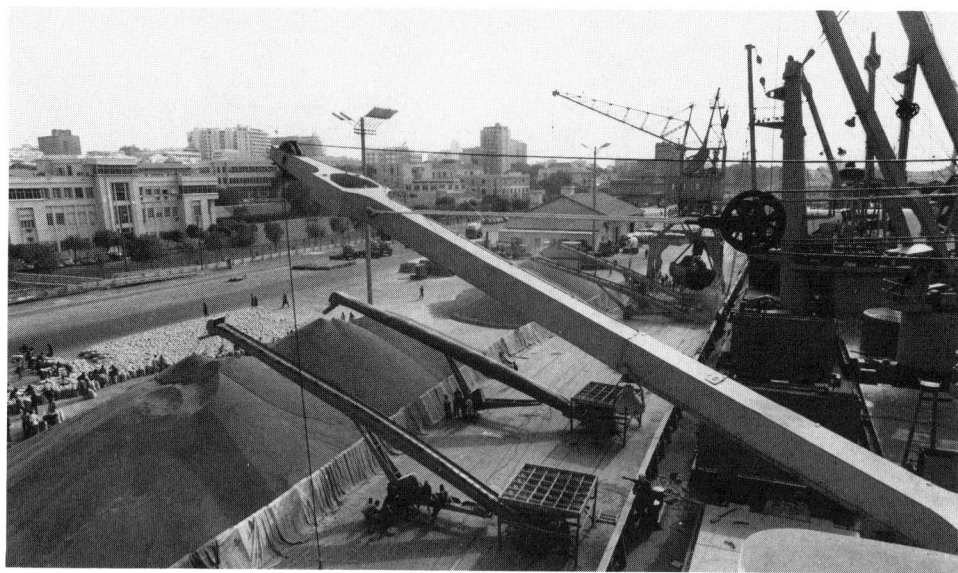

Fig. W-37. Improving the world food situation involves both short-run and long-run arrangements. The short-run: grain reserves for droughts, floods, and similar emergencies. The long-run: population control and self-help programs through the application of science and technology.

The above picture shows U.S. sorghum grain unloaded at the docks in Dakar (Africa). (Courtesy, Agency for International Development, Washington, D.C.)

Fig. W-38. PRODUCING THE NATION'S FOOD

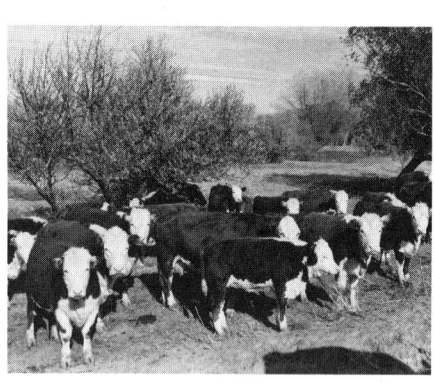

BEEF ON THE HOOF
(Courtesy, Union Pacific Railroad Co., Omaha, Neb.)

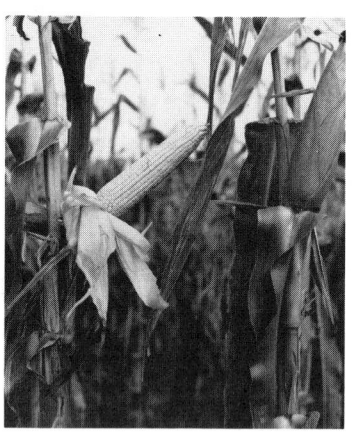

GROWING CORN
(Courtesy, USDA)

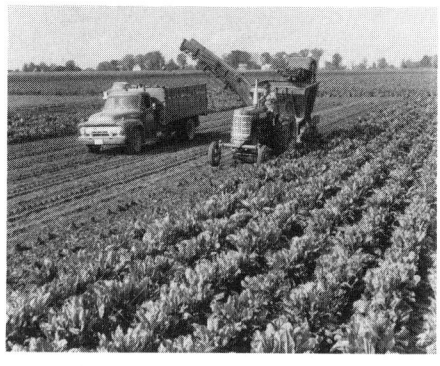

HARVESTING SUGAR BEETS
(Courtesy, J. C. Allen & Son, West Lafayette, Ind.)

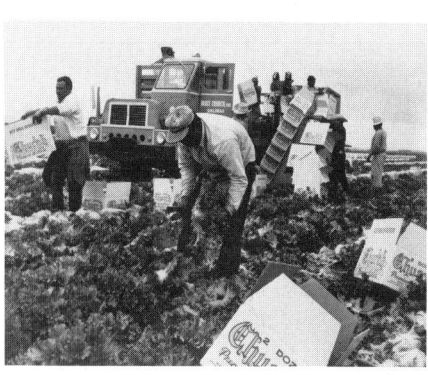

PACKING LETTUCE
(Courtesy, California Iceberg Lettuce Commission, San Rafael, Calif.)

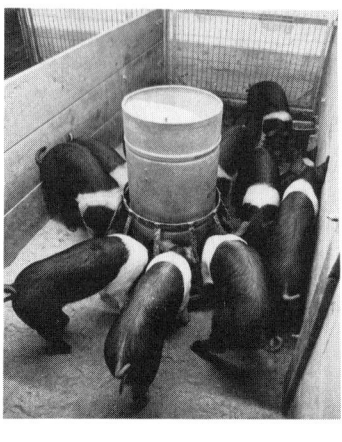

PIGS TO PORK
(Courtesy, National Hog Farmer, St. Paul, Minn.)

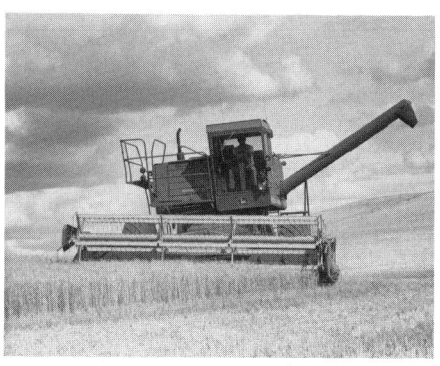

CUTTING WHEAT
(Courtesy, Henry Fisher, Oakesdale, Wash.)

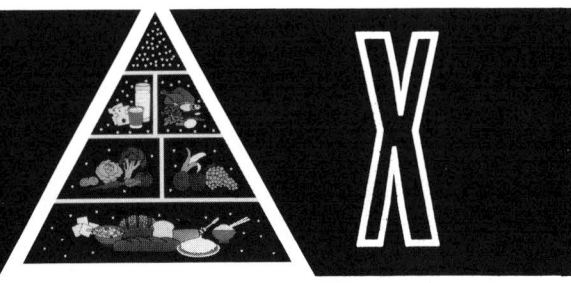

XANTHINE

An intermediate in the metabolism of purines. It was first isolated from gallstones. It occurs in animal organs, yeast, potatoes, coffee, and tea.

XANTHOMA

A benign flat yellow tumor, containing a deposit of fatty substance, commonly located on the inner side of the lower eyelid.

XANTHOPHYLL

While it is one of the most widespread naturally occurring carotenoid alcohols, it does not possess any vitamin A activity. Xanthophyll is a yellow pigment, which can be (1) isolated from certain natural products, and (2) produced synthetically.

Feeds that contain large amounts of xanthophylls produce a deep yellow color in the beak, skin, and shank of yellow-skinned breeds of chickens. The consumer associates this pigmentation with quality and, in many cases, is willing to pay a premium price for a bird of this type. Also, processors of egg yolks are frequently interested in producing dark-colored yolks to maximize coloration of egg noodles and other food products. The latter can be accomplished by adding about 60 mg of xanthophyll per kilogram of diet. In recognition of these consumer preferences, many producers add ingredients that contain xanthophylls to poultry rations.

Rich natural sources of xanthophyll follow:

Feedstuff	Xanthophyll Content
	(mg/kg)
Marigold petal meal	7,000
Algae, common, dried	2,000
Alfalfa juice protein, 40% protein	800
Alfalfa meal, 20% protein	240

(Also see ZEAXANTHIN.)

XEROPHTHALMIA

The term describing keratinization and cloudiness of the cornea caused by a vitamin A deficiency. Xerophthalmia occurs most frequently in undernourished infants and children in India, the Middle East, Southeast Asia, and parts of Africa and South America, in areas where the diet is lacking in whole milk, butter, and green or yellow vegetables. Vitamin A should be administered immediately to persons with xerophthalmia in order to arrest the disease and prevent the loss of sight.

(Also see BLINDNESS DUE TO VITAMIN A DEFICIENCY; DEFICIENCY DISEASES, Table D-1 Major Dietary Deficiency Diseases; and VITAMIN A, section headed "Deficiency Symptoms.")

XEROSIS

Abnormal dryness of the skin or front of the eye.

XYLITOL ($C_5H_{12}O_5$)

Xylitol is a sugar alcohol. The aldehyde group (C = O) of the pentose sugar—5-carbon sugar—xylose is replaced by a hydroxyl group (OH). It can be made from birchwood chips, berries, leaves and mushrooms. Xylitol is commercially produced in Finland from birchwood chips hydrolyzed by acid to xylose. In the body, xylitol is formed as an intermediate during the formation of xylulose. Ingested xylitol is also converted to xylulose. Xylulose then enters the pentose-phosphate cycle of carbohydrate metabolism.

Xylitol tastes almost as sweet as sucrose, table sugar; additionally, it has a cool taste when dissolved in the mouth due to its negative heat of solution. Furthermore, xylitol cannot be metabolized by the acid producing bacteria of the mouth which cause tooth decay. Indeed, some clinical trials have demonstrated a marked reduction in tooth decay through the use of xylitol. Xylitol is approved by the FDA for use in special dietary foods, and some chewing gums are sweetened, in part, with it. However, a British study suggested that xylitol causes cancer in laboratory animals. This places the future use of xylitol in foods in question.

Xylitol is absorbed slowly from the intestine. Hence, the consumption of large quantities may cause an osmotic diarrhea.

(Also see SWEETENING AGENTS.)

XYLOSE (WOOD SUGAR; $C_5H_{10}O_5$)

A 5-carbon—pentose—sugar widely distributed in plant material such as maple wood, cherry wood, straw, cottonseed hulls, corncobs, and peanut shells. It is one of the most abundant plant sugars in the world. However, it is of little or no importance as an energy source for the body. Xylose is not found in its free state in nature but rather as xylan—a polysaccharide built from numerous units of xylose. The sweet-tasting alcohol of xylose, known as xylitol, has been approved by the FDA for use in special dietary foods. Also xylose is employed as a diagnostic aid for the detection of malabsorption. Urinary excretion of less than 4.5 g in 5 hours following ingestion of a 25 g load suggests decreased absorptive capacity.

(Also see CARBOHYDRATE[S], Table C-6, Classification of Carbohydrates and section headed "Monosaccharides.")

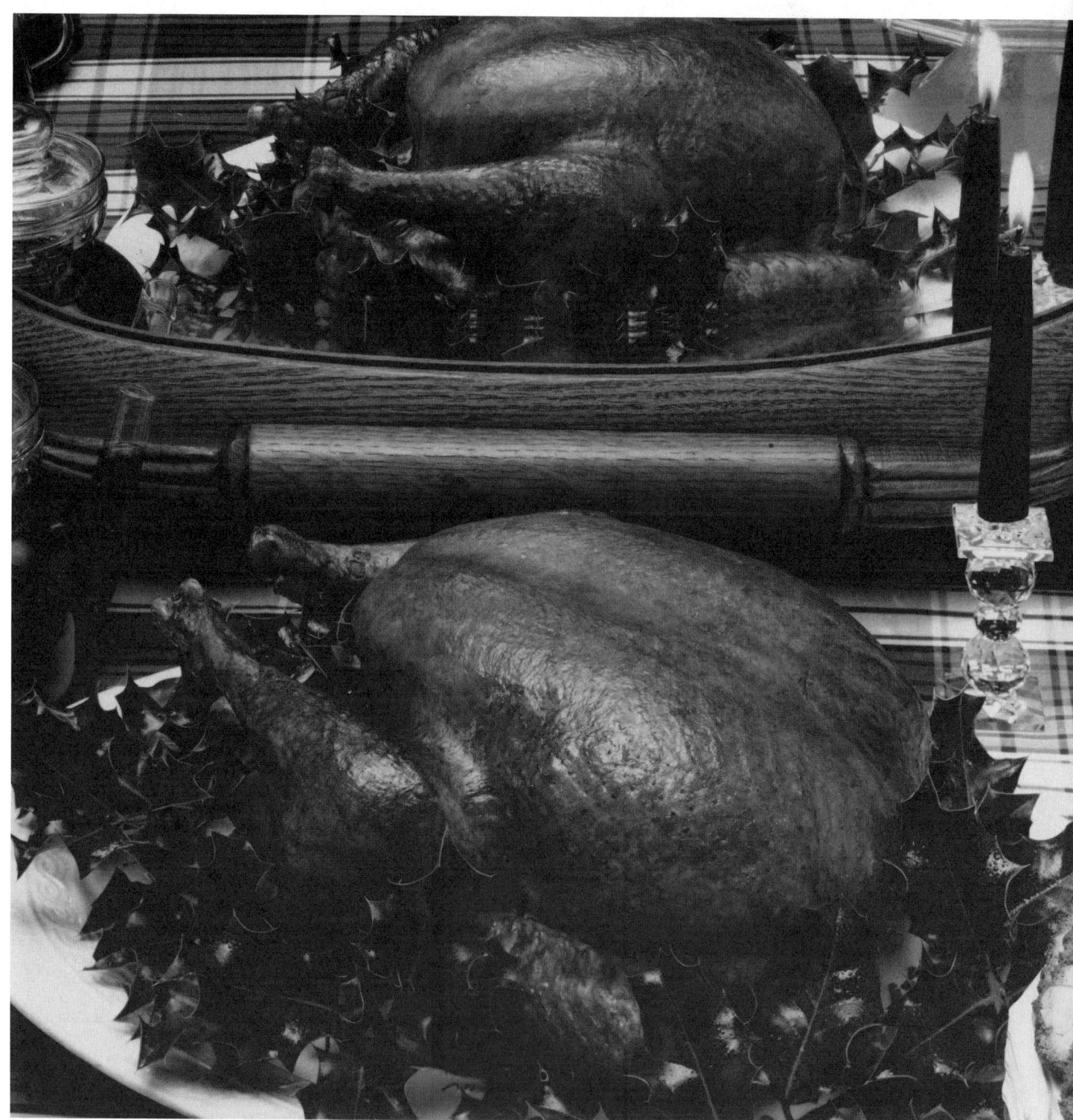

Fig. X-1. Roast turkey, a good source of amino acids. Poultry, which embraces a wide variety of birds of several species, appears more frequently in the diet of people throughout the world than any other type of meat. (Courtesy, National Turkey Federation, Reston, Va.)

YAM BEAN (MANIOC BEAN; POTATO BEAN; TURNIP BEAN) *Pachyrrhizus erosus; P. tuberosus*

These climbing vines, which are tropical legumes, are grown mainly for their edible tubers. Hence, the various common names contain both the word bean and the names of other more popular tuberous plants. The major characteristics of *P. erosus* and *P. tuberosus* are very similar, except that the bean pods of the latter are not eaten because they have irritating hairs. Therefore, the name yam bean will be the sole designation used in the rest of this article. Fig. Y-1 shows a typical yam bean.

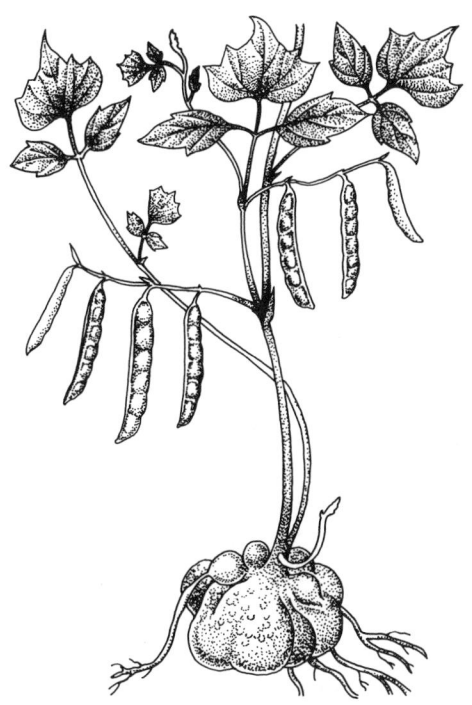

Fig. Y-1. The yam bean, a leguminous plant which has an edible tuber.

ORIGIN AND HISTORY. Various species of yam beans are native to a wide area extending from northern South America to Mexico. The Spanish took these plants to the Philippines during the 16th century. Since then, they have been adopted as crops throughout the tropics of the world.

PRODUCTION. Most of the crop comes from the humid tropical areas of western Pacific and Southeast Asia. Statistics on production are not available.

Yam beans, unlike many other tropical tubers, are grown from seeds. In the Orient, the young plants are trained to climb bamboo trellises. About 10 months are required for the production of mature tubers, which are harvested by plowing or pulling them from the ground. The average yield of tubers is about 8,000 lb per acre (*8,960 kg/ha*).

PROCESSING. The tubers of the plant are rarely processed, although starch is sometimes extracted by washing the grated tubers on a screen.

PREPARATION. Raw yam bean tubers have a crisp texture and are good when served diced or sliced in a salad. The tubers may also be boiled, fried, or roasted. The immature pods of *P. erosus* may be cooked and eaten like snap beans.

CAUTION: The mature seeds and leaves of yam beans should not be consumed, because they contain a harmful agent that is not known to be destroyed by cooking.

NUTRITIONAL VALUE. The nutrient compositions of various forms of yam bean are given in Food Composition Table F-21.

Some noteworthy observations regarding the nutrient composition of yam bean follow:

1. Compared to Irish potatoes, yam bean tubers have a higher water content and are lower in calories, protein and vitamin C. However, the protein-to-calorie ratios are about the same (2.8 g per 100 kcal) for both tubers. This means that yam bean tubers may be a fair source of protein for adults, providing that sufficient quantities are consumed.

2. Yam bean tubers are low in minerals and vitamins. Hence, they should be eaten with foods that supply these essential nutrients.

YAUPON (CASSINA)

The leaves of the yaupon are used as a tea substitute. It is a holly (*Ilex cassine*) which grows in the southern United States. The Indians attributed many virtues to the tea, and allowed only men to drink it. Yaupon tea contains caffeine.

YEAST

Fungi, of which three types are used commercially in the food industry: *Brewers' yeast*, a by-product from the brewing of beer and ale; *dried yeast*, used in leavened breads; and *torula yeast*, cultured as a foodstuff for man and animals, as a source of protein, minerals, B vitamins, and unidentified factors.

(Also see BREADS AND BAKING, section headed "Breads Leavened with Yeast and Other Microorganisms"; BREWERS' YEAST; and TORULA YEAST.)

YEAST EXTRACT

A preparation of the water-soluble fraction of autolysed (self-digested) yeast, valuable both as a rich source of the B vitamins and for its strong savory flavor. Yeast is allowed to autolyse, extracted with hot water, and concentrated by evaporation.

YEAST FERMENTATION, BOTTOM

This refers to fermentation during the manufacture of beer with a yeast that sinks to the bottom of the tank. Most beers are produced this way. Ale, porter, and stout are the principal beers produced by top fermentation.

YOGURT

A fermented milk product prepared from lowfat milk, skim milk, or whole milk. After fermentation, the yogurt may be mixed with other ingredients such as nonfat dry milk solids, vegetable gums, flavoring, or fruit preserves.

(Also see MILK AND MILK PRODUCTS.)

YOLK INDEX

This is an expression of egg quality—freshness—in terms of the spherical nature of the yolk. It is derived by measuring the height and width of the yolk. As the egg deteriorates, the index decreases.

(Also see EGGS, section headed, "Physical Characteristics of the Egg and Grading.")

YORKSHIRE PUDDING

This is a quick bread made with flour, milk and eggs, and either cooked in the pan underneath the roast of beef, or in separate muffin tins, with the meat drippings poured into the cups first. It is a first cousin to the popover.

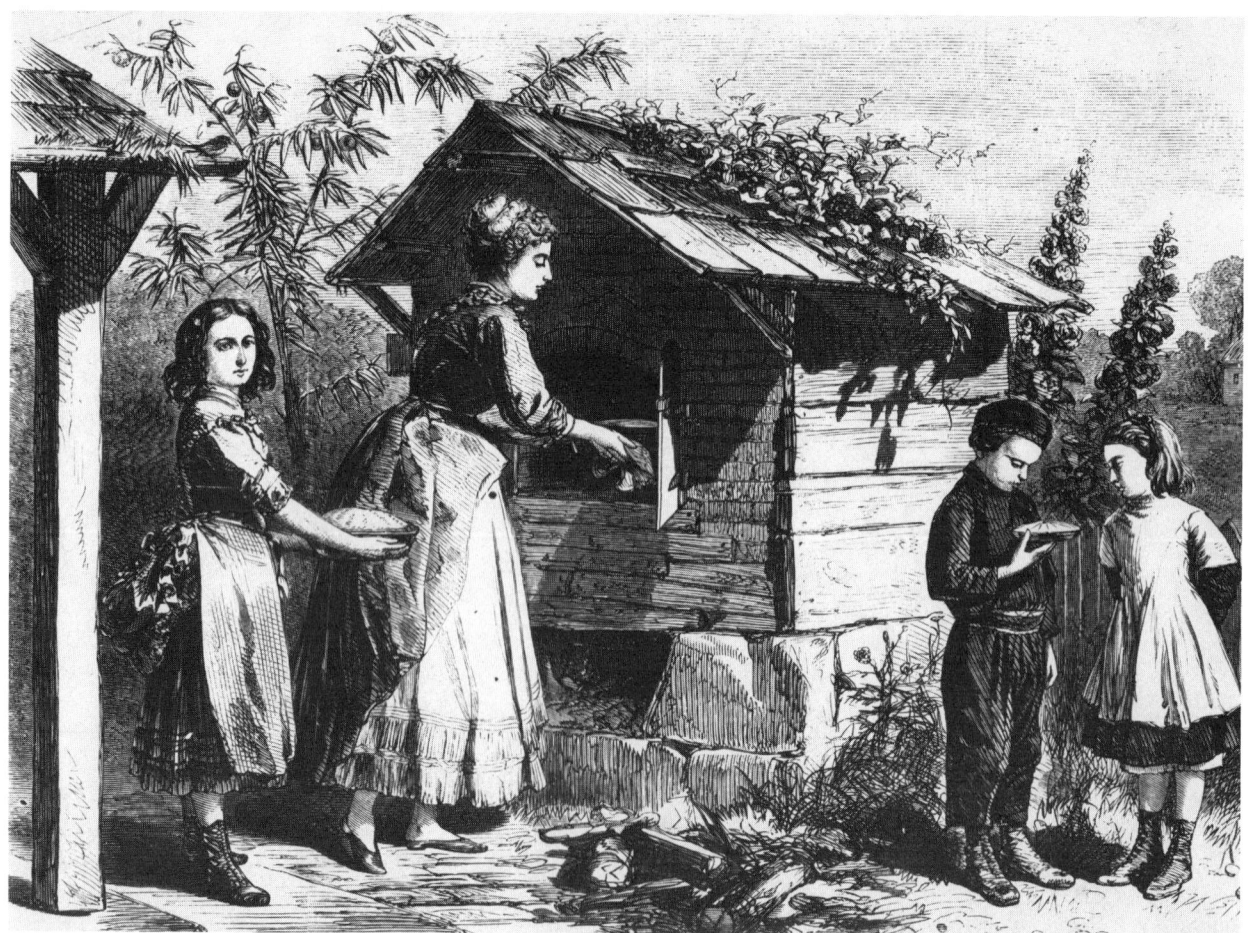

Fig. Y-2. Baking-day, 1870. (Courtesy, The Bettmann Archive, New York, N.Y.)

ZANTE CURRANT

This fruit is not a currant, but is actually a raisin; it is made from black Corinth grapes that are only about one-quarter of the size of an ordinary raisin and look like a dried black-currant. The name *Zante* was given to the raisin because it was first produced on a large scale on the island of Zante in the southeastern part of Greece. Now, they are also produced in Australia.

Zante currants have a tart, tangy flavor and are commonly used in baked products such as coffee cakes and hot cross buns.

(Also see RAISIN[S].)

ZEAXANTHIN

It is a carotenoid alcohol, and the pigment of yellow corn. However, it possesses no vitamin A activity. Zeaxanthin is widespread in nature and occurs together with xanthophyll.

(Also see XANTHOPHYLL.)

ZEDOARY ROOT

An aromatic root from one of two plants of the East Indies which belongs to the ginger family. Zedoary is a GRAS (generally recognized as safe) natural flavor additive.

ZEIN

A protein derived from corn. It lacks the essential amino acids lysine and tryptophan. Commercially, zein is extracted from corn gluten meal with alcohol. In the food industry, its prime use is as an edible coating for foodstuffs such as nut meats and candy. In manufacturing, it has a variety of uses: plastics, paper coatings, adhesives, shellac substitute, printing, laminated board, and microencapsulation.

(Also see CORN; and PROTEIN[S].)

ZEN MACROBIOTIC DIET

This phrase encompasses both a diet and a philosophy of life. Zen refers to meditation, and macrobiotic suggests a tendency to prolong life. The Zen philosophy is hundreds of years old; its beginnings may be traced back to India around 470 A.D. From India, the Zen philosophy moved to China in about 520 A.D., but it was not introduced into Japan until the 1100s and 1200s. Zen seeks to discipline the mind so that an individual comes into touch with the inner workings of his body—a "larger awareness" that cannot be taught. In the United States, the Zen philosophy and the Zen cooking—claimed traditional for the ancient Zen Japanese—was popularized by a Japanese named Georges Ohsawa, who coined the term macrobiotic.

According to the macrobiotic plan, there are ten diets or stages of the same diet. In order to live a happy, harmonious life, the follower progresses from the lowest dietary stage, −3, to the highest or +7. As the macrobiotic follower progresses, desserts, fruits and salads, animal foods, soup, and vegetables, in that order, are eliminated and replaced by increased amounts of cereal grains in the diet. Therefore, only certain stages are pure vegetarian diets, though meat is considered undesirable. All dietary stages encourage the restriction of fluid intake. Furthermore, fluid restriction is encouraged if an individual perspires. Table Z-1 lists the ten stages of the Zen macrobiotic diet and the percentage of food from the different sources.

TABLE Z-1
TEN STAGES OF THE ZEN MACROBIOTIC DIET,[1] FROM LOWEST TO HIGHEST

	Foods					
Stage No.	Cereal Grains	Vege-tables	Soup	Animal	Fruits and Salads	Desserts
	◄ ———————— (%) ———————— ►					
−3	10	30	10	30	15	5
−2	20	30	10	25	10	5
−1	30	30	10	20	10	
+1	40	30	10	20		
+2	50	30	10	10		
+3	60	30	10			
+4	70	20	10			
+5	80	20				
+6	90	10				
+7	100					

[1]All ten stages discourage the drinking of liquids.

The foods used at the different stages seek to establish a balance between foods classified as yang (the male principle) foods, and yin (the female principle) foods. The proper balance is 5 parts yin to 1 part yang. Such things as color, direction of growth, sodium and potassium level, water content, climate, taste, season, source (plant or animal), weight, and vitamin content are said to classify a food as more yang or more yin. For example, progressing from yang foods to yin foods, the following order would be observed: meat, eggs, fish, grains, vegetables, fruits, dairy products, sugar, alcohol, drugs, and chemicals. Brown rice is considered to contain a perfect balance of yang and yin. Hence, brown rice is the principal food of the diet, and the ultimate diet consists solely of brown rice. Brown rice contains no vitamin A, C, or B-12; low levels of other vitamins; low levels of calcium, iron, and other minerals; and a low-quality protein. Moreover, 2.2 lb (1 kg) of cooked brown rice would provide only 1,190 Calories (kcal) of energy—filling, but hardly adequate.

It is the overzealous individuals who persist in following the more rigid diet—high level of brown rice—who are in danger of developing serious nutritional deficiencies. Infants, children, and nursing or pregnant mothers are in particular peril. There have been reports of scurvy, anemia, hypoproteinemia (low blood protein), hypocalcemia (low blood calcium), slowed growth, rickets, loss of kidney function due to low fluid intake, and a few deaths attributed to the followers of the Zen macrobiotic diet.

(Also see VEGETARIAN DIETS.)

ZEST

The colored, oily outer layer of the peel on citrus fruits, which is also called the flavedo. It may be green due to the predominance of the pigment chlorophyll, or yellow to orange when ample amounts of carotene and xanthophyll pigments are present. The color of the zest is *not* always a good indicator of ripeness because some species of citrus fruits require cool nights for the development of the yellow and orange pigments in the peel. However, the color change from green to yellow, or from green to orange, may be induced artificially by exposing the fruit to ethylene gas in a warm room. It is noteworthy that the zest is the part of the peel that is grated and added to enhance various dishes.

(Also see FLAVEDO.)

ZINC (Zn)

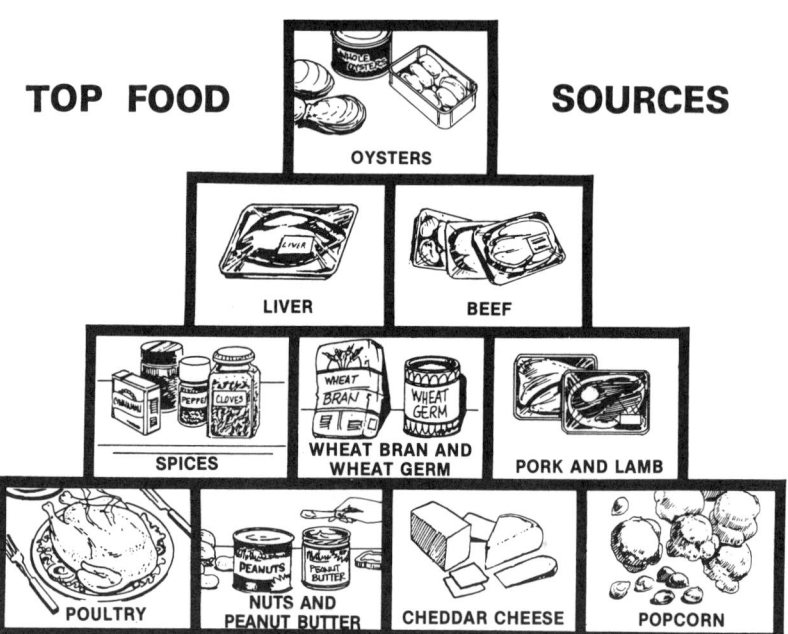

Fig. Z-1. Top food sources of zinc.

Contrary to what many people think, zinc is needed for more than covering pipes, coating wire fences, and galvanizing buckets. It is an essential element for man.

Zinc is widely distributed throughout the body, but the highest concentrations are found in the skin (the skin contains 20% of the total body zinc), hair, nails, eyes, and prostate gland. Traces occur in the liver, bones, and blood. Also, it is a constituent of enzymes involved in most major pathways. In total, the human body contains about 2.2 g of zinc —more than any other trace element except iron.

HISTORY. Zinc was first shown to be biologically important more than 100 years ago when it was found to be needed for the growth of certain bacteria. In the 1920s, it was demonstrated to be required for the growth of experimental rats. But, it wasn't until the early 1960s that zinc was shown to be an essential nutrient of man.

ABSORPTION, METABOLISM, EXCRETION. Zinc is poorly absorbed; less than 10% of dietary zinc is taken into the body, primarily in the duodenum. It appears that metallic zinc and zinc in its carbonate, sulfate, and oxide forms are all absorbed equally well. Large amounts of calcium, phytic acid, or copper inhibit zinc absorption. Cadmium appears to be a zinc antimetabolite.

After zinc is absorbed in the small intestine, it combines with plasma proteins for transport to the tissues. Relatively large amounts of zinc are deposited in bones, but these stores do not move into rapid equilibrium with the rest of the organism. The body pool of biologically available zinc appears to be small and to have a rapid turnover, as evidenced by the prompt appearance of deficiency signs in experimental animals.

Most of the zinc derived from metabolic processes is excreted in the intestine—in pancreatic, intestinal, and bile secretions. Only small amounts are excreted in the urine.

FUNCTIONS OF ZINC. Zinc is needed for normal skin, bones, and hair. It imparts *bloom* to the hair. It is a component of several different enzyme systems which are involved in digestion and respiration. Also, zinc is required for the transfer of carbon dioxide in red blood cells; for proper calcification of bones; for the synthesis and metabolism of proteins and nucleic acids; for the development and functioning of reproductive organs; for wound and burn healing; for the functioning of insulin; and for normal taste acuity (the ability to taste accurately).

DEFICIENCY SYMPTOMS. The most common cause of zinc deficiency is an unbalanced diet, although other factors may be responsible. For example, the consumption of alcohol may precipitate a zinc deficiency by flushing stored zinc out of the liver and into the urine.

Lack of zinc in the human diet has been studied in detail in Egypt and Iran, where the major constituent of the diet is an unleavened bread prepared from low extraction wheat flour. The phytate present in the flour limits the availability of zinc in these diets, with the result that the requirements for the element are not satisfied. Zinc-response has also been observed in young children from middle-class homes in the United States who consume less than an ounce (28 g) of meat per day.

Zinc deficiency is characterized by loss of appetite, stunted growth in children, skin changes, small sex glands in boys, loss of taste sensitivity, lightened pigment in hair (dull hair), white spots on the fingernails, and delayed healing of wounds. In the Middle East, pronounced zinc deficiency in man has resulted in hypogonadism and dwarfism. In pregnant animals, experimental zinc deficiency has resulted in malformation and behavioral disturbances in the offspring—a finding which suggests that the same thing may happen to human fetuses.

INTERRELATIONSHIPS. Zinc is involved in many relationships: in the metabolism of carbohydrates, fats, proteins, and nucleic acids; in interference with the utilization of copper, iron, and other trace minerals, when there are excess dietary levels of zinc; in protection against the toxic effects of cadmium, when there is ample dietary zinc; in reduced absorption, when there are high dietary levels of calcium, phosphorus, and copper.

RECOMMENDED DAILY ALLOWANCE OF ZINC.
Studies have shown that, in healthy adults, equilibrium or positive balance is obtained with intakes of 12.5 mg of zinc per day when this intake is derived from a mixed diet. This has been accepted as a minimum requirement, as the balance studies did not take into account sweat and skin losses.

The National Academy of Sciences, National Research Council, recommended daily zinc allowances are given in the section on MINERAL(S), Table M-25, Mineral Table.

The recommended daily allowances are predicated on the consumption of a mixed diet containing animal products. Diets that supply sufficient animal protein usually also furnish enough zinc, but vegetarian diets may be somewhat low.

The RDA recommended zinc allowances of the National Academy of Sciences, National Research Council, 10th edition, 1989, are as follows:

Infants, birth to 1 year, 5 mg; children, 1 to 10 years, 10 mg; males, 11 to 51+ years, 15 mg; females, 11 to 51+ years, 12 mg; pregnant females, 15 mg; lactating females, first 6 months, 19 mg; lactating females, second 6 months, 16 mg.

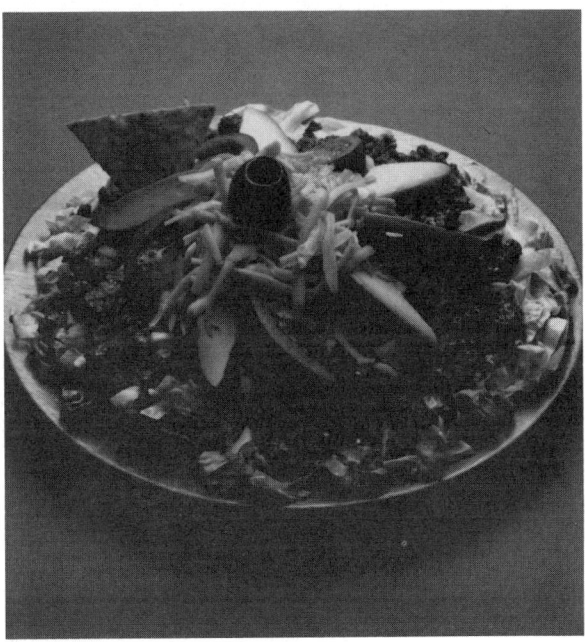

Fig. Z-2. Beef tostada. Both beef and spices are good sources of zinc. (Courtesy, California Iceberg Lettuce Commission, Monterey, Calif.)

• **Zinc intake in average U.S. diet**—The average zinc content of mixed diets consumed by the American adult has been reported to be 12.7 mg/day, but vegetarian and low-protein diets may provide less.

TOXICITY. Toxicity of zinc in man occurs with the ingestion of 2 g or more. Zinc sulfate, taken in these amounts, produces acute gastrointestinal irritation and vomiting. However, zinc has been administered to patients in tenfold excess of the dietary allowances for months and years without adverse reactions. But there is evidence that excessive intakes of zinc may aggravate marginal copper deficiency. For the latter reason, the continuous taking of zinc supplements of more than 15 mg/day, in addition to the dietary intake, should not be done without medical supervision.

Toxicity of zinc is characterized by anemia, depressed growth, stiffness, hemorrhages in bone joints, bone resorption, depraved appetite, and in severe cases, death. The anemia appears to result from an interference with iron and copper utilization because addition of these two elements can overcome the anemia caused by excessive zinc.

Zinc poisoning may result from eating foods that have been stored in galvanized containers.

SOURCES OF ZINC.
Human colostrum (the first secretion of a woman after childbirth) is a good source of zinc.

The zinc content of most municipal drinking water is negligible.

Groupings by rank of common food sources of zinc are given in the section on MINERAL(S), Table M-25, Mineral Table.

For additional sources and more precise values of zinc, see Food Composition Table F-21.

NOTE WELL: The biological availability of zinc in different foods varies widely; meats and seafoods are much better sources of available zinc than vegetables. Zinc availability is adversely affected by phytates (found in whole grains and beans), high calcium, oxalates (in rhubarb and spinach), high fiber, copper (from drinking water conveyed in copper piping), and EDTA (an additive used in certain canned foods).

(Also see MINERAL[S], Table M-25.

ZOLLINGER-ELLISON SYNDROME

Frequently, this disease produces malabsorption. It is caused by the development of a gastrin-secreting tumor in the pancreas or duodenal wall, which stimulates excessive, continued gastric secretion. This oversecretion by the stomach acidifies and dilutes the intestinal contents, leading to major disturbances in fat digestion and absorption, primarily due to the inactivation of the enzyme, pancreatic lipase. Other factors contributing to malabsorption include (1) alteration in the chemical nature of bile salts, reducing their effectiveness; (2) structural and function changes in the intestinal lining; and (3) hypermotility. Eventually, multiple peptic ulcers develop due to the excessive secretion of the hormone, gastrin. Total gastrectomy seems to be the therapy of choice.

ZWITTERION

The term used to describe the property of amino acids, when ionized in solution, to behave either as an acid or a base depending on the need of the solution in which they are present. This capacity makes amino acids good buffer substances.

ZYMASE

The name which is sometimes applied to the mixture of enzymes in yeast that change sugar to alcohol during fermentation.

ZYMOGENS

These are inactive forms of enzymes—proenzymes. Zymogens convert to active enzymes under the influence of various agents such a pH changes or other enzymes. Examples of zymogens are some of the enzymes involved in the digestion of protein. Trypsinogen and pepsinogen are both zymogens secreted into the intestine by the pancreas where they are converted to the active enzymes trypsin and pepsin, respectively.

ZYMOMETER

An instrument which is employed to measure the degree of fermentation of a fermenting liquid.

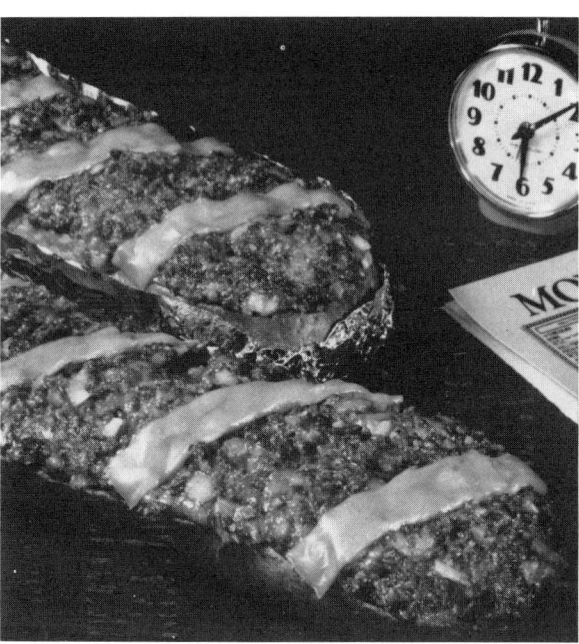

(Courtesy, Carnation, Los Angeles, Calif.)

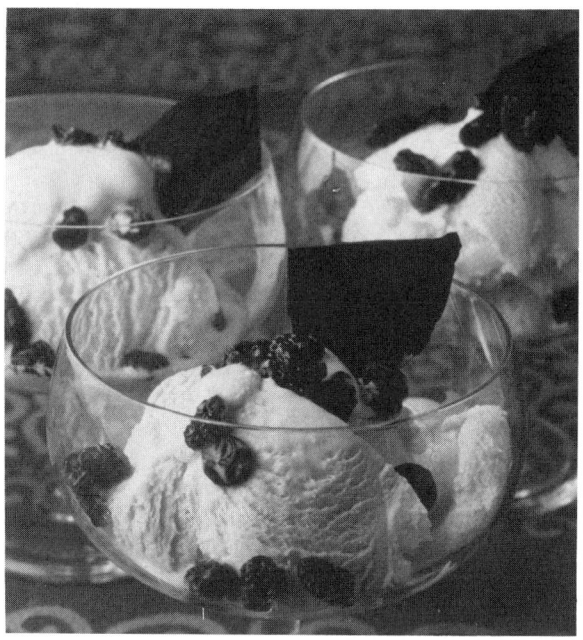

(Courtesy, Phil Siegel/Ketchum, San Francisco, Calif.)

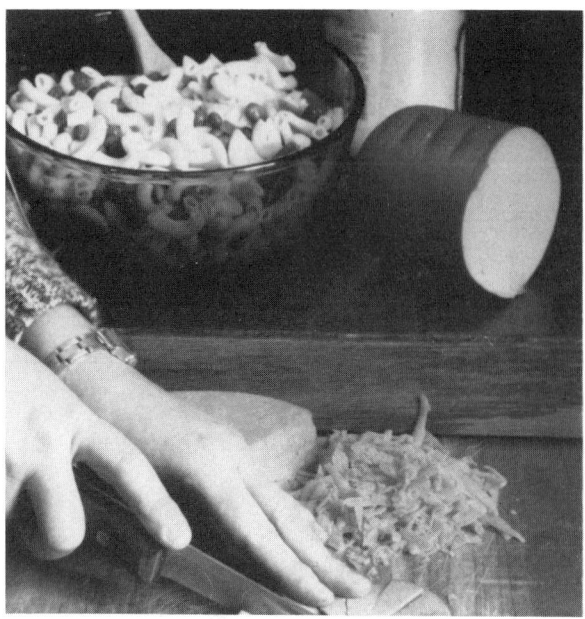

(Courtesy, University of Minnesota, St. Paul, Minn.)

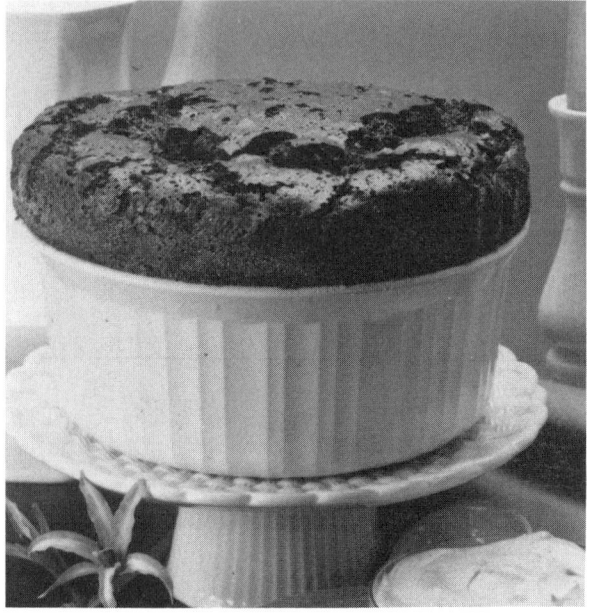

(Courtesy, Hershey Foods Corp., Hershey, Pa.)

Fig. Z-3. A balanced diet, along with an adventure in good eating, is best achieved by consuming a variety of foods.

B

C

F

J

K

L

M

O

P